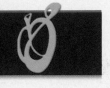

BRAUNWALD'S

Heart Disease

A Textbook of Cardiovascular Medicine

Cover and Spine Illustration:

Fused myocardial perfusion and CT coronary angiography images in a patient with hypertrophic cardiomyopathy presenting with chest pain. The images demonstrate a large area of ischemia in the distribution of the left anterior descending coronary artery and an occluded diagonal branch.

Courtesy of Drs. Marcelo F. DiCarli and Mouaz H. Al-Mallah, Brigham and Women's Hospital, Boston, Massachusetts.

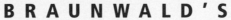

BRAUNWALD'S
Heart Disease

A Textbook of Cardiovascular Medicine

EIGHTH EDITION   **VOLUME 2**

EDITED BY

Peter Libby, MD
Mallinckrodt Professor of Medicine
Harvard Medical School
Chief, Cardiovascular Division
Brigham and Women's Hospital
Boston, Massachusetts

Robert O. Bonow, MD
Max and Lilly Goldberg Distinguished Professor of Cardiology
Northwestern University Feinberg School of Medicine
Chief, Division of Cardiology
Co-Director, Bluhm Cardiovascular Institute
Northwestern Memorial Hospital
Chicago, Illinois

Douglas L. Mann, MD
Don W. Chapman Chair
Professor of Medicine and Molecular Physiology and Biophysics
Chief, Section of Cardiology
Baylor College of Medicine
St. Luke's Episcopal Hospital
Texas Heart Institute
Houston, Texas

Douglas P. Zipes, MD
Distinguished Professor
Professor Emeritus of Medicine, Pharmacology, and Toxicology
Director Emeritus, Division of Cardiology and the Krannert Institute of Cardiology
Indiana University School of Medicine
Indianapolis, Indiana

FOUNDING EDITOR AND E-DITION EDITOR

Eugene Braunwald, MD, MD(Hon), ScD(Hon), FRCP
Distinguished Hersey Professor of Medicine
Harvard Medical School
Chairman, TIMI Study Group
Brigham and Women's Hospital
Boston, Massachusetts

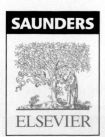

SAUNDERS

ELSEVIER

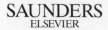

1600 John F. Kennedy Boulevard
Suite 1800
Philadelphia, PA 19103-2899

BRAUNWALD'S HEART DISEASE: A Textbook of Cardiovascular Medicine, Eighth Edition

Two-volume set	978-1-4160-4107-8
Single volume	978-1-4160-4106-1
Two-volume e-dition	978-1-4160-4105-4
Single volume e-dition	978-1-4160-4104-7
International edition	978-0-8089-2385-5
Online edition	978-1-4160-4103-0

Notice

Knowledge and best practice in this field are constantly changing. As new research and experience broaden our knowledge, changes in practice, treatment, and drug therapy may become necessary or appropriate. Readers are advised to check the most current information provided (i) on procedures featured or (ii) by the manufacturer of each product to be administered, to verify the recommended dose or formula, the method and duration of administration, and contraindications. It is the responsibility of the practitioners, relying on their own experience and knowledge of the patient, to make diagnoses, to determine dosages and the best treatment for each individual patient, and to take all appropriate safety precautions. To the fullest extent of the law, neither the Publisher nor the Editors assume any liability for any injury and/or damage to persons or property arising out of or related to any use of the material contained in this book.

The Publisher

Library of Congress Cataloging-in-Publication Data
Braunwald's heart disease : a textbook of cardiovascular medicine / Peter Libby . . . [et al.].—8th ed.
    p. ; cm.
Includes bibliographical references and index.
ISBN 978-1-4160-4106-1
1. Heart—Diseases. 2. Cardiology. I. Libby, Peter. II. Title: Heart disease.
[DNLM: 1. Heart Diseases. 2. Cardiovascular Diseases. WG 210 B825 2008]
RC681.H36 2008
616.1′2—dc22
                          2007009890

Executive Publisher: Natasha Andjelkovic
Developmental Editor: Anne Snyder
Publishing Services Manager: Frank Polizzano
Senior Project Manager: Robin E. Hayward
Multimedia Producer: David Wisner
Design Direction: Steve Stave

Printed in the United States of America.

Last digit is the print number: 9 8 7 6 5 4 3 2

To:

Beryl, Oliver, and Brigitte

Pat, Rob, and Sam

Laura, Stephanie, Jonathan, and Erica

Joan, Debra, Jeffrey, and David

Contributors

Stephan Achenbach, MD
Professor of Medicine, Department of Cardiology, University of Erlangen, Erlangen, Germany
Computed Tomography of the Heart

Philip A. Ades, MD
Professor of Medicine, University of Vermont College of Medicine; Director, Cardiac Rehabilitation and Prevention, Fletcher-Allen Health Care, Burlington, Vermont
Exercise and Sports Cardiology

Elliott M. Antman, MD
Professor of Medicine, Harvard Medical School; Senior Investigator, TIMI Study Group, and Director, Samuel A. Levine Cardiac Unit, Brigham and Women's Hospital, Boston, Massachusetts
ST-Elevation Myocardial Infarction: Pathology, Pathophysiology, and Clinical Features; ST-Elevation Myocardial Infarction: Management

Donald S. Baim, MD
Chief Medical and Scientific Officer, Boston Scientific Corporation, Natick, Massachusetts
Percutaneous Coronary and Valvular Intervention

Gary J. Balady, MD
Professor of Medicine, Boston University School of Medicine; Director, Preventive Cardiology, Boston Medical Center, Boston, Massachusetts
Exercise and Sports Cardiology

Arthur J. Barsky, MD
Professor of Psychiatry, Harvard Medical School; Director of Psychiatric Research, Brigham and Women's Hospital, Boston, Massachusetts
Psychiatric and Behavioral Aspects of Cardiovascular Disease

Joshua A. Beckman, MD, MSc
Assistant Professor of Medicine, Harvard Medical School; Director, Cardiovascular Fellowship Program, Brigham and Women's Hospital, Boston, Massachusetts
Diabetes Mellitus, the Metabolic Syndrome, and Atherosclerotic Vascular Disease

Michael A. Bettmann, MD
Professor of Radiology, Wake Forest University School of Medicine; Vice Chair, Department of Radiology, Wake Forest University Baptist Medical Center, Winston-Salem, North Carolina
The Chest Radiograph in Cardiovascular Disease

Robert O. Bonow, MD
Max and Lilly Goldberg Distinguished Professor of Cardiology, Northwestern University Feinberg School of Medicine; Chief, Division of Cardiology, and Co-Director, Bluhm Cardiovascular Institute, Northwestern Memorial Hospital, Chicago, Illinois
Nuclear Cardiology; Cardiac Catheterization; Care of Patients with End-Stage Heart Disease; Valvular Heart Disease; Guidelines: Management of Valvular Heart Disease

Eugene Braunwald, MD, MD(Hon), ScD(Hon), FRCP
Distinguished Hersey Professor of Medicine, Harvard Medical School; Chairman, TIMI Study Group, Brigham and Women's Hospital, Boston, Massachusetts
ST-Elevation Myocardial Infarction: Pathology, Pathophysiology, and Clinical Features; Unstable Angina and Non-ST Elevation Myocardial Infarction

Hugh Calkins, MD
Professor of Medicine, Johns Hopkins University School of Medicine; Director, Electrophysiology, Johns Hopkins Hospital, Baltimore, Maryland
Hypotension and Syncope

Christopher P. Cannon, MD
Associate Professor of Medicine, Harvard Medical School; TIMI Study Group, Cardiovascular Division, Brigham and Women's Hospital, Boston, Massachusetts
Approach to the Patient with Chest Pain; Unstable Angina and Non-ST Elevation Myocardial Infarction

John M. Canty, Jr., MD
Albert and Elizabeth Rekate Professor of Medicine and Chief of Cardiovascular Medicine, University at Buffalo School of Medicine and Biomedical Sciences, The State University of New York, Buffalo, New York
Coronary Blood Flow and Myocardial Ischemia

John D. Carroll, MD
Professor of Medicine, Division of Cardiology, University of Colorado Health Sciences Center; Director, Cardiac and Vascular Center, and Director, Interventional Cardiology, University of Cardiology Hospital, Denver, Colorado
Clinical Assessment of Heart Failure

Agustin Castellanos, MD
Professor of Medicine, University of Miami Leonard M. Miller School of Medicine; Director, Clinical Electrophysiology, Jackson Memorial Hospital, Miami, Florida
Cardiac Arrest and Sudden Cardiac Death

Bernard R. Chaitman, MD
Professor of Medicine and Director of Cardiovascular Research, St. Louis University School of Medicine; Attending Physician, Division of Cardiology, St. Louis University Hospital, St. Louis, Missouri
Exercise Stress Testing

Danny Chu, MD
Assistant Professor, Baylor College of Medicine; Staff
  Physician, Michael E. DeBakey VA Medical Center,
  Houston, Texas
  Traumatic Heart Disease

Heidi M. Connolly, MD
Professor of Medicine, Mayo Clinic College of Medicine;
  Consultant, Cardiovascular Diseases and Internal
  Medicine, Saint Marys Hospital, Rochester Methodist
  Hospital, Rochester, Minnesota
  Echocardiography

Rebecca B. Costello, PhD
Nutrition Scientist, Office of Dietary Supplements,
  National Institutes of Health, Bethesda, Maryland
  *Complementary and Alternative Approaches to
  Management of Patients with Heart Disease*

Mark A. Creager, MD
Professor of Medicine, Harvard Medical School; Simon C.
  Fireman Scholar in Cardiovascular Medicine and
  Director, Vascular Center, Brigham and Women's
  Hospital, Boston, Massachusetts
  *Diabetes Mellitus, the Metabolic Syndrome, and
  Atherosclerotic Vascular Disease; Peripheral Arterial
  Diseases*

Werner G. Daniel, MD
Professor of Medicine and Chair, Department of
  Cardiology, University of Erlangen, Erlangen, Germany
  Computed Tomography of the Heart

Charles J. Davidson, MD
Professor of Medicine, Northwestern University Feinberg
  School of Medicine; Chief, Cardiac Catheterization
  Laboratories, Northwestern Memorial Hospital, Chicago,
  Illinois
  Cardiac Catheterization

Vasken Dilsizian, MD
Professor of Medicine and Radiology, University of
  Maryland School of Medicine; Director of
  Cardiovascular Nuclear Medicine and Cardiac Positron
  Emission Tomography, University of Maryland Medical
  Center, Baltimore, Maryland
  Nuclear Cardiology

Stefanie Dimmeler, PhD
Professor of Molecular Cardiology, University of Frankfurt
  Medical School, Frankfurt, Germany
  *Emerging Therapies and Strategies in the Treatment of
  Heart Failure*

Pamela S. Douglas, MD
Ursula Geller Professor of Research in Cardiovascular
  Diseases and Chief, Division of Cardiovascular
  Medicine, Duke University Medical Center, Durham,
  North Carolina
  Cardiovascular Disease in Women

Kim A. Eagle, MD
Albion Walter Hewlett Professor of Internal Medicine,
  University of Michigan Medical School; Chief, Clinical
  Cardiovascular Medicine, University of Michigan Health
  System, Ann Arbor, Michigan
  *Anesthesia and Noncardiac Surgery in Patients with
  Heart Disease*

Andrew C. Eisenhauer, MD
Assistant Professor of Medicine, Harvard Medical School;
  Director, Interventional Cardiovascular Medicine
  Service, Brigham and Women's Hospital, Boston,
  Massachusetts
  *Endovascular Treatment of Noncoronary Obstructive
  Vascular Disease*

Linda L. Emanuel, MD, PhD
Professor of Medicine and Director of the Buehler Center
  on Aging, Health & Society, Northwestern University
  Feinberg School of Medicine, Chicago, Illinois
  Care of Patients with End-Stage Heart Disease

James C. Fang, MD
Associate Professor of Medicine, Case Western Reserve
  University School of Medicine; Associate Chief of
  Clinical Affairs and Medical Director of Heart Failure,
  Transplant, and Circulatory Assistance, University
  Hospital/Case Medical Center, Cleveland, Ohio
  *The History and Physical Examination: An Evidence-
  Based Approach*

Stacy D. Fisher, MD
Director, Cardiac Education for Internal Medicine
  Residency, Johns Hopkins/Sinai Hospital of Baltimore,
  Baltimore, Maryland
  *Cardiovascular Abnormalities in HIV-Infected
  Individuals*

Thomas Force, MD
Professor of Medicine, Jefferson Medical College, Thomas
  Jefferson University; Clinical Director, Center for
  Translational Medicine, Thomas Jefferson University
  Hospital, Philadelphia, Pennsylvania
  The Cancer Patient and Cardiovascular Disease

Lee A. Fleisher, MD
Robert D. Dripps Professor of Anesthesiology and Critical
  Care and Professor of Medicine, University of
  Pennsylvania School of Medicine; Chair, Department of
  Anesthesiology and Critical Care, University of
  Pennsylvania Health System, Philadelphia,
  Pennsylvania
  *Anesthesia and Noncardiac Surgery in Patients with
  Heart Disease*

Apoor S. Gami, MD
Assistant Professor of Medicine, Division of
  Cardiovascular Diseases, Mayo Clinic, Rochester,
  Minnesota
  Sleep Apnea and Cardiovascular Disease

J. Michael Gaziano, MD, MPH
Associate Professor of Medicine, Harvard Medical School;
  Chief, Division of Aging, Brigham and Women's
  Hospital; Director, Massachusetts Veterans Epidemiology
  and Research Information Center (MAVERIC), Boston
  Veterans Affairs Healthcare System, Boston,
  Massachusetts
  *Global Burden of Cardiovascular Disease; Primary and
  Secondary Prevention of Coronary Heart Disease*

Jacques Genest, MD
Professor of Medicine, McGill University Faculty of
  Medicine; Chief, Department of Cardiology, McGill
  University Health Center, Montreal, Quebec, Canada
  Lipoprotein Disorders and Cardiovascular Disease

Bernard J. Gersh, MD, DPhil
Professor of Medicine, Mayo Clinic College of Medicine; Consultant in Cardiovascular Diseases and Internal Medicine and Associate Chair of Academic Affairs and Faculty Development, Division of Cardiovascular Diseases, Mayo Clinic, Rochester, Minnesota
Chronic Coronary Artery Disease

Ary L. Goldberger, MD
Professor of Medicine, Harvard Medical School; Associate Director of Interdisciplinary Medicine and Biotechnology and Director of the Margaret and H. A. Rey Institute for Nonlinear Dynamics in Physiology and Medicine, Boston, Massachusetts
Electrocardiography

Samuel Z. Goldhaber, MD
Professor of Medicine, Harvard Medical School; Senior Staff Cardiologist, Director of the Venous Thromboembolism Research Group, and Director of the Anticoagulation Service, Brigham and Women's Hospital, Boston, Massachusetts
Pulmonary Embolism

Larry B. Goldstein, MD
Professor of Medicine, Division of Neurology, Duke University School of Medicine; Director, Center for Cerebrovascular Disease, Duke University Medical Center; Durham VA Medical Center, Durham, North Carolina
Prevention and Management of Stroke

Richard J. Gray, MD
Medical Director, Sutter Pacific Heart Centers, California Pacific Medical Center, San Francisco, California
Medical Management of the Patient Undergoing Cardiac Surgery

William J. Groh, MD, MPH
Associate Professor of Medicine, Krannert Institute of Cardiology, Indiana University School of Medicine, Indianapolis, Indiana
Neurological Disorders and Cardiovascular Disease

Joshua M. Hare, MD
Louis Lemberg Professor of Medicine, Professor of Cellular and Molecular Pharmacology, Chief of Cardiology, and Director of the Interdisciplinary Stem Cell Institute, University of Miami Leonard M. Miller School of Medicine, Miami, Florida
The Dilated, Restrictive, and Infiltrative Cardiomyopathies

David L. Hayes, MD
Professor of Medicine, Mayo Clinic College of Medicine; Chair, Division of Cardiovascular Diseases, Mayo Clinic, Rochester, Minnesota
Cardiac Pacemakers and Cardioverter-Defibrillators

Otto M. Hess, MD
Professor of Cardiology, Swiss Cardiovascular Center, University Hospital, Bern, Switzerland
Clinical Assessment of Heart Failure

L. David Hillis, MD
Daniel W. Foster Distinguished Chair in Internal Medicine and Vice-Chair of Medicine, University of Texas Southwestern Medical Center, Dallas, Texas
Toxins and the Heart

Mark A. Hlatky, MD
Professor of Health Research and Policy and Professor of Cardiovascular Medicine, Stanford University School of Medicine, Stanford, California
Economics and Cardiovascular Disease

Gary S. Hoffman, MD
Professor of Medicine, Cleveland Clinic Lerner College of Medicine of Case Western Reserve University; Harold C. Schott Chair of Rheumatic and Immunologic Diseases, Cleveland Clinic, Cleveland, Ohio
Rheumatic Diseases and the Cardiovascular System

David R. Holmes, Jr., MD
Professor of Medicine, Mayo Clinic College of Medicine; Consultant, St. Marys Hospital, Mayo Clinic, Rochester, Minnesota
Primary Percutaneous Coronary Intervention in the Management of Acute Myocardial Infarction

Eric M. Isselbacher, MD
Associate Professor of Medicine, Harvard Medical School; Associate Director of the Heart Center and Co-Director of the Thoracic Aortic Center, Massachusetts General Hospital, Boston, Massachusetts
Diseases of the Aorta

Suraj Kapa, MD
Physician, Mayo Clinic College of Medicine, Rochester, Minnesota
Cardiovascular Manifestations of Autonomic Disorders

Norman M. Kaplan, MD
Clinical Professor of Internal Medicine, University of Texas Southwestern Medical Center at Dallas; Attending Physician, Parkland Memorial Hospital, Dallas, Texas
Systemic Hypertension: Mechanisms and Diagnosis; Systemic Hypertension: Therapy

Adolf W. Karchmer, MD
Professor of Medicine, Harvard Medical School; Chief, Division of Infectious Diseases, Beth Israel Deaconess Medical Center, Boston, Massachusetts
Infective Endocarditis

Irwin Klein, MD
Professor of Medicine and Cell Biology, New York University School of Medicine; Associate Chair, Department of Medicine, North Shore University Hospital, Manhasset, New York
Endocrine Disorders and Cardiovascular Disease

Barbara A. Konkle, MD
Professor of Medicine and of Pathology and Laboratory Medicine and Director of the Penn Comprehensive Hemophilia and Thrombosis Program, University of Pennsylvania School of Medicine, Philadelphia, Pennsylvania
Hemostasis, Thrombosis, Fibrinolysis, and Cardiovascular Disease

Ronald M. Krauss, MD
Adjunct Professor, Department of Nutritional Sciences, University of California, Berkeley, Berkeley; Senior Scientist and Director, Atherosclerosis Research, Children's Hospital Oakland Research Institute, Oakland, California
Nutrition and Cardiovascular Disease

x **Mitchell W. Krucoff, MD**
Professor of Medicine, Division of Cardiology, Duke
University School of Medicine; Director, CU Devices
Unit; Director, ECG Core Lab, Duke Clinical Research
Institute, Duke University Medical Center, Durham,
North Carolina
*Complementary and Alternative Approaches to
Management of Patients with Heart Disease*

Harlan M. Krumholz, MD
Harold J. Hines, Jr. Professor of Medicine and
Epidemiology and Public Health, Yale University School
of Medicine; Director, Center for Outcomes Research
and Evaluation, Yale-New Haven Hospital, New Haven,
Connecticut
Clinical Decision-Making in Cardiology

Gary E. Lane, MD
Assistant Professor of Medicine, Mayo Clinic College of
Medicine; Director, Cardiac Catheterization Laboratory,
St. Luke's Hospital, Mayo Clinic, Jacksonville, Florida
*Primary Percutaneous Coronary Intervention in the
Management of Acute Myocardial Infarction*

Richard A. Lange, MD
E. Cowles Andrus Professor of Cardiology and Chief of
Clinical Cardiology, Johns Hopkins Hospital, Baltimore,
Maryland
Toxins and the Heart

Cheng-Han Lee, MD, PhD
Department of Pathology and Laboratory Medicine,
University of British Columbia Faculty of Medicine;
Vancouver General Hospital, Vancouver, British
Columbia, Canada
Primary Tumors of the Heart

Thomas H. Lee, MD
Professor of Medicine, Harvard Medical School; Network
President, Partners Healthcare System, Boston,
Massachusetts
*Measurement and Improvement of Quality of
Cardiovascular Care; Guidelines: Electrocardiography;
Guidelines: Exercise Stress Testing; Guidelines: Use of
Echocardiography; Guidelines: Nuclear Cardiology;
Guidelines: Appropriateness Guidelines: Cardiovascular
Magnetic Resonance; Guidelines: Appropriateness
Guidelines: Cardiac Computed Tomography; Guidelines:
Coronary Arteriography; Guidelines: Management of
Heart Failure; Guidelines: Ambulatory
Electrocardiographic and Electrophysiologic Testing;
Guidelines: Cardiac Pacemakers and Cardioverter-
Defibrillators; Guidelines: Atrial Fibrillation; Guidelines:
Treatment of Hypertension; Approach to the Patient
with Chest Pain; Guidelines: Primary Percutaneous
Coronary Intervention in Acute Myocardial Infarction;
Guidelines: Unstable Angina and Non–ST Elevation
Myocardial Infarction; Guidelines: Chronic Stable
Angina; Guidelines: Percutaneous Coronary and
Valvular Intervention; Guidelines: Management of
Valvular Heart Disease; Guidelines: Infective
Endocarditis; Guidelines: Pregnancy and Heart Disease;
Guidelines: Reducing Cardiac Risk with Noncardiac
Surgery*

Martin M. LeWinter, MD
Professor of Medicine and Molecular Physiology and
Biophysics, University of Vermont College of Medicine;
Attending Cardiologist, Fletcher Allen Health Care,
Burlington, Vermont
Pericardial Diseases

Peter Libby, MD
Mallinckrodt Professor of Medicine, Harvard Medical
School; Chief, Cardiovascular Division, Brigham and
Women's Hospital, Boston, Massachusetts
*The Vascular Biology of Atherosclerosis; Risk Factors for
Atherothrombotic Disease; Lipoprotein Disorders and
Cardiovascular Disease; Diabetes Mellitus, the
Metabolic Syndrome, and Atherosclerotic Vascular
Disease; Peripheral Arterial Diseases*

Steven E. Lipshultz, MD
Professor and Chair, Department of Pediatrics, University
of Miami, Leonard M. Miller School of Medicine,
Miami, Florida
*Cardiovascular Abnormalities in HIV-Infected
Individuals*

Peter P. Liu, MSc, MD
Heart & Stroke/Polo Chair and Professor of Medicine,
Toronto General Research Institute, University Health
Network; Heart & Stroke/Richard Lewar Centre of
Excellence in Cardiovascular Research, Toronto,
Ontario, Canada
Myocarditis

Brian F. Mandell, MD, PhD
Professor of Medicine, Cleveland Clinic Lerner College of
Medicine of Case Western Reserve University; Vice
Chairman of Medicine for Education and Staff,
Rheumatic and Immunologic Disease, Center for
Vasculitis Care and Research, Cleveland Clinic,
Cleveland, Ohio
Rheumatic Diseases and the Cardiovascular System

Douglas L. Mann, MD
Don W. Chapman Chair and Professor of Medicine and
Molecular Physiology and Biophysics; Chief, Section of
Cardiology, Baylor College of Medicine; St. Luke's
Episcopal Hospital, Texas Heart Institute, Houston,
Texas
*Pathophysiology of Heart Failure; Management of Heart
Failure Patients with Reduced Ejection Fraction;
Emerging Therapies and Strategies in the Treatment of
Heart Failure*

JoAnn E. Manson, MD, DrPH
Professor of Medicine and Elizabeth F. Brigham Professor
of Women's Health, Harvard Medical School; Chief,
Division of Preventive Medicine, Brigham and Women's
Hospital, Boston, Massachusetts
*Primary and Secondary Prevention of Coronary Heart
Disease*

Daniel B. Mark, MD, MPH
Professor of Medicine, Division of Cardiology, Duke
University School of Medicine; Director, Outcomes
Research Group, Duke Clinical Research Institute,
Durham, North Carolina
Economics and Cardiovascular Disease

Barry J. Maron, MD
Director, The Hypertrophic Cardiomyopathy Center,
  Minneapolis Heart Institute Foundation, Minneapolis,
  Minnesota; Adjunct Professor of Medicine, Tufts
  University School of Medicine, Tufts–New England
  Medical Center, Boston, Massachusetts
  Hypertrophic Cardiomyopathy

Kenneth L. Mattox, MD
Professor of Surgery, Baylor College of Medicine; Chief of
  Surgery and Chief of Staff, Ben Taub General Hospital,
  Houston, Texas
  Traumatic Heart Disease

Patrick M. McCarthy, MD
Heller-Sacks Professor of Surgery, Northwestern
  University Feinberg School of Medicine; Chief, Division
  of Cardiothoracic Surgery, Co-Director, Bluhm
  Cardiovascular Institute, Northwestern Memorial
  Hospital, Chicago, Illinois
  Surgical Management of Heart Failure

Peter A. McCullough, MD, MPH
Consultant Cardiologist and Chief, Division of Preventive
  Medicine, William Beaumont Hospital, Royal Oak,
  Michigan
  *Interface Between Renal Disease and Cardiovascular
  Illness*

Vallerie V. McLaughlin, MD
Associate Professor of Medicine, University of Michigan
  Medical School; Director, Pulmonary Hypertension
  Program, University of Michigan Health System, Ann
  Arbor, Michigan
  Pulmonary Hypertension

Bruce McManus, MD, PhD
Professor of Pathology and Laboratory Medicine,
  University of British Columbia Faculty of Medicine;
  Director of the James Hogg iCapture Centre and
  Scientific Director of the Heart Centre, St. Paul's
  Hospital, Providence Health, Vancouver, British
  Columbia, Canada
  Primary Tumors of the Heart

John M. Miller, MD
Professor of Medicine, Krannert Institute of Cardiology,
  Indiana University School of Medicine, Indianapolis,
  Indiana
  *Diagnosis of Cardiac Arrhythmias; Therapy for Cardiac
  Arrhythmias*

David M. Mirvis, MD
Professor of Preventive Medicine, University of Tennessee
  Health Science Center, Memphis, Tennessee
  Electrocardiography

David A. Morrow, MD
Assistant Professor of Medicine, Harvard Medical School;
  Brigham and Women's Hospital, Boston, Massachusetts
  *Chronic Coronary Artery Disease; Guidelines: Chronic
  Stable Angina*

Robert J. Myerburg, MD
Professor of Medicine, Division of Cardiology, University
  of Miami School of Medicine; Jackson Memorial
  Hospital, Miami, Florida
  Cardiac Arrest and Sudden Cardiac Death

Elizabeth G. Nabel, MD
Director, National Heart, Lung, and Blood Institute,
  National Institutes of Health, Bethesda, Maryland
  *Principles of Cardiovascular Molecular Biology and
  Genetics*

Yoshifumi Naka, MD, PhD
Associate Professor of Surgery, Columbia University
  College of Physicians and Surgeons; Director, Cardiac
  Transplantation and Mechanical Circulatory Support
  Program, New York–Presbyterian Hospital, Columbia
  University Medical Center, New York, New York
  Assisted Circulation in the Treatment of Heart Failure

Carlo Napolitano, MD, PhD
Senior Scientist, Molecular Cardiology Laboratories,
  IRCCS Fondazione Salvatore Maugeri, Pavia, Italy
  Genetics of Cardiac Arrhythmias

Richard W. Nesto, MD
Associate Professor of Medicine, Harvard Medical School,
  Boston; Chair, Department of Cardiovascular Medicine,
  Lahey Clinic Medical Center, Burlington, Massachusetts
  Diabetes and Heart Disease

L. Kristin Newby, MD, MHS
Associate Professor of Medicine, Division of
  Cardiovascular Medicine, Duke University School of
  Medicine; Duke University Medical Center, Durham,
  North Carolina
  Cardiovascular Disease in Women

Patrick T. O'Gara, MD
Associate Professor of Medicine, Harvard Medical School;
  Director of Clinical Cardiology and Vice Chair of
  Medicine, Brigham and Women's Hospital, Boston,
  Massachusetts
  *The History and Physical Examination: An Evidence-
  Based Approach*

Jae K. Oh, MD
Professor of Medicine, Mayo Clinic College of Medicine;
  Consultant of Cardiovascular Diseases, Co-Director of
  Echocardiography Laboratory, Director of
  Echocardiography Core Laboratory, Mayo Clinic,
  Rochester, Minnesota
  Echocardiography

Jeffrey E. Olgin, MD
Associate Professor in Residence, Chief of Cardiac
  Electrophysiology, and Melvin M. Schienman Chair in
  Electrophysiology, University of California, San
  Francisco, School of Medicine, San Francisco,
  California
  Specific Arrhythmias: Diagnosis and Treatment

Lionel H. Opie, MD, DPhil
Professor of Medicine, Faculty of Health Sciences, The
  Hatter Institute for Cardiology Research, University of
  Cape Town, Cape Town, South Africa
  Mechanisms of Cardiac Contraction and Relaxation

Catherine M. Otto, MD
J. Ward Kennedy-Hamilton Endowed Professor of
  Cardiology, Director of Cardiology Fellowship Programs,
  and Associate Director of Echocardiography, University
  of Washington School of Medicine, Seattle, Washington
  Valvular Heart Disease

xii **Dudley Pennell, MD**
Professor of Cardiology, Imperial College London; Director,
Cardiovascular Magnetic Resonance Unit, Royal
Brompton Hospital, London, United Kingdom
Cardiovascular Magnetic Resonance

Jeffrey J. Popma, MD
Associate Professor of Medicine, Harvard Medical School;
Director, Interventional Cardiology, Brigham and
Women's Hospital, Boston, Massachusetts
*Coronary Arteriography and Intravascular Imaging;
Percutaneous Coronary and Valvular Intervention*

Silvia G. Priori, MD, PhD
Associate Professor of Cardiology, University of Pavia;
Director, Molecular Cardiology, IRCCS Fondazione
Salvatore Maugeri, Pavia, Italy
Genetics of Cardiac Arrhythmias

Reed E. Pyeritz, MD, PhD
Professor of Medicine and Genetics, University of
Pennsylvania School of Medicine, Philadelphia,
Pennsylvania
*General Principles of Genetic Factors in Cardiovascular
Disease; Genetic Factors in Myocardial Disease*

B. Soma Raju, MD
Professor of Cardiology, Care Institute of Medical
Sciences; Chair, Division of Cardiology, Care Hospital,
Hyderabad, India
Rheumatic Fever

Margaret M. Redfield, MD
Professor of Medicine, Mayo Clinic College of Medicine;
Director, Mayo Heart Failure Clinic, Rochester,
Minnesota
Heart Failure with Normal Ejection Fraction

Andrew N. Redington, MD
Professor of Pediatrics, University of Toronto Faculty of
Medicine; Head of Cardiology, Hospital for Sick
Children, Toronto, Ontario, Canada
Congenital Heart Disease

Frederic S. Resnic, MD
Assistant Professor of Medicine, Harvard Medical School;
Director, Cardiac Catheterization Laboratory, Brigham
and Women's Hospital, Boston, Massachusetts
Percutaneous Coronary and Valvular Intervention

Stuart Rich, MD
Professor of Medicine, University of Chicago Pritzker
School of Medicine; Center for Pulmonary
Hypertension, University of Chicago Medical Center,
Chicago, Illinois
Pulmonary Hypertension

Paul M. Ridker, MD, MPH
Eugene Braunwald Professor of Medicine, Harvard
Medical School; Director, Center for Cardiovascular
Disease Prevention, Brigham and Women's Hospital,
Boston, Massachusetts
*Risk Factors for Atherothrombotic Disease; Primary and
Secondary Prevention of Coronary Heart Disease*

Dan M. Roden, MD
Professor of Medicine and Pharmacology; Director, Oates
Institute for Experimental Therapeutics; Assistant Vice-
Chancellor for Personalized Medicine, Vanderbilt
University School of Medicine, Nashville, Tennessee
The Principles of Drug Therapy

Eric A. Rose, MD
Professor of Surgery, Columbia University College of
Physicians and Surgeons; Director of Surgical Service
and Surgeon-in-Chief, New York–Presbyterian Hospital,
Columbia University Medical Center, New York, New
York
Assisted Circulation in the Treatment of Heart Failure

Michael Rubart, MD
Assistant Professor of Pediatrics, Herman B. Wells Center
for Pediatric Research, Indiana University School of
Medicine, Indianapolis, Indiana
*Genesis of Cardiac Arrhythmias: Electrophysiological
Considerations*

Andrew I. Schafer, MD
E. Hugh Luckey Distinguished Professor of Medicine and
Chair, Department of Medicine, Weill Medical College
of Cornell University; Physician-in-Chief, New York-
Presbyterian Hospital, Weill Cornell Medical Center,
New York, New York
*Hemostasis, Thrombosis, Fibrinolysis, and
Cardiovascular Disease*

Heinz-Peter Schultheiss, MD
Department of Cardiology and Pneumology, Charité–
University Medicine Berlin, Campus Benjamin Franklin,
Berlin, Germany
Myocarditis

Janice B. Schwartz, MD
Clinical Professor of Medicine, University of California,
San Francisco, School of Medicine; Director of
Research, Jewish Home, San Francisco, California
Cardiovascular Disease in the Elderly

Peter J. Schwartz, MD
Professor and Chair, Department of Cardiology, University
of Pavia; Chief, Coronary Care Unit, IRCCS Fondazione
Policlinico S. Matteo, Pavia, Italy
Genetics of Cardiac Arrhythmias

Christine E. Seidman, MD
Thomas W. Smith Professor of Medicine and Genetics,
Harvard Medical School; Director, Cardiovascular
Genetics Center, Brigham and Women's Hospital,
Boston, Massachusetts
*General Principles of Genetic Factors in Cardiovascular
Disease; Genetic Factors in Myocardial Disease*

Jonathan G. Seidman, PhD
Henrietta B. and Frederick H. Bugher Professor of
Cardiovascular Genetics, Department of Genetics,
Harvard Medical School, Boston, Massachusetts
Genetic Factors in Myocardial Disease

Dhun H. Sethna, MD
Associate Director of Cardiology, Almeda County Medical
Center, Oakland, California
*Medical Management of the Patient Undergoing Cardiac
Surgery*

Daniel Simon, MD
Herman K. Hellerstein Professor of Medicine, Case
Western Reserve University School of Medicine; Chief of
Cardiovascular Medicine, Director of the Heart and
Vascular Institute, University Hospitals of Cleveland/
Case Medical Center, Cleveland, Ohio
*Hemostasis, Thrombosis, Fibrinolysis, and
Cardiovascular Disease*

Jeffrey F. Smallhorn, MBBS
Professor of Pediatrics, University of Alberta Faculty of
Medicine and Dentistry; Head, Section of
Echocardiography Laboratory, Stollery Children's
Hospital, Edmonton, Alberta, Canada
Congenital Heart Disease

Virend K. Somers, MD, DPhil
Professor of Medicine, Division of Cardiovascular
Diseases, Mayo Clinic College of Medicine; Consultant,
Cardiovascular Diseases, Mayo Clinic, Rochester,
Minnesota
*Sleep Apnea and Cardiovascular Disease;
Cardiovascular Manifestations of Autonomic Disorders*

John R. Teerlink, MD
Associate Professor of Medicine, University of California,
San Francisco, School of Medicine; Director of Heart
Failure, Director of Clinical Echocardiography, San
Francisco Veterans Affairs Medical Center, San
Francisco, California
Diagnosis and Management of Acute Heart Failure

Judith Therrien, MD
Assistant Professor of Medicine, McGill University Faculty
of Medicine; Cardiologist, Sir Mortimer B. Davis Jewish
General Hospital, Montreal, Quebec, Canada
Congenital Heart Disease

Paul D. Thompson, MD
Professor of Medicine, University of Connecticut School of
Medicine; Director of Cardiology, Henry Low Heart
Center, Hartford Hospital, Hartford, Connecticut
Exercise-Based, Comprehensive Cardiac Rehabilitation

Zoltan G. Turi, MD
Professor of Medicine, Robert Wood Johnson Medical
School, University of Medicine and Dentistry of New
Jersey; Director of the Structural Heart Disease Program,
Director of the Cooper Vascular Center, Cooper
University Hospital, Camden, New Jersey
Rheumatic Fever

James E. Udelson, MD
Associate Professor of Medicine and Radiology, Tufts
University School of Medicine; Associate Chief of
Cardiology, Director of Nuclear Cardiology, and Co-
Director of the Heart Failure Service, Tufts-New
England Medical Center, Boston, Massachusetts
Nuclear Cardiology; Guidelines: Nuclear Cardiology

Ronald G. Victor, MD
Clinical Professor of Medicine, University of Texas
Southwestern Medical School; Chief of Hypertension,
Norman and Audrey Kaplan Chair in Hypertension,
University of Texas Southwestern Medical Center,
Dallas, Texas
Systemic Hypertension: Mechanisms and Diagnosis

John H. K. Vogel, MD
Former Chair, Cardiology, Santa Barbara Cottage Hospital;
Former President, American Heart Association, Santa
Barbara County, Santa Barbara, California
*Complementary and Alternative Approaches to
Management of Patients with Heart Disease*

Matthew J. Wall, Jr., MD
Professor, Michael E. DeBakey Department of Surgery,
Baylor College of Medicine; Deputy Chief of Surgery and
Chief of Cardiothoracic Surgery, Ben Taub General
Hospital, Houston, Texas
Traumatic Heart Disease

Carole A. Warnes, MD
Professor of Medicine, Mayo Clinic College of Medicine;
Consultant in Cardiovascular Diseases and Internal
Medicine, Pediatric Cardiology; Director, Adult
Congenital Heart Disease Clinic; Dean, Mayo School of
Continuing Medical Education, Mayo Clinic, Rochester,
Minnesota
Pregnancy and Heart Disease

Gary D. Webb, MD
Professor of Medicine, University of Pennsylvania School
of Medicine; Director, Philadelphia Adult Congenital
Heart Center, University of Pennsylvania Health System,
Children's Hospital of Philadelphia, Philadelphia,
Pennsylvania
Congenital Heart Disease

Christopher J. White, MD
Chairman, Department of Cardiology, Ochsner Clinic
Foundation, New Orleans, Louisiana
*Endovascular Treatment of Noncoronary Obstructive
Vascular Disease*

Lawson R. Wulsin, MD
Professor of Psychiatry and Family Medicine, University
of Cincinnati College of Medicine; Director, Family
Medicine Psychiatry Training Program, University
Hospital, Cincinnati, Ohio
*Psychiatric and Behavioral Aspects of Cardiovascular
Disease*

Clyde W. Yancy, MD
Medical Director, Baylor Heart and Vascular Institute;
Chief, Cardiothoracic Transplantation, Baylor University
Medical Center at Dallas, Dallas, Texas
Heart Disease in Varied Populations

Andreas M. Zeiher, MD
Professor of Cardiology and Chair, Department of
Medicine, University of Frankfurt, Frankfurt, Germany
*Emerging Therapies and Strategies in the Treatment of
Heart Failure*

Douglas P. Zipes, MD
Distinguished Professor; Professor Emeritus of Medicine,
Pharmacology, and Toxicology; and Director Emeritus,
Division of Cardiology and the Krannert Institute of
Cardiology, Indiana University School of Medicine,
Indianapolis, Indiana
*Genesis of Cardiac Arrhythmias: Electrophysiological
Considerations; Diagnosis of Cardiac Arrhythmias;
Therapy for Cardiac Arrhythmias; Cardiac Pacemakers
and Cardioverter-Defibrillators; Specific Arrhythmias:
Diagnosis and Treatment; Hypotension and Syncope;
Cardiovascular Disease in the Elderly; Neurological
Disorders and Cardiovascular Disease*

Contributors

The currents of contemporary cardiovascular disease run swiftly, broadly, and deeply. The Eighth Edition of *Braunwald's Heart Disease: A Textbook of Cardiovascular Medicine,* presented here, serves as the hub of a learning system designed to help physicians and students at all levels, from trainees to highly specialized practitioners, confront the challenge of staying abreast of this rapidly evolving field.

We intend *Heart Disease* to constitute the "core curriculum," an up-to-date, comprehensive, and authoritative ready reference for all practitioners. We strove to make this Eighth Edition an information source of practical clinical utility, grounded in the rapidly expanding evidence base that informs our practice. As in the previous editions of *Heart Disease,* we present the scientific underpinnings that govern cardiovascular pathophysiology and provide a rational basis for understanding therapeutics and management of cardiovascular diseases encountered in clinical practice.

Since the preparation of the last edition of *Heart Disease* much has changed, a reflection of the rapid pace of progress in our specialty. The results of manifold new clinical trials have become available in ways that in many cases profoundly affect our management strategies and practice. Novel therapeutics, both pharmacological and device-based, provide new management options. In the last few years we have not only witnessed striking advances in therapeutics but encountered challenges in the application of drug therapies and cardiovascular devices ranging from drug-eluting stents to implantable devices. The constant change and complexities in therapeutics and management strategies render obsolete textbooks published only a few years ago.

Other rapid shifts are under way in the prevalence of cardiovascular disease. In recent years cardiovascular specialists could congratulate themselves that the epidemic of cardiovascular disease had declined, based on the progress in our specialty. Current demographic trends suggest, however, that the scourge of cardiovascular disease, rather than waning, may indeed be increasing in the years to come. The aging of the population will increase the overall burden of cardiovascular disease in society, even as age-adjusted rates of cardiovascular mortality plateau or decline. We also need to confront a renewed upswing of cardiovascular risk linked to the worldwide epidemic of obesity, insulin resistance, and diabetes rooted in over-nutrition and declining physical activity. This gathering of cardiovascular risk increasingly threatens to extend the burden of cardiovascular disease to developing as well as Western societies. Thus, we cannot presume that the toll of cardiovascular disease will continue to ebb, highlighting the urgency of tools such as the *Heart Disease* Learning System that aim to help the clinician remain abreast of the constantly changing landscape of cardiovascular disease.

We have thoroughly revised this new edition to reflect these multiple changes. Thirty of eighty-nine chapters are entirely new. Thus, more than one third of the Eighth Edition represents completely new material. There are 43 new authors, comparing the Eighth to the Seventh Edition of *Heart Disease.* All of the chapters carried over from the Seventh Edition have undergone extensive revision to update them and heighten their utility. A full description of the changes introduced in this Eighth Edition exceeds the scope of this Preface. Among the major changes, Douglas L. Mann, MD, has joined the editorial team and overseen a recasting of the entire section devoted to heart failure and chapters relating to myocardial disease. As heart failure represents the leading cause of admissions of patients covered by Medicare to hospitals, and comprises an ever-increasing fraction of our patient population given the success of acute interventions, the fresh approach to this important topic should be welcome to readers. In particular, new chapters focus on acute heart failure and heart failure with preserved systolic function, two timely and challenging issues in clinical practice.

Given the growing potential of genetics and expanding knowledge of cardiovascular genetics, Christine E. Seidman, MD, and Jonathan G. Seidman, PhD, have joined the author list of *Heart Disease* and provide a thorough revision with Reed E. Pyeritz, MD, PhD, of the chapter on cardiovascular genetics and an entirely new chapter on the genetics of myocardial disease, complemented by online supplements. A new chapter on evidence-based physical examination has replaced the traditional recitation and cataloguing of signs and symptoms of cardiovascular disease. We are grateful to James C. Fang, MD, and Patrick T. O'Gara, MD, for taking on the assignment of preparing this entirely new approach to the foundation of clinical evaluation, the physical examination. Heidi M. Connolly, MD, and Jae K. Oh, MD, have prepared a new chapter on echocardiography that provides in-depth discussion of the current state-of-the-art applications of this versatile imaging modality for virtually all forms of cardiac disease. A new chapter on stroke by Larry B. Goldstein, MD, highlights what a cardiovascular practitioner needs to know about prevention and treatment of stroke and illustrates the extra-cardiac extensions of contemporary cardiology practice. A new chapter on sleep disorders likewise acknowledges the importance of an integrated multi-system approach to the management of our patients with cardiovascular disease. A new chapter on complementary and alternative approaches to cardiovascular disease reflects the growing interest in this area in patients and doctors alike. For similar reasons, we have added a new chapter on sports cardiology.

The Eighth Edition of *Heart Disease* contains 2275 illustrations, in full color where appropriate, as well as 600 tables. The CD-ROM packaged with the book contains all the figures and tables from the book, available to download to PowerPoint® to facilitate the use of these abundant materials for teaching. We hope thus to multiply the communication value of the content offered by the experts who contributed to *Heart Disease.*

As noted above, we conceive of *Heart Disease* as a family of learning tools intended to help the reader surmount the swift change in cardiovascular knowledge. To keep pace with the rapid evolution of our specialty between editions, we have approached *Heart Disease* as a living book. The *Heart Disease* website personally edited and updated by Eugene Braunwald, MD, on a weekly basis provides the readers of *Heart Disease* with a pulse of progress in cardiovascular medicine on an ongoing and contemporaneous basis. The many special features of the website, such as weekly updates, late-breaking clinical trials, hot-off-the-press topics, abstracts, and focused reviews, in addition to the searchability and functionality of the online medium, offer the interested reader the wealth and breadth of current information that no other online resource in cardiology can provide.

We intend the growing family of *Heart Disease* companion volumes to address the breadth and depth of cardiovascular medicine. Several companions are currently in print, many published or revised in the last few years. Other companions in production or the planning stages include topics such as arrhythmology and lipidology, and mechanical circulatory support will emerge in the coming years. Noteworthy additions to the family of *Heart Disease* companions include a new volume on hypertension edited by Henry R. Black, MD, and William J. Elliott, MD, PhD; an entirely revised and updated version of *Cardiovascular Therapeutics* edited by Elliott M. Antman, MD; a comprehensive volume on vascular medicine edited by Mark A. Creager, MD, Victor J. Dzau, MD, and Joseph Loscalzo, MD, PhD; and a volume on cardiac nursing edited by Debra K. Moser, DNSc, RN, and Barbara Riegel, DNSc, RN. Readers of *Heart Disease* who wish to deepen their knowledge of specific areas can turn to the companion volumes as a convenient source, bearing the hallmark of clinical utility with a clinical evidence foundation and scientific basis common to the *Heart Disease* mission. The companions are intended to complement the core curriculum of this *Heart Disease* volume. In response to the growing importance of imaging in cardiovascular practice, atlases of the emerging and established imaging technologies are currently in preparation under editorial direction of Robert O. Bonow, MD. Finally, a new edition of the *Heart Disease Review and Assessment* book is under way, to help trainees prepare for the certification examinations in the specialty of cardiovascular diseases.

These various key components of the *Heart Disease* Learning System, assembled in a personalized way to meet the needs of each practitioner, should help one navigate the rapidly flowing stream of cardiovascular knowledge. We hope that the readers will find *Heart Disease* and its associated learning tools useful in their quest to stay abreast of this ever-evolving field.

PETER LIBBY
ROBERT O. BONOW
DOUGLAS L. MANN
DOUGLAS P. ZIPES
2007

Adapted from the First Edition

Preface

Cardiovascular disease is the greatest scourge affecting the industrialized nations. As with previous scourges—bubonic plague, yellow fever, and smallpox—cardiovascular disease not only strikes down a significant fraction of the population without warning but also causes prolonged suffering and disability in an even larger number. In the United States alone, despite recent encouraging declines, cardiovascular disease is still responsible for almost 1 million fatalities each year and more than half of all deaths; almost 5 million persons afflicted with cardiovascular disease are hospitalized each year. The cost of these diseases in terms of human suffering and of material resources is almost incalculable. Fortunately, research focusing on the causes, diagnosis, treatment, and prevention of heart disease is moving ahead rapidly.

In order to provide a comprehensive, authoritative text in a field that has become as broad and deep as cardiovascular medicine, I chose to enlist the aid of a number of able colleagues. However, I hoped that my personal involvement in the writing of about half of the book would make it possible to minimize the fragmentation, gaps, inconsistencies, organizational difficulties, and impersonal tone that sometimes plague multiauthored texts.

Since the early part of the 20th century, clinical cardiology has had a particularly strong foundation in the basic sciences of physiology and pharmacology. More recently, the disciplines of molecular biology, genetics, developmental biology, biophysics, biochemistry, experimental pathology, and bioengineering have also begun to provide critically important information about cardiac function and malfunction. Although *Heart Disease: A Textbook of Cardiovascular Medicine* is primarily a clinical treatise and not a textbook of fundamental cardiovascular science, an effort has been made to explain, in some detail, the scientific bases of cardiovascular diseases.

EUGENE BRAUNWALD
1980

Contents

Part I ▪ Fundamentals of Cardiovascular Disease 1

CHAPTER 1
Global Burden of Cardiovascular Disease 1
J. Michael Gaziano

CHAPTER 2
Heart Disease in Varied Populations 23
Clyde W. Yancy

CHAPTER 3
Economics and Cardiovascular Disease 35
Mark A. Hlatky • Daniel B. Mark

CHAPTER 4
Clinical Decision-Making in Cardiology 41
Harlan M. Krumholz

CHAPTER 5
Measurement and Improvement of Quality of Cardiovascular Care 49
Thomas H. Lee

CHAPTER 6
The Principles of Drug Therapy 57
Dan M. Roden

Part II ▪ Molecular Biology and Genetics 67

CHAPTER 7
Principles of Cardiovascular Molecular Biology and Genetics 67
Elizabeth G. Nabel

CHAPTER 8
General Principles of Genetic Factors in Cardiovascular Disease 85
Reed E. Pyeritz • Christine E. Seidman

CHAPTER 9
Genetics of Cardiac Arrhythmias 101
Silvia G. Priori • Carlo Napolitano • Peter J. Schwartz

CHAPTER 10
Genetic Factors in Myocardial Disease 111
Jonathan G. Seidman • Reed E. Pyeritz • Christine E. Seidman

Part III ▪ Evaluation of the Patient 125

CHAPTER 11
The History and Physical Examination: An Evidence-Based Approach 125
James C. Fang • Patrick T. O'Gara

CHAPTER 12
Electrocardiography 149
David M. Mirvis • Ary L. Goldberger

  ⚫ GUIDELINES: Electrocardiography 190
    Thomas H. Lee

CHAPTER 13
Exercise Stress Testing 195
Bernard R. Chaitman

  ⚫ GUIDELINES: Exercise Stress Testing 220
    Thomas H. Lee

CHAPTER 14
Echocardiography 227
Heidi M. Connolly • Jae K. Oh

  ⚫ GUIDELINES: Use of Echocardiography 314
    Thomas H. Lee

CHAPTER 15
The Chest Radiograph in Cardiovascular Disease 327
Michael A. Bettmann

CHAPTER 16
Nuclear Cardiology 345
James E. Udelson • Vasken Dilsizian • Robert O. Bonow

  ⚫ GUIDELINES: Nuclear Cardiology 389
    Thomas H. Lee • James E. Udelson

CHAPTER 17
Cardiovascular Magnetic Resonance 393
Dudley Pennell

  ⚫ GUIDELINES: Appropriateness Guidelines: Cardiovascular Magnetic Resonance 412
    Thomas H. Lee

CHAPTER 18
Computed Tomography of the Heart   415
Stephan Achenbach • Werner G. Daniel

● GUIDELINES: Appropriateness Guidelines: Cardiac
Computed Tomography   436
Thomas H. Lee

CHAPTER 19
Cardiac Catheterization   439
Charles J. Davidson • Robert O. Bonow

CHAPTER 20
Coronary Arteriography and Intravascular
Imaging   465
Jeffrey J. Popma

● GUIDELINES: Coronary Arteriography   501
Thomas H. Lee

Part IV ■ Heart Failure   509

CHAPTER 21
Mechanisms of Cardiac Contraction and
Relaxation   509
Lionel H. Opie

CHAPTER 22
Pathophysiology of Heart Failure   541
Douglas L. Mann

CHAPTER 23
Clinical Assessment of Heart Failure   561
Otto M. Hess • John D. Carroll

CHAPTER 24
Diagnosis and Management of Acute Heart
Failure   583
John R. Teerlink

CHAPTER 25
Management of Heart Failure Patients with
Reduced Ejection Fraction   611
Douglas L. Mann

CHAPTER 26
Heart Failure with Normal Ejection
Fraction   641
Margaret M. Redfield

● GUIDELINES: Management of Heart Failure   657
Thomas H. Lee

CHAPTER 27
Surgical Management of Heart Failure   665
Patrick M. McCarthy

CHAPTER 28
Assisted Circulation in the Treatment of
Heart Failure   685
Yoshifumi Naka • Eric A. Rose

CHAPTER 29
Emerging Therapies and Strategies in the
Treatment of Heart Failure   697
Stefanie Dimmeler • Douglas L. Mann •
Andreas M. Zeiher

CHAPTER 30
Care of Patients with End-Stage Heart
Disease   717
Linda L. Emanuel • Robert O. Bonow

Part V ■ Arrhythmias, Sudden Death,
and Syncope   727

CHAPTER 31
Genesis of Cardiac Arrhythmias:
Electrophysiological Considerations   727
Michael Rubart • Douglas P. Zipes

CHAPTER 32
Diagnosis of Cardiac Arrhythmias   763
John M. Miller • Douglas P. Zipes

CHAPTER 33
Therapy for Cardiac Arrhythmias   779
John M. Miller • Douglas P. Zipes

● GUIDELINES: Ambulatory Electrocardiographic and
Electrophysiological Testing   823
Thomas H. Lee

CHAPTER 34
Cardiac Pacemakers and
Cardioverter-Defibrillators   831
David L. Hayes • Douglas P. Zipes

● GUIDELINES: Cardiac Pacemakers and
Cardioverter-Defibrillators   854
Thomas H. Lee

CHAPTER 35
Specific Arrhythmias: Diagnosis and
Treatment   863
Jeffrey E. Olgin • Douglas P. Zipes

● GUIDELINES: Atrial Fibrillation   923
Thomas H. Lee

CHAPTER 36
Cardiac Arrest and Sudden Cardiac
Death   933
Robert J. Myerburg • Agustin Castellanos

CHAPTER 37

Hypotension and Syncope 975
Hugh Calkins • Douglas P. Zipes

Part VI ▪ Preventive Cardiology 985

CHAPTER 38

The Vascular Biology of Atherosclerosis 985
Peter Libby

CHAPTER 39

Risk Factors for Atherothrombotic Disease 1003
Paul M. Ridker • Peter Libby

CHAPTER 40

Systemic Hypertension: Mechanisms and Diagnosis 1027
Ronald G. Victor • Norman M. Kaplan

CHAPTER 41

Systemic Hypertension: Therapy 1049
Norman M. Kaplan

 GUIDELINES: Treatment of Hypertension 1068
Thomas H. Lee

CHAPTER 42

Lipoprotein Disorders and Cardiovascular Disease 1071
Jacques Genest • Peter Libby

CHAPTER 43

Diabetes Mellitus, the Metabolic Syndrome, and Atherosclerotic Vascular Disease 1093
Joshua A. Beckman • Peter Libby • Mark A. Creager

CHAPTER 44

Nutrition and Cardiovascular Disease 1107
Ronald M. Krauss

CHAPTER 45

Primary and Secondary Prevention of Coronary Heart Disease 1119
J. Michael Gaziano • JoAnn E. Manson • Paul M. Ridker

CHAPTER 46

Exercise-Based, Comprehensive Cardiac Rehabilitation 1149
Paul D. Thompson

CHAPTER 47

Complementary and Alternative Approaches to Management of Patients with Heart Disease 1157
John H. K. Vogel • Rebecca B. Costello • Mitchell W. Krucoff

Part VII ▪ Atherosclerotic Cardiovascular Disease 1167

CHAPTER 48

Coronary Blood Flow and Myocardial Ischemia 1167
John M. Canty, Jr.

CHAPTER 49

Approach to the Patient with Chest Pain 1195
Christopher P. Cannon • Thomas H. Lee

CHAPTER 50

ST-Elevation Myocardial Infarction: Pathology, Pathophysiology, and Clinical Features 1207
Elliott M. Antman • Eugene Braunwald

CHAPTER 51

ST-Elevation Myocardial Infarction: Management 1233
Elliott M. Antman

CHAPTER 52

Primary Percutaneous Coronary Intervention in the Management of Acute Myocardial Infarction 1301
Gary E. Lane • David R. Holmes, Jr.

 GUIDELINES: Primary Percutaneous Coronary Intervention in Acute Myocardial Infarction 1314
Thomas H. Lee

CHAPTER 53

Unstable Angina and Non-ST Elevation Myocardial Infarction 1319
Christopher P. Cannon • Eugene Braunwald

 GUIDELINES: Unstable Angina and Non-ST Elevation Myocardial Infarction 1344
Thomas H. Lee

CHAPTER 54

Chronic Coronary Artery Disease 1353
David A. Morrow • Bernard J. Gersh

 GUIDELINES: Chronic Stable Angina 1405
Thomas H. Lee • David A. Morrow

CHAPTER 55
Percutaneous Coronary and Valvular Intervention 1419
Jeffrey J. Popma • Donald S. Baim • Frederic S. Resnic

GUIDELINES: Percutaneous Coronary and Valvular Intervention 1449
Thomas H. Lee

CHAPTER 56
Diseases of the Aorta 1457
Eric M. Isselbacher

CHAPTER 57
Peripheral Arterial Diseases 1491
Mark A. Creager • Peter Libby

CHAPTER 58
Prevention and Management of Stroke 1515
Larry B. Goldstein

CHAPTER 59
Endovascular Treatment of Noncoronary Obstructive Vascular Disease 1523
Andrew C. Eisenhauer • Christopher J. White

CHAPTER 60
Diabetes and Heart Disease 1547
Richard W. Nesto

Part VIII ▪ Diseases of the Heart, Pericardium, and Pulmonary Vasculature Bed 1561

CHAPTER 61
Congenital Heart Disease 1561
Gary D. Webb • Jeffrey F. Smallhorn • Judith Therrien • Andrew N. Redington

CHAPTER 62
Valvular Heart Disease 1625
Catherine M. Otto • Robert O. Bonow

GUIDELINES: Management of Valvular Heart Disease 1693
Thomas H. Lee • Robert O. Bonow

CHAPTER 63
Infective Endocarditis 1713
Adolf W. Karchmer

GUIDELINES: Infective Endocarditis 1734
Thomas H. Lee

CHAPTER 64
The Dilated, Restrictive, and Infiltrative Cardiomyopathies 1739
Joshua M. Hare

CHAPTER 65
Hypertrophic Cardiomyopathy 1763
Barry J. Maron

CHAPTER 66
Myocarditis 1775
Peter P. Liu • Heinz-Peter Schultheiss

CHAPTER 67
Cardiovascular Abnormalities in HIV-Infected Individuals 1793
Stacy D. Fisher • Steven E. Lipshultz

CHAPTER 68
Toxins and the Heart 1805
Richard A. Lange • L. David Hillis

CHAPTER 69
Primary Tumors of the Heart 1815
Bruce McManus • Cheng-Han Lee

CHAPTER 70
Pericardial Diseases 1829
Martin M. LeWinter

CHAPTER 71
Traumatic Heart Disease 1855
Matthew J. Wall, Jr. • Danny Chu • Kenneth L. Mattox

CHAPTER 72
Pulmonary Embolism 1863
Samuel Z. Goldhaber

CHAPTER 73
Pulmonary Hypertension 1883
Stuart Rich • Vallerie V. McLaughlin

CHAPTER 74
Sleep Apnea and Cardiovascular Disease 1915
Apoor S. Gami • Virend K. Somers

Part IX ▪ Cardiovascular Disease in Special Populations 1923

CHAPTER 75
Cardiovascular Disease in the Elderly 1923
Janice B. Schwartz • Douglas P. Zipes

CHAPTER 76
Cardiovascular Disease in Women   1955
L. Kristin Newby • Pamela S. Douglas

CHAPTER 77
Pregnancy and Heart Disease   1967
Carole A. Warnes

⬤ GUIDELINES: Pregnancy and Heart Disease   1979
Thomas H. Lee

CHAPTER 78
Exercise and Sports Cardiology   1983
Gary J. Balady • Philip A. Ades

CHAPTER 79
Medical Management of the Patient Undergoing Cardiac Surgery   1993
Richard J. Gray • Dhun H. Sethna

CHAPTER 80
Anesthesia and Noncardiac Surgery in Patients with Heart Disease   2013
Lee A. Fleisher • Kim A. Eagle

⬤ GUIDELINES: Reducing Cardiac Risk with Noncardiac Surgery   2028
Thomas H. Lee

Part X ▪ Cardiovascular Disease and Disorders of Other Organs   2033

CHAPTER 81
Endocrine Disorders and Cardiovascular Disease   2033
Irwin Klein

CHAPTER 82
Hemostasis, Thrombosis, Fibrinolysis, and Cardiovascular Disease   2049
Barbara A. Konkle • Daniel Simon • Andrew I. Schafer

CHAPTER 83
Rheumatic Fever   2079
B. Soma Raju • Zoltan G. Turi

CHAPTER 84
Rheumatic Diseases and the Cardiovascular System   2087
Brian F. Mandell • Gary S. Hoffman

CHAPTER 85
The Cancer Patient and Cardiovascular Disease   2105
Thomas Force

CHAPTER 86
Psychiatric and Behavioral Aspects of Cardiovascular Disease   2119
Lawson R. Wulsin • Arthur J. Barsky

CHAPTER 87
Neurological Disorders and Cardiovascular Disease   2135
William J. Groh • Douglas P. Zipes

CHAPTER 88
Interface Between Renal Disease and Cardiovascular Illness   2155
Peter A. McCullough

CHAPTER 89
Cardiovascular Manifestations of Autonomic Disorders   2171
Suraj Kapa • Virend K. Somers

Disclosure Index   DI-1

Index   I-1

PART VII

Atherosclerotic Cardiovascular Disease

CHAPTER **48**

Control of Coronary Blood Flow, 1167
Determinants of Myocardial Oxygen Consumption, 1167
Determinants of Coronary Vascular Resistance, 1171

Physiological Assessment of Coronary Artery Stenoses, 1177
Stenosis Pressure-Flow Relation, 1177
Interrelationship among Distal Coronary Pressure, Flow and Stenosis Severity, 1178
Concept of Maximal Perfusion and Coronary Reserve, 1178
Pathophysiological States Affecting Microcirculatory Coronary Flow Reserve, 1182

Coronary Collateral Circulation, 1183

Metabolic and Functional Consequences of Ischemia, 1184
Irreversible Injury and Myocyte Death, 1184
Reversible Ischemia and Perfusion-Contraction Matching, 1185

Future Perspectives, 1191

References, 1193

Coronary Blood Flow and Myocardial Ischemia

John M. Canty, Jr.

The coronary circulation is unique in that it is responsible for generating the arterial pressure that is required to perfuse the systemic circulation and yet, at the same time, has its own perfusion impeded during the systolic portion of the cardiac cycle. Because myocardial contraction is closely connected to coronary flow and oxygen delivery, the balance between oxygen supply and demand is a critical determinant of the normal beat to beat function of the heart. When this relationship is acutely disrupted by diseases affecting coronary blood flow, the resulting imbalance can immediately precipitate a vicious cycle, whereby ischemia-induced contractile dysfunction precipitates hypotension and further myocardial ischemia. Thus, a knowledge of the regulation of coronary blood flow, determinants of myocardial oxygen consumption, and the relationship between ischemia and contraction is essential for understanding the pathophysiological basis and management of many cardiovascular disorders.[1]

CONTROL OF CORONARY BLOOD FLOW

There are pronounced systolic and diastolic coronary flow variations throughout the cardiac cycle with coronary arterial inflow out of phase with venous outflow (Fig. 48-1).[2] Systolic contraction increases tissue pressure, redistributes perfusion from the subendocardial to the subepicardial layers of the heart, and impedes coronary arterial inflow which reaches a nadir. At the same time, systolic compression reduces the diameter of intramyocardial microcirculatory vessels (arterioles, capillaries, and venules) and increases coronary venous outflow, which peaks during systole. During diastole, coronary arterial inflow increases with a transmural gradient that favors perfusion to the subendocardial vessels. At this time, coronary venous outflow falls.

Determinants of Myocardial Oxygen Consumption

In contrast to most other vascular beds, myocardial oxygen extraction is near-maximal at rest, averaging approximately 75 percent of arterial oxygen content.[3] The ability to increase oxygen extraction as a means to increase oxygen delivery is limited to circumstances associated with sympathetic activation and acute subendocardial ischemia. Nevertheless, coronary venous oxygen tension (P_VO_2) can only decrease from 25 to approximately 15 torr. Because of the high resting oxygen extraction, increases in myocardial oxygen consumption ($M\dot{V}O_2$) are primarily met by proportional increases in coronary flow and oxygen delivery (Fig. 48-2). In addition to coronary flow, oxygen delivery is directly determined by arterial oxygen content. This is equal to the product of hemoglobin concentration and arterial oxygen saturation plus a small amount of oxygen dissolved in plasma that is directly related to PaO_2. Thus, for any given flow level, anemia results in proportional reductions in oxygen delivery, whereas the nonlinear oxygen dissociation curve results in relatively small reductions in oxygen content until PaO_2 falls to the steep portion of the oxygen dissociation curve (below 50 torr).

The major determinants of myocardial oxygen consumption are heart rate, systolic pressure (or myocardial wall stress), and left ventricular (LV) contractility. A twofold increase in any of these individual

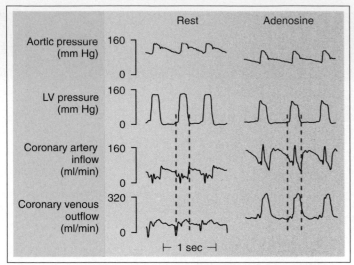

FIGURE 48–1 Phasic coronary arterial inflow and venous outflow at rest and adenosine vasodilation. Arterial inflow primarily occurs during diastole. During systole (dotted vertical lines), arterial inflow declines as venous outflow peaks, reflecting the compression of microcirculatory vessels during systole. After adenosine administration, the phasic variations in venous outflow are more pronounced. (*Modified from Canty JM Jr, Brooks A: Phasic volumetric coronary venous outflow patterns in conscious dogs. Am J Physiol 258:H1457, 1990.*)

CH 48

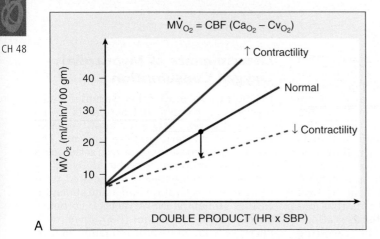

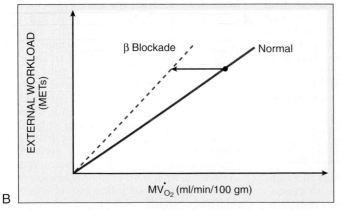

FIGURE 48–2 Fick equation and the relationship between heart rate (HR)–systolic pressure (SBP) double product and myocardial oxygen consumption ($M\dot{V}O_2$). **A,** Increases in $M\dot{V}O_2$ are primarily met by increases in coronary flow and linearly related to the double product. Twofold increases in HR, SBP, or contractility each result in approximately 50 percent increases in myocardial oxygen consumption. **B,** Beta blockade allows the same external workload to be accomplished at a lower cardiac workload ($M\dot{V}O_2$) by reducing the double product and myocardial contractility. CaO_2 = coronary arterial oxygen content; CBF = coronary blood flow; CvO_2 = coronary venous oxygen content.

determinants of oxygen consumption requires an approximately 50 percent increase in coronary flow. Experimentally, the systolic pressure volume area is proportional to myocardial work and linearly related to myocardial oxygen consumption. The basal myocardial oxygen requirements needed to maintain critical membrane function are low (approximately 15 percent of resting oxygen consumption) and the cost of electrical activation is trivial when mechanical contraction ceases during diastolic arrest (as with cardioplegia) and diminishes during ischemia (see Fig. 21-23).

Coronary Autoregulation

Regional coronary blood flow remains constant as coronary artery pressure is reduced below aortic pressure over a wide range when the determinants of myocardial oxygen consumption are kept constant.[4] This phenomenon is termed *autoregulation* (Fig. 48-3). When pressure falls to the lower limit of autoregulation, coronary resistance arteries are maximally vasodilated to intrinsic stimuli and flow becomes pressure-dependent, resulting in the onset of subendocardial ischemia. Resting coronary blood flow under normal hemodynamic conditions averages 0.7 to 1.0 ml/min/gm and can increase between four and fivefold during vasodilation.[5] The ability to increase flow above resting values in response to pharmacological vasodilation is termed *coronary reserve*. Flow in the maximally vasodilated heart is dependent on coronary arterial pressure. Maximum perfusion and coronary reserve are reduced when the diastolic time available for subendocardial perfusion is decreased (tachycardia) or the compressive determinants of diastolic perfusion (preload) are increased. Coronary reserve is also diminished by anything that increases resting flow, including increases in the hemodynamic determinants of oxygen consumption (systolic pressure, heart rate, and contractility) and reductions in arterial oxygen supply (anemia and hypoxia). Thus, circumstances can develop that precipitate subendocardial ischemia in the presence of normal coronary arteries.[1] Although initial studies have suggested that the lower pressure limit of autoregulation is 70 mm Hg, studies in conscious dogs in the basal state have shown that coronary flow can be autoregulated to mean coronary pressures as low as 40 mm Hg (diastolic pressures of 30 mm Hg).[4] These coronary pressure levels are similar to those recorded in humans without symptoms of ischemia, distal to chronic coronary occlusions, using pressure wire micromanometers. The lower autoregulatory pressure limit increases during tachycardia because of an increase in flow requirements, as well as a reduction in the time available for perfusion.[6]

Figure 48-4 illustrates important transmural variations in the lower autoregulatory pressure limit, which result in increased vulnerability of the subendocardium to ischemia.[1] Subendocardial flow primarily occurs in diastole and begins to decrease below a mean coronary pressure of 40 mm Hg.[4] In contrast, subepicardial flow occurs throughout the cardiac cycle and is maintained until coronary pressure falls below 25 mm Hg. This difference is primarily related to the increased oxygen consumption in the subendocardium, which requires a higher resting flow level, and to the more pronounced effects of systolic contraction on subendocardial vasodilator reserve.[1] The transmural difference in the lower autoregulatory pressure limit results in vulnerability of the subendocardium to ischemia at reduced pressures distal to a coronary stenosis. Although there is no pharmacologically recruitable flow reserve during ischemia in the normal coronary circulation,[7] reductions in coronary flow below the lower limit of autoregulation can occur in the presence of pharmacologically recruitable coronary flow reserve under certain circumstances.[8]

Endothelium-Dependent Modulation of Coronary Tone

Epicardial arteries do not normally contribute significantly to coronary vascular resistance, yet arterial diameter is modulated by a wide variety of paracrine factors that can be released from platelets, as well as circulating neurohormonal agonists, neural tone, and local control through vascular shear stress.[9] The most common factors related to cardiovascular disease are summarized in Table 48-1 (see Fig. 48-e1 on website). The net effect of many of these agonists is critically dependent on whether a functional endothelium is present. Furchgott and Zawadzki originally demonstrated that acetylcholine normally dilates arteries via an endothelium-dependent relaxing factor that was later identified to be nitric oxide (NO).[10] This binds to guanylyl

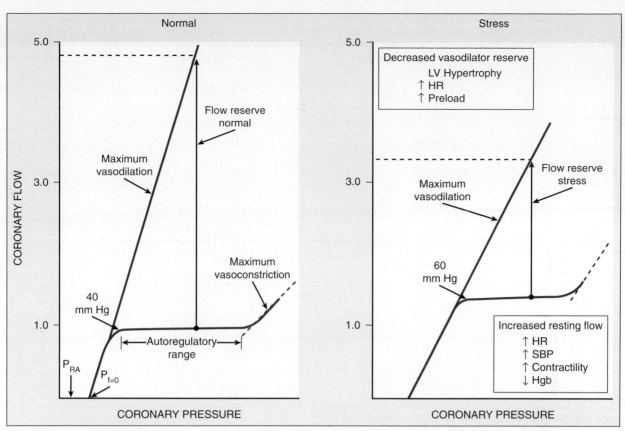

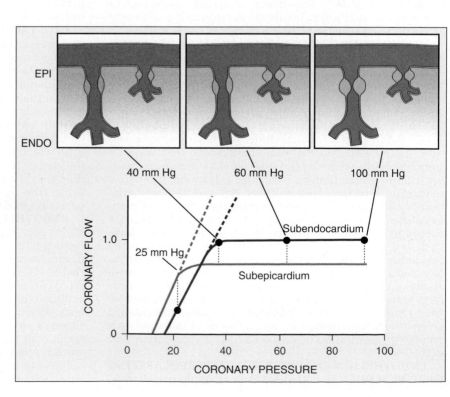

FIGURE 48–3 Autoregulatory relationship under basal conditions and following metabolic stress (e.g., tachycardia). The normal heart maintains coronary blood flow constant **(left panel)** as regional coronary pressure is varied over a wide range when the global determinants of oxygen consumption are kept constant (red lines). Below the lower autoregulatory pressure limit (approximately 40 mm Hg), subendocardial vessels are maximally vasodilated and myocardial ischemia develops. During vasodilation (blue lines), flow increases four to five times above resting values at a normal arterial pressure. Coronary flow ceases at a pressure higher than right atrial pressure (P_{RA}), called zero flow pressure ($P_{f=0}$), which is the effective back pressure to flow in the absence of coronary collaterals. Following stress **(right panel)**, factors that increase the compressive determinants of coronary resistance, or reduce the time available for perfusion, reduce maximum vasodilated flow. In addition, increases in myocardial oxygen demand or reductions in arterial oxygen content increase resting flow. These changes reduce coronary flow reserve, the ratio between dilated and resting coronary flow, and cause ischemia to develop at higher coronary pressures. LV = left ventricular; HR = heart rate; SBP = systolic blood pressure; Hgb = hemoglobin.

FIGURE 48–4 Transmural variations in coronary autoregulation and myocardial metabolism. Increased vulnerability of the subendocardium (ENDO; red) versus subepicardium (EPI; gold) to ischemia reflects the fact that autoregulation is exhausted at a higher coronary pressure (40 versus 25 mm Hg). This is the result of increased resting flow and oxygen consumption in the subendocardium and an increased sensitivity to systolic compressive effects, because subendocardial flow only occurs during diastole. Subendocardial vessels become maximally vasodilated before those in the subepicardium as coronary artery pressure is reduced. These transmural differences can be increased further during tachycardia or during conditions with elevated preload, which reduce maximum subendocardial perfusion.

CH 48

Coronary Blood Flow and Myocardial Ischemia

TABLE 48–1 Endothelium-Dependent and Net Direct Effects of Neural Stimulation, Autocoids, and Vasodilators on Coronary Tone in Isolated Conduit and Coronary Resistance Arteries

Substance	Endothelium-Dependent	Normal Response	Atherosclerosis
Acetylcholine			
Conduit	Nitric oxide	Net dilation	Constriction
Resistance	Nitric oxide, EDHF	Dilation	Attenuated dilation
Norepinephrine			
Alpha$_1$		Constriction	Constriction
Beta$_2$	Nitric oxide	Dilation	Attenuated dilation
Platelets			
Thrombin	Nitric oxide	Dilation	Constriction
Serotonin			
Conduit	Nitric oxide	Constriction	Constriction
Resistance	Nitric oxide	Dilation	Constriction
ADP	Nitric oxide	Dilation	Attenuated dilation
Thromboxane	Endothelin	Constriction	Constriction
Paracrine Agonists			
Bradykinin	Nitric oxide, EDHF	Dilation	Attenuated dilation
Histamine	Nitric oxide	Dilation	Attenuated dilation
Substance P	Nitric oxide	Dilation	Attenuated dilation
Endothelin (ET)			
ET-1	Nitric oxide	Net constriction	Increased constriction
Vasodilators			
Adenosine		Dilation	Dilation
Dipyridamole		Dilation	Dilation
Papaverine		Dilation	Dilation
Nitroglycerin		Dilation	Dilation

ADP=adenosine diphosphate; EDHF=endothelium-dependent hyperpolarizing factor.

cyclase and increases cyclic guanosine monophosphate (cGMP), resulting in vascular smooth muscle relaxation. When the endothelium is removed, the dilation to acetylcholine is converted to vasoconstriction, reflecting the effect of muscarinic vascular smooth muscle contraction. Subsequent studies have demonstrated that coronary artery resistance arteries also exhibit endothelial modulation of diameter and that the response to physical forces such as shear stress, as well as paracrine mediators, vary with resistance vessel size.[11] The major endothelium-dependent biochemical pathways involved in regulating coronary epicardial and resistance artery diameter are as follows.

NITRIC OXIDE (ENDOTHELIUM-DERIVED RELAXING FACTOR, EDRF). NO is produced in endothelial cells by the enzymatic conversion of L-arginine to citrulline via type III NO synthase. This reaction is controlled by calcium and calmodulin and is dependent on molecular oxygen, nicotinamide adenine dinucleotide phosphate, reduced form (NADPH), tetrahydrobiopterin, adenosine diphosphate (ADP), flavin adenine dinucleotide, and flavin mononucleotide. Endothelial NO diffuses abluminally into vascular smooth muscle, where it binds to guanylate cyclase, increasing cGMP production and causing relaxation through a reduction in intracellular calcium. NO-mediated vasodilation is enhanced by cyclical or pulsatile changes in coronary shear stress. Chronic upregulation of NO synthase occurs in response to episodic increases in coronary flow, such as during exercise training, which also potentiates the relaxation to various endothelium-dependent vasodilators. NO-mediated vasodilation is impaired in many disease states and in patients with one or more risk factors for coronary artery disease (CAD). This occurs via inactivation of NO by superoxide anion generated in response to oxidative stress. Such inactivation is the hallmark of impaired NO-mediated vasodilation in atherosclerosis, hypertension, and diabetes.

ENDOTHELIUM-DEPENDENT HYPERPOLARIZING FACTOR (EDHF). Endothelium-dependent hyperpolariza-

tion is an additional mechanism for selected agonists (e.g., bradykinin), as well as shear stress-induced vasodilation, in the human coronary microcirculation. EDHF is produced by the endothelium, hyperpolarizes vascular smooth muscle, and dilates arteries by opening calcium-activated potassium channels. Although the exact biochemical species of EDHF is still unclear, it appears to be a metabolite of arachidonic acid metabolism produced by the cytochrome P-450 epoxygenase pathway. The most prominent candidates are epoxyeicosatrienoic acid and endothelium-derived hydrogen peroxide.

PROSTACYCLIN. Metabolism of arachidonic acid via cyclooxygenase can also produce prostacyclin, which is a coronary vasodilator when administered exogenously. There is evidence that prostacyclin contributes to tonic coronary vasodilation in humans. Nevertheless, blocking the actions of vasodilator prostaglandins using inhibitors of cyclooxygenase fails to alter flow during ischemia distal to a stenosis or limit oxygen consumption in response to increases in metabolism, suggesting that inhibition may be overcome by other compensatory vasodilator pathways.[9] In contrast to the native resistance vasculature, vasodilator prostaglandins are very important determinants of coronary collateral vessel tone, and blocking cyclooxygenase reduces collateral perfusion in dogs.

ENDOTHELIN (ET). The endothelins (ET-1, ET-2, and ET-3) are peptide endothelium-dependent constricting factors. ET-1 is a potent constrictor derived from the enzymatic cleavage of a larger precursor molecule (pre-pro–endothelin) via endothelin-converting enzyme. In contrast to the rapid vascular smooth muscle relaxation and recovery characteristic of endothelium-derived vasodilators (NO, EDHF, and prostacyclin), the constriction to ET is prolonged. Changes in ET levels are largely mediated through transcriptional control and produce longer-term changes in coronary vasomotor tone. The effects of ET are mediated by binding to both ET-A and ET-B receptors. ET-A–mediated constriction is caused by the activation of protein kinase C in vascular smooth muscle. ET-B–mediated constriction is less pronounced and counterbalanced by prominent ET-B–mediated endothelium-dependent NO production and vasodilation. ET is not involved in regulating coronary blood flow in the normal heart but can modulate vascular tone when circulating concentrations increase in pathophysiological states such as heart failure.

Determinants of Coronary Vascular Resistance

The resistance to coronary blood flow can be divided into three major components, as summarized in Figure 48-5.[5] Under normal circumstances, there is no measurable pressure drop in the epicardial arteries, indicating negligible conduit resistance (R_1). With the development of hemodynamically significant epicardial artery narrowing (more than 50 percent diameter reduction), the fixed conduit artery resistance begins to contribute an increasing component to total coronary resistance and, when severely narrowed (more than 90 percent), may reduce resting flow.

The second component of coronary resistance (R_2) is dynamic and primarily arises from microcirculatory resistance arteries and arterioles. This is distributed throughout the myocardium across a broad range of microcirculatory resistance vessel size (20 to 200 µm in diameter) and changes in response to physical forces (intraluminal pressure and shear stress), as well as the metabolic needs of the tissue. There is normally little resistance contributed by coronary venules and capillaries and their resistance remains fairly constant during changes in vasomotor tone. Even in the maximally vasodilated heart, capillary resistance accounts for no more than 20 percent of the microvascular resistance.[12] Thus, a twofold increase in capillary density would only increase maximal myocardial perfusion by approximately 10 percent. Minimal coronary vascular resistance of the microcirculation is primarily determined by the size and density of arterial resistance vessels and results in substantial coronary flow reserve in the normal heart.

The third component, or compressive resistance (R_3), varies with time throughout the cardiac cycle and is related to cardiac contraction and systolic pressure development within the left ventricle. In heart failure, compressive effects from elevated ventricular diastolic pressure also impede perfusion via passive compression of microcirculatory vessels by elevated extravascular tissue pressure during diastole. Increases in preload effectively raise the normal back pressure to coronary flow above coronary venous pressure levels.[8] Compressive effects are most prominent in the subendocardium and are discussed in greater detail later.

Extravascular Compressive Resistance (R_3)

During systole, cardiac contraction raises extravascular tissue pressure to values equal to LV pressure at the subendocardium while it falls to values near pleural pressure at the subepicardium.[3] This produces a time-varying reduction in the

driving pressure for coronary flow caused by a vascular waterfall mechanism that impedes blood flow to the subendocardium. Although this paradigm can explain variations in systolic coronary inflow, it is not able to account for the increase in coronary venous systolic outflow. To explain both impaired inflow and accelerated venous outflow, Hoffman and Spaan have proposed the concept of the intramyocardial pump.[8] In this model, the microcirculatory vessels are compressed during systole and the deformation leads to a capacitive discharge of blood, which accelerates flow from the microcirculation into the coronary venous system (Fig. 48-6). At the same time, the upstream capacitive discharge impedes systolic coronary arterial inflow. Although this explains the phasic variations in coronary arterial inflow and venous outflow, as well as its transmural distribution in systole, vascular capacitance cannot explain compressive effects related to elevated tissue pressure during diastole. Thus, components of intramyocardial capacitance, compressive changes in resistance, and time-varying driving pressure are all likely to contribute to the compressive determinants of phasic coronary blood flow.

Transmural Variations in Minimum Coronary Resistance (R_2)

Although the subendocardium is the most vulnerable region of the myocardium to ischemia,[1] it is protected by a transmural gradient in arteriolar and capillary density, which are

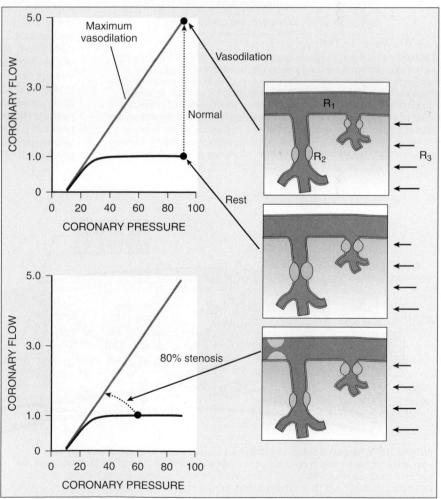

FIGURE 48–5 Schematic of components of coronary vascular resistance with and without a coronary stenosis. R_1 is epicardial conduit artery resistance, which is normally insignificant; R_2 is resistance secondary to metabolic and autoregulatory adjustments in flow and occurs in arterioles and resistance arteries; and R_3 is the time-varying compressive resistance that is higher in subendocardial than subepicardial layers. In the normal heart, $R_2 > R_3 \gg R_1$. The development of a proximal stenosis or pharmacological vasodilation reduces arteriolar resistance (R_2). In the presence of a severe epicardial stenosis, $R_1 > R_3 > R_2$.

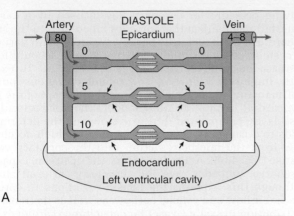

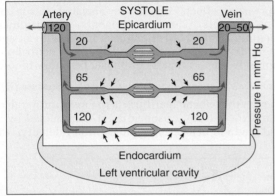

FIGURE 48-6 Effects of systolic contraction on transmural perfusion. During systole **(B)**, cardiac contraction increases intramyocardial tissue pressure surrounding compliant arterioles and venules. This results in a concealed arterial "backflow" that reduces systolic inflow in the epicardial artery, as depicted in Figure 48-1. Compression of venules accelerates venous outflow. Compressive effects during diastole **(A)** are related to tissue pressures that decrease from the subendocardium to subepicardium. At diastolic LV pressures greater than 20 mm Hg, preload determines the effective back pressure to coronary diastolic perfusion. *(Modified from Hoffman JIE, Baer RW, Hanley FL, et al: Regulation of transmural myocardial blood flow. J Biomech Eng 107:2, 1985.)*

higher than in subepicardial regions and increase subendocardial perfusion in the diastolic arrested heart. Because of this vascular gradient, transmural flow during maximal pharmacological vasodilation of the beating heart is uniform. When heart rate increases during tachycardia in the maximally vasodilated heart, there are pronounced reductions in subendocardial perfusion, whereas there is little change in maximal subepicardial perfusion. This results in a progressive fall in the endocardial to epicardial flow ratio and increases the subendocardial vulnerability to ischemia.

Coronary vascular resistance in the maximally vasodilated heart is also pressure dependent. This largely reflects passive distention of arterial resistance vessels. As a result, the instantaneous value of coronary resistance obtained at a normal coronary distending pressure will be lower than that at a reduced pressure. The curvilinearity of the coronary pressure flow relationship is prominent at reduced pressures (less than 50 mm Hg) and can lead to underestimation of the physiological significance of coronary stenoses derived from distal coronary pressure measurements during vasodilation, because these indices assume that the pressure-flow relationship is linear.[13]

The precise determinants of coronary driving pressure continue to be controversial. Earlier investigations demonstrated that coronary flow could stop at diastolic pressures as high as 40 to 50 mm Hg when vasomotor tone was present, suggesting that the back pressure to flow was governed by a vascular waterfall, resulting in critical closure of arteriolar vessels.[8] These were probably overestimates because of capacitive effects but, during constant pressure perfusion of the coronary circulation, the pressure axis intercept with vasomotor tone present is considerably higher than right atrial or diastolic LV pressure. This has been termed *zero flow pressure* ($P_{f=0}$) and can decrease to values of approximately 10 mm Hg during vasodilation. The back pressure to coronary flow becomes dependent on LV diastolic pressure when preload is elevated above 20 mm Hg. This has a very profound effect on subendocardial perfusion at reduced pressures encountered distal to coronary artery stenoses, as well as in the failing heart.

Structure and Function of the Coronary Microcirculation

The schematics in Figures 48-4 and 48-5 suggest a fairly localized site for the control of coronary vascular resistance that is useful for conceptualizing the major determinants of coronary vascular resistance. In fact, individual coronary resistance arteries are a longitudinally distributed network and in vivo studies of the coronary microcirculation have demonstrated considerable spatial heterogeneity of specific resistance vessel control mechanisms (Fig. 48-7).[9,11] Each resistance vessel needs to dilate in an orchestrated fashion to meet the needs of the downstream vascular bed, which is frequently removed from the site of resistance artery control. This can be accomplished independently of metabolic signals by sensing physical forces such as intraluminal flow (shear stress–mediated control) or intraluminal pressure changes (myogenic control). Epicardial arteries (more than 400 μm in diameter) serve a conduit artery function, with diameter primarily regulated by shear stress, and contribute little pressure drop (less than 5 percent) over a wide range of coronary flow. Coronary resistance vessels can be divided into resistance arteries (100 to 400 μm), which regulate their tone in response to local shear stress and luminal pressure changes (myogenic response), and arterioles (smaller than 100 μm),

FIGURE 48-7 Transmural distribution of coronary resistance vessels—major vasodilatory and vasoconstrictor mechanisms in epicardial conduit arteries and different sites of the microcirculation. The epicardial conduit arteries arborize into subepicardial and subendocardial resistance arteries. Intramural penetrating resistance arteries are unique in that they are removed from subendocardial metabolic stimuli and theoretically are more dependent on regulating their tone in response to shear stress and luminal pressure as mechanisms to produce dilation in response to changes in metabolism of the distal subendocardial arteriolar plexus. See text for further discussion. NEβ2 = beta2 adrenergic; NEα1 = alpha1 adrenergic; Ach = acetylcholine; TXA2 = thromboxane A2; 5-HT = serotonin; ET = endothelin; EDHF = endothelium-dependent hyperpolarizing factor; NO = nitric oxide; KATP = ATP-dependent potassium channel. *(Modified from Duncker DJ, Bache RJ: Regulation of coronary vasomotor tone under normal conditions and during acute myocardial hypoperfusion. Pharmacol Ther 86:87, 2000.)*

which are sensitive to changes in local tissue metabolism and directly control perfusion of the low-resistance coronary capillary bed. Capillary density of the myocardium averages 3500/mm², resulting in an average intercapillary distance of 17 μm, and is greater in the subendocardium than the subepicardium.

Under resting conditions, most of the pressure drop in the microcirculation arises in resistance arteries between 50 and 200 μm, with little pressure drop occurring across capillaries and venules at normal flow levels (Fig. 48-8A).[12] Following pharmacological vasodilation with dipyridamole, resistance artery vasodilation minimizes the precapillary pressure drop in arterial resistance vessels. At the same time, there is an increased pressure drop and redistribution of resistance to venular vessels, in which smooth muscle relaxation is limited and the already low resistance is fairly fixed.

There is considerable heterogeneity in microcirculatory vasodilation during physiological adjustments in flow. For example, as pressure is reduced during autoregulation, dilation is primarily accomplished by arterioles smaller than 100 μm, whereas larger resistance arteries tend to constrict because of the reduction in perfusion pressure (see Fig. 48-8B).[14] In contrast, metabolic vasodilation results from a more uniform vasodilation of resistance vessels of all sizes (see Fig. 48-8C).[15] Similar inhomogeneity in resistance vessel dilation occurs in response to endothelium-dependent agonists as well as pharmacological vasodilators.

A unique component of subendocardial coronary resistance vessels are the transmural penetrating arteries that course from the epicardium to the subendocardial plexus.[9] These vessels are removed from the metabolic stimuli that develop when ischemia is confined to the subendocardium. As a result, local control from altered shear stress and myogenic relaxation to local pressure become very critical determinants of diameter in this "upstream" resistance segment. Even during maximal vasodilation, this segment creates an additional longitudinal component of coronary vascular resistance that must be traversed before the arteriolar microcirculation is reached. Because of this greater longitudinal pressure drop, the microcirculatory pressures in subendocardial coronary arterioles are lower than in the subepicardial arterioles.

Intraluminal Physical Forces Regulating Coronary Resistance

Because much of the coronary resistance vasculature can be upstream from the effects of metabolic mediators of control, local vascular control mechanisms are critically important in orchestrating adequate regional tissue perfusion to the distal microcirculation. There is a differential expression of mechanisms among different sizes and classes of coronary resistance vessels, which coincides with their function.

MYOGENIC REGULATION. The myogenic response refers to the ability of vascular smooth muscle to oppose changes in coronary arteriolar diameter. Thus, vessels relax when distending pressure is decreased and constrict when distending pressure is elevated (Fig. 48-9A). Myogenic tone is a property of vascular smooth muscle and occurs across a large size range of coronary resistance arteries in animals[16] as well as in humans.[17] Although the cellular mechanism is uncertain, it is dependent on vascular smooth muscle calcium entry, perhaps through stretch-activated L-type Ca²⁺ channels, eliciting cross-bridge

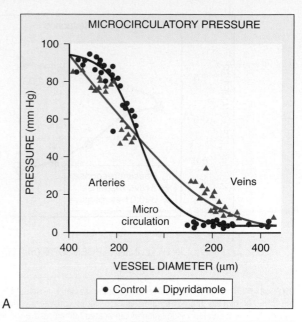
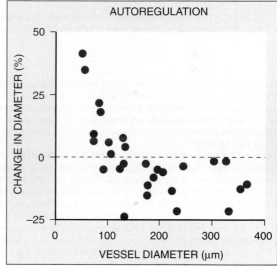
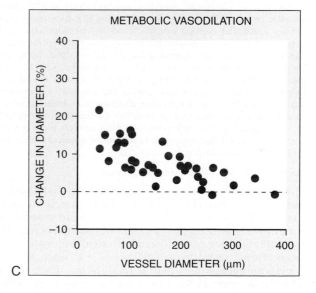

FIGURE 48-8 Microcirculatory pressure profile and local resistance changes to physiological stimuli in subepicardial vessels. **A,** Under resting conditions, most of the pressure drop to flow arises from resistance arteries and arterioles. Following dipyridamole vasodilation, there is a redistribution of microcirculatory resistance, with a greater pressure drop occurring across postcapillary venules that do not alter their resistance. **B,** Heterogeneous arterial microvessel response during autoregulation. A reduction in pressure to 38 mm Hg elicited dilation in arterioles smaller than 100 μm, whereas larger arteries tended to constrict passively from the reduction in distending pressure. **C,** Homogeneous vasodilation of resistance arteries during increases in myocardial oxygen consumption. There is dilation in all microvascular resistance arteries that is greatest in vessels smaller than 100 μm. (**A** modified from Chilian WM, Layne SM, Klausner EC, et al: Redistribution of coronary microvascular resistance produced by dipyridamole. Am J Physiol 256: H383, 1989; **B** modified from Kanatsuka H, Lamping KG, Eastham CL, et al: Heterogeneous changes in epimyocardial microvessel size during graded coronary stenosis. Evidence of the microvascular site for autoregulation. Circ Res 66:389, 1990; **C** modified from Kanatsuka H, Lamping KG, Eastham CL, et al: Comparison of the effects of increased myocardial oxygen consumption and adenosine on the coronary microvascular resistance. Circ Res 65:1296, 1989.)

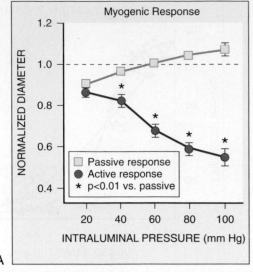

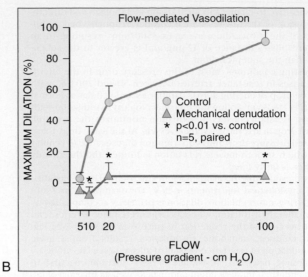

FIGURE 48–9 Effects of physical forces on coronary diameter in isolated human coronary resistance arteries (nominal diameter, 100 μm). **A,** As distending pressure is reduced from 100 mm Hg, there is progressive vasodilation consistent with myogenic regulation. Myogenic dilation reaches the maximum passive diameter of the vessel at 20 mm Hg. **B,** Flow-mediated vasodilation in cannulated human resistance arteries. As the pressure gradient across the isolated vessel is increased, intraluminal flow rises and causes progressive dilation that is abolished by removing the endothelium. Similar flow-mediated dilation occurs in most arterial vessels, including the coronary conduit arteries. (**A** modified from Miller FJ, Dellsperger KC, Gutterman DD: Myogenic constriction of human coronary arterioles. Am J Physiol 273:H257, 1997. Used with permission of the American Physiological Society; **B** modified from Miura H, Wachtel RE, Liu Y, et al: Flow-induced dilation of human coronary arterioles: Important role of Ca²⁺-activated K⁺ channels. Circulation 103:1992, 2001.)

activation. The resistance changes arising from the myogenic response tend to bring local coronary flow back to the original level. Myogenic regulation has been postulated to be one of the important mechanisms of the coronary autoregulatory response and, in vivo, appears to primarily occur in arterioles smaller than 100 μm (e.g., during autoregulation; see Fig. 48-8B).[14]

FLOW-MEDIATED RESISTANCE ARTERY CONTROL. Coronary resistance arteries and arterioles also regulate their diameter in response to changes in local shear stress (see Fig. 48-9B). Flow-induced dilation in isolated coronary arterioles was originally demonstrated by Kuo and colleagues.[11,18] They found this to be endothelium-dependent and mediated by NO, because it could be abolished with an L-arginine analogue. In contrast, isolated atrial vessels from patients undergoing cardiac surgery exhibit flow-mediated vasodilation that is mediated by EDHF.[19] The disparity with animal studies may reflect age or species variability in the relative importance of EDHF versus NO in the coronary circulation. The mechanisms also appear to vary as a function of vessel size, with studies in pigs demonstrating that hyperpolarization regulates epicardial conduit arteries[20] and NO predominates in the resistance vasculature.[18] Finally, EDHF may represent a compensatory pathway that is normally inhibited by NO and becomes upregulated in acquired disease states, in which NO-mediated vasodilation is impaired.[19] Despite the variability in isolated vessels, blocking NO synthase with an L-arginine analogue in the coronary circulation of humans reduces vasodilation to pharmacological endothelium-dependent agonists and attenuates flow increases during metabolic vasodilation, demonstrating that NO-mediated vasodilatation plays a role in determining physiological vascular tone in some segments of the coronary resistance vasculature.[21]

Metabolic Mediators of Coronary Resistance

Despite increasing knowledge regarding the distribution of coronary microvascular resistance, there is still no consensus regarding specific mediators of metabolic vasodilation. Coronary resistance in any segment of the microcirculation represents the integration of local physical factors (e.g., pressure and flow), vasodilator metabolites (e.g., adenosine, PO_2, and pH), autocoids, and neural modulation. Each of these mechanisms contributes to net coronary vascular smooth muscle tone, which may ultimately be controlled by opening and closing vascular smooth muscle ATP-sensitive K⁺ (K⁺-ATP) channels. There is considerable redundancy in the available local control mechanisms.[9] Because of this, blocking single mechanisms fails to alter coronary autoregulation

or metabolic flow regulation at normal coronary pressures. This redundancy can, however, be unmasked by stressing the heart and evaluating flow regulation at reduced pressures distal to a coronary stenosis at rest or during exercise.[9] Some of the candidates proposed and their role in metabolic resistance control and ischemia-induced vasodilation are summarized here.[3]

ADENOSINE. There has been a longstanding interest in the role of adenosine as a metabolic mediator of resistance artery control. It is released from cardiac myocytes when the rate of ATP hydrolysis exceeds its synthesis during ischemia. Its production and release also increase with myocardial metabolism. Adenosine has an extremely short half-life (less than 10 seconds) caused by its rapid inactivation by adenosine deaminase. It binds to A2 receptors on vascular smooth muscle, increases cyclic adenosine monophosphate (cAMP), and opens intermediate calcium-activated potassium channels.[22] Adenosine has a differential effect on coronary resistance arteries, primarily dilating vessels smaller than 100 μm.[15] Although adenosine has no direct effect on larger resistance arteries and conduit arteries, these dilate through endothelium-dependent vasodilation from the concomitant increases in local shear stress as arteriolar resistance falls.[23] Despite the attractiveness of adenosine as a local metabolic control mechanism, there is now substantial in vivo experimental data to demonstrate convincingly that it is not required for adjusting coronary flow to increases in metabolism or autoregulation.[24] It may, however, contribute to vasodilation during hypoxia as well as during acute exercise-induced myocardial ischemia distal to a stenosis.[9]

ATP-SENSITIVE K⁺ CHANNELS. Coronary vascular smooth muscle K⁺-ATP channels are tonically active, contributing to coronary vascular tone under resting conditions. Preventing K⁺-ATP channel opening with glibenclamide causes constriction of arterioles smaller than 100 μm, reduces coronary flow, and accentuates myocardial ischemia distal to a coronary stenosis by overcoming intrinsic vasodilatory mechanisms.[9] The K⁺-ATP channels can modulate both the coronary metabolic and autoregulatory responses. It is a potentially attractive mechanism, because many of the other candidates for metabolic flow regulation (e.g., adenosine, NO, beta$_2$ adrenoreceptors, and prostacyclin) are ultimately affected by blocking this pathway. Nevertheless, it is likely that K$^+$-ATP channel opening is a common effector rather than sensor of metabolic activity or of autoregulatory adjustments in flow. It is also possible that the reductions in coronary flow observed after blocking K$^+$-ATP channel vasodilation are pharmacological, caused by vasoconstriction of the microcirculation that overcomes intrinsic vasodilatory stimuli, as seen when other potent vasoconstrictors (e.g., endothelin or vasopressin) are administered at pharmacological doses.

HYPOXIA. Although a potent coronary vasodilatory stimulus, the role of local PO$_2$ in the regulation of arteriolar tone remains unresolved. Coronary flow increases in proportion to reductions in arterial oxygen content (reduced PO$_2$ or anemia) and there is a twofold increase in perfused capillary density in response to hypoxia.[3] Nevertheless, studies demonstrating a direct effect of oxygen on metabolic or autoregulatory adjustments are lacking and the vasodilatory response to reduced arterial oxygen delivery may simply reflect the close coupling between myocardial metabolism and flow.

ACIDOSIS. Arterial hypercapnea and acidosis (PCO$_2$) are potent stimuli that have been demonstrated to produce coronary vasodilation independent of hypoxia. Whereas their precise role in the local regulation of myocardial perfusion remains unclear, it seems reasonable that some of the vasodilation occurring with increased myocardial metabolism could arise from increased myocardial CO$_2$ production and tissue acidosis in the setting of acute ischemia.[3]

Neural Control of Coronary Conduit and Resistance Arteries

Sympathetic and vagal nerves innervate coronary conduit arteries and segments of the resistance vasculature. Neural stimulation affects tone through mechanisms that alter vascular smooth muscle as well as by stimulating the release of NO from the endothelium. Diametrically opposite effects can occur in the presence of risk factors that impair endothelium-dependent vasodilation. Their actions in normal and pathophysiological states are summarized in Table 48-1.

CHOLINERGIC INNERVATION. Resistance arteries dilate to acetylcholine, resulting in increases in coronary flow. In conduit arteries, acetylcholine normally causes mild coronary vasodilation. This reflects the net action of a direct muscarinic constriction of vascular smooth muscle counterbalanced by an endothelium-dependent vasodilation caused by direct stimulation of NOS and an increased flow-mediated dilation from concomitant resistance vessel vasodilation. The response in humans with atherosclerosis or risk factors for CAD is distinctly different. The resistance vessel dilation to acetylcholine is attenuated and the reduction in flow-mediated NO production leads to net epicardial conduit artery vasoconstriction, which is particularly prominent in stenotic segments (Fig. 48-10A).

SYMPATHETIC INNERVATION. Under basal conditions, there is no resting sympathetic tone in the heart and thus there is no effect of denervation on resting perfusion. During sympathetic activation, coronary tone is modulated by norepinephrine released from myocardial sympathetic nerves, as well as by circulating norepinephrine and epinephrine.[3,25] In conduit arteries, sympathetic stimulation leads to alpha$_1$ constriction as well as beta$_2$-mediated vasodilation. The net effect is to dilate epicardial coronary arteries. This dilation is potentiated by concomitant flow-mediated vasodilation from metabolic vasodilation of coronary resistance vessels. When NO-mediated vasodilation is impaired, alpha$_1$ constriction predominates and can dynamically increase stenosis severity in asymmetrical lesions where

the stenosis is compliant. This is one of the mechanisms that can provoke ischemia during sympathetic activation from cold pressor testing (see Fig. 48-10B).

The effects of sympathetic activation on myocardial perfusion and coronary resistance vessel tone are complex and dependent on the net actions of beta$_1$-mediated increases in myocardial oxygen consumption (resulting from increases in the determinants of myocardial oxygen consumption), direct beta$_2$-mediated coronary vasodilation, and alpha$_1$-mediated coronary constriction. Under normal conditions, exercise-induced beta$_2$-adrenergic "feed forward" dilation predominates, resulting in a higher flow relative to the level of myocardial oxygen consumption.[24] This neural control mechanism produces transient vasodilation before the buildup of local metabolites during exercise and prevents the development of subendocardial ischemia during abrupt changes in demand. After nonselective beta blockade, sympathetic activation unmasks alpha$_1$-mediated coronary artery constriction. Although flow is mildly decreased, oxygen delivery is maintained by increased oxygen extraction and a reduction in coronary venous PO$_2$ at similar levels of cardiac workload. Intense alpha$_1$-adrenergic constriction can overcome intrinsic stimuli for metabolic vasodilation to result in ischemia in the presence of pharmacological vasodilator reserve.[25] The role of pre- and postsynaptic alpha$_2$ responses is controversial. They appear to have a less significant role in controlling flow. This partly reflects the competing effects of presynaptic alpha$_2$ receptor stimulation, leading to reduced vasoconstriction by inhibiting norepinephrine release.

Paracrine Vasoactive Mediators and Coronary Vasospasm

There are a large number of paracrine factors that can affect coronary tone in normal and pathophysiological states that are unrelated to normal coronary circulatory control. The most important of these are summarized in Table 48-1 (see Fig. 48-e1 on website). Many of these agonists are released in epicardial artery thrombi after activation of the thrombotic cascade from plaque rupture. These can have important effects in modulating epicardial tone in regions near eccentric ulcerated plaques that are still responsive to stimuli that alter smooth muscle relaxation and constriction, leading to dynamic functional stenosis behavior. Many of these mediators exert differential effects on vasomotion, which are dependent on vessel size (conduit arteries versus resistance arteries) as well as on the presence of a functionally normal endothelium, because they stimulate the release of NO and EDHF.

Serotonin released from activated platelets causes vasoconstriction in normal and atherosclerotic conduit arteries and can increase the functional severity of a dynamic coronary stenosis through superimposed vasospasm. In contrast, it dilates coronary resistance vessels (smaller than 100 μm) and increases coronary flow through the endothelium-dependent release of NO. In atherosclerosis or circumstances in which NO production is impaired, the direct effects on smooth muscle predominate and the response of the microcirculation is converted to vasoconstriction. As a result, serotonin release generally exacerbates ischemia in CAD.

Thromboxane A$_2$ is a potent vasoconstrictor that is a product of endoperoxide metabolism and released during platelet aggregation. It produces vasoconstriction of conduit arteries as well as isolated coronary resistance vessels and can accentuate acute myocardial ischemia.

Adenosine diphosphate (ADP) is another platelet-derived vasodilator that relaxes coronary microvessels as well as conduit arteries. It is mediated by NO and abolished by removing the endothelium.

Thrombin normally leads to vasodilation in vitro that is endothelial-dependent and mediated by the release of prostacyclin as well as NO. In vivo, it also releases thromboxane A$_2$, leading to vasoconstriction in epicardial stenoses where endothelium-dependent vasodilation is impaired. In the coronary resistance vasculature, it acts as an endothelium-dependent vasodilator and increases coronary flow.

CORONARY VASOSPASM. Coronary spasm results in transient functional occlusion of a coronary artery that is reversible with nitrate vasodilation. It most commonly occurs in the setting of a coronary stenosis, leading to dynamic stenosis behavior, and can dissociate the

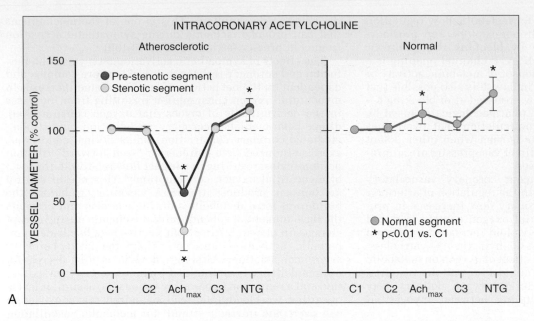

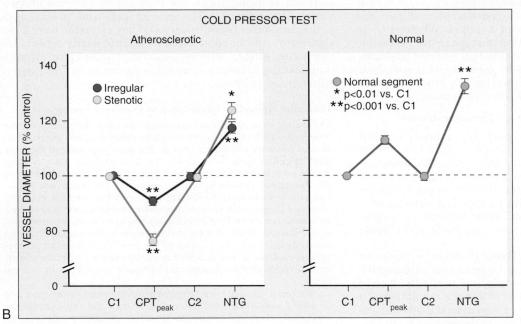

FIGURE 48–10 Differential conduit artery diameter responses in normal and atherosclerotic epicardial arteries.
A, Acetylcholine. In normal arteries, acetylcholine elicits vasodilation but there is vasoconstriction in the atherosclerotic artery, which is particularly pronounced in the stenosis **B,** Cold pressor testing. Activation of sympathetic tone normally leads to net epicardial dilation but there is vasoconstriction in proximal and stenotic coronary segments in patients with atherosclerosis. C = control; Ach = acetylcholine; CPT = cold pressor test; NTG = nitroglycerin. *(A modified from Ludmer PL, Selwyn AP, Shook TL, et al: Paradoxical vasoconstriction induced by acetylcholine in atherosclerotic coronary arteries. N Engl J Med 315:1046, 1986. Adapted with permission in 2006; B modified from Nabel EG, Ganz P, Gordon JB, et al: Dilation of normal and constriction of atherosclerotic coronary arteries caused by the cold pressor test. Circulation 77:43, 1988).*

in vitro as well as reduced vasodilatory responses. An increased propensity to coronary vasospasm can be elicited by administering corticosteroids to mimic chronic stress pharmacologically.[27]

Pharmacological Vasodilation

The effects of pharmacological vasodilators on coronary flow reflect direct actions on vascular smooth muscle tone as well as secondary adjustments in coronary resistance artery tone (see Table 48-1). Flow-mediated dilation amplifies the vasodilatory response, whereas autoregulatory adjustments can overcome vasodilation in a segment of the microcirculation and restore flow to normal.

NITROGLYCERIN. Nitroglycerin dilates epicardial conduit arteries and small coronary resistance arteries but does not increase coronary blood flow in the normal heart. The latter observation reflects the fact that transient arteriolar vasodilation is overcome by autoregulatory escape, which returns coronary resistance to control levels.[28] Although nitroglycerin does not increase coronary blood flow in the normal heart, it can produce vasodilation of large coronary resistance arteries that improves the distribution of perfusion to the subendocardium when flow-mediated[9] NO-dependent vasodilation is impaired. It can also improve subendocardial perfusion by reducing LV end-diastolic pressure through systemic venodilation in heart failure. Similarly, coronary collateral vessels dilate in response to nitroglycerin, and the reduction in collateral resistance can improve regional perfusion in some settings.

ADENOSINE. Adenosine dilates coronary arteries through activation of A2 receptors on vascular smooth muscle and is independent of the endothelium in coronary arterioles isolated from humans with heart disease.[22] Experimentally, there is a differential sensitivity of the microcirculation to adenosine with the direct effects related to resistance vessel size and primarily restricted to vessels smaller than 100 μm.[15] Larger upstream resistance arteries dilate via an NO-dependent mechanism from the increase in shear stress. Thus, in states in which endothelium-dependent vasodilation is impaired, maximal coronary flow responses to intravenous or intracoronary adenosine may be reduced in the absence of a stenosis[29] and can be increased

effects on perfusion from anatomical stenosis severity. In coronary disease, it is likely that endothelial disruption plays a role in focal vasospasm. In this setting, the normal vasodilation from autocoids and sympathetic stimulation is converted into a vasoconstrictor response because of the lack of competing endothelium-dependent vasodilation. Nevertheless, although impaired endothelium-dependent vasodilation is a permissive factor for vasospasm, it is not causal, and a trigger is required (e.g., thrombus formation or sympathetic activation).

The mechanisms responsible for variant angina with normal coronary arteries, or Prinzmetal angina, are less clear. Data from animal models have indicated that there may be sensitization of intrinsic vasoconstrictor mechanisms.[26] Rho, a GTP-binding protein, can sensitize vascular smooth muscle to calcium by inhibiting myosin phosphatase activity through an effector protein called Rho kinase. Coronary arteries demonstrate supersensitivity to vasoconstrictor agonists in vivo and by interventions that improve NO-mediated vasodilation, such as lowering low-density lipoprotein (LDL) levels.[30] Various single-dose adenosine A2 receptor agonists are currently in late phase clinical trials; these may afford more prolonged vasodilation and circumvent the need to infuse adenosine continuously for myocardial perfusion imaging (see Chap. 16).

DIPYRIDAMOLE. Dipyridamole produces vasodilation by inhibiting the myocyte reuptake of adenosine released from cardiac myocytes. It therefore has actions and mechanisms similar to those of adenosine, with the exception that the vasodilation is more prolonged. It can be reversed via the administration of the nonspecific adenosine receptor blocker aminophylline.

PAPAVERINE. Papaverine is a short-acting coronary vasodilator that was the first agent used for intracoronary vasodilation. It causes vascular smooth muscle relaxation by inhibiting phosphodiesterase and increasing cAMP. Following bolus injection, it has a rapid onset of action but the vasodilation is more prolonged than after adenosine (approximately 2 minutes). Its actions are independent of the endothelium.

Right Coronary Artery Flow

Although the general concepts of coronary flow regulation developed for the left ventricle apply to the right ventricle, there are differences related to the extent of the right coronary artery supply to the right ventricular free wall. This has been studied in dogs, in which the right coronary artery is a nondominant vessel.[31] In terms of coronary flow reserve, arterial pressure supplying the right coronary substantially exceeds right ventricular pressure minimizing the compressive determinants of coronary reserve. Right ventricular oxygen consumption is lower than that in the left ventricle, and coronary venous oxygen saturations are higher than in the left coronary circulation. Because of these differences, autoregulation of flow in the right coronary artery is not as constant as in the left. Because there is considerable oxygen extraction reserve, coronary flow decreases as pressure is reduced and oxygen delivery is maintained by increased extraction. These differences appear specific to the right ventricular free wall and, in humans, in whom the right coronary artery supplies a large amount of the left ventricle, factors affecting flow regulation to the LV myocardium are likely to predominate.

PHYSIOLOGICAL ASSESSMENT OF CORONARY ARTERY STENOSES

The physiological assessment of stenosis severity is a critical component of the management of patients with obstructive epicardial CAD.[32] Whereas epicardial artery stenoses arising from atherosclerosis increase coronary resistance and reduce maximal myocardial perfusion, it is increasingly apparent that abnormalities in coronary microcirculatory control also contribute to eliciting myocardial ischemia in many patients. As a result, difficulties arise when attempting to assess the physiological significance of a given coronary stenosis using angiographic quantitation or functional quantitation alone. A comprehensive approach would be able to separate the independent role of stenosis resistance from abnormalities in microcirculatory resistance vessel control because the latter would necessitate medical therapy and not be amenable to revascularization of the epicardial coronary arteries. Although not yet widely used, the technology to accomplish this by simultaneously assessing coronary flow and distal coronary pressure using intracoronary transducers is currently available for clinical care.[33]

The angiographically visible epicardial coronary arteries are normally able to accommodate large increases in coronary flow without producing any significant pressure drop and thus serve a conduit function to the coronary resistance vasculature. This changes dramatically in CAD, in which the epicardial artery resistance becomes dominant. This fixed component of resistance increases with stenosis severity and limits maximal myocardial perfusion.

As a starting point, it is helpful to consider the idealized relationship between stenosis severity, pressure drop, and flow that has been validated in animals as well as humans studied in circumstances in which diffuse atherosclerosis and risk factors that can impair microcirculatory resistance vessel control are minimized.[32] Figure 48-11 summarizes the major determinants of stenosis energy losses. The relationship between pressure drop across a stenosis and coronary flow for stenoses between 30 and 90 percent diameter reduction can be described using the Bernoulli principle. The total pressure drop across a stenosis is governed by three hydrodynamic factors—viscous losses, separation losses, and turbulence, although the latter is usually a relatively minor component of pressure loss. The single most important determinant of stenosis resistance for any given level of flow is the minimum lesional cross-sectional area within the stenosis.[34] Because resistance is inversely proportional to the square of the cross-sectional area, small dynamic changes in luminal area caused by thrombi or vasomotion in asymmetrical lesions (where vascular smooth muscle can relax or constrict in a portion of the stenosis) lead to major changes in the stenosis pressure-flow relationship and reduce maximal perfusion during vasodilation. Separation losses determine the curvilinearity or "steepness" of the stenosis pressure-flow relationship and become increasingly important as stenosis severity and/or flow rate increases. Stenosis length and changes in cross-sectional area distal to the stenosis are relatively minor determinants of resistance for most coronary lesions.

Diffuse abluminal outward remodeling with thickening of the arterial wall is common in coronary atherosclerosis but does not alter the pressure-flow characteristics of the stenosis for a given intraluminal geometry. In contrast, diffuse inward remodeling effectively reduces minimal lesion area along the length of the vessel and can underestimate stenosis severity using relative diameter measurements as well as contribute to a significant longitudinal pressure drop that can reduce maximum perfusion. Diffuse inward remodeling can cause measurements of relative stenosis severity to underestimate the physiological effects of the diffuse narrowing on myocardial perfusion.[32]

Stenosis resistance varies exponentially with reductions in minimum lesional cross-sectional area (Fig. 48-12). It is also flow-dependent and varies with the square of the flow or flow velocity. As a result, the instantaneous stenosis resistance increases during vasodilation. This is particularly important in determining the stenosis pres-

CH 48

Coronary Blood Flow and Myocardial Ischemia

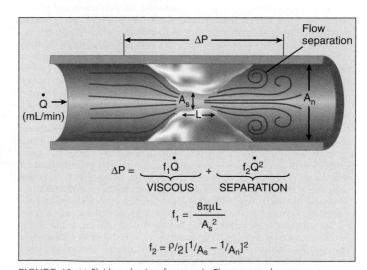

FIGURE 48–11 Fluid mechanics of a stenosis. The pressure drop across a stenosis can be predicted by the Bernoulli equation. It is inversely related to the minimum stenosis cross-sectional area and varies with the square of the flow rate as stenosis severity increases. ΔP = pressure drop; $\dot{Q}$ = flow; f_1 = viscous coefficient; f_2 = separation coefficient; A_s = area of the stenosis; A_n = area of the normal segment; L = stenosis length; μ = viscosity of blood; ρ = density of blood.

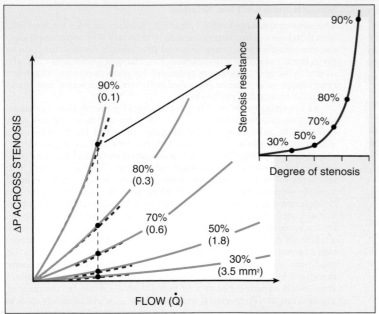

FIGURE 48–12 Curvilinearity of the pressure-flow relationship as stenosis severity increases. The relationship between pressure drop across the stenosis and flow for percent diameter narrowing of 30, 50, 70, 80, and 90 percent is calculated on the basis of a proximal reference internal diameter of 3 mm (area, 7.1 mm²). Measurements in parentheses are minimal lesional cross-sectional areas. Instantaneous resistance is the slope of the pressure-flow curve (dashed red line) and, for a given stenosis, increases as flow rate rises. At levels of resting flow (dashed vertical line), the stenosis resistance increases exponentially as stenosis severity rises (solid red line in inset). *(Modified from Klocke FJ: Measurements of coronary blood flow and degree of stenosis: Current clinical implications and continuing uncertainties. J Am Coll Cardiol 1:31, 1983.)*

sure-flow behavior for severely narrowed arteries and leads to a situation in which small reductions in luminal area result in large reductions in poststenotic coronary pressure and maximum coronary perfusion as stenosis severity increases.

Interrelationship among Distal Coronary Pressure, Flow, and Stenosis Severity

Because maximum myocardial perfusion is ultimately determined by the coronary pressure distal to a stenosis, it is helpful to place the epicardial stenosis pressure flow relationship into the context of the coronary autoregulatory and vasodilated coronary pressure flow relationships, as depicted in Figure 48-13. The effects of a stenosis on resting and vasodilated flow as a function of percentage diameter reduction when diffuse intraluminal narrowing is absent and coronary microcirculatory resistance is normal is summarized in Figure 48-13A. Because of coronary autoregulation, flow remains constant as stenosis severity increases and resting perfusion is inadequate to distinguish hemodynamically severe stenoses. In contrast, the maximally vasodilated pressure-flow relationship is much more sensitive to detect increases in stenosis severity. There is normally substantial coronary flow reserve and flow can increase approximately five times the resting flow values. Very little increase in epicardial conduit artery resistance (R_1) develops until stenosis severity reaches a 50 percent diameter reduction (see Fig. 48-13B). As a result, there is no significant pressure drop across a stenosis or stenosis-related alteration in maximal myocardial perfusion until stenosis severity exceeds a 50 percent diameter reduction (75 percent cross-sectional area). As stenosis severity increases further, the curvilinear coronary pressure flow relationship steepens and increases in stenosis resistance are accompanied by concomitant increases in the pressure drop (ΔP) across the stenosis. This reduces distal coronary pressure, the major determinant of perfusion to the microcirculation, and maximum vasodilated flow decreases (see Fig. 48-13C). Above a value of 70 percent diameter reduction, small increases in stenosis severity are accompanied by large increases in stenosis pressure drop, large reductions in distal coronary pressure, and large reductions in maximal vasodilated perfusion of the microcirculation. A critical stenosis, one in which subendocardial flow reserve is completely exhausted at rest, usually develops when stenosis severity exceeds 90 percent. Under these circumstances, pharmacological vasodilation of subepicardial resistance vessels results in a further

reduction in distal coronary pressure that actually reduces subendocardial flow, leading to a "transmural steal" phenomenon.

Concept of Maximal Perfusion and Coronary Reserve

Gould originally proposed the concept of coronary reserve over 30 years ago.[32] With technological advances, it has become possible to characterize this in humans using invasive catheter-based measurements of intracoronary pressure and flow (Fig. 48-14) as well as with noninvasive imaging of myocardial perfusion with positron emission tomography (PET), single-photon emission tomography (SPECT) and, more recently, cardiac magnetic resonance (CMR) (see Chaps. 16 and 17). With physiologically based approaches to quantify perfusion and coronary pressure, it has also become increasingly apparent that abnormalities in coronary microcirculatory control contribute to the functional significance of isolated epicardial artery stenoses in many patients with CAD. There are currently three major indices used to quantify coronary flow reserve: absolute; relative, and fractional. These are compared in Figure 48-15, and the relative advantages and limitations of each of the currently used indices are discussed here.

ABSOLUTE FLOW RESERVE. Initial approaches to assess functional stenosis severity focused on assessing the relative increase in flow following ischemic vasodilation (reactive hyperemic response following transient occlusion of the coronary artery) or pharmacological vasodilation of the microcirculation with intracoronary papaverine, adenosine, or intravenous dipyridamole. Absolute flow reserve can be quantified using intracoronary Doppler velocity or thermodilution flow measurements, as well as by quantitative approaches to image absolute tissue perfusion based on PET. It is expressed as the ratio of maximally vasodilated flow to the corresponding resting flow value in a specific region of the heart and quantifies the ability of flow to increase above the resting value (see Fig. 48-15A). Clinically important reductions in maximum flow correlating with stress-induced ischemia on SPECT are generally associated with absolute flow reserve values below 2.[33] Absolute flow reserve is not only altered by factors that affect maximal coronary flow (e.g., stenosis severity, impaired microcirculatory control, arterial pressure, heart rate) but also by the corresponding resting flow value. Resting flow can vary with hemoglobin content, baseline hemodynamics, and the resting oxygen extraction. As a result, reductions in absolute flow reserve can arise from inappropriate elevations in resting coronary flow as well as from reductions in maximal perfusion.

In the absence of diffuse atherosclerosis or LV hypertrophy, absolute flow reserve in conscious humans is similar to measurements in animals and averages four to five times the value at rest. There is also fairly good reduplication of the idealized relationship between stenosis severity and absolute flow reserve in patients with isolated one- or two-vessel CAD (Fig. 48-16A) with intracoronary vasodilation. In contrast, in patients with risk factors such as hypercholesterolemia and no significant coronary luminal narrowing, values of absolute flow reserve using PET are lower than in normals, reflecting microcirculatory impairment in flow or attenuated vasodilator responsiveness.[35] Recent cross-sectional studies of asymptomatic patients have demonstrated an inverse relationship between coronary artery calcification as a marker of subclinical atherosclerosis and quantitative measures of coronary flow reserve with CMR.[36] Thus, abnormalities in the coronary microcirculation as

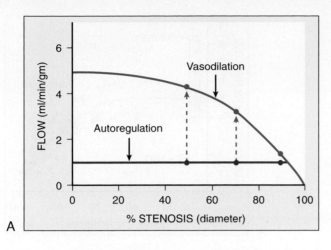

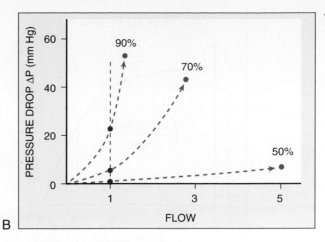

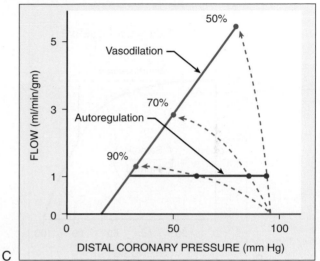

FIGURE 48–13 Interrelationship among stenosis flow reserve **(A)**, the stenosis pressure-flow relationship **(B)**, and autoregulation **(C)**. Red circles depict resting flow and blue circles maximal vasodilation for stenoses of 50, 70, and 90 percent diameter reduction. There is very little pressure drop across a 50 percent stenosis, and distal coronary pressure and vasodilated flow remain near normal. In contrast, a 90 percent stenosis critically impairs flow, because the steep pressure flow relationship causes a marked reduction in distal coronary pressure. See text for further discussion.

well as uncertainty in stenosis geometry or diffuse atherosclerosis leads to considerably more variability of the observed relationship between stenosis severity and absolute flow reserve in patients with more extensive disease (see Fig 48-16B). A significant limitation of absolute flow reserve measurements is that the importance of an epicardial stenosis cannot be dissociated from functional abnormalities in the microcirculation that are common in patients (e.g., hypertrophy and impaired endothelium-dependent vasodilation).

RELATIVE FLOW RESERVE. Relative coronary flow reserve measurements are the cornerstone of noninvasive identification of hemodynamically important coronary stenoses using nuclear perfusion imaging

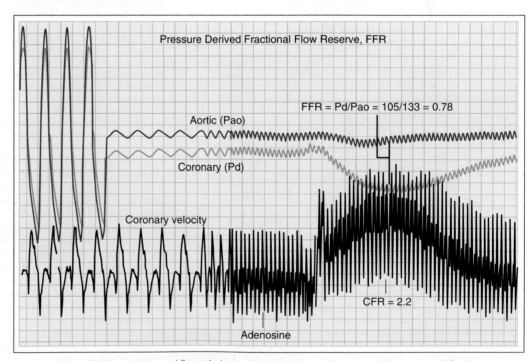

FIGURE 48–14 Coronary pressure and flow velocity tracings in a patient with an intermediate stenosis. Following intracoronary adenosine, flow velocity transiently increases and mean distal coronary pressure (Pd) falls. Absolute coronary flow reserve (CFR) is the ratio of peak flow to resting flow. Fractional flow reserve (FFR) is the ratio of Pd/Pao (distal coronary pressure divided by mean aortic pressure).

CH 48

Coronary Blood Flow and Myocardial Ischemia

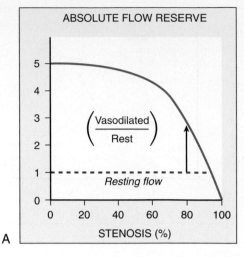

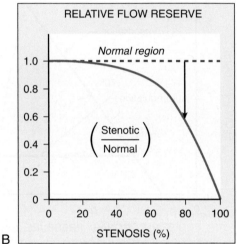

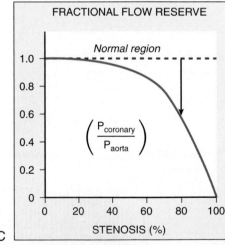

FIGURE 48–15 Absolute flow reserve, relative flow reserve, and fractional flow reserve. **A,** Absolute flow reserve is the ratio of coronary flow during vasodilation to the resting value. It can be obtained with invasive measurements of intracoronary flow velocity or quantitative kinetic perfusion measurements with positron emission tomography. **B,** Relative flow reserve compares maximal vasodilated flow in a stenotic region with an assumed normal region in the same heart and is most commonly measured with perfusion imaging during stress. **C,** Fractional flow reserve is conceptually similar to relative flow reserve and assesses maximal flow indirectly from coronary pressure measurements distal to a stenosis during vasodilation. Neither relative flow reserve nor fractional flow reserve can identify the contribution of abnormalities in microcirculatory resistance control to the development of myocardial ischemia.

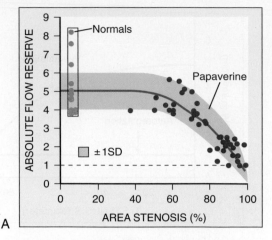

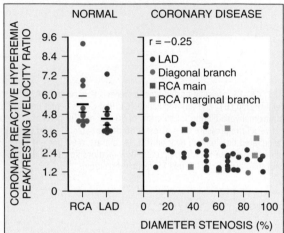

FIGURE 48–16 Absolute coronary flow reserve as a function of stenosis severity in patients. **A,** Idealized absolute flow reserve following intracoronary vasodilation in single-vessel disease without hypertrophy demonstrates a good correlation with values predicted theoretically **B,** Absolute flow reserve assessed using intraoperative epicardial Doppler flow measurements following reactive hyperemia to a 20-second occlusion. Among all vessels, there is a poor relationship with stenosis severity. This reflects variability in stenosis severity with visual interpretation as well as abnormal microcirculatory responses to ischemia and multiple risk factors for impaired endothelial function. LAD = left anterior descending artery; RCA = right coronary artery. (**A** modified from Wilson RF, Marcus ML, White CW: Prediction of the physiologic significance of coronary arterial lesions by quantitative lesion geometry in patients with limited coronary artery disease. Circulation 75:723, 1987; **B** modified from White CW, Wright CB, Doty DB, et al: Does visual interpretation of the coronary arteriogram predict the physiologic importance of a coronary stenosis? N Engl J Med 310:819, 1984. Adapted with permission in 2006).

(see Chap. 16). In this approach, relative differences in regional perfusion (per gram of tissue) are assessed during maximal pharmacological vasodilation or maximal exercise stress and expressed as a fraction of flow to normal regions of the heart (see Fig. 48-15B). This has the advantage of comparing perfusion differences under the same hemodynamic conditions and thus is relatively insensitive to variations in mean arterial pressure and heart rate. An alternative invasive approach uses absolute flow reserve measurements and derives relative flow reserve by dividing measurements in a stenotic vessel by those in remote normally perfused territories.[33] This appears to provide outcome-based results similar to those of fractional flow reserve and minimizes uncertainties regarding the exact value for coronary venous pressure. A minimum threshold value of 0.8 has been proposed to identify a significant stenosis based on invasive flow velocity measurements.[33]

Although widely used to identify hemodynamically significant stenoses, there are significant limitations in using imaging to quantify relative flow reserve. First, conventional SPECT imaging requires a normal reference segment within the left ventricle for comparison. Because of this, relative flow reserve measurements cannot accurately quantify stenosis severity when diffuse abnormalities in flow reserve related to either balanced multivessel CAD or impaired microcirculatory vasodilation are present. Large differences in relative vasodilated flow are required to detect SPECT perfusion differences because nuclear tracers become diffusion-limited and their myocardial uptake fails to increase proportionally with increases in vasodilated flow. As a result, differences in tracer deposition underestimate the actual relative difference in perfusion. This limitation can be overcome with PET tracers of perfusion and appropriate kinetic modeling. Finally, whereas prognostic data related to the perfusion deficit size are available, there are no imaging studies evaluating the quantitative severity of the stress or vasodilated flow reduction as a continuous outcome measure although, conceptually, this should be similar to fractional flow reserve.

FRACTIONAL FLOW RESERVE. Considerable focus has turned toward invasive point of care approaches that employ pressure measurements distal to a coronary stenosis as an indirect index of stenosis severity (see Fig. 48-14).[33] This technique, pioneered by Pijls, is based upon the principal that the distal coronary pressure measured during vasodilation is directly proportional to maximum vasodilated perfusion (see Fig. 48-15C). Fractional flow reserve (FFR) is an indirect index determined by measuring the driving pressure for microcirculatory flow distal to the stenosis (distal coronary pressure minus coronary venous pressure) relative to the coronary driving pressure available in the absence of a stenosis (mean aortic pressure minus coronary venous pressure). The approach assumes linearity of the vasodilated pressure-flow relationship (which is known to be curvilinear at reduced coronary pressure[13]) and usually assumes that coronary venous pressure is zero. This results in the simplified clinical FFR index of mean distal coronary pressure/mean aortic pressure (Pd/Pao). Although derived, the measurements are conceptually similar to those of relative coronary flow reserve because they only rely on minimum mean coronary pressure measurements during intracoronary vasodilation and compare stenotic with normal regions (assumed to equal 1) under similar hemodynamic conditions. They are attractive in that they can immediately assess the physiological significance of an intermediate stenosis to help guide decisions regarding coronary intervention and are unaffected by alterations in resting flow. Similarly, because they only require vasodilated coronary pressure measurements, FFR can be used to assess the functional effects of a residual lesion after percutaneous coronary intervention (PCI; see Chap. 55). A significant advantage of FFR is that there is now considerable prognostic information[13,33] including recent data indicating that FFR measurements greater than 0.75 are associated with excellent outcomes with deferred rather than prophylactic intervention.

A significant limitation of FFR is that it cannot assess abnormalities in microcirculatory flow reserve. The measurements are also critically dependent on achieving maximal pharmacological vasodilation (underestimating stenosis severity if vasodilation is submaximal). In addition, ignoring the back pressure to coronary flow by assuming that venous pressure is equal to zero and ignoring curvilinearity of the diastolic pressure-flow relationship will cause the FFR to underestimate the physiological significance of a stenosis.[13] Finally, inserting the guidewire across a stenosis can artifactually overestimate stenosis severity caused by the reduction in effective intralesional area when there is diffuse disease, when it is placed in small branch vessels, or in assessing a severe stenosis. Despite these limitations and its invasive nature, FFR is currently the most direct way to assess the physiological significance of individual coronary lesions.

STENOSIS PRESSURE-FLOW RELATION. The availability of high-fidelity pressure and flow measurements on a single wire has now facilitated the development of approaches to assess the stenosis pressure-flow relationship as well as abnormalities in microcirculatory reserve by determining FFR and absolute coronary flow reserve simultaneously. When assessed together, these measurements

have the potential to identify circumstances in which mixed abnormalities, stenosis and microcirculation, contribute to the net physiological significance of a stenosis (Fig. 48-17). In a more recent approach, the instantaneous relationship between flow and pressure drop across the stenosis can be obtained at the time of PCI. Although this has not been widely validated, it may afford a more accurate approach to assess coronary stenoses independent of the microcirculation.[33]

ADVANTAGES AND LIMITATIONS OF CORONARY FLOW RESERVE MEASUREMENTS. Assessing qualitative perfusion differences with noninvasive imaging is useful because relative perfusion deficit size is an important determinant of prognosis. The clinical role of invasive measurements quantifying stenosis severity continues to evolve. Measurements of FFR are the most widely available and are

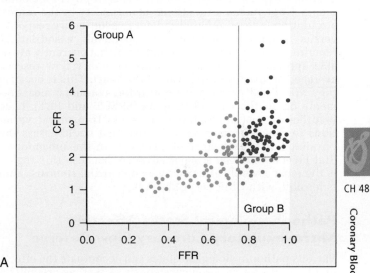

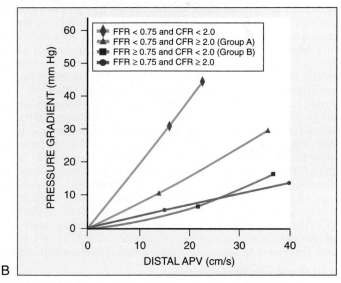

FIGURE 48–17 Characterization of coronary stenosis severity with simultaneous measurements of intracoronary pressure and flow. **A,** Vertical line represents a threshold fractional flow reserve (FFR) of 0.75 and the horizontal line predicts a threshold coronary flow reserve (CFR) of 2. Group A depicts patients with significant stenoses by FFR who have relatively preserved microvascular function and a CFR higher than 2. Group B depicts patients with microcirculatory impairment or submaximal vasodilation in whom CFR is limited but FFR is not reduced. **B,** Instantaneous stenosis pressure-flow relations corresponding to the four groups depicted in **A.** APV = average pressure gradient–flow velocity *(Modified from Meuwissen M, Chamuleau S, Siebes M, et al: Role of variability in microvascular resistance on fractional flow reserve and coronary blood flow velocity reserve in intermediate coronary lesions. Circulation 103:184, 2001.)*

particularly attractive in clinical circumstances associated with intermediate severity lesions. Although prognostic data supporting the usefulness of direct assessment of stenosis flow reserve with intracoronary approaches used in conjunction with PCI continue to emerge, there are currently no Class I indications for its use.[33]

The major assumption common to all flow reserve measurements is that the pharmacological vasodilator used consistently achieves maximal vasodilation of the resistance vasculature in normals as well as in patients with atherosclerotic disease and impaired endothelial function. The reductions in absolute flow reserve in humans with angiographically insignificant stenoses (see Fig. 48-16B) as well as variability in quantitative perfusion measurements with normal epicardial arteries and coronary risk factors indicates that this may not always be the case. The extent that this is related to a structural abnormality in the microcirculation (e.g., caused by regional hypertrophy or vascular remodeling) versus a functional abnormality in the microcirculation (altered microcirculatory vasodilatory response versus impaired endothelium-dependent vasodilation) remains unclear. A second limitation is that currently available approaches can only measure coronary flow reserve averaged across the entire wall of the heart. This is because they are based on invasive epicardial coronary measurements or, in the case of imaging (SPECT and PET), have insufficient spatial resolution to assess transmural variations in flow. An imaging technique that could assess the physiological significance of a stenosis in the subendocardial layers would be a major advance, because this region is the most severely affected by an epicardial stenosis. This is feasible with CMR (see Chap. 17).

Pathophysiological States Affecting Microcirculatory Coronary Flow Reserve

Various pathophysiological states can accentuate the effects of a fixed-diameter coronary stenosis as well as precipitate subendocardial ischemia during stress in the presence of normal coronary arteries. Thus, it is important to incorporate measurements of stenosis severity with abnormalities of coronary resistance vessel control. In the former case, treatment will be directed at the epicardial stenosis, whereas in the latter, medical therapies designed to improve abnormalities in resistance vessel control will be required. The prognostic importance of abnormalities in coronary resistance vessel control is underscored by emerging data in women evaluated for chest pain felt to be of ischemic origin. Abnormalities in coronary flow reserve and endothelium-dependent vasodilation are common in women with insignificant coronary disease and can be accompanied by metabolic ischemia, assessed by magnetic resonance imaging (MRI) spectroscopy (see Chap. 17) and they negatively affect prognosis.[37] The two most common factors affecting microcirculatory resistance control independently of coronary stenosis severity in patients are LV hypertrophy and impaired NO-mediated resistance vessel vasodilation.

Left Ventricular Hypertrophy

The effects of hypertrophy on coronary flow reserve are complex and need to be thought of in terms of the absolute flow level (e.g., measured with an intracoronary Doppler probe) as well as the flow per gram of myocardium. With acquired hypertrophy, resting flow per gram of myocardium remains constant, but the increase in LV mass necessitates an increase in the absolute level of resting flow (ml/min) through the coronary artery.[38] In terms of maximal perfusion, acquired hypertrophy does not result in vascular proliferation and coronary resistance vessels remain unchanged (Fig. 48-18). Because maximum absolute flow (ml/min) remains unchanged, maximum perfusion per gram of myocardium falls. The net effect is that coronary flow reserve at any given coronary arterial pressure is reduced and inversely related to the

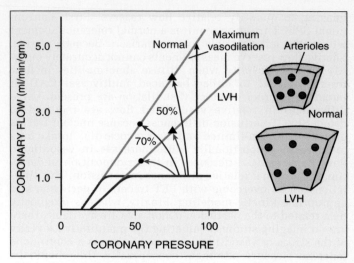

FIGURE 48–18 Effects of left ventricular hypertrophy (LVH) on maximal coronary flow. With acquired LVH, myocardial mass increases without proliferation of the microcirculatory resistance arteries (right side). Because the maximal absolute flow per minute during vasodilation remains unchanged, the maximum flow per gram of tissue falls inversely with the change in LV mass. In contrast, whereas the resting flow per gram of myocardium remains constant with hypertrophy, the increase in LV mass requires a higher absolute resting flow. The net effect of these opposing actions is to decrease coronary flow reserve at any coronary pressure. As a result of the reduction in microcirculatory reserve in the absence of a coronary stenosis, the functional significance of a 50 percent stenosis (triangles) in the hypertrophied heart could approach a more severe stenosis (in the example, 70 percent, circles) in normal myocardium. This can even result in ischemia with normal coronary arteries during stress.

change in LV mass. For example, in the absence of a change in mean aortic pressure, a twofold increase in LV mass, as is associated with severe LV hypertrophy, can reduce coronary flow reserve in a nonstenotic artery from 4 to 2 ml/min/g. This will increase the functional severity of any anatomical degree of coronary artery narrowing and can even precipitate subendocardial ischemia with normal coronary arteries.

Some degree of LV hypertrophy is common in patients with CAD and it likely contributes to reductions in coronary flow reserve that are independent of stenosis severity. The actual coronary flow reserve in hypertrophy will be critically dependent on the underlying cause of hypertrophy and its effects on coronary driving pressure. A similar degree of hypertrophy caused by untreated systemic hypertension will have a higher coronary flow reserve than in aortic stenosis, in which mean arterial pressure remains normal. Similarly, when hypertrophy is from systolic hypertension and increased pulse pressure caused by reduced aortic compliance, the accompanying reduction in diastolic pressure can lower coronary reserve.

Impaired Endothelium-Dependent Vasodilation

Measurements of coronary flow reserve in humans with risk factors for atherosclerosis are systematically lower than normals without coronary risk factors and underscore the importance of abnormalities in microvascular control in determining coronary flow reserve. Much of this may reflect abnormal local resistance vessel control via impaired endothelial-dependent vasodilation arising from NO inactivation associated with risk factors for CAD. Kuo and colleagues have demonstrated that dietary hypercholesterolemia in swine markedly attenuates the dilation of coronary arterioles in response to shear stress as well as pharmacological agonists that stimulate NO synthase in the absence of epicardial stenoses (Fig. 48-19).[39] This was reversed with L-arginine, suggesting that it reflects impaired NO synthesis or availability.

Abnormalities in NO-mediated vasodilation in vivo are functionally significant and impair the ability of the heart to autoregulate coronary blood flow. Figure 48-20 shows the effects of inhibiting NO on the coronary autoregulatory relationship in normal dogs.[40] Although resting blood flow is not altered, there is a marked increase in the coronary pressure at which intrinsic autoregulatory adjustments become exhausted, with flow beginning to decrease at a distal coronary pressure of 60 versus 45 mm Hg, approximately similar to the shift occurring in response to a twofold increase in heart rate. In vivo

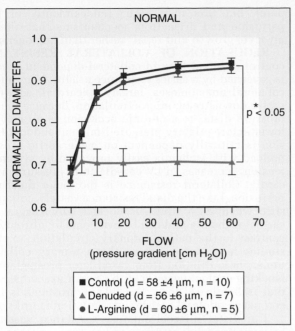

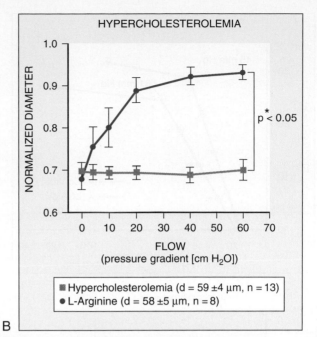

FIGURE 48–19 Flow-mediated vasodilation in coronary resistance arteries is abolished by dietary hypercholesterolemia in swine. **A,** In normal arterioles, increased flow (pressure gradient) elicits vasodilation that, similar to human vessels, is abolished by removing the endothelium (denuded). **B,** In animals with dietary hypercholesterolemia but no significant epicardial stenosis, flow-mediated vasodilation of arterioles is abolished. It was restored by administering L-arginine to increase NO production. *(Modified from Kuo L, Davis MJ, Cannon MS, et al: Pathophysiological consequences of atherosclerosis extend into the coronary microcirculation: Restoration of endothelium-dependent responses by L-arginine. Circ Res 70:465, 1992.)*

microcirculatory studies have demonstrated that there is an inability of resistance arteries to dilate maximally in response to shear stress.[23] This likely reflects excess resistance in the transmural penetrating arteries, which are upstream of metabolic stimuli for vasodilation and extremely dependent on shear stress as a stimulus for local vasodilation. These abnormalities amplify the functional effects of a coronary stenosis, resulting in the development of subendocardial ischemia at a lower workload.[41]

These observations in animals with impaired NO production appear to be relevant to pathophysiological states associated with impaired endothelium-dependent vasodilation in humans. For example, coronary flow reserve is markedly reduced in the absence of a coronary stenosis in familial hypercholesterolemia,[35] and improving endothelial function by lowering elevated LDL levels with statins produces a delayed improvement in coronary flow reserve in normal and stenotic arteries and also ameliorates clinical signs of myocardial ischemia.[30] Impaired NO-mediated vasodilation likely affects the regulation of myocardial perfusion in other disease states in which endothelium-dependent vasodilation is impaired.

CORONARY COLLATERAL CIRCULATION

Following a total coronary occlusion, residual perfusion to the myocardium persists through native coronary collateral channels that open when an intercoronary pressure gradient between the source and recipient vessel develops. In animals, the native collateral flow during occlusion is less than 10 percent of the resting flow levels and is insufficient to maintain tissue viability for longer than 20 minutes. In the absence of coronary collaterals, coronary pressure during balloon angioplasty occlusion falls to similar pressures (10 to 20 mm Hg). There is tremendous individual variability in the function of coronary collaterals among patients with chronic stenoses. Ischemia does not develop during PCI balloon occlusion when fractional flow reserve (based on coronary wedge pressure during occlusion minus venous pressure) is greater than 0.25.[33] Thus, collaterals can proliferate to the point where they are sufficient to maintain resting perfusion and sometimes prevent stress-induced ischemia at submaximal cardiac workloads.

ARTERIOGENESIS AND ANGIOGENESIS. Proliferation of coronary collaterals occurs in response to repetitive stress-induced ischemia as well as the development of transient interarterial pressure gradients between the source and recipient vessel through a process termed *arteriogenesis*.[42] Resting distal coronary pressure consistently falls as stenosis severity exceeds 70 percent and the resultant interarterial pressure gradient increases endothelial shear stress in preexisting collaterals smaller than 200 μm in diameter. This causes progressive enlargement of collaterals through a process dependent on physical forces, growth factors (particularly vascular endothelial growth factor, VEGF) and ultimately mediated via NO synthase.[43] Thus, patients with impaired NO-mediated vasodilation may also have a limited ability to develop coronary collaterals in response to a chronic coronary stenosis.

Most functional collateral flow arises from arteriogenesis in existing epicardial anastomoses that enlarge into mature vessels that can reach 1 to 2 mm in diameter. Collateral perfusion can also originate from de novo vessel growth, or angiogenesis, which refers to the sprouting of smaller, capillary-like structures from preexisting blood vessels. These vessels may provide nutritive collateral flow when they develop in the border between ischemic and nonischemic regions. Capillary angiogenesis may also occur within the ischemic region and can reduce the intercapillary distance for oxygen exchange. Nevertheless, because capillary resistance is already a small component of microcirculatory resistance, increases in capillary density in the absence of changes in arteriolar resistance will not significantly increase myocardial perfusion.

There is currently great interest in experimental interventions to improve collateral flow (e.g., recombinant growth factors, in vivo gene transfer, and endothelial progenitor cells). Although many interventions have been demonstrated to cause favorable angiogenesis of capillaries and improve myocardial function, few interventions have increased arteriogenesis in mature collaterals and randomized human clinical trials have been disappointing.[44] Part

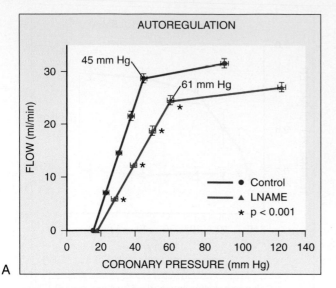

A

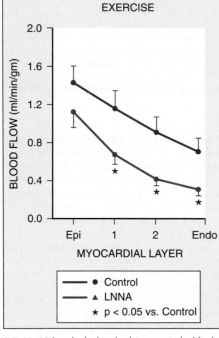

B

FIGURE 48–20 Impaired microcirculatory control with abnormal NO-mediated endothelium-dependent resistance artery dilation. **A,** Effects of blocking nitric oxide synthase (NOS) with the L-arginine analogue LNAME in chronically instrumented dogs. There is an increase in the lower autoregulatory pressure limit, resulting in the onset of ischemia at a coronary pressure of 61 mm Hg versus 45 mm Hg under normal conditions that occurred without a change in heart rate. **B,** Transmural perfusion before and after blocking NO-mediated dilation with LNNA in exercising dogs subjected to a coronary stenosis. Although coronary pressure and hemodynamics were similar, blood flow was lower in each layer of the heart after blocking NOS and not overcome by metabolic dilator mechanisms during ischemia. Collectively, these experimental data support the notion that abnormalities in endothelium-dependent vasodilation can amplify the functional effects of a coronary stenosis. Endo = endocardium; Epi = epicardium; LNAME = N^G-nitro-L-arginine methyl ester; LNNA = N^G-nitro-L-arginine. (*A modified from Smith TP Jr, Canty JM Jr: Modulation of coronary autoregulatory responses by nitric oxide: Evidence for flow-dependent resistance adjustments in conscious dogs. Circ Res 73:232, 1993; B modified from Duncker DJ, Bache RJ: Inhibition of nitric oxide production aggravates myocardial hypoperfusion during exercise in the presence of a coronary artery stenosis. Circ Res 74:629, 1994.*)

of this may arise from the fact that no intervention has resulted in measurable increases in maximum vasodilated myocardial perfusion or coronary flow reserve indices, the sine qua non of functional collateral formation. Improvements in myocardial function have been used as an end-point, but this may occur independently of increased perfusion and arise from mechanisms that alter cardiac myocyte growth and repair rather than angiogenesis.[45]

REGULATION OF COLLATERAL RESISTANCE. The control of blood flow to collateral-dependent myocardium is governed by a series resistance arising from interarterial collateral anastomoses, largely epicardial, as well as the native downstream microcirculation. Because the coronary pressure distal to a chronic occlusion is already near the lower autoregulatory pressure limit, subendocardial perfusion is critically dependent on mean aortic pressure and preload with ischemia easily provoked by systemic hypotension, increases in LV end-diastolic pressure, and tachycardia. Collateral resistance is the major determinant of perfusion. Like the distal resistance vessels, collaterals constrict when NO synthesis is blocked, which aggravates myocardial ischemia and can be overcome by nitroglycerin.[9] In contrast to the native coronary circulation, experimental studies have demonstrated that coronary collaterals are under tonic dilation from vasodilator prostaglandins, and blocking cyclooxygenase with aspirin exacerbates myocardial ischemia in dogs. The role of prostanoids in human coronary collateral resistance regulation is unknown.

The distal microcirculatory resistance vasculature in collateral-dependent myocardium appears to be regulated by mechanisms similar to those present in the normal circulation but is characterized by impaired endothelium-dependent vasodilation as compared with normal vessels. The extent that these microcirculatory abnormalities alter the normal metabolic and coronary autoregulatory responses in collateral dependent myocardium is unknown.

METABOLIC AND FUNCTIONAL CONSEQUENCES OF ISCHEMIA

Because oxygen delivery to the heart is closely coupled to coronary blood flow, a sudden cessation of regional perfusion following a thrombotic coronary occlusion quickly leads to the cessation of aerobic metabolism, depletion of creatine phosphate, and the onset of anaerobic glycolysis. This is followed by the accumulation of tissue lactate, a progressive reduction in tissue ATP levels, and an accumulation of catabolites, including those of the adenine nucleotide pool. As ischemia continues, tissue acidosis develops and there is an efflux of potassium into the extracellular space. Subsequently, ATP levels fall below those required to maintain critical membrane function, resulting in the onset of myocyte death.

Irreversible Injury and Myocyte Death

The temporal evolution and extent of irreversible tissue injury after coronary occlusion is variable and dependent on transmural location, residual coronary flow, and the hemodynamic determinants of oxygen consumption. Irreversible myocardial injury begins after 20 minutes of coronary occlusion in the absence of significant collaterals.[46] Irreversible injury begins in the subendocardium and progresses as a wavefront over time, from the subendocardial layers to the subepicardial layers (Fig. 48-21). This reflects the higher oxygen consumption in the subendocardium and the redistribution of collateral flow to the outer layers of the heart by the compressive determinants of flow at reduced coronary pressure. In experimental infarction, the entire subendocardium is irreversibly injured within 1 hour of occlusion and the transmural progression of infarction is largely completed within 4 to 6 hours after coronary occlusion. Factors that increase myocardial oxygen consumption (e.g., tachycardia) or reduce oxygen delivery (e.g., anemia, arterial hypotension) accelerate the progression of irreversible injury. In contrast, repetitive reversible ischemia or angina prior to an occlusion can reduce irreversible injury through preconditioning.[47]

The magnitude of residual coronary flow through collaterals or through a subtotal coronary occlusion is the most important determinant of the actual time course of irreversible injury in patients with chronic CAD. The relationship between infarct size and the area at risk of ischemia during a total occlusion is inversely related to collateral flow. When subendocardial collateral flow is more than approximately 30 percent of resting flow values, it prevents infarction after periods of ischemia lasting longer than 1 hour. More moderate subendocardial ischemia from a subtotal occlusion (e.g., flow reduced by no more than 50 percent) can persist for at least 5 hours without producing significant irreversible injury.[48] This explains the fact that signs and symptoms of ischemia can be present for long periods without producing significant myocardial necrosis. It also explains the observation that late coronary reperfusion with ongoing ischemia can salvage myocardium beyond the 6-hour time limit predicted from experimental models of infarction.

Cell death arises from two distinct mechanisms in myocardial infarction. Reperfusion immediately causes myocyte necrosis and sarcolemmal disruption, with the leakage of cell contents into the extracellular space. The injury is further amplified by the reentry of leukocytes into the area of injury. At later time points, myocytes initially salvaged can undergo programmed cell death or apoptosis, which can contribute to further delayed myocardial injury. Apoptosis is a coordinated involution of myocytes that circumvents the inflammation associated with necrotic cell death. Because apoptosis is an energy-dependent process, cells can be forced to switch to a necrotic pathway if energy levels are depleted below critical levels. Thus, determining the relative importance of each mechanism in myocardial infarction can be problematic and continues to be controversial.

Reversible Ischemia and Perfusion-Contraction Matching

Reversible ischemia is considerably more frequent than irreversible injury. Supply-induced ischemia can arise from transient coronary occlusion resulting from coronary vasospasm or transient thrombosis in a critically stenosed coronary artery, producing transmural ischemia similar to that present at the onset of infarction. Demand-induced ischemia arises from an inability to increase flow in response to increases in myocardial oxygen consumption in which ischemia predominantly affects the subendocardium. These have fundamentally different effects on myocardial diastolic relaxation, with supply-induced ischemia increasing LV compliance and demand-induced ischemia reducing it. There is a fairly stereotypical sequence of physiological changes that develop during an episode of spontaneous transmural ischemia (Fig. 48-22; see Fig. 48-e1 on website). Coronary occlusion results in an immediate fall in coronary venous oxygen saturation, with a reduction in ATP production. This causes a decline in regional contraction within several beats reaching dyskinesis within 1 minute. As regional contraction ceases, there is a reduction in global LV contractility (dP/dt), a progressive rise in LV end-diastolic pressure, and a fall in

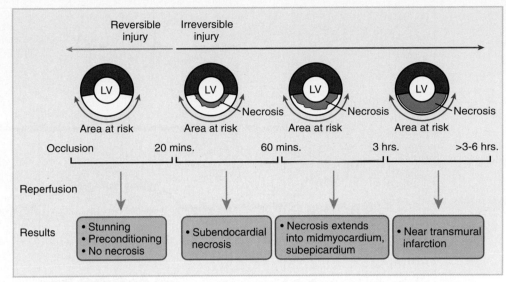

FIGURE 48-21 Wave front of necrosis in infarction in the absence of collaterals. Total occlusions shorter than 20 minutes do not cause irreversible injury but can cause myocardial stunning as well as precondition the heart and protect it against recurrent ischemic injury. Irreversible injury begins after 20 minutes and progresses as a wavefront from endocardium to epicardium. After 60 minutes, the inner third of the left ventricular (LV) wall is irreversibly injured. After 3 hours, there is a subepicardial rim of tissue remaining with the transmural extent of infarction completed between 3 and 6 hours after occlusion. The most important factor delaying the progression of irreversible injury is the magnitude of collateral flow, which is primarily directed to the outer layers of the heart. (*Modified from Kloner RA, Jennings RB: Consequences of brief ischemia: Stunning, preconditioning, and their clinical implications: Part 1. Circulation 104:2981, 2001.*)

systolic pressure. The magnitude of the systemic hemodynamic changes varies with the severity of ischemia as well as the amount of the left ventricle subjected to ischemia. Significant electrocardiographic ST changes develop within 2 minutes as efflux of potassium into the extracellular space reaches a critical level. Symptoms of chest pain are variable and usually the last event to occur in the evolution of ischemia. On restoring perfusion, the sequence is reversed with resolution of chest pain occurring before hemodynamic changes resolve, but regional contraction can remain depressed, reflecting the development of stunned myocardium. A similar temporal sequence of events occurs during exercise-induced ischemia, although the time frame of evolution can be more protracted because ischemia primarily occurs in the subendocardium. Because of the temporal delay in the development of angina and other factors, many episodes of ST depression are symptomatically silent. It is also likely that very brief episodes of ischemia, as reflected by more sensitive indices, such as reduced regional contraction or elevations in end-diastolic pressure, can be electrocardiographically silent.

ACUTE PERFUSION-CONTRACTION MATCHING DURING SUBENDOCARDIAL ISCHEMIA. When coronary pressure distal to a stenosis falls below the lower limit of autoregulation, flow reserve is exhausted, resulting in the onset of subendocardial ischemia. In this case, reductions in subendocardial flow are closely coupled to reductions in regional contractile function of the heart as measured by sensitive approaches, such as regional wall thickening. There is a relatively linear relationship between relative reductions in subendocardial blood flow and relative reductions in regional wall thickening at rest[4] and during tachycardia,[6] as well as during exercise-induced dysfunction distal to a critical stenosis (Fig. 48-23).[49,50] This forms the basis for using regional myocardial function as an index of the severity of subendocardial ischemia during stress imaging.

SHORT-TERM HIBERNATION. In steady-state ischemia, the close matching between perfusion and contraction leads to a reduced regional oxygen consumption and energy uptake, a phenomenon termed *short-term hibernation.*[48] This reestablishes a balance between supply and demand, as reflected by regeneration of creatine phosphate and ATP with the resolution of lactate production, despite persistent hypoperfusion. Short-term hibernation is an extremely tenuous state and small increases in the determinants of myocardial oxygen demand precipitate further ischemia and a rapid deterioration in function and metabolism. Thus, the ability of short-term hibernation to prevent necrosis is limited by the severity and duration of ischemia, with irreversible injury developing frequently after periods of more than 24 hours.[51]

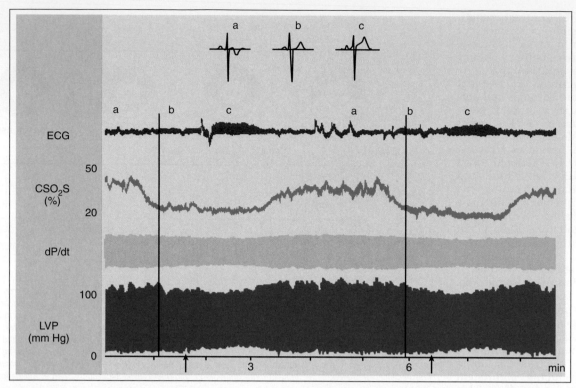

FIGURE 48–22 Physiological changes during two episodes of spontaneous asymptomatic ischemia in a patient with an acute coronary syndrome. High-speed electrocardiographic tracings depict the baseline electrocardiogram (ECG; a), pseudonormalization of T waves in early ischemia (b), and ST elevation with late ischemia (c). A primary reduction in coronary flow is depicted by the sudden fall in coronary venous oxygen saturation (CSO_2S). Shortly thereafter, left ventricular (LV) dP/dt falls, reflecting regional contractile dysfunction (solid vertical lines). Within 1 minute, LV end-diastolic pressure begins to rise (arrows) and is associated with a reduction in systolic pressure. Significant ST elevation begins after the rise in LV end-diastolic pressure c). On spontaneous resolution of ischemia (rise in CSO_2S), the changes resolve. Each episode lasted 2 minutes and was not associated with chest pain. LVP = left ventricular pressure. *(Modified from Chierchia S, Brunelli C, Simonetti I, et al: Sequence of events in angina at rest: Primary reduction in coronary flow. Circulation 61:759, 1980.)*

CH 48

Functional Consequences of Reversible Ischemia (see Fig. 16-29)

There are various late consequences of ischemia after normal myocardial perfusion is reestablished. These reflect acute as well as delayed effects on regional function, as well as protection of the heart from subsequent ischemic episodes. In the most chronic state, they result in hibernating myocardium, characterized by chronic contractile dysfunction and regional cellular mechanisms that downregulate contractile and metabolic function of the heart so as to protect it from irreversible injury. The complex interplay among these entities is summarized in Figure 48-24. Clinically, it is difficult to separate all the various mechanisms involved in contributing to ischemia-induced viable dysfunctional myocardium because they may all coexist to some extent in the same heart. They can, however, be separated experimentally, and the important features and mechanisms from basic studies are summarized here.

MYOCARDIAL PRECONDITIONING AND POSTCONDITIONING. Brief reversible ischemia preceding a prolonged coronary occlusion reduces myocyte necrosis, a phenomenon termed *acute preconditioning*.[47,52] Because acute infarction is frequently preceded by angina, preconditioning is an endogenous mechanism that can delay the evolution of irreversible myocardial injury. Acute preconditioning can be induced pharmacologically using adenosine A1 receptor stimulation as well as various pharmacological agonists that stimulate protein kinase C or open K^+-ATP channels. It has been demonstrated in humans during angioplasty with reduced subjective and objective ischemia during successive coronary occlusions as an endpoint. Preconditioning also develops on a chronic basis (delayed preconditioning) and, once induced, persists for up to 4 days.[53]

It reduces myocardial infarct size and protects the heart from ischemia-induced stunning. The mechanisms of chronic preconditioning involve protein synthesis, with upregulation of the inducible form of NO synthase (iNOS), cyclooxygenase (COX-2), and opening of the *mitochondrial* K^+-ATP channel. A final protective mechanism, *myocardial postconditioning*, refers to the ability to cause cardiac protection by producing intermittent ischemia or administering pharmacological agonists at the time of reperfusion. It is a relatively new observation and, although less extensively studied, has a greater potential to affect irreversible injury because it can be induced after myocardial ischemia is established rather than requiring pretreatment.[47]

STUNNED MYOCARDIUM. Myocardial function normalizes rapidly after single episodes of ischemia lasting less than 2 minutes. As ischemia increases in duration and/or severity, there is a temporal delay in the recovery of function that occurs, despite the fact that blood flow has been restored. Heyndrickx and associates were the first to demonstrate that regional myocardial function remained depressed for up to 6 hours after resolution of ischemia following a 15-minute occlusion in the absence of tissue necrosis, a phenomenon called "stunned myocardium" (Fig. 48-25).[52] A defining feature of isolated myocardial stunning is that function remains depressed while resting myocardial perfusion is normal. Thus, there is a dissociation of the usual close relationship between subendocardial flow and function. Stunned myocardium also occurs after demand-induced ischemia. For example, exercise-induced ischemia can result in depressed regional function distal to a coronary stenosis for hours after perfusion is restored, and repetitive ischemia can lead to cumulative stunning. Prolonged sublethal ischemia as in short-term hibernation

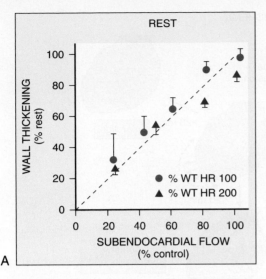

A

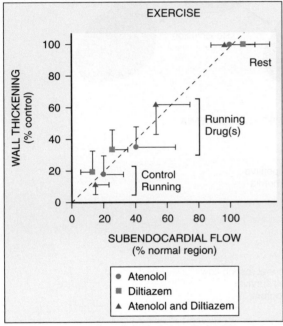

B

FIGURE 48–23 Perfusion contraction matching during acute ischemia. Relative reductions in function (regional wall thickening) are proportional to the relative reduction in subendocardial flow measured with microspheres in conscious dogs. This relationship is maintained over a wide range of heart rates during autoregulation (**A**) as well as during exercise with a fixed coronary stenosis (**B**). In the latter case, medical interventions that ameliorate ischemia improve both subendocardial flow and wall thickening during exercise. HR = heart rate. (**A** *modified from Canty JM Jr: Coronary pressure-function and steady-state pressure-flow relations during autoregulation in the unanesthetized dog. Circ Res 63:821, 1988, and Canty JM Jr, Giglia J, Kandath D: Effect of tachycardia on regional function and transmural myocardial perfusion during graded coronary pressure reduction in conscious dogs. Circulation 82:1815,1990;* **B** *modified from Matsuzaki M, Gallagher KB, Kemper WS, et al: Sustained regional dysfunction produced by prolonged coronary stenosis: Gradual recovery after reperfusion. Circulation 68:170, 1983.*)

leads to stunning on restoration of perfusion that may take up to a week to resolve in the absence of necrosis and may be an important cause of reversibly dysfunctional myocardium in the setting of an acute reduction in flow associated with an acute coronary syndrome.[54] Stunned myocardium is also responsible for postoperative pump dysfunction following cardiopulmonary bypass. Finally, areas of stunned myocardium can coexist with irreversibly injured myocardium and contribute to time-dependent improvements in function following myocardial infarction.

Acutely stunned myocardium is clinically important to recognize because contractile function normalizes during stimulation with various inotropic agents, including beta-adrenergic agonists. In contrast to other dysfunctional states, function will spontaneously normalize within 1 week, provided that there is no recurrent ischemia. If repetitive reversible ischemia develops before function normalizes, it can lead to a state of persistent dysfunction or chronic stunning. The cellular mechanism of stunning likely involves free radical–mediated myocardial injury and reduced myofilament calcium sensitivity.[55]

CHRONIC HIBERNATING MYOCARDIUM. Viable dysfunctional myocardium can be broadly defined as any region that directionally improves contractile function after coronary revascularization.[56,57] This broad definition of reversible dyssynergy includes three distinct categories with fairly diverse pathophysiological mechanisms that are summarized in Table 48-2. Complete normalization of function is the rule after acute ischemia but the exception in chronically dysfunctional myocardium. Brief occlusions or prolonged moderate ischemia (short-term hibernation) result in postischemic stunning in the absence of infarction, with complete functional recovery occurring rapidly within hours or no more than 1 week after reperfusion.[54,55] The time course of improvement is roughly dependent on the duration and severity of the ischemic episode. Reversible dyssynergy with delayed functional improvement can also occur from structural remodeling of the heart that is independent of ischemia or a coronary stenosis (e.g., remote myocardial remodeling in heart failure or the reduced infarct volume that occurs over the initial weeks following coronary reperfusion). The latter conditions can be readily identified when the clinical setting, coronary anatomy, and assessment of myocardial perfusion are taken into account. Many clinical studies have evaluated the presence of contractile reserve during dobutamine administration as a predictor of functional recovery. Although this identifies the likelihood of functional recovery (see Chap. 14), it cannot distinguish the diverse pathophysiological states underlying reversible dyssynergy. Understanding the cause may be important to the extent that it affects the time course and magnitude of functional recovery after revascularization in patients with ischemic heart failure.[57]

Chronic segmental dysfunction arising from repetitive episodes of ischemia (frequently clinically silent) is common and present in at least one coronary distribution in over 60 percent of patients with ischemic cardiomyopathy (Fig. 48-26).[58] When resting flow relative to a remote region is normal in dysfunctional myocardium distal to a stenosis, the region is chronically stunned. In contrast, when relative resting flow is reduced in the absence of symptoms or signs of ischemia, hibernating myocardium is present. Although there has previously been controversy over whether flow is normal or reduced at rest, both entities exist in patients and represent extremes in the spectrum of adaptive and maladaptive responses to chronic reversible ischemia. Viability studies are primarily required to distinguish infarction from hibernating myocardium because the myocardium is always viable when the resting flow is normal.[51]

It was originally thought that hibernating myocardium arose from a primary reduction in flow similar to experimental models of prolonged moderate ischemia and short-term hibernation. Whereas this is a plausible mechanism for the development of hibernating myocardium in association with an acute coronary syndrome, experimental studies have subsequently demonstrated that delayed subendocardial infarction is the rule rather than the exception when moderate flow reductions are maintained for more than 24 hours.[51] Many patients with hibernating myocardium present with LV dysfunction rather than symptomatic

CH 48

Coronary Blood Flow and Myocardial Ischemia

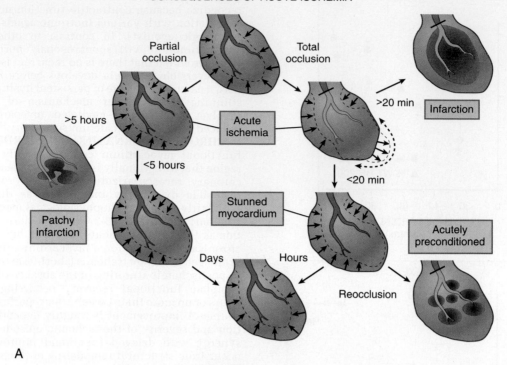

Partial occlusion

Total occlusion

Acute ischemia

>20 min → Infarction

>5 hours

<5 hours

<20 min

Patchy infarction

Stunned myocardium

Days

Hours

Reocclusion

Acutely preconditioned

A

CONSEQUENCES OF CHRONIC REPETITIVE ISCHEMIA

↓ Flow reserve

Chronically stunned myocardium

↓ Flow reserve

Chronically hibernating myocardium

Repetitive ischemia

Normal resting flow
Cell survival
Program

↑ Apoptosis
↓ β adrenergic signaling
Inhomogeneity in innervation

Reduced resting flow

Degeneration

Adaptation

Heart failure
Progressive fibrosis

Adapted to ischemia
Vulnerable to lethal arrhythmias

B

FIGURE 48–24 Effects of ischemia on left ventricular (LV) function and irreversible injury. The ventriculograms illustrate contractile dysfunction (dashed lines and arrows). **A,** Consequences of acute ischemia. A brief total occlusion (right) or a prolonged partial occlusion (caused by an acute high-grade stenosis, left) leads to acute contractile dysfunction proportional to the reduction in blood flow. Irreversible injury begins after 20 minutes following a total occlusion but is delayed for up to 5 hours following a partial occlusion (or with significant collaterals) caused by short-term hibernation. When reperfusion is established before the onset of irreversible injury, stunned myocardium develops and the time required for recovery of function is proportional to the duration and severity of ischemia. With prolonged ischemia, stunning in viable myocardium coexists with subendocardial infarction and accounts for reversible dysfunction. Brief episodes of ischemia preceding prolonged ischemia elicits protection against infarction (acute preconditioning). **B,** Effects of chronic repetitive ischemia on function distal to a stenosis. As stenosis severity increases, coronary flow reserve decreases and the frequency of reversible ischemia increases. Reversible repetitive ischemia initially leads to chronic preconditioning against infarction and stunning (not shown). Subsequently, there is a gradual progression from contractile dysfunction with normal resting flow (chronically stunned myocardium) to contractile dysfunction with depressed resting flow (hibernating myocardium). This transition is related to the physiological significance of a coronary stenosis and can occur in a time period as short as 1 week or develop chronically in the absence of severe angina. The cellular response during the progression to chronic hibernating myocardium is variable, with some patients exhibiting successful adaptation with little cell death and fibrosis and others developing degenerative changes difficult to distinguish from subendocardial infarction. See text for further discussion.

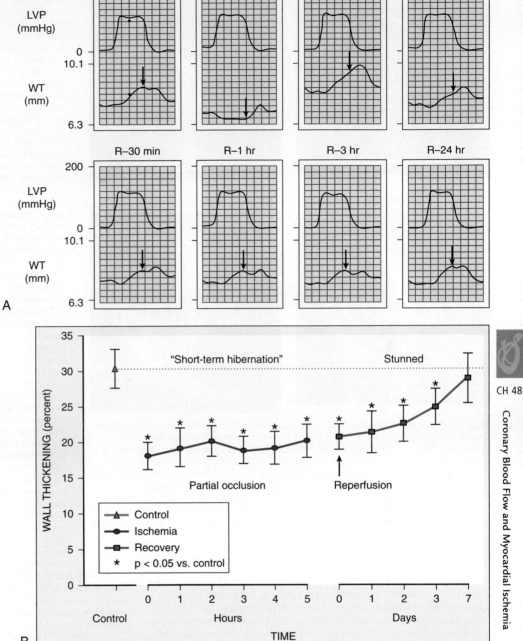

FIGURE 48–25 Stunned myocardium. **A,** Myocardial stunning following a brief total occlusion (OCCL.). Wall thickening (WT) measured by ultrasonic crystals is dyskinetic, with systolic thinning during occlusion. After reperfusion (R), function is completely normal after 24 hours. **B,** Myocardial stunning following a prolonged partial occlusion. During acute ischemia (red circles), there is short-term hibernation reflecting an acute match between reduced flow, wall thickening, and metabolism. With reperfusion (blue squares), wall thickening remains depressed and gradually returns to normal after 1 week. LVP = left ventricular pressure. (*A* modified from Heyndrickx GR, Baig H, Nellens P, et al: Depression of regional blood flow and wall thickening after brief coronary occlusions. Am J Physiol 234:H653, 1978. Used with permission of the American Physiological Society; *B* modified from Matsuzaki M, Gallagher KP, Kemper WS, et al: Sustained regional dysfunction produced by prolonged coronary stenosis: Gradual recovery after reperfusion. Circulation 68:170, 1983.)

TABLE 48–2	Viable Dysfunctional Myocardium: Patterns of Contractile Reserve, Resting Perfusion, and Temporal Recovery of Function after Revascularization			
Parameter	**Contractile Reserve**	**Resting Flow**	**Extent of Functional Recovery**	**Time Course of Recovery**
Transient Reversible Ischemia				
Postischemic stunning	Present	Normal	Normalizes	<24 hr
Short-term hibernation	Present	Normal	Normalizes	<7 days
Chronic Repetitive Ischemia				
Chronic hibernating myocardium	Variable	Reduced	Improves	Up to 12 mo
Chronic stunning	Present	Normal	Improves	Days to weeks
Structural Remodeling				
Subendocardial infarction	Variable	Reduced	Variable	Weeks
Remodeled, tethered myocardium	Present	Normal	Improves	Months

Ventriculogram

FDG

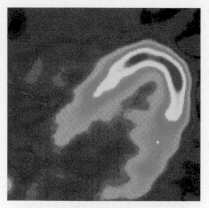

Resting flow

Vasodilated flow

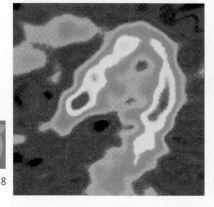
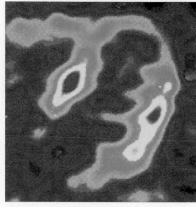

FIGURE 48–26 Hibernating myocardium in humans with a chronic LAD occlusion and collateral dependent myocardium. The RAO tracings of the left ventriculogram shows anterior akinesis (upper left). Transaxial PET scans illustrate $^{13}NH_3$ flow measurements at rest (lower left) and following pharmacological vasodilation with dipyridamole (lower right). Quantitative perfusion measurements showed LAD flow to be critically impaired. Viability (following an oral glucose load) is identified by increased ^{18}F-2-deoxyglucose (FDG) uptake in the anterior wall (upper right). LAD = left anterior descending artery; PET = position emission tomography; RAO = right anterior oblique. (See also Chap. 6.) *(Modified from Vanoverschelde J-LJ, Wijns W, Depre C, et al: Mechanisms of chronic regional postischemic dysfunction in humans: New insights from the study of noninfarcted collateral-dependent myocardium. Circulation 87:1513, 1993.)*

ischemia. Serial studies in animals have now demonstrated that the reductions in relative resting flow are a consequence rather than a cause of the contractile dysfunction.[59,60] This paradigm, relevant to chronic coronary disease, was proposed after studies in pigs with a slowly progressive left anterior descending artery (LAD) stenosis demonstrated that dysfunction with normal resting flow consistent with chronic stunning precedes the development of hibernating myocardium after 3 months (Fig. 48-27).[56] The progression from chronically stunned myocardium (with normal resting flow) to hibernating myocardium (with reduced flow) is related to the functional significance of the chronic stenosis supplying the region and is probably a reflection of its propensity to develop repetitive supply or demand-induced ischemia. This progression can develop in as little as 1 week after placement of a critical stenosis that exhausts coronary flow reserve.[61] As regional dysfunction progresses from chronically stunned to hibernating myocardium, the myocyte takes on regional characteristics similar to those from an explanted heart with advanced failure. Normally perfused remote zone cardiac myocytes can be normal or take on structural alterations similar to the dysfunctional region. Some of the major cellular responses are summarized here.

APOPTOSIS, MYOCYTE LOSS, AND MYOFIBRILLAR LOSS. The frequency of focal myocyte death from apoptosis varies during the development of viable dysfunctional myocardium and thus is probably responsible for the variability in the frequency of apoptosis when analyzing biopsies from patients.[62,63] Experimentally, apoptosis is particularly prominent during the transition from chronically stunned to hibernating myocardium, at which time there is a loss of approximately 30 percent of the regional myocytes (Fig. 48-28).[64] The myocyte loss results in compensatory regional myocyte hypertrophy to maintain approximately normal wall thickness. Vanoverschelde and colleagues have previously described light and ultrastructural characteristics of hibernating myocardium from transmural biopsies, which are characterized by small increases in interstitial connective tissue, myofibrillar loss (myolysis), increased glycogen deposition, and minimitochondria.[65] Experimental animal models of hibernating myocardium also develop these structural changes in as little as 2 weeks but they are also present in remote, normally perfused regions of the heart.[61,66] Global cellular changes have also been reported in patients in the absence of a stenosis, suggesting that the structural changes are probably the result of chronically elevated preload. Thus, although cellular dedifferentiation had been emphasized as a mechanism of adaptation, the ultrastructural changes are probably not causally related to the regional responses to ischemia in hibernating myocardium.[51,57]

CELL SURVIVAL AND ANTIAPOPTOTIC PROGRAM IN RESPONSE TO REPETITIVE ISCHEMIA. There is variability in the regulation of cell survival pathways in response to repetitive ischemia. Some studies have demonstrated upregulation of cardioprotective mechanisms in response to repetitive reversible ischemia, which may be operative in minimizing myocyte cell death and fibrosis in the chronic setting.[67] An interesting mechanism potentially linking altered metabolism and protection is the regional downregulation of glycogen synthase kinase-3β, which can ameliorate cell death and also explain the increased tissue glycogen in hibernating myocardium.[68] In some studies, antiapoptotic and stress proteins such as HSP-70 have been found to be upregulated following repetitive ischemia, whereas increased proapoptotic proteins and a profile of progressive cell death and fibrosis have been reported in human biopsies of patients with hibernating myocardium by others.[63] It is likely that the variability among studies reflects the frequency and severity of ischemia as well as the complexity of the temporal expression of adaptive and maladaptive responses in myocardium subjected to chronic repetitive ischemia.

METABOLISM AND ENERGETICS IN HIBERNATING MYOCARDIUM. Once adapted, the metabolic and contractile response of hibernating myocardium appears to be dissociated from external determinants of workload. As a result, submaximal increases in oxygen consumption can occur without immediately leading to subendocardial ischemia.[69] Experimentally, the hibernating myocardial region appears to operate over a lower range of the normal myocardial supply-demand relationship in a fashion similar to that of the nonischemic failing heart. Although glycogen content is increased, maximum rates of glucose uptake during insulin stimulation are not altered. In addition, creatine phosphate and ATP levels are not regionally altered, contrasting with the depressed ATP levels in stunning. Recently, studies of isolated mitochondria from swine with hibernating myocardium have demonstrated a downregulation of energy uptake and oxygen consumption.[70]

INHOMOGENEITY IN SYMPATHETIC INNERVATION, BETA-ADRENERGIC RESPONSES, AND SUDDEN DEATH. The contractile response of hibernating myocardium is blunted and partially related to a regional downregulation in beta-adrenergic adenylyl cyclase coupling, similar to that found globally in advanced heart failure.[71] This may be related to local norepinephrine overflow because the presynaptic uptake of norepinephrine is reduced when assessed using nuclear tracers such as ^{11}C-hydroxyephedrine.[72] The resultant inhomogeneity in myocardial sympathetic nerve function may be one of the reasons responsible for the vulnerability of experimental hibernating myocardium to develop lethal ventricular arrhythmias and ventricular fibrillation.[73] Thus, normalizing electrical instability as well as improving contractile dysfunction may account for the profound impact of revascularization on survival when hibernating myocardium is present.[57]

SUCCESSFUL ADAPTATION VERSUS DEGENERATION IN HIBERNATING MYOCARDIUM. There is considerable divergence among studies regarding the pathology of reversibly dyssynergic hibernating myocardium. At one extreme, some investigators believe that it is destined to undergo irreversible myocyte death, which is supported by data showing large amounts of fibrosis (more than 30 percent of the tissue), markedly abnormal high-energy phosphate metabolism, and retrospective analysis suggesting that the degree of fibrosis is related to the duration of hibernating myocardium.[63] At the other extreme, there are circumstances in which fibrosis is not a prominent feature with normal myocardial energetics at rest, suggesting that hibernating myocardium can be sustained for long periods without progressive degeneration.[73,74] The factors that determine the path to progressive structural degeneration versus adaptation are currently unknown but may be modulated by the superimposed neurohormonal activation, elevation in cytokine levels associated with advanced clinical heart failure, and structural degeneration that arises from small reductions in coronary flow reserve below the threshold required to maintain myocyte viability.

FUTURE PERSPECTIVES

There has been considerable progress in our mechanistic understanding of the coronary circulation and myocardial ischemia in health and disease but important gaps remain in our knowledge as well as the translation of this to clinical care. First, although advances have occurred in characterizing the physiology of the coronary microcirculation, the mechanisms of metabolic control and coronary autoregulation are still incompletely understood. There is a need for better incorporation of abnormalities of coronary microcirculatory control into the management of patients with CAD because, in some circumstances, these may be as important as epicardial coronary artery stenoses in determining prognosis. Second, although considerable basic and clinical investigation has been directed at developing angiogenic interventions to ameliorate ischemia, all the promising basic studies have failed to be translated to positive clinical trials. Incorporating quantitative approaches to assess myocardial perfusion during pharmacological vasodilation would better define the most promising interventions that could increase blood flow in a meaningful fashion. Advances in imaging that allow perfusion to be assessed in the subendocardial layers, as well as reliable quantitation of flow or flow reserve on a vessel-specific basis, would also significantly advance our ability to detect early disease that is functionally significant. Finally, we require a better understanding of the role of spontaneous episodes of ischemia in the development of chronic adaptations to ischemia, such as preconditioning and hibernating myocardium, as well as the maladaptive response of hibernating myocardium to lethal ventricular arrhythmias. These substrates may precede the development of severe LV dysfunction, and identifying inhomogeneity in myocardial sympathetic innervation arising from reversible ischemia or the onset of myocyte loss from apoptosis, for example, may help develop an approach to identify regional inhomogeneity that may lead to a substrate for arrhythmogenesis. Although much progress has been made, there is still much more to learn.

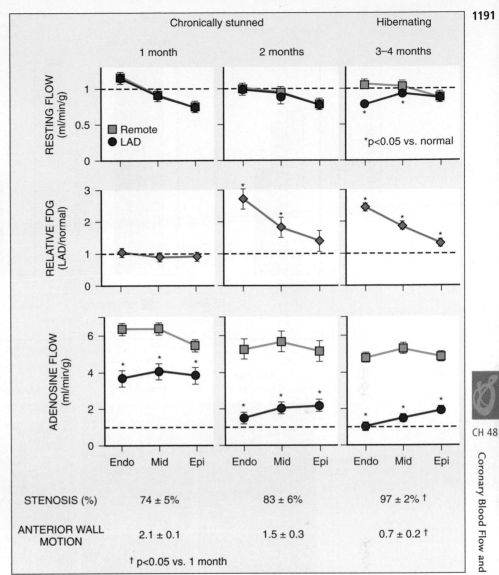

FIGURE 48–27 Progression from chronically stunned to hibernating myocardium as stenosis severity increases in swine with viable dysfunctional myocardium from a chronic LAD stenosis. Transmural flow measurements (microspheres) at rest and adenosine vasodilation are shown, along with regional FDG uptake (fasting conditions). Below are the angiographic stenosis severity and anterior wall motion score (3, normal; 2, mild hypokinesis; 1, severe hypokinesis). As stenosis severity increases over time, there is a reduction in vasodilated flow (adenosine) to the LAD region. Initially, there is anterior hypokinesis, with normal resting flow consistent with chronically stunned myocardium. After 3 months, the stenosis progresses to occlusion with collateral dependent myocardium. Subendocardial flow is critically reduced and there is a reduction in resting flow to the inner two thirds of the LAD myocardium. At this time, hibernating myocardium is present and there is no evidence of infarction. The temporal progression of abnormalities demonstrate that chronic stunning precedes the development of hibernating myocardium. In contrast to short-term hibernation resulting from acute ischemia, the reduction in resting flow is a consequence, rather than a cause, of the contractile dysfunction. Endo = endocardium; Epi = epicardium; FDG = ^{18}F-2-deoxyglucose; LAD = left anterior descending artery. (*Modified from Fallavollita JA, Canty JM Jr: Differential ^{18}F-2-deoxyglucose uptake in viable dysfunctional myocardium with normal resting perfusion: Evidence for chronic stunning in pigs. Circulation 99:2798, 1999.*)

CH 48

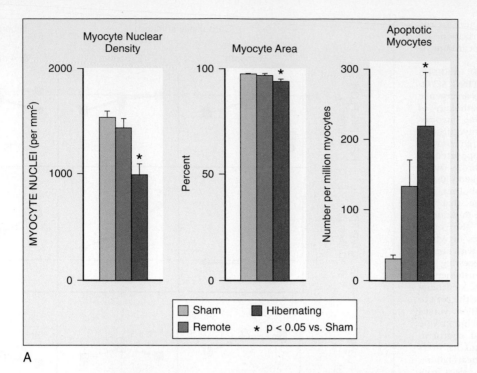

A

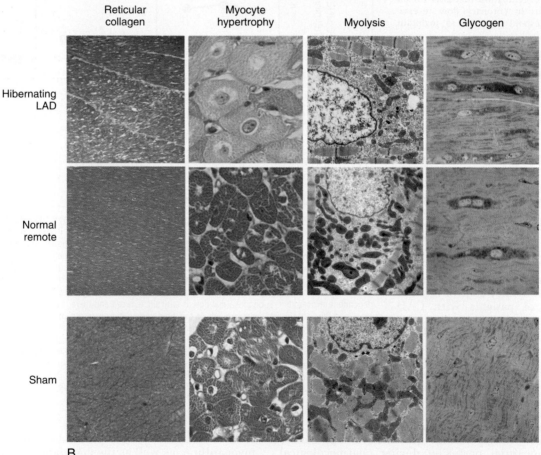

B

FIGURE 48–28 Apoptosis, hypertrophy, and myocyte cellular morphology in hibernating myocardium. Data in hibernating LAD regions are compared with remote regions as well as with LAD regions from normal animals. **A,** The progression from chronically stunned to hibernating myocardium is accompanied by regional apoptosis induced myocyte loss. There is about a 30 percent reduction in myocyte nuclear number without significant fibrosis, because the myocyte area is nearly normal. **B,** Myocyte cellular changes in hibernating myocardium. The increased myocyte loss results in compensatory myocyte cellular hypertrophy in hibernating myocardium. Whereas reticular collagen is regionally increased (about 2 percent), there is no evidence of infarction. The electron microscopic characteristics of hibernating myocardium demonstrate myofibrillar loss, an increased number of small mitochondria, and increased glycogen content. Although these are markedly different from normal myocardium (sham), biopsies of normal remote, nonischemic segments show similar morphological changes, indicating that these structural abnormalities are not directly related to ischemia nor are they the cause of regional contractile dysfunction. LAD = left anterior descending artery. (*A* from Lim H, Fallavollita JA, Hard R, et al: Profound apoptosis-mediated regional myocyte loss and compensatory hypertrophy in pigs with hibernating myocardium. Circulation 100:2380, 1999; *B* from Canty JM, Fallavollita JA: Hibernating myocardium. J Nucl Cardiol 12:104, 2005.)

REFERENCES

Control of Coronary Blood Flow

1. Hoffman JIE: Transmural myocardial perfusion. Prog Cardiovasc Dis 29:429, 1987.
2. Canty JM Jr, Brooks A: Phasic volumetric coronary venous outflow patterns in conscious dogs. Am J Physiol 258:H1457, 1990.
3. Feigl EO: Coronary physiology. Physiol Rev 63:1, 1983.
4. Canty JM Jr: Coronary pressure-function and steady-state pressure-flow relations during autoregulation in the unanesthetized dog. Circ Res 63:821, 1988.
5. Klocke FJ: Coronary blood flow in man. Prog Cardiovasc Dis 19:117, 1976.
6. Canty JM Jr, Giglia J, Kandath D: Effect of tachycardia on regional function and transmural myocardial perfusion during graded coronary pressure reduction in conscious dogs. Circulation 82:1815, 1990.
7. Canty JM Jr, Smith TP, Jr: Adenosine-recruitable flow reserve is absent during myocardial ischemia in unanesthetized dogs studied in the basal state. Circ Res 76:1079, 1995.
8. Hoffman JIE, Spaan JAE: Pressure-flow relations in coronary circulation. Physiol Rev 70:331, 1990.
9. Duncker DJ, Bache RJ: Regulation of coronary vasomotor tone under normal conditions and during acute myocardial hypoperfusion. Pharmacol Ther 86:87, 2000.
10. Furchgott RF, Zawadzki JV: The obligatory role of endothelial cells in the relaxation of arterial smooth muscle by acetylcholine. Nature 288:373, 1980.
11. Kuo L, Davis MJ, Chilian WM: Longitudinal gradients for endothelium-dependent and -independent vascular responses in the coronary microcirculation. Circulation 92:518, 1995.
12. Chilian WM, Layne SM, Klausner EC, et al: Redistribution of coronary microvascular resistance produced by dipyridamole. Am J Physiol 256:H383, 1989.
13. Spaan JA, Piek JJ, Hoffman JIE, et al: Physiological basis of clinically used coronary hemodynamic indices. Circulation 113:446, 2006.
14. Kanatsuka H, Lamping KG, Eastham CL, et al: Heterogeneous changes in epimyocardial microvascular size during graded coronary stenosis. Evidence of the microvascular site for autoregulation. Circ Res 66:389, 1990.
15. Kanatsuka H, Lamping KG, Eastham CL, et al: Comparison of the effects of increased myocardial oxygen consumption and adenosine on the coronary microvascular resistance. Circ Res 65:1296, 1989.
16. Kuo L, Davis MJ, Chilian WM: Myogenic activity in isolated subepicardial and subendocardial coronary arterioles. Am J Physiol 255:H1558, 1988.
17. Miller FJ, Dellsperger KC, Gutterman DD: Myogenic constriction of human coronary arterioles. Am J Physiol 273:H257, 1997.
18. Kuo L, Davis MJ, Chilian WM: Endothelium-dependent, flow-induced dilation of isolated coronary arterioles. Am J Physiol 259:H1063, 1990.
19. Miura H, Wachtel RE, Liu Y, et al: Flow-induced dilation of human coronary arterioles: Important role of Ca^{2+}-activated K^+ channels. Circulation 103:1992, 2001.
20. Dube S, Canty JM Jr: Shear-stress induced vasodilation in porcine coronary conduit arteries is independent of nitric oxide release. Am J Physiol 280:H2581, 2001.
21. Quyyumi AA, Dakak N, Andrews NP, et al: Contribution of nitric oxide to metabolic coronary vasodilation in the human heart. Circulation 92:320, 1995.
22. Sato A, Terata K, Miura H, et al: Mechanism of vasodilation to adenosine in coronary arterioles from patients with heart disease. Am J Physiol Heart Circ Physiol 288:H1633, 2005.
23. Jones CJ, Kuo L, Davis MJ, et al: Role of nitric oxide in the coronary microvascular responses to adenosine and increased metabolic demand. Circulation 91:1807, 1995.
24. Tune JD, Richmond KN, Gorman MW, et al: Control of coronary blood flow during exercise. Exp Biol Med 227:238, 2002.
25. Heusch G, Baumgart D, Camici P, et al: α-Adrenergic coronary vasoconstriction and myocardial ischemia in humans. Circulation 101:689, 2000.
26. Konidala S, Gutterman DD: Coronary vasospasm and the regulation of coronary blood flow. Prog Cardiovasc Dis 46:349, 2004.
27. Hizume T, Morikawa K, Takaki A, et al: Sustained elevation of serum cortisol level causes sensitization of coronary vasoconstricting responses in pigs in vivo. A possible link between stress and coronary vasospasm. Circ Res 99:767, 2006.

Pharmacological Vasodilation

28. Jones CJH, Kuo L, Davis MJ, et al: In vivo and in vitro vasoactive reactions of coronary arteriolar microvessels to nitroglycerin. Am J Physiol 271:H461, 1996.
29. Jones CJH, Kuo L, Davis MJ, et al: Role of nitric oxide in the coronary microvascular responses to adenosine and increased metabolic demand. Circulation 91:1807, 1995.
30. Guethlin M, Kasel AM, Coppenrath K, et al: Delayed response of myocardial flow reserve to lipid-lowering therapy with fluvastatin. Circulation 99:475, 1999.
31. Zong P, Tune JD, Downey HF: Mechanisms of oxygen demand/supply balance in the right ventricle. Exp Biol Med (Maywood) 230:507, 2005.

Physiological Assessment of Coronary Artery Stenosis

32. Gould KL: Coronary Artery Stenosis. New York, Elsevier Science; 1991.
33. Kern MJ, Lerman A, Bech JW, et al: Physiological Assessment of Coronary Artery Disease in the Cardiac Catheterization Laboratory. A Scientific Statement From the American Heart Association Committee on Diagnostic and Interventional Cardiac Catheterization, Council on Clinical Cardiology. Circulation 114:1321, 2006.
34. Klocke FJ: Measurements of coronary blood flow and degree of stenosis: Current clinical implications and continuing uncertainties. J Am Coll Cardiol 1:31, 1983.
35. Yokoyama I, Ohtake T, Momomura S, et al: Reduced coronary flow reserve in hypercholesterolemic patients without overt coronary stenosis. Circulation 94:3232, 1996.

36. Wang L, Jerosch-Herold M, Jacobs DR Jr, et al: Coronary artery calcification and myocardial perfusion in asymptomatic adults: The MESA (Multi-Ethnic Study of Atherosclerosis). J Am Coll Cardiol 48:1018, 2006.
37. Buchthal SD, den Hollander JA, Merz CN, et al: Abnormal myocardial phosphorus-31 nuclear magnetic resonance spectroscopy in women with chest pain but normal coronary angiograms. N Engl J Med 342:829, 2000.
38. Bache RJ: Effects of hypertrophy on the coronary circulation. Prog Cardiovasc Dis 31:403, 1988.
39. Kuo L, Davis MJ, Cannon MS, et al: Pathophysiological consequences of atherosclerosis extend into the coronary microcirculation: Restoration of endothelium-dependent responses by L-arginine. Circ Res 70:465, 1992.
40. Smith TP Jr, Canty JM, Jr: Modulation of coronary autoregulatory responses by nitric oxide: Evidence for flow-dependent resistance adjustments in conscious dogs. Circ Res 73:232, 1993.
41. Duncker DJ, Bache RJ: Inhibition of nitric oxide production aggravates myocardial hypoperfusion during exercise in the presence of a coronary artery stenosis. Circ Res 74:629, 1994.

Coronary Collateral Circulation

42. Schaper W, Ito WD: Molecular mechanisms of coronary collateral vessel growth. Circ Res 79:911, 1996.
43. Matsunaga T, Warltier DC, Weihrauch DW, et al: Ischemia-induced coronary collateral growth is dependent on vascular endothelial growth factor and nitric oxide. Circulation 102:3098, 2000.
44. Simons M: Angiogenesis: Where do we stand now? Circulation 111:1556, 2005.
45. Suzuki G, Lee TC, Fallavollita JA, et al: Adenoviral gene transfer of FGF-5 to hibernating myocardium improves function and stimulates myocytes to hypertrophy and reenter the cell cycle. Circ Res 96:767, 2005.

Metabolic and Functional Consequences of Ischemia

46. Kloner RA, Jennings RB: Consequences of brief ischemia: Stunning, preconditioning, and their clinical implications: Part 1. Circulation 104:2981, 2001.
47. Downey JM, Cohen MV: Reducing infarct size in the setting of acute myocardial infarction. Prog Cardiovasc Dis 48:363, 2006.
48. Heusch G: Hibernating myocardium. Physiol Rev 78:1055, 1998.
49. Gallagher KP, Matsuzaki M, Osakada G, et al: Effect of exercise on the relationship between myocardial blood flow and systolic wall thickening in dogs with acute coronary stenosis. Circ Res 52:716, 1983.
50. Matsuzaki M, Guth B, Tajimi T, et al: Effect of the combination of diltiazem and atenolol on exercise-induced regional myocardial ischemia in conscious dogs. Circulation 72:233, 1985.
51. Heusch G, Schulz R, Rahimtoola SH: Myocardial hibernation: A delicate balance. Am J Physiol Heart Circ Physiol 288:H984, 2005.
52. Kloner RA, Jennings RB: Consequences of brief ischemia: Stunning, preconditioning, and their clinical implications: Part 2. Circulation 104:3158, 2001.
53. Bolli R: The late phase of preconditioning. Circ Res 87:972, 2000.
54. Matsuzaki M, Gallagher KP, Kemper WS, et al: Sustained regional dysfunction produced by prolonged coronary stenosis: Gradual recovery after reperfusion. Circulation 68:170, 1983.
55. Bolli R, Marban E: Molecular and cellular mechanisms of myocardial stunning. Physiol Rev 79:609, 1999.
56. Canty JM Jr, Fallavollita JA: Chronic hibernation and chronic stunning: A continuum. J Nucl Cardiol 7:509, 2000.
57. Canty JM, Fallavollita JA: Hibernating myocardium. J Nucl Cardiol 12:104, 2005.
58. Vanoverschelde J-LJ, Wijns W, Depre C, et al: Mechanisms of chronic regional postischemic dysfunction in humans: New insights from the study of noninfarcted collateral-dependent myocardium. Circulation 87:1513, 1993.
59. Fallavollita JA, Perry BJ, Canty JM, Jr: ^{18}F-2-deoxyglucose deposition and regional flow in pigs with chronically dysfunctional myocardium: Evidence for transmural variations in chronic hibernating myocardium. Circulation 95:1900, 1997.
60. Fallavollita JA, Canty JM, Jr: Differential ^{18}F-2-deoxyglucose uptake in viable dysfunctional myocardium with normal resting perfusion: Evidence for chronic stunning in pigs. Circulation 99:2798, 1999.
61. Thomas SA, Fallavollita JA, Borgers M, et al: Dissociation of regional adaptations to ischemia and global myolysis in an accelerated swine model of chronic hibernating myocardium. Circ Res 91:970, 2002.
62. Dispersyn GD, Borgers M, Flameng W: Apoptosis in chronic hibernating myocardium: Sleeping to death? Cardiovasc Res 45:696, 2000.
63. Elsasser A, Vogt AM, Nef H, et al: Human hibernating myocardium is jeopardized by apoptotic and autophagic cell death. J Am Coll Cardiol 43:2191, 2004.
64. Lim H, Fallavollita JA, Hard R, et al: Profound apoptotis-mediated regional myocyte loss and compensatory hypertrophy in pigs with hibernating myocardium. Circulation 100:2380, 1999.
65. Vanoverschelde J-L, Wijns W, Borgers M, et al: Chronic myocardial hibernation in humans. From bedside to bench. Circulation 95:1961, 1997.
66. Thijssen VL, Borgers M, Lenders M-H, et al: Temporal and spatial variations in structural protein expression during the progression from stunned to hibernating myocardium. Circulation 110:3313, 2004.
67. Depre C, Vatner SF: Mechanisms of cell survival in myocardial hibernation. Trends Cardiovasc Med 15:101, 2005.
68. Kim SJ, Peppas A, Hong SK, et al: Persistent stunning induces myocardial hibernation and protection: flow/function and metabolic mechanisms. Circ Res 92:1233, 2003.
69. Fallavollita JA, Malm BJ, Canty JM, Jr: Hibernating myocardium retains metabolic and contractile reserve despite regional reductions in flow, function, and oxygen consumption at rest. Circ Res 92:48, 2003.

CH 48

Coronary Blood Flow and Myocardial Ischemia

1194

70. McFalls EO, Sluiter W, Schoonderwoerd K, et al: Mitochondrial adaptations within chronically ischemic swine myocardium. J Mol Cell Cardiol 41:980, 2006.

71. Iyer V, Canty JM Jr: Regional desensitization of β-adrenergic receptor signaling in swine with chronic hibernating myocardium. Circ Res 97:789, 2005.

72. Luisi AJ, Jr, Suzuki G, deKemp R, et al: Regional ¹¹C-hydroxyephedrine retention in hibernating myocardium: Chronic inhomogeneity of sympathetic innervation in the absence of infarction. J Nucl Med 46:1368, 2005.

73. Canty JM, Jr, Suzuki G, Banas MD, et al: Hibernating myocardium: Chronically adapted to ischemia but vulnerable to sudden death. Circ Res 94:1142, 2004.

74. Dispersyn GD, Ramaekers FCS, Borgers M: Clinical pathophysiology of hibernating myocardium. Coron Artery Dis 12:381, 2001.

75. Heyndrickx GR, Baig H, Nellens P, et al: Depression of regional blood flow and wall thickening after brief coronary occlusions. Am J Physiol 234:H653, 1978.

CH 48

CHAPTER 49

Causes of Acute Chest Pain, 1195
Initial Assessment, 1197
Markers of Myocardial Injury, 1197

Initial Risk Stratification, 1200
Clinical History, 1200
The Physical Examination, 1200
The Electrocardiogram, 1201
Decision Aids, 1201

Immediate Management, 1202
Chest Pain Protocols and Units, 1202
Early Noninvasive Testing, 1202

References, 1204

Approach to the Patient with Chest Pain

Christopher P. Cannon and Thomas H. Lee

Acute chest pain is one of the most common reasons for presentation to the Emergency Department (ED)—accounting for approximately 7 million ED visits per year in the United States. This presentation suggests acute coronary syndrome (ACS); however, only 15 to 25 percent of patients with acute chest pain actually have ACS after diagnostic evaluation.[1-3] The difficulty is to discriminate patients with ACS from those with noncardiac chest pain.[4-6] A missed diagnosis of ACS occurs in approximately 2 percent of patients and has substantial consequences: the short-term mortality for patients with acute myocardial infarction (MI) who are mistakenly discharged from the ED increases twofold over that expected were they admitted.[1] The legal costs that result from missed diagnoses of MI represent the largest category of losses from emergency medicine malpractice litigation.[7] For patients with low risks of complications, however, these concerns must be balanced against the costs and inconvenience that accompany admission to the hospital, and the risks of complications from tests and procedures with a low probability of improving patient outcomes.

Several advances in recent years have enhanced the accuracy and efficiency of the evaluation of patients with acute chest pain.[2] These advances include better blood markers for myocardial injury (see Chap. 50)[8]; decision aids to stratify patients according to their risks of complications; early and even immediate exercise testing[4] and radionuclide scanning for lower risk patient subsets[9]; emerging use of multislice computerized tomography for anatomical evaluation for coronary artery disease,[10] and use of chest pain units[5] and critical pathways for efficient and rapid evaluation of lower risk patients.[11]

CAUSES OF ACUTE CHEST PAIN

As noted earlier, in a typical population of patients presenting for evaluation of acute chest pain in EDs, about 15 to 25 percent have acute MI or unstable angina.[12] A small percentage have other life-threatening problems, such as pulmonary embolism or acute aortic dissection, but most are discharged without a diagnosis or with a diagnosis of a noncardiac condition. These noncardiac conditions include musculoskeletal syndromes, disorders of abdominal viscera including gastroesophageal reflux disease, and psychological conditions (Table 49-1).

MYOCARDIAL ISCHEMIA OR INFARCTION. The most common serious cause of acute chest discomfort is myocardial ischemia or infarction (see Chaps. 48, 50, and 53), which occurs when the myocardial oxygen supply is inadequate compared to myocardial oxygen demand. Myocardial ischemia usually occurs in the setting of coronary atherosclerosis but may also reflect dynamic components of coronary vascular resistance. Coronary spasm can occur in normal coronary arteries, or, in patients with coronary disease, near atherosclerotic plaques and in smaller coronary arteries (see Chap. 48). Other, less common causes of impaired coronary blood flow include syndromes that compromise the orifices of the coronary arteries or the arteries themselves, such as syphilitic aortitis, arteritides, aortic dissection, myocardial bridges, or congenital abnormalities of the coronary arteries (see Chap. 20).

Ischemic chest pain also can result from any disease process that causes occlusion of a coronary artery, such as thrombosis arising at the site of a ruptured atherosclerotic plaque. Other potential causes include coronary artery emboli such as may occur in patients with infectious or noninfectious endocarditis, or thrombus in the left atrium or left ventricle.

Myocardial ischemia can result from conditions that cause a mismatch between the perfusion pressure within the coronary arteries and myocardial oxygen demand, such as aortic stenosis, aortic regurgitation, or hypertrophic cardiomyopathy. Increases in heart rate can markedly exacerbate ischemia in such patients because, even as oxygen demand rises, myocardial perfusion falls because of a reduction in the proportion of time that the heart is in diastole, thereby decreasing the available time for coronary perfusion. Other clinical conditions can worsen oxygen delivery and/or raise oxygen need, although they generally cause myocardial ischemia and chest pain only when accompanied by coronary atherosclerosis. Such conditions include anemia, sepsis, and thyrotoxicosis.

The classic manifestation of ischemia is angina, which is usually described as a heavy chest pressure or squeezing, a "burning" feeling, or difficulty breathing. The discomfort often radiates to the left shoulder, neck, or arm. It typically builds in intensity over a period of a few minutes. The pain may begin with exercise or psychological stress, but ACS most commonly occurs without obvious precipitating factors.

"Atypical" descriptions of chest pain reduce the likelihood that the symptoms represent myocardial ischemia or injury. The American College of Cardiology and the American Heart Association (ACC/AHA) guidelines list the following as pain descriptions that are *not* characteristic of myocardial ischemia[11]:

- Pleuritic pain (i.e., sharp or knife-like pain brought on by respiratory movements or cough)
- Primary or sole location of discomfort in the middle or lower abdominal region
- Pain that may be localized at the tip of one finger, particularly over the left ventricular apex

TABLE 49-1		Common Causes of Acute Chest Pain	
System	Syndrome	Clinical Description	Key Distinguishing Features
Cardiac	Angina	Retrosternal chest pressure, burning, or heaviness; radiating occasionally to neck, jaw, epigastrium, shoulders, or left arm	Precipitated by exercise, cold weather, or emotional stress; duration <2-10 minutes.
	Rest or unstable angina	Same as angina, but may be more severe	Typically <20 minutes; lower tolerance for exertion
	Acute myocardial infarction	Same as angina, but may be more severe	Sudden onset, usually lasting 30 minutes or longer. Often associated with shortness of breath, weakness, nausea, vomiting
	Pericarditis	Sharp, pleuritic pain aggravated by changes in position; highly variable duration	Pericardial friction rub
Vascular	Aortic dissection	Excruciating, ripping pain of sudden onset in anterior of chest, often radiating to back	Marked severity of unrelenting pain; usually occurs in setting of hypertension or underlying connective tissue disorder such as Marfan syndrome
	Pulmonary embolism	Sudden onset of dyspnea and pain, usually pleuritic with pulmonary infarction	Dyspnea, tachypnea, tachycardia, and signs of right heart failure
	Pulmonary hypertension	Substernal chest pressure, exacerbated by exertion	Pain associated with dyspnea and signs of pulmonary hypertension
Pulmonary	Pleuritis and/or pneumonia	Pleuritic pain, usually brief, over involved area	Pain pleuritic and lateral to midline, associated with dyspnea
	Tracheobronchitis	Burning discomfort in midline	Midline location, associated with coughing
	Spontaneous pneumothorax	Sudden onset of unilateral pleuritic pain, with dyspnea	Abrupt onset of dyspnea and pain
Gastrointestinal	Esophageal reflux	Burning substernal and epigastric discomfort, 10-60 minutes in duration	Aggravated by large meal and postprandial recumbency; relieved by antacid
	Peptic ulcer	Prolonged epigastric or substernal burning	Relieved by antacid or food
	Gallbladder disease	Prolonged epigastric right upper quadrant pain	Unprovoked or following meal
	Pancreatitis	Prolonged, intense epigastric and substernal pain	Risk factors including alcohol, hypertriglyceridemia, and medications
Musculoskeletal	Costochondritis	Sudden onset of intense fleeting pain	May be reproduced by pressure over affected joint; occasional patients have swelling and inflammation over costochondral joint
	Cervical disc disease	Sudden onset of fleeting pain	May be reproduced with movement of neck
	Trauma or strain	Constant pain	Reproduced by palpation or movement of chest wall or arms
Infectious	Herpes zoster	Prolonged burning pain in dermatomal distribution	Vesicular rash, dermatomal distribution
Psychological	Panic disorder	Chest tightness or aching, often accompanied by dyspnea and lasting 30 minutes or more, unrelated to exertion or movement	Patient may have other evidence of emotional disorder

CH 49

- Pain reproduced with movement or palpation of the chest wall or arms
- Constant pain that persists for many hours
- Very brief episodes of pain that last a few seconds or less
- Pain that radiates into the lower extremities

However, data from large populations of patients with acute chest pain indicate that ACS occurs in patients with atypical symptoms with sufficient frequency that no single factor should be used to exclude the diagnosis of acute ischemic heart disease.[2] In particular, women may report symptoms of myocardial ischemia and/or infarction differently from typical symptoms in men (see Chap. 76).

PERICARDIAL DISEASE. The visceral surface of the pericardium is insensitive to pain, as is most of the parietal surface. Therefore, noninfectious causes of pericarditis (such as uremia) (see Chap. 70) usually cause little or no pain. In contrast, infectious pericarditis nearly always involves surrounding pulmonary pleura, so that patients typically experience pleuritic pain with breathing, coughing, and changes in position. Swallowing may induce the pain because of the proximity of the esophagus to the posterior heart. Because the central diaphragm receives its sensory supply from the phrenic nerve, and the phrenic nerve arises from the third to fifth cervical segments of the

spinal cord, pain from infectious pericarditis is frequently felt in the shoulders and neck. Involvement of the more lateral diaphragm can lead to symptoms in the upper abdomen and back, creating confusion with pancreatitis or cholecystitis. Pericarditis occasionally causes a steady, crushing substernal pain that resembles that of acute myocardial infarction.[13]

VASCULAR DISEASE. Acute aortic dissection (see Chap. 56) usually causes sudden onset of excruciating, ripping pain, the location of which reflects the site and progression of the dissection. Ascending aortic dissections tend to manifest with pain in the midline of the anterior chest, and posterior descending aortic dissections manifest with pain in the back of the chest. Aortic dissections usually occur in the presence of risk factors that include hypertension, pregnancy, atherosclerosis, and other conditions that lead to degeneration of the aortic media, such as Marfan and Ehlers-Danlos syndromes.

Pulmonary emboli (see Chap. 72) may be asymptomatic but often cause sudden onset of dyspnea and pleuritic chest pain. Massive pulmonary emboli tend to cause severe and persistent substernal pain, attributed to distention of the pulmonary artery. Smaller emboli that lead to pulmonary infarction can cause lateral pleuritic chest pain. Hemodynamically significant pulmonary emboli may cause hypotension, syncope, and signs of right heart failure. Pulmonary hypertension (see Chap. 73) can cause chest pain similar to angina pectoris, presumably because of right heart hypertrophy and ischemia.

PULMONARY. Pulmonary conditions that cause chest pain usually produce dyspnea and pleuritic symptoms, the location of which reflects the site of pulmonary disease. Tracheobronchitis tends to be associated with a burning midline pain, whereas pneumonia can produce pain over the involved lung. The pain of a pneumothorax is sudden in onset and is usually accompanied by dyspnea.

GASTROINTESTINAL. Irritation of the esophagus by acid reflux can produce a burning discomfort that is exacerbated by alcohol, aspirin, and some foods. Symptoms often are worsened by a recumbent position and relieved by sitting upright and by acid-reducing therapies. Esophageal spasm can produce a squeezing chest discomfort similar to that of angina.[14] Mallory-Weiss tears of the esophagus can occur in patients who have had prolonged vomiting episodes. Chest pain caused by ulcer disease usually occurs 60 to 90 minutes after meals and is typically relieved rapidly by acid-reducing therapies. This pain is usually epigastric in location but can radiate into the chest and shoulders. Cholecystitis produces a wide range of pain syndromes and usually causes right upper quadrant abdominal pain. Chest and back pain due to cholecystitis is not unusual, however. The pain is often described as aching or colicky. Pancreatitis typically causes an intense aching epigastric pain that may radiate to the back. Relief through acid-reducing therapies is limited.

MUSCULOSKELETAL AND OTHER CAUSES. Chest pain can arise from musculoskeletal disorders involving the chest wall, such as costochondritis, by conditions affecting the nerves of the chest wall, such as cervical disc disease, Herpes zoster, or following heavy exercise. Musculoskeletal syndromes causing chest pain are often elicited by direct pressure over the affected area or by movement of the patient's neck. The pain itself can be fleeting, or a dull ache that lasts for hours. Panic syndrome is a major cause of chest discomfort among ED patients.[19] The symptoms typically include chest tightness, often accompanied by shortness of breath and a sense of anxiety, and generally lasting 30 minutes or more.

CLINICAL EVALUATION. When evaluating patients with acute chest pain, the clinician must address a series of issues related to prognosis and immediate management. Even before trying to arrive at a definite diagnosis, high-priority questions include the following:

- *Clinical stability:* Does the patient need immediate treatment for circulatory collapse or respiratory insufficiency?
- *Immediate prognosis:* If the patient is currently clinically stable, what is the risk that the patient has a life-threatening condition, such as an ACS, pulmonary embolism, or aortic dissection?
- *Safety of triage options:* If the risks of life-threatening conditions are low, would it be safe to discharge the patient for outpatient management, or should the patient have further testing and/or observation to guide management?

Initial Assessment

The evaluation of the patient with acute chest pain actually begins before the physician sees the patient, and its effectiveness depends on the actions of office staff and other nonphysician personnel. Guidelines from the ACC/AHA[11] (see Guidelines section of Chap. 53) emphasize that patients with symptoms consistent with ACS should *not* be evaluated solely over the telephone but should be referred to

facilities that allow evaluation by a physician and the recording of a 12-lead electrocardiogram (ECG).[11,15] These guidelines also recommend strong consideration of immediate referral to an ED or a specialized chest pain unit for patients with suspected ACS with chest discomfort at rest for more than 20 minutes, hemodynamic instability, or recent syncope or presyncope. Transport as a passenger in a private vehicle is considered an acceptable alternative to an emergency vehicle only if the wait would lead to a delay of greater than 20 to 30 minutes.

The National Heart Attack Alert Program guidelines[16] recommend that patients with the following chief complaints should have immediate assessment by triage nurses and should be referred for further evaluation:

- Chest pain, pressure, tightness, or heaviness; pain that radiates to neck, jaw, shoulders, back, or one or both arms
- Indigestion or "heartburn"; nausea and/or vomiting associated with chest discomfort
- Persistent shortness of breath
- Weakness, dizziness, lightheadedness, loss of consciousness

EXAMINATION. If the patient does not need immediate intervention because of circulatory collapse or respiratory insufficiency, the physician's assessment should begin with a clinical history that captures the characteristics of pain, the time of onset, and the duration of symptoms and an examination that emphasizes vital signs and cardiovascular status. This evaluation should focus on screening for the most common life-threatening conditions: acute MI, pulmonary embolism, and acute aortic dissection (see Table 49-1). Although not shown to assist in risk stratification, information on coronary risk factors can help clinicians in the assessment of whether a patient has coronary artery disease.[17] Younger patients have a lower risk of ACS but should be screened with greater care for histories of recent cocaine use (see Chap. 68).[18,19]

ELECTROCARDIOGRAM. The most important single source of data, the ECG, should be obtained within 10 minutes after presentation in patients with ongoing chest discomfort and as rapidly as possible in patients who have a history of chest discomfort consistent with ACS but whose discomfort has resolved by the time of evaluation, to identify patients who might benefit from primary angioplasty or thrombolytic therapy.[15] When the ECG shows ST segment or T wave abnormalities that suggest the presence of ischemia and are not known to be old, discharging the patient home without further evaluation is hazardous both clinically and legally. The prevalence of acute MI is 80 percent among patients with 1 mm or more of new ST segment elevation and 20 percent among patients with ST segment depression or T wave inversion not known to be old. However, if the ECG does not show changes consistent with ischemia, the risk of acute MI is about 4 percent among patients with a history of coronary artery disease and 2 percent among patients with no such history.[2] Failure to perform an ECG is one of the most important factors in malpractice losses related to patients with acute chest pain, followed by failure to interpret the ECG correctly.[2]

Markers of Myocardial Injury

For patients with a moderate or high probability of ACS, physicians usually perform assays of markers of myocardial injury such as the cardiac troponins T or I (cTnT or cTnI) or creatine kinase MB isoenzyme (CK-MB). Many hospital laboratories perform these tests on a "stat" basis, and point-of-care ("bedside") assays for these markers are now widely available; thus, results can often guide initial management decisions (see Chap. 50).

Studies of the diagnostic performance of cTnI or cTnT or CK-MB indicate that when any of these test findings are abnormal, the patient has a high likelihood of having an ACS (Tables 49-2 and 49-3).[20] The more challenging issues in the interpretation of these test findings during the initial evaluation of acute chest pain are (1) the frequency and causes of false-positive results; (2) the prognostic implications of abnormal test results; and (3) the interpretation of single values of these tests, such as are available during the initial evaluation of acute chest pain.

DIAGNOSTIC PERFORMANCE. Studies of the major assays used to evaluate patients with acute chest pain (CK-MB, cTnI, and cTnT) indicate that with serial sampling, these agents all have excellent sensitivity for detection of acute MI.[8,20-23] Cardiac troponin abnormalities persist for several days after myocardial injury; hence, after 24 hours from symptom onset, these assays are significantly more sensitive than CK-MB.[8] The oldest of these three assays, CK-MB, provides the benchmark against which the other two are evaluated. Published data indicate that CK-MB mass has a clinical sensitivity for acute myocardial infarction of approximately 97 percent and specificity of 90 percent.[8,24]

Creatine Kinase MB Isoenzyme. The dissemination of the radioimmunoassay for CK-MB (versus the older activity assay and electrophoretic assays) has greatly reduced false-positive rates; measured CK-MB with the mass assay can be reliably assumed to represent true CK-MB. However, noncardiac muscle frequently has trace amounts of true CK-MB, and these amounts are increased in patients with conditions that cause chronic muscle destruction and regeneration, such as muscular dystrophy, high-performance athletics (e.g., marathon running), or rhabdomyolysis.[25] CK-MB elevations are particularly common in ED patients, who have higher rates of histories of alcohol abuse or trauma.

Troponins. Different genes encode troponins T and I in cardiac muscle, slow skeletal muscle, and fast skeletal muscle; hence, the assays for cardiac troponins are more specific than CK-MB for myocardial injury. Assessment of the diagnostic performance of the cardiac troponin assays is complicated by the known limitations of the "gold standard" CK-MB assay, to which troponins are compared. Using combinations of clinical criteria including CK-MB data, cardiac troponins have had good, but not perfect, sensitivity (approximately 85 percent) for detecting acute MIs.[20] cTnI and cTnT reportedly have a lower specificity for MI than the traditional CK-MB assays, but these findings likely result from the greater sensitivity for smaller degrees of myocardial damage than that detectable by CK-MB assays. Use of the 99th percentile as the cut point for a positive test has been proposed for the definition of myocardial infarction,[26] and recently validated[27] meta-analyses have shown that the diagnostic performance with the two cardiac troponins appears similar.[28]

Because of the high specificity of cardiac troponins for myocardium, "false-positive" elevations usually represent myocardial damage from causes other than coronary artery disease. Such damage may occur with myopericarditis, trauma, congestive heart failure,[29] pulmonary embolus,[30] and sepsis. Elevated levels of cardiac troponins have been reported in patients with renal disease and connective tissue diseases.[31,32] In patients with a clinical history suggestive of ACS, even slight elevations of cTnI and cTnT can identify patients with an increased risk of complications who benefit from aggressive management strategies (see Chap. 52).[33] Several of the rapid bedside assays for cTnT and cTnI using whole blood samples yield results agree closely with serum cTnT concentrations measured by the standard enzyme immunoassay.[34-36] However, calibration of the point-of-care assay results with laboratory-based assays is important to avoid confusion, especially if the assay and cut points differ between the two assays.[34] If such confusion can be avoided, use of point-of-care assays have been shown to reduce the "vein-to-brain" time, and thus potentially improve triage and clinical decision-making.[37]

OTHER MARKERS. Serum myoglobin is a smaller molecule and diffuses through interstitial fluids more rapidly after cell death than the larger CK and troponin molecules; therefore, it becomes abnormal as early as 30 minutes after myocardial injury. However, myoglobin is not specific to myocardial tissue, so false-positive rates in ED populations are high.[8]

Many patients presenting with ACS have elevated concentrations of inflammatory biomarkers such as C-reactive protein, serum amyloid A, myeloperoxidase, or interleukin 6 (IL-6), including those without evidence of myocyte necrosis.[38] To date, no study has identified exact decision cut points, or shown an incremental benefit on an admission

---

TABLE 49-2	Likelihood That Signs and Symptoms Represent an Acute Coronary Syndrome		
Feature	**High Likelihood (Any of the Following)**	**Intermediate Likelihood (Absence of High-Likelihood Features and Presence of Any of the Following)**	**Low Likelihood (Absence of High- or Intermediate-Likelihood Features but May Have Any of the Following)**
History	• Chest or left arm pain or discomfort as chief symptom reproducing prior documented angina • Known history of coronary artery disease, including myocardial infarction	• Chest or left arm pain or discomfort as chief symptom • Age >70 years • Male sex • Diabetes mellitus	• Probable ischemic symptoms in absence of any of the intermediate-likelihood characteristics • Recent cocaine use
Examination	• Transient mitral regurgitation, hypotension, diaphoresis, pulmonary edema, or rales	• Extracardiac vascular disease	• Chest discomfort reproduced by palpation
Electrocardiogram	• New, or presumably new, transient ST segment deviation (≥0.05 mV) or T wave inversion (≥0.2 mV) with symptoms	• Fixed Q waves • Abnormal ST segments or T waves not documented to be new	• T wave flattening or inversion in leads with dominant R waves • Normal ECG
Cardiac markers	• Elevated cardiac TnI, TnT, or CK-MB	• Normal	• Normal

CK-MB = Creatine kinase MB isoenzyme; ECG = electrocardiogram; TnI = troponin I; TnT = troponin T.
From Fleet RP, Dupuis G, Marchand A, et al: ACC/AHA 2002 guideline update for the management of patients with unstable angina and non–ST-segment elevation myocardial infarction: Summary article. A report of the American College of Cardiology/American Heart Association Task Force on Practice Guidelines (Committee on the Management of Patients With Unstable Angina). Circulation 106:1893, 2002.

TABLE 49–3	Short-Term Risk of Death or Nonfatal Myocardial Ischemia in Patients with Unstable Angina		
Feature	High Likelihood (Any of the Following)	Intermediate Likelihood (Absence of High-Likelihood Features and Presence of Any of the Following)	Low Likelihood (Absence of High- or Intermediate-Likelihood Features but May Have Any of the Following)
History	• Accelerating tempo of ischemic symptoms in preceding 48 hours	• Prior MI, peripheral or cerebrovascular disease, or CABG; prior aspirin use	
Character of pain	• Prolonged ongoing (>20 minutes) rest pain	• Prolonged (>20 min) rest angina, now resolved, with moderate or high likelihood of coronary artery disease • Rest angina (<20 min) or relieved with rest or sublingual NTG	• New-onset or progressive Canadian Cardiovacular System Class III or IV angina the past 2 weeks without prolonged (>20 min) rest pain but with moderate or high likelihood of coronary artery disease
Clinical findings	• Pulmonary edema, most likely due to ischemia • New or worsening mitral regurgitation murmur • S_3 or new/worsening rales • Hypotension, bradycardia, tachycardia • Age >75 years	• Age >70 years	
Electrocardiogram	• Angina at rest with transient ST segment changes >0.05 mV • Bundle-branch block, new or presumed new • Sustained ventricular tachycardia	• T wave inversions >0.2 mV • Pathological Q waves	• Normal or unchanged ECG during an episode of chest discomfort
Cardiac markers	• Elevated (e.g., TnT or TnI >0.1 ng/ml)	• Slightly elevated (e.g., TnT >0.01 but <0.1 ng/ml)	• Normal

CABG = coronary artery bypass grafting; ECG = electrocardiogram; MI = myocardial infarction; NTG = nitroglycerin; TnI = troponin I; TnT = troponin T.
From Fleet RP, Dupuis G, Marchand A, et al: ACC/AHA 2002 guideline update for the management of patients with unstable angina and non–ST-segment elevation myocardial infarction: Summary article. A report of the American College of Cardiology/American Heart Association Task Force on Practice Guidelines (Committee on the Management of Patients with Unstable Angina). Circulation 106:1893, 2002.

or treatment strategy based on these new markers, so the clinical utility of these observations remains uncertain.

Ischemia-modified albumin (IMA) has been approved by the U.S. Food and Drug Administration for clinical use.[39] The albumin cobalt binding test for detection of IMA is based on the observation that the affinity of the N-terminus of human albumin for cobalt is reduced in patients with myocardial ischemia. Reduced albumin cobalt binding also occurs in patients with spontaneous coronary ischemia.[40] However, as for the other markers, the clinical specificity of IMA, in the broad population of patients with chest pain and suspected ACS, remains an area for further investigation.

Prognostic Implications of Test Results. Abnormal levels of CK-MB, cTnI, and cTnT predict increased risk of complications (see Tables 49-2 and 49-3).[21,28,41,42] Even if patients do not have CK-MB elevations, cTnI and cTnT aid early risk stratification in patients with acute chest pain, particularly those without ST segment elevation.[23] The prognostic value of cTnI seems to be comparable to that of cTnT in patients with unstable angina.[28]

Test Performance of Single Assays. Although high sensitivities and specificities for diagnosis of myocardial injury can be achieved for several assays through serial sampling, the diagnostic performance of a single value of any of these tests is not nearly as good. A single CK-MB value in ED patients with acute chest pain has a sensitivity for detecting acute MI of 34 percent and a specificity of 88 percent[43]; a single value of cTnI has a sensitivity of about 40 percent.[44]

The diagnostic performance of single values of these tests depends considerably on the time elapsed since the onset of symptoms. For example, a single CK-MB mass or troponin drawn within 4 hours of the onset of symptoms has a sen-

sitivity of less than 25 percent. However, single values of CK-MB mass and troponins that are drawn more than 12 hours after the onset of symptoms have sensitivities for myocardial infarction in the range of 70 to 90 percent.[8]

INTERPRETATION OF TESTS: RELATION BETWEEN PRETEST PROBABILITY AND POSTTEST PROBABILITY. As is true of most tests in medicine, results should be interpreted in the context of the patient's overall probability of having the diagnosis of interest. Thus, a normal result on a test or series of tests in a patient with a high clinical probability of ACS does not exclude this diagnosis, although it raises the question of whether any myocardial injury may have occurred several days previously. Similarly, an abnormal test result in a patient with a low probability of coronary disease does not necessarily mean that the patient has had myocardial injury but should prompt a reassessment of the patient's clinical data.

To formalize such analyses, cardiac markers can be interpreted in a Bayesian framework in which pretest probabilities are modified by test results (Fig. 49-1). These calculations of posttest probabilities assume that the sensitivity and specificity of serial sampling of CK-MB mass values, for example, in patients presenting within 24 hours of the onset of symptoms are about 95 percent (see Fig. 49-1A). In contrast, the impact of single CK-MB mass results on patients' probabilities of coronary disease is quite modest (see Fig. 49-1B).

TESTING STRATEGY. The 2007 National Academy of Clinical Biochemistry (NACB) Practice Guidelines recommend measurement of biomarkers of cardiac injury in patients with symptoms that suggest ACS (Table 49-4).[8,11]

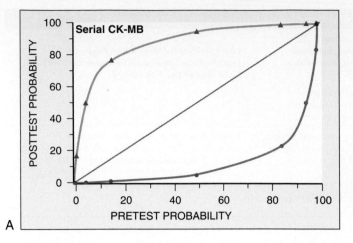

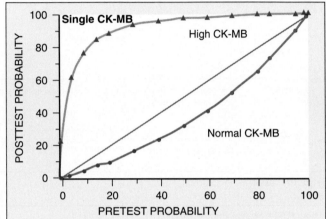

FIGURE 49–1 Effect of serial CK-MB results **(A)** and single CK-MB values **(B)** on the probability of acute myocardial infarction. The pretest probabilities, as marked along the x axis, can be derived through use of computerized algorithms, personal experience, or analysis of published data. Posttest probabilities are plotted on the y axis. The curves correspond to posttest probabilities of infarction with normal (red) or elevated (blue) CK-MB results, assuming a 95 percent sensitivity and 95 percent specificity for serial sampling of CK-MB levels and a sensitivity of 56 percent and a specificity of 98 percent for single CK-MB mass values greater than 5 ng/ml at admission. CK-MB = creatine kinase MB isoenzyme.

Furthermore, patients with very low probability of ACS should not undergo measurement of biomarkers because of the possibility that false-positive results will lead to unnecessary hospitalizations, tests, procedures, and their complications.[8]

The ACC/AHA and NACB guidelines recommend cTnI or cTnT as the preferred first-line markers, but note that CK-MB (by mass assay) is an acceptable alternative. The preference for cardiac troponins reflects the greater specificity of these markers compared with CK-MB and the prognostic value of troponin elevations in the presence of normal CK-MB levels. If the initial set of markers is negative in patients who have presented within the first 6 hours of the onset of pain, the guidelines recommend that another sample be drawn in the next 6 to 12 hours.

INITIAL RISK STRATIFICATION

For patients with chest pain, the initial risk stratification focuses on the safety of various triage and testing options. These options include the following:

- Immediate treatment of ST elevation MI with primary percutaneous coronary intervention or thrombolytic agents

- Admission to a coronary care or other intensive care unit
- Admission to a "step-down" telemetry unit
- Admission to an observation or "chest pain" unit
- Further data collection in the ED, for example by immediate exercise testing or radionuclide imaging
- Discharge to home

The decision among these options is made on the basis of information from the history, physical examination, ECG, and, for patients with suspected ACS, one or more sets of biomarkers for myocardial injury. Key factors suggesting a high likelihood of having ACS and a high risk of short-term complications from ACS include prolonged or accelerating ischemic symptoms, evidence of congestive heart failure on physical examination, electrocardiographic abnormalities consistent with ischemia that are not known to be old, and elevated markers for myocardial injury (see Tables 49-2 and 49-3).

Clinical History

Other factors from the history contribute to risk stratification in addition to the assessment of whether the patient's symptoms are consistent with myocardial ischemia, and whether the duration and pattern of symptoms suggest an elevated risk for complications (see Tables 49-2 and 49-3). A history of myocardial infarction is associated not only with a high risk of obstructive coronary disease but also with an increased likelihood of multivessel disease. Women with suspected ACS less often have epicardial coronary artery disease than do men with similar clinical presentations; such disease, when present, tends to be less severe (see Chap. 76).[45,46] Older patients, particularly beyond 70 years of age, have a higher risk for coronary disease and higher risk for adverse outcomes.[47]

Information on traditional risk factors, especially diabetes, can help identify high-risk patients among those with ACS.[48,49] However, risk factor data have relatively little value in the diagnosis of patients with acute ischemia after consideration of other data from the history, ECG, and cardiac markers.[3] Thus, ACC/AHA guidelines recommend that these data should *not* be used to determine whether a patient should be admitted.[11] Similarly, the guidelines note that a family history of premature coronary disease is *not* a useful indicator of diagnosis or prognosis for patients with acute chest pain.

The Physical Examination

The initial examination of patients with acute chest pain is directed toward identifying potential precipitating causes of myocardial ischemia (e.g., uncontrolled hypertension), important comorbid conditions (e.g., chronic obstructive pulmonary disease), and evidence of hemodynamic complications (e.g., congestive heart failure, new mitral regurgitation, or hypotension).[11] In addition to vital signs, examination of the peripheral vessels should include assessment of the presence of bruits or absent pulses that suggest extracardiac vascular disease.

For patients whose clinical presentations do not suggest myocardial ischemia, the search for noncoronary causes of chest pain should focus first on potentially life-threatening issues (aortic dissection, pulmonary embolism), and then turn to the possibility of other cardiac (e.g., pericarditis) and noncardiac (e.g., esophageal discomfort) diagnoses. Aortic dissection is suggested by blood pressure or pulse disparities or a new murmur of aortic regurgitation accompanied by back or midline anterior chest pain. Differences in breath sounds in the presence of acute dyspnea and pleuritic chest pain raise the possibility of pneumothorax. Tachycardia,

TABLE 49–4 National Academy of Clinical Biochemistry Recommendations for Use of Biochemical Markers for Risk Stratification in ACS

Class I

1. Patients with suspected ACS should undergo early risk stratification based on an integrated assessment of symptoms, physical examination findings, ECG findings, and biomarkers (Level of Evidence: C).
2. A cardiac troponin is the preferred marker for risk stratification and, if available, should be measured in all patients with suspected ACS. In patients with a clinical syndrome consistent with ACS, a maximal (peak) concentration exceeding the 99th percentile of values for a reference control group should be considered indicative of increased risk of death and recurrent ischemic events (Level of Evidence: A).
3. Blood should be obtained for testing on hospital presentation followed by serial sampling with timing of sampling based on the clinical circumstances. For most patients, blood should be obtained for testing at hospital presentation, and at 6 to 9 hours (Level of Evidence: B).

Class IIa

4. Measurement of hs-CRP may be useful, in addition to a cardiac troponin, for risk assessment in patients with a clinical syndrome consistent with ACS. The benefits of therapy based on this strategy remain uncertain (Level of Evidence: A).
5. Measurement of B-type natriuretic peptide (BNP) or N-terminal pro-BNP (NT-proBNP) may be useful, in addition to a cardiac troponin, for risk assessment in patients with a clinical syndrome consistent with ACS. The benefits of therapy based on this strategy remain uncertain (Level of Evidence: A).

Class IIb

6. Measurement of markers of myocardial ischemia, in addition to cardiac troponin and ECG, may aid in excluding ACS in patients with a low clinical probability of myocardial ischemia (Level of Evidence: C).
7. A multi-marker strategy that includes measurement of two or more pathobiologically diverse biomarkers in addition to a cardiac troponin, may aid in enhancing risk stratification in patients with a clinical syndrome consistent with ACS. BNP and hs-CRP are the biomarkers best studied using this approach. The benefits of therapy based on this strategy remain uncertain (Level of Evidence: C).
8. Early repeat sampling of cardiac troponin (e.g., 2 to 4 hours after presentation) may be appropriate if tied to therapeutic strategies (Level of Evidence: C).

Class III

Biomarkers of necrosis should not be used for routine screening of patients with low clinical probability of ACS (Level of Evidence: C).

ACS = acute coronary syndrome; ECG = electrocardiogram.

Reproduced with permission from Morrow DA, Cannon CP, Jesse RL, et al. National Academy of Clinical Biochemistry Laboratory medicine practice guidelines: Clinical characteristics and utilization of biochemical markers in acute coronary syndromes. Circulation (in press).

CH 49

Approach to the Patient with Chest Pain

tachypnea, and an accentuated pulmonic component of the second heart sound (P_2) may be the major manifestations of pulmonary embolism on physical examination.

The Electrocardiogram

The ECG provides critical information for both diagnosis and prognosis (see Tables 49-2 and 49-3), particularly when a tracing is obtained during episodes of pain. New persistent or transient ST segment abnormalities (>0.05 mV) that develop during a symptomatic episode at rest and resolve when the symptoms resolve strongly suggest acute ischemia and severe coronary disease. Nonspecific ST segment and T wave abnormalities are usually defined as lesser amounts of ST segment deviation or T wave inversion of less than or equal to 0.3 mV and are less helpful in risk stratification. A completely normal ECG does not exclude the possibility of ACS; in about 1 to 6 percent of such patients with acute chest pain, the pain evolves into an acute MI, and up to 15 percent have unstable angina. Yet, patients with a normal or near-normal ECG have a better prognosis than patients with clearly abnormal ECGs at presentation.[1,3]

The availability of a prior ECG improves diagnostic accuracy and reduces the rate of admission for patients with abnormal baseline tracings. Serial ECG tracings improve the clinician's ability to diagnose acute MI, particularly if combined with serial measurement of cardiac biomarkers.[57] Continuous ECG monitoring to detect ST-segment shifts is technically feasible but makes an uncertain contribution to patient management.[11]

Decision Aids

Multivariate algorithms have been developed and prospectively validated with the goal of improving the stratification of risk in patients with acute chest pain. These algorithms can be used to estimate the probability for individual patients of acute myocardial infarction, acute ischemic heart disease,

or the risk of major cardiac complications.[2] These algorithms have been used mainly to identify patients who are at low risk for complications and who therefore do not require admission to the hospital or coronary care unit.

A prospectively validated algorithm for prediction of risk of complications requiring intensive care unit care is presented as a flow chart in Figure 49-2.[17] In this algorithm, patients with suspected myocardial infarction on their ECGs are immediately classified as having a high risk (approximately 16 percent) of major complications within the next 72 hours. Patients whose ECGs are consistent with ischemia but not infarction are then classified as intermediate (approximately 8 percent) or high risk for complications, depending on the presence or absence of clinical risk factors—including systolic blood pressure below 100 mm Hg, bilateral rales heard above the bases, and known unstable ischemic heart disease (defined as worsening of previously stable angina, a new onset of angina after infarction or after a coronary revascularization procedure, or pain that was the same as that associated with a prior MI). These same risk factors serve to stratify patients without ischemic changes on their ECGs.

Validated algorithms for prediction of acute ischemic heart disease and the risks and benefits of thrombolytic therapy have been incorporated into computerized reports of ECGs to help clinicians make decisions about admission and to help them assess the risks and benefits of using thrombolytic therapy in individual cases.[50] A recent study, however failed, to show that such annotation improves triage or medical decision-making.[51]

Prospective trials indicate that these algorithms have little effect in the routine clinical practice of clinicians who have not received training in their use.[52] Among the reasons that practicing physicians do not use algorithms are that they are too busy, are unsure of their value, or are concerned about the legal and clinical consequences of inappropriately discharging patients who are subsequently found to have had MI.[2]

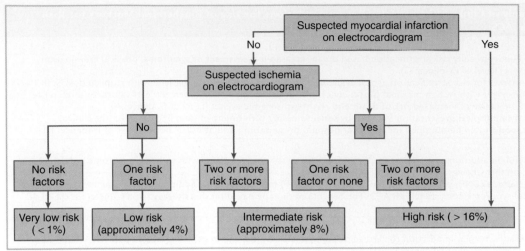

FIGURE 49–2 Derivation and validation of four groups into which patients can be categorized according to risk of major cardiac events within 72 hours after admission. See text for the risk factors considered. *(From Goldman L, Cook EF, Johnson PA, et al: Prediction of the need for intensive care in patients who come to emergency departments with acute chest pain. N Engl J Med 334:1498, 1996.)*

IMMEDIATE MANAGEMENT

The ACC/AHA guidelines suggest an approach to the immediate management of patients with possible ACS that integrates information from the history, physical examination, 12-lead ECG, and initial cardiac marker tests to assign patients to four categories: noncardiac diagnosis, chronic stable angina, possible ACS, and definite ACS (Fig. 49-3).[11] In this algorithm, patients with ST elevation are triaged immediately for reperfusion therapy, according to ACC/AHA guidelines for acute MI. Patients with ACS who have ST or T wave changes, ongoing pain, positive cardiac markers, or hemodynamic abnormalities should be admitted to hospital for management of acute ischemia. Cost-effectiveness analyses support triage of such patients to the coronary care unit for their initial care.[53] For patients with possible or definite ACS who do not have diagnostic ECGs and whose initial serum cardiac markers are within normal limits, observation in a chest pain unit or other nonintensive care facility is appropriate.

Chest Pain Protocols and Units

The main elements of a typical chest pain critical pathway are included in the bottom part of Figure 49-3. According to the ACC/AHA recommendations,[11] patients with a low risk of acute coronary syndrome or associated complications can be observed for 4 to 8 hours while undergoing electrocardiographic monitoring and serial measurement of cardiac markers. Patients who develop evidence of ischemia or other indicators of increased risk should be admitted to the coronary care unit for further management. Patients who do not develop recurrent pain or other predictors of increased risk can be triaged for early noninvasive testing (see later) either before or after discharge.

To enhance the efficiency and reliability of implementation of such chest pain protocols, many hospitals triage low-risk patients with chest pain to special chest pain units.[5,54,55] These units are often adjacent to or in EDs but are sometimes located elsewhere in the hospital. In most such units, the rate of MI has been about 1 to 2 percent. These units have proved safe and cost-saving sites of care for low-risk patients.[54,55] Chest pain units are also sometimes used for intermediate-risk patients, such as patients with a prior history of coronary disease but no other high-

risk predictors. In one community-based randomized trial, patients with unstable angina and an overall intermediate risk of complications had similar outcomes and lower costs if they were triaged to a chest pain unit versus conventional hospital management.[54]

Early Noninvasive Testing

TREADMILL ELECTROCARDIOGRAPHY. A major goal of the initial short period of observation of low-risk patients in chest pain units is to determine whether performance of exercise testing or other noninvasive tests is safe. Treadmill exercise electrocardiography is an inexpensive test that is available at many hospitals 7 days per week and beyond traditional laboratory hours, and prospective data indicate that early exercise test results provide reliable prognostic information for low-risk patient populations. Most studies have used the Bruce or modified Bruce treadmill protocol. One study found that, among low-risk patients who had exercise testing within 48 hours of presentation for acute chest pain, the 6-month event rate among 195 patients with a negative test was 2 percent, in contrast to a rate of 15 percent among patients with a positive or equivocal test result.[56] A more recent study also documented the safety of this approach in 3000 consecutive patients.[4]

Studies have shown that patients who have a low clinical risk of complications can safely undergo exercise testing within 6 to 12 hours after presentation at the hospital or even immediately.[4] In general, protocols for early or immediate exercise testing exclude patients with electrocardiographic findings consistent with ischemia not known to be old, ongoing chest pain, or evidence of congestive heart failure. Analyses of pooled data suggest that the prevalence of coronary disease in populations undergoing early exercise testing averages about 5 percent, and that the rate of adverse events is negligible.[4] The AHA has issued an Advisory Statement regarding indications and contraindications for exercise on electrocardiographic stress testing in the ED (Table 49-5).[57]

IMAGING TESTS. Stress echocardiography or radionuclide scans are the preferred noninvasive testing modalities for patients who cannot undergo treadmill electrocardiographic testing because of physical disability or who have ECGs that do lend themselves to interpretation. Imaging technologies are less readily available and more expensive than exercise electrocardiography but have increased sensitivity for detection of coronary disease and the ability to quantify the extent of and localize jeopardized myocardium. High-risk rest perfusion scans are associated with an increased risk of major cardiac complications, whereas patients with low-risk scans have low 30-day cardiac event rates (<2 percent).[58,59]

In addition to stress imaging studies to detect provokable ischemia, rest radionuclide scans also can help determine whether a patient's symptoms represent myocardial ischemia. In a multicenter prospective randomized trial of 2475 adult ED patients with chest pain or other symptoms suggestive of acute cardiac ischemia and with normal or non-

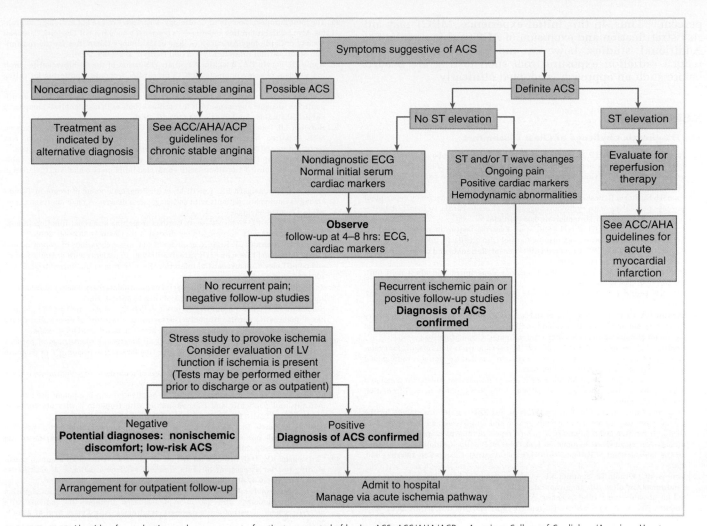

FIGURE 49–3 Algorithm for evaluation and management of patients suspected of having ACS. ACC/AHA/ACP = American College of Cardiology/American Heart Association/American College of Physicians; ACS = acute coronary syndrome; ECG = electrocardiogram; LV = left ventricular. (From Braunwald E, Antman EM, Beasley JW, et al: ACC/AHA guideline update for the management of patients with unstable angina and non-ST-segment elevation myocardial infarction—Summary article 2002: A report of the American College of Cardiology/American Heart Association Task Force on Practice Guidelines. [Committee on the Management of Patients with Unstable Angina]. Circulation 106:1893, 2002.)

TABLE 49–5	Indications and Contraindications for Exercise Electrocardiographic Testing in the Emergency Department

Requirements before exercise electrocardiographic testing that should be considered in the Emergency Department setting:
- Two sets of cardiac enzymes at 4-hr intervals should be normal
- ECG at the time of presentation and preexercise 12-lead ECG shows no significant abnormality
- Absence of rest ECG abnormalities that would preclude accurate assessment of the exercise ECG
- From admission to the time that results are available from the second set of cardiac enzymes: patient asymptomatic, lessening chest pain symptoms, or persistent atypical symptoms
- Absence of ischemic chest pain at the time of exercise testing

Contraindications to exercise electrocardiographic testing in the Emergency Department setting:
- New or evolving ECG abnormalities on the rest tracing
- Abnormal cardiac enzymes
- Inability to perform exercise
- Worsening or persistent ischemic chest pain symptoms from admission to the time of exercise testing
- Clinical risk profiling indicating imminent coronary angiography is likely

ECG = electrocardiogram.

diagnostic initial ECG results, patients were randomly assigned to receive either the usual evaluation strategy or the usual strategy supplemented with results from acute resting myocardial perfusion imaging.[9] The availability of scan results did not influence management of patients with acute MI or unstable angina, but reduced rates of hospitalization for patients without acute cardiac ischemia who underwent scanning from 52 to 42 percent.[9]

Echocardiography can also be used with and without stress to detect wall-motion abnormalities consistent with myocardial ischemia.[60,61] The presence of induced or baseline regional wall motion abnormalities correlates with a worse prognosis. Cost-effectiveness analyses indicated that radionuclide imaging, stress echocardiography, and prompt coronary angiography may all be appropriate for diagnosing coronary artery disease in some subgroups of patients,[62] but guidelines recommend exercise electrocardiography as the preferred first-line test.[11]

Multidetector computerized tomography (MDCT) has recently been evaluated in a single center study of chest pain patients presenting to the ED. Of 103 consecutive patients, 14 had ACS. On MDCT, absence of significant coronary artery stenosis or the presence of nonsignificant coronary atherosclerotic plaque (41 of 103 patients) accurately excluded ACS with a negative predictive value of 100 percent.[10] Thus, in this initial experience, MDCT may aid risk stratification and exclusion of ACS in this population. Additional studies, however, and newer techniques to reduce radiation exposure from such testing are needed before such an approach is adopted clinically.

REFERENCES

The Diagnostic Challenge of Chest Discomfort

1. Pope JH, Aufderheide TP, Ruthazer R, et al: Missed diagnoses of acute cardiac ischemia in the emergency department. N Engl J Med 342:1163-70, 2000.
2. Lee TH, Goldman L. Evaluation of the patient with acute chest pain. N Engl J Med 342:1187-95, 2000.
3. Pope JH, Ruthazer R, Beshansky JR, et al: Clinical features of emergency department patients presenting with symptoms suggestive of acute cardia ischemia: A multicenter study. J Thromb Thrombolysis 6:63-74, 1998.
4. Amsterdam EA, Kirk JD, Diercks DB, et al: Exercise testing in chest pain units: Rationale, implementation, and results. Cardiol Clin 23:503-16, 2005.
5. Blomkalns AL, Gibler WB: Chest pain unit concept: Rationale and diagnostic strategies. Cardiol Clin 23:411-21, 2005.
6. Jaffe AS: Use of biomarkers in the emergency department and chest pain unit. Cardiol Clin 23:453-65, 2005.
7. Boie ET: Initial evaluation of chest pain. Emerg Med Clin North Am 23:937-57, 2005.
8. Morrow DA, Cannon CP, Jesse RL, et al: National Academy of Clinical Biochemistry Laboratory medicine practice guidelines: Clinical characteristics and utilization of biochemical markers in acute coronary syndromes. Circulation (in press).
9. Udelson JE, Beshansky JR, Ballin DS, et al: Myocardial perfusion imaging for evaluation and triage of patients with suspected acute cardiac ischemia: A randomized controlled trial. JAMA 288:2693-700, 2002.
10. Hoffmann U, Nagurney JT, Moselewski F, et al: Coronary multidetector computed tomography in the assessment of patients with acute chest pain. Circulation 114:2251-60, 2006.
11. Braunwald E, Antman EM, Beasley JW, et al: ACC/AHA guideline update for the management of patients with unstable angina and non-ST-segment elevation myocardial infarction-2002: Summary Article: A report of the American College of Cardiology/American Heart Association Task Force on Practice Guidelines (Committee on the Management of Patients With Unstable Angina). Circulation 106:1893-900, 2002.
12. Kontos MC, Ornato JP, Schmidt KL, et al: Incidence of high-risk acute coronary syndromes and eligibility for glycoprotein IIb/IIIa inhibitors among patients admitted for possible myocardial ischemia. Am Heart J 143:70-5, 2002.
13. Spodick DH: Acute pericarditis: Current concepts and practice. JAMA 289:1150-3, 2003.
14. Eslick GD: Noncardiac chest pain: Epidemiology, natural history, health care seeking, and quality of life. Gastroenterol Clin North Am 33:1-23, 2004.
15. Antman EM, Anbe DT, Armstrong PW, et al: ACC/AHA guidelines for the management of patients with ST-elevation myocardial infarction—executive summary. A report of the American College of Cardiology/American Heart Association Task Force on Practice Guidelines (Writing Committee to revise the 1999 guidelines for the management of patients with acute myocardial infarction). J Am Coll Cardiol 44:671-719, 2004.
16. National Heart Attack Alert Program Coordinating Committee—60 Minutes to Treatment Working Group. Emergency department: Rapid identification and treatment of patients with acute myocardial infarction. Ann Emerg Med 23:311-329, 1994.
17. Goldman L, Cook EF, Johnson PA, et al: Prediction of the need for intensive care in patients who come to emergency departments with acute chest pain. N Engl J Med 334:1498-504, 1996.
18. Walker NJ, Sites FD, Shofer FS, Hollander JE: Characteristics and outcomes of young adults who present to the emergency department with chest pain. Acad Emerg Med 8:703-8, 2001.
19. Lange RA, Hillis LD: Cardiovascular complications of cocaine use. N Engl J Med 345:351-8, 2001.

Biomarkers of Ischemia/Infarction

20. Newby LK, Storrow AB, Gibler WB, et al: Bedside multimarker testing for risk stratification in chest pain units: The chest pain evaluation by creatine kinase-MB, myoglobin, and troponin I (CHECKMATE) study. Circulation 103:1832-7, 2001.
21. Westerhout CM, Fu Y, Lauer MS, et al: Short- and long-term risk stratification in acute coronary syndromes: The added value of quantitative ST-segment depression and multiple biomarkers. J Am Coll Cardiol 48:939-47, 2006.
22. Kontos MC, Fritz LM, Anderson FP, et al: Impact of the troponin standard on the prevalence of acute myocardial infarction. Am Heart J 146:446-52, 2003.
23. Newby LK, Roe MT, Chen AY, et al: Frequency and clinical implications of discordant creatine kinase-MB and troponin measurements in acute coronary syndromes. J Am Coll Cardiol 47:312-8, 2006.
24. Christenson RH, Duh SH, Apple FS, et al: Toward standardization of cardiac troponin I measurements part II: Assessing commutability of candidate reference materials and harmonization of cardiac troponin I assays. Clin Chem 52:1685-92, 2006.
25. Leers MP, Schepers R, Baumgarten R. Effects of a long-distance run on cardiac markers in healthy athletes. Clin Chem Lab Med 44:999-1003, 2006.

26. The Joint European Society of Cardiology/American College of Cardiology committee. Myocardial infarction redefined—a consensus document of The Joint European Society of Cardiology/American College of Cardiology Committee for the redefinition of myocardial infarction. J Am Coll Cardiol 36:959-69, 2000.
27. Apple FS, Parvin CA, Buechler KF, et al: Validation of the 99th percentile cutoff independent of assay imprecision (CV) for cardiac troponin monitoring for ruling out myocardial infarction. Clin Chem 51:2198-200, 2005.
28. Olatidoye AG, Wu AH, Feng YJ, Waters D: Prognostic role of troponin T versus troponin I in unstable angina pectoris for cardiac events with meta-analysis comparing published studies. Am J Cardiol 81:1405-10, 1998.
29. Horwich TB, Patel J, MacLellan WR, Fonarow GC: Cardiac troponin I is associated with impaired hemodynamics, progressive left ventricular dysfunction, and increased mortality rates in advanced heart failure. Circulation 108:833-8, 2003.
30. Giannitsis E, Muller-Bardorff M, Kurowski V, et al: Independent prognostic value of cardiac troponin T in patients with confirmed pulmonary embolism. Circulation 102:211-7, 2000.
31. Khan NA, Hemmelgarn BR, Tonelli M, et al: Prognostic value of troponin T and I among asymptomatic patients with end-stage renal disease: A meta-analysis. Circulation 112:3088-96, 2005.
32. Abbas NA, John RI, Webb MC, et al: Cardiac troponins and renal function in nondialysis patients with chronic kidney disease. Clin Chem 51:2059-66, 2005.
33. Morrow DA, Cannon CP, Rifai N, et al: Ability of minor elevations of troponin I and T to predict benefit from an early invasive strategy in patients with unstable angina and non-ST elevation myocardial infarction: Results from a randomized trial. JAMA 2001;286:2405-12, 2001.
34. Kost GJ, Tran NK. Point-of-care testing and cardiac biomarkers: The standard of care and vision for chest pain centers. Cardiol Clin 23:467-90, 2005.
35. Saadeddin S, Habbab M, Siddieg H, et al: Reliability of the rapid bedside whole-blood quantitative cardiac troponin T assay in the diagnosis of myocardial injury in patients with acute coronary syndrome. Med Sci Monit 10:MT43-6, 2004.
36. Hamm CW, Goldmann BU, Heeschen C, et al: Emergency room triage of patients with acute chest pain by means of rapid testing for cardiac troponin T or troponin I. N Engl J Med 1997;337:1648-53.
37. Azzazy HM, Christenson RH: Cardiac markers of acute coronary syndromes: Is there a case for point-of-care testing? Clin Biochem 35:13-27, 2002.
38. Morrow DA, Rifai N, Antman EM, et al: C-reactive protein is a potent predictor of mortality independently and in combination with troponin T in acute coronary syndromes: A TIMI 11A substudy. J Am Coll Cardiol 31:1460-65, 1998.
39. Peacock F, Morris DL, Anwaruddin S, et al: Meta-analysis of ischemia-modified albumin to rule out acute coronary syndromes in the emergency department. Am Heart J 152:253-62, 2006.
40. Christenson RH, Duh SH, Sanhai WR, et al: Characteristics of an albumin cobalt binding test for assessment of acute coronary syndrome patients: A multicenter study. Clin Chem 47:464-70, 2001.
41. Roe MT, Peterson ED, Pollack CV, Jr., et al: Influence of timing of troponin elevation on clinical outcomes and use of evidence-based therapies for patients with non-ST-segment elevation acute coronary syndromes. Ann Emerg Med 45:355-62, 2005.
42. Oldgren J, Wallentin L, Grip L, et al: Myocardial damage, inflammation and thrombin inhibition in unstable coronary artery disease. Eur Heart J 24:86-93, 2003.
43. Lee TH, Weisberg MC, Cook EF, et al: Evaluation of creatine kinase and creatine kinase-MB for diagnosing myocardial infarction. Clinical impact in the emergency room. Arch Intern Med 147:115-21, 1987.
44. Polanczyk CA, Lee TH, Cook EF, et al: Cardiac troponin I as a predictor of major cardiac events in emergency department patients with acute chest pain. J Am Coll Cardiol 32:8-14, 1998.

Early Management of Patients With Chest Discomfort

45. Mueller C, Neumann FJ, Roskamm H, et al: Women do have an improved long-term outcome after non-ST-elevation acute coronary syndromes treated very early and predominantly with percutaneous coronary intervention: A prospective study in 1,450 consecutive patients. J Am Coll Cardiol 40:245-50, 2002.
46. Glaser R, Herrmann HC, Murphy S, et al: Benefit of invasive strategy for women with acute coronary syndromes: Observations form the TACTICS-TIMI 18 Trial. J Am Coll Cardiol 39:313A, 2002.
47. Bach RG, Cannon CP, Weintraub WS, et al: The effect of routine, early invasive management on outcome for elderly patients with non-ST-segment elevation acute coronary syndromes. Ann Intern Med 141:186-95, 2004.
48. Roffi M, Chew DP, Mukherjee D, et al: Platelet glycoprotein IIb/IIIa inhibitors reduce mortality in diabetic patients with non-ST-segment-elevation acute coronary syndromes. Circulation 104:2767-2771, 2001.
49. Brosnan R, Newby LK: Acute coronary syndromes in patients with diabetes mellitus: Diagnosis, prognosis, and current management strategies. Curr Cardiol Rep 5:296-302, 2003.
50. Selker HP, Beshansky JR, Griffith JL, et al: Use of the acute cardiac ischemia time-insensitive predictive instrument (ACI-TIPI) to assist with triage of patients with chest pain or other symptoms suggestive of acute cardiac ischemia. A multicenter, controlled clinical trial. Ann Intern Med 129:845-55, 1998.
51. Westfall JM, Van Vorst RF, McGloin J, Selker HP: Triage and diagnosis of chest pain in rural hospitals: Implementation of the ACI-TIPI in the High Plains Research Network. Ann Fam Med 4:153-8, 2006.
52. Lee TH, Pearson SD, Johnson PA, et al: Failure of information as an intervention to modify clinical management. A time-series trial in patients with acute chest pain. Ann Intern Med 122:434-7, 1995.
53. Tosteson AN, Goldman L, Udvarhelyi IS, Lee TH. Cost-effectiveness of a coronary care unit versus an intermediate care unit for emergency department patients with chest pain. Circulation 94:143-50, 1996.

CH 49

54. Farkouh ME, Smars PA, Reeder GS, et al: A clinical trial of a chest-pain observation unit for patients with unstable angina. Chest Pain Evaluation in the Emergency Room (CHEER) Investigators. N Engl J Med 339:1882-8, 1998.

55. Gomez MA, Anderson JL, Karagounis LA, et al: For the ROMIO Study Group: An emergency department-based protocol for rapidly ruling out myocardial ischemia reduces hospital time and expense: Results of a randomized study (ROMIO). J Am Coll Cardiol 28:25-33, 1996.

56. Polanczyk CA, Johnson PA, Hartley LH, et al: Clinical correlates and prognostic significance of early negative exercise tolerance test in patients with acute chest pain seen in the hospital emergency department. Am J Cardiol 81:288-92, 1998.

57. Stein RA, Chaitman BR, Balady GJ, et al: Safety and utility of exercise testing in emergency room chest pain centers: An advisory from the Committee on Exercise, Rehabilitation, and Prevention, Council on Clinical Cardiology, American Heart Association. Circulation 102:1463-7, 2000.

58. Kontos MC, Schmidt KL, McCue M, et al: A comprehensive strategy for the evaluation and triage of the chest pain patient: A cost comparison study. J Nucl Cardiol 10:284-90, 2003.

59. Kontos MC, Tatum JL: Imaging in the evaluation of the patient with suspected acute coronary syndrome. Cardiol Clin 23:517-30, 2005.

60. Fleischmann KE, Goldman L, Robiolio PA, et al: Echocardiographic correlates of survival in patients with chest pain. J Am Coll Cardiol 23:1390-6, 1994.

61. Colon PJ, 3rd, Mobarek SK, Milani RV, et al: Prognostic value of stress echocardiography in the evaluation of atypical chest pain patients without known coronary artery disease. Am J Cardiol 81:545-51, 1998.

62. Garber AM, Solomon NA: Cost-effectiveness of alternative test strategies for the diagnosis of coronary artery disease. Ann Intern Med 130:719-28, 1999.

CH 49

Approach to the Patient with Chest Pain

CHAPTER 50

Changing Patterns in Clinical
Care, 1207

Improvements in Outcome, 1207

Pathology, 1209
Plaque, 1209
Heart Muscle, 1211

Pathophysiology, 1216
Left Ventricular Function, 1216
Ventricular Remodeling, 1218
Pathophysiology of Other Organ
Systems, 1219

Clinical Features, 1220
Predisposing Factors, 1220
History, 1221
Physical Examination, 1222
Laboratory Findings, 1224

References, 1230

ST-Elevation Myocardial Infarction: Pathology, Pathophysiology, and Clinical Features

Elliott M. Antman and Eugene Braunwald

The *pathological* diagnosis of myocardial infarction (MI) requires evidence of myocyte cell death as a consequence of prolonged ischemia. Characteristic findings include coagulation necrosis and contraction band necrosis, often with patchy areas of myocytolysis at the periphery of the infarct. During the acute phase of MI, the majority of myocyte loss in the infarct zone occurs via coagulation necrosis and proceeds to inflammation, phagocytosis of necrotic myocytes, and repair eventuating in scar formation.

The *clinical* diagnosis of MI requires an integrated assessment of the history with some combination of indirect evidence of myocardial necrosis using biochemical, electrocardiographic, and imaging modalities (Table 50-1). The sensitivity and specificity of the clinical tools for diagnosing MI vary considerably and change at varying times after the onset of the infarction.

Epidemiological reports from the World Heath Organization and American Heart Association beginning in the late 1950s required the presence of at least two of the following for the diagnosis of myocardial infarction: characteristic symptoms, electrocardiographic changes, and a typical rise and fall in biochemical markers.[1] This epidemiological approach was then generally adopted in routine clinical practice, although the rigor with which clinicians apply the electrocardiographic and biochemical criteria for infarction varies considerably.

Since the original epidemiological efforts, considerable advances have occurred in the electrocardiographic and biochemical aspects of the definition of infarction. The electrocardiographic criteria for MI were codified, and scoring systems were developed for estimation of infarct size.[2] Biochemical assays became available for markers more specific for cardiac damage. These include mass assays for the MB fraction of creatine kinase (CK) and immunoassays for cardiac-specific troponins. The cardiac-specific troponin assays have nearly absolute myocardial tissue specificity and have become the preferred biomarker for diagnosing MI. Advances in the techniques for diagnosing MI were the impetus for a consensus document published jointly by several prominent cardiac societies around the world.[2] The main features of the revised definition of MI are summarized in Table 50-2. The revised definition of MI has important implications not only for clinical care of patients but also for tracking epidemiological trends, public policy, and clinical trials.[3,4] The paradigm shift to cardiac-specific troponins as the markers of choice for the diagnosis of MI requires new cutoff values for cardiac injury. The term *normal range* has been replaced by *upper reference limit*, defined as the 99th percentile of a normal reference control group.[5]

As discussed later, the contemporary approach to patients presenting with ischemic discomfort is to consider that they are experiencing an acute coronary syndrome. The 12-lead electrocardiogram (ECG) is pivotal for segregating patients into those presenting with ST-segment elevation, the subject of Chapters 50 through 51, and those presenting without ST-segment elevation, the subject of Chapter 53. Although the revised definition of MI has greater impact on the non-ST-segment elevation end of the acute coronary syndrome spectrum (i.e., distinction between unstable angina and non-ST-segment elevation MI), the issues are also pertinent to discussion of ST-segment elevation myocardial infarction (STEMI).

CHANGING PATTERNS IN CLINICAL CARE

Despite impressive advances in diagnosis and management over the past four decades, STEMI continues to be a major public health problem in the industrialized world and is becoming an increasingly important problem in developing countries (see Chap. 1).[6] In the United States, nearly 1 million patients a year suffer from an acute MI.[7] More than 1 million patients with suspected acute MI are admitted yearly to coronary care units in the United States.[7] Of particular concern from a global perspective are projections that the burden of disease in developing countries will become similar to those now afflicting developed countries.[6] Given the wide disparity of available resources to treat STEMI in developing countries, major efforts are necessary on an international level to strengthen primary prevention programs at the community level.[8,9]

IMPROVEMENTS IN OUTCOME

Mortality from STEMI has declined steadily in several population groups since 1960.[10,11] This drop in mortality appears to result from a fall in the incidence of STEMI (replaced in part by an increase in the rate of unstable angina/non-ST-segment elevation MI[12]) and a fall in the case fatality rate once STEMI has occurred.[13]

Several phases in the management of patients have contributed to the decline in mortality from STEMI.[14] The "clinical observation phase" of coronary care consumed the first half of the 20th century and focused on a detailed recording of physical and laboratory findings, with little active treatment for the infarction. The "coronary care unit phase" began in the mid-1960s and was notable for detailed analysis and vigorous management of cardiac arrhythmias. The "high-technology phase" was ushered in by the introduction of the pulmonary artery balloon flotation catheter, setting the stage for bedside hemodynamic monitoring and more precise hemodynamic management. The modern "reperfusion era" of coronary care was introduced by intracoronary and then intravenous fibrinolysis, increased use of aspirin, and development of primary percutaneous coronary intervention (PCI) (see Chap. 52).

Driven in large part by the need for cost-saving measures, contemporary care of patients with STEMI has entered an "evidence-based coronary care phase" and is increasingly influenced by managed care systems and guidelines for clinical practice (see Guidelines).[15,15a,16]

LIMITATIONS OF CURRENT THERAPY. Despite the gratifying success of medical therapy for STEMI, several observations indicate considerable room for improvement. The short-term mortality rate of patients with STEMI who receive aggressive pharmacological reperfusion therapy as part of a randomized trial is in the range of 6.5 to 7.5 percent,[17] whereas observational data bases suggest that the mortality rate in STEMI patients in the community is 15 to 20 percent.[18] In part, this difference relates to the selection of patients without serious comorbidities for clinical trials.

Advanced age consistently emerges as one of the principal determinants of mortality in patients with STEMI.[19] Cardiac catheterization and other invasive procedures are being performed more commonly

at some point during hospitalization in elderly patients with STEMI. Nevertheless, evidence suggests that the greatest reductions in mortality for elderly patients derive from those strategies employed during the first 24 hours, a time frame in which prompt and appropriate use of life-saving reperfusion therapy has paramount importance, emphasizing the need to extend advances in drug therapy for STEMI to the elderly.[16] Clinical trial data from studies of fibrinolysis show that the elderly (75 years old or older) continue to suffer a mortality rate four times that of younger patients (Fig. 50-1).

Considerable variation exists in practice patterns for management of patients with STEMI.[20] Mortality rates for STEMI are lower in hospitals with a high clinical volume, a high rate of invasive procedures, and

TABLE 50–1	Aspects of Diagnosis of Myocardial Infarction by Different Techniques
Pathology	Myocardial cell death
Biochemistry	Markers of myocardial cell death recovered from blood samples
Electrocardiography	Evidence of myocardial ischemia (ST and T wave abnormalities) Evidence of loss of electrically functioning cardiac tissue (Q waves)
Imaging	Reduction or loss of tissue perfusion Cardiac wall motion abnormalities

Modified from Alpert JS, et al: Definition of myocardial infarction—A global consensus document of The Joint ESC/ACC/AHA/WHF/WHO Task Force for the Redefinition of Myocardial Infarction, 2007 (in press).

TABLE 50–2	Revised Definition of Myocardial Infarction (MI)

Criteria for Acute, Evolving, or Recent MI
Either of the following criteria satisfies the diagnosis for acute, evolving, or recent MI:
1. Typical rise and/or fall of biochemical markers of myocardial necrosis with at least one of the following:
   a) Ischemic symptoms
   b) Development of pathological Q waves in the ECG
   c) ECG changes indicative of ischemia (ST segment elevation or depression)
   d) Imaging evidence of new loss of viable myocardium or new regional wall motion abnormality
2. Pathological findings of an acute myocardial infarction

Criteria for Healing or Healed Myocardial Infarction
Any one of the following criteria satisfies the diagnosis for healing or healed myocardial infarction:
1. Development of new pathological Q waves in serial ECGs. The patient may or may not remember previous symptoms. Biochemical markers of myocardial necrosis may have normalized depending on the length of time that has passed since the infarction developed.
2. Pathological findings of a healed or healing infarction

CK = creatine kinase; ECG = electrocardiogram.

From Alpert JS, et al: Definition of myocardial infarction—a global consensus document of The Joint ESC/ACC/AHA/WHF/WHO Task Force for the Redefinition of Myocardial Infarction, 2007 (in press).

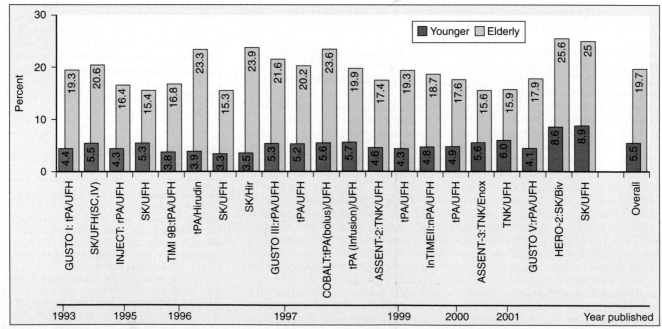

FIGURE 50–1 Mortality rates in ST-segment elevation myocardial infarction patients receiving fibrinolysis, stratified by age. The bars show the mortality at 30 to 35 days in elderly (75 years old or older) and younger (younger than 75 years old) patients who were treated with a fibrinolytic agent, aspirin, and an antithrombin in a series of randomized trials beginning in 1993; of note, the absolute mortality rates have remained relatively stable over 1.5 decades. The pooled data show a mortality rate of 19.7 percent in the elderly versus 5.5 percent in the young (odds ratio 4.37; 95 percent CI 4.16 to 4.58). (*From Ahmed S, Antman EM, Murphy SA, et al: Poor outcomes after fibrinolytic therapy for ST-segment elevation myocardial infarction: Impact of age (a meta-analysis of a decade of trials). J Thromb Thrombolysis 21:119, 2006.*)

a top ranking in quality reports (see Chap. 52). Conversely, mortality rates are higher when STEMI patients are not cared for by a cardiovascular specialist.[21,22] Variation has also been observed in the treatment patterns of certain population subgroups with STEMI, notably women and blacks.[23]

PATHOLOGY

Almost all MIs result from coronary atherosclerosis, generally with superimposed coronary thrombosis. Nonatherogenic forms of coronary artery disease are discussed later in this chapter, and causes of STEMI without coronary atherosclerosis are shown in Table 50-3.

Before the fibrinolytic era, clinicians typically divided patients with MI into those suffering a Q-wave and those suffering a non-Q-wave infarct on the basis of evolution of the pattern on the ECG over several days. The term *Q-wave infarction* was frequently considered to be virtually synonymous with *transmural infarction*, whereas *non-Q-wave infarctions* were often referred to as *subendocardial infarctions*. Contemporary studies using cardiac magnetic resonance imaging indicate that the development of a Q-wave on the ECG is determined more by the size of the infarct than the depth of mural involvement.[24] A more suitable framework that puts STEMI in perspective along with unstable angina/non-ST-elevation MI (UA/NSTEMI) based on pathophysiology is referred to as the *acute coronary syndromes* (Fig. 50-2).

Plaque

During the natural evolution of atherosclerotic plaque, especially that which is lipid laden, an abrupt and catastrophic transition can occur, characterized by plaque disruption (see Chap. 38).[25] Some patients have a systemic predisposition to plaque disruption that is independent of traditional risk factors.[26] Plaque disruption exposes substances that promote platelet activation and aggregation, thrombin generation, and ultimately thrombus formation.[27,28] The resultant thrombus interrupts blood flow and leads to an imbalance between oxygen supply and demand and, if this imbalance is severe and persistent, to myocardial necrosis (Fig. 50-3).

COMPOSITION OF PLAQUES. At autopsy, the atherosclerotic plaques of patients who died of STEMI are composed primarily of fibrous tissue of varying density and cellularity with superimposed thrombus. Calcium, lipid-laden foam cells, and extracellular lipid each constitute 5 to 10 percent of the remaining area. The atherosclerotic plaques that are associated with thrombosis and a total occlusion, located in infarct-related vessels, are generally more complex and irregular than those in vessels not associated with STEMI. Histological studies of these lesions often reveal plaque rupture or erosion. Coronary arterial thrombi responsible for STEMI are approximately 1 cm in length in most cases; adhere to the luminal surface of an artery; and contain platelets, fibrin, erythrocytes, and leukocytes (Fig. 50-4). The composition of the thrombus may vary at differ-

TABLE 50–3	Causes of Myocardial Infarction without Coronary Atherosclerosis

Coronary Artery Disease Other than Atherosclerosis
Arteritis
  Luetic
  Granulomatous (Takayasu disease)
  Polyarteritis nodosa
  Mucocutaneous lymph node (Kawasaki) syndrome
  Disseminated lupus erythematosus
  Rheumatoid spondylitis
  Ankylosing spondylitis
 	
Trauma to coronary arteries
  Laceration
  Thrombosis
  Iatrogenic
  Radiation (radiation therapy for neoplasia)
 	
Coronary mural thickening with metabolic disease or intimal proliferative disease
  Mucopolysaccharidoses (Hurler disease)
  Homocystinuria
  Fabry disease
  Amyloidosis
  Juvenile intimal sclerosis (idiopathic arterial calcification of infancy)
  Intimal hyperplasia associated with contraceptive steroids or with the postpartum period
  Pseudoxanthoma elasticum
  Coronary fibrosis caused by radiation therapy
 	
Luminal narrowing by other mechanisms
  Spasm of coronary arteries (Prinzmetal angina with normal coronary arteries)
  Spasm after nitroglycerin withdrawal
  Dissection of the aorta
  Dissection of the coronary artery
	Emboli to Coronary Arteries
	Infective endocarditis
	Nonbacterial thrombotic endocarditis
	Prolapse of mitral valve
	Mural thrombus from left atrium, left ventricle, or pulmonary veins
	Prosthetic valve emboli
	Cardiac myxoma
	Associated with cardiopulmonary bypass surgery and coronary arteriography
	Paradoxical emboli
	Papillary fibroelastoma of the aortic valve ("fixed embolus")
	Thrombi from intracardiac catheters or guidewires
	
	Congenital Coronary Artery Anomalies
	Anomalous origin of left coronary from pulmonary artery
	Left coronary artery from anterior sinus of Valsalva
	Coronary arteriovenous and arteriocameral fistulas
	Coronary artery aneurysms
	
	Myocardial Oxygen Demand-Supply Disproportion
	Aortic stenosis, all forms
	Incomplete differentiation of the aortic valve
	Aortic insufficiency
	Carbon monoxide poisoning
	Thyrotoxicosis
	Prolonged hypotension
	Takotsubo cardiomyopathy
	
	Hematological (in situ Thrombosis)
	Polycythemia vera
	Thrombocytosis
	Disseminated intravascular coagulation
	Hypercoagulability, thrombosis, thrombocytopenic purpura
	
	Miscellaneous
	Cocaine abuse
	Myocardial contusion
	Myocardial infarction with normal coronary arteries
	Complication of cardiac catheterization

Modified from Cheitlin MD, McAllister HA, de Castro CM: Myocardial infarction without atherosclerosis. JAMA 231:951, 1975. Copyright 1975, American Medical Association.

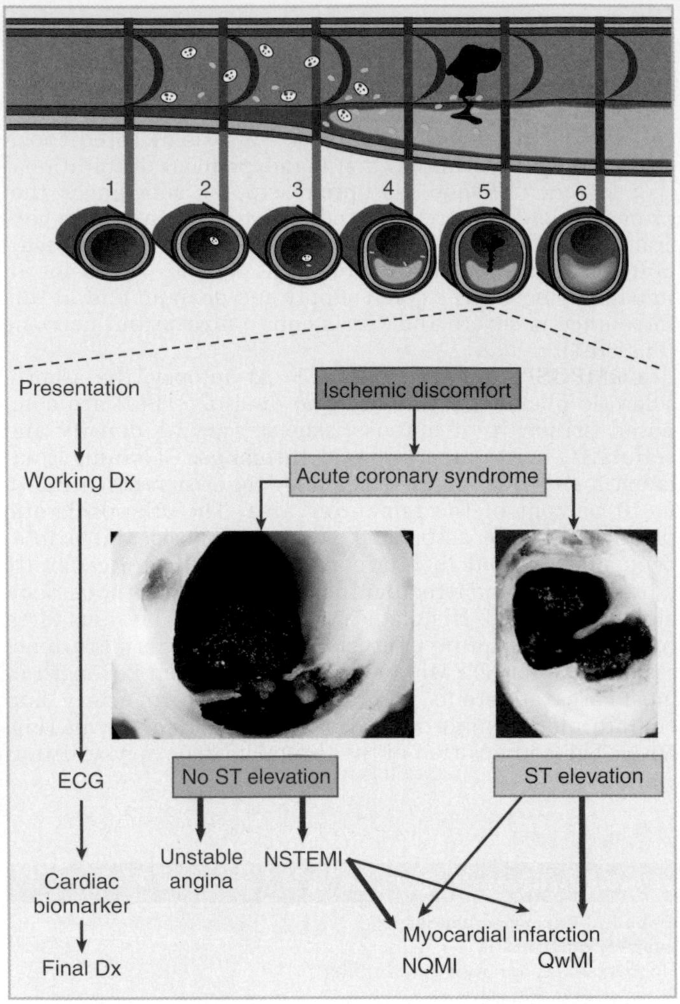

FIGURE 50–2 Acute coronary syndromes. The longitudinal section of an artery depicts the "timeline" of atherogenesis from (1) a normal artery, to (2) lesion initiation and accumulation of extracellular lipid in the intima, to (3) the evolution to the fibrofatty stage, to (4) lesion progression with procoagulant expression and weakening of the fibrous cap. An acute coronary syndrome develops when the vulnerable or high-risk plaque undergoes disruption of the fibrous cap (5); disruption of the plaque is the stimulus for thrombogenesis. Thrombus resorption may be followed by collagen accumulation and smooth muscle cell growth (6). Following disruption of a vulnerable or high-risk plaque, patients experience ischemic discomfort resulting from a reduction of flow through the affected epicardial coronary artery. The flow reduction may be caused by a completely occlusive thrombus **(bottom half, right side)** or subtotally occlusive thrombus **(bottom half, left side).** Patients with ischemic discomfort may present with or without ST-segment elevation on the electrocardiogram (ECG). Of patients with ST-segment elevation, most ultimately develop a Q-wave MI (QwMI), whereas a few develop a non-Q-wave MI (NQMI). Patients who present without ST-segment elevation are suffering from either unstable angina or a non-ST-segment elevation MI (NSTEMI), a distinction that is ultimately made on the presence or absence of a serum cardiac marker such as CK-MB or a cardiac troponin detected in the blood. Most patients presenting with NSTEMI ultimately develop an NQMI on the ECG; a few may develop a QwMI. The spectrum of clinical presentations ranging from unstable angina through NSTEMI and STEMI are referred to as the acute coronary syndromes. CK-MB = MB isoenzyme of creatine kinase; Dx = diagnosis; NQMI = non-Q-wave myocardial infarction; QwMI = Q-wave myocardial infarction. (See Fig. 53-3.) *(Modified with permission from Libby P: Circulation 104:365, 2001; Hamm CW, Bertrand M, Braunwald E: Lancet 358:1533, 2001; and Davies MJ: Heart 83:361, 2000 with permission from the BMJ Publishing Group and Antman EM, Anbe DT, Armstrong PW, et al: ACC/AHA Guidelines for the Management of Patients with ST-Elevation Myocardial Infarction: A report of the American College of Cardiology/American Heart Association Task Force on Practice Guidelines (Committee to Revise the 1999 Guidelines for the Management of Patients with Acute Myocardial Infarction). American College of Cardiology Web site, 2006. (www.acc.org/clinical/guidelines/stemi/index.pdf). Accessed 6/21/06.)*

ent levels: A white thrombus is composed of platelets, fibrin, or both, and a red thrombus is composed of erythrocytes, fibrin, platelets, and leukocytes. Early thrombi are usually small and nonocclusive and are composed predominantly of platelets.

PLAQUE FISSURING AND DISRUPTION. Atherosclerotic plaques considered prone to disruption overexpress metalloproteinase enzymes such as collagenase, gelatinase, and stromelysin that degrade components of the protective extracellular matrix.[29] Activated macrophages and mast cells abundant at the site of atheromatous erosions and plaque disruption in patients who died of STEMI can elaborate these proteinases. In addition to these structural aspects of vulnerable or high-risk plaques, stresses induced by intraluminal pressure, coronary vasomotor tone, tachycardia (cyclic stretching and compression), and disruption of nutrient vessels combine to produce plaque disruption at the margin of the fibrous cap near an adjacent, less involved segment of the coronary artery wall (shoulder region of plaque).[30] A number of key physiological variables such as systolic blood pressure, heart rate, blood viscosity, endogenous tissue plasminogen activator (t-PA) activity, plasminogen activator inhibitor-1 (PAI-1) levels, plasma cortisol levels, and plasma epinephrine levels exhibit circadian and seasonal variations and increase at times of stress. They act in concert to produce a heightened propensity to plaque disruption and coronary thrombosis, yielding the clustering of STEMI in the early morning hours, especially in the winter and after natural disasters.[31]

Acute Coronary Syndromes

When plaque disruption occurs, a sufficient quantity of thrombogenic substances is exposed, and the coronary artery lumen may become obstructed by a combination of platelet aggregates, fibrin, and red blood cells that may produce an extensive thrombus filling a large segment of the infarct-related artery (see Fig. 50-4). An adequate collateral network that prevents necrosis from occurring can result in clinically silent episodes of coronary occlusion. Disruption of plaques is now considered to underlie most acute coronary syndromes (ACS) (see Fig. 50-2).[16] Characteristically, such completely occlusive thrombi lead to a large zone of necrosis involving the full or nearly full thickness of the ventricular wall in the myocardial bed subtended by the affected coronary artery and typically produce ST elevation on the ECG (see Figs. 50-2 and 50-3). Infarction alters the sequence of depolarization ultimately reflected as changes in the QRS.[32] The most characteristic change in the QRS that develops in the majority of patients initially presenting with ST elevation is the evolution of Q waves in the leads overlying the infarct zone—leading to the term *Q-wave infarction* (see Fig. 50-2).[33] In the minority of patients presenting with ST elevation, no Q waves develop, but other abnormalities of the QRS complex are frequently seen, such as diminution in R wave height and notching or splintering of the QRS. Patients presenting without ST elevation are initially diagnosed as suffering either from unstable angina or NSTEMI (see Fig. 50-2 and Chap. 53).

The ACS spectrum concept, organized around a common pathophysiological substrate, furnishes a useful framework for developing therapeutic strategies.[15] Patients presenting with persistent ST-segment elevation are candidates for reperfusion therapy (either pharmacological or catheter based) to restore flow in the occluded epicardial infarct-related artery. ACS patients presenting without ST-segment elevation are not candidates for pharmacological reperfusion but should receive antiischemic therapy, followed by PCI. All patients with ACS should receive antithrombin therapy and antiplatelet therapy regardless of the presence or absence of ST-segment elevation. Thus the 12-lead ECG remains at the center of the decision pathway for management of patients with ACS to distinguish between presentations with ST elevation and without ST elevation (see Fig. 50-2).[12] Prognostic considerations must take into account other important factors, such as whether the ECG abnormality is caused by a first infarct versus subsequent infarct, the location of infarction (anterior versus inferior), infarct size, and demographic factors such as patient age.[15]

Heart Muscle

Gross Pathology

On gross inspection, myocardial infarction can be divided into two major types: transmural infarcts, in which myocardial necrosis involves the full thickness (or nearly full thickness) of the ventricular wall, and subendocardial (nontransmural) infarcts, in which the necrosis involves the subendocardium, the intramural myocardium, or both without extending all the way through the ventricular wall to the epicardium (Fig. 50-5).

An occlusive coronary thrombosis appears to be far more common when the infarction is transmural and localized to the distribution of a single coronary artery (see Fig. 50-4). Nontransmural infarctions, however, frequently occur in the presence of severely narrowed but still patent coronary arteries. Patchy nontransmural infarction may arise from fibrinolysis or PCI of an originally occlusive thrombus with restoration of blood flow *before* the wave front of necrosis has extended from the subendocardium across the full thickness of the ventricular wall (see Fig. 50-3).

THE FIRST HOURS. Gross alterations of the myocardium are difficult to identify until at least 6 to 12 hours have elapsed following the onset of necrosis (Fig. 50-6). However, a variety of histochemical stains can be used to identify zones of necrosis that can be discerned after only 2 to 3 hours. Tissue slices of suspected infarct sites are immersed in a solution of triphenyltetrazolium chloride (TTC), which stains viable myocardium brick red (because of preserved dehydrogenase enzymes that form a red formazan precipitate) and leaves the infarcted region pale as a result of failure of uptake of the vital dye (see Fig. 50-5). The nitroblue tetrazolium (NBT) staining technique can similarly distinguish viable zones of myocardium, which stain dark blue, from necrotic areas of myocardium that therefore remain uncolored and identifiable. Other approaches include autofluorescence staining; immunohistochemical analysis; and, more recently, special DNA staining techniques to identify apoptotic bodies in myocardial sections.[34,35]

THE FIRST DAYS. Initially, the myocardium in the affected region may appear pale and slightly swollen. Eighteen to 36 hours after the onset of the infarct, the myocardium is tan or reddish purple (because of trapped

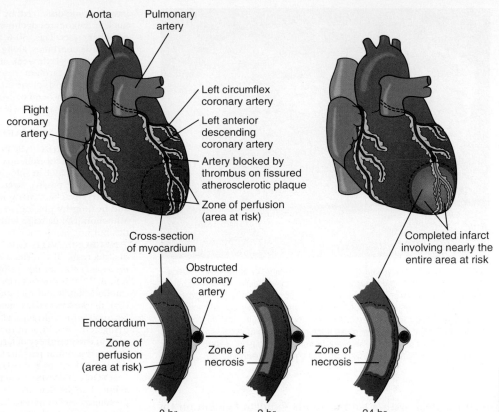

FIGURE 50-3 Schematic representation of the progression of myocardial necrosis after coronary artery occlusion. Necrosis begins in a small zone of the myocardium beneath the endocardial surface in the center of the ischemic zone. This entire region of myocardium (dashed outline) depends on the occluded vessel for perfusion and is the area at risk. A narrow zone of myocardium immediately beneath the endocardium is spared from necrosis because it can be oxygenated by diffusion from the ventricle. *(From Schoen FJ: The heart.* In *Kumar V, Abbas AK, Fausto N [eds]: Robbins & Cotran Pathologic Basis of Disease. 7th ed. Philadelphia, WB Saunders, 2005, p 678.)*

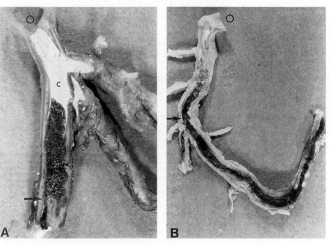

FIGURE 50-4 Thrombus propagation. **A,** Left anterior descending coronary artery cut open longitudinally, showing a dark stagnation thrombosis propagating upstream from the initiating rupture/platelet-rich thrombus at the arrow. In this case the thrombus has propagated proximally up to the nearest major side branch (the first diagonal branch). **B,** The right coronary artery cut open longitudinally, showing a huge stagnation thrombosis propagating downstream from the initiating rupture/platelet-rich thrombus at the arrow. Unlike upstream thrombus propagation, downstream propagation may, as in this case, occlude major side branches. c = contrast medium injected postmortem; O = coronary ostium. *(From Falk E: Coronary thrombosis: Pathogenesis and clinical manifestations. Am J Cardiol 68:28B, 1991.)*

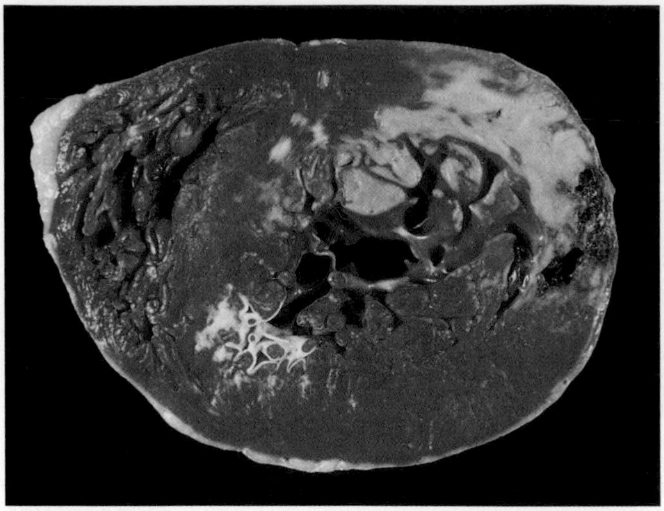

FIGURE 50–5 Acute myocardial infarction, predominantly of the posterolateral left ventricle, demonstrated histochemically by a lack of staining by the triphenyltetrazolium chloride (TTC) stain in areas of necrosis. The staining defect is caused by the enzyme leakage that follows cell death. The myocardial hemorrhage at one edge of the infarct was associated with cardiac rupture, and the anterior scar **(lower left)** was indicative of old infarct. *(Specimen oriented with posterior wall at top.)* *(From Schoen FJ: The heart. In Kumar V, Abbas AK, Fausto N [eds]: Robbins & Cotran Pathologic Basis of Disease. 7th ed. Philadelphia, WB Saunders, 2005, p 579.)*

erythrocytes), with a serofibrinous exudate evident on the epicardium in transmural infarcts. These changes persist for approximately 48 hours; the infarct then turns gray, and fine yellow lines, secondary to neutrophilic infiltration, appear at its periphery. This zone gradually widens and during the next few days extends throughout the infarct.

THE FIRST WEEKS. Eight to 10 days after infarction, the thickness of the cardiac wall in the area of the infarct is reduced as necrotic muscle is removed by mononuclear cells. The cut surface of an infarct of this age is yellow, surrounded by a reddish purple band of granulation tissue that extends through the necrotic tissue by 3 to 4 weeks. Commencing at this time and extending over the next 2 to 3 months, the infarcted area gradually acquires a gelatinous, ground-glass, gray appearance, eventually converting into a shrunken, thin, firm scar, which whitens and firms progressively with time (see Figs. 50-5 and 50-6).[36]

Histological and Ultrastructural Changes

LIGHT MICROSCOPY

In some infarcts a pattern of wavy myocardial fibers may be seen as early as 1 to 3 hours after onset, especially at the periphery of the infarct (Fig. 50-7; also see Fig. 50-6). It is hypothesized that wavy fibers result from the stretching and buckling of noncontractile fibers as forces are transmitted to them from adjacent viable contractile fibers.[36] After 8 hours, edema of the interstitium becomes evident, as do increased fatty deposits in the muscle fibers, along with infiltration of neutrophilic polymorphonuclear leukocytes and red blood cells. Muscle cell nuclei become pyknotic and then undergo karyolysis, and small blood vessels undergo necrosis.

By 24 hours, there is clumping of the cytoplasm and loss of cross-striations, with appearance of focal hyalinization and irregular cross-bands in the involved myocardial fibers. The nuclei become pyknotic and sometimes even disappear. The myocardial capillaries in the involved region dilate, and polymorphonuclear leukocytes accumulate, first at the periphery and then in the center of the infarct. During the first 3 days, the interstitial tissue becomes edematous and red blood cells may extravasate (see Fig. 50-6). Generally, on about the fourth day after infarction, removal of necrotic fibers by macrophages begins, again commencing at the periphery (see Figs. 50-6 and 50-7). Later, lymphocytes, macrophages, and fibroblasts infiltrate between myocytes, which become fragmented. At 8 days, the necrotic muscle fibers

have become dissolved; by about 10 days, the number of polymorphonuclear leukocytes declines, and granulation tissue first appears at the periphery (see Figs. 50-6 and 50-7). Ingrowth of blood vessels and fibroblasts continues, along with removal of necrotic muscle cells, until the fourth to sixth week after infarction, by which time much of the necrotic myocardium resorbs. This process continues along with increasing fibrosis of the infarcted area. By the sixth week, the infarcted area has usually been converted into a firm connective tissue scar with interspersed intact muscle fibers (see Figs. 50-6 and 50-7).

PATTERNS OF MYOCARDIAL NECROSIS

COAGULATION NECROSIS. Coagulation necrosis results from severe, persistent ischemia and is usually present in the central region of infarcts, which results in the arrest of muscle cells in the relaxed state and the passive stretching of ischemic muscle cells. The myofibrils are stretched, many with nuclear pyknosis, vascular congestion, and healing by phagocytosis of necrotic muscle cells (see Fig. 50-6). Mitochondrial damage with prominent amorphous (flocculent) densities but no calcification is evident.

NECROSIS WITH CONTRACTION BANDS. This form of myocardial necrosis, also termed *contraction band necrosis* or *coagulative myocytolysis*, results primarily from severe ischemia followed by reflow.[36,37] It is characterized by hypercontracted myofibrils with contraction bands and mitochondrial damage, frequently with calcification, marked vascular congestion, and healing by lysis of muscle cells. Necrosis with contraction bands is caused by increased Ca^{2+} influx into dying cells, resulting in the arrest of cells in the contracted state. It is seen in the periphery of large infarcts and is present to a greater extent in nontransmural than in transmural infarcts. The entire infarct may show this form of necrosis after reperfusion (see Fig. 50-7).[38]

MYOCYTOLYSIS. Ischemia without necrosis generally causes no acute changes that are visible by light microscopy. However, severe prolonged ischemia can cause myocyte vacuolization, often termed *myocytolysis*. Prolonged severe ischemia, which is potentially reversible, causes cloudy swelling, as well as hydropic, vascular, and fatty degeneration.

ELECTRON MICROSCOPY

In experimental infarction, the earliest ultrastructural changes in cardiac muscle following ligation of a coronary artery, noted within 20 minutes, consist of reduction in the size and number of glycogen granules; intracellular edema; and swelling and distortion of the transverse tubular system, sarcoplasmic reticulum, and mitochondria (see Fig. 50-6).[39] These early changes are reversible. Changes after 60 minutes of occlusion include myocyte swelling; swelling and internal disruption of mitochondria; development of amorphous, flocculent aggregation and margination of nuclear chromatin; and relaxation of myofibrils. After 20 minutes to 2 hours of ischemia, changes in some cells become irreversible and there is progression of these alterations; additional changes include indistinct tight junctions at the intercalated discs, swollen sacs of the sarcoplasmic reticulum at the level of the A band, greatly enlarged mitochondria with few cristae, thinning and fractionation of myofilaments, disappearance of the heterochromatin, rarefaction of the euchromatin and peripheral aggregation of chromatin in the nucleus, disorientation of myofibrils, and clumping of mitochondria.[36]

APOPTOSIS

An additional pathway of myocyte death involves apoptosis, or programmed cell death. In contrast to coagulation necrosis, myocytes undergoing apoptosis exhibit shrinkage of cells, fragmentation of DNA, and phagocytosis but without the usual cellular infiltrate indicative of inflammation (Fig. 50-8).[34] The role of apoptosis in the setting of MI is less well understood than that of classical coagulation necrosis. Apoptosis may occur shortly after the onset of myocardial ischemia. However, the major impact of apoptosis appears to be on late myocyte loss and ventricular remodeling after MI.[40]

MODIFICATION OF PATHOLOGICAL CHANGES BY REPERFUSION

When reperfusion of myocardium undergoing the evolutionary changes from ischemia to infarction occurs sufficiently early (i.e., within 15 to 20 minutes), it can successfully prevent necrosis from developing. Beyond this early stage, the number of salvaged myocytes and therefore the amount of salvaged myocardial tissue (area of necrosis/area at risk) relates directly to the length of time of total coronary artery occlusion,

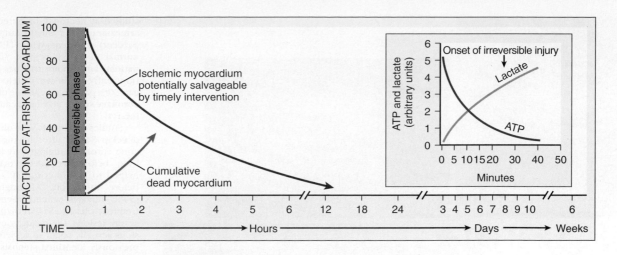

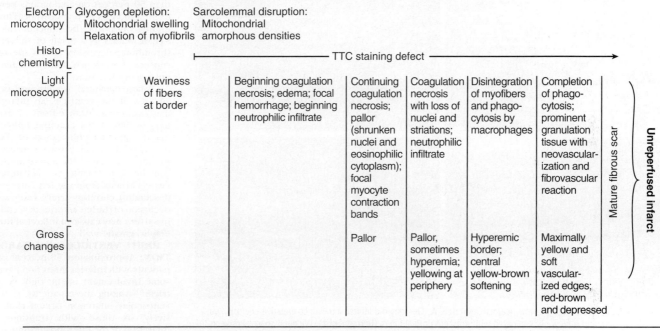

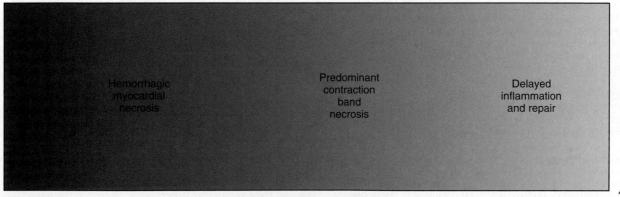

FIGURE 50–6 Temporal sequence of early biochemical, ultrastructural, histochemical, and histological findings after onset of myocardial infarction. **Top,** Schematics of the time frames for early and late reperfusion of the myocardium supplied by an occluded coronary artery. For approximately 1/2 hour after the onset of even the most severe ischemia, myocardial injury is potentially reversible; after that there is progressive loss of viability that is complete by 6 to 12 hours. The benefits of reperfusion (both early and late) are greatest when it is achieved early, with progressively smaller benefits occurring as reperfusion is delayed. Note the alterations in the temporal sequence in the reperfused infarct. The pattern of pathological findings following reperfusion is variable depending on the timing of reperfusion, prior infarction, and collateral flow. ATP = adenosine triphosphate; TTC = triphenyltetrazolium chloride. (*From Schoen FJ: The heart.* In *Kumar V, Abbas AK, Fausto N [eds]: Robbins & Cotran Pathologic Basis of Disease. 7th ed. Philadelphia, WB Saunders, 2005, p 581.*)

the level of myocardial oxygen consumption, and the collateral blood flow (Fig. 50-9; also see Fig. 50-8).[39] Typically reperfused infarcts show a mixture of necrosis, hemorrhage within zones of irreversibly injured myocytes, coagulative necrosis with contraction bands, and distorted architecture of the cells in the reperfused zone (Fig. 50-10).[39] After reperfusion, mitochondria in nonviable myocytes may develop deposits of calcium phosphate. Reperfusion of infarcted myocardium also accelerates the washout of intracellular proteins, producing an exaggerated and early peak value of substances such as CK-MB and cardiac-specific troponin T and I (see Fig. 50-6).[41]

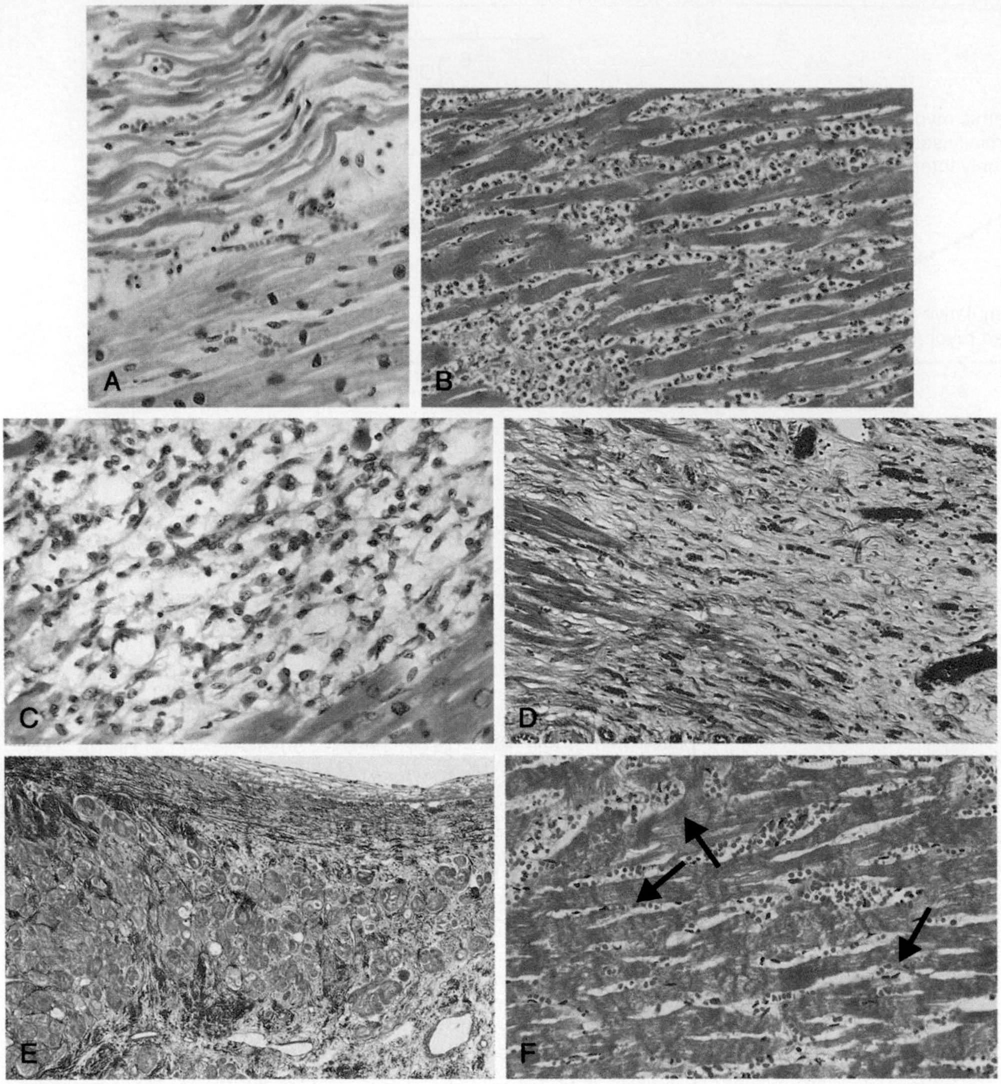

FIGURE 50–7 Microscopic features of myocardial infarction. **A,** One-day-old infarct showing coagulative necrosis, wavy fibers with elongation, and narrowing, compared with adjacent normal fibers **(lower right).** Widened spaces between the dead fibers contain edema fluid and scattered neutrophils. **B,** Dense polymorphonuclear leukocytic infiltrate in an area of acute myocardial infarction of 3 to 4 days' duration. **C,** Nearly complete removal of necrotic myocytes by phagocytosis (≈7 to 10 days). **D,** Granulation tissue with a rich vascular network and early collagen deposition, approximately 3 weeks after infarction. **E,** Well-healed myocardial infarct with replacement of the necrotic fibers by dense collagenous scar. A few residual cardiac muscle cells are present. (In **D** and **E,** collagen is highlighted as blue in this Masson trichrome stain.) **F,** Myocardial necrosis with hemorrhage and contraction bands, visible as dark bands spanning some myofibers (arrows). This is the characteristic appearance of markedly ischemic myocardium that has been reperfused. *(From Schoen FJ: The heart. In Kumar V, Abbas AK, Fausto N [eds]: Robbins & Cotran Pathologic Basis of Disease. 7th ed. Philadelphia, WB Saunders, 2005, p 680.)*

CORONARY ANATOMY AND LOCATION OF INFARCTION

Angiographic studies performed in the earliest hours of STEMI have revealed approximately a 90 percent incidence of total occlusion of the infarct-related vessel.[42] Recanalization from spontaneous thrombolysis, as well as attrition caused by some mortality among those patients with total occlusion, diminishes angiographic total occlusion in the period following the onset of MI. Pharmacological fibrinolysis and percutaneous coronary intervention markedly increase the proportion of patients with a patent infarct-related artery early after STEMI.

A STEMI with transmural necrosis typically occurs distal to an acutely totally occluded coronary artery with thrombus superimposed on a ruptured plaque. The converse is not the case, however, in that chronic total occlusion of a coronary artery does not always cause MI. Collateral blood flow and other factors such as the level of myocardial metabolism, presence and location of stenoses in other coronary arteries, rate of development of the obstruction, and quantity of myocardium supplied by the obstructed vessel all influence the viability of myocardial cells distal to the occlusion. In many series of patients

studied at necropsy or by coronary arteriography, a small number (5 percent) of patients with STEMI have normal coronary vessels. In these patients an embolus that has lysed, a transiently occlusive platelet aggregate, or a prolonged episode of severe coronary spasm may have caused the infarct.

Studies of patients who ultimately develop STEMI after having undergone coronary angiography at some time before its occurrence have helped to clarify coronary anatomy before infarction. Although high-grade stenoses, when present, more frequently lead to STEMI than do less severe lesions, the majority of occlusions actually occur in vessels with a previously identified stenosis of less than 50 percent on angiograms performed months to years earlier. This finding supports the concept that STEMI occurs as a result of sudden thrombotic occlusion at the site of rupture of previously nonobstructive but lipid-rich plaques.

When collateral vessels perfuse an area of the ventricle, an infarct may occur at a distance from a coronary occlusion. For example, following the gradual obliteration of the lumen of the right coronary artery, the inferior wall of the left ventricle can be kept viable by collateral vessels arising from the left anterior descending coronary artery. Later, an occlusion of the left anterior descending artery may cause an infarct of the diaphragmatic wall.

RIGHT VENTRICULAR INFARCTION. Approximately 50 percent of patients with inferior infarction have some involvement of the right ventricle.[43] Among these patients, right ventricular infarction occurs exclusively in those with transmural infarction of the inferoposterior wall and the posterior portion of the septum. Right ventricular infarction almost invariably develops in association with infarction of the adjacent septum and inferior left ventricular walls, but isolated infarction of the right ventricle is seen in 3 to 5 percent of autopsy-proven cases of MI (Fig. 50-11).

Right ventricular infarction occurs less commonly than would be anticipated from the frequency of atherosclerotic lesions involving the right coronary artery. This discrepancy probably can be explained by the lower oxygen demands of the right ventricle because right ventricular infarcts occur more commonly in conditions associated with increased right ventricular oxygen needs such as pulmonary hypertension and right ventricular hypertrophy. Moreover, the intercoronary collateral system of the right ventricle is richer than that of the left, and the thinness of the right ventricular wall allows the chamber to derive some nutrition from the blood within the right ventricular cavity. Therefore the right ventricle can sustain long periods of ischemia but still demonstrate excellent recovery of contractile function after reperfusion.[44]

ATRIAL INFARCTION. This can be seen in up to 10 percent of patients with STEMI if PR-segment displacement is used as the criterion for atrial infarction. Although isolated atrial infarction is observed in 3.5 percent of autopsies of patients with STEMI, it often occurs in conjunction with ventricular infarction and can cause rupture of the atrial wall.[45] This type of infarct is more common on the right side than on the left side, occurs more frequently in the atrial appendages than in the lateral or posterior walls of the atrium, and can result in thrombus formation. The difference in incidence between right and left atrial infarction might be explained by the considerably higher oxygen content of left atrial blood. Atrial infarction is frequently accompanied by atrial arrhythmias.[46] It has also been linked to reduced secretion of atrial natriuretic peptide and a low cardiac output syndrome when right ventricular infarction coexists.

COLLATERAL CIRCULATION IN ACUTE MYOCARDIAL INFARCTION (see Chaps. 48 and 54)

The coronary collateral circulation is particularly well developed in patients with (1) coronary occlusive disease, especially with the reduction of the luminal cross-sectional area by more than 75 percent in one or more major vessels; (2) chronic hypoxia, as occurs in cases of severe anemia, chronic obstructive pulmonary disease, and cyanotic congenital heart disease; and (3) left ventricular hypertrophy.

The magnitude of coronary collateral flow is one of the principal determinants of infarct size. Indeed, patients with abundant collaterals can commonly have totally occluded coronary arteries without evidence of infarction in the distribution of that artery; thus the survival of the myocardium distal to such occlusions depends in large measure on collateral blood flow. Even if collateral perfusion existing at the time of coronary occlusion does not prevent infarction, it may still exert a beneficial effect by preventing the formation of a left ventricular aneurysm. It is likely that the presence of a high-grade stenosis (90 percent), possibly with periods of intermittent total occlusion, permits the development of collaterals that remain only as potential conduits until a total occlusion occurs or recurs. Total occlusion then brings these channels into full operation.[47]

NONATHEROSCLEROTIC CAUSES OF ACUTE MYOCARDIAL INFARCTION

Numerous pathological processes other than atherosclerosis can involve the coronary arteries and result in STEMI (see Table 50-3). For example, coronary arterial occlusions can result from embolization of a coronary artery. The causes of coronary embolism are numerous: infective endocarditis and nonbacterial thrombotic endocarditis (see Chap. 63), mural thrombi, prosthetic valves, neoplasms, air that is introduced at the time of cardiac surgery, and calcium deposits from manipulation of calcified valves at operation. In situ thrombosis of coronary arteries can occur secondary to chest wall trauma (see Chap. 71).

A variety of inflammatory processes can be responsible for coronary artery abnormalities, some of which mimic atherosclerotic disease and may predispose to true atherosclerosis. Epidemiological evidence suggests that viral infections, particularly with Coxsackie B virus, may be an uncommon cause of MI. Viral illnesses precede MI occasionally in young persons who are later shown to have normal coronary arteries.

Syphilitic aortitis can produce marked narrowing or occlusion of one or both coronary ostia, whereas Takayasu arteritis can result in obstruction of the coronary arteries. Necrotizing arteritis, polyarteritis nodosa, mucocutaneous lymph node syndrome (Kawasaki disease), systemic lupus erythematosus (see Chap. 84), and giant cell arteritis can cause coronary occlusion. Therapeutic levels of mediastinal radiation can cause coronary arteriosclerosis, with subsequent infarction. MI can also result from coronary arterial involvement in patients with amyloidosis (see Chap. 64), Hurler syndrome, pseudoxanthoma elasticum, and homocystinuria.

As cocaine abuse has become more common, reports of MI after the use of cocaine have appeared with increasing frequency (see Chap. 68). Cocaine can cause MI in patients with normal coronary arteries, preexisting MI, documented coronary artery disease, or coronary artery spasm.

MYOCARDIAL INFARCTION WITH ANGIOGRAPHICALLY NORMAL CORONARY VESSELS

Patients with STEMI and normal coronary arteries tend to be young with relatively few coronary risk factors, except that they often have a history of cigarette smoking (see Table 50-3). Usually they have no history of angina pectoris before the infarction. The infarction in these patients is usually not preceded by any prodrome, but the clinical, laboratory, and ECG features of STEMI are otherwise indistinguishable from those present in the overwhelming majority of patients with STEMI who have classic obstructive atherosclerotic coronary artery disease.

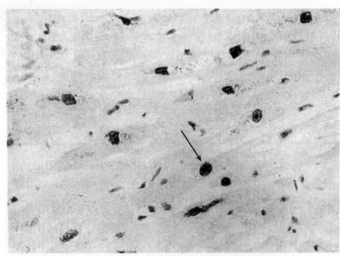

FIGURE 50–8 Apoptosis in ST-segment elevation myocardial infarction. Myocytes at the infarct border in this specimen demonstrate nuclear staining by the nick-end labeling technique (arrow) suggesting that they have undergone apoptosis (original magnification ×250). *(From Vargas SO, Sampson BA, Schoen FJ: Pathologic detection of early myocardial infarction: A critical review of the evolution and usefulness of modern techniques. Mod Pathol 12:635, 1999.)*

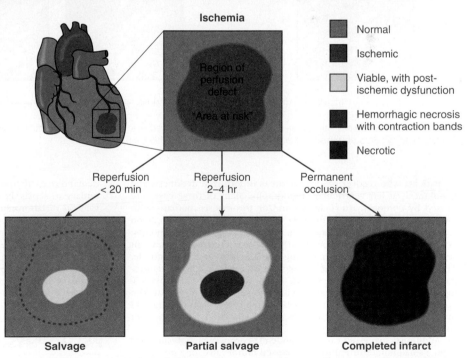

FIGURE 50–9 Consequences of reperfusion at various times after coronary adhesion. In this example, the midportion of the left anterior descending coronary artery is occluded and a large zone of ischemic myocardium develops—the "area at risk." Reperfusion in less than 20 minutes does not result in permanent tissue loss, but there may be a period of contractile dysfunction of the reperfused myocardium—a condition referred to as "stunning." Later reperfusion results in hemorrhagic necrosis with contraction bands. Permanent occlusion results in necrosis of myocardium. *(From Schoen FJ: The heart. In Kumar V, Abbas AK, Fausto N [eds]: Robbins & Cotran Pathologic Basis of Disease. 7th ed. Philadelphia, WB Saunders, 2005, p 682.)*

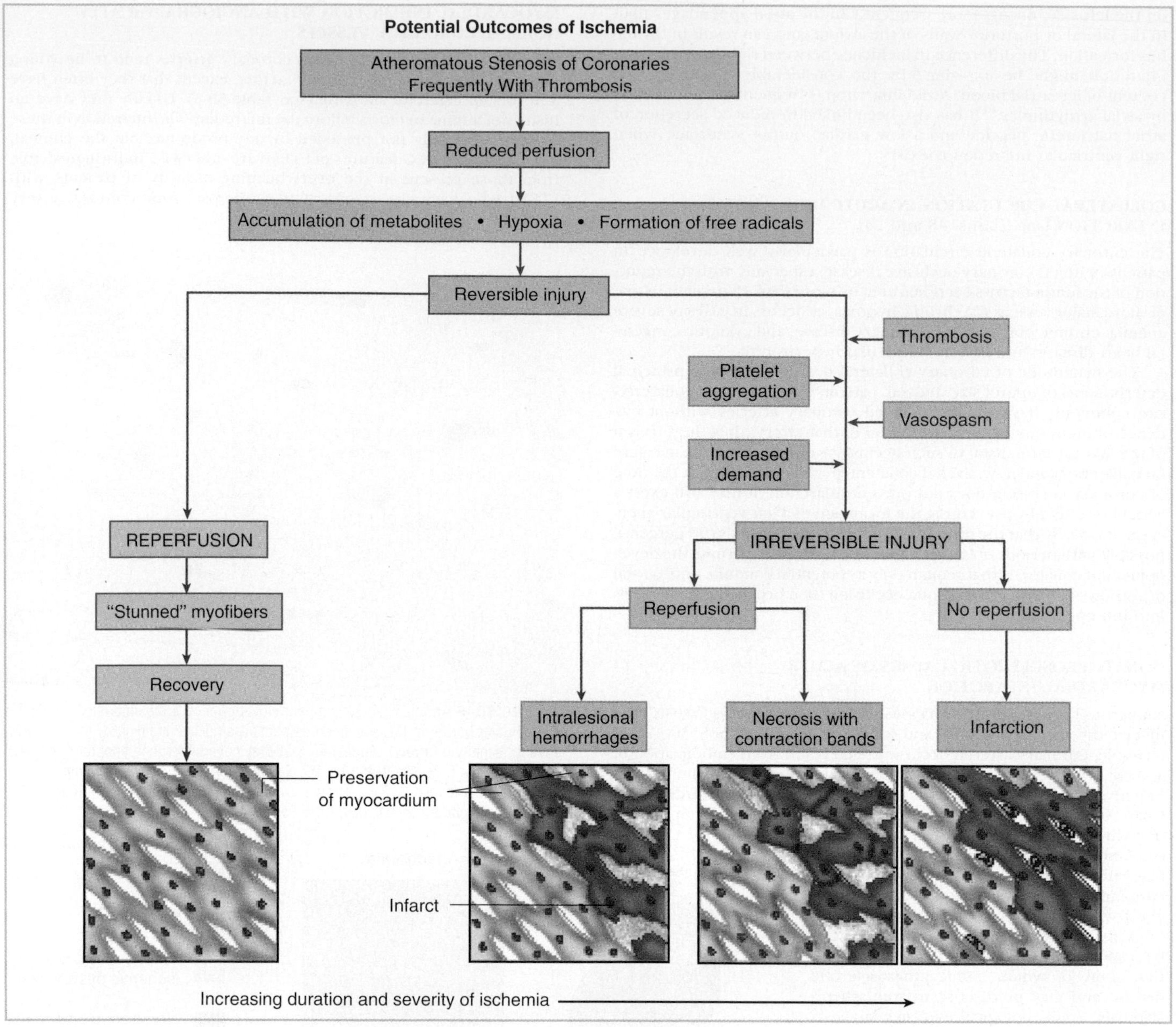

Potential Outcomes of Ischemia

FIGURE 50–10 Several potential outcomes of reversible and irreversible ischemic injury to the myocardium. *(From Schoen FJ: The heart. In Cotran RS, Kumar V, Robbins SL [eds]: Pathologic Basis of Disease. 5th ed. Philadelphia, WB Saunders, 1994, p 538.)*

Patients who recover often have areas of localized dyskinesis and hypokinesis at left ventricular angiography. Many of these cases are caused by coronary artery spasm and/or thrombosis, perhaps with underlying endothelial dysfunction or small plaques inapparent on coronary angiography. The transient left ventricular apical ballooning syndrome (takotsubo cardiomyopathy) is characterized by transient wall-motion abnormalities involving the LV apex and midventricle. This syndrome occurs in the absence of obstructive epicardial coronary disease and can mimic STEMI.[48] Typically, an episode of psychologic stress precedes presentation with takotsubo cardiomyopathy. The etiology is not clear, but experts believe that catecholamine-mediated myocardial stunning and microvascular dysfunction play important roles.

Additional suggested causes include (1) coronary emboli (perhaps from a small mural thrombus, a prolapsed mitral valve, or a myxoma); (2) coronary artery disease in vessels too small to be visualized by coronary arteriography or coronary arterial thrombosis with subsequent recanalization; (3) a variety of hematological disorders causing in situ thrombosis in the presence of normal coronary arteries (polycythemia vera, cyanotic heart disease with polycythemia, sickle cell anemia, disseminated intravascular coagulation, thrombocytosis, and thrombotic thrombocytopenic purpura); (4) augmented oxygen demand (e.g., thyrotoxicosis, amphetamine use); (5) hypotension secondary to sepsis, blood loss, or pharmacological agents; and (6) anatomical variations such as anomalous origin of a coronary artery (see Chaps. 20 and 61), coronary arteriovenous fistula (see Chap. 61), or a myocardial bridge (see Chap. 20).

PROGNOSIS. The long-term outlook for patients who have survived a STEMI with angiographically normal coronary vessels on arteriography appears brighter than for patients with STEMI and obstructive coronary artery disease. After recovery from the initial infarct, recurrent infarction, heart failure, and death are unusual in patients with normal coronary arteries. Indeed, most of these patients have normal exercise ECGs and only a minority develop angina pectoris.

PATHOPHYSIOLOGY

Left Ventricular Function

Systolic Function

Upon interruption of antegrade flow in an epicardial coronary artery, the zone of myocardium supplied by that vessel (see Fig. 50-9) immediately loses its ability to shorten and

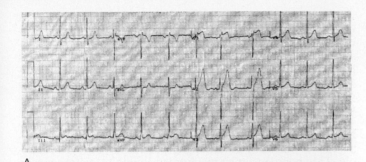

A

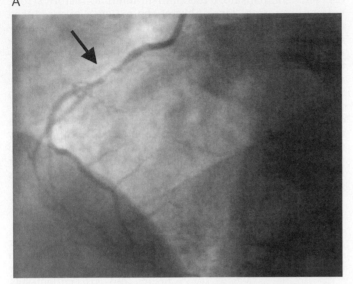

B

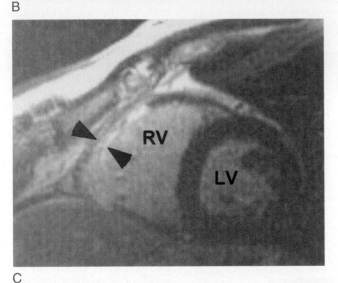

C

FIGURE 50–11 A 47-year-old man with no prior history of cardiac disease presented to an outside hospital describing "an awesome feeling that just sat in my chest" associated with bilateral arm weakness. The initial electrocardiogram **(A)** revealed ST-segment elevation in the right precordial leads and to a lesser extent in the inferior leads. The patient was treated with fibrinolytic therapy and transferred for catheterization. Angiography revealed a tight stenosis of a proximal nondominant right coronary artery **(B,** arrow) without significant disease in the left coronary artery. Contrast-enhanced cardiac magnetic resonance imaging **(C)** demonstrated delayed hyperenhancement consistent with injury of the right ventricle (RV) with distinct involvement of the right ventricular free wall (arrowheads), sparing the left ventricle (LV), as well as the right ventricular apex. The patient remained hemodynamically stable throughout his hospital course and was discharged home. *(From Finn AV, Antman EM: Images in clinical medicine. Isolated right ventricular infarction. N Engl J Med 349:1636, 2003.)*

perform contractile work. Four abnormal contraction patterns develop in sequence: (1) dyssynchrony, that is, dissociation in the time course of contraction of adjacent segments; (2) hypokinesis, reduction in the extent of shortening; (3) akinesis, cessation of shortening; and (4) dyskinesis, paradoxical expansion, and systolic bulging.[49,50] Hyperkinesis of the remaining normal myocardium initially accompanies dysfunction of the infarcting segment. The early hyperkinesis of the noninfarcted zones likely results from acute compensations including increased activity of the sympathetic nervous system and the Frank-Starling mechanism. A portion of this compensatory hyperkinesis is ineffective work because contraction of the noninfarcted segments of myocardium causes dyskinesis of the infarct zone. Increased motion of the noninfarcted region subsides within 2 weeks of infarction, during which time some degree of recovery often occurs in the infarct region as well, particularly if reperfusion of the infarcted area occurs and myocardial stunning diminishes.

Patients with STEMI often also show reduced myocardial contractile function in noninfarcted zones. This may result from previous obstruction of the coronary artery supplying the noninfarcted region of the ventricle and loss of collaterals from the freshly occluded infarct-related vessel, a condition that has been termed *ischemia at a distance*.[51] Conversely, the presence of collaterals developing before STEMI may allow for greater preservation of regional systolic function in an area of distribution of the occluded artery and improvement in left ventricular ejection fraction early after infarction.

If a sufficient quantity of myocardium undergoes ischemic injury (see Fig. 50-9), left ventricular pump function becomes depressed; cardiac output, stroke volume, blood pressure, and peak dP/dt decline[50]; and end-systolic volume increases. The degree to which end-systolic volume increases is perhaps the most powerful hemodynamic predictor of mortality following STEMI.[52] Paradoxical systolic expansion of an area of ventricular myocardium further decreases left ventricular stroke volume. As necrotic myocytes slip past each other, the infarct zone thins and elongates, especially in patients with large anterior infarcts, leading to infarct expansion. As the ventricle dilates during the first few hours to days after infarction, regional and global wall stress increase according to Laplace's law. In some patients a vicious circle of dilation begetting further dilation ensues. The degree of ventricular dilation, which depends closely on infarct size, patency of the infarct-related artery,[53] and activation of the renin-angiotensin-aldosterone system (RAAS), can be favorably modified by inhibitors of this system, even in the absence of symptomatic left ventricular dysfunction.[54]

With time, edema and cellular infiltration and ultimately fibrosis increase the stiffness of the infarcted myocardium back to and beyond control values. Increasing stiffness in the infarcted zone of myocardium improves left ventricular function because it prevents paradoxical systolic wall motion (dyskinesia).

The likelihood of developing clinical symptoms such as dyspnea and ultimately a shocklike state correlate with specific parameters of left ventricular function. The earliest abnormality is a ventricular stiffness in diastole (see later), which can be observed with infarcts that involve only a small portion of the left ventricle on angiographic examination. When the abnormally contracting segment exceeds 15 percent, the ejection fraction may decline and elevations of left ventricular end-diastolic pressure and volume occur. The risk of developing physical signs and symptoms of left ventricular failure also increase proportionally to increasing areas of abnormal left ventricular wall motion.[50] Clinical heart failure accompanies areas of abnormal contraction exceeding 25 percent, and cardiogenic shock, often fatal, accompanies loss of more than 40 percent of the left ventricular myocardium.

Unless infarct extension occurs, some improvement in wall motion takes place during the healing phase, as recovery of function occurs in initially reversibly injured (stunned) myocardium (see Fig. 50-9). Regardless of the age of the infarct, patients who continue to demonstrate abnormal wall motion of 20 to 25 percent of the left ventricle will likely manifest hemodynamic signs of left ventricular failure, with its attendant poor prognosis for long-term survival.

Diastolic Function

The diastolic properties of the left ventricle (see Chap. 26) change in infarcted and ischemic myocardium. These alterations associate with a decrease in the peak rate of decline in left ventricular pressure [peak (–)dP/dt], an increase in the time constant of the fall in left ventricular pressure, and an initial rise in left ventricular end-diastolic pressure. Over several weeks, end-diastolic volume increases and diastolic pressure begins to fall toward normal. As with impairment of systolic function, the magnitude of the diastolic abnormality appears to relate to the size of the infarct.

Circulatory Regulation

Patients with STEMI have abnormality in circulatory regulation. The process begins with an anatomical or functional obstruction in the coronary vascular bed, which results in regional myocardial ischemia and, if the ischemia persists, in infarction (Fig. 50-12). If the infarct is of sufficient size, it depresses overall left ventricular function so that left ventricular stroke volume falls and filling pressures rise. A marked depression of left ventricular stroke volume ultimately lowers aortic pressure and reduces coronary perfusion pressure; this condition may intensify myocardial ischemia and thereby initiate a vicious circle (see Fig. 50-12). Systemic inflammation secondary to the infarction process leads to the release of cytokines that contribute to vasodilation and a fall in systemic vascular resistance.[55]

The inability of the left ventricle to empty normally also leads to an increased preload; that is, it dilates the well-perfused, normally functioning portion of the left ventricle. This compensatory mechanism tends to restore stroke volume to normal levels, but at the expense of a reduced ejection fraction. The dilation of the left ventricle also elevates ventricular afterload, however, because Laplace's law dictates that at any given arterial pressure, the dilated ventricle must develop a higher wall tension. This increased afterload not only depresses left ventricular stroke volume but also elevates myocardial oxygen consumption, which in turn intensifies myocardial ischemia. When regional myocardial dysfunction is limited and the function of the remainder of the left ventricle is normal, compensatory mechanisms, especially hyperkinesis of the nonaffected portion of the ventricle, sustain overall left ventricular function. If a large portion of the left ventricle becomes necrotic, pump failure occurs.

Ventricular Remodeling

As a consequence of STEMI, the changes in left ventricular size, shape, and thickness involving both the infarcted and the noninfarcted segments of the ventricle described earlier occur and are collectively referred to as *ventricular remodeling*, which can in turn influence ventricular function and prognosis. A combination of changes in left ventricular dilation and hypertrophy of residual noninfarcted myocardium causes remodeling. After the size of infarction, the two most important factors driving the process of left ventricular dilation are ventricular loading conditions and infarct artery patency (Fig. 50-13).[56,57] Elevated ventricular pressure contributes to increased wall stress and the risk of infarct expansion, and a patent infarct artery accelerates myocardial scar formation and increases tissue turgor in the infarct zone, reducing the risk of infarct expansion and ventricular dilation.

INFARCT EXPANSION. An increase in the size of the infarcted segment, known as *infarct expansion*, is defined as "acute dilation and thinning of the area of infarction not explained by additional myocardial necrosis."[58] Infarct expansion appears to be caused by (1) a combination of slippage between

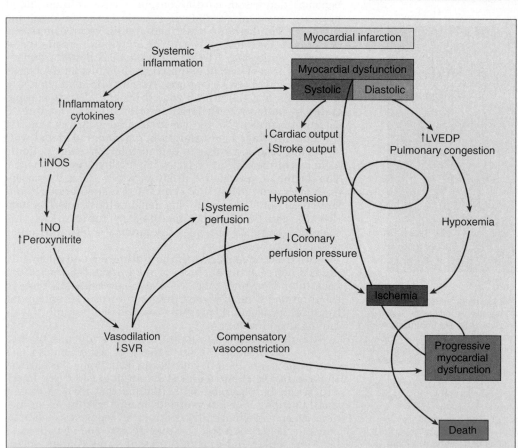

FIGURE 50–12 Classic shock paradigm is shown in black. The influence of the inflammatory response syndrome initiated by a large myocardial infarction is illustrated in red. LVEDP = left ventricular end-diastolic pressure; SVR = systemic vascular resistance. (*From Hochman J: Cardiogenic shock complicating acute myocardial infarction: Expanding the paradigm. Circulation 107:2998, 2003.*)

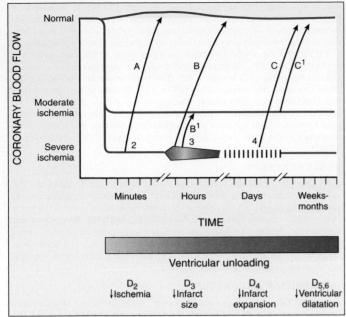

FIGURE 50–13 Therapeutic maneuvers in various stages of ischemia and infarction. Severely ischemic tissue **(2)** may be reperfused, thereby averting myocardial infarction **(A)**. Infarcting tissue **(3)** may be reperfused, leading to sparing of myocardial tissue **(B)**. If blood flow is restored only in part B, the myocardium may remain noncontractile, although viable (i.e., hibernating). After completion of the infarct **(4)**, late reperfusion **(C)** may still be useful. Mechanical reperfusion of moderately ischemic myocardium **(C¹)** may restore contractility of hibernating myocardium to normal. Ventricular unloading may be useful throughout the preinfarct and postinfarct periods. Unloading may reduce ischemia (D₂), infarct size (D₃), infarct expansion (D₄), and ventricular dilatation (D₅,₆). *(From Braunwald E, Pfeffer MA: Ventricular enlargement and remodeling following acute myocardial infarction: Mechanisms and management. Am J Cardiol 68:4D, 1991.)*

muscle bundles, reducing the number of myocytes across the infarct wall; (2) disruption of the normal myocardial cells; and (3) tissue loss within the necrotic zone.[58] It is characterized by disproportionate thinning and dilation of the infarct zone before formation of a firm, fibrotic scar. The degree of infarct expansion appears to be related to the preinfarction wall thickness, with existing hypertrophy possibly protecting against infarct thinning. The apex is the thinnest region of the ventricle and an area of the heart that is particularly vulnerable to infarct expansion. Infarction of the apex secondary to occlusion of the left anterior descending coronary artery causes the radius of curvature at the apex to increase, exposing this normally thin region to a marked elevation in wall stress.

Infarct expansion is associated with both a higher mortality and a higher incidence of nonfatal complications, such as heart failure and ventricular aneurysm. Infarct expansion is best recognized echocardiographically as elongation of the noncontractile region of the ventricle. When expansion is severe enough to cause symptoms, the most characteristic clinical finding is deterioration of systolic function associated with new or louder gallop sounds and new or worsening pulmonary congestion.

VENTRICULAR DILATION. Although infarct expansion plays an important role in the ventricular remodeling that occurs early following myocardial infarction, remodeling is also caused by dilation of the viable portion of the ventricle, commencing immediately after STEMI and progressing for months or years thereafter (see Fig. 50-13). Dilation may be accompanied by a shift of the pressure-volume curve of the left ventricle to the right, resulting in a larger left ventricular volume at any given diastolic pressure. This dilation of the noninfarct zone can be viewed as a compen-

satory mechanism that maintains stroke volume in the face of a large infarction. STEMI places an extra load on the residual functioning myocardium, a burden that presumably is responsible for the compensatory hypertrophy of the uninfarcted myocardium. This hypertrophy could help to compensate for the functional impairment caused by the infarct and may be responsible for some of the hemodynamic improvement seen in the months after infarction in some patients.

EFFECTS OF TREATMENT. Ventricular remodeling after STEMI can be affected by several factors, the first of which is infarct size (see Figs. 50-9 and 50-13). Acute reperfusion and other measures to restrict the extent of myocardial necrosis limit the increase in ventricular volume after STEMI. The second factor is scar formation in the infarct. Glucocorticosteroids and nonsteroidal antiinflammatory agents given early after MI can cause scar thinning and greater infarct expansion, whereas inhibitors of the RAAS attenuate ventricular enlargement (see Fig. 50-13).[29] Additional beneficial consequences of inhibition of angiotensin II that may contribute to myocardial protection include attenuation of endothelial dysfunction and direct antiatherogenic effects.[59] Inhibition of aldosterone action reduces collagen deposition and decreases the development of ventricular arrhythmias.[60]

Pathophysiology of Other Organ Systems

PULMONARY FUNCTION

Changes in pulmonary gas exchange, ventilation, and distribution of perfusion occur with STEMI. An inverse relationship exists between arterial oxygen tension and pulmonary artery diastolic pressure. This suggests that increased pulmonary capillary hydrostatic pressure leads to interstitial edema, which results in arteriolar and bronchiolar compression that ultimately causes perfusion of poorly ventilated alveoli with resultant hypoxemia (see Chap. 22). In addition to hypoxemia, there is a fall in diffusing capacity. Hyperventilation often occurs in patients with STEMI and may cause hypocapnia and respiratory alkalosis, particularly in restless, anxious patients with pain.

INCREASE IN INTERSTITIAL WATER. Pulmonary extravascular (interstitial) water content, left ventricular filling pressure, and the clinical signs and symptoms of left ventricular failure correlate. The increase in pulmonary extravascular water may be responsible for the alterations in pulmonary mechanics observed in patients with STEMI (i.e., reduction of airway conductance; pulmonary compliance; forced expiratory volume and midexpiratory flow rate; and an increase in closing volume, which is presumably related to the widespread closure of small, dependent airways during the first 3 days after STEMI). Ultimately, severe increases in extravascular water may lead to pulmonary edema.

REDUCTION OF VITAL CAPACITY. Virtually all lung volume indices—total lung capacity, functional residual capacity, and residual volume, as well as vital capacity—fall during STEMI. These reductions correlate with the elevations of left-sided filling pressures and are most probably caused by increases in pulmonary extravascular water. Increased pulmonary venous pressure also results in redistribution of pulmonary blood flow from the bases to the apices of the lung in patients with STEMI, altering the relationship between ventilation and perfusion. At follow-up examination 3 to 25 weeks after STEMI, however, the ventilation-perfusion relationship has usually returned to normal or almost so.

REDUCTION OF AFFINITY OF HEMOGLOBIN FOR OXYGEN. In patients with MI, particularly when complicated by left ventricular failure or cardiogenic shock, the affinity of hemoglobin for oxygen falls (i.e., the P50 is increased). The increase in P50 results from increased levels of erythrocyte 2,3-diphosphoglycerate (2,3-DPG), which constitutes an important compensatory mechanism, responsible for an estimated 18 percent increase in oxygen release from oxyhemoglobin in patients with cardiogenic shock.

ENDOCRINE FUNCTION

PANCREAS. Hyperglycemia and impaired glucose tolerance are common in patients with STEMI (see Chap. 60). Although the absolute levels of blood insulin are often in the normal range, they are usually inappropriately low for the level of blood sugar, and there may be relative insulin resistance as well. Patients with cardiogenic shock often demonstrate marked hyperglycemia and depressed levels of circulating insulin. Abnormalities in insulin secretion and the resultant impaired glucose tolerance appear due to a reduction in pancreatic blood flow as a consequence of splanchnic vasoconstriction accompanying severe left ventricular failure. In addition, increased activity of the sympathetic nervous system with augmented circulating catecholamines inhibits insulin secretion and augments glycogenolysis, also contributing to the elevation of blood sugar.

Glucose appears to be a more favorable energy source than free fatty acids for the ischemic myocardium by permitting ATP generation by anaerobic glycolysis.[61] Because hypoxic heart muscle derives a considerable portion of its energy from the metabolism of glucose (see Chap. 21) and because insulin is essential for the uptake of glucose by the myocardium, insulin deficiency has clear deleterious effects. These metabolic considerations, combined with epidemiological observations that diabetic patients have a markedly worse prognosis, have served as the foundation for efforts to more aggressively administer insulin-glucose infusions to diabetic patients with STEMI.[62,63]

ADRENAL MEDULLA. Excessive secretion of catecholamines produces many of the characteristic signs and symptoms of STEMI. The plasma and urinary catecholamine levels peak during the first 24 hours after the onset of chest pain, with the greatest rise in plasma catecholamine secretion occurring during the first hour after the onset of STEMI. These high levels of circulating catecholamines in patients with STEMI correlate with the occurrence of serious arrhythmias and result in an increase in myocardial oxygen consumption, both directly and indirectly, as a consequence of catecholamine-induced elevation of circulating free fatty acids. The concentration of circulating catecholamines correlates with the extent of myocardial damage and incidence of cardiogenic shock, as well as both early and late mortality rates.

Circulating catecholamines enhance platelet aggregation; when this occurs in the coronary microcirculation, the release of the potent local vasoconstrictor thromboxane A_2 may further impair cardiac perfusion. The marked increase in sympathetic activity associated with STEMI serves as the foundation for beta-adrenergic receptor blocker regimens in the acute phase.

ACTIVATION OF THE RENIN-ANGIOTENSIN-ALDOSTERONE SYSTEM. Noninfarcted regions of the myocardium appear to exhibit activation of the tissue renin-angiotensin system with increased angiotensin II production. Both locally and systemically generated angiotensin II can stimulate the production of various growth factors, such as platelet-derived growth factor and transforming growth factor-beta, that promote compensatory hypertrophy in the noninfarcted myocardium, as well as control the structure and tone of the infarct-related coronary and other myocardial vessels. Additional potential actions of angiotensin II that have a more negative impact on the infarction process include release of endothelin, PAI-1, and aldosterone, which may cause vasoconstriction, impaired fibrinolysis, and increased sodium retention, respectively.

NATRIURETIC PEPTIDES. The peptides atrial natriuretic factor (ANF) and N-terminal pro-ANF are released from cardiac atria in response to elevation of atrial pressure. Brain natriuretic peptide (BNP) and its precursor N-terminal pro-BNP are secreted by human atrial and ventricular myocardium. Given the larger mass of ventricular rather than atrial myocardium, the total amount of mRNA for BNP is higher in the ventricles than the atria.[64] Natriuretic peptides are released early after STEMI, peaking at about 16 hours. Evidence exists that natriuretic peptides released from the left ventricle during STEMI originate both from the infarcted myocardium, as well as viable noninfarcted myocardium.[65] The rise in BNP and N-terminal pro-BNP after STEMI correlates with infarct size and regional wall motion abnormalities.[66] Patients with anterior infarction, lower cardiac index, and more significant congestive heart failure after STEMI have higher levels of N-terminal pro-BNP and BNP and such elevations correlate with a worse prognosis.[67-71]

Measurement of natriuretic peptides can provide useful information both early and late in the course of STEMI. Patients with elevated levels 6 hours after the onset of symptoms have a marked increase in mortality even after adjusting for other known prognostic indicators.[72] Conversely, patients with persistently elevated levels at 3 to 4 weeks after STEMI have an increased risk of cardiac-related mortality over the ensuing 5 to 10 years.[73]

ADRENAL CORTEX. Plasma and urinary 17-hydroxycorticosteroids and ketosteroids, as well as aldosterone, rise markedly in patients with STEMI. Their concentrations correlate directly with the peak level oft

serum CK, implying an association between the stress imposed by larger infarcts and greater secretion of adrenal steroids. The magnitude of the elevation of cortisol correlates with infarct size and mortality. Glucocorticosteroids also contribute to impaired glucose tolerance.

THYROID GLAND. Although patients with STEMI are generally euthyroid clinically, there is evidence of a transient decrease in serum triiodothyronine (T_3) levels, a fall that is most marked on about the third day after the infarct. This fall in T_3 is usually accompanied by a rise in reverse T_3, with variable changes or no change in thyroxine (T_4) and thyroid-stimulating hormone (TSH) levels. The alteration in peripheral T_4 metabolism appears to correlate with infarct size and may be mediated by the rise in endogenous levels of cortisol that accompanies STEMI.

RENAL FUNCTION

Both prerenal azotemia and acute renal failure can complicate the marked reduction of cardiac output that occurs in cardiogenic shock. On the other hand, an increase in circulating atrial natriuretic peptide occurs following STEMI, which is correlated with the severity of left ventricular failure. An increase in natriuretic peptide is also found when right ventricular infarction accompanies inferior wall infarction, suggesting that this hormone may play a role in the hypotension that accompanies right ventricular infarction.

HEMATOLOGICAL FUNCTION

PLATELETS. STEMI generally occurs in the presence of extensive coronary and systemic atherosclerotic plaques, which may serve as the site for the formation of platelet aggregates, a sequence that has been suggested as the initial step in the process of coronary thrombosis, coronary occlusion, and subsequent MI. Circulating platelets are hyperaggregable in patients with STEMI. Platelets from STEMI patients have an increased propensity for aggregation locally in the area of a disrupted plaque and also release vasoactive substances.[74]

HEMOSTATIC MARKERS. Elevated levels of serum fibrinogen degradation products, an end-product of thrombosis, as well as release of distinctive proteins when platelets are activated, such as platelet factor 4 and beta-thromboglobulin, have been reported in some patients with STEMI. Fibrinopeptide A, a protein released from fibrin by thrombin, is a marker of ongoing thrombosis and is increased during the early hours of STEMI. Marked elevation of hemostatic markers such as FPA, TAT, and F1.2 is associated with an increased risk of mortality in STEMI patients (see Chap. 82). The interpretation of the coagulation tests in patients with STEMI may be complicated by elevated blood levels of catecholamines, concomitant shock, and/or pulmonary embolism, conditions that are all capable of altering various tests of platelet and coagulation function. Additional factors that affect coagulation tests in STEMI include the type and dosage of antithrombotic agents and reperfusion of the infarct artery.

LEUKOCYTES. Leukocytosis usually accompanies STEMI in proportion to the magnitude of the necrotic process, elevated glucocorticoid levels, and possibly inflammation in the coronary arteries. The magnitude of elevation of the leukocyte count associates with in-hospital mortality after STEMI.[75] Activation of neutrophils may produce important intermediates, such as leukotriene B_4 and reactive oxygen species, which have important microcirculatory effects.

BLOOD VISCOSITY. Clinical and epidemiological studies suggest that several hemostatic and hemorheological factors (e.g., fibrinogen, factor VII, plasma viscosity, hematocrit, red blood cell aggregation, total white blood cell count) participate in the pathophysiology of atherosclerosis and also play an integral role in acute thrombotic events. An increase in blood viscosity also occurs in patients with STEMI. During the first few days after infarction, this is mainly attributable to hemoconcentration, but later the increases in plasma viscosity and red blood cell aggregation correlate with elevated serum concentrations of alpha$_2$-globulin and fibrinogen, components of the acute phase response to tissue necrosis also responsible for the elevated sedimentation rate characteristic of STEMI. The high values of blood viscosity indices occur most frequently in patients with complications such as left ventricular failure, cardiogenic shock, and thromboembolism.

CLINICAL FEATURES

Predisposing Factors

The risk factors for atherosclerotic coronary artery disease are discussed in Chapter 39.

In up to half of patients with STEMI, a precipitating factor or prodromal symptoms can be identified. Evidence suggests that unusually heavy exercise (particularly in fatigued or habitually inactive patients) and emotional stress can precipitate STEMI.[31] Such infarctions could result from marked increases in myocardial oxygen consumption in the presence of severe coronary arterial narrowing.[76-78]

Accelerating angina and rest angina, two patterns of unstable angina, may culminate in STEMI (see Fig. 50-2). Noncardiac surgical procedures have also been noted as precursors of STEMI. Perioperative risk stratification and the use of beta blockers may reduce the likelihood of STEMI and cardiac-related mortality (see Chap. 80).[79] Reduced myocardial perfusion secondary to hypotension (e.g., hemorrhagic or septic shock) and increased myocardial oxygen demands caused by aortic stenosis, fever, tachycardia, and agitation can also be responsible for myocardial necrosis. Other factors reported as predisposing to STEMI include respiratory infections; hypoxemia of any cause; pulmonary embolism; hypoglycemia; administration of ergot preparations; use of cocaine; sympathomimetics; serum sickness; allergy; and, on rare occasion, wasp stings. In patients with Prinzmetal angina (see Chap. 53), STEMI may develop in the territory of the coronary artery that repeatedly undergoes spasm. Rarely, munition workers exposed to high concentrations of nitroglycerin develop MI when they are withdrawn from this exposure, suggesting that it is caused by vasospasm.

CIRCADIAN PERIODICITY. The time of onset of STEMI has a pronounced circadian periodicity, with peak incidence of events between 6 AM and noon.[80] Circadian rhythms affect many physiological and biochemical variables; the early morning hours are associated with rises in plasma catecholamines and cortisol and increases in platelet aggregability. Interestingly, the characteristic circadian peak was *absent* in patients receiving beta blocker or aspirin before their presentation with STEMI. The concept of "triggering" a STEMI is a complex one and likely involves the superimposition of multiple factors such as time of day, season, and the stress of natural disasters.[31]

History

PRODROMAL SYMPTOMS. Despite advances in the laboratory detection of STEMI, the patient's history remains crucial to establishing a diagnosis. The prodrome is usually characterized by chest discomfort, resembling classic angina pectoris, but it occurs at rest or with less activity than usual and can therefore be classified as unstable angina. However, it is often not disturbing enough to induce patients to seek medical attention, and if they do, they may not be hospitalized. A feeling of general malaise or frank exhaustion often accompanies other symptoms preceding STEMI. Women may present differently from men (see Chap. 76).

NATURE OF THE PAIN. The pain of STEMI varies in intensity; in most patients, it is severe and in some instances intolerable. The pain is prolonged, usually lasting for more than 30 minutes and frequently for a number of hours. The discomfort is described as constricting, crushing, oppressing, or compressing; often the patient complains of a sensation of a heavy weight or a squeezing in the chest. Although the discomfort is typically described as a choking, viselike, or heavy pain, it can also be characterized as a stabbing, knifelike, boring, or burning discomfort. The pain is usually retrosternal in location, spreading frequently to both sides of the anterior chest, with predilection for the left side. Often the pain radiates down the ulnar aspect of the left arm, producing a tingling sensation in the left wrist, hand, and fingers. Some patients note only a dull ache or numbness of the wrists in association with severe substernal or precordial discomfort. In some instances the pain of STEMI may begin in the epigastrium and simulate a variety of abdominal disorders, a fact that often causes STEMI to be misdiagnosed as "indigestion." In other patients, the discomfort of STEMI radiates to the shoulders, upper extremities, neck, jaw, and interscapular region, again usually favoring the left side. In patients with preexisting angina pectoris, the pain of infarction usually resembles that of angina with respect to location. However, it is generally much more severe, lasts longer, and is not relieved by rest and nitroglycerin.

The pain of STEMI may have subsided by the time the physician first encounters the patient (or the patient reaches the hospital), or it may persist for many hours. Opiates, in particular morphine, usually relieve the pain. Both angina pectoris and the pain of STEMI are thought to arise from nerve endings in ischemic or injured, but not necrotic, myocardium. Thus in cases of STEMI, stimulation of nerve fibers in an ischemic zone of myocardium surrounding the necrotic central area of infarction probably gives rise to the pain.

The pain often disappears suddenly and completely when blood flow to the infarct territory is restored. In patients in whom reocclusion occurs after fibrinolysis, pain recurs if the initial reperfusion has left viable myocardium. Thus what has previously been thought of as the "pain of infarction," sometimes lasting for many hours, probably represents pain caused by ongoing ischemia. The recognition that pain implies ischemia and not infarction heightens the importance of seeking ways to relieve the ischemia, for which the pain is a marker. This finding suggests that the clinician should *not* be complacent about ongoing cardiac pain under any circumstances. In some patients, particularly the elderly, diabetic patients, and heart transplantation recipients, STEMI manifests clinically not by chest pain but rather by symptoms of acute left ventricular failure and chest tightness or by marked weakness or frank syncope. Diaphoresis, nausea, and vomiting may accompany these symptoms.

OTHER SYMPTOMS. Nausea and vomiting may occur, presumably because of activation of the vagal reflex or stimulation of left ventricular receptors as part of the Bezold-Jarisch reflex. These symptoms occur more commonly in patients with inferior STEMI than in those with anterior STEMI. Moreover, nausea and vomiting are common side effects of opiates. When the pain of STEMI is epigastric in location and is associated with nausea and vomiting, the clinical picture can easily be confused with that of acute cholecystitis, gastritis, or peptic ulcer. Occasionally, a patient complains of diarrhea or a violent urge to defecate during the acute phase of STEMI. Other symptoms include feelings of profound weakness, dizziness, palpitations, cold perspiration, and a sense of impending doom. On occasion, symptoms arising from an episode of cerebral embolism or other systemic arterial embolism herald a STEMI. Chest discomfort may not accompany these symptoms.

Differential Diagnosis

The pain of STEMI may simulate that of acute pericarditis (see Chap. 70), which is usually associated with some pleuritic features: It is aggravated by respiratory movements and coughing and often involves the shoulder, ridge of the trapezius, and neck. An important feature that distinguishes pericardial pain from ischemic discomfort is that ischemic discomfort does not radiate to the trapezius ridge, a characteristic site of radiation of pericardial pain.[81] Pleural pain is usually sharp, knifelike, and aggravated in a cyclical fashion by each breath, which distinguishes it from the deep, dull, steady pain of STEMI. Pulmonary embolism (see Chap. 72) generally produces pain laterally in the chest, is often pleuritic in nature, and may be associated with hemoptysis. The pain caused by acute aortic dissection (see Chap. 56) is usually localized to the center of the chest, is extremely severe and described by the patient as a "ripping" or "tearing" sensation, is at its maximal intensity shortly after onset, persists for many hours, and often radiates to the back or lower extremities. Often one or more major arterial pulses are absent. Pain arising from the costochondral and chondrosternal articulations may be associated with localized swelling and redness; it is usually sharp and "darting" and is characterized by marked localized tenderness. Episodes of retrosternal discomfort induced by peristalsis in patients with increased esophageal stiffness and also episodes of sustained esophageal contraction can mimic the pain of STEMI.[82]

SILENT STEMI AND ATYPICAL PRESENTATION. Nonfatal STEMI can be unrecognized by the patient and discovered only on subsequent routine electrocardiographic or postmortem examinations. Of these unrecognized infarctions, approximately half are truly silent, with the patients unable to recall any symptoms whatsoever. The other half of patients with so-called *silent infarction* can recall an event characterized by symptoms compatible with acute infarction when leading questions are posed after the electrocardiographic abnormalities are discovered. Unrecognized or silent infarction occurs more commonly in patients without antecedent angina pectoris and in patients with diabetes and hypertension.[83] Silent STEMI is often followed by silent ischemia (see Chap. 54). The prognoses of patients with silent and symptomatic presentations of STEMI appear quite similar.

Atypical presentations of STEMI include the following: (1) heart failure (i.e., dyspnea without pain beginning de novo or worsening of established failure); (2) classic angina pectoris without a particularly severe or prolonged episode; (3) atypical location of the pain; (4) central nervous system manifestations, resembling those of stroke, secondary to a sharp reduction in cardiac output in a patient with cerebral arteriosclerosis; (5) apprehension and nervousness; (6) sudden mania or psychosis; (7) syncope; (8) overwhelming weakness; (9) acute indigestion; and (10) peripheral embolization.

Physical Examination

GENERAL APPEARANCE. Patients suffering STEMI often appear anxious and in considerable distress. An anguished facial expression is common, and—in contrast to patients with severe angina pectoris, who often lie, sit, or stand still, recognizing that all forms of activity increase the discomfort—some patients suffering STEMI may be restless and move about in an effort to find a comfortable position. They often massage or clutch their chests and frequently describe their pain with a clenched fist held against the sternum (the Levine sign, named after Dr. Samuel A. Levine). In patients with left ventricular failure and sympathetic stimulation, cold perspiration and skin pallor may be evident; they typically sit or are propped up in bed, gasping for breath. Between breaths, they may complain of chest discomfort or a feeling of suffocation. Cough productive of frothy, pink, or blood-streaked sputum is common.

Patients in cardiogenic shock often lie listlessly, making few, if any, spontaneous movements. The skin is cool and clammy, with a bluish or mottled color over the extremities, and there is marked facial pallor with severe cyanosis of the lips and nailbeds. Depending on the degree of cerebral perfusion, the patient in shock may converse normally or may evidence confusion and disorientation.

HEART RATE. The heart rate can vary from a marked bradycardia to a rapid regular or irregular tachycardia, depending on the underlying rhythm and the degree of left ventricular failure. Most commonly, the pulse is rapid and regular initially (sinus tachycardia at 100 to 110 beats/min), slowing as the patient's pain and anxiety are relieved; premature ventricular beats are common, occurring in more than 95 percent of patients evaluated within the first 4 hours after the onset of symptoms.

BLOOD PRESSURE. The majority of patients with uncomplicated STEMI are normotensive, although the reduced stroke volume accompanying the tachycardia can cause declines in systolic and pulse pressures and elevation of diastolic pressure. Among previously normotensive patients, a hypertensive response is occasionally seen during the first few hours, with the arterial pressure exceeding 160/90 mm Hg, presumably as a consequence of adrenergic discharge secondary to pain, anxiety, and agitation. It is common for previously hypertensive patients to become normotensive without treatment after STEMI, although many of these previously hypertensive patients eventually regain their elevated levels of blood pressure, generally 3 to 6 months after infarction. In patients with massive infarction, arterial pressure falls acutely because of left ventricular dysfunction and venous pooling secondary to administration of morphine and/or nitrates; as recovery occurs, the arterial pressure tends to return to preinfarction levels.

Patients in cardiogenic shock by definition have systolic pressures below 90 mm Hg and evidence of end-organ hypoperfusion. However, hypotension alone does not necessarily signify cardiogenic shock because some patients with inferior infarction with Bezold-Jarisch reflex activation may also transiently have systolic blood pressure below 90 mm Hg. Their hypotension eventually resolves spontaneously, although the process can be accelerated by intravenous atropine (0.5 to 1 mg) and assumption of the Trendelenburg position. Other patients who are initially only slightly hypotensive may demonstrate gradually falling blood pressures with progressive reduction in cardiac output over several hours or days as they develop cardiogenic shock as a consequence of increasing ischemia and extension of infarction (see Fig. 50-12). Evidence of autonomic hyperactivity is common, varying in type with the location of the infarction. At some time in their initial presentation, more than half of patients with inferior STEMI have evidence of excess parasympathetic stimulation, with hypotension, bradycardia, or both, whereas about half of patients with anterior STEMI show signs of sympathetic excess, having hypertension, tachycardia, or both.[84]

TEMPERATURE AND RESPIRATION. Most patients with extensive STEMI develop fever, a nonspecific response to tissue necrosis, within 24 to 48 hours of the onset of infarction. Body temperature often begins to rise within 4 to 8 hours after the onset of infarction, and rectal temperature may reach 38.3° to 38.9° C (101° to 102° F). Fever usually resolves by the fourth or fifth day after infarction.

The respiratory rate may be slightly elevated soon after the development of STEMI; in patients without heart failure, it results from anxiety and pain because it returns to normal with treatment of physical and psychological discomfort. In patients with left ventricular failure, the respiratory rate correlates with the severity of failure; patients with pulmonary edema may have respiratory rates exceeding 40 per minute. However, the respiratory rate is not necessarily elevated in patients with cardiogenic shock. Cheyne-Stokes (periodic) respiration may occur in elderly individuals with cardiogenic shock or heart failure, particularly after opiate therapy or in the presence of cerebrovascular disease.

JUGULAR VENOUS PULSE. The jugular venous pulse usually fails to show any abnormalities. The *a* wave may be prominent in patients with pulmonary hypertension secondary to left ventricular failure or reduced compliance. In contrast, right ventricular infarction (whether or not it accompanies left ventricular infarction) often results in marked jugular venous distention and, when it is complicated by necrosis or ischemia of right ventricular papillary muscles, tall c-v waves of tricuspid regurgitation are evident. Patients with STEMI and cardiogenic shock usually have elevated jugular venous pressure. In patients with STEMI, hypotension, and hypoperfusion (findings that may resemble those of patients with cardiogenic shock) but who have flat neck veins, it is likely that the depression of left ventricular performance may relate, at least in part, to hypovolemia. The differentiation can be made only by assessing left ventricular performance using echocardiography or by measuring left ventricular filling pressure with a pulmonary artery flotation catheter.

CAROTID PULSE. Palpation of the carotid arterial pulse provides a clue to the left ventricular stroke volume; a small pulse suggests a reduced stroke volume, whereas a sharp, brief upstroke is often observed in patients with mitral regurgitation or ruptured ventricular septum with a left-to-right shunt. Pulsus alternans reflects severe left ventricular dysfunction.

THE CHEST. Moist rales are audible in patients who develop left ventricular failure and/or a reduction of left ventricular compliance with STEMI. Diffuse wheezing can present in patients with severe left ventricular failure. Cough with hemoptysis, suggesting pulmonary embolism with infarction, can also occur. In 1967 Killip proposed a prognostic classification scheme on the basis of the presence and severity of rales detected in patients presenting with STEMI.[85] Class I patients are free of rales and a third heart sound. Class II patients have rales but only to a mild to moderate degree (<50 percent of lung fields) and may or may not have an S_3. Patients in class III have rales in more than half of each lung field and frequently have pulmonary edema. Finally, class IV patients are in cardiogenic shock. Despite overall improvement in mortality rate in each class, compared with data observed during the original development of the classification scheme, the classification scheme remains useful today as evidenced by data from large MI trials of STEMI patients.[17]

Cardiac Examination

Despite severe symptoms and extensive myocardial damage, the findings on examination of the heart may be quite unremarkable in patients with STEMI.

PALPATION. Palpation of the precordium may yield normal findings, but in patients with transmural STEMI, it more commonly reveals a presystolic pulsation, synchronous with an audible fourth heart sound, reflecting a vigorous left atrial contraction filling a ventricle with reduced compliance. In the presence of left ventricular systolic dysfunction, an outward movement of the left ventricle can be palpated in early diastole, coincident with a third heart sound.

AUSCULTATION (see Chap. 11)

HEART SOUNDS

The heart sounds, particularly the first sound, are frequently muffled and occasionally inaudible immediately after the infarct, and their intensity increases during convalescence. A soft first heart sound may also reflect prolongation of the P-R interval. Patients with marked ventricular dysfunction and/or left bundle branch block may have paradoxical splitting of the second heart sound.

A fourth heart sound is almost universally present in patients in sinus rhythm with STEMI but has limited diagnostic value because it is commonly audible in most patients with chronic ischemic heart disease and is recordable,

although not often audible, in many normal subjects older than 45 years.

A third heart sound in patients with STEMI usually reflects severe left ventricular dysfunction with elevated ventricular filling pressure. It is caused by rapid deceleration of transmitral blood flow during protodiastolic filling of the left ventricle and is usually heard in patients with large infarctions. This sound is detected best at the apex, with the patient in the left lateral recumbent position. A third heart sound may be caused not only by left ventricular failure but also by increased inflow into the left ventricle, as occurs when mitral regurgitation or ventricular septal defect complicates STEMI. Third and fourth heart sounds emanating from the left ventricle are heard best at the apex; in patients with right ventricular infarcts, these sounds can be heard along the left sternal border and increase on inspiration.

MURMURS

Systolic murmurs, transient or persistent, are commonly audible in patients with STEMI and generally result from mitral regurgitation secondary to dysfunction of the mitral valve apparatus (papillary muscle dysfunction, left ventricular dilation). A new, prominent, apical holosystolic murmur, accompanied by a thrill, may represent rupture of a head of a papillary muscle. The findings in cases of rupture of the interventricular septum are similar, although the murmur and thrill are usually most prominent along the left sternal border and may be audible at the right sternal border as well. The systolic murmur of tricuspid regurgitation (caused by right ventricular failure because of pulmonary hypertension and/or right ventricular infarction or by infarction of a right ventricular papillary muscle) is also heard along the left sternal border. It is characteristically intensified by inspiration and is accompanied by a prominent c-v wave in the jugular venous pulse and a right ventricular fourth sound.

FRICTION RUBS

Pericardial friction rubs may be heard in patients with STEMI, especially those sustaining large transmural infarctions.[86] Rubs are notorious for their evanescence and hence are probably even more common than reported. Although friction rubs can be heard within 24 hours or as late as 2 weeks after the onset of infarction, most commonly they are noted on the second or third day. Occasionally, in patients with extensive infarction, a loud rub can be heard for many days. Patients with STEMI and a pericardial friction rub may have a pericardial effusion on echocardiographic study, but only rarely cause the classic electrocardiographic changes of pericarditis. Delayed onset of the rub and the associated discomfort of pericarditis (as late as 3 months postinfarction) are characteristic of the now rare postmyocardial infarction (Dressler) syndrome.

Pericardial rubs are most readily audible along the left sternal border or just inside the point of maximal impulse. Loud rubs may be audible over the entire precordium and even over the back. Occasionally, only the systolic portion of a rub is heard; it can be confused with a systolic murmur, and the diagnosis of rupture of the ventricular septum or mitral regurgitation may be incorrectly considered.

OTHER FINDINGS

FUNDI. Hypertension, diabetes, and generalized atherosclerosis commonly accompany STEMI, and because these conditions can produce characteristic changes in the fundus, a funduscopic examination may provide information concerning the underlying vascular status; this is particularly useful in patients unable to provide a detailed history.

ABDOMEN. In patients with STEMI, particularly in an inferior location with diaphragmatic irritation, the pain may be localized to the epigastrium or the right upper quadrant. Pain in the abdomen associated with nausea, vomiting, restlessness, and even abdominal distention is often interpreted by patients as a sign of "indigestion," resulting in self-medication with antacids, and it can suggest an acute abdominal process to the physician. Right heart failure, characterized by hepatomegaly and a positive abdominojugular reflux, is unusual in patients with acute left ventricular infarction but does occur in patients with severe and prolonged left ventricular failure or right ventricular infarction.

EXTREMITIES. Coronary atherosclerosis is often associated with systemic atherosclerosis, and therefore patients with STEMI may have a history of intermittent claudication and demonstrate physical findings of peripheral vascular disease (see Chap. 57). Thus diminished peripheral arterial pulses, loss of hair, and atrophic skin in the lower extremities may be noted in patients with coronary artery disease. Peripheral edema is a manifestation of right ventricular failure and, like congestive hepatomegaly, is unusual in patients with acute left ventricular infarction. Cyanosis of the nailbeds is common in patients with severe left ventricular failure and is particularly striking in patients with cardiogenic shock.

NEUROPSYCHIATRIC FINDINGS. Except for the altered mental status that occurs in patients with STEMI who have a markedly reduced cardiac output and cerebral hypoperfusion, the findings on neurological examination are normal unless the patient has suffered cerebral embolism secondary to a mural thrombus. The coincidence between these two conditions can be explained by systemic hypotension caused by STEMI precipitating a cerebral infarction and the converse, as well as by mural emboli from the left ventricle causing cerebral emboli.

Patients with STEMI often exhibit alterations of the emotional state including intense anxiety, denial, and depression. Medical staff caring for STEMI patients must be sensitive to changes in the patient's emotional state; a calm, professional atmosphere, with thorough explanations of equipment and prognosis, can help alleviate the distress associated with STEMI.

CH 50

Laboratory Findings

Serum Markers of Cardiac Damage

The classic World Health Organization (WHO) criteria for the diagnosis of MI require that at least two of the following three elements be present: a history of ischemic-type chest discomfort, evolutionary changes on serially obtained ECG tracings, and a rise and fall in serum cardiac markers.[87] Considerable variability in the pattern of presentation of MI exists with respect to these three elements, as exemplified by the following statistics. ST-segment elevation and Q waves on the ECG, two features that are highly indicative of MI, are seen in only about half of MI cases on presentation. Approximately one fourth of patients with MI do not present with classic chest pain, and the event would go unrecognized unless an ECG were recorded fortuitously in temporal proximity to the infarction or permanent pathological Q waves are seen on later tracings. Nondiagnostic ECGs are recorded in approximately half of patients presenting to emergency departments with chest pain suspicious for MI who ultimately are shown to have an MI. Among patients admitted to the hospital with a chest pain syndrome, less than 20 percent are subsequently diagnosed as having had an MI. In the majority of patients, therefore, clinicians must obtain serum cardiac marker measurements at periodic intervals to either establish or exclude the diagnosis of MI; such measurements can also be useful for a rough quantitation of the size of infarction.

The availability of serum cardiac markers with markedly enhanced sensitivity for myocardial damage enables clinicians to diagnose MI in approximately an additional one third of patients who would not have fulfilled criteria for MI in the past.[88] The increased use of more sensitive biomarkers of MI combined with more precise imaging techniques has necessitated establishment of new criteria for MI (see Table 50-2). As a consequence of the enhanced sensitivity for detection of smaller infarcts using cardiac specific troponins, clinicians now face a new set of issues: More

patients are discharged with a diagnosis of MI rather than UA; lifestyle and insurance implications need to be considered; and epidemiological studies, tracking the incidence of MI over time, must account for the improved ability to diagnose MI in more contemporary patient cohorts.[2,89]

Although these considerations apply directly to patients on the UA/NSTEMI end of the ACS spectrum (see Chap. 53), a general discussion of cardiac biomarkers is contained in this chapter because there is overlap of the scientific aspects of the pathophysiological concepts and assay methodology when biomarkers are used to evaluate STEMI patients. It should be emphasized that clinicians should not wait for the results of biomarker assays to initiate treatment for the STEMI patient. As discussed in Chapter 51, there is a time urgency for reperfusion in STEMI and the 12-lead ECG is the diagnostic tool that should be used to initiate such strategies.

Necrosis compromises the integrity of the sarcolemmal membrane that is compromised and intracellular macromolecules (serum cardiac markers) begin to diffuse into the cardiac interstitium and ultimately into the microvasculature and lymphatics in the region of the infarct (Fig. 50-14 and Table 50-4).[90,91] The rate of appearance of these macromolecules in the peripheral circulation depends on several factors including intracellular location, molecular weight, local blood and lymphatic flow, and the rate of elimination from the blood.[90,92]

CREATINE KINASE. Serum CK activity exceeds the normal range within 4 to 8 hours after the onset of STEMI and declines to normal within 2 to 3 days (see Fig. 50-13). Although the peak CK occurs on average at about 24 hours, peak levels occur earlier in patients who have had reperfusion as a result of the administration of fibrinolytic therapy or mechanical recanalization (as well as in patients with early spontaneous fibrinolysis). Because reperfusion influences the time-activity curve of serum CK, and because reperfusion itself influences infarct size, reperfusion confounds estimation of infarct size by enzyme analysis (Fig. 50-15).[41]

Although elevation of the serum CK concentration is a sensitive enzymatic detector of STEMI that is routinely available in most hospitals,[93] important drawbacks include false-positive results in patients with muscle disease, alcohol intoxication, diabetes mellitus, skeletal muscle trauma, vigorous exercise, convulsions, intramuscular injections, thoracic outlet syndrome, and pulmonary embolism.[93]

CREATINE KINASE ISOENZYMES. Three isoenzymes of CK exist (MM, BB, and MB). Extracts of brain and kidney contain predominantly the BB isoenzyme; skeletal muscle contains principally MM but does contain some MB (1 to 3 percent); and cardiac muscle contains both MM and MB isoenzymes. The MB isoenzymes of CK can also be present in minor quantities in the small intestine, tongue, diaphragm, uterus, and prostate. Strenuous exercise, particularly in trained long-distance runners or professional athletes, can cause elevation of both total CK and CK-MB.[94] Because CK-MB can be detected in the blood of healthy subjects, the cutoff value for abnormal elevation of CK-MB is usually set a few units above the upper reference limit for a given laboratory (see Fig. 50-14).[93] Although small quantities of CK-MB isoenzyme occur in tissues other than the heart, elevated levels of CK-MB may be considered, for practical purposes, to be the result of MI (except in the case of trauma or surgery on the aforementioned organs).

Creatine kinase MB is analyzed in most laboratories by highly sensitive and specific enzyme immunoassays that utilize monoclonal antibodies directed against CK-MB.[93] Mass assays report results in nanograms per milliliter rather than units per milliliter and have been confirmed to be more accurate than CK-MB activity assays, especially in patients presenting within 4 hours of the onset of STEMI. It has been proposed that a ratio (relative index) of CK-MB mass to CK activity of about 2.5 is indicative of a myocardial rather than a skeletal source of the CK-MB elevation. Although this ratio may be satisfied by many patients with STEMI, it is inaccurate in several circumstances: (1) when high levels of total CK are present because of skeletal muscle injury (a large quantity of CK-MB must be released from the myocardium to satisfy criteria); (2) when chronic skeletal muscle injury releases large amounts of CK-MB; and (3) when total CK measurements are within the normal reference range for the laboratory and CK-MB is elevated (possibly indicating that a microinfarction has occurred). Patients with minimally elevated CK-MB and normal CK have a prognosis that is generally worse than that for patients with suspected MI but no CK-MB elevation.

Clinicians should not rely on measurements of CK and CK-MB at a single time but instead should evaluate the temporal rise and fall of serial values; skeletal muscle release of CK-MB generally remains elevated for a longer time than myocardial release of CK-MB and produces a "plateau" pattern of CK-MB values over several days, in contrast to the shorter time course of skeletal muscle CK-MB elevation, as depicted in Figure 50-14. Of note, because cardiac-specific troponins I and T (cTnI and cTnT) (see Fig. 50-15 and Tables 50-2 and 50-3) accurately distinguish skeletal from cardiac muscle damage, the troponins are now considered the preferred biomarker for diagnosing MI.[91]

In addition to STEMI secondary to coronary obstruction, other forms of injury to cardiac muscle, such as those resulting from myocarditis, trauma, cardiac catheterization, shock, and cardiac surgery, may also produce elevated serum CK-MB levels.[93] These latter causes of elevation of serum CK-MB values can usually be readily distinguished from STEMI by the clinical setting.

CREATINE KINASE ISOFORMS. Isoforms of the MM and MB isoenzymes have been identified.[95] Certain isoforms can appear in the blood quite rapidly, perhaps as soon as 1 hour, after the onset of infarction (see Fig. 50-14). However, with the increased availability of assays for the cardiac-specific troponins, measurement of CK isoforms has little, if any, important clinical role.[91]

MYOGLOBIN. This monomeric heme protein is released into the circulation from injured myocardial cells and can be detected within a few hours after the onset of infarction (see Table 50-3 and Fig. 50-14). Peak levels of serum myoglobin are reached considerably earlier (1 to 4 hours) than peak values of serum CK. Because of its lack of cardiac specificity, an isolated measurement of myoglobin within the first 4 to 8 hours after the onset of chest discomfort in patients with a nondiagnostic ECG should not be relied on to make the diagnosis of MI but should be supplemented by a more cardiac-specific marker such as cTnI or cTnT (see Table 50-3).[41,91,96]

CARDIAC-SPECIFIC TROPONINS. The troponin complex consists of three subunits that regulate the calcium-mediated contractile process of striated muscle. These include troponin C, which binds Ca²⁺; troponin I

CH 50

ST-Elevation Myocardial Infarction: Pathology, Pathophysiology, and Clinical Features

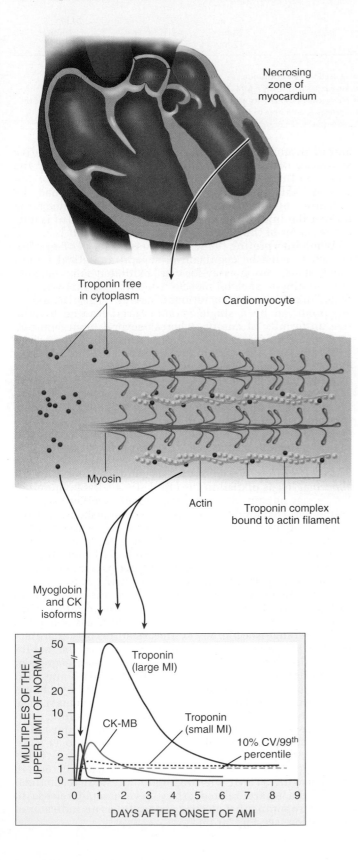

FIGURE 50-14 The zone of necrosing myocardium is shown at the top of the figure, followed in the middle portion of the figure by a diagram of a cardiomyocyte that is in the process of releasing biomarkers. After disruption of the sarcolemmal membrane of the cardiomyocyte, the cytoplasmic pool of biomarkers is released first (left-most arrow in bottom portion of figure). Markers such as myoglobin and CK isoforms are rapidly released, and blood levels rise quickly above the cutoff limit. This is then followed by a more protracted release of biomarkers from the disintegrating myofilaments that may continue for several days (three-headed arrow). Cardiac troponin levels rise to about 20 to 50 times the upper reference limit (the 99th percentile of values in a reference control group) in patients who have a "classic" acute myocardial infarction (MI) and sustain sufficient myocardial necrosis to result in abnormally elevated levels of the MB fraction of creatine kinase (CK-MB). Clinicians can now diagnose episodes of microinfarction by sensitive assays that detect cardiac troponin elevations above the upper reference limit, even though CK-MB levels may still be in the normal reference range (not shown). CV = coefficient of variation. *(Modified from Antman EM: Decision making with cardiac troponin tests. N Engl J Med 346:2079, 2002 and Jaffe AS, Babiun L, Apple FS: Biomarkers in acute cardiac disease: The present and the future. J Am Coll Cardiol 48:1, 2006.)*

TABLE 50–4	Biomarkers for the Evaluation of Patients with ST-Elevation Myocardial Infarction			
Biomarker	Molecular Weight (D)	Range of Times to Initial Elevation (hr)	Mean Time to Peak Elevations (Nonreperfused)	Time to Return to Normal Range
Frequently Used in Clinical Practice				
MB-CK	86,000	3-12	24 hr	48-72 hr
cTnI	23,500	3-12	24 hr	5-10 d
cTnT	33,000	3-12	12 hr-2 d	5-14 d
Infrequently Used in Clinical Practice				
Myoglobin	17,800	1-4	6-7 hr	24 hr
MB-CK tissue isoform	86,000	2-6	18 hr	Unknown
MM-CK tissue isoform	86,000	1-6	12 hr	38 hr

*Increased sensitivity can be achieved with sampling every 6 or 8 hr.

†Multiple assays available for clinical use—clinicians should be familiar with the cutoff value used in their institution.

cTnI = cardiac troponin I; cTnT = cardiac troponin T; MB-CK = MB isoenzyme of creatine kinase (CK); MM-CK = MM isoenzyme of CK.

Modified from Antman EM, Anbe DT, Armstrong PW, et al: ACC/AHA Guidelines for the Management of Patients with ST-Elevation Myocardial Infarction: a report of the American College of Cardiology/American Heart Association Task Force on Practice Guidelines (Committee to Revise the 1999 Guidelines for the Management of Patients with Acute Myocardial Infarction). American College of Cardiology Web site, 2006. (www.acc.org/clinical/guidelines/stemi/index.pdf). Accessed 6/21/06.

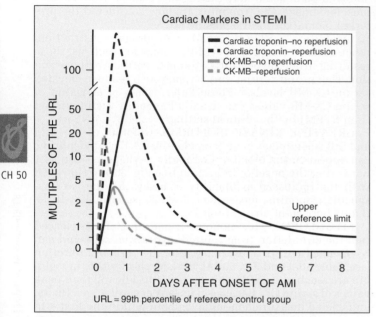

FIGURE 50–15 The kinetics of release of creatine kinase MB (CK-MB) and cardiac troponin in patients who do not undergo reperfusion are shown in the solid blue and red curves as multiples of the upper reference limit (URL). When patients with ST-segment elevation myocardial infarction (STEMI) undergo reperfusion, as depicted in the dashed blue and red curves, the cardiac biomarkers are detected sooner, rise to a higher peak value, but decline more rapidly, resulting in a smaller area under the curve and limitation of infarct size. AMI = acute myocardial infarction. (Modified from Antman EM, Anbe DT, Armstrong PW, et al: ACC/AHA Guidelines for the Management of Patients with ST-Elevation Myocardial Infarction: A report of the American College of Cardiology/American Heart Association Task Force on Practice Guidelines (Committee to Revise the 1999 Guidelines for the Management of Patients with Acute Myocardial Infarction). American College of Cardiology Web site, 2006. (www.acc.org/clinical/guidelines/stemi/index.pdf). Accessed 6/21/06.

(TnI), which binds to actin and inhibits actin-myosin interactions; and troponin T (TnT), which binds to tropomyosin, thereby attaching the troponin complex to the thin filament. Although the majority of TnT is incorporated in the troponin complex, approximately 6 percent is dissolved in the cytosol; about 2 to 3 percent of TnI is found in a cytosolic pool. Following myocyte injury, the initial release of cTnT and cTnI is from the cytosolic pool, followed subsequently by release from the structural (myofilament-bound) pool (see Fig. 50-14).[2]

Although both TnT and TnI are present in cardiac and skeletal muscle, they are encoded by different genes and their amino acid sequence differs. This permits the production of antibodies that are specific for the cardiac form (cTnT

and cTnI) and has led to the development of quantitative assays for cTnT and cTnI that have been approved by the Food and Drug Administration for clinical use (see Fig. 50-14 and Table 50-4).[90] Several studies have confirmed the reliability of these new quantitative assays for detecting myocardial injury, and measurement of cTnT or cTnI is now at the center of the new diagnostic criteria for MI.[2]

When interpreting the results of assays for cTnT or cTnI, clinicians must be cognizant of several analytical issues. The first-generation assay for cTnT exhibited some nonspecific binding to skeletal muscle troponin, but this was corrected in subsequent generations of assays.[97] The cTnT assays are produced by a single manufacturer, leading to relative uniformity of cutoffs, whereas several manufacturers produce cTnI assays. When cardiac troponins are released from myocytes, there is a mixture of free cTnT and free cTnI along with a complex of the I-C-T components that is further degraded to a complex of I-C and free cTnT (Fig. 50-16).[98,99] Evidence exists that the release pattern of troponin complexes and degradation into various troponin fragments may affect the results of various commercial assays (especially for cTnI) and may in the future be useful to gain insight into pathophysiological events such as ischemia and reperfusion.[100]

Cutoff Values. Variations in the cutoff concentration for abnormal levels of cTnI in the clinically available immunoassays may be caused in part by different specificities of the antibodies used for detecting free and complexed cTnI. Thus when using the measurement of cTnI for diagnosing STEMI, clinicians should apply the cutoff values for the particular assay used in their laboratory.[96] For both cTnT and cTnI, the definition of an abnormally increased level is a value exceeding that of 99 percent of a reference control group.[2]

Furthermore, whereas CK-MB usually increases 10- to 20-fold above the upper limit of the reference range, cTnT and cTnI typically increase more than 20 times above the reference range (see Fig. 50-14). These features of the cardiac-specific troponin assays provide an improved signal-to-noise ratio, enabling the detection of even minor degrees of myocardial necrosis. In patients with MI, cTnT and cTnI first begin to rise above the upper reference limit by 3 hours from the onset of chest pain. Because of a continuous release from a degenerating contractile apparatus in necrotic myocytes, elevations of cTnI may persist for 7 to 10 days after MI; elevations of cTnT may persist for up to 10 to 14 days. The prolonged time course of elevation of cTnT and cTnI is advantageous for the late diagnosis of MI (see Fig. 50-14). Patients with STEMI who undergo successful recanalization of the infarct-related artery have a rapid release of cardiac troponins that also may be useful as an indicator of reperfusion (see Fig. 50-15).[15]

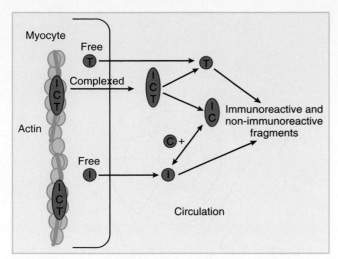

FIGURE 50–16 The troponin T-I-C complex of the thin filament is released from damaged myocytes in various molecular forms. The T-I-C complex appears in the blood and degrades first into the I-C complex (the predominant form of cTnI in blood) and free TnT. The I-C complex further degrades into free troponin subunits and fragments of intact subunits (both immunoreactive and nonimmunoreactive). A small proportion of troponin I and T and fragments is also found in the cytoplasm. Troponin I can exist in either oxidized or reduced forms, or up to two phosphorylations. *(From Wu AHB: Analytical issues for the clinical use of cardiac troponin. In Morrow DA [ed]: Cardiovascular Biomarkers: Pathophysiology and Disease Management. Totowa, NJ, Humana Press, 2006, p 29.)*

Troponin versus CK-MB. When comparing the diagnostic efficiency of the cardiac troponins versus CK-MB for MI, it is important to bear in mind that the troponin assays can probably detect episodes of myocardial necrosis that are below the detection limit of the current CK-MB assays, leading to a number of "false-positive" cases of troponin elevations if CK-MB is used as the reference standard or, conversely, false-negative cases of CK-MB elevation if troponin is used as the reference standard. From a clinical perspective, it is desirable to have diagnostic tests for MI with increased sensitivity to increase the number of MI cases identified and increased specificity to reduce the number of cases incorrectly diagnosed and treated for MI. The prognostic value of the troponins is independent of other risk factors such as age and ECG abnormalities, as well as the measurement of older biomarkers such as CK-MB.[90]

RECOMMENDATIONS FOR MEASUREMENT OF SERUM MARKERS

It seems reasonable for clinicians to measure either cTnT or cTnI in all patients with suspected MI. From a cost-effectiveness perspective, it is unnecessary to measure both a cardiac-specific troponin and CK-MB. Routine diagnosis of MI can be accomplished within 12 hours using CK-MB, cTnT, or cTnI by obtaining measurements approximately every 8 to 12 hours (see Tables 50-2 and 50-4). Retrospective diagnosis or diagnosis of MI in the presence of skeletal muscle injury is more readily accomplished with cTnT or cTnI. With increasing familiarity of clinicians with assays for the cardiac-specific troponins, it is anticipated that they will supersede assays for CK-MB not only for the diagnosis of MI but also for assessment of reperfusion, reinfarction, and estimation of infarct size.[91,41]

OTHER LABORATORY MEASUREMENTS

SERUM LIPIDS (see Chap. 42). These are often determined in patients with STEMI. However, the results may be misleading because numerous factors that can alter the values are operating at the time of the patient's admission to the hospital. Serum triglycerides are affected by caloric intake, intravenous glucose, and recumbency.

During the first 24 to 48 hours after admission, total cholesterol and high-density lipoprotein (HDL) cholesterol remain at or near baseline values but generally fall precipitously after that. The fall in HDL cholesterol after STEMI is greater than the fall in total cholesterol; thus the ratio of total cholesterol to HDL cholesterol is no longer useful for risk assessment unless measured early after MI. A lipid profile should be obtained on all STEMI patients who are admitted within 24 to 48 hours of symptoms. The success of lipid-lowering therapy in primary and secondary prevention studies and evidence that hypolipidemic therapy improves endothelial function and inhibits thrombus formation[101] indicate that early management of serum lipids in patients hospitalized for STEMI is advisable.[15,102] For patients admitted beyond 24 to 48 hours, more accurate determinations of serum lipid levels are obtained about 8 weeks after the infarction has occurred.

HEMATOLOGICAL FINDINGS. The elevation of the white blood cell count usually develops within 2 hours after the onset of chest pain, reaches a peak 2 to 4 days after infarction, and returns to normal in 1 week; the peak white blood cell count usually ranges between 12 and 15×10^3/ml but occasionally rises to as high as 20×10^3/ml in patients with large STEMI. Often there is an increase in the percentage of polymorphonuclear leukocytes and a shift of the differential count to band forms. An epidemiological association has been reported, indicating a worse angiographic appearance of culprit lesions and increased risk of adverse clinical outcomes the higher the white blood cell count is at presentation with an acute coronary syndrome.[75,103]

The erythrocyte sedimentation rate (ESR) is usually normal during the first day or two after infarction, even though fever and leukocytosis may be present. It then rises to a peak on the fourth or fifth day and may remain elevated for several weeks. The increase in the ESR does not correlate well with the size of the infarction or with the prognosis. The hematocrit often increases during the first few days after infarction as a consequence of hemoconcentration. An elevated C-reactive protein (CRP) level appears to identify patients presenting with STEMI, with worse angiographic appearance of the infarct artery and a greater likelihood of developing heart failure.[104-106]

The hemoglobin value at presentation with STEMI powerfully and independently predicts major cardiovascular events.[107] Of note is a J-shaped relationship between baseline hemoglobin values and clinical events. Cardiovascular mortality increases progressively as the presenting hemoglobin value falls below 14 to 15 gm/dl; conversely, it also rises as the hemoglobin level increases above 17 gm/dl. The increased risk from anemia probably relates to diminished tissue delivery of oxygen, while the increased risk with polycythemia may be related to an increase in blood viscosity.[107]

Electrocardiography (see Chap. 12)

In the majority of patients with STEMI, some change can be documented when serial ECGs are compared. However, many factors limit the ability of the ECG to diagnose and localize MI: the extent of myocardial injury, the age of the infarct, its location, the presence of conduction defects, the presence of previous infarcts or acute pericarditis, changes in electrolyte concentrations, and the administration of cardioactive drugs. Changes in the ST segment and T wave are quite nonspecific and may occur in a variety of conditions including stable and unstable angina pectoris, ventricular hypertrophy, acute and chronic pericarditis, myocarditis, early repolarization, electrolyte imbalance, shock, and metabolic disorders and following the administration of digitalis. Serial ECGs may be of considerable aid in differentiating these conditions from STEMI. Transient changes favor angina or electrolyte disturbances, whereas persistent changes argue for infarction if other causes such as shock, administration of digitalis, and persistent metabolic disorders can be eliminated. Nevertheless, serial standard 12-lead ECGs remain a potent and extremely useful method for the detection and localization of MI.[108] Analysis of the constellation of ECG leads showing ST elevation may also be useful for identifying the site of occlusion in the infarct artery (Fig. 50-17).[33,108] The extent of ST deviation on the ECG, location of infarction, and QRS duration correlate with risk of adverse outcomes.[109] Even when left bundle branch block is present on the ECG, MI can be diagnosed when striking ST-segment deviation is present beyond that which can be explained by the conduction defect.[108,110] In addition to the diagnostic and prognostic information contained within the 12-lead ECG, it also provides valuable noninva-

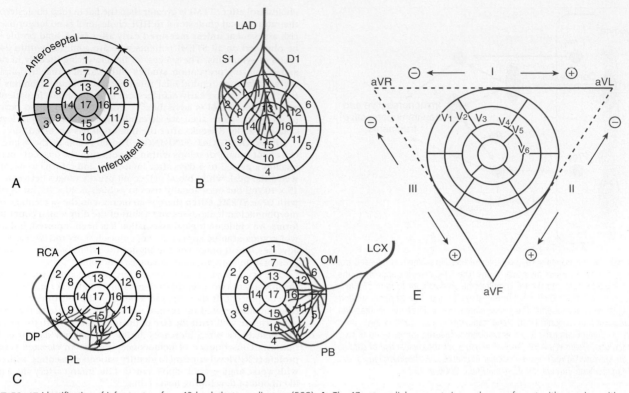

FIGURE 50–17 Identification of infarct artery from 12-lead electrocardiogram (ECG). **A,** The 17 myocardial segments in a polar map format with superimposition of the arterial supply provided by the left anterior descending artery (LAD) **(B)**, right coronary artery (RCA) **(C)**, and left circumflex artery (LCX) **(D)**. **E,** The position of the standard ECG leads relative to the polar map. The infarct artery can be deduced by identifying the leads that show ST elevation and referencing that information to **A-D.** For example, ST elevation seen most prominently in the leads overlying segments 1, 2, 7, 8, 13, 14, and 17 indicates that the LAD is the infarct artery. D_1 = first diagonal; DP = posterior descending; OM = obtuse marginal; PB = posterobasal; PL = posterolateral; S_1 = first septal. *(From Bayes-de-Luna A, Wagner G, Birnbaum Y, et al: A new terminology for the left ventricular walls and location of myocardial infarcts that present Q wave based on the standard of cardiac magnetic resonance imaging. Circulation 114:1755, 2006.)*

sive information about the success of reperfusion for STEMI (see Chap. 51).[108,111,112]

Although general agreement exists on electrocardiographic and vectorcardiographic criteria for the recognition of infarction of the anterior and inferior myocardial walls, less agreement pertains to criteria for lateral and posterior infarcts; in this area, even the terminology can be confusing. A consensus group has recommended elimination of the term "posterior" and suggests using "lateral" to be consistent with current understanding of the segmental anatomy of the heart as it sits in the thorax.[33] Patients with an abnormal R wave in V_1 (0.04 second in duration and/or R/S ratio ≥1 in the absence of preexcitation or right ventricular hypertrophy) with inferior or lateral Q waves have an increased incidence of isolated occlusion of a dominant left circumflex coronary artery without collateral circulation; such patients have a lower ejection fraction, increased end-systolic volume, and higher complication rate than patients with inferior infarction because of isolated occlusion of the right coronary artery.

Although most patients bear the ECG changes from an infarction for the rest of their lives, particularly if they evolve Q waves, in a substantial minority the typical changes disappear, Q waves regress, and the ECG can even return to normal after a number of years. Under many circumstances, Q-wave patterns simulate MI. Conditions that may mimic the electrocardiographic features of MI by producing a pattern of "pseudoinfarction" include ventricular hypertrophy, conduction disturbances, preexcitation, primary myocardial disease, pneumothorax, pulmonary embolus, amyloid heart disease, primary and metastatic tumors of the heart, traumatic heart disease, intracranial hemorrhage, hyperkalemia, pericarditis, early repolarization, and cardiac sarcoidosis.

Q-WAVE AND NON-Q-WAVE INFARCTION. As noted earlier, the presence or absence of Q waves on the surface ECG does not reliably distinguish between transmural and nontransmural (subendocardial) MI.[24] Q waves on the ECG signify abnormal electrical activity but are not synonymous with irreversible myocardial damage. Also, the absence of Q waves may simply reflect the insensitivity of the standard 12-lead ECG, especially in zones of the left ventricle supplied by the left circumflex artery (see Fig. 50-17). Angiographic studies in MI patients without ST-segment elevation show a higher incidence of subtotal occlusion of the culprit coronary vessel and greater collateral flow to the infarct zone. Observational data suggest that MI without ST-segment elevation occurs more commonly in elderly patients and patients with a prior MI.

ISCHEMIA AT A DISTANCE. Patients with new Q waves and ST-segment elevation diagnostic for STEMI in one territory often have ST-segment depression in other territories. These additional ST-segment changes, which imply a poor prognosis, are caused either by ischemia in a territory other than the area of infarction, termed *ischemia at a distance*, or by reciprocal electrical phenomena. A good deal of attention has been directed to associated ST-segment depression in the anterior leads, when it occurs in patients with acute inferior STEMI. However, despite the clinical importance of differentiation among causes of anterior ST-segment depression in such patients, including anterior ischemia, inferolateral wall infarction, and true reciprocal changes, such a differentiation cannot be made reliably by electrocardiographic or even vectorcardiographic techniques. Although precordial ST-segment depression associates more commonly with extensive infarction of the lateral, or inferior septal segments, rather than anterior wall subendocardial ischemia, imaging techniques such as echocardiography are necessary to ascertain whether an anterior wall motion abnormality is present.[113]

RIGHT VENTRICULAR INFARCTION. ST-segment elevation in right precordial leads (V_1, V_3R-V_6R) is a relatively sensitive and specific sign of right ventricular infarction.[108,114] Occasionally, ST-segment elevation in leads V_2 and V_3 results from acute right ventricular infarction; this appears to occur only when the injury to the left inferior wall is minimal (see Fig. 50-11).[115-117] Usually, the concurrent inferior wall injury suppresses this anterior ST-segment elevation resulting from right ventricular injury. Likewise, right ventricular infarction appears to reduce the anterior ST-segment depression often observed with inferior wall myocardial infarction. A QS or QR pattern in leads V_3R and/or V_4R also suggests right ventricular myocardial necrosis but has less predictive accuracy than ST-segment elevation in these leads.

Imaging

ROENTGENOGRAPHY (see Chap. 15)

The initial chest roentgenogram in patients with STEMI is almost invariably a portable film obtained in the emergency department or coronary care unit. When present, prominent pulmonary vascular markings on the roentgenogram reflect elevated left ventricular end-diastolic pressure, but significant temporal discrepancies can occur because of what have been termed *diagnostic lags* and *posttherapeutic lags*. Up to 12 hours can elapse before pulmonary edema accumulates after ventricular filling pressure has become elevated. The posttherapeutic phase lag represents a longer time interval; up to 2 days are required for pulmonary edema to resorb and the radiographic signs of pulmonary congestion to clear after ventricular filling pressure has returned toward normal. The degree of congestion and the size of the left side of the heart on the chest film are useful for defining groups of patients with STEMI who are at increased risk of dying after the acute event.

ECHOCARDIOGRAPHY (see Chap. 14)

TWO-DIMENSIONAL ECHOCARDIOGRAPHY. The relative portability of echocardiographic equipment makes this technique ideal for the assessment of patients with MI hospitalized in the coronary care unit or even in the emergency department before admission.[113] In patients with chest pain compatible with MI but with a nondiagnostic ECG, the finding on echocardiography of a distinct region of disordered contraction can be helpful diagnostically because it supports the diagnosis of myocardial ischemia. Echocardiography can also help evaluate patients with chest pain and a nondiagnostic ECG who are suspected of having an aortic dissection. The identification of an intimal flap consistent with an aortic dissection is a critical observation because it represents a major contraindication to fibrinolytic therapy (see Chap. 56). However, echocardiography has poor sensitivity for detection of the intimal flaps compared with other imaging modalities such as CT angiography.

Areas of abnormal regional wall motion are observed almost universally in patients with MI, and the degree of wall motion abnormality can be categorized with a semi-quantitative wall motion score index. Of note, abnormal wall motion is less often noted echocardiographically when the infarction is small and the age of regional wall motion abnormality cannot always be determined. Left ventricular function estimated from two-dimensional echocardiograms correlates well with measurements from angiography and is useful in establishing prognosis after MI.[113] Furthermore, the early use of echocardiography can aid in the early detection of potentially viable but stunned myocardium (contractile reserve), residual provocable ischemia, patients at risk for the development of congestive heart failure after MI, and mechanical complications of MI.[113]

Although transthoracic imaging is adequate in most patients, occasional patients have poor echo windows, especially if they are undergoing mechanical ventilation. In such patients, transesophageal echocardiography can be safely performed and can be useful in evaluating ventricular septal defects and papillary muscle dysfunction.[15]

Doppler techniques allow assessment of blood flow in the cardiac chambers and across cardiac valves. Used in conjunction with echocardiography, it can help detect and assess the severity of mitral or tricuspid regurgitation after STEMI. Identification of the site of acute ventricular septal rupture, quantification of shunt flow across the resulting defect, and assessment of acute cardiac tamponade are also possible.[15]

OTHER IMAGING MODALITIES

COMPUTED TOMOGRAPHY (see Chap. 18). This technique can provide useful cross-sectional information in patients with MI. In addition to the assessment of cavity dimensions and wall thickness, left ventricular aneurysms can be detected, and, of particular importance in patients with STEMI, intracardiac thrombi can be identified. Although cardiac computed tomography is a less convenient technique, it probably is more sensitive for thrombus detection than is echocardiography.

MAGNETIC RESONANCE IMAGING (see Chap. 17). In addition to localizing and sizing the area of infarction, magnetic resonance imaging techniques permit early recognition of MI and can provide an assessment of the severity of the ischemic insult. This modality is attractive because of its ability to assess perfusion of infarcted and noninfarcted tissue, as well as of reperfused myocardium; to identify areas of jeopardized but not infarcted myocardium; to identify myocardial edema, fibrosis, wall thinning, and hypertrophy; to assess ventricular chamber size and segmental wall motion; and to identify the temporal transition between ischemia and infarction.[118] It has limited application during the acute phase, however, because of the need to transport patients with MI to the magnetic resonance imaging facility but, as discussed later, is an extremely useful imaging technique during the subacute and chronic phase of MI.

Contrast-enhanced cardiac MRI (CMR) can detect myocardial infarction accurately. The transmural extent of late gadolinium enhancement in regions of dysfunctional myocardium accurately predicts the likelihood of contractile recovery after successful restoration of coronary flow from mechanical revascularization.[119] Numerous clinical studies have also demonstrated high sensitivity of late gadolinium enhancement ("delayed hyperenhancement") of CMR in detecting small amounts of myonecrosis. In patients with a prior MI, estimation of the size of the periinfarct zone by CMR using the delayed enhancement technique provides incremental prognostic value beyond left ventricular volumes and ejection fraction (Fig. 50-18).[120] Beyond detecting infarction, this imaging technique can characterize the presence and size of microvascular obstruction from infarction, which portends an adverse clinical outcome postinfarction.[121] Clinically unrecognized myocardial scar detected by late gadolinium enhancement imaging is associated with high risk of adverse cardiac events in patients with signs and symptoms of coronary artery disease but without a history of infarction.[122]

NUCLEAR IMAGING (see Chap. 16). Radionuclide angiography, perfusion imaging, infarct-avid scintigraphy, and positron emission tomography have been used to evaluate patients with STEMI.[123] Nuclear cardiac imaging techniques can be useful for detecting MI; assessing infarct size, collateral flow, and jeopardized myocardium; determining the effects of the infarct on ventricular function; and establishing prognosis of patients with STEMI.[123] However, the necessity of moving a critically ill patient from the coronary care

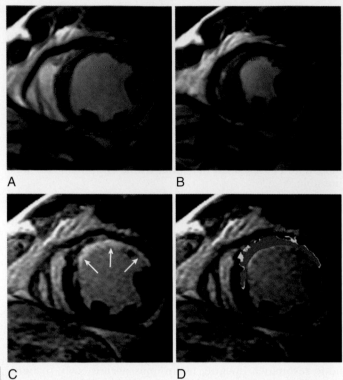

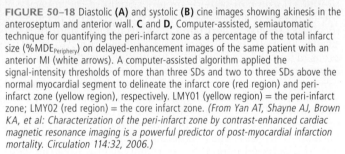

A   B

C   D

CH 50

FIGURE 50–18 Diastolic **(A)** and systolic **(B)** cine images showing akinesis in the anteroseptum and anterior wall. **C** and **D,** Computer-assisted, semiautomatic technique for quantifying the peri-infarct zone as a percentage of the total infarct size (%MDE$_{Periphery}$) on delayed-enhancement images of the same patient with an anterior MI (white arrows). A computer-assisted algorithm applied the signal-intensity thresholds of more than three SDs and two to three SDs above the normal myocardial segment to delineate the infarct core (red region) and peri-infarct zone (yellow region), respectively. LMY01 (yellow region) = the peri-infarct zone; LMY02 (red region) = the core infarct zone. *(From Yan AT, Shayne AJ, Brown KA, et al: Characterization of the peri-infarct zone by contrast-enhanced cardiac magnetic resonance imaging is a powerful predictor of post-myocardial infarction mortality. Circulation 114:32, 2006.)*

unit to the nuclear medicine department limits practical application unless a portable gamma camera is available. Cardiac radionuclide imaging for the diagnosis of MI should be restricted to special limited situations in which the triad of clinical history, ECG findings, and serum marker measurements is unavailable or unreliable.

ESTIMATION OF INFARCT SIZE

ELECTROCARDIOGRAPHY. Interest in limiting infarct size, in large part because of the recognition that the quantity of myocardium infarcted has important prognostic implications, has focused attention on the accurate determination of MI size. The sum of ST-segment elevations measured from multiple precordial leads correlates with the extent of myocardial injury in patients with anterior MI.[108] QRS scoring systems and planar or vectorcardiographic techniques to estimate infarct size also exist. Although they demonstrate good correlations with infarct size at autopsy and with enzymatic estimates, most patients do not require formal sizing of infarcts by electrocardiographic technique. A relationship between the number of ECG leads showing ST-segment elevation and mortality rate exists, however: Patients with 8 or 9 of 12 leads with ST-segment elevation have 3 to 4 times the mortality of those with only 2 or 3 leads with ST-segment elevation. The duration of ischemia time as estimated from continuous ST-segment monitoring is correlated with infarct size, the ratio of infarct size to area at risk, and the extent of regional wall motion abnormality observed subsequently.[124]

SERUM CARDIAC MARKERS. To estimate infarct size by analysis of serum cardiac markers, it is necessary to account for the quantity of the marker lost from the myocardium, its volume of distribution, and its release ratio.[125] Serial measurements of proteins released by necrotic myocardium are helpful in determining MI size. Clinically, the peak CK or CK-MB provides an approximate estimate of infarct size and is widely used prognostically. In the prefibrinolytic era, quantification of the cumulative release of CK or CK-MB correlated with other techniques for estimating infarct size in vivo, as well as with the area of necrosis at autopsy. However, as noted earlier, coronary artery reperfusion dramatically changes the wash-out kinetics of CK and other markers from myocardium, resulting in early and exaggerated peak levels and limiting the usefulness of such curves as a measure of infarct size. Measuring a cardiac-specific troponin level several days after STEMI, even in cases of successful reperfusion, may provide a reliable estimate of infarct size because such late troponin measurements reflect delayed release from the myofilament-bound pool in damaged myocytes.[41]

NONINVASIVE IMAGING TECHNIQUES. Echocardiography (see Chap. 14), radionuclide scintigraphy (see Chap. 16),[123] computed tomography (see Chap. 18), and magnetic resonance imaging (see Chap. 17) have all been utilized for the experimental and clinical assessment of infarct size. Infarct-avid scintigraphy and myocardial perfusion imaging have been used to quantify infarct size. Tomography has improved on planar techniques employing technetium-99m pyrophosphate to image MI.[126] Contrast-enhanced magnetic resonance imaging has been helpful in demonstrating the regional heterogeneity of infarction patterns in patients with persistently occluded infarct arteries versus those with successfully reperfused vessels.[127]

REFERENCES

Changing Definitions and Patterns of Care

1. Luepker RV, Apple FS, Christenson RH, et al: Case definitions for acute coronary heart disease in epidemiology and clinical research studies: A statement from the AHA Council on Epidemiology and Prevention; AHA Statistics Committee; World Heart Federation Council on Epidemiology and Prevention; the European Society of Cardiology Working Group on Epidemiology and Prevention; Centers for Disease Control and Prevention; and the National Heart, Lung, and Blood Institute. Circulation 108:2543, 2003.
2. Alpert JS, et al: Definition of myocardial infarction—a global consensus document of The Joint ESC/ACC/AHA/WHF/WHO Task Force, 2007 (in press).
3. Chew DP, Bhatt DL, Lincoff AM, et al: Clinical end point definitions after percutaneous coronary intervention and their relationship to late mortality: An assessment by attributable risk. Heart 92:945, 2006.
4. Zahger D, Hod H, Gottlieb S, et al: Influence of the new definition of acute myocardial infarction on coronary care unit admission, discharge diagnosis, management and outcome in patients with non-ST elevation acute coronary syndromes: A national survey. Int J Cardiol 106:164, 2006.
5. Apple FS, Parvin CA, Buechler KF, et al: Validation of the 99th percentile cutoff independent of assay imprecision (CV) for cardiac troponin monitoring for ruling out myocardial infarction. Clin Chem 51:2198, 2005.
6. Yusuf S, Vaz M, Pais P: Tackling the challenge of cardiovascular disease burden in developing countries. Am Heart J 148:1, 2004.
7. American Heart Association: Heart Disease and Stroke Statistics—2007 Update. Circulation 115:69, 2007.
8. Marshall T: Evaluating national guidelines for prevention of cardiovascular disease in primary care. J Eval Clin Pract 11:452, 2005.
9. Yusuf S, Hawken S, Ounpuu S, et al: Effect of potentially modifiable risk factors associated with myocardial infarction in 52 countries (the INTERHEART study): Case-control study. Lancet 364:937, 2004.
10. Goldberg RJ, Glatfelter K, Burbank-Schmidt E, et al: Trends in community mortality due to coronary heart disease. Am Heart J 151:501, 2006.
11. Kamalesh M, Subramanian U, Ariana A, et al: Similar decline in post-myocardial infarction mortality among subjects with and without diabetes. Am J Med Sci 329:228, 2005.
12. Anderson JL, Adams CD, Antman EM, et al: ACC/AHA 2007 guidelines for the management of patients with unstable angina/non-ST-elevation myocardial infarction: A report of the American College of Cardiology/American Heart Association Task Force on Practice Guidelines (Writing Committee to Revise the 2002 Guidelines for the Management of Patients With Unstable Angina/Non-ST-Elevation Myocardial Infarction). J Am Coll Cardiol 2007 (in press).

13. Ergin A, Muntner P, Sherwin R, He J: Secular trends in cardiovascular disease mortality, incidence, and case fatality rates in adults in the United States. Am J Med 117:219, 2004.

14. Braunwald E, Antman EM: Evidence-based coronary care. Ann Intern Med 126:551, 1997.

15. Antman EM, Anbe DT, Armstrong PW, et al: ACC/AHA Guidelines for the Management of Patients with ST-Elevation Myocardial Infarction: A report of the American College of Cardiology/American Heart Association Task Force on Practice Guidelines (Committee to Revise the 1999 Guidelines for the Management of Patients with Acute Myocardial Infarction). American College of Cardiology Web Site, 2006. (www.acc.org/clinical/guidelines/stemi/index.pdf). Accessed 6/21/06.

15a. Antman EM, Hand M, Armstrong PW, et al: July 2007 focused update of the ACC/AHA 2004 guidelines for the management of patients with ST-elevation myocardial infarction: a report of the American College of Cardiology/American Heart Association Task Force on Practice Guidelines. J Am Coll Cardiol 2007 (in press).

16. Boersma E, Mercado N, Poldermans D, et al: Acute myocardial infarction. Lancet 361:847, 2003.

17. Antman EM, Morrow DA, McCabe CH, et al: Enoxaparin versus unfractionated heparin with fibrinolysis for ST-elevation myocardial infarction. N Engl J Med 354:1477, 2006.

18. Canto JG, Rogers WJ, Chandra NC, et al: The association of sex and payer status on management and subsequent survival in acute myocardial infarction. Arch Intern Med 162:587, 2002.

19. Ahmed S, Antman EM, Murphy SA, et al: Poor outcomes after fibrinolytic therapy for ST-segment elevation myocardial infarction: Impact of age (a meta-analysis of a decade of trials). J Thromb Thrombolysis 21:119, 2006.

20. Krumholz HM, Chen J, Rathore SS, et al: Regional variation in the treatment and outcomes of myocardial infarction: Investigating New England's advantage. Am Heart J 146:242, 2003.

21. Dorsch MF, Lawrance RA, Sapsford RJ, et al: An evaluation of the relationship between specialist training in cardiology and implementation of evidence-based care of patients following acute myocardial infarction. Int J Cardiol 96:335, 2004.

22. Birkhead JS, Weston C, Lowe D: Impact of specialty of admitting physician and type of hospital on care and outcome for myocardial infarction in England and Wales during 2004-5: Observational study. BMJ 332:1306, 2006.

23. Jani SM, Montoye C, Mehta R, et al: Sex differences in the application of evidence-based therapies for the treatment of acute myocardial infarction: The American College of Cardiology's Guidelines Applied in Practice projects in Michigan. Arch Intern Med 166:1164, 2006.

24. Moon JC, De Arenaza DP, Elkington AG, et al: The pathologic basis of Q-wave and non-Q-wave myocardial infarction: A cardiovascular magnetic resonance study. J Am Coll Cardiol 44:554, 2004.

Pathology

25. Ohtani T, Ueda Y, Mizote I, et al: Number of yellow plaques detected in a coronary artery is associated with future risk of acute coronary syndrome: Detection of vulnerable patients by angioscopy. J Am Coll Cardiol 47:2194, 2006.

26. Wasserman EJ, Shipley NM: Atherothrombosis in acute coronary syndromes: Mechanisms, markers, and mediators of vulnerability. Mt Sinai J Med 73:431, 2006.

27. Malek AM, Alper SL, Izumo S: Hemodynamic shear stress and its role in atherosclerosis. JAMA 282:2035, 1999.

28. Rosenberg RD, Aird WC: Vascular-bed–specific hemostasis and hypercoagulable states. N Engl J Med 340:1555, 1999.

29. Ertl G, Frantz S: Healing after myocardial infarction. Cardiovasc Res 66:22, 2005.

30. Kher N, Marsh JD: Pathobiology of atherosclerosis—a brief review. Semin Thromb Hemost 30:665, 2004.

31. Kloner RA: Can we trigger an acute coronary syndrome? Heart 92:1009, 2006.

32. Gurm HS, Topol EJ: The ECG in acute coronary syndromes: New tricks from an old dog. Heart 91:851, 2005.

33. Bayes-de-Luna A, Wagner G, Birnbaum Y, et al: A new terminology for the left ventricular walls and location of myocardial infarcts that present Q wave based on the standard of cardiac magnetic resonance imaging. Circulation 114:1755, 2006.

34. Takemura G, Fujiwara H: Role of apoptosis in remodeling after myocardial infarction. Pharmacol Ther 104:1, 2004.

35. Schwarz K, Simonis G, Yu X, et al: Apoptosis at a distance: Remote activation of caspase-3 occurs early after myocardial infarction. Mol Cell Biochem 281:45, 2006.

36. Schoen FJ: The heart. In Kumar V, Abbas AK, Fausto N (eds): Robbins & Cotran Pathologic Basis of Disease. 7th ed. Philadelphia, WB Saunders, 2005.

37. Achour H, Boccalandro F, Felli P, et al: Mechanical left ventricular unloading prior to reperfusion reduces infarct size in a canine infarction model. Catheter Cardiovasc Interv 64:182, 2005.

38. Pasotti M, Prati F, Arbustini E: The pathology of myocardial infarction in the pre- and post-interventional era. Heart 92:1552, 2006.

39. Vargas SO, Sampson BA, Schoen FJ: Pathologic detection of early myocardial infarction: A critical review of the evolution and usefulness of modern techniques. Mod Pathol 12:635, 1999.

40. Elsasser A, Vogt AM, Nef H, et al: Human hibernating myocardium is jeopardized by apoptotic and autophagic cell death. J Am Coll Cardiol 43:2191, 2004.

41. Giannitsis E, Katus HA: Biomarkers of necrosis for risk assessment and management of ST-elevation myocardial infarction. In Morrow DA (ed): Cardiovascular Biomarkers: Pathophysiology and Disease Management. Totowa, NJ, Humana Press, 2006, pp 119-128.

42. DeWood MA, Spores J, Notske R, et al: Prevalence of total coronary occlusion during the early hours of transmural myocardial infarction. N Engl J Med 303:897, 1980.

43. Ozdemir K, Altunkeser BB, Icli A, et al: New parameters in identification of right ventricular myocardial infarction and proximal right coronary artery lesion. Chest 124:219, 2003.

44. Popescu BA, Antonini-Canterin F, Temporelli PL, et al: Right ventricular functional recovery after acute myocardial infarction: Relation with left ventricular function and interventricular septum motion. GISSI-3 echo substudy. Heart 91:484, 2005.

45. Neven K, Crijns H, Gorgels A: Atrial infarction: a neglected electrocardiographic sign with important clinical implications. J Cardiovasc Electrophysiol 14:306, 2003.

46. Tjandrawidjaja MC, Fu Y, Kim DH, et al: Compromised atrial coronary anatomy is associated with atrial arrhythmias and atrioventricular block complicating acute myocardial infarction. J Electrocardiol 38:271, 2005.

47. Fujita M, Nakae I, Kihara Y, et al: Determinants of collateral development in patients with acute myocardial infarction. Clin Cardiol 22:595, 1999.

48. Bybee KA, Kara T, Prasad A, et al: Systematic review: Transient left ventricular apical ballooning: A syndrome that mimics ST-segment elevation myocardial infarction. Ann Intern Med 141:858, 2004.

Pathophysiology

49. Swan HJ, Forrester JS, Diamond G, et al: Hemodynamic spectrum of myocardial infarction and cardiogenic shock. A conceptual model. Circulation 45:1097, 1972.

50. Forrester JS, Wyatt HL, Da Luz PL, et al: Functional significance of regional ischemic contraction abnormalities. Circulation 54:64, 1976.

51. Schuster EH, Bulkley BH: Ischemia at a distance after acute myocardial infarction: A cause of early postinfarction angina. Circulation 62:509, 1980.

52. White HD, Norris RM, Brown MA, et al: Left ventricular end-systolic volume as the major determinant of survival after recovery from myocardial infarction. Circulation 76:44, 1987.

53. Sadanandan S, Buller C, Menon V, et al: The late open artery hypothesis—a decade later. Am Heart J 142:411, 2001.

54. McMurray J, Solomon S, Pieper K, et al: The effect of valsartan, captopril, or both on atherosclerotic events after acute myocardial infarction: An analysis of the Valsartan in Acute Myocardial Infarction Trial (VALIANT). J Am Coll Cardiol 47:726, 2006.

55. Hochman JS: Cardiogenic shock complicating acute myocardial infarction: Expanding the paradigm. Circulation 107:2998, 2003.

56. Pfeffer JM, Pfeffer MA, Fletcher PJ, Braunwald E: Progressive ventricular remodeling in rat with myocardial infarction. Am J Physiol 260:H1406, 1991.

57. Guo X, Saini HK, Wang J, et al: Prevention of remodeling in congestive heart failure due to myocardial infarction by blockade of the renin-angiotensin system. Expert Rev Cardiovasc Ther 3:717, 2005.

58. Weisman HF, Bush DE, Mannisi JA, et al: Cellular mechanisms of myocardial infarct expansion. Circulation 78:186, 1988.

59. Schmermund A, Lerman LO, Ritman EL, Rumberger JA: Cardiac production of angiotensin II and its pharmacologic inhibition: Effects on the coronary circulation. Mayo Clin Proc 74:503, 1999.

60. Pitt B, White H, Nicolau J, et al: Eplerenone reduces mortality 30 days after randomization following acute myocardial infarction in patients with left ventricular systolic dysfunction and heart failure. J Am Coll Cardiol 46:425, 2005.

Clinical Features

61. Sack MN, Yellon DM: Insulin therapy as an adjunct to reperfusion after acute coronary ischemia: A proposed direct myocardial cell survival effect independent of metabolic modulation. J Am Coll Cardiol 41:1404, 2003.

62. Devos P, Chiolero R, Van den Berghe G, Preiser JC: Glucose, insulin and myocardial ischaemia. Curr Opin Clin Nutr Metab Care 9:131, 2006.

63. Meier JJ, Deifuss S, Klamann A, et al: Plasma glucose at hospital admission and previous metabolic control determine myocardial infarct size and survival in patients with and without type 2 diabetes: The Langendreer Myocardial Infarction and Blood Glucose in Diabetic Patients Assessment (LAMBDA). Diabetes Care 28:2551, 2005.

64. Kragelund C, Omland T: Biology of the natriuretic peptides. In Morrow DA (ed): Cardiovascular Biomarkers: Pathophysiology and Disease Management. Totowa, NJ, Humana Press, 2006, pp 347-372.

65. Abdullah SM, De Lemos JA: Natriuretic peptides in acute and chronic coronary artery disease. In Morrow DA (ed): Cardiovascular Biomarkers: Pathophysiology and Disease Management. Totowa, NJ, Humana Press, 2006, pp 409-425.

66. Cochet A, Zeller M, Cottin Y, et al: The extent of myocardial damage assessed by contrast-enhanced MRI is a major determinant of N-BNP concentration after myocardial infarction. Eur J Heart Fail 6:555, 2004.

67. Stein BC, Levin RI: Natriuretic peptides: Physiology, therapeutic potential, and risk stratification in ischemic heart disease. Am Heart J 135:914, 1998.

68. de Lemos JA, Morrow DA, Bentley JH, et al: The prognostic value of B-type natriuretic peptide in patients with acute coronary syndromes. N Engl J Med 345:1014, 2001.

69. Morrow DA, Braunwald E: Future of biomarkers in acute coronary syndromes: Moving toward a multimarker strategy. Circulation 108:250, 2003.

70. Tapanainen JM, Lindgren KS, Makikallio TH, et al: Natriuretic peptides as predictors of non-sudden and sudden cardiac death after acute myocardial infarction in the beta-blocking era. J Am Coll Cardiol 43:757, 2004.

71. Squire IB, Orn S, Ng LL, et al: Plasma natriuretic peptides up to 2 years after acute myocardial infarction and relation to prognosis: An OPTIMAAL substudy. J Card Fail 11:492, 2005.

72. Mega JL, Morrow DA, De Lemos JA, et al: B-type natriuretic peptide at presentation and prognosis in patients with ST-segment elevation myocardial infarction: An ENTIRE-TIMI-23 substudy. J Am Coll Cardiol 44:335, 2004.

73. Suzuki S, Yoshimura M, Nakayama M, et al: Plasma level of B-type natriuretic peptide as a prognostic marker after acute myocardial infarction: A long-term follow-up analysis. Circulation 110:1387, 2004.
74. Brener SJ: Insights into the pathophysiology of ST-elevation myocardial infarction. Am Heart J 151:S4, 2006.
75. Sabatine MS, Morrow DA, Cannon CP, et al: Relationship between baseline white blood cell count and degree of coronary artery disease and mortality in patients with acute coronary syndromes: A TACTICS-TIMI 18 (Treat Angina with Aggrastat and determine Cost of Therapy with an Invasive or Conservative Strategy-Thrombolysis in Myocardial Infarction 18 trial) substudy. J Am Coll Cardiol 40:1761, 2002.
76. Kloner RA: Natural and unnatural triggers of myocardial infarction. Prog Cardiovasc Dis 48:285, 2006.
77. U.S. Department of Health and Human Services: Centers for Disease Control and Prevention. The Health Consequences of Involuntary Exposure to Tobacco Smoke: A report of the Surgeon General—executive summary. (http://www.cdc.gov/tobacco). Accessed 6/30/06.
78. Lichtenstein AH, Appel LJ, Brands M, et al: Diet and lifestyle recommendations revision 2006: A scientific statement from the American Heart Association Nutrition Committee. Circulation 114:82, 2006.
79. Fleisher LA, Beckman JA, Brown KA, et al: ACC/AHA 2006 guideline update on perioperative cardiovascular evaluation for noncardiac surgery: Focused update on perioperative beta-blocker therapy: A report of the American College of Cardiology/American Heart Association Task Force on Practice Guidelines (Writing Committee to Update the 2002 Guidelines on Perioperative Cardiovascular Evaluation for Noncardiac Surgery) developed in collaboration with the American Society of Echocardiography, American Society of Nuclear Cardiology, Heart Rhythm Society, Society of Cardiovascular Anesthesiologists, Society for Cardiovascular Angiography and Interventions, and Society for Vascular Medicine and Biology. J Am Coll Cardiol 47:2343, 2006.
80. Singh JP, Muller JE: Triggers to acute coronary syndromes. *In* Theroux P (ed): Acute Coronary Syndromes: A Companion to Braunwald's Heart Disease. Philadelphia, WB Saunders, 2003, pp 108-118.
81. Spodick DH: Pericardial complications of myocardial infarction. *In* Francis GS, Alpert JS (eds): Coronary Care. 2nd ed. Boston, Little, Brown & Company, 1995, pp 333-341.
82. Balaban DH, Yamamoto Y, Liu J, et al: Sustained esophageal contraction: A marker of esophageal chest pain identified by intraluminal ultrasonography. Gastroenterology 116:29, 1999.
83. Davis TM, Fortun P, Mulder J, et al: Silent myocardial infarction and its prognosis in a community-based cohort of type 2 diabetic patients: The Fremantle Diabetes Study. Diabetologia 47:395, 2004.
84. Lombardi F, Sandrone G, Spinnler MT, et al: Heart rate variability in the early hours of an acute myocardial infarction. Am J Cardiol 77:1037, 1996.
85. Killip T III, Kimball JT: Treatment of myocardial infarction in a coronary care unit. A two year experience with 250 patients. Am J Cardiol 20:457, 1967.
86. Sugiura T, Nakamura S, Kudo Y, et al: Clinical factors associated with persistent pericardial effusion after successful primary coronary angioplasty. Chest 128:798, 2005.
87. Tunstall-Pedoe H, Kuulasmaa K, Amouyel P, et al: Myocardial infarction and coronary deaths in the World Health Organization MONICA Project. Registration procedures, event rates, and case-fatality rates in 38 populations from 21 countries in four continents. Circulation 90:583, 1994.
88. Ravkilde J, Horder M, Gerhardt W, et al: Diagnostic performance and prognostic value of serum troponin T in suspected acute myocardial infarction. Scand J Clin Lab Invest 53:677, 1993.
89. Roger VL, Killian JM, Weston SA, et al: Redefinition of myocardial infarction: Prospective evaluation in the community. Circulation 114:790, 2006.
90. Antman EM: Decision making with cardiac troponin tests. N Engl J Med 346:2079, 2002.
91. Jaffe AS, Babuin L, Apple FS: Biomarkers in acute cardiac disease: The present and the future. J Am Coll Cardiol 48:1, 2006.
92. Penttila K, Koukkunen H, Halinen M, et al: Myoglobin, creatine kinase MB isoforms and creatine kinase MB mass in early diagnosis of myocardial infarction in patients with acute chest pain. Clin Biochem 35:647, 2002.
93. Apple FS, Quist HE, Doyle PJ, et al: Plasma 99th percentile reference limits for cardiac troponin and creatine kinase MB mass for use with European Society of Cardiology/American College of Cardiology consensus recommendations. Clin Chem 49:1331, 2003.
94. Apple FS: Tissue specificity of cardiac troponin I, cardiac troponin T and creatine kinase-MB. Clin Chim Acta 284:151, 1999.
95. Roberts R, Kleiman NS: Earlier diagnosis and treatment of acute myocardial infarction necessitates the need for a 'new diagnostic mind-set'. Circulation 89:872, 1994.
96. Morrow DA, Cannon CP, Jesse RL, et al: National Academy of Clinical Biochemistry Laboratory Medicine Practice Guidelines: Clinical characteristics and utilization of biochemical markers in acute coronary syndromes. Circulation 115:e356, 2007.
97. Aviles RJ, Askari AT, Lindahl B, et al: Troponin T levels in patients with acute coronary syndromes, with or without renal dysfunction. N Engl J Med 346:2047, 2002.
98. Wu AHB: Analytical issues for the clinical use of cardiac troponin. *In* Morrow DA (ed): Cardiovascular Biomarkers: Pathophysiology and Disease Management. Totowa, NJ, Humana Press, 2006, pp 17-40.
99. Labugger R, Organ L, Collier C, et al: Extensive troponin I and T modification detected in serum from patients with acute myocardial infarction. Circulation 102:1221, 2000.
100. Jaffe AS, Van Eyk JE: Degradation of cardiac troponins: Implications for clinical practice. *In* Morrow DA (ed): Cardiovascular Biomarkers: Pathophysiology and Disease Management. Totowa, NJ, Humana Press, 2006, pp 161-174.
101. Wolfrum S, Jensen KS, Liao JK: Endothelium-dependent effects of statins. Arterioscler Thromb Vasc Biol 23:729, 2003.
102. Smith SC Jr, Allen J, Blair SN, et al: AHA/ACC guidelines for secondary prevention for patients with coronary and other atherosclerotic vascular disease: 2006 update: Endorsed by the National Heart, Lung, and Blood Institute. Circulation 113:2363, 2006.
103. Barron HV, Cannon CP, Murphy SA, et al: Association between white blood cell count, epicardial blood flow, myocardial perfusion, and clinical outcomes in the setting of acute myocardial infarction: A thrombolysis in myocardial infarction 10 substudy. Circulation 102:2329, 2000.
104. Berton G, Cordiano R, Palmieri R, et al: C-reactive protein in acute myocardial infarction: Association with heart failure. Am Heart J 145:1094, 2003.
105. Sano T, Tanaka A, Namba M, et al: C-reactive protein and lesion morphology in patients with acute myocardial infarction. Circulation 108:282, 2003.
106. Ziakas A, Gavrilidis S, Giannoglou G, et al: In-hospital and long-term prognostic value of fibrinogen, CRP, and IL-6 levels in patients with acute myocardial infarction treated with thrombolysis. Angiology 57:283, 2006.
107. Sabatine MS, Morrow DA, Giugliano RP, et al: Association of hemoglobin levels with clinical outcomes in acute coronary syndromes. Circulation 111:2042, 2005.
108. Zimetbaum PJ, Josephson ME: Use of the electrocardiogram in acute myocardial infarction. N Engl J Med 348:933, 2003.
109. Manes C, Pfeffer MA, Rutherford JD, et al: Value of the electrocardiogram in predicting left ventricular enlargement and dysfunction after myocardial infarction. Am J Med 114:99, 2003.
110. Pope JH, Ruthazer R, Kontos MC, et al: The impact of electrocardiographic left ventricular hypertrophy and bundle branch block on the triage and outcome of ED patients with a suspected acute coronary syndrome: A multicenter study. Am J Emerg Med 22:156, 2004.
111. Feldman LJ, Coste P, Furber A, et al: Incomplete resolution of ST-segment elevation is a marker of transient microcirculatory dysfunction after stenting for acute myocardial infarction. Circulation 107:2684, 2003.
112. De Luca G, Ernst N, van't Hof AW, et al: Preprocedural Thrombolysis in Myocardial Infarction (TIMI) flow significantly affects the extent of ST-segment resolution and myocardial blush in patients with acute anterior myocardial infarction treated by primary angioplasty. Am Heart J 150:827, 2005.
113. Cheitlin MD, Armstrong WF, Aurigemma GP, et al: ACC/AHA/ASE 2003 guideline update for the clinical application of echocardiography: A report of the American College of Cardiology/American Heart Association Task Force on Practice Guidelines (ACC/AHA/ASE Committee to Update the 1997 Guidelines for the Clinical Application of Echocardiography). American College of Cardiology web site, 2006. (www.acc.org/clinical/guidelines/echo/index.pdf). Accessed 6/26/06.
114. Lopez-Sendon J, Coma-Canella I, Alcasena S, et al: Electrocardiographic findings in acute right ventricular infarction: Sensitivity and specificity of electrocardiographic alterations in right precordial leads V4R, V3R, V1, V2, and V3. J Am Coll Cardiol 6:1273, 1985.
115. Geft IL, Shah PK, Rodriguez L, et al: ST elevations in leads V1 to V5 may be caused by right coronary artery occlusion and acute right ventricular infarction. Am J Cardiol 53:991, 1984.
116. Acikel M, Yilmaz M, Bozkurt E, et al: ST segment elevation in leads V1 to V3 due to isolated right ventricular branch occlusion during primary right coronary angioplasty. Catheter Cardiovasc Interv 60:32, 2003.
117. Finn AV, Antman EM: Images in clinical medicine. Isolated right ventricular infarction. N Engl J Med 349:1636, 2003.
118. Pohost GM, Hung L, Doyle M: Clinical use of cardiovascular magnetic resonance. Circulation 108:647, 2003.
119. Kim RJ, Wu E, Rafael A, et al: The use of contrast-enhanced magnetic resonance imaging to identify reversible myocardial dysfunction. N Engl J Med 343:1445, 2000.
120. Yan AT, Shayne AJ, Brown KA, et al: Characterization of the peri-infarct zone by contrast-enhanced cardiac magnetic resonance imaging is a powerful predictor of post-myocardial infarction mortality. Circulation 114:32, 2006.
121. Hombach V, Grebe O, Merkle N, et al: Sequelae of acute myocardial infarction regarding cardiac structure and function and their prognostic significance as assessed by magnetic resonance imaging. Eur Heart J 26:549, 2005.
122. Kwong RY, Chan AK, Brown KA, et al: Impact of unrecognized myocardial scar detected by cardiac magnetic resonance imaging on event-free survival in patients presenting with signs or symptoms of coronary artery disease. Circulation 113:2733, 2006.
123. Klocke FJ, Baird MG, Bateman TM, et al: ACC/AHA/ASNC guidelines for the clinical use of cardiac radionuclide imaging: A report of the American College of Cardiology/American Heart Association Task Force on Practice Guidelines (ACC/AHA/ASNC Committee to Revise the 1995 Guidelines for the Clinical Use of Radionuclide Imaging). American College of Cardiology Web Site, 2006. (http://www.acc.org/clinical/guidelines/radio/index.pdf). Accessed 6/21/06.
124. Krucoff MW, Johanson P, Baeza R, et al: Clinical utility of serial and continuous ST-segment recovery assessment in patients with acute ST-elevation myocardial infarction: Assessing the dynamics of epicardial and myocardial reperfusion. Circulation 110:e533, 2004.
125. Adams JE III, Abendschein DR, Jaffe AS: Biochemical markers of myocardial injury. Is MB creatine kinase the choice for the 1990s? Circulation 88:750, 1993.
126. Kopecky SL, Aviles RJ, Bell MR, et al: A randomized, double-blinded, placebo-controlled, dose-ranging study measuring the effect of an adenosine agonist on infarct size reduction in patients undergoing primary percutaneous transluminal coronary angioplasty: The ADMIRE (AmP579 Delivery for Myocardial Infarction REduction) study. Am Heart J 146:146, 2003.
127. Kwong RY, Yucel EK: Cardiology patient pages. Computed tomography scan and magnetic resonance imaging. Circulation 108:e104, 2003.

ST-Elevation Myocardial Infarction: Management

Elliott M. Antman

Management in the Emergency
  Department, 1234
Reperfusion Therapy, 1239
Coronary Fibrinolysis, 1241
Catheter-Based Reperfusion
  Strategies, 1249
Selection of Reperfusion
  Strategy, 1249
Antithrombin and Antiplatelet
  Therapy, 1251

Hospital Management, 1256
Coronary Care Units, 1256
Pharmacological Therapy, 1258

**Hemodynamic
Disturbances, 1264**
Hemodynamic Assessment, 1264
Left Ventricular Failure, 1267
Cardiogenic Shock, 1269
Right Ventricular Infarction, 1271
Mechanical Causes of Heart
  Failure, 1272

Arrhythmias, 1275
Ventricular Arrhythmias, 1277
Bradyarrhythmias, 1279
Supraventricular
  Tachyarrhythmias, 1281
Other Complications, 1282
Left Ventricular Thrombus and
  Arterial Embolism, 1285
Convalescence, Discharge, and Post-
  Myocardial Infarction Care, 1286
Risk Stratification after STEMI, 1286
Secondary Prevention of Acute
  Myocardial Infarction, 1289

References, 1292

Although considerable advances have been made in the process of care for patients with ST-elevation myocardial infarction (STEMI),[1] room for improvement exists, especially in special populations such as the elderly, women, and members of ethnic minority groups.[2-8] Patients who experience STEMI while hospitalized for another medical problem have a marked increase in morbidity and mortality compared with patients admitted with a STEMI from the community.[9]

It is useful to organize a discussion of the phases of management of STEMI along the chronology of the interface of clinicians with the patient. Primary and secondary prevention of STEMI are discussed in Chapter 45. Treatment at the time of onset of STEMI (prehospital issues, initial recognition and management in the emergency department, reperfusion), hospital management (medications, arrhythmics, complications, preparation for discharge), and secondary prevention of STEMI are discussed in this chapter. Chapter 52 discusses percutaneous coronary intervention (PCI) in patients with STEMI.

PREHOSPITAL CARE. The prehospital care of patients with suspected STEMI is a crucial element bearing directly on the likelihood of survival. Most deaths associated with STEMI occur within the first hour of its onset and are usually caused by ventricular fibrillation (see Chap. 36). Accordingly, the importance of the immediate implementation of definitive resuscitative efforts and of rapidly transporting the patient to a hospital cannot be overemphasized. Major components of the delay from the onset of symptoms consistent with acute myocardial infarction (MI) to reperfusion include the following[1]: (1) the time for the patient to recognize the seriousness of the problem and seek medical attention; (2) prehospital evaluation, treatment, and transportation; (3) the time for diagnostic measures and initiation of treatment in the hospital (e.g., "door-to-needle" time for patients receiving a thrombolytic agent and "door-to-balloon" time for patients undergoing a catheter-based reperfusion strategy); and (4) the time from initiation of treatment to restoration of flow (Fig. 51-1).

Patient-related factors that correlate with a longer time to the decision to seek medical attention include older age; female gender; African American race; low socioeconomic status; low emotional or somatic awareness; history of angina, diabetes, or both; consulting a spouse or other relative; and consulting a physician.[10-12] Health care professionals should heighten the level of awareness of patients at risk for STEMI (e.g., those with hypertension, diabetes, history of angina pectoris).[1] They should review and reinforce with patients and their families the need to seek urgent medical attention for a pattern of symptoms including chest discomfort, extreme fatigue, and dyspnea, especially if accompanied by diaphoresis, lightheadedness, palpita-

tions, or a sense of impending doom.[10-12] Although many patients shun such discussions and tend to minimize the likelihood of ever needing emergency cardiac treatment, emphasis should be placed on the prevention and treatment of potentially fatal arrhythmias, as well as salvage of the jeopardized myocardium by reperfusion, for which time is crucial. Patients should also be instructed in the proper use of sublingual nitroglycerin and to call 911 emergency services if the ischemic-type discomfort persists for more than 5 minutes.[13]

EMERGENCY MEDICAL SERVICES (EMS) SYSTEMS. These have three major components: emergency medical dispatch, first response, and EMS ambulance response. Ongoing efforts to shorten the time to treatment of patients with STEMI include improvement in the medical dispatch component by expanding 911 coverage, providing automated external defibrillators to first responders, placing automated external defibrillators in critical public locations, and greater coordination of EMS ambulance response.[14,15] Well-equipped ambulances and helicopters staffed by personnel trained in the acute care of the STEMI patient allow definitive therapy to commence while the patient is being transported to the hospital (Table 51-1). To be used effectively, they must be placed strategically within a community, and excellent radio communication systems must be available. These units should be equipped with battery-operated monitoring equipment, a DC defibrillator, oxygen, endotracheal tubes and suction apparatus, and commonly used cardiovascular drugs. Radiotelemetry systems that allow transmission of the electrocardiographic signal to a medical control officer are highly desirable to facilitate triage of STEMI patients and are becoming increasingly available in many communities (Fig. 51-2). Observations of simple variables such as age, heart rate, and blood pressure permit initial classification of patients into high- or low-risk subgroups.[16]

In addition to prompt defibrillation, the efficacy of prehospital care appears to

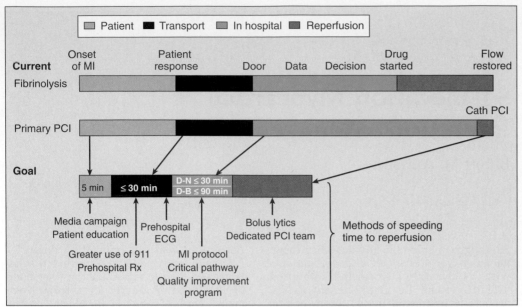

FIGURE 51–1 Major components of time delay between onset of infarction and restoration of flow in the infarct-related artery. Plotted sequentially from left to right are the time for patients to recognize symptoms and seek medical attention, transportation to the hospital, in-hospital decision-making and implementation of reperfusion strategy, and time for restoration of flow once the reperfusion strategy has been initiated. The time to initiate fibrinolytic therapy is the "door-to-needle" (D-N) time; this is followed by the period of time required for pharmacological restoration of flow. More time is required to move the patient to the catheterization laboratory for a percutaneous coronary intervention (PCI) procedure, referred to as the "door-to-balloon" (D-B) time, but restoration of flow in the epicardial infarct-related artery occurs promptly after PCI. **Bottom,** Various methods for speeding the time to reperfusion are shown, along with the goals for the time intervals for the various components of the time delay. ECG = electrocardiogram; MI = myocardial infarction. *(Modified from Antman EM, Anbe DT, Armstrong PW, et al: ACC/AHA guidelines for the management of patients with ST-elevation myocardial infarction: A report of the American College of Cardiology/American Heart Association Task Force on Practice Guidelines (Committee to Revise the 1999 Guidelines for the Management of Patients with Acute Myocardial Infarction) (www.acc.org/clinical/guidelines/stemi/index.pdf.). Accessed 4/19/06.*

CH 51

depend on several factors including early relief of pain with its deleterious physiological sequelae, reduction of excessive activity of the autonomic nervous system, and abolition of prelethal arrhythmias such as ventricular tachycardia. However, these efforts must not inhibit rapid transfer to the hospital (see Fig. 51-2).

PREHOSPITAL FIBRINOLYSIS. Several randomized trials have evaluated the potential benefits of prehospital versus in-hospital fibrinolysis. Although none of the individual trials showed a significant reduction in mortality with prehospital-initiated thrombolytic therapy, there was a generally consistent observation of benefit from earlier treatment, and a meta-analysis of all the available trials demonstrated a 17 percent reduction in mortality.[17] The CAPTIM trial reported a trend toward a lower rate of mortality among STEMI patients receiving prehospital fibrinolysis as compared with primary PCI, especially if patients were treated within 2 hours of the onset of symptoms.[18,19] Several registry reports provide additional support for the benefit of prehospital lysis.[20,21]

Several factors must be weighed when communities consider whether their ambulances and emergency transport vehicles should have the capability to initiate fibrinolytic therapy. The greatest reduction in mortality is observed when reperfusion can be initiated within 60 to 90 minutes of the onset of symptoms.[1] Streamlining of emergency department triage practices so that treatment can be started within 30 minutes, when coupled with the 15- to 30-minute transport time that is common in most urban centers, may be more cost effective than equipping all ambulances to administer prehospital fibrinolytic therapy (see Fig. 51-2).[1] The latter would require extensive training of personnel (see Table 51-1), installation of computer-assisted electro-

cardiography or systems for radio transmission of the electrocardiogram (ECG) signal to a central station, and stocking of medicine kits with the necessary drug supplies. In selected communities where transport delays may be 60 to 90 minutes or longer and experienced personnel are available on ambulances, prehospital fibrinolytic therapy is beneficial.[22] Therefore prehospital fibrinolysis is reasonable in settings in which physicians are present in the ambulance or there is a well-organized EMS system with full-time paramedics, capability for obtaining and transmitting 12-lead ECG readings from the field, and online medical command to authorize prehospital fibrinolysis.[23-25]

Management in the Emergency Department

When evaluating patients in the emergency department, physicians must confront the difficult task of rapidly identifying patients who require urgent reperfusion therapy, triaging lower-risk patients to the appropriate facility within the hospital, and not discharging patients inappropriately while avoiding unnecessary admissions. A history of ischemic-type discomfort and the initial 12-lead ECG are the primary tools for screening patients with acute coronary syndromes in the emergency department.[26] More extensive use of prehospital 12-lead electrocardiographic recordings might facilitate triage of STEMI patients in the emergency department.[27] ST segment elevation on the ECG of a patient with ischemic discomfort highly suggests thrombotic occlusion of an epicardial coronary artery, and its presence should serve as the trigger for a well-rehearsed sequence of rapid assessment of the patient for contraindications to fibrinolysis and initiation of a reperfusion strategy (Tables 51-2 and 51-3).[1] Because the 12-lead ECG is at the center of the decision pathway for initiation of reperfusion therapy, it should be obtained promptly (≤10 minutes) in patients presenting with ischemic discomfort.[1]

Because lethal arrhythmias can occur suddenly in patients with STEMI, all patients should be attached to a bedside ECG monitor and intravenous access obtained for infusion of 5 percent dextrose in water. If the initial ECG reading shows ST segment elevation of 1 mm or more in at least two contiguous leads or a new or presumably new left bundle branch block, the patient should be evaluated immediately for a reperfusion strategy. Critical factors to be considered when selecting a reperfusion strategy include (1) the time elapsed since the onset of symptoms, (2) the risk associated with STEMI, (3) the risk of administering fibrinolysis, and (4) the time required to initiate an invasive strategy (Table 51-2). Debate about which form of reperfusion therapy is superior remains controversial, and it will be discussed in depth later.

TABLE 51–1 | Reperfusion Checklist for Evaluation of the STEMI Patient

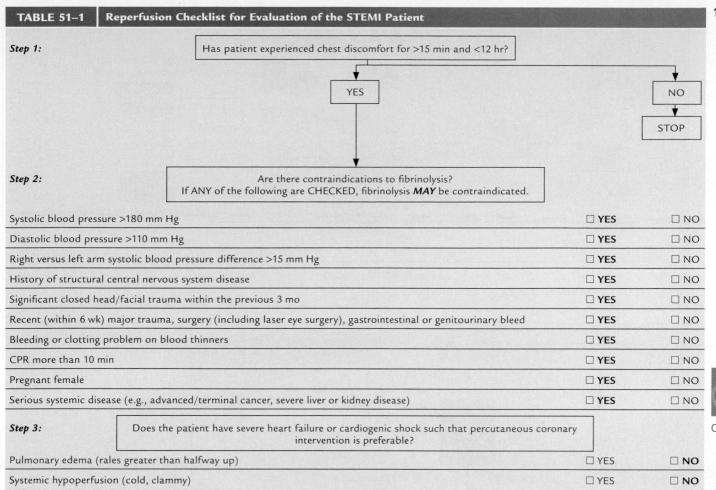

Step 1: Has patient experienced chest discomfort for >15 min and <12 hr? YES / NO / STOP		
Step 2: Are there contraindications to fibrinolysis? If ANY of the following are CHECKED, fibrinolysis *MAY* be contraindicated.		
Systolic blood pressure >180 mm Hg	☐ **YES**	☐ NO
Diastolic blood pressure >110 mm Hg	☐ **YES**	☐ NO
Right versus left arm systolic blood pressure difference >15 mm Hg	☐ **YES**	☐ NO
History of structural central nervous system disease	☐ **YES**	☐ NO
Significant closed head/facial trauma within the previous 3 mo	☐ **YES**	☐ NO
Recent (within 6 wk) major trauma, surgery (including laser eye surgery), gastrointestinal or genitourinary bleed	☐ **YES**	☐ NO
Bleeding or clotting problem on blood thinners	☐ **YES**	☐ NO
CPR more than 10 min	☐ **YES**	☐ NO
Pregnant female	☐ **YES**	☐ NO
Serious systemic disease (e.g., advanced/terminal cancer, severe liver or kidney disease)	☐ **YES**	☐ NO
Step 3: Does the patient have severe heart failure or cardiogenic shock such that percutaneous coronary intervention is preferable?		
Pulmonary edema (rales greater than halfway up)	☐ YES	☐ **NO**
Systemic hypoperfusion (cold, clammy)	☐ YES	☐ **NO**

CPR = cardiopulmonary resuscitation; STEMI = ST-elevation myocardial infarction.

From Antman EM, Anbe DT, Armstrong PW, et al: ACC/AHA guidelines for the management of patients with ST-elevation myocardial infarction: A report of the American College of Cardiology/American Heart Association Task Force on Practice Guidelines (Committee to Revise the 1999 Guidelines for the Management of Patients with Acute Myocardial Infarction) (www.acc.org/clinical/guidelines/stemi/index.pdf). Accessed 4/19/06.

Given the importance of time to reperfusion,[28] the concept of medical system goals has arisen. Benchmarks for medical systems to use when assessing the quality of their performance are a door-to-needle time of less than or equal to 30 minutes for initiation of fibrinolytic therapy and a door-to-balloon time of less than or equal to 90 minutes for percutaneous coronary perfusion (see Fig. 52-2).[1,29] With increasing sophistication of EMS systems, it is possible to initiate the process of evaluation/implementation of a reperfusion strategy even before the patient arrives in the emergency department. For those patients transported by ambulance, the medical system goals can be restated as an EMS-to-needle time of less than or equal to 30 minutes for initiation of fibrinolysis and an EMS-to-balloon time of less than or equal to 90 minutes for initiation of PCI (see Fig. 51-2).[1,30] An intriguing proposal that may also facilitate care of patients with STEMI is the development of regionalized centers for care of patients with acute ischemic heart disease.[15] Implementation of such "centers of excellence" requires a coordinated commitment of multiple components of the health care system—a formidable challenge, but one that many authorities believe is a vital step toward improvement of care of patients with STEMI.[15]

Patients with an initial ECG reading that reveals new or presumably new ST segment depression and/or T wave inversion, although not considered candidates for fibrinolytic therapy, should be treated as though they are suffering from MI without ST elevation or unstable angina (a distinc-

tion to be made subsequently after scrutiny of serial ECGs and serum cardiac marker measurements) (see Chap. 53).

In patients with a clinical history suggestive of STEMI (see Chap. 50) and an initial nondiagnostic ECG reading (i.e., no ST segment deviation or T wave inversion), serial tracings should be obtained while the patients are being evaluated in the emergency department. Emergency department staff can be alerted to the sudden development of ST segment elevation by periodic visual inspection of the bedside ECG monitor, by continuous ST segment recording, or by auditory alarms when the ST segment deviation exceeds programmed limits. Decision aids such as computer-based diagnostic algorithms, identification of high-risk clinical indicators, rapid determination of cardiac serum markers, two-dimensional echocardiographic screening for regional wall motion abnormalities, and myocardial perfusion imaging have greatest clinical utility when the ECG reading is nondiagnostic. In an effort to improve the cost-effectiveness of care of patients with a chest pain syndrome, nondiagnostic ECG reading, and low suspicion of MI but in whom the diagnosis has not been entirely excluded, many medical centers have developed critical pathways that involve a coronary observation unit with a goal of ruling out MI in less than 12 hours.[31]

General Treatment Measures

ASPIRIN. This agent is not only useful for the primary prevention of vascular events (see Chap. 45) but is also effec-

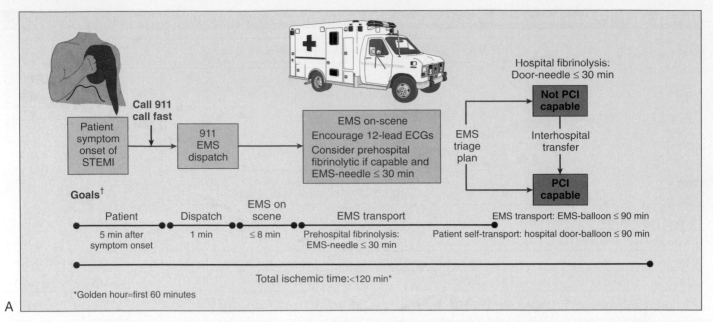

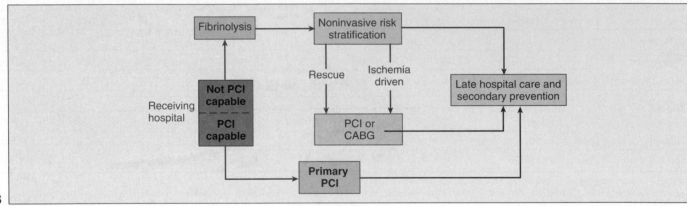

FIGURE 51–2 Options for transportation of ST-elevation myocardial infarction (STEMI) patients and initial reperfusion treatment. Reperfusion in patients with STEMI can be accomplished by the pharmacological (fibrinolysis) or catheter-based (primary percutaneous coronary intervention [PCI]) approaches. Implementation of these strategies varies based on the mode of transportation of the patient and capabilities at the receiving hospital. **A,** Patient transported by emergency medical services (EMS) after calling 911. Transport time to the hospital is variable from case to case, but the goal is to keep total ischemic time less than 120 minutes. Three possibilities exist. (1) If EMS has fibrinolytic capability and the patient qualifies for therapy, prehospital fibrinolysis should be started within 30 minutes of EMS arrival on scene. (2) If EMS is not capable of administering prehospital fibrinolysis and the patient is transported to a non-PCI capable hospital, the hospital door-to-needle time should be less than or equal to 30 minutes for patients in whom fibrinolysis is indicated. (3) If EMS is not capable of administering prehospital fibrinolysis and the patient is transported to a PCI-capable hospital, the hospital door-to-balloon time should be less than or equal to 90 minutes.

Interhospital transfer: It is also appropriate to consider emergency interhospital transfer of the patient to a PCI-capable hospital for mechanical revascularization if (1) there is a contraindication to fibrinolysis; (2) PCI can be initiated promptly (≤90 minutes after the patient presented to the initial receiving hospital or less than or equal to 60 minutes compared to when fibrinolysis could be initiated at the initial receiving hospital; (3) fibrinolysis is administered and is unsuccessful (i.e., "rescue PCI"). Secondary nonemergency interhospital transfer can be considered for recurrent ischemia **(B).**

Patient self-transport: Patient self-transportation is discouraged. If the patient arrives at a non-PCI-capable hospital, the door-to-needle time should be 30 minutes or less. If the patient arrives at a PCI-capable hospital, the door-to-balloon time should be 90 minutes or less. The treatment options and time recommendations after first hospital arrival are the same.

B, For patients who receive fibrinolysis, noninvasive risk stratification is recommended to identify the need for rescue PCI (failed fibrinolysis) or ischemia driven PCI. Regardless of the initial method of reperfusion treatment, all patients should receive late hospital care and secondary prevention of ST-elevation myocardial infarction (STEMI).

†The medical system goal is to facilitate rapid recognition and treatment of patients with STEMI such that door-to-needle (or EMS-to-needle) for initiation of fibrinolytic therapy can be achieved within 30 minutes or that door-to-balloon (or EMS-to-balloon) or PCI can be achieved within 90 minutes. These goals should not be understood as "ideal" times, but rather the longest times that should be considered acceptable for a given system. Systems that are able to achieve even more rapid times for treatment of patients with STEMI should be encouraged. CABG = coronary artery bypass grafting. (*Modified from Armstrong PW, Collen D, Antman E: Fibrinolysis for acute myocardial infarction: The future is here and now. Circulation 107:2533, 2003; and Antman EM, Anbe DT, Armstrong PW, et al: ACC/AHA guidelines for the management of patients with ST-elevation myocardial infarction: A report of the American College of Cardiology/American Heart Association Task Force on Practice Guidelines [Committee to Revise the 1999 Guidelines for the Management of Patients with Acute Myocardial Infarction] [www.acc.org/clinical/guidelines/stemi/index.pdf]. Accessed 4/19/06.*)

tive across the entire spectrum of acute coronary syndromes and forms part of the initial management strategy for patients with suspected STEMI. The pharmacology of aspirin is presented in Chapter 82. The goal of aspirin treatment is to quickly block formation of thromboxane A_2 in platelets by cyclooxygenase inhibition. Because low doses (40 to 80 mg) take several days to achieve full antiplatelet effect, at least 162 to 325 mg should be administered acutely in the emergency department.[1] To achieve therapeutic blood levels rapidly, the patient should chew the tablet to promote buccal absorption rather than absorption through the gastric mucosa.

TABLE 51–2	Assessment of Reperfusion Options for STEMI Patients

Step 1: | Assess time and risk.

- Time since onset of symptoms
- Risk of STEMI
- Risk of fibrinolysis
- Time required for transport to a skilled PCI laboratory

Step 2: | Determine if fibrinolysis or invasive strategy is preferred.

- *If presentation is <3 hr and there is no delay to an invasive strategy, there is no preference for either strategy.*

Fibrinolysis is generally preferred if:
- Early presentation (≤3 hr from symptom onset and delay to invasive strategy) (see below)
- Invasive strategy is not an option
  - Catheterization laboratory occupied or not available
  - Vascular access difficulties
  - Lack of access to a skilled PCI laboratory*†
- Delay to invasive strategy
  - Prolonged transport
  - (Door-to-Balloon)–(Door-to-Needle) more than 1 hr‡§
  - Medical contact-to-balloon or door-to-balloon more than 90 min

An invasive strategy is generally preferred if:
- Skilled PCI lab is available with surgical backup
  - Skilled PCI lab is available, defined by†‡:
  - Medical contact-to-balloon or door-to-balloon less than 90 min
  - (Door-to-balloon)–(door-to-needle) less than 1 hr‡
- High risk from STEMI
  - Cardiogenic shock
  - Killip class ≥3
- Contraindications to fibrinolysis including increased risk of bleeding and ICH
- Late presentation
  - Symptom onset was more than 3 hr ago
- Diagnosis of STEMI is in doubt

*Operator experience > a total of 75 primary PCI cases/yr.

†Team experience > a total of 36 primary PCI cases/yr.

‡Applies to fibrin-specific agents.

§This calculation implies that the estimated delay to the implementation of the invasive strategy is >1 hr versus initiation of fibrinolytic therapy immediately.

ICH = intracranial hemorrhage; PCI = percutaneous coronary intervention; STEMI = ST-elevation myocardial infarction.

From Antman EM, Anbe DT, Armstrong PW, et al: ACC/AHA guidelines for the management of patients with ST-elevation myocardial infarction: A report of the American College of Cardiology/American Heart Association Task Force on Practice Guidelines (Committee to Revise the 1999 Guidelines for the Management of Patients with Acute Myocardial Infarction) (www.acc.org/clinical/guidelines/stemi/index.pdf). Accessed 4/19/06.

TABLE 51–3	Contraindications and Cautions for Fibrinolytic Use in STEMI*

Absolute Contraindications
- Any prior intracranial hemorrhage
- Known structural cerebral vascular lesion (e.g., arteriovenous malformation)
- Known malignant intracranial neoplasm (primary or metastatic)
- Ischemic stroke within 3 mo EXCEPT acute ischemic stroke within 3 hr
- Suspected aortic dissection
- Active bleeding or bleeding diathesis (excluding menses)
- Significant closed head or facial trauma within 3 mo

Relative contraindications
- History of chronic severe poorly controlled hypertension
- Severe uncontrolled hypertension on presentation (SBP >180 Hg or DBP >110 Hg)†
- History of prior ischemic stroke >3 mo dementia, or known intracranial pathology not covered in contraindications
- Traumatic or prolonged (>10 min) CPR or major surgery (<3 wk)
- Recent (within 2-4 wk) internal bleeding
- Noncompressible vascular punctures
- For streptokinase/anistreplase: prior exposure (>5 days ago) or prior allergic reaction to these agents
- Pregnancy
- Active peptic ulcer
- Current use of anticoagulants: the higher the INR, the higher the risk of bleeding

*Viewed as advisory for clinical decision-making and may not be all-inclusive or definitive.

†Could be an absolute contraindication in low-risk patients with myocardial infarction.

CPR = cardiopulmonary resuscitation; DBP = diastolic blood pressure; INR = international normalized ratio; SBP = systolic blood pressure; STEMI = ST-elevation myocardial infarction.

From Antman EM, Anbe DT, Armstrong PW, et al: ACC/AHA guidelines for the management of patients with ST-elevation myocardial infarction: A report of the American College of Cardiology/American Heart Association Task Force on Practice Guidelines (Committee to Revise the 1999 Guidelines for the Management of Patients with Acute Myocardial Infarction) (www.acc.org/clinical/guidelines/stemi/index.pdf). Accessed 4/19/06.

CH 51

ST-Elevation Myocardial Infarction: Management

(by either increasing supply or decreasing demand) have a functional analgesic effect.

Analgesics. Although a wide variety of analgesic agents has been used to treat the pain associated with STEMI including meperidine, pentazocine, and morphine, morphine remains the drug of choice, except in patients with well-documented morphine hypersensitivity. Four to 8 mg should be administered intravenously, and doses of 2 to 8 mg repeated at intervals of 5 to 15 minutes until the pain is relieved or evident toxicity—hypotension, depression of respiration, or severe vomiting—precludes further administration of the drug. In some patients, remarkably large cumulative doses of morphine (2 to 3 mg/kg) may be required and are usually tolerated.

The reduction of anxiety resulting from morphine diminishes the patient's restlessness and the activity of the autonomic nervous system, with a consequent reduction of the heart's metabolic demands. The beneficial effect of morphine in patients with pulmonary edema is unequivocal and may be related to several factors including peripheral arterial and venous dilation (particularly among patients with excessive sympathoadrenal activity), reduction of the work of breathing, and slowing of heart rate secondary to combined withdrawal of sympathetic tone and augmentation of vagal tone.

Hypotension following the administration of nitroglycerin and morphine can be minimized by maintaining the patient in a supine position and elevating the lower extremities if systolic arterial pressure declines below 100 mm Hg. Such positioning is undesirable in the presence of pulmo-

CONTROL OF CARDIAC PAIN. Analgesia is an important element of management of STEMI patients in the emergency department. Often there is a tendency to underdose the patient for fear of obscuring response to antiischemic or reperfusion therapy. This should be avoided because pain contributes to the heightened sympathetic activity that is particularly prominent during the early phase of STEMI. Control of cardiac pain is typically accomplished with a combination of nitrates, analgesics (e.g., morphine), oxygen, and beta-adrenoceptor receptor blockers (referred to hereafter as *beta blockers*). Similar pharmacological principles apply in the coronary care unit, where many of the therapies discussed herein should continue after initial dosing in the emergency department. Because the pain associated with STEMI is related to ongoing ischemia, many interventions that act to improve the oxygen supply-demand relationship

nary edema, but morphine rarely produces hypotension under these circumstances. The concomitant administration of atropine in doses of 0.5 to 1.5 mg intravenously may be helpful in treating eventual excessive vagomimetic effects of morphine, particularly when hypotension and bradycardia are present before it is administered.[1] Respiratory depression is an unusual complication of morphine in the presence of severe pain or pulmonary edema, but as the patient's cardiovascular status improves, impairment of ventilation may supervene. It can be treated with naloxone, in doses of 0.1 to 0.2 mg intravenously initially, repeated after 15 minutes if necessary. Nausea and vomiting may be troublesome side effects of large doses of morphine and can be treated with a phenothiazine.

Nitrates. By virtue of their ability to enhance coronary blood flow by coronary vasodilation and to decrease ventricular preload by increasing venous capacitance, sublingual nitrates are indicated for most patients with an acute coronary syndrome. At present, the only groups of patients with STEMI in whom sublingual nitroglycerin should *not* be given are those with inferior MI and suspected right ventricular infarction[32] or marked hypotension (systolic pressure <90 mm Hg), especially if accompanied by bradycardia.

Once it is ascertained that hypotension is not present, a sublingual nitroglycerin tablet should be administered and the patient observed for improvement in symptoms or change in hemodynamics. If an initial dose is well tolerated and appears to be of benefit, further nitrates should be administered, with monitoring of the vital signs. Even small doses can produce sudden hypotension and bradycardia, a reaction that can be life-threatening but usually easily reversed with intravenous atropine if recognized quickly. Long-acting oral nitrate preparations should be avoided in the early course of STEMI because of the frequently changing hemodynamic status of the patient. In patients with a prolonged period of waxing and waning chest pain, intravenous nitroglycerin may be of benefit in controlling symptoms and correcting ischemia, but frequent monitoring of blood pressure is required.

Beta Blockers. These drugs relieve pain, reduce the need for analgesics in many patients, and reduce infarct size and life-threatening arrhythmias. Avoiding early intravenous blockade in patients presenting in Killip Class II or greater is important, however, because of the risk of precipitating cardiogenic shock.[33,34] A popular and relatively safe protocol for the use of a beta blocker in this situation is as follows. (1) Patients with heart failure (rales >10 cm up from diaphragm), hypotension (blood pressure <90 mm Hg), bradycardia (heart rate <60 beats/min), or heart block (PR interval >0.24 sec) are first excluded. (2) Metoprolol is given in three 5-mg intravenous boluses. (3) Patients are observed for 2 to 5 minutes after each bolus, and if the heart rate falls below 60 beats/min or systolic blood pressure falls below 100 mm Hg, no further drug is given. (4) If hemodynamic stability continues 15 minutes after the last intravenous dose, the patient is begun on oral metoprolol, 50 mg every 6 hours for 2 days, then switched to 100 mg twice daily. An infusion of an extremely short-acting beta blocker, esmolol (50 to 250 mg/kg/min), may be useful in patients with relative contraindications to beta blockade in whom heart rate slowing is considered highly desirable.

Oxygen. Hypoxemia can occur in patients with STEMI and usually results from ventilation-perfusion abnormalities that are sequelae of left ventricular failure; pneumonia and intrinsic pulmonary disease are additional causes of hypoxemia. Treating all patients hospitalized with STEMI with oxygen for at least 24 to 48 hours is common practice on the basis of the empirical assumption of hypoxia and evidence that increased oxygen in the inspired air may

protect ischemic myocardium. However, this practice may not be cost-effective. Augmentation of the fraction of oxygen in the inspired air does not elevate oxygen delivery significantly in patients who are not hypoxemic. Furthermore, it may increase systemic vascular resistance and arterial pressure and thereby lower cardiac output slightly.

In view of these considerations, arterial oxygen saturation can be estimated by pulse oximetry (an increasingly available technology), and oxygen therapy can be omitted if it is normal. On the other hand, oxygen should be administered to patients with STEMI when arterial hypoxemia is clinically evident or can be documented by measurement (e.g., SaO_2 <90 percent).[1] In these patients, serial arterial blood gas measurements can be employed to follow the efficacy of oxygen therapy. The delivery of 2 to 4 liters/min of 100 percent oxygen by mask or nasal prongs for 6 to 12 hours is satisfactory for most patients with mild hypoxemia. If arterial oxygenation is still depressed on this regimen, the flow rate may have to be increased, and other causes for hypoxemia should be sought. In patients with pulmonary edema, endotracheal intubation and positive-pressure controlled ventilation may be necessary.

Limitation of Infarct Size

Infarct size is an important determinant of prognosis in patients with STEMI. Patients who succumb from cardiogenic shock generally exhibit either a single massive infarct or a small to moderate-sized infarct superimposed on multiple prior infarctions.[35] Survivors with large infarcts frequently exhibit late impairment of ventricular function, and the long-term mortality rate is higher than for survivors with small infarcts, who tend not to develop cardiac decompensation.

In view of the prognostic importance of infarct size, the concept that modification of infarct size is possible has attracted a great deal of experimental and clinical attention (see Chap. 50, Fig. 50-9).[28,36] Efforts to limit the size of the infarct have been divided among several different (sometimes overlapping) approaches: (1) early reperfusion, (2) reduction of myocardial energy demands, (3) manipulation of sources of energy production in the myocardium, and (4) prevention of reperfusion injury. Despite the many advances in reperfusion therapy for STEMI, practical clinical decision-making in the case of individual patients is complex. Persistent uncertainties about the risk (bleeding)-benefit balance in elderly patients and those arriving late after the onset of symptoms appear to be the major factors explaining the underuse of reperfusion for STEMI in routine practice.[37]

DYNAMIC NATURE OF INFARCTION. STEMI is a dynamic process that does not occur instantaneously but evolves over hours. The fate of jeopardized, ischemic tissue can be affected favorably by interventions that restore myocardial perfusion, reduce microvascular damage in the infarct zone, reduce myocardial oxygen requirements, inhibit accumulation of or facilitate washout of noxious metabolites, augment the availability of substrate for anaerobic metabolism, or blunt the effects of mediators of injury that compromise the structure and function of intracellular organelles and constituents of cell membranes. Strong evidence in experimental animals and suggestive evidence in patients indicate that ischemic preconditioning, a form of endogenous protection against STEMI (see Chap. 21), before sustained coronary occlusion decreases infarct size and is associated with a more favorable outcome, with decreased risk of extension of infarction and recurrent ischemic events. Brief episodes of ischemia in one coronary vascular bed may precondition myocardium in a remote zone, attenuating the size of infarction in the latter when sustained coronary occlusion occurs.[38]

The perfusion of the myocardium in the infarct zone appears to be reduced maximally immediately following coronary occlusion. Up to one third of patients develop spontaneous recanalization of an occluded infarct-related artery beginning at 12 to 24 hours. This delayed spontaneous reperfusion may improve left ventricular function because it improves healing of infarcted tissue, prevents ventricular remodeling, and reperfuses hibernating myocardium. However, to *maximize* the amount of salvaged myocardium by *accelerating* the process of reperfusion and also implementing it in those patients who would otherwise have an occluded infarct-related artery, the strategies of pharmacologically induced and catheter-based reperfusion of the infarct vessel have been developed (Fig. 51-3) (see Chap. 52). An overarching concept that applies to all methods of reperfusion is the critical importance of time. Mortality reduction from STEMI is greatest the earlier the infarct artery is reperfused.[39]

Additional factors that may contribute to limitation of infarct size in association with reperfusion include relief of coronary spasm, prevention of damage to the microvasculature, improved systemic hemodynamics (augmentation of coronary perfusion pressure and reduced left ventricular end-diastolic pressure), and development of collateral circulation. The prompt implementation of measures designed to protect ischemic myocardium and support myocardial perfusion may provide sufficient time for the development of anatomical and physiological compensatory mechanisms that limit the ultimate extent of infarction (see Chap. 50, Figs. 50-3 and 50-9). Interventions designed to protect ischemic myocardium during the initial event may also reduce the incidence of extension of infarction or early reinfarction.

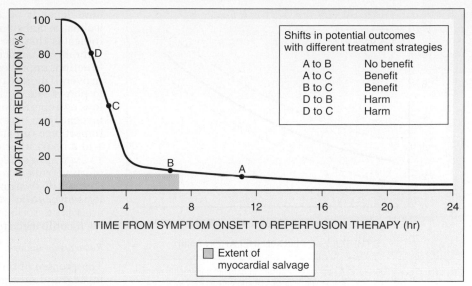

FIGURE 51–3 Mortality reduction as a benefit of reperfusion therapy is greatest in the first 2 to 3 hours after the onset of symptoms of acute myocardial infarction (MI), most likely a consequence of myocardial salvage. The exact duration of this critical early period may be modified by several factors, including the presence of functioning collateral coronary arteries, ischemic preconditioning, myocardial oxygen demands, and duration of sustained ischemia. After this early period, the magnitude of the mortality benefit is much reduced, and as the mortality reduction curve flattens, time to reperfusion therapy is less critical. The magnitude of the benefit will depend on how far up the curve the patient can be shifted. The benefit of a shift from points A or B to point C would be substantial, but the benefit of a shift from point A to point B would be small. A treatment strategy that delays therapy during the early critical period, such as patient transfer for percutaneous coronary intervention (PCI), would be harmful (shift from point D to point C or point B). *(Modified from Gersh BJ, Stone GW, White HD, Homes DR Jr: Pharmacological facilitation of primary percutaneous coronary intervention for acute myocardial infarction: Is the slope of the curve the shape of the future? JAMA 293:979, 2005.)*

ROUTINE MEASURES FOR INFARCT SIZE LIMITATION. Although reperfusion of ischemic myocardium is the most important technique for limiting infarct size, several routine measures to accomplish this goal are applicable to all patients with STEMI, whether or not reperfusion therapy is prescribed. The treatment strategies discussed in this section can be initiated in the emergency department and then continued in the coronary care unit.

It is important to maintain an optimal balance between myocardial oxygen supply and demand so that as much as possible of the jeopardized zone of the myocardium surrounding the most profoundly ischemic zones of the infarct can be salvaged. During the period before irreversible injury has occurred, myocardial oxygen consumption should be minimized by maintaining the patient at rest, physically and emotionally, and by using mild sedation and a quiet atmosphere that may lower heart rate, a major determinant of myocardial oxygen consumption. If the patient was receiving a beta blocker at the time the clinical manifestations of the infarction commenced, the drug should be continued unless a specific contraindication is noted, such as left ventricular systolic failure or bradyarrhythmia. Marked sinus bradycardia (heart rate ≤50 beats/min) and the frequently coexisting hypotension should be treated with postural maneuvers (the Trendelenburg position) to increase central blood volume and atropine and electrical pacing, but not with isoproterenol. On the other hand, the routine administration of atropine, with the resultant increase in heart rate, to patients without serious bradycardia is contraindicated. All forms of tachyarrhythmias require prompt treatment because they increase myocardial oxygen needs.[1]

Congestive heart failure should be treated promptly. Given their multiple beneficial actions in STEMI patients, inhibitors of the renin-angiotensin-aldosterone system are indicated in the treatment of congestive heart failure associated with STEMI unless the patient is hypotensive. Inotropic agents such as isoproterenol that increase myocardial oxygen consumption should be avoided.

As discussed earlier, arterial oxygenation should be restored to normal in patients with hypoxemia, such as occurs in patients with chronic pulmonary disease, pneumonia, or left ventricular failure. Oxygen-enriched air should be administered to patients with hypoxemia, and bronchodilators and expectorants should be used when indicated. Severe anemia, which can also extend the area of ischemic injury, should be corrected by the cautious administration of packed red blood cells, accompanied by a diuretic if there is any evidence of left ventricular failure. Associated conditions, particularly infections and the accompanying tachycardia, fever, and elevated myocardial oxygen needs, require immediate attention.

Systolic arterial pressure should not be allowed to deviate by more than approximately 25 to 30 mm Hg from the patient's usual level unless marked hypertension had been present before the onset of STEMI. It is likely that each patient has an optimal range of arterial pressure; as coronary perfusion pressure deviates from this level, the unfavorable balance between oxygen supply (which is related to coronary perfusion pressure) and myocardial oxygen demand (which is related to ventricular wall tension) that ensues increases the extent of ischemic injury.

Reperfusion Therapy

GENERAL CONCEPTS. Although late spontaneous reperfusion occurs in some patients, thrombotic occlusion persists in the majority of patients with STEMI while the

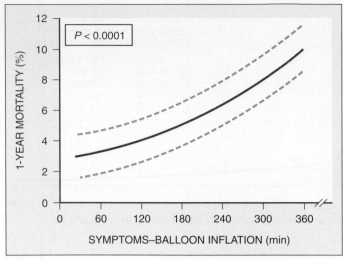

FIGURE 51–4 Importance of time to reperfusion in patients undergoing primary percutaneous coronary intervention (PCI) for ST-elevation myocardial infarction (STEMI). This plot is based on the pooled data from 1791 patients undergoing primary PCI for STEMI. After adjusting for baseline risk, there is a curvilinear relationship between the time elapsed from the onset of symptoms to balloon inflation and the rate of mortality at 1 year. For every 30-minute delay from onset of symptoms to primary PCI, there is an 8 percent increase in the relative risk of 1-year mortality. Flanking curves indicate 95% confidence intervals. *(From De Luca G, Suryapranata H, Ottervanger JP, et al: Time-delay to treatment and mortality in primary angioplasty for acute myocardial infarction: Every minute counts. Circulation 109:1223, 2004.)*

CH 51

myocardium is undergoing necrosis.[40] Timely reperfusion of jeopardized myocardium represents the most effective way of restoring the balance between myocardial oxygen supply and demand.[40] When fibrinolysis is administered, the extent of protection appears to be related directly to the rapidity with which reperfusion is implemented after the onset of coronary occlusion.[40] Evidence exists to suggest that the extent of myocardial salvage when reperfusion is achieved with PCI (including stent deployment) is less time-dependent than that for fibrinolysis.[36] The mechanisms underlying the therapy-dependent influence of time-to-treatment on myocardial salvage are not clear but probably include restoration of full antegrade flow in the infarct artery with PCI and decreasing efficacy of fibrinolytic agents as coronary thrombi mature with the passage of time.[36] Analyses adjusting for baseline risk, however, demonstrate a statistically significant increase in mortality with progressive delays between the onset of symptoms and PCI.[41,42] Each 30-minute delay from symptom onset to PCI increases by 8 percent the relative risk (RR) of 1-year mortality (Fig. 51-4).[43]

In some patients, particularly those with cardiogenic shock, tissue damage occurs in a "stuttering" manner rather than abruptly, a condition that might more properly be termed *subacute infarction*. This concept of the nature of the infarction process, as well as the observation that the incidence of complications of STEMI in both the early and late postinfarction periods is a function of infarct size, underscores the need for careful history-taking to ascertain whether the patient appears to have had repetitive cycles of spontaneous reperfusion and reocclusion. "Fixing" the time of onset of the infarction process in such patients can be difficult. In such patients with waxing and waning ischemic discomfort, a rigid time interval from the first episode of pain should not be used when determining whether a patient is "outside the window" for benefit from acute reperfusion therapy.

PATHOPHYSIOLOGY OF MYOCARDIAL REPERFUSION. Prevention of cell death by the restoration of blood flow depends on the severity and duration of preexisting ischemia. Substantial experimental and clinical evidence indicates that the earlier blood flow is restored, the more favorably influenced are recovery of left ventricular systolic function, improvement in diastolic function, and reduction in overall mortality.[44] Collateral coronary vessels also appear to play a role in the resultant left ventricular function following reperfusion.[45] They provide sufficient perfusion of myocardium to retard cell death and are probably of greater importance in patients having reperfusion later rather than 1 to 2 hours after coronary occlusion.

Even after successful reperfusion and despite the absence of irreversible myocardial damage, a period of postischemic contractile dysfunction can occur—a phenomenon referred to as *myocardial stunning*.[46] Periods of myocardial stunning are well described in experimental animals but have also been confirmed in STEMI patients using PCI.[47,48]

Reperfusion Injury

The process of reperfusion, although beneficial in terms of myocardial salvage, may come at a cost because of a process known as *reperfusion injury*. Several types of reperfusion injury have been observed in experimental animals. These consist of (1) lethal reperfusion injury—a term referring to reperfusion-induced death of cells that were still viable at the time of restoration of coronary blood flow; (2) vascular reperfusion injury—progressive damage to the microvasculature such that there is an expanding area of no reflow and loss of coronary vasodilatory reserve; (3) stunned myocardium—salvaged myocytes display a prolonged period of contractile dysfunction following restoration of blood flow because of abnormalities of intracellular metabolism leading to reduced energy production; and (4) reperfusion arrhythmias—bursts of ventricular tachycardia and on occasion ventricular fibrillation that occur within seconds of reperfusion.[49] The available evidence suggests that vascular reperfusion injury, stunning, and reperfusion arrhythmias can all occur in patients with STEMI. The concept of lethal reperfusion injury of potentially salvageable myocardium remains controversial, both in experimental animals and in patients.[49]

Reperfusion increases the cell swelling that occurs with ischemia. Reperfusion of the myocardium in which the microvasculature is damaged leads to the creation of a hemorrhagic infarct (see Chap. 50, Fig. 50-6). Fibrinolytic therapy appears more likely to produce hemorrhagic infarction than catheter-based reperfusion. Although concern has been raised that this hemorrhage may lead to extension of the infarct, this does not appear to be the case. Histological study of patients not surviving in spite of successful reperfusion has revealed hemorrhagic infarcts, but this hemorrhage usually does not extend beyond the area of necrosis.[50]

PROTECTION AGAINST REPERFUSION INJURY. A variety of adjunctive approaches may protect the myocardium against injury that occurs after reperfusion: (1) preservation of microvascular integrity by using antiplatelet agents and antithrombins to minimize embolization of atheroembolic debris; (2) prevention of inflammatory damage; and (3) metabolic support of the ischemic myocardium.[49] The effectiveness of agents directed against reperfusion injury rapidly declines the later they are administered after reperfusion[51]; eventually, no beneficial effect is detectable in animal models after 45 to 60 minutes of reperfusion has elapsed.

An alternative approach to protection against reperfusion injury is called *postconditioning*, which involves introducing brief, repetitive episodes of ischemia alternating with reperfusion. This appears to activate a number of cellular protective mechanisms centering around prosurvival kinases.[52] Many of these protective kinases are also activated during ischemic preconditioning. Clinical studies in STEMI patients undergoing PCI have provided evidence that postconditioning protects the human heart and is associated with a reduction in infarct size and improvement in myocardial perfusion (Fig. 51-5).[53]

Reperfusion Arrhythmias

Transient sinus bradycardia occurs in many patients with inferior infarcts at the time of acute reperfusion; it is most often accompanied by some degree of hypotension. This combination of hypotension and bradycardia with a sudden increase in coronary flow has been ascribed to the activation of the Bezold-Jarisch reflex.[54] Premature ventricular contractions, accelerated idioventricular rhythm, and nonsustained ventricular tachycardia are also seen commonly following successful reperfusion. Although some investigators have postulated that early afterdepolarizations participate in the genesis of reperfusion ventricular arrhythmias, early afterdepolarizations are present both during ischemia and during reperfusion and are therefore unlikely to be involved in the development of reperfusion ventricular tachycardia or fibrillation.

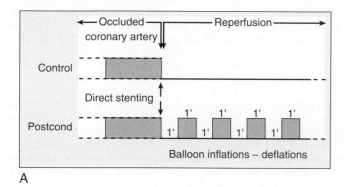

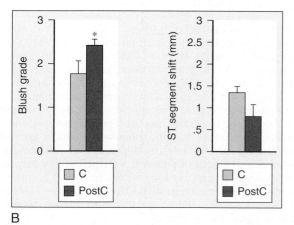

B

FIGURE 51–5 **A,** Postconditioning in ST-elevation myocardial infarction (STEMI). Experimental protocol in a clinical study of postconditioning. All patients underwent reperfusion of the occluded coronary artery by direct stenting. After reflow, control patients underwent no further intervention. In postconditioned patients, within 1 minute after direct stenting, the angioplasty balloon was reinflated 4 times during 1 minute (with a 1-minute intervening period). Thereafter, the angioplasty procedure was completed similarly in all patients. Black boxes indicate periods of ischemia. **B,** Blush grade and ST-segment shift during reperfusion. The blush grade was significantly higher in postconditioned (PostC) than in control hearts (C). At 48 hours after percutaneous transluminal coronary angioplasty (PTCA), maximal ST-segment elevation was reduced in the postconditioned group ($p = 0.09$). (From Staat P, Rioufol G, Piot C, et al: Postconditioning the human heart. Circulation 112: 2143, 2005.)

When present, rhythm disturbances may actually be a marker of successful restoration of coronary flow. However, although reperfusion arrhythmias have a high sensitivity for detecting successful reperfusion, the high incidence of identical rhythm disturbances in patients without successful coronary artery reperfusion limits their specificity for detection of restoration of coronary blood flow. In general, clinical features are poor markers of reperfusion, with no single clinical finding or constellation of findings being reliably predictive of angiographically demonstrated coronary artery patency.[1]

Although reperfusion arrhythmias may show a temporal clustering at the time of restoration of coronary blood flow in patients with successful fibrinolysis, the overall incidence of such arrhythmias appears to be similar in patients not receiving a thrombolytic agent who may develop these arrhythmias as a consequence of spontaneous coronary artery reperfusion or the evolution of the infarct process itself. These considerations, as well as the fact that the brief "electrical storm" occurring at the time of reperfusion is generally innocuous, indicate that no prophylactic antiarrhythmic therapy is necessary when fibrinolytics are prescribed.

Late Establishment of Patency of the Infarct Vessel

It has been suggested that improved survival and ventricular function after successful reperfusion are not caused entirely by limitation of infarct size. Poorly contracting or noncontracting myocardium in a zone that is supplied by a stenosed infarct-related artery with slow antegrade perfusion may still contain viable myocytes. This situation is referred to as *hibernating myocardium,*[55] and its function can be improved by PCI to augment flow in the infarct-related artery.

SUMMARY OF EFFECTS OF MYOCARDIAL REPERFUSION. Rupture of an unstable plaque in the culprit vessel produces complete occlusion of the infarct-related coronary artery. STEMI occurs with the ensuing development of left ventricular dilation and ultimate death through a combination of pump failure and electrical instability (Fig. 51-6; see also Chap. 50, Fig. 50-12). Early reperfusion shortens the duration of coronary occlusion, minimizes the degree of ultimate left ventricular dysfunction and dilation, and reduces the probability that the STEMI patient will develop pump failure or malignant ventricular tachyarrhythmias. Late reperfusion of stenosed infarct arteries may restore contractile function in hibernating myocardium.

Coronary Fibrinolysis

Many years elapsed between the first report of intracoronary clot lysis in an experimental animal and the widespread use of fibrinolytic agents in patients with STEMI. With publication of the first GISSI trial of more than 11,000 patients in 1986, in which intravenous streptokinase was shown to significantly reduce mortality in patients treated within 6 hours of the onset of symptoms, the use of fibrinolytic therapy in cases of STEMI was established.[1] It is now clear that fibrinolysis recanalizes thrombotic occlusion associated with STEMI, and restoration of coronary flow reduces infarct size and improves myocardial function and survival over both the short and the long terms.[56] The majority of the mortality benefit seen at 10-year follow-up in the GISSI trial was obtained before hospital discharge because no survival difference was seen in fibrinolysed and control patients discharged alive except for those treated within the first hour after onset of symptoms.[57]

INTRACORONARY FIBRINOLYSIS. In contemporary practice, intracoronary fibrinolysis has little place because instrumented patients are more likely to be treated by PCI (see Chap. 52).

CH 51

ST-Elevation Myocardial Infarction: Management

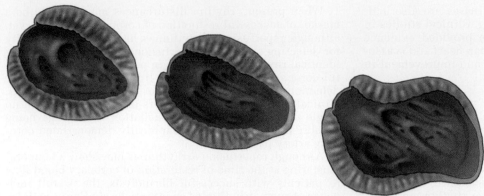

FIGURE 51-6 Remodeling of left ventricle after ST-elevation myocardial infarction (STEMI). **Left,** Apical STEMI (white zone of left ventricle). Over time, the infarct zone elongates and thins. Progressive remodeling of the left ventricle occurs **(center and right),** ultimately converting the left ventricle from an oval shape to a spherical shape. Pharmacological and catheter-based reperfusion strategies for STEMI have a favorable impact on this process by minimizing the extent of myocardial necrosis **(left)** through prompt restoration of flow in the epicardial infarct vessel. *(Modified from McMurray JJV, Pfeffer MA (eds): Heart Failure Updates. London, Martin Dunitz, 2003.)*

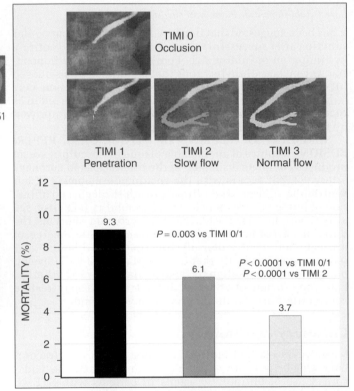

FIGURE 51-7 Correlation of TIMI flow grade and mortality. A pooled analysis of data from 5498 patients in several angiographic trials of reperfusion for ST-elevation myocardial infarction (STEMI) showed a gradient of mortality when the angiographic findings were stratified by TIMI flow grade. Patients with TIMI 0 or TIMI 1 flow had the highest rate of mortality; TIMI 2 flow was associated with an intermediate rate of mortality; and the lowest rate of mortality was observed in patients with TIMI 3 flow. TIMI = Thrombosis In Myocardial Infarction. *(Dr. Michael Gibson, personal communication.)*

Intravenous Fibrinolysis

TIMI FLOW GRADE. To provide a level of standardization for comparison of the various regimens, most investigators describe the flow in the infarct vessel according to the Thrombolysis In Myocardial Infarction (TIMI) trial grading system: grade 0, complete occlusion of the infarct-related artery; grade 1, some penetration of the contrast material beyond the point of obstruction but without perfusion of the distal coronary bed; grade 2, perfusion of the entire infarct vessel into the distal bed but with delayed flow compared with a normal artery; and grade 3, full perfusion of the infarct vessel with normal flow.[58,59] When evaluating reports of angiographic studies of fibrinolytic agents, it must be kept in mind that only in studies in which a pretreatment coronary arteriogram documents occlusion of the culprit vessel can the term *recanalization* be applied if flow is restored. If the status of the culprit vessel is not known before treatment, one can only ascertain the *patency rate* of the vessel at the moment the contrast material is injected. This snapshot in time does not reflect the fluctuating status of flow in the infarct vessel that characteristically undergoes repeated cycles of patency and reocclusion, as has been documented angiographically and by continuous ST segment monitoring.

Issues of the fluctuating nature of patency of the infarct-related artery notwithstanding, the majority of angiographic studies of reperfusion regimens for STEMI used an assessment of the TIMI flow grade at 90 or preferably 60 minutes after the start of fibrinolytic therapy.[60] TIMI grade 3 flow is far superior to grade 2 in terms of infarct size reduction and both short-term and long-term mortality benefit.[61] Therefore TIMI grade 3 flow should be considered to be the goal when assessing flow in the epicardial infarct artery (Fig. 51-7).[61]

THE TIMI FRAME COUNT. In an effort to provide a more quantitative statement of the briskness of coronary blood flow in the infarct artery and also to account for differences in the size and length of vessels (e.g., left anterior descending versus right coronary artery) and interobserver variability, Gibson and coworkers[62] developed the *TIMI frame count*—a simple count of the number of angiographic frames elapsed until the contrast material arrives in the distal bed of the vessel of interest. This objective and quantitative index of coronary blood flow independently predicts in-hospital mortality from STEMI and also discriminates patients with TIMI grade 3 flow into low- and high-risk groups.[62] Using the TIMI frame count, Gibson and coworkers[63] determined that the following were univariate predictors of delayed coronary blood flow following fibrinolytic administration: a greater percentage diameter stenosis; a decreased minimum lumen diameter; a greater percentage of the culprit artery distal to stenosis; and the presence of delayed achievement of patency, a culprit artery location in the left coronary circulation, pulsatile flow (i.e., reversible flow in systole), or intraluminal thrombus. The TIMI frame count can also be used to quantitate coronary blood flow (cc per second) calculated at

$$21 \div (\text{observed TIMI frame count}) \times 1.7$$

(based on Doppler velocity wire data showing that normal flow equals 1.7 cm^3 per second, which is proportional to 21 frames). Calculated coronary perfusion relates to mortality for patients treated with fibrinolytics or primary PCI (Fig. 51-8).

MYOCARDIAL PERFUSION. Despite intense interest in the development of reperfusion regimens that normalize flow in the epicardial infarct-related artery, the real goal of reperfusion in patients with STEMI is to improve myocardial perfusion in the infarct zone. Of course, myocardial perfusion cannot be improved adequately without restoration of flow in the occluded infarct-related artery. However, even patients with TIMI grade 3 flow may not achieve adequate myocardial perfusion, especially if there is a great delay between the onset of symptoms and restoration of epicardial flow.[64] The two major impediments to normalization of myocardial perfusion are microvascular damage (Fig. 51-9)[65] and reperfusion injury.[61] Obstruction of the distal microvasculature in the downstream bed of the infarct-related artery is caused by platelet microemboli and thrombi.[66] Microembolization of platelet aggregates may actually be exacerbated by fibrinolysis via the exposure of clot-bound thrombin, an extremely potent platelet agonist. Spasm can also occur in the microvasculature because of the release of substances from activated platelets. Reperfusion injury results in cellular edema, free radical formation, and calcium overload. In addition, cytokine activation leads to neutrophil accumulation and inflammatory mediators that contribute to tissue injury.

Several techniques can evaluate the adequacy of myocardial perfusion. Electrocardiographic ST segment resolution strongly predicts outcome in STEMI patients but is a better predictor of an occluded than of a patent infarct-related artery.[67,68] Absence of early ST segment resolution after angiographically successful primary PCI identifies patients with a higher risk of left ventricular dysfunction and mortality, presumably because of microvascular damage in the infarct zone. Thus the 12-lead ECG is a marker of the biological integrity of myocytes in the infarct zone and can reflect inadequate myocardial perfusion even in the presence of TIMI grade 3 flow.[69-71] ST-segment resolution in combination with cardiac biomarkers (troponins, natriuretic peptides) provides powerful prognostic information early in the management of STEMI patients.[72] Given the dynamic nature of coronary occlusion, it has been proposed that continuous ST segment monitoring is more informative than static 12-lead ECG recordings, but practical limitations have prevented continuous ST monitoring in widespread clinical application.[73] Defects in perfusion patterns seen with myocardial contrast echocardiography correlate with regional wall motion abnormalities and lack of myocardial viability on dobutamine stress echocardiography. A practical limitation to myocardial contrast echocardiography is the need for intracoronary injection of echo contrast, although this can be circumvented by the availability of new echo contrast agents that can be injected intravenously. Doppler flow wire studies, magnetic resonance imaging, and nuclear imaging with positron emission tomography can also define abnormalities of myocardial perfusion.

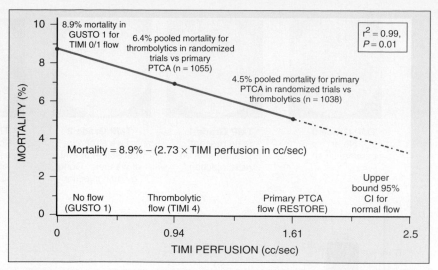

$$\text{Mortality} = 8.9\% - (2.73 \times \text{TIMI perfusion in cc/sec})$$

$r^2 = 0.99$, $P = 0.01$

FIGURE 51–8 Relationship between coronary blood flow and mortality rate in patients with acute myocardial infarction. CI = confidence interval; PTCA = percutaneous transluminal coronary angioplasty; TIMI = Thrombosis In Myocardial Infarction. *(From Gibson CM: Primary angioplasty, rescue angioplasty, and new devices. In Hennekens CH [ed]: Clinical Trials in Cardiovascular Disease: A Companion to Braunwald's Heart Disease. Philadelphia, Saunders, 1999, p 194.)*

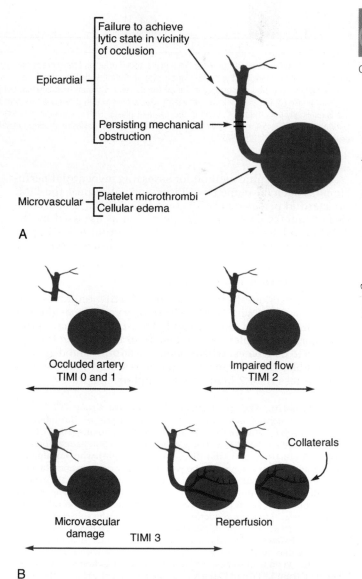

FIGURE 51–9 Patterns of response to fibrinolysis. **A,** Failure of epicardial reperfusion can occur because of failure to induce a lytic state or because of mechanical factors at the site of occlusion. Failure of microvascular reperfusion is caused by a combination of platelet microthrombi followed by endothelial swelling and myocardial edema ("no reflow"). **B,** Fibrinolysis may fail because of persistent occlusion of the epicardial infarct-related artery (TIMI grades 0 and 1), patency of an epicardial artery in the presence of impaired (TIMI grade 2) flow, or microvascular occlusion in the presence of angiographically normal (TIMI grade 3) flow. Successful reperfusion requires a patent artery with an intact microvascular network. Conversely, reperfusion may occur despite an occluded epicardial artery because of the presence of collateral arteries. TIMI = Thrombosis In Myocardial Infarction. *(From Davies CH, Ormerod OJ: Failed coronary thrombolysis. Lancet 351:1191, 1998.)*

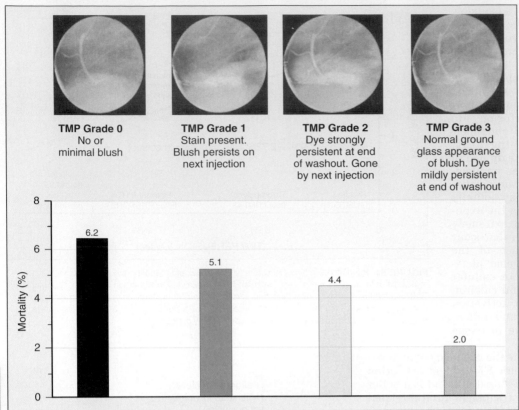

TMP Grade 0
No or
minimal blush

TMP Grade 1
Stain present.
Blush persists on
next injection

TMP Grade 2
Dye strongly
persistent at end
of washout. Gone
by next injection

TMP Grade 3
Normal ground
glass appearance
of blush. Dye
mildly persistent
at end of washout

FIGURE 51–10 Relationship between TIMI myocardial perfusion (TMP) grade and mortality. TMP grade 0 or no perfusion of the myocardium is associated with the highest rate of mortality. If the stain of the myocardium is present (grade 1), mortality is also high. A reduction in mortality is seen if the dye enters the microvasculature but is still persistent at the end of the washout phase (grade 2). The lowest mortality rate is observed in those patients with normal perfusion (grade 3) where the dye is minimally persistent at the end of the washout phase. TIMI = Thrombosis In Myocardial Infarction. *(From Gibson CM, Cannon CP, Murphy SA, et al: Relationship of TIMI myocardial perfusion grade to mortality after administration of thrombolytic drugs. Circulation 101:125, 2000.)*

An angiographic method for assessing myocardial perfusion has been developed by Gibson and colleagues: the TIMI myocardial perfusion (TMP) grade (Fig. 51-10).[74] Abnormalities of increasing myocardial perfusion as assessed by the TIMI correlate with mortality risk even after adjusting for the presence of TIMI grade 3 flow or a normal TIMI frame count.[74]

Effect of Fibrinolytic Therapy on Mortality

Early intravenous fibrinolysis undoubtedly improves survival in patients with STEMI.[1] Mortality varies considerably depending on the patients included for study and the adjunctive therapies employed. The benefit of fibrinolytic therapy appears to be greatest when agents are administered as early as possible, with the most dramatic results when the drug is given less than 2 hours after symptoms begin.[75]

The Fibrinolytic Therapy Trialists' Collaborative Group (FTT) performed a comprehensive overview of nine trials of thrombolytic therapy, each of which enrolled more than 1000 patients (Fig. 51-11).[44] The database for the FTT overview consisted of 58,600 patients including 6177 (10.5 percent) who died, 564 (1 percent) who sustained a stroke, and 436 (0.7 percent) who sustained major noncerebral bleeds. The absolute mortality rates for the control and fibrinolytic groups stratified by presenting features are shown in Figure 51-11. The overall results indicated an 18 percent reduction in short-term mortality, but as much as a 25 percent reduction in mortality for the subset of 45,000 patients with ST segment elevation or bundle branch block. Two trials, LATE and EMERAS, viewed together provide evidence that a mortality reduction may still be observed in patients treated with thrombolytic agents between 6 and 12 hours from the onset of ischemic symptoms. The data from LATE and EMERAS and the FTT overview form the basis

for extending the window of treatment with fibrinolytics up to 12 hours from the onset of symptoms. Boersma and colleagues pooled the trials in the FTT overview, two smaller studies with data on time to randomization, and 11 additional trials of more than 100 patients.[75] Patients were divided into six time categories from symptom onset to randomization. A nonlinear relationship of treatment benefit to time was observed, with the greatest benefit occurring in the first 1 to 2 hours from the onset of symptoms (Fig. 51-12).[75]

The mortality effect of fibrinolytic therapy in elderly patients is of considerable interest and controversy. Although patients older than 75 years of age were initially excluded from randomized trials of fibrinolytic therapy, they now constitute about 15 percent of the patients studied in contemporary megatrials of fibrinolysis and about 35 percent of patients analyzed in registries of STEMI patients.[76,77] Barriers to initiation of therapy in older patients with STEMI include a protracted period of delay in seeking medical care, a lower incidence of ischemic discomfort and greater incidence of atypical symptoms and concomitant illnesses, and an increased incidence of nondiagnostic ECG readings.[1] Younger patients with STEMI achieve a slightly greater relative reduction in mortality compared with elderly patients, but the higher absolute mortality in the elderly results in similar absolute mortality reductions. Thus there was a 26 percent decrease in mortality in patients who were younger than 55 years of age (11 lives saved per 1000 with thrombolytic therapy) and a 4 percent reduction in mortality in patients older than 75 years of age (10 lives saved per 1000 treated) (see Fig. 51-11).[78] Data from a Swedish national registry in patients 75 years of age or older with a first STEMI support the use of fibrinolysis in the elderly in that there was a 13 percent RR reduction ($p = 0.001$) in the composite of mortality and cerebral bleeding at 1 year compared with no fibrinolysis (Fig. 51-13).[79]

Other important baseline characteristics that have an impact on the mortality effect of fibrinolytic therapy include the vital signs at presentation and the presence of diabetes mellitus (see Fig. 51-11 and Chapter 60). For example, there was an 18 percent decrease in mortality for patients presenting with a systolic pressure less than 100 mm Hg (62 lives saved per 1000 treated), compared with a 12 percent reduction in mortality for patients with a systolic pressure of 175 mm Hg or more (10 lives saved per 1000 treated). Patients with a history of diabetes mellitus experienced a mortality reduction of 21 percent (37 lives saved per 1000 treated), compared with a mortality reduction of 15 percent (15 lives saved per 1000 treated) in patients without a history of diabetes.

A number of models have been developed to integrate the many clinical variables that affect a patient's mortality risk before administration of fibrinolytic therapy. A convenient, simple, bedside risk-scoring system for predicting 30-day mortality at presentation for fibrinolytic-eligible patients with STEMI was developed by Morrow and associates using the InTIME-II trial database (Fig. 51-14).[80,81] However, modeling of mortality risk cannot cover all clinical scenarios and should not substitute for clinical judgment in individual cases. For example, patients with inferior STEMI who might otherwise be considered to have a low risk of mortality and for whom many physicians have questioned the benefits of fibrinolytic therapy might be in a much higher mortality risk subgroup if their inferior infarction is associated with right ventricular infarction, precordial ST segment depression, or ST segment elevation in the lateral precordial leads.

The short-term survival benefit enjoyed by patients who receive fibrinolytic therapy is maintained over the 1- to 10-year follow-up.[57] Room for improvement remains, however, given reports of reocclusion rates of the infarct-related artery as high as 10 percent in hospital and up to 30 percent by 3 months,[82] and reinfarction rates as high as 9.5 percent within 6 weeks in fibrinolytic-treated patients.[83] As discussed later, advances in adjunctive antiplatelet and antithrombin therapies have led to reductions in the rate of reinfarction after fibrinolysis for STEMI.

Comparison of Fibrinolytic Agents (see Chap. 82)

Some comparative features of the approved fibrinolytic agents for intravenous therapy are presented in Table 51-4.

The tissue plasminogen activator (t-PA) molecule contains the following five domains: finger, epidermal growth factor, kringle 1 and kringle 2, and serum protease (Fig. 51-15).[84] In the absence of fibrin, t-PA is a weak plasminogen activator; fibrin provides a scaffold on

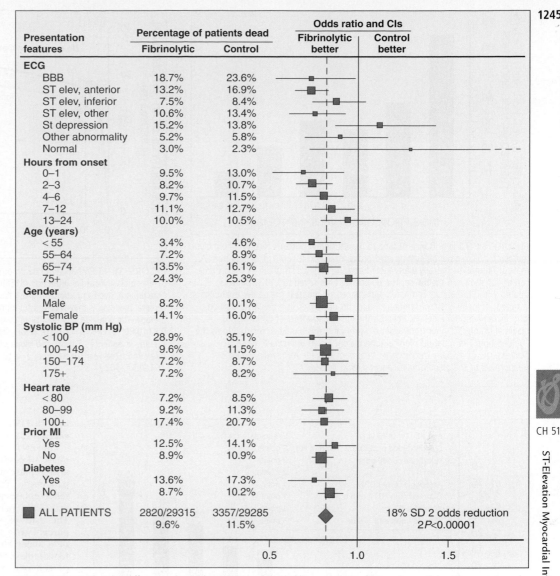

Presentation features	Percentage of patients dead		Odds ratio and CIs	
	Fibrinolytic	Control	Fibrinolytic better	Control better
ECG				
BBB	18.7%	23.6%		
ST elev, anterior	13.2%	16.9%		
ST elev, inferior	7.5%	8.4%		
ST elev, other	10.6%	13.4%		
St depression	15.2%	13.8%		
Other abnormality	5.2%	5.8%		
Normal	3.0%	2.3%		
Hours from onset				
0–1	9.5%	13.0%		
2–3	8.2%	10.7%		
4–6	9.7%	11.5%		
7–12	11.1%	12.7%		
13–24	10.0%	10.5%		
Age (years)				
< 55	3.4%	4.6%		
55–64	7.2%	8.9%		
65–74	13.5%	16.1%		
75+	24.3%	25.3%		
Gender				
Male	8.2%	10.1%		
Female	14.1%	16.0%		
Systolic BP (mm Hg)				
< 100	28.9%	35.1%		
100–149	9.6%	11.5%		
150–174	7.2%	8.7%		
175+	7.2%	8.2%		
Heart rate				
< 80	7.2%	8.5%		
80–99	9.2%	11.3%		
100+	17.4%	20.7%		
Prior MI				
Yes	12.5%	14.1%		
No	8.9%	10.9%		
Diabetes				
Yes	13.6%	17.3%		
No	8.7%	10.2%		
ALL PATIENTS	2820/29315 9.6%	3357/29285 11.5%		18% SD 2 odds reduction 2P<0.00001

0.5   1.0   1.5

FIGURE 51–11 Mortality differences during days 0 to 35 subdivided by presentation features in a collaborative overview of results from nine trials of thrombolytic therapy. The absolute mortality rates are shown for fibrinolytic and control groups in the center portion of the figure for each of the clinical features at presentation listed on the left side of the figure. The ratio of the odds of death in the fibrinolytic group to that in the control group is shown for each subdivision (colored squares), along with its 99 percent confidence interval (horizontal line). The summary OR at the bottom of the figure corresponds to an 18 percent proportional reduction in 35-day mortality and is highly statistically significant. This translates to a reduction of 18 deaths per 1000 patients treated with thrombolytic agents. BBB = bundle branch block; BP = blood pressure; CI = confidence interval; ECG = electrocardiogram; MI = myocardial infarction; SD = standard deviation. *(From Fibrinolytic Therapy Trialists' [FTT] Collaborative Group: Indications for fibrinolytic therapy in suspected acute myocardial infarction: Collaborative overview of mortality and major morbidity results from all randomized trials of more than 1000 patients. Lancet 343:311, 1994. Copyright by The Lancet Ltd.)*

which t-PA and plasminogen are held in such a way that the catalytic efficiency for plasminogen activation of t-PA is increased many-fold. Plasma clearance of t-PA is mediated to a varying degree by residues in each of the domains except the serine protease domain, which is responsible for the enzymatic activity of t-PA. The accelerated dose regimen of t-PA over 90 minutes produces more rapid thrombolysis than the standard 3-hour infusion of t-PA. The recommended dosage regimen for t-PA is a 15-mg intravenous bolus followed by an infusion of 0.75 mg/kg (maximum 50 mg) over 30 minutes, followed by an infusion of 0.5 mg/kg (maximum 35 mg) over 60 minutes.

Modifications of the basic t-PA structure have been made to yield a group of third-generation fibrinolytics (see Fig. 51-15 and Table 51-4). A common feature among the third-generation fibrinolytics is prolonged plasma clear-

ance, allowing them to be administered as a bolus rather than the bolus and double-infusion technique by which accelerated-dose t-PA is administered.[84]

RETEPLASE. This is a recombinant deletion mutant form of t-PA lacking the finger, epidermal growth factor, and kringle 1 domains, as well as the carbohydrate side chains (see Fig. 51-15 and Table 51-4).

The GUSTO III trial compared the 10 + 10 unit regimen of reteplase with accelerated t-PA in 15,059 patients.[85] The 30-day mortality rate was 7.47 percent in the reteplase group and 7.24 percent in the t-PA group corresponding to an absolute difference of 0.23 percent with a 95 percent confidence interval of −0.66 to +1.1 percent. The results of GUSTO III did not demonstrate superiority of reteplase over t-PA, and, using a 1 percent absolute difference as a boundary for equivalence, the mortality results also do not formally demonstrate equivalence.[86,87] The intracranial hemorrhage rate was 0.91 percent with reteplase and

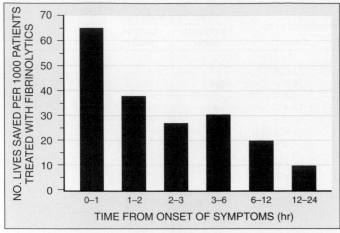

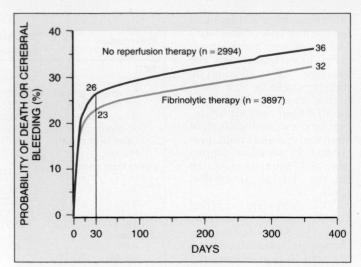

FIGURE 51–12 Importance of time to reperfusion in patients receiving fibrinolytic therapy for ST segment elevation myocardial infarction (STEMI). The data from 22 trials of fibrinolytic therapy were pooled and the findings stratified by the six time categories shown in the figure. The number of lives saved per 1000 patients treated with fibrinolytics compared with placebo is greatest the earlier treatment is initiated after the onset of symptoms, and this decreases in a nonlinear fashion with incremental time delays. Because the life-saving effect of fibrinolysis is maximal in the first hour from onset of symptoms, this has been referred to as the "golden hour" for pharmacological reperfusion. (From Boersma E, Maas AC, Deckers JW, et al: Early thrombolytic treatment in acute myocardial infarction: Reappraisal of the golden hour. Lancet 348:771, 1996.)

FIGURE 51–13 Probability of death or cerebral bleeding in elderly patients with ST-elevation myocardial infarction (STEMI). Patients older than 75 years of age entered in a Swedish national registry had significantly lower rates of death or cerebral bleeding if they received fibrinolytic therapy compared with no reperfusion therapy. The adjusted relative risk of death or cerebral bleeding through 1 year was 0.87 (0.80 to 0.94; p = 0.001). (From Stenestrand U, Wallentin L: Fibrinolytic therapy in patients 75 years and older with ST-segment-elevation myocardial infarction: One-year follow-up of a large prospective cohort. Arch Intern Med 163:965, 2003.)

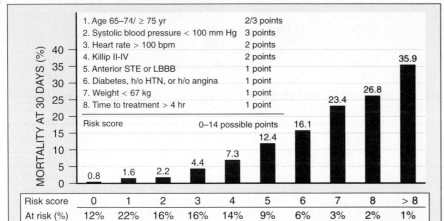

FIGURE 51–14 TIMI risk score for STE myocardial infarction predicting 30-day mortality. h/o = history of; HTN = hypertension; LBBB = left bundle branch block; STE = ST segment elevation; TIMI = Thrombosis In Myocardial Infarction. (From Morrow DA, Antman EM, Charlesworth A, et al: The TIMI risk score for ST elevation myocardial infarction: A convenient, bedside, clinical score for risk assessment at presentation: An In TIME II substudy. Circulation 102:2031, 2000.)

in both TIMI 10B and another large phase II clinical trial called ASSENT 1.[90]

ASSENT 2 was a randomized, double-blind, phase III equivalence trial comparing single bolus tenecteplase with accelerated dose t-PA in 16,949 patients.[91] The 30-day mortality rate with tenecteplase was 6.179 percent and with t-PA it was 6.151 percent (p = 0.0059 for equivalence). The rate of intracranial hemorrhage was 0.93 percent with tenecteplase and 0.94 percent with t-PA. Major bleeding occurred in 4.66 percent of tenecteplase-treated patients compared with 5.94 percent of t-PA-treated patients (p = 0.0002). There was no specific subgroup of patients in whom tenecteplase or t-PA was significantly better, with the exception of patients treated after 4 hours from the onset of symptoms, among whom the mortality rate was 7.0 percent with tenecteplase and 9.2 percent with t-PA (p = 0.018).

OTHER FIBRINOLYTIC AGENTS. *Urokinase* is used on rare occasion as an intracoronary infusion (6000 IU/min) to an average cumulative dose of 5,000,000 IU to lyse intracoronary thrombi that are believed to be responsible for an evolving STEMI.

Anistreplase, usually administered in a dose of 30 mg over 2 to 5 minutes intravenously, has a side-effect profile similar to that of streptokinase, a patency profile similar to that of conventional-dose t-PA, and a mortality benefit similar to that of streptokinase or t-PA (double-chain form, duteplase). The lack of any compelling advantages (other than bolus administration) and costs higher than streptokinase have relegated anistreplase to an extremely infrequently prescribed drug for STEMI in the United States.

Staphylokinase is a highly fibrin-specific plasminogen activator that requires priming on the surface of a clot. A pegylated, recombinant form of staphylokinase has been shown to yield TIMI grade 3 flow rates similar to those obtained with t-PA.[92]

Effect on Left Ventricular Function

Although precise measurements of infarct size would be an ideal endpoint for clinical reperfusion studies, such measures have proven impractical. Attempts to use left ventricular ejection fraction as a surrogate for infarct size have not

0.87 percent with t-PA. The secondary composite endpoint of net clinical benefit (death or disabling stroke) was 7.89 percent with reteplase and 7.91 percent with accelerated t-PA. Although GUSTO III did not fulfill formal criteria for equivalence of reteplase and t-PA, many clinicians consider the two agents to be therapeutically similar and consider the double-bolus method of administration of reteplase to be an advantage over t-PA.

TENECTEPLASE. Tenecteplase is a mutant of t-PA with specific amino acid substitutions in the kringle 1 domain and protease domain introduced to decrease plasma clearance, increase fibrin specificity, and reduce sensitivity to plasminogen activator inhibitor-1 (see Fig. 51-15 and Table 51-4). The phase II angiographic dose-ranging studies TIMI 10A and TIMI 10B helped to define the optimum dose of tenecteplase with respect to efficacy.[88,89] An analysis comparing the weight-adjusted dose of tenecteplase compared with TIMI grade 3 flow indicated that a dose of 0.53 mg/kg was optimal for achieving high rates of TIMI grade 3 flow.[89] The safety of tenecteplase was evaluated

TABLE 51–4	Comparison of Approved Fibrinolytic Agents			
	Streptokinase	**Alteplase**	**Reteplase**	**TNK-t-PA**
Dose	1.5 MU in 30-60 min	Up to 100 mg in 90 min (based on weight)	10 U × 2 (30 min apart) each over 2 min	30-50 mg based on weight*
Bolus administration	No	No	Yes	Yes
Antigenic	Yes	No	No	No
Allergic reactions (hypotension most common)	Yes	No	No	No
Systemic fibrinogen depletion	Marked	Mild	Moderate	Minimal
90-min patency rates (%)	≈50	≈75	≈75	≈75[†]
TIMI grade 3 flow (%)	32	54	60	63
Cost per dose (U.S. $)[‡]	568	2750	2750	2750 for 50 mg

*Armstrong PW, Collen D: Circulation 103:2862, 2001.
[†]Cannon CP, Gibson CM, McCabe CH, et al: Circulation 98:2805, 1998.
[‡]Medical Economics Staff: 2001 Drug Topics Red Book. 105th ed. Montvale, NJ, Medical Economics Company, 2001.
TIMI = Thrombolypsis In Myocardial Infarction; TNK = tentecteplase.
From Antman EM, Anbe DT, Armstrong PW, et al: ACC/AHA guidelines for the management of patients with ST-elevation myocardial infarction: A report of the American College of Cardiology/American Heart Association Task Force on Practice Guidelines (Committee to Revise the 1999 Guidelines for the Management of Patients with Acute Myocardial Infarction). (www.acc.org/clinical/guidelines/stemi/index.pdf). Accessed 4/19/06.

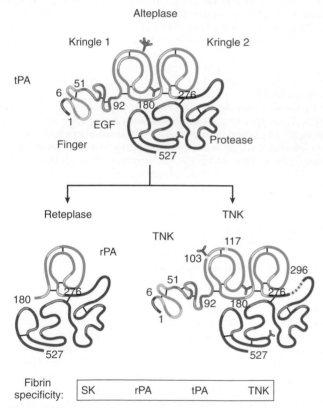

FIGURE 51–15 Molecular structure of alteplase (tPA), reteplase (rPA), and tenecteplase (TNK). Streptokinase (SK) is the least fibrin-specific thrombolytic agent in clinical use; the progressive increase in relative fibrin specificity for the various thrombolytics is shown at the bottom. *(Modified from Brener SJ, Topol EJ: Third-generation thrombolytic agents for acute myocardial infarction. In Topol EJ [ed.]: Acute Coronary Syndromes. New York, Marcel Dekker, 1998, p 169.)*

smaller volumes and better preserved ventricular shape have an improved survival. The myocardial salvage index, defined as the difference between an initial perfusion defect (e.g., by sestamibi scintigraphy) and final perfusion defect, is a useful means for comparing the effectiveness of reperfusion therapies.[93]

As with survival, improvement in global left ventricular function is related to the time of fibrinolytic treatment, with greatest improvement occurring with earliest therapy.[1] Greater improvement in left ventricular function has been reported with anterior than with inferior infarcts.[94]

Complications of Fibrinolytic Therapy

Recent (<1 year) exposure to streptococci or streptokinase produces some degree of antibody-mediated resistance to streptokinase (and anistreplase) in most patients. Although this is of clinical consequence only rarely, it is recommended that patients not receive streptokinase for STEMI if they have been treated with a streptokinase product within the past year. Bleeding complications are, of course, most common and potentially the most serious. Most bleeding is relatively minor with all agents, with more serious episodes occurring in patients requiring invasive procedures.[95] Intracranial hemorrhage is the most serious complication of fibrinolytic therapy; its frequency varies with the clinical characteristics of the patient and the fibrinolytic agent prescribed (Fig. 51-16).[1]

There have been reports of an "early hazard" with fibrinolytic therapy, that is, an excess of deaths in the first 24 hours in fibrinolytic-treated patients compared with control subjects (especially in elderly patients treated more than 12 hours).[44] However, this excess early mortality is more than offset by the deaths prevented beyond the first day, culminating in an 18 percent (range, 13 to 23 percent) reduction in mortality by 35 days.[44] The mechanisms responsible for this early hazard are not clear but are probably multiple, including an increased risk of myocardial rupture (particularly in the elderly), fatal intracranial hemorrhage,[96] inadequate myocardial reperfusion resulting in pump failure and cardiogenic shock,[97] and possible reperfusion injury of reperfused myocardium. Reports of more unusual complications such as splenic rupture, aortic dissection, and cholesterol embolization have also appeared.

been productive because little difference is seen in ejection fraction between treatment groups that show a significant difference in mortality. Methods of assessing left ventricular function, such as end-systolic volume or quantitative echocardiography, are more revealing because patients with

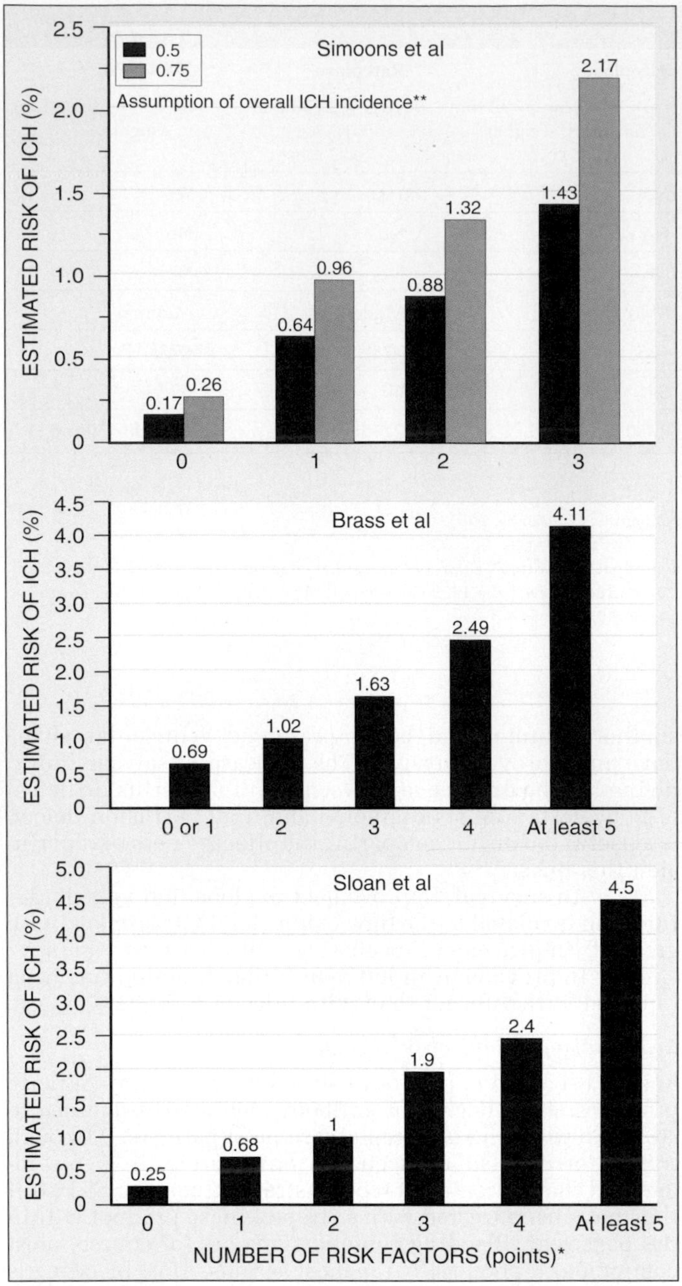

FIGURE 51–16 Estimation of risk of intracranial hemorrhage (ICH) with fibrinolysis. The number of risk factors is the sum of the points based on criteria established in the studies shown. Although the exact risk factors varied among the studies, common risk factors across all the studies include increased age, low body weight, and hypertension on admission. If the overall incidence of ICH is assumed to be 0.75 percent, patients without risk factors who receive streptokinase have a 0.26 percent probability of ICH. The risk is 0.96, 1.32, and 2.17 percent in patients with one, two, or three risk factors, respectively. See references for further discussion. *(Data from Simoons et al: Lancet 342:1523, 1993; Brass et al: Stroke 31:1802, 2000; Sloan et al: J Am Coll Cardiol:37(Suppl A):372A, 2001.)*

Recommendations for Fibrinolytic Therapy

NET CLINICAL BENEFIT OF FIBRINOLYSIS. Perhaps one of the most important messages from all of the available evidence is that fibrinolytic therapy is underutilized in patients with STEMI.[98] Hesitancy in prescribing a fibrinolytic agent is often the result of uncertainty about the risk of bleeding. Patients with a higher baseline risk of mortality are more likely to benefit from fibrinolytic therapy. Against the mortality benefit associated with fibrinolytic therapy must be weighed the excess risk of stroke. A useful concept that incorporates the benefits and risks of fibrinolytic therapy in a single composite endpoint is net clinical benefit. Thus composite endpoints such as death or nonfatal stroke; death/nonfatal MI/nonfatal major bleed may be used to compare various pharmacological reperfusion regimens.[76,85,91]

CHOICE OF AGENT. Analysis of the net clinical benefit and cost-effectiveness of one agent versus another does not easily yield recommendations for treatment because clinicians must weigh the risk of mortality and the risk of intracranial hemorrhage when confronting a fibrinolytic-eligible patient with STEMI; additional considerations may be the constraints placed on physicians' therapeutic decision-making by the health care system in which they are practicing. In the subgroup of patients presenting within 4 hours of symptom onset, the speed of reperfusion of the infarct vessel is of paramount importance, and a high-intensity fibrinolytic regimen such as accelerated t-PA is the preferred treatment, except in those individuals in whom the risk of death is low (e.g., a young patient with a small inferior MI) and the risk of intracranial hemorrhage is increased (e.g., acute hypertension), in whom streptokinase and accelerated t-PA are approximately equivalent choices. For those patients presenting between 4 and 12 hours after the onset of chest discomfort, the speed of reperfusion of the infarct vessel is of lesser importance, and therefore streptokinase and accelerated t-PA are generally equivalent options, given the difference in costs. Of note, for those patients presenting between 4 and 12 hours from symptom onset with a low mortality risk but an increased risk of intracranial hemorrhage (e.g., elderly patients with inferior MI, systolic pressure >100 mm Hg, and heart rate <100 beats/min), streptokinase is probably preferable to t-PA because of cost considerations if fibrinolytic therapy is prescribed at all in such patients.

In those patients considered appropriate candidates for fibrinolysis and in whom t-PA would have been selected as the agent of choice in the past, we believe clinicians should now consider using a bolus fibrinolytic such as reteplase or tenecteplase. The rationale for this recommendation is that bolus fibrinolysis has the advantage of ease of administration, a lower chance of medication errors (and the associated increase in mortality when such medication errors occur), and less noncerebral bleeding and also offers the potential for prehospital treatment.[99,100]

LATE THERAPY. No mortality benefit was demonstrated in the LATE and EMERAS trials when fibrinolytics were routinely administered to patients between 12 and 24 hours, although we believe it is still reasonable to consider fibrinolytic therapy in appropriately selected patients with persistent symptoms and ST elevation on the ECG beyond 12 hours. Persistent chest pain late after the onset of symptoms correlates with a higher incidence of collateral or antegrade flow in the infarct zone and is therefore a marker for patients with viable myocardium that might be salvaged. Because elderly patients treated with fibrinolytic agents more than 12 hours after the onset of symptoms are at increased risk of cardiac rupture, it is our practice to restrict late fibrinolytic administration to patients younger than 65 years of age with ongoing ischemia, especially those with large anterior infarctions. The elderly patient with ongoing ischemic symptoms but presenting late (>12 hours) is probably better managed with PCI (see Chap. 52) than with fibrinolytic therapy.

Before the institution of fibrinolytic therapy, consideration should be given to the patient's need for intravascular catheterization, as would be required for the placement of an arterial pressure monitoring line, a pulmonary artery catheter for hemodynamic monitoring, or a temporary transvenous pacemaker. If any of these are required, ideally they should be placed as expeditiously as possible *before* infusion of the fibrinolytic agent. If such procedures require an additional delay of more than 30 minutes, they should be deferred as long as possible after fibrinolytic therapy is begun. In the early hours after institution of fibrinolytic therapy, such catheterization should be performed only if crucial to the patient's survival, and then sites where excessive bleeding can be controlled should be chosen (e.g., subclavian vein catheterization should be avoided).

As noted earlier, all patients with suspected STEMI should receive aspirin (160 to 325 mg) regardless of the fibrinolytic agent prescribed. Aspirin should be continued indefinitely. The issues surrounding antithrombin therapy as an adjunct to thrombolysis are complex and are discussed in detail in a subsequent section.

Catheter-Based Reperfusion Strategies (see also Chap. 52)

Reperfusion of the infarct artery can also be achieved by a catheter-based strategy. This approach has evolved from passage of a balloon catheter over a guidewire to now include potent antiplatelet therapy (intravenous glycoprotein [GP] IIb/IIIa inhibitors, thienopyridines) and coronary stents.[1] When PCI is used in lieu of fibrinolytic therapy, it is referred to as direct or primary PCI. When fibrinolysis has failed to reperfuse the infarct vessel or a severe stenosis is present in the infarct vessel, a rescue PCI can be performed. A more conservative approach of elective PCI can be used to manage STEMI patients only when spontaneous or exercise-provoked ischemia occurs, whether or not they have received a previous course of fibrinolytic therapy.

SURGICAL REPERFUSION. Despite the extensive improvement in intraoperative preservation with cardioplegia and hypothermia and numerous surgical techniques (see Chap. 79), it is not logistically possible to provide surgical reperfusion in a timely fashion. Therefore patients with STEMI who are candidates for reperfusion routinely receive either fibrinolysis or PCI. However, about 10 to 20 percent of STEMI patients are currently referred for coronary artery bypass grafting (CABG) for one of the following indications: persistent or recurrent chest pain despite fibrinolysis or PCI, high-risk coronary anatomy (e.g., left main stenosis) discovered at catheterization, or a complication of STEMI such as ventricular septal rupture or severe mitral regurgitation caused by papillary muscle dysfunction. Patients with STEMI with continued severe ischemic and hemodynamic instability are likely to benefit from emergency revascularization. PCI with stenting as needed is the preferable technique when revascularization is needed in the first 48 to 72 hours following STEMI; surgery should be reserved for patients in whom PCI has been unsuccessful or whose anatomy dictates the need for CABG, such as patients with left main or extensive multivessel coronary artery disease.

Patients undergoing successful fibrinolysis but with important residual stenoses, who on anatomical grounds are more suitable for surgical revascularization than for PCI, have undergone CABG with quite low rates of mortality (about 4 percent) and morbidity, *provided* that they are operated on more than 24 hours from STEMI; those patients requiring urgent or emergency CABG within 24 to 48 hours of STEMI have mortality rates between 12 and 15 percent.[101] When surgery is performed under urgent conditions with active and ongoing ischemia or cardiogenic shock, the operative mortality rate rises steeply.

Selection of Reperfusion Strategy

Despite strong evidence in the literature that prompt use of reperfusion therapy improves survival of STEMI patients,

room for improvement exists because reperfusion therapy is underutilized and often not administered soon after presentation.[1] Considerable controversy exists about the optimum form of reperfusion therapy.[1] An important factor that continues to fuel this controversy is the dynamic and rapidly changing evidence base regarding the best approach to reperfusion for patients with STEMI. With respect to pharmacological reperfusion, new fibrinolytic agents, modified dosing regimens, and combinations of adjunctive treatments have produced a continuous process of refinement and improvement in medical measures to restore flow in the infarct artery (Fig. 51-17). From the perspective of PCI, improvements in catheterization laboratory facilities, new forms of stents, and distal embolization protection devices have dramatically improved the efficacy and safety of PCI for patients with STEMI (see Chap. 52). Improvements in pharmacological and PCI-based reperfusion strategies rapidly make prior studies less relevant to contemporary practice. In addition, progressive reductions in mortality from STEMI have made it increasingly difficult to conduct clinical trials of a practical size. Investigators frequently use composite endpoints that combine mortality with nonfatal events such as recurrent MI, recurrent ischemia, or target vessel revascularization. Finally, the outcomes in patients treated with primary PCI vary with the experience of the operator and the center. High-volume operators and centers can consistently achieve better outcomes in STEMI patients.[102]

In a pooled analysis of 23 randomized trials comparing PCI versus fibrinolysis for STEMI over both the short and the long terms, PCI was superior to fibrinolysis for almost all of the endpoints analyzed.[103] However, the absolute risk difference between the two reperfusion strategies varied depending on the endpoint; this translates into a wide range of patients who need to be treated (or who are harmed) to prevent one event using PCI as compared with fibrinolysis as the reperfusion strategy for patients with STEMI.

Several issues should be considered in selecting the type of reperfusion therapy:

1. *Time from the onset of symptoms to initiation of reperfusion therapy:* This is an important predictor of infarct size and patient outcome. Although infarct size is one factor that affects patient outcomes, others include the coexistence of obstructions in non–infarct-related coronary arteries; the level of electrical stability of the myocardium; the extent of left ventricular remodeling; and the number of medications prescribed following STEMI, as well as the patient's response to them. Thus for patients treated by fibrinolysis or PCI, time from the onset of symptoms is an important predictor of mortality, underscoring the need for prompt reperfusion, whichever strategy is selected (see Figs. 51-1 and 51-2).[1]

2. *Risk of STEMI:* Patients presenting with cardiogenic shock have an improved 1-year survival chance if they are treated with an early revascularization strategy (PCI and/or coronary artery bypass grafting as indicated).[104] Patients at highest risk of mortality from STEMI account for the majority of deaths from STEMI (see Fig. 51-14). Accordingly, the mortality benefit associated with PCI is largest in patients who are at highest risk of mortality; the mortality benefit of PCI decreases progressively as the patient's risk of mortality from STEMI decreases, such that the mortality advantage of PCI is no longer evident among patients whose 30-day mortality rate is estimated to be between 2 and 3 percent if treated with fibrinolytic therapy.[105]

3. *Risk of bleeding:* In patients with an increased risk of bleeding, particularly intracranial hemorrhage, therapeutic decision-making strongly favors a PCI-based reperfusion strategy (see Fig. 51-16).[106] If PCI is unavail-

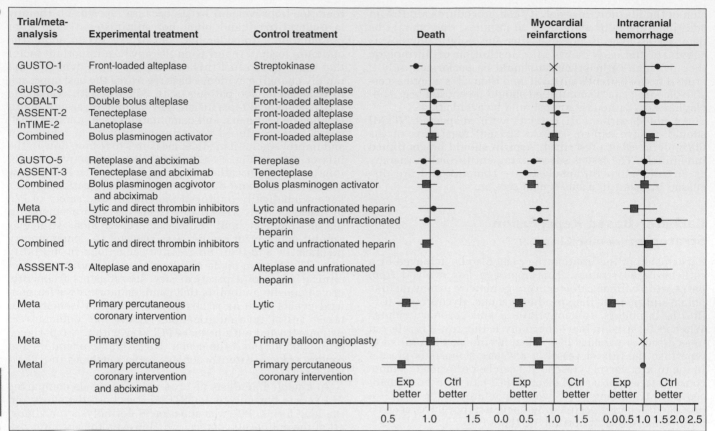

Trial/meta-analysis	Experimental treatment	Control treatment	Death	Myocardial reinfarctions	Intracranial hemorrhage
GUSTO-1	Front-loaded alteplase	Streptokinase			
GUSTO-3	Reteplase	Front-loaded alteplase			
COBALT	Double bolus alteplase	Front-loaded alteplase			
ASSENT-2	Tenecteplase	Front-loaded alteplase			
InTIME-2	Lanetoplase	Front-loaded alteplase			
Combined	Bolus plasminogen activator	Front-loaded alteplase			
GUSTO-5	Reteplase and abciximab	Rereplase			
ASSENT-3	Tenecteplase and abciximab	Tenecteplase			
Combined	Bolus plasminogen acgivotor and abciximab	Bolus plasminogen activator			
Meta	Lytic and direct thrombin inhibitors	Lytic and unfractionated heparin			
HERO-2	Streptokinase and bivalirudin	Streptokinase and unfractionated heparin			
Combined	Lytic and direct thrombin inhibitors	Lytic and unfractionated heparin			
ASSSENT-3	Alteplase and enoxaparin	Alteplase and unfrationated heparin			
Meta	Primary percutaneous coronary intervention	Lytic			
Meta	Primary stenting	Primary balloon angioplasty			
Metal	Primary percutaneous coronary intervention and abciximab	Primary percutaneous coronary intervention	Exp better / Ctrl better	Exp better / Ctrl better	Exp better / Ctrl better

0.5 1.0 1.5   0.0 0.5 1.0 1.5   0.00.51.01.52.02.5

FIGURE 51–17 Relative treatment effect associated with several acute reperfusion modalities in patients presenting with ST-elevation myocardial infarction (STEMI). Data are odds ratios and 95 percent confidence intervals. Ctrl = control. *(Modified from Boersma E, Mercado N, Poldermans, et al: Acute myocardial infarction. Lancet 361:851, 2003.)*

able, then the benefit of pharmacological reperfusion should be balanced against the risk of bleeding. A decision analysis suggests that when no PCI is available, fibrinolytic therapy should still be favored over no reperfusion treatment until the risk of a life-threatening bleed exceeds 4 percent. For patients who are not candidates for acute reperfusion because of lack of availability of PCI and contraindications to fibrinolysis, aspirin and antithrombin therapy can be prescribed.

Thus every effort should be made to provide reperfusion therapy even in clinical circumstances in which there is a perceived increase in the risk of bleeding. Arrangements for urgent primary PCI should be made for patients with a constellation of advanced age, low body weight, and hypertension on presentation because of the substantially increased risk of intracranial hemorrhage with fibrinolytic therapy. When the estimated delay to implementation of primary PCI is substantial (>90 minutes), fibrinolysis (with a fibrin-specific agent) may be preferable to no reperfusion therapy in such patients when the risk from the STEMI is high (e.g., anterior infarction with hemodynamic compromise). In the setting of absolute contraindications to fibrinolysis (see Table 51-3) and lack of access to PCI facilities, antithrombin therapy and antiplatelet therapy should be prescribed because of the small but finite chance (10 percent) of restoration of TIMI grade 3 flow in the infarct vessel and decreasing the chance of thrombotic complications of STEMI.[107]

4. *Time required for transportation to a skilled PCI center:* The greatest operational impediment to routine implementation of a PCI reperfusion strategy is the delay required for transportation to a skilled PCI center (see Figs. 51-1 and 51-2).[15] Although several trials reported that referral to a PCI center was superior to fibrinolysis administered in a local hospital, such studies were conducted in dedicated health care systems with extremely short transportation and door-to-balloon times at the PCI centers.[108-110] Evidence exists to suggest that if the delay to implementation of primary PCI is greater than 1 hour, the mortality advantage compared with administration of a fibrin-specific agent is lost.[1]

Circumstances in which fibrinolysis or PCI is the preferred reperfusion strategy are summarized in Table 51-2. The assessment of reperfusion options for STEMI is a two-step process. Step one involves the integrated assessment of the time since onset of symptoms (see Figs. 51-1, 51-2, 51-3, and 51-4), risk of STEMI (see Fig. 51-14), risk of bleeding if fibrinolysis were to be administered (see Fig. 51-16), and time required for transportation to a skilled PCI center (see Fig. 51-4 and Chap. 52). The complexities of clinical medicine do not permit the decision-making to be reduced to a simple equation or "one-size-fits-all" approach to selection of the reperfusion strategy.[110a] Instead, for step two, it is best to conceive of circumstances in which fibrinolysis is generally preferred and those in which an invasive strategy is generally preferred.

Fibrinolysis is the preferred reperfusion strategy under circumstances in which there is no ready access to a skilled PCI facility (prolonged transportation time, catheterization laboratory occupied, only inexperienced operator/team is available), PCI is not technically feasible (vascular access difficulties), or the decision-making favors initiation of lysis rather than risking the delay to PCI (door-to-balloon time >90 minutes, the difference between door-to-balloon time and prompt initiation of lysis with a fibrin-specific agent [door-to-needle time] >1 hour). When the patient presents very early after the onset of symptoms (<3 hours), either fibrinolysis or PCI is acceptable, but in most clinical circumstances fibrinolysis is preferred because of the anticipated delay to PCI, which would put the patient at risk of a substantial amount of myocardium.

An invasive strategy is generally preferred, the greater the risk. This risk may be from the STEMI itself (cardiogenic shock, Killip Class ≥ II) or from bleeding if fibrinolysis were prescribed. When a skilled PCI operator/team is available and can implement an invasive strategy without undue delay (door-to-balloon time <90 minutes or within 1 hour of the time a fibrinolytic agent could be administered), it is preferable to take the STEMI patient to the catheterization laboratory rather than administer fibrinolysis. Because of the increased risk of intracranial hemorrhage with fibrinolysis with advanced age, the elderly patient is probably better treated with PCI, provided there is no excessive delay. As coronary thrombi mature over time, they become increasingly resistant to fibrinolysis. Thus PCI is the preferred reperfusion strategy if more than 3 hours have elapsed from the onset of symptoms, again assuming there is no significant delay in the anticipated time to balloon inflation (see Fig. 51-4). Finally, when the diagnosis is in doubt, an invasive strategy is clearly the preferred strategy because it not only provides key diagnostic information regarding the patient's symptoms but does so without the risk of intracranial hemorrhage associated with fibrinolysis.

Antithrombin and Antiplatelet Therapy

Antithrombin Therapy

The rationale for administering antithrombin therapy acutely in STEMI patients includes prevention of deep venous thrombosis, pulmonary embolism, ventricular thrombus formation, and cerebral embolization. In addition, establishing and maintaining patency of the infarct-related artery, whether or not a patient receives fibrinolytic therapy, is another common rationale for antithrombin therapy in cases of STEMI (Fig. 51-18).

EFFECT ON MORTALITY. Randomized trials in STEMI patients conducted in the prefibrinolytic era showed that the risks of pulmonary embolism, stroke, and reinfarction were reduced in patients who received intravenous heparin,

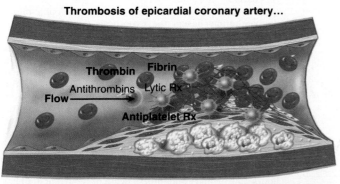

Thrombosis of epicardial coronary artery...

...the cause of STEMI

FIGURE 51–18 Pharmacological dissolution of thrombus in infarct-related artery. This figure shows a schematic view of a longitudinal section of an infarct-related artery at the level of the obstructive thrombus. Following rupture of a vulnerable plaque **(bottom center)**, the coagulation cascade is activated, ultimately leading to the deposition of fibrin strands (blue curvilinear arcs); platelets are activated and begin to aggregate (transition from flat discs representing inactive platelets to green spiked ball elements representing activated and aggregating platelets). The mesh of fibrin strands and platelet aggregates obstructs flow (normally moving from left to right) in the infarct-related artery; this would correspond to TIMI grade 0 on angiography. Pharmacological reperfusion is a multipronged approach consisting of fibrinolytic agents that digest fibrin, antithrombins that prevent the formation of thrombin and inhibit the activity of thrombin that is formed, and antiplatelet therapy. STEMI = ST-elevation myocardial infarction; TIMI = Thrombosis In Myocardial Infarction. (*Courtesy of Luke Wells, The Exeter Group.*)

providing the support for prescription of heparin to STEMI patients not treated with fibrinolytic therapy. With the introduction of the fibrinolytic era and, importantly, after the publication of the ISIS-2 trial,[111] the situation became more complicated because of strong evidence of a substantial mortality reduction with aspirin alone and confusing and conflicting data regarding the risk-benefit ratio of heparin used as an adjunct to aspirin or in combination with aspirin and a fibrinolytic agent. For every 1000 patients treated with heparin compared with aspirin alone, there are five fewer deaths ($p = 0.03$) and three fewer recurrent infarctions ($p = 0.04$), at the expense of three more major bleeds ($p = 0.001$).[112]

OTHER EFFECTS. A number of angiographic studies have examined the role of heparin therapy in establishing and maintaining patency of the infarct-related artery in patients with STEMI. Comparison of these trials is difficult because of potentially important differences in study design including whether aspirin was administered along with heparin, the fibrinolytic agent that was administered, and variations in the time of diagnostic coronary arteriography. Although the evidence favoring the use of heparin for enhancing patency of the infarct artery when a fibrin-specific fibrinolytic agent is prescribed is not conclusive, the suggestion of a mortality benefit and amelioration of the pattern of left ventricular thrombus (less protuberant) that develops after STEMI indicates it is prudent to use heparin for at least 48 hours after fibrinolysis and to maintain an activated partial thromboplastin time (aPTT) target of one-and-a-half to two times that of control.[1,113]

Although heparin may induce thrombocytopenia through an immunological mechanism, this is seen only rarely, probably occurring in only 2 to 3 percent of patients.[114] The most serious complication of antithrombotic therapy is bleeding, especially intracranial hemorrhage, when fibrinolytic agents are prescribed. Major hemorrhagic events occur more frequently in patients of low body weight, advanced age, female gender, marked prolongation of the aPTT (>90 to 100 seconds), and the performance of invasive procedures.[113] Frequent monitoring of the aPTT (facilitated by use of a bedside testing device) reduces the risk of major hemorrhagic complications in patients treated with heparin. It should be noted, however, that during the first 12 hours following fibrinolytic therapy, the aPTT may be elevated from the fibrinolytic agent alone (particularly if streptokinase is administered), making it difficult to accurately interpret the effects of a heparin infusion on the patient's coagulation status.

New Antithrombotic Agents

Potential disadvantages of unfractionated heparin include dependency on antithrombin III for inhibition of thrombin activity, sensitivity to platelet factor 4, inability to inhibit clot-bound thrombin, marked interpatient variability in therapeutic response, and the need for frequent aPTT monitoring. In an effort to circumvent these disadvantages of unfractionated heparin, there has been interest in the development of novel antithrombotic compounds.[115]

HIRUDIN AND BIVALIRUDIN. Direct thrombin inhibitors such as hirudin or bivalirudin have not been shown to reduce mortality compared with heparin when used as adjuncts to fibrinolysis.[116] Although recurrent MI is reduced by 25 to 30 percent compared with heparin, this benefit is primarily observed during the period of administration of the direct thrombin inhibitor and decreases in magnitude over time. In addition, both hirudin and bivalirudin have been associated with higher rates of major bleeding versus heparin when used with fibrinolytic agents.[116]

LOW-MOLECULAR-WEIGHT HEPARINS. Advantages of low-molecular-weight heparins include a stable, reliable anticoagulant effect, high bioavailability, permitting administration via the subcutaneous route, and a high antiXa-to-antiIIa ratio, producing blockade of the coagulation cascade in an upstream location, resulting in a marked decrement in thrombin generation. Compared with unfractionated heparin, the rate of early (60 to 90 minutes) reperfusion of the infarct artery, either assessed angiographically or by noninvasive means, is not enhanced by administration of a low-molecular-weight heparin.[117-119] However, the rates of reocclusion of the infarct artery, reinfarction, or recurrent ischemic events appear to be reduced by low-molecular-weight heparins.

The CREATE Investigators studied the effects of the low-molecular-weight heparin reviparin compared with placebo in 15,570 patients with STEMI, 73 percent of whom received a fibrinolytic (predominantly a non–fibrin-specific agent).[120] The primary composite outcome of death, recurrent MI, or stroke was reduced by 13 percent both at 7 days ($p = 0.005$) and 30 days ($p = 0.001$) with reviparin. The AMI-SK investigators reported that ST resolution at 90 and 180 minutes, as well as angiographic patency, was improved in streptokinase-treated STEMI patients who received enoxaparin compared with placebo.[118] These observations support the concepts that antithrombin therapy is a useful adjunct to a pharmacological reperfusion regimen and that low-molecular-weight heparins are clinically effective in STEMI.[121,122]

The ASSENT-3 trial compared unfractionated heparin with enoxaparin (30 mg intravenous bolus followed by subcutaneous injections of 1 mg/kg every 12 hours until hospital discharge).[123] The composite endpoint of 30-day mortality, in-hospital reinfarction, or in-hospital refractory ischemia was reduced from 15.4 percent with unfractionated heparin to 11.4 percent with enoxaparin (RR, 0.74; 95 percent CI, 0.63 to 0.87). The rate of intracranial hemorrhage was similar with unfractionated heparin versus enoxaparin (0.93 percent versus 0.88 percent; $p = 0.98$). The ASSENT-3 PLUS study compared the same unfractionated heparin and enoxaparin regimens but initiated therapy in the prehospital setting.[124] The composite endpoint of 30-day mortality, in-hospital reinfarction, or in-hospital refractory ischemia was reduced from 17.4 percent with unfractionated heparin to 14.2 percent with enoxaparin ($p = 0.08$). Of concern, however, was the increased rate of intracranial hemorrhage observed in ASSENT-3 PLUS: 1 percent with unfractionated heparin versus 2.2 percent with enoxaparin ($p = 0.05$). The increase in intracranial hemorrhage in ASSENT-3 PLUS was seen predominantly in patients older than 75 years of age: 0.8 percent with unfractionated heparin versus 6.7 percent with enoxaparin ($p = 0.01$).

The ExTRACT-TIMI 25 trial tested in a double-blind, double-dummy design the hypothesis that a strategy of enoxaparin administered for the duration of the index hospitalization was superior to the conventional antithrombin strategy of unfractionated heparin for 48 hours after fibrinolysis.[76] The enoxaparin dosing strategy was adjusted according to the patient's age and renal function. For patients younger than 75 years of age, enoxaparin (or matching placebo) was to be given as a fixed, 30-mg intravenous bolus followed 15 minutes later by a subcutaneous injection of 1 mg per kilogram, with injections administered every 12 hours. For patients at least 75 years of age, the intravenous bolus was eliminated and the subcutaneous dose was reduced to 0.75 mg per kilogram every 12 hours. The primary endpoint of death or recurrent nonfatal MI through 30 days occurred in 12 percent of patients in the unfractionated heparin group and 9.9 percent of those in the enoxaparin group (17 percent reduction in RR; $p < 0.001$). Nonfatal reinfarction occurred in 4.5 percent of the patients receiving unfractionated heparin and 3 percent of those receiving enoxaparin (33 percent reduction in RR; $p < 0.001$); 7.5 percent of patients given unfractionated heparin died, as did 6.9 percent of those given enoxaparin ($p = 0.11$). The composite of death, nonfatal reinfarction, or urgent revascularization occurred in 14.5 percent of patients given unfractionated heparin and 11.7 percent of those given enoxaparin ($p < 0.001$); major bleeding occurred in 1.4 percent and 2.1 percent, respectively ($p < 0.001$) (Fig. 51-19). The composite of death, nonfatal reinfarction, or nonfatal intracranial hemorrhage (a

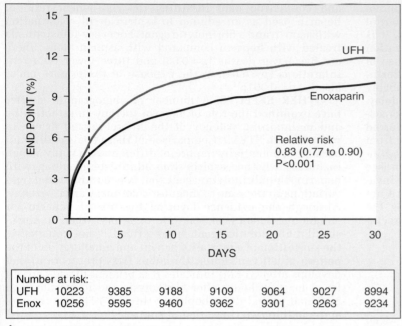

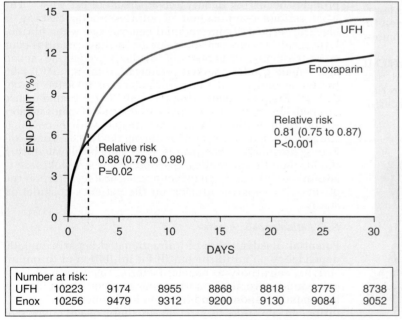

FIGURE 51–19 Comparison of enoxaparin with unfractionated heparin as adjunctive therapy in ST-elevation myocardial infarction (STEMI) patients receiving fibrinolysis. **A,** The rate of the primary endpoint (death or nonfatal myocardial infarction) at 30 days was significantly lower in the enoxaparin (Enox) group than in the unfractionated heparin (UFH) group (9.9 versus 12 percent, $p < 0.001$ by the log-rank test). The dashed vertical line indicates the comparison at day 2 (direct pharmacological comparison), at which time a trend in favor of enoxaparin was seen. **B,** The rate of the main secondary endpoint (death, nonfatal myocardial infarction, or urgent revascularization) at 30 days was significantly lower in the Enox group than in the UFH group (11.7 versus 14.5 percent, $p < 0.001$ by the log-rank test). The difference was already significant at 48 hours (6.1 percent in the UFH group versus 5.3 percent in the Emox group, $p = 0.02$ by the log-rank test). The interval shown is the time (in 24-hour intervals) from randomization to an event or the last follow-up visit. *(From Antman EM, Morrow DA, McCabe CH, et al: Enoxaparin versus unfractionated heparin with fibrinolysis for ST-elevation myocardial Infarction. N Engl J Med 354: 1477, 2006.)*

measure of net clinical benefit) occurred in 12.2 percent of patients given unfractionated heparin and 10.1 percent of those given enoxaparin ($p < 0.001$).[76]

FACTOR Xa ANTAGONISTS. The OASIS-6 trial evaluated the specific factor Xa antagonist fondaparinux (2.5 mg subcutaneously) in 12,092 patients with STEMI.[125] The trial design compared fondaparinux given for 8 days versus placebo in patients when the treating physician felt unfractionated heparin was not indicated (stratum I) and versus unfractionated heparin for 48 hours when the treating physician felt heparin was indicated (stratum II). The primary endpoint, death or reinfarction, occurred in 14 percent of placebo patients and 11.2 percent of fondaparinux patients in stratum I (HR 0.79; 0.68 to 0.92), and in 8.7 percent of unfractionated heparin patients and 8.3 percent of fondaparinux patients (HR 0.96; 0.81 to 1.13). Thus fondaparinux was superior to placebo (stratum I) but yielded similar results to those achieved with unfractionated heparin (stratum II). The outcome of patients in stratum II who underwent PCI tended to be worse when fondaparinux was used compared with unfractionated heparin, probably because of an increased risk of catheter thrombosis when fondaparinux is administered without coadministration of another antithrombin that has anti IIa activity. Severe hemorrhage occurred in 1.3 percent of control patients and 1 percent of fondaparinux patients through 9 days ($p = 0.13$).

RECOMMENDATIONS FOR ANTITHROMBIN THERAPY

Given the pivotal role thrombin plays in the pathogenesis of STEMI, antithrombotic therapy remains an important intervention (see Fig. 51-18). A regimen of intravenous unfractionated heparin bolus at 60 U/kg to a maximum of 4000 U, followed by an initial infusion of 12 U/kg/hr to a maximum of 1000 U/hr given for 48 hours has established efficacy in patients receiving fibrinolytic therapy. However, infusions of unfractionated heparin are cumbersome to administer and provide unreliable levels of anticoagulation requiring frequent measurements of aPTT to adjust the infusion rate. Thus it is clinically quite attractive to identify alternatives to the standard unfractionated heparin regimen.[115]

A lesson learned from both ExTRACT-TIMI 25 and OASIS 6 is that more prolonged administration of an antithrombin for the duration of the index hospitalization is beneficial compared with the prior practice of administering unfractionated heparin only for 48 hours unless clear-cut indications for continued anticoagulation were present. Given the superiority of a strategy of enoxaparin throughout the index hospitalization compared with unfractionated heparin for 48 hours, coupled with the ease of subcutaneous administration, and the smooth transition between the medical phase of management and PCI phase of management of STEMI (because enoxaparin can be used to support interventional procedures), enoxaparin is now the preferred antithrombin to support fibrinolysis. The benefits of enoxaparin over unfractionated heparin are evident regardless of the type of fibrinolytic administered (streptokinase or fibrin-specific) and across a wide range of patient subgroups. An initial intravenous bolus of 30 mg should be administered, followed by subcutaneous injections of 1 mg/kg every 12 hours for patients younger than age 75; for patients age 75 and older the initial intravenous bolus should be omitted and the maintenance dose should be 0.75 mg/kg every 12 hours; if the estimated creatinine clearance is less than 30 ml/min, the maintenance dose should be 1 mg/kg every 24 hours.

The role of fondaparinux in patients with STEMI is uncertain. As anticipated, fondaparinux was superior to placebo in OASIS 6. However, contemporary practice involves the administration of an antithrombin to STEMI patients, so a comparison to placebo is of limited clinical relevance. Although the convenience of once-daily subcutaneous injections of fondaparinux may be attractive compared with unfractionated heparin, the need for coadministration of an additional antithrombin with

antiIIa activity if a PCI is performed in a patient treated with fondaparinux complicates its use. Further information regarding the appropriate dosing of additional antithrombins along with fondaparinux in the catheterization laboratory, as well as additional information regarding the benefits and risks of fondaparinux across a broad range of fibrinolytics, is necessary before its role in the management of STEMI can be properly established.

In patients with known heparin-induced thrombocytopenia, it is reasonable to consider bivalirudin as a useful alternative to heparin to be used in conjunction with streptokinase. Dosing according to the HERO 2 regimen (a bolus of 0.25 mg/kg followed by an intravenous infusion of 0.5 mg/kg/hr for the first 12 hours and 0.25 mg/kg/hr for the subsequent 36 hours) is recommended but with a reduction in the infusion rate if the aPTT is greater than 75 seconds within the first 12 hours.[126] (Bivalirudin is currently indicated only for anticoagulation in patients with unstable angina who are undergoing percutaneous coronary angioplasty, but in view of the limited alternatives available to clinicians when treating patients with heparin-induced thrombocytopenia, the recommendation noted earlier should be considered.)

For patients who are referred for CABG, the preferred antithrombin is unfractionated heparin. When an alternative antithrombin has been used, it should be discontinued prior to surgery with a sufficiently long interval to avoid double anticoagulation when the patient enters the operating room and receives unfractionated heparin.

Antiplatelet Therapy

Platelets play a major role in the response to disruption of a coronary artery plaque, especially in the early phase of thrombus formation (Fig. 51-20).[127] Platelets are also activated in response to fibrinolysis, and platelet-rich thrombi are more resistant to fibrinolysis than are fibrin and erythrocyte-rich thrombi (see Fig. 51-18).[128] Thus there is a sound scientific basis for inhibiting platelet aggregation in *all* STEMI patients, regardless of whether a fibrinolytic agent is prescribed. Comprehensive overviews of randomized trials of antiplatelet therapy have summarized the overwhelming evidence of benefit of antiplatelet therapy for a wide range of vascular disorders.[129] In patients at risk for STEMI, patients with a documented prior STEMI, and patients in the acute phase of STEMI, there is a 22 percent reduction in the odds of the composite endpoint of death, nonfatal recurrent infarction, and nonfatal stroke with antiplatelet therapy (Fig. 51-21). Not unexpectedly, the absolute benefits are greatest in those patients at highest baseline risk. Although several antiplatelet regimens have been evaluated, the agent most extensively tested has been aspirin, and this is also the drug for which the most compelling evidence of benefit exists.

The ISIS-2 study was the largest trial of aspirin in STEMI patients; it provides the single strongest piece of evidence that aspirin reduces mortality in STEMI patients.[111] In contrast to the observations of a time-dependent mortality effect of fibrinolytic therapy, the mortality reduction with aspirin was similar in patients treated within 4 hours (25 percent reduction in mortality), between 5 and 12 hours (21 percent reduction), and between 13 and 24 hours (21 percent reduction). There was an overall 23 percent reduction in mortality from aspirin in ISIS-2 that was largely additive to the 25 percent reduction in mortality from streptokinase, so patients receiving both therapies experienced a 42 percent reduction in mortality.[111] The mortality reduction was as high as 53 percent in those patients who received both aspirin and streptokinase within 6 hours of symptoms. Of particular interest was the finding that the combination of streptokinase and aspirin reduced mortality *without* increasing the risk of stroke or hemorrhage.

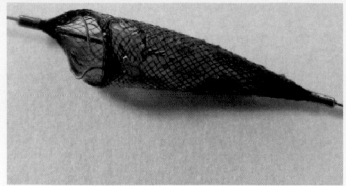

A

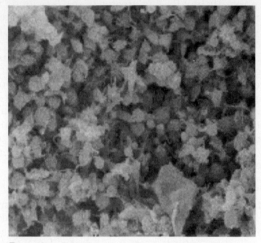

B

FIGURE 51–20 Importance of platelet aggregation early in ST-elevation myocardial infarction (STEMI). A 46-year-old man presented with STEMI resulting from occlusion of the right coronary artery. At the time of primary percutaneous coronary intervention, which was performed within 90 minutes of the onset of symptoms, a nonocclusive distal protection filter was placed downstream from the obstruction in the infarct artery. Macroscopically **(A)** the obstructing thrombus was white. Scanning electron microscopy at high (×2000) magnification **(B)** showed a platelet-rich thrombus without fibrin or erythrocytes. This case emphasizes the important role of platelet activation and aggregation early after the onset of disruption of a coronary artery plaque and underscores the necessity for antiplatelet therapy in STEMI patients. *(Modified from Beygui F, Collet JP, Nagaswami C, et al: Images in cardiovascular medicine. Architecture of intracoronary thrombi in ST-elevation acute myocardial infarction: Time makes the difference. Circulation 113: e 21, 2006.)*

Obstructive arterial thrombi that are platelet-rich are resistant to fibrinolysis and have an increased tendency to produce reocclusion after initial successful reperfusion in patients with STEMI. Despite the inhibition of cyclooxygenase by aspirin, platelet activation continues to occur through thromboxane A_2–independent pathways, leading to platelet aggregation and increased thrombin formation. The addition of other antiplatelet agents to aspirin has been proven to benefit patients with STEMI. Inhibitors of the P_2Y_{12} ADP receptor help prevent activation and aggregation of platelets. The addition of the P_2Y_{12} inhibitor clopidogrel to background treatment with aspirin to STEMI patients in the CLARITY-TIMI 28 trial reduced the risk of clinical events (death, reinfarction, stroke) and in patients receiving fibrinolytic therapy and prevented reocclusion of a successfully reperfused infarct artery (Fig. 51-22).[130] An ST Resolution (STRes) ECG substudy from the CLARITY-TIMI 28 trial provided insight into the mechanism of the benefit of clopidogrel in STEMI (Fig. 51-23).[131] There was no difference in the rate of complete STRes between the clopidogrel and placebo groups at 90 minutes (38.4 percent vs. 36.6 percent at 90 minutes).

When patients were stratified by STRes category, treatment with clopidogrel resulted in greater benefit among those with evidence of early STRes, with greater odds of an open artery at late angiography in patients with partial (odds ratio [OR] 1.4, $p = 0.04$) or complete (OR 2, $p = 0.001$) STRes, but no improvement in those with no STRes at 90 min (OR 0.89, $p = 0.48$) (p for interaction 0.003) (Fig. 51-23A). Clopidogrel was also associated with a significant reduction in the odds of an in-hospital death or MI in patients who achieved partial (OR 0.30, $p = 0.003$) or complete STRes at 90 minutes (OR 0.49, $p = 0.056$), whereas clinical benefit was not apparent in patients who had no STRes (OR 0.98, $p = 0.95$) (p for interaction 0.027) (Fig. 51-23B). Thus it appears that clopidogrel did not increase the rate of complete opening of occluded infarct arteries when fibrinolysis was administered but was highly effective in preventing reocclusion of an initially reperfused infarct artery. An analysis of patients who underwent PCI in the CLARITY-TIMI 28 trial showed that pretreatment with clopidogrel significantly reduced the incidence of cardiovascular death, MI, or stroke following PCI (34 [3.6 percent] versus 58 [6.2 percent]; adjusted OR, 0.54 [95 percent CI, 0.35-0.85]; $p = 0.008$).[132] Pretreatment with clopidogrel also reduced the incidence of MI or stroke prior to PCI (37 [4 percent] versus 58 [6.2 percent]; OR, 0.62 [95 percent CI, 0.40 to 0.95]; $p = 0.03$). There was no significant excess in the rates of TIMI major or minor bleeding (18 [2 percent] versus 17 [1.9 percent]; $p = 0.99$).

In the COMMIT trial, 45,852 patients with suspected MI were randomized to clopidogrel 75 mg/day (without a loading dose) or placebo in addition to aspirin 162 mg/day (see Fig. 51-22).[133] The patients in the clopidogrel group had a lower rate of the composite endpoint of death, reinfarction, or stroke (9.2 percent versus 10.1 percent; $p = 0.002$). They also had a significantly lower rate of death (7.5 percent versus 8.1 percent; $p = 0.03$). No excess of bleeding with clopidogrel occurred in this trial.

COMBINATION PHARMACOLOGICAL REPERFUSION. Several studies evaluated the combination of GP IIb/IIIa inhibitors and fibrinolytics.[60,134] The first series of trials combined full doses of thrombolytic agents with IIb/IIIa inhibitors.[135-138] Although these initial trials provided proof of the concept that the addition of an intravenous GP IIb/IIIa inhibitor enhanced the efficacy of a full dose of a fibrinolytic agent, unacceptably high rates of major bleeding were observed.

The combination of a reduced dose of a fibrinolytic agent and IIb/IIIa inhibitor was tested in a subsequent series of trials.[60,139-143] The rates of TIMI grade 3 flow at 60 and 90 minutes were only slightly higher with combination reperfusion compared with full-dose fibrinolytic monotherapy. These trials generally showed improved myocardial perfusion reflected in enhanced ST segment resolution and faster angiographic frame counts.[139,141,142,144]

The GUSTO V trial tested half-dose reteplase (5 U and 5 U) and full-dose abciximab compared with full-dose reteplase (10 U and 10 U) in 16,588 patients in the first 6 hours of STEMI.[145] Thirty-day mortality rates were similar in the two treatment groups (5.9 percent versus 5.6 percent). However, nonfatal reinfarction and other complications of MI were reduced in the group receiving combination reperfusion therapy. Although the rates of intracranial hemorrhage were the same in the two treatment groups (0.6 percent), moderate to severe bleeding was significantly increased from 2.3 percent to 4.6 percent with combination reperfusion therapy ($p < 0.001$). This excess bleeding risk appeared to be limited to patients older than 75 years of age. The greatest mortality benefit was observed in those patients who presented with anterior MI.

The ASSENT-3 trial randomized 6095 patients with STEMI to full-dose tenecteplase with unfractionated heparin

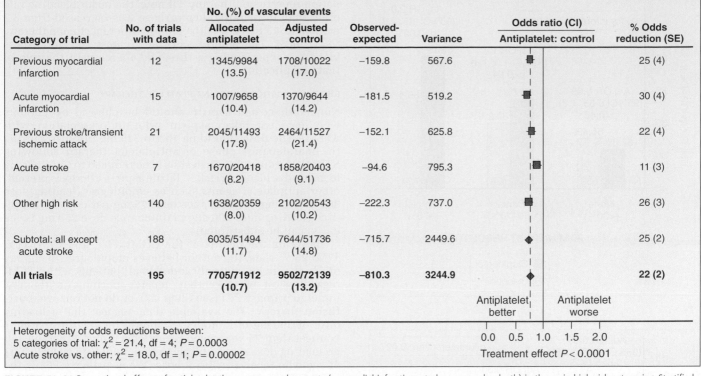

Category of trial	No. of trials with data	No. (%) of vascular events		Observed-expected	Variance	Odds ratio (CI) Antiplatelet: control	% Odds reduction (SE)
		Allocated antiplatelet	Adjusted control				
Previous myocardial infarction	12	1345/9984 (13.5)	1708/10022 (17.0)	−159.8	567.6		25 (4)
Acute myocardial infarction	15	1007/9658 (10.4)	1370/9644 (14.2)	−181.5	519.2		30 (4)
Previous stroke/transient ischemic attack	21	2045/11493 (17.8)	2464/11527 (21.4)	−152.1	625.8		22 (4)
Acute stroke	7	1670/20418 (8.2)	1858/20403 (9.1)	−94.6	795.3		11 (3)
Other high risk	140	1638/20359 (8.0)	2102/20543 (10.2)	−222.3	737.0		26 (3)
Subtotal: all except acute stroke	188	6035/51494 (11.7)	7644/51736 (14.8)	−715.7	2449.6		25 (2)
All trials	**195**	**7705/71912 (10.7)**	**9502/72139 (13.2)**	**−810.3**	**3244.9**		**22 (2)**

Antiplatelet better | Antiplatelet worse

0.0 0.5 1.0 1.5 2.0

Treatment effect P< 0.0001

Heterogeneity of odds reductions between:
5 categories of trial: χ^2 = 21.4, df = 4; P = 0.0003
Acute stroke vs. other: χ^2 = 18.0, df = 1; P = 0.00002

FIGURE 51–21 Proportional effects of antiplatelet therapy on vascular events (myocardial infarction, stroke, or vascular death) in the main high-risk categories. Stratified ratio of odds of an event in treatment groups to that in control groups is plotted for each group of trials (square) along with its 99 percent confidence interval (horizontal line). Meta-analysis of results for all trials (and 95 percent confidence interval) is represented by a diamond. *(From Antithrombotic Trialists' Collaboration: Collaborative meta-analysis of randomised trials of antiplatelet therapy for prevention of death, myocardial infarction, and stroke in high-risk patients. BMJ 324:71, 2002.)*

FIGURE 51–22 Impact of addition of clopidogrel to aspirin (ASA) in ST-elevation myocardial infarction (STEMI) patients. **A,** Effects of the addition of clopidogrel in patients receiving fibrinolysis for STEMI. Patients in the clopidogrel group (N = 1752) had a 36 percent reduction in the odds of dying, sustaining a recurrent infarction, or having an occluded infarct artery compared to the placebo group (N = 1739) in the CLARITY-TIMI 28 trial. *(Modified from Sabatine MS, Cannon CP, Gibson, CM, et al: Addition of clopidogrel to aspirin and fibrinolytic therapy for myocardial infarction with ST-segment elevation. N Engl J Med 352:1179, 2005.)* **B,** Effect of the addition of clopidogrel on in-hospital mortality after STEMI. These time-to-event curves show a 0.6 percent reduction in mortality in the group receiving clopidogrel plus aspirin (N = 22,961) compared with placebo plus aspirin (N = 22,891) in the COMMIT trial. *(Modified from Chen ZM, Jiang LX, Chen YP, et al: Addition of clopidogrel to aspirin in 45,852 patients with acute myocardial infarction: Randomised placebo-controlled trial. Lancet 366:1607, 2005.)*

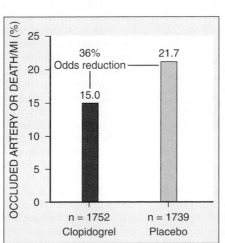

A

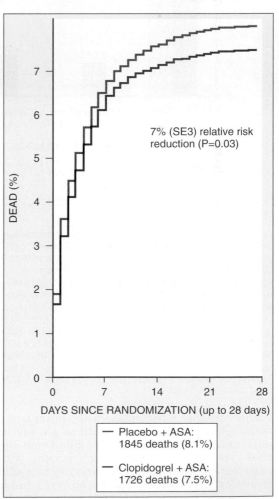

7% (SE3) relative risk reduction (P=0.03)

DEAD (%)

DAYS SINCE RANDOMIZATION (up to 28 days)

— Placebo + ASA: 1845 deaths (8.1%)
— Clopidogrel + ASA: 1726 deaths (7.5%)

B

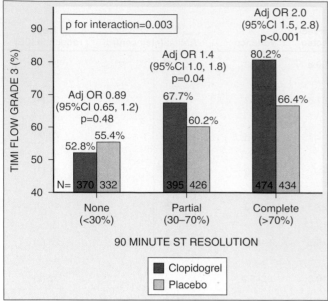

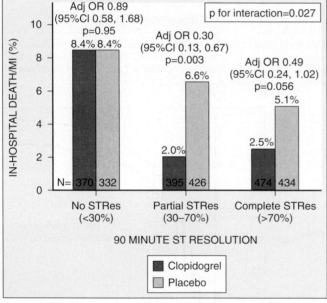

CH 51

FIGURE 51–23 Effect of clopidogrel when added to aspirin (ASA) in ST-elevation myocardial infarction (STEMI) patients. **A,** In the ST Resolution (STRes) Substudy from the CLARITY-TIMI 28 Trial, the rate of Thrombolysis In Myocardial Infarction (TIMI) flow grade 3 at late angiography (median 84 hours) was significantly improved in patients who received clopidogrel and achieved either partial or complete STRes at 90 minutes (*p* = 0.003 for interaction between STRes category and treatment). **B,** The rates of in-hospital cardiovascular death or myocardial infarction (MI) were significantly lower in patients who received clopidogrel and achieved either partial or complete STRes at 90 minutes (*p* = 0.027 for interaction between STRes category and treatment.) CI = confidence interval; OR = odds ratio. MI = myocardial infarction. *(From Scirica BM, Sabatine MS, Morrow DA, et al: The role of clopidogrel in early and sustained arterial patency after fibrinolysis for ST-segment elevation myocardial infarction: The ECG CLARITY-TIMI 28 Study. J Am Coll Cardiol 48: 37, 2006.)*

versus full-dose tenecteplase with enoxaparin or half-dose tenecteplase plus abciximab (with weight-adjusted reduced-dose unfractionated heparin).[123] Similar to the GUSTO V trial, combination reperfusion therapy with half-dose tenecteplase and abciximab was not associated with a reduction in 30-day mortality; however, in-hospital reinfarction and refractory ischemia were reduced with combi-

nation reperfusion therapy. Of note, the major bleeding rate other than intracranial hemorrhage was increased from 2.2 percent to 4.3 percent with combination reperfusion therapy (*p* = 0.0005). The elderly were at greatest risk for excess bleeding, experiencing a threefold increase in the rate of that complication.

RECOMMENDATIONS FOR ANTIPLATELET THERAPY

Nonenteric-coated aspirin should be chewed by patients who have not taken aspirin prior to presentation with STEMI. The dose should be 162 to 325 mg initially. During the maintenance phase of antiplatelet therapy following STEMI, the dose of aspirin should be reduced to 75 to 162 mg to minimize bleeding risk.[146] If true aspirin allergy is present, other antiplatelet agents such as clopidogrel (loading dose 300 to 600 mg; maintenance dose 75 mg per day) or ticlopidine (loading dose 500 mg; maintenance dose 250 mg twice daily) can be substituted.

Based on the results of the COMMIT[133] and CLARITY-TIMI 28[130] trials, the author believes clopidogrel 75 mg/day orally should be routinely added to all patients with STEMI regardless of whether they receive fibrinolytic therapy, undergo primary PCI (see Chap. 52), or do not receive reperfusion therapy. The available data suggest that a loading dose of 300 mg of clopidogrel should be given to patients younger than 75 years who receive fibrinolytic therapy, but no loading dose should be given to patients at least 75 years of age who receive a fibrinolytic. When primary PCI is the mode of reperfusion therapy, an oral loading dose of 300 to 600 mg of clopidogrel should be administered prior to stent implantation (see Chap. 52).[147]

In selected patients (anterior MI, age younger than 75 years, and low risk for bleeding), combination reperfusion therapy with abciximab and half-dose reteplase or tenecteplase may be considered for prevention of reinfarction and other complications of STEMI,[1,145] although this should not be undertaken with the expectation of a reduction in mortality. Combination pharmacological reperfusion therapy with abciximab and half-dose reteplase or tenecteplase should not be given to patients older than 75 years of age because of an increased risk of intracranial hemorrhage. A discussion of the use of GP IIb/IIIa inhibitors as part of a preparatory regimen in patients for whom PCI is planned (i.e., facilitated PCI) is found in Chapter 52.

HOSPITAL MANAGEMENT

Coronary Care Units

Deaths from primary ventricular fibrillation in patients with STEMI have been prevented because the coronary care unit (CCU) allows continuous monitoring of cardiac rhythm by highly trained nurses with the authority to initiate immediate treatment of arrhythmias in the absence of physicians, and because of the specialized equipment (defibrillators, pacemakers) and drugs available. Although all of these benefits can be achieved for patients scattered throughout the hospital, the clustering of patients with STEMI in the CCU has greatly improved the efficient use of the trained personnel, facilities, and equipment. With increasing emphasis on hemodynamic monitoring and treatment of the serious complications of STEMI with such modalities as pharmacological or catheter-based reperfusion therapy, afterload reduction, and intraaortic balloon counterpulsation, the presence of a CCU and experienced teams of physicians has assumed even greater importance. As reperfusion strategies including fibrinolytic therapy and PCI are used more routinely in STEMI patients, facilities in which patients can undergo diagnostic and therapeutic angiographic procedures are being integrated into an expanded structure of a coronary care team.[15,148,149]

At the same time, the value of CCUs for patients with uncomplicated STEMI has been questioned and restudied.[1] With increasing attention directed to the limitations of resources and to the economic impact of intensive care, efforts have been made to select patients likely to benefit from hospitalization in a CCU. The ECG reading, on presentation, particularly in conjunction with previous tracings and an immediate general clinical assessment, can be useful both for predicting which patients will have the diagnosis of STEMI confirmed and for identifying low-risk patients who may require less intensive care. Analysis of the quality of pain can help identify low-risk patients. Patients without a history of angina pectoris or MI presenting with pain that is sharp or stabbing and pleuritic, positional, or reproduced by palpation of the chest wall are extremely unlikely to be experiencing STEMI.[150] Computer-guided decision protocols are being developed to aid clinicians in identifying those STEMI patients who require admission to the CCU as opposed to a less intensive hospital ward.[37,151]

Contemporary CCUs typically have equipment available for noninvasive monitoring of single or multiple ECG leads, cardiac rhythm, ST segment deviation, arterial pressure, and arterial oxygen saturation. Computer algorithms for detection and analysis of arrhythmias are superior to visual surveillance by skilled CCU staff. However, even the most sophisticated ECG monitoring systems are susceptible to artifacts because of patient movement or noise on the signal from poor skin preparation when monitoring electrodes are applied. Noninvasive monitoring of arterial blood pressure using a sphygmomanometric cuff that undergoes cycles of inflation and deflation at programmed intervals is suitable for the majority of patients admitted to a CCU. Invasive arterial monitoring is preferred in patients with a low output syndrome under circumstances in which inotropic therapy is initiated for severe left ventricular failure.

The CCU remains the appropriate hospital unit for patients with complicated infarctions (e.g., hemodynamic instability, recurrent arrhythmias) and those patients requiring intensive nursing care for devices such as an intraaortic balloon pump. STEMI patients with an uncomplicated status, such as those without a history of previous infarction, persistent ischemic-type discomfort, congestive heart failure, hypotension, heart block, or hemodynamically compromising ventricular arrhythmias, can be safely transferred out of the CCU within 24 to 36 hours. In patients with a complicated STEMI, the duration of the CCU stay should be dictated by the need for "intensive" care; that is, hemodynamic monitoring, close nursing supervision, intravenous vasoactive drugs, and frequent changes in the medical regimen.

For patients with a low risk of mortality from STEMI, the clinician should consider admission to an intermediate care facility (see later) equipped with simple ECG monitoring and resuscitation equipment.[1] This strategy has proven cost-effective and may reduce CCU use by one third, shorten hospital stays, and have no deleterious effect on patients' recovery. Intermediate care units for low-risk STEMI patients can also be appealing to patients who stand to gain little benefit from the high staffing, intense activity, and elaborate technology available in current CCUs (with their attendant high costs) and who may be disturbed by that activity and equipment.

General Measures

The CCU staff must be sensitive to patient concerns about mortality, prognosis, and future productivity. A calm, quiet atmosphere and the "laying on of hands" with a gentle but confident touch help allay anxiety and reduce sympathetic

tone, ultimately leading to a reduction in hypertension, tachycardia, and arrhythmias.[1] To reduce the risk of nausea and vomiting early after infarction and to reduce the risk of aspiration, during the first 4 to 12 hours after admission patients should receive either nothing by mouth or a clear liquid diet (see Table 51-5). Subsequently, a diet with 50 to 55 percent of calories from complex carbohydrates and up to 30 percent from mono- and unsaturated fats should be given. The diet should be enriched in foods that are high in potassium, magnesium, and fiber but low in sodium (Table 51-5).

The results of laboratory tests obtained in the CCU should be scrutinized for any derangements potentially contributing to arrhythmias, such as hypoxemia, hypovolemia, disturbances of acid-base balance or of electrolytes, and drug toxicity. Oxazepam, 15 to 30 mg orally four times a day, is useful to allay the anxiety that is common in the first 24 to 48 hours (see Table 51-5). Delirium can be provoked by medications frequently used in the CCU, including antiarrhythmic drugs, H_2 blockers, narcotics, and beta blockers. Potentially offending agents should be discontinued in patients with an abnormal mental status. Haloperidol, a butyrophenone, can be used safely in patients with STEMI beginning with a dose of 2 mg intravenously for mildly agitated patients and 5 to 10 mg for progressively more agitated patients. Hypnotics, such as temazepam, 15 to 30 mg, or an equivalent, should be provided as needed for sleep. Dioctyl sodium sulfosuccinate, 200 mg daily, or another stool softener should be used to prevent constipation and straining (see Table 51-5).

"Coronary precautions" that do *not* appear to be supported by evidence from clinical research include the avoidance of iced fluids, hot beverages, caffeinated beverages, rectal examinations, and back rubs.[1]

PHYSICAL ACTIVITY. In the absence of complications, patients with STEMI need not be confined to bed for more than 12 hours and, unless they are hemodynamically compromised, they may use a bedside commode shortly after admission (see Table 51-5). Progression of activity should be individualized depending on the patient's clinical status, age, and physical capacity.

In patients without hemodynamic compromise, early ambulation, including dangling the feet on the side of the bed, sitting in a chair, standing, and walking around the bed, does not cause important changes in heart rate, blood pressure, or pulmonary wedge pressure. Although heart rate increases slightly (usually by less than 10 percent), pulmonary wedge pressures fall slightly as the patient assumes the upright posture for activities. Early ambulatory activities are rarely associated with any symptoms, and when symptoms do occur, they generally are related to hypotension. Thus when Levine and Lown proposed the "armchair" treatment of STEMI in the 1950s, they were undoubtedly correct that stress to the myocardium is less in the upright position. As long as blood pressure and heart rate are monitored, early ambulation offers considerable psychological and physical benefit without any clear medical risk.

INTERMEDIATE CORONARY CARE UNIT

Patients with STEMI are at risk for late in-hospital mortality from recurrent ischemia or infarction, hemodynamically significant ventricular arrhythmias, and severe congestive heart failure after discharge from the CCU. Therefore continued surveillance in intermediate CCUs (also called *step-down units*) is justifiable. Risk factors for mortality in the hospital after discharge from the CCU include significant congestive heart failure evidenced by persistent sinus tachycardia for more than 2 days and rales in greater than one third of the lung fields; recurrent ventricular tachycardia and ventricular fibrillation; atrial fibrillation or flutter while

CH 51

ST-Elevation Myocardial Infarction: Management

TABLE 51–5	**Sample Admitting Orders for the STEMI Patient**

1. Condition: Serious

2. IV: NS on D_5W to keep vein open. Start a second IV if IV medication is being given. This may be saline lock.

3. Vital signs: every 1.5 hr until stable, then every 4 hr and as needed. Notify physician if HR is <60 beats/min or > 100 beats/min, BP is <100 mm Hg systolic or >150 mm Hg systolic, respiratory rate is <8 or >22.

4. Monitor: Continuous ECG monitoring for dysrhythmia and ST segment deviation

5. Diet: NPO except for sips of water until stable. Then start 2 gm sodium/day, low saturated fat (<7% of total calories/day), low cholesterol (<200 mg/day) diet, such as total lifestyle change (TLC) diet

6. Activity: Bedside commode and light activity when stable

7. Oxygen: Continuous oximetry monitoring. Nasal cannula at 2 liters/min when stable for 6 hr, reassess for oxygen need (i.e., O_2 saturation of <90%) and consider discontinuing oxygen.

8. Medications:
   a. Nitroglycerin (NTG)
     1. Use sublingual NTG 0.4 mg every 5 min as needed for chest discomfort.
     2. Intravenous NTG for CHF, hypertension, or persistent ischemia.
   b. Aspirin (ASA; acetylsalicylic acid)
     1. If ASA not given in the emergency department (ED), chew nonenteric-coated ASA* 162-325 mg.
     2. If ASA has been given, start daily maintenance of 75-162 mg daily; may use enteric coated for gastrointestinal protection.
   c. Beta blocker
     1. If not given in the ED, assess for contraindication (i.e., bradycardia and hypotension); continue daily assessment to ascertain eligibility for beta blocker.
     2. If given in the ED, continue daily dose and optimize as dictated by heart rate and blood pressure.
   d. Angiotensin-converting enzyme (ACE) inhibitor
     1. Start ACE inhibitor orally in patients with pulmonary congestion or LVEF <40 percent if the following are absent: hypotension (SBP <100 mm Hg or <30 mm Hg below baseline) or known contraindications to this class of medications.
   e. Angiotensin receptor blocker (ARB)
     1. Start ARB orally in patients who are intolerant of ACE inhibitors and with either clinical or radiological signs of heart failure or LVEF <40 percent.
   f. Pain medications
     1. IV morphine sulfate 2-4 mg with increments of 2-8 mg IV at 5- to 15-min intervals as needed to control pain.
   g. Anxiolytics (based on a nursing assessment)
   h. Daily stool softener

*Although some trials have used enteric-coated ASA for initial dosing, more rapid buccal absorption occurs with nonenteric-coated formulations.

BP = blood pressure; CHF = coronary heart failure; ECG = electrocardiogram; HR = heart rate; IV = intravenous; NS = normal saline; NPO = nil per os (nothing by mouth); STEMI = ST-elevation myocardial infarction.

Modified from Antman EM, Anbe DT, Armstrong PW, et al: ACC/AHA guidelines for the management of patients with ST-elevation myocardial infarction: A report of the American College of Cardiology/American Heart Association Task Force on Practice Guidelines (Committee to Revise the 1999 Guidelines for the Management of Patients with Acute Myocardial Infarction). (www.acc.org/clinical/guidelines/stemi/index.pdf). Accessed 4/19/06.

CH 51

in the CCU; intraventricular conduction delays or heart block; anterior location of infarction; and recurrent episodes of angina with marked electrocardiographic ST-segment abnormalities at low activity levels.

The availability of intermediate care units may also be helpful in identifying those patients who remain free of complications and are suitable candidates for early discharge from the hospital. Aggressive reperfusion protocols with angioplasty or fibrinolytics can reduce the length of hospital stay.[152] In patients who are believed to have undergone successful reperfusion, the *absence* of early sustained ventricular tachyarrhythmias, hypotension, or heart failure, coupled with a well-preserved left ventricular ejection fraction, predicts a low risk of late complications in-hospital.[153] Such patients are suitable candidates for discharge from the hospital in less than 5 days from the onset of symptoms.

Following STEMI, patients are often eager for information, in need of reassurance, confused by misinformation and prior impressions, capable of counterproductive denial, and simply frightened. Intermediate care facilities provide ideal settings and ample opportunities to begin the rehabilitation process.[154] The capacity for the early detection of problems following STEMI and the social and educational benefits of grouping such patients together strongly argue for continued utilization of intermediate CCUs. Furthermore, the economic advantage of grouping such patients together for sharing of skilled personnel and resources outweighs any questions raised by the lack of a clear consensus regarding reduced mortality. An additional potential advantage is the facilitation of patient education in a group setting with lectures and audiovisual programs.

Pharmacological Therapy

Beta Blockers (see Chaps. 53 and 54)

The effects of beta blockers in the treatment of patients with STEMI can be divided into those that are immediate (when the drug is given early in the course of infarction) and those that are long term (secondary prevention), when the drug is initiated sometime after infarction. The immediate intravenous administration of beta blockers reduces cardiac index, heart rate, and blood pressure.[155] The net effect is a reduction in myocardial oxygen consumption per minute and per beat. Favorable effects of acute intravenous administration of beta-adrenoceptor blockers on the balance of myocardial oxygen supply and demand are reflected in reductions in chest pain, in the proportion of patients with threatened infarction who actually evolve STEMI, and in the development of ventricular arrhythmias.[156] Because beta-adrenergic blockade diminishes circulating levels of free fatty acids by antagonizing the lipolytic effects of catecholamines and because elevated levels of fatty acids augment myocardial oxygen consumption and probably increase the incidence of arrhythmias, these metabolic actions of beta-blocking agents may also benefit the ischemic heart.

More than 52,000 patients have been randomized in clinical trials studying beta-adrenergic blockade in acute MI. These trials cover a range of beta blockers and were largely conducted in the era before reperfusion strategies were developed for STEMI. The available data in the pre-reperfusion era suggested there were favorable trends toward a reduction in mortality, reinfarction, and cardiac arrest. However, in the reperfusion era the addition of a beta blocker to fibrinolytic therapy was not associated with a reduction in mortality but was helpful in reducing the rate of recurrent ischemic events.[157] Concern arose regarding the potential risk of provoking cardiogenic shock if early intravenous followed by oral beta-adrenergic blockade was routinely administered to all patients with STEMI.[156] The largest trial testing beta blockade in patients with acute MI was COMMIT, which randomized 45,852 patients within 24 hours of MI to metoprolol given as sequential intravenous boluses of 5 mg up to 15 mg followed by 200 mg per day orally or placebo.[33] There was no difference in the rate of the composite endpoint death, reinfarction, or cardiac arrest in the metoprolol group (9.4 percent) compared with the placebo group (9.9 percent). However, significant reductions occurred in reinfarction and episodes of ventricular fibrillation in the metoprolol group, translating into 5 fewer events for each of these endpoints per 1000 patients treated.[33] Yet there were 11 more episodes of cardiogenic shock in the metoprolol group per 1000 patients treated. The risk of developing cardiogenic shock (which was recorded as part of the COMMIT protocol

in contrast to earlier studies) was greatest in those patients presenting with moderate to severe left ventricular dysfunction (Killip Class II or greater).

Combining the results of the low-risk patients from COMMIT with the data from earlier trials on overview of the effects of early intravenous therapy followed by oral beta blocker therapy can be seen (Fig. 51-24). There is a 13 percent reduction in all-cause mortality (7 lives saved per 1000 patients treated), 22 percent reduction in reinfarction (5 fewer events per 1000 patients treated), and a 15 percent reduction in ventricular fibrillation or cardiac arrest (5 fewer events per 1000 patients treated).[33] In order to achieve these benefits safely, it is important to avoid the early administration of beta blockers to patients with relative contraindications as outlined in Table 51-6.

RECOMMENDATIONS. Given the evidence of benefits of early beta-adrenergic blockade in STEMI, patients without a contraindication (see Table 51-6), irrespective of administration of concomitant fibrinolytic therapy or performance of primary PCI, should promptly receive oral beta blockers. It is also reasonable to promptly administer intravenously beta blockers to STEMI patients, especially if a tachyarrhythmia or hypertension is present.[1] We use metoprolol 5 mg intravenously every 2 to 5 minutes for three doses provided the heart rate does not fall below 60 beats/min and the systolic blood pressure does not drop below 100 mm Hg. Oral maintenance dosing is initiated with metoprolol, 50 mg every 6 hours for 2 days and then 100 mg twice daily.

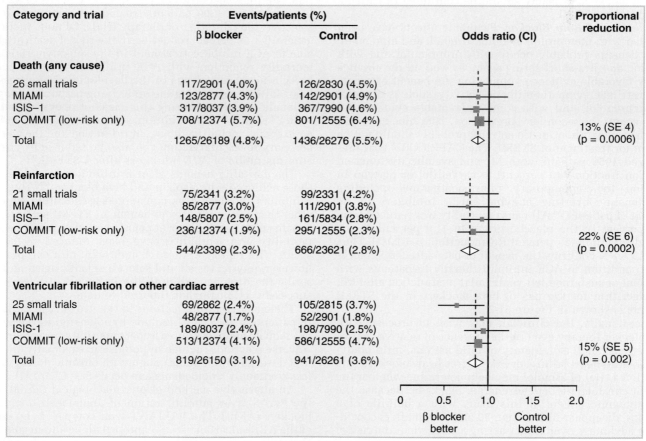

FIGURE 51–24 Meta-analysis of effects of intravenous then oral-blocker therapy on death, reinfarction, and cardiac arrest during the scheduled treatment periods in 26 small randomized trials, MIAMI, ISIS-1, and the low-risk subset of COMMIT. For COMMIT, data are included only for patients who presented with systolic blood pressure of more than 105 mm Hg, heart rate of more than 65 beats/min, and Killip Class I (as in MIAMI7). Five small trials included in the ISIS-1 report did not have any data on reinfarction. In the ISIS-1 trial, data on reinfarction in hospital were available for the last three quarters of the study, involving 11,641 patients. Odds ratios (ORs) in each (black squares with area proportional to number of events) comparing outcome in patients allocated β-blocker to that in patients allocated control, along with 99 percent confidence intervals (CIs) (horizontal line). Overall OR and 95 percent CI plotted by diamond, with value and significance given alongside. *(From Chen ZM, Pan HC, Chen YP, et al: Early intravenous then oral metoprolol in 45,852 patients with acute myocardial infarction: Randomised placebo-controlled trial. Lancet 366:1622, 2005.)*

TABLE 51-6	Contraindications to Beta-Adrenoceptor Blocker Therapy in Acute Myocardial Infarction
Heart rate < 60 beats/min	
Systolic arterial pressure <100 mm Hg	
Moderate or severe left ventricular failure	
Signs of peripheral hypoperfusion	
PR interval >0.24 sec	
Second- or third-degree atrioventricular block	
Severe chronic obstructive pulmonary disease	
History of asthma	
Severe peripheral vascular disease	
Insulin-dependent diabetes mellitus	

Beta blockers are especially helpful in patients in whom STEMI is complicated by persistent or recurrent ischemic pain, progressive or repetitive serum enzyme elevations suggestive of infarct extension, or tachyarrhythmias early after the onset of infarction. If adverse effects of beta blockers develop or if patients present with complications of infarction that are contraindications to beta blockade such as heart failure or heart block, the beta blocker should be withheld. Unless there are contraindications (see Table 51-6), beta blockade probably should be continued in patients who develop STEMI.

Selection of Beta Blocker. Favorable effects have been reported with metoprolol, atenolol, timolol, and alprenolol; these benefits probably occur with propranolol and with esmolol, an ultra-short-acting agent, as well. In the absence of any favorable evidence supporting the benefit of agents with intrinsic sympathomimetic activity, such as pindolol and oxprenolol, and with some unfavorable evidence for these agents in secondary prevention, beta blockers with intrinsic sympathomimetic activity probably should not be chosen for treatment of STEMI. The CAPRICORN trial randomized 1959 patients with MI and systolic dysfunction (ejection fraction <40 percent) to carvedilol or placebo in addition to contemporary pharmacotherapy including angiotensin-converting enzyme (ACE) inhibitors in 98 percent of patients.[158] All-cause mortality was reduced from 15.3 percent in the placebo group to 11.9 percent in the carvedilol group (23 percent RR reduction; $p = 0.031$). Thus CAPRICORN confirms the benefit of beta-adrenergic blockade in addition to ACE inhibitor therapy in patients with transient or sustained left ventricular dysfunction after MI. An algorithm for the use of beta blockers in the STEMI patients is shown in Figure 51-25.

Occasionally, the clinician may wish to proceed with beta blocker therapy even in the presence of relative contraindications, such as a history of mild asthma, mild bradycardia, mild heart failure, or first-degree heart block. In this situation a trial of esmolol may help determine whether the patient can tolerate beta-adrenergic blockade. Because the hemodynamic effects of this drug, with a half-life of 9 minutes, disappear in less than 30 minutes, it offers considerable advantage over longer-acting agents when the risk of a beta blocker complication is relatively high.

Inhibition of the Renin-Angiotensin-Aldosterone System

The rationale for inhibition of the renin-angiotensin-aldosterone system (RAAS) includes experimental and clinical evidence of a favorable impact on ventricular remodeling, improvement in hemodynamics, and reductions in conges-

tive heart failure.[159] Unequivocal evidence from randomized, placebo-controlled mortality trials shows that ACE inhibitors reduce the rate of mortality from STEMI. These trials can be grouped into two categories. The first consisted of *selected* MI patients for randomization on the basis of features indicative of increased mortality such as left ventricular ejection fraction less than 40 percent, clinical signs and symptoms of congestive heart failure,[160] anterior location of infarction,[161] and abnormal wall motion score index (Fig. 51-26).[162] The second group were *unselective* trials that randomized all patients with MI provided they had a minimum systolic pressure of approximately 100 mm Hg (ISIS-4,[163] GISSI-3,[164] CONSENSUS II,[165] and Chinese Captopril Study) (Fig. 51-27). With the exception of the SMILE trial,[161] all of the selective trials initiated ACE inhibitor therapy between 3 and 16 days after MI and maintained it for 1 to 4 years, whereas the unselective trials all initiated treatment within the first 24 to 36 hours and maintained it for only 4 to 6 weeks.

A consistent survival benefit was observed in all of the trials already noted, except for CONSENSUS II, the one study that utilized an intravenous preparation early in the course of MI.[165] An estimate of the mortality benefit of ACE inhibitors in the unselective, short duration of therapy trials was 5 per 1000 patients treated.[166,167] Analysis of these unselective short-term trials indicates that approximately one third of the lives saved occurred within the first 1 to 2 days. Certain subgroups, such as patients with anterior infarction, showed proportionately greater benefit from early administration (11 lives saved per 1000) of ACE inhibitors. Not unexpectedly, greater survival benefits of 42 to 76 lives saved per 1000 patients treated were obtained in the *selective,* long duration of therapy trials. Of note, there was generally a 20 percent reduction in the risk of death attributable to ACE inhibitor treatment in the selective trials. The mortality reduction with ACE inhibitors is accompanied by significant reductions in the development of congestive heart failure, supporting the underlying pathophysiological rationale for administering this class of drugs in patients with STEMI.[160,162,164] In addition, some data suggest that ischemic events including recurrent infarction and the need for coronary revascularization can also be reduced by chronic administration of ACE inhibitors after a STEMI.[168]

The mortality benefits of ACE inhibitors are additive to those achieved with aspirin and beta blockers.[164] Thus ACE inhibitors should not be considered a substitute for these other therapies with proven benefit in STEMI patients. The benefits of ACE inhibition appear to be a class effect because mortality and morbidity have been reduced by several agents. To replicate these benefits in clinical practice, however, physicians should select a specific agent and prescribe the drug according to the protocols utilized in the successful clinical trials reported to date.

The major *contraindications* to the use of ACE inhibitors in patients with STEMI include hypotension in the setting of adequate preload, known hypersensitivity, and pregnancy. Adverse reactions include hypotension, especially after the first dose, and intolerable cough with chronic dosing; much less commonly, angioedema can occur (see Chap. 41).

An alternative method of pharmacological inhibition of the RAAS is by administration of angiotensin-2 receptor blockers (ARBs). The VALIANT trial compared the effects of the ARB valsartan versus captopril alone and in combination with captopril on mortality in patients with acute MI complicated by left ventricular systolic dysfunction and/or heart failure.[169] Patients were randomized within 10 days of MI to valsartan (20 mg initially, titrated to 160 mg twice daily); valsartan added to captopril (20 mg and 6.25 mg initially, titrated to 80 mg twice daily and 50 mg three times daily); or captopril (6.25 mg initially, titrated to 50 mg three

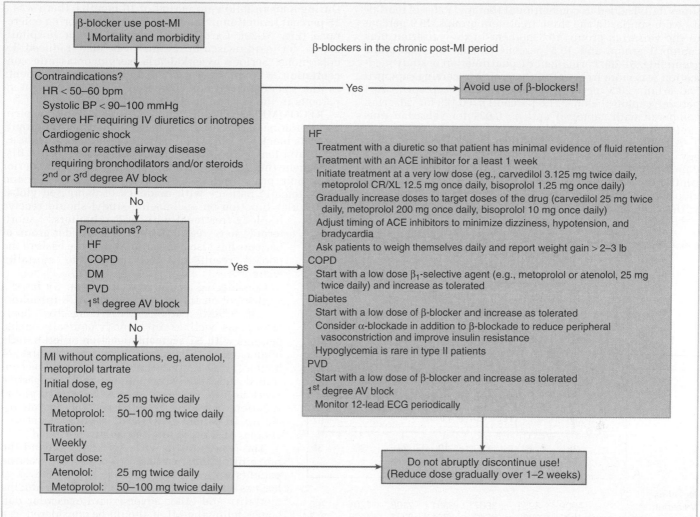

FIGURE 51–25 Algorithm for use of beta blockers in the treatment of patients with ST segment elevation myocardial infarction. ACE = angiotensin-converting enzyme; AV = atrioventricular; COPD = chronic obstructive pulmonary disease; DM = diabetes mellitus; ECG = electrocardiogram; HF = heart failure; MI = myocardial infarction; PVD = peripheral vascular disease. *(From Gheorghiade M, Goldstein S: Beta-blockers in the post-myocardial infarction patient. Circulation 106:394, 2002.)*

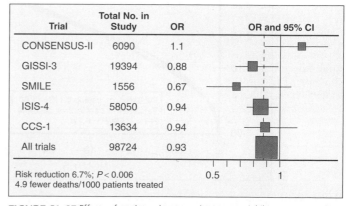

FIGURE 51–26 Effect of angiotensin-converting enzyme inhibitors on mortality after myocardial infarction: Results from the long-term trials. OR = odds ratio; CI = confidence interval. *(From Gornik H, O'Gara PT: Adjunctive medical therapy. In Manson JE, Buring JE, Ridker PM, Gaziano JM [eds]: Clinical Trials in Heart Disease: A Companion to Braunwald's Heart Disease. Philadelphia, Elsevier/ Saunders, 2004, p 114.)*

FIGURE 51–27 Effects of angiotensin-converting enzyme inhibitors on mortality after myocardial infarction: results from the short-term trials. OR = odds ratio; CI = confidence interval. *(From Gornik H, O'Gara PT: Adjunctive medical therapy. In Manson JE, Buring JE, Ridker PM, Gaziano JM [eds]: Clinical Trials in Heart Disease: A Companion to Braunwald's Heart Disease. Philadelphia, Elsevier/ Saunders, 2004, p. 114.)*

times daily) added to conventional therapy. Rates of mortality were similar in the three treatment groups: 19.9 percent in the valsartan group, 19.3 percent in the valsartan plus captopril group, and 19.5 percent in the captopril alone group (Fig. 51-28). Permanent discontinuation of study medication was more frequent in the groups receiving captopril (valsartan, 20.5 percent; valsartan plus captopril, 23.4 percent; captopril alone, 21.6 percent; $p = 0.129$ for valsartan compared with captopril and $p = 0.021$ for valsartan plus captopril versus captopril alone).

Aldosterone blockade is another pharmacological strategy for inhibition of the RAAS. The EPHESUS trial randomized 6642 patients with acute MI complicated by left ventricular dysfunction and heart failure to the selective aldosterone blocker eplerenone or placebo in conjunction with contemporary postinfarction pharmacotherapy.[170]

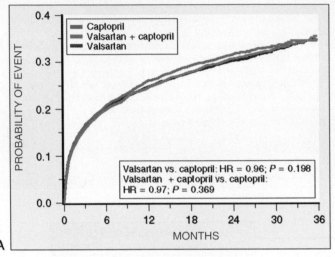

A

No. at risk

Valsartan	4909	3921	3667	3391	2188	1204	290
Valsartan and captopril	4885	3887	3646	3391	2221	1185	313
Captopril	4909	3896	3610	3355	2155	1148	295

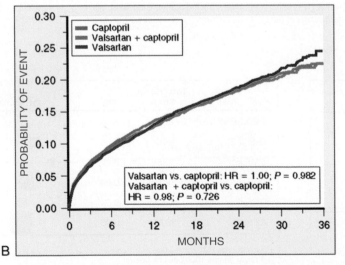

B

No. at risk

Valsartan	4909	4464	4272	4007	2648	1437	357
Valsartan and captopril	4885	4414	4265	3994	2648	1435	382
Captopril	4909	4428	4241	4018	2635	1432	364

FIGURE 51–28 Effects of an angiotensin-converting enzyme inhibitor (captopril), angiotensin receptor blocker (valsartan), or the combination after myocardial infarction. The Kaplan-Meier estimates of **(A)** mortality and **(B)** cardiovascular death, reinfarction, or hospitalization for heart failure, by treatment in the VALIANT trial are depicted. HR = hazard ratio. *(From Pfeffer M, McMurray JJ, Velasquez EJ, et al: Effects of valsartan relative to captopril in patients with myocardial infarction complicated by heart failure and or left ventricular dysfunction. N Engl J Med 349:1893, 2003.)*

During a mean follow-up period of 16 months, there was a 15 percent reduction in the RR of mortality favoring eplerenone (Fig. 51-29). Cardiovascular mortality or hospitalization for cardiovascular events was also reduced by eplerenone. Serious hyperkalemia (serum potassium concentration ≥6 mmol/liter) occurred in 5.5 percent of patients in the eplerenone group compared with 3.9 percent of patients in the placebo group ($p = 0.002$).

RECOMMENDATIONS. After administration of aspirin and initiation of reperfusion strategies and, where appropriate, beta blockade, *all* STEMI patients should be considered for inhibition of the RAAS. Although there is little disagreement that high-risk STEMI patients (elderly, anterior infarction, prior infarction, Killip Class II or greater, and asymptomatic patients with evidence of depressed global ventricular function on an imaging study) should receive life-long treatment with ACE inhibitors,[171] short-term (4 to 6 weeks) therapy to a broader group of patients has also been proposed on the basis of the pooled results of the unselective mortality trials.[163]

Considering all the available data, we favor a strategy of an initial trial of oral ACE inhibitors in all STEMI patients with congestive heart failure, as well as in hemodynamically stable patients with ST segment elevation or left bundle branch block, commencing within the first 24 hours.[167,172] ACE inhibition therapy should be continued indefinitely in patients with congestive heart failure, evidence of a reduction in global function, or a large regional wall motion abnormality. In patients without these findings at discharge, ACE inhibitors can be discontinued.

The results of the VALIANT trial expand the range of options available to clinicians treating patients with STEMI. Because the ARB was at least as effective as the ACE inhibitor in reducing mortality and other adverse cardiovascular outcomes following MI, it should be considered as a clinically effective alternative to captopril.[173] The choice between ACE inhibition and angiotensin receptor blockade following STEMI should be based on physician experience with the agents, patient tolerability, safety, convenience, and cost. Finally, based on experience from the EPHESUS study, long-term aldosterone blockade with eplerenone 25 mg/day initially and then titrated to 50 mg/day for high-risk patients following STEMI (ejection fraction ≤40 percent, clinical heart failure, diabetes mellitus) should be considered. Given the small but definite increase in the risk of serious hypokalemia when aldosterone blockade is prescribed, particularly when other measures for inhibition of the RAAS are used concurrently, periodic monitoring of the serum potassium level should be undertaken.[174]

Nitrates (see Chap. 54)

Sublingual nitroglycerin rarely opens occluded coronary arteries. However, in patients with STEMI, the potential for reductions in ventricular filling pressures, wall tension, and cardiac work coupled with improvement in coronary blood flow, especially in ischemic zones, and antiplatelet effects make nitrates a logical and attractive pharmacological intervention.[1]

In patients with STEMI the administration of nitrates reduces pulmonary capillary wedge pressure and systemic arterial pressure, left ventricular chamber volume, infarct size, and the incidence of mechanical complications. As with other inter-

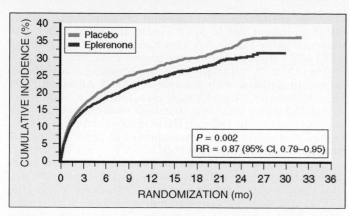

No. at risk

Placebo	3313	2754	2580	2388	2013	1494	995	558	247	77	2	0	0
Eplerenone	3319	2816	2680	2504	2096	1564	1061	594	273	91	0	0	0

FIGURE 51–29 Effect of a selective aldosterone receptor blocker (eplerenone) after myocardial infarction. The Kaplan-Meier estimates of the rate of death from cardiovascular causes or hospitalization for cardiovascular events in the EPHESUS trial are depicted. CI = confidence interval; RR = relative risk. *(From Pitt B, Remme W, Zannad F, et al: Eplerenone, a selective aldosterone blocker, in patients with left ventricular dysfunction after myocardial infarction (abstract). N Engl J Med 348:14, 2003.)*

ventions to spare ischemic myocardium in cases of STEMI, intravenous nitroglycerin appears to be of greatest benefit in patients treated earliest after the onset of symptoms.

CLINICAL TRIAL RESULTS. In the prefibrinolytic era, 10 randomized trials of acute administration of intravenous nitroglycerin (or nitroprusside, another nitric oxide donor) collectively enrolled 2042 patients. A meta-analysis of these trial results showed a reduction in mortality of 35 percent associated with nitrate therapy.[175]

In the fibrinolytic era, two megatrials of nitrate therapy have been conducted: GISSI-3[164] and ISIS-4.[163] In GISSI-3, there was no independent effect of nitrates on short-term mortality.[164] Similarly, in ISIS-4, no effect of a mononitrate on 35-day mortality was observed. A pooled analysis of more than 80,000 patients treated with nitrate-like preparations intravenously or orally in 22 trials revealed a mortality rate of 7.7 percent in the control group, which was reduced to 7.4 percent in the nitrate group. These data are consistent with a small treatment effect of nitrates on mortality such that 3 to 4 fewer deaths would occur for every 1000 patients treated.[163]

NITRATE PREPARATIONS AND MODE OF ADMINISTRATION. Intravenous nitroglycerin can be administered safely to patients with evolving STEMI as long as the dose is titrated to avoid induction of reflex tachycardia or systemic arterial hypotension. Patients with inferior wall infarction are particularly sensitive to an excessive fall in preload, particularly if concurrent right ventricular infarction is present.[1] In such cases, nitrate-induced venodilation could impair cardiac output and reduce coronary block flow, thus worsening myocardial oxygenation rather than improving it.

A useful regimen employs an initial infusion rate of 5 to 10 mg/min with increases of 5 to 20 mg/min until the mean arterial blood pressure is reduced by 10 percent of its baseline level in normotensive patients and by 30 percent for hypertensive patients, but in no case below a systolic pressure of 90 mm Hg. Alternatively, nitroglycerin can be administered as a sustained-release oral preparation (30 to 60 mg/day) or as an ointment (1 to 3 inches every 6 to 8 hours for patients with a systolic pressure >120 mm Hg). Nitroglycerin can also be given sublingually at doses of 0.3 to 0.6 mg. This route can be more hazardous because the rate of absorption is difficult to control and arterial pressure may decline precipitously.

ADVERSE EFFECTS. Clinically significant methemoglobinemia has been reported to occur during administration of intravenous nitroglycerin. Although uncommon, this problem is seen when unusually large doses of nitrates are administered. It is important not only for its potential to cause symptoms of lethargy and headache but also because elevated methemoglobin levels can impair the oxygen-carrying capacity of blood, potentially exacerbating ischemia. Dilation of the pulmonary vasculature supplying poorly ventilated lung segments may produce a ventilation-perfusion mismatch.

Tolerance to intravenous nitroglycerin (as manifested by increasing nitrate requirements) develops in many patients, often as soon as 12 hours after the infusion is started. Despite the theoretical and demonstrated benefit of sulfhydryl agents in diminishing tolerance, their use has not become widespread.

RECOMMENDATIONS FOR NITRATES IN PATIENT WITH STEMI. Nitroglycerin is indicated for the relief of persistent pain and as a vasodilator in patients with infarction associated with left ventricular failure. In the absence of recurrent angina or congestive heart failure, we do not routinely prescribe them for STEMI patients. Higher-risk patients such as those with large transmural infarctions, especially of the anterior wall, have the most to gain from nitrates in terms of reduction of ventricular remodeling, and we therefore routinely use intravenous nitrates for 24 to 48 hours in such patients. There is no clear benefit to empirical long-term cutaneous or oral nitrates in the asymptomatic patient, and we therefore do not prescribe nitrates beyond the first 48 hours unless angina or ventricular failure is present.

Calcium Antagonists (see Chap. 54)

Despite sound experimental and clinical evidence of an antiischemic effect, calcium antagonists have *not* been found to be helpful in the acute phase of STEMI, and concern has been raised in several systematic overviews about an increased risk of mortality when they are prescribed on a routine basis. A distinction should be made between the dihydropyridine type of calcium antagonists (e.g., nifedipine) and the nondihydropyridine calcium antagonists (e.g., verapamil and diltiazem).

NIFEDIPINE. In multiple trials involving more than 5000 patients, the immediate-release preparation of nifedipine has not resulted in any reduction in infarct size, prevention of progression to infarction, control of recurrent ischemia, or lowering of mortality rate. When trials of the immediate-release form of nifedipine are pooled in a meta-analysis, evidence suggests a dose-related increased risk of in-hospital mortality (especially at a dose >80 mg of nifedipine), although post-hospital mortality does not appear to be increased in nifedipine-treated patients. Nifedipine does not appear to be helpful in conjunction with either fibrinolytic therapy or beta blockade.[176] Thus we do not recommend the use of immediate-release nifedipine early in the treatment of STEMI. No trials of the sustained-release preparations of nifedipine in patients with STEMI have been reported to date.

VERAPAMIL AND DILTIAZEM. When administered during the acute phase of STEMI, these drugs have not had any demonstrated favorable effect on infarct size or other important endpoints in patients with STEMI, with the exception of control of supraventricular arrhythmias.[177] The INTERCEPT trial compared 300 mg of diltiazem with placebo in patients who received fibrinolytic therapy for STEMI.[178] Diltiazem did not reduce the cumulative occurrence of cardiac death, nonfatal reinfarction, or refractory ischemia during a 6-month follow-up.

Based on the available data, we do *not* recommend the routine use of either verapamil or diltiazem in patients with STEMI. Verapamil and diltiazem can be given for relief of ongoing ischemia or slowing of a rapid ventricular response in atrial fibrillation in patients for whom beta blockers are ineffective or contraindicated.[1] Their use should be avoided in patients with Killip Class II or greater hemodynamic findings.

CH 51

ST-Elevation Myocardial Infarction: Management

MAGNESIUM. Patients with STEMI may have a total body deficit of magnesium because of a low dietary intake, advanced age, or prior diuretic use. They may also acquire a functional deficit of available magnesium caused by trapping of free magnesium in adipocytes, as soaps are formed when free fatty acids are released by catecholamine-induced lipolysis with the onset of infarction.

Because of the risk of cardiac arrhythmias when electrolyte deficits are present in the early phase of infarction, all patients with STEMI should have a serum magnesium measurement on admission. We advocate repleting magnesium deficits to maintain a serum magnesium level of 2 mEq/liter or more. In the presence of hypokalemia (<4 mEq/liter) during the course of treatment of STEMI, the serum magnesium level should be rechecked and repleted if necessary because it is often difficult to correct a potassium deficit in the presence of a concurrent magnesium deficit. Episodes of torsades de pointes should be treated with 1 to 2 gm of magnesium delivered as a bolus over about 5 minutes. Between 1980 and 2002, 68,684 patients were studied in a series of 14 randomized trials. On the basis of the totality of available evidence and current coronary care practice, there is no indication for the routine administration of intravenous magnesium to patients with STEMI at any level of risk.[179]

GLUCOSE CONTROL DURING STEMI (see also Chap. 60). During the acute phase of STEMI there is an increase in catecholamine levels in both the blood and ischemic myocardium. Insulin levels remain low, whereas cortisol, glucagon, and free fatty acid levels increase. These factors may contribute to an elevation of the blood glucose level, which should be measured routinely on admission to the coronary care unit. An infusion of insulin is recommended to normalize blood glucose levels in STEMI patients with a complicated course.[1] Given the evidence of tight glucose control in critically ill patients, it is also reasonable to administer an insulin infusion to hyperglycemic STEMI patients even if they have an uncomplicated course.[1,180]

It was proposed that routine administration of infusions of glucose-insulin-potassium (GIK) to STEMI patients would reduce mortality. A series of small trials, the majority of which were performed in the pre-reperfusion era along with some in the setting of fibrinolysis or PCI, suggested that GIK infusions were indeed of benefit. However, the CREATE-ECLA investigators randomized 20,201 STEMI patients (83 percent of whom received reperfusion therapy) to GIK or placebo and found no evidence of a mortality benefit (30-day mortality 9.7 percent in control patients and 10 percent in GIK patients).[181] Thus in the contemporary era of management of STEMI patients in which other life-saving therapies (reperfusion, aspirin, ACE inhibitors) are administered, there appears to be no benefit to the routine use of GIK infusions.

INTRAAORTIC BALLOON COUNTERPULSATION. From a theoretical standpoint, intraaortic balloon counterpulsation might be expected to limit infarct size for several reasons. In experimental animals, intraaortic balloon counterpulsation decreases preload, increases coronary blood flow, and improves cardiac performance. No definitive information is available indicating that intraaortic balloon counterpulsation alters the prognosis in patients with relatively uncomplicated STEMI, especially in the context of other proven mortality-reducing therapies used in contemporary clinical practice. Intraaortic balloon pumping should be reserved for hemodynamically compromised patients and for those with refractory ischemia. Although noninvasive external forms of counterpulsation have been developed, these approaches have not undergone rigorous study in patients with STEMI.

OTHER AGENTS. Several adjunctive pharmacotherapies have been investigated to prevent inflammatory damage in the infarct zone.[182] Trials with antibodies against the CD11/CD18 leukocyte adhesion receptor did not show a reduction in infarct size.[183,184] Pexelizumab, a monoclonal antibody against the C5 component of complement, had no effect on infarct size in STEMI patients treated either with fibrinolytics or PCI.[185,186] It also had no effect on mortality in STEMI patients treated with primary PCI.[186a]

The AMISTAD II trial was a dose-ranging study of adenosine in patients with anterior STEMI.[94] Although high-dose adenosine (70 μg/kg/min infusion for 3 hours) was associated with a reduction in infarct size, neither high- nor low-dose adenosine reduced the primary composite clinical endpoint of death or the development of heart failure at 6 months compared with placebo.[51]

Contrary to earlier beliefs that the heart is a terminally differentiated organ without the capacity to regenerate, evidence now exists that human cardiac myocytes divide after STEMI and stem cells can promote regeneration of cardiac tissue. These observations open up the possibility of myocardial replacement therapy after STEMI (see Chap. 29).[187]

HEMODYNAMIC DISTURBANCES

Hemodynamic Assessment

In patients with clinically uncomplicated STEMI, invasive hemodynamic monitoring is not necessary because the status of the circulation can be assessed by clinical evaluation. This ordinarily consists of monitoring of heart rate and rhythm, repeated measurement of systemic arterial pressure by cuff, obtaining chest radiographs to detect heart failure, repeated auscultation of the lung fields for pulmonary congestion, measurement of urine flow, examination of the skin and mucous membranes for evidence of the adequacy of perfusion, and arterial sampling for pO_2, pCO_2, and pH when hypoxemia or metabolic acidosis is suspected.

In contrast, in patients with STEMI whose ventricular contractile performance is not normal, as evidenced by clinical signs and symptoms of heart failure, it is important to assess the degree of hemodynamic compromise to initiate therapy with drugs such as vasodilators and diuretics. In the past, central venous or right atrial pressure was used to gauge the degree of left ventricular failure in patients with STEMI. However, this technique is fraught with error because central venous pressure actually reflects right rather than left ventricular function. Right ventricular function and therefore systemic venous pressure may be normal or nearly so in patients with significant left ventricular failure. Conversely, patients with right ventricular failure caused by right ventricular infarction or pulmonary embolism may exhibit elevated right atrial and central venous pressures despite normal left ventricular function. Low values for right atrial and central venous pressures imply hypovolemia, whereas elevated right atrial pressures usually result from right ventricular failure secondary to left ventricular failure, pulmonary hypertension, or right ventricular infarction, or less commonly from tricuspid regurgitation or pericardial tamponade.

Major advances in the management of STEMI have resulted from the hemodynamic monitoring that has become widespread in CCUs (Table 51-7). This often consists of both an intraarterial catheter and a pulmonary artery catheter for measurement of pulmonary artery, pulmonary artery occlusive (equivalent to pulmonary wedge), and right atrial pressures, and cardiac output by thermodilution. In patients with hypotension, a Foley catheter provides accurate and continuous measurement of urine output.

NEED FOR INVASIVE MONITORING. The use of invasive hemodynamic monitoring is based on the following principal factors:
1. Difficulty in interpreting clinical and radiographic findings of pulmonary congestion even after a

TABLE 51-7	Indications for Hemodynamic Monitoring in Patients with STEMI

Management of complicated acute myocardial infarction
  Hypovolemia versus cardiogenic shock
  Ventricular septal rupture versus acute mitral regurgitation
  Severe left ventricular failure
  Right ventricular failure

Refractory ventricular tachycadia

Differentiating severe pulmonary disease from left ventricular failure

Assessment of cardiac tamponade

Assessment of therapy in *selected* individuals
  Afterload reduction in patients with severe left ventricular failure
  Inotropic agent therapy
  Beta-blocker therapy
  Temporary pacing (ventricular versus atrioventricular)
  Intraaortic balloon counterpulsation
  Mechanical ventilation

STEMI = ST-elevation myocardial infarction.
From Gore JM, Zwernet PL: Hemodynamic monitoring of acute myocardial infarction. *In* Francis GS, Alpert JS (eds): Modern Coronary Care. Boston, Little, Brown, 1990, p 138.

TABLE 51-8	Hemodynamic Classifications of Patients with Acute Myocardial Infarction		
A. Based on Clinical Examination		**B. Based on Invasive Monitoring**	
Class	Definition	Subset	Definition
I	Rales and S_3 absent	I	Normal hemodynamics PCWP < 18, CI > 2.2
II	Crackles, S_3 gallop, elevated jugular venous pressure	II	Pulmonary congestion PCWP > 18, CI > 2.2
III	Frank pulmonary edema	III	Peripheral hypoperfusion PCWP < 18, CI < 2.2
IV	Shock	IV	Pulmonary congestion and peripheral hypoperfusion PCWP > 18, CI < 2.2

CI = cardiac index; PCWP = pulmonary capillary wedge pressure.
A, Modified from Killip T, Kimball J: Treatment of myocardial infarction in a coronary care unit. A two year experience with 250 patients. Am J Cardiol 20:457, 1967; and **B,** From Forrester J, Diamond G, Chatterjee K, et al: Medical therapy of acute myocardial infarction by the application of hemodynamic subsets. N Engl J Med 295:1356, 1976.

thorough review of noninvasive studies such as an echocardiogram.
2. Need for identifying noncardiac causes of arterial hypotension, particularly hypovolemia.
3. Possible contribution of reduced ventricular compliance to impaired hemodynamics, requiring judicious adjustment of intravascular volume to optimize left ventricular filling pressure.
4. Difficulty in assessing the severity and sometimes even determining the presence of lesions such as mitral regurgitation and ventricular septal defect when the cardiac output or the systemic pressures are depressed.
5. Establishing a baseline of hemodynamic measurements and guiding therapy in patients with clinically apparent pulmonary edema or cardiogenic shock.
6. Underestimation of systemic arterial pressure by the cuff method in patients with intense vasoconstriction.

The prognosis and the clinical status of patients with STEMI relate to both the cardiac output and the pulmonary artery wedge pressure. Patients with normal cardiac output after STEMI have a low expected chance of mortality; prognosis worsens as cardiac output declines. Patients with intraventricular conduction defects, atrioventricular (AV) block, or both after anterior infarction have lower cardiac indices and higher pulmonary capillary wedge pressures than do patients without these conduction disturbances. On the other hand, patients with these conduction defects and inferior STEMI usually do not demonstrate such hemodynamic abnormalities.

PULMONARY ARTERY PRESSURE MONITORING. Patients most likely to benefit from pulmonary artery catheter monitoring include those whose STEMI is complicated by (1) hypotension that is not easily corrected by fluid administration; (2) hypotension in the presence of congestive heart failure; (3) hemodynamic compromise severe enough to require intravenous vasopressors or vasodilators or intraaortic balloon counterpulsation; (4) mechanical lesions (or suspected ones) such as cardiac tamponade, severe mitral regurgitation, and a ruptured ventricular septum; and (5) right ventricular infarction.[32] Other indications for hemodynamic monitoring include assessment of the effects of mechanical ventilation, differentiating pulmonary disease from left ventricular failure as the cause of hypoxemia, and management of septic shock (see Table 51-7).[1]

Before inserting a pulmonary artery catheter into a patient with STEMI, the physician must believe that the potential benefit of the information to be obtained outweighs any potential risks. Major complications from pulmonary artery catheters are not common (about 3 to 5 percent of cases), but severe problems can occur including sepsis, pulmonary infarction, and pulmonary artery rupture. Minimized duration of catheterization and strict adherence to aseptic techniques can diminish risk. Catheter-related bloodstream infections can also be reduced by using antiseptic-impregnated catheters.[188]

Accurate determination of hemodynamics by clinical assessment is difficult in critically ill patients. The use of a pulmonary artery catheter thus often leads to important changes in therapy. Of note, reports exist that rates of complications and mortality may be higher in patients who undergo pulmonary artery catheterization, although such patients are often at higher risk initially. These observations emphasize the importance of patient selection, meticulous technique, and correct interpretation of the data obtained.

Hemodynamic Abnormalities

In 1976 Swan, Forrester, and their associates measured the cardiac output and wedge pressure simultaneously in a large series of patients with acute MI and identified four major hemodynamic subsets of patients (Table 51-8): (1) patients with normal systemic perfusion and without pulmonary congestion (normal cardiac output and normal wedge pressure); (2) patients with normal perfusion and pulmonary congestion (normal cardiac output and elevated wedge pressure); (3) patients with decreased perfusion but without pulmonary congestion (reduced cardiac output and normal wedge pressure); and (4) patients with decreased perfusion and pulmonary congestion (reduced cardiac output and elevated wedge pressure). This classification, which overlaps with a crude clinical classification proposed earlier by Killip and Kimball (Table 51-9), has proved to be quite useful, but it should be noted that patients frequently pass from one category to another with therapy and sometimes apparently even spontaneously.

HEMODYNAMIC SUBSETS. These are usually reflected in the patient's clinical status. Hypoperfusion usually becomes evident clinically when the cardiac index falls below approximately 2.2 liters/min/m^2, whereas pulmonary congestion is noted when the wedge pressure exceeds approximately 20 mm Hg. However, approximately 25

TABLE 51-9	Hemodynamic Patterns for Common Clinical Conditions				
	Chamber Pressure (mg Hg)				
Cardiac Condition	RA	RV	PA	PCW	CI
Normal	0-6	25/0-6	25/0-12	6-12	≥2.5
AMI without LVF	0-6	25/0-6	30/12-18	≤18	≥2.5
AMI with LVF	0-6	30-40/0-6	30-40/18-25	>18	>2.0
Biventricular failure	>6	50-60/>6	50-60/25	18-25	>2.0
RVMI	12-20	30/12-20	30/12	≤12	<2.0
Cardiac tamponade	12-16	25/12-16	25/12-16	12-16	<2.0
Pulmonary embolism	12-20	50-60/12-20	50-60/12	<12	<2.0

AMI = acute myocardial infarction; CI = cardiac index; LVF = left ventricular failure; PA = pulmonary artery; PCW = pulmonary capillary wedge; RA = right atrium; RV = right ventricle; RVMI = right ventricular myocardial infarction.

From Gore JM, Zwernet PL: Hemodynamic monitoring of acute myocardial infarction. *In* Francis GS, Alpert JS (eds): Modern Coronary Care. Boston, Little, Brown, 1990, pp 139-164.

CH 51

percent of patients with cardiac indices less than 2.2 liters/min/m² and 15 percent of patients with elevated pulmonary capillary wedge pressures are not recognized clinically. Discrepancies in hemodynamic and clinical classification of patients with STEMI arise for a variety of reasons. Patients may exhibit "phase lags" as clinical pulmonary congestion develops or resolves, symptoms secondary to chronic obstructive pulmonary disease may be confused with those resulting from pulmonary congestion, or longstanding left ventricular dysfunction may mask signs of hypoperfusion secondary to compensatory vasoconstriction.

The hemodynamic findings shown in Tables 51-8 and 51-9 allow for rational approaches to therapy. The goals of hemodynamic therapy are to maintain ventricular performance, support blood pressure, and protect jeopardized myocardium. Because these goals occasionally may be at cross-purposes, recognition of the hemodynamic profile, as assessed clinically or as available from hemodynamic monitoring, is required before optimal therapeutic interventions can be designed along the lines discussed later.

HYPOTENSION IN THE PREHOSPITAL PHASE. During the prehospital phase of STEMI, invasive hemodynamic monitoring is not feasible and therapy should be guided by frequent clinical assessment and measurement of arterial pressure by cuff, with the recognition that intense vasoconstriction can provide a falsely low pressure measured by this method. Hypotension associated with bradycardia often reflects excessive vagotonia. Relative or absolute hypovolemia is often present when hypotension occurs with a normal or rapid heart rate, particularly among patients receiving diuretics just prior to the occurrence of infarction. Marked diaphoresis, reduction of fluid intake, or vomiting during the period preceding and accompanying the onset of STEMI may all contribute to the development of hypovolemia. Even if the effective vascular volume is normal, relative hypovolemia may be present because ventricular compliance is reduced in cases of STEMI and a left ventricular filling pressure as high as 20 mm Hg may be necessary to provide an optimal preload.

MANAGEMENT. In the absence of rales involving more than one third of the lung fields, the patient should be put in the reverse Trendelenburg position, and in patients with sinus bradycardia and hypotension, atropine should be administered (0.3 to 0.6 mg IV repeated at 3- to 10-minute intervals up to 2 mg). If these measures do not correct the hypotension, normal saline should be administered intravenously, beginning with a bolus of 100 ml followed by 50-ml increments every 5 minutes. The patient should be observed and the infusion stopped when the systolic pressure returns to approximately 100 mm Hg, if the patient becomes dyspneic, or if pulmonary rales develop or increase. Because of the poor correlation between left ventricular filling pressure and mean right atrial pressure, assessment of systemic (even central) venous pressure is of limited value as a guide to fluid therapy.

Administration of positive inotropic agents is indicated during the prehospital phase if systemic hypotension persists despite correction of hypovolemia and excessive vagotonia. In the absence of invasive hemodynamic monitoring, assessment of peripheral vascular resistance must be based on clinical observations. If cutaneous vasoconstriction is present, therapy with dobutamine, which stimulates cardiac contractility without unduly accelerating heart rate and which does not increase the impedance to ventricular outflow, may be helpful. In hypotensive patients with STEMI with clinical evidence of vasodilation, an uncommon circumstance, phenylephrine hydrochloride is preferable, although this agent, which increases coronary and peripheral vascular tone, should be used with caution.

HYPOVOLEMIC HYPOTENSION. Recognition of hypovolemia is of particular importance in hypotensive patients with STEMI because of the hazard it poses and because of the improvement in circulatory dynamics that can be achieved so readily and safely by augmentation of vascular volume. Because hypovolemia is often occult, it is frequently overlooked in the absence of invasive hemodynamic monitoring. Hypovolemia may be absolute, with low left ventricular filling pressure (8 mm Hg), or relative, with normal (8 to 12 mm Hg) or even modestly increased (13 to 18 mm Hg) left ventricular filling pressures. Because of the reduction of left ventricular compliance that occurs with acute ischemia and infarction, left ventricular filling pressures between 13 and 18 mm Hg, although above the upper limits of normal, may actually be suboptimal.

Exclusion of hypovolemia as the cause of hypotension requires the documentation of a reduced cardiac output despite left ventricular filling pressure exceeding 18 mm Hg. If, in a hypotensive patient, the pulmonary capillary wedge pressure (ordinarily measured as the pulmonary artery occlusive pressure) is below this level, fluid challenge should be carried out as described earlier. If hypovolemia is documented or suspected, the fluid replaced should resemble the fluid lost. Thus when a low hematocrit complicates STEMI, infusion of packed red blood cells or whole blood is the treatment of choice.[189] On the other hand, crystalloid or colloid solutions should be administered when the hematocrit is normal or elevated.

Hypotension caused by right ventricular infarction may be confused with that caused by hypovolemia because both are associated with a low, normal, or minimally elevated left ventricular filling pressure. The findings and management of right ventricular infarction are discussed elsewhere in this chapter.

THE HYPERDYNAMIC STATE. When infarction is not complicated by hemodynamic impairment, no therapy other than general supportive measures and treatment of arrhythmias is necessary. However, if the hemodynamic profile is of the hyperdynamic state—that is, elevation of sinus rate, arterial pressure, and cardiac index, occurring singly or together in the presence of a normal or low left ventricular filling pressure—and if other causes of tachycardia such as fever, infection, and pericarditis can be excluded, treatment with beta blockers is indicated. Presumably, the increased heart rate and blood pressure are the result of inappropriate activation of the sympathetic nervous system, possibly secondary to augmented release of catecholamines, pain and anxiety, or some combination of these.

Left Ventricular Failure

Left ventricular dysfunction is the single most important predictor of mortality following STEMI (Fig. 51-30).[173,190] In patients with STEMI, either systolic dysfunction alone or both systolic and diastolic dysfunction can occur. Left ventricular diastolic dysfunction leads to pulmonary venous hypertension and pulmonary congestion, whereas systolic dysfunction is principally responsible for a depression of cardiac output and of the ejection fraction. Clinical manifestations of left ventricular failure become more common as the extent of the injury to the left ventricle increases. In addition to infarct size, other important predictors of the development of symptomatic left ventricular dysfunction include advanced age and diabetes.[190] Mortality increases in association with the severity of the hemodynamic deficit.

THERAPEUTIC IMPLICATIONS. Classification of patients with STEMI by hemodynamic subsets has therapeutic relevance. As already noted, patients with normal wedge pressures and hypoperfusion often benefit from infusion of fluids because the peak value of stroke volume is usually not attained until left ventricular filling pressure reaches 18 to 24 mm Hg. However, a low level of left ventricular filling pressure does not imply that left ventricular damage is necessarily slight. Such patients may be relatively hypovolemic and/or may have suffered a right ventricular infarct with or without severe left ventricular damage.

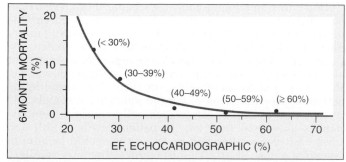

FIGURE 51–30 Impact of left ventricular function on survival following myocardial infarction. The curvilinear relationship between left ventricular ejection fraction (EF) for patients treated in the fibrinolytic era is shown. Among patients with a left ventricular EF below 40 percent, the rate of mortality is markedly increased at 6 months. Thus interventions such as thrombolysis, aspirin, and angiotensin-converting enzyme inhibitors should be of considerable benefit in patients with acute myocardial infarction to minimize the amount of left ventricular damage and interrupt the neurohumoral activation seen with congestive heart failure. *(Modified from Volpi A, De VC, Franzosi MG, et al: Determinants of 6-month mortality in survivors of myocardial infarction after thrombolysis. Results of the GISSI-2 data base. The Ad Hoc Working Group of the Gruppo Italiano per lo Studio della Sopravvivenza nell'Infarto Miocardico (GISSI)-2 Data Base. Circulation 88:416, 1993.)*

The relationship between ventricular filling pressure and cardiac index when preload is increased by an infusion of saline or dextran can provide valuable hemodynamic information, in addition to that obtained from baseline measurements. For example, the ventricular function curve rises steeply (marked increase in cardiac index, small increase in filling pressure) in patients with normal left ventricular function and hypovolemia, whereas the curve rises gradually or remains flat in those patients with a combination of hypovolemia and depressed cardiac function. Invasive hemodynamic monitoring is essential to guide therapy of patients with severe left ventricular failure (pulmonary capillary wedge pressure >18 mm Hg *and* cardiac index <2.5 liters/min/m²). Although positive inotropic agents can be useful, they do not represent the initial therapy of choice in patients with STEMI. Instead, heart failure is managed most effectively first by reduction of ventricular preload and then, if possible, by lowering of afterload. Arrhythmias can contribute to hemodynamic compromise and should be treated promptly in patients with left ventricular failure.

HYPOXEMIA. Patients with STEMI complicated by congestive heart failure characteristically develop hypoxemia caused by a combination of pulmonary vascular engorgement (and in some cases pulmonary interstitial edema), diminished vital capacity, and respiratory depression from narcotic analgesics. Hypoxemia can impair the function of ischemic tissue at the margin of the infarct and thereby contribute to establishing or perpetuating the vicious circle (see Chap. 50, Fig. 50-12). The ventilation-perfusion mismatch that results in hypoxemia requires careful attention to ventilatory support. Increasing fractions of inspired oxygen (F_IO_2) via face mask should be used initially, but if the oxygen saturation of the patient's blood cannot be maintained above 85 to 90 percent on 100 percent F_IO_2, strong consideration should be given to endotracheal intubation with positive-pressure ventilation. The improvement of arterial oxygenation and hence myocardial oxygen supply may help to restore ventricular performance. Positive end-expiratory pressure may diminish systemic venous return and reduce effective left ventricular filling pressure. This may require reduction in the amount of positive end-expiratory pressure, normal saline infusions to maintain left ventricular filling pressure, adjustment of the rate of infusion of vasodilators such as nitroglycerin, or some combination of these. Because myocardial ischemia frequently occurs during the return to unsupported spontaneous breathing, weaning should be accompanied by observation for signs of ischemia and is potentially facilitated by a period of intermittent mandatory ventilation or pressure support ventilation before extubation.

DIURETICS. Mild heart failure in patients with STEMI frequently responds well to diuretics such as furosemide, administered intravenously in doses of 10 to 40 mg, repeated at 3- to 4-hour intervals if necessary. The resultant reduction of pulmonary capillary pressure reduces dyspnea, and the lowering of left ventricular wall tension that accompanies the reduction of left ventricular diastolic volume diminishes myocardial oxygen requirements and may lead to improvement of contractility and augmentation of the ejection fraction, stroke volume, and cardiac output. The reduction of elevated left ventricular filling pressure may also enhance myocardial oxygen delivery by diminishing the impedance to coronary perfusion attributable to elevated ventricular wall tension. It may also improve arterial oxygenation by reducing pulmonary vascular congestion.

The intravenous administration of furosemide reduces pulmonary vascular congestion and pulmonary venous pressure within 15 minutes, before renal excretion of sodium and water has occurred; presumably this action results from a direct dilating effect of this drug on the systemic arterial bed. It is important not to reduce left ventricular filling pressure much below 18 mm Hg, the lower range associated with optimal left ventricular performance in STEMI, because this may reduce cardiac output further and cause arterial hypotension. Excessive diuresis may also result in hypokalemia, with its attendant risk of digitalis intoxication.

AFTERLOAD REDUCTION. Myocardial oxygen requirements depend on left ventricular wall stress, which in turn is proportional to the product of peak developed left ventricular pressure, volume, and wall thickness. Vasodilator therapy is recommended in patients with STEMI complicated by (1) heart failure unresponsive to treatment with diuretics, (2) hypertension, (3) mitral regurgitation, or (4) ventricular septal defect. In these patients, treatment with vasodilator agents increases stroke volume and may reduce myocardial oxygen requirements and thereby lessen ischemia. Hemodynamic monitoring of systemic arterial and, in many cases, pulmonary capillary wedge (or at least pulmonary artery) pressure and cardiac output in patients treated with these agents is important. Improvement of cardiac performance and energetics requires three simultaneous effects: (1) reduction of left ventricular afterload, (2) avoidance of excessive systemic arterial hypotension to maintain effective coronary perfusion pressure, and (3) avoidance of excessive reduction of ventricular filling pressure with consequent diminution of cardiac output. In general, pulmonary capillary wedge pressure should be maintained at approximately 20 mm Hg and arterial pressure above 90/60 mm Hg in patients who were normotensive before developing the STEMI.

Vasodilator therapy is particularly useful when STEMI is complicated by mitral regurgitation or rupture of the ventricular septum. In such patients, vasodilators alone or in combination with intraaortic balloon counterpulsation can sometimes serve as a "holding maneuver" and provide hemodynamic stabilization to permit definitive catheterization and angiographic studies to be carried out and to prepare the patient for early surgical intervention. Because of the precarious state of patients with complicated infarction and the need for meticulous adjustment of dosage, therapy is best initiated with agents that can be administered intravenously and that have a short duration of action, such as nitroprusside, nitroglycerin, or isosorbide dinitrate. After initial stabilization, the medication of choice is generally an ACE inhibitor, but long-acting nitrates given by mouth, sublingually, or by ointment can also be useful.

Nitroglycerin. This drug has been shown in animal experiments to be less likely than nitroprusside to produce a "coronary steal" (i.e., to divert blood flow from the ischemic to the nonischemic zone). Therefore apart from consideration of its routine use in STEMI patients discussed earlier, it may be a particularly useful vasodilator in patients with STEMI complicated by left ventricular failure. Ten to 15 mg/min is infused and the dose is increased by 10 mg/min every 5 minutes until (1) the desired effect (improvement of hemodynamics or relief of ischemic chest pain) is achieved or (2) a decline in systolic arterial pressure to 90 mm Hg, or by more than 15 mm Hg, has occurred. Although both nitroglycerin and nitroprusside lower systemic arterial pressure, systemic vascular resistance, and the heart rate-systolic blood pressure product, the reduction of left ventricular filling pressure is more prominent with nitroglycerin because of its relatively greater effect than nitroprusside on venous capacitance vessels. Nevertheless, in patients with severe left ventricular failure, cardiac output often increases despite the reduction in left ventricular filling pressure produced by nitroglycerin.

Oral Vasodilators. The use of oral vasodilators in the treatment of chronic congestive heart failure is discussed in Chapter 25. In patients with STEMI and persistent heart failure, long-term inhibition of the RAAS should be carried out. This reduced ventricular load decreases the remodeling of the left ventricle that occurs commonly in the period after STEMI and thereby reduces the development of heart failure and risk of death.[191]

DIGITALIS (see Chap. 25). Although digitalis increases the contractility and the oxygen consumption of normal hearts, when heart failure is present the diminution of heart size and wall tension frequently results in a net reduction of myocardial oxygen requirements. In animal experiments, it fails to improve ventricular performance immediately following experimental coronary occlusion, but salutary effects are elicited when it is administered several days later. The absence of early beneficial effects may be caused by the inability of ischemic tissue to respond to digitalis or the already maximal stimulation of contractility of the normal heart by circulating and neuronally released catecholamines.

Although the issue is still controversial, arrhythmias can be increased by digitalis glycosides when they are given to patients in the first few hours after the onset of STEMI, particularly in the presence of hypokalemia. Also, undesirable peripheral systemic and coronary vasoconstriction can result from the rapid intravenous administration of rapidly acting glycosides such as ouabain.

Administration of digitalis to patients with STEMI in the hospital phase should generally be reserved for the management of supraventricular tachyarrhythmias such as atrial flutter and fibrillation and of heart failure that persists despite treatment with diuretics, vasodilators, and beta-adrenoceptor agonists. There is no indication for its use as an inotropic agent in patients without clinical evidence of left ventricular dysfunction, and it is too weak an inotropic agent to be relied on as the principal cardiac stimulant in patients with overt pulmonary edema or cardiogenic shock.

BETA-ADRENERGIC AGONISTS. When left ventricular failure is severe, as manifested by marked reduction of cardiac index (<2 liters/min/m^2), and pulmonary capillary wedge pressure is at optimal (18 to 24 mm Hg) or excessive (>24 mm Hg) levels despite therapy with diuretics, beta-adrenergic agonists are indicated. Although isoproterenol is a potent cardiac stimulant and improves ventricular performance, it should be avoided in STEMI patients. It also causes tachycardia and augments myocardial oxygen consumption and lactate production; in addition, it reduces coronary perfusion pressure by causing systemic vasodilation, and in animal experiments it increases the extent of experimentally induced infarction. Norepinephrine also increases myocardial oxygen consumption because of its peripheral vasoconstrictor, as well as positive inotropic actions.

Dopamine and dobutamine (see Chap. 24) can be particularly useful in patients with STEMI and reduced cardiac output, increased left ventricular filling pressure, pulmonary vascular congestion, and hypotension. Fortunately, the potentially deleterious alpha-adrenergic vasoconstrictor effects exerted by dopamine occur only at higher doses than those required to increase contractility. The vasodilating actions of dopamine on renal and splanchnic vessels and its positive inotropic effects generally improve hemodynamics and renal function. In patients with STEMI and severe left ventricular failure, this drug should be administered at a dose of 3 μg/kg/min while pulmonary capillary wedge and systemic arterial pressures as well as cardiac output are monitored. The dose can be increased stepwise to 20 μg/kg/min to reduce pulmonary capillary wedge pressure to approximately 20 mm Hg and elevate cardiac index to exceed 2 liters/min/m^2. It must be recognized, however, that doses exceeding 5 μg/kg/min activate peripheral alpha receptors and cause vasoconstriction.

Dobutamine has a positive inotropic action comparable to that of dopamine but a slightly less positive chronotropic effect and less vasoconstrictor activity. In patients with STEMI, dobutamine improves left ventricular performance without augmenting enzymatically estimated infarct size. It can be administered in a starting dose of 2.5 μg/kg/min and increased stepwise to a maximum of 30 μg/kg/min. Both dopamine and dobutamine must be given carefully and with constant monitoring of the ECG, systemic arterial pressure, and pulmonary artery or pulmonary artery occlusive pressure and, if possible, with frequent measurements of cardiac output. The dose must be reduced if the heart rate exceeds 100 to 110 beats/min, if supraventricular or ventricular tachyarrhythmias occur, or if ST segment deviations increase.

OTHER POSITIVE INOTROPIC AGENTS. Milrinone is a noncatecholamine, nonglycoside, phosphodiesterase inhibitor with inotropic and vasodilating actions. It is useful in selected patients whose heart failure persists despite treatment with diuretics, who are not hypotensive, and who are likely to benefit from both an enhancement in contractility and afterload reduction. Milrinone should be given as a loading dose of 0.5 μg/kg/min over 10 minutes, followed by a maintenance infusion of 0.375 to 0.75 μg/kg/min.

Cardiogenic Shock

Cardiogenic shock is the most severe clinical expression of left ventricular failure and is associated with extensive damage to the left ventricular myocardium in more than 80 percent of STEMI patients in whom it occurs; the remainder have a mechanical defect such as ventricular septal or papillary muscle rupture or predominant right ventricular infarction.[193,194] In the past, cardiogenic shock has been reported to occur in up to 20 percent of patients with STEMI, but estimates from recent large trials and observational databases report an incidence rate in the range of 7 percent.[193] This low-output state is characterized by elevated ventricular filling pressures, low cardiac output, systemic hypotension, and evidence of vital organ hypoperfusion (e.g., clouded sensorium, cool extremities, oliguria, acidosis). Patients with cardiogenic shock caused by STEMI are more likely to be older, to have a history of a prior MI or congestive heart failure, and to have sustained an anterior infarction at the time of development of shock. Of note, although the incidence of cardiogenic shock in patients with STEMI has been relatively stable since the mid-1970s, the short-term mortality rate has decreased from 70 to 80 percent in the 1970s to 50 to 60 percent in the 1990s.[195] Cardiogenic shock is the cause of death in about 60 percent of patients dying after fibrinolysis for STEMI.[104,196]

PATHOLOGICAL FINDINGS. At autopsy, more than two thirds of patients with cardiogenic shock demonstrate stenosis of 75 percent or more of the luminal diameter of all three major coronary vessels, usually including the left anterior descending coronary artery.[197] Almost all patients with cardiogenic shock are found to have thrombotic occlusion of the artery supplying the major region of recent infarction, with loss of about 40 percent of the left ventricular mass.[193] Patients who die as a consequence of cardiogenic shock often have "piecemeal" necrosis—that is, progressive myocardial necrosis from marginal extension of their infarct into an ischemic zone bordering on the infarction. This is generally associated with persistent elevation of cardiac biomarkers. Such extensions and focal lesions are probably in part the result of the shock state itself. Early deterioration in left ventricular function secondary to apparent extension of infarction may, in some cases, result from expansion of the necrotic zone of myocardium without actual extension of the necrotic process. Hydrodynamic forces that develop during ventricular systole can disrupt necrotic myocardial muscle bundles, with resultant expansion and thinning of the akinetic zone of myocardium, which in turn results in deterioration of overall left ventricular function.

Other causes of cardiogenic shock in patients with STEMI include mechanical defects such as rupture of the ventricular septum, a papillary muscle, or free wall with tamponade; right ventricular infarction; or marked reduction of preload caused by conditions such as hypovolemia.[1]

PATHOPHYSIOLOGY. The shock state in patients with STEMI appears to be the result of a vicious circle, demonstrated in Figure 50-12.

DIAGNOSIS. Cardiogenic shock is characterized by marked and persistent (>30 minutes) hypotension with systolic arterial pressure less than 80 mm Hg and a marked reduction of cardiac index (generally <1.8 liters/min/m²) in the face of elevated left ventricular filling pressure (pulmonary capillary wedge pressure >18 mm Hg). Spurious estimates of left ventricular filling pressure based on measurements of the pulmonary artery wedge pressure can occur in the presence of marked mitral regurgitation, in which the tall V wave in the left atrial (and pulmonary artery wedge) pressure tracing elevates the mean pressure above left ventricular end-diastolic pressure. Accordingly, mitral regurgitation and other mechanical lesions such as ventricular septal defect, ventricular aneurysm, and pseudoaneurysm must be excluded before the diagnosis of cardiogenic shock caused by impairment of left ventricular function can be established. Mechanical complications should be suspected in any patient with STEMI in whom circulatory collapse occurs.[193] Immediate hemodynamic, angiographic, and echocardiographic evaluations are necessary in patients with cardiogenic shock. It is important to exclude mechanical complications because primary therapy of such lesions usually requires immediate operative treatment with intervening support of the circulation by intraaortic balloon counterpulsation.

MEDICAL MANAGEMENT

When the aforementioned mechanical complications are not present, cardiogenic shock is caused by impairment of left ventricular function. Although dopamine or dobutamine usually improves the hemodynamics in these patients, unfortunately neither appears to improve hospital survival significantly. Similarly, vasodilators have been used in an effort to elevate cardiac output and to reduce left ventricular filling pressure. However, by lowering the already markedly reduced coronary perfusion pressure, myocardial perfusion can be compromised further, accelerating the vicious circle illustrated in Figure 50-12. Vasodilators may nonetheless be used in conjunction with intraaortic balloon counterpulsation and inotropic agents in an effort to increase cardiac output while sustaining or elevating coronary perfusion pressure.

The systemic vascular resistance is usually elevated in patients with cardiogenic shock, but occasionally resistance is normal and in a few cases vasodilation actually predominates.[200] When systemic vascular resistance is not elevated (i.e., <1800 dynes/sec/cm⁵) in patients with cardiogenic shock, norepinephrine, which has both alpha- and beta-adrenergic agonist properties (in doses ranging from 2 to 10 μg/min), can be employed to increase diastolic arterial pressure, maintain coronary perfusion, and improve contractility. Norepinephrine should be used only when other means including balloon counterpulsation fail to maintain arterial diastolic pressure above 50 to 60 mm Hg in a previously normotensive patient. The use of alpha-adrenergic agents such as phenylephrine and methoxamine is contraindicated in patients with cardiogenic shock (unless systemic vascular resistance is inordinately low). Inspired by the observation that many patients with shock have a low systemic vascular resistance, inhibitors of nitric oxide synthase were evaluated as potential additions to the management of cardiogenic shock but have not proven to be useful.[201]

INTRAAORTIC BALLOON COUNTERPULSATION

Intraaortic balloon counterpulsation is used in the treatment of STEMI in three groups of patients: (1) those whose conditions are hemodynamically unstable and in whom support of the circulation is required for the performance of cardiac catheterization and angiography carried out to assess lesions that are potentially correctable surgically or by angioplasty; (2) those with cardiogenic shock that is unresponsive to medical management; and (3) rarely, those with persistent ischemic pain that is unresponsive to treatment with inhalation of 100 percent oxygen, beta-adrenergic blockade, and nitrates. Unfortunately, among patients with cardiogenic shock, improvement is often only temporary and "balloon dependence" commonly develops. Patients with cardiogenic shock treated with this modality can be successfully weaned from the supporting system only occasionally. Counterpulsation alone does not improve overall survival in patients either with or without a surgically remediable mechanical lesion.

COMPLICATIONS. Complications occur infrequently but include damage to or perforation of the aortic wall, ischemia distal to the site of insertion of the balloon in the femoral artery, thrombocytopenia, hemolysis, renal emboli, and mechanical failure such as rupture of the balloon. Patients at highest risk include those with peripheral vascular disease; the elderly; and women, particularly if they are small. These factors should be taken into consideration before institution of intraaortic balloon counterpulsation. Because of the potential for vascular bleeding complications, there has been a reluctance to use intraaortic pumps in patients who have undergone fibrinolytic therapy. However, despite the increased bleeding risk, because of the poor outcome among patients with shock following thrombolysis (usually ineffective thrombolysis), this modality should be considered in selected patients who are candidates for an aggressive approach to revascularization.

REVASCULARIZATION

Of the five therapies frequently used to treat patients with cardiogenic shock (vasopressors, intraaortic balloon counterpulsation, fibrinolysis, PCI, and CABG), the first two are useful temporizing maneuvers. Surgical treatment in patients with cardiogenic shock (aside from correcting mechanical abnormalities) may involve bypassing occluded, as well as severely obstructed nonoccluded vessels. Occlusion of one major vessel can cause left ventricular dysfunction and hypotension, which can then lead to hypoperfusion and ischemia of myocardium subserved by the other diseased vessels. Left ventricular function can be improved by relief of this ischemia with revascularization.

The SHOCK study evaluated early revascularization for the treatment of patients with MI complicated by cardiogenic shock. Patients with shock caused by left ventricular failure complicating STEMI were randomized to emergency revascularization ($n = 152$), accomplished by either CABG or angioplasty, or initial medical stabilization ($n = 150$). In 86 percent of patients in both groups, intraaortic balloon counterpulsation was performed. The primary endpoint was all-cause mortality at 30 days; a secondary endpoint was mortality at 6 months. At 30 days, the overall mortality rate was 46.7 percent in the revascularization group, not significantly different from the 56 percent mortality rate observed in the medical therapy group ($p = 0.11$). Subgroups of patients in the SHOCK trial that showed particular benefit from the early revascularization strategy (i.e., reduced 6-month mortality) were those who were younger than 75 years of age, had a prior MI, and were randomized less than 6 hours from onset of infarction.[202] Long-term survival improved significantly in patients with cardiogenic shock who underwent early revascularization (Fig. 51-31).[104]

RECOMMENDATIONS. We recommend assessment of patients on an individualized basis to determine their desire for aggressive care and overall candidacy for further treatment (e.g., age, mental status, comorbidities). Patients who are potential candidates for revascularization should then rapidly receive intraaortic balloon counterpulsation and be referred for coronary arteriography. Those with suitable anatomy should be revascularized as completely as possible with PCI and/or CABG.[1,104,194] Encouraging initial experience has been reported with a percutaneous left ventricular assist device as a bridge to a revascularization procedure (see Chap. 28).[203] In appropriately selected patients, emergency cardiac transplantation has also been used successfully to manage cardiogenic shock.

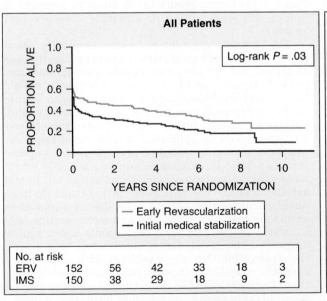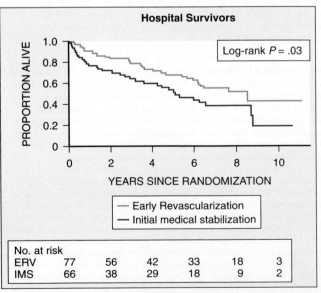

FIGURE 51–31 Impact of revascularization in patients in SHOCK trial. Among all patients, the survival rates in the early revascularization (ERV) and initial medical stabilization (IMS) groups, respectively, were 41.4 versus 28.3 percent at 3 years and 32.8 versus 19.6 percent at 6 years. With exclusion of 8 patients with aortic dissection, tamponade, or severe mitral regurgitation identified shortly after randomization, the survival curves remained significantly different ($p = 0.02$), with a 14 percent absolute difference at 6 years. Among hospital survivors, the survival rates in the ERV and IMS groups, respectively, were 78.8 versus 64.3 percent at 3 years and 62.4 versus 44.4 percent at 6 years. *(From Hochman JS, Sleeper LA, Webb JG, Dzavik V, et al: Early revascularization and long-term survival in cardiogenic shock complicating acute myocardial infarction. JAMA 295:2511, 2006.)*

Right Ventricular Infarction

Right ventricular infarction can have a range of clinical presentations from mild right ventricular dysfunction through cardiogenic shock.[1] A characteristic hemodynamic pattern (Fig. 51-32) has been observed in patients with clinically significant right ventricular infarction, which frequently accompanies inferior left ventricular infarction or rarely occurs in isolated form. Right-heart filling pressures (central venous, right atrial, and right ventricular end-diastolic pressures) are elevated, whereas left ventricular filling pressure is normal or only slightly raised; right ventricular systolic and pulse pressures are decreased, and cardiac output is often markedly depressed. Rarely, this disproportionate elevation of right-sided filling pressure causes right-to-left shunting through a patent foramen ovale. This possibility should be considered in patients with right ventricular infarction who have unexplained systemic hypoxemia. The finding of an elevation in atrial natriuretic factor level in patients with this condition has led to the suggestion that abnormally high levels of this peptide might be in part responsible for the hypotension seen in patients with right ventricular infarction. Of note, the same protective effect of ischemic preconditioning that has been described in cases of infarction of the left ventricle has also been reported in patients with infarction of the right ventricle.[204]

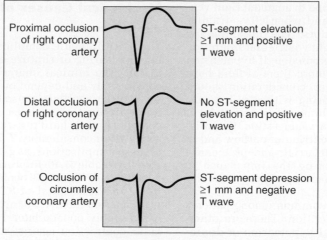

Proximal occlusion of right coronary artery		ST-segment elevation ≥1 mm and positive T wave
Distal occlusion of right coronary artery		No ST-segment elevation and positive T wave
Occlusion of circumflex coronary artery		ST-segment depression ≥1 mm and negative T wave

Clinical findings:
   Shock with clear lungs, elevated JVP
   Kussmaul sign

Hemodynamics:
   Increased RA pressure (y descent)
   Square root sign in RV tracing

ECG:
   ST elevation in R sided leads

Echo:
   Depressed RV function

Management:
   Maintain RV preload
   Lower RV afterload (PA---PCW)
   Restore AV synchrony
   Inotropic support
   Reperfusion

FIGURE 51–32 Right ventricular infarction: clinical features and management. Patients with hemodynamically significant right ventricular infarction present with shock but clear lungs and elevated JVP. ST elevation exists in right-sided ECG leads with variation in the repolarization pattern depending on the infarct artery and the location of the occlusion. **Bottom right,** Management recommendations. AV = atrioventricular; ECG = electrocardiogram; Echo = echocardiogram; JVP = jugular venous pressure; PA = pulmonary artery; PCW = pulmonary capillary wedge; RA = right atrial; RV = right ventricular. *(Modified from Wellens HJ: The value of the right precordial leads of the electrocardiogram. N Engl J Med 340:381, 1999 and Antman EM, Anbe DT, Armstrong PW, et al: ACC/AHA guidelines for the management of patients with ST-elevation myocardial infarction: A report of the American College of Cardiology/American Heart Association Task Force on Practice Guidelines (Committee to Revise the 1999 Guidelines for the Management of Patients with Acute Myocardial Infarction) (www.acc.org/clinical/guidelines/stemi/index.pdf). Accessed 4/19/06.*

DIAGNOSIS

Many patients with the combination of normal left ventricular filling pressure and depressed cardiac index have right ventricular infarcts (with accompanying inferior left ventricular infarcts). The hemodynamic picture may superficially resemble that seen in patients with pericardial disease (see Chap. 70). It includes elevated right ventricular filling pressure; steep, right atrial y descent; and an early diastolic drop and plateau (resembling the square root sign) in the right ventricular pressure tracing. Moreover, the Kussmaul sign (an increase in jugular venous pressure with inspiration) and pulsus paradoxus (a fall in systolic pressure of greater than 10 mm Hg with inspiration) may be present in patients with right ventricular infarction (see Fig. 51-32).[205] In fact, the Kussmaul sign in the setting of inferior STEMI highly predicts right ventricular involvement.

The ECG can provide the first clue that right ventricular involvement is present in the patient with inferior STEMI (see Fig. 51-32). Most patients with right ventricular infarction have ST segment elevation in lead V_4R (right precordial lead in V_4 position).[206] Transient elevation of the ST segment in any of the right precordial leads can occur with right ventricular MI, and the presence of ST segment elevation of 0.1 mV or more in any one or combination of leads V_4R, V_5R, and V_6R in patients with the clinical picture of acute MI is highly sensitive and specific for the diagnosis of right ventricular MI. Wellens has emphasized that in addition to

noting the presence or absence of convex upward ST elevation in V_4R, clinicians should determine whether the T wave is positive or negative—such distinctions help distinguish proximal versus distal occlusion of the right coronary artery versus occlusion of the left circumflex artery (see Fig. 51-32).[207] Elevation of the ST segments in leads V_1 through V_4 caused by right ventricular infarction can be confused with elevation caused by anteroseptal infarction. Although the elevated ST segments are oriented anteriorly in both cases, the frontal plane can provide important clues—the ST segments are oriented to the right in right ventricular infarction (e.g., +120 degrees), whereas they are oriented to the left in anteroseptal infarction (e.g., –30 degrees).

ECHOCARDIOGRAPHY AND RADIONUCLIDE ANGIOGRAPHY. Echocardiography is helpful in the differential diagnosis because in right ventricular infarction, in contrast to pericardial tamponade, little or no pericardial fluid accumulates. The echocardiogram shows abnormal wall motion of the right ventricle, as well as right ventricular dilation and depression of right ventricular ejection fraction.[205] Magnetic resonance imaging can also aid recognition of right ventricular infarction.[208] Serial studies have shown that some degree of recovery of an initially depressed right ventricular ejection fraction is the rule with right ventricular infarction, to a greater degree than with left ventricular ejection fraction.[205]

HEMODYNAMICS. Loss of atrial transport in patients with right ventricular infarction can result in marked reductions in stroke volume and arterial blood pressure. Disproportionate elevation of the right-sided filling pressure is the hemodynamic hallmark of right ventricular infarction. Therefore ventricular pacing may fail to increase cardiac output, and atrioventricular sequential pacing may be required.

TREATMENT

Because of their ability to reduce preload, medications routinely prescribed for left ventricular infarction may produce profound hypotension in patients with right ventricular infarction.[205] In patients with hypotension caused by right ventricular MI, hemodynamics can be improved by a combination of expanding plasma volume to augment right ventricular preload and cardiac output and, when left ventricular failure is present, arterial vasodilators.[1] The initial therapy for hypotension in patients with right ventricular infarction should almost always be volume expansion. If hypotension has not been corrected after 1 or more liters of fluid have been administered briskly, however, consideration should be given to hemodynamic monitoring with a pulmonary artery catheter because further volume infusion may be of little use and may produce pulmonary congestion. Vasodilators reduce the impedance to left ventricular outflow and in turn left ventricular diastolic, left atrial, and pulmonary (arterial) pressures, thereby lowering the impedance to right ventricular outflow and enhancing right ventricular output.

Right ventricular infarction is common among patients with inferior left ventricular infarction. Therefore otherwise unexplained systemic arterial hypotension or diminished cardiac output, or marked hypotension in response to small doses of nitroglycerin in patients with inferior infarction, should lead to the prompt consideration of this diagnosis. In view of the importance of atrial transport, patients requiring pacing should have atrial or atrioventricular sequential pacing.[209] Successful reperfusion of the right coronary artery significantly improves right ventricular mechanical function and lowers in-hospital mortality in patients with right ventricular infarction.[210] Replacement of the tricuspid valve and repair of the valve with annuloplasty rings have been carried out in the treatment of severe tricuspid regurgitation secondary to right ventricular infarction.

CH 51

Mechanical Causes of Heart Failure

FREE WALL RUPTURE

The most dramatic complications of STEMI are those that involve tearing or rupture of acutely infarcted tissue (Fig. 51-33).[1] The clinical characteristics of these lesions vary considerably and depend on the site of rupture, which may involve the papillary muscles, interventricular septum, or free wall of either ventricle. The overall incidence of these complications is hard to assess because clinical and autopsy series differ considerably.[211] The comparative clinical profile of these complications, as gathered from different studies, is shown in Table 51-10. Rupture of the free wall of the infarcted ventricle (see Fig. 51-33) occurs in up to 10 percent of patients dying in the hospital of STEMI.[212] Thinness of the apical wall, marked intensity of necrosis at the terminal end of the blood supply, poor collateral flow, the shearing effect of muscular contraction against an inert and stiffened necrotic area, and aging of the myocardium with laceration of the myocardial microstructure may all promote rupture.[213]

CLINICAL CHARACTERISTICS. The following are some features that characterize this serious complication of STEMI.[214]

1. Occurs more frequently in elderly patients and possibly more frequently in women than in men with infarction.
2. Appears to be more common in hypertensive than in normotensive patients.
3. Occurs more frequently in the left than in the right ventricle and seldom occurs in the atria.
4. Usually involves the anterior or lateral walls of the ventricle in the area of the terminal distribution of the left anterior descending coronary artery.
5. Is usually associated with a relatively large transmural infarction involving at least 20 percent of the left ventricle.
6. Occurs between 1 day and 3 weeks, but most commonly 1 to 4 days, after infarction.
7. Is usually preceded by infarct expansion—that is, thinning and a disproportionate dilation within the softened necrotic zone.[213]
8. Most commonly results from a distinct tear in the myocardial wall or a dissecting hematoma that perforates a necrotic area of myocardium (see Fig. 51-33).
9. Usually occurs near the junction of the infarct and the normal muscle.
10. Occurs less frequently in the center of the infarct, but when rupture occurs here, it is usually during the second rather than the first week after the infarct.
11. Rarely occurs in a greatly thickened ventricle or in an area of extensive collateral vessels.
12. Most often occurs in patients without previous infarction.

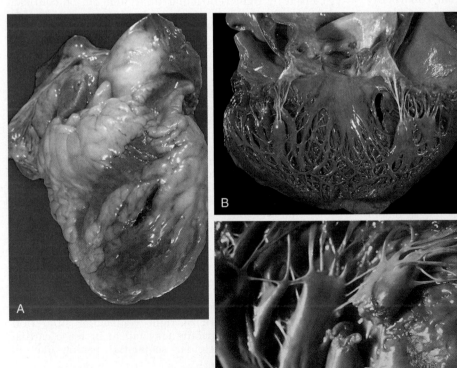

FIGURE 51–33 Cardiac rupture syndromes complicating ST-elevation myocardial infarction (STEMI). **A,** Anterior myocardial rupture in an acute infarct (arrow). **B,** Rupture of the ventricular septum (arrow). **C,** Complete rupture of a necrotic papillary muscle. *(From Schoen FJ: The heart. In Kumar V, Abbas AK, Fausto N [eds]: Robbins & Cotran Pathologic Basis of Disease. 7th ed. Philadelphia, Saunders, 2005.)*

13. There is no evidence that the intensity of anticoagulation influences the occurrence of rupture.
14. Occurs more commonly in patients who received reperfusion therapy with a fibrinolytic versus PCI.[1]

Rupture of the free wall of the left ventricle usually leads to hemopericardium and death from cardiac tamponade. Occasionally, rupture of the free wall of the ventricle occurs as the first clinical manifestation in patients with undetected or silent MI, and then it may be considered a form of "sudden cardiac death" (see Chap. 36).

The course of rupture varies from catastrophic, with an acute tear leading to immediate death, to subacute, with nausea, hypotension, and pericardial type of discomfort being the major clinical clues to its presence. Survival depends on the recognition of this complication, on hemodynamic stabilization of the patient—usually with inotropic agents and/or intraaortic balloon pump—and most importantly on prompt surgical repair.[1]

PSEUDOANEURYSM. Incomplete rupture of the heart may occur when organizing thrombus and hematoma, together with pericardium, seal a rupture of the left ventricle and thus prevent the development of hemopericardium (Fig. 51-34). With time, this area of organized thrombus and pericardium can become a pseudoaneurysm (false aneurysm) that maintains communication with the cavity of the left ventricle. In contrast to true aneurysms, which always contain some myocardial elements in their walls, the walls of pseudoaneurysms are composed of organized hematoma and pericardium and lack any elements of the original myocardial wall. Pseudoaneurysms can become quite large,

even equaling the true ventricular cavity in size, and they communicate with the left ventricular cavity through a narrow neck. Frequently, pseudoaneurysms contain significant quantities of old and recent thrombi, superficial portions of which can cause arterial emboli. Pseudoaneurysms can drain off a portion of each ventricular stroke volume exactly as do true aneurysms. The diagnosis of pseudoaneurysm can usually be made by echocardiography and contrast angiography, although at times differentiation between true aneurysm and pseudoaneurysm can be difficult by any imaging technique.[215]

DIAGNOSIS. The rupture usually presents with sudden profound shock, often rapidly leading to pulseless electrical activity caused by pericardial tamponade. Immediate pericardiocentesis confirms the diagnosis and relieves the pericardial tamponade, at least momentarily. If the patient's condition is relatively stable, echocardiography may help in establishing the diagnosis of tamponade.[1] Under the most favorable conditions, cardiac catheterization can be carried out, not necessarily to confirm the diagnosis of rupture but to delineate the coronary anatomy. This is helpful so that, in addition to ventricular repair, CABG can be performed in patients in whom high-grade obstructive lesions are present. In patients in whom hemodynamics are critically compromised, establishment of the diagnosis should be followed immediately by surgical resection of the necrotic and ruptured myocardium with primary reconstruction (Fig. 51-35). When rupture is subacute and a pseudoaneurysm is suspected or present, prompt elective surgery is indicated because rupture of the pseudoaneurysm occurs relatively frequently.

CH 51

ST-Elevation Myocardial Infarction: Management

TABLE 51-10	Characteristics of Ventricular Septal Rupture (VSR), Rupture of the Ventricular Free Wall, and Papillary Muscle Rupture		
Characteristic	**VSR**	**Rupture of Ventricular Free Wall**	**Papillary Muscle Rupture**
Incidence	1-3% without reperfusion therapy, 0.2-0.34% with fibrinolytic therapy, 3.9% among patients with cardiogenic shock	0.8-6.2%, Fibrinolytic therapy does not reduce risk; primary PTCA seems to reduce risk	About 1% (posteromedial more frequent than anterolateral papillary muscle)
Time course	Bimodal peak; within 24 h and 3-5 days; range 1-14 days	Bimodal peak; within 24 h and 3-5 days; range 1-14 days	Bimodal peak; within 24 h and 3-5 days; range 1-14 days
Clinical manifestations	Chest pain, shortness of breath hypotension	Anginal, pleuritic, or pericardial chest pain, syncope, hypotension, arrhythmia, nausea, restlessness, hypotension, sudden death	Abrupt onset of shortness of breath and pulmonary edema; hypotension
Physical findings	Harsh holosystolic murmur, thrill (+), S_3, accentuated second heart sound, pulmonary edema, RV and LV failure, cardiogenic shock	Jugular venous distention (29% of patients), pulsus paradoxus (47%), electromechanical dissociation, cardiogenic shock	A soft murmur in some cases, no thrill, variable signs of RV overload, severe pulmonary edema, cardiogenic shock
Echocardiographic findings	VSR, left-to-right shunt on color flow Doppler echocardiography through the ventricular septum, pattern of RV overload	>5 mm pericardial effusion not visualized in all cases; layered, high-acoustic echoes within the pericardium (blood clot); direct visualization of tear; signs of tamponade	Hypercontractile LV, torn papillary muscle or chordae tendineae, flail leaflet, severe MR on color flow Doppler echocardiography
Right-heart catheterization	Increase in oxygen saturation from the RA to RV, large V waves	Ventriculography insensitive, classic signs of tamponade not always present (equalization of diastolic pressures among the cardiac chambers)	No increase in oxygen saturation from the RA to RV, large V waves,* very high pulmonary-capillary wedge pressures

*Large V waves are from the pulmonary capillary wedge pressure.

LV = left ventricle/left ventricular; MR = mitral regurgitation; PTCA = percutaneous transluminal coronary angioplasty; RA = right atrium; RV = right ventricle/right ventricular.

From Antman EM, Anbe DT, Armstrong PW et al: ACC/AHA guidelines for the management of patients with ST-elevation myocardial infarction: A report of the American College of Cardiology/American Heart Association Task Force on Practice Guidelines (Committee to Revise the 1999 Guidelines for the Management of Patients with Acute Myocardial Infarction). (www.acc.org/clinical/guidelines/stemi/index.pdf) Accessed 4/19/06.

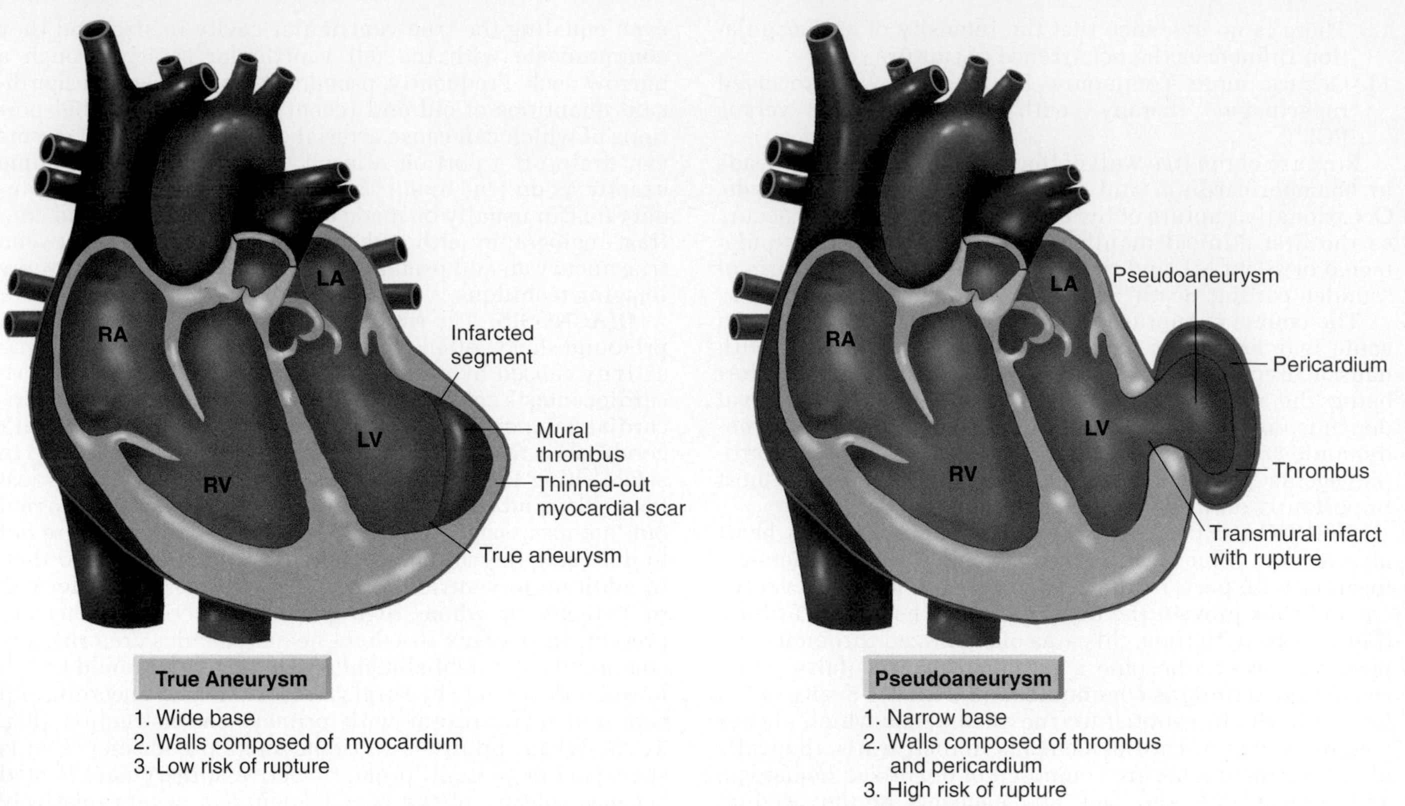

True Aneurysm
1. Wide base
2. Walls composed of myocardium
3. Low risk of rupture

Pseudoaneurysm
1. Narrow base
2. Walls composed of thrombus and pericardium
3. High risk of rupture

FIGURE 51–34 Differences between a pseudoaneurysm and a true aneurysm. LA = left atrium; LV = left ventricle; RA = right atrium; RV = right ventricle. *(From Shah PK: Complications of acute myocardial infarction. In Parmley W, Chatterjee K [eds]: Cardiology. Philadelphia, JB Lippincott, 1987.)*

RUPTURE OF THE INTERVENTRICULAR SEPTUM (see Table 51-10)

Clinical features associated with an increased risk of rupture of the interventricular septum include lack of development of a collateral network, advanced age, hypertension, anterior location of infarction, and possibly fibrinolysis.[211] Rupture of the interventricular septum after STEMI confers a high 30-day mortality.[1,216] The perforation can range in length from one to several centimeters (see Fig. 51-33). It can be a direct through-and-through opening or more irregular and serpiginous. The size of the defect determines the magnitude of the left-to-right shunt and the extent of hemodynamic deterioration, which in turn affects the likelihood of survival.[211] As in rupture of the free wall of the ventricle, transmural infarction underlies rupture of the ventricular septum. Rupture of the septum with an anterior infarction tends to be apical in location, whereas inferior infarctions are associated with perforation of the basal septum and with a worse prognosis than those in an anterior location. In contrast with rupture of the free wall, rupture of the ventricular septum more often associates with complete heart block, right bundle branch block, or atrial fibrillation.[217] Virtually all patients have multivessel coronary artery disease, with the majority exhibiting lesions in all of the major vessels. The likelihood of survival depends on the degree of impairment of ventricular function and the size of the defect.[211]

A ruptured interventricular septum is characterized by the appearance of a new harsh, loud holosystolic murmur that is heard best at the lower left sternal border and that is usually accompanied by a thrill.[1] Biventricular failure generally ensues within hours to days. The defect can also be recognized by echocardiography with color flow Doppler imaging (Fig. 51-36) or insertion of a pulmonary artery balloon catheter to document the left-to-right shunt. Catheter placement of an umbrella-shaped device within the ruptured septum has been reported to stabilize the conditions of critically ill patients with acute septal rupture after STEMI.

RUPTURE OF A PAPILLARY MUSCLE

Partial or total rupture of a papillary muscle is a rare but often fatal complication of transmural MI (see Fig. 51-33).[218] Inferior wall infarction can lead to rupture of the posteromedial papillary muscle, which occurs more commonly than rupture of the anterolateral muscle, a consequence of anterolateral MI. Rupture of a right ventricular papillary muscle is rare but can cause massive tricuspid regurgitation and right ventricular failure. Complete transection of a left ventricular papillary muscle is incompatible with life because the sudden massive mitral regurgitation that develops cannot be tolerated. Rupture of a portion of a papillary muscle, usually the tip or head of the muscle, resulting in severe, although not necessarily overwhelming, mitral regurgitation, is much more frequent and is not immediately fatal (Fig. 51-37). Unlike rupture of the ventricular septum, which occurs with large infarcts, papillary muscle rupture occurs with a relatively small infarction in approximately one half of the cases seen. The extent of coronary artery disease in these patients sometimes is modest as well. In a small number of patients, rupture of more than one cardiac structure is noted clinically or at postmortem examination; all possible combinations of rupture of the free left ventricular wall, the interventricular septum, and papillary muscles have been described.[219]

As with patients who have a ruptured ventricular septal defect, those with papillary muscle rupture manifest a new holosystolic murmur and develop increasingly severe heart failure. In both conditions the murmur may become softer or disappear as arterial pressure falls. Mitral regurgitation

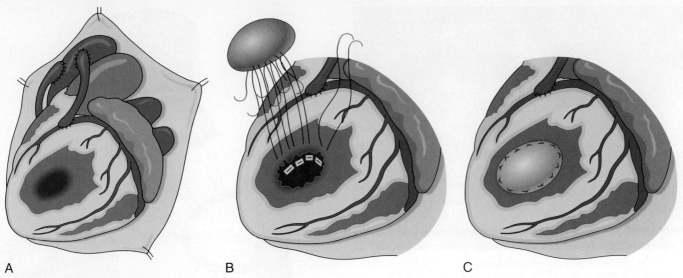

FIGURE 51–35 Management of free wall rupture. **A,** Typically, the rupture site is within a larger area of necrotic muscle. **B,** After débridement, pledgeted sutures are placed inside the ventricle and through a tailored prosthetic patch. **C,** The patch is then secured to the free wall. *(Courtesy of Dr. David Adams, Mt. Sinai Hospital, New York.)*

due to partial or complete rupture of a papillary muscle can be promptly recognized echocardiographically.[1] Color flow Doppler imaging is particularly helpful in distinguishing acute mitral regurgitation from a ventricular septal defect in the setting of STEMI (see Table 51-10).[1] Therefore an echocardiogram should be obtained immediately on any patient in whom the diagnosis is suspected because hemodynamic deterioration can ensue rapidly. Echocardiography also often permits differentiation of papillary muscle rupture from other, generally less severe forms of mitral regurgitation that occur with STEMI.

DIFFERENTIATION BETWEEN VENTRICULAR SEPTAL RUPTURE AND MITRAL REGURGITATION

It may be difficult, on clinical grounds, to distinguish between acute mitral regurgitation and rupture of the ventricular septum in patients with STEMI who suddenly develop a loud systolic murmur. This differentiation can be made most readily by color flow Doppler echocardiography. In addition, a right-heart catheterization with a balloon-tipped catheter can readily distinguish between these two complications. Patients with ventricular septal rupture demonstrate a "step-up" in oxygen saturation in blood samples from the right ventricle and pulmonary artery compared with those from the right atrium. Patients with acute mitral regurgitation lack this step-up; they may demonstrate tall C-V waves in both the pulmonary capillary and pulmonary arterial pressure tracings.

Invasive monitoring, which is essential in these patients, also allows for the critically important assessment of ventricular function.[1] Right and left ventricular filling pressures (right atrial pressure and pulmonary capillary wedge pressure) dictate fluid administration or the use of diuretics, whereas measurements of cardiac output and mean arterial pressure are obtained for calculation of systemic vascular resistance as a guide for vasodilator therapy. Unless systolic pressure is below 90 mm Hg, this therapy, generally using nitroglycerin or nitroprusside, should be instituted as soon as possible once hemodynamic monitoring is available. This may be critically important for stabilizing the patient's condition in preparation for further diagnostic studies and surgical repair. If vasodilator therapy is not tolerated or if it fails to achieve hemodynamic stabil-

ity, intraaortic balloon counterpulsation should be rapidly instituted.

SURGICAL TREATMENT

Operative intervention is most successful in patients with STEMI and circulatory collapse when a surgically correctable mechanical lesion such as ventricular septal defect or mitral regurgitation can be identified and repaired. In such patients, the circulation should at first be supported by intraaortic balloon pulsation and a positive inotropic agent such as dopamine or dobutamine in combination with a vasodilator, unless the patient is hypotensive. Surgery should not be delayed in patients with a correctable lesion who agree to an aggressive management strategy and require pharmacological and/or mechanical (counterpulsation) support. Such patients frequently develop a serious complication—infection, adult respiratory distress syndrome, extension of the infarct, or renal failure—if surgery is delayed. Surgical survival is predicted by early operation, short duration of shock, and mild degrees of right and left ventricular impairment. When the hemodynamic status of a patient with one of these mechanical lesions complicating STEMI remains stable after the patient has been weaned from pharmacological and/or mechanical support, it may be possible to postpone the operation for 2 to 4 weeks to allow some healing of the infarct to occur. Surgical repair involves correction of mitral regurgitation, insertion of a prosthetic mitral valve repair, or closure of a ventricular septal defect, usually accompanied by coronary revascularization (Figs. 51-38 and 51-39).[1]

ARRHYTHMIAS

The genesis, diagnosis, and management of arrhythmias are presented in Part 5. The role of arrhythmias in complicating the course of patients with STEMI and the prevention and treatment of these arrhythmias in this setting are discussed here and summarized in Table 51-11.

The incidence of arrhythmias is higher in patients the earlier they are seen after the onset of symptoms. Many serious arrhythmias develop before hospitalization, even before the patient is monitored. Some abnormality of cardiac

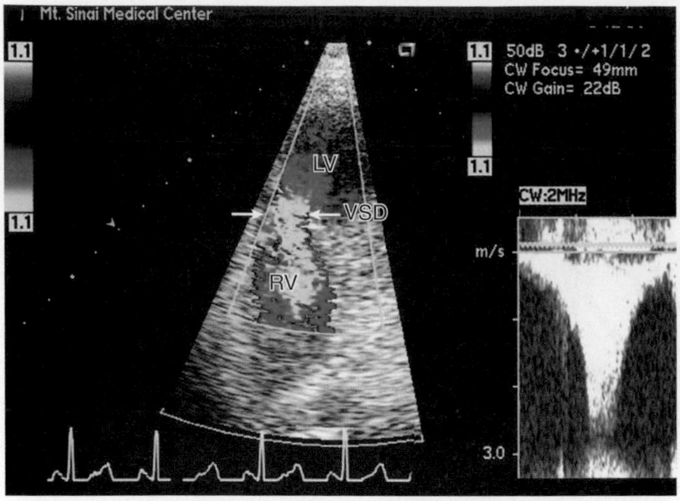

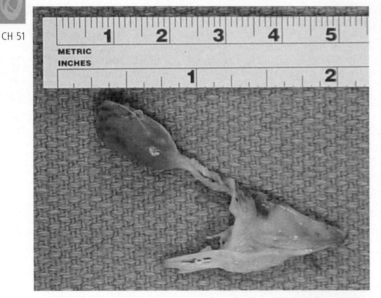

FIGURE 51–36 Two-dimensional echocardiography in an elderly female patient with a ventricular septal defect (VSD) that developed after an ST-elevation myocardial infarction (STEMI) caused by occlusion of the left anterior descending coronary artery. Close-up of ventricular septum in apical four-chamber view **(left)** demonstrates turbulent systolic color flow Doppler across large VSD. Continuous wave Doppler **(right)** demonstrates systolic flow across VSD. LV = left ventricle; RV = right ventricle; VSD = ventricular septal defect. *(From Kamran M, Attari M, Webber G: Images in cardiovascular medicine. Ventricular septal defect complicating an acute myocardial infarction. Circulation 112:e337-338, 2005.)*

FIGURE 51–37 Surgical specimen showing papillary muscle **(top left)**, chordae, and anterior mitral leaflet **(bottom right)** from a patient who had partial rupture of the papillary muscle and underwent mitral valve replacement for severe mitral regurgitation after ST-elevation myocardial infarction. *(Courtesy of John Byrne, MD, Brigham and Women's Hospital, Boston.)*

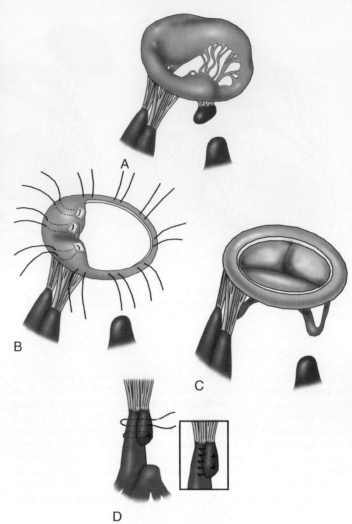

FIGURE 51–38 Surgical management of mitral regurgitation caused by ruptured papillary muscle. **A,** Acute papillary muscle rupture results in severe mitral regurgitation caused by leaflet and commissural prolapse. Mitral valve replacement is usually necessary. **B,** Mitral débridement with retention of the unruptured commissural and leaflet segment is performed to preserve partial annular papillary continuity. **C,** Mitral valve replacement is then performed. **D,** Occasionally, mitral valve repair can be performed by transfer of a papillary head to a nonruptured segment. *(Courtesy of Dr. David Adams, Mt. Sinai Hospital, New York.)*

rhythm also occurs in the majority of patients with STEMI treated in CCUs. Patients seen very early during the course of STEMI almost invariably exhibit evidence of increased activity of the autonomic nervous system. Thus sinus bradycardia, sometimes associated with AV block, and hypotension reflect augmented vagal activity.

MECHANISM OF ARRHYTHMIAS. A leading hypothesis for a major mechanism of arrhythmias in the acute phase of coronary occlusion is reentry caused by inhomogeneity of the electrical characteristics of ischemic myocardium.[220] The cellular electrophysiological mechanisms for reperfusion arrhythmias appear to include washout of various ions such as lactate and potassium and toxic metabolic substances that have accumulated in the ischemic zone.

HEMODYNAMIC CONSEQUENCES. Patients with significant left ventricular dysfunction have a relatively fixed stroke volume and depend on changes in heart rate to alter cardiac output. However, there is a narrow range of heart rate over which the cardiac output is maximal, with significant reductions occurring at both faster and slower rates. Thus all forms of bradycardia and tachycardia can depress the cardiac output in patients with STEMI. Although the optimal rate insofar as cardiac output is concerned may exceed 100 beats/min, it is important to consider that heart rate is one of the major determinants of myocardial oxygen consumption and that at more rapid heart rates, myocardial energy needs can be elevated to levels that adversely affect ischemic myocardium. Therefore in patients with STEMI, the optimal rate is usually lower, in the range of 60 to 80 beats/min.

A second factor to consider in assessing the hemodynamic consequences of a particular arrhythmia is the loss of the atrial contribution to ventricular preload. Studies in

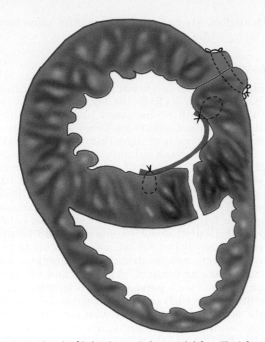

FIGURE 51-39 Repair of ischemic ventricular septal defect. The infarct typically involves a free wall and septum. Repair of the defect is performed through an incision in the ventricular wall infarct. The septal defect is closed with a prosthetic patch, and a second patch is used to close the incision in the free wall. *(Courtesy of Dr. David Adams, Mt. Sinai Hospital, New York.)*

patients without STEMI have demonstrated that loss of atrial transport decreases left ventricular output by 15 to 20 percent. In patients with reduced diastolic left ventricular compliance of any cause (including STEMI), however, atrial systole is of greater importance for left ventricular filling. In patients with STEMI, atrial systole boosts end-diastolic volume by 15 percent, end-diastolic pressure by 29 percent, and stroke volume by 35 percent.

Ventricular Arrhythmias (see Chap. 35)

Ventricular Premature Complexes

Before the widespread use of reperfusion therapy, aspirin, beta blockers, and intravenous nitrates in the management of STEMI, it was believed that frequent ventricular premature complexes (VPCs) (>5 per minute), VPCs with multiform configuration, early coupling (the "R-on-T" phenomenon), and repetitive patterns in the form of couplets or salvos presaged ventricular fibrillation. It is now clear, however, that such "warning arrhythmias" are present in as many patients who do not develop fibrillation as those who do. Several reports have shown that primary ventricular fibrillation (see later) occurs without antecedent warning arrhythmias and may even develop in spite of suppression of warning arrhythmias.[1] Both primary ventricular fibrillation and VPCs, especially R-on-T beats, occur during the early phase of STEMI, when considerable heterogeneity of electrical activity is present. Although R-on-T beats expose this heterogeneity and can precipitate ventricular fibrillation in a small minority of patients, the ubiquitous nature

CH 51

ST-Elevation Myocardial Infarction: Management

TABLE 51-11	Cardiac Arrhythmias and Their Management During Acute Myocardial Infarction		
Category	**Arrhythmia**	**Objective of Treatment**	**Therapeutic Options**
1. Electrical instability	Ventricular premature beats	Correction of electrolyte deficits and increased sympathetic tone	Potassium and magnesium solutions, beta blocker
	Ventricular tachycardia	Prophylaxis against ventricular fibrillation, restoration of hemodynamic stability	Antiarrhythmic agents; cardioversion/defibrillation
	Ventricular fibrillation	Urgent reversion to sinus rhythm	Defibrillation; bretylium tosylate
	Accelerated idioventricular rhythm	Observation unless hemodynamic function is compromised	Increase sinus rate (atropine, atrial pacing); antiarrhythmic agents
	Nonparoxysmal atrioventricular junctional tachycardia	Search for precipitating causes (e.g., digitalis intoxication); suppress arrhythmia only if hemodynamic function is compromised	Atrial overdrive pacing; antiarrhythmic agents; cardioversion relatively contraindicated if digitalis intoxication present
2. Pump failure/ excessive sympathetic stimulation	Sinus tachycardia	Reduce heart rate to diminish myocardial oxygen demands	Antipyretics; analgesics; consider beta blocker unless congestive heart failure present; treat latter if present with anticongestive measures (diuretics, afterload reduction)
	Atrial fibrillation and/or atrial flutter	Reduce ventricular rate; restore sinus rhythm	Verapamil, digitalis glycosides; anticongestive measures (diuretics, afterload reduction); cardioversion; rapid atrial pacing (for atrial flutter)
	Paroxysmal supraventricular tachycardia	Reduce ventricular rate; restore sinus rhythm	Vagal maneuvers; verapamil, cardiac glycosides, beta-adrenergic blockers; cardioversion; rapid atrial pacing
3. Bradyarrhythmias and conduction disturbances	Sinus bradycardia	Acceleration of heart rate only if hemodynamic function is compromised	Atropine; atrial pacing
	Junctional escape rhythm	Acceleration of sinus rate only if loss of atrial "kick" causes hemodynamic compromise	Atropine; atrial pacing
	Atrioventricular block and intraventricular block		Insertion of pacemaker

Modified from Antman EM, Rutherford JD (eds): Coronary Care Medicine: A Practical Approach. Boston. Martinus Nijhoff Publishing, 1986. p 78.

of VPCs in patients with STEMI and the extremely infrequent nature of ventricular fibrillation in the current era of STEMI management produce unacceptably low sensitivity and specificity of ECG patterns observed on monitoring systems for identifying patients at risk of ventricular fibrillation.

MANAGEMENT. Since the incidence of ventricular fibrillation in patients with STEMI seen in CCUs over the past 3 decades appears to be declining, the prior practice of prophylactic suppression of ventricular premature beats with antiarrhythmic drugs no longer is necessary and its use may actually increase the risk of fatal bradycardic and asystolic events.[221] Therefore we pursue a conservative course when VPCs are observed in STEMI patients and do not routinely prescribe antiarrhythmic drugs but instead determine whether recurrent ischemia or electrolyte or metabolic disturbances are present.[1] When, at the inception of an infarction, VPCs accompany sinus tachycardia, augmented sympathoadrenal stimulation is often a contributing factor and can be treated by beta-adrenergic blockade. In fact, early administration of an intravenous beta blocker is effective in reducing the incidence of ventricular fibrillation in cases of evolving MI.

ACCELERATED IDIOVENTRICULAR RHYTHM. This arrhythmia is seen in up to 20 percent of patients with STEMI. It occurs frequently during the first 2 days, with about equal frequency in anterior and inferior infarctions. Most episodes are of short duration. Accelerated idioventricular rhythm is often observed shortly after successful reperfusion has been established. However, the frequent occurrence of this rhythm in patients without reperfusion limits their reliability as markers of restoration of patency of the infarct-related coronary artery.[1] In contrast to rapid ventricular tachycardia, accelerated idioventricular rhythm is thought not to affect prognosis, and we do not routinely treat accelerated idioventricular rhythms.

Ventricular Tachycardia

Nonsustained runs of ventricular tachycardia do not appear to be associated with an increased mortality risk, either during hospitalization or over the first year. Ventricular tachycardia occurring late in the course of STEMI is more common in patients with transmural infarction and left ventricular dysfunction, is likely to be sustained, usually induces marked hemodynamic deterioration, and is associated with increased rates of both hospital mortality and long-term mortality.

MANAGEMENT. Because hypokalemia can increase the risk of developing ventricular tachycardia, low serum potassium levels should be identified quickly after a patient's admission for STEMI and should be treated promptly. We strive to maintain the serum potassium level above 4.5 mEq/liter and serum magnesium level above 2 mEq/liter. Rapid abolition of sustained ventricular tachycardia in patients with STEMI is mandatory because of its deleterious effect on pump function and because it frequently deteriorates into ventricular fibrillation. After reversion to sinus rhythm, every effort should be made to correct underlying abnormalities such as hypoxia, hypotension, acid-base or electrolyte disturbances, and digitalis excess. Although no definitive data are available, it is a common clinical practice to continue maintenance infusions of antiarrhythmic drugs for several days after an index episode of ventricular tachycardia and to discontinue the drug and either observe the patient for recurrence or perform a diagnostic electrophysiology study. Patients with recurrent or refractory ventricular tachycardia should be considered for specialized procedures such as implantation of antitachycardia devices or surgery. Occasionally, urgent attempts at revascularization with angioplasty or CABG help control refractory ventricular tachycardia.

Ventricular Fibrillation

Ventricular fibrillation can occur in three settings in hospitalized patients with STEMI. (Its occurrence as a mechanism of sudden death is discussed in Chap. 36.) *Primary* ventricular fibrillation occurs suddenly and unexpectedly in patients with no or few signs or symptoms of left ventricular failure. Although primary ventricular fibrillation occurred in up to 10 percent of patients hospitalized with STEMI several decades ago, analyses suggest that its incidence has declined. *Secondary* ventricular fibrillation is often the final event of a progressive downhill course with left ventricular failure and cardiogenic shock. So-called *late* ventricular fibrillation develops more than 48 hours after STEMI and frequently but not exclusively occurs in patients with large infarcts and ventricular dysfunction. Patients with intraventricular conduction defects and anterior wall infarction, patients with persistent sinus tachycardia, atrial flutter, or fibrillation early in the clinical course, and patients with right ventricular infarction who require ventricular pacing are at higher risk for suffering late in-hospital ventricular fibrillation than are patients without these features.

PROGNOSIS. The effect of primary ventricular fibrillation on prognosis continues to be debated.[222] The MILIS study, conducted in the pre-reperfusion era, suggested that it does not have an adverse effect on hospital mortality, whereas the GISSI investigators reporting observations in large cohorts of thrombolysis-treated patients, suggested there was an excess mortality caused by primary ventricular fibrillation during the hospital phase but not thereafter.[223] Now, with the availability of amiodarone and implantable cardioverter-defibrillators, the prognosis of late ventricular fibrillation is improving and is probably driven more by residual ventricular function and recurrent ischemia than by the arrhythmic risk per se (see Chap. 34).

PROPHYLAXIS. Lidocaine prophylaxis to prevent primary ventricular fibrillation is no longer advised. Hypokalemia associates with the risk of ventricular fibrillation in the CCU.[1] Although it has not been conclusively shown that correction of hypokalemia to a level of 4.5 mEq/liter actually reduces the incidence of ventricular fibrillation, our experience suggests that this probably is protective and of little risk. Despite the lack of a consistent relationship between hypomagnesemia and ventricular fibrillation, magnesium deficits may still link to risk of ventricular fibrillation because intracellular magnesium levels are reduced in patients with STEMI and are not adequately reflected by serum measurements. For these reasons, and because it is often difficult to repair a potassium deficit without administering supplemental magnesium, we routinely replete magnesium to a level of 2 mEq/liter. The only situation in which we might consider prophylactic lidocaine (bolus of 1.5 mg/kg followed by 20 to 50 µg/kg/min) would be the unusual circumstance in which a patient within the first 12 hours of a STEMI must be managed in a facility where cardiac monitoring is not available and equipment for prompt defibrillation is not readily accessible.

MANAGEMENT (see Chaps. 33 and 35). Treatment for ventricular fibrillation consists of an unsynchronized electrical countershock with at least 200 to 300 joules, implemented as rapidly as possible.[1] When ventricular fibrillation occurs outside an intensive care unit, resuscitative efforts are much less likely to be successful, primarily because the time interval between the onset of the episode and institution of definitive therapy tends to be prolonged. Failure of electrical countershock to restore an effective cardiac rhythm is almost always caused by rapidly recurrent ventricular tachycardia or ventricular fibrillation, by electromechanical dissociation, or, rarely, by electrical asystole.

Successful interruption of ventricular fibrillation or prevention of refractory recurrent episodes can also be facilitated by administration of intravenous amiodarone. When synchronous cardiac electrical activity is restored by countershock but contraction is ineffective (i.e., pulseless electrical activity), the usual underlying cause is extensive myocardial ischemia or necrosis or rupture of the ventricular free wall or septum. If rupture has not occurred, intracardiac administration of calcium gluconate or epinephrine may promote restoration of an effective heartbeat. We do *not* usually administer bicarbonate injections to correct acidosis because of the high osmotic load they impose and the fact that hyperventilation of the patient is probably a more suitable means of clearing the acidosis.

Bradyarrhythmias (see Chap. 34 and 35)

Sinus Bradycardia

Sinus bradycardia occurs commonly during the early phases of STEMI, particularly in patients with inferior and posterior infarction.[1] On the basis of data obtained in experimental infarction and from some clinical observations, the increased vagal tone that produces sinus bradycardia during the early phase of STEMI may actually be protective, perhaps because it reduces myocardial oxygen demands. Thus the acute mortality rate appears similar in patients with sinus bradycardia as in those without this arrhythmia.

MANAGEMENT. Isolated sinus bradycardia, unaccompanied by hypotension or ventricular ectopy, should be observed rather than treated initially. In the first 4 to 6 hours after infarction, if the sinus rate is extremely slow (<40 to 50 beats/min) and associated with hypotension, intravenous atropine in doses of 0.3 to 0.6 mg every 3 to 10 minutes (with a total dose not exceeding 2 mg) can be administered to bring the heart rate up to approximately 60 beats/min.

Atrioventricular and Intraventricular Block

Ischemic injury can produce conduction block at any level of the atrioventricular (AV) or intraventricular conduction system. Such blocks can occur in the AV node and the bundle of His, producing various grades of AV block; in either main bundle branch, producing right or left bundle branch block; and in the anterior and posterior divisions of the left bundle, producing left anterior or left posterior (fascicular) divisional blocks. Disturbances of conduction can, of course, occur in various combinations. Clinical features of proximal and distal AV conduction disturbances in patients with STEMI are summarized in Table 51-12.

FIRST-DEGREE ATRIOVENTRICULAR BLOCK. First-degree AV block generally does not require specific treatment. Beta blockers and calcium antagonists (other than nifedipine) prolong AV conduction and may be responsible for first-degree AV block as well. However, discontinuation of these drugs in the setting of STEMI has the potential of increasing ischemia and ischemic injury. Therefore it is our practice not to decrease the dosage of these drugs unless the PR interval is greater than 0.24 second. Only if higher-degree block or hemodynamic impairment occurs should these agents be stopped. If the block is a manifestation of excessive vagotonia and is associated with sinus bradycardia and hypotension, administration of atropine, as already outlined, may be helpful. Continued electrocardiographic monitoring is important in such patients in view of the possibility of progression to higher degrees of block.

SECOND-DEGREE ATRIOVENTRICULAR BLOCK. First-degree and type I second-degree AV blocks do not appear to affect survival, are most commonly associated with occlusion of the right coronary artery, and are caused by ischemia of the AV node (see Table 51-12). Specific therapy is not required in patients with second-degree AV block of the type I variety when the ventricular rate exceeds 50 beats/min and premature ventricular contractions, heart failure, and bundle branch block are absent. However, if these complications develop or if the heart rate falls below approximately 50 beats/min and the patient is symptomatic, immediate treatment with atropine (0.3 to 0.6 mg) is indicated; temporary pacing systems are almost never needed in the management of this arrhythmia.

Type II second-degree block usually originates from a lesion in the conduction system below the bundle of His (see Table 51-12). Because of its potential for progression to complete heart block, type II second-degree AV block should be treated with a temporary external or transvenous demand pacemaker with the rate set at approximately 60 beats/min.[1]

COMPLETE (THIRD-DEGREE) ATRIOVENTRICULAR BLOCK. Complete AV block can occur in patients with either anterior or inferior infarction. Complete heart block in patients with inferior infarction usually results from an intranodal or supranodal lesion and develops gradually, often progressing from first-degree or type I second-degree block. The escape rhythm is usually stable without asystole and often junctional, with a rate exceeding 40 beats/min and a narrow QRS complex in 70 percent of cases and a slower rate and wide QRS in the others. This form of complete AV block is often transient, may be responsive to pharmacological antagonism of adenosine with methylxanthines,[224] and resolves in the majority of patients within a few days (see Table 51-12).

In patients with anterior infarction, third-degree AV block often occurs suddenly, 12 to 24 hours after the onset of infarction, although it is usually preceded by intraventricular block and often type II (not first-degree or type I) AV block. Such patients have unstable escape rhythms with wide QRS complexes and rates less than 40 beats/min; ventricular asystole may occur quite suddenly. In patients with anterior infarction, AV block usually develops as a result of extensive septal necrosis that involves the bundle branches. The high rate of mortality in this group of patients with slow idioventricular rhythm and wide QRS complexes is the consequence of extensive myocardial necrosis resulting in severe left ventricular failure and often shock (see Table 51-12).

Patients with inferior infarction often have concomitant ischemia or infarction of the AV node secondary to hypoperfusion of the AV node artery. However, the His-Purkinje system usually escapes injury in such individuals. Patients with inferior STEMI who develop AV block usually have lesions in both right and left anterior descending coronary arteries. Likewise, patients with inferior STEMI and AV block have larger infarcts and more depressed right ventricular and left ventricular function than do patients with inferior infarct and no AV block. As already noted, junctional escape rhythms with narrow QRS complexes occur commonly in this setting.

Although data suggest that complete AV block is *not* an independent risk factor for mortality, whether temporary transvenous pacing per se improves survival of patients with anterior STEMI remains controversial. Some investigators contend that ventricular pacing is useless when employed to correct complete AV block in patients with anterior infarction in view of the poor prognosis in this group regardless of therapy. However, pacing may protect against transient hypotension with its attendant risks of extending infarction and precipitating malignant ventricular tachyarrhythmias. Also, pacing protects against asys-

TABLE 51–12	Atrioventricular (AV) Conduction Disturbances in Acute Myocardial Infarction	
	Location of AV Conduction Disturbance	
	Proximal	*Distal*
Site of block	Intranodal	Infranodal
Site of infarction	Inferoposterior	Anteroseptal
Compromised arterial supply	RCA (90%), LCX (10%)	Septal perforators of LAD
Pathogenesis	Ischemia, necrosis, hydropic cell swelling, excess parasympathetic activity	Ischemia, necrosis, hydropic cell swelling
Predominant type of AV nodal block	First-degree (PR > 200 msec) Mobitz type I second-degree	Mobitz type II second-degree Third-degree
Common premonitory features of third-degree AV block	(a) First–second-degree AV block (b) Mobitz I pattern	(a) Intraventricular conduction block (b) Mobitz II pattern
Features of escape rhythm following third-degree block (a) Location (b) QRS width (c) Rate (d) Stability of escape rhythm	(a) Proximal conduction system (His bundle) (b) <0.12/sec* (c) 45-60/min but may be as low as 30/min (d) Rate usually stable; asystole uncommon	(a) Distal conduction system (bundle branches) (b) >0.12/sec (c) Often <30/min (d) Rate often unstable with moderate to high risk of ventricular asystole
Duration of high-grade AV block	Usually transient (2-3 days)	Usually transient but some form of AV conduction disturbance and/or intraventricular defect may persist
Associated mortality rate	Low unless associated with hypotension and/or congestive heart failure	High because of extensive infarction associated with power failure or ventricular arrhythmias
Pacemaker therapy (a) Temporary (b) Permanent	(a) Rarely required; may be considered for bradycardia associated with left ventricular power failure, syncope, or angina (b) Almost never indicated because conduction defect is usually transient	(a) Should be considered in patients with anteroseptal infarction and acute bifascicular block (b) Indicated for patients with high-grade AV block with block in His-Purkinje system and those with transient advanced AV block and associated bundle branch block

*Some studies suggest that a wide QRS escape rhythm (>0.12 sec) following high-grade AV block in inferior infarction is associated with a worse prognosis.

LAD = left anterior descending coronary artery; LCX = left circumflex coronary artery; RCA = right coronary artery.

Modified from Antman EM. Rutherford JD: Coronary Care Medicine: A Practical Approach. Boston, Martinus Nijhoff, 1986; and Dreifus LS, Fisch C, Griffin JC, et al: Guidelines for implantation of cardiac pacemakers and antiarrhythmia devices. J Am Coll Cardiol 18:1, 1991. Reprinted with permission from the American College of Cardiology.

CH 51

tole, a particular hazard in patients with anterior infarction and infranodal block. Improved survival with pacing probably occurs in only a small fraction of patients with complete AV block and anterior wall infarcts because the extensive destruction of the myocardium that almost invariably accompanies this condition results in a high mortality rate, even in paced patients. Given these considerations, an extremely large series of patients would be required to demonstrate the small reduction of mortality that might be achieved by pacing. The absence of data supporting such an effect, however, by no means excludes the possibility that it may be present.

Pacing is not usually necessary in patients with inferior wall infarction and complete AV block that is often transient in nature, but it is indicated if the ventricular rate is slow (<40 to 50 beats/min), if ventricular arrhythmias or hypotension is present, or if pump failure develops; atropine is only rarely of value in these patients. Only when complete heart block develops in less than 6 hours after the onset of symptoms is atropine likely to abolish the AV block or cause acceleration of the escape rhythm. In such cases the AV block is more likely to be transient and related to increases in vagal tone, rather than the more persistent block seen later in the course of STEMI, which generally requires cardiac pacing.

Intraventricular Block

The right bundle branch and the left posterior division have a dual blood supply from the left anterior descending and right coronary arteries, whereas the left anterior division is supplied by septal perforators originating from the left anterior descending coronary artery. Not all conduction blocks observed in patients with STEMI can be considered to be complications of infarcts because almost half are already present at the time the first ECG is recorded, and they may represent antecedent disease of the conduction system.[225] Compared with patients without conduction defects, STEMI patients with bundle branch blocks have more comorbid conditions; are less likely to receive therapies such as thrombolytics, aspirin, and beta blockers; and have an increased in-hospital mortality rate.[226] In the prefibrinolytic era, studies of intraventricular conduction disturbances (i.e., block within one or more of the three subdivisions [fascicles] of the His-Purkinje system [the anterior and posterior divisions of the left bundle and the right bundle]) had been reported to occur in 5 to 10 percent of patients with STEMI. More recent series in the fibrinolytic era suggest that intraventricular blocks occur in about 2 to 5 percent of patients with MI.[227] Investigators performing primary PCI for STEMI have reported an association between new-onset bundle branch block and abnormal myocardial perfusion even if epicardial flow is restored.[228]

ISOLATED FASCICULAR BLOCKS. Isolated left anterior divisional block is unlikely to progress to complete AV block. Mortality is increased in these patients, although not as much as in patients with other forms of conduction block. The posterior fascicle is larger than the anterior fascicle, and, in general, a larger infarct is required to block it. As a consequence, mortality is markedly increased. Complete AV block is not a frequent complication of either form of isolated divisional block.

RIGHT BUNDLE BRANCH BLOCK. This conduction defect alone can lead to AV block because it is often a new lesion, associated with anteroseptal infarction. Isolated right bundle branch block is associated with an increased mortality risk in patients with anterior STEMI even if complete AV block does not occur, but this appears to be the case only if it is accompanied by congestive heart failure.

BIFASCICULAR BLOCK. The combination of right bundle branch block with either left anterior or posterior divisional block or the combination of left anterior and posterior divisional blocks (i.e., left bundle branch block) is known as *bidivisional* or *bifascicular block*. If new block occurs in two of the three divisions of the conduction system, the risk of developing complete AV block is quite high. Mortality is also high because of the occurrence of severe pump failure secondary to the extensive myocardial necrosis required to produce such an extensive intraventricular block.[227] Patients with intraventricular conduction defects, particularly right bundle branch block, account for the majority of patients who develop ventricular fibrillation late in their hospital stay. However, the high rate of mortality in these patients occurs even in the absence of high-grade AV block and appears to be related to cardiac failure and massive infarction rather than to the conduction disturbance.[227]

Preexisting bundle branch block or divisional block is less often associated with the development of complete heart block in patients with STEMI than are conduction defects acquired during the course of the infarct. Bidivisional block in the presence of prolongation of the P-R interval (first-degree AV block) may indicate disease of the third subdivision rather than of the AV node and is associated with a greater risk of complete heart block than if first-degree AV block is absent.

Complete bundle branch block (either left or right), the combination of right bundle branch block and left anterior divisional (fascicular) block, and any of the various forms of trifascicular block are all more often associated with anterior than with inferoposterior infarction. All these forms are more frequent with large infarcts and in older patients and have a higher incidence of other accompanying arrhythmias than is seen in patients without bundle branch block.

Use of Pacemakers in Patients with Acute
Myocardial Infarction (see Chap. 34)

TEMPORARY PACING. Just as is the case for complete AV block, transvenous ventricular pacing has not resulted in statistically demonstrable improvement in prognosis among patients with STEMI who develop intraventricular conductions defects. However, temporary pacing is advisable in some of these patients because of the high risk of developing complete AV block. This includes patients with new bilateral (bifascicular) bundle branch block (i.e., right bundle branch block with left anterior or posterior divisional block and alternating right and left bundle branch block); first-degree AV block adds to this risk. Isolated new block in only one of the three fascicles even with P-R pro-

longation and preexisting bifascicular block and normal P-R interval poses somewhat less risk; these patients should be monitored closely, with insertion of a temporary pacemaker deferred unless higher degree AV block occurs.

Noninvasive external temporary cardiac pacing is possible routinely in conscious patients and is acceptable to many but not all patients despite the discomfort. Used in a standby mode, it is virtually free of complications and contraindications and provides an important alternative to transvenous endocardial pacing.[1] Once it is clinically evident that continuous pacing is required, external pacing, which is generally not well tolerated for more than minutes to hours, should be replaced by a temporary transvenous pacemaker.

ASYSTOLE. The presence of apparent ventricular asystole on monitor displays of continuously recorded ECGs may be misleading because the rhythm may actually be fine ventricular fibrillation. Because of the predominance of ventricular fibrillation as the cause of cardiac arrest in this setting, initial therapy should include electrical countershock, even if definitive electrocardiographic documentation of this arrhythmia is not available. In the rare instance in which asystole can be documented to be the responsible electrophysiological disturbance, immediate transcutaneous pacing (or stimulation with a transvenous pacemaker if one is already in place) is indicated.[1]

PERMANENT PACING. The question of the advisability of permanent pacemaker insertion is complicated because not all sudden deaths in STEMI patients with conduction defects are caused by high-grade AV block. A high incidence of late ventricular fibrillation occurs in CCU survivors with anterior STEMI complicated by either right or left bundle branch block. Therefore ventricular fibrillation rather than asystole caused by failure of AV conduction and infranodal pacemakers could be responsible for late sudden death.

Long-term pacing is often helpful when complete heart block persists throughout the hospital phase in a patient with STEMI, when sinus node function is markedly impaired, or when type II second- or third-degree block occurs intermittently.[1] When high-grade AV block is associated with newly acquired bundle branch block or other criteria of impairment of conduction system function, prophylactic long-term pacing may be justified as well. Additional considerations that drive a decision to insert a permanent pacemaker include whether the patient is a candidate for an implantable cardioverter-defibrillator or has severe heart failure that might be improved with biventricular pacing (see Chap. 34).

Supraventricular Tachyarrhythmias
(see Chap. 35)

SINUS TACHYCARDIA. This arrhythmia is typically associated with augmented sympathetic activity and may provoke transient hypertension or hypotension. Common causes are anxiety, persistent pain, left ventricular failure, fever, pericarditis, hypovolemia, pulmonary embolism, and the administration of cardioaccelerator drugs such as atropine, epinephrine, or dopamine; rarely, it occurs in patients with atrial infarction. Sinus tachycardia is particularly common in patients with anterior infarction, especially if there is significant accompanying left ventricular dysfunction. It is an undesirable rhythm in patients with STEMI because it results in an augmentation of myocardial oxygen consumption, as well as a reduction in the time available for coronary perfusion, thereby intensifying myocardial ischemia and/or external myocardial necrosis. Persistent sinus tachycardia can signify persistent heart failure and under these circumstances connotes poor prognosis and excess

CH 51

ST-Elevation Myocardial Infarction: Management

mortality. An underlying cause should be sought and appropriate treatment instituted, such as analgesics for pain; diuretics for heart failure; oxygen, beta blockers, and nitroglycerin for ischemia; and aspirin for fever or pericarditis.

Administration of beta-adrenoceptor blocking agents, in the dosage and manner described elsewhere in this chapter, may be helpful in the treatment of sinus tachycardia, particularly when this arrhythmia is a manifestation of a hyperdynamic circulation, which is seen particularly in young patients with an initial STEMI without extensive cardiac damage. Beta blockade is contraindicated, however, in patients in whom the sinus tachycardia is a manifestation of hypovolemia or of pump failure, the latter reflected by a systolic arterial pressure below 100 mm Hg, rales involving more than one third of the lung fields, a pulmonary capillary wedge pressure exceeding 20 to 25 mm Hg, or a cardiac index below approximately 2.2 liters/min/m^2. A possible exception to this is a patient in whom persistent ischemia is believed to be the cause or the result of tachycardia—cautious administration of an ultra-short-acting beta blocker such as esmolol (25 to 200 μg/kg/min) can be tried to ascertain the patient's response to slowing of the heart rate.

ATRIAL FLUTTER AND FIBRILLATION. Atrial flutter is usually transient, and in patients with STEMI it is typically a consequence of augmented sympathetic stimulation of the atria, often occurring in patients with left ventricular failure, pulmonary emboli in whom the arrhythmia intensifies hemodynamic deterioration, or atrial infarction (see Table 51-11).

As with atrial premature complexes and atrial flutter, fibrillation is usually transient and tends to occur in patients with left ventricular failure but also occurs in patients with pericarditis and ischemic injury to the atria and right ventricular infarction.[229] The increased ventricular rate and the loss of the atrial contribution to left ventricular filling result in a significant reduction in cardiac output. Atrial fibrillation during STEMI is associated with increased mortality and stroke, particularly in patients with anterior wall infarction.[229] However, because it is more common in patients with clinical and hemodynamic manifestations of extensive infarction and a poor prognosis, atrial fibrillation is probably a marker of poor prognosis, with only a small independent contribution to increased mortality.

Management. Atrial flutter and fibrillation in patients with STEMI are treated in a manner similar to these conditions in other settings (see Chap. 33). Patients with recurrent episodes of atrial fibrillation should be treated with oral anticoagulants (to reduce the risk of stroke), even if sinus rhythm is present at the time of hospital discharge, because no antiarrhythmic regimen can be relied on to be completely effective in suppressing atrial fibrillation. In the absence of contraindications, patients should receive a beta blocker after STEMI; in addition to their several other beneficial effects, these agents are helpful in slowing the ventricular rate, should atrial fibrillation recur.

Other Complications

Recurrent Chest Discomfort

Evaluation of postinfarction chest discomfort is sometimes complicated by previous abnormalities on the ECG and a vague description of the discomfort by the patient, who either may be exquisitely sensitive to fleeting discomfort or may deny a potential recrudescence of symptoms. The critical task for clinicians is to distinguish recurrent angina or infarction from nonischemic causes of discomfort that might be caused by infarct expansion, pericarditis, pulmonary embolism, and noncardiac conditions. Important diagnostic maneuvers include a repeat physical examination,

repeat ECG reading, and assessment of the response to sublingual nitroglycerin, 0.4 mg. (The use of noninvasive diagnostic evaluation for recurrent ischemia in patients whose symptoms appear only with moderate levels of exertion is discussed elsewhere in this chapter.)

RECURRENT ISCHEMIA AND INFARCTION. The incidence of postinfarction angina without reinfarction is reduced in patients undergoing primary PCI for STEMI compared with fibrinolysis.[103] More effective antiplatelet and antithrombin therapies significantly reduce the rate of recurrent ischemic events after fibrinolysis, to a range similar to that reported for primary PCI.[130,76] When accompanied by ST and T wave changes in the same leads where Q waves have appeared, it may be caused by occlusion of an initially patent vessel, reocclusion of an initially recanalized or stented vessel, or coronary spasm.

DIAGNOSIS. *Extension* of the original zone of necrosis or *reinfarction* in a separate myocardial zone can be a difficult diagnosis, especially within the first 24 hours after the index event. It is more convenient to refer to both extension and reinfarction collectively under the more general term *recurrent infarction.* Serum cardiac markers may remain elevated from the initial infarction, and it may not be possible to distinguish the ECG changes that are part of the normal evolution after the index infarction from those caused by recurrent infarction. Within the first 18 to 24 hours following the initial infarction, when serum cardiac markers may not have returned to the normal range, recurrent infarction should be strongly considered when there is repeat ST segment elevation on the ECG. Although pericarditis remains a possibility in such patients, the two can usually be distinguished by the presence of a rub and lack of responsiveness to nitroglycerin in patients with pericardial discomfort. Beyond the first 24 hours, recurrent infarction can be diagnosed either by re-elevation of the cardiac markers or the appearance of new Q waves on the ECG reading.[1] Reinfarction is more common in patients with diabetes mellitus and those with a previous MI. The predominant angiographic predictors of reinfarction in patients undergoing primary PCI include a final coronary stenosis greater than 30 percent, post-PCI coronary dissection, and post-PCI intracoronary thrombus. Diabetic patients and those with advanced Killip class are more likely to experience reinfarction.[230]

PROGNOSIS. Regardless of whether postinfarction angina is persistent or limited, its presence is important because the short-term morbidity rate is higher among such patients; mortality is increased if the recurrent ischemia is accompanied by ECG changes and hemodynamic compromise.[1,76] Recurrent infarction (caused in many cases by reocclusion of the infarct-related coronary artery) carries serious adverse prognostic information because it is associated with twofold to fourfold higher rates of in-hospital complications (congestive heart failure, heart block) and early and long-term mortality.[231] Presumably, the higher mortality rate is related to the larger mass of myocardium whose function becomes compromised.

Management. As with the acute phase of treatment of STEMI, algorithms for management of patients with recurrent ischemic discomfort at rest center on the 12-lead ECG (Fig. 51-40). Patients with ST segment re-elevation should be referred for urgent catheterization and PCI; repeat fibrinolysis can be considered if PCI is not available. Insertion of an intraaortic balloon pump may help stabilize the patient while other procedures are being arranged. For patients believed to have recurrent ischemia who do not have evidence of hemodynamic compromise, an attempt should be made to control symptoms with sublingual or intravenous nitroglycerin and intravenous beta blockade to slow the heart rate to 60 beats/min. When hypotension, congestive

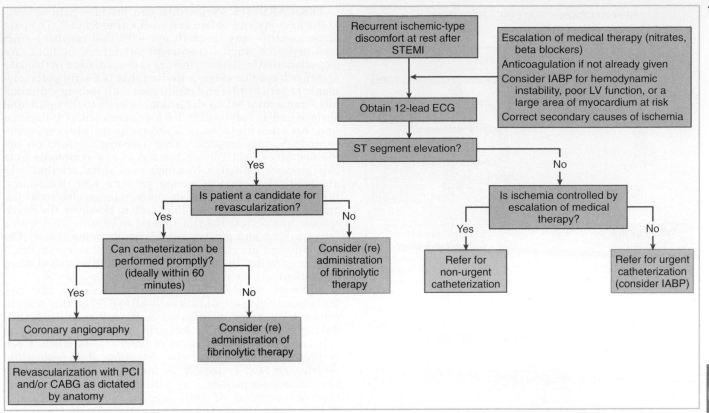

FIGURE 51–40 Algorithm for management of ischemia/infarction after ST-elevation myocardial infarction (STEMI). CABG = coronary artery bypass grafting; ECG = electrocardiogram; IABP = intraaortic balloon pump; LV = left ventricular; PCI = percutaneous coronary intervention. *(Modified from Antman EM, Anbe DT, Armstrong PW, et al: ACC/AHA guidelines for the management of patients with ST-elevation myocardial infarction: A report of the American College of Cardiology/American Heart Association Task Force on Practice Guidelines [Committee to Revise the 1999 Guidelines for the Management of Patients with Acute Myocardial Infarction]. www.acc.org/clinical/guidelines/stemi/index.pdf. Accessed 4/19/06.)*

heart failure, or ventricular arrhythmias develop during recurrent ischemia, urgent catheterization and revascularization are indicated.

Prior studies failed to show any benefit of a strategy of *routine* referral for catheterization and revascularization, either early or after a delay of 1 or 2 days. It should be realized, however, that those studies were conducted in an era in which the catheterization equipment was less technologically advanced than it is today and glycoprotein IIb/IIIa inhibitors and stents were not part of the interventionist's armamentarium. However, contemporary trials that compared primary PCI with PCI performed as soon as possible after a preparatory pharmacologic regimen had been administered, have not shown such a *facilitated PCI* approach to be more effective than primary PCI, and there are even suggestions of increased mortality because of excess bleeding in the facilitated PCI group (Fig. 51-41).[95,232]

The de facto practice in many centers currently is to pursue a routine invasive strategy after a delay of several hours (e.g., at least 12 hours) following fibrinolysis for STEMI. Although no large-scale randomized trials have been conducted in the contemporary era to support such a practice, the author finds it quite persuasive because of the consistent, encouraging findings from a series of small trials.[232-236] Lower rates of death, recurrent ischemic events, or target vessel revascularization has been reported in patients treated with routine PCI after fibrinolysis as compared with a conservative strategy of medical therapy with referral for PCI when symptoms recurred.[232] The expanded use of PCI beyond rescue PCI, referred to by Dauerman and Sobel as *pharmacoinvasive recanalization,* is in need of more vigorous testing but holds considerable promise for

reducing rates of mortality and morbidity after STEMI.[237-240] The concept of a pharmacoinvasive approach to STEMI (fibrinolysis followed by a routine delayed PCI) is especially appealing because it overcomes the delay to implementation of primary PCI and utilizes the pharmacological and mechanical approaches in an integrated rather than competitive fashion (see Fig. 51-41).

Finally, with increasing use of PCI in the management of patients with STEMI, clinicians should be alert to the problem of stent thrombosis as a cause of recurrent ischemia. Stent thrombosis can occur acutely (hours to days after deployment of a stent) or in a more subacute fashion (many months after deployment of a stent) (see Chap. 55).

PERICARDIAL EFFUSION AND PERICARDITIS (see Chap. 70)

PERICARDIAL EFFUSION. Effusions are generally detected echocardiographically, and their incidence varies with technique, criteria, and laboratory expertise. Especially sensitive techniques such as magnetic resonance imaging may detect epicardial effusions in two thirds of STEMI patients.[241] Effusions are more common in patients with anterior STEMI and with larger infarcts and when congestive failure is present. The majority of pericardial effusions that occur following STEMI do not cause hemodynamic compromise; when tamponade occurs, it is usually caused by ventricular rupture or hemorrhagic pericarditis. The reabsorption rate of a postinfarction pericardial effusion is slow, with resolution often taking several months. The presence of an effusion does not indicate that pericarditis is present; although they may occur together, the majority of effusions occur without other evidence of pericarditis.

REPERFUSION STRATEGIES FOR STEMI

Pharmacologic ←→ [?] ←→ PCI

Widely available
Quickly administered
Less effective
Bleeding risk

Limited availability
Treatment delay
More effective
Bleeding risk lower

A

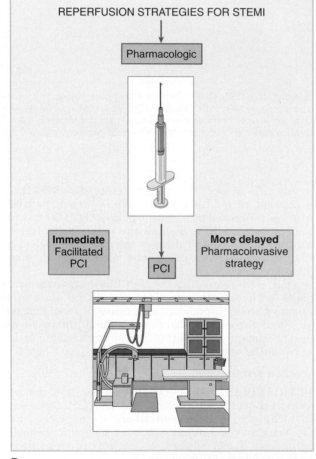

REPERFUSION STRATEGIES FOR STEMI

Pharmacologic

Immediate
Facilitated
PCI

PCI

More delayed
Pharmacoinvasive
strategy

B

FIGURE 51–41 Comparison of various approaches to reperfusion in ST-elevation myocardial infarction (STEMI). **A,** This strategy chooses between pharmacological and mechanical reperfusion for STEMI. The advantages and disadvantages of each approach are outlined at the bottom. **B,** A strategy in which all eligible patients receive pharmacological reperfusion, which is universally available and quickly administered, followed by percutaneous coronary intervention (PCI). If the PCI is routinely performed shortly after a preparatory pharmacological regimen, it is referred to as *facilitated PCI*, whereas if it is routinely performed after a delay of several hours, it is referred to as a *pharmacoinvasive approach.*

PERICARDITIS. Pericarditis can produce pain as early as the first day and as late as 6 weeks after STEMI. The pain of pericarditis may be confused with that resulting from postinfarction angina, recurrent infarction, or both. An important distinguishing feature is the radiation of the pain to either trapezius ridge, a finding that is nearly pathognomonic of pericarditis and rarely seen with ischemic discomfort. Transmural MI, by definition, extends to the epicardial surface and is responsible for local pericardial inflammation. An acute fibrinous pericarditis (pericarditis epistenocardiaca) occurs commonly after transmural infarction, but the majority of patients do not report any symptoms from this process. Although transient pericardial friction rubs are relatively common among patients with transmural infarction within the first 48 hours, pain or electrocardiographic changes occur much less often. However, the development of a pericardial rub appears to be correlated with a larger infarct and greater hemodynamic compromise. The discomfort of pericarditis usually becomes worse during a deep inspiration, but it can be relieved or diminished when the patient sits up and leans forward.

Although anticoagulation clearly increases the risk for hemorrhagic pericarditis early after STEMI, this complication has not been reported with sufficient frequency during heparinization or following fibrinolytic therapy to warrant absolute prohibition of such agents when a rub is present. Nevertheless, the detection of a pericardial effusion on ECG is usually an indication for discontinuation of anticoagulation. In patients in whom continuation or initiation of anticoagulant therapy is strongly indicated (such as during cardiac catheterization or following coronary angioplasty), heightened monitoring of clotting parameters and observation for clinical signs of possible tamponade are necessary. Late pericardial constriction caused by anticoagulant-induced hemopericardium has been reported.

Treatment of pericardial discomfort consists of aspirin, but usually in higher doses than prescribed routinely following infarction—doses of 650 mg orally every 4 to 6 hours may be necessary. Nonsteroidal antiinflammatory agents and steroids should be avoided because they may interfere with myocardial scar formation.[1,241a,241b]

DRESSLER SYNDROME. Also known as the *postmyocardial infarction syndrome,* Dressler syndrome usually occurs 1 to 8 weeks after infarction. Dressler cited an incidence of 3 to 4 percent of all MI patients in 1957, but the incidence has decreased dramatically since that time. Clinically, patients with Dressler syndrome present with malaise, fever, pericardial discomfort, leukocytosis, an elevated sedimentation rate, and a pericardial effusion. At autopsy, patients with this syndrome usually demonstrate localized fibrinous pericarditis containing polymorphonuclear leukocytes. The cause of this syndrome is not clearly established, although the detection of antibodies to cardiac tissue has raised the notion of an immunopathological process. Treatment is with aspirin, 650 mg, as often as every 4 hours. Glucocorticosteroids and nonsteroidal antiinflammatory agents are best avoided in patients with Dressler syndrome within 4 weeks of STEMI because of their potential to impair infarct healing, cause ventricular rupture,[242] and increase coronary vascular resistance. Aspirin in large doses is effective.

VENOUS THROMBOSIS AND PULMONARY EMBOLISM

Almost all peri-MI pulmonary emboli originate from thrombi in the veins of the lower extremities; much less commonly, they originate from mural thrombi overlying an area of right ventricular infarction. Bed rest and heart failure predispose to venous thrombosis and subsequent pulmonary embolism, and both of these factors occur commonly in patients with STEMI, particularly those with large infarcts. At a time when patients with STEMI were routinely subjected to prolonged periods of bed rest, significant pulmonary embolism was found in more than 20 percent of patients with STEMI coming to autopsy, and massive pulmonary embolism accounted for 10 percent of deaths from MI. In contemporary practice, with early mobilization and the widespread use of low-dose anticoagulant prophylaxis, especially using low-molecular-weight heparins, pulmonary embolism has become an uncommon cause of death in patients with STEMI. When pulmonary embolism does occur in patients with STEMI, management is generally along the lines described for noninfarction patients (see Chap. 72).

LEFT VENTRICULAR ANEURYSM

The term *left ventricular aneurysm* (often termed *true aneurysm*) is generally reserved for a discrete, dyskinetic area of the left ventricular wall with a broad neck (to differentiate it from pseudoaneurysm caused by a contained myocardial rupture). Dyskinetic or akinetic areas of the left ventricle are far more common than true aneurysms after STEMI; such poorly contracting segments are referred to as *regional wall motion abnormalities*.[243] True left ventricular aneurysms probably develop in less than 5 percent of all patients with STEMI and perhaps somewhat more frequently in patients with transmural infarction (especially anterior).[50] The wall of the true aneurysm is thinner than the wall of the rest of the left ventricle (see Fig. 51-34), and it is usually composed of fibrous tissue, as well as necrotic muscle, occasionally mixed with viable myocardium.

PATHOGENESIS. Aneurysm formation presumably occurs when intraventricular tension stretches the noncontracting infarcted heart muscle, thus producing infarct expansion, a relatively weak, thin layer of necrotic muscle, and fibrous tissue that bulges with each cardiac contraction. With the passage of time, the wall of the aneurysm becomes more densely fibrotic, but it continues to bulge with systole, causing some of the left ventricular stroke volume during each systole to be ineffective.

When an aneurysm is present after anterior STEMI, there is generally a total occlusion of a poorly collateralized left anterior descending coronary artery. An aneurysm is rarely seen with multivessel disease when there are either extensive collaterals or a nonoccluded left anterior descending artery. Aneurysms usually range from 1 to 8 cm in diameter. They occur approximately four times more often at the apex and in the anterior wall than in the inferoposterior wall. The overlying pericardium is usually densely adherent to the wall of the aneurysm, which may even become partially calcified after several years. True left ventricular aneurysms (in contrast to pseudoaneurysms) rarely rupture soon after development. Late rupture, when the true aneurysm has become stabilized by the formation of dense fibrous tissue in its wall, almost never occurs.

DIAGNOSIS. The presence of persistent ST segment elevation in an electrocardiographic area of infarction, classically thought to suggest aneurysm formation, actually indicates a large infarct with a regional wall motion abnormality but does not necessarily imply an aneurysm. The diagnosis of aneurysm is best made noninvasively by an echocardiographic study,[245] by magnetic resonance imaging, or at the time of cardiac catheterization by left ventriculography. With the loss of shortening from the area of the aneurysm, the remainder of the ventricle must be hyperkinetic in order to compensate. With relatively large aneurysms, complete compensation is impossible. The stroke volume falls, or, if it is maintained, it is at the expense of an increase in end-diastolic volume, which in turn leads to increased wall tension and myocardial oxygen demand.

Heart failure may ensue, and angina may appear or worsen.

PROGNOSIS AND TREATMENT. Left ventricular aneurysm confers a mortality up to six times higher than in patients without aneurysms, even when compared with that in patients with comparable left ventricular ejection fraction. Death in these patients is often sudden and presumably related to the high incidence of ventricular tachyarrhythmias that occur with aneurysms.[244] Aggressive management of STEMI, including prompt reperfusion, may diminish the incidence of ventricular aneurysms. Surgical aneurysmectomy generally is successful only if there is relative preservation of contractile performance in the nonaneurysmal portion of the left ventricle (Fig. 51-42). In such circumstances, when the operation is performed for worsening heart failure or angina, operative mortality is relatively low and clinical improvement can be expected.[246] Because of the importance of maintaining as normal a left ventricular shape as possible, several surgical techniques for ventricular reconstruction have been developed and may be combined with the general approach shown in Figure 51-42.[247] Because of the risk of mural thrombosis and systemic embolization, we favor long-term oral anticoagulation with warfarin in patients with a left ventricular aneurysm after STEMI.

Left Ventricular Thrombus and Arterial Embolism

Endocardial inflammation during the acute phase of infarction probably provides a thrombogenic surface for clots to form in the left ventricle. With extensive transmural infarction of the septum, however, mural thrombi may overlie infarcted myocardium in both ventricles. The incidence of

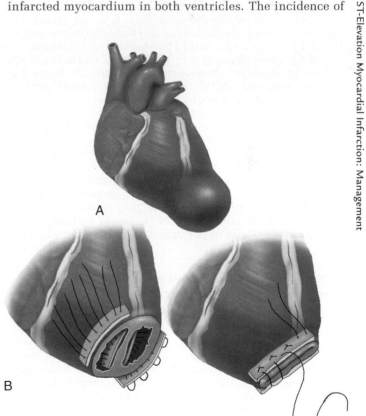

FIGURE 51–42 Surgical management of ventricular aneurysm. **A,** In this case, the aneurysm is located at the apex. **B,** The aneurysmal segment is resected and felt pledget strips are used to reinforce interrupted suture closure of the apex. **C,** Completed repair partially restores apical geometry. *(Courtesy of Dr. David Adams, Division of Cardiac Surgery, Mt. Sinai Hospital, New York.)*

left ventricular thrombus formation after STEMI appears to have dropped from about 20 to 5 percent with more aggressive use of antithrombotic strategies.[248] Prospective studies have suggested that patients who develop a mural thrombus early (within 48 to 72 hours of infarction) have an extremely poor early prognosis,[249] with a high rate of mortality from the complications of a large infarction (shock, reinfarction, rupture, and ventricular tachyarrhythmia), rather than emboli from the left ventricular thrombus.

Although a mural thrombus adheres to the endocardium overlying the infarcted myocardium, superficial portions of it can become detached and produce systemic arterial emboli. Although estimates vary on the basis of patient selection, about 10 percent of mural thrombi result in systemic embolization.[249] Echocardiographically detectable features that suggest a given thrombus is more likely to embolize include increased mobility and protrusion into the ventricular chamber, visualization in multiple views, and contiguous zones of akinesis and hyperkinesis.

MANAGEMENT. Data from previous trials with limited sample size suggested that anticoagulation (intravenous heparin or high-dose subcutaneous heparin) reduced the development of left ventricular *thrombi* by 50 percent, but, because of the low event rate, it was not possible to demonstrate a reduction in the incidence of *systemic embolism.* Fibrinolysis reduces the rate of thrombus formation and the character of the thrombi so that they are less protuberant. Of note, however, the data from fibrinolytic trials are difficult to interpret because of the confounding effect of antithrombotic therapy with heparin. Recommendations for anticoagulation vary considerably, and fibrinolysis has precipitated fatal embolization. Nevertheless, anticoagulation for 3 to 6 months with warfarin is advocated for many patients with demonstrable mural thrombi.[1,250]

On the basis of the available data, it is our practice to recommend anticoagulation (intravenous heparin to elevate the aPTT to one and a half to two times that of control, followed by a minimum of 3 to 6 months of warfarin) in the following clinical situations: (1) an embolic event has already occurred, or (2) the patient has a large anterior infarction whether or not a thrombus is visualized echocardiographically. We are also inclined to follow the same anticoagulation practice in patients with infarctions other than in the anterior distribution if a thrombus or large wall motion abnormality is detected. Aspirin, although probably not capable of affecting thrombus size in most patients, may prevent further platelet deposition on existing thrombi and also is protective against recurrent ischemic events. It should be prescribed in conjunction with warfarin to patients who are candidates for long-term anticoagulation therapy on the basis of the indications discussed earlier.

Convalescence, Discharge, and Post-Myocardial Infarction Care

TIMING OF HOSPITAL DISCHARGE. The timing of discharge from the hospital is variable. As noted earlier, patients who have undergone aggressive reperfusion protocols and have no significant ventricular arrhythmias, recurrent ischemia, or congestive heart failure have been safely discharged in less than 5 days. More commonly, discharge occurs 5 or 6 days after admission for patients who experience no complications, who can be followed readily at home, and whose family setting is conducive to convalescence. Most complications that would preclude early discharge occur within the first day or two of admission; therefore patients suitable for early discharge can be identified early during the hospitalization.[251] Several controlled trials and many uncontrolled trials of early discharge after STEMI

have failed to show any increase in risk in patients appropriately selected for early discharge. The decision regarding timing of discharge in the patients with uncomplicated STEMI should take into account the patient's psychological state after STEMI, the adequacy of the dose titration for essential drugs such as beta blockers and inhibitors of the RAAS, and the availability and timing of follow-up with visiting nurses and the patient's primary care physician.[154] For patients who have experienced a complication, discharge is deferred until their condition has been stable for several days and it is clear that they are responding appropriately to necessary medications such as antiarrhythmic agents, vasodilators, or positive inotropic agents or that they have undergone the appropriate work-up for recurrent ischemia.

COUNSELING. Before discharge from the hospital, all patients should receive detailed instruction concerning physical activity. Initially, this should consist of ambulation at home but avoidance of isometric exercise such as lifting; several rest periods should be taken daily. In addition, the patient should be given fresh nitroglycerin tablets and instructed in their use (see Chap. 54) and should receive careful instructions about the use of any other medications prescribed. As convalescence progresses, graded resumption of activity should be encouraged (see Chaps. 46 and 78). Many approaches have been utilized, ranging from formal rigid guidelines to general advice advocating moderation and avoidance of any activity that evokes symptoms. Sexual counseling is often overlooked during recovery from STEMI and should also be included as part of the educational process. Such counseling should begin early after STEMI and should include the recommendation that sexual activity be resumed after successful completion of either early submaximal or later symptom-limited exercise stress testing.[1]

Some evidence indicates that behavioral alteration is possible after recovery from STEMI and that this may improve prognosis. A cardiac rehabilitation program with supervised physical exercise and an educational component has been recommended for most STEMI patients after discharge. Although the overall clinical benefit of such programs continues to be debated, there is little question that most people derive considerable knowledge and psychological security from such interventions, and they continue to be endorsed by experienced clinicians.[1] Meta-analyses of randomized trials of medically supervised rehabilitation programs versus usual care that were conducted in an era before widespread use of beta-adrenoceptor blockers and aggressive reperfusion strategies have shown a reduction in cardiovascular death but no change in the incidence of nonfatal reinfarction. Given the relationship between depression and STEMI, interest has arisen in psychosocial intervention programs in the convalescent phase of STEMI (see Chap. 86).[252,253] Psychosocial intervention programs can decrease symptoms of depression and are a useful adjunct to standard cardiac rehabilitation programs after STEMI; however, they do not have a significant impact on the risk of mortality or recurrent MI after STEMI.[254]

Risk Stratification after STEMI

The process of risk stratification following STEMI occurs in several stages: initial presentation, in-hospital course (CCU, intermediate care unit), and at the time of hospital discharge. The tools used to form an integrated assessment of the patient consist of baseline demographic information; serial ECGs and serum cardiac marker measurements; hemodynamic monitoring data; a variety of noninvasive tests; and, if performed, the findings at cardiac catheterization (Fig. 51-43).[1]

CH 51

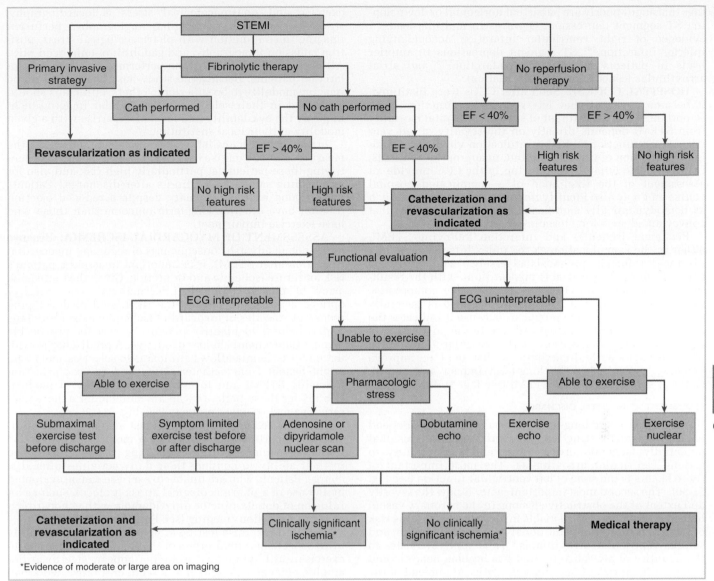

FIGURE 51–43 Algorithm for catheterization and revascularization after ST-elevation myocardial infarction (STEMI). The algorithm shows the treatment paths for patients who initially undergo a primary invasive strategy, receive fibrinolytic therapy, or do not undergo reperfusion therapy for STEMI. Patients who have not undergone a primary invasive strategy and have no high-risk features should undergo functional evaluation using one of the noninvasive tests shown. When clinically significant ischemia (evidence of moderate or large area of ischemia by imaging) is detected, patients should undergo catheterization and revascularization as indicated; if no clinically significant ischemia is detected, medical therapy is prescribed post-STEMI. cath = catheterization; ECG = electrocardiogram; echo = echocardiography; EF = ejection fraction. *(From Antman EM, Anbe DT, Armstrong PW, et al: ACC/AHA guidelines for the management of patients with ST-elevation myocardial infarction: A report of the American College of Cardiology/American Heart Association Task Force on Practice Guidelines [Committee to Revise the 1999 Guidelines for the Management of Patients with Acute Myocardial Infarction] (www.acc.org/clinical/guidelines/stemi/index.pdf). Accessed 4/19/06.)*

INITIAL PRESENTATION. Certain demographic and historical factors portend a poor prognosis in patients with STEMI, including female gender, age greater than 70 years, a history of diabetes mellitus, prior angina pectoris, and previous MI (see Fig. 51-13).[1] Diabetes mellitus, in particular, appears to confer a threefold to fourfold increase in risk (see Chap. 60). Whether this is caused by accelerated atherosclerosis or some other characteristic induced by the diabetic state (such as a larger infarct size) is unclear. (Surviving diabetic patients also experience a more complicated post-MI course including a greater incidence of postinfarction angina, infarct extension, and heart failure.[1])

In addition to playing a central role in the decision pathway for management of patients with STEMI based on the presence or absence of ST segment elevation, the 12-lead ECG carries important prognostic information.[227] Mortality is greater in patients experiencing anterior wall STEMI than

after inferior STEMI, even when corrected for infarct size. Patients with right ventricular infarction complicating inferior infarction, as suggested by ST segment elevation in V₄R, have a greater mortality rate than patients sustaining an inferior infarction without right ventricular involvement.[205,255] Patients with multiple leads showing ST elevation and a high sum of ST segment elevation have an increased mortality rate, especially if their infarct is anterior in location.[255] Patients whose ECG demonstrates persistent advanced heart block (e.g., type II, second-degree, or third-degree AV block) or new intraventricular conduction abnormalities (bifascicular or trifascicular) in the course of a STEMI have a worse prognosis than do patients without these abnormalities. The influence of high degrees of heart block is particularly important in patients with right ventricular infarction because such patients have a markedly increased mortality risk. Other electrocardiographic findings that augur poorly are persistent horizontal or downsloping ST segment depression, Q waves in multiple leads,[256] evidence of right ventricular infarction accompanying inferior infarction,[205] ST segment depressions in anterior leads in patients with inferior infarction,[255] and atrial arrhythmias (especially atrial fibrillation).

HOSPITAL COURSE. Soon after CCUs were instituted, it became apparent that left ventricular function is an important early determinant of survival. Hospital mortality from STEMI depends directly on the severity of left ventricular dysfunction.[153] Risk stratification via clinical findings; estimation of infarct size; and, in appropriate patients, invasive hemodynamic monitoring in the CCU provide an assessment of the likelihood of a complicated hospital course and may also identify important abnormalities, such as hemodynamically significant mitral regurgitation, that convey an adverse long-term prognosis (see Table 51-8).

Recurrent ischemia and infarction following STEMI, either in the same location as the index infarction or "at a distance," influence prognosis adversely.[231] Poor prognosis comes from the loss of viable myocardium, with the resulting larger area of infarction creating a greater compromise in ventricular function. Postinfarction angina generally connotes a less favorable prognosis because it indicates the presence of jeopardized myocardium. In the current era of aggressive revascularization, early postinfarction angina often leads to early interventions that tend to improve outcome, diminishing the long-term impact and significance of angina early after STEMI (see Fig. 51-41B).[257]

ASSESSMENT AT HOSPITAL DISCHARGE

Both short-term and long-term survival after STEMI depend on three factors: resting left ventricular function, residual potentially ischemic myocardium, and susceptibility to serious ventricular arrhythmias. The most important of these factors is the state of left ventricular function (see Fig. 51-30).[1] The second most important factor is how the severity and extent of the obstructive lesions in the coronary vascular bed perfusing residual viable myocardium affect the risk of recurrent infarction, additional myocardial damage, and serious ventricular arrhythmias.[1] Thus survival relates to the quantity of myocardium that has become necrotic and the quantity at risk of becoming necrotic. At one end of the spectrum, the prognosis is best for the patient with normal intrinsic coronary vessels whose completed infarction constitutes a small fraction (5 percent) of the left ventricle as a consequence of a coronary embolus and who has no jeopardized myocardium. At the other extreme is the patient with a massive infarct with left ventricular failure whose residual viable myocardium is perfused by markedly obstructed vessels. Progression of atherosclerosis or lowering of perfusion pressure in these vessels impairs the function and viability of the residual myocardium on which left ventricular function depends. Revascularization may reduce the threat to the jeopardized myocardium even in such a patient. The third risk factor, the susceptibility to serious arrhythmias, is reflected in ventricular ectopic activity and other indicators of electrical instability, such as reduced heart rate variability or baroreflex sensitivity and an abnormal signal-averaged ECG. All of these identify patients at increased risk of death.

ASSESSMENT OF LEFT VENTRICULAR FUNCTION. Left ventricular ejection fraction may be the most easily assessed measurement of left ventricular function and is extremely useful for risk stratification (see Fig. 51-30). However, imaging of the left ventricle at rest may not distinguish adequately among infarcted, irreversibly damaged, and stunned or hibernating myocardium. To circumvent this difficulty, various techniques have been investigated to assess the extent of residual viable myocardium including

exercise and pharmacological stress echocardiography, stress radionuclide ventricular angiography, perfusion imaging in conjunction with pharmacological stress, positron emission tomography, and gadolinium-enhanced MRI. All of these techniques can be performed safely in postinfarction patients. Because no study has clearly shown one imaging modality to be superior to others, clinicians should be guided in their selection of ventricular imaging technique by the availability and level of expertise with a given modality at their local institution.[258]

In patients with low left ventricular ejection fraction, the measurement of exercise capacity is useful for further identifying those patients at particularly high risk and also for establishing safe exercise limits after discharge.[1] Patients with a good exercise capacity despite a reduced ejection fraction have a better long-term outcome than those who have exercise impairment.

ASSESSMENT OF MYOCARDIAL ISCHEMIA. Because of the potent adverse consequences of recurrent myocardial infarction after STEMI, it is important to assess a patient's risk for future ischemia and infarction. Given the increasing array of pharmacological, interventional, and surgical options available to modify the likelihood of developing recurrent episodes of myocardial ischemia, most clinicians find it helpful to identify patients at risk for provocable myocardial ischemia before discharge. A predischarge evaluation for ischemia allows clinicians to select patients who might benefit from catheterization and revascularization following STEMI and to assess the adequacy of medical therapy for those patients who are suitable for a more conservative management strategy (see Fig. 51-43).

Exercise Testing. An exercise test also offers the clinician an opportunity to formulate a more precise exercise prescription and is helpful in boosting patients' confidence in their ability to conduct their daily activities after discharge. Patients who are unable to exercise can be evaluated by the use of a pharmacological stress protocol, such as an infusion of dobutamine or dipyridamole with echocardiography or perfusion imaging (see Fig. 51-43).

Treadmill exercise testing after STEMI has traditionally utilized a submaximal protocol that requires the patient to exercise until symptoms of angina appear, electrocardiographic evidence of ischemia is seen, or a target workload (≈5 metabolic equivalents) has been reached (see Chap. 13). It has been proposed that symptom-limited exercise tests can be safely performed before discharge in patients with an uncomplicated postinfarction course in-hospital.[259] Variables derived from exercise tests after STEMI that have been evaluated for their ability to predict the occurrence of death or recurrent nonfatal infarction include the development and magnitude of ST segment depression, the development of angina, exercise capacity, and the systolic blood pressure response during exercise.

ASSESSMENT FOR ELECTRICAL INSTABILITY. After STEMI, patients are at greatest risk for the development of sudden cardiac death caused by malignant ventricular arrhythmias over the course of the first 1 to 2 years.[1,260] Several techniques have been proposed to stratify patients into those who are at increased risk of sudden death following STEMI: measurement of Q-T dispersion (variability of Q-T intervals between ECG leads), ambulatory ECG recordings for detection of ventricular arrhythmias (Holter monitoring), invasive electrophysiological testing, recording a signal-averaged ECG (a measure of delayed, fragmented conduction in the infarct zone), and measuring heart rate variability (beat-to-beat variability in R-R intervals) or baroreflex sensitivity (slope of a line relating beat-to-beat change in sinus rate in response to alteration of blood pressure), but these have not proved sufficiently useful to recommend their use in routine practice.

Despite the increased risk of arrhythmic events following STEMI in patients who are found to have abnormal results on one or more of the noninvasive tests described earlier, several points should be emphasized. The low positive predictive value (<30 percent) for the noninvasive screening tests limits their usefulness when viewed in isolation. Although the predictive value of screening tests can be improved by combining several of them together, the therapeutic implications of an increased risk profile for arrhythmic events have not been established. The mortality reductions achievable with the general use of beta blockers, ACE inhibitors, aspirin, and revascularization when appropriate after infarction, coupled with concerns about the efficacy and safety of antiarrhythmic drugs and the cost of implanted defibrillators, leave considerable uncertainty about the therapeutic implications of an abnormal noninvasive test for electrical instability in an asymptomatic patient. Additional data on patient outcomes when clinicians act on the results of an abnormal finding are required before definitive recommendations can be made for asymptomatic patients.[1] The management of patients with sustained, hemodynamically compromising arrhythmias is discussed in Chapters 33 to 35.

PROPHYLACTIC ANTIARRHYTHMIC THERAPY. Although it has been recognized for decades that antiarrhythmic therapy can control atrial and ventricular arrhythmias effectively in many patients, reviews of clinical trials following STEMI have reported an increased risk of mortality with type I drugs. The most notable postinfarction trial in this area was the Cardiac Arrhythmia Suppression Trial (CAST), which tested whether encainide, flecainide, or moricizine for suppression of ventricular arrhythmias detected on ambulatory electrocardiographic monitoring would reduce the risk of cardiac arrest and death over the long term. Both the first phase of the trial (encainide or flecainide versus placebo) and the second phase of the trial (moricizine versus placebo) were stopped prematurely because of increased mortality in the active treatment groups. The mechanism of the increased risk after STEMI remains a subject of investigation, but one hypothesis that has been put forth is an adverse interaction between recurrent ischemia and the presence of an antiarrhythmic drug because the risk of death or cardiac arrest was greater in patients with a non-Q-wave acute MI than with Q-wave MI. Sodium channel blockade by antiarrhythmics may exacerbate electrophysiological differences between subepicardial and subendocardial zones of myocardium, rendering the latter more susceptible to ischemic injury.

Subsequent to CAST, another postinfarction prophylactic antiarrhythmic drug trial was undertaken with oral D-sotalol (Survival With ORal D-sotalol, or SWORD). SWORD also was stopped prematurely after enrollment of only 3121 of a planned 6400 patients because statistical evidence of increased mortality emerged in the active treatment group. The Canadian Amiodarone Myocardial Infarction Trial (CAMIAT) showed that amiodarone reduced the frequency of ventricular premature depolarization in patients with recent MI; this correlated with a reduction in arrhythmic death or resuscitation from ventricular fibrillation.[261] However, 42 percent of patients discontinued amiodarone during maintenance therapy in CAMIAT because of intolerable side effects. The European Amiodarone Myocardial Infarction Trial (EMIAT) showed a reduction in arrhythmic death after MI in patients with depressed left ventricular function, but there was no reduction in total mortality or other cardiovascular-related mortality.[262]

RECOMMENDATIONS. At this time, the *routine* use of antiarrhythmic agents (including amiodarone) cannot be recommended. Given the data cited earlier on the protective effects of beta blockers against sudden death and the ability of aspirin to reduce the risk of reinfarction, it is unclear that additional mortality reductions would be achieved by the empirical addition of amiodarone in the patient who is convalescing from a STEMI and is free of symptomatic sustained ventricular arrhythmias.

Several trials that included post-STEMI patients in the study population have shown significant mortality reductions in patients randomized to implantable cardioverter/defibrillator (ICD) implantation versus conventional medical therapy (see Chap. 34). At present, the selection of STEMI patients who are candidates for ICD implantation is based on the algorithm in Figure 51-44.

Secondary Prevention of Acute Myocardial Infarction (see Chap. 45)

The concept of secondary prevention of reinfarction and death after recovery from a STEMI has been investigated actively for several decades. Problems in proving the efficacy of various interventions have been related both to the ineffectiveness of certain strategies and to the difficulty in proving a benefit as mortality and morbidity have improved after STEMI. Nevertheless, patients who survive the initial course of STEMI still have considerable risk of recurrent events rendering imperative efforts to reduce this risk.

LIFE-STYLE MODIFICATION. Efforts to improve survival and the quality of life after MI that relate to life-style modification of known risk factors are considered in Chapter 45. Of these, cessation of smoking and control of hypertension are probably most important. Within 2 years of quitting smoking, the risk of a nonfatal MI in former smokers falls to a level similar to that in patients who never smoked.

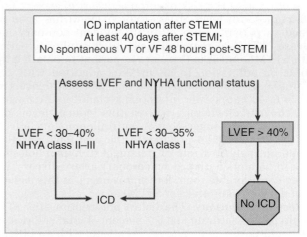

FIGURE 51–44 Algorithm for implantation of an implantable cardioverter-defibrillator (ICD) in ST-elevation myocardial infarction (STEMI) patients without ventricular fibrillation (VF) or sustained ventricular tachycardia (VT) more than 48 hours after STEMI. The appropriate management path is based on measurement of left ventricular ejection fraction (LVEF). EF measurements obtained 3 days or less after STEMI should be repeated before proceeding with the algorithm. Patients with EF less than 30 to 40 percent at least 40 days post-STEMI are referred for insertion of an ICD if they are in New York Heart Association (NYHA) Class II-III. Patients with a more depressed LVEF less than 30 to 35 percent are referred for ICD implantation even if they are NYHA Class I because of their increased risk of sudden cardiac death. Patients with preserved left ventricular function (LVEF > 40 percent) do not receive an ICD and are treated with medical therapy post-STEMI. *(Modified from Zipes DP, Camm AJ, Borggrefe M, et al: ACC/AHA/ESC 2006 guidelines for management of patients with ventricular arrhythmias and the prevention of sudden cardiac death: A report of the American College of Cardiology/American Heart Association Task Force and the European Society of Cardiology Committee for Practice Guidelines [Writing Committee to Develop Guidelines for Management of Patients with Ventricular Arrhythmias and the Prevention of Sudden Cardiac Death]. Developed in collaboration with the European Rhythm Association and the Heart Rhythm Society. Circulation 114: e385-484, 2006.)*

Being hospitalized for a STEMI is a powerful motivation for patients to cease cigarette smoking, and this is an ideal time to encourage that clearly beneficial and highly cost-effective life-style change. Smoking cessation intervention should therefore be a routine part of the discharge planning post-STEMI for all smokers. It is also an ideal time to begin to treat hypertension, counsel patients to achieve optimal body weight, and consider various strategies to improve the patient's lipid profile.[1]

DEPRESSION. Physicians caring for patients following a STEMI need to be sensitive to the prevalence of major depression after infarction. This problem is an independent risk factor for mortality. In addition, lack of an emotionally supportive network in the patient's environment after discharge is associated with an increased risk of mortality and recurrent cardiac events.[1] The precise mechanisms relating depression and lack of social support to worse prognosis after STEMI are not clear, but one possibility is lack of adherence to prescribed treatments, a behavior that has been shown to be associated with increased risk of mortality after infarction.[1] Evidence exists that a comprehensive rehabilitation program utilizing primary health care personnel who counsel patients and make home visits favorably affects the clinical course of patients after infarction and reduces the rate of rehospitalization for recurrent ischemia and infarction. A supportive physician attitude can also have a positive impact on the rate of return to work after STEMI.[254]

MODIFICATION OF LIPID PROFILE. Compelling evidence now exists that an increased cholesterol level, and most importantly an increased low-density lipoprotein (LDL) cholesterol level, is associated with an increased risk of coronary heart disease (see Chaps. 42 and 45). On the basis of this observation and the finding that lowering cholesterol reduces the risk of coronary heart disease, a target LDL cholesterol level of less than 70 mg/dl has been suggested in patients with clinically evident coronary heart disease.[263] This recommendation clearly applies to patients with STEMI, and it is therefore important to obtain a lipid profile on admission in all patients admitted with acute infarction. (It should be recalled that cholesterol levels may fall 24 to 48 hours after infarction.) In addition to lowering LDL cholesterol, therapy with statins reduces levels of C-reactive protein, suggesting an antiinflammatory effect.[264] Surveys of physician practice in the past have revealed a disappointingly low rate of treatment of hypercholesterolemia in patients with proven coronary artery disease, indicating considerable room for improvement in this aspect of secondary prevention after STEMI.

Recommendations. The dietary prescription after STEMI should be low saturated fat (<7 percent of total calories) and low cholesterol (<200 mg/day).[265] Patients with an LDL cholesterol level greater than 100 mg/dl should be discharged on statin therapy with the goal of reducing the LDL level to less than 70 mg/dl (see Chaps. 42 and 45). It is also reasonable to prescribe statin therapy to patients recovering from STEMI whose LDL cholesterol level is either unknown or is less than 100 mg/dl.[1] For many patients recovering from an acute MI, a low high-density lipoprotein cholesterol level is their primary lipid abnormality. See Chapters 42 and 45 for discussion of the management of dyslipidemia.

ANTIPLATELET AGENTS (see also Chap. 82). On the basis of the compelling data from the Antiplatelet Trialists' Collaboration of a 22 percent reduction in the risk of recurrent infarction, stroke, or vascular death in high-risk vascular patients receiving prolonged antiplatelet therapy in the absence of a true aspirin allergy, all STEMI patients should receive 75 to 162 mg of aspirin daily indefinitely.[129,146] Additional benefits of long-term aspirin that can accrue in the STEMI patient are an increased likelihood of patency of the infarct artery and smaller infarcts if recurrent MI does

take place. Patients with true aspirin allergy can be treated with clopidogrel (75 mg once daily) on the basis of experience from patients with unstable angina/non–ST segment elevation MI (UA/NSTEMI) (see Chap. 53). Given the results of the CLARITY-TIMI 28[130] and COMMIT[133] trials, as well as experience with clopidogrel in UA/NSTEMI, the author favors adding clopidogrel (75 mg/day) to aspirin in patients discharged after a STEMI. The optimum duration of treatment needs further study, but it seems reasonable to continue clopidogrel for at least 1 year after STEMI and maintain aspirin treatment indefinitely.

INHIBITION OF THE RENIN-ANGIOTENSIN-ALDOSTERONE SYSTEM. The rationale for inhibition of this neurohormonal axis after STEMI was discussed earlier. To prevent late remodeling of the left ventricle and also to decrease the likelihood of recurrent ischemic events, we advocate indefinite therapy with an ACE inhibitor to all patients with clinically evident congestive heart failure, a moderate decrease in global ejection fraction, or a large regional wall-motion abnormality, even in the face of a normal global ejection fraction. Once the STEMI patient is discharged from the hospital, the evidence based on long-term management of patients with chronic coronary artery disease is the most relevant for long-term decision-making. Based on the results of the HOPE and EUROPA trials, we advocate indefinite treatment with an ACE inhibitor in all STEMI patients with an ejection fraction less than 40 percent or diabetes regardless of ejection fraction, provided no contraindications exist.[266-268] As discussed earlier, the VALIANT trial results suggest that valsartan may be used as an alternative to an ACE inhibitor for long-term management of patients with left ventricular dysfunction after STEMI.[169]

BETA-ADRENERGIC BLOCKERS. Meta-analyses of trials from the prethrombolytic era involving more than 24,000 patients who received beta blockers in the convalescent phase of STEMI have shown a 23 percent reduction in long-term mortality.[1] When beta blockade is initiated early (6 hours) in the acute phase of infarction and continued in the chronic phase of treatment, some of the benefit may result from a reduction in infarct size. In the majority of patients who have beta blockade initiated during the convalescent phase of STEMI, however, reduction in long-term mortality is probably caused by a combination of an antiarrhythmic effect (prevention of sudden death) and prevention of reinfarction. Beta blockade over the long term is also effective for reducing the rate of mortality in patients who have undergone revascularization.[269]

Given the well-documented benefits of beta blocker therapy, it is disturbing that this form of therapy continues to be underutilized, especially in high-risk groups such as the elderly.[1] Patients with a relative contraindication to beta blockers (moderate heart failure, bradyarrhythmias) should undergo a monitored trial of therapy in the hospital. The dosage should be sufficient to blunt the heart rate response to stress or exercise. Much of the impact of beta blockers in preventing mortality occurs in the first weeks; treatment should commence as soon as possible. Evidence exists that programs providing physician feedback improve adherence to guidelines such as those noted earlier for prescription of beta-adrenoceptor blockers after acute MI.[269]

Some controversy exists as to how long patients should be treated. The collective data from five trials providing information on long-term follow-up of beta-adrenoceptor blockers after infarction suggest that therapy should be continued for at least 2 to 3 years.[1] At that time, if the beta blocker is well tolerated and if there is no reason to discontinue therapy, such therapy probably should be continued in most patients.

Not all patients derive the same benefit from beta blocker therapy. The cost-effectiveness of treatment in medium- or high-risk persons compares very favorably with that of many other accepted interventions, such as CABG, angioplasty, and lipid-lowering therapy. In patients with an extremely good prognosis (first acute MI, good ventricular function, no angina, negative stress test result, and no complex ventricular ectopy) among whom a mortality rate of approximately 1 percent per year can be anticipated, beta blockers would have a smaller impact on survival. However, it is our preference to prescribe beta blockers to such patients for whatever postinfarction benefit is achieved and also to have them as part of the patient's usual regimen should MI recur at an unpredictable time in the future.

NITRATES. Although these agents are suitable for management of specific conditions after STEMI, such as recurrent angina or as part of a treatment regimen for congestive heart failure, little evidence indicates that they reduce mortality over the long term when prescribed on a routine basis to all patients with infarction.[1]

ANTICOAGULANTS. At least three theoretical reasons exist for anticipating that anticoagulants might be beneficial in the long-term management of patients after STEMI. (1) Because the coronary occlusion responsible for the STEMI is often caused by a thrombus, anticoagulants might be expected to halt progression, slow progression, or prevent the development of new thrombi elsewhere in the coronary arterial tree. (2) Anticoagulants might be expected to diminish the formation of mural thrombi and resultant systemic embolization. (3)

Anticoagulants might be expected to reduce the incidence of venous thrombosis and pulmonary embolization.

After several decades of evaluation, the weight of evidence now suggests that anticoagulants have a favorable effect on late mortality, stroke, and reinfarction among patients hospitalized with STEMI (Table 51-13). Given the complexities of combining long-term therapy with warfarin alone with antiplatelet therapy, clinicians must weigh the need for warfarin based on established indications for anticoagulation and the risk of bleeding. An algorithm to guide decision-making is given in Figure 51-45.

CALCIUM ANTAGONISTS. At present, we do not recommend the routine use of calcium antagonists for secondary prevention of infarction. A possible exception is a patient who cannot tolerate a beta blocker because of adverse effects on bronchospastic lung disease but who has wellpreserved left ventricular function; such patients may be candidates for a rate-slowing calcium antagonist such as diltiazem or verapamil.

HORMONE THERAPY (see also Chap. 76). The decision to prescribe hormone therapy is often a complex one that involves the desire to suppress postmenopausal symptoms versus the risks of breast and endometrial cancer and vascular events. Despite improvement in lipid profiles, hormone therapy with estrogen plus progestin in postmenopausal

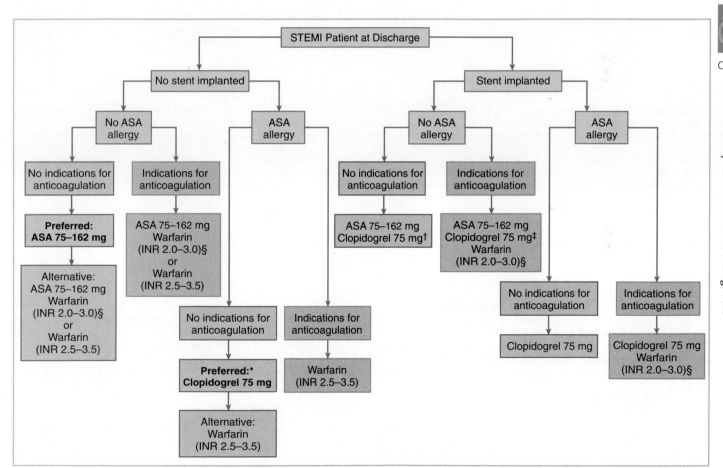

FIGURE 51–45 Algorithm for antithrombotic therapy at hospital discharge after ST-elevation myocardial ischemia (STEMI). *Clopidogrel is preferred over warfarin because of an increased risk of bleeding and low patient compliance in warfarin trials. †For 12 months. ‡Discontinue clopidogrel 1 month after implantation of a bare metal stent or several months after implantation of a drug-eluting stent (3 months after sirolimus and 6 months after paclitaxel) because of the potential increased risk of bleeding with warfarin and two antiplatelet agents. Continue ASA and warfarin long term if warfarin is indicated for other reasons such as atrial fibrillation, LV thrombus, cerebral emboli, or extensive regional wall motion abnormality. §An INR of 2 to 3 is acceptable with tight control, but the lower end of this range (2.0 to 2.5) is preferable. The combination of antiplatelet therapy and warfarin may be considered in patients younger than 75 years of age, with low bleeding risk, who can be monitored reliably. ASA = acetylsalicylic acid; INR = international normalized ratio; LV = left ventricular. *(Modified from Antman EM, Anbe DT, Armstrong PW, et al: ACC/AHA guidelines for the management of patients with ST-elevation myocardial infarction: A report of the American College of Cardiology/American Heart Association Task Force on Practice Guidelines [Committee to Revise the 1999 Guidelines for the Management of Patients with Acute Myocardial Infarction]) (www.acc.org/clinical/guidelines/stemi/index.pdf). Accessed 4/19/06.*

TABLE 51–13 | **Aspirin vs. Warfarin Therapy after ST-Elevation Myocardial Infarction (STEMI)**

Study	Study Design	Drugs Used	ASA	Second Arm	Third Arm
STEMI-Specific Trials					
WARIS II*	Randomized Open label N = 3630 FU = Mean 4 yr	ASA monotherapy vs. warfarin monotherapy vs. warfarin + ASA	160 mg daily	Dosed to target INR 2.8-4.2	Dosed to target INR 2.0-2.5 + ASA 75 mg daily
APRICOT II†	Randomized Open label N = 308 FU = 3 mo	ASA monotherapy vs. warfarin + ASA	If TIMI grade 3 post 48 hr UFH then 160 mg initially and then 80 mg daily	Dosed to target INR 2-3 if TIMI 3 post 48 hr UFH + 160 mg initially and then 80 mg daily	N/A
Trials Not Specific to STEMI					
ASPECT II‡	Randomized Open label N = 999 FU = 26 mo	ASA monotherapy vs. warfarin monotherapy vs. warfarin + ASA	80 mg daily	Dosed to target INR 3-4	Dosed to target INR 2-2.5 + ASA 80 mg daily
CHAMP§	Randomized Open label N = 5059 FU = median 2.7 yr	ASA monotherapy vs. warfarin + ASA	162 mg daily	Dosed to target INR 1.5-2.5 + 81 mg ASA daily	N/A
CARS¶	Randomized Blinded N = 8803 FU = 33 mo Median = 14 mo	ASA monotherapy vs. warfarin 1 mg + ASA	160 mg daily (avg INR @ wk 4 = 1.02)	1 mg + 80 mg ASA (avg INR @ wk 4 = 1.05)	N/A

*Hurlen M, Abdelnoor M, Smith P, et al: Warfarin, aspirin, or both after myocardial infarction. N Eng J Med 347:969, 2002.

†Brouwer MA, van den Bergh PJ, Aengevaeren WR, et al: Aspirin plus coumarin versus aspirin alone in the prevention of reocclusion after fibrinolysis for acute myocardial infarction: Results of the Antithrombotics in the Prevention of Reocclusion In Coronary Thrombolysis (APRICOT)-2 Trial. Circulation 106:659, 2002.

‡Van Es RF, Jonker JJ, Verheugt FW, et al: Aspirin and coumadin after acute coronary syndromes (the ASPECT-2 study): A randomised controlled trial. Lancet 360:109, 2002.

§Fiore LD, Ezekowitz MD, Brophy MT, et al: Department of Veterans Affairs Cooperative Studies Program Clinical Trial comparing combined warfarin and aspirin with aspirin alone in survivors of acute myocardial infarction: Primary results of the CHAMP study. Circulation 105:557, 2002.

¶O'Connor CM, Gattis WA, Hellkamp AS, et al: Comparison of two aspirin doses on ischemic stroke in post-myocardial infarction patients in the warfarin (Coumadin) Aspirin Reinfarction Study (CARS). Am J Cardiol 88:541, 2001.

**Reported as number of events per 100 person-years of follow-up.

ASA = acetylsalicylic acid (aspirin); FU = follow-up; INR = international normalized ratio; MI = myocardial infarction; N/A = not applicable; STEMI = ST-elevation myocardial infarction; TIMI = Thrombosis In Myocardial Infarction; Tx = treatment; UA = unstable angina; UFH = unfractionated heparin.

Modified from Antman EM, et al: ACC/AHA Guidelines for the Management of Patients with ST-Elevation Myocardial Infarction. 2004 (http://www.acc.org/clinical/guidelines/stemi/index.htm).

CH 51

women with established coronary heart disease does not prevent recurrent coronary events and is associated with significantly increased risk of coronary and venous thromboembolic events.[1] At present, we recommend not starting hormone therapy with estrogen plus progestin after STEMI and discontinuing it in postmenopausal women after STEMI.

ANTIOXIDANTS. Dietary supplementation with omega-3 polyunsaturated fatty acids has been associated with a reduction in coronary heart disease death and nonfatal reinfarction in patients within 3 months of a MI.[270] Vitamin E (300 mg/day) does not confer any significant clinical benefit, however.[270]

NONSTEROIDAL ANTI-INFLAMMATORY DRUGS (NSAIDs). Evidence has emerged that COX-2 selective drugs and NSAIDs that have varying COX-1 : COX-2 inhibitory ratios promote a prothrombotic state, and their use is associated with an increased risk of atherothrombotic events.[271] Given the increased risk of atherothrombosis related to the index STEMI event, the desire not to interfere with the beneficial pharmacological actions of low-dose aspirin post-

STEMI, and reports of increased mortality and reinfarction when they are used after MI, the author strongly urges clinicians to avoid prescribing NSAIDs to patients recovering from STEMI.[272] If NSAIDs must be prescribed for pain relief, the lowest dose required to control symptoms should be administered for the shortest period of time required.[271,273]

REFERENCES

Patient Characteristics That Influence Management Strategy

1. Antman EM, Anbe DT, Armstrong PW, et al: ACC/AHA guidelines for the management of patients with ST-elevation myocardial infarction: A report of the American College of Cardiology/American Heart Association Task Force on Practice Guidelines (Committee to Revise the 1999 Guidelines for the Management of Patients with Acute Myocardial Infarction) (www.acc.org/clinical/guidelines/stemi/index.pdf). Accessed 4/19/06.

2. Ahmed S, Antman EM, Murphy SA, et al: Poor outcomes after fibrinolytic therapy for ST-segment elevation myocardial infarction: Impact of age (a meta-analysis of a decade of trials). J Thromb Thrombolysis 21:119-129, 2006.

3. Duchateau FX, Ricard-Hibon A, Devaud ML, Burnod A, Mantz J: Does aging influence quality of care for acute myocardial infarction in the prehospital setting? Elderly patients with acute myocardial infarction. Am J Emerg Med 24:512, 2006.

Patients	Endpoints	Results		
		ASA Alone	**Warfarin Alone**	**ASA + Warfarin**
Age < 75 yr Hospitalized for acute MI **% STEMI = 71.8**	Death, nonfatal reinfarction, or thromboembolic stroke	20%	16.7% ($p = 0.03$ vs. ASA)	15% ($p = 0.001$ vs. ASA)
	Major, nonfatal bleeding ($p < 0.001$)	0.17%	0.68%	0.57%
Age ≤ 76 yr Acute ST MI ≤ 6 yr prior to thrombolytic Tx **% STEMI = 100**	Reooclusion (TIMI ≤ 2) ($p < 0.02$)	28%	N/A	15%
	Total occlusion (TIMI 0-1) ($p < 0.02$)	20%		9%
	Revascularization ($p < 0.01$)	31%		13%
	Reinfarction ($p < 0.05$)	8%		2%
	Event-free survival rate* ($p < 0.01$)	66%		86%
	Bleeding (TIMI major and minor ($p = NS$)	3%		5%
Acute MI or UA within preceding 8 wk	Death, MI, or stroke ($p = 0.02479$)	9%	5%	5%
	Major bleeding	1%	1%	2%
	Minor bleeding ($p < 0.0001$) Almost 20% of the warfarin and combined group discontinued therapy; 40% in therapeutic range	5%	8%	15%
Acute MI within preceding 14 days prior to enrollment	Death ($p = 0.76$)	17.3%	N/A	17.6%
	Recurrent MI ($p = 0.78$)	13.1%		13.3%
	Stroke ($p = 0.52$)	3.5%		3.1%
	Major bleeding ($p = 0.001$)	0.72**		1.2**
Age 21-85 yr (82% <70 yr) MI 3-21 days (mean 9.6 days) prior to enrollment	Ischemic stroke ($p = 0.0534$)	0.6%	N/A	1.1%

CH 51

ST-Elevation Myocardial Infarction: Management

4. Karha J, Topol EJ: Primary percutaneous coronary intervention vs. fibrinolytic therapy for acute ST-elevation myocardial infarction in the elderly. Am J Geriatr Cardiol 15:19-21, 2006.
5. Alexander KP, Newby LK, Armstrong PW, Cannon CP, Gibler WB, Rich MW, Van de Werf F, White HD, Weaver WD, Naylor MD, Gore JM, Krumholz HM, Ohman EM: Acute coronary care in the elderly. Part 2: ST-segment elevation myocardial infarction. A Statement for Healthcare Professionals from the Acute Cardiac Care Subcommittee, Council on Clinical Cardiology, American Heart Association; Endorsed by the Society of Geriatric Cardiology. Circulation 115:2570-2589, 2007.
6. Iribarren C, Tolstykh I, Somkin CP, Ackerson LM, Brown TT, Scheffler R, Syme L, Kawachi I: Sex and racial/ethnic disparities in outcomes after acute myocardial infarction: a cohort study among members of a large integrated health care delivery system in northern California. Arch Intern Med 165:2105-2113, 2005.
7. Simon T, Mary-Krause M, Cambou JP, Hanania G, Gueret P, Lablanche JM, Blanchard D, Genes N, Danchin N: Impact of age and gender on in-hospital and late mortality after acute myocardial infarction: increased early risk in younger women: results from the French nation-wide USIC registries. Eur Heart J 27:1282-1288, 2006.
8. Gold LD, Krumholz HM: Gender differences in treatment of heart failure and acute myocardial infarction: a question of quality or epidemiology? Cardiol Rev 14:180-186, 2006.
9. Maynard C, Lowy E, Rumsfeld J, Sales AE, Sun H, Kopjar B, Fleming B, Jesse RL, Rusch R, Fihn SD: The prevalence and outcomes of in-hospital acute myocardial infarction in the department of veterans affairs health system. Arch Intern Med 166:1410-1416, 2006.

Rapid Triage and Early Care

10. Mensah GA, Hand MM, Antman EM, Ryan J, TJ, Schriever R, Smith J, SC, Jacobs AK: Recommendations for the establishment of ideal systems of care to increase the number of ST-segment elevation myocardial infarction patients with timely access to primary percutaneous coronary interventions: the patient and public perspective. Circulation, in press. 2007.
11. Robertson RM, Taubert KA: Warning signs for heart attack and stroke: what more can we do? J Cardiopulm Rehabil 25:40-42, 2005.
12. Moser DK, Kimble LP, Alberts MJ, Alonzo A, Croft JB, Dracup K, Evenson KR, Go AS, Hand MM, Kothari RU, Mensah GA, Morris DL, Pancioli AM, Riegel B, Zerwic JJ: Reducing delay in seeking treatment by patients with acute coronary syndrome and stroke: a scientific statement from the American Heart Association Council on cardiovascular nursing and stroke council. Circulation 114:168-182, 2006.
13. National Heart Lung and Blood Institute. Act in time to heart attack signs. Accessed on: 4/16/06. Available at: www.nhlbi.nih.gov/actintime.
14. Hallstrom AP, Ornato JP, Weisfeldt M, Travers A, Christenson J, McBurnie MA, Zalenski R, Becker LB, Schron EB, Proschan M: Public-access defibrillation and survival after out-of-hospital cardiac arrest. N Engl J Med 351:637-646, 2004.
15. Jacobs AK, Antman EM, Ellrodt G, Faxon DP, Gregory T, Mensah GA, Moyer P, Ornato J, Peterson ED, Sadwin L, Smith SC: Recommendation to develop strategies to increase the number of ST-segment-elevation myocardial infarction patients with timely access to primary percutaneous coronary intervention. Circulation 113:2152-2163, 2006.
16. Morrow DA, Antman EM, Giugliano RP, Cairns R, Charlesworth A, Murphy SA, de Lemos JA, McCabe CH, Braunwald E: A simple risk index for rapid initial triage of patients with ST-elevation myocardial infarction: an InTIME II substudy. Lancet 358:1571-1575, 2001.
17. Morrison LJ, Verbeek PR, McDonald AC, Sawadsky BV, Cook DJ: Mortality and prehospital thrombolysis for acute myocardial infarction: A meta-analysis. JAMA 283:2686-2692, 2000.
18. Bonnefoy E, Lapostolle F, Leizorovicz A, Steg G, McFadden EP, Dubien PY, Cattan S, Boullenger E, Machecourt J, Lacroute JM, Cassagnes J, Dissait F, Touboul P: Primary angioplasty versus prehospital fibrinolysis in acute myocardial infarction: a randomised study. Lancet 360:825-829, 2002.
19. Steg PG, Bonnefoy E, Chabaud S, Lapostolle F, Dubien PY, Cristofini P, Leizorovicz A, Touboul P: Impact of time to treatment on mortality after prehospital fibrinolysis or primary angioplasty: data from the CAPTIM randomized clinical trial. Circulation 108:2851-2856, 2003.
20. Danchin N, Blanchard D, Steg PG, Sauval P, Hanania G, Goldstein P, Cambou JP, Gueret P, Vaur L, Boutalbi Y, Genes N, Lablanche JM: Impact of prehospital thrombolysis for acute myocardial infarction on 1-year outcome: results from the French Nationwide USIC 2000 Registry. Circulation 110:1909-1915, 2004.
21. Bjorklund E, Stenestrand U, Lindback J, Svensson L, Wallentin L, Lindahl B: Prehospital thrombolysis delivered by paramedics is associated with reduced time delay and mortality in ambulance-transported real-life patients with ST-elevation myocardial infarction. Eur Heart J 27:1146-1152, 2006.
22. Pedley DK, Bissett K, Connolly EM, Goodman CG, Golding I, Pringle TH, McNeill GP, Pringle SD, Jones MC: Prospective observational cohort study of time saved by prehospital thrombolysis for ST elevation myocardial infarction delivered by paramedics. BMJ 327:22-26, 2003.
23. Swor R, Hegerberg S, McHugh-McNally A, Goldstein M, McEachin CC: Prehospital 12-Lead ECG: Efficacy or Effectiveness? Prehosp Emerg Care 10:374-377, 2006.
24. Morrison LJ, Brooks S, Sawadsky B, McDonald A, Verbeek PR: Prehospital 12-lead electrocardiography impact on acute myocardial infarction treatment times and mortality: a systematic review. Acad Emerg Med 13:84-89, 2006.

25. Ortolani P, Marzocchi A, Marrozzini C, Palmerini T, Saia F, Serantoni C, Aquilina M, Silenzi S, Baldazzi F, Grosseto D, Taglieri N, Cooke RM, Bacchi-Reggiani ML, Branzi A: Clinical impact of direct referral to primary percutaneous coronary intervention following pre-hospital diagnosis of ST-elevation myocardial infarction. Eur Heart J 27:1550-1557, 2006.
26. Diercks DB, Kirk JD, Lindsell CJ, Pollack CV, Jr., Hoekstra JW, Gibler WB, Hollander JE: Door-to-ECG time in patients with chest pain presenting to the ED. Am J Emerg Med 24:1-7, 2006.
27. Garvey JL, MacLeod BA, Sopko G, Hand MM: Pre-hospital 12-lead electrocardiography programs: a call for implementation by emergency medical services systems providing advanced life support—National Heart Attack Alert Program (NHAAP) Coordinating Committee; National Heart, Lung, and Blood Institute (NHLBI); National Institutes of Health. J Am Coll Cardiol 47:485-491, 2006.
28. Gibson CM: Time is myocardium and time is outcomes. Circulation 104:2632-2634, 2001.
29. Bradley EH, Herrin J, Wang Y, McNamara RL, Radford MJ, Magid DJ, Canto JG, Blaney M, Krumholz HM: Door-to-drug and door-to-balloon times: where can we improve? Time to reperfusion therapy in patients with ST-segment elevation myocardial infarction (STEMI). Am Heart J 151:1281-1287, 2006.
30. Van de Werf F, Ardissino D, Betriu A, Cokkinos DV, Falk E, Fox KA, Julian D, Lengyel M, Neumann FJ, Ruzyllo W, Thygesen C, Underwood SR, Vahanian A, Verheugt FW, Wijns W: Management of acute myocardial infarction in patients presenting with ST-segment elevation. The Task Force on the Management of Acute Myocardial Infarction of the European Society of Cardiology. Eur Heart J 24:28-66, 2003.
31. Meyer MC, Mooney RP, Sekera AK: A critical pathway for patients with acute chest pain and low risk for short-term adverse cardiac events: role of outpatient stress testing. Ann Emerg Med 47:435 e1-e3, 2006.
32. Chockalingam A, Gnanavelu G, Subramaniam T, Dorairajan S, Chockalingam V: Right ventricular myocardial infarction: presentation and acute outcomes. Angiology 56:371-376, 2005.
33. Chen ZM, Pan HC, Chen YP, Peto R, Collins R, Jiang LX, Xie JX, Liu LS: Early intravenous then oral metoprolol in 45,852 patients with acute myocardial infarction: randomised placebo-controlled trial. Lancet 366:1622-1632, 2005.
34. Sabatine MS: Something old, something new: beta blockers and clopidogrel in acute myocardial infarction. Lancet 366:1587-1589, 2005.
35. Ellis TC, Lev E, Yazbek NF, Kleiman NS: Therapeutic strategies for cardiogenic shock, 2006. Curr Treat Options Cardiovasc Med 8:79-94, 2006.
36. Schomig A, Ndrepepa G, Mehilli J, Schwaiger M, Schuhlen H, Nekolla S, Pache J, Martinoff S, Bollwein H, Kastrati A: Therapy-dependent influence of time-to-treatment interval on myocardial salvage in patients with acute myocardial infarction treated with coronary artery stenting or thrombolysis. Circulation 108:1084-1088, 2003.
37. Alter DA, Ko DT, Newman A, Tu JV: Factors explaining the under-use of reperfusion therapy among ideal patients with ST-segment elevation myocardial infarction. Eur Heart J 27:1539-1549, 2006.
38. Hausenloy DJ, Yellon DM: Survival kinases in ischemic preconditioning and post-conditioning. Cardiovasc Res 70:240-253, 2006.
39. Gersh BJ, Stone GW, White HD, Holmes DR, Jr: Pharmacological facilitation of primary percutaneous coronary intervention for acute myocardial infarction: is the slope of the curve the shape of the future? JAMA 293:979-986, 2005.
40. Faxon DP: Early reperfusion strategies after acute ST-segment elevation myocardial infarction: the importance of timing. Nat Clin Pract Cardiovasc Med 2:22-28, 2005.
41. De Luca G, Suryapranata H, Zijlstra F, van't Hof AW, Hoorntje JC, Gosselink AT, Dambrink JH, de Boer MJ: Symptom-onset-to-balloon time and mortality in patients with acute myocardial infarction treated by primary angioplasty. J Am Coll Cardiol 42:991-997, 2003.
42. Jackson G: Primary angioplasty in acute myocardial infarction—the preferred option, but time is of the essence. Int J Clin Pract 60:379, 2006.
43. De Luca G, Suryapranata H, Ottervanger JP, Antman EM: Time delay to treatment and mortality in primary angioplasty for acute myocardial infarction: every minute of delay counts. Circulation 109:1223-1225, 2004.
44. Fibrinolytic Therapy Trialists' Collaborative Group. Indications for fibrinolytic therapy in suspected acute myocardial infarction: collaborative overview of early mortality and major morbidity results from all randomised trials of more than 1000 patients. Lancet 343:311-322, 1994.
45. Leong-Poi H, Coggins MP, Sklenar J, Jayaweera AR, Wang XQ, Kaul S: Role of collateral blood flow in the apparent disparity between the extent of abnormal wall thickening and perfusion defect size during acute myocardial infarction and demand ischemia. J Am Coll Cardiol 45:565-572, 2005.
46. Serra V, de Isla LP, Ferro MP, Rodrigo JL, Almeria C, Fernandez-Ortiz A, Garcia-Rubira JC, Zamorano J, Macaya C: Identification of stunned myocardium with parametric imaging-based, quantitative myocardial contrast echocardiography after acute myocardial infarction. Am J Cardiol 96:167-172, 2005.
47. Couvreur N, Lucats L, Tissier R, Bize A, Berdeaux A, Ghalch B: Differential effects of postconditioning on myocardial stunning and infarction: a study in conscious dogs and anesthetized rabbits. Am J Physiol Heart Circ Physiol 291:H1345-H1350, 2006.
48. Gerber BL, Wijns W, Vanoverschelde JL, Heyndrickx GR, De Bruyne B, Bartunek J, Melin JA: Myocardial perfusion and oxygen consumption in reperfused noninfarcted dysfunctional myocardium after unstable angina: direct evidence for myocardial stunning in humans. J Am Coll Cardiol 34:1939-1946, 1999.
49. Cannon RO: 3rd. Mechanisms, management and future directions for reperfusion injury after acute myocardial infarction. Nat Clin Pract Cardiovasc Med 2:88-94, 2005.
50. Vargas SO, Sampson BA, Schoen FJ: Pathologic detection of early myocardial infarction: a critical review of the evolution and usefulness of modern techniques. Mod Pathol 12:635-645, 1999.
51. Kloner RA, Forman MB, Gibbons RJ, Ross AM, Alexander RW, Stone GW: Impact of time to therapy and reperfusion modality on the efficacy of adenosine in acute myocardial infarction: the AMISTAD-2 trial. Eur Heart J 27:2400-2405, 2006.
52. Vinten-Johansen J, Yellon DM, Opie LH: Postconditioning: a simple, clinically applicable procedure to improve revascularization in acute myocardial infarction. Circulation 112:2085-2088, 2005.
53. Staat P, Rioufol G, Piot C, Cottin Y, Cung TT, L'Huillier I, Aupetit JF, Bonnefoy E, Finet G, Andre-Fouet X, Ovize M: Postconditioning the human heart. Circulation 112:2143-2148, 2005.
54. Goldstein JA, Lee DT, Pica MC, Dixon SR, O'Neill WW: Patterns of coronary compromise leading to bradyarrhythmias and hypotension in inferior myocardial infarction. Coron Artery Dis 16:265-274, 2005.
55. Voon WC, Chen YW, Hsu CC, Lai WT, Sheu SH: Q-wave regression after acute myocardial infarction assessed by Tl-201 myocardial perfusion SPECT. J Nucl Cardiol 11:165-170, 2004.
56. Boersma E, Mercado N, Poldermans D, Gardien M, Vos J, Simoons ML: Acute myocardial infarction. Lancet 361:847-858, 2003.

Reperfusion Therapies

57. Franzosi MG, Santoro E, De Vita C, Geraci E, Lotto A, Maggioni AP, Mauri F, Rovelli F, Santoro L, Tavazzi L, Tognoni G: Ten-year follow-up of the first megatrial testing thrombolytic therapy in patients with acute myocardial infarction: results of the Gruppo Italiano per lo Studio della Sopravvivenza nell'Infarto-1 study. The GISSI Investigators. Circulation 98:2659-2665, 1998.
58. TIMI Study Group: The Thrombolysis in Myocardial Infarction (TIMI) trial. Phase I findings. N Engl J Med 312:932-936, 1985.
59. Chesebro JH, Knatterud G, Roberts R, Borer J, Cohen LS, Dalen J, Dodge HT, Francis CK, Hillis D, Ludbrook P, et al: Thrombolysis in Myocardial Infarction (TIMI) Trial, Phase I: A comparison between intravenous tissue plasminogen activator and intravenous streptokinase. Clinical findings through hospital discharge. Circulation 76:142-154, 1987.
60. Antman EM, Giugliano RP, Gibson CM, McCabe CH, Coussement P, Kleiman NS, Vahanian A, Adgey AA, Menown I, Rupprecht HJ, Van der Wieken R, Ducas J, Scherer J, Anderson K, Van de Werf F, Braunwald E: Abciximab facilitates the rate and extent of thrombolysis: results of the thrombolysis in myocardial infarction (TIMI) 14 trial. The TIMI 14 Investigators. Circulation 99:2720-2732, 1999.
61. Gibson CM: Has my patient achieved adequate myocardial reperfusion? Circulation 108:504-507, 2003.
62. Gibson CM, Murphy SA, Rizzo MJ, Ryan KA, Marble SJ, McCabe CH, Cannon CP, Van de Werf F, Braunwald E: Relationship between TIMI frame count and clinical outcomes after thrombolytic administration. Thrombolysis In Myocardial Infarction (TIMI) Study Group. Circulation 99:1945-1950, 1999.
63. Gibson CM, Murphy S, Menown IB, Sequeira RF, Greene R, Van de Werf F, Schweiger MJ, Ghali M, Frey MJ, Ryan KA, Marble SJ, Giugliano RP, Antman EM, Cannon CP, Braunwald E: Determinants of coronary blood flow after thrombolytic administration. TIMI Study Group. Thrombolysis in Myocardial Infarction. J Am Coll Cardiol 34:1403-1412, 1999.
64. Gibson CM, Murphy SA, Kirtane AJ, Giugliano RP, Cannon CP, Antman EM, Braunwald E: Association of duration of symptoms at presentation with angiographic and clinical outcomes after fibrinolytic therapy in patients with ST-segment elevation myocardial infarction. J Am Coll Cardiol 44:980-987, 2004.
65. Angeja BG, de Lemos J, Murphy SA, Marble SJ, Antman EM, Cannon CP, Braunwald E, Gibson CM: Impact of diabetes mellitus on epicardial and microvascular flow after fibrinolytic therapy. Am Heart J 144:649-656, 2002.
66. Kirtane AJ, Vafai JJ, Murphy SA, Aroesty JM, Sabatine MS, Cannon CP, Gibson CM: Angiographically evident thrombus following fibrinolytic therapy is associated with impaired myocardial perfusion in STEMI: a CLARITY-TIMI 28 substudy. Eur Heart J 2006.
67. Schroder R: Prognostic impact of early ST-segment resolution in acute ST-elevation myocardial infarction. Circulation 110:e506-e510, 2004.
68. Krucoff MW, Johanson P, Baeza R, Crater SW, Dellborg M: Clinical utility of serial and continuous ST-segment recovery assessment in patients with acute ST-elevation myocardial infarction: assessing the dynamics of epicardial and myocardial reperfusion. Circulation 110:e533-e539, 2004.
69. Bainey KR, Senaratne MP: Is the outcomes of early ST-segment resolution after thrombolytic therapy in acute myocardial infarction always favorable? J Electrocardiol 38:354-360, 2005.
70. Brodie BR, Stuckey TD, Hansen C, VerSteeg DS, Muncy DB, Moore S, Gupta N, Downey WE: Relation between electrocardiographic ST-segment resolution and early and late outcomes after primary percutaneous coronary intervention for acute myocardial infarction. Am J Cardiol 95:343-348, 2005.
71. Gibson CM, Karha J, Giugliano RP, Roe MT, Murphy SA, Harrington RA, Green CL, Schweiger MJ, Miklin JS, Baran KW, Palmeri S, Braunwald E, Krucoff MW: Association of the timing of ST-segment resolution with TIMI myocardial perfusion grade in acute myocardial infarction. Am Heart J 147:847-852, 2004.
72. Bjorklund E, Jernberg T, Johanson P, Venge P, Dellborg M, Wallentin L, Lindahl B: Admission N-terminal pro-brain natriuretic peptide and its interaction with admission troponin T and ST segment resolution for early risk stratification in ST elevation myocardial infarction. Heart 92:735-740, 2006.
73. Terkelsen CJ, Norgaard BL, Lassen JF, Poulsen SH, Gerdes JC, Sloth E, Gotzsche LB, Romer FK, Thuesen L, Nielsen TT, Andersen HR: Potential significance of spontaneous and interventional ST-changes in patients transferred for primary percutaneous coronary intervention: observations from the ST-MONitoring in Acute Myocardial Infarction study (The MONAMI study). Eur Heart J 27:267-275, 2006.
74. Angeja BG, Gunda M, Murphy SA, Sobel BE, Rundle AC, Syed M, Asfour A, Borzak S, Gourlay SG, Barron HV, Gibbons RJ, Gibson CM: TIMI myocardial perfusion

grade and ST segment resolution: association with infarct size as assessed by single photon emission computed tomography imaging. Circulation 105:282-285, 2002.

75. Boersma E, Maas AC, Deckers JW, Simoons ML: Early thrombolytic treatment in acute myocardial infarction: reappraisal of the golden hour. Lancet 348:771-775, 1996.

76. Antman EM, Morrow DA, McCabe CH, Murphy SA, Ruda M, Sadowski Z, Budaj A, Lopez-Sendon JL, Guneri S, Jiang F, White HD, Fox KA, Braunwald E: Enoxaparin versus unfractionated heparin with fibrinolysis for ST-elevation myocardial infarction. N Engl J Med 354:1477-1488, 2006.

77. Rich MW: Epidemiology, clinical features, and prognosis of acute myocardial infarction in the elderly. Am J Geriatr Cardiol 15:7-11; quiz 12, 2006.

78. White HD: Thrombolytic therapy in the elderly. Lancet 356:2028-2030, 2000.

79. Stenestrand U, Wallentin L: Fibrinolytic therapy in patients 75 years and older with ST-segment-elevation myocardial infarction: one-year follow-up of a large prospective cohort. Arch Intern Med 163:965-971, 2003.

80. Morrow DA, Antman EM, Charlesworth A, Cairns R, Murphy SA, de Lemos JA, Giugliano RP, McCabe CH, Braunwald E: TIMI risk score for ST-elevation myocardial infarction: A convenient, bedside, clinical score for risk assessment at presentation: An intravenous nPA for treatment of infarcting myocardium early II trial substudy. Circulation 102:2031-2037, 2000.

81. Morrow DA, Antman EM, Parsons L, de Lemos JA, Cannon CP, Giugliano RP, McCabe CH, Barron HV, Braunwald E: Application of the TIMI risk score for ST-elevation MI in the National Registry of Myocardial Infarction 3. JAMA 286:1356-1359, 2001.

82. Brouwer MA, van den Bergh PJ, Aengevaeren WR, Veen G, Luijten HE, Hertzberger DP, van Boven AJ, Vromans RP, Uijen GJ, Verheugt FW: Aspirin plus coumarin versus aspirin alone in the prevention of reocclusion after fibrinolysis for acute myocardial infarction: results of the Antithrombotics in the Prevention of Reocclusion In Coronary Thrombolysis (APRICOT)-2 Trial. Circulation 106:659-665, 2002.

83. Aversano T, Aversano LT, Passamani E, Knatterud GL, Terrin ML, Williams DO, Forman SA: Thrombolytic therapy vs primary percutaneous coronary intervention for myocardial infarction in patients presenting to hospitals without on-site cardiac surgery: a randomized controlled trial. JAMA 287:1943-1951, 2002.

84. Llevadot J, Giugliano RP, Antman EM: Bolus fibrinolytic therapy in acute myocardial infarction. JAMA 286:442-449, 2001.

85. The Global Use of Strategies to Open Occluded Coronary Arteries—GUSTO III—Investigators. A comparison of reteplase with alteplase for acute myocardial infarction. N Engl J Med 337:1118-1123, 1997.

86. Ware JH, Antman EM: Equivalence trials. N Engl J Med 337:1159-1161, 1997.

87. White HD: Thrombolytic therapy and equivalence trials. J Am Coll Cardiol 31:494-496, 1998.

88. Cannon CP, McCabe CH, Gibson CM, Ghali M, Sequeira RF, McKendall GR, Breed J, Modi NB, Fox NL, Tracy RP, Love TW, Braunwald E: TNK-tissue plasminogen activator in acute myocardial infarction. Results of the Thrombolysis in Myocardial Infarction (TIMI) 10A dose-ranging trial. Circulation 95:351-356, 1997.

89. Cannon CP, Gibson CM, McCabe CH, Adgey AA, Schweiger MJ, Sequeira RF, Grollier G, Giugliano RP, Frey M, Mueller HS, Steingart RM, Weaver WD, Van de Werf F, Braunwald E: TNK-tissue plasminogen activator compared with front-loaded alteplase in acute myocardial infarction: results of the TIMI 10B trial. Thrombolysis in Myocardial Infarction (TIMI) 10B Investigators. Circulation 98:2805-2814, 1998.

90. Van de Werf F, Cannon CP, Luyten A, Houbracken K, McCabe CH, Berioli S, Bluhmki E, Sarelin H, Wang-Clow F, Fox NL, Braunwald E: Safety assessment of single-bolus administration of TNK tissue-plasminogen activator in acute myocardial infarction: the ASSENT-1 trial. The ASSENT-1 Investigators. Am Heart J 137:786-791, 1999.

91. Assessment of the Safety and Efficacy of a New Thrombolytic Investigators. Single-bolus tenecteplase compared with front-loaded alteplase in acute myocardial infarction: the ASSENT-2 double-blind randomised trial. Lancet 354:716-722, 1999.

92. Armstrong PW, Burton J, Pakola S, Molhoek PG, Betriu A, Tendera M, Bode C, Adgey AA, Bar F, Vahanian A, Van de Werf F: Collaborative Angiographic Patency Trial Of Recombinant Staphylokinase (CAPTORS II). Am Heart J 146:484-488, 2003.

93. Ndrepepa G, Kastrati A, Schwaiger M, Mehilli J, Markwardt C, Dibra A, Dirschinger J, Schomig A: Relationship between residual blood flow in the infarct-related artery and scintigraphic infarct size, myocardial salvage, and functional recovery in patients with acute myocardial infarction. J Nucl Med 46:1782-1788, 2005.

94. Ross AM, Gibbons RJ, Stone GW, Kloner RA, Alexander RW: A randomized, double-blinded, placebo-controlled multicenter trial of adenosine as an adjunct to reperfusion in the treatment of acute myocardial infarction (AMISTAD-II). J Am Coll Cardiol 45:1775-1780, 2005.

95. ASSENT-4 PCI Investigators. Primary versus tenecteplase-facilitated percutaneous coronary intervention in patients with ST-segment elevation acute myocardial infarction (ASSENT-4 PCI): randomised trial. Lancet 367:569-578, 2006.

96. Gore JM, Granger CB, Simoons ML, Sloan MA, Weaver WD, White HD, Barbash GI, Van de Werf F, Aylward PE, Topol EJ, et al: Stroke after thrombolysis. Mortality and functional outcomes in the GUSTO-I trial. Global Use of Strategies to Open Occluded Coronary Arteries. Circulation 92:2811-2818, 1995.

97. Kleiman NS, Terrin M, Mueller H, Chaitman B, Roberts R, Knatterud GL, Solomon R, McMahon RP, Braunwald E: Mechanisms of early death despite thrombolytic therapy: experience from the Thrombolysis in Myocardial Infarction Phase II (TIMI II) study. J Am Coll Cardiol 19:1129-1135, 1992.

98. Cohen M, Gensini GF, Maritz F, Gurfinkel EP, Huber K, Timerman A, Santopinto J, Corsini G, Terrosu P, Joulain F: The role of gender and other factors as predictors of not receiving reperfusion therapy and of outcome in ST-segment elevation myocardial infarction. J Thromb Thrombolysis 19:155-161, 2005.

99. Van de Werf F, Barron HV, Armstrong PW, Granger CB, Berioli S, Barbash G, Pehrsson K, Verheugt FW, Meyer J, Betriu A, Califf RM, Li X, Fox NL: Incidence and predictors of bleeding events after fibrinolytic therapy with fibrin-specific agents: a comparison of TNK-tPA and rt-PA. Eur Heart J 22:2253-2261, 2001.

100. Giugliano RP, Antman EM: Caeteris paribus—all things being equal. Eur Heart J 22:2221-2223, 2001.

101. Voisine P, Mathieu P, Doyle D, Perron J, Baillot R, Raymond G, Metras J, Dagenais F: Influence of time elapsed between myocardial infarction and coronary artery bypass grafting surgery on operative mortality. Eur J Cardiothorac Surg 29:319-323, 2006.

102. Kereiakes DJ, Antman EM: Clinical guidelines and practice: in search of the truth. J Am Coll Cardiol 48:1129-1135, 2006.

103. Keeley EC, Boura JA, Grines CL: Primary angioplasty versus intravenous thrombolytic therapy for acute myocardial infarction: a quantitative review of 23 randomised trials. Lancet 361:13-20, 2003.

104. Hochman JS, Sleeper LA, Webb JG, Dzavik V, Buller CE, Aylward P, Col J, White HD: Early revascularization and long-term survival in cardiogenic shock complicating acute myocardial infarction. JAMA 295:2511-2515, 2006.

105. Kent DM, Schmid CH, Lau J, Selker HP: Is primary angioplasty for some as good as primary angioplasty for all? J Gen Intern Med 17:887-894, 2002.

106. Grzybowski M, Clements EA, Parsons L, Welch R, Tintinalli AT, Ross MA, Zalenski RJ: Mortality benefit of immediate revascularization of acute ST-segment elevation myocardial infarction in patients with contraindications to thrombolytic therapy: a propensity analysis. JAMA 290:1891-1898, 2003.

107. The GUSTO Angiographic Investigators. The effects of tissue plasminogen activator, streptokinase, or both on coronary-artery patency, ventricular function, and survival after acute myocardial infarction. N Engl J Med 329:1615-1622, 1993.

108. Widimsky P, Budesinsky T, Vorac D, Groch L, Zelizko M, Aschermann M, Branny M, St'asek J, Formanek P: Long distance transport for primary angioplasty vs immediate thrombolysis in acute myocardial infarction. Final results of the randomized national multicentre trial—PRAGUE-2. Eur Heart J 24:94-104, 2003.

109. Andersen HR, Nielsen TT, Rasmussen K, Thuesen L, Kelbaek H, Thayssen P, Abildgaard U, Pedersen F, Madsen JK, Grande P, Villadsen AB, Krusell LR, Haghfelt T, Lomholt P, Husted SE, Vigholt E, Kjaergard HK, Mortensen LS: A comparison of coronary angioplasty with fibrinolytic therapy in acute myocardial infarction. N Engl J Med 349:733-742, 2003.

110. Dalby M, Bouzamondo A, Lechat P, Montalescot G: Transfer for primary angioplasty versus immediate thrombolysis in acute myocardial infarction: a meta-analysis. Circulation 108:1809-1814, 2003.

110a. Pinto SD, Kirtane AJ, Nallamothu BK, et al: Hospital delays in reperfusion for ST-elevation myocardial infarction: Implications when selecting a reperfusion strategy. Circulation 114:2019-2025, 2006.

Anticoagulant and Antiplatelet Strategies

111. ISIS-2—Second International Study of Infarct Survival—Collaborative Group. Randomised trial of intravenous streptokinase, oral aspirin, both, or neither among 17,187 cases of suspected acute myocardial infarction: ISIS-2. Lancet 2:349-360, 1988.

112. Morrow DA: Heparin and low-molecular-weight heparin. In Manson JE, Buring JE, Ridker PM, Gaziano JM (eds): Clinical Trials in Heart Disease; a Companion to Braunwald's Heart Disease. 2nd ed. Philadelphia, Elsevier Saunders, 2004, pp 45-65.

113. Menon V, Berkowitz SD, Antman EM, Fuchs RM, Hochman JS: New heparin dosing recommendations for patients with acute coronary syndromes. Am J Med 110:641-650, 2001.

114. Keeling D, Davidson S, Watson H: The management of heparin-induced thrombocytopenia. Br J Haematol 133:259-269, 2006.

115. Antman EM: The search for replacements for unfractionated heparin. Circulation 103:2310-2314, 2001.

116. Bittl JA, White HD, Antman EM: Direct thrombin inhibitors. In Manson JE, Buring JE, Ridker PM, Gaziano JM (eds): Clinical Trials in Heart Disease; a Companion to Braunwald's Heart Disease. 2nd ed. Philadelphia, Elsevier Saunders, 2004, pp 83-96.

117. Ross AM, Molhoek P, Lundergan C, Knudtson M, Draoui Y, Regalado L, Le Louer V, Bigonzi F, Schwartz W, de Jong E, Coyne K: Randomized comparison of enoxaparin, a low-molecular-weight heparin, with unfractionated heparin adjunctive to recombinant tissue plasminogen activator thrombolysis and aspirin: second trial of Heparin and Aspirin Reperfusion Therapy (HART II). Circulation 104:648-652, 2001.

118. Simoons M, Krzeminska-Pakula M, Alonso A, Goodman S, Kali A, Loos U, Gosset F, Louer V, Bigonzi F: Improved reperfusion and clinical outcome with enoxaparin as an adjunct to streptokinase thrombolysis in acute myocardial infarction. The AMI-SK study. Eur Heart J 23:1282-1290, 2002.

119. Antman EM, Louwerenburg HW, Baars HF, Wesdorp JC, Hamer B, Bassand JP, Bigonzi F, Pisapia G, Gibson CM, Heidbuchel H, Braunwald E, Van de Werf F: Enoxaparin as adjunctive antithrombin therapy for ST-elevation myocardial infarction: results of the ENTIRE-Thrombolysis in Myocardial Infarction (TIMI) 23 Trial. Circulation 105:1642-1649, 2002.

120. Yusuf S, Mehta SR, Xie C, Ahmed RJ, Xavier D, Pais P, Zhu J, Liu L: Effects of reviparin, a low-molecular-weight heparin, on mortality, reinfarction, and strokes in patients with acute myocardial infarction presenting with ST-segment elevation. JAMA 293:427-435, 2005.

121. White H: Further evidence that antithrombotic therapy is beneficial with streptokinase: improved early ST resolution and late patency with enoxaparin. Eur Heart J 23:1233-1237, 2002.

122. Eikelboom JW, Quinlan DJ, Mehta SR, Turpie AG, Menown IB, Yusuf S: Unfractionated and low-molecular-weight heparin as adjuncts to thrombolysis in aspirin-

treated patients with ST-elevation acute myocardial infarction: a meta-analysis of the randomized trials. Circulation 112:3855-3867, 2005.

123. Assessment of the Safety and Efficacy of a New Thrombolytic Regimen A-, Investigators. Efficacy and safety of tenecteplase in combination with enoxaparin, abciximab, or unfractionated heparin: the ASSENT-3 randomised trial in acute myocardial infarction. Lancet 358:605-613, 2001.

124. Wallentin L, Goldstein P, Armstrong PW, Granger CB, Adgey AA, Arntz HR, Bogaerts K, Danays T, Lindahl B, Makijarvi M, Verheugt F, Van de Werf F: Efficacy and safety of tenecteplase in combination with the low-molecular weight heparin enoxaparin or unfractionated heparin in the prehospital setting: the Assessment of the Safety and Efficacy of a New Thrombolytic Regimen (ASSENT)-3 PLUS randomized trial in acute myocardial infarction. Circulation 108:135-142, 2003.

125. Yusuf S, Mehta SR, Chrolavicius S, Afzal R, Pogue J, Granger CB, Budaj A, Peters RJ, Bassand JP, Wallentin L, Joyner C, Fox KA: Effects of fondaparinux on mortality and reinfarction in patients with acute ST-segment elevation myocardial infarction: the OASIS-6 randomized trial. JAMA 295:1519-1530, 2006.

126. White H: Thrombin-specific anticoagulation with bivalirudin versus heparin in patients receiving fibrinolytic therapy for acute myocardial infarction: the HERO-2 randomised trial. Lancet 358:1855-1863, 2001.

127. Beygui F, Collet JP, Nagaswami C, Weisel JW, Montalescot G: Images in cardiovascular medicine. Architecture of intracoronary thrombi in ST-elevation acute myocardial infarction: time makes the difference. Circulation 113:e21-e23, 2006.

128. Serebruany VL, Malinin AI, Callahan KP, Binbrek A, Van de Werf F, Alexander JH, Granger CB, Gurbel PA: Effect of tenecteplase versus alteplase on platelets during the first 3 hours of treatment for acute myocardial infarction: the Assessment of the Safety and Efficacy of a New Thrombolytic Agent (ASSENT-2) platelet substudy. Am Heart J 145:636-642, 2003.

129. Antithrombotic Trialists' Collaboration. Collaborative meta-analysis of randomised trials of antiplatelet therapy for prevention of death, myocardial infarction, and stroke in high risk patients. BMJ 324:71-86, 2002.

130. Sabatine MS, Cannon CP, Gibson CM, Lopez-Sendon JL, Montalescot G, Theroux P, Claeys MJ, Cools F, Hill KA, Skene AM, McCabe CH, Braunwald E: Addition of clopidogrel to aspirin and fibrinolytic therapy for myocardial infarction with ST-segment elevation. N Engl J Med 352:1179-1189, 2005.

131. Scirica BM, Sabatine MS, Morrow DA, Gibson CM, Murphy SA, Wiviott SD, Giugliano RP, McCabe CH, Cannon CP, Braunwald E: The role of clopidogrel in early and sustained arterial patency after fibrinolysis for ST-segment elevation myocardial infarction: the ECG CLARITY-TIMI 28 Study. J Am Coll Cardiol 48:37-42, 2006.

132. Sabatine MS, Cannon CP, Gibson CM, Lopez-Sendon JL, Montalescot G, Theroux P, Lewis BS, Murphy SA, McCabe CH, Braunwald E: Effect of clopidogrel pretreatment before percutaneous coronary intervention in patients with ST-elevation myocardial infarction treated with fibrinolytics: the PCI-CLARITY study. JAMA 294:1224-1232, 2005.

133. Chen ZM, Jiang LX, Chen YP, Xie JX, Pan HC, Peto R, Collins R, Liu LS: Addition of clopidogrel to aspirin in 45,852 patients with acute myocardial infarction: randomised placebo-controlled trial. Lancet 366:1607-1621, 2005.

134. Eisenberg MJ, Jamal S: Glycoprotein IIb/IIIa inhibition in the setting of acute ST-segment elevation myocardial infarction. J Am Coll Cardiol 42:1-6, 2003.

135. Kleiman NS, Ohman EM, Califf RM, George BS, Kereiakes D, Aguirre FV, Weisman H, Schaible T, Topol EJ: Profound inhibition of platelet aggregation with monoclonal antibody 7E3 Fab after thrombolytic therapy. Results of the Thrombolysis and Angioplasty in Myocardial Infarction (TAMI) 8 Pilot Study. J Am Coll Cardiol 22:381-389, 1993.

136. Ohman EM, Kleiman NS, Gacioch G, Worley SJ, Navetta FI, Talley JD, Anderson HV, Ellis SG, Cohen MD, Spriggs D, Miller M, Kereiakes D, Yakubov S, Kitt MM, Sigmon KN, Califf RM, Krucoff MW, Topol EJ: Combined accelerated tissue-plasminogen activator and platelet glycoprotein IIb/IIIa integrin receptor blockade with Integrilin in acute myocardial infarction. Results of a randomized, placebo-controlled, dose-ranging trial. IMPACT-AMI Investigators. Circulation 95:846-854, 1997.

137. Ronner E, van Kesteren HA, Zijnen P, Altmann E, Molhoek PG, van der Wieken LR, Cuffie-Jackson CA, Neuhaus KL, Simoons ML: Safety and efficacy of eptifibatide vs placebo in patients receiving thrombolytic therapy with streptokinase for acute myocardial infarction; a phase II dose escalation, randomized, double-blind study. Eur Heart J 21:1530-1536, 2000.

138. The PARADIGM Investigators. Combining thrombolysis with the platelet glycoprotein IIb/IIIa inhibitor lamifiban: results of the Platelet Aggregation Receptor Antagonist Dose Investigation and Reperfusion Gain in Myocardial Infarction (PARADIGM) trial. J Am Coll Cardiol 32:2003-2010, 1998.

139. Strategies for Patency Enhancement in the Emergency Department—SPEED—Group. Trial of abciximab with and without low-dose reteplase for acute myocardial infarction. Circulation 101:2788-2794, 2000.

140. Brener SJ, Zeymer U, Adgey AA, Vrobel TR, Ellis SG, Neuhaus KL, Juran N, Ivanc TB, Ohman EM, Strony J, Kitt M, Topol EJ: Eptifibatide and low-dose tissue plasminogen activator in acute myocardial infarction: the integrilin and low-dose thrombolysis in acute myocardial infarction (INTRO AMI) trial. J Am Coll Cardiol 39:377-386, 2002.

141. Giugliano RP, Roe MT, Harrington RA, Gibson CM, Zeymer U, Van de Werf F, Baran KW, Hobbach HP, Woodlief LH, Hannan KL, Greenberg S, Miller J, Kitt MM, Strony J, McCabe CH, Braunwald E, Califf RM: Combination reperfusion therapy with eptifibatide and reduced-dose tenecteplase for ST-elevation myocardial infarction: results of the integrilin and tenecteplase in acute myocardial infarction (INTEGRITI) Phase II Angiographic Trial. J Am Coll Cardiol 41:1251-1260, 2003.

142. Ohman EM, Van de Werf F, Antman EM, Califf RM, de Lemos JA, Gibson CM, Oliverio RL, Harrelson L, McCabe C, DiBattiste P, Braunwald E: Tenecteplase and tirofiban in ST-segment elevation acute myocardial infarction: results of a randomized trial. Am Heart J 150:79-88, 2005.

143. Roe MT, Green CL, Giugliano RP, Gibson CM, Baran K, Greenberg M, Palmeri ST, Crater S, Trollinger K, Hannan K, Harrington RA, Krucoff MW: Improved speed and stability of ST-segment recovery with reduced-dose tenecteplase and eptifibatide compared with full-dose tenecteplase for acute ST-segment elevation myocardial infarction. J Am Coll Cardiol 43:549-556, 2004.

144. de Lemos JA, Antman EM, Gibson CM, McCabe CH, Giugliano RP, Murphy SA, Coulter SA, Anderson K, Scherer J, Frey MJ, Van Der Wieken R, Van de Werf F, Braunwald E: Abciximab improves both epicardial flow and myocardial reperfusion in ST-elevation myocardial infarction. Observations from the TIMI 14 trial. Circulation 101:239-243, 2000.

145. Topol EJ: Reperfusion therapy for acute myocardial infarction with fibrinolytic therapy or combination reduced fibrinolytic therapy and platelet glycoprotein IIb/IIIa inhibition: the GUSTO V randomised trial. Lancet 357:1905-1914, 2001.

146. Peters RJ, Mehta SR, Fox KA, Zhao F, Lewis BS, Kopecky SL, Diaz R, Commerford PJ, Valentin V, Yusuf S: Effects of aspirin dose when used alone or in combination with clopidogrel in patients with acute coronary syndromes: observations from the Clopidogrel in Unstable angina to prevent Recurrent Events (CURE) study. Circulation 108:1682-1687, 2003.

In-Hospital Care of Myocardial Infarction

147. Smith SC, Jr., Feldman TE, Hirshfeld JW, Jr., Jacobs AK, Kern MJ, King SB, III., Morrison DA, O'Neill WW, Schaff HV, Whitlow PL, Williams DO: ACC/AHA/SCAI 2005 guideline update for percutaneous coronary intervention: a report of the American College of Cardiology/American Heart Association Task Force on Practice Guidelines (ACC/AHA/SCAI Writing Committee to Update the 2001 Guidelines for Percutaneous Coronary Intervention). American College of Cardiology Web Site. Accessed on: 7/24/06. Available at: http://www.acc.org/clinical/guidelines/percutaneous/update/index.pdf.

148. Henry TD, Unger BT, Sharkey SW, Lips DL, Pedersen WR, Madison JD, Mooney MR, Flygenring BP, Larson DM: Design of a standardized system for transfer of patients with ST-elevation myocardial infarction for percutaneous coronary intervention. Am Heart J 150:373-384, 2005.

149. Waters RE, 2nd, Singh KP, Roe MT, Lotfi M, Sketch MH, Jr., Mahaffey KW, Newby LK, Alexander JH, Harrington RA, Califf RM, Granger CB: Rationale and strategies for implementing community-based transfer protocols for primary percutaneous coronary intervention for acute ST-segment elevation myocardial infarction. J Am Coll Cardiol 43:2153-2159, 2004.

150. Anderson JL, Adams CD, Antman EM, et al: ACC/AHA 2007 guidelines for the management of patients with unstable angina and non-ST-elevation myocardial infarction: A report of the American College of Cardiology/American Heart Association Task Force on Practice Guidelines (Writing Committee to Revise the 2002 Guidelines for the Management of Patients With Unstable Angina/Non-ST-Elevation Myocardial Infarction). J Am Coll Cardiol, in press. 2007.

151. Pope JH, Selker HP: Diagnosis of acute cardiac ischemia. Emerg Med Clin North Am 21:27-59, 2003.

152. Spencer FA, Lessard D, Gore JM, Yarzebski J, Goldberg RJ: Declining length of hospital stay for acute myocardial infarction and postdischarge outcomes: a community-wide perspective. Arch Intern Med 164:733-740, 2004.

153. Peterson ED, Shaw LJ, Califf RM: Risk stratification after myocardial infarction. Ann Intern Med 126:561-582, 1997.

154. Antman EM, Kuntz KM: The length of the hospital stay after myocardial infarction. N Engl J Med 342:808-810, 2000.

155. Gheorghiade M, Goldstein S: Beta-blockers in the post-myocardial infarction patient. Circulation 106:394-398, 2002.

156. Freemantle N, Cleland J, Young P, Mason J, Harrison J: Beta blockade after myocardial infarction: systematic review and meta regression analysis. BMJ 318:1730-1777, 1999.

157. The TIMI Study Group. Comparison of invasive and conservative strategies after treatment with intravenous tissue plasminogen activator in acute myocardial infarction. Results of the thrombolysis in myocardial infarction (TIMI) phase II trial. N Engl J Med 320:618-627, 1989.

158. Dargie HJ: Effect of carvedilol on outcome after myocardial infarction in patients with left-ventricular dysfunction: the CAPRICORN randomised trial. Lancet 357:1385-1390, 2001.

159. Pfeffer MA: Left ventricular remodeling after acute myocardial infarction. Annu Rev Med 46:455-466, 1995.

160. The Acute Infarction Ramipril Efficacy—AIRE—Study Investigators. Effect of ramipril on mortality and morbidity of survivors of acute myocardial infarction with clinical evidence of heart failure. Lancet 342:821-828, 1993.

161. Ambrosioni E, Borghi C, Magnani B: The effect of the angiotensin-converting-enzyme inhibitor zofenopril on mortality and morbidity after anterior myocardial infarction. The Survival of Myocardial Infarction Long-Term Evaluation (SMILE) Study Investigators. N Engl J Med 332:80-85, 1995.

162. Kober L, Torp-Pedersen C, Carlsen JE, Bagger H, Eliasen P, Lyngborg K, Videbaek J, Cole DS, Auclert L, Pauly NC: A clinical trial of the angiotensin-converting-enzyme inhibitor trandolapril in patients with left ventricular dysfunction after myocardial infarction. Trandolapril Cardiac Evaluation (TRACE) Study Group. N Engl J Med 333:1670-1676, 1995.

163. ISIS-4 Collaborative Group. ISIS-4: a randomised factorial trial assessing early oral captopril, oral mononitrate, and intravenous magnesium sulphate in 58,050 patients with suspected acute myocardial infarction. Lancet 345:669-685, 1995.

164. Gruppo Italiano per lo Studio della Sopravvivenza nell'infarto Miocardico. GISSI-3: effects of lisinopril and transdermal glyceryl trinitrate singly and together on 6-week mortality and ventricular function after acute myocardial infarction. Lancet 343:1115-1122, 1994.

165. Swedberg K, Held P, Kjekshus J, Rasmussen K, Ryden L, Wedel H: Effects of the early administration of enalapril on mortality in patients with acute myocardial

infarction. Results of the Cooperative New Scandinavian Enalapril Survival Study II (CONSENSUS II). N Engl J Med 327:678-684, 1992.

166. ACE Inhibitor Myocardial Infarction Collaborative Group. Indications for ACE inhibitors in the early treatment of acute myocardial infarction: systematic overview of individual data from 100,000 patients in randomized trials. Circulation 97:2202-2212, 1998.

167. Pfeffer MA: ACE inhibitors in acute myocardial infarction: patient selection and timing. Circulation 97:2192-2194, 1998.

168. Rutherford JD, Pfeffer MA, Moye LA, Davis BR, Flaker GC, Kowey PR, Lamas GA, Miller HS, Packer M, Rouleau JL, et al: Effects of captopril on ischemic events after myocardial infarction. Results of the Survival and Ventricular Enlargement trial. SAVE Investigators. Circulation 90:1731-1738, 1994.

169. Pfeffer MA, McMurray JJ, Velazquez EJ, Rouleau JL, Kober L, Maggioni AP, Solomon SD, Swedberg K, Van de Werf F, White H, Leimberger JD, Henis M, Edwards S, Zelenkofske S, Sellers MA, Califf RM: Valsartan, captopril, or both in myocardial infarction complicated by heart failure, left ventricular dysfunction, or both. N Engl J Med 349:1893-1906, 2003.

170. Pitt B, Remme W, Zannad F, Neaton J, Martinez F, Roniker B, Bittman R, Hurley S, Kleiman J, Gatlin M: Eplerenone, a selective aldosterone blocker, in patients with left ventricular dysfunction after myocardial infarction. N Engl J Med 348:1309-1321, 2003.

171. Lindsay HS, Zaman AG, Cowan JC: ACE inhibitors after myocardial infarction: patient selection or treatment for all? Br Heart J 73:397-400, 1995.

172. Pfeffer MA, Greaves SC, Arnold JM, Glynn RJ, LaMotte FS, Lee RT, Menapace FJ, Jr., Rapaport E, Ridker PM, Rouleau JL, Solomon SD, Hennekens CH: Early versus delayed angiotensin-converting enzyme inhibition therapy in acute myocardial infarction. The healing and early afterload reducing therapy trial. Circulation 95:2643-2651, 1997.

173. Tokmakova M, Solomon SD: Inhibiting the renin-angiotensin system in myocardial infarction and heart failure: lessons from SAVE, VALIANT and CHARM, and other clinical trials. Curr Opin Cardiol 21:268-272, 2006.

174. Pitt B: Aldosterone blockade in patients with systolic left ventricular dysfunction. Circulation 108:1790-1794, 2003.

Adjunctive and Experimental Therapies

175. Gornik H, O'Gara PT: Adjunctive Medical Therapy. In Manson JE, Buring JE, Ridker PM, Gaziano JM (eds): Clinical Trials in Heart Disease; a Companion to Braunwald's Heart Disease. Philadelphia, Elsevier/Saunders, 2004, pp 109-128.

176. Report of The Holland Interuniversity Nifedipine/Metoprolol Trial Research Group. Early treatment of unstable angina in the coronary care unit: a randomised, double blind, placebo controlled comparison of recurrent ischaemia in patients treated with nifedipine or metoprolol or both. Br Heart J 56:400-413, 1986.

177. The Danish Study Group on Verapamil in Myocardial Infarction. Verapamil in acute myocardial infarction. Eur Heart J 5:516-528, 1984.

178. Boden WE, van Gilst WH, Scheldewaert RG, Starkey IR, Carlier MF, Julian DG, Whitehead A, Bertrand ME, Col JJ, Pedersen OL, Lie KI, Santoni JP, Fox KM: Diltiazem in acute myocardial infarction treated with thrombolytic agents: a randomised placebo-controlled trial. Incomplete Infarction Trial of European Research Collaborators Evaluating Prognosis post-Thrombolysis (INTERCEPT). Lancet 355:1751-1756, 2000.

179. MAGIC Investigators: Early administration of intravenous magnesium to high-risk patients with acute myocardial infarction in the Magnesium in Coronaries (MAGIC) Trial: a randomised controlled trial. Lancet 360:1189-1196, 2002.

180. Clement S, Braithwaite SS, Magee MF, Ahmann A, Smith EP, Schafer RG, Hirsch IB: Management of diabetes and hyperglycemia in hospitals. Diabetes Care 27:553-591, 2004.

181. Mehta SR, Yusuf S, Diaz R, Zhu J, Pais P, Xavier D, Paolasso E, Ahmed R, Xie C, Kazmi K, Tai J, Orlandini A, Pogue J, Liu L: Effect of glucose-insulin-potassium infusion on mortality in patients with acute ST-segment elevation myocardial infarction: the CREATE-ECLA randomized controlled trial. JAMA 293:437-446, 2005.

182. Falati S, Liu Q, Gross P, Merrill-Skoloff G, Chou J, Vandendries E, Celi A, Croce K, Furie BC, Furie B: Accumulation of tissue factor into developing thrombi in vivo is dependent upon microparticle P-selectin glycoprotein ligand 1 and platelet P-selectin. J Exp Med 197:1585-1598, 2003.

183. Baran KW, Nguyen M, McKendall GR, Lambrew CT, Dykstra G, Palmeri ST, Gibbons RJ, Borzak S, Sobel BE, Gourlay SG, Rundle AC, Gibson CM, Barron HV: Double-blind, randomized trial of an anti-CD18 antibody in conjunction with recombinant tissue plasminogen activator for acute myocardial infarction: limitation of myocardial infarction following thrombolysis in acute myocardial infarction (LIMIT AMI) study. Circulation 104:2778-2783, 2001.

184. Faxon DP, Gibbons RJ, Chronos NA, Gurbel PA, Sheehan F: The effect of blockade of the CD11/CD18 integrin receptor on infarct size in patients with acute myocardial infarction treated with direct angioplasty: the results of the HALT-MI study. J Am Coll Cardiol 40:1199-1204, 2002.

185. Granger CB, Mahaffey KW, Weaver WD, Theroux P, Hochman JS, Filloon TG, Rollins S, Todaro TG, Nicolau JC, Ruzyllo W, Armstrong PW: Pexelizumab, an anti-C5 complement antibody, as adjunctive therapy to primary percutaneous coronary intervention in acute myocardial infarction: the COMplement inhibition in Myocardial infarction treated with Angioplasty (COMMA) trial. Circulation 108:1184-1190, 2003.

186. Mahaffey KW, Granger CB, Nicolau JC, Ruzyllo W, Weaver WD, Theroux P, Hochman JS, Filloon TG, Mojcik CF, Todaro TG, Armstrong PW: Effect of pexelizumab, an anti-C5 complement antibody, as adjunctive therapy to fibrinolysis in acute myocardial infarction: the COMPlement inhibition in myocardial infarction treated with thromboLytics (COMPLY) trial. Circulation 108:1176-1183, 2003.

186a. APEX AMI Investigators; Armstrong PW, Granger CB, Adams PX, et al: Pexelizumab for acute ST-elevation myocardial infarction in patients undergoing primary percutaneous coronary intervention: A randomized controlled trial. JAMA 297:91-92, 2007.

187. Melo LG, Ward CA, Dzau VJ: Gene therapies for cardiovascular diseases: where we are and where we are going. In Antman EM (ed): Cardiovascular Therapeutics. Philadelphia, W.B. Saunders, 2006, in press.

Complications of Myocardial Infarction

188. Osma S, Kahveci SF, Kaya FN, Akalin H, Ozakin C, Yilmaz E, Kutlay O: Efficacy of antiseptic-impregnated catheters on catheter colonization and catheter-related bloodstream infections in patients in an intensive care unit. J Hosp Infect 62:156-162, 2006.

189. Nikolsky E, Aymong ED, Halkin A, Grines CL, Cox DA, Garcia E, Mehran R, Tcheng JE, Griffin JJ, Guagliumi G, Stuckey T, Turco M, Cohen DA, Negoita M, Lansky AJ, Stone GW: Impact of anemia in patients with acute myocardial infarction undergoing primary percutaneous coronary intervention: analysis from the Controlled Abciximab and Device Investigation to Lower Late Angioplasty Complications (CADILLAC) Trial. J Am Coll Cardiol 44:547-553, 2004.

190. Weir RA, McMurray JJ, Velazquez EJ: Epidemiology of heart failure and left ventricular systolic dysfunction after acute myocardial infarction: prevalence, clinical characteristics, and prognostic importance. Am J Cardiol 97:13F-25F, 2006.

191. Udelson JE, Patten RD, Konstam MA: New concepts in post-infarction ventricular remodeling. Rev Cardiovasc Med 4 Suppl 3:S3-S12, 2003.

192. White HD, Aylward PE, Huang Z, Dalby AJ, Weaver WD, Barvik S, Marin-Neto JA, Murin J, Nordlander RO, van Gilst WH, Zannad F, McMurray JJ, Califf RM, Pfeffer MA: Mortality and morbidity remain high despite captopril and/or Valsartan therapy in elderly patients with left ventricular systolic dysfunction, heart failure, or both after acute myocardial infarction: results from the Valsartan in Acute Myocardial Infarction Trial (VALIANT). Circulation 112:3391-3399, 2005.

193. Holmes DR, Jr: Cardiogenic shock: a lethal complication of acute myocardial infarction. Rev Cardiovasc Med 4:131-135, 2003.

194. Okuda M: A multidisciplinary overview of cardiogenic shock. Shock 25:557-570, 2006.

195. Palmeri ST, Lowe AM, Sleeper LA, Saucedo JF, Desvigne-Nickens P, Hochman JS: Racial and ethnic differences in the treatment and outcome of cardiogenic shock following acute myocardial infarction. Am J Cardiol 96:1042-1049, 2005.

196. Babaev A, Frederick PD, Pasta DJ, Every N, Sichrovsky T, Hochman JS: Trends in management and outcomes of patients with acute myocardial infarction complicated by cardiogenic shock. JAMA 294:448-454, 2005.

197. Webb JG, Lowe AM, Sanborn TA, White HD, Sleeper LA, Carere RG, Buller CE, Wong SC, Boland J, Dzavik V, Porway M, Pate G, Bergman G, Hochman JS: Percutaneous coronary intervention for cardiogenic shock in the SHOCK trial. J Am Coll Cardiol 42:1380-1386, 2003.

198. Sanborn TA, Sleeper LA, Webb JG, French JK, Bergman G, Parikh M, Wong SC, Boland J, Pfisterer M, Slater JN, Sharma S, Hochman JS: Correlates of one-year survival inpatients with cardiogenic shock complicating acute myocardial infarction: angiographic findings from the SHOCK trial. J Am Coll Cardiol 42:1373-1379, 2003.

199. Verges B, Zeller M, Desgres J, Dentan G, Laurent Y, Janin-Manificat L, L'Huillier I, Rioufol G, Beer JC, Makki H, Rochette L, Gambert P, Cottin Y: High plasma N-terminal pro-brain natriuretic peptide level found in diabetic patients after myocardial infarction is associated with an increased risk of in-hospital mortality and cardiogenic shock. Eur Heart J 26:1734-1741, 2005.

200. Hochman JS: Cardiogenic shock complicating acute myocardial infarction: expanding the paradigm. Circulation 107:2998-3002, 2003.

201. Effect of tilarginine acetate in patients with acute myocardial infarction and cardiogenic shock: The TRIUMPH Randomized Control Trial. JAMA. 2007. Accessed on: 4/3/07. Available as epub ahead of print 2007 March 26.

202. Hochman JS, Sleeper LA, Webb JG, Sanborn TA, White HD, Talley JD, Buller CE, Jacobs AK, Slater JN, Col J, McKinlay SM, LeJemtel TH: Early revascularization in acute myocardial infarction complicated by cardiogenic shock. SHOCK Investigators. Should We Emergently Revascularize Occluded Coronaries for Cardiogenic Shock. N Engl J Med 341:625-634, 1999.

203. Merhi W, Dixon SR, O'Neill WW, Hanzel GS, McCullough PA: Percutaneous left ventricular assist device in acute myocardial infarction and cardiogenic shock. Rev Cardiovasc Med 6:118-123, 2005.

204. Inoue K, Ito H, Kitakaze M, Kuzuya T, Hori M, Iwakura K, Nishikawa N, Higashino Y, Fujii K, Minamino T: Antecedent angina pectoris as a predictor of better functional and clinical outcomes in patients with an inferior wall acute myocardial infarction. Am J Cardiol 83:159-163, 1999.

205. Pfisterer M: Right ventricular involvement in myocardial infarction and cardiogenic shock. Lancet 362:392-394, 2003.

206. Zimetbaum PJ, Josephson ME: Use of the electrocardiogram in acute myocardial infarction. N Engl J Med 348:933-940, 2003.

207. Wellens HJ: The value of the right precordial leads of the electrocardiogram. N Engl J Med 340:381-383, 1999.

208. Ibrahim T, Schwaiger M, Schomig A: Images in cardiovascular medicine. Assessment of isolated right ventricular myocardial infarction by magnetic resonance imaging. Circulation 113:e78-e79, 2006.

209. Jacobs AK, Leopold JA, Bates E, Mendes LA, Sleeper LA, White H, Davidoff R, Boland J, Modur S, Forman R, Hochman JS: Cardiogenic shock caused by right ventricular infarction: a report from the SHOCK registry. J Am Coll Cardiol 41:1273-1279, 2003.

210. Manoharan G, De Bruyne B: Right ventricular myocardial infarction. Heart 91:e40, 2005.

211. Birnbaum Y, Fishbein MC, Blanche C, Siegel RJ: Ventricular septal rupture after acute myocardial infarction. N Engl J Med 347:1426-1432, 2002.

212. Sugiura T, Nagahama Y, Nakamura S, Kudo Y, Yamasaki F, Iwasaka T: Left ventricular free wall rupture after reperfusion therapy for acute myocardial infarction. Am J Cardiol 92:282-284, 2003.

213. Lesser JR, Johnson K, Lindberg JL, Reed J, Tadavarthy SM, Virmani R, Schwartz RS: Images in cardiovascular medicine. Myocardial rupture, microvascular obstruction, and infarct expansion: elucidation by cardiac magnetic resonance. Circulation 108:116-117, 2003.

214. Birnbaum Y, Chamoun AJ, Anzuini A, Lick SD, Ahmad M, Uretsky BF: Ventricular free wall rupture following acute myocardial infarction. Coron Artery Dis 14:463-470, 2003.

215. Reynen K, Strasser RH: Images in clinical medicine. Impending rupture of the myocardial wall. N Engl J Med 348:e3, 2003.

216. Crenshaw BS, Granger CB, Birnbaum Y, Pieper KS, Morris DC, Kleiman NS, Vahanian A, Califf RM, Topol EJ: Risk factors, angiographic patterns, and outcomes in patients with ventricular septal defect complicating acute myocardial infarction. GUSTO-I (Global Utilization of Streptokinase and TPA for Occluded Coronary Arteries) Trial Investigators. Circulation 101:27-32, 2000.

217. Figueras J, Cortadellas J, Soler-Soler J: Comparison of ventricular septal and left ventricular free wall rupture in acute myocardial infarction. Am J Cardiol 81:495-497, 1998.

218. Birnbaum Y, Chamoun AJ, Conti VR, Uretsky BF: Mitral regurgitation following acute myocardial infarction. Coron Artery Dis 13:337-344, 2002.

219. Liuzzo JP, Shin YT, Choi C, Patel S, Braff R, Coppola JT: Simultaneous papillary muscle avulsion and free wall rupture during acute myocardial infarction. Intra-aortic balloon pump: a bridge to survival. J Invasive Cardiol 18:135-140, 2006.

220. Carmeliet E: Cardiac ionic currents and acute ischemia: from channels to arrhythmias. Physiol Rev 79:917-1017, 1999.

221. Yadav AV, Zipes DP: Prophylactic lidocaine in acute myocardial infarction: resurface or reburial? Am J Cardiol 94:606-608, 2004.

222. Henriques JP, Gheeraert PJ, Ottervanger JP, de Boer MJ, Dambrink JH, Gosselink AT, van 't Hof AW, Hoorntje JC, Suryapranata H, Zijlstra F: Ventricular fibrillation in acute myocardial infarction before and during primary PCI. Int J Cardiol 105:262-266, 2005.

223. Volpi A, Cavalli A, Santoro L, Negri E: Incidence and prognosis of early primary ventricular fibrillation in acute myocardial infarction—results of the Gruppo Italiano per lo Studio della Sopravvivenza nell'Infarto Miocardico (GISSI-2) database. Am J Cardiol 82:265-271, 1998.

224. Altun A, Kirdar C, Ozbay G: Effect of aminophylline in patients with atropine-resistant late advanced atrioventricular block during acute inferior myocardial infarction. Clin Cardiol 21:759-762, 1998.

Prognosis Post Myocardial Infarction

225. Di Chiara A: Right bundle branch block during the acute phase of myocardial infarction: modern redefinitions of old concepts. Eur Heart J 27:1-2, 2006.

226. Wong CK, Stewart RA, Gao W, French JK, Raffel C, White HD: Prognostic differences between different types of bundle branch block during the early phase of acute myocardial infarction: insights from the Hirulog and Early Reperfusion or Occlusion (HERO)-2 trial. Eur Heart J 27:21-28, 2006.

227. Petrina M, Goodman SG, Eagle KA: The 12-lead electrocardiogram as a predictive tool of mortality after acute myocardial infarction: current status in an era of revascularization and reperfusion. Am Heart J 152:11-18, 2006.

228. Suzuki M, Sakaue T, Tanaka M, Hirose E, Saeki H, Matsunaka T, Hiramatsu S, Kazatani Y: Association between right bundle branch block and impaired myocardial tissue-level reperfusion in patients with acute myocardial infarction. J Am Coll Cardiol 47:2122-2124, 2006.

229. Kober L, Swedberg K, McMurray JJ, Pfeffer MA, Velazquez EJ, Diaz R, Maggioni AP, Mareev V, Opolski G, Van de Werf F, Zannad F, Ertl G, Solomon SD, Zelenkofske S, Rouleau JL, Leimberger JD, Califf RM: Previously known and newly diagnosed atrial fibrillation: A major risk indicator after a myocardial infarction complicated by heart failure or left ventricular dysfunction. Eur J Heart Fail 2006.

230. De Luca G, Ernst N, van't Hof AW, Ottervanger JP, Hoorntje JC, Gosselink AT, Dambrink JH, de Boer MJ, Suryapranata H: Predictors and clinical implications of early reinfarction after primary angioplasty for ST-segment elevation myocardial infarction. Am Heart J 151:1256-1259, 2006.

231. Gibson CM, Karha J, Murphy SA, James D, Morrow DA, Cannon CP, Giugliano RP, Antman EM, Braunwald E: Early and long-term clinical outcomes associated with reinfarction following fibrinolytic administration in the Thrombolysis in Myocardial Infarction trials. J Am Coll Cardiol 42:7-16, 2003.

232. Steg PG, Danchin N: WEST: new data on the integration of early thrombolysis and mechanical intervention in the early management of STEMI. Eur Heart J 27:1511-1512, 2006.

233. Scheller B, Hennen B, Hammer B, Walle J, Hofer C, Hilpert V, Winter H, Nickenig G, Bohm M: Beneficial effects of immediate stenting after thrombolysis in acute myocardial infarction. J Am Coll Cardiol 42:634-641, 2003.

234. Zeymer U, Uebis R, Vogt A, Glunz HG, Vohringer HF, Harmjanz D, Neuhaus KL: Randomized comparison of percutaneous transluminal coronary angioplasty and medical therapy in stable survivors of acute myocardial infarction with single vessel disease: a study of the Arbeitsgemeinschaft Leitende Kardiologische Krankenhausarzte. Circulation 108:1324-1328, 2003.

235. Fernandez-Aviles F, Alonso JJ, Castro-Beiras A, Vazquez N, Blanco J, Alonso-Briales J, Lopez-Mesa J, Fernandez-Vazquez F, Calvo I, Martinez-Elbal L, San Roman JA, Ramos B: Routine invasive strategy within 24 hours of thrombolysis versus ischaemia-guided conservative approach for acute myocardial infarction with ST-segment elevation (GRACIA-1): a randomised controlled trial. Lancet 364:1045-1053, 2004.

236. Armstrong PW: A comparison of pharmacologic therapy with/without timely coronary intervention vs. primary percutaneous intervention early after ST-elevation myocardial infarction: the WEST (Which Early ST-elevation myocardial infarction Therapy) study. Eur Heart J 27:1530-1538, 2006.

237. Dauerman HL, Sobel BE: Synergistic treatment of ST-segment elevation myocardial infarction with pharmacoinvasive recanalization. J Am Coll Cardiol 42:646-651, 2003.

238. O'Neill WW: "Watchful waiting" after thrombolysis: it's time for a re-evaluation. J Am Coll Cardiol 42:17-19, 2003.

239. Dauerman HL: The early days after ST-segment elevation acute myocardial infarction: reconsidering the delayed invasive approach. J Am Coll Cardiol 42:420-423, 2003.

240. McKay RG: Evolving strategies in the treatment of acute myocardial infarction in the community hospital setting. J Am Coll Cardiol 42:642-645, 2003.

241. Hombach V, Grebe O, Merkle N, Waldenmaier S, Hoher M, Kochs M, Wohrle J, Kestler HA: Sequelae of acute myocardial infarction regarding cardiac structure and function and their prognostic significance as assessed by magnetic resonance imaging. Eur Heart J 26:549-557, 2005.

241a. Timmers L, Sluijter JP, Verlaan CW, et al: Cyclooxygenase-2 inhibition increases mortality, enhauces left ventricular remodeling, and impairs systolic function after myocardial infarction in the pig. Circulation 115:326-332, 2007.

241b. Jugdutt BI: Cyclooxygenase inhibition and adverse remodeling during healing after myocardial infarction. Circulation 115:288-291, 2007.

242. Reinecke H, Wichter T, Weyand M: Left ventricular pseudoaneurysm in a patient with Dressler's syndrome after myocardial infarction. Heart 80:98-100, 1998.

243. Cheitlin MD, Armstrong WF, Aurigemma GP, Beller GA, Bierman FZ, Davis DL, Douglas PS, Faxon DP, Gillam LD, Kimball TR, Kussmaul WG, Pearlman AS, Philbrick JT, Rakowski H, Thys DM: ACC/AHA/ASE 2003 guideline update for the clinical application of echocardiography: a report of the American College of Cardiology/American Heart Association Task Force on Practice Guidelines (ACC/AHA/ASE Committee to Update the 1997 Guidelines for the Clinical Application of Echocardiography). 2003. Accessed on: 4/19/06. Available at: American College of Cardiology Web Site. Available at: www.acc.org/clinical/guidelines/echo/index.pdf.

244. Abildstrom SZ, Ottesen MM, Rask-Madsen C, Andersen PK, Rosthoj S, Torp-Pedersen C, Kober L: Sudden cardiovascular death following myocardial infarction: the importance of left ventricular systolic dysfunction and congestive heart failure. Int J Cardiol 104:184-189, 2005.

245. Madias JE, Ashtiani R, Agarwal H, Narayan VK, Win M, Sinha A: Diagnosis of ventricular aneurysm and other severe segmental left ventricular dysfunction consequent to a myocardial infarction in the presence of right bundle branch block: ECG correlates of a positive diagnosis made via echocardiography and/or contrast ventriculography. Ann Noninvasive Electrocardiol 10:53-59, 2005.

246. Ohara K: Current surgical strategy for post-infarction left ventricular aneurysm—from linear aneurysmecomy to Dor's operation. Ann Thorac Cardiovasc Surg 6:289-294, 2000.

247. Marchenko AV, Cherniavsky AM, Volokitina TL, Alsov SA, Karaskov AM: Left ventricular dimension and shape after postinfarction aneurysm repair. Eur J Cardiothorac Surg 27:475-480; discussion 480, 2005.

248. Rehan A, Kanwar M, Rosman H, Ahmed S, Ali A, Gardin J, Cohen G: Incidence of post myocardial infarction left ventricular thrombus formation in the era of primary percutaneous intervention and glycoprotein IIb/IIIa inhibitors. A prospective observational study. Cardiovasc Ultrasound 4:20, 2006.

249. Barbera S, Hillis LD: Echocardiographic Recognition of Left Ventricular Mural Thrombus. Echocardiography 16:289-295, 1999.

250. Hirsh J, Fuster V, Ansell J, Halperin JL: American Heart Association/American College of Cardiology Foundation guide to warfarin therapy. Circulation 107:1692-1711, 2003.

251. Newby LK, Califf RM, Guerci A, Weaver WD, Col J, Horgan JH, Mark DB, Stebbins A, Van de Werf F, Gore JM, Topol EJ: Early discharge in the thrombolytic era: an analysis of criteria for uncomplicated infarction from the Global Utilization of Streptokinase and t-PA for Occluded Coronary Arteries (GUSTO) trial. J Am Coll Cardiol 27:625-632, 1996.

252. Jaffe AS, Krumholz HM, Catellier DJ, Freedland KE, Bittner V, Blumenthal JA, Calvin JE, Norman J, Sequeira R, O'Connor C, Rich MW, Sheps D, Wu C: Prediction of medical morbidity and mortality after acute myocardial infarction in patients at increased psychosocial risk in the Enhancing Recovery in Coronary Heart Disease Patients (ENRICHD) study. Am Heart J 152:126-135, 2006.

253. Alter DA, Chong A, Austin PC, Mustard C, Iron K, Williams JI, Morgan CD, Tu JV, Irvine J, Naylor CD: Socioeconomic status and mortality after acute myocardial infarction. Ann Intern Med 144:82-93, 2006.

254. Mendes de Leon CF, Czajkowski SM, Freedland KE, Bang H, Powell LH, Wu C, Burg MM, DiLillo V, Ironson G, Krumholz HM, Mitchell P, Blumenthal JA: The effect of a psychosocial intervention and quality of life after acute myocardial infarction: the Enhancing Recovery in Coronary Heart Disease (ENRICHD) clinical trial. J Cardiopulm Rehabil 26:9-13; quiz 14-5, 2006.

255. Birnbaum Y, Drew BJ: The electrocardiogram in ST elevation acute myocardial infarction: correlation with coronary anatomy and prognosis. Postgrad Med J 79:490-504, 2003.

256. Wong CK, Gao W, Raffel OC, French JK, Stewart RA, White HD: Initial Q waves accompanying ST-segment elevation at presentation of acute myocardial infarction and 30-day mortality in patients given streptokinase therapy: an analysis from HERO-2. Lancet 367:2061-2067, 2006.

257. Kernis SJ, Harjai KJ, Stone GW, Grines LL, Boura JA, Yerkey MW, O'Neill W, Grines CL: The incidence, predictors, and outcomes of early reinfarction after primary

CH 51

angioplasty for acute myocardial infarction. J Am Coll Cardiol 42:1173-1177, 2003.

258. Klocke FJ, Baird MG, Bateman TM, Berman DS, Carabello BA, Cerqueira MD, DeMaria AN, Kennedy JW, Lorell BH, Messer JV, O'Gara PT, Russell RO, Jr., St. John Sutton MG, Udelson JE, Verani MS, Williams KA: ACC/AHA/ASNC guidelines for the clinical use of cardiac radionuclide imaging: a report of the American College of Cardiology/American Heart Association Task Force on Practice Guidelines (ACC/AHA/ASNC Committee to Revise the 1995 Guidelines for the Clinical Use of Radionuclide Imaging). American College of Cardiology Web Site, Accessed on: 4/19/06. Available at: Available at: http://www.acc.org/clinical/guidelines/radio/index.pdf.

259. Gibbons RJ, Balady GJ, Bridker JT, Chaitman BR, Fletcher GF, Froelicher VF, Mark DB, McCallister BD, Mooss AN, O'Reilly MG, Winters WJ, Jr: ACC/AHA 2002 guideline update for exercist testing: a report of the American College of Cardiology/American Heart Association Task Force on Practice Guidelines (Committee on Exercise Testing). 2002. American College of Cardiology Web site. Available at: www.acc.org/clinical/guidelines/exercise/dirIndex.htm. 2002.

260. Zipes DP, Camm AJ, Borggrefe M, Buxton AE, Chaitman B, Fromer M, Gregoratos G, Klein G, Moss AJ, Myerburg RJ, Priori SG, Quinones MA, Roden DM, Silka MJ, Tracy C, Smith SC, Jr., Jacobs AK, Adams CD, Antman EM, Anderson JL, Hunt SA, Halperin JL, Nishimura R, Ornato JP, Page RL, Riegel B, Blanc JJ, Budaj A, Dean V, Deckers JW, Despres C, Dickstein K, Lekakis J, McGregor K, Metra M, Morais J, Osterspey A, Tamargo JL, Zamorano JL: ACC/AHA/ESC 2006 Guidelines for Management of Patients With Ventricular Arrhythmias and the Prevention of Sudden Cardiac Death: a report of the American College of Cardiology/American Heart Association Task Force and the European Society of Cardiology Committee for Practice Guidelines (writing committee to develop Guidelines for Management of Patients With Ventricular Arrhythmias and the Prevention of Sudden Cardiac Death): developed in collaboration with the European Heart Rhythm Association and the Heart Rhythm Society. Circulation 114:e385-e484, 2006.

261. Cairns JA, Connolly SJ, Roberts R, Gent M: Randomised trial of outcome after myocardial infarction in patients with frequent or repetitive ventricular premature depolarisations: CAMIAT. Canadian Amiodarone Myocardial Infarction Arrhythmia Trial Investigators. Lancet 349:675-682, 1997.

Secondary Prevention of Myocardial Infarction

262. Julian DG, Camm AJ, Frangin G, Janse MJ, Munoz A, Schwartz PJ, Simon P: Randomised trial of effect of amiodarone on mortality in patients with left-ventricular dysfunction after recent myocardial infarction: EMIAT. European Myocardial Infarct Amiodarone Trial Investigators. Lancet 349:667-674, 1997.

263. Smith SC, Jr., Allen J, Blair SN, Bonow RO, Brass LM, Fonarow GC, Grundy SM, Hiratzka L, Jones D, Krumholz HM, Mosca L, Pasternak RC, Pearson T, Pfeffer MA, Taubert KA: AHA/ACC guidelines for secondary prevention for patients with coronary and other atherosclerotic vascular disease: 2006 update: endorsed by the National Heart, Lung, and Blood Institute. Circulation 113:2363-2372, 2006.

264. Mega JL, Morrow DA, Cannon CP, Murphy S, Cairns R, Ridker PM, Braunwald E: Cholesterol, C-reactive protein, and cerebrovascular events following intensive and moderate statin therapy. J Thromb Thrombolysis 22:71-76, 2006.

265. Lichtenstein AH, Appel LJ, Brands M, Carnethon M, Daniels S, Franch HA, Franklin B, Kris-Etherton P, Harris WS, Howard B, Karanja N, Lefevre M, Rudel L, Sacks F, Van Horn L, Winston M, Wylie-Rosett J: Diet and lifestyle recommendations revision 2006: a scientific statement from the American Heart Association Nutrition Committee. Circulation 114:82-96, 2006.

266. Yusuf S, Sleight P, Pogue J, Bosch J, Davies R, Dagenais G: Effects of an angiotensin-converting-enzyme inhibitor, ramipril, on cardiovascular events in high-risk patients. The Heart Outcomes Prevention Evaluation Study Investigators. N Engl J Med 342:145-153, 2000.

267. Fox KM: Efficacy of perindopril in reduction of cardiovascular events among patients with stable coronary artery disease: randomised, double-blind, placebo-controlled, multicentre trial (the EUROPA study). Lancet 362:782-788, 2003.

268. Doubeni C, Bigelow C, Lessard D, Spencer F, Yarzebski J, Gore J, Gurwitz J, Goldberg R: Trends and outcomes associated with angiotensin-converting enzyme inhibitors. Am J Med 119:616 e9-e16, 2006.

269. Fonarow GC: Beta-blockers for the post-myocardial infarction patient: current clinical evidence and practical considerations. Rev Cardiovasc Med 7:1-9, 2006.

270. Gruppo Italiano per lo Studio della Sopravvivenza nell'Infarto miocardico. Dietary supplementation with n-3 polyunsaturated fatty acids and vitamin E after myocardial infarction: results of the GISSI-Prevenzione trial. Lancet 354:447-455, 1999.

271. Antman EM, DeMets D, Loscalzo J: Cyclooxygenase inhibition and cardiovascular risk. Circulation 112:759-770, 2005.

272. Gislason GH, Jacobsen S, Rasmussen JN, Rasmussen S, Buch P, Friberg J, Schramm TK, Abildstrom SZ, Kober L, Madsen M, Torp-Pedersen C: Risk of death or reinfarction associated with the use of selective cyclooxygenase-2 inhibitors and nonselective nonsteroidal antiinflammatory drugs after acute myocardial infarction. Circulation 113:2906-2913, 2006.

273. Autman EM, Bennett JS, Daugherty A, et al: Use of nonsteroidal antiinflammatory drugs: Au update for clinicians: A scientific statement from the American Heart Association. Circulation 115:1634-1642, 2007.

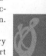

CH 51

ST-Elevation Myocardial Infarction: Management

Primary Percutaneous Coronary Intervention in the Management of Acute Myocardial Infarction

Gary E. Lane and David R. Holmes, Jr.

Randomized Trials Comparing Primary Angioplasty with Thrombolysis, 1301
Advantages of the Primary Percutaneous Coronary Intervention Strategy, 1302
Temporal Dynamics of Reperfusion Therapy, 1303
Challenging Groups of Patients, 1305

Modern Catheter-Based Reperfusion Techniques, 1307
Glycoprotein IIb/IIIa Inhibition, 1307
Primary Stent Implantation, 1308

Developments in Reperfusion Therapy Science, 1308
Distal Embolization, 1308
Pharmacological Interventions, 1309
Mechanical Myocardial Protection, 1309
Myocardial Regeneration, 1309
Combining Percutaneous Coronary Intervention and Thrombolytic Therapy, 1309

Conducting Primary Percutaneous Coronary Intervention Reperfusion Therapy, 1310

Future Directions, 1311

References, 1311

Guidelines, 1314

The restoration of blood flow to ischemic myocardium has been established as the preeminent objective for treatment of patients with acute myocardial infarction. Primary angioplasty or percutaneous coronary intervention (PCI) has evolved through continued innovation of the method and dissemination to an expanding proportion of patients. This chapter examines the evidence favoring a primary PCI strategy, modern application of the technique, and emerging evidence in reperfusion science. Historically, the transition from intracoronary to intravenous thrombolysis has led to an expansion of reperfusion therapy. Several centers have successfully practiced primary balloon angioplasty in an attempt to overcome the limitations of thrombolytic therapy and provide a reperfusion alternative to patients with thrombolysis contraindications. (See also Chaps. 51 and 53.)

RANDOMIZED TRIALS COMPARING PRIMARY ANGIOPLASTY WITH THROMBOLYSIS

Three randomized trials, published simultaneously in 1993, provided a stimulus for expanded application and investigation of the primary angioplasty strategy. The largest ($N = 395$) of these trials, the Primary Angioplasty in Myocardial Infarction (PAMI) trial, achieved reperfusion success in 97 percent (94 percent thrombolysis in myocardial infarction 3 flow [TIMI-3 flow]) within 60 minutes in the angioplasty group.[1] Although there was no significant improvement in left ventricular function during rest or exercise at 6-week follow-up, there was a trend for a reduction of in-hospital mortality (2.6 versus 6.5 percent, $P = 0.06$) in the angioplasty group in comparison with tissue plasminogen activator (t-PA). There was a significant reduction in combined death or reinfarction (5.1 versus 12 percent, $P = 0.02$) and intracranial hemorrhage (0 versus 2.0 percent, $P = 0.05$) with angioplasty. Patients classified as "not low risk" (age older than 70 years, anterior infarction or heart rate more than 100 beats/min) had a lower mortality rate (2.0 versus 10.4 percent, $P = 0.01$) with angioplasty.

Evidence favoring the primary angioplasty strategy was derived from the PCAT (Primary Coronary Angioplasty Trialists) meta-analysis[2] of 10 randomized trials (conducted from 1989 to 1996). Primary balloon angioplasty significantly reduced 30-day mortality (4.4 versus 6.5 percent, $P = 0.02$; 34 percent risk reduction) and the combination of death plus reinfarction (7.2 versus 11.9 percent, $P < 0.001$, 40 percent risk reduction). These effects were not significantly affected by the thrombolytic regimen. Primary angioplasty was also associated with a reduction in total stroke (0.7 versus 2.0 percent, $P = 0.007$) and a marked decrease in hemorrhagic stroke (0.1 versus 1.1 percent, $P < 0.001$).

A follow-up study from the PCAT investigators has revealed that 26 lives were saved/1000 patients treated with a primary angioplasty strategy.[3] This beneficial effect persists at 6 months (Fig. 52-1). A similar reduction in the estimated relative risk of death or reinfarction was noted across each of the major clinical subgroups analyzed, but the absolute benefits were greater in proportion to baseline risk.

These studies were done before the adoption of more advanced PCI techniques. More recent trials have compared thrombolysis with catheter-based reperfusion using stents and glycoprotein (GP) IIb/IIIa receptor inhibitors. For example, the Stent versus Thrombolysis for Occluded Coronary Arteries in Patients with Acute Myocardial Infarction (STOPAMI) trial compared patients reperfused with a stent plus abciximab with patients receiving t-PA.[4] Scintigraphic infarct size was significantly reduced in the PCI group because of a larger salvage index. In addition, the composite endpoint of death, reinfarction, and stroke was lower in the stent group (8.5 versus 23.2 percent at 6 months, $P = 0.02$).

A quantitative review by Keeley and colleagues[5] has combined the previous trials from the PCAT analysis with 13 more recent investigations (1997 to 2202), in which stents were used in 12 of 13 and GP IIb/IIIa inhibitors in 7 of 13 trials. Of the total group ($N = 7739$), most patients (76 percent) randomized to thrombolytic therapy received t-PA. The summary results (Fig. 52-2) ($N = 7437$) delineated a significant reduction in death, reinfarction, stroke, and hemorrhagic stroke for patients treated with primary PCI. Major hemorrhage (5 versus 7 percent, $P = 0.032$) was the only endpoint increased in the PCI patients. The benefit was similar, irrespective of the thrombolytic regimen. The survival advantage for primary PCI over thrombolysis (20 lives saved for every 1000 patients treated) is similar to the magnitude of benefit for thrombolysis compared to placebo.[6] Long-term (6 months) outcomes in several trials have been persistently favorable for the PCI patients.

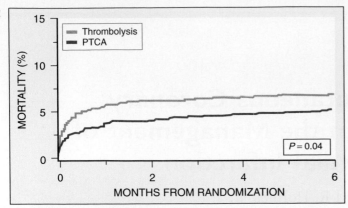

FIGURE 52–1 Mortality over 6 months from Primary Coronary Angioplasty Trialists (PCAT) analysis of 11 randomized trials.[3]

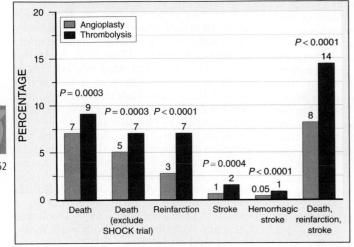

FIGURE 52–2 Short-term clinical outcomes of patients in 23 randomized trials of primary angioplasty versus thrombolysis.[5]

CH 52

TABLE 52–1	Thrombolysis in Myocardial Infarction (TIMI) Flow Grade Classification System[9]
Flow Grade	**Definition**
0	No perfusion. There is no antegrade flow beyond the point of occlusion.
1	Penetration without perfusion. Contrast material passes beyond the area of obstruction but fails to opacify the entire coronary bed distal to the obstruction for the duration of the cineangiographic filming sequence.
2	Partial perfusion. Contrast material passes across the obstruction and opacifies the coronary distal to the obstruction. However, the rate of entry of contrast material into the vessel distal to the obstruction and/or its rate of clearance from the distal bed (or both) is perceptibly slower than its flow into or clearance from comparable areas not perfused by the previously occluded vessel.
3	Complete perfusion. Antegrade flow into the bed distal to the obstruction occurs as promptly as antegrade flow into the bed proximal to the obstruction, and clearance of contrast material from the involved bed is as rapid as clearance from an uninvolved bed in the same vessel or the opposite artery.

TABLE 52–2	Thrombolysis in Myocardial Infarction (TIMI) Myocardial Perfusion Grades[9]
Perfusion Grade	**Definition**
0	Minimal or no myocardial blush is seen.
1	Dye stains the myocardium; this stain persists on the next injection.
2	Dye enters the myocardium but washes out slowly so that the dye is strongly persistent at the end of the injection.
3	There is normal entrance and exit of the dye in the myocardium so that dye is mildly persistent at the end of the injection.

Advantages of the Primary Percutaneous Coronary Intervention Strategy

Beyond outcome data, catheter-based reperfusion offers additional merits.

SUPERIOR RESTORATION OF FLOW. There is a critical link between early establishment of TIMI-3 flow (Table 52-1) with myocardial salvage and survival. Primary PCI attains TIMI-3 flow in more than 90 percent of patients.[6] In contrast, less than 65 percent of patients receiving a fibrin-specific lytic agent achieve this reperfusion benchmark. Primary PCI efficacy is sustained in the late stages of infarction, whereas thrombolysis effectiveness declines significantly within a few hours of symptom onset. This discrepancy provides a theoretical basis for the incremental improvement in outcomes with primary PCI.

Modification of pharmacological reperfusion using a reduced dose lytic agent and addition of a GP IIb/IIIa inhibitor has resulted in higher TIMI-3 flow rates.[7] This combination therapy was tested in the GUSTO-V and ASSENT-3 trials. Despite a decrease in early ischemic events (including reinfarction), there was no reduction in 30-day or 1-year mortality compared with standard lytic therapy. Combination therapy also increased the risk of hemorrhage (including intracranial) in elderly patients.[7]

Despite restoration of epicardial flow, many patients exhibit suboptimal myocardial perfusion. This has been demonstrated by several techniques, including angiogra-phy, myocardial contrast echocardiography, magnetic resonance imaging, scintigraphic methods, and Doppler flow wire measurements.[8] Epicardial flow has been more precisely quantitated using the TIMI frame count, and angiographic assessments of perfusion have been introduced, including the TIMI myocardial perfusion grade (Table 52-2) and blush score.[9] The implication of inadequate perfusion, despite adequate flow, is depicted in Figure 52-3.[10] Mortality, infarct size, and complications are all increased with impaired perfusion.

A profound reduction in perfusion, the "no-reflow" phenomenon, indicates severely impaired function of the microvasculature within the distribution of the infarct. A multitude of factors may contribute to microvascular dysfunction, including embolization of platelet thrombi or plaque-derived particulate matter, vasoconstriction, calcium overload, and reperfusion injury processes leading to neutrophil adhesion, endothelial dysfunction, and edema.[8]

Although a substantial proportion of patients exhibit impaired perfusion (as many as 80 percent)[10] after successful restoration of infarct artery flow, there appears to be more preserved microvascular perfusion among patients undergoing primary PCI. Analysis of ST segment resolution during infarction provides a simple surrogate for monitoring myocardial perfusion. In a study of thrombolytic ($N = 851$) and primary angioplasty ($N = 528$) reperfusion, ST

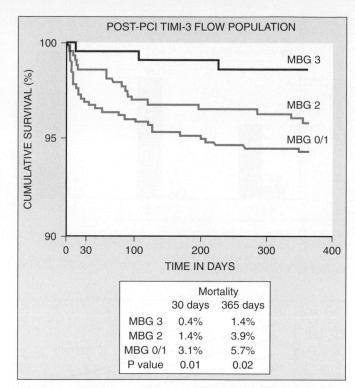

POST-PCI TIMI-3 FLOW POPULATION

	Mortality	
	30 days	365 days
MBG 3	0.4%	1.4%
MBG 2	1.4%	3.9%
MBG 0/1	3.1%	5.7%
P value	0.01	0.02

FIGURE 52–3 Cumulative survival according to final myocardial blush grade in patients from the Controlled Abciximab and Device Investigation to Lower Late Angioplasty Complications (CADILLAC) trial with post-PCI TIMI-3 flow. Mortality was increased with lower (abnormal) blush scores, despite normal epicardial flow.[10] MBG = myocardial blush grade; PCI = percutaneous coronary intervention; TIMI-3 = Thrombolysis in Myocardial Infarction 3.

resolution was accelerated in the latter group, which correlated with an improved outcome.[11] In two trials comparing primary stenting and thrombolysis, 1 to 2 weeks after treatment, the tissue myocardial perfusion grade was higher with stenting at angiography, which correlated with greater myocardial salvage and a lower mortality in the stent group.[12]

TREATMENT OF THE INCITING PATHOBIOLOGY IN ACUTE MYOCARDIAL INFARCTION. Reperfusion therapy (especially thrombolysis) targets the thrombotic intracoronary event that occurs in most myocardial infarctions. However, dynamic factors apart from thrombus, including plaque rupture, intramural hemorrhage, dissection, and spasm, are effectively treated with catheter-based reperfusion and may partially explain the advantage of primary PCI over thrombolysis.

After successful thrombolysis, a significant residual stenosis (50 percent) remains in more than 90 percent of patients.[13] Among patients in the TIMI trials, the composite of death, reinfarction, and congestive heart failure was higher with a residual stenosis, more than 50 percent (7.8 versus 2.8 percent, $P = 0.03$). Treatment of the stenosis during primary angioplasty appears to lower the risk of recurrent ischemic events. In a meta-analysis of randomized trials, reinfarction was reduced to 3 percent with primary angioplasty compared with 7 percent for thrombolytic therapy ($P < 0.0001$).[5] In-hospital reinfarction more than doubles 30-day and long-term (2-year) mortality.[14] Reocclusion occurs in 25 to 30 percent of patients after successful thrombolysis. After primary balloon angioplasty, reocclusion ranges from 5 to 16.7 percent and decreases further with stenting, to 0 to 6 percent.[15]

ANATOMICAL DEFINITION AND RISK STRATIFICATION. The angiographic and hemodynamic data obtained

at the time of emergency catheterization impart valuable decision-facilitating information and more precise risk stratification. Angiography defines the coronary anatomy in patients with equivocal or uninterruptible electrocardiographic changes. After urgent coronary angiography, a subset of patients will require emergent coronary bypass surgery for severe multivessel or left main coronary artery disease. Mechanical complications can also be identified during cardiac catheterization. An additional subset of patients exhibits spontaneous reperfusion without a significant residual stenosis and avoids the hazards of reperfusion therapy, including the hemorrhagic risks of thrombolysis.[7]

A primary PCI strategy allows stratification of patients into a low-risk group (age 70 years, left ventricular ejection fraction, LVEF, higher than 0.45, one- or two-vessel disease, successful angioplasty, no persistent arrhythmias) who can be discharged after 3 days with reduced costs and similar survival compared with longer hospitalization (7 days).[16] Using somewhat different criteria, more than 60 percent of patients fall into a low-risk category based on the Zwolle risk index (includes age, anterior infarction, Killip class, ischemic time, multivessel disease, post-PCI TIMI flow), with a mortality of 0.1 percent at 2 days and 0.2 percent between 3 and 10 days, allowing discharge 48 hours after primary PCI.[17]

REDUCTION IN MECHANICAL COMPLICATIONS OF INFARCTION. Treatment with primary angioplasty appears to reduce infarct rupture. In a combined meta-analysis of the GUSTO-I and PAMI-I/II trials, primary angioplasty resulted in an 86 percent reduction in the risk of mechanical complications compared with patients undergoing thrombolysis.[18] There was a significant reduction in acute mitral regurgitation (0.31 versus 1.73 percent, $P < 0.001$) and ventricular septal defects (0.0 versus 0.47 percent, $P < 0.001$). In a multivariate analysis of 1375 patients, treatment with primary angioplasty was independently associated with a lower risk of free wall rupture.[19]

COMPLICATIONS OF REPERFUSION THERAPY. Intracranial hemorrhage may be fatal in half to two thirds of patients and remains a devastating peril of thrombolytic therapy.[7] In a comparative analysis, the risk of intracranial hemorrhage was found to be 1 percent with thrombolysis and 0.05 percent with PCI.[5] As noted earlier, major bleeding complications were increased with PCI compared with thrombolysis (7 versus 5 percent, $P = 0.032$). However, these hemorrhages usually occur at the access site and were found to decrease in later trials.

Temporal Dynamics of Reperfusion Therapy

Rapid reperfusion of the infarct artery leading to myocardial salvage has remained the rationale for early reperfusion. The survival benefit of thrombolytic reperfusion therapy decreases with increasing delay in treatment.[7] There is an inherent delay in initiation of primary PCI reperfusion compared with thrombolysis. Despite the identified advantages and trial evidence favoring a primary PCI strategy, considerable controversy still surrounds the relative time-dependent efficacy of this approach.

Examination of primary angioplasty ($N = 27,080$) in the NRMI-2 database has revealed that the adjusted odds of hospital mortality did not increase significantly with increasing time from symptom onset to balloon inflation (ischemic time) but mortality did increase with a door to balloon time (treatment interval) longer than 2 hours.[20] One large study ($N = 2635$) has demonstrated increasing major adverse cardiac events rates with increasing presentation delay for thrombolysis but relatively stable event rates over time for primary angioplasty.[21] A mechanistic difference in reperfusion efficacy was illustrated by the

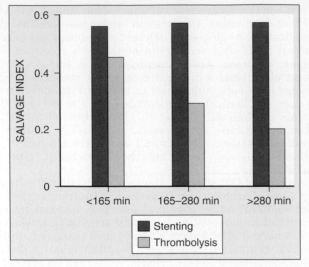

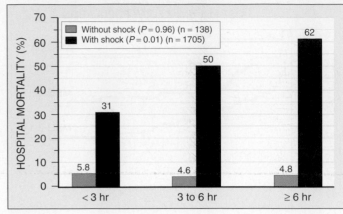

FIGURE 52–5 In-hospital mortality by time to reperfusion (symptom onset) in patients with and without shock. In this study, after adjustment for baseline variables, reperfusion time was a significant predictor of mortality in patients with shock but not in patients without shock.[23]

FIGURE 52–4 Median of myocardial salvage index according to tertiles of time to treatment interval. There was a time-dependent decrease of the salvage index in the thrombolysis group ($P = 0.03$) but not in the stenting group ($P = 0.59$).[22]

study of Schomig and associates, who demonstrated a consistent degree of myocardial salvage with primary PCI (stenting), despite increasing ischemic time.[22] Conversely, myocardial salvage achieved by thrombolysis declines markedly with increasing ischemic time, leading to a larger apparent advantage from primary PCI with later treatment (Fig. 52-4).

These data and other information have led to the consideration that the benefit of primary PCI is less time-dependent. Primary PCI attains a consistent and high reperfusion efficacy, but achievement of TIMI-3 flow decreases as treatment is delayed with thrombolysis.[6] In patients receiving thrombolysis, the complications of intracranial hemorrhage and myocardial rupture occur more frequently with longer treatment delays.[23,24] A primary PCI strategy reduces myocardial rupture and nearly eliminates intracranial hemorrhage. The enhanced patency achieved with later PCI may also enhance survival via positive effects on ventricular remodeling, augmenting electrical stability and providing a conduit for collateral flow in patients with multivessel disease.[25]

Clearly, the earliest possible restoration of blood flow into the infarct artery is desirable. In an analysis of primary PCI in 1843 patients reported by Brodie and colleagues, ischemic time was important for survival in patients with shock but independent of mortality in patients without shock (Fig. 52-5).[23] De Luca and associates have found that mortality in 1791 patients undergoing primary PCI (1994 to 2001) increases linearly according to ischemic time in high-risk but not in low-risk patients.[26] The data set was analyzed further to determine an overall continuous relationship between ischemic time and 1-year mortality. The risk of 1-year mortality increased by 7.5 percent for each 30-minute delay.[27]

The relative significance of reperfusion delay with primary PCI has been explored using linear regression analysis of data obtained from the randomized trials[5] of primary PCI and thrombolysis. Nallamothu and colleagues have reported that the two reperfusion strategies became equivalent with regard to short-term mortality after a PCI-related time delay (door to balloon time minus door to needle time) of 62 minutes.[28] The time equivalence for the composite endpoint of death, reinfarction, and stroke was 93 minutes. Equipoise in mortality was not noted for patients receiving streptokinase.[29] This analysis formed a basis for the American College of Cardiology/American Heart Association (ACC/AHA) guideline that thrombolysis should be initiated if the anticipated PCI delay is longer than 1 hour.[7] A subsequent analysis of these trials has determined that the mortality benefit for primary PCI is maintained until the PCI-related delay reaches 110 minutes.[30] By using the thrombolysis mortality as a proxy for mortality risk, multiple linear regression was used to determine the decrease in primary PCI survival benefit from PCI-related delay adjusted for risk (Fig. 52-6).[31] This demonstrates that a longer delay might be justified in high-risk patients. In contrast, longer delays may have less prognostic importance in low-risk patients and, as noted earlier, delay may not significantly increase mortality in this group.[23,26] Finally, a recent analysis of

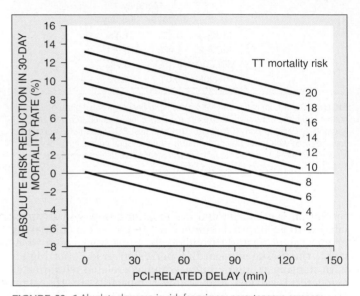

FIGURE 52–6 Absolute decrease in risk for primary percutaneous coronary intervention (PCI) over thrombolytic therapy (TT) after adjustment for TT mortality risk and PCI-related delay (risk-time benefit relation). Each line was computed from the equation $y = 0.82(TT) - 0.047(PCI\ delay) - 1.6$, which was derived from multiple regression analysis after setting mortality risk in the TT arm from 2 to 20 percent.[31]

individual patient data from 22 randomized trials has indicated that a lower mortality with primary PCI is maintained regardless of treatment delay, although the mortality reduction is significantly less with increasing delays.[32] (See later, "Late Presentation of Patients," for information on the recently reported Occluded Artery Trial [OAT].)

LOGISTIC CHALLENGE OF EFFECTIVE REPERFUSION THERAPY. Despite analytical considerations, the selection of reperfusion therapy (especially with a short ischemic time) remains a complex and controversial decision. Local factors, patient risk, and temporal dynamics must be considered. In facilities able to provide on-site primary PCI, expeditious application clearly provides the best opportunity for survival. However, only approximately 25 percent of U.S. hospitals have the capacity for primary PCI.[33] The advantage of primary PCI and an apparent prolonged temporal margin of benefit have created a foundation for expanding catheter-based reperfusion by transfer to capable centers.

A meta-analysis[34] of 6 trials comparing transfer (less than 3 hours) for primary PCI versus immediate thrombolysis

($N = 3750$) has identified a 42 percent reduction ($P < 0.001$) of the combined endpoint of death, reinfarction, and stroke. There were significant reductions in reinfarction (68 percent, $P < 0.001$) and stroke (56 percent, $P = 0.015$), with a trend for reduction in mortality (19 percent, $P = 0.08$). Notably, the PCI-related delay in these trials was 67 to 103 minutes.

The polarity of reperfusion strategy is exemplified by the findings of two trials in this meta-analysis. The DANAMI-2 randomized 1129 patients at referral hospitals to on-site thrombolysis or transport for PCI (PCI delay over thrombolysis was 67 minutes).[35] There was reduction in the composite endpoint of death, reinfarction, and stroke (8.5 versus 14.2 percent, $P = 0.002$), primarily because of less reinfarction (1.9 versus 6.2 percent, $P < 0.001$). Rescue PCI occurred in only 1.9 percent, and 4 percent of screened patients were considered unable to tolerate transport. During transport, concurrent preparation for PCI allowed a minimal delay in the treatment interval (shorter than 15 minutes) compared with a group presenting at the interventional center.

Alternatively, the CAPTIM trial ($N = 840$) compared the earliest possible initiation of thrombolysis with direct transport for PCI.[36] A physician initiated thrombolysis on site. The composite endpoint (death, reinfarction, stroke) occurred in 6.2 percent with PCI and 8.2 percent with prehospital thrombolysis ($P = 0.29$). In patients randomized within 2 hours, there was a trend for mortality reduction (2.2 versus 5.7 percent, $P = 0.058$) with prehospital thrombolysis.[37] Cardiogenic shock occurred less frequently with thrombolysis in this early group (1.3 versus 5.3 percent, $P < 0.032$). Notably, in the thrombolytic group, rescue PCI occurred in 26 percent and, by day 30, 70 percent underwent PCI.

The DANAMI-2 trial illustrates the benefits of a primary PCI strategy in a well-organized system despite time for transfer. On the other hand, physician-initiated prehospital thrombolysis when administered early in the ischemic interval with rescue PCI support may provide similar benefits for a subset of patients. Practically, a physician-supervised system of prehospital thrombolysis is not feasible in most communities and only a minority of patients present within 2 to 3 hours of the onset of their symptoms.[7,20]

Other factors should be considered with early presentation (shorter than 3 hours). Patients with contraindications to thrombolysis and those with cardiogenic shock should be transported for PCI. Higher risk patients (e.g., anterior infarction, elderly, hemodynamic compromise) also experience a larger benefit from catheter-based reperfusion, and the TIMI risk score can identify this group.[38] Patients at higher risk for intracranial hemorrhage from thrombolysis will also accrue less hazard from primary PCI.

Patients with 2- to 3-hour or longer presentation delays will be better served by a primary PCI strategy if transfer and/or reperfusion can be accomplished promptly. Despite ACC/AHA recommendations for a treatment interval (door to balloon) of less than 90 minutes, another study from NRMI-3/4 on patients transferred for PCI has determined a median door to balloon time of 180 minutes, with only 4.2 percent treated within 90 minutes.[39] The distinct advantage for a primary PCI strategy has generated considerable national and international momentum to provide timely access to this treatment for a greater proportion of patients.[33] Clinical trials have demonstrated the feasibility of rapid transport for primary PCI. Early assessment using prehospital 12-lead electrocardiogram (ECG) acquisition can allow efficient triage and advance preparation at the PCI center, with a considerable reduction in the treatment interval. However, there are several impediments to widespread application, especially in the United States, including lack

of prehospital ECG capability (10 percent in the United States),[33] economic impact on providers, organizational issues, regulatory policies involving certification, interpretation of performance metrics, and the political dynamics of achieving a broad consensus. Nevertheless, a geographic study has determined that nearly 80 percent of the adult U.S. population lives within 60 minutes of a PCI-capable hospital.[40] A recent AHA initiative is a step forward to implement timely reperfusion via primary PCI in the United States.[33]

An alternative approach to increasing the availability of primary PCI reperfusion involves increasing the number of hospitals providing this therapy. Experienced operators have performed primary PCI successfully in hospitals without on-site cardiac surgery. A randomized trial (C-PORT) has compared primary PCI with thrombolysis at 11 hospitals without on-site cardiac surgery ($N = 451$).[41] The composite primary endpoint (death, reinfarction, stroke) was significantly reduced at 6 weeks and 6 months (12.4 versus 19.9 percent, $P = 0.03$) with primary PCI without a complication requiring emergency surgery.

Although the risk of an interventional complication in the infarct artery is low, ACC/AHA guidelines have specified conduct of primary PCI at a hospital with cardiac surgery as a class IA recommendation.[7,25] A small percentage of patients will require emergency surgery for left main or complex multivessel disease and mechanical infarct complications. In a large multicenter registry, 2.1 percent of patients undergoing primary PCI ($N = 2014$) required emergency bypass surgery.[42] The indications for surgery included unsuccessful revascularization with ongoing ischemia (48 percent), extensive coronary disease (27 percent), PCI complications with ischemia or hemodynamic instability (14 percent), and mechanical complications (11 percent). There is concern regarding maintenance of institutional and operator experience, which may affect outcome. According to ACC/AHA guidelines, primary PCI without on-site surgery may be considered by experienced personnel (operator, 75 PCIs/year; institution, 36 primary PCIs/year) (class IID recommendation) with a proven plan for rapid transport to a surgery center.[7,25]

Challenging Groups of Patients

THROMBOLYTIC-INELIGIBLE PATIENTS. A significant proportion (25 to 30 percent) of patients presenting with ST elevation (or left bundle branch block, LBBB) infarction who are eligible do not receive reperfusion therapy. In the Global Registry of Acute Coronary Surgery (GRACE) 2084 patients presenting within 12 hours of the onset of ST elevation infarction, thrombolytic contraindications were present in 15 percent and, overall, 30 percent of eligible patients did not receive reperfusion therapy.[43] Correlates of the latter group included those with prior bypass surgery, diabetes, history of congestive failure, and age older than 75 years. There remains a bias against thrombolysis, particularly for the elderly. Patients with clear-cut and relative contraindications to thrombolysis are at higher risk for death.[44]

Although a large randomized trial documenting a benefit for primary PCI in patients with contraindications to thrombolysis is not available, a hypothetical comparison with placebo using data from 30 trials has indicated that primary PCI would reduce the risk of death by 44 percent ($P < 0.00001$).[45] By using a propensity analysis adjusted for patients (presenting in less than 12 hours) with contraindications to thrombolysis in the NRMI database ($N = 7810$), those undergoing immediate revascularization were at lower risk for hospital mortality (10.9 versus 20.1 percent; odds ratio, OR, 0.48; 95 percent confidence interval, CI, 0.56 to 0.75).[44] Primary PCI also achieved significant myocardial salvage and a favorable 6-month mortality in a group of patients ineligible for thrombolysis.[46]

Primary PCI can be applied to most higher risk patients who are not ideal candidates for thrombolytic therapy. The contraindications to primary angioplasty are limited to patients who cannot receive heparin, aspirin, or thienopyridines, documented life-threatening contrast allergy, or lack of vascular access.

PATIENTS IN CARDIOGENIC SHOCK. Multiple observational series of patients undergoing balloon angioplasty in cardiogenic shock have demonstrated improved hemodynamic status and suggested enhanced survival.[47] In contrast, thrombolysis appears less effective when administered to patients in shock.[47] Although thrombolysis[48] may provide a survival benefit for patients, increasing rates of PCI (28 to 54 percent) and declining rates of lytic use (20 to 6 percent) were associated with declining mortality (60 to 48 percent, $P < 0.001$) for 25,311 shock patients in the NRMI database from 1995 to 2004.[49] In this propensity-adjusted multivariable analysis, primary PCI was associated with a significant reduction in hospital mortality (OR, 0.46; 95 percent CI, 0.40 to 0.53).

The SHOCK trial randomized 302 patients to an early (within 12 hours shock onset, 36 hours of infarction onset) revascularization strategy (PCI, 63 percent; bypass surgery 38 percent) or medical stabilization (thrombolysis, 63 percent) with delayed revascularization, if appropriate.[50] Intraaortic balloon pump support was recommended (86 percent) in both groups. A significant survival advantage for early revascularization was noted at 6 months and 1 year but not at the 30-day primary endpoint (Fig. 52-7). The 30-day mortality was significantly lower with early revascularization for patients younger than 75 year. (41 versus 57 percent, $P < 0.05$). There was no benefit for the 56 patients older than 75 years, but an imbalance of baseline characteristics may have been present in this small group.[7,50] Furthermore, in the larger SHOCK registry, hospital mortality was significantly lower in elderly patients selected for early revascularization (48 versus 81 percent, $P = 0.0003$) and similar to that of younger patients (45 versus 61 percent, $P = 0.002$).[51] With exclusion of early deaths and covariate-adjusted modeling, the relative risk with revascularization was 0.46 (95 percent CI, 0.28 to 0.75; $P = 0.002$) for age of 75 years and 0.76 (95 percent CI, 0.59 to 0.99; $P = 0.045$) for age younger than 75 years. Rapid reperfusion is critical for survival and a large benefit (132 lives saved/1000 treated) is realized at 1 year.[50] Early revascularization is clearly recommended for patients younger than 75 years and suitable for many clinically selected elderly patients.[7]

The survival of 82 patients undergoing PCI in the SHOCK trial was 50 percent at 1 year.[52] One-year mortality was 38 percent with TIMI-3, 55 percent with TIMI-2, and 100 percent with TIMI 0-1 flow after PCI. The PCI success rate was 76 percent. Stents (34 percent) and GP IIb/IIIa inhibitors (32 percent) were used in the minority during the study period (1993 to 1998). A prospective registry of 96 shock patients has indicated that the use of stents and abciximab increases TIMI-3 flow rates and long-term survival.[53]

Most cardiogenic shock patients have multivessel disease (81 percent in SHOCK).[47,52,54] Survival rates for PCI and bypass surgery in the early revascularization arm were similar, although patients undergoing bypass surgery had more extensive coronary disease and a higher prevalence of diabetes.[54] There was a trend for improved 30-day survival in bypass surgery patients with complete revascularization (63 versus 17 percent, $P = 0.07$). Only 13 percent of PCI patients underwent a multivessel procedure, with a 1-year survival of 20 percent compared with 55 percent with single-vessel PCI. The role of modern multivessel PCI compared with emergency bypass surgery deserves further investigation.

Despite the improved survival of shock patients with revascularization, the mortality remains significant. Further improvement may result from advances in the process of reperfusion and therapy for the complex shock hemodynamic derangement. This is being approached by suppression of the inflammatory expression of inducible nitric oxide synthetase and ensuing inappropriate vasodilation with an inhibitor, tilarginine (L-NMMA).[55]

ELDERLY PATIENTS. The elderly patient population sustains a significant majority of the fatalities associated with myocardial infarction. Aging of the cardiovascular system can limit cardiac reserve and complicate the management of myocardial injury.

Although the relative benefit of thrombolytic therapy is diminished in the elderly, the higher overall mortality results in a greater absolute mortality reduction, as noted in a meta-analysis of major trials.[56] Despite this evidence, age predicts failure to use reperfusion therapy. Observations from the Medicare and NRMI data bases have indicated no benefit or possible harm for this group with thrombolysis, especially in patients older than 75 to 80 years.[56] Apprehension regarding the risk of intracranial hemorrhage remains, and the cumulative risk factors for this complication are more common in the elderly population. Elderly patients undergoing thrombolysis have more than a threefold risk of free wall rupture compared with no reperfusion or primary PCI.[57]

In contrast, Medicare patients undergoing primary angioplasty ($N = 2038$) exhibited a lower 30-day (8.7 versus 11.9 percent, $P = 0.001$) and 1-year (14.4 versus 17.6 percent, $P = 0.001$) mortality compared with thrombolysis ($N = 18,645$). For patients older than 75 years in the NRMI-2 registry, the combined endpoint of death and nonfatal stroke was significantly higher in patients treated with t-PA compared with primary angioplasty (18.4 versus 14.6 percent, $P = 0.001$).[56] In the PCAT analysis of 10 randomized trials, primary angioplasty was more effective in reducing 30-day mortality in patients over age 70 years compared with younger patients.[21]

A small randomized trial ($N = 87$) comparing streptokinase with primary PCI has demonstrated a striking reduction (9 versus 29 percent, $P = 0.01$) in the primary endpoint (death, reinfarction, stroke) and considerable reduction in 30-day (7 versus 22 percent, $P = 0.04$) and 1-year mortality (11 versus 29 percent, $P = 0.03$) with angioplasty in patients older than 75 years.[58] The recently presented results of the Senior PAMI trial randomized 481 lytic-eligible (no prior cerebrovascular accident, blood pressure lower than 180/100 mm Hg, no shock, less than 12 hours) patients (age greater than 70 years) to thrombolysis or primary PCI plus abciximab.[59] Primary PCI achieved TIMI-3 flow in 86 percent, and 21 percent of lytic patients underwent urgent catheterization within 12 hours. In-hospital recurrent ischemia (4.8 versus 31 percent, $P = 0.0001$), reinfarction (1.2 versus 4.4 percent, $P = 0.032$) and the 30-day endpoint of death, reinfarction, and stroke (11.6 versus 18 percent, $P = 0.05$) were significantly reduced with primary PCI. Intracranial hemorrhage (1.3 versus 0 percent, $P = 0.11$) was a hazard of lytic therapy. A marked reduction in the primary endpoint (7.7 versus 17 percent, $P < 0.01$) was evident in the

CH 52

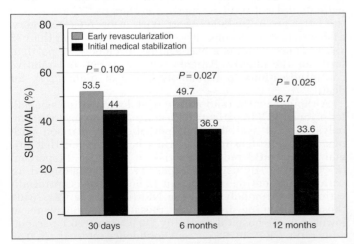

FIGURE 52-7 The temporal relation to survival for patients randomized in the SHOCK trial by treatment strategy.[50]

prestratified 70- to 80-year age group. However, no benefit was seen for patients older than 80 years ($N = 130$; primary endpoint, 22 versus 22 percent). In this trial, primary PCI was advantageous primarily by reducing recurrent ischemic events and intracranial hemorrhage. The more elderly patients may do poorly with either reperfusion strategy. A small randomized trial ($N = 120$) of primary angioplasty in low-risk patients, age 80 years, also did not detect a benefit over conservative therapy during a 3-year period.[60] In these "ultra"-elderly patients, management must include consideration of functional status and comorbid conditions.

PATIENTS WITH PRIOR CORONARY BYPASS SURGERY. Prior coronary bypass surgery independently predicts mortality in patients with acute myocardial infarction. The large thrombus burden often present in occluded vein grafts may resist the action of lytic agents. In the GUSTO-I trial, thrombolysis achieved TIMI-3 flow in bypass grafts in only 32 percent of patients.[61]

Primary PCI yields better results, although the technique is less effective than in native coronary arteries (TIMI-3 flow 87 versus 93 percent, $P = 0.024$ in the PAMI trials).[62] One-year mortality was markedly increased in patients undergoing vein graft primary PCI compared with native arteries (20 versus 6 percent, $P < 0.001$). In a review of 57 patients (1984 to 2003), vein graft patency was identified in only 64 percent at 1 year after primary PCI, but was increased in those who underwent stenting at 5-year follow-up (80 versus 45 percent, $P = 0.053$).[63]

In addition to more extensive thrombus, vein graft PCI is often complicated by graft ectasia, limited runoff, atherosclerotic debris, and an increased risk of embolization. Distal protection methodology is clearly indicated as an adjunct for PCI of stenotic vein grafts.[25,61] Further investigation is desirable to determine the efficacy of these devices and the role of thrombectomy in this small segment (3 percent of the PAMI trial population)[62] of patients presenting for primary PCI.

LATE PRESENTATION OF PATIENTS. In the NRMI data base, nearly one third of patients with acute infarction (ST elevation or new LBBB) presented more than 12 hours after symptom onset.[44] Thrombolytic therapy in this group does not significantly improve survival.[7] Guidelines restrict recommendations for reperfusion with PCI to late presentation patients (12 to 24 hours) with persistent ischemic symptoms, heart failure, and hemodynamic or electrical instability.[7]

A report from NRMI-2 has indicated an improved hospital outcome with less recurrent ischemia, reinfarction, and death (3.4 versus 5.6 percent, $P < 0.001$) for late-presentation patients undergoing PCI. Although invasive therapy was associated with lower risk features, a strong trend for reduced mortality with PCI remained after subject matching by multivariate propensity analysis (OR, 0.73; 95 percent CI, 0.53 to 1.01).[64] Data from small randomized trials evaluating the effect of PCI more than 12 hours after MI are conflicting and inconclusive.[65] Recently, the BRAVE-2 trial ($N = 365$) evaluated immediate PCI in asymptomatic patients 12 to 24 hours after symptom onset.[66] Scintigraphic infarct size was significantly smaller in PCI patients (8 versus 13 percent, $P < 0.001$). Death, reinfarction, and stroke were insignificantly reduced with PCI at 30 days (4.4 versus 6.6 percent, $P = 0.37$). Notably, at initial angiography, TIMI grades 1 to 3 flow were present in 50 percent of patients and collateral flow was seen in 44 percent of patients with TIMI grade 0.

Beyond myocardial salvage, additional benefit may be realized with an open infarct artery by favorable effects on remodeling, electrical stability, and collateral supply.[25] Infarct artery patency is a predictor of survival after infarction.[14] The recently reported Occluded Artery Trial (OAT) compared PCI to optimal medical therapy in a randomized study of 2166 stable patients with ACS with total occlusion

of the infarct related artery from 3 to 28 days after presentation. The invasive therapy did not lessen death or heart failure in 4 years of observation, and was associated with a trend toward increased reinfarction. These new data suggest that PCI should be used with caution in stable patients who present 3 days and later following onset of acute MI.[65]

MODERN CATHETER-BASED REPERFUSION TECHNIQUES

Glycoprotein IIb/IIIa Inhibition

A strong theoretical basis supports GP IIb/IIIa inhibition during catheter-based reperfusion therapy. Antagonism of platelet aggregation may "passivate" the unstable, mechanically injured, atherosclerotic arterial wall, avert thrombus formation on acutely deployed stents, and prevent microembolization with subsequent no reflow. These agents reduce ischemic events and mortality after PCI.[25] Abciximab may improve microvascular perfusion and administration has been associated with early ST segment resolution and smaller infarctions after primary PCI.[67,68]

Eight randomized trials ($N = 3949$) have been conducted examining the effect of abciximab as an adjunctive therapy during primary PCI.[68] Adverse events (except stent thrombosis) were not significantly reduced in the largest trial (Controlled Abciximab and Device Investigation to Lower Late Angioplasty Complications, CADILLAC),[69] perhaps reflecting the low-risk profile of enrolled patients.[67] A meta-analysis of these trials has demonstrated reduction of 30-day reinfarction and long term (6- to 12-month) mortality, with no significant increase in major bleeding complications (Fig. 52-8).[68]

Survival is improved when the infarct artery is patent with TIMI-3 flow prior to primary PCI.[70] In the ADMIRAL trial, those patients receiving abciximab prior to catheterization laboratory arrival attained substantially more benefit than later treatment.[71] A meta-analysis (six trials, $N = 931$) of patients receiving GP IIb/IIIa inhibitors (abciximab, tirofiban) has revealed that drug administration at initial contact (emergency department or ambulance) compared with initiation at the time of PCI results in a higher TIMI-3 flow rate prior to PCI (20.3 versus 12.2 percent, $P < 0.001$) and trends for a reduction in mortality (3.4 versus 4.7 percent) and reinfarction.[71] Validation of this form of "facilitated" PCI awaits randomized trial data.

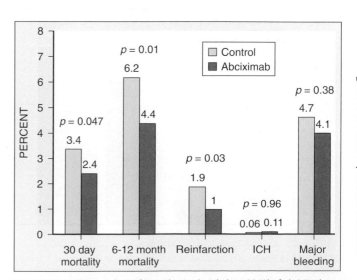

FIGURE 52–8 Meta-analysis of 8 randomized trials ($N = 3949$) of abciximab therapy for patients with ST-elevation MI undergoing primary PCI. ICH = intracranial hemorrhage.[68]

Beyond temporal considerations, future refinements may include intracoronary application. A significant reduction in major adverse cardiac events at 30 days was seen in patients with TIMI 0/1 flow with an intracoronary bolus of abciximab compared with standard intravenous therapy (12 versus 28 percent, $P < 0.002$, $N = 273$).[72] Current information suggests that abciximab should be used with primary PCI, especially in high-risk patients.[7,68] Although tirofiban and eptifibatide have been investigated, there is a lack of randomized trial data supporting adjunctive use during primary PCI.

Primary Stent Implantation

Stents are an essential component of modern PCI procedures. The initial concerns regarding the safety of stent implantation in the presence of intracoronary thrombus have abated. Several randomized trials have been conducted comparing primary stenting with primary balloon angioplasty. In the largest trial (CADILLAC), primary stenting or balloon angioplasty was compared (without abciximab) in 1080 patients.[69] TIMI-3 flow was achieved in 95 percent of both groups, with no significant difference in mortality or reinfarction, but ischemic target vessel revascularization (TVR) at 6 months was significantly lower with stenting (8.3 versus 15.7 percent, $P < 0.001$). The rate of ischemic TVR was also less with stenting when compared with patients (40 percent) who had an optimal result (stenosis less than 30 percent without dissection) with balloon angioplasty (9.1 versus 19.1 percent, $P = 0.003$).[73]

A meta-analysis ($N = 4120$) of published trials has confirmed the advantage of stent deployment (Fig. 52-9).[74] The composite incidence of major adverse events at 6 to 12 months is significantly reduced (OR, 0.52; 95 percent CI, 0.44 to 0.62) without a significant difference in mortality or reinfarction, again principally secondary to a reduction in TVR (OR, 0.43; 95 percent CI, 0.36 to 0.52) (see Fig. 52-9). The 5-year follow-up of the PAMI trials has reported a notable trend for lower mortality with stenting (10 versus 13 percent, $P = 0.058$).[75]

Despite the rapid incorporation of drug-eluting stent technology into standard interventional practice, there is a paucity of randomized trial data regarding its use during primary PCI. There are concerns regarding increased thrombogenicity of drug-eluting stent use in acute myocardial infarction. One small published randomized trial ($N = 175$) demonstrated a reduction in 8-month TVR (7 versus 20 percent, $P = 0.01$) and no stent thrombosis with the sirolimus-eluting stent.[76] Three recently presented trials compared the use of drug-eluting stents with bare metal stents for primary PCI. At 1 year, patients receiving the sirolimus-eluting stent experienced less TVR in both the TYPHOON ($N = 712$; 5.6 versus 13.4 percent, $P < 0.001$)[77] and SESAMI ($N = 423$; 5 versus 13.1 percent, $P < 0.01$)[78] trials. In contrast, no significant benefit was identified with the paclitaxel-eluting stent in the PASSION trial ($N = 620$).[79] In none of these three trials did stent thrombosis increase with the drug-eluting stent. More data from larger trials should be available in the near future regarding the use of this advance in acute infarction.

DEVELOPMENTS IN REPERFUSION THERAPY SCIENCE

Considerable investigational effort continues into the pathophysiology and therapeutics of reperfusion science. The impact of methodology for the protection of microvasculature and myocyte protection or regeneration continues to evolve.

Distal Embolization (see Chap. 55)

The common occurrence of impaired myocardial perfusion and its consequences, despite normal epicardial flow after reperfusion, have been highlighted.[10] Although numerous mechanisms may be involved, distal embolization identified by angiography during primary angioplasty was noted in 15.2 percent of patients in the Zwolle trial.[80] Procedural success (TIMI-3 flow) and perfusion (blush score) were reduced with embolization and associated with larger infarct size, lower ejection fraction, and substantially higher 5-year mortality (44 versus 9 percent, $P < 0.001$).

Several small investigations have demonstrated feasibility and suggested efficacy for mechanical protection of the microvasculature.[81] The use of distal protection devices during PCI of stenotic vein grafts yields a large benefit.[25,61] When used during primary PCI in native arteries, visible debris is obtained in nearly 75 percent of patients.[82] Despite the intuitive advantage of this approach, the EMERALD trial ($N = 501$) showed no improvement in ST segment resolution or infarct size using a distal balloon occlusion and aspiration device.[82] A lack of benefit on coronary flow velocity and infarct size was also reported in the PROMISE trial ($N = 200$) of the filter wire device.[83] Possible explanations for failure of distal protection include time delay for device use, embolization during device deployment, inability to protect side branches, incomplete capture of debris, overall small embolic burden, and greater significance of nonembolic mechanisms causing microcirculatory dysfunction.

Thrombectomy prior to primary PCI has also been tested.[81] Several smaller studies have reported improved myocardial perfusion and ST segment resolution using various thrombectomy devices. However, a preliminary report from the AiMI trial ($N = 480$) has indicated that routine use of rheolytic thrombolysis with the AngioJet device (catheter-based thrombectomy system) prior to primary PCI results in a larger infarct size (12.5 versus 9.8 percent, $P = 0.02$) and a disturbing trend for a higher 6-month mortality (5 versus 2.1 percent, $P = 0.06$).[84]

No current evidence supports the routine use of thrombectomy or distal protection devices during primary PCI. Improved devices, combined use, or selective use (possibly with complicated ruptured plaques or large thrombus burden) may justify these methods after further investigation.

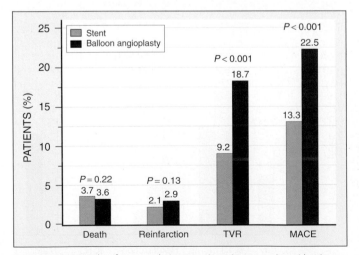

FIGURE 52–9 Results of meta-analysis comparing primary stenting with primary balloon angioplasty. MACE = major adverse cardiac events including death, reinfarction, and target vessel revascularization (TVR) *(stroke in CADILLAC and Stent-PAMI trials)*.[74]

Pharmacological Interventions

Many pharmacological adjuncts designed to preserve the myocardial cell or treat the microvascular derangement have been proposed and investigated. Research has focused on inflammatory mediators, impaired intracellular metabolism, microvascular damage, including endothelial dysfunction, and reperfusion injury.[8] Despite promising experimental data, clinical trials have largely failed to demonstrate significant myocardial salvage or improved outcomes.

Metabolic modulation using glucose-insulin-potassium (GIK) treatment was tested in a 20,201-patient trial in which 83 percent received reperfusion therapy.[85] GIK infusion had a neutral effect on mortality, cardiac arrest, reinfarction, and cardiogenic shock. Inhibition of intracellular calcium overload was tested with the sodium-calcium exchange inhibitor, Caldaret. No overall reduction in infarct size was noted in 387 patients undergoing primary PCI, although there was some evidence for a positive effect with anterior infarction and TIMI 0 to 1 flow.[86] A larger trial is forthcoming.

Attempts to reduce the inflammatory response with an antibody against the CD18 adhesion receptor were not effective. In the COMplement inhibition in Myocardial infarction treated with Angioplasty (COMMA) trial, a monoclonal antibody against C5 complement (pexelizumab) did not reduce the primary endpoint of infarct size in 814 primary PCI patients.[87] However, 6-month mortality was significantly reduced (3.2 versus 7.4 percent, $P < 0.02$) and pexelizumab is being tested in the larger APEX MI trial.

Adenosine preserves energy stores and has antiinflammatory and antiplatelet effects. Although overall clinical outcomes were not significantly improved in the AMISTAD II trial, infarct size was reduced in the high-dose (70 μg/kg/min) group and this correlated with fewer adverse clinical events.[88] Nicorandil has shown favorable effects on microvascular integrity and myocardial viability in conjunction with reperfusion therapy.[89] This drug has multiple effects as an ADP-sensitive IK^{ATP} channel opener with nitrate properties that suppresses reactive oxygen species formation. Further investigation of these agents appears warranted.

Mechanical Myocardial Protection

Myocardial temperature influences infarct size in experimental preparations. Several cooling devices using an inferior vena cava catheter have been developed to induce systemic hypothermia in an attempt to attenuate myocardial necrosis in patients undergoing reperfusion therapy. Trials conducted in patients undergoing primary PCI showed no overall reduction in infarct size.[90] However, secondary analysis did identify a significant reduction in anterior wall infarct size for patients who were cooled to a target core temperature lower than 35°C before first balloon inflation. Trials continue to evaluate this process.

Hyperbaric oxygen therapy can reduce injury and improve healing of ischemic tissue. The TherOx AO system (TherOx, Irvine, Calif) produces aqueous oxygen that is mixed with the patient's blood, leading to a PO_2 of 600 to 800 mm Hg. The hyperoxemic blood can be delivered through a subselective coronary infusion catheter. In the AMIHOT randomized trial of 269 primary PCI patients, no significant reduction in infarct size or improvement in ST-segment resolution was demonstrated with a 90-minute intracoronary infusion of hyperoxemic blood.[90] Again, on secondary analysis, favorable effects on these parameters were seen in anterior infarcts and for those presenting within 6 hours of symptom onset. Further investigations are planned to verify these observations.

Myocardial Regeneration (see Chap. 29)

Interest has emerged in cellular therapy as a method of myocardial repair after infarction. This has principally involved intracoronary infusion of bone marrow–derived cells, usually days after infarction. Several small trials have demonstrated safe application with improved ejection fraction and decreased infarct size.[91] However, recent larger trials ($N = 60$-100) have shown conflicting results. There is also controversy regarding the mechanism of improvement, which may involve transdifferentiation, angiogenesis, and/or paracrine effects. Exploration of the mechanisms, mode of application, timing and potential benefits before widespread clinical use will require considerable further investigation.

Combining Percutaneous Coronary Intervention and Thrombolytic Therapy

RESCUE PERCUTANEOUS CORONARY INTERVENTION. Despite an increasing proportion of the infarct population undergoing primary PCI, the majority of patients receive thrombolytic reperfusion therapy. There is a relative paucity of data regarding the value of rescue PCI for patients who fail to reperfuse after thrombolysis. This is reflective of the later stage, higher risk profile of patients with failed thrombolysis and complex management related to the uncertainty of lytic success, with possible need for transfer to enable rescue procedures. An early randomized trial ($N = 151$) in anterior infarction has identified a reduction in the 30-day combined endpoint of death and heart failure (6.4 versus 16.6 percent, $P = 0.05$). In a pooled analysis of several small trials, early heart failure was reduced and there was an improved 1-year survival with moderate to large infarctions.[92]

More recent investigations include the Middlesbrough Early Revascularization to Limit INfarction (MERLIN) trial, which randomized 307 patients with less than a 50 percent reduction in ST segment elevation 60 minutes after streptokinase to rescue PCI or conservative therapy.[93] There was no significant difference in the primary endpoint of mortality. Subsequent revascularization (6.5 versus 20.1 percent, $P < 0.01$) was less with rescue PCI (stents, 50 percent; GP IIb/IIIa inhibitors, 3 percent) but more strokes were seen in the PCI group (4.6 versus 0.6 percent, $P < 0.03$). Notably, with routine GP IIb/IIIa inhibition, stent-based rescue PCI results in more myocardial salvage compared with balloon angioplasty ($N = 181$, salvage index 0.35 versus 0.25, $P = 0.005$).[94] The recently published REACT trial randomized 427 patients with failed thrombolysis (less than 50 percent ST segment elevation reduction at 90 minutes) to conservative treatment, repeat thrombolysis, or rescue PCI (stents, 88 percent).[95] Although there was no mortality difference, the 6-month event-free survival was greater with rescue PCI (84.6 versus 70.1 percent for conservative and 68.7 percent for repeat lysis, $P = 0.004$).

The inaccuracy of the noninvasive determination of the status of infarct artery perfusion remains an important limitation of this approach. Use of clinical features, baseline/60-minute biomarkers, and ST-segment resolution in combination as a predictive instrument may improve accuracy.[96] It is best to maintain a high index of clinical suspicion and refer patients early for angiography, before hemodynamic compromise.[92] Current guidelines[25] recommend rescue PCI for patients with shock and heart failure, with less evidence for electrical instability or persistent ischemia. However, the results of recent investigations support the use of this approach in patients with evidence of continued ischemia.[95]

FACILITATED PERCUTANEOUS CORONARY INTERVENTION. The parallel nascent development of thrombolytic reperfusion therapy and transluminal revascularization in the catheterization laboratory has invited combined application for acute myocardial infarction in an effort to optimize the arterial lumen and reduce the risk of recurrent ischemia events. However, several trials conducted more than a decade ago have demonstrated an adverse outcome for immediate angioplasty after thrombolysis with more bleeding, recurrent ischemia, bypass surgery, and death.[7] This hazard was presumed to originate from lytic-induced enhanced platelet activation and/or extensive intramural hemorrhage. Yet, advanced angioplasty techniques have improved the safety of the procedure in this setting. In a multivariate analysis of the patients in the TIMI-10B (TNK versus t-PA) and TIMI-14 (reduced-dose t-PA and/or abciximab) trials, those undergoing adjunctive or delayed intervention (more than 60 percent stents) had a lower risk of 30-day mortality and/or reinfarction compared with patients with successful thrombolysis (TIMI-3 flow at 90 minutes) without intervention.[97]

A further impetus for pursuing a pharmacoinvasive approach has emerged from data demonstrating improved survival in high risk patients who exhibit spontaneous reperfusion (TIMI-3 flow) prior to primary PCI.[70] Conceptually, attaining effective early restoration of myocardial blood flow for patients presenting within the 2- to 3-hour presentation interval might shift the reperfusion benefit toward enhanced myocardial salvage and improved outcomes, especially in transfer patients. This information has stimulated further development of the synergistic concept of facilitated angioplasty achieving the speed advantage of pharmacological reperfusion while allowing the security of mechanical bailout and "definitive" treatment of the arterial lumen.

Pilot studies using full or reduced dose lytic drugs with or without GP IIb/IIIa inhibition have confirmed the feasibility of achieving increased TIMI-3 flow rates at initial angiography. The largest published trial of facilitated PCI (ASSENT-4) randomized 1667 patients (less than 6-hour symptom duration) to primary PCI or primary PCI preceded by full-dose tenecteplase.[98] Despite higher pre-PCI TIMI-3 flow rates (43 versus 15 percent, $P < 0.001$) in the group with lytic therapy, the trial was prematurely discontinued because of increased hospital mortality in the facilitated group (6 versus 3 percent, $P = 0.01$). Furthermore, the primary endpoint (death, heart failure, or shock within 90 days) was higher with facilitated PCI (19 versus 13 percent, $P = 0.0045$). There were also significantly more strokes (1.8 versus 0 percent, $P < 0.0001$) and ischemic complications (reinfarction, 6 versus 4 percent, $P = 0.03$) in the facilitated PCI group. The large FINESSE trial has compared early abciximab versus reduced-dose reteplase plus abciximab versus abciximab at PCI and continues to enroll patients. Notably, the BRAVE trial ($N = 253$) compared half-dose reteplase and abciximab versus abciximab alone before PCI and did not demonstrate a difference in infarct size or clinical outcomes.[99]

A recent meta-analysis of 17 facilitated PCI trials (including ASSENT-4) has indicated that although facilitated PCI results in more than a twofold increase in initial TIMI-3 flow, post-PCI flow rates do not differ (89 versus 88 percent) compared with primary PCI.[100] Mortality (5 versus 3 percent, $P = 0.04$), TVR (4 versus 1 percent, $P = 0.01$), major bleeding (7 versus 5 percent, $P = 0.01$), and stroke (1.1 versus 0.3 percent, $P = 0.0008$) were all significantly greater with facilitated PCI. Adverse outcomes were confined to patients receiving lytic drugs, whereas GP IIb/IIIa inhibition alone was not harmful.

The hemorrhagic lytic hazards (local arterial, myocardial, and cerebral damage) and temporal realities (delayed presentation, protracted thrombolytic action) apparently do not interact in a favorable manner with this approach. Despite modern progress, current evidence does not justify combining thrombolytic therapy with immediate PCI.

ADJUNCTIVE PERCUTANEOUS CORONARY INTERVENTION AFTER SUCCESSFUL THROMBOLYSIS. As noted, a significant residual stenosis is found in most infarct arteries after successful thrombolysis.[13] Reinfarction after thrombolysis is associated with a large increase in mortality and is an unpredictable event.[14] Early trials evaluating routine balloon angioplasty hours to days after successful thrombolysis did not demonstrate a benefit on reinfarction, left ventricular function, or survival.[7] Patients with spontaneous or provokable ischemia after thrombolysis have less recurrent infarction or ischemia after undergoing PCI.[25] Therefore, guidelines have recommended proceeding with PCI in post-thrombolysis patients with recurrent infarction, provokable ischemia, or shock and to consider it strongly (class IIa) in patients with heart failure, LVEF = 0.40, or serious ventricular arrhythmias.[25]

The improvements in PCI practice and technique have allowed reconsideration of the routine approach to patients after successful thrombolysis.[97] For instance in the TIMI 4, 10B, and 17 trials, PCI after thrombolysis reduced the risk of reinfarction and 2-year mortality.[14] In the GRACIA-1 trial, 500 patients were randomized to angiography and PCI with stenting and abciximab 6 to 24 hours after thrombolysis or to an ischemia-guided conservative approach. Infarct artery stenting occurred in 80 percent of the invasive group and 20 percent with the ischemia-guided strategy. At 1 year, the invasive patients had a reduced incidence of the primary endpoint of death, reinfarction, or revascularization (9 versus 21 percent, $P = 0.0008$). Unplanned revascularization during hospitalization provoked by spontaneous ischemia was five times higher with the conservative approach.[101] Although this trial was not powered to detect a survival advantage, it demonstrates that modern PCI as part of the commonly practiced post-thrombolysis invasive strategy can safely benefit the patients.

CONDUCTING PRIMARY PERCUTANEOUS CORONARY INTERVENTION REPERFUSION THERAPY

In treating acute myocardial infarction, the prime objective of achieving the most expeditious and complete infarct artery reperfusion has been confirmed by scientific and clinical evidence.

Coordinated regional emergency infarct care policy and cooperation will significantly affect the treatment interval.[33] Triage and activation of the reperfusion team should begin with first medical contact. Shifting acquisition of the ECG and interpretation from the emergency department to the prehospital setting can markedly reduce the door to balloon time.[33] A network protocol incorporating both interventional and pharmacological (prehospital initiation) reperfusion may be successful in some communities.[102] However, a simple algorithm for selective reperfusion is complex in most circumstances because of heterogeneous patient factors and local availability of resources.[7,33] In the NRMI-4 registry, greater hospital specialization with primary PCI was associated with shorter door to balloon times and lower hospital mortality.[103] It appears that exclusive use of primary PCI reperfusion will improve clinical outcomes.

In an institution, a primary interventional strategy requires a multidisciplinary commitment. On hospital arrival, evaluation should proceed in a swift and thorough manner, using precise protocols and prompt communication to allow quick entry into the catheterization laboratory. Comorbid evaluation should focus on vascular disease, allergies, risk factors for anticoagulation, renal function, possible pregnancy, and functional status. Infarct care should be initiated (including aspirin, heparin, and beta blockade or nitrates, if indicated). There has been no randomized trial evaluating IV beta blockade in primary PCI patients. Observational studies have suggested that beta blockade for primary PCI patients may have a favorable effect on mortality and reduce the risk of ventricular tachycardia or fibrillation during the procedure.[104] Caution is warranted regarding IV beta blocker administration in patients with a marginal hemodynamic status because of the excess risk of cardiogenic shock identified in the large ($N = 45,852$) COMMIT trial.[105]

The catheterization laboratory must provide ongoing intensive medical care. Comprehensive protocols provide a dedicated environment, in which events and complications are vigilantly anticipated. In most circumstances, primary PCI is more complicated than an elective procedure. The operator must tailor the approach to the environment of acute infarction.

Heparin remains the standard antithrombin agent used during primary PCI. Trials evaluating bivalirudin are ongoing. In the recent OASIS-6 trial, use of the factor Xa inhibitor fondaparinux during primary PCI resulted in more guide catheter thrombosis and abrupt closure.[106]

Preparation of both femoral access sites is a facile precautionary step. Attention should be paid to the presence of collateral flow during initial angiography to guide intervention in the infarct artery. Angiography of the infarct artery can be performed with a guide catheter. Care should be taken to maintain the guidewire in the main vessel with advancement through the occlusion. If guidewire positioning does not result in reperfusion and adequate visualization, an appropriately sized balloon catheter should be advanced and inflated to allow early reperfusion. There should be attention to development of transient reperfusion arrhythmias or hypotension. With adequate visualization, direct stenting may be considered unless a bifurcation lesion or heavy calcification is present. A small randomized trial ($N = 206$) has indicated that compared with balloon predilation, direct stenting results in improved ST segment resolution.[107] Bifurcation lesions are problematic during primary PCI. Side branches were frequently (29 percent) covered by a stent at the target lesion in the main vessel among 276 consecutive patients in a recent report.[108] Acute side branch occlusion occurred in 12.5 percent. Bifurcation stenting in the setting of acute myocardial infarction is a significant risk factor for stent thrombosis.[109]

Distal embolization and impaired myocardial perfusion remain important limitations of reperfusion therapy. Routine use of current thrombectomy or distal protection devices cannot be justified. Angiographic or intravascular ultrasound predictive characteristics may allow selective use of these devices.[81] If distal embolization or no-reflow occurs during the intervention, intracoronary administration of vasodilator agents has been used to improve myocardial perfusion. In a recent small ($N = 40$) study, intracoronary nitroprusside injection achieved better angiographic tissue myocardial perfusion compared with adenosine or verapamil.[110] In some cases, the onset of no-reflow can result in profound hemodynamic deterioration. Intracoronary epinephrine has been used to improve flow significantly in patients with refractory no-reflow and may be an appropriate treatment for patients who are hypotensive.[111] These agents are preferably administered distally in the epicardial vessels.

Multivessel disease is encountered in 40 to 65 percent of patients with acute myocardial infarction.[112] Multiple complex coronary lesions, as characterized by thrombus, ulceration, irregularity or impaired flow, have been identified in 40 percent of patients with acute infarction and may reflect a systemic process affecting widespread vulnerable plaques.[113] The presence of multiple complex plaques is associated with more recurrent ischemic events.

The conventional approach to the infarct patient with multivessel disease has incorporated urgent surgery, staged angioplasty, late surgery, or noninvasive evaluation after reperfusion. The advent of modern angioplasty technology has allowed consideration for multivessel revascularization at the time of the primary procedure. However, the current ACC/AHA guideline recommends that PCI of the noninfarct artery should be avoided in patients without hemodynamic compromise.[7,25] There is a lack of randomized investigative trials examining multivessel PCI at the time of the acute procedure. In a series of 820 primary PCI patients, at 1 year, those with multivessel disease experienced more major adverse cardiac events (31 versus 13 percent, $P < 0.001$) and a higher mortality (12 versus 3.2 percent, $P < 0.001$).[112] Multivessel PCI ($N = 152$; performed within the initial procedure [$n = 26$], or staged) was associated with higher rates of reinfarction (13 versus 2.8 percent, $P < 0.001$) and major adverse cardiac events (40 versus 28 percent, $P = 0.006$) compared with primary PCI restricted to the infarct artery. Alternatively, a report from the Mayo Clinic has evaluated outcomes of patients undergoing multivessel PCI within 7 days of ST elevation and non–ST elevation infarction. Despite a higher prevalence of adverse prognostic indicators, multivessel PCI, and infarct, artery-only PCI patients experienced a similar 1-year survival and freedom from infarction or TVR.[114] Controversy continues regarding the approach to the patient with multivessel disease, and more investigation is needed.

The benefits of rapid reperfusion are amplified in cardiogenic shock. A high clinical suspicion for mechanical complications should lead to hemodynamic, ventriculographic, or echocardiographic evaluation. Intra-aortic balloon pump counterpulsation is an essential component of cardiogenic shock therapy and should be initiated before or during PCI. The interventional team should continually review outcomes and modify processes incorporating advances derived from investigation into the dynamic field of reperfusion therapy.

FUTURE DIRECTIONS

Nearly three decades of evidence-based progress have verified the merits of a primary interventional reperfusion strategy. Perhaps the greatest incremental benefit in the future will result from implementation of logistical modifications that enable more patients to undergo primary PCI expeditiously. Technical refinements may facilitate application in patients with challenging anatomy or with risk factors for microcirculatory dysfunction. Further analysis and development of stent technology has the potential to enhance the safety and durability of the procedure. Investigation into pharmacological and mechanical methods of myocyte preservation may augment myocardial salvage. The continued evolution of myocardial regeneration therapy also holds promise.

REFERENCES

Patient Selection for Primary Percutaneous Revascularization

1. Grines CL, Browne KF, Marco J, et al: A comparison of immediate angioplasty with thrombolytic therapy for acute myocardial infarction. The Primary Angioplasty in Myocardial Infarction Study Group. N Engl J Med 328:673, 1993.

2. Weaver WD, Simes RJ, Betriu A, et al: Comparison of primary coronary angioplasty and intravenous thrombolytic therapy for acute myocardial infarction: A quantitative review. JAMA 278:2093, 1997.

3. Grines C, Patel A, Zijlstra F, et al: Primary coronary angioplasty compared with intravenous thrombolytic therapy for acute myocardial infarction: Six-month follow-up and analysis of individual patient data from randomized trials. Am Heart J 145:47, 2003.

4. Schomig A, Kastrati A, Dirschinger J, et al: Coronary stenting plus platelet glycoprotein IIb/IIIa blockade compared with tissue plasminogen activator in acute myocardial infarction. Stent versus Thrombolysis for Occluded Coronary Arteries in Patients with Acute Myocardial Infarction Study Investigators. N Engl J Med 343:385, 2000.

5. Keeley EC, Boura JA, Grines CL: Primary angioplasty versus intravenous thrombolytic therapy for acute myocardial infarction: A quantitative review of 23 randomised trials. Lancet 361:13, 2003.

6. Grines CL, Serruys P, O'Neill WW: Fibrinolytic therapy: Is it a treatment of the past? Circulation 107:2538, 2003.

7. Antman EM, Anbe DT, Armstrong PW, et al: ACC/AHA guidelines for the management of patients with ST-elevation myocardial infarction: A report of the American College of Cardiology/American Heart Association Task Force on Practice Guidelines (Committee to Revise the 1999 Guidelines for the Management of Patients with Acute Myocardial Infarction). Circulation 110:e82, 2004.

8. Prasad A, Gersh BJ: Management of microvascular dysfunction and reperfusion injury. Heart 91:1530, 2005.

9. Gibson CM, Schomig A: Coronary and myocardial angiography: Angiographic assessment of both epicardial and myocardial perfusion. Circulation 109:3096, 2004.

10. Costantini CO, Stone GW, Mehran R, et al: Frequency, correlates, and clinical implications of myocardial perfusion after primary angioplasty and stenting, with and without glycoprotein IIb/IIIa inhibition, in acute myocardial infarction. J Am Coll Cardiol 44:305, 2004.

11. Zeymer U, Schroder R, Machnig T, et al: Primary percutaneous transluminal coronary angioplasty accelerates early myocardial reperfusion compared to thrombolytic therapy in patients with acute myocardial infarction. Am Heart J 146:686, 2003.

12. Dibra A, Mehilli J, Dirschinger J, et al: Thrombolysis in myocardial infarction myocardial perfusion grade in angiography correlates with myocardial salvage in patients with acute myocardial infarction treated with stenting or thrombolysis. J Am Coll Cardiol 42:925, 2003.

13. Llevadot J, Giugliano RP, McCabe CH, et al: Degree of residual stenosis in the culprit coronary artery after thrombolytic administration (Thrombolysis In Myocardial Infarction [TIMI] trials). Am J Cardiol 85:1409, 2000.

14. Gibson CM, Karha J, Murphy SA, et al: Early and long-term clinical outcomes associated with reinfarction following fibrinolytic administration in the Thrombolysis in Myocardial Infarction trials. J Am Coll Cardiol 42:7, 2003.

15. Wilson SH, Bell MR, Rihal CS, et al: Infarct artery reocclusion after primary angioplasty, stent placement, and thrombolytic therapy for acute myocardial infarction. Am Heart J 141:704, 2001.

16. Grines CL, Marsalese DL, Brodie B, et al: Safety and cost-effectiveness of early discharge after primary angioplasty in low risk patients with acute myocardial infarction. PAMI-II Investigators. Primary Angioplasty in Myocardial Infarction. J Am Coll Cardiol 31:967, 1998.

17. De Luca G, Suryapranata H, van't Hof AW, et al: Prognostic assessment of patients with acute myocardial infarction treated with primary angioplasty: Implications for early discharge. Circulation 109:2737, 2004.

18. Kinn JW, O'Neill WW, Benzuly KH, et al: Primary angioplasty reduces risk of myocardial rupture compared to thrombolysis for acute myocardial infarction. Cathet Cardiovasc Diagn 42:151, 1997.

19. Moreno R, Lopez-Sendon J, Garcia E, et al: Primary angioplasty reduces the risk of left ventricular free wall rupture compared with thrombolysis in patients with acute myocardial infarction. J Am Coll Cardiol 39:598, 2002.

Timing of Interventions

20. Cannon CP, Gibson CM, Lambrew CT, et al: Relationship of symptom-onset-to-balloon time and door-to-balloon time with mortality in patients undergoing angioplasty for acute myocardial infarction. JAMA 283:2941, 2000.

21. Zijlstra F, Patel A, Jones M, et al: Clinical characteristics and outcome of patients with early (<2 h), intermediate (2-4 h) and late (>4 h) presentation treated by primary coronary angioplasty or thrombolytic therapy for acute myocardial infarction. Eur Heart J 23:550, 2002.

22. Schomig A, Ndrepepa G, Mehilli J, et al: Therapy-dependent influence of time-to-treatment interval on myocardial salvage in patients with acute myocardial infarction treated with coronary artery stenting or thrombolysis. Circulation 108:1084, 2003.

23. Brodie BR, Stuckey TD, Muncy DB, et al: Importance of time-to-reperfusion in patients with acute myocardial infarction with and without cardiogenic shock treated with primary percutaneous coronary intervention. Am Heart J 145:708, 2003.

24. Newby LK, Rutsch WR, Califf RM, et al: Time from symptom onset to treatment and outcomes after thrombolytic therapy. GUSTO-1 Investigators. J Am Coll Cardiol 27:1646, 1996.

25. Smith SC, Jr., Feldman TE, Hirshfeld JW, Jr., et al: ACC/AHA/SCAI 2005 Guideline Update for Percutaneous Coronary Intervention—summary article: A report of the American College of Cardiology/American Heart Association Task Force on Practice Guidelines (ACC/AHA/SCAI Writing Committee to Update the 2001 Guidelines for Percutaneous Coronary Intervention). Circulation 113:156, 2006.

26. De Luca G, Suryapranata H, Zijlstra F, et al: Symptom-onset-to-balloon time and mortality in patients with acute myocardial infarction treated by primary angioplasty. J Am Coll Cardiol 42:991, 2003.

27. De Luca G, Suryapranata H, Ottervanger JP, et al: Time delay to treatment and mortality in primary angioplasty for acute myocardial infarction: Every minute of delay counts. Circulation 109:1223, 2004.

28. Nallamothu BK, Bates ER: Percutaneous coronary intervention versus fibrinolytic therapy in acute myocardial infarction: Is timing (almost) everything? Am J Cardiol 92:824-826, 2003.

29. Nallamothu BK, Antman EM, Bates ER: Primary percutaneous coronary intervention versus fibrinolytic therapy in acute myocardial infarction: Does the choice of fibrinolytic agent impact on the importance of time-to-treatment? Am J Cardiol 94:772, 2004.

30. Betriu A, Masotti M: Comparison of mortality rates in acute myocardial infarction treated by percutaneous coronary intervention versus fibrinolysis. Am J Cardiol 95:100, 2005.

31. Tarantini G, Razzolini R, Ramondo A, et al: Explanation for the survival benefit of primary angioplasty over thrombolytic therapy in patients with ST-elevation acute myocardial infarction. Am J Cardiol 96:1503, 2005.

32. Boersma E: Does time matter? A pooled analysis of randomized clinical trials comparing primary percutaneous coronary intervention and in-hospital fibrinolysis in acute myocardial infarction patients. Eur Heart J 27:779, 2006.

33. Jacobs AK, Antman EM, Ellrodt G, et al; American Heart Association's Acute Myocardial Infarction Advisory Working Group: Recommendation to develop strategies to increase the number of ST-segment-elevation myocardial infarction patients with timely access to primary percutaneous coronary intervention. Circulation 113:2152, 2006.

34. Dalby M, Bouzamondo A, Lechat P, et al: Transfer for primary angioplasty versus immediate thrombolysis in acute myocardial infarction: A meta-analysis. Circulation 108:1809, 2003.

35. Andersen HR, Nielsen TT, Rasmussen K, et al: A comparison of coronary angioplasty with fibrinolytic therapy in acute myocardial infarction. N Engl J Med 349:733, 2003.

36. Bonnefoy E, Lapostolle F, Leizorovicz A, et al: Primary angioplasty versus prehospital fibrinolysis in acute myocardial infarction: A randomised study. Lancet 360:825, 2002.

37. Steg PG, Bonnefoy E, Chabaud S, et al: Impact of time to treatment on mortality after prehospital fibrinolysis or primary angioplasty: Data from the CAPTIM randomized clinical trial. Circulation 108:2851, 2003.

38. Thune JJ, Hoefsten DE, Lindholm MG, et al: Simple risk stratification at admission to identify patients with reduced mortality from primary angioplasty. Circulation 112:2017, 2005.

39. Nallamothu BK, Bates ER, Herrin J, et al: Times to treatment in transfer patients undergoing primary percutaneous coronary intervention in the United States: National Registry of Myocardial Infarction (NRMI)-3/4 analysis. Circulation 111:761, 2005.

40. Nallamothu BK, Bates ER, Wang Y, et al: Driving times and distances to hospitals with percutaneous coronary intervention in the United States: Implications for prehospital triage of patients with ST-elevation myocardial infarction. Circulation 113:1189, 2006.

41. Aversano T, Aversano LT, Passamani E, et al: Thrombolytic therapy vs primary percutaneous coronary intervention for myocardial infarction in patients presenting to hospitals without on-site cardiac surgery: A randomized controlled trial. JAMA 287:1943, 2002.

42. Moscucci M, O'Donnell M, Share D, et al: Frequency and prognosis of emergency coronary artery bypass grafting after percutaneous coronary intervention for acute myocardial infarction. Am J Cardiol 92:967, 2003.

43. Eagle KA, Goodman SG, Avezum A, et al: Practice variation and missed opportunities for reperfusion in ST-segment-elevation myocardial infarction: Findings from the Global Registry of Acute Coronary Events (GRACE). Lancet 359:373, 2002.

Outcomes Post Primary PCI

44. Grzybowski M, Clements EA, Parsons L, et al: Mortality benefit of immediate revascularization of acute ST-segment elevation myocardial infarction in patients with contraindications to thrombolytic therapy: A propensity analysis. JAMA 290:1891, 2003.

45. Massel D. Primary angioplasty in acute myocardial infarction: Hypothetical estimate of superiority over aspirin or untreated controls. Am J Med 118:113, 2005.

46. Kastrati A, Mehilli J, Nekolla S, et al: A randomized trial comparing myocardial salvage achieved by coronary stenting versus balloon angioplasty in patients with acute myocardial infarction considered ineligible for reperfusion therapy. J Am Coll Cardiol 43:734, 2004.

47. Lane GE, Holmes DR: The modern strategy for cardiogenic shock. In Cannon CP (ed): Management of Acute Coronary Syndromes. Totowa, NJ, Humana Press, 2003, pp 603-652.

48. French JK, Feldman HA, Assmann SF, et al: Influence of thrombolytic therapy, with or without intra-aortic balloon counterpulsation, on 12-month survival in the SHOCK trial. Am Heart J 146:804, 2003.

49. Babaev A, Frederick PD, Pasta DJ, et al: Trends in management and outcomes of patients with acute myocardial infarction complicated by cardiogenic shock. JAMA 294:448, 2005.

50. Hochman JS, Sleeper LA, White HD, et al: One-year survival following early revascularization for cardiogenic shock. JAMA 285:190, 2001.

51. Dzavik V, Sleeper LA, Cocke TP, et al: Early revascularization is associated with improved survival in elderly patients with acute myocardial infarction complicated by cardiogenic shock: A report from the SHOCK Trial Registry. Eur Heart J 24:828, 2003.

52. Webb JG, Lowe AM, Sanborn TA, et al: Percutaneous coronary intervention for cardiogenic shock in the SHOCK trial. J Am Coll Cardiol 42:1380, 2003.

53. Chan AW, Chew DP, Bhatt DL, et al: Long-term mortality benefit with the combination of stents and abciximab for cardiogenic shock complicating acute myocardial infarction. Am J Cardiol 89:132, 2002.

54. White HD, Assmann SF, Sanborn TA, et al: Comparison of percutaneous coronary intervention and coronary artery bypass grafting after acute myocardial infarction complicated by cardiogenic shock: Results from the Should We Emergently Revascularize Occluded Coronaries for Cardiogenic Shock (SHOCK) trial. Circulation 112:1992, 2005.

55. Hochman JS: Cardiogenic shock complicating acute myocardial infarction: Expanding the paradigm. Circulation 107:2998, 2003.

56. Mehta RH, Granger CB, Alexander KP, et al: Reperfusion strategies for acute myocardial infarction in the elderly: Benefits and risks. J Am Coll Cardiol 45:471, 2005.

57. Bueno H, Martinez-Selles M, Perez-David E, et al: Effect of thrombolytic therapy on the risk of cardiac rupture and mortality in older patients with first acute myocardial infarction. Eur Heart J 26:1705, 2005.

58. de Boer MJ, Ottervanger JP, van't Hof AW, et al: Reperfusion therapy in elderly patients with acute myocardial infarction: A randomized comparison of primary angioplasty and thrombolytic therapy. J Am Coll Cardiol 39:1723, 2002.

59. Grines C: Senior PAMI: A prospective randomized trial of primary angioplasty and thrombolytic therapy in elderly patients with acute myocardial infarction. Presented at Transcatheter Cardiovascular Therapeutics, Washington, DC, October 19, 2005.

60. Minai K, Horie H, Takahashi M, et al: Long-term outcome of primary percutaneous transluminal coronary angioplasty for low-risk acute myocardial infarction in patients older than 80 years: A single-center, open, randomized trial. Am Heart J 143:497, 2002.

61. de Feyter PJ: Percutaneous treatment of saphenous vein bypass graft obstructions: A continuing obstinate problem. Circulation 107:2284, 2003.

62. Nguyen TT, O'Neill WW, Grines CL, et al: One-year survival in patients with acute myocardial infarction and a saphenous vein graft culprit treated with primary angioplasty. Am J Cardiol 91:1250, 2003.

63. Brodie BR, VerSteeg DS, Brodie MM, et al: Poor long-term patient and graft survival after primary percutaneous coronary intervention for acute myocardial infarction due to saphenous vein graft occlusion. Catheter Cardiovasc Interv 65:504, 2005.

64. Elad Y, French WJ, Shavelle DM, et al: Primary angioplasty and selection bias inpatients presenting late (>12 h) after onset of chest pain and ST elevation myocardial infarction. J Am Coll Cardiol 39:826, 2002.

65. Hochman JS, Lamas GA, Buller CE, et al: Coronary intervention for persistent occlusion after myocardial infarction. N Engl J Med 355:2395, 2006.

66. Schomig A, Mehilli J, Antoniucci D, et al: Mechanical reperfusion in patients with acute myocardial infarction presenting more than 12 hours from symptom onset: A randomized controlled trial. JAMA 293:2865, 2005.

Adjunctive Therapies

67. Antoniucci D, Rodriguez A, Hempel A, et al: A randomized trial comparing primary infarct artery stenting with or without abciximab in acute myocardial infarction. J Am Coll Cardiol 42:1879, 2003.

68. De Luca G, Suryapranata H, Stone GW, et al: Abciximab as adjunctive therapy to reperfusion in acute ST-segment elevation myocardial infarction: A meta-analysis of randomized trials. JAMA 293:1759, 2005.

69. Stone GW, Grines CL, Cox DA, et al: Comparison of angioplasty with stenting, with or without abciximab, in acute myocardial infarction. N Engl J Med 346:957, 2002.

70. De Luca G, Ernst N, Zijlstra F, et al: Preprocedural TIMI flow and mortality in patients with acute myocardial infarction treated by primary angioplasty. J Am Coll Cardiol 43:1363, 2004.

71. Montalescot G, Borentain M, Payot L, et al: Early vs late administration of glycoprotein IIb/IIIa inhibitors in primary percutaneous coronary intervention of acute ST-segment elevation myocardial infarction: A meta-analysis. JAMA 292:362, 2004.

72. Wohrle J, Grebe OC, Nusser T, et al: Reduction of major adverse cardiac events with intracoronary compared with intravenous bolus application of abciximab in patients with acute myocardial infarction or unstable angina undergoing coronary angioplasty. Circulation 107:1840, 2003.

73. Cox DA, Stone GW, Grines CL, et al: Outcomes of optimal or "stent-like" balloon angioplasty in acutemyocardial infarction: The CADILLAC trial. J Am Coll Cardiol 42:971, 2003.

74. Zhu MM, Feit A, Chadow H, et al: Primary stent implantation compared with primary balloon angioplasty for acute myocardial infarction: A meta-analysis of randomized clinical trials. Am J Cardiol 88:297, 2001.

75. Mehta RH, Harjai KJ, Cox DA, et al: Comparison of coronary stenting versus conventional balloon angioplasty on five-year mortality in patients with acute myocardial infarction undergoing primary percutaneous coronary intervention. Am J Cardiol 96:901, 2005.

76. Valgimigli M, Percoco G, Malagutti P, et al: Tirofiban and sirolimus-eluting stent vs abciximab and bare-metal stent for acute myocardial infarction: A randomized trial. JAMA 293:2109, 2005.

77. Spaulding C, Henry P, Teiger E, et al: Final results of the TYPHOON study: A mulitcenter randomized trial comparing the use of sirolimus-eluting stents to bare metal stents in primary angioplasty for acute myocardial infarction. J Am Coll Cardiol 47:50B, 2006.

78. Menichilli M: Randomised trial of Sirolimus stent vs bare metal stent in acute myocardial infarction (SESAMI). Presented at Paris Course on Revascularization, Paris, May 15, 2006.

79. Dirksen M: PASSION: Randomized comparison of paclitaxel-eluting stent versus conventional stent in STEMI. Presented at the Annual Scientific Session of the American College of Cardiology, Atlanta, March 13, 2006.

80. Henriques JP, Zijlstra F, Ottervanger JP, et al: Incidence and clinical significance of distal embolization during primary angioplasty for acute myocardial infarction. Eur Heart J 23:1112, 2002.

81. Limbruno U, De Caterina R: EMERALD, AIMI, and PROMISE: Is there still a potential for embolic protection in primary PCI? Eur Heart J 27:1139, 2006.

82. Stone GW, Webb J, Cox DA, et al: Distal microcirculatory protection during percutaneous coronary intervention in acute ST-segment elevation myocardial infarction: A randomized controlled trial. JAMA 293:1063, 2005.

83. Gick M, Jander N, Bestehorn HP, et al: Randomized evaluation of the effects of filter-based distal protection on myocardial perfusion and infarct size after primary percutaneous catheter intervention in myocardial infarction with and without ST-segment elevation. Circulation 112:1462, 2005.

84. Ali A: Is thrombectomy of benefit in any patients with STEMI? Long-term and subset data from AiMI. Presented at Transcatheter Cardiovascular Therapeutics, Washington, DC, October 20, 2005.

85. Mehta SR, Yusuf S, Diaz R, et al: Effect of glucose-insulin-potassium infusion on mortality in patients with acute ST-segment elevation myocardial infarction: The CREATE-ECLA randomized controlled trial. JAMA 293:437, 2005.

86. Tzivoni D: Reduction of infarct size and improved left ventricular function with IV Caldaret (MCC-135) in patients with ST elevation myocardial infarction undergoing PCI. Presented at the Annual Scientific Session of the American College of Cardiology, New Orleans, March 7, 2004.

87. Granger CB, Mahaffey KW, Weaver WD, et al: Pexelizumab, an anti-C5 complement antibody, as adjunctive therapy to primary percutaneous coronary intervention in acute myocardial infarction: The COMplement inhibition in Myocardial infarction treated with Angioplasty (COMMA) trial. Circulation 108:1184, 2003.

88. Ross AM, Gibbons RJ, Stone GW, et al: A randomized, double-blinded, placebo-controlled multicenter trial of adenosine as an adjunct to reperfusion in the treatment of acute myocardial infarction (AMISTAD-II). J Am Coll Cardiol 45:1775, 2005.

89. Ono H, Osanai T, Ishizaka H, et al: Nicorandil improves cardiac function and clinical outcome in patients with acute myocardial infarction undergoing primary percutaneous coronary intervention: Role of inhibitory effect on reactive oxygen species formation. Am Heart J 148:E15, 2004.

90. Dixon SR: Infarct angioplasty: Beyond stents and glycoprotein IIb/IIIa inhibitors. Heart 91(Suppl 3):iii2, 2005.

91. Serruys PW: Fourth Annual American College of Cardiology International Lecture: A journey in the interventional field. J Am Coll Cardiol 47:1754, 2006.

"Rescue" and "Facilitated" PCI

92. Holmes DR Jr, Coreh BJ, Ellie SC: Rescue percutaneous coronary intervention after failed fibrinolytic therapy: Have expectations been met? Am Heart J 151:779, 2006.

93. Sutton AG, Campbell PG, Graham R, et al: A randomized trial of rescue angioplasty versus a conservative approach for failed fibrinolysis in ST-segment elevation myocardial infarction: The Middlesbrough Early Revascularization to Limit INfarction (MERLIN) trial. J Am Coll Cardiol 44:287, 2004.

94. Schomig A, Ndrepepa G, Mehilli J, et al: A randomized trial of coronary stenting versus balloon angioplasty as a rescue intervention after failed thrombolysis in patients with acute myocardial infarction. J Am Coll Cardiol 44:2073, 2004.

95. Gershlick AH, Stephens-Lloyd A, Hughes S, et al: Rescue angioplasty after failed thrombolytic therapy for acute myocardial infarction. N Engl J Med 353:2758, 2005.

96. French JK, Ramanathan K, Stewart JT, et al: A score predicts failure of reperfusion after fibrinolytic therapy for acute myocardial infarction. Am Heart J 145:508, 2003.

97. Schweiger MJ, Cannon CP, Murphy SA, et al: Early coronary intervention following pharmacologic therapy for acute myocardial infarction (the combined TIMI 10B-TIMI 14 experience). Am J Cardiol 88:831, 2001.

98. Assessment of the Safety and Efficacy of a New Treatment Strategy with Percutaneous Coronary Intervention (ASSENT-4 PCI) investigators: Primary versus tenecteplase-facilitated percutaneous coronary intervention in patients with ST-segment elevation acute myocardial infarction (ASSENT-4 PCI): Randomised trial. Lancet 367:569, 2006.

99. Kastrati A, Mehilli J, Schlotterbeck K, et al: Early administration of reteplase plus abciximab vs abciximab alone in patients with acute myocardial infarction referred for percutaneous coronary intervention: A randomized controlled trial. JAMA 291:947, 2004.

100. Keeley EC, Boura JA, Grines CL: Comparison of primary and facilitated percutaneous coronary interventions for ST-elevation myocardial infarction: Quantitative review of randomised trials. Lancet 367:579, 2006.

101. Fernandez-Aviles F, Alonso JJ, Castro-Beiras A, et al: Routine invasive strategy within 24 hours of thrombolysis versus ischaemia-guided conservative approach for acute myocardial infarction with ST-segment elevation (GRACIA-1): A randomised controlled trial. Lancet 364:1045, 2004.

102. Kalla K, Christ G, Karnik R, et al: Implementation of guidelines improves the standard of care: The Viennese registry on reperfusion strategies in ST-elevation myocardial infarction (Vienna STEMI registry). Circulation 113:2398, 2006.

103. Nallamothu BK, Wang Y, Magid DJ, et al: Relation between hospital specialization with primary percutaneous coronary intervention and clinical outcomes in ST-

segment elevation myocardial infarction: National Registry of Myocardial Infarction-4 analysis. Circulation 113:222, 2006.

104. Faxon DP: Beta-blocker therapy and primary angioplasty: What is the controversy? J Am Coll Cardiol 43:1788, 2004.

105. Chen ZM, Pan HC, Chen YP, et al: Early intravenous then oral metoprolol in 45,852 patients with acute myocardial infarction: Randomised placebo-controlled trial. Lancet 366:1622, 2005.

106. Yusuf S, Mehta SR, Chrolavicius S, et al: Effects of fondaparinux on mortality and reinfarction in patients with acute ST-segment elevation myocardial infarction: The OASIS-6 randomized trial. JAMA 295:1519, 2006.

107. Loubeyre C, Morice MC, Lefevre T, et al: A randomized comparison of direct stenting with conventional stent implantation in selected patients with acute myocardial infarction. J Am Coll Cardiol 39:15, 2002.

108. Kralev S, Poerner TC, Basorth D, et al: Side branch occlusion after coronary stent implantation in patients presenting with ST-elevation myocardial infarction: Clinical impact and angiographic predictors. Am Heart J 151:153, 2006.

109. Ong AT, Hoye A, Aoki J, et al: Thirty-day incidence and six-month clinical outcome of thrombotic stent occlusion after bare-metal, sirolimus, or paclitaxel stent implantation. J Am Coll Cardiol 45:947, 2005.

110. Hendler A, Aronovich A, Kaluski E, et al: Optimization of myocardial perfusion after primary coronary angioplasty following an acute myocardial infarction. Beyond TIMI 3 flow. J Invasive Cardiol 18:32, 2006.

111. Skelding KA, Goldstein JA, Mehta L, et al: Resolution of refractory no-reflow with intracoronary epinephrine. Catheter Cardiovasc Interv 57:305, 2002.

112. Corpus RA, House JA, Marso SP, et al: Multivessel percutaneous coronary intervention in patients with multivessel disease and acute myocardial infarction. Am Heart J 148:493, 2004.

113. Goldstein JA, Demetriou D, Grines CL, et al: Multiple complex coronary plaques in patients with acute myocardial infarction. N Engl J Med 343:915, 2000.

114. Chen LY, Lennon RJ, Grantham JA, et al: In-hospital and long-term outcomes of multivessel percutaneous coronary revascularization after acute myocardial infarction. Am J Cardiol 95:349, 2005.

 GUIDELINES *Thomas H. Lee*

Primary Percutaneous Coronary Intervention in Acute Myocardial Infarction

The American College of Cardiology and American Heart Association (ACC/AHA) published comprehensive guidelines on percutaneous coronary interventions (PCIs) in 2006.[1] The new guidelines include recommendations regarding several specific issues relevant to primary PCI. These issues were also addressed in prior ACC/AHA guidelines on acute myocardial infarction[3] and unstable angina.[4]

As with other ACC/AHA guidelines, these use the standard ACC/AHA classification system for indications:

Class I: Conditions for which there is evidence and/or general agreement that the test is useful and effective

Class II: Conditions for which there is conflicting evidence and/or a divergence of opinion about the usefulness or efficacy of performing the test

CH 52

Class IIa: Weight of evidence or opinion is in favor of usefulness or efficacy

Class IIb: Usefulness or efficacy is less well established by evidence or opinion

Class III: Conditions for which there is evidence and/or general agreement that the test is not useful or effective and in some cases may be harmful

Three levels are used to rate the evidence on which recommendations have been based. Level A recommendations are derived from data from multiple randomized clinical trials, level B recommendations are derived from a single randomized trial or nonrandomized studies, and level C recommendations are based on the consensus opinion of experts.

PRIMARY PERCUTANEOUS CORONARY INTERVENTION VERSUS FIBRINOLYSIS FOR ACUTE TRANSMURAL MYOCARDIAL INFARCTION

The ACC/AHA guidelines support the use of PCI as an alternative to fibrinolysis for patients with acute ST-elevation myocardial infarction (STEMI) with new or presumably new left bundle branch block on the electrocardiogram (ECG) within the first 12 hours after the onset of symptoms, and afterward if such symptoms continue (Table 52G-1). The procedure should be performed by a highly experienced operator in a high-volume facility as rapidly as possible. Time from symptom onset to reperfusion is a critical predictor of outcome. The guidelines recommend a goal of balloon inflation (door to balloon time) of less than 90 minutes from presentation. Mortality risk increases significantly with each 15-minute delay between time of hospital arrival and restoration of thrombolysis in myocardial infarction 3 (TIMI-3) flow.

PCI is endorsed for a longer period (up to 36 hours after the onset of infarction) for patients who present in cardiogenic shock if they are younger than 75 years (and may be reasonable for older patients) and the procedure can be performed within 18 hours of the onset of shock.

The guidelines do not support the use of PCI for non–infarct-related arteries at the time of acute myocardial infarction (AMI) and for patients who are asymptomatic after receiving fibrinolytic therapy within 12 hours.

Primary PCI should be performed in fibrinolytic-ineligible patients who present with STEMI within 12 hours of symptom onset, and may be reasonable up to 24 hours after symptom onset in patients with severe heart failure, hemodynamic or electrical instability, or evidence of persistent ischemia (Table 52G-2).

PERCUTANEOUS CORONARY INTERVENTION AFTER FIBRINOLYSIS

Performance of coronary angiography and PCI soon after failed fibrinolysis (rescue PCI) can improve infarct-related artery patency and long-term outcomes in select patients (Table 52G-3). The guidelines note that a major impediment to rescue PCI is the difficulty in accurately identifying patients in whom fibrinolytic therapy has not restored antegrade coronary flow.

Coronary angiography and PCI are commonly performed after successful fibrinolysis in all age groups, even though this strategy has not been studied extensively in clinical trials. Therefore, the ACC/AHA guidelines support relatively conservative use of angiography and PCI for patients after fibrinolysis. It is considered appropriate for patients with objective evidence of recurrent infarction or ischemia and is also given support for patients with cardiogenic shock or hemodynamic instability.

Facilitated PCI, a strategy of planned PCI immediately after an initial pharmacological regimen that includes fibrinolytic therapy and/or a glycoprotein (GP) IIb/IIIa inhibitor, may be performed in higher risk patients when PCI is not immediately available and bleeding risk is low (see Table 52G-3).

PERCUTANEOUS CORONARY INTERVENTION LATER DURING HOSPITALIZATION

The guidelines support use of PCI after the immediate treatment of AMI in reaction to clinical evidence of ischemia and for persistent hemodynamic instability (Table 52G-4; see Table 52G-3). The ACC/AHA task force did not provide much support for use of PCI for routine care of patients who were clinically stable. Given the current data, with the exception of patients presenting with cardiogenic shock, use of PCI post-STEMI should be determined by clinical need without special consideration for age. The presence of prior MI places the patient in a higher risk subset and should be considered in the PCI decision.

TABLE 52G–1 · ACC/AHA General and Specific Considerations for Performance of Percutaneous Coronary Intervention (PCI) for Acute ST-Elevation Myocardial Infarction (STEMI) as an Alternative to Fibrinolysis

Class	Indication	Level of Evidence
Class I (indicated)	If immediately available, primary PCI should be performed in patients with STEMI (including true posterior MI) or MI with new or presumably new left bundle branch block who can undergo PCI of the infarct artery within 12 hr of symptom onset, if performed in a timely fashion by operators skilled in the procedure at a high-volume facility with an appropriate laboratory environment.	A
	Primary PCI should be performed as quickly as possible, with a goal of a medical contact to balloon or door to balloon time within 90 min.	B
	Primary PCI should be performed for patients younger than 75 yr with ST elevation or presumably new left bundle branch block who develop shock within 36 hr of MI and are suitable for revascularization that can be performed within 18 hr of shock, unless further support is futile because of the patient's wishes or contraindications or unsuitability for further invasive care.	A
	Primary PCI should be performed in patients with severe congestive heart failure and/or pulmonary edema (Killip class 3) and onset of symptoms within 12 hr. The medical contact to balloon or door to balloon time should be as short as possible (i.e., goal within 90 min).	B
Class IIa (good supportive evidence)	Primary PCI is reasonable for selected patients 75 yr or older with ST elevation or left bundle branch block or who develop shock within 36 hr of MI and are suitable for revascularization that can be performed within 18 hr of shock; patients should have good prior functional status, be suitable for revascularization, and agree to invasive care.	B
	It is reasonable to perform primary PCI for patients with onset of symptoms within the prior 12 to 24 hr and one or more of the following: Severe congestive heart failure Hemodynamic or electrical instability Evidence of persistent ischemia	C
Class IIb (weak supportive evidence)	The benefit of primary PCI for STEMI patients eligible for fibrinolysis when performed by an operator who performs fewer than 75 PCI procedures/yr (or fewer than 11 PCIs for STEMI/yr) is not well established.	C
Class III (not indicated)	Elective PCI should not be performed in a non–infarct-related artery at the time of primary PCI of the infarct-related artery in patients without hemodynamic compromise.	C
	Primary PCI should not be performed in asymptomatic patients more than 12 hr after onset of STEMI who are hemodynamically and electrically stable.	C

ACC/AHA = American College of Cardiology/American Heart Association; MI = myocardial infarction; PCI = percutaneous coronary intervention; STEMI = ST-elevation myocardial infarction.

TABLE 52G–2 · ACC/AHA Guidelines for Performance of Percutaneous Coronary Intervention (PCI) for Acute ST-Elevation Myocardial Infarction (STEMI) in Fibrinolytic-Ineligible Patients

Class	Indication	Level of Evidence
Class I (indicated)	Primary PCI should be performed in fibrinolytic-ineligible patients who present with STEMI within 12 hr of symptom onset.	C
Class IIa (good supportive evidence)	Primary PCI may reasonably be performed for fibrinolytic-ineligible patients with onset of symptoms within the prior 12 to 24 hr and one or more of the following: Severe congestive heart failure Hemodynamic or electrical instability Evidence of persistent ischemia	C

ACC/AHA = American College of Cardiology/American Heart Association; PCI = percutaneous coronary intervention; STEMI = ST-elevation myocardial infarction.

TABLE 52G–3 · ACC/AHA Guidelines for Performance of Percutaneous Coronary Intervention (PCI) after Failed Fibrinolysis for Acute ST-Elevation Myocardial Infarction (Rescue PCI)

Class	Indication	Level of Evidence
Class I (indicated)	Rescue PCI should be performed in patients younger than 75 yr with ST elevation or left bundle branch block who develop shock within 36 hr of MI and are suitable for revascularization that can be performed within 18 hr of shock, unless further support is futile because of the patient's wishes or contradictions/unsuitability for further invasive care.	B
	Rescue PCI should be performed in patients with severe congestive heart failure and/or pulmonary edema (Killip class 3) and onset of symptoms within 12 hr.	B
Class IIa (good supportive evidence)	Rescue PCI is reasonable for selected patients 75 yr or older with ST elevation or left bundle branch block or who develop shock within 36 hr of MI and are suitable for revascularization that can be performed within 18 hr of shock. Patients with good prior functional status who are suitable for revascularization and agree to invasive care may be selected for such an invasive strategy.	B
	It is reasonable to perform rescue PCI for patients with one or more of the following: Hemodynamic or electrical instability Evidence of persistent ischemia	C
Class III (not indicated)	Rescue PCI in the absence of one or more of the above Class I or IIa indications is not recommended.	C

ACC/AHA = American College of Cardiology/American Heart Association; MI = myocardial infarction; PCI = percutaneous coronary intervention.

TABLE 52G–4	ACC/AHA Guidelines for Performance of Percutaneous Coronary Intervention after Successful Fibrinolysis or for Patients Not Undergoing Primary Reperfusion for Acute ST-Elevation Myocardial Infarction	
Class	**Indication**	**Level of Evidence**
Class I (indicated)	In patients whose anatomy is suitable, PCI should be performed when there is objective evidence of recurrent MI.	C
	In patients whose anatomy is suitable, PCI should be performed for moderate or severe spontaneous or provocable myocardial ischemia during recovery from STEMI.	B
	In patients whose anatomy is suitable, PCI should be performed for cardiogenic shock or hemodynamic instability.	B
Class IIa (good supportive evidence)	It is reasonable to perform routine PCI in patients with left ventricular ejection fraction ≦0.40, heart failure, or serious ventricular arrhythmias.	C
	It is reasonable to perform PCI when there is documented clinical heart failure during the acute episode, even though subsequent evaluation shows preserved left ventricular function (left ventricular ejection fraction >0.40).	C
Class IIb (weak supportive evidence)	PCI might be considered as part of an invasive strategy for fibrinolytic therapy.	C
	Facilitated PCI might be performed as a reperfusion strategy in higher risk patients when PCI is not immediately available and bleeding risk is low.	B

ACC/AHA = American College of Cardiology/American Heart Association; MI = myocardial infarction; PCI = percutaneous coronary intervention; STEMI = ST-elevation myocardial infarction.

CH 52

TABLE 52G–5	Operator and Institutional Considerations for Primary PCI for Acute ST-Elevation Myocardial Infarction (STEMI)	
Class	**Indication**	**Level of Evidence**
Class I (indicated)	Primary PCI for STEMI should be performed by experienced operators who do more than 75 elective PCI procedures/yr and, ideally, at least 11 PCI procedures for STEMI/yr. These procedures are best performed in institutions with on-site emergency cardiac surgery services that perform more than 400 elective PCIs and more than 36 primary PCI procedures for STEMI/yr.	B
Class IIb (weak supportive evidence)	The benefit of primary PCI for STEMI patients eligible for fibrinolysis when performed by an operator who performs fewer that 75 procedures/yr (or fewer than 11 PCIs for STEMI/yr) is not well established.	C
	Primary PCI for patients with STEMI might be considered in hospitals without on-site cardiac surgery, provided that appropriate planning for program development has been accomplished, including appropriately experienced physician operators (see Class I indication), an experienced catheterization team on call 24 hr a day, 7 days a week, a well-equipped catheterization laboratory, and a proven plan for rapid transport to a cardiac surgery operating room in a nearby hospital with appropriate hemodynamic support capability for transfer.	B
Class III (not indicated)	Primary PCI should not be performed in hospitals without on-site cardiac surgery and without a proven plan for rapid transport to a cardiac surgery operating room in a nearby hospital or without appropriate hemodynamic support capability for transfer.	C

MI = myocardial infarction; PCI = percutaneous coronary intervention; STEMI = ST-elevation myocardial infarction.

ADJUNCTIVE MEDICAL THERAPIES

In addition to the standard medical therapies recommended for patients undergoing elective PCI (Table 55G-6), the ACC/AHA guidelines indicate that it is reasonable to administer abciximab as early as possible for patients undergoing emergency PCI for STEMI. The guidelines were less supportive of the use of treatment with eptifibatide or tirofiban or the use of low-molecular-weight heparin as an alternative to unfractionated heparin.

OPERATOR AND INSTITUTIONAL VOLUMES

Elective PCI and primary PCI for STEMI are different, although related, disciplines. Operator experience in elective PCI is not sufficient to confer expertise in primary PCI for STEMI, given that aspects of pro-

cedural conduct are unique to primary PCI for STEMI. Fully functional institutional systems are even more important for PCI for STEMI than for elective PCI for attaining good outcomes.

The guidelines indicate that primary PCI for STEMI should be performed by experienced operators who do more than 75 elective PCI procedures per year and at least 11 PCI procedures for STEMI per year in a surgical center in which more than 400 elective PCIs and more than 36 primary PCI procedures for STEMI are performed each year (Table 52G-5).

PERCUTANEOUS CORONARY INTERVENTION WITHOUT ON-SITE CARDIAC SURGERY

The use of cardiac surgical backup for PCI has become less formal because of low rates of complications requiring emergency cardiac surgery. Some institutions use off-site surgical backup. However, the guidelines note the greater risk associated with emergency PCI and describe specific volume thresholds and institutional systems for hospitals providing this service without cardiac surgical backup.

The guidelines stipulate that primary PCI for STEMI be performed without on-site cardiac surgery only by experienced higher-volume operators (more than 75 elective and more than 11 emergency PCIs for STEMI annually). Other requirements include an experienced catheterization team on call 24 hours a day, 7 days a week, a well-equipped catheterization laboratory, and a proven plan for rapid transport to a cardiac surgery operating room in a nearby hospital with appropriate hemodynamic support capability for transfer (see Table 52G-5).

References

1. Smith SC, Jr., Feldman TE, Hirshfeld JW, Jr., et al: ACC/AHA/SCAI 2005 guideline update for percutaneous coronary intervention: A report of the American College of Cardiology/American Heart Association Task Force on Practice Guidelines (ACC/AHA/SCAI Writing Committee to Update the 2001 Guidelines for Percutaneous Coronary Intervention). J Am Coll Cardiol 47:e1, 2006.
2. Smith SC Jr, Dove JT, Jacobs AK, et al: ACC/AHA guidelines of percutaneous coronary interventions (revision of the 1993 PTCA guidelines)—executive summary. A report of the American College of Cardiology/American Heart Association Task Force on Practice Guidelines (committee to revise the 1993 guidelines for percutaneous transluminal coronary angioplasty). J Am Coll Cardiol 37:2215, 2001.
3. Antman EM, Anbe DT, Armstrong PW, et al: ACC/AHA guidelines for the management of patients with ST-elevation myocardial infarction: A report of the American College of Cardiology/American Heart Association Task Force on Practice Guidelines (Committee to Revise the 1999 Guidelines for the Management of Patients with Acute Myocardial Infarction). Circulation 110:e82, 2004.
4. Braunwald E, Antman EM, Beasley JW, et al: ACC/AHA 2002 guideline update for the management of patients with unstable angina and non-ST-segment elevation myocardial infarction—summary article: A report of the American College of Cardiology/American Heart Association task force on practice guidelines (Committee on the Management of Patients With Unstable Angina). J Am Coll Cardiol 40:1366, 2002.

Unstable Angina and Non-ST Elevation Myocardial Infarction

Christopher P. Cannon and Eugene Braunwald

Definition and Classification, 1319
Definition, 1319
Classification, 1319

Pathophysiology, 1319
Thrombosis, 1320
Platelet Activation and
  Aggregation, 1320
Coronary Vasoconstriction, 1322
Progressive Mechanical
  Obstruction, 1322
Secondary Unstable Angina, 1322

Clinical Presentation, 1322
Clinical Examination, 1322
Electrocardiogram, 1322
Cardiac Necrosis Markers for
  Diagnosis of NSTEMI, 1322
Laboratory Tests, 1323
Coronary Arteriographic
  Findings, 1323

Risk Stratification, 1323
Methods of Risk Stratification, 1324

Medical Therapy, 1326
General Measures, 1326

**Treatment Strategies and
Interventions, 1333**
Timing of an Invasive Strategy, 1334
Summary: Indications for Invasive
  versus Conservative Management
  Strategies, 1334
Other Therapies, 1335
Summary: Acute Management of
  UA/NSTEMI, 1336

Prinzmetal Variant Angina, 1337
Mechanisms, 1338
Clinical and Laboratory
  Findings, 1338
Management, 1338
Prognosis, 1339

References, 1340

Guidelines, 1344

Each year some 1.3 million patients have unstable angina or non-ST elevation myocardial infarction (UA/NSTEMI), a condition also referred to as non-ST elevation acute coronary syndrome (NSTE-ACS).[1] Acute total occlusion of a coronary artery usually causes STEMI (Chap. 50), whereas UA/NSTEMI usually results from severe obstruction, but not total occlusion, of the culprit coronary artery.

DEFINITION AND CLASSIFICATION

Definition

The definition of unstable angina is largely based on the clinical presentation.[49] *Stable angina pectoris* typically manifests as a deep, poorly localized chest or arm discomfort (rarely described as pain), reproducibly precipitated by physical exertion or emotional stress, and relieved within 5 to 15 minutes by rest and/or sublingual nitroglycerin (see Chap. 54). In contrast, *unstable* angina is defined as angina pectoris (or equivalent type of ischemic discomfort) with at least one of three features: (1) occurring at rest (or minimal exertion) and usually lasting >20 minutes (if not interrupted by nitroglycerin administration); (2) being severe and described as frank pain, and of new onset (i.e., within 1 month; and (3) occurring with a crescendo pattern (i.e., more severe, prolonged, or frequent than previously).[2] Of this group, approximately one half will have evidence of myocardial necrosis on the basis of elevated cardiac serum markers, such as creatine kinase isoenzyme (CK)-MB, and/or troponin T or I, and thus have a diagnosis of NSTEMI.

Classification

Because UA/NSTEMI comprises such a heterogeneous group of patients, classification schemes based on clinical features are useful. A clinical classification of UA/NSTEMI, presented by one of the authors (Table 53-1)[3] has been found to be a useful means of stratifying risk.[4] Patients fall into three groups according to the clinical circumstances of the acute ischemic episode: primary unstable angina, secondary angina (e.g., with angina related to obvious precipitating factors such as anemia), and post-MI unstable angina. Patients are also classified according to the severity of the ischemia (see Table 53-1). This classification predicts coronary thrombus at angiography, or in atherectomy specimens, as well as prognosis.[4]

An etiologic approach has been proposed.[5] Five pathophysiological processes may contribute to the development of UA/NSTEMI (Fig. 53-1). These include (1) plaque rupture or erosion with superimposed nonocclusive thrombus (by far the most common cause of UA/NSTEMI); (2) dynamic obstruction (i.e., coronary spasm of an epicardial artery, as in Prinzmetal angina or constriction of the small muscular coronary arteries), (3) progressive mechanical obstruction, (4) inflammation, and (5) secondary unstable angina, related to increased myocardial oxygen demand or decreased supply (e.g., anemia). Individual patients may have several of these processes coexisting as the cause of their episode of UA/NSTEMI. As noted subsequently, several new serum markers can serve as effective tools in identifying these pathophysiological processes, and in predicting outcome—forming the foundation of a "multimarker strategy" for evaluation and risk stratification (Fig. 53-2).[6]

PATHOPHYSIOLOGY

The pathophysiology of UA/NSTEMI involves a broad timeline with three phases rather than an isolated ischemic event. Traditionally, attention focused only on the acute phase of UA/NSTEMI, whereas the pathophysiology may actually begin several decades before the acute clinical event, and then may span more than 20 years afterward. The acute event, which usually involves thrombus formation at the site of a ruptured or eroded atherosclerotic plaque, is currently referred to as "atherothrombosis" (see Chap. 38), a term that is replacing "atherosclerosis" because it more fully describes the pathophysiology of the disease that involves both progression and disruption of the atheroma and superimposed thrombosis.

The acute ischemia in UA/NSTEMI can also result from an increase in myocardial oxygen demand (e.g., precipitated by tachycardia or hypertension) and/or by a reduc-

Class	Definition	Death or MI to One Year* (%)
Severity		
Class I:	New onset of severe angina or accelerated angina; no rest pain	7.3
Class II:	Angina at rest within past month but not within preceding 48 hr (angina at rest, subacute)	10.3
Class III:	Angina at rest within 48 hr (angina at rest, subacute)	10.8[†]
Clinical Circumstances		
A. (Secondary Angina)	Develops in the presence of extracardiac condition that intensifies myocardial ischemia	14.1
B. (Primary Angina):	Develops in the absence of extracardiac condition	8.5
C. (Post Infarction Angina):	Develops within 2 wk after acute myocardial infarction	18.5[‡]
Intensity of treatment	Patients with unstable angina may also be divided into three groups depending on whether unstable angina occurs (1) in the absence of treatment for chronic stable angina; (2) during treatment for chronic stable angina; or (3) despite maximal antiischemic drug therapy. There three groups that may be designated subscripts 1, 2, and 3, respectively.	
ECG changes	Patients with unstable angina may be further divided into those with or without transient ST-T wave changes during pain.	

TABLE 53–1 Braunwald Clinical Classification of UA/NSTEMI

*Data from TIMI III Registry: Scirica BM, et al: Am J Cardiol 90:821-826, 2002.
[†]$p = 0.057$
[‡]$p < 0.001$.
UA/NSTEMI = unstable angina/non-ST elevation myocardial infarction.
From Braunwald E: Unstable angina: A classification. Circulation 80:410-4, 1989.

CH 53

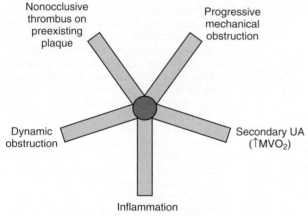

FIGURE 53–1 Schematic representation of the causes of unstable angina (UA). MVO_2 = myocardial O_2 consumption. (Reproduced from Braunwald E: Unstable angina: An etiologic approach to management. Circulation 98:2219-22, 1998.)

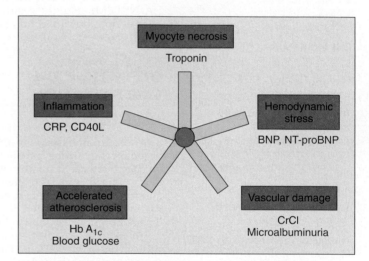

FIGURE 53–2 A multimarker strategy for evaluation of the etiology and prognosis of UA/NSTEMI. Many new markers have recently been identified that can help assess the etiology of a given patient's UA/NSTEMI event. In addition, these now have been seen to be independent markers of an adverse prognosis. BNP = B-type natriuretic peptide; CD40L = CD40 ligand; CrCl = creatinine clearance; Hb A_{1c} = hemoglobin A_{1c}; CRP = C-reactive protein; UA/NSTEMI = unstable angina or non-ST elevation myocardial infarction. (Adapted with permission from Morrow DA, Braunwald E: Circulation. 108:250-2, 2003.)

tion in supply (e.g., due to reduction in coronary lumen diameter by platelet-rich thrombi, vasospasm, or hypotension). Rapid progression of the underlying coronary artery disease can also occur in some patients. A sequence of events has been documented in UA/NSTEMI, in which there is first a reduction in coronary sinus oxygen saturation (signifying a reduction in coronary blood flow), then ST segment depression, followed by chest discomfort, and elevations in blood pressure and/or heart rate.

Thrombosis

The central role of coronary artery thrombosis (see also Chaps. 38 and 82) in the pathogenesis of UA/NSTEMI is supported by six sets of observations: (1) at autopsy, thrombi usually localize at the site of a ruptured or eroded coronary plaque (Fig. 53-3)[7]; (2) coronary atherectomy specimens demonstrate a high incidence of thrombotic lesions as compared with those obtained from stable angina patients; (3) coronary angioscopy frequently visualizes thrombus in UA/NSTEMI[8]; (4) Coronary angiography has demonstrated ulceration or irregularities suggesting a ruptured plaque, and/or thrombus in many patients (Fig. 53-4)[9]; (5) elevation

of several markers of platelet activity and fibrin formation supports ongoing thrombosis[10,11]; and (6) the improvement in the clinical outcome by antithrombotic therapy.

Platelet Activation and Aggregation

Platelets play a key role in the transformation of a stable atherosclerotic plaque to an unstable lesion (Fig. 53-5) (see also Chap. 82). Rupture or ulceration of an atherosclerotic plaque often exposes the subendothelial matrix (e.g., collagen and tissue factor) to circulating blood. The first step is *platelet adhesion* via platelet glycoprotein (GP) Ib binding to von Willebrand factor and GP VI binding to collagen. *Platelet activation* ensues which leads to (1) a shape change in the platelet (from a smooth discoid shape to a spiculated form, which increases the surface area on which thrombin

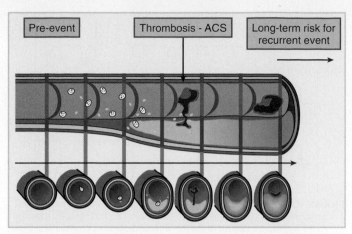

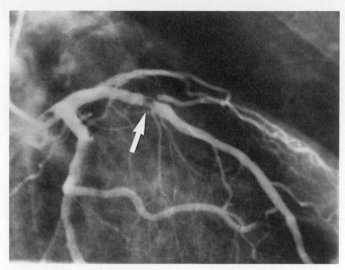

FIGURE 53–3 Atherothrombosis: a generalized and progressive process. This "time-line" depiction of the development of atherothombosis in a coronary vessel emphasizes the long-term nature of this disease. There are three phases of the disease from the perspective of the ACS event: the process of atheroma development up to the time of ACS, the acute manifestation of ACS, and the long-term risk of recurrent events. ACS = acute coronary syndrome. (See also Fig. 50-2.) *(Adapted from Libby P: Circulation 104:365, 2001, with permission.)*

FIGURE 53–4 Coronary artery thrombus in a patient with unstable angina. A 60-year-old man presented with prolonged rest pain and transient anterior ST elevations. Coronary angiography shows an irregular hazy filling defect in the left anterior descending artery at the level of the second diagonal branch (arrow). Contrast medium surrounds the globular thrombus, which extends into the diagonal branch.

generation can occur); (2) degranulation of the platelet alpha and dense granules, releasing thromboxane A$_2$, serotonin, and other platelet aggregatory and chemoattractant agents; and (3) increased expression of GP IIb/IIIa on the platelet surface and a conformational change in GP IIb/IIIa that enhances affinity for fibrinogen. The final step is *platelet aggregation* (i.e., the formation of the platelet plug). Fibrinogen binds to the activated platelet GP IIb/IIIa, creating a growing platelet aggregate.

Secondary Hemostasis

Simultaneously with formation of the platelet plug, the plasma coagulation system is activated. Tissue factor triggers most coronary artery thrombosis. (See Chap. 38 and 82.) Ultimately, factor X is activated (to factor Xa), which leads to generation of thrombin (factor IIa), which plays a central role in arterial thrombosis: (1) thrombin converts fibrinogen to fibrin; (2) thrombin powerfully stimulates platelet aggregation; and (3) it activates factor XIII, which leads to cross-linking and stabilization of the fibrin clot. Thrombin molecules are incorporated into coronary thrombi and can form the nidus of rethrombosis.

Coronary Vasoconstriction

There are three settings in which the process of dynamic coronary

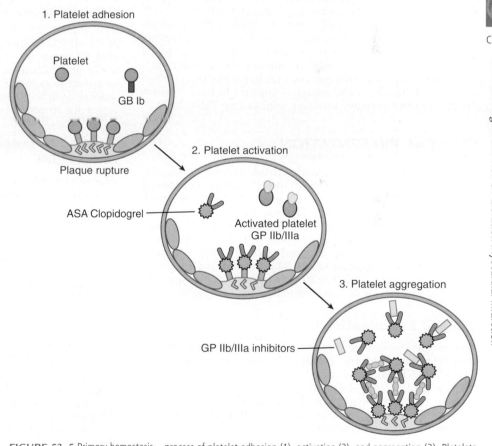

FIGURE 53–5 Primary hemostasis—process of platelet adhesion (1), activation (2), and aggregation (3). Platelets initiate thrombosis at the site of a ruptured plaque: the first step is platelet adhesion (1) via the glycoprotein Ib receptor in conjunction with von Willebrand factor. This is followed by platelet activation (2), which leads to a shape change in the platelet, degranulation of the alpha and dense granules, and expression of GP IIb/IIIa receptors on the platelet surface with activation of the receptor, such that it can bind fibrinogen. The final step is platelet aggregation (3), in which fibrinogen (or von Willebrand factor) binds to the activated GP IIb/IIIa receptors of two platelets. Aspirin (ASA) and clopidogrel act to decrease platelet activation (see text for details), whereas the GP IIb/IIIa inhibitors inhibit the final step of platelet aggregation. GP = glycoprotein. (See also Fig. 82-8.)

CH 53

Unstable Angina and Non-ST Elevation Myocardial Infarction

obstruction is identified: (1) Prinzmetal variant angina[13] (see later); (2) coronary vasoconstriction causing "microcirculatory angina" results from constriction of the small intramural coronary resistance vessels (see Chaps. 48 and 76); and (3) (the most common) local vasoconstrictors released from platelets, serotonin and thromboxane A_2, as well as those present within the thrombus, such as thrombin. A dysfunctional coronary endothelium with reduced production of nitric oxide and increased release of endothelin can also lead to vasoconstriction. Adrenergic stimuli, cold immersion, cocaine, or mental stress[14] can also cause coronary vasoconstriction.

Progressive Mechanical Obstruction

The fourth etiology of UA/NSTEMI results from progressive luminal narrowing. This is most commonly seen in the setting of restenosis following percutaneous coronary intervention (PCI) (see Chap. 55). However, angiographic and atherectomy studies in non-PCI patients have shown progressive luminal narrowing of the culprit vessel related to rapid cellular proliferation.[15]

Secondary Unstable Angina

This form of unstable angina results from an imbalance in myocardial oxygen supply and demand caused by conditions extrinsic to the coronary arteries in patients with prior coronary stenosis.[3,4] Conditions that increase oxygen demand include tachycardia (e.g., atrial fibrillation with rapid ventricular response), fever, thyrotoxicosis, hyperadrenergic states, and elevations of left ventricular afterload such as hypertension or aortic stenosis. Secondary unstable angina can also occur because of impaired oxygen delivery, as occurs in anemia, hypoxemia, and hyperviscosity states, or hypotension. Secondary angina appears to have a worse prognosis than primary unstable angina (see Table 53-1).[4]

CLINICAL PRESENTATION

Women present more often with unstable angina, comprising 30-45 percent of patients with unstable angina in several studies compared with 25 to 30 percent of patients with NSTEMI and approximately 20 percent of patients with STEMI.[16] In comparison to the latter, patients with unstable angina also have higher rates of prior MI, angina, previous coronary revascularization, and extracardiac vascular disease.[16] Indeed, approximately 80 percent of patients with UA/NSTEMI have a history of cardiovascular disease and most have evidence of prior coronary risk factors.[17]

Clinical Examination

The physical examination may be unremarkable or may support the diagnosis of cardiac ischemia. Signs that suggest that UA/NSTEMI involves a large fraction of the left ventricle include diaphoresis, pale cool skin, sinus tachycardia, a third or fourth heart sound, and basilar rales on lung examination. Rarely, the severity of left ventricular dysfunction causes hypotension.

Electrocardiogram

In UA/NSTEMI, ST depression (or transient ST elevation) and T wave changes occur in up to 50 percent of patients.[18,19] New (or presumably new) ST segment deviation is a specific and important measure of ischemia and prognosis. Traditionally, ST depression has only been considered significant if it is ≥0.1 mV—as occurs in 20 to 25 percent of patients.

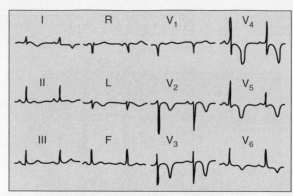

FIGURE–53-6 Electrocardiogram (ECG) showing deep symmetrical anterolateral T wave inversion without ST segment deviation. Such ECG findings are frequently associated with critical stenosis of the left anterior descending coronary artery and are a useful marker in patients at high-risk of subsequent death or myocardial infarction. *(Reproduced from Haines et al: Am J Cardiol 52:14-8, 1983, with permission.)*

However, an additional 20 percent of patients will present with 0.05 mV ST depression,[18] and they can have an adverse prognosis approaching that of patients with 0.1 mV ST depression.[18] Transient (i.e., <20 minutes) ST elevation, which occurs in approximately 10 percent of patients, portends the worst prognosis in UA/NSTEMI. T wave changes are sensitive but not as specific for acute ischemia, unless they are marked (>0.3 mV) (Fig. 53-6).

Continuous ECG Monitoring

Continuous ECG monitoring serves two purposes in UA/NSTEMI: (1) to identify arrhythmias; (2) to identify recurrent ST segment deviation indicative of ischemia. For the latter goal, clinical trials have used high-fidelity Holter monitors to detect ST segment deviation, which is a strong marker of adverse outcome,[20] even when used in conjunction with troponins and clinical variables.

Cardiac Necrosis Markers for Diagnosis of NSTEMI

Among patients presenting with symptoms consistent with UA/NSTEMI, elevations of markers of myocardial necrosis (i.e. CK-MB, troponin T or I) identify patients with the diagnosis of NSTEMI.[21] With the use of troponins, which are more sensitive than CK-MB, a greater percentage of patients are classified as having NSTEMI, which is associated with a worse prognosis.[22,23]

Although the appropriate cut point to define an elevated troponin has engendered controversy, growing consensus has focused on use of the 99th percentile of a normal population of subjects[21] and not greater than a 10 percent coefficient of variation, a measure of reproducibility of the assay. Low-level elevation of cardiac troponin is associated with a higher risk of death or recurrent ischemic events.[23]

Because each assay differs, each hospital needs to review the specific cut points defined by the assay used.[24] Point-of-care tests can have a positive versus negative result or provide a quantitative result, although the sensitivity and diagnostic accuracy of some of these tests have only recently matched the accuracy of current-generation laboratory-based assays.

Despite increasingly accurate assays, apparent false-positive troponin elevations have been found in patients later found at coronary angiography not to have epicardial stenoses.[25] These elevations may be the result of an alternative diagnosis, such as congestive heart failure, in which troponin elevations in the absence of coronary artery disease (CAD) is associated with an adverse prognosis.[26] An analysis from TACTICS-TIMI 18 also raised a cautionary note that these troponin elevations should not be discarded as simply a false positive. Patients presenting with UA/NSTEMI, who had elevations of troponin but no apparent coronary artery disease on angiography, had a significantly worse prognosis than those who were troponin negative without coro-

Laboratory Tests

A chest x-ray may be useful in identifying pulmonary congestion or edema, which would be more likely in patients with NSTEMI involving a significant proportion of the left ventricle or in those with known left ventricular dysfunction. The presence of congestion confers an adverse prognosis.

Obtaining a serum lipid panel including low-density lipoprotein and high-density lipoprotein cholesterol, is useful in identifying important, treatable risk factors for coronary atherothombosis. Because serum cholesterol levels fall as much as 30 to 40 percent beginning 24 hours following UA/NSTEMI or STEMI, they should be measured at the time of initial presentation. If only a later sample is obtained, the clinician should be aware that this low-density lipoprotein (LDL) value likely may be as much as 30 to 40 percent lower than the patient's actual baseline. Other circulating markers of increased risk are discussed subsequently. Evaluation for other secondary causes of UA/NSTEMI,[3] may also be appropriate in selected patients (e.g., assessing thyroid function in patients who present with UA/NSTEMI and persistent tachycardia).

Noninvasive Testing

In the management of UA/NSTEMI, noninvasive testing is used (1) at presentation, usually in the emergency department to diagnose the presence or absence of coronary artery disease (in patients with low likelihood of coronary disease) (see Chap. 49); (2) after hospitalization and medical therapy has begun, to evaluate the extent of residual ischemia, and to guide further therapy as part of an "early conservative" strategy; (3) to evaluate left ventricular function; and (4) to estimate prognosis (i.e., risk stratification). Certain results from noninvasive tests portend high risk of future cardiac events in patients with UA, MI, and stable coronary artery disease. The markers of high risk are either evidence of ischemia on stress testing or left ventricular dysfunction (either at rest or stress induced).

The need for angiography and revascularization for patients who had a strongly positive stress test (i.e., evidence of ischemia) has long been assumed to be necessary and has been utilized in the conservative arms of most randomized trials.[28,29] The safety of early stress testing in patients with UA/NSTEMI has been debated, but evidence from the several trials has suggested pharmacological, or symptom-limited stress testing is safe after a period of at least 24 to 48 hours of stabilization.[30] Contraindications to stress testing are a recent recurrence of rest pain, especially if it is associated with ECG changes or other signs of instability (hemodynamic or arrhythmic).

The merits of various modalities of stress testing have been compared in relatively small series of patients (see also Chaps. 13 and 51). Stress myocardial perfusion imaging with sestamibi or stress echocardiographic imaging has slightly more sensitivity than ECG stress testing alone and has shown greater prognostic value, but is generally cost effective only in higher risk patients. A recommended approach is to individualize the choice based on patient characteristics, local availability, and expertise in interpretation. For most patients ECG stress testing is recommended if the ECG lacks significant ST segment abnormalities. If ST abnormalities exist, then perfusion or echo imaging is recommended. Exercise testing is generally recommended unless the patient cannot walk sufficiently to achieve a significant workload—in which case pharmacological stress testing provides an alternative.

Coronary Arteriographic Findings

The extent of coronary disease among patients with UA/NSTEMI enrolled in the invasive arm of TACTICS-TIMI 18, who systematically underwent angiography, was: 34 percent had significant obstruction (>50 percent luminal diameter stenosis) of three vessels; 28 percent had two vessel disease; 26 percent had single vessel disease; and 13 percent had no coronary stenosis >50 percent.[29] Approximately 5 to 10 percent had left main stem stenosis >50 percent.[29] Registries of unselected UA/NSTEMI patients have reported similar findings. Women and non-whites with UA/NSTEMI have less extensive coronary disease than their counterparts,[16] whereas patients with NSTEMI have more extensive disease than those who present with unstable angina.[16,31]

Women and non-whites comprise a larger proportion of patients with symptoms of UA/NSTEMI without epicardial coronary disease—suggesting either a difficulty in making a firm diagnosis of UA/NSTEMI in these groups and/or a different pathophysiological mechanism for their clinical presentation (see also Chap. 76).[16] Approximately one third of patients with UA/NSTEMI without a critical epicardial obstruction have impaired coronary flow assessed angiographically—suggesting a pathophysiological role for coronary microvascular dysfunction. The short-term prognosis is excellent in this group of patients.[32]

The culprit lesion in UA/NSTEMI typically exhibits an eccentric stenosis with scalloped or overhanging edges and a narrow neck (see also Chap. 20).[9] These angiographic findings may represent disrupted atherosclerotic plaque, thrombus, or a combination. Features suggesting thrombus include globular intraluminal masses with a rounded or polypoid shape (see Fig. 53-4).[9] "Haziness" of a lesion has been used as an angiographic marker of possible thrombus, but this finding is less specific. Patients with angiographically visualized thrombus have impaired coronary flow and worse clinical outcomes, compared to those without thrombus. Patients with UA/NSTEMI have impaired coronary flow as measured by the TIMI flow grade or frame count, and TIMI myocardial perfusion grade—especially those with an elevated troponin level,[31] which is independently associated with adverse outcomes.

Angioscopy and Intravascular Ultrasound

Greater definition of the culprit lesion has been possible using angioscopy, where "white" (platelet-rich) thrombi are frequently observed, as opposed to "red" thrombi, more often seen in patients with acute ST elevation MI. Although useful for research purposes, it is not generally available for routine clinical care. Intravascular ultrasound examination identified more echolucent plaques and fewer calcified lesions among patients with unstable versus stable angina.

RISK STRATIFICATION

PATHOPHYSIOLOGY OF LONG-TERM RISK FOLLOWING ACUTE CORONARY SYNDROME. An important concept that has emerged regarding the long-term outcome following an ACS event is that the risk of recurrent ischemic events links to multifocal lesions other than the culprit lesion responsible for the ACS event. Studies of coronary anatomy using angiography, intravascular coronary ultrasound,[33] or angioscopy,[8] have shown multiple active plaques in addition to the culprit lesion (Fig. 53-7). Thus, as aggressive interventional approaches are used to successfully treat the culprit lesion, the remaining plaques often provoke

Multiple "vulnerable" plaques detected in non-culprit segments 1–7

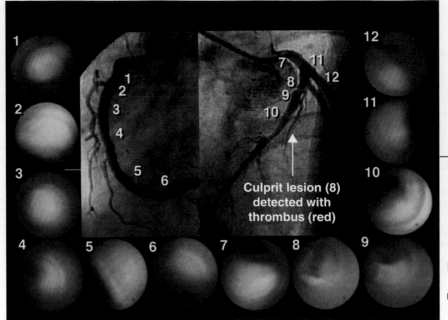

Culprit lesion (8) detected with thrombus (red)

Multiple "vulnerable" plaques detected in non-culprit segments 10–12

FIGURE 53–7 Evidence of multiple "vulnerable" plaques in acute coronary syndrome. This figure shows angiographic and angioscopic images of 58-year-old male with anterior myocardial infarction. The culprit lesion is seen in the proximal left anterior descending artery at site 8. However, other segments of the artery, which appear normal on the coronary angiogram, demonstrate at angioscopy the presence of vulnerable plaques (sites 10-12 and 1, 3, 4, 7). *(Adapted from Asakura M, et al: J Am Coll Cardiol 37:1284-8, 2001.)*

CH 53

recurrent events. The percentage of patients with more than one active plaque on angiography was related to an increasing baseline C-reactive protein (CRP) level.[33] These findings provide an important pathophysiological link between inflammation, more diffuse active coronary disease, and recurrent cardiac events in the months to years following a clinical ACS event.

NATURAL HISTORY. Patients with UA have lower short-term mortality (1.7 percent at 30 days) than those with NSTEMI or STEMI, whereas the mortality risk of the two types of MI is similar (5.1 percent for each type).[19] The early mortality risk in ACS is related to the extent of myocardial damage and resulting hemodynamic compromise.[34] In contrast, long-term outcomes—both for mortality and nonfatal events, is actually *worse* for patients with either UA or NSTEMI compared with STEMI.[19] This finding likely results from the older age, greater extent of coronary disease, and prior MI and comorbidities—such as diabetes and impaired renal function—in patients with UA/NSTEMI versus STEMI.

Methods of Risk Stratification

Because patients with UA/NSTEMI are a heterogeneous group, with a prognosis that ranges from one with an excellent outcome with modest adjustments in therapeutic regimen to one in which the risk of death or MI is high, requiring intensive treatment. Accordingly, risk stratification plays a central role in the evaluation and management of patients with this condition. Specific subgroups of patients, identified by clinical features, electrocardiographic findings and/or cardiac (or vascular) markers are at higher risk of adverse outcomes (Table 53-2). Furthermore, these groups appear to derive greater benefit from aggressive antithrombotic and/or interventional therapies (see later). Clinical predictors can also assist triage of patients. Those determined to be at highest risk should be admitted to the coronary care unit, whereas those at intermediate or lower risk may be admitted to a monitored bed on a cardiac step-

TABLE 53–2	Clinical Indicators of Increased Risk in UA/NSTEMI

History
Advanced age (>70 yr)
Diabetes mellitus
Post–myocardial infarction angina
Prior peripheral vascular disease
Prior cerebrovascular disease

Clinical Presentation
Braunwald class II or III (acute or subacute rest pain)
Braunwald class B (secondary unstable angina)
Heart failure/hypotension
Multiple episodes of pain within 24 hr

ECG
ST segment deviation ≥0.05 mV
T wave inversion ≥0.3 mV
Left bundle branch block

Cardiac Markers
Increased troponin T or I or creatine kinase-MB
Increased C-reactive protein or white blood cell count
Increased B-type natriuretic peptide
Elevated creatinine
Elevated glucose or hemoglobin A_1C

Angiogram
Thrombus
Multivessel disease
Left ventricular dysfunction

UA/NSTEMI = unstable angina/non-ST elevation myocardial infarction.

down unit. Patients sometimes referred to as "low risk," and those who are at low likelihood of having ACS, can be evaluated and managed in emergency department observation units or chest pain centers (see Chap. 49).

Clinical Variables

The aforementioned classification of unstable angina[3] (see Table 53-1) has proved clinically useful in several studies for identifying high-risk patients, notably those with ongoing or recurrent rest pain, post-MI unstable angina, and/or secondary unstable angina.[4]

HIGH-RISK CLINICAL SUBGROUPS. Increasing age is associated with a significant increase in adverse outcomes in patients with UA/NSTEMI.[35] Diabetic patients with UA/NSTEMI are at approximately 50 percent higher risk than nondiabetics (see also Chap. 60).[36] Patients with extracardiac vascular disease (i.e., those with either cerebrovascular disease or peripheral arterial vascular disease) also appear to have approximately 50 percent higher rates of death or recurrent ischemic events compared with patients without previous peripheral or cerebrovascular disease, even after controlling for other differences in baseline characteristics (see also Chap. 57).[37,38] As with STEMI, patients with UA/NSTEMI who present with evidence of congestive heart failure (Killip Class >II) have an increased risk of death.[39]

Risk Assessment by ECG

The admission ECG is useful in predicting long-term adverse outcomes. In the TIMI III Registry of patients with UA/NSTEMI, independent predictors of 1-year death or MI included left bundle branch block (risk ratio 2.8); ST segment deviation >0.05 mV (risk ratio 2.45); both $p < 0.001$.[18] There appears to be a gradient of risk based on the degree of ST segment deviation.[40]

Risk Assessment by Cardiac Markers

CK-MB AND THE TROPONINS. Patients with NSTEMI, defined as associated with an elevated biomarker of necrosis, CK-MB, or troponin, have a worse long-term prognosis than those with UA.[22,23,41] Beyond just a positive versus negative test result, there is a linear relation between the level of troponin T or I in the blood and subsequent risk of death—the higher the troponin level, the higher the mortality risk.[41] On the other hand, a higher risk of MI (or recurrent MI) was observed with *lower* degrees of troponin elevation in several studies; thus the overall rate of death or MI is equally high among patients with low or higher troponin values.[23,42,43]

C-REACTIVE PROTEIN

Among the growing list of additional markers that appear to be useful in assessing patients with UA/NSTEMI, CRP holds considerable promise. Elevated levels of high sensitivity (hs) CRP relate to increased risk of death, MI, and/or need for urgent revascularization.[42] Of note, because CRP is an acute-phase reactant, it is known to be elevated by an ACS. Thus, "elevated" levels of CRP in patients with ACS are approximately five times higher than for stable patients.[44-46] Among patients with negative troponin I at baseline who overall had a 14-day mortality of only 1.5 percent, CRP was able to discriminate a high- and low-risk group: mortality for patients with an elevated CRP was 5.8 percent versus 0.4 percent for patients without elevated CRP.[45] When using both CRP and troponin T, mortality could be stratified from 0.4 percent for patients with both markers negative, 4.7 percent if either CRP or troponin were positive, to 9.1 percent if both were positive.[45] Multiple other studies have yielded similar results.[42,47,48] Of note, however, CRP has not yet been shown in the setting of UA/NSTEMI to predict a differential benefit of a therapy.[49]

CRP measured after stabilization post-ACS strongly predicts outcome after 3 to 12 months.[46,50] Study of other inflammatory markers has offered consistent evidence of an association between systemic inflammation and recurrent adverse events, including serum amyloid A,[51] monocyte chemoattractant protein (MCP)-1,[52] and interleukin-6.[52,53] These studies indicate that inflammation is related to the instability of patients and an increased risk of recurrent cardiac events.

WHITE BLOOD CELL COUNT

Another, even simpler and universally available marker of inflammation is the white blood cell (WBC) count. Several studies of patients with acute MI,[54] and more recently with UA/NSTEMI,[48,54,55] have observed that patients with elevated WBC counts have higher risk of mortality and recurrent MI. This association was independent of CRP,[48] suggest-

ing that no one marker, such as CRP, captures all the information regarding the influence of inflammation on outcomes.

MYELOPEROXIDASE

Myeloperoxidase (MPO) is a heme protein expressed by leukocytes that generates hypochlorous acid, a potent pro-oxidant. One case-control study found an association of MPO levels with the presence of angiographically documented CAD, independent of other cardiovascular risk factors and of WBC count.[56] In patients presenting to the emergency department with chest pain,[57] and in patients with UA/NSTEMI, MPO serum levels predict increased risk for subsequent death or MI, independent of other risk factors and other cardiac markers.[58] as well as mortality alone in other populations.[59] Elevations of MPO have been seen throughout the coronary vasculature in patients with UA/NSTEMI.[60] Thus, MPO may be a marker of inflammation, but also suggests a direct role of leukocyte activation in the pathophysiology of vascular inflammation and ACS.

B-TYPE NATRIURETIC PEPTIDE

B-type natriuretic peptide (BNP) is a neurohormone that is synthesized in ventricular myocardium and released in response to increased wall stress. It has many actions including natriuresis, vasodilation, inhibition of sympathetic nerve activity, and inhibition of the renin-angiotensin-aldosterone system. BNP has usefulness as a diagnostic and prognostic marker among patients with congestive heart failure,[61] and in patients with acute MI.[62] BNP has prognostic value across the full spectrum of patients with ACS, including those with UA/NSTEMI: In OPUS-TIMI 16, patients with elevated levels of BNP (>80 pg/ml) or Ntpro BNP had a two- to threefold higher risk of death by 10 months.[63] This finding was confirmed in the TIMI 11 and TACTICS-TIMI 18 trials.[64,65] Together, these data suggest that measurement of BNP in patients presenting with UA/NSTEMI adds importantly to our current tools for risk stratification.

CREATININE

Another simple tool for risk stratification is the use of creatinine and/or calculation of creatinine clearance. Several recent studies have found that elevated creatinine is associated with an adverse prognosis.[66,67] The risk appears to be independent of other standard risk factors, such as troponin elevation. This factor may also play a role in decreased drug clearance, indicating the need for adjustment of doses of medications such as low-molecular-weight heparin (LMWH).[68]

GLUCOSE

Elevated admission glucose values predicts adverse outcomes among diabetic patients with acute MI as compared with those without hyperglycemia (see also Chap. 60).[69] Recent studies have extended this association even to patients without known diabetes.[70] This association applies to patients with either STEMI or UA/NSTEMI and does not depend on other baseline risk factors.[71] A similar association of poor glycemic control, as measured by hemoglobin A_{1c} has emerged from other studies.[72] Thus, in patients with UA/NSTEMI, a higher baseline glucose level at the time of presentation predicts significantly higher long-term mortality, independent of a history of diabetes, and is a risk factor that may be modifiable with aggressive treatment.

COMBINED RISK ASSESSMENT SCORES

Integrating all of the above factors, several groups have developed comprehensive risk scores that use clinical variables and findings from the ECG and/or from serum cardiac markers.[73-75] The TIMI Risk score identified seven independent risk factors: age >65 years, >3 risk factors for CAD, documented coronary artery disease at catheterization, ST deviation >0.5 mm, >2 episodes of angina in last 24 hours, ASA within prior week, and elevated cardiac markers. Use of this scoring system was able to risk-stratify patients across a 10-fold gradient of risk, from 4.7 percent to 40.9 percent ($p < 0.001$) (Fig. 53-8A).[74] More importantly, this risk score predicts the response to several of the therapies in UA/NSTEMI: patients with higher TIMI risk scores had significant reductions in events when treated with enoxaparin as compared with unfractionated heparin,[74] with a GP IIb/IIIa inhibitor as compared with placebo,[76] and with an invasive versus conservative strategy (see Fig. 53-8B).[29,77] The Global Registry of Acute Coronary Events (GRACE). Registry identified factors that were associated independently with increased mortality; the most important baseline determinants of higher mortality were increased age, Killiip class, increased heart rate, lower systolic blood pressure, ST-segment depression, signs of heart failure, cardiac arrest at presentation, and elevated serum creatinine

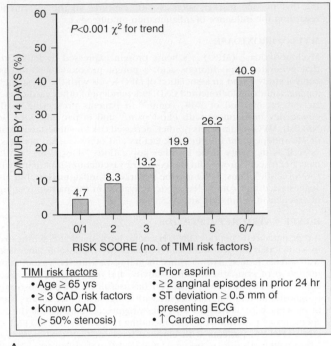

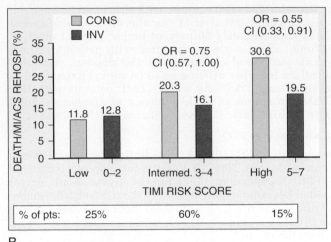

A

B

FIGURE 53–8 **A,** Thrombolysis in myocardial ischemia (TIMI) risk score for unstable angina or non-ST elevation myocardial infarction (UA/NSTEMI). The risk factors are shown below and the risk of death (D), myocardial infarction (MI), or urgent revascularization (UR) is shown along the vertical axis. **B,** Use of the TIMI risk score for UA/NSTEMI to predict the benefit of an early invasive strategy. In a prospectively defined analysis, the TIMI risk score was applied in the Treat Angina with Aggrastat and determine Cost of Therapy with an Invasive or Conservative Strategy (TACTICS)-TIMI 18 trial. As shown, 75 percent of patients had a risk score of 3 or higher, and in these patients a significant benefit of an invasive strategy was observed. ACS = acute coronary syndrome; CAD = coronary artery disease; CI = confidence interval; CONS = conservative; ECG = electrocardiogram; INV = invasive; OR = odds ratio. (**A,** *Adapted from Antman EM, Cohen M, Bernink PJLM, et al: The TIMI risk score for unstable angina/non-ST elevation MI: A method for prognostication and therapeutic decision-making. JAMA 284:835, 2000;* **B,** *data from Cannon CP, Weintraub WS, Demopoulos LA, et al: Comparison of early invasive and conservative strategies in patients with unstable coronary syndromes treated with the glycoprotein IIb/IIIa inhibitor tirofiban. N Engl J Med 344:1879, 2001.*)

CH 53

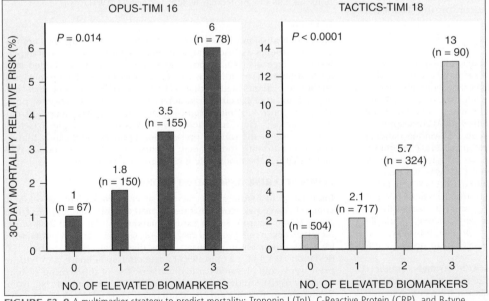

FIGURE 53–9 A multimarker strategy to predict mortality: Troponin I (TnI), C-Reactive Protein (CRP), and B-type natriuretic peptide (BNP) as determinants of 30-day mortality in UA/NSTEMI. (*Adapted from Sabatine MS, Morrow DA, de Lemos JA, et al: Multimarker approach to risk stratification in non-ST elevation acute coronary syndromes. Circulation.105:1760-63, 2002.*)

or cardiac marker enzymes. With the ever-growing number of new cardiac markers (see earlier), comprehensive risk scores will likely include these new markers as they become more widely available in clinical practice, as shown in one study using three markers in a "multimarker strategy" for evaluation (Fig. 53-9).

MEDICAL THERAPY

General Measures

Patients with UA/NSTEMI if at high risk should be admitted to an intensive (cardiac) care unit, or if at low or intermediate risk to a monitored bed. In these settings, continuous ECG monitoring (i.e., telemetry) is used to detect cardiac arrhythmias.

Bed rest is usually prescribed initially for patients with UA/NSTEMI. Ambulation as tolerated is permitted if the patient has been stable without recurrent chest discomfort for at least 12 to 24 hours or following revascularization. Supplemental oxygen is frequently administered to patients with UA/NSTEMI, but its usefulness has not been documented. It is advisable to provide supplemental oxygen only to patients with cyanosis, extensive rales and/or when arterial O_2 saturation, measured by oximetry, declines below 92 percent.

Relief of chest pain is an initial goal of treatment. In patients with persistent pain despite therapy with nitrates and beta blockers (see later), morphine sulfate 1 to 4 mg intravenously is usually administered. Contraindications

Anticoagulants

HEPARIN

Anticoagulation, traditionally with unfractionated heparin (UFH) is a cornerstone of therapy for patients with UA/NSTEMI.[89] A meta-analysis showed a trend toward a 33 percent reduction in death or MI comparing UFH plus aspirin versus aspirin alone.[129] Variability in the anticoagulant effects of UFH, so-called "heparin resistance," is thought to result from the heterogeneity of unfractionated heparins and to the neutralization of heparin by circulating plasma factors and by proteins released by activated platelets.[130] Clinically, frequent monitoring of the anticoagulant response using activated partial thromboplastin time (APTT) is recommended with titrations made according to a standardized nomogram aiming for an APTT of 50 to 70 seconds (Table 53-4). Based on available data, the current ACC/AHA Guidelines recommend a weight adjusted dosing of UFH (60 U/kg bolus and 12 U/kg/hr infusion), frequent monitoring of APTT (every 6 hours until in the target range and every 12 to 24 hours thereafter), and titration of UFH using a standardized nomogram (example in Table 53-4) with a target range of APTT between 1.5 to 2 times control or approximately 50 and 70 seconds. Adverse effects include bleeding, especially when APTT is elevated, and heparin-induced thrombocytopenia, which is more common with longer durations of treatment (see Chap. 82).[131]

LOW-MOLECULAR-WEIGHT HEPARIN (LMWH)

LMWHs have been widely tested as a means of improving on anticoagulation with UFH. These agents combine factor IIa and factor Xa inhibition and thus inhibit both the action and generation of thrombin.[132] LMWH has several potential advantages over UFH: First, its greater anti-factor Xa activity inhibits thrombin generation more effectively. LMWH also induces a greater release of tissue factor pathway inhibitor than does UFH, and it is not neutralized by platelet factor 4.[132] LMWH causes thrombocytopenia at a lower rate than UFH.[133] Its high bioavailability allows for subcutaneous administration. Finally, LMWH binds less avidly to plasma proteins and thus has a more consistent anticoagulant effect in relation to the dose administered, and monitoring of the level of anticoagulation is not necessary. However, LMWHs are more affected by renal dysfunction than UFH, and the dose should be reduced in patients with a creatinine clearance <30 mL/min. Also, in the event of bleeding, the anticoagulant effect of UFH can be reversed more effectively with protamine.

LMWH (plus aspirin) has proved effective compared with aspirin alone, leading to a 66 percent reduction in the odds of death or MI.[129] In comparisons of all LMWHs versus UFH, no significant difference was observed.[129] On the other hand, early trials with enoxaparin showed a 20 percent reduction in death, MI, and/or recurrent ischemia, compared with UFH.[134,135] In the two most recent trials, enoxaparin was found to be noninferior to UFH.[136,137] In a meta-analysis of all trials in UA/NSTEMI, enoxaparin yielded a statistically significant 9 percent reduction in the odds of death or MI at 30 days (95 percent CI, 0.83 to 0.99) (Fig. 53-15).[135] A prospective analysis of the A to Z trial showed that enoxaparin provided significant benefit over UFH in patients managed conservatively (who are typically on heparin/LMWH for at least 48 hours) but not in those managed invasively (who are taken to the catheterization laboratory within 48 hours and have their heparin discontinued thereafter).[138] Treatment with enoxaparin was not associated with an excess of major bleeding, but increases in minor bleeding have been observed.[135]

One study of 438 patients with UA/NSTEMI directly compared two LMWHs—enoxaparin and tinzaparin. The primary composite endpoint, death, MI or recurrent angina at 7 days was significantly lower

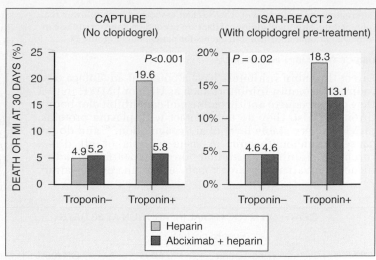

FIGURE 53–14 Benefit of abciximab in the CAPTURE trial of patients with refractory unstable angina treated with angioplasty in those with positive versus negative troponin T at study entry **(left panel).** Benefit of abciximab versus placebo even after patients undergoing percutaneous coronary intervention (PCI) were pretreated with 600 mg of clopidogrel **(right panel).** CAPTURE = c7E3 AntiPlatelet Therapy in Unstable Refractory angina; ISAR-REACT 2 = Intracoronary Stenting and Antithrombotic: Regimen Rapid Early Action for Coronary Treatment 2; MI = myocardial infarction. *(Data from Hamm CW, et al: N Engl J Med 340:1623-9, 1999; and Kastrati A, et al: JAMA 295:1531-1538, 2006.)*

TABLE 53–4	Standardized Nomogram for Titration of Heparin*	
APTT (sec)[†]	Change	IV Infusion (U/kg/hr)
<35	70 U/kg bolus	+3
35-49	35 U/kg bolus	+2
50-70	0	0
71-90	0	−2
>100	Hold infusion for 30 min	−3

*Initial Dose: 60 U/kg bolus and 12 U/kg/hr infusion.
[†]APTT should be checked and infusion adjusted at 6, 12, 24 hr post–initiation of heparin, daily thereafter, and 4-6 hr after any adjustment in dose.
APTT = activated partial thromboplastin time.
From Becker et al: Am Heart J 137:59-71, 1999.

in the enoxaparin group: 12.3 percent versus 21.1 percent in the tinzaparin group (*p* = 0.015).[139] The 2002 update of the ACC/AHA UA/NSTEMI Guideline made a Class IIa recommendation that enoxaparin is preferred over UFH.[2] The standard dose of enoxaparin is 1 mg/kg subcutaneously every 12 hours, with dosing only once daily for patients with a creatinine clearance <30 ml/min.

FONDAPARINUX

Fondaparinux is a synthetic pentasaccharide that is an indirect Xa inhibitor that requires antithrombin for its action. The OASIS-5 trial compared fondaparinux, administered at a relatively low dose, 2.5 mg subcutaneously, once daily with standard-dose enoxaparin in 20,078 patients with high-risk UA/NSTEMI. The rates of death, MI, or refractory ischemia throughout the first 9 days were similar with fondaparinux and enoxaparin (5.9 percent versus 5.8 percent), meeting the prespecified hypothesis of noninferiority (Fig. 53-16).[140] Of importance, however, the rate of major bleeding was almost 50 percent lower in the fondaparinux arm (2.2 percent versus 4.1 percent, *p* < 0.001).[140] By 30 days, mortality was significantly lower in the fondaparinux arm (2.9 percent versus 3.5 percent, *p* = 0.02). However, in the subset of patients undergoing PCI, fondaparinux was associated with more than a threefold increased risk of catheter-related thrombi, something also observed in patients with STEMI treated with fondaparinux.[141] Supplemental UFH at the time of catheterization appeared to minimize the risk of this complication. Thus, fondaparinux appears to be a new alternative for patients with UA/NSTEMI associated with a lower risk of bleeding, although additional data are needed on appropriate use of other/additional antithrombin agents for patients undergoing PCI.

DIRECT THROMBIN INHIBITORS

Direct thrombin inhibitors have a potential advantage over indirect thrombin inhibitors such as UFH or LMWH in that they do not require antithrombin and can inhibit clot-bound thrombin; also they do not interact with plasma proteins, provide a very stable level of anticoagulation,[130] and do not cause thrombocytopenia. A meta-analysis of all direct thrombin inhibitors studied through 2001, including hirudin, bivalirudin, argatroban, efegatran, or inogatran,

showed a modest 9 percent reduction in death or MI at 30 days, favoring the direct thrombin inhibitor over unfractionated heparin.[142] The only current U.S. Food and Drug Administration–approved indication for lepirudin and argatroban is for anticoagulation in patients with heparin-induced thrombocytopenia (HIT) and associated thromboembolic disease.

Bivalirudin has recently been studied in UA/NSTEMI. The Acute Catheterization and Urgent Intervention Triage Strategy (ACUITY) trial randomized 13,819 patients with UA/NSTEMI to one of three treatments: UFH or enoxaparin plus a GP IIb/IIIa inhibitor, bivalirudin plus a GP IIb/IIIa inhibitor, or bivalirudin alone. Patients were managed with an early invasive strategy; The primary endpoint was the composite of death, myocardial infarction, unplanned revascularization for ischemia, and major bleeding at 30 days.[143] No differences were observed in the direct comparison of the anticoagulants: i.e., between bivalirudin plus GP IIb/IIIa inhibitor and UFH/enoxaparin plus a GP IIb/IIIa inhibitor, with rates of 11.8 percent versus 11.7 percent for the efficacy endpoint, and 5.3 percent versus 5.7 percent for major bleeding. For the bivalirudin alone group, when compared with the group receiving UFH/enoxaparin

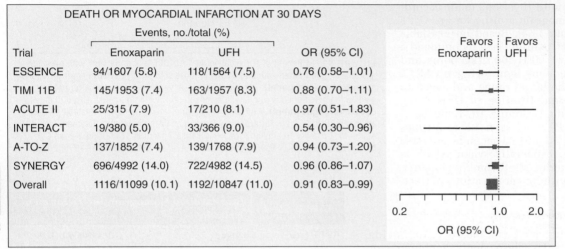

DEATH OR MYOCARDIAL INFARCTION AT 30 DAYS

Trial	Events, no./total (%) Enoxaparin	UFH	OR (95% CI)
ESSENCE	94/1607 (5.8)	118/1564 (7.5)	0.76 (0.58–1.01)
TIMI 11B	145/1953 (7.4)	163/1957 (8.3)	0.88 (0.70–1.11)
ACUTE II	25/315 (7.9)	17/210 (8.1)	0.97 (0.51–1.83)
INTERACT	19/380 (5.0)	33/366 (9.0)	0.54 (0.30–0.96)
A-TO-Z	137/1852 (7.4)	139/1768 (7.9)	0.94 (0.73–1.20)
SYNERGY	696/4992 (14.0)	722/4982 (14.5)	0.96 (0.86–1.07)
Overall	1116/11099 (10.1)	1192/10847 (11.0)	0.91 (0.83–0.99)

FIGURE 53–15 Meta-analysis of randomized trials of enoxaparin versus unfractionated heparin (UFH). CI = confidence interval; ACUTE II = Antithrombotic Combination Using Tirofiban and Enoxaparin II; A-to-Z = Aggrastat-to-Zocor study; ESSENCE = Efficacy and Safety of Subcutaneous Enoxaparin in Non-Q-Wave Coronary Events; INTERACT = Integrilin and Enoxaparin Randomized Assessment of Acute Coronary Syndrome Treatment; OR = odds ratio; SYNERGY = Superior Yield of the New Strategy of Enoxaparin, Revascularization and Glycoprotein IIb/IIIa inhibitors; TIMI 11B = Thrombolysis in Myocardial infarction 11B. *(Reproduced from Petersen JL, et al: JAMA 292:89-96, 2004.)*

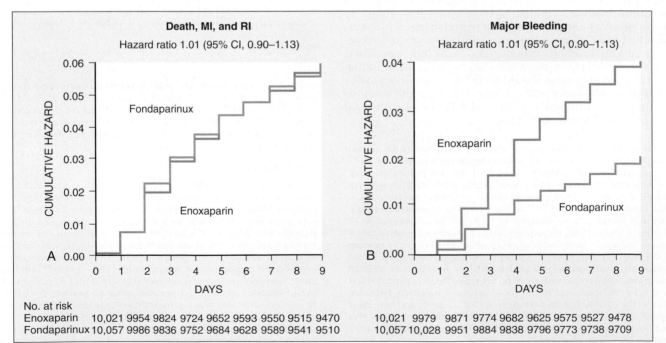

FIGURE 53–16 Effects of fondaparinux as compared with enoxaparin in the OASIS 5 trial. **A** shows equivalent rates of death, myocardial infarction (MI), or refractory ischemia (RI) to day 9; **B** shows a nearly 50 percent reduction in major bleeding that appeared to be associated with a reduction in 6-month mortality. OASIS = Organization to Assess Strategies for Ischemic Syndromes. *(Reproduced from Yusuf S, et al: N Engl J Med. 354(14):1464-76, 2006.)*

plus a GP IIb/IIIa inhibitor, there were no differences in the efficacy endpoint, but a lower rate of bleeding (3.0 percent versus 5.7 percent, $p < 0.001$.[143] Thus, the substitution of bivalirudin as the anticoagulant among patients receiving supplemental GP IIb/IIIa inhibitors did not change efficacy or safety outcomes, but the strategy of bivalirudin alone was associated with less bleeding than the combination of a GP IIb/IIIa inhibitor with either UFH or enoxaparin.

ORAL ANTICOAGULATION

Several trials have examined oral anticoagulation with warfarin following ACS, with the rationale that prolonged treatment might extend the benefit of early anticoagulation with an antithrombin agent (e.g., UFH, LMWH). Although initial large trials failed to show a significant benefit of long-term warfarin plus aspirin versus aspirin alone,[144] subsequent trials suggested that if a sufficient degree of anticoagulation were achieved, a benefit accrued from the combination of aspirin plus warfarin.[145-147] In the largest study, 4930 patients with ACS within the prior 8 weeks were randomized to warfarin alone (target international normalized ratio (INR) of 2.8 to 4.2), aspirin alone (160 mg daily), or aspirin (75 mg daily), combined with warfarin (target INR of 2.0 to 2.5).[145] During an average of 4 years of follow-up, the rate of death, MI, or thromboembolic cerebral stroke occurred in 20.0 percent of patients receiving aspirin alone, 16.7 percent of patients receiving warfarin ($p = 0.03$), and 15.0 percent of patients receiving warfarin and aspirin ($p = 0.001$).[145] Rates of major bleeding were 0.62 percent per treatment-year in both groups receiving warfarin and 0.17 percent in patients receiving aspirin ($p < 0.001$). Thus, the combination of aspirin plus warfarin was more effective than aspirin alone for long-term secondary prevention.

However, given the similar benefit seen with clopidogrel plus aspirin over aspirin alone, the lack of need for monitoring of the INR, and the frequent use of PCI and stenting in the patient population in whom the need for clopidogrel is well established, the clinical use of aspirin plus warfarin is limited. Among patients *without a coronary stent* but with another indication for warfarin, such as chronic atrial fibrillation or severe left ventricular dysfunction who are at high risk of systemic embolization, the combination of aspirin plus warfarin would be preferable as the long-term antithrombotic strategy.[148] The combination of all three agents has not been tested prospectively to date but might be associated with a high bleeding risk during long-term therapy. Use of all three agents together is sometimes needed among patients with atrial fibrillation or other strong indications for warfarin (e.g., stenting). In such patients, the ACC/AHA Guidelines recommend use of low-dose aspirin (75 to 81 mg daily), warfarin (titrated meticulously to an INR of 2.0 to 2.5), and use of clopidogrel for as short a time as recommended for the type of stent placed.[149] Research is ongoing to identify alternative oral anticoagulants, including oral direct thrombin inhibitors and factor Xa inhibitors in place of coumadin, to avoid the need for monitoring the INR.

FIBRINOLYTIC THERAPY FOR UA/NSTEMI

No benefit of fibrinolysis in UA/NSTEMI has been observed; the rates of both recurrent MI and intracranial hemorrhage were *higher* with tissue plasminogen activator treatment versus placebo in this population.[28] The proposed mechanism for adverse effect of fibrinolysis in UA/NSTEMI is a prothrombotic effect of fibrinolysis. Fibrinolytic agents can activate platelets, and the dissolution of the fibrin clot exposes clot-bound thrombin, which is enzymatically active and can lead to clot formation. Because most patients with UA/NSTEMI have a patent culprit artery, these prothrombotic forces can lead to progression of the thrombus to total occlusion, thereby causing a new MI (as was observed in TIMI IIIB).[28] In contrast, in STEMI, the culprit vessel is totally occluded and can only improve with fibrinolysis. Accordingly, fibrinolytic therapy is not indicated in UA/NSTEMI.

TREATMENT STRATEGIES AND INTERVENTIONS

Two general approaches to the use of cardiac catheterization and revascularization in UA/NSTEMI exist: an early invasive strategy, involving routine early cardiac catheterization and revascularization with percutaneous coronary intervention (PCI) or coronary bypass grafting (CABG) depending on the coronary anatomy. The other is a more conservative approach with initial medical management with catheterization and revascularization only for recurrent ischemia either at rest or on a noninvasive stress test. To date, ten randomized trials have studied the relative merits of these two strategies. The first three and the most recent trial did not demonstrate a significant difference; however, six trials have shown a significant benefit of an early invasive therapy (Fig. 53-17).[29,150,151]

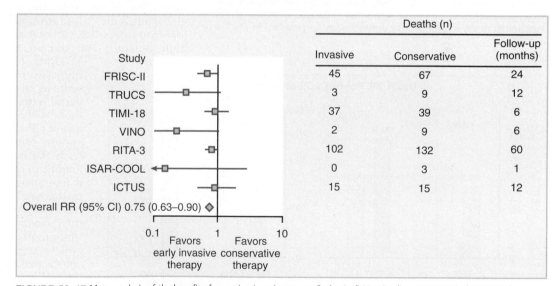

FIGURE 53–17 Meta-analysis of the benefit of a routine invasive versus "selective" invasive (i.e., conservative) strategy for patients with unstable angina or NSTEMI on the rate of death, myocardial infarction, or rehospitalization through follow-up. FRISC-II = Fragmin and Fast Revascularization During Instability in Coronary Disease; ICTUS = Invasive Versus Conservative Treatment in Unstable Coronary Syndromes Investigators; ISAR-COOL = Intracoronary Stenting With Antithrombotic Regimen Cooling Off; RITA-3 = Randomized Intervention Trial of Unstable Angina; RR = risk ratio; TACTICS TIMI-18 = Treat Angina With Aggrastat and Determine the Cost of Therapy With an Invasive or Conservative Strategy—Thrombolysis in Myocardial Infarction; TRUCS = Treatment of Refractory Unstable Angina in Geographically Isolated Areas Without Cardiac Surgery; VINO = Value of First Day Coronary Angiography/Angioplasty in Evolving Non-ST-Segment Elevation Myocardial Infarction. *(Reproduced with permission from Bavry AA, et al: J Am Coll Cardiol 48:1319-25, 2006.)*

FRISC II showed a large difference in the rate of revascularization between the invasive versus conservative strategies because of strict criteria for catheterization. The rate of death or MI at 6 months was significantly lower in the invasive versus the conservative group, 9.4 percent versus 12.1 percent, $p = 0.031$.[150] At 1 year there was a significant reduction in mortality in the invasive versus the conservative groups (2.2 percent and 3.9 percent, respectively, $p = 0.016$).[150] Additional analyses showed greater benefit of the invasive strategy in higher risk groups identified by ST segment depression on the admission ECG or troponin T greater than or equal to 0.01 ng per dl.[34] In a five-year follow-up overall death or MI was lower with an invasive strategy, but the mortality advantage observed earlier was not seen in the group as a whole; mortality was significantly reduced in high-risk groups, but not in those with low risk.[152]

In the TACTICS-TIMI 18 trial, the rate of death, MI, or rehospitalization for ACS at 6 months fell from 19.4 percent in the conservative group to 15.9 percent in the early invasive group; $p = 0.025$.[29] Death or nonfatal MI declined significantly at 30 days and at 6 months. In patients with a troponin I level >0.1 ng per mL, there was a relative 39 percent risk reduction in the primary endpoint with the invasive versus conservative strategy ($p < .001$), whereas patients with a negative troponin had similar outcomes with either strategy (Fig. 53-18).[23] Using the TIMI risk score, there was significant benefit of the early invasive strategy in intermediate- (score, 3 to 4) and high-risk patients (5 to 7); whereas low-risk (0 to 2) patients had similar outcomes when managed with either strategy.[29] Interestingly, the invasive strategy has proved cost-effective, with the estimated cost per year of life gained for the invasive strategy of $12,739 in TACTICS-TIMI 18.[153]

The Randomized Intervention Trial of Unstable Angina (RITA-3) trial also demonstrated a benefit of an early invasive strategy, with a 34 percent reduction in the primary endpoint of death, MI, or refractory angina at 4 months; this benefit was driven primarily by a reduction in refractory angina.[154] Yet by 5 years there was a significantly lower cardiovascular mortality rate in the early invasive arm.[155] The most recent trial, examined an invasive versus conservative approach in 1200 patients. All patients received aspirin, enoxaparin, abciximab for PCI, and intensive statin therapy. At 1 year there was no significant difference in the rate of the primary endpoint, death, MI, or rehospitalization for angina.[156] During the index hospitalization, there was a higher rate of MI in the invasive arm, although this trial used a definition of MI that included any elevation of any biomarker following PCI, and thus had a much higher periprocedural MI rate compared with earlier trials. In contrast, the risk of nonprocedure-related MI tended to be lower (relative risk [RR] 0.80; 95 percent CI, 0.46 to 1.34) and the invasive arm showed a significantly lower risk of rehospitalization (RR 0.68; 95 percent CI, 0.47 to 0.98). A meta-analysis of contemporary trials has confirmed an overall significant reduction in death, MI, or rehospitalization and of matality during follow-up (see Fig. 53-17).[157]

Indications for Invasive versus Conservative Management Strategies

Based on multiple randomized trials, an early invasive strategy is now recommended in patients with UA/NSTEMI with ST segment changes and/or positive troponin on admission or that evolves over the next 24 hours. In addition, other high-risk indicators, such as recurrent ischemia or evidence of congestive heart failure, are indications for an early invasive strategy.[2] An early invasive approach appears warranted in those with cardiogenic shock, based on studies in acute MI.[161] An early invasive strategy is also advised in those who present with UA/NSTEMI within 6 months of a prior PCI, in whom restenosis may be frequent. Benefit of an early invasive approach also applies to patients with prior CABG.[162]

Timing of an Invasive Strategy

The Intracoronary Stenting with Antithrombotic Regimen Cooling-Off (ISAR-COOL) trial found a benefit of an immediate invasive strategy with an average time from randomization to catheterization of only 2 hours, compared with a delayed invasive strategy (average time to catheterization, 4 days).[110] A second study compared an immediate invasive approach (but without GP IIb/IIIa inhibition) with a strategy that included early GP IIb/IIIa inhibition followed by catheterization within 24 to 48 hours. This study did not find an improvement in the immediate invasive approach as compared with an early invasive strategy.[158] Similarly, two observational studies of the timing of angiography failed to find any major differences in outcomes among patients who underwent protocol-mandated catheterization within the first 12 hours versus 12 to 24 versus 24 to 48 hours.[159,160] Additional trials are ongoing to evaluate the optimal timing of an invasive approach, but based on available information the optimal timing appears to be within the first 48 hours of presentation.

Percutaneous Coronary Intervention

PCI is an effective means of reducing coronary obstruction, improving acute ischemia, and improving regional and global left ventricular function in patients with UA/NSTEMI (see also Chap. 52). Current angiographic success rates are high, generally >95 percent, although the presence of UA/NSTEMI or visualized thrombus can increase the risk of acute complications such as abrupt closure or MI (as compared with patients with stable angina or those without visualized thrombus) Thus, use of GP IIb/IIIa inhibitors, clopidogrel, and/or other antithrombotic drugs in such patients improves both acute and long-term outcomes following PCI. Use of drug-eluting stents reduces the risk of restenosis.[163] Recent studies, however, have emphasized the risk of late stent thrombosis following drug-eluting stent implantation, especially when clopidogrel is stopped.[164] This observation has emphasized the need for effective long-term (likely 2 or more years) dual antiplatelet therapy in these patients (see Chap. 55).

Percutaneous Coronary Intervention versus Coronary Artery Bypass Grafting

When revascularization is required in patients with UA/NSTEMI, the choice is between PCI and CABG. More than eight

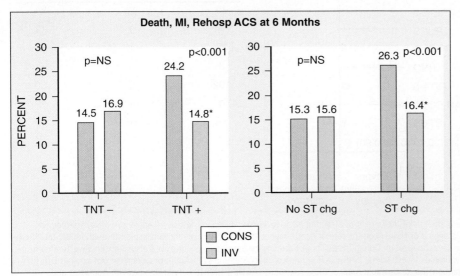

FIGURE 53–18 Risk stratification with troponin T (TnT) or ST segment changes to determine the benefit of an early invasive (INV) versus conservative (CON) strategy in the TACTICS-TIMI 18 trial. ACS = acute coronary syndrome; MI = myocardial infarction. (Data from Cannon CP, et al: N Engl J Med 344:1879-87, 2001.)

trials have compared PCI and CABG in patients with ischemic heart disease, many of whom had UA/NSTEMI. The results of these trials are reviewed in Chapter 54. Based on the results of these trials, CABG is recommended for patients with disease of the left main coronary artery and multivessel disease and impaired left ventricular function. For other patients, either PCI or CABG may be suitable: PCI is associated with a slightly lower initial morbidity and mortality than CABG, but a higher rate of repeat procedures, whereas CABG is associated with more effective relief of angina.

Other Therapies

Angiotensin-Converting Enzyme Inhibitors and Angiotensin Receptor Blockers

For acute treatment, three large trials showed a 0.5 percent absolute mortality benefit of early (initiated within 24 hours) angiotensin-converting enzyme (ACE) inhibitor therapy in patients with acute MI.[78,79] However, the ISIS-4 study showed no benefit in patients without ST elevation.[79] Long-term use of ACE inhibition does prevent recurrent ischemic events and mortality in a broad population of patients now including those with any evidence of CAD (see also Chap. 51).[165,166] Notably, captopril or enalapril reduced recurrent MI and the need for revascularization in the SAVE and SOLVD trials,[167,168] a not observations confirmed using ramipril and perindopril in the HOPE and EUROPA trials,[165,166] These results suggest an anti-ischemic effect of this entire class of agents. Although the PEACE trial did not show any benefit with trandolapril, this may have been because the patients were at relatively low risk at baseline due to more intensive statin therapy and coronary revascularization.[169]

Angiotensin receptor blockers can be substituted for ACE inhibitors based on the Valsartan in Acute Myocardial Infarction Trial (VALIANT) trial, that showed equivalent outcomes in post MI patients between captopril and valsartan.[170] These agents are also indicated in patients who cannot tolerate ACE inhibitors.

Lipid-Lowering Therapy

Long-term treatment with lipid-lowering therapy, especially with statins, has shown benefit in patients following acute MI and unstable angina (see also Chaps. 42 and 51).[171] In the Long-Term Intervention with Pravastatin in Ischemic Disease (LIPID) trial, a prespecified subgroup of more than 3200 UA patients, pravastatin therapy led to a significant 26 percent reduction in total mortality ($p = 0.004$).[172] When initiated in-hospital at the time of an ACS, studies have found improved long-term treatment rates.[173] Trials testing the clinical benefit of early initiation of statin therapy post-ACS have found early reductions in recurrent ischemic events.[174]

Over a longer period of follow-up, in the PROVE-IT TIMI 22 trial, intensive lipid-lowering therapy with atorvastatin 80 mg resulted in a 16 percent reduction in the primary endpoint and a 25 percent reduction in death, MI, or urgent revascularization compared with moderate lipid-lowering therapy with pravastatin 40 mg.[175] A benefit emerged after only 30 days post-ACS,[176] highlighting the importance of early initiation of intensive statin therapy post-ACS (Fig. 53-19). The average LDLs achieved in the two arms were 62 mg/dl and 95 mg/dl, respectively. Based in part on these results, the Adult Treatment Panel III of the National Cholesterol Education Program issued an update in which they recommended a new optional therapeutic LDL goal of <70 mg/dl in high-risk patients with coronary heart disease, such as those with a history of an acute coronary syndrome.[177] There have been three additional trials of intensive statin therapy, one in ACS and two in stable coronary artery disease patients, which have been analyzed by meta-analysis, showing a highly significant 16 percent reduction in coronary death or MI with intensive versus standard statin therapy (Fig. 53-20).[178]

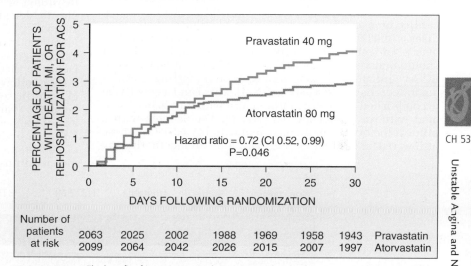

Number of patients at risk							
2063	2025	2002	1988	1969	1958	1943	Pravastatin
2099	2064	2042	2026	2015	2007	1997	Atorvastatin

FIGURE 53–19 The benefit of intensive statin therapy initiated early after acute coronary syndrome (ACS) in the PROVE IT–TIMI 22 trial. A significant reduction in events is seen in the first 30 days. CI = confidence interval; MI = myocardial infarction. *(Reproduced from Ray KK, et al: J Am Coll Cardiol 46:1405-10, 2005.)*

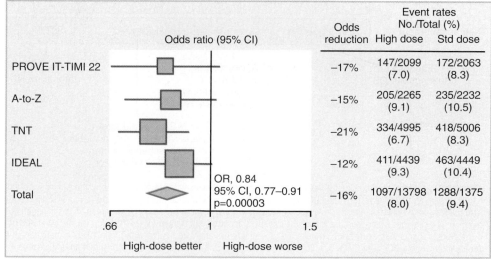

FIGURE 53–20 Meta-analysis of trials of intensive versus standard statin therapy, showing a highly significant 16 percent reduction in the risk of coronary death or myocardial infarction ($p < 0.0001$). A-to-Z = Aggrastat-to-Zocor trial; IDEAL = Incremental Decrease in End Points Through Aggressive Lipid-Lowering trial; PROVEIT–Time-22 = Pravastatin or Atorvastatin Evaluation and Infection Therapy–Thrombolysis In Myocardial Infarction-22 trial; TNT = Treating to New Targets trial. *(Reproduced from Cannon CP, et al: J Am Coll Cardiol 48(3):438-45, 2006.)*

CH 53

Intraaortic Balloon Pump Counterpulsation

Intraaortic balloon pump (IABP) counterpulsation is a very effective means of increasing diastolic coronary blood flow and reducing left ventricular afterload, which act in concert to reduce ischemia (Chap. 51). IABP counterpulstation is usually reserved for patients with UA/NSTEMI who are refractory to maximal medical therapy and those with hemodynamic compromise who are awaiting cardiac catheterization, or those identified to have very high-risk coronary anatomy (e.g., left main stenosis) as a bridge to PCI or CABG. No randomized trials are available to document its benefit, but this method can effectively stabilize patients with refractory ischemia. However, an analysis of 12,730 MI patients (NSTEMI and STEMI) with cardiogenic shock found that increased use of IABP counterpulstation was associated with lower mortality.[179]

Summary: Acute Management of UA/NSTEMI

The evaluation of patients with UA/NSTEMI begins with the clinical history, ECG testing, and measurement of cardiac biomarkers to assess (1) the likelihood of coronary disease and (2) the patient's risk of death or recurrent cardiac events. Patients with a low likelihood of having UA/NSTEMI should undergo a "diagnostic pathway" evaluation via serial ECGs, cardiac biomarkers, and early stress testing to evaluate for coronary disease (Fig. 53-21). This can frequently be accomplished in an observation/chest pain unit in or associated with an emergency department. For patients with a clinical history strongly consistent with UA/NSTEMI, those at low risk should be treated with antithrombotic therapy with aspirin, clopidogrel, an antithrombin, beta blockers, and nitrates. An early conservative strategy is adequate in low-risk patients. For high-risk patients (e.g., those with positive troponin, ST-segment changes, TIMI Risk Score >3), GP IIb/IIIa inhibition (thus, four antithrombotic agents) should be added to the aforementioned medications, and an early invasive strategy is preferred (see Fig. 53-21).

Long-Term Secondary Prevention Following UA/NSTEMI

The time of hospital discharge following UA/NSTEMI affords a "teachable moment" for the patient,[180] when the physician and staff can review and optimize the medical regimen for long-term treatment. Risk factor modification is critical and includes discussions with the patient (as appropriate to their risk factors) on the importance of smoking cessation, achieving optimal weight, exercise, following appropriate diet, good blood pressure control, tight control of hyperglycemia in diabetic patients, and intensive statin therapy (Table 53-5).

Five classes of drugs that have improved outcomes following UA/NSTEMI in large randomized trials should be instituted for long-term treatment. Each agent may contribute to long-term clinical stability in different ways: statins[175,178,181] and ACE inhibitors[182] are recommended for long-term treatment that may facilitate plaque stabilization and progression. Beta blockers are indicated for anti-ischemic therapy and may help decrease "triggers" for MI during follow-up. For antiplatelet therapy, the combination of aspirin and clopidogrel for at least a year confers benefit[101,103] and likely prevents or decreases the severity of any thrombosis that occurs if a plaque were to rupture. Longer duration may be appropriate in patients at high risk of recurrent ischemic events[183] and is generally recommended in patients with drug-eluting stents. Smoking cessation programs involving counseling, the use of nicotine patches or gum, the anxiolytic agent bupropion, and/or the recently approved acetylcholine partial agonist varenicline should be encouraged strongly.[184] Exercise-based cardiac rehabilitation programs coupled with education on weight control, diet, and drug adherence are also advisable. Thus, a multifactorial approach to long-term medical therapy can address the various components of atherothrombosis.

Registry Experience

A major problem identified in clinical practice is that a large proportion of patients do not receive guideline-recommended therapies. Many large registries, in the United States and worldwide, have documented that only 80 to 85 percent of patients received aspirin.[153,185,186] One analysis did observe a slight improvement in utilization of recommended therapies after widespread dissemination and education of national guidelines, but rates of treatment were still suboptimal.[187] These data suggest that in addition to guideline develop-

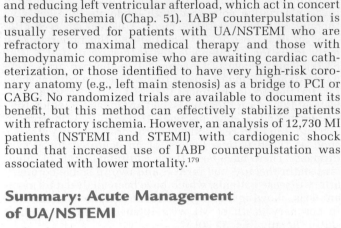
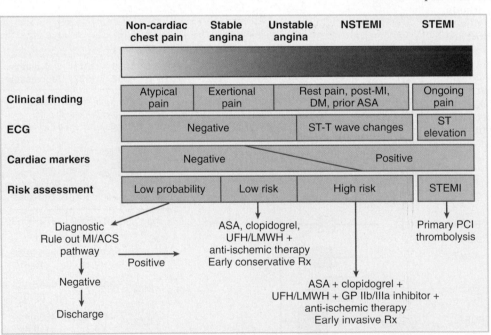

FIGURE 53–21 Algorithm for risk stratification and treatment of patients with UA/NSTEMI. Using the clinical history of the type of pain and medical history, the ECG, and cardiac markers, one can identify patients who have a low likelihood of UA/NSTEMI, for whom a diagnostic "rule-out MI or acute coronary syndrome (ACS)" is warranted. If this is negative, the patient is discharged home, and if positive, the patient is admitted and treated for UA/NSTEMI. On the other end of the spectrum, patients with acute ongoing pain and ST segment elevation are treated with thrombolysis or percutaneous coronary intervention (PCI) (see Chap. 52). For those with UA/NSTEMI, all patients are treated with standard treatment with aspirin, clopidogrel, unfractionated or low molecular weight heparin (LMWH) and antiischemic therapy with beta blockers and nitrates. Risk stratification is used to identify patients at medium to high risk, for whom aggressive treatment with GP IIb/IIIa inhibition and an early invasive strategy is warranted. For patients at low risk, standard treatment is likely sufficient, and a more conservative approach could be expected to be equivalent in outcomes to a more invasive one. ASA = aspirin; DM = diabetes mellitus; ECG = electrocardiogram; MI = myocardial infarction; Rx = treatment; STEMI = ST elevation myocardial infarction.

TABLE 53-5	Cardiac Checklist for UA/NSTEMI*

Cardiac Checklist—ADMISSION

Admit Date: _____

Patient Name: _____
(First Name)   (Middle Initial)   (Last Name)

Brief History: _____

Medications:
1. Aspirin... ☐
2. Clopidogrel... ☐
3. Heparin, LMWH, or other anticoagulant)................. ☐
4. GP IIb/IIIa inhibitor.. ☐
5. Beta blocker... ☐
6. Nitrate... ☐
7. ACE inhibitor.. ☐

Interventions:
8. Cath/revascularization for recurrent ischemia or in
   intermediate- and high-risk patients..................... ☐

Risk Factor Modification:
9. Cholesterol—check and treat as needed.................. ☐
10. Treat other risk factors (e.g., smoking) .... ☐

Cardiac Checklist—DISCHARGE

Admit Date: _____

Patient Name: _____
(First Name)   (Middle Initial)   (Last Name)

Brief History: _____

Medications:
1. Aspirin (low dose)... ☐
2. Clopidogrel... ☐
3. Statin (high-dose).. ☐
4. ACE inhibitor.. ☐
5. Beta blocker... ☐

Interventions:
6. LDL controlled to goal...................................... ☐
7. Blood pressure controlled.................................. ☐
8. Diabetes controlled... ☐
9. Smoking cessation counseling (if applicable)............ ☐
10. Cardiac rehabilitation/life style change................. ☐

*These simple lists serve as reminders of guideline-recommended therapies, such as aspirin, clopidogrel, heparin, or LMWH, etc. This "cardiac checklist" could be used in two ways: physicians could keep a copy on a small index card in their pocket or in their personal digital assistant (PDA)—and run down the list when writing admission orders for patients, or it could be used in developing standard orders for UA/NSTEMI—either printed order sheets or computerized orders. See text for details of specific indications and contraindications for medications.

ACE = angiotensin-converting enzyme; cath = cathetenzation; GP = glycoprotein; LDL = low-density lipoprotein; LMWH = low-molecular-weight heparin.

CH 53

ment and education, there is a need for specific tools to improve implementation of guideline recommendations on a patient-by-patient basis. Most importantly, lack of adherence to the guidelines is associated with adverse outcomes.[188-190] Patients at high risk for recurrent events (the elderly and patients with diabetes mellitus, renal dysfunction, and heart failure) were less likely to receive guideline-recommended therapies than were lower-risk patients.[191]

Critical Pathways and Continuous Quality Improvement

Critical pathways and/or the process of Continuous Quality Improvement (CQI) are means of trying to improve care.[192,193] Critical pathways are standardized protocols for the management of specific diseases (e.g., ACS) that aim to optimize and streamline patient care.[192,194] In general, these pathways involve having standardized order sets, (or computerized ones), and/or simple pocket cards, reminders, or checklists of the appropriate therapies (see Table 53-5). The process of implementation of pathways generally involves physician and nursing education, including presentations at grand rounds, "in services," and other educational meetings throughout the institution to the relevant caregivers. Another key part of an overall CQI effort is to monitor performance—that is, utilization of guideline-recommended therapies.

Critical Pathways Improve Outcomes

There are now several well-conducted studies showing that use of critical pathways can improve quality of care. The Cardiac Hospitalization Atherosclerosis Management Program (CHAMP) program involved staff who assisted the physicians to ensure that all the patients were treated with appropriate guideline-recommended therapies. This measure improved the use of therapies such as aspirin at the time of hospital discharge, from 78 percent up to 92 percent. Importantly, at 1 year follow-up the CHAMP program was able to increase utilization further—up to 94 percent of patients.[195] The same improvement in was seen for beta blocker, ACE inhibitor, and statin use.

The American College of Cardiology–sponsored Guidelines Applied in Practice (GAP) Program has also provided

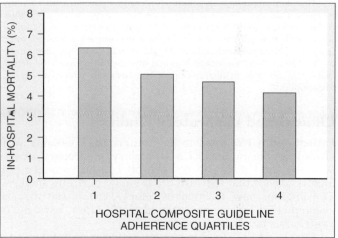

FIGURE 53–22 Association between hospital guideline adherence and in-hospital mortality. *(Adapted with permission from Peterson ED, et al: JAMA 295:1912-20, 2006.)*

important multicenter data supporting the efficacy of critical pathways.[196] Lower mortality is associated with better compliance with use of guideline recommended therapies (Fig. 53-22). In the GAP program, patients in whom the clinical records showed that the pathways and tools had been used had the highest rates of treatment with the recommended therapies.[196] This observation demonstrated that having tools available for clinicians to use as reminders can improve the use of indicated therapies. Most importantly, significantly lower mortality was observed in patients after institution of the GAP project.[197]

PRINZMETAL VARIANT ANGINA

In 1959, Prinzmetal and colleagues described a syndrome of ischemic pain that occurred at rest and not with exertion, accompanied by ST segment elevation.[13] This syndrome, known as Prinzmetal or "variant" angina, may be associated with acute MI, ventricular tachycardia, or fibrillation, as well as with sudden death. Here we refer to this condition as Prinzmetal variant angina (PVA). Incidence of PVA has always been greater in Japan, but across the world the incidence appears to have fallen over the past two decades; this decline is related to more aggressive use of calcium antagonists for hypertension.[198]

Mechanisms

The original hypothesis of Prinzmetal and colleagues was that variant angina results from transient increases in coronary vasomotor tone or vasospasm. The focal vasospasm in PVA should not be confused with generalized vasoconstriction of both the large and small coronary vessels, a normal response to stimuli such as cold exposure; the latter response is much less intense.

The precise mechanisms have not been established, but a systemic alteration in nitric oxide production or an imbalance between endothelium-derived relaxing and contracting factors may prevail.[199] Enhanced phospholipase C (PLC) activity has also been documented. Because PLC (through activating the inositol triphosphate pathway) mobilizes Ca^{2+} from intracellular stores, it may enhance contraction of smooth muscle cells.[200] An inflammatory etiology is supported by the finding of elevated levels of serum hs-CRP in these patients.[201] Polymorphisms of the alpha$_2$ presynaptic and the postsynaptic beta$_2$ receptor are associated with PVA in a known population.[202]

Histological findings in patients undergoing coronary atherectomy suggest that repetitive coronary vasospasm may provoke vascular injury and lead to the formation of neointimal hyperplasia at the initial site of spasm, leading to rapid progression of coronary stenosis in some patients.[203] Imaging with iodine-123-labeled metaiodobenzylguanidine (^{123}I-MIBG) has demonstrated regional myocardial sympathetic denervation in the area of distribution of the vessel in which vasospasm developed.[204]

CH 53

Clinical and Laboratory Findings

Patients with PVA tend to be younger than patients with chronic stable angina or UA secondary to coronary atherosclerosis, and many do not exhibit classic coronary risk factors except that they are often heavy cigarette smokers. The anginal pain is often extremely severe and may be accompanied by syncope, related to AV block, asystole, or ventricular tachyarrhythmias.[205-207]

Attacks of PVA tend to cluster between midnight and 8 AM,[208] and sometimes occur in clusters of two or three within 30 to 60 minutes. Although exercise capacity is generally well preserved in patients with PVA, some patients experience typical pain and ST segment elevations not only at rest but also during or after exertion. Patients with PVA and severe fixed coronary obstruction may have a combination of fixed-threshold, exertion-induced angina with ST segment depression and episodes of angina at rest with ST segment elevation. Some patients appear to have a distinct relation between emotional distress and episodes of coronary vasospasm, in agreement with studies suggesting that sympathovagal imbalance may precipitate spasm in patients with PVA. In rare cases, PVA develops after coronary artery bypass surgery, and occasionally it appears to be a manifestation of a generalized vasospastic disorder associated with migraine and/or Raynaud phenomenon. PVA can also occur in association with aspirin-induced asthma and administration of 5-fluorouracil and cyclophosphamide.[209]

ELECTROCARDIOGRAPHY. The key to the diagnosis of PVA lies in the detection of episodic ST segment elevation with pain (Fig. 53-23).[210-212] Many patients exhibit multiple episodes of asymptomatic ST segment elevation (silent ischemia). ST segment deviations may be present in any leads. Transient conduction disturbances may occur during episodes of ischemia.[213] Myocardial cell damage may occur in the absence of persistent ECG changes in patients with prolonged attacks of PVA. Q wave MI caused by coronary artery spasm in the absence of angiographically demonstrable obstructive CAD has been well documented.[214]

Exercise testing in patients with PVA can yield variable responses. Approximately equal numbers of patients show ST segment depression, no change in ST segments during exercise, or ST segment elevation. These changes reflect the presence of underlying fixed CAD in some patients, the absence of significant lesions in others, and the provocation of spasm by exercise in the remainder. Ambulatory ECG monitoring or the use of a telephone transmitter may be helpful in capturing ST segment elevations during symptomatic episodes.[215]

CORONARY ARTERIOGRAPHY. Spasm of a proximal coronary artery with resultant transmural ischemia and abnormalities in left ventricular function are the diagnostic hallmarks of PVA (see Fig. 53-23).[210,211] Patients with no or mild fixed coronary obstruction tend to experience a more benign course than patients with associated severe obstructive lesions.[216] The vasospastic process almost always involves large segments of the epicardial vessels at a single site, but at different times other sites may be involved. The right coronary artery is the most frequent site, followed by the left anterior descending coronary artery.[215]

PROVOCATIVE TESTS
Ergonovine

Several provocative tests for coronary spasm have been developed. Of these, the ergonovine test is the most sensitive. Ergonovine maleate, an ergot alkaloid that stimulates both alpha-adrenergic and serotonergic receptors and, therefore, exerts a direct constrictive effect on vascular smooth muscle, can induce coronary artery spasm.[215]

When administered intravenously in doses ranging from 0.05 to 0.40 mg, ergonovine provides a sensitive and specific test for provoking coronary artery spasm. The majority of patients who have a response to ergonovine do so at a dose of less than 0.20 mg.[215] In low doses, and in carefully controlled clinical situations, ergonovine is a relatively safe drug, but prolonged coronary artery spasm precipitated by ergonovine may cause MI. Occasionally, conduction disturbances (heart block, asystole) or severe tachyarrhythmias develop. Because of these hazards, it is recommended that ergonovine be administered only to patients in whom coronary arteriography has demonstrated normal or nearly normal coronary arteries and in gradually increasing doses, beginning with a very low dose. Intracoronary nitrates and calcium antagonists are usually effective in providing prompt relief from drug-induced spasm. Absolute contraindications to ergonovine testing include pregnancy, severe hypertension, severe left ventricular dysfunction, moderate to severe aortic stenosis, and high-grade left main coronary artery stenosis.

Acetylcholine

Stimulation of acetylcholine receptors produces a uniform endothelium-dependent dilation of normal coronary vessels of all sizes but leads to vasoconstriction when endothelial function is impaired. In patients with PVA, intracoronary injections of acetylcholine can induce severe coronary spasm and reproduce the clinical syndrome.[217] This focal spasm should not be confused with the mild diffuse constriction that acetylcholine induces in patients with abnormal coronary endothelium. Acetylcholine is infused over a 1-minute period into a coronary artery in incremental doses of 10, 25, 50, and 100 µg, and doses should be separated by 5-minute intervals.

Histamine, dopamine, and serotonin can also induce coronary artery spasm. Hyperventilation can also provoke episodes of PVA.[218] Exercise, the cold pressor test, and induced alkalosis can all cause coronary spasm in patients with PVA, but none of these tests is as sensitive as ergonovine or acetylcholine.

Management

Patients with PVA should be urged strongly to stop smoking. The mainstay of therapy is a calcium antagonist alone or in combination with long-acting nitrates. There are several important differences between the optimal management of

PVA and that of classic (stable and unstable) angina.

1. Patients with both PVA and classic angina usually respond well to nitrates; sublingual or intravenous nitroglycerin often abolishes attacks of PVA promptly, and long-acting nitrates are useful in preventing attacks. Calcium antagonists have proved extremely effective in preventing the coronary artery spasm of PVA,[198,219] and they should ordinarily be prescribed in maximally tolerated doses on a long-term basis. Because calcium antagonists act through a different mechanism than nitrates, these two classes of drugs may have additive vasodilatory effects. All first- and second-generation calcium antagonists have similar (approximately 90 percent) efficacy in producing relief of symptoms, and they also suppress asymptomatic ischemia. In rare instances, a patient responds to only one of these agents—even less commonly, the simultaneous administration of two or even three calcium antagonists is required. Some patients need extremely high doses, although side effects are increased. A rebound of symptoms may occur when calcium antagonist therapy is discontinued.

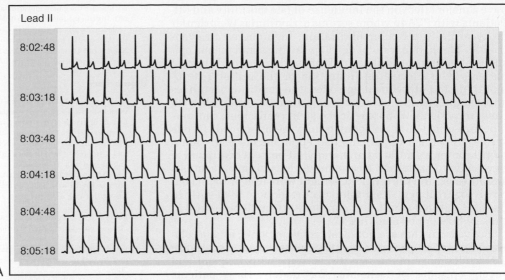

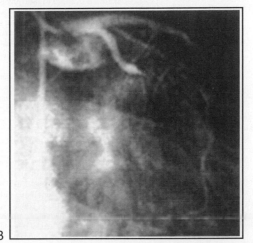

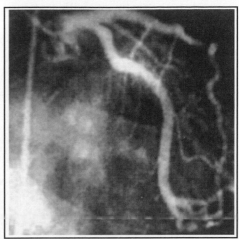

FIGURE 53–23 Findings in a 39-year-old man with Prinzmetal angina. **A,** During an episode of angina, transient ST segment elevation (in lead II) was noted on continuous telemetry. **B,** Hyperventilation-induced total occlusion of the proximal left circumflex artery (visible on angiography from the right anterior oblique caudal view). **C,** Spasm that resolved with the administration of intracoronary nitroglycerine and diltiazem. The patient's symptoms were controlled with oral nitrates and calcium channel blockade during a follow-up of 2 years. *(From Chen HSV, Pinto DS: Prinzmetal angina. N Engl J Med 349:e1, 2003.)*

2. Response to beta blockade in patients with PVA varies.[220] Some, particularly those with associated fixed lesions, exhibit a reduction in the frequency of exertion-induced angina caused primarily by augmentation of myocardial O_2 requirements. In others, however, nonselective beta blockers may actually be detrimental because blockade of $beta_2$ receptors, which subserve coronary dilation, allows unopposed alpha receptor–mediated coronary vasoconstriction to occur; in these patients, the duration of episodes of vasospastic angina may be prolonged by beta blockers.

3. Prazosin, a selective alpha adrenoreceptor blocker, may also have value in patients with PVA.[221] Nicorandil, a vasodilator that influences coronary arterial tone by acting through potassium channel activation, appears to be effective for the treatment of vasospastic angina.[222]

4. Aspirin, helpful in unstable angina, may theoretically increase the severity of ischemic episodes in patients with PVA because it inhibits biosynthesis of the naturally occurring coronary vasodilator prostacyclin. Estradiol supplementation has also been tested with some promise in women.[223]

5. PCI and occasionally CABG may be helpful in patients with PVA and discrete, proximal fixed obstructive lesions.[224] However, spasm may develop at a site different from the initial stenosis; therefore, calcium antagonists should be continued for at least 6 months following successful revascularization. PCI and CABG are contraindicated in patients with isolated coronary artery spasm without accompanying fixed obstructive disease.

6. Patients who have experienced ischemia-associated ventricular fibrillation who continue to manifest ischemia despite maximal medical treatment should receive an implantable cardioverter-defibrillator.[225]

Prognosis

Many patients with PVA pass through an acute, active phase, with frequent episodes of angina and cardiac events during the first 6 months after diagnosis. In a series of 277 patients with a median follow-up of 7.5 years, recurrent angina was common (39 percent), but cardiac death and MI were relatively infrequent and occurred in 3.5 and 6.5 percent of patients, respectively.[226] The extent and severity of the underlying CAD and the activity or the tempo of the syndrome have a major effect on the incidence of late mortality and MI. Patients with PVA in whom serious arrhythmias (ventricular tachycardia, ventricular fibrillation, high-degree atrioventricular block, or asystole) develop during spontaneous episodes of pain have a higher risk of sudden death.[227] In most patients who survive an infarction or the initial 3- to 6-month period of frequent episodes, the condition stabilizes and symptoms and cardiac events tend to diminish with time. In patients who experience such remissions, cautious tapering of calcium antagonists may be attempted. In one series, 16 percent of patients had spontaneous remission 3 months after withdrawal of therapy, 44 percent continued to have symptoms despite treatment with calcium antagonists and nitrates, and the other 40 percent were free of angina but receiving treatment. Remission occurred more frequently in patients without significant coronary artery stenoses and in those who stopped smoking.[228]

For reasons that are not clear, some patients, after a relatively quiescent period of months or even years, experience a recrudescence of vasospastic activity with frequent and severe episodes of ischemia. Fortunately, these patients respond to retreatment with calcium antagonists and nitrates.

REFERENCES

Epidemiology and Pathophysiology

1. American Heart Association: 2006 Heart and Stroke Statistical Update. American Heart Association, 2006: www.amheart.org.
2. Braunwald E, Antman EM, Beasley JW, et al: ACC/AHA guideline update for the management of patients with unstable angina and non-ST segment elevation myocardial infarction-2002: Summary Article: A report of the American College of Cardiology/American Heart Association Task Force on Practice Guidelines (Committee on the Management of Patients with Unstable Angina). Circulation 106:1893-900, 2002.
3. Braunwald E: Unstable angina: A classification. Circulation 80:410-4, 1989.
4. Scirica BM, Cannon CP, McCabe CH, et al: Prognosis in the Thrombolysis in Myocardial Ischemia III Registry according to the Braunwald unstable angina pectoris classification. Am J Cardiol 90:821-826, 2002.
5. Braunwald E: Unstable angina: An etiologic approach to management. Circulation 98:2219-22, 1998.
6. Morrow DA, Braunwald E: Future of biomarkers in acute coronary syndromes: Moving toward a multimarker strategy. Circulation 108:250-2, 2003.
7. Davies MJ: The composition of coronary-artery plaques. N Engl J Med 336:1312-1314, 1997.
8. Asakura M, Ueda Y, Yamaguchi O, et al: Extensive development of vulnerable plaques as a pan-coronary process in patients with myocardial infarction: An angioscopic study. J Am Coll Cardiol 37:1284-8, 2001.
9. The TIMI IIIA Investigators. Early effects of tissue-type plasminogen activator added to conventional therapy on the culprit lesion in patients presenting with ischemic cardiac pain at rest. Results of the Thrombolysis in Myocardial Ischemia (TIMI IIIA) Trial. Circulation 87:38-52, 1998.
10. Kennon S, Price CP, Mills PG, et al: The central role of platelet activation in determining the severity of acute coronary syndromes. Heart 89:1253-4, 2003.
11. Serebruany VL, Glassman AH, Malinin AI, et al: Enhanced platelet/endothelial activation in depressed patients with acute coronary syndromes: Evidence from recent clinical trials. Blood Coagul Fibrinolysis 14:563-567, 2003.
12. Storey RF, May JA, Heptinstall S: Potentiation of platelet aggregation by heparin in human whole blood is attenuated by P_2Y_{12} and P_2Y_1 antagonists but not aspirin. Thromb Res 115:301-7, 2005.
13. Prinzmetal M, Kennamer R, Merliss R, et al: A variant form of angina pectoris. Am J Med 27:375, 1959.
14. Strike PC, Steptoe A: Systematic review of mental stress-induced myocardial ischaemia. Eur Heart J 24:690-703, 2003.
15. Kaski JC: Rapid coronary artery disease progression and angiographic stenosis morphology. Ital Heart J 1:21-5, 2000.
16. Hochman JS, Tamis JE, Thompson TD, et al: Sex, clinical presentation, and outcome in patients with acute coronary syndromes. Global Use of Strategies to Open Occluded Coronary Arteries in Acute Coronary Syndromes IIb Investigators [see comments]. N Engl J Med 341:226-32, 1999.
17. Khot UN, Khot MB, Bajzer CT, et al: Prevalence of conventional risk factors in patients with coronary heart disease. JAMA 290:898-904, 2003.
18. Cannon CP, McCabe CH, Stone PH, et al: The electrocardiogram predicts one-year outcome of patients with unstable angina and non-Q wave myocardial infarction: Results of the TIMI III Registry ECG Ancillary Study. J Am Coll Cardiol 30:133-140, 1997.
19. Savonitto S, Ardissino D, Granger CB, et al: Prognostic value of the admission electrocardiogram in acute coronary syndromes. JAMA 281:707-13, 1999.
20. Goodman SG, Fitchett D, Armstrong PW, et al: Randomized evaluation of the safety and efficacy of enoxaparin versus unfractionated heparin in high-risk patients with non-ST segment elevation acute coronary syndromes receiving the glycoprotein IIb/IIIa inhibitor eptifibatide. Circulation 107:238-244, 2003.
21. The Joint European Society of Cardiology/American College of Cardiology committee. Myocardial infarction redefined—a consensus document of The Joint European Society of Cardiology/American College of Cardiology Committee for the redefinition of myocardial infarction. J Am Coll Cardiol 36:959-69, 2000.

Biomarkers

22. Kleiman N, Lakkis N, Cannon C, et al: Prospective analysis of creatine kinase muscle-brain fraction and comparison with troponin T to predict cardiac risk and benefit of an invasive strategy in patients with non-ST elevation acute coronary syndromes. J Am Coll Cardiol 40:1044-1050, 2002.
23. Morrow DA, Cannon CP, Rifai N, et al: Ability of minor elevations of troponin I and T to predict benefit from an early invasive strategy in patients with unstable angina and non-ST elevation myocardial infarction: Results from a randomized trial. JAMA 286:2405-2412, 2001.
24. Morrow DA, Rifai N, Sabatine MS, et al: Evaluation of the AccuTnI cardiac troponin I assay for risk assessment in acute coronary syndromes. Clin Chem 49:1396-8, 2003.
25. Fleming SM, O'Byrne L, Finn J, et al: False-positive cardiac troponin I in a routine clinical population. Am J Cardiol 89:1212-5, 2002.
26. Horwich TB, Patel J, MacLellan WR, Fonarow GC: Cardiac troponin I is associated with impaired hemodynamics, progressive left ventricular dysfunction, and increased mortality rates in advanced heart failure. Circulation 108:833-8, 2003.
27. Dokainish H, Pillai M, Murphy S, et al: Prognostic implications of elevated troponin in patients with suspected acute coronary syndromes but no epicardial coronary disease. J Am Coll Cardiol 45:19-24, 2005.
28. The TIMI IIIB Investigators. Effects of tissue plasminogen activator and a comparison of early invasive and conservative strategies in unstable angina and non-Q-wave myocardial infarction: Results of the TIMI IIIB Trial. Circulation 89:1545-56, 1994.
29. Cannon CP, Weintraub WS, Demopoulos LA, et al: Comparison of early invasive and conservative strategies in patients with unstable coronary syndromes treated with the glycoprotein IIb/IIIa inhibitor tirofiban. N Engl J Med 344:1879-87, 2001.
30. Karha J, Cannon CP, Murphy S, et al: Safety of stress testing following an acute coronary syndrome. Am J Cardiol 94:1534-6, 2004.
31. Wong GC, Morrow DA, Murphy S, et al: Elevations in troponin T and I are associated with abnormal tissue level perfusion: A TACTICS-TIMI 18 Substudy. Circulation 106:202-207, 2002.
32. Roe MT, Harrington RA, Prosper DM, et al: Clinical and therapeutic profile of patients presenting with acute coronary syndromes who do not have significant coronary artery disease. The Platelet Glycoprotein IIb/IIIa in Unstable Angina: Receptor Suppression Using Integrilin Therapy (PURSUIT) Trial Investigators. Circulation 102:1101-6, 2000.
33. Zairis MN, Papadaki OA, Manousakis SJ, et al: C-reactive protein and multiple complex coronary artery plaques in patients with primary unstable angina. Atherosclerosis 164:355-9, 2002.
34. Lindahl B, Diderholm E, Lagerqvist B, et al: Mechanisms behind the prognostic value of troponin T in unstable coronary artery disease: A FRISC II substudy. J Am Coll Cardiol 38:979-86, 2001.

Management

35. Bach RG, Cannon CP, Weintraub WS, et al: The effect of routine, early invasive management on outcome for elderly patients with non-ST segment elevation acute coronary syndromes. Ann Intern Med 141:186-95, 2004.
36. Roffi M, Chew DP, Mukherjee D, et al: Platelet glycoprotein IIb/IIIa inhibitors reduce mortality in diabetic patients with non-ST-segment-elevation acute coronary syndromes. Circulation 104:2767-2771, 2001.
37. Cotter G, Cannon CP, McCabe CH, et al: Prior peripheral arterial disease and cerebrovascular disease are independent predictors of adverse outcome in patients with acute coronary syndromes: Are we doing enough? Results from the Orbofiban in Patients with Unstable Coronary Syndromes-Thrombolysis In Myocardial Infarction (OPUS-TIMI) 16 study. Am Heart J 145:622-7, 2003.
38. Januzzi JL, Buros J, Cannon CP, Braunwald E, on behalf of the TACTICS-TIMI 18 Investigators: Peripheral arterial disease, acute coronary syndromes, and early invasive management: The TACTICS-TIMI 18 Trial. Clin Cardiol 28:238-242, 2005.
39. Khot UN, Jia G, Moliterno DJ, et al: Prognostic importance of physical examination for heart failure in non-ST-elevation acute coronary syndromes: The enduring value of Killip classification. JAMA 290:2174-81, 2003.
40. Westerhout CM, Fu Y, Lauer MS, et al: Short- and long-term risk stratification in acute coronary syndromes: The added value of quantitative ST-segment depression and multiple biomarkers. J Am Coll Cardiol 48:939-47, 2006.
41. Antman EM, Tanasijevic MJ, Thompson B, et al: Cardiac-specific troponin I levels to predict the risk of mortality in patients with acute coronary syndromes. N Engl J Med 335:1342-49, 1996.
42. James SK, Armstrong P, Barnathan E, et al: Troponin and C-reactive protein have different relations to subsequent mortality and myocardial infarction after acute coronary syndrome: A GUSTO-IV substudy. J Am Coll Cardiol 41:916-24, 2003.
43. Kastrati A, Mehilli J, Neumann FJ, et al: Abciximab in patients with acute coronary syndromes undergoing percutaneous coronary intervention after clopidogrel pretreatment: The ISAR-REACT 2 randomized trial. JAMA 295:1531-8, 2006.
44. Ridker PM, Rifai N, Rose L, et al: Comparison of C-reactive protein and low-density lipoprotein cholesterol levels in the prediction of first cardiovascular events. N Engl J Med 347:1557-65, 2002.

45. Morrow DA, Rifai N, Antman EM, et al: C-reactive protein is a potent predictor of mortality independently and in combination with troponin T in acute coronary syndromes: A TIMI 11A substudy. J Am Coll Cardiol 31:1460-5, 1998.
46. Ridker PM, Cannon CP, Morrow D, et al: C-reactive protein levels and outcomes after statin therapy. N Engl J Med 352:20-8, 2005.
47. Lenderink T, Boersma E, Heeschen C, et al: Elevated troponin T and C-reactive protein predict impaired outcome for 4 years in patients with refractory unstable angina, and troponin T predicts benefit of treatment with abciximab in combination with PTCA. Eur Heart J 24:77-85, 2003.
48. Sabatine MS, Morrow DA, Cannon CP, et al: Relationship between baseline white blood cell count and degree of coronary artery disease and mortality in patients with acute coronary syndromes: A TACTICS-TIMI 18 (Treat Angina with Aggrastat and determine Cost of Therapy with an Invasive or Conservative Strategy—Thrombolysis in Myocardial Infarction 18 Trial)substudy. J Am Coll Cardiol 40:1761-8, 2002.
49. Heeschen C, Hamm CW, Bruemmer J, Simoons ML, for the Chimeric c7E3 AntiPlatelet Therapy in Unstable angina REfractory to standard treatment trial (CAPTURE) Investigators: Predictive value of C-reactive protein and troponin T in patients with unstable angina: A comparative analysis. J Am Coll Cardiol 35:1535-42, 2000.
50. Morrow DA, de Lemos JA, Sabatine MS, et al: Clinical relevance of C-reactive protein during follow-up of patients with acute coronary syndromes in the Aggrastat-to-Zocor Trial. Circulation 114:281-8, 2006.
51. Morrow DA, Rifai N, Antman EM, et al: Serum amyloid A predicts early mortality in acute coronary syndromes: A TIMI 11A study. J Am Coll Cardiol 35:358-362, 2000.
52. de Lemos JA, Morrow DA, Sabatine MS, et al: Association between plasma levels of monocyte chemoattractant protein-1 and long-term clinical outcomes in patients with acute coronary syndromes. Circulation 107:690-5, 2003.
53. Lindmark E, Diderholm E, Wallentin L, Siegbahn A: Relationship between interleukin 6 and mortality in patients with unstable coronary artery disease: Effects of an early invasive or noninvasive strategy. JAMA 286:2107-13, 2001.
54. Cannon CP, McCabe CH, Wilcox RG, et al., for the OPUS-TIMI 16 Investigators: Association of white blood cell count with increased mortality in acute myocardial infarction and unstable angina pectoris. Am J Cardiol 87:636-639, 2001.
55. Mueller C, Neumann FJ, Roskamm H, et al: Women do have an improved long-term outcome after non-ST-elevation acute coronary syndromes treated very early and predominantly with percutaneous coronary intervention: A prospective study in 1450 consecutive patients. J Am Coll Cardiol 40:245-50, 2002.
56. Zhang R, Brennan ML, Fu X, et al: Association between myeloperoxidase levels and risk of coronary artery disease. JAMA 286:2136-42, 2001.
57. Brennan ML, Penn MS, Van Lente F, et al: Prognostic value of myeloperoxidase in patients with chest pain. N Engl J Med 349:1595-604, 2003.
58. Baldus S, Heeschen C, Meinertz T, et al: Myeloperoxidase serum levels predict risk in patients with acute coronary syndromes. Circulation 108(12):1440-5, 2003.
59. Kalantar-Zadeh K, Brennan ML, Hazen SL. Serum myeloperoxidase and mortality in maintenance hemodialysis patients. Am J Kidney Dis 48:59-68, 2006.
60. Buffon A, Biasucci LM, Liuzzo G, et al: Widespread coronary inflammation in unstable angina. N Engl J Med 347:5-12, 2002.
61. Dao Q, Krishnaswamy P, Kazanegra R, et al: Utility of B-type natriuretic peptide in the diagnosis of congestive heart failure in an urgent-care setting. J Am Coll Cardiol 37:379-85, 2001.
62. Richards AM, Nicholls MG, Yandle TG, et al: Plasma N-terminal pro-brain natriuretic peptide and adrenomedullin: New neurohormonal predictors of left ventricular function and prognosis after myocardial infarction. Circulation 97:1921-9, 1998.
63. de Lemos JA, Morrow DA, Bentley JH, et al: The prognostic value of B-type natriuretic peptide in patients with acute coronary syndromes. N Engl J Med 345:1014-21, 2001.
64. Omland T, de Lemos JA, Morrow DA, et al: Prognostic value of N-terminal pro-atrial and pro-brain natriuretic peptide in patients with acute coronary syndromes. Am J Cardiol 89:463-465, 2002.
65. Morrow DA, de Lemos JA, Sabatine MS, et al: Evaluation of B-type natriuretic peptide for risk assessment in unstable angina/non-ST-elevation myocardial infarction: B-type natriuretic peptide and prognosis in TACTICS-TIMI 18. J Am Coll Cardiol 41:1264-72, 2003.
66. Januzzi JL, Cannon CP, DiBattiste PM, et al: Effects of renal insufficiency on early invasive management in patients with acute coronary syndromes (The TACTICS-TIMI 18 Trial). Am J Cardiol 90:1246-9, 2002.
67. Gibson CM, Pinto DS, Murphy SA, et al: Association of creatinine and creatinine clearance on presentation in acute myocardial infarction with subsequent mortality. J Am Coll Cardiol 42:1535-43, 2003.
68. Becker RC, Spencer FA, Gibson M, et al: Influence of patient characteristics and renal function on factor Xa inhibition pharmacokinetics and pharmacodynamics after enoxaparin administration in non-ST-segment elevation acute coronary syndromes. Am Heart J 143:753-9, 2002.
69. Malmberg K, Norhammar A, Wedel H, Ryden L: Glycometabolic state at admission: Important risk marker of mortality in conventionally treated patients with diabetes mellitus and acute myocardial infarction: Long-term results from the Diabetes and Insulin-Glucose Infusion in Acute Myocardial Infarction (DIGAMI) study. Circulation 99:2626-32, 1999.
70. Pinto DS, Skolnick A, Kirtane AJ, et al: U-shaped relationship of blood glucose with adverse outcomes among patients with ST-segment elevation myocardial infarction. J Am Coll Cardiol 46:178-180, 2005.
71. Bhadriraju S, Ray KK, DeFranco AC, et al: Association between blood glucose and long-term mortality in patients with acute coronary syndromes in the OPUS-TIMI 16 trial. Am J Cardiol 97:1573-7, 2006.
72. Tenerz A, Nilsson G, Forberg R, et al: Basal glucometabolic status has an impact on long-term prognosis following an acute myocardial infarction in non-diabetic patients. J Intern Med 254:494-503, 2003.
73. Boersma E, Pieper KS, Steyerberg EW, et al: Predictors of outcome in patients with acute coronary syndromes without persistent ST-segment elevation. Results from an international trial of 9461 patients. Circulation 101:2557-67, 2000.
74. Antman EM, Cohen M, Bernink PJ, et al: The TIMI risk score for unstable angina/non-ST elevation MI: A method for prognostication and therapeutic decision making. JAMA 284:835-42, 2000.
75. Granger CB, Goldberg RJ, Dabbous O, et al: Predictors of hospital mortality in the global registry of acute coronary events. Arch Intern Med 163:2345-53, 2003.
76. Morrow DA, Antman EM, Snapinn SM, et al: An integrated clinical approach to predicting the benefit of tirofiban in non-ST elevation acute coronary syndromes: Application of the TIMI risk score for UA/NSTEMI in PRISM-PLUS. Eur Heart J 23:223-229, 2002.
77. James SK, Lindback J, Tilly J, et al: Troponin-T and N-terminal pro-B-type natriuretic peptide predict mortality benefit from coronary revascularization in acute coronary syndromes: A GUSTO-IV substudy. J Am Coll Cardiol 48:1146-54, 2006.
78. Gruppo Italiano per lo Studio della Sopravvivenza nell'Infarto Miocardico. GISSI-3: effect of lisinopril and trasdermal glyceryl trinitrate singly and together on 6-week mortality and ventricular function after acute myocardial infarction. Lancet 343:1115-1122, 1994.
79. ISIS-4 Collaborative Group. ISIS-4: Randomized factorial trial assessing early oral captopril, oral mononitrate, and intravenous magnesium sulphate in 58,050 patients with suspected acute myocardial infarction. Lancet 345:669-685, 1995.
80. Gottlieb SO, Weisfeldt ML, Ouyang P, et al: Effect of the addition of propranolol to therapy with nifedipine for unstable angina: A randomized, double-blind, placebo-controlled trial. Circulation 73:331-7, 1986.
81. The Holland Interuniversity Nifedipine/Metoprolol Trial (HINT) Research Group. Early treatment of unstable angina in the coronary care unit: A randomised, double blind, placebo controlled comparison of recurrent ischaemia in patients treated with nifedipine or metoprolol or both. Br Heart J 56:400-13, 1986.
82. Yusuf S, Peto R, Lewis J, et al: Beta-blockade during and after myocardial infarction: An overview of the randomized trials. Prog Cardiovasc Dis 27:335-71, 1985.
83. Shivkumar K, Schultz L, Goldstein S, Gheorghiade M: Effects of propranolol in patients entered in the Beta Blocker Heart Attack Trial with their first myocardial infarction and persistent electrocardiographic ST-segment depression. Am Heart J 135:261-7, 1998.
84. Gibson RS, Boden WE, Theroux P, et al: Diltiazem and reinfarction in patients with non-Q wave myocardial infarction. Results of a double-blind, randomized, multicenter trial. N Engl J Med 315:423-429, 1986.
85. The Danish Study Group on Verapamil in Myocardial Infarction. Effect of verapamil on mortality and major events after acute infarction (The Danish Verapamil Infarction Trial II- DAVIT II). Am J Cardiol 66:779, 1990.
86. The Multicenter Diltiazem Postinfarction Trial Research Group. The effect of diltiazem on mortality and reinfarction after myocardial infarction. N Engl J Med 319:385-92, 1998.
87. Packer M, O'Connor CM, Ghali JK, et al: Effect of amlodipine on morbidity and mortality in severe chronic heart failure. N Engl J Med 335:1107-14, 1996.
88. Cohn JN, Ziesche S, Smith R, et al: Effect of the calcium antagonist felodipine as supplementary vasodilator therapy in patients with chronic heart failure treated with enalapril: V-HeFT III. Vasodilator-Heart Failure Trial (V-HeFT) Study Group. Circulation 96:856-63, 1997.

Antiplatelet and Anticoagulant Use

89. Theroux P, Ouimet H, McCans J, et al: Aspirin, heparin or both to treat unstable angina. N Engl J Med 1988;319:1105-11, 1998.
90. The RISC Group: Risk of myocardial infarction and death during treatment with low-dose aspirin and intravenous heparin in men with unstable coronary artery disease. Lancet 336:827-30, 1990.
91. Antithrombotic Trialists' Collaboration. Collaborative meta-analysis of randomised trials of antiplatelet therapy for prevention of death, myocardial infarction, and stroke in high risk patients. BMJ 324:71-86, 2002.
92. Topol EJ, Easton D, Harrington RA, et al: Randomized, double-blind, placebo-controlled, international trial of the oral IIb/IIIa antagonist lotrafiban in coronary and cerebrovascular disease. Circulation 108:399-406, 2003.
93. Peters RJ, Mehta SR, Fox KA, et al: Effects of aspirin dose when used alone or in combination with clopidogrel in patients with acute coronary syndromes: Observations from the Clopidogrel in Unstable angina to prevent Recurrent Events (CURE) study. Circulation 108:1682-7, 2003.
94. Eikelboom JW, Hirsh J, Weitz JI, et al: Aspirin-resistant thromboxane biosynthesis and the risk of myocardial infarction, stroke, or cardiovascular death in patients at high risk for cardiovascular events. Circulation 105:1650-1655, 2002.
95. Gum PA, Kottke-Marchant K, Welsh PA, et al: A prospective, blinded determination of the natural history of aspirin resistance among stable patients with cardiovascular disease. J Am Coll Cardiol 41:961-5, 2003.
96. Frelinger AL, 3rd, Furman MI, Linden MD, et al: Residual arachidonic acid-induced platelet activation via an adenosine diphosphate-dependent but cyclooxygenase-1- and cyclooxygenase-2-independent pathway: A 700-patient study of aspirin resistance. Circulation 113:2888-96, 2006.
97. Gum PA, Kottke-Marchant K, Poggio ED, et al: Profile and prevalence of aspirin resistance in patients with cardiovascular disease. Am J Cardiol 88:230-5, 2001.
98. Mirkhel A, Peyster E, Sundeen J, et al: Frequency of aspirin resistance in a community hospital. Am J Cardiol 98:577-9, 2006.
99. Goto S, Tamura N, Eto K, et al: Functional significance of adenosine 5'-diphosphate receptor (P_2Y_{12}) in platelet activation initiated by binding of von Willebrand factor

to platelet GP Ib alpha induced by conditions of high shear rate. Circulation 105:2531-6, 2002.

100. Clopidogrel in Unstable Angina to Prevent Recurrent Events Trial Investigators: Effects of clopidogrel in addition to aspirin in patients with acute coronary syndromes without ST-segment elevation. N Engl J Med 345:494-502, 2001.
101. Steinhubl SR, Berger PB, Mann JT, 3rd, et al: Early and sustained dual oral antiplatelet therapy following percutaneous coronary intervention: A randomized controlled trial. JAMA 288:2411-20, 2002.
102. Bhatt DL, Bertrand ME, Berger PB, et al: Meta-analysis of randomized and registry comparisons of ticlopidine with clopidogrel after stenting. J Am Coll Cardiol 39:9-14, 2002.
103. Yusuf S, Mehta SR, Zhao F, et al: Early and late effects of clopidogrel in patients with acute coronary syndromes. Circulation 107:966-72, 2003.
104. Mehta SR, Yusuf S, Peters RJ, et al: Effects of pretreatment with clopidogrel and aspirin followed by long-term therapy in patients undergoing percutaneous coronary intervention: The PCI-CURE study. Lancet 358:527-33, 2001.
105. Sabatine MS, Cannon CP, Gibson CM, et al: Effect of clopidogrel pretreatment before percutaneous coronary intervention in patients with ST-elevation myocardial infarction treated with fibrinolytics: The PCI-CLARITY study. JAMA 294:1224-32, 2005.
106. Smith SC, Jr., Feldman TE, Hirshfeld JW, Jr., et al: ACC/AHA/SCAI 2005 Guideline Update for Percutaneous Coronary Intervention-Summary Article: A Report of the American College of Cardiology/American Heart Association Task Force on Practice Guidelines (ACC/AHA/SCAI Writing Committee to Update the 2001 Guidelines for Percutaneous Coronary Intervention). J Am Coll Cardiol 47:216-35, 2006.
107. Fox KA, Mehta SR, Peters R, et al: Benefits and risks of the combination of clopidogrel and aspirin in patients undergoing surgical revascularization for non-ST-elevation acute coronary syndrome: The Clopidogrel in Unstable angina to prevent Recurrent ischemic Events (CURE) Trial. Circulation 110:1202-8, 2004.
108. Cannon CP: What is the Optimal timing of clopidogrel in acute coronary syndromes. Crit Path Cardiol 4:46-50, 2005.
109. Montalescot G, Sideris G, Meuleman C, et al: A randomized comparison of high clopidogrel loading doses in patients with non-ST-segment elevation acute coronary syndromes: The ALBION (Assessment of the Best Loading Dose of Clopidogrel to Blunt Platelet Activation, Inflammation, and Ongoing Necrosis) trial. J Am Coll Cardiol 48:931-8, 2006.
110. Neumann FJ, Kastrati A, Pogatsa-Murray G, et al: Evaluation of prolonged antithrombotic pretreatment ("cooling-off" strategy) before intervention in patients with unstable coronary syndromes: A randomized controlled trial. JAMA 290:1593-9, 2003.

111. Patti G, Colonna G, Pasceri V, et al: Randomized trial of high loading dose of clopidogrel for reduction of periprocedural myocardial infarction in patients undergoing coronary intervention: Results from the ARMYDA-2 (Antiplatelet therapy for Reduction of MYocardial Damage during Angioplasty) study. Circulation 111:2099-106, 2005.
112. Gurbel PA, Bliden KP, Zaman KA, et al: Clopidogrel loading with eptifibatide to arrest the reactivity of platelets: Results of the Clopidogrel Loading With Eptifibatide to Arrest the Reactivity of Platelets (CLEAR PLATELETS) study. Circulation 111:1153-9, 2005.
113. Gurbel PA, Bliden KP, Hayes KM, et al: The relation of dosing to clopidogrel responsiveness and the incidence of high post-treatment platelet aggregation in patients undergoing coronary stenting. J Am Coll Cardiol 45:1392-6, 2005.
114. Matetzky S, Shenkman B, Guetta V, et al: Clopidogrel resistance is associated with increased risk of recurrent atherothrombotic events in patients with acute myocardial infarction. Circulation 109:3171-5, 2004.
115. Wiviott SD, Antman EM: Clopidogrel resistance: A new chapter in a fast-moving story. Circulation 109:3064-7, 2004.
116. Wiviott SD, Antman EM, Winters KJ, et al: Randomized comparison of prasugrel (CS-747, LY640315), a novel thienopyridine P_2Y_{12} antagonist, with clopidogrel in percutaneous coronary intervention: Results of the Joint Utilization of Medications to Block Platelets Optimally (JUMBO)-TIMI 26 trial. Circulation 111:3366-73, 2005.
117. Husted S, Emanuelsson H, Heptinstall S, et al: Pharmacodynamics, pharmacokinetics, and safety of the oral reversible P_2Y_{12} antagonist AZD6140 with aspirin in patients with atherosclerosis: A double-blind comparison to clopidogrel with aspirin. Eur Heart J 27:1038-47, 2006.
118. Wiviott SD, Antman EM, Gibson CM, et al: Evaluation of prasugrel compared with clopidogrel in patients with acute coronary syndromes: Design and rationale for the TRial to assess Improvement in Therapeutic Outcomes by optimizing platelet InhibitioN with prasugrel Thrombolysis In Myocardial Infarction 38 (TRITON-TIMI 38). Am Heart J 152:627-35, 2006.
119. Boersma E, Harrington RA, Moliterno DJ, et al: Platelet glycoprotein IIb/IIIa inhibitors in acute coronary syndromes: A meta-analysis of all major randomised clinical trials. Lancet 359:189-98, 2002.
120. Hamm CW, Heeschen C, Goldmann B, et al: Benefit of abciximab in patients with refractory unstable angina in relation to serum troponin T levels. N Engl J Med 340:1623-9, 1999.
121. Heeschen C, Hamm CW, Goldmann B, et al: Troponin concentrations for stratification of patients with acute coronary syndromes in relation to therapeutic efficacy of tirofiban. Lancet 354:1757-62, 1999.
122. Morrow DA, Sabatine MS, Cannon CP, Theroux P: Benefit of tirofiban among patients treated without coronary intervention: Application of the TIMI Risk Score for Unstable Angina and Non-ST Elevation MI in PRISM-PLUS. Circulation 104 (Suppl. II):II-782, 2001.
123. Topol EJ, Yadav JS: Recognition of the importance of embolization in atherosclerotic vascular disease. Circulation 101:570-80, 2000.
124. Peterson ED, Pollack CV, Jr., Roe MT, et al: Early use of glycoprotein IIb/IIIa inhibitors in non-ST-elevation acute myocardial infarction: Observations from the National Registry of Myocardial Infarction 4. J Am Coll Cardiol 42:45-53, 2003.
125. Stone GW, McLaurin BT, Cox DA, et al: ACUITY: Timing of glycoprotein IIb/IIIa inhibition for patients with acute coronary syndromes. JAMA 297:591-602, 2007.
126. Giugliano RP, Newby LK, Harrington RA, et al: The early glycoprotein IIb/IIIa inhibition in non-ST-segment elevation acute coronary syndrome (EARLY ACS) trial: A randomized placebo-controlled trial evaluating the clinical benefits of early front-loaded eptifibatide in the treatment of patients with non-ST-segment elevation acute coronary syndrome—study design and rationale. Am Heart J 149:994-1002, 2005.
127. Scirica BM, Cannon CP, Cooper R, et al: Drug-induced thrombocytopenia and thrombosis: evidence from patients receiving an oral glycoprotein IIb/IIIa inhibitor in the Orbofiban in Patients with Unstable coronary Syndromes—(OPUS-TIMI 16) trial. J Thromb Thrombolysis 22:95-102, 2006.
128. Cannon CP, McCabe CH, Wilcox RG, et al: Oral glycoprotein IIb/IIIa inhibition with orbofiban in patients with unstable coronary syndromes (OPUS-TIMI 16) trial. Circulation 102:149-156, 2000.
129. Eikelboom JW, Anand SS, Malmberg K, et al: Unfractionated heparin and low-molecular-weight heparin in acute coronary syndrome without ST elevation: A meta-analysis. Lancet 355:1936-42, 2000.
130. Rich JD, Maraganore JM, Young E, et al: Heparin resistance in acute coronary syndromes. J Thromb Thrombolysis 23:93-100, 2007.
131. Warkentin TE, Kelton JG: Temporal aspects of heparin-induced thrombocytopenia. N Engl J Med 344:1286-92, 2001.
132. Hirsh J, Warkentin TE, Shaughnessy SG, et al: Heparin and low-molecular-weight heparin: Mechanisms of action, pharmacokinetics, dosing, monitoring, efficacy, and safety. Chest 119:64S-94S, 2001.
133. Warkentin TE, Levine MN, Hirsh J, et al: Heparin-induced thrombocytopenia in patients treated with low-molecular-weight heparin or unfractionated heparin. N Engl J Med 332:1330-1335, 1995.
134. Antman EM, McCabe CH, Gurfinkel EP, et al: Enoxaparin prevents death and cardiac ischemic events in unstable angina/non-Q-wave myocardial infarction : Results of the Thrombolysis In Myocardial Infarction (TIMI) 11B trial. Circulation 100:1593-601, 1999.
135. Petersen JL, Mahaffey KW, Hasselblad V, et al: Efficacy and bleeding complications among patients randomized to enoxaparin or unfractionated heparin for antithrombin therapy in non-ST-segment elevation acute coronary syndromes: A systematic overview. JAMA 292:89-96, 2004.
136. Blazing MA, de Lemos JA, White HD, et al: Safety and efficacy of enoxaparin vs unfractionated heparin in patients with non-ST-segment elevation acute coronary syndromes who receive tirofiban and aspirin: A randomized controlled trial. JAMA 292:55-64, 2004.
137. Ferguson JJ, Califf RM, Antman EM, et al: Enoxaparin vs unfractionated heparin in high-risk patients with non-ST-segment elevation acute coronary syndromes managed with an intended early invasive strategy: Primary results of the SYNERGY randomized trial. JAMA 292:45-54, 2004.
138. de Lemos JA, Blazing MA, Wiviott SD, et al: Enoxaparin versus unfractionated heparin in patients treated with tirofiban, aspirin and an early conservative initial management strategy: Results from the A phase of the A-to-Z trial. Eur Heart J 25:1688-94, 2004.
139. Michalis LK, Katsouras CS, Papamichael N, et al: Enoxaparin versus tinzaparin in non-ST-segment elevation acute coronary syndromes: The EVET trial. Am Heart J 146:304-10, 2003.
140. Yusuf S, Mehta SR, Chrolavicius S, et al: Comparison of fondaparinux and enoxaparin in acute coronary syndromes. N Engl J Med 354:1464-76, 2006.
141. Yusuf S, Mehta SR, Chrolavicius S, et al: Effects of fondaparinux on mortality and reinfarction in patients with acute ST-segment elevation myocardial infarction: The OASIS-6 randomized trial. JAMA 295:1519-30, 2006.
142. Direct Thrombin Inhibitor Trialists' Collaborative Group: Direct thrombin inhibitors in acute coronary syndromes: Principal results of a meta-analysis based on individual patients' data. Lancet 359:294-302, 2002.
143. Stone GW, McLaurin BT, Cox DA, et al: Bivalirudin for patients with acute coronary syndromes. N Engl J Med 355:2203-16, 2006.
144. Fiore LD, Ezekowitz MD, Brophy MT, et al: Department of Veterans Affairs Cooperative Studies Program clinical trial comparing combined warfarin and aspirin with aspirin alone in survivors of acute myocardial infarction: Primary results of the CHAMP Study. Circulation 105:557-63, 2002.
145. van Es RF, Jonker JJC, Verheugt FWA, et al., for the Antithrombotics in the Secondary Prevention of Events in Coronary Thrombosis-2 (ASPECT-2) Research Group. Aspirin and Coumadin after acute coronary syndromes (the ASPECT-2 study): A randomised controlled trial. Lancet 360:109-13, 2002.
146. Hurlen M, Abdelnoor M, Smith P, et al: Warfarin, aspirin, or both after myocardial infarction. N Engl J Med 347:969-74, 2002.
147. Brouwer MA, van den Bergh PJ, Aengevaeren WR, et al: Aspirin plus coumarin versus aspirin alone in the prevention of reocclusion after fibrinolysis for acute myocardial infarction: Results of the Antithrombotics in the Prevention of Reocclusion In Coronary Thrombolysis (APRICOT)-2 Trial. Circulation 106:659-65, 2002.
148. Loh E, Sutton MS, Wun CC, et al: Ventricular dysfunction and the risk of stroke after myocardial infarction. N Engl J Med 336:1916, 1997.

Invasive and Noninvasive Strategies

149. Antman EM, Anbe DT, Armstrong PW, et al: ACC/AHA guidelines for the management of patients with ST-elevation myocardial infarction—executive summary. A report of the American College of Cardiology/American Heart Association Task Force on Practice Guidelines (Writing Committee to revise the 1999 guidelines for the management of patients with acute myocardial infarction). J Am Coll Cardiol 44:671-719, 2004.

150. FRagmin and Fast Revascularisation during InStability in Coronary artery disease Investigators. Invasive compared with non-invasive treatment in unstable coronary artery disease: FRISC II prospective randomised multicentre study. Lancet 354:708-15, 1999.
151. Fox KA, Goodman SG, Klein W, et al: Management of acute coronary syndromes. Variations in practice and outcome; findings from the Global Registry of Acute Coronary Events (GRACE). Eur Heart J 23:1177-89, 2002.
152. Lagerqvist B, Husted S, Kontny F, et al: 5-year outcomes in the FRISC-II randomised trial of an invasive versus a non-invasive strategy in non-ST-elevation acute coronary syndrome: A follow-up study. Lancet 368:998-1004, 2006.
153. Mahoney EM, Jurkovitz CT, Chu H, et al: Cost and cost-effectiveness of an early invasive versus conservative strategy for the treatment of unstable angina and non-ST elevation myocardial infarction. JAMA 288:1851-8, 2002.
154. Fox KA, Poole-Wilson PA, Henderson RA, et al: Interventional versus conservative treatment for patients with unstable angina or non-ST-elevation myocardial infarction: The British Heart Foundation RITA 3 randomised trial. Randomized Intervention Trial of unstable Angina. Lancet 360:743-51, 2002.
155. Fox KAA, Poole-Wilson P, Clayton TC, et al: 5-Year outcome of an interventional strategy in non-ST-elevation acute coronary syndrome: The British Heart Foundation RITA 3 randomised trial. Lancet 366:914-20, 2005.
156. de Winter RJ, Windhausen F, Cornel JH, et al: Early invasive versus selectively invasive management for acute coronary syndromes. N Engl J Med 353:1095-104, 2005.
157. Bavry AA, Kumbhani DJ, Rassi AN, et al: Benefit of early invasive therapy in acute coronary syndromes: A meta-analysis of contemporary randomized clinical trials. J Am Coll Cardiol 48:1319-25, 2006.
158. van't Hof AW, de Vries ST, Dambrink JH, et al: A comparison of two invasive strategies in patients with non-ST elevation acute coronary syndromes: Results of the Early or Late Intervention in unStable Angina (ELISA) pilot study. 2b/3a upstream therapy and acute coronary syndromes. Eur Heart J 24:1401-5, 2003.
159. McCullough PA, Gibson CM, DiBattiste PM, et al: Timing of angiography and revascularization in acute coronary syndromes: An analysis from the TACTICS-TIMI 18 trial. J Interv Cardiol 81-86, 2004.
160. Ryan JW, Peterson ED, Chen AY, et al: Optimal timing of intervention in non-ST-segment elevation acute coronary syndromes: Insights from the CRUSADE (Can Rapid risk stratification of Unstable angina patients Suppress ADverse outcomes with Early implementation of the ACC/AHA guidelines) Registry. Circulation 112:3049-57, 2005.
161. Hochman JS, Sleeper LA, Webb JG, et al: Early revascularization in acute myocardial infarction complicated by cardiogenic shock. N Engl J Med 341:625-34, 1999.
162. Kugelmass AD, Sadanandan S, Cannon CP, et al: Early invasive strategy improves outcomes in acute coronary syndrome patients with prior CABG: Results from TACTICS-TIMI 18. Circulation 104 (Suppl. II):II-548, 2001.
163. Moses JW, Leon MB, Popma JJ, et al: Sirolimus-eluting stents versus standard stents in patients with stenosis in a native coronary artery. N Engl J Med 349:1315-23, 2003.
164. Iakovou I, Schmidt T, Bonizzoni E, et al: Incidence, predictors, and outcome of thrombosis after successful implantation of drug-eluting stents. JAMA 293:2126-30, 2005.
165. Yusuf S, Sleight P, Pogue J, et al: Effects of an angiotensin-converting-enzyme inhibitor, ramipril, on cardiovascular events in high-risk patients. N Engl J Med 342:145-53, 2000.
166. Fox KM. Efficacy of perindopril in reduction of cardiovascular events among patients with stable coronary artery disease: Randomised, double-blind, placebo-controlled, multicentre trial (the EUROPA study). Lancet 362:782-8, 2003.
167. Rutherford JD, Pfeffer MA, Moye LA, et al: Effects of captopril on ischemic events after myocardial infarction. Results of the Survival and Ventricular Enlargement Trial. Circulation 90:1731-1738, 1994.
168. The SOLVD Investigators: Effect of enalapril on survival in patients with reduced left ventricular ejection fractions and congestive heart failure. N Engl J Med 325:293-302, 1991.
169. Braunwald E, Domanski MJ, Fowler SE, et al: Angiotensin-converting-enzyme inhibition in stable coronary artery disease. N Engl J Med 351:2058-68, 2004.
170. Pfeffer MA, McMurray JJ, Velazquez EJ, et al: Valsartan, captopril, or both in myocardial infarction complicated by heart failure, left ventricular dysfunction, or both. N Engl J Med 349:1893-906, 2003.
171. Heart Protection Study Collaborative Group: MRC/BHF Heart Protection Study of cholesterol lowering with simvastatin in 20,536 high-risk individuals: A randomised placebo controlled trial. Lancet 360:7-22, 2002.
172. Tonkin AM, Colquhoun D, Emberson J, et al: Effects of pravastatin in 3260 patients with unstable angina: Results from the LIPID study. Lancet 356:1871-5, 2000.
173. Smith CS, Cannon CP, McCabe CH, et al: Early initiation of lipid-lowering therapy for acute coronary syndromes improves compliance with guideline recommendations: Observations from the orbobifan in patients with unstable coronary syndromes (OPUS-TIMI 16) Trial. Am Heart J 149:444-50, 2005.
174. Hulten E, Jackson JL, Douglas K, et al: The effect of early, intensive statin therapy on acute coronary syndrome: A meta-analysis of randomized controlled trials. Arch Intern Med 166:1814-21, 2006.
175. Cannon CP, Braunwald E, McCabe CH, et al: Intensive versus moderate lipid lowering with statins after acute coronary syndromes. N Engl J Med 350:1495-1504, 2004.
176. Ray KK, Cannon CP, McCabe C, et al: Early and late benefits of high-dose Atorvastatin in patients with acute coronary syndromes: Results from the PROVE IT-TIMI 22 Trial. J Am Coll Cardiol 46:1405-10, 2005.
177. Grundy SM, Cleeman JI, Merz CNB, et al: Implications of Recent Clinical Trials for the National Cholesterol Education Program Adult Treatment Panel III Guidelines. Circulation 110:227-39, 2004.
178. Cannon CP, Steinberg BA, Murphy SA, et al: Meta-analysis of cardiovascular outcomes trials comparing intensive versus moderate statin therapy. J Am Coll Cardiol 48:438-45, 2006.
179. Chen EW, Canto JG, Parsons LS, et al: Relation between hospital intra-aortic balloon counterpulsation volume and mortality in acute myocardial infarction complicated by cardiogenic shock. Circulation 108:951-7, 2003.
180. Fonarow GC: In-hospital initiation of statins: Taking advantage of the 'teachable moment'. Cleve Clin J Med 70:502, 504-6, 2003.
181. Baigent C, Keech A, Kearney PM, et al: Efficacy and safety of cholesterol-lowering treatment: Prospective meta-analysis of data from 90,056 participants in 14 randomised trials of statins. Lancet 366:1267-78, 2005.
182. Heart Outcomes Prevention Evaluation Study Investigators. Effects of ramipril on cardiovascular and microvascular outcomes in people with diabetes mellitus: Results of the HOPE study and MICRO-HOPE substudy. Lancet 355:253-9, 2000.
183. Bhatt DL, Fox KA, Hacke W, et al: Clopidogrel and aspirin versus aspirin alone for the prevention of atherothrombotic events. N Engl J Med 354:1706-7, 2006.
184. Tonstad S, Tonnesen P, Hajek P, et al: Effect of maintenance therapy with varenicline on smoking cessation: A randomized controlled trial. JAMA 296:64-71, 2006.
185. Hasdai D, Behar S, Wallentin L, et al: A prospective survey of the characteristics, treatments and outcomes of patients with acute coronary syndromes in Europe and the Mediterranean basin: The Euro Heart Survey of Acute Coronary Syndromes (Euro Heart Survey ACS). Eur Heart J 23:1190-201, 2002.
186. Hoekstra JW, Pollack CV, Jr., Roe MT, et al: Improving the care of patients with non-ST-elevation acute coronary syndromes in the emergency department: The CRUSADE initiative. Acad Emerg Med 9:1146-55, 2002.
187. Scirica BM, Cannon CP, Gibson CM, et al: Assessing the effect of publication of clinical guidelines on the management of unstable angina and non-ST-elevation myocardial infarction in the TIMI III (1990-93) and the GUARANTEE (1995-96) registries. Crit Path Cardiol 1:151-160, 2002.
188. Giugliano RP, Lloyd-Jones DM, Camargo CA, Jr., et al: Association of unstable angina guideline care with improved survival. Arch Intern Med 160:1775-80, 2000.
189. Peterson ED, Parsons LS, Pollack CV, et al: Variation in AMI care quality across 1085 US hospitals and its association with hospital mortality rates. Circulation 106 (suppl II):II-722, 2002.
190. Peterson ED, Roe MT, Mulgund J, et al: Association between hospital process performance and outcomes among patients with acute coronary syndromes. JAMA 295:1912-20, 2006.
191. Roe MT, Peterson ED, Newby LK, et al: The influence of risk status on guideline adherence for patients with non-ST-segment elevation acute coronary syndromes. Am Heart J 151:1205-13, 2006.
192. Cannon CP, O'Gara PT: Goals, design and implementation of critical pathways in cardiology. *In* Cannon CP, O'Gara PT (eds): Critical Pathways in Cardiology. Philadelphia, Lippincott, Williams and Wilkins, 2001, pp 3-6.
193. Califf RM, Peterson ED, Gibbons RJ, et al: Integrating quality into the cycle of therapeutic development. J Am Coll Cardiol 40:1895-901, 2002.
194. Cannon CP, Hand MH, Bahr R, et al: Critical pathways for management of patients with acute coronary syndromes: An assessment by the National Heart Attack Alert Program. Am Heart J 143:777-89, 2002.
195. Fonarow GC, Gawlinski A, Moughrabi S, Tillisch JH: Improved treatment of coronary heart disease by implementation of a Cardiac Hospitalization Atherosclerosis Management Program (CHAMP). Am J Cardiol 87:819-22, 2001.
196. Mehta RH, Montoye CK, Gallogly M, et al: Improving quality of care of acute myocardial infarction: The Guideline Applied in Practice (GAP) Initiative in Southeast Michigan. JAMA 287:1269-1276, 2002.
197. Eagle KA, Montoye CK, Riba AL, et al: Guideline-based standardized care is associated with substantially lower mortality in medicare patients with acute myocardial infarction: The American College of Cardiology's Guidelines Applied in Practice (GAP) Projects in Michigan. J Am Coll Cardiol 46:1242-8, 2005.

Vasospasm

198. Sueda S, Kohno H, Fukuda H, Uraoka T: Did the widespread use of long-acting calcium antagonists decrease the occurrence of variant angina? Chest 124:2074-8, 2003.
199. Mayer S, Hillis LD: Prinzmetal's variant angina. Clin Cardiol 21:243-6, 1998.
200. Okumura K, Osanai T, Kosugi T, et al: Enhanced phospholipase C activity in the cultured skin fibroblast obtained from patients with coronary spastic angina: Possible role for enhanced vasoconstrictor response. J Am Coll Cardiol 36:1847-52, 2000.
201. Hung MJ, Cherng WJ, Yang NI, et al: Relation of high-sensitivity C-reactive protein level with coronary vasospastic angina pectoris in patients without hemodynamically significant coronary artery disease. Am J Cardiol 96:1484-90, 2005.
202. Park JS, Zhang SY, Jo SH, et al: Common adrenergic receptor polymorphisms as novel risk factors for vasospastic angina. Am Heart J 151:864-9, 2006.
203. Suzuki H, Kawai S, Aizawa T, et al: Histological evaluation of coronary plaque in patients with variant angina: relationship between vasospasm and neointimal hyperplasia in primary coronary lesions. J Am Coll Cardiol 33:198-205, 1999.
204. Sakata K, Miura F, Sugino H, et al: Assessment of regional sympathetic nerve activity in vasospastic angina: Analysis of iodine 123-labeled metaiodobenzylguanidine scintigraphy. Am Heart J 133:484-9, 1997.
205. Onaka H, Hirota Y, Shimada S, et al: Clinical observation of spontaneous anginal attacks and multivessel spasm in variant angina pectoris with normal coronary arteries: Evaluation by 24-hour 12-lead electrocardiography with computer analysis. J Am Coll Cardiol 27:38-44, 1996.
206. Hung M-J, Cheng CW, Yang NI, al. E. Coronary vasospasm-induced acute coronary syndrome complicated by life-threatening cardia arrhythmias in patients without

hemodynamically significant coronary artery disease. Int J Cardiol 117:37-44, 2007.

207. Yuksel UD, Celik T, Iyisoy A, et al:. Polymorphic ventricular tachycardia induced by coronary vasospasm: A malignant case of variant angina. Int J Cardiol, 2006. E-pubahead of print, Nov. 22, 2006.

208. Kawano H, Motoyama T, Yasue H, et al: Endothelial function fluctuates with diurnal variation in the frequency of ischemic episodes in patients with variant angina. J Am Coll Cardiol 40:266-70, 2002.

209. Matsuguchi T, Araki H, Nakamura N, et al: Prevention of vasospastic angina by alcohol ingestion: Report of 2 cases. Angiology 39:394-400, 1988.

210. Raxwal V, Gupta K: Images in cardiovascular medicine. Coronary artery spasm. Circulation 113:e689-90, 2006.

211. Chen HS, Pinto DS: Images in clinical medicine. Prinzmetal's angina. N Engl J Med 349:e1, 2003.

212. Wang K, Asinger RW, Marriott HJ. ST-segment elevation in conditions other than acute myocardial infarction. N Engl J Med 349:2128-35, 2003.

213. Unverdorben M, Haag M, Fuerste T, et al: Vasospasm in smooth coronary arteries as a cause of asystole and syncope. Cathet Cardiovasc Diagn 41:430-4, 1997.

214. Lip GY, Gupta J, Khan MM, Singh SP: Recurrent myocardial infarction with angina and normal coronary arteries. Int J Cardiol 51:65-71, 1995.

215. Pepine CJ, el-Tamimi H, Lambert CR: Prinzmetal's angina (variant angina). Heart Dis Stroke 1:281-6, 1992.

216. Crea F: Variant angina in patients without obstructive coronary atherosclerosis: a benign form of spasm. Eur Heart J 17:980-2, 1996.

217. Hirano Y, Ueharfa H, Nakamura H, et al: Diagnosis of vasospastic angina: Comparison of hyperventilation and cold-pressor stress echocardiography, and coronary angiography with intracoronary injection of acetylcholine. Int J Cardiol 116:331-337, 2007.

218. Nakao K, Ohgushi M, Yoshimura M, et al: Hyperventilation as a specific test for diagnosis of coronary artery spasm. Am J Cardiol 80:545-9, 1997.

219. Antman E, Muller J, Goldberg S, et al: Nifedepine therapy for coronary artery spasm. Experience in 127 patients. N Engl J Med 302:1269-73, 1980.

220. De Cesare N, Cozzi S, Apostolo A, et al: Facilitation of coronary spasm by propranolol in Prinzmetal's angina: Fact or unproven extrapolation? Coron Artery Dis 5:323-30, 1994.

221. Tzivoni D, Keren A, Benhorin J, et al: Prazosin therapy for refractory variant angina. Am Heart J 105:262-6, 1983.

222. Kaski JC: Management of vasospastic angina—role of nicorandil. Cardiovasc Drugs Ther 9 Suppl 2:221-7, 1995.

223. Kawano H, Motoyama T, Hirai N, et al: Estradiol supplementation suppresses hyperventilation-induced attacks in postmenopausal women with variant angina. J Am Coll Cardiol 37:735-40, 2001.

224. Tanabe Y, Itoh E, Suzuki K, et al: Limited role of coronary angioplasty and stenting in coronary spastic angina with organic stenosis. J Am Coll Cardiol 39:1120-6, 2002.

225. Meisel SR, Mazur A, Chetboun I, et al: Usefulness of implantable cardioverter-defibrillators in refractory variant angina pectoris complicated by ventricular fibrillation in patients with angiographically normal coronary arteries. Am J Cardiol 89:1114-6, 2002.

226. Bory M, Pierron F, Panagides D, et al: Coronary artery spasm in patients with normal or near normal coronary arteries. Long-term follow-up of 277 patients. Eur Heart J 17:1015-21, 1996.

227. Shimokawa H, Nagasawa K, Irie T, et al: Clinical characteristics and long-term prognosis of patients with variant angina. A comparative study between western and Japanese populations. Int J Cardiol 18:331-49, 1998.

228. Tashiro H, Shimokawa H, Koyanagi S, Takeshita A: Clinical characteristics of patients with spontaneous remission of variant angina. Jpn Circ J 57:117-22, 1993.

GUIDELINES *Thomas H. Lee*

Unstable Angina and Non-ST Elevation Myocardial Infarction

CH 53

American College of Cardiology/American Heart Association (ACC/AHA) guidelines for the management of unstable angina and non-ST elevation myocardial infarction (UA/NSTEMI) were published in 2000[1] and updated just 2 years later because of rapid progress in clinical research in this area.[2] An AHA scientific statement published in 2005 offered practical approaches for implementing the guidelines.[3]

Recommendations made in these guidelines that are relevant to the initial evaluation of the patient with acute chest pain are included in the text of Chapter 49. Other recommendations relevant to this topic have been published in guidelines for the use of percutaneous coronary interventions (PCI), summarized in the appendix to Chapter 52.

As with other ACC/AHA guidelines, these use the standard ACC/AHA classification system for indications:

Class I: Conditions for which there is evidence and/or general agreement that the test is useful and effective

Class II: Conditions for which there is conflicting evidence and/or a divergence of opinion about the usefulness or efficacy of performing the test

Class IIa: Weight of evidence or opinion is in favor of usefulness or efficacy

Class IIb: Usefulness or efficacy is less well established by evidence or opinion

Class III: Conditions for which there is evidence and/or general agreement that the test is not useful or effective and in some cases may be harmful

Three levels are used to rate the evidence on which recommendations have been based. Level A recommendations are derived from data from multiple randomized clinical trials, level B recommendations are derived from a single randomized trial or nonrandomized studies, and level C recommendations are based on the consensus opinion of experts.

EARLY RISK STRATIFICATION AND MANAGEMENT

The ACC/AHA guidelines describe a framework for classification of patients into groups at high, intermediate, and low risk for complications on the basis of early clinical data (Table 53G-1). (Details of the components of the initial clinical evaluation and management of the patient with possible acute ischemic heart disease are given in Chapter

49.) Of note is the recommendation that a cardiac-specific troponin is the preferred biomarker of myocardial injury and that biomarkers of injury should be sampled within 6 hours and then again at 6 to 12 hours from the onset of symptoms (Table 53G-2). The guidelines consider evidence to be somewhat favorable (Class IIa) for use of an early marker of cardiac injury such as myoglobin or creatine kinase muscle and brain (CK-MB) subforms in patients who present early after the onset of symptoms but are less encouraging of other tests.

The ACC/AHA guidelines recommend admission to hospital for patients with definite acute coronary syndromes and any of the following:

- Ongoing pain
- Positive cardiac markers
- New ST segment deviations
- New deep T wave inversions
- Hemodynamic abnormalities
- Positive stress test

For patients with possible acute coronary syndrome and negative cardiac markers, early stress testing is recommended; this testing can be performed on an outpatient basis for lower risk patients.

HOSPITAL CARE

The guidelines recommend that patients admitted for acute coronary syndromes with continuing discomfort or hemodynamic instability, or both, be hospitalized for at least 24 hours in a coronary care unit characterized by a nurse-to-patient ratio sufficient to provide continuous rhythm monitoring and rapid resuscitation and defibrillation should it be necessary. Patients who do not have continuing discomfort or hemodynamic instability can be admitted to a step-down unit.

When a patient with high-risk acute coronary syndrome is admitted, treatment should be initiated with aspirin, a beta blocker, antithrombin therapy, and a glycoprotein IIb/IIIa inhibitor unless contraindications exist (Fig. 53G-1). Clinicians should choose between an early invasive strategy, including prompt angiography and revascularization if appropriate, and an early conservative strategy, in which patients are stabilized with medical therapy and angiography is performed if patients have recurrent symptoms or ischemia, heart failure, or serious arrhythmias. Patients managed according to the early con-

TABLE 53G–1	American College of Cardiology/American Heart Association System for Risk Stratification of Patients with Unstable Angina		
Feature	High Risk *At Least One of the Following Features*	Intermediate Risk *No High-Risk Feature but Must Have One of the Following*	Low Risk *No High- or Intermediate-Risk Feature but May Have Any of the Following Features*
History	Accelerating tempo of ischemic symptoms in preceding 48 hr	Prior MI, peripheral or cerebrovascular disease, or CABG, prior aspirin use	
Character of pain	Prolonged ongoing (>20 min) rest pain	Prolonged rest angina, now resolved, with moderate or high likelihood of CAD Rest angina < 20 min or relieved with rest or sublingual NTG	New-onset or progressive CCS Class III or IV angina the past 2 wk without prolonged rest pain but with moderate or high likelihood of CAD
Clinical findings	Pulmonary edema, most likely caused by ischemia New or worsening MR murmur S_3 or new worsening rales Hypotension, bradycardia, tachycardia Age > 75 yr	Age > 70 yr	
ECG	Angina at rest with transient ST segment changes > 0.05 mV Bundle branch block, new or presumed new Sustained ventricular tachycardia	T wave inversions > 0.2 mV Pathological Q waves	Normal or unchanged ECG during an episode of chest discomfort
Cardiac markers	Elevated	Slightly elevated	Normal

CABG = coronary artery bypass graft; CAD = coronary artery disease; CCS = Canadian Cardiovascular Society; ECG = electrocardiogram; MI = myocardial infarction; MR = mitral regurgitation; NTG = nitroglycerin.

TABLE 53G–2	American College of Cardiology/American Heart Association Guidelines for Data Collection for Early Risk Stratification	
Class	Indication	Level of Evidence
Class I (indicated)	A determination should be made in all patients with chest discomfort of the likelihood of acute ischemia caused by CAD as high, intermediate, or low.	C
	Patients who present with chest discomfort should undergo early risk stratification that focuses on anginal symptoms, physical findings, ECG findings, and biomarkers of cardiac injury.	B
	A 12-lead ECG should be obtained immediately (within 10 min) in patients with ongoing chest discomfort and as rapidly as possible in patients who have a history of chest discomfort consistent with ACS but whose discomfort has resolved by the time of evaluation.	C
	Biomarkers of cardiac injury should be measured in all patients who present with chest discomfort consistent with ACS. A cardiac-specific troponin is the preferred marker, and, if available, it should be measured in patients with negative cardiac markers within 6 hr of the onset of pain; another sample should be drawn in the 6- to 12-hr time frame (e.g., at 9 hr after the onset of symptoms).	C
Class IIa (good supportive evidence)	For patients who present within 6 hr of the onset of symptoms, an early marker of cardiac injury (e.g., myoglobin or CK-MB subforms) should be considered in addition to a cardiac troponin.	C
Class IIb (weak supportive evidence)	C-reactive protein (CRP) and other markers of inflammation should be measured.	B
Class III (not indicated)	Total CK (without MB), aspartate aminotransferase (AST, SGOT), beta-hydroxybutyric dehydrogenase, and/or lactate dehydrogenase should be the markers for the detection of myocardial injury in patients with chest discomfort suggestive of ACS.	C

ACS = acute coronary syndrome; AST = aspartate aminotransferase; CAD = coronary artery disease; CK-MB = creatine kinase muscle and brain fraction; ECG = electrocardiogram; SGOT = serum glutamic-oxaloacetic transaminase.

servative strategy should undergo an assessment of left ventricular function and a stress test; they should also undergo angiography if they are found to have an ejection fraction below 40 percent or if they have an intermediate- or high-risk exercise test result.

Patients admitted with acute coronary syndromes should be placed at bed rest with electrocardiographic monitoring (Table 53G-3). Supplemental oxygen is not recommended for routine use by the guidelines because of lack of evidence for benefit; instead, it should be used when patients have cyanosis or respiratory distress. Medical therapy should include nitrates and, in the absence of contraindications, beta block-

ers. If contraindications to beta blockers exist, patients with recurrent ischemia can be treated with a nondihydropyridine calcium antagonist (e.g., verapamil or diltiazem). Morphine sulfate should be used for patients whose condition is not controlled with nitrates or when patients have pulmonary congestion, severe agitation, or both. An angiotensin-converting enzyme (ACE) inhibitor should be started if hypertension persists despite antiischemic therapy or if patients have left ventricular systolic dysfunction or diabetes. The guidelines consider use of immediate-release dihydropyridine calcium antagonists in the absence of a beta blocker inappropriate (Class III).

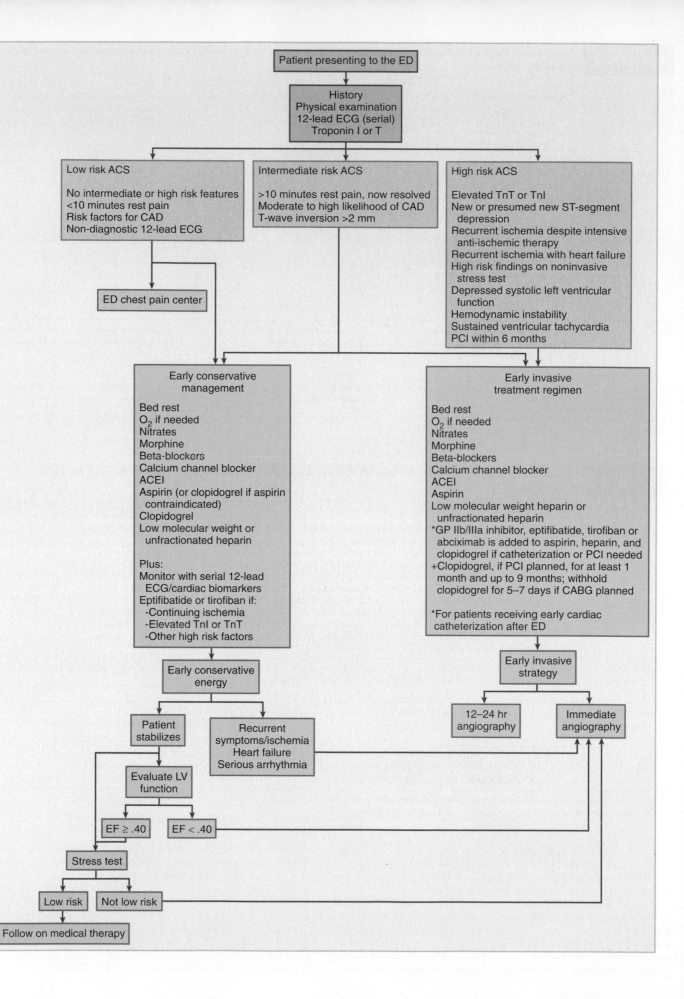

Patient presenting to the ED

History
Physical examination
12-lead ECG (serial)
Troponin I or T

Low risk ACS

No intermediate or high risk features
<10 minutes rest pain
Risk factors for CAD
Non-diagnostic 12-lead ECG

Intermediate risk ACS

>10 minutes rest pain, now resolved
Moderate to high likelihood of CAD
T-wave inversion >2 mm

High risk ACS

Elevated TnT or TnI
New or presumed new ST-segment
    depression
Recurrent ischemia despite intensive
    anti-ischemic therapy
Recurrent ischemia with heart failure
High risk findings on noninvasive
    stress test
Depressed systolic left ventricular
    function
Hemodynamic instability
Sustained ventricular tachycardia
PCI within 6 months

ED chest pain center

Early conservative management

Bed rest
O_2 if needed
Nitrates
Morphine
Beta-blockers
Calcium channel blocker
ACEI
Aspirin (or clopidogrel if aspirin
    contraindicated)
Clopidogrel
Low molecular weight or
    unfractionated heparin

Plus:
Monitor with serial 12-lead
    ECG/cardiac biomarkers
Eptifibatide or tirofiban if:
    -Continuing ischemia
    -Elevated TnI or TnT
    -Other high risk factors

Early invasive treatment regimen

Bed rest
O_2 if needed
Nitrates
Morphine
Beta-blockers
Calcium channel blocker
ACEI
Aspirin
Low molecular weight heparin or
    unfractionated heparin
*GP IIb/IIIa inhibitor, eptifibatide, tirofiban or
    abciximab is added to aspirin, heparin, and
    clopidogrel if catheterization or PCI needed
+Clopidogrel, if PCI planned, for at least 1
    month and up to 9 months; withhold
    clopidogrel for 5–7 days if CABG planned

*For patients receiving early cardiac
    catheterization after ED

Early conservative energy

Early invasive strategy

Patient stabilizes

Recurrent symptoms/ischemia
Heart failure
Serious arrhythmia

12–24 hr angiography

Immediate angiography

Evaluate LV function

EF ≥ .40

EF < .40

Stress test

Low risk

Not low risk

Follow on medical therapy

Class	Indication	Level of Evidence
TABLE 53G–3	**American College of Cardiology/American Heart Association Recommendations for Antiischemic Therapy**	
Class I (indicated)	Bed rest with continuous ECG monitoring for ischemia and arrhythmia detection in patients with ongoing rest pain	C
	NTG, sublingual tablet or spray, followed by intravenous administration, for the immediate relief of ischemia and associated symptoms	C
	Supplemental oxygen for patients with cyanosis or respiratory distress; finger pulse oximetry or arterial blood gas determination to confirm adequate arterial oxygen saturation (SaO$_2$ greater than 90%) and continued need for supplemental oxygen in the presence of hypoxemia	C
	Morphine sulfate intravenously when symptoms are not immediately relieved with NTG or when acute pulmonary congestion and/or severe agitation is present	C
	A beta blocker, with the first dose administered intravenously if there is ongoing chest pain, followed by oral administration. in the absence of contraindications	B
	In patients with continuing or frequently recurring ischemia when beta blockers are contraindicated, a nondihydropyridine calcium antagonist (e.g., verapamil or diltiazem) as initial therapy in the absence of severe LV dysfunction or other contraindications	B
	An ACEI when hypertension persists despite treatment with NTG and a beta blocker in patients with LV systolic dysfunction or CHF and in ACS patients with diabetes	B
Class IIa (good supportive evidence)	Oral long-acting calcium antagonists for recurrent ischemia in the absence of contraindications and when beta blockers and nitrates are fully used	C
	An ACEI for all post-ACS patients	B
	Intraaortic balloon pump (IABP) counterpulsation for severe ischemia that is continuing or recurs frequently despite intensive medical therapy or for hemodynamic instability in patients before or after coronary angiography	C
Class IIb (weak supportive evidence)	Extended-release form of nondihydropyridine calcium antagonists instead of a beta blocker	B
	Immediate-release dihydropyridine calcium antagonists in the presence of a beta blocker	B
Class III (not indicated)	NTG or other nitrate within 24 hr of sildenafil (Viagra) use	C
	Immediate-release dihydropyridine calcium antagonists in the absence of a beta blocker	A

ACEI = angiotensin-converting enzyme inhibitor; ACS = acute coronary syndrome; CHF = congestive heart failure; ECG = electrocardiographic; LV = left ventricular; NTG = nitroglycerin; SaO$_2$ = oxygen saturation in arterial blood.

CH 53

Recommendations for use of antithrombotic therapy were revised considerably to reflect more recent research in the 2002 update to the guidelines, leading to an expanded role for clopidogrel and more complex tactics for use of platelet glycoprotein IIb/IIIa inhibitors.[2] Aspirin continues to be recommended for initial therapy, but the 2002 guidelines describe Class I indications for clopidogrel for patients who are unable to take aspirin, for patients in whom an early noninterventional approach is planned, and for patients in whom percutaneous coronary intervention (PCI) is planned (Table 53G-4). Clopidogrel should be withheld for 5 to 7 days before elective coronary artery bypass grafting (CABG). The guidelines also recommend anticoagulation with low-molecular-weight or unfractionated heparin in addition to antiplatelet therapy.

Glycoprotein IIb/IIIa inhibitors are considered clearly indicated (Class I) in the 2002 guidelines when percutaneous intervention (PCI) is planned for patients receiving aspirin and heparin. If such patients are already receiving heparin, aspirin, and clopidogrel, the ACC/AHA task force considered evidence less conclusive but still generally supportive for addition of a glycoprotein IIb/IIIa inhibitor (Class IIa indication; see Table 53G-4). These agents also received some support for use in high-risk subsets of patients with acute coronary syndromes, even if an invasive strategy is not planned (Class IIa), but the task force thought evidence was generally not favorable for their use in patients without continuing ischemia or other high-risk features. Abciximab was considered inappropriate in patients for whom PCI is not planned.

LATER RISK STRATIFICATION AND MANAGEMENT

The ACC/AHA guidelines support early stress testing in low-risk patients (see Table 53G-1 for risk category definition); for intermediate-risk patients, stress testing can be performed after they have been free of ischemia and heart failure for a minimum of 2 to 3 days (Table 53G-5). The first choice in noninvasive tests is exercise electrocardiography; imaging technologies and pharmacological stress tests should be used for subsets of patients for whom exercise electrocardiography would be expected to have a high likelihood of providing inadequate data. Data from noninvasive tests can be used to stratify patients into high-, intermediate-, and low-risk groups (Table 53G-6). The guidelines endorse prompt angiography without noninvasive risk stratification for patients who are not readily stabilized by intensive medical therapy.

The guidelines recommend an early invasive strategy for patients with acute coronary syndromes and high-risk indicators from their clinical data or noninvasive testing (Table 53G-7). In the absence of such high-risk indicators, the guidelines consider either an early conservative or early invasive strategy to be reasonable. The guidelines also provide some support for use of an early invasive strategy in patients with repeated episodes of suspected acute coronary syndrome without clear evidence for ischemia.

For patients who require coronary revascularization, the principles for choosing between coronary CABG and PCI are similar to those

FIGURE 53G-1 Integrated ACC/AHA guidelines—diagnostic and treatment strategies in the emergency department (ED) for patients with acute coronary syndromes and subsequent management. ACS = acute coronary syndrome; ECG = electrocardiogram; CAD = coronary artery disease; CABG = coronary artery bypass grafting; ACEI = angiotensin-converting enzyme inhibitor; LV = left ventricular; EF = ejection fraction; TnT = troponin T; TnI = troponin I; PCI = percutaneous intervention. *(Modified from Gibler WB, Cannon CP, Blomkalns AL, et al: Practical implementation of the guidelines for unstable angina/non-ST-segment elevation myocardial infarction in the emergency department: A scientific statement from the American Heart Association Council on Clinical Cardiology (Subcommittee on Acute Cardiac Care), Council on Cardiovascular Nursing, and Quality of Care and Outcomes Research Interdisciplinary Working Group, in Collaboration With the Society of Chest Pain Centers. Circulation 111:2699, 2005; and from Braunwald E, Antman EM, Beasley JW, et al: ACC/AHA 2002 guideline update for the management of patients with unstable angina and non-ST-segment elevation myocardial infarction—summary article: A report of the American College of Cardiology/American Heart Association task force on practice guidelines [Committee on the Management of Patients With Unstable Angina]. J Am Coll Cardiol 40:1366, 2002.)*

Unstable Angina and Non-ST Elevation Myocardial Infarction

TABLE 53G-4	American College of Cardiology/American Heart Association Guidelines for Antiplatelet and Anticoagulation Therapy	
Class	Indication	Level of Evidence
Class I (indicated)	Antiplatelet therapy should be initiated promptly. ASA should be administered as soon as possible after presentation and continued indefinitely.	A
	Clopidogrel should be administered to hospitalized patients who are unable to take ASA because of hypersensitivty or major gastrointestinal intolerance.	A
	In hospitalized patients in whom an early noninterventional approach is planned, clopidogrel should be added to ASA as soon as possible on admission and administered for at least 1 mo and for up to 9 mo.	B
	In patients for whom a PCI is planned, clopidogrel should be started and continued for at least 1 mo and up to 9 mo in patients who are not at high risk for bleeding.	B
	In patients taking clopidogrel in whom elective CABG is planned, the drug should be withheld for 5 to 7 d.	B
	Anticoagulation with subcutaneous LMWH or intravenous UFH should be added to antiplatelet therapy with ASA and/or clopidogrel.	A
	A platelet GP IIb/IIa antagonist should be administered, in addition to ASA and heparin, to patients in whom catheterization and PCI are planned. The GP IIb/IIa antagonist may also be administered just prior to PCI.	A
Class IIa (good supportive evidence)	Eptifibatide or tirofiban should be administered, in addition to ASA and LMWH or UFH, to patients *with* continuing ischemia, elevated troponin, or other high-risk features in whom an invasive management strategy is *not* planned.	A
	Enoxaparin is preferable to UFH as an anticoagulant in patients with UA/NSTEMI, unless CABG is planned within 24 hr.	A
	A platelet GP IIb/IIa antagonist should be administered to patients already receiving heparin, ASA, *and* *clopidogrel* in whom catheterization and PCI are planned. The GP IIb/IIIa antagonist may also be administered just prior to PCI.	B
Class IIb (weak supportive evidence)	Eptifibatide or tirofiban, in addition to ASA and LMWH or UFH, should be administered to patients *without* continuing ischemia who have no other high-risk features and in whom PCI is *not* planned.	A
Class III (not indicated)	Intravenous fibrinolytic therapy in patients without acute ST-segment elevation, a true posterior MI, or a presumed new left bundle branch block.	A
	Abciximab administration in patients in whom PCI is not planned.	A

ASA = acetylsalicylic acid (aspirin); CABG = coronary artery bypass graft; GP = glycoprotein; LMWH = low-molecular-weight heparin; MI = myocardial infarction; PCI = percutaneous coronary intervention; UA/NSTEMI = unstable angina or non-ST-elevation myocardial infarction; UFH = unfractionated heparin.

CH 53

TABLE 53G-5	American College of Cardiology/American Heart Association Guidelines for Risk Stratification in Patients with Acute Coronary Syndromes	
Class	Indication	Level of Evidence
Class I (indicated)	Noninvasive stress testing in low-risk patients (see Table 53G-1) who have been free of ischemia at rest or with low-level activity and of CHF for a minimum of 12 to 24 hr.	C
	Noninvasive stress testing in patients at intermediate risk who have been free of ischemia at rest or with low-level activity and of CHF for a minimum of 2 or 3 d.	C
	Choice of stress test based on the resting ECG, ability to perform exercise, local expertise, and technologies available. Treadmill exercise is suitable in patients able to exercise in whom the ECG is free of baseline ST segment abnormalities, bundle branch block, LV hypertrophy, intraventricular conduction defect, paced rhythm, preexcitation, and digoxin effect.	C
	An imaging modality is added in patients with resting ST segment depression (greater than or equal to 0.10 mV), LV hypertrophy, bundle branch block, intraventricular conduction defect, preexcitation, or digoxin who are able to exercise. In patients undergoing a low-level exercise test, imaging modality may add sensitivity.	B
	Pharmacological stress testing with imaging when physical limitations (e.g., arthritis, amputation, severe peripheral vascular disease, severe COPD, general debility) preclude adequate exercise stress.	B
	Prompt angiography without noninvasive risk stratification for failure of stabilization with intensive medical treatment.	B
Class IIa (good supportive evidence)	A noninvasive test (echocardiogram or radionuclide angiogram) to evaluate LV function in patients with definite ACS who are not scheduled for coronary arteriography and left ventriculography.	C
Class IIb (weak supportive evidence)	None	
Class III (not indicated)	None	

ACS = acute coronary syndrome; CHF = congestive heart failure; COPD = chronic obstructive pulmonary disease; ECG = electrocardiogram; LV = left ventricular.

TABLE 53G-6	American College of Cardiology/American Heart Association Noninvasive Risk Stratification

High Risk (>3% Annual Mortality Rate)
1. Severe resting LV dysfunction (LVEF < 0.35)
2. High-risk treadmill score (score ≤ −11)
3. Severe exercise LV dysfunction (exercise LVEF < 0.35)
4. Stress-induced large perfusion defect (particularly if anterior)
5. Stress-induced multiple perfusion defects of moderate size
6. Large, fixed perfusion defect with LV dilation or increased lung uptake (thallium-201)
7. Stress-induced moderate perfusion defect with LV dilation or increased lung uptake (thallium-201)
8. Echocardiographic wall motion abnormality (involving > two segments) developing at a low dose of dobutamine (≤ 10 mg/kg/min) or at a low heart rate (< 120 beats/min)
9. Stress echocardiographic evidence of extensive ischemia

Intermediate Risk (1-3% Annual Mortality Rate)
1. Mild/moderate resting LV dysfunction (LVEF 0.35-0.49)
2. Intermediate-risk treadmill score (−11 < score < 5)
3. Stress-induced moderate perfusion defect without LV dilation or increased lung intake (thallium-201)
4. Limited stress echocardiographic ischemia with a wall motion abnormality only at higher doses of dobutamine involving two segments or less

Low Risk (<1% Annual Mortality Rate)
1. Low-risk treadmill score (score ≥ 5)
2. Normal or small myocardial perfusion defect at rest or with stress
3. Normal stress echocardiographic wall motion or no change of limited resting wall motion abnormalities during stress

LV = left ventricular; LVEF = left ventricular ejection fraction.
From Gibbons RJ, Chatterjee K, Daley J, et al: ACC/AHA/ACP-ASIM guidelines for the management of patients with chronic stable angina. J Am Coll Cardiol 33:2092, 1999.

used for patients with chronic stable angina. The guidelines recommend CABG over PCI for patients with significant left main coronary artery disease and for patients with multivessel disease and diminished ejection fraction or diabetes (Tables 53G-8 and 53G-9). CABG and PCI are both considered appropriate for patients with one- or two-vessel disease without proximal left anterior descending (LAD) coronary artery disease but who have large areas of myocardium in jeopardy (see Table 53G-9). The guidelines provided some support for revascularization with CABG or PCI for patients with proximal LAD disease alone (Class IIa) but do not recommend revascularization for patients without proximal LAD disease or those who have only small amounts of ischemia detected by noninvasive testing.

HOSPITAL DISCHARGE AND POSTHOSPITAL DISCHARGE CARE

The ACC/AHA guidelines emphasize the importance of aggressive risk factor modification and teaching of patients about management of ischemic episodes. Class I indications for pharmacological therapy include the following:

Aspirin 75 to 325 mg/d in the absence of contraindications

Clopidogrel 75 mg/d in the absence of contraindications when aspirin is not tolerated

The combination of aspirin and clopidogrel for 9 months after UA/NSTEMI

Beta blockers in the absence of contraindications

Lipid-lowering agents and diet with low-density lipoprotein (LDL) cholesterol level greater than 130 mg/dl

Lipid-lowering agents if the LDL cholesterol level after diet is greater than 100 mg/dl

ACE inhibitors for patients with heart failure, left ventricular dysfunction, hypertension, or diabetes

CH 53

TABLE 53G-7	American College of Cardiology/American Heart Association Guidelines for Early Conservative versus Invasive Strategies	
Class	**Indication**	**Level of Evidence**

Class I (indicated)	An early invasive strategy in patients with UA/NSTEMI and any of the following high-risk indicators:
	  Recurrent angina or ischemia at rest or with low-level activities despite intensive antiischemic therapy
	  Elevated TnT or TnI
	  New or presumably new ST segment depression
	  Recurrent angina or ischemia with CHF symptoms, and S₃ gallop, pulmonary edema, worsening rales, or new or worsening MR
	  High-risk finding on noninvasive stress testing
	  Depressed LV systolic function (e.g., EF less than 0.40 on noninvasive study)
	  Hemodynamic instability
	  Sustained ventricular tachycardia
	  PCI within 6 mo
	  Prior CABG
		A

	In the absence of these findings, either an early conservative or an early invasive strategy in hospitalized patients without contraindications for revascularzation.	B
Class IIa (good supportive evidence)	An early invasive strategy in patients with repeated presentations for ACS despite therapy and without evidence for ongoing ischemia or high risk	C
Class IIb (weak supportive evidence)		
Class III (not indicated)	Coronary angiography in patients with extensive comorbidities (e.g., liver or pulmonary failure, cancer) in whom the risks of revascularization are not likely to outweigh the benefits	C
	Coronary angiography in patients with acute chest pain and a low likelihood of ACS	C
	Coronary angiography in patients who do not consent to revascularization regardless of the findings	C

ACS = acute coronary syndrome; CABG = coronary artery bypass graft; CHF = congestive heart failure; EF = ejection fraction; LV = left ventricular; MR = mitral regurgitation; PCI = percutaneous coronary intervention; TnI = troponin I; TnT = troponin T; UA/NSTEMI = unstable angina or non-ST-elevation myocardial infarction.

TABLE 53G–8	American College of Cardiology/American Heart Association Guidelines for Revascularization with Percutaneous Coronary Intervention and Coronary Artery Bypass Graft in Patients with Unstable Angina or Non-ST-Elevation Myocardial Infarction	
Class	**Indication**	**Level of Evidence**
Class I (indicated)	CABG for patients with significant left main CAD	A
	CABG for patients with three-vessel disease; the survival benefit is greater in patients with abnormal LV function (EF less than 0.50)	A
	CABG for patients with two-vessel disease with significant proximal left anterior descending CAD and either abnormal LV function (EF less than 0.50) or demonstrable ischemia on noninvasive testing	A
	PCI or CABG for patients with one- or two-vessel CAD without significant proximal left anterior descending CAD but with a large area of viable myocardium and high-risk criteria on noninvasive testing	B
	PCI for patients with multivessel coronary disease with suitable coronary anatomy, with normal LV function and without diabetes	A
	Intravenous platelet GP IIb/IIIa inhibitor in patients with UA/NSTEMI undergoing PCI	A
Class IIa (good supportive evidence)	Repeat CABG for patients with multiple saphenous vein graft (SVG) stenoses, especially when there is significant stenosis of a graft that supplies the LAD	C
	PCI for focal SVG lesions or multiple stenoses in poor candidates for reoperative surgery	C
	PCI or CABG for patients with one- or two-vessel CAD without significant proximal left anterior descending CAD but with a moderate area of viable myocardium and ischemia on noninvasive testing	B
	PCI or CABG for patients with one-vessel disease with significant proximal left anterior descending CAD	B
	CABG with the internal mammary artery for patients with multivessel disease and treated diabetes mellitus	B
Class IIb (weak supportive evidence)	PCI for patients with two- or three-vessel disease with significant proximal left anterior descending CAD, with treated diabetes or abnormal LV function, and with anatomy suitable for catheter-based therapy	B
Class III (not indicated)	PCI or CABG for patients with one- or two-vessel CAD without significant proximal left anterior descending CAD or with mild symptoms or symptoms that are unlikely to be caused by myocardial ischemia or who have not received an adequate trial of medical therapy and who have no demonstrable ischemia on noninvasive testing	C
	PCI or CABG for patients with insignificant coronary stenosis (less than 50% diameter)	C
	PCI in patients with significant left main coronary artery disease who are candidates for CABG	B

CABG = coronary artery bypass graft; CAD = coronary artery disease; EF = ejection fraction; GP = glycoprotein; LAD = left anterior descending; LV = left ventricular; PCI = percutaneous coronary intervention; UA/NSTEMI = unstable angina or non-ST-elevation myocardial infarction.

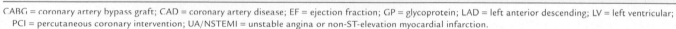

TABLE 53G–9	American College of Cardiology/American Heart Association Guidelines for Mode of Coronary Revascularization for Unstable Angina or Non-ST-Elevation Myocardial Infarction			
Extent of Disease		**Treatment**	**Appropriateness Class**	**Level of Evidence**
Left main disease (≥50% stenosis), candidate for CABG		CABG	I	A
		PCI	III	C
Left main disease, not candidate for CABG		PCI	IIb	C
Three-vessel disease with EF < 0.50		CABG	I	A
Multivessel disease including proximal LAD with EF < 0.50 or treated diabetes		CABG	I	A
		PCI	IIb	B
Multivessel disease with EF > 0.50 and without diabetes		PCI	I	A
One- or two-vessel disease without proximal LAD but with large areas of myocardial ischemia or high-risk criteria on noninvasive testing		CABG or PCI	I	B
One-vessel disease with proximal LAD		CABG or PCI	IIa	B
One- or two-vessel disease without proximal LAD with small area of ischemia or no ischemia on noninvasive testing		CABG or PCI	III*	C
Insignificant coronary stenosis		CABG or PCI	III	C

*Class = I if severe angina persists despite medical therapy.
CABG = coronary artery bypass graft; EF = ejection fraction; LAD = left anterior descending; PCI = percutaneous coronary intervention.

Special Groups

The guidelines indicate that women with acute coronary syndromes should be managed according to the same principles as men, using the same indications for noninvasive tests and treatments. For elderly patients, the guidelines recommend that physicians consider the patient's overall health, comorbidities, cognitive status, and life expectancy as choices are made regarding aggressiveness of management.

For patients with diabetes, the guidelines recommend CABG with internal mammary artery grafts over PCI for diabetic patients with multivessel disease who require revascularization; otherwise, management decisions should be similar to those made for nondiabetics. The task force noted that the use of stents, particularly with abciximab, may provide more favorable results in diabetics but that further data are needed before this approach can be routinely recommended.

For patients with acute coronary syndromes who have previously undergone CABG, the guidelines recommend a lower threshold for angiography because of the many potential causes of ischemia. The guidelines support the use of imaging with stress testing for patients who have previously had CABG (Class IIa indication).

Calcium antagonists and nitrates are recommended for patients with chest pain after cocaine use and for patients with clinical syndromes consistent with coronary spasm. In patients who have used cocaine, coronary angiography is recommended for patients whose ST segments remain elevated after such medical treatment.

References

1. Braunwald E, Antman EM, Beasley JW, et al: ACC/AHA guidelines for the management of patients with unstable angina and non-ST-segment elevation myocardial infarction. A report of the American College of Cardiology/American Heart Association Task Force on Practice Guidelines (Committee on the Management of Patients With Unstable Angina). J Am Coll Cardiol 36:970, 2000.
2. Braunwald E, Antman EM, Beasley JW, et al: ACC/AHA 2002 guideline update for the management of patients with unstable angina and non-ST-segment elevation myocardial infarction—summary article: A report of the American College of Cardiology/American Heart Association task force on practice guidelines (Committee on the Management of Patients With Unstable Angina). J Am Coll Cardiol 40:1366, 2002.
3. Gibler WB, Cannon CP, Blomkalns AL, et al: Practical implementation of the guidelines for unstable angina/non-ST-segment elevation myocardial infarction in the emergency department: A scientific statement from the American Heart Association Council on Clinical Cardiology (Subcommittee on Acute Cardiac Care), Council on Cardiovascular Nursing, and Quality of Care and Outcomes Research Interdisciplinary Working Group, in Collaboration With the Society of Chest Pain Centers. Circulation 111:2699, 2005.

CHAPTER 54

Chronic Coronary Artery Disease

David A. Morrow and Bernard J. Gersh

Magnitude of the Problem, 1353

Stable Angina Pectoris, 1353
Clinical Manifestations, 1353
Differential Diagnosis of Chest
  Pain, 1354
Physical Examination, 1355
Pathophysiology, 1355
Noninvasive Testing, 1356
Catheterization, Angiography, and
  Coronary Arteriography, 1359
Natural History of Angina Pectoris
  and Risk Stratification, 1360
Medical Management, 1362
Pharmacological Management, 1367
Percutaneous Coronary
  Intervention, 1379
Coronary Artery Bypass Surgery, 1380

Other Manifestations of
Coronary Artery Disease, 1395
Prinzmetal (Variant) Angina, 1395
Chest Pain with Normal Coronary
  Arteriogram, 1395
Silent Myocardial Ischemia, 1396
Heart Failure in Ischemic Heart
  Disease, 1397
Cardiac Transplantation–Associated
  Coronary Arteriopathy, 1400

References, 1401

Guidelines, 1405

Chronic coronary artery disease (CAD) is most commonly caused by obstruction of the coronary arteries by atheromatous plaque (the pathogenesis of atherosclerosis is described in Chap. 38). Factors that predispose to this condition are discussed in Chapter 39, the control of coronary blood flow in Chapter 48, acute myocardial infarction in Chapters 50 and 51, and unstable angina in Chapter 53; sudden cardiac death, another significant consequence of CAD, is presented in Chapter 36.

The clinical presentations of CAD are highly variable. Chest discomfort is usually the predominant symptom in chronic (stable) angina, unstable angina, Prinzmetal (variant) angina, microvascular angina, and acute myocardial infarction. However, syndromes of CAD also occur in which ischemic chest discomfort is absent or not prominent, such as asymptomatic (silent) myocardial ischemia, congestive heart failure, cardiac arrhythmias, and sudden death. Obstructive CAD also has many nonatherosclerotic causes, including congenital abnormalities of the coronary vessels, myocardial bridging, coronary arteritis in association with the systemic vasculitides, and radiation-induced coronary disease. Myocardial ischemia and angina pectoris may also occur in the absence of obstructive CAD, as in the case of aortic valve disease (see Chap. 62), hypertrophic cardiomyopathy (see Chap. 65), and idiopathic dilated cardiomyopathy (see Chap. 64). Moreover, CAD may coexist with these other forms of heart disease.

MAGNITUDE OF THE PROBLEM

The importance of CAD in contemporary society is attested to by the almost epidemic number of persons afflicted (see Chap. 1). It is estimated that 13,200,000 Americans have CAD, 6,500,00 of whom have angina pectoris and 7,200,000 have had myocardial infarction.[1] Based on data from the Framingham Heart Study, the lifetime risk of developing symptomatic CAD after age 40 is 49 percent for men and 32 percent for women. In 2003, CAD accounted for 53 percent of all deaths caused by cardiovascular disease and was the single most frequent cause of death in American men and women, resulting in more than one in five deaths in the United States.[1] Approximately every 26 seconds, someone in the United States will suffer a coronary event, and approximately every 60 seconds a coronary event will result in a fatal outcome.[1] The economic cost of CAD in the United States in 2006 has been estimated at $142.5 billion.[1] Ischemic heart disease is now the leading cause of death worldwide, and it is expected that the rate of CAD will only accelerate in the next decade; contributory factors include aging of the population, alarming increases in the worldwide prevalence of obesity, type 2 diabetes, and the metabolic syndrome, as well as a rise in cardiovascular risk factors in younger generations.[2] The World Health Organization has estimated that by 2020, the global number of deaths from CAD will have risen from 7.2 million in 2002 to 11.1 million.[3]

STABLE ANGINA PECTORIS

Clinical Manifestations

CHARACTERISTICS OF ANGINA (see Chap. 11). Angina pectoris is a discomfort in the chest or adjacent areas caused by myocardial ischemia. It is usually brought on by exertion and is associated with a disturbance in myocardial function, without myocardial necrosis. Heberden's initial description of angina as conveying a sense of "strangling and anxiety" is still remarkably pertinent. Other adjectives frequently used to describe this distress include viselike, constricting, suffocating, crushing, heavy, and squeezing. In other patients, the quality of the sensation is more vague and described as a mild pressure-like discomfort, an uncomfortable numb sensation, or a burning sensation. The site of the discomfort is usually retrosternal, but radiation is common and usually occurs down the ulnar surface of the left arm; the right arm and the outer surfaces of both arms may also be involved. Epigastric discomfort alone or in association with chest pressure is not uncommon. Anginal discomfort above the mandible or below the epigastrium is rare. Anginal equivalents (i.e., symptoms of myocardial ischemia other than angina), such as dyspnea, faintness, fatigue, and eructations, are common, particularly in the elderly. A history of abnormal exertional dyspnea may be an early indicator of CAD even when angina is absent or no evidence of ischemic heart disease can be found on the electrocardiogram (ECG). Dyspnea at rest or with exertion may be a manifestation of severe ischemia, leading to increases in left ventricular (LV) filling pressure.[4] Nocturnal angina should raise the suspicion of sleep apnea (see Chap. 74).

The typical episode of angina pectoris usually begins gradually and reaches its maximum intensity over a period of minutes before dissipating. It is unusual for angina pectoris to reach its maximum severity within seconds, and it is characteristic that patients with angina usually prefer to rest, sit, or stop walking during episodes. Chest discomfort while walking in the cold, uphill, or after a meal is suggestive of angina. Features suggesting the absence of angina pectoris include pleuritic pain, pain localized to the tip of one finger, pain reproduced by movement or palpation of the chest wall or arms, and constant pain lasting many hours or, alternatively, very brief episodes of pain lasting seconds. Pain radiating into the lower extremities is also a highly unusual manifestation of angina pectoris.

Typical angina pectoris is relieved within minutes by rest or the use of nitroglycerin. The response to the latter is often a useful diagnostic tool, although it should be remembered that esophageal pain and other syndromes may also respond to nitroglycerin. A delay of more than 5 to 10 minutes before relief is obtained by rest and nitroglycerin suggests that the symptoms are either not caused by ischemia or are caused by severe ischemia, as with acute myocardial infarction or unstable angina. The phenomenon of first-effort or warm-up angina is used to describe the ability of some patients in whom angina develops with exertion to continue subsequently at the same or even greater level of exertion without symptoms after an intervening period of rest. This attenuation of myocardial ischemia observed with repeated exertion has been postulated to be caused by ischemic preconditioning and appears to require preceding ischemia of at least moderate intensity to induce the warm-up phenomenon.

GRADING OF ANGINA PECTORIS. A system of grading the severity of angina pectoris proposed by the Canadian Cardiovascular Society has gained widespread acceptance (see Table 11-1).[5] The system is a modification of the New York Heart Association (NYHA) functional classification but allows patients to be categorized in more specific terms. Other grading systems include a specific activity scale developed by Goldman and associates and an anginal score developed by Califf and colleagues. The Goldman scale is based on the metabolic cost of specific activities and appears to be valid when used by both physicians and nonphysicians. The anginal score of Califf and coworkers integrates the clinical features and tempo of angina together with ST and T wave changes on the ECG and offers independent prognostic information beyond that provided by age, gender, LV function, and coronary angiographic anatomy. A limitation of all these grading systems is their dependence on accurate patient observation and patients' widely varying tolerance for symptoms. Functional estimates based on the Canadian Cardiovascular Society criteria have shown a reproducibility of only 73 percent and still did not correlate well with objective measures of exercise performance.

MECHANISMS. The mechanisms of cardiac pain and the neural pathways involved are poorly understood. It is presumed that angina pectoris results from ischemic episodes that excite chemosensitive and mechanoreceptive receptors in the heart. Stimulation of these receptors results in the release of adenosine, bradykinin, and other substances that excite the sensory ends of the sympathetic and vagal afferent fibers. The afferent fibers traverse the nerves that connect to the upper five thoracic sympathetic ganglia and upper five distal thoracic roots of the spinal cord. Impulses are transmitted by the spinal cord to the thalamus and hence to the neocortex. Data from animal studies have identified the vanilloid receptor-1 (VR_1), an important sensor for somatic nociception, to be present on the sensory nerve endings of the heart and have suggested that VR_1 functions as a transducer of myocardial tissue ischemia.[6] Within the spinal cord, cardiac sympathetic afferent impulses may converge with impulses from somatic thoracic structures, which may be the basis for referred cardiac pain—for example, to the chest. In comparison, cardiac vagal afferent fibers synapse in the nucleus tractus solitarius of the medulla and then descend to excite the upper cervical spinothalamic tract cells, which may contribute to the anginal pain experienced in the neck and jaw. Positron emission tomography (PET) imaging of the brain in subjects with silent ischemia has suggested that failed transmission of signals from the thalamus to the frontal cortex may contribute to this phenomenon, along with impaired afferent signaling, such as that caused by autonomic neuropathy. Experimental observations with VR_1 knockout mice have suggested that ischemia-induced activation of VR_1 triggers a cardioprotective response that may be necessary for ischemic preconditioning.[7]

Differential Diagnosis of Chest Pain

ESOPHAGEAL DISORDERS. Common disorders that may simulate or coexist with angina pectoris are gastroesophageal reflux and disorders of esophageal motility, including diffuse spasm and nutcracker esophagus, which is characterized by high-amplitude peristaltic contractions and vigorous achalasia. To compound the difficulty in distinguishing between angina and esophageal pain, both may be relieved by nitroglycerin. However, esophageal pain is often relieved by milk, antacids, foods or, occasionally, warm liquids.

ESOPHAGEAL MOTILITY DISORDERS. Esophageal motility disorders are not uncommon in patients with retrosternal chest pain of unclear cause and should be specifically excluded or confirmed, if possible. In addition to chest pain, most such patients have dysphagia. Both CAD and esophageal disease are common clinical entities that may coexist. Diagnostic evaluation for an esophageal disorder may be indicated in patients with CAD who have a poor symptomatic response to antianginal therapy in the absence of documentation of severe ischemia or in patients with persistent symptoms, despite adequate coronary revascularization.

BILIARY COLIC. Although visceral symptoms are a common association of myocardial ischemia (particularly acute inferior myocardial infarction; see Chap. 50), cholecystitis and related hepatobiliary disorders may also mimic ischemia and should always be considered in patients with atypical chest discomfort, particularly those with diabetes. The pain is steady, usually lasts 2 to 4 hours, and subsides spontaneously, without any symptoms between attacks. It is generally most intense in the right upper abdominal area but may also be felt in the epigastrium or precordium. This discomfort is often referred to the scapula, may radiate around the costal margin to the back, or may in rare cases be felt in the shoulder and suggest diaphragmatic irritation.

COSTOSTERNAL SYNDROME. In 1921, Tietze first described a syndrome of local pain and tenderness, usually limited to the anterior chest wall and associated with swelling of costal cartilage. This condition causes pain that can resemble angina pectoris. The full-blown Tietze syndrome (i.e., pain associated with tender swelling of the costochondral junctions) is uncommon, whereas costochondritis causing tenderness of the costochondral junctions (without swelling) is relatively common. Pain on palpation of these joints is a useful clinical sign. Local pressure should be applied routinely to the anterior chest wall during examination of a patient with suspected angina pectoris. In addition, costochondritis is usually well localized. Although palpation of the chest wall often reproduces pain in patients with various musculoskeletal conditions, it should be appreciated that chest wall tenderness may also be associated with and does not exclude symptomatic CAD.

OTHER MUSCULOSKELETAL DISORDERS. Cervical radiculitis may be confused with angina. This condition may occur as a constant ache, sometimes resulting in a sensory deficit. The pain may be related to motion of the neck, just as motion of the shoulder triggers attacks of pain from bursitis. Occasionally, pain mimicking angina can be caused by compression of the brachial plexus by the cervical ribs, and tendinitis or bursitis involving the left shoulder may also cause angina-like pain. Physical examination may also detect pain brought about by movement of an arthritic shoulder or a calcified shoulder tendon.

OTHER CAUSES OF ANGINA-LIKE PAIN. Acute myocardial infarction is usually associated with prolonged (longer than 30 minutes), severe pain occurring at rest that, apart from duration, intensity, and precipitants, may be similar to stable angina pectoris. It is associated with characteristic electrocardiographic changes and the release of cardiac markers (see Chap. 50). Unstable angina is a severe form of angina that is characterized by an accelerated pattern and/or occurrence at rest (see Chap. 53). The classic symptom of aortic dissection is a severe, often sharp pain that radiates to the back (see Chap. 56).

Severe pulmonary hypertension may be associated with exertional chest pain with the characteristics of angina pectoris and, indeed, this pain is thought to be caused by right ventricular ischemia that develops during exertion (see Chap. 73). Other associated symptoms include exertional dyspnea, dizziness, and syncope. Associated findings on physical examination, such as parasternal lift, a palpable and loud pulmonary component of the second sound, and right ventricular hypertrophy on the ECG, are usually readily recognized.

Pulmonary embolism is initially characterized by dyspnea as the cardinal symptom, but chest pain may also be present (see Chap. 72). Pleuritic pain suggests pulmonary infarction and a history of exacerbation of the pain with inspiration, along with a pleural friction rub, usually helps distinguish it from angina pectoris.

The pain of acute pericarditis (see Chap. 70) may at times be difficult to distinguish from angina pectoris. However, pericarditis tends to occur in younger patients and the diagnosis depends on the combination of chest pain not relieved by rest or nitroglycerin, exacerbation by movement, deep breathing, and lying flat, a pericardial friction rub which may be evanescent, and electrocardiographic changes.

Physical Examination

Many patients with chronic CAD present with normal physical findings and thus the single best clue to the diagnosis of angina is the clinical history. Nonetheless, careful examination may reveal the presence of risk factors for coronary atherosclerosis or the consequences of myocardial ischemia.

GENERAL EXAMINATION. Inspection of the eyes may reveal a corneal arcus and examination of the skin may show xanthomas. In patients with heterozygous familial hypercholesterolemia (in whom CAD is common), the presence of a corneal arcus increases with age and, in some studies, correlates positively with levels of cholesterol and low-density lipoprotein (LDL) as well as with the prognosis. Xanthelasma, in which lipid deposits are intracellular, appears to be promoted by increased levels of triglycerides and a relative deficiency of high-density lipoprotein (HDL). The presence of xanthelasma is a strong marker of dyslipidemia and often of a family history of cardiovascular disease. Retinal arteriolar changes are common in patients with CAD and diabetes mellitus or hypertension.

Blood pressure may be chronically elevated or may rise acutely (along with the heart rate) during an angina attack. Changes in blood pressure may precede and precipitate or follow (and be caused by) angina.

The association between peripheral vascular disease and CAD is strong and well documented.[8] This association is not confined to patients with symptomatic or clinically overt peripheral vascular disease or CAD, but is also seen in asymptomatic subjects with a reduced ankle-brachial blood pressure index or evidence of early carotid disease on ultrasonography. The presence of carotid and peripheral arterial disease on palpation and auscultation increases the likelihood that chest discomfort of unclear origin is caused by CAD, and indicates that these are markers of an adverse cardiovascular prognosis.[9]

CARDIAC EXAMINATION. The physical findings of hypertrophic cardiomyopathy (see Chap. 65) or aortic valve disease (see Chap. 62) suggest that angina may be caused by conditions other than (or in addition to) CAD. It is often helpful to examine the heart during an episode of pain because ischemia may produce transient LV dysfunction with a third heart sound and pulmonary rales detectable on physical examination.[10] If massage of the carotid sinus produces pain relief, the pain is probably anginal. A displaced ventricular impulse, particularly if dyskinetic, is a sign of significant LV systolic dysfunction.

Transient apical systolic murmurs are common in CAD and have been attributed to reversible papillary muscle dysfunction secondary to transient myocardial ischemia. These murmurs are more prevalent in patients with extensive CAD, especially those with prior myocardial infarction and LV dysfunction, and may indicate an adverse prognosis.

Pathophysiology

Angina pectoris results from myocardial ischemia, caused by an imbalance between myocardial O_2 requirements and myocardial O_2 supply. The former may be elevated by increases in heart rate, LV wall stress, and contractility (see Chap. 48); the latter is determined by coronary blood flow and coronary arterial O_2 content (Fig. 54-1).

Angina Caused by Increased Myocardial O_2 Requirements

In this condition, sometimes termed *demand angina*, the myocardial O_2 requirement increases in the face of a constant and usually restricted O_2 supply. The increased requirement commonly stems from norepinephrine release by adrenergic nerve endings in the heart and vascular bed, a physiological response to exertion, emotion, or mental stress. Of great importance to the myocardial O_2 requirement is the rate at which any task is carried out. Hurrying is particularly likely to precipitate angina, as are efforts involving motion of the hands over the head. Mental and emotional stress may also precipitate angina, presumably by increased hemodynamic and catecholamine responses to stress, increased adrenergic tone, and reduced vagal activity. The combination of physical exertion and emotion in association with sexual activity commonly precipitates angina pectoris. Anger may produce constriction of coronary arteries with preexisting narrowing, without necessarily affecting O_2 demand. Other precipitants of angina include physical exertion after a heavy meal and the excessive metabolic demands imposed by chills, fever, thyrotoxicosis, tachycardia from any cause, and hypoglycemia.

Angina Caused by Transiently Decreased O_2 Supply

Evidence has suggested that not only unstable angina but also chronic stable angina may be caused by transient reductions in O_2 supply as a consequence of coronary vasoconstriction, a condition sometimes termed *supply angina* and caused by dynamic stenosis. In the presence of organic stenoses, platelet thrombi and leukocytes may elaborate vasoconstrictor substances, such as serotonin and thromboxane A_2. Also, endothelial damage in atherosclerotic coronary arteries may result in decreased production of vasodilator substances and an abnormal vasoconstrictor response to exercise and other stimuli. A variable threshold of myocardial ischemia in patients with chronic stable angina may be caused by dynamic changes in peristenotic smooth muscle tone and also by constriction of arteries distal to the stenosis.

In rare patients without organic obstructing lesions, severe dynamic obstruction occurring at rest alone can cause myocardial ischemia and result in angina (see Prinzmetal [Variant] Angina, Chap. 53). On the other hand,

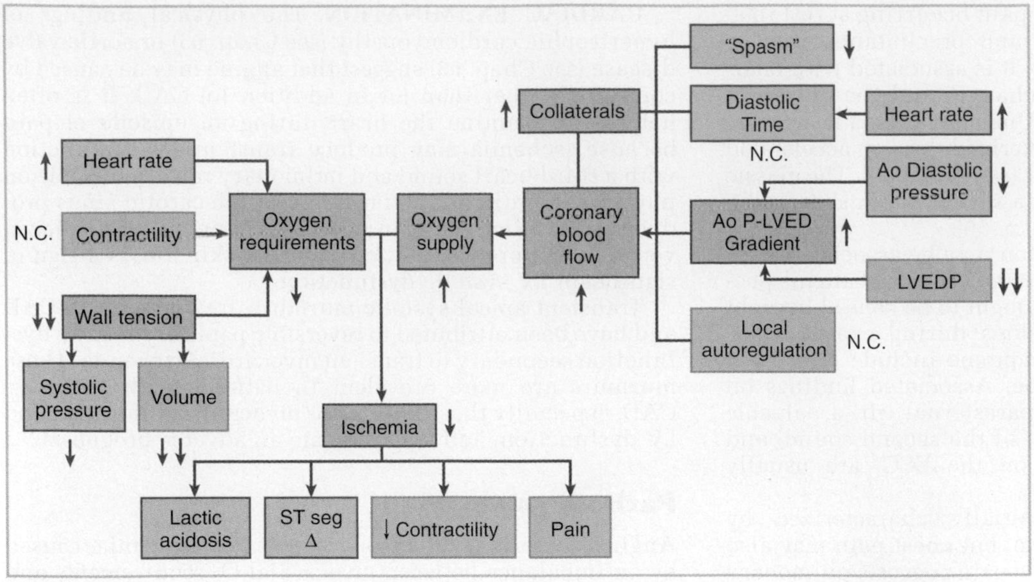

FIGURE 54–1 Factors influencing the balance between myocardial O_2 requirement **(left)** and supply **(right)**. Arrows indicate effects of nitrates. In relieving angina pectoris, nitrates exert favorable effects by reducing O_2 requirements and increasing supply. Although a reflex increase in heart rate would tend to reduce the time for coronary flow, dilation of collaterals and enhancement of the pressure gradient for flow to occur as the left ventricular end-diastolic pressure (LVEDP) falls tend to increase coronary flow. Ao P-LVED = aortic pressure–left ventricular end-diastolic; N.C. = no change. *(From Frishman WH: Pharmacology of the nitrates in angina pectoris. Am J Cardiol 56:8I-13I, 1985.)*

in patients with severe fixed obstruction to coronary blood flow, only a minor increase in dynamic obstruction is necessary for blood flow to fall below a critical level and cause myocardial ischemia.

FIXED-THRESHOLD COMPARED WITH VARIABLE-THRESHOLD ANGINA. In patients with fixed-threshold angina precipitated by increased O_2 demands with few if any dynamic (vasoconstrictor) components, the level of physical activity required to precipitate angina is relatively constant. Characteristically, these patients can predict the amount of physical activity that will precipitate angina—for example, walking up exactly two flights of stairs at a customary pace. When tested on a treadmill or bicycle, the pressure-rate product (the so-called double product), a correlate of the myocardial O_2 requirement) that elicits angina and/or electrocardiographic evidence of ischemia is relatively constant.

Most patients with variable-threshold angina have atherosclerotic coronary arterial narrowing, but dynamic obstruction caused by vasoconstriction plays an important role in causing myocardial ischemia. These patients typically have good days, when they are capable of substantial physical activity, as well as bad days, when even minimal activity can cause clinical and/or electrocardiographic evidence of myocardial ischemia or angina at rest. They often complain of a circadian variation in angina that is more common in the morning. Angina on exertion and sometimes even at rest may be precipitated by cold temperature, emotion, and mental stress.

Postprandial angina may be a marker of severe multivessel CAD. The mechanism has not been explained, but it may be caused by redistribution of coronary blood flow away from the territory supplied by severely stenosed vessels. Some evidence has indicated that this phenomenon is more prominent after high-carbohydrate than high-fat meals.

MIXED ANGINA. The term *mixed angina* has been proposed by Maseri and colleagues to describe the many patients who fall between the two extremes of fixed-threshold and variable-threshold angina.

The pathophysiological and clinical correlations of ischemia in patients with stable CAD may have important implications for the selection of antiischemic agents, as well as for their timing. The greater the contribution from increased myocardial O_2 requirements to the imbalance between supply and demand, the greater the likelihood that beta-blocking agents will be effective, whereas nitrates and calcium channel blocking agents, at least hypothetically, are likely to be especially effective in episodes caused primarily by coronary vasoconstriction. The finding that, in most patients with chronic stable angina, an increase in myocardial O_2 requirement precedes episodes of ischemia—that is, that they have demand angina—argues in favor of beta blockers as essential therapeutic agents.

Noninvasive Testing

Biochemical Tests

In patients with chronic stable angina, metabolic abnormalities that are risk factors for the development of CAD are frequently detected. These abnormalities include hypercholesterolemia and other dyslipidemias (see Chap. 42), carbohydrate intolerance, and insulin resistance. Moreover, chronic kidney disease is strongly associated with the risk of atherosclerotic vascular disease (see Chap. 88).[11] All patients with established or suspected CAD warrant biochemical evaluation of total cholesterol, LDL cholesterol, HDL cholesterol, triglyceride, serum creatinine (estimated glomerular filtration), and fasting blood glucose levels.

Several other biochemical markers have been shown to be associated with higher risk of future cardiovascular events (see Chap. 39). Measurement of lipoprotein(a) and other lipid elements that are particularly atherogenic, such as apoprotein B and small dense LDLs, appear to add prognostic information to the measurement of total cholesterol and LDL,[12] and may be considered as a secondary target for therapy in patients who have achieved therapeutic targets for LDL; however, no consensus has been reached regarding routine measurement.[13] Similarly, lipoprotein-associated phospholipase A_2 (Lp-PLA2) has been associated with the risk of coronary heart disease as well as recurrent events independent of traditional risk factors.[14] An assay for Lp-PLA2 is available for clinical use but has not been incorporated into guidelines for routine risk assessment. Homocysteine has also been linked to atherogenesis and correlates with the risk of CAD; however, in aggregate, prospective studies have supported at most a modest increase in risk associated with elevated homocysteine levels and have not consistently demonstrated a relationship independent of traditional risk factors or other biochemical markers. Therefore, general screening for elevated homocysteine levels is not recommended.[15]

Advances in understanding regarding the pathobiology of atherothrombosis (see Chap. 38) have generated intense interest in inflammatory biomarkers as noninvasive indicators of underlying atherosclerosis and cardiovascular risk. High-sensitivity measurement of the acute-phase protein C-reactive protein (hsCRP) has shown a strong and consistent relationship to the risk of incident cardiovascular events.[16] The prognostic value of hsCRP is additive to traditional risk factors, including lipid screening.[17] Measurement of hsCRP in patients judged at intermediate risk by global risk assessment (10 to 20 percent risk of coronary heart disease [CHD]/10 years) may help direct further evaluation and therapy in the primary prevention of CHD (see Chap. 39) and may be useful as an independent marker of prognosis in patients with established CAD.[18] Other biomarkers of inflammation, such as myeloperoxidase, soluble CD40 ligand, and metalloproteinases, remain under study as markers of underlying athersclerosis.[19]

Blood levels of cardiac markers of necrosis (e.g., cardiac troponin) are normal in patients with chronic stable angina, which serves to differentiate them from patients with acute myocardial infarction. Novel biomarkers of myocardial ischemia are currently under study and may ultimately prove valuable in the noninvasive detection of ischemia in patients with stable CAD.[20] For example, the plasma concentration of brain natriuretic peptide (BNP) increases in response to spontaneous or provoked ischemia.[21] Although BNP and N-terminal pro-BNP may not have sufficient specificity to aid in the diagnosis of stable CAD, their concentration is associated with the risk of future cardiovascular events in those at risk for and with established CAD.[22]

Resting Electrocardiogram

The resting ECG (see Chap. 12) is normal in approximately half of patients with chronic stable angina pectoris, and even patients with severe CAD may have a normal tracing at rest. A normal resting ECG suggests the presence of normal resting LV function and is an unusual finding in a patient with an extensive previous infarction. The most common electrocardiographic abnormalities in patients with chronic CAD are nonspecific ST-T wave changes with or without abnormal Q waves. In addition to myocardial ischemia, other conditions that can produce ST-T wave abnormalities include LV hypertrophy and dilation, electrolyte abnormalities, neurogenic effects, and antiarrhythmic drugs. In patients with known CAD, however, the occurrence of ST-T wave abnormalities on the resting ECG may correlate with the severity of the underlying heart disease. This association may explain the adverse association of ST-T wave changes with prognosis in these patients. In contrast, a normal resting ECG is a more favorable long-term prognostic sign in patients with suspected or definite CAD.

Interval ECGs may reveal the development of Q wave infarctions that have gone unrecognized clinically. Various conduction disturbances, most frequently left bundle branch block and left anterior fascicular block, may occur in patients with chronic stable angina, and they are often associated with impairment of LV function and reflect multivessel disease and previous myocardial damage. Hence, such conduction disturbances are an indicator of a relatively poor prognosis.[10] Abnormal Q waves are relatively specific but insensitive indicators of previous myocardial infarction. Various arrhythmias, especially ventricular premature beats, may be present on the ECG, but they too have low sensitivity and specificity for CAD. LV hypertrophy on the ECG suggests a poor prognosis in patients with chronic stable angina. This finding suggests the presence of underlying hypertension, aortic stenosis, hypertrophic cardiomyopathy, or prior myocardial infarction (MI) with remodeling and warrants further evaluation, such as echocardiography to assess LV size, wall thickness, and function.

During an episode of angina pectoris, the ECG becomes abnormal in 50 percent or more of patients with normal resting ECGs. The most common finding is ST segment depression, although ST segment elevation and normalization of previous resting ST-T wave depression or inversion (pseudonormalization) may develop. Ambulatory electrocardiographic monitoring has shown that many patients with symptomatic myocardial ischemia also have episodes of silent ischemia that would otherwise go unrecognized during normal daily activities. Although this form of electrocardiographic testing provides a quantitative estimate of the frequency and duration of ischemic episodes during routine activities, its sensitivity for detecting CAD is less than that of exercise electrocardiography.

Noninvasive Stress Testing (see Chaps. 13, 14, and 16)

Noninvasive stress testing can provide useful and often indispensable information to establish the diagnosis and estimate the prognosis in patients with chronic stable angina.[23] However, the indiscriminate use of such tests may provide limited incremental information beyond that provided by the physician's detailed and thoughtful clinical assessment. Appropriate application of noninvasive tests requires consideration of bayesian principles, which state that the reliability and predictive accuracy of any test are defined not only by its sensitivity and specificity but also by the prevalence of disease (or pretest probability) in the population under study. A reasonable estimate of the pretest probability of CAD may be made on clinical grounds (Table 54-1).

Noninvasive testing should be performed only if the incremental amount of information provided by a test is likely to alter the planned management strategy. The value of noninvasive stress testing is greatest when the pretest likelihood is intermediate because the test result is likely to have the greatest effect on the posttest probability of CAD and, hence, on clinical decision-making.

EXERCISE ELECTROCARDIOGRAPHY (see Chap. 13)

Diagnosis of Coronary Artery Disease. The exercise ECG is particularly helpful in patients with chest pain syndromes who are considered to have a moderate probability of CAD and in whom the resting ECG is normal, provided that they are capable of achieving an adequate workload.[23] Although the incremental diagnostic value of exercise testing is limited in patients in whom the estimated prevalence of CAD is high or low, the test provides useful additional information about the degree of functional limitation in both groups of patients and about the severity of ischemia and prognosis in patients with a high pretest probability of CAD. Interpretation of the exercise test should include consideration of the exercise capacity (duration and metabolic equivalents) and clinical, hemodynamic, and electrocardiographic responses.[23]

Influence of Antianginal Therapy. Antianginal pharmacological therapy reduces the sensitivity of exercise testing as a screening tool. A negative exercise test result in patients receiving antianginal drugs does not exclude significant and possibly severe CAD. Therefore, if the purpose of the exercise test is to diagnose ischemia, it should be performed, if possible, in the absence of antianginal medications. Two or 3 days is required for patients receiving long-acting beta blockers. Unless the patient has severe angina, sublingual nitroglycerin for 1 or 2 days is likely to be sufficient to control symptoms if other therapy is withdrawn. For long-acting nitrates, calcium antagonists, and short-

TABLE 54–1	Pretest Likelihood of Coronary Artery Disease in Symptomatic Patients According to Age and Gender*					
	Nonanginal Chest Pain		Atypical Angina		Typical Angina	
Age (yr)	Men	Women	Men	Women	Men	Women
30-39	4	2	34	12	76	26
40-49	13	3	51	22	87	55
50-59	20	7	65	31	93	73
60-69	27	14	72	51	94	86

*Each value represents the percentage with significant coronary artery disease at coronary angiography.

From Gibbons RJ, Abrams J, Chatterjee K, et al: ACC/AHA 2002 guideline update for the management of patients with chronic stable angina: A report of the American College of Cardiology/American Heart Association Task Force on Practice Guidelines (Committee to update the 1999 guidelines for the management of patients with chronic stable angina). © 2002 American College of Cardiology and American Heart Association (http://www.acc.org/clinical/guidelines/stable/stable.pdf).

TABLE 54–2	Sensitivity and Specificity of Stress Testing*		
Modality	Total Patients	Sensitivity†	Specificity†
Exercise ECG	24,047	0.68	0.77
Exercise SPECT	5,272	0.88	0.72
Adenosine SPECT	2,137	0.90	0.82
Exercise echocardiography	2,788	0.85	0.81
Dobutamine echocardiography	2,582	0.81	0.79

*Without correction for referral bias.
†Weighted average pooled across individual trials.
ECG = electrocardiogram; SPECT = single-photon emission computed tomography.
Data from Gibbons RJ, Abrams J, Chatterjee K, et al: ACC/AHA guideline update for the management of patients with chronic stable angina: A report of the American College of Cardiology/American Heart Association Task Force on Practice Guidelines (Committee to update the 1999 guidelines for the management of patients with chronic stable angina). © 2002 American College of Cardiology and American Heart Association. (Available at www.acc.org/clinical/guidelines/stable/stable.pdf.)

acting beta blockers, discontinuing use of the medications the day before testing usually suffices if the purpose of the exercise test is to identify safe levels of daily activity or the extent of functional disability.

NUCLEAR CARDIOLOGY TECHNIQUES (see Chap. 16)

Stress Myocardial Perfusion Imaging. Exercise perfusion imaging with simultaneous electrocardiographic testing is superior to exercise electrocardiography alone in detecting CAD, in identifying multivessel disease, in localizing diseased vessels, and in determining the magnitude of ischemic and infarcted myocardium. Exercise single-photon emission computed tomography (SPECT) yields an average sensitivity and specificity of 88 and 72 percent, respectively (ranges, 71 to 98 percent and 36 to 92 percent, respectively) compared with 68 percent sensitivity and 77 percent specificity for exercise electrocardiography alone (Table 54-2).[10] Referral bias may account, in part, for the low specificity of many studies, and the few studies that have adjusted for referral bias report a specificity higher than 90 percent.[10] Perfusion imaging is also valuable for detecting myocardial viability in patients with regional or global LV dysfunction, with or without Q waves, and provides important information in regard to prognosis in all patients.

Stress myocardial scintigraphy is particularly helpful in the diagnosis of CAD in patients with abnormal resting ECGs and in those in whom ST segment responses cannot be interpreted accurately, such as patients with repolarization abnormalities caused by LV hypertrophy, those with left bundle branch block, and those receiving digitalis. Because stress myocardial perfusion imaging is a relatively expensive test (three to four times the cost of an exercise ECG), stress myocardial perfusion scintigraphy should *not* be used as a screening test in patients in whom the prevalence of CAD is low, because most abnormal tests will yield false-positive results, and a regular exercise ECG should always be considered first in patients with chest pain and a normal resting ECG for screening and detection of CAD.[10]

Pharmacological Nuclear Stress Testing. For patients unable to exercise adequately, especially the elderly and patients with peripheral vascular disease, pulmonary disease, arthritis, or a previous stroke, pharmacological vasodilator stress with dipyridamole or adenosine may be used.[10] In most nuclear cardiology laboratories, such patients account for approximately 40 percent of those referred for perfusion imaging. Although the diagnostic accuracy of pharmacological vasodilator stress perfusion imaging is comparable to that achieved with exercise perfusion imaging (see Table 54-2),[10] treadmill testing is preferred for patients who are capable of exercising because the exercise component of the test provides additional diagnostic and prognostic information, including ST segment changes, effort tolerance and symptomatic response, and heart rate and blood pressure response. Vasodilator stress agents are also used with PET to diagnose CAD and determine CAD and its severity (see Chap. 16).

STRESS ECHOCARDIOGRAPHY (see Chap. 14).

Two-dimensional echocardiography is useful in the evaluation of patients with chronic CAD because it can assess global and regional LV function under basal conditions and during ischemia, as well as detecting LV hypertrophy and associated valve disease. Stress echocardiography may be performed using exercise or pharmacological stress and allows for the detection of regional ischemia by identifying new areas of wall motion disorders. Adequate images can be obtained in more than 85 percent of patients, and the test is highly reproducible. Numerous studies have shown that exercise echocardiography can detect the presence of CAD with an accuracy similar to that of stress myocardial perfusion imaging and superior to exercise electrocardiography alone (see Table 54-2). Stress echocardiography is also valuable in localizing and quantifying ischemic myocardium. As with perfusion imaging, stress echocardiography also provides important prognostic information about patients with known or suspected CAD. Pharmacological stress, such as with dobutamine, should be used in patients unable to exercise, those unable to achieve adequate heart rates with exercise, and those in whom the quality of the echocardiographic images during or immediately after exercise is poor.

Stress echocardiography is an excellent alternative to nuclear cardiology procedures. Limitations imposed by poor visualization of endocardial borders in a sizable subset of patients have been reduced by newer contrast-assisted and imaging technological modalities (see Chap. 14).[24,25] Although less expensive than nuclear perfusion imaging, stress echocardiography is more expensive than and not as widely available as exercise electrocardiography.

CLINICAL APPLICATION OF NONINVASIVE TESTING

Gender Differences in the Diagnosis of CAD (see Chap. 76). On the basis of earlier studies that indicated a much higher frequency of false-positive stress test results in women than in men, it is generally accepted that electrocardiographic stress testing is not as reliable in women. However, the prevalence of CAD in women in the patient populations under study was low, and the lower positive predictive value of exercise ECG in women can be accounted for, in large part, on the basis of bayesian principles (see Table 54-1).[23] Once men and women are stratified appropriately according to the pretest prevalence of disease, the results of stress testing are similar, although the specificity is probably slightly less in women.[23] Exercise imaging modalities have greater diagnostic accuracy than exercise electrocardiography in men and women.[23]

IDENTIFICATION OF PATIENTS AT HIGH RISK. When applying noninvasive tests to the diagnosis and management of CAD, it is useful to grade the results as negative, indeterminate, positive, not high risk, and positive, high risk. The criteria for high-risk findings on stress electrocardiography, myocardial perfusion imaging, and stress echocardiography are listed in Table 54-3.

Regardless of the severity of symptoms, patients with high-risk noninvasive test results have a high likelihood of CAD and, if they have no obvious contraindications to revascularization, should undergo coronary arteriography. Such patients, even if asymptomatic, are at risk for left main or triple-vessel CAD, and many have impaired LV function. In contrast, patients with clearly negative exercise test results, regardless of symptoms, have an excellent prognosis that cannot usually be improved by revascularization. If they do not have serious symptoms, coronary arteriography is generally not indicated.

ASYMPTOMATIC PERSONS. Exercise testing in asymptomatic individuals without known CAD is generally not recommended.[23] Exercise testing may be appropriate for asymptomatic individuals with diabetes mellitus who plan to begin vigorous exercise,[26] for those with evidence of myocardial ischemia on ambulatory electrocardiographic monitoring, or for those with severe coronary calcifications on electron beam computed tomography (CT).[10]

Chest Roentgenography (see Chap. 15)

The chest roentgenogram is usually within normal limits in patients with chronic stable angina, particularly if they have a normal resting ECG and have not experienced a myocardial infarction. If cardiomegaly is present, it is indicative of severe CAD with previous myocardial infarction, preexisting hypertension, or an associated nonischemic condition such as concomitant valvular heart disease or cardiomyopathy.

Computed Tomography (see Chap. 18)

Electron beam and now multislice cardiac CT has emerged as a highly sensitive method for detecting coronary calcification which is diagnostic of coronary atherosclerosis. This is being used at some centers as a screening technique for

TABLE 54–3	Risk Stratification Based on Noninvasive Testing

High Risk (>3% Annual Mortality Rate)
1. Severe resting left ventricular dysfunction (LVEF < 0.35)
2. High-risk treadmill score (score ≤ −11)
3. Severe exercise left ventricular dysfunction (exercise LVEF < 0.35)
4. Stress-induced large perfusion defect (particularly if anterior)
5. Stress-induced multiple perfusion defects of moderate size
6. Large, fixed perfusion defect with LV dilation or increased lung uptake (thallium-201)
7. Stress-induced moderate perfusion defect with LV dilation or increased lung uptake (thallium-201)
8. Echocardiographic wall motion abnormality (involving more than two segments) developing at low dose of dobutamine (≤10 μg/kg/min) or at a low heart rate (<120 beats/min)
9. Stress echocardiographic evidence of extensive ischemia

Intermediate Risk (1-3% Annual Mortality Rate)
1. Mild/moderate resting left ventricular dysfunction (LVEF = 0.35-0.49)
2. Intermediate-risk treadmill score (−11 < score < 5)
3. Stress-induced moderate perfusion defect without LV dilation or increased lung intake (thalium-201)
4. Limited stress echocardiographic ischemia with a wall motion abnormality only at higher doses of dobutamine involving two segments or less

Low Risk (<1% Annual Mortality Rate)
1. Low-risk treadmill score (score ≥ 5)
2. Normal or small myocardial perfusion defect at rest or with stress*
3. Normal stress echocardiographic wall motion or no change of limited resting wall motion abnormalities during stress*

*Although the published data are limited, patients with these findings will probably not be at low risk in the presence of either a high-risk treadmill score or severe resting left ventricular dysfunction (LVEF < 0.35).

LV = left ventricular, LVEF = LV ejection fraction.

From Gibbons RJ, Abrams J, Chatterjee K, et al: ACC/AHA 2002 guideline update for the management of patients with chronic stable angina: A report of the American College of Cardiology/American Heart Association Task Force on Practice Guidelines (Committee to update the 1999 guidelines for the management of patients with chronic stable angina). © 2002 American College of Cardiology and American Heart Association (http://www.acc.org/clinical/guidelines/stable/stable.pdf).

CAD. The calcium score is a quantitative index of total coronary artery calcium detected by CT, and this score has been shown to be a good marker of the total coronary atherosclerotic burden.[27] However, the relationship of the coronary calcium score to subsequent cardiac events in asymptomatic persons has not been fully established.[28] Although coronary calcification is a highly sensitive (approximately 90 percent) finding in patients who have CAD, the specificity for identifying patients with obstructive CAD is low (approximately 50 percent). In view of this limitation and the potential consequences of expensive and unnecessary testing as the result of false-positive results, CT is currently *not* recommended as a routine approach for screening for obstructive CAD.[10] Moreover, in patients with known or suspected CAD, exercise testing is preferable to CT imaging for determining the extent of CAD, the presence of ischemia, and indications for coronary angiography. Selective screening of individuals at intermediate risk of CAD events may be appropriate to intensify risk factor modification.[29] The results of ongoing investigations will guide future recommendations regarding the role of this technique in the assessment and management of CAD.

In addition to application for detection of coronary calcification, CT technology may also evolve to enable reliable noninvasive coronary angiography. Preliminary evidence with newer multislice spiral CT technology in conjunction with aggressive beta blockade to reduce the heart rate during imaging has shown promise for the detection of obstructive CAD in the major epicardial arteries; however, at present, it is limited by a high number of false-positive and nonevaluable results.[30]

Cardiac Magnetic Resonance Imaging (see Chap. 17)

Cardiac magnetic resonance imaging (CMR) is established as a valuable clinical tool for imaging the aorta and cerebral and peripheral arterial vasculature and is emerging as a versatile noninvasive cardiac imaging modality that has multiple applications for patients with CAD.[31] At present, the clinical use of CMR for myocardial viability assessment is growing based on evidence demonstrating its ability to predict functional recovery after percutaneous or surgical revascularization and its very good correlation with PET.[32,33] Pharmacological stress perfusion imaging with CMR also compares favorably with other methods and is being used clinically in some centers, particularly for individuals who present limitations for the use of other imaging modalities. In these patients, CMR also offers accurate characterization of LV function. New techniques are likely to lead to further improvements in magnetic resonance imaging as a tool for stress testing.[34]

Because of its ability to visualize arteries in three dimensions and differentiate tissue constituents, CMR has received intense interest as a potential, but as yet clinically unproven, method to characterize arterial atheroma and assess vulnerability to rupture on the basis of compositional analysis.[31] Characterization of arterial plaque has been achieved in the aorta and carotid arteries in humans and has been shown to be predictive of subsequent vascular events.[35] Initial studies evaluating CMR coronary angiography in humans have demonstrated its ability to detect stenoses in the proximal and middle segments of major epicardial vessels or surgical bypass grafts,[36] as well as to characterize congenital coronary anomalies (see Chap. 61).

Catheterization, Angiography, and Coronary Arteriography

The clinical examination and noninvasive techniques described earlier are extremely valuable in establishing the diagnosis of CAD and are indispensable to an overall assessment of patients with this condition. Currently, however, definitive diagnosis of CAD and precise assessment of its anatomical severity still require cardiac catheterization and coronary arteriography (see Chaps. 19 and 20). In patients with chronic stable angina pectoris referred for coronary arteriography, approximately 25 percent each have single-, double-, or triple-vessel disease (i.e., more than 70 percent luminal diameter narrowing). Five to 10 percent have obstruction of the left main coronary artery and, in approximately 15 percent, no critical obstruction is detectable. Newer invasive techniques such as intravascular ultrasonography (IVUS) provide a cross-sectional view of the coronary artery and have substantially enhanced the detection and quantification of coronary atherosclerosis, as well as the potential to characterize the vulnerability of coronary atheroma (see Chap. 20).[37] Studies incorporating both coronary angiography and IVUS have demonstrated that the severity of CAD may be underestimated by angiography alone. CT coronary angiography is evolving as a noninvasive tool for this purpose as well.

Coronary angiographic findings differ between patients presenting with acute MI and those with chronic stable angina. Patients with unheralded myocardial infarction have fewer diseased vessels, fewer stenoses and chronic occlusions, and less diffuse disease than chronic stable angina patients, suggesting that the pathophysiological substrate and propensity for thrombosis differ between these

CH 54

Chronic Coronary Artery Disease

two groups of patients. In patients with chronic angina who have a history of prior infarction, total occlusion of at least one major coronary artery is more common than in those without such a history.

CORONARY ARTERY ECTASIA AND ANEURYSMS. Patulous aneurysmal dilation involving most of the length of a major epicardial coronary artery is present in approximately 1 to 3 percent of patients with obstructive CAD at autopsy or angiography. This angiographic lesion does not appear to affect symptoms, survival, or incidence of MI. Most coronary artery ectasia and/or aneurysms are caused by coronary atherosclerosis (50 percent), and the rest are caused by congenital anomalies and inflammatory diseases, such as Kawasaki disease. Coronary artery aneurysms have also been reported as occurring more frequently in chronic users of cocaine.[38] Despite the absence of overt obstruction, 70 percent of patients with multivessel fusiform coronary artery ectasia or aneurysms have demonstrated evidence of cardiac ischemia based on cardiac lactate levels during ergometry and atrial pacing.

Coronary ectasia should be distinguished from discrete coronary artery aneurysms, which are almost never found in arteries without severe stenosis, are most common in the left anterior descending coronary artery, and are usually associated with extensive CAD. These discrete atherosclerotic coronary artery aneurysms do not appear to rupture and their resection is not warranted.

CORONARY COLLATERAL VESSELS (see Chap. 20). Provided that they are of adequate size, collaterals may protect against myocardial infarction when total occlusion occurs. In patients with abundant collateral vessels, myocardial infarct size is smaller than in patients without collaterals, and total occlusion of a major epicardial artery may not lead to LV dysfunction. In patients with chronic occlusion of a major coronary artery but without infarction, collateral-dependent myocardial segments show nearly normal baseline blood flow and O_2 consumption, but severely limited flow reserve. This finding helps explain the ability of collaterals to protect against resting ischemia but not against exercise-induced angina.

MYOCARDIAL BRIDGING. Bridging of coronary arteries (see Chap. 20) is observed at coronary angiography at a rate of less than 5 percent in otherwise angiographically normal coronary arteries and ordinarily does not constitute a hazard.[39] Occasionally, compression of a portion of a coronary artery by a myocardial bridge can be associated with clinical manifestations of myocardial ischemia during strenuous physical activity and may even result in myocardial infarction or initiate malignant ventricular arrhythmias.[39] The functional consequences of myocardial bridging may be better characterized with the use of IVUS and intracoronary Doppler measurements.[39]

LEFT VENTRICULAR FUNCTION. LV function can be assessed by means of biplane contrast ventriculography (see Chap. 20). Global abnormalities of LV systolic function are reflected by elevations in LV end-diastolic and end-systolic volumes and depression of the ejection fraction. These changes are, however, nonspecific and can occur in many forms of heart disease. Abnormalities of regional wall motion (e.g., hypokinesis, akinesia, dyskinesia) are more characteristic of CAD. Ventricular relaxation, as reflected in the early diastolic ventricular filling rate, may be impaired at rest in patients with chronic CAD. Diastolic filling becomes even more abnormal (slowed) during exercise, when ischemia intensifies. In patients with chronic stable angina, the frequency of elevated LV end-diastolic pressure and reduced cardiac output at rest, generally attributed to abnormal LV dynamics, increases with the number of vessels exhibiting critical narrowing and with the number of prior infarctions. LV end-diastolic pressure may be elevated secondary to reduced ventricular compliance, LV systolic failure, or a combination of these two processes. Left ventriculography is useful for determining the presence and severity of mitral valve regurgitation.

CORONARY BLOOD FLOW AND MYOCARDIAL METABOLISM. Cardiac catheterization can also document abnormal myocardial metabolism in patients with chronic stable angina. With a catheter in the coronary sinus, arterial and coronary venous lactate measurements are obtained at rest and after suitable stress, such as the infusion of isoproterenol or pacing-induced tachycardia. Because lactate is a byproduct of anaerobic glycolysis, its production by the heart and subsequent appearance in coronary sinus blood is a reliable sign of myocardial ischemia.

Studies of coronary flow reserve (maximum flow divided by resting flow) and endothelial function are frequently abnormal in patients with CAD and chronic stable angina and may play an important role in determining the functional significance of a stenosis or detecting microvascular dysfunction in those without obstructive epicardial disease. These techniques are discussed in Chapter 48.

Natural History of Angina Pectoris and Risk Stratification

Data from the Framingham Study, obtained before the widespread use of aspirin, beta blockers, and aggressive modification of risk factors, have shown that the average annual mortality rate of patients with chronic stable angina is 4 percent.[10] The combination of these treatments has improved prognosis. In 1995, data from a 15-year follow-up of middle-aged men with prevalent CAD indicated an annual mortality rate of 1.7 to 3 percent and an annual rate of major ischemic events of 1.4 to 2.4 percent. Similar rates have also been observed in more recent clinical trials.[40] Clinical, noninvasive, and invasive tools are useful for refining the estimate of risk for the individual patient with stable angina. Moreover, noninvasively acquired information is valuable in identifying patients who are candidates for invasive evaluation with cardiac catheterization.

CLINICAL CRITERIA. A composite risk score based on multiple clinical variables (e.g., age, gender, diabetes, previous myocardial infarction, nature of the chest pain) may be strongly predictive of the presence of severe CAD (triple-vessel or left main CAD) and thus provide a strong indication for angiography (Fig. 54-2). A number of studies have attested to the adverse prognostic effect of congestive heart failure (based on a clinical history and/or the presence of cardiomegaly on chest radiography), previous MI, hypertension, and advanced age in patients with stable angina pectoris.[10] The severity of angina, especially the tempo of intensification, and the presence of dyspnea[4] are also important predictors of outcome.

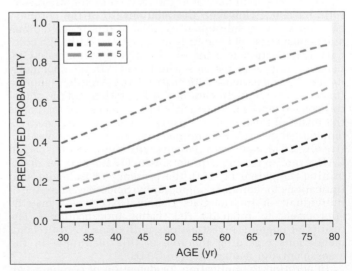

FIGURE 54–2 Nomogram showing the probability of severe (triple-vessel or left main) coronary artery disease based on a five-point clinical score assigned on the basis of clinical variables: male gender, typical angina, history and electrocardiographic evidence of myocardial infarction, and diabetes. *(Modified from Hubbard BL, Gibbons RJ, Lapyre AC, et al: Identification of severe coronary artery disease using simple clinical parameters. Arch Intern Med 152:309, 1992.)*

NONINVASIVE TESTING (see Chaps. 13, 14, and 16)

Exercise Electrocardiography. The prognostic importance of the treadmill exercise test was determined by several observational studies in the 1980s and early 1990s. One of the most important and consistent predictors is the maximal exercise capacity, regardless of whether it is measured by exercise duration or workload achieved or whether the test was terminated because of dyspnea, fatigue, or angina.[4] After adjustment for age, the peak exercise capacity measured in metabolic equivalents is among the strongest predictors of mortality in men with cardiovascular disease.[41] Other factors with a poor prognosis identified in individual series of patients with chronic stable angina are delineated in Table 54-3.

Stress Nuclear Myocardial Perfusion Imaging (see Chap. 16). The prognostic value of myocardial perfusion imaging is now well established. In particular, the ability of myocardial perfusion SPECT to identify patients at low (less than 1 percent), intermediate (1 to 5 percent), or high (more than 5 percent) risk for future cardiac events is valuable in patient management decisions. The prognostic data obtained from myocardial perfusion SPECT are incremental over clinical and treadmill exercise data for predicting future cardiac events. In patients with normal SPECT imaging findings, the annual risk of death or myocardial infarction is less than 1 percent.

Echocardiography. Echocardiographic assessment of LV function is one of the most valuable aspects of noninvasive imaging. Such testing is not necessary for all patients with angina pectoris and, in patients with a normal ECG and no previous history of myocardial infarction, the likelihood of preserved LV systolic function is high. In contrast, in patients with a history of myocardial infarction, ST-T wave changes, or conduction defects or Q waves on the ECG, LV function should be measured with echocardiography or an equivalent technique. The presence or absence of inducible regional wall motion abnormalities and the response of the ejection fraction to exercise or pharmacological stress appear to provide incremental prognostic information to the data provided by the resting echocardiogram. Moreover, a negative stress test portends a low risk for future events (less than 1 percent/person-year).

ANGIOGRAPHIC CRITERIA. The independent impact of multivessel disease and left ventricular dysfunction and their interaction on the prognosis of patients with CAD is well established (Fig. 54-3). The adverse effects of impaired ventricular function on prognosis are more pronounced as the number of stenotic vessels increases.[10] Although several indices have been used to quantify the extent of severity of CAD, the simple classification of disease into single-, double-, triple-vessel, or left main CAD is the most widely used and is effective. Additional prognostic information is provided by the severity of obstruction and its location, whether proximal or distal. The concept of the gradient of risk is illustrated in Figure 54-4. Studies of treated symptomatic patients have revealed that if only one of the three major coronary arteries has more than 50 percent stenosis, the annual mortality rate is approximately 2 percent. The importance to survival of the quantity of myocardium that is jeopardized is reflected in the observation that an obstructive lesion proximal to the first septal perforating branch of the left anterior descending coronary artery was associated with a 5-year survival rate of 90 percent in comparison with 98 percent for patients with more distal lesions.

High-grade lesions of the left main coronary artery or its equivalent, as defined by severe proximal left anterior descending and proximal left circumflex CAD, are particularly life-threatening. Mortality in medically treated patients has been reported to be 29 percent at 18 months and 43 percent at 5 years. Survival is better for patients with 50 to 70 percent stenosis (1- and 3-year survival rates of 91 and 66 percent, respectively) than for patients with a left main coronary artery stenosis more than 70 percent (1- and 3-year survival rates of 72 and 41 percent, respectively). Furthermore, a number of characteristics found at catheterization or on noninvasive examination are predictors

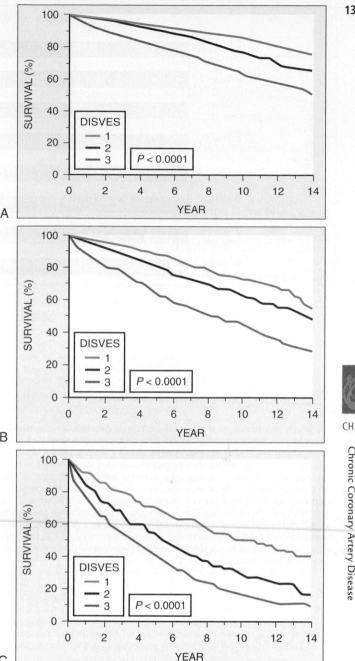

FIGURE 54–3 Graphs showing survival for medically treated Coronary Artery Surgery Study (CASS) patients. **A,** Patients with single-, double-, or triple-vessel disease and an ejection fraction of 0.50 to 1.00 stratified by the number of diseased vessels (DISVES). **B,** Patients with single-, double-, or triple-vessel disease and an ejection fraction of 0.35 to 0.49 stratified by the number of diseased vessels. **C,** Patients with single-, double-, or triple-vessel disease and an ejection fraction of ≤0.34 stratified by the number of diseased vessels. (*A to C, From Emond M, Mock MB, Davis KB, et al: Long-term survival of medically treated patients in the Coronary Artery Surgery Study [CASS] Registry. Circulation 90:2651, 1994.*)

of an adverse prognosis in patients with 70 percent or more left main coronary artery stenosis, including chest pain at rest, ST-T wave changes on the resting ECG, cardiomegaly on chest radiography, a history of congestive heart failure, and the presence of LV dysfunction at catheterization.

Limitations of Angiography. The pathophysiological significance of coronary stenoses lies in their impact on resting and exercise-induced blood flow and in their potential for plaque rupture, with superimposed thrombotic occlusion. It is generally accepted that a stenosis of more than 60 percent of the luminal diameter is hemody-

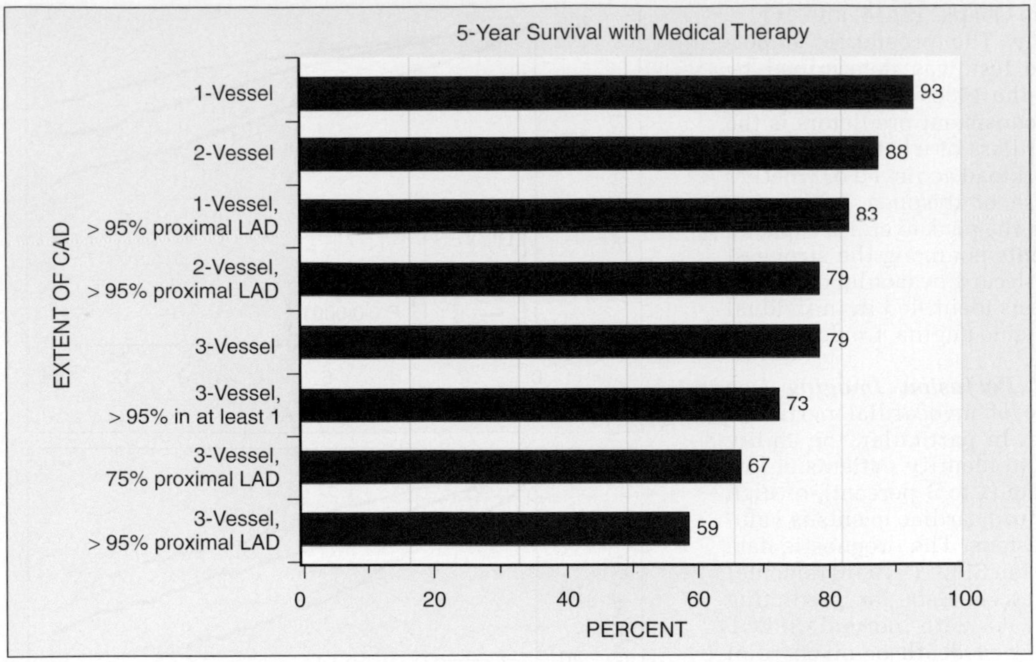

5-Year Survival with Medical Therapy

EXTENT OF CAD

	PERCENT
1-Vessel	93
2-Vessel	88
1-Vessel, > 95% proximal LAD	83
2-Vessel, > 95% proximal LAD	79
3-Vessel	79
3-Vessel, > 95% in at least 1	73
3-Vessel, 75% proximal LAD	67
3-Vessel, > 95% proximal LAD	59

FIGURE 54–4 Angiographic extent of coronary artery disease (CAD) and subsequent survival with medical therapy. A gradient of mortality risk is established based on the number of diseased vessels and the presence and severity of disease of the proximal left anterior descending (LAD) artery. *(Data from Califf RM, Armstrong PW, Carver JR, et al: Task Force 5: Stratification of patients into high-, medium-, and low-risk subgroups for purposes of risk factor management. J Am Coll Cardiol 27:964, 1996.)*

CH 54

namically significant in that it may be responsible for a reduction in exercise-induced myocardial blood flow that causes angina and ischemia. The immediate functional significance of obstruction of intermediate severity (approximately 50 percent diameter stenosis) is less well established. Coronary angiography is not a reliable indicator of the functional significance of stenosis, nor is it sensitive to the presence of thrombus. Moreover, the coronary angiographic determinants of the severity of stenosis are based on a decrease in the caliber of the lumen at the site of the lesion relative to adjacent reference segments, which are considered, often erroneously, to be relatively free of disease. This approach may lead to significant underestimation of the severity and extent of atherosclerosis.[42]

The most serious limitation to the routine use of coronary angiography for prognosis in patients with chronic stable angina is its inability to identify which coronary lesions can be considered to be at high risk, or vulnerable, for future events, such as myocardial infarction or sudden death. Although it is widely accepted that myocardial infarction is the result of thrombotic occlusion at the site of plaque rupture or erosion (see Chaps. 38 and 50), it is clear that it is not necessarily the plaque causing the most severe stenosis that subsequently ruptures. Lesions causing mild obstructions can rupture, thrombose, and occlude, thereby leading to myocardial infarction and sudden death. Approaches to quantifying the extent of coronary disease, inclusive of nonobstructive lesions, appear to offer additional prognostic information.[43] In contrast, arteries with severe preexisting stenoses may proceed to clinically silent complete occlusion, often without infarction, presumably because of the formation of collaterals as the ischemia gradually becomes more severe.

In summary, angiographic documentation of the extent of CAD provides useful information toward assessment of the patient's risk of death and future ischemic events and is an indispensable step in the selection of patients for coronary revascularization, particularly if the interaction between the anatomical extent of disease, left ventricular function, and the severity of ischemia is taken into account. However, angiography is not helpful in predicting the site of subsequent plaque rupture or erosion that can precipitate myocardial infarction or sudden cardiac death. Additional tools that improve the imaging of coronary atheroma (e.g., IVUS) or the functional assessment of a stenosis (Doppler determination of coronary flow reserve) may be helpful in deciding on the flow-limiting significance of a specific lesion and the need for coronary revascularization. Characterization of the atheroma using CT or CMR remains under evaluation but is not yet a routine clinical tool.

Medical Management

Comprehensive management of chronic stable angina has five aspects: (1) identification and treatment of associated diseases that can precipitate or worsen angina; (2) reduction of coronary risk factors; (3) application of general and nonpharmacological methods, with particular attention to adjustments in life style; (4) pharmacological management; and (5) revascularization by percutaneous catheter-based techniques or by coronary bypass surgery. Although discussed individually in this chapter, all five of these approaches must be considered, often simultaneously, in each patient. Of the medical therapies, three (aspirin, angiotensin-converting enzyme [ACE] inhibition, and effective lipid lowering) have been shown to reduce mortality and morbidity in patients with chronic stable angina and preserved LV function. Other therapies such as nitrates, beta blockers, and calcium antagonists have been shown to improve symptomatology and exercise performance but their effect, if any, on survival in patients with stable angina has not been demonstrated.

In stable patients with LV dysfunction following myocardial infarction, evidence has consistently indicated that ACE inhibitors and beta blockers reduce both mortality and the risk of repeat infarction, and these agents are recommended in such patients, with or without chronic angina, along with aspirin and lipid-lowering drugs.

TREATMENT OF ASSOCIATED DISEASES. Several common medical conditions that can increase myocardial O_2 demand or reduce O_2 delivery may contribute to the onset of new angina pectoris or the exacerbation of previously stable angina. These conditions include anemia, marked weight gain, occult thyrotoxicosis, fever, infections, and tachycardia. Cocaine, which can cause acute coronary spasm and myocardial infarction, is discussed in Chapter 68. In patients with CAD, heart failure, by causing cardiac dilation, mitral regurgitation, or tachyarrhythmias (including sinus tachycardia), can increase myocardial O_2 need, along with an increase in the frequency and severity of angina. Identification and treatment of these conditions are critical to the management of chronic stable angina.

Reduction of Coronary Risk Factors

HYPERTENSION (see Chaps. 40, 41, and 45). Epidemiological links between increased blood pressure and CAD severity and mortality are well established.[44] For individuals aged 40 to 70 years, the risk of ischemic heart disease doubles for each 20-mm Hg increment in systolic blood pressure across the entire range of 115 to 185 mm Hg.[45] Hypertension predisposes to vascular injury, accelerates the development of atherosclerosis, increases myocardial O_2 demand, and intensifies ischemia in patients with preexisting obstructive coronary vascular disease. Although the relationship between hypertension and CAD is linear,[45] LV hypertrophy is a stronger predictor of myocardial infarction and CAD death than the actual degree of increase in blood pressure. A meta-analysis of clinical trials of treatment of mild to moderate hypertension has shown a statistically significant 16 percent reduction in CAD events and mortality in patients receiving antihypertensive therapy. This treatment effect is nearly twice as great in older compared with younger persons. It is logical to extend these observations about the benefits of antihypertensive therapy to patients with established CAD.[46] Moreover, the number of individuals treated to avoid one death is lower in subjects with established cardiovascular disease. Therefore, blood pressure control is an essential aspect of the management of patients with chronic stable angina with a goal of less than 140/90 or less than 130/80 mm Hg for patients with concomitant diabetes or chronic kidney disease.[47]

CIGARETTE SMOKING. This remains one of the most powerful risk factors for the development of CAD in all age groups (see Chap. 39). In patients with angiographically documented CAD, cigarette smokers have a higher 5-year risk of sudden death, myocardial infarction, and all-cause mortality than those who have stopped smoking. Moreover, smoking cessation lessens the risk of adverse coronary events in patients with established CAD.[48] Cigarette smoking may be responsible for aggravating angina pectoris other than through the progression of atherosclerosis. It may increase myocardial O_2 demand and reduce coronary blood flow by means of an alpha-adrenergically mediated increase in coronary artery tone and thereby cause acute ischemia. Smoking cessation is one of the most effective and certainly the least expensive approach to the prevention of disease progression in native vessels and bypass grafts. Strategies for smoking cessation are discussed in Chapter 46.

MANAGEMENT OF DYSLIPIDEMIA (see Chap. 42). Clinical trials in patients with established atherosclerotic vascular disease have demonstrated a significant reduction in subsequent cardiovascular events in patients with a wide range of serum cholesterol and LDL cholesterol levels treated with 3-hydroxy-3-methylglutaryl coenzyme A (HMG-CoA) reductase inhibitors (statins).[49] In aggregate, angiographic trials of cholesterol lowering in patients with chronic CAD, many of whom had chronic stable angina, have shown that the effects on coronary obstruction are modest and in striking contrast with the substantive reduction in cardiovascular events, suggesting that atherosclerosis regression is not the primary mechanism of benefit. Several, but not all, studies have shown that statins significantly improve endothelium-mediated responses in the coronary and systemic arteries of patients with hypercholesterolemia or known atherosclerosis. Nonetheless, in one angiographic trial using IVUS, open-label intensive statin therapy was associated with regression of coronary atherosclerotic burden in patients with angiographic CAD.[50]

Lipid-lowering with statins has been shown to reduce circulating levels of C-reactive protein, decrease thrombogenicity, and favorably alter the collagen and inflammatory components of arterial atheroma; these effects do not appear to correlate well with the change in serum LDL cholesterol level and suggest antiatherothrombotic properties of statins.[51] These properties contribute to improvement in blood flow, reduction in inducible myocardial ischemia, and reduction in coronary events in patients treated with statins.

Results from secondary prevention trials of patients with a history of chronic stable angina, unstable angina, or previous myocardial infarction have provided convincing evidence that effective lipid-lowering therapy significantly improves overall survival and reduces cardiovascular mortality in patients with CAD. The National Cholesterol Education Program Guidelines (see Chaps. 42 and 45) advocate

cholesterol-lowering therapy for all patients with CAD or extracardiac atherosclerosis to LDL levels below 100 mg/dl, and these guidelines have been adopted in recommendations from the American College of Cardiology/American Heart Association (ACC/AHA).[10,47] Moreover, the Heart Protection Study has demonstrated an improvement in survival and reduction in future coronary events with statin therapy in those with diabetes, or cerebrovascular or peripheral vascular disease, as well as in those with established CAD, regardless of their baseline levels of cholesterol.[49] In addition, results from two trials of intensive versus moderate dose statin therapy in patients with stable CAD have provided evidence for a reduction in major cardiovascular events with more aggressive lipid lowering therapy to an LDL concentration of less than 100 mg/dL (Fig. 54-5).[52,53] These findings are also supported by conclusive findings from patients with a recent acute coronary syndrome,[54] and have led to the recommendation that it is reasonable to treat to an achieved LDL concentration of less than 70 mg/dL in all patients with CAD (see Chap. 45).[47]

Low HDL Cholesterol. Patients with established CAD and low levels of HDL cholesterol represent a subgroup at considerable risk for future coronary events.[55] Low HDL levels are often associated with obesity, hypertriglyceridemia, and insulin resistance and often signify the presence of small lipoprotein remnants and small, dense, LDL particles that are thought to be particularly atherogenic (see Chap. 42). Therapy has focused on diet and exercise, as well as on LDL cholesterol reduction, in patients with a concomitant increase in LDL cholesterol levels. The Veterans Affairs High-Density Lipoprotein Cholesterol Intervention Trial (VA-HIT) Study Group demonstrated the efficacy of gemfibrozil treatment in patients with low HDL cholesterol (40 mg/dl or lower) without elevations in LDL cholesterol (140 mg/dl or lower) or triglyceride levels (mean, 160 mg/dl). Gemfibrozil resulted in a 6 percent increase in HDL cholesterol and a 31 percent decrease in triglyceride levels, and these changes were associated with a 24 percent reduction in death, nonfatal myocardial infarction, and stroke. Emerging therapies aimed at promoting reverse cholesterol transport and/or interfering with HDL metabolism to raise the concentration of HDL or the related apolipoprotein A-I (the main protein in HDL) are under investigation.[56] Results of a randomized trial of torcetrapib, a cholesteryl ester transfer protein (CETP) inhibitor, in patients with coronary disease showed a 61 percent increase in HDL cholesterol and 20 percent relative decrease in LDL cholesterol, but no significant decrease in the progression of atherosclerosis.[56a] An increase in blood pressure observed with torcetrapib may explain the excess in deaths and ischemic events observed in a larger randomized clinical outcomes trial with this agent, which was stopped prematurely.[56b] However, it is not known whether there are other unexpected adverse effects specific to this molecule or its drug class.

Dyslipidemia after Myocardial Revascularization. In patients who have undergone coronary artery bypass grafting (CABG), elevation of the LDL cholesterol level is a risk factor for the development of saphenous vein graft occlusive disease, as well as progression of atherosclerosis in the native coronary arteries. Lipid-lowering therapy reduces mortality and acute coronary events in patients who have undergone surgical or percutaneous revascularization, and therapy for dyslipidemia should be given to these patients and to all patients with chronic CAD.

MANAGEMENT OF DIABETES MELLITUS (see Chaps. 43, 45, and 60). Patients with diabetes mellitus are at significantly higher risk of atherosclerotic vascular disease. Although the favorable impact of control of glycemia on microvascular complications of diabetes is clear,

CH 54

Chronic Coronary Artery Disease

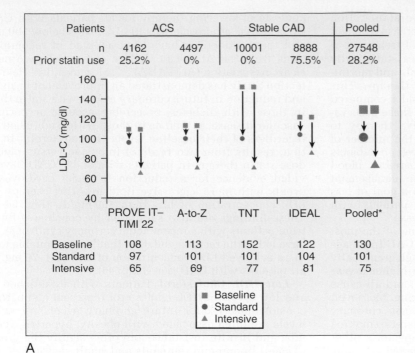

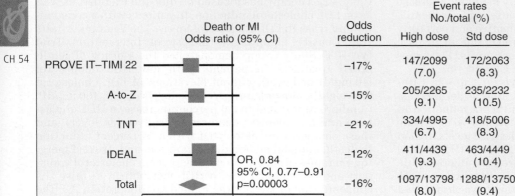

A

B

FIGURE 54–5 Pooled evaluation of intensive versus standard statin therapy for patients with established coronary artery disease in the Pravastatin or Atorvastatin Evaluation and Infection Therapy Trial (PROVE-IT–TIMI 22; Atorvastatin 80 mg daily versus pravastatin 40 mg daily), Aggrastat-to-Zocor Trial (A-to-Z; simvastatin 40 mg daily for 30 days followed by 80 mg daily versus placebo for 4 months, followed by simvastatin 20 mg daily), Treat to New Targets Trial (TNT; atorvastatin 80 mg daily versus atorvastatin 10 mg daily), and Incremental Decrease in Endpoints Through Aggressive Lipid-Lowering Trial (IDEAL; atorvastatin 80 mg daily versus simvastatin 20 mg daily). Intensive statin therapy was associated with significantly lower achieved levels of low-density lipoprotein cholesterol, LDL-C **(A)** and a 16% lowering of the risk of death or myocardial infarction, MI **(B)**. ACS = acute coronary syndrome; CAD = coronary artery disease; CI = confidence interval; OR = odds ratio. *(From Cannon CP, Steinberg BA, Murphy SA, et al: Meta-analysis of cardiovascular outcomes trials comparing intensive versus moderate statin therapy. J Am Coll Cardiol 48:438, 2006.)*

the effect on macrovascular complications (including CAD) is unclear. During a mean follow-up of 17 years in participants in the Diabetes Control and Complications Trial, patients with type 1 diabetes assigned to intensive glycemic therapy were at lower risk of cardiovascular complications.[57] In an analysis of a secondary endpoint of the Prospective Pioglitazone Clinical Trial in Macrovascular Events Trial (PROACTIVE), treatment of patients with type 2 diabetes with the oral hypoglycemic agent pioglitazone reduced the risk of death, non-fatal MI, or stroke.[58] Caution is raised regarding interpretation of this finding from PROACTIVE on controlling hyperglycemia given the neutral result of the trial with respect to its primary endpoint and effects of pioglitazone on metabolic elements other than blood glucose. Management of hypercholesterolemia and hypertension are

particularly important in patients with type 2 diabetes.[57]

ESTROGEN REPLACEMENT. A large data base derived from observational studies has suggested a protective effect of hormone replacement therapy for postmenopausal women. However, the major randomized, controlled primary and secondary prevention trials have shown no cardiovascular benefit from hormone replacement therapy. Thus, in view of the collective data from randomized clinical trials, it is *not* advised that hormone replacement therapy be initiated or continued for secondary cardiovascular prevention in women with CAD.[10,47]

EXERCISE (see Chap. 46). The conditioning effect of exercise on skeletal muscles allows a greater workload at any level of total-body O_2 consumption. By decreasing the heart rate at any level of exertion, a higher cardiac output can be achieved at any level of myocardial O_2 consumption. The combination of these two effects of exercise conditioning permits patients with chronic stable angina to increase physical performance substantially following institution of a continuing exercise program.[59]

Most of the information about the physiological effects of exercise and their effect on prognosis in patients with CAD has come from studies on patients entered into cardiac rehabilitation programs, many of whom previously sustained a myocardial infarction. Less information is available on the benefits of exercise in patients with chronic stable CAD, but nine small randomized studies with a total of 980 patients have consistently demonstrated improved effort tolerance, O_2 consumption, and quality of life in patients undergoing exercise training.[10] Randomized trials evaluating symptom reduction and objective measures of ischemia in patients with stable CAD are few, with most supporting a reduction in symptoms or evidence of ischemia, such as with myocardial perfusion imaging.[10,59] One randomized trial of exercise training compared with angioplasty in 101 patients with stable angina showed fewer hospitalizations and revascularization procedures in those allocated to regular exercise.[60] Others have demonstrated a striking and direct relationship between the intensity of exercise and favorable changes in the morphology of obstructive lesions on angiography, as well as favorable effects on vascular endothelial function thought to be mediated through the expression and phosphorylation of endothelial nitric oxide synthase.[61] Whether exercise accelerates the development of collateral vessels in patients with chronic CAD is unclear.

Exercise is safe if begun under supervision and increased gradually[59] and, if survivors of myocardial infarction can be used as a yardstick, it is probably cost-effective. The psychological benefits of exercise are difficult to evaluate. However, a single nonrandomized study has demonstrated significant improvement in well-being scores and positive affect scores, as well as a reduction in disability scores, in patients in a structured exercise program. Patients who are involved in exercise programs are also more likely to be health conscious, to pay attention to diet and weight, and to discontinue cigarette smoking. For all these reasons, patients should be urged to participate in regular exercise programs, usually walking, in conjunction with their drug therapy.[10,59]

INFLAMMATION (see Chaps. 38, 39, and 45). Atherothrombosis has been identified as an inflammatory disease. Moreover, markers of systemic inflammation, of which high-sensitivity C-reactive protein is the most extensively studied, have identified patients with established vascular disease who are at higher risk for death and future ischemic events. Inflammation has now been identified as a potential target for therapeutic intervention in patients with CAD.[62] For example, additional analyses from the Cholesterol and Recurrent Events (CARE) trial and the Air Force/Texas Coronary Atherosclerosis Prevention Study (AFCAPS/TexCAPS) are among the many studies that have demonstrated lowering of circulating levels of hsCRP after treatment with statins. Moreover, results from two studies have indicated that achieving lower levels of hsCRP with statin therapy in patients 1 month after an acute coronary syndrome is associated with better long-term prognosis.[63,64] These findings lend support to the hypothesis that statins are effective in modifying the risk associated with evidence of systemic inflammation and that inflammatory markers may complement LDL measurement in monitoring the efficacy of statin therapy. Other established preventive interventions, as well as novel therapeutic strategies, may also have antiinflammatory effects that could target inflammation. Aspirin, ACE inhibitors, thiazolidinediones, thienopyridines, and fibric acid derivatives are among those agents that have been shown to exert antiinflammatory or immunoregulatory actions.[62] Additional research is needed to clarify whether inflammation is a viable target for risk reduction in patients with stable CAD.

Additional Pharmacotherapy for Secondary Prevention

ASPIRIN (see Chaps. 45 and 82). A meta-analysis of 140,000 patients in 300 studies has confirmed the prophylactic benefit of aspirin in men and women with angina pectoris, previous MI, or stroke and after bypass surgery. In a Swedish trial of men and women with chronic stable angina, 75 mg of aspirin in conjunction with the beta blocker sotalol conferred a 34 percent reduction in acute myocardial infarction and sudden death. In a smaller study confined to men with chronic stable angina but without a history of myocardial infarction, 325 mg of aspirin on alternate days reduced the risk of myocardial infarction by 87% during 5 years of follow-up. Therefore, administration of aspirin daily is advisable in patients with chronic stable angina but without contraindications to this drug.[10,47] Dosing at 75 to 162 mg daily appears to have comparable effects for secondary prevention with dosing at 160 to 325 mg daily[65] and appears to be associated with lower bleeding risk. Therefore, aspirin 75 to 162 mg daily is preferred for secondary prevention in the absence of recent intracoronary stenting.[47] Although warfarin has proved beneficial in patients after MI, no evidence supports the use of chronic anticoagulation in patients with stable angina.

CLOPIDOGREL. Another orally acting class of agents that blocks platelet aggregation is the thienopyridine derivatives, including clopidogrel. Clopidogrel may be substituted for aspirin in patients with aspirin hypersensitivity or those who cannot tolerate aspirin (see Chap. 82).[47] In a randomized comparison between clopidogrel and aspirin in patients with established atherosclerotic vascular disease (the Clopidogrel versus Aspirin in Patients at Risk of Ischaemic

Events [CAPRIE] trial), treatment with clopidogrel resulted in a modest 8.7 percent relative reduction in the risk of vascular death, ischemic stroke, or myocardial infarction ($P = 0.043$) over 2 years. Studies evaluating the addition of clopidogrel to aspirin in patients with non-ST elevation acute coronary syndromes or after percutaneous coronary intervention[66] have indicated robust risk reductions. However, the Clopidogrel for High Atherothrombotic Risk and Ischemic Stabilization Management and Avoidance (CHARISMA) trial has shown no overall benefit of the addition of clopidogrel to aspirin with respect to the primary endpoint of cardiovascular death, MI, or stroke over a median of 28 months (6.8 versus 7.3 percent; $P = 0.22$) in patients with clinically evident cardiovascular disease ($N = 12,153$) or multiple risk factors ($N = 3284$).[67] Subgroup analyses from the trial have demonstrated a 1 percent lower risk of these events (6.9 versus 7.9 percent; $P = 0.046$) with the addition of clopidogrel to aspirin for those with established vascular disease, supporting a hypothesis of a potential modest benefit from clopidogrel in patients with established CAD taking aspirin.[67]

BETA BLOCKERS. The value of beta blockers in reducing death and recurrent myocardial infarction in patients who have experienced a myocardial infarction is well established (see Chap. 51), as is their usefulness in the treatment of angina. Moreover, patients receiving beta blockers for hypertension are more likely to present with stable angina rather than MI as their first manifestation of CAD.[68] Whether these drugs are also of value in preventing infarction and sudden death in patients with chronic stable angina without previous infarction is uncertain and, despite at least one observational study suggesting lower mortality in the patients who were taking beta blockers,[69] there have been no controlled trials against placebo. However, there is no reason to assume that the favorable effects of beta blockers on ischemia and perhaps on arrhythmias should not apply to patients with chronic stable angina pectoris. Therefore, it is sensible to use these drugs when angina, hypertension, or both are present in patients with chronic CAD and when these drugs are well tolerated.

ACE INHIBITORS. Although ACE inhibitors are not indicated for the treatment of angina, these drugs appear to have important benefits in reducing the risk of future ischemic events in some patients with cerebrovascular disease (CVD). An unexpected finding from randomized trials of ACE inhibitors in postinfarction and other patients with ischemic and nonischemic causes of LV dysfunction was the striking reduction in incidence of subsequent ischemic events such as myocardial infarction, unstable angina, and the need for coronary revascularization procedures. The potentially beneficial effects of ACE inhibitors include reductions in LV hypertrophy, vascular hypertrophy, progression of atherosclerosis, plaque rupture, and thrombosis, in addition to a potentially favorable influence on myocardial O_2 supply and demand relationships, cardiac hemodynamics, and sympathetic activity. ACE inhibitors enhance coronary endothelial vasomotor function in patients with CAD. In addition, in vitro experiments have shown that angiotensin II induces inflammatory changes in human vascular smooth muscle cells, and treatment with ACE inhibitors can reduce signs of inflammation in animal models of atherosclerosis.[62]

Two trials have provided strong evidence supporting the therapeutic benefit of ACE inhibitors in patients with normal LV function and absence of heart failure (Fig. 54-6). In the Heart Outcomes Protection Evaluation (HOPE) study, ramipril significantly decreased the risk of the primary composite endpoint of cardiovascular death, myocardial infarction, and stroke from 17.7 to 14.1 percent (relative risk reduction of 22 percent; $P < 0.001$) compared with placebo in 9297 patients with atherosclerotic vascular disease or diabetes mellitus. In addition, the European Trial on Reduction of Cardiac Events with Perindopril in stable CAD (EUROPA) provided additional convincing support for the benefit of ACE inhibitors, with a 20 percent relative reduction in the risk of cardiovascular death, MI or cardiac arrest in 13,655 patients with stable CAD in the absence of heart failure.[70] In contrast, trandolapril, administered to a target dose of 4 mg daily, showed no effect on the risk of cardiovascular death, MI, or coronary revascularization (21.9 versus 22.5 percent; $P = 0.43$) in 8290 patients with stable CAD and preserved LV function receiving intensive preventive therapy, usually including revascularization and lipid-lowering agents (see Fig. 54-6).[40] Notably, in patients with evidence of renal dysfunction (estimated glomerular filtration rate lower than 60 ml/min/1.73 m^2), trandolapril was associated with lower all-cause mortality.[71] Hence, ACE inhibitors are recommended for all patients with CAD with left ventricular dysfunction and for those with hypertension, diabetes, or chronic kidney disease.[47] ACE inhibitors may be considered for optional use in all other patients with normal LV ejection fraction and cardiovascular risk

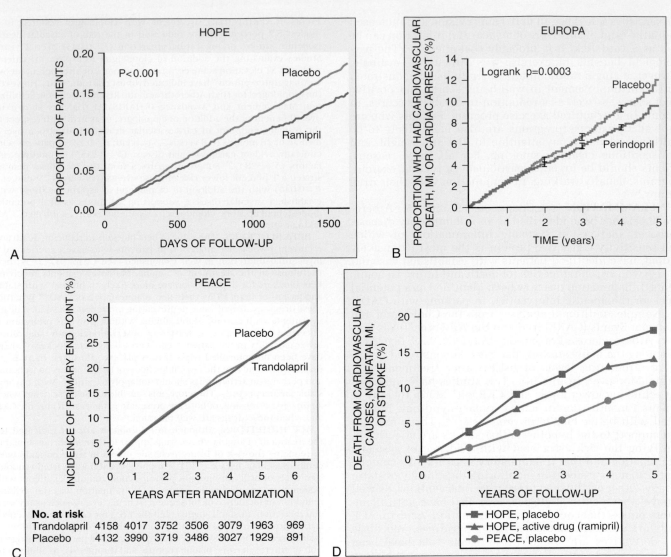

FIGURE 54-6 Kaplan-Meier time-to-event curves for the primary endpoint of three large randomized, placebo-controlled trials of angiotensin-converting enzyme inhibitors for patients at high risk for or with established cardiovascular disease without heart failure. **A,** Cumulative incidence of cardiovascular death, myocardial infarction [MI], or stroke with ramipril versus placebo among patients in the Heart Outcomes Protection Evaluation (HOPE) Trial. **B,** Cumulative incidence of cardiovascular death, MI, or cardiac arrest with perindopril or placebo in the European Trial on the Reduction of Cardiac Events with Perindopril in Stable Coronary Artery Disease (EUROPA Trial). **C,** Cumulative incidence of cardiovascular death, MI, or coronary revascularization in the Prevention of Events with Angiotensin-Converting Enzyme Inhibition (PEACE) trial. **D,** Comparison of cardiovascular death, MI, or stroke in the HOPE and PEACE trials. The cumulative incidence of major cardiovascular events was lower in patients treated with placebo in PEACE than in the patients treated with ramipril in HOPE. (**A,** *From HOPE Study Investigators: Effects of an angiotensin-converting enzyme inhibitor, ramipril, on cardiovascular events in high risk patients. N Engl J Med 342:145, 2000;* **B,** *from EUROPA Investigators: Efficacy of perindopril in reduction of cardiovascular events among patients with stable coronary artery disease: Randomized double-blind, placebo-controlled, multicenter trial [the EUROPA study]. Lancet 363:782, 2003;* **C,** *from PEACE Trial Investigators: Angiotensin-converting enzyme inhibition in stable coronary artery disease. N Engl J Med 351:2058, 2004.)*

factors that are well controlled in whom revascularization has been performed.[47]

ANTIOXIDANTS (see Chap. 45). Oxidized LDL particles are strongly linked to the pathophysiology of atherogenesis, and descriptive, prospective cohort, and case-control studies have suggested that a high dietary intake of antioxidant vitamins (A, C, and beta-carotene) and flavonoids (polyphenolic antioxidants), naturally present in vegetables, fruits, tea, and wine, is associated with a decrease in CAD events. Clinical data have also suggested that supplementation of vitamin E and C slows atherosclerosis progression assessed by carotid intima-media thickness.[72] However, the Heart Protection Study Collaborative Group enrolled more than 20,000 individuals with established atherosclerotic vascular disease or diabetes mellitus and found no reduction in all-cause mortality, myocardial infarction, or other vascular events with supplementation of vitamin E, vitamin C, and beta-carotene versus matched placebo during 5 years of follow-up.[73] Moreover, supplements combining folic acid and vitamins B_6 and B_{12} did not reduce the risk of major cardiovascular events in two large randomized trials of therapy to lower homocysteine in patients with vascular disease.[74,75] Thus, based on current evidence, there is no basis for recommending

that individuals take supplemental folate, vitamin E, vitamin C, or beta-carotene for the purpose of treating CAD.[10,47]

Counseling and Changes in Life Style

The psychosocial issues faced by a patient who develops chronic stable angina for the first time are similar to, although usually less intense than, those experienced by a patient with an acute myocardial infarction. Depressive symptoms are strongly associated with health status as reported by the patient, including the burden of symptoms and overall quality of life, independently of LV function and the presence of provokable ischemia. In addition, the association between depressive symptoms and CAD may reflect a causal relationship between the former and atherothrombosis. Depressive symptoms are associated with higher levels of circulating biomarkers of inflammation.[76] In conjunction with counseling, treatment with a selective serotonin reuptake inhibitor appears to be safe and effective in managing depression in patients with acute coronary syndromes and may be expected to be safe in patients with stable CAD.[77] Thus, efforts to evaluate and treat depression in patients with CAD is an important element of their overall management. Moreover, psychosocial stress at work, home, or both is associated with an increased risk of myocardial infarction and may be a target for preventive interventions.[78]

An important aspect of the physician's role is to counsel patients with respect to dietary habits, goals for physical activity,[79] the types of work they can do, and their leisure activities. Certain changes in life style may be helpful, such as modifying strenuous activities if they constantly and repeatedly produce angina. A history of CAD and stable angina is not inconsistent with the ability to continue to exert themselves, which is important not only in regard to recreational activities and life style but also for patients in whom some physical exertion is required in their employment. However, isometric activities such as weight lifting and other activities such as snow shoveling, which involves an energy expenditure between 60 and 65 percent of peak oxygen consumption, and cross-country or downhill skiing are undesirable. In addition, some activities expose the individual to the detrimental effects of cold on the O_2 demand and supply relationship, and these activities should also be avoided whenever possible.

Eliminating or reducing the factors that precipitate anginal episodes is of obvious importance. Patients learn their usual threshold by trial and error. Patients should avoid sudden bursts of activity, particularly after long periods of rest, after meals, and in cold weather. Both chronic and unstable angina exhibit a circadian rhythm characterized by a lower angina threshold shortly after arising. Therefore, morning activities such as showering, shaving, and dressing should be done at a slower pace and, if necessary, with the use of prophylactic nitroglycerin. The stress of sexual intercourse is approximately equal to that of climbing one flight of stairs at a normal pace or any activity that induces a heart rate of approximately 120 beats/min. With proper precautions (i.e., commencing more than 2 hours postprandially and taking an additional dose of a short-acting beta blocker 1 hour before and nitroglycerin 15 minutes before), most patients with chronic stable angina are able to continue satisfactory sexual activity. Although it is desirable to minimize the number of bouts of angina, an occasional episode is not to be feared. Indeed, unless patients occasionally reach their angina threshold, they may not appreciate the extent of their exercise capacity. Patients with stable CAD may use sildenafil but not in conjunction with nitrates.[80]

Pharmacological Management

Nitrates

MECHANISM OF ACTION. Even though the clinical effectiveness of amyl nitrite in angina pectoris was first described in 1867 by Brunton, organic nitrates are still the drugs most commonly used in the treatment of patients with this condition. The action of these agents is to relax vascular smooth muscle. The vasodilator effects of nitrates are evident in systemic (including coronary) arteries and veins, but they appear to be predominant in the venous circulation. The venodilator effect reduces ventricular preload, which in turn reduces myocardial wall tension and O_2 requirements. The action of nitrates in reducing preload and afterload makes them useful in the treatment of heart failure (see Fig. 54-1), as well as angina pectoris. By reducing the heart's mechanical activity, volume, and O_2 consumption, nitrates increase exercise capacity in patients with ischemic heart disease, thereby allowing a greater total-body workload to be achieved before the angina threshold is reached. In patients with stable angina, nitrates improve exercise tolerance and time to ST segment depression during treadmill exercise tests. When used in combination with calcium-channel blockers and/or beta blockers, the antianginal effects appear greater.[10]

EFFECTS ON THE CORONARY CIRCULATION (Table 54-4). Nitroglycerin causes dilation of epicardial stenoses. These stenoses are often eccentric lesions, and nitroglycerin causes relaxation of the smooth muscle in the wall of the coronary artery that is not encompassed by plaque. Even a small increase in a narrowed arterial lumen can produce a significant reduction in resistance to blood flow across obstructed regions. Nitrates may also exert a beneficial effect in patients with impaired coronary flow reserve by alleviating the vasoconstriction caused by endothelial dysfunction.

TABLE 54–4	Effects of Antianginal Agents on Indices of Myocardial Oxygen Supply and Demand*							
		Beta-Adrenoceptor Blockers				**Calcium Antagonists**		
		ISA		**Cardioselective**				
Index	**Nitrates**	*No*	*Yes*	*No*	*Yes*	*Nifedipine*	*Verapamil*	*Diltiazem*
Supply								
Coronary resistance								
Vascular tone	↓↓	↑	0	↑	0↑	↓↓↓	↓↓↓	↓↓↓
Intramyocardial diastolic tension	↓↓↓	↑	0	↑	↑	↓↓	0↑	0
Coronary collateral circulation	↑	0	0	0	0	↑	0	↑
Duration of diastole	0 (↓)	↑↑↑	0↓	↑↑↑	↑↑↑	0↑ (↓↓)	↑↑↑ (↓)	↑↑ (↓)
Demand								
Intramyocardial systolic tension								
Preload	↓↓↓	↑	0	↑	↑	↓0	↑0↓	0↓
Afterload (peripheral vascular resistance)	↓	↑	↑	↑↑	↑	↓↓	↓	↓
Contractility	0 (↑)	↓↓↓	↓	↓↓↓	↓↓↓	↓ (↑↑)†	↓↓(↑)†	↓(↑)†
Heart rate	0 (↑)	↓↓↓	0↓	↓↓↓	↓↓↓	0 (↑↑)	↓↓ (↑)	↓↓ (↑)

*↑ = Increase; ↓ = decrease; 0 = little or no definite effect. The number of arrows represents the relative intensity of effect. Symbols in parentheses indicate reflex-mediated effects.

†Effect of calcium entry on left ventricular contractility, as assessed in the intact animal model. The net effect on left ventricular performance is variable, because it is influenced by alterations in afterload, reflex cardiac stimulation, and the underlying state of the myocardium.

ISA = intrinsic sympathomimetic activity.

From Shub C, Vlietstra RE, McGoon MD: Selection of optimal drug therapy for the patient with angina pectoris. Mayo Clin Proc 60:539, 1985.

REDISTRIBUTION OF BLOOD FLOW. Nitroglycerin causes redistribution of blood flow from normally perfused to ischemic areas, particularly in the subendocardium.[81] This redistribution may be mediated in part by an increase in collateral blood flow and in part by lowering of ventricular diastolic pressure, thereby reducing subendocardial compression. Nitroglycerin appears to reduce coronary vascular resistance preferentially in viable myocardium with ischemia, as detected by SPECT imaging.[82] In patients with chronic stable angina responsive to nitroglycerin, topical nitroglycerin under resting conditions alters myocardial perfusion by preferentially increasing flow to areas of reduced perfusion, with little or no change in global myocardial perfusion.

ANTITHROMBOTIC EFFECTS. Stimulation of guanylate cyclase by nitric oxide (NO) results in inhibitory action on platelets in addition to vasodilation. Although the antithrombotic effects of intravenous nitroglycerin have been demonstrated in patients with unstable angina and in those with chronic stable angina, the clinical significance of these actions is not clear.[83]

CELLULAR MECHANISM OF ACTION. Nitrates have the ability to cause vasodilation, regardless of whether the endothelium is intact. After entering the vascular smooth muscle cell, nitrates are converted to reactive NO or *S*-nitrosothiols, which activate intracellular guanylate cyclase to produce cyclic guanosine monophosphate (cGMP), which in turn triggers smooth muscle relaxation and antiplatelet aggregator effects (Fig. 54-7). Evidence now exists that the biotransformation of nitroglycerin occurs via mitochondrial aldehyde dehydrogenase and that inhibition of this enzyme may contribute to the development of tolerance.[84] Although the aggregate evidence supports the release of NO as the major cellular mechanism of action of oral nitrates, experimental data have raised challenges to this conclusion. In particular, the arterial vasodilatory effects of nitroglycerin in vitro depend at least in part on endothelial calcium-activated potassium channels.[85]

POTENTIAL FOR ADVERSE EFFECTS OF LONG-TERM ADMINISTRATION. Experimental data have raised questions regarding potentially competing long-term effects of oral nitrates. Multiple animal experiments have demonstrated that extended exposure to nitrates can impair endothelial-dependent vasodilation through the generation of free radical species.[86] However, in an animal model of hypercholesterolemia, large doses of a nitrate had endothelial protective effects and attenuated the increase in intima-media thickness.[87] Long-term studies in humans are necessary to determine the clinical relevance of these findings.[86]

TYPES OF PREPARATIONS AND ROUTES OF ADMINISTRATION

Nitroglycerin administered sublingually remains the drug of choice for the treatment of acute angina episodes and for the prevention of angina (Table 54-5). Because sublingual administration avoids first-pass hepatic metabolism, a transient but effective concentration of the drug rapidly appears in the circulation. The half-life of nitroglycerin itself is brief and it is rapidly converted to two inactive metabolites, both of which are found in the urine. Within 30 to 60 minutes, hepatic breakdown has abolished the hemodynamic and clinical effects. The usual sublingual dose is 0.3 to 0.6 mg, and most patients respond within 5 minutes to one or two 0.3-mg tablets. If symptoms are not relieved by a single dose, additional doses of 0.3 mg may be taken at 5-minute intervals, but no more than 1.2 mg should be used within a 15-minute period. The development of tolerance (see later) is rarely a problem with intermittent use. Sublingual nitroglycerin is especially useful when taken prophylactically shortly before undertaking physical activities that are likely to cause angina. When used for this purpose, it may prevent angina for up to 40 minutes.

ADVERSE REACTIONS. Adverse reactions are common and include headache, flushing, and hypotension. The last is rarely severe, but in some patients with volume depletion and in an upright posture, nitrate-induced hypotension is accompanied by a paradoxical bradycardia, consistent with a vasovagal or vasodepressor response. This reaction is more common in the elderly, who are less able to tolerate hypovolemia. Administration of nitrates before or soon after a meal, particularly in patients with a tendency toward postprandial hypotension, may augment venous pooling, preload reduction, and extent of the fall in blood pressure after the meal. In addition, the partial pressure of O_2 in arterial blood may fall after large doses of nitroglycerin because of a ventilation-perfusion imbalance caused by inability of the pulmonary vascular bed to constrict in areas of alveolar hypoxia, thereby leading to perfusion of less hypoxic tissues. Methemoglobinemia is a rare complication of very large doses of nitrates; commonly used doses of nitrates cause small elevations of methemoglobin levels that are probably not of clinical significance.

PREPARATIONS

Nitroglycerin Tablets. Nitroglycerin tablets tend to lose their potency, especially if exposed to light, and should thus

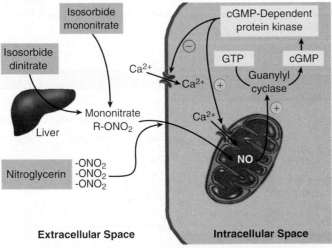

FIGURE 54–7 Mechanism of action of nitrates. Evidence exists that biotransformation of mononitrates occurs through the action of mitochondrial aldehyde reductase, producing nitric oxide (NO). NO activates soluble guanylyl cyclase, resulting in increased production of cyclic guanosine monophosphate (cGMP). The second messenger cGMP reduces cytoplasmic calcium (Ca^{2+}) by inhibiting inflow and stimulating mitochondrial uptake of calcium, thus mediating the relaxation of smooth muscle cells and causing vasodilation. Isosorbide dinitrate is metabolized by the liver, whereas the liver is bypassed by mononitrates. GTP = guanosine triphosphate. R-ONO₂ = mononitrate. (*Modified from Gori T, Parker JD: Nitrate tolerance: A unifying hypothesis. Circulation 106:2510, 2002; and Opie LH: Drugs for the Heart. 4th ed. Philadelphia, WB Saunders, 1995, p 33.*)

TABLE 54–5	Recommended Dosing Regimens for Long-Term Nitrate Therapy	
Preparation of Agent	**Dose**	**Schedule**
Nitroglycerin*		
Ointment	0.5-2 inches	Two or three times daily
Buccal or transmucosal	1-3 mg	Three times daily
Transdermal patch	0.2-0.8 mg/hr	q 24 hr; remove at bedtime for 12-14 hr
Sublingual tablet	0.3-0.6 mg	As needed, up to three doses 5 min apart
Spray	1-2 sprays	As needed, up to three doses 5 min apart
Oral sustained release	2.5-6.5 mg	Two or three times daily[†]
Isosorbide Dinitrate*		
Oral	10-40 mg	Two or three times daily
Oral sustained release	80-120 mg	Once or twice daily (eccentric schedule)
Isosorbide 5-Mononitrate		
Oral	20 mg	Twice daily (given 7-8 hr apart)
Oral sustained release	30-240 mg	Once daily

*A 10- to 12-hour nitrate-free interval is recommended.
[†]Very limited data available on efficacy.

be kept in dark containers. Other nitrate preparations are available in sublingual, buccal, oral, spray, and ointment forms (see Table 54-5). An oral nitroglycerin spray that dispenses metered, aerosolized doses of 0.4 mg may be better absorbed than the sublingual form in patients with dry mucosal membranes. It can also be quickly sprayed onto or under the tongue. For prophylaxis, the spray should be used 5 to 10 minutes before angina-provoking activities.

Isosorbide Dinitrate. This drug is an effective antianginal agent but has low bioavailability after oral administration. It undergoes hepatic metabolism rapidly, and marked variation in plasma concentrations may be seen after oral administration. It has two metabolites, one with potent vasodilator action, that are cleared less rapidly than the parent drug and excreted unchanged in the urine. It is available in tablets for sublingual use, in chewable form, in tablets for oral use, and in sustained-release capsules.

Partial or complete nitrate tolerance (see later) develops with regimens of isosorbide dinitrate when it is administered as 30 mg three or four times daily. A dosage schedule should be adopted that allows a 10- to 12-hour nitrate-free interval. If the drug is administered on a three times/day schedule (e.g., at 8 AM, 1 PM, and 6 PM), the antianginal benefit lasts for approximately 6 hours, and the magnitude of the antianginal benefit decreases with each successive dose.

Isosorbide 5-Mononitrate. This active metabolite of the dinitrate is completely bioavailable with oral administration because it does not undergo first-pass hepatic metabolism, and it is efficacious in the treatment of chronic stable angina. Plasma levels of isosorbide 5-mononitrate reach their peak between 30 minutes and 2 hours after ingestion, and the drug has a plasma half-life of 4 to 6 hours. A single 20-mg tablet still exhibits activity 8 hours after administration. Tolerance has not been demonstrated with once-daily or eccentric dosing intervals but does occur with a twice-daily dosing regimen at 12-hour intervals. The only sustained-release preparation of isosorbide 5-mononitrate is Imdur, which is given once daily in a dosage of 30 to 240 mg. Presumably, this preparation avoids tolerance by providing a sufficiently low nitrate level or a duration of action of 12 hours or less. Once-daily dosing of oral nitrates improves compliance and may offer better efficacy in reducing angina.[88]

Topical Nitroglycerin

1. *Ointment.* Nitroglycerin ointment (15 mg/inch) is efficacious when applied (most commonly to the chest) in strips of 0.5 to 2.0 inches. The delay in onset of action is approximately 30 minutes. Because this form of the drug is effective for 4 to 6 hours, it is particularly useful in patients with severe angina or unstable angina who are confined to bed and chair. Nitroglycerin ointment may also be used prophylactically after retiring by patients with nocturnal angina. Skin permeability increases with increased hydration, and absorption is also enhanced if the paste is covered with plastic with edges taped to the skin.
2. *Transdermal Patches.* Application of silicone gel or polymer matrix impregnated with nitroglycerin results in absorption for 24 to 48 hours at a rate determined by various methods of preparation of the patch, including a semipermeable membrane placed between the drug reservoir and the skin. The release rate of the patches varies from 0.1 to 0.8 mg/hr. Relatively low doses (0.1 to 0.2 mg/hr) may not produce sufficient plasma and tissue concentrations to sustain consistent, effective antianginal effects. Transdermal nitroglycerin therapy has been shown to increase exercise duration and maintain antiischemic effects for 12 hours after patch application throughout 30 days of therapy, without significant evidence of nitrate tolerance or rebound phenomena, provided that the patch is not applied for more than 12 out of 24 hours.

Nitrate Tolerance

A major problem with the use of nitrates is the development of nitrate tolerance, which has been demonstrated with all forms of nitrate administration delivering continuous, relatively stable blood levels of the drug. Although nitrate tolerance is rapid in onset, renewed responsiveness is easily established after a short nitrate-free interval. The problem of tolerance applies to all nitrate preparations; it is particularly important in patients with chronic stable angina pectoris, as opposed to those receiving short-acting courses of nitrates (e.g., with unstable angina and myocardial infarction). Nitrate tolerance appears to be limited to the capacitance and resistance vessels and has not been noted in the large conductance vessels, including the epicardial coronary arteries and radial arteries, despite continuous administration of nitroglycerin for 48 hours.

MECHANISMS. Several mechanisms of nitrate tolerance have been proposed. Evidence has supported the hypothesis that increased generation of vascular superoxide anion ($\cdot O_2^-$) is central to the process.[89] There are multiple possible contributors to generation of oxygen free radicals, including the effects of nitroglycerin on endothelial nitric oxide synthase (NOS uncoupling) and counterregulatory neurohormonal activation. There are a number of consequences of increased superoxide anion formation; these include plausible links to many of the proposed mechanisms of nitrate tolerance: (1) plasma volume expansion and neurohormonal activation; (2) impaired biotransformation of nitrates to NO; and (3) decreased end-organ responsiveness to NO.[89]

MANAGEMENT. The primary strategy to manage nitrate tolerance is to prevent it by providing a nitrate-free interval. The optimal interval is unknown, but with patches or ointment of nitroglycerin or preparations of isosorbide dinitrate or isosorbide 5-mononitrate, a 12-hour off-period is recommended. There are mixed data as to whether angiotensin receptor blockers may attenuate nitrate tolerance.[90]

NITRATE WITHDRAWAL. A common form of nitrate withdrawal (rebound) is observed in patients whose angina is intensified after discontinuation of large doses of long-acting nitrates. In this situation, patients may also have heightened sensitivity to constrictor stimuli. The potential for rebound can be modified by adjusting the dose and timing of administration in addition to the use of other antianginal drugs.

Interaction with Sildenafil

The combination of nitrates and sildenafil may cause serious, prolonged, and potentially life-threatening hypotension. Nitrate therapy is an absolute contraindication to the use of sildenafil, and vice versa. Patients who wish to take sildenafil should be aware of the serious nature of this adverse drug interaction and be warned about taking sildenafil within 24 hours of any nitrate preparation, including short-acting sublingual nitroglycerin tablets.

Beta-Adrenoceptor Blocking Agents

Beta-adrenoceptor blocking drugs (beta blockers) constitute a cornerstone of therapy for angina pectoris. In addition to their antiischemic properties, beta blockers are effective antihypertensives (see Chap. 41) and antiarrhythmics (see Chap. 33). They have also been shown to reduce mortality and reinfarction in patients after myocardial infarction (see Chap. 51) and to reduce mortality in patients with heart failure (see Chap. 25). This combination of actions makes them extremely useful in the management of chronic stable angina. A number of studies have shown that beta blockers, in doses that are generally well tolerated, reduce the frequency of anginal episodes and raise the anginal threshold, both when given alone and when added to other antianginal agents.

The beneficial actions of these drugs depends on their ability to cause competitive inhibition of the effects of neuronally released and circulating catecholamines on beta adrenoceptors (Table 54-6). Beta blockade reduces myocardial O_2 requirements, primarily by slowing the heart rate; the slower heart rate in turn increases the fraction of the

Chronic Coronary Artery Disease

TABLE 54–6	Physiological Actions of Beta-Adrenergic Receptors	
Organ	**Receptor Type**	**Response to Stimulus**
Heart		
SA node	Beta₁	Increased heart rate
Atria	Beta₁	Increased contractility and conduction velocity
AV node	Beta₁	Increased automaticity and conduction velocity
His-Purkinje system	Beta₁	Increased automaticity and conduction velocity
Ventricles	Beta₁	Increased automaticity, contractility, and conduction velocity
Arteries		
Peripheral	Beta₂	Dilation
Coronary	Beta₂	Dilation
Carotid	Beta₂	Dilation
Other	Beta₁	Increased insulin release Increased liver and muscle glycogenolysis
Lungs	Beta₂	Dilation of bronchi
Uterus	Beta₂	Smooth muscle relaxation

AV = atrioventricular; SA = sinoatrial.

From Abrams J: Medical therapy of stable angina pectoris. *In* Beller G, Braunwald E (eds): Chronic Ischemic Heart Disease. Atlas of Heart Disease. Vol 5. Philadelphia, WB Saunders 1995, p 7.19.

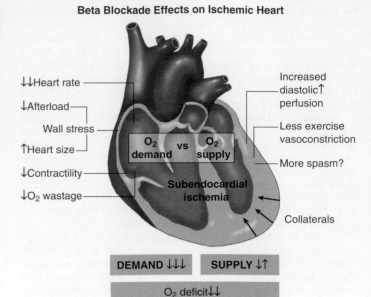

Beta Blockade Effects on Ischemic Heart

FIGURE 54–8 Effects of beta blockade on the ischemic heart. Beta blockade has a beneficial effect on ischemic myocardium unless (1) the preload rises substantially, as in left-sided heart failure, or (2) vasospastic angina is present, in which case spasm may be promoted in some patients. Note the suggestion that beta blockade diminishes exercise-induced vasoconstriction. (*Modified from Opie LH: Drugs for the Heart. 4th ed. Philadelphia, WB Saunders, 1995, p 6.*)

cardiac cycle occupied by diastole, with a corresponding increase in the time available for coronary perfusion (Fig. 54-8; see also Table 54-4). These drugs also reduce exercise-induced increases in blood pressure and limit exercise-induced increases in contractility. Thus, beta blockers reduce myocardial O_2 demand primarily during activity or excitement, when surges of increased sympathetic activity occur. In the face of impaired myocardial perfusion, the effects of beta blockers on myocardial O_2 demand may critically and favorably alter the imbalance between supply and demand, thereby resulting in the elimination of ischemia.

Beta blockers may reduce blood flow to most organs by means of the combination of unopposed alpha-adrenergic vasoconstriction and beta₂ receptor blockade (Table 54-7). Complications are relatively minor but, in patients with peripheral vascular disease, the reduction in blood flow to skeletal muscles with the use of nonselective beta blockers may reduce maximal exercise capacity. In patients with preexisting LV dysfunction, beta blockade may increase ventricular volume and thereby enhance O_2 demand.

Characteristics of Different Beta Blockers

SELECTIVITY. Two major subtypes of beta receptors, designated beta₁ and beta₂, are present in different proportions in different tissues. Beta₁ receptors predominate in the heart, and stimulation of these receptors leads to an increase in heart rate, atrioventricular (AV) conduction, and contractility, release of renin from juxtaglomerular cells in the kidneys, and lipolysis in adipocytes. Beta₂ stimulation causes bronchodilation, vasodilation, and glycogenolysis. Nonselective beta-blocking drugs (e.g., propranolol, nadolol, penbutolol, pindolol, sotalol, timolol, carteolol) block both beta₁ and beta₂ receptors, whereas cardioselective beta blockers (e.g., acebutolol, atenolol, betaxolol, bisoprolol, esmolol, metoprolol) block beta₁ receptors while having less effect on beta₂ receptors. Thus, cardioselective beta blockers reduce myocardial O_2 requirements while tending not to block bronchodilation, vasodilation, or glycogenolysis. However, as the doses of these drugs are increased, this cardioselectivity diminishes. Because cardioselectivity is only relative, the use of cardioselective beta blockers in doses sufficient to control angina may still cause bronchoconstriction in some susceptible patients. Nevertheless, beta blockers are relatively well tolerated in most patients with obstructive pulmonary disease.[91]

Some beta blockers also cause vasodilation. Such drugs include labetalol (an alpha-adrenergic blocking agent and beta₂ agonist; see

Chap. 41), carvedilol (with alpha- and beta₁-blocking activity), and bucindolol (a nonselective beta blocker that causes direct [non–alpha-adrenergic mediated] vasodilation).

ANTIARRHYTHMIC ACTIONS (see Chap. 33). Beta blockers have antiarrhythmic properties as a direct effect of their ability to block sympathoadrenal myocardial stimulation, which in certain situations may be arrhythmogenic.

INTRINSIC SYMPATHOMIMETIC ACTIVITY. Beta blockers with intrinsic sympathomimetic activity (ISA), such as acebutolol, bucindolol, carteolol, celiprolol, penbutolol, and pindolol, are partial beta agonists that also produce blockade by shielding beta receptors from more potent beta agonists. Pindolol and acebutolol produce low-grade beta stimulation when sympathetic activity is low (at rest), whereas these partial agonists behave more like conventional beta blockers when sympathetic activity is high. Agents with ISA may not be as effective as those without this property in reducing the heart rate or the frequency, duration, and magnitude of ambulatory ST segment changes or in increasing the duration of exercise in patients with severe angina.

POTENCY. Potency can be measured by the ability of beta blockers to inhibit the tachycardia produced by isoproterenol. All drugs are considered in reference to propranolol, which is given a value of 1.0 (see Table 54-7). Timolol and pindolol are the most potent agents, and acebutolol and labetalol are the least potent.

LIPID SOLUBILITY. The hydrophilicity or lipid solubility of beta blockers is a major determinant of their absorption and metabolism. The lipid-soluble (lipophilic) beta blockers propranolol, metoprolol, and pindolol are readily absorbed from the gastrointestinal tract, are metabolized predominantly by the liver, have a relatively short half-life, and usually require administration twice or more daily to achieve continuing pharmacological effects. If metoprolol or propranolol is administered intravenously, a much higher concentration reaches the bloodstream, and therefore intravenous dosing has much greater potency than oral dosing does. The water-soluble (hydrophilic) beta blockers (e.g., atenolol, sotalol, nadolol) are not as readily absorbed from the gastrointestinal tract, are not as extensively metabolized, have relatively long plasma half-lives, and can be administered once daily. Water-soluble beta blockers are usually eliminated unchanged by the kidneys. Lipid-soluble agents are often preferable in patients with significant renal dysfunction for whom clearance of water-soluble agents is reduced. Greater lipid solubility is associated with greater penetration to the central nervous system and may contribute to side effects (e.g., lethargy, depression, hallucinations) that are not clearly related to beta-blocking activity.

ALPHA-ADRENOCEPTOR BLOCKING ACTIVITY. The alpha-blocking potency of labetalol (approximately 10 percent that of phentolamine) is approximately 20 percent of its beta-blocking potency (see Table 54-7). Labetalol's combined alpha- and beta-blocking effects make it a particularly useful antihypertensive agent (see Chap. 41), and it is especially so in patients with hypertension and angina. The major side effects of labetalol are postural hypotension and retrograde ejaculation. Carvedilol is a newer beta blocker that also possesses alpha-adrenergic blocking activity with an alpha$_1$-to-beta blocking ratio of approximately 1:10.

GENETIC POLYMORPHISMS. The metabolism of metoprolol, carvedilol, and propranolol may be influenced by genetic polymorphisms or other medications.[92] The oxidative metabolism of metoprolol occurs primarily through the cytochrome P-450 enzyme CYP2D6 and exhibits the debrisoquin type of genetic polymorphism; poor hydroxylators or metabolizers (10 percent of whites or less) have significant prolongation of the elimination half-life of the drug in comparison to extensive hydroxylators or metabolizers. Thus, angina might be controlled by a single daily dose of metoprolol in poor metabolizers, whereas extensive metabolizers require the same dose two or three times daily. If a patient exhibits an exaggerated clinical response (e.g., extreme bradycardia) following the administration of metoprolol, propranolol, or other lipid-soluble beta blockers, it may be the result of prolongation of the elimination half-life because of slow oxidative metabolism. Metabolism of metoprolol may also be altered by drugs that interact with CYP2D6.[92] Preliminary evidence has raised the possibility of differences in survival in patients with unstable coronary disease treated with beta blockers based on polymorphisms of the beta$_2$-adrenergic receptor (*ADRB2*).[93]

EFFECTS ON SERUM LIPID LEVELS. Beta blocker therapy (with agents lacking ISA) usually causes no significant changes in total or LDL cholesterol levels but increases triglyceride and reduces HDL cholesterol levels. The most commonly studied drug has been propranolol, which can increase plasma triglyceride concentrations by 20 to 50 percent and reduce HDL cholesterol levels by 10 to 20 percent. Increasing beta$_1$ selectivity is associated with lesser effects on lipid levels. Adverse effects on the lipid profile may be more frequent with nonselective than with beta$_1$-selective blockers. The effects of these changes in serum lipid levels by long-term administration of beta blockers must be considered when this therapy is begun or maintained for hypertension or angina.

DOSAGE. For optimal results, the dosage of a beta blocker should be carefully adjusted. In the case of atenolol, it is useful to start with a dose of 50 mg once daily. The usual effective dosage is 50 to 100 mg daily; however, some patients benefit from up to 200 mg daily. In the case of metoprolol, it is often preferable from a perspective of the patient's compliance to use an extended-release formulation, which may be started at a dose of 100 mg once daily. Other beta blockers should be started at comparable doses. Efficacy is determined by the effect on heart rate and symptoms and, when these are unclear, the effect on exercise performance can be evaluated by treadmill exercise testing. The resting heart rate should be reduced to between 50 and 60 beats/min, and an increase of less than 20 beats/min should occur with modest exercise (e.g., climbing one flight of stairs). Therapy with beta blockers needs to be individualized and requires repeated clinical evaluation during the initial period of drug administration.

ADVERSE EFFECTS AND CONTRAINDICATIONS. Most of the adverse effects of beta blockers occur as a consequence of the known properties of these drugs and include cardiac effects (e.g., severe sinus bradycardia, sinus arrest, AV block, reduced LV contractility), bronchoconstriction, fatigue, mental depression, nightmares, gastrointestinal upset, sexual dysfunction, intensification of insulin-induced hypoglycemia, and cutaneous reactions (Table 54-8; see also Table 54-6). Lethargy, weakness, and fatigue may be caused by reduced cardiac output or may arise from a direct effect on the central nervous system. Bronchoconstriction results from blockade of beta$_2$ receptors in the tracheobronchial

tree. As a consequence, asthma and chronic obstructive lung disease may be considered as relative contraindications to beta blockers, even to beta$_1$-selective agents.[91]

In patients who already have impaired LV function, congestive heart failure may be intensified, an effect that can be counteracted in part by the use of digitalis or diuretics. Beginning therapy with a very low dose (e.g., metoprolol XL, 25 mg daily, for 2 weeks in patients with NYHA functional Class II) and then gradually increasing the dose over the course of several weeks has been shown to be well tolerated and beneficial in patients with idiopathic dilated cardiomyopathy and those with heart failure caused by ischemic heart disease (see Chap. 25). This approach is recommended when using beta blockers in patients with angina and heart failure.[94]

Beta blockers should be prescribed with caution for patients with cardiac conduction disease involving the sinus node or AV conduction system. In patients with symptomatic conduction disease, beta blockers are contraindicated unless a pacemaker is in place. In patients with asymptomatic sinus node dysfunction or first-degree AV block, beta blockers may be tolerated, but their administration requires careful observation. Pindolol, because of its ISA activity, may be preferable in this situation. Blockade of noncardiac beta$_2$ receptors inhibits catecholamine-induced glycogenolysis, so noncardioselective beta blockers can impair the defense to insulin-induced hypoglycemia. Nevertheless, beta blockers are generally well tolerated in patients with diabetes mellitus. Moreover, carvedilol has been shown to exhibit modest insulin-sensitizing properties and can relieve some manifestations of the metabolic syndrome.[95] Blockade of beta$_2$ receptors also inhibits the vasodilating effects of catecholamines in peripheral blood vessels and leaves the constrictor (alpha-adrenergic) receptors unopposed, thereby enhancing vasoconstriction. Noncardioselective beta blockers may precipitate episodes of Raynaud phenomenon in patients with this condition and may cause uncomfortable coldness in the distal extremities. Reduced flow to the limbs may occur in patients with peripheral vascular disease.

Abrupt withdrawal of beta-adrenoceptor blocking agents after prolonged administration can result in increased total ischemic activity in patients with chronic stable angina. This increased ischemia may be caused by a return to the previously high levels of myocardial O$_2$ demand while the underlying atherosclerotic process has progressed, but a rebound phenomenon resulting in increased beta-adrenergic sensitivity probably occurs in some patients. Occasionally, such withdrawal can precipitate unstable angina and may, in rare cases, even provoke myocardial infarction. Chronic beta blocker therapy can be safely discontinued by slowly withdrawing the drug in a stepwise manner over the course of 2 to 3 weeks. If abrupt withdrawal of beta blockers is required, patients should be instructed to reduce exertion and manage angina episodes with sublingual nitroglycerin and/or substitute a calcium antagonist.

Calcium Antagonists

The critical role of calcium ions in the normal contraction of cardiac and vascular smooth muscle is discussed in Chapter 21. Calcium antagonists (see Chap. 41) are a heterogeneous group of compounds that inhibit calcium ion movement through slow channels in cardiac and smooth muscle membranes by noncompetitive blockade of voltage-sensitive L-type calcium channels.[96] The three major classes of calcium antagonists are the dihydropyridines (nifedipine is the prototype), the phenylalkylamines (verapamil is the prototype), and the modified benzothiazepines (diltiazem is the prototype). Amlodipine and felodipine are additional dihydropyridines that are among the most commonly used

TABLE 54–7 | **Pharmacokinetics and Pharmacology of Some Beta-Adrenoceptor Blockers**

Characteristic	Atenolol	Metoprolol/XL	Nadolol	Pindolol	Propranolol/LA	Timolol	Acebutolol
Extent of absorption (%)	~50	>95	~30	>90	>90	>90	~70
Extent of bioavailability (% of dose)	~40	~50/77	~30	~90	~30/20	75	~50
Beta-blocking plasma concentration	0.2-0.5 µg/ml	50-100 ng/ml	50-100 ng/ml	50-100 ng/ml	50-100 ng/ml	50-100 ng/ml	0.2-2.0 µg/ml
Protein binding (%)	<5	12	~30	57	93	~10	30-40
Lipophilicity*	Low	Moderate	Low	Moderate	High	Low	Low
Elimination half-life (hr)	6-9	3-7	14-25	3-4	3.5 to 6/8-11	3-4	3-4†
Drug accumulation in renal disease	Yes	No	Yes	No	No	No	Yes‡
Route of elimination	RE (mostly unchanged	HM	RE	RE (40% unchanged and HM)	HM	RE (20% unchanged and HM)	HM‡
Beta blocker potency ratio (propranolol = 1)	1.0	1	1.0	6.0	1	6.0	0.3
Adrenergic-receptor blocking activity	β_1¶	β_1¶	β_1/β_2	β_1/β_2	β_1/β_2	β_1/β_2	β_1¶
Intrinsic sympathetic activity	0	0	0	+	0	0	+
Membrane-stabilizing activity	0	0	0	+	++	0	+
Usual maintenance dose	50-100 mg/d	50-100 mg b.i.d.-q.i.d./ 50-400 mg/d	40-80 mg/d	10-40 mg/d (b.i.d.-t.i.d.)	80-320 mg/d (b.i.d.-t.i.d.)/ 80-160 mg/d	10-30 mg b.i.d.	200-600 mg b.i.d.
FDA-approved indications: Hypertension	Yes	Yes/Yes	Yes	Yes	Yes/Yes	Yes	Yes
Angina	Yes	Yes/Yes	Yes	No	Yes/Yes	No	No
Post-MI	Yes	Yes/No	No	No	Yes/No	Yes	No
Heart failure	No	Yes/Yes	No	No	No/No	No	No

*Determined by the distribution ratio between octanol and water.
†Half-life of the active metabolite, diacetolol, is 12 to 15 hours.
‡Acebutolol is mainly eliminated by the liver, but its major metabolite, diacetolol, is excreted by the kidney.
§Rapid metabolism by esterases in the cytosol of red blood cells.
¶Beta₁ selectivity is maintained at lower doses, but beta₂ receptors are inhibited at higher doses.
FDA = U.S. Food and Drug Administration; HM = hepatic metabolism; MI = myocardial infarction; ND = no data; RE = renal excretion.

calcium antagonists in the United States. The two predominant effects of calcium antagonists result from blocking the entry of calcium ions and slowing recovery of the channel. Phenylalkylamines have a marked effect on recovery of the channel and thereby exert depressant effects on cardiac pacemakers and conduction, whereas dihydropyridines, which do not impair channel recovery, have little effect on the conduction system.

MECHANISM OF ACTION. The efficacy of calcium antagonists in patients with angina pectoris is related to the reduction in myocardial O_2 demand and the increase in O_2 supply that they induce (see Table 54-4). The latter effect is particularly important in patients with conditions in which a prominent vasospastic or vasoconstrictor component may be present, such as Prinzmetal (variant) angina (see Chap. 53), variable-threshold angina, and angina related to impaired vasodilator reserve of small coronary arteries. Calcium antagonists may be effective on their own or in combination with beta-adrenoceptor blockers

and nitrates in patients with chronic stable angina. Several calcium antagonists are effective for the treatment of angina pectoris (Table 54-9). Each relaxes vascular smooth muscle in the systemic arterial and coronary arterial beds. In addition, blockade of the entry of calcium into myocytes results in a negative inotropic effect, which is counteracted to some extent by peripheral vascular dilation and by activation of the sympathetic nervous system in response to drug-induced hypotension. However, the negative inotropic effect must be taken into consideration in patients with significant LV dysfunction.

With a rapid onset of action and metabolism by the liver, calcium antagonists have a limited bioavailability of between 13 and 52 percent and a half-life of between 3 and 12 hours. Amlodipine and felodipine are exceptions in that both drugs have long half-lives and may be administered once daily. In the case of some of the other calcium antagonists (e.g., nifedipine and diltiazem), sustained-release preparations have been shown to be effective.

ANTIATHEROGENIC ACTION. Hyperlipidemia-induced changes in the permeability of smooth muscle cells to calcium may play a role in atherogenesis; thus, the hypothesis that calcium antagonists might

Labetalol	Bisoprolol	Betaxolol	Carteolol	Penbutolol	Carvedilol	Esmolol (IV)	Sotalol
>90	>90	>90	>90	100	ND	ND	ND
~25	80	90	85	100	~30	100	>90
0.7-3.0 µg/ml	0.01-0.1 µg/ml	20-50 ng/ml	40-160 ng/ml	ND	ND	0.15-2.0 µg/ml	ND
~50	30	50-60	23-30	80-98	95-98	55	0
Low	Moderate	Moderate	Low	High	High	Low	Low
~6	7-15	12-22	5-7	17-26	6-10	4.5 min	12
No	Yes	Yes	Yes	Yes	No	No	Yes
HM	HM 50%; RE 50%	HM	RE	HM	HM	§	RE
0.3	10	4	10	1	10	0.02	0.3
$\beta_1/\beta_2/\alpha_1$	β_1¶	β_1¶	β_1/β_2	β_1/β_2	$\beta_1/\beta_2/\alpha_1$	β_1¶	β_1/β_2
0	0	0	+	+	0	0	0
0	0	0	0	0	+	0	0
100-400 mg b.i.d.	5-20 mg/d	5-20 mg/d	2.5-10 mg/d	10-40 mg/d	3.125-50 mg/ b.i.d.	Bolus of 500 µg/kg; infusion at 50-200 µg/ kg/min	80-160 mg b.i.d.
Yes	Yes	Yes	Yes	Yes	Yes	Yes	No
No	No	No	No	No	No	No	No
No	No	No	No	No	No	Yes	No
No	No	No	No	No	Yes	No	No

CH 54

Chronic Coronary Artery Disease

inhibit atherogenesis has been explored since the 1970s but has not yet achieved consensus. Experimental work with calcium channel blockers, in particular with more lipophilic second-generation agents such as amlodipine, have demonstrated improved endothelial function, inhibition of smooth muscle cell proliferation, migration, and ameliorated unfavorable membrane alterations.[10,97] In a randomized trial in patients with established CAD, treatment with amlodipine, compared with placebo, was associated with less progression of carotid atherosclerosis measured by intima-medial thickness; however, no difference was detected in the progression of coronary atherosclerosis. Moreover, evidence regarding both first- and subsequent-generation agents with respect to lesion progression and restenosis remains mixed,[98] with an aggregate result that maintains the possibility that calcium antagonists may have some role in atheroprotection.

FIRST-GENERATION CALCIUM ANTAGONISTS

NIFEDIPINE. Nifedipine, a dihydropyridine, is a particularly effective dilator of vascular smooth muscle and is a more potent vasodilator than diltiazem or verapamil. Although its in vitro actions on myocardium and specialized cardiac tissue are similar to those of other agents, the concentration required to reproduce effects on these tissues is not reached in vivo because of the early appearance of its powerful vasodilating effects. Thus, in clinical practice, the potential negative chronotropic, inotropic, and dromotropic (on AV conduction) effects of nifedipine are seldom a problem, with the exception that nifedipine has been reported to worsen heart failure in patients with preexisting chronic congestive heart failure.

The beneficial effects of nifedipine in the treatment of angina result from its capacity to reduce myocardial O_2 requirements because of its afterload-reducing effect and to increase myocardial O_2 delivery as a result of its dilating action on the coronary vascular bed (see Table 54-4). Oral nifedipine in capsule form exerts hypotensive effects within

20 minutes of administration. This immediate-release formulation is no longer recommended because of concerns regarding adverse events. An extended-release formulation using the gastrointestinal therapeutic system of drug delivery (see Table 54-9) is designed to deliver 30, 60, or 90 mg of nifedipine in a single daily dose at a relatively constant rate over a 24-hour period and is useful for the treatment of chronic stable angina, Prinzmetal angina, and hypertension. Steady-state plasma levels are typically achieved within 48 hours of initiation. The efficacy of the extended-release preparation, either alone or in conjunction with beta blockers, in reducing episodes of angina and ischemia on ambulatory monitoring has been documented.

Adverse Effects. These occur in 15 to 20 percent of patients and require discontinuation of medication in about 5 percent. Most adverse effects are related to systemic vasodilation and include headache, dizziness, palpitations, flushing, hypotension, and leg edema (unrelated to heart failure). Gastrointestinal side effects, including nausea, epigastric pressure, and vomiting, are noted in approximately 5 percent of patients. In rare cases, in patients with extremely severe fixed coronary obstructions, nifedipine aggravates angina, presumably by lowering arterial pressure excessively, with subsequent reflex tachycardia. For this reason, combined treatment of angina with nifedipine and a beta blocker is particularly effective and superior to nifedipine alone. Most adverse effects are reduced by the use of extended-release preparations.

Several clinical case-control studies of hypertension and associated reviews have suggested that short-acting nifedipine may cause an increase in mortality. The randomized, placebo controlled ACTION (A Coronary disease Trial Investigating Outcome with Nifedipine gastrointestinal therapeutic system [GITS]) trial allocated 7665 patients with stable angina, most of whom were receiving beta blockers, to nifedipine GITS or placebo for a median of 4.9 years. The primary results demonstrated no difference in the rate of death, myocardial infarction, refractory angina, new heart failure, stroke, or peripheral revascularization. Long-acting nifedipine should be considered an effective and safe antianginal drug for the treatment of symptomatic patients with chronic CAD who are already receiving beta blockers, with or without nitrates. Short-acting nifedipine should ordinarily be avoided.

Because of its potent vasodilator effects, nifedipine is contraindicated in patients who are hypotensive or have

TABLE 54-8	Candidates for Use of Beta-Blocking Agents for Angina

Ideal Candidates
Prominent relationship of physical activity to attacks of angina
Coexistent hypertension
History of supraventricular or ventricular arrhythmias
Previous myocardial infarction
Left ventricular systolic dysfunction
Mild to moderate heart failure symptoms
  (NYHA functional Classes II, III)
Prominent anxiety state

Poor Candidates
Asthma or reversible airway component in chronic lung disease
  patients
Severe left ventricular dysfunction with severe heart failure symptoms
  (NYHA functional Class IV)
History of severe depression
Raynaud phenomenon
Symptomatic peripheral vascular disease
Severe bradycardia or heart block
Brittle diabetes

NYHA = New York Heart Association.
Modified from Abrams JA: Medical therapy of stable angina pectoris. *In* Beller G, Braunwald E (eds): Chronic Ischemic Heart Disease. Atlas of Heart Disease. Vol. 5. Philadelphia, WB Saunders, 1995. p 7.22.

TABLE 54-9	Pharmacokinetics of Some Calcium Antagonists Used for Angina Pectoris			
Characteristic	Diltiazem/SR	Nicardipine	Nifedipine/SR	
Usual adult dose	IV: 0.25 mg/kg bolus, then 5-15 mg/hr Oral: 30-90 mg t.i.d.-q.i.d. SR: 60-180 mg b.i.d. CD: 120-480 mg/d	IV: 3-15 mg/hr Oral: 20-40 mg t.i.d. SR: 30-60 mg b.i.d.	Oral: 10-30 mg t.i.d. SR: 90 mg/d	
Extent of absorption (%)	80-90	100	90	
Extent of bioavailability (%)	40-70	30	65-75/86	
Onset of action	IV: 3 min Oral: 30-60 min	IV: 1 min Oral: 20 min	20 min	
Time to peak serum concentration (hr)	2-3/6-11	0.5-2.0	0.5/6	
Therapeutic serum levels (ng/ml)	50-200	30-50	25-100	
Elimination half-life (hr)	3.5/5-7	2.0-4.0	2.0-5.0	
Elimination	60% metabolized by liver; remainder excreted by kidneys	High first-pass hepatic metabolism	High first-pass hepatic metabolism	
Heart rate	↓	↑	↑↑	
Peripheral vascular resistance	↓	↓↓↓	↓↓↓	
FDA-approved indications	IR	SR		IR	SR
Hypertension	No	Yes	Yes†	No	Yes
Angina	Yes	Yes	Yes	Yes	Yes
Coronary spasm	Yes	No	No	Yes	Yes

*Half-life of 4.5 to 12 hours with multiple dosing; may be prolonged in the elderly.
†The sustained-release formulation may be preferred for hypertension.
CD = combination drug; CR = controlled release; IR = immediate release; ND = no data; SR = sustained release; U.S. FDA = Food and Drug Administration.

severe aortic valve stenosis and in patients with unstable angina who are not simultaneously receiving a beta blocker in whom reflex-mediated increases in the heart rate may be harmful. Nifedipine (or a second-generation dihydropyridine) is the calcium antagonist of choice in patients with sinus bradycardia, sick sinus syndrome, or AV block, particularly if a beta-adrenoceptor blocking agent is administered concurrently and additional drug therapy for angina is indicated. This recommendation is based on the observation that in doses used clinically, nifedipine has fewer negative effects on myocardial contractility, heart rate, and AV conduction than verapamil or diltiazem.

Nifedipine interacts significantly with prazosin (resulting in excessive hypotension), cimetidine, and phenytoin (resulting in increased bioavailability of nifedipine). In patients with Prinzmetal angina, abrupt cessation of nifedipine therapy may result in a rebound increase in the frequency and duration of attacks (see Chap. 53).

VERAPAMIL. Verapamil dilates systemic and coronary resistance vessels and large coronary conductance vessels. It slows the heart rate and reduces myocardial contractility. This combination of actions results in a reduction in myocardial O_2 requirement, which is the basis for the drug's efficacy in the management of chronic stable angina.

Verapamil reduces the frequency of angina and prolongs exercise tolerance in patients with symptomatic chronic CAD, and the combination of verapamil and a beta blocker provides clinical benefit that is additive. When evaluated in the International Verapamil-Trandolapril Study (INVEST), a strategy combining sustained-release verapamil and trandolapril compared with atenolol and a diuretic for the treatment of patients with hypertension and CAD showed equivalent outcomes with respect to death, MI, or stroke.[99] Despite the marked negative inotropic effects of verapamil in isolated cardiac muscle preparations, changes in contractility are modest in patients with normal cardiac function. However, in patients with cardiac dysfunction, verapamil may reduce cardiac output, increase LV filling pressure, and cause clinical heart failure. In clinically useful doses, verapamil inhibits calcium influx into specialized cardiac cells, sometimes causing slowing of the heart rate and AV conduction. Therefore, it is contraindicated for patients with preexisting AV nodal disease or sick sinus syndrome, congestive heart failure, and suspected digitalis or quinidine toxicity.

The usual starting dose of verapamil for oral administration is 40 to 80 mg three times daily to a maximal dose of 480 mg daily (see Table 54-9). Sustained-release preparations of verapamil are available, and starting doses are 120 to 240 mg twice daily, with a usual optimal dosage range of 240 to 360 mg daily.

Verapamil interacts significantly with several other drugs. Intravenous verapamil should generally not be used together with a beta blocker (given intravenously or orally), nor should a beta blocker be administered intravenously in patients receiving oral verapamil. Both drugs can be administered orally but with caution in view of the potential for the development of bradyarrhythmias and negative inotropic effects. The bioavailability of verapamil is increased by cimetidine and carbamazepine, whereas verapamil may increase plasma levels of cyclosporine and digoxin and may be associated with excessive hypotension in patients receiving quinidine or prazosin. Hepatic enzyme inducers such as phenobarbital may reduce the effects of verapamil. Verapamil should not be administered in conjunction with the antiarrhythmic drug dofetilide.

Adverse effects of verapamil are noted in approximately 10 percent of patients and relate to systemic vasodilation (hypotension and facial flushing), gastrointestinal symptoms (constipation and nausea), and central nervous system reactions, such as headache and dizziness. A rare side effect is gingival hyperplasia, which appears after 1 to 9 months of therapy.

DILTIAZEM. Diltiazem's actions are intermediate between those of nifedipine and verapamil. In clinically

Verapamil/SR		Amlodipine	Felodipine	Isradipine	Nisoldipine
IV: 0.075-0.15 mg/kg Oral: 80-120 mg t.i.d.-q.i.d. SR: 180-480 mg/d		Oral: 2.5-10 mg/d	Oral SR: 2.5-10 mg/d	Oral CR: 2.5-10 mg b.i.d.	Oral SR: 10-40 mg/d
90		>90	>90	>90	ND
20-35		60-90	20	25	5
IV: 2-5 min Oral: 30 min		0.5-1.0 hr	2 hr	20 min	1-3 hr
IV: 3-5 min Oral: 1-2; SR: 7-9		6-12	2-5	1.5	6-12
80-300		5-20	1-5	2-10	ND
3.0-7.0*		30-50	11-16	8	7-12
85% eliminated by first-pass hepatic metabolism		Hepatic	High first-pass hepatic metabolism	High first-pass hepatic metabolism	Hepatic
↓		0	↑	0	0
↓↓		↓↓↓	↓↓↓	↓↓↓	↓↓↓
IR	SR				
Yes	Yes	Yes	Yes	Yes	Yes
Yes	No	Yes	No	No	Yes
Yes	No	Yes	No	No	No

useful doses, its vasodilator effects are less profound than those of nifedipine, and its cardiac depressant action, on the sinoatrial and AV nodes and myocardium, is less than that of verapamil. This profile may explain the remarkably low incidence of adverse effects of diltiazem. Diltiazem is a systemic vasodilator that lowers arterial pressure at rest and during exertion and increases the workload required to produce myocardial ischemia, but it may also increase myocardial O_2 delivery. Although this drug causes little vasodilation of epicardial coronary arteries under basal conditions, it may enhance perfusion of the subendocardium distal to a flow-limiting coronary stenosis; it also blocks exercise-induced coronary vasoconstriction. In patients with chronic stable angina receiving maximally tolerated doses of diltiazem, the heart rate is significantly reduced at rest, but no effect on peak blood pressure is achieved during exercise, and the duration of symptom-limited treadmill exercise is prolonged.

Several sustained-release formulations of diltiazem are available for once-daily treatment of systemic hypertension and angina pectoris. The usual starting dosage of sustained-release formulations is 120 mg once daily up to a typical maintenance dosage of 180 to 360 mg once daily. The maximum effect on blood pressure may not be observed until 14 days after starting therapy.

Diltiazem is a highly effective antianginal agent. Atenolol and diltiazem have similar efficacy in increasing nonischemic exercise duration in patients with variable-threshold angina and act primarily by slowing the resting heart rate. High doses (mean dose, 340 mg) have been shown to be a relatively safe addition to maximally tolerated doses of isosorbide dinitrate and a beta blocker and cause increases in exercise tolerance and resting and exercise LV ejection fractions. Major side effects are similar to those of the other calcium channel blockers and are related to vasodilation, but they are relatively infrequent, particularly if the dosage does not exceed 240 mg daily. As is the case with verapamil, diltiazem should be prescribed with caution for patients with sick sinus syndrome or AV block. In patients with preexisting LV dysfunction, diltiazem may exacerbate or precipitate heart failure.

Diltiazem interacts with other drugs, including beta-adrenergic blocking agents (causing enhanced negative inotropic, chronotropic, and dromotropic effects), flecainide, and cimetidine (which increases the bioavailability of diltiazem), and diltiazem has been associated with increased plasma levels of cyclosporine, carbamazepine, and lithium carbonate. Diltiazem may cause excessive sinus node depression if administered with disopyramide and may reduce digoxin clearance, especially in patients with renal failure.

SECOND-GENERATION CALCIUM ANTAGONISTS

The second-generation calcium antagonists (e.g., nicardipine, isradipine, amlodipine, felodipine) are mainly dihydropyridine derivatives, with nifedipine being the prototypical agent. Considerable experience has also accumulated with nimodipine, nisoldipine, and nitrendipine. These agents differ in potency, tissue specificity, and pharmacokinetics and, in general, are potent vasodilators because of greater vascular selectivity than that seen with the first-generation antagonists (e.g., verapamil, nifedipine, diltiazem).

AMLODIPINE. This agent, which is less lipid soluble than nifedipine, has a slow, smooth onset and ultralong duration of action (plasma half-life of 36 hours). It causes marked coronary and peripheral dilation and may be useful in the treatment of patients with angina accompanied by hypertension. It may be used as a once-daily hypotensive or antianginal agent. In a series of randomized placebo-controlled studies in patients with stable exercise-induced angina pectoris, amlodipine was shown to be effective and well tolerated. In two trials in patients with established CAD, amlodipine reduced the risk of major cardiovascular events. Amlodipine has little, if any, negative inotropic action and may be especially useful in patients with chronic angina and LV dysfunction.

The usual dosage of amlodipine is 5 to 10 mg once daily. Downward adjustment of the starting dose is appropriate for patients with liver disease and the elderly. Significant changes in blood pressure are typically not evident until 24 to 48 hours after initiation. Steady-state serum levels are achieved at 7 to 8 days.

NICARDIPINE. This drug has a half-life similar to that of nifedipine (2 to 4 hours), but appears to have greater vascular selectivity. Nicardipine may be used as an antianginal and antihypertensive agent and requires administration three times daily, although a sustained-release formulation is available for twice-daily dosing in hypertension. For chronic stable angina pectoris, it appears to be as effective as verapamil or diltiazem, and its efficacy is enhanced when combined with a beta blocker.

FELODIPINE AND ISRADIPINE. In the United States, both drugs are approved by the U.S. Food and Drug Administration (FDA) for the treatment of hypertension but not for angina pectoris. One study has documented similar efficacy between felodipine and nifedipine in patients with chronic stable angina. Felodipine has also been reported to be more vascular selective than nifedipine and to have a mild positive inotropic effect as a result of calcium channel agonist properties. Isradipine has a longer half-life than nifedipine and demonstrates greater vascular sensitivity.

Other Pharmacological Agents

RANOLAZINE Ranolazine is a piperazine derivative that was approved in 2006 in the United States for use in patients with chronic stable angina in conjunction with beta blockers, calcium antagonists, or nitrates.[100] Ranolazine is unique among currently approved antianginals in that its antiischemic effects are achieved without a clinically meaningful change in heart rate or blood pressure.[101] The mechanism of action of this agent remains under investigation. When studied at high concentrations in in vitro experiments, ranolazine was shown to shift myocardial substrate uptake from fatty acid to glucose and thus was considered to be a potential metabolic agent. However, subsequent studies at concentrations of ranolazine consistent with doses tested in clinical trials have suggested that ranolazine exerts favorable effects on ischemia through a reduction in calcium overload in the ischemic myocyte via inhibition of the late sodium current (I_{Na}).[100] In animal models of ischemia and reperfusion, ranolazine preserves tissue levels of adenosine triphosphate, improves myocardial contractile function, and reduces the extent of irreversible myocardial injury measured by biomarkers of necrosis and by electron microscopy.

A sustained-release formulation of ranolazine has been studied in three randomized placebo-controlled clinical trials and has improved exercise performance and increased the time to ischemia during exercise treadmill testing when used as monotherapy or when used in combination with the most frequently used doses of atenolol, amlodipine, or diltiazem.[102] Ranolazine also decreases angina frequency and nitroglycerin use when used in combination with a beta blocker or calcium channel blocker.[102]

When studied in a randomized, blinded, placebo-controlled trial of 6560 patients with non-ST elevation acute coronary syndrome, ranolazine, administered for an average of approximately 1 year, did not add to standard therapy for the secondary prevention of major cardiovascular events. However, ranolazine reduced the incidence of recurrent ischemia, in particular worsening angina, in a significantly more diverse population with established CAD than studied previously with ranolazine.[102a]

The half-life of the sustained release formulation of ranolazine is approximately 7 hours. A steady state is generally achieved within 3 days of dosing twice daily. Ranolazine is metabolized primarily through the cytochrome P-450 (CYP3A4) pathway and thus the plasma concentration is increased if administered in combination with moderate (e.g., diltiazem) or strong (e.g., ketoconazole and macrolide antibiotic)

inhibitors of this system. Verapamil increases the absorption of ranolazine by inhibition of P-glycoprotein. Plasma concentrations of simvastatin are increased approximately twofold after administration of ranolazine.

Ranolazine should be started as 500 mg twice daily and may be increased to a maximum of 1000 mg twice daily in patients with persistent angina. The most commonly reported adverse effects in clinical studies are nausea, generalized weakness, and constipation. Dizziness has also been reported, as has a small dose-related increase in the corrected QT interval, an average of 2 to 5 milliseconds in the dosage range of 500 to 1000 mg twice daily.[100] The electrophysiologic effects of ranolazine include inhibition of the delayed rectifier current and inhibition of I_{Na}; the net effect is to shorten action potential duration and suppress early afterdepolarizations.[103] Thus, ranolazine does not have the electrophysiological profile that has been observed with QT-prolonging drugs associated with torsades de pointes. Ranolazine is contraindicated in patients with preexisting QT prolongation, receiving other QT-prolonging medications, or with hepatic impairment, which has been associated with a steeper relationship between ranolazine and the QTc.

There was no adverse trend in the incidence of symptomatic documented arrhythmias, all-cause mortality, or sudden cardiac death with ranolazine in the randomized trial of 6560 patients with recent acute coronary syndromes. A significant reduction in the incidence of arrhythmias detected on 7 days of Holter monitoring with ranolazine compared with placebo in this study suggests possible anti-arrhythmic actions of the agent that may warrant additional investigation.[102a]

NICORANDIL.* Nicorandil is a nicotinamide ester that dilates peripheral and coronary resistance vessels via action on ATP-sensitive potassium channels and possesses a nitrate moiety that promotes systemic venous and coronary vasodilation.[104] As a result of these dual actions, nicorandil reduces preload and afterload and results in an increase in coronary blood flow. In addition to these effects, nicorandil may have cardioprotective actions mediated through the activation of potassium channels.

Nicorandil has antianginal efficacy similar to beta blockers, nitrates, and calcium channel blockers. In a recent randomized clinical trial ($N = 5126$), nicorandil reduced the risk of cardiac death, myocardial infarction, or hospital admission for angina (hazard ratio, 0.83; $P = 0.014$) compared with placebo when added to standard antianginal therapy.[105]

IVABRADINE.* Ivabradine is a specific and selective inhibitor of the I_f ion channel, the principal determinant of the sinoatrial node pacemaker current.[106] Ivabradine reduces the spontaneous firing rate of sinoatrial pacemaker cells and thus slows heart rate through a mechanism that is not associated with negative inotropic effects. Ivabradine reduces peak heart rate during exercise and increases the time to limiting angina compared with placebo,[107] and is equivalent to atenolol with respect to exercise performance and time to ischemia (ST segment depression) in patients with stable angina undergoing exercise treadmill testing.[108]

FASUDIL.* Fasudil is an orally available inhibitor of rho kinase, an intracellular signaling molecule that participates in vascular smooth muscle contraction. Fasudil was shown to increase the time to ischemia in a study of 84 patients with CAD undergoing exercise treadmill testing.[109]

METABOLIC AGENTS.* Agents aimed at increasing the metabolic efficiency of cardiac myocytes have also been studied in patients with chronic stable angina. Partial inhibitors of fatty acid oxidation appear to shift myocardial metabolism to more oxygen-efficient pathways. Trimetazidine and perhexiline are agents that have been shown to inhibit fatty acid metabolism and to reduce the frequency of angina without hemodynamic effects in patients with chronic stable angina.[110]

Other Considerations of Medical Management of Angina Pectoris

RELATIVE ADVANTAGES OF BETA BLOCKERS AND CALCIUM ANTAGONISTS (Table 54-10). The choice between a beta blocker and a calcium channel antagonist as initial therapy in patients with chronic stable angina is controversial because both classes of agents are effective in relieving symptoms and reducing ischemia.[10] Trials comparing beta blockers and calcium antagonists have not shown any difference in the rate of death or myocardial

---

*Has not been approved by the FDA at the time of this writing.

TABLE 54-10	Recommended Drug Therapy* in Patients Who Have Angina in Conjunction with Other Medical Conditions
Clinical Condition	**Recommended Drug†**
Cardiac Arrhythemia or Conduction Disturbance	
Sinus bradycardia	Nifedipine or amlodipine
Sinus tachycardia (not caused by cardiac failure)	Beta blocker
Supraventricular tachycardia	Beta blocker (verapamil)
Atrioventricular block	Nifedipine or amlodipine
Rapid atrial fibrillation	Verapamil or beta blocker
Ventricular arrhythmia	Beta blocker
Left Ventricular Dysfunction	
Heart failure	Beta blocker
Miscellaneous Medical Conditions	
Systemic hypertension	Beta blocker (calcium antagonist)
Severe preexisting headaches	Beta blocker (verapamil or diltiazem)
COPD with bronchospasm or asthma	Nifedipine, amlodipine, verapamil, or diltiazem
Hyperthyroidism	Beta blocker
Raynaud syndrome	Nifedipine or amlodipine
Claudication	Calcium antagonist
Severe depression	Calcium antagonist

*Calcium antagonist versus beta blocker.
†Alternatives in parentheses.
COPD = chronic obstructive pulmonary disease.

infarction,[10] although in some studies beta blockers appeared to have greater clinical efficacy and less frequent discontinuation because of side effects. Because long-term administration of beta blockers has been demonstrated to prolong life in patients after acute myocardial infarction and in the treatment of hypertension, it is reasonable to consider beta blockers over calcium antagonists as the agents of choice in treating patients with chronic stable angina.[10] However, it must be recognized that beta blockers (without ISA) increase serum triglyceride levels and decrease HDL cholesterol levels, with uncertain long-term consequences. In addition, these drugs may produce fatigue, depression, and sexual dysfunction. In contrast, although calcium antagonists do not show these adverse effects, their long-term administration has *not* been shown to improve long-term survival after acute myocardial infarction. However, diltiazem is apparently effective in preventing severe angina and early reinfarction after non-Q-wave infarction. Verapamil reduces reinfarction rates in patients post-MI and, when combined with trandolapril, achieves similar outcomes to atenolol together with a diuretic for the treatment of patients with hypertension and CAD.

The choice of drug with which to initiate therapy is influenced by a number of clinical factors (see Table 54-10)[10]:

1. Calcium antagonists are the preferred agents in patients with a history of asthma or chronic obstructive lung disease with wheezing on clinical examination, in whom beta blockers, even relatively selective agents, are contraindicated. Consideration to a trial of beta blockers should be given if the patient has a history of prior MI.

2. Nifedipine (long-acting), amlodipine, and nicardipine are the calcium antagonists of choice in patients with chronic stable angina and sick sinus syndrome, sinus bradycardia, or significant AV conduction disturbances, whereas beta blockers and verapamil should be used only with great caution in such patients. In patients with symptomatic conduction disease, neither a beta blocker nor a calcium channel blocker should be used unless a pacemaker is in place. If a beta blocker

is required in patients with asymptomatic evidence of conduction disease, pindolol, which has the greatest ISA, is useful. In the case of calcium channel blockers in patients with conduction system disease, nifedipine or nicardipine is preferable to verapamil and diltiazem, but careful observation for deterioration of conduction is mandatory.

3. Calcium antagonists are clearly preferred for patients with suspected Prinzmetal (variant) angina (see Chap. 53); beta blockers may even aggravate angina under these circumstances.

4. Calcium antagonists may be preferred over beta blockers in patients with significant, symptomatic peripheral arterial disease because the latter may cause peripheral vasoconstriction.

5. Beta blockers should usually be avoided in patients with a history of significant depressive illness and should be prescribed cautiously for patients with sexual dysfunction, sleep disturbance, nightmares, fatigue, or lethargy.

6. The presence of moderate to severe LV dysfunction in patients with angina limits the therapeutic options. The beneficial effects of beta blockers on survival in patients with LV dysfunction after myocardial infarction, coupled with their beneficial effects on survival and LV performance in patients with heart failure,[111] have established beta blockers as the drug class of choice for the treatment of angina in patients with LV dysfunction, with or without symptoms of heart failure, together with ACE inhibitors, diuretics, and digitalis. If angina persists despite beta blockade and nitrates, amlodipine can be administered. Verapamil, nifedipine, and diltiazem should be avoided.

7. Short-acting nifedipine should not be used because the reflex-mediated tachycardia may aggravate ischemia.

8. Hypertensive patients with angina pectoris do well with either beta blockers or calcium antagonists because both agents have antihypertensive effects. However, beta blockers are the preferred initial agent for treating angina in such patients, as noted earlier, and an ACE inhibitor should be strongly considered for all patients with CAD with hypertension.

COMBINATION THERAPY. The combination of a beta blocker, calcium antagonist, and long-acting nitrate is widely used in the management of chronic stable angina. When adrenergic blockers and calcium antagonists are used together in the treatment of angina pectoris, several issues should be considered:

1. The addition of a beta blocker enhances the clinical effect of nifedipine and other dihydropyridines.

2. In patients with moderate or severe LV dysfunction, sinus bradycardia, or AV conduction disturbances, combination therapy with calcium antagonists and beta blockers should be avoided or should be initiated with caution. In patients with AV conduction system disease, the preferred combination is a long-acting dihydropyridine and a beta blocker. The negative inotropic effects of calcium antagonists are not usually a problem in combined therapy with low doses of beta blockers but can become significant with higher doses. With such doses, amlodipine is the calcium antagonist of choice, but it should be used cautiously.

3. The combination of a dihydropyridine and a long-acting nitrate (without a beta blocker) is not an optimal combination because both are vasodilators.

Approach to Patients with Chronic Stable Angina

This approach is as follows:

1. Identify and treat precipitating factors, such as anemia, uncontrolled hypertension, thyrotoxicosis, tachyarrhythmias, uncontrolled congestive heart failure, and concomitant valvular heart disease.

2. Initiate risk factor modification, physical exercise, diet, and life-style counseling. Initiate therapy with an HMG-CoA reductase inhibitor, as needed, to reduce the LDL cholesterol level to at least below 100 mg/dl.

3. Initiate pharmacotherapy with aspirin and a beta blocker. Initiate an ACE inhibitor in all patients with an LV ejection fraction 40 percent or lower and in those with hypertension, diabetes, or chronic kidney disease. In addition, an ACE inhibitor should be considered for all other patients.

4. Use sublingual nitroglycerin for alleviation of symptoms and for prophylaxis.

5. If angina occurs more than two or three times weekly, the next step is addition of a calcium antagonist or long-acting nitrate via dosing schedules to prevent nitrate tolerance. The decision to add a calcium antagonist or long-acting nitrate is not based entirely on the frequency and severity of symptoms. The need to treat concomitant hypertension or the presence of LV dysfunction and symptoms of heart failure may be an indication for the use of one of these agents, even in patients in whom episodes of symptomatic angina are infrequent.

6. If angina persists despite two antianginal agents (a beta blocker with a long-acting nitrate preparation or a calcium antagonist), add a third antianginal agent.

7. Coronary angiography, with a view to considering coronary revascularization, is indicated in patients with refractory symptoms or ischemia despite optimal medical therapy. It should also be carried out in patients with high-risk noninvasive test results (see Table 54-3) and in those with occupations or life styles that require a more aggressive approach.

Other Therapies

SPINAL CORD STIMULATION. An option for patients with refractory angina who are not candidates for coronary revascularization is spinal cord stimulation using a specially designed electrode inserted into the epidural space.[112] The beneficial effects of neuromodulation on pain via this technique are based on the gate theory, in which stimulation of axons in the spinal cord that do not transmit pain to the brain will reduce input to the brain from axons that do transmit pain. Irrespective of the mechanism, several observational studies have reported success rates of up to 80 percent in terms of reducing the frequency and severity of angina. What is less easily explained is an apparent antiischemic effect of this technique. In a small randomized trial in patients with angina and CAD not amenable to percutaneous coronary intervention (PCI), spinal cord stimulation was associated with similar symptom relief and long-term quality of life compared with CABG.[113] Mortality was lower after 6 months in those treated with spinal stimulation and comparable at 5 years between the two groups. Exercise capacity was better in the CABG group. Randomized placebo-controlled trials are impossible to perform, and this approach should be reserved for patients in whom all other treatment options have been exhausted.

ENHANCED EXTERNAL COUNTERPULSATION. The use of enhanced external counterpulsation (EECP) is another alternative treatment of refractory angina.[114] EECP is generally administered as 35 1-hour treatments over 7 weeks. Observational data have suggested that EECP reduces the frequency of angina and the use of nitroglycerin and improves exercise tolerance and quality of life, and that the responses can last for up to 2 years.[114,115] In a randomized, double-blind, sham-controlled study of EECP for patients with chronic stable angina, active counterpulsation was associated with an increase in time to ST-segment depression during exercise testing and a reduction in angina, as well as an improvement in health-related quality of life that extended to at least 1 year. There are no definitive data that EECP reduces the extent of ischemia determined by myocardial perfusion imaging.

The mechanisms underlying the effects of EECP are poorly understood. Possible mechanisms include the following: (1) durable hemodynamic changes that reduce myocardial O_2 demand; (2) improvement in myocardial perfusion caused by the capacity of increased transmyocardial pressure to open collaterals; and (3) the elaboration of various substances that improve endothelial function and vascular remodeling caused by augmented flow through the arterial vascular bed.[116] Finally, the possibility of placebo effects should be recognized; most of the evidence demonstrating favorable effects of EECP is from uncontrolled studies, and data from sham-controlled studies are few.

CHELATION. Randomized trials have shown no benefit, and these agents may be harmful. They have no place in the management of acute or chronic CAD.

Percutaneous Coronary Intervention (see Chap. 55)

PCI, which includes percutaneous transluminal coronary angioplasty (PTCA), stenting, and related techniques, represents an important therapeutic option in the management of chronic stable angina. The practice of interventional cardiology has changed radically with increased operator experience, improved adjunctive pharmacotherapy, and advances in technology, including drug-eluting stents, distal protection devices, and devices directed at specific technical issues (e.g., thrombectomy and atherectomy catheters).[117] In line with more frequent use of percutaneous intervention for complex and/or multivessel CAD, the number of coronary interventions increased by 326 percent from 1987 to 2003.[1] In 2003, approximately 84 percent of patients undergoing coronary angioplasty received one or more intracoronary stents.[1] Despite these advances, it must be appreciated that a dilatable lesion represents an isolated target, whereas atherosclerosis is frequently a diffuse or multifocal process. Thus, PCI is but one aspect of a comprehensive therapeutic strategy that should vigorously address the risk factors for CAD.

PATIENT SELECTION. Improved technology and increasing operator experience have continued to expand the pool of patients with both single-vessel and multivessel disease who are candidates for PCI. Factors that need to be considered in patient selection include the following:

1. The need for mechanical revascularization (surgical or catheter based) as opposed to intensification of medical therapy, including stringent risk factor modification.
2. The likelihood of successful catheter-based revascularization based on the angiographic characteristics of the lesion. Equally important are factors such as vessel size, extent of calcification, tortuosity, and relationships to side branches (see Chap. 55).
3. The risk and potential consequences of acute failure of PCI, which are a function, in part, of the coronary artery anatomy (multivessel and/or diffuse disease), the percentage of viable myocardium at risk, and underlying LV function.
4. The likelihood of restenosis, which has been associated with clinical (e.g., diabetes, prior restenosis) and angiographic factors (small-vessel diameter, long lesion length, total occlusion, and saphenous vein graft disease).
5. The need for complete revascularization based on the extent of CAD, volume of myocardium in the distribution of the narrowed artery(ies), severity of ischemia, and presence or absence of LV dysfunction.
6. The presence of comorbid conditions and the suitability of the patient for surgery.
7. Patient preference.

Patients with chronic stable angina who are ideal for PCI are those with significant symptoms despite intensive medical therapy, who are at low risk for complications, and in whom the likelihood of technical success is high—no history of congestive heart failure and an ejection fraction greater than 40 percent. Although these characteristics

define the ideal candidate, excellent technical and clinical results can still be obtained in many patients who do not fulfill these ideal criteria; newer technologies have substantially expanded the pool of suitable candidates and, during the last 5 years, most revascularization procedures in the United States and the United Kingdom were PCI as opposed to CABG.[1]

Features associated with an increased risk for PCI failure include advanced age, female gender, unstable angina, congestive heart failure, left main coronary artery–equivalent disease, and multivessel CAD.[118] Diabetes mellitus in patients with multivessel disease has been associated with increased periprocedural ischemic complications and late mortality in comparison with patients without diabetes. Patients with impaired renal function, particularly those with diabetes, are also at increased risk for periprocedural morbidity and, in particular, contrast agent nephropathy.[119]

EARLY OUTCOME. Continued improvement in the technical aspects of PCI (predominantly coronary stenting), as well as increasing operator experience, has had a favorable impact on the rate of primary success and the rate of reductions in complications.[118] Current expectations for PCI are an overall procedural success rate of at least 90 percent with a mortality of less than 1 percent, rate of Q wave myocardial infarction of less than 1.5 percent, and rate of emergency bypass surgery of 1 to 2 percent. Outcomes in specific challenging subgroups of patients, such as those with chronic total occlusions or left main coronary stenosis, are discussed in Chapter 55.

LONG-TERM OUTCOME. Long-term outcome after PCI is well characterized, with LV function, extent of coronary disease, diabetes, renal function, and the patient's age being the major determinants of mortality risk, and restenosis at the site of intervention being a major contributor to recurrent ischemia and the need for subsequent procedures. The introduction of bare metal and drug-eluting coronary stents (see Chap. 55) has dramatically reduced the incidence of restenosis compared with balloon angioplasty.

RESTENOSIS AND LATE STENT THROMBOSIS (see Chap. 55)

Comparisons Between PCI and Medical Therapy

Randomized clinical trials comparing PCI with medical therapy are few in number, have involved fewer than 5000 patients (in total). Most have enrolled patients with predominantly single-vessel disease, and were completed prior to routine use of coronary stenting and enhanced adjunctive pharmacotherapy. In aggregate, the results of these trials have supported superior control of angina, improved exercise capacity, and improved quality of life in patients treated with angioplasty compared with medical therapy (Fig. 54-9).[120] No randomized trial to date has demonstrated a reduction in death or myocardial infarction with PCI compared with medical therapy for patients with chronic stable angina. To the contrary, the second Randomized Intervention Treatment of Angina (RITA-2) investigators observed an excess of death and periprocedural myocardial infarction with angioplasty compared with medical therapy (6.3 versus 3.3 percent; $P = 0.02$); it is worthy of note that 62 percent of the patients enrolled in RITA-2 had multivessel CAD. In patients with stable single- or double-vessel CAD and mild symptoms (asymptomatic or Canadian Cardiovascular Society class I or II angina) and preserved LV function, medical therapy, including aggressive lipid lowering, provided similar results to angioplasty with respect to a composite of cardiovascular death, need for (repeat) revascularization, myocardial infarction, or worsening angina resulting in hospitalization. Results of the Clinical Outcomes Utilization Revascularization and Aggressive DruG Evaluation (COURAGE) trial, in which 2287 patients with myocardial ischemia and significant coronary disease were randomly assigned to undergo PCI with optimal medical therapy or optimal medical therapy alone, showed that PCI did not reduce the risk of death or MI over a median 4.6 years of follow-up (hazard ratio 1.05; 95 percent confidence interval 0.87 to 1.27; $P = 0.62$) (Fig. 54-10).[121] In contrast to previous trials, 94 percent of patients in the PCI group received at least one stent, and background medical therapy in both treatment groups included aggressive risk-factor modification. Notably, the rate of death or MI was similar with PCI or medical therapy alone in the subgroups of patients with multivessel disease and diabetes mellitus.[121] Similar results were observed in elderly patients enrolled in the Trial of Invasive versus Medical therapy in the Elderly (TIME) trial (see Fig. 54-e1 on website).

Based on the best available data from randomized trials, it appears reasonable to pursue a strategy of initial medical therapy for most patients with chronic stable angina and Canadian Cardiovascular Society class I or II symptoms and to reserve revascularization for those with persistent and/or more severe symptoms despite optimal medical

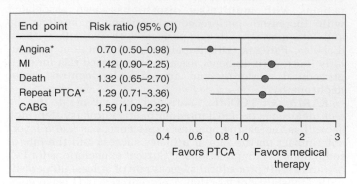

End point	Risk ratio (95% CI)
Angina*	0.70 (0.50–0.98)
MI	1.42 (0.90–2.25)
Death	1.32 (0.65–2.70)
Repeat PTCA*	1.29 (0.71–3.36)
CABG	1.59 (1.09–2.32)

0.4   0.6 0.8 1.0   2   3

Favors PTCA   Favors medical
                           therapy

FIGURE 54–9 Relative risk of recurrent cardiac events with percutaneous transluminal coronary angioplasty (PTCA) versus medical therapy from meta-analysis of six randomized trials (*N* = 1904). Compared with medical therapy, angioplasty reduced the relative risk of recurrent angina by 30 percent. Randomized trials have not included sufficient numbers of patients for informative estimates of the effect of angioplasty on myocardial infarction (MI), death, or subsequent revascularization; however, trends in the available data do not favor angioplasty. These trials do not reflect the widespread use of coronary stenting. *Test for heterogeneity, *P* < 0.0001. CABG = coronary artery bypass grafting; CI = confidence interval. (*From Bucher HC, Hengstler P, Schindler C, et al: Percutaneous transluminal coronary angioplasty versus medical therapy for treatment of non-acute coronary heart disease: A meta-analysis of randomised controlled trials. BMJ 321:73, 2000.*)

CH 54

therapy or those with high-risk criteria on noninvasive testing, such as inducible ischemia involving a moderate or large territory of myocardium.[10]

PCI in Specific Subgroups of Patients with Chronic Stable Angina

DIABETES MELLITUS. Patients with diabetes are at substantially higher risk for complications after PCI (see Chap. 60). Possible explanations for the higher rate of adverse outcomes include an altered vascular biological response in diabetic patients to balloon injury and rapid progression of disease in nondilated segments. The diabetic atherosclerotic milieu is characterized by a procoagulant state, decreased fibrinolytic activity, increased proliferation, and inflammation. Restenosis is more frequent in diabetic patients, as is disease progression. For this reason, CABG, which bypasses most of the vessel instead of a specific lesion, may offer a better intermediate- to long-term outcome.[122] The optimal revascularization strategy (CABG versus PCI) for patients with diabetes and multivessel disease bears further study in the era of drug-eluting stents, which have been shown to reduce restenosis substantially, including in patients with diabetes.[123,124] Moreover, the role of revascularization for patients with diabetes mellitus who are either asymptomatic with a positive stress test or have mild stable myocardial ischemia compared with aggressive pharmacological therapy is currently under investigation in the Bypass Angioplasty Revascularization Investigation 2 Diabetes trial.[125]

LEFT VENTRICULAR DYSFUNCTION. Despite advances in interventional cardiology, LV dysfunction remains independently associated with higher in-hospital and long-term mortality after PCI. Specifically, in patients with stable CAD and estimated ejection fractions of 40 percent or less, 41 to 49, and 50 percent or higher in the National Heart, Lung, and Blood Institute (NHLBI) Dynamic Registry, mortality at 1 year after PCI was 11.0, 4.5, and 1.9 percent, respectively.[126]

WOMEN AND OLDER PATIENTS. Specific issues related to PCI in women and older adults are discussed in Chapters 75 and 76.

PREVIOUS CORONARY BYPASS GRAFTING. CABG and PCI are often considered competitive procedures, but it is more appropriate to view them as complementary. An increasing number of patients who have had CABG and later have recurrent ischemia undergo revascularization with PCI. Technical aspects and procedural outcomes of PCI in venous bypass grafts are discussed in Chapter 55.

Coronary Artery Bypass Surgery

In 1964, Garrett, Dennis, and DeBakey first used CABG as a "bailout" procedure. Widespread use of the technique by Favoloro and Johnson and their respective collaborators followed in the late 1960s. Use of the internal mammary artery (IMA) graft was pioneered by Kolessov in 1967 and by Green and colleagues in 1970.

The annual number of coronary bypass operations in the United States rose steadily between 1979 and 1997, increasing by 227 percent over that period. In 2003, approximately 268,000 patients underwent coronary bypass surgery; a decline of 26 percent since 1997 that may be attributed in part to the growth of the use of PCI.[1] Nevertheless, CABG remains one of the most frequently performed operations in the United States, resulting in the expenditure of almost $50 billion annually. CABG provides excellent short- and intermediate-term results in the management of stable CAD; its long-term results are affected by failure of venous grafts. Long-term data with totally arterial surgical revascularization are few.

Technical Considerations

When a decision has been reached to proceed with CABG, administration of beta blockers, nitrates, and calcium antagonists is continued until surgery. It is crucial to minimize perioperative damage and protect the myocardium. The most commonly used method involves a

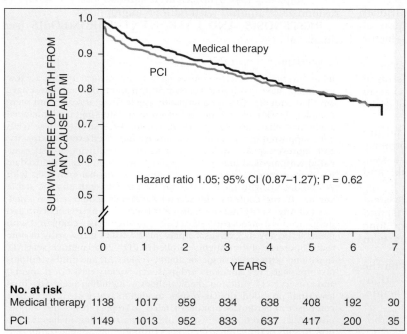

FIGURE 54–10 Outcome in 2287 patients with objective evidence of myocardial ischemia and significant coronary artery disease enrolled in the Clinical Outcomes Utilization Revascularization and Aggressive DruG Evaluation (COURAGE) trial and randomized to percutaneous coronary intervention (PCI) and optimal medical therapy or optimal medical therapy alone (Medical therapy). No difference in the primary endpoint of death from any cause or myocardial infarction was observed between the two treatment groups. (*From Boden WE, O'Rourke RA, Teo KK, et al: Optimal medical therapy with or without PCI for stable coronary disease. N Engl J Med 356:1503, 2007.*)

Hazard ratio 1.05; 95% CI (0.87–1.27); P = 0.62

No. at risk								
Medical therapy	1138	1017	959	834	638	408	192	30
PCI	1149	1013	952	833	637	417	200	35

single period of aortic cross clamping, with intermittent infusion of cold cardioplegia solution. Technical modifications of traditional CABG, using more limited incisions, eliminating cardiopulmonary bypass (CPB), or both, have been aimed at reducing the morbidity associated with this major surgery. It has been estimated that in 2004 at least 20 percent of CABG operations were performed off-pump[127] and that this proportion is increasing. Other technical factors include the selection and method of preparation of bypass conduits, use of sutureless anastomotic devices, and the method of cardioplegia, if used.

Minimally Invasive CABG

Less invasive or minimally invasive approaches may be divided into four major categories based on the approach and use of CPB. Port access CABG is performed using limited incisions with femoral-femoral CPB and cardioplegic arrest. Port access technology has also now enabled totally endoscopic robotically assisted CABG (TECAB) to be performed on the arrested heart.[128] Off-pump CABG is performed using a standard median sternotomy, with generally small skin incisions, and stabilization devices to reduce motion of the target vessels while anastomoses are performed without CPB. Finally, minimally invasive direct coronary artery bypass (MIDCAB) is performed through a left anterior thoracotomy without CPB. Thus, off-pump approaches to CABG include both off-pump CAB (OPCAB) and MIDCAB techniques (Fig. 54-11).

The potential advantages of the minimally invasive approaches include reduced postoperative patient discomfort, minimized risk of wound infection, and shorter recovery times.[129] The avoidance of CPB may mitigate the risk of bleeding, systemic thromboembolism, renal insufficiency, myocardial stunning, stroke, and damaging neurological effects of bypass, particularly in the elderly and in patients with heavily calcified aortas.[130] Amelioration of the systemic inflammatory response that occurs after CABG using CPB is viewed as an additional advantage that may affect these clinical outcomes. The learning curve of minimally invasive CABG has led to reports of early graft failure. It should be emphasized that with conventional surgical techniques, the early patency rates of an IMA graft are excellent (98.7 percent in one large series). Short-term clinical and angiographic outcomes have suggested that the less invasive techniques can be used to achieve results comparable to those of traditional CABG. As the development of newer positioning and stabilizing devices has enabled bypassing of all coronary territories during OPCAB, the ultimate success of these nontraditional approaches to CABG will depend on long-term graft patency.[127,129]

In addition, novel approaches to coronary revascularization may also include CABG with PCI by combining a minimally invasive coronary bypass surgical procedure on the left anterior descending coronary artery with PCI on the remaining vessels. Further experience is needed to clarify appropriate selection criteria and to determine whether this strategy offers important advantages over multivessel bypass surgery alone.[131]

PORT ACCESS CABG. An innovative approach to coronary revascularization is the port access method, which uses small thoracotomy ports for cardiac manipulation; CPB is established by groin cannulation and an intraaortic balloon clamp for occlusion of the aorta. The two largest single-center series and the first report of the Port Access International Registry, which documented the results of 555 bypass procedures, were encouraging. Data comparing port access with traditional CABG are few but have indicated similar short-term outcomes.[132] Limitations to the use of this technique include atherosclerotic involvement of the aortic arch, high cost, long operating times caused by technically very demanding surgery, and the risk of aortic dissection.[132] As a result, the port access approach is currently not widely used. However, port access technology has enabled TECAB to be performed and may increase in use if this new approach becomes more widely adopted.[128]

MINIMALLY INVASIVE DIRECT CABG. MIDCAB is performed through a limited left thoracotomy on the beating heart (off-pump), most commonly with grafting of the left internal thoracic artery to the left anterior descending artery. Studies of early angiographic patency have shown rates (98 percent) comparable to those of traditional CABG.[133] Accumulation of operator experience appears to reduce perioperative adverse events. In a randomized trial comparing MIDCAB with stenting for treatment of isolated left anterior descending (LAD) artery disease, the rate of death or myocardial infarction was similar between the two groups (3 percent with stenting versus 6 percent with MIDCAB; $P = 0.5$; $N = 220$). The need for repeated revascularization during the following 6 months was significantly higher in patients treated with coronary stenting (29 versus 8 percent; $P = 0.003$).[134] In this trial, early reoperation for graft failure was necessary in 3 percent of patients and conversion to a full sternotomy was necessary in 5 percent. All grafts were patent at 6 months.[134] Five-year follow-up showed a trend toward lower rates of death or MI in patients who were initially stented and a significant reduction in the need for revascularization and fewer symptoms in those who were allocated to MIDCAB.[135]

Limitations include the requirement that the patient can tolerate single-lung ventilation and that the operation be generally limited to revascularization of the LAD territory because of lesser accessibility of the left circumflex and right coronary arteries. The latter limitation may be successfully addressed by combined MIDCAB of the LAD artery with revascularization of other diseased arteries by PCI.[131] This approach has been evaluated predominantly in small observational studies; the benefit of so-called integrated coronary revascularization compared with established strategies remains to be studied adequately.

OFF-PUMP CABG. An alternative approach to revascularization on the beating heart is OPCAB, entailing a conventional median sternotomy and mechanical suction stabilizing systems. This combination enhances surgical exposure compared with MIDCAB and is particularly useful if multivessel bypass grafting is contemplated. Most surgeons consider only hemodynamic instability or poor quality target vessels as contraindications.[129] Although poor patency rates in some series have highlighted the value of intraoperative confirmation of graft patency, it is possible to achieve excellent results with angiographic patency rates as high as 99 percent at hospital discharge at 1 month and as high as 95 percent at 6 months.[127,136]

Meta-analyses of observational and randomized trials of OPCAB versus CPB[136,137] have demonstrated that although at least similar out-

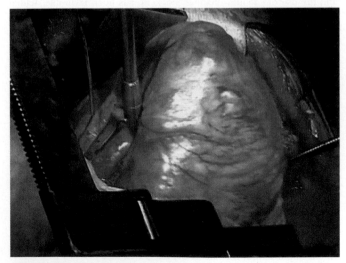

FIGURE 54–11 Off-pump coronary artery bypass grafting performed using a standard median sternotomy and a stabilization device to reduce motion of the target vessel while the anastomosis is performed without cardiopulmonary bypass. *(Courtesy of Dr. Tomislav Mihaljevic while at Brigham & Women's Hospital, Boston.)*

comes can be achieved, to date there is no clear advantage of OPCAB over CPB with respect to mortality or major morbidity. Nevertheless, postoperative complications appear to be reduced with OPCAB, along with nonsignificant trends toward lower rates of death, MI, or stroke.[130] Generally consistent findings across randomized and observational data sets have included comparable completeness of revascularization, reductions in blood loss and/or transfusion requirements, fewer wound infections, less postoperative atrial fibrillation, lower indices of myocardial injury, shorter duration of mechanical ventilation, and earlier hospital discharge with OPCAB.[137,138] Although trends toward neurocognitive benefits are evident, important reductions in stroke or long-term cognitive impairment with OPCAB versus traditional CABG have not yet been consistently demonstrated.[139] Intraoperative conversion from OPCAB to CPB appears to be on the order of 8%.[140]

CARDIOPLEGIA. Favorable outcomes with respect to postoperative ventricular function are in large part dependent on optimal intraoperative myocardial protection.[141] Early cardioplegic techniques relied on cold crystalloid to initiate and maintain intraoperative cardiac arrest. However, blood cardioplegia facilitates myocardial aerobic metabolism, preserves myocardial high-energy phosphate stores, and reduces lactate production compared with crystalloid cardioplegia.[142] Enhancement of cardioplegia has included using metabolic substrates, use of warm (37°C) or tepid (29°C) induction of cardioplegic arrest and alternative delivery such as retrograde and/or antegrade, and continuous versus intermittent cardioplegia. Novel approaches with separate administration of additives such as sodium-hydrogen exchange inhibitors, L-arginine, insulin, or adenosine as additional myocardial protectants are under study. Acadesine, an agent that increases adenosine concentration, has been reported to reduce mortality associated with postperfusion myocardial infarction.[143] Future advances may stem from ongoing investigation of the mediators of myocardial injury during cardioplegia and the impact of cardioplegic alternatives.

In patients with satisfactory preoperative cardiac function, a wide range of techniques have produced excellent results. In contrast, in patients with depressed LV function (both acutely and chronically), it is easier to demonstrate a benefit with more specialized protocols, including the use of sanguineous cardioplegic techniques, with or without substrate enhancement, and blood cardioplegia.[141]

VENOUS CONDUITS. The saphenous vein is used mainly for distal branches of the right and circumflex coronary arteries and for sequential grafts to these vessels and diagonal branches (see Figs. 54-e2 and 54-e3 on website). In emergency situations, many surgeons prefer the saphenous vein to the IMA, because the saphenous vein can be harvested and grafted more rapidly. When the greater saphenous vein is not available, the lesser saphenous vein and upper extremity veins, usually the cephalic or basilic, may be used. However, arm vein grafts are not as effective as IMA or saphenous vein grafts. Endoscopic harvesting of the saphenous vein provides improved cosmetic results and may reduce morbidity compared with open harvesting. Few data are available; however, these have indicated similar macroscopic quality of minimally invasively harvested veins.[144] Cryopreserved homologous saphenous vein grafts and glutaraldehyde-treated umbilical veins have been used, but the patency rates are not optimal, and these veins should therefore be used only when there are no other alternatives.

Recently developed aortic-saphenous vein graft connectors have enabled surgeons to create the proximal anastomosis without the use of side-biting aortic clamps that may contribute to aortic injury and perioperative stroke. Early experience with sutureless connectors has suggested high rates of stenosis during the first 6 months after placement; thus, although these devices have potential for substantial expansion of use in conjunction with minimally invasive CABG, additional experience and long-term data are needed to clarify their role.[145]

INTERNAL MAMMARY ARTERY BYPASS GRAFTS. The IMA, also known as the internal thoracic artery, is usually remarkably free of atheroma, especially in patients younger than 65 years. When it is grafted to a coronary artery (see Fig. 54-e4 on website), it appears to be virtually immune to the development of intimal hyperplasia, which is almost universally seen in aortocoronary vein grafts, and the functional (endothelium-dependent vasodilatory) capacity of the artery remains intact. The diameter of the IMA graft is usually a closer match to that of the recipient coronary artery than the diameter of a saphenous vein.

The current standard for bypass grafting advocates routine use of the left IMA for grafting the LAD coronary artery, with supplemental saphenous vein grafts to other vessels. Although the benefits of a single IMA graft over a saphenous vein graft alone are not in dispute,[146] the superiority of bilateral IMA grafts over a single IMA graft and one saphenous vein graft is less well accepted.[147] Initial enthusiasm for the use of bilateral IMA grafts was tempered by a higher rate of postoperative complications, including bleeding, wound infection, and prolonged ventilatory support.[148] Wound infection, which has been of particular concern, remains modest in frequency (less than 3 percent), except in patients who are obese or diabetic or those who require prolonged ventilatory support. Subsequent series have shown that bilateral versus single IMA grafting is associated with lower rates of recurrent angina pectoris, reoperation, and myocardial infarction and improved survival in nonrandomized studies and, in some series, the risk of wound infection does not differ substantially from that with single IMA grafts. The increased technical demands and longer operative times of bilateral IMA grafting have also been a barrier to more widespread adoption but may be overcome if evidence supporting a survival advantage continues to accumulate.[149]

Complications. Inadequate flow rates with evidence of myocardial ischemia in the perioperative period are rare after IMA grafts to the LAD coronary artery or its diagonal branches. Perioperative spasm is the presumed cause and can be managed by the administration of sodium nitroprusside or a combination of glyceryl trinitrate and verapamil.

OTHER CONDUITS. The success of IMA grafts has stimulated interest in the use of other arterial conduits, particularly in patients who are younger, diabetic, or hyperlipidemic or in whom the saphenous veins are unsuitable or unavailable. Options for arterial grafts include the radial, right gastroepiploic, inferior epigastric and, very rarely, the subscapular, intercostal, splenic, left gastric, and gastroduodenal arteries. Initial enthusiasm for use of the radial artery was blunted by reports of high reocclusion rates. More recent experience, in which attention has been paid to avoiding spasm by minimizing manipulation and the use of calcium channel blockers, has been favorable. Radial arterial grafts may be associated with fewer perioperative complications and thus are preferable to the right IMA as a second arterial graft.[150] Total arterial revascularization using both IMAs and free radial or alternative arterial grafts has also gained interest. A randomized trial comparing grafting using the left IMA plus additional venous grafts with total arterial revascularization detected no differences in the number of vessels grafted, time on CPB, or postoperative complications but at a mean follow-up of 12 months, patients managed with total arterial revascularization were less likely to have recurrent angina or to require additional revascularization.[151]

The right gastroepiploic artery can be harvested by extending the median sternotomy incision toward the umbilicus. It is frequently placed as a graft to the right coronary artery, but both the circumflex and LAD coronary arteries can be grafted with this conduit. Results have demonstrated excellent patency rates, but there is a paucity of data on long-term results. Bovine IMA, Dacron, and polytetrafluoroethylene (PTFE) grafts have also been used with lower patency (approximately 50 to 60 percent) over the mid term. These grafts should only be used as a last resort.

DISTAL VASCULATURE. The state of the distal coronary vasculature is important for the fate of bypass grafts. Late patency of grafts is related to coronary arterial runoff as determined by the diameter of the coronary artery into which the graft is inserted, size of the distal vascular bed, and severity of coronary atherosclerosis distal to the site of insertion of the graft. The highest graft patency rates are found when the lumina of the vessels distal to the graft insertion are larger than 1.5 mm in diameter, perfuse a large vascular bed, and are free of atheroma obstructing more than 25 percent of the vessel lumen. For saphenous veins, optimal patency rates are achieved with a lumen of 2.0 mm or larger.

Surgical Outcomes

The patient population undergoing CABG has been changing over time, particularly with the wider use of PCI. In comparison with the 1970s, patients undergoing CABG today are older, include a higher percentage of women, and are sicker, in that a greater proportion have unstable angina, triple-vessel disease, previous coronary revascularization with either CABG or PCI, LV dysfunction, and comorbid conditions, including hypertension, diabetes, and peripheral vascular disease. Despite the increasing risk profile of this population, outcomes with CABG have generally remained stable or have improved.[152]

OPERATIVE MORTALITY. Risk factors for death following coronary artery surgery may be separated into five categories: (1) preoperative factors related to CAD, including recent acute myocardial infarction, hemodynamic instability, LV dysfunction, extensive CAD, the presence of left main CAD, and severe or unstable angina; (2) preoperative factors related to the aggressiveness of the arteriosclerotic process, as reflected in associated carotid or peripheral vascular disease; (3) preoperative biological factors (older age at surgery, diabetes mellitus, comorbidities, including pulmonary and renal disease, and perhaps female gender); (4) intraoperative factors (intraoperative ischemic damage and failure to use IMA grafts); and (5) environmental or institutional factors, including the specific surgeon and treatment protocols used.[153] Of these factors, several variables have consistently emerged as the most potent predictors of mortality after CABG: (1) age; (2) urgency of operation; (3) prior cardiac surgery; (4) LV function; (5) percent stenosis of the left main coronary artery; and (6) number of epicardial vessels with significant disease.

In-hospital mortality after isolated CABG was characterized by a steady decline from 1967 to the 1980s. Despite a shift toward higher risk demographics, early mortality continued to decline in the 1990s.[154] Specifically, during the period from 1990 to 1999, unadjusted mortality through 30 days after CABG in the United States fell by 0.9 percent (23.1 percent relative decrease; $P < 0.0001$). Mortality among the 503,478 CABG-only operations recorded in the Society of Thoracic Surgeons (STS) data base between 1997 and 1999 was 3.05 percent.[152] In 2005, the cumulative mortality for CABG-only operations in the STS data base was approximately 2.2 percent.[155] Moreover, with increasingly wide scrutiny of procedural results, it has become recognized that absolute rates of morbidity and mortality might not provide a fair basis for comparing institutions and individuals, unless patients' characteristics are considered. Several models have been developed and refined with the objective of predicting perioperative mortality.[156] Application of such models have demonstrated even greater declines in CABG mortality over the past decade when adjusted for changes in risk profile.[154]

Perioperative Complications

Perioperative morbidity (see Chap. 79) has increased because of a larger fraction of higher risk patients. Major morbidity (e.g., death, stroke, renal failure, reoperation, prolonged ventilation, sternal infection) occurred in 13.4 percent through 30 days among the 503,478 CABG-only operations recorded in the Society of Thoracic Surgeons data base between 1997 and 1999.[152]

MYOCARDIAL INFARCTION. Perioperative MI, particularly if associated with hemodynamic or arrhythmic complications or preexisting LV dysfunction, has a major adverse effect on early and late

prognosis. The reported incidence varies widely (0 to more than 10 percent), in large part because of heterogeneous diagnostic criteria, with an average of 3.9 percent (median, 2.9 percent).[157] Elevation of the myocardial creatine kinase-MB (CK-MB) isoenzyme level more than five times the upper limit of normal is commonly considered diagnostic of myocardial infarction in this setting. Data from a prospectively performed study of routine monitoring of CK-MB postoperatively has shown CK-MB to be independently associated with mortality.[158] Predictors of perioperative myocardial infarction in the Coronary Artery Surgery Study (CASS) were female gender, severe perioperative angina pectoris, severe stenosis of the left main coronary artery, and triple-vessel disease. It is possible that mortality associated with perioperative myocardial infarction may be reduced with acadesine, an experimental agent that increases the concentration of adenosine in ischemic tissue.[143]

RESPIRATORY COMPLICATIONS. Most patients are extubated within 6 to 8 hours after undergoing CABG. Prolonged mechanical ventilation (longer than 24 hours) is necessary in 5 to 6 percent of first-time CABGs and 10 to 11 percent of reoperations.[159] The cause is multifactorial and includes the presence of preexisting pulmonary disease and numerous perioperative factors related directly to anesthesia, level of consciousness, CPB, incisional pain, chest tube placement, and occasionally phrenic nerve damage. Severe chronic obstructive pulmonary disease, as defined by a forced expiratory volume in 1 second (FEV$_1$) of less than 50 percent or an FEV$_1$/forced vital capacity (FVC) ratio less than 0.70, is associated with a high incidence of postoperative pulmonary complications (29 percent) and a near doubling of long-term mortality, even in the absence of other major medical comorbid conditions.[160] The LV ejection fraction is also an important determinant of prolonged ventilation.

BLEEDING. Impaired hemostasis and bleeding complications are an inherent risk of CABG. Reoperation for bleeding is required in 2 to 6 percent of patients and is associated with a nearly threefold higher in-hospital mortality. CPB causes derangement of the intrinsic coagulation and fibrinolytic systems in addition to impairing platelet function. The risk of bleeding is increased with age, a smaller body surface area, duration of CPB, reoperation, bilateral internal thoracic artery grafts, and preoperative use of heparin, aspirin, and fibrinolytic agents.[161] Bleeding may be reduced with aprotinin and lysine analogues, such as aminocaproic acid and tranexamic acid. Use of clopidogrel within 5 days of CABG is associated with a significantly increased risk of bleeding and the need for transfusion.[162] Present guidelines advocate discontinuation of clopidogrel at least 5 days prior to CABG, whenever possible.

WOUND INFECTIONS. Major perioperative wound complications, especially mediastinitis and/or wound dehiscence, occur in 1 to 4 percent of patients and are associated with significant morbidity as well as higher mortality.[163] This risk is substantially increased in those undergoing reoperation and by the use of double IMA grafts, particularly in diabetic patients, and is markedly increased in obese patients. Preventive measures include careful skin preparation, increased attention to sterility in the perioperative environment, and preoperative use of antimicrobial agents. Other factors that may decrease perioperative infection include strict control of glucose in patients with diabetes and the avoidance of unnecessary blood transfusion in view of the immunosuppressive effect of the latter. Successful management of deep sternal wound infection involves prompt recognition and aggressive débridement with muscle flap closure.

POSTOPERATIVE HYPERTENSION. Hypertension can occur in up to one third of patients postoperatively. The mechanisms are unclear but may be related to increased levels of circulating catecholamines and other humoral factors in addition to vasoconstriction secondary to activation of the renin-angiotensin system. Control of postoperative hypertension is important to prevent myocardial ischemia, cardiac failure, and perioperative bleeding.

CEREBROVASCULAR COMPLICATIONS. Neurological abnormalities following cardiac surgery are dreaded complications and are associated with higher long-term mortality.[164] Postulated mechanisms include emboli from atherosclerosis of the aorta or other large arteries, emboli possibly from the CPB machine circuit and its tubing, and intraoperative hypotension, particularly in patients with preexisting hypertension.[165] Type I injury is associated with major neurological deficits, stupor, and coma, and type II injury is characterized by a deterioration in intellectual function and memory. The incidence of neurological abnormalities is variably estimated, depending on how the deficits are defined. The incidence of stroke reported in the Northern New England Cardiovascular Disease Study Group data base between 1992 to 2001 was 1.6 percent and has been documented as higher in prospective studies (1.5 to 5 percent).[164] Studies aimed at careful evaluation of neurological deficits report more frequent neurological sequelae; type I deficits have been documented in 6 percent of patients early after CABG, with short-term cognitive decline in 33 to 83 percent. A prospective long-term study using sophisticated neurocognitive testing revealed cognitive decline in 53 percent of patients at the time of hospital discharge, 36 percent at 6 weeks, and 24 percent at 6 months.[130] In regard to the neurological sequelae of CPB (including stroke, delirium, and neurocognitive dysfunction), older age, in addition to other comorbid conditions (particularly diabetes), associated with atherosclerosis, and intraoperative manipulation of the aorta are the more powerful predictors. In most, but not all, studies, atherosclerosis of the proximal aorta has also been a strong predictor of stroke, as has the use of an intraaortic balloon pump.[166] Mild hypothermia in the intra- and perioperative periods may improve neurocognitive function after CABG.[167]

ATRIAL FIBRILLATION. This arrhythmia is one of the most frequent complications of CABG. It occurs in up to 40 percent of patients, primarily within 2 to 3 days. In the early postoperative period, rapid ventricular rates and loss of atrial transport may compromise systemic hemodynamics, increase the risk of embolization, and lead to a significant increase in the duration and cost of the hospital stay, and it is associated with a twofold to threefold increase in postoperative stroke. Older age, hypertension, prior atrial fibrillation, and congestive heart failure are associated with higher risk of developing atrial fibrillation after cardiac surgery.[168] Prior statin therapy may be associated with less frequent postoperative atrial fibrillation.[169]

Prophylactic use of beta blockers reduces the frequency of postoperative atrial fibrillation; these should be administered routinely before and after CABG to patients without contraindications. Amiodarone is also effective in prophylaxis against postoperative atrial fibrillation and may be considered in patients at high risk for developing this dysrhythmia (see Chap. 79). Off-pump techniques may be associated with less frequent postoperative atrial fibrillation.[130,140] Up to 80 percent of patients spontaneously revert to sinus rhythm within 24 hours without treatment other than digoxin or other agents used for controlling the ventricular rate. In a randomized trial of patients with postoperative atrial fibrillation that had resolved prior to discharge, there was no detectable benefit of extended antiarrhythmic therapy beyond a short course of 1 week.[170] Most patients return to sinus rhythm by 6 weeks after surgery.

BRADYARRHYTHMIAS AND CONDUCTION DISTURBANCES. The incidence of postoperative bradyarrhythmias requiring permanent pacemaker implantation was 0.8 percent in a series of 1614 consecutive patients discharged from the hospital after coronary bypass surgery. Predictive factors were preoperative left bundle branch block, concomitant LV aneurysmectomy, and older age. Most patients continued to require permanent pacemaker support during follow-up.

RENAL DYSFUNCTION. The incidence of renal failure requiring dialysis after CABG remains low (0.5 to 1.0 percent) but is associated with significantly greater morbidity and mortality. A decline in renal function defined by a postoperative serum creatinine level higher than 2.0 mg/dl or an increase of more than 0.7 mg/dl is more frequent (7 to 8 percent). Predictors of postoperative renal dysfunction include advanced age, diabetes, preexisting renal dysfunction, and heart failure.[171] Patients with preoperative renal dysfunction and a serum creatinine level higher than 2.5 mg/dl appear to be at increased risk of the need for hemodialysis and may be candidates for alternative approaches to revascularization or prophylactic dialysis. A randomized trial of *N*-acetylcysteine for the prevention of development of renal dysfunction in 295 patients undergoing CABG showed no difference compared with placebo.[172]

RETURN TO EMPLOYMENT. Return to full employment has been variable (35 to 80 percent) but is as high as 80 percent in those who were employed prior to undergoing CABG. Patients who undergo CABG take approximately 6 weeks longer to return to work than those who are treated with PCI; however, long-term employment is similar (more than 80 percent) in patients treated with CABG or PCI. Factors that adversely affect the prospects of patients for returning to work include advanced age, postoperative angina, job satisfaction prior to surgery, and a period of unemployment or disability before surgery.

PATENCY OF VENOUS GRAFTS. Experimental studies and observations in patients have suggested that the development of disease in venous aortocoronary artery bypass grafts occurs in several phases. The occlusion rate, which is high in the first year, decreases substantially between the first and sixth years. Between 6 and 10 years after surgery, the attrition rate for grafts increases again. Early occlusion (before hospital discharge) occurs in 8 to 12 percent of venous grafts and, by 1 year, 15 to 30 percent of vein grafts have become occluded. After the first year, the annual occlusion rate is 2 percent and rises to approximately 4 percent annually between years 6 and 10. At 10 years, approximately 50 percent of vein grafts have become occluded, and significant atherosclerosis is present in the substantial proportion of grafts remaining patent, with significant stenoses in 20 to 40 percent.[173] Patency rates with IMA grafts are superior. Predictors of graft occlusion include small target vessel diameter and patient risk factors, such as high LDL and low HDL cholesterol levels, prior myocardial infarction, male gender, and active smoking. Failure of venous bypass grafts is associated with a greater than twofold higher risk of death, myocardial infarction or need for additional revascularization procedures.[173]

Early Phase (First Month). Technical factors that may cause thrombotic closure at the proximal or distal anastomoses include kinking because of excessive length, tension from insufficient length, poor graft flow, and inadequate distal runoff. Surgical manipulation of the saphenous vein during harvesting and preparation prior to grafting play key roles in initiating the sequence of endothelial damage, with subsequent platelet and fibrin deposition leading to thrombosis.

Intermediate Phase (1 Month to 1 Year). Vein grafts that have been implanted in the arterial circulation for 1 month to 1 year are subject to substantial endothelial denudation and proliferation and to migration of medial cells to the intima. Migration of vascular smooth muscle cells through the internal elastic lamina into the intima may also occur.[174] This initial phase of rapid proliferation is followed after several months by a marked increase in the connective tissue matrix, which further increases intimal and medial thickness. This accelerated process of intimal hyperplasia and thickening is an early stage of atherosclerotic plaque formation and is believed to occur because of interaction between platelets and macrophages and endothelial damage. If the proliferation is severe and localized, as may occur at the site of anastomosis between the grafts and the recipient artery, total occlusion can occur within 1 year.

Late Phase (Beyond 1 Year). Some investigators believe that the development of atherosclerosis in vein grafts, as in native arteries, represents a continuum, starting from platelet deposition and advancing to smooth muscle cell proliferation and finally to lipid incorporation into the plaque. By 10 years, nearly half of venous grafts patent at 5 years have become occluded. Beyond the first year, particularly after 3 to 5 years, the histological appearance of occluded or obstructed coronary bypass grafts is consistent with atherosclerosis. Late graft atherosclerosis is often characterized by an extensive thrombotic burden and marked friability of the lesions; the resultant intermittent distal embolization in turn complicates repeat revascularization procedures, either by PCI or reoperation.

Determination of Graft Patency. Although angiography is the most frequently used method for the determination of vein graft patency, the diffuseness of the atherosclerotic process, which in many patients decreases the luminal diameter of the entire vessel, may lead to an underestimation of the severity of a more focal lesion. Alternative approaches to the evaluation of vein graft patency that are being investigated include contrast-enhanced CT (see Chap.

CH 54

18),[175] phase contrast magnetic resonance angiography (see Chap. 17),[176] fluorescent imaging techniques, and transcutaneous ultrasonographic and magnetic resonance measurements of angiographic flow.

ARTERIAL GRAFT PATENCY. Comparative morphological and angiographic studies of IMA and saphenous vein bypass grafts that have been implanted long-term have shown that accelerated atherosclerosis occurs commonly in saphenous vein grafts but is extremely rare in IMA grafts. Several possible explanations may be offered for the superiority of the IMA graft. The media of the artery may derive nourishment from the lumen as well as from the vasa vasorum, and the internal elastic lamina of the IMA is uniform. Moreover, the finding that the endothelium of the IMA produces significantly more prostacyclin than that of the saphenous vein may explain the more pronounced endothelium-dependent relaxation and may allow flow-dependent autoregulation to occur. Fibrointimal proliferation occasionally develops in IMA grafts, and the resultant narrowing may be a factor in late graft closure.

Clinical and angiographic outcomes are superior when IMA grafts are used compared with venous grafts. In one series, IMA grafts had patency rates of 95, 88, and 83 percent at 1, 5, and 10 years, respectively. Although comparable at 1 year, these rates are significantly higher than those observed for venous grafts at 5 and 10 years. For example, in the VA cooperative studies trial, the patency of venous and IMA grafts at 10 years was 61 versus 85 percent respectively.[177] Excellent long-term results have also been achieved with use of the right IMA as a free or sequential graft. Consistent with these angiographic findings, patients receiving an IMA graft have a decreased risk of short-term and long-term major cardiac events, including death, myocardial infarction, and reoperations, and this clinical advantage persists for up to 20 years. Radial artery grafts are similarly associated with superior patency to venous grafts at 1 year (91.8 versus 86.4 percent).[178]

PROGRESSION OF DISEASE IN NONGRAFTED ARTERIES. Disease progression, defined as worsening of a preexisting lesion or the appearance of a new diameter narrowing of 50 percent or greater, can occur at a rate of 20 to 40 percent over 5 to 10 years in nongrafted native vessels. The rate of disease progression appears highest in arterial segments already showing evidence of disease, and it is between three and six times higher in grafted native coronary arteries than in nongrafted native vessels. These data have suggested that bypassing an artery with minimal disease, even if initially successful, may ultimately be harmful to patients, who incur both the risk of graft closure and the increased risk of accelerated obstruction of native vessels. Lesions in the native vessel that are long (more than 10 mm) and more than 70 percent in diameter are at increased risk of progressing to total occlusion.[179]

EFFECTS OF THERAPY ON VEIN GRAFT OCCLUSION AND NATIVE VESSEL PROGRESSION. Measures aimed at enhancing long-term patency are generally directed at delaying the overall process of atherosclerosis, and thus they may have several additional benefits. Secondary preventive therapy, in particular lipid-lowering treatment, is important to reducing the risk of failure of venous grafts. Chronic anticoagulant therapy has *not* been shown convincingly to alter outcomes. Other novel approaches, such as pretreatment of venous grafts to increase resistance to atherothrombosis, have not been definitively evaluated.

Antiplatelet Therapy. Several trials have demonstrated the efficacy of aspirin therapy when started 1, 7, or 24 hours preoperatively, but the benefit is lost when aspirin is started more than 48 hours postoperatively. Aspirin, 80 to 325 mg daily, should be continued indefinitely. The addition of dipyridamole or warfarin in conventional doses has not been shown definitively to provide added benefit.[180] Although the effects of clopidogrel on graft patency have not been studied specifically, it is likely to be at least as effective as aspirin and is recommended in those who have an allergy to aspirin or who have had a recent acute coronary syndrome.[181]

Lipid-lowering Therapy. Three randomized trials of lipid-lowering therapy have shown a favorable impact on the development of graft

disease.[180] The rationale for lowering lipid levels in patients with CAD was extended to postoperative patients with at least one patent vein graft and LDL cholesterol concentrations between 130 and 175 mg/dl in the Post-Coronary Artery Bypass Graft Trial. Patients who received aggressive treatment with lovastatin and, if needed, cholestyramine to decrease LDL cholesterol to less than 100 mg/dl, in comparison with moderate therapy resulting in an LDL cholesterol level of 134 mg/dl, had a lower rate of progressive atherosclerosis in grafts (27 versus 39 percent; $P < 0.001$) and a lower rate of repeat revascularization procedures over a 4-year period. Similar benefits are achieved with other lipid-lowering therapies, including colestipol, niacin, and gemfibrozil.

Smoking Cessation. Strong evidence from the Coronary Artery Surgery Study (CASS) randomized trial and other series has indicated that continued smoking after bypass surgery increases mortality, recurrence rate of angina, need for repeat hospitalization, and repeat revascularization procedures. Not unexpectedly, continued smoking has been associated with angiographic progression of graft disease.

OTHER TREATMENTS. A randomized, blinded, placebo-controlled trial of edifoligide, a decoy of the E2F transcription factor family that participates in the regulation of smooth muscle cell proliferation for the prevention of vein graft failure, has shown no benefit compared with placebo.[182] With the potential for improvement in transfection techniques and greater knowledge regarding the participants in cellular signaling, interest in gene therapy of venous bypass grafts remains active.

Patient Selection

Indications for CABG consist of the need for improvement in the quality and/or duration of life.[183] Patients whose angina is not adequately controlled by medical management or who have unacceptable side effects with such management should be considered for coronary revascularization. The decision to perform PCI or CABG is based partly on coronary anatomy, LV function, other medical comorbidities that may affect the patient's risk for either procedure, and patient preference.[122] Technological developments have enlarged the pool of patients with single-vessel or multivessel disease amenable to PCI.[184] However, most patients with triple-vessel or double-vessel disease with LAD involvement undergo CABG.[122] For patients who are suitable for PCI and who do not fulfill the criteria of anatomy requiring surgery (e.g., left main CAD or severe triple-vessel disease and LV dysfunction), PCI is generally the procedure of choice. However, if medical therapy has failed (i.e., the symptoms are severe or sufficient to impair quality of life), and the patient is not a good candidate for initial or repeat PCI, CABG should be strongly considered. This procedure is also indicated for patients with CAD, regardless of symptoms, in whom survival is likely to be prolonged, and for patients in whom noninvasive testing suggests high risk (Table 54-11).

In making the decision about revascularization, it is important to assess the patient's prognosis and how it may be affected by surgery. The key initial step is to stratify patients into categories of risk with continued medical therapy based on an analysis of clinical, noninvasive and, in some patients, angiographic variables. This process defines the indications for revascularization over medical therapy and, by implication, the indications for coronary angiography in patients with chronic stable angina, as well as which modality of revascularization (PCI or surgery) is preferable.[10]

The four major determinants of risk in CAD are the extent of ischemia, the number of vessels diseased, LV function, and the electrical substrate. The major effect of coronary revascularization is on ischemia, and the magnitude of the benefit compared with that of medical therapy is enhanced with LV dysfunction, particularly in the presence of reversibly ischemic jeopardized myocardium. In this context, patients can be risk-stratified according to the expected benefit of revascularization versus medical therapy. Patients

TABLE 54–11	Impact of Coronary Bypass Surgery on Survival*			
Category of Risk	Number of Vessels Diseased	Severity of Ischemia	Ejection Fraction	Results of Surgery on Survival
Mild	2 3	Mild	>0.50	Unchanged[†] Unchanged[†]
Moderate	2 3	Moderate to severe	>0.50	Unchanged[†] Improved[†]
	2 3	Mild	<0.50	Unchanged[†] Improved[‡]
Severe	2 3	Moderate to severe	<0.50	Improved[‡] Improved[‡]

*In subsets of patients studied in the Coronary Artery Surgery Study (CASS) randomized trial and registry studies.

[†]Randomized trial.

[‡]Survival improved with surgery versus medicine. In the European Coronary Surgery Trial, patients with double-vessel disease and involvement of the proximal left anterior descending coronary artery had improved survival with surgery irrespective of left ventricular function.

with more extensive and severe CAD have an increasing magnitude of benefit from CABG over medical therapy (Figs. 54-12 and 54-13; Table 54-12). Selection of patients for surgery is based on clinical, angiographic, and noninvasive testing characteristics that may be considered markers or, in some cases, surrogates of the three major predictors—ischemia, LV function, and, to a lesser extent, arrhythmia. Other factors that must always be considered in the decision are general health and noncoronary comorbid conditions.

The appropriate use of invasive cardiovascular procedures is undergoing increasing scrutiny. It is therefore reassuring to note that in studies of coronary angiography and bypass surgery, less than 4 percent of bypass procedures are considered inappropriate, using criteria from an international panel.[183]

Results

In 1972, a committee of the AHA indicated that the most widely accepted indication for surgical revascularization was "significant disability from moderate to severe angina pectoris, unresponsive to optimal medical care." More than three decades later, with the development of PCI and improvements both in medical therapy of CAD and in CABG, the realization that CABG prolongs survival in subgroups of patients with minimal or mild to moderate symptoms has shifted the emphasis toward ischemia instead of symptoms alone as the target for coronary revascularization. Severe ischemia and/or reversible LV dysfunction provides a window of opportunity for improving survival (in comparison to medical therapy) that has resulted in an increase in the frequency of CABG in patients with unstable angina and in survivors of acute myocardial infarction. LV dysfunction, initially a relative contraindication for surgery, has become a major indication. Nonetheless, severe symptoms or even moderate symptoms that interfere with the quality of life, despite adequate medical therapy, remain as firm an indication for coronary revascularization (PCI or CABG) as they were for CABG three decades ago.

RELIEF OF ANGINA. CABG is highly effective in providing complete relief from angina in some patients and improvement in the severity of symptoms in most of the remainder.[183] For example, in a series of patients who received saphenous vein grafts alone, approximately 90 percent were free of angina at 1 year. In the following 4 years, the recurrence rate was approximately 3 percent/year and 5 percent/year thereafter. Approximate rates of freedom from angina were 78 percent at 5 years, which decreased to 52 and 23 percent at

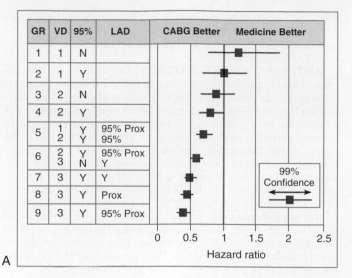

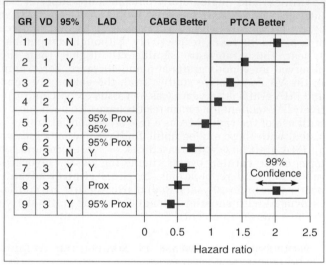

FIGURE 54–12 A, Adjusted hazard (mortality) ratios comparing coronary artery bypass grafting (CABG) and medical therapy for nine coronary anatomy severity groups (GR) according to the number of vessels diseased (VD), the presence or absence of a 95 percent proximal stenosis (95%), and involvement of the left anterior descending coronary artery (LAD). **B,** Adjusted hazard (mortality) ratios comparing CABG and percutaneous transluminal coronary angioplasty (PTCA) for nine coronary anatomy groups according to the number of vessels diseased, the presence or absence of a 95 percent proximal stenosis, and LAD involvement. In patients with the least severe categories of disease, 5-year survival appears to be better with PTCA (single-vessel disease without proximal stenosis and without LAD involvement), whereas for patients with triple-vessel disease and higher grade, more complex, double-vessel disease, a survival benefit is noted with surgery. For other subsets of patients with double-vessel disease, no difference in survival was seen in those treated with CABG or PTCA, and many of these patients are probably similar to those included in the randomized trials. *(Data from the Duke University data base; A and B, from Jones RH, Kesler K, Phillips HR III, et al: Long-term survival benefits of coronary artery bypass grafting and percutaneous transluminal angioplasty in patients with coronary artery disease. J Thorac Cardiovasc Surg 111:1013, 1996.)*

10 and 15 years, respectively. Trials in which the contemporary practice of using one or more arterial grafts was prevalent have demonstrated similar or superior rates of freedom from angina during short-term and mid-term follow-up.[185] The major randomized trials all have demonstrated greater relief of angina, better exercise performance, and a lower requirement for antianginal medications for surgically versus medically treated patients 5 years postoperatively. Beyond 5 years, differences in symptoms between patients initially treated medically and surgically are diminished, in part because of the high crossover rate from medical to surgical therapy in patients with continued symptoms and progression of disease in vein grafts and in non-bypassed vessels in the surgical group. In the bypass surgery arms of

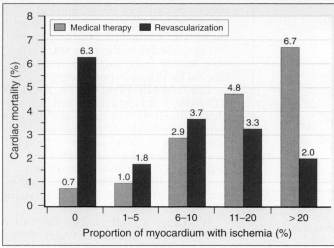

FIGURE 54–13 Rate of cardiac death in patients treated with medical therapy versus revascularization, stratified by the proportion of ischemic myocardium on stress nuclear imaging. A total of 10,627 consecutive patients without prior myocardial infarction or revascularization were followed for a mean of 1.6 years after exercise or adenosine myocardial perfusion imaging. Patients with moderate to severe ischemia who underwent percutaneous or surgical coronary revascularization within 60 days of stress imaging had lower mortality than those treated with medical therapy ($P < 0.0001$). However, those patients with no or mild ischemia had no survival advantage with revascularization. *(From Hachamovitch R, Hayes SW, Friedman JD, et al: Comparison of the short-term survival benefit associated with revascularization compared with medical therapy in patients with no prior coronary artery disease undergoing stress myocardial perfusion single photon emission computed tomography. Circulation 107:2900, 2003.)*

	Effects of Coronary Artery Bypass Grafting on Survival*	
TABLE 54–12		
Subgroup	Medical Treatment Mortality Rate (%)	P Value for CABG Surgery versus Medical Treatment
Vessel Disease		
One vessel	9.9	0.18
Two vessels	11.7	0.45
Three vessels	17.6	<0.001
Left main artery	36.5	0.004
No LAD Disease		
One or two vessels	8.3	0.88
Three vessels	14.5	0.02
Left main artery	45.8	0.03
Overall	12.3	0.05
LAD Disease Present		
One or two vessels	14.6	0.05
Three vessels	19.1	0.009
Left main artery	32.7	0.02
Overall	18.3	0.001
LV Function		
Normal	13.3	<0.001
Abnormal	25.2	0.02
Exercise Test Status		
Missing	17.4	0.10
Normal	11.6	0.38
Abnormal	16.8	<0.001
Severity of Angina		
Class 0, I, II	12.5	0.005
Class III, IV	22.4	0.001

*Systematic overview of the effect of coronary artery bypass grafting (CABG) versus medical therapy on survival based on data from seven randomized trials comparing a strategy of initial CABG surgery with one of initial medical therapy. Subgroup results at 5 years are shown.

LAD = left anterior descending artery; LV = left ventricular.

From Yusuf S, Zucker D, Peduzzi P, et al: Effect of coronary artery bypass surgery on survival: Overview of 10-year results from randomized trials by the Coronary Artery Bypass Surgery Trialists Collaboration. Lancet 344:563, 1994.

randomized trials of PCI and CABG,[183] recurrent angina pectoris was reported in 21.5 to 34 percent of patients at a follow-up ranging from 2 to 3 years, but (Canadian Cardiovascular Society classification) grade III or IV angina was present in only 6 percent at 2.5 years. The reoperation rate for recurrence of symptoms has been reported to be in the range of 6 to 8 percent per year. Independent predictors of recurrence of angina are female gender, obesity, preoperative hypertension, and lack of use of the IMA as a conduit. In patients with triple-vessel disease undergoing coronary bypass surgery, the completeness of revascularization is a significant determinant of the relief of symptoms at 1 year and over a 5-year period.[184]

In summary, after 5 years, approximately 75 percent of surgically treated patients can be predicted to be free of an ischemic event, sudden death, occurrence of myocardial infarction, or recurrence of angina; about 50 percent remain free for approximately 10 years and about 15 percent for 15 or more years. Symptomatic improvement is best maintained in patients with the most complete revascularization.

EFFECTS ON SURVIVAL. Current clinical practice has been shaped by three major randomized trials of CABG compared with medical therapy that enrolled patients between 1972 and 1984: the Veterans Affairs (VA) Trial, the European Cardiac Society Study (ECSS), and the National Institutes of Health–supported CASS (Fig. 54-14).[183] The evidence base comprised data from 2649 patients participating in these and several smaller trials. It has provided a wealth of important information but has several important limitations with respect to application to current practice because the risk profile of patients referred for surgery, as well as the available surgical and medical interventions, have evolved substantially. In particular, these trials antedated the widespread use of one or two IMAs. As a result, the extent of the completeness of coronary revascularization, graft patency rates, and perioperative mortality fall far short of current expectations and reflect, in part, the initial learning experience of coronary bypass surgery. Moreover, although the patients allocated to initial CABG had a sig-

nificantly lower mortality at 5, 7, and 10 years, 41 percent of the patients assigned to medical treatment had undergone CABG by 10 years (so-called crossovers).

The results of the trials of surgical versus medical therapy have generally been highly consistent, and thus the major points guiding clinical practice may still be drawn from a meta-analysis of the results. In each of the trials, a survival benefit of CABG emerged during mid-term follow-up (2 to 6 years), but this advantage eroded during long-term follow-up and remained statistically significant only in the ECSS. Considered together, the results of these trials support a 4.1 percent absolute reduction in long-term mortality (10 years) with CABG ($P = 0.03$). Subgroup analyses have revealed several high-risk criteria that identify patients who are likely to sustain a more substantial survival benefit: (1) left main CAD; (2) single- or double-vessel disease with proximal LAD disease; (3) LV systolic dysfunction; and (4) a composite evaluation that indicates high risk, including severity of symptoms, high-risk exercise tolerance test, history of prior myocardial infarction, and the presence of ST depression on the resting ECG.

The most recent randomized data comparing CABG with medical therapy are from the Asymptomatic Cardiac Ischemia Pilot (ACIP) study of 558 patients. This trial of angina-guided versus angina plus ischemia-guided medical therapy (using ambulatory monitoring) in comparison to revascularization by PTCA (92 patients) or CABG (79 patients) enrolled relatively low-risk patients. After 2 years of follow-up, mortality was significantly lower in patients assigned to routine revascularization (1.1 versus 6.6 and 4.4 percent for the two

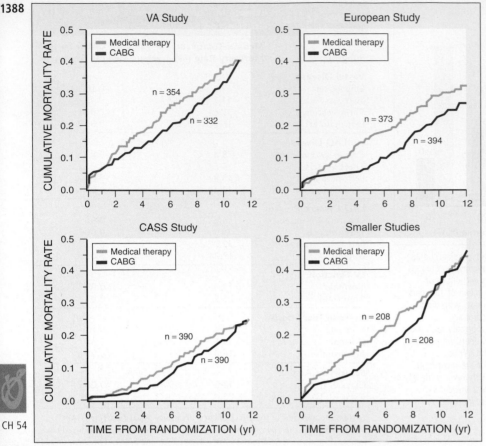

FIGURE 54–14 Survival curves of three large randomized trials and four smaller studies combined. CABG = coronary artery bypass grafting. *(From Eagle KA, Guyton RA, Davidoff R, et al: ACC/AHA guidelines for coronary artery bypass graft surgery: A report of the American College of Cardiology/American Heart Association Task Force on Practice Guidelines [Committee to Revise the 1991 Guidelines for Coronary Artery Bypass Graft Surgery]. American College of Cardiology/American Heart Association. J Am Coll Cardiol 34:1262, 1999.)*

medical groups [$p < 0.02$]), and rates of death or myocardial infarction were 12.1 percent (angina-guided medical therapy), 8.9 percent (ischemia-guided medical therapy), and 4.7 percent (coronary revascularization) ($P < 0.04$). Although this trial was designed as a pilot study and the number of patients was relatively small, the observed risk reductions were statistically significant and suggest that the benefits of revascularization in the context of current revascularization technique may be greater than previously appreciated. The trial was not designed to assess differences between PTCA and bypass surgery.

Taken together, the results of all the trials and registries indicate that the sicker the patient—based on the severity of symptoms or ischemia, age, the number of vessels diseased, and the presence of LV dysfunction—the greater the benefit of surgical over medical therapy on survival (see Figs. 54-12 and 54-13 and Table 54-12). CABG prolongs survival in patients with significant left main CAD irrespective of symptoms, in patients with multivessel disease and impaired LV function, and in patients with triple-vessel disease that includes the proximal LAD coronary artery, irrespective of LV function. Surgical therapy has also been demonstrated to prolong life in patients with double-vessel disease and LV dysfunction, particularly those with proximal narrowing of one or more coronary arteries and in the presence of severe angina. Although no study has documented a survival benefit with surgical treatment in patients with single-vessel disease, some evidence has indicated that such patients, who have impaired LV function, have a poor long-term survival with medical therapy. Patients with

angina or evidence of ischemia at a low or moderate level of exercise, especially those with obstruction of the proximal left anterior descending coronary artery, may benefit from coronary revascularization by PCI or bypass surgery.

LEFT MAIN CORONARY ARTERY STENOSIS. It is widely agreed that surgical treatment improves survival in patients with left main coronary artery obstruction or its equivalent. The CASS Registry has demonstrated that the superiority of revascularization is equivalent in symptomatic and asymptomatic patients with disease affecting the left main coronary artery.

Whether a left main–equivalent anatomy exists that has a natural history similar to that of left main CAD is uncertain. The condition in question may consist of disease in the proximal portions of both the LAD and left circumflex coronary arteries. It is likely that significant left main coronary disease has an ominous nature because a single event (rupture of a single plaque) can cause infarction of a very large quantity of myocardium. Consequently, although combined disease of the proximal left anterior descending and circumflex coronary arteries does identify a subgroup of high-risk patients, the prognosis is not as poor as it is for patients with left main CAD. Nevertheless, patients with combined stenoses of 70 percent or greater in the LAD coronary artery, before the first septal perforating branch, and in the proximal circumflex coronary artery, before the first obtuse marginal branch, who have impaired ventricular function also have improved survival and less angina following surgical revascularization than if they are treated medically, particularly in the face of LV dysfunction. The median survival of surgically treated patients with left main–equivalent disease is 13.1 versus 6.2 years for those medically treated.

EFFECT ON SUBSEQUENT MYOCARDIAL INFARCTION. The major randomized trials of patients with mild to moderate angina have suggested that the likelihood of occurrence of myocardial infarction after 5 to 10 years of follow-up is similar in medically and surgically treated patients. In both the VA study and CASS, the major benefit of surgery on myocardial infarction does not appear to be mediated by a decrease in the frequency of myocardial infarction but by a decrease in the case-fatality rate of patients who subsequently have infarction. Potential explanations are that previous bypass surgery results in smaller infarcts caused by distal occlusions and that the bypass may enhance myocardial perfusion distal to the obstructing lesion.

Patients with Depressed Left Ventricular Function

Depressed LV function is one of the most powerful predictors of perioperative and late mortality. In the New York State CABG registry, an ejection fraction less than or equal to 25 percent was associated with 6.5 percent in-hospital mortality compared with 1.4 percent in those with an ejection fraction greater than 40 percent.[186] In the Society of Thoracic Surgeons data base, the mean ejection fraction in approximately 136,330 patients undergoing initial coronary bypass in 1999 was 0.51, and approximately 25 percent had an ejection fraction of less than

0.45.[154] Moreover, as the population ages and the proportion undergoing reoperation increases, the number of patients with preoperative LV dysfunction and clinical heart failure will increase. In the CABG Patch trial confined to patients with an ejection fraction of 0.35 or less, perioperative mortality was 3.5 percent for patients without clinical signs of heart failure versus 7.7 percent for those with NYHA classes I to IV heart failure.

Although the effect of a reduced ejection fraction on operative mortality cannot be eliminated, careful attention to intraoperative metabolic, inotropic, and mechanical support, including preoperative intraaortic balloon counterpulsation in some patients, may decrease perioperative mortality in comparison with the mortality rates expected from prediction models. In addition to advances in myocardial protection for those undergoing CABG with CPB, off-pump approaches to CABG may also lead to improved surgical outcomes in this high-risk population.[187] Thus, in experienced centers, the in-hospital mortality for patients with severe LV dysfunction is less than 4 percent.

The powerful effect of the preoperative ejection fraction on late survival emphasizes that currently, the presence of LV dysfunction, in association with viable myocardium, has changed from a relative contraindication to coronary bypass to a strong indication. This shift in focus has been caused by the realization that viable dysfunctional myocardium may improve after coronary revascularization.[188] Indeed, the most striking survival benefits of CABG, as well as symptomatic and functional improvements, are shown by patients with seriously impaired left ventricular function in whom the prognosis of medical therapy is poor.[189] In patients with a history of congestive heart failure and multivessel (particularly triple-vessel) disease, coronary bypass surgery may also reduce the incidence of sudden cardiac death. Although preoperative LV dysfunction creates the potential for significant benefit, the perioperative risk should not be underestimated, particularly in the setting of clinical congestive heart failure.[190] Selection of patients with viable myocardium supplied by a reasonable target vessel(s) for grafting appears critical when considering CABG for patients with severe LV dysfunction.[188]

MYOCARDIAL HIBERNATION (see Chap. 48). Improvement in survival and LV function following CABG depends on successful reperfusion of viable but noncontractile or poorly contracting myocardium. Two related pathophysiological conditions have been described to explain reversible ischemic contractile dysfunction: (1) myocardial stunning—prolonged but temporary postischemic ventricular dysfunction without myocardial necrosis; and (2) myocardial hibernation—persistent LV dysfunction when myocardial perfusion is chronically reduced (or repetitively stunned) but sufficient to maintain the viability of tissue.[191] The reduction in myocardial contractility in hibernating myocardium conserves metabolic demands and may be protective, but more prolonged and severe hibernation may lead to severe ultrastructural abnormalities, irreversible loss of contractile units, and apoptosis.

Hibernating myocardium can cause abnormal systolic or diastolic ventricular function, or both. The predominant clinical feature of myocardial ischemia in these patients may not be angina but dyspnea secondary to increased LV diastolic pressure. Symptoms of heart failure resulting from chronic LV dysfunction may be inappropriately ascribed to myocardial necrosis and scarring when the symptoms may, in fact, be reversed after the chronic ischemia is relieved by coronary revascularization.[192]

Detection of Hibernating Myocardium (see Chaps. 14, 16, and 17). Several clinical markers may be used to determine the likelihood that a dysfunctional myocardial segment is viable or nonviable (Table 54-13). The presence of angina and the absence of Q waves on the ECG or a history of prior myocardial infarction are useful clues. A severe reduction in the diastolic wall thickness of dysfunctional LV segments is indicative of scarring. On the other hand, akinetic or dyskinetic segments with preserved diastolic wall thickness may represent a mixture of scarred and viable myocardium. A useful strategy for the assessment of dysfunctional segments has been developed (Fig. 54-15). Although a number of imaging tools may be used for this assessment, the most readily available in most settings is low-dose dobutamine echocardiography[193] (see Chap. 14). PET (see Chap. 16) has emerged as an excellent method for demonstrating viable myocardium in patients with impaired LV function.[194] In comparative studies, PET has yielded the highest predictive accuracy of all imaging modalities in detecting dysfunctional myocardium that will improve after revascularization. However, the high cost, technical difficulty, and need for a cyclotron continue to limit this technique's widespread applicability. Contrast-enhanced

TABLE 54–13	Markers of Viable Myocardium	
Clinical Indicator	**Diagnostic Test**	**Alternative Test**
Diastolic wall thickness	Echo	CT, MRI
Systolic wall thickening	Echo	CT, MRI, gated SPECT
Regional wall motion	Echo	CT, MRI, gated SPECT
Regional blood flow	SPECT	PET, MRI
Myocardial metabolism	PET	SPECT
Cell membrane integrity	SPECT	PET
Contractile reserve	Dobutamine, Echo	Angiography, CT, MRI

CT = computed tomography; Echo = echocardiography; MRI = magnetic resonance imaging; PET = positron emission tomography; SPECT = single-photon emission computed tomography.

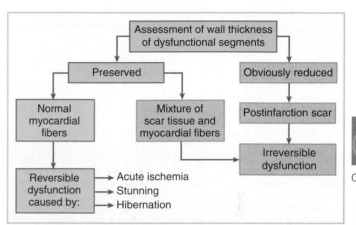

FIGURE 54–15 Flow diagram illustrating the practical assessment of noncontractile segments of myocardial wall potentially recoverable by revascularization procedures. An obviously reduced wall thickness is indicative of a postinfarction scar. Absence of contractile function in segments of the ventricular wall with preserved wall thickness may be caused by different mechanisms. An acute ischemic cause can be excluded by the administration of sublingual nitrates. Stunning can be excluded by repeating the ventricular wall motion study several days after the last ischemic episode. Hibernating myocardium should be distinguished from a mixture of scar tissue and viable myocardial cells. *(From Maseri A: Ischemic Heart Disease: A Rational Basis for Clinical Practice and Clinical Research. New York, Churchill Livingstone, 1995.)*

CMR is emerging as a valuable alternative technique for assessment of myocardial viability.[195] Thallium-201 rest-redistribution imaging continues to exist as an alternative (see Chap. 16).

Prognostic Implications of Identifying Viable Myocardium. A growing body of evidence has indicated that the detection of viable myocardium in patients with CAD and LV dysfunction not only identifies those in whom improvement in cardiac function is likely after revascularization, but also identifies a group of high-risk patients in whom revascularization improves survival (Fig. 54-16).[194] Studies with PET, thallium-201, and dobutamine echocardiography have uniformly demonstrated that patients with LV dysfunction and evidence of hibernating myocardium have a high mortality rate during medical therapy and appear to have a better outcome with revascularization.[196] All these studies have limitations, including a small number of patients, the retrospective nature of the analysis, and lack of a randomized control group.[188] However, the consistency of the findings has been striking. Viability assessment is also helpful in the selection of patients for revascularization because patients selected for revascularization on the basis of an imaging study demonstrating myocardial viability have lower operative mortality and a higher long-term survival rate than those with no evidence of important myocardial viability or those in whom a viability assessment is not performed.[197]

The mechanisms for improved survival after revascularization in patients with hibernating myocardium in these retrospective studies

CH 54

Chronic Coronary Artery Disease

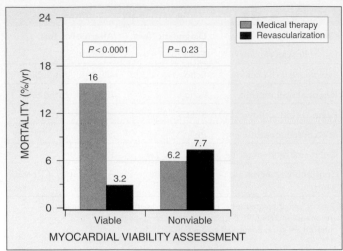

FIGURE 54–16 Meta-analysis of observational studies examining late survival with revascularization versus medical therapy for patients with coronary artery disease and left ventricular dysfunction. Analysis of results from 24 studies (N = 3088) demonstrated that revascularization is associated with a significant reduction in annual mortality compared with medical therapy in patients with myocardial viability. No advantage of revascularization was detected in patients without myocardial viability. *(Modified from Allman KC, Shaw LJ, Hachamovitch R, et al: Myocardial viability testing and impact of revascularization on prognosis in patients with coronary artery disease and left-ventricular dysfunction: A meta-analysis. J Am Coll Cardiol 39:1151, 2002.)*

CH 54

may be related to improvement in LV function. However, it is likely that other factors are also operative, including reductions in LV remodeling, the propensity for serious arrhythmias, and the likelihood of a future fatal acute ischemic event. Prospective trials are needed to provide definitive evidence about whether myocardial viability testing identifies patients with LV dysfunction in whom revascularization improves survival and quality of life.

Surgical Treatment in Special Groups

WOMEN (see Chap. 76). Women are less likely than men to be referred for coronary angiography and subsequent revascularization. In some studies, gender-based differences in referral for revascularization are explained fully by clinical factors. Moreover, it has not been established whether gender-based differences represent inappropriately less consideration of referrals for women, inappropriately more consideration of referrals for men, or both.[198] In comparison with men, women who undergo CABG are sicker, as defined by age, comorbid conditions, severity of angina, and history of congestive heart failure.[199] In-hospital mortality and perioperative morbidity after CABG has remained, on average, two times higher in women compared with men.[200] However, when adjusted for the greater risk profile of women referred for CABG, short-term mortality rates as well as long-term outcomes are similar to those for men in most, but not all, studies.[200] The independent predictors of long-term prognosis in women are similar to those in men and include older age, previous coronary bypass surgery, previous myocardial infarction, and diabetes.

An excess risk of short-term mortality reported in younger women undergoing CABG in two studies has not been well explained.[199] Smaller vessel size (as a function of smaller body surface area), a higher incidence of LV hypertrophy, and hypertensive heart disease have been raised as potential contributors to higher surgical risk in women. However, these differences are reasonably expected to be more important in older women; the pathophysiological bases for the observed difference in younger women compared with men require further exploration.[199]

With generally similar long-term outcomes after surgical revascularization, gender should not be a significant factor in decisions regarding whether to offer CABG.[199] Newer technical approaches such as OPCAB may be particularly advantageous to women.

YOUNGER PATIENTS. Patients 35 years of age or younger who undergo CABG usually have hyperlipidemia and other major risk factors for CAD. Despite the severity of the underlying disease and the rapidity of the atherosclerotic process, CABG is associated with excellent actuarial survival rates of 94 percent at 5 years and 85 percent at 10 years. Nonetheless, in the CASS Registry, patients younger than 35 years had markedly impaired survival over a 15-year period in comparison with an age- and gender-matched U.S. population. This impaired survival is probably the result of progression of premature atherosclerotic disease, the presence of multiple risk factors, and the development of progressive vein graft disease.

OLDER PATIENTS (see Chap. 75). A demographic tide in combination with marked improvement in perioperative care and in the outcomes of CABG has resulted in a burgeoning population of elderly patients with extensive disease undergoing such surgery. The number of individuals older than 75 years of age in the United States is expected to quadruple in the next 50 years, with cardiovascular disease being the leading cause of morbidity and mortality in this population. Many such individuals are likely to become candidates for CABG.[201]

Older patients are sicker than their younger counterparts in that they have a greater frequency of comorbid conditions, including peripheral vascular and cerebrovascular disease, more extensive triple-vessel and left main CAD, and a higher frequency of LV dysfunction and history of congestive heart failure.[183] Not unexpectedly, these differences are translated into higher perioperative mortality and complication rates, with a sharp increase in the slope of the curve relating mortality to age seen in patients older than 70 years. Despite these differences, in-hospital mortality for the elderly has declined over time to 7 to 9 percent in those undergoing CABG only and has been reported to be as low as 3 to 4 percent in the subgroup of octogenarians without significant medical comorbidities. Perioperative morbidity is higher in the elderly, with high rates of low-output syndrome, stroke, gastrointestinal complications, wound infection, and postoperative atrial fibrillation.[183] Given marked variation in the outcomes in older patients undergoing revascularization, decisions should be based on individual risk and needs assessment.[202]

RENAL DISEASE. Cardiovascular disease is the major cause of mortality in patients with end-stage renal disease (ESRD) and accounts for 54 percent of deaths (see Chap. 88). Patients with ESRD, as well as those with less severe renal insufficiency, have numerous risk factors that not only accelerate the development of CAD but also complicate its medical management. These risk factors include diabetes, hypertension with LV hypertrophy, systolic and diastolic dysfunction, abnormal lipid metabolism, anemia, and increased homocysteine levels. Therefore, mild or more severe renal dysfunction is prevalent in as many as 50 percent of patients presenting for CABG.[203] Coronary revascularization with PCI or CABG is feasible and well documented in patients with ESRD, but the mortality and complication rates are increased. Patients with milder degrees of renal insufficiency who are not dependent on dialysis are also at higher risk of major perioperative complications, longer recovery times, and lower rates of short- and mid-term survival.[203,204] Observational data have suggested that in patients on chronic dialysis, CABG is the preferred strategy for revascularization over PCI. However, randomized data are few, and 30-day mortality in patients with ESRD undergoing CABG ranges from 9 to as high as 20 percent.

PATIENTS WITH DIABETES (see Chap. 60). In comparison with age-matched nondiabetic patients, diabetic patients with angiographically proven CAD are more likely to be women with evidence of peripheral vascular disease and a higher number of coronary occlusions. Diabetes is an important independent predictor of mortality among patients undergoing surgical revascularization.[205] However, the benefit of CABG versus medical therapy is maintained in patients with diabetes, with a significant 44 percent relative reduction in mortality provided by surgery. Patients with diabetes have smaller distal vessels judged to be poorer targets for bypass grafting. Nevertheless, the patency of arterial and venous grafts appears similar in diabetics and nondiabetic patients. In the absence of new data to the contrary, patients with diabetes and multivessel disease who are at acceptable surgical risk should be considered as candidates for surgical revascularization.

Coronary Bypass Surgery in Patients with Associated Vascular Disease

Management of patients with combined CAD and peripheral vascular disease involving the carotid arteries, the abdominal aorta, or the vessels of the lower extremities presents many challenges. Combined disease is becoming increasingly frequent as the population of patients under consideration for CABG ages and as technical improvements allow the application of coronary revascularization to ever more complex cases.

IMPACT OF COMBINED CAD AND PERIPHERAL VASCULAR DISEASE. Clinically apparent CAD occurs frequently in patients with peripheral vascular disease. In patients undergoing peripheral vascular surgery, late outcomes are dominated by cardiac causes of morbidity and mortality. Conversely, in patients with CAD, the presence of peripheral vascular disease, even if asymptomatic, is associated with an adverse prognosis, presumably because of the greater total atherosclerotic burden borne by these patients.

Because patients with CAD and peripheral atherosclerosis tend to be older and have more widespread vascular disease and end-organ damage than patients without peripheral atherosclerosis, the perioperative mortality and morbidity consequent to CABG are high and the late outcome is not as favorable.[206] In the Northern New England Cardiovascular data base, in-hospital mortality after CABG was 2.4-fold greater in patients with peripheral vascular disease than in those without it, particularly for patients with lower extremity disease. Diffuse atheroembolism is a particularly serious complication of CABG in patients with peripheral vascular disease and aortic atherosclerosis. It is a major cause of perioperative death, stroke, neurocognitive dysfunction, and multiorgan dysfunction after CABG.

Peripheral vascular disease is also a strong marker of an adverse long-term outcome. For example, in the Northern New England Cardiovascular data base, the 5-year mortality was approximately twofold greater in patients with peripheral vascular disease than in those without it, even after adjusting for other comorbid conditions, which are more frequent in patients with peripheral vascular disease. Nevertheless, given the diffuse nature of coronary disease in patients with peripheral vascular disease, there may be advantages to surgical coronary revascularization rather than PCI in many such patients.[207]

CAROTID ARTERY DISEASE. In patients with stable CAD and carotid artery disease in whom carotid endarterectomy is planned, exercise stress testing and consideration of coronary revascularization can ordinarily be performed after the carotid surgery. The prevalence of significant carotid disease in an increasingly older population being considered for CABG is high; approximately 20 percent have a stenosis of 50 percent or greater, 6 to 12 percent have a stenosis of 80 percent or greater, and the percentage is higher in patients with left main CAD.[208] In patients for whom surgical treatment is considered for both carotid artery disease and CAD, the merits of a combined versus a staged approach have been debated. Neither strategy has been demonstrated to be unequivocally superior to the other, and an individualized approach, depending on the patient's initial condition, severity of symptoms, anatomy of the coronary and carotid vessels, and individual institutional experience, is most appropriate. Preoperative or simultaneous carotid stenting is under investigation as an alternative approach to combined carotid endarterectomy and CABG.

MANAGEMENT OF PATIENTS WITH ASSOCIATED VASCULAR DISEASE (see Chap. 57). Patients with severe or unstable CAD requir-

ing revascularization can be categorized into two groups according to the severity and instability of the accompanying vascular disease. When the noncoronary vascular procedures are elective, they can generally be postponed until the cardiac symptoms have stabilized, either by intensive medical therapy or by revascularization. A combined procedure is necessary in patients with both unstable CAD and an unstable vascular condition, such as frequent recurrent transient ischemic attacks[209] or a rapidly expanding abdominal aortic aneurysm. In some patients in this category, PCI offers the potential for stabilizing the patient's cardiac condition before proceeding with a definitive vascular repair. A problem is posed by the use of clopidogrel after stenting; this will increase bleeding unless surgery is performed at least 5 days after discontinuation of clopidogrel.

PATIENTS REQUIRING REOPERATION. Currently, approximately 12 percent of coronary artery procedures are reoperations and, in some centers, particularly tertiary care centers, the proportion is increasing rapidly and accounts for 20 percent of all CABG operations.[183] The major indication for reoperation is late disease of saphenous vein grafts. An added factor underlying recurrent symptoms is progression of disease in native vessels between the first and second operations. Several series have emphasized the sicker preoperative status of patients undergoing reoperation, including older age, more serious comorbidity, associated valvular heart disease, and a greater prevalence of LV dysfunction and greater extent of ischemic jeopardized myocardium.[210]

Not unexpectedly, the mortality associated with reoperation is significantly higher than that of initial bypass procedures. In the 1997 data base of the Society of Thoracic Surgeons, the mortality in 99,810 patients undergoing an elective first CABG procedure was 1.7 versus 5.2 percent for elective reoperations. For patients undergoing first operations, mortality was 2.6 percent for urgent and 6 percent for emergency procedures in comparison with 7.4 and 13.5 percent, respectively, in patients undergoing repeat bypass surgery. Indications for reoperation have not been defined by randomized trials, but in general, the same principles that apply to patients with initial disease should be followed.

Summary of Indications for Coronary Revascularization

1. Certain anatomical subsets of patients are candidates for CABG, regardless of the severity of symptoms or LV dysfunction. Such patients include those with significant left main CAD and most patients with triple-vessel disease that includes the proximal LAD coronary artery, especially those with LV dysfunction (ejection fraction less than 50 percent). Patients with chronic stable angina and double-vessel CAD with significant proximal disease of the LAD, and either LV dysfunction or high-risk findings on noninvasive testing, should also be considered for CABG.[10]

2. The benefits of CABG are well documented in patients with LV dysfunction and multivessel disease, regardless of symptoms. In patients whose dominant symptom is heart failure without severe angina, the benefits of coronary revascularization are less well defined, but this approach should be considered in patients who also have evidence of severe ischemia (regardless of angina symptoms), particularly in the presence of a significant extent of potentially viable dysfunctional (hibernating) myocardium.[183]

3. The primary objective of coronary revascularization in patients with single-vessel disease is relief of significant symptoms or objective evidence of severe ischemia. For most of these patients, PCI is the revascularization modality of choice.

4. In patients with angina who are not considered to be at high risk, survival is similar for surgery, PCI, and medical management.

5. All the indications discussed earlier relate to the potential benefits of surgery over medical therapy on survival. Coronary revascularization with PCI or CABG is highly efficacious in relieving symptoms and may be considered for patients with moderate to severe ischemic symptoms who are not controlled by and/or are dissatisfied with medical therapy, even if they are not in a high-risk subset. For such patients, the optimal method of revascularization is selected on the basis of LV function and arteriographic findings and the likelihood of technical success.

Comparisons Between PCI and CABG

OBSERVATIONAL STUDIES. Catheter-based revascularizations in most comparative studies have been limited mainly to PTCA and the findings were largely consistent.[183] Over a period of 1 to 5 years, the rates of mortality and nonfatal infarction were not significantly different between patients revascularized with CABG versus PTCA, but recurrent events, including angina pectoris and the need for repeat revascularization procedures, were significantly more frequent in the PTCA than the CABG group, largely as a consequence of incomplete revascularization and restenosis. However, several subgroups of patients who may derive a survival benefit from CABG compared to PTCA have been identified. These include patients with LV dysfunction, probably because of the ability to achieve more complete revascularization with the CABG. In addition, CABG provided a survival benefit compared with PTCA when proximal LAD stenosis (more than 70 percent) was present.

More recent studies have included patients undergoing stenting. In an analysis of approximately 60,000 patients with multivessel CAD treated with coronary stenting or CABG and recorded in the New York State Registry between 1997 and 2000, CABG was found to be associated with higher survival after adjustment for medical comorbidities in patients with two or more diseased vessels, with or without involvement of the LAD.[211] Nevertheless, the similarity of the unadjusted rates of survival highlights the role of clinical judgment in selecting the optimal therapy for the individual patient and the ability to achieve good outcomes in appropriately selected patients with two-vessel disease, particularly without involvement of the proximal LAD.[122,211]

Randomized Trials

PCI VERSUS CABG IN PATIENTS WITH SINGLE-VESSEL DISEASE. Both the Lausanne and Medicine, Angioplasty, or Surgery Study (MASS) trials were limited to patients with isolated disease of the proximal LAD coronary artery. The RITA investigators also published results for the subset of patients (45 percent) who had single-vessel disease. The results of these small trials were consistent in that over 2 to 3 years, the rates of mortality and myocardial infarction were similar in the two treatment arms, as was improvement in symptoms, but at the cost of more frequent reintervention in patients treated with PTCA. At least one trial has now compared minimally invasive direct CABG to stenting for patients with isolated stenosis in the proximal LAD.[134] Results from this small study (N = 220) were similar to those of prior trials. Although patients treated with CABG were less likely to have recurrent symptoms or undergo repeat revascularization, there was no detectable difference in the risk of death or myocardial infarction with PCI versus CABG (3 versus 6 percent; P = 0.5).

These results suggest that PCI and CABG are both highly effective in preventing symptoms in patients with single-vessel disease, with similar long-term survival. Moreover, technological advances in PCI since PTCA was developed (e.g., use of stents—first bare metal and more recently drug-eluting) have achieved reductions in the frequency of reintervention for patients undergoing these procedures.

MULTIVESSEL DISEASE. At least nine published studies have compared PCI with CABG in patients with multivessel disease. Despite the heterogeneity of the trials in regard to design, methods, and the patient population enrolled, the results are generally comparable and provide a consistent perspective of CABG and PCI in selected patients with multivessel disease. A major limitation is that these trials, except for the Arterial Revascularization Therapy Study (ARTS) and the Argentine randomized trial of PTCA versus CAB surgery in multivessel disease (ERACI II), were conducted before the widespread use of stents and other advances in PCI technology, as well as newer adjunctive therapy, such as clopidogrel and glycoprotein IIb/IIIa platelet inhibition. Also, these trials lacked an aggressive approach to lipid lowering in both groups of patients. In RITA, the Argentine randomized stent study (ERACI), ARTS, and the French Monocentric trials, the ability to achieve equivalent degrees of revascularization in the two groups was an inclusion criterion. Moreover, most patients entered into the trials had well-preserved LV function. Therefore, patients enrolled in these trials were at relatively low risk, with predominantly double-vessel disease and normal LV ejection fraction—that is, a high proportion of patients in whom CABG surgery had *not* been previously shown to be superior to medical therapy in regard to survival. Thus, one would not expect a significant mortality difference between PCI and CABG, particularly with the relatively small sample size of the trials.[10]

The Bypass Angioplasty Revascularization Investigation (BARI) trial enrolled 1829 patients with multivessel disease in the United States and Canada. This trial is the largest of the completed randomized trials of PTCA and bypass surgery and the only trial with sufficient statistical power to detect a substantial mortality difference. At 5 years, overall survival rates were not different between the two groups (89.3 percent with CABG and 86.3 percent with PTCA; P = 0.19), nor was any difference noted in the incidence of myocardial infarction. An initially unexpected finding, but one that has subsequently been reinforced by ARTS and observational data, was that patients with previously treated diabetes who underwent PTCA had a 5-year mortality of 34.5 versus 19.4 percent for those who underwent CABG (P = 0.003; Fig. 54-17). This advantage of CABG over PTCA for patients with diabetes became more robust by 7 years of follow-up. More rapid progression of atherosclerosis and high rates of restenosis in patients undergoing percutaneous revascularization are largely responsible for this difference. It is possible that the introduction of drug-eluting stents and more aggressive medical therapy of diabetes will reduce or eliminate this advantage of CABG over PCI in patients with diabetes.[212]

NONFATAL OUTCOMES. Review of the nonfatal outcomes in the randomized trials has revealed some differences between CABG and

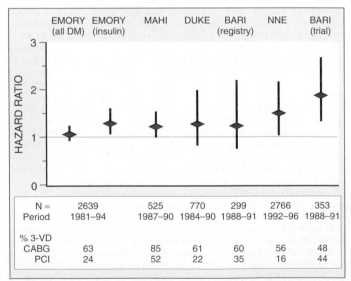

FIGURE 54–17 Five- to six-year survival after coronary artery bypass grafting (CABG) versus percutaneous coronary intervention (PCI) in patients with diabetes mellitus (DM) and multivessel coronary artery disease. Data from both observational and randomized studies show trends toward survival or superior survival with CABG. All hazard ratios are adjusted, with the exception of the data from the Mid America Heart Institute (MAHI). BARI = Bypass-Angioplasty Revascularization Investigation; NNE = Northern New England data base study; 3-VD = triple-vessel coronary artery disease. *(Modified from Niles NW, McGrath PD, Malenka D, et al: Survival of patients with diabetes and multivessel coronary artery disease after surgical or percutaneous revascularization: Results of a large regional prospective study. J Am Coll Cardiol 37:1008, 2001.)*

PCI. In each of the studies, CABG was initially associated with greater improvement in angina, which appears to be proportional to the more complete revascularization in patients with multivessel disease. Moreover, as anticipated from the observational data, repeat revascularization procedures were more frequent after PCI. This difference was less in the ARTS trial, in which repeat revascularization through 1 year was performed in only 16.9 percent of patients in the stented group (Fig. 54-18), contrasting with 38 percent within 2 years after angioplasty in RITA-1. In the ERACI II study, results were similar to those in the ARTS trial, with only 16.8 percent of patients who had PCI with stenting requiring repeat revascularization in follow-up versus 4.8 percent of CABG patients. However, in the BARI trial, other measures of procedural success, including indices of the quality of life, cognitive function, and return to employment, were similar between PTCA and CABG.

Another consistent but not unexpected finding was the lower in-hospital cost for patients undergoing PCI. This initial cost advantage was sustained at 1 year in ARTS. However, the need for recurrent hospitalization and repeat revascularization procedures over the long term contributed to an increase in postdischarge cost in the PCI arms, resulting in similar overall cost over 3 to 5 years in BARI and a diminished cost advantage at 3 years in ARTS.[213] A major determinant of lower cost is the presence of double-vessel disease; in comparison, patients with congestive heart failure, comorbid conditions, or diabetes are likely to accrue higher cost regardless of the procedure.

Choosing Between PCI and CABG

Medical management of chronic CAD involves a reduction in reversible risk factors, counseling in life-style alteration, treatment of conditions that intensify angina, and pharmacological management of ischemia. When an unacceptable level of angina persists despite medical management, the patient has troubling side effects from the antiischemic drugs, and/or exhibits a high-risk result on noninvasive testing, the coronary anatomy should be defined to allow selection of the appropriate technique for revascularization.[183] After elucidation of the coronary anatomy, selection of the technique of revascularization is made as follows (Fig. 54-19 and Table 54-14; see Figs. 54-17 and 54-18):

SINGLE-VESSEL DISEASE. In patients with single-vessel disease in whom revascularization is deemed necessary and the lesion is anatomically suitable, PCI is generally preferred over bypass surgery.

MULTIVESSEL DISEASE. The first step is to decide whether a patient falls into the category of those who were included in randomized trials comparing PCI and CABG. Most of the patients included in these trials were at lower

TABLE 54–14	Comparison of Revascularization Strategies in Multivessel Disease
Advantages	**Disadvantages**
Percutaneous Coronary Intervention	
Less invasive	Restenosis
Shorter hospital stay	High incidence of incomplete revascularization
Lower initial cost	
Easily repeated	Relative inefficacy in patients with severe left ventricular dysfunction
Effective in relieving symptoms	Less favorable outcome in diabetics
	Limited to specific anatomical subsets
Coronary Artery Bypass Graft Surgery	
Effective in relieving symptoms	Cost
Improved survival in certain subsets	Morbidity
Ability to achieve complete revascularization	
Wider applicability (anatomical subsets)	

Modified from Faxon DP: Coronary angioplasty for stable angina pectoris. *In* Beller G, Braunwald E (eds): Chronic Ischemic Heart Disease. Atlas of Heart Disease. Vol 5. Philadelphia, WB Saunders, 1995, p 9.15.

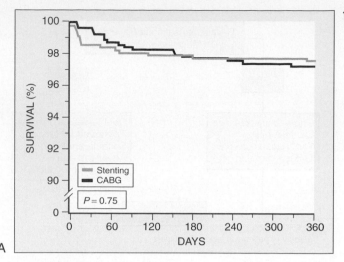

A,

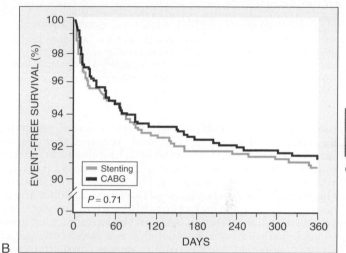

B,

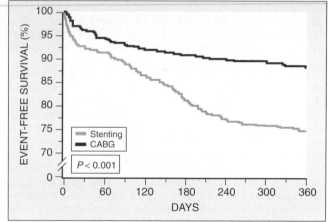

C,

CH 54

Chronic Coronary Artery Disease

FIGURE 54–18 Outcomes from 1205 patients with multivessel coronary artery disease randomly assigned to undergo percutaneous revascularization with coronary stenting or coronary artery bypass grafting (CABG) in the Arterial Revascularization Therapies Study (ARTS). One year after the revascularization procedure, rates of death, myocardial infarction, and cerebrovascular events were not statistically different between the two revascularization strategies. However, patients undergoing initial stenting were more likely to require repeat revascularization. **A,** Actuarial survival in the stenting versus CABG groups. **B,** Kaplan-Meier estimates of survival free of myocardial infarction or cerebrovascular events. **C,** Kaplan-Meier estimates of survival free of myocardial infarction, cerebrovascular events, or repeated revascularization. *(From Serruys PW, Unger F, Sousa JE, et al: Comparison of coronary artery bypass surgery and stenting for the treatment of multivessel disease. N Engl J Med 344:1117, 2001.)*

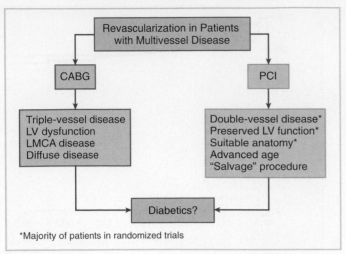

FIGURE 54–19 Indications for coronary revascularization with bypass surgery (CABG) or percutaneous coronary intervention (PCI) in patients with multivessel disease. The combination of triple-vessel disease and left ventricular (LV) dysfunction and/or left main coronary artery (LMCA) disease is primarily surgical, whereas most patients entered into the randomized trials were suitable for angioplasty on the basis of double-vessel disease, preserved LV dysfunction, and suitable anatomy. Diabetics should be treated individually.

risk, as defined by double-vessel disease and well-preserved LV function. Moreover, several trials required that equivalent degrees of revascularization be achievable by both techniques. Most patients with chronically occluded coronary arteries were excluded and, of those who were clinically eligible, approximately two thirds were excluded for angiographic reasons. The lack of any difference in late mortality and myocardial infarction between the two treatment arms in such patients indicates that PCI is a reasonable initial strategy, provided that the patient accepts the distinct possibility of symptom recurrence and need for repeat revascularization. Patients with a single localized lesion in each affected vessel and preserved LV function fare best with PCI. Additional anatomical factors, such as the presence of severe proximal LAD disease, should also be considered and weigh in favor of surgery (see Fig. 54-12).

NEED FOR COMPLETE REVASCULARIZATION. Complete revascularization is an important goal in patients with LV dysfunction and/or multivessel disease.[214] The major advantage of CABG surgery over PCI is its greater ability to achieve complete revascularization, particularly in patients with triple-vessel disease. In most of these patients, particularly those with chronic total coronary occlusion, LV dysfunction, or left main CAD, CABG is the procedure of choice. In patients with borderline LV function (ejection fraction between 0.40 and 0.50) and milder degrees of ischemia, PCI may provide adequate revascularization, even if it is not complete anatomically.

In many patients, either method of revascularization is suitable. Other factors to be considered include the following:

1. Access to a high-quality team and operator (surgeon or interventional cardiologist)
2. Patient preference—some patients are reluctant to remain at risk for symptom recurrence and reintervention; such patients are better candidates for surgical treatment. Other patients are attracted by the less invasive nature and more rapid recovery from PCI; these patients prefer to have PCI as their initial revascularization with the idea of undergoing CABG if symptoms persist and/or an excellent revascularization has not been achieved

3. Advanced patient age and comorbidity—frail, very elderly patients and those with comorbid conditions are often better candidates for PCI
4. Younger patient age—PCI is also often preferable in younger patients (younger than 50 years) with the expectation that they may require CABG at some time in the future and that PCI will postpone the need for surgery; this sequence may be preferable to two operations. Patient preference is a pivotal aspect of the decision to perform PCI or CABG in these patient groups.

PCI AND CABG IN DIABETIC PATIENTS (see Chap. 60). The poorer outcomes after PCI than after CABG in treated diabetic patients in the BARI trial, together with similar findings in the ARTS trial, have raised concern about whether all diabetic patients with multivessel disease should be treated surgically. This important issue has significant economic implications. Further analysis has suggested that treatment of diabetic patients can be individualized, as in nondiabetic patients.[205]

One point of debate is related to the patient selection criteria for enrollment into the trials. In the BARI Registry, in which patients were treated according to the preference of the individual physician, and in two large data base studies, poorer outcomes were noted for both CABG and PTCA in diabetics versus nondiabetics but, among diabetics, no survival difference was noted between PTCA and CABG.[122] Similar trends were noted in two large community studies. Diabetic patients as a group in the BARI trial had a greater prevalence of triple-vessel disease, LV dysfunction, and a history of congestive heart failure. It is noteworthy that in the Emory University study of diabetic patients, approximately 85 percent of those with triple-vessel disease underwent bypass surgery, whereas the use of PTCA and CABG was similar among those with double-vessel disease. A plausible explanation for the differences in results in the registry and data base studies compared with the randomized trials is that in the latter, sicker diabetic patients with triple-vessel disease and LV dysfunction, by design, were treated equally with bypass surgery and PTCA, whereas in clinical practice, such patients are referred appropriately for surgery.[122] Consistent with this notion, earlier data base studies have suggested that 3- to 5-year survival after CABG in the higher risk subgroups is superior to that obtained with PCI.

The therapeutic implications of these observations are evident. The revascularization strategy in diabetic patients should be based on the number of vessels diseased, lesion-related technical factors, the caliber of the distal vessels, and the presence or absence of LV dysfunction. Most of the comparisons between PCI and CABG described earlier involved balloon angioplasty or bare metal stents. No comparisons between PCI using drug-eluting stents and CABG are currently available. Because the major disadvantage of PCI prior to the development of drug-eluting stents has been the high rate of restenosis, which has now been substantially reduced, the fraction of patients referred for PCI is increasing, with a corresponding reduction in those referred for CABG. The choice between PCI with drug-eluting stents and CABG will likely revolve around the ability of each procedure to achieve complete revascularization in any given patient.[125,205,215]

Other Surgical Procedures for Ischemic Heart Disease

CABG may be combined with surgical procedures aimed at correction of atherosclerotic disease elsewhere in the cardiovascular system, correction of mechanical complications of myocardial infarction (mitral regurgitation or ventricular septal defect), LV aneurysms, and concomitant valvular heart disease. Not unexpectedly, morbidity and mortality are correspondingly increased because of the added complexity of the procedure and, in many patients who require these other procedures, the presence of underlying LV dysfunction (see later).

TRANSMYOCARDIAL LASER REVASCULARIZATION. Transmyocardial laser revascularization (TMLR) is performed by placing a laser on the epicardial surface of the left ventricle, exposed through a lateral thoracotomy, and creating small channels from the epicardial to endocardial surfaces. TMLR has been reported to improve symptoms in patients with refractory angina; however, the mechanism and magnitude of benefit remain uncertain.[216] The initial assumption was that laser-mediated channels would provide a network of functional connections between the LV cavity and the ischemic myocardium. Subsequent observations demonstrating closure of the channels within hours or days despite apparent relief of symptoms have led to alternative explanations for the apparent clinical success of the procedure. These explanations include improved perfusion by stimulation of angiogenesis, a placebo effect, and an anesthetic effect mediated by the destruction of sympathetic nerves carrying pain-sensitive afferent fibers or periprocedural infarction. The failure of two sham-controlled trials of percutaneous laser myocardial revascularization to show any benefit has highlighted the impact of placebo effect in response to laser myocardial revascularization.[216] On the basis of data from the randomized trials, it would appear that the widespread use of TMLR as a stand-alone method cannot be justified. Because of the perioperative morbidity associated with surgical TMLR, careful selection of patients is necessary.[217]

OTHER MANIFESTATIONS OF CORONARY ARTERY DISEASE

Prinzmetal (Variant) Angina

See Chapter 53.

Chest Pain with Normal Coronary Arteriogram

The syndrome of angina or angina-like chest pain with a normal coronary arteriogram, often termed *syndrome X* (to be differentiated from metabolic syndrome X, characterized by abdominal obesity, hypertriglyceridemia, low HDL cholesterol, insulin resistance, hyperinsulinemia, and hypertension), is an important clinical entity that should be distinguished from classic ischemic heart disease caused by obstructive CAD. Patients with chest pain and normal coronary arteriograms may represent as many as 10 to 20 percent of those undergoing coronary arteriography because of clinical suspicion of angina. The cause(s) of the syndrome is not conclusively defined and is likely not homogeneous. However, vascular dysfunction and myocardial metabolic abnormalities have been implicated.[218] True myocardial ischemia, reflected in the production of lactate by the myocardium during exercise or pacing, is present in some of these patients; however, others have no metabolic evidence for ischemia as the cause of their discomfort. The incidence of coronary calcification on multislice CT scanning is significantly higher than that of normal controls (53 versus 20 percent) but lower than that in patients with angina secondary to obstructive CAD (96 percent). The prognosis of patients with angina and normal or near-normal coronary angiography is generally more favorable than that for those with angina caused by obstructive coronary atherosclerosis. However, observational data have indicated that their outcome is not as uniformly excellent as suggested by early cohort studies.[219,220]

It has been postulated that the syndrome of angina pectoris with normal coronary arteries reflects a number of conditions. Included in syndrome X are patients with endothelial dysfunction or microvascular dysfunction or spasm in whom angina may be the result of ischemia.[218] This condition is frequently termed *microvascular angina*. In others, chest discomfort without ischemia may be caused by abnormal pain perception or sensitivity.[221] Also, IVUS studies have demonstrated anatomical and physiological heterogeneity of syndrome X, with a spectrum ranging from normal coronary arteries to vessels with intimal thickening and

atheromatous plaque but without critical obstructions.[218] It is likely that some patients with syndrome X have a combination of pathobiological contributors. In addition, it is difficult to distinguish patients with syndrome X in whom chest pain is caused by ischemia from patients with noncardiac pain. Behavioral or psychiatric disorders may be evident.

MICROVASCULAR DYSFUNCTION (INADEQUATE VASODILATOR RESERVE). Patients with chest pain, angiographically normal coronary arteries, and no evidence of large-vessel spasm, even after an acetylcholine challenge, may demonstrate an abnormally decreased capacity to reduce coronary resistance and increase coronary flow in response to stimuli such as exercise, adenosine, dipyridamole, and atrial pacing.[222] These patients also have an exaggerated response of small coronary vessels to vasoconstrictor stimuli and an impaired response to intracoronary papaverine. Abnormal endothelium-dependent vasoreactivity has been associated with regional myocardial perfusion defects on SPECT and PET imaging.[223] It has been reported that patients with syndrome X also have impaired vasodilator reserve in forearm vessels and airway hyperresponsiveness, which suggests that the smooth muscle of systemic arteries and other organs may be affected in addition to that of the coronary circulation.

Endothelial dysfunction and endothelial cell activation, reported in patients with syndrome X, may participate in the release of cellular adhesion molecules, proinflammatory cytokines, and constricting mediators that induce changes in the arterial wall, resulting in microvascular dysfunction and higher risk for future development of obstructive CAD.[218] Patients with syndrome X have been observed to have higher levels of circulating intercellular adhesion molecule-1, vasoconstrictor endothelin-1, and inflammatory marker hsCRP; moreover, the level of hsCRP appears to correlate with the severity of symptoms and burden of ischemic electrocardiographic changes.[224]

EVIDENCE FOR ISCHEMIA. Despite general acceptance that microvascular and/or endothelial dysfunction is present in many patients with syndrome X, whether ischemia is in fact the putative cause of the symptoms in these patients is not clear. Studies of transmyocardial production of lactate have generated mixed results.[218] The development of LV dysfunction and electrocardiographic or scintigraphic abnormalities during exercise in some of these patients supports an ischemic cause. However, stress echocardiography with dobutamine detects regional contraction abnormalities consistent with ischemia in a subset of patients. More sensitive techniques, such as perfusion analysis with MRI, have demonstrated that subendocardial perfusion abnormalities, in particular, may be associated with syndrome X.

ABNORMAL PAIN PERCEPTION. The lack of definitive evidence of ischemia in some patients with syndrome X has focused attention on alternative nonischemic causes of cardiac-related pain, including a decreased threshold for pain perception—the so-called sensitive heart syndrome.[221] This hypersensitivity may result in an awareness of chest pain in response to stimuli such as arterial stretch or changes in heart rate, rhythm, or contractility. A sympathovagal imbalance with sympathetic predominance in some of these patients has also been postulated. At the time of cardiac catheterization, some patients with syndrome X are unusually sensitive to intracardiac instrumentation, with typical chest pain being consistently produced by direct right atrial stimulation and saline infusion. Measurements of regional cerebral blood flow at rest and during chest pain have suggested differential handling of afferent stimuli between patients with syndrome X and those with obstructive CAD.[225]

Clinical Features

The syndrome of angina or angina-like chest pain with normal epicardial arteries occurs more frequently in women, many of whom are premenopausal, whereas obstructive CAD is found more commonly in men and postmenopausal women.[218] Fewer than half of patients with syndrome X have typical angina pectoris; most have various forms of atypical chest pain. Although the features are frequently atypical, the chest pain may nonetheless be severe and disabling. The condition may have markedly adverse effects on the quality of life, employment, and use of health care resources.

In some patients with minimal or no CAD, an exaggerated preoccupation with personal health is associated with the chest pain, and panic disorder may be responsible in a proportion of such patients. Up to two thirds of patients with chest pain and normal coronary arteries have been observed to have psychiatric disorders. Others have reported that the incidence of obstructive CAD is extremely low in patients with atypical chest pain who are anxious and/or depressed. The association between syndrome X and insulin resistance warrants further study.

PHYSICAL AND LABORATORY EXAMINATION. Abnormal physical findings reflecting ischemia, such as a precordial bulge, gallop sound, and the murmur of mitral regurgitation, are uncommon in syndrome X. The resting ECG may be normal, but nonspecific ST-T wave abnormalities are often observed, sometimes occurring in association with the chest pain. Approximately 20 percent of patients with chest pain and normal coronary arteriograms have positive exercise tests. However, many patients with this syndrome do not complete the exercise test because of fatigue or mild chest discomfort. LV function is usually normal at rest and during stress, unlike the situation in obstructive CAD, in which function often becomes impaired during stress.

PROGNOSIS. Important prognostic information on patients with angina and normal or near-normal coronary arteriograms has been obtained from the CASS Registry. In patients with an ejection fraction of 0.50 or more, the 7-year survival rate was 96 percent for patients with a normal arteriogram and 92 percent for those whose arteriographic study revealed mild disease (50 percent luminal stenosis). Thus, long-term survival of patients with anginal chest pain and normal coronary angiograms is generally excellent, markedly better than in patients with obstructive CAD. Clinical indicators of worse prognosis may be evident. Some but not all studies have indicated that an ischemic response to exercise is associated with increased mortality.[219] Moreover, in women with angina and no obstructive CAD enrolled in the Women's Ischemic Syndrome Evaluation (WISE), persistence of symptoms was associated with a more than two-fold higher risk of cardiovascular events.[226] Such patients may be appropriate candidates for formal studies of vascular function and aggressive risk factor modification.[218] (See also Chap. 76.)

MANAGEMENT. In patients with angina-like chest pain syndrome and normal epicardial coronary arteries, noncardiac causes, such as esophageal abnormalities, should be considered. In patients with syndrome X in whom ischemia can be demonstrated by noninvasive stress testing, a trial of antiischemic therapy with nitrates, calcium channel blockers, and beta blockers is logical, but the response to this therapy is variable. Perhaps because of the heterogeneity of this population, studies testing these antianginal therapies have produced conflicting results.[218] For example, beta blockers may be most effective in patients with syndrome X who also have evidence of increased sympathetic nervous activity (e.g., tachycardia and reduced heart rate variability). Sublingual nitroglycerin has shown paradoxical effects on blood flow and exercise tolerance in some studies and beneficial effects in others. Alpha blockers have been demonstrated to be ineffective. Observational studies of calcium antagonists have in general shown disappointing results with respect to amelioration of symptoms.[218]

ACE inhibitors have favorable effects on endothelial function, vascular remodeling, and sympathetic tone that may be relevant to the pathophysiology of syndrome X. Preliminary data studying ACE inhibitors in this population are promising. Similarly, estrogen has been shown to attenuate normal coronary vasomotor responses to acetylcholine, increase coronary blood flow, and potentiate endothelium-dependent vasodilation in postmenopausal women. Studies of estrogen replacement in postmenopausal women with syndrome X have shown improvement in symptoms and/or exercise performance; however, the role of exogenous estrogen in treatment of this group remains in question. Aimed at the altered somatic and visceral pain perception in many patients with syndrome X, imipramine (50 mg) and structured psychological intervention have been reported to be helpful in some.[218]

Silent Myocardial Ischemia

The prognostic importance and the mechanisms of silent ischemia have been the subject of considerable interest for almost 30 years. Patients with silent ischemia have been stratified into three categories by Cohn and associates.[227] The first and least common form, type I silent ischemia, occurs in totally asymptomatic patients with obstructive CAD, which may be severe. These patients do not experience angina at any time; indeed, some type I patients do not even experience pain in the course of myocardial infarction. Epidemiological studies of sudden death (see Chap. 36), as well as clinical and postmortem studies of patients with silent myocardial infarction and studies of patients with chronic angina pectoris, have suggested that many patients with extensive coronary artery obstruction never experience angina pectoris in any of its recognized forms (stable, unstable, or variant). These patients with type I silent ischemia may be considered to have a defective anginal warning system. Type II silent ischemia is the form that occurs in patients with documented previous myocardial infarction.

The third and much more frequent form, designated type III silent ischemia, occurs in patients with the usual forms of chronic stable angina, unstable angina, and Prinzmetal angina. When monitored, patients with this form of silent ischemia exhibit some episodes of ischemia that are associated with chest discomfort and other episodes that are not—that is, episodes of silent (asymptomatic) ischemia. The total ischemic burden in these patients refers to the total period of ischemia, both symptomatic and asymptomatic.

AMBULATORY ELECTROCARDIOGRAPHY. The use of ambulatory electrocardiographic monitoring has led to a greater appreciation of the high frequency of type III silent ischemia, occurring in up to one third of patients with stable angina treated with appropriate therapy.[227] It has become apparent that anginal pain underestimates the frequency of significant cardiac ischemia.[228]

The role of myocardial O_2 demand in the genesis of myocardial ischemia has been evaluated by measuring the heart rate and blood pressure changes preceding silent ischemic events during ambulatory studies. In one series, 92 percent of all episodes were silent, and 60 to 70 percent were preceded by significant increases in heart rate or blood pressure. The circadian variations in heart rate and blood pressure also paralleled the increase in silent ischemic events. This and other studies have suggested that increases in myocardial O_2 demand have a significant role in the genesis of silent ischemia, but in other patients reductions in myocardial O_2 supply may make an important contribution to the initiation of both symptomatic and asymptomatic episodes. The mechanisms underlying the development of ischemia, as detected by ambulatory electrocardiographic and exercise testing, may be different, and, in patients in the ACIP study, concordance between the ambulatory ECG and SPECT was only 50 percent. For identification of silent ischemia, the two techniques probably complement each other.

Transient ST segment depression of 0.1 mV or more that lasts longer than 30 seconds is a rare finding in normal subjects. Patients with known CAD show a strong correlation between such transient ST segment depression and independent measurements of impaired regional myocardial perfusion and ischemia, determined by rubidium-82 uptake as measured by PET. In patients with type III silent ischemia, perfusion defects occur in the same myocardial regions during symptomatic and asymptomatic episodes of ST segment depression.

Type III silent ischemia is extremely common. Analysis of ambulatory electrocardiographic recordings among patients with CAD who had both symptomatic and silent myocardial ischemia has shown that 85 percent of ambulant ischemic episodes occur without chest pain and 66 percent of angina reports were unaccompanied by ST segment depression. Their frequency is such that it has been suggested that overt angina pectoris is merely the "tip of the ischemic iceberg." In patients with stable CAD enrolled 1 to 6 months after hospitalization for an acute ischemic event, only 15 percent had angina with exercise,

CH 54

but 28 percent had ST segment depression and 41 percent had reversible myocardial perfusion defects on thallium scintigraphy. Episodes of silent ischemia have been estimated to be present in approximately one third of all treated patients with angina, although a higher prevalence has been reported in diabetics.[229] Episodes of ST segment depression, symptomatic and asymptomatic, exhibit a circadian rhythm and are more common in the morning. Asymptomatic nocturnal ST segment changes are almost invariably an indicator of double- or triple-vessel CAD or left main coronary artery stenosis.

Pharmacological agents that reduce or abolish episodes of symptomatic ischemia (e.g., nitrates, beta blockers, calcium antagonists) also reduce or abolish episodes of silent ischemia.[227]

MECHANISMS OF SILENT ISCHEMIA. It is not clear why some patients with unequivocal evidence of ischemia do not experience chest pain, whereas others are symptomatic. Differences in both peripheral and central neural processing of pain have been proposed as important factors underlying silent ischemia. PET imaging of cerebral blood flow during painful versus silent ischemia has pointed toward differences in handling of afferent signals by the central nervous system. Specifically, overactive gating of afferent signals in the thalamus may reduce the cortical activation necessary for perception of pain from the heart. Autonomic neuropathy has also been implicated as a reason for reduced sensation of pain during ischemia. Although increased release of endorphins may play a role in some patients with silent ischemia, the results of clinical studies are mixed.[227] Some researchers have suggested that antiinflammatory cytokines are at play in reducing inflammatory processes that may participate in the genesis of cardiac pain.

PROGNOSIS. Although some controversy remains, ample evidence has supported the view that episodes of myocardial ischemia, regardless of whether they are symptomatic or asymptomatic, are of prognostic importance in patients with CAD.[227,230] In asymptomatic patients (type I), the presence of exercise-induced ST segment depression has been shown to predict a fourfold to fivefold increase in cardiac mortality in comparison with patients without this finding. Similarly, in patients with stable angina or prior myocardial infarction, the presence of inducible ischemia evident by ST depression or perfusion abnormalities during exercise testing is associated with unfavorable outcomes, regardless of whether symptoms are present.[231] The strength of this association is greatest when the ischemia is found to occur at a low workload. Several studies evaluating the prognostic implications of silent ischemia on ambulatory monitoring in patients with stable angina (type III) have demonstrated that the presence of myocardial ischemia on the ambulatory ECG, whether silent or symptomatic, is also associated with an adverse cardiac outcome. Moreover, in the ACIP study, in patients treated medically, myocardial ischemia detected by the ambulatory ECG and by an abnormal exercise treadmill test result were each independently associated with adverse cardiac outcomes. However, other studies have not detected a relationship between silent ischemia on ambulatory monitoring and subsequent hard outcomes.

Nevertheless, when the subgroup of patients with ischemia on stress testing is considered, silent ischemia on Holter monitoring is also a significant predictor of subsequent death or myocardial infarction. In addition, patients with ischemia on the ambulatory ECG are more likely to have multivessel CAD, severe proximal stenoses, and a greater frequency of complex lesion morphology, including intracoronary thrombus, ulceration, and eccentric lesions, than patients without evidence of ischemia on ambulatory monitoring. The presence of severe and complex CAD may partly explain the apparent independent effect of silent ischemia during ambulatory monitoring on prognosis.

Substantial improvements in technology have made long-term ambulatory monitoring for ischemia more convenient and reliable with respect to data quality.[232] Nevertheless, whether the incremental prognostic information provided by adding an ambulatory ECG to a standard stress test justifies the cost of using this modality as a tool for widespread screening remains to be determined, but it is unlikely. The exercise ECG can identify most patients likely to have significant ischemia during their daily activities and remains the most important screening test for significant CAD. Many patients with type I silent ischemia have been identified because of an asymptomatic positive exercise ECG obtained following myocardial infarction. In such patients, with a defective anginal warning system, it is reasonable to assume

that asymptomatic ischemia has a significance similar to that of symptomatic ischemia and that their management with respect to disease modifying preventive therapy, coronary angiography, and revascularization should be similar.

MANAGEMENT. Drugs that are effective in preventing episodes of symptomatic ischemia (e.g., nitrates, calcium antagonists, beta blockers) are also effective in reducing or eliminating episodes of silent ischemia.[227] A number of studies have shown that beta blockers reduce the frequency, duration, and severity of silent ischemia in a dose-dependent fashion. For example, in the Atenolol Silent Ischemia Study Trial (ASIST), 4 weeks of atenolol therapy decreased the number of ischemic episodes detected on ambulatory ECG (from 3.6 to 1.7; $P < 0.001$) and also the average duration (from 30 to 16.4 minutes/48 hours; $P < 0.001$). Coronary revascularization is also effective in reducing the rate of both angina and ambulatory ischemia. In the ACIP pilot study, 57 percent of patients treated with revascularization were free of ischemia at 1 year, compared with 31 and 36 percent in the "ischemia-" and "angina-guided" strategies, respectively ($P < 0.0001$). Aggressive secondary prevention with lipid-lowering therapy has also been shown to reduce ischemia on ambulatory monitoring.

Although suppression of ischemia in patients with asymptomatic ischemia appears to be a worthwhile objective, whether treatment should be guided by symptoms or by ischemia as reflected by the ambulatory ECG has not been established. In a study of bisoprolol, nifedipine, and a combination of the two, patients achieving complete eradication of ischemia, symptomatic and asymptomatic, were less likely to suffer death, myocardial infarction, or angina requiring revascularization. Similarly, amelioration of all symptomatic and asymptomatic ischemia in the ASIST trial conferred an advantage with respect to the primary endpoint of death, resuscitated ventricular tachycardia or ventricular fibrillation, myocardial infarction, unstable angina, revascularization, or worsening angina. However, in the ACIP trial, no differences in outcome were detected between the groups allocated to ischemia-guided versus angina-guided therapy. In contrast, the early benefits of revascularization on ischemia were associated with improved clinical outcomes. Specifically, the rate of death or myocardial infarction was 12.1 percent in the angina-guided strategy, 8.8 percent in the ischemia-guided strategy, and 4.7 percent in the revascularization strategy, and a strong reduction was also seen in recurrent hospitalizations and the revascularization strategies. Patients who continue to suffer silent ischemia after revascularization may be at increased risk for recurrent cardiac events compared with those who are free of any ischemia.[233]

Heart Failure in Ischemic Heart Disease

Currently, the leading cause of heart failure in developed countries is CAD.[234] In the United States, CAD and its complications account for two thirds to three fourths of all cases of heart failure. In many patients, the progressive nature of heart failure reflects the progressive nature of the underlying CAD. The term *ischemic cardiomyopathy* is used for the clinical syndrome in which one or more of the pathophysiological features just discussed result in LV dysfunction and heart failure symptoms.[235] This condition is the predominant form of heart failure related to CAD. Additional complications of CAD that may become superimposed on ischemic cardiomyopathy and precipitate heart failure are the development of LV aneurysm and mitral regurgitation caused by papillary muscle dysfunction.

In 1970, Burch and colleagues first used the term *ischemic cardiomyopathy* to describe the condition in which CAD results in severe myocardial dysfunction, with clinical manifestations often indistinguishable from those of primary dilated cardiomyopathy (see Chap. 64). Symptoms of heart failure caused by ischemic myocardial dysfunction and hibernation, diffuse fibrosis, or multiple infarctions, alone or in combination, may dominate the clinical picture of CAD. In some patients with chronic CAD, angina may be the principal clinical manifestation at one time, but later this symptom diminishes or even disappears as heart failure becomes more prominent. Other patients with ischemic cardiomyopathy have no history of angina or myocardial infarction (type I silent ischemia), and it is in this subgroup that ischemic cardiomyopathy is most often confused with dilated cardiomyopathy.

It is important to recognize hibernating myocardium in patients with ischemic cardiomyopathy because symptoms resulting from chronic LV dysfunction may be incorrectly thought to result from necrotic and scarred myocardium rather than from a reversible ischemic process.[236] Hibernating myocardium may be present in patients with known or suspected CAD with a degree of cardiac dysfunction or heart failure not readily accounted for by previous myocardial infarctions.

The outlook for patients with ischemic cardiomyopathy treated medically is poor, and revascularization or cardiac transplantation may be considered.[188] The prognosis is particularly poor for patients in whom ischemic cardiomyopathy is caused by multiple myocardial infarctions, in those with associated ventricular arrhythmias, and in those with extensive amounts of hibernating myocardium. However, this last group of patients, whose heart failure, even if severe, is caused by large segments of reversibly dysfunctional but viable myocardium, appear to have a significantly better prognosis after revascularization. Revascularization in this group also significantly relieves heart failure symptoms. Thus, the key to management of patients with ischemic cardiomyopathy is to assess the extent of residual viable myocardium with a view to coronary revascularization of viable myocardium. Patients with little or no viable myocardium in whom heart failure is secondary to extensive myocardial infarction and/or fibrosis should be managed in a manner similar to those with dilated cardiomyopathy (see Chaps. 25 and 64). Their prognosis is poor.

Additional, more rigorous, adequately sized observational studies and randomized controlled trials are needed to determine the efficacy of revascularization versus medical therapy and to define the role of viability testing. Three such studies are underway—the Surgical Treatment for Ischemic Heart Failure (STICH) trial, the Heart Failure Revascularization Trial (HEART), and the PET and Recovery Following Revascularization-2 (PARR-2) study.[188]

Left Ventricular Aneurysm

LV aneurysm is usually defined as a segment of the ventricular wall that exhibits paradoxical (dyskinetic) systolic expansion. Chronic fibrous aneurysms interfere with ventricular performance principally through loss of contractile tissue. Aneurysms made up largely of a mixture of scar tissue and viable myocardium or of thin scar tissue also impair LV function by a combination of paradoxical expansion and loss of effective contraction.[237] False aneurysms (pseudoaneurysms) represent localized myocardial rupture in which the hemorrhage is limited by pericardial adhesions, and have a mouth that is considerably smaller than the maximal diameter (Fig. 54-20). True and false aneurysms may coexist, although the combination is extremely rare.

The frequency of LV aneurysms depends on the incidence of transmural myocardial infarction and congestive heart failure in the population studied. LV aneurysms and the need for aneurysmectomy have declined dramatically during the last 5 to 10 years in concert with the expanded use of acute reperfusion therapy in evolving myocardial infarction. More than 80 percent of LV aneurysms are located anterolaterally near the apex. They are often associated with total occlusion of the LAD coronary artery and a poor collateral blood supply. Approximately 5 to 10 percent of aneurysms are located posteriorly. Three fourths of patients with aneurysms have multivessel CAD.

Almost 50 percent of patients with moderate or large aneurysms have symptoms of heart failure, with or without associated angina, approximately 33 percent have severe angina alone, and approximately 15 percent have symptomatic ventricular arrhythmias that may be intractable and life threatening. Mural thrombi are found in almost half of patients with chronic LV aneurysms and can be detected by angiography and two-dimensional echocardiography (see Chap. 14). Systemic embolic

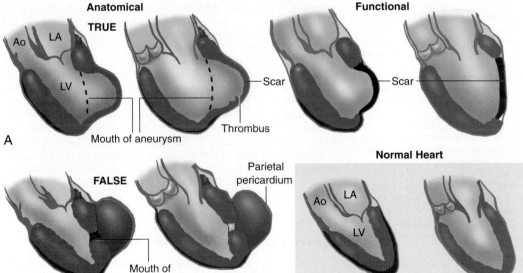

Left Ventricular Aneurysm in Coronary Heart Disease

Anatomical

Functional

TRUE

Ao — LA

LV

Scar

Scar

Thrombus

A — Mouth of aneurysm

FALSE

Parietal pericardium

Normal Heart

Ao — LA

LV

Mouth of aneurysm

B — Systole — Diastole — Systole — Diastole

FIGURE 54–20 Hearts in systole and diastole with true and false anatomical and functional left ventricular (LV) aneurysms and healed myocardial infarction. A normal heart in systole and diastole is shown for comparison **(inset). A,** A true anatomical left ventricular aneurysm protrudes during both systole and diastole, has a mouth that is as wide as or wider than the maximal diameter, has a wall that was formerly the wall of the left ventricle, and is composed of fibrous tissue with or without residual myocardial fibers. A true aneurysm may or may not contain thrombus and almost never ruptures once the wall is healed. **B,** A false anatomical left ventricular aneurysm protrudes during both systole and diastole, has a mouth that is considerably smaller than the maximal diameter of the aneurysm and represents a myocardial rupture site, has a wall made up of parietal pericardium, almost always contains thrombus, and often ruptures. A functional left ventricular aneurysm protrudes during ventricular systole but not during diastole and consists of fibrous tissue with or without myocardial fibers. Ao = aorta; LA = left atrium. *(From Cabin HS, Roberts WC: Left ventricular aneurysm, intraaneurysmal thrombus, and systemic embolus in coronary heart disease. Chest 77:586, 1980.)*

events in patients with thrombi and LV aneurysm tend to occur early after myocardial infarction. In patients with chronic LV aneurysm (documented at least 1 month after infarction), subsequent systemic emboli were extremely uncommon (0.35/100 patient-years in patients not receiving anticoagulants).

DETECTION. Clues to the presence of aneurysm include persistent ST segment elevations on the resting ECG (in the absence of chest pain) and a characteristic bulge of the silhouette of the left ventricle on a chest roentgenogram. Marked calcification of the LV silhouette may be present. These findings, when clear-cut, are relatively specific, but they have limited sensitivity. Radionuclide ventriculography and two-dimensional echocardiography can demonstrate LV aneurysm more readily; the latter is also helpful in distinguishing between true and false aneurysms based on the demonstration of a narrow neck in relation to cavity size in the latter. Color-flow echocardiographic imaging is useful in establishing the diagnosis because flow "in and out" of the aneurysm as well as abnormal flow within the aneurysm can be detected, and subsequent pulsed Doppler imaging can reveal a "to-and-fro" pattern with characteristic respiratory variation in the peak systolic velocity. CMR may be emerging as the preferred noninvasive technique for the preoperative assessment of ventricular shape, thinning, and resectability.[238]

LEFT VENTRICULAR ANEURYSMECTOMY. True LV aneurysms do not rupture, and operative excision is carried out to improve the clinical manifestations, most often heart failure but sometimes also angina, embolization, and life-threatening tachyarrhythmias.[237] Coronary revascularization is frequently performed along with aneurysmectomy, especially in patients in whom angina accompanies heart failure.

A large LV aneurysm in a patient with symptoms of heart failure, particularly if angina pectoris is also present, is an indication for surgery. The operative mortality rate for LV aneurysmectomy is approximately 8 percent (ranging from 2 to 19 percent), with rates as low as 3 percent reported in more recent series.[239] Risk factors for early death include poor LV function, triple-vessel disease, recent myocardial infarction, presence of mitral regurgitation, and intractable ventricular arrhythmias.[239] The presence of angina pectoris instead of dyspnea as the dominant preoperative symptom is associated with lower operative mortality. Surgery carries a particularly high risk in patients with severe heart failure, a low-output state, and akinesis of the interventricular septum, as assessed echocardiographically. Akinesis or dyskinesia of the posterior basal segment of the left ventricle and significant right coronary artery stenoses are additional risk factors.

Risk factors for late mortality following survival from surgery include incomplete revascularization, impaired systolic function of the basal segments of the ventricle and septum not involved by the aneurysm, the presence of a large aneurysm with a small quantity of residual viable myocardium, and the presence of severe cardiac failure as the initial feature.

Improvement in LV function has been reported in survivors of resection of LV aneurysms. Anterior ventricular restoration has the potential to reverse adverse remodeling, realign contractile fibers, and decrease ventricular wall stress. By removing the abnormal mechanical burden, LV aneurysmectomy has been associated with late improvement in overall systolic function and improvement in the performance of regional nonischemic myocardium in zones remote from the LV aneurysm, in addition to improvement in measures of LV relaxation and cardiovascular neuroregulatory mechanisms A concomitant improvement in exercise performance and clinical symptoms may also occur, particularly in patients who have undergone complete revascularization. In one series of 285 patients, 67 percent of patients undergoing ventricular reconstruction had an improvement in symptoms, with a survival of 82 percent at 5 years.[237]

Newer surgical approaches to the repair of LV aneurysms are designed to restore normal LV geometry by using an alternative method of epicardial closure and/or an endocardial patch to divide the area of the aneurysm from the remainder of the ventricular cavity (Fig. 54-21). Favorable clinical and hemodynamic results following the use of these newer techniques have been reported, with 5-year survival rates ranging from 73 to 87.5 percent and a corresponding improvement in hemodynamics and clinical symptoms.[239] In one series, 88 percent of patients treated with the endoaneurysmorrhaphy technique were in NYHA Class I or II after a mean follow-up of approximately 3.5 years.

The value of surgical therapy, including surgical ventricular restoration, for patients with ischemic cardiomyopathy is being tested in the ongoing Surgical Treatment for Ischemic Heart Failure (STICH) trial.

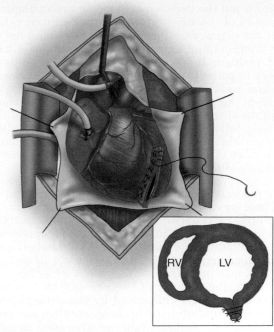

FIGURE 54–21 Linear repair technique used in left ventricular (LV) aneurysm repair. The aneurysm walls are closed in a vertical line between two layers of Teflon felt. Two layers of interrupted horizontal mattress sutures are reinforced with two layers of running sutures. RV = right ventricle. *(From Glower DD, Lowe JE: Left ventricular aneurysm. In Cohn LC, Edmunds LH [eds]: Cardiac Surgery in the Adult. New York, McGraw-Hill, 2003, p 597.)*

CH 54

Chronic Coronary Artery Disease

Mitral Regurgitation Secondary to Coronary Artery Disease

Mitral regurgitation is an important cause of heart failure in some patients with CAD. Rupture of a papillary muscle or the head of a papillary muscle usually causes severe acute mitral regurgitation in the course of acute myocardial infarction (see Chap. 62). The cause of chronic mitral regurgitation in patients with CAD is multifactorial and the geometric determinants are complex; these include papillary muscle dysfunction from ischemia and fibrosis in conjunction with a wall motion abnormality and changes in ventricular shape in the region of the papillary muscle and/or dilation of the mitral annulus.[240] Enlargement of the mitral annulus at end-systole is asymmetrical, with lengthening primarily involving the posterior annular segments and leading to prolapse of leaflet tissue tethered by the posterior papillary muscle and restriction of leaflet tissue attached to the anterior leaflet. Most patients with chronic CAD and mitral regurgitation have suffered a previous MI. Clinical features that help identify mitral regurgitation secondary to papillary muscle dysfunction as the cause of acute pulmonary edema or of milder symptoms of left-sided failure include a loud systolic murmur and demonstration of a flail mitral valve leaflet on echocardiography.

In some patients with severe mitral regurgitation into a small, unprepared left atrium, the murmur may be unimpressive or inaudible. Doppler echocardiography is helpful in assessing the severity of the regurgitation (see Chap. 14). As in mitral regurgitation of other causes, the left atrium is not usually greatly enlarged unless mitral regurgitation has been present for more than 6 months. The ECG is nonspecific, and most patients have angiographic evidence of multivessel CAD.

MANAGEMENT. In patients with severe mitral regurgitation, the indications for surgical correction, usually in association with CABG, are fairly clear-cut. Mitral valve repair, as opposed to mitral replacement, is the procedure of choice, but the decision is based on the anatomical characteristics of the structures forming the mitral valve apparatus, the urgency of the need for surgery, and the severity of LV dysfunction. A more complex and frequently encountered problem involves the indications for mitral valve surgery in patients undergoing CABG in whom the severity of mitral regurgitation is moderate.[240] The decision is based partly on the presence or absence of structural abnormalities of the mitral apparatus and the amenability of the valve to repair. Intraoperative transesophageal echocardiography is invaluable in assessing the severity of regurgitation, the reparability of the valve, and the success of the integrity of the repair after discontinuation of CPB.

The mortality associated with combined CABG and mitral valve placement in the 2005 Society of Thoracic Surgeons data base was approximately 10 percent. For bypass surgery and mitral valve repair, mortality from 1995 to 2005 was 7 percent overall, including emergency and reoperative procedures.[155] Predictors of early mortality include the need for replacement versus repair (in some but not all series) but, in addition, may include other variables such as age, comorbid conditions, the urgency of surgery, and LV function. Late results are strongly influenced by the pathophysiological mechanisms underlying mitral regurgitation and are poorer in patients with regurgitation resulting from annular dilation or restrictive leaflet motion than in patients with chordal or papillary muscle rupture. It is encouraging that despite the relatively high operative mortality, late survival of hospital survivors is excellent. In patients with very poor LV function and dilation of the mitral annulus, mitral regurgitation can intensify the severity of LV failure. In such patients, the risk of surgery is high and the long-term benefit is not established,[241] and a trial of intensive medical therapy, including afterload reduction, beta blockade, and biventricular pacing (see Chap. 25) may be worthwhile, because favorable remodeling may reduce the severity of mitral regurgitation. For those patients undergoing CABG, the procedural risks associated with combined CABG and mitral valve repair may outweigh the benefit of reduced mitral regurgitation in those at highest perioperative risk.[242]

Cardiac Arrhythmias

In some patients with CAD, cardiac arrhythmias are the dominant clinical manifestation of the disease. Various degrees and forms of ventricular ectopic activity are the most common arrhythmias in patients with CAD, but serious ventricular arrhythmias may be a major component of the clinical findings in other subgroups. The clinical presentation of arrhythmias and their management in patients with CAD are discussed in Chapters 32 and 33.

Nonatheromatous Coronary Artery Disease

Although atherosclerosis is by far the most important cause of CAD, other conditions may also be responsible. The most common causes of nonatheromatous CAD resulting in myocardial ischemia are the syndrome of angina-like pain with normal coronary arteriograms (i.e., so-called syndrome X) and Prinzmetal angina (see Chap. 53).

Nonatheromatous CAD may result from other diverse abnormalities, including congenital abnormalities in the origin or distribution of the coronary arteries (see Chaps. 20 and 61). The most important of these abnormalities are anomalous origin of a coronary artery (usually the left) from the pulmonary artery, origin of both coronary arteries from either the right or the left sinus of Valsalva, and coronary arteriovenous fistula.[243] An anomalous origin of the left main coronary artery or right coronary artery from the aorta, with subsequent coursing between the aorta and pulmonary trunk, is a rare and sometimes fatal coronary arterial anomaly. Coronary anomalies are reported to cause between 12 and 19 percent of sports-related deaths in U.S. high school and college athletes and account for one third of cardiac anomalies in military recruits with nontraumatic sudden death.[244]

MYOCARDIAL BRIDGING. This cause of systolic compression of the LAD coronary artery is a well-recognized angiographic phenomenon of questionable clinical significance.[245]

CONNECTIVE TISSUE DISORDERS. Several inherited connective tissue disorders are associated with myocardial ischemia (see Chap. 8), including Marfan syndrome (causing aortic and coronary artery dissection), Hurler syndrome (causing coronary obstruction), homocystinuria (causing coronary artery thrombosis), Ehlers-Danlos syndrome (causing coronary artery dissection), and pseudoxanthoma elasticum (causing accelerated CAD). Kawasaki disease, the mucocutaneous lymph node syndrome), may cause coronary artery aneurysms and ischemic heart disease in children.

SPONTANEOUS CORONARY DISSECTION. This is a rare cause of myocardial infarction and sudden cardiac death.[246] Chronic dissection manifested as congestive heart failure has been described. In one series, approximately 75 percent of cases were diagnosed at autopsy and 75 percent occurred in women, half of which were associated with a postpartum state. Some cases are associated with atherosclerosis. Hypertension has been postulated as a cause of multivessel spontaneous coronary dissection in some patients and, in others, no obvious cause has been identified. In the acute phase, thrombolytic therapy may be dangerous, but early angiography may identify patients who could benefit from stenting or bypass surgery. In survivors of spontaneous coronary artery dissection, the subsequent 3-year mortality was 20 percent, but complete healing as defined angiographically may lead to a favorable outcome without intervention.

CORONARY VASCULITIS. This condition, resulting from connective tissue diseases or autoimmune forms of vasculitis, including polyarteritis nodosa, giant cell (temporal) arteritis, and scleroderma, has been well described (see Chap. 84). Coronary arteritis is seen at autopsy in about 20 percent of patients with rheumatoid arthritis but is rarely associated with clinical manifestations. The incidence of CAD is increased in women with systemic lupus erythematosus (SLE). In SLE patients, CAD has been attributed to a vasculitis, immune complex-mediated endothelial damage, and coronary thrombosis from antiphospholipid antibodies, as well as accelerated atherosclerosis. Giant coronary artery aneurysm associated with SLE is an unusual manifestation that has been associated with the development of acute myocardial infarction, despite therapy. The antiphospholipid syndrome, characterized by arterial and venous thrombosis and associated with the presence of antiphospholipid antibodies, may be associated with myocardial infarction, angina, and diffuse LV dysfunction.

TAKAYASU ARTERITIS. In rare cases (see Chap. 84), this condition is associated with angina, myocardial infarction, and cardiac failure in patients younger than 40 years of age. Coronary blood flow may be decreased by involvement of the ostia or proximal segments of the coronary arteries, but disease in distal coronary segments is rare.[247] The average age at onset of symptoms is 24 years, and the event-free survival rate 10 years after diagnosis is approximately 60 percent. Luetic aortitis may also produce myocardial ischemia by causing coronary ostial obstruction.

POSTMEDIASTINAL IRRADIATION. The occurrence of CAD and morbid cardiac events in young persons after mediastinal irradiation is highly suggestive of a cause and effect relationship.[248] Pathological changes include adventitial scarring and medial hypertrophy with severe intimal atherosclerotic disease. Radiation injury may be latent and may not be manifested clinically for many years after therapy. Contributory factors include higher doses than those currently administered and the presence of cardiac risk factors.[249] Among patients without risk factors who receive an intermediate total dose of 30 and 40 Gy, the risk of cardiac death and myocardial infarction is low.

Myocardial ischemia not caused by coronary atherosclerosis can also result from embolism from infective endocarditis (see Chap. 63), implanted prosthetic cardiac valves (see Chap. 62), calcified aortic valves, mural thrombi, and primary cardiac tumors (see Chap. 69).

COCAINE (see Chap. 68). Because of its widespread use, cocaine has become a well-documented cause of chest pain, myocardial infarction, and sudden cardiac death.[250] In a population-based study of sudden death in persons 20 to 40 years old in Olmsted County over a 30-year period, a high prevalence of cocaine abuse was observed in the more recent cohort of young adults who died suddenly. The principal effects of cocaine are mediated by alpha-adrenergic stimulation, which causes an increase in myocardial O_2 demand and a reduction in O_2 supply because of coronary vasoconstriction.

Cardiac Transplantation–Associated Coronary Arteriopathy

See Chapters 27 and 38.

REFERENCES

1. American Heart Association: Heart Disease and Stroke Statistics—2006 Update. Dallas, American Heart Association, 2006.
2. Bonow RO, Smaha LA, Smith SC Jr, et al: World Heart Day 2002: The international burden of cardiovascular disease: Responding to the emerging global epidemic. Circulation 106:1602, 2002.
3. American Heart Association: International cardiovascular disease statistics. Dallas, American Heart Association, 2006.

Stable Angina Pectoris

4. Abidov A, Rozanski A, Hachamovitch R, et al: Prognostic significance of dyspnea in patients referred for cardiac stress testing. N Engl J Med 353:1889, 2005.
5. Dagenais GR, Armstrong PW, Theroux P, Naylor CD: Revisiting the Canadian Cardiovascular Society grading of stable angina pectoris after a quarter of a century of use. Can J Cardiol 18:941, 2002.
6. Pan HL, Chen SR: Sensing tissue ischemia: Another new function for capsaicin receptors? Circulation 110:1826, 2004.
7. Wang L, Wang DH: TRPV1 gene knockout impairs postischemic recovery in isolated perfused heart in mice. Circulation 112:3617, 2005.
8. Hirsch AT, Haskal ZJ, Hertzer NR, et al: ACC/AHA 2005 Practice Guidelines for the management of patients with peripheral arterial disease (lower extremity, renal, mesenteric, and abdominal aortic): A collaborative report from the American Association for Vascular Surgery/Society for Vascular Surgery, Society for Cardiovascular Angiography and Interventions, Society for Vascular Medicine and Biology, Society of Interventional Radiology, and the ACC/AHA Task Force on Practice Guidelines (Writing Committee to Develop Guidelines for the Management of Patients With Peripheral Arterial Disease): Endorsed by the American Association of Cardiovascular and Pulmonary Rehabilitation; National Heart, Lung, and Blood Institute; Society for Vascular Nursing; TransAtlantic Inter-Society Consensus; and Vascular Disease Foundation. Circulation 113:e463, 2006.
9. Feringa HH, Bax JJ, van Waning VH, et al: The long-term prognostic value of the resting and postexercise ankle-brachial index. Arch Intern Med 166:529, 2006.
10. Gibbons RJ, Abrams J, Chatterjee K, et al: ACC/AHA 2002 guideline update for the management of patients with chronic stable angina—summary article: A report of the American College of Cardiology/American Heart Association Task Force on practice guidelines (Committee on the Management of Patients With Chronic Stable Angina). J Am Coll Cardiol 41:159, 2003.
11. Meisinger C, Doring A, Lowel H: Chronic kidney disease and risk of incident myocardial infarction and all-cause and cardiovascular disease mortality in middle-aged men and women from the general population. Eur Heart J 27:1245, 2006.

Noninvasive Testing

12. Walldius G, Jungner I: Rationale for using apolipoprotein B and apolipoprotein A-I as indicators of cardiac risk and as targets for lipid-lowering therapy. Eur Heart J 26:210, 2005.
13. Grundy SM: Low-density lipoprotein, non-high-density lipoprotein, and apolipoprotein B as targets of lipid-lowering therapy. Circulation 106:2526, 2002.
14. O'Donoghue M, Morrow DA, Sabatine MS, et al: Lipoprotein-associated phospholipase A2 and its association with cardiovascular outcomes in patients with acute coronary syndromes in the PROVE IT-TIMI 22 (PRavastatin Or atorVastatin Evaluation and Infection Therapy-Thrombolysis In Myocardial Infarction) trial. Circulation 113:1745, 2006.
15. Smith SC Jr, Milani RV, Arnett DK, et al: Atherosclerotic Vascular Disease Conference: Writing Group II: Risk factors. Circulation 109:2613, 2004.
16. Ridker PM: Clinical application of C-reactive protein for cardiovascular disease detection and prevention. Circulation 107:363, 2003.
17. Ridker PM, Rifai N, Rose L, et al: Comparison of C-reactive protein and low-density lipoprotein cholesterol levels in the prediction of first cardiovascular events. N Engl J Med 347:1557, 2002.
18. Pearson TA, Mensah GA, Alexander RW, et al: Markers of inflammation and cardiovascular disease: application to clinical and public health practice: A statement for healthcare professionals from the Centers for Disease Control and Prevention and the American Heart Association. Circulation 107:499, 2003.
19. Heeschen C: Beyond C-reactive protein: Novel markers of vascular inflammation. In Morrow DA (ed): Cardiovascular Biomarkers: Pathophysiology and Disease Management. Totowa, NJ, Humana Press, 2006, pp 277-294.
20. Morrow DA, de Lemos JA, Sabatine MS, Antman EM: The search for a biomarker of cardiac ischemia. Clin Chem 49:537, 2003.
21. Sabatine MS, Morrow DA, de Lemos JA, et al: Acute changes in circulating natriuretic peptide levels in response to myocardial ischemia. J Am Coll Cardiol 44:1988, 2004.
22. Wang TJ, Larson MG, Levy D, et al: Plasma natriuretic peptide levels and the risk of cardiovascular events and death. N Engl J Med 350:655, 2004.
23. Gibbons RJ, Balady GJ, Bricker JT, et al: ACC/AHA 2002 guideline update for exercise testing: summary article: A report of the American College of Cardiology/American Heart Association Task Force on Practice Guidelines (Committee to Update the 1997 Exercise Testing Guidelines). Circulation 106:1883, 2002.
24. Vlassak I, Rubin DN, Odabashian JA, et al: Contrast and harmonic imaging improves accuracy and efficiency of novice readers for dobutamine stress echocardiography. Echocardiography 19:483, 2002.
25. Voigt JU, Exner B, Schmiedehausen K, et al: Strain-rate imaging during dobutamine stress echocardiography provides objective evidence of inducible ischemia. Circulation 107:2120, 2003.
26. Albers AR, Krichavsky MZ, Balady GJ: Stress testing in patients with diabetes mellitus: Diagnostic and prognostic value. Circulation 113:583, 2006.
27. Budoff MJ, Diamond GA, Raggi P, et al: Continuous probabilistic prediction of angiographically significant coronary artery disease using electron beam tomography. Circulation 105:1791, 2002.
28. Chen J, Krumholz HM: How useful is computed tomography for screening for coronary artery disease? Screening for coronary artery disease with electron-beam computed tomography is not useful. Circulation 113:125; discussion 125, 2006.
29. Budoff MJ, Achenbach S, Blumenthal RS, et al: Assessment of coronary artery disease by cardiac computed tomography. A scientific statement from the American Heart Association Committee on Cardiovascular Imaging and Intervention, Council on Cardiovascular Radiology and Intervention, and Committee on Cardiac Imaging, Council on Clinical Cardiology. Circulation 114:1761, 2006.
30. Garcia MJ, Lessick J, Hoffmann MHK, for the CATSCAN Study Investigators: Accuracy of 16-Row Multidetector Computed Tomography for the Assessment of Coronary Artery Stenosis. JAMA 296:403, 2006.
31. Fuster V, Kim RJ: Frontiers in cardiovascular magnetic resonance. Circulation 112:135, 2005.
32. Klein C, Nekolla SG, Bengel FM, et al: Assessment of myocardial viability with contrast-enhanced magnetic resonance imaging: Comparison with positron emission tomography. Circulation 105:162, 2002.
33. Gerber BL, Garot J, Bluemke DA, et al: Accuracy of contrast-enhanced magnetic resonance imaging in predicting improvement of regional myocardial function in patients after acute myocardial infarction. Circulation 106:1083, 2002.
34. Kuijpers D, Ho KY, van Dijkman PR, et al: Dobutamine cardiovascular magnetic resonance for the detection of myocardial ischemia with the use of myocardial tagging. Circulation 107:1592, 2003.
35. Moody AR, Murphy RE, Morgan PS, et al: Characterization of complicated carotid plaque with magnetic resonance direct thrombus imaging in patients with cerebral ischemia. Circulation 107:3047, 2003.
36. Langerak SE, Vliegen HW, Jukema JW, et al: Value of magnetic resonance imaging for the noninvasive detection of stenosis in coronary artery bypass grafts and recipient coronary arteries. Circulation 107:1502, 2003.

Coronary Angiography

37. Nicholls SJ, Tuzcu EM, Sipahi I, et al: Intravascular ultrasound in cardiovascular medicine. Circulation 114:e55, 2006.
38. Satran A, Bart BA, Henry CR, et al: Increased prevalence of coronary artery aneurysms among cocaine users. Circulation 111:2424, 2005.
39. Mohlenkamp S, Hort W, Ge J, Erbel R: Update on myocardial bridging. Circulation 106:2616, 2002.

Risk Stratification

40. Braunwald E, Domanski MJ, Fowler SE, et al: Angiotensin-converting-enzyme inhibition in stable coronary artery disease. N Engl J Med 351:2058, 2004.
41. Myers J, Prakash M, Froelicher V, et al: Exercise capacity and mortality among men referred for exercise testing. N Engl J Med 346:793, 2002.
42. Schoenhagen P, Nissen S: Understanding coronary artery disease: Tomographic imaging with intravascular ultrasound. Heart 88:91, 2002.
43. Bigi R, Cortigiani L, Colombo P, et al: Prognostic and clinical correlates of angiographically diffuse non-obstructive coronary lesions. Heart 89:1009, 2003.

Management of Risk Factors

44. Chobanian AV, Bakris GL, Black HR, et al: The Seventh Report of the Joint National Committee on Prevention, Detection, Evaluation, and Treatment of High Blood Pressure: The JNC 7 report. JAMA 289:2560, 2003.
45. Lewington S, Clarke R, Qizilbash N, et al: Age-specific relevance of usual blood pressure to vascular mortality: A meta-analysis of individual data for one million adults in 61 prospective studies. Lancet 360:1903, 2002.
46. Psaty BM, Lumley T, Furberg CD, et al: Health outcomes associated with various antihypertensive therapies used as first-line agents: A network meta-analysis. JAMA 289:2534, 2003.
47. Smith SC Jr, Allen J, Blair SN, et al: AHA/ACC guidelines for secondary prevention for patients with coronary and other atherosclerotic vascular disease: 2006 update: Endorsed by the National Heart, Lung, and Blood Institute. Circulation 113:2363, 2006.
48. Critchley JA, Capewell S: Mortality risk reduction associated with smoking cessation in patients with coronary heart disease: A systematic review. JAMA 290:86, 2003.
49. Heart Protection Study Collaborative Group: MRC/BHF Heart Protection Study of cholesterol lowering with simvastatin in 20,536 high-risk individuals: A randomised placebo-controlled trial. Lancet 360:7, 2002.
50. Nissen SE, Nicholls SJ, Sipahi I, et al: Effect of very high-intensity statin therapy on regression of coronary atherosclerosis: The ASTEROID trial. JAMA 295:1556, 2006.
51. Ray KK, Cannon CP: The potential relevance of the multiple lipid-independent (pleiotropic) effects of statins in the management of acute coronary syndromes. J Am Coll Cardiol 46:1425, 2005.
52. LaRosa JC, Grundy SM, Waters DD, et al: Intensive lipid lowering with atorvastatin in patients with stable coronary disease. N Engl J Med 352:1425, 2005.
53. Pedersen TR, Faergeman O, Kastelein JJ, et al: High-dose atorvastatin vs usual-dose simvastatin for secondary prevention after myocardial infarction: The IDEAL study: A randomized controlled trial. JAMA 294:2437, 2005.
54. Cannon CP, Braunwald E, McCabe CH, et al: Intensive versus moderate lipid lowering with statins after acute coronary syndromes. N Engl J Med 350:1495, 2004.
55. Ansell BJ, Watson KE, Fogelman AM, et al: High-density lipoprotein function: Recent advances. J Am Coll Cardiol 46:1792, 2005.

CH 54

Chronic Coronary Artery Disease

56. Duffy D, Rader DJ: Emerging therapies targeting high-density lipoprotein metabolism and reverse cholesterol transport. Circulation 113:1140, 2006.

56a. Nissen SE, Tardif JC, Nicholls SJ, et al: Effect of torcetrapib on the progression of coronary atherosclerosis. N Engl J Med 356:1304-1316, 2007.

56b. Tall AR: CETP inhibitors to increase HDL cholesterol levels. N Engl J Med 356:1364-1366, 2007.

57. Nathan DM, Cleary PA, Backlund JY, et al: Intensive diabetes treatment and cardiovascular disease in patients with type 1 diabetes. N Engl J Med 353:2643, 2005.

58. Dormandy JA, Charbonnel B, Eckland DJ, et al: Secondary prevention of macrovascular events in patients with type 2 diabetes in the PROactive Study (PROspective pioglitAzone Clinical Trial In macroVascular Events): A randomised controlled trial. Lancet 366:1279, 2005.

59. Thompson PD, Buchner D, Pina IL, et al: Exercise and physical activity in the prevention and treatment of atherosclerotic cardiovascular disease. Circulation 107:3109, 2003.

60. Hambrecht R, Walther C, Mobius-Winkler S, et al: Percutaneous coronary angioplasty compared with exercise training in patients with stable coronary artery disease: A randomized trial. Circulation 109:1371, 2004.

61. Hambrecht R, Adams V, Erbs S, et al: Regular physical activity improves endothelial function in patients with coronary artery disease by increasing phosphorylation of endothelial nitric oxide synthase. Circulation 107:3152, 2003.

62. Libby P, Aikawa M: Stabilization of atherosclerotic plaques: New mechanisms and clinical targets. Nat Med 8:1257, 2002.

63. Ridker PM, Cannon CP, Morrow D, et al: C-reactive protein levels and outcomes after statin therapy. N Engl J Med 352:20, 2005.

64. Morrow DA, de Lemos JA, Sabatine MS, et al: Clinical relevance of C-reactive protein during follow-up of patients with acute coronary syndromes in the Aggrastat-to-Zocor Trial. Circulation 114:281, 2006.

65. Antithrombotic Trialists' Collaboration: Collaborative meta-analysis of randomised trials of antiplatelet therapy for prevention of death, myocardial infarction, and stroke in high-risk patients. BMJ 324:71, 2002.

66. Steinhubl SR, Berger PB, Mann JT 3rd, et al: Early and sustained dual oral antiplatelet therapy following percutaneous coronary intervention: A randomized controlled trial. JAMA 288:2411, 2002.

67. Bhatt DL, Fox KA, Hacke W, et al: Clopidogrel and aspirin versus aspirin alone for the prevention of atherothrombotic events. N Engl J Med 354:1706, 2006.

68. Go AS, Iribarren C, Chandra M, et al: Statin and beta-blocker therapy and the initial presentation of coronary heart disease. Ann Intern Med 144:229, 2006.

69. Bunch TJ, Muhlestein JB, Bair TL, et al: Effect of beta-blocker therapy on mortality rates and future myocardial infarction rates in patients with coronary artery disease but no history of myocardial infarction or congestive heart failure. Am J Cardiol 95:827, 2005.

70. Fox KM: Efficacy of perindopril in reduction of cardiovascular events among patients with stable coronary artery disease: Randomised, double-blind, placebo-controlled, multicentre trial (the EUROPA study). Lancet 362:782, 2003.

71. Solomon SD, Rice MM, Jablonski KA, et al: Renal function and effectiveness of angiotensin-converting enzyme inhibitor therapy in patients with chronic stable coronary disease in the Prevention of Events with ACE inhibition (PEACE) trial. Circulation 114:26, 2006.

72. Salonen RM, Nyyssonen K, Kaikkonen J, et al: Six-year effect of combined vitamin C and E supplementation on atherosclerotic progression: The Antioxidant Supplementation in Atherosclerosis Prevention (ASAP) Study. Circulation 107:947, 2003.

73. Heart Protection Study Collaborative Group: MRC/BHF Heart Protection Study of antioxidant vitamin supplementation in 20,536 high-risk individuals: A randomised placebo-controlled trial. Lancet 360:23, 2002.

74. Lonn E, Yusuf S, Arnold MJ, et al: Homocysteine lowering with folic acid and B vitamins in vascular disease. N Engl J Med 354:1567, 2006.

75. Bonaa KH, Njolstad I, Ueland PM, et al: Homocysteine lowering and cardiovascular events after acute myocardial infarction. N Engl J Med 354:1578, 2006.

76. Empana JP, Sykes DH, Luc G, et al: Contributions of depressive mood and circulating inflammatory markers to coronary heart disease in healthy European men: The Prospective Epidemiological Study of Myocardial Infarction (PRIME). Circulation 111:2299, 2005.

77. Glassman AH, O'Connor CM, Califf RM, et al: Sertraline treatment of major depression in patients with acute MI or unstable angina. JAMA 288:701, 2002.

78. Rosengren A, Hawken S, Ounpuu S, et al: Association of psychosocial risk factors with risk of acute myocardial infarction in 11119 cases and 13648 controls from 52 countries (the INTERHEART study): Case-control study. Lancet 364:953, 2004.

79. Lichtenstein AH, Appel LJ, Brands M, et al: Diet and lifestyle recommendations revision 2006: A scientific statement from the American Heart Association Nutrition Committee. Circulation 114:82, 2006.

80. Kostis JB, Jackson G, Rosen R, et al: Sexual dysfunction and cardiac risk (the Second Princeton Consensus Conference). Am J Cardiol 96:85M, 2005.

Pharmacological Management of Angina Pectoris

81. Bottcher M, Madsen MM, Randsbaek F, et al: Effect of oral nitroglycerin and cold stress on myocardial perfusion in areas subtended by stenosed and nonstenosed coronary arteries. Am J Cardiol 89:1019, 2002.

82. Tadamura E, Mamede M, Kubo S, et al: The effect of nitroglycerin on myocardial blood flow in various segments characterized by rest-redistribution thallium SPECT. J Nucl Med 44:745, 2003.

83. Munzel T, Mulsch A, Kleschyov A: Mechanisms underlying nitroglycerin-induced superoxide production in platelets: Some insight, more questions. Circulation 106:170, 2002.

84. Chen Z, Zhang J, Stamler JS: Identification of the enzymatic mechanism of nitroglycerin bioactivation. Proc Natl Acad Sci U S A 99:8306, 2002.

85. Gruhn N, Boesgaard S, Eiberg J, et al: Effects of large conductance Ca$^{(2+)}$-activated K$^{(+)}$ channels on nitroglycerin-mediated vasorelaxation in humans. Eur J Pharmacol 446:145, 2002.

86. Gori T, Parker JD: Long-term therapy with organic nitrates: The pros and cons of nitric oxide replacement therapy. J Am Coll Cardiol 44:632, 2004.

87. Muller S, Laber U, Mullenheim J, et al: Preserved endothelial function after long-term eccentric isosorbide mononitrate despite moderate nitrate tolerance. J Am Coll Cardiol 41:1994, 2003.

88. Kardas P: Comparison of once-daily versus twice-daily oral nitrates in stable angina pectoris. Am J Cardiol 94:213, 2004.

89. Gori T, Parker JD: Nitrate tolerance: A unifying hypothesis. Circulation 106:2510, 2002.

90. Hirai N, Kawano H, Yasue H, et al: Attenuation of nitrate tolerance and oxidative stress by an angiotensin II receptor blocker in patients with coronary spastic angina. Circulation 108:1446, 2003.

91. Egred M, Shaw S, Mohammad B, et al: Under-use of beta-blockers in patients with ischaemic heart disease and concomitant chronic obstructive pulmonary disease. QJM 98:493, 2005.

92. Flockhart DA, Tanus-Santos JE: Implications of cytochrome P450 interactions when prescribing medication for hypertension. Arch Intern Med 162:405, 2002.

93. Lanfear DE, Jones PG, Marsh S, et al: Beta$_2$-adrenergic receptor genotype and survival among patients receiving beta-blocker therapy after an acute coronary syndrome. JAMA 294:1526, 2005.

94. Ko DT, Hebert PR, Coffey CS, et al: Adverse effects of beta-blocker therapy for patients with heart failure: A quantitative overview of randomized trials. Arch Intern Med 164:1389, 2004.

95. Bakris GL, Fonseca V, Katholi RE, et al: Metabolic effects of carvedilol vs metoprolol in patients with type 2 diabetes mellitus and hypertension: A randomized controlled trial. JAMA 292:2227, 2004.

96. Grossman E, Messerli FH: Calcium antagonists. Prog Cardiovasc Dis 47:34, 2004.

97. The ENCORE Investigators: Effect of nifedipine and cerivastatin on coronary endothelial function in patients with coronary artery disease: The ENCORE I Study (Evaluation of Nifedipine and Cerivastatin On Recovery of coronary Endothelial function). Circulation 107:422, 2003.

98. Dens JA, Desmet WJ, Coussement P, et al: Long-term effects of nisoldipine on the progression of coronary atherosclerosis and the occurrence of clinical events: The NICOLE study. Heart 89:887, 2003.

99. Pepine CJ, Handberg EM, Cooper-DeHoff RM, et al: A calcium antagonist vs a non-calcium antagonist hypertension treatment strategy for patients with coronary artery disease. The International Verapamil-Trandolapril Study (INVEST): A randomized controlled trial. JAMA 290:2805, 2003.

100. Chaitman BR: Ranolazine for the treatment of chronic angina and potential use in other cardiovascular conditions. Circulation 113:2462, 2006.

101. Rousseau MF, Pouleur H, Cocco G, Wolff AA: Comparative efficacy of ranolazine versus atenolol for chronic angina pectoris. Am J Cardiol 95:311, 2005.

102. Chaitman BR, Pepine CJ, Parker JO, et al: Effects of ranolazine with atenolol, amlodipine, or diltiazem on exercise tolerance and angina frequency in patients with severe chronic angina: A randomized controlled trial. JAMA 291:309, 2004.

102a. Morrow DA, Scirica BM, Karwatowska-Prokopczuk E, et al: Effects of ranolazine on recurrent cardiovascular events in patients with non-ST-elevation acute coronary syndromes: The MERLIN-TIMI 36 Randomized Trial. JAMA 297:1775, 2007.

103. Antzelevitch C, Belardinelli L, Zygmunt AC, et al: Electrophysiological effects of ranolazine, a novel antianginal agent with antiarrhythmic properties. Circulation 110:904, 2004.

104. Simpson D, Wellington K: Nicorandil: A review of its use in the management of stable angina pectoris, including high-risk patients. Drugs 64:1941, 2004.

105. Walker A, McMurray J, Stewart S, et al: Economic evaluation of the impact of nicorandil in angina (IONA) trial. Heart 92:619, 2006.

106. DiFrancesco D, Camm JA: Heart rate lowering by specific and selective I(f) current inhibition with ivabradine: A new therapeutic perspective in cardiovascular disease. Drugs 64:1757, 2004.

107. Borer JS, Fox K, Jaillon P, Lerebours G: Antianginal and antiischemic effects of ivabradine, an I(f) inhibitor, in stable angina: A randomized, double-blind, multi-centered, placebo-controlled trial. Circulation 107:817, 2003.

108. Tardif JC, Ford I, Tendera M, et al: Efficacy of ivabradine, a new selective I(f) inhibitor, compared with atenolol in patients with chronic stable angina. Eur Heart J 26:2529, 2005.

109. Vicari RM, Chaitman B, Keefe D, et al: Efficacy and safety of fasudil in patients with stable angina: a double-blind, placebo-controlled, phase 2 trial. J Am Coll Cardiol 46:1803, 2005.

110. Morrow DA, Givertz MM: Modulation of myocardial energetics: Emerging evidence for a therapeutic target in cardiovascular disease. Circulation 112:3218, 2005.

111. Gheorghiade M, Colucci WS, Swedberg K: Beta-blockers in chronic heart failure. Circulation 107:1570, 2003.

112. Yang EH, Barsness GW, Gersh BJ, et al: Current and future treatment strategies for refractory angina. Mayo Clin Proc 79:1284, 2004.

113. Ekre O, Eliasson T, Norrsell H, et al: Long-term effects of spinal cord stimulation and coronary artery bypass grafting on quality of life and survival in the ESBY study. Eur Heart J 23:1938, 2002.

114. Bonetti PO, Holmes DR Jr, Lerman A, Barsness GW: Enhanced external counterpulsation for ischemic heart disease: What's behind the curtain? J Am Coll Cardiol 41:1918, 2003.

115. Soran O, Kennard ED, Kfoury AG, Kelsey SF: Two-year clinical outcomes after enhanced external counterpulsation (EECP) therapy in patients with refractory

CH 54

angina pectoris and left ventricular dysfunction (report from The International EECP Patient Registry). Am J Cardiol 97:17, 2006.

116. Akhtar M, Wu GF, Du ZM, et al: Effect of external counterpulsation on plasma nitric oxide and endothelin-1 levels. Am J Cardiol 98:28, 2006.

Percutaneous Coronary Intervention

117. Sousa JE, Costa MA, Tuzcu EM, et al: New frontiers in interventional cardiology. Circulation 111:671, 2005.

118. Wu C, Hannan EL, Walford G, et al: A risk score to predict in-hospital mortality for percutaneous coronary interventions. J Am Coll Cardiol 47:654, 2006.

119. Herzog CA, Ma JZ, Collins AJ: Comparative survival of dialysis patients in the United States after coronary angioplasty, coronary artery stenting, and coronary artery bypass surgery and impact of diabetes. Circulation 106:2207, 2002.

120. Katritsis DG, Ioannidis JP: Percutaneous coronary intervention versus conservative therapy in nonacute coronary artery disease: A meta-analysis. Circulation 111:2906, 2005.

121. Boden WE, O'Rourke RA, Teo KK, et al: Optimal medical therapy with or without PCI for stable coronary disease. N Engl J Med 356:1503, 2007.

122. Gersh BJ, Frye RL: Methods of coronary revascularization—things may not be as they seem. N Engl J Med 352:2235, 2005.

123. Dangas G, Moses JW: Is surgery preferred for the diabetic with multivessel disease? Debate on revascularization strategy for diabetic patients with multivessel coronary artery disease. Circulation 112:1507; discussion, 1514, 2005.

124. King SB 3rd: Is surgery preferred for the diabetic with multivessel disease? Surgery is preferred for the diabetic with multivessel disease. Circulation 112:1500; discussion, 1514, 2005.

125. Sobel BE, Frye R, Detre KM: Burgeoning dilemmas in the management of diabetes and cardiovascular disease: Rationale for the Bypass Angioplasty Revascularization Investigation 2 Diabetes (BARI 2D) Trial. Circulation 107:636, 2003.

126. Keelan PC, Johnston JM, Koru-Sengul T, et al: Comparison of in-hospital and one-year outcomes in patients with left ventricular ejection fractions ≤40%, 41% to 49%, and ≥50% having percutaneous coronary revascularization. Am J Cardiol 91:1168, 2003.

Coronary Artery Bypass Surgery

127. Keenan TD, Abu-Omar Y, Taggart DP: Bypassing the pump: Changing practices in coronary artery surgery. Chest 128:363, 2005.

128. Argenziano M, Katz M, Bonatti J, et al: Results of the prospective multicenter trial of robotically assisted totally endoscopic coronary artery bypass grafting. Ann Thorac Surg 81:1666; discussion, 1674, 2006.

129. Verma S, Fedak PW, Weisel RD, et al: Off-pump coronary artery bypass surgery: Fundamentals for the clinical cardiologist. Circulation 109:1206, 2004.

130. Sellke FW, DiMaio JM, Caplan LR, et al; American Heart Association: Comparing on-pump and off-pump coronary artery bypass grafting: Numerous studies but few conclusions: A scientific statement from the American Heart Association council on cardiovascular surgery and anesthesia in collaboration with the interdisciplinary working group on quality of care and outcomes research. Circulation 111:2858, 2005.

131. Vassiliades TA Jr, Douglas JS, Morris DC, et al: Integrated coronary revascularization with drug-eluting stents: Immediate and seven-month outcome. J Thorac Cardiovasc Surg 131:956, 2006.

132. Dogan S, Graubitz K, Aybek T, et al: How safe is the port access technique in minimally invasive coronary artery bypass grafting? Ann Thorac Surg 74:1537, 2002.

133. Oliveira SA, Lisboa LA, Dallan LA, et al: Minimally invasive single-vessel coronary artery bypass with the internal thoracic artery and early postoperative angiography: Midterm results of a prospective study in 120 consecutive patients. Ann Thorac Surg 73:505, 2002.

134. Diegeler A, Thiele H, Falk V, et al: Comparison of stenting with minimally invasive bypass surgery for stenosis of the left anterior descending coronary artery. N Engl J Med 347:561, 2002.

135. Thiele H, Oettel S, Jacobs S, et al: Comparison of bare-metal stenting with minimally invasive bypass surgery for stenosis of the left anterior descending coronary artery: A 5-year follow-up. Circulation 112:3445, 2005.

136. Parolari A, Alamanni F, Polvani G, et al: Meta-analysis of randomized trials comparing off-pump with on-pump coronary artery bypass graft patency. Ann Thorac Surg 80:2121, 2005.

137. Wijeysundera DN, Beattie WS, Djaiani G, et al: Off-pump coronary artery surgery for reducing mortality and morbidity: Meta-analysis of randomized and observational studies. J Am Coll Cardiol 46:872, 2005.

138. Puskas JD, Williams WH, Duke PG, et al: Off-pump coronary artery bypass grafting provides complete revascularization with reduced myocardial injury, transfusion requirements, and length of stay: A prospective randomized comparison of two hundred unselected patients undergoing off-pump versus conventional coronary artery bypass grafting. J Thorac Cardiovasc Surg 125:797, 2003.

139. Al-Ruzzeh S, George S, Bustami M, et al: Effect of off-pump coronary artery bypass surgery on clinical, angiographic, neurocognitive, and quality of life outcomes: Randomised controlled trial. BMJ 332:1365, 2006.

140. Jones RH: The year in cardiovascular surgery. J Am Coll Cardiol 47:2094, 2006.

141. Onorati F, De Feo M, Mastroroberto P, et al: Determinants and prognosis of myocardial damage after coronary artery bypass grafting. Ann Thorac Surg 79:837, 2005.

142. Guru V, Omura J, Alghamdi AA, et al: Is blood superior to crystalloid cardioplegia? A meta-analysis of randomized clinical trials. Circulation 114:I331, 2006.

143. Mangano DT, Miao Y, Tudor IC, Dietzel C: Post-reperfusion myocardial infarction: Long-term survival improvement using adenosine regulation with acadesine. J Am Coll Cardiol 48:206, 2006.

144. Aziz O, Athanasiou T, Panesar SS, et al: Does minimally invasive vein harvesting technique affect the quality of the conduit for coronary revascularization? Ann Thorac Surg 80:2407, 2005.

145. Kachhy RG, Kong DF, Honeycutt E, et al: Long-term outcomes of the symmetry vein graft anastomosis device: a matched case-control analysis. Circulation 114:I425, 2006.

146. Dabal RJ, Goss JR, Maynard C, Aldea GS: The effect of left internal mammary artery utilization on short-term outcomes after coronary revascularization. Ann Thorac Surg 76:464, 2003.

147. Nishida H, Tomizawa Y, Endo M, Kurosawa H: Survival benefit of exclusive use of in situ arterial conduits over combined use of arterial and vein grafts for multiple coronary artery bypass grafting. Circulation 112:I299, 2005.

148. Baskett RJ, Cafferty FH, Powell SJ, et al: Total arterial revascularization is safe: Multicenter ten-year analysis of 71,470 coronary procedures. Ann Thorac Surg 81:1243, 2006.

149. Lytle BW, Blackstone EH, Sabik JF, et al: The effect of bilateral internal thoracic artery grafting on survival during 20 postoperative years. Ann Thorac Surg 78:2005; discussion, 2012, 2004.

150. Zacharias A, Habib RH, Schwann TA, et al: Radial artery conduits in coronary artery bypass grafting: Current perspective. J Thorac Cardiovasc Surg 130:232, 2005.

151. Muneretto C, Negri A, Manfredi J, et al: Safety and usefulness of composite grafts for total arterial myocardial revascularization: A prospective randomized evaluation. J Thorac Cardiovasc Surg 125:826, 2003.

152. Shroyer AL, Coombs LP, Peterson ED, et al: The Society of Thoracic Surgeons: 30-day operative mortality and morbidity risk models. Ann Thorac Surg 75:1856, 2003.

153. Cram P, Rosenthal GE, Vaughan-Sarrazin MS: Cardiac revascularization in specialty and general hospitals. N Engl J Med 352:1454, 2005.

154. Ferguson TB Jr, Hammill BG, Peterson ED, et al: A decade of change—risk profiles and outcomes for isolated coronary artery bypass grafting procedures, 1990-1999: A report from the STS National Database Committee and the Duke Clinical Research Institute. Society of Thoracic Surgeons. Ann Thorac Surg 73:480, 2002.

155. Society of Thoracic Surgeons: Cumulative Mortality for CABG-only Operations, 2005 (http://www.sts.org/sections/stsnationaldatabase/html).

156. Shahian DM, Blackstone EH, Edwards FH, et al: Cardiac surgery risk models: A position article. Ann Thorac Surg 78:1868, 2004.

157. Nalysnyk L, Fahrbach K, Reynolds MW, et al: Adverse events in coronary artery bypass graft (CABG) trials: A systematic review and analysis. Heart 89:767, 2003.

158. Ramsay J, Shernan S, Fitch J, et al: Increased creatine kinase MB level predicts postoperative mortality after cardiac surgery independent of new Q waves. J Thorac Cardiovasc Surg 129:300, 2005.

159. Serrano N, Garcia C, Villegas J, et al: Prolonged intubation rates after coronary artery bypass surgery and ICU risk stratification score. Chest 128:595, 2005.

160. Leavitt BJ, Ross CS, Spence B, et al: Long-term survival of patients with chronic obstructive pulmonary disease undergoing coronary artery bypass surgery. Circulation 114:I430, 2006.

161. Karthik S, Grayson AD, McCarron EE, et al: Reexploration for bleeding after coronary artery bypass surgery: Risk factors, outcomes, and the effect of time delay. Ann Thorac Surg 78:527; discussion, 534, 2004.

162. Mehta RH, Roe MT, Mulgund J, et al: Acute clopidogrel use and outcomes in patients with non-ST-segment elevation acute coronary syndromes undergoing coronary artery bypass surgery. J Am Coll Cardiol 48:281, 2006.

163. Toumpoulis IK, Anagnostopoulos CE, Derose JJ Jr, Swistel DG: The impact of deep sternal wound infection on long-term survival after coronary artery bypass grafting. Chest 127:464, 2005.

164. Dacey LJ, Likosky DS, Leavitt BJ, et al: Perioperative stroke and long-term survival after coronary bypass graft surgery. Ann Thorac Surg 79:532; discussion, 537, 2005.

165. Samuels MA: Can cognition survive heart surgery? Circulation 113:2784, 2006.

166. Bar-Yosef S, Anders M, Mackensen GB, et al: Aortic atheroma burden and cognitive dysfunction after coronary artery bypass graft surgery. Ann Thorac Surg 78:1556, 2004.

167. Boodhwani M, Rubens FD, Wozny D, et al: Predictors of early neurocognitive deficits in low-risk patients undergoing on-pump coronary artery bypass surgery. Circulation 114:I461, 2006.

168. Sedrakyan A, Zhang H, Treasure T, Krumholz HM: Recursive partitioning-based preoperative risk stratification for atrial fibrillation after coronary artery bypass surgery. Am Heart J 151:720, 2006.

169. Marin F, Pascual DA, Roldan V, et al: Statins and postoperative risk of atrial fibrillation following coronary artery bypass grafting. Am J Cardiol 97:55, 2006.

170. Izhar U, Ad N, Rudis E, et al: When should we discontinue antiarrhythmic therapy for atrial fibrillation after coronary artery bypass grafting? A prospective randomized study. J Thorac Cardiovasc Surg 129:401, 2005.

171. Eriksen BO, Hoff KR, Solberg S: Prediction of acute renal failure after cardiac surgery: Retrospective cross-validation of a clinical algorithm. Nephrol Dial Transplant 18:77, 2003.

172. Burns KE, Chu MW, Novick RJ, et al: Perioperative N-acetylcysteine to prevent renal dysfunction in high-risk patients undergoing cabg surgery: A randomized controlled trial. JAMA 294:342, 2005.

173. Halabi AR, Alexander JH, Shaw LK, et al: Relation of early saphenous vein graft failure to outcomes following coronary artery bypass surgery. Am J Cardiol 96:1254, 2005.

174. Tsui JC, Dashwood MR: Recent strategies to reduce vein graft occlusion: A need to limit the effect of vascular damage. Eur J Vasc Endovasc Surg 23:202, 2002.

175. Stein PD, Beemath A, Skaf E, et al: Usefulness of 4-, 8-, and 16-slice computed tomography for detection of graft occlusion or patency after coronary artery bypass grafting. Am J Cardiol 96:1669, 2005.

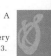

176. Stauder NI, Scheule AM, Hahn U, et al: Perioperative monitoring of flow and patency in native and grafted internal mammary arteries using a combined MR protocol. Br J Radiol 78:292, 2005.

177. Goldman S, Zadina K, Moritz T, et al: Long-term patency of saphenous vein and left internal mammary artery grafts after coronary artery bypass surgery: Results from a Department of Veterans Affairs Cooperative Study. J Am Coll Cardiol 44:2149, 2004.

178. Desai ND, Cohen EA, Naylor CD, Fremes SE: A randomized comparison of radial-artery and saphenous-vein coronary bypass grafts. N Engl J Med 351:2302, 2004.

179. Pond KK, Martin GV, Every N, et al: Predictors of progression of native coronary narrowing to total occlusion after coronary artery bypass grafting. Am J Cardiol 91:971, 2003.

180. Okrainec K, Platt R, Pilote L, Eisenberg MJ: Cardiac medical therapy in patients after undergoing coronary artery bypass graft surgery: A review of randomized controlled trials. J Am Coll Cardiol 45:177, 2005.

181. Stein PD, Schunemann HJ, Dalen JE, Gutterman D: Antithrombotic therapy in patients with saphenous vein and internal mammary artery bypass grafts: The Seventh ACCP Conference on Antithrombotic and Thrombolytic Therapy. Chest 126:600S, 2004.

182. Alexander JH, Hafley G, Harrington RA, et al: Efficacy and safety of edifoligide, an E2F transcription factor decoy, for prevention of vein graft failure following coronary artery bypass graft surgery: PREVENT IV: A randomized controlled trial. JAMA 294:2446, 2005.

183. Eagle KA, Guyton RA, Davidoff R, et al: ACC/AHA 2004 guideline update for coronary artery bypass graft surgery: A report of the American College of Cardiology/American Heart Association Task Force on Practice Guidelines (Committee to Update the 1999 Guidelines for Coronary Artery Bypass Graft Surgery). Circulation 110:e340, 2004.

184. Ng AT, Serruys PW: Complete revascularization: Coronary artery bypass graft surgery versus percutaneous coronary intervention. Circulation 114:249, 2006.

185. Unger F, Serruys PW, Yacoub MH, et al: Revascularization in multivessel disease: Comparison between two-year outcomes of coronary bypass surgery and stenting. J Thorac Cardiovasc Surg 125:809, 2003.

186. Topkara VK, Cheema FH, Kesavaramanujam S, et al: Coronary artery bypass grafting in patients with low ejection fraction. Circulation 112:I344, 2005.

187. Antunes PE, de Oliveira JM, Antunes MJ: Coronary surgery with non-cardioplegic methods in patients with advanced left ventricular dysfunction: Immediate and long-term results. Heart 89:427, 2003.

188. Chareonthaitawee P, Gersh BJ, Araoz PA, Gibbons RJ: Revascularization in severe left ventricular dysfunction: The role of viability testing. J Am Coll Cardiol 46:567, 2005.

189. Lytle BW: The role of coronary revascularization in the treatment of ischemic cardiomyopathy. Ann Thorac Surg 75:S2, 2003.

190. Gibbons RJ, Chareonthaitawee P, Bailey KR: Revascularization in systolic heart failure: A difficult decision. Circulation 113:180, 2006.

191. Klocke FJ. Resting blood flow in hypocontractile myocardium: Resolving the controversy. Circulation 112:3222, 2005.

192. Carr JA, Haithcock BE, Paone G, et al: Long-term outcome after coronary artery bypass grafting in patients with severe left ventricular dysfunction. Ann Thorac Surg 74:1531, 2002.

193. Zaglavara T, Pillay T, Karvounis H, et al: Detection of myocardial viability by dobutamine stress echocardiography: Incremental value of diastolic wall thickness measurement. Heart 91:613, 2005.

194. Tarakji KG, Brunken R, McCarthy PM, et al: Myocardial viability testing and the effect of early intervention in patients with advanced left ventricular systolic dysfunction. Circulation 113:230, 2006.

195. Selvanayagam JB, Kardos A, Francis JM, et al: Value of delayed-enhancement cardiovascular magnetic resonance imaging in predicting myocardial viability after surgical revascularization. Circulation 110:1535, 2004.

196. Rizzello V, Poldermans D, Schinkel AF, et al: Long-term prognostic value of myocardial viability and ischaemia during dobutamine stress echocardiography in patients with ischaemic cardiomyopathy undergoing coronary revascularisation. Heart 92:239, 2006.

197. Kleikamp G, Maleszka A, Reiss N, et al: Determinants of mid- and long-term results in patients after surgical revascularization for ischemic cardiomyopathy. Ann Thorac Surg 75:1406, 2003.

198. Stramba-Badiale M, Fox KM, Priori SG, et al: Cardiovascular diseases in women: A statement from the policy conference of the European Society of Cardiology. Eur Heart J 27:994, 2006.

199. Jacobs AK: Women, ischemic heart disease, revascularization, and the gender gap: What are we missing? J Am Coll Cardiol 47:S63, 2006.

200. Blankstein R, Ward RP, Arnsdorf M, et al: Female gender is an independent predictor of operative mortality after coronary artery bypass graft surgery: Contemporary analysis of 31 Midwestern hospitals. Circulation 112:I323, 2005.

201. Kurlansky PA, Williams DB, Traad EA, et al: Arterial grafting results in reduced operative mortality and enhanced long-term quality of life in octogenarians. Ann Thorac Surg 76:418, 2003.

202. Peterson ED, Alexander KP, Malenka DJ, et al: Multicenter experience in revascularization of very elderly patients. Am Heart J 148:486, 2004.

203. Cooper WA, O'Brien SM, Thourani VH, et al: Impact of renal dysfunction on outcomes of coronary artery bypass surgery: Results from the Society of Thoracic Surgeons National Adult Cardiac Database. Circulation 113:1063, 2006.

204. Hillis GS, Croal BL, Buchan KG, et al: Renal function and outcome from coronary artery bypass grafting: Impact on mortality after a 2.3-year follow-up. Circulation 113:1056, 2006.

205. Flaherty JD, Davidson CJ: Diabetes and coronary revascularization. JAMA 293:1501, 2005.

206. Hannan EL, Wu C, Bennett EV, et al: Risk stratification of in-hospital mortality for coronary artery bypass graft surgery. J Am Coll Cardiol 47:661, 2006.

207. O'Rourke DJ, Quinton HB, Piper W, et al: Survival in patients with peripheral vascular disease after percutaneous coronary intervention and coronary artery bypass graft surgery. Ann Thorac Surg 78:466; discussion, 470, 2004.

208. Naylor AR, Mehta Z, Rothwell PM, Bell PR: Carotid artery disease and stroke during coronary artery bypass: A critical review of the literature. Eur J Vasc Endovasc Surg 23:283, 2002.

209. Zacharias A, Schwann TA, Riordan CJ, et al: Operative and 5-year outcomes of combined carotid and coronary revascularization: Review of a large contemporary experience. Ann Thorac Surg 73:491, 2002.

210. Sabik JF 3rd, Blackstone EH, Gillinov AM, et al: Occurrence and risk factors for reintervention after coronary artery bypass grafting. Circulation 114:I454, 2006.

Comparisons Between PCI and CABG

211. Hannan EL, Racz MJ, Walford G, et al: Long-term outcomes of coronary-artery bypass grafting versus stent implantation. N Engl J Med 352:2174, 2005.

212. Barsness GW, Gersh BJ, Brooks MM, Frye RL: Rationale for the revascularization arm of the Bypass Angioplasty Revascularization Investigation 2 Diabetes (BARI 2D) Trial. Am J Cardiol 97:31G, 2006.

213. Legrand VM, Serruys PW, Unger F, et al: Three-year outcome after coronary stenting versus bypass surgery for the treatment of multivessel disease. Circulation 109:1114, 2004.

214. Hannan EL, Racz M, Holmes DR, et al: Impact of completeness of percutaneous coronary intervention revascularization on long-term outcomes in the stent era. Circulation 113:2406, 2006.

215. Ong AT, Serruys PW, Mohr FW, et al: The SYNergy between percutaneous coronary intervention with TAXus and cardiac surgery (SYNTAX) study: Design, rationale, and run-in phase. Am Heart J 151:1194, 2006.

Other Surgical Procedures

216. Saririan M, Eisenberg MJ: Myocardial laser revascularization for the treatment of end-stage coronary artery disease. J Am Coll Cardiol 41:173, 2003.

217. Bridges CR, Horvath KA, Nugent WC, et al: The Society of Thoracic Surgeons practice guideline series: Transmyocardial laser revascularization. Ann Thorac Surg 77:1494, 2004.

Other Manifestations of Coronary Artery Disease

218. Bugiardini R, Bairey Merz CN: Angina with "normal" coronary arteries: A changing philosophy. JAMA 293:477, 2005.

219. Johnson BD, Shaw LJ, Buchthal SD, et al: Prognosis in women with myocardial ischemia in the absence of obstructive coronary disease: Results from the National Institutes of Health-National Heart, Lung, and Blood Institute-Sponsored Women's Ischemia Syndrome Evaluation (WISE). Circulation 109:2993, 2004.

220. Bugiardini R: Women, 'non-specific' chest pain, and normal or near-normal coronary angiograms are not synonymous with favourable outcome. Eur Heart J 27:1387, 2006.

221. Valeriani M, Sestito A, Le Pera D, et al: Abnormal cortical pain processing in patients with cardiac syndrome X. Eur Heart J 26:975, 2005.

222. Handberg E, Johnson BD, Arant CB, et al: Impaired coronary vascular reactivity and functional capacity in women: Results from the NHLBI Women's Ischemia Syndrome Evaluation (WISE) Study. J Am Coll Cardiol 47:S44, 2006.

223. Schindler TH, Nitzsche E, Magosaki N, et al: Regional myocardial perfusion defects during exercise, as assessed by three dimensional integration of morphology and function, in relation to abnormal endothelium dependent vasoreactivity of the coronary microcirculation. Heart 89:517, 2003.

224. Cosin-Sales J, Pizzi C, Brown S, Kaski JC: C-reactive protein, clinical presentation, and ischemic activity in patients with chest pain and normal coronary angiograms. J Am Coll Cardiol 41:1468, 2003.

225. Rosen SD, Paulesu E, Wise RJ, Camici PG: Central neural contribution to the perception of chest pain in cardiac syndrome X. Heart 87:513, 2002.

226. Johnson BD, Shaw LJ, Pepine CJ, et al: Persistent chest pain predicts cardiovascular events in women without obstructive coronary artery disease: Results from the NIH-NHLBI-sponsored Women's Ischaemia Syndrome Evaluation (WISE) study. Eur Heart J 27:1408, 2006.

227. Cohn PF, Fox KM, Daly C: Silent myocardial ischemia. Circulation 108:1263, 2003.

228. Stern S: Symptoms other than chest pain may be important in the diagnosis of "silent ischemia," or "the sounds of silence." Circulation 111:e435, 2005.

229. Gazzaruso C, Solerte SB, De Amici E, et al: Association of the metabolic syndrome and insulin resistance with silent myocardial ischemia in patients with type 2 diabetes mellitus. Am J Cardiol 97:236, 2006.

230. Sajadieh A, Nielsen OW, Rasmussen V, et al: Prevalence and prognostic significance of daily-life silent myocardial ischaemia in middle-aged and elderly subjects with no apparent heart disease. Eur Heart J 26:1402, 2005.

231. Elhendy A, Schinkel AF, van Domburg RT, et al: Comparison of late outcome in patients with versus without angina pectoris having reversible perfusion abnormalities during dobutamine stress technetium-99m sestamibi single-photon emission computed tomography. Am J Cardiol 91:264, 2003.

232. Enseleit F, Duru F: Long-term continuous external electrocardiographic recording: A review. Europace 8:255, 2006.

233. Zellweger MJ, Weinbacher M, Zutter AW, et al: Long-term outcome of patients with silent versus symptomatic ischemia six months after percutaneous coronary intervention and stenting. J Am Coll Cardiol 42:33, 2003.

CH 54

234. Gheorghiade M, Sopko G, DeLuca L et al: Navigating the crossroads of coronary artery disease and heart failure. Circulation 114:1202, 2006.
235. Felker GM, Shaw LK, O'Connor CM: A standardized definition of ischemic cardiomyopathy for use in clinical research. J Am Coll Cardiol 39:210, 2002.
236. Carluccio E, Biagioli P, Alunni G, et al: Patients with hibernating myocardium show altered left ventricular volumes and shape, which revert after revascularization: Evidence that dyssynergy might directly induce cardiac remodeling. J Am Coll Cardiol 47:969, 2006.
237. Mickleborough LL, Merchant N, Ivanov J, et al: Left ventricular reconstruction: Early and late results. J Thorac Cardiovasc Surg 128:27, 2004.
238. Mickleborough LL, Merchant N, Provost Y, et al: Ventricular reconstruction for ischemic cardiomyopathy. Ann Thorac Surg 75:S6, 2003.
239. Lundblad R, Abdelnoor M, Svennevig JL: Repair of left ventricular aneurysm: Surgical risk and long-term survival. Ann Thorac Surg 76:719, 2003.
240. Borger MA, Alam A, Murphy PM, et al: Chronic ischemic mitral regurgitation: Repair, replace or rethink? Ann Thorac Surg 81:1153, 2006.
241. Wu AH, Aaronson KD, Bolling SF, et al: Impact of mitral valve annuloplasty on mortality risk in patients with mitral regurgitation and left ventricular systolic dysfunction. J Am Coll Cardiol 45:381, 2005.
242. Kang DH, Kim MJ, Kang SJ, et al: Mitral valve repair versus revascularization alone in the treatment of ischemic mitral regurgitation. Circulation 114:I499, 2006.

243. Rigatelli G, Docali G, Rossi P, Bandello A: Validation of a clinical-significance-based classification of coronary artery anomalies. Angiology 56:25, 2005.
244. Eckart RE, Scoville SL, Campbell CL, et al: Sudden death in young adults: A 25-year review of autopsies in military recruits. Ann Intern Med 141:829, 2004.
245. Alegria JR, Herrmann J, Holmes DR Jr, et al: Myocardial bridging. Eur Heart J 26:1159, 2005.
246. Egred M, Viswanathan G, Davis GK: Myocardial infarction in young adults. Postgrad Med J 81:741, 2005.
247. Endo M, Tomizawa Y, Nishida H, et al: Angiographic findings and surgical treatments of coronary artery involvement in Takayasu arteritis. J Thorac Cardiovasc Surg 125:570, 2003.
248. Byrd BF 3rd, Mendes LA: Cardiac complications of mediastinal radiotherapy. The other side of the coin. J Am Coll Cardiol 42:750, 2003.
249. Hull MC, Morris CG, Pepine CJ, Mendenhall NP: Valvular dysfunction and carotid, subclavian, and coronary artery disease in survivors of hodgkin lymphoma treated with radiation therapy. JAMA 290:2831, 2003.
250. Jones JH, Weir WB: Cocaine-associated chest pain. Med Clin North Am 89:1323, 2005.

GUIDELINES · *Thomas H. Lee and David A. Morrow*

Chronic Stable Angina

The American College of Cardiology and the American Heart Association (ACC/AHA) updated guidelines for management of patients with stable chest pain syndromes and known or suspected ischemic heart disease in 2002.[1] Populations addressed by these guidelines include patients with "ischemic equivalents" such as dyspnea or arm pain with exertion and patients with ischemic heart disease who have become asymptomatic including those who have undergone revascularization procedures. Patients with unstable ischemic syndromes are not included in these guidelines but are instead addressed in guidelines summarized in appendices to Chapter 53. As with other ACC/AHA guidelines, indications for interventions are classified into the following four groups:

Class I—for generally accepted indications

Class IIa—when indications are controversial, but the weight of evidence is supportive

Class IIb—when usefulness or efficacy is less well established

Class III—when there is consensus against the usefulness of the intervention

The guidelines use a convention for rating levels of evidence on which recommendations have been based, as follows:

Level A—derived from data from multiple randomized clinical trials

Level B—derived from a single randomized trial or nonrandomized studies

Level C—based on the consensus opinion of experts

OVERVIEW

The ACC/AHA guidelines emphasize the importance of detailed symptom history, focused physical examination, and directed risk-factor assessment for patients presenting with chest pain. These data are to be used by the clinician to estimate the probability of significant coronary artery disease as low, intermediate, or high. For patients with a low probability of coronary disease (e.g., ≤5 percent), cardiovascular interventions should be limited, whereas noncardiac causes of chest pain should be evaluated (Fig. 54G-1). Recommended initial tests are summarized in Table 54G-1. Routine use of chest radiographs or electron-beam computed tomography (CT) is not recommended.[2]

For patients with an intermediate or high probability of coronary disease, the clinician should exclude unstable ischemic syndromes and conditions that might exacerbate or cause angina. If these are not present, then noninvasive testing should be considered to refine the diagnostic assessment of patients with an intermediate probability of coronary disease and to perform risk stratification for patients with a high probability of coronary disease (Fig. 54G-2).

CH 54

The ACC/AHA guidelines do not mandate exercise testing in all such patients. Pharmacological imaging studies are recommended for patients who are unable to exercise. Exercise imaging studies are recommended for patients who have had previous coronary revascularization or whose resting electrocardiograms (ECGs) are uninterpretable. Imaging studies are also supported when the clinical evaluation and exercise ECGs have not provided sufficient information to guide management. If the results of noninvasive studies suggest a high risk for complications of coronary heart disease, then coronary angiography and revascularization should be considered.

The treatment algorithm recommended by the ACC/AHA guidelines emphasizes the importance of patient education about coronary disease; prevention of ischemia through use of nitrates, beta blockers, and calcium blockers; and prevention of progression of atherosclerosis through risk factor management (Fig. 54G-3).

The ACC/AHA guidelines require clarity from the clinician in defining the critical issues for the individual patient. For patients with a chest pain complaint of uncertain etiology, the dominant question may be whether coronary artery disease is present or absent (diagnosis). For patients with known or strongly suspected coronary disease, the focus is likely to be on the patient's risk. In these guidelines a specific test may be considered an appropriate option for addressing one or the other of these issues.

The guidelines clearly differentiate between indications for the same tests for the purpose of diagnosis and risk stratification. For example, exercise ECGs are discouraged for establishing diagnosis in patients with a high clinical probability of coronary artery disease on the basis of age, gender, and symptoms (class IIb indication). However, exercise ECGs are strongly supported as a class I indication when used to assess prognosis in this same patient population. Thus interpretation of these guidelines demands rigorous definition of the clinical question at hand.

DIAGNOSIS

Noninvasive Studies

Exercise Electrocardiography. Exercise testing is considered most valuable for diagnosis when the patient's other clinical data suggest an intermediate probability of coronary disease. The ACC/AHA guidelines support the use of exercise ECGs for such patients unless their baseline ECGs show abnormalities likely to render the exercise tracing uninterpretable (Table 54G-2). However, exercise ECGs were considered appropriate for patients with complete right bundle branch block or less than 1 mm of

Chronic Coronary Artery Disease

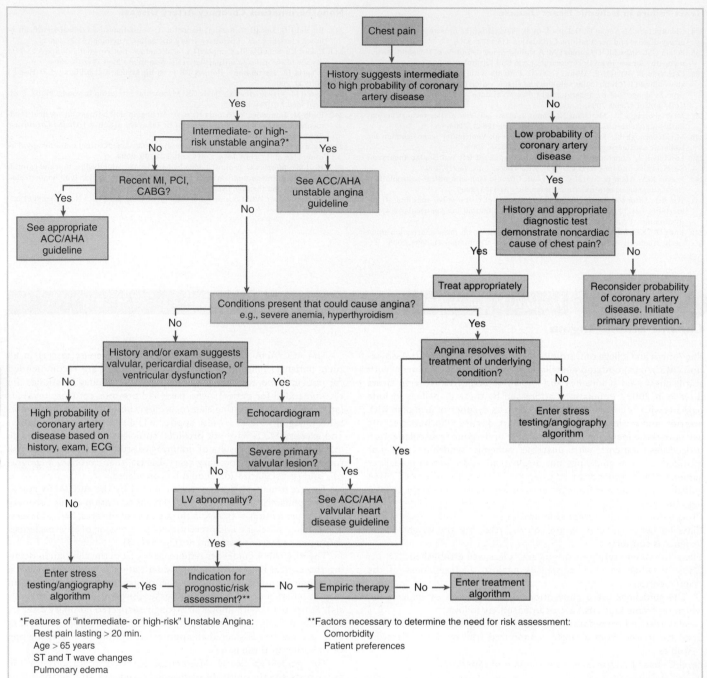

FIGURE 54G–1 Approach to the clinical assessment of chest pain. ACC = American College of Cardiology; AHA = American Heart Association; CABG = coronary artery bypass grafting; ECG = electrocardiogram; LV = left ventricular; MI = myocardial infarction; PCI = percutaneous coronary intervention. *(From ACC/AHA 2002 guideline update for the management of patients with chronic stable angina: A report of the American College of Cardiology/American Heart Association Task Force on Practice Guidelines [Committee to Update the 1999 Guidelines for the Management of Patients with Chronic Stable Angina]. Copyright 2002, American College of Cardiology Foundation and the American Heart Association, p 8.)*

ST depression at rest. Use of the exercise test was considered of uncertain value (class IIb) for patients with high or low pretest probability of coronary disease or those who had less than 1 mm of ST depression and were either using digoxin or had ECG evidence of left ventricular hypertrophy.

Echocardiography. The ACC/AHA guidelines state that "most patients undergoing a diagnostic evaluation for angina do not need an echocardiogram." Echocardiograms are supported to evaluate systolic murmurs suggestive of aortic stenosis or hypertrophic cardiomyopathy and for evaluation of the extent of ischemia when the study can be obtained within 30 minutes after the end of an ischemic episode (Table 54G-3). However, routine use of echocardiography for patients with a normal ECG, no history of myocardial infarction, and no evidence of structural heart disease is considered inappropriate (class III).

Stress Imaging Studies. The ACC/AHA guidelines recommend stress imaging as opposed to exercise ECG in (1) patients who have complete left bundle branch block, electronically paced ventricular rhythm, preexcitation (Wolff-Parkinson-White) syndrome, and other such ECG conduction abnormalities; (2) patients who have more than 1 mm of ST segment depression at rest including those with left ventricular hypertrophy or taking drugs such as digitalis; (3) patients who are unable to exercise to a level high enough to give meaningful results on exercise ECGs; and (4) patients with coronary disease who have undergone prior revascularization, in whom localization of ischemia and establishing the significance of lesions is important.

The guidelines specify that exercise stress testing is preferable to pharmacological stress testing when the patient can exercise to develop

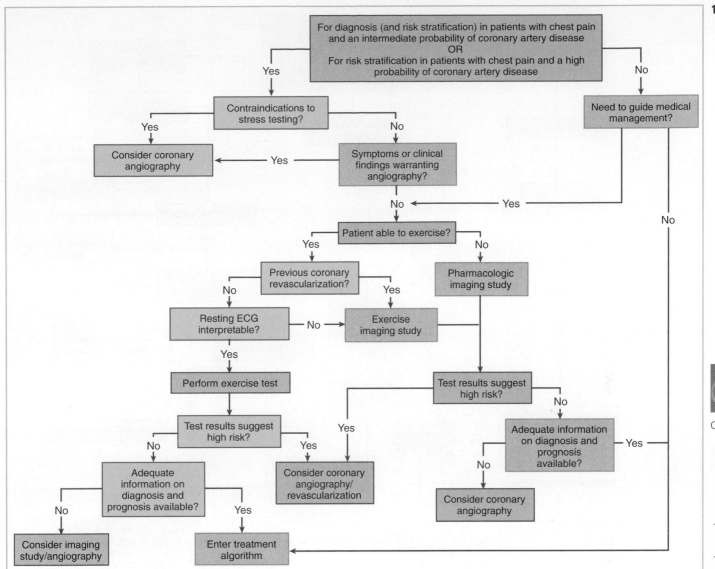

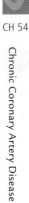

FIGURE 54G–2 Stress testing and angiography in patients with chest pain. ECG = electrocardiogram. *(From ACC/AHA 2002 guideline update for the management of patients with chronic stable angina: A report of the American College of Cardiology/American Heart Association Task Force on Practice Guidelines [Committee to Update the 1999 Guidelines for the Management of Patients with Chronic Stable Angina]. Copyright 2002, American College of Cardiology Foundation and the American Heart Association, p 9.)*

TABLE 54G–1	ACC/AHA Guidelines for Routine Clinical Testing in Patients with Chronic Stable Angina	
Class	**Indication**	**Evidence***
I (indicated)	1. Rest ECG in patients without an obvious noncardiac cause of chest pain	B
	2. Rest ECG during an episode of chest pain	B
	3. Chest radiograph in patients with signs or symptoms of congestive heart failure, valvular heart disease, pericardial disease, or aortic dissection/aneurysm	B
	4. Hemoglobin	C
	5. Fasting glucose	C
	6. Fasting lipid panel	C
IIa (good supportive evidence)	Chest radiograph in patients with signs or symptoms of pulmonary disease	B
IIb (weak supportive evidence)	1. Chest radiograph in other patients	C
	2. Electron-beam CT	B
III (not indicated)	None	

*See guidelines text for definitions of level of evidence.
ACC = American College of Cardiology; AHA = American Heart Association; ECG = electrocardiogram.

CH 54

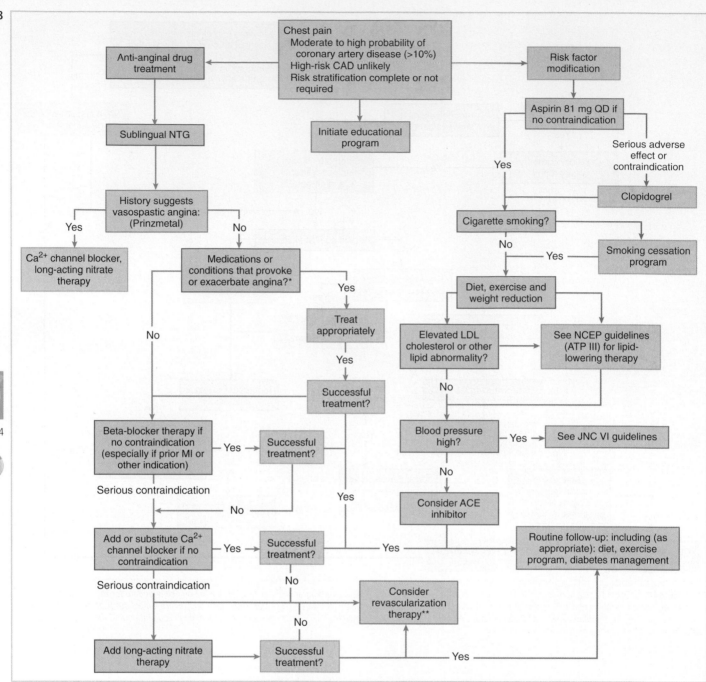

FIGURE 54G–3 Approach to the treatment of chest pain. CAD = coronary artery disease; JNC = Joint National Committee; MI = myocardial infarction; NCEP = National Cholesterol Education Program; NTG = nitroglycerin. *Conditions that exacerbate or provoke angina are medications (vasodilators, excessive thyroid replacement, and vasoconstrictors); other cardiac problems (tachyarrhythmias, bradyarrhythmias, valvular heart disease, especially aortic stenosis); and other medical problems (hypertrophic cardiomyopathy, profound anemia, uncontrolled hypertension, hyperthyroidism, hypoxemia). **At any point in this process, based on coronary anatomy, severity of anginal symptoms, and patient preferences, it is reasonable to consider evaluation for coronary revascularization. Unless a patient is documented to have left main, triple-vessel, or double-vessel coronary artery disease with significant stenosis of the proximal left anterior descending coronary artery, there is no demonstrated survival advantage associated with revascularization in low-risk patients with chronic stable angina; thus medical therapy should be attempted in most patients before considering percutaneous coronary intervention or coronary artery bypass grafting. *(From ACC/AHA 2002 guideline update for the management of patients with chronic stable angina: A report of the American College of Cardiology/American Heart Association Task Force on Practice Guidelines [Committee to Update the 1999 Guidelines for the Management of Patients with Chronic Stable Angina]. Copyright 2002, American College of Cardiology Foundation and the American Heart Association, p 10.)*

an appropriate level of cardiovascular stress (e.g., 6 to 12 minutes). Tables 54G-4 and 54G-5 summarize the appropriate indications for stress imaging in patients who are and who are not able to exercise, respectively. As is the case with exercise ECGs, these tests are considered most useful for diagnosis in patients with an intermediate probability of disease.

The guidelines comment on the choice among stress imaging technologies. They conclude that dobutamine perfusion imaging has

significant limitations compared with dipyridamole or adenosine perfusion imaging because it does not provoke as great an increase in coronary flow. Therefore the guidelines recommend that dobutamine be used to provoke ischemia for perfusion imaging only when patients have contraindications to the other agents. In contrast, dobutamine is the agent of choice for pharmacological stress echocardiography because it enhances myocardial contractile performance and wall motion, which can be directly observed by echocardiography.

TABLE 54G-2 ACC/AHA Guidelines for Diagnosis of Obstructive CAD with Exercise ECG Testing without an Imaging Modality

Class	Indication	Evidence*
I (indicated)	Patients with an intermediate pretest probability of CAD based on age, gender, and symptoms including those with complete right bundle branch block or <1 mm of ST depression at rest (exceptions are listed in classes II and III)	B
IIa (good supportive evidence)	Patients with suspected vasospastic angina	C
IIb (weak supportive evidence)	1. Patients with a high pretest probability of CAD by age, gender, and symptoms 2. Patients with a low pretest probability of CAD by age, gender, and symptoms 3. Patients taking digoxin whose ECG has <1 mm of baseline ST segment depression 4. Patients with ECG criteria for LVH and <1 mm of baseline ST segment depression	B B B B

III (not indicated)	1. Patients with the following baseline ECG abnormalities:
	   a. Preexcitation (Wolff-Parkinson-White) syndrome
	   b. Electronically paced ventricular rhythm
	   c. >1 mm of ST depression at rest
	   d. Complete left bundle branch block
	2. Patients with an established diagnosis of CAD because of prior myocardial infarction or coronary angiography; however, testing can assess functional capacity and prognosis
		
		B
		B
		B
		B

*See guidelines text for definitions of level of evidence.
ACC = American College of Cardiology; AHA = American Heart Association; CAD = coronary artery disease; ECG = electrocardiogram; LVH = left ventricular hypertrophy.

TABLE 54G-3 ACC/AHA Guidelines for Echocardiography for Diagnosis of Cause of Chest Pain in Patients with Suspected Chronic Stable Angina Pectoris

Class	Indication	Evidence*
I (indicated)	1. Patients with systolic murmur suggestive of aortic stenosis or hypertrophic cardiomyopathy 2. Evaluation of extent (severity) of ischemia (e.g., LV segmental wall motion abnormality) when the echocardiogram can be obtained during pain or within 30 min after its abatement	C C
IIa (good supportive evidence)		
IIb (weak supportive evidence)	Patients with a click or murmur to diagnose mitral valve prolapse	C
III (not indicated)	Patients with a normal ECG, no history of myocardial infarction, and no signs or symptoms suggestive of heart failure, valvular heart disease, or hypertrophic cardiomyopathy	C

*See guidelines text for definitions of level of evidence.
ACC = American College of Cardiology; AHA = American Heart Association; ECG = electrocardiogram; LV = left ventricular.

Specific Patient Subsets. Although treadmill ECG testing is less accurate for diagnosis in women than in men, the guidelines note that the diagnostic performance of imaging technologies is also compromised by technical issues (e.g., breast tissue) in women. Therefore the guidelines conclude that "there currently are insufficient data to justify replacing standard exercise testing with stress imaging in the initial evaluation of women."

The ACC/AHA guidelines discourage use of noninvasive testing for coronary disease with and without imaging for asymptomatic patients. No class I and class IIa indications exist for exercise testing of asymptomatic patients, and there is just one class IIb indication (weak support): asymptomatic patients with possible myocardial ischemia on ambulatory ECG monitoring or with severe coronary calcification on electron-beam CT scanning. Myocardial perfusion imaging testing also receives only weak support (class IIb) for asymptomatic patients who, despite the recommendations of guidelines, had undergone exercise ECGs and who had an intermediate-risk or high-risk Duke treadmill score or an inadequate exercise ECG.

Coronary Angiography

Coronary angiography is a necessary step in the management of patients for whom revascularization with percutaneous coronary intervention (PCI) or coronary artery bypass grafting (CABG) is likely to be beneficial because of a high risk for complications with medical therapy alone. Thus the ACC/AHA guidelines support coronary angiography for diagnosis in patients with angina who have survived sudden death (Table 54G-6). The guidelines consider coronary angiography to be possibly indicated (class IIa) when patients with chest pain have contraindications to noninvasive testing or such testing is inadequate or likely to be inadequate to guide management.

The committee thought that noninvasive and clinical data are usually sufficient to establish or exclude the diagnosis of coronary disease and that coronary angiography should rarely be used for this purpose. The guidelines assert that coronary angiography is "generally not indicated" for diagnosis in asymptomatic patients. They offer only weak support (class IIb) for coronary angiography to establish a definitive diagnosis for patients with recurrent hospitalization for chest pain.

RISK STRATIFICATION

The ACC/AHA guidelines emphasize the following four factors that predict survival for patients with coronary artery disease: (1) left ventricular function; (2) anatomical extent and severity of coronary atherosclerosis; (3) presence of recent plaque rupture; and (4) the patient's general health and noncoronary comorbidity.

Assessment of Left Ventricular Function

The guidelines consider assessment of left ventricular function with either echocardiography or radionuclide angiography appropriate (class I) in patients with symptoms or signs of heart failure, a history of prior myocardial infarction, or pathological Q waves on ECG. Echo-

TABLE 54G–4	ACC/AHA Guidelines for Cardiac Stress Imaging as the Initial Test for Diagnosis in Patients with Chronic Stable Angina Who Are Able to Exercise	
Class	**Indication**	**Evidence***
I (indicated)	1. Exercise myocardial perfusion imaging or exercise echocardiography in patients with an intermediate pretest probability of CAD who have one of the following baseline ECG abnormalities:	
	a. Preexcitation (Wolff-Parkinson-White) syndrome	B
	b. >1 mm of ST depression at rest	B
	2. Exercise myocardial perfusion imaging or exercise echocardiography in patients with prior revascularization (either PCI or CABG)	B
	3. Adenosine or dipyridamole myocardial perfusion imaging in patients with an intermediate pretest probability of CAD and one of the following baseline ECG abnormalities:	
	a. Electronically paced ventricular rhythm	C
	b. Left bundle branch block	B
IIa (good supportive evidence)		
IIb (weak supportive evidence)	1. Exercise myocardial perfusion imaging or exercise echocardiography in patients with a low or high probability of CAD who have one of the following baseline ECG abnormalities:	
	a. Preexcitation (Wolff-Parkinson-White) syndrome	B
	b. >1 mm of ST depression	B
	2. Adenosine or dipyridamole myocardial perfusion imaging in patients with a low or high probability of CAD and one of the following baseline ECG abnormalities:	
	a. Electronically paced ventricular rhythm	C
	b. Left bundle branch block	B
	3. Exercise myocardial perfusion imaging or exercise echocardiography in patients with an intermediate probability of CAD who have one of the following:	
	a. Digoxin use with <1 mm ST depression on the baseline ECG	B
	b. LVH with <1 mm ST depression on the baseline ECG	B
	4. Exercise myocardial perfusion imaging, exercise echocardiography, adenosine or dipyridamole myocardial perfusion imaging, or dobutamine echocardiography as the initial stress test in a patient with a normal rest ECG who is not taking digoxin	B
	5. Exercise or dobutamine echocardiography in patients with left bundle branch block	C
III (not indicated)		

*See guidelines text for definitions of level of evidence.

ACC = American College of Cardiology; AHA = American Heart Association; CABG = coronary artery bypass grafting; CAD = coronary artery disease; ECG = electrocardiogram; LVH = left ventricular hypertrophy; PCI = percutaneous coronary intervention.

CH 54

TABLE 54G–5	ACC/AHA Guidelines for Cardiac Stress Imaging as the Initial Test for Diagnosis in Patients with Chronic Stable Angina Who Are Unable to Exercise	
Class	**Indication**	**Evidence***
I (indicated)	1. Adenosine or dipyridamole myocardial perfusion imaging or dobutamine echocardiography in patients with an intermediate pretest probability of CAD	B
	2. Adenosine or dipyridamole myocardial perfusion imaging or dobutamine echocardiography in patients with prior revascularization (either PCI or CABG)	B
IIa (good supportive evidence)		
IIb (weak supportive evidence)	1. Adenosine or dipyridamole myocardial perfusion imaging or dobutamine echocardiography in patients with a low or high probability of CAD in the absence of electronically paced ventricular rhythm or left bundle branch block	B
	2. Adenosine or dipyridamole myocardial perfusion imaging in patients with a low or a high probability of CAD and one of the following baseline ECG abnormalities:	
	a. Electronically paced ventricular rhythm	C
	b. Left bundle branch block	B
	3. Dobutamine echocardiography in patients with left bundle branch block	C
III (not indicated)		

*See guidelines text for definitions of level of evidence.

ACC = American College of Cardiology; AHA = American Heart Association; CAD = coronary artery disease; PCI = percutaneous coronary intervention; CABG = coronary artery bypass grafting; ECG = electrocardiogram.

cardiography is also considered appropriate for patients with mitral regurgitation to assess its severity and etiology and for patients with complex ventricular arrhythmias to assess left ventricular function. However, the guidelines note that a normal ECG correlates strongly with normal left ventricular function at rest and therefore do not endorse echocardiography as a routine test for patients with a normal ECG, no history of myocardial infarction, and no symptoms or signs of congestive heart failure. They also do not support routine periodic echocardiography for stable patients in whom no new change in therapy is contemplated.

Noninvasive Tests for Ischemia

Exercise testing is recommended for assessment of prognosis for all patients with an intermediate or high probability of coronary artery

TABLE 54G–6	ACC/AHA Guidelines for Coronary Angiography to Establish a Diagnosis in Patients with Suspected Angina Including Those with Known CAD Who Have a Significant Change in Anginal Symptoms	
Class	**Indication**	**Evidence***
I (indicated)	Patients with known or possible angina pectoris who have survived sudden cardiac death	B
IIa (good supportive evidence)	1. Patients with an uncertain diagnosis after noninvasive testing in whom the benefit of a more certain diagnosis outweighs the risk and cost of coronary angiography	C
	2. Patients who cannot undergo noninvasive testing because of disability, illness, or morbid obesity	C
	3. Patients with an occupational requirement for a definitive diagnosis	C
	4. Patients who by virtue of young age at onset of symptoms, noninvasive imaging, or other clinical parameters are suspected of having a nonatherosclerotic cause for myocardial ischemia (coronary artery anomaly, Kawasaki disease, primary coronary artery dissection, radiation-induced vasculopathy)	C
	5. Patients in whom coronary artery spasm is suspected and provocative testing may be necessary	C
	6. Patients with a high pretest probability of left main or triple-vessel CAD	C
IIb (weak supportive evidence)	1. Patients with recurrent hospitalization for chest pain in whom a definite diagnosis is judged necessary	C
	2. Patients with an overriding desire for a definitive diagnosis and intermediate or high probability of CAD	C
III (not indicated)	1. Patients with significant comorbidity in whom the risk of coronary arteriography outweighs the benefit of the procedure	C
	2. Patients with an overriding personal desire for a definitive diagnosis and a low probability of CAD	C

*See guidelines text for definitions of level of evidence.
ACC = American College of Cardiology; AHA = American Heart Association; CAD = coronary artery disease.

disease, except those with ECG abnormalities that compromise interpretation of the exercise tracing and those for which the information is unlikely to alter management (Table 54G-7). The committee directly addressed the issue of whether the additional information provided by imaging technologies might make them preferable tests for risk stratification but concluded the greater costs of these tests could not be justified for most patients. Therefore the guidelines endorse a stepwise approach in which the exercise ECG is used as the initial test in patients who are not taking digoxin, have a normal rest ECG, and are able to exercise.

The ACC/AHA guidelines support use of stress testing with either echocardiographic or radionuclide imaging to identify the severity of ischemia in patients who have ECG abnormalities precluding interpretation of the exercise tracing and for patients in whom the functional significance of coronary lesions will guide management (Tables 54G-8 and 54G-9). Dipyridamole or adenosine myocardial perfusion imaging is recommended for patients with left bundle branch block or electronically paced ventricular rhythms because of higher rates of false-positive septal perfusion defects with exercise than with either dipyridamole or adenosine. Relatively few data exist on the performance of dobutamine echocardiography in this setting, so this approach is not endorsed by the guidelines for patients with left bundle branch block or electronically paced ventricular rhythms. Stress imaging studies are also supported for assessment of the functional significance of coronary lesions in planning PCI.

The guidelines discourage use of noninvasive testing for risk stratification of patients who have no symptoms of coronary disease. No class I or class IIa indications exist for use of cardiac stress imaging as an initial test for risk stratification. Supporting evidence is considered weak for use of cardiac stress imaging for asymptomatic patients with severe coronary calcification on electron-beam CT or who had undergone an exercise ECG and had inadequate tests or intermediate- or high-risk Duke treadmill scores.

Coronary Angiography

In the ACC/AHA guidelines, the decision to proceed to coronary angiography should be based on symptomatic status and risk stratification derived from clinical data and noninvasive test results. The guidelines define noninvasive findings that predict a high (>3 percent), intermediate (1 to 3 percent), and low (<1 percent) expected annual mortality

rate (Table 54G-10). Coronary angiography for risk stratification and as a prelude to intervention is endorsed for patients with high-risk criteria, as well as those with disabling chronic stable angina despite medical therapy or other clinical characteristics suggesting high risk (Table 54G-11). The committee considered evidence to be generally supportive (class IIa) for coronary angiography for patients with milder angina in the setting of left ventricular dysfunction even if they do not have high-risk criteria on noninvasive testing; for asymptomatic patients with high-risk criteria; and for patients whose risk status is uncertain despite noninvasive testing.

Conversely, coronary angiography is discouraged (class III) for patients who have mild angina and no evidence of ischemia on noninvasive testing or would not undergo revascularization. Only weak support (class IIb) exists for coronary angiography for patients with mild angina and good left ventricular function in the absence of high-risk criteria on noninvasive testing, for patients with severe angina whose symptoms were controlled with medical therapy, or for patients with mild angina but unacceptable side effects to adequate medical therapy.

TREATMENT

ACC/AHA guidelines for medical therapy of patients with chronic stable angina are oriented toward preventing myocardial infarction and death and reducing symptoms. When coronary revascularization has been shown to extend life, it is the recommended approach, but in many settings there are a variety of reasonable options including medical therapy, PCI, and CABG. Cost-effectiveness and patient preference are considered important components of the decision-making process.

The guidelines assert that the goal of treatment of patients with chronic stable angina should be the complete or nearly complete elimination of anginal chest pain and return to normal activities, with minimal side effects. They recommend that the initial treatment of the patient should include all the elements in the following mnemonic:
A = Aspirin and antianginal therapy
B = Beta blocker and blood pressure
C = Cigarette smoking and cholesterol
D = Diet and diabetes
E = Education and exercise

TABLE 54G–7 ACC/AHA Guidelines for Exercise Testing Risk Assessment and Prognosis in Patients with an Intermediate or High Probability of CAD

Class	Indication	Evidence*
I (indicated)	1. Patients undergoing initial evaluation (exceptions are listed below in classes IIb and III) 2. Patients after a significant change in cardiac symptoms	B C
IIa (good supportive evidence)		

IIb (weak supportive evidence)	1. Patients with the following ECG abnormalities:
	  a. Preexcitation (Wolff-Parkinson-White) syndrome
	  b. Electronically paced ventricular rhythm
	  c. >1 mm of ST depression at rest
	  d. Complete left bundle branch block
	2. Patients who have undergone cardiac catheterization to identify ischemia in the distribution of coronary lesion of borderline severity
	3. Postrevascularization patients who have a significant change in anginal pattern suggestive of ischemia
		
		B
		B
		B
		B
		C
		
		C

III (not indicated)	Patients with severe comorbidity likely to limit life expectancy or prevent revascularization	C

*See guidelines text for definitions of level of evidence.
ACC = American College of Cardiology; AHA = American Heart Association; ECG = electrocardiogram.

TABLE 54G–8 ACC/AHA Guidelines for Cardiac Stress Imaging as the Initial Test for Risk Stratification of Patients with Chronic Stable Angina Who Are Able to Exercise

Class	Indication	Evidence*
I (indicated)	1. Exercise myocardial perfusion imaging or exercise echocardiography to identify the extent, severity, and location of ischemia in patients who do not have left bundle branch block or an electronically paced ventricular rhythm and who either have an abnormal rest ECG or are using digoxin 2. Dipyridamole or adenosine myocardial perfusion imaging in patients with left bundle branch block or electronically paced ventricular rhythm 3. Exercise myocardial perfusion imaging or exercise echocardiography to assess the functional significance of coronary lesions (if not already known) in planning PCI	B B B
IIa (good supportive evidence)		
IIb (weak supportive evidence)	1. Exercise or dobutamine echocardiography in patients with left bundle branch block 2. Exercise, dipyridamole, or adenosine myocardial perfusion imaging, or exercise or dobutamine echocardiography as the initial test in patients who have a normal rest ECG and who are not taking digoxin	C B
III (not indicated)	1. Exercise myocardial perfusion imaging in patients with left bundle branch block 2. Exercise, dipyridamole, or adenosine myocardial perfusion imaging, or exercise or dobutamine echocardiography in patients with severe comorbidity likely to limit life expectation or prevent revascularization	C C

*See guidelines text for definitions of level of evidence.
ACC = American College of Cardiology; AHA = American Heart Association; ECG = electrocardiogram; PCI = percutaneous coronary intervention.

TABLE 54G–9 ACC/AHA Guidelines for Cardiac Stress Imaging as the Initial Test for Risk Stratification of Patients with Chronic Stable Angina Who Are Unable to Exercise

Class	Indication	Evidence*
I (indicated)	1. Dipyridamole or adenosine myocardial perfusion imaging or dobutamine echocardiography to identify the extent, severity, and location of ischemia in patients who do not have left bundle branch block or electronically paced ventricular rhythm 2. Dipyridamole or adenosine myocardial perfusion imaging in patients with left bundle branch block or electronically paced ventricular rhythm 3. Dipyridamole or adenosine myocardial perfusion imaging or dobutamine echocardiography to assess the functional significance of coronary lesions (if not already known) in planning PCI	B B B
IIa (good supportive evidence)		
IIb (weak supportive evidence)	Dobutamine echocardiography in patients with left bundle branch block	C
III (not indicated)	Dipyridamole or adenosine myocardial perfusion imaging or dobutamine echocardiography in patients with severe comorbidity likely to limit life expectation or prevent revascularization	C

*See guidelines text for definitions of level of evidence.
ACC = American College of Cardiology; AHA = American Heart Association; PCI = percutaneous coronary intervention.

Pharmacological Therapy

The guidelines emphasize the importance of aspirin and beta blockers for patients with coronary disease in the absence of contraindications (Table 54G-12). Absolute contraindications to beta blockers include severe bradycardia; preexisting high degree of atrioventricular block, sick sinus syndrome; and severe, unstable left ventricular failure. Relative contraindications to beta blockers include asthma and bronchospastic disease, severe depression, and peripheral vascular disease. The guidelines note that most patients with diabetes tolerate beta blockers, although these drugs should be used with caution in patients who require insulin.

Angiotensin-converting enzyme (ACE) inhibitors are recommended (class I indication) for patients with diabetes and/or left ventricular systolic dysfunction, and evidence is considered good for their use in other patients with coronary disease (class IIa). The guidelines recommend that nitrates and/or calcium antagonists should be used for symptom control but indicate that short-acting dihydropyridine calcium antagonists should be avoided. Low-density lipoprotein cholesterol (LDL-C) should be controlled with a target of less than 100 mg/dl (see "Risk Reduction" later). Further reduction of LDL-C to less than 70 mg/dl is reasonable (class IIa).

Several recommendations about pharmacological therapy may be altered in future revisions of these guidelines because of subsequent research providing insight into the effects of these agents. For example, evidence is considered weak for anticoagulation with warfarin in addition to aspirin; since these guidelines were published, a randomized trial has shown that the combination of warfarin and aspirin was superior to aspirin alone in preventing future events but at the price of a higher rate of bleeding complications.[3] Use of dipyridamole or chelation therapy is discouraged.

For asymptomatic patients with known coronary disease (e.g., patients with prior myocardial infarction), the guidelines recommend aspirin and beta blockers in the absence of contraindications and the use of lipid-lowering therapies and ACE inhibitors as described earlier.

Risk Reduction

For patients with chronic stable angina, the ACC/AHA guidelines support intensive management of risk factors including hypertension, cigarette smoking, diabetes, LDL-C, and obesity (Table 54G-13). The

TABLE 54G–10	ACC/AHA Guideline Criteria for Noninvasive Risk Stratification

High Risk (>3% Annual Mortality Rate)
1. Severe resting left ventricular dysfunction (LVEF < 0.35)
2. High-risk treadmill score (score ≤ −11)
3. Severe exercise LV dysfunction (exercise LVEF < 0.35)
4. Stress-induced large perfusion defect (particularly if anterior)
5. Stress-induced multiple perfusion defects of moderate size
6. Large, fixed perfusion defect with LV dilation or increased lung uptake (thallium-201)
7. Stress-induced moderate perfusion defect with LV dilation or increased lung uptake (thallium-201)
8. Echocardiographic wall motion abnormality (involving >2 segments) developing at low dose of dobutamine (≤10 mg/kg/min) or at a low heart rate (<120 beats/min)
9. Stress echocardiographic evidence of extensive ischemia

Intermediate Risk (1-3% Annual Mortality Rate)
1. Mild/moderate resting LV dysfunction (LVEF = 0.35-0.49)
2. Intermediate-risk treadmill score (−11 < score < 5)
3. Stress-induced moderate perfusion defect without LV dilation or increased lung intake (thallium-201)
4. Limited stress echocardiographic ischemia with a wall motion abnormality only at higher doses of dobutamine involving ≥2 segments

Low Risk (<1% Annual Mortality Rate)
1. Low-risk treadmill score (score ≥ 5)
2. Normal or small myocardial perfusion defect at rest or with stress*
3. Normal stress echocardiographic wall motion or no change of limited resting wall motion abnormalities during stress*

*Although the published data are limited, patients with these findings will probably not be at low risk in the presence of either a high-risk treadmill score or severe resting left ventricular dysfunction (LVEF < 0.35).

ACC = American College of Cardiology; AHA = American Heart Association; LV = left ventricular; LVEF = LV ejection fraction.

From ACC/AHA 2002 guideline update for the management of patients with chronic stable angina: A report of the American College of Cardiology/American Heart Association Task Force on Practice Guidelines (Committee to Update the 1999 Guidelines for the Management of Patients with Chronic Stable Angina). 2002, American College of Cardiology Foundation and the American Heart Association.

CH 54

Chronic Coronary Artery Disease

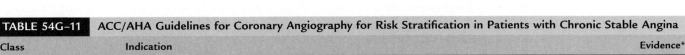

TABLE 54G–11	ACC/AHA Guidelines for Coronary Angiography for Risk Stratification in Patients with Chronic Stable Angina	
Class	**Indication**	**Evidence***
I (indicated)	1. Patients with disabling (Canadian Cardiovascular Society [CCS] classes III and IV) chronic stable angina despite medical therapy	B
	2. Patients with high-risk criteria on noninvasive testing regardless of anginal severity	B
	3. Patients with angina who have survived sudden cardiac death or serious ventricular arrhythmia	B
	4. Patients with angina and symptoms and signs of CHF	C
	5. Patients with clinical characteristics that indicate a high likelihood of severe CAD	C
IIa (good supportive evidence)	1. Patients with significant LV dysfunction (ejection fraction<0.45), CCS class I or II angina, and demonstrable ischemia but no high-risk criteria on noninvasive testing	C
	2. Patients with inadequate prognostic information after noninvasive testing	C
	3. Patients with high-risk criteria suggesting ischemia on noninvasive testing	C
IIb (weak supportive evidence)	1. Patients with CCS class I or II angina, preserved LV function (ejection fraction >0.45), but no high-risk criteria on noninvasive testing	C
	2. Patients with CCS class III (not indicated) or IV angina, which with medical therapy improves to class I or II	C
	3. Patients with CCS class I or II angina but intolerance (unacceptable side effects) to adequate medical therapy	C
III (not indicated)	1. Patients with CCS class I or II angina who respond to medical therapy and who have no evidence of ischemia on noninvasive testing	C
	2. Patients who prefer to avoid revascularization	C

*See guidelines text for definitions of level of evidence.

ACC = American College of Cardiology; AHA = American Heart Association; CAD = coronary artery disease; CHF = congestive heart failure; LV = left ventricular.

TABLE 54G–12 ACC/AHA Guidelines for Pharmacotherapy for Chronic Stable Angina

Class	Indication	Evidence*
I (indicated)	1. Aspirin in the absence of contraindications	A
	2. Beta blockers as initial therapy in the absence of contraindications in patients with prior myocardial infarction or without prior myocardial infarction	A,B
	3. ACE inhibitor in all patients with CAD who also have diabetes and/or LV systolic dysfunction	A
	4. LDL-lowering therapy in patients with documented or suspected CAD and LDL cholesterol >130 mg/dl, with a target LDL of <100 mg/dl	A
	5. Sublingual nitroglycerin or nitroglycerin spray for the immediate relief of angina	B
	6. Calcium antagonists† or long-acting nitrates as initial therapy for reduction of symptoms when beta blockers are contraindicated	B
	7. Calcium antagonists† or long-acting nitrates in combination with beta blockers when initial treatment with beta blockers is not successful	B
	8. Calcium antagonists† and long-acting nitrates as a substitute for beta blockers if initial treatment with beta blockers leads to unacceptable side effects	C
IIa (good supportive evidence)	1. Clopidogrel when aspirin is absolutely contraindicated	B
	2. Long-acting nondihydropyridine calcium antagonists† instead of beta blockers as initial therapy	B
	3. In patients with documented or suspected CAD and LDL cholesterol 100-129 mg/dl, several therapeutic options are available:	B
	a. Lifestyle and/or drug therapies to lower LDL to <100 mg/dl; further reduction to <70 mg/dl is reasonable	
	b. Weight reduction and increased physical activity in persons with the metabolic syndrome	
	c. Institution of treatment of other lipid or nonlipid risk factors; consider use of nicotinic acid or fibric acid for elevated triglycerides or low HDL cholesterol	
	4. ACE inhibitor in patients with CAD or other vascular disease	B
IIb (weak supportive evidence)	Low-intensity anticoagulation with warfarin in addition to aspirin	B
III (not indicated)	1. Dipyridamole	B
	2. Chelation therapy	B

*See guidelines text for definitions of level of evidence.
†Short-acting dihydropyridine calcium antagonists should be avoided.
ACC = American College of Cardiology; AHA = American Heart Association; ACE = angiotensin-converting enzyme; CAD = coronary artery disease; LDL = low-density lipoprotein; LV = left ventricular.

TABLE 54G–13 ACC/AHA Guidelines for Treatment of Risk Factors

Class	Indication	Evidence*
I (indicated)	1. Treatment of hypertension according to Joint National Conference VI guidelines	A
	2. Smoking cessation therapy	B
	3. Management of diabetes	C
	4. Comprehensive cardiac rehabilitation program (including exercise)	B
	5. LDL-lowering therapy in patients with documented or suspected CAD and LDL cholesterol ≥130 mg/dl, with a target LDL of <100 mg/dl	A
	6. Weight reduction in obese patients in the presence of hypertension, hyperlipidemia, or diabetes mellitus	C
IIa (good supportive evidence)	1. In patients with documented or suspected CAD and LDL cholesterol 100-129 mg/dl, several therapeutic options are available:	B
	a. Lifestyle and/or drug therapies to lower LDL to <100 mg/dl; further reduction to below 70 mg/dl is reasonable	B
	b. Weight reduction and increased physical activity in persons with the metabolic syndrome	B
	c. Institution of treatment of other lipid or nonlipid risk factors; consider use of nicotinic acid or fibric acid for elevated triglycerides or low HDL cholesterol	B
	2. Therapy to lower non-HDL cholesterol in patients with documented or suspected CAD and triglycerides >200 mg/dl, with a target non-HDL cholesterol <130 mg/dl	B
	3. Weight reduction in obese patients in the absence of hypertension, hyperlipidemia, or diabetes mellitus	C
IIb (weak supportive evidence)	1. Folate therapy in patients with elevated homocysteine levels	C
	2. Identification and appropriate treatment of clinical depression to improve CAD outcomes	C
	3. Intervention directed at psychosocial stress reduction	C
III (not indicated)	1. Initiation of hormone replacement therapy in postmenopausal women for the purpose of reducing cardiovascular risk	A
	2. Vitamins C and E supplementation	A
	3. Chelation therapy	C
	4. Garlic	C
	5. Acupuncture	C
	6. Coenzyme Q	C

*See guidelines text for definitions of level of evidence.
ACC = American College of Cardiology; AHA = American Heart Association; CAD = coronary artery disease; HDL = high-density lipoprotein; LDL = low-density lipoprotein.

TABLE 54G–14 Specific Goals for Risk Reduction Strategies in Patients with Chronic Stable Angina

Risk Factor/Strategy	Goal
Smoking	Complete cessation
Blood pressure	<140/90 or 130/80 mm Hg if heart failure, renal insufficiency, or diabetes
Lipid management	Primary goal: LDL < 100 mg/dl; further reduction of LDL-C to <70 mg/dl is reasonable (class IIa) Secondary goal: If triglycerides ≥200 mg/dl, then non-HDL should be <130 mg/dl
Physical activity	Minimum goal: 30 min 3 or 4 d/wk Optimal goal: daily
Weight management	BMI 18.5-24.9 kg/m^2
Diabetes management	HbA1c < 7%
Antiplatelet agents/anticoagulants	All patients: indefinite use of aspirin 75-325 mg/d if not contraindicated. Consider clopidogrel as an alternative if aspirin is contraindicated. Manage warfarin to international normalized ratio = 2.0 to 3.0 in patients after myocardial infarction when clinically indicated or for those not able to take aspirin or clopidogrel
ACE inhibitors	Start and continue indefinitely in all patients with LV ejection fraction ≤40% and in those with hypertension, diabetes, or chronic kidney disease, unless contraindicated. Consider chronic therapy for all other patients with coronary or other vascular disease unless contraindicated. Use as needed to manage blood pressure or symptoms in all other patients
Beta blockers	Start in all postmyocardial infarction and acute patients (arrhythmia, LV dysfunction, inducible ischemia) at 5-28 days. Continue 6 mo minimum. Observe usual contraindications. Use as needed to manage angina, rhythm, or blood pressure in all patients

ACE = angiotensin-converting enzyme; BMI = body mass index; HbA1c = hemoglobin A1c; CHF = congestive heart failure; LDL = low-density lipoprotein; LV = left ventricular.

TABLE 54G–15 ACC/AHA Guidelines for Revascularization with PCI and CABG in Patients with Stable Angina

Class	Indication	Evidence*
I (indicated)	1. CABG for patients with significant left main coronary disease	A
	2. CABG for patients with triple-vessel disease. The survival benefit is greater in patients with abnormal LV function (ejection fraction <0.50)	A
	3. CABG for patients with double-vessel disease with significant proximal LAD CAD and either abnormal LV function (ejection fraction <50%) or demonstrable ischemia on noninvasive testing	A
	4. PCI for patients with double- or triple-vessel disease with significant proximal LAD CAD, who have anatomy suitable for catheter-based therapy and normal LV function and who do not have treated diabetes	B
	5. PCI or CABG for patients with single- or double-vessel CAD without significant proximal LAD CAD but with a large area of viable myocardium and high-risk criteria on noninvasive testing	B
	6. CABG for patients with single- or double-vessel CAD without significant proximal LAD CAD who have survived sudden cardiac death or sustained ventricular tachycardia	C
	7. In patients with prior PCI, CABG or PCI for recurrent stenosis associated with a large area of viable myocardium or high-risk criteria on noninvasive testing	C
	8. PCI or CABG for patients who have not been successfully treated by medical therapy and can undergo revascularization with acceptable risk	B
IIa (good supportive evidence)	1. Repeat CABG for patients with multiple saphenous vein graft stenoses, especially when there is significant stenosis of a graft supplying the LAD; it may be appropriate to use PCI for focal saphenous vein graft lesions or multiple stenoses in poor candidates for reoperative surgery	C
	2. Use of PCI or CABG for patients with single- or double-vessel CAD without significant proximal LAD disease but with a moderate area of viable myocardium and demonstrable ischemia on noninvasive testing	B
	3. Use of PCI or CABG for patients with single-vessel disease with significant proximal LAD disease	B
IIb (weak supportive evidence)	1. Compared with CABG, PCI for patients with double- or triple-vessel disease with significant proximal LAD CAD, who have anatomy suitable for catheter-based therapy and who have treated diabetes or abnormal LV function	B
	2. Use of PCI for patients with significant left main coronary disease who are not candidates for CABG	C
	3. PCI for patients with single- or double-vessel CAD without significant proximal LAD CAD who have survived sudden cardiac death or sustained ventricular tachycardia	C
III (not indicated)	1. Use of PCI or CABG for patients with single- or double-vessel CAD without significant proximal LAD CAD, who have mild symptoms that are unlikely due to myocardial ischemia, or who have not received an adequate trial of medical therapy and a. have only a small area of viable myocardium Or b. have no demonstrable ischemia on noninvasive testing	C
	2. Use of PCI or CABG for patients with borderline coronary stenoses (50-60% diameter in locations other than the left main coronary artery) and no demonstrable ischemia on noninvasive testing	C
	3. Use of PCI or CABG for patients with insignificant coronary stenosis (<50% diameter)	C
	4. Use of PCI in patients with significant left main coronary artery disease who are candidates for CABG	B

*See guidelines text for definitions of level of evidence.

ACC = American College of Cardiology; AHA = American Heart Association; CAD = coronary artery disease; CABG = coronary artery bypass grafting; LAD = left anterior descending [coronary artery]; LV = left ventricular; PCI = percutaneous coronary intervention.

guidelines support use of pharmacological therapy for patients with LDL levels greater than 130 mg/dl, with a target of 100 mg/dl. For patients with coronary disease who have an LDL of 100 to 129 mg/dl, the guidelines consider several options reasonable (class IIa) including life-style modifications or drug therapies.

In changes from prior guidelines, initiation of hormone therapy for the purpose of reducing cardiovascular risk is considered inappropriate (class III), as is use of vitamins C and E supplementation, chelation therapy, garlic, acupuncture, and coenzyme Q for this purpose. Evidence to support interventions based on lipoprotein(a) and homocysteine levels are considered inconclusive.

Specific goals for key risk reduction interventions are summarized in Table 54G-14.

Revascularization

ACC/AHA guidelines for revascularization with PCI or CABG for patients with chronic stable angina focus on improvement of survival for patients with high clinical risk of mortality on medical therapy and on controlling symptoms in patients who have an inadequate quality of life on medical therapy. Recommendations include the use of CABG for patients with significant left main coronary artery disease and in

patients with triple-vessel disease, particularly in those with abnormal left ventricular function (Table 54G-15). PCI and CABG are supported for patients with double- and triple-vessel coronary disease and who do not have treated diabetes. Revascularization is also supported for patients with single- or double-vessel coronary disease who have a large area of viable myocardium and high-risk criteria on noninvasive testing.

The guidelines discourage use of PCI or CABG for single- or double-vessel coronary disease without significant proximal left anterior descending (LAD) coronary artery disease if they have mild symptoms or have not received an adequate trial of medical therapy, particularly if noninvasive testing data indicate either that they have only a small area of viable myocardium or have no demonstrable ischemia on noninvasive testing. PCI for patients with diabetes is considered a second-choice strategy compared with CABG.

For asymptomatic patients, the guidelines for revascularization with PCI or CABG are identical to those for other patients with chronic stable angina (see Table 54G-15), except that the following indications that were considered class IIa are regarded as weaker (class IIb) in asymptomatic patients:

Use of PCI or CABG for patients with single- or double-vessel CAD without significant proximal LAD disease but with a moderate area

TABLE 54G–16	ACC/AHA Guidelines for Echocardiography, Treadmill Exercise Testing, Stress Radionuclide Imaging, Stress Echocardiography Studies, and Coronary Angiography During Patient Follow-up	
Class	**Indication**	**Evidence***
I (indicated)	1. Chest radiograph for patients with evidence of new or worsening CHF	C
	2. Assessment of LV ejection fraction and segmental wall motion by echocardiography or radionuclide imaging in patients with new or worsening CHF or evidence of intervening myocardial infarction by history or ECG	C
	3. Echocardiography for evidence of new or worsening valvular heart disease	C
	4. Treadmill exercise test for patients without prior revascularization who have a significant change in clinical status, are able to exercise, and do not have any of the ECG abnormalities listed in No. 5	C
	5. Stress radionuclide imaging or stress echocardiography procedures for patients without prior revascularization who have a significant change in clinical status and are unable to exercise or have one of the following ECG abnormalities: a. Preexcitation (Wolff-Parkinson-White) syndrome b. Electronically paced ventricular rhythm c. >1 mm of ST depression at rest d. Complete left bundle branch block	C
	6. Stress radionuclide imaging or stress echocardiography procedures for patients who have a significant change in clinical status and required a stress imaging procedure on their initial evaluation because of equivocal or intermediate-risk treadmill results	C
	7. Stress radionuclide imaging or stress echocardiography procedures for patients with prior revascularization who have a significant change in clinical status	C
	8. Coronary angiography in patients with marked limitation of ordinary activity (CCS class III) despite maximal medical therapy	C
IIa (good supportive evidence)		
IIb (weak supportive evidence)	Annual treadmill exercise testing in patients who have no change in clinical status, can exercise, have none of the ECG abnormalities listed in class I No. 5, and have an estimated annual mortality rate >1%	C
III (not indicated)	1. Echocardiography or radionuclide imaging for assessment of LV ejection fraction and segmental wall motion in patients with a normal ECG, no history of myocardial infarction, and no evidence of CHF	C
	2. Repeat treadmill exercise testing in <3 yr in patients who have no change in clinical status and an estimated annual mortality rate <1% on their initial evaluation, as demonstrated by one of the following: a. Low-risk Duke treadmill score (without imaging) b. Low-risk Duke treadmill score with negative imaging c. Normal LV function and a normal coronary angiogram d. Normal LV function and insignificant CAD	C
	3. Stress imaging or echocardiograph procedures for patients who have no change in clinical status and a normal rest ECG, are not taking digoxin, are able to exercise, and did not require a stress imaging or echocardiographic procedure on their initial evaluation because of equivocal or intermediate-risk treadmill results	C
	4. Repeat coronary angiography in patients with no change in clinical status, no change on repeat exercise testing or stress imaging, and insignificant CAD on initial evaluation	

*See guidelines text for definitions of level of evidence.

ACC = American College of Cardiology; AHA = American Heart Association; CAD = coronary artery disease; CCS = Canadian Cardiovascular Society; CHF = congestive heart failure; ECG = electrocardiogram; LV = left ventricular.

of viable myocardium and demonstrable ischemia on noninvasive testing

Use of PCI or CABG for patients with single-vessel disease with significant proximal LAD disease

Alternative Therapies

The guidelines do not consider alternative therapies to be sufficiently supported by evidence to warrant a class I indication for patients with chronic stable angina. Surgical laser transmyocardial revascularization is given a class IIa indication, and enhanced external counterpulsation and spinal cord stimulation are given class IIb indications.

PATIENT FOLLOW-UP

The ACC/AHA guidelines recommend that patients with chronic stable angina should have follow-up evaluations every 4 to 12 months during the first year of therapy; subsequently, annual evaluations are recommended if the patient is stable and reliable enough to call when angina symptoms become worse or other symptoms occur. The guidelines urge restraint in the use of routine testing in follow-up of patients with chronic stable angina if they have not had a change in clinical status (Table 54G-16). All of the class I indications for testing are for patients who have had a significant change in clinical status, except for the use of coronary angiography for patients with marked limitations of ordinary activity despite maximal medical therapy.

References

1. Gibbons RJ, Abrams J, Chatterjee K, et al: ACC/AHA 2002 guideline update for the management of patients with chronic stable angina: A report of the American College of Cardiology/American Heart Association Task Force on Practice Guidelines (Committee to Update the 1999 Guidelines for the Management of Patients with Chronic Stable Angina). 2002 (www.acc.org/clinical/guidelines/stable/stable.pdf).
2. O'Rourke RA, Brundage BH, Froelicher VF, et al: American College of Cardiology/American Heart Association Expert Consensus Document on electron-beam computed tomography for the diagnosis and prognosis of coronary artery disease. Circulation 102:126-140, 2000.
3. Hurlen M, Abdelnoor M, Smith P, et al: Warfarin, aspirin, or both after myocardial infarction. N Engl J Med 347:969-974, 2002.

Percutaneous Coronary and Valvular Intervention

Jeffrey J. Popma, Donald S. Baim,* and Frederic S. Resnic

Indications for Percutaneous Coronary Intervention, 1419
Patient-Specific Considerations for Percutaneous Coronary Intervention, 1421

Vascular Access, 1423
Vascular Access Complications, 1424
Vascular Closure Devices, 1424

Coronary Devices, 1424
Balloon Angioplasty, 1425
Coronary Atherectomy, 1425
Thrombectomy and Aspiration Devices, 1425
Embolic Protection Devices, 1425
Coronary Stents, 1428
Drug-Eluting Stents, 1429

Antiplatelet Agents, 1436

Antithrombin Agents, 1437

Outcomes Following Percutaneous Coronary Intervention, 1437
Outcomes Benchmarking and Quality Assurance, 1441

Percutaneous Valvular Intervention, 1441
Mitral Valvuloplasty, 1441
Percutaneous Mitral Valve Repair, 1442
Aortic Valvuloplasty, 1442
Percutaneous Aortic Valve Replacement, 1444

Future Directions, 1446

References, 1446

Guidelines, 1449

The use of percutaneous coronary intervention (PCI) to treat ischemic coronary artery disease (CAD) has expanded dramatically over the past three decades. In the absence of left main or diffuse multivessel CAD, PCI is often the preferred method of revascularization in the United States for most patients with ischemic CAD. The estimated 1,000,000 PCI procedures performed annually in the United States now exceeds the number of coronary bypass operations performed each year,[1] although the annual number of PCI procedures may also have peaked because of the effectiveness of risk factor modification and prevention restenosis with drug-eluting-stents. Key enablers of the expanded use of PCI in patients with complex CAD include progressive improvements in equipment design (e.g., catheters with lower profile and enhanced deliverability), adjunctive pharmacological strategies (e.g., thienopyridine derivatives, glycoprotein IIb/IIIa [GP IIb/IIIa] inhibitors, and direct thrombin inhibitors), and better patient selection (e.g., hemodynamic support devices in "ultra" high-risk patients).[2] Percutaneous valvular intervention has also expanded beyond balloon dilation of the aortic and mitral valves over this period to include more definitive percutaneous techniques that can provide an alternative to aortic and mitral valve repair and replacement. "Hybrid" procedures for the treatment of coronary and valvular heart disease have been performed with collaboration of interventional cardiologists and cardiac surgeons.[3,4]

This chapter reviews the developments that led to current approaches for PCI, outlines the indications and clinical considerations for the selection of patients for PCI, discusses the current array of coronary devices, antithrombotic therapy, and vascular closure devices used for PCI, and details the short- and long-term outcomes of PCI. This chapter also considers the emerging opportunities in percutaneous treatment of valvular heart disease.

PERCUTANEOUS CORONARY INTERVENTION

Coronary balloon angioplasty, or percutaneous transluminal coronary angioplasty (PTCA), was first performed by Andreas Gruentzig in 1977 using a fixed-wire balloon catheter. The procedure was initially limited to the fewer than 10% of patients with symptomatic CAD who had a single, focal, noncalcified lesion of a proximal coronary vessel. As equipment design and operator experience evolved over the next decade, the use of PCI expanded to include an increasing spectrum of coronary anatomy including multivessel disease, total occlusions, diseased saphenous vein grafts (SVGs), and patients with acute ST segment elevation myocardial infarction (STEMI), among other complexities.[5,6] Two limitations prevented the widespread use of balloon angioplasty for CAD: abrupt closure of the treated vessel occurred in 5 to 8 percent of cases and required emergency coronary artery bypass graft (CABG) surgery in 3 to 5 percent of patients, and restenosis resulted in symptom recurrence in 30 percent of patients within the ensuing 6 to 9 months.

New coronary devices were developed in the late 1980s to improve on the limitations associated with balloon angioplasty. Coronary stents were designed to scaffold the inner arterial wall to prevent early and late vascular remodeling. Directional, rotational, and extraction atherectomy devices removed atherosclerotic plaque and were developed as stand-alone therapy or to be used in combination with coronary stents (Fig. 55-1). By early 2000, a number of other devices were developed to protect the distal circulation from atherothrombotic embolization (i.e., embolic protection devices) and to remove large thrombi from within the vessel and prevent distal embolization (i.e., aspiration and thrombectomy catheters). The term *percutaneous coronary intervention* encompasses the broad array of the balloons, stents, and adjunct devices required to perform a safe and effective percutaneous revascularization.

INDICATIONS FOR PERCUTANEOUS CORONARY INTERVENTION

The major value of percutaneous or surgical coronary revascularization is the relief of symptoms and signs of ischemic CAD (see also Chap. 54 and the guidelines in Chaps. 54 and 55).[7] PCI may reduce mortality and subsequent MI risk when compared with medical therapy in unstable patients, but these events require concomitant systemic therapies aimed at reducing the extent of atherosclerosis, such as lipid-lowering therapy, hypertension control, and smoking cessation. In contrast, CABG surgery prolongs life in certain anatomical subsets, such as in patients with left main disease, three-vessel CAD, or left anterior

---

*At the time that Dr. Baim prepared this chapter he was a Professor of Medicine at Harvard Medical School and Senior Physician at Brigham and Women's Hospital. Since then he has assumed the position of Chief Medical and Scientific Officer at Boston Scientific Company and serves as an Adjunct Professor of Medicine at Harvard Medical School.

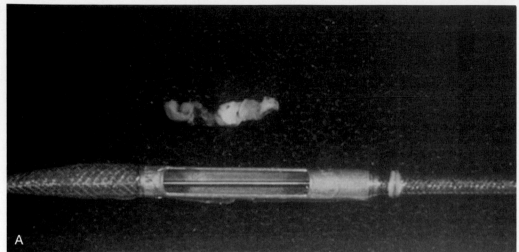

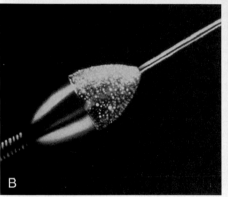

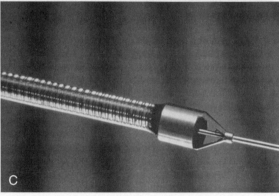

FIGURE 55–1 Atherectomy devices. **A,** Directional coronary atherectomy device with macroscopic tissue resection. **B,** Rotational atherectomy device. **C,** Transluminal extraction catheter.

large area of viable myocardium as determined by noninvasive testing.[7] Patients with recurrent symptoms while receiving medical therapy are candidates for revascularization even if they have a higher risk for an adverse outcome with revascularization.[7] Patients with Class II to IV symptoms should not undergo revascularization without noninvasive evidence of myocardial ischemia or a trial of medical therapy, particularly if only a small region of myocardium is at risk, the likelihood of success is low, or the chance of complications is high.

PATIENTS WITH UNSTABLE ANGINA OR NON-ST SEGMENT MI (see Chaps. 52 and 53). Cardiac catheterization and coronary revascularization in moderate- to high-risk patients who present with unstable angina (UA) or non-ST segment MI (NSTEMI) may improve the prognosis and reduced the rate of reinfarction.[10] A meta-analysis of seven trials that included 9212 patients suggested that the overall rate of death or MI was reduced from 14.4 percent in patients assigned to the selective invasive group to 12.2 percent in patients assigned to the routine invasive group ($p = 0.001$).[11] There was a significant reduction in MI alone in patients assigned to the routine invasive group (9.4 percent in selective invasive patients compared with 7.3 percent in the routine invasive group; $p < 0.001$), and this effect was most pronounced in patients with elevated cardiac biomarker levels.[11] Although death and myocardial infarction was slightly higher during the initial 30 days after a routine invasive approach, this was offset by reductions in death and MI following the procedure (11.0 percent versus 7.4 percent in routine invasive approach; $p < 0.001$).[11] At the end of follow-up, the routine invasive strategy reduced severe angina by 33 percent and rehospitalization by 34 percent.[11]

In a subsequent randomized study, 1200 patients with NSTEMI received maximal therapy that included aspirin, enoxaparin for 48 hours, clopidogrel, lipid-lowering therapy, and abciximab at the time of PCI and were assigned to an invasive strategy or to a more conservative (selectively invasive) strategy for revascularization.[12] The 1-year primary endpoint, a composite of death, nonfatal MI, or rehospitalization, occurred in 22.7 percent in the group assigned to early invasive management and 21.2 percent in the group assigned to selectively invasive management ($p = 0.33$). Although MI was significantly more frequent in the group assigned to early invasive management (15.0 percent versus 10.0 percent, $p = 0.005$), rehospitalization was less frequent in the group assigned to invasive management (7.4 percent versus 10.9 percent, $p = 0.04$).[12] These trial results underscore the importance of maximal medical therapy in the period before revascularization in patients with acute coronary syndromes.

descending artery disease with involvement of one or two additional vessels, irrespective of left ventricular function. The risks and benefits of coronary revascularization need careful review with the patient and family members, and the relative options of PCI, CABG, or continued medical therapy should be discussed before performance of these procedures. A joint task by the American College of Cardiology and American Heart Association has published guidelines for the performance of PCI and CABG.[8]

ASYMPTOMATIC PATIENTS OR THOSE WITH MILD ANGINA. Asymptomatic patients or those who have only mild symptoms are generally best treated with medical therapy, unless one or more high-grade lesions subtend a moderate to large area of viable myocardium, the patient prefers to maintain an aggressive life style or has a high-risk occupation, and the procedure can be performed with a high chance of success and low likelihood of complications.[7] Coronary revascularization should not be performed in patients with absent or mild symptoms if only a small area of myocardium is at risk, if no objective evidence of ischemia can be found, or if the likelihood of success is low or the chance of complications is high.[7] Although one recent analysis of intermediate lesions has reported excellent intermediate-term outcomes after sirolimus-eluting stent placement,[9] there is no evidence that preemptive PCI of a hemodynamically insignificant "vulnerable plaque" prevents subsequent MI.

PATIENTS WITH MODERATE TO SEVERE ANGINA (see Chap. 54). Patients with Canadian Cardiovascular Society (CCS) Class II to IV angina, particularly those who are refractory to medical therapy, can benefit from coronary revascularization, provided that the lesion subtends a moderate to

Current guidelines suggest that an early invasive strategy should be pursued in patients with recurrent ischemia despite therapy, elevated tropinin levels, new ST depression, new or worsening symptoms of congestive heart failure, depressed left ventricular function, hemodynamic instability, sustained ventricular tachycardia, or a recent PCI or CABG.[7]

PATIENTS WITHOUT OPTIONS FOR REVASCULARIZATION. Patients who suffer from substantial angina, yet are poor candidates for conventional revascularization, have limited therapeutic options. These patients generally have either a single, proximal vessel occlusion that subtends a large amount of myocardium or they have undergone one or more prior CABG surgeries with stenoses or occlusions of the SVGs poorly suited for conventional repeat revascularization. "Limited options" patients compose approximately 4 to 12 percent of those undergoing coronary angiography; a larger percentage of patients (20 to 30 percent) have incomplete revascularization due to unsuitable coronary anatomy using surgical or percutaneous techniques.

Creation of new blood vessels in the ischemic tissue using laser injury, also known as therapeutic angiogenesis, may provide symptom relief in these patients. Both surgical and percutaneous approaches have been used to improve regional blood flow to the ischemic myocardium in these patients, although these strategies vary with respect to the depth of myocardial injury, the laser-tissue interactions, the presence or absence of guidance, and the number of channels created. No therapy has yet proved efficacious in blinded clinical trials. Enhanced external counterpulsation support may provide improvement of angina in patients with refractory ischemia,[13,14] although the mechanism of benefit using this technique is not clear.[15]

Patient-Specific Considerations for Percutaneous Coronary Intervention

Assessment of the potential risks and benefits of PCI must address five fundamental patient-specific risk factors: extent of jeopardized myocardium, baseline lesion morphology, underlying cardiac function (including left ventricular function, rhythm stability and coexisting valvular heart disease), presence of renal dysfunction, and preexisting medical comorbidities that render the patient at higher risk for PCI. Each of these factors contributes independently to the risk and benefit attributable to PCI. Proper planning for a PCI procedure requires careful attention to each of these factors.

EXTENT OF JEOPARDIZED MYOCARDIUM. The proportion of viable myocardium subtended by the treated coronary artery is the principal consideration in assessing the acute risk of the PCI procedure.[7,8,16,17] PCI interrupts coronary blood flow for a period of seconds to minutes, and the ability of the patient to hemodynamically tolerate a sustained coronary occlusion depends on both the extent of "downstream" viable myocardium and the presence and grade of collaterals to the ischemic region. Although the risk for abrupt closure has been reduced substantially with the availability of coronary stents, when other procedural complications develop, such as a large side-branch occlusion, distal embolization, perforation, or no-reflow, there may be rapid clinical deterioration that is proportionate to the extent of jeopardized myocardium. In the unlikely event that out-of-hospital stent thrombosis develops, the clinical sequelae of the episode relates to the extent of myocardium subtended by the occluded stent.[18] Predictors for the occurrence of cardiovascular collapse with a failed PCI include the percentage of myocardium at risk, preangioplasty percent diameter stenosis, multivessel CAD, and the presence of diffuse disease.[7]

Whether complete revascularization in patients with multivessel CAD should be performed in a single or staged setting remains controversial. In patients presenting with STEMI, revascularization of only the culprit infarct-related artery is generally recommended,[7] unless there is ongoing cardiogenic shock because of jeopardized myocardium in other regions. Current practice defers addition revascularizations for 3 to 7 days in this circumstance. In other non-acute situations, the number of vessels treated in a single setting will depend on whether procedural complications have occurred, the length of time required for additional vessel treatment, the underlying renal function, and the general ability of the patient to tolerate long procedures. Staged procedures can be safely performed up to 4 to 8 weeks after the initial procedure.[19]

BASELINE LESION MORPHOLOGY. Several angiographic findings increase the technical complexity of PCI and elevate the risk for acute and long-term complications. Although coronary stents have reduced the need for emergency coronary bypass surgery from 3 to 8 percent with balloon angioplasty to less than 1 percent with the availability of coronary stents, they have not eliminated the risk for periprocedural MI, stent thrombosis, or distal embolization and "no reflow." Vessel patency and lesion complexity remain important predictors of outcome in patients undergoing coronary stent placement (Table 55-1).[20] Recent reviews of registry data have confirmed the impact of high risk lesion features on procedural success rates and the risk of short and long-term complications.[20,21]

Chronic Total Occlusions. Coronary occlusions occur in 50 percent of patients with severe (>70 percent stenosis) CAD and are the most important factor leading to the referral of patients to coronary bypass surgery rather than PCI.[22] Successful guidewire recanalization of total coronary occlusions depends on the occlusion duration and on the presence of bridging collaterals, occlusion length greater than 15 mm, and the absence of a "nipple" to guide wire advancement. Although newer guidance technologies have been used to recanalize refractory occlusions,[23] better guidewires and wire techniques have accounted for much of the improvement in crossing success over recent years.[24-26] Once

CH 55

Percutaneous Coronary and Valvular Intervention

TABLE 55–1	SCAI Lesion Classification System for Risk Assessment

Type I Lesion (Highest Success Expected; Lowest Risk)
(1) Does not meet criteria for ACC/AHA C lesion
(2) Patent

Type II Lesions
(1) Meets any of these criteria for ACC/AHA C lesion
    Diffuse (greater than 2 cm length)
    Excessive tortuosity of proximal segment
    Extremely angulated segments greater than 90 degrees
    Inability to protect major side branches
    Degenerated vein grafts with friable lesions
(2) Patent

Type III Lesions
(1) Does not meet criteria for ACC/AHA C Lesion
(2) Occluded

Type IV Lesions (Lowest Success Expected; Highest Risk)
(1) Meets any of these criteria for ACC/AHA C lesion
    Diffuse (greater than 2 cm length)
    Excessive tortuosity of proximal segment
    Extremely angulated segments greater than 90 degrees
    Inability to protect major side branches
    Degenerated vein grafts with friable lesions
(2) Occluded

ACC/AHA = American College of Cardiology/American Heart Association; SCAI = Society for Coronary Angiography and Interventions.
Modified from Krone R, Shaw R, Klein L, Block P, Anderson H, Weintraub W, et al. Evaluation of the American College of Cardiology/American Heart Association and the Society for Coronary Angiography and Interventions lesion classification system in the current "stent era" of coronary interventions (from the ACC-National Cardiovascular Data Registry). Am J Cardiol 92(4):389-94, 2003.

the chronic total occlusion has been crossed, drug-eluting stents may be used to reduce late clinical recurrence.[27,28]

Saphenous Vein Grafts. Saphenous vein grafts (SVGs) interventions compose approximately 8 percent of PCI procedures and pose an increased risk of postprocedural MI caused by atheroembolization that occurs during PCI.[29] When no reflow occurs, SVG administration of arterial vasodilators may improve the flow into the distal native circulation, but there is still a substantial increased risk for death and myocardial infarction.[30] More extensive SVG degeneration and bulkier lesions (larger estimated plaque volume) are associated with higher complication rates than SVGs that have less extensive disease.[29] In the setting of "high-risk" SVG anatomy, alternative approaches using the native coronary artery should be pursued whenever possible.[7] Lower rates of restenosis in SVG lesions are found after coronary stent placement than after balloon angioplasty. Although drug-eluting stents may provide even lower angiographic restenosis rates,[31,32] the sirolimus-eluting stent is poorly suited to SVGs larger than 4.5 mm in diameter and large, and bare metal stents are preferred in this setting.

Bifurcation Lesions. Optimal management of lesions involving both branches of a coronary bifurcation remains controversial. "Snowplowing" of plaque into the adjacent parent vessel or side branch is a major limitation of conventional balloon angioplasty. Atheroablative devices, such as directional atherectomy, have only partially reduced this risk. Risk stratification for bifurcation PCI includes assessment of the extent of atherosclerotic disease in both vessels, estimation of the relative vessel size and distribution in the parent vessel and side branch, and determination of the orientation of the vessels to one another. Stent placement in one vessel rather than in both the parent vessel and side branch is generally preferred, but when there is extensive disease in both vessels, a number of strategies have been used, including simultaneous kissing stents and "crush," culotte, and T stenting (Fig. 55-2). Drug-eluting stents appear to reduce restenosis compared with bare metal stents, but when recurrence develops in patients treated with a drug-eluting stent, it generally occurs at the origin of the side branch.[33] Irrespective of the bifurcation strategy used, a final "kissing" balloon inflation in the parent vessel and side branch should be performed.[34] Newly developed bifurcating coronary stents are currently in clinical trials with promising initial results.[35,36]

Lesion Calcification. The presence of extensive coronary calcification poses unique challenges for PCI because calcium in the vessel wall leads to irregular and inflexible lumens, and makes the delivery of guidewires, balloons, and stents much more challenging. Extensive coronary calcification also renders the vessel wall rigid, necessitating higher balloon inflation pressures to obtain complete stent expansion, and, on occasion, leading to "undilatable" lesions that resist any achievable balloon expansion pressure. Rotational atherectomy effectively ablates vessel wall calcification and facilitates stent delivery and complete stent expansion (Figs. 55-3 and 55-4).

Thrombus. Conventional angiography has poor sensitivity for the detection of coronary thrombus, but the presence of a large, angiographically apparent coronary thrombus heightens risk for procedural complications. Large coronary thrombi may fragment and embolize during PCI, or may extrude through gaps between stent struts placed in the vessel, risking lumen compromise or thrombus propagation and acute thrombosis of the treated vessel. In addition, large coronary thrombi can embolize to other coronary branches or vessels, or dislodge and compromise the cerebral or other vascular beds.

UNDERLYING CARDIAC FUNCTION. Left ventricular function is an important predictor of outcome during PCI. For each 10 percent decrement in resting left ventricular ejection fraction, the risk of in-hospital mortality following PCI increases by approximately twofold.[37] Associated valvular disease or ventricular arrhythmias further increases the risk for PCI in the setting of left ventricular dysfunction. Intraaortic balloon pump support may be useful when there is severe compromise of left ventricular function (i.e., ejection fraction <35 percent) or when the PCI target lesion supplies a substantial portion of viable myocardium.[7,38] Percutaneous cardiopulmonary support devices that do not effectively reduce left ventricular pressures have been replaced by percutaneous left ventricular assist devices that are positioned in the left atrium (e.g., TandemHeart, CardiacAssist Inc., Pittsburgh, PA)[39,40] or directly in the left ventricle (Impella LP 2.5, Abiomed Inc., Danvers, MA).[40-42] These devices permit ultra-high risk PCI without the risk of hemodynamic collapse during the procedure.

RENAL INSUFFICIENCY. The morbidity and mortality associated with PCI relates directly to the extent of baseline renal disease (see also Chap. 88). Patients with evidence of

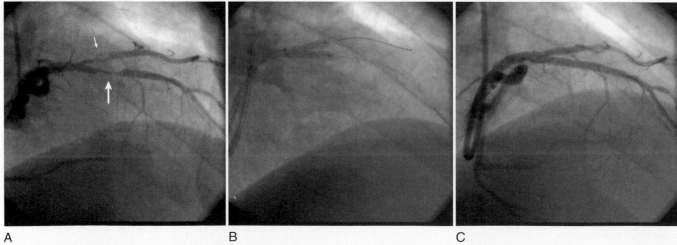

A **B** **C**

FIGURE 55–2 Bifurcation lesion treated with simultaneous kissing stents. **A,** A complex bifurcation lesion involves both the left anterior descending artery (large arrow) and its diagonal branch (small arrow). **B,** After predilation with balloons in both branches, simultaneous inflation of two 3.0-mm × 18-mm CYPHER stents (Cordis Corp., Warren, NJ) in the left anterior descending and diagonal branches is performed. **C,** Following postdilation of both branches with simultaneous inflations to expand the stents, an excellent angiographic result is obtained.

mild renal dysfunction have a 20 percent higher risk of death at 1 year following PCI than patients with preserved renal function.[43-46] Renal dysfunction following contrast administration during angiography may relate to either contrast-induced nephropathy (CIN), cholesterol embolization syndrome (see Chaps. 57 and 88), or both. The risk of CIN is dependent on the dose of the contrast agents used, hydration status at the time of the procedure, preexisting renal function of the patient, age, hemodynamic stability, anemia, and diabetes,[43,47] and the risk for cholesterol embolization syndrome relates to catheter manipulation in an ascending or descending atherosclerotic aorta that releases cholesterol crystals.[48] Although the risk of hemodialysis is less than 3 percent in cases of uncomplicated CIN, the in-hospital mortality in the setting of hemodialysis exceeds 30 percent.[49] Mild renal dysfunction following PCI may increase the risk of death up to fourfold at 1 year following PCI compared with patients with preserved renal function.[43,44,46,49]

ASSOCIATED MEDICAL CO-MORBIDITIES. A number of preexisting medical conditions may increase short- or long-term risks of PCI and should be considered when evaluating the risks, benefits, and strategic approach for patients undergoing PCI. Diabetic patients have higher recurrence rates with bare metal stents,[50] and a long-term survival benefit was shown in diabetic patients undergoing coronary bypass surgery compared with multivessel balloon angioplasty (see Chap. 60).

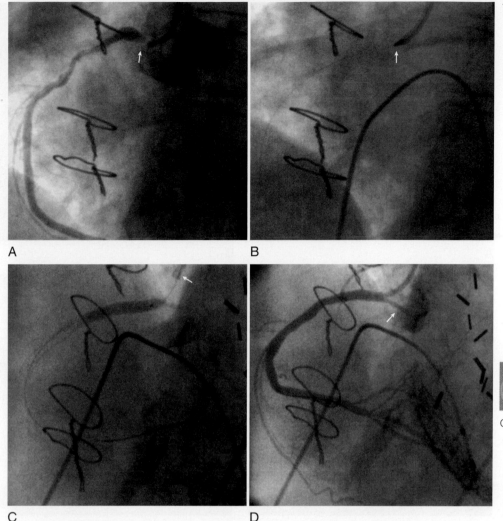

FIGURE 55–3 Rotational atherectomy of an ostial right coronary artery stenosis. **A,** A heavily calcified stenosis of the ostium of the right coronary artery (arrow) precludes conventional balloon angioplasty and stent placement. **B,** A 1.25-mm rotational atherectomy burr (arrow) was advanced to ablate the calcium in the ostium. An additional 1.50-mm rotational atherectomy burr was also used to further ablate the calcific plaque. **C,** After balloon predilation using a 2.5 mm balloon, a 3.50-mm × 23-mm CYPHER stent (Cordis Corp, Warren, NJ) was advanced and inflated to 16 atm. Note the guiding catheter is withdrawn (small arrow) to allow stent placement just at the origin of the right coronary artery. **D,** An excellent final angiographic result is obtained with no residual stenosis. Note the free reflux of contrast from the right coronary artery ostium after stent placement (arrow).

Whether the surgical survival benefit persists compared with patients undergoing multivessel drug-eluting stent placement is the subject of ongoing study.

A bleeding diathesis or need for chronic warfarin therapy may preclude the patient from tolerating long-term combination aspirin and clopidogrel therapy after drug-eluting stent placement, thereby placing the patient at higher risk for stent thrombosis.[51] The need for discontinuation of dual antiplatelet therapy prior to impending noncardiac surgery soon after stent implantation may also predispose to stent thrombosis. In each of these circumstances, bare metal stent placement may be the preferred approach, particularly if the surgery can be deferred for 6 to 8 weeks after stent placement.[52]

VASCULAR ACCESS

The most frequently used vascular access sites for PCI include the common femoral artery, the brachial artery, and, more recently, the radial artery (see Chap. 20). The femoral approach (either right- or left-sided) is the most commonly used vascular access site, and provides the advantages of large vessel size (typically 6 to 8 mm diameter) and the ability to accommodate larger (>6 Fr) sheath sizes including intraaortic balloon pump catheters. In addition, because of the typically straight path from the femoral artery to the ascending aorta, the femoral approach provides excellent guide catheter support and manipulability and access to the venous system through the adjacent femoral vein. The presence of severe peripheral arterial disease, peripheral vascular bypass grafts, and requirement for immobilization following the procedure limits the use of the femoral approach in some patients.

The brachial arterial approach was historically used as the principle alternative to femoral access. However, because the brachial artery provides the only circulation to the forearm and hand (i.e., it is a functional end-artery), any compromise of the brachial artery can lead to severe ischemic complications of the hand. The radial arterial approach has gained in popularity as an alternative to femoral access in patients without significant peripheral vascular disease, particularly in obese patients in whom direct compression of the radial artery reduces vascular complications.[53-55] The

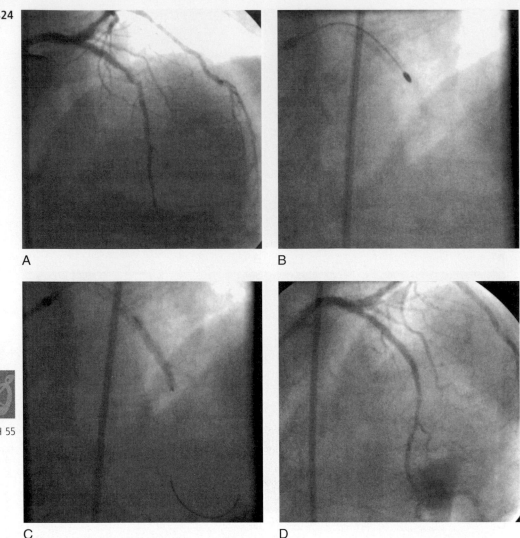

FIGURE 55-4 Rotational atherectomy of an undilatable left anterior descending artery. **A,** A heavily calcified diffuse lesion in the left anterior descending artery is generally considered undilatable using conventional balloon techniques. **B,** A 1.5-mm rotational atherectomy burr revolving at 160,000 rpm is advanced to ablate the calcified lesion. **C,** A 3.0-mm × 28-mm stent can then be advanced across the blockage and inflated to 16 atm. It is unlikely that full stent expansion could have occurred without pretreatment with rotational atherectomy. **D,** The final angiographic result shows no residual stenosis and normal flow into the distal vessel.

to an increased risk of serious vascular complications following PCI include age, female gender, vascular sheath size, low body mass index, renal insufficiency, and degree of anticoagulation during the procedure.[54,58] The location of the entry point for transfemoral access predicts the risk and type of vascular complication. If the access site is above the level of the inguinal ligament, the risk of retroperitoneal hemorrhage is substantially increased.[59,60] If the access site is distal to the femoral bifurcation, pseudoaneurysms (0.4 percent) and arteriovenous fistulas (0.2 percent) may occur.[61] Major vascular complications of the femoral approach include limb-threatening ischemia (0.1 percent) and retroperitoneal hemorrhage (0.4 percent), which itself increases the risk of death 2- to 10-fold in the first 30 days following the PCI procedure.[62,63]

Vascular Closure Devices

Vascular access closure devices were introduced in the mid-1990s as a new way of managing the access site following femoral access procedures. Vascular closure devices reduce the time to ambulation, increase patient comfort following PCI, and provide efficiencies of patient flow in the catheterization laboratory.

Currently approved vascular closure devices fall into three categories. Sealant devices include collagen- and thrombin-based systems that leave no mechanical anchor inside or outside the vessel. Mechanical closure devices include suture-mediated and nitinol clip-based systems, and provide immediate secure closure to the vessel. Hybrid closure devices, such as the dissolvable AngioSeal device (St. Jude Medical, Minneapolis, MN), use a combination of collagen sealant with an internal mechanical closure to effect rapid hemostasis. Although each device has proved relatively safe and effective, little comparative data permits evaluation of the relative risks and benefits of each device. Two recent meta-analyses concluded that vascular closure devices do not lower the risk of vascular complications,[64,65] but infections may occur more often with suture-based closure devices and occlusions are found more often with hybrid devices.

radial approach provides direct access to the ascending aorta and the unique advantage of allowing immediate mobilization following PCI. The small size of the radial artery limits the size of guiding catheters used during PCI (typically 5F or 6F for women and 7F for men). Transradial access is associated with a generally lower rate (2 percent) of vascular complications, however, the procedure is associated with an asymptomatic loss of radial artery patency in 3 percent of cases.[56] An Allen test is essential prior to the performance of radial artery catheterization. Tortuosity of the brachiocephalic trunk may limit the use of the approach in less than 10 percent of interventions.[53-55]

Vascular Access Complications

Vascular access site complications occur after 3 to 7 percent of PCIs and lead to significantly increased length of hospital stay, total costs, and morbidity and mortality.[57] Complications range from relatively minor access site hematomas to life-threatening retroperitoneal bleeds requiring emergent blood transfusion to damage to the vasculature requiring prompt surgical intervention. Factors predisposing patients

CORONARY DEVICES

Over the past three decades, steady improvements in the equipment used for coronary revascularization (e.g., reductions in device profile and improvements in catheter flexibility) have been supplemented with the introduction of periodic "transformational technology," such as coronary stents and, more recently, drug-eluting stents that have extended the scope and breadth of clinical practice. The type of lesions amenable to PCI has become progressively more complex over this period, and the outcomes associated with the use of these devices have progressively improved. A brief overview of the currently available coronary devices follows.

Balloon Angioplasty

Balloon angioplasty expands the coronary lumen by stretching and tearing the atherosclerotic plaque and vessel wall and, to a lesser extent, by redistributing atherosclerotic plaque along its longitudinal axis. Elastic recoil of the stretched vessel wall generally leaves a 30 to 35 percent residual diameter stenosis, and the vessel expansion can result in propagating coronary dissections leading to abrupt vessel closure in 5 to 8 percent of patients. Although stand-alone balloon angioplasty is rarely used other than for very small (<2.25 mm) vessels, balloon angioplasty remains integral to PCI for predilating lesions before stent placement, deploying coronary stents, and further expanding stents after deployment.

Most of the enhancements in balloon technology relate to the development of low-profile (deflated diameter <0.7 mm) balloons that are more trackable through tortuous anatomy, and noncompliant balloons that can inflate to pressures in excess of 20 atm without overexpansion or rupture. A modification of balloon angioplasty includes a focused-force dilation in which a scoring blade or guidewire external to the balloon concentrates dilating force and resists balloon slippage during inflation. The Cutting Balloon (Boston Scientific, Natick, MA) and the FX Minirail (Abbott Vascular, Redwood City, CA) are focused-force balloon angioplasty systems that are currently used in a small minority (less than 5 percent) of PCIs.

Coronary Atherectomy

Atherectomy refers to removal (rather than simple displacement) of the obstructing atherosclerotic plaque. By removal of plaque or improving lesion wall compliance in calcified or fibrotic lesions, atherectomy can provide a larger final minimal lumen diameter than achieved by balloon angioplasty alone. Atherectomy was performed in 30 percent of interventional procedures between 1992 and 1994, but its use fell dramatically with the availability of coronary stents. Fewer than 5 percent of current procedures involve the use of atherectomy devices, most often rotational atherectomy in combination with coronary stents.

Directional Coronary Atherectomy. Directional coronary atherectomy (DCA) (Abbott Vascular, Santa Rosa, CA) uses a rotating cup-shaped blade within a windowed cylinder to directionally excise plaque (average total weight approximately 20 mg) from the vessel wall. This tissue removal and subsequent mechanical dilation with balloon angioplasty provides a larger acute lumen than balloon angioplasty alone, although a substantial amount of atherosclerotic plaque remains even after aggressive DCA. Clinical trials showed that effective use of DCA produced a modest (roughly 30%) reduction in restenosis compared to balloon angioplasty alone. A randomized study showed no benefit of DCA plus stenting over stenting alone in patients with complex anatomy. In current practice, DCA is used in <1 percent of patients with noncalcified bifurcation lesions involving a large branch or in the ostium of the left anterior descending artery.

Rotational Coronary Atherectomy. Rotational coronary atherectomy (RA) (Boston Scientific, Natick, MA) removes the atheromatous plaque by the abrasion of inelastic calcified plaque using microscopic (20 to 50 microns) diamond chips on the surface of a rapidly rotating (160,000 rpm) olive-shaped atherectomy burr. This abrasion generates 2- to 5-micron microparticles that pass through the coronary microcirculation for removal by the reticuloendothelial system. Burrs travel over a specialized 0.009-inch guidewire and are available in diameters ranging from 1.25 to 2.50 mm. In the setting of severe calcification, smaller (1.25 mm) burrs can be initially used followed by larger burrs in 0.25 to 0.50 mm increments up to 70 percent of the reference vessel diameter. Aggressive RA techniques do not provide a restenosis advantage over more conservative methods, and tend to increase acute procedural complications. Rotational atherectomy does not appear to reduce restenosis compared to balloon angioplasty in noncalcified vessels.[66] Current use of RA is reserved for ostial and heavily calcified lesions that cannot be dilated with balloon PTCA or those that prevent delivery of coronary stents (see Figs. 55-3 and 55-4). RA is generally limited to abrasion of superficial calcification with a single 1.5 or 1.75 mm burr to improve lesion compliance (plaque modification) before the lesion is treated definitively by balloon dilation and stent placement. RA is currently used in less than 5 to 10 percent of PCI procedures.

Thrombectomy and Aspiration Devices

The Angiojet rheolytic thrombectomy catheter (Possis Medical, Inc., Minneapolis, MN) was introduced as a dedicated device for thrombus removal through the dissolution and aspiration of the thrombus. High-speed saline jets within the tip of the catheter create intense local suction via the Venturi effect, pulling surrounding blood, thrombus, and saline into the lumen of the catheter opening, propelling the debris proximally through the catheter lumen. Rheolytic thrombectomy was superior to a prolonged intraluminal urokinase infusion in patients with a large thrombus,[67] but its routine use in patients with ST segment elevation MI was not associated with improvement in myocardial infarction size using single photon emission computed tomography (SPECT) imaging and may have caused more complications.[68] Rheolytic thrombectomy may still be useful in clinical practice when there is a large angiographic thrombus in a native vessel or saphenous vein graft.

Newer lower profile aspiration catheters that use 6F guiding catheters have been developed as alternatives to rheolytic thrombectomy in patients with thrombus-containing lesions (Fig. 55-5).[69-71] These techniques may be slightly less effective (particularly against partially organized thrombus) than the rheolytic thrombectomy, although the risk of distal particulate embolization and device trauma in smaller vessels may be less with these aspiration catheters.

Embolic Protection Devices

The advent of embolic protection systems has reduced the risk of postprocedural adverse events following SVG and selective native vessel PCI.[72] Although embolization of atherosclerotic debris was not considered a major complication during the early years of native coronary balloon angioplasty, it is now recognized as one potential cause of distal myocardial necrosis after PCI, particularly in friable SVG lesions. Distal embolization causes postprocedural cardiac enzyme elevation in nearly 20 percent of cases after SVG PCI, and this enzyme elevation is associated with substantial morbidity and mortality. Numerous additional occlusive and filter-based distal protection systems, as well as

CH 55

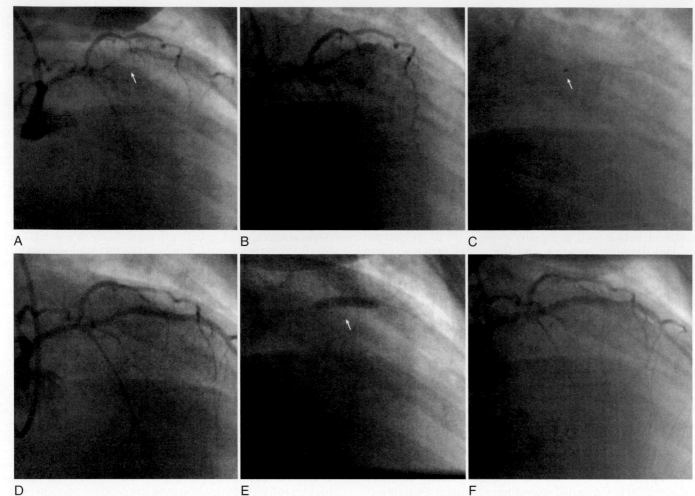

FIGURE 55–5 Aspiration thrombectomy for STEMI. A thrombotic occlusion of the proximal left anterior descending artery is shown (**A,** arrow). There is minimal improvement in flow following a 2.5-mm balloon inflation with the suspicion of thrombus precluding flow (**B).** An Export catheter is used to remove the thrombus (**C),** and anterograde flow is reestablished and the thrombus is removed (**D).** A 3.0 mm drug-eluting stent was placed (**E),** resulting in no residual stenosis and TIMI 3 flow into the distal vessel (**F).** TIMI$_3$ = Thrombolysis in Myocardial Infarction trial 3.

novel proximal occlusion devices, have undergone evaluation and approval for use in SVG interventions.[73-75] Despite their potential benefit in preventing thromboembolization in patients with STEMI, none of the embolic protection devices has reduced myocardial infarction size with primary intervention, possibly relating to the high profile of the devices.[76,77] Embolic protection devices fall into three broad categories: distal occlusion devices, distal embolic filters, and proximal occlusion devices.

DISTAL OCCLUSION DEVICES. Two distal occlusion devices are available for clinical use. The Guardwire(Medtronic Vascular, Santa Rosa, CA) is a low-pressure balloon mounted on a hollow guidewire shaft. The device is passed across the target lesion and inflated with a saline contrast admixture to occlude flow; the debris liberated by intervention remains trapped in the stagnant column of blood and is aspirated using a specially designed aspiration catheter before the occlusion balloon is deflated to restore antegrade flow (Fig. 55-6).[74] Compared to SVG intervention without distal occlusion, use of the Guardwire reduced 30-day major adverse clinical events (from 16.9 to 9.6 percent; $p < 0.01$) and no-reflow (from 8.3 to 3.3 percent; $p < 0.01$) (Fig. 55-7).[74] The Triactive Device (Kensey-Nash, Exton, PA) proved noninferior to other occlusion devices but has the advantage of having a continuous aspiration catheter and more rapid balloon inflation and deflation using CO_2 rather than saline for balloon inflation.[75] The major disadvantage of both of these devices is that blood flow is stopped during SVG intervention while the balloons are inflated.

EMBOLIC PROTECTION FILTERS. Distal filters are advanced across the target lesion in their smaller collapsed state, and a retaining sheath is withdrawn, allowing the filters to open and expand against the vessel wall. The filters then remain in place to catch any liberated embolic material larger than the filter pore size (usually 120 to 150 microns) during intervention.[78] At the end of the intervention, the filters are collapsed using a sheath, and the captured embolic material is removed from the body.[73] This type of device has the advantages of maintaining antegrade flow during the procedure and allowing intermittent contrast injection to visualize underlying anatomy, but it has the potential disadvantage of allowing the component of debris with a diameter less than the filter pore size to pass. The FilterWire (Boston Scientific, Natick, MA) was noninferior to the Guardwire distal occlusion in one randomized trial.[73] Newer filter devices with reduced crossing profiles and more efficient capture of embolic debris have been developed (Figs. 55-8 and 55-9).[79,80]

PROXIMAL OCCLUSION DEVICES. The third type of embolic protection device occludes flow into the vessel using a balloon on the tip of or just beyond the tip of the guiding catheter. Two proximal occlusion devices are currently in use: the Proxis catheter (St Jude Medical, Minneaoplis MN)[81] and Kerberos embolic protection system (Kerberos, Sunnyvale, CA).[82] With such inflow occlusion, retrograde flow generated by distal collaterals or infusion through a "rinsing" catheter can propel any liberated debris back into the lumen of the guiding catheter. These approaches have the potential advantage of providing embolic protection even before the first wire crosses the target lesion.

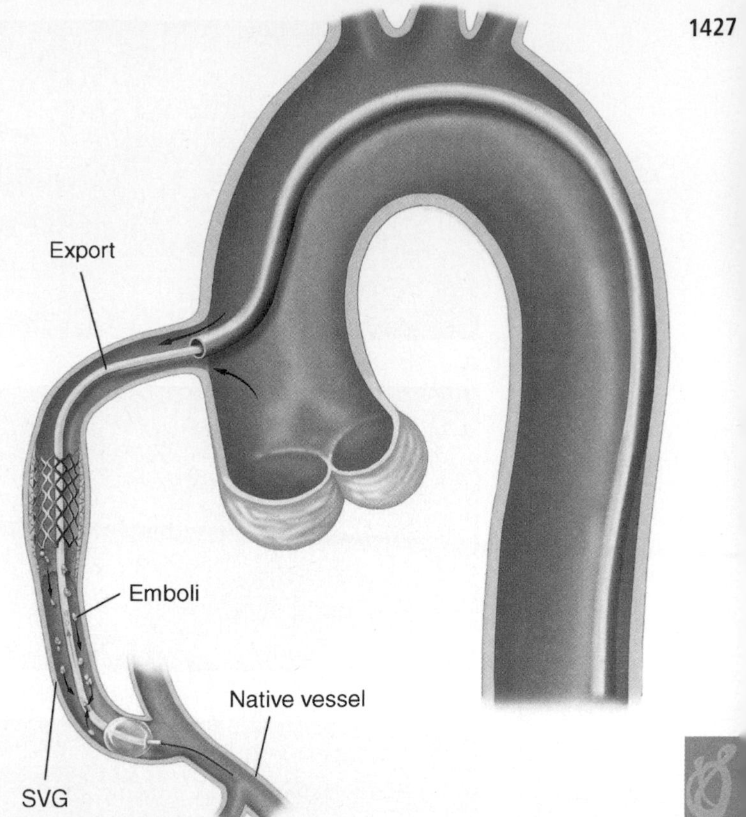

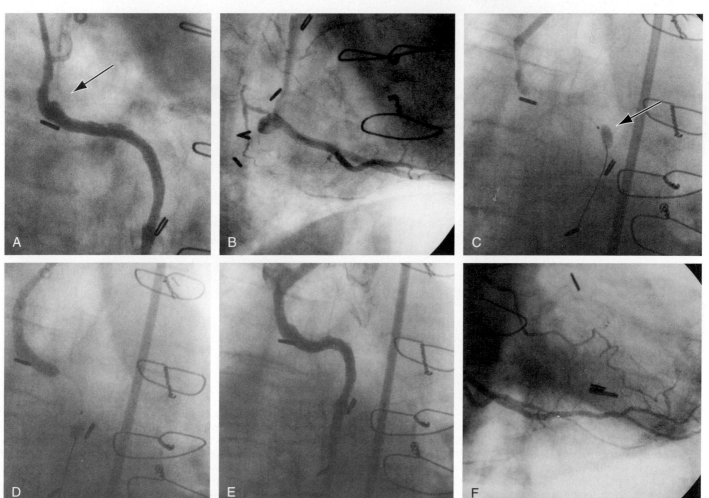

FIGURE 55–6 Key components of the Guardwire Distal protection balloon (Medtronic Vascular, Santa Rosa, CA). The Guardwire device is advanced through the saphenous vein graft (SVG) into a distal portion of the SVG that is free of significant stenosis. The occlusion balloon is inflated and, after demonstration of the occlusion, stent placement is performed within the SVG. At the end of stent deployment, an Export catheter is advanced and approximately 40 ml of blood and particulate matter are removed. *(From Baim D, Wahr D, George B, et al: Randomized trial of a distal embolic protection device during percutaneous intervention of saphenous vein aorto-coronary bypass grafts. Circulation 105[11]:1285-90, 2000.)*

Export

Emboli

Native vessel

SVG

FIGURE 55–7 Saphenous vein graft (SVG) percutaneous intervention with the Guardwire balloon (Medtronic Vascular, Santa Rosa, CA). Distal profusion **(A)** shows a degenerated SVG to the posterior descending artery with a diffuse stenosis in the proximal segment of the SVG (arrow). **B,** Normal distal perfusion of the SVG with demonstration of secondary and tertiary branches. Positioning of the Guardwire balloon in the distal portion of the SVG **(C,** arrow) and a 4.0-mm stent in the proximal SVG **(D)** resulted in minimal residual stenosis **(E)** and no evidence of distal embolization **(F).**

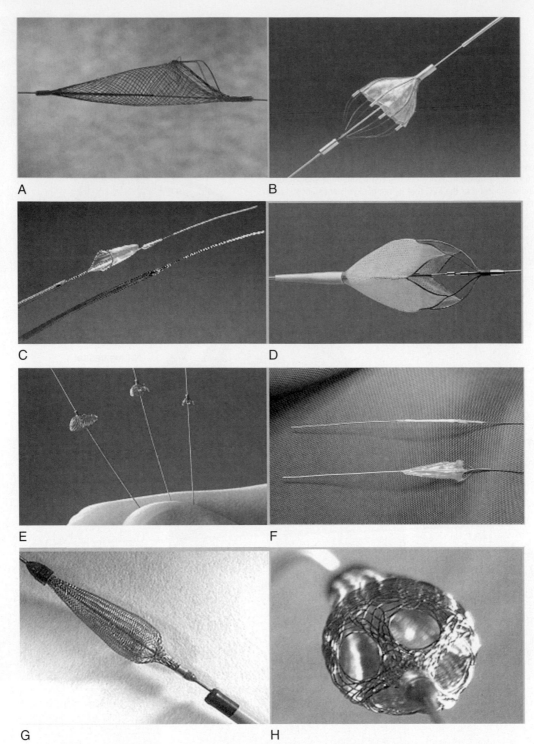

FIGURE 55-8 Filters for distal protection. **A,** The Spider Filter (ev3, Minneapolis, MN); **B,** Angioguard Device (Cordis, Warren, NJ); **C,** EPI Filterwire (Boston Scientific, Natick, MA); **D,** Accunet device (Guidant, Santa Clara, CA); **E,** MedNova (Abbott, Chicago, IL); **F,** Rubicon Filter (Boston Scientific, Natick, MA); **G** and **H,** The Interceptor Filter (Medtronic Vascular, Santa Rosa, CA) in longitudinal view **(G)** and axial view **(H).**

Coronary Stents

Coronary stents have emerged as the predominant form of PCI and are currently used in more than 90 percent of PCI procedures worldwide. Coronary stents scaffold arterial dissection flaps, thereby lowering the incidence of vessel closure and need for emergency CABG surgery, and lessen the frequency of restenosis, because of their effect on preventing arterial constriction that is the primary mechanism

of restenosis with balloon angioplasty and atherectomy. Despite late clinical improvements compared with balloon angioplasty, restenosis after coronary stent placement occurs in some patients due to excessive intimal hyperplasia within the stent. A number of second-generation balloon-expandable stents were introduced between 1997 and 2003, varying in metallic composition (i.e., cobalt chromium or layered metals versus solid 316 L stainless steel), strut design, stent length, delivery and deployment system, and

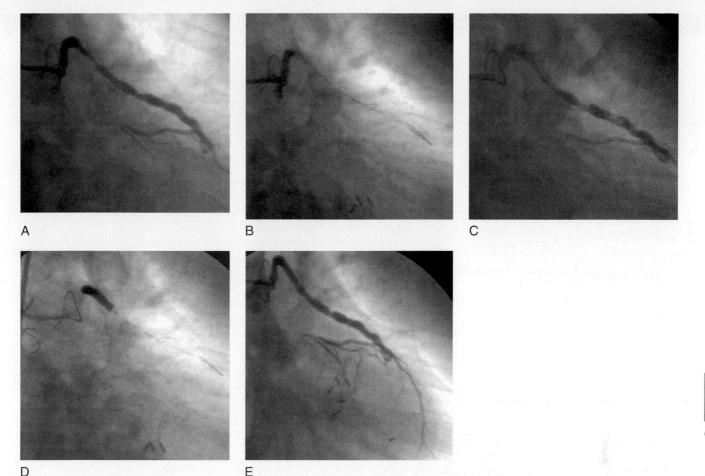

FIGURE 55–9 Saphenous vein graft (SVG) percutaneous intervention with Filterwire distal protection. **A,** A degenerated SVG to the left anterior descending artery has a stenosis in its proximal segment. **B,** The Filterwire (Boston Scientific, Natick, MA) is positioned across the stenosis and deployed against the wall of the SVG. **C,** Flow is shown through the SVG. **D,** A stent is deployed in the proximal segment of the SVG. **E,** The Filterwire is removed, and there is excellent flow into the distal SVG without evidence of distal embolization.

arterial surface coverage, among other factors. These modifications enhanced flexibility and ease of delivery of the stent, while also improving vessel scaffolding and side branch access.

The early use of coronary stents was limited by high (3 to 5 percent) subacute thrombosis rates, despite aggressive antithrombotic therapy with aspirin (>325 mg daily), dipyridamole (225 mg daily), periprocedural low-molecular-weight dextran, and an uninterrupted transition from intravenous heparin to oral warfarin. Subacute thrombosis produced profound clinical consequences, resulting in an untoward outcome (e.g., death, MI, or emergency revascularization) in virtually every such patient. Lower frequencies of subacute stent thrombosis (roughly 0.5 percent) have resulted from use of high-pressure stent deployment, and with a drug regimen that includes aspirin and a thienopyridine (e.g., clopidogrel) started just after stent placement.

While bare metal coronary stents reduce the incidence of angiographic and clinical restenosis compared to balloon angioplasty (Table 55-2), angiographic restenosis (follow-up diameter stenosis >50 percent) still occurs in 20 to 30% of patients and clinical restenosis (recurrent angina due to restenosis in the treated segment) develops in 10 to 15 percent of patients in the first year after treatment.[50,83] Restenosis with bare metal coronary stents occurs more often in patients with small vessels, long lesions, and in patients with diabetes mellitus, among other factors (Table 55-3).[50] Adjunctive pharmacological therapy has not prevented restenosis after stent placement, although cilostazol or oral rapamycin has modestly reduced the occurrence of bare metal stent restenosis.

Several mechanical treatments for in-stent restenosis were attempted, including balloon redilation, removal of in-stent hyperplasia by means of atherectomy, and repeat bare metal stenting. Brachytherapy using beta or gamma sources did modestly improve this outcome for in-stent restenosis (Table 55-4),[84,85] but brachytherapy has several limitations, including the requirement for a radiation therapist, a tendency for late "catch-up" restenosis, and inhibition of endothelialization that markedly increased the risk of thrombosis if another stent was implanted in the same vessel segment. Brachytherapy was inferior to drug-eluting stent placement in two randomized studies.[86,87]

Drug-Eluting Stents

Drug-eluting stents were developed in the early 2000s to provide sustained local delivery of an antiproliferative agent at the site of vessel wall injury. The three components of current drug-eluting stents are the balloon expandable stent, a durable or resorbable polymer coating that provides sustained drug delivery, and the pharmacological agent employed to limit intimal hyperplasia (Table 55-5).

Drug-eluting stents have proven efficacy in patients with focal, de novo (Table 55-6)[88-92] and "workhorse" lesions that include reference vessel diameters between 2.5 mm

TABLE 55–2 | **Early and Late Outcome In Randomized Trials of Coronary Stent Placement Versus Balloon PTCA**

Variable	Stress[1]		Benestent[2]		Benestent II[3]		Rest[4]		Saved[5]		Tosca[6]	
	PTCA	Stent	PTCA	Stent	PTCA	Stent	PTCA	Stent	PTCA	Stent	PTCA	Stent
Lesion type	De Novo, Native		De Novo, Native		De Novo, Native		Restenotic, Native		SVGs		Chronic Occlusion	
Years of entry	1991-1993		1991-1993		1995-1996		1991-1996		1993-1995		1996-1997	
Number of patients	202	205	257	259	410	413	176	178	107	108	208	202
Baseline factors												
Mean age, years	60	60	58	57	59	50	60	59	66	66	58	58
Women, %	27	17	18	20	20	23	18	20	21	18	20	16
Diabetes mellitus	16	15	6	7	11	13	15	20	36	23	18	15
Unstable angina,%	48	47	NA	NA	40	45	22	17	77	82	25	24
Multivessel disease, %	32	36	NA	NA	NA	NA	32	33	NA	NA	NA	NA
Angiographic success, %	92.6	99.5	98.1	96.9	99	99	93.2	98.9	86	97	NA	NA
Clinical success, %	89.6	96.1	91.1	92.7	95	96	100	100	69	92	87.9	94.6
Reference diameter, mm	2.99	3.03	3.01	2.99	2.93	2.96	3.04	3.01	3.19	3.18	3.53	3.61
Final % stenosis	35	19	33	22	8	7	30	6	32	12	38	27
Stent use, %	6.9	96.1	5.1	94.6	13.4	96.6	6.8	98.9	7.0	97	9.6	96
Early complications	0-14 Days		In Hospital		1 Month		In Hospital		In Hospital		In Hospital	
Death, %	1.5	0	0	0	0.2	0	0.6	1.1	2	2	0	0
Q-wave Infarction, %	3.0	2.9	0.8	1.9	1.0	1.2	0.6	2.8	1	2	NR	NR
Emergency CABG, % CK-MB Elevation >3×	4.0	2.4	1.6	1.9	0.5	0.7	0.6	1.1	4	2	0	0.5
Late clinical outcome	15-240 Days		7 Months		12 Months		6 Months		240 Days		180 days	
Death, %	0	1.5	0.4	0.8	1.0	1.0	1.1	1.1	9	7	0	0
Q-wave MI	0.5	1.0	1.6	2.7	1.5	1.9	0.6	2.8	4	5	NR	NR
Revascularization,%	15.4	10.2	NA	NA	NA	NA	NA	NA	NA	NA	15.4	8.4[+]
Repeat PTCA	11.4	9.8	20.6	10.0	15.6	9.4	26.6	10.3	16	13	14.4	6.9
CABG follow-up	4.5	2.4	2.3	3.1	1.5	1.9	0.6	2.2	12	7	1.4	1.5
Angiography												
Restenosis, %	42.1	31.6	32	22	31	16	32	18	47	36	70	55[+++]
Follow-up MLD	1.56	1.74	1.73	1.82	1.66	1.89	1.85	2.04	1.49	1.73	1.23	1.49
Follow-up % stenosis	49	42	43	38	17	17	47	30	51	46	61	53
Any bleeding complication	4.0	7.3	3.1	13.5	1.0	1.2	1.1	11.2	5	17	NR	NR

[+] = p < 0.05; [++] = p < 0.01; [+++] p < 0.005; [++++] p < 0.001.

CABG = coronary artery bypass graft; CK-MB = creative kinase isoenzyme; MI = myocardial infarction; MLD = minimal lumen diameter; NA = not available; NR = not recorded; PTCA = percutaneous transluminal coronary angioplasty; SVG = saphenous vein graft.

From Fischman DL, Leon MB, Baim DS, et al: A randomized comparison of coronary-stent placement and balloon angioplasty in the treatment of coronary artery disease. N Engl J Med 331; 496, 1994; Serruys PW, de Jaegere P, Kiemeneij F, et al: A comparison of balloon-expandable-stent implantation with balloon angioplasty in patients with coronary artery disease. Benestent Study Group N Engl J Med 331:489, 1994; Serruys PW, van Hout B, Bonnier H, et al: Randomised comparison of implantation of heparin-coated stents with balloon angioplasty in selected patients with coronary artery disease (Benestent II). Lancet 352:673, 1998; Erbel R, Haude M, Hopp HW, et al: Coronary-artery stenting compared with balloon angioplasty for restenosis after initial balloon angioplasty. N Engl J Med 339:1672, 1998; Savage MP, Douglas JS, Fischman DL: Stent placement compared with balloon angioplasty for obstructed coronary bypass grafts. Saphenous Vein De Novo Trial Investigators N Engl J Med 337:740, 1997; Buller CE, Dzavik V, Carere RG, et al: Primary stenting versus balloon angioplasty in occluded coronary arteries: The Total Occlusion Study of Canada (TOSCA). Circulation 100;236, 1999.

and 3.5 mm and lesion lengths between 15 and 30 mm (Table 55-7).[93-97] Additional randomized trials and registries have also demonstrated the benefit of drug-eluting stents in patients with long (>20 mm length) (Table 55-8)[98-101] and small (<2.5 mm) vessels (Table 55-9),[102-105] chronic total occlusions (Table 55-10),[27,106-110] SVG and internal mammary disease (Table 55-11),[31,111-116] in-stent restenosis (Table 55-12),[86,87,117-120] and in patients with STEMI (Table 55-13).[121-123] With the expanded follow-up of patients receiving drug-eluting stents, it has become apparent that drug-eluting stent placement requires extended (up to 1 year) therapy with the combination of aspirin and clopidogrel to prevent stent thrombosis.[51] Moreover, even after 1 year, there is an infrequent (0.2 to 0.6 percent) annual rate of very late stent thrombosis,[124] warranting a careful discussion of the risk, benefits, and alternative therapies in candidates for PCI.

SIROLIMUS-ELUTING STENTS. The CYPHER (Cordis, Warren, NJ) stent contains sirolimus, a naturally occurring immunosuppressive agent that causes cytostatic inhibition of cell proliferation. Sirolimus is released from a biostable polymer that releases sirolimus over a 30-day period. The CYPHER stent received Conformité Européenne Mark approval in Europe in April 2002, and approval by the U.S. Food and Drug Administration (FDA) in the United States in May 2003.

The pivotal SIRIUS Trial included 1058 patients with workhorse lesions who were randomized to treatment with a sirolimus-eluting stent or a bare metal stent.[93] The primary clinical endpoint of 8-month target-vessel failure, composed of target vessel revascularization, death, or MI, was reduced from 21 percent in patients treated with bare metal stents to 8.6 percent in patients with sirolimus-eluting stents ($p < 0.001$). Angiographic restenosis rates were also lower in patients assigned to treatment with the sirolimus-eluting stents within the stent (35.4 percent with bare metal stents versus 3.2 percent with sirolimus-eluting stents; $p < 0.001$) and within the treated segment including 5 mm proximal and distal margins (36.3 percent with bare metal stents versus 8.9 percent with sirolimus-eluting stents; $p < 0.001$).[93] Target vessel revascularization was reduced from 16.6 percent in bare metal stents to 4.1 percent in sirolimus-eluting stents ($p < 0.001$).[93] Reduction in intimal hyperplasia endured for at least 2 years after the procedure (Fig. 55-10).[125]

PACLITAXEL-ELUTING STENTS. The TAXUS stent (Boston Scientific, Natick, MA) is composed of a stainless steel stent platform, a polyolefin polymer derivative, and the microtubular stabilizing agent paclitaxel that has antiinflammatory effects while also inhibiting both cell migration and division. Paclitaxel release is completed within 30 days of implantation, although a substantial portion (>90%) of the paclitaxel remains within the polymer indefinitely. The pivotal TAXUS-IV trial randomly assigned 1314 patients with single de novo coronary lesions to either a TAXUS stent or an identical-appearing bare metal stent.[98] The ischemia-driven target-vessel revascularization at 9 months was reduced from 11.3 to 3 percent and remained significantly reduced at 12 months (from 17.1 to 7.1 percent) in patients with the paclitaxel-eluting stents ($p < 0.001$). The rate of binary angiographic restenosis was reduced both within the stent (24.4 percent with bare metal stents versus 5.5 percent with the paclitaxel-eluting stent; $p < 0.001$) and within the treated segment including 5 mm proximal and distal margins (26.6 percent and 7.9 percent, respectively; $p < 0.001$).

ZOTAROLIMUS-ELUTING STENTS. Zotarolimus (previously known as ABT-578) is another rapamycin analogue released from a phosphorylcholine (PC)-coated stent that has been evaluated using the Endeavor stent (Medtronic Vascular, Santa Rosa, CA) and the Zomaxx stent (Abbott Vascular, Redwood City, CA). In the Endeavor-II trial, 1197 patients were assigned to treatment with the Endeavor

Text continues on p. 1436.

TABLE 55–3	Factors Predictive of Restenosis after Coronary Stenting

Clinical Factors

Angina pattern prior to presentation
  Unstable angina
  ST segment elevation myocardial infarction
Prior recurrence
Early symptom recurrence after stent placement (<3 months)
Diabetes mellitus
End-stage renal disease
Elevated C-reactive protein

Anatomical Factors

Proximal left anterior descending artery
Smaller reference vessel diameters
Long lesion length
Diffuse pattern of restenosis
Total coronary occlusion
Saphenous vein graft

Procedural Factors

Higher post-procedural diameter stenosis
Smaller final lumen diameter
Smaller acute gain
Stent length

TABLE 55–4	Late Outcome In Randomized Trials of Radiation Brachytherapy for the Prevention of In-Stent Restenosis									
	Scripps[1]		Wrist[2]		Gamma-1[3]		Start[84]		Inhibit[85]	
Variable	Ir-192	PL	Ir-192	PL	Ir-192	PL	Sr-90	PL	P-32	PL
Number of patients	26	29	65	65	131	121	244	232	166	166
Baseline factors:										
Mean age, years	70	69	63	62	58	61	61	61	62	61
Women, %	27	24	34	28	25.2	26.6	32	37	30	27
Diabetes mellitus	27	41	39	45	31.3	31.4	31	32	33	27
Lesion length, mm	12.9	11.9	28.8	26.7	19	20.3	16.3	16.0	16.9	17.9
Reference diameter, mm	2.88	2.78	2.71	2.72	2.69	2.73	2.76	2.77	2.68	2.71
MLD, mm										
Baseline	1.10	1.03	0.94	0.81	0.98	0.96	0.98	0.98	1.01	0.95
Final	2.82	2.88	2.23	2.25	2.09	2.12	1.94	1.94	1.92	1.96
Follow-up	2.43[+]	1.85	2.03[++++]	1.24	1.47	1.31	1.65[++++]	1.41	1.54[+]	1.38
% Diameter stenosis										
Baseline	62	62	65	70	63.3	64.6	64.2	64.2	61.9	65.2
Final	7	5	19	20	23.9	24.5	31.4	30.7	29.6	28.5
Follow-up	17[+]	54	30[++++]	57	45.6	53.2	41.7[++++]	50.1	43.3[+++]	51.3
Restenosis rate, %	17[+]	54	22[++++]	60	32.4[+]	55.3	28.8[++++]	45.2	26[++++]	52
Stent thrombosis, %	1	0	9.2	3.5	6.3	1.6		0.4	3	1
Follow-up period, mo	6 months		12 months		9 months		8 months		290 days	
TLR, %	12[+]	45	23.0[++++]	63.1	24.4[++]	42.1	13.9[++++]	24.9	8[++++]	26
Late clinical events, %	19[+]	62	35.3[++++]	67.6	28.2[+]	43.8	19.1[+]	28.7	12[++++]	28
Death	0	3	6.2	6.2	3.1	0.8	1.3	0.5	3	2
Q wave MI	4	0	0	0	4.6	2.5	0	0	2	0

[+] = $p < 0.05$; [++] = $p < 0.01$; [+++] $p < 0.005$; [++++] $p < 0.001$.

CABG = coronary artery bypass graft; Ir = Iridium; MI = myocardial infarction; MLD = minimal lumen diameter; P = phosphorus; PCI = percutaneous coronary intervention; PL = placebo; Sr = strontium-90; TLR = target lesion revascularization.

From Teirstein P, Massullo V, Jani S, et al: Catheter-based radiotherapy to inhibit restenosis after coronary stenting. N Engl J Med 336:1697, 1997; Waksman R, White R, Chan R, et al: Intracoronary gamma-radiation therapy after angioplasty inhibits recurrence in patients with in-stent restenosis. Circulation 101:2130, 2000; Leon M, Teirstein P, Moses J, et al: Localized intracoronary gamma radiation therapy to inhibit the recurrence of restenosis after stenting. N Engl J Med 344:250, 2001.

TABLE 55–5 | Design Characteristics of Drug-Eluting Stent Programs

Type of Stent	Stent Platform	Stent Material	Polymer Coating	Drug Elution	Clinical Trials
CYPHER	Bx velocity	Stainless steel	Durable co-polymer: Polyethylene-co-vinyl acetate (PEVA) and poly-*n*-butyl methacrylate (PBMA)	Sirolimus	SIRIUS
TAXUS	NIR stent Express-II Liberte	Stainless steel	Polyolefin polymer derivative	Paclitaxel	TAXUS
ENDEAVOR	Driver	Cobalt chromium	Phosphorylcholine	Zotarolimus	ENDEAVOR
Xience	Vision	Cobalt chromium	Durable fluoropolymer	Everolimus	SPIRIT
CoStar	CoStar	Cobalt chromium	Poly-lactic co-glycolic acid resorbable polymer	Paclitaxel	PISCES
Zomaxx	Trimax	Stainless steel–tantalum alloy	Phosphorylcholine	Zotarolimus	Zomaxx

TABLE 55–6 | Drug-Eluting Stent Comparative Studies in Patients with Focal Lesions

Lesion Complexity	Stent Type	N	Length, mm	RVD, mm	DM, %	FU, mo	Binary Restenosis, % In Segment	In Stent	Late Lumen Loss, mm In Segment	In Stent	FU, mo	TLR, %	Death, %	MI, %	MACE, %
RAVEL[88]	BMS	118	9.61	2.64	21	6	NA	26.6+++	NA	0.80+++	12	22.8	1.69	1.69	28.8+++
	SES	120	9.56	2.60	16		NA	0	NA	−0.01		0.0	1.66	0.83	5.8
TAXUS-I[89]	BMS	30	11.89	2.94	13	6	NA	10	NA	0.71++	12	10	0	0	10
	PES	31	10.70	2.99	23		NA	0	NA	0.36		0.0	0	0	3.0
SPIRIT-I[90]	BMS	29	10.9	2.71	10	12	NA	NA	0.59+++	0.84+++	12	21.4	0.0a	0.0	21.4
	EES	27	10.1	2.61	11		NA	NA	0.14	0.24		7.7	0.0a	7.6	15.4
ENDEAVOR I[91]	ZES	100	10.9	2.96	16	12	5.4	5.4	0.43	0.61	12	2.0	0.0	1.0	2.0

aCardiac death

+p < 0.05; ++p < 0.01; +++p < 0.001 treatment versus control

BMS = bare metal stent; DM = diabetes mellitus; EES = everolimus-eluting stent; FU = follow-up; MACE = major adverse cardiac events; MI = myocardial infarction; N = number; NA = not available; PES = paclitaxel-eluting stent; RVD = reference vessel diameter; SES = sirolimus-eluting stent; TLR = target lesion revascularization; ZES = zotarolimus eluting stent.

TABLE 55–7 | Drug-Eluting Stent Comparative Studies in Patients with Intermediate-Risk Lesions[a]

Lesion Complexity	Stent Type	N	Length, mm	RVD, mm	DM, %	FU, mo	Binary Restenosis, % In Lesion	In Stent	Late Lumen Loss, mm In Lesion	In Stent	FU, mo	TLR, %	Death, %	MI, %	MACE, %
SIRIUS[93]	BMS	525	14.4	2.81	28.0	6	36.3+++	35.4+++	0.81+++	1.00+++	9	16.6+++	0.6	3.2	18.9+++
	SES	533	14.4	2.79	25.0		8.9	3.2	0.24	0.17		4.10	5.9	2.8	7.1
E SIRIUS[95]	BMS	177	15.1	2.51	27.0	8	42.3+++	41.7+++	0.24+++	1.05+++	9	20.9+++	0.6	2.3	22.6+++
	SES	175	14.9	2.60	19.0		5.9	3.9	0.19	0.80		4.0	1.1	4.6	8.0
C SIRIUS[96]	BMS	50	12.6	2.62	24.0	8	52.3+++	45.5+++	0.79+++	1.02+++	9	18.0+	0.0	4.0	18.0+
	SES	50	14.5	2.65	24.0		2.3	0.0	0.12	0.12		4.0	0.0	2.0	4.0
TAXUS IV[94]	BMS	652	13.4	2.75	25.0	9	26.6+++	24.4+++	0.61+++	0.92+++	9	11.3+++	1.1b	3.7	15.0+++
	PES	662	13.4	2.75	23.4		7.9	5.5	0.23	0.39		3.0	1.4b	3.5	8.5
ENDEAVOR II[97]	BMS	599	14.38	2.76	22.0	8	35.0+++	33.5+++	0.72+++	1.03+++	9	11.8+++	0.5	3.9	14.4+++
	ZES	598	14.05	2.74	18.0		13.2	9.4	0.36	0.61		4.6	1.2	2.7	7.3
SPIRIT II[92]	PES	77	13.2	2.82	24	6	5.8	3.5	0.15	0.37	6	6.5	1.3b	2.6	6.5
	EES	223	13.0	2.70	23		3.4	1.3	0.07	0.12		2.7	0.0b	0.9	2.7

aIntermediate risk lesions are defined as those with a reference diameter between 2.5 and 3.5 mm and lesion lengths between 15 and 30 mm.

bCardiac death.

+p < 0.05; ++p < 0.01; +++p < 0.001 treatment versus control.

BMS = Bare metal stent; DM = diabetes mellitus; EES = everolimus-eluting stent; FU = follow-up; MACE = major adverse cardiac events; MI = myocardial infarction; N = number; NA = not available; PES = paclitaxel-eluting stent; RVD = reference vessel diameter; SES = sirolimus-eluting stent; TLR = target lesion revascularization; ZES = zotarolimus eluting stent.

CH 55

| TABLE 55–8 | Drug-Eluting Stent Comparative Studies in Patients with Long (>20 mm) Lesions |

Lesion Complexity	Stent Type	N	Length, mm	RVD, mm	DM, %	FU, mo	Binary Restenosis, % In Segment	In Stent	Late Lumen Loss, mm In Segment	In Stent	FU, mo	Late Clinical Follow-up TLR, %	Death, %	MI, %	MACE, %
TAXUS V[98]	BMS	579	17.2	2.69	29.9	9	33.9[+++]	31.9[+++]	0.60[+++]	0.90[+++]	9	15.7[+++]	0.9[a]	4.6	21.2[++]
	PES	577	17.3	2.68	31.7		18.9	13.7	0.33	0.49		8.6	0.5[a]	5.4	15.0
TAXUS VI[99]	BMS	227	20.32	2.77	22.0	9	35.7[+++]	32.9[+++]	0.66[+++]	0.99[+++]	9	18.9[+++]	0.9[a]	6.2	22.5
	PES	219	20.94	2.81	17.8		12.4	9.1	0.24	0.39		6.8	0.0[a]	8.2	16.4
Long DES II[100]	SES	250	33.9	2.84	32.8	6	3.3[+++]	2.9[+++]	0.24[+++]	0.09[+++]	9	2.4[+]	0.8	8.8	12.0
	PES	250	34.5	2.82	33.6		14.6	11.7	0.61	0.45		7.2	0.0	10.8	17.2
Kim et al[101]	BMS	177	32.0	3.10	32.2	6	42.5[+++]	40.6[+++]	1.02[+++]	1.35[+++]	9	19.2[+++]	0.6	8.5	26.6[+++]
	SES	184	36.0	2.73	31.0		9.3	7.6	0.14	0.26		3.8	1.1	8.7	13.0
	PES	166	36.3	2.90	31.9		21.3	16.0	0.56	0.78		6.0	0.6	9.6	15.7
CORPAL II[1]	TES	52	NA	NA	NA	6	NA	22.0	NA	0.78	15	15.0	1.92	1.92	NA
	SES	56	NA	NA	NA		NA	18.0	NA	0.48		11.0	0.0	0.0	NA

[a]Cardiac death.
*p < 0.05; ++p < 0.01; +++p < 0.001 treatment versus control.
[1]Delgado A, et al: CORPAL II Trial results presented at the American Heart Association Annual Scientific Sessions, Chicago, IL, November 2006.
BMS = bare metal stent; DM = diabetes mellitus; EES = everolimus-eluting stent; FU = follow-up; MACE = major adverse cardiac events; MI = myocardial infarction; N = number; NA = not available; PES = paclitaxel-eluting stent; RVD = reference vessel diameter; SES = sirolimus-eluting stent; TES = tacrolimus eluting stent; TLR = target lesion revascularization.

| TABLE 55–9 | Drug-Eluting Stent Comparative Studies in Patients with Small (<2.5 mm) Vessels |

Lesion Complexity	Stent Type	N	Length, mm	RVD, mm	DM, %	FU, mo	Binary Restenosis, % In Segment	In Stent	Late Lumen Loss, mm In Segment	In Stent	FU, mo	Late Clinical Follow-up TLR, %	Death, %	MI, %	MACE, %
REALITY[103]	SES	684	16.96	2.40	27.3	8	9.6	7	0.04[+++]	0.09[+++]	12	6	1.5	5.1	10.7
	PES	669	17.31	2.40	28.7		11.1	8.3	0.16	0.31		6.1	1	6	11.4
SVELTE[104]	BMS	323	14.4	2.42	30	8	39.0[+++]	38.0[+++]	0.76[+++]	0.97[+++]	8	13.2[+++]	1.2**	3.1**	15.2[++]
	SES	101	14.5	2.36	26.7		6.3	3.2	0.20	0.22		0	3	3	5.4
	SES*	350	14.6	2.41	27.1		11.6	3.9	0.27	0.16		4.6	1.4	2.8	7.8
SES-SMART[102]	BMS	128	10.66	2.17	29.7	8	53.1[+++]	49.1[+++]	0.69[+++]	0.9[+++]	8	21.1[++]	1.6	7.8[+]	31.3[+++]
	SES	129	13.01	2.22	19.4		9.8	4.9	0.16	0.16		7	0	1.6	9.3
ISAR-SMART 3[105]	SES	180	12.9	2.44	NA	6-8	11.4[+]	8[+]	0.13[+++]	0.25[+++]	12	6.6[++]	1.7	3.9	NA
	PES	180	11.7	2.40	NA		19	14.9	0.34	0.56		14.7	2.2	3.3	NA

*CYPHER control from SIRIUS trial.
**Clinical follow-up at 12 months.
+p < 0.05; ++p < 0.01; +++p < 0.001 treatment versus control.
BMS = bare metal stent; DM = diabetes mellitus; FU = follow-up; MACE = major adverse cardiac events; MI = myocardial infarction; N = number; NA = not available; PES = paclitaxel-eluting stent; RVD = reference vessel diameter; SES = sirolimus-eluting stent; TLR = target lesion revascularization.

| TABLE 55–10 | Drug-Eluting Stent Comparative Studies in Patients with Chronic Total Occlusions |

Lesion Complexity	Stent Type	N	Length, mm	RVD, mm	DM, %	FU, mo	Binary Restenosis, % In Segment	In Stent	Late Lumen Loss, mm In Segment	In Stent	FU, mo	Late Clinical Follow-up TLR, %	Death, %	MI, %	MACE, %
PRISON II[109]	BMS	100	16.3	2.60	16	6	41[+++]	36[+++]	0.64[+++]	1.09[+++]	6	19[+++]	0	3	20[+++]
	SES	100	16	2.53	10		11	7	−0.07	0.05		4	0	2	4
SCANDSTENT[108]	BMS	63	22.8	NA	21	6	38[+++]	38[+++]	0.99[+++]	1.07[+++]	7	33.3[+++]	0	1.6	34.9[+++]
	SES	64	27.5	NA	19		0	0	−0.05	−0.05		0	0	0	4.7
Hoye et al[106]	BMS	28	12.7	NA	7.1	6	NA	NA	NA	NA	12	NA	NA	NA	17.9[+]
	SES	56	11.3	NA	14.3		NA	9.1[+]	NA	0.13		NA	NA	NA	3.6
Nakamura et al[110]	BMS	120	32.5	3.32	33	6	NA	32[+++]	NA	1.36[+++]	12	23[+++]	0	3	42[+++]
	SES	60	35	3.12	33		NA	2	NA	0.08		2	0	0	3
Jang et al[107]	SES	107	36.5	2.9	26	6	NA	9.4[+]	NA	0.4[+]		3.7	0	0*	3.7[+]
	PES	29	28	3.1	21		NA	28.6	NA	0.8		6.9	3.4	0*	10.3
Werner et al[27]	BMS	82	NA	2.66	30	6	55[+++]	NA	1.26[+++]	NA	12	53.4[+++]	3.3	0	56.7[+++]
	PES	82	NA	2.59	35		11.7	NA	0.24	NA		10	0	0	13.3

*Q wave MI.
+p < 0.05; ++p < 0.01; +++p < 0.001 treatment versus control.
BMS = bare metal stent; DM = diabetes mellitus; FU = follow-up; MACE = major adverse cardiac events; MI = myocardial infarction; N = number; NA, not available; PES = paclitaxel-eluting stent; RVD = reference vessel diameter; SES = sirolimus-eluting stent; TLR = target lesion revascularization.

TABLE 55–11 **Drug Eluting Stent Comparative Studies in Patients with Saphenous Vein Graft Disease**

Lesion Complexity	Stent Type	N (lesions)	Length, mm	RVD, mm	DM, %	FU, mo	Binary Restenosis, %		Late Lumen Loss, mm		FU, mo	Late Clinical Follow-up			
							In Segment	In Stent	In Segment	In Stent		TLR (TVR), %	Death, %	MI, %	MACE, %
RRISC[116]	BMS	37 (49)	16.2	3.34	13.5	6	32.6[+]	30.6[+]	0.56[+]	0.56[+++]	6	21.6[+]	0.0	0.0	29.7
	SES	38 (47)	18.6	3.28	15.8		13.6	11.3	0.56	0.56		5.3	2.6	2.6	15.8
Lee et al [31]	BMS	84	NA	2.96	24.0	9	NA	NA	NA	0.29[++]	9	(37)[+]	4.0[+]	20.0[+]	37.0[+]
	DES	139	NA	2.94	23.0		NA	NA	NA	0.08		(10)	1.0	4.0	10.0
Wöhrle et al[115]	BMS	26	12.4	3.00	30.8	6	34.6[+]	34.6[+]	0.81	1.05[+]	12	(34.6)	3.84		38.46[+]
	PES	13	12.1	3.04	23.1		0.0	0.0	0.10	0.23		(7.69)	0.0		7.69
Chu et al[113]	BMS	57	18.8	4.1	40.0	NA	NA	NA	NA	NA	12	7.0	7.0	0.0	18.0
	SES	48	17.6	4.0	46.0		NA	NA	NA	NA		6.0	6.0	4.0	21.0
Chu et al[112]	SES	47	NA	NA	31.9	NA	NA	NA	NA	NA	6	2.1	4.3	8.5	8.5
	PES	42	NA	NA	35.7		NA	NA	NA	NA		2.6	5.3	10.5	10.5
Hoffman et al[114]	BMS	60	10.8	3.06	28.0	6	NA	33[+]	1.05[+]	1.06[+]	6	22.0[+]	NA	NA	37.0[+]
	PES	60	11.8	3.05	25.0		NA	12	0.63	0.61		6.0	NA	NA	15.0
Buch et al[a111]	BMS	39	NA	NA	NA	NA	NA	NA	NA	NA	6	10.0	5.1	5.1	15.4
	DES	30	NA	NA	NA		NA	NA	NA	NA		3.3	6.7	12.8	10.0

[a]Internal mammary grafts.

[+]$p < 0.05$; [++]$p < 0.01$; [+++]$p < 0.001$ treatment versus control.

BMS = bare metal stent; DES = drug-eluting stent; DM = diabetes mellitus; FU = follow-up; MACE = major adverse cardiac events; MI = myocardial infarction; N = number; NA = not available; PES = paclitaxel-eluting stent; RVD = reference vessel diameter; SES = sirolimus-eluting stent; TLR = target lesion revascularization; TVR = target vessel revascularization; ZES = zotarolimus eluting stent.

TABLE 55–12 **Drug-Eluting Stent Comparative Studies in Patients with In-Stent Restenosis**

Lesion Complexity	Stent Type	N	Length, mm	RVD, mm	DM, %	FU, mo	Binary Restenosis, %		Late Lumen Loss, mm		FU, mo	Late Clinical Follow-up			
							In Segment	In Stent (injured segment)	In Segment	In Stent (injured segment)		TLR, (TVR) %	Death, %	MI, %	MACE, %
SISR[86]	Brach	125	16.76	2.62	29.6	6	29.5	17.1	0.33	0.23	9	19.2[++]	0	0	19.2[+]
	SES	259	17.22	2.64	33.3		19.8	18.1	0.27	0.33		8.5	0	2.7	10
TAXUS V ISR[87]	Brach	201	15.0	2.61	30.3	9	31.2[+++]	(20.1)[+++]	0.22	(0.11)[+++]	9	20.1[+++]	0.5	4.6	20.1[+]
	PES	195	15.9	2.68	40		14.5	7	0.13	0.25		7.9	0	3.7	11.5
RIBS-II[119]	SES	76	16.9	2.66	38	9	11.0[+++]	7.0[+++]	0.13[+++]	0.11[+++]	12	(10.5)[++]	3.9	2.6	11.8[++]
	BA	74	15.7	2.68	31		39	(39)	0.69	(0.69)		(29.7)	4.1	2.7	31.1
Li, et al[120]	SES	36	20.5	2.85	19.4	7	5.6[+]	13.9[+]	0.14[++]	0.14[++]	7	8.3	0	NA	8.3
	PES	18	25.7	2.94	22.2		27.8	44.4	0.75	0.87		22.2	0	NA	22.2

[+]$p < 0.05$; [++]$p < 0.01$; [+++]$p < 0.001$ treatment versus control.

BMS = bare metal stent; DM = diabetes mellitus; EES = everolimus-eluting stent; FU = follow-up; MACE = major adverse cardiac events; MI = myocardial infarction; N = number; NA = not available; PES = paclitaxel-eluting stent; RVD = reference vessel diameter; SES = sirolimus-eluting stent; TLR = target lesion revascularization; TVR = target vessel revascularization; ZES = zotarolimus eluting stent.

TABLE 55–13 | Drug Eluting Stent Comparative Studies in Patients with ST Segment Elevation Myocardial Infarction

Lesion Complexity	Stent Type	N	Length, mm	RVD, mm	DM, %	FU, mo	Binary Restenosis, %		Late Lumen Loss, mm		Late Clinical Follow-up				
							In Segment	In Stent	In Segment	In Stent	FU, mo	TLR, (TVR), %	Death, %	MI, %	MACE, %
TYPHOON[122]	BMS	357	NA	2.84	17.1	8	20.3+	20.3+++	0.56+++	0.83+++	12	(13.4)+++	2.2	1.4	14.8+++
	SES	355	NA	2.78	15.5		7.1	3.5	0.17	0.14		(5.6)	2.3	1.1	7.5
PASSION[123]	BMS	309	10-19	3.20	12	NA	NA	NA	NA	NA	12	7.8	6.5	2	12.8
	PES	310	10-19	3.13	10		NA	NA	NA	NA		5.3	4.6	1.7	8.8
STRATEGY[a121]	BMS	88	13.1	2.33	12	8	36++	28++	NA	0.6+++	8	20++	9	9	32+
	SES	87	13	2.27	17		11	7.5	NA	−0.22		6	8	7	18
SESAMI[b]	BMS	160	NA	NA	24	12	21.3+	NA	NA	NA	12	11.2+	NA	NA	16.8+
	SES	160	NA	NA	18		9.3	NA	NA	NA		4.3	NA	NA	6.8
MISSION[c]	BMS	158	NA	NA	NA	9	NA	22.8+++	0.68+++	NA	12	(13.3)++	2.7	9.3	NA
	SES	158	NA	NA	NA		NA	3.8	0.12	NA		(5.1)	1.3	5.7	NA
HAAMU-STENT[d]	BMS	82	NA	NA	8.5	NA	NA	NA	NA	0.73+++	12	(11.0)	4.9	4.9	17
	PES	82	NA	NA	21.0		NA	NA	NA	0.26		(3.7)	9.8	1.2	13

[a]Single high-dose bolus tirofiban and sirolimus stent versus abciximab and bare metal stent in myocardial infarction.

[b]Menichelli M, et al: SESAMI trial results presented at the EuroPCR, Paris, France, May 2006.

[c]van der Hoeven BL, et al: Mission Trial results presented at the American Heart Association Annual Scientific Sessions, Chicago, IL, November 2006.

[d]Tierala I, et al: HAAMU-Stent Trial results presented at the Transcatheter Cardiovascular Therapeutics meeting, Washington, DC, October 2006.

+$p < 0.05$; ++$p < 0.01$; +++$p < 0.001$ treatment versus control.

BMS = bare metal stent; DM = diabetes mellitus; EES = everolimus-eluting stent; FU = follow-up; MACE = major adverse cardiac events; MI = myocardial infarction; N = number; NA = not available; PES = paclitaxel-eluting stent; RVD = reference vessel diameter; SES = sirolimus-eluting stent; TLR = target lesion revascularization; ZES = zotarolimus-eluting stent.

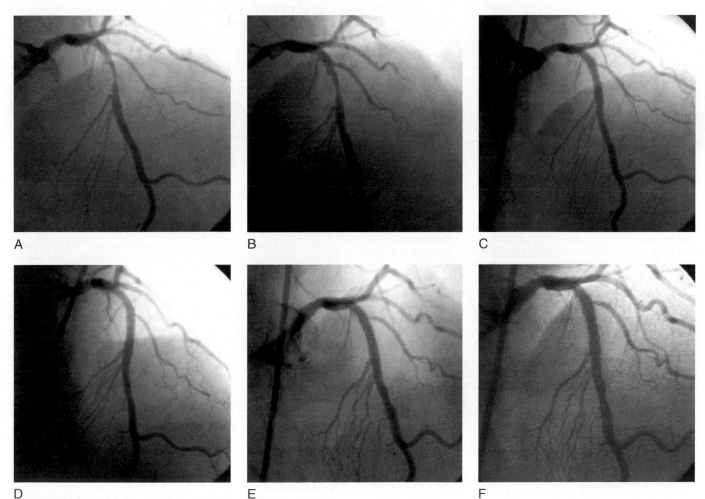

FIGURE 55–10 First-in-human CYPHER stent implantation. **A,** A focal stenosis is shown in the mid-left anterior descending artery, **B,** A CYPHER sirolimus-eluting stent (Cordis Corp., Warren, NJ) is positioned across the stenosis. **C,** There is excellent initial angiographic result and no residual stenosis. Follow-up angiography was performed at 4 months **(D),** 1 year **(E),** and 2 years **(F)** after the procedure without evidence of lumen renarrowing. *(Courtesy of Eduardo Sousa, São Paulo, Brazil.)*

CH 55

Percutaneous Coronary and Valvular Intervention

zotarolimus-eluting PC polymer-coated stent or the same bare metal stent but without the drug or the polymer coating.[97] The 9-month primary endpoint of target vessel failure was reduced from 15.1 percent with the bare metal stent to 7.9 percent with the Endeavor ($p = 0.0001$).[97] In-stent late loss was reduced from 1.03 mm to 0.61 mm in patients treated with the Endeavor stent ($p < 0.001$) and the rate of in-segment restenosis was reduced from 35 percent to 13.2 percent with the Endeavor stent ($p < 0.0001$).[97] The ENDEAVOR-III trial compared the latter stent to CYPHER in a 436 patient study (3:1 randomization) and failed to meet the primary endpoint of noninferior in-segment late loss at 8 months (0.34 with zotarolimus-eluting stents versus 0.13 mm with sirolimus-eluting stents) with higher late loss (0.60 and 0.15 mm, respectively, $p < 0.001$). There was no significant difference in target lesion revascularization between the two groups (6.3 percent and 3.5 percent, respectively, $p = 0.34$).[126] The Zomaxx program was stopped after slightly higher late lumen loss was found with this stent design in the Zomaxx-I trial.

EVEROLIMUS-ELUTING STENT. The Xience stent program (Abbot Vascular, Santa Rosa, CA) using the cobalt chromium Vision stent, a durable fluoropolymer, and everolimus, which is a rapamycin analogue that has both immunosuppressive and antiproliferative effects. Based on initial studies that evaluated use of an absorbable poly-L-lactic acid (PLA) polymer,[127] the SPIRIT program has shown reduction in late lumen loss comparable to the CYPHER stent.[90,92] A pivotal SPIRIT III randomized trial comparing the everolimus-eluting Vision stent to the TAXUS stent in >1000 patients is ongoing.

COSTAR PROGRAM. The CoStar stent (Conor Medsystems, Menlo Park, CA) is composed of a cobalt chromium stent with 492 drug reservoirs spaced over its 16 mm that are coated with a bioresorbable poly-lactic co-glycolic acid (PLGA) polymer that elutes paclitaxel over a 10- to 30-day period. The CObalt Chromium STent with Antiproliferative for Restenosis (COSTAR-II) trial compared 8-month clinical outcomes of patients treated with CoStar stent with the Taxus stent. At 8 months, patients treated with the CoStar stent had significantly higher MACE rate (11.0 percent) than patients treated with the Taxus stent (6.9 percent; p = 0.005). This difference was largely due to more frequent target vessel revascularization in patients treated with the CoStar stent (8.1 percent) compared with the Taxus stent (4.3 percent; p = 0.002). There were no differences in the occurrence of cardiac death (0.5 percent for the CoStar stent vs. 0.7 percent for the Taxus stent; p = 0.541) or new MI (3.4 percent vs. 2.4 percent, respectively; p = 0.24) (Personal communications, Mitchell W. Krucoff, EuroPCR, Barcelona, May 2007).

ANTIPLATELET AGENTS (see also Chap. 82)

CH 55

ASPIRIN. Aspirin irreversibly inhibits cyclooxygenase and thus blocks the synthesis of thromboxane A_2, a vasoconstricting agent that promotes platelet aggregation. Aspirin substantially reduces periprocedural MI caused by thrombotic occlusions compared with placebo and has been established as a standard for all patients undergoing PCI. Although the minimum effective aspirin dosage in the setting of PCI remains uncertain, patients on daily chronic aspirin therapy should receive 75 to 325 mg aspirin before PCI.[7] Patients not on daily aspirin regimens should receive 162 to 325 mg aspirin before PCI.[7] The inhibitory effect of aspirin occurs within 60 minutes, and its effect on platelets lasts for up to 7 days after discontinuation. Although current practice guidelines for patients who receive a drug-eluting stent recommend aspirin, 325 mg, and clopidogrel, 75 mg, daily therapy for 3 (sirolimus-eluting stents) or 6 months (paclitaxel-eluting stents) after drug-eluting stent placement,[7] this higher dose of aspirin is associated with a 50 percent higher bleeding risk than the lower 81 mg aspirin dose. Accordingly, many clinicians reduce the aspirin dose to 81 mg daily within 7 to 30 days after PCI and continue this indefinitely for secondary prevention.

THIENOPYRIDINE DERIVATIVES. Thienopyridine derivatives cause irreversible platelet inhibition because of their effects on the P_2Y_{12} adenosine diphosphate (ADP) receptor that can activate the GP IIb/IIIa complex. Because aspirin and thienopyridine derivatives have distinct mechanisms of action, their combination inhibits platelet aggregation to a greater extent than either agent alone. The combination of aspirin and clopidogrel (or previously, ticlopidine) was essential for 14 to 28 days to prevent stent thrombosis after bare metal stent placement. The combination of aspirin and clopidogrel also reduces death, MI, and urgent revascularization within 9 months in patients with NSTEMI and UA and in those undergoing elective PCI.[7] Recent studies have suggested that a loading dose of 600 mg rather than 300 mg of clopidogrel results in more rapid (<2 hours) platelet inhibition[129-132] and improved clinical outcomes.[133] Additional clopidogrel loading with 300 mg or 600 mg may also be used in patients on chronic maintenance clopidogrel therapy.[134] The need for pretreatment with clopidogrel is more controversial, balancing improved clinical outcomes with the potential risk for bleeding, should CABG surgery be needed (see also Chap. 51). Current guidelines recommend a 300 mg loading dose of clopidogrel at least 6 hours before PCI.[7]

Current guidelines suggest that in the absence of risk factors for bleeding, clopidogrel therapy should continue for 12 months after drug-eluting stent placement. Prolonged thienopyridine therapy not only reduces late stent thrombosis but also prevents MI by thrombi that complicate plaques remote from the initial intervention. Indefinite aspirin and clopidogrel therapy is recommended in patients receiving brachytherapy and higher doses (150 mg daily) of chronic clopidogrel are recommended in those patients in whom stent thrombosis may be catastrophic, such as patients with unprotected left main artery disease or those with the last remaining vessel if there is a less than 50 percent inhibition of platelet aggregation.[7]

GLYCOPROTEIN (GP) IIB/IIIA INHIBITORS. Thrombin and collagen are potent platelet agonists that can cause ADP and serotonin release and activate GP IIb/IIIa fibrinogen receptors on the platelet surface. Functionally active GP IIb/IIIa serves in the "final common pathway" of platelet aggregation by binding fibrinogen and other adhesive proteins that bridge adjacent platelets. There are three GP IIb/IIIa inhibitors approved for clinical use.

The monoclonal antibody abciximab irreversibly binds to platelets—leaving little circulating abciximab after administration. Abciximab reduces events in patients with acute coronary syndromes, including STEMI, and in patients undergoing elective stent placement. In higher risk populations, such as diabetics and those with non-STEMI, abciximab reduces late mortality rates, presumably by mechanisms that are unrelated to the occurrence of periprocedural myocardial necrosis. Addition of abciximab reduced clinical events in patients with acute coronary syndromes when given in addition to clopidogrel, 600 mg, particularly in patients with elevated troponin levels.[135] Abciximab can be safely administered in patients with renal insufficiency, and platelet infusions can reverse the effect of this agent.

Eptifibatide is a cyclic peptide derivative that reversibly binds GP IIb/IIIa. A double eptifibatide bolus, 180 µg/kg boluses 10 minutes apart, and infusion dose, 2.0 µg/kg/min for 18 to 24 hours, results in sufficient platelet inhibition to prevent ischemic events in patients undergoing PCI. Addition of eptifibatide to clopidogrel, 600 mg loading dose, also results in incremental platelet inhibition.[136] A reduction of the eptifibatide infusion to 1 µg/kg/min is necessary in patients with a creatinine clearance <50 ml per minute. Platelet transfusions do not reverse the platelet inhibition with eptifibatide.

Tirofiban, a peptidomimetic small molecule, has also undergone evaluation for its adjunctive benefit during PCI but is inferior to abciximab for the prevention of ischemic events during PCI. Subsequent studies have suggested that the tirofiban bolus dose given in this study may not have produced optimal anticoagulation during PCI, and larger bolus doses can improve the inhibition of platelet aggregation but have not been tested in clinical studies. Tirofiban is generally used for patients with acute coronary syndrome before PCI or initiation of optimal medical therapy.

The GP IIb/IIIa inhibitors, in particular abciximab and eptifibatide, have demonstrated benefit in improving clinical outcomes within the first 30 days after PCI, and are particularly useful in patients with troponin-positive acute coronary syndromes. These agents have primarily reduced ischemic complications, including non-Q-wave MI and recurrent ischemia. There is no consistent evidence that the GP IIb/IIIa inhibitors reduce the frequency of late restenosis. Bleeding is the major risk of GP IIb/IIIa inhibitors, and a downward adjustment of the unfractionated heparin dose is recommended. GP IIb/IIIa inhibitors are recommended in patient with NSTEMI and unstable angina who are not pretreated with clopidogrel, and it is reasonable to administer to patients who have a troponin-positive NSTEMI who have also been pretreated with clopidogrel.[135] GP IIb/IIIa administration is also reasonable in patients with STEMI, and abciximab is preferred over eptifibatide or tirofiban in this setting.[7]

ANTITHROMBIN AGENTS

Unfractionated heparin (see also Chap. 82) is the most commonly used thrombin inhibitor during PCI. "Near-patient" activated clotting time (ACT) monitoring has facilitated heparin dose titration during PCI, and retrospective studies with balloon angioplasty have related the ACT value to clinical outcome after PCI. An ACT in the range of 350 to 375 seconds provided the lowest composite ischemic event rate, although any level of ACT >200 seconds had no further reductions in ischemic complications with concomitant use of GP IIb/IIIa inhibitors. A more recent study failed to correlate ischemic outcomes with the level of anticoagulation achieved with unfractionated heparin during coronary stent placement.[137] Weight-adjusted heparin dosing regimens of 50 to 70 IU/kg help to avoid "overshooting" the ACT. Sufficient unfractionated heparin should be administered during PCI to achieve an ACT around 300 seconds if no GP IIb/IIIa inhibitor is given, and more than 200 seconds if GP IIb/IIIa inhibitors are given. Routine use of intravenous heparin after PCI is no longer indicated. Early sheath removal is encouraged when the ACT falls to less than 150 to 180 seconds.

LOW-MOLECULAR-WEIGHT HEPARIN (see also Chap. 82). Enoxaparin is considered a reasonable alternative to unfractionated heparin in patients with non-ST segment elevation acute coronary syndromes undergoing PCI,[7] but difficulty monitoring the levels of anticoagulation in the event that PCI is performed has limited its clinical use at many centers. The Superior Yield of the New Strategy of Enoxaparin, Revascularization and Glycoprotein IIb/IIIa Inhibitors (SYNERGY) trial prospectively randomized 10,027 high-risk patients with non-ST segment elevation acute coronary syndrome with an intended early invasive strategy to treatment with subcutaneous enoxaparin or intravenous unfractionated heparin.[138] The 30-day primary efficacy outcome, a composite clinical endpoint of all-cause death or nonfatal MI, occurred in 14 percent of patients assigned to enoxaparin and 14.5 percent of patients assigned to unfractionated heparin. More TIMI (Thrombolysis in Myocardial Infarction) major bleeding was observed in patients treated with enoxparin (9.1 percent versus 7.6 percent; $p = 0.008$). The bleeding risk was highest in those patients who received "crossover" therapy with unfractionated heparin and enoxaparin. When enoxaparin is given before PCI, empirical dose algorithms have been designed to guide additional anticoagulation therapy during PCI. If the last dose of enoxaparin was less than 8 hours before PCI, no additional antithrombin is needed. If the last dose of enoxaparin was given between 8 and 12 hours, a 0.3 mg per kg bolus of intravenous enoxaparin should be given.[139] If the dose was administrated more than 12 hours before PCI, conventional anticoagulation therapy is indicated.

BIVALIRUDIN. Bivalirudin is a direct thrombin inhibitor that has been used as an alternative to unfractionated heparin in patients undergoing PCI. Bivalirudin generally causes fewer bleeding complications than unfractionated heparin due to its shorter (25 minutes) and more predictable bioavailability. Bivalirudin is also accessible to clot-bound thrombin because its anticoagulant effect does not depend on binding with antithrombin. Bivalirudin was not inferior to the combination of unfractionated heparin and a GP IIb/IIIa inhibitor in one trial of 6010 "low-risk" patients.[140] In a larger study of 13,819 patients with UA and NSTEMI, bivalirudin alone was compared with bivalirudin with a GP IIb/IIIa inhibitor and heparin with a GP IIb/IIIa inhibitor. Using a composite ischemia endpoint of death, MI, or unplanned revascularization for ischemia and major bleeding to determine net clinical benefit, bivalirudin alone, as compared with heparin plus a GP IIb/IIIa inhibi-

tor, showed noninferiority in the composite ischemia endpoint (7.8 percent and 7.3 percent, respectively; $p = 0.32$) and significantly reduced rates of major bleeding (3.0 percent versus 5.7 percent; $p < 0.001$) resulting in a better net clinical outcome endpoint (10.1 percent versus 11.7 percent; $p = 0.02$.[141] Bivalirudin is considered a reasonable alternative to unfractionated heparin in low-risk patients undergoing PCI[7] and may reduce bleeding complications in higher risk patients with unstable angina and NSTEMI. Its relative value in patients with STEMI is currently under evaluation.

SPECIFIC FACTOR Xa INHIBITORS. Fondaparinux is a pentasaccharide that has specific anti-Xa activity without effects on Factor IIa and may have less bleeding when used for the treatment of patients with acute coronary syndromes. The OASIS-5 trial randomly assigned 20,078 patients with acute coronary syndromes to receive either fondaparinux (2.5 mg daily) or enoxaparin (1 mg/kg of body weight twice daily) for a mean of 6 days.[142] The occurrence of the 9-day primary study endpoint (death, MI, or refractory ischemia) was similar in the two groups (5.8 percent with fondaparinux and 5.7 percent with enoxaparin), although the risk of major bleeding at 9 days was markedly lower with fondaparinux (2.2 percent) than with enoxaparin (4.1 percent; $p < 0.001$).[142] This reduction in bleeding was accompanied by an improvement in late mortality in patients treated with fondaparinux. Potential limitations of this approach are the relative long half-life of fondaparinux and the need for adjunct anticoagulation with heparin during PCI to avoid the occurrence of catheter thrombi.

OUTCOMES FOLLOWING PERCUTANEOUS CORONARY INTERVENTION

Procedural success and complication rates are used to measure outcomes after PCI. Early (<30 day) success (e.g., relief of angina, freedom from death, MI, and urgent revascularization) generally relates to the safety and effectiveness of the initial procedure, whereas late (30 days to 1 year) success (e.g., freedom from recurrence of angina, target vessel revascularization, MI, or death) depends on both clinical restenosis and progressive atherosclerosis at remote sites.[7] Substantial improvements in coronary devices (e.g., drug-eluting stents), adjunct anticoagulation used during PCI (e.g, ADP antagonists, GP IIb/IIIa inhibitors, direct thrombin inhibitors), and secondary prevention after PCI (e.g., therapy with lipid-lowering agents, beta adrenergic blockers, antiplatelet drugs) have markedly improved early and late clinical outcomes following PCI over time[143,144] (Fig. 55-11; Table 55-14).

EARLY CLINICAL OUTCOME. Anatomical (or angiographic) success after PCI is defined as the attainment of residual diameter stenosis less than 50 percent, which is generally associated with at least a 20 percent improvement in diameter stenosis and relief of ischemia. With the widespread use of coronary stents, the angiographic criterion for success is a 20 percent stenosis or less when stents are used.[7] Procedural success is defined as angiographic success without the occurrence of major complications (death, MI, or CABG surgery) within 30 days of the procedure. Clinical success is defined as procedural success without the need for urgent repeat PCI or surgical revascularization within the first 30 days of the procedure.[7] A number of clinical, angiographic, and technical variables predict risk of procedural failure in patients undergoing PCI (Table 55-15). Major complications include death, MI, or stroke and minor complications include transient ischemic attacks, vascular complications, contrast-induced nephropathy, and a number of angiographic complications.[7]

Mortality. Although mortality after PCI is rare (less than 1 percent), it is higher in the setting of STEMI, cardiogenic shock, and in patients who develop an occlusion with poor left ventricular function.[7] A number of risk factors for early mortality after PCI have been identified (Table 55-16).

Myocardial Infarction. Periprocedural MI is one of the most common complications of PCI. Two classification

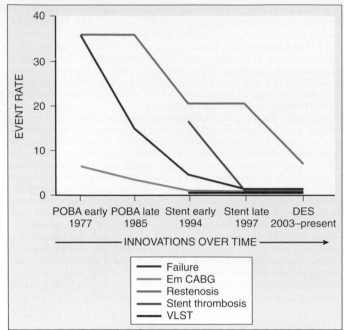

FIGURE 55–11 Changing outcomes with the introduction of new iterations of coronary revascularization devices over time. Over the last 30 years, percutaneous coronary intervention has undergone progressive improvements in success, safety, and durability. Em CABG = emergency coronary bypass graft surgery; DES = drug-eluting stent; POBA = plain old balloon angioplasty; VLST = very late stent thrombosis. *(Courtesy of Donald Baim, MD.)*

systems have been used to classify MI after PCI. Most clinical device trials have used the World Health Organization (WHO) classification system that defines MI as a total creatine kinase (CK) elevation more than two times normal in association with the elevation of the CK-MB isoform. Using this definition, periprocedural MI occurs after 1 to 2 percent of PCI procedures. Larger infarcts following PCI correlate with angiographic complications, such as loss of a major side-branch, prolonged no-reflow or severe vessel dissection, and associate strongly with long-term mortality. The second definition is more commonly used with evaluations of adjunct pharmacological agents by the FDA and defines MI as an elevation in CK-MB three times normal or higher after the procedure. In clinical practice, asymptomatic CK-MB elevations (<5× the upper normal limits) occur following 3 to 11 percent of technically successful PCI, and have little apparent clinical consequence. Larger degrees of myonecrosis (CK-MB >5× upper normal limits) predict higher 1-year mortality rates and should be considered a periprocedural MI.[7] Many of these clinically silent infarcts may reflect a higher atherosclerotic burden in patients who suffer such events or subtle effects on ventricular function. Troponin T and I elevations occur more commonly than CK-MB elevations, but their prognostic significance over those of the CK-MB elevation is not known.

Urgent Revascularization. Emergent or urgent CABG surgery following PCI is now uncommon and, in the era of coronary stents, results from catastrophic complications during PCI, such as coronary perforation or severe dissection and abrupt closure. Chest pain after PCI is relatively common and its evaluation requires an immediate 12-lead electrocardiogram (ECG).[7] Recurrent ischemia following PCI manifested by chest pain, electrocardiographic abnormalities, and elevation of cardiac biomarkers may occurred as a result of acute or subacute stent thrombosis, residual dissections, plaque prolapse, side-branch occlusion, or thrombus at the treatment site, or may relate to residual

disease not treated with the initial procedure. In the presence of suspect recurrent ischemia, coronary arteriography is the most expeditious way to identify the cause of the residual ischemia.

Angiographic Complications. A number of complications may occur during PCI and, depending on their severity and duration, may result in periprocedural MI. In coronary dissections that extend deeper into the media or adventitia or begin to compromise the true lumen of the vessel, clinical ischemia may develop (Fig. 55-12). Whereas most intraprocedural dissections can be treated promptly with stenting, significant residual dissections of the treated artery occur in 1.7 percent of patients. These residual dissections raise the risk of postprocedure MI, need for emergent CABG surgery, and stent thrombosis and increase mortality three-fold.[145] In addition to barotrauma-induced dissections, guiding catheter dissections represent another mechanism for disrupting the coronary vessel and compromising distal flow.

Coronary perforation develops in 0.2 to 0.5 percent of patients undergoing PCI and is more common with atheroablative devices and hydrophilic wires than with balloon angioplasty or with conventional guidewires. Depending on the rate of flow through the vessel perforation, cardiac tamponade and hemodynamic collapse can occur within minutes, requiring immediate recognition and treatment of the perforation. Strategies for controlling coronary perforations include reversal of intraprocedural anticoagulation and prolonged inflation (up to 10 minutes) of an oversized balloon at low pressure at the site of the perforation to encourage sealing of the tear in the vessel. Management strategies for perforations include the use of perfusion balloons, which provide for a small amount of distal perfusion, and use of polytetrafluoroethylene (PTFE)-covered stents, which may control free perfusions, in addition to decompression of the pericardial pressure with prompt pericardiocentesis. Approximately one-third of cases of PCI-associated coronary artery perforation require emergent cardiac surgery.[146,147]

"No-reflow" is defined as reduced anterograde perfusion in the absence of a flow-limiting stenosis, and occurs in up to 2 to3 percent of PCI procedures, typically occurring during interventions on degenerated SVGs and during acute myocardial infarction interventions.[30,148] No-reflow is likely caused by distal embolization of atheromatous and thrombotic debris dislodged by balloon inflation or stent implantation. Once it occurs, no-reflow can cause severe short- and long-term consequences including a fivefold increased risk of periprocedural MI and threefold increased risk of death.[30] Although numerous pharmacological strategies have been used to treat no-reflow, their efficacy in reducing the frequency of subsequent adverse events remains debated.

STENT THROMBOSIS. With the routine use of high-pressure stent postdilation and dual antiplatelet therapy following stent implantation, the rate of stent thrombosis has declined to approximately 1 percent within the first year after stenting.[149] A number of clinical, angiographic, and procedural factors predispose to its occurrence (Table 55-17). Lesion-specific factors that increase the likelihood of stent thrombosis include a residual dissection at the margin of the stent, impaired flow into or out of the stent, small stent diameters (<3 mm), long stent lengths, and treatment of an acute myocardial infarction, among other factors. Patient noncompliance with dual antiplatelet therapy, resistance to the antiplatelet effects of aspirin and clopidogrel, and hypercoagulability may also play important roles in the development of stent thrombosis.[150,151]

The timing of the stent thrombosis is defined as acute (<24 hours), subacute (24 hours to 30 days), late (30 days to 1 year), and very late (after 1 year).[152] Traditional definitions

TABLE 55–14	In-Hospital Outcomes Associated with Percutaneous Intervention Over Time							
Variable	NHLBI-I[a]	NHLBI-II[a]	STRESS PTCA Arm[b]	BOAT PTCA Arm[c]	Benestent II PTCA Arm[d]	DYNAMIC Registry All PCI[e]	ACC-NCDR Registry[144]	DEScover Registry[143]
Years of entry	1977-1981	1985-1986	1991-1993	1994-1995	1995-1996	1997-1998	1998-2000	2005
Number of patients	1,155	1,802	203	492	413	1,559	100,292	6,509
Baseline Factors								
Mean age, years	54	58	60	58	50	62.1	64	63
Women, %	25	26	27	24	23	32.1	34	31
diabetes mellitus	9	14	16	14	13	25.8	26	31
Acute coronary syndrome, %	37	49	48	NA	45	42.8	62	52
Multivessel disease, %	25	53	32	NA	NA	54.1	59	43
Angiographic success, %	68	91	92.6	NA	99	93.7	95	98.4
Procedure success, %	61	78	89.6	87	96	92.0	92	98.2
Early complications			7.9	3.3	7.0	4.9	4	3.2
Death, %	1.2	1.0	1.5	0.4	0	1.9	1	0.5
Q wave	4.9	4.3	3.0	1.2	1.2	NR	0	1.1
Infarction, %								
EmergencyCABG, %	5.8	3.4	4.0	2.0	0.7	1.5	2	0.07
Late clinical outcome	5 years	5 years	8 months	12 months	12 months	NA	NA	12 months
Any event			23.8	31.1	23.2	NA	NA	5.2
Death, %	4.9	8.3	0	1.6	1.0	NA	NA	3.1
Q wave MI	9.7	9.1	0.5	1.6	1.9	NA	NA	2.1
Revascularization,%	32.1	38.8	15.4	19.7	18.9	NA	NA	
Repeat PTCA	22.5	30.9	11.4	NA	9.4	NA	NA	8.4
CABG	15.5	13.4	4.5	NA	1.9	NA	NA	1.4

CABG = coronary artery bypass graft; MI = myocardial infarction; NR = not reported; PTCA = percutaneous transluminal coronary angioplasty.

Modified from Hirshfeld, et al: with permission.

[a]Detre K, Holubkov R, Kelsey S, et al: Percutaneous transluminal coronary angioplasty in 1985-1986 and 1977-1981. The National Heart, Lung, and Blood Institute Registry. N Engl J Med 318:265, 1988.

[b]Fischman D, Leon M, Baim D, et al: A randomized comparison of coronary-stent placement and balloon angioplasty in the treatment of coronary artery disease. Stent Restenosis Study Investigators. N Engl J Med 331:496, 1994.

[c]Baim D, Cutlip D, Sharma S, et al: Final results of the Balloon vs Optimal Atherectomy Trial (BOAT). Circulation 97:322, 1998.

[d]Serruys P, van Hout B, Bonnier H, et al: Randomized comparison of implantation of heparin-coated stents with balloon angioplasty in selected patients with coronary artery disease (Benestent II). Lancet 352:673, 1998.

[e]Williams D, Holubkov R, Yeh W, et al: Percutaneous coronary intervention in the current era compared with 1985-1986: The National Heart, Lung, and Blood Institute Registries. Circulation 102:2945, 2000

TABLE 55–15	Variables Associated with Early Failure and Complications Following Percutaneous Coronary Intervention

Clinical Variables

Women
Advanced age
Diabetes mellitus
Unstable or CCS Class IV angina
Congestive heart failure
Cardiogenic shock
Renal insufficiency
Preprocedural instability requiring intraaortic balloon pump support
Preprocedural elevation of C-reactive protein
Multivessel CAD

Anatomical Variables

Multivessel CAD
Left main artery disease
Thrombus
SVG intervention
ACC/AHA types B2 and C lesion morphology
Chronic total coronary occlusion

Procedural Factors

A higher final percent diameter stenosis
Smaller minimal lumen diameter
Presence of a residual dissection or trans-stenotic pressure gradient

ACC/AHA = American College of Cardiology/American Heart Association; CAD = coronary artery disease; CCS = Canadian Cardiovascular Society; SVG = saphenous vein graft.

TABLE 55–16	Factors Associated with Early Mortality Following Percutaneous Coronary Intervention (PCI)

Clinical Variables

Advanced age
Female gender
Diabetes mellitus
Chronic lung disease
Prior myocardial infarction
Impairment of left ventricular function
Renal dysfunction
Cardiogenic shock
Salvage, urgent, or emergent PCI

Anatomical Variables

Multivessel coronary artery disease
Left main artery disease
Proximal left anterior descending artery disease
Large area of myocardium at risk
PCI of artery supplying collaterals to large artery
Higher SCAI lesion classification

Modified from Smith SC, Jr., Feldman TE, Hirshfeld JW, Jr., et al: ACC/AHA/SCAI 2005 guideline update for percutaneous coronary intervention: A report of the American College of Cardiology/American Heart Association Task Force on Practice Guidelines (ACC/AHA/SCAI Writing Committee to Update the 2001 Guidelines for Percutaneous Coronary Intervention). J Am Coll Cardiol 47(1): e1-121, 2006; and Shaw R, Anderson H, Brindis R, et al: Development of a risk adjustment mortality model using the American College of Cardiology–National Cardiovascular Data Registry (ACC-NCDR) experience: 1998-2000. J Am Coll Cardiol 39(7):1104-12, 2002.

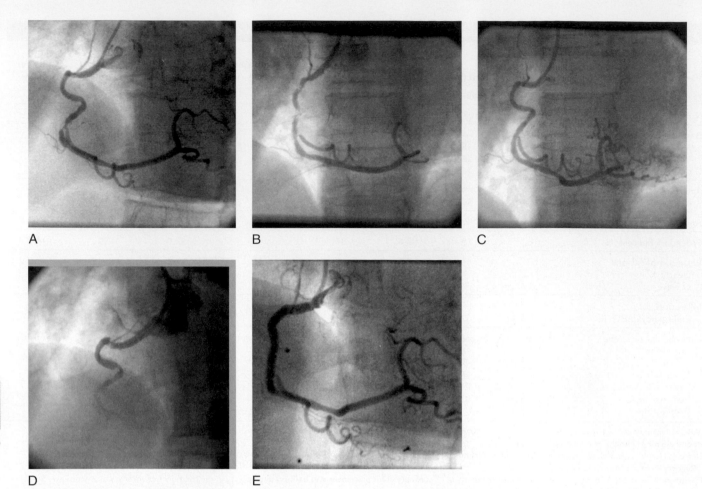

FIGURE 55–12 Abrupt closure following coronary stent placement. **A,** An extremely tortuous right coronary artery has a stenosis in its mid-portion, **B,** After crossing with a coronary guidewire, there is marked straightening of the vessel. **C,** After a stent is placed and the guidewire is removed, there is an excellent result. **D,** Abrupt closure develops because of a guide catheter dissection, resulting in typical chest pain and ST segment elevation. **E,** Coronary stents are placed to "bail out" the severe coronary dissection and normal flow is reestablished to the vessel. Without the availability of coronary stents, it is highly likely that coronary artery bypass graft surgery would have been needed to reverse the abrupt closure event.

TABLE 55–17	Variables Associated with Stent Thrombosis

Clinical Variables
Acute myocardial infarction
Clopidogrel noncompliance and discontinuation
Clopidogrel bioavailability
Diabetes mellitus
Renal failure
Congestive heart failure
Prior radiation brachytherapy

Anatomical Variables
Long lesions
Smaller vessels
Multivessel disease
Acute myocardial infarction
Bifurcation lesions

Procedural Factors
Stent underexpansion
Incomplete wall apposition
Residual inflow and outflow disease
Margin dissections
Crush technique
Overlapping stent
Polymer materials

of stent thrombosis have included only those episodes associated with an acute coronary syndrome and angiographic or pathological demonstration of thrombosis within the stent or its margins. The Academic Research Consortium has proposed new criteria for documentation of all possible stent thrombosis in clinical studies, including the categories of definite stent thrombosis, probable stent thrombosis, and possible stent thrombosis (Table 55-18).

Recent reports suggest an incremental risk (0.2 to 0.5 percent per year) of very late stent thrombosis occurring 1 year or more after drug-eluting stent implantation.[124,153] Inhibition of endothelialization caused by the potent antiproliferative effect of the drugs delivered by drug-eluting stents (DES) may significantly prolong the period of risk for patients to develop stent thrombosis.[154] Although concerning, these events have not yet been shown to cause a significant increase in late morbidity or mortality, likely owing to the benefits of DES in reducing the need for repeat revascularization procedures, and the avoidance of the complications associated with the development of in-stent restenosis. Ongoing evaluation of the long-term safety of DES has engendered intense investigation, with efforts focused on determining whether patient and lesion-specific risk factors, such as insensitivity to aspirin or thienopyridine derivatives may contribute, whether these risks are device- or drug-specific phenomena, and whether prolonged dual antiplatelet therapy may ameliorate these risks.

TABLE 55–18	Academic Research Consortium (ARC) Stent Thrombosis Definitions

Event	Definition

Definite	Angiographic confirmation:
	   TIMI 0 with occlusion originating in or within 5 mm of stent in the presence of a thrombus *or*
	   TIMI flow grade 1, 2, or 3 originating in or within 5 mm of stent in the presence of a thrombus *and* ≥1 of the following criteria < 48 hours:
	     New acute onset of ischemic symptoms at rest (typical chest pain with duration >20 minutes)
	     New ischemic electrocardiographic changes suggestive of acute ischemia
	     Typical rise and fall in cardiac biomarkers
	Pathological confirmation:
	   Evidence of recent thrombus within the stent determined at autopsy or via examination of tissue retrieved following thrombectomy

Probable	Any unexplained death within the first 30 days Irrespective of the time after the index procedure, any myocardial infarction which is related to documented acute ischemia in the territory of the implanted stent without angiographic confirmation of stent thrombosis and in the absence of any other cause
Possible	Any unexplained death >30 days after intracoronary stenting

TIMI = Thrombolysis in Myocardial Infarction.
Modified from Mavei L, Hsieh WH, Massaro JM, et al: Stent thrombosis in randomized clinical trials of drug eluting stents. N Engl J Med 356:1020-1029, 2007.

The not infrequent scenario of a patient requiring noncardiac surgery in the weeks following PCI can markedly increase the risk of stent thrombosis. Studies of outcomes in patients undergoing noncardiac surgery soon after bare metal stent PCI have documented stent thrombosis occurring in up to 8 percent of patients in the first 2 weeks following PCI, with risks declining to baseline rates by 8 weeks.[52] This increased risk likely results from the frequent cessation of thienopyridine therapy before surgery, as well as the hypercoagulable state in the perioperative period.

LATE CLINICAL OUTCOMES. Ischemic events within the first year after PCI result from one of three processes. Lumen renarrowing that requires repeat revascularization (i.e., target lesion revascularization [TLR]) occurs in 20 to 30 percent of patients undergoing balloon angioplasty because of reparative arterial constriction, also known as "negative remodeling." Clinical restenosis after stent implantation is less common (10 to 20 percent) and is attributable to intimal hyperplasia within the stent. Clinical recurrence caused by restenosis is least common (3 to 5 percent) after drug-eluting stent placement because of focal tissue growth within the stent or at its margins. A second cause of clinical events after PCI is the progression of coronary atherosclerosis at a site remote from that treated earlier by PCI. Death and MI can also result from sudden rupture of a plaque that is remote from the site of the initial intervention.

These processes can be partially distinguished by the timing of their occurrence. Clinical restenosis resulting from lumen renarrowing at the site of PCI generally develops within the first 6 to 9 months after PCI, whereas death and MI due to plaque instability may occur at any point after PCI at a low, but constant risk (1 to 2 percent risk per year). Predictors of higher risk of all-cause late mortality include advanced age, reduced left ventricular function, congestive heart failure, diabetes mellitus, number of diseased vessels, inoperable disease, or severe comorbid conditions. A 95 percent 10-year survival rate can be expected in patients with single-vessel CAD and an 80 percent survival rate after PCI can be achieved in those with multivessel CAD.

Outcomes Benchmarking and Quality Assurance

Along with CABG surgery, PCI ranks among the most studied of all procedures in the United States. National structured outcomes registries such as the National Heart Lung and Blood Institute (NHLBI) dynamic registry and the American College of Cardiology National Cardiovascular Data Repository (ACC-NCDR) provide contemporary risk-adjusted outcomes benchmarking to hundreds of participating institutions. Participants in such national, regional, or statewide outcomes reporting initiatives can compare their risk-adjusted clinical outcomes with institutions of similar patient mix and size. The detailed nature of these datasets, in which the data collected spans the range of patient clinical characteristics, lesions descriptors, and device level information, provides centers with a comprehensive comparison of their practice patterns and outcomes compared with peer institutions. Current guidelines recommend that all centers performing PCI participate in a prospective quality assessment and outcomes registry.[7]

PERCUTANEOUS VALVULAR INTERVENTION

Percutaneous valve dilation has been used as an alternative to surgical repair or replacement in selected patients with symptomatic valvular stenosis, particularly of the mitral valve. Mitral valvuloplasty is a safe and effective alternative to surgical repair in selected patients with mitral stenosis, whereas aortic valvuloplasty provides only short-term palliation and should be reserved for inoperable patients with degenerative calcific aortic stenosis. The indications and contraindications for mitral and aortic valvuloplasty are reviewed in detail elsewhere (see Chap. 62 and its guidelines). This chapter focuses on the technical issues, patient selection, and outcomes associated with mitral and aortic valvuloplasty, as well as the emerging areas of percutaneous mitral valve repair and percutaneous aortic valve replacement.

Mitral Valvuloplasty

Percutaneous mitral valvuloplasty (PMV) (see also Chaps. 62 and 83) was first performed in 1984 as an alternative to surgical mitral valve commissurotomy in patients with rheumatic mitral stenosis. Subsequent reports confirmed the immediate and long-term benefits of this procedure, which is now widely used for that condition (particularly in developing countries where rheumatic fever and valvular heart disease continue to be endemic). PMV can use several approaches, most commonly transvenous or antegrade, using a transseptal puncture to gain access to the left atrium. A balloon catheter is then floated across the mitral valve into the left ventricle using either two simultaneous-inflated cylindrical balloons (18 to 20 mm diameters), or a single Inoue balloon, which is a self-positioning, pressure-distensible dumbbell-shaped balloon that locks itself into the stenotic mitral orifice and progressively dilates the orifice to 25 to 28 mm by increasing the inflation volume (Fig. 55-13). Stepwise dilation minimizes the risk of mitral leaflet injury and mitral regurgitation. A percutaneous mechanical valve dilator has also been used, and it has the advantage of resterilization and reuse in developing countries.

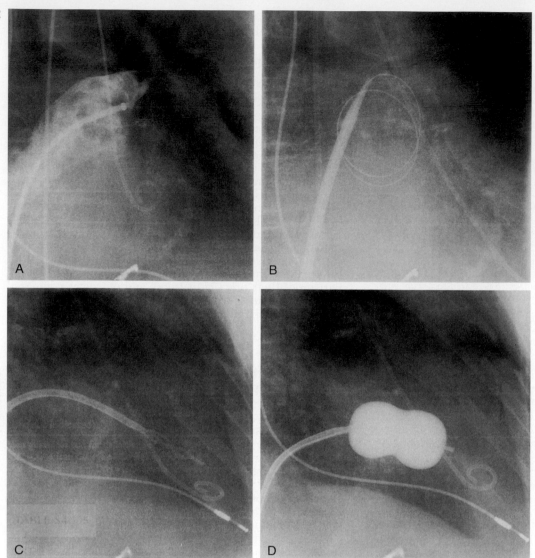

A

B

C

D

FIGURE 55–13 Mitral valvuloplasty. After transseptal puncture, a Mullins sheath is advanced into the left atrium, as demonstrated by contrast injection (**A**). An Inoue guidewire is coiled in the left atrium and an Inoue dilator is advanced across the intraatrial septum (**B**). Advancement of the Inoue balloon dilation catheter into the left ventricle (**C**) and inflation (**D**) resulted in a successful procedure. *(Courtesy of Andrew Eisenhauer, MD.)*

Patients with fewer than two risk factors for early restenosis (echocardiographic score >8, left ventricular end-diastolic pressure >10 mm Hg, or NYHA functional Class IV) had a predicted 5-year event-free survival rate of 60 to 84 percent, whereas patients with two or three risk factors had a predicted 5-year event-free survival rate of only 13 to 41 percent.

Percutaneous Mitral Valve Repair

Unlike rheumatic mitral stenosis, the treatment of mitral regurgitation has remained the exclusive province of cardiac surgery until recently. Repair of the regurgitant mitral valve yields better results than replacement by using a combination of annuloplasty (to reduce the posterior annular circumference and the septal-lateral mitral dimension), removal of excess leaflet tissue, and Alfieri edge-to-edge repair.[155]

Several techniques are under investigation to replicate these surgical procedures using percutaneous methods (Fig. 55-14).[156] A small clip applied during transseptal catheterization (MitraClip, eValve, Mountain View, CA) effects the edge-to-edge repair. A feasibility trial has been completed with favorable safety and efficacy,[157] and a randomized study known as the EVEREST II trial comparing the procedure to surgical repair has begun. Attempts to replicate surgical annuloplasty have mostly centered on the coronary sinus, which lies outside of and roughly in the same plane with the posterior mitral annulus. Attempts to placate or straighten the coronary sinus, in an effort to reduce mitral regurgitation, are just entering clinical trials,[158] whereas others have only preclinical information available.[159,160] The evolution of this new form of catheter-based intervention will raise important considerations relating to training, patient selection, and the appropriate comparison groups.[161]

Aortic Valvuloplasty

Calcific aortic stenosis has become the most frequent cause of acquired valvular heart disease in Western countries. Unlike mitral stenosis, in which the problem is commissural fusion, rigid valve lesions are the causative factor in acquired calcific stenosis. Percutaneous aortic valvuloplasty (PAV) fractures the calcified aortic leaflets, thereby increasing

Serial hemodynamic measurements, alone or in combination with echocardiography, evaluate the result achieved with PMV. An immediate improvement in left atrial mean pressure (and reduction of the transmittal gradient) should occur, with a gradual decrease in pulmonary artery pressure and an increase in cardiac output. Criteria for termination of the procedure include[1] a mitral valve area larger than 1 cm^2 per square meter of body surface area,[2] complete opening of at least one commissure, or the appearance of an increment in mitral regurgitation.[3] Transesophageal echocardiography performed during the procedure may guide the transseptal puncture in patients with obscure cardiac landmarks or skeletal deformity. Echocardiography can also assess the prognosis after PMV by semiquantitatively scoring leaflet mobility, valvular and subvalvular thickening, and valvular calcification. Successful PMV has an estimated 5-year mortality rate of 24 percent and an estimated 5-year event rate (i.e., mitral valve replacement, repeat valvuloplasty, or death from cardiac causes) of nearly 50 percent. Multivariable predictors of late events after PMV include a high mitral valve echocardiographic score, an elevated left ventricular end-diastolic pressure, and a worse New York Heart Association (NYHA) functional class ($p = 0.04$).

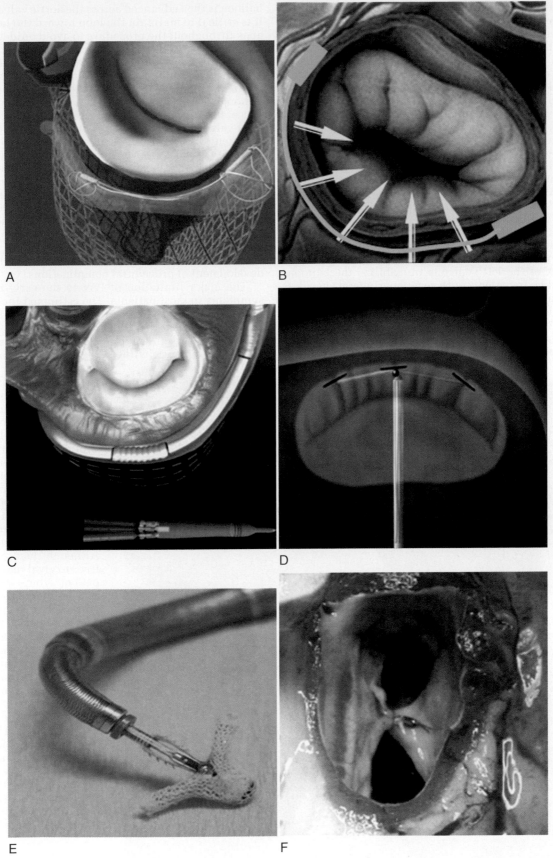

FIGURE 55–14 Percutaneous devices for correction of mitral regurgitation. The Cardiac Dimensions Carillon (Cardiac Dimensions, Inc., Kirkland, WA) **(A)**; the Edwards Viking (Edwards Life Sciences, Irvine, CA) **(B)**; and the Viacor device (Viacor, Inc., Wilmington, MA) **(C)**—all utilize the proximity of the coronary sinus to the posterior mitral annulus to effect a simulated annuloplasty. Other devices such as Mitralign (Mitralign, Inc., Tewksbury, MA) **(D)** perform direct mitral annuloplasty using a percutaneous approach to the ventricular aspect of the annulus. Edge-to-edge approximation of the A$_2$ and P$_2$ portions of the mitral valve is achieved by either deployment of an eValve clip **(E)** or direct suture (Edwards Milano II, **F**). *(Reproduced from Davidson MJ, White JK, Baim DS: Percutaneous therapies for valvular heart disease. Cardiovasc Pathol 15:123, 2006.)*

their flexibility, and somewhat dilating the surrounding aorta (Fig. 55-15). When the annulus recoils and the leaflets recalcify, even the modest hemodynamic improvements afforded by this procedure rapidly abate (over days to weeks). These issues limit the long-term clinical benefit associated with PAV for calcific aortic stenosis. Therefore, PAV is generally reserved for adult patients with critical calcific aortic stenosis who have severe medical comorbidities that preclude aortic valve replacement. Extenuating factors include cardiogenic shock, as a "bridge" to definitive surgical correction, or in patients with severe left ventricular dysfunction (i.e., "low flow, low gradient") who have an uncertain hemodynamic response to aortic valve replacement. In the absence of these indications, definitive aortic valve replacement rather than PAV should be performed, even in elderly patients.[162-164] PAV in patients with congenital aortic stenosis is discussed in Chapters 61 and 62.

The retrograde femoral arterial approach has been the most frequently used for PAV. After crossing the aortic valve with a guidewire, an extra-stiff 0.038-inch wire is inserted into the apex of the left ventricle to stabilize the balloon during inflation. In patients with severe peripheral vascular disease, a brachial approach or anterograde approach using a transseptal puncture can be used to pass a long wire through the left ventricle, across the aortic valve, and into the descending aorta. The interatrial septum is then dilated with a peripheral balloon, and an Inoue mitral valvuloplasty

balloon is then advanced across the aortic valve and inflated. It is critical to maintain the loop toward the left ventricular apex throughout the procedure to avoid guidewire injury to the anterior mitral leaflet, and rapid ventricular pacing (220 beats/min) may help reduce antegrade output and prevent ejection of the balloon during inflation. The transaortic valve gradient should fall immediately after the procedure, although little change may be noted in cardiac output. After successful dilation, 25 to 47 percent of patients will obtain a final valve area larger than 1 cm^2, whereas 22 to 39 percent of patients fail to achieve a valve area above 0.7 cm^2. Hospital mortality after PAV varies from 3.5 to 13.5 percent of patients and at least one in-hospital complication develops in 20 to 25 percent of patients, including the need for vascular access repair, embolic cerebrovascular events, aortic regurgitation, and with the use of oversized balloons, rupture of the aortic ring). Predictors of procedural mortality include the patient's age, NYHA class, concomitant CAD, congestive heart failure, lower initial left ventricular systolic pressure, smaller final aortic valve area, lower baseline cardiac output, and the development of procedural complications.

The major limitation of PAV is the early recurrence of symptoms in most patients. The estimated incidence of late restenosis is 36 to 80 percent in the first year. Determinants of late outcomes after PAV were studied in 205 patients undergoing this procedure. The event-free survival rate, defined as survival without recurrent symptoms, repeated valvuloplasty, or aortic valve replacement, was 18 percent over the 24-month follow-up (range, 1 to 47 months). Significant predictors of event-free survival included the left ventricular ejection fraction, left ventricular and aortic systolic pressure before PAV, and percent reduction in the aortic valve pressure gradient; the pulmonary capillary wedge pressure was inversely associated with event-free survival. Although the predicted event-free survival rate for the entire patient group was 50 percent at 1 year and 25 percent at 2 years, the probability of event-free survival at 1 year varied between 23 and 65 percent when patients were stratified according to three independent predictors: aortic systolic pressure, pulmonary capillary wedge pressure, and percent reduction in the peak aortic valve gradient. The best long-term results after valvuloplasty occurred among patients who should also have had excellent long-term results after aortic valve replacement. Repeat PAV for symptom recurrence may also be useful.[163]

Percutaneous Aortic Valve Replacement

New devices are under development for the percutaneous replacement of the stenotic

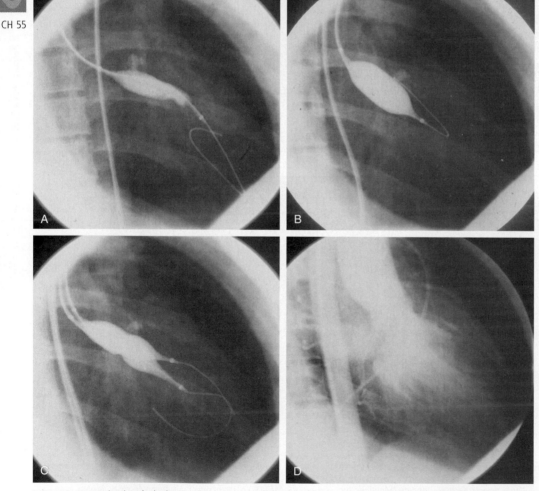

FIGURE 55–15 Aortic valvuloplasty. A 16 mm aortic valvuloplasty balloon is inflated across the aortic valve (A) and exchanged for a 24 mm balloon (B) because of a persistent gradient. To further improve the aortic gradient, two 16 mm valvuloplasty balloons are advanced across the aortic valve (C). Because of the relative oversizing of the balloons in relation to the aortic ring, aortic regurgitation results (D).

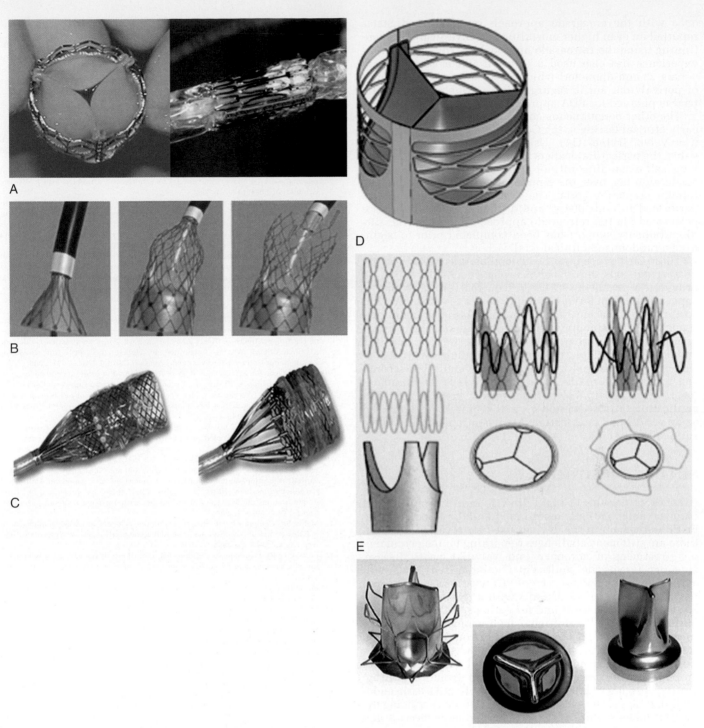

FIGURE 55–16 Percutaneous aortic valve devices and concepts. **A,** The Cribier-Edwards valve (Edwards Life Sciences, Irvine, CA) consists of three equine pericardial leaflets fixed to a balloon-expandable steel stent. It is hand-crimped over a delivery balloon prior to deployment. **B,** The Corevalve system (Corevalve, Inc., Irvine, CA) is a self-expanding nitinol cage housing three porcine pericardial leaflets. Devices in preclinical development include the Sadra self-expanding Lotus valve (Sadra Medical, Inc., Campbell, CA) **(C)**, the Aortx valve **(D)**, the Bonhoeffer valve **(E)**, and the eNitinol thin-membrane PercValve **(F)**. *(Reproduced from Davidson MJ, White JK, Baim DS: Percutaneous therapies for valvular heart disease. Cardiovasc Pathol 15:123, 2006.)*

aortic valve (Fig. 55-16). Unlike surgical replacement, the diseased aortic leaflets remain in place, and a preliminary balloon aortic valvuloplasty is performed. A prosthesis consisting of a balloon- or self-expanding stent into which a functional pericardial valve is sewn, is advanced into the aortic orifice over a heavy-duty guidewire. Deployment of the stent within the diseased valve then allows the new pericardial leaflets to begin functioning.

The first procedure was performed by Cribier in April 2002 using the Cribier-Edwards valve (Edwards, Irvine, CA) via an antegrade transseptal approach[165] and his series of 36 attempted placements was reported recently.[166] The aortic valve area increased from 0.6 to 1.7 cm^2, although roughly one half of the patients had 2+ perivalvular aortic regurgitation and there were a total of seven in-hospital deaths from various complications. Attempts to reproduce this experience with the antegrade approach in the United States reported an even higher mortality, and investigation is continuing using the retrograde approach.[167] This more recent experience has also used a larger diameter stent (26 mm versus 23 mm diameter) which has reduced the incidence of perivalvular aortic regurgitation. A subsequent pivotal trial is planned for FDA approval in the United States.

The other percutaneous aortic valve that has undergone early clinical testing is the CoreValve Revalving procedure (CoreValve, Irvine, CA). Using this percutaneous aortic valve, the pericardial leaflets are mounted within a 50 mm–long self-expanding nitinol stent that extends from the aortic annulus, over the sinuses of Valsalva, and into the tubular ascending aorta. The first clinical procedure was performed in mid-2004,[168] and a pilot registry of 40 cases performed via the retrograde approach during partial cardiopulmonary support has been completed prior to beginning a randomized clinical trial.

These early procedures have demonstrated the feasibility of percutaneous aortic valve replacement and ability to provide an excellent aortic orifice area (~1.7 cm^2) that is superior to that of PAV and similar to the results of surgical aortic valve replacements. The ongoing issues of stable and accurate placement, prevention of perivalvular aortic regurgitation, and minimizing insertion site trauma from the current devices (19 to 21F, 6 to 8 mm in diameter) will continue to be addressed by these devices and other second-generation counterparts. For patients who are not candidates for surgical aortic valve replacement, however, further application of this technology will require both improved acute results and demonstrated valve durability akin to the surgical procedure.

CH 55

FUTURE DIRECTIONS

After three decades of rapid growth and dissemination of coronary interventional techniques, and the associated dramatic refinement in the devices used for revascularization, there are still many challenges remaining for the percutaneous treatment of coronary and valvular heart disease. Ongoing large-scale multicenter randomized trials will assess the safety and efficacy of PCI with DES as compared with CABG surgery for patients with unprotected left main coronary artery stenosis and for patients with diabetes and multivessel CAD.[169] Additional technologies are currently in clinical testing for the treatment of complex bifurcation stenosis, using dedicated bifurcation stent systems. In addition, novel approaches for chronic total occlusions are an area of intense investigation. Continued evolution of drug-eluting design will attempt to optimize effective early endothelialization of the stented segment without sacrificing the long-term benefits of DES in terms of reducing target lesion revascularization. Determination of the optimal duration of antiplatelet therapy following DES deployments requires further study. Bioabsorbable stents, produced from bioerodable polymers or magnesium alloys, show promise as a mechanism of providing short-term scaffolding to prevent abrupt closure of the vessel and leaving nothing permanent in the vessel wall after 6 months, thereby potentially reducing the risks of stent thombosis.[170] Early investigations into myocardial regeneration following acute myocardial infarction using percutaneous delivery of autologous stem cell or progenitor cell lines has generated great interest in the potential of such therapies to improve myocardial recovery (see Chap. 29). Continued refinement of ventricular support devices offers hope for myocardial recovery in the setting of severe myocardial dysfunction. The entire arena of percutaneous valvular repair and replacement is undergoing active innovation and investigation.

Acknowledgments

The authors acknowledge Richard E. Kuntz, MD, for his prior contribution to this chapter and Faisal Khan, MD, and Alexandra Almonacid, MD, for their contributions to this work.

REFERENCES

Indications for Revascularization

1. Thom T, Haase N, Rosamond W, et al: Heart disease and stroke statistics—2006 update: A report from the American Heart Association Statistics Committee and Stroke Statistics Subcommittee. Circulation 113(6):e85-151, 2006.
2. Popma J, Kuntz R, Baim D: A decade of improvement in the clinical outcomes of percutaneous coronary intervention for multivessel coronary artery disease. Circulation 106(13):1592-4, 2002.
3. Byrne JG, Leacche M, Unic D, et al: Staged initial percutaneous coronary intervention followed by valve surgery ("hybrid approach") for patients with complex coronary and valve disease. J Am Coll Cardiol 45(1):14-8, 2005.
4. Murphy GJ, Bryan AJ, Angelini GD: Hybrid coronary revascularization in the era of drug-eluting stents. Ann Thorac Surg 78:1861-7, 2004.
5. Holmes D, Selzer F, Johnston J, et al: Modeling and risk prediction in the current era of interventional cardiology: A report from the National Heart, Lung, and Blood Institute Dynamic Registry. Circulation 107(14):1871-6, 2003.
6. Keeley EC, Boura JA, Grines CL: Primary angioplasty versus intravenous thrombolytic therapy for acute myocardial infarction: A quantitative review of 23 randomised trials. Lancet 361(9351):13-20, 2003.
7. Smith SC, Jr., Feldman TE, Hirshfeld JW, Jr., et al: ACC/AHA/SCAI 2005 guideline update for percutaneous coronary intervention: A report of the American College of Cardiology/American Heart Association Task Force on Practice Guidelines (ACC/AHA/SCAI Writing Committee to Update the 2001 Guidelines for Percutaneous Coronary Intervention). J Am Coll Cardiol 47(1):e1-121, 2006.
8. Eagle KA, Guyton RA, Davidoff R, et al: ACC/AHA 2004 guideline update for coronary artery bypass graft surgery: A report of the American College of Cardiology/American Heart Association Task Force on Practice Guidelines (Committee to Update the 1999 Guidelines for Coronary Artery Bypass Graft Surgery). Circulation 110(14):e340-437, 2004.
9. Moses JW, Stone GW, Nikolsky E, et al: Drug-eluting stents in the treatment of intermediate lesions: Pooled analysis from four randomized trials. J Am Coll Cardiol 47(11):2164-71, 2006.
10. Braunwald E, Antman E, Beasley J, et al: ACC/AHA 2002 guideline update for the management of patients with unstable angina and non-ST segment elevation myocardial infarction—summary article: A report of the American College of Cardiology/American Heart Association task force on practice guidelines (Committee on the Management of Patients with Unstable Angina). J Am Coll Cardiol 40(7):1366-74, 2002.
11. Mehta SR, Cannon CP, Fox KA, et al: Routine vs selective invasive strategies in patients with acute coronary syndromes: A collaborative meta-analysis of randomized trials. JAMA 293:2908-17, 2005.
12. de Winter RJ, Windhausen F, Cornel JH, et al: Early invasive versus selectively invasive management for acute coronary syndromes. N Engl J Med 353:1095-104, 2005.
13. Shea ML, Conti CR, Arora RR: An update on enhanced external counterpulsation. Clin Cardiol 28:115-8, 2005.
14. Cohn PF: Enhanced external counterpulsation for the treatment of angina pectoris. Prog Cardiovasc Dis 49:88-97, 2006.
15. Nichols WW, Estrada JC, Braith RW, et al: Enhanced external counterpulsation treatment improves arterial wall properties and wave reflection characteristics in patients with refractory angina. J Am Coll Cardiol 48:1208-14, 2006.
16. Gibbons RJ, Abrams J, Chatterjee K, et al: ACC/AHA 2002 guideline update for the management of patients with chronic stable angina—summary article: A report of the American College of Cardiology/American Heart Association Task Force on Practice Guidelines (Committee on the Management of Patients with Chronic Stable Angina). Circulation 107(1):149-58, 2003.
17. Silber S, Albertsson P, Aviles FF, et al: Guidelines for percutaneous coronary interventions. The Task Force for Percutaneous Coronary Interventions of the European Society of Cardiology. Eur Heart J 26(8):804-47, 2005.
18. Moreno R, Fernandez C, Hernandez R, et al: Drug-eluting stent thrombosis: Results from a pooled analysis including 10 randomized studies. J Am Coll Cardiol 45(6):954-9, 2005.
19. Nikolsky E, Halabi M, Roguin A, et al: Staged versus one-step approach for multivessel percutaneous coronary interventions. Am Heart J 143(6):1017-26, 2002.

Patient-Specific Considerations for Percutaneous Coronary Intervention

20. Krone R, Shaw R, Klein L, et al: Evaluation of the American College of Cardiology/American Heart Association and the Society for Coronary Angiography and Interventions lesion classification system in the current "stent era" of coronary interventions (from the ACC-National Cardiovascular Data Registry). Am J Cardiol 92(4):389-94, 2003.
21. Singh M, Rihal CS, Lennon RJ, et al: Comparison of Mayo Clinic risk score and American College of Cardiology/American Heart Association lesion classification in the prediction of adverse cardiovascular outcome following percutaneous coronary interventions. J Am Coll Cardiol 44:357-61, 2004.
22. Christofferson RD, Lehmann KG, Martin GV, et al: Effect of chronic total coronary occlusion on treatment strategy. Am J Cardiol 95:1088-91, 2005.

23. Baim DS, Braden G, Heuser R, et al: Utility of the Safe-Cross-guided radiofrequency total occlusion crossing system in chronic coronary total occlusions (results from the Guided Radio Frequency Energy Ablation of Total Occlusions Registry Study). Am J Cardiol 94:853-8, 2004.

24. Saito S, Tanaka S, Hiroe Y, et al: Angioplasty for chronic total occlusion by using tapered-tip guidewires. Catheter Cardiovasc Interv 59:305-11, 2003.

25. Stone GW, Reifart NJ, Moussa I, et al: Percutaneous recanalization of chronically occluded coronary arteries: A consensus document: Part II. Circulation 112:2530-7, 2005.

26. Stone GW, Kandzari DE, Mehran R, et al: Percutaneous recanalization of chronically occluded coronary arteries: A consensus document: Part I. Circulation 112:2364-72, 2005.

27. Werner GS, Krack A, Schwarz G, et al: Prevention of lesion recurrence in chronic total coronary occlusions by paclitaxel-eluting stents. J Am Coll Cardiol 44(12):2301-6, 2004.

28. Migliorini A, Moschi G, Vergara R, et al: Drug-eluting stent-supported percutaneous coronary intervention for chronic total coronary occlusion. Catheter Cardiovasc Interv 67(3):344-8, 2006.

29. Giugliano GR, Kuntz RE, Popma JJ, et al: Determinants of 30-day adverse events following saphenous vein graft intervention with and without a distal occlusion embolic protection device. Am J Cardiol 95(2):173-7, 2005.

30. Resnic FS, Wainstein M, Lee MK, et al: No-reflow is an independent predictor of death and myocardial infarction after percutaneous coronary intervention. Am Heart J 145(1):42-6, 2003.

31. Lee MS, Shah AP, Aragon J, et al: Drug-eluting stenting is superior to bare metal stenting in saphenous vein grafts. Catheter Cardiovasc Interv 66(4):507-11, 2005.

32. Ge L, Iakovou I, Sangiorgi GM, et al: Treatment of saphenous vein graft lesions with drug-eluting stents: Immediate and midterm outcome. J Am Coll Cardiol 45(7):989-94, 2005.

33. Colombo A, Moses JW, Morice MC, et al: Randomized study to evaluate sirolimus-eluting stents implanted at coronary bifurcation lesions. Circulation 109(10):1244-9, 2004.

34. Ge L, Airoldi F, Iakovou I, et al: Clinical and angiographic outcome after implantation of drug-eluting stents in bifurcation lesions with the crush stent technique: Importance of final kissing balloon post-dilation. J Am Coll Cardiol 46:613-20, 2005.

35. Lefevre T, Ormiston J, Guagliumi G, et al: The Frontier stent registry: Safety and feasibility of a novel dedicated stent for the treatment of bifurcation coronary artery lesions. J Am Coll Cardiol 46(4):592-8, 2005.

36. Ikeno F, Kim YH, Luna J, et al: Acute and long-term outcomes of the novel side access (SLK-View) stent for bifurcation coronary lesions: A multicenter nonrandomized feasibility study. Catheter Cardiovasc Interv 67(2):198-206, 2006.

37. Shaw RE, Anderson HV, Brindis RG, et al: Development of a risk adjustment mortality model using the American College of Cardiology–National Cardiovascular Data Registry (ACC-NCDR) experience: 1998-2000. J Am Coll Cardiol 39(7):1104-12, 2002.

38. Santa-Cruz RA, Cohen MG, Ohman EM: Aortic counterpulsation: A review of the hemodynamic effects and indications for use. Catheter Cardiovasc Interv 67(1):68-77, 2006.

39. Aragon J, Lee MS, Kar S, Makkar RR: Percutaneous left ventricular assist device: "TandemHeart" for high-risk coronary intervention. Catheter Cardiovasc Interv 65(3):346-52, 2005.

40. Lee MS, Makkar RR: Percutaneous left ventricular support devices. Cardiol Clin 24(2):265-75, 2006.

41. Gemmato CJ, Forrester MD, Myers TJ, et al: Thirty-five years of mechanical circulatory support at the Texas Heart Institute: An updated overview. Tex Heart Inst J 32(2):168-77, 2005.

42. Henriques JP, Remmelink M, Baan J, Jr., et al: Safety and feasibility of elective high-risk percutaneous coronary intervention procedures with left ventricular support of the Impella Recover LP 2.5. Am J Cardiol 97(7):990-2, 2006.

43. McCullough P: Outcomes of contrast-induced nephropathy: Experience in patients undergoing cardiovascular intervention. Catheter Cardiovasc Interv 67(3):335-43, 2006.

44. Stigant C, Izadnegahdar M, Levin A, et al: Outcomes after percutaneous coronary interventions in patients with CKD: Improved outcome in the stenting era. Am J Kidney Dis 45(6):1002-9, 2005.

45. Keeley EC, Kadakia R, Soman S, et al: Analysis of long-term survival after revascularization in patients with chronic kidney disease presenting with acute coronary syndromes. Am J Cardiol 92(5):509-14, 2003.

46. Ix JH, Mercado N, Shlipak MG, et al: Association of chronic kidney disease with clinical outcomes after coronary revascularization: The Arterial Revascularization Therapies Study (ARTS). Am Heart J 149(3):512-9, 2005.

47. Dangas G, Iakovou I, Nikolsky E, et al: Contrast-induced nephropathy after percutaneous coronary interventions in relation to chronic kidney disease and hemodynamic variables. Am J Cardiol 95(1):13-9, 2005.

48. Fukumoto Y, Tsutsui H, Tsuchihashi M, et al: The incidence and risk factors of cholesterol embolization syndrome, a complication of cardiac catheterization: A prospective study. J Am Coll Cardiol 42(2):211-6, 2003.

49. Rihal CS, Textor SC, Grill DE, et al: Incidence and prognostic importance of acute renal failure after percutaneous coronary intervention. Circulation 105(19):2259-64, 2002.

50. Cutlip D, Chauhan M, Baim D, et al: Clinical restenosis after coronary stenting: perspectives from multicenter clinical trials. J Am Coll Cardiol 40(12):2082-9, 2002.

51. Iakovou I, Schmidt T, Bonizzoni E, et al: Incidence, predictors, and outcome of thrombosis after successful implantation of drug-eluting stents. JAMA 293(17):2126-30, 2005.

52. Wilson SH, Fasseas P, Orford JL, et al: Clinical outcome of patients undergoing non-cardiac surgery in the two months following coronary stenting. J Am Coll Cardiol 42(2):234-40, 2003.

Vascular Access

53. Archbold RA, Robinson NM, Schilling RJ: Radial artery access for coronary angiography and percutaneous coronary intervention. BMJ 329(7463):443-6, 2004.

54. Cox N, Resnic FS, Popma JJ, et al: Comparison of the risk of vascular complications associated with femoral and radial access coronary catheterization procedures in obese versus nonobese patients. Am J Cardiol 94(9):1174-7, 2004.

55. Agostoni P, Biondi-Zoccai GG, de Benedictis ML, et al: Radial versus femoral approach for percutaneous coronary diagnostic and interventional procedures: Systematic overview and meta-analysis of randomized trials. J Am Coll Cardiol 44(2):349-56, 2004.

56. Bazemore E, Mann JT, 3rd: Problems and complications of the transradial approach for coronary interventions: A review. J Invasive Cardiol 17(3):156-9, 2005.

57. Kugelmass AD, Cohen DJ, Brown PP, et al: Hospital resources consumed in treating complications associated with percutaneous coronary interventions. Am J Cardiol 97(3):322-7, 2006.

58. Piper WD, Malenka DJ, Ryan TJ, Jr., et al: Predicting vascular complications in percutaneous coronary interventions. Am Heart J 145(6):1022-9, 2003.

59. Farouque HM, Tremmel JA, Raissi SF, et al: Risk factors for the development of retroperitoneal hematoma after percutaneous coronary intervention in the era of glycoprotein IIb/IIIa inhibitors and vascular closure devices. J Am Coll Cardiol 45:363-8, 2005.

60. Ellis SG, Bhatt D, Kapadia S, et al: Correlates and outcomes of retroperitoneal hemorrhage complicating percutaneous coronary intervention. Catheter Cardiovasc Interv 67:541-5, 2006.

61. Meyerson SL, Feldman T, Desai TR, et al: Angiographic access site complications in the era of arterial closure devices. Vasc Endovascular Surg 36(2):137-44, 2002.

62. Rao SV, O'Grady K, Pieper KS, et al: Impact of bleeding severity on clinical outcomes among patients with acute coronary syndromes. Am J Cardiol 96(9):1200-6, 2005.

63. Eikelboom JW, Mehta SR, Anand SS, et al: Adverse impact of bleeding on prognosis in patients with acute coronary syndromes. Circulation 114(8):774-82, 2006.

64. Nikolsky E, Mehran R, Halkin A, et al: Vascular complications associated with arteriotomy closure devices in patients undergoing percutaneous coronary procedures: A meta-analysis. J Am Coll Cardiol 44(6):1200-9, 2004.

65. Lasic Z, Nikolsky E, Kesanakurthy S, Dangas G: Vascular closure devices: A review of their use after invasive procedures. Am J Cardiovasc Drugs 5(3):185-200, 2005.

Coronary Devices

66. Mauri L, Reisman M, Buchbinder M, et al: Comparison of rotational atherectomy with conventional balloon angioplasty in the prevention of restenosis of small coronary arteries: Results of the Dilatation vs Ablation Revascularization Trial Targeting Restenosis (DART). Am Heart J 145(5):847-54, 2003.

67. Kuntz R, Baim D, Cohen D, et al: A trial comparing rheolytic thrombectomy with intracoronary urokinase for coronary and vein graft thrombus (the Vein Graft AngioJet Study [VeGAS 2]). Am J Cardiol 89(3):326-30, 2002.

68. Ali A, Cox D, Dib N, et al: Rheolytic thrombectomy with percutaneous coronary intervention for infarct size reduction in acute myocardial infarction: 30-Day results from a multicenter randomized study. J Am Coll Cardiol 48(2):244-52, 2006.

69. Siddiqui DS, Choi CJ, Tsimikas S, Mahmud E. Successful utilization of a novel aspiration thrombectomy catheter (Pronto) for the treatment of patients with stent thrombosis. Catheter Cardiovasc Interv 67:894-9, 2006.

70. Silva-Orrego P, Colombo P, Bigi R, et al: Thrombus aspiration before primary angioplasty improves myocardial reperfusion in acute myocardial infarction: The DEAR-MI (Dethrombosis to Enhance Acute Reperfusion in Myocardial Infarction) study. J Am Coll Cardiol 48:1552-9, 2006.

71. Burzotta F, Trani C, Romagnoli E, et al: A pilot study with a new, rapid-exchange, thrombus-aspirating device in patients with thrombus-containing lesions: The Diver C.E. study. Catheter Cardiovasc Interv 67:887-93, 2006.

72. Mauri L, Rogers C, Baim DS: Devices for distal protection during percutaneous coronary revascularization. Circulation 113(22):2651-6, 2006.

73. Stone GW, Rogers C, Hermiller J, et al: Randomized comparison of distal protection with a filter-based catheter and a balloon occlusion and aspiration system during percutaneous intervention of diseased saphenous vein aorto-coronary bypass grafts. Circulation 108(5):548-53, 2003.

74. Baim D, Wahr D, George B, et al: Randomized trial of a distal embolic protection device during percutaneous intervention of saphenous vein aorto-coronary bypass grafts. Circulation 105(11):1285-90, 2002.

75. Carrozza JP, Jr., Mumma M, Breall JA, et al: Randomized evaluation of the TriActiv balloon-protection flush and extraction system for the treatment of saphenous vein graft disease. J Am Coll Cardiol 46(9):1677-83, 2005.

76. Stone GW, Webb J, Cox DA, et al: Distal microcirculatory protection during percutaneous coronary intervention in acute ST-segment elevation myocardial infarction: A randomized controlled trial. JAMA 293(9):1063-72, 2005.

77. Kuntz RE, Rogers C, Baim DS: Percutaneous coronary intervention-induced emboli during primary PCI for STEMI: Too little, too much, or too late? Am Heart J 150(1):4-6, 2005.

78. Rogers C, Huynh R, Seifert PA, et al: Embolic protection with filtering or occlusion balloons during saphenous vein graft stenting retrieves identical volumes and sizes of particulate debris. Circulation 109:1735-40, 2004.

79. Young JJ, Kereiakes DJ, Rabinowitz AC, et al: A novel, low-profile filter-wire (Interceptor) embolic protection device during saphenous vein graft stenting. Am J Cardiol 95:511-4, 2005.

80. Dixon SR, Mann JT, Lauer MA, et al: A randomized, controlled trial of saphenous vein graft intervention with a filter-based distal embolic protection device: TRAP trial. J Interv Cardiol 18:233-41, 2005.

81. Mauri L, Rogers C, Baim DS: Devices for distal protection during percutaneous coronary revascularization. Circulation 113:2651-2656, 2006.

82. Webb JG, Vaderah S, Hamburger J, et al: Proximal protection during saphenous vein graft angioplasty: The Kerberos embolic protection system. Catheter Cardiovasc Interv 64:383-6, 2005.

83. Cutlip DE, Chhabra AG, Baim DS, et al: Beyond restenosis: Five-year clinical outcomes from second-generation coronary stent trials. Circulation 110(10):1226-30, 2004.

84. Popma J, Suntharalingam M, Lansky A, et al: Randomized trial of 90Sr/90Y beta-radiation versus placebo control for treatment of in-stent restenosis. Circulation 106(9):1090-6, 2002.

85. Waksman R, Raizner A, Yeung A, et al: Use of localised intracoronary beta radiation in treatment of in-stent restenosis: the INHIBIT randomised controlled trial. Lancet 359(9306):551-7, 2002.

Drug-Eluting Stents

86. Holmes DR, Jr., Teirstein P, Satler L, et al: Sirolimus-eluting stents vs vascular brachytherapy for in-stent restenosis within bare-metal stents: The SISR randomized trial. JAMA 295(11):1264-73, 2006.

87. Stone GW, Ellis SG, O'Shaughnessy CD, et al: Paclitaxel-eluting stents vs vascular brachytherapy for in-stent restenosis within bare-metal stents: the TAXUS V ISR randomized trial. JAMA 295:1253-63, 2006.

88. Morice M, Serruys P, Sousa J, et al: A randomized comparison of a sirolimus-eluting stent with a standard stent for coronary revascularization. N Engl J Med 346(23):1773-80, 2002.

89. Grube E, Silber S, Hauptmann K, et al: TAXUS I: six- and twelve-month results from a randomized, double-blind trial on a slow-release paclitaxel-eluting stent for de novo coronary lesions. Circulation 107(1):38-42, 2003.

90. Tsuchida K, Piek J, Neuman F: One-year results of a durable polymer everolimus-eluting stent in de novo coronary narrowings (the SPIRIT FIRST trial). EuroInterv 1:266-272, 2005.

91. Meredith I, Ormiston J, Whitbourn R: First-in-human study of the Endeavor ABT-578-eluting phosphorylcholine-encapsulated stent system in de novo native coronary artery lesions: Endeavor I Trial. EuroInterv 2:157-164, 2005.

92. Serruys P, Ruygrok P, Neuzner J: A randomized comparison of an everolimus-eluting coronary stent with a paclitaxel-eluting coronary stent: The SPIRIT II Trial. EuroInterv 2:286-294, 2006.

93. Moses JW, Leon MB, Popma JJ, et al: Sirolimus-eluting stents versus standard stents in patients with stenosis in a native coronary artery. N Engl J Med 349(14):1315-23, 2003.

94. Stone GW, Ellis SG, Cox DA, et al: A polymer-based, paclitaxel-eluting stent in patients with coronary artery disease.[see comment]. N Engl J Med 350(3):221-31, 2004.

95. Schofer J, Schluter M, Gershlick AH, et al: Sirolimus-eluting stents for treatment of patients with long atherosclerotic lesions in small coronary arteries: Double-blind, randomised controlled trial (E-SIRIUS). Lancet 362:1093-9, 2003.

96. Schampaert E, Cohen EA, Schluter M, et al: The Canadian study of the sirolimus-eluting stent in the treatment of patients with long de novo lesions in small native coronary arteries (C-SIRIUS). J Am Coll Cardiol 43:1110-5, 2004.

97. Fajadet J, Wijns W, Laarman G, et al: Randomized, double-blind, multicenter study of the Endeavor zotarolimus-eluting phosphorylcholine-encapsulated stent for treatment of native coronary artery lesions: Clinical and angiographic results of the ENDEAVOR II trial. Circulation 114(8):798-806, 2006.

98. Stone GW, Ellis SG, Cannon L, et al: Comparison of a polymer-based paclitaxel-eluting stent with a bare metal stent in patients with complex coronary artery disease: A randomized controlled trial. JAMA 294:1215-23, 2005.

99. Dawkins KD, Grube E, Guagliumi G, et al: Clinical efficacy of polymer-based paclitaxel-eluting stents in the treatment of complex, long coronary artery lesions from a multicenter, randomized trial: Support for the use of drug-eluting stents in contemporary clinical practice. Circulation 112:3306-13, 2005.

100. Kim YH, Park SW, Lee SW, et al: Sirolimus-eluting stent versus paclitaxel-eluting stent for patients with long coronary artery disease. Circulation 114:2148-53, 2006.

101. Kim YH, Park SW, Lee CW, et al: Comparison of sirolimus-eluting stent, paclitaxel-eluting stent, and bare metal stent in the treatment of long coronary lesions. Catheter Cardiovasc Interv 67:181-7, 2006.

102. Ardissino D, Cavallini C, Bramucci E, et al: Sirolimus-eluting vs uncoated stents for prevention of restenosis in small coronary arteries: A randomized trial. JAMA 292:2727-34, 2004.

103. Morice MC, Colombo A, Meier B, et al: Sirolimus- vs. paclitaxel-eluting stents in de novo coronary artery lesions: The REALITY trial: A randomized controlled trial [see comment]. JAMA 295(8):895-904, 2006.

104. Meier B, Sousa E, Guagliumi G, et al: Sirolimus-eluting coronary stents in small vessels. Am Heart J 151:1019.e1-7, 2006.

105. Mehilli J, Dibra A, Kastrati A, et al: Randomized trial of paclitaxel- and sirolimus-eluting stents in small coronary vessels. Eur Heart J 27:260-6, 2006.

106. Hoye A, Tanabe K, Lemos PA, et al: Significant reduction in restenosis after the use of sirolimus-eluting stents in the treatment of chronic total occlusions. J Am Coll Cardiol 43:1954-8, 2004.

107. Jang JS, Hong MK, Lee CW, et al: Comparison between sirolimus- and paclitaxel-eluting stents for the treatment of chronic total occlusions. J Invasive Cardiol 18:205-8, 2006.

108. Kelbaek H, Helqvist S, Thuesen L, et al: Sirolimus versus bare metal stent implantation in patients with total coronary occlusions: Subgroup analysis of the Stenting Coronary Arteries in Non-Stress/Benestent Disease (SCANDSTENT) trial. Am Heart J 152:882-6, 2006.

109. Suttorp MJ, Laarman GJ, Rahel BM, et al: Primary Stenting of Totally Occluded Native Coronary Arteries II (PRISON II): A randomized comparison of bare metal stent implantation with sirolimus-eluting stent implantation for the treatment of total coronary occlusions. Circulation 114(9):921-8, 2006.

110. Nakamura S, Muthusamy TS, Bae JH, et al: Impact of sirolimus-eluting stent on the outcome of patients with chronic total occlusions. Am J Cardiol 95:161-6, 2005.

111. Buch AN, Xue Z, Gevorkian N, et al: Comparison of outcomes between bare metal stents and drug-eluting stents for percutaneous revascularization of internal mammary grafts. Am J Cardiol 98:722-4, 2006.

112. Chu WW, Kuchulakanti PK, Wang B, et al: Efficacy of sirolimus-eluting stents as compared to paclitaxel-eluting stents for saphenous vein graft intervention. J Interv Cardiol 19:121-5, 2006.

113. Chu WW, Rha SW, Kuchulakanti PK, et al: Efficacy of sirolimus-eluting stents compared with bare metal stents for saphenous vein graft intervention. Am J Cardiol 97:34-7, 2006.

114. Hoffmann R, Pohl T, Koster R, et al: Implantation of paclitaxel-eluting stents in saphenous vein grafts. Clinical and angiographic follow-up results from a multicentre study. Heart 93:331-4, 2007. Epub Aug 29, 2006.

115. Wöhrle J, Nusser T, Kestler HA, et al: Comparison of the slow-release polymer-based paclitaxel-eluting Taxus-Express stent with the bare-metal Express stent for saphenous vein graft interventions [Record Supplied By Publisher]. Clin Res Cardiol 96:70-6, 2007. Epub Dec 8, 2006.

116. Vermeersch P, Agostoni P, Verheye S, et al: Randomized double-blind comparison of sirolimus-eluting stent versus bare-metal stent implantation in diseased saphenous vein grafts: Six-month angiographic, intravascular ultrasound, and clinical follow-up of the RRISC Trial. J Am Coll Cardiol 48:2423-31, 2006.

117. Mishra S, Wolfram RM, Torguson R, et al: Comparison of effectiveness and safety of drug-eluting stents versus vascular brachytherapy for saphenous vein graft in-stent restenosis. Am J Cardiol 97:1303-7, 2006.

118. Liistro F, Fineschi M, Angioli P, et al: Effectiveness and safety of sirolimus stent implantation for coronary in-stent restenosis: The TRUE (Tuscany Registry of Sirolimus for Unselected In-Stent Restenosis) Registry. J Am Coll Cardiol 48:270-5, 2006.

119. Alfonso F, Perez-Vizcayno MJ, Hernandez R, et al: A randomized comparison of sirolimus-eluting stent with balloon angioplasty in patients with in-stent restenosis: Results of the Restenosis Intrastent: Balloon Angioplasty versus Elective Sirolimus-Eluting Stenting (RIBS-II) trial. J Am Coll Cardiol 47:2152-60, 2006.

120. Li JJ, Xu B, Yang YJ, et al: A comparison of angiographic and clinical outcomes after sirolimus-eluting versus paclitaxel-eluting stents for the treatment of in-stent restenosis. Chin Med J 119:1059-64, 2006.

121. Valgimigli M, Percoco G, Malagutti P, et al: Tirofiban and sirolimus-eluting stent vs abciximab and bare-metal stent for acute myocardial infarction: A randomized trial. JAMA 293:2109-17, 2005.

122. Spaulding C, Henry P, Teiger E, et al: Sirolimus-eluting versus uncoated stents in acute myocardial infarction. N Engl J Med 355:1093-104, 2006.

123. Laarman GJ, Suttorp MJ, Dirksen MT, et al: Paclitaxel-eluting versus uncoated stents in primary percutaneous coronary intervention. N Engl J Med 355:1105-13, 2006.

124. Ong A, McFadden E, Regar E, et al: Late angiographic stent thrombosis (LAST) events with drug-eluting stents. J Am Coll Cardiol 45(12):2088-92, 2005.

125. Sousa J, Costa M, Abizaid A, et al: Sirolimus-eluting stent for the treatment of in-stent restenosis: A quantitative coronary angiography and three-dimensional intravascular ultrasound study. Circulation 107(1):24-7, 2003.

126. Kandzari DE, Leon MB: Overview of pharmacology and clinical trials program with the zotarolimus-eluting endeavor stent. J Interv Cardiol 19:405-13, 2006.

127. Costa RA, Lansky AJ, Mintz GS, et al: Angiographic results of the first human experience with everolimus-eluting stents for the treatment of coronary lesions (the FUTURE I trial). Am J Cardiol 95(1):113-6, 2005.

128. Serruys PW, Sianos G, Abizaid A, et al: The effect of variable dose and release kinetics on neointimal hyperplasia using a novel paclitaxel-eluting stent platform: The Paclitaxel In-Stent Controlled Elution Study (PISCES). J Am Coll Cardiol 46(2):253-60, 2005.

129. Cuisset T, Frere C, Quilici J, et al: Benefit of a 600-mg loading dose of clopidogrel on platelet reactivity and clinical outcomes in patients with non-ST-segment elevation acute coronary syndrome undergoing coronary stenting. J Am Coll Cardiol 48:1339-45, 2006.

130. von Beckerath N, Taubert D, Pogatsa-Murray G, et al: Absorption, metabolization, and antiplatelet effects of 300-, 600-, and 900-mg loading doses of clopidogrel: Results of the ISAR-CHOICE (Intracoronary Stenting and Antithrombotic Regimen: Choose Between 3 High Oral Doses for Immediate Clopidogrel Effect) Trial. Circulation 112:2946-50, 2005.

131. Montalescot G, Sideris G, Meuleman C, et al: A randomized comparison of high clopidogrel loading doses in patients with non-ST-segment elevation acute coronary syndromes: The ALBION (Assessment of the Best Loading Dose of Clopidogrel to Blunt Platelet Activation, Inflammation and Ongoing Necrosis) trial. J Am Coll Cardiol 48:931-8, 2006.

132. Hochholzer W, Trenk D, Frundi D, et al: Time dependence of platelet inhibition after a 600-mg loading dose of clopidogrel in a large, unselected cohort of candidates for percutaneous coronary intervention. Circulation 111:2560-4, 2005.

CH 55

133. Patti G, Colonna G, Pasceri V, et al: Randomized trial of high loading dose of clopidogrel for reduction of periprocedural myocardial infarction in patients undergoing coronary intervention: Results from the ARMYDA-2 (Antiplatelet therapy for Reduction of MYocardial Damage during Angioplasty) study. Circulation 111:2099-106, 2005.

134. Kastrati A, von Beckerath N, Joost A, et al: Loading with 600 mg clopidogrel in patients with coronary artery disease with and without chronic clopidogrel therapy. Circulation 110:1916-9, 2004.

135. Kastrati A, Mehilli J, Neumann FJ, et al: Abciximab in patients with acute coronary syndromes undergoing percutaneous coronary intervention after clopidogrel pretreatment: The ISAR-REACT 2 randomized trial. JAMA 295:1531-8, 2006.

136. Gurbel PA, Bliden KP, Zaman KA, et al: Clopidogrel loading with eptifibatide to arrest the reactivity of platelets: Results of the Clopidogrel Loading With Eptifibatide to Arrest the Reactivity of Platelets (CLEAR PLATELETS) study. Circulation 111:1153-9, 2005.

137. Brener SJ, Bhatt DL, Moliterno DJ, et al: Revisiting optimal anticoagulation with unfractionated heparin during coronary stent implantation. Am J Cardiol 92:1468-71, 2003.

138. Ferguson JJ, Califf RM, Antman EM, et al: Enoxaparin vs unfractionated heparin in high-risk patients with non-ST-segment elevation acute coronary syndromes managed with an intended early invasive strategy: Primary results of the SYNERGY randomized trial. JAMA 292:45-54, 2004.

139. Bhatt D, Lee B, Casterella P, et al: Safety of concomitant therapy with eptifibatide and enoxaparin in patients undergoing percutaneous coronary intervention: Results of the Coronary Revascularization Using Integrilin and Single bolus Enoxaparin Study. J Am Coll Cardiol 41(1):20-5, 2003.

140. Lincoff A, Bittl J, Harrington R, et al: Bivalirudin and provisional glycoprotein IIb/IIIa blockade compared with heparin and planned glycoprotein IIb/IIIa blockade during percutaneous coronary intervention: REPLACE-2 randomized trial. JAMA 289(7):853-63, 2003.

141. Stone G, McLaurin B, Cox D, et al: Bivalirudin for patients with acute coronary syndromes. N Engl J Med 355(21):2203-16, 2006.

142. Yusuf S, Mehta SR, Chrolavicius S, et al: Comparison of fondaparinux and enoxaparin in acute coronary syndromes. N Engl J Med 354:1464-76, 2006.

Outcomes Following Percutaneous Coronary Intervention

143. Williams DO, Abbott JD, Kip KE: Outcomes of 6906 patients undergoing percutaneous coronary intervention in the era of drug-eluting stents: Report of the DEScover Registry. Circulation 114:2154-62, 2006.

144. Anderson H, Shaw R, Brindis R, et al: A contemporary overview of percutaneous coronary interventions. The American College of Cardiology–National Cardiovascular Data Registry (ACC-NCDR). J Am Coll Cardiol 39(7):1096-103, 2002.

145. Biondi-Zoccai GG, Agostoni P, Sangiorgi GM, et al: Incidence, predictors, and outcomes of coronary dissections left untreated after drug-eluting stent implantation. Eur Heart J 27(5):540-6, 2006.

146. Javaid A, Buch AN, Satler LF, et al: Management and outcomes of coronary artery perforation during percutaneous coronary intervention. Am J Cardiol 98:911-4, 2006.

147. Ramana RK, Arab D, Joyal D, et al: Coronary artery perforation during percutaneous coronary intervention: Incidence and outcomes in the new interventional era. J Invasive Cardiol 17:603-5, 2005.

148. Harding SA: The role of vasodilators in the prevention and treatment of no-reflow following percutaneous coronary intervention. Heart 92:1191-3, 2006.

149. Cutlip D, Baim D, Ho K, et al: Stent thrombosis in the modern era: A pooled analysis of multicenter coronary stent clinical trials. Circulation 103(15):1967-71, 2001.

150. Wenaweser P, Dorffler-Melly J, Imboden K, et al: Stent thrombosis is associated with an impaired response to antiplatelet therapy. J Am Coll Cardiol 45:1748-52, 2005.

151. Park DW, Park SW, Park KH, et al: Frequency of and risk factors for stent thrombosis after drug-eluting stent implantation during long-term follow-up. Am J Cardiol 98:352-6, 2006.

152. Cutlip DE: Academic Research Consortium presented at Transcatheter Cardiovascular Therapeutics, Washington, DC, October 2006.

153. Bavry AA, Kumbhani DJ, Helton TJ, et al: Late thrombosis of drug-eluting stents: A meta-analysis of randomized clinical trials. Am J Med 119:1056-61, 2006.

154. Joner M, Finn AV, Farb A, et al: Pathology of drug-eluting stents in humans: Delayed healing and late thrombotic risk. J Am Coll Cardiol 48(1):193-202, 2006.

Percutaneous Valvular Intervention

155. Kherani AR, Cheema FH, Casher J, et al: Edge-to-edge mitral valve repair: The Columbia Presbyterian experience. Ann Thorac Surg 78(1):73-6, 2004.

156. Davidson MJ, White JK, Baim DS: Percutaneous therapies for valvular heart disease. Cardiovasc Pathol 15:123-9, 2006.

157. Feldman T, Wasserman HS, Herrmann HC, et al: Percutaneous mitral valve repair using the edge-to-edge technique: Six-month results of the EVEREST Phase I Clinical Trial. J Am Coll Cardiol 46(11):2134-40, 2005.

158. Webb JG, Harnek J, Munt BI, et al: Percutaneous transvenous mitral annuloplasty: Initial human experience with device implantation in the coronary sinus. Circulation 113(6):851-5, 2006.

159. Liddicoat JR, Mac Neill BD, Gillinov AM, et al: Percutaneous mitral valve repair: A feasibility study in an ovine model of acute ischemic mitral regurgitation. Catheter Cardiovasc Interv 60(3):410-6, 2003.

160. Kaye DM, Byrne M, Alferness C, Power J: Feasibility and short-term efficacy of percutaneous mitral annular reduction for the therapy of heart failure-induced mitral regurgitation. Circulation 108(15):1795-7, 2003.

161. Vassiliades TA, Jr., Block PC, Cohn LH, et al: The clinical development of percutaneous heart valve technology: A position statement of the Society of Thoracic Surgeons (STS), the American Association for Thoracic Surgery (AATS), and the Society of Cardiovascular Angiography and Intervention (SCAI). Catheter Cardiovasc Interv 65(1):73-9, 2005.

162. Vahanian A, Palacios IF: Percutaneous approaches to valvular disease. Circulation 109(13):1572-9, 2004.

163. Agarwal A, Kini AS, Attanti S, et al: Results of repeat balloon valvuloplasty for treatment of aortic stenosis in patients aged 59 to 104 years. Am J Cardiol 95(1):43-7, 2005.

164. Bonow RO, Carabello BA, Chatterjee K, et al: ACC/AHA 2006 guidelines for the management of patients with valvular heart disease: A report of the American College of Cardiology/American Heart Association Task Force on Practice Guidelines (writing Committee to Revise the 1998 guidelines for the management of patients with valvular heart disease) developed in collaboration with the Society of Cardiovascular Anesthesiologists endorsed by the Society for Cardiovascular Angiography and Interventions and the Society of Thoracic Surgeons. J Am Coll Cardiol 48(3):e1-148, 2006.

165. Cribier A, Eltchaninoff H, Tron C, et al: [Percutaneous artificial heart valves: From animal experimentation to the first human implantation in a case of calcified aortic stenosis]. Arch Mal Coeur Vaiss 96(6):645-52, 2003.

166. Cribier A, Eltchaninoff H, Tron C, et al: Treatment of calcific aortic stenosis with the percutaneous heart valve: Mid-term follow-up from the initial feasibility studies: The French experience. J Am Coll Cardiol 47(6):1214-23, 2006.

167. Webb JG, Chandavimol M, Thompson CR, et al: Percutaneous aortic valve implantation retrograde from the femoral artery. Circulation 113(6):842-50, 2006.

168. Grube E, Laborde JC, Zickmann B, et al: First report on a human percutaneous transluminal implantation of a self-expanding valve prosthesis for interventional treatment of aortic valve stenosis. Catheter Cardiovasc Interv 66(4):465-9, 2005.

Future Directions

169. Ong AT, Serruys PW, Mohr FW, et al: The SYNergy between percutaneous coronary intervention with TAXus and cardiac surgery (SYNTAX) study: Design, rationale, and run-in phase. Am Heart J 151:1194-204, 2006.

170. Ormiston JA, Webster MW, Armstrong G: First-in-human implantation of a fully bioabsorbable drug-eluting stent: The BVS poly-L-lactic acid everolimus-eluting coronary stent [epub ahead of print]. Catheter Cardiovasc Interv 69:128-131, 2007.

171. Shaw R, Anderson H, Brindis R, et al: Development of a risk adjustment mortality model using the American College of Cardiology–National Cardiovascular Data Registry (ACC-NCDR) experience: 1998-2000. J Am Coll Cardiol 39(7):1104-12, 2002.

GUIDELINES *Thomas H. Lee*

Percutaneous Coronary and Valvular Intervention

The American College of Cardiology/American Heart Association (ACC/AHA) updated its guidelines for percutaneous coronary interventions (PCIs) in 2006.[1] Since the previous guidelines were published in 2001,[2] the introduction of coronary stents and other devices has broadened the scope of patients who can be approached by PCI, and coronary stenting has become the dominant final therapy in patients undergoing PCI.

The updated guidelines cover the use of PCI in various settings. This appendix focuses on recommendations relevant to the use of PCI for stable ischemic heart disease and for unstable angina with ST-elevation myocardial infarction (UA/NSTEMI). Recommendations for

PCI in the setting of acute ST-elevation myocardial infarction (STEMI) are summarized in the appendix to Chapter 52. Guidelines for percutaneous valvular interventions, published by the ACC/AHA in 2006,[3] are summarized in the appendix to Chapter 62.

As with other ACC/AHA guidelines, these use the standard ACC/AHA classification system for indications:

Class I: Conditions for which there is evidence and/or general agreement that the test is useful and effective

Class II: Conditions for which there is conflicting evidence and/or a divergence of opinion about the usefulness or efficacy of performing the test

Class IIa: Weight of evidence or opinion is in favor of usefulness or efficacy

Class IIb: Usefulness or efficacy is less well established by evidence/opinion

Class III: Conditions for which there is evidence and/or general agreement that the test is not useful or effective and in some cases may be harmful

Three levels are used to rate the evidence on which recommendations have been based. Level A recommendations are derived from data from multiple randomized clinical trials, level B recommendations are derived from a single randomized trial or nonrandomized studies, and level C recommendations are based on the consensus opinion of experts.

INDICATIONS

Earlier PCI guidelines[2] made recommendations based on the number of diseased vessels. The current guidelines assume that the operator can perform single-vessel or multivessel PCI with a high likelihood of initial success and low risk. Thus, they are based on the patient's clinical condition, specific coronary lesion morphology and anatomy, left ventricular function, and associated medical conditions.

Medical therapy and aggressive risk factor reduction is the starting point for most patients without symptoms or mild angina. However, for patients with mild or moderate ischemia and few symptoms, revascularization with PCI or coronary artery bypass grafting (CABG) is considered reasonable across a range of indications (Table 55G-1). PCI is considered inappropriate when the amount of viable myocardium at risk is small, when symptoms are unlikely to be caused by ischemia, or when there is a high risk of complications.

For patients with more severe angina, the threshold for performing PCI is lower (Table 55G-2). PCI is considered appropriate for patients with single-vessel or multivessel disease if a moderate or large area of viable myocardium is at risk, the procedure has a high likelihood of success, and the risk of complications is low. PCI is considered inap-

propriate in the absence of these indications or for patients with significant left main disease who are candidates for CABG.

For patients who have undergone CABG, the guidelines support an aggressive approach to detecting and addressing ischemia detected less than 30 days after surgery (Table 55G-3). Usually, such early ischemia represents graft failure, often related to thrombosis, which can be corrected with PCI. If feasible, PCI of offending stenoses in both bypass grafts and native vessels should be attempted, particularly if intracoronary stents can be deployed successfully. When ischemia occurs 1 to 12 months after surgery, the cause is usually perianastomotic graft stenosis, which also responds well to PCI. Ischemia occurring more than 1 year postoperatively usually reflects the development of new stenoses in graft conduits and/or native vessels that may be amenable to PCI. The guidelines note that PCI for chronic vein occlusions is characterized by lower success and higher complication rates, and thresholds for PCI are therefore higher when patients have ischemia more than 1 year after CABG.

The guidelines acknowledge substantial variability in outcomes of PCI in different populations, with particular attention to poorer outcomes in elderly patients and those with diabetes mellitus. The committee concluded that much of the increase in adverse outcomes in these patient groups, as well as in women, is because of comorbidities; thus, with rare exception, separate recommendations for subgroups defined by gender and age were not developed.

UNSTABLE ANGINA AND NON-ST ELEVATION MYOCARDIAL INFARCTION

Two different treatment strategies, early conservative and early invasive, have evolved for patients with UA/NSTEMI (see Fig. 53G-1). In the early conservative strategy, coronary angiography is reserved for patients with evidence of recurrent ischemia (angina at rest or with minimal activity or dynamic ST segment changes) or a strongly positive

TABLE 55G-1	ACC/AHA Recommendations for Percutaneous Coronary Interventions in Patients with Asymptomatic Ischemia or CCS Class I or II Angina	
Class	**Indication**	**Level of Evidence**
Class IIa (good supportive evidence)	PCI is reasonable in patients with asymptomatic ischemia or CCS Class I or II angina who have one or more significant lesions in one or two coronary arteries suitable for PCI with a high likelihood of success and a low risk of morbidity. The vessels to be dilated must subtend a moderate to large area of viable myocardium or be associated with a moderate to severe degree of ischemia on noninvasive testing.	B
	PCI is reasonable for patients with asymptomatic ischemia or CCS Class I or II angina and recurrent stenosis after PCI with a large area or viable myocardium or high-risk criteria on noninvasive testing.	C
	Use of PCI is reasonable in patients with asymptomatic ischemia or CCS Class I or II angina with significant left main CAD (greater than 50% diameter stenosis) who are candidates for revascularization but are not eligible for CABG.	B
Class IIb (weak supportive evidence)	The effectiveness of PCI is not well established for patients with asymptomatic ischemia or CCS Class I or II angina who have two- or three-vessel disease with significant proximal left anterior descending CAD who are otherwise eligible for CABG with one arterial conduit and who have treated diabetes or abnormal left ventricular function.	B
	PCI might be considered for patients with asymptomatic ischemia or CCS Class I or II angina with nonproximal left anterior descending CAD that subtends a moderate area of viable myocardium and demonstrates ischemia on noninvasive testing.	C
Class III (not indicated)	PCI is not recommended in patients with asymptomatic ischemia or CCS Class I or II angina who do not meet the criteria as listed under the Class II recommendations or who have one or more of the following: Only a small area of viable myocardium risk No objective evidence of ischemia Lesions that have a low likelihood of successful dilation Mild symptoms that are unlikely to be caused by myocardial ischemia Factors associated with increased risk of morbidity or mortality Left main disease and eligibility of CABG Insignificant disease (less than 50% coronary stenosis)	C

ACC/AHA = American College of Cardiology/American Heart Association; CABG = coronary artery bypass grafting; CAD = coronary artery disease; CCS = Canadian Cardiovascular Society; PCI = percutaneous coronary intervention.

TABLE 55G–2	ACC/AHA Recommendations for Percutaneous Coronary Interventions in Patients with CCS Class III Angina	
Class	Indication	Level of Evidence
Class IIa (good supportive evidence)	It is reasonable that PCI be performed in patients with CCS Class III angina and single-vessel or multivessel CAS who are undergoing medical therapy and who have one or more significant lesions in one or more coronary arteries suitable for PCI with a high likelihood of success and low risk of morbidity or mortality.	B
	It is reasonable that PCI be performed in patients with CCS Class III angina with single-vessel or multivessel CAD who are not undergoing medical therapy with focal saphenous vein graft lesions or multiple stenoses who are poor candidates for reoperative surgery.	C
	Use of PCI is reasonable in patients with CCS Class III angina with significant left main CAD (greater than 50% diameter stenosis) who are candidates for revascularization but are not eligible for CABG.	B
Class IIb (weak supportive evidence)	PCI may be considered in patients with CCS Class III angina with single-vessel or multivessel CAD who are undergoing medical therapy and who have one or more lesions to be dilated with a reduced likelihood of success.	B
	PCI may be considered in patients with CCS Class III angina and no evidence of ischemia on noninvasive testing or who are undergoing medical therapy and two- or three-vessel CAD with significant proximal left anterior descending CAD and treated diabetes or abnormal left ventricular function.	B
Class III (not indicated)	PCI is not recommended for patients with CCS Class III angina with single-vessel or multivessel CAD, no evidence of myocardial injury or ischemia on objective testing, and no trial of medical therapy, or who have one of the following: Only a small area of myocardium at risk. All lesions or culprit lesion to be dilated with morphology that conveys a low likelihood of success A high risk of procedure-related morbidity or mortality Insignificant disease (less than 50% coronary stenosis) Significant left main CAD and candidacy for CABG	C

ACC/AHA = American College of Cardiology/American Heart Association; CABG = coronary artery bypass grafting; CAD = coronary artery disease; CCS = Canadian Cardiovascular Society; PCI = percutaneous coronary intervention.

TABLE 55G–3	ACC/AHA Recommendations for Percutaneous Coronary Interventions in Patients with Prior Coronary Artery Bypass Surgery	
Class	Indication	Level of Evidence
Class I (indicated)	When technically feasible, PCI should be performed in patients with early ischemia (usually within 30 days) after CABG.	B
	It is recommended that distal embolic protection devices be used when technically feasible in patients undergoing PCI to saphenous vein grafts.	B
Class IIa (good supportive evidence)	PCI is reasonable in patients with ischemia that occurs 1 to 3 years after CABG and who have preserved left ventricular function with discrete lesions in graft conduits.	B
	PCI is reasonable in patients with disabling angina secondary to new disease in a native coronary circulation after CABG. (If angina is not typical, objective evidence of ischemia should be obtained.)	B
Class IIb (weak supportive evidence)	PCI is reasonable in patients with diseased vein grafts more than 3 years after CABG.	B
	PCI is reasonable when technically feasible in patients with a patent left internal mammary artery graft and clinically significant obstructions in other vessels.	C
Class III (not indicated)	PCI is not recommended in patients with prior CABG for chronic total vein graft occlusions.	B
	PCI is not recommended in patients who have multiple target lesions with prior CABG and multivessel disease, failure of multiple saphenous vein grafts, and impaired left ventricular function unless repeat CABG poses excessive risk because of severe comorbid conditions.	B

ACC/AHA = American College of Cardiology/American Heart Association; CABG = coronary artery bypass grafting; CAD = coronary artery disease; PCI = percutaneous coronary intervention.

stress test despite vigorous medical therapy. In the early invasive strategy, patients without clinically obvious contraindications to coronary revascularization are routinely recommended for coronary angiography and angiographically directed revascularization, if possible. Following the ACC/AHA guidelines for UA/NSTEMI published in 2002,[4] the 2006 PCI guidelines recommend an early invasive strategy for select high-risk patients without serious comorbidities. These include patients with recurrent ischemia despite intensive antiischemic therapy, elevated troponin levels, new ST segment depression, heart failure symptoms or new or worsening mitral regurgitation, depressed left ventricular systolic function, hemodynamic instability, sustained ventricular tachycardia, PCI within the previous 6 months, or prior CABG (Table 55G-4). For UA/NSTEMI patients without these high-risk features, PCI is not recommended for those with single- or multivessel CAD and no trial of medical therapy, or one or more of the following:

a small area of myocardium at risk; lesions with morphology indicating a low likelihood of success; high risk of procedure-related morbidity or mortality, insignificant disease (less than 50 percent coronary stenosis), or significant left main coronary artery disease (CAD) and candidacy for CABG.

ADJUNCTIVE TECHNOLOGIES

Intravascular ultrasonography can be used to assess the need for PCI or facilitate deployment of coronary stents, but the guidelines do not consider it necessary for all stent procedures (Table 55G-5). The guidelines recommend that intravascular ultrasonography be considered (Class IIa) to assess the adequacy of stent deployment, determine the mechanism of stent restenosis and select appropriate therapy, evalu-

TABLE 55G–4	ACC/AHA Recommendations for Percutaneous Coronary Interventions in Patients with Unstable Angina or Non-ST Elevation Myocardial Infarction	
Class	**Indication**	**Level of Evidence**
Class I (indicated)	An early invasive PCI strategy is indicated for patients with UA/NSTEMI who have no serious comorbidity and coronary lesions amenable to PCI. Patients must have any of the following high-risk features: Recurrent ischemia despite intensive antiischemic therapy Elevated troponin level New ST segment depression Heart failure symptoms or new or worsening mitral regurgitation Depressed left ventricular systolic function Hemodynamic instability Sustained ventricular tachycardia PCI within 6 mo Prior CABG	A
Class IIa (good supportive evidence)	It is reasonable to perform PCI in patients with UA/NSTEMI and single-vessel or multivessel CAD who are undergoing medical therapy with focal saphenous vein graft lesions or multiple stenoses who are poor candidates for reoperative surgery.	C
	In the absence of high-risk features associated with UA/NSTEMI, it is reasonable to perform PCI in patients with amenable lesions and no contraindication for PCI with either an early invasive or early conservative strategy.	B
	Use of PCI is reasonable in patients with UA/NSTEMI with significant left main CAD (greater than 50% diameter stenosis) who are candidates for revascularization but are not eligible for CABG.	B
Class IIb (weak supportive evidence)	In the absence of high-risk features associated with UA/NSTEMI, PCI may be considered in patients with single-vessel or multivessel CAD who are undergoing medical therapy and who have one or more lesions to be dilated with reduced likelihood of success.	B
	PCI may be considered in patients with UA/NSTEMI who are undergoing medical therapy who have two- or three-vessel disease, significant proximal left anterior descending CAD, and treated diabetes or abnormal left ventricular function.	B
Class III (not indicated)	In the absence of high-risk features associated with UA/NSTEMI, PCI is not recommended for patients with UA/NSTEMI who have single-vessel or multivessel CAD and no trial of medical therapy, or who have one or more of the following: Only a small area of myocardium at risk All lesions or culprit lesion to be dilated with morphology that conveys low likelihood of success A high risk of procedure-related morbidity or mortality Insignificant disease (less than 50% coronary stenosis) Significant left main CAD and candidacy for CABG	C

ACC/AHA = American College of Cardiology/American Heart Association; CABG = coronary artery bypass grafting; CAD = coronary artery disease; PCI = percutaneous coronary intervention; UA/NSTEMI = unstable angina/non-ST elevation myocardial infarction.

CH 55

ate coronary obstruction at a location difficult to image by angiography, assess suboptimal angiographic results after PCI, and guide the use of directional coronary atherectomy.

The guidelines present a relatively narrow role for Doppler ultrasound and fractional flow reserve for the assessment of the physiological effects of intermediate coronary stenosis (30 to 70 percent luminal narrowing) in patients with angina symptoms, but they are dubious about its value for assessing the severity of angiographic disease in patients with a positive, unequivocal, noninvasive functional study.

MANAGEMENT ISSUES

Recommendations for the use of medications in patients undergoing PCI electively and with acute myocardial infarction are summarized in Table 55G-6. Antiplatelet therapy with aspirin and clopidogrel are considered Class I indications for all patients, whereas warfarin is inappropriate except in patients with other indications for this medication. Glycoprotein IIb/IIIa inhibitors are considered clearly appropriate for patients with UA/NSTEMI undergoing PCI without clopidogrel administration, but less clearly so (Class II) for UA/NSTEMI patients undergoing PCI with clopidogrel administration, or for STEMI or elective PCI patients. Unfractionated heparin is considered appropriate during PCI; bivalirudin or argatroban may be used for patients with heparin-induced thrombocytopenia. The role of low-molecular-weight heparin has not yet been resolved.

In addition to medications, aggressive risk factor reduction is an essential component of secondary prevention. As outlined in the latest AHA/ACC guidelines for secondary prevention for patients with coronary and other atherosclerotic vascular disease,[5] this includes aggressive control of serum lipid levels, in some cases to a low-density lipoprotein level (LDL) of 70 mg/dl or below, control of blood pressure, diabetes management, abstinence from tobacco, weight control, regular exercise, and yearly vaccination against influenza. Participation in a cardiac rehabilitation program is also strongly encouraged.

During long-term follow-up of patients after PCI, the guidelines do not endorse routine exercise testing of asymptomatic patients. The ACC/AHA practice guidelines for exercise testing[6] favor selective evaluation in patients considered to be at particularly high risk, such as those with decreased left ventricular function, multivessel CAD, proximal left anterior descending disease, previous sudden death, diabetes mellitus, left main disease, hazardous occupations, and suboptimal PCI results. If patients are symptomatic, the guidelines recommend that they undergo stress imaging studies to localize disease.

RESTENOSIS

Restenosis reflects a complex pathophysiology that involves postangioplasty recoil, neointimal proliferation, and residual coronary stenosis. Although widespread use of stents has minimized the incidence of recoil, restenosis caused by neointimal proliferation and residual coro-

TABLE 55G–5 ACC/AHA Recommendations for Use of Adjunctive Technology* with Percutaneous Coronary Interventions

Class	Indication	Level of Evidence
Intravascular Ultrasound Imaging		
Class IIa (good supportive evidence)	IVUS is reasonable for the following:	
	Assessment of the adequacy of deployment of coronary stents, including extent of stent apposition and determination of minimum luminal diameter with the stent	B
	Determination of the mechanism of stent restenosis (inadequate expansion versus neointimal proliferation) and to enable selection of appropriate therapy (vascular brachytherapy versus repeat balloon expansion)	B
	Evaluation of coronary obstruction at a location difficult to image by angiography in a patient with a suspected flow-limiting stenosis	C
	Assessment of a suboptimal angiographic result after PCI	C
	Establishment of the presence and distribution of coronary calcium in patients for whom adjunctive rotational atherectomy is contemplated	C
	Determination of plaque location and circumferential distribution for guidance of directional coronary atherectomy	B
Class IIb (weak supportive evidence)	IVUS may be considered for the following:	C
	Determination of the extent of atherosclerosis in patients with characteristic anginal symptoms and positive functional study with no focal stenoses or mild CAD on angiography	
	Preinterventional assessment of lesional characteristics and vessel dimensions as a means to select an optimal revascularization device	
	Diagnosis of coronary disease after cardiac transplantation	
Class III (not indicated)	IVUS not recommended when the angiographic diagnosis is clear and no interventional treatment is planned	C
Fractional Flow Reserve and Coronary Vasodilatory Reserve		
Class IIa (good supportive evidence)	Reasonable to use intracoronary physiological measurements (Doppler ultrasound, fractional flow reserve) to assess effects of intermediate coronary stenoses (30% to 70% luminal narrowing) in patients with anginal symptoms; coronary pressure or Doppler velocimetry may be useful alternatives to performing noninvasive functional testing to determine whether intervention is warranted	B
Class IIb (weak supportive evidence)	Intracoronary physiological measurements may be considered for evaluation of success of PCI in restoring flow reserve and to predict risk of restenosis	C
	Intracoronary physiological measurements may be considered for evaluation of patients with anginal symptoms without an apparent angiographic culprit lesion	C
Class III (not indicated)	Routine assessment with intracoronary physiological measurements (e.g., Doppler ultrasound or fractional flow reserve) to assess severity of angiographic disease in patients with a positive, unequivocal noninvasive functional study not recommended	C

*Intracoronary ultrasound imaging, flow velocity, and pressure.
ACC/AHA = American College of Cardiology/American Heart Association; CAD = coronary artery disease; IVUS = intravascular ultrasound; PCI = percutaneous coronary intervention.

nary stenosis remains a major limitation of PCI. In subsets of patients in whom trial data suggest efficacy, a drug-eluting stent should be considered as an alternative to a bare metal stent to prevent restenosis.

According to the guidelines, among patients who develop restenosis following percutaneous transluminal coronary angioplasty (PTCA) or PTCA with an atheroablative device, repeat coronary intervention with a coronary stent is reasonable if anatomical features are appropriate (Table 55G-7).

The substantial increase in coronary stenting has led to a proportional increase in in-stent restenosis. The guidelines suggest that reasonable approaches to the treatment of in-stent restenosis include repeat PCI with a drug-eluting stent and brachytherapy. However, results of a large randomized trial that appeared after the guidelines had been published indicate that sirolimus-eluting stents result in superior clinical and angiographic outcomes compared with vascular brachytherapy for the treatment of restenosis with a bare metal stent.[7]

INSTITUTIONAL AND OPERATOR COMPETENCE

The updated guidelines give considerable attention to institutional and physician-specific factors associated with better outcomes and

lower complication rates. Citing an ACC Training Statement,[8] the guidelines recommend that physicians undergo a 3-year comprehensive cardiac training program with 12 months of training in diagnostic catheterization during which the trainee performs 300 diagnostic catheterizations, including 200 as the primary operator. Interventional training requires a fourth year of training, including more than 250 interventional procedures but not more than 600, a level that is also required for physicians to be eligible for the American Board of Internal Medicine certifying examination in interventional cardiology.[9]

The guidelines favor performance of PCI by higher volume operators, defined as those performing more than 75 procedures per year at high-volume centers, defined as those in which more than 400 procedures are performed each year (Table 55G-8). Despite technical improvements that have decreased the intensity of surgical backup coverage for PCI at many institutions, the guidelines continue to recommend that elective PCI should not be performed in facilities without on-site cardiac surgery, except in underserved areas that are geographically far removed from major centers.

Institutions must have a system for quality measurement and improvement that includes valid peer review. The guidelines recommend that quality assessment reviews take into consideration risk adjustment, statistical power, and national benchmark statistics. They should also include tabulation of adverse event rates for comparison with benchmark values and case review of complicated procedures and some uncomplicated procedures.

CH 55

Percutaneous Coronary and Valvular Intervention

TABLE 55G-6	ACC/AHA Recommendations for Pharmacological Management of Patients Undergoing Percutaneous Coronary Interventions	
Class	**Indication**	**Level of Evidence**

Oral Antiplatelet Therapy

Class	Indication	Level of Evidence
Class I (indicated)	Patients already taking daily chronic aspirin therapy should take 75 to 325 mg of aspirin before the PCI procedure is performed.	A
	Patients not already taking daily chronic aspirin therapy should be given 300 to 325 mg of aspirin at least 2 hr and preferably 24 hr before the PCI procedure is performed.	C
	After the PCI procedure, in patients with neither aspirin resistance, allergy, nor increased risk of bleeding, aspirin 325 mg daily should be given for at least 1 mo after bare-metal stent implantation, 3 mo after sirolimus-eluting stent implantation, and 6 mo after paclitaxel-eluting stent implantation, after which daily chronic aspirin use should be continued indefinitely at a dose of 75 to 162 mg.	B
	A loading dose of clopidogrel should be administered before PCI is performed.	A
	An oral loading dose of 300 mg, administered at least 6 hr before the procedure, has the best established evidence of efficacy.	B
	In patients who have undergone PCI, clopidogrel 75 mg daily should be given for at least 1 mo after bare-metal stent implantation (unless the patient is at increased risk of bleeding; then it should be given for a minimum of 2 wk), 3 mo after sirolimus stent implantation, and 6 mo after paclitaxel stent implantation, and ideally up to 12 mo in patients who are not at high risk of bleeding.	B
Class IIa (good supportive evidence)	If clopidogrel is given at the time of procedure, supplementation with GP IIb/IIIa receptor antagonists can be beneficial to facilitate earlier platelet inhibition than with clopidogrel alone.	B
	For patients with an absolute contraindication to aspirin, it is reasonable to give a 300 mg loading dose of clopidogrel, administered at least 6 hr before PCI, and/or GP IIb/IIIa antagonists, administered at the time of PCI.	C
	When a loading dose of clopidogrel is administered, a regimen of more than 300 mg is reasonable to achieve higher levels of antiplatelet activity more rapidly, but the efficacy and safety compared with a 300-mg loading dose are less established.	C
	It is reasonable that patients undergoing brachytherapy be given daily clopidogrel 75 mg indefinitely and daily aspirin 75 to 325 mg indefinitely unless there is significant risk for bleeding.	C
Class IIb (weak supportive evidence)	In patients in whom subacute thrombosis may be catastrophic or lethal (unprotected left main, bifurcating left main, or last patent coronary vessel), platelet aggregation studies may be considered and the dose of clopidogrel increased to 150 mg/d if less than 50% inhibition of platelet aggregation is demonstrated.	C

Glycoprotein IIb/IIIa Inhibitors

Class	Indication	Level of Evidence
Class I (indicated)	In patients with UA/NSTEMI undergoing PCI without clopidogrel administration, a GP IIb/IIIa inhibitor (abciximab, eptifibatide, or tirofiban) should be administered.	A
Class IIa (good supportive evidence)	In patients with UA/NSTEMI undergoing PCI with clopidogrel administration, it is reasonable to administer a GP IIb/IIIa inhibitor (abciximab, eptifibatide, or tirofiban).	B
	In patients with STEMI undergoing PCI, it is reasonable to administer abciximab as early as possible.	B
	In patients undergoing elective PCI with stent placement, it is reasonable to administer a GP IIb/IIIa inhibitor (abciximab, eptifibatide, or tirofiban).	B
Class IIb (weak supportive evidence)	In patients with STEMI undergoing PCI, treatment with eptifibatide, or tirofiban may be considered.	C

Antithrombotic Therapy

Class	Indication	Level of Evidence
Class I (indicated)	Unfractionated heparin should be administered to patients undergoing PCI.	C
	For patients with heparin-induced thrombocytopenia, it is recommended that bivalirudin or argatroban be used to replace heparin.	B
Class IIa (good supportive evidence)	It is reasonable to use bivalirudin as an alternative to unfractionated heparin and GP IIb/IIIa antagonists in low-risk patients undergoing elective PCI.	B
	Low-molecular-weight heparin is a reasonable alternative to unfractionated heparin in patients with UA/NSTEMI undergoing PCI.	B
Class IIb (weak supportive evidence)	Low-molecular-weight heparin may be considered as an alternative to unfractionated heparin in patients with STEMI undergoing PCI.	B

ACC/AHA = American College of Cardiology/American Heart Association; CAD = coronary artery disease; GP = glycoprotein; PCI = percutaneous coronary intervention; STEMI = ST-elevation myocardial infarction; UA/NSTEMI = unstable angina/non-ST elevation myocardial infarction.

CH 55

TABLE 55G–7	ACC/AHA Recommendations for the Prevention and Management of Restenosis Following Percutaneous Coronary Intervention	
Class	Indication	Level of Evidence
Prevention Class I (indicated)	A drug-eluting stent (DES) should be considered as an alternative to a bare metal stent in subsets of patients in whom trial data suggests efficacy.	A
Class IIb (weak supportive evidence)	A DES may be considered for use in anatomical settings in which the usefulness, effectiveness, and safety have not been fully documented in published trials.	C
Management Class IIa (good supportive evidence)	Patients who develop restenosis after PTCA or PTCA with atheroablative devices are reasonable candidates for repeat coronary intervention with intracoronary stents if anatomical factors are appropriate.	B
Class IIa (good supportive evidence)	It is reasonable to perform repeat PCI for in-stent restenosis with a DES or new DES for patients who develop in-stent restenosis if anatomical factors are appropriate.	B
Class IIa (good supportive evidence)	Brachytherapy can be useful as a safe and effective treatment for in-stent restenosis.	A

ACC/AHA = American College of Cardiology/American Heart Association; PCI = percutaneous coronary intervention; PTCA = percutaneous transluminal coronary angioplasty.

Percutaneous Coronary and Valvular Intervention

TABLE 55G–8	ACC/AHA Recommendations for Percutaneous Coronary Intervention Institutional and Operator Volumes at Centers with On-Site Cardiac Surgery	
Class	Indication	Level of Evidence
Quality Assurance Class I (indicated)	Institutions performing PCI should establish an ongoing mechanism for valid peer review of its quality and outcomes at the level of the individual practitioner and the entire program. Quality assessment reviews should take risk adjustment, statistical power, and national benchmark statistics into consideration, and include both tabulation of adverse event rates for comparison with benchmark values and case review of complicated and some uncomplicated procedures.	C
	Institutions that perform PCI should participate in a recognized PCI data registry to benchmark its outcomes against current national norms.	C
Operator and Institutional Volumes Class I (indicated)	Elective PCI should be performed by operators with acceptable annual volume (at least 75 procedures/yr) at high-volume centers (more than 400 procedures/yr) with on-site cardiac surgery	B
	Elective PCI should be performed by operators and institutions whose historical and current risk-adjusted outcomes statistics are comparable to those reported in contemporary national data registries.	C
Class IIa (good supportive evidence)	It is reasonable for operators with acceptable volume (at least 75 PCI procedures/yr) to perform PCI at low-volume centers (200 to 400 procedures/yr) with on-site cardiac surgery.	B
	It is reasonable for low-volume operators (fewer than 75 PCI procedures/yr) to perform PCI at high-volume centers (more than 400 procedures/yr) with on-site cardiac surgery. Ideally, operators with an annual procedure volume less than 75/yr should only work at institutions with an activity level of more than 600 procedures/yr and develop a defined mentoring relationship with a highly experienced operator (annual procedural volume of 150 procedures/yr or more).	B
Class III (not indicated)	It is not recommended that elective PCI be performed by low-volume operators (fewer that 75 procedures/yr) at low-volume centers (200 to 400 procedures/yr) with or without on-site cardiac surgery. An institution with a volume of fewer than 200 procedures/yr, unless in a region that is underserved because of geography, should carefully consider whether it should continue to offer this service.	B
Role of On-Site Cardiac Surgical Backup Class I (indicated)	Elective PCI should be performed by operators with acceptable annual volume (at least 75 procedures/yr) at high-volume centers (more than 400 procedures/yr) that provide immediately available on-site emergency cardiac surgical services.	B
Class III (not indicated)	Elective PCI should not be performed at institutions that do not provide on-site cardiac surgery.	C

ACC/AHA = American College of Cardiology/American Heart Association; PCI = percutaneous coronary intervention.

1456 References

1. Smith SC Jr, Feldman TE, Hirshfeld JW, et al: ACC/AHA/SCAI 2005 guideline update for percutaneous coronary intervention—summary article: A report of the American College of Cardiology/American Heart Association Task Force on Practice Guidelines. Circulation 113:156, 2006.

2. Smith SC, Jr., Dove JT, Jacobs AK, et al: ACC/AHA guidelines of percutaneous coronary interventions (revision of the 1993 PTCA guidelines)—executive summary. A report of the American College of Cardiology/American Heart Association Task Force on Practice Guidelines (committee to revise the 1993 guidelines for percutaneous transluminal coronary angioplasty). J Am Coll Cardiol 37:2215, 2001.

3. Bonow RO, Carabello BA, Kanu C, et al: ACC/AHA 2006 guidelines for the management of patients with valvular heart disease: A report of the American College of Cardiology/American Heart Association Task Force on Practice Guidelines (writing committee to revise the 1998 Guidelines for the Management of Patients With Valvular Heart Disease): Developed in collaboration with the Society of Cardiovascular Anesthesiologists: Endorsed by the Society for Cardiovascular Angiography and Interventions and the Society of Thoracic Surgeons. Circulation 114:e84, 2006.

4. Braunwald E, Antman EM, Beasley JW, et al: ACC/AHA 2002 guideline update for the management of patients with unstable angina and non-ST-segment elevation myocardial infarction—summary article: A report of the American College of Cardiology/ American Heart Association task force on practice guidelines (Committee on the Management of Patients With Unstable Angina). J Am Coll Cardiol 40:1366, 2002.

5. Smith SC Jr, Allen J, Blair SN, et al: AHA/ACC guidelines for secondary prevention for patients with coronary and other atherosclerotic vascular disease: 2006 update: Endorsed by the National Heart, Lung, and Blood Institute. Circulation 113:2363, 2006.

6. Gibbons RJ, Balady GJ, Bricker JT, et al: ACC/AHA 2002 guideline update for exercise testing: Summary article: A report of the American College of Cardiology/American Heart Association Task Force on Practice Guidelines (Committee to Update the 1997 Exercise Testing Guidelines). Circulation 106:1883, 2002.

7. Holmes DR Jr, Teirstein P, Satler L, et al: Sirolimus-eluting stents vs vascular brachytherapy for in-stent restenosis within bare-metal stents: The SISR randomized trial. JAMA 295:1264, 2006.

8. Hirshfeld JW Jr, Banas JS Jr, Brundage BH, et al: American College of Cardiology training statement on recommendations for the structure of an optimal adult interventional cardiology training program: A report of the American College of Cardiology task force on clinical expert consensus documents. J Am Coll Cardiol 34:2141, 1999.

9. American Board of Internal Medicine: Subspecialty Policies for Interventional Cardiology. American Board of Internal Medicine 2005 (http://www.abim.org/cert/policies_aqic.shtm).

CH 55

CHAPTER 56

The Normal Aorta, 1457

Examination of the Aorta, 1458

Aortic Aneurysms, 1458
Abdominal Aortic Aneurysms, 1458
    Management, 1461
Thoracic Aortic Aneurysms, 1464
    Management, 1467

Aortic Dissection, 1469
Diagnostic Techniques, 1474
Management, 1479
    Immediate Medical
        Management, 1479
    Definitive Therapy, 1480
    Long-Term Therapy and Late
        Follow-Up, 1482
Atypical Aortic Dissection, 1483
Aortic Trauma, 1486
Aortic Atheroembolic Disease, 1486

Acute Aortic Occlusion, 1486

Aortoarteritis Syndromes, 1486
Bacterial Infections of the
    Aorta, 1486

Primary Tumors of the
Aorta, 1487

References, 1487

Diseases of the Aorta

Eric M. Isselbacher

THE NORMAL AORTA

FUNCTION

The aorta is the largest and strongest artery in the body, carrying roughly 200 million liters of blood through the body in an average lifetime. Three layers compose the aorta: the thin inner layer, or *intima;* a thick middle layer, or *media;* and a somewhat thin outer layer, the *adventitia* (see Chap. 38). The strength of the aorta lies in the media, which is composed of laminated but intertwining sheets of elastic tissue arranged in a spiral manner that affords maximal tensile strength. Indeed, as thin as it is, experimentally the aortic wall can withstand the pressure of thousands of millimeters of mercury without bursting. In contrast to smaller muscular arteries, the aortic media contains multiple layers of elastic laminae (see Chap. 38). It is this tremendous accretion of elastic tissue that gives the aorta not only tensile strength but also distensibility and elasticity, which serve a vital circulatory role. The endothelium-lined aortic intima is a thin, delicate layer and is easily traumatized. The adventitia contains mainly collagen and carries the important vasa vasorum, which nourishes the outer half of the aortic wall, including much of the media.

Ventricular systole distends the aorta by the force of the blood ejected from the left ventricle. In this manner, part of the kinetic energy generated by the contracting left ventricle is converted into potential energy stored in the aortic wall. Then, during diastole, this potential energy is transformed back into kinetic energy as the aortic walls recoil and propel the blood in the aortic lumen distally into the arterial bed. Thus, the aorta plays an essential role in maintaining forward circulation of the blood in diastole after it is delivered into the aorta by the left ventricle during systole. The pulse wave itself, with its milking effect, is transmitted along the aorta to the periphery at a speed of about 5 msec. This speed is much faster than the velocity of the intraluminal blood itself, which travels at only 40 to 50 cm/sec.

The systolic pressure developing within the aorta is a function of the volume of blood ejected into the aorta, the compliance or distensibility of the aorta, and resistance to blood flow. This resistance depends primarily on the tone of the peripheral muscular arteries and arterioles and, to a slight extent, on the inertia of the column of blood in the aorta when systole commences.

In addition to its conductance and pumping functions, the aorta also plays a role in indirectly controlling systemic vascular resistance and heart rate. Pressure-responsive receptors, analogous to those in the carotid sinus, lie in the ascending aorta and aortic arch and send afferent signals to the vasomotor center in the brain stem by way of the vagus nerves. An increase in intraaortic pressure causes reflex bradycardia and a reduction in systemic vascular resistance, whereas a decrease in intraaortic pressure increases the heart rate and vascular resistance.

ANATOMICAL CONSIDERATIONS

The aorta is divided anatomically into thoracic and abdominal components. The thoracic aorta is further divided into the *ascending, arch,* and *descending* segments, and the abdominal aorta consists of *suprarenal* and *infrarenal* segments.

The ascending aorta is approximately 5 cm long and has two distinct segments. The lower segment is the *aortic root,* which begins at the level of the aortic valve and extends to the sinotubular junction. This portion of the ascending aorta is the widest and measures about 3.5 cm. The bases of the aortic leaflets are supported by the aortic root, from which the three sinuses of Valsalva bulge outward to allow for full excursion of the aortic valve leaflets during systole. In addition, the two coronary artery trunks arise from these sinuses of Valsalva. The upper tubular segment of the ascending aorta begins at the sinotubular junction and rises to join the aortic arch. Normally, the ascending aorta sits just to the right of midline, with its proximal portion lying within the pericardial cavity. The arch of the aorta gives rise to all the brachiocephalic arteries. From the ascending aorta, the arch courses slightly leftward in front of the trachea and then proceeds posteriorly to the left of the trachea and esophagus. The pulmonary artery bifurcation and right pulmonary artery lie inferior to the arch, as does the left lung.

The descending thoracic aorta begins in the posterior mediastinum to the left of the vertebral column and gradually courses in front of the vertebral column as it descends, where it lies immediately behind the esophagus. Distally, it passes through the diaphragm, usually at the level of the 12th thoracic vertebra.

The point at which the aortic arch joins the descending aorta is called the *aortic isthmus.* The aorta is especially vulnerable to trauma at this site because it is here that the relatively mobile portion of the aorta—the ascending aorta and arch—becomes relatively fixed to the thoracic cage by the pleural reflections, the paired intercostal arteries, and the left subclavian artery. Coarctations of the aorta also localize to this region. The abdominal aorta continues from the thoracic aorta, gives rise to the mesenteric and renal arteries, and ends at its bifurcation into common iliac arteries at the level of the fourth lumbar vertebra.

Aging of the Aorta

As discussed, the elastic properties of the aorta contribute crucially to its normal function. However, the elasticity and distensibility of the aorta decline with age. Such changes occur even in normal healthy adults. The loss of elasticity and aortic compliance probably accounts for the increase in pulse pressure commonly seen in elderly persons and accompanies slow but progressive dilatation of the aorta. This loss of aortic elasticity with aging is accelerated among persons with hypertension, hypercholesterolemia, or coronary artery disease, as compared with control subjects. Conversely, among healthy athletes, aortic elasticity is higher than in their age-matched controls.

Histologically, the aging aortic wall exhibits fragmentation of elastin with a concomitant increase in collagen that results in an increased collagen-to-elastin ratio, which contributes to the loss of aortic distensibility observed physiologically. Experimental animal data suggest that impairment of vasa vasorum flow to the aortic wall results in stiffening of the aorta with similar histological changes and may, therefore, be one cause of the degenerative changes seen with age.

In animals, loss of aortic distensibility directly affects the mechanical performance of the left ventricle, with increases noted in left ventricular systolic pressure and wall tension and in end-diastolic pressure and volume. Reduced aortic compliance causes a 20 to 40 percent increase in myocardial oxygen consumption to maintain a given stroke volume. Over time, the changes in aortic compliance seen with age may cause clinically important alternations in cardiac function.

EXAMINATION OF THE AORTA

Unless the aorta is abnormally enlarged, the only location in which it can be palpated is the abdomen. The ease with which it can be felt depends largely on body habitus and pulse pressure: It is readily felt in thin individuals. Auscultation is usually unrevealing in patients with aortic diseases, except for occasional bruits at sites of narrowing of the aorta or its arterial branches. Diseases of the aortic root and proximal ascending aorta sometimes involve the aortic valve, with resultant aortic regurgitation that may be detectable on auscultation. Regurgitant murmurs secondary to root dilatation rather than primary valvular disease are often loudest along the right rather than the left sternal border.

Chest radiography is a valuable and simple procedure for assessing the aorta. Normally, the ascending aorta is not visible on the direct posterior-anterior chest radiograph. The aorta appears as a "knob" in the superior mediastinum just to the left of the vertebral column. The lateral border of the descending thoracic aorta can often be found to the left of the spine. On the lateral chest radiograph, the aortic root and proximal ascending aorta are visible as an indistinct shadow in the middle of the mediastinum arising from the base of the heart. The left anterior oblique projection best demonstrates the ascending aorta and arch.

A number of imaging modalities are available for diagnostic examination of the aorta, including aortography, computed tomography (CT), magnetic resonance imaging (MRI), and both transthoracic echocardiography (TTE) and transesophageal echocardiography (TEE). The respective usefulness of these imaging modalities is discussed here in the context of specific aortic diseases.

CH 56

AORTIC ANEURYSMS

The term *aortic aneurysm* refers to a pathological dilatation of the normal aortic lumen involving one or several segments. One useful criterion defines aortic aneurysm as a permanent localized dilatation of the aorta having a diameter at least 1.5 times that of the expected normal diameter of that given aortic segment, although no definition is universally accepted. Aneurysms are usually described in terms of their location, size, morphological appearance, and origin. The morphology of an aortic aneurysm is typically either *fusiform,* which is the more common shape, or *saccular.* A fusiform aneurysm has a fairly uniform shape, with symmetrical dilatation that involves the full circumference of the aortic wall. Saccular aneurysms, on the other hand, have more localized dilatation that appears as an outpouching of only a portion of the aortic wall. In addition, the aorta may have a *pseudoaneurysm* or *false aneurysm,* which is not actually an aneurysm at all, but rather a well-defined collection of blood and connective tissue outside the vessel wall. This defect may result from a contained rupture of the aortic wall.

The presence of an aortic aneurysm may be a marker of more diffuse aortic disease. Overall, up to 13 percent of all patients in whom an aortic aneurysm is diagnosed have multiple aneurysms, with 25 to 28 percent of those with thoracic aortic aneurysms having concomitant abdominal aortic aneurysms. For this reason, a patient in whom an aortic aneurysm is discovered should undergo examination of the entire aorta for the possible presence of other aneurysms.

Abdominal Aortic Aneurysms

Abdominal aortic aneurysms are much more common than thoracic aortic aneurysms. Age is an important risk factor. The incidence of abdominal aortic aneurysm rises rapidly after 55 years of age in men and 70 years of age in women, and abdominal aortic aneurysms occur 5 to 10 times more frequently in men than in women. Men 65 years of age and older screened by ultrasonography have a prevalence of abdominal aortic aneurysms of 5 percent. The true prevalence of abdominal aortic aneurysms is difficult to determine because there may be as much as a 10-fold variation depending on the diagnostic criteria, the imaging modality used, and the age, gender distribution, and baseline risk of the population examined. Nevertheless, the incidence of abdominal aneurysms appears to have increased fourfold over the past three decades. Some of the increase may reflect more widespread screening than in the past and more frequent use of abdominal CT scanning, which may reveal aortic aneurysms as incidental findings, for other diagnostic purposes. However, these data likely reflect, at least in part, a true increase in disease incidence.

The large majority of abdominal aortic aneurysms arise below the renal arteries and are known as *infrarenal aneurysms.* Only a small minority, known as *suprarenal aneurysms,* arise between the level of the diaphragm and the renal arteries. As a result of flow disturbance through the aneurysmal aortic segment, blood may stagnate along the walls and thus allow the formation of mural thrombus. Such thrombus, as well as atherosclerotic debris, may embolize and compromise the circulation of distal arteries. However, rupture poses the major risk of abdominal aortic aneurysms. When rupture does occur, 80 percent rupture into the retroperitoneum, which may contain the rupture; whereas most of the remainder rupture into the peritoneal cavity and cause uncontrolled hemorrhage and rapid circulatory collapse.

ETIOLOGY AND PATHOGENESIS

A number of risk factors favor the development of aneurysms. Smoking most strongly associates with abdominal aortic aneurysms followed by male gender, age, hypertension, hyperlipidemia, and atherosclerosis. The duration of smoking is associated with the risk of abdominal aortic aneurysm but, interestingly, the amount smoked (when controlling for the duration of smoking) is not.[1] Smoking also increases the risks of aneurysm expansion and rupture as well as the risk associated with aneurysm repair. Men are 10 times more likely than women to have an abdominal aortic aneurysm of 4.0 cm or greater.[2] However, women with aneurysms have a risk of rupture significantly higher than men. Those with a family history (first-degree relative) of abdominal aortic aneurysm have an increased risk; siblings of those affected have a 19 percent risk—compared with the 2 to 5 percent risk in the general population.[3] In addition, those with familial aneurysms tend to be younger and have higher rates of rupture than those with sporadic aneurysms. Given the results of pedigree analysis and the fact that single gene defects have not yet been identified, the increased risk is probably polygenic.

The aortic wall resists expansion because of the strength of its extracellular matrix, notably elastin and collagen. Degradation of these structural proteins, because of any of a number of factors, in turn weakens the aortic wall and allows aneurysms to develop. As the aorta then widens, tension in the vessel wall rises in accordance with Laplace law, which states that tension is proportional to the product of pressure and radius. Further widening results in even greater wall tension, which in turn leads to acceleration of aneurysm enlargement. A vicious cycle ensues in which the dilatation often progresses rapidly.

Classically, atherosclerosis has been considered the underlying cause of abdominal aortic aneurysms. The infrarenal abdominal aorta is most affected by the atherosclerotic process and is similarly the most common site of abdominal aneurysm formation; only a fraction of abdominal aortic aneurysms are suprarenal, and these tend to arise as an extension of a thoracic (thoracoabdominal) aneurysm. The atherosclerotic process less often involves the thoracic aorta. Atherosclerotic disease of the aorta may produce either stenotic obstruction, a process that tends to be confined to the infrarenal abdominal aorta, or aneurysmal dilatation; why one process should predominate over the other in any given individual, however, is unknown.

Although aortic atherosclerosis clearly contributes to the process, ongoing research supports a multifactorial pathogenesis of abdominal aortic aneurysms. Genetic, environmental, hemodynamic, and immunological factors all appear to play a role in the development and progressive growth of aneurysms. Although it was once thought that atherosclerotic and inflammatory abdominal aortic aneurysms were distinct conditions, it now appears that they actually share a common underlying pathophysiology, with inflammatory aneurysms simply representing an extreme of atherosclerotic aneurysms.[3a]

Inflammation within the aortic wall may promote the degradation of the extracellular matrix. There is histological evidence of inflammatory infiltrates—in particular macrophages and T lymphocytes—within the media and adventitia of aneurysms. These findings may represent a primary inflammatory response whose stimuli are unknown. Infection is one possible causal factor, with a number of studies identifying viral or bacterial antigens within aneurysm wall tissue. Whatever the stimuli, the macrophages and T lymphocytes produce proteolytic enzymes that degrade aortic elastin, collagen, and other matrix proteins. It should be noted, however, that there is also some competing protein synthesis, so ultimately the process is one of a dynamic balance between protein degradation and synthesis that leads to remodeling of the aortic wall. T lymphocytes may induce smooth muscle cell apoptosis within the aneurysm wall. Because smooth muscle cells produce elastin and collagen, the loss of cellularity may lead to impaired maintenance and repair of the extracellular matrix in the face of ongoing degradation (see Chap. 38).

Matrix metalloproteinases are zinc- and calcium-dependent enzymes that are produced by smooth muscle and inflammatory cells, and several of these proteinases may participate in abdominal aortic aneurysm formation. Indeed, certain matrix metalloproteinases can degrade elastin and collagen, primary components of the aortic extracellular matrix. The levels of some matrix metalloproteinases (e.g., MMP-2, MMP-8, MMP-9, MMP-14) rise significantly in the walls of aneurysms compared with control aortas. In one study, the levels of MMP-9 messenger RNA expression was fourfold higher in large (5.0 to 6.9 cm) than in small (3.0 to 4.9 cm) aneurysms. Circulating levels of MMP-9 are elevated in at least 50 percent of patients with abdominal aortic aneurysms, and levels decrease after open or endovascular aneurysm repair. A recent study of ruptured aneurysms revealed that levels of MMP-8 and -9 were significantly higher at the site of rupture than in the corresponding unruptured wall, suggesting that an increase in collagen breakdown may be a precursor to rupture.[4] The evidence linking the matrix metalloproteinases to aneurysm formation is, however, more than just circumstantial. In fact, in an experimental mouse model of aneurysm formation in which MMP-2 and MMP-9-levels are increased, both MMP-2- and MMP-9-deficient mice resisted aneurysm formation.[5] Reduced levels of metalloproteinase inhibitors, known as TIMPs (tissue inhibitors of metalloproteinases), in the walls of aneurysms may promote matrix breakdown by MMPs as well.

Pharmacological inhibition of proteolysis might slow the growth of aneurysms in humans. The tetracyclines weakly inhibit matrix metalloproteinases through a mechanism unrelated to their antibiotic activity. In animal models of abdominal aortic aneurysms, treatment with either doxycycline or tetracycline derivatives without antibiotic activity has reduced aortic wall production of MMP-9, led to preservation of medial elastin, and reduced aneurysmal expansion. In one murine model, doxycycline administration reduced aneurysm growth by 33 to 66 percent at circulating doxycycline levels similar to those achieved in humans at standard doses.[6] The early data in human trials is encouraging. Curci and colleagues found that preoperative treatment with oral doxycycline resulted in a fivefold reduction in the amount of MMP-9 expressed within aneurysm wall tissue resected at surgery.[7] A multicenter group led by Robert Thompson has reported a phase II trial demonstrating the safety of prolonged 6-month administration of doxycycline (100 mg twice daily) to subjects with abdominal aortic aneurysms. Their findings also showed that therapy gradually reduces plasma MMP-9 levels.[8] In a relatively small trial of 92 subjects, roxithromycin therapy for 28 days reduced the rate of aneurysm expansion by 44 percent in the first year, although by only 5 percent in the second

year of follow-up.[9] *Chlamydia pneumoniae* may contribute to the inflammatory process underlying aneurysm formation. Because doxycycline is effective in the treatment of *C. pneumoniae* infection as well, this may provide another mechanism by which the drug might slow aneurysm expansion.

More recently, there is evidence that HMG-CoA reductase inhibitors may protect against aneurysms. In a murine aneurysm model, treatment with simvastatin reduced MMP-9 expression and increased TIMP-1 expression, and was associated with preservation of medial elastin and vascular smooth muscle cells. Importantly, in both hypercholesterolemic and normal mice, simvastatin therapy suppressed the development of experimental aortic aneurysms.[10] Indeed, in humans undergoing elective abdominal aneurysm repair, preoperative therapy with a variety of statins is associated with a decrease in MMP-9 levels in the aortic wall.[11] Clinical trials are underway, and early reports are promising (see later).

In addition to the matrix metalloproteinases, several other proteinases, including plasminogen activators, serine elastases, and cathepsins, may contribute to the formation of aneurysms. Cathepsins S and K are potent elastases overexpressed in human atheromas. Increased levels of cathepsin S have been demonstrated in both atherosclerotic plaques and aneurysms. Alternatively, in humans a lower level of cystatin C, an endogenous cathepsin S inhibitor, is associated with larger aneurysms and a faster rate of growth.[12]

More recently, abdominal aortic aneurysm tissue has been found to have a high level of c-Jun N-terminal kinase (JNK), an enzyme that increases degradation and reduces synthesis of the extracellular matrix. Importantly, in an in vivo murine model, selective inhibition of JNK not only prevented aneurysm development but also caused regression of established aneurysms.[13]

CLINICAL MANIFESTATIONS. Most abdominal aortic aneurysms are asymptomatic and are discovered incidentally on routine physical examination or on imaging studies ordered for other indications. Younger patients (50 years old or younger), however, are several times more likely to be symptomatic at the time of diagnosis. Among these patients, pain is the most frequent complaint and is usually located in the hypogastrium or lower part of the back. The pain is usually steady, has a gnawing quality, and may last for hours to days at a time. In contrast to musculoskeletal back pain, movement does not affect aneurysm pain, although patients may be more comfortable in certain positions, such as with the legs drawn up.

RUPTURED ANEURYSM. The development of new or worsening pain, often of sudden onset, may herald expansion or impending rupture of an aneurysm. This pain is characteristically constant, severe, and located in the back or lower part of the abdomen, sometimes with radiation into the groin, buttocks, or legs. Actual rupture is associated with abrupt onset of back pain along with abdominal pain and tenderness. Most patients have a palpable, pulsatile abdominal mass, and many are hypotensive when initially seen. However, this familiar triad of abdominal/back pain, a pulsatile abdominal mass, and hypotension—recognized as pathognomonic of a ruptured abdominal aortic aneurysm—is seen in as few as one-third of cases. A ruptured aneurysm may mimic other acute abdominal conditions, such as renal colic, diverticulitis, or a gastrointestinal hemorrhage, and may, therefore, be initially misdiagnosed in as many as 30 percent of cases.

Patients who suffer rupture of an abdominal aortic aneurysm (Fig. 56-1) are critically ill. Hemorrhagic shock and its complications may ensue rapidly. Retroperitoneal hemorrhage may be signaled by hematomas in the flanks and groin. Rupture into the abdominal cavity may result in abdominal distention, whereas rupture into the duodenum is manifested as massive gastrointestinal hemorrhage.

PHYSICAL EXAMINATION. Many aneurysms can be detected on physical examination, although even large aneurysms may be difficult or impossible to detect in obese individuals. When palpable, a pulsatile mass extending variably from the xiphoid process to the umbilicus may be appreciated. Because of difficulty in distinguishing the abdominal aorta from surrounding structures by palpation, the size of an aneurysm tends to be overestimated on physical examination. Moreover, it may be difficult to differentiate a tortuous, ectatic aorta from true aneurysmal dilatation. Aneurysms are often sensitive to palpation and may be quite tender if rapidly expanding or about to rupture. Although tender aneurysms should be examined cautiously, no risk is known to be associated with palpation of the abdominal aorta.

Associated occlusive arterial disease is sometimes present in the femoral pulses and distal pulses in the legs and feet. Bruits arising from associated narrowed arteries can be heard over the aneurysm. Occasionally, an arteriovenous fistula is formed by spontaneous rupture into

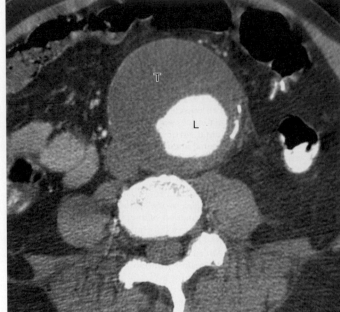

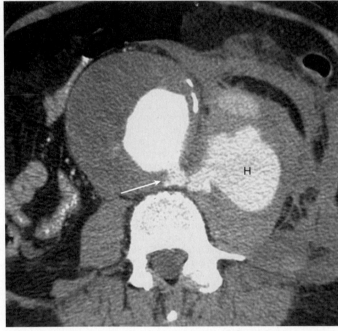

FIGURE 56–1 A, Axial contrast-enhanced computed tomography scan of the abdomen revealing a 6.8 cm infrarenal abdominal aortic aneurysm. The lumen of the aneurysm (L) is narrowed by extensive mural thrombus (T). **B,** A similar computed tomography scan of the same aneurysm immediately following its rupture (arrow) into the retroperitoneum. The high-attenuation material extending from the aneurysm into the left perirenal space is consistent with a contained hematoma (H).

the inferior vena cava, iliac vein, or renal vein and can cause a syndrome of hemodynamic collapse and acute high-output cardiac failure.

DIAGNOSIS AND SIZING. Several diagnostic imaging modalities are currently used for detecting, sizing, and serially monitoring abdominal aortic aneurysms, as well as for precise definition of the aortic anatomy preoperatively. Abdominal ultrasonography is perhaps the most practical way to screen for abdominal aortic aneurysms. It can visualize an aneurysm in the transverse and longitudinal planes, has a sensitivity of 87 to 99 percent (depending on the segment involved),

and can accurately define aneurysm size to within ±0.3 cm, but it is limited by less reliable measurements of the suprarenal aorta and significant interobserver variability. Its major advantages are that it is relatively inexpensive, is noninvasive, and does not require the use of a contrast agent. However, because ultrasonography is limited in its ability to visualize the cephalic or pelvic extent of disease or define the associated mesenteric and renal arterial anatomy, it is insufficient for planning operative repair.

Computed tomography is an extremely accurate method for both diagnosing aortic aneurysms (Fig. 56-2A) and sizing them to within ±0.2 cm. CT has an advantage over ultrasonography in that it can better define the shape and extent of the aneurysm as well as the local anatomical relation of the visceral and renal vessels. Its disadvantages are that the procedure is more expensive and less widely available than ultrasonography, and it also requires the use of ionizing radiation and intravenous contrast. Although CT may be less practical than ultrasonography as a screening tool, its high accuracy in sizing aneurysms makes it an excellent modality for serially monitoring changes in aneurysm size. It is important to note that CT measurements of aneurysm size tend to be larger than ultrasonographic measurements by an average of 0.27 cm. Spiral (helical) CT, which permits three-dimensional display of the aorta and its branches, provides more comprehensive evaluation of the anatomy of an abdominal aortic aneurysm and information regarding renal, mesenteric, or iliac arterial occlusive disease and thus may suffice for preoperative evaluation of abdominal aneurysms (see Fig. 56-2B).

Magnetic resonance angiography (MRA) is also an alternative for the preoperative evaluation of aortic aneurysms. On conventional spin-echo MRI, flowing blood appears as a signal void, but with the use of MRA, blood has a bright appearance and vessels can be visualized in a projective fashion, similar to traditional angiography. Because tomographic images are reconstructed to create a three-dimensional image, the aorta can be visualized from a series of projections to facilitate appreciation of anatomical relationships. MRA is extremely accurate in determining aneurysm size, and it correctly defines the proximal extent of disease and iliofemoral involvement in more than 80 percent of cases.

Aortography may underestimate aneurysm size in the presence of nonopacified mural thrombus lining the aneurysm walls, but it remains an excellent technique for defining the suprarenal extent of the aneurysm and any associated renal, mesenteric, or iliofemoral arterial disease. Its disadvantages are that it is expensive, it is an invasive procedure with inherent risks, and it requires the use of intraarterial contrast and ionizing radiation. Preoperative aortography is now used only in selected cases because CT and MRA provide sufficient information in most cases.

Many practitioners currently recommend the use of screening ultrasonography only for patients at high risk—in particular, those with a family history of abdominal aortic aneurysm or those older than 60 years who have a history of smoking or hypertension. However, an important, but not fully resolved, issue is the potential usefulness of routine screening of asymptomatic patients for the presence of abdominal aneurysms. The largest and most definitive trial to date is the recent report of the Multicentre Aneurysm Screening Study Group, which provides a 4-year cost-effective analysis based on the results of a controlled trial in which a population-based sample of 67,800 men (aged 65 to 74 years) were randomized to an invitation to ultrasonography screening or to a control group not offered screening.[14] Eighty percent accepted the invitation for screening. Men found to have an abdominal aortic aneurysm of 3 cm or greater were followed with serial ultrasonographic scans for a mean of 4 years. Surgery was considered when the diameter reached 5.5 cm or greater, grew more than 1 cm per year, or became tender. There were 65 deaths related to the aneurysm in the invited group, compared with 113 in the control group, yielding an estimated risk reduction of 42 percent. After 4 years, the cost was estimated to be $57,000 per quality-adjusted life year gained; it was expected to fall to $14,200 at 10 years. Screening of 710 subjects was required to prevent one death. The authors conclude that at 4 years, the cost-effectiveness of screening for abdominal aortic aneurysm is acceptable and is likely to become increasingly favorable over time. However, one important question left unanswered by this study is the cost-effectiveness of screening women for abdominal aneurysms. Another British study addressed the potential usefulness of repeated screening for abdominal aneurysms.[15] The investigators followed 223 65-year-old men who had abdominal aortic diameters of less than 2.6 cm at baseline with repeated ultrasonographic evaluations at 5 and 12 years. None of those who survived the 12-year interval had any

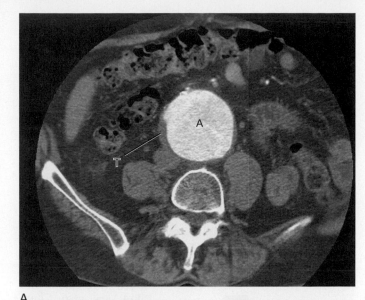

A

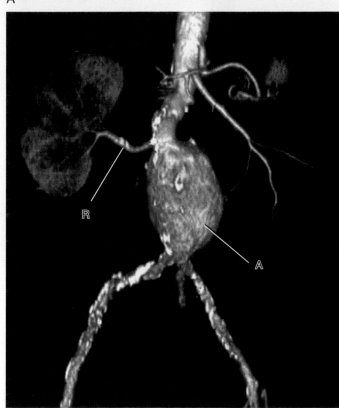

B

FIGURE 56-2 A, Axial contrast-enhanced computed tomography (CT) scan showing a 7.2 cm juxtarenal abdominal aortic aneurysm (A) lined with mural thrombus (T). **B,** Three-dimensional shaded-surface display of the same CT scan. This anteroposterior projection demonstrates that the aneurysm (A) is juxtarenal and displays its anatomical relation to surrounding structures, including the right renal arteries (R) proximally and the aortic bifurcation distally. The left renal artery and left kidney are absent.

clinically significant increase in the mean aortic diameter, and none of those who died did so from a ruptured abdominal aneurysm. The authors conclude that a normal ultrasonogram at age 65 effectively excludes the risk of a clinically significant aneurysm for life.

The U.S. Preventive Services Task Force (USPSTF) recently reviewed the data and concluded the evidence sufficient to prompt them now to recommend one-time screening for abdominal aortic aneurysm by ultrasonography in men age 65 to 75 years who have ever smoked

(current and former smokers).[16] Many experts also recommend screening those with a family history (first-degree relative) of abdominal aneurysm.

NATURAL HISTORY. The paramount concern in managing abdominal aortic aneurysms is their tendency to rupture. Mortality from rupture is quite high: Among the participants in the United Kingdom Small Aneurysm Trial who suffered a ruptured abdominal aneurysm, 25 percent died before reaching a hospital and 51 percent died in the hospital without undergoing surgery. The operative mortality rate for the 13 percent undergoing surgery was 46 percent (compared with 4 to 6 percent for elective surgery), yielding an overall 30-day survival of just 11 percent.[17] To prevent the associated mortality, surgical repair is the therapy of choice for aneurysms considered to be at significant risk of rupture.

It is well established that the risk of rupture increases with aneurysm size. The United Kingdom Small Aneurysm Trial found that aneurysms smaller than 4.0 cm have a 0.3 percent annual risk of rupture, those 4.0 to 4.9 cm have a 1.5 percent annual risk of rupture, and those 5.0 to 5.9 cm have a 6.5 percent annual risk of rupture.[17] For aneurysms 6.0 to 6.9 cm the risk of rupture is 10 percent, which then rises sharply to 33 percent for aneurysms 7.0 cm or larger.[18] Although abdominal aneurysms are less prevalent among women than among men, when present they rupture three times more frequently among women and at a smaller aortic diameter (mean diameter of 5.0 cm among women versus 6.0 cm among men). Rupture is also more common among current smokers and those with hypertension.[17]

Because 80 percent of abdominal aortic aneurysms expand over time, with as many as 15 to 20 percent expanding rapidly (>0.5 cm/yr), the risk of rupture may concomitantly increase with time. Accordingly, the ability to predict rates of aortic aneurysm expansion would be useful in estimating the risk of future rupture. Although the mean rate of abdominal aortic aneurysm expansion is thought to approximate 0.4 cm per year, the rates of expansion within a population are extremely variable. Expansion rates even vary within one individual over time, as would be expected given the "vicious cycle" of aneurysm growth explained earlier. Baseline aneurysm size is perhaps the best predictor of aneurysm expansion rate, with larger aneurysms expanding more rapidly than smaller ones, probably as a consequence of the Laplace law. A rapid rate of expansion apparently also predicts aneurysm rupture, especially abdominal aneurysms 5.0 cm or greater in diameter. Many surgeons consider both large size and rapid expansion to be indications for repair.

Management

SURGICAL TREATMENT. The goal of treating abdominal aortic aneurysms is to prolong life by preventing rupture. The decision to operate must weigh the natural history of the aneurysm and life expectancy of the patient against the anticipated morbidity and mortality of the proposed surgical procedure. Operative mortality is 4 to 6 percent overall for elective aneurysm repair and as low as 2 percent in low-risk patients. However, operative mortality rises to 19 percent for urgent aortic repair and reaches 50 percent for repair of a ruptured aneurysm. Aneurysm size remains the primary indicator for repair of asymptomatic aneurysms, and for many years there has been debate on the minimum aneurysm diameter that necessitates surgery. Two recent large-scale clinical trials have investigated this very question. The United Kingdom Small Aneurysm Trial[19] randomized 1090 patients aged 60 to 76 years with small aortic aneurysms (diameter 4.0 to 5.5 cm) to either early elective surgery or regular ultrasonographic surveillance. They found no long-term difference in survival between the early-surgery group and the surveillance group, although after 8 years, total mortality was slightly lower in the early-surgery group. However, because the operative mortality rate in this trial was 5.8 percent, some practitioners have questioned whether there may have been a survival benefit from early surgery had the operative mortality rate been lower. A similar trial known as the Aneurysm Detection and Management (ADAM) Veterans Affairs Cooperative Study[20] has suggested otherwise. In ADAM, 1136 patients with small asymptomatic aneurysms (diameter 4.0 to 5.4 cm) were randomized to undergo immediate surgical repair or surveillance at 6-month intervals by ultrasonography or CT scanning. Despite a remarkably low operative mortality rate of 2.1 percent, after a mean follow-up of 5 years there was no difference in survival between the two groups. Collectively, these trials suggest that surgery is not indicated in most instances for patients with asymptomatic aneurysms less than 5.5 cm in size. However, it should be recognized that the subjects randomized to the surveillance arms of these trials have careful clinical follow-up with both medical management and regular surveillance imaging to monitor the aneurysm. Such careful follow-up does not always take place in general practice settings outside a trial. Another important limitation is that these two study populations consisted almost entirely of men (United Kingdom Small Aneurysm Trial, 78 percent; ADAM, 99 percent), and because the risk of aneurysm rupture is greater and occurs at smaller diameters in women than in men, these results may well not apply equally to women.[21] Indeed, recognizing that aneurysms tend to rupture at smaller sizes in women than in men, the Joint Council of the American Association for Vascular Surgery and Society for Vascular Surgery has formally recommended that women undergo elective repair at an aortic diameter of 4.5 to 5.0 cm.[22]

Surgical repair of abdominal aortic aneurysms consists of opening of the aneurysm and insertion of a synthetic prosthesis, usually fabricated of Dacron or expanded polytetrafluoroethylene (Gore-Tex). Sometimes, a simple tube graft is all that is necessary, although frequently the operation must be carried distally into one or both of the iliac arteries to excise the aneurysm completely. In the case of large aneurysms, much of the aneurysm wall may be left in situ ("intrasaccular approach of Creech"), thereby reducing the need for extensive dissection and thus decreasing aortic cross-clamping time.

A less invasive alternative to open surgery for repair of abdominal aortic aneurysms is the use of percutaneously implanted, expanding endovascular stent-grafts (Figs. 56-3 and 56-4; see also Chap. 59). The device consists of a collapsible prosthetic tube graft that is inserted remotely (e.g., via the femoral artery), advanced transluminally across the aneurysm under fluoroscopic guidance, and then secured at both its proximal and distal ends with an expandable stent attachment system. For aortic aneurysm repair, the stent-graft bridges the region of the aneurysm, thereby excluding it from the circulation while allowing aortic blood flow to continue distally through the prosthetic stent-graft lumen. In some cases, stent-grafts are bifurcated, with two arms on the distal end designed to extend into the common iliac arteries when these vessels are aneurysmal as well. The rate of successful stent-graft implantation in several series over the past decade has ranged from 78 to 99 percent, with several recent large series reporting rates of 98 percent. Despite these promising results, only 30 to 60 percent of patients with abdominal aortic aneurysms have aneurysm anatomy suitable for endovascular repair. One of the major technical difficulties associated with the stent-graft technique that has yet to be overcome is the frequent occurrence of *endoleaks*,

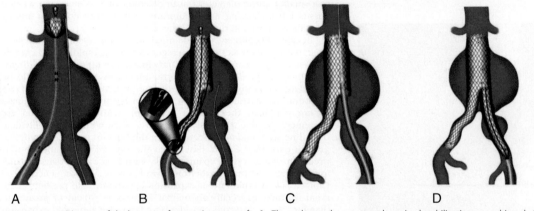

FIGURE 56–3 Diagram of deployment of an aortic stent graft. **A,** The catheter placement and proximal stabilization are achieved via right femoral access. **B,** The body and right limb of the stent graft are positioned and deployed. **C,** The cannula for deployment of the left limb of the graft is placed via left femoral access. **D,** The left limb of the graft is deployed, completing the endovascular repair of the aortic aneurysm with left iliac involvement. *(Courtesy of Medtronics Corporation.)*

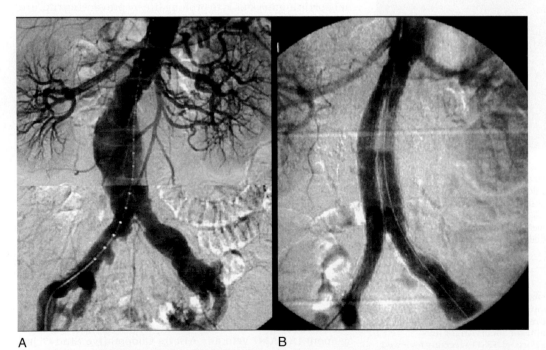

FIGURE 56–4 Angiographic views of an infrarenal abdominal aortic aneurysm with bi-iliac involvement treated by stent grafting before **(A)** and following **(B)** deployment of the aortic stent graft. *(Courtesy of Edwin Graveraux, M.D., Brigham and Women's Hospital, Boston.)*

which are seen angiographically as persistent contrast flow into the aneurysm sac because of failure to completely exclude the aneurysm from the aortic circulation. Such endoleaks, if left untreated, may leave the patient at continued risk for aneurysm expansion or rupture, and often necessitate secondary interventions.

The long-term outcome of endovascular stent-graft repair versus open surgical repair remains uncertain. Recently, however, several randomized controlled trials have begun to define the short- and mid-term outcomes. The Dutch Randomized Endovascular Aneurysm Management (DREAM) Trial Group compared open repair with endovascular repair in 345 patients with an abdominal aneurysm 5 cm or larger in diameter who were suitable candidates for either technique. The 30-day operative mortality was significantly lower in the endovascular-repair group than in the open-repair group, at 1.2 percent and 4.6 percent, respectively.[23] The Endovascular Aneurysm Repair (EVAR) trial randomized 1082 patients (similar to those just mentioned) and found a significant and nearly identical reduction in operative mortality: 1.7 percent in the endovascular-repair group versus 4.7 percent in the open-repair group.[24] Collectively, these trials generated enthusiasm because they demonstrated a clear early mortality advantage for endovascular repair.

Despite their favorable early success rates, longitudinal studies of endovascular stent-graft repair have reported failure rates of approximately 3 percent per year (1 percent for rupture and 2 percent for conversion to open repair), compared with failure rates of 0.3 percent for open repair.[25] Not surprisingly, then, the mid-term outcomes have been far less encouraging. Indeed, in the DREAM trial, the two-year cumulative survival rates were actually no different for endovascular versus open repair, at 89.7 and 89.6 percent, respectively.[26] In the EVAR trial, although there was, at 4 years, a persistent reduction in aneurysm-related deaths in the endovascular stent-graft group (4 percent versus 7 percent; $p = 0.04$), there was no difference between the two groups in all-cause mortality.[27] These trials indicate that endovascular aneurysm repair offers no clear late advantage over open repair among those who are good candidates for either procedure. Therefore, at present, the use of stent-grafts for endovascular repair of abdominal aortic aneurysms has generally been limited to a subset of patients: typically older patients or those at high operative risk.

ASSESSING OPERATIVE RISK. Because patients with abdominal aortic aneurysms in almost all cases have atherosclerosis, their high likelihood of concomitant coronary, renal, and cerebrovascular arterial disease significantly increases the risk of major vascular surgery (see Chap. 80). Indeed, one-half of all perioperative deaths from aneurysm repair result from myocardial infarction. In addition, in one study, routine coronary arteriography in patients undergoing aneurysm repair revealed severe revascularizable coronary artery disease in 18 percent of all patients, including an 8 percent incidence in patients without prior symptoms of coronary ischemia.[28] Among those with angiographically significant coronary artery disease, about one-half have multivessel disease.

Several studies have demonstrated that cardiac scintigraphy is an effective means of identifying patients at highest risk for perioperative ischemic events. Patients with reversible perfusion defects in multiple segments of myocardium are at highest risk, and it is in this subgroup that coronary angiography is likely to be most helpful. The safety of nuclear imaging with pharmacological stress in such patients has been well established. Although exercise scintigraphy is also a useful screening method, many patients with vascular disease fail to achieve an adequate heart rate because of limited exercise capacity. Other useful techniques for preoperative evaluation of myocardial ischemia include dobutamine stress echocardiography and electrocardiographic exercise testing in patients with a normal baseline electrocardiogram and adequate exercise tolerance.

Selective preoperative evaluation to identify the presence and severity of coronary artery disease in patients with clinical markers of coronary artery disease has been widely advocated, and some investigators further suggest screening those with strong cardiac risk factors despite the absence of clinical evidence of coronary artery disease. Although patients found to have significant revascularizable coronary artery disease are presumed to benefit from preoperative coronary revascularization with selective coronary artery bypass surgery or angioplasty, this conclusion remains unproved. Data available from nonrandomized studies of patients with significant coronary artery disease undergoing vascular surgery demonstrate lower mortality for those who have undergone coronary bypass surgery. Furthermore, a randomized study demonstrated that the long-term outcome of patients with combined peripheral vascular disease and high-risk coronary artery disease is improved by coronary artery revascularization in patients with three-vessel coronary disease. As is the case for coronary artery bypass surgery, no data are yet available to confirm that preoperative percutaneous coronary revascularization for significant coronary stenoses decreases the risk from major vascular surgery.

In addition to such preoperative screening and potential coronary revascularization, the use of perioperative invasive hemodynamic monitoring and careful perioperative surveillance for evidence of ischemia may further reduce operative risk secondary to cardiac ischemic events. Furthermore, myocardial ischemia and perhaps myocardial infarction may be prevented by using beta-adrenergic blockers perioperatively.

LATE SURVIVAL. A review of late survival following abdominal aortic aneurysm repair among nearly 2500 patients revealed 1-, 5-, and 10-year survival rates of 93, 63, and 40 percent, respectively.

MEDICAL MANAGEMENT. Risk factor modification is fundamental in the medical management of abdominal aortic aneurysms. Most patients with abdominal aortic aneurysms are cigarette smokers, and given the increased risk of aneurysm rupture among active smokers, the habit must be discontinued. Hypertension should be carefully controlled. Beta blockers have long been considered an important therapy for reducing the risk of aneurysm expansion and rupture, and both animal and human studies support such a role. Propranolol delays the development of aneurysms in a mouse model prone to spontaneous aortic aneurysms. Interestingly, it appears that the drug's efficacy in this model may have been independent of reductions in blood pressure or diminution of the rate of left ventricular ejection (dP/dt) and, instead, may have resulted from changes in connective tissue metabolism and the structure of the aortic wall. In humans, the data are mixed. Several trials have shown that treatment with propranolol has no significant impact on the rate of growth of smaller aneurysms (less than 4 cm in diameter), but decreases the rate of growth of larger aneurysms (4.0 to 5.0 cm in diameter, or larger) by 50 percent or more.[29] Therefore, beta blockers should be recommended for patients with larger aneurysms who are managed medically.

Hypercholesterolemia, if present, should be treated. As already mentioned, experimental data suggest that HMG-CoA reductase inhibitor (statin) therapy may protect even aneurysm patients with normal cholesterol. In a recent nonrandomized study of 130 patients with abdominal aortic aneurysms, investigators compared the rate of aneurysm growth among those treated with and not treated with statins. At 2 years, the mean aneurysm size increased significantly (from 4.5 cm to 5.3 cm) among those not treated with statins, whereas the mean aneurysm size did not increase at all (from 4.6 cm to 4.5 cm) among those treated with statins ($p < 0.001$).[30] Although we must certainly await randomized controlled trials to confirm such findings, this compelling report suggests that statins may contribute to the prevention and management of abdominal aneurysms.

Following an abdominal aortic aneurysm 4.0 cm in size or larger requires careful routine follow-up to detect either rapid expansion (>0.5 cm/yr) or an increase in size to 5.5 cm or larger—either of which is an indication for surgery. CT scanning every 6 months, perhaps as frequently as every 3 months for those at higher risk, has been advocated for follow-up in such patients. CT scanning is preferable to ultrasonography for monitoring aneurysm growth because CT measurements of aneurysm size are more accurate.

Thoracic Aortic Aneurysms

Thoracic aortic aneurysms are much less common than aneurysms of the abdominal aorta. Thoracic aneurysms are classified by the portion of aorta involved (i.e., the ascending, arch, or descending thoracic aorta). This anatomical distinction is important because the etiology, natural history, and treatment of thoracic aneurysms differ for each of these segments. In modern series, aneurysms of the ascending aorta occur most commonly (60 percent), followed by aneurysms of the descending aorta (40 percent), whereas arch aneurysms (10 percent) and thoracoabdominal aneurysms (10 percent) occur less often. *Thoracoabdominal aortic aneurysm* refers to descending thoracic aneurysms that extend distally to involve the abdominal aorta. Sometimes, the entire aorta may be ectatic, with localized aneurysms seen at sites in both the thoracic and abdominal aorta.

ETIOLOGY AND PATHOGENESIS. Aneurysms of the ascending thoracic aorta most often result from cystic medial degeneration (or cystic medial necrosis). Histologically, cystic medial degeneration has the appearance of smooth muscle cell drop-out and elastic fiber degeneration, with the presence in the media of cystic spaces filled with mucoid material. Although these changes occur most frequently in the ascending aorta, some cases may involve the entire aorta. The histological changes lead to weakening of the aortic wall, which in turn results in the formation of a fusiform aneurysm. Such aneurysms often involve the aortic root and may consequently result in aortic regurgitation: The term *annuloaortic ectasia* (Fig. 56-5) is often used to describe this condition (see later).

Cystic medial necrosis occurs to some extent with aging and is accelerated by hypertension. At younger ages, cystic medial degenera-

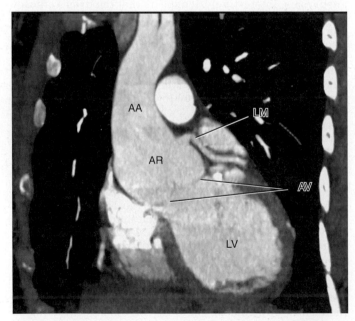

FIGURE 56–5 A contrast-enhanced computed tomography scan with three-dimensional reconstruction in the coronal projection in a woman with Marfan syndrome and annuloaortic ectasia. Note the bulbous, pear-shaped appearance of the 5.1 cm aortic root (AR), and the less pronounced dilatation of the proximal ascending thoracic aorta (AA). The aorta tapers to a normal diameter proximal to the aortic arch. The aortic valve leaflets (AV), left main coronary artery (LM), and left ventricle (LV) are readily visualized on this high-resolution 64-slice multidetector CT angiogram.

tion is classically associated with Marfan syndrome and can be associated with other connective tissue disorders as well, such as Ehlers-Danlos syndrome. Marfan syndrome (see Chap. 8) is an autosomal dominant heritable disorder of connective tissue caused by mutations in the genes for fibrillin-1, a protein that is the major component of microfibrils of elastin. These mutations result in a decrease in the amount of elastin in the aortic wall, together with a loss of elastin's normally highly organized structure. As a consequence, from an early age, a marfanoid aorta exhibits markedly abnormal elastic properties and increased systemic pulse wave velocities—over time the aorta exhibits progressively increasing degrees of stiffness and dilatation. More recently, the Johns Hopkins group has demonstrated that beyond its structural role, fibrillin-1 appears to regulate the cytokine TGF-β, and leads to excessive TGF-β signaling that, in turn, contributes to progressive aortic root enlargement. In a mouse model of Marfan syndrome, mice with fibrillin-1 mutations and aortic root enlargement were treated with a polyclonal TGF-β neutralizing antibody. Treatment resulting in reduced elastic fiber fragmentation and reduced TGF-β signaling in the aortic media, as well as the arrest of aortic growth. There is now evidence that the angiotensin-1 antagonist losartan, which also limits TGF-β action, prevents aortic aneurysms in the mouse model of Marfan syndrome.[31]

Cystic medial degeneration also occurs in patients with ascending thoracic aortic aneurysms who do not have overt connective tissue disorders. Some patients who have annuloaortic ectasia and proven cystic medial degeneration without the classic phenotypic manifestations of Marfan syndrome may have a variation, or *forme fruste,* of Marfan syndrome. Indeed, increasing evidence suggests that many of these patients also have a genetic mutation that may account for cystic medial degeneration. Although cases of thoracic aortic aneurysms in the absence of overt connective tissue disorders may be sporadic, they are often familial in nature and are now referred to as the *familial thoracic aortic aneurysm syndrome.*

Analysis of a large database of patients treated at Yale-New Haven Hospital identified those with a familial pattern of thoracic aortic aneurysms and compared them with both sporadic cases and those with Marfan syndrome. At least 19 percent of patients had a family history of a thoracic aortic aneurysm. The mean age of presentation for patients with familial syndromes was 57 years, which was significantly younger than sporadic cases (64 years) but older than Marfan syndrome cases (25 years). Most pedigrees suggested an autosomal dominant mode of inheritance, but some suggested a recessive mode and possibly X-linked inheritance as well.[32] Investigation of the families of 158 patients referred for surgical repair or thoracic aortic aneurysms or dissections found that first-degree relatives of probands had a higher risk (risk ratio [RR] 1.8 for fathers and sisters, RR 10.9 for brothers) of thoracic aortic aneurysms or sudden death compared with control subjects.[33]

Milewicz and colleagues have identified a mutation on 3p24.2-25 that can cause both isolated and familial thoracic aortic aneurysms. Although there appears to be dominant inheritance, there is marked variability in the expression and penetrance of the disorder, such that some inherit and pass on the gene but show no manifestation. Pathological evaluation of the aorta in these families reveals cystic medial degeneration.[34] Two subsequent studies of familial thoracic aortic aneurysm syndromes successfully mapped the mutations to at least two different chromosomal loci, but some families mapped to neither of these, suggesting additional loci. Most recently, mutations in transforming growth factor-beta receptor type II have been associated with some cases of familial thoracic aortic aneurysms.[35] As more families are studied, the extent of genetic heterogeneity is likely to become more evident. Indeed, the fact that there is such variable expression and penetrance suggests that this may be a polygenic condition.

Some cases of ascending thoracic aortic aneurysms are associated with an underlying bicuspid aortic valve (see Chap. 62). In fact, the risks of aortic dilatation, aneurysm, and dissection increase significantly among those with a bicuspid aortic valve. Historical teaching attributed such aneurysms to "poststenotic dilatation" of the ascending aorta, but the data suggest otherwise. Fifty-two percent of young people with normally functioning bicuspid aortic valves have echocardiographic evidence of aortic dilatation. Dilatation occurs most frequently at the level of the tubular portion of the ascending aorta (44 percent), but the 20 percent have dilatation at the level of sinuses. In a community sample, Nkomo and colleagues demonstrated that bicuspid aortic valve is associated with a dilated aorta regardless of the presence or absence of hemodynamically significant valve dysfunction.[36]

Cystic medial degeneration appears to underlie the aortic aneurysms associated with bicuspid aortic valve. Indeed, 75 percent of patients with bicuspid aortic valve undergoing aortic valve replacement surgery have biopsy-proven significant cystic medial necrosis of the ascending aorta, compared with only 14 percent of patients with tricuspid aortic valves undergoing similar surgery.[37] Inadequate production of fibrillin-1 during embryogenesis may result in both the bicuspid aortic valve and a weakened aortic wall.[38] Fibrillin-1 content is reduced in bicuspid aortic valve aortas compared with that seen in aortas of those with healthy or diseased tricuspid aortic valves, independent of valve function and patient age, whereas elastin and collagen content are similar, suggesting aortic dilatation results from a congenital deficiency of fibrillin-1. Moreover, MMP-2 activity is increased twofold in bicuspid aortic valve aortas, whereas MMP-9 activity is similar.[39] No single gene responsible for bicuspid aortic valve has yet been identified, and it is likely genetically heterogeneous. Moreover, in one study, 48 percent of patients with bicuspid valves had aortic dimensions equal to those of control subjects, so it appears that not all have increased risk.

The mechanisms underlying thoracic aortic aneurysms in the setting of tricuspid aortic valves appear to differ. In contradistinction to those with bicuspid aortic valves, aneurysms associated with tricuspid aortic valves have normal levels of MMP-2 activity and increased activity of MMP-9. Whereas aneurysms associated with bicuspid aortic valves have little inflammatory infiltrate and preserved elastin content, those with tricuspid aortic valves show evidence of significant elevation of the macrophage marker CD68 and reduced elastin content.[40] A recent study of genomic DNA from aortic tissue or blood found that the frequency of the MMP-9 8202A/G polymorphism was significantly higher in patients with thoracic aortic aneurysms and aortic dissection, with an odds ratio approaching 5,[41] and in a murine model MMP-9 gene deletion attenuated thoracic aortic aneurysm formation.[42]

ATHEROSCLEROSIS. Atherosclerotic aneurysms infrequently occur in the ascending aorta and, when they do, tend to associate with diffuse aortic atherosclerosis. Aneurysms in the aortic arch are often contiguous with aneurysms of the ascending or descending aorta. They may be caused by atherosclerotic disease, cystic medial degeneration, and syphilis or other infections. The predominant cause of aneurysms of the descending thoracic aorta is atherosclerosis. These aneurysms tend to originate just distal to the origin of the left subclavian artery and may be either fusiform or saccular. The pathogenesis of such atherosclerotic aneurysms in the thoracic aorta may resemble that of abdominal aneurysms but this has not been extensively examined.

SYPHILIS. Syphilis was once a common cause of ascending thoracic aortic aneurysm, but today it has become a rarity in most major medical centers as a result of aggressive antibiotic treatment of the disease in its early stages. The latent period from initial spirochetal infection to aortic complications may range from 5 to 40 years but is most commonly 10 to 25 years. During the secondary phase of the disease, spirochetes directly infect the aortic media, most commonly involving the ascending aorta. The infection and attendant inflammatory response destroys the muscular and elastic medial elements, which undergo replacement by fibrous tissue that frequently calcifies. Weakening of the aortic wall from medial destruction results in progressive aneurysmal dilatation. In addition, the infection may spread into the aortic root, and the subsequent root dilation may result in aortic regurgitation.

INFECTIOUS AORTITIS. Infectious aortitis is a rare cause of aortic aneurysm that can result from a primary infection of the aortic wall causing aortic dilation with the formation of fusiform or saccular aneurysms. More commonly, infected, or mycotic, aneurysms arise secondarily from an infection occurring in a preexisting aneurysm of another cause. When an infected aneurysm involves the ascending aorta, it is often the consequence of direct spread from aortic valve bacterial endocarditis.

Several other causes of thoracic aortic aneurysms are discussed in detail elsewhere in this or other chapters, including giant cell arteritis (see Chap. 84), aortic trauma (see Chap. 71), and aortic dissection (see later). Note that the clinical features, natural history, and treatment of thoracic aneurysms discussed here apply specifically to nondissecting thoracic aortic aneurysms.

CLINICAL MANIFESTATIONS. At least one half of patients with thoracic aortic aneurysms are asymptomatic at the time of diagnosis, with such aneurysms typically discovered as incidental findings on a routine physical examination, chest radiograph, or CT scan. When patients

do experience symptoms, the symptoms tend to reflect either a vascular consequence of the aneurysm or a local mass effect. Vascular consequences include aortic regurgitation from dilation of the aortic root, often associated with secondary congestive heart failure, or distal thromboembolism. A local mass effect from an ascending or arch aneurysm may cause superior vena cava syndrome as a result of obstruction of venous return via compression of the superior vena cava or innominate vein. Aneurysms of the arch or descending aorta may compress the trachea (Fig. 56-6) or main stem bronchus and produce tracheal deviation, wheezing, cough, dyspnea (with symptoms that may be positional), hemoptysis, or recurrent pneumonitis. Compression of the esophagus can produce dysphagia, and compression of the recurrent laryngeal nerve can cause hoarseness. Chest pain or back pain occurs in 25 percent of cases of nondissecting aneurysms and result from direct compression of other intrathoracic structures of the chest wall, or from erosion into adjacent bone. Typically, such pain is steady, deep, boring, and at times severe.

As with abdominal aortic aneurysms, the most worrisome consequence of thoracic aneurysms is leakage or rupture. Rupture is accompanied by the dramatic onset of excruciating pain, often in the region where less severe pain had previously existed. Rupture occurs most commonly into the left intrapleural space or the mediastinum and is manifested as hypotension. Less often, an aneurysm of the descending thoracic aorta ruptures into the adjacent esophagus (an aortoesophageal fistula), which causes life-threatening hematemesis. Acute aneurysm expansion, which may herald rupture, can cause similar pain. Thoracic aneurysms can also be accompanied by aortic dissection, as discussed in detail subsequently.

DIAGNOSIS AND SIZING. Many thoracic aneurysms are readily visible on chest radiographs (Fig. 56-7) and are characterized by widening of the mediastinal silhouette,

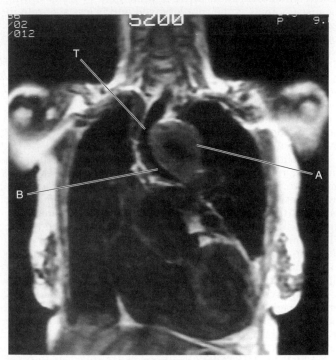

FIGURE 56–6 Magnetic resonance imaging scan in the coronal projection of a large thoracic aortic aneurysm in an elderly woman with dyspnea and cough. In this view, the markedly dilated aortic arch (A) is compressing the trachea (T) and causing rightward tracheal deviation. The aneurysm is also compressing the left main stem bronchus (B). In addition, all four cardiac chambers are dilated, consistent with the patient's known idiopathic dilated cardiomyopathy.

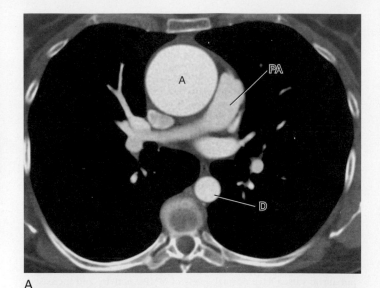

FIGURE 56–7 Chest radiograph of a patient with a very large aneurysm of the ascending thoracic aorta. Evident are both marked widening of the mediastinum and an abnormal aortic contour.

enlargement of the aortic knob, or displacement of the trachea from the midline. Unfortunately, smaller aneurysms, especially saccular ones, may not be evident on the chest radiograph; therefore, this technique cannot exclude the diagnosis of aortic aneurysm.

Aortography had long been the preferred modality for the preoperative evaluation of thoracic aortic aneurysms and for precise definition of the anatomy of the aneurysm and great vessels. However, as is the case for abdominal aortic aneurysms, CT and MRA now suffice in most cases to define both aortic and branch vessel anatomy. Either contrast-enhanced CT scanning (Fig. 56-8) or MRI very accurately detect and size thoracic aortic aneurysms. When aneurysms involve the aortic root, MRA is preferable to CT scanning because CT images the root less well and is less accurate in sizing its diameter. When patients have a tortuous thoracic aorta, which is often the case among the elderly, one should use caution in using axial images to measure the aortic diameter. The axial images often cut through the descending aorta off-axis, resulting in a falsely large aortic diameter. When the axial data are reconstructed into three-dimensional images (i.e., CT angiography), one can measure the tortuous aorta in true cross-section and obtain an accurate diameter. Such three-dimensional imaging should then always be used to follow such patients over time.

Transthoracic echo is an excellent modality for imaging the aortic root, which is important for patients with Marfan syndrome, but it does not image the middle or distal ascending aorta well in many cases and is particularly limited in its ability to image the descending thoracic aorta. Therefore, among patients other than those with Marfan syndrome, TTE should not be used for diagnosing thoracic aneurysms. Transesophageal echocardiography can image almost the entire thoracic aorta quite well and has become widely used for detection of aortic dissection. However, given that TEE is a semi-invasive procedure, CT and MR are usually preferred imaging techniques in the evaluation of nondissecting thoracic aneurysms. The advantages and disadvantage of each imaging modality are discussed later in greater detail.

NATURAL HISTORY. Defining the natural history of thoracic aortic aneurysms has been challenging because both the etiology and the location of a thoracic aneurysm can affect its rate of growth and propensity for dissection or rupture. During the recent decades in which it has been routine to image aneurysms serially to document growth

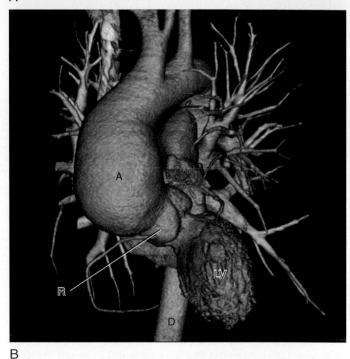

FIGURE 56–8 **A,** An axial contrast-enhanced computed tomography scan of the chest at the level of the right pulmonary artery demonstrating a 5.6 cm ascending thoracic aortic aneurysm (A).The descending aorta (D) is normal in caliber at 2.1 cm. Also evident is the main pulmonary artery (PA). **B,** A three-dimensional shaded-surface display of the same computed tomography scan. This anteroposterior projection demonstrates that the aneurysm (A) involves the ascending thoracic aorta and extends to the innominate artery. However, the aortic root (R) is spared and remains normal in diameter. The aortic arch vessels have a bovine configuration. Also evident is the left ventricle (LV).

and size, surgery has typically been performed when aneurysms have been large enough to be considered at high risk for rupture. Those patients whose large aneurysms have been managed without surgery are often elderly or have significant comorbidities, thereby increasing their mortality irrespective of the aneurysm.

Perhaps the best data currently available on the natural history of thoracic aortic aneurysms come from a longitudinal study recently reported from Yale-New Haven Hospital in which 304 patients with thoracic aortic aneurysms at least 3.5 cm in size were followed for a mean of more than 31 months.[43] The mean rate of growth for all thoracic aneurysms was 0.1 cm/yr. The rate of growth was significantly greater for aneurysms of the descending aorta (0.19 cm/yr), however, than for those of the ascending aorta (0.07 cm/yr). In addition, dissected thoracic aneurysms grew significantly more rapidly (0.14 cm/yr) than did nondissected ones (0.09 cm/yr), and patients with Marfan syndrome also had higher growth rates. The mean rate of rupture or dissection was only 2 percent per year for aneurysms less than 5 cm in diameter, rose slightly to 3 percent per year for aneurysms 5.0 to 5.9 cm, but increased sharply to 7 percent per year for aneurysms 6.0 cm or larger. In a multivariate logistic regression analysis of the predictors of dissection or rupture, the relative risk associated with an aneurysm diameter of 5.0 to 5.9 cm was 2.5; with an aneurysm diameter of 6.0 cm or larger, 5.2; with Marfan syndrome, 3.7; and with female gender, 2.9. In addition, concomitant vascular disease or abdominal aortic aneurysm were univariate predictors of both dissection/rupture and mortality. Other natural history studies focused on thoracic and thoracoabdominal aneurysms have found that the odds of rupture are increased by chronic obstructive pulmonary disease (COPD) (RR, 3.6), advanced age (RR, 2.6/decade), and aneurysm-related pain (RR, 2.3).

As with abdominal aneurysms, initial size is an important predictor of the rate of thoracic aneurysm growth. In one series of patients with thoracic aortic aneurysms followed by serial CT scanning or MRI, the mean linear expansion rate was 2.6 mm/year. The expansion rate correlated with baseline thoracic aneurysm diameter (i.e., aortic diameter <4.0 cm: 0.20 cm/yr; 4.0 to 4.9 cm: 0.23 cm/yr; 5.0 to 5.9 cm: 0.36 cm/yr; >6.0 cm: 0.56 cm/yr). Unfortunately, even when controlling for initial aneurysm size, substantial variation was still seen in individual aneurysm growth rates, thus rendering such mean growth rates of little value in predicting aneurysm growth for a given patient. Fortunately, it is rare that aneurysms 4.0 cm or smaller at baseline show rapid growth.

Rupture or acute dissection are the major complications of thoracic aortic aneurysms and can be fatal. Fewer than one half of patients with rupture may arrive at the hospital alive; mortality at 6 hours is 54 percent and at 24 hours reaches 76 percent.

Management

SURGICAL TREATMENT. The optimal timing of surgical repair of thoracic aortic aneurysms remains uncertain for several reasons. First, as noted earlier, the data available on the natural history of thoracic aneurysms are limited, especially with respect to the outcomes of surgical intervention. Second, with the high incidence of coexisting cardiovascular disease in this population, many patients die of other cardiovascular diseases before their aneurysms ever rupture. Significant risks are associated with thoracic aortic surgery, particularly in the arch and descending aorta, which in many cases may outweigh the potential benefits of aortic repair.

When aneurysms of the ascending thoracic aorta reach 5.5 cm or larger, and when aneurysms of the descending thoracic aorta reach 6.0 cm or larger, or perhaps 7.0 cm or larger in patients at high operative risk, surgery is recommended. Indications for surgery in patients with smaller aneurysms include a rapid rate of expansion, associated significant aortic regurgitation, or the presence of aneurysm-related symptoms. In patients with Marfan syndrome, bicuspid aortic valve, or a familial thoracic aortic aneurysm syndrome, given their higher risk of dissection and rupture, we often recommend repair of ascending thoracic aneurysms when they reach only 5.0 cm in size. Surgery can be considered even sooner (e.g., 4.5 cm) in Marfan syndrome patients at especially high risk, such as those with rapid and

progressive aortic dilation, those with a family history of Marfan syndrome plus aortic dissection, or women planning pregnancy. Finally, if patients require aortic valve replacement for a dysfunctional bicuspid valve, we recommend replacement of the ascending aorta if its diameter is 4 cm or larger, given that they are now recognized to be at high risk for postoperative aortic dissection. Of course, the aggressiveness with which surgical repair is undertaken in any case should be appropriately influenced by the general condition of the individual patient.

Cardiopulmonary bypass is necessary for the removal of ascending aortic aneurysms, and partial bypass to support the circulation distal to the aneurysm while the aortic site being repaired is cross-clamped is often advisable when resecting descending thoracic aortic aneurysms. Thoracic aortic aneurysms are generally resected and replaced with a prosthetic sleeve of appropriate size. The use of a composite graft consisting of a Dacron tube with a prosthetic aortic valve sewn into one end (known as a *composite aortic repair* or the *Bentall procedure*) is generally the method of choice in treating ascending thoracic aneurysms involving the root and associated with significant aortic regurgitation. The valve and graft are sewn directly into the aortic annulus, and the coronary arteries are then reimplanted into the Dacron aortic graft (Fig. 56-9). The operative risk for mortality ranges from 1 to 5 percent, depending on the patient population.[44] For patients with structurally normal aortic valve leaflets whose aortic regurgitation is secondary to dilatation of the root, it may be possible to repair the native valve either by reimplanting it within a Dacron graft or by remodeling of the aortic root. By avoiding valve replacement, it is expected that this procedure, when successful, will eliminate the long-term risks associated with a prosthetic valve and reduce the risk for repeat valve surgery. In a series by David and colleagues of 151 patients with aortic root aneurysms who underwent valve-sparing surgery, 67 percent had mild or no aortic regurgitation during the first 8 years of follow-up, with only 2 percent developing severe aortic regurgitation.[45]

When younger patients have a dilated aortic root but the aortic valve cannot be spared, an alternative to a composite aortic graft is a pulmonary autograft (the *Ross procedure*). This involves replacing the patient's native aortic valve and root with the patient's own pulmonary root, which is transplanted into the aortic position. The pulmonary root is then replaced with a cryopreserved homograft root. Another surgical alternative to a composite graft is the use of cryopreserved aortic allografts (cadaveric aortic root and proximal ascending aorta). However, these approaches are generally not favored because their durability is often limited by late autograft root dilation and late structural valvular deterioration, respectively.[46]

Aneurysms of the aortic arch can be successfully excised surgically, but the procedure remains particularly challenging. Neurological damage is a major cause of morbidity and mortality from aortic arch repair and typically results from embolization of atherosclerotic debris or as a consequence of global ischemic injury during antegrade circulatory arrest. The brachiocephalic vessels must be removed from the aortic arch before its resection and then reimplanted into the prosthetic tube graft arch after its interposition. Traditionally, the surgical procedure involved removing and then reimplanting the brachiocephalic vessels en bloc (i.e., as an island of native aortic tissue containing the three branch vessels), after which normal cerebral perfusion is restored. More recently, however, several novel surgical techniques have been introduced to reduce the hypothermic circulatory arrest times and embolic events by placing a multilimbed prosthetic arch graft, to which each arch vessel is, in turn, anastomosed individually (Fig. 56-10).

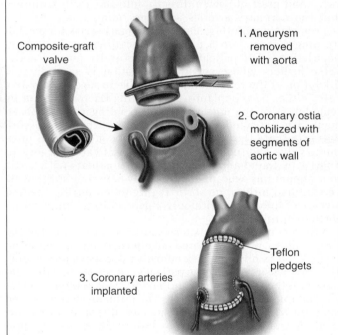

Giant aneurysm

Level of annulus

Composite-graft valve

1. Aneurysm removed with aorta

2. Coronary ostia mobilized with segments of aortic wall

3. Coronary arteries implanted

Teflon pledgets

FIGURE 56–9 Technique for the composite graft replacement of an aneurysm of the ascending aorta. **Top,** The aneurysm is shown involving the sinuses of Valsalva. The patient is maintained on total cardiopulmonary bypass. **Bottom,** The composite graft is shown, with a low-profile, tilting disc aortic prosthesis attached to its inferior end. (1) The aneurysm is resected with the native aortic valve. (2) The coronary ostia have been excised and mobilized with a button of aortic wall. (3) The composite graft has been secured in place with Teflon felt reinforcement for the suture line. The coronary artery ostia are then reimplanted directly into the graft.

Three methods of cerebral protection have been used for aortic arch surgery. The traditional method has been the use of profound hypothermic circulatory arrest with arrest of cerebral perfusion. The hypothermia is intended to reduce the cerebral metabolic rate by cooling to 10°C to 13°C. The simplicity of the technique, however, is offset by the high incidence of stroke and temporary neurological dysfunction. In 1990, the use of retrograde cerebral perfusion via a superior vena cava cannula was introduced as an adjunct for cerebral protection during hypothermic arrest. It was originally suggested that this technique would improve outcomes by providing nutrients and oxygen to the brain and to flush out both air and particulate matter from the cerebral and carotid arteries that would otherwise embolize. More

extensive studies have shown that there is, in fact, no metabolic benefit to the brain from retrograde cerebral perfusion, and several studies have shown no improvement in outcomes. More recently, the technique of selective antegrade cerebral perfusion has been introduced, in which perfusion cannulas inserted directly into the cerebral vessels allow perfusion of the brain through all but brief periods during the procedure. Indeed, the use of the multilimbed prosthetic aortic graft makes selective antegrade cerebral perfusion easier and more effective. This technique allows for a longer time of safe circulatory arrest, which is of greater importance in more complex arch procedures. Additional strategies have also been recently introduced, such as antegrade cerebral perfusion via cannulation of the right axillary or subclavian artery and the use of a trifurcated graft anastomosed to the brachiocephalic arteries.[47] The available data suggest that selective antegrade cerebral perfusion does not reduce the risk of stroke but does significantly reduce the incidence of temporary neurological dysfunction.[48] Historically, for aortic arch repair, the rates of mortality and stroke were as high as 6 to 20 percent and 4 to 11 percent, respectively, but with the use of these modern techniques in experienced hands, the rates are as low as 4 percent and 2 percent, respectively.[49]

Many of the patients undergoing surgical repair of a thoracic aortic aneurysm have multiple aortic segments involved. Such widespread aneurysmal dilatation of the aorta presents a particular challenge to the surgeon and often precludes surgery. Although it is possible to successfully replace virtually the entire diseased thoracic aorta, attempts to replace the ascending, arch, and descending thoracic aorta in one surgery carry increased risks. An alternative strategy is the use of a staged procedure, known as the "elephant trunk" technique, in which the ascending aorta and arch are replaced initially, whereas the descending aorta is replaced at a later date. Use of the elephant trunk technique has been shown to facilitate such extensive surgical procedures, yet operative mortality is as high as 12 percent.[50] A promising new staged hybrid approach has been recently introduced, which begins with an elephant trunk followed by endovascular stent-grafting (see later) to treat the descending thoracic aorta.[51] The outcomes of this technique are under investigation.

Elective surgical repair of ascending and descending thoracic aortic aneurysms in large centers is associated with mortality rates of 3 to 10 percent and 5 to 14 percent, respectively. Major complications include stroke and hemorrhage. A catastrophic complication of resection of descending thoracic aortic aneurysms is postoperative paraplegia secondary to interruption of the blood supply to the spinal cord. The incidence of paraplegia has been as high as 13 to 17 percent, but in most modern series is 5 to 6 percent. A number of methods have been proposed to reduce the likelihood of paraplegia, although none has proved to be consistently safe and effective. One of the more promising techniques involves regional hypothermic protection of the spinal cord with epidural cooling during surgical repair of the aorta, which has reduced the frequency of spinal cord complications to 3 percent (compared with a historical control of 20 percent) in one large series. The use of cerebrospinal fluid drainage was similarly shown to reduce the rate of paraplegia to 3 percent in a randomized trial by Coselli and colleagues.[52] Other important techniques that may also reduce the risk of spinal cord injury include the reimplantation of patent critical intercostal arteries, the use of intraoperative somatosensory- or motor-evoked potential monitoring, and maintenance of distal aortic perfusion during surgery with the use of atriofemoral (left heart) bypass to the distal aorta during the proximal anastomosis. Controlled trials might better clarify the efficacy of such techniques.

An alternative approach to the surgical management of descending thoracic aneurysms is the use of a transluminally placed endovascular stent-graft (see Chap. 59). This technique has the advantage of being far less invasive than surgery with potentially fewer postoperative complications and a lower morbidity rate. However, the aortic anatomy has to be favorable (adequate proximal and distal landing zones), so not all patients are reasonable candidates for stent-grafting. A recent multicenter prospective nonrandomized phase II study of the GORE TAG thoracic aortic endoprosthesis was conducted at 17 academic centers and enrolled 142 selected patients. Device implantation was successful in 98%. The 30-day event rates for stroke, temporary or permanent paraplegia, and death were 3 percent, 3 percent, and 2 percent, respectively, which were far lower than event rates in an open surgical control population.[53] The device has been recently approved for clinical use, and its use is rapidly growing. Unfortunately, the curvilinear nature of the ascending aorta and arch makes application of similar techniques to aneurysms of these proximal aortic segments far more challenging. Nevertheless, there are efforts to apply hybrid techniques to arch aneurysms as well, beginning with debranching the arch using a trifurcated graft from the ascending thoracic aorta to the brachioce-phalic arteries, followed by endovascular stent-grafting of the arch aneurysm.[54]

Complications of associated atherosclerosis, such as myocardial infarction, cerebrovascular accidents, and renal failure, often arise under the massive physiological stress of aortic surgery. The most frequent causes of early postoperative death are myocardial infarction, congestive heart failure, stroke, renal failure, hemorrhage, respiratory failure, and sepsis. Advanced age, emergency surgery, prolonged aortic cross-clamp time, extent of the aneurysm, diabetes, prior aortic surgery, aneurysm symptoms, and intraoperative hypotension are the most important factors determining perioperative morbidity and mortality. Many patients with atherosclerotic aneurysms are heavy smokers, and pulmonary complications following surgery are common. The left lung may be severely traumatized by compression during resection of large aneurysms of the descending thoracic aorta, a complication that can seriously jeopardize the patient's survival, particularly in the setting of underlying pulmonary disease.

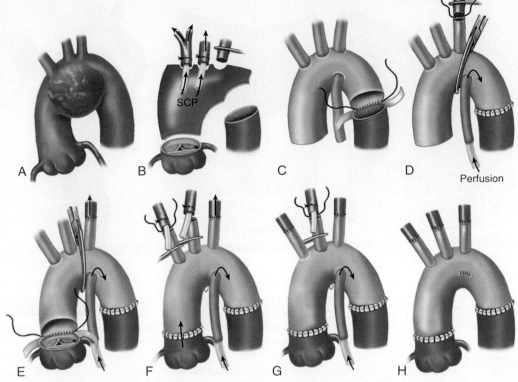

FIGURE 56–10 A-H, Surgical technique for total arch replacement with a branched aortic graft. Following initiation of circulatory arrest, the aneurysm is transected in the ascending aorta and where it meets the proximal descending aorta. The branched graft is anastomosed at its distal end. The graft proximal to the fourth limb is clamped and perfusion is restored through this limb to the distal circulation. The third limb is anastomosed to the left subclavian artery and flow to this vessel is restored. Then, the proximal end of the graft is anastomosed to the stump of the ascending aorta, flow is restored to the remaining arch vessels, and the fourth branch is then resected. *(Adapted from Kazui T, Washiyama N, Muhammad BAH, et al: Improved results of atherosclerotic arch aneurysm operations with a refined technique. J Thorac Cardiovasc Surg 121:491, 2001.)*

CH 56

Diseases of the Aorta

MEDICAL MANAGEMENT. The long-term impact of medical therapy on aneurysm growth and survival in patients with typical atherosclerotic thoracic aneurysms has not been examined. However, a study of the efficacy of beta blockers in adult patients with Marfan syndrome (see Chap. 8) found that therapy significantly slowed the rate of aortic dilatation, reduced adverse clinical endpoints (death, aortic dissection, aortic regurgitation, aortic root larger than 6 cm), and significantly lowered mortality. Although the study examined only the effect of beta blockade in patients with Marfan syndrome, it follows logically that medical therapy to reduce dP/dt and control blood pressure is essential to the treatment of thoracic aortic aneurysms, both for patients with smaller aneurysms being monitored serially and for patients who have undergone aortic aneurysm repair. There is also the possibility that losartan may slow the growth of aortic aneurysms in Marfan syndrome (see earlier); a randomized trial of losartan versus beta blockers is underway.

AORTIC DISSECTION

Acute aortic dissection is an uncommon but potentially catastrophic illness that occurs with an incidence of approximately 2.9/100,000/yr with at least 7000 cases per year in the United States.[55] Early mortality is as high as 1 percent per hour if untreated, but survival may be improved substantially by the timely institution of appropriate medical and/or surgical therapy. Prompt clinical recognition and definitive diagnostic testing are essential in the management of patients with aortic dissection.

Aortic dissection is believed to begin with the formation of a tear in the aortic intima that directly exposes an underlying diseased medial layer to the driving force (or pulse pressure) of intraluminal blood (Fig. 56-11A). This blood penetrates the diseased medial layer and cleaves the media longitudinally, thereby dissecting the aortic wall. Driven by persistent intraluminal pressure, the dissection process extends a variable length along the aortic wall, typically antegrade (driven by the forward force of aortic blood flow) but sometimes retrograde from the site of the intimal tear. The blood-filled space between the dissected layers of the aortic wall becomes the false lumen. Shear forces may lead to further tears in the intimal flap (the inner portion of the dissected aortic wall) and produce exit sites or additional entry sites for blood flow into the false lumen. Distention of the false lumen with blood may cause the intimal flap to bow into the true lumen and thereby narrow its caliber and distort its shape.

Alternatively, aortic dissection may begin with rupture of the vasa vasorum within the aortic media; that is, with the development of an intramural hematoma (see Fig. 56-11B). Local hemorrhage then secondarily ruptures through the intimal layer and creates the intimal tear and aortic dissection. Because in autopsy series as many as 13 percent of aortic dissections do not have an identifiable intimal tear, at least in a minority of cases independent medial hemorrhage does appear to be the primary cause of dissection. One might argue that the lack of an intimal tear in these patients indicates they do not, in fact, have classic aortic dissection but rather have intramural hematoma of the aorta, a closely related condition (see later).

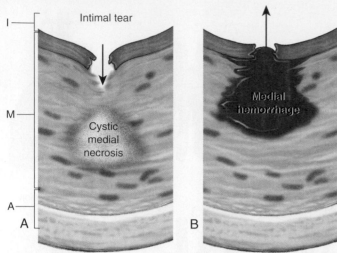

FIGURE 56–11 Proposed mechanisms of initiation of aortic dissection. A = adventitia; I = intima; M = media.

TABLE 56–1	Commonly Used Classification Systems to Describe Aortic Dissection
Type	**Site of Origin and Extent of Aortic Involvement**
DeBakey	
Type I	Originates in the ascending aorta, propagates at least to the aortic arch and often beyond it distally
Type II	Originates in and is confined to the ascending aorta
Type III	Originates in the descending aorta and extends distally down the aorta or, rarely, retrograde into the aortic arch and ascending aorta
Stanford	
Type A	All dissections involving the ascending aorta, regardless of the site of origin
Type B	All dissections not involving the ascending aorta
Descriptive	
Proximal	Includes DeBakey types I and II or Stanford type A
Distal	Includes DeBakey type III or Stanford type B

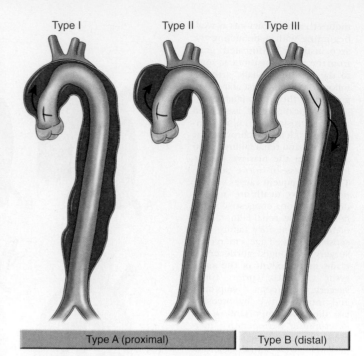

FIGURE 56–12 Commonly used classification systems for aortic dissection. *(Refer to Table 56-1 for definitions.)*

CLASSIFICATION. Most classification schemes for aortic dissection are based on the fact that the vast majority of aortic dissections originate in one of two locations: (1) the ascending aorta, within several centimeters of the aortic valve; and (2) the descending aorta, just distal to the origin of the left subclavian artery at the site of the ligamentum arteriosum. Sixty-five percent of intimal tears occur in the ascending aorta, 20 percent in the descending aorta, 10 percent in the aortic arch, and 5 percent in the abdominal aorta.

Three major classification systems are used to define the location and extent of aortic involvement, as defined in Table 56-1 and depicted in Figure 56-12: (1) DeBakey types I, II, and III; (2) Stanford types A and B; and (3) the anatomical categories "proximal" and "distal." All three schemes share the same basic principle of distinguishing aortic dissections with and without ascending aortic involvement for prognostic and therapeutic reasons; in general, surgery is indicated for dissections involving the ascending aorta, whereas medical management is reserved for dissections without ascending aortic involvement. Accordingly, because both DeBakey types I and II involve the ascending aorta, they are grouped together for simplicity in the Stanford (type A) and anatomical (proximal) classification systems, irrespective of the site of intimal tear. Less experienced clinicians will sometimes misclassify as type A those dis-

sections that begin in the aortic arch and progress distally, but because the ascending aorta is not involved, such cases should, in fact, be classified as type B. Aortic dissections confined to the abdominal aorta, although quite uncommon, are best categorized as type B or distal dissections. Proximal or type A dissections occur in about two thirds of cases, with distal dissections composing the remaining one third.

In addition to its location, aortic dissection is also classified according to its duration, defined as the length of time from symptom onset to medical evaluation. The mortality from dissection and its risk of progression decrease progressively over time, which makes therapeutic strategies for longstanding aortic dissections quite different from those seen acutely. A dissection present less than 2 weeks is defined as "acute," whereas those present 2 weeks or more are defined as "chronic" because the mortality curve for untreated aortic dissections begins to level off at 75 to 80 percent at 2 weeks. At diagnosis, the large majority of aortic dissections are acute.

ETIOLOGY AND PATHOGENESIS. Cystic medial degeneration, as described earlier, is the chief predisposing factor in aortic dissection. Therefore, any disease process or other condition that undermines the integrity of the elastic or muscular components of the media predisposes the aorta to dissection. Cystic medial degeneration is an intrinsic feature of several hereditary defects of connective tissue, most notably Marfan and Ehlers-Danlos (see Chap. 8) syndromes, and is also common among patients with bicuspid aortic valve. In addition to their propensity for thoracic aortic aneurysms, patients with Marfan syndrome are indeed at high risk for aortic dissection, especially proximal dissection, at a relatively young age. In fact, Marfan syndrome accounts for 5 percent of all aortic dissections.[56]

In the absence of Marfan syndrome, histologically classic cystic medial degeneration occurs in only a minority of cases of aortic dissection. Nevertheless, the degree of medial degeneration found in most other cases of aortic dissection still tends to be qualitatively and quantitatively much greater than expected as part of the aging process. Although the cause of such medial degeneration remains unclear, advanced age and hypertension appear to be two of the most important factors.

The peak incidence of aortic dissection is in the sixth and seventh decades of life, with men affected twice as often as women. About three quarters of patients with aortic dissection have a history of hypertension. A bicuspid aortic valve is a well-established risk factor for proximal aortic dissection and occurs in 5 to 7 percent of aortic dissections. As is the case with ascending thoracic aortic aneurysms, the risk of aortic dissection appears to be independent of the severity of the bicuspid valve stenosis. Certain other congenital cardiovascular abnormalities predispose the aorta to dissection, including coarctation of the aorta and Turner syndrome. Rarely, aortic dissection complicates arteritis involving the aorta (see Chap. 84), particularly giant cell arteritis. A number of reports describe aortic dissection in association with cocaine abuse, typically among young, black, and hypertensive men. However, cocaine abuse likely accounts for less than 1 percent of cases of aortic dissection and the mechanisms by which it causes dissection remain speculative.[57]

An unexplained relation exists between pregnancy and aortic dissection (see Chap. 77). About one-quarter of all aortic dissections in women younger than 40 years occur during pregnancy, typically in the third trimester and also occasionally in the early postpartum period. The increases in blood volume, cardiac output, and blood pressure seen in late pregnancy may contribute to the risk, although this explanation cannot account for postpartum occurrence. Women with Marfan syndrome and a dilated aortic root are at particular risk for acute aortic dissection during pregnancy, and in some cases, diagnosis of Marfan syndrome is first made when such women are evaluated for peripartum aortic dissection.

Direct trauma to the aorta may also cause aortic dissection. Blunt trauma tends to cause localized tears, hematomas, or frank aortic transection (see Chap. 71) and only rarely causes classic aortic dissection. Iatrogenic trauma is associated with true aortic dissection and accounts for 5 percent of cases.[58] Both intraarterial catheterization and the insertion of intraaortic balloon pumps may induce aortic dissection, probably from direct trauma to the aortic intima. Cardiac surgery also entails a very small risk (0.12 to 0.16 percent) of acute aortic dissection. The majority of these dissections are discovered intraoperatively and are repaired at that time, although 20 percent are detected only after a delay. In addition, aortic dissection sometimes occurs late (months to years) after cardiac surgery; in fact, as many as 18 percent of those with acute aortic dissection have had prior cardiac surgery. Of cardiac surgical patients, those undergoing aortic valve replacement have the highest risk for aortic dissection as a late complication. The association with aortic valve surgery may occur because many such patients had surgery to replace dysfunctional bicuspid aortic valves. As discussed earlier, cystic medial degeneration often accompanies this condition and can predispose them to subsequent dissection. This association argues for an aggressive approach in replacing even a mildly dilated ascending aorta at the time of bicuspid aortic valve replacement, as discussed earlier.

Clinical Manifestations

SYMPTOMS. Much of the data presented regarding the clinical manifestations of aortic dissection are from older clinical series, as well as from a more recent series from the International Registry of Acute Aortic Dissection (IRAD), which studied 464 consecutive patients with acute aortic dissection from 12 international referral centers.[56] By far, the most common initial symptom of acute aortic dissection

is pain, which is found in up to 96 percent of cases, whereas the large majority of those without pain are found to have chronic dissections. The pain is typically severe and of sudden onset and is as severe at its inception as it ever becomes, in contrast to the pain of myocardial infarction, which usually has a crescendo-like onset and is not as intense. In fact, the pain of aortic dissection may be all but unbearable in some instances and force the patient to writhe in agony, fall to the ground, or pace restlessly in an attempt to gain relief. Several features of the pain should arouse suspicion of aortic dissection. The quality of the pain as described by the patient is often morbidly appropriate to the actual event, with adjectives such as "tearing," "ripping," "sharp," and "stabbing" frequently used in more than one half the cases. In fact, it is not uncommon to hear descriptors that are collectively almost diagnostic of aortic dissection, but quite unlike the symptoms of myocardial ischemia or infarction, such as someone "stabbed me in the chest with a knife" or "hit me in the back with an ax."

Another important characteristic of the pain of aortic dissection is its tendency to migrate from its point of origin to other sites, generally following the path of the dissection as it extends through the aorta. However, such migratory pain is described in as few as 17 percent of cases. The location of pain may be quite helpful in suggesting the location of the aortic dissection because localized symptoms tend to reflect involvement of the underlying aorta. Spittell and colleagues found that when the location of chest pain was anterior only (or if the most severe pain was anterior), more than 90 percent of patients had involvement of the ascending aorta. Conversely, when the chest pain was interscapular only (or when the most severe pain was interscapular), more than 90 percent of patients had involvement of the descending thoracic aorta (i.e., DeBakey type I or III). The presence of any pain in the neck, throat, jaw, or face strongly predicted involvement of the ascending aorta, whereas pain anywhere in the back, abdomen, or lower extremities strongly predicted involvement of the descending aorta.[59] In rare cases, the presenting pain is only pleuritic in nature caused by acute pericarditis that results from hemorrhage into the pericardial space from the dissected ascending aorta. In such cases, the underlying diagnosis may be overlooked if one does not search for other symptoms or signs that might suggest the presence of aortic dissection.

Less common symptoms at initial evaluation, occurring with or without associated chest pain, include congestive heart failure (7 percent), syncope (13 percent), cerebrovascular accident (6 percent), ischemic peripheral neuropathy, paraplegia, and cardiac arrest or sudden death. The presence of acute congestive heart failure in this setting is almost invariably caused by severe aortic regurgitation induced by a proximal aortic dissection (discussed later). Patients with syncope have a higher rate of mortality than those without syncope and are more likely to have cardiac tamponade or stroke. However, when the complications of cardiac tamponade and stroke are excluded, syncope alone does not increase mortality.[60] On occasion, a patient presents with acute chest pain, and the initial imaging study reveals hemopericardium yet fails to demonstrate an aortic dissection. In such a scenario, unless another diagnosis, such as tumor metastatic to the pericardium, is evident, one must still suspect the presence of acute aortic dissection (or contained aortic rupture). Ideally, such a patient would be taken presumptively to the operating room or, at the very least, would immediately undergo additional imaging with other modalities to confirm the diagnosis.[61]

PHYSICAL FINDINGS. Although extremely variable, findings on physical examination generally reflect the location of aortic dissection and the extent of associated cardiovascular involvement. In some cases, physical findings alone may be sufficient to suggest the diagnosis, whereas in other cases, such pertinent physical findings may be subtle or absent, even in the presence of extensive aortic dissection. Hypertension is seen in 70 percent of patients with distal aortic dissection but in only 36 percent with proximal dissection. Hypotension, on the other hand, occurs much more commonly among those with proximal than those with distal aortic dissection (25 and 4 percent, respectively). True hypotension is usually the result of cardiac tamponade, acute severe aortic regurgitation, intrapleural rupture, or intraperitoneal rupture. Dissection involving the brachiocephalic vessels may result in pseudohypotension, an inaccurate measurement of blood pressure caused by compromise or occlusion of the brachial arteries.

The physical findings most typically associated with aortic dissection—pulse deficits, the murmur of aortic regurgitation, and neurological manifestations—are more characteristic of proximal than of distal dissection. Reduced or absent pulses in patients with acute chest pain strongly suggests the presence of aortic dissection. Such pulse abnormalities are present in about 30 percent of proximal aortic dissections and occur throughout the arterial tree, but occur in only 15 percent of distal dissections, where they usually involve the femoral or left subclavian artery. Impaired pulses, and similarly, visceral ischemia, result from extension of the dissection flap into a branch artery with compression of the true lumen by the false channel (Fig. 56-13), which diminishes blood flow in the aortic true lumen because of narrowing or obliteration by the distended false lumen (occurring most commonly in the descending or abdominal aorta); impaired pulses may also result from proximal obstruction of flow caused by a mobile portion of the intimal flap overlying the branch vessel's orifice. Whichever the cause, the pulse deficits in aortic dissection may be transient, secondary to decompression of the false lumen by distal reentry into the true lumen or secondary to movement of the intimal flap away from the occluded orifice.

Aortic regurgitation is an important feature of proximal aortic dissection, with the murmur of aortic regurgitation detected in one-third of cases. When present in patients with distal dissection, aortic regurgitation generally antedates the dissection and may be the result of preexisting dilation of the aortic root from the underlying aortic pathological condition, such as cystic medial degeneration. The murmur of aortic regurgitation may wax and wane, the intensity varying directly with the height of the arterial blood pressure. Depending on the severity of the regurgitation, other peripheral signs of aortic regurgitation may be present, such as collapsing pulses and a wide pulse pressure. In some cases, however, congestive heart failure secondary to severe acute aortic regurgitation may occur with little or no murmur and no peripheral signs of aortic runoff.

The acute aortic regurgitation associated with proximal aortic dissection, which occurs in one half to two thirds of such cases, may result from any of several mechanisms (Fig. 56-14). First, the dissection may dilate the aortic root, thereby widening the sinotubular junction from which the aortic leaflets hang so that the leaflets are unable to coapt properly in diastole (incomplete closure). Second, the dissection may extend into the aortic root and detach one or more aortic leaflets from their commissural attachments at the sinotubular junction, thereby resulting in diastolic leaflet prolapse. Not infrequently, both incomplete closure and leaflet prolapse are present at the same time. Finally, in the setting of an extensive or circumferential intimal tear the unsupported intimal flap may prolapse into the left ventricular outflow tract, occasionally appearing as frank intimal intussusception, and produce severe aortic regurgitation.

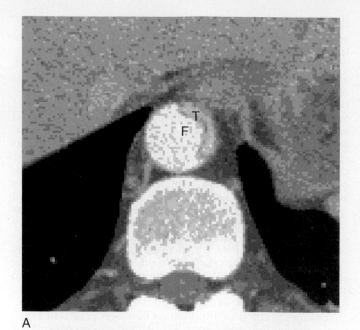

A

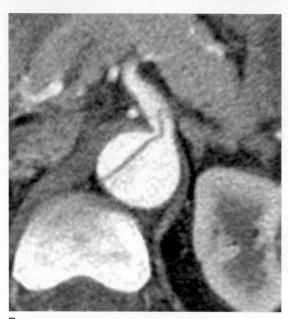

B

FIGURE 56–13 Mechanisms of compromised perfusion of branch arteries due to aortic dissection. **A,** The branch artery still originates from the true lumen, but the true lumen (T) is markedly compressed by the false lumen (F) throughout the cardiac cycle, resulting in low pressure and reduced flow within the true lumen and its branches. **B,** The intimal flap of the aortic dissection extends into the ostium of a branch artery, potentially narrowing or obstructing it.

Neurological manifestations occur in as many as 6 to 19 percent of all aortic dissections and accompany proximal dissection more frequently. Cerebrovascular accidents may occur in 3 to 6 percent when the innominate or left common carotid arteries are directly involved. Less often, patients may have altered consciousness or even coma. When spinal artery perfusion is compromised, ischemic spinal cord damage may produce paraparesis or paraplegia.

In a small minority, about 1 to 2 percent of cases, a proximal dissection flap may involve the ostium of a coronary artery and cause acute myocardial infarction. Because most proximal dissections arise above the right sinus of Valsalva, retrograde extension into the aortic root more often affects the right coronary artery than the left, which explains why

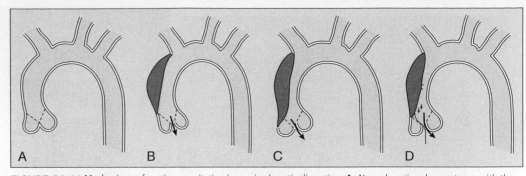

FIGURE 56–14 Mechanisms of aortic regurgitation in proximal aortic dissection. **A,** Normal aortic valve anatomy, with the leaflets suspended (dotted lines) from the sinotubular junction. **B,** A type A dissection dilates the ascending aorta, which in turn widens the sinotubular junction from which the aortic leaflets hang so that the leaflets are unable to coapt properly in diastole (incomplete closure). Aortic regurgitation (arrow) results. **C,** A type A dissection extends into the aortic root and detaches an aortic leaflet from its commissural attachment to the sinotubular junction. Diastolic leaflet prolapse results. **D,** In the setting of an extensive or circumferential intimal tear, the unsupported intimal flap may prolapse across the aortic valve and into the left ventricular outflow tract and prevent normal leaflet coaptation.

these myocardial infarctions tend to be inferior in location. Unfortunately, when secondary myocardial infarction does occur, its symptoms may complicate the clinical picture by obscuring symptoms of the primary aortic dissection. Most worrisome is the possibility that in the setting of electrocardiographic evidence of myocardial infarction, the underlying aortic dissection may go unrecognized. Moreover, the consequences of such a misdiagnosis in the era of thrombolytic therapy can be catastrophic, with an early mortality rate of 71 percent (many from cardiac tamponade) among patients with aortic dissection treated with thrombolysis. It remains essential that when evaluating patients with acute myocardial infarction, particularly inferior infarctions, one carefully considers the possibility of an underlying aortic dissection before thrombolytic or anticoagulant therapy is instituted. Although some physicians feel reassured that performing a chest radiograph before the institution of thrombolysis is adequate to exclude the diagnosis of dissection, studies have shown it is not sufficient.

Extension of aortic dissection into the abdominal aorta can cause other vascular complications. Compromise of one or both renal arteries occurs in about 5 to 8 percent and can lead to renal ischemia or frank infarction and, eventually, severe hypertension and acute renal failure. Mesenteric ischemia and infarction—occasional and potentially lethal complications of abdominal dissection—occur in 3 to 5 percent of cases. In addition, aortic dissection may extend into the iliac arteries and cause diminished femoral pulses (12 percent) and acute lower extremity ischemia. If in such cases the associated chest pain is minimal or absent, the absent pulse and ischemic peripheral neuropathy may be mistaken for a peripheral embolic event.

Additional clinical manifestations of aortic dissection include the presence of small pleural effusions, seen more commonly on the left side. The effusion typically arises secondary to an inflammatory reaction around the involved aorta, but in some cases larger effusions may result from hemothorax caused by a transient rupture or leak from a descending dissection. Several rarely encountered clinical manifestations of aortic dissection include hoarseness, upper airway obstruction, rupture into the tracheobronchial tree with hemoptysis, dysphagia, hematemesis from rupture into the esophagus, superior vena cava syndrome, pulsating neck masses, Horner syndrome, and unexplained fever. Other rare findings associated with the presence of a continuous murmur include rupture of the aortic dissection into the right atrium, into the right ventricle, or into the left atrium with secondary congestive heart failure. A variety of conditions can mimic aortic dissection, including myocardial infarction or ischemia, pericarditis, pulmonary embolism, acute aortic regurgitation without dissection, nondissecting thoracic or abdominal aortic aneurysms, or mediastinal tumors.

Because of the variable extent of aortic, branch vessel, and cardiac involvement occurring with aortic dissection, the signs and symptoms associated with the condition occur sporadically. Consequently, the presence or absence of aortic dissection cannot be diagnosed accurately in most cases on the basis of symptoms and clinical findings alone. In one series, of all aortic dissections (without a known diagnosis), the initial clinical diagnosis was aortic dissection in only 62 percent, and the other 38 percent of patients were initially thought to have myocardial ischemia, congestive heart failure, nondissecting aneurysms of the thoracic or abdominal aorta, symptomatic aortic stenosis, pulmonary embolism, and so on. Among this 38 percent in whom aortic dissection went undiagnosed at initial evaluation, nearly two thirds of patients had their aortic dissection detected incidentally while undergoing a diagnostic procedure for other clinical questions, and in nearly one third, the aortic dissection remained undiagnosed until necropsy. Given the clinical challenge that detection of aortic dissection presents, physicians should remain vigilant for any risk factors, symptoms, and signs consistent with aortic dissection if a timely diagnosis is to be made.

LABORATORY FINDINGS. Chest radiography is included in the discussion of clinical manifestations of aortic dissection rather than the discussion of diagnostic techniques because an abnormal incidental finding on a routine chest radiograph may first raise clinical suspicion of aortic dissection (Fig. 56-15). Moreover, although chest radiography may help support a diagnosis of suspected aortic dissection, the findings are nonspecific and rarely diagnostic. The results of chest radiography therefore add to the other available clinical data used in deciding whether suspicion of aortic dissection warrants proceeding to a more definitive diagnostic study.

The most common abnormality seen on a chest radiograph in cases of aortic dissection is widening of the aortic silhouette, which appears in 81 to 90 percent of cases. Less often, nonspecific widening of the superior mediastinum is seen. If calcification of the aortic knob is present, separation of the intimal calcification from the outer aortic soft tissue border by more than 1.0 cm—the "calcium sign"—is suggestive, although not diagnostic, of aortic dissection. Comparison of the current chest radiograph with a previous study may reveal acute changes in the aortic or mediastinal silhouettes that would otherwise have gone unrecognized. Pleural effusions are common, typically occur on the left side, and are more often associated with dissection involving the descending aorta. Although the majority of patients with aortic dissection have one or more of these radiographic abnormalities, the remainder, up to 12 percent, have chest radiographs that appear unremarkable. Therefore, a normal chest radiograph can never exclude the presence of aortic dissection.

Electrocardiographic findings in patients with aortic dissection are nonspecific. One third of electrocardiograms show changes consistent with left ventricular hypertrophy,

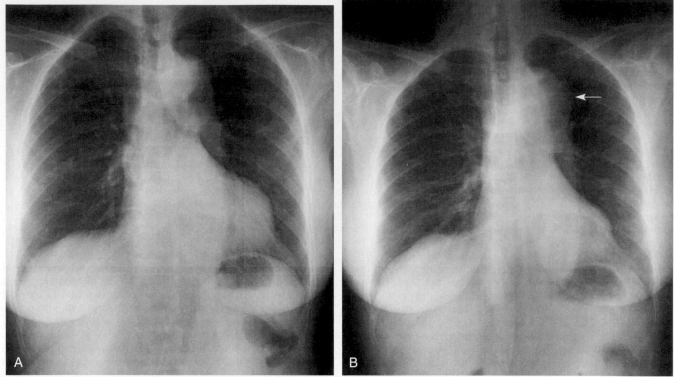

FIGURE 56–15 Chest radiograph of a patient with aortic dissection. **A,** The patient's baseline study from 3 years prior to admission, with a normal-appearing aorta. **B,** The chest radiograph on admission, which is remarkable for the interval enlargement of the aortic knob (arrow). The patient was found to have a proximal aortic dissection. *(From Isselbacher EM: Aortic dissection. In Creager MA [ed]: Atlas of Vascular Disease. 2nd ed. Philadelphia, Current Medicine, 2003.)*

whereas another one third are normal. Nevertheless, obtaining an electrocardiogram is diagnostically important for two reasons: (1) in cases of aortic dissection, nonspecific chest pain and the absence of ischemic ST segment and T wave abnormalities on electrocardiogram may argue against the diagnosis of myocardial ischemia and thereby prompt consideration of other chest pain syndromes, including aortic dissection, and (2) in patients with proximal dissection, the electrocardiogram may reveal acute myocardial infarction when the dissection flap has involved a coronary artery.

Currently, there are no reliable biomarkers that are diagnostic of aortic dissection, although a number or markers are under investigation. However, recent studies have shown that a markedly elevated D-dimer level may indicate acute aortic dissection. In a series comparing 94 consecutive patients with aortic dissection and 94 controls, a D-dimer of >400 ng/ml had a sensitivity of 99 percent and a specificity of 34 percent. Moreover, D-dimer levels correlated with the anatomical extent of the dissection and with in-hospital mortality.[62] This suggests that D-dimer levels may be useful as a screening test in the emergency department, with elevated levels prompting at least clinical consideration, if not diagnostic investigation, of possible aortic dissection.

Diagnostic Techniques

Once suspected on clinical grounds, it is essential to confirm the diagnosis of aortic dissection both promptly and accurately. The modalities currently available for this purpose include aortography, contrast-enhanced CT, MRI, and TTE or TEE. Each modality has certain advantages and disadvantages with respect to diagnostic accuracy, speed, convenience, risk, and cost, but none is appropriate in all situations.

When comparing the four imaging modalities, one must begin by considering what diagnostic information is needed. First and foremost, the study must confirm or refute the diagnosis of aortic dissection. Second, it must determine whether the dissection involves the ascending aorta (i.e., proximal or type A) or is confined to the descending aorta or arch (i.e., distal or type B). Third, if possible, it should identify a number of the anatomical features of the dissection, including its extent, the sites of entry and reentry, the presence of thrombus in the false lumen, branch vessel involvement by the dissection, the presence and severity of aortic regurgitation, the presence or absence of pericardial effusion, and any coronary artery involvement by the intimal flap. Unfortunately, no single imaging modality provides all of this anatomical detail. The choice of diagnostic modalities should, therefore, be guided by the clinical scenario and by targeting information that will best assist in patient management.

AORTOGRAPHY. Retrograde aortography was the first accurate diagnostic technique for evaluating suspected aortic dissection. The diagnosis of aortic dissection is based on direct angiographic signs, including visualization of two lumina or an intimal flap (considered diagnostic), as in Figure 56-16, or on indirect signs (considered suggestive), such as deformity of the aortic lumen, thickening of the aortic walls, branch vessel abnormalities, and aortic regurgitation.

Aortography had long been considered the diagnostic standard for the evaluation of aortic dissection because for several decades it was the only accurate method of diagnosing aortic dissection antemortem, although its true sensitivity could not be defined. However, the more recent introduction of alternative diagnostic modalities has shown that aortography is not as sensitive as previously thought. Prospective studies have found that for the diagnosis of

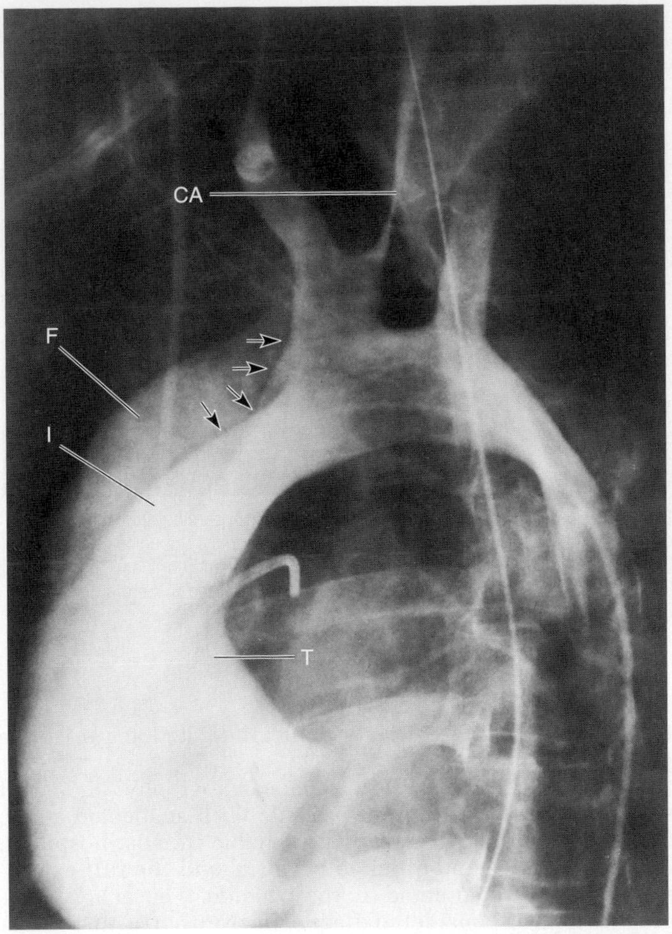

FIGURE 56–16 Aortogram in the left oblique view demonstrating proximal aortic dissection and its associated cardiovascular complications. The true lumen (T) and false lumen (F) are separated by the intimal flap (I), which is faintly visible as a radiolucent line following the contour of the pigtail catheter. The true lumen is better opacified than the false lumen, and two planes of the intimal flap can be distinguished (arrows). The branch vessels are opacified, along with marked narrowing of the right carotid artery (CA), which suggests that its lumen is compromised by the dissection. (From Isselbacher EM: Aortic dissection. In Creager MA [ed.]: Atlas of Vascular Disease. 2nd ed. Philadelphia, Current Medicine, 2003.)

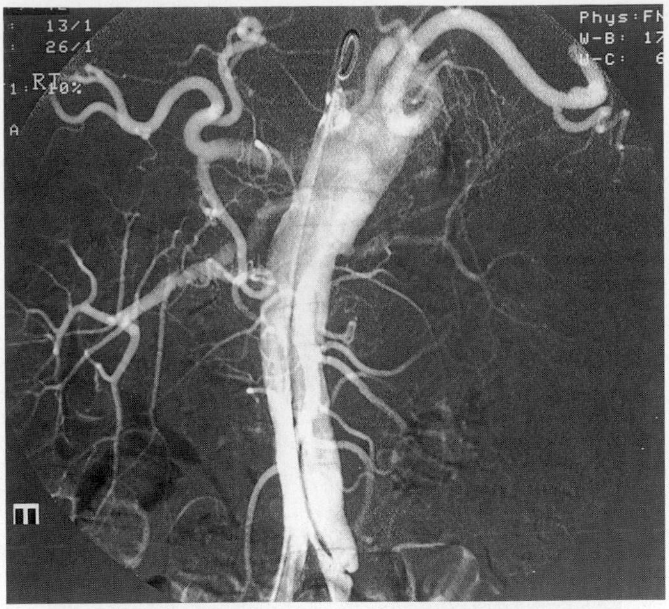

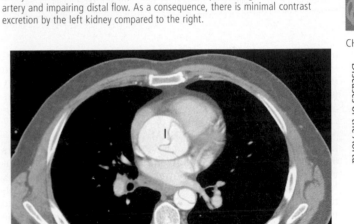

FIGURE 56–17 Digital subtraction angiogram of the abdominal aorta, in a patient with a distal thoracic aortic dissection, to assess the status of renal perfusion. This study confirmed the presence of an intimal flap extending down into the left common iliac artery. The celiac axis, superior mesenteric artery, and right renal artery are widely patent and fill from the true lumen. The left renal artery fills from the false lumen, with the intimal flap involving the ostium of the artery and impairing distal flow. As a consequence, there is minimal contrast excretion by the left kidney compared to the right.

FIGURE 56–18 Computed tomography (CT) for diagnosing aortic dissection. Shown is a contrast-enhanced spiral CT scan of the chest at the level of the right pulmonary artery showing an intimal flap (I) in both the ascending and descending thoracic aorta separating the two lumina in a type B aortic dissection. (Reprinted with permission from Isselbacher EM: Aortic dissection. In Creager MA [ed]: Atlas of Vascular Disease. 2nd ed. Philadelphia, Current Medicine, 2003.)

aortic dissection, the sensitivity of aortography is 88 percent and falls to only 77 percent when the definition of aortic dissection includes intramural hematoma with noncommunicating dissection. The specificity of aortography is 94 percent. False-negative aortograms occur because of thrombosis of the false lumen, equal and simultaneous opacification of both the true and false lumina, or the presence of an intramural hematoma.

Important advantages of aortography include its ability to delineate the extent of the aortic dissection, including branch vessel involvement (Fig. 56-17). It is also useful in detecting some of the major complications of aortic dissection, such as the presence of aortic regurgitation, and is often useful in revealing patency of the coronary arteries. In addition to the limited sensitivity of aortography, other disadvantages are the inherent risks of the invasive procedure, the risks associated with the use of contrast material, and the time needed to complete the study, both in assembling an angiography team and the long duration of the procedure. Finally, aortography requires that potentially unstable patients travel to the angiography suite.

COMPUTED TOMOGRAPHY. In contrast-enhanced CT scanning, aortic dissection is diagnosed by the presence of two distinct aortic lumina, either visibly separated by an intimal flap (Fig. 56-18) or distinguished by a differential rate of contrast opacification. Spiral (helical) CT scanning, which is now used routinely, permits three-dimensional display of the aorta and its branches (Fig. 56-19) and has improved the accuracy of CT in diagnosing aortic dissection, as well as in defining anatomical features. Several series have found that spiral CT scanning has both a sensitivity and specificity for acute aortic dissection of 96 to 100 percent (see Chap. 18).

Computed tomography scanning has the advantage that, unlike aortography, it is noninvasive, although it does require the use of an intravenous contrast agent. Most hospitals are equipped with a readily accessible CT scanner

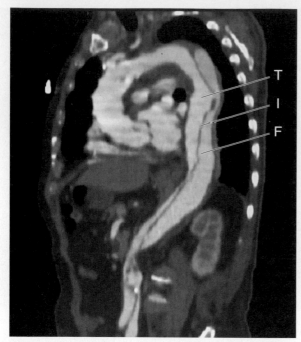

FIGURE 56–19 Computed tomography (CT) for diagnosing aortic dissection. Shown is a contrast-enhanced spiral CT scan of the chest at the level of the pulmonary artery showing an intimal flap (I) in the descending thoracic aorta separating the two lumina in a type B aortic dissection. F = false lumen; T = true lumen.

CH 56

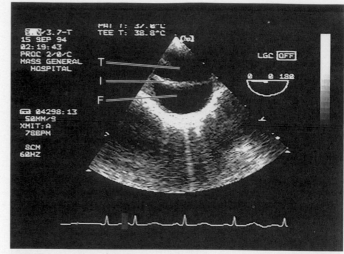

FIGURE 56–20 Cross-sectional transesophageal echocardiogram of the descending thoracic aorta demonstrating aortic dissection. The aorta is dilated. Evident is an intimal flap (I) dividing the true lumen (T) anteriorly and the false lumen (F) posteriorly. The true lumen fills during systole and is therefore seen bowing slightly into the false lumen in this systolic image.

available on an emergency basis. CT is also helpful in identifying the presence of thrombus in the false lumen and in detecting pericardial effusion. The use of CT angiography (three-dimensional reconstruction of axial CT data) permits assessment of branch vessel compromise in both the thoracic and abdominal segments.

MAGNETIC RESONANCE IMAGING. MRI has particular appeal for diagnosing aortic dissection because it is entirely noninvasive and does not require the use of intravenous contrast material or ionizing radiation. Furthermore, MRI produces high-quality images in the transverse, sagittal, and coronal planes, as well as in a left anterior oblique view that displays the entire thoracic aorta in one plane (see Chap. 17). The availability of these multiple views facilitates the diagnosis of aortic dissection and determination of its extent and in many cases reveals the presence of branch vessel involvement.

Magnetic resonance imaging has both a sensitivity and a specificity of approximately 98 percent. Furthermore, use of the cine-MRI technique in a subset of these patients showed 85 percent sensitivity for detecting aortic regurgitation. Intravenous administration of gadolinium yields a magnetic resonance angiogram, which defines the patency of aortic branch vessels. Still, MRI does have a number of disadvantages. It is contraindicated in patients with pacemakers or implantable defibrillators and certain types of vascular clips. MRI provides only limited images of branch vessels (unless gadolinium is used) and does not consistently identify the presence of aortic regurgitation. In most hospitals, magnetic resonance scanners are not readily available on an emergency basis. Many patients with aortic dissection are hemodynamically unstable, often intubated or receiving intravenous antihypertensive medications with arterial pressure monitoring, but magnetic resonance scanners limit the presence of many monitoring and support devices in the imaging suite and also limit patient accessibility during the lengthy study. Understandably, concern for the safety of unstable patients has led many physicians to conclude that

the use of MRI is relatively contraindicated for unstable patients.

ECHOCARDIOGRAPHY. Echocardiography is well suited for the evaluation of patients with suspected aortic dissection because it is readily available in most hospitals, it is noninvasive and quick to perform, and the full examination can be completed at the bedside. The echocardiographic finding considered diagnostic of an aortic dissection is the presence of an undulating intimal flap within the aortic lumen that separates the true and false channels. Reverberations and other artifacts can cause linear echodensities within the aortic lumen that mimic aortic dissection. To distinguish an intimal flap definitively from such artifacts, the flap should be identified in more than one view, it should have motion independent of that of the aortic walls or other cardiac structures, and a differential in color Doppler flow patterns should be noted between the two lumina. In cases in which the false lumen is thrombosed, displacement of intimal calcification or thickening of the aortic wall may suggest aortic dissection.

TRANSTHORACIC ECHOCARDIOGRAPHY. Transthoracic echocardiography has a sensitivity of 59 to 85 percent and a specificity of 63 to 96 percent for the diagnosis of aortic dissection. Such poor sensitivity significantly limits the general usefulness of this technique. Furthermore, image quality is often adversely affected by obesity, emphysema, mechanical ventilation, or small intercostal spaces.

TRANSESOPHAGEAL ECHOCARDIOGRAPHY. The proximity of the esophagus to the aorta enables TEE to overcome many of the limitations of transthoracic imaging and permits the use of higher frequency ultrasonography, which provides better anatomical detail (Figs. 56-20 and 56-21). The examination is generally performed at the bedside with the patient under sedation or light general anesthesia and typically requires 10 to 15 minutes to complete. The procedure does not require arterial access nor intravenous contrast or ionizing radiation. Relative contraindications include known esophageal disease such as strictures or tumors. The incidence of important side effects (such as hypertension, bradycardia, bronchospasm, or rarely, esophageal perforation) is much less than 1 percent. One important disadvantage of TEE is its limited ability to visualize the distal ascending aorta and proximal arch because of interposition of the air-filled trachea and main stem bronchus.

The results of large prospective studies have demonstrated that the sensitivity of TEE for aortic dissection is 98 to 99 percent, whereas the sensitivity for detecting an intimal tear (Fig. 56-22) is 73 percent. TEE detects both aortic regurgitation and pericardial effusion in 100 percent of cases. The specificity of TEE for the diagnosis of aortic dissection is less well defined but is likely in the range of 94 to 97 percent. Among patients with suspected aortic dissection, the diagnosis is excluded in as many as two thirds of cases, which yields a group of patients with a chest pain syndrome of unknown origin. Among patients determined not to have aortic dissection, TEE identifies alternative cardiovascular diagnoses (e.g., other aortic abnormalities or evidence of acute myocardial infarction or ischemia) in 66 to 73 percent.

Selecting an Imaging Modality

Each of the four imaging modalities has particular advantages and disadvantages. In selecting among them, one must consider the accuracy as well as the safety and availability of each test. Given their extremely high sensitivity and specificity and ability to provide three-dimensional images, CT angiography and MRA are considered the current standards for evaluating aortic dissection. The four imaging modalities described earlier differ in their ability to detect complications associated with dissection, so the specific diagnostic information sought by the treating physician and/or surgeon should have a bearing on the procedure chosen.

Both the accessibility of imaging studies and the time required to complete them are key considerations, given the high rate of early mortality associated with unoperated proximal aortic dissection. Aortography can be performed only rarely on an emergency basis, because it often requires assembly of an angiography team and is subject to the risks associated with an invasive procedure and use of a contrast agent. MRI is also generally unavailable on an emergency basis and poses the risk of limited patient monitoring and accessibility during the lengthy procedure. CT scanning is

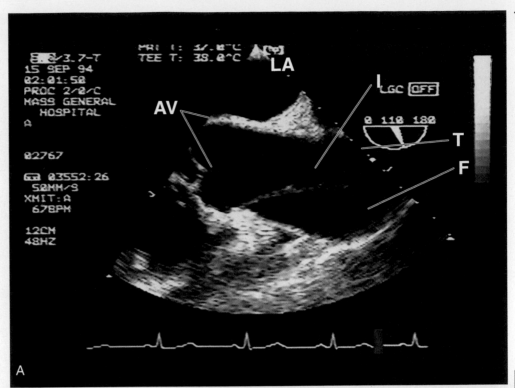

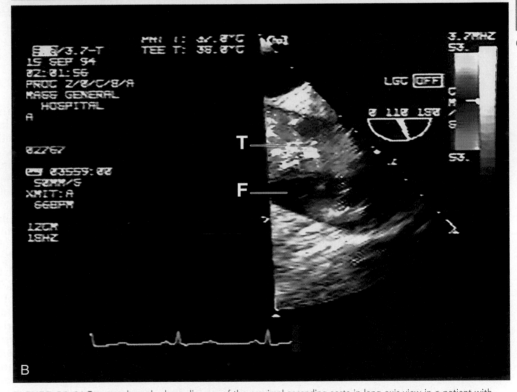

FIGURE 56–21 Transesophageal echocardiogram of the proximal ascending aorta in long-axis view in a patient with proximal aortic dissection. **A,** The left atrium (LA) is closest to the transducer. The aortic valve (AV) is seen on the left in this view, with the ascending aorta extending to the right. Within the proximal aorta is an intimal flap (I) that originates just at the level of the sinotubular junction above the right sinus of Valsalva. The true lumen (T) and the false lumen (F) are separated by the intimal flap. **B,** The addition of color flow Doppler in the same view confirms the presence of two distinct lumina. The true lumen (T) fills completely with brisk blood flow (bright blue color), simultaneously, minimal retrograde flow (dark orange) is seen in the false lumen (F).

more readily available in most emergency departments and is quickly completed. TEE is also readily available in most larger centers and can be completed quickly at the bedside, which makes it ideal for evaluating unstable patients. Among the centers in the IRAD, CT was used most often (63

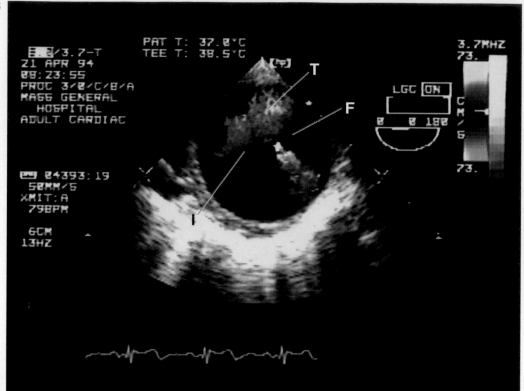

FIGURE 56-22 Cross-sectional transesophageal echocardiogram of a descending aortic dissection demonstrating a site of intimal tear. Blood flow (in orange) is evident in the true lumen (T) during systole, while a narrow jet of high-velocity blood (in blue) crosses into the false lumen (F) through a tear in the intimal flap (I).

whereas others are content to assess the coronary arteries intraoperatively. Two types of coronary artery involvement must be considered in the setting of aortic dissection. The first is acute proximal coronary narrowing or occlusion as a result of the dissection itself, often caused by occlusion of the coronary ostia by the intimal flap. The second is the possible presence of chronic atherosclerotic coronary artery disease, which, although generally independent of the dissection process, may complicate its surgical management.

In some cases, coronary involvement by the intimal flap is self-evident if the electrocardiogram shows evidence of acute myocardial ischemia or infarction. Should this acute process not be clinically evident, however, TEE can effectively define the patency of the proximal coronary arteries in a majority of cases. Aortography may also reveal such coronary artery involvement. More comprehensive evaluation requires the performance of coronary angiography; however, this study may be risky in patients with aortic dissection and often prolongs the time to aortic repair by several hours. Moreover, catheterization of the coronary arteries is sometimes unsuccessful in patients with proximal dissection and a dilated root, in which case the added procedural delay offers no potential benefit. In addition, such proximal coronary obstructions can usually be readily identified at the time of surgery.

Chronic coronary artery disease is seen in about one fourth of patients with aortic dissection. Identifying the presence of this underlying coronary disease is beyond the capability of any of the four imaging modalities discussed earlier. The impact of unrecognized coronary artery disease on outcome is not certain. Among patients in whom unrecognized coronary artery disease was discovered at autopsy, none died of coronary ischemia but several died of aortic rupture in one series. Moreover, in 122 consecutive patients undergoing emergency aortic repair, patients who had preoperative angiography and those who did not had similar in-hospital mortality.[64] Accordingly, we and others recommend avoiding preoperative coronary angiography unless a specific indication exists, such as a known history of coronary artery disease, prior coronary artery bypass grafting, or the presence of ischemic electrocardiographic changes. Conversely, others have reported good outcomes when performing combined aortic repair and coronary artery bypass grafting in patients with underlying coronary artery disease and, therefore, argue that all stable patients with acute proximal dissection should undergo preoperative coronary angiography. While the debate continues unresolved, the trend in the literature has been a retreat from the routine performance of coronary angiography in cases of acute aortic dissection.

percent) as the imaging study of first choice, with TEE performed first about half as often (32 percent).[63] Aortography and MRI were rarely used as the initial imaging modality (4 percent and 1 percent, respectively).

In a setting in which all these imaging modalities are available, CT should be considered first in the evaluation of suspected aortic dissection in light of its accuracy, safety, speed, and convenience. When CT identifies a type A aortic dissection, the patient may be taken directly to the operating room, where TEE can then be performed to assess the anatomy and competence of the aortic valve without unduly delaying surgery. However, in cases of suspected aortic dissection in which aortic valve disease is suspected or the patient is unstable, TEE may be the initial procedure of choice.

Despite its relative disadvantages, aortography still plays an important role when clear definition of the anatomy of the branch vessels is essential for management. Aortography should also be considered when a definitive diagnosis is not made by one or more of the other imaging modalities.

In the final analysis, each institution must determine its own best diagnostic approach to the evaluation of suspected aortic dissection and base it on available human and material resources and the speed with which they can be mobilized. The level of skill and experience of those who carry out each diagnostic procedure should also enter into the choice of diagnostic modality.

The Role of Coronary Angiography

The importance of assessing the status of coronary artery patency before surgical repair of acute aortic dissection continues to be controversial. Some surgeons believe that obtaining this information before surgery is essential,

Management

Therapy for aortic dissection aims to halt progression of the dissecting hematoma because lethal complications arise not from the intimal tear itself but rather from the subsequent course taken by the dissecting aorta, such as vascular compromise or aortic rupture. Without treatment, aortic dissection has a high mortality rate. In a collective review of long-term survival in patients with untreated aortic dissection, more than 25 percent of all patients died within the first 24 hours after the onset of dissection, more than 50 percent died within the first week, more than 75 percent died within 1 month, and more than 90 percent died within 1 year.

Definitive surgical therapy was pioneered by DeBakey and colleagues in the early 1950s. Its purpose is to excise the intimal tear, obliterate the false channel by oversewing the aortic edges, reconstitute the aorta directly or with the interposition of a synthetic graft, and in the case of proximal dissection, restore aortic valve competence either by resuspension of the displaced aortic leaflets or by prosthetic aortic valve replacement.

Aggressive medical treatment of aortic dissection was first advocated by Wheat and colleagues in the 1960s. The authors established reduction of systolic blood pressure and diminution of the rate of left ventricular ejection (dP/dt) as the two primary goals of pharmacological therapy. Originally introduced for patients too ill to withstand surgery, medical therapy is now the initial treatment for virtually all patients with aortic dissection before definitive diagnosis and furthermore serves as the primary long-term therapy in a subset of patients, particularly those with distal dissections.

Immediate Medical Management

All patients strongly suspected of having acute aortic dissection should immediately be placed in an acute care setting for hemodynamic stabilization and monitoring of blood pressure, cardiac rhythm, and urine output. An arterial line should be placed, preferably in the right arm so that it remains functional during surgery when the aorta is cross-clamped. However, in cases in which the blood pressure on the left exceeds that on the right, the arterial line should be placed on the left. In patients with a lower likelihood of dissection who are hemodynamically stable, an automatic blood pressure cuff should suffice.

BLOOD PRESSURE REDUCTION. Initial therapeutic goals include the elimination of pain and reduction of systolic blood pressure to 100 to 120 mm Hg (mean of 60 to 75 mm Hg) or the lowest level commensurate with adequate vital organ (cardiac, cerebral, renal) perfusion. Beta-blocking agents should be administered simultaneously, regardless of whether pain or systolic hypertension is present. The use of long-acting medications should be avoided in patients who are surgical candidates because they may complicate intraoperative arterial pressure management. Pain, which may itself exacerbate hypertension and tachycardia, should be promptly treated with intravenous morphine sulfate.

For the acute reduction of arterial pressure, the potent vasodilator sodium nitroprusside is effective. It is initially infused at 20 µg/min with the dosage titrated upward, as high as 800 µg/min, according to the blood pressure response. When used alone, however, sodium nitroprusside can actually cause an increase in dP/dt, which in turn may potentially contribute to propagation of the dissection. Therefore, concomitant beta-blocking treatment is essential. For those patients with acute or chronic renal insufficiency, intravenous fenoldopam may be preferable to sodium nitroprusside.

To reduce dP/dt acutely, an intravenous beta blocker should be administered in incremental doses until evidence of satisfactory beta blockade is noted, usually indicated by a heart rate of 60 to 80 beats/min in the acute setting. Because propranolol was the first generally available beta blocker, it has been used most widely in treating aortic dissection. However, it is believed that other noncardioselective beta blockers are equally effective. Propranolol should be administered in intravenous doses of 1 mg every 3 to 5 minutes until the desired effect is achieved, although the maximum initial dose should not exceed 0.15 mg/kg (or approximately 10 mg). To maintain adequate beta blockade, as evidenced by the heart rate, additional propranolol should be given intravenously every 4 to 6 hours, or administered as a continuous infusion.

Labetalol, which acts as both an alpha- and a beta-adrenergic receptor blocker, can be especially useful in the setting of aortic dissection because it effectively lowers both dP/dt and arterial pressure. The initial dose of labetalol is 20 mg, administered intravenously over a 2-minute period, followed by additional doses of 40 to 80 mg every 10 to 15 minutes (up to a maximum total dose of 300 mg) until the heart rate and blood pressure have been controlled. Maintenance dosing can then be achieved with a continuous intravenous infusion starting at 2 mg/min and titrating up to 5 to 10 mg/min.

The ultra-short-acting beta blocker esmolol may be particularly useful in patients with labile arterial pressure, especially if surgery is planned, because use of this drug can be abruptly discontinued if necessary. It is administered as a 500 µg/kg intravenous bolus followed by continuous infusion at 50 µg/kg/min and titrated up to 200 µg/kg/min. Esmolol can also be useful as a means to test beta blocker safety and tolerance in patients with a history of obstructive pulmonary disease who may be at uncertain risk for bronchospasm from beta blocker administration. In such patients, a cardioselective beta blocker, such as atenolol or metoprolol, can be considered.

When contraindications exist to the use of beta blockers—including severe sinus bradycardia, second- or third-degree atrioventricular block, congestive heart failure, or bronchospasm—other agents to reduce arterial pressure and dP/dt should be considered. Calcium channel antagonists, which are effective in managing hypertensive crisis, are used on occasion in the treatment of aortic dissection. The combined vasodilator and negative inotropic effects of both diltiazem and verapamil make these agents well suited for the treatment of aortic dissection. Moreover, these agents may be administered intravenously. Nifedipine has the advantage that it can be given immediately by the sublingual route while other medications are being prepared. A key limitation of nifedipine, however, is that it has little negative chronotropic or inotropic effect.

Refractory hypertension may result when a dissection flap compromises one or both of the renal arteries, thereby causing the release of large amounts of renin. In this situation, the most efficacious antihypertensive may be the intravenous angiotensin-converting enzyme (ACE) inhibitor enalaprilat, which is administered initially in doses of 0.625 to 1.25 mg every 6 hours and then titrated upward if necessary to a maximum of 5 mg every 6 hours.

In the event that a patient with suspected aortic dissection has significant hypotension, rapid volume expansion should be considered, given the possible presence of cardiac tamponade or aortic rupture. Before initiating aggressive treatment of such hypotension, however, the possibility of *pseudohypotension,* which occurs when arterial pressure is being measured in an extremity where the circulation is selectively compromised by the dissection, should be carefully excluded. If vasopressors are absolutely required for refractory hypotension, norepinephrine (Levophed) or phenylephrine (Neo-Synephrine) is preferred. Dopamine should be reserved for improving renal perfusion and used only at very low doses, given that it may raise dP/dt.

Once appropriate medical therapy has been initiated and the patient is sufficiently stabilized, a definitive diagnostic study should be promptly undertaken. If a patient remains unstable, TEE is preferred because it can be performed at the bedside in the emergency department or intensive care unit, thereby allowing both monitoring and therapeutic intervention to continue uninterrupted. When a patient with a strongly suspected dissection becomes extremely unstable, aortic rupture or cardiac tamponade is likely and the patient should go directly to the operating room rather than delaying surgery for diagnostic imaging. In such situations, intraoperative TEE can be used both to confirm the diagnosis and to guide surgical repair.

MANAGEMENT OF CARDIAC TAMPONADE. Cardiac tamponade frequently complicates acute proximal aortic dissection and is one of the most common mechanisms of death in these patients. It is often the cause of hypotension when patients have aortic dissection, and pericardiocentesis is commonly performed in this setting in an effort to stabilize patients while they await definitive surgical repair. In a retrospective series, however, we found that pericardiocentesis may be harmful rather than beneficial in this setting because it can precipitate hemodynamic collapse and death rather than stabilize the patient as intended. Seven patients in this series were relatively stable initially (six hypotensive, one normotensive). Three of four who underwent successful pericardiocentesis died suddenly between 5 and 40 minutes after the procedure because of acute pulseless electrical activity. In contrast, none of the three patients without pericardiocentesis died before surgery. It may be that in such patients, the increase in intraaortic pressure that follows pericardiocentesis causes a closed communication between the false lumen and pericardial space to reopen, thereby leading to recurrent hemorrhage and lethal cardiac tamponade.

Therefore, when a patient with acute aortic dissection complicated by cardiac tamponade is relatively stable, the risks of pericardiocentesis probably outweigh the benefits and *every effort should be made to proceed as urgently as possible to the operating room for direct surgical repair of the aorta with intraoperative drainage of the hemopericardium.* However, when patients have pulseless electrical activity or marked hypotension, an attempt to resuscitate the patient with pericardiocentesis is warranted and may indeed be successful. A prudent strategy in such cases is to aspirate only enough pericardial fluid to raise blood pressure to the lowest acceptable level.

Definitive Therapy

Despite minor variations from center to center, a reasonable consensus regarding definitive therapy for aortic dissection has evolved over the past several decades. All practitioners agree that surgical therapy is superior to medical therapy for acute proximal dissection. With even limited progression of a proximal dissection, patients may suffer the potentially devastating consequences of aortic rupture or cardiac tamponade, acute aortic regurgitation, or neurological compromise. Thus, by controlling this risk, immediate surgical repair promises a better outcome. Occasional patients with proximal dissection who refuse surgery or for whom surgery is contraindicated (e.g., by age or prior debilitating illness) may be treated successfully with medical therapy with a 30-day survival rate of up to 42 percent.[56]

Patients suffering acute distal aortic dissection, on the other hand, are at much lower risk of early death from complications of the dissection than are those with proximal dissection. Because patients with distal dissection tend to be older and have a relatively increased prevalence of advanced atherosclerosis or cardiopulmonary disease, their surgical risk is often considerably higher. A large retrospective series involving patients from both Duke and Stanford universities has, by multivariate analysis, shown that medical therapy provides an outcome equivalent to that of surgical therapy in patients with uncomplicated distal dissection. As a consequence, medical therapy for such patients is favored. An important exception is that when distal dissection is complicated by vital organ or limb ischemia, uncontrolled pain, and rapid expansion, medical therapy yields poor results and surgery is, therefore, recommended.

Patients with chronic aortic dissection have, through self-selection, survived the early period of highest mortality, and whether treated medically or surgically, their subsequent hospital survival rate is approximately 90 percent. Accordingly, medical therapy is recommended for the management of all stable patients with chronic proximal and distal dissection, again unless complicated by rupture, aneurysm formation, aortic regurgitation, arterial occlusion, or extension or recurrence of dissection.

SURGICAL MANAGEMENT. Generally advocated indications for definitive surgical therapy are summarized in Table 56-2. Surgical candidacy should be determined whenever possible at the start of the patient's evaluation because this option guides the selection of diagnostic studies. Preoperative mortality in patients with acute dissection ranges from 3 percent when surgery is expedited to as high as 20 percent when the preoperative evaluation is prolonged. These data reinforce the need for prompt diagnosis and repair to prevent even minimal progression of the dissection, which might lead to further complications. Surgical risk for all patients is increased by age, comorbid disease, aneurysm leakage, cardiac tamponade, shock, cerebrovascular accident, or mesenteric, renal, or myocardial ischemia.[65]

The usual objectives of definitive surgical therapy include resection of the most severely damaged segment of aorta, excision of the intimal tear when possible, and obliteration of entry into the false lumen by suturing of the edges of the dissected aorta both proximally and distally. After the diseased segment containing the intimal tear is resected, typically a segment of the ascending aorta in proximal dissections or the proximal descending aorta in distal dissections, aortic continuity is then reestablished by interposing a prosthetic sleeve graft between the two ends of the aorta (Fig. 56-23).

Importantly, several studies have demonstrated that the immediate and long-term survival of patients treated surgically was not significantly affected by failure to excise the intimal tear. Some patients with proximal dissection have an intimal tear located in the aortic arch. Because surgical

TABLE 56–2	Indications for Definitive Surgical and Medical Therapy in Aortic Dissection

Surgical

Treatment of choice for acute proximal dissection

Treatment for acute distal dissection complicated by the following:
  Progression with vital organ compromise
  Rupture or impending rupture (e.g., saccular aneurysm formation)
  Retrograde extension into the ascending aorta
  Dissection in Marfan syndrome

Medical

Treatment of choice for uncomplicated distal dissection

Treatment for stable, isolated arch dissection

Treatment of choice for stable chronic dissection (uncomplicated dissection manifesting 2 weeks or later after onset)

several groups suggest that even these challenging lesions can be resected with favorable results.

When aortic regurgitation complicates aortic dissection, simple decompression of the false lumen is sometimes all that is required to allow resuspension of the aortic leaflets and restoration of valvular competence. More often, however, preservation of the aortic valve requires approximation of the two layers of dissected aortic wall and resuspension of the commissures with pledgeted sutures. In this setting, the use of intraoperative TEE may be particularly helpful to the surgeon in guiding aortic valve repair.[67] This resuspension technique has had favorable results with a fairly low incidence of recurrent aortic regurgitation in long-term follow-up. Preserving the aortic valve in this fashion may avoid the complications associated with prosthetic valve replacement, especially the requirement for oral anticoagulation, which may pose an added risk in patients prone to future aortic rupture.

Prosthetic aortic valve replacement is sometimes necessary—either because attempts at valve repair are unsuccessful or in the setting of preexisting valvular disease or Marfan syndrome. Many surgeons are aggressive about replacing the aortic valve if it appears that even moderate aortic regurgitation will remain after the leaflets are resuspended and choose to avoid the risk of having to replace the aortic valve at some later date in a second operation through a diseased aorta. When the proximal aorta is fragile or badly torn, most surgeons use a composite prosthetic graft (described earlier) for replacement of both the ascending aorta and the aortic valve together. The operative procedure for aortic dissection is technically demanding. The wall of the diseased aorta is often friable, and the repair must be performed with meticulous care. Use of Teflon felt to buttress the wall and prevent sutures from tearing through the fragile aorta is essential (see Fig. 56-23).

Complications. Bleeding, infection, pulmonary failure, and renal insufficiency constitute the most common early complications of surgical therapy. Spinal cord ischemia with paraplegia caused by inadvertent interruption of the blood supply from the anterior spinal or intercostal arteries is an uncommon but dreaded consequence of descending thoracic aortic repair. Late complications include progressive aortic regurgitation if the aortic valve has not been replaced, localized aneurysm formation, and recurrent dissection at the original site or at a secondary site. With modern operative techniques, 30-day surgical survival rates for proximal and distal dissections are 74 and 69 percent, respectively.[56]

NEWER SURGICAL TECHNIQUES. As a modification of more standard operative techniques, many surgeons now use tissue glues to appose permanently the dissected aortic layers to both eliminate the false lumen and to strengthen friable aortic tissue to improve the anastomoses. After resection of the diseased aortic segment, this glue is used in place of pledgeted sutures to seal the false lumen of the aortic stumps, before implantation of the Dacron prosthesis. The glue not only hardens and reinforces the fragile dissected aortic tissue but may also simplify the operation, facilitate resuspension of the aortic valve, and potentially reduce the incidence of late aortic root aneurysm formation.[68] Although some reports have shown favorable morbidity and mortality with the use of these new techniques, others suggest that glue use may result in late complications of tissue necrosis,[69] particularly if the glue is used improperly. Before wide adoption of the use of tissue glue, a direct comparison with standard operative techniques is needed.

ENDOVASCULAR TECHNIQUES. One of the more promising avenues of investigation is the use of endovascular techniques for treating high-risk patients with aortic dissection. For example, because patients with renal or visceral artery compromise from dissection have had operative mortality rates exceeding 50 percent, alternative management strategies are desirable. Several endovascular techniques have been used in many centers to manage patients with acute distal vascu-

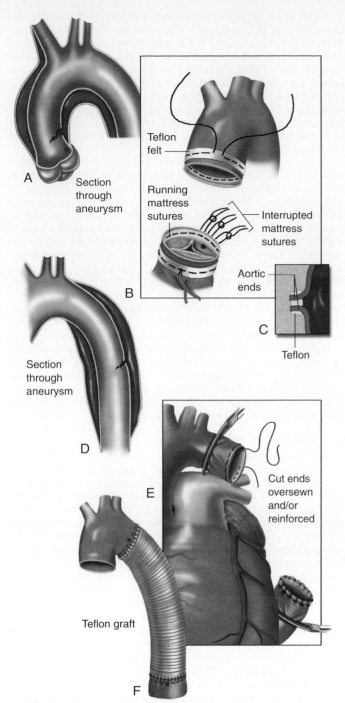

FIGURE 56–23 Several steps in the surgical repair of proximal (**A, B,** and **C**) and distal (**D, E,** and **F**) aortic dissections. **A** and **D,** Dissections and intimal tears. **B,** The aorta has been transected, and the ends of the aorta have been oversewn to obliterate the false lumen and buttressed with Teflon felt to prevent the sutures from tearing through the fragile tissue. **C,** The aortic ends are brought together in such a way that the Teflon is again used to reinforce the suture line between the two ends of the aorta and between the aorta and a sleeve graft, if such a graft is necessary for reconstitution of the aorta. **E,** Resection of a distal dissection, with a Teflon graft interposed in **F.** (*D, E,* and *F* from Austen WG, DeSanctis RW: Surgical treatment of dissecting aneurysm of the thoracic aorta. N Engl J Med 272:1314, 1965.)

repair of the arch may increase the morbidity and mortality associated with the procedure and because resection of the tear may not necessarily improve mortality,[66] many surgeons elect not to repair the arch if the sole purpose of surgery is resection of the intimal tear. However, with improvements in surgical technique during the last decade,

lar complications of aortic dissection. The first is balloon fenestration of the intimal flap, which involves crossing an intact intimal flap with a wire, passing a balloon-tipped catheter over the wire, and then expanding the balloon to tear a hole in the intimal flap. The hole acts as a site of reentry to allow blood to flow from the false into the true lumen, thereby decompressing the distended false lumen. The second technique involves percutaneous stenting of an affected arterial branch whose flow has been compromised by the dissection process. In comparing our recent 10-year experience with a previously reported 30-year experience, we found that current methods of peripheral vascular intervention have reduced the overall mortality of dissection-associated branch vessel occlusion from 51 percent to 23 percent.[70] In the large IRAD series of acute aortic dissection, 3.2 percent of patients were treated with percutaneous fenestration procedures.[56]

More recently, intraluminal stent-grafts placed percutaneously by the transfemoral catheter technique have been introduced as a potential alternative to aortic repair. This procedure aims to close the site of entry into the false lumen (intimal tear), decompress and promote thrombosis of the false lumen, and relieve any obstruction of branch vessels that may accompany the dissection. This approach may reduce the morbidity and mortality of aortic dissection and reduce the risk of subsequent aneurysm formation. Comparisons of the use of stent-graft placement with standard surgical repair in a group of 24 patients with subacute or chronic type B aortic dissection and a patent false lumen,[71] showed no procedural complications occurred among the 12 patients undergoing stent-graft treatment, and when compared with the surgical group, the stent-graft group had a significantly shorter hospital stay, lower rate of morbidity, and lower 1-year postprocedural mortality rate. Insertion of stent-grafts in the descending thoracic aortas of 19 patients with acute aortic dissection and a patent false lumen who suffered from obstruction of branch vessels, acute aortic rupture, or persistent back pain[72] showed successful endovascular stent-graft deployment was successful in all cases, with complete thrombosis of the false lumen in 79 percent and partial thrombosis in the remaining 21 percent. Restoration of flow to ischemic arterial branches with relief of corresponding symptoms occurred in 76 percent of obstructed branches. The results of these two series are extremely promising, but larger studies with more patients and longer follow-up will be required before stent-graft therapy becomes an accepted therapy for aortic dissection. A randomized trial (the INSTEAD trial) to compare the 2-year outcome of endovascular stenting versus medical therapy for uncomplicated distal dissections is well underway in Europe.[73]

DEFINITIVE MEDICAL MANAGEMENT. As discussed earlier, stable patients with uncomplicated acute distal dissection should undergo medical management (see Table 56-2) given that the 30-day survival rate for those with distal dissection treated medically is 92 percent.[56] However, surgery (or percutaneous intervention) clearly must be performed in cases of rupture or impending rupture, vital organ compromise, an inability to control pain, or retrograde progression of a type B dissection into the ascending aorta. Because of the extreme difficulty to surgically repair the aortic arch when it is involved by the dissection, medical therapy is also usually advocated for type B dissections that either originate in the arch or extend retrograde into the arch. Operative therapy is again reserved for patients with serious complications. Medical therapy is also generally recommended for patients with chronic aortic dissection, whether proximal or distal, unless late complications of the dissection, such as aortic regurgitation or localized aneurysm formation, necessitate surgery.

Severe hypertension is relatively common during the period of hospitalization after acute aortic dissection and may occur even in patients without a history of significant hypertension. In the past, some practitioners have argued that such refractory hypertension should be considered an indication for aortic repair because it might increase the risk of early complications. Our retrospective analysis, however, found that although almost two-thirds of our patients with distal dissections required the administration of four or more antihypertensive medications to control refractory hypertension early in their hospitalization, there was no increase in adverse events as compared with patients

without such hypertension, and surgery is generally not necessary in this setting.[74] The etiology for this hypertensive response is unclear but it may reflect a marked increase in sympathetic tone triggered by the severe inflammation of the aortic wall that accompanies dissection. Renal ischemia rarely causes hypertension, so in the absence of a fall in urine output or a rise in serum creatinine, renal artery imaging is typically not necessary. Furthermore, the severe hypertension usually improves 5 to 7 days after onset of the aortic dissection, allowing a reduction in antihypertensive therapy.

When patients with type B aortic dissection are managed medically, in addition to the reduction in dP/dt and heart rate, a second goal is to monitor the patient vigilantly for any evidence of branch arterial compromise, with the most lethal consequence being mesenteric ischemia. Unfortunately, the clinical features of mesenteric ischemia may be subtle initially and therefore go unrecognized, and by the time they have become clinically obvious, organ damage may be irreversible. Adding to the challenge of this condition, in as many as half such cases,[75] imaging studies such as urgent CT scanning may show patent mesenteric vessels arising from the true lumen with no evidence of the dissection flap extending into the branches. However, often a large false lumen is distended with blood and compresses a small true lumen throughout most of the cardiac cycle, markedly reducing antegrade flow through the true lumen to the mesenteric vessels and resulting in nonobstructive ischemia (see Fig. 56-13). In this setting, a strong clinical suspicion and a low threshold for surgical or percutaneous intervention are the keys to preventing a catastrophic outcome.

Long-Term Therapy and Late Follow-up

Late follow-up of patients leaving the hospital with treated aortic dissection shows an actuarial survival rate not much worse than that of individuals of comparable age without dissection. No significant differences are seen among discharged patients when comparing proximal versus distal dissection, acute versus chronic dissection, or medical versus surgical treatment. Five-year survival rates for all these groups (among discharged patients) are typically 75 to 82 percent. Thus, the initial success of surgical or medical therapy is usually sustained on long-term follow-up. Late complications include aortic regurgitation, recurrent dissection, and aneurysm formation or rupture. The presence of a persistently patent false lumen is one of the strongest predictors of adverse late outcomes, including more rapid aortic dilatation, a greater likelihood of requiring subsequent aortic surgery, and late mortality.

Long-term medical therapy to control hypertension and reduce dP/dt is indicated for all patients who have sustained an aortic dissection, regardless of whether their in-hospital definitive treatment was surgical or medical. Indeed, one study found that late aneurysm rupture after aortic dissection was 10 times more common in patients with poorly controlled hypertension than in those with controlled blood pressure, which dramatically demonstrates the importance of aggressive lifelong antihypertensive therapy. Systolic blood pressure should be maintained at or below 130 mm Hg. The preferred agents are beta blockers or, if contraindicated, other agents with a negative inotropic as well as a hypotensive effect, such as verapamil or diltiazem. ACE inhibitors and angiotensin receptor blockers are attractive antihypertensive agents for treating aortic dissection and may be of particular benefit in patients with some degree of renal ischemia as a consequence of the dissection. Pure vasodilators, such as dihydropyridine calcium channel antagonists or hydralazine, may cause an increase in dP/dt and should therefore be used only in conjunction with adequate beta blockade.

Up to 29 percent of late deaths following surgery result from rupture of either the dissecting aneurysm or another aneurysm at a remote site. The incidence of subsequent aneurysm formation at a site remote from the surgical repair is 17 to 25 percent, with these remote aneurysms accounting for many of the rupture-related deaths. Many such aneurysms occur from dilatation of the residual false lumen in the more distal aortic segments not resected at the time of surgery. Because the dissected aneurysm wall is relatively thin and consists of only the outer half of the original aortic wall, these aneurysms rupture more frequently than do typical atherosclerotic thoracic aneurysms. Thus, an aggressive approach to treating such late-appearing aneurysms may be indicated.

The high incidence of late aneurysm formation and rupture emphasizes both the diffuse nature of the aortic disease process in this population and the tremendous importance of careful follow-up. The primary goal of long-term surveillance is the early detection of aortic lesions that might require subsequent surgical intervention, such as the appearance of new aneurysms or rapid aneurysm expansion, progression or recurrence of dissection, aortic regurgitation, or peripheral vascular compromise.

Follow-up evaluation of patients after aortic dissection should include serial aortic imaging with CT, MRI, or TEE. We generally prefer CT for serially monitoring of these patients because it is completely noninvasive and provides excellent anatomical detail that may be exceedingly helpful in evaluating interval changes. Patients are at highest risk immediately after hospitalization and during the first 2 years, with the risk progressively declining thereafter. It is therefore important to have more frequent early follow-up; for example, patients can be seen and imaged at 1, 3, and 6 months initially and then return every 6 months for 2 years, after which time they can often be re-imaged at 12-month intervals, depending on the given patient's risk.

Atypical Aortic Dissection

In aortic dissection as classically described, two other diseases of the aorta are closely related, *intramural hematoma* of the aorta and *penetrating atherosclerotic ulcer* of the aorta. These two conditions share with aortic dissection many of the predisposing risk factors and initial symptoms, and indeed, both may lead to either classic aortic dissection or aortic rupture. In light of their clinical similarities, it is appropriate to consider classic aortic dissection and its variants collectively among the "acute thoracic aortic syndromes," a category that also includes traumatic aortic transection and rupture, contained rupture (pseudoaneurysm), or acute expansion of thoracic aortic aneurysms.

INTRAMURAL HEMATOMA. Intramural hematoma is an acute aortic syndrome that is essentially a hemorrhage contained within the medial layer of the aortic wall but—unlike classic aortic dissection—without an evident tear in the intima or active communication between the hematoma and the aortic lumen. Hence, some practitioners have termed it *aortic dissection without intimal rupture.* The actual causes of intramural hematoma remain debatable. Historically, it has been presumed that intramural hematoma results from rupture of the vasa vasorum within the aortic wall. Others have argued, however, that the hematoma results from a tear in the intima (too small to visualize) that permits transient blood flow from the lumen into the aortic wall, which then thromboses to form a hematoma rather than a false lumen. The hematoma can be localized or discrete, but more often the hemorrhage extends for a variable distance by dissecting along the outer media beneath the adventitia.

Clinically, intramural hematoma can be indistinguishable from true aortic dissection. The risk factors, signs, and symptoms associated with intramural hematoma resemble those seen in classic aortic dissection, and it is therefore impossible to predict on clinical grounds (without an imaging study) whether a patient with suspected aortic dissection has a classic aortic dissection or intramural hematoma. Indeed, a significant minority—historically 10 percent to 17 percent—of apparent aortic dissection cases are diagnosed as intramural hematoma. Furthermore, many of the acute complications of aortic dissection such as aortic regurgitation rupture into the pericardium, pleural and pericardial effusions, and branch vessel occlusion also occur with intramural hematoma, raising the question of whether intramural hematoma is just a morphological variant of aortic dissection or a distinct clinical entity with a different course and prognosis.

On axial imaging studies (i.e., CT, MRI, and TEE) intramural hematoma appears as a crescentic or sometimes circumferential thickening of the aortic wall, with no evidence of flow within the hematoma. The appearance of the thickened wall, especially in the ascending aorta, is often subtle on TEE, so the reader must be vigilant when clinical suspicion is high. CT scanning is the modality that best demonstrates the intramural hematoma. On a non-contrast-enhanced CT scan (see Fig. 56-24B) it appears as a continuous, crescentic, high-attenuation area along the aortic wall without evidence of an intimal tear, false lumen, or associated intimal atherosclerotic ulcer. This first examination is followed by a contrast-enhanced CT scan (Fig. 56-24A), which demonstrates failure of the intramural hematoma to enhance (appearing as a darker crescentic thickening of the aortic wall), thereby excluding communication with the aortic lumen. In some cases, it may be challenging to distinguish intramural hematoma from aortic dissection with thrombosis of the false lumen or from mural thrombus within an aortic aneurysm. With an intramural hematoma, however, the aortic lumen retains its overall size and round shape, unlike the case with aortic dissection or a thrombus-lined aneurysm.

Conversely, intramural hematoma is often not detected by catheter-based contrast aortography, because this technique images the aortic lumen itself—which, in this case, appears normal—and not the aortic wall where the abnormality lies. During the years that contrast aortography was the standard imaging technique for suspected aortic dissection, intramural hematomas often went clinically unrecognized. In fact, the sensitivity of aortography for detecting intramural hematoma is as low as 19 percent; therefore, although a negative aortogram can exclude the presence of classic aortic dissection, it does not reliably exclude the important variant of intramural hematoma.

Although intramural hematoma is now recognized as pathoanatomically distinct from classic aortic dissection, its natural history is still debated. When followed with serial imaging studies, it can have four possible courses: the hematoma may persist (although its thickness may change); it may be reabsorbed, so that the appearance of the aortic wall returns to normal; it may lead to an aortic aneurysm; or it may convert to a classic aortic dissection, with the development of a typical intimal flap and flow in a false lumen.

In the 1990s, several retrospective reports described the outcomes of intramural hematoma, but the study samples were small. A recent review of 160 patients from 11 studies reporting outcomes of aortic intramural hematoma found that proximal intramural hematoma was associated with a mortality rate of 47 percent when managed medically compared with 24 percent when managed surgically.[76] On the other hand, distal intramural hematoma was associated

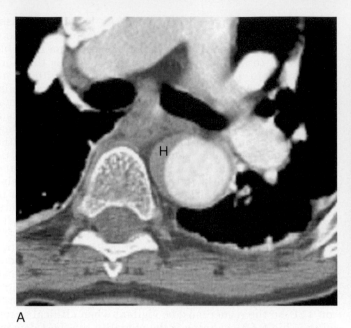
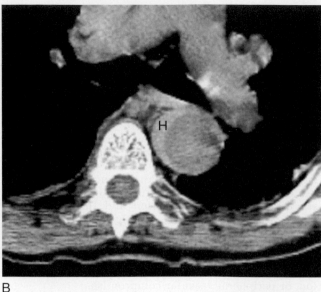

FIGURE 56–24 Intramural hematoma of the descending thoracic aorta. **A,** An axial contrast-enhanced computed tomography (CT) scan at the level of the pulmonary artery demonstrating crescentic dark thickening of the aortic wall (H) that does not enhance, confirming the presence of an intramural hematoma. Note that neither the size nor the shape of the aortic lumen is distorted the way it would typically be in the presence of a classic aortic dissection. **B,** On a non-contrast-enhanced CT scan there is crescentic thickening of the aortic wall that is of increased density (H) compared with blood in the lumen, consistent with an intramural hematoma of the aorta.

CH 56

with a mortality rate of 13 percent with medical management compared with 15 percent with surgical repair. These rates are similar to those for classic aortic dissection as reported by the IRAD[56]: 58 percent for proximal aortic dissection when managed medically compared with 26 percent when managed surgically, and 11 percent for distal aortic dissection with medical management compared with 31 percent with surgical repair. Consequently, most treatment centers currently accept a general management strategy for aortic intramural hematoma similar to that used for classic aortic dissection: proximal aortic involvement is treated surgically and distal aortic involvement is managed medically. Physicians should have a low threshold for proceeding to surgery in patients with distal disease if symptoms persist or evidence of progression is seen, however. Medical management should, therefore, include serial imaging studies to monitor progression or regression of the intramural hematoma.

Several recent reports have suggested that the outcomes associated with proximal intramural hematoma may be more benign than with classic aortic dissection, with a large proportion of patients surviving with medical therapy alone. For example, Song and coworkers[77] reported in-hospital mortality rates for medically managed proximal and distal intramural hematoma of only 7 percent and 1 percent, respectively, both of which are substantially lower than the rates of 47 percent and 13 percent, respectively, previously reported.

How can such dramatic differences be reconciled? The samples studied may not be comparable. In fact, in Song's series, 29 percent of apparent aortic dissection cases were diagnosed as intramural hematoma, a proportion about double what other investigators have reported. This series may have identified and included more subtle cases of intramural hematoma, which would go undetected in other hospitals and which are likely to be associated with a lower risk of progression or rupture. There may be a continuum of risk for intramural hematoma rather than an absolute risk. The morphological features that distinguish intramural hematoma from classic aortic dissection, such as the absence of a patent false lumen, suggest that intramural hematomas

are somewhat less likely to rupture. However, factors that increase aortic wall stress, such as large aortic diameters and thick hematomas, could increase the risk of rupture or dissection. Indeed, one recent study of acute intramural hematoma[78] found that a maximum aortic diameter 50 mm or larger independently predicted progression, whereas in another study of patients with distal intramural hematoma managed medically,[79] both a maximum aortic diameter of 40 mm or larger and a maximum aortic wall thickness of 10 mm or larger independently predicted progression. These findings confirm that some patients with intramural hematoma may be at considerably lower risk than others, suggesting that baseline differences in patient characteristics could substantially influence outcomes. However, until further studies help to better define those patients at very low risk, we still recommend the strategy of routine aortic surgery for proximal intramural hematoma.[80]

PENETRATING ATHEROSCLEROTIC ULCER. Penetrating atherosclerotic ulcer, first defined in the modern literature in 1986, is an ulceration of an atherosclerotic lesion of the aorta that penetrates the internal elastic lamina and allows hematoma formation within the media of the aortic wall (Fig. 56-25). Although such ulcerations usually occur in the descending thoracic aorta, they may also localize in the arch or rarely in the ascending aorta. The hematoma that results from a penetrating atherosclerotic ulcer usually remains localized or extends several centimeters in length, but a classic false lumen typically does not develop. However, some cases of intramural hematoma of the aorta may, in fact, result from small penetrating atherosclerotic ulcers that have escaped detection on imaging studies but are later identified at the time of surgery.

Atherosclerotic aortic ulcers penetrate through the media in one quarter of cases to cause aortic pseudoaneurysms or less often through the adventitia to cause transmural aortic rupture. Rarely, a penetrating atherosclerotic ulcer may progress to an extensive classic aortic dissection. Over time, penetrating atherosclerotic ulcers frequently lead to the late formation of saccular or fusiform aortic aneurysms. Patients in whom penetrating atherosclerotic ulcers develop tend to be elderly with a history of hypertension and smoking. The majority have evidence of other atherosclerotic cardiovascular disease and as many as one half also have a history of an abdominal or thoracic aortic aneurysm. Initial symptoms include chest and back pain similar to that of aortic dissection, and most patients have hypertension at initial evaluation. However, because penetrating atherosclerotic ulcers tend to be localized, the vascular compromise or aortic regurgitation that often complicates aortic dissection does not develop.

Chest radiographs often demonstrate a dilated descending thoracic aorta as well as left-sided or bilateral pleural effusions. Aortography had been the diagnostic standard for detecting a penetrating atherosclerotic ulcer, with the lesion appearing as a contrast-filled outpouching in the descending aorta in the absence of an intimal flap or false lumen. However, penetrating atherosclerotic ulcers are now particularly well visualized with the use of CT or MRA (Fig. 56-26), in which the lesion appears as a focal ulceration with thickening of the aortic wall and is consistent with an associated intramural hematoma. TEE may identify the presence of a culprit atherosclerotic ulcer in the setting of a visible intramural hematoma, but making the diagnosis is more difficult than with the above-mentioned imaging modalities.

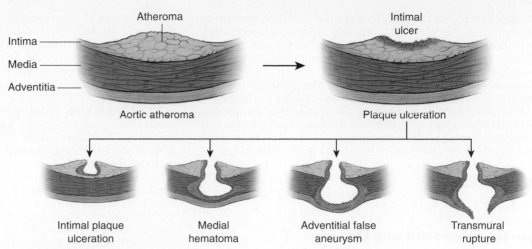

FIGURE 56–25 Evolution of a penetrating atherosclerotic ulcer of the aorta. Once an intimal ulcer has formed, it may then progress to a variable depth. Penetration through the intima causes a medial hematoma, whereas penetration through the media leads to the formation of a pseudoaneurysm, and perforation through the adventitial layer results in aortic rupture. *(From Stanson AW, Kazmier FJ, Hollier LH, et al: Penetrating atherosclerotic ulcers of the thoracic aorta: Natural history and clinicopathological correlations. Ann Vasc Surg 1:15, 1986.)*

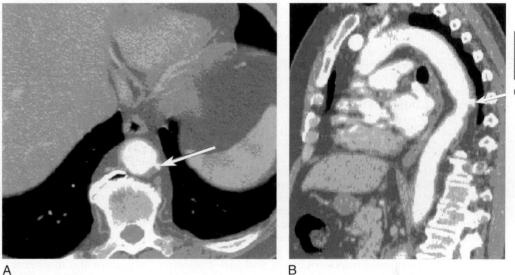

FIGURE 56–26 Contrast-enhanced CT scan through the distal descending aorta demonstrating the presence of a penetrating atherosclerotic ulcer. **A,** An axial image showing a small discrete ulcer (arrow) penetrating the aortic intima and producing a very localized hematoma within the aortic wall. **B,** Computed tomography angiogram in the same patient showing how the ulcer (arrow) projects out from the lumen of the distal descending aorta.

The natural history of a penetrating atherosclerotic ulcer remains largely unclear, and likely differs significantly between patients presenting with symptoms (i.e., acute aortic syndrome) versus without symptoms (i.e., an incidental finding). Coady and colleagues found that the risk of rupture and 1-year mortality is greater among patients with penetrating atherosclerotic ulcer than among those with aortic dissection.[81] At present, no consensus prevails regarding definitive treatment strategy. Certainly, patients who are hemodynamically unstable or who have evidence of pseudoaneurysm formation or transmural rupture should undergo urgent surgical repair. Continued or recurrent pain, distal embolization, and progressive aneurysmal dilation are also indications for surgery. However, it remains unclear if otherwise stable patients with distal penetrating atherosclerotic ulcers should undergo surgery or can be safely managed medically, as in the case of classic aortic dissection. In one study of 26 patients with penetrating athero-

sclerotic ulcer,[82] there was no difference in the 1- or 5-year survival between surgical and medical management strategies, suggesting that surgery may not improve the otherwise poor prognosis. Transluminal placement of an endovascular stent-graft may become a lower risk alternative to surgery in such patients.

Ganaha and coworkers[83] examined the outcomes of 31 patients with penetrating atherosclerotic ulcers, of whom 17 were managed medically, whereas 8 underwent surgical repair and the other 6 underwent stent-grafting for evidence of aortic rupture or impending rupture. Importantly, there was no significant difference in early survival among the three strategies. The authors compared patients with a progressive in-hospital course—defined as aortic rupture, hematoma expansion, or appearance of a distinct false lumen—to those with a stable course. Uncontrolled pain and an enlarging pleural effusion were both highly predictive of a progressive course. CT findings associated with a progressive rather than a stable course included maximum diameter of the ulcer (21 mm and 12 mm, respectively), maximum depth of the ulcer (14 mm and 7 mm, respectively), and an ulcer located in the proximal one third of the descending aorta rather than more distal. Using these various markers, about one half of the patients in their study would have been considered low-risk for a progressive course. We recommend treating patients with such uncomplicated conditions with antihypertensive medications and close monitoring with serial imaging studies, similar to the management of a patient with a distal aortic dissection.

Aortic Trauma

See Chapter 71.

Aortic Atheroembolic Disease

See Chapter 57.

ACUTE AORTIC OCCLUSION

Acute aortic occlusion is an infrequent, but potentially catastrophic, condition with an early mortality rate of 31 to 52 percent. It is caused by either embolic occlusion of the infrarenal aorta at the bifurcation, known as a "saddle embolus," or acute thrombosis of the abdominal aorta. At least 95 percent of aortic emboli originate from the left side of the heart, typically as a thrombus from the left atrium secondary to atrial fibrillation, particularly in the setting of rheumatic mitral stenosis, or from the left ventricle secondary to myocardial infarction, aneurysm, or dilated cardiomyopathy. Less common cardiac sources of emboli include atrial myxoma, prosthetic valve thrombus, and acute bacterial or fungal endocarditis. Primary thrombosis accounts for the remaining 35 to 92 percent of acute aortic occlusions. Seventy-five to 80 percent of thrombotic aortic occlusions occur in the setting of underlying severe aortoiliac occlusive disease and are frequently precipitated by a low-flow state secondary to heart failure or dehydration.

Acute aortic occlusion is in most cases heralded by the sudden onset of excruciating bilateral lower extremity pain, usually radiating from the midportion of the thigh distally and associated with weakness, numbness, and paresthesias. Nonclassic manifestations include sudden onset of bilateral lower extremity weakness, severe hypertension from renal artery involvement, and abdominal pain from mesenteric ischemia. Persistent ischemia may lead to myonecrosis with secondary hypotension, hyperkalemia, myoglobinuria, and acute tubular necrosis. If perfusion is not reestablished within hours, death usually ensues.

DIAGNOSIS. Physical examination reveals cold pale extremities that are cyanotic and often exhibit a mottled, reticulated, and reddish blue appearance that may progress to the blue-black color of gangrene. Pulses are notably absent below the abdominal aorta, and capillary refill is absent. Signs of ischemic neuropathy are present and include symmetrical weakness, loss of all modalities of sensation (usually with demarcation at the level of the midthigh), and diminished or absent deep tendon reflexes. When neurological symptoms predominate, patients are often mistakenly thought to have spinal cord infarction or compression and their ischemic symptoms may initially be overlooked. In fact, as many as 11 to 17 percent of such patients first undergo neurological or neurosurgical evaluation before the vascular cause is recognized.

The diagnosis of acute aortic occlusion is confirmed by aortography. Although some practitioners suggest that all stable patients should undergo the procedure, others advise

prompt surgical intervention without angiography if the diagnosis is strongly suspected because added delays increase the likelihood of irreversible ischemic damage to the limbs. Aortography is desirable in the presence of concomitant abdominal pain, hypertension, or anuria to evaluate the possibility of renal and mesenteric arterial involvement.

MANAGEMENT. Once a clinical diagnosis of acute aortic occlusion is made, intravenous heparin therapy should be initiated while the patient awaits immediate surgery. A saddle embolus can be removed by using Fogarty balloon-tipped catheters inserted through a transfemoral arterial approach under local anesthesia. If the embolus cannot be retrieved with Fogarty catheters, removal by direct transabdominal aortotomy is undertaken. Patients with thrombotic occlusion generally undergo either direct aortic reconstruction or revascularization with aortofemoral or axillofemoral bypass. The operative mortality rate for acute aortic occlusion is 31 to 40 percent and as high as 85 percent among patients with severe left ventricular dysfunction or a hypercoagulable state. Limb salvage rates are as high as 98 percent. Lifelong anticoagulant therapy is necessary after surgery in almost all cases to prevent recurrent emboli.

AORTOARTERITIS SYNDROMES

See Chapter 84.

Bacterial Infections of the Aorta

Infected aortic aneurysms are rare, with as few as one case per year reported from large medical centers. In an effort to avoid confusion with infections truly of fungal origin, the term *infected aneurysm* has gradually replaced the original designation, *mycotic aneurysm,* used by Osler to define localized dilatation in the wall of the aorta caused by sepsis. Although saccular aneurysms are seen most commonly, infections can also cause fusiform and false aneurysms. In a minority of cases, infection may arise in a preexistent aortic aneurysm, typically atherosclerotic ones. Rarely, one may encounter nonaneurysmal bacterial aortitis.

PATHOGENESIS. Aortic infection can arise by several mechanisms. A septic embolus from bacterial endocarditis was once the most common cause but has become rare in the era of effective antibiotic treatment of septicemia. Contiguous spread of infection from adjacent sites can also occur infrequently. The most common cause of an infected aneurysm is direct deposition of circulating bacteria in a diseased, atherosclerotic, or traumatized aortic intima, after which organisms penetrate the aortic wall through breaches in intimal integrity to cause microbial arteritis. In some cases, aortic infections occur in patients with impaired immunity as a consequence of chronic disease, immunosuppressive therapy, or immune deficiency, whereas in other cases, the infection is introduced from distant surgical sites or via intraaortic catheterization procedures.

MICROBIOLOGY. Although virtually any organism can infect the aorta, certain bacteria seem to have a proclivity for this site. *Staphylococcus aureus* and *Salmonella* species are consistently the most frequently identified organisms.[84] *Salmonella* commonly infects atherosclerotic arteries but can also adhere to a normal aortic wall and directly penetrate an intact intima. Other gram-positive organisms, particularly *Pneumococcus,* and gram-negative organisms can also cause infected aortic aneurysms. *Pseudomonas, Bacteroides fragilis, Campylobacter fetus, Neisseria gonorrhoeae,* and fungal infections occur less often. Aortic infections with unusual organisms now occur with increasing frequency in the overtly immunocompromised population.

CLINICAL MANIFESTATIONS. Most patients with infected aortic aneurysm are febrile, with extremely high fevers and rigors being common. Symptoms can arise from localized expansion of an infected aneurysm, which is palpable in as many as 50 percent of patients and almost always tender. A tender and pulsatile abdominal mass in a febrile patient should therefore be considered an infected aneurysm until proved otherwise.

Leukocytosis and an elevated erythrocyte sedimentation rate are present in most cases. When positive, blood cultures are helpful in suggesting the diagnosis and identifying the pathogen. In any patient with persistent fever and documented *Salmonella* bacteremia, an arterial source of infection should be considered. The absence of positive blood cultures, however, does not exclude the diagnosis of infected aortic aneurysm, because cultures can be negative in 25 percent of cases.

Although abdominal ultrasonography may identify the presence of an aortic aneurysm, CT scanning is superior in demonstrating associated pathological findings suggestive of an infectious cause. Sometimes the aorta is normal in size when bacterial aortitis is first evaluated, however, so lack of aneurysmal dilation does not exclude the diagnosis. In such cases, if a patient's fever, leukocytosis, and pain persist, follow-up imaging should be performed because the aorta can rapidly dilate during the course of the infection. Aortography can also make the diagnosis and is sometimes performed preoperatively to assist in surgical planning.

The natural history of infected aortic aneurysms is that of expansion and eventual rupture, with extremely rapid progression. *Salmonella* and other gram-negative infections have a greater tendency to early rupture and death. Overall mortality from infected aortic aneurysms is more than 50 percent, despite advances in therapy.

MANAGEMENT. Infected aortic aneurysms require treatment with intravenous antibiotics and most often surgical excision. The standard surgical approach involves resection of the infected aneurysm and infected retroperitoneal tissue, oversewing of the native aorta as stumps, and restoration of distal perfusion by placement of an extra-anatomical bypass graft tunneled through unaffected tissue planes to avoid placing a graft in a contaminated region. Antibiotic therapy must be continued postoperatively for at least 6 weeks. Several reports suggest that in selected patients with localized infection and no gross pus, an effective and simpler surgical approach is in situ reconstruction of the aorta with a prosthetic graft[85] or cryopreserved arterial allograft.[86]

PRIMARY TUMORS OF THE AORTA

Primary tumors of the aorta are quite rare, although as a result of improvements in noninvasive imaging techniques, the frequency of reports of such tumors has increased significantly over the past two decades. Most are diagnosed in the seventh to eighth decades of life. The thoracic aorta and abdominal aorta are involved with equal frequency. In several cases, aortic tumors have appeared in association with previously inserted Dacron aortic grafts. Histologically, sarcomas constitute the majority of primary aortic tumors, with the malignant fibrous histiocytoma subtype being especially common.

The majority of primary aortic tumors arise in the intima and grow along the intimal surface and into the aortic lumen to form polypoid masses (often with superimposed thrombus), but they tend to not invade the aortic wall. Intimal tumors may be characterized by symptoms of vascular obstruction from narrowing of the aortic lumen or, more typically, by signs and symptoms of peripheral embo-

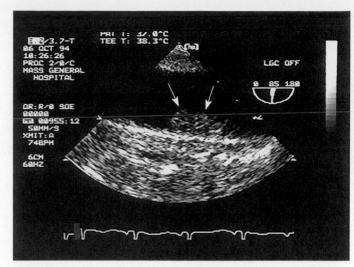

FIGURE 56-27 Transesophageal echocardiogram in a long-axis view of the descending thoracic aorta demonstrating a primary tumor of the aorta (arrows) protruding into the lumen. The tumor, 3.5 cm in length, involves the intimal layer but does not appear to be invading any farther into the aortic wall.

lization identical to those of atherothrombotic emboli.[87] Emboli are commonly a mixture of tumor and thrombus, and the correct diagnosis may remain obscure until histological analysis of an embolectomy specimen is completed. Less commonly, aortic tumors arise in the medial or adventitial layers of the aortic wall. Such tumors tend to not invade the aortic lumen but, instead, behave as aggressive mass lesions and cause constitutional symptoms or back pain.

Because primary aortic tumors are uncommon and their features are nonspecific, the diagnosis is rarely considered before surgical exploration or necropsy. However, several imaging modalities can be helpful in suggesting the diagnosis. Aortography demonstrates narrowing of the lumen or an intraluminal filling defect in the presence of an intimal tumor, but it may be negative if the tumor is adventitial. CT scanning can detect intimal tumors but may not easily differentiate these masses from protruding atheromas. MRI may better define both the tumor anatomy and the extent of invasion. Finally, the ability of TEE to image the aortic intima may make it especially useful in the detection of intimal tumors of the thoracic aorta (Fig. 56-27).

Treatment of primary aortic tumors has met with little success. Because the majority of patients initially have metastatic disease, surgical approaches are often only palliative, to prevent further embolization. Many patients die secondary to the consequences of multiple emboli to vital organs. Of those undergoing surgical therapy, most die within days to months postoperatively.

REFERENCES

Epidemiology of Aortic Disease

1. Singh K, Bonaa KH, Jacobsen BK, et al: Prevalence of and risk factors for abdominal aortic aneurysms in a population-based study: The Tromso Study. Am J Epidemiol 154:236-244, 2001.
2. Lederle FA, Johnson GR, Wilson SE, et al: Abdominal aortic aneurysm in women. J Vasc Surg 34:122-126, 2001.
3. Ogata T, MacKean GL, Cole CW, et al: The lifetime prevalence of abdominal aortic aneurysms among siblings of aneurysm patients is eightfold higher than among siblings of spouses: An analysis of 187 aneurysm families in Nova Scotia, Canada. J Vasc Surg 42:891-897, 2005.

Pathophysiology of Aortic Disease

3a. Shimizu K, Mitchell RN, Libby P: Inflammation and cellular immune responses in abdominal aortic aneurysms. Review. Arterioscler Thromb Vasc Biol 26:987-994, 2006.

4. Wilson WR, Anderton M, Schwalbe EC, et al: Matrix metalloproteinase-8 and -9 are increased at the site of abdominal aortic aneurysm rupture. Circulation 113:438-445, 2006.

5. Longo GM, Xiong W, Greiner TC, et al: Matrix metalloproteinases 2 and 9 work in concert to produce aortic aneurysms. J Clin Invest 110:625-632, 2002.

6. Prall AK, Longo M, Mayhan WG, et al: Doxycycline in patients with abdominal aortic aneurysms and in mice: Comparison of serum levels and effect on aneurysm growth in mice. J Vasc Surg 35:923-929, 2002.

7. Curci JA, Mao D, Bohner DG, et al: Preoperative treatment with doxycycline reduces aortic wall expression and activation of matrix metalloproteinases in patients with abdominal aortic aneurysms. J Vasc Surg 31:325-342, 2000.

8. Baxter BT, Pearce WH, Waltke EA, et al: Prolonged administration of doxycycline in patients with small asymptomatic abdominal aortic aneurysms: Report of a prospective (phase II) multicenter study. J Vasc Surg 36:1-12, 2002.

9. Vammen S, Lindholt JS, Ostergaard L, et al: Randomized double-blind trial of roxithromycin for prevention of abdominal aortic aneurysm expansion. Br J Surg 88:1066-1072, 2001.

10. Steinmetz EF, Buckley C, Shames ML, et al: Treatment with simvastatin suppresses the development of experimental abdominal aortic aneurysms in normal and hypercholesterolemic mice. Ann Surg 241:92-101, 2005.

11. Wilson WR, Evans J, Bell PR, Thompson MM: HMG-CoA reductase inhibitors (statins) decrease MMP-3 and MMP-9 concentrations in abdominal aortic aneurysms. Eur J Vasc Endovasc Surg 30:259-262, 2005.

12. Lindholt JS, Erlandsen EJ, Henneberg EW: Cystatin C deficiency is associated with the progression of small abdominal aortic aneurysms. Br J Surg 88:1472-1475, 2001.

13. Yoshimura K, Aoki H, Ikeda Y: Regression of abdominal aortic aneurysm by inhibition of c-Jun N-terminal kinase. Nature Medicine 11:1330-1338, 2005.

Diagnosis and Detection of Aortic Disease

14. Multicentre Aneurysm Screening Study Group: Multicentre aneurysm screening study (MASS): Cost-effectiveness analysis of screening for abdominal aortic aneurysms based on four year results from a randomised controlled trial. BMJ 325:1135-1141, 2002.

15. Crow P, Shaw E, Earnshaw JJ, et al: A single normal ultrasonographic scanning at age 65 years rules out significant aneurysm disease for life in men. Br J Surg 88:941-944, 2001.

16. U.S. Preventive Services Task Force: Screening for abdominal aortic aneurysm: Recommendation statement. Ann Int Med 142:198-202, 2005.

17. Brown LC, Powell JT: Risk factors for aneurysm rupture in patients kept under ultrasound surveillance. UK Small Aneurysm Trial Participants. Ann Surg 230:289-296, 1999.

18. Lederle FA, Johnson GR, Wilson SE, et al: Rupture rate of large abdominal aortic aneurysms in patients refusing or unfit for elective repair. JAMA 287:2968-2972, 2002.

Management of AAA

19. The United Kingdom Small Aneurysm Trial Participants: Long-term outcomes of immediate repair compared with surveillance of small abdominal aortic aneurysms. N Engl J Med 346:1445-1452, 2002.

20. Lederle FA, Wilson ES, Johnson GR, et al: Immediate repair compared with surveillance of small abdominal aortic aneurysms. N Engl J Med 346:1437-1444, 2002.

21. Thompson RW: Detection and management of small aortic aneurysms. N Engl J Med 346:1484-1486, 2002.

22. Brewster DC, Cronenwett JL, Hallett JW Jr, et al: Guidelines for the treatment of abdominal aortic aneurysms. Report of a subcommittee of the Joint Council of the American Association for Vascular Surgery and Society for Vascular Surgery. J Vasc Surg 37:1106-1117, 2003.

23. Prinssen M, Verhoeven EL, Buth J, et al: Dutch Randomized Endovascular Aneurysm Management (DREAM) Trial Group. A randomized trial comparing conventional and endovascular repair of abdominal aortic aneurysms. N Engl J Med 351:1607-1618, 2004.

24. Greenhalgh RM, Brown LC, Kwong GP, et al: Comparison of endovascular aneurysm repair with open repair in patients with abdominal aortic aneurysm (EVAR trial 1), 30-day operative mortality results: Randomised controlled trial. Lancet 364:843-848, 2004.

25. Lederle FA. Abdominal aortic aneurysm-open versus endovascular repair. N Engl J Med 351:1677-1679, 2004.

26. Blankensteijn JD, de Jong SE, Prinssen M, et al: Dutch Randomized Endovascular Aneurysm Management (DREAM) Trial Group. Two-year outcomes after conventional or endovascular repair of abdominal aortic aneurysms. N Engl J Med 352:2398-2405, 2005.

27. EVAR trial participants: Endovascular aneurysm repair versus open repair in patients with abdominal aortic aneurysm (EVAR trial 1): Randomised controlled trial. Lancet 365:2179-2186, 2005.

28. Kioka Y, Tanabe A, Kotani Y, et al: Review of coronary artery disease in patients with infrarenal abdominal aortic aneurysm. Circ J 66:1110-1112, 2002.

29. The Propranolol Aneurysm Trial Investigators: The propranolol for small abdominal aortic aneurysms: Results of a randomized trial. J Vasc Surg 35:72-79, 2002.

30. Sukhija R, Aronow WS, Sandhu R, et al: Mortality and size of abdominal aortic aneurysm at long-term follow-up of patients not treated surgically and treated with and without statins. Am J Cardiol 97:279-280, 2006.

31. Habashi JP, Judge DP, Holm TM, et al: Losartan, an AT1 antagonist, prevents aortic aneurysm in a mouse model of Marfan syndrome. Science 312:117-121, 2006.

Thoracic Aortic Aneurysms

32. Coady MA, Davis RR, Roberts M, et al: Familial patterns of thoracic aortic aneurysms. Arch Surg 134:361-367, 1999.

33. Biddinger A, Rocklin M, Coselli J, Milewicz DM: Familial thoracic aortic dilatations and dissections: A case control study. J Vasc Surg 25:506-511, 1997.

34. Milewicz DM, Chen H, Park E-S, et al: Reduced penetrance and variable expressivity of familial thoracic aortic aneurysms/dissections. Am J Cardiol 82:474-479, 1998.

35. Pannu H, Fadulu VT, Chang J, et al: Mutations in transforming growth factor-beta receptor type II cause familial thoracic aortic aneurysms and dissections. Circulation 112:513-520, 2005.

36. Nkomo VT, Enriquez-Sarano M, Ammash NM, et al: Bicuspid aortic valve associated with aortic dilatation: A community-based study. Arterioscler Thromb Vasc Biol 23:351-356, 2003.

37. de Sa M, Moshkovitz Y, Butany J, David TE: Histologic abnormalities of the ascending aorta and pulmonary trunk in patients with bicuspid aortic valve disease: Clinical relevance to the Ross procedure. J Thorac Cardiovasc Surg 118:588-596, 1999.

38. Huntington K, Hunter AG, Chan KL: A prospective study to assess the frequency of familial clustering of congenital bicuspid aortic valve. J Am Coll Cardiol 30:1809-1812, 1997.

39. Fedak PW, de Sa MP, Verma S, et al: Vascular matrix remodeling in patients with bicuspid aortic valve malformations: Implications for aortic dilatation. J Thorac Cardiovasc Surg 126:797-806, 2003.

40. LeMaire SA, Wang X, Wilks JA, et al: Matrix metalloproteinases in ascending aortic aneurysms: Bicuspid versus trileaflet aortic valves. J Surg Res 123:40-48, 2005.

41. Chen L, Wang X, Carter SA, et al: A single nucleotide polymorphism in the matrix metalloproteinase 9 gene (-8202A/G) is associated with thoracic aortic aneurysms and thoracic aortic dissection. J Thorac Cardiovasc Surg 131:1045-1052, 2006.

42. Ikonomidis JS, Barbour JR, Amani Z, et al: Effects of deletion of the matrix metalloproteinase 9 gene on development of murine thoracic aortic aneurysms. Circulation 112(9 Suppl):I242-I248, 2005.

43. Davies RR, Goldstein LJ, Coady MA, et al: Yearly rupture or dissection rates for thoracic aortic aneurysms: Simple prediction based on size. Ann Thorac Surg 73:17-28, 2002.

44. Hagl C, Strauch JT, Spielvogel D, et al: Is the Bentall procedure for ascending aorta or aortic valve replacement the best approach for long-term event-free survival? Ann Thorac Surg 76:698-703, 2003.

45. David TE, Ivanov J, Armstrong S, et al: Aortic valve-sparing operations in patients with aneurysms of the aortic root or ascending aorta. Ann Thorac Surg 74:S1758-S1761, 2002.

46. Isselbacher EM: Contemporary reviews in cardiovascular medicine: Thoracic and abdominal aortic aneurysms. Circulation 111:816-828, 2005.

47. Spielvogel D, Strauch JT, Minanov OP, et al: Aortic arch replacement using a trifurcated graft and selective cerebral antegrade perfusion. Ann Thorac Surg 74:S1810-S1814, 2002.

48. Hagl C, Ergin MA, Galla JD, et al: Neurologic outcome after ascending aorta-aortic arch operations: Effect of brain protection technique in high-risk patients. J Thorac Cardiovasc Surg 121:1107-1121, 2001.

49. Kazui T, Washiyama N, Muhammad BAH, et al: Improved results of atherosclerotic arch aneurysm operations with a refined technique. J Thorac Cardiovasc Surg 121:491-499, 2001.

50. LeMaire SA, Carter SA, Coselli JS: The elephant trunk technique for staged repair of complex aneurysms of the entire thoracic aorta. Ann Thorac Surg 81:1561-1569, 2006.

51. Greenberg RK, Haddad F, Svensson L, et al: Hybrid approaches to thoracic aortic aneurysms: The role of endovascular elephant trunk completion. Circulation 112:2619-2626, 2005.

52. Coselli JS, LeMaire SA, Koksoy C, et al: Cerebrospinal fluid drainage reduces paraplegia after thoracoabdominal aortic aneurysm repair: Results of a randomized clinical trial. J Vasc Surg 35:631-639, 2002.

53. Makaroun MS, Dillavou ED, Kee ST, et al: Endovascular treatment of thoracic aortic aneurysms: Results of the phase II multicenter trial of the GORE TAG thoracic endoprosthesis. J Vasc Surg 41:1-9, 2005.

54. Carrel TP, Do DD, Triller J, Schmidli J: A less invasive approach to completely repair the aortic arch. Ann Thorac Surg 80:1475-1478, 2005.

Aortic Dissection

55. Meszaros I, Morocz J, Szlavi J, et al: Epidemiology and clinicopathology of aortic dissection: A population-based longitudinal study over 27 years. Chest 117:1271-1278, 2000.

56. Hagan PG, Nienaber CA, Isselbacher EM, et al: International Registry of Acute Aortic Dissection (IRAD): New insights into an old disease. JAMA 283:897-903, 2000.

57. Eagle KA, Isselbacher EM, DeSanctis W: Cocaine-related aortic dissection in perspective. Circulation 105:1529-1530, 2002.

58. Januzzi JL, Sabatine MS, Eagle KA, et al: Iatrogenic aortic dissection. Am J Cardiol 89:623-626, 2002.

59. Spittell PC, Spittell JA, Jr., Joyce JW, et al: Clinical features and differential diagnosis of aortic dissection: Experience with 236 cases (1980 through 1990). Mayo Clin Proc 68:642-651, 1993.

60. Nallamothu BK, Mahta RH, Saint S, et al: Syncope in acute aortic dissection: Diagnostic, prognostic, and clinical implications. Am J Med 133:468-471, 2002.

61. Kim MH, Eagle KA, Isselbacher EM: Bayesian persuasion. Circulation 100:e68-e72, 1999.

62. Ohlmann P, Faure A, Morel O, et al: Diagnostic and prognostic value of circulating D-dimers in patients with acute aortic dissection. Crit Care Med 34:1358-1364, 2006.

63. Moore AG, Eagle KA, Bruckman D, et al: Choice of computed tomography, transesophageal echocardiography, magnetic resonance imaging, and aortography in acute aortic dissection: International Registry of Acute Aortic Dissection (IRAD). Am J Cardiol 89:1235-1238, 2002.

64. Penn MS, Smedira N, Lytle B, Brener SJ: Does coronary angiography before emergency aortic surgery affect in-hospital mortality? J Am Coll Cardiol 35:889-894, 2000.

65. Trimarchi S, Nienaber CA, Rampoldi V, et al: Contemporary results of surgery in acute type A aortic dissection: The International Registry of Acute Aortic Dissection experience. J Thorac Cardiovasc Surg 129:112-122, 2005.

66. Sabik JF, Lytle BW, Blackstone EH, et al: Long-term effectiveness of operations for ascending aortic dissections. J Thorac Cardiovasc Surg 119:946-962, 2000.

67. Movsowitz HD, Levine RA, Hilgenberg AD, Isselbacher EM: Transesophageal echocardiographic description of the mechanisms of aortic regurgitation in acute type A aortic dissection: Implications for aortic valve repair. J Am Coll Cardiol 36:884-890, 2000.

68. Bavaria JE, Brinster DR, Gorman RC, et al: Advances in the treatment of acute type a dissection: An integrated approach, Ann Thorac Surg 74:S1848-S1852, 2002.

69. Kazui T, Washiyama N, Bashar AHM, et al: Role of biologic glue repair of proximal aortic dissection in the development of early and midterm re-dissection of the aortic root. Ann Thorac Surg 72:509-514, 2001.

70. Lauterbach SE, Cambria RP, Brewster DC, et al: Contemporary management of aortic branch compromise resulting from acute aortic dissection. J Vasc Surg 33:1185-1192, 2001.

71. Nienaber CA, Fattori R, Lund G, et al: Nonsurgical reconstruction of thoracic aortic dissection by stent-graft placement. N Engl J Med 340:1539-1545, 1999.

72. Dake MD, Kato N, Mitchell RS, et al: Endovascular stent-graft placement for the treatment of acute aortic dissection. N Engl J Med 340:1546-1552, 1999.

73. Nienaber CA, Zannetti S, Barbieri B, et al: INvestigation of STEnt grafts in patients with type B Aortic Dissection: Design of the INSTEAD trial—a prospective, multicenter, European randomized trial. Am Heart J 149:592-599, 2005.

74. Januzzi JL, Sabatine MS, Choi JC, et al: Refractory systemic hypertension following type B aortic dissection. Am J Cardiol 88:686-688, 2001.

Other Aortic Syndromes

75. Neri E, Sassi S, Massetti M, et al: Nonocclusive intestinal ischemia in patients with acute aortic dissection. J Vasc Surg 36:738-745, 2002.

76. Sawhney NS, DeMaria AN, Blanchard DG: Aortic intramural hematoma: An increasingly recognized and potentially fatal entity. Chest 120:1340-1346, 2001.

77. Song J-K, Kim H-S, Song JM, et al: Outcomes of medically treated patients with aortic intramural hematoma. Am J Med 113:181-187, 2002.

78. Kaji S, Nishigami K, Akasaka T, et al: Prediction of progression or regression of type A intramural hematoma by computed tomography. Circulation 100(Suppl II): II281-II286, 1999.

79. Sueyoshi E, Imada T, Sakamoto I, et al: Analysis of predictive factors for progression of type B aortic intramural hematoma with computed tomography. J Vasc Surg 35:1179-1183, 2002.

80. Isselbacher EM: Intramural hematoma of the aorta: Should we let down our guard? Am J Med 113:244-246, 2002.

81. Coady MA, Rizzo JA, Hammond GL, et al: Penetrating ulcer of the thoracic aorta: What is it? How do we recognize it? How do we manage it? J Vasc Surg 27:1006-1015, 1998.

82. Tittle SL, Lynch RJ, Cole PE, et al: Midterm follow-up of penetrating ulcer and intramural hematoma of the aorta. J Thorac Cardiovasc Surg 123:1051-1059, 2002.

83. Ganaha F, Miller DC, Sugimoto K, et al: Prognosis of aortic intramural hematoma with and without penetrating atherosclerotic ulcer: A clinical and radiological analysis. Circulation 106:342-348, 2002.

84. Muller BT, Wegener OR, Grabitz K, et al: Mycotic aneurysms of the thoracic and abdominal aorta and iliac arteries: Experience with anatomic and extra-anatomic repair in 33 cases. J Vasc Surg 33:106-113, 2001.

85. Oderich GS, Panneton JM, Bower TC, et al: Infected aortic aneurysms: Aggressive presentation, complicated early outcome, and durable results. J Vasc Surg 34:900-908, 2001.

86. Leseche G, Castier Y, Petit M-D, et al: Long-term results of cryopreserved arterial allograft reconstruction in infected prosthetic grafts and mycotic aneurysms of the abdominal aorta. J Vasc Surg 34:616-622, 2001.

87. Bohner H, Luther B, Braunstein S, et al: Primary malignant tumors of the aorta: Clinical presentation, treatment, and course of different entities. J Vasc Surg 38:1430-1433, 2003.

CH 56

Diseases of the Aorta

CHAPTER 57

Epidemiology, 1491

Risk Factors for Peripheral Arterial
Disease, 1491

Pathophysiology of Peripheral Arterial
Disease, 1493
Skeletal Muscle Structure and Metabolic
    Function, 1494

Clinical Presentation, 1494
Symptoms, 1494
Physical Findings, 1495
Categorization, 1495

Testing for Peripheral Arterial
Disease, 1496
Segmental Pressure Measurement and
    Ankle/Brachial Indices, 1496
Ankle/Brachial Index, 1496
Treadmill Exercise Testing, 1497
Duplex Ultrasound Imaging, 1498
Magnetic Resonance Angiography, 1498
Computed Tomographic Angiography, 1499
Contrast Angiography, 1499

Prognosis, 1499

Treatment, 1500
Risk Factor Modification, 1500
Smoking Cessation, 1500
Treatment of Diabetes, 1501
Blood Pressure Control, 1501
Antiplatelet Therapy, 1502
Pharmacotherapy, 1502
Exercise Rehabilitation, 1504

Percutaneous Transluminal Angioplasty
and Stents, 1504
Peripheral Arterial Surgery, 1505
Algorithm for Treatment of the Symptomatic
    Leg, 1505

Vasculitis, 1505

Thromboangiitis Obliterans, 1505
Pathology and Pathogenesis, 1505
Clinical Presentation, 1506
Diagnosis, 1506
Treatment, 1506

Takayasu Arteritis and Giant Cell
Arteritis, 1507

Fibromuscular Dysplasia, 1507

Popliteal Artery Entrapment
Syndrome, 1507

Acute Limb Ischemia, 1507
Prognosis, 1507
Pathogenesis, 1508
Diagnostic Tests, 1508
Treatment, 1508

Atheroembolism, 1509
Pathogenesis, 1509
Clinical Presentation, 1510
Diagnostic Tests, 1510
Treatment, 1511

References, 1511

Peripheral Arterial Diseases

Mark A. Creager and Peter Libby

The term *peripheral arterial disease* (PAD) generally refers to a disorder that obstructs the blood supply to the lower or upper extremities. It is most commonly caused by atherosclerosis but may also result from thrombosis, embolism, vasculitis, fibromuscular dysplasia, or entrapment. The term *peripheral vascular disease* has less specificity because it encompasses a group of diseases affecting blood vessels including not only PAD but also other atherosclerotic conditions such as renal artery disease and carotid artery disease, as well as vasculitides, vasospasm, venous thrombosis, venous insufficiency, and lymphatic disorders.

Traditionally, cardiologists have devoted most of their efforts to the diagnosis and treatment of arterial disease of the coronary tree. Although cardiology training and practice often accord a place to diseases of the aorta, focus on the disease of the peripheral arteries has lagged. PAD strongly correlates with risk of major cardiovascular events because it frequently associates with coronary and cerebral atherosclerosis. Moreover, symptoms of PAD including intermittent claudication jeopardize quality of life and independence for many patients. In contrast to coronary artery afflictions, PAD is commonly underdiagnosed and undertreated. Thus practitioners of cardiology have increasing interest in the diagnosis and management of PAD. This chapter provides a framework for the approach to the diagnosis and management of the patient with PAD.

EPIDEMIOLOGY

The prevalence of PAD varies depending on the population studied, the diagnostic method used, and whether symptoms are included to derive estimates. Most epidemiological studies have used a noninvasive measurement, the ankle/brachial index (ABI), to diagnose PAD. The ABI is the ratio of the ankle-to-brachial systolic blood pressure and is described in greater detail later in this chapter. In relatively large population-based studies conducted in the United States, Europe, and the Middle East, the prevalence of PAD based on abnormal ABI ranged from 3.6 to 29 percent (Table 57-1).[1-4] PAD is present in approximately 4 percent of persons 40 years of age and older but in 15 to 20 percent of those 65 years and older. PAD prevalence is greater in men than in women in some studies. The prevalence of PAD is greater in blacks than non-Hispanic whites.[5] In the Multi-Ethnic Study of Atherosclerosis (MESA), the odds for developing PAD were 1.47 times higher in blacks than non-Hispanic whites, whereas it was less than 0.5 in Hispanics and Chinese.[6] These aggregate data indicate that some 8 to 10 million individuals in the United States have PAD.

Questionnaires specifically designed to elicit symptoms of intermittent claudication can assess the prevalence of symptomatic disease in these populations. Estimates have varied depending on the age and gender of the population but generally indicate that only 10 to 30 percent of patients with PAD have symptoms of claudication. Overall, the estimated prevalence of claudication ranges from 1 to 4.5 percent of a population typically older than 40 years of age.[4,7] The prevalence and incidence of claudication increase with age and are greater in men than in women in most but not all studies (Fig. 57-1).[1,4,7,8] Less information is available regarding the incidence of critical limb ischemia, but it is estimated at 400 to 450 per million population per year.[4] The incidence of amputation ranges from 112 to 250 per million population per year.

RISK FACTORS FOR PERIPHERAL ARTERIAL DISEASE (see also Chap. 39)

The well-known modifiable risk factors associated with coronary atherosclerosis also contribute to atherosclerosis of the

TABLE 57–1 | **Prevalence of Peripheral Arterial Disease**

Study/Location	No.	Population Age (yr)	Prevalence (%)
San Diego	613	38-82	11.7
The Jerusalem Lipid Research Clinic Prevalence Study	1592	≥35	4.6
The Edinburgh Artery Study	1592	55-74	9.0
The Cardiovascular Health Study	5084	≥65	12.4
The Rotterdam Study	7715	≥55	19.1
The Limburg PAOD Study 3650	3650	40-78	12.4
The Strong Heart Study	4549	45-74	5.3
The PARTNERS Program	6979	50-69*; ≥70	29
German Epidemiologic Trial on ABI	6880	≥65	19.8
The Framingham Offspring Study	3313	≥40	3.6
NHANES	2174	≥40 ≥70	4.3 14.5

*Age 50-69 plus diabetes or cigarette smoking.

ABI = ankle/brachial index; NHANES = National Health and Nutrition Examination Survey; PAOD = peripheral arterial occlusive disease.

CH 57

TABLE 57–2 | **Risk of Peripheral Arterial Disease in Persons with Modifiable Risk Factors**

Risk Factor	Odds Ratio
Cigarette smoking	2.0-2.7
Diabetes mellitus	1.9-4.0
Hypertension	1.3-2.2
Hypercholesterolemia (per 10 mg/dl increase in total cholesterol)	1.05-1.10
Fibrinogen	2.2-2.5
C-reactive protein	2.1-2.8
Hyperhomocysteinemia	1.7-6.8

peripheral circulation. Cigarette smoking, diabetes mellitus, dyslipidemia, and hypertension increase the risk of PAD (Table 57-2).[9] Data derived from several observational studies (including the Edinburgh Artery Study, the Framingham Heart Study, and the Cardiovascular Health Study) indicate a twofold to threefold increase in the risk of developing PAD in smokers.[1,4,10] Approximately 84 to 90 percent of patients with claudication are current or ex-smokers.[11] Progression of disease to critical limb ischemia and limb loss is more likely to occur in patients who continue to smoke than in those who stop. Smoking can even increase the risk of developing PAD more than it does coronary artery disease. Current smoking dose-dependently correlates with the presence of PAD in both men and women, and smoking cessation lowers PAD risk.[12] Patients with diabetes mellitus often have extensive and severe PAD and a greater propensity for arterial calcification.[13,14] Involvement of the femoral and popliteal arteries resembles that of nondiabetic persons, but distal disease affecting the tibial and peroneal arteries occurs more frequently. The risk of developing PAD increases twofold to fourfold in patients with diabetes mellitus.[10] Among patients with PAD, diabetic patients are more likely to have an amputation than nondiabetic patients.

Abnormalities in lipid metabolism also associate with an increased prevalence of PAD. Elevations in total or low-density lipoprotein (LDL) cholesterol increase the risk of developing PAD and claudication in some studies but not in others.[10,15] The odds ratio for developing claudication in the Framingham Heart Study was 1.2 for each 40 mg/dl increase in total cholesterol.[16] Analysis of a cohort of patients participating in a Lipid Research Clinic protocol, however, found no association between LDL cholesterol and PAD based on a multiple logistic regression model that included cigarette smoking, blood pressure, glucose, and obesity.[1] Hypertriglyceridemia independently predicts risk for PAD.[10,17,18] Some, but not all epidemiological studies have found a link between hypertension and PAD.[19] The risk of developing PAD and intermittent claudication increases progressively with the burden of contributing factors. In the Framingham study the probability of claudication in a 70-year-old man whose only risk factor was smoking versus nonsmoking was 2.5 versus 0.8 percent per 4 years. In a 70-year-old male smoker who was also hypertensive, hypercholesterolemic, and diabetic, the risk increased to 24 percent per 4 years (Fig. 57-2).[16] Similar observations apply to women.

Contemporary views of atherogenesis emphasize a role for inflammation as a link between risk factors and the formation and complication of lesions. Strong evidence supports the concept that the pathobiology of PAD involves inflammation, as in the coronary circulation. Classic studies associated high levels of fibrinogen with risk not only of coronary events but also with the development of PAD. Current analyses suggest that adjustment for the trigger of the acute phase response interleukin-6, or for inflammatory markers such as C-reactive protein (CRP), eliminates the risk for PAD associated with fibrinogen.[20] Thus the elevated fibrinogen levels in PAD may reflect inflammation as much or more than a procoagulant effect. Considerable evidence links leukocytes, the crucial cellular mediators of the inflammatory response, and the development of PAD. Levels of the soluble forms of leukocyte adhesion molecules correlate with the development and extent of PAD and with the

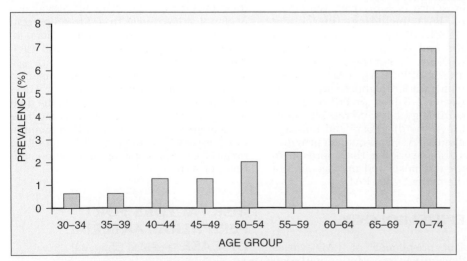

FIGURE 57–1 Age-related prevalence of intermittent claudication derived from large population-based studies. *(From Dormandy JA, Rutherford RB: Management of peripheral arterial disease (PAD). Norgren L, Hiatt WR, Dormandy JA, et al: Inter-Society Consensus for the Management of Peripheral Arterial Disease (TASC II). Eur J Vasc Endovasc Surg 33:S1-S75, 2007.)*

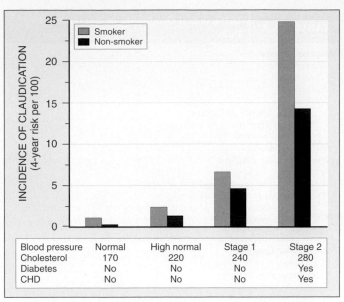

Blood pressure	Normal	High normal	Stage 1	Stage 2
Cholesterol	170	220	240	280
Diabetes	No	No	No	Yes
CHD	No	No	No	Yes

FIGURE 57–2 The incidence of intermittent claudication in the Framingham Heart Study in smokers and nonsmokers is compounded by an increased burden of risk factors. CHD = coronary heart disease. *(From Murabito JM, D'Agostino RB, Silbershatz H, Wilson WF: Intermittent claudication: A risk profile from the Framingham Heart Study. Circulation 96:44, 1997.)*

risk of complications.[21-25] Levels of CRP and of monocytes in peripheral blood independently associate with PAD, consistent with a role for innate immunity and chronic inflammation in its pathogenesis.[24,26] Inflammation provides the mechanistic link between many of the common risk factors for atherosclerosis and the pathophysiological processes in the arterial wall that lead to PAD. Ongoing studies will determine whether biomarkers of inflammation add to traditional risk factors in gauging susceptibility to PAD.

PATHOPHYSIOLOGY OF PERIPHERAL ARTERIAL DISEASE

Pathophysiological considerations in patients with PAD must take into account the balance of circulatory supply of nutrients to the skeletal muscle and the oxygen and nutrient demand of the skeletal muscle (Table 57-3). Intermittent claudication occurs when skeletal muscle oxygen demand during effort exceeds blood oxygen supply and results from activation of local sensory receptors by accumulation of lactate or other metabolites. Patients with intermittent claudication may have single or multiple occlusive lesions in the arteries supplying the limb. Blood flow and leg oxygen consumption are normal at rest, but the obstructive lesions limit blood flow and oxygen delivery so that the metabolic needs of the exercising muscle during exercise outstrip the available supply of oxygen and nutrients. Patients with critical limb ischemia typically have multiple occlusive lesions that often affect proximal and distal limb arteries. As a result, even the resting blood supply diminishes and cannot meet the nutritional needs of the limb.

FACTORS REGULATING BLOOD SUPPLY (see also Chap. 48)

The primary determinant of inadequate blood supply to the extremity is a flow-limiting lesion of a conduit artery. Flow through an artery is directly proportional to perfusion pressure and inversely proportional to the vascular resistance. If atherosclerosis causes a stenosis, flow through the artery is reduced, as described in the Poiseuille equation, in which

TABLE 57–3	Pathophysiological Considerations in Peripheral Arterial Disease

Factors Regulating Blood Supply to Limb
Flow-limiting lesion (stenosis severity, inadequate collateral vessels)

Impaired vasodilation (decreased nitric oxide and reduced responsiveness to vasodilators)

Accentuated vasoconstriction (thromboxane, serotonin, angiotensin II, endothelin, norepinephrine)

Abnormal rheology (reduced red blood cell deformability, increased leukocyte adhesivity, platelet aggregation, microthrombosis, increased fibrinogen)

Altered Skeletal Muscle Structure and Function
Axonal denervation of skeletal muscle

Loss of type II, glycolytic fast twist fibers

Impaired mitochondrial enzymatic activity

$$Q = \frac{\Delta P \pi r^4}{8 \eta l}$$

where ΔP is the pressure gradient across the stenosis, r is the radius of the residual lumen, η is blood viscosity, and l is the length of the vessel affected by the stenosis. As the severity of a stenotic lesion increases, flow becomes progressively reduced. The pressure gradient across the stenosis increases in a nonlinear manner, emphasizing the importance of a stenosis at high blood flow rates. Usually, a blood pressure gradient exists at rest if the stenosis reduces the lumen diameter by more than 50 percent because as distorted flow develops, there is loss of kinetic energy. A stenosis that does not cause a pressure gradient at rest may cause a gradient during exercise, when blood flow rises consequent to higher cardiac output and vascular resistance decreases. Thus as flow through a stenosis increases, distal perfusion pressure is not maintained. Also, as the metabolic demand of exercising muscle outstrips its blood supply, local metabolites including adenosine, nitric oxide, potassium, and hydrogen ion accumulate and peripheral resistance vessels dilate. This results in a further drop of perfusion pressure because the stenosis limits flow. In addition, intramuscular pressure rises during exercise and may exceed the arterial pressure distal to an occlusion, causing blood flow to cease. Flow through collateral blood vessels can usually meet the resting metabolic needs of the skeletal muscle tissue but does not suffice during exercise.

Functional abnormalities in vasomotor reactivity may also interfere with blood flow. Vasodilator capability of both conduit and resistance vessels is less in patients with peripheral atherosclerosis. Normally, arteries dilate in response to pharmacological and biochemical stimuli such as acetylcholine, serotonin, thrombin, or bradykinin, as well as to shear stress induced by increases in blood flow. This vasodilator response results from the release of biologically active substances from the endothelium, particularly nitric oxide (see Chap. 48). The vascular relaxation of a conduit vessel that occurs after a flow stimulus, such as that induced by exercise, may assist the delivery of blood to exercising muscles in healthy persons. Endothelium-dependent vasodilation subsequent to flow or pharmacological stimuli is impaired in the atherosclerotic femoral arteries and calf resistance vessels of patients with PAD. This failure of vasodilation might prevent an increase in nutritive blood supply to exercising muscle because endothelium-derived nitric oxide can contribute to hyperemic blood volume after an ischemic stimulus. It is not known whether vasodilator function with respect to prostacyclin, adenosine, or ion-channels is abnormal in atherosclerotic peripheral arteries. Endogenous vasoconstrictor substances such as prostanoids and other lipid mediators, thrombin, serotonin, angiotensin II, endothelin, and norepinephrine may interfere with vasodilation.

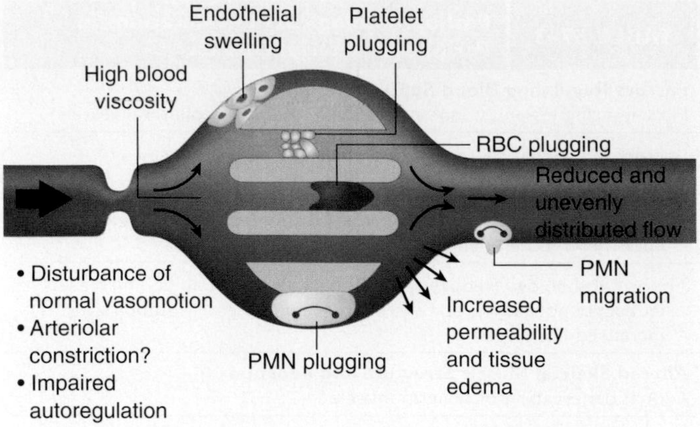

High blood viscosity

Endothelial swelling

Platelet plugging

RBC plugging

Reduced and unevenly distributed flow

PMN migration

- Disturbance of normal vasomotion
- Arteriolar constriction?
- Impaired autoregulation

PMN plugging

Increased permeability and tissue edema

FIGURE 57–3 Schematic representation of potential pathophysiological mechanisms that lead to microvascular obstruction in patients with critical limb ischemia. PMN = polymorphonuclear leukocyte; RBC = red blood cell. *(From Brevetti G, Corrado S, Marone VD, et al: Microcirculation and tissue metabolism in peripheral arterial disease. Clin Hemorheol Microcirc 21:245, 1999.)*

TABLE 57–4	Differential Diagnosis of Exertional Leg Pain

Vascular Causes
  Atherosclerosis
  Thrombosis
  Embolism
  Vasculitis
    Thromboangiitis obliterans
    Takayasu arteritis
    Giant cell arteritis
  Aortic coarctation
  Fibromuscular dysplasia
  Irradiation
  Endofibrosis of the external iliac artery
  Extravascular compression
    Arterial entrapment (e.g., popliteal artery entrapment, thoracic outlet syndrome)
  Adventitial cysts

Nonvascular Causes
  Lumbosacral radiculopathy
    Degenerative arthritis
    Spinal stenosis
    Herniated disc
  Arthritis
    Hips, knees
  Venous insufficiency
  Myositis
  McArdle syndrome

CH 57

Abnormalities in the microcirculation contribute to the pathophysiology of critical limb ischemia. Patients with severe limb ischemia have a reduced number of perfused skin capillaries. Other potential causes of decreased capillary perfusion in this condition include reduced red blood cell deformability, increased leukocyte adhesivity, platelet aggregates, fibrinogen, microvascular thrombosis, excessive vasoconstriction, and interstitial edema (Fig. 57-3). Intravascular pressure may also decrease because of precapillary arteriolar dilation caused by locally released vasoactive metabolites.[27]

Skeletal Muscle Structure and Metabolic Function

Electrophysiological and histopathological examination has found evidence of partial axonal denervation of the skeletal muscle in legs affected by PAD. Preservation of type I, oxidative slow twitch fibers exists, but there is a loss of type II, or glycolytic fast twitch fibers in the skeletal muscle of patients with PAD.[8] The loss of type II fibers correlates with decreased muscle strength and reduced exercise capacity. In skeletal muscle distal to PAD, there is a shift to anaerobic metabolism earlier during exercise and it persists longer after cessation of exercise. Patients with claudication have increased lactate release and accumulation of acylcarnitines during exercise, indicative of ineffective oxidative metabolism.[28] Moreover, mitochondrial respiratory activity and phosphocreatine and adenosine triphosphate recovery time decrease in the calf muscles of PAD patients as assessed after submaximal exercise by ^{31}P magnetic resonance spectroscopy.[29,30]

CLINICAL PRESENTATION

Symptoms

The cardinal symptoms of PAD include intermittent claudication and rest pain. The term *claudication* is derived from the Latin word *claudicare*, "to limp." Intermittent claudication refers to a pain, ache, sense of fatigue, or other discomfort that occurs in the affected muscle group with exercise, particularly walking, and resolves with rest. The location of the symptom often relates to the site of the most proximal stenosis. Buttock, hip, or thigh claudication typically occurs in patients with obstruction of the aorta and iliac arteries.

Calf claudication characterizes femoral or popliteal artery stenoses. The gastrocnemius muscle consumes more oxygen during walking than other muscle groups in the leg and hence causes the most frequent symptom reported by patients. Ankle or pedal claudication occurs in patients with tibial and peroneal artery disease. Similarly, stenoses of the subclavian, axillary, or brachial arteries may cause shoulder, biceps, or forearm claudication, respectively. Symptoms should resolve several minutes after cessation of effort. Calf and thigh pain that occurs at rest, such as nocturnal cramps, should not be confused with claudication and is not a symptom of PAD. The history obtained from persons reporting claudication should note the walking distance, speed, and incline that precipitate claudication. This baseline assessment evaluates disability and provides an initial qualitative measure with which to determine stability, improvement, or deterioration during subsequent encounters with the patient. Symptoms other than claudication can limit functional capacity.[31] Patients with PAD walk more slowly and have less walking endurance than patients who do not have PAD.[32,33]

Several questionnaires have been developed to assess the presence and severity of claudication. The Rose Questionnaire was developed initially to diagnose both angina and intermittent claudication in epidemiological surveys. It questions whether the patient develops pain in either calf with walking and whether the pain occurs at rest, while walking at an ordinary or hurried pace, or when walking uphill. Several modifications to this questionnaire include the Edinburgh Claudication Questionnaire and the San Diego Claudication Questionnaire,[34,35] both of which are more sensitive and specific in comparison to a physician's diagnosis of intermittent claudication based on walking distance, walking speed, and nature of symptoms. Another validated instrument, the Walking Impairment Questionnaire, asks a series of questions and develops a point score based on walking distance, walking speed, and the nature of the symptoms.[36]

Symptoms resembling limb claudication occasionally result from nonatherosclerotic causes of arterial occlusive disease (Table 57-4). Several of these are discussed later in the chapter and include arterial embolism, vasculitides such as thromboangiitis obliterans, Takayasu arteritis, giant cell arteritis, aortic coarctation, fibromuscular dysplasia, irradiation, endofibrosis of the external iliac artery, or extravascular compression caused by arterial entrapment or adventitial cyst (see Chap. 84). Several nonvascular causes of exertional leg pain should be considered in patients who present with symptoms suggestive of intermittent claudication (see Table 57-4). Lumbosacral radiculopathy resulting from degenerative joint disease, spinal stenosis, and herniated discs can cause pain in the buttock, hip, thigh, calf, and/or foot with walking, often after short distances or even with standing. The term *neurogenic pseudoclaudication* has been used to describe this symptom. Lumbosacral spine disease and PAD both preferentially affect the elderly and hence may coexist in the same individual. Arthritis of the hips and knees also provokes leg pain with walking. Typically, the pain localizes to the affected joint and can be elicited on physical examination through palpation and range-of-motion maneuvers. Exertional compartment syndrome is most often seen in athletes with large calf muscles. Increased tissue pressure during exercise limits microvascular flow and results in calf pain or tightness. Symptoms improve after cessation of exercise. Rarely, skeletal muscle disorders such as myositis can cause exertional leg pain. Muscle tenderness, an abnormal neuromuscular examination finding, elevated skeletal muscle enzyme levels, and a normal pulse examination finding should distinguish myositis from PAD. McArdle syndrome, in which there is a deficiency of skeletal muscle phosphorylase, can cause symptoms mimicking the claudication of PAD. Patients with chronic venous insufficiency sometimes report leg discomfort with exertion, which is designated *venous claudication*. Venous hypertension during exercise increases arterial resistance in the affected limb and limits blood flow. In the case of venous insufficiency, elevated extravascular pressure caused by interstitial edema further diminishes capillary perfusion. A physical examination demonstrating peripheral edema, venous stasis pigmentation, and occasionally venous varicosities will identify this unusual cause of exertional leg pain.

Symptoms may occur at rest in patients with critical limb ischemia. Typically, patients complain of pain or paresthesias in the foot or toes of the affected extremity. This discomfort worsens on leg elevation and improves with leg dependency, as might be anticipated by the effect of gravity on perfusion pressure. The pain can be particularly severe at sites of skin fissuring, ulceration, or necrosis. Often the skin is sensitive and even the weight of bedclothes or sheets elicits pain. Patients may sit on the edge of the bed and dangle their legs to alleviate the discomfort. Patients with ischemic or diabetic neuropathy can experience little or no pain despite the presence of severe ischemia.

Critical limb and digital ischemia can result from arterial occlusions other than those caused by atherosclerosis. These include conditions such as thromboangiitis obliterans, vasculitides such as systemic lupus erythematosus or scleroderma, vasospasm, atheromatous embolism, and acute arterial occlusion caused by thrombosis or embolism (see later). Acute gouty arthritis, trauma, and sensory neuropathies such as those caused by diabetes mellitus, lumbosacral radiculopathies, and complex regional pain syndrome (previously known as reflex sympathetic dystrophy) can cause foot pain. Leg ulcers also occur in patients with venous insufficiency and sensory neuropathies, particularly those related to diabetes. These ulcers are easily distinguished from arterial ulcers. The venous ulcer usually localizes near the medial malleolus and has an irregular border and a pink base with granulation tissue. Venous ulcers produce milder pain than arterial ulcers. Neurotrophic ulcers occur where there is pressure or trauma,

usually on the sole of the foot. These ulcers are deep, frequently infected, and usually not painful because of the loss of sensation.

Physical Findings

The complete cardiovascular examination includes palpation of pulses and auscultation of accessible arteries for bruits. Pulse abnormalities and bruits increase the likelihood of PAD.[37] Readily palpable pulses in healthy individuals include the brachial, radial, and ulnar arteries of the upper extremities and the femoral, popliteal, dorsalis pedis, and posterior tibial arteries of the lower extremities. The aorta can also be palpated in asthenic persons. A decreased or absent pulse provides insight into the location of arterial stenoses. For example, a normal right femoral pulse but absent left femoral pulse suggests the presence of left iliofemoral arterial stenosis. A normal femoral artery pulse but absent popliteal artery pulse would indicate a stenosis in the superficial femoral artery or proximal popliteal artery. Similarly, disease of the anterior and posterior tibial arteries can be inferred when the popliteal artery pulse is present but the dorsalis pedis and posterior tibial pulses, respectively, are not palpable. Bruits often indicate accelerated blood flow velocity and flow disturbance at sites of stenosis. A stethoscope should be used to auscultate the supraclavicular and infraclavicular fossae for evidence of subclavian artery stenosis; the abdomen, flank, and pelvis for evidence of stenoses in the aorta and its branch vessels; and each groin for evidence of femoral artery stenoses. Pallor can be elicited on the soles of the feet of some patients with PAD by performing a maneuver in which the feet are elevated above the level of the heart and the calf muscles are exercised by repeated dorsiflexion and plantar flexion of the ankle. The legs are then placed in the dependent position and the time to the onset of hyperemia and venous distention is measured. Each of these variables depends on the rate of blood flow, which in turn reflects the severity of stenosis and adequacy of collateral vessels.

The legs of patients with chronic aortoiliac disease may show muscle atrophy. Additional signs of chronic low-grade ischemia include hair loss, thickened and brittle toenails, smooth and shiny skin, and subcutaneous fat atrophy of the digital pads. Patients with severe limb ischemia have cool skin and may also have petechiae, persistent cyanosis or pallor, dependent rubor, pedal edema resulting from prolonged dependency, skin fissures, ulceration, or gangrene. Arterial ulcers typically have a pale base with irregular borders and usually involve the tips of the toes or the heel of the foot, or they develop at sites of pressure (Fig. 57-4). These ulcers vary in size and may be as small as 3 to 5 mm.

Categorization

Classification of patients with PAD depends on the severity of the symptoms and abnormalities detected on physical examination. Categorization of the clinical manifestations of PAD improves communication among professionals caring for these patients and provides a structure for defining guidelines for therapeutic interventions. Fontaine described one widely used scheme that classified patients in one of four stages progressing from asymptomatic to critical limb ischemia (Table 57-5). Several professional vascular societies have adopted a contemporary, more descriptive classification that includes asymptomatic patients, three grades of claudication, and three grades of critical limb ischemia ranging from rest pain alone to minor and major tissue loss (Table 57-6).[38]

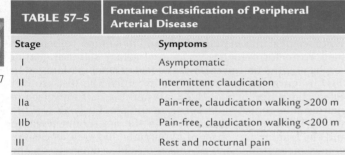

FIGURE 57–4 The typical arterial ulcer is a discrete, circumscribed, necrotic ulcer located on the great toe.

TABLE 57–5	Fontaine Classification of Peripheral Arterial Disease
Stage	**Symptoms**
I	Asymptomatic
II	Intermittent claudication
IIa	Pain-free, claudication walking >200 m
IIb	Pain-free, claudication walking <200 m
III	Rest and nocturnal pain
IV	Necrosis, gangrene

TABLE 57–6		Clinical Categories of Chronic Limb Ischemia
Grade	**Category**	**Clinical Description**
	0	Asymptomatic, not hemodynamically correct
I	1	Mild claudication
	2	Moderate claudication
	3	Severe claudication
II	4	Ischemic rest pain
	5	Minor tissue loss: nonhealing ulcer, focal gangrene with diffuse pedal ulcer
III	6	Major tissue loss extending above transmetatarsal level, functional foot no longer salvageable

Modified from Rutherford RB, Baker JD, Ernst C, et al: Recommended standards for reports dealing with lower extremity ischemia: Revised version. J Vasc Surg 26:517, 1997.

TESTING FOR PERIPHERAL ARTERIAL DISEASE

Segmental Pressure Measurement and Ankle/Brachial Indices

The measurement of systolic blood pressure along selected segments of each extremity furnishes one of the most useful and simplest noninvasive tests to evaluate the presence and severity of stenoses in the peripheral arteries. In the lower extremities, pneumatic cuffs are placed on the upper and lower portions of the thigh, the calf, above the ankle, and often over the metatarsal area of the foot. Likewise, for the upper extremity, pneumatic cuffs are placed on the upper arm over the biceps, on the forearm below the elbow, and at the wrist. Systolic blood pressure at each respective limb segment can be measured by first inflating the pneumatic cuff to suprasystolic pressure and then determining the pressure at which blood flow occurs during cuff deflation. The onset of flow can be assessed by placing a Doppler ultrasound flow probe over an artery distal to the cuff. In the lower extremities, it is most convenient to place the Doppler probe on the foot over the posterior tibial artery as it courses inferior and posterior to the medial malleolus or over the dorsalis pedis artery on the dorsum of the metatarsal arch. In the upper extremities, the Doppler probe can be placed over the brachial artery in the antecubital fossa or over the radial and ulnar arteries at the wrist.

Left ventricular contraction imparts kinetic energy to blood, which is maintained throughout the large and medium-sized vessels. Systolic blood pressure in the more distal vessels may be higher than in the aorta and proximal vessels because of amplification and reflection of blood pressure waves. A stenosis can cause loss of pressure energy as a result of increased frictional forces and flow disturbance at the site of the stenosis. Approximately 90 percent of the cross-sectional area of the aorta must be narrowed before a pressure gradient develops. In smaller vessels, such as the iliac and femoral arteries, a 70 to 90 percent decrease in cross-sectional area will cause a resting pressure gradient sufficient to decrease systolic blood pressure distal to the stenosis. Taking into consideration the precision of this noninvasive method and the variability in blood pressure over even short periods of time, a blood pressure gradient in excess of 20 mm Hg between successive cuffs is generally used as evidence of arterial stenosis in the lower extremity, whereas a 10 mm Hg gradient indicates a stenosis between sequential cuffs in the upper extremity. Systolic blood pressure in the toes and fingers approximates 60 percent of the systolic blood pressure at the ankle and wrist, respectively, as pressure diminishes further in the smaller distal vessels.

Figure 57-5 gives examples of leg segmental pressure measurements in a patient with bilateral calf claudication. In the right leg, there are pressure gradients between the upper and lower thigh and between the calf and ankle. These gradients indicate stenoses in the superficial femoral artery and in the tibioperoneal arteries. In the left leg, pressure gradients between the upper and lower thigh, between the lower thigh and calf, and between the calf and ankle indicate stenoses in the superficial femoral and popliteal arteries and in the tibioperoneal arteries.

Ankle/Brachial Index

Determination of the ABI furnishes a simplified application of leg segmental blood pressure measurements readily used at the bedside (see Fig. 57-5). This index is the ratio of the systolic blood pressure measured at the ankle to the systolic blood pressure measured at the brachial artery. A pneumatic cuff placed around the ankle is inflated to suprasystolic pressure and subsequently deflated, while the onset of flow is detected with a Doppler ultrasound probe placed over the dorsalis pedis and posterior tibial arteries, thus denoting ankle systolic blood pressure. Brachial artery systolic pressure can be assessed in a routine manner, using either a stethoscope to listen for the first Korotkoff sound or a Doppler probe to listen for the onset of flow during cuff deflation. The normal ABI should be 1 or greater. However,

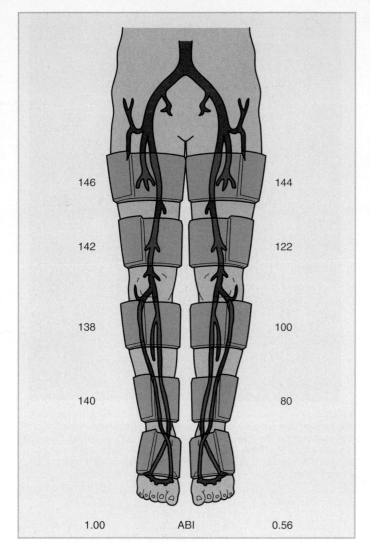

FIGURE 57–5 Segmental pressure measurements in a patient with left calf intermittent claudication. Brachial artery systolic pressure in each arm equals 140. Pressure gradient is present between the left upper and lower thigh cuffs, lower thigh and calf cuffs, and calf and ankle cuffs consistent with multisegmental disease affecting the femoral-popliteal and tibial arteries. The left ankle brachial index is 0.56, which is abnormal. The segmental pressure measurements and ankle brachial index in the right leg are normal.

Treadmill exercise testing serves to evaluate the clinical significance of peripheral arterial stenoses and to provide objective evidence of the patient's walking capacity. The initial claudication distance is defined as the point at which symptoms of claudication first develop, and the absolute claudication distance is when the patient can no longer continue walking because of severe leg discomfort. This standardized and more objective measurement of walking capacity supplements the patient's history and thus provides a quantitative assessment of the patient's disability, as well as a metric for monitoring therapeutic interventions.

Treadmill exercise protocols use a motorized treadmill that incorporates fixed or progressive speeds and angles of incline. A fixed workload test usually maintains a constant grade of 12 percent and speed of 1.5 to 2 miles per hour. A progressive, or graded, treadmill protocol typically maintains a constant speed of 2 miles per hour while the grade is gradually increased by 2 percent every 2 to 3 minutes. Reproducibility of repeated treadmill test results is reportedly better with progressive than with constant grade protocols.[40]

Treadmill testing provides a means to determine whether arterial stenoses contribute to the patient's symptoms of exertional leg pain. During exercise, blood flow through a stenosis increases as vascular resistance falls in the exercising muscle. According to Poiseuille's law, described previously, the pressure gradient across the stenosis increases in direct proportion to flow. Thus ankle and brachial systolic blood pressures are measured under resting conditions before treadmill exercise, within 1 minute after exercise, and repeatedly until baseline values are reestablished. Normally, the blood pressure increase that occurs during exercise should be the same in both upper and lower extremities, maintaining a constant ABI of 1 or greater. In the presence of peripheral arterial stenoses, the ABI decreases because the increase in blood pressure that is observed in the arm is not matched by a comparable increase in ankle blood pressure. A 25 percent or greater decrease in ABI after exercise in a patient whose walking capacity is limited by claudication is considered diagnostic, implicating PAD as a cause of the patient's symptoms.

Many patients with PAD also have coronary atherosclerosis. The addition of cardiac monitoring to the exercise protocol may provide adjunctive information regarding the presence of myocardial ischemia. A workload sufficient to increase myocardial oxygen demand and provoke myocardial ischemia may not be achieved in patients whose exercise capacity is limited by claudication. Nonetheless, electrocardiographic changes, particularly during low levels of treadmill exercise, may provide evidence of severe coronary artery disease.

PULSE VOLUME RECORDING

The pulse volume recording graphically illustrates the volumetric change in a segment of the limb that occurs with each pulse. Plethysmographic instruments, typically using strain gauges or pneumatic cuffs, are used to transduce volumetric changes in the limb, which can be displayed on a graphic recorder. These transducers are strategically placed along the limb to record the pulse volume in its different segments, such as the thigh, calf, ankle, metatarsal region, and toes or the upper arm, forearm, and fingers. The normal pulse volume contour is influenced by both local arterial pressure and vascular wall distensibility and resembles a blood pressure waveform. It consists of a sharp systolic upstroke, rising rapidly to a peak, a dicrotic notch, and a concave downslope that drops off gradually toward the baseline. The contour of the pulse wave changes distal to a stenosis. Loss of the dicrotic notch, a slower rate of rise, a more rounded peak, and a slower descent occur. The amplitude becomes lower with increasing severity of disease, and the pulse wave may not be recordable at all in the critically ischemic limb. Segmental analysis of the pulse wave may indicate

CH 57

Peripheral Arterial Diseases

recognizing the variability intrinsic to sequential blood pressure measurements, an ABI of less than 0.90 is considered abnormal and is 90 to 95 percent sensitive and 98 to 100 percent specific for angiographically verified peripheral arterial stenosis.[4] The ABI is often used to gauge the severity of PAD. Patients with symptoms of leg claudication often have ABIs ranging from 0.5 to 0.8, and patients with critical limb ischemia usually have an ABI of less than 0.5. The ABI correlates inversely with walking distance and speed. Less than 40 percent of patients whose ABI is less than 0.40 can complete a 6-minute walk.[39] In patients with skin ulcerations, an ankle pressure of less than 55 mm Hg would predict poor ulcer healing. One limitation of leg blood pressure recordings is that they cannot be used reliably in patients with calcified vessels, as might occur in persons with diabetes mellitus or renal insufficiency. The calcified vessel cannot be compressed during inflation of the pneumatic cuff, and therefore the Doppler probe indicates continuous blood flow even when the mercury manometer records pressure in excess of 250 mm Hg.

the location of an arterial stenosis, which is likely to be sited in the artery between normal and abnormal pulse volume recordings. The pulse volume wave also provides information regarding the integrity of blood flow when blood pressure measurements cannot be accurately obtained because of noncompressible vessels.

DOPPLER ULTRASONOGRAPHY

Continuous wave and pulsed wave Doppler systems transmit and receive high-frequency ultrasound signals. The Doppler frequency shift caused by moving red blood cells varies directly with the velocity of blood flow. Typically, the perceived frequency shift is between 1 and 20 kHz and is within the audible range of the human ear. Therefore placement of a Doppler probe along an artery enables the examiner to hear whether blood flow is present and the vessel is patent. Processing and graphically recording the Doppler signal permits a more detailed analysis of the frequency components.

Doppler instruments can be used without or with gray scale imaging to evaluate an artery for the presence of stenoses. The Doppler probe is positioned at approximately a 60-degree angle over the common femoral, superficial femoral, popliteal, dorsalis pedis, and posterior tibial arteries. The normal Doppler waveform has three components: a rapid forward flow component during systole, a transient flow reversal during early diastole, and a slow antegrade component during late diastole. The Doppler waveform becomes altered if the probe is placed distal to an arterial stenosis and is characterized by deceleration of systolic flow, loss of the early diastolic reversal, and diminished peak frequencies. Arteries in a limb with critical ischemia may not show any Doppler frequency shift. As with pulse volume recordings, a change from a normal to an abnormal Doppler waveform as the artery is interrogated more distally provides inferential evidence of the location of a stenosis.

Duplex Ultrasound Imaging

Duplex ultrasound imaging provides a direct, noninvasive means of assessing both the anatomical characteristics of peripheral arteries and the functional significance of arterial stenoses. The methodology incorporates gray scale B-mode ultrasound imaging, pulsed Doppler velocity measurements, and color coding of the Doppler-shift information (Fig. 57-6). Real-time ultrasonography scanners emit and receive high-frequency sound waves, typically ranging from 2 to 10 mHz, to construct an image. The acoustic properties of the vascular wall differ from those of the surrounding tissue, enabling them to be imaged easily. Atherosclerotic plaque may be present and visible on gray scale images. Pulsed wave Doppler systems emit ultrasound beams at precise times and can therefore sample the reflected ultrasound waves at specific depths, enabling the examiner to determine the blood flow velocity within the lumen of the artery. By positioning the pulsed Doppler beam at a known angle, the examiner can calculate blood flow velocity according to the following equation:

$$Df = 2VF\cos\theta/C$$

where Df is the frequency shift, V is the velocity, F is the frequency of the transmitted sound, θ is the angle between the transmitted sound and the velocity vector, and C is the velocity of sound and tissue. For optimal measurements, the angle of the pulsed Doppler beam should be less than 60 degrees. With color Doppler, the frequency shift information within the entire field sampled by the ultrasound beam can be superimposed on the gray scale image. This provides a composite real-time display of flow velocity within the vessel.

Color-assisted duplex ultrasound imaging is an effective means of localizing peripheral arterial stenoses (Fig. 57-7). Normal arteries have laminar flow, with the highest velocity at the center of the artery. The corresponding color image is usually homogeneous, with relatively constant hue and intensity. In the presence of an arterial stenosis, blood flow velocity increases through the narrowed lumen. As the velocity increases, there is progressive desaturation of the

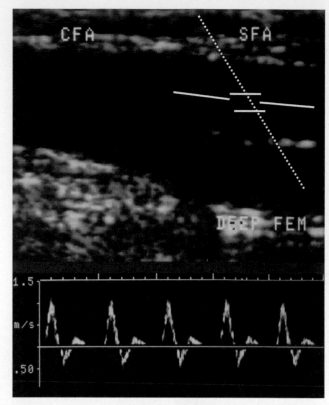

FIGURE 57–6 Duplex ultrasonogram of the common femoral artery bifurcation into the superficial and deep femoral arteries. The **upper image** shows a normal gray-scale image of the artery in which the intima is not thickened and the lumen is widely patent. The **lower image** is a recording of the pulse Doppler velocity sampled from the superficial femoral artery. The triphasic profile is apparent, the envelope is thin, and the peak systolic velocity is within normal limits.

color display, and flow disturbance distal to the stenosis causes changes in hue and color. Pulsed Doppler velocity measurements can be made along the length of the artery, particularly at areas of flow abnormalities suggested by the color image. A twofold or greater increase in peak systolic velocity at the site of an atherosclerotic plaque indicates a 50 percent or greater diameter stenosis (see Fig. 57-7). A threefold increase in velocity suggests 75 percent or greater stenosis. An occluded artery generates no Doppler signal. Using contrast angiography as a reference standard, duplex ultrasound imaging for identifying sites of arterial stenoses has approximately a 95 percent specificity and an 80 to 90 percent sensitivity.[41,42]

Magnetic Resonance Angiography

Magnetic resonance angiography (MRA) can noninvasively visualize the aorta and the peripheral arteries (see Chaps. 17 and 56). A detailed description of the instrumentation and technique is beyond the scope of this chapter. The resolution of the vascular anatomy with gadolinium-enhanced MRA approaches that of conventional contrast digital subtraction angiography (Fig. 57-8). Comparative studies have reported excellent interobserver agreement and sensitivities of 93 to 100 percent and specificity of 96 to 100 percent for the aorta, iliac, femoropopliteal, and tibioperoneal arteries.[42-45] Currently, MRA's greatest utility is for evaluating symptomatic patients to assist decision-making before endovascular and surgical intervention or in patients at risk for renal, allergic, or other complications during conventional angiography.

Computed Tomographic Angiography

Computed tomographic angiography (CTA) uses intravenous administration of radiocontrast material to opacify and visualize the aorta and peripheral arteries (see Chap. 18). New computed tomography scanners use multidetector technology to acquire cross-sectional images. This advance permits imaging of peripheral arteries with excellent spatial resolution over a relatively short period of time and using reduced amounts of radiocontrast (Fig. 57-9).[46,47] Images can be displayed in three dimensions and rotated to optimize visualization of arterial stenoses. Compared with conventional contrast angiography, the sensitivity and specificity for stenoses greater than 75 percent reported for CTA using

multiple detector technology are 94 to 100 percent and 98 to 100 percent, respectively.[46,48-50] CTA offers an advantage over MRA in that it can be used in patients with stents, metal clips, and pacemakers, although it also has the disadvantage of requiring radiocontrast and ionizing radiation.

Contrast Angiography (see Chap. 59)

Conventional angiography, using a radioiodinated or other contrast agent, can aid the evaluation of the arterial anatomy prior to a revascularization procedure. It still has occasional utility when the diagnosis is in doubt. Most contemporary angiography laboratories use digital subtraction techniques following intraarterial administration of contrast material to enhance resolution. Evaluation of the aorta and the peripheral arteries generally uses retrograde transfemoral catheterization. Injection of the radiocontrast material into the aorta permits visualization of the aorta and iliac arteries, and injection of contrast material into the iliofemoral segment of the involved leg permits optimal visualization of the femoral, popliteal, tibial, and peroneal arteries (Fig. 57-10). In patients with aortic occlusion, catheterization of the femoral arteries is not feasible. The aorta can be approached by brachial or axillary artery cannulation or, if necessary, directly by a translumbar approach.

PROGNOSIS

Patients with PAD have an increased risk for adverse cardiovascular events as well as the risk of limb loss and impaired quality of life.[7,9,51] Patients with PAD frequently have concomitant coronary artery disease and cerebrovascular disease.[4,7] The relative prevalence of each of these manifestations of atherosclerosis depends, in part, on the diagnostic criteria used to establish their diagnosis. Patients with abnormal ABIs are twofold to fourfold more likely than those with normal ABIs to have a history of myocardial infarction, angina, congestive heart failure, or cerebrovascular ischemia.[4,7] Coronary calcium scores and carotid artery intima-media thickness are greater in patients with PAD than those without PAD.[52] Angiographically significant coronary artery disease occurs in approximately 60 to 80

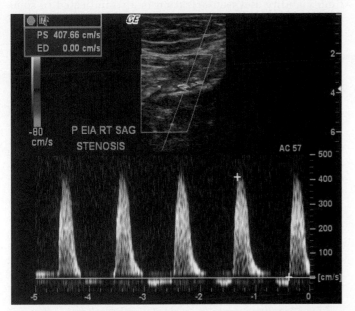

FIGURE 57–7 Duplex ultrasonogram of the external iliac artery. The **upper image** shows a color image of the artery in which there is heterogeneity and desaturation of color indicative of high-velocity flow through a stenosis. The **lower image** is a recording of the pulse Doppler velocity sampled from the right external iliac artery. The peak velocity of 350 cm/sec is elevated. These features are consistent with a significant stenosis.

CH 57

Peripheral Arterial Diseases

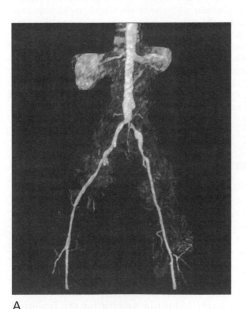

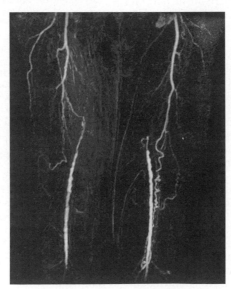

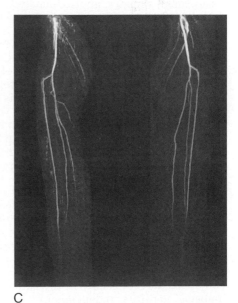

A   B   C

FIGURE 57–8 Gadolinium-enhanced two-dimensional magnetic resonance angiogram of the aorta and both legs, extending from the thighs to above the ankle. **A,** Aortoiliac atherosclerosis with stenosed left common iliac artery. **B,** Bilateral superficial femoral artery occlusion with reconstitution of the distal portion of the right and left superficial femoral arteries. **C,** The anterior tibial, posterior tibial, and peroneal arteries, which are patent in each leg.

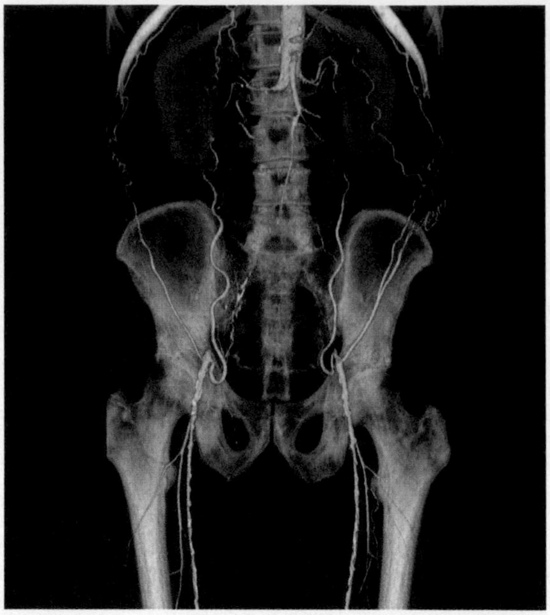

FIGURE 57-9 Computed tomographic angiogram of a patient with complete occlusion of the aorta and both iliac arteries. Reconstitution of the common femoral arteries is present. *(Courtesy of the 3D and Image Processing Center of Brigham and Women's Hospital, Boston.)*

CH 57

percent of patients with PAD.[7] Also, 15 to 25 percent of patients with PAD have significant carotid artery stenoses as detected by duplex ultrasonography. Two international registries have detected a high coprevalence of coronary artery disease and cerebrovascular disease in patients with PAD. In the Reduction in Atherothrombosis for Continued Health (REACH) registry, 62 percent of patients had either or both coronary and cerebrovascular disease.[53] Approximately 28 percent of the patients with PAD had a history of myocardial infarction, 30 percent had angina, 16 percent had a prior stroke, and 15 percent had a prior transient ischemic attack. In the AGATHA (A Global Atherothrombosis Assessment) registry, approximately 50 percent of patients with PAD had established coronary artery disease and 50 percent had prior stroke, transient ischemic attack, or carotid artery revascularization.[54] The specificity of an abnormal ABI to predict future cardiovascular events is approximately 90 percent.[55] The risk of death from cardiovascular causes increases 2.5- to 6-fold in patients with PAD, and their annual mortality rate is 4.3 to 4.9 percent.[4,7] The risk of death is greatest in those with the most severe PAD, and mortality correlates with decreasing ABI (Fig. 57-11).[56,57] Approximately 25 percent of patients with critical limb ischemia die within 1 year, and the 1-year mortality rate among patients who have undergone amputation for PAD may be as high as 45 percent.[4]

Approximately 25 percent of patients with claudication develop worsening symptoms. Moreover, mobility loss occurs more commonly in patients with PAD than in those without PAD, even among patients who do not have classic symptoms of claudication.[31] Clinical progression to critical limb ischemia occurs in 7.5 to 8 percent of patients with claudication in the first year after diagnosis and in approximately 2.2 percent each year thereafter.[58] Both smoking and diabetes mellitus independently predict progression of disease.[4,7] Of patients with PAD, the risk of amputation in those with diabetes mellitus is at least 12-fold higher than in nondiabetic persons.[59]

TREATMENT

The goals of treatment for PAD include reduction in cardiovascular morbidity and mortality, as well as improvement in quality of life by decreasing symptoms of claudication, eliminating rest pain, and preserving limb viability.[60,61] Therapeutic considerations, therefore, include risk factor modification by life-style measures and pharmacological therapy to reduce the risk of adverse cardiovascular events, such as myocardial infarction, stroke, and death. Symptoms of claudication can improve with pharmacotherapy or exercise rehabilitation. Optimal management of critical limb ischemia often includes endovascular interventions or surgical reconstruction to improve blood supply and maintain limb viability. Revascularization is also indicated in some patients with disabling symptoms of claudication that persist despite exercise therapy and pharmacotherapy.[4,7]

Risk Factor Modification (see Chaps. 42 and 45)

Lipid-lowering therapy reduces the risk of adverse cardiovascular events in patients with coronary artery disease. Secondary prevention trials with statins documented reduced risk of nonfatal myocardial infarction or death from coronary artery disease by 24 to 34 percent (see Chap. 42). The Heart Protection Study found that lipid-lowering therapy with simvastatin reduced the risk of adverse cardiovascular outcomes by 25 percent in patients with atherosclerosis including more than 6700 patients with PAD (Fig. 57-12).[62] The National Cholesterol Education Program Adult Treatment Panel III designated PAD a "coronary risk equivalent," hence the current recommendations for lipid-lowering therapy in patients with PAD. Such patients should receive diet and drug therapy to achieve a target LDL cholesterol level of 100 mg/dl or less.[7,63] Gemfibrozil reduced coronary events in men with coronary heart disease and low high-density lipoprotein (HDL) cholesterol.[64] Fenofibrate did not reduce coronary events in patients with diabetes.[65] It is not known whether niacin or fibrates improve cardiovascular outcome in patients with PAD.

Several clinical trials have found that lipid-lowering therapy with diet, niacin, binding resins, or clofibrate reduces the progression of femoral artery atherosclerosis. In one study the addition of probucol to cholestyramine did not affect femoral atherosclerosis.[66] Several older studies suggest that lipid-lowering therapy can reduce the incidence or severity of claudication.[67,68] Prospective trials have found that statins improve walking distance in patients with PAD.[69-71] In the Treatment of Peripheral Atherosclerotic Disease with Moderate or Intensive Lipid Lowering (TREADMILL) trial, atorvastatin (80 mg) increased pain-free walking distance by more than 60 percent compared with an 38 percent increase with placebo (Fig. 57-13).[70] Two additional trials support these findings.[69,71] Also, patients treated with statins have superior leg functioning as assessed by walking speed and distance compared with those not so treated.[72]

Smoking Cessation

Prospective trials examining the benefits of smoking cessation are lacking. However, observational evidence unequivocally supports the notion that cigarette smoking increases the risk of atherosclerosis and its clinical sequelae. Nonsmokers with PAD have lower rates of myocardial infarction and mortality than those who have smoked or continue to smoke, and PAD patients who discontinue smoking have approximately twice the 5-year survival rate of those who continue to smoke.[11] Smoking cessation also lowers the risk of developing critical limb ischemia. In addition to frequent physician advice, pharmacological interventions that are effective in promoting smoking cessation include nicotine replacement therapy, bupropion, and varenicline.[73,74]

Treatment of Diabetes

(see Chaps. 43 and 60)

Aggressive treatment of diabetes decreases the risk for microangiopathic events such as nephropathy and retinopathy; however, only limited data support the benefit of aggressive treatment of diabetes on the clinical manifestations of atherosclerosis (see Chap. 43). In the Diabetes Control and Complications Trial (DCCT), which involved patients with type I diabetes mellitus, a 13-year follow-up analysis found that intensive insulin therapy, as compared with usual care, reduced the risk of cardiovascular events by 42 percent.[75] Also, after 6 years, the rate of growth of carotid intima-media thickness was less in the intensive treatment group, indicating a favorable effect on atherosclerosis progression.[76] The United Kingdom Prospective Diabetes Study (UKPDS) of patients with type II diabetes mellitus found that intensive treatment with sulfonylureas or insulin was associated with a 16 percent reduction in myocardial infarction, a finding of borderline statistical significance, and a trend for a decrease in the incidence of death or amputation from PAD.[77] The ProActive (Prospective Pioglitazone Clinical Trial in Cardiovascular Events) Study assessed the effect of pioglitazone versus placebo on a broad range of cardiovascular endpoints in patients with type II diabetes and established atherosclerosis including coronary artery disease, cerebrovascular disease, and PAD and found no significant benefit of pioglitazone on the primary outcome.[78] However, there was a significant reduction in the risk of a composite secondary endpoint consisting of all-cause mortality, nonfatal myocardial infarction, and stroke. Current guidelines recommend that patients with PAD and diabetes be treated with glucose-lowering agents to achieve a hemoglobin A_{1C} of less than 7 percent.[7]

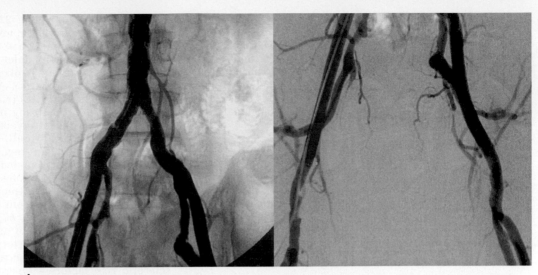

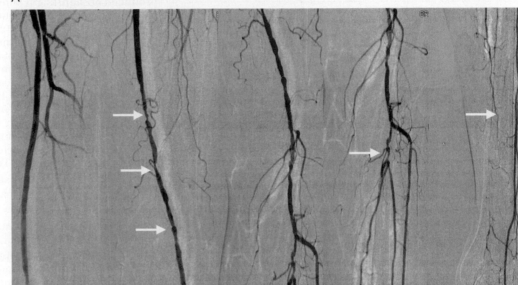

FIGURE 57–10 Angiogram of a patient with disabling left calf claudication. **A,** The aorta and bilateral common iliac arteries are patent. **B,** The left superficial femoral artery has multiple stenotic lesions (arrows). Significant stenosis of the left tibioperoneal trunk and left posterior tibial artery exists (arrows).

CH 57
Peripheral Arterial Diseases

Blood Pressure Control

Antihypertensive therapy reduces the risk of stroke, coronary artery disease, and vascular death. In the Appropriate Blood Pressure Control in Diabetes (ABCD) trial, intensive blood pressure control to levels approximating 128/75 mm Hg substantially reduced cardiovascular events as compared with moderate blood pressure control in patients with PAD.[79] It is not known whether antihypertensive therapy limits the progression of PAD. Treatment of hypertension might decrease perfusion pressure to extremities already compromised by peripheral arterial stenoses. In addition, concern has been raised regarding the potential adverse affects of beta-adrenergic receptor blockers on peripheral blood flow and symptoms of claudication or critical limb ischemia. Beta-adrenergic blocking agents worsen claudication in some trials but not in others. A meta-analysis that included 11 studies of beta-blocker therapy, as compared with placebo, in patients with intermittent claudication found no significant impairment on walking capacity.[80] Beta-blocking drugs reduce the risk of myocardial infarction and death in patients with coronary artery disease, a problem affecting many patients with PAD. Thus if clinically indicated for other conditions, these drugs should not be withheld in patients with PAD. The balance of evidence supports treatment of hypertension in patients with PAD according to established clinical guidelines (see Chap. 41 and its guidelines).[81]

Angiotensin-converting enzyme (ACE) inhibitors reduce cardiovascular events in patients with atherosclerosis. In the Heart Outcomes Prevention Evaluation (HOPE) study, the ACE inhibitor ramipril decreased the risk for vascular death, myocardial infarction, or stroke by 22 percent. Forty-four percent of the patients enrolled in the HOPE trial had evidence of PAD as manifested by an ABI less than 0.9. Ramipril reduced cardiovascular events in the patients with PAD to a comparable degree as in those without PAD (Fig. 57-14).[82] Current guidelines recommend that patients with PAD and hypertension be treated with blood pressure–lowering agents to achieve a target blood pressure of less than 140/90 mm Hg or to less than 130/80 mm Hg in patients with diabetes.[7]

Antiplatelet Therapy

Substantial evidence supports the use of antiplatelet agents to reduce adverse cardiovascular outcomes in patients with atherosclerosis. A meta-analysis that included approximately 135,000 high-risk patients with atherosclerosis including those with acute and prior myocardial infarction, stroke, or transient cerebrovascular ischemia and other high-risk groups including those with PAD found that anti-

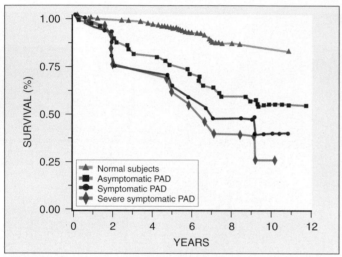

FIGURE 57-11 Survival rates of patients with peripheral arterial disease (PAD) derived from a population-based study. PAD was diagnosed by measuring the ankle/brachial index. Just the presence of PAD, even in the absence of symptoms, was associated with decreased survival. Survival was poorest in patients with symptoms. *(From Criqui M, Langer RD, Fronek A, et al: Mortality over a period of 10 years in patients with peripheral arterial disease. N Engl J Med 326:381, 1992.)*

platelet therapy yielded a 22 percent odds reduction for subsequent vascular death, myocardial infarction, or stroke (see Chap. 82).[62] Among the 9214 patients with PAD included in this analysis, antiplatelet therapy reduced the risk of myocardial infarction, stroke, or death by 22 percent (Fig. 57-15).[62] The Clopidogrel vs. Aspirin in Patients at Risk for Ischemic Events (CAPRIE) trial compared clopidogrel with aspirin in terms of efficacy in preventing ischemic events in patients with recent myocardial infarction, recent ischemic stroke, or PAD. Overall, there was an 8.7 percent relative risk reduction for myocardial infarction, ischemic stroke, or cardiovascular death in the group treated with clopidogrel.[83] Notably, among the 6452 patients in the PAD subgroup, clopidogrel treatment reduced adverse cardiovascular events by 23.8 percent (Fig. 57-16). The CHARISMA trial compared the efficacy of dual antiplatelet therapy with clopidogrel plus aspirin to aspirin alone in patients with established coronary artery disease, cerebrovascular disease, or PAD, as well as patients with multiple atherosclerotic risk factors.[84] Overall, dual antiplatelet therapy produced no significant benefit compared with aspirin alone on the primary efficacy endpoint that was a composite of myocardial infarction, stroke, or cardiovascular death. Current guidelines recommend that patients with PAD be treated with an antiplatelet drug such as aspirin or clopidogrel.[7] Oral anticoagulation with warfarin is not recommended to reduce cardiovascular events in patients with PAD because it is no more effective than antiplatelet therapy and confers a higher risk of bleeding. Antiplatelet therapy also prevents occlusion in the peripheral circulation after revascularization procedures. Of approximately 3000 patients with peripheral arterial procedures previously analyzed by the Antiplatelet Trialists' Collaboration, the odds reduction for arterial or graft occlusion by antiplatelet therapy, primarily aspirin or aspirin plus dipyridamole, was 43 percent.

Pharmacotherapy

The development of effective pharmacotherapy for treating symptoms of PAD has lagged substantially behind drug treatment for coronary artery disease. Published consensus guidelines for conducting clinical trials of pharmacological agents for treatment of patients with PAD should provide common ground for the objective evaluation of new drugs.[85]

Most studies of vasodilator therapy have failed to demonstrate any efficacy in patients with intermittent claudication. Several pathophysiological explanations may account for the failure of vasodilator therapy in patients with PAD. During exercise, resistance vessels distal to a stenosis dilate in response to ischemia. Vasodilators would have minimal, if any, effect on these endogenously dilated vessels but would decrease resistance in other vessels and create a relative steal phenomenon, reducing blood flow and perfusion pressure to the affected leg. Moreover, in contrast to their effects on myocardial oxygen consumption in patients with coronary artery disease

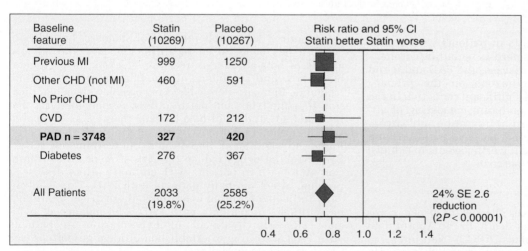

FIGURE 57-12 Relative risk of adverse cardiovascular events in participants in the Heart Protection Study based on treatment with statin or placebo. Included in this study were 6700 patients with peripheral arterial disease (PAD) including 3748 patients who had no prior coronary heart disease (CHD), in whom there was an approximate 24 percent risk reduction of vascular events. CI = confidence interval; CVD = cardiovascular disease; MI = myocardial infarction; SE = standard error. *(From MRC/BHF: Heart Protection Study of cholesterol lowering with simvastatin in 20,536 high-risk individuals: A randomized placebo-controlled trial. Lancet 360:7, 2002.)*

(because of afterload reduction), vasodilators do not reduce skeletal muscle oxygen demand.

In the United States the Food and Drug Administration has approved two drugs, pentoxifylline (Trental) and cilostazol (Pletal), for treating claudication in patients with PAD. Additional drugs have been approved by licensing bodies in Europe, Asia, and South America. Pentoxifylline is a xanthine derivative used to treat patients with intermittent claudication. Its action is thought to be mediated via its hemorheological properties including its ability to decrease blood viscosity and improve erythrocyte flexibility. It may have antiinflammatory and antiproliferative effects. Two meta-analyses of randomized placebo-controlled trials of pentoxifylline found that it increased initial claudication distance by approximately 20 to 30 m and absolute claudication distance by approximately 45 to 50 m.[86,87] Cilostazol is a quinoline derivative that inhibits phosphodiesterase III, thereby decreasing cyclic adenosine monophosphate degradation and increasing its concentration in platelets and blood vessels. Although cilostazol inhibits platelet aggregation and causes vasodilation in experimental animals, its mechanism of action in patients with PAD is not known. Several trials have reported that cilostazol improves absolute claudication distance by 40 to 50 percent as compared with placebo (Fig. 57-17).[88] Quality of life measures, assessed by the Medical Outcomes Scale (SF-36) and Walking Impairment Questionnaire, also demonstrated improvement. One study also found that absolute walking distance improves more with cilostazol than with either pentoxifylline or placebo, with the latter two having equivalent efficacy.[89] An advisory from the U.S. Food and Drug Administration (FDA) stated that cilostazol should not be used in patients with congestive heart failure because other phosphodiesterase III inhibitors have been shown to decrease survival in these patients. The effect of cilostazol on cardiac morbidity and mortality is not known.

Other classes of drugs have been studied or are currently under investigation for treatment of either claudication or critical limb ischemia. These include statins, ACE inhibitors, serotonin (5HT-2) antagonists, calcium channel blockers, L-arginine, carnitine derivatives, vasodilator prostaglandins, and angiogenic growth factors. As noted previously, three trials have found that statins improve walking distance in patients with PAD.[69-71] One recent study reported that the ACE inhibitor ramipril improved maximal claudication time.[90] Naftidrofuryl, a serotonin-antagonist, has been reported to have improved symptoms of claudication in some trials and is currently available for use in Europe.[91,92] In several preliminary trials, selective serotonin-2a antagonists have not been effective in improving claudication distance.[93,94] L-Arginine, the precursor for endothelium-derived nitric oxide,[95,96] has not proven useful for improving PAD symptoms.[97] Propionyl L-carnitine, a cofactor for fatty acid metabolism, has been reported to improve claudication, particularly in patients whose baseline maximum walking distance is less than 250 m.[98,99] Therapy with vasodilator prostaglandins has been investigated in patients with intermittent claudication and in those with critical limb ischemia. Intravenous administration of prostaglandin E1 (PGE1) or its precursor and oral administration of prostacyclin analogues[95,100-103] have also failed to show consistent benefit in appropriately powered studies.

The therapeutic use of angiogenic growth factors has engendered considerable enthusiasm. Administration of basic fibroblast growth factor and vascular endothelial growth factor as protein or gene therapy increases collateral blood vessel development, capillary number, and blood flow in experimental models of hind limb ischemia.[104,105] Despite initial enthusiasm from preliminary studies, the results of the few placebo-controlled clinical trials in patients with either claudication or critical limb ischemia that have evaluated angiogenic growth factors such as vascular endothelial growth factor have been disappointing.[106] Other studies, with angiogenic factors such as hepatocyte growth factor and hypoxia-inducible factor 1α are in progress.

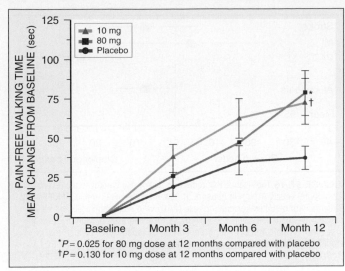

*P = 0.025 for 80 mg dose at 12 months compared with placebo
†P = 0.130 for 10 mg dose at 12 months compared with placebo

FIGURE 57–13 In the TREADMILL Study, lipid-lowering therapy with atorvastatin improved pain-free walking time in patients with intermittent claudication. (From Mohler ER III, Hiatt WR, Creager MA: Cholesterol reduction with atorvastatin improves walking distance in patients with arterial artery disease. Circulation 108:1481, 2003.)

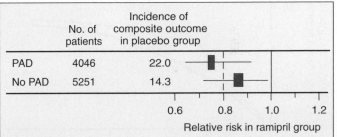

FIGURE 57–14 The relative risk of adverse cardiovascular events in the patients with and without peripheral arterial disease (PAD) according to treatment with the angiotensin-converting enzyme inhibitor ramipril in the Heart Outcomes Prevention Evaluation (HOPE) study. (Modified from Yusuf S, Sleight P, Pogue J, et al: Effects of an angiotensin-converting enzyme inhibitor, ramipril, on cardiovascular events in high-risk patients. The Heart Outcomes Prevention Evaluation Study Investigators [published erratum appears in N Engl J Med 342:748, 2000]. N Engl J Med 342:145, 2000.)

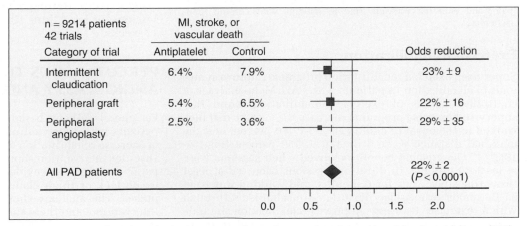

FIGURE 57–15 The effect of antiplatelet therapy on cardiovascular events in patients with peripheral arterial disease (PAD) based on the Antiplatelet Trialists' Collaboration. The odds ratios are shown for patients with claudication, infrainguinal bypass grafts, and percutaneous transluminal angioplasty. MI = myocardial infarction. (From Antithrombotic Trialists' Collaboration: Collaborative meta-analysis of randomised trials of antiplatelet therapy for prevention of death, myocardial infarction, and stroke in high risk patients. BMJ 324:71, 2002.)

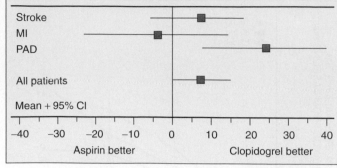

FIGURE 57–16 The relative risk reduction in adverse cardiovascular events in the Clopidogrel versus Aspirin in Patients at Risk for Ischemic Events (CAPRIE) study. Patients with peripheral arterial disease (PAD) who received placebo had a 24 percent risk reduction compared with those receiving aspirin. MI = myocardial infarction. *(From CAPRIE Steering Committee: A randomised, blinded trial of clopidogrel versus aspirin in patients at risk of ischaemic events (CAPRIE). Lancet 348:1329, 1996.)*

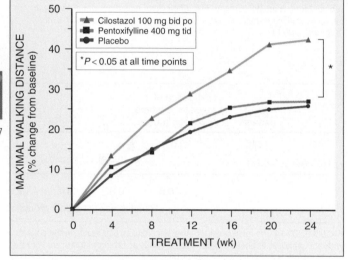

FIGURE 57–17 The effect of cilostazol, compared with pentoxifylline and placebo, on maximal walking distance. *(From Dawson DL, Cutler BS, Hiatt WR, et al: A comparison of cilostazol and pentoxifylline for treating intermittent claudication. Am J Med 109:523, 2000.)*

One study found that intramuscular administration of bone marrow–derived mononuclear cells to induce angiogenesis improved ABI, rest pain, and pain-free walking time in patients with chronic limb ischemia.[105]

Exercise Rehabilitation

Supervised exercise rehabilitation programs improve symptoms of claudication in patients with PAD. Meta-analyses of controlled studies of exercise rehabilitation found that supervised exercise programs increase the average distance walked to the onset of claudication by 180 percent and the maximal distance walked by 120 to 150 percent (Fig. 57-18).[107,108] The greatest benefit occurred when sessions were at least 30 minutes in duration, sessions occurred at least three times per week for 6 months, and walking was used as the mode of exercise. Postulated mechanisms through which exercise training improves claudication include formation of collateral vessels and improvement in endothelium-dependent vasodilation, hemorheology, muscle metabolism, and walking efficiency.[109,110] Studies in experimental models of hind limb ischemia have suggested that regular exercise increases the development of collateral

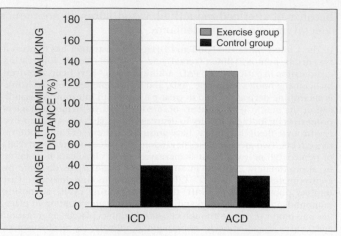

FIGURE 57–18 The effect of supervised exercise training on peak treadmill exercise time in patients with intermittent claudication. ACD = absolute claudication difference; ICD = initial claudication distance. *(Modified from Gardner AW, Poehlman ET: Exercise rehabilitation programs for the treatment of claudication pain. A meta-analysis. JAMA 274:975, 1995.)*

blood vessels.[109] Exercise increases the expression of angiogenic factors, particularly in hypoxic tissue.[111,112] Exercise training may improve endothelium-dependent vasodilation in patients with PAD, as it does in patients with coronary atherosclerosis.[113-116] Improvement in calf blood flow has not been demonstrated consistently in patients with claudication after exercise training, although one study found that maximal calf blood flow increased commensurate with improvement in walking distance.[109,117] To date, no imaging studies have demonstrated increased collateral blood vessels after exercise training in patients with PAD.

The benefits of exercise training in patients with PAD may result from changes in skeletal muscle function, such as increased muscle mitochondrial enzyme activity, ATP production rate, and lactate production. In patients with PAD, improvement in exercise performance is associated with a decrease in plasma and skeletal muscle short-chain acylcarnitine concentrations, which indicate improvement in oxidative metabolism, and an increase in peak oxygen consumption.[8] Training may also enhance biomechanical performance, enabling patients to walk more efficiently with less energy expenditure. Current guidelines recommend that patients with intermittent claudication undergo supervised exercise rehabilitation as initial therapy. Supervised exercise training should consist of 30- to 45-minute sessions, at least three times per week, for a minimum of 12 weeks.[7]

PERCUTANEOUS TRANSLUMINAL ANGIOPLASTY AND STENTS (see Chap. 59)

Peripheral catheter-based interventions are indicated for patients with lifestyle-limiting claudication despite a trial of exercise rehabilitation or pharmacotherapy.[4,7] Also, endovascular intervention should be considered in symptomatic patients and clinical evidence of inflow disease, as manifest by buttock or thigh claudication and diminished femoral pulses. The anatomy should be suitable for endovascular intervention, and there should be a reasonable likelihood of symptomatic improvement with minimal risk. Endovascular intervention is also indicated in patients with critical limb ischemia whose anatomy is amenable to catheter-based therapy. In patients with both inflow and outflow lesions, the inflow lesions should be treated first.[7] Endovascular intervention is not indicated for lesions detected in the asymptomatic patient. Initial success rates and durability of endovascular interventions relate to the morphology of the lesions and the clinical features of the patients. Long-term patency is greater in large versus small arteries, short versus long stenosis/occlusions, and single versus multiple lesions. Patency rates are less in patients with diabetes or renal insufficiency. More information regarding the indications and efficacy of peripheral catheter-based interventions can be found in Chapter 59.

Peripheral Arterial Surgery

Surgical revascularization is generally indicated to improve quality of life in patients with disabling claudication on maximal medical therapy and to relieve rest pain and preserve limb viability in patients with critical limb ischemia not amenable to percutaneous interventions. The specific operation must take into account the anatomical location of the arterial lesions and the presence of comorbid conditions. The surgical procedure is planned after identification of the arterial obstruction by imaging, ensuring that there is sufficient arterial inflow to and outflow from the graft to maintain patency. A preoperative evaluation to assess the risk of vascular surgery should be performed because many of these patients have coexisting coronary artery disease. Guidelines for this evaluation exist (see Chap. 80 and its guidelines).[118]

Aorta-bifemoral bypass is the most frequent operation for patients with aortoiliac disease. Typically, a knitted or woven prosthesis made of Dacron or polytetrafluoroethylene (PTFE) is anastomosed proximally to the aorta and distally to each common femoral artery. Occasionally, the iliac artery is used for the distal anastomosis to maintain antegrade flow into at least one hypogastric artery.

Extra-anatomic surgical reconstructive procedures for aortoiliac disease include axillo-bifemoral bypass, iliobifemoral bypass, and femoral-femoral bypass. These bypass grafts, made of Dacron or PTFE, circumvent the aorta and iliac arteries and are generally used in high-risk patients with critical limb ischemia. Long-term patency rates are inferior to those of aorto-bifemoral bypass procedures. Five-year patency rates for axillo-bifemoral bypass operations range from 50 to 70 percent, and for femoral-femoral bypass grafts from 70 to 80 percent.[7] The operative mortality rate for extra-anatomic bypass procedures is 3 to 5 percent, reflecting, in part, the serious comorbid conditions and advanced atherosclerosis of many of the patients who undergo these procedures.

Reconstructive surgery for infrainguinal arterial disease includes femoral-popliteal and femoral-tibial or femoral-peroneal artery bypass. In situ or reversed autologous saphenous veins or synthetic grafts made of PTFE are used for the infrainguinal bypass. Patency rates for autologous saphenous vein bypass grafts exceed those with PTFE grafts.[4,7] Also, patency rates are better for grafts in which the distal anastomosis is placed in the popliteal artery above the knee as compared with below the knee.[4] Five-year primary patency rates for femoral-popliteal reconstruction in patients with claudication are approximately 80 percent and 75 percent for autogenous vein grafts or PTFE grafts, respectively, and in patients with critical limb ischemia are approximately 65 percent and 45 percent, respectively. For femoral-below-knee bypass including tibioperoneal artery reconstruction, the 5-year patency rates for saphenous vein grafts in patients with claudication or critical limb ischemia are comparable with those for femoral-popliteal above-knee grafts and range from 60 to 80 percent. The 5-year patency rate for PTFE grafts in the infrapopliteal position is considerably inferior, approximating 65 percent in patients with claudication and 33 percent in patients with critical limb ischemia. The operative mortality rate for infrainguinal bypass operations is 1 to 2 percent.

Graft stenoses can result from technical errors at the time of surgery, such as retained valve cuffs or intimal flap or valvotome injury; from fibrous intimal hyperplasia, usually within 6 months of surgery; or from atherosclerosis, usually occurring within the vein graft at least 1 to 2 years after surgery. Institution of graft surveillance protocols using color-assisted duplex ultrasonography has enabled the identification of graft stenoses, prompting graft revision and avoiding complete graft failure.[7] Graft outcome is improved as a result of routine ultrasonographic surveillance. Also, antithrombotic agents including antiplatelet drugs and coumarin derivatives improve graft patency. Several studies have suggested that antiplatelet drugs may be more effective in preserving synthetic grafts, whereas coumarin derivatives may be more effective for vein bypass grafts.[119,120]

Algorithm for Treatment of the Symptomatic Leg

A management algorithm for treating symptomatic PAD is illustrated in Figure 57-19.

VASCULITIS

See Chapter 84.

THROMBOANGIITIS OBLITERANS

Thromboangiitis obliterans (TAO) is a segmental vasculitis that affects the distal arteries, veins, and nerves of the upper and lower extremities. It typically occurs in young persons who smoke. A patient with characteristics of TAO was described initially by von Winiwater in 1879.[121] Leo Buerger coined the term *thromboangiitis obliterans* and described its pathology in 11 amputated limbs.[121]

Pathology and Pathogenesis

Thromboangiitis obliterans primarily affects the medium and small vessels of the arms including the radial, ulnar, palmar, and digital arteries, as well as their counterparts in the legs including the tibial, peroneal, plantar, and digital arteries. Involvement can extend to the cerebral, coronary, renal, mesenteric, aortoiliac, and pulmonary arteries.[121] The pathological findings include an occlusive, highly cellular thrombus incorporating polymorphonuclear leukocytes, microabscesses, and occasionally multinucleated giant cells.[122] The inflammatory infiltrate can also affect the vascular wall, but the internal elastic membrane remains intact. In the chronic phase of the disease, the thrombus becomes organized and the vascular wall becomes fibrotic.

The precise cause of TAO is not known. Tobacco use or exposure is present in virtually all patients. Potential immunological mechanisms include increased cellular sensitivity to type I and type III collagen or the presence of antiendothelial cell antibodies. CD4 T cells have been identified in cellular infiltrates of vessels of patients with TAO.[123,124] The prevalence of anticardiolipin antibodies may be increased, particularly among the more severely affected patients.[125] Decreased endothelium-dependent vasodilation to acetylcholine can occur in both affected and unaffected limbs of patients with TAO, raising the possibility that reduced bioavailability of nitric oxide contributes to the disorder.[126]

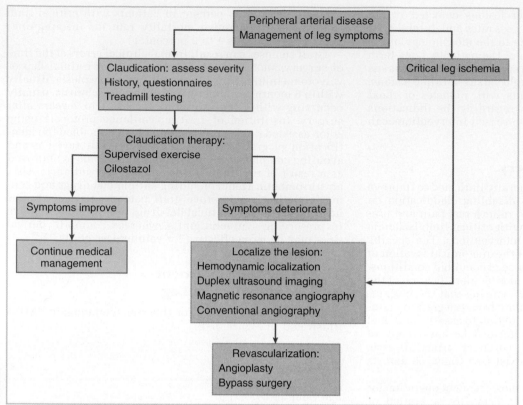

FIGURE 57–19 Management algorithm for the treatment of symptomatic peripheral arterial disease. *(From Hiatt WR: Medical management of peripheral arterial disease and claudication. N Engl J Med 344;1608, 2001.)*

Clinical Presentation

The prevalence of TAO is greater in Asia than in North America or Western Europe. In the United States, TAO occurs in approximately 13 per 100,000 population.[122] Most patients with TAO develop symptoms before 45 years of age, and 75 to 90 percent are men. Patients can have claudication of the hands, forearms, feet, or calves. Most patients with TAO present with rest pain and digital ulcerations. Often, more than one extremity is affected. Raynaud phenomenon occurs in approximately 45 percent of patients, and superficial thrombophlebitis, which may be migratory, occurs in approximately 40 percent of patients. The risk of amputation within 5 years is approximately 25 percent.[127]

The radial, ulnar, dorsalis pedis, and posterior tibial pulses may be absent if the corresponding vessel is involved. The clinical characteristics of critical limb ischemia and ischemic digital ulcerations are described earlier in this chapter. The Allen test result is abnormal in two thirds of patients.[122] To perform the Allen test, both radial and ulnar arteries are compressed while the hand is clenched and then opened. This maneuver causes palmar blanching. Release of compression from either pulse should normally produce palmar erythema if the palmar arches are patent. If these are occluded, pallor persists on the side where compression is maintained. The distal aspects of the extremities may have discrete, tender, erythematous, subcutaneous cords, indicating a superficial thrombophlebitis.

Diagnosis

No specific laboratory tests other than biopsy can diagnose TAO. Therefore most tests are performed to exclude other diseases that might have similar clinical presentations including autoimmune diseases such as scleroderma or sys-temic lupus erythematosus, hypercoagulable states, diabetes, or acute arterial occlusion caused by embolism. Acute phase indicators such as the erythrocyte sedimentation rate or C-reactive protein are usually normal. Serum immunological markers including antinuclear antibodies and rheumatoid factor should not be present, and serum complement levels should be normal. If clinically indicated, a proximal source of embolism should be excluded by cardiac and vascular ultrasonography or by computed tomography (CT), magnetic resonance, or conventional arteriography. Arteriography of an affected limb supports the diagnosis of TAO if there is segmental occlusion of small and medium-size arteries, absence of atherosclerosis, and corkscrew collateral vessels circumventing the occlusion (Fig. 57-20). These same findings, however, can occur in patients with scleroderma, systemic lupus erythematosus, mixed connective tissue disease, and antiphospholipid antibody syndrome. The pathognomonic test is a biopsy showing the classic pathological findings. This procedure is rarely indicated, and biopsy sites may fail to heal because of severe ischemia. The diagnosis, therefore, usually depends on an age of onset younger than 45 years; a history of tobacco use; physical examination demonstrating distal limb ischemia; exclusion of other diseases; and, if necessary, angiographic demonstration of typical lesions.

Treatment

The cornerstone of treatment is cessation of tobacco use. Patients without gangrene who stop smoking rarely require amputation.[121,127,128] In contrast, one or more amputations may ultimately be required in 40 to 45 percent of those patients with TAO who continue to smoke.

Several drugs can benefit patients with TAO. The prostacyclin analogue iloprost, administered 6 hours per day for 28 days, was more effective than aspirin in relieving rest pain and healing ulcers.[129] In a multicenter trial, however, oral iloprost administered for 8 weeks had no greater effect than placebo in healing ulcers, although there was somewhat more effective relief of pain at low doses.[130] Cyclophosphamide improved symptoms but not the angiographic appearance of TAO in one study.[131] Nonrandomized studies of therapeutic angiogenesis with autologous bone marrow mononuclear cells have reported improvements in pain and ulcer healing.[132,133] Vascular reconstructive surgery is usually not a viable option because of the segmental nature of this disease and involvement of distal vessels. An autogenous saphenous vein bypass graft can be considered if a target vessel for the distal anastomosis is available. Long-term patency rates are better in ex-smokers than in smokers.[134]

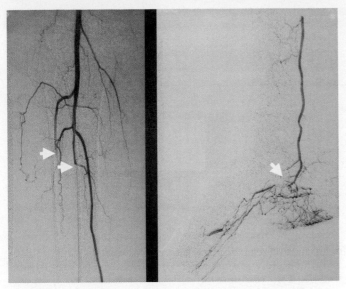

FIGURE 57-20 Angiogram of a young woman with thromboangiitis obliterans. The **left panel** demonstrates occlusion of the anterior tibial and peroneal arteries (arrows). The **right panel** demonstrates an occlusion of the distal portion of the posterior tibial artery (arrow) with bridging collateral vessels.

TAKAYASU ARTERITIS AND GIANT CELL ARTERITIS

See Chapter 84.

FIBROMUSCULAR DYSPLASIA

Fibromuscular dysplasia is a disease of medium-sized and large arteries. It typically affects the renal and carotid arteries. It may affect the arteries supplying the leg, particularly the iliac arteries and less so the femoral, popliteal, tibial, and peroneal arteries.[135] Fibromuscular dysplasia is a rare cause of either intermittent claudication or critical limb ischemia. Fibromuscular dysplasia most often occurs in young Caucasian women but can occur at any age in both genders. The histopathology is characterized by fibroplasia that most often affects the media but can involve the intima or adventitia. The histological classification of fibromuscular dysplasia includes the medial subtypes, medial fibroplasia, perimedial hyperplasia, and medial hyperplasia, as well as intimal fibroplasia and adventitial hyperplasia.[8,135] Depending on the histopathological type, stenosis results from hyperplasia of fibrous or muscular components of the vessel wall. Angiography demonstrates a beaded appearance of arteries affected by medial and perimedial fibroplasia and focal or tubular stenosis in arteries affected by intimal fibroplasia. Percutaneous transluminal angioplasty is indicated for treatment of symptomatic patients.

POPLITEAL ARTERY ENTRAPMENT SYNDROME

Popliteal artery entrapment syndrome is an uncommon cause of intermittent claudication. It occurs when an anatomical variation in the configuration or insertion of the medial head of the gastrocnemius muscle compresses the popliteal artery.[136] The popliteus muscle can also compress the popliteal artery and cause this syndrome. Popliteal artery entrapment is bilateral in approximately one third of affected patients. It should be suspected when a young,

typically athletic, person presents with claudication. The majority of cases are men. Potential consequences include popliteal artery thrombosis, embolism, or aneurysm formation.

The peripheral pulse examination may be normal unless provocative maneuvers are performed. Walking or repeated ankle dorsiflexion and plantar flexion maneuvers may cause attenuation or disappearance of pedal pulses and a decrease in the ABI in patients with popliteal artery entrapment. Imaging studies such as duplex ultrasound, CT or MRA, or conventional angiography performed at rest and during ankle flexion maneuvers are indicated to confirm the diagnosis. Magnetic resonance and CT imaging will also provide information about the relationship of the gastrocnemius muscle to the popliteal artery.

Treatment of popliteal artery entrapment syndrome involves release of the popliteal artery. This may require division and reattachment of the medial head of the gastrocnemius muscle. Occasionally, surgical bypass of the popliteal artery is required if it is occluded.

ACUTE LIMB ISCHEMIA

Acute limb ischemia occurs when an arterial occlusion suddenly reduces blood flow to the arm or leg. The metabolic needs of the tissue outstrip perfusion, placing limb viability in jeopardy. The clinical presentation of patients with acute limb ischemia relates to the location of the arterial occlusion and the resulting decrease in blood flow. Depending on the severity of ischemia, patients may note disabling claudication or pain at rest. Pain may develop over a short period and is manifest in the affected extremity distal to the site of obstruction. It is not necessarily confined to the foot or toes, or hand or fingers, as is usually the case in chronic limb ischemia. Concurrent ischemia of peripheral nerves causes sensory loss and motor dysfunction.

The physical findings can include absence of pulses distal to the occlusion, cool skin, pallor, delayed capillary return and venous filling, diminished or absent sensory perception, and muscular weakness or paralysis. This constellation of symptoms and signs is often recalled as the five Ps: *pain, pulselessness, pallor, paresthesias,* and *paralysis*.

Prognosis

Comorbid cardiovascular disorders are usually found in patients who present with acute limb ischemia and may even be responsible for the event. Therefore long-term prognosis is limited in this population.[4] The 5-year survival rate after acute limb ischemia caused by thrombosis approximates 45 percent and after embolism is less than 20 percent.[137] The 1-month survival rate in persons older than 75 years of age with acute limb ischemia approximates 40 percent.[138] The risk of limb loss depends on the severity of the ischemia and the elapsed time before a revascularization procedure is undertaken.

A classification scheme that takes into consideration the severity of ischemia and the viability of the limb, along with related neurological findings and Doppler signals, has been developed by the Society for Vascular Surgery and the International Society for Cardiovascular Surgery (Table 57-7).[38] A viable limb, category I, is not immediately threatened, has neither sensory nor motor abnormalities, and has blood flow detectable by Doppler. Threatened viability, category II, indicates that the severity of ischemia will cause limb loss unless the blood supply is restored promptly. The category is subdivided into marginally and immediately threatened limbs, the latter characterized by pain, sensory deficits, and muscular weakness. Doppler interrogation cannot detect

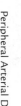

TABLE 57–7 Clinical Categories of Acute Limb Ischemia (Modified from the SVS/ISCVS Classification)

Category	Description/Prognosis	Findings		Doppler Signals	
		Sensory loss	*Muscle weakness*	*Arterial*	*Venous*
I. Viable	Not immediately threatened	None	None	A udible	Audible
II. Threatened					
a. Marginally	Salvageable if promptly treated	Minimal (toes) or none	None	(Often) inaudible	Audible
b. Immediately	Salvageable with immediate revascularization	More than toes, rest pain	Mild, moderate	(Usually) inaudible	Audible
III. Irreversible	Major tissue loss or permanent nerve damage inevitable	Profound, anesthetic	Profound, paralysis (rigor)	Inaudible	Inaudible

SVS = Society for Vascular Surgery; ISCVS = International Society for Cardiovascular Surgery.
Modified from Rutherford RB, Baker JD, Ernst C, et al: Recommended standards for reports dealing with lower extremity ischemia: Revised version. J Vasc Surg 26:517, 1997.

arterial blood flow. Irreversible limb ischemia leading to tissue loss and requiring amputation, category III, is characterized by loss of sensation, paralysis, and the absence of Doppler-detected blood flow in both arteries and veins distal to the occlusion.

Pathogenesis

The causes of acute limb ischemia include arterial embolism, thrombosis in situ, dissection, and trauma. Most arterial emboli arise from thrombotic sources in the heart. Atrial fibrillation complicating valvular heart disease, congestive heart failure, coronary artery disease, and hypertension accounts for approximately 50 percent of cardiac emboli to the limbs. Other sources include rheumatic or prosthetic cardiac valves, ventricular thrombus resulting from myocardial infarction or left ventricular aneurysm, paradoxical embolism of venous thrombi through the intraatrial or intraventricular communications, and cardiac tumors such as left atrial myxomas. Aneurysms of the aorta or peripheral arteries may harbor thrombi, which subsequently embolize to more distal arterial sites, usually lodging at branch points where the artery decreases in size.

Thrombosis in situ occurs in atherosclerotic peripheral arteries, infrainguinal bypass grafts, peripheral artery aneurysms, and normal arteries of patients with hypercoagulable states. In patients with peripheral atherosclerosis, thrombosis in situ may complicate plaque rupture, causing acute arterial occlusion and limb ischemia, in a manner analogous to that which occurs in coronary arteries in patients with acute myocardial infarction. Thrombosis complicating popliteal artery aneurysms is a much more common complication than rupture and may account for 10 percent of cases of acute limb ischemia in elderly men.[4,139] One of the most common causes of acute limb ischemia is thrombotic occlusion of an infrainguinal bypass graft, as discussed previously. Acute thrombotic occlusion of a normal artery is unusual but may occur in patients with acquired thrombophilic disorders such as antiphospholipid antibody syndrome, heparin-induced thrombocytopenia, disseminated intravascular coagulation, and myeloproliferative diseases.[140] Limited evidence indicates that inherited thrombophilic disorders such as activated protein C resistance (Factor V Leiden), prothrombin G20210 gene mutation, or deficiencies of antithrombin III, protein C and S, increase the risk of acute peripheral arterial thrombosis.[141,142]

Diagnostic Tests

The history and physical examination usually establish the diagnosis of acute limb ischemia. Time available for diagnostic tests is often limited, and diagnostic tests should not delay urgent revascularization procedures if limb viability is immediately threatened. The pressure in the affected limb and corresponding ABI can be measured if flow is detectable by Doppler ultrasonography. A Doppler probe can be used to detect the presence of blood flow in peripheral arteries, particularly when pulses are not palpable. Color-assisted duplex ultrasonography can determine the site of occlusion. It is particularly applicable to evaluate the patency of infrainguinal bypass grafts. Magnetic resonance imaging, CT, and conventional contrast arteriography can demonstrate the site of occlusion and provide an anatomical guide for revascularization.

Treatment

Analgesic medications should be administered to reduce pain. For patients with acute leg ischemia, the bed should be positioned such that the feet are lower than chest level, thereby increasing limb perfusion pressure via gravitational effects. This can be accomplished by putting blocks under the posts at the head of the bed. Efforts should be made to reduce pressure on the heels, on bony prominences, and between the toes by appropriate placement of soft material on the bed, such as sheepskin, and between the toes, such as lamb's wool. The room should be kept warm to prevent cold-induced cutaneous vasoconstriction.

Heparin is administered intravenously as soon as the diagnosis of acute limb ischemia is made. The dose should be sufficient to increase the partial thromboplastin time by 1.5 to 2.5 times control values to prevent thrombus propagation or recurrent embolism. Whether low-molecular-weight heparin would be as effective as unfractionated heparin in patients with acute limb ischemia is unknown.

Revascularization is indicated when the viability of the limb is threatened or when symptoms of ischemia persist. Options for revascularization include intraarterial thrombolytic therapy, percutaneous mechanical thrombectomy, or surgical revascularization. Catheter-directed intraarterial thrombolysis is an initial treatment option for patients presenting with either category I or II acute limb ischemia, if there is no contraindication to thrombolysis.[143] Catheter-based thrombolysis can also be considered for patients who are considered a high risk for surgical intervention. Long-term patency after thrombolysis is greater in patients with category I and II critical limb ischemia than in those with category III, in native arteries than in grafts, and in vein grafts than in prosthetic grafts.[144] Identification and repair of a graft stenosis after successful thrombolysis improves long-term graft patency.[144,145] Thrombolytic regimens have employed streptokinase, urokinase, recombinant tissue plasminogen activator, and reteplase. The duration of catheter-based thrombolytic therapy should generally not exceed

48 hours to achieve optimal benefit and limit the risk of bleeding. Percutaneous, catheter-based, mechanical thrombectomy, using devices that apply hydrodynamic forces or use rotating baskets, can be used alone or in addition to pharmacological thrombolysis to treat patients with acute limb ischemia.[146,147]

Surgical thromboembolectomy is not commonly used anymore but is occasionally employed in patients whose acute limb ischemia is caused by systemic embolism.[148] Surgical reconstruction, bypassing the occluded area, is an option for restoring blood flow to an ischemic limb. These techniques were discussed previously in this chapter.

Five prospective randomized trials, comprising 1283 patients, have compared the benefits and risks of thrombolysis and surgical reconstruction in patients presenting with acute limb ischemia (Table 57-8).[149] The Surgery versus Thrombolysis for Ischemia of the Lower Extremity (STILE) trial compared thrombolysis with either recombinant tissue plasminogen activator or urokinase to surgery after native artery or graft occlusion in patients with limb ischemia of less than 6 months' duration. The trial was stopped prematurely after enrollment of 393 patients. The composite outcome of death, ongoing or recurrent ischemia, major amputation, and major morbidity occurred in 62 percent of the group randomized to thrombolysis compared with 36 percent of those randomized to surgery. Of those patients who had symptoms for less than 14 days, however, amputation-free survival at 6 months was greater in the patients treated with thrombolysis than in those treated with surgery.[150] In the Thrombolysis or Peripheral Arterial Study (TOPAS), intraarterial thrombolysis with urokinase was compared to surgery in 554 patients with acute limb ischemia of less than 14 days. Amputation-free survival at 6 and 12 months was 72 and 65 percent, respectively, in the thrombolysis group and 75 and 70 percent, respectively, in the surgery group.[151] Taken together, the findings from these trials would suggest that catheter-based thrombolysis is an appropriate initial option in patients with category I and IIA acute limb ischemia of less than 7 days' duration, whereas surgical revascularization would be more appropriate for those with category IIB and early III acute limb ischemia and in those whose symptoms have been present for more than 7 days (Fig. 57-21).

ATHEROEMBOLISM

Atheroembolism refers to the occlusion of arteries resulting from detachment and embolization of atheromatous debris including fibrin, platelets, cholesterol crystals, and calcium fragments. Other terms include *atherogenic embolism* and *cholesterol embolism*. Atheroemboli originate most frequently from shaggy, protruding atheromas of the aorta and less frequently from atherosclerotic branch arteries. The atheroemboli typically occlude small downstream arteries and arterioles of the extremities, brain, eye, kidneys, or mesentery.[152,153] The prevalence of atheroembolism in the general population is not known. Most affected individuals are males who are older than 60 years of age with clinical evidence of atherosclerosis.

Pathogenesis

The risk of atheroembolism is greatest in patients with aortic atherosclerosis characterized by large protruding atheromas (Fig. 57-22). There is a strong association between

CH 57

Peripheral Arterial Diseases

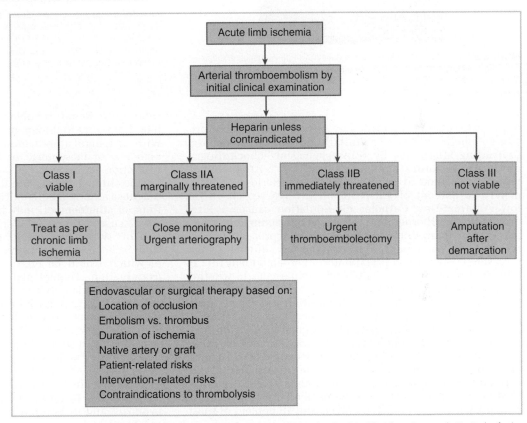

FIGURE 57–21 Management algorithm for the treatment of acute limb ischemia. *(Modified from Dormandy JA, Rutherford RB: Management of peripheral arterial disease (PAD). TASC Working Group. J Vasc Surg 31:S1, 2000.)*

TABLE 57–8	Comparison of Catheter-Directed Thrombolysis and Surgical Revascularization in Treatment of Limb Ischemia						
		Catheter Directed Thrombolysis			Surgical Revascularization		
Study	Results at	Patients	Limb Salvage (%)	Mortality (%)	Patients	Limb Salvage (%)	Mortality (%)
Rochester	12 mo	57	82	16	57	82	42
STILE[150]	6 mo	248	88	6	144	89	8
TOPAS[151]	12 mo	272	85	20	272	86	17

STILE = Surgery versus Thrombolysis for Ischemia of the Lower Extremity; TOPAS = Thrombolysis Or Peripheral Arterial Study.
Modified from Norgren L, Hiatt WR, Dormandy JA, et al: Inter-Society Consensus for the Management of Peripheral Arterial Disease (TASC II). J Vasc Surg 45:S5-S67, 2007.

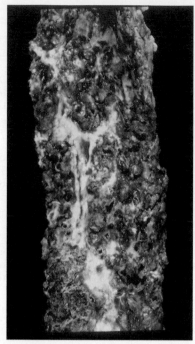

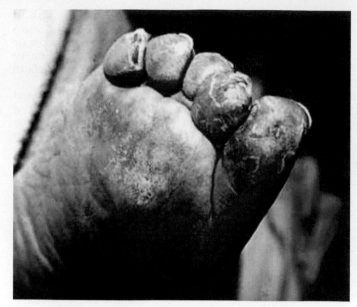

FIGURE 57–23 Atheroemboli to the foot, or "blue toe syndrome." Cyanotic discoloration of the toes, with localized areas of violaceous discoloration, exists. *(Modifed from Beckman JA, Creager MA: Peripheral arterial disease: Clinical evaluation. In MA Creager, Dzau VJ, Loscalzo J (eds): Vascular Medicine: A Companion to Braunwald's Heart Disease. Philadelphia, Elsevier, 2006, p 259.)*

FIGURE 57–22 Atherosclerotic aorta of a patient with atheroemboli. Multiple, protruding, shaggy atheromas with superimposed mural thrombi are shown. *(Courtesy of R.N. Mitchell, MD, PhD, Department of Pathology, Brigham and Women's Hospital, Boston.)*

CH 57

large aortic plaques identified by ultrasonography and previous embolic disease.[152] Similarly, identification of large protruding atheromas by transesophageal echocardiography predicts future embolic events.[152,154,155] Atheroemboli typically occlude arterioles and small arteries. Approximately 50 percent of atheroemboli involve vessels in the lower extremities. Catheter manipulation causes a large proportion of atheroemboli, affecting approximately 1 to 2 percent of patients undergoing endovascular procedures.[153,156] Similarly, surgical manipulation of the aorta during cardiac or vascular operations precipitates atheroembolism in 2 to 3 percent of patients.[157] Controversy remains as to whether anticoagulants or thrombolytic drugs contribute to atheroembolism.[155,158,159] In the Stroke Prevention and Atrial Fibrillation (SPAF) study, atheroembolism occurred in 0.7 percent per patient-year in those patients assigned to adjusted-dose warfarin.[160] In the French Study of Aortic Plaques in Stroke Group, no patient receiving warfarin developed clinical evidence of atheroembolism.[154] Muscle biopsies at the time of coronary artery bypass surgery in patients with recent myocardial infarction detected atheroemboli in 14 percent of patients who received thrombolysis and 10 percent of those who did not.[161]

Clinical Presentation

The most notable clinical features of atheroembolism to the extremities include painful cyanotic toes, resulting in the appellation *blue-toe syndrome* (Fig. 57-23). Livedo reticularis occurs in approximately 50 percent of patients. Local areas of erythematous or violaceous discoloration may be present on the lateral aspects of the feet, soles, and calves. Other findings include digital and foot ulcerations, nodules, purpura, and petechiae. Pedal pulses are typically present because the emboli tend to lodge in the more distal digital arteries and arterioles. Symptoms and signs indicating additional organ involvement with atheroemboli should be sought. Fundoscopy can visualize Hollenhorst plaques in patients with visual loss secondary to retinal ischemia or

infarction. Renal involvement manifested by increased blood pressure and azotemia commonly occurs in patients with peripheral atheroemboli. Patients also sometimes have evidence of mesenteric or bladder ischemia and splenic infarction.

The clinical setting and findings are usually sufficient to diagnose atheroembolism. However, some of the manifestations of atheroemboli may be present with other diseases. As discussed previously, critical limb ischemia occurs in patients with severe peripheral atherosclerosis, and acute limb ischemia is a consequence of thromboembolism, each of which would be characterized by an abnormal pulse examination. Hypersensitivity vasculitides secondary to connective tissue diseases, infections, drugs, polyarteritis nodosa, or cryoglobulinemia, for example, may manifest with multisystem organ damage and cutaneous findings of purpura, ulcers, and digital ischemia similar to those findings that result from atheroemboli (see Chap. 84). Procoagulant disorders such as antiphospholipid antibody syndrome, heparin-induced thrombocytopenia, and myeloproliferative disorders such as essential thrombocythemia can cause digital artery thrombosis with resultant digital ischemia, cyanosis, and ulceration.

Diagnostic Tests

Laboratory studies that are consistent with atheroembolism include an elevated erythrocyte sedimentation rate, eosinophilia, and eosinophiluria. Other findings may include anemia, thrombocytopenia, hypocomplementemia, and azotemia. Imaging of the aorta with transesophageal echocardiography, MRA, or CT may identify sites of severe atherosclerosis and shaggy atheroma indicative of a source for atheroemboli. The only definitive test for atheroembolism is pathological confirmation by skin or muscle biopsy. Pathognomonic findings include elongated needle-shaped clefts in small arteries, which are caused by cholesterol crystals, often accompanied by inflammatory infiltrates composed of lymphocytes and possibly giant cells and eosinophils, intimal thickening, and perivascular fibrosis.

Treatment

No definitive treatment exists for atheroembolism. Analgesics should be administered for pain. Local foot care should be provided as described previously for patients with acute limb ischemia. It may be necessary to excise or amputate necrotic areas.

Patients with this condition are subject to recurrent atheroembolic events. Risk factor modification, such as lipid-lowering therapy with statins and smoking cessation, can have favorable effects on overall outcome from atherosclerosis, but it is not established whether such intervention will prevent recurrent atheroembolism. The use of antiplatelet drugs to prevent recurrent atheroembolism remains controversial.[158] Administering antiplatelet agents even in the absence of strong clinical evidence of efficacy is reasonable, however, because the agents will prevent other adverse cardiovascular events in patients with atherosclerosis. The use of warfarin also engenders controversy, and some investigators have even suggested that anticoagulants precipitate atheroemboli.[158] Others have found that warfarin reduces atheroembolic events, particularly in patients with mobile aortic atheroma.[155,159] The use of corticosteroids to treat atheroembolism also remains controversial.[158]

Surgical removal of the source should be considered in patients with atheroembolism, particularly in those in whom it recurs. Surgical procedures include excision and replacement of affected portions of the aorta, endarterectomy, and bypass operations. Operative intervention is targeted to the site of the aorta, iliac, or femoral arteries where there is aneurysm formation or obvious shaggy friable atherosclerotic plaque. Often, the aorta is diffusely affected by severe atherosclerosis and it is not possible to identify the precise segment that is responsible for atheroembolism. In addition, many of these patients are elderly and have coexisting coronary artery disease, which increases the risk of major vascular operations. Endovascular placement of stents and stent grafts to prevent recurrent atheroembolism has been reported in several small case series.[153]

REFERENCES

PAD Epidemiology and Risk Factors

1. Criqui MH: Peripheral arterial disease—epidemiological aspects. Vasc Med 6:3-7, 2001.
2. Diehm C, Schuster A, Allenberg JR, et al: High prevalence of peripheral arterial disease and co-morbidity in 6880 primary care patients: Cross-sectional study. Atherosclerosis 172:95-105, 2004.
3. Selvin E, Erlinger TP: Prevalence of and risk factors for peripheral arterial disease in the United States: Results from the National Health and Nutrition Examination Survey, 1999-2000. Circulation 110:738-743, 2004.
4. Norgren L, Hiatt WR, Dormandy JA, et al: Inter-Society Consensus for the Management of Peripheral Arterial Disease (TASC II). J Vasc Surg 45:S5-S67, 2007.
5. Criqui MH, Vargas V, Denenberg JO, et al: Ethnicity and peripheral arterial disease: The San Diego Population Study. Circulation 112:2703-2707, 2005.
6. Allison MA, Criqui MH, McClelland RL, et al: The effect of novel cardiovascular risk factors on the ethnic-specific odds for peripheral arterial disease in the Multi-Ethnic Study of Atherosclerosis (MESA). J Am Coll Cardiol 48:1190-1197, 2006.
7. Hirsch AT, Haskal ZJ, Hertzer NR, et al: ACC/AHA 2005 guidelines for the management of patients with peripheral arterial disease (lower extremity, renal, mesenteric, and abdominal aortic): Executive summary a collaborative report from the American Association for Vascular Surgery/Society for Vascular Surgery, Society for Cardiovascular Angiography and Interventions, Society for Vascular Medicine and Biology, Society of Interventional Radiology, and the ACC/AHA Task Force on Practice Guidelines (Writing Committee to Develop Guidelines for the Management of Patients With Peripheral Arterial Disease) endorsed by the American Association of Cardiovascular and Pulmonary Rehabilitation; National Heart, Lung, and Blood Institute; Society for Vascular Nursing; TransAtlantic Inter-Society Consensus; and Vascular Disease Foundation. J Am Coll Cardiol 47:1239-1312, 2006.
8. Virmani R, Burke AP, Taylor AJ: Congenital malformations of the vasculature. In Creager MA, Dzau VJ, Loscalzo J (eds): Vascular Medicine: A Companion to Braunwald's Heart Disease. Philadelphia, Elsevier, 2006, pp 934-960.
9. Criqui MH, Ninomiya J: The epidemiology of peripheral arterial disease. In MA Creager, Dzau VJ, Loscalzo J (eds): Vascular Medicine: A Companion to Braunwald's Heart Disease. Philadelphia, Elsevier, 2006, pp 223-238.
10. Doyle J, Creager MA: Pharmacotherapy and behavioral intervention for peripheral arterial disease. Rev Cardiovasc Med 4:18-24, 2003.
11. Lu JT, Creager MA: The relationship of cigarette smoking to peripheral arterial disease. Rev Cardiovasc Med 5:189-193, 2004.
12. He Y, Jiang Y, Wang J, et al: Prevalence of peripheral arterial disease and its association with smoking in a population-based study in Beijing, China. J Vasc Surg 44:333-338, 2006.
13. Marso SP, Hiatt WR: Peripheral arterial disease in patients with diabetes. J Am Coll Cardiol 47:921-929, 2006.
14. Aboyans V, Criqui MH, Denenberg JO, et al: Risk factors for progression of peripheral arterial disease in large and small vessels. Circulation 113:2623-2629, 2006.
15. Ridker PM, Stampfer MJ, Rifai N: Novel risk factors for systemic atherosclerosis: A comparison of C-reactive protein, fibrinogen, homocysteine, lipoprotein(a), and standard cholesterol screening as predictors of peripheral arterial disease. JAMA 285:2481-2485, 2001.
16. Murabito JM, D'Agostino RB, Silbershatz H, Wilson WF: Intermittent claudication. A risk profile from The Framingham Heart Study. Circulation 96:44-49, 1997.
17. Wattanakit K, Folsom AR, Selvin E, et al: Risk factors for peripheral arterial disease incidence in persons with diabetes: The Atherosclerosis Risk in Communities (ARIC) Study. Atherosclerosis 180:389-397, 2005.
18. Cheng SW, Ting AC, Wong J: Lipoprotein (a) and its relationship to risk factors and severity of atherosclerotic peripheral vascular disease. Eur J Vasc Endovasc Surg 14:17-23, 1997.
19. Olin JW: Hypertension and peripheral arterial disease. Vasc Med 10:241-246, 2005.
20. Tzoulaki I, Murray GD, Lee AJ, et al: C-reactive protein, interleukin-6, and soluble adhesion molecules as predictors of progressive peripheral atherosclerosis in the general population: Edinburgh Artery Study. Circulation 112:976-983, 2005.
21. Barani J, Nilsson JA, Mattiasson I, et al: Inflammatory mediators are associated with 1-year mortality in critical limb ischemia. J Vasc Surg 42:75-80, 2005.
22. Brevetti G, Schiano V, Chiariello M: Cellular adhesion molecules and peripheral arterial disease. Vasc Med 11:39-47, 2006.
23. Pradhan AD, Rifai N, Ridker PM: Soluble intercellular adhesion molecule-1, soluble vascular adhesion molecule-1, and the development of symptomatic peripheral arterial disease in men. Circulation 106:820-825, 2002.
24. Wildman RP, Muntner P, Chen J, et al: Relation of inflammation to peripheral arterial disease in the national health and nutrition examination survey, 1999-2002. Am J Cardiol 96:1579-1583, 2005.
25. Owens CD, Ridker PM, Belkin M, et al: Elevated C-reactive protein levels are associated with postoperative events in patients undergoing lower extremity vein bypass surgery. J Vasc Surg 45:2-9, 2007.
26. Nasir K, Guallar E, Navas-Acien A, et al: Relationship of monocyte count and peripheral arterial disease: Results from the National Health and Nutrition Examination Survey 1999-2002. Arterioscler Thromb Vasc Biol 25:1966-1971, 2005.

PAD Pathophysiology

27. Brevetti G, Corrado S, Martone VD, et al: Microcirculation and tissue metabolism in peripheral arterial disease. Clin Hemorheol Microcirc 21:245-254, 1999.
28. Hiatt WR, Brass EP: Pathophysiology of intermittent claudication. In Creager MA, Dzau VJ, Loscalzo J (eds): Vascular Medicine: A Companion to Braunwald's Heart Disease. Philadelphia, Elsevier, 2006, pp 239-247.
29. Pipinos II, Shepard AD, Anagnostopoulos PV, et al: Phosphorus 31 nuclear magnetic resonance spectroscopy suggests a mitochondrial defect in claudicating skeletal muscle. J Vasc Surg 31:944-952, 2000.
30. Kemp GJ, Roberts N, Bimson WE, et al: Mitochondrial function and oxygen supply in normal and in chronically ischemic muscle: A combined 31P magnetic resonance spectroscopy and near infrared spectroscopy study in vivo. J Vasc Surg 34:1103-1110, 2001.

Clinical Assessment of PAD

31. McDermott MM, Liu K, Greenland P, et al: Functional decline in peripheral arterial disease: associations with the ankle brachial index and leg symptoms. JAMA 292:453-461, 2004.
32. McDermott MM, Fried L, Simonsick E, et al: Asymptomatic peripheral arterial disease is independently associated with impaired lower extremity functioning: The women's health and aging study. Circulation 101:1007-1012, 2000.
33. McDermott MM, Liu K, Guralnik JM, et al: The ankle brachial index independently predicts walking velocity and walking endurance in peripheral arterial disease. J Am Geriatr Soc 46:1355-1362, 1998.
34. Leng GC, Fowkes FG: The Edinburgh Claudication Questionnaire: An improved version of the WHO/Rose Questionnaire for use in epidemiological surveys. J Clin Epidemiol 45:1101-1109, 1992.
35. Criqui MH, Denenberg JO, Bird CE, et al: The correlation between symptoms and non-invasive test results in patients referred for peripheral arterial disease testing. Vasc Med 1:65-71, 1996.
36. Coyne KS, Margolis MK, Gilchrist KA, et al: Evaluating effects of method of administration on Walking Impairment Questionnaire. J Vasc Surg 38:296-304, 2003.
37. Khan NA, Rahim SA, Anand SS, et al: Does the clinical examination predict lower extremity peripheral arterial disease? JAMA 295:536-546, 2006.
38. Rutherford RB, Baker JD, Ernst C, et al: Recommended standards for reports dealing with lower extremity ischemia: revised version. J Vasc Surg 26:517-538, 1997.
39. McDermott MM, Greenland P, Liu K, et al: The ankle brachial index is associated with leg function and physical activity: The Walking and Leg Circulation Study. Ann Intern Med 136:873-883, 2002.
40. Chaudhry H, Holland A, Dormandy J: Comparison of graded versus constant treadmill test protocols for quantifying intermittent claudication. Vasc Med 2:93-97, 1997.

41. Pemberton M, London NJ: Colour flow duplex imaging of occlusive arterial disease of the lower limb. Br J Surg 84:912-919, 1997.

42. Visser K, Hunink MG: Peripheral arterial disease: gadolinium-enhanced MR angiography versus color-guided duplex US—a meta-analysis. Radiology 216:67-77, 2000.

43. Nelemans PJ, Leiner T, de Vet HC, van Engelshoven JM: Peripheral arterial disease: meta-analysis of the diagnostic performance of MR angiography. Radiology 217:105-14, 2000.

44. Ouwendijk R, Kock MC, Visser K, et al: Interobserver agreement for the interpretation of contrast-enhanced 3D MR angiography and MDCT angiography in peripheral arterial disease. AJR Am J Roentgenol 185:1261-1267, 2005.

45. Ouwendijk R, de Vries M, Pattynama PM, et al: Imaging peripheral arterial disease: A randomized controlled trial comparing contrast-enhanced MR angiography and multi-detector row CT angiography. Radiology 236:1094-1103, 2005.

46. Rubin GD, Schmidt AJ, Logan LJ, Sofilos MC: Multi-detector row CT angiography of lower extremity arterial inflow and runoff: Initial experience. Radiology 221:146-158, 2001.

47. Flohr TG, Schaller S, Stierstorfer K, et al: Multi-detector row CT systems and image-reconstruction techniques. Radiology 235:756-773, 2005.

48. Rubin GD: MDCT imaging of the aorta and peripheral vessels. Eur J Radiol 45(Suppl 1):S42-49, 2003.

49. Martin ML, Tay KH, Flak B, et al: Multidetector CT angiography of the aortoiliac system and lower extremities: A prospective comparison with digital subtraction angiography. A J R Am J Roentgenol 180:1085-1091, 2003.

50. Willmann JK, Baumert B, Schertler T, et al: Aortoiliac and lower extremity arteries assessed with 16-detector row CT angiography: Prospective comparison with digital subtraction angiography. Radiology 236:1083-1093, 2005.

51. Belch JJ, Topol EJ, Agnelli G, et al: Critical issues in peripheral arterial disease detection and management: a call to action. Arch Intern Med 163:884-892, 2003.

52. McDermott MM, Liu K, Criqui MH, et al: Ankle-brachial index and subclinical cardiac and carotid disease: The multi-ethnic study of atherosclerosis. Am J Epidemiol 162:33-41, 2005.

53. Cacoub P: Control of Cardiovascular Risk Factors in the REACH Registry. Presented at AHA Scientific Sessions 2006.

54. Fowkes FG, Low LP, Tuta S, Kozak J: Ankle-brachial index and extent of atherothrombosis in 8891 patients with or at risk of vascular disease: results of the international AGATHA study. Eur Heart J 27:1861-1867, 2006.

Prognosis and Management of PAD

55. Doobay AV, Anand SS: Sensitivity and specificity of the ankle-brachial index to predict future cardiovascular outcomes: A systematic review. Arterioscler Thromb Vasc Biol 25:1463-1469, 2005.

56. O'Hare AM, Katz R, Shlipak MG, et al: Mortality and cardiovascular risk across the ankle-arm index spectrum: Results from the Cardiovascular Health Study. Circulation 113:388-393, 2006.

57. Resnick HE, Lindsay RS, McDermott MM, et al: Relationship of high and low ankle brachial index to all-cause and cardiovascular disease mortality: The Strong Heart Study. Circulation 109:733-739, 2004.

58. Leng GC, Lee AJ, Fowkes FG, et al: Incidence, natural history and cardiovascular events in symptomatic and asymptomatic peripheral arterial disease in the general population. Int J Epidemiol 25:1172-1181, 1996.

59. Centers for Disease Control and Prevention (CDC): Diabetes-related amputations of lower extremities in the Medicare population—Minnesota, 1993-1995. MMWR Morb Mortal Wkly Rep 47:649-652, 1998.

60. Gornik HL, Creager MA: Medical treatment of peripheral arterial disease. In Creager MA, Dzau VJ, Loscalzo J (eds): Vascular Medicine: A Companion to Braunwald's Heart Disease. Philadelphia, Elsevier, 2006, pp 239-247.

61. Murabito JM, Evans JC, Nieto K, et al: Prevalence and clinical correlates of peripheral arterial disease in the Framingham Offspring Study. Am Heart J 143:961-965, 2002.

62. Heart Protection Study Collaborative Group: MRC/BHF Heart Protection Study of cholesterol lowering with simvastatin in 20,536 high-risk individuals: A randomised placebo-controlled trial. Lancet 360:7-22, 2002.

63. Executive Summary of The Third Report of The National Cholesterol Education Program (NCEP) Expert Panel on Detection, Evaluation, and Treatment of High Blood Cholesterol In Adults (Adult Treatment Panel III). JAMA 285:2486-2497, 2001.

64. Robins SJ, Collins D, Wittes JT, et al: Relation of gemfibrozil treatment and lipid levels with major coronary events: VA-HIT: A randomized controlled trial. JAMA 285:1585-1591, 2001.

65. Keech A, Simes RJ, Barter P, et al: Effects of long-term fenofibrate therapy on cardiovascular events in 9795 people with type 2 diabetes mellitus (the FIELD study): Randomised controlled trial. Lancet 366:1849-1861, 2005.

66. Walldius G, Erikson U, Olsson AG, et al: The effect of probucol on femoral atherosclerosis: The Probucol Quantitative Regression Swedish Trial (PQRST). Am J Cardiol 74:875-883, 1994.

67. Buchwald H, Bourdages HR, Campos CT, et al: Impact of cholesterol reduction on peripheral arterial disease in the Program on the Surgical Control of the Hyperlipidemias (POSCH). Surgery 120:672-679, 1996.

68. Pedersen TR, Kjekshus J, Pyorala K, et al: Effect of simvastatin on ischemic signs and symptoms in the Scandinavian simvastatin survival study (4S). Am J Cardiol 81:333-335, 1998.

69. Aronow WS, Nayak D, Woodworth S, Ahn C: Effect of simvastatin versus placebo on treadmill exercise time until the onset of intermittent claudication in older patients with peripheral arterial disease at six months and at one year after treatment. Am J Cardiol 92:711-712, 2003.

70. Mohler ER III, Hiatt WR, Creager MA: Cholesterol reduction with atorvastatin improves walking distance in patients with peripheral arterial disease. Circulation 108:1481-1486, 2003.

71. Mondillo S, Ballo P, Barbati R, et al: Effects of simvastatin on walking performance and symptoms of intermittent claudication in hypercholesterolemic patients with peripheral vascular disease. Am J Med 114:359-364, 2003.

72. McDermott MM, Guralnik JM, Greenland P, et al: Statin use and leg functioning in patients with and without lower-extremity peripheral arterial disease. Circulation 107:757-761, 2003.

73. Gonzales D, Rennard SI, Nides M, et al: Varenicline, an alpha4beta2 nicotinic acetylcholine receptor partial agonist, vs sustained-release bupropion and placebo for smoking cessation: A randomized controlled trial. JAMA 296:47-55, 2006.

74. Jorenby DE, Hays JT, Rigotti NA, et al: Efficacy of varenicline, an alpha4beta2 nicotinic acetylcholine receptor partial agonist, vs placebo or sustained-release bupropion for smoking cessation: A randomized controlled trial. JAMA 296:56-63, 2006.

75. Nathan DM, Cleary PA, Backlund JY, et al: Intensive diabetes treatment and cardiovascular disease in patients with type 1 diabetes. N Engl J Med 353:2643-2653, 2005.

76. Nathan DM, Lachin J, Cleary P, et al: Intensive diabetes therapy and carotid intima-media thickness in type 1 diabetes mellitus. N Engl J Med 348:2294-2303, 2003.

77. UK Prospective Diabetes Study (UKPDS) Group: Intensive blood-glucose control with sulphonylureas or insulin compared with conventional treatment and risk of complications in patients with type 2 diabetes (UKPDS 33). Lancet 352:837-853, 1998.

78. Dormandy JA, Charbonnel B, Eckland DJ, et al: Secondary prevention of macrovascular events in patients with type 2 diabetes in the PROactive Study (PROspective pioglitAzone Clinical Trial In macroVascular Events): A randomised controlled trial. Lancet 366:1279-1289, 2005.

79. Mehler PS, Coll JR, Estacio R, et al: Intensive blood pressure control reduces the risk of cardiovascular events in patients with peripheral arterial disease and type 2 diabetes. Circulation 107:753-756, 2003.

80. Radack K, Deck C: Beta-adrenergic blocker therapy does not worsen intermittent claudication in subjects with peripheral arterial disease. A meta-analysis of randomized controlled trials. Arch Intern Med 151:1769-1776, 1991.

81. Chobanian AV, Bakris GL, Black HR, et al: The Seventh Report of the Joint National Committee on Prevention, Detection, Evaluation, and Treatment of High Blood Pressure: The JNC 7 report. JAMA 289:2560-2572, 2003.

82. Yusuf S, Sleight P, Pogue J, et al: Effects of an angiotensin-converting-enzyme inhibitor, ramipril, on cardiovascular events in high-risk patients. The Heart Outcomes Prevention Evaluation Study Investigators. N Engl J Med 342:145-153, 2000.

83. A randomised, blinded, trial of clopidogrel versus aspirin in patients at risk of ischaemic events (CAPRIE). CAPRIE Steering Committee. Lancet 348:1329-1339, 1996.

84. Bhatt DL, Fox KA, Hacke W, et al: Clopidogrel and aspirin versus aspirin alone for the prevention of atherothrombotic events. N Engl J Med 354:1706-1717, 2006.

85. Labs KH, Dormandy JA, Jaeger KA, et al: Transatlantic Conference on Clinical Trial Guidelines in Peripheral Arterial Disease: Clinical trial methodology. Basel PAD Clinical Trial Methodology Group. Circulation 100:e75-81, 1999.

86. Hood SC, Moher D, Barber GG: Management of intermittent claudication with pentoxifylline: Meta-analysis of randomized controlled trials. CMAJ 155:1053-1059, 1996.

87. Girolami B, Bernardi E, Prins MH, et al: Treatment of intermittent claudication with physical training, smoking cessation, pentoxifylline, or nafronyl: A meta-analysis. Arch Intern Med 159:337-345, 1999.

88. Regensteiner JG, Ware JE Jr, McCarthy WJ, et al: Effect of cilostazol on treadmill walking, community-based walking ability, and health-related quality of life in patients with intermittent claudication due to peripheral arterial disease: Meta-analysis of six randomized controlled trials. J Am Geriatr Soc 50:1939-1946, 2002.

89. Dawson DL, Cutler BS, Hiatt WR, et al: A comparison of cilostazol and pentoxifylline for treating intermittent claudication. Am J Med 109:523-530, 2000.

90. Ahimastos AA, Lawler A, Reid CM, et al: Brief communication: ramipril markedly improves walking ability in patients with peripheral arterial disease: a randomized trial. Ann Intern Med 144:660-664, 2006.

91. Barradell LB, Brogden RN: Oral naftidrofuryl. A review of its pharmacology and therapeutic use in the management of peripheral occlusive arterial disease. Drugs Aging 8:299-322, 1996.

92. Kieffer E, Bahnini A, Mouren X, Gamand S: A new study demonstrates the efficacy of naftidrofuryl in the treatment of intermittent claudication. Findings of the Naftidrofuryl Clinical Ischemia Study (NCIS). Int Angiol 20:58-65, 2001.

93. Hiatt WR, Hirsch AT, Cooke JP, et al: Randomized trial of AT-1015 for treatment of intermittent claudication. A novel 5-hydroxytryptamine antagonist with no evidence of efficacy. Vasc Med 9:18-25, 2004.

94. Norgren L, Jawien A, Matyas L, et al: Sarpogrelate, a 5-hT2A receptor antagonist in intermittent claudication. A phase II European study. Vasc Med 11:75-83, 2006.

95. Boger RH, Bode-Boger SM, Thiele W, et al: Restoring vascular nitric oxide formation by L-arginine improves the symptoms of intermittent claudication in patients with peripheral arterial occlusive disease. J Am Coll Cardiol 32:1336-1344, 1998.

96. Oka RK, Szuba A, Giacomini JC, Cooke JP: A pilot study of L-arginine supplementation on functional capacity in peripheral arterial disease. Vasc Med 10:265-274, 2005.

97. Maxwell AJ, Anderson BE, Cooke JP: Nutritional therapy for peripheral arterial disease: a double-blind, placebo-controlled, randomized trial of HeartBar. Vasc Med 5:11-19, 2000.

98. Brevetti G, Diehm C, Lambert D: European multicenter study on propionyl-L-carnitine in intermittent claudication. J Am Coll Cardiol 34:1618-1624, 1999.

99. Hiatt WR, Regensteiner JG, Creager MA, et al: Propionyl-L-carnitine improves exercise performance and functional status in patients with claudication. Am J Med 110:616-622, 2001.

100. Belch JJ, Bell PR, Creissen D, et al: Randomized, double-blind, placebo-controlled study evaluating the efficacy and safety of AS-013, a prostaglandin E1 prodrug, in patients with intermittent claudication. Circulation 95:2298-2302, 1997.

101. Lievre M, Morand S, Besse B, et al: Oral Beraprost sodium, a prostaglandin I(2) analogue, for intermittent claudication: A double-blind, randomized, multicenter controlled trial. Beraprost et Claudication Intermittente (BERCI) Research Group. Circulation 102:426-431, 2000.

102. Mohler ER III, Hiatt WR, Olin JW, et al: Treatment of intermittent claudication with beraprost sodium, an orally active prostaglandin I2 analogue: A double-blinded, randomized, controlled trial. J Am Coll Cardiol 41:1679-1686, 2003.

103. Prostanoids for chronic critical leg ischemia. A randomized, controlled, open-label trial with prostaglandin E1. The ICAI Study Group. Ischemia Cronica degli Arti Inferiori. Ann Intern Med 130:412-421, 1999.

104. Baumgartner I, Pieczek A, Manor O, et al: Constitutive expression of phVEGF165 after intramuscular gene transfer promotes collateral vessel development in patients with critical limb ischemia. Circulation 97:1114-1123, 1998.

105. Tateishi-Yuyama E, Matsubara H, Murohara T, et al: Therapeutic angiogenesis for patients with limb ischaemia by autologous transplantation of bone-marrow cells: A pilot study and a randomised controlled trial. Lancet 360:427-435, 2002.

106. Rajagopalan S, Mohler ER III, Lederman RJ, et al: Regional angiogenesis with vascular endothelial growth factor in peripheral arterial disease: A phase II randomized, double-blind, controlled study of adenoviral delivery of vascular endothelial growth factor 121 in patients with disabling intermittent claudication. Circulation 108:1933-1938, 2003.

107. Gardner AW, Poehlman ET: Exercise rehabilitation programs for the treatment of claudication pain. A meta-analysis. JAMA 274:975-980, 1995.

108. Leng GC, Fowler B, Ernst E: Exercise for intermittent claudication. Cochrane Database Syst Rev:CD000990, 2000.

109. Stewart KJ, Hiatt WR, Regensteiner JG, Hirsch AT: Exercise training for claudication. N Engl J Med 347:1941-1951, 2002.

110. Brass EP, Hiatt WR, Green S: Skeletal muscle metabolic changes in peripheral arterial disease contribute to exercise intolerance: a point-counterpoint discussion. Vasc Med 9:293-301, 2004.

111. Hoppeler H: Vascular growth in hypoxic skeletal muscle. Adv Exp Med Biol 474:277-286, 1999.

112. Gustafsson T, Puntschart A, Kaijser L, et al: Exercise-induced expression of angiogenesis-related transcription and growth factors in human skeletal muscle. Am J Physiol 276:H679-85, 1999.

113. Hambrecht R, Wolf A, Gielen S, et al: Effect of exercise on coronary endothelial function in patients with coronary artery disease. N Engl J Med 342:454-460, 2000.

114. Hambrecht R, Fiehn E, Weigl C, et al: Regular physical exercise corrects endothelial dysfunction and improves exercise capacity in patients with chronic heart failure. Circulation 98:2709-2715, 1998.

115. Brendle DC, Joseph LJ, Corretti MC, et al: Effects of exercise rehabilitation on endothelial reactivity in older patients with peripheral arterial disease. Am J Cardiol 87:324-329, 2001.

116. Hambrecht R, Adams V, Erbs S, et al: Regular physical activity improves endothelial function in patients with coronary artery disease by increasing phosphorylation of endothelial nitric oxide synthase. Circulation 107:3152-3158, 2003.

117. Gardner AW, Katzel LI, Sorkin JD, et al: Exercise rehabilitation improves functional outcomes and peripheral circulation in patients with intermittent claudication: A randomized controlled trial. J Am Geriatr Soc 49:755-762, 2001.

118. Fleisher LA, Beckman JA, Brown KA, et al: ACC/AHA 2006 guideline update on perioperative cardiovascular evaluation for noncardiac surgery: Focused update on perioperative beta-blocker therapy: A report of the American College of Cardiology/American Heart Association Task Force on Practice Guidelines (Writing Committee to Update the 2002 Guidelines on Perioperative Cardiovascular Evaluation for Noncardiac Surgery): Developed in collaboration with the American Society of Echocardiography, American Society of Nuclear Cardiology, Heart Rhythm Society, Society of Cardiovascular Anesthesiologists, Society for Cardiovascular Angiography and Interventions, and Society for Vascular Medicine and Biology. Circulation 113:2662-2674, 2006.

119. Dorffler-Melly J, Buller HR, Koopman MM, Prins MH: Antithrombotic agents for preventing thrombosis after infrainguinal arterial bypass surgery. Cochrane Database Syst Rev:CD000536, 2003.

120. Dorffler-Melly J, Koopman MM, Adam DJ, et al: Antiplatelet agents for preventing thrombosis after peripheral arterial bypass surgery. Cochrane Database Syst Rev: CD000535, 2003.

Thromboangiitis Obliterans (Buerger's Disease)

121. Olin JW: Thromboangiitis obliterans (Buerger's disease). In MA Creager, Dzau VJ, Loscalzo J (eds): Vascular Medicine: A Companion to Braunwald's Heart Disease. Philadelphia, Elsevier, 2006, pp 641-656.

122. Olin JW: Thromboangiitis obliterans (Buerger's disease). N Engl J Med 343:864-869, 2000.

123. Lee T, Seo JW, Sumpio BE, Kim SJ: Immunobiologic analysis of arterial tissue in Buerger's disease. Eur J Vasc Endovasc Surg 25:451-457, 2003.

124. Eichhorn J, Sima D, Lindschau C, et al: Antiendothelial cell antibodies in thromboangiitis obliterans. Am J Med Sci 315:17-23, 1998.

125. Maslowski L, McBane R, Alexewicz P, Wysokinski WE: Antiphospholipid antibodies in thromboangiitis obliterans. Vasc Med 7:259-264, 2002.

126. Makita S, Nakamura M, Murakami H, et al: Impaired endothelium-dependent vasorelaxation in peripheral vasculature of patients with thromboangiitis obliterans (Buerger's disease). Circulation 94:II211-215, 1996.

127. Cooper LT, Tse TS, Mikhail MA, et al: Long-term survival and amputation risk in thromboangiitis obliterans (Buerger's disease). J Am Coll Cardiol 44:2410-2411, 2004.

128. Olin JW, Shih A: Thromboangiitis obliterans (Buerger's disease). Curr Opin Rheumatol 18:18-24, 2006.

129. Fiessinger JN, Schafer M: Trial of iloprost versus aspirin treatment for critical limb ischaemia of thromboangiitis obliterans. The TAO Study. Lancet 335:555-557, 1990.

130. Oral iloprost in the treatment of thromboangiitis obliterans (Buerger's disease): A double-blind, randomised, placebo-controlled trial. The European TAO Study Group. Eur J Vasc Endovasc Surg 15:300-307, 1998.

131. Saha K, Chabra N, Gulati SM: Treatment of patients with thromboangiitis obliterans with cyclophosphamide. Angiology 52:399-407, 2001.

132. Durdu S, Akar AR, Arat M, et al: Autologous bone-marrow mononuclear cell implantation for patients with Rutherford grade II-III thromboangiitis obliterans. J Vasc Surg 44:732-739, 2006.

133. Koshikawa M, Shimodaira S, Yoshioka T, et al: Therapeutic angiogenesis by bone marrow implantation for critical hand ischemia in patients with peripheral arterial disease: A pilot study. Curr Med Res Opin 22:793-798, 2006.

134. Sasajima T, Kubo Y, Inaba M, et al: Role of infrainguinal bypass in Buerger's disease: An eighteen-year experience. Eur J Vasc Endovasc Surg 13:186-192, 1997.

Other Peripheral Arterial Syndromes

135. Slovut DP, Olin JW: Fibromuscular dysplasia. N Engl J Med 350:1862-1871, 2004.

136. Rigberg DA, Freischlag JA, Machleder HE: Vascular compression syndromes. In Creager MA, Dzau VJ, Loscalzo J (eds): Vascular Medicine: A Companion to Braunwald's Heart Disease. Philadelphia, Elsevier, 2006, pp 920-933.

137. Aune S, Trippestad A: Operative mortality and long-term survival of patients operated on for acute lower limb ischaemia. Eur J Vasc Endovasc Surg 15:143-146, 1998.

138. Braithwaite BD, Davies B, Birch PA, et al: Management of acute leg ischaemia in the elderly. Br J Surg 85:217-220, 1998.

139. Ascher E, Markevich N, Schutzer RW, et al: Small popliteal artery aneurysms: Are they clinically significant? J Vasc Surg 37:755-760, 2003.

140. Greaves M: Acquired thrombophilia. Vasc Med 9:215-218, 2004.

141. Walker ID: Inherited thrombophilia. Vasc Med 9:219-221, 2004.

142. Bauer KA: Inherited and acquired hypercoagulable states. In Loscalzo J, Schafer AI (eds): Thrombosis and Hemorrhage. 3rd ed. Philadelphia, Lippincott Williams & Wilkins, 2003, pp 648-84.

143. Ouriel K: Acute arterial occlusion. In Creager MA, Dzau VJ, Loscalzo J (eds): Vascular Medicine: A Companion to Braunwald's Heart Disease. Philadelphia, Elsevier, 2006, pp 669-676.

144. Thrombolysis in the management of lower limb peripheral arterial occlusion—a consensus document. J Vasc Interv Radiol 14:S337-349, 2003.

145. Semba CP, Murphy TP, Bakal CW, et al: Thrombolytic therapy with use of alteplase (rt-PA) in peripheral arterial occlusive disease: Review of the clinical literature. The Advisory Panel. J Vasc Interv Radiol 11:149-161, 2000.

146. Ouriel K: Acute arterial occlusion. Curr Treat Options Cardiovasc Med 2:255-264, 2000.

147. Kasirajan K, Gray B, Beavers FP, et al: Rheolytic thrombectomy in the management of acute and subacute limb-threatening ischemia. J Vasc Interv Radiol 12:413-421, 2001.

148. Dormandy J, Heeck L, Vig S: Acute limb ischemia. Semin Vasc Surg 12:148-153, 1999.

149. Berridge DC, Kessel D, Robertson I: Surgery versus thrombolysis for acute limb ischaemia: Initial management. Cochrane Database Syst Rev:CD002784, 2002.

150. Results of a prospective randomized trial evaluating surgery versus thrombolysis for ischemia of the lower extremity. The STILE trial. Ann Surg 220:251-266; discussion 66-68, 1994.

151. Ouriel K, Veith FJ, Sasahara AA: A comparison of recombinant urokinase with vascular surgery as initial treatment for acute arterial occlusion of the legs. Thrombolysis or Peripheral Arterial Surgery (TOPAS) Investigators. N Engl J Med 338:1105-1111, 1998.

152. Tunick PA, Kronzon I: Atheroembolism. In Creager MA, Dzau VJ, Loscalzo J (eds): Vascular Medicine: A Companion to Braunwald's Heart Disease. Philadelphia, Elsevier, 2006, pp 677-687.

153. Liew YP, Bartholomew JR: Atheromatous embolization. Vasc Med 10:309-326, 2005.

154. Atherosclerotic disease of the aortic arch as a risk factor for recurrent ischemic stroke. The French Study of Aortic Plaques in Stroke Group. N Engl J Med 334:1216-1221, 1996.

155. Ferrari E, Vidal R, Chevallier T, Baudouy M: Atherosclerosis of the thoracic aorta and aortic debris as a marker of poor prognosis: benefit of oral anticoagulants. J Am Coll Cardiol 33:1317-1322, 1999.

156. Fukumoto Y, Tsutsui H, Tsuchihashi M, et al: The incidence and risk factors of cholesterol embolization syndrome, a complication of cardiac catheterization: A prospective study. J Am Coll Cardiol 42:211-216, 2003.

157. Kolh PH, Torchiana DF, Buckley MJ: Atheroembolization in cardiac surgery. The need for preoperative diagnosis. J Cardiovasc Surg (Torino) 40:77-81, 1999.

158. Smyth JS, Scoble JE: Atheroembolism. Curr Treat Options Cardiovasc Med 4:255-265, 2002.

1514

159. Dressler FA, Craig WR, Castello R, Labovitz AJ: Mobile aortic atheroma and systemic emboli: efficacy of anticoagulation and influence of plaque morphology on recurrent stroke. J Am Coll Cardiol 31:134-138, 1998.

160. Blackshear JL, Zabalgoitia M, Pennock G, et al: Warfarin safety and efficacy in patients with thoracic aortic plaque and atrial fibrillation. SPAF TEE Investigators. Stroke Prevention and Atrial Fibrillation. Transesophageal echocardiography. Am J Cardiol 83:453-455, A9, 1999.

161. Blankenship JC, Butler M, Garbes A: Prospective assessment of cholesterol embolization in patients with acute myocardial infarction treated with thrombolytic vs conservative therapy. Chest 107:662-668, 1995.

CHAPTER 58

Medical Therapy for Stroke
Prevention, 1515
Platelet Antiaggregants, 1515
Anticoagulation, 1516
HMG-CoA Reductase Inhibitors
   (Statins), 1517
Antihypertensives, 1518

Management of Acute Ischemic
Stroke, 1519
Intravenous rt-PA, 1519
Endovascular Therapy, 1520
Other Measures for Stroke
   Treatment, 1521
Stroke after Percutaneous Coronary
   Interventions and Thrombolytic
   Treatment for Myocardial
   Infarction, 1522

References, 1522

Prevention and Management of Stroke

Larry B. Goldstein

Each year, more than 700,000 Americans have strokes and more than 150,000 die, making stroke the country's third leading cause of death.[1] More than 25 percent of stroke survivors older than age 65 are disabled 6 months later. Stroke disproportionately affects minority populations, and more than 60 percent of stroke-related deaths occur in women. Although advancing age is a major risk factor for stroke, more than one third of strokes occur in persons younger than age 65, and even children can be affected. Although many of the risk factors for stroke overlap with those of cardiac and peripheral vascular disease (i.e., the concept of global risk), it is critical to recognize that stroke represents a variety of conditions and can reflect a diverse set of pathophysiological processes and that specific therapeutic interventions can confer levels of benefit and risk that differ from other forms of vascular disease. This discussion focuses on therapeutic interventions for stroke prevention and treatment of particular relevance to cardiologists. The American Stroke Association/American Heart Association provide detailed, current evidence-based guidelines for the Primary Prevention of Ischemic Stroke,[2] Prevention of Ischemic Stroke in Patients with Prior Stroke or TIA,[3] and for the Early Management of Patients with Ischemic Stroke.[4,5]

MEDICAL THERAPY FOR STROKE PREVENTION

Approximately 70 percent of strokes are first cardiovascular events, making primary prevention of paramount importance.[1] Prevention of recurrent events is also critical as 15 percent of survivors will have a second stroke within 1 year and 30 percent will do so within 5 years. The period soon after the stroke is associated with the highest rate of recurrence. The risk of ischemic stroke after a transient ischemic attack (TIA, a condition frequently misdiagnosed and defined as a "brief episode of neurological dysfunction caused by a focal disturbance of brain or retinal ischemia, with clinical symptoms typically lasting less than 1 hour and without radiological evidence of infarction") is as high as 10.5 percent over 90 days (with the highest risk over the first week).[3] The risks and benefits of therapeutic interventions for stroke may differ for primary and secondary stroke prevention.

Platelet Antiaggregants

Primary Prevention

The use of platelet antiaggregants for primary stroke prevention needs to be considered in the context of the patient's global risk for cardiovascular events and stroke. No evidence indicates that platelet antiaggregants reduce the risk of stroke in persons at low risk.[2]

The benefit of aspirin for primary prophylaxis outweighs its associated risk of bleeding complications among persons with a 10-year risk of coronary heart events of 6 to 10 percent, but there is no evidence of a reduction in stroke risk even in these patients (predominantly men), and aspirin is not recommended for this purpose.[2] Although the Women's Health Study found no reduction in its prespecified primary endpoint (nonfatal MI, nonfatal stroke, or cardiovascular death) with aspirin (100 mg on alternate days), there was a 17 percent reduction in the risk of stroke, albeit with an increase in the risk of bleeding[6] (see also Chap. 45). This benefit was primarily in women at increased stroke risk because of the presence of other risk factors (e.g., hypertension, diabetes). As a result, aspirin may be considered in women whose risk of stroke is sufficiently high to outweigh its associated bleeding risk.[2] No evidence of a benefit in reducing the risk of a first stroke with any other platelet antiaggregant exists.

Secondary Prevention

Aspirin (lowest effective dose compared with placebo is 50 mg/day) lowers by approximately 18 percent the risk of recurrent stroke in persons with a noncardioembolic ischemic stroke.[3] Sustained-release dipyridamole (200 mg twice daily) is as efficacious as aspirin in reducing the risk of recurrent stroke caused by focal brain or retinal ischemia, with a further significant reduction (≈37 percent) when the two drugs are combined.[3,7] Aspirin/sustained release dipyridamole is available in the United States in a fixed-dose combination (25 mg aspirin plus 200 mg dipyridamole) that is given twice daily. Cardiologists are often concerned that dipyridamole might increase the risk of cardiac ischemia, but clinical trials have not substantiated this reservation. Cardiologists are also concerned that the total dose of aspirin (50 mg/day), although effective for secondary stroke prophylaxis, is below the dose shown to be effective for cardiac prophylaxis. To address this potential limitation of fixed-combination aspirin dipyridamole, a small additional dose of aspirin can be added (e.g., 81 mg/day).[7]

Clopidogrel monotherapy given to patients with a history of MI, stroke, or symptomatic peripheral arterial disease reduces by 8.7 percent the combined risk of MI, stroke, or vascular death as compared with aspirin.[3] Although based on a potentially underpowered subgroup analysis, there is no evidence of a significant reduction in stroke among those with prior stroke.[3] No reduction occurred in a composite endpoint of MI, stroke, or cardiovascular death in patients with cardiovascular disease (including stroke) or multiple risk factors with aspirin plus clopidogrel as compared with aspirin alone.[8] When tested directly in patients with stroke, the combination of aspirin and clopidogrel was associated generally with a significant increase in bleeding complications without a significant reduction in ischemic stroke.[9] Aspirin and clopidogrel as compared to cliclclogrel alone should not be used in combination for stroke prophylaxis in patients at high risk or in patients with recent stroke.[3]

Anticoagulation

Primary Prevention

The use of long-term anticoagulation to reduce the risk of a first cardiogenic embolism in patients at increased risk due to conditions such as mechanical heart valves, atrial fibrillation, and cardiomyopathy is addressed fully in Chaps. 25, 35, 62, and 82.

Secondary Prevention

The evidence supporting the use of anticoagulation for prevention of recurrent stroke in patients without atrial fibrillation or other high-risk cardiogenic sources is uncertain or suggests that the benefit does not outweigh the risk of warfarin-associated bleeding complications.

For patients with noncardioembolic stroke, the Warfarin-Aspirin Recurrent Stroke Study (WARSS) directly compared warfarin (INR 2 to 3) versus aspirin (325 mg/day).[10] An insignificant advantage was associated with aspirin treatment (17.8 percent of recurrent stroke or death for warfarin versus 16 percent for aspirin, $p = 0.25$) (Fig. 58-1). Given the increased costs and monitoring associated with warfarin, there is no reason to use this drug for this purpose.

Although based on post hoc analysis, data from WARSS was also evaluated to address the problem of aspirin failures. This term is used variably to refer to patients taking aspirin who have no measurable platelet antiaggregant effect or to patients who have a recurrent ischemic event such as stroke despite treatment. The latter definition was used in the WARSS analysis. Of the patients who had a history of stroke before the study index stroke, those taking aspirin before randomization (i.e., aspirin failures) and randomized to receive aspirin had a 31.8 percent rate of recurrent stroke as compared with a 16.9 percent rate in those who were randomized to aspirin but had not been taking aspirin before randomization (i.e., the rate of recurrent stroke was higher in those who had failed aspirin). The rate of recurrent stroke, however, was 29 percent in those who had failed aspirin and were randomized to warfarin. Therefore, based on the data from WARSS, despite a high rate of recurrent stroke in patients failing aspirin who were subsequently treated with aspirin, treatment with warfarin showed no advantage. No data show that patients failing aspirin benefit from an alternative antiplatelet regimen.

A retrospective data analysis suggested that patients with symptomatic, intracranial, large-vessel stenotic-occlusive disease benefited from warfarin as compared with aspirin.[11] This hypothesis was subsequently tested in the Warfarin-Aspirin Symptomatic Intracranial Disease (WASID) trial comparing warfarin (INR 2 to 3) with aspirin (1300 mg/day).[12] The rate of recurrent ischemic stroke, intracerebral hemorrhage, or nonstroke vascular death did not differ between the two treatment regimens (22 percent with warfarin versus 21 percent with aspirin, $p = 0.83$); however, there was a higher rate of major hemorrhages with warfarin (8.3 versus 3.2 percent, $p = 0.01$). Because of a lack of efficacy and a higher rate of bleeding complications, warfarin should generally not be used for patients with symptomatic large-vessel intracranial stenotic-occlusive disease. Angioplasty

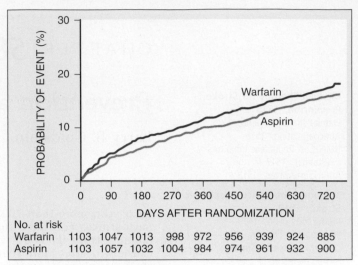

FIGURE 58–1 Kaplan-Meier analyses of the time to recurrent ischemic stroke or death according to treatment assignment. *(From Mohr JP, Thompson JL, Lazar RM, et al: A comparison of warfarin and aspirin for the prevention of recurrent ischemic stroke. N Engl J Med 345:1444, 2001.)*

and stenting for patients with this condition who fail medical therapy may also be considered; however, a prospective randomized trial comparing this approach with medical therapy has not been conducted.

Although a patent foramen ovale (PFO, with or without an atrial septal aneurysm) is found more commonly in young patients with cryptogenic stroke, optimal medical therapy for secondary stroke prophylaxis is uncertain. Randomized trials assessing the potential benefits of endovascular closure as compared with medical therapy are in progress. Uncertainty about appropriate management exists, in part, because of the unclear relationship between the presence of PFO (whether large or small and with or without an atrial septal aneurysm) and the risk of *recurrent* stroke and death. A systematic literature review of 129 articles identified 4 meeting minimal quality criteria and found, as compared with those without a PFO, no significant increase in recurrent stroke or death for those with PFO (OR 0.95, 95 percent CI 0.62 to 1.44), small PFO (OR 1.23, 95 percent CI 0.76 to 2), large PFO (OR 0.59, 95 percent CI 0.28 to 1.24), or combined PFO and atrial septal aneurysm (OR 2.10, 95 percent CI 0.86 to 5.06).[13] This finding agrees with the results of the subsequently reported PFO in Cryptogenic Stroke Study (PICSS) that found nearly identical rates of recurrent stroke or death regardless of the presence of a PFO.[14] Essentially no prospective randomized trials have compared antiplatelet and anticoagulant therapy in this setting, and PICSS found nearly identical rates of recurrent stroke or death with aspirin or warfarin in those with and without a PFO.

The various inherited (e.g., protein C, protein S, or antithrombin III deficiency; factor V Leiden; prothrombin G20210A mutation) and acquired (e.g., lupus anticoagulant, anticardiolipin or antiphospholipid antibodies) coagulopathies are more commonly associated with venous as compared with arterial thromboses (see Chap. 82).[3] Although there are clear instances in which these types of disorders are associated with ischemic stroke, particularly in children or young adults, causal relationships remain controversial. For example, in another substudy of the WARSS trial, the Antiphospholipid Antibody Stroke Study (APASS), 41 percent of 1770 subjects were positive for one or more antiphospholipid antibodies.[15] Rates of recurrent thromboembolic events were somewhat higher for those who were antiphospholipid antibody positive, but there was no differ-

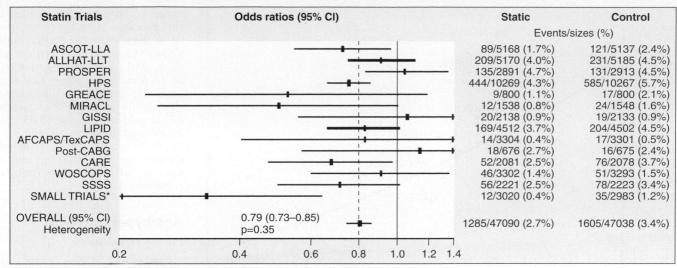

Odds ratios for all strokes in clinical trials of statins. AFCAPS/TexCAPS = Air Force Coronary Atherosclerosis Prevention Study/Texas Coronary Atherosclerosis Prevention Study; ALLHAT-LLT = Antihypertensive and Lipid-Lowering Treatment to Prevent Heart Attack Trial-Lipid Lowering Trial; ASCOT-LLA = Anglo-Scandinavian Cardiac Outcomes Trial-Lipid Lowering Arm; CARE = Cholesterol and Recurrent Events; GISSI = Gruppo Italiano per lo Studio della Sopravvivenza nell'Infarto Miocardico; GREACE = Greek Atorvastatin and Coronary-Heart Disease Evaluation; HPS = Heart Protection Study; LIPID = Long-Term Intervention with Pravastatin in Ischemic Disease; MIRACL = Myocardial Ischemia Reduction with Aggressive Cholesterol Lowering; PostCABG = Post-Coronary Artery Bypass Graft Trial; PROSPER = Prospective Study of Pravastatin in the Elderly at Risk; SSSS = Scandinavian Simvastatin Survival Study; WOSCOPS = West of Scotland Coronary Prevention Study. *Pooled odds ratios for all strokes in small trials calculated with the Mantel-Haenszel method. Small trials included: ACAPS = Asymptomatic Carotid Artery Progression Study; CARE = Cholesterol and Recurrent Events; GISSI = Gruppo Italiano per lo Studio della Sopravvivenza nell'Infarto Miocardico; HTAS = HDL-Atherosclerosis Treatment Study; KAPS = Kuopio Atherosclerosis Prevention Study; L-CAD = Lipid-Coronary Artery Disease; LRT = Lovastatin Restenosis Trial; MARS = Monitored Atherosclerosis Regression Study; PLAC = Pravastatin Limitation of Atherosclerosis in the Coronary Arteries; PMNSG = Pravastatin Multinational Study Group; PostCABG = Post-Coronary Artery Bypass Graft Trial; REGRESS = Regression Growth Evaluation Statin Study; SCAT = Simvastatin/Enalapril Coronary Atherosclerosis Trial. *(From Amarenco P, Labreuche J, Lavallee P, Touboul PJ: Statins in stroke prevention and carotid atherosclerosis: Systematic review and up-to-date meta-analysis. Stroke 35:2902, 2004.)*

ence in event rates for those antibody-positive patients who were treated with warfarin as compared with aspirin. Patients with venous thromboembolic events who are found to have an underlying coagulopathy or those with stroke or TIA otherwise fulfilling criteria for the antiphospholipid antibody syndrome (venous and arterial occlusive disease in multiple organs, miscarriages, and livedo reticularis) are appropriately treated with warfarin. Because coagulopathies (especially the generic forms listed earlier) are more commonly associated with venous thromboses, cryptogenic stroke in this setting should prompt an evaluation for sources of potential paradoxical embolism. The yield of magnetic resonance imaging of the pelvic and lower extremities is higher than with Doppler ultrasound and should be considered in patients with a presumed paradoxical embolus.[16] Those with arterial stroke and found to have only elevated antiphospholipid antibody levels may be reasonably treated with aspirin.[3]

HMG-CoA Reductase Inhibitors (Statins)

Primary Prevention

The role of statins in the management of patients with coronary heart disease or at elevated coronary heart disease (CHD) risk is addressed in Chaps. 42 and 45. Treatment of these groups of patients with statins is associated with not only a reduction in cardiac events but also a reduction in the risk of a first stroke. A meta-analysis including the results of 26 trials found a 21 percent reduction in the risk of stroke among patients with established CHD or risk (Fig. 58-2).[17] For each 10 percent LDL-cholesterol reduction, the relative risk of stroke decreases by 13 percent (Fig. 58-3).[17] Specific studies show a reduction in the risk of first stroke

with statin treatment among diabetics,[18,19] hypertensives,[20] and the elderly.[21]

Secondary Prevention

In contrast to the large amount of data showing a reduction in the risk of a first stroke in patients with CHD or at high CHD risk who are treated with a statin, until recently there has been no evidence that treatment with a statin reduces the risk of a second stroke. The Heart Protection Study (HPS) included 3280 subjects with a history of stroke (including 1820 with stroke and no history of CHD) who were treated with either a statin or placebo.[22] Among those with a prior history of stroke, statin treatment reduced by 20 percent the frequency of major vascular events (MI, stroke, revascularization procedure, or vascular death) but did not lower the risk of recurrent stroke (occurring in 10.5 percent in those treated with placebo versus 10.4 percent in those treated with the statin). Several plausible reasons exist for this lack of effect on recurrent stroke; however, the most important might be that patients were randomized an average of approximately 4 years after the index event. Most recurrent strokes occur soon (within the first few years), so those randomized in the HPS were at relatively low risk of recurrent stroke.

The Stroke Prevention with Aggressive Reduction in Cholesterol Levels (SPARCL) trial randomized more than 4700 subjects within 6 months of a noncardioembolic stroke or TIA and who had no known CHD to high-dose statin or placebo for a primary endpoint of the first occurrence of a nonfatal or fatal stroke.[23] Those randomized to high-dose statin treatment had a 16 percent relative reduction in nonfatal or fatal stroke (post hoc analysis found this overall benefit occurred despite a small increased risk of brain hemorrhage), as well as a 35 percent relative reduction in

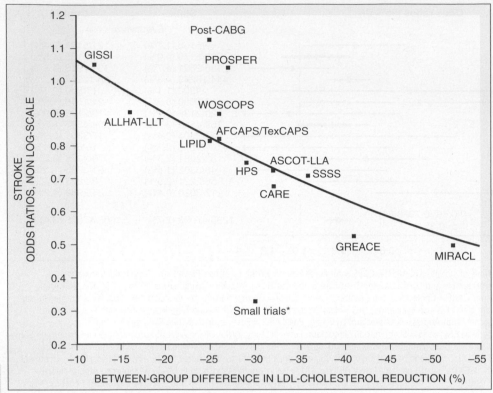

FIGURE 58–3 Relationship between odds ratios for stroke and corresponding LDL-C reduction. The regression line was plotted and weighted for the inverse variance of odds ratios. *Size-weighted combined estimates for the small trials. AFCAPS/TexCAPS = Air Force Coronary Atherosclerosis Prevention Study/Texas Coronary Atherosclerosis Prevention Study; ALLHAT-LLT = Antihypertensive and Lipid-Lowering Treatment to Prevent Heart Attack Trial-Lipid Lowering Trial; ASCOT-LLA = Anglo-Scandinavian Cardiac Outcomes Trial-Lipid Lowering Arm; CARE = Cholesterol and Recurrent Events; GISSI = Gruppo Italiano per lo Studio della Sopravvivenza nell'Infarto Miocardico; GREACE = Greek Atorvastatin and Coronary-Heart Disease Evaluation; HPS = Heart Protection Study; LIPID = Long Term Intervention with Pravastatin in Ischemic Disease; MIRACL = Myocardial Ischemia Reduction with Aggressive Cholesterol Lowering; PostCABG = Post-Coronary Artery Bypass Graft Trial; PROSPER = Prospective Study of Pravastatin in the Elderly at Risk; SSSS = Scandinavian Simvastatin Survival Study; WOSCOPS = West of Scotland Coronary Prevention Study. *(From Amarenco P, Labreuche J, Lavallee P, Touboul PJ: Statins in stroke prevention and carotid atherosclerosis: Systematic review and up-to-date meta-analysis. Stroke 35:2902, 2004.)*

CH 58

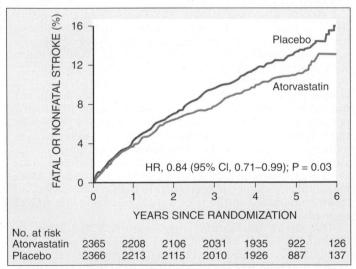

FIGURE 58–4 Kaplan-Meier curve for stroke or transient ischemic attack (TIA). The data report an intention-to-treat analysis with prespecified adjustments for geographic region, entry event, time since entry event, sex, and baseline age for the first occurrence of a fatal or nonfatal stroke or TIA. CI = confidence interval; HR = hazard ratio. *(From Amarenco P, Bogousslavsky J, Callahan A III, et al: High-dose atorvastatin after stroke or transient ischemic attack. N Engl J Med 355:549, 2006.)*

major coronary events. Added to the previous data on prevention of a first stroke, SPARCL now shows that treatment with high-dose statin can reduce the risk of recurrent stroke or TIA (Fig. 58-4). Further, the results suggest that noncardioembolic stroke be considered as a CHD risk equivalent because of the dramatic reduction in CHD events despite the subjects having no known CHD at the time of randomization.

Antihypertensives

Primary Prevention

Hypertension is one of the most important treatable risk factors for both ischemic stroke and parenchymal intracerebral hemorrhage. The Seventh Report of the Joint National Committee on Prevention, Detection, Evaluation, and Treatment of High Blood Pressure (JNC 7) provides comprehensive, evidence-based guidelines for the classification and treatment of hypertension, reiterated in the current American Stroke Association Primary Stroke Prevention Guidelines.[2,24] Both guidelines indicate that the choice of a specific antihypertensive regimen must be individualized but that the reduction in blood pressure is generally more important than the specific agent(s) used to achieve this goal. A meta-analysis of randomized controlled trials comparing antihypertensive drugs with placebo or no treatment on stroke, including more than 73,500 participants and nearly 2900 stroke events found similar risk reductions for angiotensin-converting enzyme (ACE) inhibitors (28 percent), beta-adrenergic receptor blockers (beta blockers) or diuretics (35 percent), and calcium channel antagonists (39 percent) corresponding to blood pressure reductions of 5/2, 13/6, and 10/5 mm Hg, respectively (Fig. 58-5).[25]

Secondary Prevention

Only limited data directly address the role of blood pressure treatment in secondary prevention among persons with a history of stroke or TIA. A systematic review focused on the relationship between blood pressure reduction and the secondary prevention of stroke and other vascular events and included 7 trials with a combined sample size of 15,527 participants with ischemic stroke, TIA, or intracerebral hemorrhage randomized from 3 weeks to 14 months after the index event and followed between 2 and 5 years.[26] Treatment with antihypertensive drugs was associated with significant reductions in all recurrent strokes (24 percent); nonfatal recurrent stroke (21 percent); myocardial infarction (MI, 21 percent); and all vascular events (21 percent) (Fig. 58-6). Data regarding the relative benefits of specific antihypertensive regimens for secondary stroke prevention are largely lacking. This meta-analysis found a reduction in recurrent stroke with diuretics (32 percent) and diuretics and ACE inhibitors in combination (45 percent), but not with beta blockers or ACE inhibitors used alone.[26] The overall reductions in both stroke and all vascular events were related to the degree of blood pressure lowering.

Whether there is a specific benefit of ACE inhibitors in reducing the risk of recurrent stroke also remains uncertain. The Heart Outcomes Prevention Evaluation (HOPE) study compared the effects of an ACE inhibitor with placebo in high-risk persons and found a 24 percent risk reduction in the risk of stroke, MI, or vascular death among the 1013 patients with a history of stroke or TIA.[3] Although the benefit was not considered attributable to the relatively low degree of blood pressure lowering that was achieved, this may have been related to the way in which blood pressure was measured in relation to when the drug was given. A substudy using ambulatory blood pressure monitoring found a substantial 10/4 mm Hg reduction over 24 hours and a 17/8 mm Hg reduction during nighttime. The Perindopril Protection Against Recurrent Stroke Study (PROGRESS) was specifically designed to test the effects of a blood pressure–lowering regimen including an ACE inhibitor in 6105 patients with stroke or TIA within the prior 5 years.[3] Randomization was stratified by intention to use single (the ACE inhibitor) or combination (ACE inhibitor plus the diuretic indapamide) therapy in both hypertensive (>160 mm Hg systolic or > 90 mm Hg diastolic) and nonhypertensive patients. The combination (reducing blood pressure by an average of 12/5 mm Hg) resulted in a 43 percent reduction in the risk of recurrent stroke and a 40 percent reduction in the risk of major vascular events with the effect present in both hypertensive and normotensive groups. However, there was no significant benefit of either antihypertensive given alone. The choice of a specific antihypertensive regimen should be guided by specific patient characteristics and comorbid conditions.

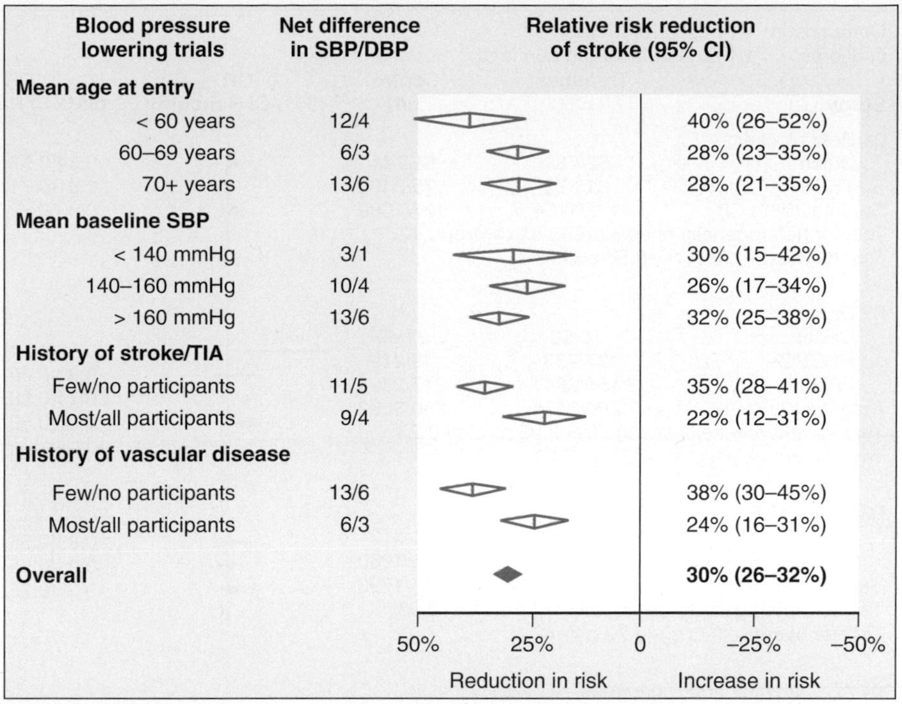

Blood pressure lowering trials	Net difference in SBP/DBP	Relative risk reduction of stroke (95% CI)
Mean age at entry		
< 60 years	12/4	40% (26–52%)
60–69 years	6/3	28% (23–35%)
70+ years	13/6	28% (21–35%)
Mean baseline SBP		
< 140 mmHg	3/1	30% (15–42%)
140–160 mmHg	10/4	26% (17–34%)
> 160 mmHg	13/6	32% (25–38%)
History of stroke/TIA		
Few/no participants	11/5	35% (28–41%)
Most/all participants	9/4	22% (12–31%)
History of vascular disease		
Few/no participants	13/6	38% (30–45%)
Most/all participants	6/3	24% (16–31%)
Overall		**30% (26–32%)**

50%   25%   0   −25%   −50%
Reduction in risk   Increase in risk

FIGURE 58–5 Randomized controlled trials comparing antihypertensive drugs with a placebo (or no treatment) by subgroup. The meta-analyses of blood pressure–lowering trials stratify into subgroups on the basis of mean age of trial participants at entry, baseline systolic blood pressure level, and whether trial participants predominantly had a history of stroke/transient ischemic attack or vascular disease. The diamonds are centered on the pooled estimate of effect and represent a 95 percent confidence interval. The solid diamond represents the pooled relative risk and 95 percent confidence interval for all contributing trials. BP = blood pressure; CI = confidence interval; DBP = diastolic blood pressure; SBP = systolic blood pressure; TIA = transient ischemic attack. *(From Lawes CM, Bennett DA, Feigin FL, Rodgers A: Blood pressure and stroke: An overview of published reviews. Stroke 35:1024, 2004.)*

CH 58

Prevention and Management of Stroke

MANAGEMENT OF ACUTE ISCHEMIC STROKE

As with acute coronary syndromes, time is of the essence in the treatment of patients with acute ischemic stroke. Stroke has a large variety of etiological causes and potential pathophysiological mechanisms that can be critical for the rational use of secondary preventive therapies, some of which were reviewed in the preceding sections. A variety of conditions may cause symptoms and signs that can be mistaken for those of a stroke. In the period immediately following the onset of ischemic symptoms, however, evaluation is aimed at determining whether the patient may be a candidate for reperfusion therapy.

Intravenous rt-PA

Intravenous rt-PA is currently the only specific treatment for acute ischemic stroke that has received approval from the FDA. The treatment is aimed at lysis of a clot occluding a cerebral artery. On the basis of the pivotal NIH-sponsored randomized clinical trial, treatment of appropriate patients is associated with an approximate 13 percent absolute (32 percent relative) increase in the proportion of patients free of disability 3 months later.[5] Benefits are similar for patients with small-penetrating artery distribution ischemic stroke and for those with occlusion of larger intracranial arteries. Although treatment is also associated with an increase in the risk of hemorrhage (6.4 percent risk of symptomatic intracerebral hemorrhage with treatment versus 0.6 percent with placebo, 2.9 percent risk of fatal hemorrhage versus 0.3 percent with placebo), the overall benefit includes these adverse events. The drug must be given within 3 hours of the onset of symptoms, which means that the patient must generally arrive at a properly equipped and organized hospital within 2 hours of symptom onset to have the necessary evaluations (including brain computed tomography [CT] scan to exclude hemorrhage or other conditions) completed. Within the 3-hour window, the sooner that treatment can be given, the greater the likelihood of a favorable response.[27] To use the drug safely, a strict protocol needs to be closely followed and patients carefully selected (Table 58-1).[5] Development of organized systems of stroke care have been advocated to rapidly perform the necessary clinical evaluations, minimize delays in treatment, make certain that other interventions associated with improved outcomes are followed, and assure that patients receive appropriate secondary prevention.[28]

Up to one third of patients may have early arterial reocclusion after intravenous thrombolysis.[5] One study has suggested that clot lysis might be assisted by concomitant exposure to ultrasound provided by transcranial Doppler,

1520

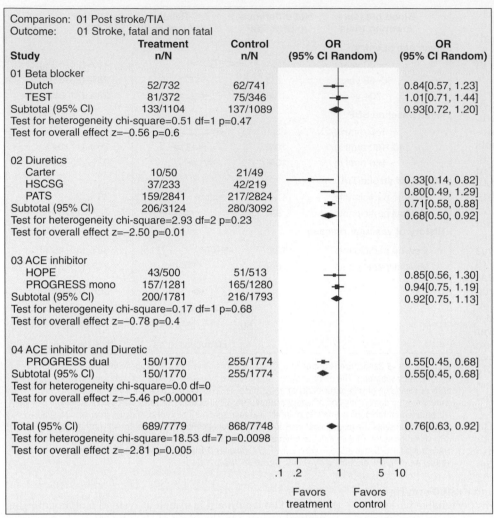

Comparison: 01 Post stroke/TIA				
Outcome: 01 Stroke, fatal and non fatal				
Study	Treatment n/N	Control n/N	OR (95% CI Random)	OR (95% CI Random)
01 Beta blocker				
Dutch	52/732	62/741		0.84[0.57, 1.23]
TEST	81/372	75/346		1.01[0.71, 1.44]
Subtotal (95% CI)	133/1104	137/1089		0.93[0.72, 1.20]
Test for heterogeneity chi-square=0.51 df=1 p=0.47				
Test for overall effect z=−0.56 p=0.6				
02 Diuretics				
Carter	10/50	21/49		0.33[0.14, 0.82]
HSCSG	37/233	42/219		0.80[0.49, 1.29]
PATS	159/2841	217/2824		0.71[0.58, 0.88]
Subtotal (95% CI)	206/3124	280/3092		0.68[0.50, 0.92]
Test for heterogeneity chi-square=2.93 df=2 p=0.23				
Test for overall effect z=−2.50 p=0.01				
03 ACE inhibitor				
HOPE	43/500	51/513		0.85[0.56, 1.30]
PROGRESS mono	157/1281	165/1280		0.94[0.75, 1.19]
Subtotal (95% CI)	200/1781	216/1793		0.92[0.75, 1.13]
Test for heterogeneity chi-square=0.17 df=1 p=0.68				
Test for overall effect z=−0.78 p=0.4				
04 ACE inhibitor and Diuretic				
PROGRESS dual	150/1770	255/1774		0.55[0.45, 0.68]
Subtotal (95% CI)	150/1770	255/1774		0.55[0.45, 0.68]
Test for heterogeneity chi-square=0.0 df=0				
Test for overall effect z=−5.46 p<0.00001				
Total (95% CI)	689/7779	868/7748		0.76[0.63, 0.92]
Test for heterogeneity chi-square=18.53 df=7 p=0.0098				
Test for overall effect z=−2.81 p=0.005				

.1 .2 1 5 10
Favors treatment / Favors control

FIGURE 58–6 Forrest plot of the effect of antihypertensive therapy in patients with prior stroke or transient ischemic attack on subsequent fatal and nonfatal stroke. ACE = angiotensin-converting enzyme; CI = confidence interval; Dutch = Dutch TIA Trial Study Group; HOPE = Heart Outcome Prevention Evaluation; HSCSG = Hypertension-Stroke Cooperative Study Group; PATS = Post-Stroke Antihypertensive Treatment Study; PROGRESS = Perindopril Protection Against Recurrent Stroke Study; TIA = transient ischemic attack. (*From Rashid P, Leonardi-Bee J, Bath P: Blood pressure reduction and secondary prevention of stroke and other vascular events: A systematic review. Stroke 34:2741, 2003.*)

CH 58

Endovascular Therapy

Catheter-based, endovascular approaches for acute reperfusion have the theoretical advantages of allowing for direct clot visualization and localized rather than systemic administration of thrombolytics, as well as the opportunity for mechanical clot disruption. However, no prospective randomized trials directly comparing endovascular therapy with intravenous rt-PA have occurred. In addition, endovascular therapy can only be accomplished in centers with immediate access to neurovascular interventionalists, is not generally feasible in patients with distal arterial occlusions, and might entail longer times to reperfusion (related to the need for access to an interventional suite, catheter placement time).

Prospective randomized data comparing intraarterial thrombolysis with nonthrombolytic medical therapy come primarily from a single clinical trial.[5] This study evaluated intraarterial thrombolysis with pro-urokinase in patients within 6 hours of angiographically proven proximal middle cerebral artery occlusion and found a significant improvement in 3-month outcome (40 percent of treated patients versus 25 percent of control patients had little or no disability), despite a trend toward an increase in symptomatic intracerebral hemorrhages (10 versus 2 percent, respectively). Pro-urokinase has not been approved by the FDA and is not currently available in the United States. Intraarterial rt-PA is commonly used for this purpose in patients who do not qualify for treatment with intravenous rt-PA (mostly commonly because of arriving at the hospital too late) and otherwise fulfill the inclusion criteria for the cited pro-urokinase trial. In addition to patients with middle cerebral artery occlusions up to 6 hours earlier, on the basis of case series data, selected patients with basilar artery occlusion up to 12 hours or longer may also be treated with this approach. Several ongoing studies are evaluating intraarterial thrombolysis with rt-PA, but the FDA has not yet approved this approach.

Mechanical clot retrieval has the theoretical advantage of avoiding the bleeding risk associated with thrombolytic drugs. The "MERCI" clot retriever was approved by the FDA for removal of blood clots from brain blood vessels (but not as a specific treatment for acute stroke). This approval was based on the results of an uncontrolled case series involving 151 enrolled (141 of whom could be treated) patients with proximal (internal carotid, middle cerebral, or vertebrobasilar) arterial occlusions within 6 hours (mean 4.3 hours to catheterization).[30] Recanalization was achieved in 48 percent of patients, 30 percent of whom died or had a second stroke or MI within 30 days. Approximately 30 percent died within 90 days, but 46 percent of those surviving at 90 days had little or no disability. Procedural complications occurred in 13 percent (6 arterial perforations, 4 arterial dissections, 3 cases of embolization to another artery, 3 subarachnoid hemorrhages, and 3 groin hematomas) with 28 percent having asymptomatic intracerebral hemorrhages and 8 percent symptomatic hemorrhages. The frequency of parenchymal hemorrhages might at first seem surprising; however, the arterial endothelium can be subject to ischemia-related damage and reperfusion of a damaged artery (with or without a thrombolytic) can lead to bleeding. This study had no concurrent controls, leaving open whether outcomes would be similar, better, or worse than with other reperfusion treatments. The approach has the same logistic limitations as endovascular thrombolytic therapy but does offer the possibility of treatment for selected patients who cannot be treated with a thrombolytic drug (e.g., patients already anticoagulated, having a recent operation or inva-

which can also be used to monitor clot dissolution.[29] A prospective trial is evaluating the usefulness of this approach.

TABLE 58–1	Characteristics of Patients with Ischemic Stroke Who Could Be Treated with r-tPA
Diagnosis of ischemic stroke causing measurable neurological deficit	
Neurological signs should not be clearing spontaneously	
Neurological signs should not be minor and isolated	
Caution should be exercised in treating a patient with major deficits	
Symptoms of stroke should not be suggestive of subarachnoid hemorrhage	
Onset of symptoms<3 hr before beginning treatment	
No head trauma or prior stroke in previous 3 mo	
No myocardial infarction in previous 3 mo	
No gastrointestinal or urinary tract hemorrhage in previous 21 days	
No major surgery in previous 14 days	
No arterial puncture at a noncompressible site in previous 7 days	
No history of previous intracranial hemorrhage	
Blood pressure not elevated (systolic > 185 mm Hg or diastolic > 110 mm Hg)	
No evidence of active bleeding or acute trauma (fracture) on examination	
Not taking an oral anticoagulant or if anticoagulant being taken, INR < 1.7	
If receiving heparin in previous 48 hr, aPTT must be in normal range	
Platelet count > 100,000 mm3	
Blood glucose concentration > 50 mg/dl (2.7 mmol/liter)	
No seizure with postictal residual neurological impairments	
CT does not show a multilobar infarction (hypodensity $^1/_3$ cerebral hemisphere)	
The patient or family understand the potential risks and benefits from treatment	

INR=international normalized ratio.
From Adams HP, Adams R, Del Zoppo G, Goldstein LB: Guidelines for the early management of patients with ischemic stroke: 2005 guidelines update. A scientific statement from the Stroke Council of the American Heart Association/American Stroke Association. Stroke 36:916, 2005.

sive procedure, or having an embolus complicating cardiac or other catheterization after the catheter sheath has been removed).

Other Measures for Stroke Treatment

Several other important questions often arise in the management of patients with acute ischemic stroke and other interventions that are generally used even without definitive supporting data.

Anticoagulation and Platelet Antiaggregant Therapy

The indications for acute anticoagulation of patients with ischemic stroke are extremely limited. The most recent American Heart Association/American Academy of Neurology guidelines reflect this view and specifically indicate that emergent anticoagulation with the goal of improving neurological outcomes or preventing early recurrent stroke is not recommended for the treatment of patients with acute ischemic stroke, that urgent anticoagulation is not recommended for treatment of patients with moderate-to-severe stroke because of a high risk of intracranial bleeding com-

plications, and that initiation of anticoagulant therapy within 24 hours of treatment with intravenously administered rt-PA is not recommended.[31] Patients with atrial fibrillation–associated stroke benefit from long-term anticoagulation unless contraindicated because of high bleeding risk (e.g., prior intracerebral hemorrhage, falls). The risk of early recurrence in patients with stroke related to atrial fibrillation is generally low (≈0.3 to 0.5 percent per day for the first 2 weeks), so the timing of the initiation of anticoagulation needs to be balanced against the risk of bleeding. Those with large strokes and those with uncontrolled hypertension are generally at highest risk of spontaneous hemorrhagic transformation of an ischemic stroke.

The use of anticoagulants in patients with stroke related to infective endocarditis is problematic. Systemic embolization occurs in 22 to 50 percent of patients with infective endocarditis with up to 65 percent of emboli affecting the central nervous system, the majority of which (90 percent) involve the middle cerebral artery.[32] No benefit for anticoagulation in patients with native valve endocarditis has been demonstrated, and it is generally not recommended for at least the first 2 weeks of antibiotic therapy in patients with stroke related to Staphylococcus aureus prosthetic valve endocarditis.[32] Of particular concern is the possible development of mycotic intracranial aneurysms. These are often multiple and can be either asymptomatic, associated with focal neurological signs, or, because they most commonly affect distal branches of the middle cerebral artery, associated with signs and symptoms of subarachnoid hemorrhage or a sterile meningitis.[32] Although CT angiography (in patients without renal insufficiency) or magnetic resonance angiography can be useful screening tests in patients with symptoms suggesting the presence of a mycotic aneurysm, because distal portions of the artery are most commonly affected, catheter angiography is the gold standard for the detection of these lesions (distal portions of the middle cerebral artery can be difficult to visualize on CT or magnetic resonance angiography). The management of patients with intracranial mycotic aneurysms is complex, with many regressing with antibiotic treatment. Depending on a variety of factors, surgical clipping or endovascular obliteration can also be considered. Anticoagulation is generally avoided in patients with known mycotic aneurysms because of their propensity to rupture.

As reflected earlier, the use of platelet antiaggregants reduces the risk of recurrent stroke in patients with a history of ischemic stroke or TIA. In the acute setting, there may be benefit from treatment with aspirin begun within 48 hours of acute ischemic stroke (antiplatelet drugs are prohibited for the first 24 hours in patients treated with intravenous rt-PA). A combined analysis of two relevant trials found that treatment with aspirin (160 mg to 325 mg daily) was associated with a small but statistically significant reduction of 9 (±3) fewer deaths or nonfatal strokes per 1000 treated patients.[31] No data have shown a benefit of any other platelet antiaggregant, given either alone or in combination, in the setting of acute ischemic stroke.

Blood Pressure Management

Management of blood pressure in the setting of acute ischemic stroke remains largely empirical.[5] Treatment of elevated blood pressure in patients who might otherwise be candidates for intravenous rt-PA differs from that of patients who are not thrombolytic candidates and follows a specific protocol.[5] Relatively aggressive treatment for elevated blood pressure is used in patients who have been treated with a thrombolytic because of an increased risk of bleeding complications associated with uncontrolled hypertension.

Several lines of evidence suggest cautious blood pressure management in non–thrombolytic-treated patients with

1522 acute ischemic stroke who do not have malignant hypertension (i.e., in patients who do not have hypertensive encephalopathy, aortic dissection, acute renal failure, acute pulmonary edema, acute MI, or blood pressures > 220/120 mm Hg).[5] Cerebral autoregulation maintains cerebral blood flow (CBF) constant despite fluctuations in systemic blood pressure. CBF is determined by the cerebral perfusion pressure (generally the mean arterial pressure, MAP) divided by cerebrovascular resistance (CVR).[33] As reflected by this relationship, decreases in MAP lead to dilation of cerebral arterioles (decreased CVR), thereby keeping CBF constant. The local acidosis that accompanies brain ischemia leads to maximal vasodilation. As a result, decreases in MAP are directly reflected in changes in local CBF (if CVR remains constant). Therefore lowering blood pressure may further compromise already ischemic brain, potentially increasing the size of the stroke. If treatment is necessary, precipitous drops should be avoided.

Stroke after Percutaneous Coronary Interventions and Thrombolytic Treatment for Myocardial Infarction

Although occurring infrequently, stroke can be a major complication of percutaneous coronary intervention (PCI). The same principles outlined for management of acute stroke in other settings are applicable. If neurological symptoms are recognized while the catheter sheath is still in place, the patient might be treated with intravenous rt-PA, provided that all of the other inclusion criteria are met and there are no other contraindications to the therapy. If symptoms are first noted after the catheter sheath has been removed, then the patient could be evaluated for catheter-based, endovascular treatment. Having a system in place is important to assure that patients having a stroke after PCI can be rapidly evaluated and treated.

Intracerebral hemorrhage following thrombolytic administration for acute MI is another serious treatment-related complication. The infusion should be stopped and heparin discontinued for any patient developing acute neurological symptoms. Because these symptoms might be due to either hemorrhage or ischemia, a brain imaging study is mandatory before proceeding with further treatment. Treatments to reduce the amount of thrombolytic-associated intracerebral hemorrhage once it has occurred are not well established. The administration of cryoprecipitate and/or fresh frozen plasma has been advocated. Those with brainstem compression related to cerebellar hemorrhage may benefit from surgical evacuation of the hematoma. Patients should be transferred to a setting with expertise in neurological intensive care as soon as feasible.

REFERENCES

CH 58

General Considerations and Guidelines for Stroke Prevention and Treatment

1. American Heart Association: Heart disease and stroke statistics—2006 update. Circulation 113:e85, 2006.
2. Goldstein LB, Adams R, Alberts MJ, et al: Primary prevention of ischemic stroke: A guideline from the American Heart Association/American Stroke Association Stroke Council. Stroke 37:1583, 2006.
3. Sacco RL, Adams R, Albers G, et al: Guidelines for prevention of stroke in patients with ischemic stroke or transient ischemic attack. A statement for healthcare professionals from the American Heart Association/American Stroke Association Council on Stroke. Stroke 37:577, 2006.
4. Adams HP, Adams RJ, Brott T, et al: Guidelines for the early management of patients with ischemic stroke: A scientific statement from the Stroke Council of the American Stroke Association. Stroke 34:1056, 2003.
5. Adams HP, Adams R, Del Zoppo G, Goldstein LB: Guidelines for the early management of patients with ischemic stroke: 2005 guidelines update. A scientific statement from the Stroke Council of the American Heart Association/American Stroke Association. Stroke 36:916, 2005.

Antiplatelet and Anticoagulant Strategies

6. Ridker PM, Cook NR, Lee I-M, et al: A randomized trial of low-dose aspirin in the primary prevention of cardiovascular disease in women. N Engl J Med 352:1293, 2005.
7. Esprit Study Group, Halkes PH, van Gijn J, et al: Aspirin plus dipyridamole versus aspirin alone after cerebral ischaemia of arterial origin (ESPRIT): Randomised controlled trial. Lancet 367:1665, 2006.
8. Bhatt DL, Fox KA, Hacke W, et al: Clopidogrel and aspirin versus aspirin alone for the prevention of atherothrombotic events. N Engl J Med 354:1706, 2006.
9. Diener H-C, Bogousslavsky J, Brass LM, et al: Aspirin and clopidogrel compared with clopidogrel alone after recent ischaemic stroke or transient ischaemic attack in high-risk patients (MATCH): Randomised, double-blind, placebo-controlled trial. Lancet 364:331, 2004.
10. Mohr JP, Thompson JLP, Lazar RM, et al: A comparison of warfarin and aspirin for the prevention of recurrent ischemic stroke. N Engl J Med 345:1444, 2001.
11. Chimowitz MI, Kokkinos J, Strong J, et al: The Warfarin-Aspirin Symptomatic Intracranial Disease study. Neurology 45:1488, 1995.
12. Chimowitz MI, Lynn MJ, Howlett-Smith H, et al: Comparison of warfarin and aspirin for symptomatic intracranial arterial stenosis. N Engl J Med 352:1305, 2005.
13. Messé SR, Silverman IE, Kizer JR, et al: Practice parameter: Recurrent stroke with patent foramen ovale and atrial septal aneurysm—Report of the Quality Standards Subcommittee of the American Academy of Neurology. Neurology 62:1042, 2004.
14. Homma S, Sacco RL, Di Tullio MR, et al: Effect of medical treatment in stroke patients with patent foramen ovale: Patent Foramen Ovale in Cryptogenic Stroke Study. Circulation 105:2625, 2002.
15. Levine SR, Brey RL, Tilley BC, et al: Antiphospholipid antibodies and subsequent thrombo-occlusive events in patients with ischemic stroke. JAMA 291:576, 2004.
16. Cramer SC, Rordorf G, Maki JH, et al: Increased pelvic vein thrombi in cryptogenic stroke—Results of the Paradoxical Emboli from Large Veins in Ischemic Stroke (PELVIS) study. Stroke 35:46, 2004.

Lipid Therapy and Stroke

17. Amarenco P, Labreuche J, Lavallee P, Touboul PJ: Statins in stroke prevention and carotid atherosclerosis. Systematic review and up-to-date meta-analysis. Stroke 35:2902, 2004.
18. Heart Protection Study Collaborative Group: MRC/BHF Heart Protection Study of cholesterol-lowering with simvastatin in 5963 people with diabetes: A randomized placebo-controlled trial. Lancet 361:2005, 2003.
19. Colhoun HM, Betteridge DJ, Durrington PN, et al: Primary prevention of cardiovascular disease with atorvastatin in type 2 diabetes in the Collaborative Atorvastatin Diabetes Study (CARDS): Multicentre randomised placebo-controlled trial. Lancet 364:685, 2004.
20. Sever PS, Dahlof B, Poulter NR, et al: Prevention of coronary and stroke events with atorvastatin in hypertensive patients who have average or lower-than-average cholesterol concentrations, in the Anglo-Scandinavian Cardiac Outcomes Trial—Lipid Lowering Arm (ASCOT-LLA): A multicentre randomised controlled trial. Lancet 361:1149, 2003.
21. Shepherd J, Blauw GJ, Murphy MB, et al: Pravastatin in elderly individuals at risk of vascular disease (PROSPER): A randomised controlled trial. Lancet 360:1623, 2002.
22. Heart Protection Study Collaborative Group: Effects of cholesterol-lowering with simvastatin on stroke and other major vascular events in 20,536 people with cerebrovascular disease or other high-risk conditions. Lancet 363:757, 2004.
23. Amarenco P, Bogousslavsky K, Callahan A III, et al: High dose atorvastatin after stroke or transient ischemic attack. N Engl J Med 355:549, 2006.

Blood Pressure Treatment and Other Interventions

24. Chobanian AV, Bakris GL, Black HR, et al: The Seventh Report of the Joint National Committee on Prevention, Detection, Evaluation, and Treatment of High Blood Pressure: The JNC 7 Report. JAMA 289:2560, 2003.
25. Lawes CMM, Bennett DA, Feigin VL, Rodgers A: Blood pressure and stroke. An overview of published reviews. Stroke 35:776, 2004.
26. Rashid P, Leonardi-Bee J, Bath P: Blood pressure reduction and secondary prevention of stroke and other vascular events—A systematic review. Stroke 34:2741, 2003.
27. Hacke W, Donnan G, Fieschi C, et al: Association of outcome with early stroke treatment: Pooled analysis of ATLANTIS, ECASS, and NINDS rt-PA stroke trials. Lancet 363:768, 2004.
28. Schwamm LH, Pancioli A, Acker JE III, et al: Recommendations for the establishment of stroke systems of care: Recommendations from the American Stroke Association's Task Force on the Development of Stroke Systems. Circulation 111:1078, 2005.
29. Alexandrov AV, Molina CA, Grotta JC, et al: Ultrasound-enhanced systemic thrombolysis for acute ischemic stroke. N Engl J Med 351:2170, 2004.
30. Smith WS, Sung G, Starkman S, et al: Safety and efficacy of mechanical embolectomy in acute ischemic stroke: Results of the MERCI trial. Stroke 36:1432, 2005.
31. Coull BM, Williams LS, Goldstein LB, et al: Anticoagulants and antiplatelet agents in acute ischemic stroke. Report of the Joint Stroke Guideline Development Committee of the American Academy of Neurology and the American Stroke Association. Neurology 59:13, 2002.
32. Baddour LM, Wilson WR, Bayer AS, et al: Infective endocarditis: Diagnosis, antimicrobial therapy, and management of complications. Circulation 111:e394, 2005.
33. Goldstein LB: Blood pressure management in patients with acute ischemic stroke. Hypertension 43:137, 2004.

CHAPTER 59

Atherosclerotic Peripheral Artery Disease, 1523
Atherosclerotic Lower Extremity Disease, 1523
Atherosclerotic Renal Artery Disease, 1532
Chronic Mesenteric Ischemia, 1535
Brachiocephalic and Subclavian Obstructive Disease, 1536
Carotid and Vertebral Disease, 1538

Obstructive Venous Disease, 1542
Lower Extremity Deep Venous Thrombosis, 1542
Central Venous Obstruction, 1543

Conclusion, 1544

References, 1544

Endovascular Treatment of Noncoronary Obstructive Vascular Disease

Andrew C. Eisenhauer and Christopher J. White

Noncoronary peripheral vascular disease encompasses a very broad range of arterial, venous, and lymphatic diseases. This chapter will focus on percutaneous, catheter-based, endovascular treatment of atherosclerotic peripheral arterial disease (upper and lower extremities, aortic arch vessels, renal, mesenteric, carotid, and vertebral arteries) and venous disease. Atherosclerotic peripheral arterial disease (PAD) is increasingly being recognized for its high prevalence and clinical importance (see Chap. 57). As the population ages, the number of people with symptomatic and asymptomatic PAD increases. Physicians and patients alike are developing more awareness of the ramifications of PAD, including its associated morbidity and increased risk of mortality. Revascularization strategies are shifting from open surgery to percutaneous, or endovascular, procedures. Percutaneous transluminal angioplasty (PTA) was initially developed as treatment for PAD. Recent improvements in technology have generally led to better and more reliable clinical results. These advances in technology have combined with patient demand for less invasive therapies and revolutionized revascularization therapies for PAD. The widespread availability of high-resolution noninvasive diagnostic imaging, capable of accurately identifying pathology and identifying arterial obstructions that are amenable to less invasive treatment, has further lowered the threshold for recommending percutaneous therapies for symptomatic PAD.

Although historically the primary method of revascularization therapy for PAD involved surgery, percutaneous catheter-based or endovascular therapies now provide patients with a less invasive and equally effective modality for the treatment of atheromatous disease in almost all vascular territories. Catheter-based interventions have assumed importance as treatment for lower and upper extremity, renal, mesenteric, cervical, and cerebral ischemia. Effective therapies for arterial aneurysmal disease and venous conditions are currently available and offer advantages over surgical treatments. The American College of Cardiology and American Heart Association updated guidelines and recommendations for the diagnosis and treatment of atherosclerotic peripheral arterial disease have been published.[1] To provide optimal therapy, clinicians must be knowledgeable about the specific disease state being managed and aware of the full range of treatment options. In complicated cases, the patient will benefit from the input of multiple vascular-related specialties.

ATHEROSCLEROTIC PERIPHERAL ARTERY DISEASE

Atherosclerotic Lower Extremity Disease

Lower extremity intermittent claudication is caused by stenosis or occlusion of the iliac, femoral-popliteal, or tibioperoneal vessels (see Chap. 57). Claudication is an exertion-related discomfort affecting specific muscle groups and is relieved with rest. Symptoms affect the muscle groups below the level of the arterial narrowing. For example, vascular blockages (occlusions or stenoses) of the iliac vessels typically cause hip, thigh, and calf pain, whereas femoral and popliteal artery obstructions cause symptoms in the calf and foot muscles. Patients with typical symptoms of intermittent claudication represent fewer than 20 percent of patients with objective evidence of PAD. The clinician must distinguish pseudoclaudication (discomfort from spinal stenosis, compartment syndromes, venous congestion, or arthritis) from claudication (Table 59-1).[2]

The initial therapy for patients with claudication should be atherosclerosis risk factor modification, antiplatelet therapy, and supervised exercise training (see Chap. 57). Because it is uncommon for patients with claudication to progress to limb-threatening ischemia, revascularization is reserved for those patients who have failed a trial of medical therapy or those with life style–limiting symptoms and favorable anatomy for revascularization. Patients with more advanced disease, such as vocation-limiting claudication or limb-threatening ischemia (rest pain, nonhealing ulcers, or gangrene) require a more aggressive approach and are considered candidates for revascularization.

The goal of therapy for patients with claudication is relief of symptoms, resulting in an increased walking distance and improvement in their quality of life. Strategically, for those with claudication, a durable revascularization solution is important, because symptoms will likely return if restenosis occurs. This is in contrast to patients with limb-threatening ischemia, in whom the goal of therapy is limb salvage. The best treatment option will offer a high success rate for restoration of pulsatile flow to the distal limb with a low procedural morbidity. Less blood flow is required to maintain tissue integrity than to heal a wound; restenosis will generally not result in recurrent limb-threatening ischemia without a subsequent reinjury to the limb. For the clinician caring for patients with lower extremity

TABLE 59–1 | **Intermittent Claudication versus Pseudoclaudication**

Parameter	Intermittent Claudication	Pseudoclaudication
Character of discomfort	Cramping, tightness, or tiredness	Same or tingling, weakness, clumsiness
Location of discomfort	Buttock, hip, thigh, calf, foot	Same
Exercise induced	Yes	Yes or no
Distance to claudication	Same each time	Variable
Occurs with standing	No	Yes
Relief	Stop walking	Often must sit or change body position

Modified from Krajewski LP, Olin J: Atherosclerosis of the aorta and the lower extremities. *In* Young JR (ed): Peripheral Vascular Diseases. Chicago, Mosby–Year Book, 1991, p. 183.

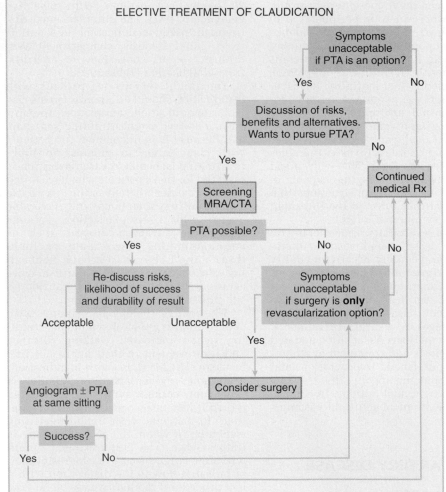

FIGURE 59–1 A strategy for aggressive treatment of claudication. The strategy is based on assessment of symptoms and frank discussion with patients about the risks and benefits of available therapies. Currently, noninvasive diagnostic imaging is used not to make a diagnosis but to ascertain the anatomical suitability for intervention and to assess the patient's procedural risk profile. CTA = computed tomography angiography; MRA = magnetic resonance angiography; PTA = percutaneous transluminal angioplasty; Rx = treatment. See also Figure 57-19 for a management scheme for life-style limiting claudication.

vascular disease, it is important to weigh improvement in functional capacity and quality of life, as well as long-term results, when considering revascularization therapy.

Basic noninvasive testing includes the ankle-brachial index (ABI). Pulse volume recordings with segmental Doppler pressures are helpful in confirming the presence of obstructive disease and estimating its level and severity (see Chap. 57). In general, lower extremity angiography is reserved for patients who meet criteria for revascularization, if suitable anatomy is found. Recent advances in axial imaging techniques (both magnetic resonance angiography, MRA, and computed tomography angiography, CTA) enable remarkable noninvasive definition of the vascular anatomy. These noninvasive angiograms will largely replace invasive diagnostic angiography as the technology advances; studies are now frequently obtained to confirm the diagnosis and help formulate a strategy and approach to revascularization. Invasive angiography is reserved for those situations in which the results from noninvasive imaging are ambiguous. For critical limb ischemia, anatomical definition is required in almost all cases to plan therapy. In the case of claudication, imaging should be performed as outlined in Figure 59-1.

The probability of clinical success and the technical approach to percutaneous revascularization will vary according to anatomic site. These aspects are best considered separately for aortoiliac, femoropopliteal, and tibioperoneal segments.

Aortoiliac Obstructive Disease

BACKGROUND. Ischemia-producing lesions (stenosis or occlusion) of the aorta and iliac vessels are most commonly atherosclerotic in origin and treatment for both sites, typically labeled "inflow vessels" to the leg, is similar. Lower extremity vascular disease frequently involves multiple levels. Patients with aortoiliac occlusive disease will often also have femoral and/or tibial disease. In patients with claudication and multilevel disease, correction of any hemodynamically significant inflow lesions may be undertaken as the first stage in revascularization. Aortoiliac revascularization will often result in symptomatic improvement by increasing inflow to the limb and thus collateral blood flow to the distal extremity.

The preferred mode of revascularization of the aortoiliac vessels has shifted from predominantly surgical to almost completely catheter-based percutaneous therapies. This change is based on the less invasive nature of PTA and the excellent rate of clinical success, which now rivals that of surgical bypass in many patients.[3] Furthermore, the primary use of stents, as opposed to balloon angioplasty alone, has become the clinical standard of care in aortoiliac vessels.

TREATMENT. Because experience has suggested that when excellent angiographic and hemodynamic results are obtained from PTA alone, patency and clinical success rates at 2 years are similar to those of stent placement, some interventionalists favor a strategy of provisional stenting, wherein stents are reserved for cases of failed balloon angioplasty. However, even with this strategy many, if not most, patients ultimately receive stents. An important meta-analysis of trials published after 1990 has suggested that both the immediate success rate (96 versus 91 percent) and the 4-year patency (77 versus 65 percent) are superior for stents versus PTA alone.[4] Longer lesions, diffuse disease, and occlusions, in particular, will benefit from primary stenting. The current guidelines recommend primary stent placement in the iliac arteries.[1] Limited or compromised runoff seems to predict higher failure rates.[5] For the subset of patients with stenotic or occlusive disease that involves the terminal aorta and compromises the origins of the common iliac arteries, the preferred therapy is placement of "kissing" balloon-expandable stents (Fig. 59-2).

Finally, with regard to the composition of the stent selected, current data suggest no advantage for self-expanding nitinol over stainless steel.[6] Balloon-expandable stents offer stronger radial force and more precise placement, whereas self-expanding stents offer flexible diameters that accommodate a tapering and sometimes tortuous vessel.

The most serious complications of endovascular aortoiliac repair remain distal embolization, with rates ranging from 4 to 7 percent,[7] and arterial perforation or rupture, which is rare. Covered stents, or stent grafts, are available for treating vessel rupture. Based on these improved outcomes, percutaneous treatment is generally attempted for short occlusions and for longer iliac stenosis or occlusions that are technically suitable (Figs. 59-3 and 59-4). Total occlusions of the abdominal aorta are more often treated surgically, although thrombolysis followed by PTA remains an option.

In summary, primary stent placement represents appropriate first-line therapy for aortoiliac obstructive disease. Stent placement offers high procedural success and durability similar to that of surgical reconstruction, with less risk and at reduced cost. In the small percentage of patients in whom patency cannot be maintained, surgery remains a feasible option. The availability of these effective, less invasive techniques has lowered the threshold at which intervention can be offered to patients with aortoiliac disease who are disabled by claudication or limb ischemia (Table 59-2).

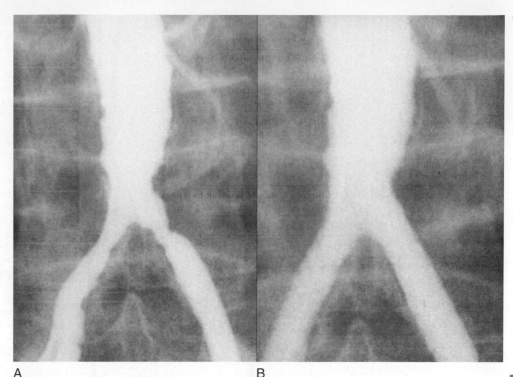

A   **B**

FIGURE 59–2 A, Baseline angiogram with bifurcation stenosis of the terminal aorta and common iliac arteries. **B,** Final angiogram after placement of "kissing" balloon-expandable stents.

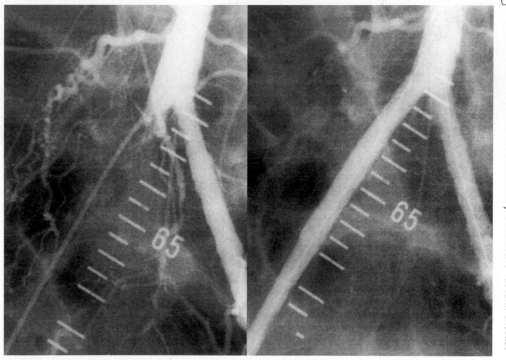

A   **B**

FIGURE 59–3 A, Occlusion of right common iliac artery. **B,** Recanalization and stent placement of right common iliac artery.

Femoropopliteal Obstructive Disease

BACKGROUND. Prior experience has shown little difference between the results of endovascular therapy for the superficial femoral artery (SFA) and popliteal artery. Accordingly, these two vessels are traditionally considered together with respect to indications and results. The SFA, particu-

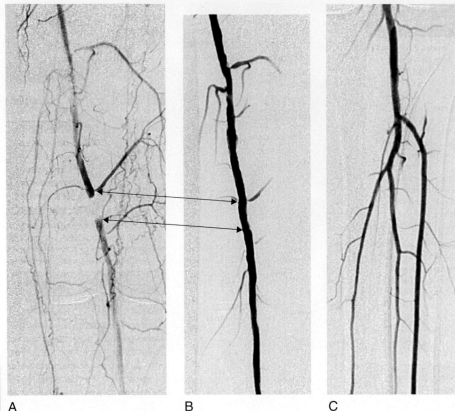

FIGURE 59–4 Result of recanalization and balloon dilation of a short-segment femoropopliteal occlusion. In **A,** a digital subtraction angiogram illustrates the area of total occlusion and compares it with that in **B,** showing the results of balloon dilation only. Both areas are indicated by the double-ended black arrows. **C,** An intact three-vessel runoff without evidence of distal embolization.

larly within the adductor canal of the thigh, has a propensity to accumulate atherosclerotic plaque. Whether this is caused by the physical stresses and flow patterns specific to this vessel (low-flow vessel, high-resistance bed), the presence of a natural collateral (the profunda femoris artery) or other factors yet to be defined is unknown. Currently, procedural success for femoropopliteal recanalization exceeds 90 percent. The advent of hydrophilic guidewires and catheters has greatly enhanced the ability to traverse femoropopliteal occlusions, which now can be successfully treated in 80 to 90 percent of cases.

Whereas hydrophilic wires and other technological advances have improved acute success, the rate of restenosis remains more than twofold that for iliac disease and far exceeds what would be expected considering the size of the SFA (mean lumen diameter, 5 to 6 mm). Various adjunct technologies have been used in an attempt to improve long-term patency. Cryotherapy, cutting balloons, and debulking devices, such as directional atherectomy, excimer laser, and rotational atherectomy, although sometimes providing a better immediate anigographic result, have not demonstrated a reduction in restenosis in any controlled comparative trials.

TREATMENT. Multiple small trials failed to demonstrate an advantage for stent placement over PTA in the femo-

TABLE 59–2		Results of Iliac Artery Stent Placement*									
Lead Author	Year	No. of Patients	Lesions Treated	No. of Patients with Occlusions (%)	Technical Success (%)	Ankle-Brachial Index Before	Ankle-Brachial Index After	Mean Lesion Length (cm)	Stent Used	Primary Patency at 2 Years (%)	Cumulative Patency at 2 Years (%)
Reyes[86]	1997	59	61	100	92	0.51	0.9	10	SES	73	88
Dyet[87]	1997	72	72	100	93	NA	NA	6.7	BES, SES	85	85
Murphy[88]	1998	65	90	31	97	0.62	0.9	5.6	BES, SES	69	80
Tetteroo[89]	1998	143	187	9	NA	0.78	NA	NA	BES	NA	71.3
Powell[90]	2000	87	210	NA	97	0.56	0.75	NA	Various	43	72
Saha[91]	2001	50	61	4	97	NA	NA	NA	BES, SES	97	100
Timaran[92]	2001	189	247	NA	97	NA	NA	NA	BES, SES	NA	—
Haulon[93]	2002	106	212	NA	100	NA	NA	NA	BES/SES	79.4	97.7
Siskin[94]	2002	42	59	8.5	95	0.68	0.99	NA	BES/SES	72	88
Mohamed[95]	2002	24	48	42	100	NA	NA	5.2	BES/SES	58	84
Reekers[96]	2002	126	143	10	100	0.67	0.92	3.3	BES	84[†]	89[†]
Funovics[97]	2002	78	94	100	96	NA	NA	6.2	Various	74.5	88.8

*Historical and contemporary results of iliac artery stent placement. The difficulty in interpreting the reports in literature is that these reports of experience include patients with widely varying degrees of disease and incorporate a variety of stent types and techniques. Nevertheless, cumulative 2-year patency is approximately 90% in most series.

†At 12 months.

BES = balloon-expandable stainless steel; SES = self-expanding stainless steel; SEN = self-expanding nitinol; SESG = self-expanding stent graft; NA = not assessed or reported.

ropopliteal vessels until a meta-analysis demonstrated that stents had superior patency at 3 years, compared with PTA, in patients with the most severe lesions—that is, those with critical limb ischemia and occlusions.[8] There is now good clinical evidence from a randomized trial that a strategy of primary stent placement in the femoropopliteal vessels yields superior patency rates and functional outcomes compared with provisional stent placement (placement of stents for failed PTA).[9] Restenosis at 1 year was reduced from 63 percent in the PTA group to 37 percent in the stent arm. Functionally, both the walking distance and ABI were significantly increased in the stent arm compared with the PTA group. These benefits accrued even though 32 percent of the PTA group crossed over and received a stent after a suboptimal balloon angioplasty result.

The use of endovascular approaches to recanalize and stent diffuse femoropopliteal disease is reemerging (Figs. 59-5 to 59-7; see Fig. 59-4). With the dramatic reduction of restenosis with drug-eluting coronary stents, there has been a strong interest in the development of stent coatings such as sirolimus for lower extremity stents. In a randomized series of long-segment SFA disease patients, the results for those receiving sirolimus-coated nitinol self-expanding stents

were no different from those in the bare metal stent control group.[10] One concern raised in this trial was a high incidence of stent fractures, which appeared to be related to restenosis.[11] So far, the results have not been encouraging, but this work remains in its preliminary stages (Table 59-3).

When weighing the risks and benefits for invasive therapy, each patient and lesion requires individual consideration. When comparing medical therapy with revascularization, quality of life measures for treatment of claudication have shown that PTA is more effective than exercise alone, with a cost-effectiveness ratio within the acceptable range.[12] If one compares surgery with PTA in patients with claudication, remembering that late patency is the key to long-term symptom relief, it has been estimated that as long as the 5-year patency rate for PTA is more than 30 percent, PTA will always be the preferred strategy.[13]

The preference for an endovascular "first" approach has also been demonstrated for patients with critical limb ischemia and femoropopliteal vascular disease.[14] In a large (N = 452) randomized trial, a surgery-first strategy was compared with PTA-first strategy with follow-up over 5 years. PTA and surgery resulted in similar outcomes for amputation-free survival and PTA was less expensive,

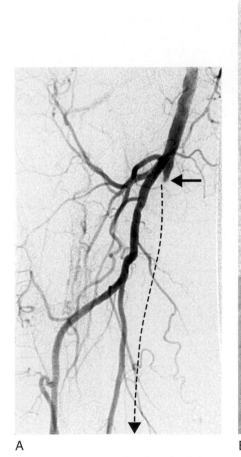
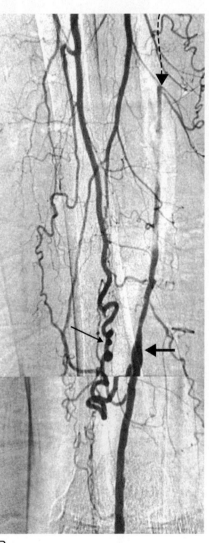
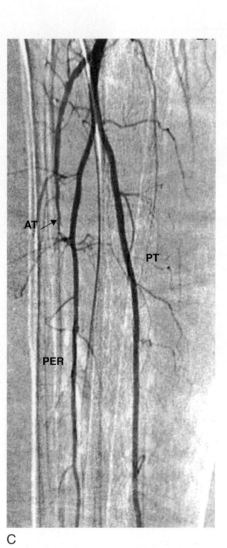

A   B   C

FIGURE 59–5 Long-segment chronic total occlusion. In contrast to the short-segment disease in Figure 59-4, this requires recanalization from the origin of the superficial femoral artery (SFA) (**A,** solid arrow) along the path of the SFA (dashed arrow) continuing to the level of the most significant collateral inflow and reconstitution of the vessel (**B**). **C,** Crural vessels, demonstrating occlusion of the anterior tibial (AT) with patent peroneal (PER) and posterior tibial (PT) runoff.

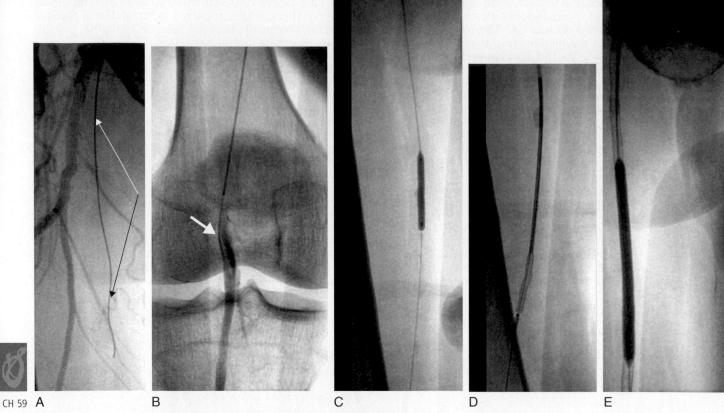

A **B** **C** **D** **E**

FIGURE 59–6 A, Recanalization of the lesion in Figure 59-5 was accomplished from the contralateral approach using a hydrophilic guidewire advanced into the occluded segment (arrows). **B,** Once the guidewire is free in the distal vessel, a small catheter is passed over the wire and a contrast agent injection is made to confirm the intravascular position (arrow). This is followed by predilation **(C),** self-expanding stent placement from distal to proximal **(D)** and, finally, postdilation to the appropriate size **(E).**

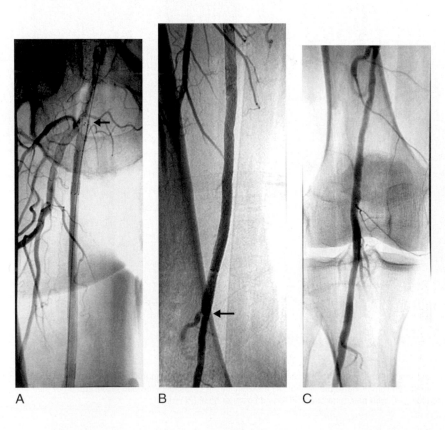

A **B** **C**

FIGURE 59–7 Recanalization of this long-segment occlusion and stenting from the origin of the superficial femoral artery (SFA) in **A** (arrow) to the level of collateral reconstitution in **B** (arrow) resulted in reconstitution of the normal distal anatomy **(C),** and return of pedal pulses, and healing of digital ulcers. Care was taken to preserve the collateral vessel ostia so that, in the event of restenosis, collateral pathways are present. This anatomy should be contrasted with total occlusion of the SFA (but short-segment disease) shown in Figure 59-4. These cases illustrate the anatomical variations that commonly occur and emphasize the difficulty in characterizing the true extent of disease in patients with total occlusions of this vessel.

TABLE 59–3 | Results of Femoropopliteal Interventions*

Lead Author	Year	No. of Patients	Lesions Treated	No. with Occlusions (%)	Technical Success (%)	Ankle-Brachial Index Before	Ankle-Brachial Index After	Mean Lesion Length (cm)	Devices Used Primarily	Primary Success (%)†	Cumulative Duration (mo)	Success (%)†	Duration (mo)
Gray[98]	1997	55	58	NA	NA	0.48	0.71	16.5	SES, BES	22	24	46	24
Martin[99]	1999	68	NA	6	100	NA	NA	NA	PTA	NA	–	57	24
Kessel[100]	1999	20	NA	–	95	0.6	1	17	SG	29	12	64	12
Conroy[101]	2000	48	61	100	100	NA	NA¶	13.5	SES, BES	47	12	79	12
Cheng[102]	2001	55	69	NA	92	NA	NA	13.8	SES, BES	53.8	24	72.1	24
Gordon[103]	2001	57	71	100	NA	0.59	0.86	14.4	SES	38.2	24	76.2	24
Scheinert[104]	2001	318	411	100	83	0.62	NA	19.4	LPTA, SEN	33.6†	12	75.9	12
Lofberg[105]	2001	92	121	47	88	NA	NA	NA	PTA	27	60	34	60
Bauermeister[106]	2001	35	NA	100	100	0.25	0.87	22	SG§	73.2	12	82.6	12
Duda[107]	2002	36	36	57	100	NA	NA	8.5	DEN/SEN	100/77	6	NA	–
Steinkamp[108]	2002	312	312	100	91.7	0.56	0.88	7.5	LPTA, SEN	61.5	24	90.2	24
Gray[109]	2002	23	NA	84	88	0.54	0.84	6.2	LPTA	33	24	75	24
Jamsen[110]	2002	173	218	NA	83.5	NA	NA	NA	PTA	25	60	4.1	60
Cho[111]	2003	40	40	100	100	0.61	0.93	NA	SEN	NA	–	NA	–
Becquemin[112]	2003	251	277	NA	90	0.52	NA	2.5	BES vs. PTA	65/67‡	12	NA	–
Jahnke[113]	2003	52	63	83	100	0.54	0.89	10.9	SG	74.1	24	83.2	24
Duda[10]	2005	57	57	65		0.61	0.87	81.5	DEN vs. SEN	20.7/17.9	18	NA	–
Schillinger[9]	2006	104	104	35	100	0.58	0.84	13.2	SEN vs. PTA	37/63	12	NA	–

*Summary of reports of femoropopliteal interventions from the literature. A wide variety of anatomical situations are represented here, including many with chronic long-segment total occlusions. Of note is that primary patency of 2 years, when reported, is considerably lower than that for iliac interventions, yet cumulative patency ranges from approximately 75% to 90%. This emphasizes the need for both postprocedure surveillance and consideration of the performance of a femoral intervention when embarking on a course of therapy.

†Clinical or objective patency.

‡Angiographic patency (<50% stenosis) in mandatory stent group vs. PTA with selective stenting group.

§Devices placed surgically.

¶Average increase of 0.26.

BES = balloon-expandable stainless steel; SES = self-expanding stainless steel; SEN = self-expanding nitinol; DEN = drug-eluting nitinol; PTA = percutaneous transluminal (balloon) angioplasty; LPTA = excimer laser-assisted PTA; SG = stent graft; NA = not assessed or reported.

leading to a recommendation that whenever possible, a PTA-first strategy be attempted.

To summarize, in many cases, either surgery or interventional techniques can ameliorate symptoms. The decision about which is the most appropriate therapy can be made by the patient and physician, taking into account the risks and discomforts of the proposed procedure, its probable durability and reproducibility, the degree to which a procedure closes the door to other therapies, the magnitude of life-style limitation, and the individual patient's tolerance for risk.

The treatment of symptomatic femoropopliteal disease should favor a percutaneous approach over an open surgical procedure; primary stent placement appears to be the preferred strategy, particularly if stent fractures can be avoided. The advent of fracture-resistant stent designs and better recanalization techniques for occlusions may further improve outcomes. The future of effective drug-eluting stents may provide enhancements, although the long-term thrombotic risks and appropriate duration of antiplatelet therapy remain uncertain.

Tibioperoneal Obstructive Disease

BACKGROUND. PAD often involves multiple levels from proximal to distal in the extremity. When disease is present in the proximal vessels, the infrapopliteal arteries often also have significant occlusive disease (anterior tibial, peroneal, and posterior tibial). Similarly, when tibioperoneal narrowing is present, proximal disease probably coexists. Rarely is a symptomatic lesion isolated to a single vessel below the knee. Revascularization strategies for below-knee lesions must take into account the extent, severity, and distribution of disease in more proximal vessels.

For patients with claudication and multilevel disease, correction of inflow obstructive disease in a proximal vessel may be sufficient for symptom relief. This differs from critical limb ischemia, in which restoration of uninterrupted (pulsatile flow) patency to at least one vessel to the foot is generally required to heal the lesion. In the absence of severe and flow-limiting proximal disease, significant disease of all three crural vessels is usually required to provoke symptomatic calf claudication or higher grades of ischemia (rest pain or tissue loss).

TREATMENT. Historically, revascularization of tibioperoneal vessels has been reserved for patients with critical limb ischemia. Endovascular approaches are rapidly replacing the traditional surgical bypass. Technological advances and the use of coronary equipment allow for routine and uncomplicated access to the infrapopliteal vessels. Numerous reports have confirmed the feasibility, safety, and efficacy of tibioperoneal PTA. Primary success rates are generally 80 to 95 percent and cumulative 2-year patency rates can approximate 75 percent (Table 59-4).[15-21] Limb salvage rates for percutaneous intervention rival those of surgical reconstruction.[19,20] PTA can also effectively salvage ischemic limbs in diabetic patients with small-vessel disease.[22,23]

For tibioperoneal PTA, focal stenoses have the best outcomes, and those patients with fewer than five separate lesions have a higher success rate. The success of endovascular therapy is measured by relief of rest pain, healing of ulcers, and avoiding amputation, not necessarily by long-term vessel patency. An underlying principle of treatment of ischemic ulcers is that it takes more oxygenated blood to heal a wound than to maintain tissue integrity.

The safe and effective revascularization of tibioperoneal vessels with the percutaneous approach in this higher risk cohort has changed the management of patients with critical limb ischemia. When anatomically feasible, a strategy of PTA first is now considered to be a reasonable and appropri-

ate strategy for revascularization in *all* patients, even those with low surgical risk for infrapopliteal bypass (Figs. 59-8 and 59-9).[14]

The changing paradigm for revascularization also relates to the indications for intervention in patients with symptomatic but less critical tibioperoneal disease. The threshold for revascularization had traditionally been very high, largely because of the risk of the surgical approach. The availability of effective and less invasive options permits a lower threshold for intervention. Specifically, in the subset of patients who claudicate solely because of infrapopliteal disease, favorable acute and intermediate-term patency and clinical results have been achieved using PTA.[20] Such a strategy should be limited to patients who have severe symptoms (Rutherford category 3) and straightforward anatomy. Infrapopliteal PTA may also help those with claudication undergoing proximal revascularization (either with surgery or PTA), with severely impaired runoff. When tibial outflow is a major determinant of long-term patency, recanalizing the runoff vessels may provide a benefit.

In summary, optimal management of patients with lower extremity arterial occlusive disease and associated symptoms requires the input of practitioners knowledgeable about the efficacy of percutaneous and surgical revascularization. A strategy of PTA first should be considered if the anatomy is favorable. The physician must provide a frank discussion of the risks, potential symptomatic benefit, and durability of the proposed intervention for the patient. For patients with claudication, little evidence suggests that early and aggressive revascularization alters the natural history of lower extremity occlusive disease. Thus, treatment should be guided by the patient's degree of functional impairment.

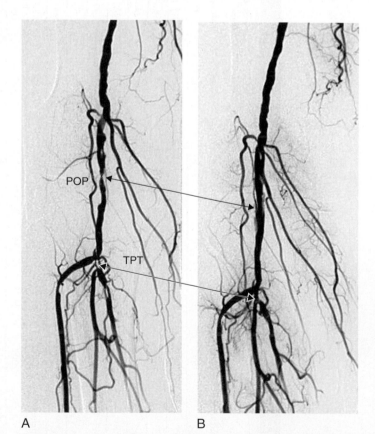

FIGURE 59-8 Intervention in tibial artery disease. **A,** Lesions in the below-knee popliteal artery (POP) and in the very short tibioperoneal trunk (TPT) **(B)** were identified and successfully treated with percutaneous transluminal angioplasty.

TABLE 59–4 | **Results of Tibioperoneal Artery Interventions***

Lead Author	Year	No. of Patients	Lesions Treated	No. with Occlusion (%)	Technical Success (%)	Ankle-Brachial Index		Mean Lesion Length (cm)	Primary Device	Primary Patency		Cumulative Patency		Event-Free Survival		Limb Salvage	
						Before	After			%	Duration (mo)	%	Duration (mo)	%	Duration (mo)	%	Duration (mo)
Sivananthan[15]	1994	38	73	24	96	NA	NA	NA	PTA	NA	–	NA	–	NA	–	NA	–
Varty[16]	1995	38	40	17	98	0.55	0.84	1	PTA	59	24	68	24	NA	–	77	12
Dorros[17]	1998	312	657	27	98	NA	NA	NA	PTA	NA	–	NA	–	NA	–	NA	–
Desgranges[18]	2000	33	NA	NA	82	NA	NA	NA	PTA	66	12	77	12	94	12	91	12
Soder[19]	2000	60	72	35	84/61†	NA	NA	NA	PTA	68/48†	10	56	18	NA	–	80	18
Dorros[20]	2001	235	529	28.9	92	NA	NA	NA	PTA	NA	–	NA	–	31	60	91	60
Tsetis[21]	2002	12	13	100	92.3	0.35	0.68	7	VPTA	NA	–	NA	–	NA	–	NA	–

*Summary of recent literature on tibial artery interventions. Most reports are reviews of single-center experience and procedural results. The 2001 report of Dorros and associates deserves special mention; it is of long-term follow-up of event-free survival and limb salvage.

†Stenosis/occlusion.

PTA = percutaneous transluminal (balloon) angioplasty; VPTA = vibrational PTA; NA = not assessed or reported.

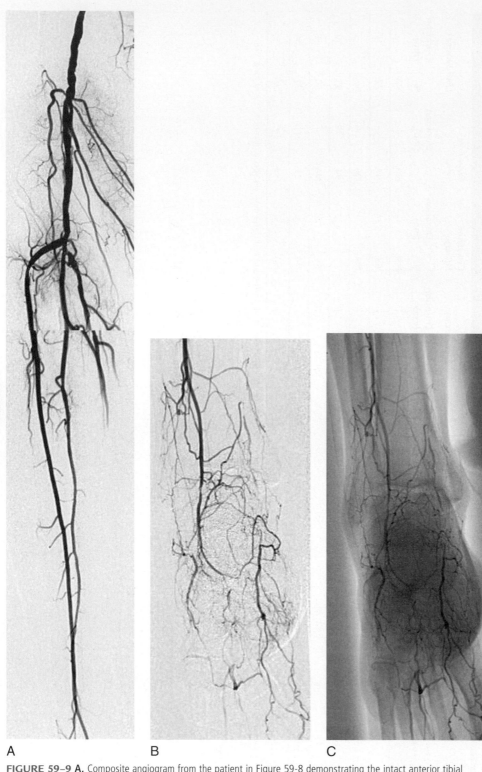

A   B   C

FIGURE 59–9 A, Composite angiogram from the patient in Figure 59-8 demonstrating the intact anterior tibial runoff in the calf. The peroneal normally attenuates by the level of the malleoli and, in this case, the posterior tibial is also occluded. **B** and **C,** Pedal circulation in both digital subtraction angiography and native views. Although "straight line" flow to the foot was reconstituted and the patient's ulcers healed, the evident diffuse small-vessel disease in the pedal vessels still places the foot in long-term jeopardy. Careful surveillance and compulsive continuing medical management are critical for this group of patients, even in the context of technical procedural success.

evidence supports a PTA-first approach in selected patients with limb-threatening ischemia and obstructive infrainguinal PAD.[14] As the short- and long-term outcomes of catheter-based interventions continue to improve, these endovascular techniques will assume an even more prominent role in the treatment of patients presenting with claudication or critical limb ischemia.

Regardless of initial treatment strategy, optimum long-term outcome requires diligent follow-up. Although surveillance strategies for surgical bypass grafts exist, we lack formal guidelines for monitoring patients following percutaneous therapy. However, there is general agreement that these individuals should undergo regular evaluation, including examination of the affected limb and performance of noninvasive testing.

Atherosclerotic Renal Artery Disease

Atherosclerosis of the renal artery resulting in renal artery stenosis (RAS) is associated with increased cardiovascular events and mortality. Assessment of a general population[24] by renal duplex ultrasound in individuals older than 65 years has revealed a 6.8 percent prevalence of RAS. The prevalence of RAS increases to 20 to 30 percent in high-risk populations (e.g., patients with known atherosclerotic vascular disease).[25] Atherosclerotic RAS is a progressive disease associated with a loss of renal mass over time despite control of hypertension. Progression of RAS to occlusion is more likely with more severe (more than 60 percent) lesions and occurs at a rate of 10 to 20 percent/year.[26]

Atherosclerotic RAS is an important cause of renal insufficiency, refractory hypertension, and cardiac destabilization syndromes (unstable angina and flash pulmonary edema). Unilateral RAS manifests clinically as a vasoconstrictor-mediated hypertension, whereas bilateral RAS causes hypertension caused by volume overload. Up to 20 percent of patients older than age 50 entering renal dialysis programs in the United States have atherosclerotic RAS (ischemic nephropathy) as the cause of their renal failure. The 2-, 5-, and 10-year survival rates were 56, 18, and 5 percent, respectively, for dialysis-dependent patients with RAS. The mortality risk depends on the severity of RAS (Table 59-5). The median survival for

Limb-threatening ischemia, in contrast, requires prompt treatment, using the modality that will provide the most complete revascularization with the lowest procedural risk. The principle of restoring straight-line pulsatile flow to the extremity affected by diffuse disease or long-segment femoropopliteal obstruction may be accomplished with traditional bypass surgery or an endovascular approach. Current

dialysis patients with atherosclerotic RAS was 25 months compared with 133 months for patients with polycystic kidney disease. Clearly, the early diagnosis of RAS and the prevention of end-stage renal disease (ESRD) are important goals.

Renal Artery Stenosis (see Chap. 40)

DIAGNOSIS. Clinical clues to the diagnosis of RAS (Table 59-6),[1] such as the onset of diastolic hypertension after the age of 55, refractory or malignant hypertension, resistant hypertension in a previously well-controlled patient, and/or an increasing serum creatinine level, should alert the clinician and prompt further diagnostic testing (Figs. 59-10 and 59-11). Imaging best diagnoses RAS. Duplex renal artery ultrasound, CTA, and MRA are all recommended as noninvasive screening tests in patients suspected of having RAS.[1] Invasive renal angiography is recommended when the clinical suspicion is high and noninvasive testing is inconclusive or inconsistent with the clinical evidence.[1] Some experts have also recommended renal angiography at the time of cardiac catheterization or peripheral vascular angiography in patients who are at increased risk for RAS. Screening modalities that are not recommended include captopril renal scintigraphy, measurement of plasma renin activity (with or without captopril stimulation), and selective renal vein renin measurements.[1]

TREATMENT. After establishing the anatomical diagnosis of renal artery stenosis, one must consider the most appropriate management. The goals of treatment include blood pressure control, preserving or improving renal function, and possibly reducing cardiovascular events and mortality. The indications for revascularization require the presence of clinical findings related to RAS with a hemodynamically significant stenosis defined by the following: (1) 50 percent diameter stenosis with a systolic translesional gradient (measured with a 5 French catheter or pressure wire) of 20 mm Hg or a mean pressure gradient of 10 mm Hg; (2) 70 percent diameter stenosis measured by quantitative angiographic methods; or (3) 70 percent diameter stenosis determined by intravascular ultrasound measurement.[27]

Although PTA alone remains the treatment of choice for fibromuscular dysplasia (FMD) lesions, primary stent placement for atherosclerotic RAS is the current standard of care (Fig. 59-12).[1] Stents are strongly believed to lead to more predictable and hemodynamically favorable results in renal revascularization. A literature survey has suggested that probable restenosis rates for renal stenting may be even lower (Table 59-7).

The strongest predictor of late renal stent patency is acute gain, or maximizing the stent lumen. Larger diameter (6-mm) renal arteries have lower restenosis rates than smaller (less than 4.5-cm) vessels.[28] Long-term (5-year) follow-up in two case series has shown primary patency rates of 79 and 84.5 percent and sec-

ondary patency rates of 92.4 and 98 percent. Almost all in-stent restenosis occurs during the first year after stent implantation, with restenosis later than 2 years an unusual occurrence.

However, in spite of technical success rates in excess of 95 percent using stents, angiographic stenosis does not

TABLE 59-5	Association of Severity of Renal Artery Stenosis (RAS) and Survival[85]
Severity of RAS (%)	**4-Year Survival**
No RAS	90
50 to 75	70
76 to 95	68
>95	48

TABLE 59-6	Clinical Predictors of Renal Artery Stenosis
Onset of hypertension in patients <30 or >55 yr old
Malignant, accelerated, or resistant hypertension
Unexplained renal dysfunction
Development of azotemia or worsening renal function after ACE inhibitor or ARB agent
Pulmonary edema
Atrophic kidney or size discrepancy between kidneys more than 1.5 cm
Multivessel coronary disease or
Peripheral arterial disease

ACE = angiotensin-converting enzyme; ARB = angiotensin receptor blocker.

CH 59

Endovascular Treatment of Noncoronary Obstructive Vascular Disease

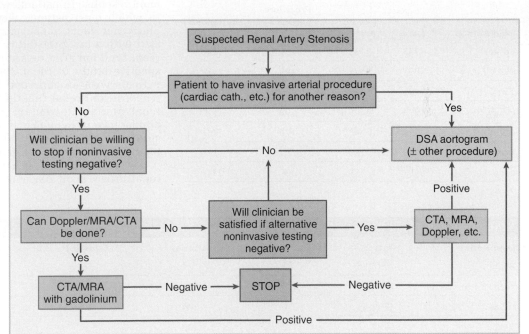

FIGURE 59-10 Approach to the anatomical evaluation of renal artery stenosis. Once stenosis is suspected, if the patient is to have another invasive arterial procedure, noninvasive imaging is deferred and a low-volume digital subtraction aortogram (DSA) is obtained at the time of that procedure. In other cases, the clinician should assess whether a negative noninvasive test would be sufficient evidence to acquit the renal arteries. If so, noninvasive testing should be performed. If not, consideration should be given to digital subtraction aortography and selective angiography. cath = catheterization; CTA = computed tomography angiography; MRA = magnetic resonance angiography. (See also Fig. 40-15.)

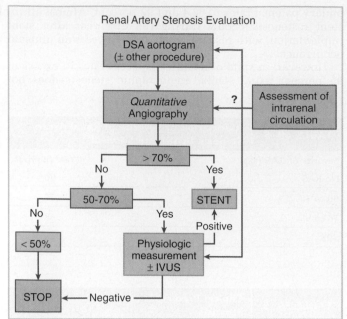

Renal Artery Stenosis Evaluation

FIGURE 59–11 Approach to the angiographic evaluation and treatment of renal artery stenosis. Once a digital subtraction aortogram (DSA) is performed confirming the presence of renovascular disease, quantitative angiography and objective evaluation of the severity of stenosis should be performed. Very severe (more than 70 percent diameter stenosis) lesions are subjected to revascularization and mild lesions (less than 50 percent diameter stenosis) are not. We believe that the intermediate lesion should be assessed with physiological evaluation and/or an additional anatomical documentation of severity, such as intravascular ultrasound (IVUS) or fractional flow reserve. The absence of translesional flow acceleration or a pressure gradient should mitigate the desire to intervene. (See also Fig. 40-15.)

CH 59

predict clinical benefit (Table 59-8). This implies that either the renal artery stenosis is not causally related to the hypertension or the successful revascularization procedure did not relieve the renal hypoperfusion. A major difficulty in predicting a treatment response in patients with renovascular disease is that they commonly have other nephrotoxic conditions that may confound their response to revascularization—diabetes, essential hypertension, atheroemboli, and medication-related insults.

PATIENT SELECTION: Analogous to the coronary technique of fractional flow reserve (FFR), the renal fractional flow reserve serves as a lesion-specific functional assessement of a renal artery stenosis. Consistent with the unpredictable clinical results, a poor correlation has been shown for RAS between quantitative angiography and hemodynamic gradients (peak, mean, and hyperemic), whereas an excellent correlation has been shown for the renal FFR and baseline pressure gradient.[29] Renal FFR determined in 17 patients with poorly controlled hypertension correlated with clinical improvement. An abnormal renal FFR (less than 0.8) predicted blood pressure improvement (86 percent) compared with a 30 percent improvement if the FFR was normal ($P = 0.04$).[30]

Brain natriuretic peptide (BNP) promotes diuresis, natriuresis, arterial vasodilation, and antagonizes the renin angiotensin system and angiotensin II, and may serve as a biomarker of response to renal revascularization. In 27 patients with uncontrolled hypertension and RAS (70 percent diameter stenosis), hypertension improved in 77 percent of those with elevated BNP levels, compared with none of the five patients with a baseline BNP level less than or equal to 80 pg/ml ($P = 0.001$). If the BNP level fell more than 30 percent after successful stent placement, 94 percent (16 of 17 patients) had improvement in their blood pressure control.[31]

The renal artery resistive index (RI), measured noninvasively by Doppler ultrasound, may also stratify patients likely to respond to renal intervention. However, there are conflicting data regarding the ability of RI to predict treatment response in patients with RAS. A retrospective study, in which most patients were treated with balloon angioplasty, not stents, has suggested that an elevated RI is associated with a low probability of improved blood pressure or renal function after revascularization.[32] However, in a prospective study of renal stent placement in 241 patients, patients with an abnormal RI experienced blood pressure response and renal functional improvement at 1 year after renal arterial intervention (Figs. 59-13 and 59-14).[33] The preponderance of evidence and scientific quality of the latter studies favors the conclusion that an elevated RI should not preclude performance of renal artery intervention.

Several clinical trials have demonstrated that successful renal artery stent placement improves or stabilizes renal

TABLE 59–7	Renal Stent Placement Outcomes			
Lead Author	Date	No. of Arteries	Procedure Success (%)	Restenosis (%)
White[114]	1997	133	99	18.8
Blum[115]	1997	74	100	11.0
Tuttle[116]	1998	148	98	14.0
Henry[117]	1999	209	99	11.4
van de Ven[118]	1999	43	90	14.0
Rocha-Singh[28]	1999	180	97	12.0
Lederman[28]	2001	358	100	21.0

TABLE 59–8	Blood Pressure Response to Renal Artery Stenting					
Lead Author	Year	Patients	Arteries	Cure (%)	Improve (%)	Benefit (%)
Blum[115]	1997	68	74	16	62	78
Tuttle[116]	1998	129	148	2	55	57
Henry[117]	1999	210	244	19	61	78
Rocha-Singh[28]	1999	150	180	6	50	56
Dorros[119]	1998	105	—	2	47	49*
White[114]	1997	100	133	NR	76	76
Lederman[28]	2001	261	NR	<1	70	70

*Dorros (1998) is a long-term (4-year) follow up.

function in patients with atherosclerotic renovascular insufficiency. Patients with renal insufficiency and hemodynamically significant RAS improved after stent placement.[34] Successful renal artery stent placement can significantly slow the progression of renal failure. Calculation of the mean slope of the reciprocal of serum creatinine values before and after stent placement has shown a fourfold slowing in the progression of renal insufficiency after renal artery stent placement. One of the best predictors of improvement in renal function following percutaneous revascularization is a rapid rate of decline in renal function, suggesting that the rapid decline in renal function reflects a more acute injury that is more likely to be reversible.[35] Alternatively, approximately 20 percent of patients who undergo renal intervention will have a decline or worsening in their renal function. One contributing factor may be atheroembolism, resulting from the trauma to the bulky aortic plaque (Fig. 59-15). Work is ongoing to adapt embolic protection for renal interventions.[36]

UNILATERAL RENAL ARTERY STENOSIS AND NEPHROPATHY. Traditional teaching holds that unilateral RAS does not cause ischemic nephropathy when the contralateral renal artery is patent. However, revascularization of unilateral RAS can improve or stabilize renal function. Two clinical trials have demonstrated improvement in overall renal function in patients with unilateral renal stenosis.[33,35] Revascularization of unilateral renal artery stenosis results in measurable improvement in the split renal function of the stenotic kidney.[37,38] Restoring flow to the stenotic kidney has reversed the hyperfiltration of the non-stenotic kidney, resulting in decreased proteinuria.[38] These data suggest that in patients with abnormal renal function, treatment of unilateral RAS may improve and/or stabilize renal function.

In summary, percutaneous treatment of renovascular disease offers a safe and effective therapy preferable to open surgical revascularization. Renal artery stenting can ameliorate hypertension and improve or stabilize renal function, and may delay the need for hemodialysis in appropriately selected patients. In addition, the advent of distal protection devices to limit atheroembolic complications may further improve safety and renal parenchymal preservation. The current recommended systematic approach to the investigation and treatment of this condition is outlined in Figures 59-10 and 59-11.

Chronic Mesenteric Ischemia

BACKGROUND. The clinical syndrome of chronic mesenteric ischemia (CMI) is surprisingly uncommon, given the high frequency of atherosclerotic disease of the aorta and the common finding of aorto-ostial stenosis of the visceral vessels.[39] The mesenteric circulation consists of the celiac trunk, the superior mesenteric artery (SMA), and inferior mesenteric artery (IMA). The rarity of the clinical syndrome probably reflects the redundancy of the visceral circulation with multiple pathways from the SMA and the IMA. Women are disproportionately affected (70 percent) and the classic presentation is postprandial abdominal discomfort and weight loss. Patients with CMI typically avoid food and usually have significant weight loss. Even in advanced cases, a number of other causes for the presence of weight

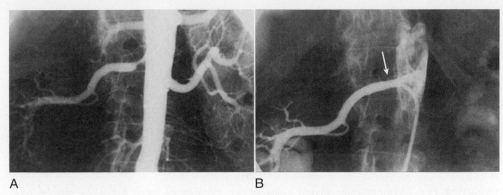

FIGURE 59–12 A, Baseline aortogram showing 70 percent diameter stenosis of right renal artery. **B,** Poststent. Note mild residual narrowing (arrow).

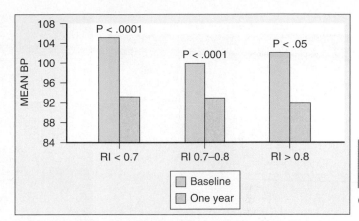

FIGURE 59–13 Blood pressure (BP) response in patients with normal resistive index (RI) less than 0.7, moderate elevation (RI = 0.7 to 0.8), and severe impairment (RI more than 0.8) at 1 year after stent placement. (Data from Zeller T, et al: Stent angioplasty of severe atherosclerotic ostial renal artery stenosis in patients with diabetes mellitus and nephrosclerosis. Catheter Cardiovasc Interv 58:510, 2003.)

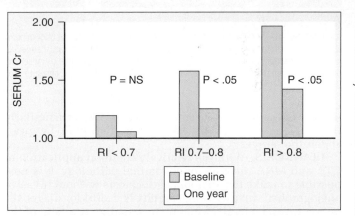

FIGURE 59–14 Renal function change in patients with normal resistive index (RI) less than 0.7, moderate elevation (RI = 0.7 to 0.8), and severe nephrosclerosis (RI more than 0.8) at 1 year after stent placement. Cr = creatinine. (Data from Zeller T, et al: Stent angioplasty of severe atherosclerotic ostial renal artery stenosis in patients with diabetes mellitus and nephrosclerosis. Catheter Cardiovasc Interv 58:510, 2003.)

loss and abdominal pain are often entertained before intestinal angina comes into focus as the diagnosis of exclusion. Evidence of significant obstruction of two or more of these vessels is often found when classic symptoms and endoscopy suggest bowel ischemia, although single-vessel disease,

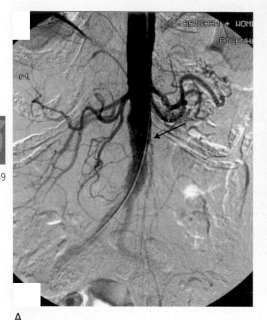

FIGURE 59–15 **A,** Baseline selective right renal angiogram. Note normal cortical vessels. **B,** Poststent. Note "absence" of distal filling because of atheroembolization.

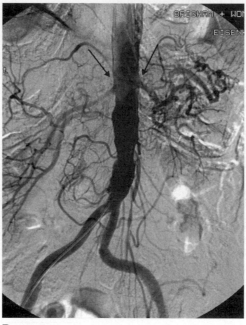

FIGURE 59–16 Visceral angiogram from a patient with postprandial abdominal pain, weight loss, and abdominal bruits. Note that this projection does not demonstrate the origins of the celiac or superior mesenteric arteries although in **A,** early in the run, the thin arrow indicates a stenosis at the origin of the inferior mesenteric artery. A later frame, **B,** shows the origins of the renal arteries (arrows); although potentially not seen in absolute profile, they appear unobstructed.

circumvents the need for general anesthesia and the operative trauma associated with open surgery and may result in a lower acute mortality and morbidity.[43,44]

Because of the relative infrequency of this disease, there are no comparative trials of surgery versus endovascular treatment for CMI. Interpretation of the literature, which has reported successful case series of both surgical and interventional treatment, is confounded by the obvious case selection and other inherent biases. Interventional treatment offers a clear alternative for the management of chronic visceral ischemia that may have advantages over surgery, especially in those patients with advanced age or additional increased risk of morbidity and mortality (see Fig. 59-17).

The single largest series of endovascular therapy for CMI was recently reported, with a technical success rate of 96 percent and symptom relief in 88 percent of 59 patients (79 vessels).[45] At a mean follow-up of 38 ± 15 months, 17 percent had recurrence of symptoms but none developed acute mesenteric ischemia, and all underwent successful revascularization without complication. Follow-up was achieved in 90 percent of the patients and 90 percent of the vessels with angiographic CT, conventional angiography, or Duplex ultrasound, showing an in-stent restenosis rate of 29 percent.

In summary, although there are no prospective controlled data comparing outcomes of balloon angioplasty versus stent placement for the treatment of mesenteric arterial stenoses, studies have suggested that endovascular stent placement confers superior immediate and long-term results, better than balloon angioplasty alone, for which stent revascularization should be the percutaneous treatment of choice.

usually of the SMA, can sometimes cause CMI, particularly if collateral connections have been disrupted by prior abdominal surgery.

DIAGNOSIS. With the relatively common application of CTA and MRA imaging for abdominal pathology, it is now possible to make the anatomical diagnosis without invasive angiography.[40] Invasive angiography is useful for diagnosis, but requires a lateral aortogram to visualize the ostia of the mesenteric vessels (Figs. 59-16 and 59-17). When the symptoms are typical, the anatomical findings severe, and the alternative pathological explanations few, the diagnosis is confirmed and revascularization is in order. As might be expected, however, this patient group has a high incidence of coronary artery disease and the surgical mortality and morbidity ranges from 5 to 8 percent, with the highest incidence of complications occurring in patients older than 70 years.[41,42]

TREATMENT. Obstructions of the visceral vessels resemble those of the renal arteries, and the technical considerations for PTA and stent placement are similar to those for renal artery intervention. The endovascular approach

Brachiocephalic and Subclavian Obstructive Disease

BACKGROUND. Once considered relatively rare, brachiocephalic and subclavian artery obstructions have received increased attention because of the use of internal mammary conduits for coronary bypass surgery. Asymptomatic difference in systolic arm pressures (10 mm Hg) is the most common presentation of brachiocephalic or subclavian stenosis. Subclavian steal syndrome arises because of reversal of flow in the vertebral artery as blood is shunted to the upper extremity circulation. Vertebrobasilar symptoms of dizziness, syncope, and vertigo are most common,

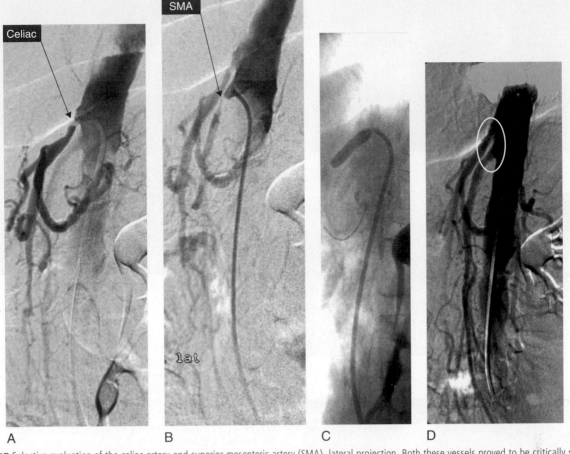

FIGURE 59–17 Selective evaluation of the celiac artery and superior mesenteric artery (SMA), lateral projection. Both these vessels proved to be critically stenosed (**A** and **B**) and were treated interventionally (**C**), restoring wide patency to both, as outlined in **D**. The patient's symptoms abated, and she began to gain weight.

along with upper extremity claudication of the ipsilateral limb. In coronary subclavian steal, there is reversal of flow within the left internal mammary artery because of proximal subclavian stenosis. These patients often come to clinical attention with myocardial ischemia. Although conservative therapy offers some clinical improvement, it usually requires relief of the anatomical obstruction.[46]

TREATMENT. Balloon angioplasty for subclavian artery stenosis was described in the early 1980s, with subsequent reports showing that acute success and patency rates at follow-up are comparable to those of surgery. Furthermore, there was a low rate of complications and infrequent mortality. There was initial concern about the potential for distal embolization and stroke, uncertain long-term patency, and difficulty in treating total occlusions. With continued improvements in anesthetic and operative technique, short hospital stays, and early discharge, many practitioners continue to regard surgery as the standard against which endovascular methods must be compared.

Clinical data regarding long-term patency of the subclavian and brachiocephalic vessels are limited (Fig. 59-18). An evaluation of the reports of surgery versus angioplasty and stenting of this condition has been published, compiling technical success (the ability to perform the planned procedure yielding target lesion revascularization and survival to discharge), patient death, stroke, and patency of the treated segment. There was no uniformity or standardization for evaluation or reporting of complications in the studies in which stenting was performed, but adverse events were reported in approximately 6 percent of patients.[47]

Similarly, the overall incidence of postprocedure complications, such as vascular access bleeding, hemorrhage, pseudoaneurysm, transfusion, or contrast-mediated transient renal insufficiency, is not known. Technical success has been reported in 97 percent of cases. No strokes or deaths occurred. Follow-up data were available in about two thirds of cases at a mean duration of 16.8 months. Occlusion or restenosis was found in less than 10 percent.[47] Additional reports of subclavian stent placement have continued to suggest that perioperative strokes are uncommon and the results are favorable.[48] There have been some concerns not only about long-term patency but also about durability of the stent because of wire fracture at the site of flexion and compression.

One of the largest series reviewed 115 patients with subclavian disease who were treated percutaneously.[49] Successful revascularization was achieved in 98 percent of patients. There were no periprocedural deaths, one patient had a transient ischemic attack from the left vertebral artery, and two patients had emboli, one to the renal and one to the mesenteric arteries. All three patients recovered completely from these events. Whereas patency rates were significantly higher at 1 year in the stent group compared with those only treated with angioplasty (95 versus 76 percent), by 4 years of follow-up there was more restenosis in the stent patients.[49]

In summary, it is unlikely, because of the relative infrequency of this disease, that a large well-designed trial will compare surgical and interventional treatment of patients with brachiocephalic and subclavian disease. At present,

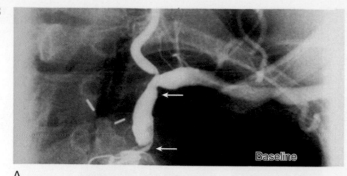

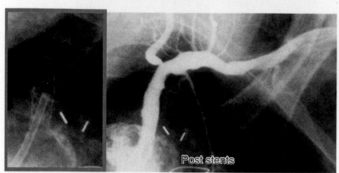

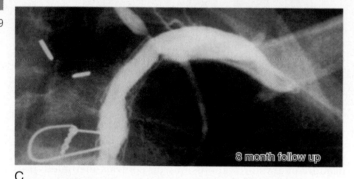

FIGURE 59–18 **A,** Baseline angiogram of a left subclavian artery with a tight proximal stenosis and a moderate stenosis just proximal to the vertebral artery. **B,** After placement of two balloon-expandable stents. Note position of stents in inset. **C,** Follow-up angiogram at 8 months, with patent stents.

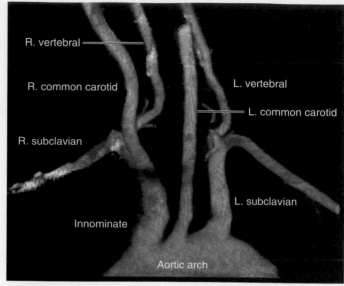

FIGURE 59–19 Computed tomography angiogram of aortic arch and arch vessels.

experience and examination of the literature support the consideration of a primary percutaneous approach in most patients with symptomatic obstructive disease.

Carotid and Vertebral Disease

Carotid Artery Disease

BACKGROUND. Slightly more than half of the 731,000 strokes annually in the United States result from extracranial atherosclerotic carotid artery disease. Stroke is the leading cause of disability and the third leading cause of death after coronary artery disease and cancer in the United States (see Chap. 58). Atherosclerotic extracranial carotid artery disease usually results in symptoms caused by embolic events. In contrast to acute coronary syndromes, a minority of ischemic strokes are caused by thrombotic occlusion.

The two internal carotid arteries and two vertebral arteries come together at the base of the skull to form the circle of Willis, which is an ideal anastomotic network. In theory,

a single vessel could supply the circulatory needs of the entire brain. However, although a circle of Willis is present in every brain, there is a huge amount of individual variability, and fewer than half are complete.

Cerebrovascular events are classified as transient ischemic attacks (TIAs) if they completely resolve within 24 hours, or as strokes if they cause a deficit lasting longer than 24 hours. Patients with a TIA have a 1 in 20 (5 percent) chance of stroke within 30 days, and almost 25 percent will have a recurrent cerebrovascular event within 1 year. Hemispheric symptoms refer to a single carotid distribution, typically causing contralateral hemiparesis or hemiparesthesia, aphasia, and/or ipsilateral monocular blindness (amaurosis fugax). Nonhemispheric symptoms include dysarthria, diplopia, vertigo, syncope, and/or transient confusion.

NONINVASIVE IMAGING. Doppler ultrasound of the carotid arteries is cost-effective, accurate, and reproducible. Blood flow velocity measurements are translated into estimates of lesion severity that have clinical relevance. There is controversy regarding the ability of ultrasound imaging to serve as the sole imaging criteria for selecting patients for carotid revascularization.[50,51] One trial has suggested that although ultrasound is an excellent screening tool, its accuracy in a community setting is not sufficient to replace angiography.[52] MRA and CTA are being used to image the extracranial carotid arteries and intracerebral vessels (Fig. 59-19).[53,54] The images can be reconstructed into noninvasive angiograms that have the advantage of depicting the circle of Willis with excellent resolution and clarity.

INVASIVE ANGIOGRAPHY. All the revascularization trials that have informed carotid artery treatment decisions have used angiographic criteria for patient selection. Digital subtraction angiography (DSA) is the gold standard for the diagnosis of vascular pathology of the aortic arch, cervical, and cerebral vessels (Fig. 59-20). Invasive angiography can cause adverse events, including a 0.5 percent stroke rate.[55]

SURGICAL TREATMENT. Treatment of carotid artery disease aims to prevent disabling stroke and death. All therapies should be judged ultimately on their ability to achieve these endpoints rather than surrogates. For revascularization to benefit patients, the strokes *prevented* by the procedure must exceed the strokes *caused.* Similarly, procedure-related mortality cannot obliterate the late benefit of surgery. This concept is important, because the longer

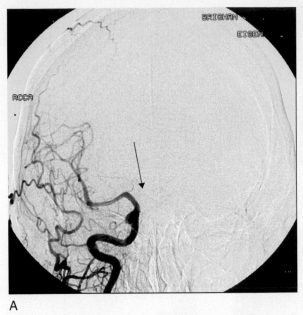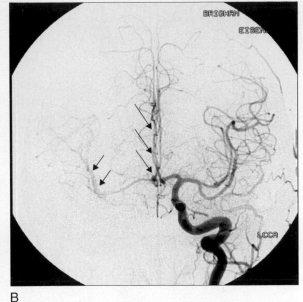

FIGURE 59–20 Corresponding anteroposterior (Townes) views of the right **(A)** and left **(B)** intracranial carotid angiograms. **A,** Perfusion of the right middle cerebral territory only; no flow is seen into the anterior cerebral vessel, the expected location of which is delineated by the arrow. **B,** Injection of the left carotid artery, demonstrating filling of both hemispheres, including the right anterior cerebral (three long arrows) and middle cerebral (two short arrows) territories.

TABLE 59–9	Carotid Surgery Versus Medical Therapy Trials		
Trial (Success Rate)	**Medical Risk of Stroke (%)**	**CEA Risk of Stroke (%)**	**Perioperative 30-day Stroke and Death (%)**
NASCET (70–99%)	25.1	8.9	5.8
NASCET (50–69%)	16.2	11.3	7.1
ECST (70–99%)	16.8	10.3	7.5
ACAS (>60%)	11	5.1	2.3
ACST (>60%)	11	3.8	3.1

CEA = carotid endarterectomy; NASCET = North American Symptomatic Carotid Endarterectomy Trial; ECST = European Carotid Surgery Trial; ACAS = Asymptomatic Carotid Atherosclerosis Study; ACST = Asymptomatic Carotid Surgery Trial:

patients live after a revascularization procedure, the greater the benefit they will enjoy. Very old or very ill patients may not live long enough to justify placing them at risk of a procedure-related death.

Carotid endarterectomy (CEA) is an established surgical procedure for stroke prevention in patients with extracranial carotid artery disease (Table 59-9). Randomized controlled trials in selected populations have demonstrated benefit in symptomatic (more than 50 percent) and asymptomatic (60 percent) patients for stroke prevention with CEA compared with medical therapy.[56-59]

The applicability of these surgical trial results to daily patient outcomes has generated controversy.[60,61] The American Heart Association (AHA) expert consensus panel has suggested indications for CEA that include good surgical risk candidates with symptoms related to more than 50 percent stenosis, and asymptomatic patients with more than 80 percent stenosis, if the perioperative risk of stroke and death does not exceed 3 percent for asymptomatic patients, 6 percent for symptomatic patients, or 10 percent for repeat CEA.[62]

CATHETER-BASED TREATMENT. Carotid artery stent (CAS) placement has evolved over the past 20 years to become an accepted method for treating selected patients (Fig. 59-21). Self-expanding stents are used to avoid stent deformation and compression. Concern over the potential release of atheroemboli has led to the development of several

emboli protection systems, including the following: (1) distal balloon occlusion with aspiration[63]; (2) proximal occlusion with aspiration[64]; and (3) distal filter systems.[65]

Several large contemporary, non-randomized, prospective registry studies (e.g., BEACH, ARCHeR, SECuRITY) have investigated the safety and efficacy of CAS with embolic protection in symptomatic and asymptomatic patients at increased risk for surgical treatment.[66-70] All these trials have met their targets for safety and efficacy (Fig. 59-22).

The Stenting and Angioplasty with Protection in Patients at High Risk for Endarterectomy (SAPPHIRE) was a randomized controlled trial that compared CAS with distal emboli protection to CEA in patients at increased risk for CEA.[71] A total of 747 patients were entered into the trial, with 159 randomized to CAS with distal protection and 151 randomized to CEA. An additional 406 patients were refused surgery and were treated in a stent registry, whereas only 7 patients were refused CAS and were treated in a surgery registry.

In the randomized patients, the 30-day incidence of stroke, death, and myocardial infarction was lower for CAS patients (4.8 percent) than for CEA patients (9.6 percent; $P = 0.14$). The CEA group also had an excess of cranial nerve injuries (5.3 percent), which were not seen in the CAS group. The 1-year combined endpoint for the CAS group was 12 percent compared with 20.1 percent ($P = 0.048$) in the CEA group (Fig. 59-23). This trial met the criteria for noninferior-

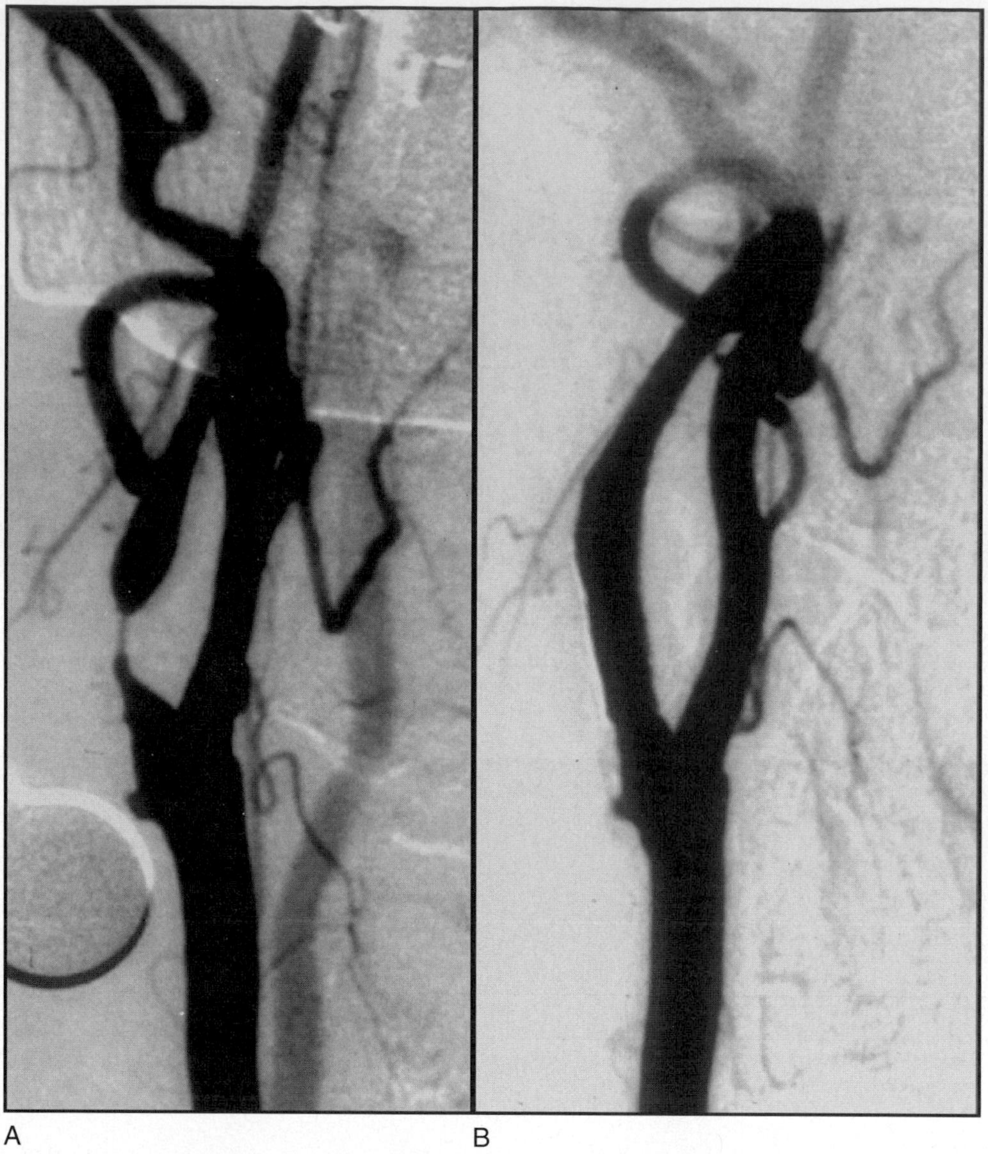

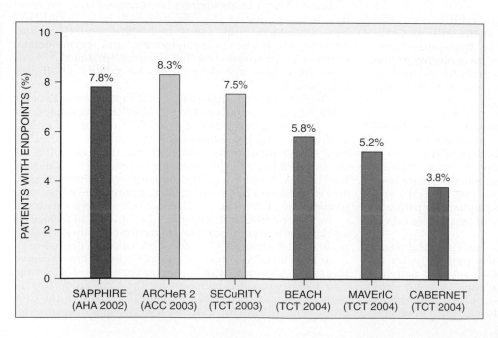

FIGURE 59–21 A, Baseline selective carotid angiogram showing critical stenosis of the internal carotid artery. The external carotid is identified as the vessel that gives off branches. **B,** Following stent deployment.

FIGURE 59–22 Bar graph showing 30-day composite endpoint (stroke, death, myocardial infarction) for U.S. carotid stent trials.[66-71]

ity and led to the first U.S. Food and Drug Administration (FDA) approval of a carotid stent. This randomized trial provides compelling evidence that CAS with distal protection is the procedure of choice for patients at increased risk for carotid surgery.

However, the results of two randomized trials of CEA versus CAS in patients not necessarily at high surgical risk have also been published. The Endarterectomy versus Stenting in Patients with Symptomatic Severe Carotid Stenosis (EVA-3S) trial compared CAS with various techniques and variable cerebral embolic protection with CEA; the results have shown statistically lower rates of stroke and death at 6 months in the endarterectomy group.[72,73] This trial was carried out by experienced vascular surgeons and relatively inexperienced interventionalists and used a much wider variety of techniques for CAS than other trials. Similarly, the 30-day results of the Stent-Supported Percutaneous Angioplasty versus Endarterectomy of the Carotid Artery versus Endarterectomy (SPACE) trial did not demonstrate noninferiority of carotid stenting compared with endarterectomy. The rate of ipsilateral stroke or death was 6.84 percent among patients who underwent carotid stenting, compared with 6.38 percent among those who had endarterectomy.[74] The results did not achieve statistical significance for endarterectomy, although the trial was stopped early when it became clear that further enrollment would not alter the result.[75] These two trials reflect the current controversies in carotid revascularization and are likely to be viewed both supportively and skeptically, depending on the bias of the reader. The moderate viewpoint is that the short-term results of both techniques are not wildly different and that much still remains to be learned about their safe and effective applications.

In summary, current indications for carotid artery stent placement are for symptomatic (diameter more than 50 percent) and asymptomatic (80 percent) stenoses in patients at increased risk for carotid surgery who are anatomically good candidates for CAS (Table 59-10). Currently, patients who do not meet high surgical risk criteria (Table 59-11) should be offered surgery[76] or participation in a clinical trial. Trials are continuing to enroll low surgical risk patients, prophylactic medical therapy is improving and, as always, the best patient care will continue to require knowledge, skill, and the judicious application by the physician.

Vertebral Artery Disease

BACKGROUND. Humans can tolerate well ligature of one of the two vertebral arteries, making the clinical presentation of vertebrobasilar insufficiency infrequent. Atherosclerotic occlusive disease of the origin of both vertebral arteries is the most common clinical lesion found; however, other combinations of carotid, subclavian, and innominate stenoses can compromise the posterior circulation and precipitate symptoms of vertebrobasilar insufficiency. In patients presenting with symptoms of cerebrovascular disease, 40 percent will have evidence of at least vertebral stenosis and 10 percent will have a vertebral occlusion.[77] Of those with posterior circulation symptoms (e.g., dizziness, ataxia, drop attacks, or diplopia), 35 percent will have a stroke within 5 years.[78]

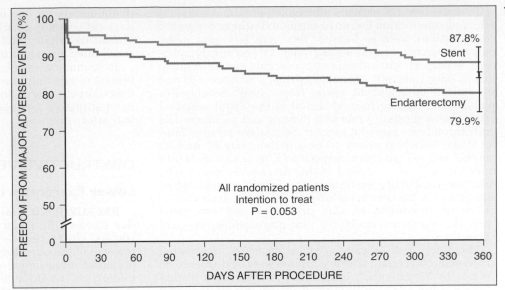

FIGURE 59–23 One-year outcome for freedom from major adverse events showing superiority for carotid stent over carotid surgery in randomized patients by intention to treat in the SAPPHIRE trial.[71]

CH 59

TABLE 59–10	Increased Risk of Complications for Carotid Stent Placement
· Tortuous aortic arch	
· Platelet or clotting disorder	
· Difficult vascular access	
· Lesion or vessel calcification	
· Visible thrombus	

TABLE 59–11	Factors Associated with Increased Risk for Carotid Artery Surgery
Anatomical criteria	
High cervical or intrathoracic lesion	
Prior neck surgery or radiation therapy	
Contralateral carotid artery occlusion	
Prior ipsilateral carotid endarterectomy	
Contralateral laryngeal nerve palsy	
Tracheostoma	
Medical comorbidities	
Age > 80 yr	
Class III/IV congestive heart failure	
Class III/IV angina pectoris	
Left main coronary disease	
Two- or three-vessel coronary artery disease	
Need for open heart surgery	
Ejection fraction ≤ 30%	
Recent myocardial infarction	
Severe chronic obstructive lung disease	

TREATMENT. Although initial treatment with platelet inhibitors and anticoagulants is warranted, arch and four-vessel studies (CTA, MRA, or DSA) are indicated if symptoms continue despite medical management. Surgical therapy is difficult and associated with significant perioperative morbidity.[79] Transection of the vertebral artery above the stenosis and reimplantation into the ipsilateral subclavian or carotid artery, vertebral artery endarterectomy, or vein patch angioplasty are the commonly used surgical techniques for treatment of this disease.

Endovascular Treatment of Noncoronary Obstructive Vascular Disease

In one series, 174 patients undergoing proximal vertebral artery reconstruction had no in-hospital deaths and reported complications were as follows: recurrent laryngeal nerve palsy, 2 percent; Horner's syndrome, 15 percent; lymphocele, 4 percent; chylothorax, 0.5 percent; and immediate thrombosis, 1 percent. Secondary patency rates were 95 and 91 percent at 5 and 10 years, respectively. Seventy-five patients undergoing reconstruction of the distal vertebral artery had a mortality rate of 4 percent and an immediate graft thrombosis rate of 8 percent. Secondary patency rates for distal vertebral artery reconstruction were 87 and 82 percent at 5 and 10 years, respectively. Although mortality rates for surgical treatment of this disease are acceptable, excessive morbidity restricts this technique from widespread use in the treatment of vertebral artery disease. Percutaneous treatment of this disease is not associated with the excessive morbidity that accompanies surgical correction.

The safety and efficacy of stent placement in treating atherosclerotic vertebral artery disease were evaluated in 38 vessels in 32 patients.[80] Indications for revascularization included diplopia ($n = 4$), blurred vision ($n = 4$), dizziness ($n = 23$), transient ischemic attacks ($n = 4$), drop attack ($n = 1$), gait disturbance ($n = 1$), headache ($n = 2$), and asymptomatic critical stenosis ($n = 1$). Success (less than 20 percent residual diameter stenosis, without stroke or death) was achieved in all 32 patients (100 percent; Fig. 59-24). One patient experienced a TIA 1 hour after the procedure. At follow-up (mean 10.6 months), all patients (100 percent) were alive and 31 of 32 (97 percent) were asymptomatic. One patient (3 percent) had in-stent restenosis at 3.5 months and underwent successful balloon angioplasty. Concern about the risk of distal embolization of debris makes debulking devices

inappropriate for use in the cerebral circulation. Because the most common location for vertebral artery stenoses is at or near its origin from the subclavian artery, considerable recoil often accompanies PTA alone.

In summary, endoluminal stenting of vertebral artery lesions is safe and effective, with a durable result, as evidenced by the low recurrence rate. Primary stent placement is an attractive treatment option for atherosclerotic vertebral artery disease.

OBSTRUCTIVE VENOUS DISEASE

Lower Extremity Deep Venous Thrombosis

BACKGROUND. Unlike atherosclerotic arterial obstructive disease, the major presenting obstructive element in venous obstruction is thrombus. Thus, dissolution or removal of the offending thrombus is the most evident goal of interventions for extremity venous thrombosis. However, underlying the thrombus is almost always a predisposing factor such as a hypercoagulable state, external obstruction, venous stricture, scarring, or indwelling foreign body. As a result, the treatment of venous thrombosis includes not only the removal of thrombus but also an attempt to correct the underlying cause.

TREATMENT. For most patients, anticoagulation and/or thrombolytic therapy are the mainstays of therapy (see Chaps. 72 and 82). Both systemic and catheter-directed thrombolysis have achieved some success (Fig. 59-25). Mechanical thrombectomy, balloon venoplasty, and stenting have all been reported, but evidence supporting the use of catheter-directed therapy is limited.

Because of the suggestions of a reduction in the incidence of postthrombotic syndrome with lysis compared with anticoagulation alone and of reduced major bleeding, catheter-directed therapy seems reasonable for patients at higher risk for systemic lysis complications and for those who have a large thrombus burden and/or a high risk of developing a postthrombotic syndrome. In addition, more interventional concepts are emerging. There have been reports of experience with rheolytic thrombectomy[81] and mechanical clot disruption. Additional experience with stents has suggested that in cases in which there is residual venous obstruction from scarring or external compression, relief of that obstruction with self-expanding stents may be important to maintain venous patency and prevent recurrent thrombosis. This is particularly true when the initial insult, such as an indwelling port infusion catheter, has been removed. Balloon venoplasty is also increasingly used to provide temporary relief of venous obstruction to facilitate the placement of transvenous pacing and/or defibrillator leads.

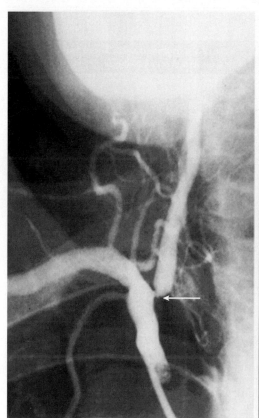 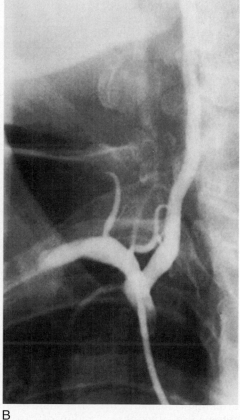

A   B

FIGURE 59-24 A, Angiogram of a tight stenosis at the ostium of the right vertebral artery (arrow). **B,** After balloon-expandable stent placement.

In summary, the mainstay of venous thrombosis of the extremities is anticoagulation. However, the selective application of catheter-based thrombolysis, thrombectomy, and venous stenting to relieve symptoms and help prevent postphlebitic syndromes is appropriate based on individual circumstances.

Central Venous Obstruction

Superior Vena Cava Syndrome

BACKGROUND. Superior vena cava (SVC) syndrome results from the obstruction of the blood flow in the superior vena cava (see Chap. 85). Pathological processes from contiguous structures can compress or directly invade the SVC. Superimposed venous thrombosis may contribute to the development of SVC syndrome in up to 50 percent of patients. Historically, SVC syndrome was most frequently caused by direct tumor compression. Currently, the use of indwelling venous access catheters, coupled with the improved survival of chemotherapy patients, is increasing the occurrence of nonmalignant SVC syndrome in patients who have been cured of their cancers. The explosion in the use of the automatic implantable cardioverter-defibrillator (ICD) and sophisticated multilead pacing systems has increased the incidence and recognition of this condition.

PERCUTANEOUS TREATMENT. Medical and surgical options for the treatment of superior vena cava obstruction are well established and reviewed in **Chapter 85.** Since the initial description of successful percutaneous treatment of SVC syndrome in the adult, the use of angioplasty alone has been limited by a high rate of initial failure and early restenosis caused by recoil of the highly elastic SVC wall. Stenting therefore quickly gained acceptance in this area of vascular intervention after it was first reported in the 1980s. Over 300 cases of SVC stenting have been documented in the literature since then.

Stenting in malignant SVC syndrome results in rapid improvement of symptoms. Patients report almost immediate resolution of headache, visual disturbances, and other central nervous system symptoms. Dyspnea, cough, and edema usually resolve within 1 to 3 days but occasionally may take up to 1 week. Stenting results in complete resolution of symptoms in most patients with malignant SVC syndrome. In the largest series, 76 consecutive patients with SVC syndrome were treated with stents and compared with historical controls of patients treated with radiation. Procedural success was 100 percent and all patients had improvement of symptoms within 48 hours. Ninety percent of patients treated with a stent had no symptoms of SVC obstruction at the time of death, compared with 12 percent of patients treated with radiation.[82] The recurrence rate of SVC syndrome after percutaneous intervention has been reported to vary widely, occurring in up to 45 percent of patients. This is likely because recurrence can be a result of various mechanisms. Acute stent thrombosis can develop shortly after stent placement in patients on insufficient anticoagulation or antiplatelet therapy; tumor ingrowth through stent struts, intimal hyperplasia, or fibrous scarring can

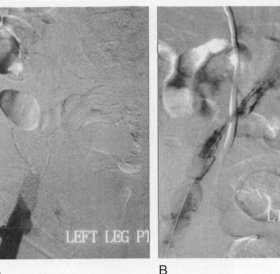

occur. Stent length oversizing may prevent recurrence of SVC syndrome caused by stent edge overgrowth. However, it may increase the risk of SVC stent thrombosis or restenosis. Patients with total SVC occlusion have the highest recurrence rate of SVC syndrome but repeated procedures in these patients are uniformly successful with additional stent placement, angioplasty, and/or thrombolysis, alone or in combination.[83]

In the developed world, SVC syndrome of nonmalignant cause (benign SVC syndrome) is usually iatrogenic in origin, most frequently caused by indwelling intravenous catheters and pacing leads. Complications of pacemaker lead placement, such as venous thrombosis and stenosis, occur in up to 30 percent of patients. Only a few patients become symptomatic, however, but the presence of multiple leads, retention of severed lead(s), and previous lead infection may increase risk of SVC syndrome. The largest series of percutaneous therapy in benign SVC syndrome included 16 patients. Ten patients had SVC syndrome caused by the indwelling catheter, two caused by the pacemaker wire, and one each caused by goiter, fibrous mediastinitis, heart-lung transplantation, and spontaneous thrombosis. The patency rate in 13 patients followed for a mean of 17 months was 85 percent.[84] Similar results can be expected in patients with SVC syndrome associated with central venous infusion catheters. Ideally, interventional treatment should also include removal of the inciting lead or catheter.

In summary, superior vena cava stenting is a low-risk procedure that provides fast and long-lasting symptomatic relief in malignant caval obstruction, often in combination with chemotherapy or radiation, to provide patients with the benefits of life prolongation and effective symptom control. In patients with SVC syndrome of nonmalignant cause, based on mid-term follow-up results, stenting is the treatment of choice (Fig. 59-26). Surgical therapy should be reserved for patients with benign SVC syndrome refractory to percutaneous therapy. Only a few patients are likely to become truly refractory, because most patients with recurrent SVC syndrome can be treated successfully with repeated percutaneous intervention.

FIGURE 59–25 Venogram of the left femoral vein after gaining access at the popliteal vein with ultrasound guidance. The patient is lying face down on the table to allow access to the popliteal vein. **A,** Baseline shows occlusion of the left femoral. **B,** Multiholed catheter across the venous occlusion; adminstration of lytic agents is started. **C,** 4 hours after lysis following percutaneous transluminal angioplasty and placement of a self-expanding stent to restore patency.

CH 59

Endovascular Treatment of Noncoronary Obstructive Vascular Disease

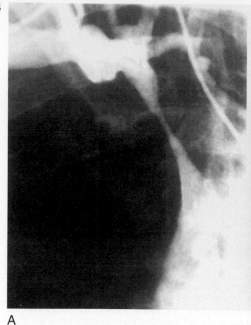
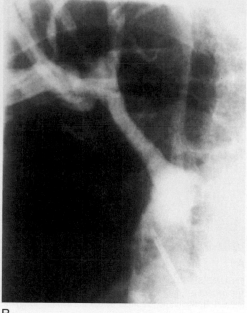

A B

FIGURE 59–26 Superior vena cava (SVC) syndrome and its treatment. **A,** Baseline venogram shows a tight stenosis of the SVC, which was crossed with a 0.035-inch guidewire from the femoral vein. The stenosis was predilated with a balloon and a large self-expanding stent was then placed to overcome recoil. **B,** Final venogram.

CH 59

CONCLUSION

Although the specific tools and techniques vary, the theme of endovascular intervention is similar across many vascular territories. In general, vascular stenting has become the mainstay of percutaneous revascularization for relief of symptoms. The challenge for the future will be to continue to improve the long-term durability of endovascular therapy and to explore its potential for preventing the complications of progressive vascular disease.

REFERENCES

1. Hirsch AT, Haskal ZJ, Hertzer NR, et al; American Association for Vascular Surgery; Society for Vascular Surgery; Society for Cardiovascular Angiography and Interventions; Society for Vascular Medicine and Biology; Society of Interventional Radiology; ACC/AHA Task Force on Practice Guidelines; American Association of Cardiovascular and Pulmonary Rehabilitation; National Heart, Lung, and Blood Institute; Society for Vascular Nursing; TransAtlantic Inter-Society Consensus; Vascular Disease Foundation: ACC/AHA 2005 guidelines for the management of patients with peripheral arterial disease (lower extremity, renal, mesenteric, and abdominal aortic): Executive summary a collaborative report from the American Association for Vascular Surgery/Society for Vascular Surgery, Society for Cardiovascular Angiography and Interventions, Society for Vascular Medicine and Biology, Society of Interventional Radiology, and the ACC/AHA Task Force on Practice Guidelines (Writing Committee to Develop Guidelines for the Management of Patients With Peripheral Arterial Disease) endorsed by the American Association of Cardiovascular and Pulmonary Rehabilitation; National Heart, Lung, and Blood Institute; Society for Vascular Nursing; TransAtlantic Inter-Society Consensus; and Vascular Disease Foundation. J Am Coll Cardiol 47:1239, 2006.

Peripheral Arterial Revascularization

2. Krajewski LP, Olin J: Atherosclerosis of the aorta and the lower extremities. In Young JR (ed): Peripheral Vascular Diseases. Chicago, Mosby–Year Book, 1991, p 183.
3. St. Goar FG, Joye JD, Laird JR: Percutaneous arterial aortoiliac intervention. J Interv Cardiol 14:533, 2001.
4. Bosch JL, Hunink MG: Meta-analysis of the results of percutaneous transluminal angioplasty and stent placement for aortoiliac occlusive disease. Radiology 204:87, 1994.
5. Timaran CH, Ohki T, Gargiulo NJ 3rd, et al: Iliac artery stenting in patients with poor distal runoff: Influence of concomitant infrainguinal arterial reconstruction. J Vasc Surg 38:479; discussion, 484, 2003.
6. Ponec D: Cordis Randomized Iliac Stent Project (CRISP). Presented at the 28th Annual Society of Interventional Radiology Meeting. Salt Lake City, March 27-April 1, 2003.
7. Henry M, Amor M, Ethevenot G, et al: Percutaneous endoluminal treatment of iliac occlusions: Long-term follow-up in 105 patients. J Endovasc Surg 5:228, 1998.

8. Muradin GS, Bosch JL, Stijnen T, Hunink MG.: Balloon dilation and stent implantation for treatment of femoropopliteal arterial disease: Meta-analysis. Radiology 221:137, 2001.
9. Schillinger M, Sabeti S, Loewe C, et al: Balloon angioplasty versus implantation of nitinol stents in the superficial femoral artery. N Engl J Med 354:1879, 2006.
10. Duda SH, Bosiers M, Lammer J, et al: Sirolimus-eluting versus bare nitinol stent for obstructive superficial femoral artery disease: The SIROCCO II trial. J Vasc Interv Radiol 16:331, 2005.
11. Scheinert D, Scheinert S, Sax J, et al: Prevalence and clinical impact of stent fractures after femoropopliteal stenting. J Am Coll Cardiol 45:312, 2005.
12. de Vries SO, Visser K, de Vries JA, et al: Intermittent claudication: Cost-effectiveness of revascularization versus exercise therapy. Radiology 222:25, 2002.
13. Hunink MG, Wong JB, Donaldson MC, et al: Revascularization for femoropopliteal disease. A decision and cost-effectiveness analysis. JAMA 274:165, 1995.
14. Adam DJ, Beard JD, Cleveland T, et al: Bypass versus angioplasty in severe ischaemia of the leg (BASIL): Multicentre, randomised controlled trial. Lancet 366:1925, 2005.
15. Sivananthan UM, Browne TF, Thorley PJ, Rees MR: Percutaneous transluminal angioplasty of the tibial arteries. Br J Surg 81:1282, 1994.
16. Varty K, Bolia A, Naylor AR, et al: Infrapopliteal percutaneous transluminal angioplasty: A safe and successful procedure. Eur J Vasc Endovasc Surg 9:341, 1995.
17. Dorros G, Jaff MR, Murphy KJ, Mathiak L: The acute outcome of tibioperoneal vessel angioplasty in 417 cases with claudication and critical limb ischemia. Cathet Cardiovasc Diagn 45:251, 1998.
18. Desgranges P, Kobeiter K, d'Audiffret A, et al: Acute occlusion of popliteal and/or tibial arteries: The value of percutaneous treatment. Eur J Vasc Endovasc Surg 20:138, 2000.
19. Soder HK, Manninen HI, Jaakkola P, et al: Prospective trial of infrapopliteal artery balloon angioplasty for critical limb ischemia: Angiographic and clinical results. J Vasc Interv Radiol 11:1021, 2000.
20. Dorros G, Jaff MR, Dorros AM, et al: Tibioperoneal (outflow lesion) angioplasty can be used as primary treatment in 235 patients with critical limb ischemia: Five-year follow-up. Circulation 104:2057, 2001.
21. Tsetis DK, Michalis LK, Rees MR, et al: Vibrational angioplasty in the treatment of chronic infrapopliteal arterial occlusions: preliminary experience. J Endovasc Ther 9:889, 2002.
22. Faglia E, Mantero M, Caminiti M, et al: Extensive use of peripheral angioplasty, particularly infrapopliteal, in the treatment of ischaemic diabetic foot ulcers: Clinical results of a multicentric study of 221 consecutive diabetic subjects. J Intern Med 252:225, 2002.
23. Faglia E, Dalla Paola L, Clerici G, et al: Peripheral angioplasty as the first-choice revascularization procedure in diabetic patients with critical limb ischemia: Prospective study of 993 consecutive patients hospitalized and followed between 1999 and 2003. Eur J Vasc Endovasc Surg 29:620, 2005.

Renal Artery Disease

24. Hansen KJ, Edwards MS, Craven TE, et al: Prevalence of renovascular disease in the elderly: A population-based study. J Vasc Surg 36:443, 2002.
25. Weber-Mzell D, Kotanko P, Schumacher M, et al: Coronary anatomy predicts presence or absence of renal artery stenosis. A prospective study in patients undergoing cardiac catheterization for suspected coronary artery disease. Eur Heart J 23:1684, 2002.

26. Safian RD, Textor SC: Renal-artery stenosis. N Engl J Med 344:431, 2001.

27. Rundback JH, Sacks D, Kent KC, et al; AHA Councils on Cardiovascular Radiology, High Blood Pressure Research, Kidney in Cardiovascular Disease, Cardio-Thoracic and Vascular Surgery, and Clinical Cardiology, and the Society of Interventional Radiology FDA Device Forum Committee. American Heart Association: Guidelines for the reporting of renal artery revascularization in clinical trials. American Heart Association. Circulation 106:1572, 2002.

28. Lederman R, Mendelsohn FO, Santos R, et al: Primary renal artery stenting: Characteristics and outcomes after 363 procedure. Am Heart J 142:314, 2001.

29. Subramanian R, White CJ, Rosenfield K, et al: Renal fractional flow reserve: A hemodynamic evaluation of moderate renal artery stenoses. Catheter Cardiovasc Interv 64:480, 2005.

30. Mitchell J, Subramanian R, Stewart R, et al: Pressure-derived renal fractional flow reserve with clinical outcomes following intervention [abstract]. Catheter Cardiovasc Interv 65:135, 2005.

31. Silva JA, Chan AW, White CJ, et al: Elevated brain natriuretic peptide predicts blood pressure response after stent revascularization in patients with renal artery stenosis. Circulation 111:328, 2005.

32. Radermacher J, Chavan A, Bleck J, et al: Use of Doppler ultrasonography to predict the outcome of therapy for renal-artery stenosis. N Engl J Med 344:410, 2001.

33. Zeller T, Frank U, Muller C, et al: Predictors of improved renal function after percutaneous stent-supported angioplasty of severe atherosclerotic ostial renal artery stenosis. Circulation 108:2244, 2003.

34. Watson P, Hadjipetrou P, Cox SV, et al: Effect of renal artery stenting on renal function and size in patients with atherosclerotic renovascular disease. Circulation 102:1671, 2000.

35. Muray S, Martin M, Amoedo ML, et al: Rapid decline in renal function reflects reversibility and predicts the outcome after angioplasty in renal artery stenosis. Am J Kidney Dis 39:60, 2002.

36. White CJ: Catheter-based therapy for atherosclerotic renal artery stenosis. Circulation 113:1464, 2006.

37. Leertouwer TC, Derkx FH, Pattynama PM, et al: Functional effects of renal artery stent placement on treated and contralateral kidneys. Kidney Int 62:574, 2002.

38. La Batide-Alanore A, Azizi M, Froissart M, et al: Split renal function outcome after renal angioplasty in patients with unilateral renal artery stenosis. J Am Soc Nephrol 12:1235, 2001.

Mesentenc Ischemia

39. Hansen KJ, Wilson DB, Craven TE, et al: Mesenteric artery disease in the elderly. J Vasc Surg 40:45, 2004.

40. Chow LC, Chan FP, Li KC: A comprehensive approach to MR imaging of mesenteric ischemia. Abdom Imaging 27:507, 2002.

41. Park WM, Cherry KJ Jr, Chua HK, et al: Current results of open revascularization for chronic mesenteric ischemia: A standard for comparison. J Vasc Surg 35:853, 2002.

42. Leke MA, Hood DB, Rowe VL, et al: Technical consideration in the management of chronic mesenteric ischemia. Am Surg 68:1088, 2002.

43. Cognet F, Ben Salem D, Dranssart M, et al: Chronic mesenteric ischemia: Imaging and percutaneous treatment. Radiographics 22:863; discussion, 879, 2002.

44. Matsumoto AH, Angle JF, Spinosa DJ, et al: Percutaneous transluminal angioplasty and stenting in the treatment of chronic mesenteric ischemia: Results and long-term follow-up. J Am Coll Surg 194(Suppl 1):S22, 2002.

45. Silva JA, White CJ, Collins TJ, et al: Endovascular therapy for chronic mesenteric ischemia. J Am Coll Cardiol 47:944, 2006.

Great Artery and Carotid Intervention

46. Eisenhauer AC: Subclavian and innominate revascularization: Surgical therapy versus catheter-based intervention. Curr Interv Cardiol Rep 2:101, 2000.

47. Eisenhauer AC, Shaw JA: Atherosclerotic subclavian artery disease and revascularization. In Abella G (ed): Peripheral Vascular Disease. Basic Diagnostic and Therapeutic Approaches. Philadelphia, Lippincott Williams & Wilkins, 2004, pp 283-294.

48. Amor M, Eid-Lidt G, Chati Z, Wilentz JR: Endovascular treatment of the subclavian artery: Stent implantation with or without predilatation. Catheter Cardiovasc Interv 63:364, 2004.

49. Schillinger M, Haumer M, Schillinger S, et al: Risk stratification for subclavian artery angioplasty: Is there an increased rate of restenosis after stent implantation? J Endovasc Ther 8:550, 2001.

50. Angelini P: Is angiography the gold standard to establish the severity of a carotid lesion? Does duplex doppler ultrasound compete with it? Catheter Cardiovasc Interv 52:16, 2001.

51. Rothwell PM: For severe carotid stenosis found on ultrasound, further arterial evaluation prior to carotid endarterectomy is unnecessary: The argument against. Stroke 34:1817; discussion, 1819, 2003.

52. Qureshi AI, Suri MF, Ali Z, et al: Role of conventional angiography in evaluation of patients with carotid artery stenosis demonstrated by Doppler ultrasound in general practice. Stroke 32:2287, 2001.

53. Back MR, Wilson JS, Rushing G, et al: Magnetic resonance angiography is an accurate imaging adjunct to duplex ultrasound scan in patient selection for carotid endarterectomy. J Vasc Surg 32:429; discussion, 439, 2000.

54. Johnston DC, Eastwood JD, Nguyen T, Goldstein LB: Contrast-enhanced magnetic resonance angiography of carotid arteries: Utility in routine clinical practice. Stroke 33:2834, 2002.

55. Fayed AM, White CJ, Ramee SR, et al: Carotid and cerebral angiography performed by cardiologists: Cerebrovascular complications. Catheter Cardiovasc Interv 55:277, 2002.

56. North American Symptomatic Carotid Endarterectomy Trial Collaborators: Beneficial effect of carotid endarterectomy in symptomatic patients with high-grade carotid stenosis. N Engl J Med 325:445, 1991.

57. Barnett HJ, Taylor DW, Eliasziw M, et al: Benefit of carotid endarterectomy in patients with symptomatic moderate or severe stenosis. North American Symptomatic Carotid Endarterectomy Trial Collaborators. N Engl J Med 339:1415, 1998.

58. Executive Committee for the Asymptomatic Carotid Atherosclerosis Study (ACAS): Endarterectomy for asymptomatic carotid artery stenosis. JAMA 273:1421, 1995.

59. Halliday A, Mansfield A, Marro J, et al; MRC Asymptomatic Carotid Surgery Trial (ACST) Collaborative Group: Prevention of disabling and fatal strokes by successful carotid endarterectomy in patients without recent neurological symptoms: Randomised controlled trial. Lancet 363:1491, 2004.

60. Wennberg D, Lucas FL, Birkmeyer JD, et al: Variation in carotid endarterectomy mortality in the Medicare population. JAMA 279:1278, 1998.

61. Rothwell PM, Slattery J, Warlow CP: A systematic review of the risks of stroke and death caused byendarterectomy for symptomatic carotid stenosis. Stroke 27:260, 1996.

62. Biller J, Feinberg WM, Castaldo JE, et al: Guidelines for carotid endarterectomy: A statement for healthcare professionals from a Special Writing Group of the Stroke Council, American Heart Association. Circulation 97:501, 1998.

63. Henry M, Amor M, Henry I, et al: Carotid stenting with cerebral protection: First clinical experience using the PercuSurge GuardWire system. J Endovasc Surg 6:321, 1999.

64. Grunwald IQ, Dorenbeck U, Axmann C, et al: (Proximal protection systems using carotid artery stent.) Radiologe 44:998, 2004.

65. Muller-Hulsbeck S, Jahnke T, Liess C, et al: Comparison of various cerebral protection devices used for carotid artery stent placement: An in vitro experiment. J Vasc Interv Radiol 14:613, 2003.

66. Gray W: Two-year composite endpoint results for the Archer Trials: Acculink for revascularization of carotids in high risk patients. Am J Cardiol 94(Suppl 6A): 62E, 2004.

67. Gray WA: A cardiologist in the carotids. J Am Coll Cardiol 43:1602, 2004.

68. White C, Iyer SS, Hopkins LN, et al: Carotid stenting with distal protection in high surgical risk patients: The BEACH trial 30 day results. Catheter Cardiovasc Interv 67:503, 2006.

69. Whitlow P: Security: More good data for protected carotid stenting in high-risk surgical patients. Available at: http://www.medscape.com/viewarticle/461721_print.

70. Ramee S, Higashida R: Evaluation of the Medtronic self-expanding carotid stent system with distal protection in the treatment of carotid artery stenosis. Am J Cardiol 94(Suppl 6A):61E, 2004.

71. Yadav JS, Wholey MH, Kuntz RE, et al; Stenting and Angioplasty with Protection in Patients at High Risk for Endarterectomy Investigators: Protected carotid-artery stenting versus endarterectomy in high-risk patients. N Engl J Med 351:1493, 2004.

72. Mas JL, Chatellier G, Beyssen B, et al: Endarterectomy versus stenting in patients with symptomatic severe carotid stenosis. N Engl J Med 355:1660, 2006.

73. Furlan AJ: Carotid-artery stenting—case open or closed? N Engl J Med 355:1726, 2006.

74. SPACE Collaborative Group; Ringleb PA, Allenberg J, Bruckmann H, et al: 30-day results from the SPACE trial of stent-protected angioplasty versus carotid endarterectomy in symptomatic patients: a randomised non-inferiority trial. Lancet 368:1239, 2006.

75. Naylor AR: SPACE: Not the final frontier. Lancet 368:1215, 2006.

76. Coward LJ, Featherstone RL, Brown MM: Safety and efficacy of endovascular treatment of carotid artery stenosis compared with carotid endarterectomy. A Cochrane systematic review of the randomized evidence. Stroke 36:905, 2005.

77. Hass WK, Fields WS, North RR, et al: Joint study of extracranial arterial occlusion. II. Arteriography, techniques, sites, and complications. JAMA 203:961, 1968.

78. Cartlidge NE, Whisnant JP, Elveback LR: Carotid and vertebral-basilar transient cerebral ischemic attacks. A community study, Rochester, Minnesota. Mayo Clin Proc 52:117, 1977.

79. Kline RA, Berguer R: Vertebral artery reconstruction. Ann Vasc Surg 7:497, 1993.

80. Jenkins JS, White CJ, Ramee SR, et al: Vertebral artery stenting. Catheter Cardiovasc Interv 54:1, 2001.

81. Kasirajan K, Gray B, Beavers FP, et al: Rheolytic thrombectomy in the management of acute and subacute limb-threatening ischemia. J Vasc Interv Radiol 12:413, 2001.

Superior Vena Cava Syndrome

82. Nicholson AA, Ettles DF, Arnold A, et al: Treatment of malignant superior vena cava obstruction: Metal stents or radiation therapy. J Vasc Interv Radiol 8:781, 1997.

83. Schifferdecker B, Shaw JA, Piemonte TC, Eisenhauer AC: Nonmalignant superior vena cava syndrome: Pathophysiology and management. Catheter Cardiovasc Interv 65:416, 2005.

84. Kee ST, Kinoshita L, Razavi MK, et al: Superior vena cava syndrome: treatment with catheter-directed thrombolysis and endovascular stent placement. Radiology 206:187, 1998.

General

85. Conlon PJ, Little MA, Pieper K, Mark DB: Severity of renal vascular disease predicts mortality in patients undergoing coronary angiography. Kidney Int 60:1490, 2001.

86. Reyes R, et al: Treatment of chronic iliac artery occlusions with guide wire recanalization and primary stent placement. J Vasc Interv Radiol 8:1049, 1997.

CH 59

Endovascular Treatment of Noncoronary Obstructive Vascular Disease

1546

87. Dyet JF: Endovascular stents in the arterial system—Current status. Clin Radiol 52:83, 1997.

88. Murphy TP, Khwaja AA, Webb MS: Aortoiliac stent placement in patients treated for intermittent claudication. J Vasc Interv Radiol 9:421, 1998.

89. Tetteroo E, et al: Randomised comparison of primary stent placement versus primary angioplasty followed by selective stent placement in patients with iliac artery occlusive disease. Dutch iliac stent trial study group. Lancet 351:1153, 1998.

90. Powell RJ, et al: The durability of endovascular treatment of multisegment iliac occlusive disease. J Vasc Surg 31:1178, 2000.

91. Saha S, et al: Stenting for localised arterial stenoses in the aorto-iliac segment. Eur J Vasc Endovasc Surg 22:37, 2001.

92. Timaran CH, et al: External iliac and common iliac artery angioplasty and stenting in men and women. J Vasc Surg 34:440, 2001.

93. Haulon S, et al: Percutaneous reconstruction of the aortoiliac bifurcation with the "kissing stents" technique: Long-term follow-up in 106 patients. J Endovasc Ther 9:363, 2002.

94. Siskin GP, et al: Results of iliac artery stent placement in patients younger than 50 years of age. J Vasc Interv Radiol 13:785, 2002.

95. Mohamed F, et al: Outcome of "kissing stents" for aortoiliac atherosclerotic disease, including the effect on the non-diseased contralateral iliac limb. Cardiovasc Intervent Radiol 25:472, 2002.

96. Reekers JA, et al: Results of a European multicentre iliac stent trial with a flexible balloon expandable stent. Eur J Vasc Endovasc Surg 24:511, 2002.

97. Funovics MA, et al: Predictors of long-term results after treatment of iliac artery obliteration by transluminal angioplasty and stent deployment. Cardiovasc Intervent Radiol 25:397, 2002.

98. Gray BH, et al: High incidence of restenosis/reocclusion of stents in the percutaneous treatment of long-segment superficial femoral artery disease after suboptimal angioplasty. J Vasc Surg 25:74, 1997.

99. Martin DR, et al: Percutaneous transluminal angioplasty of infrainguinal vessels. Ann Vasc Surg 13:184, 1999.

100. Kessel DO, et al: Endovascular stent-grafts for superficial femoral artery disease: Results of 1-year follow up. J Vasc Interv Radiol 10:289, 1999.

101. Conroy RM, et al: Angioplasty and stent placement in chronic occlusion of the superficial femoral artery: Technique and results. J Vasc Interv Radiol 11:1009, 2000.

102. Cheng SW, Ting AC, Wong J: Endovascular stenting of superficial femoral artery stenosis and occlusions: Results and risk factor analysis. Cardiovasc Surg 9:133, 2001.

103. Gordon IL, et al: Three-year outcome of endovascular treatment of superficial femoral artery occlusion. Arch Surg 136:221, 2001.

104. Scheinert D, et al: Excimer laser-assisted recanalization of long, chronic superficial femoral artery occlusions. J Endovasc Ther 8:150, 2001.

105. Lofberg AM, et al: Percutaneous transluminal angioplasty of the femoropopliteal arteries in limbs with chronic critical lower limb ischemia. J Vasc Surg 34:114, 2001.

106. Bauermeister G: Endovascular stent-grafting in the treatment of superficial femoral artery occlusive disease. J Endovasc Ther 8:315, 2001.

107. Duda SH, et al: Sirolimus-eluting stents for the treatment of obstructive superficial femoral artery disease: Six-month results. Circulation 106:1505, 2002.

108. Steinkamp HJ, et al: Short (1-10 cm) superficial femoral artery occlusions: Results of treatment with excimer laser angioplasty. Cardiovasc Intervent Radiol 25:388, 2002.

109. Gray BH, et al: Complex endovascular treatment for critical limb ischemia in poor surgical candidates: A pilot study. J Endovasc Ther 9:599, 2002.

110. Jamsen TS, et al: Long-term outcome of patients with claudication after balloon angioplasty of the femoropopliteal arteries. Radiology 225:345, 2002.

111. Cho L, et al: Superficial femoral artery occlusion: Nitinol stents achieve better flow and reduce the need for medications than balloon angioplasty alone. J Invasive Cardiol 15:198, 2003.

112. Becquemin JP, et al: Systematic versus selective stent placement after superficial femoral artery balloon angioplasty: A multicenter prospective randomized study. J Vasc Surg 37:487, 2003.

113. Jahnke T, et al: Hemobahn stent-grafts for treatment of femoropopliteal arterial obstructions: midterm results of a prospective trial. J Vasc Interv Radiol 14:41, 2003.

114. White CJ, et al: Renal artery stent placement: Utility in lesions difficult to treat with balloon angioplasty. J Am Coll Cardiol 30:1445, 1997.

115. Blum U, et al: Treatment of ostial renal-artery stenoses with vascular endoprostheses after unsuccessful balloon angioplasty. N Engl J Med 336:459, 1997.

116. Tuttle KR, et al: Treatment of atherosclerotic ostial renal artery stenosis with the intravascular stent. Am J Kidney Dis 32:611, 1998.

117. Henry M, et al: Stents in the treatment of renal artery stenosis: Long-term follow-up. J Endovasc Surg 6:42, 1999.

118. van de Ven PJ, et al: Arterial stenting and balloon angioplasty in ostial atherosclerotic renovascular disease: A randomised trial. Lancet 353:282, 1999.

119. Dorros G, et al: Four-year follow-up of Palmaz-Schatz stent revascularization as treatment for atherosclerotic renal artery stenosis. Circulation 98:642, 1998.

CH 59

CHAPTER 60

Scope of the Problem, 1547

Medical Therapy of Acute
Coronary Syndromes, 1548
Antiplatelet Drugs, 1549
Aspirin, 1549
Glycoprotein IIb/IIIa Blockers, 1550
Beta-Adrenergic Blocking
   Agents, 1551
Angiotensin-Converting Enzyme
   Inhibitors, 1551
Insulin, 1552

Heart Failure, 1553
Overview, 1553
Diabetes-Specific Factors Related to
   CHF, 1554
CHF Caused by Diabetes, 1555
Other Causes of CHF in
   Diabetes, 1555

Reducing the Risk of Heart
Failure in Diabetes, 1556
Glycemic Control, 1556
Medical Therapy to Treat or Prevent
   Heart Failure in Diabetic
   Patients, 1556

Treating Diabetes in Patients
with CHD, ACS, or CHF, 1557
Medical Therapy, 1557
Coronary Revascularization, 1557

References, 1558

Diabetes and Heart Disease

Richard W. Nesto

SCOPE OF THE PROBLEM

People with diabetes have an increased prevalence of atherosclerosis and coronary heart disease (CHD) and experience higher morbidity and mortality after acute coronary syndrome and myocardial infarction (MI) than people without diabetes (Fig. 60-1). Analysis of data collected for the Organization to Assess Strategies for Ischemic Syndromes (OASIS) Registry, showed that diabetes significantly increased all-cause death and the incidence of new MI, stroke, and heart failure during a 2-year mean follow-up in patients who were hospitalized for unstable angina or non-Q-wave MI.[1] A similar study of patients hospitalized with a confirmed MI, found that diabetes was associated with an adjusted hazard ratio for mortality of 1.7 (95 percent confidence interval [CI] 1.2 to 2.3) compared with patients without diabetes and no previous MI.[2] Diabetes also appears to be a major cause of the higher rate of both short- and long-term mortality observed in women hospitalized with acute MI compared to men.[3] In general, diabetes confers as much additional risk as having had a previous MI, and the number of cardiovascular events associated with diabetes is growing. In New York City over the decade from 1989 to 1999, the percentage of all acute MIs occurring in patients with diabetes increased from 21 percent to 36 percent, and the number of hospital days associated with MI increased 51 percent despite a reduction in the number of hospital days associated with MI in the overall population.[4] Similarly, a recent examination of the reasons for the dramatic decline in CHD mortality in the United Kingdom since 1981 noted that decreased mortality occurred despite adverse trends in obesity, physical activity, and diabetes. Over the 19 years of the study, diabetes increased 66 percent, resulting in approximately 2900 diabetes-related additional CHD deaths.[5]

In the past, at least part of the increased cardiovascular risk associated with diabetes resulted from a failure to apply standard clinical measures known to improve outcome following cardiovascular events in patients without diabetes. For example, patients with diabetes were frequently denied beta blockers post-MI because of concern that use of these drugs could mask hypoglycemia and compromise glycemic control. Recent evidence suggests that MI patients with diabetes may actually have a better response to standard treatments than patients without diabetes. In a large registry study in Germany, total hospital mortality of diabetic patients hospitalized for MI declined from 29 percent in 1999 to 17 percent in 2001, and mortality within 24 hours of admission fell from 16 percent to 4 percent over the same period.[6] This reduction was associated with increased use of therapeutic approaches (e.g., coronary angiography, stenting, antiplatelet therapy) in diabetic patients during this period. Similarly, a study that compared invasive and noninvasive strategies for treatment of unstable coronary artery disease (CAD) in diabetic and nondiabetic patients noted that invasive treatment resulted in a greater benefit in diabetic (odds ratio [OR] = 0.61) versus nondiabetic patients

(OR = 0.72), although mortality and reinfarction after 12 months were still higher in diabetics, regardless of treatment.[7] A retrospective analysis of data from diabetic patients with ST-segment elevation myocardial infarction (STEMI) treated with reteplase or the combination of reteplase and abciximab showed that—although combination therapy significantly reduced the incidence of reinfarction, recurrent ischemia, and urgent revascularization—diabetic patients continued to have a worse outcome from MI than nondiabetic patients.[8]

Traditional CHD risk factors such as hypertension, dyslipidemia, and excess weight and obesity cluster in patients with impaired glucose tolerance or diabetes (see discussion of metabolic syndrome in Chap. 43), but this clustering cannot account for all of the increased risk in these patients (Fig. 60-2). In addition to the traditional risk factors associated with CHD and heart failure, a number of diabetes-specific risk factors contribute to the increased morbidity and mortality of CAD. For example, patients with diabetes have lipid-rich atherosclerotic plaque that is more vulnerable to rupture than plaque found in patients without diabetes.[9,10] Analysis of carotid plaques taken from diabetic patients undergoing endarterectomy indicates that they contain more inflammatory cell types and inflammatory markers and have a higher lipid content than plaques from nondiabetic patients. This enhanced vascular inflammatory reaction may result from overexpression of receptor for advanced glycation end products (RAGE), which correlates linearly with hemoglobin A1c (HbA1C) levels.[11] RAGE can enhance matrix metalloproteinase activity that can destabilize plaques. Additionally, platelets harvested from patients with diabetes exhibit enhanced aggregation and increased expression of activation-dependent adhesion molecules, such as glycoprotein (GP) IIb/IIIa and CD40 ligand, factors which contribute to thrombus formation.[12,13]

Changes in vascular function may also contribute to the poorer outcomes in diabetes. No reflow following successful percutaneous recanalization of an infarct-related coronary artery occurs more commonly in the presence of diabetes and/or

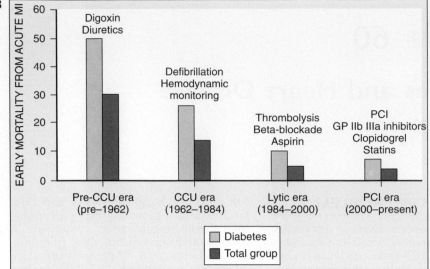

FIGURE 60–1 People with diabetes have an increased prevalence of atherosclerosis and coronary heart disease and experience higher morbidity and mortality after acute coronary syndrome and myocardial infarction than people without diabetes. CCU = coronary care unit; GP = glycoprotein; PCI = percutaneous coronary intervention. *(Adapted from Braunwald E: Cardiovascular medicine at the turn of the millennium: Triumphs, concerns, and opportunities. New Engl J Med 337:1360-1369, 1997.)*

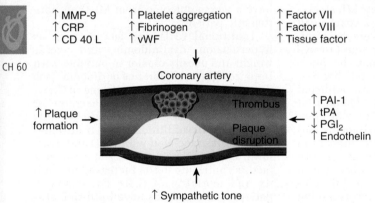

FIGURE 60–2 Traditional coronary heart disease risk factors such as hypertension, dyslipidemia, and excess weight and obesity cluster in patients with impaired glucose tolerance or diabetes, but this clustering cannot account for all of the increased risk in these patients. CD 40 L = CD 40 ligand; CRP = C-reactive protein; MMP = matrix metalloproteinase; PAI-1 = plasmin activator inhibitor type 1; PGI_2 = prostacyclin; tPA = tissue type plasminogen activator; vWF = von Willebrand factor.

patients include hypertension, left ventricular hypertrophy, and valvular heart disease. Although diabetes is an important risk factor for CHF, it rarely occurs independently and, in fact, appears to act synergistically with other risk factors.

The emerging recognition that CHD involves a proinflammatory state suggests that the increased plasma C-reactive protein levels seen in people with diabetes reflect increased risk.[20] Other diabetes-specific changes that occur include diabetic cardiomyopathy, which impairs myocardial performance and renders the myocardium more susceptible to and less able to recover from ischemia, and diabetic autonomic neuropathy, which results in sympathovagal imbalance and contributes to cardiovascular mortality.[21] Advanced glycation end products (AGEs) may contribute to many of these diabetes-specific changes (see Chap. 43).

MEDICAL THERAPY OF ACUTE CORONARY SYNDROMES

A history of diabetes is important in determining the treatment of patients during and following an acute MI. However, patients with acute coronary syndromes (ACS) commonly have undiagnosed diabetes and impaired glucose metabolism. A study of 3266 patients scheduled for coronary angiography found a prevalence of previously undiagnosed diabetes of nearly 18 percent.[22] Patients with acute MI have an even higher percentage (25 to 31 percent) of previously undiagnosed diabetes.[23]

The negative relation between diabetes and the prognosis after MI extends to patients with elevated blood glucose at the time of admission. Several studies have shown this relation. For example, 1664 consecutively hospitalized patients with an acute MI were categorized by history of diabetes and by whether they had a blood glucose concentration greater than 198 mg/dl (Fig. 60-3).[24] The patients who had a history of diabetes or who were hyperglycemic had a significantly elevated risk of in-hospital mortality compared with those without either condition. In a similar study, patients with acute hyperglycemia, defined as plasma glucose >198 mg/dl, on admission for acute MI had a higher in-hospital mortality rate than normoglycemic patients (16 percent versus 6 percent; $p < 0.001$) regardless of diabetes status.[25] In those patients who received percutaneous coronary intervention (PCI), hyperglycemia was also associated with a higher incidence of no reflow during PCI (21 percent versus 12 percent; $p < 0.001$). In a study that compared plasma glucose at admission and fasting plasma glucose within 8 hours of admission as predictors of 30-day mortality in nondiabetic patients admitted for acute MI, fasting plasma glucose was shown to be the better predictor of mortality.[26] The OR for 30-day mortality of patients with a normal admission plasma glucose but an elevated fasting plasma glucose was 9.6 compared to patients with normal admission and fasting plasma glucose levels (Fig. 60-4). The equivalent OR for patients with elevated plasma glucose at admission but normal fasting glucose was 0.71. In both diabetic and nondiabetic patients, plasma glucose at time of admission correlates with creatinine kinase activity, an index of myocardial damage.[27] The greater degree of myocardial damage experienced by patients with hyperglycemia undoubtedly contributes to the lower post-MI survival rate in these patients.

hyperglycemia and may contribute to left ventricular dysfunction. No reflow in this circumstance probably results from platelet-endothelial cell interactions that impair microvascular function and decrease myocardial blood flow. Patients with diabetes have increased levels of plasminogen activator inhibitor type 1 (PAI-1) in plasma and in atheromas.[14,15] Elevated tissue PAI-1 could decrease fibrinolysis, increase thrombus formation, and accelerate plaque formation. Other vascular changes, including increased endothelin activity and reduced prostacyclin and nitric oxide activity, lead to abnormal control of blood flow.[16,17]

Diabetes also increases the risk of heart failure. Patients with diabetes are two to five times more likely to develop heart failure than those without diabetes,[18] and, following development of heart failure, diabetic patients have higher mortality and heart failure-related morbidity.[19] Diabetic and nondiabetic subjects share fundamental causes of heart failure. In both groups, previous MI and the resultant loss of contracting myocardium cause most chronic congestive heart failure (CHF). Other contributors to CHF in diabetic

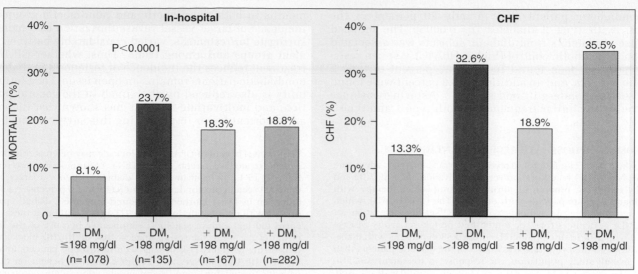

FIGURE 60–3 The negative relation between diabetes mellitus (DM) and the prognosis after MI extends to patients with elevated blood glucose at the time of admission. CHF = congestive heart failure. (**Left panel** *adapted from Wahab NN, Cowden EA, Pearce NJ, on behalf of the ICONs Investigators: Is blood glucose an independent predictor of mortality in acute myocardial infarction in the thrombolytic era? J Am Coll Cardiol 40:1748-1754, 2002.*)

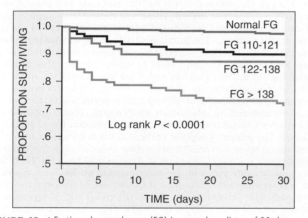

FIGURE 60–4 Fasting plasma glucose (FG) is a good predictor of 30-day mortality in nondiabetic patients admitted for acute MI. (*Adapted from Suleiman M, Hammerman H, Boulos M, et al: Fasting glucose is an important independent risk factor for 30-day mortality in patients with acute myocardial infarction: A prospective study. Circulation 111:754-760, 2005.*)

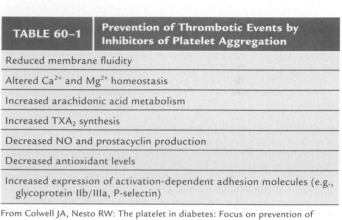

TABLE 60–1	Prevention of Thrombotic Events by Inhibitors of Platelet Aggregation
Reduced membrane fluidity	
Altered Ca^{2+} and Mg^{2+} homeostasis	
Increased arachidonic acid metabolism	
Increased TXA_2 synthesis	
Decreased NO and prostacyclin production	
Decreased antioxidant levels	
Increased expression of activation-dependent adhesion molecules (e.g., glycoprotein IIb/IIIa, P-selectin)	

From Colwell JA, Nesto RW: The platelet in diabetes: Focus on prevention of ischemic events. Diabetes Care 26:2181-2188, 2003.

The presence of the metabolic syndrome worsens outcome following an MI. In a group of 633 consecutive, unselected patients hospitalized for MI, 46 percent were found to meet the National Cholesterol Education Adult Treatment Panel III criteria for diagnosis of metabolic syndrome.[28] In multivariate analysis, the presence of metabolic syndrome was a strong independent predictor of heart failure. Based on predictive analysis of the components of the metabolic syndrome, hyperglycemia was the major determinant.

Antiplatelet Drugs

Studies have consistently shown that patients with either type 1 or type 2 diabetes have enhanced platelet aggregation in response to a variety of agonists.[12] Enhanced aggregability results in part from increased production of thromboxane, altered calcium and magnesium homeostasis, and increased expression of activation-dependent adhesion molecules. Endothelial dysfunction, characterized by decreased production of nitric oxide and prostacyclin, is common in diabetic individuals and enhances platelet aggregation and adhesiveness in vivo.[12] Thus, agents directed at inhibiting platelet aggregation in vivo consistently reduce the incidence of thrombotic events in nondiabetic and diabetic individuals (Table 60-1).

Aspirin

In the Early Treatment of Diabetic Retinopathy Study (ETDRS), patients with type 1 or type 2 diabetes randomly assigned to aspirin, 650 mg/day, had a significantly lowered risk of MI without incurring an increase in the risk of vitreous or retinal bleeding, even in patients with retinopathy.[29] The Hypertension Optimal Treatment (HOT) trial confirmed this benefit in 1501 diabetic subjects who experienced a significant 15 percent reduction in cardiovascular events and a 36 percent reduction in MI while being treated with aspirin, 75 mg/day.[29] This cardiovascular benefit resembled that seen in the nondiabetic cohort. The American Diabetes Association currently recommends enteric-coated aspirin (81 to 325 mg/day) for (1) secondary prevention in men and women with diabetes and evidence of macrovascular disease and (2) primary prevention in persons with type 1 or type 2 diabetes and additional coronary risk factors.[29]

Recently the issue of aspirin resistance has been addressed in the diabetic patient.[20-32] A study that compared platelet response to aspirin in patients with type 2 diabetes and nondiabetics demonstrated that aspirin, 150 mg, taken for 1 week reduced platelet adhesiveness in 69 percent of the nondiabetic patients but in only 29 percent of the patients with type 2 diabetes ($p = 0.0006$). The reduced response of platelets from diabetic subjects was associated with poor metabolic control (higher HbA1C). Aspirin resistance has also been found in 19 to 22 percent of type 2 diabetic patients, and an additional 16.9 percent were found to be semiresponders in one study.[31-32] Aspirin resistance occurred with similar frequency in both type 1 and type 2 diabetic patients.[32]

ADENOSINE DIPHOSPHATE RECEPTOR ANTAGONISTS

Ticlopidine and clopidogrel irreversibly block platelet adenosine diphosphate (ADP) receptors, preventing activation of GP IIb/IIIa and thereby inhibiting binding of fibrinogen. Antiplatelet therapy with clopidogrel benefits patients with diabetes. The CAPRIE trial, which compared outcomes in patients with non-ST-segment elevation MI (NSTEMI), ischemic stroke, or established peripheral artery disease treated with aspirin or clopidogrel, enrolled 3866 patients with diabetes.[33] Although the event rate was higher in the diabetic patients than in the overall study population, the response to treatment was also better. The event rate for the primary endpoint (vascular death, ischemic stroke, MI, or rehospitalization for ischemia or bleeding) was 17.7 percent for diabetic patients treated with aspirin and 15.6 percent for those randomized to clopidogrel, a significant relative risk reduction of 12.5 percent.

The Clopidogrel in Unstable Angina to Prevent Recurrent Events (CURE) study tested clopidogrel plus aspirin against aspirin alone in patients with unstable angina or non-Q-wave MI. After 9 months the incidence of the primary composite endpoint (cardiovascular death, nonfatal MI, or stroke) was reduced in the clopidogrel plus aspirin group by 20 percent.[34] Subgroup analysis showed that this effect extended to the patients with diabetes.

In the Clopidogrel for the Reduction of Events During Observation (CREDO) trial, 2116 patients who were undergoing elective PCI or were deemed to have a high likelihood of PCI were randomized to receive either a 300 mg clopidogrel loading dose 24 hours before the procedure followed by 75 mg/day for 28 days or placebo.[35] Both groups received aspirin. The endpoint of the study was 1-year incidence of the composite of death, MI, or stroke. In the clopidogrel treatment arm, 27.5 percent of the patients were diabetic. A subanalysis showed that a benefit of clopidogrel for reducing the risk of the endpoint was present in the nondiabetic group (relative risk reduction [RRR] = 32 percent; 95 percent CI 47.8 to 0.060) but did not extend to patients with diabetes specifically (RRR = 11.2 percent; 95 percent CI 46.2 to 46.8).

Glycoprotein IIb/IIIa Blockers

These potent antiplatelet agents have improved outcomes in patients with unstable angina and non-Q-wave infarction and have reduced the incidence of acute ischemic events by 35 to 50 percent in patients undergoing PCI.[36] At least one of the GP IIb/IIIa inhibitors, abciximab, reduced long-term mortality.[37] In general, these agents appear to have equal or better efficacy in diabetic than nondiabetic patients, although most studies lack sufficient power to evaluate this interaction fully.

Four placebo-controlled trials of the use of GP IIb/IIIa blockade during PCI included detailed outcome data for the diabetic subgroups.[36] Three studies (the Evaluation of c7E3 for Prevention of Ischemic Complications [EPIC], Evaluation in PTCA to Improve Long-term Outcome with abciximab GP IIb/IIIa blockade [EPILOG], and Evaluation of Platelet Inhibition in STENTing [EPISTENT]) evaluated abciximab, and the fourth (Enhanced Suppression of the Platelet IIb/IIIa Receptor with Integrilin Therapy [ESPRIT]) tested eptifibatide. The magnitude of the reduction in acute ischemic events (death, MI, or urgent revascularization occurring within 30 days) in the active treatment group compared with the placebo group was similar in both diabetic (21 to 67 percent reduction) and nondiabetic patients (30 to 51 percent reduction). This treatment effect was durable, as indicated by the similar reductions in death or MI at 6

months in both the diabetic and nondiabetic groups. The incidence of target vessel revascularization at 6 months, a surrogate for restenosis, varied considerably between treatment groups and among trials. Thus, whether GP IIb/IIIa treatment reduces the incidence of restenosis in diabetic or nondiabetic patients remains an open issue. Long-term mortality is also reduced by abciximab in the general population, and multivariate analysis has shown that diabetes is an important factor in predicting this survival benefit.[37]

The survival benefit of GP IIb/IIIa blockade may be greater in diabetic patients treated with stents. In EPISTENT, 1-year mortality was reduced from 4.1 to 1.2 percent in stented, diabetic patients, a larger benefit than that seen in the nondiabetic group (1.9 to 1.0 percent).[38] A similar reduction in 1-year mortality was found in stented, diabetic patients treated with eptifibatide in the ESPRIT trial.[39] Although these differences did not achieve statistical significance because of the limited power of the study, the results suggest that GP IIb/IIIa blockade neutralizes the mortality risk usually seen in diabetic patients following PCI. GP IIb/IIIa blockers also confer a survival benefit on diabetic patients treated for non-ST-segment elevation acute coronary syndromes (ACS). A meta-analysis of six major studies involving 6458 diabetic patients showed a reduction in 30-day mortality from 6.2 percent in the placebo group to 4.8 percent in the treated group ($p = 0.007$).[40] No benefit was seen in the 23,072 nondiabetic patients.

Although the efficacy of GP IIb/IIIa blockade had been demonstrated in retrospective diabetic subsets of clinical trials, until recently no data from a large, randomized trial of these agents in diabetic patients was available. The Intracoronary Stenting and Antithrombotic Regimen: Is Abciximab a Superior Way to Eliminate Elevated Thrombotic Risk in Diabetics (ISAR-SWEET) study addressed this deficit by recruiting 701 diabetic patients with CAD who underwent an elective PCI with bare metal stents after pretreatment (>2 hours prior to the procedure) with clopidogrel, 600 mg.[41] After pretreatment, the patients were randomized to abciximab (0.25 mg/kg bolus, followed by 0.125 µg/kg/min [maximum of 10 µg/min] infusion for 12 hours) or placebo. The primary endpoint of the study was composite incidence of death or MI at 1 year. The secondary endpoint was frequency of angiographic restenosis (diameter of stenosis = 50 percent). There was no significant difference in the two treatment groups with regard to the primary endpoint. In contrast, the incidence of angiographic restenosis was 28.9 percent in the abciximab group and 37.8 percent in patients treated with placebo ($p = 0.01$). These findings suggest that abciximab reduces the risk of restenosis in diabetic patients who receive bare metal stents.

A recent study has also assessed the efficacy of the GP IIb/IIIa blocker eptifibatide in 2064 high-risk patients, defined by age, diabetes, elevated cardiac markers, and recent STEMI or unstable angina, and low-risk patients undergoing nonurgent coronary stent implantation.[42] In both risk groups, patients were randomized to eptifibatide or placebo. After 1 year of treatment, the composite endpoint of death or MI was seen in 15.9 percent of the placebo patients and 8 percent of the eptifibatide patients in the high-risk group. In contrast, the primary endpoint occurred in 9 percent of the placebo patients and 8.1 percent of the eptifibatide patients in the low-risk group. Thus, the greatest benefit of eptifibatide therapy during stent placement is seen in the high-risk patients.

Part of the increased risk of thrombotic events in diabetic patients stems from their altered platelet function, including altered arachidonic acid metabolism and increased expression of activation-dependent adhesion molecules such as GP IIb/IIIa, resulting in enhanced platelet aggregation.[12] This diabetic thrombocytopathy may explain, in part, the greater effect of GP IIb/IIIa blockers in diabetic patients compared with nondiabetic patients. GP IIb/IIIa blockade may also improve microvascular dysfunction in ACS patients,[43] although the mechanism of this platelet-endothelial interaction has not yet been elucidated.

DIRECT THROMBIN INHIBITORS

Bivalirudin, a synthetic analogue of hirudin, an anticoagulant that is found in the saliva of the medicinal leech, directly inhibits thrombin by specifically binding to both the catalytic site and the anion-binding sites of circulating and clot-bound thrombin, thus inhibiting the cleavage of fibrinogen into fibrin monomers. In the Randomized Evaluation in PCI Linking Angiomax to reduced Clinical Events (REPLACE-2) trial, 6010 patients undergoing urgent or elective PCI received intravenous

CH 60

bivalirudin (0.75 mg/kg bolus, 1.75 mg/kg /hour for the duration of PCI) with provisional GP IIb/IIIa inhibition or heparin (65 U/kg bolus) with planned GP IIb/IIIa inhibition.[44,45] Both groups also received daily aspirin and a thienopyridine for at least 30 days after the PCI. The primary outcome measures were incidence of death, MI, or repeat vascularization within 6 months and death by 12 months after enrollment. The diabetic subgroup of REPLACE-2 consisted of 1624 diabetic patients.[45] Compared with nondiabetic patients, diabetic patients had higher mortality at 1 year (3.06 percent versus 1.85 percent; p = 0.004). There was no difference in the incidence of short-term or long-term ischemic events among the diabetic patients in the two treatment arms, suggesting that bivalirudin is equally effective in diabetic and nondiabetic patients. Patients treated with bivalirudin and provisional GP IIb/IIIa inhibitors experienced a significant reduction in minor bleeding events.

Beta-Adrenergic Blocking Agents

Beta-adrenergic blocking agents (beta blockers) reduce mortality and reinfarction in patients with MI and have recently become a routinely accepted treatment in the diabetic subgroup of this population. In the past, the use of beta blockers was sometimes avoided in diabetic patients because of the potential of these drugs to mask hypoglycemic symptoms, precipitate glucose intolerance, inhibit the release of insulin, adversely affect the plasma lipid profile, and precipitate development of diabetes in patients with CAD who were not previously diabetic.[46] However, several studies of diabetic patients treated with beta blockers following MI indicate that use of these drugs reduces mortality and may provide benefit that exceeds that seen in nondiabetic patients. In a recent retrospective, population-based Canadian study that used the Saskatchewan Health Databases to assess outcome in diabetic patients who were admitted for MI, use of beta blockers within 30 days of discharge was associated with fewer deaths than in a control cohort that had not used beta blockers (18.5 percent versus 38.5 percent (p < 0.001) although there was no improvement in survival in a multivariate analysis.[47] A more definitive answer regarding the use of beta blockers in the diabetic population will be provided by the The PeriOperative Ischemic Evaluation (POISE) trial.[48] This clinical outcomes trial that compares the efficacy of metoprolol and placebo for reducing cardiovascular events following noncardiac surgery has already recruited 6300 patients, 30 percent of whom have diabetes.

The metabolic issues associated with early-generation beta blockers may not apply to the noncardioselective beta blocker carvedilol that, in addition to being an antiarrhythmic drug, is also an alpha-1 blocker with antiinflammatory and antioxidant properties.[49] In the Glycemic Effects in Diabetes Mellitus: Carvdeilol-Metoprolol Comparison in Hypertensives (GEMINI) trial, patients with documented type 2 diabetes and hypertension who were taking a stable dose of either an angiotensin receptor blocker or and angiotensin-converting enzyme (ACE) inhibitor were randomized to receive either carvedilol (maximum dose 25 mg twice daily; n = 498) or metoprolol (maximum dose 200 mg twice daily; n = 737).[50] Patients were treated to a blood pressure goal and then maintained for 5 months. Although the degree of blood pressure control was similar with both beta blockers, HbA1C increased significantly with metoprolol but not with carvedilol. Similarly, insulin sensitivity increased significantly with carvedilol but not with metoprolol. These findings suggest that carvedilol may be an effective antihypertensive agent for diabetic patients when used in combination with renin-angiotensin system inhibitors.

The greater relative benefit of beta blockers in diabetic patients may derive from several factors. Beta blockers can help restore sympathovagal balance in diabetic patients with autonomic neuropathy and may decrease fatty acid

utilization within the myocardium, thus reducing oxygen demand. However, despite the continuing growth of evidence regarding their efficacy and safety in the diabetic patient, beta blockers continue to be underprescribed in this group.[51]

Angiotensin-Converting Enzyme Inhibitors

ACE inhibitors reduce infarct size, limit ventricular remodeling, improve survival after myocardial infarction, and may be of particular benefit in patients with diabetes.[52] A post hoc analysis of one thrombolytic trial (Grupo Italiano per lo Studio della Sopravivenza nell'Infarto Miocardico-3 [GISSI-3]) revealed that early administration of lisinopril in the setting of acute MI reduced 6-week and 6-month mortality comparatively more in diabetic versus nondiabetic patients (30 versus 5 percent reduction at 6 weeks and 20 versus 0 percent at 6 months).[53] Another retrospective analysis, the Trandolapril Cardiac Evaluation (TRACE) study, compared the effect of oral trandolapril versus placebo in anterior MI in patients with and without diabetes.[54] Patients with diabetes experienced a greater relative improvement in survival over 5 years of follow-up than the nondiabetic cohort. Furthermore, ACE inhibition reduced by nearly 50 percent the risk of sudden death, reinfarction, and progression of CHF in patients with diabetes. In a more recent retrospective study, 2179 patients admitted for treatment of acute MI were divided into diabetic (24 percent) and nondiabetic patients, and 1-year mortality was compared in the two groups based on whether they had received ACE inhibitors.[55] In both the diabetic and nondiabetic patients, those receiving ACE inhibitors were older and sicker at admission to the study. Despite their poorer baseline health, diabetic patients who received ACE inhibitors had significantly less mortality after 1 year than diabetics who did not receive ACE inhibitors (16.2 percent and 18.8 percent, respectively), a benefit that was not seen in the nondiabetic patients.

The effects of renin-angiotensin system stimulation can also be blocked with angiotensin II receptor blockers (ARBs). Several large clinical trials have examined the effects of these agents on mortality and cardiovascular outcomes in high-risk patients, including patients with diabetes. In the Valsartan in Acute Myocardial Infarction (VALIANT) trial, patients were randomized to receive valsartan (20 mg titrated to a maximum of 160 mg twice daily), captopril (6.5 mg titrated to 50 mg three times a day), or a combination of the two drugs (valsartan 80 mg twice daily, captopril 50 mg three times a day) within 10 days of an acute MI.[56] The study included 3400 patients with diabetes. After a median of 24.7 months of follow-up, mortality in the three treatment arms was the same in the overall population of the study. Similarly, there was no difference in the effectiveness of the three treatment arms in terms of death from any cause or cardiovascular events in the diabetic patients.

In a subsequent retrospective analysis of the VALIANT data, outcomes were analyzed by diabetes status at presentation.[57] Patients were grouped into three categories: previously known diabetes, newly diagnosed diabetes at randomization, and no known diabetes. At 1 year after enrollment, patients with previously known and newly diagnosed diabetes had a similar increased adjusted risk of mortality (HR = 1.43 and 1.50, respectively) and cardiovascular events (HR = 1.37 and 1.34, respectively). The poor prognosis of patients with newly diagnosed diabetes suggests that metabolic abnormalities preceding onset of frank diabetes contribute to adverse outcomes.

In the Candesartan in Heart failure Assessment of Reduction in Mortality and morbidity (CHARM) trial, 7600 patients with left ventricular ejection fractions of <40 percent (28 percent with diabetes) were randomly assigned to receive candesartan titrated to 32 mg every day or placebo for at least 2 years.[58] The primary outcome of the study was all-cause mortality. During the follow-up period, 23 percent of the patients in the candesartan group and 25 percent in the placebo group died from any cause (covariate adjusted HR 0.91; p = 0.32). The lower mortality in the candesartan group was primarily attributable to fewer cardiovascular deaths with candesartan. The relative reductions in risk were similar among patients with or without a history of diabetes.

The development of diabetes was a predefined secondary outcome of the CHARM trial that was assessed in 5436 patients with heart failure, irrespective of ejection fraction, who did not have a diagnosis of diabetes at entry into the trial. Of the patients treated with candesartan, 6.0 percent developed diabetes during follow-up as compared with 7.4 percent in the placebo group ($p = 0.020$), indicating that this ARB may prevent diabetes in patients with heart failure.[59]

Many factors may explain the particular benefits of ACE inhibitors and ARBs in diabetic patients with acute MI. These agents can prevent or limit remodeling of the ventricle, particularly when administered early in the course of acute MI, reduce recurrent ischemic events, and restore sympathovagal imbalance. ACE inhibitors and ARBs may also improve endothelial function in diabetes, promote fibrinolysis by suppression of PAI-1 expression, and decrease insulin resistance.[60] In the Heart Outcomes Prevention Evaluation (HOPE) study, ramipril significantly reduced the rates of MI, stroke, and cardiovascular death in diabetic subjects with or without a prior history of CAD or CHF over a 5-year period when compared with placebo.[61]

Insulin

Although it is well established that hyperglycemia at the time of admission for an MI increases the risk of in-hospital mortality regardless of diabetic status,[62] recent studies have also shown that hyperglycemia increases the risk of mortality during cardiopulmonary bypass[63] (Fig. 60-5) and that the curve representing risk of adverse events as a function of blood glucose concentration is U-shaped, with risk also increasing with hypoglycemia.[64] The value of baseline plasma glucose levels and short-term changes in plasma glucose as predictors of longer term mortality has also been examined.[65] In an analysis of data from 1469 patients with acute MI, both admission blood glucose levels and failure to reduce glucose levels after 24 hours were significant predictors of 30- and 180-day mortality in nondiabetic patients (Fig. 60-6).

Following MI, the blood glucose level may increase in proportion to infarct size and hemodynamic stress in nondiabetic patients as a result of catecholamine, glucagon,

cortisol, and growth hormone release. These hormones may create "transient" insulin resistance, with serum glucose returning to normal at discharge. In some cases, a very high admission glucose level out of proportion to infarct size indicates previously undiagnosed diabetes.

Risk of events may also be increased in subjects with prediabetic states. In the Whitehall Study, 17,869 male civil servants were followed for 33 years and outcomes were correlated with baseline measurements of blood glucose taken 2 hours after an oral glucose load (2hBG).[66] In these subjects, the HR for CHD mortality increased as a linear function of 2hBG for all values of 2hBG above 83 mg/dl. Within the 2hBG range 83 to 200 mg/dl, the age-adjusted HR for CHD was 3.62 (95 percent CI: 2.3 to 5.6).

Aggressive control of plasma glucose levels during the treatment of myocardial ischemia in diabetic patients can improve outcomes. In the Diabetes and Insulin-Glucose Infusion in Acute Myocardial Infarction (DIGAMI) study, 620 diabetic patients with acute MI were randomly assigned to either intensive insulin therapy (insulin-glucose infusion for 24 hours, followed by subcutaneous insulin injection for at least 3 months) or a standard glycemic control strategy.[67] Those receiving the intensive insulin regimen had a lower blood glucose level during the first hour (9.6 versus 11.7 mmol/liter, $p < 0.01$) and at discharge (8.2 versus 9.0 mmol/liter, $p < 0.01$) than the control group. During the first year of follow-up, a significant reduction in mortality was seen in the intensive insulin group compared with the conventionally treated group (19 versus 26 percent, $p < 0.027$). Mortality remained lower in the intensive control group through 3.4 years than in the conventional care group (33 versus 44 percent, $p < 0.011$).[68] Predictors of mortality were age, history of CHF, diabetes duration, admission glucose, and admission HbA1C level. The subgroup whose diabetes had been managed with diet or oral hypoglycemic drugs before infarction enjoyed the greatest survival benefit.

A recent follow-up to DIGAMI, DIGAMI 2, a prospective, randomized, open-label trial, compared outcomes of acute MI in patients with either type 1 or type 2 diabetes treated with three glycemic control strategies following acute MI: group 1 received acute insulin-glucose infusion followed by long-term glucose control ($n = 474$); group 2 received insulin-glucose infusion followed by conventional glucose control ($n = 473$); group 3 received routine metabolic management ($n = 306$).[69] All patients were followed for a median of 2.1 years. All-cause mortality (primary endpoint) did not differ between groups 1 and 2 and groups 2 and 3. There were no significant differences among the 3 groups in nonfatal reinfarctions and strokes. The lack of effect of long-term insulin treatment on outcomes may be at least partially explained by the fact that 14 percent of the patients in the conventional treatment group received insulin-glucose infusions in violation of the protocol and as many as 41 percent had extra glucose injections. As a result, the blood glucose levels in all 3 groups were not significantly different following treatment.

The value of intensive metabolic control for improving outcomes has recently been examined in two settings. In a study comparing perioperative outcomes of diabetic patients undergoing coronary artery bypass grafting (CABG) who were treated with continuous insulin infusion or intermittent subcutaneous insulin, insulin infusion significantly reduced mortality compared with subcutaneous insulin treatment (2.5 percent versus 5.3 percent, $p < 0.0001$).[70] Although no placebo group was reported, mortality in the insulin infusion group was significantly less than predicted by Society of Thoracic Surgeons' risk model. In a randomized trial in a medical intensive care unit (ICU), 1200 patients (16.9 percent diabetics) received insulin infusion to maintain blood glucose within a range of 80 to 110 mg/dl or insulin injection when plasma glucose exceeded 215 mg/dl.[71] Intensive glycemic control with insulin infusion did not reduce mortality but significantly reduced morbidity by preventing renal damage, accelerating removal of mechanical ventilation, and hastening discharge from the ICU and hospital.

Infusion of glucose-insulin-potassium (GIK) solution, originally used in the 1960s and 1970s as a polarizing agent to maintain electrical stability, is regaining favor as a method to influence myocardial metabolism positively during treatment of MI, coronary revascularization procedures, and CABG. A meta-analysis of nine studies including 1932 patients conducted between 1965 and 1987 concluded that GIK infusion reduced in-hospital mortality from 21 to 16.1 percent.[72] However,

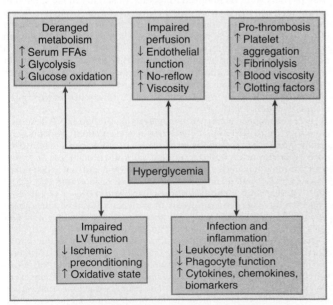

FIGURE 60–5 Schematic representation of factors that contribute to increased risk of mortality during cardiopulmonary bypass in patients with hyperglycemia. FFAs = free fatty acids; LV = left ventricular.

only two of the studies were double-blinded, and no information about diabetic patients was provided. In a prospective, randomized, open-label study of GIK infusion in 940 patients undergoing percutaneous transluminal coronary angioplasty (PTCA) for an acute MI, no mortality benefit was seen in the GIK group compared with the placebo group.[73] Although there seemed to be a benefit in the diabetic subgroup, in which GIK infusion reduced mortality from 12.2 to 4 percent, the small size of the subgroup and the small number of deaths prevented this effect from reaching statistical significance. In diabetic patients undergoing elective CABG, GIK infusion beneficially influenced metabolism, as indicated by an elimination of myocardial extraction of nonesterified fatty acids and an increase in myocardial uptake of lactate and glucose.[74] A comparison of CABG outcomes in diabetic patients ($n = 141$) prospectively randomized to receive GIK solution to maintain tight glycemic control during surgery or receiving standard therapy (intermittent subcutaneous insulin) has also been reported.[75] GIK patients had lower serum glucose levels during the immediate postoperative period (138 versus 260 mg/dl; $p < 0.0001$), a lower incidence of atrial fibrillation (16.6 versus 42 percent; $p = 0.0017$), and a shorter postoperative length of hospitalization (6.5 versus 9.2 days; $p = 0.003$). Although there was no difference in the two treatment arms in 30-day mortality, patients treated with GIK had a significant survival advantage over a 2-year period following surgery. Further prospective studies are necessary to determine the long-term effect of GIK infusion in diabetic patients treated for MI or ACS.

A number of mechanisms have been proposed to explain the proposed benefit of GIK infusion during treatment of MI and ACS. The ability of GIK to attenuate the rise in free fatty acids (FFAs) that is seen during MI is thought to shift myocardial oxidative metabolism from FFAs to glucose oxidation, a metabolic process that is more efficient (i.e., produces more adenosine triphosphate per mole of O_2).[76] The net effect of these changes in metabolism is reduction of cellular injury from ischemia and reperfusion and improved postischemic function. The validity of this conclusion has recently been questioned based on the results of animal studies demonstrating that the protection from ischemic myocardial damage associated with increased glucose and insulin levels was not related to changes in cardiac efficiency or coupling of glucose oxidation to glycolysis.[77]

The benefit of GIK in the setting of MI may also be a result of direct effects of insulin (Fig. 60-7). Administration of both GIK and insulin alone have been shown to have antiinflammatory and profibrinolytic effects during MI that could protect the myocardium.[78,79] Additionally, insulin may limit damage of the myocardium by attenuating apoptosis, thus promoting cell survival during reperfusion.[80]

HEART FAILURE

Overview

Congestive heart failure (CHF) is the pathophysiological state in which the heart is unable to maintain cardiac output sufficient to meet the metabolic needs of the body. CHF and its attendant morbidity and mortality continue to be a growing problem in the United States. Although MI and hypertension are the most common risk factors associated with CHF, diabetes mellitus is also a strong and independent risk factor. Novel metabolic factors reflecting insulin resistance (e.g., increased fasting proinsulin) have also been found to be predictive of development of CHF.[81]

In a recent, large retrospective cohort study, 8231 patients with type 2 diabetes and 8845 age- and gender-matched controls without CHF were followed for 6 years to estimate the new CHF incidence rate.[82] During this period, the incidence rate of CHF per 1000 person-years was 30.9 in type 2 diabetics versus 12.4 for nondiabetics for a rate ratio of 2.5 (95 percent CI 2.3 to 2.7). The difference in rate of development of CHF between persons with and without diabetes was much greater in the younger age groups. For example, in the <45 years age group, the incidence rate of CHF in persons with diabetes was 11 times greater than in nondiabetic subjects.

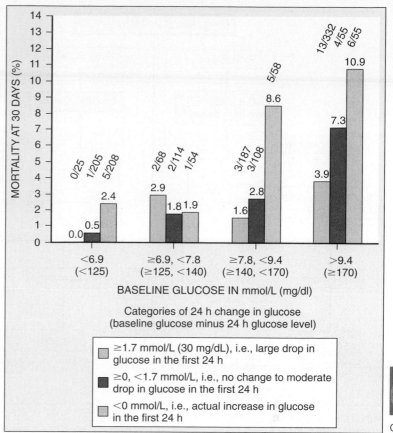

FIGURE 60–6 Blood glucose levels significantly predict mortality in nondiabetic patients. *(Adapted from Goyal A, Mahaffey KW, Garg J, et al: Prognostic significance of the change in glucose level in the first 24 hours after acute myocardial infarction: Results from the CARDINAL study. Eur Heart J 27:1289-1297, 2006.)*

CH 60

Diabetes and Heart Disease

The incidence of heart failure in elderly (>65 years old) patients with diabetes who were not in managed care was estimated in a study of a cohort of Medicare beneficiary claims from 1994 to 1999.[83] Of the 151,738 beneficiaries identified as having diabetes, 22.3 percent had diabetes at the beginning of the study. The subsequent rate of development of CHF among beneficiaries who did not have CHF in 1994 was 12.6 per 100-person years. Mortality during the study period among elderly patients who developed CHF was 44.9 percent compared with 24.0 percent of patients who remained free of CHF.

Not only are diabetic patients at higher risk for CHF, but those who develop CHF have a worse prognosis than nondiabetic individuals with CHF. In retrospective studies of data from the Beta-Blocker Evaluation of Survival Trial (BEST) and the Studies of Left Ventricular Dysfunction (SOLVD) trial, diabetes was independently associated with an increase in all-cause mortality ($RR = 1.33$ to 1.37) in patients with ischemic cardiomyopathy but not in those with nonischemic etiology of CHF.[84,85] This finding suggests that diabetes and ischemic heart disease interact to accelerate the progression of myocardial dysfunction. Similarly, a multivariable Cox regression model analysis of data from the Candesartan in Heart Failure: Assessment of Reduction in Mortality (CHARM) trial identified diabetes as a significant predictor of cardiovascular death or CHF hospitalization ($RR = 1.59$; 95 percent CI 1.43 to 1.74).[86]

The increased incidence of CHF and its poorer prognosis in diabetic patients compared with those without diabetes suggest that there are alterations in the underlying myocardium of the diabetic patient that render it more susceptible to ischemia and less able to recover after an ischemic insult (Fig. 60-8). Over the years, substantial evidence has accumulated that a specific, "true" diabetic cardiomyopathy dis-

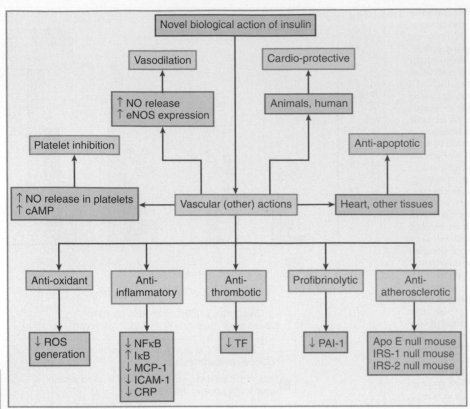

FIGURE 60–7 Novel biological effects of insulin. CRP = C-reactive protein; cAMP = cyclic adenosine monophosphate; E-NOS = endothelial NO synthase; IκB = inhibitor of NFκB; MCP = monocyte chemotactic protein; NFκB = nuclear factor kappa B; NO = nitric oxide; PAI-1 = plasmin activator inhibitor type 1; ROS = reactive oxygen species. *(Adapted from Dandona P, Aljada A, Chaudhuri A, et al: Metabolic syndrome: A comprehensive perspective based on interactions between obesity, diabetes, and inflammation. Circulation 111:1448-1454, 2005.)*

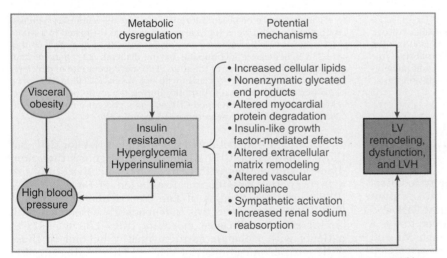

FIGURE 60–8 Alterations of the myocardium in the diabetic patient may render it more susceptible to ischemia and less able to recover after an ischemic insult. LV = left ventricle; LVH = left ventricular hypertrophy. *(Adapted from Rutter MK, Parise H, Benjamin EJ, et al: Impact of glucose intolerance and insulin resistance on cardiac structure and function: Sex-related differences in the Framingham Heart Study. Circulation 107:448-454, 2003.)*

tinct from ischemic injury exists. In an analysis of the combined Framingham Study cohort and Framingham Offspring Study cohort, gender-specific linear regression analysis was used to assess the contribution of diabetes and glucose intolerance to age-adjusted echocardiographic parameters in more than 4500 men and women.[87] Across the range of glucose tolerances from normal to known diabetes, there was a significant trend for greater left ventricular wall thickness and left ventricular mass, larger left ventricular

end-diastolic volume, and greater left atrial size, particularly in women. The exact cause of the cardiac dysfunction directly attributable to diabetes is difficult to isolate because other comorbidities of diabetes, such as hypertension, coronary atherosclerosis, and microvascular dysfunction, can independently impair myocardial performance.

DIABETES-SPECIFIC FACTORS RELATED TO CHF

ADVANCED GLYCATION PRODUCTS (AGES). AGEs accumulate in tissue exposed to hyperglycemia as a result of a nonenzymatic reaction between reducing sugars and proteins and are implicated in the morphological changes that occur in the diabetic heart.[88] Accumulation of AGE-modified extracellular matrix results in loss of elasticity of the vessel wall that could interfere with myocardial function. Serum levels of circulating AGEs and their soluble receptor are also correlated with the severity of nephropathy in type 2 diabetic patients.[89] The presence of AGEs may explain the clinical observation that diabetic patients can develop CHF as a result of diastolic dysfunction in the absence of hypertension or increased wall thickness, or both.

MYOCARDIAL CALCIUM HANDLING. Abnormalities in myocardial calcium (Ca^2) handling may also contribute to abnormal cardiac mechanics in the diabetic heart. Insulin-dependent diabetes impairs sarcoplasmic reticular Ca^{2+} pump activity, which slows Ca^2 removal from the cytoplasm in diastole.[90] This abnormality may contribute to the increased diastolic stiffness characteristic of diabetic cardiomyopathy. Diabetes-related changes in troponin T, the contractile regulatory protein of the thin myofilament, may also be a factor in both diastolic and systolic dysfunction.

MYOCARDIAL METABOLISM. The direct effects of hyperglycemia and insulin resistance on myocardial cellular metabolism may contribute to chronic left ventricular dysfunction (cardiomyopathy) in diabetes. Type 2 diabetes has complex effects on the energy metabolism of the heart and altered energy substrate supply and utilization may explain some of the morphological changes seen in the diabetic heart.[91,92] The heart uses nonesterified (or "free") fatty acids as its primary energy source during aerobic perfusion at normal workloads but increasingly relies on glycolysis and pyruvate oxidation during periods of ischemia or increased work. The diabetic heart may have an exaggerated impairment of glycolytic adenosine triphosphate (ATP) generation during ischemia because of reduced glucose transport into cardiac myocytes. Accumulated triglycerides and FFAs in myocytes can also result in changes in gene expression that are associated with contractile dysfunction that also contribute to the development of diabetic cardiomyopathy.[93,94]

CORONARY MICROCIRCULATION. Diabetic patients not only suffer more severe and diffuse CAD,[95] but also, as noted previously, the structure and function of the coronary microcirculation may be abnormal in diabetes and contribute to the development of CHF. Endothelial dysfunction, characterized by reduced synthesis or bioavailability of the potent vasodilator nitric oxide, commonly occurs in the diabetic coronary vasculature during diabetes and may lead to abnormal control of blood flow **(see also Chap.43)**. Resting coronary blood flow in diabetic subjects is normal or even slightly elevated despite endothelial dysfunction.[96] However, a reduced capacity of the myocardial circulation to vasodilate with stimulation is seen with diabetes. This abnormal myocardial blood flow response during stimulation improves with increased glycemic control.[97]

The angiogenic response to ischemia also appears to be abnormal in diabetes.[98] Diabetic patients have impaired formation of coronary collateral circulation in response to ischemia compared with normal subjects, a finding that might contribute to diabetic cardiomyopathy and poor prognosis following MI. A study of samples from the left ventricular wall of patients with diabetes demonstrated that diabetes is associated with decreased expression of the receptor for vascular endothelial growth factor (VEGF) and a downregulation of VEGF signal transduction, factors that may contribute to impaired angiogenesis.[99]

FAILURE OF ISCHEMIC PRECONDITIONING. Ischemic preconditioning refers to the observation that short periods of transient ischemia protect the myocardium against subsequent, longer ischemic insults. Evidence of this protective effect has been shown in animal experiments[100] and in human myocardial biopsy samples.[101] Diabetes as well as hyperglycemia in the absence of diabetes appears to eliminate ischemic preconditioning in human myocardium.[101,102] The opening of myocardial adenosine triphosphate (ATP)-sensitive potassium (K_{ATP}) channels is an essential factor in ischemic preconditioning and the use of sulfonylureas, which block K_{ATP} channels, by type 2 diabetic patients has created controversy to be discussed in more detail later.

CHF Caused by Diabetes

DIABETIC CARDIOMYOPATHIES. CHF in diabetes can result from a direct effect of diabetes on cardiac muscle per se or as a result of conventional risk factors exacerbated by diabetes. Autopsy and biopsy samples of cardiac muscle from diabetic patients with CHF display a variety of morphological changes, including myocyte hypertrophy, myofibril depletion, interstitial fibrosis, increased microvascular basement membrane thickness, increased matrix and basement membrane within arteriolar walls, and intramyocardial microangiopathy.[103] These lesions are not specific to diabetes, and all can be found to some degree in cardiomyopathy of other etiologies. However, the coexistence of diabetes and other risk factors for cardiomyopathy can amplify the pathology. For example, in endomyocardial specimens from patients with diabetes, ultrastructural changes, including capillary basement membrane thickening and interstitial and myocardial fibrosis, are accentuated by coexisting hypertension.

Fibrosis is a key feature of the heart of diabetic patients, even when cardiac disease is not evident. Increased levels of collagen and changes in left ventricular diastolic function have been detected in patients with type 1 or type 2 diabetes.[104] Changes in left ventricular function can occur even in patients with well-controlled type 2 diabetes. In a study that used magnetic resonance imaging to compare left ventricular function in 12 asymptomatic, normotensive, newly diagnosed type 2 diabetic patients and 12 control subjects, the diabetic patients had normal left ventricular mass and systolic function but all measures of left ventricular diastolic function were reduced compared with those in the control group.[105]

Other Causes of CHF in Diabetes

Coronary Heart Disease

As already noted, diabetes is a major risk factor for acute MI. Following an acute MI, the presence of diabetes increases the risk of developing new CHF.[1] The OASIS registry, which provided long-term data on 8013 patients with unstable coronary syndromes, showed that diabetes increases the risk of developing new CHF after hospitalization for unstable angina or non-Q-wave MI by 82 percent ($p = 0.001$).[1] Diabetic patients with a history of CHD had a considerably higher risk. The reasons diabetes increases the incidence of CHF following an acute MI are not fully understood, but several factors may contribute. Because diabetic patients may have a decreased awareness of pain or an atypical pre-

sentation of symptoms during an acute MI, they often delay treatment, resulting in more extensive and severe ischemic myocardial damage. In some cases, these patients have unrecognized or silent MI, creating a myocardial substrate predisposed to develop CHF. However, the increased incidence of CHF in diabetes cannot be accounted for solely by more extensive or severe myocardial infarctions. After correction of data to account for differences in infarct size and baseline risk factors, CHF still occurs much more often in patients with diabetes than in those without the disease.

REMODELING FOLLOWING MYOCARDIAL INFARCTION

Following an MI, the heart undergoes short- and long-term adaptation in response to the loss of contractile function, a process that is accentuated in persons with diabetes. Immediately after an acute MI, diabetic patients have less compensatory increase in contractility of noninfarcted myocardium than nondiabetic patients. This deficit persists over time, resulting in less compensation for the loss of stroke volume than in the nondiabetic heart. For example, left ventricular size increases less in diabetic patients than in nondiabetic patients during the 2 years following an MI, a difference that is associated with a twofold higher incidence of CHF in the diabetic cohort.[106] The failure of the diabetic myocardium to remodel appropriately is probably caused by a combination of factors associated with diabetic cardiomyopathy, including reduced heart muscle metabolism, insufficient glucose transport, endothelial dysfunction, impaired control of myocardial blood flow, and left ventricular fibrosis resulting in impaired filling, and diabetic autonomic dysfunction.[107]

HYPERTENSION

Diabetes and hypertension often occur together and this combination amplifies the morphological changes seen in diabetic cardiomyopathy (Table 60-2). In the United Kingdom Prospective Diabetic Study (UKPDS), systolic blood pressure associated strongly with the incidence of nonfatal CHF.[108] For each 10 mm Hg increase in systolic blood pressure, the risk of CHF increased by 12 per cent. In the treatment phase of the study, 1148 hypertensive type 2 diabetic patients received either tight control (target blood pressure <150/85 mm Hg) or less tight control of blood pressure (target blood pressure <180/105 mm Hg). After a median follow-up period of 8.4 years, the average blood pressure achieved in the two treatment groups was 144/82 mm Hg in the tight control group and 154/87 mm Hg in the less tight group. This small difference in average blood pressure was associated with a large difference in the incidence of CHF, which fell by 56 percent in the tight control group compared with the less tight control group. In the tight control group, a

TABLE 60–2	Pathophysiologic Changes in Diabetic Cardiomyopathy
Sympathetic nervous system activation	
Renin-angiotensin system activation	
Increased risk of arrhythmias	
Increased NaCl and H_2O retention	
Decreased vascular compliance	
Elevated endothelin levels (in diabetes)	
Loss of "dipping" nocturnal BP pattern	
Increased free fatty acid levels	
Increased LVH/mass via myocyte hypertrophy	
Powerful contributor to nephropathy	

BP=blood pressure; LVH=left ventricular hypertrophy.

similar benefit was seen regardless of the antihypertensive agent used.

The Antihypertensive and Lipid-Lowering Treatment to Prevent Heart Attack Trial (ALLHAT) addressed the issue of whether a certain class of antihypertensive drugs might more effectively reduce the incidence of CHF in hypertensive diabetic patients.[109] In ALLHAT, a calcium channel blocker (amlodipine) or an ACE inhibitor (lisinopril) was compared with a thiazide diuretic (chlorthalidone) as first-line therapy based on their ability to prevent cardiovascular events in 33,357 hypertensive subjects, 36 percent of whom were diabetic at baseline. During the average 4.9-year follow-up, the incidence of new-onset CHF in the diabetic patients was significantly lower in the group receiving thiazide diuretic than in either of the other treatment groups. This finding is in contrast to that of the Second Australian National Blood Pressure Study, which had few diabetic patients and showed no treatment-dependent difference in the incidence of CHF.[110]

REDUCING THE RISK OF HEART FAILURE IN DIABETES

Glycemic Control

CH 60

Poor glycemic control increases the risk of developing heart failure in diabetes. Two studies clearly illustrate the relation between glycemic control and the incidence of CHF in diabetes. In a group of 48,858 diabetic subjects with no history of heart failure followed for a median period of 2.2 years after measurement of HbA1C levels, the incidence of hospitalizations for CHF or death related to CHF was correlated with baseline HbA1C in the diabetic cohort.[111] The association was stronger in men than in women. Each absolute 1 percent increase in HbA1C was associated with a 12 percent increase in CHF in men after adjustment for other factors, including use of ACE inhibitors, beta blockers, and incidence of MI during the follow-up period. In women, a 1 percent increase in HbA1C was associated with a 4 percent increase in CHF. A similar, although steeper, relation was found in 4585 participants with type 2 diabetes in the UKPDS.[112] During the 7.5- to 12.5-year follow-up period, each absolute 1 percent increase in average HbA1C was associated with a 16 percent increase in CHF ($p = 0.021$). These studies suggest that tight glycemic control might reduce the incidence of CHF and, because no threshold was identified, the target HbA1C levels should be as close to normal as possible.

Medical Therapy to Treat or Prevent Heart Failure in Diabetic Patients

The goals of treatment of left ventricular dysfunction and heart failure in diabetic patients are the same as those in nondiabetic patients: relief of pulmonary congestion, slowing the progression of the disease, and prolonging survival. In general, drug therapies for heart failure have similar, if not better, efficacy in diabetic patients than in those without the disease.

Beta-Adrenergic Blocking Agents

As noted earlier when discussing ACS, beta blockers reduce mortality and reinfarction in diabetic patients post-MI. These benefits also extend to diabetic patients with CHF, regardless of severity.[113-117] The mortality benefit in patients with heart failure has been seen with nonselective beta blockers (e.g., bucindolol[113,117]), with cardioselective beta blockers (e.g., metoprolol[114]), and with a nonselective beta blocker that also blocks alpha$_1$-adrenergic receptors (carvedilol[115,118]). Beta blockers with intrinsic sympathomi-

metic activity, such as pindolol, may be contraindicated in patients with CHF, particularly in diabetic patients. Carvedilol may offer advantages in diabetic patients because of its favorable effects on insulin sensitivity and plasma lipid profile as well as its ability to dilate the peripheral vasculature. In the Carvedilol Or Metoprolol European Trial (COMET), patients with New York Heart Association (NYHA) Class II to IV CHF randomly received either carvedilol or metoprolol for a mean of 5 years.[118] All-cause mortality was reduced by 17 percent in the carvedilol group compared with the metoprolol group. A similar benefit of carvedilol was seen in the 24 percent of the study population who were diabetic at baseline.

Angiotensin-Converting Enzyme Inhibitors

ACE inhibitors clearly and convincingly reduce the morbidity and mortality associated with left ventricular dysfunction, but early clinical trials lacked sufficient power to address rigorously the question of whether these benefits extended to patients with diabetes and CHF. Several more recent studies have addressed these questions and have shown that, indeed, ACE inhibitors are effective for CHF in diabetic patients.[119]

In GISSI-3, lisinopril reduced 6-week and 6-month mortality in the diabetic subgroup when treatment was started within 24 hours of an acute MI, but it did not affect the incidence of CHF or other signs of left ventricular dysfunction.[119] In the TRACE study, patients with an enzyme-confirmed acute MI and left ventricular dysfunction (left ventricular ejection fraction <35 percent) present 2 to 6 days after the MI randomly received either the ACE inhibitor trandolapril or matching placebo.[119] In the diabetic group, trandolapril reduced the rate of progression to severe CHF by 62 percent ($p < 0.001$), a benefit not seen in treated patients without diabetes.

ANGIOTENSIN II RECEPTOR BLOCKERS

Angiotensin II receptor blockers (ARBs) have demonstrated rough equivalence to ACE inhibitors in preventing morbidity and mortality associated with CHF in three major clinical trials.[120-122] The benefit may be smaller in the diabetic cohort, however.[121,122] Two studies of the ARB losartan suggest that this pharmacological class may prevent CHF in type 2 diabetes. In the Reduction in Endpoints in NIDDM with the Angiotensin II Antagonist Losartan (RENAAL) study, type 2 diabetic patients with nephropathy and no history of CHF received either losartan or placebo in addition to conventional antihypertensive therapy.[123] Treatment with losartan not only slowed the progression of kidney failure during the 4-year study, but also reduced the incidence of CHF by 32 percent ($p < 0.005$). In the Losartan Intervention For Endpoint Reduction (LIFE) study, 1195 diabetic patients with hypertension and signs of left ventricular hypertrophy were randomly assigned either losartan or atenolol as the primary antihypertensive agent and were observed for an average of 4.7 years.[124] Not only was the incidence of the primary composite endpoint (cardiovascular death, MI, or stroke) reduced but hospitalizations for CHF also fell by 41 percent ($p < 0.013$).

ARBs are well tolerated and have an excellent safety record. In contrast to ACE inhibitors, the incidence of cough with ARB treatment is no higher than in patients treated with placebo, and angioedema occurs rarely. Despite these advantages, ARBs should probably be reserved for patients who are unable to tolerate ACE inhibition until the results of clinical studies clearly demonstrate superiority or equivalence to ACE inhibitors for the treatment of CHF. Currently, only valsartan and candesartan are approved for the treatment of CHF.

ALDOSTERONE ANTAGONISTS

Aldosterone was traditionally thought to contribute to the pathophysiology of CHF only through its action to increase sodium retention and potassium excretion. However, aldosterone may also directly stimulate the production of inflammatory mediators, cause myocardial fibrosis, and promote endothelial dysfunction and vascular stiffening.[125,126] Evidence of the benefit of blocking aldosterone receptors was presented in the results of the Eplerenone Post-Acute Myocardial Infarction Heart Failure Efficacy and Survival Study (EPHESUS).[127] In EPHESUS, the mineralocorticoid-selective aldosterone antagonist eplerenone was added to optimal therapy (ACE inhibition 87 percent, beta blockade 75 percent, diuretics 60 percent, and aspirin 88 percent) in patients who had suffered a recent MI with documented reduction in left ventricular ejection fraction and symptoms of CHF. Treatment with eplerenone reduced the composite risk of cardiovascular death or hospitalization for cardiovascular causes by 13 percent compared to placebo ($p < 0.002$). A similar degree of benefit was observed in diabetic patients, who constituted 32 percent of the total population of patients, but the study was not powered to evaluate the effect fully in this subgroup.

TREATING DIABETES IN PATIENTS WITH CHD, ACS, OR CHF

Medical Therapy

Sulfonylureas

In the 1970s, data emerged suggesting that patients with type 2 diabetes treated with the sulfonylurea tolbutamide had an increased risk of cardiovascular mortality and CAD compared with similar patients treated with insulin.[100] The sulfonylureas induce insulin release by blocking K^+-ATP channels in pancreatic β cells. The discovery that K^+-ATP channels also exist in the myocardium and that blocking them with sulfonylureas prevented ischemic preconditioning, a cardioprotective mechanism, and attenuated coronary vasodilation in animal models suggested that these drugs might contribute to ischemic injury in diabetic patients. However, the results reported in the UKPDS argue strongly against a proischemic class effect of sulfonylureas. This prospective, randomized trial assessed the impact of tight glycemic control using a variety of treatment strategies on the incidence and severity of microvascular and macrovascular complications in newly diagnosed diabetes.[128] Patients treated with chlorpropamide or glibenclamide had a rate of MI and sudden death over the 10-year follow-up similar to that of patients treated with insulin. In a more recent study, treatment of newly diagnosed type 2 diabetic patients with glyburide was actually associated with a lower risk of cardiovascular events including CHF than treatment with rosiglitazone but had a higher cumulative incidence of treatment failure after 5 years (34 percent versus 15 percent).[129]

Diabetes attenuates or eliminates ischemic preconditioning in the human heart and certain sulfonylureas may further inhibit this phenomenon.[101,102] The discovery that cardiac and vascular K^+-ATP channels are structurally distinct from pancreatic beta cell channels stimulated studies that described differences in specificity of sulfonylureas for receptor subtypes. Pharmacokinetic differences among the sulfonylureas may have important implications for the treatment of diabetes in patients with CHD.[130] Despite this complication, sulfonylureas are widely used, given the benefits of improved glycemic control for preventing diabetes-related microvascular complications. The potential risks, benefits, and adverse events of individual sulfonylureas should be considered before choosing a specific drug for a particular patient.

Thiazolidinediones

Thiazolidinediones (TZDs) decrease glucose levels in type 2 diabetes by increasing the insulin sensitivity of target tissues and also induce a wide variety of nonglycemic effects mediated through activation of the PPAR-γ nuclear receptor that may benefit the cardiovascular system.[131,132] In the Prospective Pioglitazone Clinical Trial in Macrovascular Events (PROactive Study), treatment with pioglitazone significantly reduced the composite endpoint of all-cause mortality, nonfatal MI, and stroke compared to placebo in high-risk patients with type 2 diabetes over a 34.5 month follow-up.[133] Similarly, in the Diabetes Reduction Assessment with Ramapril and Rosiglitazone Medication (DREAM) trial, treatment with rosiglitazone significantly reduced the incidence of the composite endpoint of type 2 diabetes or death

in patients with impaired glucose tolerance or elevated fasting glucose compared to placebo (HR = 0.40; 95 percent CI 0.35-0.46) and increased the likelihood of regression to normoglycemia.[134] In both PROactive and DREAM, nonfatal CHF was more common in patients treated with TZDs, presumably because of reversible fluid retention rather than loss of myocardial function. The substantial benefits of TZDs for the reduction of macrovascular events associated with diabetes and prevention of onset of diabetes in susceptible patients outweighs the risk of treatable fluid retention. None of the TZDs are recommended for use in patients with NYHA Class III or IV CHF.

Metformin

Metformin (dimethylbiguanide) lowers blood glucose both by increasing insulin sensitivity and by decreasing hepatic glucose output and has been shown to have benefit for reducing mortality in type 2 diabetic patients compared with sulfonylurea monotherapy.[135,136] In addition to improved glycemic control, beneficial properties of metformin include weight reduction and favorable effects on lipid parameters and the fibrinolytic pathway.

The effectiveness of metformin as a treatment for type 2 diabetic patients with CHF was assessed in a recent survey of the Saskatchewan Health databases. Patients who were taking oral antidiabetic agents and who also had diagnosed CHF ($n = 1833$) were identified. Comparison of outcomes in patients grouped by antidiabetic therapy more than 2.5 years indicated that metformin, given as either monotherapy or in combination, resulted in significantly fewer deaths than sulfonylurea monotherapy (HR = 0.70 and 0.61, respectively).[137] Interpretation of the data was limited by lack of data regarding glycemic control and severity of CHF.

Lactic acidosis is a rare but potentially life-threatening complication of metformin use, with a reported incidence of about 0.03 cases per 1000 patient-years of use and with a fatality rate of about 50 percent and is seen more commonly in patients with renal insufficiency or with tissue hypoperfusion and hypoxemia.[138] Because patients with CHF are at higher risk for hypoperfusion or hypoxemia, the use of metformin is contraindicated in those patients who require pharmacological treatment of CHF. The degree of lactic acidosis associated with metformin is controversial, however. A recent Cochran database review of 206 comparative trials and cohort studies of metformin concluded that there is no evidence from prospective comparative trials or observational cohort studies that metformin is associated with an increased risk of lactic acidosis or increased level of lactate compared to other antihyperglycemic treatments when prescribed under study conditions.[139]

Coronary Revascularization

Percutaneous Transluminal Coronary Angioplasty

Large-scale trials have generally not shown a benefit of aggressive revascularization after thrombolytic therapy for acute MI. Similar considerations apply to diabetic patients. Although diabetic and nondiabetic patients have similar rates of initial angioplasty success, diabetic patients have higher restenosis rates after PTCA and worse long-term outcomes.[140,141] Although stenting has reduced restenosis rates in both diabetic and nondiabetic patients, diabetic patients have smaller lumina in the stented vessels and a significantly higher restenosis rate (55 versus 20 percent; $p < 0.001$) within 4 months of the procedure, despite similar baseline and procedural characteristics.[142] The mechanism underlying the increased restenosis rate in diabetes after coronary intervention is unclear. A variety of metabolic and anatomical abnormalities associated with diabetes and greater degree of plaque burden may all contribute to vessel restenosis in diabetic patient.[140]

Although the introduction of drug-eluting stents has reduced the need for target lesion revascularization in diabetic patients, the rate of restenosis of drug-eluting stents in diabetic patients is still higher than in patients without diabetes.[140] It should be noted that the total number of diabetic patients included in studies of drug-eluting stents has been small, and the studies specifically excluded patients with multivessel disease.[143]

Coronary Artery Bypass Graft Surgery

Most studies comparing outcomes in diabetic and nondiabetic patients undergoing CABG surgery show an increased risk of postoperative death, 30-day and long-term mortality, and an increased need for subsequent reoperation in the diabetic population.[140] Although diabetic patients have a worse risk profile, tend to be older, and have more extensive CAD and poorer left ventricular function than do nondiabetic patients, their higher long-term mortality does not depend entirely on these factors and continues to diverge from that of nondiabetic patients during long-term follow-up—a difference that probably reflects accelerated disease progression in both bypassed and untreated coronary vessels.

In the Bypass Angioplasty Revascularization Investigation (BARI) trial, diabetic patients who received CABG had a 15 percent absolute survival advantage compared to balloon-only PCI.[140] However, 5-year mortality was higher in diabetic patients than in nondiabetic patients. CABG significantly reduced mortality after MI in diabetic patients compared with angioplasty, whereas no such protective effect of CABG was noted in nondiabetic patients who had an MI.

Coronary Artery Bypass Graft Versus Percutaneous Transluminal Coronary Angioplasty

In general, randomized trials comparing PTCA with CABG have reported similar outcomes. However, in patients with diabetes, CABG may provide better outcomes than standard PTCA, especially in patients with three-vessel disease.[140] In the BARI trial, diabetic patients with multivessel disease randomly assigned to CABG had a higher survival rate at 5 years than diabetic patients assigned to PTCA (81 versus 66 percent; $p < 0.003$). The benefit of CABG accrued primarily to patients receiving internal mammary artery conduits.

Diabetic patients undergoing stenting for multivessel disease may also have a worse outcome than those undergoing CABG. In the Arterial Revascularization Therapy Study (ARTS), the 208 patients with diabetes who underwent percutaneous revascularization had a lower 1-year survival (63 percent) than those undergoing CABG (84 percent).[140] In contrast, no difference was detected in the Veterans Affairs Angina With Extremely Serious Operative Mortality Evaluation (AWESOME) study between diabetic patients who underwent PTCA (54 percent with stents) and those who underwent CABG.[140] Survival was similar in the two groups at 30 days, 6 months, and 36 months.

CARDIOVASCULAR AUTONOMIC NEUROPATHY (See Chap. 89)

Cardiovascular autonomic neuropathy (CAN) is a common form of diabetic neuropathy that contributes to the morbidity and mortality associated with both type 1 and type 2 diabetes.[144] The majority of patients with CAN present with complaints of postural hypotension, resting tachycardia, exercise intolerance, or painless MI or infarction. The risk for CAN depends on the duration of diabetes and the degree of glycemic control and tends to parallel the development of other end-organ disease related to diabetes such as retinopathy, nephropathy, and vasculopathy.[144] Signs and symptoms of CAN often occur relatively late in the natural history of this complication. Because reliable and quantitative noninvasive methods to assess autonomic function have become available, the diagnosis of CAN may now precede the development of symptoms. Most clinicians regard CAN as a major complication of type 1 diabetes because the challenge of managing this complication often dominates the care of these patients. CAN tends to be less fully expressed in patients with type 2 diabetes, who are typi-

cally older and have a wider variety of comorbid conditions. In recognition of the importance of CAN, the American Diabetes Association has recently issued guidelines for the diagnosis, prevention, and management of diabetic neuropathies, including CAN.[145]

REFERENCES

Epidemiology of Diabetic Heart Disease

1. Malmberg K, Yusuf S, Gerstein HC, et al: Impact of diabetes on long-term prognosis in patients with unstable angina and non-Q-wave myocardial infarction: Results of the OASIS (Organization to Assess Strategies for Ischemic Syndromes) Registry. Circulation 102:1014, 2000.
2. Mukamal KJ, Nesto RW, Cohen MC, et al: Impact of diabetes on long-term survival after acute myocardial infarction: Comparability of risk with prior myocardial infarction. Diabetes Care 24:1422, 2001.
3. Jiang SL, Ji XP, Zhao YX, et al: Predictors of in-hospital mortality difference between male and female patients with acute myocardial infarction: Am J Cardiol 98:100, 2006.
4. Fang J, Alderman MH: Impact of the increasing burden of diabetes on acute myocardial infarction in New York City. Diabetes 55:768, 2006.
5. Unal B, Critchley JA, Capewell S: Explaining the decline in coronary heart disease mortality in England and Wales between 1981 and 2000. Circulation 109:1101, 2004.
6. Schnell O, Doering W, Schafer O, et al: Intensification of therapeutic approaches reduces mortality in diabetic patients with acute myocardial infarction. Diabetes Care 27:455-460, 2004.
7. Norhammar A, Malmberg K, Diderholm D, et al: Diabetes mellitus: The major risk factor in unstable coronary artery disease even after consideration of the extent of coronary artery disease and benefits of revascularization. J Am Coll Cardiol 43:585, 2004.
8. Gurm HS, Lincoff AM, Lee D, et al: Outcome of acute ST-segment elevation myocardial infarction in diabetics treated with fibrinolytic or combination reduced fibrinolytic therapy and platelet glycoprotein IIb/IIIa inhibition. Lessons from the GUSTO V trial. J Am Coll Cardiol 43:542, 2004.
9. Moreno PR, Murcia AM, Palacios AF, et al: Coronary composition and macrophage infiltration in atherectomy specimens from patients with diabetes mellitus. Circulation 102:2180, 2000.

Pathophysiology of Diabetic Heart Disease

10. Marfella R, D'Amico M, Esposito K, et al: The ubiquitin-proteasome system and inflammatory activity in diabetic atherosclerotic plaques : Effects of rosiglitazone treatment. Diabetes 55:622, 2006.
11. Cipollone F, Iezzi A, Fazia M, et al: The receptor RAGE as a progression factor amplifying arachidonate-dependent inflammatory and proteolytic response in human atherosclerotic plaques: Role of glycemic control. Circulation 108:1070, 2003.
12. Colwell JA, Nesto RW: The platelet in diabetes: Focus on prevention of ischemic events. Diabetes Care 26:2181, 2003.
13. Varo N, Vincent D, Libby P, et al: Elevated plasma levels of the atherogenic mediator soluble CD40 ligand in diabetic patients: A novel target of thiazolidinediones. Circulation 107:2644, 2003.
14. Sobel BE, Woodcock-Mitchell J, Schneider DJ, et al: Increased plasminogen activator inhibitor type 1 in coronary artery atherectomy specimens from type 2 diabetic compared with nondiabetic patients: A potential factor predisposing to thrombosis and its persistence. Circulation 97:2213, 1998.
15. Pandolfi A, Cetrullo D, Polishuck R, et al: Plasminogen activator inhibitor type 1 is increased in the arterial wall of type II diabetic subjects. Arterioscler Thromb Vasc Biol 21:1378, 2001.
16. Cosentino F, Eto M, De Paolis P, et al: High glucose causes upregulation of cyclooxygenase-2 and alters prostanoid profile in human endothelial cells: Role of protein kinase C and reactive oxygen species. Circulation 107:1017, 2003.
17. Cardillo C, Campia U, Bryant MB, et al: Increased activity of endogenous endothelin in patients with type II diabetes mellitus. Circulation 106:1783, 2002.
18. Nichols GA, Hillier TA, Erbey JR, et al: Congestive heart failure in type 2 diabetes: Prevalence, incidence, and risk factors. Diabetes Care 24:1614, 2001.
19. Shindler DM, Kostis JB, Yusuf S, et al: Diabetes mellitus, a predictor of morbidity and mortality in the Studies of Left Ventricular Dysfunction (SOLVD) Trials and Registry. Am J Cardiol 77:1017, 1996.
20. King DE, Mainous AG, Buchanan TA, Pearson WS: C-reactive protein and glycemic control in adults with diabetes. Diabetes Care 26:1535, 2003.
21. Vinik AI, Maser RE, Mitchell BD, et al: Diabetic autonomic neuropathy. Diabetes Care 26:1553, 2003.
22. Taubert G, Winkelmann BR, Schleiffer T, et al: Prevalence, predictors, and consequences of unrecognized diabetes mellitus in 3266 patients scheduled for coronary angiography. Am Heart J 145:285, 2003.

Diabetes and Acute Myocardial Infarction

23. Norhammar A, Tenerz A, Nilsson G, et al: Glucose metabolism in patients with acute myocardial infarction and no previous diagnosis of diabetes mellitus: A prospective study. Lancet 359:2140, 2002.
24. Wahab NN, Cowden EA, Pearce NJ, et al: Is blood glucose an independent predictor of mortality in acute myocardial infarction in the thrombolytic era? J Am Coll Cardiol 40:1748, 2002.
25. Ishihara M, Kojima S, Sakamoto T, et al: Acute hyperglycemia is associated with adverse outcome after acute myocardial infarction in the coronary intervention era. Am Heart J 150:814, 2005.
26. Suleiman M, Hammerman H, Boulos M, et al: Fasting glucose is an important independent risk factor for 30-day mortality in patients with acute myocardial infarction: A prospective study. Circulation 111:754, 2005.

27. Meir JJ, Deifuss S, Klamann A, et al: Plasma glucose at hospital admission and previous metabolic control determine myocardial infarct size and survival in patients with and without type 2 diabetes. Diabetes Care 28:2551, 2005.

28. Zeller M, Steg PG, Ravisy J, et al: Prevalence and impact of metabolic syndrome on hospital outcomes in acute myocardial infarction. Arch Int Med 165:1192, 2005.

Therapy of Heart Disease in Diabetic Patients

29. Colwell JA: Antiplatelet agents for the prevention of cardiovascular disease in diabetes mellitus. Am J Cardiovasc Drugs 4:87, 2004.

30. Watala C, Golanski J, Pluta J, et al: Reduced sensitivity of platelets from type 2 diabetic patients to acetylsalicylic acid (aspirin)—its relation to metabolic control. Thromb Res 113:97, 2004.

31. Fateh-Moghadam S, Plockinger U, Cabeze N, et al: Prevalence of aspirin resistance in patients with type 2 diabetes. Acta Diabetol 42:99, 2005.

32. Mehta SS, Silver RJ, Aaronson A, Goldfine AB: Comparison of aspirin resistance in type 1 versus type 2 diabetes mellitus. Am J Cardiol 97:567, 2006.

33. Hirsh J, Bhatt DL: Comparative benefits of clopidogrel and aspirin in high-risk patient populations. Lessons from the CAPRIE and CURE studies. Arch Intern Med 164:2106, 2004.

34. Yusuf S, Zhao F, Mehta SR, et al: Effects of clopidogrel in addition to aspirin in patients with acute coronary syndromes without ST-segment elevation. N Engl J Med 345:494, 2001.

35. Steinhubl SR, Berger PB, Mann JT, et al: Early and sustained dual oral antiplatelet therapy following percutaneous coronary intervention: A randomized controlled study. JAMA 288:2411, 2002.

36. Lincoff AM: Important triad in cardiovascular medicine: Diabetes, coronary intervention, and platelet glycoprotein IIb/IIIa receptor blockade. Circulation 107:1556, 2003.

37. Kereiakes DJ, Lincoff AM, Anderson KM, et al: Abciximab survival advantage following percutaneous coronary intervention is predicted by clinical risk profile. Am J Cardiol 90:628, 2002.

38. Topol EJ, Mark DB, Lincoff AM, et al: Outcomes at 1 year and economic implications of platelet glycoprotein IIb/IIIa blockade in patients undergoing coronary stenting: Results from a multicentre randomised trial. EPISTENT Investigators. Evaluation of Platelet IIb/IIIa Inhibitor for Stenting. Lancet 354:2019, 1999.

39. Labinaz M, Madan M, O'Shea JO, et al: Comparison of one-year outcomes following coronary artery stenting in diabetic versus nondiabetic patients (from the Enhanced Suppression of the Platelet IIb/IIIa Receptor With Integrilin Therapy [ESPRIT] trial). Am J Cardiol 90:585, 2002.

40. Roffi M, Chew DP, Mukherjee D, et al: Platelet glycoprotein IIb/IIIa inhibitors reduce mortality in diabetic patients with non-ST-segment-elevation acute coronary syndromes. Circulation 104:2767, 2001.

41. Mehilli J, Kastrati A, Schühlen, H, et al: Randomized clinical trial of abciximab in diabetic patients undergoing elective percutaneous coronary interventions after treatment with a high loading dose of clopidogrel. Circulation 110:3627, 2004.

42. Puma JA, Banko LT, Pieper KS, et al: Clinical characteristics predict benefits from eptifibatide therapy during coronary stenting: Insights from the Enhanced Suppression of the Platelet IIb/IIIa Receptor with Integrillin Therapy (ESPIRIT) trial. J Am Coll Cardiol 47:715, 2006.

43. Heitzer T, Ollmann I, Koke K, et al: Platelet glycoprotein IIb/IIIa receptor blockade improves vascular nitric oxide bioavailability in patients with coronary artery disease. Circulation 108:536, 2003.

44. Lincoff Am, Kleiman NS, Kereiakes DJ, et al: Long-term efficacy of bivalidurin and provisional glycoprotein IIb/IIIa blockade vs heparin and planned glycoprotein IIb/IIIa blockade during percutaneous coronary revascularization. REPLACE-2 randomized trial. JAMA 292:696, 2004.

45. Gurm HS, Sarembock IJ, Kereiakes DJ, et al: Use of bivalirudin during percutaneous coronary intervention in patients with diabetes mellitus: An analysis from the Randomized Evaluation in Percutaneous Coronary Intervention Linking Angiomax to Reduced Clinical Events (REPLACE)-2 trial: J Am Coll Cardiol 45:1932, 2005.

46. Cooper-Dehoff R, Cohen JD, Bakris GL, et al: Predictors of development of diabetes mellitus in patients with coronary artery disease taking antihypertensive medications (findings from the International VErapamil SR-Trandolapril Study [INVEST]). Am J Cardiol 98:890, 2006.

47. McDonald CG, Majumdar SR, Mahon JL, Johnson JA: The effectiveness of beta blockers after myocardial infarction in patients with type 2 diabetes. Diabetes Care 28:2113, 2005.

48. Devereaux PJ, Yang H, Guyatt GH, et al: Rationale, design, and organization of the PeriOperative Ischemic Evaluation (POISE) trial: A randomized controlled trial of metoprolol versus placebo in patients undergoing noncardiac surgery. Am Heart J 152:223, 2006.

49. Kopecky SL: Effecet of beta blockers, particularly carvedilol, on reducing the risk of events after acute myocardial infarction. Am J Cardiol 98:1115, 2006.

50. Bakris GL, Fonseca V, Katholi RE, et al: Metabolic effects of carvedilol vs metoprolol in patients with type 2 diabetes mellitus and hypertension. A randomized controlled trial. JAMA 292:2227, 2004.

51. Brogan GX, Peterson ED, Mulgund J, Bhatt DL, et al: Treatment disparities in the care of patients with and without diabetes presenting with non-ST-segment elevation acute coronary syndromes. Diabetes Care 29:9, 2006.

52. Nesto RW, Zarich S: Acute myocardial infarction in diabetes mellitus: Lessons learned from ACE inhibition. Circulation 97:12, 1998.

53. Zuanetti G, Latini R, Maggioni AP, et al: Effect of the ACE inhibitor lisinopril on mortality in diabetic patients with acute myocardial infarction: Data from the GISSI-3 study. Circulation 96:4239, 1997.

54. Gustafsson I, Torp-Pedersen C, Køber L, et al: Effect of the angiotensin-converting enzyme inhibitor trandolapril on mortality and morbidity in diabetic patients with left ventricular dysfunction after acute myocardial infarction. Trace Study Group. J Am Coll Cardiol 34:83, 1999.

55. Gottlieb S, Leor J, Shotan A, et al: Comparison of effectiveness of angiotensin-converting enzyme inhibitors after acute myocardial infarction in diabetic versus nondiabetic patients. Am J Cardiol 92:1020, 2003.

56. Pfeffer MA, McMurray JJV, Velazquez EJ, et al: Valsartan, captopril, or both in myocardial infarction complicated by heart failure, left ventricular dysfunction, or both. N Eng J Med 349:1893, 2003.

57. Aguilar D, Solomon SD, Kober L, et al: Newly diagnosed and previously known diabetes mellitus and 1-year outcomes of acute myocardial infarction: The Valsartan in Acute Myocardial Infarction (VALIANT) trial. Circulation 110:1572, 2004.

58. Pfeffer MA, Swedberg K, Granger CB, et al: Effects of candesartan on mortality and morbidity in patients with chronic heart failure: The CHARM-Overall programme. Lancet 362:759, 2003.

59. Yusuf S, Ostergren JB, Gerstein HC, et al: Effects of candesartan in the development of a new diagnosis of diabetes mellitus in patients with heart failure. Circulation 112:48, 2005.

60. McFarlane SI, Kumar A, Sowers JR: Mechanisms by which angiotensin-converting enzyme inhibitors prevent diabetes and cardiovascular disease. Am J Cardiol 91:30H, 2003.

61. Heart Outcomes Prevention Evaluation (HOPE) study investigators: Effects of ramipril on cardiovascular and microvascular outcomes in people with diabetes mellitus: Results of the HOPE study and MICRO-HOPE substudy. Lancet 355:253, 2000.

62. Foo K, Cooper J, Deaner A, et al: A single serum glucose measurement predicts adverse outcomes across the whole range of acute coronary syndromes. Heart 89:512, 2003.

63. Doenst T, Wijeysundera D, Karkouti K, et al: Hyperglycemia during cardiopulmonary bypass is an independent risk factor for mortality in patients undergoing cardiac surgery. J Thorac Cardiovasc Surg 131:11, 2006.

64. Pinto DS, Skolnick AH, Kirtane AJ, et al: U-shaped relationship of blood glucose with adverse outcomes among patients with ST-segment elevation myocardial infarction. J Am Coll Cardiol 46:178, 2005.

65. Goyal A, Mahaffey KW, Garg J, et al: Prognostic significance of the change in glucose level in the first 24 h after acute myocardial infarction: Results from the CARDINAL study. Eur Heart J 27:1289, 2006.

66. Brunner EJ, Shipley MJ, Witte DR, et al: Relation between blood glucose and coronary mortality over 33 years in the Whitehall study. Diabetes Care 29:26, 2006.

Insulin Therapy in Diabetic Patients With Heart Disease

67. Malmberg K, Ryden L, Efendic S, et al: Randomized trial of insulin-glucose infusion followed by subcutaneous insulin treatment in diabetic patients with acute myocardial infarction (DIGAMI study): Effects on mortality at 1 year. J Am Coll Cardiol 26:57, 1995.

68. Malmberg K, Norhammar A, Wedel H, et al: Glycometabolic state at admission: Important risk marker of mortality in conventionally treated patients with diabetes mellitus and acute myocardial infarction: Long-term results from the Diabetes and Insulin-Glucose Infusion in Acute Myocardial Infarction (DIGAMI) study. Circulation 99:2626, 1999.

69. Malmberg K, Ryden L, Wedel H, et al: Intense metabolic control by means of insulin in patients with diabetes mellitus and acute myocardial infarction (DIGAMI 2): Effects on mortality and morbidity. Eur Heart J 26:650-661, 2005.

70. Furnary AP, Gao G, Grunkemeier GL, et al: Continuous insulin infusion reduces mortality in patients with diabetes undergoing coronary artery bypass grafting. J Thorac Cardiovasc Surg 125:1007, 2003.

71. Van den Berghe G, Wilmer A, Hermans G, et al: Intensive insulin therapy in the medical ICU. N Engl J Med 354:449, 2006.

72. Fath-Ordoubadi F, Beatt KJ: Glucose-insulin-potassium therapy for treatment of acute myocardial infarction: An overview of randomized placebo-controlled trials. Circulation 96:1152, 1997.

73. van der Horst IC, Zijlstra F, van't Hof AW, et al: Glucose-insulin-potassium infusion inpatients treated with primary angioplasty for acute myocardial infarction: The glucose-insulin-potassium study: A randomized trial. J Am Coll Cardiol 42:784, 2003.

74. Lazar HL, Chipkin S, Philippides G, et al: Glucose-insulin-potassium solutions improve outcomes in diabetics who have coronary artery operations. Ann Thorac Surg 70:145, 2000.

75. Lazar HL, Chipkin SR, Fitzgerald CA, et al: Tight glycemic control in diabetic coronary artery graft patients improves perioperative outcomes and decreases recurrent ischemic events. Circulation 109:1497, 2004.

76. Apstein CS: The benefits of glucose-insulin-potassium for acute myocardial infarction (and some concerns). J Am Coll Cardiol 42:792, 2003.

77. Wang P, Lloyd SG, Chatham JC: Impact of high glucose/high insulin and dichloroacetate treatment on carbohydrate oxidation and functional recovery after low-flow ischemia and reperfusion in the isolated perfused rat heart. Circulation 111:2066, 2005.

78. Chaudhuri A, Janicke D, Wilson MF, et al: Anti-inflammatory and profibrinolytic effect of insulin in acute ST-segment-elevation myocardial infarction. Circulation 109:849, 2004.

79. Dandona P, Mohanty P, Chaudhuri A, et al: Insulin infusion in acute illness. J Clin Invest 115:2069, 2005.

80. Sack MN, Yellon DM: Insulin infusion as an adjunct to reperfusion after acute coronary ischemia. A proposed direct myocardial cell survival effect independent of metabolic modulation. J Am Coll Cardiol 41:1404, 2003.

Heart Failure in Diabetic Patients

81. Ingelsson E, Arnlov J, Sundstrom J, et al: Novel metabolic risk factors for heart failure. J Am Coll Cardiol 46:2054, 2005.

82. Nichols GA, Gullio CM, Koro CE, et al: The incidence of congestive heart failure in type 2 diabetes: An update. Diabetes Care 27:1879, 2004.

83. Bertoni AG, Hundley WG, Massing MW, et al: Heart failure prevalence, incidence, and mortality in the elderly with diabetes. Diabetes Care 27:699, 2004.

84. Dries DL, Sweitzer NK, Drazner MH, et al: Prognostic impact of diabetes mellitus in patients with heart failure according to the etiology of left ventricular systolic dysfunction. J Am Coll Cardiol 38:421, 2001.

85. Domanski M, Krause-Steinrauf H, et al: The effect of diabetes on outcomes of patients with advanced heart failure in the BEST trial. J Am Col Cardiol 42:914, 2003.

86. Pocock SJ, Wang, D, Pfeffer MA, et al: Predictors of mortality and morbidity in patients with chronic heart failure. Eur Heart J 27:65, 2006.

87. Rutter MK, Parise H, Benjamin EJ, et al: Impact of glucose intolerance and insulin resistance on cardiac structure and function: Sex-related differences in the Framingham Heart Study. Circulation 107:448, 2003.

88. Zieman S, Kass D: Advanced glycation end product cross-linking: Pathophysiologic roles and therapeutic target in cardio vascular disease. Congest Heart Fail 10:144-149, 2004.

89. Tan KC, Shiu SW, Chow WS, et al: Association between serum levels of soluble receptor for advanced glycation end products and circulating advanced glycation end products in type 2 diabetes. Diabetologica 49:2756, 2006.

90. Belke DD, Dillmann WH: Altered cardiac calcium handling in diabetes. Curr Hypertens Rep 6:424, 2004.

91. Taegtmeyer H, McNulty P, Young ME: Adaptation and maladaptation of the heart in diabetes: Part I. Circulation 105:1727, 2002.

92. Young ME, McNulty P, Taegtmeyer H: Adaptation and maladaptation of the heart in diabetes: Part II. Circulation 105:1861, 2002.

93. Sharma S, Adrogue JV, Golfman L, et al: Intramyocardial lipid accumulation in the failing human heart resembles the lipotoxic rat heart. FASEB J 18:1692, 2004.

94. Peterson HR, Herrero P, Schechtman KB, et al: Effect of obesity and insulin resistance on myocardial substrate metabolism and efficiency in young women. Circulation 109:2191, 2004.

95. Ledru F, Ducimetiere P, Battaglia S, et al: New diagnostic criteria for diabetes and coronary artery disease: Insights from an angiographic study. J Am Coll Cardiol 37:1543, 2001.

96. McDonagh PF, Hokama JY: Microvascular perfusion and transport in the diabetic heart. Microcirculation 7:163, 2000.

97. Schindler TH, Facta AD, Prior JO, et al: Improvement of coronary vascular dysfunction on type 2 diabetic patients with euglycemic control. Heart 93:345, 2007.

98. Martin A, Komada MR, Sane DC: Abnormal angiogenesis in diabetes mellitus. Med Res Rev 23:117, 2003.

99. Sasso FC, Torella D, Carbonara O, et al: Increased vascular endothelial growth factor expression but impaired vascular endothelial growth factor receptor signaling in the myocardium of type 2 diabetic patients with chronic coronary heart disease. J Am Coll Cardiol 46:827, 2005.

100. Grover GJ, Garlid KD: ATP-sensitive potassium channels: A review of their cardioprotective pharmacology. J Mol Cell Cardiol 32:677, 2000.

101. Ghosh S, Standen NB, Galinianes M: Failure to precondition pathological human myocardium. J Am Coll Cardiol 37:711, 2001.

102. Ishihara M, Inoue I, Kawagoe T, et al: Diabetes mellitus prevents ischemic preconditioning in patients with a first acute anterior wall myocardial infarction. J Am Coll Cardiol 38:1007, 2001.

103. Fonarow GC, Srikanthan P: Diabetic cardiomyopathy. Endocrinol Metab Clin North Am 35:575, 2006.

104. Picano E: Diabetic cardiomyopathy. The importance of being earliest. J Am Coll Cardiol 42:454, 2003.

105. Diamant M, Lamb HJ, Groeneveld Y, et al: Diastolic dysfunction is associated with altered myocardial metabolism in asymptomatic normotensive patients with well-controlled type 2 diabetes mellitus. J Am Coll Cardiol 42:328, 2003.

106. Solomon SD, St. John Sutton M, Lamas GA, et al: Ventricular remodeling does not accompany the development of heart failure in diabetic patients after myocardial infarction. Circulation 106:1251, 2002.

107. Standl E, Schnell O: A new look at the heart in diabetes mellitus: From ailing to failing. Diabetologia 43:1455, 2000.

108. Deedwania PC: Diabetes and hypertension, the deadly duet: Importance, therapeutic strategy, and selection of drug therapy. Cardiol Clin 23:139, 2005.

109. The ALLHAT Officers and Coordinators for the ALLHAT Collaborative Research Group. Major outcomes in high-risk hypertensive patients randomized to angiotensin-converting enzyme inhibitor or calcium channel blocker vs. diuretic: The Antihypertensive and Lipid-Lowering Treatment to Prevent Heart Attack Trial (ALLHAT) 288:2981, 2002.

110. Wing LM, Reid CM, Ryan P, et al: A comparison of outcomes with angiotensin-converting—enzyme inhibitors and diuretics for hypertension in the elderly. N Engl J Med 348:583, 2003.

111. Iribarren C, Karter AJ, Go AS, et al: Glycemic control and heart failure among adult patients with diabetes. Circulation 103:2668, 2001.

112. Stratton IM, Adler AI, Neil HA, et al: Association of glycaemia with macrovascular and microvascular complications of type 2 diabetes (UKPDS 35): Prospective observational study. BMJ 321:405, 2000.

Management of Heart Disease in Diabetic Patients

113. Beta-blocker Evaluation of Survival Trial Investigators. A trial of the beta-blocker bucindolol in patients with advanced chronic heart failure. N Engl J Med 344:1659, 2001.

114. Hjalmarson A, Goldstein S, Fagerberg B, et al: Effects of controlled-release metoprolol on total mortality, hospitalizations, and well-being in patients with heart failure: The Metoprolol CR/XL Randomized Intervention Trial in congestive heart failure (MERIT-HF). JAMA 283:1295, 2000.

115. Packer M, Coats AJ, Fowler MB, et al: Effect of carvedilol on survival in severe chronic heart failure. N Engl J Med 344:1651, 2001.

116. Packer M, Fowler MB, Roecker EB, et al: Effect of carvedilol on the morbidity of patients with severe chronic heart failure: Results of the carvedilol prospective randomized cumulative survival (COPERNICUS) study. Circulation 106:2194, 2002.

117. Domanski M, Krause-Steinrauf H, Deedwania P, et al: The effect of diabetes on outcomes of patients with advanced heart failure in the BEST trial. J Am Coll Cardiol 42:914, 2003.

118. Poole-Wilson PA, Swedberg K, Cleland JG, et al: Comparison of carvedilol and metoprolol on clinical outcomes in patients with chronic heart failure in the Carvedilol Or Metoprolol European Trial (COMET): Randomised controlled trial. Lancet 362:7, 2003.

119. Nesto RW: Pharmacological treatment and prevention of heart failure in the diabetic patient. Rev Cardiovasc Med 5:1, 2004.

120. Pitt B, Poole-Wilson PA, Segal R, et al: Effect of losartan compared with captopril on mortality in patients with symptomatic heart failure: Randomised trial-The Losartan Heart Failure Survival Study ELITE II. Lancet 355:1582, 2000.

121. Cohn JN, Tognoni G: A randomized trial of the angiotensin-receptor blocker valsartan in chronic heart failure. N Engl J Med 345:1667, 2001.

122. Pfeffer MA, Swedberg K, Granger CB, et al: Effects of candesartan on mortality and morbidity in patients with chronic heart failure: The CHARM-Overall programme. Lancet 362:759, 2003.

123. Brenner BM, Cooper ME, de Zeeuw D, et al: Effects of losartan on renal and cardiovascular outcomes in patients with type 2 diabetes and nephropathy. N Engl J Med 345:861, 2001.

124. Lindholm LH, Ibsen H, Dahlof B, et al: Cardiovascular morbidity and mortality in patients with diabetes in the Losartan Intervention For Endpoint reduction in hypertension study (LIFE): A randomised trial against atenolol. Lancet 359:1004, 2002.

125. Stier CT Jr., Chander PN, Rocha R: Aldosterone as a mediator in cardiovascular injury. Cardiol Rev 10:97, 2002.

126. Weber KT: Aldosterone in congestive heart failure. N Engl J Med 345:1689, 2001.

127. Pitt B, Remme W, Zannad F, et al: Eplerenone, a selective aldosterone blocker, in patients with left ventricular dysfunction after myocardial infarction. N Engl J Med 348:1309, 2003.

128. UK Prospective Diabetes Study (UKPDS) group: Intensive blood-glucose control with sulphonylureas or insulin compared with conventional treatment and risk of complications in patients with type 2 diabetes (UKPDS 33). Lancet 352:837, 1998.

129. Kahn SE, Hafner SM, Heise MA, et al: Gylcemic durability of rosiglitazone, metformin, or glyburide monotherapy. N Engl J Med 355:2427, 2006.

130. Quast U, Stephan D, Bleger S, Russ U: The impact of ATP-sensitive K+ channel subtype selectivity of insulin secretagogues for the coronary vasculature and myocardium. Diabetes 53(Suppl 3):S156, 2004.

131. Goldstein BJ: Differentiating members of the thiazolidinedione class: A focus on efficacy. Diabetes Metab Res Rev 18(Suppl 2):S16, 2002.

132. Nesto RW, Bell D, Bonow RO, et al: Thiazolidinedione use, fluid retention, and congestive heart failure: A consensus statement from the American Heart Association and American Diabetes Association. Circulation 108:2941, 2003.

133. Dormandy JA, Charbonnel B, Eckland DJA, et al: Secondary prevention of macrovascular events in patients with type 2 diabetes in the PROactive Study (PROspective pioglitAzone Clinical Trial in macroVascular Events): A randomized controlled trial. Lancet 366:1279, 2005.

134. Gerstein HC, Yusuf S, Bosch J, et al: Effect of rosiglitazone on the frequency of diabetes in patients with impaired glucose tolerance or impaired fasting glucose: A randomized controlled trial. Lancet 368:1096, 2006.

135. Libby P: Metformin and vascular protection: A cardiologist's view. Diabetes Metab 29:6S17, 2003.

136. Johnson JA, Majumdar SR, Simpson SH, et al: Decreased mortality associated with the use of metformin compared with sulfonylurea monotherapy in type 2 diabetes. Diabetes Care 25:2244, 2002.

137. Eurich DT, Majumdar SR, McAlister FA, et al: Improved clinical outcomes associated with metformin in patients with diabetes and heart failure. Diabetes Care 28:2345, 2005.

138. Krenz AJ, Bailey CJ: Oral antidiabetic agents: current role in type 2 diabetes mellitus. Drugs 65:385, 2005.

139. Salpeter S, Greyber E, Pasternak G, Salpeter E: Risk of fatal and nonfatal lactic acidosis with metformin use in type 2 diabetes mellitus. Cochrane Database Sys Rev CD002967, 2006.

140. Flaherty JD, Davidson CJ: Diabetes and coronary revascularization. JAMA 293:1501, 2005.

141. Kip KE, Alderman EL, Bourassa MG, et al: Differential influence of diabetes mellitus on increased jeopardized myocardium after initial angioplasty or bypass surgery: Bypass angioplasty revascularization investigation. Circulation 105:1914, 2002.

142. Reginelli JP, Bhatt DL: Why diabetics are at risk in percutaneous coronary intervention and the appropriate management of diabetics in interventional cardiology. J Invasive Cardiol 14(Suppl E):2E, 2002.

143. Lepor NE, Madyoon H, Kereiakes D: Effective and efficient strategies for coronary revascularization in the drug-eluting stent era. Rev Cardiovasc Med 3:S38, 2002.

144. Maser RE, Lenhard MJ: Review: Cardiovascular autonomic neuropathy due to diabetes mellitus: Clinical manifestations, consequences, and treatment. J Clin Endocrinol Metab 90:5896, 2005.

145. Boulton AJM, Vinik AI, Arezzo JC, et al: Diabetic neuropathies: A statement by the American Diabetes Association. Diabetes Care 28:956, 2005.

CH 60

PART VIII

Diseases of the Heart, Pericardium, and Pulmonary Vasculature Bed

CHAPTER 61

Etiology, 1563
Prevention, 1563
Anatomy and Embryology, 1563
Normal Cardiac Anatomy, 1564
Fetal and Transitional
  Circulations, 1565

Pathological Consequences of Congenital Cardiac Lesions, 1566
Congestive Heart Failure, 1566
Cyanosis, 1567
Pulmonary Hypertension, 1568
Cardiac Arrhythmias, 1570
Infective Endocarditis, 1571
Chest Pain, 1571

Evaluation of the Patient with Congenital Heart Disease, 1572
Physical Examination, 1572
Electrocardiogram, 1572
Chest Radiograph, 1572
Cardiovascular MRI, 1573
Transthoracic
  Echocardiography, 1573
Transesophageal
  Echocardiography, 1575
Three-Dimensional
  Echocardiography, 1575
Intracardiac Echocardiography, 1575
Cardiac Catheterization, 1575

Specific Cardiac Defects, 1577
Left-to-Right Shunts, 1577
Cyanotic Heart Disease, 1587
Valvular and Vascular
  Conditions, 1605
Miscellaneous Lesions, 1618

References, 1621

Congenital Heart Disease

Gary D. Webb, Jeffrey F. Smallhorn, Judith Therrien, and Andrew N. Redington

This chapter has been written for the practicing cardiologist and is compatible with the existing expert management recommendations[1-10] for the care of adult patients with congenital cardiac defects. These guidelines are available at www.cachnet. org, www.achd-library.com, and www. isaccd.org. More detailed information can be found in other sources.[11,12] *Congenital cardiovascular disease* is defined as an abnormality in cardiocirculatory structure or function that is present at birth, even if it is discovered much later. Congenital cardiovascular malformations usually result from altered embryonic development of a normal structure or failure of such a structure to progress beyond an early stage of embryonic or fetal development. The aberrant patterns of flow created by an anatomical defect may, in turn, significantly influence the structural and functional development of the remainder of the circulation. For instance, the presence in utero of mitral atresia may prohibit normal development of the left ventricle, aortic valve, and ascending aorta. Similarly, constriction of the fetal ductus arteriosus may result in right ventricular dilation and tricuspid regurgitation in the fetus and newborn, contribute importantly to the development of pulmonary arterial aneurysms in the presence of a ventricular septal defect (VSD) and absent pulmonary valve, or result in an alteration in the number and caliber of fetal and newborn pulmonary vascular resistance vessels.

Postnatal events can markedly influence the clinical presentation of a specific "isolated" malformation. Infants with Ebstein malformation of the tricuspid valve may improve dramatically as the magnitude of tricuspid regurgitation diminishes with the normal fall in pulmonary vascular resistance after birth; and infants with pulmonary atresia or severe stenosis may not become cyanotic until normal spontaneous closure of a patent ductus arteriosus (PDA) occurs. Ductal constriction many days after birth also may be a central factor in some infants in the development of coarctation of the aorta. Still later in life, patients with a VSD may experience spontaneous closure of the abnormal communication or may develop right ventricular outflow tract obstruction and/or aortic regurgitation or pulmonary vascular obstructive disease. These selected examples serve to emphasize that anatomical and physiological changes in the heart and circulation can continue indefinitely from prenatal life in association with any specific congenital cardiocirculatory lesion.

INCIDENCE. The true incidence of congenital cardiovascular malformations is difficult to determine accurately, partly because of difficulties in definition. About 0.8 percent of live births are complicated by a cardiovascular malformation. This figure does not take into account what may be the two most common cardiac anomalies: the congenital, functionally normal bicuspid aortic valve and prolapse of the mitral valve.

Specific defects can show a definite gender preponderance: PDA, Ebstein anomaly of the tricuspid valve, and atrial septal defect (ASD) are more common in females, whereas aortic valve stenosis, coarctation of the aorta, hypoplastic left heart, pulmonary and tricuspid atresia, and transposition of the great arteries (TGA) are more common in males.

Extracardiac anomalies occur in about 25 percent of infants with significant cardiac disease, and their presence may significantly increase mortality. The extracardiac anomalies are often multiple. One third of infants with both cardiac and extracardiac anomalies have some established syndrome.

ADULT PATIENT. Thanks to the great successes of pediatric cardiac care, the overall number of adult patients with congenital heart disease (CHD) is now greater than the number of pediatric cases. In 2000, there were about 485,000 American adults with moderately complex to very complex CHD. There were another 300,000 patients with simple forms of CHD, for a total population of 785,000 adult CHD patients in the United States. The 485,000 moderately to very complex patients are at significant risk of premature mortality, reoperation, or future complications of their conditions and their treatments. Many patients, especially those with moderately to very complex conditions, should see a specialist. At present, there are not enough such practitioners or facilities to always make this possible. Adult patients should have been taught in adolescence about their condition, their future outlook, and the possibility of further surgery and complications if appropriate, and they also should have been advised about their responsibilities in ensuring self-care and professional surveillance. Copies of operative reports should accompany patients being transferred for adult care, along with other key documents from the pediatric file.

Table 61-1 lists the types of patients who should be considered "simple" and suitable for community care. Tables 61-2 and 61-3 show the diagnoses for "moderately complex" and "very complex" patients. Moderately and very complex patients should be monitored throughout their lives.

CHD in the adult is not simply a continuation of the childhood experience. The patterns of many lesions change in adult life. Arrhythmias are more frequent and of a different character (see Chap. 35). Cardiac chambers often enlarge, and ventricles tend to develop systolic dysfunction. Bioprosthetic valves, prone to early failure in childhood, last longer when implanted at an older age. The comorbidities that tend to develop in adult life often become important factors needing attention. As a result, the needs of these adult CHD patients are often best met by a physician or a team familiar with both pediatric and adult cardiology issues. Congenital heart surgery and interventional catheterization procedures should be performed at centers with adequate surgical and institutional volumes of congenital heart cases at any age.

Echocardiographic studies, diagnostic heart catheterizations, electrophysiological studies, and magnetic resonance imaging (MRI) and other imaging of complex cases (see Chaps. 14 to 19) are best done where qualified staff has relevant training, experience, and equipment. Ideally, patient care should be multidisciplinary. Special cardiology and echocardiography skills are essential, but individuals with other special training, experience, and interest should also be accessible. These include congenital heart surgeons and their teams, nurses, reproductive health staff, mental health professionals, medical imaging specialists, respiratory consultants, and others.

TABLE 61–1	Types of Adult Patients with Simple Congenital Heart Disease*

Native Disease
Isolated congenital aortic valve disease
Isolated congenital mitral valve disease (except parachute valve, cleft leaflet)
Isolated patent foramen ovale or small atrial septal defect
Isolated small ventricular septal defect (no associated lesions)
Mild pulmonic stenosis

Repaired Conditions
Previously ligated or occluded ductus arteriosus
Repaired secundum or sinus venosus atrial septal defect without residua
Repaired ventricular septal defect without residua

*These patients can usually be cared for in the general medical community.
From Webb G, Williams R, Alpert J, et al: 32nd Bethesda Conference: Care of the Adult with Congenital Heart Disease, October 2-3, 2000. J Am Coll Cardiol 37:1161, 2001.

TABLE 61–2	Types of Adult Patients with Congenital Heart Disease of Moderate Severity*

Aorto-left ventricular fistulas

Anomalous pulmonary venous drainage, partial or total

Atrioventricular septal defects (partial or complete)

Coarctation of the aorta

Ebstein anomaly

Infundibular right ventricular outflow obstruction of significance

Ostium primum atrial septal defect

Patent ductus arteriosus (not closed)

Pulmonary valve regurgitation (moderate to severe)

Pulmonic valve stenosis (moderate to severe)

Sinus of Valsalva fistula/aneurysm

Sinus venosus atrial septal defect

Subvalvular or supravalvular aortic stenosis (except HOCM)

Tetralogy of Fallot

Ventricular septal defect with the following:
    Absent valve or valves
    Aortic regurgitation
    Coarctation of the aorta
    Mitral disease
    Right ventricular outflow tract obstruction
    Straddling tricuspid/mitral valve
    Subaortic stenosis

*These patients should be seen periodically at regional adult congenital heart disease centers.
HOCM = hypertrophic obstructive cardiomyopathy.
From Webb G, Williams R, Alpert J, et al: 32nd Bethesda Conference: Care of the Adult with Congenital Heart Disease, October 2-3, 2000. J Am Coll Cardiol 37:1161, 2001.

TABLE 61–3	Types of Adult Patients with Congenital Heart Disease of Great Complexity*

Conduits, valved or nonvalved

Cyanotic congenital heart (all forms)

Double-outlet ventricle

Eisenmenger syndrome

Fontan procedure

Mitral atresia

Single ventricle (also called *double inlet* or *outlet, common* or *primitive*)

Pulmonary atresia (all forms)

Pulmonary vascular obstructive diseases

Transposition of the great arteries

Tricuspid atresia

Truncus arteriosus/hemitruncus

Other abnormalities of atrioventricular or ventriculoarterial connection not included above (i.e., crisscross heart, isomerism, heterotaxy syndromes, ventricular inversion)

*These patients should be seen regularly at adult congenital heart disease centers.
From Webb G, Williams R, Alpert J, et al: 32nd Bethesda Conference: Care of the Adult with Congenital Heart Disease, October 2-3, 2000. J Am Coll Cardiol 37:1161, 2001.

Etiology

Congenital cardiac malformations can occur with mendelian inheritance directly as a result of a genetic abnormality, be strongly associated with an underlying genetic disorder (e.g., trisomy), be related directly to the effect of an environmental toxin (e.g., alcohol), or result from an interaction between multifactorial genetic and environmental influences too complex to allow a single definition of cause (e.g., CHARGE syndrome [see "Syndromes in Congenital Heart Disease" later]). The latter group is shrinking as genetic research identifies new genetic abnormalities underlying many conditions.

GENETIC. A single gene mutation can be causative in the familial forms of ASD with prolonged atrioventricular (AV) conduction; mitral valve prolapse; VSD; congenital heart block; situs inversus; pulmonary hypertension; and the syndromes of Noonan, LEOPARD, Ellis-van Creveld, and Kartagener (see "Syndromes in Congenital Heart Disease" later). The genes responsible for several defects have now been identified (e.g., long-QT syndrome, Holt-Oram syndrome, Marfan syndrome, hypertrophic cardiomyopathy, supravalvular aortic stenosis), and contiguous gene defects on the long arm of chromosome 22 underlie the conotruncal malformations of DiGeorge and velocardiofacial syndromes. At present, less than 15 percent of all cardiac malformations can be accounted for by chromosomal aberrations or genetic mutations or transmission (see Chaps. 7-9).

It is interesting, but unexplained, that several different gene defects may lead to the same cardiac malformation (e.g., AVSD). Furthermore, the finding that, with some exceptions, only one of a pair of monozygotic twins is affected by CHD indicates that most cardiovascular malformations are not inherited in a simple manner. However, this observation may have led, in the past, to an underestimation of the genetic contribution because most recent twin studies reveal more than double the incidence of heart defects in monozygotic twins but usually in only one of the pair. Family studies indicate a 2-fold to 10-fold increase in the incidence of CHD in siblings of affected patients or in the offspring of an affected parent. Malformations are often concordant or partially concordant within families. Routine fetal cardiac screening of subsequent pregnancies should be performed in such circumstances.

ENVIRONMENTAL. Maternal rubella, ingestion of thalidomide and isotretinoin early during gestation, and chronic maternal alcohol abuse are environmental insults known to interfere with normal cardiogenesis in humans. Rubella syndrome consists of cataracts; deafness; microcephaly; and, either singly or in combination, PDA, pulmonary valve and/or arterial stenosis, and ASD. Thalidomide exposure is associated with major limb deformities and, occasionally, with cardiac malformations without a predilection for a specific lesion. Tricuspid valve anomalies are associated with ingestion of lithium during pregnancy. The fetal alcohol syndrome consists of microcephaly, micrognathia, microphthalmia, prenatal growth retardation, developmental delay, and cardiac defects (often defects of the ventricular septum) in about 45 percent of affected infants.

Prevention

Physicians who deal with pregnant women should be aware of the effects of known teratogens, as well as drugs (e.g., ACE inhibition) and fetal renal development that may have a functional rather than a structural damaging influence on the fetal and newborn heart and circulation, and they should recognize that for many drugs, information about their teratogenic potential is inadequate. Similarly, appropriate radiological equipment and techniques for reducing gonadal and fetal radiation exposure should always be used to reduce the potential hazards of this likely cause of birth defects.

Detection of genetic abnormalities is becoming an increasing reality for many problems. Fetal cells are obtained from amniotic fluid or chorionic villus biopsy. Many fetuses in whom CHD is detected will undergo genetic testing, and fetal echo is frequently indicated when a chromosomal abnormality is diagnosed for other reasons. Many social, religious, and legal considerations influence whether termination of pregnancy is performed under these circumstances, but the improved outcomes for even the most complex CHDs frequently argue against the cardiac condition being used as the sole reason. Immunization of children with rubella vaccine has been one of the most effective preventive strategies against fetal rubella syndrome and its associated congenital cardiac abnormalities.

ANATOMY AND EMBRYOLOGY
Embryology

NORMAL CARDIAC DEVELOPMENT. During the first month of gestation, the primitive, straight cardiac tube is formed, comprising the sinuatrium (most cephalad), the primitive ventricle, the bulbus cordis, and the truncus arteriosus (most caudad) in series. In the second month of gestation, this tube doubles over on itself to form two parallel pumping systems, each with two chambers and a great artery. The two atria develop from the sinuatrium, the AV canal is divided by the endocardial cushions into tricuspid and mitral orifices, and the right and left ventricles develop from the primitive ventricle and bulbus cordis. Differential growth of myocardial cells causes the straight cardiac tube to bear to the right, and the bulboventricular portion of the tube doubles over on itself, bringing the ventricles side by side. Migration of the AV canal to the right and of the ventricular septum to the left serves to align each ventricle with its appropriate AV valve. At the distal end of the cardiac tube, the bulbus cordis divides into a subaortic muscular conus and a subpulmonary muscular conus; the subpulmonary conus elongates and the subaortic conus resorbs, allowing the aorta to move posteriorly and connect with the left ventricle.

ABNORMAL DEVELOPMENT. A host of anomalies can result from defects in this basic developmental pattern. Double-inlet left ventricle is observed if the tricuspid orifice does not align over the right ventricle. The various types of persistent truncus arteriosus result from failure of the truncus to divide into main pulmonary artery and aorta. Double-outlet anomalies of the right ventricle are produced by failure of either the subpulmonary or subaortic conus to resorb, whereas resorption of the subpulmonary instead of the subaortic conus may lead to TGA.

ATRIA. The primitive sinuatrium is separated into right and left atria by the down growth from its roof of the septum primum toward the AV canal, thereby creating an inferior interatrial ostium primum opening. Numerous perforations form in the anterosuperior portion of the septum primum as the septum secundum begins to develop to the right of the former. The coalescence of these perforations forms the ostium secundum. The septum secundum completely separates the atrial chambers except for a central opening—the fossa ovalis—that is covered by tissue of the septum primum, forming the valve of the foramen ovale.

Fusion of the endocardial cushions anteriorly and posteriorly divides the AV canal into tricuspid and mitral inlets. The inferior portion of the atrial septum, the superior portion of the ventricular septum, and portions of the septal leaflets of both the tricuspid and mitral valves are formed from the endocardial cushions. The integrity of the atrial septum depends on growth of the septum primum and septum secundum and proper fusion of the endocardial cushions. ASDs and various degrees of AV defect are the result of developmental deficiencies of this process.

VENTRICLES. Partitioning of the ventricles occurs as cephalic growth of the main ventricular septum results in its fusion with the endocardial cushions and the infundibular or conus septum. Defects in the ventricular septum may occur because of a deficiency of septal substance; malalignment of septal components in different planes preventing their fusion; or an overly long conus, keeping the septal components apart. Isolated defects probably result from the first mechanism, whereas the latter two appear to generate the VSDs in tetralogy of Fallot and transposition complexes.

PULMONARY VEINS. These structures arise from the primitive foregut and are drained early in embryogenesis by channels from the splanchnic plexus to the cardinal and umbilicovitelline veins. An outpouching from the posterior left atrium forms the common pulmonary vein, which communicates with the splanchnic plexus establishing pulmonary venous drainage to the left atrium. The umbilicovitelline and anterior cardinal vein communications atrophy as the common pulmonary vein is incorporated into the left atrium. Anomalous pulmonary venous connections to the umbilicovitelline (portal) venous system or to the cardinal system (superior vena cava) result from failure of the common pulmonary vein to develop or establish communications to the splanchnic plexus. Cor triatriatum results from a narrowing of the common pulmonary vein to the left atrial junction.

GREAT ARTERIES. The truncus arteriosus is connected to the dorsal aorta in the embryo by six pairs of aortic arches. Partition of the truncus arteriosus into two great arteries is a result of the fusion of tissue arising from the back wall of the vessel and the truncus septum. Rotation of the truncus coils the aortopulmonary septum and creates the normal spiral relation between aorta and pulmonary artery. Semilunar valves and their related sinuses are created by absorption and hollowing out of tissue at the distal side of the truncus ridges. Aortopulmonary septal defect and persistent truncus arteriosus represent various degrees of partitioning failure.

Although the six aortic arches appear sequentially, portions of the arch system and dorsal aorta disappear at different times during embryogenesis. The first, second, and fifth sets of paired arches regress completely. The proximal portions of the sixth arches become the right and left pulmonary arteries, and the distal left sixth arch becomes the ductus arteriosus. The third aortic arch forms the connection between internal and external carotid arteries, and the left fourth arch becomes the arterial segment between left carotid and subclavian arteries. The proximal portion of the right subclavian artery forms from the right fourth arch. An abnormality in regression of the arch system in a number of sites can produce a wide variety of arch anomalies, whereas a failure of regression usually results in a double aortic arch malformation.

CH 61

Normal Cardiac Anatomy

The key to understanding CHD is an appreciation of the segmental approach to the diagnosis of both simple and complex lesions.

CARDIAC SITUS. This refers to the status of the atrial appendages. The normal left atrial appendage is a finger-like structure with a narrow base and no guarding crista. On the other hand, the right atrial appendage is broad based and has a guarding crista and pectinate muscles. *Situs solitus* or *inversus* refers to hearts with both a morphological left and right atrium. *Situs ambiguous* refers to hearts with two morphological left or right atrial appendages. These are dealt with in the section on isomerism and have implications with regard to associated intracardiac and extracardiac abnormalities.

ATRIOVENTRICULAR CONNECTIONS. This refers to the connections between the atria and ventricles. The AV connections are said to be concordant if the morphological left atrium is connected to a morphological left ventricle via the mitral valve, with the morphological right atrium connecting to the morphological right ventricle via a tricuspid valve. They are said to be discordant in other circumstances, such as in congenitally corrected TGA (cc-TGA).

VENTRICULOARTERIAL CONNECTIONS. This refers to the connections between the semilunar valve and the ventricles. Ventriculoarterial concordance occurs when the morphological left ventricle is connected to the aorta, while the morphological right ventricle is connected to the pulmonary artery. Ventriculoarterial discordance occurs when the morphological left ventricle is connected to the pulmonary artery, with the aorta being connected to the morphological right ventricle. Double-outlet right ventricle occurs

when more than 50 percent of both great arteries are connected to the morphological right ventricle. A single-outlet heart has only one great artery connected to the heart.

ATRIA. The assignment of either a morphological left or right atrium is determined by the morphology of the atrial appendages and not by the status of the systemic or pulmonary venous drainage. Although the pulmonary veins usually drain to a morphological left atrium, and the systemic veins drain into a morphological right atrium, this is not always the case.

ATRIOVENTRICULAR VALVES. The morphological mitral valve is a bileaflet valve with the anterior leaflet in fibrous continuity with the noncoronary cusp of the aortic valve. The mitral valve leaflets are supported by two papillary muscle groups located in the anterolateral and posteromedial positions. Each papillary muscle supports the adjacent part of both valve leaflets, with considerable variation in the morphology of the papillary muscles.

The tricuspid valve is a trileaflet valve, although it can frequently be difficult to identify all three leaflets. With close inspection, the commissural chordae that arise from the papillary muscles may permit the identification of the three leaflets. The three leaflets occupy a septal anterior, superior, and inferior position. The commissures between the leaflets are the anterior septal, anterior inferior, and inferior. The papillary muscles supporting the valve leaflets arise mostly from the trabeculoseptomarginalis and its apical ramifications.

MORPHOLOGICAL RIGHT VENTRICLE. The morphological right ventricle is a triangular-shaped structure with an inlet, trabecular, and outlet component. The inlet component of the right ventricle has attachments from the septal leaflet of the tricuspid valve. Inferior to this is the moderator band, which arises at the base of the trabeculoseptomarginalis, with extensive trabeculations toward the apex of the right ventricle. The outlet component of the right ventricle consists of a fusion of three structures (i.e., the infundibular septum separating the aortic from the pulmonary valve, the ventriculoinfundibular fold separating the tricuspid valve from the pulmonary valve, and finally the anterior and posterior limbs of the trabeculoseptomarginalis).

MORPHOLOGICAL LEFT VENTRICLE. The morphological left ventricle is an elliptical-shaped structure with a fine trabecular pattern, with absent septal attachments of the mitral valve in the normal heart. It consists of an inlet portion containing the mitral valve and a tension apparatus, with an apical trabecular zone that is characterized by fine trabeculations and an outlet zone that supports the aortic valve.

SEMILUNAR VALVES. The aortic valve is a trileaflet valve with the left and right cusps giving rise to the left and right coronary arteries, respectively, with the noncoronary cusp lacking a coronary artery connection. Of note, the noncoronary cusp is in fibrous continuity with the anterior leaflet of the mitral valve. The aortic valve has a semilunar attachment to the junction of the ventricular outlet and its great arteries. The aortic cusps have a main core of fibrous tissue with endocardial linings on each surface. The cusps are thickened at the midpoint to form a nodule. The characteristics of the pulmonary valve are similar to its aortic counterpart, noting the absence of the coronary ostia arising at the superior portion of the sinuses.

AORTIC ARCH AND PULMONARY ARTERIES. In the normal heart the aortic arch usually points to the left with the first branch, the innominate artery, giving rise to the right carotid and subclavian artery. In general, the left carotid and left subclavian arteries arise separately from the aortic arch. By definition the ascending aorta is proximal to the origin of the innominate artery, with the transverse aortic arch being from the innominate artery to the origin of the left subclavian artery. The aortic isthmus is the area between the left subclavian artery and a PDA or ligamentum arteriosum.

SYSTEMIC VENOUS CONNECTIONS. In the normal heart the left and right innominate veins form the superior vena cava, which connects to the roof of the right atrium. The inferior vena cava connects to the inferior portion of the morphological right atrium, with hepatic veins joining the inferior vena cava before its insertion into the atrium. The coronary veins drain into the flow of the coronary sinus, with the latter running in the posterior AV groove and terminating in the right atrium. The inferior vena cava is guarded by the eustachian valve, which may vary in size among hearts.

PULMONARY VENOUS DRAINAGE IN THE NORMAL HEART. The pulmonary veins drain to the left-sided atrium. Usually three pulmonary veins arise from the trilobed right lung and two pulmonary veins from the bilobed left lung. The pulmonary veins drain into the left atrium in superior and inferior locations. There is a short segment of extraparenchymal pulmonary vein before disappearing into the adjacent hila of the lungs.

FETAL AND TRANSITIONAL CIRCULATIONS (Fig. 61-1)

CHD is being diagnosed with increasing frequency during fetal life. Our ability to modify the evolution of structural (by fetal intervention) and physiological (by drug therapy) heart disease is increasing. Knowledge of the changes in cardiovascular structure, function, and metabolism that occur during fetal development is more important today than at any time in the past.

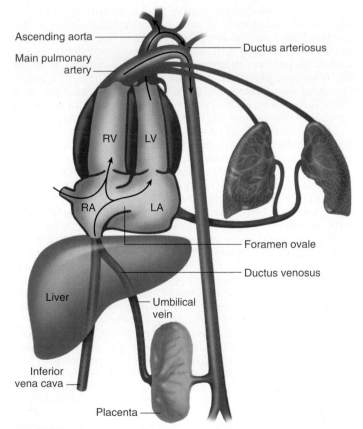

FIGURE 61-1 The fetal circulation, with arrows indicating the directions of flow. A fraction of umbilical venous blood enters the ductus venosus and bypasses the liver. This relatively highly oxygenated blood flows across the foramen ovale to the left side of the heart, preferentially perfusing the coronary arteries, head, and upper trunk. The output of the right ventricle flows preferentially across the ductus arteriosus and circulates to the placenta, as well as to the abdominal viscera and lower trunk. *(Courtesy of Dr. David Teitel.)*

FETAL CIRCULATORY PATHWAYS. Dynamic alterations occur in the circulation during the transition from fetal to neonatal life when the lungs take over the function of gas exchange from the placenta. The fetal circulation consists of parallel pulmonary and systemic pathways in contrast to the "in series" circuit of the normal postnatal circulation. Oxygenated blood returns from the placenta through the umbilical vein and enters the portal venous system. A variable amount of this stream bypasses the hepatic microcirculation and enters the inferior vena cava by way of the ductus venosus. Inferior vena caval blood is from the ductus venosus, hepatic veins, and lower body venous drainage and is partly deflected across the foramen ovale into the left atrium. Because of a streaming effect, almost all superior vena caval blood passes directly through the tricuspid valve, entering the right ventricle. Most of the blood that reaches the right ventricle bypasses the high-resistance, unexpanded lungs and passes through the ductus arteriosus into the descending aorta. The right ventricle contributes about 55 percent and the left ventricle 45 percent to the total fetal cardiac output. The major portion of blood ejected from the left ventricle supplies the brain and upper body, with lesser flow to the coronary arteries; the balance passes across the aortic isthmus to the descending aorta, where it joins with the large stream from the ductus arteriosus before flowing to the lower body and back to the placenta.

FETAL PULMONARY CIRCULATION. In fetal life, the alveoli are fluid filled, and the pulmonary arteries and arterioles have relatively thick walls and a small lumen, similar to arteries in the systemic circulation. The low pulmonary blood flow in the fetus (7 to 10 percent of the total cardiac output) is the result of high pulmonary vascular resistance. Fetal pulmonary vessels are highly reactive to changes in oxygen tension or in the pH of blood perfusing them, as well as to a number of other physiological and pharmacological influences.

EFFECTS OF CARDIAC MALFORMATIONS ON THE FETUS. Although fetal somatic growth may be unimpaired, the hemodynamic effects of many cardiac malformations can alter the development and structure of the fetal heart and circulation. For example, although lesions associated with left-to-right shunts in postnatal life rarely influence fetal cardiac size and function, regurgitant AV valves can lead to chamber dilation, hydrops, and fetal death. Ventricular obstructive lesions (e.g., aortic valve stenosis) may variably lead to hypertrophy, dilation, and failure. The secondary effects of congenital lesions are also important. Reduced flow through the left heart can result in aortic hypoplasia and coarctation. Reduced antegrade pulmonary blood flow is associated with pulmonary artery hypoplasia. These effects rarely affect the fetal circulation overtly, however, and often only become exposed as problems after birth as the ductus arteriosus closes.

FUNCTION OF THE FETAL HEART. Compared with the adult heart, the fetal and newborn heart is unique with respect to its ultrastructural appearance, its mechanical and biochemical properties, and its autonomic innervation. During late fetal and early neonatal development there is maturation of the excitation-contraction coupling process and changes in the biochemical composition of the heart's energy-utilizing myofibrillar proteins and of adenosine triphosphate and creatine phosphate energy-producing proteins. Moreover, fetal and neonatal myocardial cells are small in diameter and reduced in density so that the immature heart contains relatively more noncontractile mass (primarily mitochondria, nuclei, and surface membranes) than later in postnatal life. As a result, force generation and the extent and velocity of shortening are decreased, and stiffness and water content of ventricular myocardium are increased in the fetal and early newborn periods. The fetal heart is surrounded by fluid-filled rather than air-filled lungs. As a result, the fetal and neonatal heart has limited ability to increase cardiac output in the presence of either a volume load or a lesion that increases resistance to emptying. Ultimately, cardiac output is much more dependent on changes in heart rate, explaining why bradycardia is so poorly tolerated by the fetal circulation. Tachycardia can also rapidly lead to heart failure in the fetus, whether due to the hemodynamic issues discussed earlier or a manifestation of energy-substrate utilization.

CHANGES AT BIRTH. Inflation of the lungs at the first inspiration produces a marked reduction in pulmonary vascular resistance. The reduced extravascular pressure and increased alveolar oxygen content, as fluid is removed from the lungs and replaced by air, leads to pulmonary vasodilation and recruitment. As a result, pulmonary artery pressure falls, and pulmonary blood flow increases greatly, raising left atrial pressure and closing the flap valve of the foramen ovale. Conversely, systemic vascular resistance rises. This is related to loss of the low-resistance placental circulation and gradual closure of the ductus arteriosus. It is also related to a sudden increase in arterial blood oxygen tension, subsequent to the lack of mixing of oxygenated and deoxygenated blood that characterizes the fetal milieu. In healthy, mature infants the ductus arteriosus is profoundly constricted at 10 to 15 hours and is closed functionally by 72 hours, with total anatomical closure following within a few weeks by a process of thrombosis, intimal proliferation, and fibrosis. Preterm infants have a high incidence of persistent patency of the ductus arteriosus because of an immaturity of those mechanisms responsible for constriction.

The ductus venosus, ductus arteriosus, and foramen ovale remain potential channels for blood flow after birth. Thus persistent patency of the ductus venosus is capitalized on during balloon atrial septostomy performed via the umbilical vein. Lesions producing right or left atrial volume or pressure overload can stretch the foramen ovale and render incompetent the flap valve mechanism for its closure. Anomalies that depend on patency of the ductus arteriosus for preserving pulmonary or systemic blood flow remain latent until the ductus arteriosus constricts. A common example is the rapid intensification of cyanosis observed in infants with tetralogy of Fallot when the magnitude of pulmonary hypoperfusion is unmasked by spontaneous closure of the ductus arteriosus. Moreover, increasing evidence shows that ductal constriction is a key factor in the postnatal development of coarctation of the aorta and is clearly the most important factor governing the presentation in babies with a duct-dependent systemic circulation. The management of these conditions is discussed in the appropriate sections.

NEONATE AND INFANT. Most management decisions in patients with significant CHD occur during the first few months of life. An increase in the prenatal diagnosis of major congenital heart defects has resulted in earlier admission and intervention in the neonate with CHD. These neonates are, in general, healthier than in the past because of the administration of prostaglandins at the time of delivery, thus maintaining hemodynamic stability. With improved surgery and interventional catheterization techniques, many of these neonates undergo intervention within the first days or weeks of life. Indeed, there has been a trend toward complete repair in the neonate and young infant due to an improvement in myocardial preservation and surgical techniques. In most major cardiac centers the surgical mortality for this age group is in the range of 2 to 4 percent, which is an improvement on the results of the past, when a palliative procedure often preceded a complete repair.

CH 61

With increasing experience in this age group, the focus has now shifted from mortality to morbidity. Because the expectation is that most of these neonates and young infants will survive into their adult years, their neurodevelopmental outcome has become as important as the results of the cardiac intervention.[13] Ongoing research in this age group will provide increasing data as to the benefit of early intervention in neonates and infants with CHD.

CHILD AND ADOLESCENT. The rapid somatic growth rates of infancy and adolescence are periods of rapid hemodynamic change. Stenotic lesions that may be relatively slowly progressive throughout early childhood need more frequent surveillance during adolescence. Childhood and adolescence is a time to begin educating patients, not just their parents, about their heart disease and the responsibilities that go with it. Issues such as the need for compliance with medications, avoidance of smoking and illicit drug use, and pregnancy and contraception counseling are by no means exclusively issues of the adult with CHD and increasingly require discussion in the pediatric cardiac clinic.

Indeed, the early teenage years should be regarded as part of the transition process before transfer to adult follow-up. The whole area of the follow-up of adults with newly discovered or previously treated CHD is a burgeoning new subspecialty that will require careful planning to ensure adequate resources for the increasing number of adult "graduates" of pediatric programs. A coordinated approach with specialists in an affiliated adult congenital clinic is clearly desirable.

ADULT. Patients, and often family members, should understand their cardiac condition[14] both in terms of what has been done so far and what could happen in the future. This is important for a young patient graduating into the adult world. Patients need information and should become partners in their own care.

Potential long-term complications in adults with CHD (such as arrhythmias, ventricular failure, conduit obstruction, and endocarditis) should be explained to patients who are at relatively high risk. The possible need for future therapy—medical (antiarrhythmics, anticoagulation, heart failure therapy); catheter based (valve dilation, stents, arrhythmia ablation); or surgical (redo surgery, transplantation)—should be discussed if the patient may require them in the short or intermediate future. Day-to-day issues of concern for these young adults need to be addressed, such as exercise prescriptions,[15] driving restrictions, and traveling limitations. Many young people with CHD need advice regarding career choices, entering the work force, insurability, and life expectancy.

Many will want to start a family, and reproductive issues will need to be addressed. Discussion of appropriate contraception methods for any given patient should be offered. Counseling before conception as to the risk to the mother and the fetus for any given pregnancy should be done by specialized physicians. They will take into account the maternal cardiac anatomy, maternal functional status, maternal life expectancy, risk of CHD transmission to the offspring, and risk of premature birth. High-risk patients (e.g., Marfan with aortic root dilation, severe pulmonary hypertension, New York Heart Association [NYHA] Class III or IV, and severe aortic stenosis) must be advised against pregnancy. Intermediate-risk patients (e.g., cyanotic, mechanical valve and other warfarin [Coumadin]-requiring patients, moderate left ventricular outflow tract obstruction, moderate-to-severe left ventricular dysfunction) need to know that pregnancy, although possible, may be complicated and that they will require careful follow-up.[16,17]

Last but not least, comorbidities such as obesity, smoking, high blood pressure, diabetes, and high cholesterol level add new levels of complexity to these adults as they age and must be part of the mandate of the patient's cardiologist.

PATHOLOGICAL CONSEQUENCES OF CONGENITAL CARDIAC LESIONS

Congestive Heart Failure (see Chaps. 22 to 26)

Although the basic mechanisms of cardiac failure are similar for all ages, the common causes, time of onset, and often the approach to treatment vary with age (see Chaps. 27 to 30, 75). The development of fetal echocardiography has allowed the diagnosis of intrauterine cardiac failure. The cardinal findings of *fetal heart failure* are scalp edema, ascites, pericardial effusion, and decreased fetal movements. In *preterm infants*, especially of less than 1500 gm birth weight, persistent patency of the ductus arteriosus is the most common cause of cardiac decompensation, and other forms of structural heart disease are rare. In *full-term newborns* the earliest important causes of heart failure are the hypoplastic left heart and aortic coarctation syndromes, sustained tachyarrhythmia, cerebral or hepatic arteriovenous fistula, and myocarditis. Among the lesions commonly producing heart failure *beyond age 1 to 2 weeks,* when diminished pulmonary vascular resistance allows substantial left-to-right shunting, are VSDs and AV septal defects, TGA, truncus arteriosus, and total anomalous pulmonary venous connection. *Infants younger than 1 year* who have cardiac malformations account for 80 to 90 percent of pediatric patients who develop congestive failure. In *older children,* heart failure is often due to acquired disease or is a complication of open-heart surgical procedures. In the acquired category are rheumatic and endomyocardial diseases, infective endocarditis, hematological and nutritional disorders, and severe cardiac arrhythmias.

The distinction between left and right heart failure is less obvious in infants than in the older children or adults. Conversely, augmented filling or elevated pressure of the right ventricle in infants reduces left ventricular compliance disproportionately when compared with older children or adults and gives rise to signs of both systemic and pulmonary venous congestion.

Care of infants with heart failure must include careful consideration of the underlying structural or functional disturbance. The general aims of treatment are to achieve an increase in cardiac performance, augment peripheral perfusion, and decrease pulmonary and systemic venous congestion. In many conditions, medical management cannot control the effects of the abnormal loads imposed by a host of congenital cardiac lesions. Under these circumstances, cardiac diagnosis and interventional catheter or operative intervention may be urgently required.

Congestive heart failure is not common in adult congenital heart practice, although prevention of myocardial dysfunction is a common concern. The adult patient with CHD may develop heart failure in the presence of a substrate (e.g., myocardial dysfunction, valvular regurgitation) and a precipitant (e.g., sustained arrhythmia, pregnancy, hyperthyroidism). Patients prone to congestive failure include those with long-standing volume loads (e.g., valvular regurgitation and left-to-right shunts), those with a primary depression of myocardial function (e.g., systemic right ventricles, ventricles damaged during surgery or because of late treatment of ventricular overload). Treatment depends on a clear understanding of the elements contributing to decompensation and addressing each of the treatable components. The greatest success is achieved when the main elements can be eliminated. When this is not possible, standard palliative adult heart failure regimens are applied and may include angiotensin-converting enzyme (ACE) inhibitors,[18,19] angiotensin receptor blockers, beta blockers,[20] diuretics, resynchronization pacing,[21] transplantation,[22] and other novel therapies.

Cyanosis

DEFINITION. *Central cyanosis* refers to arterial oxygen desaturation resulting from the shunting or mixing of systemic venous blood into the arterial circulation. The magnitude of shunting/mixing and the amount of pulmonary blood flow determine the severity of desaturation.

MORPHOLOGY. Cardiac defects that result in central cyanosis can be divided into two categories: (1) those with increased pulmonary blood flow or (2) those with decreased pulmonary blood flow (Table 61-4).[1]

PATHOPHYSIOLOGY. Hypoxemia increases renal production of erythropoietin, which in turn stimulates bone marrow production of circulating red blood cells, enhancing oxygen-carrying capacity. Secondary erythrocytosis should be present in all cyanotic patients because it is a physiological response to tissue hypoxia. The improved tissue oxygenation that results from this adaptation may be sufficient to reach a new equilibrium at a higher hematocrit. However, adaptive failure can occur if the increased whole blood viscosity rises so much that it impairs oxygen delivery.

CLINICAL FEATURES

Hyperviscosity Syndrome. Erythrocytosis, by virtue of increasing whole blood viscosity, may cause hyperviscosity symptoms including headaches, faintness, dizziness, fatigue, altered mentation, visual disturbances, paresthesias, tinnitus and myalgias. Iron deficiency, a common finding in cyanotic adult patients if repeated phlebotomies or excessive bleeding occurs, may cause hyperviscosity symptoms at hematocrit levels well below 65 percent. The patient usually experiences the same hyperviscosity symptoms each time (e.g., headache, visual disturbances, fatigue), and the symptoms must be relieved by phlebotomy to qualify as hyperviscosity symptoms.

Hematological. Hemostatic abnormalities have been documented in cyanotic patients with erythrocytosis and can occur in up to 20 percent of patients. A bleeding tendency can be mild and superficial, leading to easy bruising, skin petechiae, and mucosal bleeding, or it can be moderate or life threatening with hemoptysis or intracranial, gastrointestinal, or postoperative bleeding. An elevated prothrombin and partial thromboplastin time; decreased levels of factors V, VII, VIII, and IX; qualitative and quantitative platelet disorders[23]; increased fibrinolysis; and systemic endothelial dysfunction from increased shear stress have all been implicated.[24]

Central Nervous System. Neurological complications including cerebral hemorrhage can occur secondary to hemostatic defects and can be seen in patients taking anticoagulants. Patients with right-to-left shunts may be at risk for paradoxical cerebral emboli, especially if they are iron deficient. A brain abscess should be suspected in a cyanotic patient with a new or different headache or new neurological symptoms. Air filters should be used in peripheral/central venous lines in cyanotic patients to avoid paradoxical emboli through a right-to-left shunt.

Renal. Renal dysfunction can manifest itself as proteinuria, hyperuricemia, or renal failure. Pathological studies at the level of the glomeruli show evidence of vascular abnormalities, as well as increased cellularity and fibrosis. Hyperuricemia is common and is thought to be due mainly to the decreased reabsorption of uric acid rather than to overproduction with erythrocytosis. Urate nephropathy, uric acid nephrolithiasis, and gouty arthritis may occur.

Arthritic. Rheumatological complications include gout and, especially, hypertrophic osteoarthropathy, which is thought to be responsible for the arthralgias and bone pain affecting up to one third of patients. In patients with right-to-left shunting, megakaryocytes released from the bone marrow can bypass the lung. The entrapment of megakaryocytes in the systemic arterioles and capillaries induces the release of platelet-derived growth factor, promoting local cell proliferation. New osseous formation with periostitis ensues and gives rise to arthralgia and bony pain.

Coronary Arteries. Patients with central cyanosis display dilated coronaries with no obstruction. Their level of total cholesterol is also lower than that of the general population.[25]

INTERVENTIONAL OPTIONS AND OUTCOMES

Physiological Repair. Physiological repair results in total or near-total anatomical and physiological separation of the pulmonary and systemic circulations in complex cyanotic lesions that leads to relief of cyanosis. Such procedures should be performed whenever feasible.

Palliative Surgical Intervention. Palliative surgical interventions can be performed in patients with cyanotic lesions to increase pulmonary blood flow while allowing cyanosis to persist. Palliative surgical shunts are summarized in Table 61-5. Blalock-Taussig, central, and Glenn (also called *cavopulmonary*) shunts are still in use today. Blalock-Taussig shunts seldom caused pulmonary hypertension and were less prone to causing pulmonary artery distortion. Glenn shunts have the advantage of increasing pulmonary flow without imposing a volume load on the systemic ventricle. Glenn shunts require low pulmonary artery pressures to work, and they are associated with the development over time of pulmonary arteriovenous fistulas, which can worsen cyanosis.

TABLE 61–4	Cardiac Defects Causing Central Cyanosis
Transposition of the great arteries	Ebstein's anomaly
Tetralogy of Fallot	Eisenmenger physiology
Tricuspid atresia	Critical pulmonary stenosis or atresia
Truncus arteriosus	Functionally single ventricle
Total anomalous pulmonary venous return	

Note 5 Ts and 2 Es.

TABLE 61–5	Palliative Systemic-to-Pulmonary Shunts

Arterial

Blalock-Taussig shunt (subclavian artery to PA)
  Classic—end-to-side, no or reduced ipsilateral arm pulses
  Current—side-to-side tubular grafts, preserved arm pulses

Central shunt (side-to-side tubular graft, aorta to PA)

Potts shunt (descending aorta to LPA)

Waterston shunt (ascending aorta to RPA)

Venous

Glenn shunt (SVC to ipsilateral PA without cardiac or other PA connection)

Bidirectional cavopulmonary (Glenn) shunt (end-to-side SVC to LPA and RPA shunt)

LPA = left PA; PA = pulmonary artery; RPA = right PA; SVC = superior vena cava.

Transplantation (see Chap. 27). Transplantation of heart, one or both lungs with surgical cardiac repair, and heart-lung transplantation have been performed in cyanotic patients with or without palliation who were no longer candidates for other forms of intervention. Pulmonary vascular obstructive disease precludes isolated heart transplantation. An increasing number of CHD patients with previous palliation and ventricular failure are successfully undergoing cardiac transplantation.[26] Timing of transplantation in these patients remains difficult.

OTHER MANAGEMENT

Phlebotomy. The goal of phlebotomy is symptom control. When patients have troubling symptoms of hyperviscosity, are iron replete, and are not dehydrated, removal of 250 to 500 ml of blood over 30 to 45 minutes should be performed with concomitant quantitative volume replacement. The procedure may be repeated every 24 hours until symptomatic improvement occurs or the hemoglobin level has fallen below 18 to 19 g/dl. Phlebotomy is not indicated for asymptomatic patients. The only indication for prophylactic phlebotomy is in the preoperative patient when the hematocrit is higher than 65 percent, to reduce the chances of perioperative bleeding.

Iron Replacement. If iron deficiency anemia is found or anticipated, iron supplements should be prescribed. Cyanotic patients should be helped to avoid iron deficiency, which can cause functional deterioration and is associated with an increased risk of stroke.

Bleeding Diathesis. Platelet transfusions, fresh frozen plasma, vitamin K, cryoprecipitate, and desmopressin can be used to treat severe bleeding. Given the inherent tendency to bleed, aspirin, heparin, and warfarin should be avoided in the cyanotic patient unless the risks of treatment are outweighed by the risks of nontreatment. Likewise, nonsteroidal anti-inflammatory drugs should be avoided to prevent bleeding.

Gouty Arthritis. Symptomatic hyperuricemia and gouty arthritis can be treated as needed with colchicine, probenecid, or allopurinol.

REPRODUCTIVE ISSUES. Pregnancy in cyanotic CHD (excluding Eisenmenger syndrome) results in a 32 percent incidence of maternal cardiovascular complications and a 37 percent incidence of fetal prematurity. Pregnant women with a resting oxygen saturation greater than 85 percent fare better than women with an oxygen saturation less than 85 percent.[16]

FOLLOW-UP. All cyanotic patients should be followed by a CHD cardiologist, and particular attention should be paid to the underlying heart condition; symptoms of hyperviscosity; systemic complications of cyanosis; change in exercise tolerance; change in saturation levels; and prophylaxis against endocarditis, influenza, and pneumococcal infections. In stable cyanotic patients, yearly follow-up is recommended and should include annual flu shots, periodic pneumococcal vaccination, yearly blood work (complete blood count, ferritin, clotting profile, renal function, uric acid), and regular echo Doppler studies. Home oxygen therapy may have a role in increasing oxygen saturation via its pulmonary vasodilatory effect, but clinical indications and outcomes are not clear.[27]

Pulmonary Hypertension

Pulmonary hypertension is a common accompaniment of many congenital cardiac lesions, and the status of the pulmonary vascular bed is often the principal determinant of the clinical manifestations, the course, and whether corrective treatment is feasible (see Chap. 73). Increases in pulmonary arterial pressure result from elevations of pulmonary blood flow and/or resistance, the latter sometimes caused by an increase in vascular tone but usually the result of underdevelopment and/or obstructive/obliterative structural changes within the pulmonary vascular bed. Although pulmonary hypertension usually affects the entire pulmonary vascular bed, it may occur focally. For example, unilateral pulmonary hypertension may occur in an overshunted lung (the other lung perhaps protected and fed by a cavopulmonary Glenn shunt) or in lung segments supplied by aortopulmonary collateral flow.

Pulmonary vascular resistance normally falls rapidly immediately after birth because of the onset of ventilation and subsequent release of hypoxic pulmonary vasoconstriction. Subsequently, the medial smooth muscle of pulmonary arterial resistance vessels thins gradually. This latter process is often delayed by several months in infants with large aortopulmonary or ventricular communications, at which time levels of pulmonary vascular resistance are still somewhat elevated. In patients with high pulmonary arterial pressures from birth, failure of normal growth of the pulmonary circulation may occur, and anatomical changes in the pulmonary vessels in the form of proliferation of intimal cells and intimal and medial thickening often progress, so in an older child or adult vascular resistance ultimately may become relatively fixed by obliterative changes in the pulmonary vascular bed. The causes of pulmonary vascular obstructive disease remain unknown, although increased pulmonary arterial blood pressure, elevated pulmonary venous pressure, erythrocytosis, systemic hypoxia, acidemia, and the nature of the bronchial circulation all have been implicated. Quite likely, injury to pulmonary vascular endothelial cells initiates a cascade of events that involve the release or activation of factors that alter the extracellular matrix, induce hypertrophy, cause proliferation of vascular smooth muscle cells, and promote connective tissue protein synthesis. Considered together, these may permanently alter vessel structure and function.

MECHANISMS OF DEVELOPMENT. Intimal damage appears to be related to shear stresses because endothelial cell damage occurs at high shear rates. A reduction in pulmonary arteriolar lumen size due to either thickened medial muscle or vasoconstriction increases the velocity of flow. Shear stress also increases as blood viscosity rises; therefore infants with hypoxemia and high hematocrit levels, as well as increased pulmonary blood flow, are at increased risk of developing pulmonary vascular disease. In patients with left-to-right shunts, pulmonary arterial hypertension, if not present in infancy or childhood, may never occur or may not develop until the third or fourth decade or later. Once developed, intimal proliferative changes with hyalinization and fibrosis are not reversible by repair of the underlying cardiac defect. In severe pulmonary vascular obstructive disease, arteriovenous malformations may develop and predispose to massive hemoptysis.

Most vexing is the variability among patients with the same or similar cardiac lesions in both the time of appearance and the rate of progression of their pulmonary vascular obstructive process. Although genetic influences may be operative (an example is the apparent acceleration of pulmonary vascular disease in patients with CHD and trisomy 21), evidence is now accumulating for important prenatal and postnatal modifiers of the pulmonary vascular bed that appear, at least in part, to be lesion dependent. Thus a quantitative variability exists in the pulmonary vascular bed related to the number, not just the size and wall structure, of arterial vessels within the pulmonary circulation.

Modeling of the blood vessels occurs proximal to and within terminal bronchioles (preacinar and intraacinar vessels, respectively) continuously from before birth. The intraacinar vessels, in particular, increase in size and number from late fetal life throughout childhood, with minimal muscularization of their walls. The ensuing increase in the cross-sectional area of the pulmonary arterial circulation allows the cardiac output to rise substantially without an increase in pulmonary arterial pressure. If, however, the presence of a cardiac lesion interferes with the normal growth and multiplication of these peripheral arteries, the resulting elevation of pulmonary vascular resistance may first be related to failure of the intraacinar pulmonary circulation to develop fully, and then secondarily to the morphological changes of obliterative vascular disease—medial thickening; intimal proliferation; hyalinization and fibrosis; angiomatoid and plexiform lesions; and, ultimately, arterial necrosis.

EISENMENGER SYNDROME

DEFINITION. *Eisenmenger syndrome*, a term coined by Paul Wood, is defined as pulmonary vascular obstructive disease that develops as a consequence of a large preexisting left-to-right shunt such that pulmonary artery pressures approach systemic levels and the direction of the flow becomes bidirectional or right to left. Congenital heart defects that can result in Eisenmenger syndrome include "simple" defects such as ASD, VSD, and PDA, as well as more "complex" defects such as AV septal defect, truncus arteriosus, aortopulmonary window, and univentricular heart. The high pulmonary vascular resistance is usually established in infancy (by age 2 years, except in ASD) and is sometimes present from birth.

NATURAL HISTORY OF THE UNOPERATED PATIENT. Patients with defects that allow free communication between the pulmonary and systemic circuits at the aortic or ventricular levels usually have a fairly healthy childhood and gradually become overtly cyanotic during their second or third decade. Exercise intolerance (dyspnea and fatigue) is proportional to the degree of hypoxemia or cyanosis. In the absence of complications, these patients generally have an excellent to good functional capacity up to their third decade and thereafter usually experience a slowly progressive decline in their physical abilities. Most patients survive to adulthood, with a reported 77 percent and 42 percent survival rate at 15 and 25 years of age, respectively.[28]

Congestive heart failure in patients with Eisenmenger syndrome usually occurs after 40 years of age. The most common modes of death are sudden death (≈30 percent), congestive heart failure (≈25 percent), and pulmonary hemorrhage (≈15 percent). Pregnancy, perioperative mortality after noncardiac surgery, and infectious causes (brain abscesses and endocarditis) account for most of the remainder.

CLINICAL MANIFESTATIONS. Patients can present with the following complications: those related to their cyanotic state; palpitations in nearly half the patients (atrial fibrillation/flutter in 35 percent, ventricular tachycardia in up to 10 percent); hemoptysis in about 20 percent; pulmonary thromboembolism, angina, syncope, and endocarditis

in about 10 percent each; and congestive heart failure. Hemoptysis is usually due to bleeding bronchial vessels or pulmonary infarction. Physical examination reveals central cyanosis and clubbing of the nail beds. Patients with Eisenmenger PDA can have pink nail beds on the right (>left) hand and cyanosis and clubbing of both feet, so-called "differential cyanosis." This occurs because venous blood shunts through the ductus and enters the aorta distal to the subclavian arteries. The jugular venous pressure in patients with Eisenmenger syndrome can be normal or elevated, especially with prominent v waves when tricuspid regurgitation is present. Signs of pulmonary hypertension—a right ventricular heave, palpable and loud P_2, and a right-sided S_4—are typically present. In many patients a pulmonary ejection click and a soft and scratchy systolic ejection murmur, attributable to dilation of the pulmonary trunk, and a high-pitched decrescendo diastolic murmur of pulmonary regurgitation (Graham Steell) are audible. Peripheral edema is absent until right-sided heart failure ensues.

LABORATORY INVESTIGATIONS

ELECTROCARDIOGRAPHY (ECG). Peaked P waves consistent with right atrial overload and evidence of right ventricular hypertrophy with right axis deviation are the rule. Atrial arrhythmias can be present.

CHEST RADIOGRAPHY. Dilated central pulmonary arteries with rapid tapering of the peripheral pulmonary vasculature are the radiographic hallmarks of Eisenmenger syndrome. Pulmonary artery calcification may be seen and is diagnostic of long-standing pulmonary hypertension. Eisenmenger syndrome due to VSD or PDA usually has a normal or slightly increased cardiothoracic ratio. Eisenmenger syndrome due to an ASD typically has a large cardiothoracic ratio due to right atrial and ventricular dilation, along with an inconspicuous aorta. Calcification of the duct may be seen in Eisenmenger PDA.

ECHOCARDIOGRAPHY. The intracardiac defect should be seen readily along with bidirectional shunting. A pulmonary hypertensive PDA is not easily seen. Evidence of pulmonary hypertension is found. Assessment of pulmonary right ventricular function adds prognostic value.

CARDIAC CATHETERIZATION. Cardiac catheterization not only provides direct measurement of the pulmonary artery pressure, documenting the existence of severe pulmonary hypertension, but can also allow assessment of reactivity of the pulmonary vasculature. Administration of pulmonary arterial vasodilators (O_2, nitric oxide, prostaglandin I_2 [epoprostenol]) can discriminate among patients in whom surgical repair is contraindicated and those with reversible pulmonary hypertension who may benefit from surgical repair. Radiographic contrast material may cause hypotension and worsening cyanosis and should be used cautiously.

OPEN-LUNG BIOPSY. Open-lung biopsy should be considered only when reversibility of the pulmonary hypertension is uncertain from the hemodynamic data. An expert opinion will be necessary to determine the severity of the changes, often using the Heath-Edwards classification.

INDICATIONS FOR INTERVENTION. The underlying principle of clinical management in patients with Eisenmenger syndrome is to avoid any factors that may destabilize the delicately balanced physiology. In general, an approach of nonintervention has been traditionally recommended, although research in the treatment of pulmonary hypertension may alter this approach in the future. The main interventions, therefore, are directed toward preventing complications (e.g., flu shots to reduce the morbidity of respiratory infections) or restoring the physiological balance (e.g., iron replacement for iron deficiency, antiarrhythmic management of atrial arrhythmias, diuretics for right-sided heart failure). As a general rule, the first episode of hemoptysis should be considered an indication for investigation. Bed rest is usually recommended; and, although usually self-limiting, each such episode should be regarded as potentially life threatening, and a treatable cause should

Congenital Heart Disease

be sought. When patients are severely incapacitated from severe hypoxemia or congestive heart failure, the main intervention available is lung transplantation (plus repair of the cardiac defect) or, with somewhat better results, heart-lung transplantation. This is generally reserved for individuals without contraindications who are thought to have a 1-year survival of less than 50 percent. Such assessment is fraught with difficulty because of the unpredictability of the time course of the disease and the risk of sudden death.

Noncardiac surgery should be performed only when absolutely necessary because of its high associated mortality. Eisenmenger syndrome patients are particularly vulnerable to alterations in hemodynamics induced by anesthesia or surgery, such as a minor decrease in systemic vascular resistance that can increase right-to-left shunting and possibly potentiate cardiovascular collapse. Local anesthesia should be used whenever possible. Avoidance of prolonged fasting and especially dehydration, the use of antibiotic prophylaxis when appropriate, and careful intraoperative monitoring are recommended. The choice of general versus epidural-spinal anesthesia is controversial.[29] An experienced cardiac anesthetist with an understanding of Eisenmenger syndrome physiology should administer anesthesia. Additional risks of surgery include excessive bleeding, postoperative arrhythmias, and deep venous thrombosis with paradoxical emboli. An "air filter" or "bubble trap" should be used for most intravenous lines in cyanotic patients. Early ambulation is recommended. Postoperative care in an intensive care unit setting is optimal.

Interventional Options and Outcomes

Oxygen. Supplemental nocturnal oxygen has recently been shown to have no impact on exercise capacity or on survival in adult patients with Eisenmenger syndrome.[30] Supplemental oxygen during commercial air travel is often recommended, but the scientific basis for this recommendation is lacking.

Transplantation. Lung transplant may be undertaken in association with repair of existing cardiovascular defect(s). Alternatively, heart-lung transplantation may be required if the intracardiac anatomy is not correctable. The 1-year survival rate for adults undergoing lung transplantation with primary intracardiac repair is 55 percent. The 1-year survival rate after heart-lung transplantation is 70 percent.[31] These procedures offer the best hope to individuals with end-stage CHD who are confronting death and have an intolerable quality of life.

Medical Therapy[32,33]

Prostacyclin. Two reports have been published on the use of long-term prostacyclin therapy for patients with Eisenmenger syndrome. In 20 patients (9 ASDs, 7 VSDs, 4 TGAs, 3 PDAs, 3 partial anomalous pulmonary venous drainage, and 1 aortopulmonary window), the chronic infusion of prostacyclin led to an improvement in hemodynamics after a 1-year period of therapy.[34] A subsequent study of McLaughlin and associates evaluated 33 patients with secondary forms of pulmonary hypertension, 7 of whom had CHD. In these patients mean pulmonary arterial pressure decreased by 18 percent over a mean 1-year follow-up.[35]

Endothelin Receptor Antagonists. A randomized trial of a nonselective endothelin receptor antagonist (Bosentan) in patients with Eisenmenger syndrome[36] showed that pulse oximetry was not reduced. Compared with placebo, Bosentan reduced the pulmonary vascular resistance index and pulmonary artery pressure and improved 6-minute walk and functional class. A smaller observational study of Bosentan 125 mg twice a day in nine Eisenmenger patients showed an improvement in functional class and increased and resting oxygen saturation levels.[37]

Sildenafil (Viagra) in a large double-blind, placebo-controlled study administered in varying doses to 278 patients with symptomatic pulmonary arterial hypertension of different etiologies improved the 6-minute walk distance, maintained for the 1 year of the trial; increased functional class; and modestly improved pulmonary arterial pressures and cardiac output.[38] A second randomized, placebo-controlled, double-blind crossover study of a smaller group of patients produced similar improvements.[39]

FOLLOW-UP. Patient education is critical. Avoidance of over-the-counter medications, dehydration, smoking, high-altitude exposure, and excessive physical activity should be stressed. Avoidance of pregnancy is of paramount importance. Annual flu shots and use of endocarditis prophylaxis together with proper skin hygiene (avoidance of nail biting) are recommended. A yearly assessment of complete blood cell count and uric acid, creatinine, and ferritin levels should be done to monitor treatable causes of deterioration.

Cardiac Arrhythmias (see Chaps. 31 to 35)

In teenagers and young adults, most arrhythmias (see Chap. 35) encountered are in association with previously operated CHD. Arrhythmias can be a major clinical challenge in adolescent and adult congenital heart patients. They are the most frequent reason for emergency department visits and hospital admissions, and they are usually recurrent and may worsen or become less responsive to treatment with time. Treatment may be challenging.

ATRIAL ARRHYTHMIAS. Atrial flutter and, to a lesser degree, atrial fibrillation are most common. Atrial flutter tends to reflect right atrial abnormalities, and atrial fibrillation, left atrial abnormalities. Atrial flutter in such patients is often atypical in appearance and behavior and is better called *intraatrial reentrant tachycardia*. Recognition of atrial flutter can be difficult, and the observer must be vigilant in recognizing 2 : 1 conduction masquerading as sinus rhythm. Recurrence is likely and should not necessarily be assumed to represent failure of the management strategy. The conditions in which atrial flutter is most likely are Mustard/Senning repairs of TGA, repaired or unrepaired ASDs, repaired tetralogy of Fallot, Ebstein anomaly of the tricuspid valve, and after a Fontan operation. Atrial flutter may reflect hemodynamic deterioration in patients who have had Mustard, Senning, tetralogy of Fallot, or Fontan repairs. Its arrival is usually associated with more symptoms and functional limitation.

The pharmaceutical agents most commonly used in therapy are warfarin, beta blockers, amiodarone, sotalol, propafenone, and digoxin. As a rule, patients with good ventricular function can receive sotalol or propafenone, whereas those with depressed ventricular function should receive amiodarone. Other therapies including pacemakers, ablative procedures, and innovative surgery are being both applied and refined. Sustained ventricular tachycardia or ventricular fibrillation occurs less often, usually in the setting of ventricular dilation, dysfunction, and scarring. Although sudden death is common in several conditions, the mechanism is poorly understood.

VENTRICULAR TACHYCARDIA. This arrhythmia can be seen as a manifestation of proarrhythmic effects of various agents; in patients with acute myocardial injury or infarction; and in CHD patients with severe ventricular dysfunction. In particular, sustained VT has been seen in patients with repaired tetralogy of Fallot, where it is seen as a manifestation of hemodynamic problems requiring repair; as a reflection of right ventricular dilation and dysfunction; and in relation to ventricular scarring.

CH 61

SUDDEN DEATH. In contrast to adults, children seldom die suddenly and unexpectedly of cardiovascular disease. Nonetheless, sudden death has been reported with arrhythmias, aortic stenosis, hypertrophic obstructive cardiomyopathy, primary pulmonary hypertension, Eisenmenger syndrome, myocarditis, congenital complete heart block, primary endocardial fibroelastosis, and when there are certain anomalies of the coronary arteries. Sudden death is more frequent in older patients with postoperative heart disease, particularly after atrial switch procedures, and repair of tetralogy of Fallot.

ATRIOVENTRICULAR BLOCK. First-degree AV block is commonly seen in patients with AV septal defects, Ebstein anomaly, complete TGA (D-TGA), and the older ASD patient. Complete heart block may develop in patients with cc-TGA and may develop postoperatively in these and other patients. When pacing is required, epicardial leads are usually placed in cyanotic patients. Many adult patients with CHD are prone to problems of vascular access because of prior surgeries and pacing leads.

Infective Endocarditis

Infective endocarditis complicating CHD is uncommon before 2 years of age, except in the immediate postoperative period. The list of those conditions not requiring antibiotic prophylaxis is shorter than for those requiring it and is limited to patients before and after closure of a secundum ASD, after closure of a PDA, after spontaneous closure of a muscular and sometimes perimembranous VSD, and in those with unoperated or operated anomalous pulmonary venous drainage in whom there is no residual hemodynamic abnormality.

Chest Pain

Angina pectoris is an uncommon symptom of cardiac disease in young infants and children, although it probably explains the irritability and crying during or after feeding in babies with coronary ischemia resulting from anomalous origin of the coronary artery from the pulmonary artery. In older children and young adults with severe left or right ventricular outflow tract obstruction and pulmonary hypertension, chest pain commonly follows effort and may be identical to effort angina of coronary artery disease in older adults. A sensation of chest discomfort or cardiac awareness is frequently interpreted as pain by the parents of children with cardiac arrhythmias. Careful questioning serves to identify palpitations rather than pain as the symptom and often elicits an additional history of anxiety, pallor, and sweating. Pain caused by pericarditis is commonly of acute onset and associated with fever and can be identified by specific physical, radiographic, and echocardiographic findings. Most commonly, late postoperative chest pain is musculoskeletal in origin and may be reproduced on upper extremity movement or by palpation. Finally, children and adults may suffer chest pain of nonspecific form because of anxiety, with or without hyperventilation.

SYNDROMES IN CONGENITAL HEART DISEASE

ALCAPA SYNDROME. The acronym stands for *a*nomalous *l*eft coronary *a*rtery *a*rising from the *p*ulmonary *a*rtery. It is also called *Bland-White-Garland syndrome.*

ALAGILLE SYNDROME. This is a hereditary syndrome consisting of intrahepatic cholestasis, characteristic facies, butterfly-like vertebral anomalies, and varying degrees of peripheral pulmonary artery stenoses or diffuse hypoplasia of the pulmonary artery and its branches. It is associated with a deletion in chromosome 20p.

DIGEORGE SYNDROME. This syndrome is caused by a microdeletion at chromosome 22q11, resulting in a wide clinical spectrum. It was previously referred to as "CATCH 22" syndrome, with CATCH standing for *c*ardiac defect, *a*bnormal facies, *t*hymic hypoplasia, *c*left palate, and *h*ypocalcemia. Cardiac defects include conotruncal defects such as interrupted aortic arch, tetralogy of Fallot, truncus arteriosus, and double-outlet right ventricle. This umbrella grouping also encompasses those with *velocardiofacial syndrome.*

CHARGE ASSOCIATION. This anomaly is characterized by the presence of coloboma or choanal atresia and three of the following defects: CHD, nervous system anomaly or mental retardation, genital abnormalities, ear abnormality, or deafness. Congenital heart defects seen in the CHARGE association are tetralogy of Fallot with or without other cardiac defects, AV septal defect, double-outlet right ventricle, double-inlet left ventricle, TGA, interrupted aortic arch, and others.

DOWN SYNDROME. This is the most common genetic malformation and is caused by trisomy 21. Most of the patients (95 percent) have complete trisomy of chromosome 21; some have translocation or mosaic forms. The phenotype is diagnostic (short stature, characteristic facial appearance, mental retardation, brachydactyly, atlantoaxial instability, and thyroid and white blood cell disorders). Congenital heart defects are frequent (40 percent), with AV septal defect, VSD, and PDA being the most common. Patients with Down syndrome are prone to earlier and more severe pulmonary vascular disease than otherwise expected as a result of the lesions identified. Hypothyroidism is common in later life, and patients should be screened intermittently.

ELLIS-VAN CREVELD SYNDROME. This is an autosomal recessive syndrome in which common atrium, primum ASD, and partial AV septal defects are the most common cardiac lesions.

HOLT-ORAM SYNDROME. This is an autosomal dominant syndrome consisting of radial abnormalities of the forearm and hand associated with secundum ASD (most common); VSD; or, rarely, other cardiac malformations.

LEOPARD SYNDROME. This autosomal dominant condition includes *l*entigines, *E*CG abnormalities, *o*cular hypertelorism, *p*ulmonary stenosis, *a*bnormal genitalia, *r*etardation of growth, and *d*eafness. Rarely, cardiomyopathy or complex CHD may be present.

NOONAN SYNDROME. This is an autosomal dominant syndrome, phenotypically somewhat similar to Turner syndrome but with a normal chromosomal complement. Noonan syndrome is associated with congenital cardiac anomalies, especially dysplastic pulmonary valve stenosis, pulmonary artery stenosis, and ASD. Hypertrophic cardiomyopathy is less common. Congenital lymphedema is a commonly associated anomaly that may be unrecognized.

RUBELLA SYNDROME. This is a wide spectrum of malformations caused by rubella infection early in pregnancy including cataracts, retinopathy, deafness, CHD, bone lesions, and mental retardation. The spectrum of congenital heart lesions is wide and includes pulmonary artery stenosis, PDA, tetralogy of Fallot, and VSD.

SCIMITAR SYNDROME. This is a constellation of anomalies including total or partial anomalous pulmonary venous connection (PAPVC) of the right lung to the inferior vena cava, often associated with hypoplasia of the right lung and right pulmonary artery. The lower portion of the right lung (sequestered lobe) tends to receive its arterial supply from the abdominal aorta. The name of the syndrome derives from the appearance on posteroanterior chest radiograph of the shadow formed by the anomalous pulmonary venous connection that resembles a Turkish sword, or scimitar.

SHONE COMPLEX (SYNDROME). This is an association of multiple levels of left ventricular inflow and outflow obstruction (subvalvular and valvular left ventricular outflow tract obstruction, coarctation of the aorta, and mitral stenosis [parachute mitral valve and supramitral ring]).

TURNER SYNDROME. This is a clinical syndrome due to the 45 XO karyotype in about 50 percent of cases, with various other X chromosome abnormalities comprising the remainder. There is a characteristic but variable phenotype, an association with congenital cardiac anomalies, especially postductal coarctation of the aorta and other left-sided obstructive lesions, as well as PAPVC without ASD. The female phenotype varies with the age of presentation and is somewhat similar to that of Noonan syndrome.

WILLIAMS SYNDROME. This is a congenital syndrome of heterogeneous cause, often sporadic, occasionally autosomal dominant, associated with infantile hypercalcemia, characteristic phenotype, and CHD, especially supravalvular aortic stenosis and multiple peripheral pulmonary stenoses.

CH 61

Congenital Heart Disease

EVALUATION OF THE PATIENT WITH CONGENITAL HEART DISEASE

Physical Examination

Although the advances in technology have profoundly improved our diagnostic abilities, there is still a role for detailed clinical examination in the assessment and follow-up of unoperated, palliated, and repaired CHD. The relevant findings pertaining to specific abnormalities are outlined in the appropriate sections that follow, but some general principles bear consideration (see Chap. 11).

PHYSICAL ASSESSMENT. One should assess both cardiac and visceral situs and not assume the heart will be left sided. The presence of characteristic facial or somatic features of an underlying syndrome may be a strong clue to the type of heart disease (e.g., Williams, Noonan, Down) at any age. Central cyanosis can be difficult to diagnose clinically when mild but should be actively excluded by oximetry in any patient with suspected CHD. Performing careful surveillance of the chest wall for scars is also important in older patients and adults, who do not always know or report the type and sequence of their surgical interventions. The thin chest wall of children and many young adults with CHD assists the detection of chamber enlargement by palpation, as well as the detection of systolic or diastolic thrills.

The infant or child with hemodynamically significant heart disease may show signs of failure to thrive (underweight, small, or both). The weight and height should therefore be plotted sequentially against normal growth curves appropriate to race, sex, and underlying syndrome (e.g., Down syndrome growth chart). The manifestations of "heart failure" vary with age and the underlying problem. In children, peripheral edema is rare, but intercostal recession, nasal flaring, and grunting with respiration are signs of congestive heart failure. In small children, liver size and pulsatility are an excellent barometer of cardiac function, reflecting right atrial pressure, right ventricular filling time, and diastolic dysfunction or tricuspid regurgitation. The jugular venous pressure is difficult to assess in young children but is a fundamental part of the examination of the older child, teenager, and adult.

Examination of the upper and lower limb peripheral pulses is important at any age. Delay, absence, or reduction of a pulse is an important clue to the presence of arterial obstruction and its site. The left brachial pulse is often compromised by surgery for coarctation, and blood pressure measurements should not be taken in only the left arm. Similarly, other palliative procedures (Blalock-Taussig shunt, interposition grafts) may affect either or both upper limb pulses. Assessing the femoral and carotid pulses in addition to the upper limb pulses is important in such patients. Just as in acquired disease, the pulse volume and character also provide important information regarding severity of obstructive or regurgitant left heart disease. A low-volume pulse (usually with a narrow pulse pressure) reflects a low cardiac output. Pulsus alternans signifies severe systemic ventricular dysfunction. Pulsus paradoxus points to cardiac tamponade. In adolescents and adults the jugular venous pressure examination is often important. It may give indication of cardiac decompensation, cardiac chamber hypertrophy or noncompliance, valvular regurgitation or stenosis, arrhythmia or conduction disturbance, cardiac tamponade, pericardial constriction, and other phenomena.

AUSCULTATION. The rules of auscultation also follow those developed for acquired heart disease. However, cardiac and vascular malposition may significantly affect the appreciation of heart sounds and murmurs. For example, in TGA treated by an atrial switch procedure, the aorta remains anterior to the pulmonary artery. Consequently the aortic component of the second sound can be exceptionally loud, and the pulmonary component may be virtually inaudible, making it difficult to estimate the pulmonary artery pressure clinically under such circumstances. Conversely, when there is a valved conduit between the right ventricle and pulmonary artery, the pulmonary closure sound may be extremely loud, even though the pulmonary artery diastolic pressure is low. This is because the conduit is frequently "stuck" to the chest wall, assisting sound transmission to the stethoscope placed close to it. Calcification of semilunar valves is relatively unusual in childhood and early adult life, making the differentiation of valve stenosis from subvalve or supravalve narrowing, by the presence of an ejection click, more precise in these patients. The differentiation of multiple murmurs is sometimes a challenge. Systolic and/or diastolic murmurs in an individual may have several causes, and supplementary clinical information may be required to establish their significance in some cases. Auscultating over the entire anterior and posterior chest wall is important. The continuous murmurs of aorto-aortic collateral arteries in coarctation may be audible only between the shoulder blades posteriorly, for example, and similarly the presence of a localized distal pulmonary artery stenosis or the presence of an aortopulmonary collateral artery may be detected only in a localized area of the chest wall, particularly in adults.

Electrocardiogram

The ECG (see Chap. 12) remains an important tool in the assessment of CHD. Heart rhythm and rate, as well as AV conduction, can be evaluated. The dominant theme that runs through ECGs in CHD is the prevalence of right heart disease. This often takes the form of right axis deviation along with right atrial and right ventricular hypertrophy. Right ventricular hypertrophy may reflect pulmonary hypertension, right ventricular outflow tract obstruction, or a subaortic right ventricle. Incomplete right bundle branch block often indicates right ventricular hypertrophy due to pressure (e.g., pulmonary hypertension or pulmonary stenosis) or volume (e.g., ASD) overload. Right ventricular volume overload is likely when the r′ in V_1 is less than 7 mm. Very wide QRS complexes should be seen as possible manifestations of dilated and dysfunctional ventricles, most specifically in patients with repaired tetralogy, complete right bundle branch block, and severe pulmonary regurgitation. The ECG may be uninterpretable in patients with abnormal cardiac or visceral situs unless it is clear where the leads were placed.

Atrial flutter (often in an atypical form—so-called *intraatrial reentrant tachycardia*) is much more common in young patients than is atrial fibrillation. First-degree block is often seen in AV septal defects, cc-TGA, and Ebstein anomaly. Complete heart block is most often seen in patients with cc-TGA, as well those with older VSD repairs.

Left atrial overload may reflect increased pulmonary blood flow, as well as AV valve dysfunction and myocardial failure. Left axis deviation should make one think of AV septal defect, a univentricular heart, and a hypoplastic right ventricle. Deep q waves in the left chest leads can be caused by left ventricular volume overload in a young person with aortic or mitral regurgitation. Pathological Q waves can be evidence of the anomalous origin of the left coronary from the pulmonary artery.

Chest Radiograph

The chest radiograph (see Chap. 15) is another valuable tool for the discerning physician caring for patients with con-

CH 61

genital heart defects. Although more recent technologies have rightly attracted much attention, there is value in learning how to interpret the chest radiograph. Some teaching points can be made that may anchor the interpretation of chest radiographs of some CHD patients. The following sections provide a number of clinical and radiographic differential diagnoses.

CRITERIA FOR SHUNT VASCULARITY. These include (1) uniformly distributed vascular markings with absence of the normal lower lobe vascular predominance; (2) right descending pulmonary artery diameter that exceeds 17 mm; and (3) a pulmonary artery branch that is larger than its accompanying bronchus (best noted in the right parahilar area). Prominent vascularity is apparent only if the pulmonary-to-systemic flow ratio is greater than 1.5 to 1. As a rule, cardiac enlargement usually implies a shunt greater than 2.5 to 1. Anemia, pregnancy, thyrotoxicosis, and a pulmonary AV fistula may mimic shunt vascularity.

CYANOTIC PATIENTS WITH SHUNT VASCULARITY. This group includes single ventricle with transposition, persistent truncus arteriosus, tricuspid atresia without significant pulmonary outflow obstruction, total anomalous pulmonary venous connection, double-outlet right ventricle, and a common atrium.

CYANOTIC PATIENTS WITH A VSD AND NORMAL OR DECREASED PULMONARY VASCULARITY. This group includes tetralogy of Fallot; tricuspid atresia with pulmonary stenosis; single ventricle and pulmonary stenosis; D-TGA with pulmonary stenosis; cc-TGA with pulmonary stenosis; double-outlet right ventricle with pulmonary stenosis; pulmonary atresia; and asplenia syndrome.

CAUSES OF RETROSTERNAL FILLING ON LATERAL CHEST RADIOGRAPH. These include right ventricular dilation, TGA, ascending aortic aneurysm, and noncardiovascular masses (e.g., lymphoma, thymoma, teratoma, thyroid).

CAUSES OF A STRAIGHT LEFT HEART BORDER. These include right ventricular dilation, left atrial dilation, cc-TGA, pericardial effusion, Ebstein anomaly, and congenital absence of the left pericardium.

CARDIOVASCULAR DISEASES ASSOCIATED WITH SCOLIOSIS. These include cyanotic CHD, Eisenmenger syndrome, Marfan syndrome, and occasionally mitral prolapse.

CAUSES OF LARGE CENTRAL PULMONARY ARTERIES. These include increased pulmonary flow (main pulmonary artery and branches), increased pulmonary pressure (main pulmonary artery and branches), pulmonary stenosis (main and left pulmonary artery), and idiopathic dilation of the pulmonary artery (main pulmonary artery).

SITUS SOLITUS WITH CARDIAC DEXTROVERSION. Situs solitus with cardiac dextroversion is associated with CHD in more than 90 percent of cases. Up to 80 percent have a congenitally corrected transposition with a high incidence of associated VSD, pulmonary stenosis, and tricuspid atresia. *Situs inversus with dextrocardia* carries a low incidence of CHD, whereas *situs inversus with levocardia* is virtually always associated with severe CHD.

Cardiovascular MRI

Cardiac MRI (see Chap. 17) in adolescents and adults with CHD has become of ever-increasing importance in the past decade. MRI can circumvent the echocardiographic problem of suboptimal visualization of the heart in adult patients, especially those who have had surgery. This technique can now generate information never previously available and do so more easily or more accurately than by other means. New MRI image acquisition methods are faster and provide improved temporal and spatial resolution. Major advances in hardware design, new pulse sequences, and faster image reconstruction techniques now permit rapid high-resolution imaging of complex cardiovascular anatomy. MRI can produce quantitative measures of ventricular volumes, mass, and ejection fraction. MRI can quantify blood flow in any vessel.

Cardiac MRI is of particular value when transthoracic echocardiography cannot provide the needed diagnostic information; as an alternative to diagnostic cardiac cathe-

terization; and for MRI's unique capabilities such as tissue imaging, myocardial tagging, and vessel-specific flow quantification. The value of MRI over echocardiography in the evaluation of the right ventricle is becoming increasingly appreciated. The capability of MRI to assess the right ventricle is of great importance because the right ventricle is a key component of many of the more complex CHD lesions. In addition, MRI can evaluate valve regurgitation, postoperative systemic and pulmonary venous pathways, Fontan pathways, and the great vessels. MRI should be considered the main imaging modality in adolescents and adults with repaired tetralogy of Fallot, TGA, Fontan procedure, and diseases of the aorta. In the near future, we will see real-time MRI to allow MR-guided interventional procedures and molecular imaging that will further expand MRI's capabilities.

Transthoracic Echocardiography (see Chap. 14)

FETAL ECHOCARDIOGRAPHY

General Considerations. Fetal echocardiography has graduated from being a special area of interest to some pediatric cardiologists to one of standard care. As early as 16 weeks' gestation, excellent images of the fetal cardiac structures can be obtained by the transabdominal route, along with an appreciation of cardiac and placental physiology through the use of Doppler technology. Transvaginal ultrasound is a newer approach that permits the echocardiographer to obtain images at approximately 13 to 14 weeks' gestation. Data is beginning to emerge as to the benefit of this approach, though current opinion would support a follow-up cardiac screen at 18 weeks' gestation. Although it has some application for cases with a higher risk of recurrent CHD (e.g., obstructive left-sided lesions), its accuracy has yet to be determined. This is in part because of the limited number of views that are possible due to a relatively fixed position of the transducer. Although there are specific indications for fetal echocardiographic scanning, the highest number of cases arise from anatomical or functional abnormalities detected at routine obstetrical screening. A routine anatomical screen has become a standard of care in many obstetrical practices throughout the world. As a result there has been a tremendous push by pediatric fetal echocardiographers to improve the standard of routine screening of the prenatal heart. A rapid rise has occurred in the number of abnormalities that are detected by general obstetrical ultrasonographers and subsequently referred in a timely manner to the pediatric cardiologist and echocardiographer. Nevertheless, the routine detection rate in unselected populations is still just slightly more than 50 percent.

Impact of Fetal Echocardiography. Most major structural congenital heart defects are now accurately categorized through fetal echocardiography. Once the abnormalities are identified, families and obstetrical caregivers can be counseled as to the impact of the abnormality both to the fetus and the family. Decisions appropriate to the individual family and fetus can then be made. Although termination of pregnancy is one of the consequences of prenatal diagnosis, it is not the main objective. In fact, data are starting to appear in the literature indicating that prenatal diagnosis of some major cardiac malformations has a direct impact on outcome, from a survival, morbidity, and cost outcome. This is in part due to the fact that when a prenatal diagnosis is made, subsequent caregivers are prepared for the immediate postnatal effects of the defect. For example, in hypoplastic left heart syndrome and other duct-dependent lesions, prostaglandin E_1 can be started immediately after birth, hopefully in a hospital within or attached to a pediatric cardiology facility.

Fetal echocardiography has also permitted an improved understanding of the evolution of certain congenital cardiac malformations. For example, although the fetal heart is fully formed by the time a prenatal scan is performed, tremendous growth of the cardiac structures still must occur. Therefore, in some circumstances a cardiac chamber that may appear only mildly hypoplastic at 16 weeks' gestation may be profoundly affected at the time of birth. This has a major impact on the management of the newborn as well as the counseling process at 16 weeks' gestation.

Direct Fetal Intervention. The next step is direct intervention for specific cardiac lesions. This has initially involved obstructive lesions, thus far mainly being limited to the left ventricle.[40] The rationale behind this therapy is based on the notion that the relief of obstructive outflow tract lesions will permit growth of the affected ventricle, potentially changing a neonatal pathway from univentricular to biventricular. Cardiac surgery to the fetus is also a future option, and indeed there is already a considerable amount of research on the impact of this in fetal animal models.

SEGMENTAL APPROACH TO ECHOCARDIOGRAPHY IN CONGENITAL HEART DISEASE. The following four echocardiographic steps of segmental analysis are crucial in any patient with CHD. Starting from a standard subcostal view, one should determine the position of the apex, the situs of the atria, as well as the AV and ventriculoarterial relationships.

1. Apex Position. From a standard subcostal view, determine if the apex of the heart is pointing to the right (dextrocardia), to the left (levocardia), or to the middle (mesocardia).

2. Situs of the Atria (Fig. 61-2). The right and left atria differ morphologically with regard to their appendages. A morphological right atrium has a broad right atrial appendage, whereas a morphological left atrium has a narrow left atrial appendage. Right and left atrial appendages, however, are difficult to visualize by transthoracic echocardiography, and one often has to rely on abdominal situs to determine the atrial situs. Atrial situs follows abdominal situs in about 70 to 80 percent of the cases. From a standard subcostal view with the probe pointing at a right angle to the spine, one can visualize the abdominal aorta, as well as the inferior vena cava and the spine at the back. When the aorta is to the left of the spine and the inferior vena cava to the right of the spine, there is abdominal situs solitus and, in all probability, corresponding atrial situs solitus (meaning the morphological right atrium is on the right side and the morphological left atrium is on the left side). When the aorta is to the right of the spine and the inferior vena cava is to the left of the spine, there is abdominal situs inversus and, in all probability, corresponding atrial situs inversus (morphological right atrium on the left side and morphological left atrium on the right side). When both the aorta and inferior vena cava are to the left of the spine, there is abdominal and atrial left isomerism (two morphological left atria). When both the aorta and inferior vena cava are to the right of the spine, there is abdominal and atrial right isomerism (two morphological right atria).

3. Atrioventricular Relationship. Once the situs of the atria is determined, one must assess the position of the ventricles in relation to the atria. The morphological right ventricle has four characteristic features that distinguish it from the morphological left ventricle: (1) a trabeculated apex, (2) a moderator band, (3) septal attachment of the tricuspid valve, and (4) lower (apical) insertion of the tricuspid valve. The tricuspid valve is always "attached" to the morphological right ventricle. The morphological left ventricle has the following characteristics: (1) a smooth apex, (2) no moderator band, (3) no septal attachment of the mitral valve, and (4) higher (basal) insertion of the mitral valve. The mitral valve is always "attached" to the morphological left ventricle. Once the position of the ventricles is determined, one can then establish the AV relationship. When the morphological right atrium empties into the morphological right ventricle and the morphological left atrium empties into the morphological left ventricle, there is AV concordance. When the morphological right atrium empties into the morphological left ventricle, and the morphological left atrium empties into the morphological right ventricle, there is AV discordance. When both atria empty into one ventricle (right or left), it is called a *double-inlet* (right or left) *ventricle*.

4. Ventriculoarterial Relationship. Once the AV relationship has been determined, one should assess the position of the great arteries in relation to the ventricles. The pulmonary artery can be distinguished by its early branching pattern into the left and right pulmonary arteries; the pulmonary valve is always "attached" to the pulmonary artery. Similarly, the aorta can be distinguished by its "candy cane" shape and the take-off of its three head and neck vessels (innominate, carotid, and subclavian arteries). The aortic valve is always "attached" to the aorta. Once the position of the great arteries is determined, one can then establish the ventriculoarterial relationship. When the morphological right ventricle ejects into the pulmonary artery and the morphological left ventricle ejects into the aorta, there is ventriculoarterial concordance. When the morphological right ventricle ejects into the aorta and the morphological left ventricle ejects into the pulmonary artery, there is ventriculoarterial discordance. When both great arteries exit from one ventricle (right or left), this is called a *double-outlet* (right or left) *ventricle*.

Once segmental analysis has been completed, one can then proceed to the usual echocardiographic windows to determine the nature of the specific lesions, as well as their hemodynamic relevance.

ECHOCARDIOGRAPHY IN THE NEONATE AND INFANT. Echocardiography is of immense value in differentiating between heart disease and lung disease in newborns. Indeed, it has become the standard for the diagnosis of virtually all cardiovascular malformations. Most neonates and infants are now referred directly after ultrasound study for operative repair, without intervening cardiac catheterization. It is simpler to list those lesions where it cannot be used as the sole mode of investigation before making a management deci-

CH 61

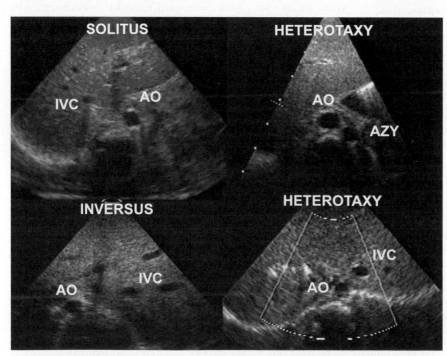

FIGURE 61–2 Montage of the different types of situs as seen by a subcostal echocardiographic scan. Note that situs solitus and inversus are just the mirror image of each other. The upper right picture is in the setting of heterotaxy with an interrupted intrahepatic inferior vena cava, with azygos continuation on the left. This is seen more frequently in left atrial isomerism. The lower right picture is also in the setting of heterotaxy with an intrahepatic inferior vena cava that is positioned closer to the aorta than in solitus or inversus. Note also the midline liver. This pattern is seen more commonly in right atrial isomerism. AO = aorta; AZY = azygos; IVC = inferior vena cava.

sion.[41] For example, in pulmonary atresia and VSD with multiple aortopulmonary collaterals, echocardiography is used as an adjunct to angiocardiography. Echocardiography provides details about the intracardiac pathology, whereas angiocardiography is necessary to delineate the sources of pulmonary blood supply. In pulmonary atresia with intact ventricular septum, the presence or absence of a right ventricular dependent coronary circulation is best assessed by angiocardiography. Apart from these two lesions, there are few other preoperative decisions that cannot be made by echocardiography alone in the newborn and infant. Postoperative management is different, particularly for those defects that are on a Fontan track where precise hemodynamic measurements are of key importance in the decision process.

Transesophageal echocardiography (TEE) is usually unnecessary for the preoperative evaluation of the neonate or infant with heart disease. This technique has now become a standard in the immediate postoperative period for the evaluation of residual anatomical or functional abnormalities. Newer techniques such as tissue Doppler and three-dimensional (3D) echocardiography are being applied to this age group and will be used more widely in the future.

ECHOCARDIOGRAPHY IN THE OLDER CHILD AND ADOLESCENT. This technique still plays a key role in the diagnosis and follow-up of the older child and adolescent with congenital or acquired heart disease. Because many of the patients underwent surgery in the neonatal or infant periods, they often have suboptimal ultrasound windows that necessitate other modes of investigation, especially magnetic resonance angiography (MRA). The application of newer technologies such as tissue Doppler and 3D echocardiography are already possible in this population and provide additional information that has thus far not been obtainable from standard techniques. For example, force-frequency relationships have been obtained in postoperative patients to try to predict optimal heart rates for maintaining maximum cardiac efficiency. On the other hand, 3D echocardiography can provide new insights into AV valve function (Fig. 61-3A and B)[42,43] that have not been possible from standard two-dimensional (2D) techniques. In the future, 3D echocardiography may replace some TEE procedures. Despite the new information from this technique, it is still limited by the quality of the transthoracic window, which is more of a problem in the older and previously repaired patient.

ECHOCARDIOGRAPHY IN THE ADULT. Advances in cardiac ultrasonography now allow comprehensive noninvasive assessment of cardiovascular structure and function in adults with CHD. Because of its widespread availability, easy use, and quick interpretation, transthoracic echocardiography remains the technique of choice for the initial diagnosis and for follow-up in adults with CHD. The general initial approach to the diagnosis of CHD by transthoracic echocardiography starts with a segmental approach to ascertain the relative position of the various cardiac chambers. Once the segmental approach has been completed, a more lesion-specific approach can then be carried out, as discussed in the individual lesion sections.

Transesophageal Echocardiography

DIAGNOSTIC ASSESSMENT. TEE offers a better 2D resolution than transthoracic echocardiography. This is especially important in adult patients with multiple previous cardiac operations, when adequate transthoracic windows are often difficult to obtain.

TEE should be used whenever transthoracic echo does not provide adequate 2D, color, or Doppler information. TEE should be considered in the setting of the conditions discussed in the following sections.

SECUNDUM ATRIAL SEPTAL DEFECT. Use TEE for assessment of device closure feasibility, measuring ASD size, assessing adequacy of margins for device anchoring, and ruling out anomalous pulmonary venous connection.

MITRAL REGURGITATION. Use TEE for preoperative evaluation of mitral valve leaflet morphology and suitability for mitral valve repair versus replacement.

EBSTEIN ANOMALY. Use TEE for preoperative assessment of tricuspid valve morphology and the potential for tricuspid valve repair.

FONTAN. Use TEE when right atrial clot is suspected on clinical grounds or by transthoracic echocardiography, or when circuit obstruction is suspected.

PRECARDIOVERSION. For any patient who is not anticoagulated, presenting with atrial flutter or fibrillation longer than 24 hours, TEE should be performed before chemical or electrical cardioversion. Patients with a Fontan circuit should undergo TEE irrespective of the duration of atrial tachyarrhythmia to rule out a right or left atrial thrombus.

GUIDANCE OF THERAPEUTIC INTERVENTION. TEE can be instrumental in helping guide therapy at the time of transcatheter or surgical procedures. TEE is particularly helpful in the following situations.

PERCUTANEOUS DEVICE CLOSURE. TEE is performed at the time of transcatheter ASD closure to assist ASD-stretched balloon sizing and device deployment, unless intracardiac echocardiography (ICE) (see later) is available.

INTRAOPERATIVE AND POSTOPERATIVE ASSESSMENT. TEE is often required for the intraoperative and postoperative assessment of the adult patient undergoing congenital cardiac surgery. It has a particular role in the intraoperative assessment of adequacy of valve repair. A TEE service by an experienced echocardiographer is an essential requirement for centers performing adult congenital cardiac surgery.

Three-Dimensional Echocardiography

DIAGNOSTIC ASSESSMENT. Three-dimensional echocardiography has advanced from the research arena to a clinical tool with the advent of transthoracic real-time systems. Although it still depends on an adequate transthoracic window, important new information can be obtained from this approach. An improved understanding of mitral valve form and function is possible (Fig. 61-4).[44] In addition, this technique can be used to improve the accuracy of left ventricular volume calculation by echocardiography.[45] Just on the horizon is a 3D real-time TEE probe that will open a whole new door for those patients with a difficult transthoracic window.

Intracardiac Echocardiography

Intracardiac echocardiography (ICE) uses lower frequency transducers that have been miniaturized and mounted into catheters capable of percutaneous insertion into the heart. ICE not only provides high-resolution 2D and hemodynamic data with full Doppler capabilities but also eliminates the need for general anesthesia, which is often required for TEE.[46]

CURRENT APPLICATIONS

PERCUTANEOUS ASD DEVICE CLOSURE. ICE supports percutaneous ASD device closure by adequately sizing the defect and assisting device positioning[47] while avoiding the need for general anesthesia.

ELECTROPHYSIOLOGICAL STUDIES. ICE assists electrophysiological procedures by guiding transseptal puncture, enabling endocardial visualization, and ensuring electrode/tissue contact at the time of ablative procedures.[48]

Cardiac Catheterization

With the development of cross-sectional echocardiography and the subsequent introduction of MRI and fast computed

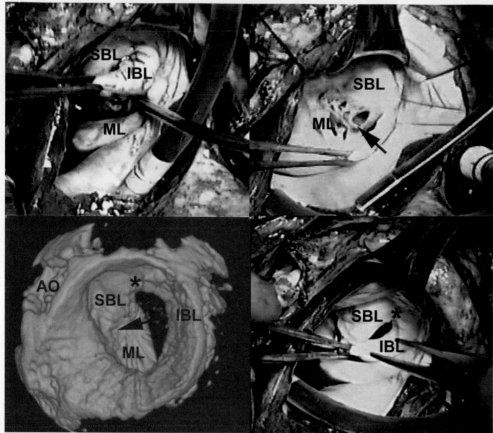

CH 61

FIGURE 61–3 A, Montage of a left atrioventricular valve (LAVV) in an atrioventricular septal defect as seen by the surgeon, as well as by the echocardiographer. The lower left panel is a reconstructed three-dimensional echocardiographic image displayed in a surgical view. Note there is fusion between the superior and mural leaflets, giving the LAVV a keyhole appearance. The surgical images are from the same patient. The upper right-hand panel shows the site of fusion between the superior and mural leaflets. The lower right-hand panel shows the residual cleft, and the upper right image shows the commissure between the inferior and mural leaflets. B, Montage of the regurgitant jets in same patient as in A. The upper left-hand image shows the site of poor coaptation during systole as seen by the echocardiographer, whereas the upper right image shows what the surgeon sees. The lower left-hand image is in the same orientation as the upper left-hand panel and shows the large regurgitant jet through the main site of poor coaptation, with some additional regurgitation between the inferior and mural commissures. The lower right-hand panel shows just the regurgitant jets with the image removed. AO = aorta, IBL = inferior bridging leaflet, ML = mural leaflet, SBL = superior bridging leaflet.

tomographic methods, truly diagnostic cardiac catheterization (see Chap. 19) is a thing of the past for both children and adults. "Diagnostic" catheterization is reserved for resolving unanswered questions from the less-invasive techniques and measuring hemodynamics. A good example of this is the assessment of major aortopulmonary collateral arteries in tetralogy of Fallot with pulmonary atresia, where their presence and distribution may be shown beautifully by MR angiography, but cardiac catheterization is required to demonstrate the presence of communications with the central pulmonary arteries and measure the pressure within them. There is no adequate substitute for cardiac catheterization to measure ventricular end-diastolic pressures or pulmonary artery pressures and resistance with the precision required to plan for, or to assess, the Fontan circulation. Furthermore, diagnostic testing may also be needed to evaluate possible coronary artery disease, especially before heart surgery.

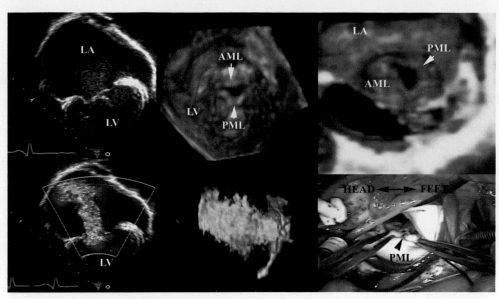

FIGURE 61–4 This montage is from a patient with a congenitally dysplastic mitral valve and significant mitral valve regurgitation. The two left-hand images show the transthoracic four-chamber view during systole. Note the large central jet of regurgitation. The upper middle panel is a real-time three-dimensional (3D) image of the mitral valve as seen from below. Note the tethered posterior leaflet. The lower middle panel shows the 3D regurgitant jet. The upper right-hand panel views the mitral valve from above. Note the poor coaptation of the two leaflets. The lower right-hand panel is the surgical view of the valve that demonstrates the tethering of the posterior leaflet. AML = anterior mitral leaflet, LA = left atrium, LV = left ventricle, PML = posterior mitral leaflet.

THERAPEUTIC CATHETERIZATION. Balloon atrial septostomy was the first catheter intervention that proved useful in treating heart disease, and it remains the standard initial palliation in many infants with D-TGA. Many transcatheter techniques are now used successfully to treat CHD: blade atrial septostomy; device or coil closure of PDA; closure of ASD and patent foramen ovale; transluminal balloon dilation of pulmonary and aortic valve stenosis; radiofrequency perforation of pulmonary valve atresia; balloon-expandable intravascular stents for right ventricular outflow tract, pulmonary artery, aortic coarctation, and other vascular stenoses; and device occlusion of unwanted collateral vessels and AV fistulas. These have all become treatments of choice in centers with these capabilities. Some are universally accepted as the standard of care (e.g., balloon pulmonary valvuloplasty), whereas debate continues for other interventions (e.g., unoperated coarctation).[49] Going along with the extraordinary expansion of interventional techniques for the treatment of structural abnormalities, ablative techniques for the treatment of tachycardias are now performed routinely in centers with congenital heart electrophysiology programs and are crucial to the management of the adult with operated and unoperated CHD, in whom arrhythmias are such a burden in terms of their morbidity, as well as a significant cause of late mortality. The indications, outcomes, and current status of each of these techniques are discussed later in detail in the sections concerning specific lesions.

SPECIFIC CARDIAC DEFECTS

Left-to-Right Shunts

ATRIAL SEPTAL DEFECT

MORPHOLOGY. Four types of ASDs or interatrial communications exist: ostium primum, ostium secundum, sinus venosus, and coronary sinus defects (Fig. 61-5A and D).

(Ostium primum is discussed in the section on AV septal defect.) Ostium secundum defects occur from either excessive resorption of the septum primum or from deficient growth of the septum secundum and are occasionally associated with anomalous pulmonary venous connection (<10 percent). Sinus venosus defect of the superior vena cava type occurs at the cardiac junction of the superior vena cava, giving rise to a superior vena cava connected to both atria, and is almost always associated with anomalous pulmonary venous connection (right >> left). Sinus venosus–inferior vena cava–type defects are very uncommon and abut the junction of the inferior vena cava, inferior to the fossa ovalis. Coronary sinus septal defects are rare and arise from an opening of its wall with the left atrium, allowing left-to-right atrial shunting.

PATHOPHYSIOLOGY. In any type of ASD, the degree of left-to-right atrial shunting depends on the size of the defect and the relative diastolic filling properties of the two ventricles. Any condition causing reduced left ventricular compliance (e.g., systemic hypertension, cardiomyopathy, myocardial infarction) or increased left atrial pressure (mitral stenosis and/or regurgitation) tends to increase the left-to-right shunt. If similar forces are present in the right heart, this will diminish the left-to-right shunt and promote right-to-left shunting.

NATURAL HISTORY. A large ASD (pulmonary artery blood flow relative to systemic blood flow [Qp/Qs] > 2.0/1.0) may cause congestive heart failure and failure to thrive in an infant or child. An undetected ASD with a significant shunt (Qp/Qs > 1.5/1.0) probably causes symptoms over time in adolescence or adulthood, and symptomatic patients usually become progressively more physically limited as they age. Effort dyspnea is seen in about 30 percent of patients by the third decade and more than 75 percent of patients by the fifth decade.[50] Supraventricular arrhythmias (atrial fibrillation or flutter) and right-sided heart failure develop by 40 years of age in about 10 percent of patients and become more prevalent with aging. Paradoxical embolism resulting in a transient ischemic attack or stroke can call the diagnosis to attention. The development of pulmo-

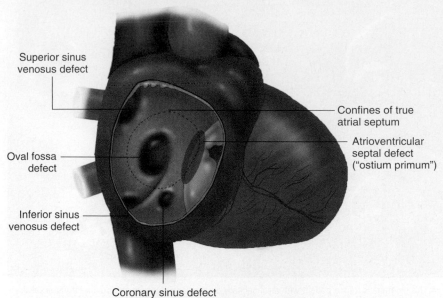

Superior sinus
venosus defect

Confines of true
atrial septum

Oval fossa
defect

Atrioventricular
septal defect
("ostium primum")

Inferior sinus
venosus defect

Coronary sinus defect

A

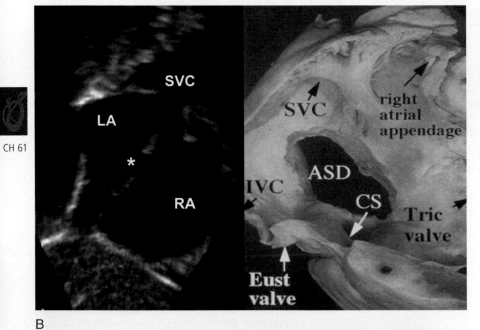

SVC

LA

*

RA

SVC

right
atrial
appendage

IVC

ASD

CS

Eust
valve

Tric
valve

B

FIGURE 61–5 A, Schematic diagram outlining the different types of interatrial shunting that can be encountered. Note that only the central defect is suitable for device closure. **B,** Subcostal right anterior oblique view of a secundum atrial septal defect (asterisk) that is suitable for device closure. The right panel is a specimen as seen in a similar view, outlining the landmarks of the defect. **C,** The left image is a transesophageal echocardiogram with color flow before device closure, whereas the right side shows postrelease of an Amplatzer device.

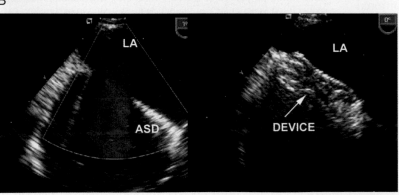

LA

LA

ASD

DEVICE

C

nary hypertension, although probably not as common as originally thought, can occur at an early age.[51] If pulmonary hypertension is severe, a second causative diagnosis should be sought. Life expectancy is clearly reduced in ASD patients, although not as severely as was quoted in earlier papers because only patients with large ASDs were reported.

CLINICAL FEATURES

Pediatrics. Most children are asymptomatic, and the diagnosis is made following the discovery of a murmur. Occasionally, increased pulmonary blood flow may be so great that congestive heart failure, recurrent chest infections, chronic wheeze, or even pulmonary hypertension may necessitate closure in infancy. Spontaneous closure of an ASD may occur within the first year of life. Even quite substantial defects diagnosed in the neonatal period (<7 mm) may reduce in size and not require later intervention. Thus in asymptomatic children with isolated secundum ASD, intervention is usually deferred so that elective device closure becomes an option if indicated.

Adults. The most common presenting symptoms in adults are exercise intolerance (exertional dyspnea and fatigue) and palpitations (typically from atrial flutter, atrial fibrillation, or sick sinus syndrome). Right ventricular failure can be the presenting symptom in older patients. The presence of cyanosis should alert one to the possibility of shunt reversal and Eisenmenger syndrome or, alternatively, to a prominent eustachian valve directing inferior vena cava flow to the left atrium via a secundum ASD or sinus venosus ASD of the inferior vena cava type.

On examination, there is "left atrialization" of the jugular venous pressure (A wave = V wave). A hyperdynamic right ventricular impulse may be felt at the left sternal border at the end of expiration or in the subxiphoid area on deep inspiration. A dilated pulmonary artery trunk may be palpated in the second left intercostal space. A wide and fixed split of S_2 is the auscultatory hallmark of ASD, although not always present. A systolic ejection murmur, usually grade 2 and often scratchy, is best heard at the second left intercostal space and a mid-diastolic rumble, from increased flow through the tricuspid valve, may be present at the left lower sternal border. When right ventricular failure occurs, a pansystolic murmur of tricuspid regurgitation is usual.

LABORATORY INVESTIGATIONS

ECG. Sinus rhythm or atrial fibrillation or flutter may be present. The QRS axis is typically rightward in secundum ASD. Negative P waves in the inferior leads indicate a low atrial pacemaker often seen in sinus venosus–superior vena cava–type defects, which are located in the area of the sinoatrial node and render it deficient. Complete right bundle branch block appears as a function of age. Tall R or R′ waves in V_1 often indicate pulmonary hypertension.

CHEST RADIOGRAPHY. The classic radiographic features are of cardiomegaly (from right atrial and ventricular enlargement), dilated central pulmonary arteries with pulmonary plethora indicating increased pulmonary flow, and a small aortic knuckle (reflecting a chronic low cardiac output state).

ECHOCARDIOGRAPHY. Transthoracic echocardiography documents the type(s) and size (defect diameter) of the ASD(s), the direction(s) of the shunt (see Fig. 61-5B), and sometimes the presence of anomalous pulmonary venous return. The functional importance of the defect can be estimated by the size of the right ventricle, the presence or absence of right ventricular volume overload (paradoxical septal motion), and the calculation of Qp/Qs. Indirect measurement of the pulmonary artery pressure can be obtained from the Doppler

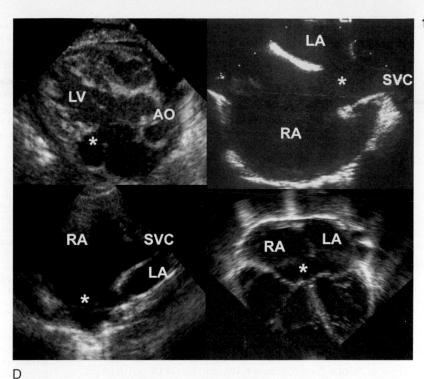

D

FIGURE 61–5, cont'd **D,** Montage of interatrial communications that are not atrial septal defects (asterisks) and therefore not suitable for device closure. The upper left is a coronary sinus defect, due to unroofing; the top right is a superior sinus venosus defect; the bottom left is an inferior sinus venosus defect; and the bottom right is an atrial septal defect in the setting of an atrioventricular septal defect. AO = aorta; ASD = atrial septal defect; CS = coronary sinus; Eust = eustachian; IVC = inferior vena cava; LA = left atrium; LV = left ventricle; RA = right atrium; SVC = superior vena cava; Tric = tricuspid.

velocity of the tricuspid regurgitation jet. TEE permits better visualization of the interatrial septum and is usually required when device closure is contemplated, partly to ensure that pulmonary venous drainage is normal. Intracardiac echo (ICE) can be used instead of TEE during device closure to help guide device insertion, reducing the fluoroscopy and procedural time and forgoing the need for general anesthesia.[52,53]

INDICATIONS FOR INTERVENTION. In asymptomatic children, the decision to intervene is based on the presence of right-sided heart dilation and a significant ASD (>5 mm) that shows no sign of spontaneous closure. Shunt fractions are now rarely measured and are reserved for "borderline" cases. Hemodynamically insignificant ASDs (Qp/Qs < 1.5) do not require closure, with the possible exception of trying to prevent paradoxical emboli in older patients after a stroke. "Significant" ASDs (Qp/Qs > 1.5, or ASDs associated with right ventricular volume overload) should be closed, especially if device closure is available and appropriate.[3,54] For patients with pulmonary hypertension (pulmonary artery pressure > $^2/_3$ systemic arterial blood pressure or pulmonary arteriolar resistance > $^2/_3$ systemic arteriolar resistance), closure can be recommended if there is a net left-to-right shunt of at least 1.5 : 1, evidence of pulmonary artery reactivity when challenged with a pulmonary vasodilator (e.g., oxygen or nitric oxide), or evidence on lung biopsy (rarely required) that pulmonary arterial changes are potentially reversible.

INTERVENTIONAL OPTIONS AND OUTCOMES

Device Closure. Device closure of secundum ASDs percutaneously under fluoroscopy and TEE or with intracardiac echo guidance[3] is the therapy of choice when appropriate (see Fig. 61-5C).[55] Indications for device closure are the same as for surgical closure, but the selection criteria are stricter.

Depending on the device, this technique is available only for patients with a secundum ASD with a stretched diameter of less than 41 mm and with adequate rims to enable secure deployment of the device. Anomalous pulmonary venous connection or proximity of the defect to the AV valves or coronary sinus or systemic venous drainage usually precludes the use of this technique. It is a safe and effective procedure in experienced hands, with major complications (e.g., device embolization, atrial perforation, thrombus formation[56]) occurring in less than 1 percent of patients and clinical closure achieved in more than 80 percent of patients. Device closure of an ASD improves functional status in symptomatic patients and exercise capacity in asymptomatic and symptomatic patients.[57] Intermediate follow-up data have proved ASD device closure to be safe and effective[58] with better preservation of right ventricular function[59] and lower complication rates than surgery.[60]

Surgery. Device closure is not an option for those with sinus venosus or ostium primum defects or with secundum defects with unsuitable anatomy. Surgical closure of ASDs can be performed by primary suture closure or using a pericardial or synthetic patch. The procedure is usually performed via a midline sternotomy, but the availability of an inframammary or minithoracotomy approach to a typical secundum ASD should be made known to cosmetically sensitive patients. Surgical mortality in the adult without pulmonary hypertension should be less than 1 percent. Surgical closure of an ASD improves functional status and exercise capacity in symptomatic patients[61] and improves (but usually does not normalize) survival and improves or eliminates congestive heart failure, especially when patients are operated on at an earlier age. However, surgical closure of ASD in adult life does not prevent atrial fibrillation/flutter or stroke, especially when patients are operated on after the age of 40 years. The role of a concomitant Cox/maze procedure in patients with a prior history of atrial flutter/fibrillation should be considered[62,63] (see Chaps. 33 and 35).

REPRODUCTIVE ISSUES. Pregnancy is well tolerated in patients after ASD closure. Pregnancy is also well tolerated in women with unrepaired ASDs, but the risk of paradoxical embolism is increased (still only to a very low risk) during pregnancy and in the postpartum period. Pregnancy is contraindicated in Eisenmenger syndrome because of the high maternal (≤50 percent) and fetal (≤60 percent) mortality.

FOLLOW-UP. Most children with isolated secundum defect can be discharged to the care of their family physician 6 months after complete closure is confirmed, no matter whether surgical or by device. After device closure, patients require 6 months of aspirin and endocarditis prophylaxis until the device endothelializes, following which, assuming there is no residual shunt, they do not require any special precautions or endocarditis prophylaxis. Patients with sinus venosus defect are at risk of developing caval and/or pulmonary vein stenosis and should be kept under intermittent review. Patients who have had surgical or device repair as adults, patients with atrial arrhythmias preoperatively or postoperatively, and patients with ventricular dysfunction should remain under long-term cardiology surveillance.

PATENT FORAMEN OVALE

ANATOMY. The foramen ovale is a tunnel-like space between the overlying septum secundum and septum primum and typically closes in 75 percent of patients at birth by fusion of the septum primum and secundum. In utero the foramen ovale is necessary for blood flow across the fetal atrial septum. Oxygenated blood from the placenta returns to the IVC, crosses the foramen ovale, and enters the systemic circulation. In about 25 percent of patients, a patent foramen ovale (PFO) persists into adulthood. PFOs may be associated with atrial septal aneurysms (a redundancy in the interatrial septum), Eustachian valves (a remnant of the sinus venosus valve), and Chiari networks (filamentous strands in the right atrium).

PATHOPHYSIOLOGY

PFOs have recently been scrutinized for their implication in the mechanism of cryptogenic stroke. Many of the basic tenets linking PFO and stroke seem plausible but have not been demonstrated. The current views may be summarized as follows. PFOs may serve as either a conduit for paradoxical embolization from the venous side to the systemic circulation or, because of their tunnel-like structure and propensity to stagnant flow, may serve as a nidus for in situ thrombus formation. Variation in PFO size, right atrial anatomy, varying hemodynamic conditions, and occurrence of venous thrombi may all contribute to the chances of paradoxical embolization. The risk of a cryptogenic stroke seems increased for larger PFOs. The presence of an interatrial septal aneurysm in combination with a PFO also increases the risk of an adverse event,[64] perhaps because of increased in situ thrombus formation in the aneurysmal sac or simply because PFOs associated with an interatrial septal aneurysm tend to be larger. Eustachian valves and a Chiari network may direct blood flow from the inferior vena cava toward the atrial septum, encouraging right to left shunting in the presence of an interatrial communication. Physiological (Valsalva maneuvers) and pathological conditions increasing right ventricular pressure will raise the right atrial pressure favoring right-to-left shunting. Finally, pelvic vein thrombi are found more frequently in young patients with cryptogenic stroke than in patients with known cause of stroke[65] and may provide the source of venous thrombi.

PFOs have also been implicated in the pathophysiology of decompression sickness (arterial gas embolism from the venous side), as well as more recently in the pathogenesis of migraine headaches.[66] Platypnea-orthodeoxia syndrome (dyspnea and arterial desaturation in the upright position, which improves when lying down) has also been attributed to the presence of a PFO.

CLINICAL IMPACT. The cause and effect relationship between PFO and cryptogenic stroke is still tentative and needs clarification. The recent body of literature would suggest a strong association, if not a causative link, especially in younger patients. Indeed, young patients with cryptogenic stroke have a significantly higher incidence of PFO (36 to 54 percent) than normal controls (15 to 25 percent). The association is more controversial in the older patient population. Older patients often have more risk factors for stroke, and the causative role of a PFO in these patients is more difficult to establish.

When a patient presents with a stroke and a PFO is discovered, the usual causes of stroke must first be eliminated. Causes are atherosclerotic risk factors (diabetes, hypertension, smoking, hypercholesterolemia); carotid artery disease; atrial fibrillation; neurovascular abnormalities; and/or prothrombotic tendencies. If after an exhaustive investigation (see later) no other cause of the stroke can be found, the PFO may be seen to have had a possible causative role. The diagnosis of a PFO as a cause of cryptogenic stroke is, at best, a diagnosis of exclusion.

INVESTIGATIONS

A PFO is usually detected by transthoracic echocardiography, transesophageal echocardiography or transcranial Doppler. Transesophageal echocardiogram is the most sensitive test, especially when performed with contrast media injected during a cough or Valsalva maneuver. A PFO is judged to be present if microbubbles are seen in the left-sided cardiac chambers within three cardiac cycles from the maximum right atrial opacification.

Screening for prothrombotic states (e.g., protein C or S deficiency, antithrombin III, or lupus anticoagulant), atrial fibrillation, significant carotid atherosclerosis by carotid Doppler imaging, and neurovascular abnormalities by brain magnetic resonance angiography must be undertaken in each patient before PFOs can be considered a possible culprit.

CH 61

THERAPEUTIC OPTIONS. Once the presumptive diagnosis of a cryptogenic stroke caused by a PFO is determined, treatment modalities to prevent recurrent events include antiplatelet or anticoagulant agents, percutaneous device closure, or surgical PFO closure. Medical therapy for secondary prevention of stroke with Coumadin or antiplatelet agents is often used as "first-line" therapy with similar efficacy, a yearly recurrence rate of about 2 percent.[67,68] Patients with PFO and atrial septal aneurysm who have had strokes seem to be at higher risk of recurrent stroke (as high as 15 percent per year), and a preventive strategy other than aspirin or Coumadin should perhaps be considered. Device closure is safe and seems effective, with a recurrence rate of stroke between 0 and 3.8 percent per year.[73] Surgical closure of PFO is usually performed when cardiac surgery is required for other reasons.

Recent nonrandomized trials comparing anticoagulation and antiplatelet treatment showed a lower risk of recurrent events with anticoagulation.[68-71] Regarding medical management, the available nonrandomized trials support anticoagulation for patients with PFO and atrial septal aneurysm, and at least antiplatelet treatment for patients with PFO without atrial septal aneurysm. The recurrence rate of stroke after transcatheter closure of PFO is lower compared with trials that used medical treatment. For patients with atrial septal aneurysm or those with recurrent cryptogenic ischemic events, closure of PFO should be considered to provide a lower recurrence rate of ischemic events and to avoid the bleeding risk associated with long-term anticoagulation.[72]

Randomized clinical trials comparing various treatment options are necessary before definitive recommendations regarding the optimal treatment of cryptogenic stroke can be made.

ATRIOVENTRICULAR SEPTAL DEFECT

TERMINOLOGY. The terms *atrioventricular septal defect, atrioventricular canal defect,* and *endocardial cushion defect* can be used interchangeably to describe this group of defects. The variable components of these lesions are explained in the following sections.

MORPHOLOGY. The basic morphology of AV septal defect is common to all types and is independent of the presence or absence of an ASD or VSD.[41,74] These common features (Figs. 61-6 and 61-7) are absence of the muscular AV septum (resulting in the AV valves being at the same level on echo); inlet/outlet disproportion (resulting in an elongated left ventricular outflow tract, the so-called goose-neck deformity); abnormal lateral rotation of the posteromedial papillary muscle; and abnormal configuration of the AV valves. The left AV valve is a trileaflet valve made of superior and inferior bridging leaflets separated by a mural leaflet. The space between the superior and inferior leaflets as they bridge the interventricular septum is called the *cleft* in the left AV valve. The bridging leaflets may be completely adherent to the crest of the interventricular septum, free floating, or attached by chordal apparatus.

PARTITIONED VERSUS COMPLETE ATRIOVENTRICULAR SEPTAL DEFECTS. A *partitioned*

orifice is one in which the superior and inferior leaflets are joined by a connecting tongue of tissue as they bridge the interventricular septum. This partitions the valve into a separate left and right orifice. A *common* AV valve orifice is one in which there is no such connecting tongue, resulting in one large orifice that encompasses the left- and right-sided components. Interatrial (ostium primum) and interventricular defects are common in AV septal defect.

The left ventricular outflow tract is elongated and predisposes to subaortic stenosis. The papillary muscles are closer together than normal. The term *unbalanced AV septal defect* refers to cases in which one ventricle is hypoplastic. This is seen more commonly in patients with heterotaxy and those with left-sided obstructive defects.

PATHOPHYSIOLOGY

NATIVE. The pathophysiology of those with an isolated shunt at atrial level (commonly referred to as a *primum ASD*) is similar to that of a large secundum ASD, with unrestricted left-to-right shunting through the primum ASD, leading to right-sided atrial and ventricular volume overload. Chronic left AV valve regurgitation may produce left-sided ventricular and atrial volume overload. Complete AV septal defect has a greater degree of left-to-right shunting from the primum ASD, as well as the nonrestrictive VSD, which triggers earlier left ventricular dilation and a greater degree of pulmonary hypertension.

AFTER CORRECTION. Residual significant left AV valve regurgitation may occur and cause significant left atrial, as well as left ventricular, dilation. Left AV valve stenosis from overzealous repair of the valve may also occur. The long, narrow left ventricular outflow tract of AV septal defect promotes left ventricular outflow tract obstruction and leads to subaortic stenosis in about 5 percent of patients.

NATURAL HISTORY. Patients with an isolated primum ASD have a course similar to that of those with large secundum ASDs, although symptoms may appear sooner when significant left AV valve regurgitation is present. Patients may be asymptomatic until their third or fourth decade, but progressive symptoms related to congestive heart failure, atrial arrhythmias, complete heart block, and variable degrees of pulmonary hypertension develop in virtually all of them by the fifth decade.

Most patients with complete AV septal defect have had surgical repair in infancy. Infants present with dyspnea, congestive heart failure, and failure to thrive. When pre-

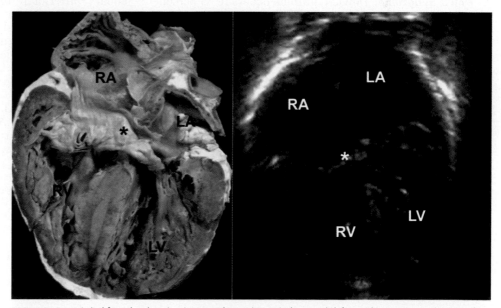

FIGURE 61–6 Apical four-chamber view in a complete atrioventricular septal defect with a common atrioventricular valve orifice **(*)**. Note the large interatrial and interventricular communications and the large free-floating superior bridging leaflet. LA = left atrium; LV = left ventricle; RA = right atrium; RV = right ventricle.

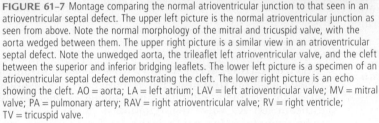

FIGURE 61–7 Montage comparing the normal atrioventricular junction to that seen in an atrioventricular septal defect. The upper left picture is the normal atrioventricular junction as seen from above. Note the normal morphology of the mitral and tricuspid valve, with the aorta wedged between them. The upper right picture is a similar view in an atrioventricular septal defect. Note the unwedged aorta, the trileaflet left atrioventricular valve, and the cleft between the superior and inferior bridging leaflets. The lower left picture is a specimen of an atrioventricular septal defect demonstrating the cleft. The lower right picture is an echo showing the cleft. AO = aorta; LA = left atrium; LAV = left atrioventricular valve; MV = mitral valve; PA = pulmonary artery; RAV = right atrioventricular valve; RV = right ventricle; TV = tricuspid valve.

CH 61

senting unrepaired, most adults have established pulmonary vascular disease. Patients with Down syndrome have a propensity to develop pulmonary hypertension at an even earlier age than do other patients with AV septal defect.

CLINICAL ISSUES

Down Syndrome. Down syndrome occurs in 35 percent of patients with AV septal defect. These patients more commonly have a complete AV septal defect with a common AV valve orifice and a large associated VSD. They often present in infancy with pulmonary hypertension. Clinical features are cardiomegaly, a right ventricular heave, and a pulmonary outflow tract murmur. If associated AV valve regurgitation exists, there is a pansystolic murmur.

Non–Down Syndrome. Clinical presentation depends on the presence and size of the ASD and the VSD and on the competence of the left AV valve. A large left-to-right shunt gives rise to symptoms of heart failure (exertional dyspnea or fatigue) or pulmonary vascular disease (exertional syncope, cyanosis). In adulthood, palpitations from atrial arrhythmias are common. Cardiac findings on physical examination for patients with an isolated shunt at atrial level are similar to those of patients with secundum ASD, with the important addition of a prominent left ventricular apex and pansystolic murmur when significant left AV valve regurgitation is present. Cases with a primum ASD and a restrictive VSD have similar findings, but with the addition of a pansystolic VSD murmur heard best at the left sternal border. Complete AV septal defects have a single S₁ (common AV valve), a mid-diastolic murmur from augmented AV valve inflow, and findings of pulmonary hypertension and/or a right-to-left shunt.

LABORATORY INVESTIGATIONS

ECG. Most patients have first-degree AV block and left axis deviation. Complete AV block and/or atrial fibrillation/flutter can be present in older patients. Partial or complete right bundle branch block is usually associated with right ventricular dilation or prior surgery.

CHEST RADIOGRAPHY. If unrepaired, this demonstrates cardiomegaly with right atrial and right ventricular prominence with increased pulmonary vascular markings. In those cases with a small interatrial communication and left AV valve regurgitation, there is cardiomegaly due to left ventricular enlargement and normal pulmonary vascular markings. Findings of Eisenmenger syndrome are also possible. When repaired, the study may be normal with sternal wires.

ECHOCARDIOGRAPHY. This has replaced angiography in assessing virtually all cases with AV septal defect.[41,74] The cardinal and common features discussed in the morphology section are readily recognized by echocardiography. In the four-chamber view the AV valve(s) appear at the same level, irrespective of the presence or absence of a VSD. The typical inferior ASD and the posteriorly positioned VSD will be sought. The degree of associated AV valve regurgitation, the left-to-right shunt, and the estimated right ventricular systolic pressure should be assessed. When using the right AV valve to assess right ventricular pressure, care must be taken to ensure that the jet is not contaminated by an obligatory left ventricle-right atrial shunt.

CARDIAC CATHETERIZATION. In general this technique has been replaced by echocardiography for the evaluation of patients with an AV septal defect. The one role it still has is in the evaluation of the patient who presents late and may have associated pulmonary vascular or coronary disease.

OPEN-LUNG BIOPSY. This should be considered only when the reversibility of pulmonary hypertension is uncertain from the hemodynamic data.

INDICATIONS FOR INTERVENTION. The patient with an unoperated or newly diagnosed AV septal defect and significant hemodynamic defects requires surgical repair. Equally, patients with persistent left AV valve regurgitation (or stenosis from previous repair) causing symptoms, atrial arrhythmia or deterioration in ventricular function, or patients with significant subaortic obstruction (a gradient ≥ 50 mm Hg at rest) require surgical intervention.[3]

In the presence of severe pulmonary hypertension (pulmonary artery pressure > ²/₃ systemic blood pressure or pulmonary arteriolar resistance > ²/₃ systemic arteriolar resistance), there must be a net left-to-right shunt of at least 1.5 : 1, evidence of pulmonary artery reactivity when challenged with a pulmonary vasodilator (e.g., oxygen, nitric oxide, and/or prostaglandins), or lung biopsy evidence that pulmonary arterial changes are potentially reversible (Heath-Edwards grade ≤ II-III) before surgical intervention can be carried out.

INTERVENTIONAL OPTIONS AND OUTCOMES

Isolated Shunt at Atrial Level (Primum Atrial Septal Defect). Pericardial patch closure of the primum ASD with concomitant suture (with or without annuloplasty) of the "cleft" left AV valve is usually performed. When left AV valve repair is not possible, replacement may be necessary. In the short term the results of repair of partial AV septal defect are similar to those following closure of secundum ASD, but sequelae of left AV ("mitral") valve regurgitation,[75,76] subaortic stenosis,[77] and AV block may develop or progress.

Complete Atrioventricular Septal Defect. The "staged approach" (pulmonary artery banding followed by intracardiac repair) has been supplanted by primary intracardiac repair in infancy. The goals of intracardiac repair are ventricular and atrial septation with adequate mitral and tricuspid reconstruction. Both single- and double-patch techniques to close ASDs and VSDs have been described with comparable results. Occasionally, left AV valve replacement is necessary when valve repair is not possible. The intermediate results of repair of complete AV septal defect are good for Down syndrome patients, as well as non–Down syndrome patients,[78,79] with similar problems as with partial AV septal defect.

REPRODUCTIVE ISSUES. Pregnancy is well tolerated in patients with complete repair and no significant residual lesions. Women in NYHA Classes I and II with unoperated, isolated primum ASD usually tolerate pregnancy well. Pregnancy is contraindicated in Eisenmenger syndrome because of the high maternal (≤50 percent) and fetal (≤60 percent) mortality.

FOLLOW-UP ISSUES. All patients require periodic follow-up by an expert cardiologist because of the possibility of postoperative complications, which include patch dehiscence or residual septal defects (1 percent), the development of complete heart block (3 percent), late atrial fibrillation/flutter, significant left AV valve dysfunction (10 percent), and subaortic stenosis (5 to 10 percent). Left AV valve regurgitation requires reoperation in at least 10 percent of patients. Subaortic stenosis develops or progresses in 5 to 10 percent of patients after repair, particularly in patients with primum ASD, especially if the left AV ("mitral") valve has been replaced. Particular attention should be paid to those patients with pulmonary hypertension preoperatively. Antibiotic prophylaxis is necessary in most patients after repair, given the common occurrence of residual "mitral" regurgitation.

ISOLATED VENTRICULAR SEPTAL DEFECT

MORPHOLOGY. The ventricular septum can be divided into three major components—inlet, trabecular, and outlet—all abutting on a small membranous septum lying just underneath the aortic valve. VSDs (Fig. 61-8) are classified into three main categories according to their location and margins (Fig. 61-9). *Muscular* VSDs are bordered entirely by myocardium and can be trabecular, inlet, or outlet in location. *Membranous* VSDs often have inlet, outlet, or trabecular extension and are bordered in part by fibrous continuity between the leaflets of an AV valve and an arterial valve. *Doubly committed* subarterial VSDs are more common in Asian patients, are situated in the outlet septum, and are bordered by fibrous continuity of the aortic and pulmonary valves. This section deals with VSDs occurring in isolation from major associated cardiac anomalies.

PATHOPHYSIOLOGY. A *restrictive* VSD is a defect that produces a significant pressure gradient between the left ventricle and the right ventricle (pulmonary/aortic systolic pressure ratio < 0.3) and is accompanied by a small (<1.4/1) shunt. A *moderately restrictive* VSD is accompanied by a moderate shunt (Qp/Qs = 1.4 to 2.2/1) with a pulmonary/aortic systolic pressure ratio less than 0.66. A large or *nonrestrictive* VSD is accompanied by a large shunt (Qp/Qs > 2.2) and a pulmonary/aortic systolic pressure ratio greater than 0.66. An *Eisenmenger* VSD has a systolic pressure ratio of 1 and Qp/Qs less than 1 : 1, a net right-to-left shunt.[3]

NATURAL HISTORY. A *restrictive* VSD does not cause significant hemodynamic derangement[80] and may close spontaneously during childhood and sometimes in adult life. Small VSDs pose an ongoing and relatively high risk of endocarditis. A perimembranous defect in an immediately subaortic position, or any doubly committed VSD, may be associated with progressive aortic regurgitation.[81] Late development of subaortic and subpulmonary stenosis (see double-chambered right ventricle), as well as the formation of a left ventricular to right atrial shunt, are well described[81] and should be excluded at follow-up. A *moderately restrictive* VSD imposes a hemodynamic burden on the left ventricle, which leads to left atrial and ventricular dilation and dysfunction as well as a variable increase in pulmonary vascular resistance. A large or nonrestrictive VSD features left ventricular volume overload early in life with a progressive rise in pulmonary artery pressure and a fall in left-to-right shunting. In turn, this leads to higher pulmonary vascular resistance and to Eisenmenger syndrome.

CLINICAL FEATURES

Pediatrics. Neonatal presentation with a murmur is increasingly frequent. Most of these patients have a restrictive defect, the murmur becoming apparent only as the pulmonary vascular resistance falls. Paradoxically, those infants with large nonrestrictive defects tend to present later. This is because equalization of pressures across the defect obviates the generation of a pansystolic murmur. Instead, pulmonary blood flow increases progressively as the pulmonary vascular resistance falls. Presentation with breathlessness, congestive heart failure, and failure to thrive in the second and third months of life are usual. At that time a pulmonary ejection murmur and a mitral rumble may be heard, reflecting increased pulmonary flow and pulmonary venous return. Cyanosis is rare in early childhood and, if present, other causes of a raised pulmonary vascular

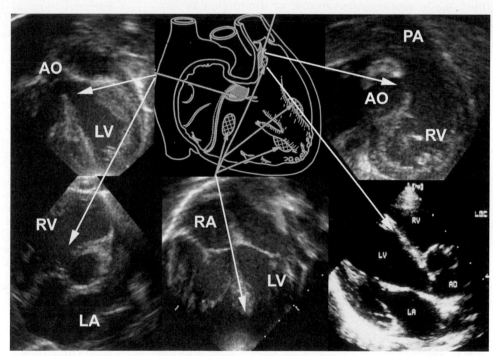

FIGURE 61–8 Montage of the different types of ventricular septal defects. The central diagram outlines the location of the various types of defects as seen from the right ventricle. The two left images show a perimembranous ventricular septal defect as seen in the five-chamber and short-axis views. Note the defect is roofed by the aorta and is next to the tricuspid valve. The bottom middle echocardiogram is a muscular apical defect. The upper right image is a right anterior oblique view in a doubly committed ventricular septal defect. The lower right is a short-axis view showing an outlet ventricular septal defect with prolapse of the right coronary cusp. AO = aorta; LV = left ventricle; PA = pulmonary artery; RA = right atrium; RV = right ventricle.

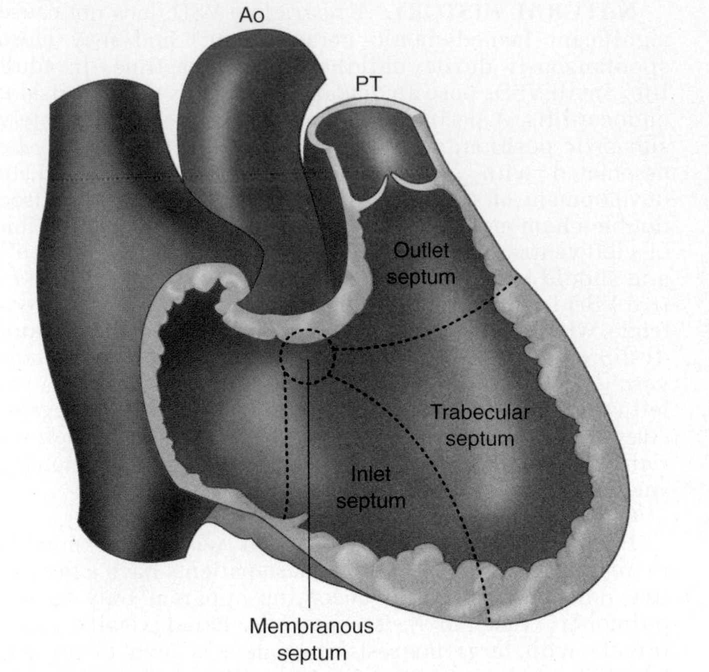

FIGURE 61–9 Four components of the ventricular septum shown here from the right ventricular aspect are now described by Anderson and associates as inlet and outlet components of the right ventricle because these areas do not correspond to septal structures as initially suggested. Ao = aorta; PT = pulmonary trunk. (*Modified from Anderson RH, Becker AE, Lucchese E, et al: Morphology of Congenital Heart Disease. Baltimore, University Park Press, 1983.*)

resistance should be excluded (e.g., mitral stenosis or coexisting lung pathology).

Medical management of the symptomatic infant is directed at improving symptoms before surgery or "buying time", while spontaneous closure, or diminution in size, occurs. Treatment with diuretics is universally accepted, and increasingly, the successful use of ACE inhibition is being reported.

Adults. Most adult patients with a small *restrictive* VSD are asymptomatic. Physical examination reveals a harsh or high-frequency pansystolic murmur, usually grade 3 to 4/6, heard with maximal intensity at the left sternal border in the 3rd or 4th intercostal space. Patients with a *moderately restrictive* VSD often present with dyspnea in adult life, perhaps triggered by atrial fibrillation. Physical examination typically reveals a displaced cardiac apex with a similar pansystolic murmur, as well as an apical diastolic rumble and third heart sound at the apex from the increased flow through the mitral valve. Patients with large *nonrestrictive* Eisenmenger VSDs present with central cyanosis and clubbing of the nail beds. Signs of pulmonary hypertension—a right ventricular heave, palpable and loud P$_2$, and a right-sided S$_4$—are typically present. A pulmonary ejection click, a soft and scratchy systolic ejection murmur, and a high-pitched decrescendo diastolic murmur of pulmonary regurgitation (Graham Steell) may be audible. Peripheral edema usually reflects right-sided heart failure.

LABORATORY INVESTIGATIONS

ECG. The ECG mirrors the size of the shunt and the degree of pulmonary hypertension. Small, *restrictive* VSDs usually produce a normal tracing. *Moderate*-sized VSDs produce a broad, notched P wave characteristic of left atrial overload, as well as evidence of left ventricular volume overload, namely deep Q and tall R waves with tall T waves in leads V$_5$ and V$_6$, and perhaps eventually atrial fibrillation. Following repair, the ECG is usually normal with right bundle branch block.

CHEST RADIOGRAPHY. The chest radiograph reflects the magnitude of the shunt, as well as the degree of pulmonary hypertension. A *moderate*-sized shunt causes signs of left ventricular dilation with some pulmonary plethora.

ECHOCARDIOGRAPHY. Transthoracic echocardiography can identify the location, size, and hemodynamic consequences of the VSD as well as any associated lesions (aortic regurgitation, right ventricular outflow tract obstruction, or left ventricular outflow tract obstruction).

CARDIAC CATHETERIZATION. Cardiac catheterization may be required when the hemodynamic significance of a VSD is questioned or when assessment of pulmonary artery pressures and resistances is necessary. In some centers therapeutic catheterization is performed for percutaneous closure (see later).

INDICATIONS FOR INTERVENTION. The presence of a significant VSD (the symptomatic patient shows a Qp/Qs > 1.5/1; pulmonary artery systolic pressure > 50 mm Hg; increased LV and LA size; or deteriorating left ventricular function) in the absence of irreversible pulmonary hypertension warrants surgical closure. If severe pulmonary hypertension (see ASD section) is present, closure is seldom feasible. Other relative indications for VSD closure include the presence of a perimembranous or outlet VSD with more than mild aortic regurgitation[82] and a history of recurrent endocarditis.

In children the presence of a nonrestrictive VSD or a smaller VSD with significant symptoms failing to respond to medication are indications for surgical or device closure. Elective surgery is usually performed between 3 and 9 months of age. Some patients have pulmonary hypertension. If pulmonary arteriolar resistance is less than 7 Wood units, closure can be safely undertaken if there is a net left-to-right shunt of at least 1.5/1, strong evidence of pulmonary reactivity when challenged with a pulmonary vasodilator (oxygen, nitric oxide), or lung biopsy evidence that pulmonary artery changes are reversible (rarely required).

INTERVENTIONAL OPTIONS AND OUTCOMES

Surgery. Surgical closure by direct suture or with a patch has been used for more than 50 years with a low perioperative mortality—even in adults—and a high closure rate. Patch leaks are not uncommon but seldom need reoperation. Late sinus node disease may occur.[83]

Device Closure. Successful transcatheter device closure of trabecular (muscular) and perimembranous VSDs has been reported. Trabecular VSDs have proven more amenable to this technique because of their relatively straightforward anatomy and muscular rim to which the device attaches well and as such results in excellent closure rates with a low procedural mortality.[84,85] Immediate, as well as short-term results, are good. The closure of perimembranous VSDs is technically more challenging due to its proximity to valve structures and requires careful patient selection.[86] It should be performed only in centers with appropriate expertise. Short-term follow-up data show complete closure in 96 percent of patients with development of aortic and/or tricuspid regurgitation or development of complete heart block in less than 5 percent of patients.[85] No long-term follow-up data are available yet.

REPRODUCTIVE ISSUES. Pregnancy is well tolerated in women with small or moderate VSDs and in women with repaired VSDs. Pregnancy is contraindicated in Eisenmenger syndrome because of high maternal (≤50 percent) and fetal (≤60 percent) mortality.

FOLLOW-UP. For patients with good to excellent functional class and good left ventricular function before surgical closure, life expectancy after surgical correction is close to normal.[83] The risk of progressive aortic regurgitation is reduced after surgery, as is the risk of endocarditis, unless a residual VSD persists. Yearly cardiac evaluation is suggested for patients with right ventricular outflow tract obstruction, left ventricular outflow tract obstruction, and aortic regurgitation not undergoing surgical repair; patients with Eisenmenger syndrome; and adults with significant atrial or ventricular arrhythmias. Cardiac surveillance is also recommended for patients who had late repair of moderate or large defects, which are often associated with left ventricular impairment and elevated pulmonary artery pressure at the time of surgery.

PATENT DUCTUS ARTERIOSUS

MORPHOLOGY. The ductus arteriosus derives from the left sixth primitive aortic arch and connects the proximal left pulmonary artery to the descending aorta, just distal to the left subclavian artery.

PATHOPHYSIOLOGY. The ductus is widely patent in the normal fetus, carrying unoxygenated blood from the right ventricle through the descending aorta to the placenta, where the blood is oxygenated. Functional closure of the ductus from vasoconstriction occurs shortly after a term birth, whereas anatomical closure from intimal proliferation and fibrosis takes several weeks to complete. Some patients have "ductus-dependent" physiology as neonates. This means their circulation depends on the ductus for pulmonary blood flow such as in severe aortic coarctation, hypoplastic left heart syndrome, and sometimes D-TGA. If spontaneous closure of the ductus occurs in such neonates, clinical deterioration and death usually follow.

Isolated PDAs, the subject of this section, are often categorized according to the degree of left-to-right shunting, which is determined by both the size and length of the duct and the difference between systemic and pulmonary vascular resistances, as follows:

- Silent: tiny PDA detected only by nonclinical means (usually echo)
- Small: continuous murmur common; Qp/Qs < 1.5/1
- Moderate: continuous murmur common; Qp/Qs = 1.5 to 2.2/1
- Large: continuous murmur present; Qp/Qs > 2.2/1
- Eisenmenger: continuous murmur absent; substantial pulmonary hypertension, differential hypoxemia, and differential cyanosis (pink fingers, blue toes)

NATURAL HISTORY

Premature Infants. Patency of a ductus arteriosus is common in a preterm infant who lacks the normal mechanisms for postnatal ductal closure because of immaturity. A PDA is thus an expected finding in a premature infant, and delayed spontaneous closure of the ductus may be anticipated if the infant does not succumb to other problems.

Full-Term Infants. In a full-term newborn, patency of a ductus is a true congenital malformation. Occasionally, some full-term newborns have persistent patency of the ductus arteriosus because their relative hypoxemia contributes to vasodilation of the channel. This includes infants born at high altitude; those with congenital malformations causing hypoxemia; or malformations in which ductal flow supplies the systemic circulation, such as hypoplastic left heart syndrome, interrupted aortic arch, or aortic coarctation.

Children and Adults. Children and adults with *silent* PDAs are detected by nonclinical means, usually echocardiography, and face virtually no long-term complications. An exception occurs if the patient's murmur is inaudible because of obesity or other somatic factors. A *small* ductus accompanied by a small shunt does not cause a significant hemodynamic derangement but may predispose to endarteritis,[87] especially when a murmur is present. A *moderate-sized* duct and shunt pose a volume load on the left atrium and ventricle with resultant left ventricular dilation and dysfunction and perhaps eventual atrial fibrillation. A *large* duct results initially in left ventricular volume overload but develops a progressive rise in pulmonary artery pressures and eventually irreversible pulmonary vascular changes by 2 years of age (Eisenmenger syndrome).

CLINICAL FEATURES

Premature Infants. Most preterm infants with a birth weight less than 1500 gm have a PDA, and about one third have a large enough shunt to cause significant cardiopulmonary deterioration. Clinical findings in these patients include bounding peripheral pulses, an infraclavicular and interscapular systolic murmur (occasionally a continuous murmur), precordial hyperactivity, hepatomegaly, and either multiple episodes of apnea and bradycardia or ventilator dependence.

Full-Term Infants, Children, and Adults. A *small* audible duct usually causes no symptoms but may rarely present as an endovascular infection. Physical examination may reveal a grade 1 or 2 continuous murmur peaking in late systole and best heard in the 1st or 2nd left intercostal space. Patients with a *moderate-sized* duct may present with dyspnea or palpitations from atrial arrhythmias. A louder continuous or "machinery" murmur in the 1st or 2nd left intercostal space is typically accompanied by a wide systemic pulse pressure from aortic diastolic runoff into the pulmonary trunk and signs of left ventricular volume overload, such as a displaced left ventricular apex and sometimes a left-sided S_3 (meaningful in adults only). With a moderate degree of pulmonary hypertension, the diastolic component of the murmur disappears, leaving a systolic murmur. Adults with a *large* uncorrected PDA eventually present with a short systolic ejection murmur, hypoxemia in the feet more than the hands (differential cyanosis), and Eisenmenger physiology.

LABORATORY INVESTIGATIONS IN PREMATURE INFANTS

ECG. This may be normal or demonstrate right or left ventricular hypertrophy or both, depending on the amount of left-to-right shunting and the degree of associated pulmonary hypertension.

CHEST RADIOGRAPHY. This may demonstrate cardiomegaly and increased pulmonary vascular markings that may be difficult to interpret in the setting of hyaline membrane disease.

ECHOCARDIOGRAPHY. This is the key to diagnosis. The ductus arteriosus can be imaged in its entirety and its size estimated. Doppler demonstrates the shunt and permits an accurate assessment of mean pulmonary artery pressure. This is achieved from calculating the mean left-to-right spectral trace and subtracting it from the mean blood pressure. Measurements of the left atrial and left ventricular size provide indirect evidence of the magnitude of left-to-right shunting.

LABORATORY INVESTIGATIONS IN FULL-TERM INFANTS, CHILDREN, AND ADULTS

ECG. The ECG reflects the size and degree of shunting occurring through the duct. A *small* duct produces a normal ECG. A *moderate* duct may show left ventricular volume overload with broad, notched P waves together with deep Q waves, tall R waves, and peaked T waves in V_5 and V_6. A *large* duct with Eisenmenger physiology produces findings of right ventricular hypertrophy.

CHEST RADIOGRAPHY. A *small* duct produces a normal chest radiograph. A *moderate*-sized duct causes moderate cardiomegaly with left-sided heart enlargement, a prominent aortic knuckle, and increased pulmonary perfusion. Ring calcification of the ductus may be seen through the soft tissue density of the aortic arch or pulmonary trunk in older adults. The large PDA produces an Eisenmenger appearance with a prominent aortic knuckle.

ECHOCARDIOGRAPHY. This determines the presence, size, and degree of shunting and the physiological consequences of the shunt. The PDA is seen with difficulty in an Eisenmenger context. A bubble study shows the communication.

INDICATIONS FOR INTERVENTION

Premature Infants. Treatment of preterm infants with a PDA varies with the magnitude of shunting and the severity of hyaline membrane disease because the ductus may contribute importantly to mortality in infants with respiratory distress syndrome. Intervention in an asymptomatic infant with a small left-to-right shunt is unnecessary because the

PDA almost invariably undergoes spontaneous closure. Those infants who demonstrate unmistakable signs of a significant ductal left-to-right shunt during the course of the respiratory distress syndrome are often unresponsive to medical measures to control congestive heart failure and require closure of the PDA to survive. These infants are best treated by pharmacological inhibition of prostaglandin synthesis with indomethacin or ibuprofen to constrict and close the ductus. Surgical ligation is required in the estimated 10 percent of infants who are unresponsive to indomethacin.

Full-Term Infants. In the clinical settings in which the ductus preserves pulmonary blood flow, the inevitable spontaneous closure of the vessel is associated with profound clinical deterioration and often death. Undesirable ductal closure may be reversed medically within the first 4 or 5 days of life by an infusion of prostaglandin E₁. By dilating the constricted ductus arteriosus, a temporary increase should occur in arterial blood oxygen tension and saturation and correction of acidemia.

Children and Adults. Closure of an isolated, clinically detectable PDA, in the absence of irreversible pulmonary hypertension, is often recommended. There is no debate about the desirability of closing a hemodynamically important PDA. There is debate about closing a PDA strictly to reduce the risk of endarteritis. The risk of endarteritis in a patient with a silent PDA is considered negligible, and closure of such ducts is seldom recommended for that reason. In the presence of severe pulmonary hypertension (see "ASD" earlier), closure is seldom indicated. Contraindications to ductal closure include irreversible pulmonary hypertension or active endarteritis.[3]

INTERVENTIONAL OPTIONS AND OUTCOMES

Transcatheter Treatment (Fig. 61-10). Over the past 20 years, the efficacy and safety of transcatheter device closure for ducts smaller than 8 mm have been established, with complete ductal closure achieved in more than 85 percent of patients by 1 year following device placement at a mortality rate of less than 1 percent.[88] In centers with appropriate resources and experience, transcatheter device occlusion should be the method of choice for ductal closure.[88,89]

Surgical Treatment. Surgical closure, by ductal ligation and/or division, has been performed for more than 50 years with a marginally greater closure rate than device closure but somewhat greater morbidity and mortality. Immediate clinical closure (no shunt audible on physical examination) is achieved in more than 95 percent of patients. Surgical closure is a low-risk procedure in children. Surgical mortality in adults is 1 to 3.5 percent and relates to the presence of pulmonary arterial hypertension and difficult ductal morphology (calcified or aneurysmal) often seen in adults. Surgical closure should be reserved for those in whom the PDA is too large for device closure or at centers without access to device closure.

REPRODUCTIVE ISSUES. Pregnancy is well tolerated in women with silent and small PDA or in patients who were asymptomatic before pregnancy. In the woman with a hemodynamically important PDA, pregnancy may precipitate or worsen heart failure. Pregnancy is contraindicated in Eisenmenger syndrome because of the high maternal (≤50 percent) and fetal (≤60 percent) mortality.

FOLLOW-UP. Patients with device occlusion or after surgical closure should be examined periodically for possible recanalization. Silent residual shunts may be found by transthoracic echocardiography.[90] The risk of late endarteritis from a clinically silent residual shunt after device implantation or surgical closure is low, and the need for endocarditis prophylaxis in such patients is uncertain. Endocarditis prophylaxis is recommended for 6 months following PDA device closure or for life if any residual defect persists. Patients with a silent PDA probably do not require endocarditis prophylaxis or follow-up.

PERSISTENT TRUNCUS ARTERIOSUS

MORPHOLOGY. Persistent truncus arteriosus is an anomaly in which a single vessel forms the outlet of both ventricles and gives rise to the systemic, pulmonary, and coronary arteries. It is always accompanied by a VSD and frequently with a right-sided aortic arch. The truncal valve is usually tricuspid but is quadricuspid in about one third of patients. Truncal valve regurgitation and truncal valve stenosis are each seen in 10 to 15 percent of patients. There can be a single coronary artery.

Truncus malformations can be classified either anatomically according to the mode of origin of pulmonary vessels from the common trunk or from a functional point of view on the basis of the magnitude of blood flow to the lungs. In the common type (type I) of truncus arteriosus, a partially separate pulmonary trunk of variable length exists and gives rise to left and right pulmonary arteries. In type II each pulmonary artery arises separately but close to the other from the posterior aspect of the truncus. In type III each pulmonary artery arises from the lateral aspect of the truncus. Less commonly, one pulmonary artery branch may be absent, with aortopulmonary collateral arteries supplying the lung that does not receive a pulmonary artery branch from the truncus.

PATHOPHYSIOLOGY. Pulmonary blood flow is governed by the size of the pulmonary arteries and the pulmonary vascular resistance. In infancy, pulmonary blood flow is usually excessive because pulmonary vascular resistance is not greatly increased. Thus, in the neonate, only minimal cyanosis is present. With time, pulmonary vascular resistance increases, relieving the left ventricular volume load but at the price of increasing cyanosis. When pulmonary vascular resistance reaches systemic levels, Eisenmenger physiology and bidirectional shunting occur. Significant truncal valve regurgitation produces a volume load on both right and left ventricles because of the biventricular origin of the truncal artery.

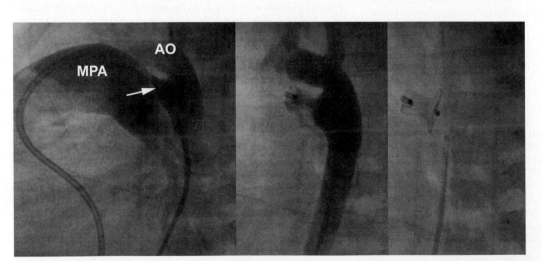

FIGURE 61-10 Montage of a patent arterial duct (arrow), before and after device occlusion. AO = aorta; MPA = main pulmonary artery.

NATURAL HISTORY. Most deaths from congestive heart failure occur before 1 year of age. Unoperated patients who survive past 1 year most likely present with established pulmonary hypertension. The prevalence of truncal valve regurgitation increases with age, causing biventricular heart failure and increasing susceptibility to endocarditis.

CLINICAL FEATURES

Pediatrics. Infants with truncus arteriosus usually present with mild cyanosis coexisting with the cardiac findings of a large left-to-right shunt. This is the result of excessive pulmonary blood flow due to a low pulmonary vascular resistance. Symptoms of heart failure and poor physical development usually appear in the first weeks or months of life. The most frequent physical findings include cardiomegaly, collapsing peripheral pulses, a loud single second heart sound, a harsh systolic murmur preceded by an ejection click, and a low-pitched mid-diastolic rumbling murmur and bounding pulses. A decrescendo diastolic murmur suggests associated truncal valve regurgitation.

DiGeorge syndrome may be seen with truncus arteriosus. Facial dysmorphism, a high incidence of extracardiac malformations (particularly of the limbs, kidneys, and intestine), atrophy or absence of the thymus gland, T-lymphocyte deficiency, and a predilection to infection also may be features of the clinical presentation.

The physical findings are different if pulmonary blood flow is restricted by a high pulmonary vascular resistance: Cyanosis is prominent, and only a short systolic murmur may be heard in association with an ejection click. Pulmonary vascular obstruction usually does not restrict pulmonary blood flow before 1 year of age.

Adults. Adults presenting with an unrepaired truncus arteriosus have Eisenmenger syndrome and its typical findings.

LABORATORY INVESTIGATIONS (UNREPAIRED)

ECG. This demonstrates biventricular hypertrophy with strain as the pulmonary resistance rises.

CHEST RADIOGRAPHY. This demonstrates cardiomegaly with prominent pulmonary arterial markings and unusually high hilar areas. A right aortic arch occurs in 50 percent of cases.

ECHOCARDIOGRAPHY (Fig. 61-11). In most cases, 2D echocardiography provides a complete diagnosis. The study should demonstrate the overriding truncal root, the origin of the pulmonary arteries, the number of truncal cusps, the origin of the coronary arteries, the functional status of the truncal valve, and VSD size.

CARDIAC CATHETERIZATION AND ANGIOGRAPHY. This is rarely necessary and in fact carries a risk of both morbidity and mortality. In general, significant arterial desaturation in the absence of branch pulmonary artery stenosis indicates that the lesion cannot be repaired.

INDICATIONS FOR INTERVENTION. Early surgical intervention is indicated in all cases within the first 2 months of life. In the presence of severe pulmonary hypertension (see ASD section), surgical intervention is usually not performed.

INTERVENTIONAL OPTIONS AND OUTCOMES. Operation consists of closure of the VSD, leaving the aorta arising from the left ventricle; excision of the pulmonary arteries

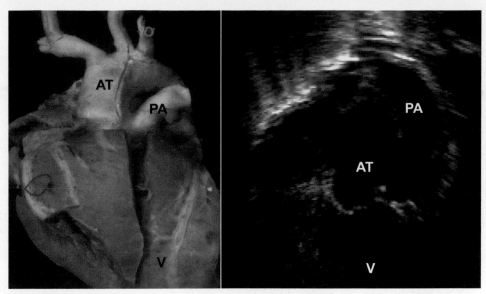

FIGURE 61-11 View of the origin of the pulmonary artery in truncus arteriosus. Note the lateral origin of the pulmonary artery. AT = ascending trunk; PA = pulmonary artery; V = ventricle.

from their truncus origin; and a valve-containing prosthetic conduit or aortic homograft valve conduit between the right ventricle and the pulmonary arteries to establish circulatory continuity.[91] Truncal valve insufficiency is a challenging problem and may require valve replacement or repair.[92]

Important risk factors for perioperative death are severe truncal valve regurgitation, interrupted aortic arch, coronary artery anomalies, and age at operation older than 100 days. Patients with only one pulmonary artery are especially prone to early development of severe pulmonary vascular disease.

REPRODUCTIVE ISSUES. Patients with a repaired truncus arteriosus and no hemodynamically important residual lesions should tolerate pregnancy well. Patients with significant conduit obstruction and/or important truncal valve regurgitation need prepregnancy counseling, with correction of the lesions before pregnancy and/or careful follow-up throughout pregnancy. Pregnancy is contraindicated in patients with Eisenmenger syndrome, given its 50 percent maternal mortality.

FOLLOW-UP. Patients operated on early (<1 year of age) generally do well. However, conduit change is often indicated within the first few years after repair as the patient outgrows its size.[91] Those cases with significant truncal valve stenosis and/or regurgitation may eventually require truncal valve replacement. Patients operated on late (>1 year of age) require careful follow-up for any signs of pulmonary hypertension progression. Endocarditis prophylaxis is required in all patients.

Cyanotic Heart Disease

TETRALOGY OF FALLOT (INCLUDING TETRALOGY WITH PULMONARY ATRESIA)

MORPHOLOGY (Figs. 61-12 and 61-13). The four components of tetralogy of Fallot are an outlet VSD, obstruction to right ventricular outflow, overriding of the aorta (<50 percent), and right ventricular hypertrophy. The fundamental abnormality contributing to each of these features is anterior and cephalad deviation of the outlet septum, which is malaligned with respect to the trabecular septum. Tetralogy may also coexist with an AV septal defect. Right ventricular outflow tract obstruction is variable. Often a

CH 61

Congenital Heart Disease

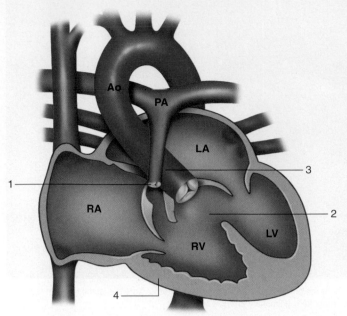

FIGURE 61–12 Diagrammatic representation of tetralogy of Fallot. 1, Pulmonary stenosis; 2, ventricular septal defect; 3, overriding aorta; 4, right ventricle hypertrophy. Ao = aorta; LA = left atrium; LV = left ventricle; PA = pulmonary artery; RA = right atrium; RV = right ventricle. *(From Mullins CE, Mayer DC: Congenital Heart Disease: A Diagrammatic Atlas. New York, Wiley-Liss, 1988.)*

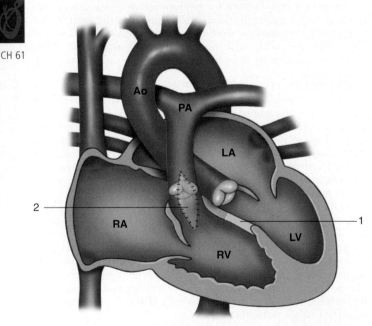

FIGURE 61–13 Diagrammatic representation of the surgical repair of tetralogy of Fallot. 1, Patch closure of ventricular septal defect; 2, right ventricular outflow/main pulmonary artery outflow patch (transannular patch). Ao = aorta; LA = left atrium; LV = left ventricle; PA = pulmonary artery; RA = right atrium; RV = right ventricle. *(From Mullins CE, Mayer DC: Congenital Heart Disease: A Diagrammatic Atlas. New York, Wiley-Liss, 1988.)*

stenotic, bicuspid pulmonary valve with supravalvular hypoplasia exists. The dominant site of obstruction is usually at the subvalve level. In some cases the outflow tract is atretic, and the heart can be diagnosed as having tetralogy of Fallot with pulmonary atresia (also known as *complex*

pulmonary atresia when major aortopulmonary collateral arteries are present). The management and outcome for patients with major aortopulmonary collateral arteries are significantly different from those with less extreme forms of tetralogy and are discussed separately at the end of this section.

Associated Anomalies. A right aortic arch occurs in about 25 percent of patients, and abnormalities of the course of the coronary arteries occur in approximately 5 percent. The most common anomaly is when the anterior descending artery originates from the right coronary artery and courses anteriorly to cross the infundibulum of the right ventricle. Absent pulmonary valve syndrome is a rare form of tetralogy in which stenosis and regurgitation of the right ventricular outflow tract is due to a markedly stenotic pulmonary valve ring with poorly formed or absent valve leaflets. The pulmonary arteries are markedly dilated or aneurysmal. This may produce airway compression at birth, a poor prognostic feature.

PATHOPHYSIOLOGY. In the absence of alternative sources of pulmonary blood flow, the degree of cyanosis reflects the severity of right ventricular outflow tract obstruction and the level of systemic vascular resistance. There is right-to-left shunting across the VSD. A tetralogy "spell" is an acute fall in arterial saturation, and it may be life threatening. Its treatment is aimed at relieving obstruction and increasing systemic resistance. Relief of hypoxia with morphine, intravenous propranolol, and systemic vasoconstriction (e.g., squatting, knee-chest position, vasoconstrictor drugs) usually reverses the cyanosis.

NATURAL HISTORY. Progressive hypoxemia in the first years of life is expected. Survival to adult life is rare without palliation or correction. The presence of additional sources of blood supply (see later) modifies the rate of progression of cyanosis and its complications.

CLINICAL FEATURES

Unoperated Patients. Variable cyanosis exists. A right ventricular impulse and systolic thrill are often palpable along the left sternal border. An early systolic ejection sound that is aortic in origin may be heard at the lower left sternal border and apex; the second heart sound is usually single. The intensity and duration of the systolic ejection murmur vary inversely with the severity of obstruction—the opposite of the relation that exists in patients with pulmonary valve stenosis. With extreme outflow tract stenosis or pulmonary atresia and during an attack of paroxysmal hypoxemia, no murmur or only a short, faint murmur may be detected. A continuous murmur faintly audible over the anterior or posterior chest reflects flow through enlarged bronchial collateral vessels.

After Surgery, Palliated. Progressive cyanosis with its complications can result from worsening right ventricular outflow tract obstruction, gradual stenosis and occlusion of palliative aortopulmonary shunts, or the development of pulmonary hypertension (sometimes seen after Waterston or Potts shunts). Progressive aortic dilation and aortic regurgitation are becoming increasingly recognized. Central cyanosis and clubbing are invariably present.

After Surgery, Repaired. After intracardiac repair, more than 85 percent of patients are asymptomatic on follow-up, although objective testing may demonstrate a marked reduction in exercise performance.[93] Palpitations from atrial and ventricular arrhythmias and exertional dyspnea from progressive right ventricular dilation secondary to chronic pulmonary regurgitation or severe residual right ventricular outflow tract obstruction occur in 10 to 15 percent of patients at 20 years after initial repair. An ascending aortic aneurysm and progressive aortic regurgitation from a dilated aortic root can also be present.[94] A parasternal right ventricular lift and a soft and delayed P₂ with a low-pitched diastolic murmur from pulmonary regurgitation may exist. A systolic ejection murmur from right ventricular outflow tract obstruction, a high-pitched diastolic murmur from aortic regurgitation, and a pansystolic murmur from a VSD patch leak may also be heard.

Tetralogy of Fallot with Pulmonary Atresia and Major Aortopulmonary Collateral Arteries. This subgroup represents one of the greatest challenges in CHD. The aim of unifocalization surgery is to amalgamate all the sources of pulmonary blood flow and establish unobstructed right ventricular-to-pulmonary artery continuity while achieving a normal pulmonary artery pressure and a closed ventricular septum. If an adequate number of segments can be unifocalized in an unobstructed fashion, then coincident intracardiac repair can be contemplated. When this is not possible, a combined interventional catheterization and surgical approach is required.[95] Balloon dilation and stenting of stenosed arteries and anastomoses can "rehabilitate" segmental supply and allow subsequent VSD closure or, if already closed, reduce right ventricular pressure.

LABORATORY INVESTIGATIONS

ECG. Right axis deviation with right ventricular and right atrial hypertrophy is common. In adults with repaired tetralogy of Fallot, a complete right bundle branch block following repair has been the rule. QRS width may reflect the degree of right ventricular dilation and, when extreme (>180 msec) or rapidly progressive, may be a risk factor for sustained ventricular tachycardia and sudden death.

CHEST RADIOGRAPHY. Characteristically, there is a normal-sized, boot-shaped heart *(coeur en sabot)* with prominence of the right ventricle and a concavity in the region of the underdeveloped right ventricular outflow tract and main pulmonary artery. The pulmonary vascular markings are typically diminished, and the aortic arch may be on the right side (25 percent). The ascending aorta is often prominent.

ECHOCARDIOGRAPHY (Fig. 61-14). A complete diagnosis can usually be established by echo-Doppler alone. The study should identify the malaligned and nonrestrictive VSD and overriding aorta (<50 percent override) and the presence and degree of right ventricular outflow tract obstruction (infundibular, valvular, and/or pulmonary arterial stenosis). Rarely, other investigations are required before corrective surgery. The exception to this rule is when there are additional sources of pulmonary blood flow. In patients with *repaired* tetralogy of Fallot, residual pulmonary stenosis and regurgitation, residual VSD, right and left ventricular sizes and function, aortic root size, and the degree of aortic regurgitation should be assessed.

CARDIAC CATHETERIZATION AND ANGIOCARDIOGRAPHY. Although echocardiography, MRA, and fast computed tomography (CT) may delineate the presence and proximal course of the pulmonary blood vessels, the preoperative assessment of tetralogy with pulmonary atresia with major aortopulmonary collateral arteries must include delineation of the arterial supply to both lungs by selective catheterization and angiography to show the course and segmental supply from the collateral arteries and central pulmonary arteries. Major aortopulmonary collateral arteries usually arise from the descending aorta at the level of the tracheal bifurcation.

MRI. The goals of MRI examination after tetralogy of Fallot repair include the quantitative assessment of left and particularly right ventricular volumes, stroke volumes, and ejection fraction; imaging of the anatomy of the right ventricular outflow tract, pulmonary arteries, aorta, and aortopulmonary collaterals; and quantifying pulmonary, aortic, and tricuspid regurgitation.

INDICATIONS FOR INTERVENTION

Children. Symptomatic infants are now repaired at any age, and elective repair in asymptomatic infants during the first 6 months is advocated by many.[96] This is often at the expense of a transannular patch enlargement of the right ventricular outflow tract, which may be a risk factor for later failure. Marked hypoplasia of the pulmonary arteries, small body size, and prematurity are relative contraindications for early corrective operation, and these patients may be successfully palliated by balloon dilation of the right ventricular outflow tract and pulmonary arteries.

Adults, Unoperated. For unoperated adults, surgical repair is still recommended because the results are gratifying and the operative risk is comparable to pediatric series provided there is no serious coexisting morbidity.

Palliated. Palliation was seldom intended as a permanent treatment strategy, and most of these patients should undergo surgical repair. In particular, palliated patients with increasing cyanosis and erythrocytosis (from gradual shunt stenosis or development of pulmonary hypertension), left ventricular dilation, or aneurysm formation in the shunt should undergo intracardiac repair with takedown of the shunt unless irreversible pulmonary hypertension has developed.

Repaired. The following situations *may* warrant intervention after repair: a residual VSD with a shunt greater than 1.5/1; residual pulmonary stenosis (either the native right ventricular outflow or valved conduit if one is present) with right ventricular systolic pressure two thirds or more of systemic pressure; or severe pulmonary regurgitation associated with substantial right ventricular dilation/dysfunction (perhaps a right ventricular diastolic volume index > 170 cc/m²),[97] exercise intolerance, or sustained arrhythmias.[3] The coexistence of substantial left ventricular dysfunction or a QRS duration ≥ 180 msec offers additional support when other indications are present. The development of major cardiac arrhythmias, most commonly atrial flutter/fibrillation or sustained ventricular tachycardia, usually reflects hemodynamic deterioration and should be

CH 61

Congenital Heart Disease

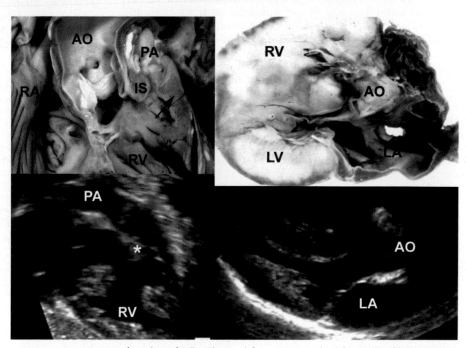

FIGURE 61–14 Montage of tetralogy of Fallot. The two left images are in the right anterior oblique view that demonstrates the anteriorly deviated infundibular septum (asterisk) and the ventricular septal defect. The arrow on the specimen points to the hypertrophied septoparietal trabeculations. The right images demonstrate the overriding aorta and the ventricular septal defect. AO = aorta; IS = infundibular septum; LA = left atrium; PA = pulmonary artery; RA = right atrium; RV = right ventricle.

treated accordingly. Surgery is occasionally necessary for significant aortic regurgitation associated with symptoms and/or progressive left ventricular dilation and for aortic root enlargement of 55 mm or more. Rapid enlargement of a right ventricular outflow tract aneurysm needs surgical attention.

INTERVENTIONAL OPTIONS

Surgery. Reparative surgery involves closing the VSD with a Dacron patch and relieving the right ventricular outflow tract obstruction. The latter may involve resection of infundibular muscle and insertion of a right ventricular outflow tract or transannular patch—a patch across the pulmonary valve annulus that disrupts the integrity of the pulmonary valve and causes important pulmonary regurgitation. When an anomalous coronary artery crosses the right ventricular outflow tract and precludes transection of the latter, an extracardiac conduit is placed between the right ventricle and pulmonary artery, bypassing the right ventricular outflow tract obstruction. A patent foramen ovale or secundum ASD may be closed. Additional treatable lesions such as muscular VSDs, PDAs, and aortopulmonary collaterals should also be addressed at the time of surgery.

Reoperation is necessary in 10 to 15 percent of patients after reparative surgery over a 20-year follow-up. For persistent right ventricular outflow tract obstruction, resection of residual infundibular stenosis or placement of a right ventricular outflow or transannular patch, with or without pulmonary arterioplasty, can be performed. Occasionally, an extracardiac valved conduit may be necessary. Pulmonary valve replacement (either homograft or xenograft) is used to treat severe pulmonary regurgitation. Concomitant tricuspid valve annuloplasty may be performed for moderate or severe tricuspid regurgitation. Concomitant cryoablation should often be performed at the time of surgery for patients with either preexisting atrial or ventricular arrhythmias.[98]

Interventional. Significant branch pulmonary artery stenosis can be managed with balloon dilation and usually stent insertion. A catheter-delivered pulmonary valve replacement is now entering clinical trials. The Bonhoeffer valve[99] is a bovine jugular venous valve mounted in a balloon dilatable stent and has been implanted in more than 100 patients, primarily those with RV-PA conduits.

INTERVENTIONAL OUTCOMES. The overall survival of patients who have had initial operative repair is excellent, provided the VSD has been closed and the right ventricular outflow tract obstruction has been relieved. A 25-year survival of 94 percent has been reported. Pulmonary valve replacement for chronic pulmonary regurgitation or right ventricular outflow tract obstruction after initial intracardiac repair can be done safely with a mortality rate of 1 percent. Pulmonary valve replacement, when performed for significant pulmonary regurgitation, leads to an improvement in exercise tolerance, as well as right ventricular dimension and function.[100] Sudden death can occur. Ventricular tachycardia can arise at the site of the right ventriculotomy, from VSD patch sutures, or from the right ventricular outflow tract. Patients at high risk for sudden death include those with right ventricular dilation and a QRS duration of 180 milliseconds or more on their ECG. Moderate to severe left ventricular dysfunction is another risk factor for sudden death.[101] The reported incidence of sudden death is approximately 5 percent, which accounts for approximately one third of late deaths over the first 20 years of follow-up.

FOLLOW-UP. All patients should have expert cardiology follow-up every 1 to 2 years.

Fontan Procedure–Requiring Lesions

The next four sections describe lesions usually or often treated with a Fontan procedure. These include tricuspid atresia, hypoplastic left heart syndrome, double-inlet ventricle, and isomerism. *Fontan procedure* has become a generic term to describe a palliative surgical procedure that redirects the systemic venous return directly to the pulmonary arteries without passing through a subpulmonary ventricle. It is performed in patients having a "functionally single" ventricle or when an intracardiac repair is not possible, even though there are two good-sized ventricles. Although undoubtedly imperfect, the Fontan circuit restores an in-series pulmonary-to-systemic circulation, removing the chronic volume load of the systemic ventricle previously supporting a parallel circuit of pulmonary and systemic circulations. The earliest iteration of the Fontan procedure was a simple "atriopulmonary" connection, whereby the right atrium or its appendage was anastomosed to the pulmonary arteries. Because of the long-term problems of atrial dilation, arrhythmia, and thrombosis, this procedure has been abandoned in favor of hemodynamically superior versions. In the early 1990s the total cavopulmonary anastomosis was introduced. This consisted of a direct, end-to-side superior cavopulmonary anastomosis (bidirectional Glenn operation) in combination with an intraatrial baffle or tube connection of the inferior vena cava to the underside of the confluent pulmonary arteries. More recently the inferior vena cava has been directed to the pulmonary arteries via an extracardiac conduit, completely excluding the atrium from the circuit. It remains to be seen whether these modifications will have the desired effect of reducing late morbidity, and all patients will require regular and careful review in special centers.

TRICUSPID ATRESIA (ABSENT RIGHT ATRIOVENTRICULAR CONNECTION)

MORPHOLOGY. *Classical tricuspid atresia* is best described as absence of the right AV connection (Figs. 61-15 and 61-16). Consequently, there must be an ASD. There is usually hypoplasia of the morphological right ventricle, which communicates to the dominant ventricle via a VSD. Patients may be subdivided into those with concordant ventriculoarterial connections and normally related great arteries (70 to 80 percent of cases) and those with discordant connections, where the aorta arises from the small right ventricle and is fed via the VSD. Associated lesions in the latter group include subaortic stenosis and aortic arch anomalies.

PATHOPHYSIOLOGY. The clinical picture and management are dominated by issues related to the ventriculoarterial connections. All patients have "mixing" of atrial blood, and thus their degree of cyanosis is governed by the amount of pulmonary blood flow and systemic venous saturations. Patients with concordant ventriculoarterial connections tend to be more cyanosed (depending on the size of the VSD), whereas those with discordant connections are pinker and tend to develop heart failure (because the unobstructed pulmonary circulation arises directly from the left ventricle). Some present with a critical reduction of systemic blood flow because of obstruction at the VSD and/or associated aortic arch anomalies and behave much like hypoplastic left heart syndrome.

LABORATORY INVESTIGATIONS

ECG. Left axis deviation, right atrial enlargement, and left ventricular hypertrophy often occur. Left atrial enlargement may be present if pulmonary flow is high.

CHEST RADIOGRAPHY. Situs solitus, levocardia, and a left-sided aortic arch usually occur. The heart size and pulmonary vascular markings vary with the amount of pulmonary blood flow. The main pulmonary trunk is inapparent. A right aortic arch exists in 25 percent of patients.

ECHOCARDIOGRAM. This establishes the full segmental diagnosis. The size of the ASD, VSD, and aortic arch all must be carefully assessed.

CARDIAC CATHETERIZATION. This is rarely required for initial diagnosis or management. It can be useful to assess the degree of subaortic stenosis (by assessing the change in left ventricle–to-aortic pressure gradient while performing an isoprenaline or dobutamine challenge) and is mandatory to measure the pulmonary artery pressure and resistance prior to venopulmonary connections.

MANAGEMENT OPTIONS. In those with concordant ventriculoarterial connections and severe cyanosis, a systemic-to-pulmonary shunt is performed in the first 6 to 8 weeks of life, and in older children, a primary bidirectional Glenn procedure can be considered. In infants with discordant arterial connections, early palliation ranges from pulmonary artery banding to reduce pulmonary blood flow when there is no subaortic narrowing to a full Norwood stage 1 procedure in those presenting with severe stenosis and a hypoplastic ascending aorta and arch.

The aim of early palliation is to prepare for a Fontan procedure. This should be performed only when there is good ventricular function, unobstructed systemic blood flow, and minimal AV valve regurgitation. Candidates for these corrective procedures must also have normal pulmonary vascular resistance and a low pulmonary resistance, a mean pulmonary artery pressure less than 15 mm Hg, and pulmonary arteries of adequate size.

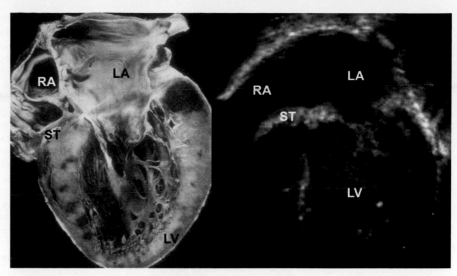

FIGURE 61–15 Apical four-chamber view in univentricular connection of left ventricular type with absent right connection (tricuspid atresia). Note the wedge of sulcus tissue in the floor of the right atrium. LA = left atrium; LV = left ventricle; RA = right atrium; ST = sulcus tissue.

HYPOPLASTIC LEFT HEART SYNDROME

DEFINITION. *Hypoplastic left heart syndrome* is a generic term used to describe a group of closely related cardiac anomalies characterized by underdevelopment of the left cardiac chambers, in association with atresia or stenosis of the aortic and/or the mitral orifices, and hypoplasia of the aorta. The term should be restricted to those with normally connected hearts with concordant AV and ventriculoarterial connections. Hypoplastic left heart syndrome (Fig. 61-17) is characterized by duct-dependent systemic blood flow and so tends to present with severe symptoms within the first week of life, as ductal constriction occurs. Untreated, the disease is almost uniformly fatal in infancy. In the past, many infants would present with severe acidemic circulatory collapse, but this is becoming less frequent as fetal ultrasound screening for cardiac anomalies becomes more generally available and successful. Fetal diagnosis allows for a planned delivery and institution of prostaglandin therapy from birth and has now been proven to reduce subsequent preoperative morbidity and perioperative mortality during the first stage of surgical repair.

PATHOPHYSIOLOGY. It remains uncertain whether hypoplastic left heart syndrome reflects a primary myocardial disease or is a consequence of a structural or hemodynamic abnormality. There is no doubt that in some patients, an apparently isolated dilated cardiomyopathy in early fetal life may evolve (as a result of a subsequent lack of left ventricular growth) into hypoplastic left heart syndrome later in gestation. Congenital structural abnormalities clearly play a significant role as well. This is exemplified by the effect of isolated valvular stenosis to produce a continuum of hypoplastic left heart syndrome to critical aortic stenosis with a normal-sized left ventricle. Therefore hypoplastic left heart syndrome is likely multifactorial in origin.

CLINICAL FEATURES. The diagnosis should be considered in any infant with the sudden onset of circulatory collapse and severe lactic acidosis. As such, it must be distinguished from neonatal sepsis and metabolic disorders. Until excluded, any child presenting in this way

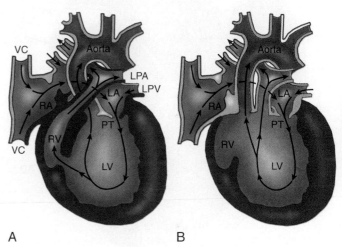

FIGURE 61–16 A, Tricuspid atresia with normally related great arteries, a small ventricular septal defect, diminutive right ventricular chamber, and narrowed outflow tract. **B,** An example of tricuspid atresia and complete transposition of the great arteries in which the left ventricular chamber is essentially a common ventricle, with the aorta arising from an infundibular component (RV) of the common ventricle. LA = left atrium; LPA = left pulmonary artery; LPV = left pulmonary vein; LV = left ventricle; PT = pulmonary trunk; RA = right atrium; RV = right ventricle; VC = vena cava. *(**A** and **B,** Modified from Edwards JE, Burchell HB: Congenital tricuspid atresia: Classification. Med Clin North Am 33:1177, 1949.)*

should be treated with prostaglandin, which may have a dramatic positive effect if there is an underlying cardiac abnormality and little effect if there is not.

LABORATORY INVESTIGATIONS

ECG. This frequently shows right axis deviation, right atrial and ventricular enlargement, and ST and T wave abnormalities in the left precordial leads.

CHEST RADIOGRAPHY. This usually shows some cardiac enlargement shortly after birth, but with clinical deterioration there may be marked cardiomegaly and increased pulmonary venous and arterial vascular markings.

ECHOCARDIOGRAPHY (Fig. 61-18). Cross-sectional echocardiography provides a full segmental diagnosis. In its classic form, the left ventricular cavity is small, with a diminutive mitral valve. The myocardium may be thinned or be of normal thickness, but the endocardium is usually thickened, consistent with endocardial fibroelastosis. There may be fistulous communications between the left ventricular cavity and the coronary arteries, a feature much more likely when the mitral valve is patent rather than atretic. The aortic root is usually diminutive, less than 4 to 5 mm in diameter at the level of the sinuses of Valsalva and narrowed in its ascending portion. The aortic arch is usually larger, but there is often a juxtaductal coarctation. The duct varies in size according to treatment, and assessment of this and the size of the interatrial communication are crucial to management. There may be profound desaturation and rapid demise (because of a combination of reduced pulmonary blood flow and pulmonary edema) in children with an intact atrial septum or restrictive patent foramen ovale.

MANAGEMENT OPTIONS. Early treatment with prostaglandin is mandatory. Those presenting in shock require

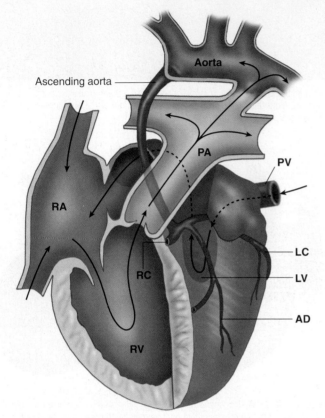

FIGURE 61–17 Hypoplastic left heart with aortic hypoplasia, aortic valve atresia, and a hypoplastic mitral valve and left ventricle. AD = anterior descending; LC = left circumflex; LV = left ventricle; PA = pulmonary artery; PV = pulmonary vein; RA = right atrium; RC = right coronary artery; RV = right ventricle. *(From Neufeld HN, Adams P Jr, Edwards JE, et al: Diagnosis of aortic atresia by retrograde aortography. Circulation 25:278, 1962.)*

paralysis, mechanical ventilation, and inotropic support. Crucial to managing these patients is maintenance of a balanced pulmonary and systemic blood flow. The cardiac output is fixed and is distributed according to the relative magnitude of the systemic and pulmonary vascular resistance. Thus measures to elevate the pulmonary resistance (by imposing hypercapnia or by alveolar hypoxia) and reduce the systemic resistance (using vasodilators) are frequently required.

Surgical Treatment. Staged surgical management now provides long-term palliation to most patients with hypoplastic left heart syndrome. The first stage, often referred to as the *Norwood procedure,* now has many versions, but its essence is the creation of an unobstructed communication between the right ventricle and an unobstructed aorta. The right ventricular to aortic connection is accomplished by direct connection between the transected proximal pulmonary trunk and ascending aorta, usually with a patch extending around the augmented aortic arch. Pulmonary blood flow is established via a systemic-to-pulmonary shunt or the more recently introduced right ventricle-to-pulmonary artery conduit. The PDA is ligated, and a large interatrial communication is created. Early results of this procedure were poor, but survival rates higher than 85 percent have recently been published. Institutional variations, the interval mortality, and those unsuitable to progress to stage 2 must also be taken into account, however, and in some centers, the preferred operation is cardiac transplantation.

Stage 2 consists of an end-to-side superior vena cava–to-pulmonary artery connection (bidirectional Glenn procedure) or a hemi-Fontan (incorporating the roof of the atrium into the pulmonary artery anastomosis). This is performed at approximately 6 months of age as an intermediate step before stage 3, a Fontan operation.

ADULT ISSUES. The survivors of the earliest attempts at staged Norwood palliation are just now entering adult life. Their issues are likely to be common to all late survivors of Fontan palliation.

DOUBLE-INLET VENTRICLE

DEFINITION. Double-inlet connection falls under the umbrella of univentricular AV connections. These hearts are defined by having more than 50 percent of each AV connection connected to a dominant ventricle. In practice this usually means the whole of one and greater than 50 percent of the alternative junction is connected to either a left or right ventricle. When there is a common junction, more than 75 percent of the junction must be connected to the dominant ventricle.

MORPHOLOGY. In about 75 percent of patients, the dominant ventricle is a left ventricle that is separated from the right ventricle by a VSD. In 20 percent the dominant ventricle is a right ventricle, and the small, incomplete ventricle is of left ventricular apical morphology. In only 5 percent of cases is there truly only one ventricle in the ventricular mass. In double-inlet left ventricle the most common ventriculoarterial connection is discordant. Thus the aorta arises from the small right ventricle and is fed via the VSD, and the generally unobstructed pulmonary artery arises from the left ventricle. Aortic and aortic arch anomalies are frequent in these patients.

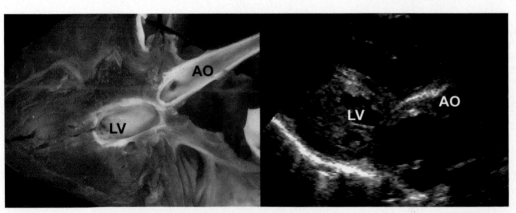

FIGURE 61–18 Long-axis view of the left ventricle and aorta in hypoplastic left heart syndrome. Note the associated endocardial fibroelastosis in the specimen. AO = aorta, LV = left ventricle.

PATHOPHYSIOLOGY. The basic circulatory physiology of *double-inlet left ventricle* is identical to that of tricuspid atresia. Common mixing of systemic and pulmonary venous blood occurs, and the blood is then ejected from the left ventricle into the pulmonary artery (with discordant connections) or aorta (with concordant connections). In the former the blood must pass through the VSD to gain egress to the aorta. Subaortic stenosis, aortic hypoplasia, and arch anomalies are therefore common. In *double-inlet right ventricle,* it is those patients with concordant ventriculoarterial connections who are at particular risk of systemic outflow obstruction. One or the other or both of the two AV valves (when present) may be stenotic, atretic, or regurgitant. Under these circumstances the integrity of the atrial septum becomes important. If there is left or right atrial outflow obstruction, a septectomy or septostomy will be required.

CLINICAL FEATURES. When there is critical reduction of systemic outflow, infants may be duct dependent and present with acidemic shock. Conversely, when pulmonary blood flow is reduced, presentation may be with severe cyanosis or with duct-dependent pulmonary blood flow. Other patients may not present in the neonatal period and will develop heart failure because of increased pulmonary blood flow. Patients undergo the same surgical algorithms as those with tricuspid atresia and so ultimately will undergo a Fontan operation. Their clinical issues are typical of any patient after this procedure.

LABORATORY INVESTIGATIONS

ECG. This is highly variable. Ventricular hypertrophy appropriate to the dominant ventricle is expected.
CHEST RADIOGRAPHY. This is similarly variable and rarely diagnostic.
ECHOCARDIOGRAPHY (Fig. 61-19). A full segmental diagnosis should be possible in all patients. Particular attention should be paid to defining AV valve anomalies and the presence and anatomy of any subaortic obstruction. This may develop, even if not present at birth, and should be part of the routine surveillance of these patients.

INDICATIONS AND OPTIONS FOR INTERVENTION.
Survival without intervention may be prolonged, but at the expense of increasing cyanosis (when there is restriction to pulmonary blood flow) or pulmonary vascular disease (when there is unrestricted pulmonary blood flow). Those born with restricted systemic blood flow require urgent surgical intervention, usually undergoing a Norwood-type repair to establish the pulmonary valve as the unobstructed systemic outflow tract. Pulmonary artery banding is only offered to those infants with pulmonary overcirculation, heart failure, and unobstructed systemic outflow. Subsequently, and sometimes as the primary procedure, a bidirectional Glenn anastomosis is performed as a prelude to a Fontan procedure.

FOLLOW-UP. These patients should be reviewed frequently and in a center conversant with the issues of the Fontan operation.

ISOMERISM

DEFINITION. For the purposes of illustrating the cardiac manifestations, isomerism describes the situation in which both atrial appendages have either left or right anatomical features (i.e., bilateral right or bilateral left atrial appendages).

MORPHOLOGY. Experts have made many attempts to describe hearts with complex abnormalities of visceral and atrial situs, whereby normal lateralization is lost. Terms such as *heterotaxy, asplenia,* and *polysplenia* fail to ade-quately describe either the visceral or cardiac manifestations with enough precision. The left atrial appendage is characterized by its tubular shape and pectinate muscles confined to the appendage. The pectinate muscles of the triangular right atrial appendage extend from its broad junction with the atrium, to extend around the vestibule or AV junction. Thus the arrangement of the atria (be it usual, mirror image, right or left isomerism) can be defined independent of the venous anatomy.

In left isomerism it is not unusual to have a biventricular AV connection, with separate AV junctions. A common junction (with an AV septal defect) is seen in approximately 30 percent of cases of left isomerism and more than 90 percent of hearts with isomerism of the right atrial appendages. Concordant ventriculoarterial connections predominate in left isomerism, and a double-outlet right ventricle with an anterior aorta is most frequently seen when there is right isomerism. The venous connections are variable. These variations significantly affect the clinical and interventional management of these patients.

ISOMERISM OF THE RIGHT ATRIAL APPENDAGES

CLINICAL FEATURES. Bilateral "right-sidedness" results in a pattern of visceral abnormalities sometimes described as asplenia syndrome. The liver is midline, both lungs are trilobed with symmetrically short bronchi on the chest radiograph, and the spleen is hypoplastic or absent. The latter mandates immunization against pneumococcal infection and continuous penicillin prophylaxis against gram-positive sepsis. The diagnosis can be inferred from the bronchial pattern on the chest radiograph but most often is established by cross-sectional echocardiography because of early presentation with severe CHD. Abdominal scanning shows ipsilateral arrangement of the aorta and an anterior inferior vena cava. The intracardiac anatomy is most often that of an AV septal defect with varying degrees of right ventricular dominance, and frequently there is an associated double-outlet right ventricle with an anterior aorta and subpulmonary stenosis or atresia. Thus cyanosis is the most common presentation. The inferior vena cava may connect to either right atrium, and superior venae cavae are often lateralized and separate. It is the pulmonary venous drainage that is crucial to the presentation and outcome of these children. By definition, the pulmonary veins are draining anomalously to one or other right atrium, but frequently this is indirect and/or obstructed. Adequate repair of the latter is fundamental to the outcome of these children, who almost uniformly ultimately require a Fontan procedure.

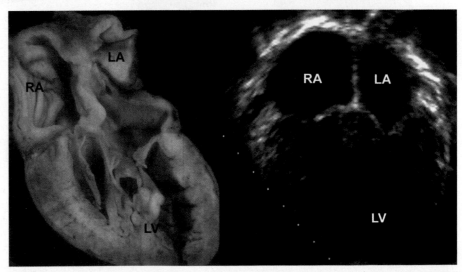

FIGURE 61–19 Apical four-chamber view in a double-inlet univentricular connection of left ventricular type with two atrioventricular valves. LA = left atrium; LV = left ventricle; RA = right atrium.

MANAGEMENT OPTIONS AND OUTCOMES. Initial palliation is usually directed toward regulating pulmonary blood flow and dealing with anomalies of pulmonary venous connection. Subsequently these patients (even when there are equal-sized ventricles) are treated along a Fontan algorithm. This is because repair of complete AV septal defect in the setting of abnormal ventriculoarterial connections is technically difficult or impossible. Thus a unilateral or bilateral superior cavopulmonary anastomosis is performed at approximately 6 months of age, followed when possible by a Fontan procedure when aged 2 to 4 years.

The long-term outcome of surgery for right isomerism, however, has been poor. Improved early palliation and a staged approach toward the Fontan procedure have led to improved results. The prognosis for these infants, particularly when there is obstruction to pulmonary venous return, must remain guarded.

ISOMERISM OF THE LEFT ATRIAL APPENDAGES

CLINICAL FEATURES. These patients have bilateral "left-sidedness." Hence they have two left lungs and bronchi, tend to have polysplenia, and frequently have malrotation of the gut. The cardiac abnormalities tend to be less severe than those of right isomerism. These patients are particularly prone to develop atrial arrhythmias because the normal sinoatrial node is a right atrial structure and is usually absent in these patients. The ECG often shows an abnormal P wave axis, or wandering pacemaker. The anatomical diagnosis is usually established by echocardiography. The abdominal great vessels are both to the right or left of the spine, as with right isomerism, but in left isomerism the vein is a posterior azygos vein that continues to connect to a left- or right-sided superior vena cava. The intrahepatic inferior vena cava is absent in 90 percent, and under these circumstances the hepatic veins drain directly to the atria. The pulmonary venous connection needs to be defined precisely before any surgical intervention. Pulmonary arteriovenous malformations are not infrequently seen in patients with left isomerism. These can lead to cyanosis in unoperated or operated patients. The intracardiac anatomy varies from essentially normal to complex. Again, AV septal defect (partial and complete) is overrepresented but with less frequent ventricular imbalance and abnormalities of ventriculoarterial connection.

MANAGEMENT OPTIONS. A biventricular repair is achieved in many more of these patients, albeit with the need for complex atrial baffle surgery to separate the systemic and pulmonary venous returns. The long-term outcome for patients with left isomerism is therefore much better than for those with right isomerism. The issues are much like those related to the type of surgery, but monitoring for arrhythmia needs to be even more intense than usual.

THE FONTAN PATIENT (Fig. 61-20)

BACKGROUND. As stated in the introduction to this section, the uncertain nature of the Fontan circulation and the frequency of its failure require that all patients should be followed regularly in a specialized center for CHD, and new symptoms should prompt early re-evaluation in such a center.

Since its description for the surgical management of tricuspid atresia in 1971, the Fontan procedure has become the definitive palliative surgical treatment when a biventricular repair is not possible. The principle is diversion of the systemic venous return directly to the pulmonary arteries without passing through a subpulmonary ventricle. Over the years, many modifications of the original procedure have been described and performed, namely, direct atriopulmonary connection, total cavopulmonary connection, and extracardiac conduit. Fenestration (5-mm diameter) of the Fontan circuit into the left atrium is sometimes performed at the time of surgery in high-risk patients, permitting right-to-left shunting and decompression of the Fontan circuit.

PATHOPHYSIOLOGY. Elevation of the central venous pressure and a reduced cardiac output (sometimes at rest[102] but always on exercise) are inevitable consequences of the Fontan procedure. Small adverse changes in ventricular function (particularly diastolic); circuit efficiency (elevated pulmonary resistance, obstruction, thrombosis); or the onset of arrhythmia all potentially lead to major symptomatic deterioration.

Although it is reasonable to describe patients after the Fontan procedure as existing in a form of chronic heart failure (since their right atrial pressure must be high), this is seldom due to marked systolic dysfunction.[103] Indeed, a small elevation in ventricular diastolic pressure may be much more harmful. Thus it may be incorrect to treat these patients with traditional heart failure medications. In a randomized, blinded placebo-controlled study, ACE inhibition failed to improve functional performance, and some indices worsened.

The more "streamlined" Fontan circulations (total cavopulmonary anastomosis, extracardiac conduit) that exclude the right atrium from the circulation have demonstrably better fluid dynamic properties and improved functional performance. Physical obstruction at surgical anastomoses, the distal pulmonary arteries, or pulmonary veins (often due to compression by a dilated

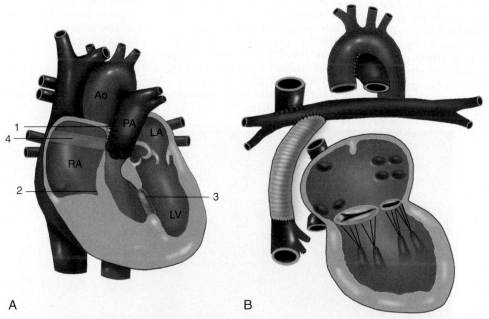

FIGURE 61-20 Modification of the Fontan operation. **A,** Direct atriopulmonary connection (1) for tricuspid valve atresia (2); ventricular septal defect, oversewn (3); patch closure of atrial septal defect (4). **B,** Extracardiac conduit made of a Dacron graft bypassing the right atrium, connecting the inferior vena cava to the inferior aspect of the right pulmonary artery. Superior vena cava is anastomosed to the superior aspect of the right pulmonary artery. Ao = aorta; LA = left atrium; LV = left ventricle; PA = pulmonary artery; RA = right atrium. (**A,** From Mullins CE, Mayer DC: Congenital Heart Disease: A Diagrammatic Atlas. New York, Wiley-Liss, 1988; **B,** from Marcelletti C: Inferior vena cava-pulmonary artery extracardiac conduit: A new form of right heart bypass. J Thorac Cardiovasc Surg 100:228, 1990.)

right atrium) all reduce circulatory efficiency, however. Similarly, elevated pulmonary arteriolar resistances have adverse effects. This is because the pulmonary vascular resistance is the single biggest contributor to impairment of venous return and elevation of venous pressure. Relatively little is known about pulmonary vascular resistance late after the procedure, but it has recently been shown to be elevated in a significant number of patients and to be reactive to inhaled nitric oxide, suggesting pulmonary endothelial dysfunction.[104]

CLINICAL FEATURES. The majority of patients (≈90 percent) present with functional class I to II at 5 years' follow-up after a Fontan procedure. Progressive deterioration of functional status with time is the rule. Supraventricular arrhythmias such as atrial tachycardia, flutter, and fibrillation are common. Physical examination in an otherwise uncomplicated patient reveals an elevated, usually nonpulsatile jugular venous pulse (10 cm above the sternal angle and needed to provide the hydrostatic pressure to drive cardiac output through the pulmonary circulation), a quiet apex, a normal S_1, and a single S_2 (the pulmonary artery having been tied off). A heart murmur should not be present, and its identification suggests the presence of systemic AV valve regurgitation or subaortic obstruction. Generalized edema and ascites may be a sign of protein-losing enteropathy (see later).

COMPLICATIONS AND SEQUELAE

Arrhythmia. Although often associated with marked symptomatic decline, atrial arrhythmias tend to reflect the consequences of the abnormalities of ventricular function and circulatory efficiency described earlier. The massively dilated right atrium after an atriopulmonary connection is commonly associated with atrial flutter and fibrillation.[105] With new-onset arrhythmia, hemodynamic abnormalities and atrial/venous thrombosis, which may develop within 2 hours of arrhythmia onset, should be actively excluded before therapy. Atrial flutter/fibrillation is common (15 to 20 percent at 5 years' follow-up) and increases with duration of follow-up. Atrial flutter/fibrillation carries significant morbidity, can be associated with profound hemodynamic deterioration, and needs prompt medical attention. The combination of atrial incisions and multiple suture lines at the time of Fontan surgery along with increased right atrial pressure and size probably explains the high incidence of atrial arrhythmias in such patients. Patients at greater risk for atrial tachyarrhythmias are those who were operated on at an older age, with poor ventricular function, systemic AV valve regurgitation, or increased pulmonary artery pressure. It has been suggested that the exclusion of the right atrium from elevated systemic venous pressure (as in total cavopulmonary connection or extracardiac conduit) leads to a decrease in the incidence of atrial arrhythmias. This apparent benefit may, however, be due exclusively to the shorter length of follow-up in this group of patients. Sinus node dysfunction and complete heart block can occur and require pacemaker insertion.

Thrombosis and Stroke. The reported incidence of thromboembolic complications in the Fontan circuit varies from 6 to 25 percent, depending on the diagnostic method used and the length of follow-up.[106] Thrombus formation may relate to the presence of supraventricular arrhythmias, right atrial dilation, right atrial "smoke," and the presence of artificial material used to construct the Fontan circuit.[106] Accordingly, a similar incidence of thrombus formation had been reported for all types of Fontan circuits. Systemic arterial embolism in patients with and without a fenestrated Fontan has also been reported. Protein C deficiency has been reported in these patients and may explain in part their propensity to thromboembolism.

Protein-Losing Enteropathy. Protein-losing enteropathy, defined as severe loss of serum protein into the intestine, occurs in 4 to 13 percent of patients after a Fontan proce-

dure.[107] Patients present with generalized edema, ascites, pleural effusion, and/or chronic diarrhea. Protein-losing enteropathy is thought to result principally from chronically elevated systemic venous pressure causing intestinal lymphangiectasia with consequent loss of albumin, protein, lymphocytes, and immunoglobulin into the gastrointestinal tract. The diagnosis is confirmed by finding low serum albumin and protein; low plasma alpha$_1$-antitrypsin level and lymphocyte counts; and, most important, a high alpha$_1$-antitrypsin stool clearance. It carries a dismal prognosis, with a 5-year survival of 46 to 59 percent.

Right Pulmonary Vein Compression/Obstruction. Right pulmonary vein obstruction/compression can occur from the enlarged right atrium or atrial baffle bulging into the left atrium and can lead to increased pulmonary artery pressure with further dilation of the right atrium. It should be sought.

Pulmonary Thromboembolism is increasingly recognized[106,108] and will elevate central venous pressure. There is continuing debate as to the role of anticoagulation, antiplatelet therapy, or both in the long-term management of these patients, but most receive some form of therapy.[109,110]

Fontan Obstruction. Stenosis or partial obstruction of the Fontan connection leads to exercise intolerance, atrial tachyarrhythmias, and right-sided heart failure. Sudden total obstruction (usually thrombotic) can present as sudden death.

Ventricular Dysfunction and Valvular Regurgitation. Progressive deterioration of systemic ventricular function, with or without progressive AV valve regurgitation, is common. Patients with morphological systemic right ventricles may fare less well than those with morphological left ventricles.

Hepatic Dysfunction. Mildly raised hepatic transaminase levels from hepatic congestion are frequent but seldom clinically important. Cirrhosis apparently due to chronic venous hypertension has been described.

Cyanosis. Worsening cyanosis may relate to worsening of ventricular function, the development of venous collateral channels draining to the left atrium, or the development of pulmonary arteriovenous malformations (especially if a classic Glenn procedure remains as part of the Fontan circulation).

LABORATORY INVESTIGATIONS

ECG. Sinus rhythm, atrial flutter, junctional rhythm, or complete heart block may be present. The QRS complex reflects the basic underlying cardiac anomaly. In patients with tricuspid atresia, left axis deviation is the norm. In patients with univentricular hearts, the conduction pattern varies widely and depends on the morphology and relative position of the rudimentary chamber.

CHEST RADIOGRAPHY. Mild bulging of the right lower heart border from a dilated right atrium is often seen in patients with an atriopulmonary connection.

ECHOCARDIOGRAPHY. The presence or absence of right atrial stasis, thrombus, patency of a fenestration, and Fontan circuit obstruction should be sought. Superior and inferior venae cavae biphasic and pulmonary artery triphasic flow patterns suggest unobstructed flow in the Fontan circuit, whereas a mean gradient between the Fontan circuit and the pulmonary artery of 2 mm Hg or more may represent significant obstruction. Assessment of the pulmonary venous flow pattern is important in detecting pulmonary vein obstruction (right pulmonary vein > left pulmonary vein) sometimes caused by an enlarged right atrium (often ≈80 × 60 mm in adults with atriopulmonary connections). Concomitant assessment of systemic ventricular function and AV valve regurgitation can be readily accomplished. TEE may be required if there is inadequate visualization of the Fontan anastomosis or to exclude thrombus in the right atrium.

DIAGNOSTIC CATHETERIZATION. Complete heart catheterization is advised if surgical reintervention is planned or if adequate assessment of the hemodynamics is not obtained by noninvasive means.

MRI. The objectives of MRI in Fontan patients include assessment of the pathways from the systemic veins to the pulmonary arteries for obstruction and thrombus; detection of Fontan baffle fenestration or leaks; evaluation of the pulmonary veins for compression; assessing systemic ventricular volume, mass, and ejection fraction; imaging of the systemic ventricular outflow tract for obstruction; and quantitative assessment of the AV and semilunar valve(s) for regurgitation, the aorta for obstruction or an aneurysm, and for aortopulmonary, systemic venous, or systemic-to-pulmonary venous collateral vessels.

MANAGEMENT OPTIONS AND OUTCOMES. Patient selection is of utmost importance and has a major impact on clinical outcome. Long-term survival in "ideal" candidates is 81 percent at 10 years, compared with 60 to 71 percent in "all comers." Death occurs mostly from congestive heart failure and atrial arrhythmias. The Fontan procedure remains a palliative, not curative, procedure. A more radical approach to the failing Fontan circulation including surgical revision of the circuit to an extracardiac conduit, in combination with a Cox/maze procedure and, frequently, simultaneous epicardial pacemaker insertion, has recently been shown to provide good early palliation.[111-113] Ultimately cardiac transplantation may be required by many of these patients.[107]

Arrhythmias. Atrial tachyarrhythmias are quite difficult to manage and should quickly raise the thought of long-term warfarin therapy. When atrial flutter/fibrillation are present, an underlying hemodynamic cause should always be sought, and, in particular, evidence for obstruction of the Fontan circuit needs to be sought. Prompt attempts should be made to restore sinus rhythm. Antiarrhythmic medications, alone or combined with an epicardial antitachycardia pacing device, and radiofrequency catheter ablation techniques have had limited success. Surgical conversion from an atriopulmonary Fontan to a total cavopulmonary connection with concomitant atrial cryoablation therapy at the time of surgery has been reported with good short-term success.[113] Epicardial pacemaker insertion for sinus node dysfunction and/or complete heart block may be necessary. Epicardial AV sequential pacing should be employed whenever possible.

Anticoagulant Therapy. The use of prophylactic long-term anticoagulation is contentious. Experts recommend that patients with a history of documented arrhythmias, fenestration in the Fontan connection, or spontaneous contrast (smoke) in the right atrium on echocardiography be anticoagulated.[109] For established thrombus, thrombolytic therapy versus surgical removal of the clot and conversion of the Fontan circuit have been described, both with high mortality rates.

Protein-Losing Enteropathy. Treatment modalities include a low-fat, high-protein, medium-chain triglyceride diet to reduce intestinal lymphatic production; albumin infusions to increase intravascular osmotic pressure; and/or the introduction of diuretics, afterload-reducing agents, and positive inotropic agents to lower central venous pressure. Most often these therapies are ineffective and should not be continued if indeed tried at all. Catheter-based interventions such as balloon dilation of pathway obstruction or creation of an atrial fenestration, as well as surgical interventions from conversion or takedown of the Fontan circuit to cardiac transplantation, have also been advocated. Other reportedly effective treatment modalities include subcutaneous heparin, octreotide treatment, and prednisone therapy. All therapies have a similar failure rate of about 50 percent.

Right Pulmonary Vein Compression/Obstruction. When hemodynamically significant, Fontan conversion to a total cavopulmonary connection or extracardiac conduit may be recommended.

Fontan Obstruction. Surgical revision of obstructed right atrium to pulmonary artery or superior and inferior venae cavae to pulmonary artery connections is recommended, usually to an extracardiac Fontan. Alternatively, balloon angioplasty with or without stenting may be used when appropriate and feasible.

Ventricular Failure and Valvular Regurgitation. ACE inhibitors are of unproven benefit, do not appear to enhance exercise capacity, and may cause clinical deterioration. Patients with systemic AV valve regurgitation may require AV valve repair or replacement. Cardiac transplantation should also be considered.

Cyanosis. In the setting of a fenestrated Fontan, surgical or preferably transcatheter closure of the fenestration can be attempted. Pulmonary arteriovenous fistulas from a classic Glenn may be improved by surgical conversion to a bidirectional Glenn connection.

FOLLOW-UP. Close and expert follow-up is recommended with particular attention to ventricular function and systemic AV valve regurgitation. The development of atrial tachyarrhythmia should instigate a search for possible obstruction at the Fontan anastomosis, right pulmonary vein obstruction, or thrombus within the right atrium.

TOTAL ANOMALOUS PULMONARY VENOUS CONNECTION

DEFINITION. This describes the situation in which all pulmonary veins fail to drain directly to the left atrium. As a result, all of the systemic and pulmonary venous return drains to the right atrium, albeit using varied routes.

MORPHOLOGY (Fig. 61-21). The anatomical varieties of total anomalous pulmonary venous connection may be subdivided, depending on the level of the abnormal drainage. The anomalous connection is most often supradiaphrag-

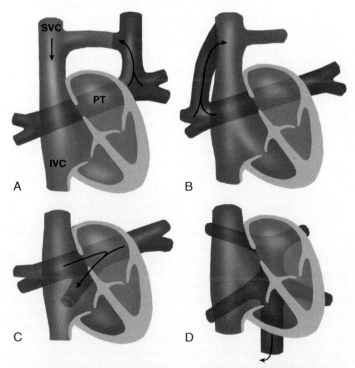

FIGURE 61–21 Anatomical types of total anomalous pulmonary venous return: supracardiac, in which the pulmonary veins drain either via the vertical vein to the anomalous vein (**A**) or directly to the superior vena cava (SVC) with the orifice close to the orifice of the azygos vein (**B**). **C**, Drainage into the right atrium via the coronary sinus. **D**, Infracardiac drainage via a vertical vein into the portal vein or the inferior vena cava (IVC). PT = pulmonary trunk. (**A** to **D**, From Stark J, deLeval M: Surgery for Congenital Heart Defects. 2nd ed. Philadelphia, WB Saunders, 1994, p 330.)

matic, connecting via a vertical vein to the left brachiocephalic vein, direct to the right atrium, to the coronary sinus, or directly to the superior vena cava. In about 10 to 15 percent the site of connection is below the diaphragm. The anomalous trunk then connects into the portal vein or one of its tributaries; the ductus venosus; or, rarely, to the hepatic or other abdominal veins.

PATHOPHYSIOLOGY. The physiological consequences and, accordingly, the clinical picture depend on the size of the interatrial communication and the magnitude of the pulmonary vascular resistance. When the interatrial communication is small, systemic blood flow is severely limited with right-sided heart failure. Obstruction to pulmonary venous return and pulmonary venous hypertension are invariably present in patients with infradiaphragmatic anomalous pulmonary venous connection.

NATURAL HISTORY. Most patients with total anomalous pulmonary venous connection have symptoms during the first year of life, and 80 percent die before 1 year of age if not treated. The presence of obstruction in the pulmonary venous pathway or at the atrial septum leads to earlier presentation. When the obstruction is severe, neonatal presentation with severe cyanosis and cardiovascular collapse may occur. This is incompatible with survival without urgent surgical intervention.

CLINICAL FEATURES. Symptomatic infants with total anomalous pulmonary venous connection present with signs of heart failure and/or cyanosis. Infants with pulmonary venous obstruction present with the early onset of severe dyspnea, pulmonary edema, cyanosis, and right-sided heart failure. When unobstructed, cyanosis may be minimal and go undetected. On auscultation there is usually a fixed, widely split second heart sound with an accentuated pulmonic component.

LABORATORY INVESTIGATIONS

ECG. This usually shows right axis deviation and right atrial and right ventricular hypertrophy.

CHEST RADIOGRAPHY. In the unrepaired patient, this usually shows cardiomegaly with increased pulmonary blood flow. The right atrium and ventricle are dilated and hypertrophied, and the pulmonary artery segment is enlarged. The so-called "figure-of-8" or "snowman" heart is due to enlargement of the heart and the presence of a dilated right superior vena cava, innominate vein, and left vertical vein.

ECHOCARDIOGRAPHY (Fig. 61-22). This usually shows marked enlargement of the right ventricle and a small left atrium. Demonstrating the entire pathway of pulmonary venous drainage is usually possible, and cardiac catheterization (which may be hazardous) is almost never performed now. An echo-free space representing the pulmonary venous confluence can usually be seen behind the left atrium. The drainage of all four pulmonary veins and their connections must be identified.

MRI. Although not often used, especially in infants, MRI may be helpful to delineate the site of connections of total anomalous pulmonary venous return, when there are multiple mixed sites, in older children, and to detect stenosis in postoperative patients.

INDICATIONS FOR INTERVENTION. Medical therapy, other than mechanical ventilation, has a limited role in the symptomatic infant, and corrective surgery should be performed as soon as possible. In asymptomatic children without pulmonary hypertension, surgery can be deferred to 3 to 6 months of age.

INTERVENTIONAL OPTIONS AND OUTCOMES. Occasionally an urgent balloon atrial septostomy is required to increase systemic blood flow before surgery. Otherwise, interventional catheterization is restricted to attempts at relieving postoperative pulmonary venous stenosis, although this is often unrewarding. Historically, surgical repair of restenosis was also disappointing. However, the sutureless

technique, whereby the pulmonary veins are opened widely into the retroatrial space, has markedly improved the results of such surgery. Adult patients have almost always had surgical repair in childhood. As a rule, they function normally and are not too prone to arrhythmias or other problems. They are seen as low- to moderate-risk adults.

FOLLOW-UP. Early follow-up should be frequent and aimed at early detection of stenosis of the pulmonary veins or the surgical anastomosis. If not present within the first year, stenosis is rare, but annual follow-up during childhood is required.

TRANSPOSITION COMPLEXES

The key anatomical feature that characterizes this group of diagnoses is ventriculoarterial discordance. This is most commonly seen in the context of AV concordance, also known as *complete transposition* or *D-TGA*. The second condition that is discussed in this section is the combination of ventriculoarterial discordance with AV discordance, commonly referred to as *congenitally corrected TGA* or *L-TGA*. More complicated arrangements are not considered here.

COMPLETE TRANSPOSITION OF THE GREAT ARTERIES

DEFINITION AND NATURAL HISTORY. This is a common and potentially lethal form of heart disease in newborns and infants. The malformation consists of the origin of the aorta from the morphological right ventricle and that of the pulmonary artery from the morphological left ventricle. Consequently, the pulmonary and systemic circulations are connected in parallel rather than the normal in-series connection. In one circuit, systemic venous blood passes to the right atrium, the right ventricle, and then to the aorta. In the other, pulmonary venous blood passes through the left atrium and ventricle to the pulmonary artery. This situation is incompatible with life unless mixing of the two circuits occurs.

Approximately two thirds of patients have no major associated abnormalities ("simple" transposition), and one third have associated abnormalities ("complex" transposition). The most common associated abnormalities are VSD and pulmonary/subpulmonary stenosis. It is increasingly being diagnosed in utero. Without treatment, about 30 percent of these infants die within the first week of life, and 90 percent die within the first year.

MORPHOLOGY. Some communication between the two circulations must exist after birth to sustain life; otherwise, unoxygenated systemic venous blood is directed inappropriately to the systemic circulation and oxygenated pulmonary venous blood is directed to the pulmonary circulation. Almost all patients have an interatrial communication, blood flow across which governs the amount of desaturation. Two thirds have a PDA, and about one third have an associated VSD.

PATHOPHYSIOLOGY. The degree of tissue hypoxia, the nature of the associated cardiovascular anomalies, and the anatomical and functional status of the pulmonary vascular bed determine the clinical course. The anatomical arrangement results in two separate and parallel circulations. The systemic arterial oxygen saturation is governed by the amount of blood exchanged between the two circulations. Infants with D-TGA are particularly susceptible to the early development of pulmonary vascular obstructive disease even in the absence of a PDA and with an intact ventricular septum.

CLINICAL FEATURES

Pediatric. Average birth weight and size of infants born with complete transposition of the great arteries are greater than normal. The usual clinical manifestations are dyspnea and cyanosis from birth, progressive hypoxemia, and congestive heart failure. The most severe cyanosis and hypoxemia are observed in infants who have only a small patent

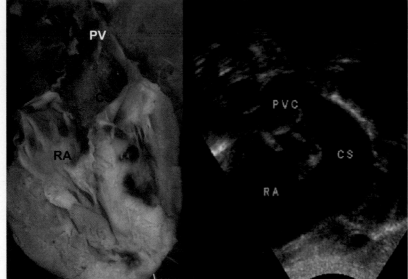

A

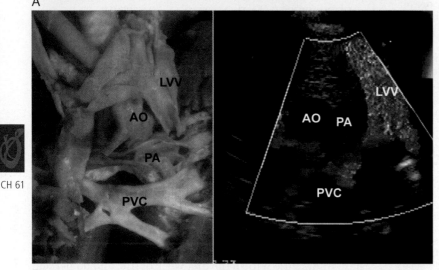

B

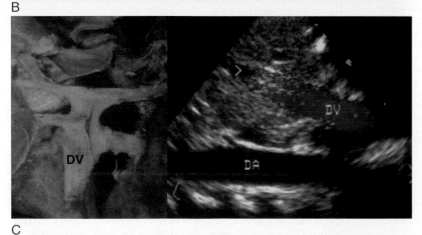

C

FIGURE 61–22 **A,** Subcostal view demonstrating total anomalous pulmonary drainage to the coronary sinus. Note the dilated coronary sinus in both images. The echocardiogram also demonstrates an associated confluence that connects to the coronary sinus. **B,** Suprasternal view demonstrating total anomalous pulmonary venous drainage to a left vertical vein. Note the direction of flow in the vertical vein that differentiates it from a left superior vena cava. **C,** Total anomalous pulmonary venous drainage below the diaphragm. The specimen shows the pulmonary veins as they enter the confluence, whereas the echocardiogram demonstrates the descending veins as they enter the liver. Note the direction of flow is away from the heart. AO = aorta; CS = coronary sinus; DA = descending aorta; DV = descending vein; LVV = left vertical vein; PA = pulmonary artery; PV = pulmonary vein; PVC = pulmonary venous confluence; RA = right atrium.

foramen ovale or ductus arteriosus and an intact ventricular septum, or in those infants with relatively reduced pulmonary blood flow because of left ventricular outflow tract obstruction. With a large PDA or large VSD, cyanosis can be minimal, and heart failure is usually the dominant problem after the first few weeks of life. Cardiac murmurs are of little diagnostic significance.

The 2D echocardiogram should establish the complete diagnosis including the coronary artery pattern. Prenatal detection is possible and favorably modifies neonatal morbidity and mortality. Ultrasound imaging has become a standard procedure to guide catheter placement and manipulation during balloon atrial septostomy and to assess the anatomical adequacy of the septostomy.

MANAGEMENT OPTIONS. Dilation of the duct by prostaglandin E_1 in the early neonatal period improves the arterial saturation by enhancing mixing. A frequent misconception is that significant mixing occurs at the ductal level. This is incorrect; the effect of prostaglandin is to increase pulmonary blood flow, and by so doing to increase left atrial pressure and increase mixing at the atrial level. This is usually as a prelude to the creation or enlargement of an interatrial communication by a balloon or blade atrial septostomy. Surgical atrial septectomy is seldom required now.

Surgery. Although balloon atrial septostomy is often life saving, it is palliative before "corrective" surgery. Atrial redirection procedures were developed in the 1950s and 1960s but were replaced by the arterial switch operation, which became widely adopted in the 1980s.[114]

Atrial Switch (Fig. 61-23). The most common surgical procedure in patients who are currently adults is the atrial switch operation. Patients will have had either a Mustard or a Senning procedure. Blood is redirected at the atrial level using a baffle made of Dacron or pericardium (Mustard operation) or atrial flaps (Senning operation), achieving physiological correction. Systemic venous return is diverted through the mitral valve into the subpulmonary left ventricle, and the pulmonary venous return is rerouted through the tricuspid valve into the subaortic right ventricle. By virtue of this repair, the morphological right ventricle is left to support the systemic circulation.

Palliative Atrial Switch. Uncommonly, in patients with a large VSD and established pulmonary vascular disease, a palliative atrial switch operation is done to improve oxygenation. The VSD is left open or enlarged at the time of atrial baffle surgery. These patients resemble patients with Eisenmenger VSDs and should be managed as such.

Arterial Switch Operation (Fig. 61-24). In this operation the arterial trunks are transected and reanastomosed to the contralateral root. If present, a VSD is closed. The coronary arteries must be transposed to the neoaorta. This is the most challenging part of the procedure and accounts for most of the mortality. Nonetheless, this rate has fallen to less than 2 percent in most large centers.[114,115] The major advantages of the arterial switch procedure, when compared with the atrial switch procedure, are restoration of the left ventricle as the systemic pump and the potential for long-term maintenance of sinus rhythm.

Follow-up studies after the arterial switch operation have demonstrated good left ventricular function and normal exercise capacity.[115,116] Potential sequelae of the operation include coronary occlusion; supravalvular pulmonary stenosis (which may be treated by either reoperation or balloon angioplasty); supravalvular aortic stenosis; and neoaortic regurgitation, usually mild.[117-119] Long-term patency and growth of the coronary arteries appear satisfactory.

Rastelli Procedure. Infants with TGA plus a VSD and left ventricular outflow tract obstruction may require an early systemic-to-pulmonary artery anastomosis when a pronounced diminution in pulmonary blood flow exists. A later corrective procedure for these patients bypasses the left ventricular outflow obstruction with an extracardiac prosthetic conduit between the right ventricle and the distal end of a divided pulmonary artery and uses an intracardiac ventricular baffle to tunnel the left ventricle to the aorta.

MANAGEMENT OUTCOMES

Atrial Switch. After atrial baffle surgery, most patients who reach adulthood are in NYHA Classes I and II, but abnormalities of ventricular filling, due to the abnormal atrial pathways, may be of more direct importance to functional capacity than right ventricular performance issues in many. Some present with symptoms of congestive heart failure (2 to 15 percent). Echocardiographic evidence of moderate or severe systemic right ventricular dysfunction is present in up to 40 percent of patients. Relative right ventricular ischemia (supply-demand mismatch) is thought to perhaps play a role in systemic right ventricular dysfunction.[120] More than mild systemic tricuspid regurgitation is present in 10 to 40 percent, both reflecting and exacerbating right ventricular dysfunction. Palpitations and near-syncope/syncope from rhythm disturbances are fairly common. Atrial flutter occurs in 20 percent of patients by 20 years of age, and sinus node dysfunction is seen in half of the patients by that time. These rhythm disturbances are a consequence of direct and indirect atrial and sinus node damage at the time of atrial baffle surgery.

A shortened life expectancy is the rule, with 70 to 80 percent survival at 20 to 30 years' follow-up. Patients with "complex" TGA in general fare much worse than those with "simple" TGA. Sudden cardiac death occurs in about 5 percent of these patients and may relate to systemic right ventricular dysfunction, the presence of atrial flutter, and pulmonary hypertension. Significant pulmonary vascular disease can develop over time and relates to older age at the time of atrial switch operation, particularly in patients with a substantial VSD, as well as in those with long-standing left-to-right shunts through a baffle leak. Superior vena cava or inferior vena cava baffle obstruction often goes undetected because collateral drainage through the azygos vein prevents systemic venous congestion. Pulmonary venous baffle obstruction causes elevated pulmonary artery pressure, and patients can present with dyspnea and pulmonary venous congestive features.

Physical examination of a patient whose condition is otherwise uncomplicated reveals a right ventricular parasternal lift, a normal S_1, a single S_2 (P_2 is not heard because of its posterior location), a pansystolic murmur from tricuspid regurgitation if present (best heard at the left lower sternal border, but not increasing with inspiration), and a right-sided S_3 when severe systemic ventricular dysfunction is present.

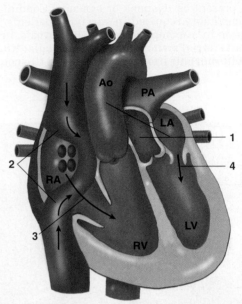

FIGURE 61–23 Diagrammatic representation of atrial switch surgery (Mustard/Senning procedure). Superior vena cava (SVC) and inferior vena cava (IVC) blood is redirected into the morphological left ventricle (LV), which pumps blood into the pulmonary artery (PA), whereas the pulmonary venous blood flow is rerouted to the morphological right ventricle (RV), which empties into the aorta (Ao). RA = right atrium; LA = left atrium; 1 = transposition of the great arteries; 2 = atrial baffles; 3 = pulmonary vein blood flow through tricuspid valve to RV; 4 = IVC and SVC blood flow through mitral valve to LV. *(From Mullins CE, Mayer DC: Congenital Heart Disease: A Diagrammatic Atlas. New York, Wiley-Liss, 1988.)*

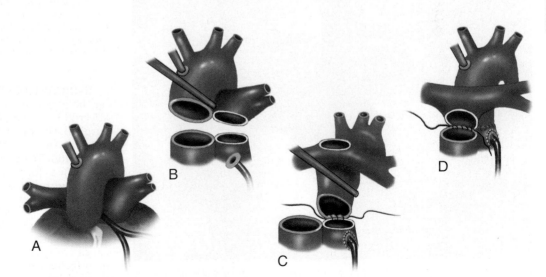

FIGURE 61–24 Complete transposition of the great arteries, corrected by a modified arterial switch operation **(A)**. The aorta and pulmonary artery are transected, and the orifices of the coronary arteries are excised with a rim of adjacent aortic wall **(B)**. The aorta is brought under the bifurcation of the pulmonary artery, and the pulmonary artery and the aorta are anastomosed without necessitating graft interposition. The coronary arteries are transferred to the pulmonary artery **(C)**. The mobilized pulmonary artery is directly anastomosed to the proximal aortic stump **(D)**. *(A to D, From Stark J, deLaval M: Surgery for Congenital Heart Defects. New York, Grune & Stratton, 1983, p 379.)*

Arterial Switch. Data on clinical presentation in adults who have undergone the arterial switch procedure are lacking because most patients have not yet reached adulthood. Clinical arrhythmia promises to be less of a problem in this group of patients.[117] Concerns about the development of supra-neopulmonary artery stenosis, ostial coronary artery disease, and progressive neoaortic valve regurgitation remain to be addressed over the long term. Cardiac examination in uncomplicated patients is normal.

Rastelli. Progressive right ventricular-to-pulmonary artery conduit obstruction can cause exercise intolerance or right ventricular angina. Left ventricular tunnel obstruction can present as dyspnea or syncope. Conduit replacement is inevitably required in surviving patients. Physical examination in uncomplicated patients reveals, in contrast to those after atrial switch, no right ventricular lift, an ejection systolic murmur from the conduit, and two components to the S_2.

LABORATORY INVESTIGATIONS

ECG. Sinus bradycardia or junctional rhythm (without a right atrial overload pattern) with evidence of marked right ventricular hypertrophy is characteristically present in patients after the atrial switch procedure. The ECG is typically normal in patients after the arterial switch procedure. The ECG typically shows right bundle branch block after a Rastelli procedure.

CHEST RADIOGRAPHY. On the posteroanterior film, a narrow vascular pedicle with an oblong cardiac silhouette ("egg on side") is typically seen in patients after the atrial switch procedure. On the lateral view, the anterior aorta is seen to fill the retrosternal space. For the arterial switch, normal mediastinal borders are present despite the Lecompte maneuver. After the Rastelli procedure, the chest radiograph is normal unless the conduit becomes calcified or a nonhomograft prosthesis is employed.

ECHOCARDIOGRAPHY. After the atrial switch procedure, parallel great arteries are the hallmark of TGA (Fig. 61-25). They are best visualized from a parasternal long-axis view (running side by side) or from a parasternal short-axis view (seen *en face*, with the aorta anterior and rightward). Qualitative assessment of systemic right ventricular function, the degree of tricuspid regurgitation, and the presence or absence of subpulmonary left ventricular obstruction (dynamic or fixed) is possible. Assessment of baffle leak or obstruction (Fig. 61-26) is best done using color and Doppler flow imaging. Normal baffle flow should be phasic in nature and vary with respiration, with a peak velocity less than 1 meter per second. After arterial switch, neoaortic valve regurgitation, supra-neopulmonary valve stenosis, and segmental wall motion abnormality from ischemia due to coronary ostial stenosis should be sought. In patients who have undergone the Rastelli operation, left ventricular-to-aorta tunnel obstruction, as well as right ventricular-to-pulmonary artery conduit degeneration (stenosis/regurgitation) must be sought.

MRI. The major role of MRI in patients with atrial switch is to evaluate the baffles and systemic right ventricular volume and ejection fraction. As a rule, MRI reports better right ventricular size and function than does echo. For patients who are claustrophobic or have a pacemaker, a computed tomographic angiogram—preferably at a pulse rate of 70 or less—will serve as a substitute. MRI can evaluate issues in arterial switch and Rastelli patients as well.

CARDIAC CATHETERIZATION. Diagnostic cardiac catheterization may be required for assessing the presence or severity of systemic/pulmonary baffle obstruction, baffle leak, and pulmonary hypertension; coronary ostial stenosis; or tunnel or conduit obstruction when not diagnosed by noninvasive means.

INDICATIONS FOR REINTERVENTION. After the *atrial switch procedure,* severe symptomatic right ventricular dysfunction may warrant surgical treatment in the form of a *two-stage arterial switch* procedure[121] or cardiac transplantation. Tricuspid valve replacement is rarely performed for severe systemic (tricuspid) AV valve regurgitation if due to a flail leaflet or cusp perforation providing right ventricular function is adequate. A baffle leak resulting in a significant left-to-right shunt (>1.5/1), any right-to-left shunt, or attributable symptoms requires surgical or transcatheter closure. Superior vena cava or inferior vena cava pathway obstruction may require intervention. Superior vena cava stenosis is usually benign, whereas inferior vena cava stenosis may have greater hemodynamic consequences, depending on the adequacy of alternative routes of venous return, usually via the azygos vein to the superior vena cava. Balloon

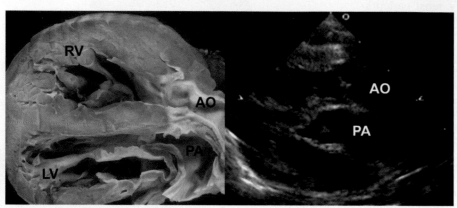

FIGURE 61–25 Parasternal long-axis view in transposition of the great arteries. Note the parallel nature of the aorta and pulmonary artery. AO = aorta; LV = left ventricle; PA = pulmonary artery; RV = right ventricle.

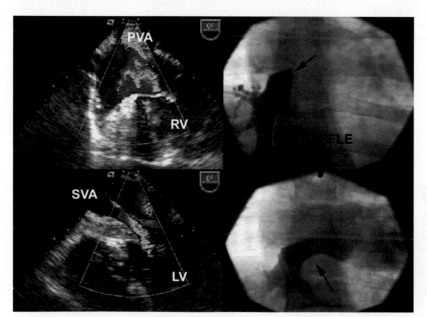

FIGURE 61–26 Montage of post-Mustard cases. The angiogram on the right upper panel shows complete obstruction of the inferior limb of the systemic venous baffle, whereas the lower right panel is the same case after stenting. The upper left image is a transesophageal echocardiogram showing the pulmonary venous baffle with some mild flow acceleration in its midpoint. The lower left panel shows the systemic venous baffle at its left ventricular end. IVC = inferior vena cava; LV = left ventricle; PVA = pulmonary venous atrium; RV = right ventricle; SVA = systemic venous atrium.

dilation of superior vena cava or inferior vena cava stenosis is an option in expert hands. Stenting usually relieves the stenosis completely.

Pathway obstruction after the Senning operation is usually more amenable to balloon dilation and stenting. Pulmonary venous obstruction, although usually seen early and reoperated on in childhood, may present in adulthood. Symptomatic bradycardia warrants permanent pacemaker implantation, whereas tachyarrhythmias may require catheter ablation, an antitachycardia pacemaker device, or medical therapy. After an atrial switch, transvenous pacing leads must traverse the upper limb of the baffle to enter the morphological left ventricle. Active fixation is required because coarse trabeculation is absent in the morphological left ventricle. Transvenous pacing should be avoided in patients with residual intracardiac communications because paradoxical emboli can occur.

After an *arterial switch procedure*, significant right ventricular outflow tract obstruction at any level (gradient > 50 mm Hg or right-to-left ventricular pressure ratio > 0.6) may require surgical or catheter augmentation of the right ventricular outflow tract.[1] Myocardial ischemia from coronary artery obstruction may require coronary artery bypass grafting, preferably with arterial conduits. Significant neoaortic valve regurgitation may warrant aortic valve replacement.

In patients who have had the *Rastelli procedure*, significant right ventricle–to-pulmonary artery conduit stenosis (>50 mm Hg withdrawal gradient or mean echo gradient) or significant regurgitation necessitates conduit replacement. Subaortic obstruction across the left ventricle–to-aorta tunnel necessitates left ventricle–to-aorta baffle reconstruction. A significant residual VSD (shunt > 1.5/1) may require surgical closure.

Patients with clinical deterioration and a palliative atrial switch should be considered for lung or heart-lung transplantation.

REINTERVENTION OPTIONS

Medical Therapy. The role of afterload reduction with ACE inhibitors to preserve systemic right ventricular function is unknown. In light of the effects of these drugs on dysfunctional systemic left ventricles, it seems logical to assume that similar beneficial effects on systemic right ventricles may occur.[18,19]

Two-Stage Arterial Switch. Patients with symptomatic, severe systemic (right) ventricular dysfunction with or without severe systemic (tricuspid) AV valve regurgitation, following an atrial switch procedure, may require consideration of a conversion procedure to an arterial switch (two-stage arterial switch) or heart transplantation. The two-stage arterial switch, or switch-conversion procedure, consists of banding the pulmonary artery in the first stage to induce subpulmonary left ventricular hypertrophy and to "train" the left ventricle to support systemic pressure. Once left ventricular systolic pressure is more than 75 percent of systemic pressure and the left ventricular mass is considered adequate, in the second stage the atrial baffles and the pulmonary band are taken down, the atrial septum is reconstructed, and the great arteries are switched, leaving the morphological left ventricle as the systemic ventricle. This procedure is still experimental in adults, with little data available to assess its short- and long-term efficacy.

Cardiac Transplantation. Heart transplantation should be considered as an alternative, given its relatively good 5- to 10-year survival.

REPRODUCTIVE ISSUES. Severe systemic ventricular dysfunction or intractable arrhythmias may be a contraindication to pregnancy, and baffle obstruction should, ideally, be relieved before pregnancy. Women who have had an atrial switch usually tolerate pregnancy well, but about 15 percent will develop worsening right ventricular function or tricuspid regurgitation during the pregnancy. In half of these cases the problem does not improve after delivery.[122]

FOLLOW-UP. Regular follow-up by physicians with special expertise in CHD is recommended.

Atrial Switch. Serial follow-up of systemic right ventricular function is warranted. MRI is best, followed by computed tomographic angiography and perhaps by special echocardiography. Asymptomatic baffle obstruction should be sought with echocardiography or MRI. Regular Holter monitoring is recommended to diagnose unacceptable bradyarrhythmias or tachyarrhythmias.

Arterial Switch. Regular follow-up with echocardiography is recommended.

Rastelli. Regular follow-up with echocardiography is warranted given the inevitability of conduit degeneration over time.

CONGENITALLY CORRECTED TRANSPOSITION OF THE GREAT ARTERIES

DEFINITION. The term *congenitally corrected transposition of the great arteries* describes hearts in which there are discordant AV connections in combination with discordant ventriculoarterial connections.

MORPHOLOGY (Fig. 61-27). cc-TGA is a rare condition, accounting for less than 1 percent of all CHD. When there is the usual atrial arrangement, systemic venous blood passes from the right atrium through a mitral valve to a left ventricle and then to the posteriorly located pulmonary artery. Pulmonary venous blood passes from the left atrium through a tricuspid valve to a left-sided right ventricle and then to an anterior, left-sided aorta. The circulation is thus "physiologically" corrected, but the morphological right ventricle supports the systemic circulation. Associated anomalies occur in up to 95 percent of patients and consist of VSD (75 percent), pulmonary or subpulmonary stenosis (75 percent), and left-sided (tricuspid and often "Ebstein-like") valve anomalies (>75 percent).

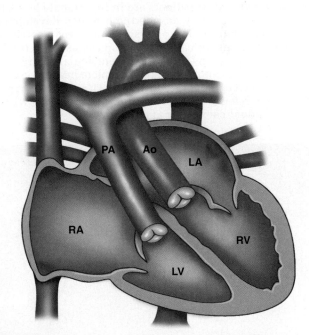

FIGURE 61–27 Diagrammatic representation of congenitally corrected transposition of the great arteries. Ao = aorta; LA = left atrium; LV = left ventricle; PA = pulmonary artery; RA = right atrium; RV = right ventricle; *(From Mullins CE, Mayer DC: Congenital Heart Disease: A Diagrammatic Atlas. New York, Wiley-Liss, 1988.)*

Because of the inherently abnormal conduction system, 5 percent of patients with cc-TGA are born with congenital complete heart block.

PATHOPHYSIOLOGY. Patients with no associated abnormalities ("isolated" cc-TGA) can exceptionally survive until the seventh or eighth decade. Progressive systemic (tricuspid) AV valve regurgitation and systemic (right) ventricular dysfunction tend to occur from the fourth decade onward, whereas atrial tachyarrhythmias are more common from the fifth decade onward.[123] In addition to those born with congenital complete heart block, acquired complete AV block continues to develop at a rate of 2 percent per year, concentrated mainly at the time of cardiac surgery. Patients with associated anomalies (VSD, pulmonary stenosis, left-sided [tricuspid] valve anomaly) often have undergone surgical palliation (systemic-to-pulmonary artery shunt for cyanosis) or repair of the associated anomalies (see Surgical Procedures), but a significant number of patients are naturally balanced by a combination of their VSD and subpulmonary left ventricular outflow tract obstruction. Although cyanosed, they often remain well, with no intervention for many years.[124]

CLINICAL FEATURES

Unoperated. Patients with no associated defects (≤5 percent) can be asymptomatic until late adulthood. Dyspnea, exercise intolerance from developing congestive heart failure, and palpitations from supraventricular arrhythmias most often arise in the fifth or sixth decade. Patients with well-balanced VSD and pulmonary stenosis can present with paradoxical emboli or cyanosis, especially if pulmonary stenosis is severe. Physical examination of a patient whose condition is otherwise uncomplicated reveals a somewhat more medial apex due to the side-by-side orientation of the two ventricles. The A_2 is often palpable in the 2nd left intercostal space due to the anterior location of the aorta. A single S_2 (A_2) is heard, with P_2 often being silent due to its variably posterior location. The murmur of an associated VSD or of left AV valve regurgitation may be heard. The murmur of pulmonary stenosis radiates upward and to the right, given the rightward direction of the main pulmonary artery. If there is complete heart block, cannon "*a* waves" with an S_1 of variable intensity are present.

VSD Patch and Left Ventricular–to–Pulmonary Artery Conduit Repair. Most patients are in functional class I at 5 to 10 years after surgery despite the common development of tricuspid regurgitation and systemic right ventricular dysfunction after surgical repair. Dyspnea, exercise intolerance, and palpitations from supraventricular arrhythmia often occur in the fourth decade. Complete heart block may complicate surgery in an additional 25 percent. Physical examination reflects the basic cardiac malformation with or without residual coexisting anomalies.

LABORATORY INVESTIGATIONS

ECG. An abnormal direction of initial (septal) depolarization from right to left causes reversal of the precordial Q wave pattern (Q waves are often present in the right precordial leads and absent in the left). First-degree AV block occurs in about 50 percent, and complete AV block occurs in up to 25 percent of patients. Atrial arrhythmias may be seen.

CHEST RADIOGRAPHY. Chest radiography characteristically reveals absence of the normal pulmonary artery segment in favor of a smooth convexity of the left supracardiac border produced by the left-sided ascending aorta. The main pulmonary trunk is medially displaced and absent from the cardiac silhouette; the right pulmonary hilum is often prominent and elevated compared with the left, producing a right-sided "waterfall" appearance.

ECHOCARDIOGRAPHY (Fig. 61-28). Echocardiography permits the identification of the basic malformation, as well as any associated anomalies. The morphological left ventricle is characterized by its smooth endocardial surface and is guarded by a bileaflet AV (mitral) valve with no direct septal attachment. The morphological right ventricle is recognized by its apical trabeculation and moderator band and is guarded by a trileaflet apically displaced AV valve (tricuspid valve) with direct attachment to the septum. The AV valves therefore show reversed offsetting, a strong clue to the diagnosis. Ebstein-like malformation of the left (tricuspid) AV valve is defined by excessive (>8 mm/m^2 BSA) apical displacement of the left (tricuspid) AV valve, with or without dysplastic features.

MRI. The major role of MRI in cc-TGA patients is to evaluate the systemic right ventricular volume and ejection fraction. It does so better than echocardiography can at present. For claustrophobic or pacemaker patients, a high-quality radionuclide angiogram with volume estimates serves as a substitute. MRI can evaluate other issues as well including conduit function and AV valve regurgitation.

CARDIAC CATHETERIZATION. This is rarely required for diagnosis but may be indicated before surgical repair to demonstrate the coronary artery anatomy, as well as ventricular end-diastolic and pulmonary artery pressures.

INDICATIONS FOR INTERVENTION AND REINTERVENTION. If moderate or severe systemic (tricuspid, left) AV valve regurgitation develops, valve replacement should be considered. Left AV valve replacement should be performed before systemic right ventricular function deteriorates, namely at an ejection fraction of 45 percent or more.[125] When tricuspid regurgitation is associated with poor systemic (right) ventricular function, the double-switch procedure should perhaps be considered.[126] Patients with end-stage symptomatic heart failure should be referred for cardiac transplantation. The presence of a hemodynamically significant VSD (Qp/Qs > 1.5/1) or residual VSD with significant native or postsurgical (conduit) pulmonary outflow tract stenosis (echo mean or catheter gradient > 50 mm Hg) may require surgical correction. Left AV valve replacement at the time of VSD and pulmonary stenosis surgery should be considered if concomitant left AV valve regurgitation is present. Pacemaker implantation is usual when complete AV block is present. The optimal pacing modality is DDD. Active fixation electrodes are required because of the lack of apical trabeculation in the morphological left ventricle. Transvenous pacing should be avoided if there are intracardiac shunts because paradoxical emboli may occur. Epicardial leads are preferred under these circumstances.

INTERVENTIONAL OPTIONS

Medical Therapy. ACE inhibitor or beta-blocker therapy for patients with systemic ventricular dysfunction may be intuitive, but the role of such agents has not yet been demonstrated.

Conduit Replacement. This is inevitably required in survivors of this type of initial surgery.

CH 61

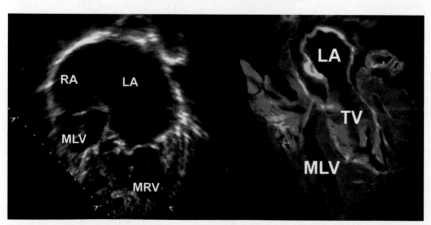

FIGURE 61–28 Four-chamber view in congenitally corrected transposition with dysplasia and displacement of the morphological left-sided tricuspid valve. LA = left atrium; MLV = morphological left ventricle; MRV = morphological right ventricle; RA = right atrium; TV = tricuspid valve.

Tricuspid Valve Replacement. For significant regurgitation, this is preferable to tricuspid valve repair.[125] Valve repair is usually unsuccessful because of the abnormal, often Ebstein-like anatomy of the valve.

Double-Switch Procedure. This procedure has been successfully performed in children. It should be considered for patients with severe tricuspid regurgitation and systemic ventricular dysfunction.[126] Its purpose is to relocate the left ventricle into the systemic circulation and the right ventricle into the pulmonary circulation, achieving physiological correction. An atrial switch procedure (Mustard or Senning), together with either an arterial switch procedure (when pulmonary stenosis is not present) or a Rastelli-type repair, the so-called Ilbawi procedure[127] (left ventricle tunneled to aorta and right ventricle–to–pulmonary artery valved conduit when VSD and pulmonary stenosis are present), can be performed after adequate left ventricular retraining, leaving the regurgitant tricuspid valve and failing right ventricle on the pulmonary side.

Cardiac Transplantation. Patients with deteriorating systemic (right) ventricular function should be treated aggressively with medical therapy but may need to be considered for transplantation.

INTERVENTIONAL OUTCOMES. After conduit repair and VSD patching, the median survival of patients reaching adulthood is 40 years. The usual causes of death are sudden (presumed arrhythmic) or, more commonly, progressive systemic right ventricular dysfunction with systemic (tricuspid) AV valve regurgitation. The major predictor of poor outcome is the presence of left AV (tricuspid) valve regurgitation. Reoperation is common (15 to 25 percent), with left AV valve replacement usually being the primary reason. Data in adults using the double-switch procedure are lacking, and this procedure should be considered experimental in this patient population.

FOLLOW-UP. All patients should have at least annual cardiology follow-up with an expert in the care of patients with congenital cardiac defects. Regular assessment of systemic (tricuspid) AV valve regurgitation by serial echocardiographic studies and systemic ventricular function by MRI or radionuclide angiography should be done. Holter recording can be useful if paroxysmal atrial arrhythmias or transient complete AV block is suspected.

DOUBLE-OUTLET RIGHT VENTRICLE

DEFINITION. The term *double-outlet right ventricle* describes hearts in which more than 50 percent of each semilunar valve arises from the morphological right ventricle. It may coexist with any form of atrial arrangement or AV connection and is independent of infundibular (conal) anatomy.

MORPHOLOGY (Fig. 61-29). Few morphological descriptors have invoked more discussion and controversy than double-outlet right ventricle. The definition given earlier is flawed but pragmatic.[128] To some extent this anatomical definition is less important than the understanding of the relationship between the great vessels and the VSD and the anatomy of the outlets to the great vessels, both of which are crucial determinants of clinical presentation and management.

CLINICAL FEATURES. Three main categories of double-outlet right ventricle exist: (1) double-outlet right ventricle with a subaortic VSD, (2) double-outlet right ventricle with a subpulmonary VSD, and (3) double-outlet right ventricle with a noncommitted VSD.

When present, the anatomy of the infundibular septum further modifies the hemodynamics. Taking double-outlet right ventricle with a *subaortic VSD* as an example, where the aorta and its semilunar valve is closest to, or overriding, the trabecular septum, anterior deviation of the outlet septum causes subpulmonary stenosis, and the clinical scenario and management algorithm are similar or identical to that of tetralogy of Fallot. Conversely, if the outlet septum is deviated posteriorly, there will be subaortic stenosis, often with a coexisting abnormality of the aortic arch. The presentation and management of this variation are therefore entirely different. If there is no deviation of the outlet septum, and no outlet obstruction, the clinical scenario will be that of a simple VSD. Double-outlet right ventricle with a *subpulmonary VSD* (Taussig-Bing anomaly) can be considered along with TGA. This is because the usual position of the pulmonary artery (posterior and leftward to the aorta) means that the streaming of deoxygenated and oxygenated blood is similar to that of transposition, even though most of the pulmonary valve is connected to the right ventricle. Anterior deviation of the outlet septum causes subaortic stenosis and aortic anomalies, and posterior deviation causes subpulmonary stenosis and limits pulmonary blood flow. It is also important to recognize double-outlet right ventricle with a *noncommitted VSD*. This defines hearts in which the VSD is remote from the outlets. Surgical management may be particularly difficult.

ASSOCIATED LESIONS. More than half of patients with double-outlet right ventricles have associated anomalies of the AV valves. Mitral valve atresia associated with a hypoplastic left ventricle is common. Ebstein anomaly of the tricuspid valve, complete AV septal defect, and overriding or straddling of either AV valve may occur.[129]

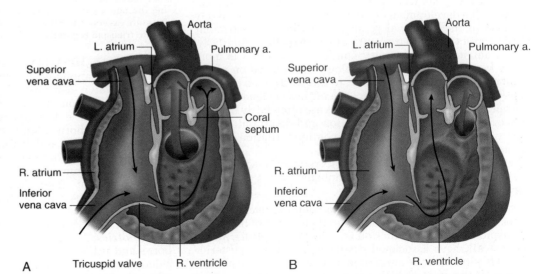

FIGURE 61–29 Double-outlet right ventricle with side-by-side relation of great arteries is illustrated in both panels. **A,** A subaortic ventricular septal defect below the crista supraventricularis favors delivery of left ventricular blood to the aorta. **B,** Subpulmonary location of the ventricular septal defect above the crista favors streaming to the pulmonary trunk. (*A and B, From Castañeda A, Jonas RA, Mayer JE, et al: Cardiac Surgery of the Neonate and Infant. Philadelphia, WB Saunders, 1994, p 446.*)

LABORATORY INVESTIGATIONS. Because of the diversity of underlying anatomies, discussion of the ECG and radiographic features is not included here.

ECHOCARDIOGRAPHY. This is the mainstay of diagnosis. The commitment of the semilunar valves to the ventricles is ascertained. When present, deviation of the outlet septum beneath a semilunar valve likely has implications for downstream development. For example, when there is subaortic stenosis, the echocardiographic examination is incomplete until abnormalities of the aorta and arch have been excluded. Preoperative evaluation must also take into account potential AV valve anomalies and straddling, in particular.

INDICATIONS FOR INTERVENTION. The goals of operative treatment are to establish left ventricle–to-aorta continuity, create adequate right ventricle–to-pulmonary continuity, and repair associated lesions. Palliative surgery is reserved for those in whom biventricular repair is not possible and in those with markedly reduced pulmonary blood flow. In the latter, an aortopulmonary shunt may be placed to temporize before complete correction. For the remainder, complete repair is now performed as a primary procedure in the majority.[130] In double-outlet right ventricle with a subaortic VSD, repair is accomplished by creating an intraventricular baffle that conducts left ventricular blood to the aorta. If there is coexisting subpulmonary stenosis, the repair is similar to that of tetralogy of Fallot. When the VSD is subpulmonary, but without subpulmonary stenosis, repair is accomplished by closure of the VSD and arterial switch. Subpulmonary stenosis is frequently present in a double-outlet right ventricle with a subpulmonary VSD. In these cases the aorta is connected to the left ventricle using an intraventricular baffle, and a right ventricle-to-pulmonary artery conduit is placed to complete the repair (Rastelli procedure). Classic surgical approaches cannot be used when the VSD is remote and uncommitted to either semilunar orifice. Occasionally the VSD can be baffled toward the aorta, but when this is not possible, the right ventricle may be used as the systemic ventricle. This requires a Mustard or Senning atrial redirection procedure, closure of the VSD, and placement of a conduit between the left ventricle and the pulmonary trunk.

INTERVENTIONAL OPTIONS AND OUTCOMES. The late follow-up of the surgical procedures described earlier (e.g., tetralogy of Fallot repair, arterial switch, Rastelli) tends to be less satisfactory when there is a double-outlet right ventricle than when performed for more classic indications.[130] The development of subaortic stenosis is more likely because of the abnormal geometry of the left ventricular outflow tract that often results after correction. Similarly, right ventricle–to-pulmonary conduit obstruction is more likely because of the spatial difficulties imposed on placement of the conduit, with respect to the position on the right ventricle and the sternum. Because of these considerations, the options for catheter interventions are often fairly limited. However, recurrent arch obstruction and distal pulmonary artery obstruction are amenable to balloon dilation with or without stenting.

FOLLOW-UP. All of these patients require at least annual review by a congenital heart cardiologist.

EBSTEIN ANOMALY

MORPHOLOGY (Fig. 61-30). The common feature in all cases of Ebstein anomaly is apical displacement of the septal tricuspid leaflet in conjunction with leaflet dysplasia. Many, but not all, have associated displacement of the posterior mural leaflet, with the anterior leaflet never being displaced. Although the anterior leaflet is never displaced apically, it may be adherent to the free wall of the right ventricle, causing right ventricular outflow tract obstruction. The displacement of the tricuspid valve results in "atrialization" (functioning as an atrial chamber) of the inflow tract of the

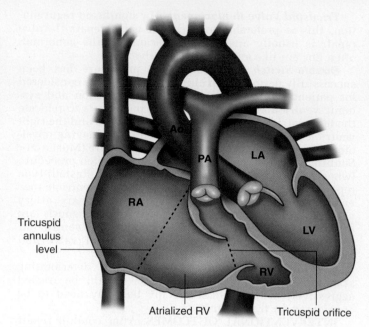

FIGURE 61–30 Diagrammatic representation of Ebstein anomaly. Ao = aorta; LA = left atrium; LV = left ventricle; RA = right atrium; RV = right ventricle; PA = pulmonary artery. *(From Mullins CE, Mayer DC: Congenital Heart Disease: A Diagrammatic Atlas. New York, Wiley-Liss, 1988.)*

right ventricle and consequently produces a variably small, functional right ventricle. Associated anomalies include patent foramen ovale or ASD in approximately 50 percent of patients; accessory conduction pathways in 25 percent (usually right sided); and, occasionally, varying degrees of right ventricular outflow tract obstruction, VSD, aortic coarctation, PDA, or mitral valve disease. Left ventricular abnormalities resembling noncompaction syndrome have also been described.[131]

PATHOPHYSIOLOGY. Varying degrees of tricuspid regurgitation (or exceptionally tricuspid stenosis) result from the abnormal tricuspid leaflet morphology with consequent further right atrial enlargement. Right ventricular volume overload from significant tricuspid regurgitation and infundibular dilation can also be present. Right-to-left shunting through a patent foramen ovale or ASD occurs if the right atrial pressure exceeds the left atrial pressure (which is often the case when severe tricuspid regurgitation is present).

NATURAL HISTORY. The natural history of patients with Ebstein anomaly depends on its severity. When the tricuspid valve deformity and dysfunction are extreme, death in utero from hydrops fetalis is the norm. When the tricuspid valve deformity is severe, symptoms usually develop in newborn infants. Patients with moderate tricuspid valve deformity and dysfunction usually develop symptoms during late adolescence or young adult life. Adults with Ebstein anomaly can occasionally remain asymptomatic throughout their life if the anomaly is mild—exceptional survival to the ninth decade has been reported.

CLINICAL ISSUES

Pediatrics. With severe tricuspid valve deformity, newborns and infants present with failure to thrive and right-sided congestive heart failure. Most other pediatric patients who present after the neonatal period remain asymptomatic until late adolescence or early adult life.

Adults. Most adult patients present with exercise intolerance (exertional dyspnea and fatigue), palpitations of supraventricular origin, or cyanosis from a right-to-left shunt at atrial level. Occasionally, a paradoxical embolus resulting in a transient ischemic attack or stroke can call attention to the diagnosis. Right-sided cardiac failure from severe tricuspid regurgitation and right ventricular dysfunction is possible. Sudden death (presumed to be arrhythmic in nature) is described. Physical examination typically reveals an unimpressive jugular venous pressure because of the large and compliant right atrium and atrialized right ventricle; a widely split S_1 with a loud tricuspid component (the "sail sound"); a widely split S_2 from the right bundle branch block; and a right-sided third heart sound. A pansystolic murmur increasing on inspiration from tricuspid regurgitation is best heard at the lower left sternal border. Cyanosis from a right-to-left shunt at the atrial level may or may not be present.

LABORATORY INVESTIGATIONS

ECG. The ECG presentation of Ebstein anomaly varies widely. Low voltage is typical. Peaked P waves in leads II and V_1 reflect right atrial enlargement. The PR interval is usually prolonged, but a short PR interval and a delta wave from early activation through an accessory pathway can be present. An rsr′ pattern consistent with right ventricular conduction delay is typically seen in lead V_1, and right bundle branch block is common in adults. Atrial flutter and fibrillation are common. The ECG may be normal.

CHEST RADIOGRAPHY. A rightward convexity from an enlarged right atrium and atrialized right ventricle coupled with a leftward convexity from a dilated infundibulum give the heart a "water bottle" appearance on chest radiograph. Cardiomegaly, highly variable in degree, is the rule. The aorta and the pulmonary trunk are inconspicuous. The pulmonary vasculature is usually normal to reduced.

ECHOCARDIOGRAPHY (Fig. 61-31). The diagnosis of Ebstein anomaly is usually made by echocardiography. Apical displacement of the septal leaflet of the tricuspid valve by 8 mm/m^2 or more, combined with an elongated sail-like appearance of the anterior leaflet, confirms the diagnosis. The size of the atrialized portion of the right ventricle (identified between the tricuspid annulus and the ventricular attachment of the tricuspid valve leaflets) and the systolic performance of the functional right ventricle can be estimated. The degree of tricuspid regurgitation (and more rarely stenosis) can be assessed. Associated defects such as ASDs, as well as the presence and direction of shunting, can also be identified.

ANGIOGRAPHY. Cardiac catheterization is required mainly when concomitant coronary artery disease is suspected and to determine if pulmonary artery pressures are elevated. When performed, selective right ventricular angiography shows the extent of tricuspid valve displacement, the size of the functional right ventricle, and configuration of its outflow tract.

MRI. This investigation can offer insights into functional right ventricular volume and function.

INDICATIONS FOR INTERVENTION. Indications for intervention include substantial cyanosis, right-sided heart failure, deteriorating functional capacity (≥Class III NYHA), and perhaps the occurrence of paradoxical emboli. Recurrent supraventricular arrhythmias not controlled by medical or ablation therapy and asymptomatic substantial cardiomegaly (cardiothoracic ratio >65 percent) are relative indications.[2]

INTERVENTIONAL OPTIONS. Tricuspid valve repair when feasible is preferable to tricuspid valve replacement. The feasibility of tricuspid valve repair depends primarily on the experience and skill of the surgeon, as well as the adequacy of the anterior leaflet of the tricuspid valve to form a monocusp valve. Tricuspid valve repair is possible when the edges of the anterior leaflet of the tricuspid valve are not severely tethered down to the myocardium and when the functional right ventricle is of adequate size (>35 percent of the total right ventricle). If the tricus-

pid valve is irreparable, valve replacement will be necessary, usually with a bioprosthetic tricuspid valve.

For "high-risk" patients (those with severe tricuspid regurgitation, an inadequate functional right ventricle [because of size or function], and/or chronic supraventricular arrhythmias), a bidirectional cavopulmonary connection can be added to reduce right ventricular preload if pulmonary artery pressures are low. Occasionally a Fontan operation may be the best option in patients with tricuspid stenosis and/or a hypoplastic right ventricle.[132] A concomitant right atrial or biatrial maze procedure at the time of surgery should be considered in patients with chronic atrial flutter/fibrillation.[133] If an accessory pathway is present, this should be mapped and obliterated either at the time of surgical repair or preoperatively in the catheter laboratory. An atrial communication, if present, should be closed. In occasional patients with a resting oxygen saturation ≥ 90 percent, and exercise intolerance due to worsening hypoxemia, closure of the PFO/ASD may be indicated without addressing the tricuspid valve itself.

With satisfactory valve repair, with or without plication of the atrialized right ventricle or bidirectional cavopulmonary connection, the medium-term prognosis is excellent. Late arrhythmias can occur.[134] With valve replacement, results are less satisfactory. Valve replacement may be necessary because of a failing bioprosthesis or a thrombosed mechanical valve.

REPRODUCTIVE ISSUES. In the absence of maternal cyanosis, right-sided heart failure, or arrhythmias, pregnancy is usually well tolerated.[135]

FOLLOW-UP. All patients with Ebstein anomaly should have regular follow-up, the frequency being dictated by the severity of their disease. Particular attention should be paid to patients with cyanosis, substantial cardiomegaly, poor right ventricular function, and recurrent atrial arrhythmias. Patients with substantial tricuspid regurgitation following tricuspid valve repair need close follow-up, as do patients with recurrent atrial arrhythmias, degenerating bioprostheses, or dysfunctional mechanical valves.

Valvular and Vascular Conditions

(see Chaps. 56, 57, and 62)

Left Ventricular Outflow Tract Lesions (Fig. 61-32)

COARCTATION OF THE AORTA. Aortic arch obstruction may be divided into (1) localized coarctation in close

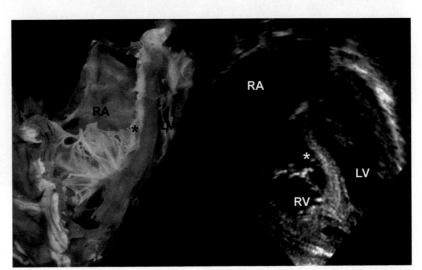

FIGURE 61–31 Apical four-chamber view in Ebstein malformation of the tricuspid valve. Note the significant displacement of the septal tricuspid valve leaflet (asterisk), with associated valve dysplasia. LV = left ventricle; RA = right atrium; RV = right ventricle.

proximity to a PDA or ligamentum, (2) tubular hypoplasia of some part of the aortic arch system, and (3) aortic arch interruption.

LOCALIZED AORTIC COARCTATION

MORPHOLOGY. This lesion consists of a localized shelf in the posterolateral aortic wall opposite the ductus arteriosus. A neonatal presentation is more often associated with a shelf plus transverse aortic arch and isthmic hypoplasia, whereas with a later presentation these areas are larger.[136]

CLINICAL FEATURES. Coarctation occurs two to five times more commonly in males, and there is a high degree of association with gonadal dysgenesis (Turner syndrome) and bicuspid aortic valve. Other common associated anomalies include VSD and mitral stenosis or regurgitation. Additional lesions have an impact on outcome.[137]

NEONATES. Rapid, severe obstruction in infancy is a prominent cause of left ventricular failure and systemic hypoperfusion. Heart failure in this setting is due to a sudden increase in left ventricular wall stress after closure of the arterial duct. Substantial left-to-right shunting across a patent foramen ovale and pulmonary venous hypertension secondary to heart failure cause pulmonary arterial hypertension. Because little or no aortic obstruction existed during fetal life, the collateral circulation in the newborn period is often poorly developed. In these infants, peripheral pulses are characteristically weak throughout the body until left ventricular function is improved with medical management; a significant pressure difference then develops between the arms and the legs, allowing detection of a pulse discrepancy. Cardiac murmurs are nonspecific in infancy and are commonly derived from associated lesions.

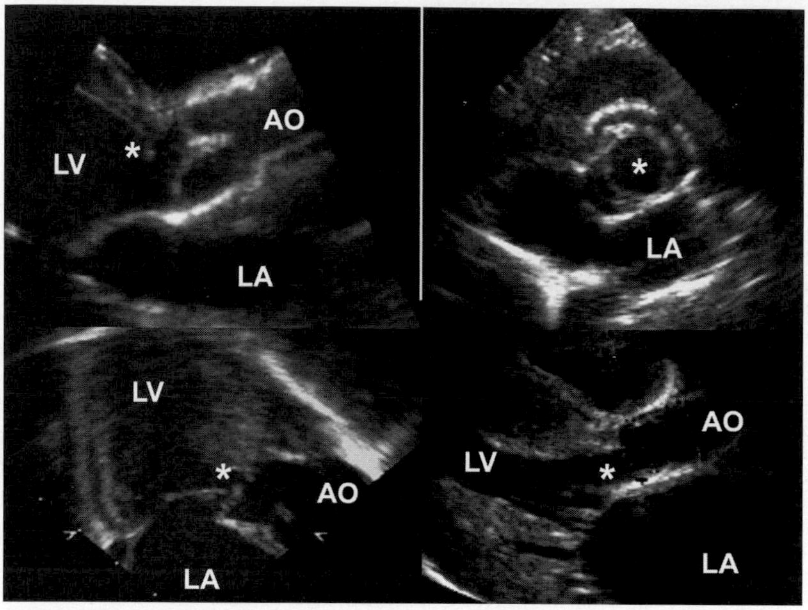

LABORATORY INVESTIGATIONS

ECG. This shows right axis deviation and right ventricular hypertrophy.

CHEST RADIOGRAPHY. This shows generalized cardiomegaly and pulmonary arterial and venous engorgement.

ECHOCARDIOGRAPHY (Fig. 61-33A). This demonstrates the posterior shelf and the degree of associated isthmic and/or transverse arch hypoplasia. Doppler echocardiography is helpful if the ductus is closed or partially restrictive and demonstrates a high-velocity jet during systole and diastole. On the other hand, if the ductus is widely patent, then the usual right-to-left shunting makes the Doppler assessment invalid because the distal pressure then reflects the high pulmonary artery pressure. With associated tubular hypoplasia, Doppler-derived gradients provide higher and less reliable values compared with those obtained by blood pressure or catheterization measurements.[138,139]

MRA. Although this is the gold standard for evaluation of the aortic arch in the older child and adult, it is usually unnecessary in the neonate and infant.[140]

FIGURE 61–32 Montage demonstrating the different types of left ventricular outflow tract obstruction (asterisks). The upper left image shows isolated fibromuscular obstruction; the upper right, stenosis due to a bicuspid aortic valve; the lower left, obstruction because of chordal apparatus from the anterior mitral leaflet; and the lower right, obstruction due to tunnel narrowing at the valve, annular, and subvalve level. AO = aorta; LA = left atrium; LV = left ventricle.

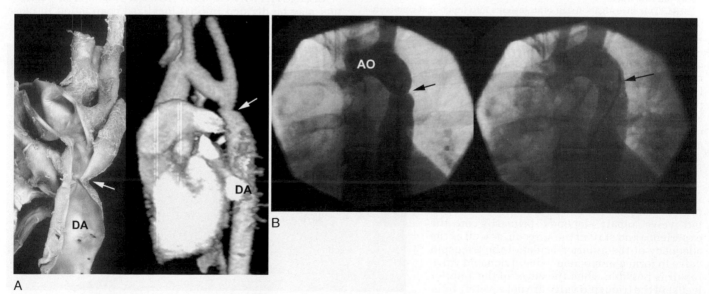

FIGURE 61–33 A, Montage of a coarctation of the aorta. The left image is a specimen that shows the site of the posterior shelf, as outlined by the arrow. The right image is from an MRI and shows the posterior shelf and some associated transverse arch hypoplasia. **B,** Angiogram of a coarctation of the aorta, before and after stenting. AO = aorta; DA = descending aorta.

MANAGEMENT. Management usually involves prostaglandin therapy in an attempt to reopen or maintain patency of a ductus arteriosus. After prostaglandin E_1 infusion to dilate the ductus arteriosus, the pressure difference may be obliterated across the site of coarctation because the fetal flow pattern is reestablished. This has the additional benefit of improving renal perfusion, which in turn helps reverse the frequently associated metabolic acidosis.

INTERVENTION. Intervention in this age group usually involves surgical relief of the obstruction with excision of the area of coarctation and extended end-to-end repair or end-to-side anastomosis with absorbable sutures to allow remodeling of the aorta with time. Subclavian flap aortoplasty, which was employed extensively in the past, is now less popular than the earlier-mentioned procedures. Experts generally believe that balloon dilation does not play a role in management in this age group because there is a lower rate of medium-term success.[141] Early surgery is associated with a lower incidence of long-term hypertension.

INFANTS AND CHILDREN

Presentation. Most infants and children with isolated coarctation are asymptomatic, with the findings of reduced femoral pulses and/or hypertension being detected during routine medical care of the pediatric patient. Heart failure is uncommon because the left ventricle has a chance to become hypertrophied, thus maintaining a normal wall stress. Complaints of headache, cold extremities, and claudication with exercise may be noted in the older child and adolescent.

A midsystolic murmur over the anterior chest, back, and spinous processes is most frequent, becoming continuous if the lumen is sufficiently narrowed to result in a high-velocity jet across the lesion throughout the cardiac cycle. Additional systolic and continuous murmurs over the lateral thoracic wall may reflect increased flow through dilated and tortuous collateral vessels, which are commonly not heard until later childhood.

LABORATORY INVESTIGATIONS

ECG. This reveals left ventricular hypertrophy of various degrees, depending on the height of arterial pressure above the obstruction and the patient's age. Coexisting right ventricular hypertrophy usually implies a complicated lesion.

CHEST RADIOGRAPHY. The characteristic posteroanterior film feature is the so-called figure-3 configuration of the proximal descending thoracic aorta due to both prestenotic and poststenotic dilation. Rib notching (unilateral or bilateral, second to ninth ribs) is present in 50 percent of cases. Rib notching is unilateral if the right or left subclavian arteries arise from the aorta distal to the coarctation. Rib notching is noted as an erosion of the undersurface of a posterior rib, usually at its outer margin, with a sclerotic margin.

ECHOCARDIOGRAPHY. This demonstrates a posterior shelf, a well-expanded isthmus and transverse aortic arch (in most cases), and a high-velocity continuous jet through the coarctation site. Interestingly, a slow upstroke on the abdominal aortic velocity profile is observed when compared with that seen in the ascending aorta.

MRI. This provides detailed information in this age group and may be performed before intervention, particularly if balloon dilation is the treatment of choice. This is the best tool for postintervention imaging and has become routine in many centers.[140]

ANGIOCARDIOGRAPHY. This is reserved for delineating the coarctation at the time of balloon dilation. Primary management in those cases with a well-expanded isthmus and transverse aortic arch invariably involves balloon dilation.

INTERVENTION. Balloon dilation is the current technique in many centers, with surgery being reserved for cases with associated arch hypoplasia. Extended end-to-end anastomosis is the currently favored surgical approach, with patch augmentation being reserved for cases with significant arch hypoplasia.

Paradoxical hypertension of short duration is often noted in the immediate postoperative period, a phenomenon much less common after balloon angioplasty. A resetting of carotid baroreceptors and increased catecholamine secretion appears to be responsible for the initial phase of postoperative systemic hypertension, with a later, second phase of prolonged elevation of systolic and particularly diastolic blood pressure related to activation of the renin-angiotensin system. A necrotizing panarteritis of the small vessels of the gastrointestinal tract of uncertain cause occasionally complicates the course of recovery.

Recoarctation. The risk of recurrent narrowing after repair of coarctation in infancy is 5 to 10 percent. Such narrowing is best screened for with Doppler ultrasonography, with MRI being the gold standard for imaging. Clinical decisions to intervene are usually based on a cuff blood pressure difference between the right arm and leg (for a left aortic arch and normal innominate artery). Although there are no hard and fast rules for absolute blood pressure difference, it has been common practice to reintervene when the blood pressure difference is more than 25 to 30 mm Hg in the presence of systemic hypertension. Although Doppler measurements can detect the presence of a recurrent obstruction, this technique provides an overestimation of the blood pressure–measured gradients due to the phenomenon of pressure recovery.[138] Recoarctation is usually addressed with balloon dilation if the obstruction is relatively localized. In the presence of long-segment narrowings, surgical intervention may be necessary, with the use of patch augmentation of the hypoplastic segment. More recently in the adolescent or adult, balloon-expandable stents have been employed with good success.[142] This has the advantage of avoiding the risk of potential neurological damage in postintervention cases that invariably have poorly developed collaterals.

Long-term Complications. In patients who survive the first 2 years of life, complications of juxtaductal coarctation are uncommon before the second or third decade.[143,144] The chief hazards to patients with coarctation result from severe hypertension and include the development of cerebral aneurysms and hemorrhage, hypertensive encephalopathy, rupture of the aorta, left ventricular failure, and infective endocarditis. Systemic hypertension in the absence of residual coarctation has been observed in resting or exercise-stressed patients postoperatively and appears to be related to the duration of preoperative hypertension.[15,145] These patients also have abnormalities of vascular reactivity, as demonstrated by flow-mediated studies.[146] Increased left ventricular mass is observed, even in the absence of a residual arm-leg gradient, with the suggestion that this may be related to an abnormal genotype.[147] Life-long observation is desirable because of the late onset of hypertension in some postoperative patients.

ADULTS. Although much of the previous material is also relevant to the adult, there are some differences in the issues faced by adult patients. *Complex coarctation* is used to describe coarctation in the presence of other important intracardiac anomalies (e.g., VSD, left ventricular outflow tract obstruction, and mitral stenosis) and is usually detected in infancy. *Simple coarctation* refers to coarctation in the absence of such lesions. It is the most common form detected de novo in adults. Associated abnormalities include bicuspid aortic valve in most cases; intracranial aneurysms (most commonly of the circle of Willis) in up to 10 percent; and acquired intercostal artery aneurysms. One definition of *significant coarctation* requires a gradient greater than 20 mm Hg across the coarctation site at angiography with or without proximal systemic hypertension. A second definition of significant coarctation requires the presence of proximal hypertension in the company of echocardiographic or angiographic evidence of aortic coarctation. If there is an extensive collateral circulation, there may be minimal or no pressure gradient and acquired aortic atresia.

Death in patients who do not undergo repair is usually due to heart failure (usually older than 30 years of age), coronary artery disease, aortic rupture/dissection, concomitant aortic valve disease, infective endarteritis/endocarditis, or cerebral hemorrhage. Of Turner syndrome patients, 35 percent have aortic coarctation.

Clinical Features. Patients can be asymptomatic, or they can present with minimal symptoms of epistaxis, headache, and leg weakness on exertion or more serious symptoms of congestive heart failure, angina, aortic stenosis, aortic dissection, or unexplained intracerebral hemorrhage. Leg claudication (pain) is rare unless there is concomitant abdominal aortic coarctation. A thorough clinical examination reveals upper limb systemic hypertension, as well as a differential systolic blood pressure of at least 10 mm Hg (brachial > popliteal artery pressure). Radial-femoral pulse delay is evident unless significant aortic regurgitation coexists. Auscultation may reveal an inter-scapular systolic murmur emanating from the coarctation site and a widespread crescendo-decrescendo systolic murmur throughout the chest wall from intercostal collateral arteries. Funduscopic examination can reveal "corkscrew" tortuosity of retinal arterioles.

Interventional Outcomes

Surgical. After surgical repair of simple coarctation, the obstruction is usually relieved, with minimal mortality (1 percent). Paraplegia due to spinal cord ischemia is uncommon (0.4 percent) and may occur in patients who do not have well-developed collateral circulation. The prevalence of recoarctation reported in the literature varies widely, from 7 to 60 percent depending on the definition used, the length of follow-up, and the age at surgery. The appropriateness of the surgical repair for a given anatomy is probably the main factor dictating the chance of recoarctation rather than the type of surgical repair itself. True aneurysm formation at the site of coarctation repair is also a well-recognized entity, with a reported incidence between 2 and 27 percent. Aneurysms are particularly common after Dacron patch aortoplasty and usually occur in the native aorta opposite the patch.[148] Late dissection at the repair site is rare, but false aneurysms, usually at the suture line, can occur. Long-term follow-up after surgical correction of coarctation of the aorta still reveals an increased incidence of premature cardiovascular disease and death.

Transcatheter. After balloon dilation (Fig. 61-33B), aortic dissection, restenosis, and aneurysm formation at the site of coarctation all have been documented. These complications may well be reduced if stents are used.[142,149] The significance of aneurysm formation is often unknown, and longer-term data are necessary.[150]

Prior hypertension resolves in up to 50 percent of patients but may recur later in life, especially if the intervention is performed at an older age. In some of these patients this may be essential hypertension, but a hemodynamic basis should be sought and blood pressure control should be attained. Systolic hypertension is also common with exercise and is not a surrogate marker for recoarctation of the aorta.[15] It may be related to residual arch hypoplasia or to increased renin and catecholamine activity from residual functional abnormalities of the precoarctation vessels. The criteria for and significance of exertional systolic hypertension are controversial.[15] Late cerebrovascular events occur, notably in those patients undergoing repair as adults and in those with residual hypertension. Endocarditis or endarteritis can occur at the coarctation site or on intracardiac lesions; and if this occurs at the coarctation site, embolic manifestations are restricted to the legs.

FOLLOW-UP. All patients should have a follow-up examination every 1 to 3 years. Particular attention should be directed toward residual hypertension; heart failure; intracardiac disease such as an associated bicuspid aortic valve, which can become stenotic or regurgitant later in life; or an ascending aortopathy sometimes seen in the presence of bicuspid aortic valve. Complications at the site of repair such as restenosis and aneurysm formation should also be sought using clinical examination, chest radiography, echocardiography, and periodic MRI or CT scanning. Patients with Dacron patch repair should probably undergo an MRI or spiral CT examination every 3 to 5 years or so to detect subclinical aneurysm formation. Hemoptysis from a leaking or ruptured aneurysm is a serious complication requiring immediate investigation and surgery. New or unusual headaches raise the possibility of berry aneurysms. Endocarditis prophylaxis is recommended for any residual turbulent flow.

AORTIC ARCH HYPOPLASIA

MORPHOLOGY. The aortic isthmus, the portion of the aorta between the left subclavian artery and the ductus arteriosus, should be narrowed in the fetus and newborn. The lumen of the aortic isthmus is about two-thirds that of the ascending and descending portions of the aorta until age 6 to 9 months, when the physiological narrowing disappears. Pathological tubular hypoplasia of the aortic arch usually is noted in the aortic isthmus and is most commonly associated with presentation of aortic coarctation in the newborn period. Despite this, in a small group of cases the arch obstruction is due primarily to tubular hypoplasia, usually involving both the aortic isthmus and transverse aortic arch (between the innominate and subclavian artery). These cases usually present early on in life with similar findings to those with a severe coarctation of the aorta. As with the latter, they are duct dependent and may also be associated with other left-sided obstructive lesions.

MANAGEMENT OPTIONS. Provided the other left-sided structures are formed well enough to sustain life, the management involves arch reconstruction with a patch, in a similar fashion to those cases undergoing a Norwood procedure for hypoplastic left heart syndrome. If the left-sided structures are hypoplastic, then palliative surgery with a Norwood procedure or cardiac transplantation are the two treatments of choice.

Complex Coarctation. In some instances the coarctation of the aorta is part of a more complex spectrum of lesions. This can be seen in cases with double-outlet right ventricle, cc-TGA, D-TGA, functionally single ventricle, truncus arteriosus, and AV septal defect. In these cases the decision process involves not only the coarctation repair but the management of the associated lesion(s). The current trend is to complete repair of the intracardiac lesion at the same time as the arch repair.

AORTIC ARCH INTERRUPTION

Aortic arch interruption is a rare and usually lethal anomaly. Unless treated surgically, almost all infants die within the first month of life. Interruptions distal to the left subclavian artery (type A) occur with almost equal frequency to interruptions distal to the left common carotid artery (type B). The right subclavian artery is of variable origin, frequently arising from the descending aortic segment distal to the interruption. The clinical presentation resembles that in tubular hypoplasia or severe coarctation of the aorta with a patent ductus arteriosus.

Virtually all patients have associated intracardiac anomalies. A patent ductus arteriosus almost always connects the main pulmonary artery with the descending aorta. Patients with interrupted aortic arch typically have either a VSD (80 to 90 percent of cases) or an aortico-pulmonary window (10 to 20 percent). Because the ductus arteriosus provides lower-body blood flow, its spontaneous constriction results in profound clinical deterioration. The latter may be temporarily managed by prostaglandin E₁ infusion. Other complex intracardiac malformations such as transposition of the great arteries, aortopulmonary window, and truncus arteriosus are common.

CLINICAL FEATURES. An association is frequent with the genetic 22q11 deletion DiGeorge syndrome. The major clinical problem is severe congestive heart failure as a consequence of volume overload of the left ventricle from an associated intracardiac left-to-right shunt and of pressure overload imposed by systemic hypertension. Absent upper and lower limb pulses, with a palpable superficial temporal pulse is a helpful clue to the diagnosis.

LABORATORY INVESTIGATIONS

ECG. This demonstrates right ventricular hypertrophy with right axis deviation and ST-T wave changes.

Chest X-ray. Cardiomegaly with increased pulmonary markings and pulmonary edema.

Echocardiography. This is the gold standard for the diagnosis of aortic arch interruption and associated lesions. The ventricular septal defect can be characterized, as can the degree of left ventricular outflow tract obstruction.

MANAGEMENT. The perioperative clinical condition of most patients can be improved by intensive medical management with mechanical ventilation, inotropic support, and prostaglandin infusion. There has been increasing success with complete primary repair in infancy as the procedure of choice. In some cases in which the left ventricular outflow tract obstruction is felt to be too severe for standard primary repair, a Norwood procedure is initially performed. This is followed by a complete repair by tunneling the left ventricle through the VSD to the new aorta and placement of a right ventricle to pulmonary artery conduit.

OUTCOME. The medium and long term outcomes are reasonable, but there may be a need for reintervention for left ventricular outflow tract obstruction and recurrent arch obstruction.[151]

SINUS OF VALSALVA ANEURYSM AND FISTULA

MORPHOLOGY. The malformation consists of a separation, or lack of fusion, between the media of the aorta and the annulus fibrosus of the aortic valve. The receiving chamber of a right aortic sinus aortocardiac fistula is usually the right ventricle, but occasionally, when the noncoronary cusp is involved, the fistula drains into the right atrium. From 5 to 15 percent of aneurysms originate in the posterior or noncoronary sinus. The left aortic sinus is seldom involved. Associated anomalies are common and include a VSD, bicuspid aortic valve, and aortic coarctation.

CLINICAL FEATURES. The deficiency in the aortic media appears to be congenital. Reports in infants are exceedingly rare and are infrequent in children because progressive aneurysmal dilation of the weakened area develops but may not be recognized until the third or fourth decade of life, when rupture into a cardiac chamber occurs.[152] A congenital aneurysm of an aortic sinus of Valsalva, particularly the right coronary sinus, is an uncommon anomaly that occurs three times more often in males. An unruptured aneurysm usually does not produce a hemodynamic abnormality. Rarely, myocardial ischemia may be caused by coronary arterial compression. Rupture is often of abrupt onset, causes chest pain, and creates continuous arteriovenous shunting and acute volume loading of both right and left heart chambers, which promptly results in heart failure. An additional complication is infective endocarditis, which may originate either on the edges of the aneurysm or on those areas in the right side of the heart that are traumatized by the jetlike stream of blood flowing through the fistula.

The presence of this anomaly should be suspected in a patient with a combination of chest pain of sudden onset; resting or exertional dyspnea; bounding pulses; and a loud, superficial, continuous murmur accentuated in diastole when the fistula opens into the right ventricle, as well as a thrill along the right or left lower sternal border. The physi-cal findings can be difficult to distinguish from those produced by a coronary arteriovenous fistula.

LABORATORY INVESTIGATIONS

ECG. This may show biventricular hypertrophy, or it may be normal.

CHEST RADIOGRAPHY. This may demonstrate generalized cardiomegaly and usually heart failure.

ECHOCARDIOGRAPHY. Studies based on 2D and pulsed Doppler echocardiography may detect the walls of the aneurysm and disturbed flow within the aneurysm or at the site of perforation. TEE may provide more precise information than the transthoracic approach.[153,154]

CARDIAC CATHETERIZATION. This reveals a left-to-right shunt at the ventricular or, less commonly, the atrial level; the diagnosis may be established definitively by retrograde thoracic aortography.

MANAGEMENT OPTIONS AND OUTCOMES. Preoperative medical management consists of measures to relieve cardiac failure and to treat coexistent arrhythmias or endocarditis, if present. At operation the aneurysm is closed and amputated, and the aortic wall is reunited with the heart, either by direct suture or with a prosthesis. All efforts should be made to preserve the aortic valve in children because patch closure of the defect combined with prosthetic valve replacement greatly increases the risk of operation in small patients. Rarely, device closure of the ruptured aneurysm has been attempted.[155]

VASCULAR RINGS

MORPHOLOGY. The term *vascular ring* is used for those aortic arch or pulmonary artery malformations that exhibit an abnormal relation with the esophagus and trachea, often causing dysphagia and/or respiratory symptoms.

Double Aortic Arch (Fig. 61-34). The most common vascular ring is produced by a double aortic arch in which both the right and left fourth embryonic aortic arches persist. In the most common type of double aortic arch, there is a left ligamentum arteriosum or occasionally a ductus arteriosus. Although both arches may be patent at the time of diagnosis, invariably the left arch distal to the left subclavian artery is atretic and is connected to the descending aorta by a fibrous remnant that completes the ring. In the setting where both arches are patent, the right arch is usually larger than the left. This usually occurs as an isolated lesion, with the respiratory symptoms being caused by tracheal compression and frequently associated laryngomalacia, usually in the neonate and young infant.

Right Aortic Arch. A right aortic arch with a left ductus or ligamentum arteriosum connecting the left pulmonary artery and the upper part of the descending aorta is the next most important vascular ring seen. Although all cases with this lesion have a vascular ring, not all cases are symptomatic. Indeed, those patients who are symptomatic usually have an associated diverticulum of Kommerrell.[156] This is a large outpouching at the distal takeoff of the left subclavian artery from the descending aorta. It is the combination of the diverticulum and the ring that causes the airway compression.

Anomalous Origin of a Right Subclavian Artery. Anomalous origin of a right subclavian artery is one of the most common abnormalities of the aortic arch. Although the aberrant right subclavian artery runs posterior to the esophagus, it does not form a vascular ring unless there is an associated right-sided ductus or ligamentum to complete the ring. During adulthood about 5 percent of patients with an aberrant right subclavian artery (and a left ductus) develop symptoms due to rigidity of the aberrant vessel.

Retroesophageal Descending Aorta. This is a rarer but more problematic type of vascular ring. In this setting there may be either an ascending left and descending right aorta or an ascending right and descending left aorta. The retro-

Congenital Heart Disease

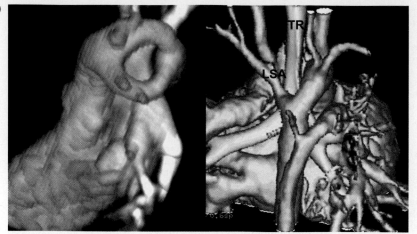

FIGURE 61-34 The left image is a three-dimensional reconstruction of a double aortic arch from an MRI, whereas the right image is from an aberrant left subclavian artery as seen by spiral CT. LSA = left subclavian artery; TR = trachea.

normal branching pattern of pulmonary arteries cannot be identified. In this setting color Doppler permits the identification of the left pulmonary artery as it arises from the right pulmonary artery and runs in a posterior and leftward direction.

MRI AND CT. MRI and CT play a major role in the evaluation of patients with a vascular ring. In fact, MRI has become the gold standard for the evaluation of the aorta and its branches. The only disadvantage for infants is that it often requires general anesthesia to achieve a successful examination. On the other hand, spiral CT is a technique that is fast and provides better definition of the affected airways. This latter technique is particularly valuable for patients with a pulmonary artery sling, where the vascular ring plays a secondary role to the airway abnormalities. The advantages of these techniques are that, unlike echocardiography, they permit a precise assessment of the more posterior vascular structures and their relationships to the esophagus and airways. These techniques are particularly valuable in the more complex forms, such as a retroesophageal descending aorta.

esophageal component of the descending aorta causes the tracheal compression, in conjunction with the left- or right-sided ligamentum.[157]

Pulmonary Artery Sling. This is usually made up of the left pulmonary artery arising from the right pulmonary artery and runs posterior to the trachea but anterior to the esophagus. This is usually seen in isolation and is associated with significant hypoplasia of the bronchial tree, which is the predominant cause of the airway symptoms.

CLINICAL FEATURES. The symptoms produced by vascular rings depend on the tightness of anatomical constriction of the trachea and esophagus and consist principally of respiratory difficulties including stridor, cyanosis (especially with feeding), and dysphagia. Not all patients with a vascular ring are symptomatic, and cases with an aberrant left subclavian artery are frequently detected at the time of evaluation for associated CHD. Although most patients with a true ring and some airway compression present early on in life, others present later on with dysphagia, with others escaping diagnosis forever.

LABORATORY INVESTIGATIONS

ECG. This appears normal unless associated cardiovascular anomalies are present.

CHEST RADIOGRAPHY. If there is evidence of a right aortic arch in a symptomatic patient, then a vascular ring should be suspected. In some instances there is evidence of some airway narrowing. The barium esophagogram is a useful screening procedure. Prominent posterior indentation of the esophagus is observed in many of the common vascular ring arrangements, although the pulmonary artery vascular sling produces an anterior indentation.

ECHOCARDIOGRAPHY. Echocardiography is a sensitive tool for evaluating the laterality of the aortic arch including a detailed assessment of the associated brachiocephalic vessels. In general if there is normal branching of the innominate artery, to the right for a left aortic arch and to the left for a right, along with the correct "sidedness" of the descending aorta, then a vascular ring can be excluded. *Most cases with a double aortic arch* have a dominant right arch, with the descending aorta appearing to dip posteriorly as it runs behind the esophagus. A patent ductus or ligamentum can usually be identified by echocardiography. When both arches are patent, a frontal plane sweep from inferior to superior demonstrates both patent arches, as well as their brachiocephalic vessels. *A right aortic arch with an aberrant left subclavian artery* is suspected when it is not possible to identify normal branching of the left-sided innominate artery. *A retroesophageal descending aorta* should be suspected when the ascending aorta and its brachiocephalic arteries are readily identified but there is difficulty in identifying the descending aorta as it traverses behind the esophagus. *A left pulmonary artery sling* is suspected when the

MANAGEMENT OPTIONS AND OUTCOMES. The severity of symptoms and the anatomy of the malformation are the most important factors in determining treatment. Patients, particularly infants, with respiratory obstruction require prompt surgical intervention. A left thoracotomy is the surgical approach in most patients with a vascular ring. For the most common vascular rings, such as a double aortic arch or aberrant left subclavian artery, the combination of a chest radiograph, barium swallow, and echocardiogram is all that is necessary before surgical intervention.

Operative repair of the double aortic arch requires division of the minor arch (usually the left) and the ligamentum. Patients with a right aortic arch and a left ductus or ligamentum arteriosum require division of the ductus or ligamentum and/or ligation and division of the left subclavian artery, which is the posterior component of the ring. Video-assisted thoracoscopy holds promise as an alternative to open thoracotomy for management.[158] In patients with a pulmonary artery vascular sling, operation consists of detachment of the left pulmonary artery at its origin and anastomosis to the main pulmonary artery directly or by way of a conduit with its proximal end brought anterior to the trachea. The addition of tracheal narrowing that requires surgical intervention adds to the mortality in this group of patients, as does the association with intracardiac malformations.[159]

CONGENITAL AORTIC VALVE STENOSIS

GENERAL CONSIDERATIONS. We deal here only with this condition in newborns and children because the adult presentation is dealt with in Chapter 52. Congenital aortic valve stenosis is a relatively common anomaly. Congenital aortic valve stenosis occurs much more frequently in males, with a gender ratio of 4:1. Associated cardiovascular anomalies have been noted in up to 20 percent of patients. PDA and coarctation of the aorta occur most frequently with aortic valve stenosis; all three of these lesions may coexist.

MORPHOLOGY. The basic malformation consists of thickening of valve tissue with various degrees of commissural fusion. The valve is most commonly bicuspid. In some patients the stenotic aortic valve is unicuspid and dome shaped, with no or one lateral attachment to the aorta at the level of the orifice. In infants and young children with severe aortic stenosis, the aortic valve annulus may be relatively underdeveloped. This lesion forms a continuum with the hypoplastic left heart syndrome and the aortic atresia and hypoplasia complexes. Secondary calcification of the valve is rare in childhood. When the obstruction is hemodynamically significant, concentric hypertrophy of the left ventricular wall and dilation of the ascending aorta occur.

NEONATAL PRESENTATION. The newborn presentation is often similar to that seen with other obstructive left-sided lesions, such as coarctation of the aorta or interrupted aortic arch. They present with heart failure and depend on ductal patency for survival. An association with varying degrees of left ventricular hypoplasia, mitral valve abnormalities, and endocardial fibroelastosis occurs frequently. With the advent of good prenatal screening, many are detected before birth, with deliveries being performed in a high-risk obstetrical unit attached to a congenital heart facility. The decision process around single versus biventricular repair is a complex one and beyond the scope of this chapter. Suffice it to say, formulas have been derived to assist the pediatric cardiologist in the decision process.[160]

Clinical Findings. Newborns generally have weak pulses throughout, signs of heart failure, and often little in the way of murmurs, despite the severe left ventricular outflow tract obstruction.

LABORATORY INVESTIGATIONS

ECG. An electrocardiogram usually shows right ventricular dominance with evidence of diffuse ST wave changes due to left ventricular strain.

CHEST RADIOGRAPHY. Chest radiography usually shows cardiomegaly due to a large right ventricle, and varying degrees of pulmonary edema.

ECHOCARDIOGRAPHY. Echocardiography is currently the diagnostic test of choice. It usually shows a poorly contracting left ventricle with varying degrees of endocardial fibroelastosis and frequently hypoplasia of the left ventricle and aortic root. Doppler assessment of gradients are often unreliable due to poor left ventricular function. The presence of right ventricular hypertension and tricuspid valve regurgitation are common associated findings.

Management. Prostaglandin therapy is instituted in this patient population to maintain the fetal circulation with retrograde ductal flow that permits coronary and cerebral perfusion. The nature of further treatment depends on whether the left ventricle and aortic root are believed to be of a sufficient size to support a biventricular repair. If so, balloon dilation is rapidly becoming the treatment of choice,[161] though surgical intervention is still preferred by some. If the left heart structures are believed to be too small to sustain life, then either cardiac transplantation or a Norwood procedure can be undertaken.[160]

PRESENTATION BEYOND THE NEWBORN PERIOD. The diagnosis is invariably made following the detection of a murmur. Occasionally heart failure ensues, usually in the first 1 to 2 months of life when there is a rapid progression of the obstruction and lack of left ventricular mass to maintain a normal wall stress. Natural history studies performed several years ago demonstrated that more rapid progression of aortic valve stenosis is more likely to happen within the first 2 years of life, following which the rate of progressive obstruction is more uniform.

Clinical Findings. In general the children are asymptomatic, having normal peripheral pulses if the stenosis is less severe and low-volume, slow-rising pulses when it progresses. Exercise fatigue and chest pain are rare complaints and occur only when the stenosis is severe. With severe stenosis there is a systolic thrill in the same area that can also be felt in the suprasternal notch and carotid arteries. Beyond the newborn period there is usually an ejection click at the apex that precedes the murmur. The second heart sound is usually normal in children. An ejection systolic murmur is heard along the left sternal border, with radiation into the right infraclavicular area. Associated aortic regurgitation may be heard.

ECG. Left ventricular hypertrophy with or without strain are the hallmark features.

CHEST RADIOGRAPHY. Overall heart size is normal, or the degree of enlargement is slight in most children with congenital aortic valve stenosis.

ECHOCARDIOGRAPHY. 2D echocardiography provides detailed information about the morphology of the valve, the left ventricular function, and the presence of associated left-sided lesions. Doppler echocardiography can be used to determine the severity of stenosis and the presence or absence of associated aortic regurgitation. Doppler provides peak instantaneous gradients that are higher than the peak-to-peak gradients determined from cardiac catheterization.[162] The importance of this lies in the fact that the natural history studies and clinical decision-making have thus far been based on peak-to-peak catheterization gradients in the infant, child, and adolescent. Valve areas are usually not calculated in this age group because there are no good data to support their use in pediatric patients. Mean gradients as derived from Doppler and catheterization correlate closely, but again, no data support their use in clinical decision-making. Some data convert the Doppler-derived mean gradients to peak to peak, with the addition of the pulse pressure as obtained from blood pressure measurements. Whatever absolute number is chosen to work with, the additional finding of left ventricular hypertrophy on ECG and echocardiography provides supportive data regarding timing for intervention. The pediatric population generally agrees that a peak-to-peak gradient of 60 mm Hg or more probably warrants intervention.

CARDIAC CATHETERIZATION. Cardiac catheterization is now rarely used to establish the site and severity of obstruction to left ventricular outflow. Instead, catheterization is undertaken when therapeutic interventional balloon aortic valvuloplasty is indicated.

Management Options. In this era, balloon dilation has almost completely replaced primary surgical valvotomy in children.

FOLLOW-UP. Follow-up studies indicate that aortic valvotomy is a safe and effective means of palliative treatment with excellent relief of symptoms. Aortic insufficiency can occasionally be progressive and require valve replacement.[163,164] Moreover, after commissurotomy, the valve leaflets remain somewhat deformed, and further degenerative changes including calcification will likely lead to significant stenosis in later years. Thus prosthetic aortic valve replacement is required in approximately 35 percent of patients within 15 to 20 years of the original operation. For those children and adolescents requiring aortic valve replacement, the surgical options include replacement with a mechanical aortic valve, an aortic homograft, or a pulmonary autograft in the aortic position. Accumulating evidence shows that the pulmonary autograft may ultimately be preferable to the aortic homograft. In the pulmonary autograft, called the *Ross procedure,* the patient's pulmonary valve is removed and used to replace the diseased aortic valve, and the right ventricular outflow tract is reconstructed with a pulmonary valve homograft.[164,165] We consider it likely that the Ross procedure may emerge as the approach of choice in the future,[166,165] although caution is necessary when applied to patients with bicuspid aortic valve and aortic regurgitation. This is due to associated aortic root dilation, which is inherent to this lesion and may complicate the long-term reliability of the Ross procedure.[167] This surgical approach can be applied from neonatal through adult life. Neither homografts nor autografts require anticoagulation.

SUBAORTIC STENOSIS

MORPHOLOGY

Discrete Fibromuscular. This lesion consists of a ridge or fibrous ring encircling the left ventricular outflow tract at varying distances from the aortic valve. The subvalvular fibrous process usually extends onto the aortic valve cusps and almost always makes contact with the ventricular aspect of the anterior mitral leaflet at its base. In other cases with fibrous discontinuity between the mitral and aortic valves, it forms more of a tunnel obstruction.

Focal Muscular. Rarely there is no fibrous element, but rather a focal muscular obstruction on the crest of the interventricular septum, which differs from cases with hypertrophic cardiomyopathy.

Hypoplasia of the Left Ventricular Outflow Tract. In some cases, valvular and subvalvular aortic stenoses coexist with hypoplasia of the aortic valve annulus and thickened valve leaflets, producing a tunnel-like narrowing of the left ventricular outflow tract. Additional findings often include a small ascending aorta.

Discrete Subaortic Stenosis and VSD. This combination is frequently encountered in the pediatric age group, with the fibromuscular component often being absent at the initial echocardiographic evaluation. The association should be suspected in VSDs with some associated anterior mala lignment of the aorta and a more acute aortoseptal angle. These hearts frequently develop subpulmonary stenosis. In a different subset of patients with aortic arch interruption and a VSD, there is muscular subaortic stenosis due to posterior deviation of the infundibular septum.

Complex Subaortic Stenosis. Various anatomical lesions other than a discrete ridge may produce subaortic stenosis. Among these are abnormal adherence of the anterior leaflet of the mitral valve to the septum and the presence in the left ventricular outflow tract of accessory endocardial cushion tissue.[168] These are frequently associated with a "cleft in the anterior mitral valve leaflet," which is to be differentiated from that seen in an AV septal defect. These types of obstruction are seen more commonly in those cases with abnormalities of the ventriculoarterial connection in association with a VSD (e.g., double-outlet right ventricle, transposition, VSD).

CLINICAL FEATURES. These types of obstruction are usually identified as secondary lesions in those cases with associated VSDs, with or without abnormalities of the ventriculoarterial connections or aortic arch obstruction. In general the substrate for left ventricular outflow tract obstruction is present, though in some cases actual physiological obstruction is absent. In other cases the patients are referred with a systolic murmur for evaluation. In cases with a gradient across their left ventricular outflow tract, there is an ejection systolic murmur heard along the lower left sternal border with the absence of an ejection click.

LABORATORY INVESTIGATIONS

ECG. In those with associated defects, the ECG reflects the major abnormality rather than the associated left ventricular outflow tract obstruction. With isolated forms of left ventricular outflow tract obstruction, there may be left ventricular hypertrophy when the obstruction is significant.

CHEST RADIOGRAPHY. This is usually unhelpful in these cases.

ECHOCARDIOGRAPHY. Echocardiography is the current standard diagnostic tool in this lesion.[169,170] Not only can it permit an accurate delineation of the mechanisms of obstruction, but it provides detailed data regarding associated lesions. In all forms the parasternal long-axis view is key to providing an accurate diagnosis. The presence of mitral aortic discontinuity, the relationship of a fibromuscular ridge to the aortic valve, the presence of accessory obstructive tissue, and the dimensions of the aortic annulus and root all are well imaged in this view. In addition, color-flow mapping permits the identification of associated aortic valve regurgitation and provides hemodynamic evidence of the site of onset of obstruction. The extension of a fibromuscular ridge onto the anterior mitral leaflet is best appreciated in the apical five-chamber view. This also provides the best site for pulsed or continuous-wave Doppler assessment of the maximum gradient across the left ventricular outflow tract. In the older patient TEE plays an important role in delineating the pathology.

CARDIAC CATHETERIZATION. This technique is no longer of importance in evaluating this lesion. Although balloon dilation has been attempted, it is generally believed that this is a surgical lesion.

MRI. In general, MRI is unnecessary unless there are problems obtaining the needed information by echocardiography.

INTERVENTIONAL OPTIONS. Surgical intervention is indicated either at the time of the repair of the underlying primary lesion or in those cases with discrete obstruction when the obstruction is severe enough to raise concerns.

Discrete Subaortic Stenosis (Fibrous and Muscular). The rate of progression is varied and may be slow.[171] In general the approach to the latter group has been to intervene when there is a mean gradient across the left ventricular outflow tract of greater than 30 mm Hg to avoid future aortic leaflet damage. Surgery involves a fibromectomy, with care to avoid damage to the aortic valve or to create a traumatic VSD. There is a recurrence rate of subaortic stenosis requiring reoperation in up to 20 percent of cases. In some cases the recurrence is in the form of a fibrous ridge, whereas in others there is acquired pathology of the aortic valve in the form of stenosis, as well as regurgitation. Reoperation may involve just repeat resection of a recurrent fibrous ridge, or it may involve surgery for the aortic valve in those cases with significant aortic regurgitation.[172]

Complex Forms of Left Ventricular Outflow Tract Obstruction and an Intact Ventricular Septum. In cases with an intact ventricular septum the indications for intervention are similar to those cases with discrete obstruction. The difference lies in the fact that the surgical approach must be modified according to the underlying pathology. Resection of any fibromuscular component or accessory tissue (provided it is not a primary support mechanism for the mitral valve); a valve-sparing Konno operation; and, in those cases with a hypoplastic aortic annulus, a classic Konno procedure with aortic valve replacement are the potential surgical options.[173]

Left Ventricular Outflow Tract Obstruction and Complex Forms of CHD. In general, surgery to the left ventricular outflow tract is part of the general repair of the lesion and is not dependent on the precise degree of obstruction across this site.

OUTCOMES. Immediate complications related to surgery include complete AV block, creation of a VSD, or mitral regurgitation from intraoperative damage to the mitral valve apparatus. Long-term complications include recurrence of fibromuscular subvalvular left ventricular outflow tract obstruction (up to 20 percent). Clinically important aortic regurgitation is not uncommon (up to 25 percent of patients). In some cases with predominant acquired aortic valve stenosis, balloon dilation has been the treatment of choice.

FOLLOW-UP. Particular attention should be paid to patients with residual or recurrent subaortic stenosis or those with an associated bicuspid aortic valve or important aortic regurgitation because they are most likely to require surgery eventually. Patients with bioprosthetic aortic valves in the aortic position (following the Konno procedure) or the pulmonary position (following the Ross-Konno procedure) need close follow-up. Endocarditis prophylaxis should be used for prosthetic valves or in the presence of any residual lesions.

SUPRAVALVULAR AORTIC STENOSIS

MORPHOLOGY. Three anatomical types of supravalvular aortic stenosis are recognized, although some patients may have findings of more than one type. Most common is the hourglass type, in which marked thickening and disorganization of the aortic media produce a constricting annular ridge at the superior margin of the sinuses of Valsalva. The membranous type is the result of a fibrous or fibromuscular semicircular diaphragm with a small central opening stretched across the lumen of the aorta. Diffuse hypoplasia of the ascending aorta characterizes the third type.

Because the coronary arteries arise proximal to the site of outflow obstruction in supravalvular aortic stenosis, they are subjected to the elevated pressure that exists within the left ventricle. These vessels are often dilated and tortuous, and premature coronary arteriosclerosis has been described. Moreover, if the free edges of some or all of the aortic cusps adhere to the site of supravalvular stenosis, coronary artery inflow may be compromised. The left ventricle may have a "ballerina foot" configuration, which can result in muscular left ventricular outflow tract obstruction, particularly when associated with significant supravalvular obstruction.

CLINICAL FEATURES. The clinical picture of supravalvular obstruction differs in major respects from that observed in the other forms of aortic stenosis. Chief among these differences is the association of supravalvular aortic stenosis with idiopathic infantile hypercalcemia, a disease that occurs in the first years of life and can be associated with deranged vitamin D metabolism.

WILLIAMS SYNDROME. The designation *supravalvular aortic stenosis syndrome, Williams syndrome,* or *Williams-Beuren syndrome* has been applied to the distinctive picture produced by the coexistence of the cardiac features in the setting of a multisystem disorder. Beyond infancy in these patients, a challenge with vitamin D- or calcium-loading tests unmasks abnormalities in the regulation of circulating 25-hydroxyvitamin D. Infants with Williams syndrome often exhibit feeding difficulties, failure to thrive, and gastrointestinal problems in the form of vomiting, constipation, and colic. The entire spectrum of clinical manifestations includes auditory hyperacusis, inguinal hernia, a hoarse voice, and a typical personality that is outgoing and engaging. Other manifestations of this syndrome include intellectual impairment, "elfin facies," narrowing of peripheral systemic and pulmonary arteries, strabismus, and abnormalities of dental development consisting of microdontia, enamel hypoplasia, and malocclusion.

Many medical conditions can complicate the course of Williams syndrome including systemic hypertension, gastrointestinal problems, and urinary tract abnormalities. In an older child or adult, progressive joint limitation and hypertonia may become a problem. Adult patients are usually handicapped by their developmental disabilities.

Williams syndrome was previously considered to be nonfamilial; however, a number of families in which parent-to-child transmission of Williams syndrome has occurred have now been identified. All of these families show a parent and child to be affected with Williams syndrome including one instance of male-to-male transmission. This supports autosomal dominant inheritance as the likely pattern, with most cases of Williams syndrome probably occurring as the result of a new mutation. New information indicates that a genetic defect for supravalvular aortic stenosis is located in the same chromosomal subunit as elastin on chromosome 7q11.23.[174] Elastin is an important component of the arterial wall, but precisely how mutations in elastin genes cause the phenotypes of supravalvular aortic stenosis is not known.

FAMILIAL AUTOSOMAL DOMINANT PRESENTATION. Occasionally the aortic anomaly and peripheral pulmonary arterial stenosis are also found in familial and sporadic forms not associated with the other features of the syndrome.[175] Affected patients have normal intelligence and are normal in facial appearance. Genetic studies suggest that when the anomaly is familial, it is transmitted as autosomal dominant with variable expression. Some family members may have peripheral pulmonary stenosis either as an isolated lesion or in combination with the supravalvular aortic anomaly.

CLINICAL FEATURES. Patients with Williams syndrome are intellectually challenged (Fig. 61-35). The typical appearance is similar to that of the elfin facies observed in the severe form of idiopathic infantile hypercalcemia and is characterized by a high prominent forehead, stellate or lacy iris patterns, epicanthal folds, underdeveloped bridge of the nose and mandible, overhanging upper lip, strabismus, and anomalies of dentition. Recognition of this distinctive appearance, even in infancy, should alert the physician to the possibility of underlying multisystem disease. In addition, a positive family history in a patient with a normal appearance and clinical signs suggesting left ventricular outflow obstruction should lead to the suspicion of either supravalvular aortic stenosis or hypertrophic obstructive cardiomyopathy.

CH 61

Congenital Heart Disease

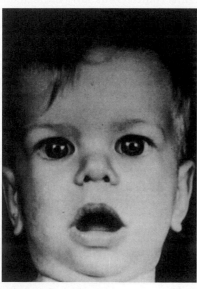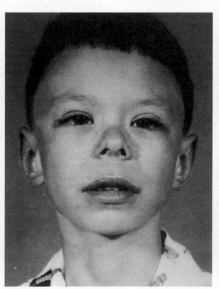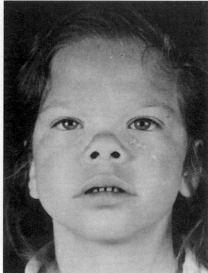

FIGURE 61–35 Typical elfin facies in three patients with supravalvular aortic stenosis. *(From Friedman WF, Kirkpatrick SE: Congenital aortic stenosis. In Adams FH, Emmanouilides GC, Riemenschneider TA, et al [eds]: Moss' Heart Disease in Infants, Children, and Adolescents. 4th ed. Baltimore, Williams & Wilkins, 1989.)*

Studies of the natural history of the principal vascular lesions in these patients—supravalvular aortic stenosis and peripheral pulmonary artery stenosis[176]—indicate that the aortic lesion is usually progressive, with an increase in the intensity of obstruction related often to poor growth of the ascending aorta. In contrast, the patients with pulmonary branch stenosis, whether associated with the aortic lesion or not, tend to show no change or a reduction in right ventricular pressure with time.[177]

With few exceptions, the major *physical findings* resemble those observed in patients with aortic valve stenosis. Among these exceptions are accentuation of aortic valve closure due to elevated pressure in the aorta proximal to the stenosis, an absent ejection click, and the especially prominent transmission of a thrill and murmur into the jugular notch and along the carotid vessels. The narrowing of the peripheral pulmonary arteries may produce a late systolic or continuous murmur heard best in the lung fields and is usually accentuated by inspiration. Another hallmark of supravalvular aortic stenosis is that the systolic pressure in the right arm is usually higher than in the left arm. This pulse disparity may relate to the tendency of a jet stream to adhere to a vessel wall (Coanda effect) and selective streaming of blood into the innominate artery.

LABORATORY INVESTIGATIONS

ECG. This usually reveals left ventricular hypertrophy when obstruction is severe. Biventricular or even right ventricular hypertrophy may be found if there is significant narrowing of peripheral pulmonary arteries.

CHEST RADIOGRAPHY. In contrast to valvular and discrete subvalvular aortic stenosis, poststenotic dilation of the ascending aorta is absent.

ECHOCARDIOGRAPHY. This is a valuable technique for localizing the site of obstruction to the supravalvular area. Most often the sinuses of Valsalva are dilated, and the ascending aorta and arch appear small or of normal size. The diameter of the aortic annulus is always greater than that of the sinotubular junction. Doppler examination determines the location of obstruction but usually overestimates the gradient compared with that obtained at cardiac catheterization. This results from the obstruction being lengthy, and the Doppler gradient is overestimated due to the phenomena of pressure recovery.

ANGIOCARDIOGRAPHY. In most cases this is necessary to define an accurate hemodynamic gradient across the left ventricular outflow tract, as well as to determine the status of the coronary arteries. Usually it also involves an assessment of the branch pulmonary arteries, as well as the brachiocephalic, renal, and mesenteric arteries, all of which can be stenotic. Because of the nature of the anatomical defect, transcatheter balloon angioplasty, with or without stenting, is not an effective treatment option.

INTERVENTIONAL OPTIONS AND OUTCOMES. Surgical intervention for supravalvular aortic stenosis has been successful in most cases with good medium- and long-term results.[178] A variety of surgical procedures may be performed, all of which are tailored to the type of pathology. The use of a Y patch, resection with end-to-end anastomosis, or a Ross procedure are the main techniques employed. Additional lesions including coronary ostial stenosis, aortic valvuloplasty, and subaortic resection may be necessary in some cases.

The cardiac prognosis is good, with some patients requiring further surgery for recurrent supravalvular stenosis.[176,179] As peripheral pulmonary artery stenosis tends to improve with time, there is a reluctance to attempt intervention, either surgical or via balloon angioplasty. Long-term behavioral and intellectual problems persist.[179]

Congenital Mitral Valve Anomalies

CONGENITAL MITRAL STENOSIS

MORPHOLOGY. Anatomical types of mitral stenosis include the parachute deformity of the valve, in which

shortened chordae tendineae converge and insert into a single large papillary muscle; thickened leaflets with shortening and fusion of the chordae tendineae; an anomalous arcade of obstructing papillary muscles; accessory mitral valve tissue; and a supravalvar circumferential ridge or "ring" of connective tissue arising at the base of the atrial aspect of the mitral leaflets. Associated cardiac defects are common including endocardial fibroelastosis, coarctation of the aorta, PDA, and left ventricular outflow tract obstruction. An association between persistence of the left superior vena cava and obstructive left-sided lesions also exists.

CLINICAL FEATURES. In most cases the findings are incidental at the time of evaluation of another left-sided obstructive lesion, such as coarctation of the aorta or aortic valve stenosis. The classic auscultatory findings seen with rheumatic mitral valve stenosis are often absent in the congenital form. Typical findings include a normal S_1, a mid-diastolic murmur with or without some presystolic accentuation, and no opening snap.

LABORATORY INVESTIGATIONS

ECG. In milder forms this is usually normal, or there may be left atrial overload, with or without right ventricular hypertrophy due to associated pulmonary hypertension.

CHEST RADIOGRAPHY. This is normal in milder forms, with evidence of pulmonary edema in those cases with more severe obstruction.

ECHOCARDIOGRAPHY. 2D echocardiography, combined with Doppler studies, usually provides a complete analysis of the anatomy and function of congenital mitral stenosis. The status of the papillary muscles is best appreciated in the precordial short-axis view. If two papillary muscles are present, they are usually closer together than is seen in the normal heart. The precordial long-axis view permits identification of a supravalvular mitral ring, as well as the degree of mobility of the valve leaflets. Color flow Doppler allows identification of the level of the obstruction, as well as the presence of mitral valve regurgitation. Pulsed or continuous-wave Doppler provides an accurate assessment of the mean gradient across the mitral valve. The advantage of the pressure half-time lies in the fact that it is independent of cardiac output, unlike the mean gradient across the mitral valve. Due to more rapid heart rates in children, the pressure half-time is of less value.

INTERVENTIONAL OPTIONS AND OUTCOMES. In asymptomatic cases clinical and echocardiographic follow-up is all that is necessary. The presence of a single papillary muscle in itself does not predict progressive stenosis.[180] If the patient starts to develop pulmonary hypertension or symptoms, surgical intervention is usually indicated. Mitral valve balloon dilation is not as successful as it is in rheumatic mitral valve stenosis.[181] Surgery usually involves removing a supramitral ring if present, splitting papillary muscles and fused chordal apparatus in those cases with more common forms of congenital mitral stenosis. In general, surgical intervention provides temporary relief, with many operated cases requiring valve replacement later in life.[182,183]

CONGENITAL MITRAL REGURGITATION
MORPHOLOGY

Isolated Congenital Mitral Valve Regurgitation. This is usually due to either an isolated cleft of the anterior mitral valve leaflet or as the result of leaflet dysplasia. In these cases there is evidence of shortened chordae in conjunction with dysplastic valve leaflets. In those with an isolated mitral valve *cleft,* the deficiency in the anterior mitral leaflet points toward the left ventricular outflow tract, unlike those cases with an AV septal defect. In general, the larger the cleft in the anterior mitral leaflet, the greater the degree of regurgitation.[183,184]

In cases with a *dysplastic* mitral valve the chordal apparatus is shortened with varying degrees of dysplasia of the leaflets. Other anatomical lesions such as mitral valve arcade resulting in regurgitation are usually part of a more generalized abnormality of the left side of the heart.

Complex Congenital Mitral Valve Regurgitation. This is seen more frequently in association with abnormalities of the ventriculoarterial connection, such as double-outlet right ventricle, transposition and VSD, and corrected transposition.[185-187] In the first two it is frequent to have a cleft in the anterior mitral valve leaflet with some chordal support apparatus that renders the valve less regurgitant than in those cases with an isolated cleft. In cc-TGA the morphological mitral valve may have an associated cleft, be dysplastic, or have multiple papillary muscles, all of which increase the tendency for it to be regurgitant.

CLINICAL FEATURES. The presence of symptoms relates to the severity of the regurgitation in cases in which the pathology is isolated to the valve. Exercise intolerance, combined with a pansystolic murmur at the apex, with or without a mid-diastolic murmur, are the cardinal clinical features.

LABORATORY INVESTIGATIONS

ECG. This is either normal or demonstrates left atrial and left ventricular hypertrophy.

CHEST RADIOGRAPHY. This demonstrates cardiomegaly predominantly involving the left ventricle and atrium.

ECHOCARDIOGRAPHY. Doppler and 2D echocardiography provide an accurate evaluation of the mechanisms and degree of valvular regurgitation. The cleft in the anterior mitral valve leaflet is best seen in the precordial short-axis view, pointing toward the left ventricular outflow tract. Patients with a dysplastic mitral valve lack mobility of the valve leaflets and have shortened chordae. Color Doppler interrogation helps in locating the site of regurgitation. The severity of regurgitation is assessed in the standard fashion. 3D echocardiography permits a comprehensive evaluation of the mechanisms of regurgitation, with additional information being obtained regarding commissural length, leaflet area, and sites of regurgitation from color flow Doppler.[188,189]

ANGIOCARDIOGRAPHY AND MRI. These procedures are seldom helpful in management planning.

INTERVENTIONAL OPTIONS AND OUTCOMES. This depends on the severity of regurgitation and its impact on left ventricular function. Surgery should not be delayed until the patients become symptomatic. Surgery involves suture of an isolated cleft, with or without associated commissuroplasties. In those cases with a dysplastic mitral valve, leaflet extension in conjunction with an annuloplasty and commissuroplasty usually results in effective control of the regurgitation in the short and medium term.[190,191] Despite this, many of these patients end up with a mitral valve replacement at some stage in the future. Attempted surgical repair, rather than replacement, is important in the pediatric age group because it permits temporary relief that allows the child to grow, such that future surgery can be done into a larger mitral annulus. When required, mitral valve replacement has had a good short- and medium-term outcome in cases in which repair is not possible.[192]

Right Ventricular Outflow Tract Lesions

PERIPHERAL PULMONARY ARTERY STENOSIS (Fig. 61-36). *Right ventricular outflow tract* is a term that applies to patients with both peripheral pulmonary artery stenosis and an intact ventricular septum. It excludes those with an associated VSD, which is dealt with in the sections on tetralogy of Fallot and pulmonary atresia with a ventricular septal defect. Also excluded is Noonan syndrome, which is dealt with in the subsequent section on pulmonary valve stenosis.

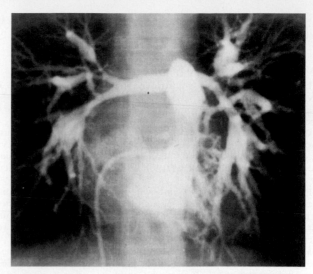

FIGURE 61–36 Right ventricular angiocardiogram showing numerous sites of peripheral pulmonic stenosis and poststenotic dilation of the peripheral pulmonic arteries.

ETIOLOGY

Rubella Syndrome. The most important cause of significant pulmonary artery stenoses producing symptoms in newborns used to be intrauterine rubella infection. Other cardiovascular malformations commonly found in association with congenital rubella include PDA, pulmonary valve stenosis, and ASD. Generalized systemic arterial stenotic lesions also may be a feature of the rubella embryopathy, which may involve large- and medium-sized vessels such as the aorta and coronary, cerebral, mesenteric, and renal arteries. Cardiovascular lesions are but one manifestation of intrauterine rubella infection because cataracts, microphthalmia, deafness, thrombocytopenia, hepatitis, and blood dyscrasias are also common. The clinical picture in infants with rubella syndrome depends on the severity of the cardiovascular lesions and the associated abnormalities.

Williams Syndrome. Peripheral pulmonary artery stenosis is also associated with supravalvular aortic stenosis in patients with Williams syndrome, which is discussed in the section on supravalvular aortic stenosis.[177]

Alagille Syndrome. Peripheral pulmonary artery stenosis is a component of this syndrome, with some cases having a *JAG1* mutation.[193]

Isolated Branch Pulmonary Artery Stenosis. This is encountered mainly in the proximal left pulmonary artery and is invariably related to a sling of ductal tissue that causes stenosis when the ductus arteriosus closes after birth. In most cases this is fairly mild, but a significant obstruction resulting in failure of distal growth of the left pulmonary artery may also be seen.

MORPHOLOGY. Apart from the isolated form mentioned earlier, the stenoses are usually diffuse and bilateral and extend into the mediastinal, hilar, and intraparenchymal pulmonary arteries.

CLINICAL FEATURES. The degree of obstruction is the principal determinant of clinical severity. The type of obstruction determines the feasibility of intervention. Most patients are asymptomatic. An ejection systolic murmur heard at the upper left sternal border and well transmitted to the axilla and back is most common. No pulmonary ejection click is heard. The pulmonic component of the second heart sound may be accentuated and is loud only if there is proximal pulmonary hypertension. A continuous murmur is often audible in patients with significant branch stenosis.

The murmurs in the lung fields are typically increased by inspiration.

LABORATORY INVESTIGATIONS

ECG. Right ventricular hypertrophy is seen when obstruction is severe. Left axis deviation with counterclockwise orientation of the frontal QRS vector is common in rubella syndrome and when there is also supravalvular aortic stenosis.

CHEST RADIOGRAPHY. Mild or moderate stenosis usually produces normal findings. Detectable differences in vascularity between regions of the lungs or dilated pulmonary artery segments are uncommon. When obstruction is bilateral and severe, right atrial and ventricular enlargement may be seen.

ECHOCARDIOGRAPHY. Echocardiography is helpful in making the diagnosis and excluding associated lesions; however, it is limited in its ability to image the distal pulmonary arteries beyond the hilum of the lung. Right ventricular pressure assessment may be predicted if there is associated tricuspid valve regurgitation.

MRI AND SPIRAL CT. These are valuable diagnostic tests because they permit a more distal evaluation of the branch pulmonary arteries. The advantage of spiral CT in young children is that it can be performed without the need for heavy sedation or even general anesthesia. Although most patients require cardiac catheterization and angiography, these other techniques are excellent for the initial evaluation and for following the progress of the lesions.

RADIONUCLIDE QUANTITATIVE LUNG PERFUSION SCAN. This is valuable in cases with unilateral stenosis to determine whether intervention is necessary. Similar flow estimates can now be obtained by MRI.

CARDIAC CATHETERIZATION AND ANGIOCARDIOGRAPHY. This permits the assessment of right ventricular pressure and the pressures in the pulmonary arterial tree. Angiocardiography is the key to precisely assessing the extent and severity of the stenoses.

INTERVENTIONAL OPTIONS AND OUTCOMES. For those cases with isolated left pulmonary artery stenosis where there is less than 30 percent of flow to the lung, balloon dilation with or without stent insertion is effective in relieving the obstruction. In those cases with more diffuse bilateral stenoses, the indications for intervention depend on the right ventricular pressure. As the natural history of diffuse peripheral pulmonary artery stenosis in Williams syndrome is one of potential regression over time, intervention is in general reserved for those cases with systemic or suprasystemic right ventricular pressure. Intervention also depends in part on the extent of the stenosis and the dilation capability of the lesions, with or without stenting.[194-196] In some cases, several attempts at dilation are required to achieve any improvement in vessel caliber. High-pressure balloons are usually necessary, but some lesions cannot be dilated even with such balloons. Recently, improved results have been reported using "cutting" balloons, which may assist dilation in an otherwise undilatable stenosis. As a rule, surgery has little to offer those patients with diffuse peripheral pulmonary artery stenoses and can indeed make the situation worse.

SUPRAVALVULAR RIGHT VENTRICULAR OUTFLOW TRACT OBSTRUCTION. Supravalvular right ventricular outflow tract obstruction seldom occurs in isolation. It can occur in tetralogy of Fallot, Williams syndrome, Noonan syndrome, VSD, or arteriohepatic dysplasia (Alagille syndrome). Supravalvular right ventricular outflow tract obstruction can progress in severity and should be monitored. Dilation of the pulmonary trunk is not a feature of subvalvular and supravalvular right ventricular outflow tract obstruction. Intervention is recommended when the peak gradient across the right ventricular outflow tract is more than 50 mm Hg at rest or when the patient is symptomatic.

PULMONARY STENOSIS WITH INTACT VENTRICULAR SEPTUM (Figs. 61-37 and 61-38). This lesion exists as a continuum, ranging from patients with isolated valvular stenosis to others in whom there is complete atresia of the pulmonary outflow tract. Two modes of presentation exist. The first presents in the neonatal period, usually with associated pathology of the tricuspid valve, right ventricle, and/or coronary arteries. The second mode of presentation is beyond the neonatal period, when the valvular stenosis is usually isolated. Some cases with severe stenosis diagnosed in utero can present with valvular atresia at the time of birth.

MORPHOLOGY. The pulmonary valve may vary from a well-formed trileaflet valve with varying degrees of commissural fusion to an imperforate membrane. If stenosis is present, the right ventricle is usually of normal size or only mildly hypoplastic. Patients with an imperforate valve and a patent infundibulum invariably have a larger right ventricular volume than patients with both infundibular and valve atresia.

CLINICAL FEATURES

Neonate with Critical Pulmonary Valve Stenosis. The neonate presents with central cyanosis due to right-to-left shunting at the atrial level and depends on a prostaglandin infusion to maintain the patency of the ductus arteriosus. Auscultatory findings include a single second heart sound; no ejection click; and a murmur that, when present, is due to tricuspid valve regurgitation.

Infant and Child. In cases beyond the newborn period the referral is usually for the assessment of a cardiac murmur. This may be detected within the first few weeks of life, more commonly at the routine 6-week postnatal visit or later. These patients usually have an ejection click and a second heart sound that moves with respiration but with a soft pulmonary component. An ejection murmur of varying intensity and duration is heard best in the pulmonary area.

Adult. Adults with isolated mild to moderate right ventricular outflow tract obstruction of any type usually have no symptoms. Patients with severe right ventricular outflow tract obstruction may present with exertional fatigue, dyspnea, lightheadedness, and chest discomfort (right ventricular

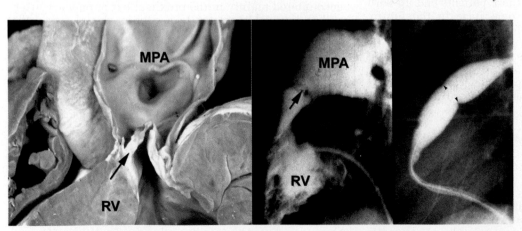

FIGURE 61–37 Montage of pulmonary valve stenosis demonstrating typical pathology (**left,** arrow) with a thickened pulmonary valve and obstruction due to commissural fusion. Note the poststenotic dilation. The angiogram demonstrates a case before (**middle,** arrow) and during (**right**) balloon dilation. MPA = main pulmonary artery; RV = right ventricle.

angina). Physical examination may reveal a prominent jugular A wave, a right ventricular lift, and possibly a thrill in the 2nd left intercostal space. Auscultation reveals a normal S_1, a single or split S_2 with a diminished P_2 (unless the obstruction is supravalvular, in which case the intensity of the P_2 is normal or increased), and a systolic ejection murmur best heard in the 2nd left intercostal space. When the pulmonary valve is thin and pliable, a systolic ejection click will be heard which decreases on inspiration. As the severity of the pulmonary stenosis progresses, the interval between S_1 and the systolic ejection click becomes shorter, S_2 becomes widely split, P_2 diminishes or disappears, and the systolic ejection murmur lengthens and peaks later in systole, often extending beyond A_2. An ejection click seldom occurs with dysplastic pulmonary stenosis. Cyanosis may be present when a patent foramen ovale or ASD permits right-to-left shunting.

Adult patients with trivial and mild valvular right ventricular outflow tract obstruction do not become worse with time. Moderate valvular right ventricular outflow tract obstruction can progress in 20 percent of unoperated patients, especially in adults because of calcification of the valve, and may require intervention. Some of these patients can also become symptomatic, particularly in later life, because of atrial arrhythmias resulting from right ventricular pressure overload and tricuspid regurgitation. Patients with severe valvular right ventricular outflow tract obstruction will have had balloon or surgical valvotomy to survive to adult life. Long-term survival in patients with repaired pulmonary valve stenosis is similar to that of the general population, with excellent to good functional class at long-term follow-up in most patients. A few patients have severe pulmonary regurgitation.

LABORATORY INVESTIGATIONS

ECG. *In the newborn* period this may show left axis deviation and left ventricular dominance in cases with significant right ventricular hypoplasia. Other patients may have a normal QRS axis. Right atrial overload is present in those with increased right atrial pressure. *In the infant, child, and adult* the findings depend on the severity of the stenosis. In milder cases the ECG should be normal. As the stenosis progresses, evidence of right ventricular hypertrophy appears. Severe stenosis is seen in the form of a tall R wave in lead V_4R or V_1 with a deep S wave in V_6. A tall QR wave in the right precordial leads with T wave inversion and ST segment depression (right ventricular "strain") reflects severe stenosis. When an rSR' pattern is observed in lead V_1 (20 percent of patients), lower right ventricular pressures are found than in patients with a pure R wave of equal amplitude. Right atrial overload is associated with moderate to severe pulmonary stenosis.

CHEST RADIOGRAPHY. *In the neonate* this demonstrates pulmonary oligemia with a prominent right heart border in those with associated tricuspid valve regurgitation. *In the infant, child, and adult* with mild or moderate pulmonary stenosis, chest radiography often shows a heart of normal size and normal pulmonary vascularity. Poststenotic dilation of the main and left pulmonary arteries is often seen. Right atrial and right ventricular enlargement are observed in patients with severe obstruction and right ventricular failure. The pulmonary vascularity is usually normal in the absence of a right-to-left atrial shunt but may be reduced in patients with severe stenosis and right ventricular failure.

ECHOCARDIOGRAPHY. Combined 2D echocardiographic and continuous-wave Doppler examination characterizes the anatomical valve abnormality and its severity and has essentially eliminated the requirement for diagnostic cardiac catheterization. Although tradition-

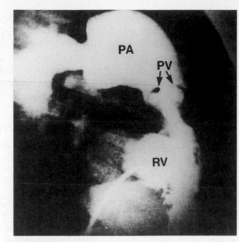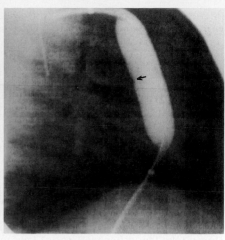

FIGURE 61–38 Right ventriculogram (RV) in the lateral projection **(left)** from a patient with valvular pulmonic stenosis. The pulmonary valve (PV) is thickened and domes in systole (arrows). Poststenotic dilation of the pulmonary artery (PA) is seen. At the right, successful balloon valvuloplasty shows almost complete disappearance of the stenotic waist (arrow). *(Courtesy of Dr. Thomas G. DiSessa.)*

ally maximum instantaneous gradients have been used to select patients for balloon valvuloplasty, recent data would suggest the contrary. Mean Doppler gradients appear to correlate better with catheter-derived peak-peak gradients, with a value of 50 mm Hg being the cutpoint for intervention.[197] Invasive studies are currently used for balloon valvuloplasty.

Right ventricular size is currently best assessed indirectly from the tricuspid annular dimension. In the absence of a VSD there is an excellent correlation between the two. Right ventricular pressure can be assessed indirectly from the tricuspid regurgitation gradient. Tricuspid valve morphology and function and the status of the interatrial septum all need to be addressed.

INTERVENTIONAL OPTIONS AND OUTCOMES

Neonate. In the neonate, prostaglandin E_1 is instituted in cases with ductal dependency. Following this, balloon dilation is performed in those with stenosis, whereas radiofrequency perforation in conjunction with dilation may be undertaken in those with pulmonary valve atresia. If relief of the obstruction is successful, then the prostaglandins are slowly weaned to determine if the right ventricle is large enough to support the circulation. If not, a systemic-to-pulmonary artery shunt is necessary early in the management. In cases with a normal-sized right ventricle, no further therapy is usually necessary in the future because there is a low recurrence rate of stenosis. Newborns with isolated pulmonary stenosis do well after relief of the stenosis.

Infant and Older Child. Balloon dilation of the pulmonary valve is the therapeutic procedure of choice with excellent short- and medium-term results.

Adults. Balloon valvuloplasty is recommended when the gradient across the right ventricular outflow tract is greater than 50 mm Hg at rest[2] or when the patient is symptomatic.

Despite the excellent survival results from the second natural history study (survival after surgical valvotomy of 95.7 percent compared with sex-matched controls of 96.6 percent), recent long-term data suggest that this patient population faces ongoing challenges. After a mean follow-up period of 33 years, 53 percent of patients had required further intervention and 38 percent had either atrial or ventricular arrhythmias.[198]

DYSPLASTIC PULMONARY VALVE STENOSIS

MORPHOLOGY. In pulmonary valve stenosis due to valvular dysplasia, the obstruction is caused not by commissural fusion but by a combination of thickened and dysplastic pulmonary valve leaflets in combination with varying degrees of supravalvular pulmonary stenosis. The supravalvular stenosis is classically at the distal part of pulmonary valve sinuses, and there is usually no poststenotic pulmonary artery dilation. This entity is associated with Noonan syndrome, which in turn may be associated with hypertrophic cardiomyopathy.

CLINICAL FEATURES. In most cases the diagnosis is made either during an evaluation of a systolic murmur or in a child with dysmorphic features who is undergoing clinical evaluation. Children with Noonan syndrome have short stature, webbed necks, and broad-shaped chests in a fashion similar to Turner syndrome. Although this syndrome does not have an associated chromosomal abnormality, it may be familial and affects both sexes equally. A unique association in the newborn is pulmonary lymphangiectasia. The auscultatory finding that differentiates the dysplastic valves from simple pulmonary valve stenosis is the lack of an ejection click. The other features of the murmur are similar to that described in pulmonary valve stenosis.

LABORATORY INVESTIGATIONS

ECG. The ECG is helpful in that patients with dysplastic pulmonary stenosis frequently have a leftward QRS axis, particularly when associated with hypertrophic cardiomyopathy. The remainder of the ECG is similar to that seen in pulmonary valve stenosis.

CHEST RADIOGRAPHY. The findings are similar to typical pulmonary valve stenosis, apart from the lack of poststenotic pulmonary trunk dilation, even in the presence of severe obstruction. In those with pulmonary lymphangiectasia the chest radiograph has a ground-glass appearance, which can be difficult to differentiate from pulmonary venous obstruction.

ECHOCARDIOGRAPHY. This demonstrates a thickened fleshy pulmonary valve, lack of poststenotic dilation, and varying degrees of supravalvular pulmonary stenosis. The associated diagnosis of hypertrophic cardiomyopathy can be confirmed or excluded. If the initial echocardiogram does not demonstrate hypertrophic cardiomyopathy, further studies should be performed throughout childhood and adolescence, particularly in cases with left axis deviation.

INTERVENTIONAL OPTIONS AND OUTCOMES

Cardiac Catheterization and Angiography. Although the results of balloon valvuloplasty are less rewarding than those with stenosis due to commissural fusion, it is worth attempting this before considering surgical intervention. Success has been varied, with many cases having some reduction in gradient that can delay surgery.

Surgical Intervention. If balloon valvuloplasty fails, then surgical intervention is indicated. This usually involves a partial valvectomy in conjunction with patch repair of the supravalvular stenosis.

Outcomes. Adequate relief of the right ventricular outflow tract obstruction results in an excellent outlook, with the greatest long-term risk factor being the presence of hypertrophic cardiomyopathy.

SUBPULMONARY RIGHT VENTRICULAR OUTFLOW TRACT OBSTRUCTION (ANOMALOUS MUSCLE BUNDLES OR A DOUBLE-CHAMBERED RIGHT VENTRICLE)

MORPHOLOGY. A double-chambered right ventricle is formed by right ventricular obstruction due to anomalous muscle bundles.[199] Although this can occur in isolation, it is more frequently part of a combination of lesions that includes right ventricular muscle bundles, a perimembranous-outlet VSD, and subaortic stenosis with or without aortic valve prolapse.

CLINICAL FEATURES. Most cases are discovered as an incidental finding during the evaluation of a VSD. In some cases there may be only an ejection systolic murmur. If the obstruction is isolated, there is an ejection systolic murmur that is heard best in the upper left sternal border. If the VSD is the predominant lesion, the right ventricular outflow

tract murmur may not be appreciated. Before the routine use of echocardiography, the diagnosis was often made during follow-up for a VSD when the pansystolic murmur decreased in intensity and a systolic ejection murmur emerged. The patients are usually pink unless there is progression of the subpulmonary stenosis in the setting of a VSD. The diagnosis may be more problematic in adults.[200]

LABORATORY INVESTIGATIONS

ECG. The ECG is similar to those with isolated pulmonary valve stenosis beyond the newborn period. In cases with a nonrestrictive VSD and mild subpulmonary stenosis, the ECG typically shows biventricular hypertrophy due to a left-to-right shunt and associated pulmonary hypertension. If the stenosis is more severe, right ventricular hypertrophy will be seen. Those with a restrictive VSD may have a normal ECG or left ventricular hypertrophy, the latter of which is replaced with right ventricular hypertrophy if the subpulmonary stenosis increases in severity.

CHEST RADIOGRAPHY. This is usually normal in those with isolated subpulmonary stenosis, whereas those with a VSD may have increased or reduced pulmonary blood flow, depending on the severity of the obstruction.

ECHOCARDIOGRAPHY. Doppler and 2D echocardiography usually provide a complete diagnosis. The level of subpulmonary obstruction is appreciated best in a combination of subcostal right anterior oblique and precordial short-axis views. These views permit the identification of the relationship of the VSD to the muscle bundles, as well as the degree of anterior malalignment of the infundibular septum in those with a VSD. The precordial short-axis view is the best position to evaluate the presence of possible subaortic stenosis and aortic cusp prolapse. Color and pulsed or continuous-wave Doppler evaluation usually allows differentiation of the VSD flow jet from that originating from the muscle bundles. This permits an accurate assessment of the hemodynamic effect of the subpulmonary obstruction.

CARDIAC CATHETERIZATION AND ANGIOCARDIOGRAPHY. This technique is rarely necessary. In older patients in whom the echocardiographic images of the subpulmonary region may be suboptimal, a combination of MRA[201] and echocardiography is all that is generally necessary.

MANAGEMENT OPTIONS AND OUTCOMES. Management is dictated by the severity of the subpulmonary stenosis and the presence of associated defects. In patients with isolated subpulmonary stenosis, surgery is indicated when the right ventricular pressure is more than 60 percent of systemic. This involves resection of the muscle bundles through the right atrium. For those cases with an associated VSD, the decision is based on the size of the VSD, the degree of associated subaortic stenosis, the presence of aortic valve prolapse, and the severity of the subpulmonary stenosis. These patients tend to have a progressive disease, so many cases that are followed conservatively for several years will eventually require surgery. In general the outcome is excellent with a low rate of recurrence after surgical resection of obstructive muscle bundles.[202] Infrequently, recurrence of the subaortic obstruction may occur.

Miscellaneous Lesions

COR TRIATRIATUM

MORPHOLOGY. In this malformation, failure of resorption of the common pulmonary vein results in a left atrium divided by an abnormal fibromuscular diaphragm into a posterosuperior chamber receiving the pulmonary veins and an anteroinferior chamber giving rise to the left atrial appendage and leading to the mitral orifice. The communication between the divided atrial chambers may be large, small, or absent, depending on the size of the opening(s) in the diaphragm, which determines the degree of obstruction to pulmonary venous return. Elevations of both pulmonary venous pressure and pulmonary vascular resistance may result in severe pulmonary artery hypertension.

CLINICAL FEATURES. Cor triatriatum may be detected as an incidental finding in a patient who has an echocardiogram for another reason. In general these represent the unobstructed form that requires no early intervention. Cases with more severe obstruction present in a fashion similar to patients with congenital pulmonary vein stenosis.

LABORATORY INVESTIGATIONS

ECG. In unobstructed cases this is normal, whereas in those with significant obstruction there is right ventricular hypertrophy due to the associated pulmonary hypertension.

CHEST RADIOGRAPHY. This may be normal in those with mild obstruction or who demonstrate pulmonary edema with significant obstruction.

ECHOCARDIOGRAPHY. The diagnosis is established by 2D echo or TEE, with further insight from 3D reconstruction.[203] The obstructive diaphragm is visualized in the parasternal long- and short-axis and four-chamber views and can be distinguished from a supravalvular mitral ring by its position superior to the left atrial appendage, which forms part of the distal chamber. Also present is diastolic fluttering of the mitral leaflets and high-velocity flow detected by Doppler examination in the distal atrial chamber and at the mitral orifice.

CARDIAC CATHETERIZATION AND ANGIOCARDIOGRAPHY. This technique is usually unnecessary with the advent of echocardiography and MRI.

MANAGEMENT OPTIONS AND OUTCOMES. Surgical resection of the membrane is the treatment of choice for patients with significant obstruction. This results in symptom relief and a reduction of pulmonary artery pressure. In general the outcome following surgery is good. With the advent of more routine echocardiography, a subset of cases with typical but nonobstructive forms has been recognized. Thus far these cases appear to remain asymptomatic, with an infrequent need for surgical intervention.

PULMONARY VEIN STENOSIS. Congenital pulmonary vein stenosis may occur as a focal stenosis at the atrial junction or generalized hypoplasia of one or more pulmonary veins. The incidence of associated cardiac malformations is extremely high including VSD, ASD, tetralogy of Fallot, tricuspid and mitral atresia, and AV septal defect. In other cases the pulmonary vein stenosis is acquired after surgical intervention for total anomalous pulmonary venous connection. Children frequently present with recurrent respiratory infections, whereas adults exhibit exercise intolerance. Pulmonary hypertension is one of the consequences of pulmonary vein stenosis, whether it is congenital or acquired. In cases with unilateral pulmonary vein stenosis, clinical symptoms are frequently absent because there is pulmonary blood flow redistribution away from the affected lung.

LABORATORY INVESTIGATIONS

ECG. The ECG is usually normal unless there is evidence of pulmonary hypertension, in which case right ventricular hypertrophy may be seen.

CHEST RADIOGRAPHY. With unilateral pulmonary vein stenosis there is oligemia of the affected lung and increased flow to the contralateral side. If the obstruction is bilateral, pulmonary edema is seen.

ECHOCARDIOGRAPHY. This can usually exclude or confirm the diagnosis of pulmonary vein stenosis. Assessment of pulmonary artery pressure from tricuspid or pulmonary valve regurgitation is possible. Doppler color flow assessment of the right- and left-sided pulmonary veins is the best screening tool. If there is evidence of turbulence or aliasing in the color flow pattern, then spectral analysis with pulsed Doppler will help confirm the diagnosis. Usually pulmonary venous flow is low velocity and phasic. If the pattern is high velocity and turbulent, there is disturbed pulmonary venous flow. Absolute Doppler gradients may or may not be helpful for two reasons. First, the absolute velocity depends on the amount of pulmonary blood flow to that segment of lung. Second, it is often difficult to obtain a parallel line

of interrogation of the pulmonary veins that will affect gradient assessment. The absolute velocity is less important than the diagnosis of pulmonary vein stenosis and its effect on pulmonary artery pressure.

MRI (Fig. 61-39). This technique has now become the gold standard for the diagnosis of pulmonary vein stenosis. This permits a detailed assessment of the pulmonary veins. Velocity assessment is now possible, though this is in the actual veins themselves rather than at the venoatrial junction, which is the site assessed by Doppler echocardiography.

CARDIAC CATHETERIZATION AND ANGIOGRAPHY. In general a combination of echocardiography and MRI makes invasive procedures unnecessary.

MANAGEMENT OPTIONS AND OUTCOMES. If the patient has unilateral pulmonary vein stenosis and normal pulmonary artery pressure, no treatment may be necessary. Continued follow-up is important because this is often a progressive disease that can subsequently affect both sides. In cases with bilateral stenoses the outlook in the past was believed to be hopeless, with a virtually 100 percent mortality. Stents usually provided only temporary relief. More recently a pericardial reflection procedure using native tissue has resulted in some early success in this lesion. This involves using native atrial tissue to form a pocket around the surgically resected stenotic region.

PARTIAL ANOMALOUS PULMONARY VENOUS CONNECTION

MORPHOLOGY. This refers to conditions in which part or all of one lung drains to a site other than the left atrium. Sinus venosus defects have PAPVC typically from the right upper and middle lobe pulmonary veins to the superior vena cava.[204] PAPVC may be directed to a left vertical vein, to the superior vena cava at the level of or above the right pulmonary artery, to the azygos vein, or to the coronary sinus. PAPVC to the inferior vena cava (scimitar syndrome) may have associated hypoplasia of the right lung, pulmonary sequestration, and abnormal collateral supply to the sequestered segment. It can be seen in some patients (<10 percent) with a secundum ASD, as well as in association with many other forms of CHD. PAPVC to the right atrium has the pulmonary veins lying in the normal position; however, there is deviation of the septum primum to the left

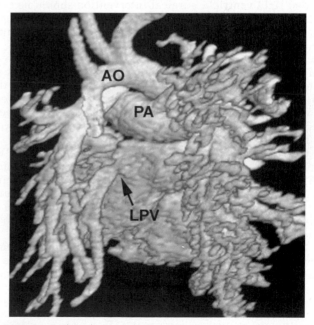

FIGURE 61–39 Three-dimensional MRI demonstrating stenosis of the left lower lobe pulmonary vein. AO = aorta; LPV = left pulmonary vein; PA = pulmonary artery.

with absence of the septum secundum. This type of lesion is seen more frequently in hearts with visceral heterotaxy.

CLINICAL FEATURES. In the absence of associated anomalies, the physiological disturbance is determined by the number of anomalous veins and their site of connection, the presence and size of an ASD, and the state of the pulmonary vascular bed. In the usual patient with isolated partial pulmonary venous connection, the hemodynamic state and physical findings are similar to those in ASD.

LABORATORY INVESTIGATIONS

ECG. In isolated cases, findings similar to a secundum ASD may be seen.

CHEST RADIOGRAPHY. Isolated cases show cardiomegaly involving the right ventricle with increased pulmonary vascular markings. In scimitar syndrome there is invariably right lung hypoplasia, with a secondary shift of the heart into the right thorax and a right-sided scimitar sign that represents the anomalous pulmonary vein.

ECHOCARDIOGRAPHY. If there is a significant left-to-right shunt, then there is right ventricular volume overload with paradoxical interventricular septal motion. A dilated coronary sinus is seen in PAPVC to the coronary sinus. In scimitar syndrome the abnormal pulmonary vein can be seen from the subcostal position during evaluation of the inferior vena cava. Associated stenosis of the pulmonary vein may exist. The suprasternal position permits identification of a left vertical vein, and in general it is possible in children to identify the number of connecting veins on that side. Abnormal venous drainage to the right superior vena cava may be more difficult to identify unless a systematic approach is undertaken. The suprasternal frontal plane view allows the identification of veins that connect just above the right pulmonary artery. Those that connect just behind the right pulmonary artery, either into the superior vena cava or the azygos, can be identified with a right anterior oblique view of the superior vena cava, whether from the subcostal position or a high right parasternal location. In adults, TEE may also be useful in detecting PAPVC.

MRI. Although TEE can be used in older patients with a poorer ultrasound window with a considerable degree of accuracy, it is less invasive to obtain the data using MRI.[205] This provides superb images of the connecting veins that can be seen more distally to their connections with the hilum of the lung. The pulmonary-to-systemic flow ratio can be calculated, obviating the need for hemodynamic evaluation. The pulmonary-to-systemic flow ratio can also be calculated by radionuclide techniques.

MANAGEMENT OPTIONS. In cases with a volume-loaded right ventricle, surgical intervention should be considered. Surgery is not necessary when a single anomalously draining vein has not produced right ventricular volume loading. Surgery is typically performed at a similar time to an ASD at approximately 3 to 5 years of age. The type of surgery depends on the location of the drainage[206] but in general consists of reconnecting the abnormal vein(s) to the left atrium, either directly in the case of a left vertical vein or via a baffle in most other instances. In scimitar syndrome occlusion of the collateral arteries may be necessary, as well as redirection of the pulmonary veins.

OUTCOMES. In general, patients with repaired PAPVC have a good outcome similar to patients with an isolated ASD. What is unclear is the exact patency rate of the veins that are reconnected or baffled back to the left atrium. Patients with scimitar syndrome fare well if the lesion is relatively isolated but do poorly if there is significant associated intracardiac pathology.

PULMONARY ARTERIOVENOUS FISTULA. Abnormal development of the pulmonary arteries and veins in a common vascular complex is responsible for this uncommon congenital anomaly. A variable number of pulmonary arteries communicate directly with branches of the pulmonary veins. Most patients have an associated Weber-Osler-Rendu syndrome; associated problems include bronchiectasis and other malformations of the bronchial tree, as well as absence of the right lower lobe. Pulmonary

AV fistulas may also complicate classic Glenn shunts used in the palliation of cyanotic CHD and are believed to be due to the absence of "hepatic factor" in the venous blood feeding the superior vena cava–pulmonary artery connection. The amount of right-to-left shunting depends on the extent of the fistulous communications and may result in cyanosis. Paradoxical emboli or a brain abscess may cause major neurological deficits. Patients with hereditary hemorrhagic telangiectasia are often anemic because of repeated blood loss and may have less obvious cyanosis because of anemia. Systolic and continuous murmurs may be audible over areas of the fistula. Rounded opacities of various sizes in one or both lungs on chest radiography may suggest the presence of the lesion.

LABORATORY INVESTIGATIONS. Echocardiography is helpful in the initial diagnostic process with the use of a saline contrast injection into a systemic vein.[207] With pulmonary arteriovenous malformations, there is early pulmonary venous return to the left atrium, but not as quickly as for patients with a patent foramen ovale or ASD and right-to-left atrial shunting. More recently, CT and MRI techniques have provided valuable diagnostic information. Pulmonary angiography reveals the site and extent of the abnormal communication.

MANAGEMENT OPTIONS. Unless the lesions are widespread throughout both lungs, surgical treatment aimed at removing the lesions with preservation of healthy lung tissue is commonly indicated to avoid the complications of massive hemorrhage, bacterial endocarditis, and rupture of arteriovenous aneurysms. Transcatheter balloon or plug or coil occlusion embolotherapy may prove to be the therapeutic procedure of choice in some patients.

CORONARY ARTERIOVENOUS FISTULA

MORPHOLOGY. A coronary arteriovenous fistula is a communication between one of the coronary arteries and a cardiac chamber or vein. The right coronary artery (or its branches) is the site of the fistula in about 55 percent of patients; the left coronary artery is involved in about 35 percent; and both coronary arteries are involved in a few. Connections between the coronary system and a cardiac chamber appear to represent persistence of embryonic intertrabecular spaces and sinusoids. Most of these fistulas drain into the right ventricle, right atrium, or the coronary sinus. Coronary to pulmonary artery fistulas are an occasional and usually incidental finding in the adult coronary angiography suite.

CLINICAL FEATURES. The shunt through the fistula is usually small, and myocardial blood flow is not compromised. Potential complications include pulmonary hypertension and congestive heart failure if a large left-to-right shunt exists, bacterial endocarditis, rupture or thrombosis of the fistula or of an associated arterial aneurysm, and myocardial ischemia distal to the fistula due to a "myocardial steal."

Most pediatric patients are asymptomatic and are referred because of a cardiac murmur that is loud, superficial, and continuous at the lower or midsternal border. The site of maximal intensity of the murmur is related to the site of drainage and is usually away from the 2nd left intercostal space—the classic site of the continuous murmur of persistent ductus arteriosus.

LABORATORY INVESTIGATIONS

ECG. This is usually normal unless there is a large left-to-right shunt.

CHEST RADIOGRAPHY. Radiographic findings are often normal and seldom show selective chamber enlargement.

ECHOCARDIOGRAPHY. Coronary artery fistulas are now recognized with a high degree of accuracy with the advent of routine coronary artery evaluation during most pediatric echocardiography examinations. A significantly enlarged feeding coronary artery can be detected, and the entire course and site of entry of the arteriovenous fistula can be traced by Doppler color flow mapping. The shunt entry site is characterized by a continuous turbulent systolic and diastolic flow pattern. Multiplane TEE also accurately defines the origin, course, and drainage site of the fistula.

CARDIAC CATHETERIZATION AND ANGIOCARDIOGRAPHY. If echocardiography demonstrates a significant coronary artery fistula, hemodynamic evaluation is warranted. Standard retrograde thoracic aortography, balloon occlusion angiography of the aortic root with a 45-degree caudal tilt of the frontal camera ("laid back" aortogram), or coronary arteriography can be used reliably to identify the size and anatomical features of the fistulous tract.

MANAGEMENT OPTIONS AND OUTCOMES.

Small fistulas have an excellent long-term prognosis. Untreated larger fistulas may predispose the individual to premature coronary artery disease in the affected vessel. Coil embolization at the time of cardiac catheterization is rapidly becoming the treatment of choice.[208] Surgical treatment is still required in some instances.[209]

REFERENCES

1. Therrien J, Warnes C, Daliento L, et al: Canadian Cardiovascular Society Consensus Conference 2001 update: Recommendations for the management of adults with congenital heart disease part III. Can J Cardiol 17:1135, 2001.
2. Therrien J, Gatzoulis M, Graham T, et al: Canadian Cardiovascular Society Consensus Conference 2001 update: Recommendations for the Management of Adults with Congenital Heart Disease—Part II. Can J Cardiol 17:1029, 2001.
3. Therrien J, Dore A, Gersony W: CCS Consensus Conference 2001 update: Recommendations for the management of adults with congenital heart disease. Part I. Can J Cardiol 17:940, 2001.
4. Deanfield J, Thaulow E, Warnes C, et al: Management of grown up congenital heart disease. Eur Heart J 24:1035, 2003.
5. Skorton DJ, Garson A Jr, Allen HD, et al: Task force 5: Adults with congenital heart disease: Access to care. J Am Coll Cardiol 37:1193, 2001.
6. Child JS, Collins-Nakai RL, Alpert JS, et al: Task force 3: Workforce description and educational requirements for the care of adults with congenital heart disease. J Am Coll Cardiol 37:1183, 2001.
7. Foster E, Graham TP Jr, Driscoll DJ, et al: Task force 2: Special health care needs of adults with congenital heart disease. J Am Coll Cardiol 37:1176, 2001.
8. Warnes CA, Liberthson R, Danielson GK, et al: Task force 1: The changing profile of congenital heart disease in adult life. J Am Coll Cardiol 37:1170, 2001.
9. Webb GD, Williams RG: Care of the adult with congenital heart disease: Introduction. J Am Coll Cardiol 37:1166, 2001.
10. Landzberg MJ, Murphy DJ Jr, Davidson WR Jr, et al: Task force 4: Organization of delivery systems for adults with congenital heart disease. J Am Coll Cardiol 37:1187, 2001.
11. Gatzoulis MA, Webb GD, Daubeney P: Diagnosis and Management of Adult Congenital Heart Disease: Philadelphia, Churchill Livingstone, 2003.
12. Robert H, Anderson EJB, Ferguson J, et al: Paediatric Cardiology. 2nd ed. Philadelphia, Churchill Livingstone, 2001.

Anatomy and Embryology

13. Wernovsky G: Current insights regarding neurological and developmental abnormalities in children and young adults with complex congenital cardiac disease. Cardiol Young 16(Suppl 1):92, 2006.
14. Dore A, de Guise P, Mercier LA: Transition of care to adult congenital heart centres: What do patients know about their heart condition? Can J Cardiol 18:141, 2002.
15. Swan L, Goyal S, Hsia C, et al: Exercise systolic blood pressures are of questionable value in the assessment of the adult with a previous coarctation repair. Heart 89:189, 2003.
16. Siu SC, Sermer M, Colman JM, et al: Prospective multicenter study of pregnancy outcomes in women with heart disease. Circulation 104:515, 2001.
17. Siu SC, Colman JM: Heart disease and pregnancy. Heart 85:710, 2001.

Pathological Consequences of Congenital Cardiac Lesions

18. Hechter SJ, Fredriksen PM, Liu P, et al: Angiotensin-converting enzyme inhibitors in adults after the Mustard procedure. Am J Cardiol 87:660, A611, 2001.
19. Lester SJ, McElhinney DB, Viloria E, et al: Effects of losartan in patients with a systemically functioning morphologic right ventricle after atrial repair of transposition of the great arteries. Am J Cardiol 88:1314, 2001.
20. Laer S, Mir TS, Behn F, et al: Carvedilol therapy in pediatric patients with congestive heart failure: A study investigating clinical and pharmacokinetic parameters. Am Heart J 143:916, 2002.
21. Rodriguez-Cruz E, Karpawich PP, Lieberman RA, Tantengco MV: Biventricular pacing as alternative therapy for dilated cardiomyopathy associated with congenital heart disease. Pacing Clin Electrophysiol 24:235, 2001.
22. Pigula FA, Gandhi SK, Ristich J, et al: Cardiopulmonary transplantation for congenital heart disease in the adult. J Heart Lung Transplant 20:297, 2001.

Cyanosis

23. Horigome H, Hiramatsu Y, Shigeta O, et al: Overproduction of platelet microparticles in cyanotic congenital heart disease with polycythemia. J Am Coll Cardiol 39:1072, 2002.
24. Oechslin E, Kiowski W, Schindler R, et al: Systemic endothelial dysfunction in adults with cyanotic congenital heart disease. Circulation 112:1106, 2005.
25. Fyfe A, Perloff JK, Niwa K, et al: Cyanotic congenital heart disease and coronary artery atherogenesis. Am J Cardiol 96:283, 2005.
26. Hosseinpour AR, Cullen S, Tsang VT: Transplantation for adults with congenital heart disease. Eur J Cardiothorac Surg 30:508, 2006.
27. Walker F, Mullen MJ, Woods SJ, Webb GD: Acute effects of 40% oxygen supplementation in adults with cyanotic congenital heart disease. Heart 90:1073, 2004.

Pulmonary Hypertension

28. Saha A, Balakrishnan KG, Jaiswal PK, et al: Prognosis for patients with Eisenmenger syndrome of various aetiology. Int J Cardiol 45:199, 1994.
29. Martin JT, Tautz TJ, Antognini JF: Safety of regional anesthesia in Eisenmenger's syndrome. Reg Anesth Pain Med 27:509, 2002.
30. Sandoval J, Aguirre JS, Pulido T, et al: Nocturnal oxygen therapy in patients with the Eisenmenger syndrome. Am J Respir Crit Care Med 164:1682, 2001.
31. Waddell TK, Bennett L, Kennedy R, et al: Heart-lung or lung transplantation for Eisenmenger syndrome. J Heart Lung Transplant 21:731, 2002.
32. Berman EB, Barst RJ: Eisenmenger's syndrome: Current management. Prog Cardiovasc Dis 45:129, 2002.
33. Granton JT, Rabinovitch M: Pulmonary arterial hypertension in congenital heart disease. Cardiol Clin 20:441, vii, 2002.
34. Rosenzweig EB, Kerstein D, Barst RJ: Long-term prostacyclin for pulmonary hypertension with associated congenital heart defects. Circulation 99:1858, 1999.
35. McLaughlin VV, Genthner DE, Panella MM, et al: Compassionate use of continuous prostacyclin in the management of secondary pulmonary hypertension: A case series. Ann Intern Med 130:740, 1999.
36. Galie N, Beghetti M, Gatzoulis MA, et al: Bosentan therapy in patients with Eisenmenger syndrome: A multicenter, double-blind, randomized, placebo-controlled study. Circulation 114:48, 2006.
37. Christensen DD, McConnell ME, Book WM, Mahle WT: Initial experience with Bosentan therapy in patients with the Eisenmenger syndrome. Am J Cardiol 94:261, 2004.
38. Galie N, Ghofrani HA, Torbicki A, et al: Sildenafil citrate therapy for pulmonary arterial hypertension. N Engl J Med 353:2148, 2005.
39. Singh TP, Rohit M, Grover A, et al: A randomized, placebo-controlled, double-blind, crossover study to evaluate the efficacy of oral sildenafil therapy in severe pulmonary artery hypertension. Am Heart J 151:851, 2006.

Cardiac Arrhythmias

40. Makikallio K, McElhinney DB, Levine JC, et al: Fetal aortic valve stenosis and the evolution of hypoplastic left heart syndrome: Patient selection for fetal intervention. Circulation 113:1401, 2006.
41. Sittiwangkul R, Ma RY, McCrindle BW, et al: Echocardiographic assessment of obstructive lesions in atrioventricular septal defects. J Am Coll Cardiol 38:253, 2001.
42. Sugeng L, Spencer KT, Mor-Avi V, et al: Dynamic three-dimensional color flow Doppler: An improved technique for the assessment of mitral regurgitation. Echocardiography 20:265, 2003.
43. Barrea C, Levasseur S, Roman K, et al: Three-dimensional echocardiography improves the understanding of left atrioventricular valve morphology and function in atrioventricular septal defects undergoing patch augmentation. J Thorac Cardiovasc Surg 129:746, 2005.
44. Sebag IA, Morgan JG, Handschumacher MD, et al: Usefulness of three-dimensionally guided assessment of mitral stenosis using matrix-array ultrasound. Am J Cardiol 96:1151, 2005.
45. van den Bosch AE, Robbers-Visser D, Krenning BJ, et al: Real-time transthoracic three-dimensional echocardiographic assessment of left ventricular volume and ejection fraction in congenital heart disease. J Am Soc Echocardiogr 19:1, 2006.
46. Zanchetta M, Onorato E, Rigatelli G, et al: Intracardiac echocardiography-guided transcatheter closure of secundum atrial septal defect: A new efficient device selection method. J Am Coll Cardiol 42:1677, 2003.
47. Jan SL, Hwang B, Lee PC, et al: Intracardiac ultrasound assessment of atrial septal defect: Comparison with transthoracic echocardiographic, angiocardiographic, and balloon-sizing measurements. Cardiovasc Intervent Radiol 24:84, 2001.
48. Bruce CJ, Friedman PA: Intracardiac echocardiography. Eur J Echocardiogr 2:234, 2001.
49. Hornung TS, Benson LN, McLaughlin PR: Catheter interventions in adult patients with congenital heart disease. Curr Cardiol Rep 4:54, 2002.

Left-to-Right Shunts

50. Campbell M: Natural history of atrial septal defect. Br Heart J 32:820, 1970.
51. Roberts KE, McElroy JJ, Wong WP, et al: BMPR2 mutations in pulmonary arterial hypertension with congenital heart disease. Eur Respir J 24:371, 2004.
52. Bartel T, Konorza T, Arjumand J, et al: Intracardiac echocardiography is superior to conventional monitoring for guiding device closure of interatrial communications. Circulation 107:795, 2003.
53. Boccalandro F, Baptista E, Muench A, et al: Comparison of intracardiac echocardiography versus transesophageal echocardiography guidance for percutaneous transcatheter closure of atrial septal defect. Am J Cardiol 93:437, 2004.

CH 61

Congenital Heart Disease

54. Attie F, Rosas M, Granados N, et al: Surgical treatment for secundum atrial septal defects in patients > 40 years old. A randomized clinical trial. J Am Coll Cardiol 38:2035, 2001.

55. Mullen MJ, Dias BF, Walker F, et al: Intracardiac echocardiography guided device closure of atrial septal defects. J Am Coll Cardiol 41:285, 2003.

56. Krumsdorf U, Ostermayer S, Billinger K, et al: Incidence and clinical course of thrombus formation on atrial septal defect and patent foramen ovale closure devices in 1,000 consecutive patients. J Am Coll Cardiol 43:302, 2004.

57. Du ZD, Hijazi ZM, Kleinman CS, et al: Comparison between transcatheter and surgical closure of secundum atrial septal defect in children and adults: Results of a multicenter nonrandomized trial. J Am Coll Cardiol 39:1836, 2002.

58. Masura J, Gavora P, Podnar T: Long-term outcome of transcatheter secundum-type atrial septal defect closure using Amplatzer septal occluders. J Am Coll Cardiol 45:505, 2005.

59. Cheung YF, Lun KS, Chau AK: Doppler tissue imaging analysis of ventricular function after surgical and transcatheter closure of atrial septal defect. Am J Cardiol 93:375, 2004.

60. Butera G, Carminati M, Chessa M, et al: Percutaneous versus surgical closure of secundum atrial septal defect: Comparison of early results and complications. Am Heart J 151:228, 2006.

61. Brochu MC, Baril JF, Dore A, et al: Improvement in exercise capacity in asymptomatic and mildly symptomatic adults after atrial septal defect percutaneous closure. Circulation 106:1821, 2002.

62. Morton JB, Sanders P, Vohra JK, et al: Effect of chronic right atrial stretch on atrial electrical remodeling in patients with an atrial septal defect. Circulation 107:1775, 2003.

63. Silversides CK, Siu SC, McLaughlin PR, et al: Symptomatic atrial arrhythmias and transcatheter closure of atrial septal defects in adult patients. Heart 90:1194, 2004.

64. Mas JL, Arquizan C, Lamy C, et al: Recurrent cerebrovascular events associated with patent foramen ovale, atrial septal aneurysm, or both. N Engl J Med 345:1740, 2001.

65. Cramer SC, Rordorf G, Maki JH, et al: Increased pelvic vein thrombi in cryptogenic stroke: Results of the Paradoxical Emboli from Large Veins in Ischemic Stroke (PELVIS) study. Stroke 35:46, 2004.

66. Beda RD, Gill EA Jr: Patent foramen ovale: Does it play a role in the pathophysiology of migraine headache? Cardiol Clin 23:91, 2005.

67. Mohr JP, Thompson JL, Lazar RM, et al: A comparison of warfarin and aspirin for the prevention of recurrent ischemic stroke. N Engl J Med 345:1444, 2001.

68. Homma S, Sacco RL, Di Tullio MR, et al: Effect of medical treatment in stroke patients with patent foramen ovale: Patent foramen ovale in Cryptogenic Stroke Study. Circulation 105:2625, 2002.

69. Cujec B, Mainra R, Johnson DH: Prevention of recurrent cerebral ischemic events in patients with patent foramen ovale and cryptogenic strokes or transient ischemic attacks. Can J Cardiol 15:57, 1999.

70. Windecker S, Wahl A, Nedeltchev K, et al: Comparison of medical treatment with percutaneous closure of patent foramen ovale in patients with cryptogenic stroke. J Am Coll Cardiol 44:750, 2004.

71. Schuchlenz HW, Weihs W, Berghold A, et al: Secondary prevention after cryptogenic cerebrovascular events in patients with patent foramen ovale. Int J Cardiol 101:77, 2005.

72. Wohrle J: Closure of patent foramen ovale after cryptogenic stroke. Lancet 368:350, 2006.

73. Martin F, Sanchez PL, Doherty E, et al: Percutaneous transcatheter closure of patent foramen ovale in patients with paradoxical embolism. Circulation 106:1121, 2002.

74. Smallhorn JF: Cross-sectional echocardiographic assessment of atrioventricular septal defect: basic morphology and preoperative risk factors. Echocardiography 18:415, 2001.

75. Ten Harkel AD, Cromme-Dijkhuis AH, Heinerman BC, et al: Development of left atrioventricular valve regurgitation after correction of atrioventricular septal defect. Ann Thorac Surg 79:607, 2005.

76. Murashita T, Kubota T, Oba J, et al: Left atrioventricular valve regurgitation after repair of incomplete atrioventricular septal defect. Ann Thorac Surg 77:2157, 2004.

77. Lim DS, Ensing GJ, Ludomirsky A, et al: Echocardiographic predictors for the development of subaortic stenosis after repair of atrioventricular septal defect. Am J Cardiol 91:900, 2003.

78. Masuda M, Kado H, Tanoue Y, et al: Does Down syndrome affect the long-term results of complete atrioventricular septal defect when the defect is repaired during the first year of life? Eur J Cardiothorac Surg 27:405, 2005.

79. Frid C, Bjorkhem G, Jonzon A, et al: Long-term survival in children with atrioventricular septal defect and common atrioventricular valvar orifice in Sweden. Cardiol Young 14:24, 2004.

80. Gabriel HM, Heger M, Innerhofer P, et al: Long-term outcome of patients with ventricular septal defect considered not to require surgical closure during childhood. J Am Coll Cardiol 39:1066, 2002.

81. Eroglu AG, Oztunc F, Saltik L, et al: Evolution of ventricular septal defect with special reference to spontaneous closure rate, subaortic ridge and aortic valve prolapse. Pediatr Cardiol 24:31, 2003.

82. Eroglu AG, Oztunc F, Saltik L, et al: Aortic valve prolapse and aortic regurgitation in patients with ventricular septal defect. Pediatr Cardiol 24:36, 2003.

83. Roos-Hesselink JW, Meijboom FJ, Spitaels SE, et al: Outcome of patients after surgical closure of ventricular septal defect at young age: Longitudinal follow-up of 22-34 years. Eur Heart J 25:1057, 2004.

84. Thanopoulos BD, Rigby ML: Outcome of transcatheter closure of muscular ventricular septal defects with the Amplatzer ventricular septal defect occluder. Heart 91:513, 2005.

85. Carminati M, Butera G, Chessa M, et al: Transcatheter closure of congenital ventricular septal defect with Amplatzer septal occluders. Am J Cardiol 96:52L, 2005.

86. Arora R, Trehan V, Kumar A, et al: Transcatheter closure of congenital ventricular septal defects: Experience with various devices. J Interv Cardiol 16:83, 2003.

87. Sadiq M, Latif F, Ur-Rehman A: Analysis of infective endarteritis in patent ductus arteriosus. Am J Cardiol 93:513, 2004.

88. Galal MO: Advantages and disadvantages of coils for transcatheter closure of patent ductus arteriosus. J Interv Cardiol 16:157, 2003.

89. Moore JW, Levi DS, Moore SD, et al: Interventional treatment of patent ductus arteriosus in 2004. Catheter Cardiovasc Interv 64:91, 2005.

90. Bennhagen RG, Benson LN: Silent and audible persistent ductus arteriosus: An angiographic study. Pediatr Cardiol 24:27, 2003.

Cyanotic Heart Disease

91. Dearani JA, Danielson GK, Puga FJ, et al: Late follow-up of 1095 patients undergoing operation for complex congenital heart disease utilizing pulmonary ventricle to pulmonary artery conduits. Ann Thorac Surg 75:399, 2003; discussion 410-391.

92. Mavroudis C, Backer CL: Surgical management of severe truncal insufficiency: Experience with truncal valve remodeling techniques. Ann Thorac Surg 72:396, 2001.

93. Graham TP Jr: Management of pulmonary regurgitation after tetralogy of Fallot repair. Curr Cardiol Rep 4:63, 2002.

94. Niwa K, Perloff JK, Bhuta SM, et al: Structural abnormalities of great arterial walls in congenital heart disease: Light and electron microscopic analyses. Circulation 103:393, 2001.

95. Mair DD, Puga FJ: Management of pulmonary atresia with ventricular septal defect. Curr Treat Options Cardiovasc Med 5:409, 2003.

96. Alexiou C, Mahmoud H, Al-Khaddour A, et al: Outcome after repair of tetralogy of Fallot in the first year of life. Ann Thorac Surg 71:494, 2001.

97. Therrien J, Provost Y, Merchant N, et al: Optimal timing for pulmonary valve replacement in adults after tetralogy of Fallot repair. Am J Cardiol 95:779, 2005.

98. Therrien J, Siu SC, Harris L, et al: Impact of pulmonary valve replacement on arrhythmia propensity late after repair of tetralogy of Fallot. Circulation 103:2489, 2001.

99. Khambadkone S, Bonhoeffer P: Percutaneous pulmonary valve implantation. Semin Thorac Cardiovasc Surg Pediatr Card Surg Annu 23-28, 2006.

100. Vliegen HW, van Straten A, de Roos A, et al: Magnetic resonance imaging to assess the hemodynamic effects of pulmonary valve replacement in adults late after repair of tetralogy of fallot. Circulation 106:1703, 2002.

101. Ghai A, Silversides C, Harris L, et al: Left ventricular dysfunction is a risk factor for sudden cardiac death in adults late after repair of tetralogy of Fallot. J Am Coll Cardiol 40:1675, 2002.

102. Senzaki H, Masutani S, Kobayashi J, et al: Ventricular afterload and ventricular work in Fontan circulation: Comparison with normal two-ventricle circulation and single-ventricle circulation with Blalock Taussig shunts. Circulation 105:2885, 2002.

103. Milanesi O, Stellin G, Colan SD, et al: Systolic and diastolic performance late after the Fontan procedure for a single ventricle and comparison of those undergoing operation at < 12 months of age and at > 12 months of age. Am J Cardiol 89:276, 2002.

104. Khambadkone S, Li J, de Leval MR, et al: Basal pulmonary vascular resistance and nitric oxide responsiveness late after Fontan-type operation. Circulation 107:3204, 2003.

105. Wong T, Davlouros PA, Li W, et al: Mechano-electrical interaction late after Fontan operation: Relation between P-wave duration and dispersion, right atrial size, and atrial arrhythmias. Circulation 109:2319, 2004.

106. Coon PD, Rychik J, Novello RT, et al: Thrombus formation after the Fontan operation. Ann Thorac Surg 71:1990, 2001.

107. Brancaccio G, Carotti A, D'Argenio P, et al: Protein-losing enteropathy after Fontan surgery: Resolution after cardiac transplantation. J Heart Lung Transplant 22:484, 2003.

108. Varma C, Warr MR, Hendler AL, et al: Prevalence of "silent" pulmonary emboli in adults after the Fontan operation. J Am Coll Cardiol 41:2252, 2003.

109. Jacobs ML, Pourmoghadam KK, Geary EM, et al: Fontan's operation: Is aspirin enough? Is Coumadin too much? Ann Thorac Surg 73:64, 2002.

110. Seipelt RG, Franke A, Vazquez-Jimenez JF, et al: Thromboembolic complications after Fontan procedures: Comparison of different therapeutic approaches. Ann Thorac Surg 74:556, 2002.

111. Deal BJ, Mavroudis C, Backer CL: Beyond Fontan conversion: Surgical therapy of arrhythmias including patients with associated complex congenital heart disease. Ann Thorac Surg 76:542, 2003; discussion 553-544.

112. Mavroudis C, Deal BJ, Backer CL: Arrhythmia surgery in association with complex congenital heart repairs excluding patients with Fontan conversion. Semin Thorac Cardiovasc Surg Pediatr Card Surg Annu 6:33, 2003.

113. Mavroudis C, Backer CL, Deal BJ, et al: Total cavopulmonary conversion and maze procedure for patients with failure of the Fontan operation. J Thorac Cardiovasc Surg 122:863, 2001.

114. Williams WG, McCrindle BW, Ashburn DA, et al: Outcomes of 829 neonates with complete transposition of the great arteries 12-17 years after repair. Eur J Cardiothorac Surg 24:1, 2003; discussion 9-10.

CH 61

115. Rehnstrom P, Gilljam T, Sudow G, Berggren H: Excellent survival and low complication rate in medium-term follow-up after arterial switch operation for complete transposition. Scand Cardiovasc J 37:104, 2003.

116. Hovels-Gurich HH, Kunz D, Seghaye M, et al: Results of exercise testing at a mean age of 10 years after neonatal arterial switch operation. Acta Paediatr 92:190, 2003.

117. Losay J, Touchot A, Serraf A, et al: Late outcome after arterial switch operation for transposition of the great arteries. Circulation 104(Suppl 1):I121, 2001.

118. Yoshizumi K, Yagihara T, Uemura H: Approach to the neoaortic valve for replacement after the arterial switch procedure in patients with complete transposition. Cardiol Young 11:666, 2001.

119. Legendre A, Losay J, Touchot-Kone A, et al: [Prevalence and diagnosis of coronary lesions after arterial switch]. Arch Mal Coeur Vaiss 96:485, 2003.

120. Hauser M, Bengel FM, Kuhn A, et al: Myocardial blood flow and flow reserve after coronary reimplantation in patients after arterial switch and Ross operation. Circulation 103:1875, 2001.

121. Daebritz SH, Tiete AR, Sachweh JS, et al: Systemic right ventricular failure after atrial switch operation: Midterm results of conversion into an arterial switch. Ann Thorac Surg 71:1255, 2001.

122. Guedes A, Mercier LA, Leduc L, et al: Impact of pregnancy on the systemic right ventricle after a Mustard operation for transposition of the great arteries. J Am Coll Cardiol 44:433, 2004.

123. Kafali G, Elsharshari H, Ozer S, et al: Incidence of dysrhythmias in congenitally corrected transposition of the great arteries. Turk J Pediatr 44:219, 2002.

124. Rutledge JM, Nihill MR, Fraser CD, et al: Outcome of 121 patients with congenitally corrected transposition of the great arteries. Pediatr Cardiol 23:137, 2002.

125. Beauchesne LM, Warnes CA, Connolly HM, et al: Outcome of the unoperated adult who presents with congenitally corrected transposition of the great arteries. J Am Coll Cardiol 40:285, 2002.

126. Duncan BW, Mee RB, Mesia CI, et al: Results of the double switch operation for congenitally corrected transposition of the great arteries. Eur J Cardiothorac Surg 24:11, 2003; discussion 19-20.

127. Ilbawi MN, Ocampo CB, Allen BS, et al: Intermediate results of the anatomic repair for congenitally corrected transposition. Ann Thorac Surg 73:594, 2002; discussion 599-600.

128. Anderson RH: Double outlet right ventricle. Eur J Cardiothorac Surg 22:853, 2002.

129. Anderson RH, McCarthy K, Cook AC: Continuing medical education. Double outlet right ventricle. Cardiol Young 11:329, 2001.

130. Brown JW, Ruzmetov M, Okada Y, et al: Surgical results in patients with double outlet right ventricle: A 20-year experience. Ann Thorac Surg 72:1630, 2001.

131. Attenhofer Jost CH, Connolly HM, Warnes CA, et al: Noncompacted myocardium in Ebstein's anomaly: Initial description in three patients. J Am Soc Echocardiogr 17:677, 2004.

132. Dearani JA, Danielson GK: Surgical management of Ebstein's anomaly in the adult. Semin Thorac Cardiovasc Surg 17:148, 2005.

133. Khositseth A, Danielson GK, Dearani JA, et al: Supraventricular tachyarrhythmias in Ebstein anomaly: Management and outcome. J Thorac Cardiovasc Surg 128:826, 2004.

134. Chauvaud SM, Brancaccio G, Carpentier AF: Cardiac arrhythmia in patients undergoing surgical repair of Ebstein's anomaly. Ann Thorac Surg 71:1547, 2001.

135. Almange C: [Ebstein anomaly and pregnancy]. Arch Mal Coeur Vaiss 95:525, 2002.

Valvular and Vascular Conditions

136. Aluquin VP, Shutte D, Nihill MR, et al: Normal aortic arch growth and comparison with isolated coarctation of the aorta. Am J Cardiol 91:502, 2003.

137. Levine JC, Sanders SP, Colan SD, et al: The risk of having additional obstructive lesions in neonatal coarctation of the aorta. Cardiol Young 11:44, 2001.

138. De Mey S, Segers P, Coomans I, et al: Limitations of Doppler echocardiography for the post-operative evaluation of aortic coarctation. J Biomech 34:951, 2001.

139. Lim DS, Ralston MA: Echocardiographic indices of Doppler flow patterns compared with MRI or angiographic measurements to detect significant coarctation of the aorta. Echocardiography 19:55, 2002.

140. Godart F, Labrot G, Devos P, et al: Coarctation of the aorta: Comparison of aortic dimensions between conventional MR imaging, 3D MR angiography, and conventional angiography. Eur Radiol 12:2034, 2002.

141. Fiore AC, Fischer LK, Schwartz T, et al: Comparison of angioplasty and surgery for neonatal aortic coarctation. Ann Thorac Surg 80:1659, 2005; discussion 1664-1655.

142. Zabal C, Attie F, Rosas M, et al: The adult patient with native coarctation of the aorta: Balloon angioplasty or primary stenting? Heart 89:77, 2003.

143. Toro-Salazar OH, Steinberger J, Thomas W, et al: Long-term follow-up of patients after coarctation of the aorta repair. Am J Cardiol 89:541, 2002.

144. von Kodolitsch Y, Aydin MA, Koschyk DH, et al: Predictors of aneurysmal formation after surgical correction of aortic coarctation. J Am Coll Cardiol 39:617, 2002.

145. O'Sullivan JJ, Derrick G, Darnell R: Prevalence of hypertension in children after early repair of coarctation of the aorta: A cohort study using casual and 24 hour blood pressure measurement. Heart 88:163, 2002.

146. de Divitiis M, Pilla C, Kattenhorn M, et al: Ambulatory blood pressure, left ventricular mass, and conduit artery function late after successful repair of coarctation of the aorta. J Am Coll Cardiol 41:2259, 2003.

147. Zadinello M, Greve G, Liu XQ, et al: Angiotensin I converting enzyme genotype affects ventricular remodelling in children with aortic coarctation. Heart 91:367, 2005.

148. Pacini D, Bergonzini M, Loforte A, et al: Aneurysms after coarctation repair associated with hypoplastic aortic arch: Surgical management through median sternotomy. Ann Thorac Surg 81:758, 2006.

149. Tzifa A, Ewert P, Brzezinska-Rajszys G, et al: Covered Cheatham-platinum stents for aortic coarctation: Early and intermediate-term results. J Am Coll Cardiol 47:1457, 2006.

150. Harrison DA, McLaughlin PR, Lazzam C, et al: Endovascular stents in the management of coarctation of the aorta in the adolescent and adult: One year follow up. Heart 85:561, 2001.

151. Suzuki T, Ohye RG, Devaney EJ, et al: Selective management of the left ventricular outflow tract for repair of interrupted aortic arch with ventricular septal defect: Management of left ventricular outflow tract obstruction. J Thorac Cardiovasc Surg 131:779, 2006.

152. Dong C, Wu QY, Tang Y: Ruptured sinus of Valsalva aneurysm: A Beijing experience. Ann Thorac Surg 74:1621, 2001.

153. Pasteuning WH, Roukema JA, van Straten AH, et al: Rapid hemodynamic deterioration because of acute rupture of an aneurysm of the sinus of Valsalva: The importance of echocardiography in early diagnosis. J Am Soc Echocardiogr 15:1108, 2002.

154. Shah RP, Ding ZP, Ng AS, Quek SS: A ten-year review of ruptured sinus of Valsalva: Clinico-pathological and echo-Doppler features. Singapore Med J 42:473, 2001.

155. Fedson S, Jolly N, Lang RM, Hijazi ZM: Percutaneous closure of a ruptured sinus of Valsalva aneurysm using the Amplatzer Duct Occluder. Catheter Cardiovasc Interv 58:406, 2003.

156. van Son JA, Konstantinov IE, Burckhard F: Kommerell and Kommerell's diverticulum. Tex Heart Inst J 29:109, 2002.

157. Philip S, Chen SY, Wu MH, et al: Retroesophageal aortic arch: Diagnostic and therapeutic implications of a rare vascular ring. Int J Cardiol 79:133, 2001.

158. Mihaljevic T, Cannon JW, del Nido PJ: Robotically assisted division of a vascular ring in children. J Thorac Cardiovasc Surg 125:1163, 2003.

159. Chiu PP, Rusan M, Williams WG, et al: Long-term outcomes of clinically significant vascular rings associated with congenital tracheal stenosis. J Pediatr Surg 41:335, 2006.

160. Lofland GK, McCrindle BW, Williams WG, et al: Critical aortic stenosis in the neonate: A multi-institutional study of management, outcomes, and risk factors. Congenital Heart Surgeons Society. J Thorac Cardiovasc Surg 121:10, 2001.

161. McCrindle BW, Blackstone EH, Williams WG, et al: Are outcomes of surgical versus transcatheter balloon valvotomy equivalent in neonatal critical aortic stenosis? Circulation 104:I152, 2001.

162. Barker PC, Ensing G, Ludomirsky A, et al: Comparison of simultaneous invasive and noninvasive measurements of pressure gradients in congenital aortic valve stenosis. J Am Soc Echocardiogr 15:1496, 2002.

163. Bacha EA, Satou GM, Moran AM, et al: Valve-sparing operation for balloon-induced aortic regurgitation in congenital aortic stenosis. J Thorac Cardiovasc Surg 122:162, 2001.

164. Ohye RG, Gomez CA, Ohye BJ, et al: The Ross/Konno procedure in neonates and infants: Intermediate-term survival and autograft function. Ann Thorac Surg 72:823, 2001.

165. Al-Halees Z, Pieters F, Qadoura F, et al: The Ross procedure is the procedure of choice for congenital aortic valve disease. J Thorac Cardiovasc Surg 123:437, 2002; discussion 441-432.

166. Williams IA, Quaegebeur JM, Hsu DT, et al: Ross procedure in infants and toddlers followed into childhood. Circulation 112(Suppl):I390, 2005.

167. Favaloro R, Stutzbach P, Gomez C, et al: Feasibility of the Ross procedure: Its relationship with the bicuspid aortic valve. J Heart Valve Dis 11:375, 2002; discussion 382.

168. Cohen L, Bennani R, Hulin S, et al: Mitral valvar anomalies and discrete subaortic stenosis. Cardiol Young 12:138, 2002.

169. Marasini M, Zannini L, Ussia GP, et al: Discrete subaortic stenosis: Incidence, morphology and surgical impact of associated subaortic anomalies. Ann Thorac Surg 75:1763, 2003.

170. Freedom RM, Yoo SJ, Russell J, et al: Thoughts about fixed subaortic stenosis in man and dog. Cardiol Young 15:186, 2005.

171. Oliver JM, Gonzalez A, Gallego P, et al: Discrete subaortic stenosis in adults: Increased prevalence and slow rate of progression of the obstruction and aortic regurgitation. J Am Coll Cardiol 38:835, 2001.

172. Stassano P, Di Tommaso L, Contaldo A, et al: Discrete subaortic stenosis: Long-term prognosis on the progression of the obstruction and of the aortic insufficiency. Thorac Cardiovasc Surg 53:23, 2005.

173. Caldarone CA: Left ventricular outflow tract obstruction: The role of the modified Konno procedure. Semin Thorac Cardiovasc Surg Pediatr Card Surg Annu 6:98, 2003.

174. Antonell A, de Luis O, Domingo-Roura X, Perez-Jurado LA: Evolutionary mechanisms shaping the genomic structure of the Williams-Beuren syndrome chromosomal region at human 7q11.23. Genome Res 15:1179, 2005.

175. Vaideeswar P, Shankar V, Deshpande JR, et al: Pathology of the diffuse variant of supravalvar aortic stenosis. Cardiovasc Pathol 10:33, 2001.

176. Eronen M, Peippo M, Hiippala A, et al: Cardiovascular manifestations in 75 patients with Williams syndrome. J Med Genet 39:554, 2002.

177. Bruno E, Rossi N, Thuer O, et al: Cardiovascular findings, and clinical course, in patients with Williams syndrome. Cardiol Young 13:532, 2003.

178. English RF, Colan SD, Kanani PM, Ettedgui JA: Growth of the aorta in children with Williams syndrome: Does surgery make a difference? Pediatr Cardiol 24:566, 2003.

179. Einfeld SL, Tonge BJ, Rees VW: Longitudinal course of behavioral and emotional problems in Williams syndrome. Am J Ment Retard 106:73, 2001.

180. Schaverien MV, Freedom RM, McCrindle BW: Independent factors associated with outcomes of parachute mitral valve in 84 patients. Circulation 109:2309, 2004.

181. McElhinney DB, Sherwood MC, Keane JF, et al: Current management of severe congenital mitral stenosis: Outcomes of transcatheter and surgical therapy in 108 infants and children. Circulation 112:707, 2005.

182. Agarwal S, Airan B, Chowdhury UK, et al: Ventricular septal defect with congenital mitral valve disease: Long-term results of corrective surgery. Indian Heart J 54:67, 2002.

183. Van Praagh S, Porras D, Oppido G, et al: Cleft mitral valve without ostium primum defect: Anatomic data and surgical considerations based on 41 cases. Ann Thorac Surg 75:1752, 2003.

184. Fraisse A, Massih TA, Kreitmann B, et al: Characteristics and management of cleft mitral valve. J Am Coll Cardiol 42:1988, 2003.

185. Fraisse A, Massih TA, Vouhe P, et al: Management and outcome of patients with abnormal ventriculo-arterial connections and mitral valve cleft. Ann Thorac Surg 74:786, 2002.

186. Fraisse A, Massih TA, Bonnet D, et al: Cleft of the mitral valve in patients with Down's syndrome. Cardiol Young 12:27, 2002.

187. Fraisse A, Le Bret E, Massih TA, et al: Intra-aortic extension of ductal tissue. J Thorac Cardiovasc Surg 123:568, 2002.

188. Macnab A, Jenkins NP, Ewington I, et al: A method for the morphological analysis of the regurgitant mitral valve using three dimensional echocardiography. Heart 90:771, 2004.

189. Macnab A, Jenkins NP, Bridgewater BJ, et al: Three-dimensional echocardiography is superior to multiplane transoesophageal echo in the assessment of regurgitant mitral valve morphology. Eur J Echocardiogr 5:212, 2004.

190. Chauvaud S: Congenital mitral valve surgery: Techniques and results. Curr Opin Cardiol 21:95, 2006.

191. Prifti E, Vanini V, Bonacchi M, et al: Repair of congenital malformations of the mitral valve: Early and midterm results. Ann Thorac Surg 73:614, 2002.

192. Erez E, Kanter KR, Isom E, et al: Mitral valve replacement in children. J Heart Valve Dis 12:25, 2003; discussion 30.

193. McElhinney DB, Krantz ID, Bason L, et al: Analysis of cardiovascular phenotype and genotype-phenotype correlation in individuals with a JAG1 mutation and/or Alagille syndrome. Circulation 106:2567, 2002.

194. Trivedi KR, Benson LN: Interventional strategies in the management of peripheral pulmonary artery stenosis. J Interv Cardiol 16:171, 2003.

195. Rothman A, Levy DJ, Sklansky MS, et al: Balloon angioplasty and stenting of multiple intralobar pulmonary arterial stenoses in adult patients. Catheter Cardiovasc Interv 58:252, 2003.

196. Rosales AM, Lock JE, Perry SB, Geggel RL: Interventional catheterization management of perioperative peripheral pulmonary stenosis: Balloon angioplasty or endovascular stenting. Catheter Cardiovasc Interv 56:272, 2002.

197. Silvilairat S, Cabalka AK, Cetta F, et al: Echocardiographic assessment of isolated pulmonary valve stenosis: Which outpatient Doppler gradient has the most clinical validity? J Am Soc Echocardiogr 18:1137, 2005.

198. Earing MG, Connolly HM, Dearani JA, et al: Long-term follow-up of patients after surgical treatment for isolated pulmonary valve stenosis. Mayo Clin Proc 80:871, 2005.

199. Alva C, Ortegon J, Herrera F, et al: Types of obstructions in double-chambered right ventricle: Mid-term results. Arch Med Res 33:261, 2002.

200. Lascano ME, Schaad MS, Moodie DS, Murphy D Jr: Difficulty in diagnosing double-chambered right ventricle in adults. Am J Cardiol 88:816, 2001.

201. Kilner PJ, Sievers B, Meyer GP, Ho SY: Double-chambered right ventricle or sub-infundibular stenosis assessed by cardiovascular magnetic resonance. J Cardiovasc Magn Reson 4:373, 2002.

202. Hachiro Y, Takagi N, Koyanagi T, et al: Repair of double-chambered right ventricle: Surgical results and long-term follow-up. Ann Thorac Surg 72:1520, 2001.

203. Roldan FJ, Vargas-Barron J, Espinola-Zavaleta N, et al: Cor triatriatum dexter: Transesophageal echocardiographic diagnosis and 3-dimensional reconstruction. J Am Soc Echocardiogr 14:634, 2001.

204. Oliver JM, Gallego P, Gonzalez A, et al: Sinus venosus syndrome: Atrial septal defect or anomalous venous connection? A multiplane transoesophageal approach. Heart 88:634, 2002.

205. Ferrari VA, Scott CH, Holland GA, et al: Ultrafast three-dimensional contrast-enhanced magnetic resonance angiography and imaging in the diagnosis of partial anomalous pulmonary venous drainage. J Am Coll Cardiol 37:1120, 2001.

206. Brown JW, Ruzmetov M, Minnich DJ, et al: Surgical management of scimitar syndrome: An alternative approach. J Thorac Cardiovasc Surg 125:238, 2003.

207. Gudavalli A, Kalaria VG, Chen X, Schwarz KQ: Intrapulmonary arteriovenous shunt: Diagnosis by saline contrast bubbles in the pulmonary veins. J Am Soc Echocardiogr 15:1012, 2002.

208. Ito T, Okubo T, Kimura M, et al: Increase in diameter of ventricular septal defect and membranous septal aneurysm formation during the infantile period. Pediatr Cardiol 22:491, 2001.

209. Kamiya H, Yasuda T, Nagamine H, et al: Surgical treatment of congenital coronary artery fistulas: 27 years' experience and a review of the literature. J Card Surg 17:173, 2002.

CHAPTER 62

Valvular Heart Disease

Catherine M. Otto and Robert O. Bonow*

Aortic Stenosis, 1625
Etiology and Pathology, 1625
Pathophysiology, 1626
Clinical Presentation, 1628
Disease Course, 1631
Management, 1633

Aortic Regurgitation, 1635
Etiology and Pathology, 1635
Chronic Aortic Regurgitation, 1636
Pathophysiology, 1636
Clinical Presentation, 1638
Disease Course, 1641
Management, 1641
Acute Aortic Regurgitation, 1645

Mitral Stenosis, 1646
Etiology, 1646
Pathophysiology, 1647
Clinical Presentation, 1649
Disease Course, 1651
Management, 1652

Mitral Regurgitation, 1657
Etiology and Pathology, 1657
Pathophysiology, 1659
Clinical Presentation, 1662
Disease Course, 1664
Management of Chronic Mitral
Regurgitation, 1665
Acute Mitral Regurgitation, 1668

Mitral Valve Prolapse
Syndrome, 1669
Etiology and Pathology, 1669
Clinical Presentation, 1670
Disease Course, 1672
Management, 1673

Tricuspid, Pulmonic, and
Multivalvular Disease, 1674
Tricuspid Stenosis, 1674
Tricuspid Regurgitation, 1675
Pulmonic Valve Disease, 1678
Multivalvular Disease, 1680

Prosthetic Cardiac Valves, 1682
Mechanical Prostheses, 1682
Tissue Valves, 1684
Hemodynamics of Valve
Replacements, 1686
Selection of an Artificial Valve, 1687

References, 1688

Guidelines, 1693

Valvular heart disease accounts for 10 to 20 percent of all cardiac surgical procedures in the United States. Although the prevalence of rheumatic valve disease now is very low in the United States and Europe because of primary prevention of rheumatic fever, an increasing number of elderly adults with age-associated calcific valve disease exists. About two thirds of all heart valve operations are for aortic valve replacement, most often for aortic stenosis (AS). Mitral valve surgery is most often performed for mitral regurgitation (MR) because most patients with mitral stenosis are treated by a percutaneous approach. In addition to patients with severe valve disease that eventually requires mechanical intervention, there is a larger group of patients with mild to moderate disease who need accurate diagnosis and appropriate medical management. Guidelines for the management of patients with valvular heart disease have been published.[1,2] Recent studies suggest that age-related calcific valve dysfunction is the end result of an active disease process, rather than an inevitable consequence of aging.

AORTIC STENOSIS

Etiology and Pathology

Obstruction to left ventricular (LV) outflow is localized most commonly at the aortic valve and is discussed in this section. However, obstruction may also occur above the valve (supravalvular stenosis) or below the valve (discrete subvalvular stenosis) (see Chap. 61), or it may be caused by hypertrophic cardiomyopathy (HCM) (see Chap. 65). Valvular AS has three principal causes: a congenital bicuspid valve with superimposed calcification, calcification of a normal trileaflet valve (e.g., "degenerative AS") and rheumatic disease (Fig. 62-1). In a recent U.S. series of 933 patients undergoing AVR for AS, a bicuspid valve was present in more than 50 percent including two thirds of those younger than 70 years old and 40 percent of those older than 70 years of age.[3]

In addition, AS may be caused by a congenital valve stenosis presenting in infancy or childhood. Rarely AS is caused by severe atherosclerosis of the aorta and aortic valve; this form of AS occurs most frequently in patients with severe hypercholesterolemia and is observed in children with homozy-gous type II hyperlipoproteinemia. Rheumatoid involvement of the valve is a rare cause of AS and results in nodular thickening of the valve leaflets and involvement of the proximal portion of the aorta. Ochronosis with alkaptonuria is another rare cause of AS.

CONGENITAL AORTIC STENOSIS (see also Chap. 61). Congenital malformations of the aortic valve may be unicuspid, bicuspid, or tricuspid, or there may be a dome-shaped diaphragm. Unicuspid valves produce severe obstruction in infancy and are the most frequent malformations found in fatal valvular AS in children younger than 1 year of age. Congenitally bicuspid valves may be stenotic with commissural fusion at birth, but more often they are not responsible for serious narrowing of the aortic orifice during childhood.[4,5]

BICUSPID AORTIC VALVE. A congenital bicuspid valve is more prevalent in men, accounting for 70 to 80 percent of cases. A subset of bicuspid aortic valve patients have familial clustering consistent with an autosomal dominant inheritance with incomplete penetrance.[4,6] In some families with bicuspid aortic valve and associated congenital anomalies, a mutation in the NOTCH1 gene has been described.[7] A bicuspid aortic valve usually functions normally in childhood. Approximately 20 percent of bicuspid valves develop severe aortic regurgitation (AR) requiring AVR between 10 and 40 years of age. Patients with a bicuspid aortic valve also are at increased risk for endocarditis (0.4 per 100,000) accounting for about 1200 deaths per year in the United States. Bicuspid valves are often associated with dilatation of the ascending aorta[4,6,8,9] related to accelerated degeneration of the aortic media[6,10] but not related to the severity of valve dysfunction per se. The risk of aortic dissection in patients with a bicuspid aortic valve is five to nine times higher than the general population.[11] However, most patients with a bicuspid valve develop calcific valve stenosis later in life, typically presenting with severe AS after 50 years of age.

Although the histopathology of calcific stenosis of a bicuspid aortic valve is no different than that of a trileaflet valve, the turbulent flow and increased leaflet stress caused by the abnormal architecture is postulated to result in accelerated valve changes, providing an explanation for the earlier average age at presentation of patients with a bicuspid, compared with trileaflet, stenotic valve.

CALCIFIC AORTIC STENOSIS. Age-related calcific (formerly termed *senile* or *degenerative*) AS of a congenital bicuspid or normal trileaflet valve is now the most common cause of AS in adults.[12] In a population-based echocardiographic study,

*Some material was provided by Eugene Braunwald, MD, who authored this chapter in previous editions.

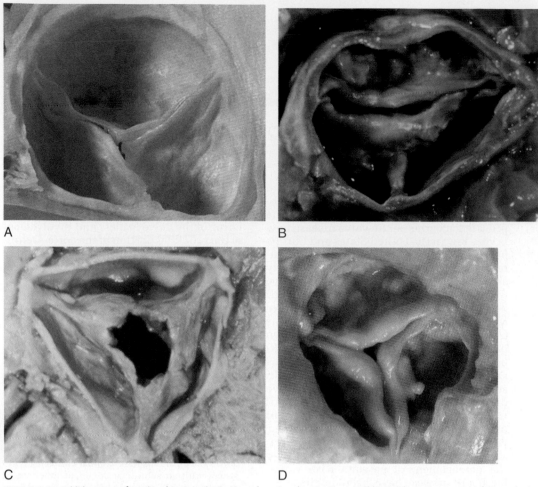

FIGURE 62–1 Major types of aortic valve stenosis. **A,** Normal aortic valve. **B,** Congenital bicuspid aortic stenosis. A false raphe is present at 6 o'clock. **C,** Rheumatic aortic stenosis. The commissures are fused with a fixed central orifice. **D,** Calcific degenerative aortic stenosis. (**A** and **D,** From Manabe H, Yutani C [eds]: Atlas of Valvular Heart Disease. Singapore, Churchill Livingstone, 1998, pp 6 and 131; **B** and **C,** Courtesy of William C. Roberts, MD.)

The risk factors for the development of calcific AS are similar to those for vascular atherosclerosis: elevated serum levels of LDL cholesterol and Lp(a), diabetes, smoking, and hypertension.[17,23,24] Calcific AS has also been linked to inflammatory markers and components of the metabolic syndrome.[25-27] Retrospective studies have linked treatment with HMG-CoA reductase (statin) medications with a lower rate of progression of calcific AS,[28-30] and this effect has been demonstrated in an animal model of hypercholesterolemia.[31] Hence there is growing consensus that "degenerative" calcific AS shares many pathophysiological features with atherosclerosis and that specific pathways might be targeted to prevent or retard disease progression.[12,17,32,33] Although no benefit was seen in a small prospective randomized trial of atorvastatin versus placebo, despite a significant lowering of serum LDL levels, in patients with relatively advanced calcific AS,[34] a subsequent prospective study in patients with less severe AS demonstrated a significant reduction in the rate of progression of aortic stenosis with rosuvastatin.[35] A prospective European trial is in progress with more than 1800 subjects randomized to simvastatin plus ezetimibe or to placebo; results will be available in the near future.

RHEUMATIC AORTIC STENOSIS. Rheumatic AS results from adhesions and fusions of the commissures and cusps and vascularization of the leaflets of the valve ring, leading to retraction and stiffening of the free borders of the cusps. Calcific nodules develop on both surfaces, and the orifice is reduced to a small round or triangular opening (see Fig. 62-1C). As a consequence, the rheumatic valve is often regurgitant, as well as stenotic. Patients with rheumatic AS invariability have rheumatic involvement of the mitral valve. With the decline in rheumatic fever in developed nations, rheumatic AS is decreasing in frequency, although it continues to be a major problem on a worldwide basis.

Pathophysiology (Fig. 62-3)

In adults with AS, outflow obstruction usually develops and increases gradually over a prolonged period. In infants and children with congenital AS, the valve orifice shows little change as the child grows, thereby intensifying the relative obstruction quite gradually. LV function can be well maintained in experimentally produced, gradually developing

2 percent of persons 65 years of age or older had frank calcific AS, whereas 29 percent exhibited age-related aortic valve sclerosis without stenosis, defined by Otto and colleagues[13] as irregular thickening of the aortic valve leaflets detected by echocardiography without significant obstruction and believed to represent a milder and/or earlier disease process. Calcific valve disease, even in the absence of valve obstruction, is associated with a 50 percent increased risk of cardiovascular death and myocardial infarction.[13-15] Although once considered to represent the result of years of normal mechanical stress on an otherwise normal valve, the evolving concept is that the disease process represents proliferative and inflammatory changes, with lipid accumulation, upregulation of angiotensin-converting enzyme (ACE) activity, and infiltration of macrophages and T lymphocytes (Fig. 62-2),[12,13,16,17] ultimately leading to bone formation[18,19] in a manner analogous to vascular calcification. Progressive calcification, initially along the flexion lines at their bases, leads to immobilization of the cusps (see Fig. 62-1D). A high prevalence of calcific AS also exists in patients with Paget disease of bone and end-stage renal disease.

Age-related calcific AS shares common risk factors with mitral annular calcification,[20,21] and the two conditions often coexist. Genetic polymorphisms have been linked to the presence of calcific AS including the vitamin D receptor, interleukin 10 alleles, and the apolipoprotein E4 allele. Familial clustering of calcific AS also has been described, suggesting a possible genetic predisposition to valve calcification.[22]

subcoronary AS in animals. In the experimental model, as well as in children and adults with chronic, severe AS, LV output is maintained by the presence of LV hypertrophy, which may sustain a large pressure gradient across the aortic valve for many years without a reduction in cardiac output, LV dilation, or the development of symptoms.

Severe obstruction to LV outflow is usually characterized by (1) an aortic jet velocity greater than 4 m/sec, (2) a mean systolic pressure gradient exceeding 40 mm Hg in the presence of a normal cardiac output, or (3) an effective aortic orifice (calculated by the continuity equation, see Chap. 14) less than approximately 1.0 cm^2 in an average-sized adult (i.e., <0.6 cm^2/m^2 of body surface area—$< \approx^1/_4$ of the normal aortic orifice of 3.0 to 4.0 cm^2). An aortic valve orifice of 1.0 to 1.5 cm^2 is considered moderate stenosis, and an orifice of 1.5 to 2.0 cm^2 is referred to as *mild stenosis* (Table 62-1). However, the degree of stenosis associated with symptom onset varies between patients and there is no single number that defines severe or critical AS in an individual patient. Clinical decisions are based on consideration of symptom status and the LV response to chronic pressure overload, in conjunction with hemodynamic severity. In some cases, additional measures of hemodynamic severity, such as stroke work loss or valvular impedance, or evaluation with changing loading conditions (e.g., dobutamine stress) or with exercise, are necessary to fully evaluate disease severity.[36]

Chronic pressure overload typically results in concentric LV hypertrophy with increased wall thickness and a normal chamber size. The increased wall thickness allows normalization of wall stress (afterload) so that LV contractile function is maintained. However, the increased myocardial cell mass and increased interstitial fibrosis results in diastolic dysfunction, which may persist even after relief of AS. Gender differences in the LV response to AS have been reported, with women more frequently exhibiting normal LV performance and a smaller, thicker-walled, concentrically hypertrophied left ventricle with diastolic dysfunction (to be discussed) and normal or even subnormal systolic wall stress. Men more frequently have eccentric LV hypertrophy, excessive systolic wall stress, systolic dysfunction, and chamber dilation.

The ventricular changes caused by chronic pressure overload are reflected in the LV and left atrial pressure waveforms and in the Doppler velocity curves. As contraction of the left ventricle becomes progressively more isometric, the LV pressure pulse exhibits a rounded, rather than flattened, summit and the Doppler velocity curve exhibits a progressively later systolic peak. The elevated LV end-diastolic pressure and the corresponding Doppler changes in LV filling, which are characteristic of severe AS, reflect delayed relaxation and eventually decreased compliance of the hypertrophied LV wall. In patients with severe AS, large

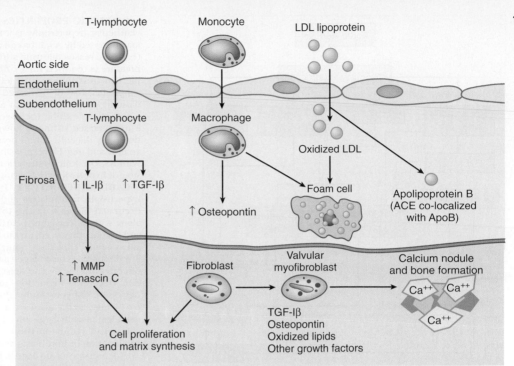

FIGURE 62–2 Potential pathway depicting calcific aortic valve disease. T-lymphocytes and macrophages infiltrate the endothelium and release cytokines, which act on valvular fibroblasts to promote cellular proliferation and extracellular matrix remodeling. A subset of valvular fibroblasts within the fibrosa layer differentiates into myofibroblasts, which possess characteristics of smooth muscle cells. Low-density lipoprotein that is taken into the subendothelial layer is oxidatively modified and taken up by macrophages to become foam cells. Angiotensin-converting enzyme (ACE) is colocalized with apolipoprotein B (ApoB) and facilitates the conversion of angiotensin II (AngII), which acts on angiotensin 1 receptors (AT-1R), expressed on valvular myofibroblasts. A subset of valvular myofibroblasts differentiates into an osteoblast phenotype that is capable of promoting calcium nodule and bone formation. *(From Freeman RV, Otto CM: Spectrum of calcific aortic valve disease: Pathogenesis, disease progression and treatment strategies. Circulation 111: 3316, 2005.)*

CH 62

a waves usually appear in the left atrial pressure pulse and in the Doppler LV filling curve because of the combination of enhanced contraction of a hypertrophied left atrium and diminished LV compliance. Atrial contraction plays a particularly important role in filling of the left ventricle in AS. It raises LV end-diastolic pressure without causing a concomitant elevation of mean left atrial pressure. This "booster pump" function of the left atrium prevents the pulmonary venous and capillary pressures from rising to levels that would produce pulmonary congestion, while at the same time maintaining LV end-diastolic pressure at the elevated level necessary for effective contraction of the hypertrophied left ventricle. Loss of appropriately timed, vigorous atrial contraction, as occurs in atrial fibrillation (AF) or atrioventricular dissociation, may result in rapid clinical deterioration in patients with severe AS.

Systemic vascular resistance also contributes to total LV afterload in adults with AS. Concurrent hypertension increases total ventricular load and may affect the evaluation of AS severity.[37] Mild pulmonary hypertension is present is about one third of adults with AS because of chronic elevation of LV end diastolic pressure; more severe pulmonary hypertension is seen in about 15 percent of AS patients.

Exercise physiology is abnormal in adults with moderate to severe AS, and even asymptomatic patients have a reduced exercise tolerance. Although cardiac output at rest is within normal limits, the normal increase in cardiac output with exercise is blunted and is mediated primarily by increased heart rate with little change in stroke volume. Even though stroke volume is unchanged, transvalvular flow rate increases due to the shortened systolic ejection period so that aortic jet velocity and transvalvular gradient increase proportionally. Prior to symptom onset, valve area increases

Valvular Heart Disease

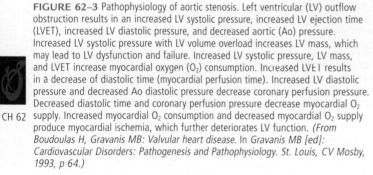

FIGURE 62–3 Pathophysiology of aortic stenosis. Left ventricular (LV) outflow obstruction results in an increased LV systolic pressure, increased LV ejection time (LVET), increased LV diastolic pressure, and decreased aortic (Ao) pressure. Increased LV systolic pressure with LV volume overload increases LV mass, which may lead to LV dysfunction and failure. Increased LV systolic pressure, LV mass, and LVET increase myocardial oxygen (O_2) consumption. Increased LVET results in a decrease of diastolic time (myocardial perfusion time). Increased LV diastolic pressure and decreased Ao diastolic pressure decrease coronary perfusion pressure. Decreased diastolic time and coronary perfusion pressure decrease myocardial O_2 supply. Increased myocardial O_2 consumption and decreased myocardial O_2 supply produce myocardial ischemia, which further deteriorates LV function. (From Boudoulas H, Gravanis MB: Valvular heart disease. In Gravanis MB [ed]: Cardiovascular Disorders: Pathogenesis and Pathophysiology. St. Louis, CV Mosby, 1993, p 64.)

slightly with exercise (by 0.2 cm² on average), but as AS becomes more severe and symptoms are imminent, valve area becomes fixed, resulting in an even greater rise in jet velocity and pressure gradient with exercise. At this point, there is an abnormal blood pressure response to exercise (rise in systolic blood pressure <10 mm Hg) signifying severe valve obstruction.

MYOCARDIAL FUNCTION IN AORTIC STENOSIS

When the aorta is suddenly constricted in experimental animals, LV pressure rises, wall stress increases significantly, and both the extent and the velocity of shortening decline. As pointed out in Chapter 22, the development of LV hypertrophy is one of the principal mechanisms by which the heart adapts to such an increased hemodynamic burden.[38] The increased systolic wall stress induced by AS leads to parallel replication of sarcomeres and concentric hypertrophy. The increase in LV wall thickness is often sufficient to counterbalance the increased pressure so that peak systolic wall tension returns to normal or remains normal if the obstruction develops slowly. An inverse correlation between wall stress and ejection fraction has been described in patients with AS. This suggests that the depressed ejection fraction and velocity of fiber shortening that occur in some patients are a consequence of inadequate wall thickening, resulting in "afterload mismatch." In others, the lower ejection fraction is secondary to a true depression of contractility; in this group, surgical treatment is less effective. Thus both increased afterload and altered contractility are operative to varying extents in depressing LV performance. In order to evaluate myocardial function in patients with AS, the ejection phase indices, such as ejection fraction and myocardial fiber shortening, should be related to the existing wall tension.

DIASTOLIC PROPERTIES (see also Chaps. 21 and 26). Although ventricular hypertrophy is a key adaptive mechanism to the pressure load imposed by AS, it has an adverse pathophysiological consequence (i.e., it increases diastolic stiffness).[38] As a result, greater intracavitary pressure is required for LV filling. Some patients with AS manifest an increase in stiffness of the left ventricle (increased chamber stiffness) simply because of increased muscle mass with no alteration in the diastolic properties of each unit of myocardium (normal muscle stiffness); others exhibit increases in both chamber and muscle stiffness. This increased stiffness, however produced, contributes to the elevation of LV diastolic filling pressure at any level of ventricular diastolic volume and may be responsible for flash pulmonary edema in patients with AS. Diastolic dysfunction may revert toward normal with regression of hypertrophy following surgical relief of AS.

CARDIAC STRUCTURE. In adults with AS, both myocardial cellular hypertrophy and relative and absolute increases in connective tissue occur. An increase in the total collagen volume of the myocardium along with increased myocardial gene expression for collagen I and III and fibronectin are related to activation of the cardiac renin angiotensin system.[39] This likely contributes to the altered diastolic properties just discussed. The collagen and fibronectin gene expression correlates directly with the LV end-diastolic pressure and inversely with the ejection fraction.[39] Reduction in renin-angiotensin activation parallels regression of hypertrophy after relief of AS.[40]

Changes in the myocardial ultrastructure in patients with severe AS include unusually large nuclei, loss of myofibrils, accumulation of mitochondria, large cytoplasmic areas devoid of contractile material, and proliferation of fibroblasts and collagen fibers in the interstitial space. The depression of myocardial function that occurs late in the course of the disease may well be related to these morphological alterations.

ISCHEMIA. In patients with AS, coronary blood flow at rest is elevated in absolute terms but is normal when corrections are made for myocardial mass.[41] Reduced coronary blood flow reserve may produce inadequate myocardial oxygenation in patients with severe AS, even in the absence of coronary artery disease. The hypertrophied LV muscle mass, the increased systolic pressure, and the prolongation of ejection all elevate myocardial oxygen consumption. The abnormally heightened pressure compressing the coronary arteries may exceed the coronary perfusion pressure, and the shortening of diastole interferes with coronary blood flow, thus leading to an imbalance between myocardial oxygen supply and demand.[42] Myocardial perfusion is also impaired by the relative decrease in myocardial capillary density as myocardial mass increases and by the elevation of LV end-diastolic pressure, which lowers the aortic-LV pressure gradient in diastole (i.e., the coronary perfusion pressure gradient). This underperfusion may be responsible for the development of subendocardial ischemia,[41] especially when oxygen demand is increased or the diastolic filling period is reduced (e.g., tachycardia, anemia, infection, pregnancy).

Myocardial ischemia in patients with severe AS and normal coronary arteries may also develop secondary to high systolic and diastolic stresses caused by inadequate ventricular hypertrophy and the reduced coronary flow reserve just described. Metabolical evidence of myocardial ischemia (i.e., lactate production) can be demonstrated when myocardial oxygen needs are stimulated by exercise or by isoproterenol in patients with AS, even in the absence of coronary artery narrowing.[43]

Clinical Presentation

Symptoms

The cardinal manifestations of acquired AS are exertional dyspnea, angina pectoris, syncope, and ultimately heart failure.[43,44] Many patients now are diagnosed before symptom onset on the basis of the finding of a systolic murmur on physical examination with confirmation of the diagnosis by echocardiography. Symptoms typically occur at age 50 to 70 years with bicuspid aortic valve stenosis and at older than age 70 years with calcific stenosis of a trileaflet valve, although even in this age group about 40 percent of AS patients have a congenital bicuspid valve.[3]

The most common clinical presentation in patients with a known diagnosis of AS who are followed prospectively is a gradual decrease in exercise tolerance, fatigue, or dyspnea on exertion. The mechanism of exertional dyspnea may be

TABLE 62-1	Classification of the Severity of Valve Disease in Adults		
	Mild	Moderate	Severe
Aortic Stenosis			
Jet velocity (m/s)	<3.0	3.0-4.0	>4.0
Mean gradient (mm Hg)*	<25	25-40	>40
Valve area (cm²)	>1.5	1.0-1.5	<1.0
Valve area index (cm²/m²)			<0.6
Mitral Stenosis			
Mean gradient (mm Hg)*	<5	5-10	>10
Pulmonary artery systolic pressure (mm Hg)	<30	30-50	>50
Valve area (cm²)	>1.5	1.0-1.5	<1.0
Aortic Regurgitation			
Qualitative			
Angiographic grade	1+	2+	3-4+
Color Doppler jet width	Central jet, width <25% of LVOT	> Mild but no signs of severe AR	Central jet, width > 65% of LVOT
Doppler vena contracta width (cm)	<0.3	0.3-0.6	>0.6
Quantitative (Cath or Echo)			
Regurgitant volume (ml/beat)	<30	30-59	≥60
Regurgitant fraction (%)	<30	30-49	≥50
Regurgitant orifice area (cm²)	<0.10	0.10-0.29	≥0.30
Additional Essential Criteria			
Left ventricular size			Increased
Mitral Regurgitation			
Qualitative			
Angiographic grade	1+	2+	3-4+
Color Doppler jet area	Small, central jet (<4 cm² or <20% LA area)	Signs of MR >mild present, but no criteria for severe MR	Vena contracta width >0.7 cm with large central MR jet (area >40% of LA area) or with a wall-impinging jet of any size, swirling in LA
Doppler vena contracta width (cm)	<0.3	0.3-0.69	≥0.7
Quantitative (Cath or Echo)			
Regurgitant volume (ml/beat)	<30	30-59	≥60
Regurgitant fraction (%)	<30	30-49	≥50
Regurgitant orifice area (cm²)	<0.20	0.2-0.39	≥0.40
Additional Essential Criteria			
Left atrial size			Enlarged
Left ventricular size			Enlarged

Right-Sided Valve Disease (Severe)
Severe tricuspid stenosis: Valve area <1.0 cm²
Severe tricuspid regurgitation: Vena contracta width >0.7 cm and systolic flow reversal in hepatic veins
Severe pulmonic stenosis: Jet velocity >4 m/sec or maximum gradient >60 mm Hg
Severe pulmonic regurgitation: Color jet fills outflow tract
Dense continuous wave Doppler signal with a steep deceleration slope

*Valve gradients are flow dependent and when used as estimates of severity of valve stenosis should be assessed with knowledge of cardiac output or forward flow across the valve.

From Bonow RO, Carabello BA, Chatterjee K, et al: ACC/AHA 2006 guidelines for the management of patients with valvular heart disease: A report of the American College of Cardiology/American Heart Association Task Force on Practice Guidelines (writing committee to revise the 1998 Guidelines for the Management of Patients with Valvular Heart Disease): Developed in collaboration with the Society of Cardiovascular Anesthesiologists: endorsed by the Society for Cardiovascular Angiography and Interventions and the Society of Thoracic Surgeons. Circulation 114:e84, 2006; Zoghbi WA, Enriquez-Sarano M, Foster E, et al: Recommendations for evaluation of the severity of native valvular regurgitation with two-dimensional and Doppler echocardiography. J Am Soc Echocardiogr 16:777, 2003.

LV diastolic dysfunction with an excessive rise in end-diastolic pressure leading to pulmonary congestive. Alternatively, exertional symptoms may be due to the limited ability to increase cardiac output with exercise. More severe exertional dyspnea with orthopnea, paroxysmal nocturnal dyspnea, and pulmonary edema reflect varying degrees of pulmonary venous hypertension. These are relatively late symptoms in patients with AS, and intervention now is typically undertaken before this disease stage.

Angina occurs in approximately two thirds of patients with severe AS (about half of whom have associated significant coronary artery obstruction).[43] It usually resembles the angina observed in patients with coronary artery disease, in that it is commonly precipitated by exertion and relieved by rest. In patients without coronary artery disease, angina results from the combination of the increased oxygen needs of the hypertrophied myocardium and the reduction of oxygen delivery secondary to the excessive compression of coronary vessels.[42] In patients with coronary artery disease, angina is caused by a combination of the epicardial coronary artery obstruction in combination with the oxygen imbalance characteristic of AS. Very rarely, angina results from calcium emboli to the coronary vascular bed.

Syncope is most commonly due to the reduced cerebral perfusion that occurs during exertion when arterial pressure declines consequent to systemic vasodilation in the presence of a fixed cardiac output. Syncope has also been attributed to malfunction of the baroreceptor mechanism in severe AS, as well as to a vasodepressor response to a greatly elevated LV systolic pressure during exercise. Premonitory symptoms of syncope are common. Exertional hypotension may also be manifested as "graying out" spells or dizziness on effort. Syncope at rest may be due to transient ventricular fibrillation, from which the patient recovers spontaneously; to transient AF with loss of the atrial contribution to LV filling, which causes a precipitous decline in cardiac output; or to transient atrioventricular block due to extension of the calcification of the valve into the conduction system.

Other late findings in patients with isolated AS include AF, pulmonary hypertension, and systemic venous hypertension. Although AS may be responsible for sudden death, this usually occurs in patients who had previously been symptomatic (see Chap. 36).

Gastrointestinal bleeding may develop in patients with severe AS, often associated with angiodysplasia (most commonly of the right colon) or other vascular malformations. This complication arises from shear stress–induced platelet aggregation with reduction in high-molecular-weight multimers of von Willebrand factor and increases in proteolytic subunit fragments.[45] These abnormalities correlate with the severity of AS and are correctable by AVR.[45,46]

Infective endocarditis is a greater risk in younger patients with milder valvular deformity than in older patients with rocklike calcific aortic deformities. Cerebral emboli resulting in stroke or transient ischemic attacks may be due to microthrombi on thickened bicuspid valves. Calcific AS may cause embolization of calcium to various organs including the heart, kidneys, and brain. Abrupt loss of vision has been reported when calcific emboli occlude the central retinal artery.[43]

Physical Examination

The key features on physical examination in patients with AS are palpation of the carotid upstroke, evaluation of the systolic murmur, assessment of splitting of the second heart sound, and examination for signs of heart failure.

The carotid upstroke directly reflects the arterial pressure waveform. The expected finding with severe AS is a slow-rising, late-peaking, low-amplitude carotid pulse, the "parvus and tardus" carotid impulse (Fig. 62-4). When present, this finding is specific for severe AS. However, many adults with AS have concurrent conditions, such as AR or systemic hypertension, that affect the arterial pressure curve, and the carotid impulse. Thus an apparently normal carotid impulse is not reliable for excluding the diagnosis of severe AS. Similarly, blood pressure is not a helpful method for evaluation of AS severity. When severe AS is present, systolic blood pressure and pulse pressures may be reduced. However, in patients with associated AR or in older patients with an inelastic arterial bed, both systolic and pulse pressures may be normal or even increased. With severe AS, radiation of the murmur to the carotids may result in a palpable thrill or carotid shudder.

The cardiac impulse is sustained and becomes displaced inferiorly and laterally with LV failure. Presystolic distention of the left ventricle (i.e., a prominent precordial a wave) is often both visible and palpable. A hyperdynamic left ventricle suggests concomitant AR and/or mitral regurgitation (MR). A systolic thrill is usually best appreciated when the patient leans forward during full expiration. It is palpated most readily in the 2nd right intercostal space or in the suprasternal notch and is frequently transmitted along the carotid arteries. A systolic thrill is quite specific, but not sensitive, for severe AS.

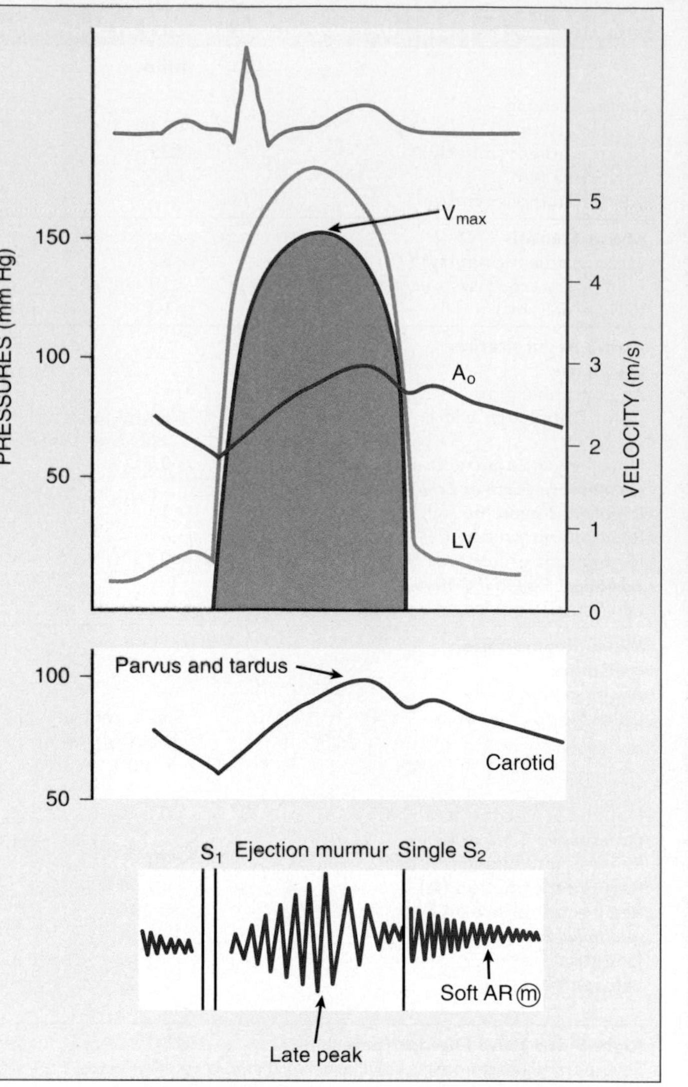

AUSCULTATION. The ejection systolic murmur of AS typically is late peaking and heard best at the base of the heart with radiation to the carotids (see Fig. 62-4). Cessation of the murmur before A2 is helpful in differentiation from a pansystolic mitral murmur. In patients with calcified aortic valves, the systolic murmur is loudest at the base of the heart, but high-frequency components may radiate to the apex (the so-called *Gallavardin phenomenon*), in which the murmur may be so prominent that it is mistaken for the murmur of MR. In general,

FIGURE 62–4 Relationship between left ventricular (LV) and aortic (Ao) pressures and the Doppler aortic stenosis velocity curve (in red) is shown. The pressure difference between the left ventricle and aorta in systole is four times the velocity squared (the Bernoulli equation). Thus a maximum velocity (V_{max}) of 4.3 m/sec corresponds to a maximum LV to Ao pressure difference of 74 mm Hg and a mean systolic gradient of 44 mm Hg. On physical examination the slow rate of rise and delayed peak in the carotid pulse (or parvus and tardus) matches the contour of the aortic pressure waveform. The murmur corresponds to the Doppler velocity curve with a harsh crescendo-decrescendo late-peaking systolic murmur, best heard at the aortic region (upper right sternal border). Often a soft high-pitched diastolic decrescendo murmur of aortic regurgitation also is appreciated.

a louder and later peaking murmur, indicates more severe stenosis. However, although a systolic murmur of grade 3 intensity or greater is relatively specific for severe AS, this finding is insensitive and many patients with severe AS have only a grade 2 murmur. High-pitched decrescendo diastolic murmurs secondary to AR are common in many patients with dominant AS.

Splitting of the second heart sound is helpful in excluding the diagnosis of severe AS because normal splitting implies the aortic valve leaflets are flexible enough to create an audible closing sound (A2). With severe AS, S2 may be single because calcification and immobility of the aortic valve make A2 inaudible, P2 is buried in the prolonged aortic ejection murmur, or prolongation of LV systole makes A2 coincide with P2. Paradoxical splitting of S2, which suggests associated left bundle branch block or LV dysfunction, may also occur. Thus in older adults, normal splitting of S2 indicates a low likelihood of severe AS. S1 is normal or soft and S4 is prominent, presumably because atrial contraction is vigorous and the mitral valve is partially closed during presystole.

In young patients with congenital AS (see Chap. 61), the flexible valve may result in an accentuated A2 so that S2 may be normally split, even with severe valve obstruction. In addition, an aortic ejection sound may be audible, due to the halting upward movement of the aortic valve. Like an audible A2, this sound is dependent on mobility of the valve cusps and disappears when they become severely calcified. Thus it is common in children and young adults with congenital AS but is rare in adults with acquired calcific AS and rigid valves.

When the left ventricle fails and the stroke volume falls, the systolic murmur of AS becomes softer; rarely, it disappears altogether. The slow rise in the arterial pulse is more difficult to recognize. Stated simply, with LV failure, the clinical picture changes from typical AS to that of severe LV failure with a low cardiac output. Thus occult AS may be a cause of intractable heart failure, and severe AS should be ruled out by echocardiography in patients with heart failure of unknown cause because operative treatment may be life saving and result in substantial clinical improvement.

DYNAMIC AUSCULTATION. The intensity of the systolic murmur varies from beat to beat when the duration of diastolic filling varies, as in AF or following a premature contraction. This characteristic is helpful in differentiating AS from MR, in which the murmur is usually unaffected. The murmur of valvular AS is augmented by squatting, which increases stroke volume. It is reduced in intensity during the strain of the Valsalva maneuver and when standing, which reduce transvalvular flow.

Echocardiography

Echocardiography is the standard approach for evaluating and following patients with AS and selecting them for operation (see also Chap. 14 and Figs. 14-38, 39, 40, 47, 48, and 49).

Echocardiographic imaging allows accurate definition of valve anatomy including the cause of AS and the severity of valve calcification and sometimes allows direct imaging of the orifice area. Echocardiographic imaging also is invaluable for evaluation of LV hypertrophy and systolic function, with calculation of ejection fraction, as well as for measurement of aortic root dimensions and detection of associated mitral valve disease.[47]

Doppler echocardiography allows measurement of the transaortic jet velocity, which is the most useful measure for following disease severity and predicting clinical outcome. Effective orifice area is calculated using the continuity equation, and mean transaortic pressure gradient can be calculated using the modified Bernoulli equation (see Fig. 14-40).[36,48,49] Both valve area and pressure gradient calculations from Doppler data have been well validated compared with invasive hemodynamics (see Fig. 62-38A) and in terms of their ability to predict clinical outcome. However, the accuracy of these measures requires an experienced laboratory with meticulous attention to technical details.

The combination of pulsed, continuous wave and color flow Doppler echocardiography is helpful in detecting and determining the severity of AR (which coexists in ≈75 percent of patients with predominant AS) and in estimating pulmonary artery pressure. In some patients, additional measures of AS severity may be necessary, such as correction for poststenotic pressure recovery, calculation of ventricular stroke work loss or valvular impedance, or transesophageal imaging of valve anatomy.[36] Evaluation of AS severity is affected by the presence of systemic hypertension so that reevaluation after blood pressure control may be necessary.[37] In patients with LV dysfunction and low cardiac output, assessing the severity of AS can be enhanced by assessing hemodynamic changes during dobutamine infusion (discussed subsequently).

Other Diagnostic Evaluation

ELECTROCARDIOGRAPHY. The principal ECG change is LV hypertrophy, which is found in approximately 85 percent of patients with severe AS. The absence of LV hyper-

trophy does not exclude the presence of critical AS, and the correlation between the absolute ECG voltages in precordial leads and the severity of obstruction is poor in adults but good in children with congenital AS. T wave inversion and ST segment depression in leads with upright QRS complexes are common. There is evidence of left atrial enlargement in more than 80 percent of patients with severe, isolated AS. AF occurs in only 10 to 15 percent of AS patients. The extension of calcific infiltrates from the aortic valve into the conduction system may cause various forms and degrees of atrioventricular and intraventricular block in 5 percent of patients with calcific AS. Such conduction defects are more common in patients who have associated mitral annular calcification.

RADIOLOGICAL FINDINGS (see Figs. 15-8 and 15-21). On chest radiography the heart is usually of normal size or slightly enlarged, with a rounding of the LV border and apex, unless regurgitation or LV failure is present and causes substantial cardiomegaly. Dilatation of the ascending aorta is a common finding, particularly in patients with a bicuspid aortic valve. Calcification of the aortic valve is found in almost all adults with hemodynamically significant AS but is rarely visible on chest radiograph, although readily detected on fluoroscopy or by cardiac computed tomography (see Fig. 18-14). The left atrium may be slightly enlarged in patients with severe AS, and there may be radiological signs of pulmonary venous hypertension. However, when left atrial enlargement is marked, the presence of associated mitral valvular disease should be suspected.

CARDIAC CATHETERIZATION AND ANGIOGRAPHY. In nearly all patients the echocardiographic examination provides the important hemodynamic information required for patient management, and cardiac catheterization now is recommended only when noninvasive tests are inconclusive, when clinical and echocardiographic findings are discrepant, and for coronary angiography prior to surgical intervention.[48,49,50] Hemodynamic or echocardiographic assessment of AS severity at rest and with dobutamine is reasonable when AS is associated with low cardiac output and impaired LV function.[1]

CHEST COMPUTED TOMOGRAPHY. In addition to assessing aortic valve calcification, chest CT is useful for evaluating aortic dilation in patients with evidence of aortic root disease by echocardiography or on chest radiography. Measurement of aortic dimensions at several levels including the sinuses of Valsalva, sinotubular junction, and ascending aorta is necessary for clinical decision making and surgical planning.

CARDIAC MAGNETIC RESONANCE (CMR) (see also Chap. 17). CMR is useful in assessing LV volume, function, and mass, especially in settings in which this information cannot be obtained readily from echocardiography. AS severity also can be quantitated by cardiac MRI, although this approach is not widely used (see Fig. 17-13).[51,52]

Disease Course

Clinical Outcome

ASYMPTOMATIC PATIENTS. The severity of outflow tract obstruction gradually increases over 10 to 15 years, so there is a long latent period during which stenosis severity is only mild to moderate and clinical outcomes are similar to age-matched normal patients.[1,43,44] In patients with mild valve thickening but no obstruction to outflow (e.g., aortic sclerosis) 16 percent will develop valve obstruction at 1 year of follow-up, but only 2.5 percent develop severe valve obstruction at an average of 8 years after the diagnosis of aortic sclerosis.[53]

Once moderate to severe stenosis is present, prognosis remains excellent as long as the patient remains asymptomatic. However, a recent retrospective study of survival in adults with severe aortic stenosis diagnosed by echocardiography emphasizes the progressive nature of the disease and the need for close follow-up.[54] Although ste-

TABLE 62–2 | **Clinical Outcomes in Prospective Studies of Asymptomatic Aortic Stenosis in Adults**

Author, Year	No. of Patients	Severity of Aortic Stenosis	Age (Yr)	Mean Follow-up	Event-Free Survival without Symptoms
Kelly et al., 1988	51	$V_{max}>3.6$ m/sec	63±8	5-25 mo	Overall: 59% at 15 mo
Pellikka et al., 1990	113	$V_{max}\geq4.0$ m/sec	40-94	20 mo	Overall: 86% at 1 yr 62% at 2 yr
Kennedy et al., 1991	66	AVA 0.7-1.2 cm²	67±10	35 mo	Overall: 59% at 4 yr
Otto et al., 1997	123	$V_{max}\geq2.6$ m/sec	63±16	2.5±1.4 yr	Overall: 93±5% at 1 yr 62±8% at 3 yr 26±10% at 5 yr *Subgroups:* $V_{max}<3$ m/sec: 84±16% at 2 yr V_{max} 3-4 m/sec: 66±13% at 2 yr $V_{max}>4$ m/sec: 21±18% at 2 yr
Rosenhek et al., 2000	128	$V_{max}>4.0$ m/sec	60±18	22±18 mo	Overall: 67±5% at 1 yr 56±55% at 2 yr 33±5% at 4 yr *Subgroups:* No or mild Ca⁺⁺: 75±9% at 4 yr Mod-severe Ca⁺⁺: 20±5% at 4 yr
Amato et al., 2001	66	AVA≤1.0 cm²	18-80 (50±15)	15±12 mo	Overall: 57% at 1 yr 38% at 2 yr *Subgroups:* AVA 0.7 cm² or greater: 72% at 2 yr AVA<0.7 cm²: 21% at 2 yr Negative exercise test: 85% at 2 yr Positive exercise test*: 19% at 2 yr
Das et al., 2005	125	AVA<1.4 cm²	56-74 (mean 65)	12 mo	Overall: 71% at 1 yr *Subgroups:* AVA 1.2 cm² or greater: 100% at 1 yr AVA 0.8 cm² or less: 46% at 1 yr No symptoms on exercise test: 89% at 1 yr Symptoms on exercise test: 49% at 1 yr
Pellikka et al., 2005	622	$V_{max}\geq4.0$ m/sec	72±11	5.4±4.0 yr	Overall: 82% at 1 yr 67% at 2 yr 33% at 5 yr

*Positive exercise test=symptoms, abnormal ST-segment response, or abnormal blood pressure response (<20 mm Hg increase) with exercise.

AVA=aortic valve area; Ca++=aortic valve calcification; Mod=moderate; V_{max}=maximum velocity

From Bonow RO, Carabello BA, Chatterjee K, et al: ACC/AHA 2006 guidelines for the management of patients with valvular heart disease: A report of the American College of Cardiology/American Heart Association Task Force on Practice Guidelines (writing committee to revise the 1998 Guidelines for the Management of Patients with Valvular Heart Disease): Developed in collaboration with the Society of Cardiovascular Anesthesiologists: endorsed by the Society for Cardiovascular Angiography and Interventions and the Society of Thoracic Surgeons. Circulation 114:e84, 2006.

nosis severity on average is more severe in symptomatic versus asymptomatic patients, there is marked overlap in all measures of severity between these two groups. Prospective studies evaluating the rate of progression to symptomatic AS in initially asymptomatic patients are summarized in Table 62-2. The strongest predictor of progression to symptoms is the Doppler aortic jet velocity. Survival free of symptoms is 84 percent at 2 years when jet velocity is less than 3 m/sec compared with only 21 percent when jet velocity is greater than 4 m/sec (Fig. 62-5).[36] In adults with severe AS (Doppler velocity >4 m/sec) event-free survival at 5 years is 75 ± 9 percent in those with little valve calcification compared with 20 ± 5 percent in those with moderate to severe valve calcification.[55,56] Retrospective studies reported some cases of sudden death in apparently asymptomatic adults with severe AS. However, more recent prospective studies suggest that sudden death in asymptomatic patients is very unlikely, with an estimated risk of less than 1 percent per year.[1,57]

SYMPTOMATIC PATIENTS. Once even mild symptoms are present, survival is poor unless outflow obstruction is relieved. Survival curves derived from older retrospective studies show that the interval from the onset of symptoms to the time of death is approximately 2 years in patients with heart failure, 3 years in those with syncope, and 5 years in those with angina. More recent series confirm this poor prognosis with an average survival of only 1 to 3 years after symptom onset.[1,55] Among symptomatic patients with severe AS, the outlook is poorest when the left ventricle has failed and the cardiac output and transvalvular gradient are both low. The risk of sudden death is high

with symptomatic severe AS, so these patients should be promptly referred for surgical intervention. In patients who do not undergo surgical intervention, recurrent hospitalizations for angina and decompensated heart failure are common.

Hemodynamic Progression

The average rate of hemodynamic progression is an annual decrease in aortic valve area of 0.12 cm²/year,[36] an increase in aortic jet velocity of 0.32 m/sec per year, and an increase in mean gradient of 7 mm Hg per year. However, the rate of progression is highly variable and difficult to predict in individual patients. In clinical studies the factors associated with more rapid hemodynamic progression include older age, more severe leaflet calcification, renal insufficiency, hypertension, smoking and hyperlipidemia. The role of genetic factors remains unclear.

Because of the variability in hemodynamic severity at symptom onset and because many patients fail to recognize symptom onset due to the insidious rate of disease progression, both exercise testing (see Table 62-2)[58,59] and serum brain natriuretic peptide (BNP) levels[60-62] have been evaluated as measures of disease progression and predictors of symptom onset. Clearly, patients who develop symptoms on treadmill exercise or who have a fall in blood pressure with exertion show evidence of severe symptomatic disease. An elevated BNP level may be helpful when symptoms are equivocal or when stenosis severity is only moderate, but the role of BNP in evaluation of disease progression has not been fully defined.

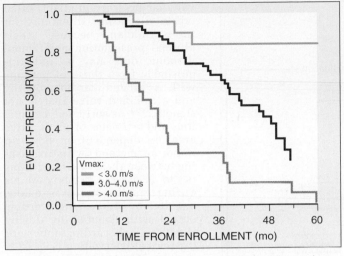

FIGURE 62–5 Natural history of asymptomatic patients with aortic stenosis. Initial aortic jet velocity (Vmax) stratifies patients according to the likelihood that symptoms requiring valve replacement will develop over time. The majority of events in this series were the onset of symptoms warranting aortic valve replacement. *(From Otto CM, Burwarsh IG, Legget ME, et al: A prospective study of asymptomatic valvular aortic stenosis: Clinical, echocardiographic, and exercise predictors of outcome. Circulation 95:2262, 1997.)*

Management

Medical Treatment

The most important principle in management of adults with AS is patient education regarding the disease course and typical symptoms.[36,63] Patients should be advised to report promptly the development of any symptoms possibly related to AS. Patients with severe AS should be cautioned to avoid vigorous athletic and physical activity. However, such restrictions do not apply to patients with mild obstruction. Evolving recommendations for infective endocarditis prophylaxis should be explained (see Chap. 63). Although medical therapy has not been shown to affect disease progression, adults with AS (as any other adult) should be evaluated and treated for conventional coronary disease risk factors, as per established guidelines.[17,34]

Echocardiography is recommended for initial diagnosis and assessment of AS severity, for assessment of LV hypertrophy and systolic function, for reevaluation in patients with changing signs or symptoms, and for reevaluation annually for severe AS, every 1-2 years for moderate AS, and every 3 to 5 years for mild AS.[1,2] Because patients may tailor their lifestyles to minimize symptoms or may ascribe fatigue and dyspnea to deconditioning or aging, they may not recognize early symptoms as important warning signals, although these symptoms often can be elicited by a careful history. Exercise testing may be helpful in apparently asymptomatic patients to detect covert symptoms, limited exercise capacity, or an abnormal blood pressure response.[1,36] Exercise stress testing should be absolutely avoided in symptomatic patients.

Symptomatic patients with severe AS are usually operative candidates because medical therapy has little to offer. However, medical therapy may be necessary in patients who are considered to be inoperable (usually because of comorbid conditions that preclude surgery). Although diuretics are beneficial when there is abnormal accumulation of fluid, they must be used with caution because hypovolemia may reduce the elevated LV end-diastolic pressure, lower cardiac output, and produce orthostatic hypotension. ACE inhibitors should be used with caution but are beneficial in treating patients with symptomatic LV systolic dysfunction who

are not candidates for surgery. They should be initiated at low doses and increased slowly to target doses, avoiding hypotension. Beta-adrenergic blockers can depress myocardial function and induce LV failure and should be avoided in patients with AS.

Atrial flutter or fibrillation occurs in less than 10 percent of patients with severe AS, perhaps because of the late occurrence of left atrial enlargement in this condition. When such an arrhythmia is observed in a patient with AS, the possibility of associated mitral valvular disease should be considered. When AF occurs, the rapid ventricular rate may cause angina pectoris. The loss of the atrial contribution to ventricular filling and a sudden fall in cardiac output may cause serious hypotension. Therefore AF should be treated promptly, usually with cardioversion. New onset AF in a previously asymptomatic patient with severe AS may be a marker of impending symptom onset.

Management of concurrent cardiac conditions, such as hypertension and coronary disease, is complicated in patients with asymptomatic AS by the concern that vasodilatory effects of medications may not be offset by a compensatory increase in cardiac output. Despite this concern, AS patients should receive appropriate treatment for concurrent disease, although medications should be started at low doses and slowly titrated upward with close monitoring of blood pressure and symptoms. Adults with asymptomatic severe AS can undergo noncardiac surgery and pregnancy with careful hemodynamic monitoring and optimization of loading conditions. However, when stenosis is very severe, elective AVR prior to noncardiac surgery or a planned pregnancy may be considered.[64]

Surgical Treatment

CHILDREN. In the adolescent or young adult with severe congenital AS, balloon aortic valvotomy is recommended in all symptomatic patients and in asymptomatic patients with a transvalvular gradient greater than 60 mm Hg or ECG ST changes at rest or with exercise. The same indications are appropriate for surgical intervention, although balloon valvotomy is probably preferable at experienced centers.[1] At surgery, simple commissural incision under direct vision usually leads to substantial hemodynamic improvement with low risk (i.e., a mortality rate of <1 percent) (see Chap. 61). Despite the salutary hemodynamic results following percutaneous or surgical valvotomy, the valve is not rendered entirely normal anatomically. The turbulent blood flow through the valve may subsequently lead to further deformation, calcification, the development of regurgitation, and restenosis after 10 to 20 years, often requiring reoperation and valve replacement later.

ADULTS. AVR is recommended in adults with symptomatic severe AS, even if symptoms are mild. AVR also is recommended for severe AS with an ejection fraction less than 50 percent and in patients with severe asymptomatic AS who are undergoing coronary bypass grafting or other heart surgery (Fig. 62-6)[1,2,65-69] In addition, AVR may be considered for severe AS when exercise testing provokes symptoms or a fall in blood pressure. In asymptomatic patients with severe AS and a low operative risk, AVR may be considered when markers of rapid disease progression are present or when AS is very severe, depending on patient preferences regarding the risk of earlier intervention versus careful monitoring with intervention promptly at symptom onset.[1] Coronary angiography should be performed before valve replacement in most adults with AS.

Surgical AVR is the procedure of choice for relief of outflow obstruction in adults with valvular AS. Surgical repair is not feasible as attempts at debridement of valve calcification have not been successful. Balloon aortic valvotomy has only a modest hemodynamic effect in patients

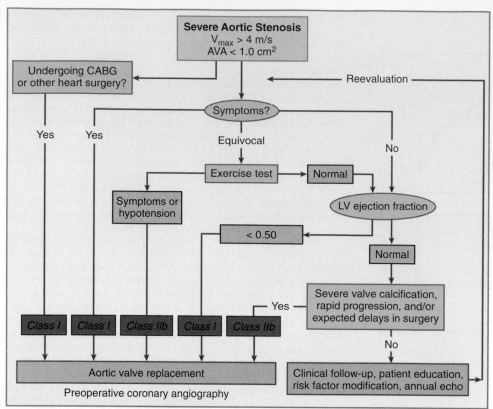

FIGURE 62-6 Management strategy for patients with severe aortic stenosis. Preoperative coronary angiography should be performed routinely as determined by age, symptoms, and coronary risk factors. Cardiac catheterization and angiography may also be helpful when there is discordance between clinical findings and echocardiography. AVA = aortic valve area, BP = blood pressure, CABG = coronary artery bypass graft surgery, LV = left ventricular, V_{max} = maximal velocity across aortic valve by Doppler echocardiography. *(From Bonow RO, Carabello BA, Chatterjee K, et al: ACC/AHA 2006 guidelines for the management of patients with valvular heart disease: a report of the American College of Cardiology/American Heart Association Task Force on Practice Guidelines (writing committee to revise the 1998 Guidelines for the Management of Patients With Valvular Heart Disease): Developed in collaboration with the Society of Cardiovascular Anesthesiologists: Endorsed by the Society for Cardiovascular Angiography and Interventions and the Society of Thoracic Surgeons. Circulation 114:e84, 2006.)*

valvular pressure gradient) often create diagnostic dilemmas for the clinician because their clinical presentation and hemodynamic data may be indistinguishable from those of patients with a dilated cardiomyopathy and a calcified valve that is not stenotic.[38,82] As aortic valve velocities and estimates of aortic valve area are dependent on flow, an important method for distinguishing between these two conditions is to reassess hemodynamics during transient increases in flow, usually by increasing cardiac output with dobutamine during Doppler echocardiography or cardiac catheterization (Fig. 62-7; see also Fig. 14-49).[77,78,83] Patients with severe AS will manifest an increase in valve gradient and no change in valve area during dobutamine, whereas those with mild or moderate AS manifest an increase in calculated valve area. Dobutamine echocardiography also provides evidence of myocardial contractile reserve, which is an important predictor of operative risk, improvement in LV function, and survival after AVR in these patients.[78,79]

RESULTS. Successful replacement of the aortic valve results in substantial clinical and hemodynamic improvement in patients with AS, AR, or combined lesions. In patients without frank LV failure, the operative risk ranges from 2 to 5 percent in most centers, and in patients younger than 70 years of age the operative risk has been reported to be as low as 1 percent. The STS National Database Committee reports an overall operative mortality rate of 4 percent in 32,968 patients undergoing isolated AVR and 6.8 percent in 32,538 patients undergoing AVR and coronary artery bypass grafting[84] (Table 62-3). Risk factors associated with a higher mortality rate include a high New York Heart Association (NYHA) class, impairment of LV function, advanced age, and the presence of associated coronary artery disease. The 10-year actuarial survival rate of hospital survivors in surgically treated patients is approximately 85 percent.[1,85-87] Risk factors for late death include higher preoperative NYHA class, advanced age, concomitant untreated coronary artery disease, preoperative impaired LV function, preoperative ventricular arrhythmias, and associated significant AR.

Although age is a determinant of risk, there is increasing experience in most surgical centers in performing AVR in symptomatic patients older than 70 or even 80 years of age with calcific AS.[80,88] The results of AVR are often quite satisfactory in this age group, with improved quality of life and survival. Surgical risk is related to the higher prevalence of comorbid conditions in older patients, rather than to age per se.[87] Therefore advanced age should not be considered a contraindication to operation. Particular attention must be directed to the adequacy of hepatic, renal, and pulmonary functions in these patients.

Symptoms of pulmonary congestion (exertional dyspnea) and of myocardial ischemia (angina pectoris) are relieved in almost all patients, and most patients will have an improvement in exercise tolerance, even if only mildly reduced prior to surgery. Hemodynamic results of AVR are also impressive; elevated end-diastolic and end-systolic volumes show significant reduction. Impaired ventricular performance returns to normal more frequently in patients with AS than in those with AR or MR. However, the finding that the strongest predictor of postoperative LV dysfunction is preoperative dysfunction[1,38,43]

with calcific AS and does not favorably impact long-term outcome. Thus balloon aortic valvotomy is not recommended as an alternate to AVR for calcific AS. In selected cases, balloon valvotomy might be reasonable as a bridge to surgery in unstable patients or as a palliative procedure when surgery is very high risk. Newer percutaneous methods for implantation of prosthetic valves in seriously ill patients who are not candidates for surgery are under development.[70] Limited clinical experience has been reported to date.[71-73]

AORTIC STENOSIS WITH LEFT VENTRICULAR DYSFUNCTION. Surgical risk is higher in patients with impaired LV function (EF < 35 percent).[74-78] However, their prognosis is extremely poor without operation, overall survival is improved with AVR, and many patients in this group have significant clinical and functional recovery following AVR.[74-79] Hence AVR should generally be offered to these patients. Even octogenarians with LV dysfunction can have improved survival after AVR, although their operative risks are higher.[74,76,80] Exceptions are patients with advanced congestive heart failure or LV dysfunction that can be related to previous myocardial infarction rather than to AS. In acutely ill patients with decompensated heart failure, nitroprusside has been reported to be safe and effective in rapidly improving hemodynamics[81] and may be used in bridging critically ill patients to AVR.

AORTIC STENOSIS WITH LOW GRADIENT AND LOW CARDIAC OUTPUT. Patients with critical AS, severe LV dysfunction, and low cardiac output (and hence a low trans-

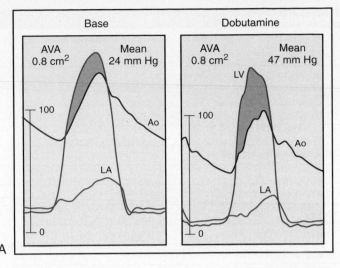

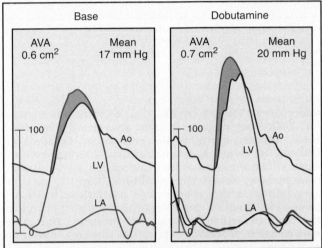

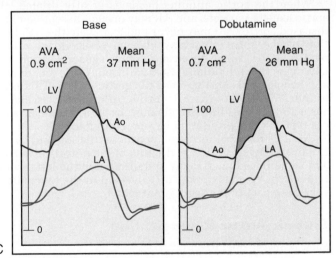

FIGURE 62-7 Hemodynamic tracings from three patients with left ventricular dysfunction, low cardiac output, and low aortic valve gradient, demonstrating three different responses to dobutamine. **A,** Increase in cardiac output and in mean aortic valve gradient from 24 to 47 mm Hg. Aortic valve area (AVA) remained 0.8 cm². This patient underwent successful valve replacement. **B,** Increase in cardiac output and minimal increase in mean pressure gradient from 17 to 20 mm Hg. The final calculated aortic valve area was 0.7 cm². The patient was found to have only minimal aortic stenosis (AS) at the time of surgery. **C,** No change in cardiac output, with decrease in mean pressure gradient from 37 to 26 mm Hg in response to dobutamine, and the test was terminated because of hypotension. The patient was found to have severe AS at the time of surgery. Ao = aortic; LA = left atrial; LV = left ventricular. *(From Nishimura RA, Grantham A, Connolly HM, et al: Low-output, low-gradient aortic stenosis in patients with depressed left ventricular systolic function: The clinical utility of the dobutamine challenge in the catheterization laboratory. Circulation 106:809, 2002.)*

suggests that patients should, if possible, be operated on before LV function becomes seriously impaired. The increased LV mass is reduced toward (but not to) normal within 18 months after AVR in patients with AS,[89] with further reduction over the next several years.[90] Coronary flow reserve[91,92] and diastolic function[89] also demonstrate considerable improvement after AVR. However, interstitial fibrosis regresses more slowly than myocyte hypertrophy so that diastolic dysfunction may persist for years after successful valve replacement.

When operation is carried out in patients with critical AS, frank LV failure, a depressed ejection fraction, or a low cardiac output (and hence a reduced transaortic pressure gradient), the operative risk is higher, and the mortality rate ranges from 8 to 20 percent, depending on the skill of the surgical team and the severity of heart failure.[75-78] Obviously, performing surgery before heart failure develops is desirable, but emergency operation, even in patients with heart failure, is sometimes life saving. In view of the extremely poor prognosis of such patients who are treated medically, unless serious comorbid conditions exist that preclude surgery, there is usually little choice but to advise immediate mechanical relief of obstruction.

In patients with AS and obstructive coronary artery disease (a relatively common combination), AVR and myocardial revascularization should be performed together.[93] Although the risk of AVR is increased when accompanied by coronary artery bypass grafting (see Table 62-3),[84] the surgical risk increases even more when severe coronary artery disease is left untreated. The ability to avoid serious myocardial ischemia in the perioperative period is a major factor that has served to reduce operative mortality in these patients. Characteristics of patients that have been shown to increase the risk of AVR, as reported in different series, are shown in Table 62-4.

There has been increasing interest in performing AVR through a very small incision, generally a transverse sternotomy, so-called "minimally invasive surgery." Although the advantages (shorter hospital stay, less tissue damage, better cosmetic results) are clear, the procedure is technically demanding and the mortality rate may actually be higher than when a standard approach is employed.[94]

AORTIC REGURGITATION

Etiology and Pathology

AR may be caused by primary disease of the aortic valve leaflets and/or the wall of the aortic root (Fig. 62-8).[95] Among patients with pure AR who undergo valve replacement, the percentage with aortic root disease has been increasing steadily during the past few decades and now represents the most common etiology and accounts for more than 50 percent of all such patients in some series.[96,97]

Valvular Disease

Primary valvular causes of AR include calcific AS in the elderly, in which some degree (usually mild) of AR is present in 75 percent of patients; infective endocarditis (see Chap. 63), in which the infection may destroy or cause perforation of a leaflet, or the vegetations may interfere with proper coaptation of the cusps; and trauma that results in a tear of the ascending aorta, in which loss of commissural support can cause prolapse of an aortic cusp. Although the most common complication of a congenitally bicuspid valve in adults is stenosis, incomplete closure and/or prolapse of a bicuspid valve may also cause isolated regurgitation or a combination of stenosis and regurgitation.[6] Rheumatic fever remains a common cause of primary disease of the aortic valve that leads to regurgitation.[96] The cusps become infiltrated with fibrous tissues and retract, a process that prevents cusp apposition during diastole and usually leads to regurgitation into the left ventricle through a defect in the center of the valve (see Fig. 62-1C). The associated fusion of the commissures may restrict the opening of the valve, resulting in combined AS and AR; some associated mitral valve involvement is also common. Progressive AR may occur in patients with a large ventricular septal defect, as well as in patients with membranous subaortic stenosis (see Chap. 61) and as a complication of percutaneous aortic

TABLE 62–3 | **Operative Mortality Rates Following Valve Replacement and Repair**

Operative Category	No.*	Operative Mortality* (%)	No.†	Operative Mortality† (%)
AVR (isolated)	26,317	4.3	32,968	4.0
MVR (isolated)	13,936	6.4	16,105	6.04
Multiple valve replacement	3,840	9.6	—	—
AVR + CAB	22,713	8.0	32,538	6.8
MVR + CAB	8,788	15.3	10,925	13.3
Multiple valve replacement + CAB	1,424	18.8		
AVR + any valve repair	938	7.4		
MVR + any valve repair	1,266	12.5		
Aortic valve repair	597	5.9		
Mitral valve repair	4,167	3.0		
Tricuspid valve repair	144	13.9		
AVR + aortic aneurysm repair	1,723	9.7		

*Modified from Jamieson WRE, Edwards FH, Schwartz M, et al: Risk stratification for cardiac valve replacement. National Cardiac Surgery Database. Ann Thorac Surg 67:943, 1999.

†Modified from Edwards FH, Peterson ED, Coombs LP, et al: Prediction of operative mortality after valve replacement surgery. J Am Coll Cardiol 37:885, 2001.

AVR=aortic valve replacement; CAB=coronary artery bypass; MVR=mitral valve replacement.

TABLE 62–4 | **Predictors of Poor Outcome after Aortic Valve Replacement for Aortic Stenosis**

Advanced age (>70 yr)

Female gender

Emergent surgery

Coronary artery disease

Previous coronary artery bypass grafting surgery

Hypertension

Left ventricular dysfunction (ejection fraction <0.45 or 0.50)

Heart failure

Atrial fibrillation

Concurrent mitral valve replacement or repair

Renal failure

Modified from Otto CM: Valvular Heart Disease. 2nd ed. Philadelphia, WB Saunders, 2004, p 227.

balloon valvotomy. Progressive regurgitation may also occur in patients with myxomatous proliferation of the aortic valve. An increasingly common cause of valvular AR is structural deterioration of a bioprosthetic valve.

Less common causes of AR include various forms of congenital AR, such as unicommissural and quadricuspid valves, or rupture of a congenitally fenestrated valve, particularly in the presence of hypertension. Other less common causes of AR occur in association with systemic lupus erythematosus; rheumatoid arthritis; ankylosing spondylitis; Jaccoud arthropathy; Takayasu disease; Whipple disease; Crohn disease; and, in the past, use of certain anorectic drugs. Isolated congenital AR is an uncommon lesion on necropsy studies but, when present, is usually associated with a bicuspid valve.

Aortic Root Disease (see also Chap. 56)

AR secondary to marked dilatation of the ascending aorta is now more common than primary valve disease in patients undergoing AVR for pure AR.[96,97] The conditions responsible for aortic root disease include age-related (degenerative) aortic dilation, cystic medial necrosis of the aorta (either isolated or associated with classic Marfan syndrome), aortic dilation related to bicuspid valves, aortic dissection, osteogenesis imperfecta, syphilitic aortitis, ankylosing spondylitis, the Behçet syndrome, psoriatic arthritis, arthritis associated with ulcerative colitis, relapsing polychondritis, reactive arthritis, giant cell arteritis, and systemic hypertension, as well as exposure to some appetite suppressant drugs.

When the aortic annulus becomes greatly dilated, the aortic leaflets separate, and AR may ensue. Dissection of the diseased aortic wall may occur and aggravate the AR. Dilation of the aortic root may also have secondary effects on the aortic valve because dilation causes tension and bowing of the individual cusps, which may thicken, retract, and become too short to close the aortic orifice. This leads to intensification of the AR, further dilating the ascending aorta and thus leading to a vicious circle in which, as is the case for MR, "regurgitation begets regurgitation."

AR, regardless of its cause, produces dilation and hypertrophy of the left ventricle, dilation of the mitral valve ring, and sometimes hypertrophy and dilation of the left atrium. Endocardial pockets frequently develop in the LV cavity at sites of impact of the regurgitant jet.

Chronic Aortic Regurgitation

Pathophysiology (Fig. 62-9)

In contrast to MR, in which a fraction of the LV stroke volume is ejected into the low-pressure left atrium, in AR the entire LV stroke volume is ejected into a high-pressure chamber (i.e., the aorta), although the low aortic diastolic pressure does facilitate ventricular emptying during early systole. In MR, especially acute MR, the reduction of wall tension (i.e., reduced afterload) allows more complete systolic emptying; in AR the increase in LV end-diastolic volume (i.e., increased preload) provides hemodynamic compensation.[1,96,98]

Severe AR may occur with a normal effective forward stroke volume and a normal ejection fraction (forward plus

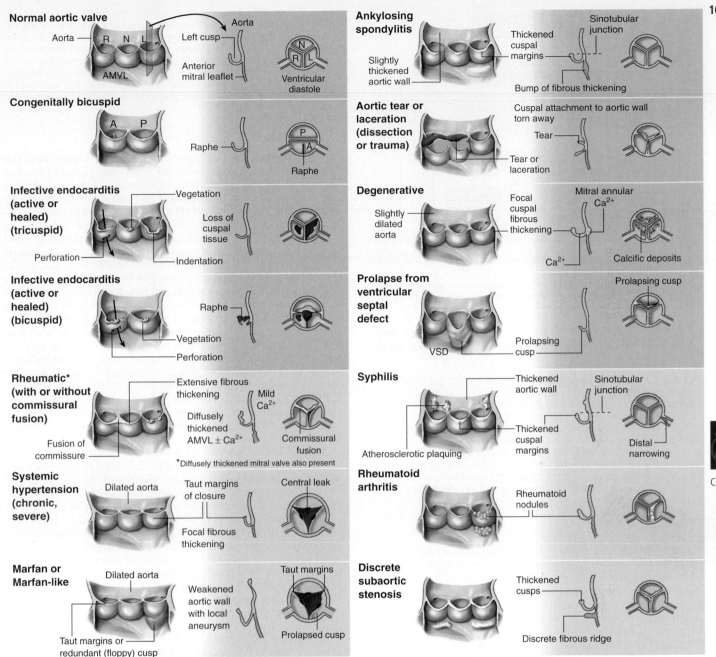

FIGURE 62–8 Diagram of various causes of pure aortic regurgitation. A = anterior; AMVL = anterior mitral valve leaflet; P = posterior; VSD = ventricular septal defect. *(From Waller BF: Rheumatic and nonrheumatic conditions producing valvular heart disease. Cardiovasc Clin 16:30, 1986.)*

regurgitant stroke volume/end-diastolic volume), together with an elevated LV end-diastolic volume, pressure, and stress (Fig. 62-10).[96,98,99] In accord with Laplace's law (which indicates that wall tension is related to the product of the intraventricular pressure and radius divided by wall thickness), LV dilation also increases the LV systolic tension required to develop any level of systolic pressure. This leads to eccentric hypertrophy, with replication of sarcomeres in series and elongation of myocytes and myocardial fibers. In compensated AR, there is sufficient wall thickening so that the ratio of ventricular wall thickness to cavity radius remains normal. This maintains or returns end-diastolic wall stress to normal levels. Thus in AR there is an increase in both preload and afterload. LV systolic function is maintained through the combination of chamber dilation and hypertrophy.[96,98] AR contrasts with AS, in which there is pressure overload (concentric) hypertrophy with replication

of sarcomeres largely in parallel and an increased ratio of wall thickness to radius, but like AS there is an increase in interstitial connective tissue.[39,89,100] In AR, LV mass is usually greatly increased (Fig. 62-11), often to levels even higher than in isolated AS. As AR persists and increases in severity over time, wall thickening fails to keep pace with the hemodynamic load and end-systolic wall stress rises. At this point, the afterload mismatch results in a decline in systolic function, and ejection fraction falls.[96,98,99]

Patients with severe chronic AR have the largest end-diastolic volumes of those with any form of heart disease (resulting in so-called *cor bovinum*). However, end-diastolic pressure is not uniformly elevated (i.e., LV compliance is often increased, see Fig. 62-10).

In the more severe cases of AR, the regurgitant flow may exceed 20 liters/min, so the total LV output at rest approaches 25 liters/min, a level that can be achieved acutely only by a

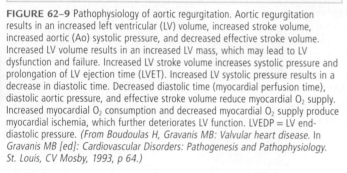

FIGURE 62–9 Pathophysiology of aortic regurgitation. Aortic regurgitation results in an increased left ventricular (LV) volume, increased stroke volume, increased aortic (Ao) systolic pressure, and decreased effective stroke volume. Increased LV volume results in an increased LV mass, which may lead to LV dysfunction and failure. Increased LV stroke volume increases systolic pressure and prolongation of LV ejection time (LVET). Increased LV systolic pressure results in a decrease in diastolic time. Decreased diastolic time (myocardial perfusion time), diastolic aortic pressure, and effective stroke volume reduce myocardial O₂ supply. Increased myocardial O₂ consumption and decreased myocardial O₂ supply produce myocardial ischemia, which further deteriorates LV function. LVEDP = LV end-diastolic pressure. *(From Boudoulas H, Gravanis MB: Valvular heart disease. In Gravanis MB [ed]: Cardiovascular Disorders: Pathogenesis and Pathophysiology. St. Louis, CV Mosby, 1993, p 64.)*

CH 62

trained endurance runner during maximal exercise. Thus the adaptive response to gradually increasing, chronic AR permits the ventricle to function as an effective high-compliance pump, handling a large stroke volume, often with little increase in filling pressure. During exercise, peripheral vascular resistance declines, and with an increase in heart rate, diastole shortens and the regurgitation per beat decreases,[1,101] facilitating an increment in effective (forward) cardiac output without substantial increases in end-diastolic volume and pressure. The ejection fraction and related ejection phase indices are often within normal limits, both at rest and during exercise, even though myocardial function, as reflected in the slope of the end-systolic pressure-volume relationship, is depressed.[102]

LEFT VENTRICULAR FUNCTION. As the left ventricle decompensates, interstitial fibrosis increases, compliance declines, and LV end-diastolic pressure and volume rise (see Fig. 62-10). In advanced stages of decompensation, left atrial, pulmonary artery wedge, pulmonary arterial, right ventricular (RV), and right atrial pressures rise and the effective (forward) cardiac output falls, at first during exercise and then at rest. The normal decline in end-systolic volume or the rise in ejection fraction fails to occur during exercise. Symptoms of heart failure, particularly those secondary to pulmonary congestion, develop.

MYOCARDIAL ISCHEMIA. When acute AR is induced experimentally, myocardial oxygen requirements rise substantially, secondary to an increase in wall tension. In patients with chronic, severe AR, total myocardial oxygen requirements are also augmented by the increase in LV mass. Because the major portion of coronary blood flow occurs during diastole, when arterial pressure is lower than normal in AR,

coronary perfusion pressure is reduced.[101] Studies in experimentally induced AR have shown a reduction in coronary flow reserve with a change in forward coronary flow from diastole to systole. The result—a combination of increased oxygen demand and reduced supply—sets the stage for the development of myocardial ischemia, especially during exercise. Thus patients with severe AR exhibit a reduction of coronary reserve, which may be responsible for myocardial ischemia and which may in turn play a role in the deterioration of LV function.

Clinical Presentation

SYMPTOMS. In patients with chronic, severe AR, the left ventricle gradually enlarges while the patient remains asymptomatic.[96,98] Symptoms of reduced cardiac reserve or myocardial ischemia develop, most often in the fourth or fifth decade and usually only after considerable cardiomegaly and myocardial dysfunction have occurred. The principal complaints of exertional dyspnea, orthopnea, and paroxysmal nocturnal dyspnea usually develop gradually. Angina pectoris is prominent late in the course; nocturnal angina may be troublesome and is often accompanied by diaphoresis that occurs when the heart rate slows and arterial diastolic pressure falls to extremely low levels. Patients with severe AR often complain of an uncomfortable awareness of the heartbeat, especially on lying down, and disagreeable thoracic pain due to pounding of the heart against the chest wall. Tachycardia, occurring with emotional stress or exertion, may cause troubling palpitations and head pounding. Premature ventricular contractions are particularly distressing because of the great heave of the volume-loaded left ventricle during the postextrasystolic beat. These complaints may be present for many years before symptoms of overt LV dysfunction develop.

PHYSICAL EXAMINATION (see also Chap. 11). In patients with chronic, severe AR, the head frequently bobs with each heartbeat (de Musset sign), and the pulses are of the "water-hammer" or collapsing type with abrupt distention and quick collapse (Corrigan pulse). The arterial pulse is often prominent and can be best appreciated by palpation of the radial artery with the patient's arm elevated. A bisferiens pulse may be present and is more readily recognized in the brachial and femoral arteries than in the carotid arteries. A variety of auscultatory findings provide confirmation of a wide pulse pressure. Traube sign (also known as "pistol shot sounds") refers to booming systolic and diastolic sounds heard over the femoral artery, Müller sign consists of systolic pulsations of the uvula, and Duroziez sign consists of a systolic murmur heard over the femoral artery when it is compressed proximally and a diastolic murmur when it is compressed distally. Capillary pulsations (i.e., Quincke sign) can be detected by pressing a glass slide on the patient's lip, by transmitting a light through the patient's fingertips, or by exerting gentle pressure on the tip of a fingernail.

Systolic arterial pressure is elevated, and diastolic pressure is abnormally low. Hill sign refers to popliteal cuff systolic pressure exceeding brachial cuff pressure by more than 60 mm Hg. Korotkoff sounds often persist to zero even though intraarterial pressure rarely falls below 30 mm Hg.[98] The point of change in Korotkoff sounds (i.e., the muffling of these sounds in phase IV) correlates with the diastolic pressure. As heart failure develops, peripheral vasoconstriction may occur and arterial diastolic pressure may rise. This finding should not be interpreted as the presence of mild AR.

The apical impulse is diffuse and hyperdynamic and is displaced laterally and inferiorly; there may be systolic retraction over the parasternal region. A rapid ventricular filling wave is often palpable at the apex. The augmented stroke volume may create a systolic thrill at the base of the heart or suprasternal notch, and over the carotid arteries.[98] In many patients, a carotid shudder is palpable.

AUSCULTATION. The PR interval may be prolonged, causing a soft S1. A2 may be normal or accentuated when AR is due to disease of the aortic root but is soft or absent when the valve is causing AR. P2 may be obscured by the early diastolic murmur. Thus S2 may be absent or single or exhibit narrow or paradoxical splitting. A systolic ejection sound, presumably related to abrupt distention of the aorta by the augmented stroke volume, is frequently audible. An S3 gallop correlates with an increased LV end-diastolic volume.[98] Its development may be a sign of impaired LV function, which is useful in identifying patients with severe AR who are candidates for surgical treatment.

The aortic regurgitant murmur, the principal physical finding of AR, is one of high frequency that begins immediately after A2. It may be distinguished from the murmur of pulmonic regurgitation by its earlier onset (i.e., immediately after A2 rather than after P2) and usually by the presence of a widened pulse pressure. The murmur is heard best with the diaphragm of the stethoscope while the patient is sitting up and leaning forward, with the breath

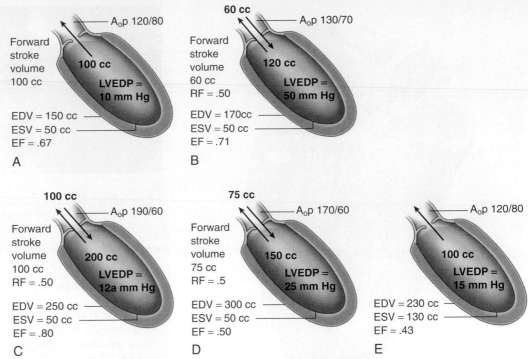

FIGURE 62–10 Hemodynamics of aortic regurgitation. **A,** Normal conditions. **B,** The hemodynamic changes that occur in severe acute aortic regurgitation. Although total stroke volume is increased, forward stroke volume is reduced. Left ventricular end-diastolic pressure (LVEDP) rises dramatically. **C,** Hemodynamic changes occurring in chronic compensated aortic regurgitation are shown. Eccentric hypertrophy produces increased end-diastolic volume (EDV), which permits an increase in total, as well as forward, stroke volume. The volume overload is accommodated, and left ventricular filling pressure is normalized. Ventricular emptying and end-systolic volume (ESV) remain normal. **D,** In chronic decompensated aortic regurgitation, impaired left ventricular emptying produces an increase in end-systolic volume and a fall in ejection fraction (EF), total stroke volume, and forward stroke volume. There is further cardiac dilation and reelevation of left ventricular filling pressure. **E,** Immediately following valve replacement, preload estimated by EDV decreases, as does filling pressure. ESV also is decreased, but to a lesser extent. The result is an initial fall in EF. Despite these changes, elimination of regurgitation leads to an increase in forward stroke volume. Aop = aortic pressure; RF = regurgitant fraction. *(From Carabello BA: Aortic regurgitation: Hemodynamic determinants of prognosis. In Cohn LH, DiSesa VJ [eds]: Aortic Regurgitation: Medical and Surgical Management. New York, Marcel Dekker, 1986.)*

held in deep exhalation. In severe AR, the murmur reaches an early peak and then has a dominant decrescendo pattern throughout diastole.

The severity of AR correlates better with the duration than with the intensity of the murmur. In mild AR, the murmur may be limited to early diastole and is typically high pitched and blowing. In severe AR, the murmur is holodiastolic and may have a rough quality. When the murmur is musical ("cooing dove" murmur), it usually signifies eversion or perforation of an aortic cusp. In patients with severe AR and LV decompensation, equilibration of aortic and LV pressures in late diastole abolishes the late diastolic component of the regurgitant murmur. When regurgitation is caused by primary valvular disease, the diastolic murmur is heard best along the left sternal border in the 3rd and 4th intercostal spaces. However, when it is caused mainly by dilation of the ascending aorta, the murmur is often more readily audible along the right sternal border.[98]

Many patients with chronic AR have a harsh systolic outflow murmur caused by the increased total LV stroke volume and ejection rate, and this often radiates to the carotid vessels. The systolic murmur is often more readily audible than the diastolic murmur. It may be higher pitched and less rasping than the murmur of AS but is often accompanied by a systolic thrill. Palpation of the carotid pulses will elucidate the cause of the systolic murmur and differentiate it from the murmur of AS.

A mid-diastolic and late diastolic apical rumble, the Austin Flint murmur, is common in severe AR and may occur in the presence of a normal mitral valve. This murmur appears to be created by rapid antegrade flow across a mitral orifice that is narrowed by the rapidly rising LV diastolic pressure caused by severe aortic reflux impinging on the anterior leaflet of the mitral valve. The Austin Flint murmur may be difficult to differentiate from that caused by mitral stenosis (MS), but the presence of an opening snap and a loud S1 in MS and the absence of these findings in AR are helpful clues. As the

LV end-diastolic pressure rises, the Austin Flint murmur commences and terminates earlier.

DYNAMIC AUSCULTATION. The diastolic murmur of AR may be accentuated when the patient sits up and leans forward or by interventions that raise the arterial pressure, such as squatting or isometric exercise. The intensity of the murmur is reduced by interventions that lower the systolic pressure, such as inhalation of amyl nitrite or the strain of the Valsalva maneuver. The Austin Flint murmur, like the murmur of AR, is augmented by isometric exercise and administration of vasopressors and is reduced by amyl nitrite inhalation.

Echocardiography

Echocardiography is helpful in identifying the cause of AR (see Figs. 14-52 and 14-53) and may demonstrate a bicuspid valve, thickening of the valve cusps, other congenital abnormalities, prolapse of the valve, a flail leaflet, or vegetation. In addition to leaflet anatomy and motion, the size and shape of the aortic root can be evaluated, although visualization of the ascending aorta is not always adequate and may require additional imaging procedures. Transthoracic imaging is usually satisfactory, but transesophageal echocardiography often provides more detail, particularly of the aortic root.

Transthoracic echocardiography is useful for the measurement of LV end-diastolic and end-systolic dimensions and volumes, ejection fraction, and mass.[101] 2D guided M-mode measurements of LV dimensions are recommended, as the high temporal resolution of this modality allows more accurate identification of endocardial borders. Care is needed to ensure measurements are not oblique and are at the same site on subsequent studies. These measurements,

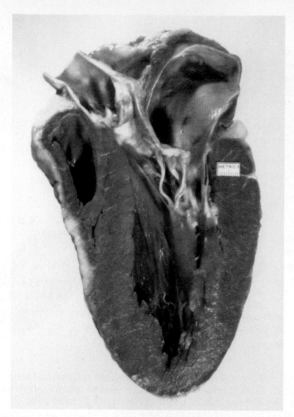

FIGURE 62–11 Heart of a young man with chronic aortic regurgitation who died suddenly, demonstrating both left ventricular dilation and marked left ventricular hypertrophy. *(Courtesy of William C. Roberts, MD.)*

CH 62

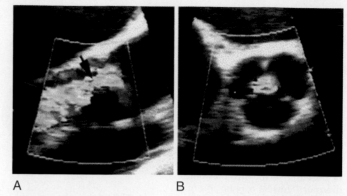

A   B

FIGURE 62–12 Transesophageal color Doppler imaging of the aortic regurgitant jet. **A,** Long-axis view. The black arrow indicates the vena contracta, the narrowest portion of the jet located at or just distal to its orifice. The width (in millimeters) of the vena contracta correlates well with volumetric measurement of regurgitant fraction and regurgitant volume. **B,** Short-axis view in the same patient. *(From Willett DL, Hall SA, Jessen ME, et al: Assessment of aortic regurgitation by transesophageal color Doppler imaging of the vena contracta: Validation against an intraoperative aortic flow probe. J Am Coll Cardiol 37:1450, 2001.)*

when made serially, are of great value in selecting the optimal time for surgical intervention.

High-frequency fluttering of the anterior leaflet of the mitral valve during diastole is an important echocardiographic finding in both acute and chronic AR. However, it does not develop when the mitral valve is rigid, as occurs with rheumatic involvement. This sign, unlike the Austin Flint murmur, occurs even in mild AR and results from the movement imparted to the anterior leaflet of the mitral valve by the jet of blood regurgitating from the aorta.

Doppler echocardiography and color flow Doppler imaging are the most sensitive and accurate noninvasive techniques in the diagnosis and evaluation of AR. They readily detect mild degrees of AR that may be inaudible on physical examination. Both the aortic regurgitant orifice size and the aortic regurgitant flow can be estimated quantitatively (Fig. 62-12)[103-105] and are strongly recommended.[1,105] These quantitative data provide the basis for the definitions of mild, moderate, and severe AR (see Table 62-1). Serial studies permit determination of the progression of AR and its effect on the left ventricle.

Other Diagnostic Evaluation

ELECTROCARDIOGRAPHY. Chronic, severe AR results in left axis deviation and a pattern of LV diastolic volume overload, characterized by an increase in initial forces (prominent Q waves in leads I, aVL, and V3 through V6) and a relatively small wave in lead V1. With the passage of time, these initial forces diminish, but the total QRS amplitude increases. The T waves may be tall and upright in the left precordial leads early in the course, but more commonly they are inverted, with ST segment depressions. An LV "strain" pattern correlates with the presence of dilation and hypertrophy. Intraventricular conduction defects occur late in the course and are usually associated with LV dysfunction. The ECG is not an accurate predictor of the severity of AR or cardiac weight. When AR is caused by an inflammatory process, prolongation of the PR interval may be present.[98]

RADIOLOGICAL FINDINGS (see Fig. 15-20). Cardiac size is a function of the duration and severity of regurgitation and the state of LV function. In acute AR, there may be minimal cardiac enlargement, but marked enlargement is a common finding in chronic AR. Typically, the left ventricle enlarges in an inferior and leftward direction, causing a significant increase in the long axis but sometimes causing little or no increase in the transverse diameter of the heart. Calcification of the aortic valve is uncommon in patients with pure AR but is often present in patients with combined AS and AR. Distinct left atrial enlargement in the absence of heart failure suggests associated mitral valve disease. Dilation of the ascending aorta is usually more marked than in AS and may involve the entire aortic arch including the aortic knob. Severe aneurysmal dilation of the aorta suggests that aortic root disease (e.g., the Marfan syndrome, cystic medial necrosis, or annuloaortic ectasia) is responsible for the AR. Linear calcifications in the wall of the ascending aorta are seen in syphilitic aortitis but are nonspecific and are observed in degenerative disease as well.

ANGIOGRAPHY. For angiographic assessment of AR, contrast material should be injected rapidly (i.e., 25 to 35 ml/sec) into the aortic root, and filming should be carried out in the right and left anterior oblique projections (see Chap. 19). Opacification may be improved by filming during a Valsalva maneuver. In acute AR, there is only a slight increase in LV end-diastolic volume, but with the passage of time both the end-diastolic volume and the thickness of the LV wall increase, usually in parallel.

RADIONUCLIDE IMAGING (see Chap. 16). In most patients, echocardiography provides the needed information regarding severity of AR and the status of the left ventricle. Radionuclide angiography is useful when echocardiographic images are suboptimal, there is a discrepancy between the clinical and the echocardiographic information, or there is a need for more precise measurement of LV ejection fraction.[1] This technique provides an accurate noninvasive assessment of the severity of AR by allowing determination of the regurgitant fraction and of the LV/RV stroke volume ratio. This measurement is nonspecific because the ratio is increased by the presence of associated MR and reduced by tricuspid regurgitation (TR) or pulmonary regurgitation. However, in the absence of these complicating lesions, an LV/RV stroke volume ratio of 2 or more denotes severe AR. Radionuclide angiography is also of value in the assessment of LV function during exercise in patients with AR.[94] Serial measurements are useful in the early detection of deterioration of LV function.

MAGNETIC RESONANCE IMAGING (see Fig. 17-12B). Cardiac MRI provides accurate measurements of regurgitant volumes and the regurgitant orifice in AR. It is the most accurate noninvasive technique for assessing LV end-systolic volume, diastolic volume, and mass (see Chap. 17). Cardiac MRI provides accurate quantitation of AR severity on the basis of the antegrade and retrograde flow volumes in the ascending aorta and is recommended when echocardiographic evaluation of regurgitation is suboptimal.[1,106]

Disease Course

Natural History of Chronic Aortic Regurgitation

Moderately severe or even severe chronic AR may be associated with a generally favorable prognosis for many years. Among asymptomatic patients with severe AR and normal LV ejection fractions, more than 45 percent remain asymptomatic with normal LV function at 10 years (Fig. 62-13), with an average rate of developing symptoms or LV systolic dysfunction less than 6 percent per year[1] (Table 62-5). The likelihood of sudden death in these asymptomatic patients is less than 0.5 percent per year. However, as is the case for AS, once the patient becomes symptomatic, the downhill course becomes rapidly progressive. Congestive heart failure, punctuated by episodes of acute pulmonary edema, and sudden death may occur, usually in previously symptomatic patients who have considerable LV dilation. Data compiled in the presurgical era indicate that without surgical treatment, death usually occurs within 4 years after the development of angina pectoris and within 2 years after the onset of heart failure. Dujardin and colleagues have confirmed these findings in the current era, demonstrating that

4-year survival without surgery in patients with NYHA Class III or IV symptoms is approximately 30 percent (Fig. 62-14).

Gradual deterioration of LV function may occur even during the asymptomatic period, and some patients may develop significant impairment of systolic function before the onset of symptoms. Numerous surgical series over the past two decades indicate that depressed LV ejection fraction is among the most important determinants of mortality after AVR, particularly when LV dysfunction is irreversible and does not improve after operation.[1] LV dysfunction is more likely to be reversible if detected early before ejection fraction becomes severely depressed, before the left ventricle becomes markedly dilated, and before significant symptoms develop; it is therefore important to intervene surgically before these changes have become irreversible.[1,96,99,107]

Management

MEDICAL TREATMENT. Recommendations for antibiotic prophylaxis for infective endocarditis have changed recently, and the majority of patients with AR are not candidates for prophylaxis (see also Chap. 63). Patients with mild or moderate AR who are asymptomatic with normal or only minimally increased cardiac size require no therapy but should be followed clinically and by echocardiography every 12 or 24 months. Asymptomatic patients with chronic, severe AR and normal LV function should be examined at intervals of approximately 6 months. In addition to clinical examination, serial echocardiographic assessments of LV size and ejection fraction should be made. Left-heart catheterization and aortography are usually not necessary but may be useful in patients whose noninvasive test results are inconclusive or discordant with clinical findings.[1] Similarly, other noninvasive tests such as radionuclide angiography or cardiac magnetic resonance have an important role primarily when echocardiographic information is not adequate. Patients with mild to moderate AR and those with severe AR with normal ejection fractions and only mild ventricular dilation may engage in aerobic forms of exercise. However, patients with AR who have limitations of cardiac reserve and/or evidence of declining LV function should not engage in vigorous sports or heavy exertion.[108] Systemic arterial diastolic hypertension, if present, should be treated because it increases the regurgitant flow; vasodi-

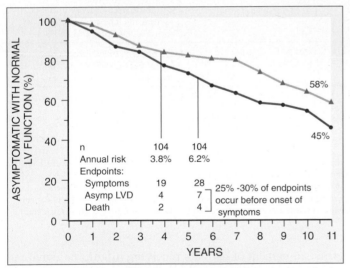

FIGURE 62–13 Natural history of chronic asymptomatic aortic regurgitation in patients with normal left ventricular (LV) ejection fraction at rest, in the series reported by Bonow and associates (blue line) and Borer and colleagues (magenta line), each enrolling 104 patients. At 11 years, 45 to 58 percent of patients remained asymptomatic with normal LV function, such that the risk of developing symptoms, LV dysfunction, or death is roughly 4 to 6 percent per year. The endpoints encountered in these series are indicated. The majority of patients who deteriorated developed symptoms leading to aortic valve replacement. However, 25 to 30 percent of the endpoints, either asymptomatic LV dysfunction (Asymp LVD) or death, occurred without warning symptoms. (Modified from Bonow RO, Lakatos E, Maron BJ, et al: Serial long-term assessment of the natural history of asymptomatic patients with chronic aortic regurgitation and normal left ventricular systolic function. Circulation 84:1625, 1991; and Borer JS, Hochreiter C, Herrold EM, et al: Prediction of indications for valve replacement among asymptomatic and minimally symptomatic patients with chronic aortic regurgitation and normal left ventricular performance. Circulation 97:525, 1998.)

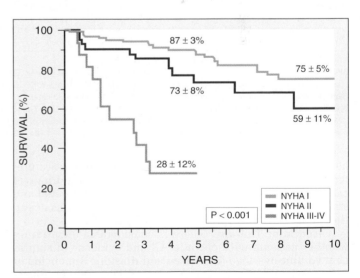

FIGURE 62–14 Survival without surgery in 242 patients with chronic aortic regurgitation, demonstrating the importance of symptoms in determining outcome. Patients with New York Heart Association (NYHA) Class III or IV symptoms had a survival of only 28 percent at 4 years. In contrast, the 10-year survival in patients in Class I was 75 percent, which was identical to that of an age-matched normal population (75 percent at 10 years). (From Dujardin KS, Enriquez-Sarano M, Schaff HV, et al: Mortality and morbidity of aortic regurgitation in clinical practice: A long-term follow-up study. Circulation 99:1851, 1999.)

TABLE 62–5 | Studies of the Natural History of Asymptomatic Aortic Regurgitation

Author, Yr	No. of Patients	Mean Follow-up (Yr)	Progression to Symptoms, Death, or LV Dysfunction, *Rate/Yr*	Progression to Asymptomatic LV Dysfunction		Mortality (No. Patients)	Comments
				(n)	*(Rate/Yr)*		
Bonow et al., 1983, 1991	104	8.0	3.8%	4	0.5%	2	Outcome predicted by LV ESD, EDD, change in EF with exercise, and rate of change in ESD and EF at rest with time
Scognamiglio et al., 1986*	30	4.7	2.1%	3	2.1%	0	3 patients developing asymptomatic LV dysfunction initially had lower PAP/ESV ratios and trend toward higher LV ESD and EDD and lower FS
Siemienczuk et al., 1989	50	3.7	4.0%	1	0.5%	0	Patients included those receiving placebo and medical dropouts in a randomized drug trial; included some patients with NYHA FC II symptoms; outcome predicted by LV ESV, EDV, change in EF with exercise, and end-systolic wall stress
Scognamiglio et al., 1994*	74	6.0	5.7%	15	3.4%	0	All patients received digoxin as part of a randomized trial
Tornos et al., 1995	101	4.6	3.0%	6	1.3%	0	Outcome predicted by pulse pressure, LV ESD, EDD, and EF at rest
Ishii et al., 1996	27	14.2	3.6%	—	—	0	Development of symptoms predicted by systolic BP, LV ESD, EDD, mass index, and wall thickness; LV function not reported in all patients
Borer et al., 1998	104	7.3	6.2%	7	0.9%	4	20% of patients in NYHA FC II; outcome predicted by initial FC II symptoms, change in LV EF with exercise, LV ESD, and LV FS
Tarasoutchi et al., 2003	72	10	4.7%	1	0.1%	0	Development of symptoms predicted by LV ESD and EDD. LV function not reported in all patients
Evangelista et al., 2005	31	7	3.6%	—	—	1	Placebo control group in 7-year vasodilator clinical trial
Average	593	6.6	4.3%	37	1.2%	(0.18%/y)	

*Two studies by same authors involved separate patient groups.

BP=blood pressure; EDD=end-diastolic dimension; EDV=end-diastolic volume; EF=ejection fraction; ESD=end-systolic dimension; ESV=end-systolic volume; FC=functional class; FS=fractional shortening; LV=left ventricular; NYHA=New York Heart Association; PAP=pulmonary artery pressure.

From Bonow RO, Carabello BA, Chatterjee K, et al: ACC/AHA 2006 guidelines for the management of patients with valvular heart disease: A report of the American College of Cardiology/American Heart Association Task Force on Practice Guidelines (writing committee to revise the 1998 Guidelines for the Management of Patients with Valvular Heart Disease): Developed in collaboration with the Society of Cardiovascular Anesthesiologists: endorsed by the Society for Cardiovascular Angiography and Interventions and the Society of Thoracic Surgeons. Circulation 114:e84, 2006.

lating agents such as nifedipine or ACE inhibitors are preferred, and beta-blocking agents should be used with great caution. AF and bradyarrhythmias are poorly tolerated and should be prevented if possible. If these arrhythmias occur, they must be treated promptly and vigorously.

Vasodilator Therapy. There is considerable uncertainty whether patients with chronic AR and evidence of significant volume overload (increased end-diastolic dimension or volume) should be considered for vasodilator therapy. Short-term studies spanning 6 months to 2 years have demonstrated beneficial hemodynamic effects of oral hydralazine, nifedipine, felodipine, and ACE inhibitors. One randomized study followed asymptomatic patients with severe AR for 6 years, comparing the effects of long-acting nifedipine (69 patients) and digoxin (74 patients) on LV function and symptoms.[109] Nifedipine delayed the need for operation: at 6 years, 85 percent of patients receiving nifedipine remained asymptomatic with normal LV ejection fraction, compared with only 65 percent of patients receiving digoxin. However, a second randomized trial compared placebo, long-acting nifedipine, and enalapril in 95 consecutive patients, who were followed up for 7 years.[110] Neither nifedipine nor enalapril reduced the development of symptoms or LV dysfunction warranting AVR compared with placebo. Moreover, neither drug significantly altered LV dimension, ejection fraction, or mass over the course of time compared with placebo. In view of this equipoise, definitive recommendations regarding the indications for long-active nifedipine or ACE inhibitors are not possible.[1]

Symptomatic Patients. AVR is the treatment of choice in symptomatic patients. Chronic medical therapy may be necessary in some patients who refuse surgery or are considered to be inoperable because of comorbid conditions. These patients should receive an aggressive heart failure regimen (see also Chap. 25) with ACE inhibitors (and perhaps other vasodilators), digoxin, diuretics, and salt restriction, but beta blockers should be avoided. Even though nitroglycerin and other nitrates are not as helpful in relieving anginal pain in patients with AR as they are in patients with coronary artery disease or AS, they are worth a try.

In patients who are candidates for surgery but who have severely decompensated LV dysfunction, vasodilator therapy may be particularly helpful in stabilizing patients while preparing for operation.[1] Such patients also respond, at least temporarily, to treatment with digitalis glycosides, salt restriction, and diuretics.

SURGICAL TREATMENT

Indications for Operation. Because of their excellent prognosis in the short and medium term, operative correction should be deferred in patients with chronic, severe AR who are asymptomatic, have good exercise tolerance, and have an ejection fraction greater than 50 percent without severe LV dilation (i.e., an end-diastolic diameter <70 mm and an end-systolic diameter <50 mm). In the absence of obvious contraindications or serious comorbidity, surgical treatment is advisable for symptomatic patients with severe AR and for asymptomatic patients with an ejection fraction less than 50 percent and severe LV dilation (end-diastolic diameter >75 mm or end-systolic diameter ≥55 mm).[1] Between these two ends of the clinical-hemodynamic spectrum are many patients in whom it may be quite difficult to balance the immediate risks of operation and the continuing risks of an implanted prosthetic valve, on the one hand, against the hazards of allowing a severe volume overload to damage the left ventricle, on the other.[96,99,107,111]

A proposed management strategy for patients with chronic severe AR is shown in Figure 62-15. Because severe symptoms (NYHA Class III or IV) and LV dysfunction with an ejection fraction less than 50 percent are independent risk factors for poor postoperative survival (Fig. 62-16), surgery should be carried out in NYHA Class II patients before severe LV dysfunction has developed.[1,98,107,111,112]

Even after successful correction of AR, patients with severe LV dysfunction may have persistent cardiomegaly and depressed LV function.[99,112,113] Such patients often exhibit histological changes in the left ventricle, including massive fiber hypertrophy and increased interstitial fibrous tissue. Therefore it is highly desirable to operate on patients before irreversible LV changes have occurred.

Because AR has complex effects on both preload and afterload, the selection of appropriate indices of ventricular contractility to identify patients for operation is challenging. The relationship between end-systolic wall stress and ejection fraction or percent fractional shortening is a useful measurement,[102] as are more load-independent measures of LV contractility. However, in the absence of such complex

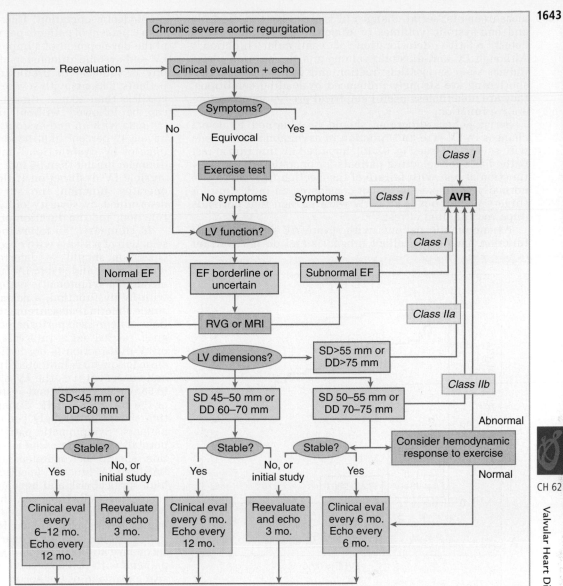

FIGURE 62–15 Management strategy for patients with chronic severe aortic regurgitation. Preoperative coronary angiography should be performed routinely as determined by age, symptoms, and coronary risk factors. Cardiac catheterization and angiography may also be helpful when there is discordance between clinical findings and echocardiography. "Stable" refers to stable echocardiographic measurements. In some centers, serial follow-up may be performed with radionuclide ventriculography or cardiac magnetic resonance rather than echocardiography to assess LV volume and systolic function. DD = end-diastolic dimension; EF = ejection fraction; RVG = radionuclide ventriculography; MRI = magnetic resonance imaging; SD = end-systolic dimension. (*From Bonow RO, Carabello BA, Chatterjee K, et al: ACC/AHA 2006 guidelines for the management of patients with valvular heart disease: a report of the American College of Cardiology/American Heart Association Task Force on Practice Guidelines (writing committee to revise the 1998 Guidelines for the Management of Patients With Valvular Heart Disease). Circulation 114:e84, 2006.*)

CH 62

Valvular Heart Disease

measurements, serial changes in ventricular end-diastolic and end-systolic volumes or dimensions can be used to detect relative deterioration of ventricular function.[99] Although LV end-diastolic volume and the ejection phase indices such as ejection fraction and ventricular fraction shortening are strongly influenced by loading conditions, they are nonetheless useful empirical predictors of postoperative function.

Serial echocardiograms should be obtained to detect changes in LV size and function in asymptomatic patients with severe AR (see Fig. 62-16). Impaired LV function at rest is the basis for selecting patients for operation; normal LV function at rest with failure of the ejection fraction to rise normally with exercise is not considered an indication for surgery per se, but is an early warning sign that portends impaired function at rest.[1,102]

Asymptomatic patients with severe AR but normal LV function have an excellent prognosis and do not warrant

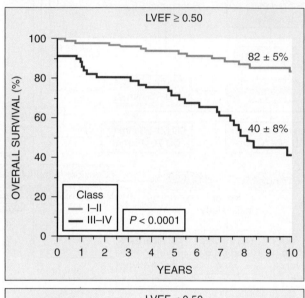

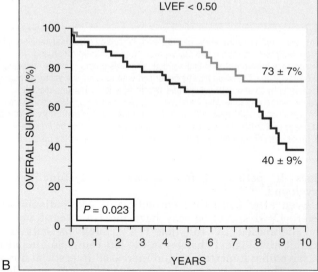

FIGURE 62–16 Long-term postoperative survival in patients with aortic regurgitation, stratified according to the severity of preoperative symptoms and preoperative left ventricular ejection fraction (LVEF). Patients with New York Heart Association (NYHA) Class III or IV symptoms experienced significantly worse survival than those with Class I or II symptoms whether the echocardiographic LVEF was higher than 0.50 **(A)** or less than 0.50 **(B)** without associated coronary artery disease. *(From Klodas E, Enriquez-Sarano M, Tajik AJ, et al: Optimizing timing of surgical correction in patients with severe aortic regurgitation: Role of symptoms. J Am Coll Cardiol 30:746, 1997.)*

prophylactic operation[1] (see Table 62-5). On average, less than 6 percent of patients per year require operation because of the development of symptoms or of LV dysfunction. The LV end-systolic dimension determined by echocardiography is valuable in predicting outcome in asymptomatic patients. Patients with severe AR and an end-systolic diameter less than 40 mm almost invariably remain stable and can be followed without immediate surgery. However, patients with an end-systolic diameter greater than 50 mm have a 19 percent likelihood per year of developing symptoms of LV dysfunction,[1] and those with an end-systolic diameter greater than 55 mm have an increased risk of irreversible LV dysfunction if they are not operated on. Postoperative function and survival in this latter group is determined by severity of symptoms, severity of LV dysfunction, and the duration of LV dysfunction.[99,107,112]

In summary, the following considerations apply to the selection of patients with chronic AR for surgical treatment. Operation should be deferred in asymptomatic patients with normal and stable LV function and should be recommended in symptomatic patients. In asymptomatic patients with LV dysfunction, a decision should be based not on a single abnormal measurement but rather on several observations of depressed performance and impaired exercise tolerance, carried out at intervals of 2 to 4 months. If evidence of LV dysfunction is borderline or inconsistent, continued close follow-up is indicated. If abnormalities are progressive and consistent (i.e., the LV ejection fraction declines to 50 to 55 percent, the LV end-systolic diameter rises to ≥55 mm, or the LV end-diastolic dimension rises to ≥75 mm, operation should be strongly considered even in asymptomatic patients.[1] Symptomatic patients with severe AR who have normal, mildly depressed, or moderately depressed LV function should be operated upon. Patients with severely impaired LV function (ejection fraction <25 percent) are at high surgical risk and have a guarded prognosis even after successful AVR. However, their outlook is also extremely poor when they receive medical therapy alone, and their management should be considered on an individual basis.

The indications for surgery in patients with severe AR secondary to aortic root disease are similar to those in patients with primary valvular disease. However, progressive expansion of the aortic root and/or a diameter greater than 50 mm by echocardiography with any degree of regurgitation in patients with a bicuspid valve and a diameter greater than 55 mm in other patients is also an indication for surgery in patients with aortic root disease.[1]

As is the case for patients with other valvular lesions, adult surgical candidates who may have underlying coronary artery disease, based on symptoms, age, gender, and risk factors, should undergo preoperative coronary arteriography. Those with coronary artery stenoses should undergo revascularization at the time of AVR.

Operative Procedures. There is growing experience with surgical aortic valve repair, which is a viable option for selected patients in experienced centers.[114-116] Occasionally, when a leaflet has been torn from its attachments to the aortic annulus by trauma, surgical repair may be possible, and in patients with AR secondary to prolapse of an aortic leaflet, aortic cusp resuspension or cusp resection may be employed. When AR is caused by leaflet perforation resulting from healed infective endocarditis, a pericardial patch can be used for repair. However, unlike patients with chronic MR, the large majority of patients with pure AR will require AVR rather than repair.

Because an increasing proportion of patients with severe, isolated AR coming to operation now have primary aortic root rather than primary valvular disease, an increasing number can be treated surgically by correcting the dilated aortic root.[4,11,117] One of two annuloplasty procedures may be employed—an encircling suture of the aorta or a subcommissural annuloplasty. Aneurysmal dilation of the ascending aorta requires excision, replacement with a graft that includes a prosthetic valve, and reimplantation of the coronary arteries. In some patients with aortic root disease, the native valve can be spared when the aortic root is replaced or repaired (Fig. 62-17).[115,117,118]

When AVR is performed in patients with severe AR, the aortic annulus is usually not as narrow as it is in patients with AS. Hence a larger prosthetic valve can be inserted, and mild postoperative obstruction to LV outflow is less of a problem than it is in some patients with AS. In general the risks and results of AVR in patients with AR are similar to those in patients with AS, with a large percentage of patients exhibiting striking improvement in symptoms. Reductions in heart size and in LV diastolic volume and mass occur in the majority of patients.[99] Exceptions are patients who are in NYHA Class III or IV heart failure and/or patients who have severe LV dysfunction preoperatively.[111,113] As is true for patients with AS, the operative risk of AVR for patients with AR depends on the general condition of the patient, the state of LV function, and the skill and experience of the surgical team. The mortality rate ranges from 3 to 8 percent in most medical centers (see Table 62-3). A late mortality of approximately 5 to 10 percent per year is observed in survivors who had marked cardiac enlargement and/or prolonged LV dysfunction preoperatively. Follow-up studies have shown both early rapid and then slower long-term reductions of LV mass, ejection fraction, myocyte hypertrophy, and ventricular fibrous content following relief of AR.[89] By extending the indications for operation to symptomatic patients with normal LV function, as well as to asymptomatic patients with LV dysfunction, both early and late results are improving.[1,112] With the continued improvement of surgical techniques and results, it will likely become possible to extend the recommendation for operative treatment to asymptomatic patients with severe regurgitation, normal LV systolic function, and only mild LV dilation. However, given the risks of operation and the long-term complications of presently available prosthetic valves, we do not believe that the time for such a policy has yet arrived.

Acute Aortic Regurgitation

Acute AR is caused most commonly by infective endocarditis, aortic dissection, or trauma. The characteristic features of acute AR are tachycardia and an increase in LV diastolic pressures. In contrast to the pathophysiological events in chronic AR just described, in which the left ventricle is able to adapt to the increased hemodynamic load, in acute AR the regurgitant volume fills a ventricle of normal size that cannot accommodate the combined large regurgitant volume and inflow from the left atrium. Because the ability of total stroke volume to rise acutely is limited, forward stroke volume declines. The sudden increase in LV filling causes the LV diastolic pressure to rise rapidly above left atrial pressure during early diastole (see Fig. 62-10),[119] causing the mitral valve to close prematurely in diastole. Premature closure of the mitral valve, together with tachycardia that also shortens diastole, reduces the time interval during which the mitral valve is open. The tachycardia may compensate for the reduced forward stroke volume, and the LV and aortic systolic pressures may exhibit little change. However, acute, severe AR may cause profound hypotension and cardiogenic shock. In light of the limited ability of the left ventricle to tolerate acute, severe AR, patients with this valvular lesion often develop clinical manifestations of sudden cardiovascular collapse including weakness, severe dyspnea, and profound hypotension secondary to the reduced stroke volume and elevated left atrial pressure. In some patients the aortic diastolic pressure equilibrates with the elevated LV diastolic pressure.

PHYSICAL EXAMINATION. Patients with acute, severe AR appear gravely ill, with tachycardia, severe peripheral vasoconstriction and cyanosis, and sometimes pulmonary congestion and edema. The

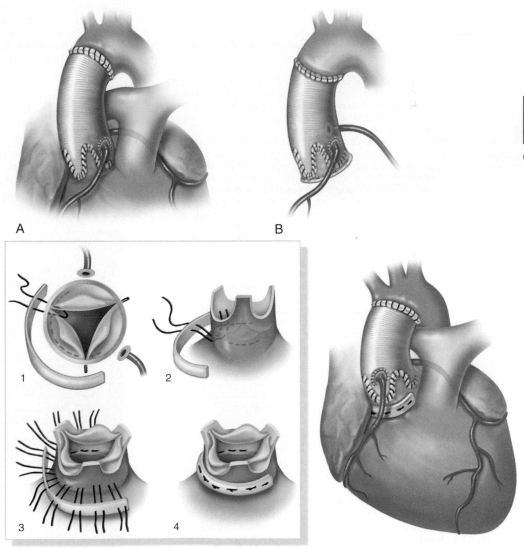

FIGURE 62–17 Repair of aortic regurgitation caused by aortic root dilation. **A,** Remodeling of the aortic root with replacement of all three aortic sinuses. **B,** Reimplantation of the aortic valve in patients with annuloaortic ectasia and aortic root aneurysm. **C** and **D,** Aortic annuloplasty in patients with annuloaortic ectasia. *(From David TE: Aortic root aneurysms: Remodeling or composite replacement? Ann Thorac Surg 64:1564, 1997.)*

peripheral signs of AR are often not impressive and certainly not as dramatic as in patients with chronic AR. Duroziez murmur, Traube sign over the peripheral arteries, and bisferiens pulses are usually absent in acute AR. The normal or only slightly widened pulse pressure may lead to serious underestimation of the severity of the valvular lesion. The LV impulse is normal or nearly so, and the rocking motion of the chest characteristic of chronic AR is not apparent. S1 may be soft or absent because of premature closure of the mitral valve,[119] and the sound of mitral valve closure in mid or late diastole is occasionally audible. However, closure of the mitral valve may be incomplete, and diastolic MR may occur. Evidence of pulmonary hypertension, with an accentuated P2, S3, and S4, is frequently present.

The early diastolic murmur of acute AR is lower pitched and shorter than that of chronic AR because as LV diastolic pressure rises, the (reverse) pressure gradient between the aorta and the left ventricle is rapidly reduced. A systolic murmur is common, resulting in "to and fro" sounds. The Austin Flint murmur is often present, but is brief and ceases when LV pressure exceeds left atrial pressure in diastole. With premature diastolic closure of the mitral valve, the presystolic portion of the Austin Flint murmur is eliminated.

ECHOCARDIOGRAPHY. In acute AR the echocardiogram reveals a dense diastolic Doppler signal with an end-diastolic velocity approaching zero, and premature closure and delayed opening of the mitral valve.[119] LV size and ejection fraction are normal. This contrasts with the findings in chronic AR, in which end-diastolic dimensions and wall motion are increased. Occasionally, with equilibration of aortic and LV pressures in diastole, premature opening of the aortic valve may be detected.

OTHER DIAGNOSTIC EVALUATION

Electrocardiography. In acute AR the ECG may or may not show LV hypertrophy, depending on the severity and duration of the regurgitation. However, nonspecific ST segment and T wave changes are common.

Radiological Findings. In acute AR, there is often evidence of marked pulmonary venous hypertension and pulmonary edema. The cardiac silhouette is usually remarkably normal, although left atrial enlargement may be present and, depending on the cause of the AR, there may be enlargement of the ascending aorta.

MANAGEMENT OF ACUTE AORTIC REGURGITATION. Because early death caused by LV failure is frequent in patients with acute, severe AR despite intensive medical management, prompt surgical intervention is indicated. Even a normal ventricle cannot sustain the burden of acute, severe volume overload. Therefore the risk of acute AR is much greater than that of chronic AR.[119] While the patient is being prepared for surgery, treatment with an intravenous positive inotropic agent (dopamine or dobutamine) and/or a vasodilator (nitroprusside) is often necessary. The agent and dosage should be selected on the basis of arterial pressure (see Chap. 25). Beta-blocking agents and intra-aortic balloon counterpulsation are contraindicated, as either lowering the heart rate or augmenting peripheral resistance during diastole can lead to rapid hemodynamic decompensation. In hemodynamically stable patients with acute AR secondary to active infective endocarditis, operation may be deferred to allow 5 to 7 days of intensive antibiotic therapy. However, AVR should be undertaken at the earliest sign of hemodynamic instability or if echocardiographic evidence of diastolic closure of the mitral valve develops.

MITRAL STENOSIS

Etiology

The predominant cause of mitral stenosis (MS) is rheumatic fever,[1,120] with rheumatic changes present in 99 percent of stenotic mitral valves excised at the time of mitral valve (MV) replacement. About 25 percent of all patients with rheumatic heart disease have isolated MS, and about 40 percent have combined MS and mitral regurgitation (MR). Multivalve involvement is seen in 38 percent of MS patients, with the aortic valve affected in about 35 percent and the tricuspid valve in about 6 percent. The pulmonic valve is rarely affected. Two thirds of all patients with rheumatic MS are female.[1] The interval between the initial episode of rheumatic fever (see Chap. 83) and clinical evidence of mitral valve obstruction is variable, ranging from a few years to more than 20 years.

Rheumatic fever results in characteristic changes of the mitral valve with the diagnostic features being thickening at the leaflet edges, fusion of the commissures, and chordal shortening and fusion (Fig. 62-18).[121] With acute rheumatic fever, there is inflammation and edema of the leaflets, with small fibrin-platelet thrombi along the leaflet contact zones. Subsequent scarring leads to the characteristic valve deformity with obliteration of the normal leaflet architecture by fibrosis, neovascularization and increased collagen and tissue cellularity. Superimposed calcification results in further dysfunction. Aschoff bodies, the pathologic hallmark of rheumatic disease, are most frequently seen in the myocardium, not the valve tissue with Aschoff bodies identified in only 2 percent of autopsied patients with chronic valve disease.[122]

These anatomical changes lead to a typical functional appearance of the rheumatic mitral valve. When the leaflets open in diastole, the relatively flexible leaflets snap into a curved shape due to restriction of motion at the leaflet tips. This diastolic "doming" is most evident in the motion of the anterior leaflet and becomes less prominent as the leaflets become more fibrotic and calcified. The symmetric fusion of the commissures results in a small central oval orifice in diastole that on pathologic specimens is shaped like a "fish mouth" or buttonhole (because the anterior leaflet is not in the physiological open position) (Fig. 62-19), With end-stage disease, the thickened leaflets may be so adherent and rigid that they cannot open or shut, reducing or rarely even abolishing the first heart sound (S1) and leading to combined MS and MR. When rheumatic fever results exclusively or predominantly in contraction and fusion of the chordae tendineae, with little fusion of the valvular commissures, dominant MR results.[121]

A debate continues about whether the anatomical changes in severe MS result from recurrent episodes of rheumatic fever, a chronic autoimmune process caused by cross-reactivity between a streptococcal protein and valve tissue (see Chap. 83) or if the constant trauma produced by the turbulent blood flow leads to progressive fibrosis, thicken-

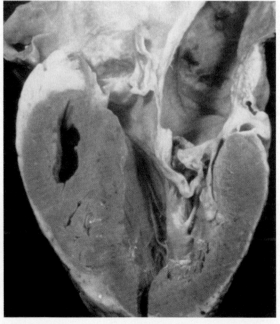

FIGURE 62–18 Rheumatic mitral stenosis. There are severe valvular changes, including marked fibrosis and calcification of the mitral valve leaflets and severe chordal thickening and fusion into pillars of fibrous tissue. (From Becker AE, Anderson RH [eds]: Cardiac Pathology: An Integrated Text and Colour Atlas. New York, Raven Press, 1983, p 4.3.)

ing, and calcification of the valve apparatus.[122,123] Evidence supporting recurrent infection as an important factor in disease progression includes the correlation between the geographic variability in the prevalence of rheumatic heart disease and the age at which patients present with severe MS. In North America and Europe, where there is approximately 1 case per 100,000 population, patients present with severe valve obstruction in the sixth decade of life. In contrast, in Africa, with a disease prevalence of 35 per 100,000,

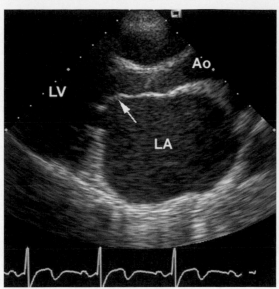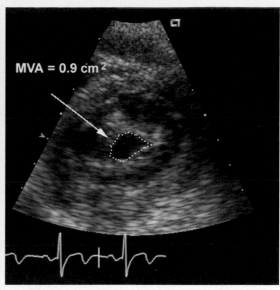

FIGURE 62–19 Parasternal long **(left)** and short axis **(right)** 2D echocardiographic views showing the characteristic findings in rheumatic mitral stenosis. Note the commissural fusion that results in doming of the leaflets in the long axis view and in a decrease in the width of the mitral orifice in the short axis view. This patient has relatively thin, flexible leaflets with little subvalvular involvement. Ao = aorta; LA = left atrium, LV = left ventricle. *(From Otto CM: Valvular Heart Disease. Elsevier, Philadelphia, 2004.)*

severe disease often is seen in teenagers. Another observation supporting the role of recurrent infection is that restenosis after mitral valvuloplasty is caused by leaflet thickening and fibrosis rather than recurrent commissural fusion.

Congenital MS is uncommon and typically is diagnosed in infancy or early childhood (see Chap. 61). MS is a rare complication of malignant carcinoid disease, systemic lupus erythematosus, rheumatoid arthritis, mucopolysaccharidoses of the Hunter-Hurler phenotype, Fabry disease, and Whipple disease. Amyloid deposits may occur on rheumatic valves and contribute to the obstruction to left atrial emptying. Methysergide therapy is an unusual but documented cause of MS. The association of atrial septal defect with rheumatic MS is called *Lutembacher syndrome* (see Chap. 61).

A number of conditions may simulate the physiology of MS: obstruction to left atrial outflow may be caused by a left atrial tumor, particularly myxoma (see Chap. 69); ball-valve thrombus in the left atrium (usually associated with MS); infective endocarditis with large vegetations (see Chap. 63); and a congenital membrane in the left atrium (i.e., cor triatriatum) (see Chap. 61). In the elderly, extensive mitral annular calcification may result in restriction of the size of the conduit for left ventricular (LV) diastolic filling, with functional MS. Mitral annular calcification extends onto the base of the mitral leaflets in some cases, in contrast to the thickening at the leaflet tips seen with rheumatic disease. Calcific MS rarely results in severe valve obstruction.

Pathophysiology

The most useful descriptor of the severity of mitral valve obstruction is the degree of valve opening in diastole, or the mitral valve orifice area. In normal adults the cross-sectional area of the mitral valve orifice is 4 to 6 cm² (see Table 62-1). When the orifice is reduced to approximately 2 cm², which is considered to represent mild MS, blood can flow from the left atrium to the left ventricle only if propelled by a small, although abnormal, pressure gradient. When the mitral valve opening is reduced to 1 cm², which is considered to represent severe MS,[120] a left atrioventricular pressure gradient of approximately 20 mm Hg (and there-

fore in the presence of a normal LV diastolic pressure, a mean left atrial pressure of ≈25 mm Hg) is required to maintain normal cardiac output at rest (Fig. 62-20; see also Fig. 19-15).

Transvalvular pressure gradient for any given valve area is a function of the square of the transvalvular flow rate.[124] Thus a doubling of flow rate quadruples the pressure gradient. The elevated left atrial pressure, in turn, raises pulmonary venous and capillary pressures, resulting in exertional dyspnea. The first bouts of dyspnea in patients with MS are usually precipitated by tachycardia resulting from exercise, pregnancy, hyperthyroidism, anemia, infection, or atrial fibrillation (AF), all of which both (1) increase the rate of blood flow across the mitral orifice resulting in further elevation of the left atrial pressure and (2) decrease the diastolic filling time resulting in a reduction in forward cardiac output.[1,120,125] Because diastole shortens proportionately more than systole as heart rate increases, the time available for flow across the mitral valve is reduced at higher heart rates. Therefore at any given stroke volume, tachycardia results in a higher instantaneous volume flow rate and a higher transmitral pressure gradient, which elevates left atrial pressures further.[1] This higher transmitral gradient, often in combination with inadequate ventricular filling (because of the shortened diastolic filling time), explains the sudden occurrence of dyspnea and pulmonary edema in previously asymptomatic patients with MS who develop AF with a rapid ventricular rate. It also accounts for the equally rapid improvement in these patients when the ventricular rate is slowed.

Atrial contraction augments the presystolic transmitral valvular gradient by approximately 30 percent in patients with MS. AF is common in patients with MS, with an increasing prevalence with age. In patients with severe MS younger than 30 years, only about 10 percent are in AF compared with about 50 percent of those older than 50 years of age. Withdrawal of atrial transport when AF develops reduces cardiac output by approximately 20 percent, often resulting in symptom onset.

Obstruction at the mitral valve level has other hemodynamic consequences, which account for many of the adverse clinical outcomes associated with this disease. Elevated left atrial pressure results in pulmonary artery hypertension

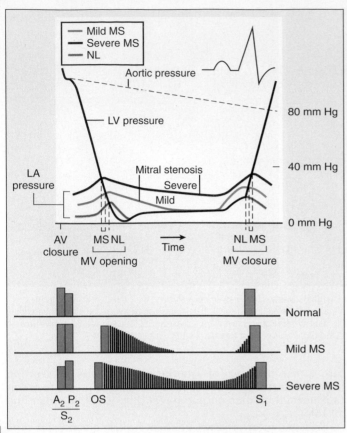

FIGURE 62–20 Schematic representation of left ventricular (LV), aortic, and left atrial (LA) pressures, showing normal relationships and alterations with mild and severe mitral stenosis (MS). Corresponding classic auscultatory signs of MS are shown at the bottom. Compared with mild MS, with severe MS the higher left atrial *v* wave causes earlier pressure crossover and earlier mitral valve (MV) opening, leading to a shorter time interval between aortic valve (AV) closure and the opening snap (OS). The higher left atrial end-diastolic pressure with severe MS also results in later closure of the mitral valve. With severe MS, the diastolic rumble becomes longer and there is accentuation of the pulmonic component (P2) of the second heart sound (S2) in relation to the aortic component (A2).

with secondary effects on the pulmonary vasculature and right heart. In addition, left atrial enlargement and stasis of blood flow is associated with an increased risk of thrombus formation and systemic embolism. Typically, the left ventricle is relatively normal, unless there is coexisting MR, with the primary abnormalities of the left ventricle being a small, underfilled chamber and paradoxical septal motion caused by right ventricular (RV) enlargement and dysfunction.

INTRACARDIAC AND INTRAVASCULAR PRESSURES

LEFT ATRIAL AND RIGHT HEART PRESSURES. In patients with MS and sinus rhythm, mean left atrial pressure is elevated (see Fig. 62-20), and the left atrial pressure curve shows a prominent atrial contraction (*a*) wave with a gradual pressure decline after mitral valve opening (*y* descent). In patients with mild to moderate MS without elevated pulmonary vascular resistance, pulmonary arterial pressure may be normal or only minimally elevated at rest but rises during exercise. However, in patients with severe MS and those in whom the pulmonary vascular resistance is significantly increased, pulmonary arterial pressure is elevated when the patient is at rest. Rarely, in patients with extremely elevated pulmonary vascular resistance, pulmonary arterial pressure may exceed systemic arterial pressure. Further elevations of left atrial and pulmonary vascular pressures occur during exercise and/or tachycardia. With moderately elevated pulmonary arterial pres-

sure (systolic pressure 30 to 60 mm Hg), RV performance is usually maintained. However, a greater elevation of pulmonary arterial pressure represents serious impedance to emptying of the right ventricle. Hence, patients with MS and severe pulmonary hypertension commonly fail to exhibit normal hyperkinesis of the right ventricle during exercise, and ultimately develop RV dysfunction and dilation at rest, with accompanying tricuspid regurgitation (TR).

LEFT VENTRICULAR DIASTOLIC PRESSURE. This pressure is normal in patients with isolated MS; however, coexisting MR, aortic valve lesions, systemic hypertension, ischemic heart disease, and cardiomyopathy may all be responsible for elevations of LV diastolic pressure. In approximately 85 percent of patients with isolated MS, the LV end-diastolic volume is within the normal range, whereas it is reduced in the remaining patients. In approximately 25 percent of patients with isolated MS, the ejection fraction and other ejection indices of systolic performance are below normal, most likely resulting in part from chronic reduction in preload and elevated afterload. Regional hypokinesis has been described, perhaps caused by extension of the scarring process from the mitral valve into the adjacent posterior basal myocardium or by associated ischemic heart disease. Leftward displacement of the interventricular septum secondary to more rapid early filling of the right ventricle may be responsible for a reduction of LV compliance (LV stiffening).[125] The LV mass is usually normal but may be slightly reduced.

The bulk of available evidence suggests that LV contractility is normal or only slightly impaired in the majority of patients with isolated MS. Most patients with MS have a normal elevation of ejection fraction and a reduction of end-systolic volume during exercise, although ejection fraction does not increase normally with exercise in a subset of patients. In these latter patients, the normal increase in LV diastolic volume during exercise fails to occur, resulting in reduced stroke volume and ejection fraction responses to exercise. Associated ischemic heart disease is not common in younger patients, but the normal increase in coronary disease prevalence with age is seen in patients with MS[1] and contributes to myocardial dysfunction in some patients.

PULMONARY HYPERTENSION. Pulmonary hypertension in patients with MS results from (1) passive backward transmission of the elevated left atrial pressure; (2) pulmonary arteriolar constriction, which presumably is triggered by left atrial and pulmonary venous hypertension (reactive pulmonary hypertension); and (3) organic obliterative changes in the pulmonary vascular bed, which may be considered to be a complication of longstanding and severe MS[123,125] (see Chap. 73). In time, severe pulmonary hypertension results in right-sided heart failure, with dilation of the right ventricle and its annulus and secondary TR and sometimes pulmonic regurgitation. These changes in the pulmonary vascular bed may also exert a protective effect; the elevated precapillary resistance makes the development of symptoms of pulmonary congestion less likely by tending to prevent blood from surging into the pulmonary capillary bed and damming up behind the stenotic mitral valve, although this protection occurs at the expense of a reduced cardiac output. In patients with severe MS, pulmonary vein-bronchial vein shunts occur. Their rupture may cause hemoptysis. Patients with severe MS manifest a reduction in pulmonary compliance, an increase in the work of breathing, and a redistribution of pulmonary blood flow from the base to the apex.

EXERCISE HEMODYNAMICS. At any given severity of stenosis, the clinical picture is dictated largely by the levels of cardiac output and pulmonary vascular resistance with exertion. The response to a given degree of mitral obstruction may be characterized at one end of the hemodynamic spectrum by a normal cardiac output and a high left atrioventricular pressure gradient or, at the opposite end of the spectrum, by a markedly reduced cardiac output and low transvalvular pressure gradient. Thus in some patients with moderate MS (mitral valve area = 1.0 to 1.5 cm²), cardiac output at rest may be normal and rises normally during exertion. However, the high transvalvular pressure gradient with exertion elevates left atrial and pulmonary capillary pressures, leading to pulmonary congestion during exertion. In contrast, in other patients with moderate MS, there is an inadequate rise in cardiac output during exertion resulting in a smaller rise in pulmonary venous pressure. In these patients, symptoms are caused by a low cardiac output rather than by pulmonary congestion. In patients with severe MS (mitral valve area <1 cm²), particularly when pulmonary vascular resistance is elevated, cardiac output is usually depressed at rest and may fail to rise at all during exertion. These patients frequently have resting weakness and fatigue secondary to a low cardiac output with both low output and pulmonary congestion symptoms with exercise.

LEFT ATRIAL CHANGES. The combination of mitral valve disease and atrial inflammation secondary to rheumatic carditis causes (1) left atrial dilation, (2) fibrosis of the atrial wall, and (3) disorganization of the atrial muscle bundles. These changes lead to disparate conduction velocities and inhomogeneous refractory periods. Premature atrial activation, caused either by an automatic focus or reentry, may stimulate the left atrium during the vulnerable period and thereby precipitate AF. The development of this arrhythmia correlates independently with the severity of the MS, the degree of left atrial dilation, and the height of the left atrial pressure. However, in recent series of patients with severe MS undergoing percutaneous balloon mitral valvotomy (BMV), the strongest predictor of AF is older age.[126,127] AF is often episodic at first but then becomes more persistent. AF per se causes diffuse atrophy of atrial muscle, further atrial enlargement, and further inhomogeneity of refractoriness and conduction. These changes, in turn, lead to irreversible AF.

Clinical Presentation

Symptoms

DYSPNEA. The most common presenting symptoms of MS are fatigue and decreased exercise tolerance.[128] Symptoms may be caused by a reduced ability to increase cardiac output normally with exercise or elevated pulmonary venous pressures and reduced pulmonary compliance. Dyspnea may be accompanied by cough and wheezing. Vital capacity is reduced, presumably owing to the presence of engorged pulmonary vessels and interstitial edema. Patients who have critical obstruction to left atrial emptying and dyspnea with ordinary activity (New York Heart Association [NYHA] Class III) generally have orthopnea as well and are at risk of experiencing attacks of frank pulmonary edema. The latter may be precipitated by effort, emotional stress, respiratory infection, fever, sexual intercourse, pregnancy, or AF with a rapid ventricular rate or other tachyarrhythmia. Indeed, pulmonary edema may be caused by any condition that increases the flow rate across the stenotic mitral valve, either because of an increase in total cardiac output or a reduction in the time available for blood flow across the mitral orifice to occur. In patients with a markedly elevated pulmonary vascular resistance, RV function is often impaired and the presentation may include symptoms and signs of right heart failure as well.[125]

MS is a slowly progressive disease, and many patients remain seemingly asymptomatic merely by readjusting their lifestyles to a more sedentary level. Usually, symptom status can be accurately assessed by a directed history, asking the patient to compare current levels of maximum exertion to specific time points in the past. Exercise testing may be useful in selected patients to determine functional status in an objective manner and may be combined with Doppler echocardiography (see later) to assess exercise hemodynamics.

HEMOPTYSIS. Hemoptysis is rare in patients with a known diagnosis of MS because intervention is performed before severe obstruction becomes chronic. When hemoptysis does occur it can be sudden and severe, caused by rupture of thin-walled, dilated bronchial veins, usually as a consequence of a sudden rise in left atrial pressure, or it may be milder with only blood-stained sputum associated with attacks of paroxysmal nocturnal dyspnea. MS patients also may have pink, frothy sputum characteristic of acute pulmonary edema with rupture of alveolar capillaries. Hemoptysis also may be caused by pulmonary infarction, a late complication of MS associated with heart failure.

CHEST PAIN. Chest pain is not a typical symptom of MS, but a small percentage, perhaps 15 percent, of patients with MS experience chest discomfort that is indistinguishable from angina pectoris. This symptom may be caused by severe RV hypertension secondary to the pulmonary vascular disease or by concomitant coronary atherosclerosis.[1]

Rarely, chest pain may be secondary to coronary obstruction caused by coronary embolization. In many patients, however, a satisfactory explanation for the chest pain cannot be uncovered even after complete hemodynamic and angiographic studies.

PALPITATIONS AND EMBOLIC EVENTS. Patients with AF often are initially diagnosed when they present with AF or an embolic event (see later).

OTHER SYMPTOMS. Compression of the left recurrent laryngeal nerve by a greatly dilated left atrium, enlarged tracheobronchial lymph nodes, and a dilated pulmonary artery may cause hoarseness (Ortner syndrome). A history of repeated hemoptysis is common in patients with pulmonary hemosiderosis. Systemic venous hypertension, hepatomegaly, edema, ascites, and hydrothorax are all signs of severe MS with elevated pulmonary vascular resistance and right-sided heart failure.

Physical Examination (see Chap. 11)

The most common findings on physical examination in patients with MS are an irregular pulse caused by AF and signs of left and right heart failure. The classical diastolic murmur and loud first heart sound are often difficult to appreciate. Patients with severe chronic MS, a low cardiac output, and systemic vasoconstriction may exhibit the so-called *mitral facies,* characterized by pinkish-purple patches on the cheeks. The arterial pulse is usually normal, but in patients with a reduced stroke volume, the pulse may be small in volume. The jugular venous pulse usually exhibits a prominent *a* wave in patients with sinus rhythm and elevated pulmonary vascular resistance. In patients with AF, the *x* descent of the jugular venous pulse disappears, and there is only one crest, a prominent *v* or *c-v* wave, per cardiac cycle. Palpation of the cardiac apex usually reveals an inconspicuous left ventricle; the presence of either a palpable presystolic expansion wave or an early diastolic rapid filling wave speaks strongly against serious MS. A readily palpable, tapping S1 suggests that the anterior mitral valve leaflet is pliable. When the patient is in the left lateral recumbent position, a diastolic thrill of MS may be palpable at the apex. Often a RV lift is felt in the left parasternal region in patients with pulmonary hypertension. A markedly enlarged right ventricle may displace the left ventricle posteriorly and produce a prominent RV apex beat that can be confused with a LV lift. A loud pulmonic closure sound (P2) may be palpable in the 2nd left intercostal space in patients with MS and pulmonary hypertension.

AUSCULTATION. The auscultatory features of MS (see Fig. 62-20) include an accentuated first heart sound (S1) with prolongation of the Q-S1 interval, correlating with the level of the left atrial pressure. Accentuation of S1 occurs when the mitral valve leaflets are flexible. It is caused, in part, by the rapidity with which LV pressure rises at the time of mitral valve closure, as well as by the wide closing excursion of the leaflets. Marked calcification and/or thickening of the mitral valve leaflets reduce the amplitude of S1, probably because of diminished motion of the leaflets. As pulmonary arterial pressure rises, closure of the pulmonic valve (P2) at first becomes accentuated and widely transmitted and can often be readily heard at both the mitral and the aortic areas. With further elevation of pulmonary arterial pressure, splitting of the second heart sound (S2) narrows because of reduced compliance of the pulmonary vascular bed, with earlier pulmonic valve closure. Finally, S2 becomes single and accentuated. Other signs of severe pulmonary hypertension include a nonvalvular pulmonic ejection sound that diminishes during inspiration, owing to dilation of the pulmonary artery; a systolic murmur of TR; a Graham Steell murmur of pulmonic regurgitation; and a fourth heart sound (S4) originating from the right ventricle. A third heart sound (S3) originating from the left ventricle is absent in patients with MS unless significant MR or AR coexists.

The opening snap (OS) of the mitral valve is caused by a sudden tensing of the valve leaflets after the valve cusps have completed their opening excursion. The OS occurs when the movement of the mitral dome into the left ventricle suddenly stops. It is most readily audible at the apex, using the diaphragm of the stethoscope. The OS can usually be differentiated from P2 because the OS occurs later, unless right bundle branch block is present. In addition, the OS usually is loudest at the apex whereas S2 is best heard at the cardiac base. The mitral valve cannot be totally rigid if it produces an OS, which is usually accompanied by an accentuated S1. Calcification confined to the tip of the mitral valve leaflets does not preclude an OS, although calcification of both the body and the tip does. The mitral OS follows A2 by 0.04 to 0.12 second; this interval varies inversely with the left atrial pressure. A short A2-OS interval is a reliable indicator of severe MS but accurate estimation of this time interval requires considerable experience.

THE DIASTOLIC MURMUR OF MITRAL STENOSIS. This murmur is a low-pitched, rumbling murmur, best heard at the apex, with the bell of the stethoscope and with the patient in the left lateral recumbent position. When this murmur is soft, it is limited to the apex, but when louder, it may radiate to the left axilla or the lower left sternal area. Although the intensity of the diastolic murmur is not closely related to the severity of stenosis, the duration of the murmur is a guide to the severity of mitral valve narrowing. The murmur persists for as long as the left atrioventricular pressure gradient exceeds approximately 3 mm Hg. The murmur usually commences immediately after the OS. In mild MS, the early diastolic murmur is brief, but in the presence of sinus rhythm it resumes in presystole. In severe MS the murmur is holodiastolic, with presystolic accentuation while sinus rhythm is maintained (see Fig. 16-20).

The diastolic rumbling murmur of MS is heard best using the bell (low-frequency setting) at the apex with the patient lying in the left lateral decubitus position. This low-pitched sound is often difficult to appreciate and may be masked by the presence of a thick chest wall, pulmonary emphysema, or a low cardiac output with a low flow rate across the mitral valve. In addition, the murmur is often localized and thus missed unless palpation is used to detect the apex of the left ventricle and to pinpoint the area at which auscultation should be carried out. In so-called "silent" MS, there is usually marked RV enlargement. Consequently, the right ventricle occupies the cardiac apex, the left ventricle is rotated posteriorly, and cardiac output is reduced so that the murmur either is not audible at all or can be heard only in the midaxillary or posterior axillary line. In addition to placing the patient in the left lateral position, auscultation of the murmur is facilitated during held expiration after having the patient increase cardiac output by walking or climbing a flight of stairs.

DYNAMIC AUSCULTATION (see also Chap. 11). The diastolic murmur and OS of MS are often reduced during inspiration and augmented during expiration, which is the opposite of what occurs when these findings are secondary to tricuspid stenosis. During inspiration, the A2-OS interval widens, and three sequential sounds (A2, P2, and OS) may be audible. Sudden standing and the resultant reduction of venous return lower the left atrial pressure and widen the A2-OS interval; this maneuver is useful in distinguishing an A2-OS combination from a split S2, which narrows on standing. In contrast, the A2-OS interval is significantly narrowed during exercise as left atrial pressure rises. The diastolic rumbling murmur of MS is reduced during the strain of a Valsalva maneuver and in any condition in which transmitral valve flow rate declines. Maneuvers such as coughing, isometric or isotonic exercise, and sudden squatting may accentuate a faint or equivocal murmur of MS.

OTHER AUSCULTATORY FINDINGS. A pansystolic murmur of TR and an S3 originating from the right ventricle may be audible in the 4th intercostal space in the left parasternal region in patients with severe MS. These signs, which are secondary to pulmonary hypertension, may be confused with the findings of MR. However, the inspiratory augmentation of the murmur and of the S3 and the prominent *v* wave in the jugular venous pulse aid in establishing that the murmur originates from the tricuspid valve. A high-pitched decrescendo diastolic murmur along the left sternal border in patients with MS and pulmonary hypertension may be audible pulmonic regurgitation (Graham Steell murmur) but often is caused by concomitant AR.

DIFFERENTIAL DIAGNOSIS. MS is a rare diagnosis in developed countries and most apical diastolic murmurs are due to other causes. In elderly patients, an apical diastolic rumble most likely is due to mitral annular calcification and 90 percent of patients with a diastolic apical murmur have no evidence of MS on echocardiography. In severe MR—indeed in any condition in which flow across a nonstenotic mitral valve is increased (such as a ventricular septal defect)—there may also be a short diastolic murmur following an S3. Left atrial myxoma may

produce auscultatory findings similar to those in rheumatic valvular MS (see Chap. 69). A diastolic rumble may also be present in some patients with HCM, caused by early diastolic flow into the hypertrophied, nondistensible left ventricle.

Echocardiography (see also Chap. 14)

Echocardiography is the most accurate approach to diagnosis and evaluation of MS.[125] Echocardiography is recommended in all patients with MS at initial presentation, for reevaluation of changing symptoms or signs, and at regular intervals (depending on disease severity) for monitoring disease progression (see Table 62-1).[1]

Imaging shows the characteristic anatomy with leaflet thickening and restriction of opening caused by symmetric fusion of the commissures, resulting in "doming" of the leaflets in diastole (see Fig. 62-19). As disease becomes more severe, thickening extends from the leaflet tips toward the base with further restriction of motion and less curvature of the leaflet in diastole. The mitral chords are variably thickening, fused, and shortened and there may be superimposed calcification of the valve apparatus (see also Figs. 14-4C, 5C, and 5D).

Mitral valve area is measured by direct planimetry from 2D short axis images and calculated by the Doppler pressure half-time method (see Figs. 14-41 and 44). The transmitral gradient is also calculated (see Fig. 14-38B) and any coexisting MR is quantitated on the basis of the accepted guidelines.[105] Evaluation of the morphology of the valve is key in predicting the hemodynamic results and outcome of percutaneous BMV. A score of 0 to 4+ is given for leaflet thickness, mobility, calcification, and chordal involvement to provide an overall score that is favorable (low) or unfavorable (high) for valvuloplasty. Other important anatomical features of the valve are the degree of anterior leaflet doming, the symmetry of commissural fusion, and the distribution of leaflet calcification.

Other key features on echocardiography are left atrial size, pulmonary artery pressures, LV size and systolic function, and RV size and systolic function. When pulmonary hypertension is present, the right ventricle is frequently dilated with reduced systolic function. TR may be secondary to RV dysfunction and annular dilation or may be caused by rheumatic involvement of the tricuspid valve. Complete evaluation of aortic valve anatomy and function is also important because the aortic valve is affected in approximately one third of patients with MS.

When transthoracic images are suboptimal, transesophageal echocardiography (TEE) is appropriate.[1] TEE is also necessary to exclude left atrial thrombus and to evaluate MR severity when percutaneous BMV is considered.[1] However, MV morphology typically is best evaluated on transthoracic imaging. With transesophageal imaging, it is rarely possible to obtain a short axis image of the valve, which is helpful in evaluation of the symmetry and calcification of the commissures. In addition, the subvalvular region often is shadowed by the more proximal valve leaflets with this approach.

In nearly all patients with MS, a detailed echocardiographic examination, including two-dimensional echocardiography (transthoracic or transesophageal), a Doppler study, and color flow Doppler imaging, provides sufficient information to develop a therapeutic plan without the need for cardiac catheterization (see later).

EXERCISE TESTING WITH DOPPLER ECHOCARDIOGRAPHY. Exercise testing is useful in many patients with MS to ascertain the level of physical conditioning and to elicit covert cardiac symptoms. The exercise test can be combined with Doppler echocardiography to assess exercise hemodynamics,[1] usually with the Doppler examination

CH 62

performed at rest after termination of exercise. Exercise Doppler testing is recommended when there is a discrepancy between resting echocardiographic findings and the severity of clinical symptoms.[1] Useful parameters on exercise testing include: (1) exercise duration, (2) blood pressure and heart rate response, (3) change in mean transmitral gradient with exercise, and (4) the increase in pulmonary pressures with exercise, compared with the expected normal changes. An exercise pulmonary systolic pressure greater than 60 mm Hg is a key decision point in management of these patients.

Other Diagnostic Evaluation

ELECTROCARDIOGRAPHY (see also Chap. 12). The electrocardiogram (ECG) is relatively insensitive for detecting mild MS, but it does show characteristic changes in moderate or severe obstruction. Left atrial enlargement (P-wave duration in lead II ≥0.12 second and/or a P-wave axis between +45 and −30 degrees) is a principal ECG feature of MS and is found in 90 percent of patients with significant MS and sinus rhythm. The ECG signs of left atrial enlargement correlate more closely with left atrial volume than with left atrial pressure and often regress following successful valvotomy. AF usually develops in the presence of pre-existing ECG evidence of left atrial enlargement and is related to the size of the chamber, the extent of fibrosis of the left atrial myocardium, the duration of atriomegaly, and the age of the patient.

Whether or not there is ECG evidence of RV hypertrophy depends largely on the height of RV systolic pressure. Approximately half of all patients with RV systolic pressures between 70 and 100 mm Hg manifest the ECG criteria for RV hypertrophy including both a mean QRS axis greater than 80 degrees in the frontal plane and an R : S ratio greater than 1 in lead V1. Other patients with this degree of pulmonary hypertension have no frank evidence of RV hypertrophy, but the R : S ratio fails to increase from the right to the midprecordial leads. When RV systolic pressure is greater than 100 mm Hg in patients with isolated or predominant MS, ECG evidence of RV hypertrophy is found quite consistently.

RADIOLOGICAL FINDINGS (see also Figs. 15-14, 15-16, and 15-17). Although their cardiac silhouette may be normal in the frontal projection, patients with hemodynamically significant MS almost invariably have evidence of left atrial enlargement on the lateral and left anterior oblique views. Extreme left atrial enlargement rarely occurs in pure MS; when it is present, MR is usually severe. Enlargement of the pulmonary artery, right ventricle, and right atrium (as well as the left atrium) is commonly seen in patients with severe MS. Occasionally, calcification of the mitral valve is evident on the chest roentgenogram, but, more commonly, fluoroscopy is required to detect valvular calcification.

Radiological changes in the lung fields indirectly reflect the severity of MS. Interstitial edema, an indication of severe obstruction, is manifested as Kerley B lines (dense, short, horizontal lines most commonly seen in the costophrenic angles). This finding is present in 30 percent of patients with resting pulmonary arterial wedge pressures less than 20 mm Hg and in 70 percent of patients with pressures greater than 20 mm Hg. Severe, longstanding mitral obstruction often results in Kerley A lines (straight, dense lines up to 4 cm in length running toward the hilum), as well as the findings of pulmonary hemosiderosis and rarely of parenchymal ossification. Pulmonary edema is seldom evident.

CARDIAC CATHETERIZATION. Catheter-based measurement of left atrial and LV pressures shows the expected hemodynamics and allows measurement of mean transmitral pressure gradient and, in conjunction with measurement of transmitral volume flow rate, calculation of valve

area using the Gorlin formula (see Chap. 19). Occasionally, diagnostic cardiac catheterization is necessary when echocardiography is nondiagnostic or results are discrepant with clinical findings. More often, these measurements now are recorded for monitoring before, during, and after percutaneous BMV. Routine diagnostic cardiac catheterization is not recommended for evaluation of MS.

Disease Course

Interval Between Acute Rheumatic Fever and Mitral Valve Obstruction

In temperate zones, such as the United States and Western Europe, patients who develop acute rheumatic fever have an asymptomatic period of approximately 15 to 20 years before symptoms of MS develop. It then takes approximately 5 to 10 years for most patients to progress from mild disability (i.e., early NYHA Class II) to severe disability (i.e., NYHA Class III or IV) (Fig. 62-21). The progression is much more rapid in patients in tropical and subtropical areas, in Polynesians, and in Alaskan Inuits. In India, critical MS may be present in children as young as 6 to 12 years old. In North America and Western Europe, however, symptoms develop more slowly and occur most commonly between the ages of 45 and 65.[1] The most likely cause for these differences are the relative prevalence of rheumatic fever, and lack of primary and secondary prevention resulting in recurrent episodes of valve scarring (see Chap. 83).

Hemodynamic Progression

Serial echocardiographic data have described the rate of hemodynamic progression in patients with mild MS.[30] The two largest series followed a combined total of 153 adults with a mean age about 60 years, for an average of slightly more than 3 years.[129,130] As in most series of MS patients, 75 percent to 80 percent were women. The initial valve area was 1.7 ± 0.6 cm^2 and the overall rate of progression was a decrease in valve area of 0.09 cm^2/yr. Approximately one third of patients showed rapid progression defined as a decrease in valve area greater than 0.1 cm^2/yr. These data apply to the older MS patients seen in developed countries. There are little data on the rate of hemodynamic progression of rheumatic MS in underdeveloped countries where the age at symptom onset is much younger.

CLINICAL OUTCOMES

Natural history data obtained in the presurgical era indicate that symptomatic patients with MS have a poor outlook with 5-year survival rates of 62 percent among patients with MS in NYHA Class III but only 15 percent among those in Class IV. Data from unoperated patients in the surgical era still report a 5-year survival rate of only 44 percent in patients with symptomatic MS who refused valvotomy (Fig. 62-22).

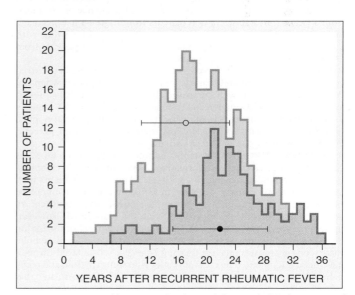

FIGURE 62–21 Interval between active rheumatic fever and clinical symptoms of valve disease in 177 patients with mitral stenosis (yellow bars) and 121 with aortic stenosis (blue bars). *(From Horstkotte D, Niehues R, Strauer BE: Pathomorphological aspects, aetiology, and natural history of acquired mitral valve stenosis. Eur Heart J 12[Suppl B]:55, 1991.)*

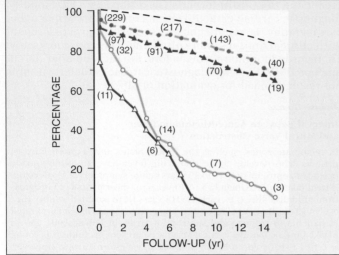

FIGURE 62–22 Natural history of 159 patients with isolated mitral stenosis (solid blue line) or mitral regurgitation (solid purple line) who were not operated on (even though the operation was indicated) compared with patients treated with valve replacement for mitral stenosis (dashed blue line) or mitral regurgitation (dashed purple line). The expected survival rate in the absence of mitral valve disease is indicated by the upper curve (dashed black line). *(From Horstkotte D, Niehues R, Strauer BE: Pathomorphological aspects, aetiology, and natural history of acquired mitral valve stenosis. Eur Heart J 12[Suppl B]:55, 1991.)*

Overall clinical outcomes are greatly improved in patients who undergo surgical or percutaneous relief of valve obstruction on the basis of current guidelines.[1] However, longevity is still shortened compared with expected for age, largely because of complications of the disease process (AF, systemic embolism, pulmonary hypertension) and side effects of therapy (e.g., prosthetic valves, anticoagulation).

COMPLICATIONS

Atrial Fibrillation

The most common complication of MS is AF. The prevalence of AF in patients with MS is related to both the severity of valve obstruction and patient age. In historical series AF was present in 17 percent of those age 21 to 30 years, 45 percent of those age 31 to 40 years, 60 percent of those age 41 to 50 years and 80 percent of those older than age 51 years. Even when stenosis is severe, the prevalence of AF is related to age. In more recent BMV studies the prevalence of AF ranged from 4 percent in a series of 600 patients from India with a mean age of 27 years and 27 percent in a series of 4832 patients from China with a mean age of 37 years to 40 percent in a series of 1024 patients from France with a mean age of 49 years.

AF may precipitate or worsen symptoms caused by loss of the atrial contribution to filling and to a short diastolic filling period when the ventricular rate is not well controlled. In addition, AF predisposes to left atrial thrombus formation and systemic embolic events. AF conveys a worse overall prognosis in MS patients than in the general population. In patients with AF and MS, 5-year survival is only 64 percent, compared with 85 percent in AF patients without MS.

SYSTEMIC EMBOLISM. Systemic embolism in patients with MS is caused by left atrial thrombus formation. Although systemic embolization most often occurs in patients with AF, 20 percent of patients with MS and a systemic embolic event are in sinus rhythm. When embolization occurs in patients in sinus rhythm, the possibility of transient AF or underlying infective endocarditis should be considered. However, up to 45 percent of patients with MS who are in normal sinus rhythm have prominent spontaneous left atrial contrast (a marker of embolic risk) seen on transesophageal imaging (see Chap. 14). Atrial thrombi have been documented in a few MS patients in sinus rhythm, and many patients with new-onset AF have left atrial thrombi. It is postulated that loss of atrial appendage contractile function, despite electrical evidence of sinus rhythm, leads to blood flow stasis and thrombus formation.

The risk of embolism correlates directly with patient age and left atrial size and inversely with the cardiac output. Before the advent of surgical treatment, this serious complication of MS developed in at least 20 percent of patients at some time during the course of their disease. Before the era of anticoagulant therapy and surgical treatment, approximately 25 percent of all fatalities in patients with mitral valve disease were secondary to systemic embolism.

Approximately half of all clinically apparent emboli are found in the cerebral vessels. Coronary embolism may lead to myocardial infarction and/or angina pectoris, and renal emboli may be responsible for the development of systemic hypertension. Emboli are recurrent and multiple in approximately 25 percent of patients who develop this complication. Rarely, massive thrombosis develops in the left atrium, resulting in a pedunculated ball-valve thrombus, which may suddenly aggravate obstruction to left atrial outflow when a specific body position is assumed or may cause sudden death. Similar consequences occur in patients with free-floating thrombi in the left atrium. These two conditions are usually characterized by variability in the physical findings, often on a positional basis. They are very hazardous and require surgical treatment, often as an emergency.

INFECTIVE ENDOCARDITIS (see also Chap. 63). MS is a predisposing factor for endocarditis in less than 1 percent of cases in clinical series of bacterial endocarditis. The estimated risk of endocarditis in patients with MS is 0.17 per 1000 patient-years, which is much lower than the risk in patients with MR or aortic valve disease.

Management

Medical Treatment

The medical management of MS is primarily directed toward (1) prevention of recurrent rheumatic fever, (2) prevention and treatment of complications of MS and (3) monitoring disease progression to allow intervention at the optimal time point.[131] Patients with MS caused by rheumatic heart disease should receive penicillin prophylaxis for beta-hemolytic streptococcal infections to prevent recurrent rheumatic fever per established guidelines (see Chap. 83). Prophylaxis for infective endocarditis is no longer recommended (see Chap. 63). Anemia and infections should be treated promptly and aggressively in patients with valvular heart disease. However, blood cultures should always be considered before beginning antibiotic therapy in patients with valve disease because the presentation of endocarditis often is mistaken for a noncardiac infection.

Anticoagulant therapy is indicated for prevention of systemic embolism in MS patients with AF (persistent or paroxysmal), any prior embolic events (even if in sinus rhythm) and in those with documented left atrial thrombus. Anticoagulation also may be considered in patients with severe MS and sinus rhythm when there is severe left atrial enlargement (diameter >55 mm) or spontaneous contrast on echocardiography. Treatment with warfarin is used to maintain the international normalized ratio (INR) between 2 and 3.[1,132]

Asymptomatic patients with mild to moderate rheumatic mitral valve disease should have a history and physical examination yearly[1] with echocardiography every 3 to 5 years for mild stenosis, every 1 to 2 years for moderate stenosis, and annually for severe stenosis. More frequent evaluation is appropriate for any change in signs or symptoms. All patients with significant MS should be advised to avoid occupations requiring strenuous exertion.

In patients with severe MS with persistent symptoms after intervention or when intervention is not possible, medical therapy with oral diuretics and the restriction of sodium intake may improve symptoms. Digitalis glycosides do not alter the hemodynamics and usually do not benefit patients with MS and sinus rhythm, but these drugs are of value in slowing the ventricular rate in patients with AF and in treating patients with right-sided heart failure. Hemoptysis is managed by measures designed to reduce pulmonary venous pressure, including sedation, assumption of the upright position, and aggressive diuresis. Beta-blocking agents and rate-slowing calcium antagonists may increase exercise capacity by reducing heart rate in patients with sinus rhythm and especially in patients with AF.[1]

TREATMENT OF ARRHYTHMIAS. AF is a frequent complication of severe MS. Management of AF in patients with MS is similar to management in patients with AF of any cause. However, it typically is more difficult to restore and maintain sinus rhythm because of pressure overload of the left atrium in conjunction with effects of the rheumatic process on atrial tissue and the conducting system.

Immediate treatment of AF includes administration of intravenous heparin followed by oral warfarin. The ventricular rate should be slowed as stated in the ACC/AHA Guidelines for management of atrial fibrillaton,[132] initially with an intravenous beta-blocker or nondihydropyridine calcium channel antagonist, followed by long-term rate control with oral doses of these agents. When these medications are ineffective or when additional rate control is necessary, digoxin or amiodarone may be considered. Digoxin alone for long-term management of AF may be considered in patients with concurrent LV dysfunction or a sedentary lifestyle. An effort should be made to reestablish sinus rhythm by a combination of pharmacological treatment and cardioversion. If cardioversion is planned in a patient who has had AF for more than 24 hours before the procedure, anticoagulation with warfarin for more than 3 weeks is indicated. Alternatively, if a transesophageal echocardiogram shows no atrial thrombus, immediate cardioversion can be carried out provided the patient is effectively anticoagulated with intravenous heparin before and during the procedure and with warfarin for at least 1 month after cardioversion. Paroxysmal AF and repeated conversions, spontaneous or induced, carry the risk of embolization. In patients who cannot be converted or maintained in sinus rhythm, digitalis should be used to maintain the ventricular rate at rest at approximately 60 beats/min. If this is not possible, small doses of a beta-blocking agent, such as atenolol (25 mg daily) or metoprolol (50 to 100 mg daily), may be added. Beta blockers are particularly helpful in preventing rapid ventricular responses that develop during exertion. Multiple repeat cardioversions are not indicated if the patient fails to sustain sinus rhythm while on adequate doses of an antiarrhythmic.

Patients with chronic AF who undergo surgical MV repair or MV replacement may undergo the maze procedure (atrial compartment operation).[133,134] More than 80 percent of patients undergoing this procedure can be maintained in sinus rhythm postoperatively and can regain normal atrial function, including a satisfactory success rate in those with significant left atrial enlargement. Early intervention with percutaneous valvotomy may prevent development of AF.[135]

Mitral Valvotomy

PERCUTANEOUS BALLOON MITRAL VALVOTOMY
(see Chap. 55)

Patients with mild to moderate MS who are asymptomatic frequently remain so for years, and clinical outcomes are similar to age-matched normal patients. However, severe or symptomatic MS is associated with poor long-term outcomes if the stenosis is not relieved mechanically (see Fig. 62-22). Percutaneous BMV is the procedure of choice for treatment of MS so that surgical intervention now is reserved for patients who require intervention and are not candidates for a percutaneous procedure.[1,136,137]

BMV is recommended in symptomatic patients with moderate to severe MS (i.e., a mitral valve area

< ≈1 cm²/m² body surface area (BSA) or <1.5 cm² in normal-sized adults) and with: favorable valve morphology, no or mild MR, and no evidence for left atrial thrombus (Fig. 62-23). Even mild symptoms, such as a subtle decrease in exercise tolerance, are an indication for intervention because the procedure relieves symptoms and improves long-term outcome with a low procedural risk. In addition, BMV is recommended for asymptomatic patients with moderate-severe MS when mitral valve obstruction has resulted in pulmonary hypertension with a pulmonary systolic pressure greater than 50 mm Hg at rest or 60 mm Hg with exercise.[1]

BMV also is reasonable in symptomatic patients who are at high risk for surgery, even when valve morphology is not ideal, including patients with restenosis after a previous BMV or previous commissurotomy,[138] who are unsuitable for surgery because of very high risk. These include very elderly, frail patients; patients with associated severe ischemic heart disease; patients in whom MS is complicated by pulmonary, renal, or neoplastic disease; women of childbearing age in whom MV replacement is undesirable; and pregnant women with MS.[139]

BMV may be considered in patients with moderate to severe MS and new onset AF and in those with "mild" MS when significant pulmonary hypertension is present (see Fig. 62-23). In this last group, it is likely that valve obstruction is the cause of pulmonary hypertension, even when stenosis severity does not meet the valve area criteria for severe obstruction. BMV also has acceptable results in patients with accompanying mild or moderate AR.

This percutaneous technique consists of advancing a small balloon flotation catheter across the interatrial septum (after transseptal puncture), enlarging the opening, advancing a large (23 to 25 mm) hourglass-shaped balloon (the

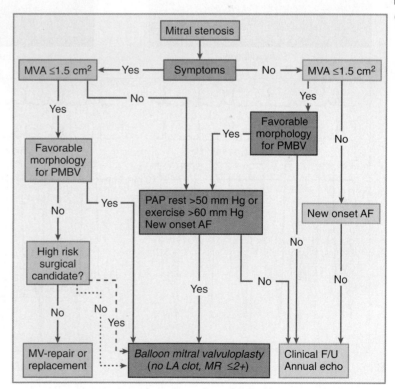

FIGURE 62–23 Management strategy for patients with mitral stenosis. AF = atrial fibrillation; MV = mitral valve; MVA = mitral valve area; PAP = pulmonary artery systolic pressure. *(Modified from Bonow RO, Carabello BA, Chatterjee K, et al: ACC/AHA 2006 guidelines for the management of patients with valvular heart disease: a report of the American College of Cardiology/American Heart Association Task Force on Practice Guidelines (writing committee to revise the 1998 Guidelines for the Management of Patients With Valvular Heart Disease). Circulation 114:e84, 2006.)*

1654 Inoue balloon), and inflating it within the orifice (Fig. 62-24).[136] Alternatively, two smaller (15 to 20 mm) side-by-side balloons across the mitral orifice may be employed. A third technique involves retrograde, nontransseptal dilation of the mitral valve in which the balloon is positioned across the mitral valve using a steerable guidewire. Because the cost of the balloon catheter is deemed high in countries with restricted financial resources, a reusable metallic valvulotome has been devised. Early results are at least as good as those achieved with balloon catheters.[140]

Commissural separation and fracture of nodular calcium appear to be the mechanisms responsible for improvement in valvular function. In several series, the hemodynamic results of BMV have been quite favorable (Fig. 62-25), with reduction of the transmitral pressure gradient from an average of approximately 18 mm Hg to 6 mm Hg, a small (average 20 percent) increase in cardiac output, and an average doubling of the calculated mitral valve area from 1 to 2 cm^2.[131,136] Results are especially impressive in younger patients without severe valvular thickening or calcification (see Fig. 62-19). Elevated pulmonary vascular resistance declines rapidly, although usually not completely.[141] The reported mortality rate has ranged from 1 to 2 percent. Complications include cerebral emboli and cardiac perforation, each in approximately 1 percent of patients, and the development of MR severe enough to require operation in another 2 percent (≈15 percent develop lesser, but still undesirable, degrees of MR). Approximately 5 percent of patients are left with a small residual atrial septal defect, but this closes or decreases in size in the majority. Rarely, the defect is large enough to cause right-sided heart failure; this complication most often is seen in conjunction with an unsuccessful mitral valvotomy.

The likelihood of hemodynamic benefit and the risk of complication with BMV are predicted by anatomical features of the stenosed valve. Rigid, thickened valves with extensive subvalvular fibrosis and calcification lead to suboptimal results.[1] One echocardiographic scoring system divides patients into 3 groups: those with a pliable, noncalcified anterior leaflet and little chordal disease (Group 1); those with a pliable, noncalcified anterior leaflet but with chordal thickening and shortening (<10 mm long) (Group 2); and those with fluoroscopic evidence of calcification of any extent of the valve apparatus (Group 3).[142] Event-free survival at 3 years is highest for Group 1 (89 percent) compared with Group 2 (78 percent) or Group 3 (65 percent).[127,142] With an alternate echocardiographic scoring system, leaflet rigidity, leaflet thickening, valvular calcification, and subvalvular disease are each scored from 0 to 4.[1,125,137] A score of 8 or less is usually associated with an excellent immediate and long-term result, whereas scores exceeding 8 are associated with less impressive results (Fig. 62-26) including the risk of development of MR. Commissural calcification also is a predictor of poor outcomes.[1,143]

Transesophageal echocardiography should be performed just prior to BMV to exclude left atrial thrombus and to confirm that MR is not moderate or severe. Transesophageal echocardiography also is appropriate for evaluation of MS severity and mitral valve morphology when

CH 62

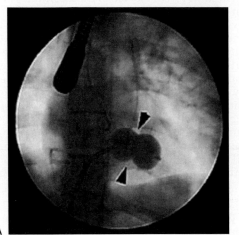
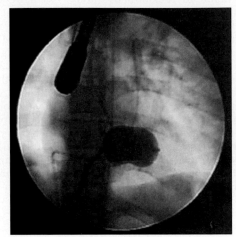

A

Early inflation   Full expansion

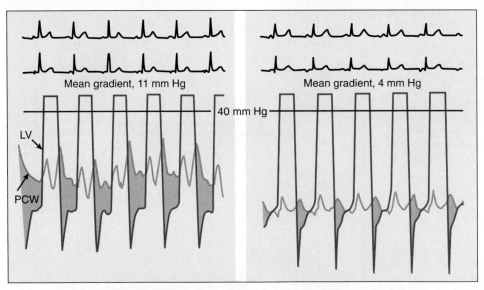

B

Before valvuloplasty   After valvuloplasty

Mean gradient, 11 mm Hg Mean gradient, 4 mm Hg

40 mm Hg

LV

PCW

FIGURE 62–24 Percutaneous balloon mitral valvotomy (BMV) for mitral stenosis using the Inoue technique. **A,** The catheter is advanced into the left atrium via the transseptal technique and guided antegrade across the mitral orifice. As the balloon is inflated, its distal portion expands first and is pulled back so that it fits snugly against the orifice. With further inflation, the proximal portion of the balloon expands to center the balloon within the stenotic orifice **(left).** Further inflation expands the central "waist" portion of the balloon **(right),** resulting in commissural splitting and enlargement of the orifice. **B,** Successful BMV results in significant increase in mitral valve area, as reflected by reduction in the diastolic pressure gradient between left ventricle (magenta) and pulmonary capillary wedge (blue) pressure, as indicated by the shaded area. (See also Chap. 55.) *(From Delabays A, Goy JJ: Images in clinical medicine: Percutaneous mitral valvuloplasty. N Engl J Med 345:e4, 2001.)*

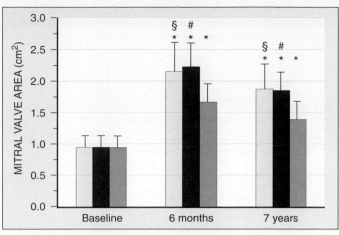

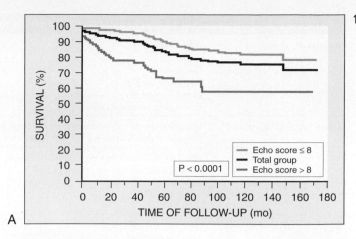

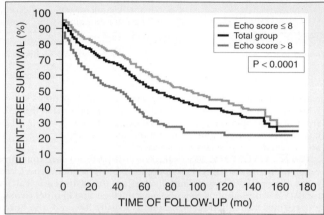

FIGURE 62–25 Mitral valve area before and 6 months and 7 years after valvotomy in a prospective, randomized trial of balloon mitral valvotomy (BMV, yellow bars), open surgical mitral commissurotomy (OMC, purple bars) and closed mitral commissurotomy (CMC, blue bars). At 6 months and 7 years, the results of BMV were equivalent to those of OMC and superior to those of CMC. *(From Farhat MB, Ayari M, Maatouk F, et al: Percutaneous balloon versus surgical closed and open mitral commissurotomy: Seven-year follow-up results of a randomized trial. Circulation 97:245, 1998.)*

transthoracic images are suboptimal, but the chordal apparatus is less well visualized compared to transthoracic imaging. During the procedure, transthoracic, transesophageal or intracardiac echocardiography is used to monitor placement of the catheters and balloon, assess hemodynamic results after each inflation, and detect complications such as MR.

In patients with favorable anatomical findings, long-term results are favorable with excellent survival rates without functional disability or need for surgery or repeat BMV.[126,127,136,144,145] A prospective randomized trial in which patients with severe MS were randomized to undergo BMV, closed surgical valvotomy, or open surgical valvotomy resulted in similar clinical results with BMV and the open surgical technique that were superior to the results of the closed surgical valvotomy.[145] After 7 years, mitral valve area was equivalent in the BMV and open surgical groups, both significantly greater than in the closed valvotomy group (see Fig. 62-25). In another randomized study that included older patients with less favorable valve morphology, compared with open surgical commissurotomy, patients randomized to BMV had a smaller increase in valve area and higher likelihood of restenosis (28 versus 18 percent at 4 years).[146] Excellent results have also been reported in children and adolescents in developing nations, where patients tend to be younger. These young patients usually have quite pliable valves, which are ideal for BMV.

SURGICAL VALVOTOMY

Three operative approaches are available for the treatment of rheumatic MS: (1) closed mitral valvotomy using a transatrial or transventricular approach; (2) open valvotomy (i.e., valvotomy carried out under direct vision with the aid of cardiopulmonary bypass, which may be combined with other repair techniques, such as leaflet resection, chordal procedures and annuloplasty when MR is present; and (3) MV replacement (Table 62-6). Surgical intervention for MS is recommended in patients with severe MS and significant symptoms (NYHA Class III or IV) when BMV is not available, BMV is contraindicated because of persistent left atrial thrombus or moderate to severe MR, or when the valve is calcified and surgical risk is acceptable. The preferred surgical approach is valve repair (open valvotomy with or without

FIGURE 62–26 Long-term survival **(A)** and event-free survival **(B)** after balloon mitral valvotomy for 879 patients who were stratified by baseline echocardiographic morphology score: 8 or less (blue line) or greater than 8 (gold line). Patients with the lower echo score had a significantly better outcome initially and over the next 12 to 13 years. *(From Palacios IF, Sanchez PL, Harrell LC, et al: Which patients benefit from percutaneous mitral balloon valvuloplasty? Prevalvuloplasty and postvalvuloplasty variables that predict long-term outcome. Circulation 105:1465, 2002.)*

additional procedures) whenever possible. Surgery also is reasonable in patients with severe MS and severe pulmonary hypertension when BMV is not possible and may be considered in patients with moderate to severe MS with recurrent embolic events despite anticoagulation.

CLOSED MITRAL VALVOTOMY. Closed mitral valvotomy is rarely used in the United States today, having been replaced by BMV, which is of greater effectiveness in patients who are candidates for closed mitral valvotomy.[144] Closed mitral valvotomy is more popular in developing nations, where the expense of open-heart surgery and even of balloon catheters for BMV is an important factor and where patients with MS are younger and therefore have more pliable valves. But even in these nations, closed mitral valvotomy is being displaced by BMV.

This procedure is performed without cardiopulmonary bypass but with the aid of a transventricular dilator. It is an effective operation, provided that MR, atrial thrombosis, or valvular calcification is not serious and that chordal fusion and shortening are not severe. Echocardiography is useful in selecting suitable candidates for this procedure by identifying patients without valvular calcification or dense fibrosis. If possible, closed mitral valvotomy should be carried out with "pump standby"; if the surgeon is unable to achieve a satisfactory result, the patient can be placed on cardiopulmonary bypass and the valvotomy carried out under direct vision or the valve replaced.

On average, the mitral valve area is increased by 1 cm², with only 20 to 30 percent of patients requiring MV replacement within 15 years.[143] The hospital mortality rate is 1 to 2 percent in experienced centers. Marked symptomatic improvement occurs in the majority of

TABLE 62–6	Approaches to Mechanical Relief of Mitral Stenosis	
Approach	**Advantages**	**Disadvantages**
Closed surgical valvotomy	Inexpensive Relatively simple Good hemodynamic results in selected patients Good long-term outcome	No direct visualization of valve Only feasible with flexible, noncalcified valves Contraindicated if MR >2+ Surgical procedure with general anesthesia
Open surgical valvotomy	Visualization of valve allows directed valvotomy Concurrent annuloplasty for MR is feasible	Best results with flexible, noncalcified valves Surgical procedure with general anesthesia

Valve replacement	Feasible in all patients regardless of extent of
	  valve calcification or severity of MR
		Surgical procedure with general anesthesia
		Effect of loss of annular-papillary muscle continuity on
		  LV function
		Prosthetic valve
		Chronic anticoagulation

Balloon mitral valvotomy	Percutaneous approach Local anesthesia Good hemodynamic results in selected patients Good long-term outcome	No direct visualization of valve Only feasible with flexible, noncalcified valves Contraindicated if MR >2+

LV=left ventricular; MR=mitral regurgitation.
From Otto CM: Valvular Heart Disease. 2nd ed. Philadelphia, WB Saunders, 2004, p 296.

CH 62

patients, and there is excellent long-term survival in patients selected with low echo scores.[137] Long-term follow-up has shown that the results are best if the operation is carried out before chronic AF and/or heart failure has occurred, and complication rates are higher when valves are calcified and/or severely thickened.[1,137]

OPEN VALVOTOMY. Most surgeons now prefer to carry out direct-vision or open valvotomy. This operation is most frequently performed in patients with MS whose mitral valves are too distorted or calcified for BMV. Cardiopulmonary bypass is established, and in order to obtain a dry, quiet heart, body temperature is usually lowered, the heart is arrested, and the aorta is occluded intermittently. Thrombi are removed from the left atrium and its appendage, and the latter is often amputated in order to remove a potential source of postoperative emboli. The commissures are incised, and, when necessary, fused chordae tendineae are separated, the underlying papillary muscle is split, and the valve leaflets are debrided of calcium. Mild or even moderate MR may be corrected using similar repair approaches as for primary MR. Left atrial and ventricular pressures are measured after bypass has been discontinued to confirm that the valvotomy has, in fact, been effective. When it has not been effective, another attempt can be made. When repair is not possible—most commonly owing to severe distortion and calcification of the valve and subvalvular apparatus with accompanying regurgitation that cannot be corrected—MV replacement should be carried out. In patients with AF, a left atrial maze or AF ablation procedure typically is done at the time of surgery to increase the likelihood of long-term sinus rhythm. Open valvotomy is feasible and successful in more than 80 percent of patients referred for this procedure, with an operative mortality of 1 percent, a rate of reoperation for MV replacement of 0 to 16 percent at 36 to 53 months, and 10-year actuarial survival rates of 81 to 100 percent.[143]

RE-STENOSIS AFTER VALVOTOMY

Mitral valvotomy, whether percutaneous or operative and whether open or closed, is palliative rather than curative, and even when successful, there is some degree of residual mitral valve dysfunction. Because the valve is not normal postoperatively, turbulent flow usually persists in the para-valvular region, and the resultant trauma may well play a role in restenosis. These changes are analogous to the gradual development of obstruction in a congenitally bicuspid aortic valve and are not usually the result of recurrent rheumatic fever. It is likely that the process of superimposed leaflet calcification and increased stiffness superimposed on the rheumatic valve is similar to the calcific changes seen in aortic valve stenosis.

On clinical grounds alone (based on the reappearance of symptoms), the incidence of "restenosis" has been estimated to range widely (from 2 to 60 percent). Recurrence of symptoms is usually not due to restenosis but may be caused by one or more of the following conditions: (1) an inadequate first operation with residual stenosis; (2) increased severity of MR, either at operation or as a consequence of infective endocarditis; (3) progression of aortic valve disease; or (4) development of coronary artery disease. True restenosis occurs in less than 20 percent of patients who are followed for 10 years.[1]

Thus in properly selected patients, mitral valvotomy, however performed—percutaneous BMV, closed or open surgical valvotomy—is a low-risk procedure that results in a significant increase in the size of the mitral orifice and favorably alters the clinical course of an otherwise progressive disease. Pulmonary arterial pressure falls promptly and decisively when mitral obstruction is effectively relieved. The majority of patients maintain clinical improvement for 10 to 15 years of follow-up. When a second procedure is required because of symptomatic deterioration, the valve is usually calcified and more seriously deformed than at the time of the first operation, and adequate reconstruction may not be possible. Accordingly, MV replacement is often necessary at that time.

Mitral Valve Replacement

MV replacement is recommended for symptomatic patients with severe MR when BMV or surgical MV repair are not possible. Most often, MV replacement is required in patients with combined MS and moderate or severe MR; in those with extensive commissural calcification, severe fibrosis, and subvalvular fusion; and in those who have undergone previous valvotomy. The operative mortality rate for isolated MV replacement ranges from 3 to 8 percent in most centers and averaged 6.04 percent in the large database of 16,105 such operations for patients with MS and/or MR reported in the Society of Thoracic Surgeons (STS) National Database[84] (see Table 62-3). Prosthetic valves are associated with increased risk because of valve deterioration and chronic anticoagulation, so the threshold for operation should be higher in patients in whom preoperative evaluation suggests that MV replacement may be required than in patients in whom valvotomy alone appears to be indicated. Generally, a mechanical valve is preferred when MV replacement for MS is necessary in patients younger than 65 years of age, particularly when AF is present because of the need for chronic anticoagulation.[1] In patients younger than age 65 who are in sinus rhythm, a mechanical valve is reasonable because of the risk of tissue valve deterioration and likely need for a second operation in the future. However, some younger patients may choose a bioprosthetic valve for lifestyle considerations, despite the risk of valve deterioration. A bioprosthetic valve is appropriate in patients who cannot take warfarin and is reasonable in patients older than 65 years of age.[1]

MV replacement is indicated in two groups of patients with MS whose valves are not suitable for valvotomy: (1) those with a mitral valve area less than 1.5 cm² in NYHA Class III or IV; and (2) those with severe MS (mitral valve area <1 cm²), NYHA Class II, and severe pulmonary hypertension (pulmonary artery systolic pressure >70 mm Hg).[1] Because the operative mortality risk may be quite high (10 to 20 percent) in patients in NYHA Class IV, operation should be carried out before patients reach this stage if possible. On the other hand, even such high-risk patients should not be denied operation unless they have comorbid conditions that preclude surgery or a satisfactory outcome.

MITRAL REGURGITATION

Etiology and Pathology

The mitral valve apparatus involves the mitral leaflets per se, chordae tendineae, papillary muscles, and mitral annulus (Fig. 62-27). Abnormalities of any of these structures may cause MR.[96,147] The major causes of MR include mitral valve prolapse (MVP), rheumatic heart disease, infective endocarditis, annular calcification, cardiomyopathy, and ischemic heart disease (Table 62-7). Specific aspects of the MVP syndrome, the most important cause of significant MR in the United States, are discussed in a separate section. Less common causes of MR include collagen vascular diseases, trauma, the hypereosinophilic syndrome, carcinoid, and exposure to certain drugs.

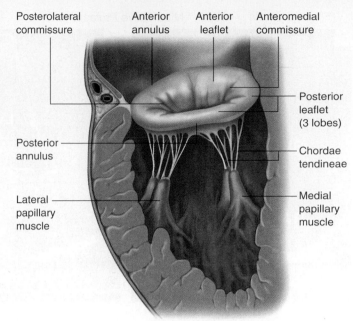

FIGURE 62–27 Continuity of the mitral apparatus and the left ventricular myocardium. Mitral regurgitation (MR) may be caused by any condition that affects the leaflets or the structure and function of the left ventricle. Similarly, a surgical procedure that disrupts the mitral apparatus in an attempt to correct MR has adverse effects on left ventricular geometry, volume, and function. *(From Otto CM: Evaluation and management of chronic mitral regurgitation. N Engl J Med 345:740, 2001.)*

CH 62

Valvular Heart Disease

TABLE 62–7	Causes of Acute and Chronic Mitral Regurgitation
Acute	**Chronic**
Mitral Annulus Disorders	***Inflammatory***
Infective endocarditis (abscess formation)	Rheumatic heart disease
Trauma (valvular heart surgery)	Systemic lupus erythematosus
Paravalvular leak caused by suture interruption (surgical technical problems or infective endocarditis)	Scleroderma
	Degenerative
Mitral Leaflet Disorders	Myxomatous degeneration of mitral valve leaflets (Barlow click-murmur syndrome, prolapsing leaflet, mitral valve prolapse)
Infective endocarditis (perforation or interference with valve closure by vegetation)	Marfan syndrome
Trauma (tear during percutaneous balloon mitral valvotomy or penetrating chest injury)	Ehlers-Danlos syndrome
Tumors (atrial myxoma)	Pseudoxanthoma elasticum
Myxomatous degeneration	Calcification of mitral valve annulus
Systemic lupus erythematosus (Libman-Sacks lesion)	***Infective***
Rupture of Chordae Tendineae	Infective endocarditis affecting normal, abnormal, or prosthetic mitral valves
Idiopathic (e.g., spontaneous)	***Structural***
Myxomatous degeneration (mitral valve prolapse, Marfan syndrome, Ehlers-Danlos syndrome)	Ruptured chordae tendineae (spontaneous or secondary to myocardial infarction, trauma, mitral valve prolapse, endocarditis)
Infective endocarditis	Rupture or dysfunction of papillary muscle (ischemia or myocardial infarction)
Acute rheumatic fever	
Trauma (percutaneous balloon valvotomy, blunt chest trauma)	Dilation of mitral valve annulus and left ventricular cavity (congestive cardiomyopathies, aneurysmal dilation of the left ventricle)
Papillary Muscle Disorders	Hypertrophic cardiomyopathy
Coronary artery disease (causing dysfunction and rarely rupture)	Paravalvular prosthetic leak
Acute global left ventricular dysfunction	***Congenital***
Infiltrative diseases (amyloidosis, sarcoidosis)	Mitral valve clefts or fenestrations
Trauma	Parachute mitral valve abnormality in association with:
Primary Mitral Valve Prosthetic Disorders	Endocardial cushion defects
Porcine cusp perforation (endocarditis)	Endocardial fibroelastosis
Porcine cusp degeneration	Transposition of the great arteries
Mechanical failure (strut fracture)	Anomalous origin of the left coronary artery
Immobilized disc or ball of the mechanical prosthesis	

From Jutzy KR, Al-Zaibag M: Acute mitral and aortic valve regurgitation. *In* Al-Zaibag M, Duran CMG (eds): Valvular Heart Disease. New York, Marcel Dekker, 1994, pp 345-362 (left column); and Haffajee CI: Chronic mitral regurgitation. *In* Dalen JE. Alpert JS (eds): Valvular Heart Disease. 2nd ed. Boston, Little, Brown, 1987, p 112 (right column).

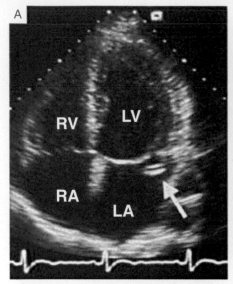

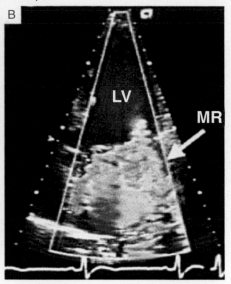

Idiopathic Dilated Cardiomyopathy

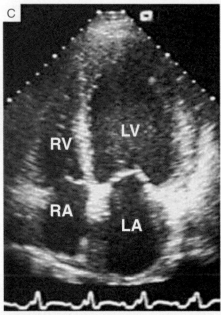

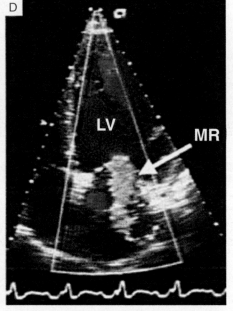

FIGURE 62–28 Echocardiographic four-chamber images in two patients with mitral regurgitation (**A** and **C**) with color Doppler images of the same patients (**B** and **D**). The top panels were obtained in a 46-year-old man with mitral valve prolapse and a partial flail posterior leaflet (arrow in **A**). The left ventricle (LV) is not dilated, but the left atrium (LA) is enlarged, and there is severe mitral regurgitation (MR). The bottom images were obtained in a patient with dilated cardiomyopathy, demonstrating left ventricular dilation, normal mitral valve leaflets, and restricted motion of the mitral leaflets leading to malcoaptation of the leaflets and moderate MR. RA = right atrium; RV = right ventricle. *(From Otto CM: Evaluation and management of chronic mitral regurgitation. N Engl J Med 345:740, 2001.)*

Abnormalities of Valve Leaflets

MR caused by involvement of the valve leaflets occurs in many situations. MR in patients with chronic rheumatic heart disease, in contrast to MS, is more frequent in men than in women. It is a consequence of shortening, rigidity, deformity, and retraction of one or both mitral valve cusps and is associated with shortening and fusion of the chordae tendineae and papillary muscles. MVP involves both leaflets and chordae and may also affect the annulus (Fig. 62-28). Infective endocarditis can cause MR by perforating valve leaflets (see Chap. 63); vegetations can prevent leaflet coaptation, and valvular retraction during the healing phase of endocarditis can cause MR. Destruction of the mitral valve leaflets can also occur in patients with penetrating and nonpenetrating trauma (see Chap. 71). MR associated with drug exposure also results from anatomical changes in the valve leaflets.[148-151]

Abnormalities of the Mitral Annulus

DILATION. In a normal adult, the mitral annulus measures approximately 10 cm in circumference. It is soft and flexible, and contraction of the surrounding LV muscle during systole causes the annular constriction that contributes importantly to valve closure. MR secondary to dilation of the mitral annulus can occur in any form of heart disease characterized by dilation of the left ventricle, especially dilated cardiomyopathy (see Fig. 62-28). LV submitral aneurysm has been reported as a cause of annular MR in sub-Saharan Africa and appears to be due to a congenital defect in the posterior portion of the annulus. Diagnosis by transesophageal echocardiography and surgical repair have been reported.

CALCIFICATION. Idiopathic (degenerative) calcification of the mitral annulus is one of the most common cardiac abnormalities found at autopsy; in most hearts it is of little functional consequence. However, when severe (see also Fig. 15-19), it may be an important cause of MR,[96,152] and in contrast to MR secondary to rheumatic fever, it is more common in women than in men. The development of degenerative calcification of the mitral annulus shares common risk factors with atherosclerosis including systemic hypertension, hypercholesterolemia, and diabetes.[20] Hence mitral annular calcification is associated with coronary and carotid atherosclerosis[21] and identifies patients at higher risk for cardiovascular morbidity and mortality.[20] Annular calcification may also be accelerated by an intrinsic defect in the fibrous skeleton of the heart, as occurs in the Marfan and Hurler syndromes. In these two latter syndromes, the mitral annulus is not only calcified but also dilated, further contributing to MR. The incidence of mitral annular calcification is also increased in patients who have chronic renal failure with secondary hyperparathyroidism. The annulus may also become thick, rigid, and calcified secondary to rheumatic involvement; when this process is severe, it also can interfere with valve closure.

With severe annular calcification, a rigid, curved bar or ring of calcium encircles the mitral orifice (see Fig. 15-19), and calcific spurs may project into the adjacent LV myocardium. The calcification may immobilize the basal portion of the mitral leaflets, preventing their normal excursion in diastole and coaptation in systole, and aggravating the MR that results from loss of the normal sphincteric action of the mitral ring. Rarely, obstruction to LV filling may occur when severe calcification encroaches on or protrudes into the mitral orifice. In patients with severe calcification, the conduction system may be invaded by calcium, leading to atrioventricular and/or intraventricular conduction defects. Calcification of the aortic valve cusps is an associated finding in approximately 50 percent of patients with severe mitral annular calcification, but this rarely causes aortic stenosis (AS). Occasionally, calcific deposits extend into the coronary arteries.

ABNORMALITIES OF THE CHORDAE TENDINEAE. Such abnormalities are important causes of MR. Lengthening and rupture of the chordae tendineae are cardinal features of the MVP syndrome[153] (see Fig. 62-28). The chordae may be congenitally abnormal; rupture may be spontaneous ("primary") or may occur as a consequence of infective endocarditis, trauma, rheumatic fever, or, rarely, osteogenesis imperfecta or relapsing polychondritis. In most patients, no cause for chordal rupture is apparent other than increased mechanical strain. Chordae to the posterior leaflet rupture more frequently than those to the anterior leaflet. Patients with idiopathic rupture of mitral chordae tendineae frequently exhibit pathological fibrosis of the papillary muscles. It is possible that the dysfunction of the papillary muscles may cause stretching and ultimately rupture of the chordae tendineae. Chordal rupture may also result from acute LV dilation, regardless of the cause. Depending on the number of chordae involved in rupture and the rate at which rupture occurs, the resultant MR may be mild, moderate, or severe and acute, subacute, or chronic.

INVOLVEMENT OF THE PAPILLARY MUSCLES. Diseases of the LV papillary muscles are a frequent cause of MR. Because these muscles are perfused by the terminal portion of the coronary vascular bed, they are particularly vulnerable to ischemia, and any disturbance in coronary perfusion may result in papillary muscle dysfunction. When ischemia is transient, it results in temporary papillary muscle dysfunction and may cause transient episodes of MR that are sometimes associated with attacks of angina pectoris or pulmonary edema.[154] When ischemia of papillary muscles is severe and prolonged, it causes papillary muscle dysfunction and scarring, as well as chronic MR. The posterior papillary muscle, which is supplied by the posterior descending branch of the right coronary artery, becomes ischemic and infarcted more frequently than does the anterolateral papillary muscle; the latter is supplied by diagonal branches of the left anterior descending coronary artery and often by marginal branches from the left circumflex artery as well. Ischemia of the papillary muscles is caused most commonly by coronary atherosclerosis, but it may also occur in patients with severe anemia, shock, coronary arteritis of any cause, or an anomalous left coronary artery. MR occurs frequently in patients with healed myocardial infarcts[155-158] and is most frequently caused by regional dysfunction of the LV myocardium at the base of a papillary muscle resulting in tethering of the mitral leaflets and incomplete leaflet coaptation. Although necrosis of a papillary muscle is a frequent complication of myocardial infarction, frank rupture is far less common; the latter is usually fatal because of the extremely severe MR that it produces (see Chap. 50). However, rupture of one or two of the apical heads of a papillary muscle results in a lesser degree of MR and thus makes survival possible, usually following surgical therapy.

Various other disorders of the papillary muscles may also be responsible for the development of MR (see Table 62-7). These include congenital malposition of the muscles; absence of one papillary muscle, resulting in the so-called *parachute mitral valve syndrome;* and involvement or infiltration of the papillary muscles by a variety of processes including abscesses, granulomas, neoplasms, amyloidosis, and sarcoidosis.

Left Ventricular Dysfunction

Ischemic LV dysfunction and dilated cardiomyopathy are important etiological factors in development of MR (see Fig. 62-28), and represent the second leading cause of MR after MVP in the United States. LV dilatation of any cause including ischemia can alter the spatial relationships between the papillary muscles and the chordae tendineae and thereby result in functional MR.[155-158]

Some degree of MR is found in approximately 30 percent of patients with coronary artery disease who are being considered for coronary artery bypass surgery. In most of these patients, MR develops from tethering of the posterior leaflet because of regional LV dysfunction. The outlook for the patient with ischemic MR is substantially worse than that for MR from other causes because of the associated LV remodeling and systolic dysfunction. There may be additional ischemic damage to the papillary muscles, dilation of the mitral valve ring, and/or loss of systolic annular contraction contributing further to MR. In most of these patients, MR is mild; however, in the small percentage with severe MR (3 percent in one large series of patients with coronary artery disease proved by coronary arteriography), it is associated with a poor prognosis.[159,160] The incidence and severity of regurgitation vary inversely with the LV ejection fraction and directly with the LV end-diastolic pressure. MR occurs in approximately 20 percent of patients following acute myocardial infarction and, even when mild, is associated with a higher risk of adverse outcomes.[161,162]

Other causes of MR, discussed in greater detail elsewhere, include obstructive HCM (see Chap. 65), the hypereosinophilic syndrome, endomyocardial fibrosis, trauma affecting the leaflets and/or papillary muscles (see Chap. 71), Kawasaki disease (see Chaps. 61 and 84), left atrial myxoma (see Chap. 69), and various congenital anomalies including cleft anterior leaflet and ostium secundum atrial septal defect (see Chap. 61).

Pathophysiology

Because the regurgitant mitral orifice is functionally in parallel with the aortic valve, the impedance to ventricular emptying is reduced in patients with MR. Consequently, MR enhances LV emptying. Almost 50 percent of the regurgitant volume is ejected into the left atrium before the aortic valve opens. The volume of MR flow depends on a combination of the instantaneous size of the regurgitant orifice and the (reverse) pressure gradient between the left ventricle and the left atrium.[1,147] Both the orifice size and the pressure gradient are labile. LV systolic pressure, and therefore the LV–left atrial gradient, depends on systemic vascular resistance, and in patients in whom the mitral annulus has normal flexibility, the cross-sectional area of the mitral annulus may be altered by many interventions. Thus increase of both preload and afterload and depression of contractility increase LV size and enlarge the mitral annulus and thereby the regurgitant orifice. When LV size is reduced by treatment with positive inotropic agents, diuretics, and particularly vasodilators, the regurgitant orifice size decreases, and the volume of regurgitant flow declines, as reflected in the height of the v wave in the left atrial pressure pulse and in the intensity and duration of the systolic murmur. Conversely, LV dilation, regardless of cause, may increase MR.

LEFT VENTRICULAR COMPENSATION. The left ventricle initially compensates for the development of acute MR in part by emptying more completely and in part by increasing preload (i.e., by use of the Frank-Starling principle). Because acute MR reduces both late systolic ventricular pressure and radius, LV wall tension declines markedly (and proportionally to a greater extent than LV pressure), permitting a reciprocal increase in both the extent and the velocity of myocardial fiber shortening, leading to a reduced end-systolic volume (Fig. 62-29). As regurgitation, particularly severe regurgitation, becomes chronic, the LV end-diastolic volume increases and the end-systolic volume returns to normal. By means of the Laplace principle (which states that myocardial wall tension is related to the product of intraventricular pressure and radius), the increased ventricular end-diastolic volume increases wall tension to normal or supranormal levels in the so-called chronic compensated stage of severe MR.[96,99] The resultant increase in LV end-diastolic volume and mitral annular diameter may create a vicious circle in which "MR begets more MR." In patients with chronic MR, both LV end-diastolic volume

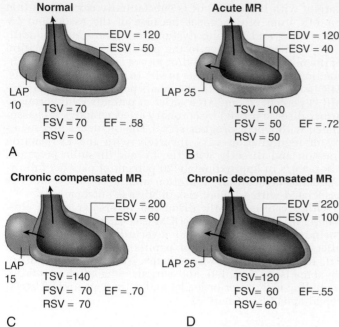

FIGURE 62–29 Three phases of mitral regurgitation (MR) are depicted and compared with normal physiology **(A)**. In acute MR **(B)**, an increase in preload and a decrease in afterload cause an increase in end-diastolic volume (EDV) and a decrease in end-systolic volume (ESV), producing an increase in total stroke volume (TSV). However, forward stroke volume (FSV) is diminished because 50 percent of the TSV regurgitates as the regurgitant stroke volume (RSV), resulting in an increase in left atrial pressure (LAP). In the chronic compensated phase **(C)**, eccentric hypertrophy has developed, and EDV is now increased substantially. Afterload has returned toward normal as the radius term of the Laplace relationship increases with the increase in EDV. Normal muscle function and a large increase in EDV permit a substantial increase in TSV from the acute phase. This, in turn, permits a normal FSV. Left atrial enlargement now accommodates the regurgitant volume at lower LAP. Ejection fraction (EF) remains greater than normal. In the chronic decompensated phase **(D)**, muscle dysfunction has developed, impairing ejection fraction, diminishing both TSV and FSV. EF, although still "normal," has decreased to 0.55, and LAP is reelevated because less volume is ejected during systole, causing a higher ESV. *(From Carabello BA: Progress in mitral and aortic regurgitation. Curr Probl Cardiol 28:553, 2003.)*

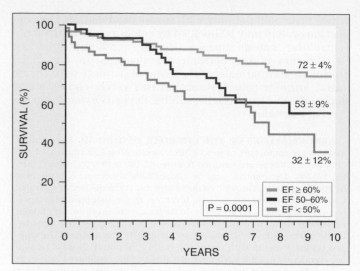

FIGURE 62–30 Late survival of patients after surgical correction of mitral regurgitation subdivided on the basis of the preoperative echocardiographic ejection fraction (EF). *(From Enriquez-Sarano M, Tajik AJ, Schaff HV, et al: Echocardiographic prediction of survival after surgical correction of organic mitral regurgitation. Circulation 90:833, 1994.)*

and mass are increased; i.e., typical volume overload (eccentric) hypertrophy develops. However, the degree of hypertrophy is often not proportionate to the degree of LV dilation, so that the ratio of LV mass to end-diastolic volume may be less than normal.[96,99,163] Nonetheless, the reduced afterload permits maintenance of ejection fraction in the normal to supranormal range. The reduced LV afterload allows a greater proportion of the contractile energy of the myocardium to be expended in shortening than in tension development and explains how the left ventricle can adapt to the load imposed by MR.

The eccentric ventricular hypertrophy that accompanies the elevated end-diastolic volume of chronic MR is secondary to new sarcomeres laid down in parallel. A shift to the right (greater volume at any pressure) occurs in the LV diastolic pressure-volume curve in patients with chronic MR. With decompensation, chamber stiffness increases, raising the diastolic pressure at any volume.

In most patients with severe primary MR, compensation is maintained for years, but in some patients the prolonged hemodynamic overload ultimately leads to myocardial decompensation.[99] End-systolic volume, preload, and afterload all rise, whereas ejection fraction and stroke volume decline. In such patients, there is evidence of neurohormonal activation[164,165] and elevation of circulating proinflammatory cytokines.[166] Plasma natriuretic peptide levels also increase in response to the volume load, more so in patients with symptomatic decompensation.[164,166]

Coronary flow rates may be increased in patients with severe MR, but the increases in myocardial oxygen consumption (MVO$_2$) are relatively modest compared with patients with AS and AR, because myocardial fiber shortening, which is elevated in patients with MR, is not one of the principal determinants of MVO$_2$. One of these determinants, mean LV wall tension, may actually be reduced in patients with MR, whereas the other two, contractility and heart rate, may be little affected. Thus patients with MR have a low incidence of clinical manifestations of myocardial ischemia compared with the much higher incidence occurring in those with AS and AR, conditions in which MVO$_2$ is greatly augmented.

ASSESSMENT OF MYOCARDIAL CONTRACTILITY IN MITRAL REGURGITATION. Because the ejection phase indices of myocardial contractility are inversely correlated with afterload, patients with early MR (with reduced LV afterload) often exhibit elevations in ejection phase indices of myocardial contractility, such as ejection fraction (EF), fractional fiber shortening (FS), and velocity of circumferential fiber shortening (VCF).[1,96,99] Many patients ultimately develop symptoms because of elevated left atrial and pulmonary venous pressures related to the regurgitant volume, and may do so with no change in these ejection phase indices, which remain elevated. However, in other patients, major symptoms reflect serious contractile dysfunction, at which time EF, FS, and mean see VCF have declined to low normal or below normal levels (see Fig. 62-29). As MR persists, the reduction in afterload, which increases myocardial fiber shortening and the earlier-mentioned ejection phase indices, is opposed by the impairment of myocardial function characteristic of severe chronic diastolic overload. However, even in patients with overt heart failure secondary to MR, the EF and FS may be only modestly reduced.[167] Therefore values in the low normal range for the ejection phase indices of myocardial performance in patients with chronic MR may actually reflect impaired myocardial function, whereas moderately reduced values (e.g., EF of 40 to 50 percent) generally signify severe, often irreversible, impairment of contractility,[168,169] identifying patients who may do poorly after surgical correction of the MR (Fig. 62-30). An EF of less than 35 percent in patients with severe MR usually represents advanced myocardial dysfunction; such patients are high operative risks and may not experience satisfactory improvement following MV replacement.

END-SYSTOLIC VOLUME. Preoperative myocardial contractility is an important determinant of the risk of operative death, of cardiac failure perioperatively, and of the level of LV function postoperatively. Therefore it is not surprising that the end-systolic pressure/volume (or stress/dimension) relation has emerged as a useful index for evaluating LV function in patients with MR.[170] Indeed, the simple measurement of end-systolic volume or diameter has been found to be a useful predictor of function and survival following mitral valve surgery.[1,96,168-170] A preoperative LV end-systolic diameter that exceeds 40 mm identifies a patient with a high likelihood of impaired LV systolic function following surgery.[1,169,170]

HEMODYNAMICS. Effective (forward) cardiac output is usually depressed in severely symptomatic patients with MR, whereas total LV output (the sum of forward and regurgitant flow) is usually elevated until quite late in the patient's course. The cardiac output achieved during exercise, not the regurgitant volume, is the principal determinant of functional capacity. The atrial contraction (a) wave in the left atrial pressure pulse is usually not as prominent in MR as in MS, but the v wave is characteristically much taller because it is inscribed during ventricular systole, when the left atrium is being filled with blood from the pulmonary veins, as well as from the left ventricle. Occasionally, backward transmission of the tall v wave into the pulmonary arterial bed may result in an early diastolic "pulmonary arterial v wave" (Fig. 62-31). In patients with pure MR, the y descent in the pulmonary capillary pressure pulse is particularly rapid as the distended left atrium empties rapidly during early diastole. However, in patients with combined MS and MR, the y descent is gradual. Although a left atrioventricular pressure gradient persisting throughout diastole signifies the presence of significant associated MS, a brief early diastolic gradient may occur in patients with isolated,

severe MR as a result of the rapid flow of blood across a normal-sized mitral orifice early in diastole, often accompanied by an early diastolic murmur at the apex.

LEFT ATRIAL COMPLIANCE

The compliance of the left atrium (and pulmonary venous bed) is an important determinant of the hemodynamic and clinical picture in patients with severe MR. Three major subgroups of patients with severe MR based on left atrial compliance have been identified and are characterized as follows:

NORMAL OR REDUCED COMPLIANCE. In this subgroup, there is little enlargement of the left atrium but marked elevation of the mean left atrial pressure, particularly of the v wave, and pulmonary congestion is a prominent symptom. Severe MR usually develops acutely, as occurs with rupture of the chordae tendineae, infarction of one of the heads of a papillary muscle, or perforation of a mitral leaflet as a consequence of trauma or endocarditis. In patients with acute MR, the left atrium initially operates on the steep portion of its pressure-volume curve with a marked rise in pressure for a small increase in volume. Sinus rhythm is usually present; after the passage of weeks or a few months, the left atrial wall becomes hypertrophied, is capable of contracting vigorously, and facilitates LV filling. The thicker atrium is less compliant than normal, which further increases the height of the v wave. Thickening of the walls of the pulmonary veins and proliferative changes in the pulmonary arteries, as well as marked elevations of pulmonary vascular resistance and pulmonary artery pressure, usually develop over the course of 6 to 12 months after the onset of acute, severe MR.

MARKEDLY INCREASED COMPLIANCE. At the opposite end of the spectrum from patients in the first group are those with severe, longstanding MR with massive enlargement of the left atrium and normal or only slightly elevated left atrial pressure. The atrial wall contains only a small remnant of muscle surrounded by fibrous tissue. Longstanding MR in these patients has altered the physical properties of the left atrial wall and thereby displaced the atrial pressure-volume curve to the right, allowing a normal or almost normal pressure to exist in a greatly enlarged left atrium. Pulmonary arterial pressure and pulmonary vascular resistance may be normal or only slightly elevated at rest. AF and a low cardiac output are almost invariably present.

MODERATELY INCREASED COMPLIANCE. This most common subgroup consists of patients between the ends of the spectrum rep-

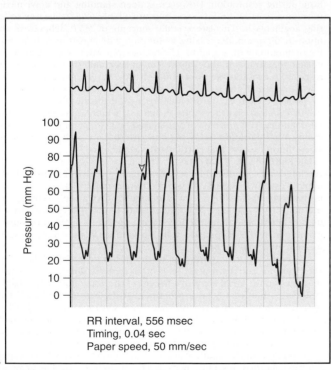

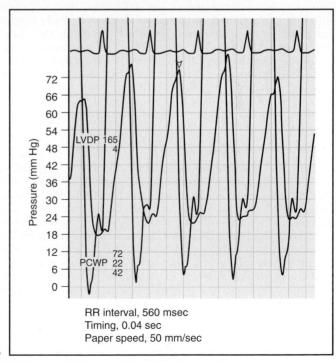

FIGURE 62–31 Hemodynamic tracings in a 45-year-old woman with acute mitral regurgitation from bacterial endocarditis. **A,** Pulmonary artery pressure. **B,** Simultaneous left ventricular diastolic pressure (LVDP) and pulmonary capillary wedge pressure (PCWP). The PCWP demonstrates a markedly elevated v wave (arrowhead, **B**) that transmits to the pulmonary artery pressure (arrowhead, **A**). *(Modified from Wisse B, Sniderman AD: Severe mitral regurgitation. N Engl J Med 343:1386, 2000.)*

resented by the first and second groups. These patients have severe, chronic MR and exhibit variable degrees of enlargement of the left atrium, associated with significant elevation of the left atrial pressure, and these two factors (in association with age) determine the likelihood that AF will ensue.

Clinical Presentation

Symptoms

The nature and severity of symptoms in patients with chronic MR are functions of a combination of inter-related factors including the severity of MR; the rate of its progression; the level of left atrial, pulmonary venous, and pulmonary arterial pressure; the presence of episodic or chronic atrial tachyarrhythmias; and the presence of associated valvular, myocardial, or coronary artery disease. Symptoms may occur with preserved LV contractile function in patients with chronic MR who have severely elevated pulmonary venous pressures or AF. In other patients, symptoms herald LV decompensation. In patients with rheumatic MR, the time interval between the initial attack of rheumatic fever and the development of symptoms tends to be longer than in those with MS and often exceeds two decades. Hemoptysis and systemic embolization are less common in patients with isolated or predominant MR than in those with MS. The development of AF affects the course adversely but perhaps not as dramatically as in MS. On the other hand, chronic weakness and fatigue secondary to a low cardiac output are more prominent features in MR.

The majority of patients with MR of rheumatic origin have only mild disability, unless regurgitation progresses as a result of chronic rheumatic activity, infective endocarditis, or rupture of the chordae tendineae. However, the indolent course of MR may be deceptive. By the time that symptoms secondary to a reduced cardiac output and/or pulmonary congestion become apparent, serious and sometimes even irreversible LV dysfunction may have developed.

In patients with severe, chronic MR who have a greatly enlarged left atrium and relatively mild left atrial hypertension (patients with increased left atrial compliance [second subgroup], described earlier), pulmonary vascular resistance does not usually rise markedly. Instead, the major symptoms, fatigue and exhaustion, are related to the depressed cardiac output. Right-sided heart failure, characterized by congestive hepatomegaly, edema, and ascites, may be prominent in patients with acute MR, elevated pulmonary vascular resistance, and pulmonary hypertension. Angina pectoris is rare unless coronary artery disease coexists.

Physical Examination (see Chap. 11)

Palpation of the arterial pulse is helpful in differentiating AS from MR, both of which may produce a prominent systolic murmur both at the base of the heart and at the apex. The carotid arterial upstroke is sharp in severe MR and delayed in AS; the volume of the pulse may be normal or reduced in the presence of heart failure. The cardiac impulse, like the arterial pulse, is brisk and hyperdynamic. It is displaced to the left, and a prominent LV filling wave is frequently palpable. Systolic expansion of the enlarged left atrium may result in a late systolic thrust in the parasternal region, which may be confused with RV enlargement.

AUSCULTATION. When chronic severe MR is caused by defective valve leaflets, S1, produced by mitral valve closure, is usually diminished. Wide splitting of S2 is common and results from the shortening of LV ejection and an earlier A2 as a consequence of reduced resistance to LV ejection. In patients with MR who have severe pulmonary hypertension, P2 is louder than A2. The abnormal increase in the flow rate across the mitral orifice during the rapid filling phase is often associated with an S3, which should not be interpreted as a feature of heart failure in these patients, and this may be accompanied by a brief diastolic rumble.

The systolic murmur is the most prominent physical finding; it must be differentiated from the systolic murmur of AS, TR, and ventricular septal defect. In most patients with severe MR, the systolic murmur commences immediately after the soft S1 and continues beyond and may obscure the A2 because of the persisting pressure difference between the left ventricle and left atrium after aortic valve closure. The holosystolic murmur of chronic MR is usually constant in intensity, blowing, high-pitched, and loudest at the apex with frequent radiation to the left axilla and left infrascapular area. However, radiation toward the sternum or the aortic area may occur with abnormalities of the posterior leaflet and is particularly common in patients with MVP involving this leaflet. The murmur shows little change even in the presence of large beat-to-beat variations of LV stroke volume, as occur in AF. This contrasts with most midsystolic (ejection) murmurs, such as in AS, which vary greatly in intensity with stroke volume and therefore with the duration of diastole. There is little correlation between the intensity of the systolic murmur and the severity of MR. Indeed, in patients with severe MR caused by LV dilation, acute myocardial infarction, or paraprosthetic valvular regurgitation, or in those who have marked emphysema, obesity, chest deformity, or a prosthetic heart valve, the systolic murmur may be barely audible or even absent, a condition referred to as "silent MR."

The murmur of MR may be holosystolic, late systolic, or early systolic. When the murmur is confined to late systole, the regurgitation is usually not severe and may be secondary to prolapse of the mitral valve or to papillary muscle dysfunction. These causes of MR are frequently associated with a normal S1 because initial closure of the mitral valve cusps may be unimpaired. The late systolic murmur of papillary muscle dysfunction is particularly variable; it may become accentuated or holosystolic during acute myocardial ischemia and often disappears when ischemia is relieved. A midsystolic click preceding a mid-to-late systolic murmur, and the response of that murmur to a number of maneuvers, helps to establish the diagnosis of MVP. Early systolic murmurs are typical of acute MR. When the left atrial v wave is markedly elevated in acute MR, the murmur may diminish or disappear in late systole as the reverse pressure gradient declines. As noted previously, a short, low-pitched diastolic murmur following S3 may be audible in patients with severe MR, even without accompanying MS.

DYNAMIC AUSCULTATION. The holosystolic murmur of MR varies little during respiration. However, sudden standing and amyl nitrite inhalation usually diminish the murmur (Table 62-8), whereas squatting augments it. The late systolic murmur of MVP behaves in the opposite direction, decreasing in duration with squatting and increasing in duration with standing. The holosystolic MR murmur is reduced during the strain of the Valsalva maneuver and shows a left-sided response (i.e., a transient overshoot that occurs six to eight beats following release of the strain). The murmur of MR is usually intensified by isometric exercise, differentiating it from the systolic murmurs of valvular AS and obstructive HCM, both of which are reduced by this intervention. The murmur of MR caused by LV dilatation decreases in intensity and duration following effective therapy with cardiac glycosides, diuretics, rest, and particularly vasodilators.

DIFFERENTIAL DIAGNOSIS. The holosystolic murmur of MR resembles that produced by a ventricular septal defect. However, the latter is usually loudest at the sternal border rather than the apex and is often accompanied by a parasternal, rather than an apical, thrill. The murmur of MR may also be confused with that of TR, but the latter is usually heard best along the left sternal border, is augmented during inspiration, and is accompanied by a prominent v wave and y descent in the jugular venous pulse.

When the chordae tendineae to the posterior leaflet of the mitral valve rupture, the regurgitant jet is often directed anteriorly, so that it impinges on the atrial septum adjacent to the aortic root and causes a systolic murmur that is most prominent at the base of the heart. This murmur can be confused with that of AS. On the other hand, when the chordae tendineae to the anterior leaflet rupture, the jet is usually directed to the posterior wall of the left atrium, and the murmur may be transmitted to the spine or even to the top of the head.

Patients with rheumatic disease of the mitral valve exhibit a spectrum of abnormalities, ranging from pure MS to pure MR. The presence of an S3, a rapid LV filling wave and LV impulse on palpation, and a soft S1 all favor predominant MR. In contrast, an accentuated S1, a prominent opening snap (OS) with a short A2-OS interval, and a soft,

TABLE 62–8 | **Effect of Various Interventions on Systolic Murmurs**

Intervention	Hypertrophic Obstructive Cardiomyopathy	Aortic Stenosis	Mitral Regurgitation	Mitral Valve Prolapse
Valsalva	↑	↓	↓	↑ or ↓
Standing	↑	↑ or unchanged	↓	↑
Handgrip or squatting	↓	↓ or unchanged	↑	↓
Supine position with legs elevated	↓	↑ or unchanged	Unchanged	↓
Exercise	↑	↑ or unchanged	↓	↑
Amyl nitrite	↑↑	↑	↓	↑
Isoproterenol	↑↑	↑	↓	↑

↑↑=markedly increased.

Modified from Paraskos JA: Combined valvular disease. *In* Dalen JE, Alpert JS, Rahimtoola SH (eds): Valvular Heart Disease. 3rd ed. Philadelphia, Lippincott Williams & Wilkins, 2000, p 332.

short systolic murmur all point to predominant MS. Elucidation of the predominant valvular lesion may be complicated by the presence of a holosystolic murmur of TR in patients with pure MS and pulmonary hypertension; this murmur may sometimes be heard at the apex when the right ventricle is greatly enlarged and may therefore be mistaken for the murmur of MR.

Echocardiography (see also Chap. 14)

Echocardiography plays a central role in the diagnosis of MR, in determining its etiology and potential for repair, and in quantifying its severity. In patients with severe MR, echocardiographic imaging shows enlargement of the left atrium and left ventricle, with increased systolic motion of both chambers. The underlying cause of the regurgitation, e.g., rupture of chordae tendineae, MVP (see Fig. 14-57), rheumatic mitral disease, a flail leaflet (see Fig. 62-28A), vegetations (see Chap. 63), and LV dilatation (see Fig. 62-28B) can often be determined on the transthoracic echocardiogram. It may also show calcification of the mitral annulus as a band of dense echoes between the mitral apparatus and the posterior wall of the heart. This technique is also useful for estimating the hemodynamic consequences of MR; in patients with LV dysfunction, end-diastolic and end-systolic volumes are increased and the ejection fraction and shortening rate may decline.

Doppler echocardiography in MR characteristically reveals a high-velocity jet in the left atrium during systole.[171] The severity of the regurgitation is reflected in the width of the jet across the valve (see Fig. 14-54) and the size of the left atrium. Qualitative assessment using either color flow Doppler imaging or pulsed techniques correlates reasonably well with angiographic methods in estimating the severity of MR. However, color flow jet areas are significantly influenced by the cause of the regurgitation and jet eccentricity, thus limiting the accuracy of this approach. Quantitative methods to measure regurgitant fraction, regurgitant volume and regurgitant orifice area have greater accuracy in comparison with angiography[168,171] (see Figs. 14-42, 43, 55, and 56), and these methods are strongly recommended (see Table 62-1).[1,105] The vena contracta, defined as the narrowest cross-sectional areas of the regurgitant jet as mapped by color flow Doppler echocardiography, also predicts the severity of MR (Fig. 62-32).[105,172] The proximal isovelocity surface area (PISA) method[171] estimates MR severity with isovelocity hemispheric shells as regurgitant flow accelerates toward the mitral orifice. Reversal of flow in the pulmonary veins during systole[168] and a high peak mitral inflow velocity are also useful signs of severe MR.

Doppler echocardiography is also an important tool to estimate the pulmonary artery systolic pressure and to

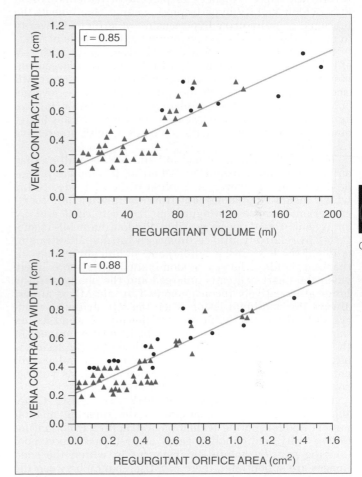

FIGURE 62–32 Linear regression plot showing good correlation between biplane vena contracta width and regurgitant volume **(top)** and regurgitant orifice area **(bottom)**. Blue triangles indicate central jets and magenta circles indicate eccentric jets. *(From Hall SA, Brickner E, Willen DL, et al: Assessment of mitral regurgitation severity by Doppler color-flow mapping of the vena contracta. Circulation 95:636, 1997.)*

determine the presence and severity of associated AR or TR.

Transesophageal echocardiography (see Chap. 14) is superior to transthoracic echocardiography in assessing the detailed anatomy of the regurgitant mitral valve and in assessing severity of MR.[173] Therefore this technique is useful when the transthoracic image is suboptimal and also when determining whether MV repair is feasible or whether

MV replacement is necessary. Three-dimensional transthoracic echocardiography and three-dimensional color Doppler[156] have also been reported to help elucidate the mechanism of MR.

Exercise echocardiography is helpful in determining severity of MR and hemodynamic abnormalities (such as pulmonary hypertension) during exercise.[1,174] This is a useful, objective means to evaluate symptoms in patients who appear to have only mild MR at rest and, alternatively, to determine functional status and dynamic changes in hemodynamics in patients who otherwise appear stable and asymptomatic.

Other Diagnostic Evaluation

ELECTROCARDIOGRAPHY. The principal ECG findings are left atrial enlargement and AF. ECG evidence of LV enlargement occurs in about one third of patients with severe MR. Approximately 15 percent of patients exhibit ECG evidence of RV hypertrophy, a change that reflects the presence of pulmonary hypertension of sufficient severity to counterbalance the hypertrophied left ventricle of MR.

RADIOLOGICAL FINDINGS. Cardiomegaly with LV enlargement, and particularly with left atrial enlargement, is a common finding in patients with chronic, severe MR (see Fig. 15-18). Although the left atrium may be severely enlarged, there is little correlation between left atrial size and pressure. Interstitial edema with Kerley B lines is frequently seen in patients with acute MR or with progressive LV failure.

In patients with combined MS and MR, overall cardiac enlargement and particularly left atrial dilation are prominent findings. However, it is often difficult to determine which lesion is predominant from the plain chest roentgenogram because distinguishing between right and LV enlargement may not be possible. Predominant MS is suggested by relatively mild cardiomegaly (principally straightening of the left cardiac border) and significant changes in the lung fields, whereas predominant MR is more likely when the heart is greatly enlarged and the changes in the lungs are relatively inconspicuous. Chronic MR is almost always the dominant lesion when the left atrium is aneurysmally dilated. Calcification of the mitral annulus, an important cause of MR in the elderly, is most prominent in the posterior third of the cardiac silhouette. The lesion is best visualized on chest films exposed in the lateral or right anterior oblique projections, in which it appears as a dense, coarse, C-shaped opacity (see Fig. 15-19).

RADIONUCLIDE ANGIOGRAPHY (see also Chap. 16). Although echocardiography is the imaging method most suited for routine evaluation of structure, function and MR severity, radionuclide gated or first pass blood pool imaging may be helpful in instances in which the echo images are suboptimal, there is a discrepancy between the clinical and the echocardiography information, or there is a need for more precise measurement of LV ejection fraction.[1]

CARDIAC MAGNETIC RESONANCE (CMR) (see also Chap. 17). CMR provides accurate measurements of regurgitant flow that correlate well with quantitative Doppler imaging.[106] It is also the most accurate noninvasive technique for measuring LV end-diastolic volume, end-systolic volume, and mass. Although detailed visualization of mitral valve structure and function is obtained more reliably with echocardiography, CMR offers a promising approach for more accurate assessment of regurgitant severity.

LEFT VENTRICULAR ANGIOGRAPHY. The prompt appearance of contrast material in the left atrium following its injection into the left ventricle indicates the presence of MR. The injection should be rapid enough to permit LV opacification but slow enough to avoid the development of premature ventricular contractions, which can induce spurious regurgitation (see Chap. 19).

The regurgitant volume can be determined from the difference between the total LV stroke volume, estimated by angiocardiography, and the simultaneous measurement of the effective forward stroke volume by the Fick method. In patients with severe MR, the regurgitant volume may approach, and even exceed, the effective forward stroke volume. Qualitative but clinically useful estimates of the severity of MR may be made by cineangiographic observation of the degree of opacification of the left atrium and pulmonary veins following the injection of contrast material into the left ventricle.

The cause of the regurgitation (e.g., prolapse of the mitral valve) and a flail leaflet can often be distinguished by angiography, but this assessment has been superseded by echocardiography in most institutions. MR secondary to rheumatic heart disease is characterized angiographically by a central regurgitant jet and by thickened leaflets that exhibit reduced motion. In regurgitation caused by other problems, particularly dilation or calcification of the mitral annulus or ruptured chordae tendineae and papillary muscles, the systolic jet may be eccentric, and the valves consist of thin filaments that display excessive motion.

Disease Course

The natural history of MR is highly variable and depends on a combination of the volume of regurgitation, the state of the myocardium, and the cause of the underlying disorder. Asymptomatic patients with mild primary MR usually remain in a stable state for many years. Severe regurgitation develops in only a small percentage of these patients, most commonly because of intervening infective endocarditis or rupture of the chordae tendineae. In patients with mild MR related to MVP, the rate of progression in severity of MR is highly variable; in most patients progression is gradual unless a ruptured chordae or flail leaflet supervenes.[168] Regurgitation tends to progress more rapidly in patients with connective tissue diseases, such as the Marfan syndrome, than in those with chronic MR of rheumatic origin. Acute rheumatic fever is a frequent cause of isolated, severe MR in adolescents in developing nations, and these patients often have a rapidly progressive course.

AF is a common arrhythmia is patients with chronic MR, associated with age and left atrial dilation, and its onset is a marker for disease progression. Patients with AF have an adverse outcome compared to patients who remain in sinus rhythm,[175-178] and development of AF is considered an indication for operative intervention, especially in patients who are candidates for MV repair.[1]

Because the natural history of severe MR has been altered greatly by surgical intervention, it is difficult now to predict the course of patients who receive medical therapy alone. However, Horstkotte and associates reported a 5-year survival of only 30 percent in patients who were candidates for operation (presumably because of symptoms) but who declined (see Fig. 62-22). Among patients with severe MR resulting from flail leaflets, the annual mortality rate is as high as 6.3 percent,[168] and at 10 years 90 percent have died or undergone surgical correction (Fig. 62-33). This latter series included many patients who were initially symptomatic or had LV dysfunction or AF, and thus might be considered to be a higher risk.

Whether patients with severe MR who are asymptomatic with normal LV function are at risk of death is a subject of debate. One long-term retrospective study demonstrated that patients with severe MR, defined quantitatively as an effective orifice area greater than 40 mm^2 (see Table 62-1), had a 4 percent per year risk of cardiac death.[172] In contrast, a second study reported the outcomes of 132 patients with severe MR followed prospectively for 5 years,[179] during which the indications for surgery were symptoms or the development of LV dysfunction (ejection fraction <0.60), LV end-systolic dimension greater than 45 mm, AF, or pulmonary hypertension. Only 2 patients in this latter study had cardiac death, both of whom met criteria for surgery but refused this intervention. However, mortality arguments aside, all studies uniformly indicate that among asymptomatic patients with initially normal LV ejection fractions, severe MR is associated with a high likelihood of requiring surgery over the next 6 to 10 years because of heart failure symptoms, LV dysfunction, or AF (see Fig. 62-33).[172,179]

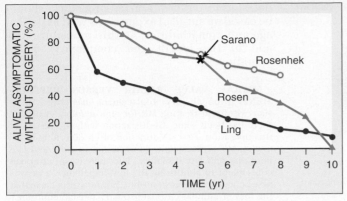

FIGURE 62–33 Four series examining the natural history of patients with severe mitral regurgitation (MR) including a series of patients with flail mitral leaflets reported by Ling and associates (magenta), many of whom were symptomatic, had atrial fibrillation, or had evidence of left ventricular (LV) dysfunction, and three series reported by Rosen et al (blue triangles), Sarano et al (black asterisk) and Rosenhek et al (gold open circles) in patients who initially were asymptomatic with normal LV function. Although the patients with flail leaflets had a steeper initial attrition rate, all series demonstrated that patients with severe MR have a high likelihood of developing symptoms or other indications for surgery over the course of 6 to 10 years. *(Modified from Ling LH, Enriquez-Sarano M, Seward JB, et al: Clinical outcome of mitral regurgitation due to flail leaflet. N Engl J Med 335:1417, 1996; Rosen SF, Borer JS, Hochreiter C, et al: Natural history of the asymptomatic patient with severe mitral regurgitation secondary to mitral valve prolapse and normal right and left ventricular performance. Am J Cardiol 74:374, 1994; Enriquez-Sarano M, Avierinos JF, Messika-Zeitoun D, et al: Quantitative determinants of the outcome of asymptomatic mitral regurgitation. N Engl J Med 352:875,2005; and Rosenhek R, Rader F, Klaar U, et al: Outcome of watchful waiting in asymptomatic severe mitral regurgitation. Circulation 113:2238, 2006.)*

Management of Chronic Mitral Regurgitation

Medical Treatment

The role of pharmacological therapy for MR remains another subject of uncertainty and some debate. Although there is no doubt that afterload reduction therapy is indicated, and indeed may be lifesaving, in patients with acute MR, the indications for such therapy in patients with chronic MR are much less clear. As afterload is not excessive in most patients with chronic MR, in whom systolic shortening is facilitated by the reduced systolic wall stress, systemic vasodilator therapy to reduce afterload further may not provide additional benefit. Acute administration of nitroprusside, nifedipine, and ACE inhibitors to severely symptomatic patients has been demonstrated to alter hemodynamics favorably in some studies, but these effects may not pertain to asymptomatic patients with preserved systolic function. Several small studies of chronic therapy with ACE inhibitors, ranging from 4 weeks to 6 months, have failed to provide evidence of hemodynamic benefit, and there are no long-term studies and no randomized trials with which to make definitive recommendations. At the present time, there is lack of convincing data that vasodilator therapy affects LV volumes or systolic function favorably in the absence of symptoms or hypertension, and current guidelines do not recommend the use of these agents for chronic therapy.[1,2] An exception would be those patients with severe chronic MR, with symptoms or LV dysfunction (or both) who are not candidates for surgery because of age or other comorbidities. These patients should receive standard, aggressive management for heart failure with ACE inhibitors and beta adrenergic blocking agents (see Chap. 25).

The accumulating experimental data suggest that beta-blocking drugs may be more beneficial than ACE inhibitors

in preserving or improving LV function.[96,165,180,181] Although conceptually attractive, at present there are no clinical data with which to justify chronic beta blocker therapy.

Antibiotic prophylaxis to prevent infective endocarditis is no longer recommended routinely in patients with MR (see Chap. 63). All patients with AF, paroxysmal or chronic, should receive chronic anticoagulation.

Surgical treatment should be considered for patients with functional disability and/or for patients with no symptoms or only mild symptoms but with progressively deteriorating LV function or progressively increasing LV dimensions as documented by noninvasive studies.[1,2] The indications for surgery are discussed subsequently.

In patients considered for surgery, two-dimensional transthoracic or transesophageal echocardiography with Doppler echocardiography and color flow Doppler imaging provide detailed assessment of mitral valve structure and function. However, left heart catheterization, LV angiocardiography, and coronary arteriography are indicated for the following: (1) in evaluating a discrepancy between echocardiographic findings and the clinical picture; (2) in detecting and assessing the severity of any associated valvular lesions; and (3) in determining the presence and assessing the extent of coronary artery disease.[1]

Surgical Treatment

Without surgical treatment, the prognosis for patients with MR and heart failure is poor (see Fig. 62-22), and hence MV repair or replacement is indicated in symptomatic patients. When operative treatment is being considered, the chronic and often slowly but relentlessly progressive nature of MR must be weighed against the immediate risks and long-term uncertainties attendant upon surgery, especially if MV replacement is required. Surgical mortality depends on the patient's clinical and hemodynamic status (particularly the function of the left ventricle); on the patient's age[182,183]; on the presence of comorbid conditions such as renal, hepatic, or pulmonary disease[86,87]; and on the skill and experience of the surgical team.[84,184,185] The decision to replace or to repair the valve (Fig. 62-34) is of critical importance, and MV repair is strongly recommended whenever possible.[1] Replacement involves the operative risk, as well as the risks of thromboembolism and anticoagulation in patients receiving mechanical prostheses, of late structural valve deterioration in patients receiving bioprostheses, and of late mortality, especially in patients with associated coronary artery disease who require coronary artery bypass grafting (see Table 62-3). Surgical mortality does not depend significantly on which of the currently used tissue or mechanical valve prostheses is selected.

Repair of the mitral valve is most often successful in (1) children and adolescents with pliable valves; (2) adults with degenerative MR secondary to MVP; (3) annular dilation; (4) papillary muscle dysfunction secondary to ischemia or rupture; (5) chordal rupture, or (6) perforation of a mitral leaflet due to infective endocarditis. These procedures are less likely to be successful in older patients with the rigid, calcified, deformed valves of rheumatic heart disease or those with severe subvalvular chordal thickening and major loss of leaflet substance, and many of these latter patients require MV replacement. Young patients in developing countries who have severe rheumatic MR in the absence of active carditis may undergo successful repair.

MV repair for degenerative MR consists of reconstruction of the valve, which usually is accompanied by a mitral annuloplasty employing a rigid or a flexible prosthetic ring (see Fig. 62-34).[186-189] Prolapsed valves causing severe MR are usually treated with resection of the prolapsing segment with plication and reinforcement of the annulus. Replacing, reimplanting, elongating, or shortening of chordae tendin-

Reduction excision of posterior leaflet

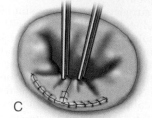

- Anterior leaflet

- Posterior leaflet

A

Reattach posterior leaflet (sliding valvuloplasty)

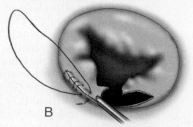

B

Repair posterior leaflet

C

Completed supported repair

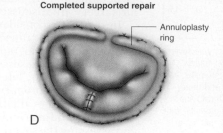

- Annuloplasty ring

D

FIGURE 62–34 Mitral valve repair (**A** to **D**) employing reduction excision and reattachment of the posterior leaflet with implantation of an annuloplasty ring. *(From Doty DB [ed]: Cardiac Surgery: Operative Technique. St. Louis, Mosby–Year Book, 1997, p 259.)*

CH 62

eae; splitting the papillary muscles; and repairing the subvalvular apparatus have been successful in selected patients with pure or predominant MR in whom subvalvular pathology contributes to the MR.[186-190] Repair of anterior, as well as posterior prolapsing leaflets, is successful in experienced centers.[190-191]

Ischemic MR secondary to regional LV dysfunction with annular dilation may be treated by annuloplasty (see Chap. 27). Annuloplasty is also successful in many patients with significant functional MR resulting from dilated cardiomyopathy.[192] Episodic MR due to transient ischemia is often eliminated by coronary revascularization, whereas moderate to severe, chronic MR secondary ischemic heart disease usually requires MV repair or replacement.[193-197] In patients undergoing coronary artery bypass surgery, some investigators recommend that concomitant MV repair should be considered for even mild MR.[198]

Intraoperative transesophageal echocardiography and Doppler is extremely useful in assessing the adequacy of MV repair.[1,199] In the minority of patients with persistent severe MR in whom the operative results are unsatisfactory, the problem can usually be corrected immediately, or, if necessary, the valve can be replaced. LV outflow tract obstruction due to systolic anterior motion of the mitral valve occurs in 5 to 10 percent of patients following MV repair for degenerative MR. The causes are not clear; but they may include excess valvular tissue with severe leaflet redundancy and/or an interventricular septum bulging into a small left ventricle. These complications may also be recognized intraoperatively by transesophageal echocardiography. Treatment with volume loading and beta-blocking agents is often helpful. The obstruction usually disappears with time; if it does not, reoperation and re-repair or MV replacement may be necessary.

Preoperative AF is an independent predictor of reduced long-term survival after MV surgery for chronic MR.[175,176,178] The persistence of AF postoperatively requires long-term anticoagulation, thereby partially nullifying the advantages of MV repair. In patients who have developed AF, whether chronic or paroxysmal, outcomes are improved if a maze procedure is performed at the time of MV repair or replacement,[133,134,200] with reduced risk of postoperative stroke. The

decision to perform a maze procedure should be based on surgical expertise as well as patient age and comorbidities, as this procedure may add to the length and complexity of the operation.

MITRAL VALVE REPAIR VERSUS REPLACEMENT. Although MV replacement has been used successfully in treating MR for almost four decades,[201] there has been some dissatisfaction with the results of this operation. First, LV function often deteriorates following MV replacement, contributing to early and late mortality and late disability. The increase in afterload consequent to abolishing the low impedance leak was first believed to be responsible, but now it is clear that the loss of annular-chordal-papillary muscle continuity (see Fig. 62-27) interferes with LV geometry, volume, and function in patients who have undergone MV replacement. This does not occur after MV repair. Indeed, animal experiments have shown convincingly that the normal function of the MV apparatus "primes" the left ventricle for normal contraction and that contraction is prevented when operation causes discontinuity of this apparatus.[96] There is evidence from animal experiments and from human patients that preservation of the papillary muscle and its chordal attachments to the mitral annulus is beneficial to postoperative LV function, after both MV reconstruction[168] and replacement. Thus preservation of these tissues, whenever possible, is now considered a critical feature of MV replacement.

A second disadvantage of MV replacement is the prosthesis itself, including the risks of thromboembolism or hemorrhage associated with mechanical prostheses, late structural deterioration of bioprostheses, and infective endocarditis with all prostheses.

For these reasons, increasing efforts are being made to repair the mitral valve whenever possible in patients with isolated or predominant MR.[1,186-189] The STS National Database Committee reports an operative mortality rate of less than 2 percent in 4584 patients undergoing isolated MV repair in 2005.[202] This compares favorably to the 6 percent operative mortality for the 4235 patients undergoing isolated MV replacement.

With growing experience in MV repair for degenerative causes of MR (including MVP and rupture of chordae tendineae) as well as for ischemic MR, the number of patients in whom valve reconstruction is carried out is increasing on a yearly basis.[1,202] In many centers in the United States, over two-thirds of all patients requiring operation for pure or predominant MR now undergo MV repair. However, in 2003 only 42 percent of patients undergoing surgery for pure MR in the STS National Cardiac Surgery Database received repair and 58 percent underwent MV replacement.[203] Although this percentage has increased to roughly 50 percent, as noted above,[202] it appears that many patients who are candidates for repair continue to receive MV replacement. MV repair is technically a more demanding procedure than is MV replacement, with a distinct learning curve for the surgeon. In addition, MR recurs after MV repair in a subset of patient with degenerative valve disease,[204] which is predicted, in part, by the presence of residual MR immediately following repair.[188] Hence there is growing emphasis of referral of patients requiring surgery for pure MR to centers of excellence in performing MV repair.[1,205]

Minimally invasive surgical techniques utilizing a small, low, asymmetrical sternotomy or anterior thoracotomy and percutaneous cardiopulmonary bypass[206,207] have been found to be less traumatic and can be employed for both MV repair and replacement. This approach has been reported to reduce cost, improve cosmetic results, and shorten the recovery time. However, it also is quite demanding technically and is successfully performed by only a minority of cardiac surgeons. There is now growing interest in the development of percutaneous approaches to MV repair[208] using either the edge-to-edge technique[209] analogous to the Alfieri surgical method[210] or the coronary sinus approach for percutaneous mitral annuloplasty.[211]

SURGICAL RESULTS. Operative mortality rates of 3 to 9 percent are now common in many centers for patients with pure or predominant MR (NYHA Class II or III) who undergo elective isolated MV replacement. The overall mortality rate is 6 percent in the STS National Database of more than 39,000 patients undergoing isolated MV replacement between 1997 and 2005, and less than 2 percent for the 28,000 patients undergoing MV repair.[202] In comparison, the operative mortality rate for isolated AVR during the same period is 3 to 4 percent. The combination of MV replacement with coronary artery bypass grafting, however, is associated with a mortality rate of 10 to 13 percent,[202] and the mortality rate is higher (up to 25 percent) in patients with severe LV dysfunction, especially when MR is secondary to myocardial ischemia, when pulmonary or renal function is impaired, or when the operation must be carried out as an emergency.[86,87] Age per se is no barrier to successful surgery; MV repair or replacement can be performed in patients older than 75 years of age if their general health status is adequate[182,183]; however, surgery in these patients has a higher risk than in younger patients. A review of Medicare data,[185] involving 684 U.S. hospitals and more than 61,000 patients, indicates that the average in-hospital mortality for isolated MV replacement in patients over the age of 65 years is 14.1 percent (20.5 percent in low-volume centers and 10.1 percent in high-volume centers).

Surgical treatment substantially improves survival in patients with symptomatic MR. Preoperative factors such as age less than 60 years, NYHA Class II, a cardiac index exceeding 2.0 liters/min/m², a LV end-diastolic pressure less than 12 mm Hg, and a normal ejection fraction and end-systolic volume all correlate with excellent immediate and long-term survival rates. Both preoperative LV ejection fraction (see Fig. 62-30) and end-systolic diameter are important predictors of short-term and long-term outcome.[168-170] Excellent outcome is anticipated in patients with end-systolic diameters less than 40 mm and ejection fractions of 60 percent or more. Intermediate outcomes are observed in patients with end-systolic diameters between 40 and 50 mm and ejection fractions between 50 and 60 percent. Poor outcomes are associated with values beyond these limits.

A large proportion of operative survivors have improved clinical status, quality of life, and exercise tolerance following MV repair or replacement. Severe pulmonary hypertension is reduced, LV end-diastolic volume and mass decrease, and coronary flow reserve increases. Depressed contractile function improves, especially if the papillary muscles and chordal attachment to the annulus remain intact. However, patients with MR who have marked LV dysfunction preoperatively sometimes remain symptomatic with depressed LV function despite a technically satisfactory surgical procedure.[168] Indeed, progressive LV dysfunction and death from heart failure may occur, presumably because LV dysfunction may be quite advanced and largely irreversible by the time patients with pure MR develop serious symptoms. Thus every effort should be made to operate on patients before they develop serious symptoms, and even asymptomatic patients with severe MR may be considered for surgery in an experienced center if there is a high likelihood (>90 percent) that the valve can be repaired successfully without residual MR.[1,168]

Even though surgical results are suboptimal in patients with MR who have developed severe symptoms or marked LV dysfunction,[1,96,168] operation is still indicated in the majority of these patients because conservative therapy has little to offer. Postoperative survival rates are lower in patients in AF than those in sinus rhythm.[169,177,178] As with patients with MS, the arrhythmia by itself does not unfavorably influence outcome, but is a marker for older age and other clinical and hemodynamic features associated with less optimal results.

The cause of MR clearly plays an important role in determining outcome following surgical treatment.[152,159,160,187-193,197,212] In patients with primary, degenerative disease of the mitral valve, MV repair or replacement has the potential to improve LV performance. However, in those with functional MR, the primary problem is disease of the LV myocardium, and prognosis is strongly influenced by the degree of LV dysfunction. MV repair or replacement in these latter patients has less beneficial effects on long-term outcome, particularly in those with ischemic MR,[159,160,193] compared to patients with degenerative MR.

Occlusive coronary artery disease coexisting with MR, but not the primary cause of MR, requires simultaneous coronary artery bypass grafting and MV repair or replacement.[213] CAD is associated with decreased perioperative and long-term postoperative survival (Fig. 62-35).

INDICATIONS FOR OPERATION. A proposed management strategy for patients with chronic severe MR is shown in Figure 62-36.[1] The threshold for surgical treatment of MR is declining for several reasons. These include the reduc-

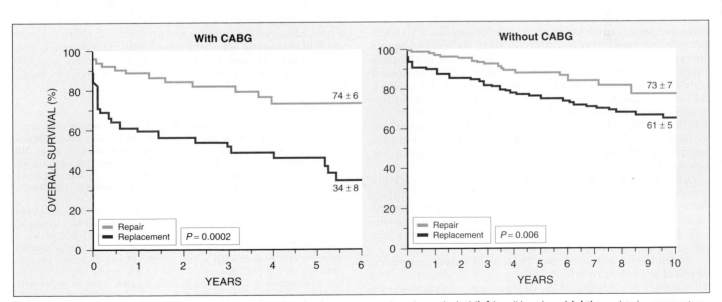

FIGURE 62–35 Plots of overall survival compared for mitral repair and replacement groups in patients who had **(left)** or did not have **(right)** associated coronary artery bypass grafting (CABG). Note that the outcome is better with repair than with replacement in both groups and that the outcome is worse in patients who underwent CABG and mitral valve replacement. *(From Enriquez-Sarano M, Schaff HV, Orszulak TA, et al: Valve repair improves the outcome of surgery for mitral regurgitation: A multivariate analysis. Circulation 91:1022, 1995.)*

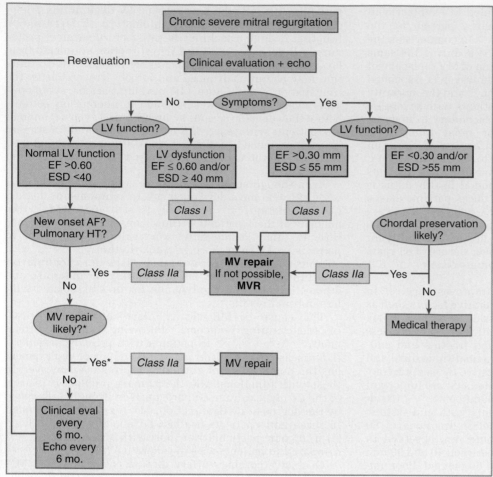

FIGURE 62–36 Management strategy for patients with chronic severe mitral regurgitation. AF = atrial fibrillation, EF = ejection fraction, ESD = end-systolic dimension, HT = hypertension, MV = mitral valve, MVR = mitral valve repair. *Mitral valve repair may be performed in asymptomatic patients with normal LV function if performed by an experienced surgical team and the likelihood of successful MV repair is greater than 90 percent. *(From Bonow RO, Carabello BA, Chatterjee K, et al: ACC/AHA 2006 guidelines for the management of patients with valvular heart disease: a report of the American College of Cardiology/American Heart Association Task Force on Practice Guidelines (writing committee to revise the 1998 Guidelines for the Management of Patients With Valvular Heart Disease): Developed in collaboration with the Society of Cardiovascular Anesthesiologists: Endorsed by the Society for Cardiovascular Angiography and Interventions and the Society of Thoracic Surgeons. Circulation 114:e84, 2006.)*

tions in operative mortality, the improvements in MV repair procedures, long-term results indicating stability of repair in experienced centers[187-189] and the recognition of the poor long-term results in many patients when MR is corrected only after a long history of symptoms, impaired LV function, AF, or pulmonary hypertension. A detailed echocardiographic examination should be carried out to assess the likelihood that MV repair, rather than MV replacement, is possible, and the difference in outcome between these procedures should be weighed when deciding whether or not to proceed.

ASYMPTOMATIC PATIENTS. Asymptomatic patients (NYHA Class I) should be considered for MV repair if they have LV systolic dysfunction (ejection fraction ≤60 percent and/or LV end-systolic diameter >40 mm).[1] It is also reasonable to consider MV repair in asymptomatic patients when AF or pulmonary hypertension is present.

A number of centers are moving toward a more aggressive surgical approach in which MV repair is recommended to all patients with severe MR, independent of symptoms or LV function. Such a recommendation should be considered only in patients with severe MR (see Table 62-1) and in centers in which the surgical experience indicates that the patient will undergo successful MV repair with a very high

degree of certainty.[1] Unfortunately, successful MV repair cannot be guaranteed, and even in the best of circumstances, with this approach some young asymptomatic patients may be subjected to the risks of prosthetic valves prematurely and unnecessarily.

When MV repair is not recommended, asymptomatic patients with normal LV function should be followed clinically and by echocardiography every 6 to 12 months. At times, a careful history and performance of an exercise test often reveal that these patients are not truly asymptomatic.[1,174]

If MV replacement is likely to be necessary, a higher threshold for clinical and hemodynamic impairment should be employed than if MV repair is contemplated, and there are few indications for MV replacement in asymptomatic patients other than LV systolic dysfunction (see Fig 62-36). Because of the higher operative mortality, older patients (older than 75 years of age) should, in general, undergo surgery only if they are symptomatic.

SYMPTOMATIC PATIENTS. Patients with severe MR and moderate or severe symptoms (NYHA Classes II, III, and IV) should generally be considered for surgery. One exception is a patient in whom the LV ejection fraction is less than 30 percent and echocardiography suggests that MV replacement will be required and that the subvalvular apparatus cannot be preserved. Because of the high risk of operation and the poor long-term results in these patients, medical therapy is usually advised, but the outcome is poor in any event. However, when MV repair appears possible, even patients with serious LV dysfunction may be considered for operation (see Fig 62-36).

Acute Mitral Regurgitation

The causes of acute MR (see Table 62-7) are diverse and represent acute manifestations of disease processes that may, under other circumstances, cause chronic MR. Especially important causes of acute MR are spontaneous rupture of chordae tendineae, infective endocarditis with disruption of valve leaflets or chordal rupture, ischemic dysfunction or rupture of a papillary muscle, and malfunction of a prosthetic valve.

Acute, severe MR causes a marked reduction of forward stroke volume, a slight reduction of end-systolic volume, and an increase in end-diastolic volume. One major hemodynamic difference between acute and chronic MR derives from the differences in left atrial compliance. Patients who develop acute, severe MR usually have a normal-sized left atrium with normal or reduced left atrial compliance. The left atrial pressure rises abruptly, which often leads to pulmonary edema, marked elevation of pulmonary vascular resistance, and right-sided heart failure.

Because the *v* wave is markedly elevated in patients with acute, severe MR, the reverse pressure gradient between the left ventricle and left atrium declines at the end of systole, and the murmur may be decrescendo rather than holosystolic, ending well before A2. It is usually lower pitched and softer than the murmur of chronic MR. A left-sided S4 is frequently found. Pulmonary hypertension, which is common in patients with acute MR, may increase the intensity of P2 and the murmurs of pulmonary regurgitation and TR may also develop along with a right-sided S4. In patients with severe, acute MR, a v wave (late systolic pressure rise) in the pulmonary artery pressure pulse (see Fig. 62-31) may rarely cause premature closure of the pulmonary valve, an early P2, and paradoxical splitting of S2. Acute MR, even if severe, often does not increase overall cardiac size, as seen on the chest roentgenogram, and may produce only mild left atrial enlargement despite marked elevation of left atrial pressure. In addition, the echocardiogram may show little increase in the internal diameter of either the left atrium or the left ventricle, but increased systolic motion of the left ventricle is prominent. Characteristic features on Doppler echocardiography are the severe jet of MR and elevation of the pulmonary artery systolic pressure.

In severe MR secondary to acute myocardial infarction, pulmonary edema, hypotension, and frank cardiogenic shock may develop. It is essential to determine the cause of the MR, which include a ruptured papillary muscle, annular dilation from severe LV dilation, and papillary muscle displacement with leaflet tethering.

MEDICAL MANAGEMENT OF ACUTE MITRAL REGURGITATION. Afterload reduction with afterload reducing agents is of particular importance in treating patients with acute MR. Intravenous nitroprusside may be lifesaving in patients with acute MR due to rupture of the head of a papillary muscle that occurs during an acute myocardial infarction. It may permit stabilization of the patient's condition and thereby allow coronary arteriography and surgery to be performed with the patient in optimal condition. In patients with acute MR who are hypotensive, an inotropic agent such as dobutamine should be administered with the nitroprusside. Intraaortic balloon counterpulsation may be necessary to stabilize the patient as preparations for surgery are made.

SURGICAL TREATMENT OF ACUTE MITRAL REGURGITATION. Emergency surgical treatment may be required for patients with acute LV failure caused by acute MR. Emergency surgery is associated with higher mortality rates than is elective surgery for chronic MR. However, unless patients with acute, severe MR and heart failure are treated aggressively, a fatal outcome is almost certain.

Acute papillary muscle rupture requires emergency surgery, with either MV repair or replacement.[214] In patients with papillary muscle dysfunction, initial treatment should consist of hemodynamic stabilization, usually with the aid of an intra-aortic balloon pump, and surgery should be considered for those patients who do not improve with aggressive medical therapy. If patients with MR can be stabilized by medical treatment, it is preferable to defer operation until 4 to 6 weeks after the infarction. Vasodilator treatment may be useful during this period. However, medical management should not be prolonged if multisystem (renal and/or pulmonary) failure develops.

Surgical mortality rates are also higher in patients with acute MR and refractory heart failure (NYHA Class IV), in those with prosthetic valve dysfunction, and in those with active infective endocarditis (of either a native or a prosthetic valve). Despite the higher surgical risks, the efficacy of early operation has been established in patients with infective endocarditis complicated by medically uncontrollable congestive heart failure and/or recurrent emboli (see Chap. 63).[212,215]

MITRAL VALVE PROLAPSE SYNDROME

Etiology and Pathology

DEFINITION. The MVP syndrome has been given many names including the systolic click-murmur syndrome, Barlow syndrome, billowing mitral cusp syndrome, myxomatous mitral valve syndrome, floppy valve syndrome, and redundant cusp syndrome.[216,217] It is a variable clinical syndrome that results from diverse pathogenic mechanisms of one or more portions of the mitral valve apparatus, valve leaflets, chordae tendineae, papillary muscle, and valve annulus. The MVP syndrome is one of the most prevalent cardiac valvular abnormalities. Using standardized echocardiographic diagnostic criteria, a community-based study showed that MVP syndrome occurs in 2.4 percent of the population.[218,219] The syndrome is twice as frequent in

females as in males. However, serious MR occurs more frequently in older males (older than 50 years) with MVP than in young females with this disorder.

The clinical and echocardiographic criteria for the diagnosis of MVP have been well established. The characteristic systolic click and mid-to-late systolic murmur is a major diagnostic criterion. The most specific echocardiographic criterion is superior displacement of one or both mitral valve leaflets by more than 2 mm above the plane of the annulus[217,219] in the long axis (see Fig. 14-57). Other echocardiographic criteria include diffuse leaflet thickening and redundancy, excessive chordal length and motion, and evidence of ruptured chords, in addition to prolapse of leaflet segments.

ETIOLOGY. A classification of MVP is shown in Table 62-9. Most frequently, MVP occurs as a primary condition that is not associated with other diseases and can be familial or nonfamilial. Familial MVP is transmitted as an autosomal trait, and several chromosomal loci have been identified.[220-222] The MVP syndrome is more prevalent in young women, who generally have a benign course, whereas severe myxomatous disease is more common in older men, who have a higher risk of complications, including the need for surgical MV repair. MVP has also been associated with many conditions, occurring quite commonly in heritable disorders of connective tissue that increase the size of the mitral leaflets and apparatus. Echocardiographic evidence of MVP is found in most patients with the Marfan syndrome (see Chap. 8) and in many of their first-degree relatives. MVP has also been associated with Ehlers-Danlos syndrome (see Chap. 8), osteogenesis imperfecta, pseudoxanthoma elasticum, periarteritis nodosa, myotonic dystrophy, von Willebrand disease, hyperthyroidism, and congenital malformations such as Ebstein anomaly of the tricuspid valve, atrial septal defect of the ostium secundum variety, the Holt-Oram syndrome, and HCM. There may be a higher incidence of MVP in patients with an asthenic habitus and various congenital thoracic deformities, including "straight back syndrome," pectus excavatum, and a shallow chest. These associations have not been proved using rigorous echocardiographic criteria, and, with the exception of connective tissue disorders, it is not clear how many of these are chance associations.

PATHOLOGY. Findings include myxomatous proliferation of the mitral valve leaflets, in which the spongiosa component of the valve (i.e., the middle layer of the leaflet

TABLE 62–9	Classification of Mitral Valve Prolapse

Mitral Valve Prolapse Syndrome
Younger age (20-50 yr)
Predominantly female
Click or click-murmur on physical examination
Thin leaflets with systolic displacement on echocardiography
Associated with low blood pressure, orthostatic hypotension, palpitations
Benign long-term course

Myxomatous Mitral Valve Disease
Older age (40-70 yr)
Predominantly male
Thickened, redundant valve leaflets
Mitral regurgitation on physical exam and echocardiography
High likelihood of progressive disease requiring mitral valve surgery

Secondary Mitral Valve Prolapse
Marfan syndrome
Hypertrophic cardiomyopathy
Ehlers-Danlos syndrome
Other connective tissue diseases

Modified from Otto CM: Valvular Heart Disease. 2nd ed. Philadelphia, WB Saunders, 2004, p 369.

between the atrialis and the ventricularis composed of loose, myxomatous material) is unusually prominent[216,217,223] and the quantity of acid mucopolysaccharide is increased.[224] Electron microscopy shows a haphazard arrangement of cells with disruption and with fragmentation of collagen fibrils. Secondary effects include fibrosis of the surface of the MV leaflets, thinning and/or elongation of the chordae tendineae, and ventricular friction lesions.

In mild cases, the valvular myxoid stroma is enlarged on histological examination, but the leaflets are grossly normal. However, with increasing quantities of myxoid stroma, the leaflets become grossly abnormal, redundant, and prolapsed. There is interchordal hooding due to leaflet redundancy that includes both the rough and clear zones of the involved leaflets. Regions of endothelial disruption are common and are possible sites of endocarditis or thrombus formation. The severity of MR depends on the extent of the prolapse. The cusps of the mitral valve, the chordae tendineae, and the annulus may all be affected by myxomatous proliferation. Degeneration of collagen and myxomatous changes within the central core of the chordae tendineae, with associated decreases in tensile strength,[153,223] are primarily responsible for chordal rupture, which often occurs and may intensify the severity of MR. Increased chordal tension resulting from the enlarged area of the valve cusps may play a contributory role. Myxomatous changes in the annulus may result in annular dilation and calcification, further contributing to the severity of MR.

Myxomatous proliferation, although most commonly affecting the mitral valve, has also been described in the tricuspid, aortic, and pulmonic valves, particularly in patients with the Marfan syndrome, and may lead to regurgitation of these valves as well as the mitral valve.

Clinical Presentation

The clinical presentations of the MVP syndrome are diverse. The condition has been observed in patients of all ages and in both sexes. Despite the overestimation of the prevalence in the population referred to earlier, MVP is the most common cause of isolated MR requiring surgical treatment in the United States[217] and the most common cardiac condition predisposing patients to infective endocarditis[225] (see Chap. 63).

Symptoms

The vast majority of patients with MVP are asymptomatic and remain so throughout their lives. Although early studies called attention to an "MVP syndrome" with a characteristic systolic nonejection click and various nonspecific symptoms, such as fatigability, palpitations, postural orthostasis, and anxiety and other neuropsychiatric symptoms, as well as symptoms of autonomic dysfunction, these associations have not been confirmed in carefully controlled studies.[217,226] How, and even whether, these symptoms relate to the presence of MVP is not clear.

Patients may complain of syncope, presyncope, palpitations, chest discomfort, and, when MR is severe, symptoms of diminished cardiac reserve. Chest discomfort may be typical of angina pectoris but is more often atypical in that it is prolonged, not clearly related to exertion, and punctuated by brief attacks or severe stabbing pain at the apex. The discomfort may be secondary to abnormal tension on papillary muscles. In patients with MVP and severe MR, the symptoms of the latter (fatigue, dyspnea, and exercise limitation) may be present. Patients with MVP may also develop symptomatic arrhythmias (to be discussed).

Physical Examination (see Chap. 11)

The body weight is often low, and the habitus may be asthenic. Blood pressure is usually normal or low; ortho-

static hypotension may be present. As already mentioned, patients with MVP have a higher than expected prevalence of "straight back syndrome," scoliosis, and pectus excavatum.[216] MR ranges from absent to severe.

AUSCULTATION

The auscultatory findings unique to the MVP syndrome are best elicited with the diaphragm of the stethoscope. The patient should be examined in the supine, left decubitus, and sitting positions. The most important finding is a nonejection systolic click at least 0.14 second after S1.[216,226,227] This can be differentiated from a systolic ejection click because it occurs after the beginning of the carotid pulse upstroke. Occasionally, multiple mid and late systolic clicks are audible, most readily along the lower left sternal border. The clicks are believed to be produced by sudden tensing of the elongated chordae tendineae and of the prolapsing leaflets. They are often, although not invariably, followed by a mid- to late crescendo systolic murmur that continues to A2. This murmur is similar to that produced by papillary muscle dysfunction, which is readily understandable because both result from mid- to late systolic MR. In general, the duration of the murmur is a function of the severity of the MR. When the murmur is confined to the latter portion of systole, MR usually is not severe. However, as MR becomes more severe, the murmur commences earlier and ultimately becomes holosystolic.

There is considerable variability of the physical findings in the MVP syndrome. Some patients exhibit both a midsystolic click and a mid-to-late systolic murmur; others present with only one of these two findings; still others have only a click on one occasion and only a murmur on another, both on a third examination, and no abnormality at all on a fourth. Conditions other than MVP that may cause midsystolic clicks include tricuspid valve prolapse, atrial septal aneurysms, and extracardiac causes.

DYNAMIC AUSCULTATION. The auscultatory findings are exquisitely sensitive to physiological and pharmacological interventions, and recognition of the changes induced by these interventions is of great value in the diagnosis of the MVP syndrome (Fig. 62-37 and see Table 62-8). The mitral valve begins to prolapse when the reduction of LV volume during systole reaches a critical point at which the valve leaflets no longer coapt; at that instant, the click occurs and the murmur

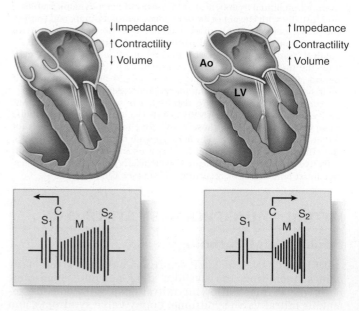

FIGURE 62–37 Dynamic auscultation in mitral valve prolapse. Any maneuver that decreases left ventricular (LV) volume (e.g., decreased venous return, tachycardia, decreased outflow impedance, increased contractility) worsens the mismatch in size between the enlarged mitral valve and LV chamber, resulting in prolapse earlier in systole and movement of the click (C) and murmur (M) toward the first heart sound (S₁). Conversely, maneuvers that increase LV volume (e.g., increased venous return, bradycardia, increased outflow impedance, decreased contractility) delay the occurrence of prolapse, resulting in movement of the click and murmur toward the second heart sound (S₂). Ao = aorta. *(Modified from O'Rourke RA, Crawford MH: The systolic click-murmur syndrome: Clinical recognition and management. Curr Probl Cardiol 1:9, 1976.)*

commences. Any maneuver that decreases LV volume, such as a reduction of impedance to LV outflow, a reduction in venous return, tachycardia, or an augmentation of myocardial contractility, results in an earlier occurrence of prolapse during systole. As a consequence, the click and onset of the murmur move closer to S1. When prolapse is severe and/or LV size is markedly reduced, prolapse may begin with the onset of systole. As a consequence, the click may not be audible, and the murmur may be holosystolic. On the other hand, when LV volume is augmented by an increase in the impedance to LV emptying, an increase in venous return, a reduction of myocardial contractility, or bradycardia, both the click and the onset of the murmur will be delayed.

During the straining phase of the Valsalva maneuver and upon sudden standing, cardiac size decreases, and both the click and the onset of the murmur occur earlier in systole. In contrast, a sudden change from the standing to the supine position, leg-raising, squatting, maximal isometric exercise, and, to a lesser extent, expiration will delay the click and the onset of the murmur. During the overshoot phase of the Valsalva maneuver (i.e., six to eight cycles following release) and with prolongation of the R-R interval, either following a premature contraction or in AF, the click and onset of the murmur are usually delayed, and the intensity of the murmur is reduced. Maneuvers that elevate arterial pressure, such as isometric exercise, increase the intensity of the click and murmur. In general, when the onset of the murmur is delayed, both its duration and intensity are diminished, reflecting a reduction in the severity of MR.

The response to several interventions may be helpful in differentiating obstructive HCM from MVP (see Chap. 65). During the strain of the Valsalva maneuver, the murmur of HCM increases in intensity, whereas the murmur of MVP becomes longer but usually not louder. The murmur of HCM becomes louder after amyl nitrite inhalation, whereas that of MVP does not. Following a premature beat, the murmur of HCM increases in intensity and duration, whereas that due to MVP usually remains unchanged or decreases.

Echocardiography (see also Chap. 14)

Echocardiography plays an essential role in the diagnosis of MVP and has been instrumental in the delineation of this syndrome[228] (Fig. 62-38, see also Fig. 14-57). To establish the

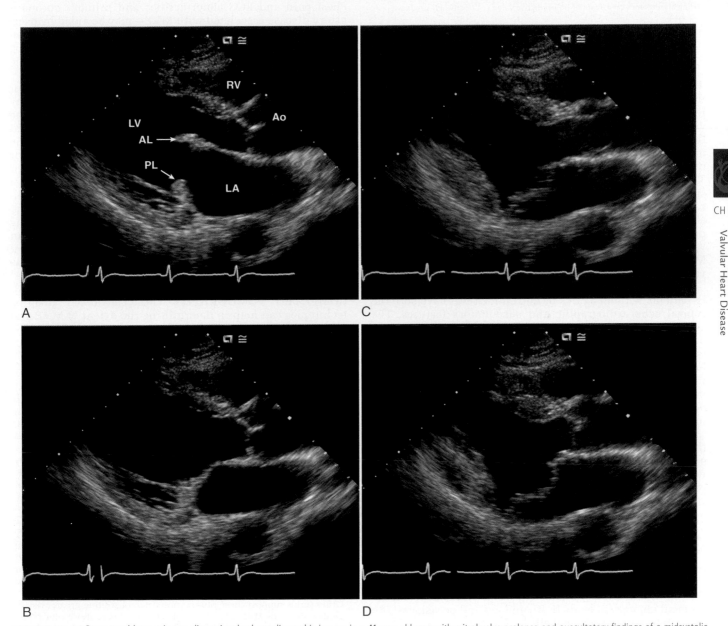

FIGURE 62–38 Parasternal long-axis two-dimensional echocardiographic images in a 41-year-old man with mitral valve prolapse and auscultatory findings of a midsystolic click and mitral regurgitation (MR). **A,** End-diastolic image. The mitral valve leaflets are severely thickened, and the anterior leaflet (AL) is elongated. **B** to **D,** Serial images from early systole to midsystole, demonstrating bileaflet prolapse. Color-flow imaging in this patient demonstrated severe MR. Patients with these findings are at increased risk of complications, such as infective endocarditis, systemic emboli, and heart failure. Ao = aorta; LA = left atrium; LV = left ventricle; PL = posterior leaflet; RV = right ventricle.

TABLE 62–10	Predictors of Clinical Outcome in Mitral Valve Prolapse			
	Survival	Valve Surgery	Arrhythmias/ Sudden Death	Endocarditis
Age	+++*	+++	–	–
Gender	++	++	–	–
Leaflet thickness or redundancy	+++	+++	++++	++++
Severity of mitral regurgitation	++++	++++	++++	++++
Systolic click	+	–	–	–
Left ventricular dilation	+	++++	++	–
Left atrial dilation	–	++	+	–

*The symbols indicate the relative predictive value of each variable for the listed clinical outcomes on a scale of no predictive value (–) to strongly predictive (++++).

From Otto CM: Valvular Heart Disease. 2nd ed. Philadelphia, WB Saunders, 2004, p 376.

CH 62

diagnosis, the two-dimensional echocardiogram must show that one or both mitral valve leaflets billow by at least 2 mm into the left atrium during systole in the long-axis view.[217,219,226] Thickening of the involved leaflet to greater than 5 mm supports the diagnosis. Findings of more severe myxomatous disease include increased leaflet area, leaflet redundancy, chordal elongation, and annular dilation. These findings, are also helpful in identifying patients at significant risk for developing severe MR or infective endocarditis (Table 62-10). The mitral annular diameter is often abnormally increased. Transesophageal echocardiography provides additional details regarding integrity of the mitral valve apparatus, such as rupture of chordae tendineae. In MR secondary to MVP, the echocardiogram also provides valuable information regarding LV size and function.

The echocardiographic findings of MVP may be observed in patients without a click or murmur. Others have both the typical echocardiographic and auscultatory features. The echocardiographic findings of MVP have been reported to occur in a large number of first-degree relatives of patients with established MVP. Two-dimensional echocardiography has also revealed prolapse of the tricuspid and aortic valves in approximately 20 percent of patients with MVP.[217] Conversely, however, prolapse of the tricuspid and aortic valves occurs uncommonly in patients without prolapse of the mitral valve.

Doppler echocardiography frequently reveals mild MR that is not always associated with an audible murmur. Moderate to severe MR is present in about two-thirds of patients with posterior leaflet prolapse and in about one-fourth of patients with anterior leaflet prolapse.[229] Severity of MR should be assessed quantitatively as previously discussed (see Table 62-1).

Other Diagnostic Evaluation

ELECTROCARDIOGRAPHY. The ECG is usually normal in asymptomatic patients with MVP. In a minority of asymptomatic patients and in many symptomatic patients, the ECG shows inverted or biphasic T waves and nonspecific ST segment changes in leads II, III, and aVf and occasionally in the anterolateral leads as well.

ARRHYTHMIAS. A spectrum of arrhythmias have been observed in patients with MVP. These include atrial and ventricular premature contractions and supraventricular

and ventricular tachyarrhythmias,[217,230] as well as bradyarrhythmias due to sinus node dysfunction or varying degrees of atrioventricular block. The mechanism of the arrhythmias is not clear. Diastolic depolarization of muscle fibers in the anterior mitral leaflet in response to stretch has been demonstrated experimentally, and the abnormal stretch of the prolapsed leaflet may be of pathogenetic significance.

Paroxysmal supraventricular tachycardia is the most common sustained tachyarrhythmia in patients with MVP and may be related to an increased incidence of left atrioventricular bypass tracts. The incidence of MVP among patients with the Wolff-Parkinson-White syndrome is increased. There is also an increased association between MVP and prolongation of the QT interval, and this association may play a role in the pathogenesis of serious ventricular arrhythmias. Patients with MVP have an increased incidence of abnormal late potentials on signal-averaged ECGs, as well as reduced heart rate variability.

STRESS SCINTIGRAPHY. The differential diagnosis between two common conditions—MVP associated with chest pain and ECG abnormalities and primary coronary artery disease associated with MVP—may be aided by exercise electrocardiography. However, myocardial perfusion scintigraphy using thallium-201 or sestamibi during pharmacological exercise stress (see Chap. 16) is more specific for diagnosing associated coronary artery disease.

ANGIOGRAPHY. Angiography is not recommended for the diagnostic evaluation of MVP. However, if angiography is performed for other indications, there are features of the left ventriculogram that are characteristic of MVP. The right anterior oblique projection is most useful for defining the posterior leaflet of the mitral valve, and the left anterior oblique projection is most useful for studying the anterior leaflet. The most helpful sign is extension of the mitral leaflet tissue inferiorly and posteriorly to the point of attachment of the mitral leaflets to the mitral annulus. Angiography may also reveal scalloped edges of the leaflets, reflecting redundancy of tissue. Other angiographic abnormalities in some patients with MVP include LV dilation, decreased systolic contraction (especially of the basal portion of the ventricle), and calcification of the mitral annulus.

MAGNETIC RESONANCE IMAGING AND CARDIAC COMPUTED TOMOGRAPHY. These advanced imaging techniques can help in determining the extent of MVP and LV function in patients with suboptimal echocardiographic examinations. CMR is also useful for evaluating presence and severity of MR.

Disease Course

The outlook for patients with MVP in general is excellent; a large majority remain asymptomatic for many years without any change in clinical or laboratory findings.[1,219,226,231] Serious complications (cardiac death, need for cardiac surgery, acute infective endocarditis, or cerebral embolic events) occur at a rate of only 1 per 100 patient years, and 4 percent of patients died during the 8 years. In contrast, one study reported a much more aggressive course in 833 patients with MVP, with a 19 percent mortality rate at 10 years and a 20 percent rate of MVP-related events, including heart failure, AF, cerebrovascular events, arterial thromboembolism, and endocarditis.[232] The apparent explanation for these latter observations is that patients with MVP could be risk stratified on the basis of several factors (Fig. 62-39).[232] The primary risk factors were moderate to severe MR and/or LV ejection fraction less than 50 percent, and secondary risk factors included mild MR, left atrial dimension 40 mm or greater, flail leaflet, and age 50 years or older. Patients with a primary risk factor had excessive mortality and morbidity, as did those with two or more secondary risk factors.[232] Other series support these observations, demonstrating greater risk of cardiac death or MVP-related complications in men, those older than 45 years old, those with holosystolic murmurs, those with severe MR,[229] and those with left atrial dimension greater than 40 mm. Other series which have reported a lower prevalence of adverse sequelae of MVP[219,233] have included relatively fewer patients with these risk

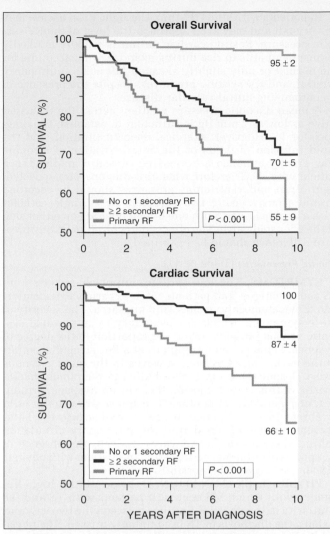

Overall Survival

- No or 1 secondary RF
- ≥ 2 secondary RF
- Primary RF

$P < 0.001$

95 ± 2
70 ± 5
55 ± 9

Cardiac Survival

- No or 1 secondary RF
- ≥ 2 secondary RF
- Primary RF

$P < 0.001$

100
87 ± 4
66 ± 10

YEARS AFTER DIAGNOSIS

FIGURE 62–39 Survival in patients with mitral valve prolapse according to categories of baseline risk factors (RFs). Primary RFs were moderate-to-severe mitral regurgitation (MR) and ejection fraction less than 0.50. Secondary RFs were mild MR, left atrium larger than 40 mm, flail leaflet, atrial fibrillation, and age older than 50 years. *(Modified from Avierinos JF, Gersh BJ, Melton LJ, et al: Natural history of asymptomatic mitral valve prolapse in the community. Circulation 106:1355, 2002.)*

factors. Variables associated with an adverse outcome are summarized in Table 62-10.

Progressive MR with gradual increase in left atrial and LV size, AF, pulmonary hypertension, and the development of congestive heart failure is the most frequent serious complication,[1,217] occurring in about 15 percent of patients over a 10- to 15-year period. Patients with the MVP syndrome are also at risk of developing infective endocarditis.[225] Both severe MR and endocarditis develop more frequently in patients with both murmurs and clicks than in those with an isolated click, in patients with thickened (greater than 5 mm) and redundant mitral valve leaflets, and in men older than 50 years (see Table 62-10). In many patients, rupture of chordae tendineae is responsible for the precipitation and/or intensification of the MR.[168,234] Infective endocarditis often aggravates the severity of MR and therefore the need for surgical treatment.

Acute hemiplegia, transient ischemic attacks, cerebellar infarcts, amaurosis fugax, and retinal arteriolar occlusions have been reported to occur more frequently in patients with the MVP syndrome, suggesting that cerebral emboli are unusually common in this condition.[217,226,232] It has been proposed that these neurological complications are associated with loss of endothelial continuity and tearing of the endocardium overlying the myxomatous valve, which initiates platelet aggregation and the formation of mural platelet-fibrin complexes. Although it has been proposed that embolization secondary to MVP may be a signifi-

cant cause for unexplained strokes in young people without cerebrovascular disease, a large case-controlled study showed no association between MVP and ischemic neurological events in persons under 45 years of age.[233]

MITRAL VALVE PROLAPSE AND SUDDEN DEATH. The relation between the MVP syndrome and sudden death is not clear. However, the best evidence suggests that MVP increases the risk of sudden death slightly,[216,217,226,235,236] especially in patients with severe MR or severe valvular deformity, and those with complex ventricular arrhythmias, QT interval prolongation, and a history of syncope and palpitations.

Management

Patients with the physical findings of MVP (and those without such findings who have been given the diagnosis) should undergo transthoracic echocardiography. This procedure also should be performed in first-degree relatives of patients with MVP.[1] The diagnosis of MVP requires definitive echocardiographic findings, and overdiagnosis and incorrect "labeling" have been a major problem with this condition. Asymptomatic patients (or those whose principal complaint is anxiety), with no arrhythmias evident on a routine extended ECG tracing and without evidence of MR, have an excellent prognosis. They should be reassured about the favorable prognosis and be encouraged to engage in normal lifestyles, but should have follow-up examinations every 3 to 5 years. This should include a two-dimensional echocardiogram and a color flow Doppler study.

Patients with a long systolic murmur may show progression of MR and should be evaluated more frequently, at intervals of approximately 12 months. Endocarditis prophylaxis is no longer recommended routinely for patients with MVP, including those with a systolic murmur and typical echocardiographic findings (see also Chap. 63).[1]

Patients with a history of palpitations, lightheadedness, dizziness, or syncope or those who have ventricular arrhythmias or QT prolongation on a routine ECG should undergo ambulatory (24-hour) ECG monitoring and/or exercise ECG to detect arrhythmias. Because of the risk, albeit very low, of sudden death, further electrophysiologic studies may be carried out to characterize arrhythmias if they exist. Beta-adrenergic blockers are useful in the treatment of palpitations secondary to frequent premature ventricular contractions and for self-terminating episodes of supraventricular tachycardia. These drugs may also be useful in the treatment of chest discomfort, both in patients with associated coronary artery disease and in those with normal coronary vessels in whom the symptoms may be due to regional ischemia secondary to MVP. Radiofrequency ablation of atrioventricular bypass tracts is useful for frequent or prolonged episodes of supraventricular tachycardia.

Aspirin should be given to patients with MVP who have had a documented focal neurological event and in whom no other cause, such as a left atrial thrombus or AF, is apparent.

Patients with MVP and severe MR should be treated similarly to other patients with severe MR and may require MV surgery. MV repair without replacement is usually possible (see Fig. 62-34).[186-188,190] Therefore the threshold for surgical treatment in these patients is lower than in patients with MR in whom MV replacement may be necessary, providing that patients are referred to a surgical team with established success in MV repair, as noted previously. The majority of all MV repairs for MR are now carried out in patients with MVP. Resection of the most deformed leaflet segment, usually the middle scallop of the posterior leaflet, and insertion of an annuloplasty ring to reduce the dilated annulus is the most commonly employed procedure. Repair of anterior leaflet prolapse is more challenging. Rupture of the chordae tendineae to the anterior leaflet can sometimes be treated by chordal transfer from the posterior leaflet. In

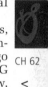

other patients, shortening of the chordae tendineae and/or papillary muscle is necessary. The average operative mortality is 2 to 3 percent,[202] and long term studies demonstrate excellent durability of MV repair in the majority of patients.[186-188] However, MR recurs in a subset of patients,[188,204] at which point it may be necessary to perform MV replacement.

Coronary arteriography is reasonable in patients with angina pectoris on effort and/or ischemic ECG changes, and especially in those with abnormalities on a stress myocardial perfusion scan. Treatment should take into account both the responsiveness of symptoms to medical management and the coronary anatomy.

Although this discussion has focused attention on complications of the MVP syndrome, it should not be forgotten that, on the whole, this is a benign condition and that the vast majority of patients with this syndrome remain asymptomatic for their entire lives and require, at most, observation every few years and reassurance.

TRICUSPID, PULMONIC, AND MULTIVALVULAR DISEASE

Tricuspid Stenosis

Etiology and Pathology

Tricuspid stenosis (TS) is almost always rheumatic in origin.[237] Other causes of obstruction to right atrial emptying are unusual and include congenital tricuspid atresia (see Chap. 61); right atrial tumors, which may produce a clinical picture suggesting rapidly progressive TS (see Chap. 69); and the carcinoid syndrome[238] (see Chap. 64), which more frequently produces TR. Rarely, obstruction to RV inflow can be due to endomyocardial fibrosis, tricuspid valve vegetations,[239] a pacemaker lead,[240] or extracardiac tumors.

The majority of patients with rheumatic tricuspid valve disease present with TR or a combination of TS and TR. Isolated rheumatic TS is uncommon and almost never occurs as an isolated lesion but generally accompanies mitral valve disease.[1,237,241] In many patients with TS, the aortic valve is also involved (i.e., trivalvular stenosis is present). TS is found at autopsy in about 15 percent of patients with rheumatic heart disease but is of clinical significance in only about 5 percent.[237] Organic tricuspid valve disease is more common in India, Pakistan, and other developing nations near the equator than in North America or Western Europe. The anatomical changes of rheumatic TS resemble those of MS, with fusion and shortening of the chordae tendineae and fusion of the leaflets at their edges, producing a diaphragm with a fixed central aperture.[237] However, valvular calcification is rare. As is the case with MS, TS is more common in women. The right atrium is often greatly dilated in TS, and its walls are thickened. There may be evidence of severe passive congestion, with enlargement of the liver and spleen.

Pathophysiology

A diastolic pressure gradient between the right atrium and ventricle—the hemodynamic expression of TS—is augmented when the transvalvular blood flow increases during inspiration or exercise and is reduced when the blood flow declines during expiration. A relatively modest diastolic pressure gradient (i.e., a mean gradient of only 5 mm Hg) is usually sufficient to elevate mean right atrial pressure to levels that result in systemic venous congestion and, unless sodium intake has been restricted or diuretics have been given, is associated with jugular venous distention, ascites, and edema.

In patients with sinus rhythm, the right atrial a wave may be very tall and may even approach the level of the RV systolic pressure. Resting cardiac output is usually markedly reduced and fails to rise during exercise. This accounts for the normal or only slightly elevated left atrial, pulmonary arterial, and RV systolic pressures, despite the presence of accompanying mitral valvular disease.

A mean diastolic pressure gradient across the tricuspid valve as low as 2 mm Hg is sufficient to establish the diagnosis of TS. However, exercise, deep inspiration, and the rapid infusion of fluids or the administration of atropine may greatly enhance a borderline pressure gradient in a patient with TS. Therefore when this diagnosis is suspected, right atrial and ventricular pressures should be recorded simultaneously, using two catheters or a single catheter with a double lumen, with one lumen opening on either side of the tricuspid valve. The effects of respiration on any pressure difference should be examined.

Clinical Presentation (Table 62-11)

SYMPTOMS. The low cardiac output characteristic of TS causes fatigue, and patients often experience discomfort due to hepatomegaly, ascites, and anasarca. The severity of these symptoms, which are secondary to an elevated systemic venous pressure, is out of proportion to the degree of dyspnea. Some patients complain of a fluttering discomfort in the neck, caused by giant a waves in the jugular venous pulse. Despite the coexistence of MS, the symptoms characteristic of this valvular lesion (i.e., severe dyspnea, orthopnea, and paroxysmal nocturnal dyspnea) are usually mild or absent in the presence of severe TS because the latter prevents surges of blood into the pulmonary circulation behind the stenotic mitral valve. Indeed, the absence of symptoms of pulmonary congestion in a patient with obvious MS should suggest the possibility of TS.

PHYSICAL EXAMINATION. Because of the high frequency with which MS occurs in patients with TS and the similarity in the physical findings between the two valvular lesions, the diagnosis of TS is commonly missed. The physical findings are mistakenly attributed to MS, which is more common and may be more obvious. Therefore a high index

TABLE 62–11	Clinical and Laboratory Features of Rheumatic Tricuspid Stenosis

History
Progressive fatigue, edema, anorexia
Minimal orthopnea, paroxysmal nocturnal dyspnea
Rheumatic fever in two thirds of patients
Female preponderance
Pulmonary edema and hemoptysis are rare

Physical Findings
Signs of multivalvular involvement
Diastolic rumble at lower left sternal border, increasing in intensity with inspiration
Often confused with mitral stenosis
Peripheral cyanosis
Neck vein distention, with prominent v waves and slow y descent
Absent right ventricular lift
Associated murmurs of mitral and aortic valve disease
Hepatic pulsation
Ascites, peripheral edema

Laboratory Findings
Electrocardiogram: tall right atrial P waves and no right ventricular hypertrophy
Chest roentgenogram: a dilated right atrium without an enlarged pulmonary artery segment
Echocardiography: diastolic doming of tricuspid valve leaflet

Modified from Ockene IS: Tricuspid valve disease. *In* Dalon JE. Alpert JS (eds): Valvular Heart Disease. 2nd ed. Boston, Little, Brown, 1987, pp 356, 390.

CH 62

of suspicion is required to detect the tricuspid valvular lesion. In the presence of sinus rhythm, the a wave in the jugular venous pulse is tall, and a presystolic hepatic pulsation is often palpable. The y descent is slow and barely appreciable. The lung fields are clear, and despite engorged neck veins and the presence of ascites and anasarca, the patient may be comfortable while lying flat. Thus the diagnosis of TS may be suspected from inspection of the jugular venous pulse in a patient with MS but without clinical evidence of pulmonary hypertension. This suspicion is strengthened when a diastolic thrill is palpable at the lower left sternal border, particularly if the thrill appears or becomes more prominent during inspiration.

The auscultatory findings of the accompanying MS are usually prominent and often overshadow the more subtle signs of TS. A tricuspid opening snap (OS) may be audible but is often difficult to distinguish from a mitral OS. However, the tricuspid OS usually follows the mitral OS and is localized to the lower left sternal border, whereas the mitral OS is usually most prominent at the apex and radiates more widely. The diastolic murmur of TS is also commonly heard best along the lower left parasternal border in the 4th intercostal space and is usually softer, higher pitched, and shorter in duration than the murmur of MS. The presystolic component of the TS murmur has a scratchy quality and a crescendo-decrescendo configuration that diminishes before S1. The diastolic murmur and OS of TS are both augmented by maneuvers that increase transtricuspid valve flow, including inspiration, the Mueller maneuver, assumption of the right lateral decubitus position, leg raising, inhalation of amyl nitrite, squatting, and isotonic exercise. They are reduced during expiration or the strain of the Valsalva maneuver and return to control levels immediately (i.e., within two to three beats) after Valsalva release.

ECHOCARDIOGRAPHY (see also Chap. 14). The echocardiographic changes of the tricuspid valve in TS resemble those observed in the mitral valve in MS. Two-dimensional echocardiography characteristically shows diastolic doming of the leaflets (especially the anterior tricuspid valve leaflet), thickening and restricted motion of the other leaflets, reduced separation of the tips of the leaflets, and a reduction in diameter of the tricuspid orifice. Transesophageal echocardiography allows added delineation of the details of valve structure. Doppler echocardiography shows a prolonged slope of antegrade flow and compares well with cardiac catheterization in the quantification of TS and in the assessment of associated TR.[242] Doppler evaluation of TS has largely replaced the need for catheterization to assess severity.[241]

OTHER DIAGNOSTIC EVALUATION

ELECTROCARDIOGRAM. In the absence of AF in a patient with valvular heart disease, TS is suggested by the presence of ECG evidence of right atrial enlargement (see Chap. 12). The P wave amplitude in leads II and V1 exceeds 0.25 mV. Because most patients with TS have mitral valvular disease, the ECG signs of biatrial enlargement are commonly found. The amplitude of the QRS complex in lead V1 may be reduced by the dilated right atrium.

RADIOLOGICAL AND ANGIOGRAPHIC FINDINGS. The key radiological finding is marked cardiomegaly with conspicuous enlargement of the right atrium (i.e., prominence of the right heart border), which extends into a dilated superior vena cava and azygos vein, but without conspicuous dilation of the pulmonary artery. The vascular changes in the lungs characteristic of mitral valvular disease may be masked, with little or no interstitial edema or vascular redistribution, but left atrial enlargement may be present.

Angiography following injection of contrast material into the right atrium and filming in the 30-degree right anterior oblique projection characteristically shows thickening and decreased mobility of the leaflets, a diastolic jet through

the constricted orifice, and thickening of the normal atrial wall.

MANAGEMENT

Although the fundamental approach to the management of severe TS is surgical treatment, intensive sodium restriction and diuretic therapy may diminish the symptoms secondary to the accumulation of excess salt and water. A preparatory period of diuresis may diminish hepatic congestion and thereby improve hepatic function sufficiently to diminish the risks of subsequent operation.

Most patients with TS have coexisting valvular disease that requires surgery. In patients with combined TS and MS, the former must not be corrected alone because pulmonary congestion or edema may ensue. Surgical treatment of TS should be carried out at the time of MV repair or replacement in patients with TS in whom the mean diastolic pressure gradient exceeds 5 mm Hg and the tricuspid orifice is less than approximately 2.0 cm². The final decision concerning surgical treatment is often made at the operating table.

Because TS is almost always accompanied by some TR, simple finger fracture valvotomy may not result in significant hemodynamic improvement but may merely substitute severe TR for TS. However, open valvotomy in which the stenotic tricuspid valve is converted into a functionally bicuspid valve may result in substantial improvement. The commissures between the anterior and septal leaflets and between the posterior and septal leaflets are opened. It is not advisable to open the commissure between the anterior and posterior leaflets for fear of producing severe TR. If open valvotomy does not restore reasonably normal valve function, the tricuspid valve may have to be replaced.[243] A large bioprosthesis is preferred to a mechanical prosthesis in the tricuspid position because of the high risk of thrombosis of the latter and the longer durability of bioprostheses in the tricuspid than in the mitral or aortic positions. The feasibility of tricuspid balloon valvuloplasty has been demonstrated, and this procedure may be combined with mitral balloon valvuloplasty.

Tricuspid Regurgitation

Etiology and Pathology (Table 62-12)

The most common cause of TR is not intrinsic involvement of the valve itself (i.e., primary TR) but rather dilation of the right ventricle and of the tricuspid annulus causing secondary (functional) TR. This may be a complication of RV failure of any cause. It is observed in patients with RV hypertension secondary to any form of cardiac or pulmonary vascular disease, most commonly mitral valve disease.[237] In general, a RV systolic pressure greater than 55 mm Hg will cause functional TR.[1] TR can also occur secondary to RV infarction,[237] congenital heart disease (see Chap. 61) (e.g., pulmonic stenosis and pulmonary hypertension secondary to Eisenmenger syndrome), primary pulmonary hypertension (see Chap. 73), and, rarely, cor pulmonale. In infants, TR may complicate RV failure secondary to neonatal pulmonary diseases and pulmonary hypertension with persistence of the fetal pulmonary circulation. In all of these cases, TR reflects the presence of, and in turn aggravates, severe RV failure. Functional TR may diminish or disappear as the right ventricle decreases in size with the treatment of heart failure. TR can also occur as a consequence of dilation of the annulus in the Marfan syndrome, in which RV dilation secondary to pulmonary hypertension is not present.

A variety of disease processes can affect the tricuspid valve apparatus directly and lead to regurgitation (primary TR). Thus organic TR may occur on a congenital basis (see Chap. 61), as part of Ebstein anomaly, in the atrioventricular canal, and when the tricuspid valve is involved in the formation of an aneurysm of the ventricular septum, or in corrected transposition of the great arteries, or it may occur as an isolated congenital lesion. Rheumatic fever may involve the tricuspid valve directly.[241] When this occurs, it usually causes scarring of the valve leaflets and/or chordae tendineae, leading to limited leaflet mobility and either iso-

TABLE 62–12	Causes and Mechanisms of Pure Tricuspid Regurgitation

CAUSES
Anatomically ABNORMAL valve
  Rheumatic
  Nonrheumatic
    Infective endocarditis
    Ebstein anomaly
    Floppy (prolapse)
    Congenital (non-Ebstein)
    Carcinoid
    Papillary muscle dysfunction
    Trauma
    Connective tissue disorders (Marfan)
    Rheumatoid arthritis
    Radiation injury
Anatomically NORMAL valve (functional)
  Elevated right ventricular systolic pressure (dilated annulus)

MECHANISMS

Condition	Leaflet Area	Annular Circumference	Leaflet Insertion
Floppy	↑	↑	Normal
Ebstein anomaly	↑	↑	Abnormal
Pulmonary/right ventricular systolic hypertension	Normal	↑	Normal
Papillary muscle dysfunction	Normal	Normal	Normal
Carcinoid	↓/Normal	Normal	Normal
Rheumatic	↓/Normal	Normal	Normal
Infective endocarditis	↓/Normal	Normal	Normal

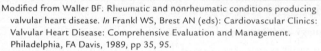

Modified from Waller BF. Rheumatic and nonrheumatic conditions producing valvular heart disease. In Frankl WS, Brest AN (eds): Cardiovascular Clinics: Valvular Heart Disease: Comprehensive Evaluation and Management. Philadelphia, FA Davis, 1989, pp 35, 95.

lated TR or a combination of TR and TS. Rheumatic involvement of the mitral, and often aortic, valves coexist.

TR or the combination of TR and TS is an important feature of the carcinoid syndrome (Fig. 62-40; see also Fig. 14-50), which leads to focal or diffuse deposits of fibrous tissue on the endocardium of the valvular cusps and cardiac chambers and on the intima of the great veins and coronary sinus[238,244] (see Chap. 64). The white, fibrous carcinoid plaques are most extensive on the right side of the heart, where they are usually deposited on the ventricular surfaces of the tricuspid valve and cause the cusps to adhere to the underlying RV wall, thereby producing TR. Endomyocardial fibrosis with shortening of the tricuspid leaflets and chordae tendineae is an important cause of TR in tropical Africa (see Chap. 64). TR may result from prolapse of the tricuspid valve caused by myxomatous changes in the valve and chordae tendineae (Fig. 62-41); prolapse of the mitral valve is usually present in these patients as well.[237] Prolapse of the tricuspid valve occurs in about 20 percent of all patients with MVP. Tricuspid valve prolapse may also be associated with atrial septal defect. Other causes of TR include penetrating and nonpenetrating trauma, dilated cardiomyopathy, infective endocarditis (particularly staphylococcal endocarditis in narcotics addicts), and following surgical excision of the tricuspid valve in patients with infective endocarditis that is unresponsive to medical management. Less common causes of TR include cardiac tumors (particularly right atrial myxoma), transvenous pacemaker leads, repeated endomyocardial biopsy in a transplanted heart, endomyocardial fibrosis, methysergide-induced valvular disease, exposure to fenfluramine-phentermine, and systemic lupus erythematosus involving the tricuspid valve.

Clinical Presentation

SYMPTOMS. In the absence of pulmonary hypertension, TR is generally well tolerated. However, when pulmonary hypertension and TR coexist, cardiac output declines, and the manifestations of right-sided heart failure become intensified. Thus the symptoms of TR result from a reduced cardiac output and from ascites, painful congestive hepatomegaly, and massive edema. Occasionally, patients have throbbing pulsations in the neck, which intensify on effort and are due to jugular venous distention; and systolic pulsations of the eyeballs have also been described. In the many patients with TR who have mitral valve disease, the symptoms of the latter usually predominate. Symptoms of pulmonary congestion may abate as TR develops, but they are replaced by weakness, fatigue, and other manifestations of a depressed cardiac output.

PHYSICAL EXAMINATION. Evidence of weight loss and cachexia, cyanosis, and jaundice are often present on inspection in patients with severe TR. AF is common. There is jugular venous distention,[237] the normal x and x' descents disappear, and a prominent systolic wave, i.e., a *c-v* wave (or *s* wave), is apparent. The descent of this wave, the y descent, is sharp and becomes the most prominent feature of the venous pulse (unless there is coexisting TS, in which case it is slowed). A venous systolic thrill and murmur in the neck may be present in patients with severe TR. The RV impulse is hyperdynamic and thrusting in quality. Systolic pulsations of an enlarged, tender liver are commonly present initially. However, in patients with chronic TR and congestive cirrhosis, the liver may become firm and nontender.[245] Ascites and edema are frequent.

Auscultation usually reveals an S3 originating from the right ventricle, which is accentuated by inspiration. When TR is associated with and secondary to pulmonary hypertension, P2 is accentuated as well. When TR occurs in the presence of pulmonary hypertension, the systolic murmur is usually high-pitched, pansystolic, and loudest in the 4th intercostal space in the parasternal region but occasionally is loudest in the subxiphoid area. When TR is mild, the murmur may be short. When TR occurs in the absence of pulmonary hypertension (e.g., in infective endocarditis or following trauma), the murmur is usually of low intensity and limited to the first half of systole. When the right ventricle is greatly dilated and occupies the anterior surface of the heart, the murmur may be prominent at the apex and difficult to distinguish from that produced by MR.

The response of the systolic murmur to respiration and other maneuvers is of considerable aid in establishing the diagnosis of TR. The murmur is characteristically augmented during inspiration (Carvallo sign). However, when the failing ventricle can no longer increase its stroke volume in the recumbent or sitting positions, the inspiratory augmentation may be elicited by standing. The murmur also increases during the Mueller maneuver (forced inspiration against a closed glottis), exercise, leg-raising, and hepatic compression. It demonstrates an immediate overshoot after release of the Valsalva strain but is reduced in intensity and duration in the standing position and during the strain of the Valsalva maneuver. Increased atrioventricular flow across the tricuspid orifice in diastole may cause a short early diastolic flow rumble in the left parasternal region following S3. Tricuspid valve prolapse, like MVP, causes nonejection systolic clicks and late systolic murmurs. However, in tricuspid valve prolapse, these findings are more prominent at the lower left sternal border. With inspiration, the clicks occur later, and the murmurs intensify and become shorter in duration.

ECHOCARDIOGRAPHY (see Fig. 14-62). The goal of echocardiography is to detect TR, estimate its severity, and assess pulmonary arterial pressure and RV function.[242] In patients with TR secondary to dilation of the tricuspid annulus, the right atrium, right ventricle, and tricuspid annulus are all usually greatly dilated on echocardiography. There is evidence of RV diastolic overload with paradoxical motion of the ventricular septum similar to that observed in atrial septal defect. Exaggerated motion and delayed closure of the tricuspid valve are evident in patients with Ebstein anomaly (see Fig. 14-112). Prolapse of the tricuspid valve due to myxomatous degeneration may be evident on echocardiography.[237] Echocardiographic indications of tricuspid valve abnormalities, especially TR by Doppler examination (see Fig. 62-40), can be detected in the majority of patients with carcinoid heart disease. In patients with TR due to endocarditis, echocardiography may reveal vegetations on the valve or a flail valve. Transesophageal echocardiography enhances detection of TR.

Doppler echocardiography is a sensitive technique for visualizing the TR jet. The magnitude of TR can be quantified using techniques similar to those used to evaluation MR (Fig. 62-42).[241,246] Contrast echocardiography also improves detection of TR and can trace regurgitant microbubbles into the inferior vena cava and hepatic veins.[241,246]

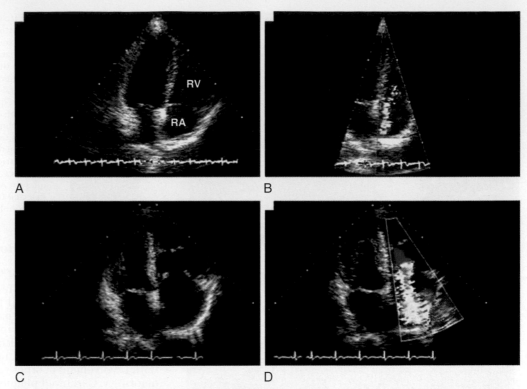

FIGURE 62–40 Tricuspid regurgitation (TR) caused by carcinoid involvement of the tricuspid valve. Serial two-dimensional echocardiograms (**A** and **C**) and color Doppler studies (**B** and **D**), separated by 3 years are shown. After 3 years, there is severe thickening and fixation of the tricuspid leaflets (**C**), leading to severe TR and associated right ventricular (RV) and right atrial (RA) enlargement. *(From Møller JE, Connolly HM, Rubin J, et al: Factors associated with progression of carcinoid heart disease. N Engl J Med 348:1005, 2003.)*

OTHER DIAGNOSTIC EVALUATION

ELECTROCARDIOGRAM. The ECG is usually nonspecific and characteristic of the lesion causing TR. Incomplete right bundle branch block, Q waves in lead V1, and AF are commonly found.

RADIOLOGICAL FINDINGS. In patients with functional TR, marked cardiomegaly is usually evident, and the right atrium is prominent. Evidence of elevated right atrial pressure may include distention of the azygos vein and the presence of a pleural effusion. Ascites with upward displacement of the diaphragm may be present. Systolic pulsations of the right atrium may be present on fluoroscopy.

HEMODYNAMIC FINDINGS. The right atrial and RV end-diastolic pressures are often elevated in TR, whether the condition is due to organic disease of the tricuspid valve or is secondary to RV systolic overload. The right atrial pressure tracing usually reveals absence of the x descent and a prominent *v* or *c-v* wave ("ventricularization" of the atrial pressure). Absence of these findings essentially excludes moderate or severe TR. As the severity of TR increases, the contour of the right atrial pressure pulse increasingly resembles that of the RV pressure pulse. A rise or no change in right atrial pressure on deep inspiration, rather than the usual fall, is a characteristic finding. Determination of the pulmonary arterial (or RV) systolic pressure may be helpful in deciding whether the TR is primary (i.e., due to disease of the valve or its supporting structures) or functional (i.e., secondary to RV dilation). A pulmonary arterial or RV systolic pressure less than 40 mm Hg favors a primary cause, whereas a pressure greater than 55 mm Hg suggests that TR is secondary.

MANAGEMENT

TR in the absence of pulmonary hypertension usually is well tolerated and may not require surgical treatment. Indeed, both human patients

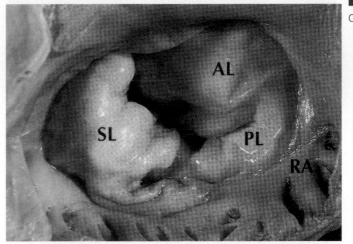

FIGURE 62–41 Tricuspid valve prolapse, viewed from the right atrium (RA). AL = anterior leaflet; PL = posterior leaflet; SL = septal leaflet. *(From Virmani R, Burke AP, Farb A: Pathology of valvular heart disease. In Rahimtoola SH [ed]: Valvular Heart Disease. In Braunwald E [series ed]: Atlas of Heart Diseases. vol 11. Philadelphia, Current Medicine, 1997, p 1.17.)*

and experimental animals with normal pulmonary arterial pressure may tolerate total excision of the tricuspid valve as long as RV systolic pressure is normal. Dilation of the right side of the heart usually occurs months or years after tricuspid valvectomy (usually carried out for acute infective endocarditis).

Surgical treatment of acquired regurgitation secondary to annular dilation was greatly improved with development of annuloplasty techniques, with or without an annuloplasty ring. At the time of mitral valve surgery in patients with TR secondary to pulmonary hypertension, the severity of the regurgitation should be assessed by palpation of the tricuspid valve. In addition, it should be determined whether the TR is secondary to pulmonary hypertension, in which case the

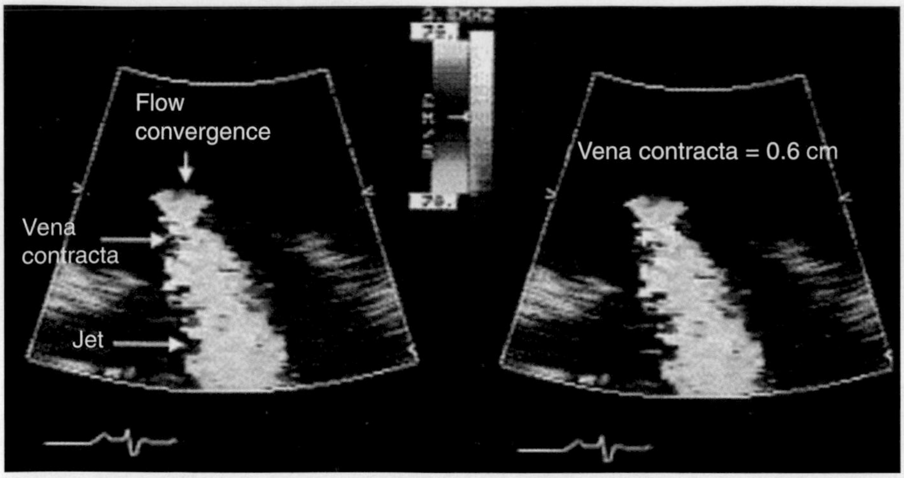

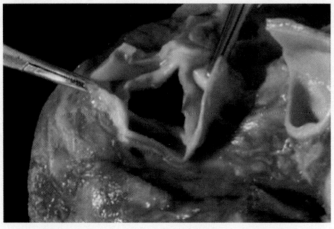

FIGURE 62–42 Tricuspid regurgitation flow visualized by color-flow Doppler echocardiography in the apical view. This defines the three components of regurgitant flow **(left)** and measurement of the width of the vena contracta **(right)**. *(From Tribouilloy CM, Enriquez-Sarano M, Bailey KR, et al: Quantification of tricuspid regurgitation by measuring the width of the vena contracta with Doppler color flow imaging: A clinical study. J Am Coll Cardiol 36:472, 2000.)*

FIGURE 62–43 Carcinoid heart disease. The pulmonary valve is viewed from above. *(From Kulke MH, Mayer RJ: Carcinoid tumors. N Engl J Med 340:858, 1999. Courtesy of James R. Stone, MD, PhD, Department of Pathology, Brigham and Women's Hospital, Boston.)*

valve is normal, or whether it is secondary to other disease processes. Patients with mild TR without annular dilation usually do not require surgical treatment;[237] pulmonary vascular pressures decline following successful mitral valve surgery, and the mild TR tends to disappear. However, even mild TR should be repaired if there is dilation of the tricuspid annulus, as the TR is likely to progress in severity if left untreated.[1,247,248] Excellent results have been reported in patients with mild to moderate TR with the use of suture annuloplasty of the posterior (unsupported) portion of the annulus. Patients with severe TR, with or without annular dilation, require valvotomy and ring annuloplasty. A surgical mortality rate of 13.9 percent has been reported (see Table 62-3).[249] Residual TR after tricuspid annuloplasty is determined principally by the degree of preoperative tricuspid leaflet tethering.[250] If these procedures do not provide a good functional result at the operating table (as assessed by transesophageal echocardiography), valve replacement using a large bioprosthesis may be required.

When organic disease of the tricuspid valve (Ebstein anomaly or carcinoid heart disease) causes TR severe enough to require surgery, valve replacement is usually needed. The risk of thrombosis of mechanical prostheses is greater in the tricuspid than in the mitral or aortic positions, presumably because pressure and flow rates are lower in the right side of the heart. For this reason, the artificial valve of choice for the tricuspid position in adults is a bioprosthesis. Anticoagulants are not required, and a graft durability of more than 10 years has been established.

In treating the difficult problem of tricuspid endocarditis in IV drug users (see Chap. 68), total excision of the tricuspid valve without immediate replacement can generally be tolerated by these patients, who usually do not have associated pulmonary hypertension. When antibiotic therapy is unsuccessful, valve replacement frequently results in reinfection or continued infection. Therefore diseased valvular tissue should be excised to eradicate the endocarditis, and antibiotic treatment can then be continued. Initially, most patients tolerate loss of the tricuspid valve without great difficulty. However, RV dysfunction usually occurs subsequently. A bioprosthetic valve may therefore be inserted 6 to 9 months after valve excision and control of the infection.

Pulmonic Valve Disease

Etiology and Pathology

PULMONIC STENOSIS. The congenital form is the most common cause of pulmonic stenosis (PS).[241] Manifestations in children and adults are discussed in Chapter 61. Rheumatic inflammation of the pulmonic valve is very uncommon, is usually associated with involvement of other valves, and rarely leads to serious deformity. Carcinoid plaques, similar to those involving the tricuspid valve, are often present in the outflow tract of the right ventricle of patients with malignant carcinoid. The plaques result in constriction of the pulmonic valve ring, retraction and fusion of the valve cusps, and either PS or the combination of PS and pulmonic regurgitation (Fig. 62-43).[238,244] Obstruction in the region of the pulmonic valve may be extrinsic to the valve apparatus and may be produced by cardiac tumors or by aneurysm of the sinus of Valsalva. Management of congenital PS focuses on balloon dilation (see Chaps. 55 and 61)

PULMONIC REGURGITATION. By far the most common cause of pulmonic regurgitation (PR) is dilation of the valve ring secondary to pulmonary hypertension (of any etiology) or to dilation of the pulmonary artery, either idiopathic or consequent to a connective tissue disorder such as the Marfan syndrome. The second most common cause of PR is infective endocarditis. Less frequently, PR is iatrogenic and is induced at the time of surgical treatment of congenital PS or tetralogy of Fallot (Fig. 62-44).[251,252] PR may also result from various lesions that directly affect the pulmonic valve. These include congenital malformations, such as absent, malformed, fenestrated, or supernumerary leaflets. These anomalies may occur as isolated lesions but more often are associated with other congenital anomalies, particularly tetralogy of Fallot, ventricular septal defect, and pulmonic valvular stenosis. Less common causes include trauma, carcinoid syndrome,[238] rheumatic involvement, injury produced by a pulmonary artery flow-directed catheter, syphilis, and chest trauma.

Clinical Presentation

Like TR, isolated PR causes RV volume overload and may be tolerated for many years without difficulty unless it complicates, or is complicated by, pulmonary hypertension. In this case, PR is usually accompanied by and aggravates RV failure. Patients with PR caused by infective endocarditis who develop septic pulmonary emboli and pulmonary hypertension often exhibit severe RV failure. In most patients, the clinical manifestations of the primary disease are severe and usually overshadow the PR, which often results only in incidental auscultatory findings.

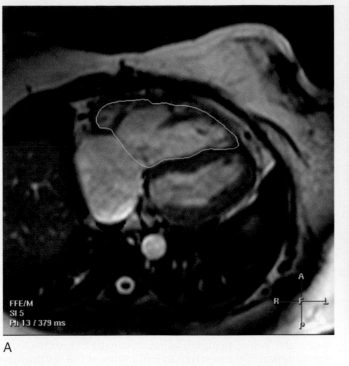

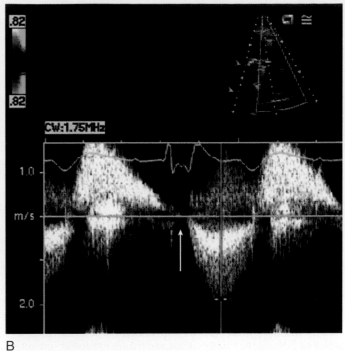

A

B

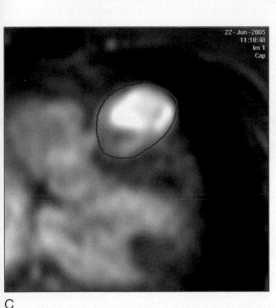

C

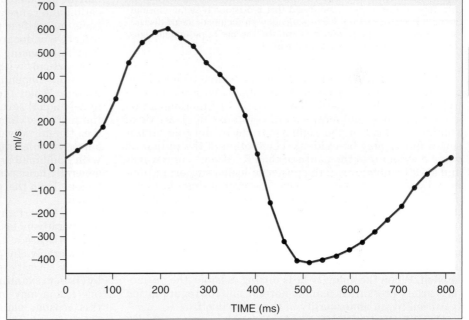

D

FIGURE 62–44 Cardiac magnetic resonance (CMR) and Doppler echocardiographic evaluation in a 40-year-old woman who underwent repair of tetralogy of Fallot as a child. She is asymptomatic but has significant right ventricular (RV) enlargement on echocardiography. **A,** RV dilation is confirmed in the CMR images, with a calculated RV end-diastolic volume of 444 ml. **B,** The Doppler tracing shows a dense signal in diastole with a steep deceleration slope that reaches the baseline before the end of diastole (arrow). **C,** Interrogation of pulmonary artery flow in the CMR phase-velocity images is performed by drawing a region of interest (red) around the pulmonary artery. **D,** Graph of the pulmonary artery flow within the region of interest indicated demonstrates both antegrade and retrograde flow. The total RV stroke volume was 245 ml with antegrade flow of 98 ml, yielding a regurgitant fraction of 67 percent.

PHYSICAL EXAMINATION. The right ventricle is hyperdynamic and produces palpable systolic pulsations in the left parasternal area, and an enlarged pulmonary artery often produces systolic pulsations in the 2nd left intercostal space. Sometimes systolic and diastolic thrills are felt in the same area. A tap reflecting pulmonic valve closure is usually easily palpable in the 2nd intercostal space in patients with pulmonary hypertension and secondary PR.

AUSCULTATION. P2 is not audible in patients with congenital absence of the pulmonic valve; however, this sound is accentuated in patients with PR secondary to pulmonary hypertension. There may be wide splitting of S2 caused by prolongation of RV ejection accompanying the augmented RV stroke volume. A nonvalvular systolic ejection click due to the sudden expansion of the pulmonary artery by the augmented RV stroke volume frequently initiates a midsystolic ejection murmur, most prominent in the 2nd left intercostal space. An S3 and S4 originating from the right ventricle are often audible, most readily in the 4th intercostal space at the left parasternal area, and are augmented by inspiration.

In the absence of pulmonary hypertension, the diastolic murmur of PR is low pitched and usually heard best at the 3rd and 4th left intercostal spaces adjacent to the sternum. The murmur commences when pressures in the pulmonary artery and right ventricle diverge, approximately 0.04 second after P2. It is diamond-shaped in configuration and brief, reaching a peak intensity when the gradient between these pressures is maximal and ending with equilibration of the pressures. The murmur becomes louder during inspiration.

The Graham Steell Murmur

When systolic pulmonary arterial pressure exceeds approximately 55 mm Hg, dilatation of the pulmonic annulus results in a high-velocity regurgitant jet that is responsible for the Graham Steell murmur of PR. (Doppler ultrasonography reveals pulmonary regurgitation at much lower pulmonary arterial pressures.) The Graham Steell murmur is a high-pitched, blowing, decrescendo murmur beginning immediately after P2 and is most prominent in the left parasternal region in the 2nd to 4th intercostal spaces. Thus although it resembles the murmur of AR, it is usually accompanied by severe pulmonary hypertension, i.e., an accentuated P2 or fused S2, an ejection sound, and a systolic murmur of TR, and not by a widened arterial pulse pressure. Sometimes a low-frequency presystolic murmur is present, i.e., a right-sided Austin Flint murmur originating from the tricuspid valve.

The Graham Steell murmur of PR secondary to pulmonary hypertension usually increases in intensity with inspiration, exhibits little change after amyl nitrite inhalation or vasopressor administration, is diminished during the Valsalva strain, and returns to baseline intensity almost immediately after release of the Valsalva strain. This murmur resembles and may be confused with the diastolic blowing murmur of AR. However, it is well established that a diastolic blowing murmur along the left sternal border in patients with rheumatic heart disease and pulmonary hypertension (even in the absence of peripheral signs of AR) is usually due to AR rather than PR.

ECHOCARDIOGRAPHY. Two-dimensional echocardiography shows RV dilation and, in patients with pulmonary hypertension, RV hypertrophy as well. RV function can be evaluated. Abnormal motion of the septum characteristic of volume overload of the right ventricle in diastole and/or septal flutter may be evident. The motion of the pulmonic valve may point to the cause of the PR. Absence of *a* waves and systolic notching of the posterior leaflet suggest pulmonary hypertension; large *a* waves indicate pulmonic stenosis. Doppler echocardiography is extremely accurate in detecting PR and in helping to estimate its severity (see Fig. 62-44; see also Fig. 14-63). Abnormal Doppler signals in the RV outflow tract with velocity sustained throughout diastole are generally observed in patients in whom PR is caused by dilation of the valve ring secondary to pulmonary hypertension. When the velocity falls during diastole, the pulmonary artery pressure is usually normal, and the regurgitation is caused by an abnormality of the valve itself.

OTHER DIAGNOSTIC EVALUATION

ELECTROCARDIOGRAM. In the absence of pulmonary hypertension, PR often results in an ECG that reflects RV diastolic overload, i.e., an rSr (or rsR) configuration in the right precordial leads. PR secondary to pulmonary hypertension is usually associated with ECG evidence of RV hypertrophy.

RADIOLOGICAL AND ANGIOGRAPHIC FINDINGS. Both the pulmonary artery and the right ventricle are usually enlarged, but these signs are nonspecific. Fluoroscopy may demonstrate pronounced pulsation of the main pulmonary artery. PR can be diagnosed by observing opacification of the right ventricle following injection of contrast material into the main pulmonary artery, but this diagnosis is made in virtually all patients with echocardiography or cardiac magnetic resonance.

CARDIAC MAGNETIC RESONANCE. CMR plays an important role in assessing pulmonary artery dilation, imaging the regurgitant jet and quantifying PR severity (see Fig. 62-44 and also Fig. 17-12A). CMR also is useful in evaluating RV dilation and systolic function.[252,253]

MANAGEMENT

PR alone is seldom severe enough to require specific treatment. Treatment of the primary condition, such as infective endocarditis, or the lesion responsible for the pulmonary hypertension, such as surgery for mitral valvular disease, often ameliorates the PR. Surgical treatment directed specifically at the pulmonic valve, such as patients with severe PR caused by surgical correction of tetralogy of Fallot,[251,253] is required only occasionally because of intractable right heart failure. Under such circumstances, valve replacement may be carried out, preferably with a porcine bioprosthesis or a pulmonary allograft.[254] There is growing experience with catheter-based approaches to pulmonic valve replacement in native pulmonic valve disease and in PR following surgical correction of congenital heart defects.[70,255,256]

Multivalvular Disease

Multivalvular involvement is caused frequently by rheumatic fever, and various clinical and hemodynamic syndromes can be produced by different combinations of valvular abnormalities. Myxomatous MR and associate pulmonary hypertension is a leading cause of concomitant TR, often with dilation of the tricuspid annulus. The Marfan syndrome and other connective tissue disorders may cause multivalve prolapse and dilation, resulting in multivalvular regurgitation. Degenerative calcification of the aortic valve may be associated with degenerative mitral annular calcification and cause AS and MR. Different pathological conditions may affect two valves in the same patient, such as infective endocarditis on the aortic valve causing AR and ischemia causing MR.

In patients with multivalvular disease, the clinical manifestations depend on the relative severities of each of the lesions. When the valvular abnormalities are of approximately equal severity, clinical manifestations produced by the more proximal (upstream) of the two valvular lesions (i.e., the mitral valve in patients with combined mitral and aortic valvular disease and the tricuspid valve in patients with combined tricuspid and mitral valvular disease) are generally more prominent than those produced by the distal lesion. Thus the proximal lesion tends to mask the distal lesion.

It is important to recognize multivalvular involvement preoperatively because failure to correct all significant valvular disease at the time of operation increases mortality considerably. In patients with multivalvular disease, the relative severity of each lesion may be difficult to estimate by clinical examination and noninvasive techniques because one lesion may mask the manifestations of the other. For this reason, patients suspected of having multivalvular involvement and who are being considered for surgical treatment should undergo careful clinical evaluation and both full Doppler echocardiographic evaluation and right- and left-cardiac catheterization and angiography. If there is any question concerning the presence of significant AS in patients undergoing mitral valve surgery, the aortic valve should be inspected because overlooking this condition can lead to a high perioperative mortality. Similarly, it is useful to palpate the tricuspid valve at the time of mitral valve surgery.

MITRAL STENOSIS AND AORTIC REGURGITATION. Approximately two-thirds of patients with severe MS have an early blowing diastolic murmur along the left sternal border with a normal pulse pressure. In about 90 percent of these patients, the murmur is due to mild or moderate AR that is usually of little clinical importance. However, approximately 10 percent of patients with MS have severe rheumatic AR,[257] which can generally be recognized by the usual clinical and laboratory signs of AR.

In keeping with the general observation that a proximal lesion may mask a distal lesion, significant AR may be missed in patients with severe MS. The widened pulse pressure, in particular, may be absent. On the other hand, MS may be missed or, conversely, may be falsely diagnosed on clinical examination of patients with obvious AR. An accentuated S1 and an opening snap in a patient with AR should suggest the possibility of mitral valvular disease. However, an Austin Flint murmur is often inappropriately considered to be the diastolic rumbling murmur of MS. These two murmurs may be distinguished at the bedside by means of amyl nitrite inhalation, which diminishes the Austin Flint murmur but augments the murmur of MS; isometric handgrip and squatting augment both the diastolic murmur of AR and the Austin Flint murmur. Echocardiography, particularly pulsed Doppler echocardiography, is of decisive value in detecting MS and MR.

Since double-valve replacement is associated with increased short-term and long-term risk,[258] balloon mitral valvotomy can be the first procedure. If this causes LV dilation, AVR can follow. Alternatively, open mitral valvotomy and AVR can be performed at the same time.[1,258]

MITRAL STENOSIS AND AORTIC STENOSIS. The left ventricle of a patient with these two lesions is usually small, stiff, and hypertrophied. When severe MS and AS coexist, the former masks many of the manifestations of the latter.[257] The cardiac output tends to be reduced more than in patients with isolated AS. The reduced cardiac output lowers both the transaortic valvular pressure gradient and the LV systolic pressure, diminishes the incidence of angina pectoris, and retards the development of aortic valvular calcification and LV hypertrophy. On the other hand, clinical manifestations associated with MS, such as pulmonary congestion and hemoptysis, AF, and systemic embolization, occur more frequently in patients with coexisting MS and AS than in those with isolated AS.

On physical examination, an S4 (which is common in patients with pure AS) is usually not present. The midsystolic murmur characteristic of AS may be reduced in intensity and duration because the stroke volume is reduced by the MS. The ECG may fail to demonstrate LV hypertrophy, but left atrial enlargement is common. The chest roentgenogram is usually typical of MS except that calcium may be present in the region of the aortic valve, and LV enlargement may occur (see Fig. 15-8). The two-dimensional and Doppler echocardiograms are of the greatest value because stenosis of both valves may be evident. However, the low cardiac output characteristic of the combined lesions may reduce the transvalvular pressure gradients estimated by Doppler echocardiography.

It is vital to recognize the presence of hemodynamically significant aortic valvular disease (i.e., AS and/or AR) preoperatively in patients who are to undergo mitral valvotomy. This procedure may be hazardous because it can impose a sudden hemodynamic load on the left ventricle that had previously been protected by the MS and may lead to acute pulmonary edema. Balloon mitral valvotomy and AVR may be the treatment of choice.

AORTIC STENOSIS AND MITRAL REGURGITATION. This combination of lesions is usually caused by rheumatic heart disease, although AS may be congenital and MR may be due to MVP. The combination of severe AS and MR is a hazardous one, but fortunately it is relatively uncommon. Obstruction to LV outflow augments the volume of MR flow, whereas the presence of MR diminishes the ventricular preload necessary for maintenance of the LV stroke volume in patients with AS.[257] The result is a reduced forward cardiac output and marked left atrial and pulmonary venous hypertension. The development of AF (due to left atrial enlargement) has an adverse hemodynamic effect in the presence of AS. The physical findings may be confusing because it may be difficult to recognize two distinct systolic murmurs. On echocardiography and roentgenography, the left atrium and ventricle are usually larger than in isolated AS. In patients with severe AS and MR, both valves must usually be treated surgically by AVR and, if possible, by MV repair.[258]

AORTIC REGURGITATION AND MITRAL REGURGITATION. This relatively frequent combination of lesions[257] may be caused by rheumatic heart disease, by prolapse of both the aortic and the mitral valves due to myxomatous degeneration, or by dilation of both annuli in patients with connective tissue disorders. The left ventricle is usually greatly dilated. The clinical features of AR usually predominate, and it is sometimes difficult to determine whether the MR is due to organic involvement of this valve or to dilation of the mitral valve ring secondary to LV enlargement. When both valvular leaks are severe, this combination of lesions is poorly tolerated. The normal mitral valve ordinarily serves as a "backup" to the aortic valve, and premature (diastolic) closure of the mitral valve limits the volume of reflux that occurs in patients with acute AR. With severe combined regurgitant lesions, regardless of the cause of the mitral lesion, blood may reflux from the aorta through both chambers of the left side of the heart into the pulmonary veins. Physical and laboratory examinations usually show evidence of both lesions. An S3 and a brisk arterial pulse are frequently present. The relative severity of each lesion can be assessed best by Doppler echocardiography and contrast angiography. This combination of lesions leads to severe LV dilation.

MR that occurs in patients with AR secondary to LV dilation often regresses following AVR alone. If severe, the MR may be corrected by annuloplasty at the time of AVR.[258] An intrinsically normal mitral valve that is regurgitant because of a dilated annulus should not be replaced.

SURGICAL TREATMENT OF MULTIVALVULAR DISEASE

Combined AVR and MV replacement is usually associated with a higher risk and poorer survival than is replacement of either of the valves alone.[260] The operative risk of double-valve replacement is about 70 percent higher than it is for single-valve replacement. The STS National Database Committee reported an overall operative mortality rate of 9.6 percent for multiple (usually double) valve replacement in 3840 patients, compared with 4.3 and 6.4 percent for isolated AVR and MV replacement, respectively[261] (see Table 62-3). The long-term survival depends strongly on the preoperative functional status. Patients operated on for combined AR and MR have poorer outcomes than patients receiving double-valve replacement for any of the other combinations of lesions, presumably because both AR and MR may produce irreversible LV damage. MV repair or balloon valvotomy in combination with AVR is preferable to double-valve replacement and should be carried out whenever possible.[249,259] Risk factors that reduce long-term survival after double-valve replacement include advanced age, higher NYHA class, lower LV ejection fraction, greater LV enlargement, and accompanying ischemic heart disease requiring coronary artery bypass grafting.

Given the higher risks, a higher threshold is required for multivalvular versus single-valve surgery. Thus patients are generally advised not to undergo multivalvular surgery until they reach late NYHA Class II or Class III, unless there is evidence of declining LV function. Despite a detailed noninvasive and invasive workup, the decision to treat more than one valve is often made by palpation or by direct inspection at the operating table.

TRIPLE-VALVE DISEASE

Hemodynamically significant disease involving the mitral, aortic, and tricuspid valves is uncommon. Patients with trivalvular disease may present in advanced heart failure with marked cardiomegaly, and surgical correction of all three valvular lesions is imperative. However, triple-valve replacement is a long and complex operation. Early in the experience with this procedure, the mortality rate was 20 percent for patients in NYHA Class III and 40 percent for patients in Class IV. More

CH 62

Valvular Heart Disease

recently, the mortality rate has declined, but, nevertheless, triple-valve replacement should be avoided if possible. In many patients with trivalvular disease, it is possible to replace the aortic valve, repair the mitral valve, and perform a tricuspid annuloplasty or valvuloplasty.

Patients who survive triple-valve replacement surgery usually show substantial clinical improvement during the early postoperative period, and postoperative catheterization studies show marked reductions in pulmonary arterial and capillary pressures. However, some patients die of arrhythmias or congestive heart failure in the late postoperative period despite three normally functioning prostheses. The cause of cardiac failure in this situation is not known, but it may be related to intraoperative myocardial ischemia, microemboli from the multiple prostheses, or continued subclinical episodes of rheumatic myocarditis.

When multiple prosthetic valves must be inserted, it is logical to select either two bioprostheses or two mechanical prostheses for the left side of the heart. If the patient is to be exposed to the hazards of anticoagulants for one mechanical prosthesis, it seems unreasonable to add the potential risks of early failure of a bioprosthesis. However, if two mechanical prostheses are selected for the left side of the heart, the use of a bioprosthesis in the tricuspid position is suggested.

PROSTHETIC CARDIAC VALVES

The first successful replacements of cardiac valves in the human were accomplished in 1960 by Nina Braunwald and colleagues, Harken and coworkers, and Starr and Edwards. Two major groups of prosthetic valves are currently available in models designed for both the atrioventricular (mitral and tricuspid) and the aortic positions: mechanical prostheses and bioprostheses (tissue valves). The major differences are related to the risk of thromboembolism (higher with mechanical valves) and the risk of structural deterioration of the prosthesis (higher with bioprostheses).

Mechanical Prostheses (Fig. 62-45)

Mechanical prosthetic valves are classified into three major groups: bileaflet, tilting-disc, and ball-cage. The bileaflet valves are the most commonly implanted mechanical valves because of their low bulk and flat profile and superior hemodynamics. The St. Jude bileaflet valve (see Fig. 62-45D), currently the most widely used prosthesis worldwide, is coated with pyrolytic carbon and has two semicircular discs that pivot between open and closed positions without the need for supporting struts.[262,263] It has favorable flow characteristics and causes a lower transvalvular pressure gradient at any outer diameter and cardiac output than the caged-ball or tilting disc valves.[264] The St. Jude valve appears to have particularly favorable hemodynamic characteristics in the smaller sizes; Therefore it is especially useful in children. Thrombogenicity in the mitral position may be less than that associated with other prosthetic valves.[264] However, as with other mechanical prostheses, lifelong anticoagulation is needed.[1] A variation of the St. Jude valve, the CarboMedics prosthesis (see Fig. 62-45E), is also a bileaflet valve composed of pyrolytic carbon with a titanium housing that can be rotated to avoid interference with disc excursion by subvalvular tissue.[265]

There are two principal tilting disc valves in current use. The Omniscience valve (see Fig. 62-45B), the successor to the Lillehei-Kaster pivoting-disc valve, consists of a titanium valve housing with a polyester knit sewing ring in which a pyrolytic disc is suspended. In the open position, the disc swings to an angle of 80 degrees, providing a large central flow orifice. A closely related valve is the Medtronic-Hall valve (see Fig. 62-45C), which has a Teflon sewing ring and titanium housing; its thin, carbon-coated pivoting disc has a central perforation that allows improved hemodynam-

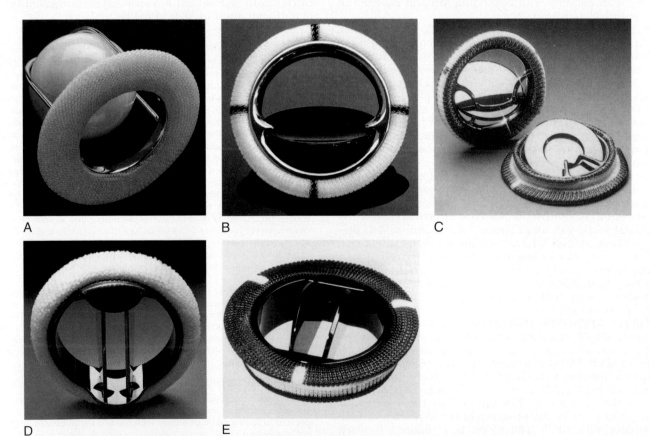

FIGURE 62–45 Mechanical heart valves. **A,** The Starr-Edwards caged-ball valve. **B,** The Omniscience valve. **C,** The Medtronic-Hall valve. **D,** The St. Jude bileaflet valve. **E,** The CarboMedics bileaflet valve. *(From Grunkemeier GL, Rahimtoola SH, Starr A: Prosthetic heart valves. In Rahimtoola SH [ed]: Valvular Heart Disease. In Braunwald E [series ed]: Atlas of Heart Diseases. vol 11. Philadelphia, Current Medicine, 1997, pp 13.4-13.6.)*

ics. Thrombogenicity appears to be quite low[264] (less than one episode per 100 patient-years in the mitral position), and mechanical performance is excellent over the long term. Both the bileaflet and the tilting-disc valves are associated with small (5-10 ml/beat) obligatory (normal) regurgitation. All have distinctive auscultatory features (Fig. 62-46).

The Starr-Edwards caged-ball valve is the oldest prosthetic valve in continuous use (Fig. 62-45A).[262,264,266] The poppet is made of silicone rubber, the cage of Stellite alloy, and the sewing ring of Teflon/polypropylene cloth. A disadvantage is its bulky cage design. Therefore the Starr-Edwards valve is not suitable for the mitral position in patients with a small LV cavity or for the aortic position in those with a small aortic annulus or those requiring a valve-aortic arch composite graft. In a small number of patients, this valve induces hemolysis, which may be greatly exaggerated and become clinically important if a perivalvular leak develops. When they are of small size, the Starr-Edwards valves may cause mild obstruction, and the incidence of thromboembolism is slightly higher than with the tilting-disc valve or bileaflet valve.[1,264,266]

Durability and Thrombogenicity

All mechanical prosthetic valves have an excellent record of durability, up to 40 years for the Starr-Edwards valve and over 25 years for the St. Jude valve.[264] In the mitral position, perivalvular regurgitation appears to occur more frequently with mechanical than with tissue valves.[267] Thrombosis and thromboembolism risks are greater with any mechanical valve in the mitral than in the aortic position, and higher doses of warfarin are generally recommended for mitral prostheses.[1] However, patients with any mechanical prosthesis, regardless of design or site of placement, require long-term anticoagulation and aspirin administration because of the hazard of thromboembolism, which is greatest in the first postoperative year. Without anticoagulants and aspirin, the incidence of thromboembolism is three- to six-fold higher than when proper doses of these medications are administered. Very rarely, thrombosis of the mechanical valve occurs. This may be a fatal event, but when nonfatal, it interferes with prosthetic valve function.

Warfarin should begin about 2 days after operation, and the international normalized ratio (INR) should be in the range of 2.0 to 3.0 for patients with the bileaflet disc and the Medtronic-Hall valve in the aortic position. The INR should be between 2.5 and 3.5 for patients at higher risk for thrombosis (e.g., AF, previous thromboembolism) as well as for patients with other mechanical valves in the aortic position and for all valves in the mitral position (see also Chap. 82).[1] This relatively conservative approach reduces the risk of anticoagulant hemorrhage but does not appear to be associated with a greater frequency of thromboembolism

than an INR of 3.0 to 4.0. Antiplatelet agents without anticoagulants do not provide adequate protection. However, the addition of aspirin, 80 to 150 mg daily, together with warfarin may reduce the risk of thromboembolism and should be given to all patients with prosthetic valves.[1] Although this approach does increase the risk of bleeding slightly,[269,270] there is a favorable risk-to-benefit profile.[269]

Prosthetic valve thrombosis should be suspected by the sudden appearance of dyspnea and muffled sounds or new murmurs on auscultation (see Fig. 62-46). This serious complication is diagnosed by transesophageal two-dimensional and Doppler echocardiography. Unless surgical risk is high, the preferred treatment for left-sided valve thrombosis is emergency surgery when NYHA Class III-IV symptoms are present or there is a large clot burden. Fibrinolytic therapy is reasonable for right-sided valve thrombosis, left-sided valve thrombosis with a small clot burden and only mild symptoms. Fibrinolytic therapy is followed by intravenous heparin, and aspirin until the INR is therapeutic..[1,270,271]

It must be recognized that (1) the administration of warfarin carries its own mortality and morbidity, i.e., serious hemorrhage, estimated at 0.2 and 2.2 episodes per 100 patient-years, respectively; and (2) despite treatment with anticoagulants, the incidence of thromboembolic complications with the best mechanical prosthesis is still about 0.2 fatal complications and 1.0 to 2.0 nonfatal complications per 100 patient-years for aortic valves and 2.0 to 3.0 nonfatal complications for mitral valves. Valve thrombosis, a particularly hazardous complication, occurs at an incidence of about 0.1 percent per year in the aortic position and 0.35 percent per year in the mitral position. Thrombosis of mechanical prostheses in the tricuspid position is quite high, and for this reason bioprostheses are preferred at this site. The incidence of embolization in patients who have experienced repeated emboli from a prosthetic valve despite anticoagulants may be reduced by replacement with a tissue valve.

Mechanical prostheses regularly cause mild hemolysis, but this is not severe enough to be of clinical importance unless the patient develops periprosthetic regurgitation.

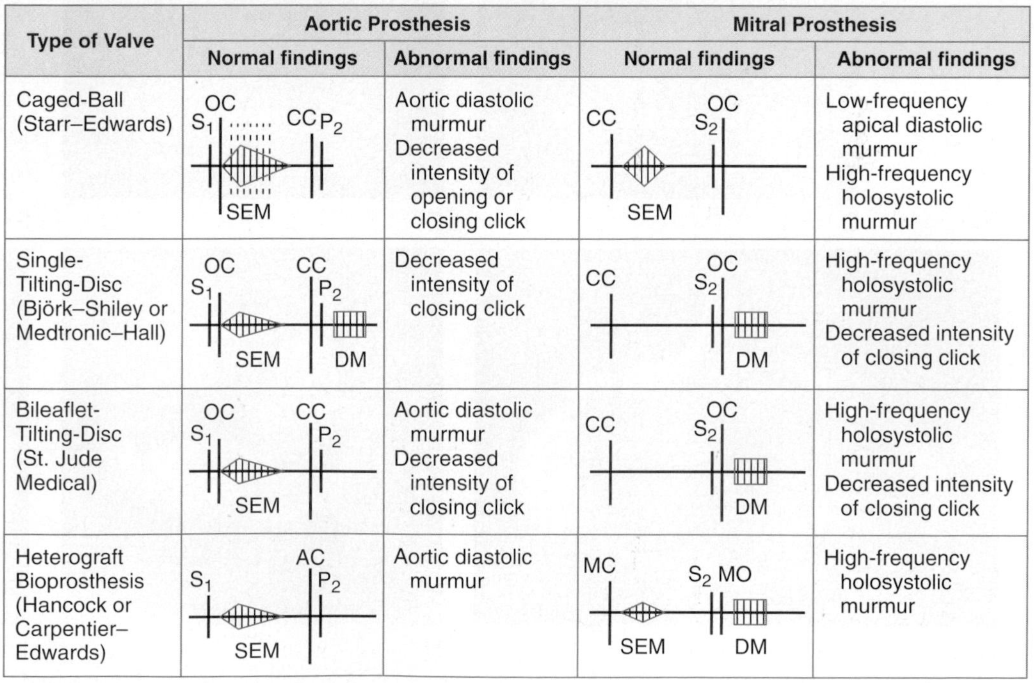

CH 62

Valvular Heart Disease

Type of Valve	Aortic Prosthesis		Mitral Prosthesis	
	Normal findings	Abnormal findings	Normal findings	Abnormal findings
Caged-Ball (Starr–Edwards)	OC ... CC P₂ / S₁ / SEM	Aortic diastolic murmur, Decreased intensity of opening or closing click	CC ... OC / S₂ / SEM	Low-frequency apical diastolic murmur, High-frequency holosystolic murmur
Single-Tilting-Disc (Björk–Shiley or Medtronic–Hall)	OC CC / S₁ P₂ / SEM DM	Decreased intensity of closing click	CC OC / S₂ / DM	High-frequency holosystolic murmur, Decreased intensity of closing click
Bileaflet-Tilting-Disc (St. Jude Medical)	OC CC / S₁ P₂ / SEM	Aortic diastolic murmur, Decreased intensity of closing click	CC OC / S₂ / DM	High-frequency holosystolic murmur, Decreased intensity of closing click
Heterograft Bioprosthesis (Hancock or Carpentier–Edwards)	AC / S₁ P₂ / SEM	Aortic diastolic murmur	MC S₂ MO / SEM DM	High-frequency holosystolic murmur

FIGURE 62–46 Auscultatory characteristics of various prosthetic valves in the aortic and mitral positions, with schematic diagrams of normal findings and descriptions of abnormal findings. AC = aortic closure; CC = closing click; DM = diastolic murmur; MC = mitral valve closure; MO = mitral opening; OC = opening click; SEM = systolic ejection murmur. (From Vongpatanasin W, Hillis LD, Lange RA: Prosthetic heart valves. N Engl J Med 335:407, 1996.)

Tissue Valves (Fig. 62-47)

Tissue valves (bioprostheses) have been developed primarily to overcome the risk of thromboembolism that is inherent in all mechanical prosthetic valves and the attendant hazards and inconvenience of permanent anticoagulant therapy.

Porcine Heterografts

Stented porcine aortic heterografts were developed for both the mitral and the aortic positions and have been in wide clinical use since 1965.[264] The semirigid stents facilitate implantation and maintain the three-dimensional relationship between the leaflets. Three porcine heterografts are widely used today.[272-273] The Hancock valve (see Fig. 62-47A) is fixed and preserved in glutaraldehyde and is mounted on a Dacron cloth-covered flexible polypropylene strut. In the smaller aortic models, the right coronary cusp is replaced by a posterior cusp from another valve to reduce obstruction resulting from the septal shelf of the valve.[273] The Carpentier-Edwards valve (see Fig. 62-47B) is pressure-fixed, preserved in glutaraldehyde, and mounted on a Teflon-covered Elgiloy strut so as to minimize the septal shelf.[273] The Medtronic Intact valve (see Fig. 62-47C) is also glutaraldehyde-treated but at a fixation pressure of zero and with toluidine in an attempt to inhibit calcium deposition.[272] The hemodynamic profiles of the porcine heterografts are similar to those of comparably sized low-profile mechanical prostheses.

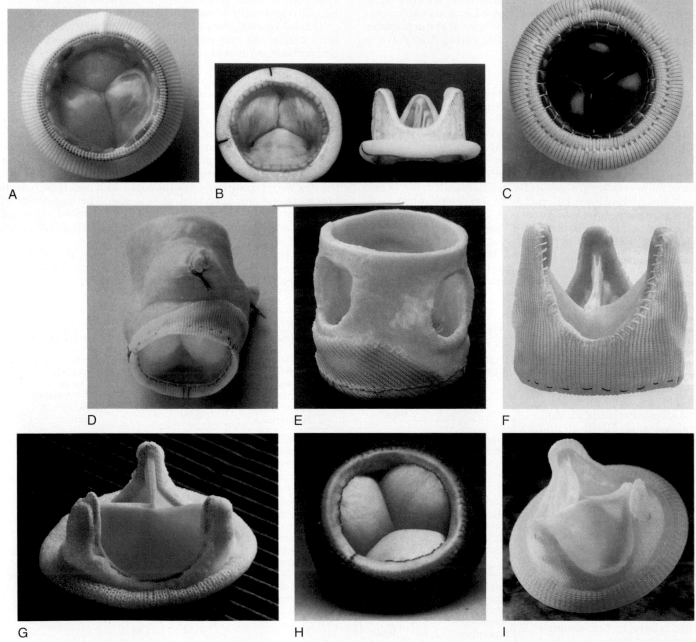

FIGURE 62–47 Bioprosthetic valves. The top row shows stented porcine valves: **A,** Hancock porcine valve; **B,** Carpentier-Edwards porcine valve; and **C,** Medtronic Intact porcine valve. The middle row shows stentless valves: **D,** Medtronic Freestyle stentless valve; **E,** Edwards Prima stentless valve; and **F,** St. Jude Medical Toronto SPV stentless valve. The bottom row shows pericardial valves: **G,** Carpentier-Edwards pericardial valve; **H,** Sorin Pericarbon pericardial valve; and **I,** Autologous pericardial valve. *(From Grunkemeier GL, Rahimtoola SH, Starr A: Prosthetic heart valves. In Rahimtoola SH [ed]: Valvular Heart Disease. In Braunwald E [series ed]: Atlas of Heart Diseases. vol 11. Philadelphia, Current Medicine, 1997, pp 13.9-13.13.)*

During the first 3 postoperative months, while the sewing ring becomes endothelialized, there is a risk of thromboembolic rate so that warfarin anticoagulation is reasonable. Thereafter, anticoagulants are not required for porcine valves in the aortic position, and the thromboembolic rate is approximately 1 to 2 episodes per 100 patient-years without these drugs.[1,264] When these valves have been placed in the mitral position in patients who are in sinus rhythm, who do not have heart failure or thrombus in the left atrium or the left atrial appendage, and who do not have a history of embolism preoperatively, anticoagulants are not needed after the first 3 postoperative months, and the thromboembolic rate is also approximately 1 to 2 episodes per 100 patient-years. This rate is comparable to that observed in patients with the St. Jude or other mechanical valves who are receiving anticoagulants and are therefore subject to the risks of hemorrhage. It is unlikely that any MV replacement can be associated with a thromboembolic rate much below 0.5 episode per 100 patient-years because some of the emboli in patients with longstanding mitral disease are derived from the left atrium rather than from the valve itself. In patients undergoing MV replacement with a bioprosthesis who have experienced a previous embolism, in whom thrombus is found in the left atrium at operation, or who remain in AF postoperatively (approximately one third of all patients receiving MV replacement), the hazard of thromboembolism and the need for anticoagulants persist. This negates the principal advantage of the tissue valves, and mechanical prostheses would appear to be preferable to bioprostheses in these patients.

The major problem with porcine bioprostheses is their limited durability (Fig. 62-48). Cuspal tears, degeneration, fibrin deposition, disruption of the fibrocollagenous structure, perforation, fibrosis, and calcification sufficiently severe to require reoperation begin to appear in some patients in the fourth or fifth postoperative year, and by 10 years the rate of primary tissue failure averages 30 percent. It then accelerates, and by 15 years postoperatively the actuarial freedom from bioprosthetic primary tissue failure has ranged from 30 percent to 60 percent in several series. Hypercholesterolemia has been shown to contribute to prosthesis calcification and degeneration,[274,275] suggesting that secondary prevention strategies may slow down this process.

Structural valve deterioration is more frequent in patients with bioprostheses in the mitral than in the aortic position,[267] presumably because of the higher closing pressure. With the passage of time, it is anticipated that many of the currently implanted valves will likely fail, especially in younger patients, and essentially all valves implanted into patients less than 60 years of age may have to be replaced ultimately. Fortunately, however, these valves usually do not fail suddenly (as is often the case for structural failure or thrombosis of mechanical prostheses). Re-replacement of a bioprosthetic valve should be carried out when significant and/or progressive structural deterioration is evident but before operation becomes an emergency. The second operation, when carried out on an elective basis, may be associated with a surgical mortality rate of 10 percent to 15 percent.

Color Doppler echocardiography with two-dimensional imaging is extremely helpful in the early detection of bioprosthetic valve malfunction. Transesophageal echocardiography is more sensitive than transthoracic imaging in detecting bioprosthetic valve deterioration. Even patients without new murmurs or other physical findings of valve dysfunction should have routine echocardiographic studies to look for early bioprosthetic valve dysfunction every year for 5 to 6 years after valve replacement and every 6 months after that.

The rate of structural valve failure is age-dependent, and is significantly lower in patients older than 65 years than in younger patients, especially in the aortic position (Fig. 62-49A). In patients over 65 years undergoing AVR with a porcine bioprosthesis, the rate of structural deterioration is less than 10 percent at 10 years.[1,267,272] Valve failure is prohibitively rapid in children and in adults under 35 to 40 years of age. Therefore bioprostheses are not advisable in these age groups. On the other hand, degeneration is rare when these valves are implanted into patients over 70 years of age.[1,273] Bioprostheses also have been reported to have extremely limited durability in patients with chronic renal failure, but recent studies have called this into question (discussed subsequently).

Prosthetic valve endocarditis is a serious, often grave illness (see Chap. 63).

STENTLESS PORCINE XENOGRAFTS. Since the stent adds to the obstruction and thereby increases stress on the leaflets, stentless valves have been developed for the aortic position (see Fig. 62-47) and are now being used increasingly, especially in patients with small aortic roots. These include the Toronto SPV stentless valve (St. Jude Medical valve), the Edwards stentless valve, and the Medtronic freestyle valve. These valves have been reported to have more

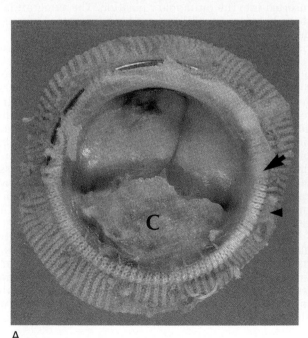

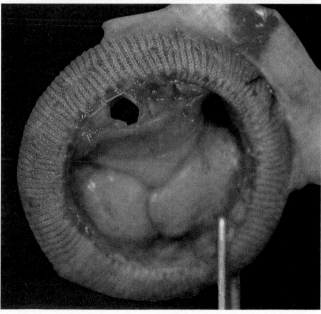

A   B

FIGURE 62–48 Structural deterioration of bioprosthetic valves. **A,** Valve failure related to mineralization and collagen degeneration. **B,** Cuspal tears and perforations. These processes may occur independently, or they may be synergistic. (**A,** From Virmani R, Burke AP, Farb A: Pathology of valvular heart disease. In Rahimtoola SH [ed]: Valvular Heart Disease. In Braunwald E [series ed]: Atlas of Heart Diseases. vol 11. Philadelphia, Current Medicine, 1997, p 1.26; **B,** from Manabe H, Yutani C [eds]: Atlas of Valvular Heart Disease. Singapore, Churchill Livingstone, 1998, p 158.)

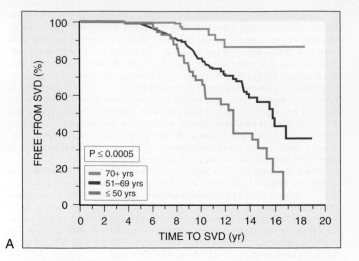

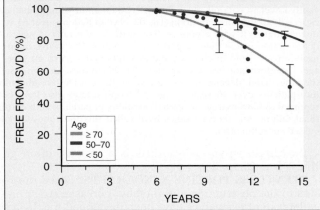

FIGURE 62–49 Estimates of freedom from structural valve deterioration (SVD) for patients undergoing porcine **(A)** and bovine pericardial **(B)** aortic valve replacement who are stratified according to age. (**A,** From Cohn LH, Collins JJ Jr, Rizzo RJ, et al: Twenty-year follow-up of the Hancock modified orifice porcine aortic valve. Ann Thorac Surg 66:S30, 1998; **B,** from Banbury MK, Cosgrove DM, White JA, et al: Age and valve size effect on the long-term durability of the Carpentier-Edwards aortic pericardial bioprosthesis. Ann Thorac Surg 72:753, 2001.)

physiologic flow and lower transvalvular gradients than stented porcine valves, with the potential for enhanced regression of LV hypertrophy and improved LV function. Although the early experience tends to confirm this, it is yet uncertain whether this translates into improved outcomes in terms of survival and long-term prosthesis durability.[276,277] It is hoped that the slightly improved hemodynamics provided by the stentless valves will translate into better valve longevity than that of valves mounted on stents.

Pericardial (Xenograft) Aortic Valves

Bovine pericardial valves, unlike porcine valves, are fabricated rather than harvested directly (see Fig. 62-47). Although the first generation of these valves had a high rate of premature structural deterioration, the current generation of stented bovine pericardial prostheses has been demonstrated to have good long-term durability that appears to be equivalent or better than that of the porcine bioprosthesis.[278] As with the stented porcine valves, the rate of structural deterioration is extremely low in individuals aged 70 years or older (see Fig. 62-49B).[279] There is a greater risk for the development of stenosis in the mitral position.

Homograft (Allograft) Aortic Valves

These are harvested from cadavers, often along with kidneys, usually within 24 hours of donor death. They are sterilized with antibiotics and cryopreserved for long periods at −196°C. They are inserted directly, usually in the aortic position, without being placed into a prosthetic stent. In the aortic position, the isolated valve is implanted in the subcoronary position, or the valve and a portion of attached aorta are implanted as a root replacement, with reimplantation of the coronary arteries into the graft. Homograft hemodynamics are superior to those of stented porcine valves and similar to those of stentless porcine valves. Like porcine xenografts, their thrombogenicity is low, but cryopreserved valves appear to have similar issues with structural deterioration,[1] with evidence that this rate is reduced with the use of freshly harvested valves, approximate matching of donor's and patient's ages, and use of the root replacement technique. The subcoronary technique is associated with higher incidence of prosthetic AR and reoperation.[280,281] In addition, the homograft valve and root is prone to severe calcification, making reoperation difficult. One possible advantage of homografts is in the avoidance of early endocarditis, and homografts are commonly employed in the treatment of aortic valve endocarditis,[282] particularly complex aortic root endocarditis, However, in randomized studies there was no benefit of homografts compared to other tissue valves in outcome after endocarditis.[283,284]

Autograft Aortic Valves

PERICARDIAL AUTOGRAFT VALVES. The patient's own pericardium is inserted into a frame on the operating table and is inserted into either the aortic or the mitral position (see Fig. 62-47I). Long-term durability appears to be excellent; in 267 patients undergoing isolated AVR, the 14-year actuarial freedom of need for re-replacement because of structural valve dysfunction was 85 percent (94 percent in patients greater than 65 years of age).

PULMONARY AUTOGRAFTS. In this operation, the Ross procedure, the patient's own pulmonary valve and adjacent main pulmonary artery are removed and used to replace the diseased aortic valve and often the neighboring aorta, with reimplantation of the coronary arteries into the graft.[285,286] A human pulmonary or aortic homograft is then inserted into the pulmonary position. The autograft is nonthrombogenic. In children and adolescents, there is evidence that the autograft grows along with the patient.[287] The risk of endocarditis is very low, anticoagulants are not required, and, perhaps most important, the long-term durability appears to be excellent. A high incidence of pulmonary homograft stenosis has been reported in some series,[288,289] which may represent a postoperative inflammatory reaction. The pulmonary artery tissue adapts to the aortic pressure and usually does not dilate.[290] However, this procedure should not be performed in patients with bicuspid valves and dilated aortic roots, as the implanted pulmonary artery tissue exposed to the higher aortic pressures may also undergo degenerative changes leading to significant dilation of the autograft.[291] A subcoronary technique, in which the pulmonary autograft is inserted without a root replacement, may circumvent this problem.[292]

The pulmonary autograft is the replacement valve of choice in children, adolescents, and younger adults who have a long (greater than 20-year) life expectancy,[287] particularly young women who wish to become pregnant. However, its use has been limited because the operation is technically much more demanding than a simple AVR. The procedure should be carried out only by experienced surgeons.

Hemodynamics of Valve Replacements

The most commonly used prosthetic valves, i.e., mechanical prostheses and stented porcine or pericardial xenografts, have an effective in vitro orifice size that is smaller than the normal valve at the same site. Unstented porcine xenografts, homografts and pulmonary autografts have larger effective valve areas than comparable stented valves, but still do not restore valve area or hemodynamics to normal. After implantation, tissue ingrowth and endothelialization reduce the size of the effective orifice even more. Therefore the prosthetic valves that are currently available must be considered to be mildly stenotic. However, postoperative hemodynamic measurements of the mechanical prostheses show reasonably good function, with effective mitral valve orifice areas averaging 1.7 to 2.0 cm^2 and mitral valve gradients of 4 to 8 mm Hg at rest. The cloth-covered Starr-Edwards valve appears to be intrinsically slightly more stenotic than the Medtronic-Hall or Omniscience tilting-disc valves. The bileaflet St. Jude and CarboMedics valves, in turn, may be slightly superior to the Medtronic-Hall or Omniscience valve. In hemodynamic studies, the stented porcine mitral valves behave in a manner similar to mechanical prosthetic valves of the same diameter. Serious hemodynamic obstruction of an artificial valve in the mitral position is quite uncommon, unless the valve (most commonly the Starr-Edwards valve) is placed into a small LV cavity or into an unusually small mitral annulus or the prosthesis chosen is of inappropriate size.

The problem of physiologic stenosis of a normally functioning prosthetic valve (often called "patient-prosthesis mismatch") may be more serious in patients who undergo AVR for AS. The annulus into which the prosthesis is inserted in these patients is usually smaller than it is in patients with AR, and the surgeon may be forced to select an artificial valve of relatively small size. As a consequence, AVR may not abolish obstruction in patients with AS, but the prosthesis-patient mismatch[261,293] may merely convert severe to mild or moderate obstruction. When the smaller models of the stented porcine xenograft or mechanical prosthesis are placed into the aortic position, effective orifice areas of about 1.1 to 1.3 cm^2 are common. In such patients, peak transvalvular gradients as high as 40 mm Hg during exercise have been recorded. Patient prosthetic mismatch adversely affects both short-term and long-term survival after valve surgery.[294,295] Mismatch can be avoided by choosing a valve with an adequate orifice area for the patient's body size. In some cases, an annular enlarging procedure may be necessary. Rarely, reoperation to correct a malfunctioning prosthesis may be necessary.

Selection of an Artificial Valve

Most comparisons of mechanical and bioprosthetic valves indicate similar overall results in terms of early and late mortality, prosthetic valve endocarditis and other complications, and the need for reoperation, at least for the first 5 years postoperatively.[296] As indicated, there appear to be no significant differences insofar as hemodynamics are concerned, except that patients with an unusually small LV cavity or mitral or aortic annulus may have better results with the low-profile (tilting-disc) St. Jude or CarboMedics prosthesis or a tissue valve. Patients with a small aortic annulus may be better candidates for unstented homografts, heterografts, or pulmonary autografts. In general, patient outcome after valve surgery is related more to preoperative factors, such as age, LV function, associated coronary artery disease, and comorbid conditions, than to the prosthesis itself.

The major task in selecting an artificial valve is to weigh the advantage of durability and the disadvantages of the risks of thromboembolism and anticoagulant treatment inherent in mechanical prostheses on the one hand with the advantage of low thrombogenicity and the disadvantage of abbreviated durability of bioprostheses on the other. Hammermeister and associates[267] compared the 15-year outcome in 575 men who were randomized to undergo MV replacement or AVR with either mechanical or a bioprosthetic valve. Patients undergoing AVR with a mechanical valve had better survival than those receiving the bioprosthesis (Fig. 62-50), principally because of the higher rate of structural deterioration of the bioprosthesis (especially in patients less than 65 years of age). Much of the increased mortality in patients receiving the tissue valve was related to reoperation (which is associated with about twice the mortality of the initial procedure). The prosthetic valve did not influence survival after MV replacement, nor the probability of developing other valve-related complications, including endocarditis, valve thrombosis, and systemic embolism. As anticipated, anticoagulant-related bleeding was higher in patients receiving mechanical valves. Patients with mechanical valves also had a higher incidence of perivalvular regurgitation in the mitral position and a trend for this complication in the aortic position. In the Edinburgh randomized trial, which also compared a mechanical with a porcine xenograft valve,[297] actuarial survival rates tended to be better and the freedom from all valve-related adverse events was significantly better with mechanical valves. Retrospective cohort analyses are in agreement with the results of these trials.[298] Therefore mechanical prostheses, usually of the bileaflet variety, are the valves of choice in the majority of patients younger than 65 years of age.

However, the following groups of patients should receive bioprostheses: (1) patients with coexisting disease who are prone to hemorrhage and who therefore tolerate anticoagulants poorly, such as those with bleeding disorders, intestinal polyposis, and angiodysplasia; (2) patients who are likely to be noncompliant with permanent anticoagulant treatment, who are unwilling to take anticoagulants on a regular basis, or who live in developing nations and cannot be monitored; (3) patients over the age of 65 years in whom bioprosthetic valves deteriorate very slowly (see Fig. 62-49), who are unlikely to outlive their bioprostheses, and who because of their age may also be at greater risk of hemorrhage while taking anticoagulants; (4) patients with a small

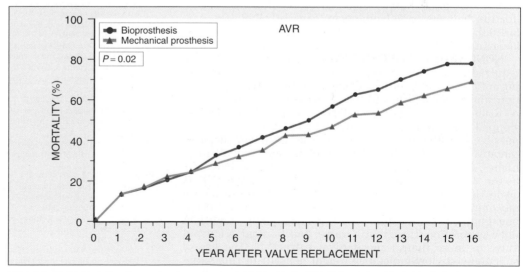

FIGURE 62–50 Mortality after aortic valve replacement (AVR) with the Björk-Shiley and porcine valves from the Department of Veterans Affairs trial. *(From Hammermeister KE, Sethi GK, Henderson WG, et al: Outcomes 15 years after valve replacement with a mechanical versus a bioprosthetic valve: Final report of the Veterans Affairs randomized trial. J Am Coll Cardiol 36:1152, 2000.)*

aortic annulus in whom an unstented (free) bioprosthetic graft may provide superior hemodynamics; and (5) younger women wishing to bear children, who require AVR.

Special Situations

PREGNANCY (see also Chap. 77). Women with artificial valves can tolerate the hemodynamic burden of pregnancy well, but the hypercoagulable state of pregnancy increases the risk of thromboembolism in pregnant patients with mechanical prostheses.[299-301] Anticoagulation must not be interrupted, although an increased risk of fatal fetal hemorrhage occurs in women in whom anticoagulants are continued. There is also a risk of fetal malformation caused by the probable teratogenic effect of warfarin. Although these problems represent rationales for the use of tissue valves in all women of childbearing age, their limited durability in young adults makes their use unacceptable. Therefore every effort should be made to defer valve replacement until after childbirth. In pregnant women with critical MS or AS, balloon valvuloplasty should be considered, and, if at all possible, MV repair instead of replacement should be undertaken for patients with MR. Women of childbearing potential who have a mechanical prosthesis should be counseled against pregnancy.

When a woman who already has a mechanical prosthetic valve becomes pregnant, the risk of fetal defects with oral anticoagulants must be balanced against the risk of inadequate anticoagulation if oral therapy is interrupted. The management of anticoagulation in pregnant women with mechanical valves is controversial. All agree that the goal is continuous, effective, monitored anticoagulation and avoidance of fetal defects. In pregnant patients who receive warfarin, oral therapy is discontinued at week 36 of gestation and replaced with continuous intravenous unfractionated heparin.[1,301,302] Heparin should be discontinued at the onset of labor but may be restarted, along with warfarin, several hours after delivery. Between weeks 1 to 36 the options include: (1) continued oral therapy with warfarin to maintain a therapeutic INR, (2) replacement of warfarin between weeks 6 and 12 (when the risk of fetal defects is highest) or (3) for the duration of pregnancy by continuous intravenous or dose adjusted SQ heparin or by dose adjusted SC low molecular weight heparin.[1] The most important management principle is to ensure that anticoagulation is not interrupted and to ensure that the dose of anticoagulation is adequate based on frequent monitoring of PTT (for intravenous or subcutaneous heparin), INR (for warfarin), or anti-Xa levels (for low-molecular-weight heparin).[299,300,303]

NONCARDIAC SURGERY. When noncardiac surgery is required in patients with prosthetic valves who are receiving anticoagulants, the risk depends on the valve type, location, and associated risk factors. In patients with an isolated AVR and no associated risk factors, the anticoagulant is stopped 1 to 3 days preoperatively and resumed as soon as possible postoperatively without the need for heparin therapy. However, when the risk of thromboembolism is higher, intravenous heparin is started when the INR falls below 2.0 and resumed postoperatively until the INR is again therapeutic. High-risk patients include those with a mechanical mitral valve prosthesis, AF, previous thromboem-bolism, LV dysfunction, hypercoagulable condition, older-generation thrombotic valve, mechanical tricuspid valve or more than 1 mechanical valve.[304-306] The use of subcutaneous low-molecular weight heparin in this situation has been advocated by some experts, but this topic represents another area of controversy.

CHILDREN AND PATIENTS RECEIVING CHRONIC HEMODIALYSIS. The high incidence of bioprosthetic valve failure in children and adolescents virtually prohibits their use in these groups. In young adults between the ages of 25 and 35 years, the failure of bioprosthetic valves is somewhat higher than it is in older adults; this serves as a relative, but not an absolute, contraindication to their use in this age group.

In children, a mechanical prosthesis (generally the St. Jude valve) with its favorable hemodynamics and established durability is preferred despite the disadvantages inherent in the need for anticoagulants in this age group. Alternatively, if an experienced surgical team is available and the patient requires an AVR, a pulmonary autograft is an excellent alternative.

Previous studies indicated a high rate of bioprosthetic structural deterioration in patients receiving chronic renal dialysis. However, several studies have reported no difference in survival of patients with a bioprosthesis or a mechanical valve, coupled with an unacceptably high rate of stroke and major bleeding in patients with the mechanical valves.[307] Current guidelines no longer recommend mechanical valves in these patients,[1] but this clearly is an area in which physician judgment is important for individual patients.

TRICUSPID POSITION. The risk of thrombosis for all valves is highest in the tricuspid position because of the lower pressures and velocity of blood flow. This complication appears to be highest for tilting-disc valves, intermediate for caged-ball valves, and lowest for bioprostheses, which are the valves of choice as tricuspid replacements. Fortunately, bioprostheses exhibit a much slower rate of mechanical deterioration in the tricuspid position than in the mitral or aortic positions.

REFERENCES

1. Bonow RO, Carabello BA, Chatterjee K, et al: ACC/AHA 2006 guidelines for the management of patients with valvular heart disease: A report of the American College of Cardiology / American Heart Association Task Force on Practice Guidelines (writing committee to revise the 1998 Guidelines for the Management of Patients with Valvular Heart Disease): Developed in collaboration with the Society of Cardiovascular Anesthesiologists: endorsed by the Society for Cardiovascular Angiography and Interventions and the Society of Thoracic Surgeons. Circulation 114:e84, 2006.
2. Vahanian A, Baumgartner H, Bax J, et al: Guidelines on the management of valvular heart disease. Eur Heart J 28:230, 2007.

Aortic Stenosis

3. Roberts WC, Ko JM: Frequency by decades of unicuspid, bicuspid, and tricuspid aortic valves in adults having isolated aortic valve replacement for aortic stenosis, with or without associated aortic regurgitation. Circulation 111:920, 2005.
4. Braverman AC, Guven H, Beardslee MA, et al: The bicuspid aortic valve. Curr Probl Cardiol 30:470, 2005.
5. Lewin MB, Otto CM: The bicuspid aortic valve: adverse outcomes from infancy to old age. Circulation 111:832, 2005.
6. Fedak PWM, Verma S, David TE: Clinical and pathophysiological implications of a bicuspid aortic valve. Circulation 106:900, 2002.
7. Garg V, Muth AN, Ransom JF, et al: Mutations in NOTCH1 cause aortic valve disease. Nature 437:270, 2005.
8. Keane MG, Wiegers SE, Plappert T, et al: Bicuspid aortic valves are associated with aortic dilatation out of proportion to coexistent valvular lesions. Circulation 102: III-35, 2000.
9. Ferencik M, Pape LA: Changes in size of ascending aorta and aortic valve function with time in patients with congenitally bicuspid aortic valves. Am J Cardiol 92:43, 2003.
10. Nataatmadja M, West M, West J, et al: Abnormal extracellular matrix protein transport associated with increased apoptosis of vascular smooth muscle cells in Marfan syndrome and bicuspid aortic valve thoracic aortic aneurysm. Circulation 100 (suppl II).II-329, 2003.
11. Borger MA, Preston M, Ivanov J, et al: Should the ascending aorta be replaced more frequently in patients with bicuspid aortic valve disease? J Thorac Cardiovasc Surg 128:677, 2004.
12. Rajamannan NM, Gersh B, Bonow RO: Calcific aortic stenosis: From bench to bedside—emerging clinical and cellular concepts. Heart 89:1, 2003.
13. Freeman RV, Otto CM: Spectrum of calcific aortic valve disease: Pathogenesis, disease progression, and treatment strategies. Circulation 111:3316, 2005.
14. Olsen MH, Wachtell K, Bella JN, et al: Aortic valve sclerosis relates to cardiovascular events in patients with hypertension (a LIFE substudy). Am J Cardiol 95:132, 2005.

15. Taylor HA, Jr., Clark BL, Garrison RJ, et al: Relation of aortic valve sclerosis to risk of coronary heart disease in African-Americans. Am J Cardiol 95:401, 2005.

16. O'Brien KD, Shavelle DM, Caulfield MT, et al: Association of angiotensin-converting enzyme with low-density lipoprotein in aortic valvular lesions and in human plasma. Circulation 106:2224, 2002.

17. Rajamannan NM, Otto CM: Targeted therapy to prevent progression of calcific aortic stenosis. Circulation 110:1180, 2004.

18. Mohler ER, Gannon F, Reynolds C, et al: Bone formation and inflammation in cardiac valves. Circulation 103:1522, 2001.

19. Rajamannan NM, Subramaniam M, Rickard D, et al: Human aortic valve calcification is associated with an osteoblast phenotype. Circulation 107:2181, 2003.

20. Fox CS, Vasan RS, Parise H, et al: Mitral annular calcification predicts cardiovascular morbidity and mortality: The Framingham Heart Study. Circulation 107:1492, 2003.

21. Jeon DS, Atar S, Brasch AV, et al: Association of mitral annulus calcification, aortic valve sclerosis and aortic root calcification with abnormal myocardial perfusion single photon emission tomography in subjects <65 years old. J Am Coll Cardiol 38:1988, 2001.

22. Probst V, Le Scouarnec S, Legendre A, et al: Familial aggregation of calcific aortic valve stenosis in the western part of France. Circulation 113:856, 2006.

23. Palta S, Pai AM, Gill K, et al: New insights into the progression of aortic stenosis: Implications for secondary prevention. Circulation 101:2497, 2000.

24. Peltier M, Trojette F, Enriquez-Sarano M, et al: Relation between cardiovascular risk factors and nonrheumatic severe calcific aortic stenosis among patients with a three-cuspid aortic valve. Am J Cardiol 91:97, 2003.

25. Galante A, Pietroiusti A, Vellini M, et al: C-reactive protein is increased in patients with degenerative aortic valvular stenosis. J Am Coll Cardiol 38:1078, 2001.

26. Katz R, Wong ND, Kronmal R, et al: Features of the metabolic syndrome and diabetes mellitus as predictors of aortic valve calcification in the Multi-Ethnic Study of Atherosclerosis. Circulation 113:2113, 2006.

27. Briand M, Lemieux I, Dumesnil JG, et al: Metabolic syndrome negatively influences progression and prognosis in aortic stenosis. J Am Coll Cardiol 47:2229, 2006.

28. Novaro GM, Tiong IY, Pearce GL, et al: Effect of hydoxymethylglutarul coenzyme A reductase inhibitors on the progression of calcific aortic stenosis. Circulation 104:2205, 2001.

29. Shavelle DM, Takasu J, Budoff MJ, et al: HMG CoA reductase inhibitor (statin) and aortic valve calcium. Lancet 359:1125, 2002.

30. Bellamy MF, Pellikka PA, Klarich KW, et al: Association of cholesterol levels, hydroxymethylglutarul coenzyme-A reductase inhibitor treatment, and progression of aortic stenosis in the community. J Am Coll Cardiol 40:1723, 2002.

31. Rajamannan NM, Subramanian M, Sebo T, et al: Atorvastatin inhibits hypercholesterolemia-induced cellular proliferation and bone matrix production in the rabbit aortic valve. Circulation 105:2660, 2002.

32. Alpert JS: Aortic stenosis: A new face for an old disease. Arch Intern Med 163:1769, 2003.

33. Chan C: Is aortic stenosis a preventable disease? J Am Coll Cardiol 42:593, 2003.

34. Cowell SJ, Newby DE, Prescott RJ, et al: A randomized trial of intensive lipid-lowering therapy in calcific aortic stenosis. N Engl J Med 352:2389, 2005.

35. Moura LM, Ramos SF, Zamorano JL, et al: Rosuvastatin Affective Aortic Valve Endothelium to slow the progression of aortic stenosis. J Am Coll Cardiol 49:554, 2007.

36. Otto CM: Valvular aortic stenosis: disease severity and timing of intervention. J Am Coll Cardiol 47:2141, 2006.

37. Kadem L, Dumesnil JG, Rieu R, et al: Impact of systemic hypertension on the assessment of aortic stenosis. Heart 91:354, 2005.

38. Carabello BA: Aortic stenosis. N Engl J Med 346:677, 2002.

39. Fielitz J, Hein S, Mitrovic V, et al: Activation of the cardiac renin-angiotensin system and increased myocardial collagen expression in human aortic valve disease. J Am Coll Cardiol 37:1443, 2001.

40. Walther T, Schubert A, Falk V, et al: Left ventricular reverse remodeling after surgical therapy for arotic stenosis: Correlation to renin-angiotensin system gene expression. Circulation 106:I-23, 2002.

41. Rajappan K, Rimoldi OE, Dutka DP, et al: Mechanisms of coronary microcirculatory dysfunction in patients with aortic stenosis and angiographically normal coronary arteries. Circulation 105:470, 2002.

42. Gould KL, Carabello BA: Why angina in aortic stenosis with normal coronary arteriograms? Circulation 107:3121, 2003.

43. Levinson GE, Alpert JS. Aortic stenosis. In Alpert JS, Dalen JE, Rahimtoola SH (eds): Valvular Heart Disease. 3rd ed. Philadelphia, Lippincott Williams & Wilkins, 2000, pp 183-211.

44. Carabello BA: Evaluation and management of patients with aortic stenosis. Circulation 105:1746, 2002.

45. Vincentelli A, Susen S, Le Tourneau T, et al: Acquired von Willebrand syndrome in aortic stenosis. N Engl J Med 349:343, 2003.

46. Pareti FI, Lattuada A, Bressi C, et al: Proteolysis of von Willebrand factor and shear stress-induced platelet aggregation in patients with aortic stenosis. Circulation 102:1290, 2000.

47. Otto CM: Valvular stenosis. In Otto CM (ed): Textbook of Clinical Echocardiography. 3rd ed. Philadelphia, Elsevier Saunders, 2004.

48. Garcia D, Pibarot P, Dumesnil JG, et al: Assessment of aortic valve stenosis severity: A new index based on the energy loss concept. Circulation 101:765, 2000.

49. Garcia D, Dumesnil JG, Durand LG, et al: Discrepancies between catheter and Doppler estimates of valve effective orific area can be predicted from the pressure recovery phenomenon: Practical implications with regard to quantification of aortic stenosis severity. J Am Coll Cardiol 41:435, 2003.

50. Chambers J, Bach D, Dumesnil J, et al: Crossing the aortic valve in severe aortic stenosis: no longer acceptable? J Heart Valve Dis 13:344, 2004.

51. John AS, Dill T, Brandt RR, et al: Magnetic resonance to assess the aortic valve area in aortic stenosis. J Am Coll Cardiol 42:519, 2003.

52. Caruthers SD, Lin SJ, Brown P, et al: Practical value of cardiac magnetic resonance imaging for clinical quantification of aortic valve stenosis: Comparison with echocardiography. Circulation 208:2236, 2003.

53. Cosmi JE, Kort S, Tunick PA, et al: The risk of the development of aortic stenosis in patients with "benign" aortic valve thickening. Arch Intern Med 162:2345, 2002.

54. Varadarajan P, Kapoor N, Bansal RC, Pai RG: Clinical profile and natural history of 453 nonsurgically managed patients with severe aortic stenosis. Ann Thorac Surg 82:2111, 2006.

55. Rosenhek R, Porenta G, Lang I, et al: Predictors of outcome in severe, asymptomatic aortic stenosis. N Engl J Med 343:611, 2000.

56. Rosenhek R, Klaar U, Schemper M, et al: Mild and moderate aortic stenosis. Natural history and risk stratification by echocardiography. Eur Heart J 25:199, 2004.

57. Pellikka PA, Sarano ME, Nishimura RA, et al: Outcome of 622 adults with asymptomatic, hemodynamically significant aortic stenosis during prolonged follow-up. Circulation 111:3290, 2005.

58. Das P, Rimington H, Chambers J: Exercise testing to stratify risk in aortic stenosis. Eur Heart J 26:1309, 2005.

59. Lancellotti P, Lebois F, Simon M, et al: Prognostic importance of quantitative exercise Doppler echocardiography in asymptomatic valvular aortic stenosis. Circulation 112:I377, 2005.

60. Bergler-Klein J, Klaar U, Heger M, et al: Natriuretic peptides predict symptom-free survival and postoperative outcome in severe aortic stenosis. Circulation 109:2302, 2004.

61. Lim P, Monin JL, Monchi M, et al: Predictors of outcome in patients with severe aortic stenosis and normal left ventricular function: role of B-type natriuretic peptide. Eur Heart J 25:2048, 2004.

62. Gerber IL, Legget ME, West TM, et al: Usefulness of serial measurement of N-terminal pro-brain natriuretic peptide plasma levels in asymptomatic patients with aortic stenosis to predict symptomatic deterioration. Am J Cardiol 95:898, 2005.

63. Baumgartner H: What influences the outcome of valve replacement in critical aortic stenosis? Heart 91:1254, 2005.

64. Christ M, Sharkova Y, Geldner G, et al: Preoperative and perioperative care for patients with suspected or established aortic stenosis facing noncardiac surgery. Chest 128:2944, 2005.

65. Amato MCM, Moffa PJ, Ramires JAF: Treatment decision in asymptomatic aortic valve stenosis: Role of exercise testing. Heart 86:381, 2001.

66. Smith WT, Ferguson TB, Jr., Ryan T, et al: Should coronary artery bypass graft surgery patients with mild or moderate aortic stenosis undergo concomitant aortic valve replacement? A decision analysis approach to the surgical dilemma. J Am Coll Cardiol 44:1241, 2004.

67. Iung B, Cachier A, Baron G, et al: Decision-making in elderly patients with severe aortic stenosis: why are so many denied surgery? Eur Heart J 26:2714, 2005.

68. Pereira JJ, Balaban K, Lauer MS, et al: Aortic valve replacement in patients with mild or moderate aortic stenosis and coronary bypass surgery. Am J Med 118:735, 2005.

69. Gillinov AM, Garcia MJ: When is concomitant aortic valve replacement indicated in patients with mild to moderate stenosis undergoing coronary revascularization? Curr Cardiol Rep 7:101, 2005.

70. Boudjemline Y, Bonhoeffer P: Steps toward percutaneous aortic valve replacement. Circulation 105:775, 2002.

71. Cribier A, Eltchaninoff H, Bash A, et al: Percutaneous transcatheter implantation of an aortic valve prosthesis for calcific aortic stenosis: First human case description. Circulation 106:3006, 2002.

72. Cribier A, Eltchaninoff H, Tron C, et al: Early experience with percutaneous transcatheter implantation of heart valve prosthesis for the treatment of end-stage inoperable patients with calcific aortic stenosis. J Am Coll Cardiol 43:698, 2004.

73. Webb JG, Candavimol M, Thompson CR, et al: Percutaneous aortic valve implantation retrograde from the femoral artery. Circulation 113:842, 2006.

74. Connolly HM, Oh JK, Schaff HV, et al: Severe aortic stenosis with low transvalvular gradient and severe left ventricular dysfunction: Result of aortic valve replacement in 52 patients. Circulation 101:1940, 2000.

75. Rahimtoola SH: Severe aortic stenosis with low systolic gradient: The good and bad news. Circulation 101:1892, 2000.

76. Pereira JJ, Lauer MS, Bashir M, et al: Survival after aortic valve replacement for severe aortic stenosis with low transvalvular gradients and severe left ventricular dysfunction. J Am Coll Cardiol 39:1356, 2002.

77. Monin JL, Monchi M, Gest V, et al: Aortic stenosis with severe left ventricular dysfunction and low transvalvular pressure gradients: Risk stratification by low-dow dobutamine echocardiography. J Am Coll Cardiol 37:2102, 2001.

78. Monin JL, Quere JP, Monchi M, et al: Low-gradient aortic stenosis: Operative risk stratification and predictors for long-term outcome. A multicenter study using dobutamine stress hemodynamics. Circulation 108:319, 2003.

79. Powell DE, Tunick PA, Rosenzweig BP, et al: Aortic valve replacement in patients with aortic stenosis and severe left ventricular dysfunction. Arch Intern Med 160:1337, 2000.

80. Jolobe O: Surgery for aortic stenosis in severely symptomatic patients older than 80 years: Experience in a single UK centre. Heart 83:583, 2000.

81. Khot UN, Novaro GM, Popovic ZB, et al: Nitroprusside in critically ill patients with left ventricular dysfunction and aortic stenosis. N Engl J Med 348:1756, 2003.

82. Zile MR, Gaasch WH: Heart failure in aortic stenosis: Improving diagnosis and treatment. N Engl J Med 348:1735, 2003.

83. Nishimura RA, Grantham A, Connolly HM, et al: Low-output, low-gradient aortic stenosis in patients with depressed left ventricular systolic function: The clinical

utility of the dobutamine challenge in the catheterization laboratory. Circulation 106:809, 2002.

84. Edwards FH, Peterson ED, Coombs LP, et al: Prediction of operative mortality after valve replacement surgery. J Am Coll Cardiol 37:885, 2001.

85. Kivdal P, Bergström R, Hörte LG, et al: Observed and relative survival after aortic valve replacement. J Am Coll Cardiol 35:747, 2000.

86. Shroyer AL, Coombs LP, Peterson ED, et al: The Society of Thoracic Surgeons: 30-day operative mortality and morbidity risk models. Ann Thorac Surg 75:1856, 2003.

87. Ambler G, Omar RZ, Royston P, et al: Generic, simple risk stratification model for heart valve surgery. Circulation 112:224, 2005.

88. Sundt TM, Bailey MS, Moon MR, et al: Quality of life after aortic valve replacement at the age of >80 years. Circulation 102:III-70, 2000.

89. Lamb HJ, Beyerbacht HP, de Roos A, et al: Left ventricular remodeling early after aortic valve replacement: Differential effects on diastolic function in aortic valve stenosis and aortic regurgitation. J Am Coll Cardiol 40:2182, 2002.

90. Khan SS, Siegel RJ, DeRobertis MA, et al: Regression of hypertrophy after Carpentier-Edwards pericardial aortic valve replacement. Ann Thorac Surg 69:531, 2000.

91. Hildek-Smtih DJR, Shapiro LM: Coronary flow reserve improves after aortic valve replacement for aortic stenosis: An adenosine transthoracic echocardiography study. J Am Coll Cardiol 36:1889, 2000.

92. Rajappan K, Rimoldi OE, Camici PG, et al: Functional changes in coronary micro-circulation after valve replacement in patients with aortic stenosis. Circulation 107:3170, 2003.

93. Gall S Jr, Lowe JE, Wolfe WG, et al: Efficacy of the internal mammary artery in combined aortic valve replacement coronary artery bypass grafting. J Thorac Surg 69:524, 2000.

94. Bouchard D, Perrault LP, Carrier M, et al: Ministernotomy for aortic valve replacement: A study of the preliminary experience. Can J Surg 43:39, 2000.

Aortic Regurgitation

95. Maurer G: Aortic regurgitation. Heart 92:994, 2006.

96. Carabello BA: Progress in mitral and aortic regurgitation. Curr Probl Cardiol 28:553, 2003.

97. Roberts WC, Ko JM, Moore TR, Jones WH III: Causes of pure aortic regurgitation in patients having isolated aortic valve replacement at a single US tertiary hospital (1993-2005). Circulation 114:442, 2006.

98. Bonow RO: Chronic aortic regurgitation. In Alpert JS, Dalen JE, Rahimtoola SH (eds): Valvular Heart Disease. 3rd ed. Philadelphia, Lippincott Williams & Wilkins, 2000, pp 245-268.

99. Rigolin VH, Bonow RO: Hemodynamic characteristics and progression to heart failure in regurgitant lesions. Heart Failure Clinics 2:453, 2007.

100. Borer JS, Truter S, Herrold EM, et al: Myocardial fibrosis in chronic aortic regurgitation: Molecular and cellular responses to volume overload. Circulation 105:1837, 2002.

101. Otto CM: Aortic regurgitation. In Otto CM (ed): Valvular Heart Disease. 2nd ed. Philadelphia, Saunders, 2004, pp 302-335.

102. Borer JS, Bonow RO: Contemporary approach to aortic and mitral regurgitation. Circulation 108:2432, 2003.

103. Tribouilloy CM, Enriquez-Sarano M, Bailey KR, et al: Assessment of severity of aortic regurgitation using the width of the vena contracta: A clinical color Doppler imaging study. Circulation 102:558, 2000.

104. Willett DL, Hall SA, Jessen ME, et al: Assessment of aortic regurgitation by trans-esophageal color Doppler imaging of the vena contracta: Validation against an intraoperative aortic flow probe. J Am Coll Cardiol 37:1450, 2001.

105. Zoghbi WA, Enriquez-Sarano M, Foster E, et al: Recommendations for evaluation of the severity of native valvular regurgitation with two-dimensional and Doppler echocardiography. J Am Soc Echocardiogr 16:777, 2003.

106. Gelfand EV, Hughes S, Hauser TH, et al: Severity of mitral and aortic regurgitation as assessed by cardiovascular magnetic resonance: optimizing correlation with Doppler echocardiography. J Cardiovasc Magn Reson 8:503, 2006.

107. Enriquez-Sarano M, Tajik AJ: Clinical practice: aortic regurgitation. N Engl J Med 351:1539, 2004.

108. Bonow RO, Cheitlin M, Crawford M, Douglas PS: 36th Bethesda Conference: Recommendations for Determining Eligibility for Competition in Athletes with Cardiovascular Abnormalties. Task Force 3: Valvular Heart Disease. J Am Coll Cardiol 14:1334, 2005.

109. Scognamiglio R, Rahimtoola SH, Fasoli G, et al: Nifedipine in asymptomatic patients with severe aortic regurgitation and normal left ventricular function. N Engl J Med 331:689, 1994.

110. Evangelista A, Tornos P, Sambola A, Permanyer-Miralda G, Soler-Soler J: Long-term vasodilator therapy in patients with severe aortic regurgitation. N Engl J Med 353:1342, 2005.

111. Borer JS: Aortic valve replacement for the asymptomatic patient with aortic regurgitation: A new piece of the strategic puzzle. Circulation 106:2637, 2002.

112. Tornos P, Sambola A, Permanyer-Miralda G, Evangelista A, Gomez Z, Soler-Soler J: Long-term outcome of surgically treated aortic regurgitation: influence of guideline adherence toward early surgery. J Am Coll Cardiol 47:1012, 2006.

113. Chaliki HP, Mohty D, Avierinos JF, et al: Outcomes after aortic valve replacement in patients with severe aortic regurgitation and markedly reduced left ventricular function. Circulation 106:2687, 2002.

114. Casselman FP, Gillinov AM, Akhrass R, et al: Intermediate-term durability of bicuspid aortic valve repair for prolapsing leaflet. Eur J Cardiothorac Surg 15:302, 1999.

115. David TE, Armstrong S, Ivanov J, et al: Results of aortic valve-sparing operations. J Thorac Cardiovasc Surg 122:39, 2001.

116. Minakata K, Schaff HV, Zehr KJ, et al: Is repair of aortic valve regurgitation a safe alternative to valve replacement? J Thorac Cardiovasc Surg 127:645, 2004.

117. Burkhart HM, Zehr KJ, Schaff HV, et al: Valve-preserving aortic root reconstruction: A comparison of techniques. J Heart Valve Dis 12:62, 2003.

118. David TE, Ivanov J, Armstrong S, et al: Aortic valve-sparing operations in patients with aneurysms of the aortic root or ascending aorta. Ann Thorac Surg 74:S1758, 2002.

119. Alpert JS: Acute aortic insufficiency. In Alpert JS, Dalen JE, Rahimtoola SH (eds): Valvular Heart Disease. 3rd ed. Philadelphia, Lippincott Williams & Wilkins, 2000, pp 269-289.

Mitral Stenosis

120. Rahimtoola SH, Durairaj A, Mehra A, et al: Current evaluation and management of patients with mitral stenosis. Circulation 106:1183, 2002.

121. Filgner CL, Reichenbach DD, Otto CM: Pathology and etiology of valvular heart disease. In Otto CM (ed): Valvular Heart Disease. 2nd ed. Philadelphia, Saunders, 2004, pp 30-33.

122. Rajamannan NM, Nealis TB, Subramaniam M, et al: Calcified rheumatic valve neoangiogenesis is associated with vascular endothelial growth factor expression and osteoblast-like bone formation. Circulation 111:3296, 2005.

123. Dalen JE, Fenster PE: Mitral stenosis. In Alpert JS, Dalen JE, Rahimtoola SH (eds): Valvular Heart Disease. 3rd ed. Philadelphia, Lippincott Williams & Wilkins, 2000. pp 75-83.

124. Grossman W: Profiles in valvular heart disease. In Baim DS, Grossman W (eds): Cardiac Catheterization, Angiography and Interventions. 6th ed. Baltimore, Lippincott Williams & Wilkins, 2000.

125. Otto CM: Mitral stenosis. In Otto CM (ed): Valvular Heart Disease. 2nd ed. Philadelphia, Saunders, 2004, pp 252-255.

126. Hernandez R, Banuelos C, Alfonso F, et al: Long-term clinical and echocardiographic follow-up after percutaneous mitral valvuloplasty with the Inoue balloon. Circulation 99:1580, 1999.

127. Iung B, Garbarz E, Michaud P, et al: Late results of percutaneous mitral commissurotomy in a series of 1024 patients. Analysis of late clinical deterioration: frequency, anatomic findings, and predictive factors. Circulation 99:3272, 1999.

128. Shaw TR, Sutaria N, Prendergast B: Clinical and haemodynamic profiles of young, middle aged, and elderly patients with mitral stenosis undergoing mitral balloon valvotomy. Heart 89:1430, 2003.

129. Sagie A, Freitas N, Padial LR, et al: Doppler echocardiographic assessment of long-term progression of mitral stenosis in 103 patients: Valve area and right heart disease. J Am Coll Cardiol 28:472, 1996.

130. Gordon SP, Douglas PS, Come PC, et al: Two-dimensional and Doppler echocardiographic determinants of the natural history of mitral valve narrowing in patients with rheumatic mitral stenosis: implications for follow-up. J Am Coll Cardiol 19:968, 1992.

131. Carabello BA: Modern management of mitral stenosis. Circulation 112:432, 2005.

132. Fuster V, Rydén LE, Cannom DS, et al: ACC/AHA/ESC 2006 Guidelines for the Management of Patients With Atrial Fibrillation-Executive Summary: A Report of the American College of Cardiology/American Heart Association Task Force on Practice Guidelines and the European Society of Cardiology Committee for Practice Guidelines (Writing Committee to Revise the 2001 Guidelines for the Management of Patients With Atrial Fibrillation): Developed in Collaboration With the European Heart Rhythm Association and the Heart Rhythm Society. Circulation 114:700, 2006.

133. Abreu Filho CAC, Lisboa LA, Dallan LA: Effectiveness of the maze procedure using cooled-tip radiofrequency ablation in patients with permanent atrial fibrillation and rheumatic mitral valve disease. Circulation 112 (suppl I):I-20, 2005.

134. Doukas G, Samani NJ, Alexiou C, et al: Left atrial radiofrequency ablation during mitral valve surgery for continuous atrial fibrillation: a randomized controlled trial. JAMA 294:2323, 2005.

135. Krasuski RA, Assar MD, Wang A, et al: Usefulness of percutaneous balloon mitral commissurotomy in preventing the development of atrial fibrillation in patients with mitral stenosis. Am J Cardiol 93:936, 2004.

136. Kang DH, Park SW, Song JK, et al: Long-term clinical and echocardiographic outcome of percutaneous mitral valvuloplasty: Randomized comparison of Inoue and double-balloon techniques. J Am Coll Cardiol 35:169, 2000.

137. Palacios IF, Sanchez PL, Harrell LC, et al: Which patients benefit from percutaneous mitral balloon valvuloplasty? Prevalvuloplasty and postvalvuloplasty variables that predict long-term outcome. Circulation 105:1465, 2002.

138. Iung B, Garbarz E, Michaud P, et al: Percutaneous mitral commissurotomy for restenosis after surgical commissurotomy: Late efficacy and implications for patient selection. J Am Coll Cardiol 35:1295, 2000.

139. de Souza JAM, Martinez EE, Ambrose JA, et al: Percutaneous balloon mitral valvuloplasty in comparison with open mitral mitral valve commissurotomy for mitral stenosis during pregnancy. J Am Coll Cardiol 37:900, 2001.

140. Cribier A, Elchaninoff H, Koning R, et al: Percutaneous mechanical mitral commissurotomy with a newly designed metallic valvulotome: Immediate results of the initial experience in 153 patients. Circulation 99:793, 1999.

141. Gomez-Hospital JA, Cequier A, Romero PV, et al: Partial improvement in pulmonary function after successful percutaneous balloon mitral valvotomy. Chest 117:643, 2000.

142. Iung B, Cormier B, Ducimetiere P, et al: Functional results 5 years after successful percutaneous mitral commissurotomy in a series of 528 patients and analysis of predictive factors. J Am Coll Cardiol 27:407, 1996.

143. Otto CM: Surgical and percutaneous intervention for mitral stenosis. In Otto CM (ed): Valvular Heart Disease. 2nd ed. Philadelphia, Saunders, 2004, pp 272-276.

144. Ben Farhat M, Ayari M, Maatzouk F, et al: Percutaneous balloon versus surgical closed and open mitral commissurotomy: Seven-year follow-up results of a randomized trial. Circulation 97:245, 1998.

145. Ben Farhat M, Betbout F, Gamra H, et al: Predictors of long-term event-free survival and of freedom from restenosis after percutaneous balloon mitral commissurotomy. Am Heart J 142:1072, 2001.

146. Cotrufo M, Renzulli A, Ismeno G, et al: Percutaneous mitral commissurotomy versus open mitral commissurotomy: a comparative study. Eur J Cardiothorac Surg 15:646, 1999.

Mitral Regurgitation

147. Otto CM: Evaluation and management of chronic mitral regurgitation. N Engl J Med 345:740, 2001.

148. Sachdev M, Miller WC, Ryan T, Jollis JG: Effect of fenfluramine-derivative diet pills on cardiac valves: a meta-analysis of observational studies. Am Heart J 144:1065, 2002.

149. Van CG, Flamez A, Cosyns B, et al: Treatment of Parkinson's disease with pergolide and relation to restrictive valvular heart disease. Lancet 363:1179, 2004.

150. Schade R, Andersohn F, Suissa S, et al: Dopamine agonists and the risk of cardiac-valve regurgitation. N Engl J Med 356:29, 2007.

151. Zanettini R, Antonini A, Gatto G, et al: Valvular heart disease and the use of dopamine agonists for the treatment of Parkinson's disease. N Engl J Med 356:39, 2007.

152. Feindel CM, Tufail Z, David TE, et al: Mitral valve surgery in patients with extensive calcification of the mitral annulus. J Thorac Cardiovasc Surg 126:777, 2003.

153. Barber JE, Ratliff NB, Cosgrove DM, et al: Myxomatous mitral valve chordae. I: Mechanical properties. J Heart Valve Dis 10:320, 2001.

154. Pierard LA, Lancellotti P: The role of ischemic mitral regurgitation in the pathogenesis of pulmonary edema. N Engl J Med 351:1627, 2004.

155. Kumanohoso T, Otsuji Y, Yoshifuku S, et al: Mechanism of higher incidence of ischemic mitral regurgitation in patients with inferior myocardial infarction: quantitative analysis of left ventricular and mitral valve geometry in 103 patients with prior myocardial infarction. J Thorac Cardiovasc Surg 125:135, 2003.

156. Kwan J, Shiota T, Agler DA, et al: Geometric differences of the mitral apparatus between ischemic and dilated cardiomyopathy with significant mitral regurgitation: real-time three-dimensional echocardiography study. Circulation 107:1135, 2003.

157. Levine RA: Dynamic mitral regurgitation—more than meets the eye. N Engl J Med 351:1681, 2004.

158. Levine RA, Schwammenthal E: Ischemic mitral regurgitation on the threshold of a solution: from paradoxes to unifying concepts. Circulation 112:745, 2005.

159. Thourani VH, Weintraub WS, Guyton RA, et al: Outcomes and long-term survival for patients undergoing mitral valve repair versus replacement: Effect of age and concomitant coronary artery bypass grafting. Circulation 108:298, 2003.

160. Dahlberg PS, Orszulak TA, Mullany CJ, et al: Late outcome of mitral valve surgery for patients with coronary artery disease. Ann Thorac Surg 76:1539, 2003.

161. Grigioni F, Enriquez-Sarano M, Zehr KJ, et al: Ischemic mitral regurgitation: long-term outcome and prognostic implications with quantitative Doppler assessment. Circulation 103:1759, 2001.

162. Bursi F, Enriquez-Sarano M, Nkomo VT, et al: Heart failure and death after myocardial infarction in the community: the emerging role of mitral regurgitation. Circulation 111:295, 2005.

163. Carabello BA: Concentric versus eccentric remodeling. J Card Fail 8 (suppl):S258, 2002.

164. Sutton TM, Stewart RAH, Gerber IL, et al: Plasma natriuretic peptide levels increase with symptoms and severity of mitral regurgitation. J Am Coll Cardiol 41:2280, 2003.

165. Tallaj J, Hankes GH, Holland M, et al: Beta1-adrenergic receptor blockade attenuates angiotensin II-mediated catecholamine release into the cardiac interstitium in mitral regurgitation. Circulation 108:225, 2003.

166. Oral H, Sivasubramanian N, Dyke DB, et al: Myocardial proinflammatory cytokine expression and left ventricular remodeling in patients with chronic mitral regurgitation. Circulation 107:831, 2003.

167. Timmis SB, Kirsh MM, Montgomery DG, Starling MR: Evaluation of left ventricular ejection fraction as a measure of pump performance in patients with chronic mitral regurgitation. Cathet Cardiovasc Intervent 49:290, 2000.

168. Enriquez-Sarano M, Schaff HV, Tajik AJ, et al: Chronic mitral regurgitation. In Alpert JS, Dalen JE, Rahimtoola SH (eds): Valvular Heart Disease. 3rd ed. Philadelphia, Lippincott Williams & Wilkins, 2000, pp 113-142.

169. Matsumura T, Ohtaki E, Tanaka K, et al: Echocardiographic prediction of left ventricular dysfunction after mitral valve repair for mitral regurgitation as an indicator to decide the optimal timing of repair. J Am Coll Cardiol 42:458, 2003.

170. Flemming MA, Oral H, Rothman ED, et al: Echocardiographic markers for mitral valve surgery to preserve left ventricular performance in mitral regurgitation. Am Heart J 140:476, 2000.

171. Heinle SK, Grayburn PA: Doppler echocardiographic assessment of mitral regurgitation. Coron Artery Dis 11:11, 2000.

172. Enriquez-Sarano M, Avierinos JF, Messika-Zeitoun D, et al: Quantitative determinants of the outcome of asymptomatic mitral regurgitation. N Engl J Med 352:875, 2005.

173. Pu M, Thomas JD, Vandervoort PM, et al: Comparison of quantitative and semi-quantitative methods for assessing regurgitation by transesophageal echocardiography. Am J Cardiol 87:66, 2001.

174. Armstrong GP, Griffin BP: Exercise echocardiographic assessment in severe mitral regurgitation. Coron Artery Dis 11:23, 2000.

175. Lim E, Barlow CW, Hosseinpour AR, et al: Influence of atrial fibrillation on outcome following mitral valve repair. Circulation 104:I-59, 2001.

176. Grigioni F, Avierinos JF, Ling LH, et al: Atrial fibrillation complicating the course of degenerative mitral regurgitation: determinants and long-term outcome. J Am Coll Cardiol 40:84, 2002.

177. Bando K, Kasegawa H, Okada Y, et al: Impact of preoperative and postoperative atrial fibrillation on outcome after mitral valvuloplasty for nonischemic mitral regurgitation. J Thorac Cardiovasc Surg 129:1032, 2005.

178. Eguchi K, Ohtaki E, Matsumura T, et al: Pre-operative atrial fibrillation as the key determinant of outcome of mitral valve repair for degenerative mitral regurgitation. Eur Heart J 26:1866, 2005.

179. Rosenhek R, Rader F, Klaar U, et al: Outcome of watchful waiting in asymptomatic severe mitral regurgitation. Circulation 113:2238, 2006.

180. Nemoto S, Hamawaki M, De Freitas G, et al: Differential effects of the angiotensin-converting enzyme inhibitor lisinopril versus the beta-adrenergic receptor blocker atenolol on hemodynamics and left ventricular contractile function in experimental mitral regurgitation. J Am Coll Cardiol 40:149, 2002.

181. Perry GJ, Wei CC, Hankes GH, et al: Angiotensin II receptor blockade does not improve left ventricular function and remodeling in subacute mitral regurgitation in the dog. J Am Coll Cardiol 39:1374, 2002.

182. DiGregorio V, Zehr KJ, Orszulak TA, et al: Results of mitral surgery in octogenarians with isolated nonrheumatic mitral regurgitation. Ann Thorac Surg 78:807, 2004.

183. Nagendran J, Norris C, Maitland A, et al: Is mitral valve surgery safe in octogenarians? Eur J Cardiothorac Surg 28:83, 2005.

184. Nowicki ER, Birkmeyer NJ, Weintraub RW, et al: Multivariable prediction of in-hospital mortality associated with aortic and mitral valve surgery in Northern New England. Ann Thorac Surg 77:1966, 2004.

185. Goodney PP, O'Connor GT, Wennberg DE, Birkmeyer JD: Do hospitals with low mortality rates in coronary artery bypass also perform well in valve replacement? Ann Thorac Surg 76:1131, 2003.

186. Gillinov AM, Cosgrove DM, Blackstone EH, et al: Durability of mitral valve repair for degenerative disease. J Thorac Cardiovasc Surg 116:734, 1998.

187. Braunberger E, Deloche A, Berregi A, et al: Very long-term results (more than 20 years) of valve repair with Carpentier's techniques in nonrheumatic mitral valve insufficiency. Circulation 104:I-8, 2001.

188. Mohty D, Orszulak TA, Schaff HV, et al: Very long-term survival and durability of mitral valve repair for mitral valve prolapse. Circulation 104:I-1, 2001.

189. Chauvand S, Fuzellier JF, Berrebi A, et al: Long-term (29 years) results of reconstructive surgery in rheumatic mitral valve insufficiency. Circulation 104:I-12, 2001.

190. Phillips MR, Daly RC, Schaff HV, et al: Repair of anterior leaflet mitral valve prolapse: Chordal replacement versus chordal shortening. Ann Thorac Surg 69:25, 2000.

191. De Bonis M, Lorusso R, Lapenna E, et al: Similar long-term results of mitral valve repair for anterior compated with posterior leaflet prolapse. J Thorac Cardiovasc Surg 131:364, 2006.

192. Bishay ES, McCarthy PM, Cosgrove DM, et al: Mitral valve surgery in patients with severe left ventricular dysfunction. Eur J Cardiothorac Surg 17:213, 2000.

193. von Oppell UO, Stemmet F, Braink J, et al: Ischemic mitral valve repair surgery. J Heart Valve Dis 9:64, 2000.

194. Gillinov AM, Wierup PN, Blackstone EH, et al: Is repair preferable to replacement for ischemic mitral regurgitation? J Thorac Cardioavasc Surg 122:1125, 2001.

195. Prifti E, Bonacchi M, Frati G, et al: Ischemic mitral valve regurgitation grade II-III: correction in patients with impaired left ventricular function undergoing simultaneous coronary revascularization. J Heart Valve Dis 10:754, 2001.

196. Lam BK, Gillinov AM, Blackstone EH, et al: Importance of moderate ischemic mitral regurgitation. Ann Thorac Surg 79:462, 2005.

197. Bax JJ, Braun J, Somer ST, et al: Restrictive annuloplasty and coronary revascularization in ischemic mitral regurgitation results in reverse left ventricular remodeling. Circulation 110(suppl II):II-103, 2004.

198. Schroder JN, Williams ML, Hata JA, et al: Impact of mitral regurgitation evaluated by intraoperative echocardiography on long-term outcomes after coronary artery bypass grafting. Circulation 112 (suppl I):I-293, 2005.

199. Click RL, Schaff HV: Intraoperative transesophageal echocardiography: 5-year prospective review of impact on surgical management. Mayo Clin Proc 75:241, 2000.

200. Nakajima H, Kobayashi J, Bando K, et al: The effect of cryo-maze procedure on early and intermediate term outcome in mitral valve disease: Case matched study. Circulation 106:I-46, 2002.

201. Remadi JP, Baron O, Roussel C, et al: Isolated mitral valve replacement with St. Jude medical prosthesis. Long-term results: A follow-up of 19 years. Circulation 103:1542, 2001.

202. Society of Thoracic Surgeons National Cardiac Surgery Database. http://www.sts.org/documents/pdf/STS-ExecutiveSummaryFall2006.pdf. Accessed December 20, 2006.

203. Savage EB, Ferguson TB, DiSesa VJ: Use of mitral valve repair: analysis of contemporary United States experience reported to the Society of Thoracic Surgeons National Cardiac Database. Ann Thorac Surg 75:820, 2003.

204. Flameng W, Herijgers P, Bogaerts K: Recurrence of mitral valve regurgitation after mitral valve repair in degenerative valve disease. Circulation 107:1609, 2003.

205. Bridgewater B, Hooper T, Munsch C, et al: Mitral repair best practice: proposed standards. Heart 92:939, 2006.

206. Greelish JP, Cohn LH, Leacche M, et al: Minimally invasive mitral valve repair suggests earlier operations for mitral valve disease. J Thorac Cardiovasc Surg 126:365, 2003.

207. Dogan S, Aybek T, Risteski P, et al: Minimally invasive port access versus conventional mitral valve surgery: prospective randomized study. Ann Thorac Surg 79:492, 2005.

208. Vassiliades TA Jr, Block PC, Cohn LH, et al: The clinical development of percutaneous heart valve technology. A position statement of the Society of Thoracic Surgeons, the American Association for Thoracic surgery, and the Society for Cardiovascular Angiography and Intervention. Endorsed by the American College of Cardiology Foundation and the American Heart Association. J Am Coll Cardiol 45:1554, 2005.

209. Feldman T, Wasserman HS, Herrmann HC, et al: Percutaneous mitral valve repair using the edge-to-edge technique: six month results of the EVEREST Phase I clinical trial. J Am Coll Cardiol 46:2134, 2005.

210. Maisano F, Caldarola A, Blasio A, De Bonis M, La Canna G, Alfieri O: Midterm results of edge-to-edge mitral valve repair without annuloplasty. J Thorac Cardiovasc Surg 126:1987, 2003.

211. Webb JG, Harnek J, Munt BI, et al: Percutaneous transvenous mitral annuloplasty: initial human experience with device implantation in the coronary sinus. Circulation 113:851, 2006.

212. Iung B, Rousseau-Paziaud J, Cormier B, et al: Contemporary results of mitral valve repair for infective endocarditis. J Am Coll Cardiol 43:386, 2004.

213. Gillinov AM, Faber C, Houghtaling PL, et al: Repair versus replacement for degenerative mitral valve disease with coexisting ischemic heart disease. J Thorac Cardioavasc Surg 125:1197, 2003.

214. Tavakoli R, Weber A, Vogt P, et al: Surgical management of acute mitral valve regurgitation due to post-infarction papillary muscle rupture. J Heart Valve Dis 11:20, 2002.

215. Zegdi R, Debieche M, Latremouille C, et al: Long-term results of mitral valve repair in active endocarditis. Circulation 111:2532, 2005.

Mitral Valve Prolapse Syndrome

216. O'Rourke RA: Syndrome of mitral valve prolapse. In Alpert JS, Dalen JE, Rahimtoola SH (eds): Valvular Heart Disease. 3rd ed. Philadelphia, Lippincott Williams & Wilkins, 2000, pp 157-182.

217. Otto CM: Mitral valve prolapse. In Otto CM (ed): Valvular Heart Disease. 2nd ed. Philadelphia, Saunders, 2004, pp 368-387.

218. Freed LA, Levy D, Levine RA, et al: Prevalence and clinical outcome of mitral-valve prolapse. N Engl J Med 241:341, 1999.

219. Freed LA, Benjamin EJ, Levy D, et al: Mitral valve prolapse in the general population : The benign nature of the echocardiographic features in the Framingham Heart Study. J Am Call Cardiol 40:1298, 2002.

220. Disse S, Abergel E, Berrebi A, et al: Mapping of a first locus for autosomal dominant myxomatous mitral-valve prolapse to chromosome 16p11.2-p12.1. Am J Hum Genet 65:1242, 1999.

221. Freed LA, Acierno JS Jr, Dai D, et al: A locus for autosomal dominant mitral valve prolapse on chromosome 11p15.4. Am J Hum Genet 72:1551, 2003.

222. Nesta F, Leyne M, Yosefy C, et al: New locus for autosomal dominant mitral valve prolapse on chromosome 13: clinical insights from genetic studies. Circulation 112:2022, 2005.

223. Becker AE, Davies MJ: Pathomorphology of mitral valve prolapse. In Boudoulas H, Wooley CF (eds): Mitral Valve: Floppy Mitral Valve, Mitral Valve Prolapse, Mitral Valvular Regurgitation. 2nd ed. Armonk, NY, Futura, 2000, pp 91-114.

224. Grande-Allen KJ, Griffin BP, Calabro A, et al: Myxomatous mitral valve chordae. II: Selective elevation of glycosaminoglycan content. J Heart Valve Dis 10:325, 2001.

225. Mylonakis E, Calderwood SB: Infective endocarditis in adults N Engl J Med 345:1318, 2001.

226. Hayek E, Gring CN, Griffin BP. Mitral valve prolapse. Lancet 365:507, 2005.

227. Fontana MF: Mitral valve prolapse and floppy mitral valve: Physical examination. In Boudoulas H, Wooley CF (eds): Mitral Valve: Floppy Mitral Valve, Mitral Valve Prolapse, Mitral Valvular Regurgitation. 2nd ed. Armonk, NY, Futura, 2000, pp 283-304.

228. Malkowski MJ, Pearson AC: The echocardiographic assessment of the floppy mitral valve: An integrated approach. In Boudoulas H, Wooley CF (eds): Mitral Valve: Floppy Mitral Valve, Mitral Valve Prolapse, Mitral Valvular Regurgitation. 2nd ed. Armonk, NY, Futura, 2000, pp 231-252.

229. Kim S, Kuroda T, Nishinaga M, et al: Relationship between severity of mitral regurgitation and prognosis of mitral valve prolapse: echocardiographic follow-up study. Am Heart J 132:348, 1996.

230. Schaal SF: Mitral valve prolapse: Cardiac arrhythmias and electrophysiological correlates. In Boudoulas H, Wooley CF (eds): Mitral Valve: Floppy Mitral Valve, Mitral Valve Prolapse, Mitral Valvular Regurgitation. 2nd ed. Armonk, NY, Futura, 2000, pp 409-430.

231. Boudoulas H, Kolibash AJ, Wooley CF: Floppy mitral valve, mitral valve prolapse, mitral valvular regurgitation: Natural history. In Boudoulas H, Wooley CF (eds): Mitral Valve: Floppy Mitral Valve, Mitral Valve Prolapse, Mitral Valvular Regurgitation. 2nd ed. Armonk, NY, Futura, 2000, pp 503-540.

232. Avierinos JF, Gersh BJ, Melton LJ, et al: Natural history of asymptomatic mitral valve prolapse in the community. Circulation 106:1355, 2002.

233. Gilon D, Buonanno FS, Joffe MM, et al: Lack of evidence of an association between mitral-valve prolapse and stroke in young patients. N Engl J Med 341:8, 1999.

234. Ling LH, Enriquez-Sarano M: Long-term outcomes of patients with flail mitral valve leaflets. Coron Artery Dis 11:3, 2000.

235. Boudoulas H, Wooley CF: Floppy mitral valve/Mitral valve prolapse: Sudden death. In Boudoulas H, Wooley CF (eds): Mitral Valve: Floppy Mitral Valve, Mitral Valve Prolapse, Mitral Valvular Regurgitation. 2nd ed. Armonk, NY, Futura, 2000, pp 431-448.

236. Corrado D, Basso C, Rizzoli G, et al: Does sports activity enhance the risk of sudden death in adolescents and young adults? J Am Coll Cardiol 42:1959, 2003.

Tricuspid, Pulmonic, and Multivalvular Disease

237. Ewy GA. Tricuspid valve disease. In Alpert JS, Dalen JE, Rahimtoola SH (eds): Valvular Heart Disease. 3rd ed. Philadelphia, Lippincott Williams & Wilkins, 2000. pp 377-392.

238. Møller JE, Connolly HM, Rubin J, et al: Factors associated with progression of carcinoid heart disease. N Engl J Med 348;1005, 2003.

239. Hagers Y, Koole M, Schoors D, Van Camp G: Tricuspid stenosis: A rare complication of pacemaker-related endocarditis. J Am Soc Echocardiogr 13:66, 2000.

240. Heaven DJ, Henein MY, Sutton R: Pacemaker lead related to tricuspid stenosis: A report of two cases. Heart 83:351, 2000.

241. Otto CM: Right-sided valve disease. In Otto CM (ed): Valvular Heart Disease. 2nd ed. Philadelphia, Saunders, 2004, pp. 415-436.

242. Ha JW, Chung N, Jang Y, Rim SJ: Tricuspid stenosis and regurgitation: Doppler and color flow echocardiography and cardiac catheterization findings. Clin Cardiol 23:51, 2000.

243. Del Campo C, Sherman JR: Tricuspid valve replacement: Results comparing mechanical and biological prostheses. Ann Thorac Surg 69:1295, 2000.

244. Simula DV, Edwards WD, Tazelaar HD, et al: Surgical pathology of carcinoid heart disease: A study of 139 valves from 75 patients spanning 20 years. Mayo Clin Proc 77:139, 2002.

245. Naschitz JE, Goldstein L, Zuckerman E, et al: Benign course of congestive cirrhosis associated with tricuspid regurgitation: Does pulsatility protect against complications of venous hypertension? J Clin Gastroenterol 30:213, 2000.

246. Tribouilloy CM, Enriquez-Sarano M, Bailey KR, et al: Quantification of tricuspid regurgitation by measuring the width of the vena contracta with Doppler color flow imaging: A clinical study. J Am Coll Cardiol 36:472, 2000.

247. McCarthy PM, Bhudia SK, Rajeswaran J, et al: Tricuspid valve repair: durability and risk factors for failure. J Thorac Cardiovasc Surg 127:674, 2004.

248. Dreyfus GD, Corbi PJ, Chan KM, Bahrami T: Secondary tricuspid regurgitation or dilatation: which should be the criteria for surgical repair? Ann Thorac Surg 79:127, 2005.

249. Jamieson WRE, Edwards FH, Schwartz M, et al: Risk stratification for cardiac valve replacement. National Cardiac Surgery Database. Ann Thorac Surg 67:943, 1999.

250. Fukuda S, Song JM, Gillinov AM, et al: Tricuspid valve tethering predicts residual tricuspid regurgitation after tricuspid annuloplasty. Circulation 111:975, 2005.

251. Discigil B, Dearani JA, Puga FJ, et al: Late pulmonary valve replacement after repair of tetralogy of Fallot. J Thorac Cardiovasc Surg 121:344, 2001.

252. Buechel ER, Dave HH, Kellenberger CJ, et al: Remodeling of the right ventricle after early pulmonary valve replacement in children with repaired tetralogy of Fallot: assessment by cardiovascular magnetic resonance. Eur Heart J 26:2721, 2005.

253. Therrien J, Provost Y, Merchant N, et al: Optimal timing for pulmonary valve replacement in adults after tetralogy of Fallot repair. Am J Cardiol 95:779, 2005.

254. Connolly HM, Schåff HV, Mullany CJ, et al: Carcinoid heart disease: Impact of pulmonary valve replacement in right ventricular function and remodeling. Circulation 106:I-51, 2002.

255. Khambadkone S, Coats L, Taylor A, et al: Percutaneous pulmonary valve implantation in humans: Results in 59 consecutive patients. Circulation 112:1189, 2005.

256. Coats L, Tsang V, Khambadkone S, et al: The potential impact of percutaneous pulmonary valve stent implantation on right ventricular outflow tract re-intervention. Eur J Cardiothorac Surg 27:536, 2005.

257. Paraskos JA: Combined valve disease. In Alpert JS, Dalen JE, Rahimtoola SH (eds): Valvular Heart Disease. 3rd ed. Philadelphia, Lippincott Williams & Wilkins, 2000, pp 291-337.

258. Gillinov AM, Blackstone EH, Cosgrove DM, et al: Mitral valve repair with aortic valve replacement in superior to double valve replacement. J Thorac Cardiovasc Surg 125:1372, 2003.

260. John S, Ravikumar E, John CN, Bashi VV: 25-year experience with 456 combined mitral and aortic valve replacement for rheumatic heart disease. Ann Thorac Surg 69:1167, 2000.

Prosthetic Cardiac Valves

261. David TE: Is prosthesis-patient mismatch a clinically relevant entity? Circulation 111:3186, 2005.

262. Murday AJ, Hochstitzky A, Mansfield J, et al: A prospective controlled trial of St. Jude versus Starr Edwards aortic and mitral valve prostheses. Ann Thorac Surg 76:66, 2003.

263. Emery RW, Erickson CA, Arom KV, et al: Replacement of the aortic valve in patients under 50 years of age: Long-term follow up of the St. Jude medical prosthesis. Ann Thorac Surg 75:1815, 2003.

264. Grunkemeier GL, Li HH, Naftel DC, et al: Long-term performance of heart valve prostheses. Curr Probl Cardiol 25:73, 2000.

265. Jamieson WR, Fradet GJ, Miyagishima RT, et al: CarboMedics mechanical prosthesis: Performance at eight years. J Heart Valve Dis 9:678, 2000.

266. Rahimtoola SH: Choice of prosthetic heart valve for adult patients. J Am Coll Cardiol 41:893, 2003.

267. Hammermeister KE, Sethi GK, Henderson WG, et al: Outcomes 15 years after valve replacement with a mechanical versus a bioprosthetic valve: Final report of the Veterans Affairs randomized trial. J Am Coll Cardiol 36:1152, 2000.

268. Laffort P, Roudaut R, Roques X, et al: Early and long-term (one-year) effects of the association of aspirin and oral anticoagulant on thrombi and morbidity after replacement of the mitral valve with the St. Jude medical prosthesis: A clinical and transesophageal echocardiographic study. J Am Coll Cardiol 35:739, 2000.

269. Massel D, Little SH: Risks and benefits of adding anti-platelet therapy to Warfarin among patients with prosthetic heart valves: A meta-analysis. J Am Coll Cardiol 37:569, 2001.

CH 62

270. Roudaut R, Lafitte S, Roudaut MF, et al: Fibrinolysis of mechanical prosthetic valve thrombosis: a single-center study of 127 cases. J Am Coll Cardiol 241:653, 2003.

271. Tong AT, Roudaut R, Ozkan M, et al: Transesophageal echocardiography improves risk assessment of thrombolysis of prosthetic valve thrombosis: results of the international PRO-TEE registry. J Am Coll Cardiol 43:77, 2004.

272. Jamieson WRE, Lemieux MD, Sullivan JA, et al: Medtronic intact porcine bioprosthesis experience to twelve years. Ann Thorac Surg 71:S278, 2001.

273. Jamieson WR, David TE, Feindel CM, et al: Performance of the Carpentier-Edwards SAV and Hancock-II porcine bioprostheses in aortic valve replacement. J Heart Valve Dis 11:424, 2002.

274. Nollert G, Miksch J, Kreuzer E, et al: Risk factors for atherosclerosis and the degeneration of pericardial valves after aortic valve replacement. J Thorac Cardiovasc Surg 126:965, 2003.

275. Farivar RS, Cohn LS: Hypercholesterolemia is a risk factor for bioprosthetic valve calcification and explantation. J Thorac Cardiovasc Surg 126:969, 2003.

276. Cohen G, Christakis GT, Joyner CD, et al: Are stentless valves hemodynamically superior to stented valves? A prospective randomized trial. Ann Thorac Surg 73:767, 2002.

277. Halstead JC, Tsui SS: Randomized trial of stentless versus stented bioprostheses for aortic valve replacement. Ann Thorac Surg 76:1338, 2003.

278. Banbury MK, Cosgrove DM, Thomas JD, et al: Hemodynamic stability during 17 years of the Carepentier-Edwards aortic pericardial bioprosthesis. Ann Thorac Surg 73:1460, 2002.

279. Banbury MK, Cosgrove DM, White JA, et al: Age and valve size effect on the long-term durability of the Carpentier-Edwards aortic pericardial bioprosthesis. Ann Thorac Surg 72:753, 2001.

280. Willems TP, Takkenberg JJM, Sterberg WE, et al: Human tissue valves in the aortic position: Determinants of reoperation and valve regurgitation. Circulation 103:1515, 2001.

281. Palka P, Harrocks S, Lange A, et al: Primary aortic valve replacement with cryopreserved aortic allograft: An echocardiographic follow-up study of 570 patients. Circulation 105:61, 2002.

282. Lytle BW, Sabik JF, Blackstone EH, et al: Reoperative cryopreserved root and ascending aorta replacement for acute aortic prosthetic valve endocarditis. Ann Thorac Surg 74:S1754, 2002.

283. Alexiou C, Langley SM, Stafford H, et al: Surgery for active culture-positive endocarditis: determinants of early and late outcome. Ann Thorac Surg 69:1448, 2000.

284. Leyh RG, Knobloch K, Hagl C, et al: Replacement of the aortic root for acute prosthetic valve endocarditis: prosthetic composite versus aortic allograft root replacement. J Thorac Cardiovasc Surg 127:1416, 2004.

285. Aklog L, Carr-White GS, Birks EJ, Yacoub MH: Pulmonary autograft versus aortic homograft for aortic valve replacement: interim results from a prospective randomized trial. J Heart Valve Dis 9:176, 2000.

286. Bohm JO, Botha CA, Hemmer W, et al: Hemodynamic performance following the Ross operation: comparison of two different techniques. J Heart Valve Dis 13:174, 2004.

287. Raja SG, Pozzi M: Ross operation in children and young adults: the Alder Hey case series. BMC Cardiovasc Disord 4:3, 2004.

288. Carr-White GS, Kilner PJ, Hon JK, et al: Incidence, location, pathology, and significance of pulmonary homograft stenosis after the Ross operation. Circulation 104: I-16, 2001.

289. Laforest I, Dumesnil JG, Briand M, et al: Hemodynamic performance at rest and during exercise after aortic replacement: Comparison of pulmonary autografts versus aortic homografts. Circulation 106:I-57, 2002.

290. Carr-White GS, Afoke A, Birks EJ, et al: Aortic root characteristics of human pulmonary autografts. Circulation 102:III-15, 2000.

291. Luciani GB, Casali G, Favaro A, et al: Fate of the aortic root late after Ross operation. Circulation 108:II-61, 2003.

292. Schmidtke C, Bechtel JF, Noetzold A, et al: Up to seven years of experience with the Ross procedure in patients >60 years of age. J Am Coll Cardiol 36:117, 2000.

293. Tasca G, Brunelli F, Cirillo M, et al: Impact of valve prosthesis-patient mismatch on left ventricular mass regression following aortic valve replacement. Ann Thorac Surg 79:505, 2005.

294. Blais C, Dumesnil JG, Baillot R, et al: Impact of valve prosthesis-patient mismatch on short-term mortality after aortic valve replacement. Circulation 108:983, 2003.

295. Pibarot P, Dumesnil JG: Prosthesis-patient mismatch: definition, clinical impact, and prevention. Heart 92:1022, 2006.

296. Seiler C: Management and follow up of prosthetic heart valves. Heart 90:818, 2004.

297. Taylor KM: The Edinburgh heart valve study. Heart 89:697, 2003.

298. Peterseim DS, Cen YY, Cheruvu S, et al: Long-term outcome after biologic versus mechanical aortic valve replacement in 841 patients. J Thorac Cardiovasc Surg 117:890, 1999.

299. Reimold SC, Rutherford JD: Clinical practice. Valvular heart disease in pregnancy. N Engl J Med 349:52, 2003.

300. Ginsberg JS, Chan WS, Bates SM, Kaatz S: Anticoagulation of pregnant women with mechanical heart valves. Arch Intern Med 163:694, 2003.

301. Elkayam U, Bitar F: Valvular heart disease and pregnancy, part II: prosthetic valves. J Am Coll Cardiol 46:403, 2005.

302. Hung L, Rahimtoola SH: Prosthetic heart valves and pregnancy. Circulation 107;1240, 2003.

303. Ansell J, Hirsh J, Poller L, et al: The pharmacology and management of the vitamin K antagonists: the Seventh ACCP Conference on Antithrombotic and Thrombolytic Therapy. Chest 126:204S, 2004.

304. Salem DN, Stein PD, Al Ahmad A, et al: Antithrombotic therapy in valvular heart disease—native and prosthetic: the Seventh ACCP Conference on Antithrombotic and Thrombolytic Therapy. Chest 126:457S, 2004.

305. Spyropoulos AC, Frost FJ, Hurley JS, et al: Costs and clinical outcomes associated with low-molecular-weight heparin vs unfractionated heparin for perioperative bridging in patients receiving long-term oral anticoagulant therapy. Chest 125:1642, 2004.

306. Kovacs MJ, Kearon C, Rodger M, et al: Single-arm study of bridging therapy with low-molecular-weight heparin for patients at risk of arterial embolism who require temporary interruption of warfarin. Circulation 110:1658, 2004.

307. Herzog CA, Ma JZ, Collins AJ: Long-term survival of dialysis patients in the United States with prosthetic heart valves: Should ACC/AHA practice guidelines on valve selection be modified? Circulation105:1336, 2002.

CH 62

Valvular Heart Disease

GUIDELINES   *Thomas H. Lee and Robert O. Bonow*

Management of Valvular Heart Disease

The American College of Cardiology and the American Heart Association (ACC/AHA) first published guidelines for the management of patients with valvular heart disease in 1998.[1] These were updated in 2006.[2] Some material from the 2006 guidelines is presented elsewhere in this book: In addition to the guidelines tables and figures in Chapter 62, guidelines for the prevention and treatment of infective endocarditis are summarized in the appendix to Chapter 63 and guidelines for the management of anticoagulation in pregnancy are included in the appendix to Chapter 77. Other recommendations for valvular heart diseases are included in ACC/AHA guidelines for the use of echocardiography,[3] ACC guidelines for assessment of athletes with cardiovascular abnormalities,[4] and guidelines from the AHA[5] and ACC on cardiovascular assessment of athletes.[4]

The guidelines emphasize that the clinical assessment should be based on the patient's symptomatic status and findings from the physical examination. Cardiac auscultation remains the most widely used method of screening for valvular heart disease. The chest radiograph and electrocardiogram (ECG), if normal, can often provide reassurance that a murmur is clinically insignificant. Echocardiography should be considered after assessment of these more routine data, and the guidelines consider echocardiography to be inappropriate for the evaluation of murmurs that experienced observers consider innocent or functional. In contrast, echocardiography is considered appropriate even in asymptomatic patients with murmurs suggesting significant valvular disease or with other signs or symptoms of cardiovascular disease (Table 62G-1), and there is emphasis on the use of Doppler echocardiography to quantify severity of valvular stenosis and regurgitation (see Table 62-1). In some cases cardiac catheterization and angiography are appropriate (Fig. 62G-1), as is exercise stress testing.

As with other ACC/AHA guidelines, these use the standard ACC/AHA classification system for indications:

Class I: Conditions for which there is evidence and/or general agreement that the test is useful and effective.

Class II: Conditions for which there is conflicting evidence and/or a divergence of opinion about the usefulness/efficacy of performing the test.

Class IIa: Weight of evidence/opinion is in favor of usefulness/efficacy.

Class IIb: Usefulness/efficacy is less well established by evidence/opinion.

Class III: Conditions for which there is evidence and/or general agreement that the test is not useful/effective and in some cases may be harmful.

TABLE 62G–1   ACC/AHA Guidelines for Echocardiography in Patients with a Cardiac Murmur

Class	Indication	Level of Evidence
Class I	Indicated for evaluation of asymptomatic patients with diastolic, continuous, holosystolic, and late systolic murmurs, murmurs associated with ejection clicks or those that radiate to the neck or back	C
	Indicated for evaluation of patients with heart murmurs and symptoms or signs of heart failure, myocardial ischemia/infarction, syncope, thromboembolism, infective endocarditis, or other clinical evidence of structural heart disease	C
	Indicated for evaluation of asymptomatic patients who have grade 3 or louder midpeaking systolic murmurs	C
Class IIa	Useful for the evaluation of asymptomatic patients with murmurs associated with other abnormal cardiac physical findings or murmurs associated with an abnormal electrocardiogram or chest radiograph	C
	Useful for patients whose symptoms and/or signs are likely noncardiac in origin but in whom a cardiac basis cannot be excluded by standard evaluation	C
Class III	Not recommended for patients with grade 2 or softer midsystolic murmurs identified as innocent or functional by an experienced observer	C

ACC/AHA = American College of Cardiology/American Heart Association.

CH 62

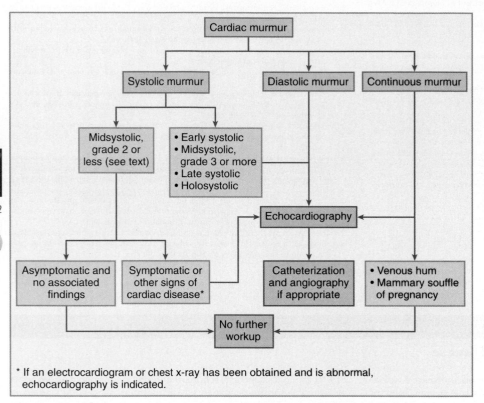

* If an electrocardiogram or chest x-ray has been obtained and is abnormal, echocardiography is indicated.

FIGURE 62G–1 Strategy for evaluating heart murmurs. *(From Bonow RO, Carabello BA, Chatterjee K, et al: ACC/AHA 2006 guidelines for the management of patients with valvular heart disease. J Am Coll Cardiol 48:e1, 2006.)*

Three levels are used to rate the evidence on which recommendations have been based. Level A recommendations are derived from data from multiple randomized clinical trials, level B recommendations are derived from a single randomized trial or nonrandomized studies, and level C recommendations are based on the consensus opinion of experts.

AORTIC STENOSIS

Doppler echocardiography is a highly appropriate test for diagnosis and assessment of aortic stenosis and for evaluation of left ventricular (LV) function in patients with this condition. The guidelines indicate that yearly echocardiograms are helpful for management of asymptomatic patients with severe aortic stenosis but recommend intervals of 1 to 2 years for asymptomatic patients with moderate aortic steno-sis and 3 to 5 years for those with mild aortic stenosis (Table 62G-2). For patients with severe aortic stenosis and low cardiac output (low-flow/low-gradient aortic steno-sis), dobutamine stress echocardiography may be a reasonable tool for evaluation.

Exercise testing of asymptomatic patients can be performed safely and may be a reasonable approach for eliciting symptoms, but it should not be performed in symptomatic patients. The guidelines stress that an experienced physician should supervise exercise tests for patients with aortic stenosis and closely monitor blood pressure and the ECG. Physical activity should not be restricted in asymptomatic patients with mild aortic stenosis. However, the Task Force on Acquired Valvular Heart Disease of the 26th Bethesda Conference recommended that patients with mild to moderate aortic stenosis avoid competitive sports with high dynamic and static muscular demands.[4]

Cardiac Catheterization. The ACC/AHA guidelines consider coronary angiography to be appropriate in patients with possible coronary artery disease, and catheterization may be necessary to assess the hemodynamic severity of stenosis in symptomatic patients when other data are not conclusive (see Table 62G-2). Catheterization is discouraged solely for the purposes of confirming information available from noninvasive tests or assessing LV function and severity of aortic stenosis in asymptomatic patients. Cardiac catheterization with infusion of dobutamine may be useful for hemodynamic evaluation in patients with low-flow/low-gradient aortic stenosis and LV dysfunction.

Aortic Valve Replacement. This procedure is considered in virtually all symptomatic patients with severe aortic stenosis, and the ACC/AHA guidelines are generally supportive (Class IIa) of this procedure for patients with moderate disease who were undergoing coronary artery bypass grafting (CABG) or surgery on the aorta or other heart valves. The guidelines are less supportive of aortic valve replacement in patients who were asymptomatic despite severe aortic stenosis (see Table 62G-2). Aortic balloon valvotomy was given qualified support as a "bridge" to surgery in hemodynamically unstable patients who could not undergo immediate aortic valve replacement or as palliation in those who cannot undergo valve replacement. It is not recommended as an alternative to aortic valve replacement except in the case

TABLE 62G–2	ACC/AHA Guidelines for Management of Patients with Aortic Valve Stenosis			
Indication	**Class I (Indicated)**	**Class IIa (Strong Supportive Evidence)**	**Class IIb (Weak Supportive Evidence)**	**Class III (Not Indicated)**
Echocardiography	For the diagnosis and assessment of AS severity **(B)** In patients with AS for the assessment of LV wall thickness, size, and function **(B)** For reevaluation of patients with known AS and changing symptoms or signs **(B)** For the assessment of changes in hemodynamic severity and LV function in patients with known AS during pregnancy **(B)** Transthoracic echocardiography is recommended for re-evaluation of asymptomatic patients: every year for severe AS; every 1 to 2 years for moderate AS; and every 3 to 5 years for mild AS **(B)**			
Exercise testing			May be considered in asymptomatic patients with AS to elicit exercise-induced symptoms and abnormal blood pressure responses **(B)**	Should not be performed in symptomatic patients with AS **(B)**
Cardiac catheterization	Coronary angiography is recommended before AVR in patients with AS at risk for CAD **(B)** Cardiac catheterization for hemodynamic measurements is recommended for assessment of severity of AS in symptomatic patients when noninvasive tests are inconclusive or when there is a discrepancy between noninvasive tests and clinical findings regarding severity of AS **(C)** Coronary angiography is recommended before AVR in patients with AS for whom a pulmonary autograft (Ross procedure) is contemplated and if the origin of the coronary arteries was not identified by noninvasive technique **(C)**			Not recommended for hemodynamic measurements for the assessment of severity of AS before AVR when noninvasive tests are adequate and concordant with clinical findings **(C)** Not recommended for hemodynamic measurements for the assessment of LV function and severity of AS in asymptomatic patients **(C)**
Low-flow/low-gradient aortic stenosis		Dobutamine stress echocardiography is reasonable for evaluation of patients with low-flow/low-gradient AS and LV dysfunction **(B)** Cardiac catheterization for hemodynamic measurements with infusion of dobutamine can be useful for evaluation of patients with low-flow/low-gradient AS and LV dysfunction **(B)**		

Continues

TABLE 62G–2 ACC/AHA Guidelines for Management of Patients with Aortic Valve Stenosis—cont'd

Indication	Class I (Indicated)	Class IIa (Strong Supportive Evidence)	Class IIb (Weak Supportive Evidence)	Class III (Not Indicated)
Aortic valve replacement	Indicated for symptomatic patients with severe AS **(B)** Indicated for patients with severe AS undergoing CABG **(C)** Indicated for patients with severe AS undergoing surgery on the aorta or other heart valves **(C)** Recommended for patients with severe AS and LV systolic dysfunction (ejection fraction <0.50) **(C)**	Reasonable for patients with moderate AS undergoing CABG or surgery on the aorta or other heart valves **(B)**	May be considered for asymptomatic patients with severe AS and abnormal response to exercise **(C)** May be considered for adults with severe asymptomatic AS and a high likelihood of rapid progression or if surgery might be delayed at the time of symptom onset **(C)** May be considered in patients undergoing CABG who have mild AS and evidence that progression may be rapid **(C)** May be considered for asymptomatic patients with extremely severe AS (aortic valve area <0.6 cm², mean gradient >60 mm Hg, and jet velocity >5 m/sec) if the expected operative mortality is ≤1% **(C)**	Not useful for the prevention of sudden death in asymptomatic patients with AS who have none of the findings listed under the Class IIa/IIb recommendations **(B)**
Aortic balloon valvotomy			May be reasonable as a bridge to surgery in hemodynamically unstable adult patients with AS who are at high risk for AVR **(C)** May be reasonable for palliation in adult patients with AS in whom AVR cannot be performed because of serious comorbid conditions **(C)**	Not recommended as an alternative to AVR in adult patients with AS; certain younger adults without valve calcification may be an exception **(B)**

ACC/AHA = American College of Cardiology/American Heart Association; AS = aortic stenosis; AVR = aortic valve replacement; CABG = coronary artery bypass grafting; CAD = coronary artery disease; LV = left ventricular.

CH 62

of some younger patients with congenital aortic stenosis without valve calcification.

AORTIC REGURGITATION

Doppler echocardiography is a highly appropriate test for the diagnosis and serial assessment of patients with aortic regurgitation (Table 62G-3). Serial echocardiography is indicated to periodically evaluate LV size and function in asymptomatic patients with severe aortic regurgitation and to re-evaluate aortic regurgitation in patients with new or changing symptoms to ensure that rapid progression is not under way. Asymptomatic patients with mild aortic regurgitation, normal LV function, and little or no LV dilation can be seen on an annual basis, and echocardiography can be performed every 2 to 3 years in the absence of changes in symptoms. However, the guidelines support echocardiography every 6 to 12 months for patients with severe aortic regurgitation and significant LV dilation, such as end-diastolic dimension greater than 60 mm. For patients with even more advanced LV dilation, echocardiography as often as every 3 months is endorsed.

Exercise testing is considered appropriate for assessment of functional capacity in patients in whom the history is not definitive, but the impact of this test on management is not otherwise strongly supported by the ACC/AHA guidelines. Cardiac magnetic resonance

(CMR) is reasonable for estimating severity of aortic regurgitation and LV volume and function in patients with equivocal echocardiograms. Radionuclide angiography is less positively endorsed as an alternative to echocardiography for assessment of LV volume and function. The ACC/AHA guidelines emphasize that there is no need for serial testing with both technologies.

Medical Therapy. The ACC/AHA guidelines consider vasodilator therapy appropriate in patients with hypertension or LV dysfunction, even those who are asymptomatic. However, the guidelines do not endorse long-term vasodilator therapy in normotensive patients with normal LV function and mild aortic regurgitation and emphasize that vasodilator therapy is not an alternative to surgery for patients who are appropriate candidates for valve replacement.

Cardiac Catheterization. Cardiac catheterization is not routinely needed to confirm the diagnosis or assess the severity of aortic regurgitation when echocardiographic studies are adequate. The most common appropriate indication for cardiac catheterization is the performance of coronary angiography as a prelude to surgery.

Aortic Valve Replacement. The ACC/AHA guidelines deem aortic valve replacement to be clearly appropriate in patients with severe (New York Heart Association [NYHA] Class III or IV) symptoms, progressive LV dilation, mild to moderate LV dysfunction, or declining exercise tolerance (see Table 62G-3). The guidelines were not supportive of surgery solely because of a decline in ejection fraction during

TABLE 62G–3	ACC/AHA Guidelines for Management of Patients with Aortic Regurgitation (AR)			
Indication	Class I (Indicated)	Class IIa (Strong Supportive Evidence)	Class IIb (Weak Supportive Evidence)	Class III (Not Indicated)
Echocardiography	Indicated to confirm the presence and severity of acute or chronic AR (B) Indicated for diagnosis and assessment of the cause of chronic AR (including valve morphology and aortic root size and morphology) and for assessment of LV hypertrophy, dimension (or volume), and systolic function (B) Indicated in patients with an enlarged aortic root to assess regurgitation and the severity of aortic dilation (B) Indicated for periodic reevaluation of LV size and function in asymptomatic patients with severe AR (B) Indicated to reevaluate mild, moderate, or severe AR in patients with new or changing symptoms (B)			
Exercise stress testing		Reasonable for patients with chronic AR for assessment of functional capacity and symptomatic response in patients with a history of equivocal symptoms (B) Reasonable for patients with chronic AR for the evaluation of symptoms and functional capacity before participation in athletic activities (C)	Exercise stress testing in patients with radionuclide angiography may be considered for assessment of LV function in asymptomatic or symptomatic patients with chronic AR (B)	
Radionuclide imaging or MRI	Radionuclide angiography or CMR is indicated for the initial and serial assessment of LV volume and function at rest in patients with AR and suboptimal echocardiograms (B)	MRI is reasonable for the estimation of AR severity in patients with unsatisfactory echocardiograms (B)		
Vasodilator therapy	Indicated for chronic therapy in patients with severe AR who have symptoms or LV dysfunction when surgery is not recommended because of additional cardiac or noncardiac factors (B)	Reasonable for short-term therapy to improve the hemodynamic profile of patients with severe heart failure symptoms and severe LV dysfunction before proceeding with AVR (C)	May be considered for long-term therapy in asymptomatic patients with severe AR who have LV dilation but normal systolic function (B)	Not indicated for long-term therapy in asymptomatic patients with mild to moderate AR and normal LV systolic function (B) Not indicated for long-term therapy in asymptomatic patients with LV systolic dysfunction who are otherwise candidates for AVR (C) Not indicated for long-term therapy in symptomatic patients with either normal LV function or mild to moderate LV systolic dysfunction who are otherwise candidates for AVR (C)

Continues

TABLE 62G–3 ACC/AHA Guidelines for Management of Patients with Aortic Regurgitation (AR)—cont'd

Indication	Class I (Indicated)	Class IIa (Strong Supportive Evidence)	Class IIb (Weak Supportive Evidence)	Class III (Not Indicated)
Cardiac catheterization with aortic root angiography and measurement of LV pressure	Indicated for assessment of severity of regurgitation, LV function, or aortic root size when noninvasive tests are inconclusive or discordant with clinical findings in patients with AR **(B)** Coronary angiography is indicated before AVR in patients at risk for CAD **(C)**			Cardiac catheterization with aortic root angiography and measurement of LV pressure is not indicated for assessment of LV function, aortic root size, or severity of regurgitation before AVR when noninvasive tests are adequate and concordant with clinical findings and coronary angiography is not necessary **(C)** Cardiac catheterization with aortic root angiography and measurement of LV pressure is not indicated for assessment of LV function and severity of regurgitation in asymptomatic patients when noninvasive tests are adequate **(C)**
Valve replacement or repair	Indicated for symptomatic patients with severe AR irrespective of LV systolic function **(B)** Indicated for asymptomatic patients with chronic severe AR and LV systolic dysfunction (ejection fraction ≤0.50) at rest **(B)** Indicated for patients with chronic severe AR while undergoing CABG or surgery on the aorta or other heart valves **(C)**	AVR is reasonable for asymptomatic patients with severe AR with normal LV systolic function (ejection fraction >0.50) but with severe LV dilation (end-diastolic dimension >75 mm or end-systolic dimension >55 mm)* **(B)**	May be considered in patients with moderate AR while undergoing surgery on the ascending aorta **(C)** May be considered in patients with moderate AR while undergoing CABG **(C)** May be considered for asymptomatic patients with severe AR and normal LV systolic function at rest (ejection fraction >0.50) when the degree of LV dilation exceeds an end-diastolic dimension of 70 mm or end-systolic dimension of 50 mm, when there is evidence of progressive LV dilation, declining exercise tolerance, or abnormal hemodynamic responses to exercise* **(C)**	Not indicated for asymptomatic patients with mild, moderate, or severe AR and normal LV systolic function at rest (ejection fraction >0.50) when degree of dilation is not moderate or severe (end-diastolic dimension <70 mm, end-systolic dimension <50 mm)* **(B)**
Bicuspid aortic valve with dilated ascending aorta	Initial transthoracic echocardiogram to assess the diameters of the aortic root and ascending aorta (B) CMR or cardiac CT when morphology of the aortic root or ascending aorta cannot be assessed accurately by echocardiography **(C)** Serial evaluation of the aortic root/ascending aorta size and morphology by echocardiography, cardiac MRI or cardiac CT on a yearly basis when dilation of the aortic root or ascending aorta is >4 cm **(C)**	Beta-adrenergic blocking agents are a reasonable option for patients with bicuspid valves and dilated aortic roots (diameter >4 cm*) who are not candidates for surgical correction and who do not have moderate to severe AR **(C)**		

CH 62

| | | Class IIa (Strong | Class IIb (Weak | |
Indication	Class I (Indicated)	Supportive Evidence)	Supportive Evidence)	Class III (Not Indicated)
	Surgery to repair the aortic root or replace the ascending aorta is indicated in patients with bicuspid aortic valves if the diameter of the aortic root or ascending aorta is >5 cm* or if the rate of increase in diameter is 0.5 cm per year or more **(C)**	Cardiac MRI or cardiac CT is reasonable in patients with bicuspid aortic valves when aortic root dilation is detected by echocardiography to further quantify severity of dilation and involvement of the ascending aorta **(B)**		
	In patients with bicuspid valves undergoing valve repair or replacement because of severe AS or AR, repair of the aortic root or replacement of the ascending aorta is indicated if the diameter of the aortic root or ascending aorta is >4.5 cm* **(C)**			

TABLE 62G–3 ACC/AHA Guidelines for Management of Patients with Aortic Regurgitation (AR)—cont'd

*Consider lower thresholds for patients of small stature of either gender.
ACC/AHA = American College of Cardiology/American Heart Association; AS = aortic stenosis; AVR = aortic valve replacement; CABG = coronary artery bypass grafting; CAD = coronary artery disease; CMR = cardiac magnetic resonance; CT = computed tomography; LV = left ventricular.

exercise. Following aortic valve repair, close follow-up is necessary to evaluate both the function of the new valve and LV function. This usually includes an echocardiogram soon after surgery to be used as a baseline. Patients should be followed clinically at 6 months, 12, months, and then yearly if the clinical course is uncomplicated. Serial postoperative echocardiograms after the initial early postoperative study are usually not indicated if the clinical course is uncomplicated. Patients with persistent LV dilation on the initial postoperative echocardiogram should be treated as would any other patient with symptomatic or asymptomatic LV dysfunction including treatment with angiotensin-converting enzyme (ACE) inhibitors and beta-adrenergic blocking agents.

BICUSPID AORTIC VALVE WITH DILATED ASCENDING AORTA

Transthoracic echocardiography should be used to initially evaluate patients with known bicuspid aortic valves. CMR or computed tomography (CT) should be used when echocardiography cannot adequately assess the aortic root or ascending aorta or to further quantify the severity of dilation and involvement of the ascending aorta. Surgical repair or replacement is indicated if the diameter of the aortic root or ascending aorta is greater than 5 cm (or smaller in patients of small stature) or if the rate of increase in diameter is 0.5 cm per year or more.

MITRAL STENOSIS

Transthoracic echocardiography is endorsed in the ACC/AHA guidelines as the first-line test for diagnosis and follow-up of patients with mitral stenosis; transesophageal echocardiography is considered to have a potential role (Class IIa) for detection of left atrial thrombus in patients being considered for percutaneous mitral balloon valvotomy or cardioversion (Table 62G-4) but not for routine evaluation of mitral valve morphology or hemodynamics unless transesophageal echocardiography has not been successful.

Medical Management. Patients with more than mild mitral stenosis should be counseled to avoid unusual physical stresses. Anticoagulation is recommended for patients with mitral stenosis if they have a history of atrial fibrillation, a prior embolic event, or left atrial thrombus. The guidelines are not strongly supportive of anticoagulation on the basis of left atrial dimension greater than 55 mm alone.

Cardiac Catheterization. The guidelines support the use of cardiac catheterization for hemodynamic evaluation when noninvasive tests are not conclusive or yield discrepant results.

Percutaneous Mitral Balloon Valvotomy. In centers with skilled operators the guidelines indicate that percutaneous mitral balloon valvotomy is the initial procedure of choice for symptomatic patients (NYHA functional Class II-IV) with moderate or severe mitral stenosis and favorable valve morphology and for asymptomatic patients with pulmonary hypertension (see Table 62G-4). It is not indicated in patients with mild mitral stenosis or those with left atrial thrombus.

Surgical Options. When possible, mitral valve repair is indicated for patients with symptomatic (NYHA functional Class II-IV) moderate or severe mitral valve stenosis when percutaneous mitral valve balloon valvotomy is not possible. Mitral valve repair may be considered in asymptomatic patients who experience recurrent embolic events despite adequate anticoagulation. Mitral valve replacement is an option when repair is not feasible.

MITRAL VALVE PROLAPSE

Recommendations on the use of echocardiography for patients with mitral valve prolapse were presented in the ACC/AHA guidelines on echocardiography. The diagnosis of mitral valve prolapse should be made by physical examination; two-dimensional and Doppler echocardiography should be used primarily for evaluation of mitral regurgitation and ventricular compensation, as well as for excluding the diagnosis of mitral valve prolapse in patients who have been given the diagnosis inappropriately (Table 62G-5). Serial use of echocardiography in stable patients with mild or no regurgitation is discouraged.

Management. Reassurance is an important element of the management of patients with mitral valve prolapse. A normal lifestyle and regular exercise are encouraged, especially in patients with mild or no symptoms and mild prolapse.

In general, asymptomatic athletes with mitral valve prolapse need not have any restrictions, but guidelines from the AHA[5] and ACC[6] recommended restriction of patients to low-intensity competitive sports (such as golf and bowling) if any of the following are present: (1) history of syncope, judged probably arrhythmogenic in origin; (2) family history of sudden death caused by mitral valve prolapse; (3) repetitive supraventricular or complex ventricular tachyarrhythmias, particularly if exacerbated by exercise; (4) moderate to severe mitral regurgitation; and (5) prior embolic event.

CH 62

Valvular Heart Disease

TABLE 62G–4 ACC/AHA Guidelines for Management of Patients with Mitral Stenosis (MS)

Indication	Class I (Indicated)	Class IIa (Strong Supportive Evidence)	Class IIb (Weak Supportive Evidence)	Class III (Not Indicated)
Echocardiography	Should be performed in patients for the diagnosis of MS, assessment of hemodynamic severity, assessment of concomitant valvular lesions, and assessment of valve morphology (to determine suitability for percutaneous mitral balloon valvotomy) **(B)** Should be performed for re-evaluation in patients with known MS and changing symptoms or signs **(B)** Should be performed to assess the hemodynamic response of the mean gradient and pulmonary artery pressure by exercise Doppler echocardiography in patients with MS when there is a discrepancy among resting Doppler echocardiographic findings, clinical findings, symptoms, and signs **(C)** Transesophageal echocardiography should be performed to assess the presence or absence of left atrial thrombus and to further evaluate the severity of MR in patients considered for percutaneous mitral balloon valvotomy **(C)** Transesophageal echocardiography should be performed to evaluate MV morphology and hemodynamics in patients when transthoracic echocardiography provides suboptimal data **(C)**	Reasonable for the re-evaluation of asymptomatic patients with MS and stable clinical findings to assess pulmonary artery pressure (for those with severe MS, every year; moderate MS, every 1 to 2 years; and mild MS, every 3 to 5 years) **(C)**		Not indicated for routine evaluation of MV morphology and hemodynamics when complete transthoracic echocardiographic data are satisfactory **(C)**
Anticoagulation therapy	Indicated in patients with MS and atrial fibrillation (paroxysmal, persistent, or permanent) **(B)** Indicated in patients with MS and a prior embolic event, even in sinus rhythm **(B)** Indicated in patients with MS with left atrial thrombus **(B)**		May be considered for asymptomatic patients with severe MS and left atrial dimension ≥55 mm by echocardiography **(B)** May be considered for patients with severe MS, an enlarged left atrium, and spontaneous contrast on echocardiography **(C)**	
Cardiac catheterization	Should be performed for hemodynamic evaluation to assess severity of MS when noninvasive tests are inconclusive or when there is discrepancy between noninvasive tests and clinical findings regarding severity of MS **(C)** Catheterization for hemodynamic evaluation including left ventriculography (to evaluate severity of MR) for patients with MS is indicated when there is a discrepancy between the Doppler-derived mean gradient and valve area **(C)**	Cardiac catheterization is reasonable to assess the hemodynamic response of pulmonary artery and left atrial pressures to exercise when clinical symptoms and resting hemodynamics are discordant **(C)** Reasonable in patients with MS to assess the cause of severe pulmonary arterial hypertension when out of proportion to severity of MS as determined by noninvasive testing **(C)**		Diagnostic cardiac catheterization is not recommended to assess MV hemodynamics when 2D and Doppler echocardiographic data are concordant with clinical findings **(C)**

CH 62

TABLE 62G-4	ACC/AHA Guidelines for Management of Patients with Mitral Stenosis (MS)—cont'd			
Indication	Class I (Indicated)	Class IIa (Strong Supportive Evidence)	Class IIb (Weak Supportive Evidence)	Class III (Not Indicated)
Percutaneous mitral balloon valvotomy	Effective for symptomatic patients (NYHA functional Class II, III, or IV), with moderate or severe MS and valve morphology favorable for percutaneous mitral balloon valvotomy in the absence of left atrial thrombus or moderate to severe MR (A) Effective for asymptomatic patients with moderate or severe MS and valve morphology that is favorable for percutaneous mitral balloon valvotomy who have pulmonary hypertension (pulmonary artery systolic pressure >50 mm Hg at rest or >60 mm Hg with exercise) in the absence of left atrial thrombus or moderate to severe MR (C)	Reasonable for patients with moderate or severe MS who have a nonpliable calcified valve, are in NYHA functional Class III-IV, and are either not candidates for surgery or are at high risk for surgery (C)	May be considered for asymptomatic patients with moderate or severe MS and valve morphology favorable for percutaneous mitral balloon valvotomy who have new-onset of atrial fibrillation in the absence of left atrial thrombus or moderate to severe MR (C) May be considered for symptomatic patients (NYHA functional Class II, III, or IV) with MV area >1.5 cm² if there is evidence of hemodynamically significant MS based on pulmonary artery systolic pressure >60 mm Hg, pulmonary artery wedge pressure of 25 mm Hg or more, or mean MV gradient >15 mm Hg during exercise (C) May be considered as an alternative to surgery for patients with moderate or severe MS who have a nonpliable calcified valve and are in NYHA Class III-IV (C)	Not indicated for patients with mild MS (C) Not indicated for patients with moderate to severe MR or left atrial thrombus (C)
Surgery	MV surgery (repair if possible) is indicated in patients with symptomatic (NYHA functional Class III-IV) moderate or severe MS when: Percutaneous mitral balloon valvotomy is unavailable (B) Percutaneous mitral balloon valvotomy is contraindicated because of left atrial thrombus despite anticoagulation or because concomitant moderate to severe MR is present (B), or the valve morphology is not favorable for percutaneous mitral balloon valvotomy in a patient with acceptable operative risk (B) MV replacement is indicated for symptomatic patients with moderate to severe MS who also have moderate to severe MR, unless valve repair is possible at the time of surgery (C)	MV replacement is reasonable for patients with severe MS and severe pulmonary hypertension (pulmonary artery systolic pressure > 60) with NYHA functional class I-II symptoms who are not considered candidates for percutaneous mitral balloon valvotomy or surgical MV repair (C)	MV repair may be considered for asymptomatic patients with moderate or severe MS who have had recurrent embolic events while receiving adequate anticoagulation and who have valve morphology favorable for repair (C)	MV repair for MS is not indicated for patients with mild MS (C) Closed commissurotomy should not be performed in patients undergoing MV repair; open commissurotomy is the preferred approach (C)

ACC/AHA = American College of Cardiology/American Heart Association; MR = mitral regurgitation; MV = mitral valve; NYHA = New York Heart Association.

TABLE 62G–5	ACC/AHA Guidelines for Management of Patients with Mitral Valve Prolapse (MVP)			
Indication	Class I (Indicated)	Class IIa (Strong Supportive Evidence)	Class IIb (Weak Supportive Evidence)	Class III (Not Indicated)
Evaluation and management of the asymptomatic patient	Echocardiography is indicated for the diagnosis of MVP and assessment of MR, leaflet morphology, and ventricular compensation in asymptomatic patients with physical signs of MVP (B)	Echocardiography can effectively exclude MVP in asymptomatic patients who have been diagnosed without clinical evidence to support the diagnosis (C) Echocardiography can be effective for risk stratification in asymptomatic patients with physical signs of MVP or known MVP (C)		Echocardiography is not indicated to exclude MVP in asymptomatic patients with ill-defined symptoms in the absence of a constellation of clinical symptoms or physical findings suggestive of MVP or a positive family history (B) Routine repetition of echocardiography is not indicated for the asymptomatic patient who has MVP and no MR or MVP and mild MR with no changes in clinical signs or symptoms (C)
Evaluation and management of the symptomatic patient	Aspirin therapy (75 to 325 mg per day) is recommended for symptomatic patients with MVP who experience cerebral transient ischemic attacks (C) In patients with MVP and atrial fibrillation, warfarin therapy is recommended for patients aged >65 or those with hypertension, MR murmur, or a history of heart failure (C) Aspirin therapy (75 to 325 mg per day) is recommended for patients with MVP and atrial fibrillation who are younger than 65 years old and have no history of MR, hypertension, or heart failure (C) In patients with MVP and a history of stroke, warfarin therapy is recommended for those with MR, atrial fibrillation, or left atrial thrombus (C)	In patients with MVP and a history of stroke, who do not have MR, atrial fibrillation or left atrial thrombus, warfarin therapy is reasonable for patients with echocardiographic evidence of thickening (≥5 mm) and/or redundancy of the valve leaflets (C) In patients with MVP and a history of stroke, aspirin therapy is reasonable for patients who do not have MR, atrial fibrillation, left atrial thrombus, or echocardiographic evidence of thickening (≥5 mm) or redundancy of the valve leaflets (C) Warfarin therapy is reasonable for patients with MVP with transient ischemic attacks despite aspirin therapy (C) Aspirin therapy (75 to 325 mg per day) can be beneficial for patients with MVP and a history of stroke who have contraindications to anticoagulants (B)	Aspirin therapy (75 to 325 mg per day) may be considered for patients in sinus rhythm with echocardiographic evidence of high-risk MVP (C)	

ACC/AHA = American College of Cardiology/American Heart Association; MR = mitral regurgitation.

Daily low-dose aspirin therapy is recommended for patients with mitral valve prolapse who have experienced transient ischemic attacks, as well as younger patients with atrial fibrillation but without mitral regurgitation, hypertension, or heart failure. Anticoagulation with warfarin is recommended for poststroke patients with mitral valve prolapse who have mitral regurgitation, atrial fibrillation, or left atrial thrombus. Warfarin is also recommended in poststroke patients with echocardiographic evidence of thickening or redundancy of the valve leaflets and those who experience recurrent transient ischemic attacks while taking aspirin.

Until recently antibiotic prophylaxis has been considered appropriate for patients with the characteristic click-murmur complex or with echocardiographic evidence of mitral prolapse with regurgitation (see summary of revised recommendations in Chapter 63 Guidelines).

MITRAL REGURGITATION

The ACC/AHA guidelines consider transthoracic echocardiography to be appropriate for diagnosis of acute or chronic mitral regurgitation, as well as for annual or semiannual surveillance of LV function in patients with severe mitral regurgitation even if asymptomatic (Table 62G-6). Serial use of chest radiographs and ECGs are considered to be of less value. In asymptomatic patients with mild mitral regurgitation and no evidence of LV dysfunction, the guidelines recommend yearly evaluations to detect worsening symptomatic status but do not support annual echocardiography. Transesophageal echocardiography is considered most appropriate for intraoperative guidance and when transthoracic studies are inadequate.

Cardiac Catheterization. Catheterization is usually performed as a prelude to surgery in patients with mitral regurgitation, or when non-

TABLE 62G–6 ACC/AHA Guidelines for Management of Patients with Mitral Regurgitation

Indication	Class I (Indicated)	Class IIa (Strong Supportive Evidence)	Class IIb (Weak Supportive Evidence)	Class III (Not Indicated)
Transthoracic echocardiography	Indicated for baseline evaluation of LV size and function, RV and left atrial size, pulmonary artery pressure, and severity of MR in any patient suspected of having MR (C) Indicated for delineation of the mechanism of MR (B) Indicated for annual or semiannual surveillance of LV function (estimated by ejection fraction and end-systolic dimension) in asymptomatic patients with moderate to severe MR (C) Indicated in patients with MR to evaluate the MV apparatus and LV function after a change in signs or symptoms (C) Indicated to evaluate LV size and function and MV hemodynamics in the initial evaluation after MV replacement or MV repair (C)	Exercise Doppler echocardiography is reasonable in asymptomatic patients with severe MR to assess exercise tolerance and the effects of exercise on pulmonary artery pressure and MR severity (C)		Not indicated for routine follow-up evaluation of asymptomatic patients with mild MR and normal LV size and systolic function (C)
Transesophageal echocardiography	Indicated for evaluation of MR patients in whom transthoracic echocardiography provides nondiagnostic information regarding severity of MR, mechanism of MR, and/or status of LV function (B) Preoperative or intraoperative transesophageal echocardiography is indicated to establish the anatomic basis for severe MR in patients in whom surgery is recommended to assess feasibility of repair and to guide repair (B)	Preoperative transesophageal echocardiography is reasonable in asymptomatic patients with severe MR who are considered for surgery to assess feasibility of repair (C)		Transesophageal echocardiography is not indicated for routine follow-up or surveillance of asymptomatic patients with native valve MR (C)
Cardiac catheterization	Left ventriculography and hemodynamic measurements are indicated when noninvasive tests are inconclusive regarding severity of MR, LV function, or the need for surgery (C) Hemodynamic measurements are indicated when pulmonary artery pressure is out of proportion to the severity of MR as assessed by noninvasive testing (C) Left ventriculography and hemodynamic measurements are indicated when there is a discrepancy between clinical and noninvasive findings regarding severity of MR (C) Coronary angiography is indicated before MV repair or MV replacement in patients at risk for CAD (C)			Left ventriculography and hemodynamic measurements are not indicated in patients with MR in whom valve surgery is not contemplated (C)
Surgery	MV surgery is recommended for the symptomatic patient with acute severe MR (B) MV surgery is beneficial for patients with chronic severe MR and NYHA functional Class II, III, or IV symptoms in the absence of severe LV dysfunction (severe LV dysfunction is defined as ejection fraction <0.30) and/or end-systolic dimension >55 mm (B)	MV repair is reasonable in experienced surgical centers for asymptomatic patients with chronic severe MR with preserved LV function (ejection fraction >0.60 and end-systolic dimension <40 mm) in whom the likelihood of successful repair without residual MR is >90% (B) MV surgery is reasonable for asymptomatic patients with chronic severe MR, preserved LV function, and new onset of atrial fibrillation (C)	MV repair may be considered for patients with chronic severe secondary MR caused by severe LV dysfunction (ejection fraction <0.30) who have persistent NYHA functional Class III-IV symptoms despite optimal therapy for heart failure, including biventricular pacing (C)	MV surgery is not indicated for asymptomatic patients with MR and preserved LV function (ejection fraction >0.60 and end-systolic dimension <40 mm) in whom significant doubt about the feasibility of repair exists (C)

CH 62

Valvular Heart Disease

Continues

		Class IIb (Weak	
		Class IIa (Strong	Supportive	Class III (Not
Indication	Class I (Indicated)	Supportive Evidence)	Evidence)	Indicated)

TABLE 62G–6 ACC/AHA Guidelines for Management of Patients with Mitral Regurgitation—cont'd

Indication	Class I (Indicated)	Class IIa (Strong Supportive Evidence)	Class IIb (Weak Supportive Evidence)	Class III (Not Indicated)
	MV surgery is beneficial for asymptomatic patients with chronic severe MR and mild to moderate LV dysfunction, ejection fraction 0.30 to 0.60, and/or end-systolic dimension ≥40 mm **(B)** MV repair is recommended over MV replacement in the majority of patients with severe chronic MR* who require surgery, and patients should be referred to surgical centers experienced in MV repair **(C)**	MV surgery is reasonable for asymptomatic patients with chronic severe MR, preserved LV function, and pulmonary hypertension (pulmonary artery systolic pressure >50 mm Hg at rest or >60 mm Hg with exercise) **(C)** MV surgery is reasonable for patients with chronic severe MR caused by a primary abnormality of the mitral apparatus and NYHA functional Class III-IV symptoms and severe LV dysfunction (ejection fraction <0.30 and/or end-systolic dimension >55 mm) in whom MV repair is highly likely **(C)**		Isolated MV surgery is not indicated for patients with mild or moderate MR **(C)**

ACC/AHA = American College of Cardiology/American Medical Association; CAD = coronary artery disease; LV = left ventricular; MR = mitral regurgitation; MV = mitral valve.

invasive tests yield discordant results or do not provide adequate information to guide management. The ACC/AHA guidelines do not consider coronary angiography routinely necessary in patients with mitral regurgitation when valve surgery is not planned.

Surgery. The guidelines consider mitral valve repair to be the operation of choice for patients with suitable valves when performed by an experienced operator. Surgery is deemed appropriate for acute symptomatic mitral regurgitation and for patients with chronic severe mitral regurgitation and symptoms of congestive heart failure, even if they have normal LV function (see Table 62G-6). Among asymptomatic patients, surgery is appropriate when there is evidence of mild or greater LV dysfunction (ejection fraction 0.30 to 0.60 and/or end-systolic dimension <40 mm).

The 2006 guidelines contain two important new recommendations regarding mitral valve repair. The first applies to asymptomatic patients with severe mitral regurgitation and normal LV function. The guidelines indicate that it is reasonable to consider mitral valve repair in such patients if they undergo surgery in experienced surgical centers in which the likelihood of successful repair without residual regurgitation is greater than 90% (a new class IIa indication). A stronger recommendation (class I) indicates that mitral valve repair is recommended over mitral valve replacement in the majority of patients who undergo surgery, and patients should be referred to surgical centers experienced in mitral valve repair.

OTHER VALVULAR DISEASE

Multiple Valve Disease. Given the large number of possible combinations and the slim evidence base for diagnosis and management, the ACC/AHA guidelines offer no specific recommendations for the management of mixed valve disease.

Tricuspid Valve Disease. Tricuspid valve repair is appropriate for correcting severe tricuspid regurgitation in patients with mitral valve disease requiring valve repair or replacement (Table 62G-7). Tricuspid valve replacement or annuloplasty is considered reasonable for patients with symptomatic severe primary tricuspid regurgitation. Annuloplasty may be considered in patients with mild to moderate tricuspid regurgitation who are undergoing surgery for mitral valve disease if they have pulmonary hypertension or dilation of the tricuspid annulus.

DRUG-RELATED VALVULAR HEART DISEASE

The use of anorectic drugs (fenfluramine and dexfenfluramine), ergotamine-like agents (ergotamine, methysergide), and at least one dopamine-receptor agonist (pergolide) have been linked with valvular disease. The ACC/AHA task force does not consider it possible to offer definitive diagnostic and treatment guidelines for patients who have received these beyond recommending discontinuation of these agents and careful periodic examinations. The guidelines recommend echocardiography as indicated and treatment dictated by the nature of the heart valve lesion.

VALVULAR DISEASE IN ADOLESCENTS AND YOUNG ADULTS

With regard to valvular disease in younger individuals, the ACC/AHA guidelines concentrate on isolated valve involvement when it is the primary anomaly. For adolescents and young adults with aortic stenosis, the guidelines recommend a lower threshold for exercise testing and cardiac catheterization to assess the risk of participation in athletics (Table 62G-8). In this population, balloon valvotomy is an effective and appropriate option. Because this procedure has little morbidity and mortality, the indications for intervention are more liberal in younger patients than in adults. The indications for management of chronic aortic regurgitation and mitral valve disease are similar to those for older adult patients. Repair of a dysfunctional tricuspid valve is indicated, along with catheterization closure of septal defect if present. Balloon valvotomy is considered an appropriate intervention for patients who are symptomatic because of pulmonic stenosis and for asymptomatic patients with a peak valve gradient greater than 50 mm.

SURGICAL CONSIDERATIONS

Numerous options are available for the surgical management of valve disease. The ACC/AHA guidelines generally favor mitral valve repair over replacement. The standard surgical approach usually entails a median sternotomy with cardiopulmonary bypass. However, numer-

TABLE 62G–7 ACC/AHA Guidelines for Management of Patients with Tricuspid Valve (TV) Disease

Indication	Class I (Indicated)	Class IIa (Strong Supportive Evidence)	Class IIb (Weak Supportive Evidence)	Class III (Not Indicated)
Surgery	Tricuspid valve repair is beneficial for severe TR in patients with MV disease requiring MV surgery (B)	Tricuspid valve replacement or annuloplasty is reasonable for severe primary TR when symptomatic (C) Tricuspid valve replacement is reasonable for severe TR secondary to diseased/abnormal tricuspid valve leaflets not amenable to annuloplasty or repair (C)	Tricuspid annuloplasty may be considered for < severe TR in patients undergoing MV surgery when there is pulmonary hypertension or tricuspid annular dilatation (C)	Tricuspid valve replacement or annuloplasty is not indicated in asymptomatic patients with TR whose pulmonary artery systolic pressure is <60 mm Hg in the presence of a normal MV (C) Tricuspid valve replacement or annuloplasty is not indicated in patients with mild primary TR (C)

ACC/AHA = American College of Cardiology/American Heart Association; MV = mitral valve; TR = tricuspid regurgitation.

TABLE 62G–8 ACC/AHA Guidelines for the Management of Valvular Heart Disease in Adolescents and Young Adults

Indication	Class I (Indicated)	Class IIa (Strong Supportive Evidence)	Class IIb (Weak Supportive Evidence)	Class III (Not Indicated)
Evaluation	A yearly ECG is recommended in the asymptomatic adolescent or young adult with AS who has a Doppler mean gradient >30 mm Hg or a peak velocity >3.5 m per second (peak gradient >50 mm Hg) and every 2 years if the echocardiographic Doppler mean gradient is ≤30 mm Hg or the peak velocity is ≤3.5 m per second (peak gradient ≤50 mm Hg) (C) Doppler echocardiography is recommended yearly in the asymptomatic adolescent or young adult with AS who has a Doppler mean gradient >30 mm Hg or a peak velocity >3.5 m per second (peak gradient >50 mm Hg) and every 2 years if the Doppler gradient is ≤30 mm Hg or the peak jet velocity is ≤3.5 m per second (peak gradient ≤50 mm Hg) (C) Cardiac catheterization for the evaluation of AS is an effective diagnostic tool in the asymptomatic adolescent or young adult when results of Doppler echocardiography are equivocal regarding severity of AS or when there is a discrepancy between clinical and noninvasive findings regarding severity of AS (C) Cardiac catheterization is indicated in the adolescent or young adult with AS who has symptoms of angina, syncope, or dyspnea on exertion if the Doppler mean gradient is >30 mm Hg or the peak velocity is >3.5 m/sec (peak gradient >50 mm Hg) (C) Cardiac catheterization is indicated in the asymptomatic adolescent or young adult with AS who develops T-wave inversion at rest over the left precordium if the Doppler mean gradient is >30 mm Hg or the peak velocity is >3.5 m/sec (peak gradient >50 mm Hg) (C)	Graded exercise testing is a reasonable diagnostic evaluation in the adolescent or young adult with AS who has a Doppler mean gradient >30 mm Hg or a peak velocity >3.5 m per second (peak gradient >50 mm Hg) if the patient is interested in athletic participation, or if the clinical findings and Doppler findings are disparate (C) Cardiac catheterization for the evaluation of AS is a reasonable diagnostic tool in the asymptomatic adolescent or young adult who has a Doppler mean gradient >40 mm Hg or a peak velocity >4 m per second (peak gradient >64 mm Hg) (C) Cardiac catheterization for the evaluation of AS is reasonable in the adolescent or young adult who has a Doppler mean gradient >30 mm Hg or a peak velocity >3.5 m per second (peak gradient >50 mm Hg) if the patient is interested in athletic participation or becoming pregnant, or if the clinical findings and the Doppler echocardiographic findings are disparate (C)		

Continues

TABLE 62G–8	ACC/AHA Guidelines for the Management of Valvular Heart Disease in Adolescents and Young Adults—cont'd			
Indication	**Class I (Indicated)**	**Class IIa (Strong Supportive Evidence)**	**Class IIb (Weak Supportive Evidence)**	**Class III (Not Indicated)**
Aortic balloon valvotomy	Indicated in the adolescent or young adult patient with AS who has symptoms of angina, syncope, or dyspnea on exertion and a catheterization peak LV-to-peak aortic gradient ≥50 mm Hg without a heavily calcified valve* **(C)** Indicated for the asymptomatic adolescent or young adult patient with AS who has a catheterization peak LV-to-peak aortic gradient >60 mm Hg* **(C)** Indicated in the asymptomatic adolescent or young adult patient with AS who develops ST or T-wave changes over the left precordium on ECG at rest or with exercise and who has a catheterization peak LV–to-aortic gradient >50 mm Hg* **(C)**	Reasonable in the asymptomatic adolescent or young adult patient with AS when catheterization peak IV-to-peak aortic gradient >50 mm Hg and the patient wants to play competitive sports or desires to become pregnant* **(C)** In the adolescent or young adult patient with AS, aortic balloon valvotomy is probably recommended over valve surgery when balloon valvotomy is possible; patients should be referred to a center with expertise in balloon valvotomy* **(C)**		Should not be performed when the asymptomatic adolescent or young adult patient with AS has a catheterization peak LV-to- peak aortic gradient <40 mm Hg without symptoms or ECG changes **(C)**
Aortic regurgitation (AR)	An adolescent or young adult with chronic severe AR with onset of symptoms of angina, syncope, or dyspnea on exertion should receive aortic valve repair or replacement **(C)** Asymptomatic adolescent or young adult patients with chronic severe AR with LV systolic dysfunction (ejection fraction <0.50) on serial studies 1 to 3 months apart should receive aortic valve repair or replacement **(C)** Asymptomatic adolescent or young adult patients with chronic severe AR with progressive LV enlargement (end-diastolic dimension >4 standard deviations above normal) should receive aortic valve repair or replacement **(C)** Coronary angiography is recommended before AVR in adolescent or young adult patients with AR in whom a pulmonary autograft (Ross operation) is contemplated when the origin of the coronary arteries has not been identified by noninvasive techniques **(C)**		An asymptomatic adolescent with chronic severe AR with moderate AS (peak LV-to-peak aortic gradient >40 mm Hg at cardiac catheterization) may be considered for aortic valve repair or replacement **(C)** An asymptomatic adolescent with chronic severe AR with onset of ST depression or T-wave inversion over the left precordium on ECG at rest may be considered for aortic valve repair or replacement **(C)**	
Mitral regurgitation (MR)	MV surgery is indicated in the symptomatic adolescent or young adult with severe congenital MR with NYHA functional Class III or IV symptoms **(C)** MV surgery is indicated in the asymptomatic adolescent or young adult with severe congenital MR and LV systolic dysfunction (ejection fraction ≤0.60) **(C)**	MV repair is reasonable in experienced surgical centers in the asymptomatic adolescent or young adult with severe congenital MR with preserved LV systolic function if the likelihood of successful repair without residual MR is >90% **(B)**	The effectiveness of MV surgery is not well established in asymptomatic adolescent or young adult patients with severe congenital MR* and preserved LV systolic function in whom valve replacement is highly likely **(C)**	
Mitral stenosis (MS)	MV surgery is indicated in adolescent or young adult patients with congenital MS who have symptoms (NYHA functional Class III or IV) and mean MV gradient >10 mm Hg on Doppler echocardiography **(C)**	MV surgery is reasonable in adolescent or young adult patients with congenital MS who have mild symptoms (NYHA functional Class II) and mean MV gradient >10 mm Hg on Doppler echocardiography **(C)**	The effectiveness of MV surgery is not well established in the asymptomatic adolescent or young adult with congenital MS and new-onset atrial fibrillation or multiple systemic emboli while receiving adequate anticoagulation **(C)**	

CH 62

TABLE 62G-8 ACC/AHA Guidelines for the Management of Valvular Heart Disease in Adolescents and Young Adults—cont'd

Indication	Class I (Indicated)	Class IIa (Strong Supportive Evidence)	Class IIb (Weak Supportive Evidence)	Class III (Not Indicated)
		MV surgery is reasonable in the asymptomatic adolescent or young adult with congenital MS with pulmonary artery systolic pressure ≥50 mm Hg and a mean MV gradient ≥10 mm Hg **(C)**		
Tricuspid valve disease	Surgery for severe TR is recommended for adolescent and young adult patients with deteriorating exercise capacity (NYHA functional Class III or IV) **(C)** Surgery for severe TR is recommended for adolescent and young adult patients with progressive cyanosis and arterial saturation <80% at rest or with exercise **(C)** Interventional catheterization closure of the atrial communication is recommended for the adolescent or young adult with TR who is hypoxemic at rest and with exercise intolerance due to increasing hypoxemia with exercise, when the tricuspid valve appears difficult to repair surgically	Surgery for severe TR is reasonable in adolescent and young adult patients with NYHA functional Class II symptoms if the valve appears to be repairable **(C)** Surgery for severe TR is reasonable in adolescent and young adult patients with atrial fibrillation **(C)**	Surgery for severe TR may be considered in asymptomatic adolescent and young adult patients with increasing heart size and a cardiothoracic ratio of more than 65% **(C)** Surgery for severe TR may be considered in asymptomatic adolescent and young adult patients with stable heart size and an arterial saturation of <85% when the tricuspid valve appears repairable **(C)** In adolescent and young adult patients with TR who are mildly cyanotic at rest but who become very hypoxemic with exercise, closure of the atrial communication by interventional catheterization may be considered when the valve does not appear amenable to repair **(C)** If surgery for Ebstein anomaly is planned in adolescents and young adult patients (tricuspid valve repair or replacement), a preoperative electrophysiological study may be considered to identify accessory pathways. If present, these may be considered for mapping and ablation either preoperatively or at the time of surgery **(C)**	
Pulmonic stenosis	An ECG is recommended for the initial evaluation of pulmonic stenosis in adolescent and young adult patients, and serially every 5 to 10 years for follow-up examinations **(C)** Transthoracic Doppler echocardiography is recommended for the initial evaluation of pulmonic stenosis in adolescent and young adult patients, and serially every 5 to 10 years for follow-up examinations **(C)** Cardiac catheterization is recommended in the adolescent or young adult with pulmonic stenosis for evaluation of the valvular gradient if the Doppler		Balloon valvotomy may be reasonable in asymptomatic adolescent and young adult patients with pulmonic stenosis and an RV-to-pulmonary artery peak-to-peak gradient 30 to 39 mm Hg at catheterization **(C)**	Diagnostic cardiac catheterization is not recommended for the initial diagnostic evaluation of pulmonic stenosis in adolescent and young adult patients **(C)** Balloon valvotomy is not recommended in asymptomatic adolescent and young adult patients with pulmonic stenosis and RV-to-pulmonary artery peak-to-peak gradient <30 mm Hg at catheterization **(C)**

Continues

TABLE 62G–8	ACC/AHA Guidelines for the Management of Valvular Heart Disease in Adolescents and Young Adults—cont'd			
Indication	Class I (Indicated)	Class IIa (Strong Supportive Evidence)	Class IIb (Weak Supportive Evidence)	Class III (Not Indicated)
	peak jet velocity is >3 m/sec (estimated peak gradient >36 mm Hg) and balloon dilation can be performed if indicated **(C)** Balloon valvotomy is recommended in adolescent and young adult patients with pulmonic stenosis who have exertional dyspnea, angina, syncope, or presyncope and an RV-to-pulmonary artery peak-to-peak gradient >30 mm Hg at catheterization **(C)** Balloon valvotomy is recommended in asymptomatic adolescent and young adult patients with pulmonic stenosis and RV-to-pulmonary artery peak-to-peak gradient >40 mm Hg at catheterization **(C)**			

*Gradients are usually obtained with patients sedated. If general anesthesia is used, the gradients may be somewhat lower.

ACC/AHA = American College of Cardiology/American Heart Association; AS = aortic stenosis; AVR = aortic valve replacement; ECG = electrocardiogram; LV = left ventricular; MV = mitral valve; RV = right ventricular; TR = tricuspid regurgitation.

CH 62

TABLE 62G–9	ACC/AHA Major Criteria for the Selection of Replacement Valves for Individuals with Valvular Heart Disease	
Class	Indication	Level of Evidence
Atrial Valve Selection		
Class I (indicated)	A mechanical prosthesis is recommended for AVR in patients with a mechanical valve in the mitral or tricuspid position.	C
	A bioprosthesis is recommended for AVR in patients of any age who will not take warfarin or who have major medical contraindications to warfarin therapy.	C
Class IIa (strong supportive evidence)	Patient preference is a reasonable consideration in the selection of aortic valve operation and valve prosthesis. A mechanical prosthesis is reasonable for AVR in patients younger than 65 years of age who do not have a contraindication to anticoagulation. A bioprosthesis is reasonable for AVR in patients younger than 65 years of age who elect to receive this valve for lifestyle considerations after detailed discussions of the risks of anticoagulation versus the likelihood that a second AVR may be necessary in the future.	C
	A bioprosthesis is reasonable for AVR in patients aged 65 years or older without risk factors for thromboembolism.	C
	Aortic valve re-replacement with a homograft is reasonable for patients with active prosthetic valve endocarditis.	C
Class IIb (weak supportive evidence)	A bioprosthesis might be considered for AVR in a woman of childbearing age.	C
Mitral Valve Selection		
Class I (indicated)	A bioprosthesis is indicated for MV replacement in a patient who will not take warfarin, is incapable of taking warfarin, or has a clear contraindication to warfarin therapy.	C
Class IIa (strong supportive evidence)	A mechanical prosthesis is reasonable for MV replacement in patients younger than 65 years of age with longstanding atrial fibrillation.	C
	A bioprosthesis is reasonable for MV replacement in patients 65 years of age or older.	C
	A bioprosthesis is reasonable for MV replacement in patients younger than 65 years of age in sinus rhythm who elect to receive this valve for life-style considerations after detailed discussions of the risks of anticoagulation versus the likelihood that a second MV replacement may be necessary in the future.	C

ACC/AHA = American College of Cardiology/American Heart Association; AVR = aortic valve replacement; MV = mitral valve.

ous alternatives are gaining acceptance. These include minimally invasive approaches such as partial sternotomy and small right thoracotomy. Percutaneous approaches to mitral valve repair,[7] pulmonary valve implantation,[8] and aortic valve replacement[9] have been conducted in small, selected series with generally successful results. Whether such catheter-based approaches gain widespread acceptance will depend on larger long-term results and advances in device technology.

When replacement is necessary, several variables influence the selection of a bioprosthetic versus a mechanical valve (Table 62G-9).

Patient preference plays an important role in determining the choice of a prosthetic valve. In the 1998 guidelines, bioprosthetic valves were considered appropriate only in patients older than 65 years for aortic valve replacement and 70 years for mitral valve replacement. The 2006 guidelines emphasize that a bioprosthesis is reasonable in patients younger than 65 years of age who elect to receive this valve for lifestyle considerations after detailed discussion of the risks of anticoagulation versus the likelihood that a second valve replacement may be necessary in the future.

TABLE 62G–10	Recommendations for Antithrombotic Therapy in Patients with Prosthetic Heart Valves*			
	Aspirin (75-100 mg)	Warfarin (INR 2-3)	Warfarin (INR 2.5-3.5)	No Warfarin
Mechanical prosthetic valves				
AVR—low risk				
<3 mo	Class I	Class I	Class IIa	
>3 mo	Class I	Class I		
AVR—high risk	Class I		Class I	
MVR	Class I		Class I	
Biological prosthetic valves				
AVR—low risk				
<3 mo	Class I	Class IIa		Class IIb
>3 mo	Class I			Class IIa
AVR—high risk	Class I	Class I		
MVR—low risk				
<3 mo	Class I	Class IIa		
>3 mo	Class I			Class IIa
MVR—high risk	Class I	Class I		

*Antithrombotic therapy must be individualized depending on a patient's clinical status. Among patients receiving warfarin, aspirin is recommended in virtually all situations. Risk factors include atrial fibrillation, left ventricular dysfunction, previous thromboembolism, and hypercoagulable condition. INR should be maintained between 2.5 and 3.5 for aortic disc valves and Starr-Edwards valves.

AVR = aortic valve replacement; INR = international normalized ratio; MVR = mitral valve replacement.

The 1998 guidelines also considered bioprosthetic valves inappropriate for patients with end-stage renal failure, especially those undergoing chronic dialysis, because of concerns of accelerated calcification of bioprosthetic valves. Subsequent randomized trials have not demonstrated a difference in outcomes between mechanical and bioprosthetic valves in these patients, and this recommendation was removed in 2006.

INTRAOPERATIVE ASSESSMENT

The ACC/AHA guidelines emphasize the importance of intraoperative transesophageal echocardiography by recommending its use during valve repair; valve replacement with a stentless xenograft, homograft, or autograft valve; or valve surgery for infective endocarditis. It may also be reasonable for all patients undergoing cardiac valve surgery. The guidelines committee recommends that institutions performing valve surgery establish consistent and credible intraoperative echocardiography programs capable of providing accurate anatomical and functional information relevant to valve operations. Given that even a generally a safe procedure such as transesophageal echocardiography has risks, preoperative screening for risk factors and obtaining informed consent should be a routine part of each intraoperative transesophageal study.

PATIENTS WITH PROSTHETIC HEART VALVES

The ACC/AHA guidelines recommend warfarin therapy for patients with mechanical valves. For aortic valve replacement patients, those with bileaflet mechanical valves and Medtronic Hall valves should maintain an international normalized ratio (INR) between 2 and 3, whereas those with Starr-Edwards valves or mechanical disc valves should maintain an INR between 2.5 and 3.5 (Table 62G-10). The same target is indicated following mitral valve replacement with a mechanical valve. Aspirin (75 to 325 mg/day) is indicated for patients who are unable to take warfarin. Low-dose aspirin (75 to 100 mg/day) is recommended in addition to warfarin for all patients with mechanical heart valves and those with biological valves who have risk factors such as atrial fibrillation, prior thromboembolism, LV dysfunction, or a hypercoagulable condition. Clopidogrel may be considered for those who cannot take aspirin.

"Bridging" Therapy. Antithrombotic medications must sometimes be interrupted in patients with mechanical valve prostheses for noncardiac surgery, invasive procedures, or dental care. In patients at low risk of thrombosis, warfarin should be stopped 48 to 72 hours before the procedure and started no more than 24 hours after the procedure

(Table 62G-11). The ACC/AHA guidelines indicate that the use of heparin is usually unnecessary in patients at low risk of thrombosis, defined as those with a bileaflet mechanical aortic valve prosthesis with no risk factors. They recommend bridging anticoagulant therapy for the higher-risk individuals including those with a mechanical mitral or tricuspid prosthesis or those with an mechanical aortic prosthesis who have risk factors such as atrial fibrillation, a recent thrombosis or embolus, LV dysfunction, an older-generation thrombogenic valve, and those with demonstrated thrombotic problems when previously off therapy. The recommended bridging therapy is intravenous unfractionated heparin (class I), but subcutaneous doses of unfractionated heparin or low-molecular weight heparin may also be considered (class IIb).

Prosthetic Valve Thrombosis. Emergency surgery is reasonable for patients with a thrombosed left-sided prosthetic valve and moderate to severe symptoms (NYHA Class III-IV) or a large clot burden. Fibrinolytic therapy may considered in patients with less severe symptoms, smaller clot burdens, or when surgery is high risk or unavailable (Table 62G-12).

Follow-up. After prosthetic valve implantation, asymptomatic patients should be seen 2 to 4 weeks after hospital discharge and then at 1-year intervals (Table 62G-13). Routine annual echocardiograms are not indicated in the absence of changes in clinical status. All patients should also receive primary and secondary prevention measures to reduce the risk of future cardiovascular events.

Patients who do not improve after receiving a prosthetic heart valve or who later show deterioration of functional capacity should undergo appropriate testing to determine the cause. Patients with postoperative LV systolic dysfunction, even if it is asymptomatic, should receive standard medical therapy for systolic heart failure indefinitely, even if systolic function or symptoms improve.

EVALUATION AND MANAGEMENT OF CORONARY ARTERY DISEASE IN PATIENTS WITH VALVULAR HEART DISEASE

Concomitant coronary artery disease (CAD) is common in patients with valvular disease. Because of the impact of untreated CAD on perioperative and long-term postoperative survival, preoperative identification of CAD is of great importance in patients with aortic or mitral stenosis, as well as those with aortic regurgitation. Thus in symptomatic patients and/or those with LV dysfunction, the guidelines recommend preoperative coronary angiography in men aged 35 years and older, premenopausal women older than age 35 years with coronary risk factors, and postmenopausal women* (Table 62G-14).

TABLE 62G–11 ACC/AHA Recommendations for Bridging Therapy in Patients with Mechanical Valves Who Require Interruption of Warfarin Therapy for Noncardiac Surgery, Invasive Procedures, or Dental Care

Class I (Indicated)	Class IIa (Strong Supportive Evidence)	Class IIb (Weak Supportive Evidence)	Class III (Not Indicated)
In patients at low risk of thrombosis, defined as those with a bileaflet mechanical AVR with no risk factors,* it is recommended that warfarin be stopped 48 to 72 hr before the procedure (so that the INR falls to <1.5) and restarted within 24 hr after the procedure. Heparin is usually unnecessary **(B)**	It is reasonable to give fresh frozen plasma to patients with mechanical valves who require interruption of warfarin therapy for emergency noncardiac surgery, invasive procedures, or dental care. Fresh frozen plasma is preferable to high-dose vitamin K₁ **(B)**	In patients at high risk of thrombosis (see earlier), therapeutic doses of subcutaneous UFH (15 000 U every 12 hr) or LMWH (100 U per kg every 12 hr) may be considered during the period of a subtherapeutic INR **(B)**	In patients at high risk of thrombosis (see earlier), therapeutic doses of subcutaneous UFH (15 000 U every 12 hr) or LMWH (100 U per kg every 12 hr) may be considered during the period of a subtherapeutic INR **(B)**
In patients at high risk of thrombosis, defined as those with any mechanical MV replacement or a mechanical AVR with any risk factor, therapeutic doses of intravenous UFH should be started when the INR falls below 2 (typically 48 hr before surgery), stopped 4 to 6 hr before the procedure, restarted as early after surgery as bleeding stability allows, and continued until the INR is again therapeutic with warfarin therapy **(B)**			

*Risk factors include atrial fibrillation, previous thromboembolism, LV dysfunction, hypercoagulable conditions, older-generation thrombogenic valves, mechanical tricuspid valves, or more than 1 mechanical valve.

ACC/AHA = American College of Cardiology/American Hospital Association; AVR = aortic valve replacement; INR = international normalized ratio; LMWH = low-molecular-weight heparin; MV = mitral valve; UFH = unfractionated heparin.

CH 62

TABLE 62G–12 ACC/AHA Guidelines for Management of Thrombosis of Prosthetic Heart Valves

Class I (Indicated)	Class IIa (Strong Supportive Evidence)	Class IIb (Weak Supportive Evidence)	Class III (Not Indicated)
Transthoracic and Doppler echocardiography is indicated in patients with suspected prosthetic valve thrombosis to assess hemodynamic severity **(B)** Transesophageal echocardiography and/or fluoroscopy is indicated in patients with suspected valve thrombosis to assess valve motion and clot burden **(B)**	Emergency operation is reasonable for patients with a thrombosed left-sided prosthetic valve and NYHA functional Class III-IV symptoms **(C)** Emergency operation is reasonable for patients with a thrombosed left-sided prosthetic valve and a large clot burden **(C)** Fibrinolytic therapy is reasonable for patients with thrombosed right-sided prosthetic heart valves with NYHA Class III-IV symptoms or a large clot burden **(C)**	Fibrinolytic therapy may be considered as a first-line therapy for patients with a thrombosed left-sided prosthetic valve, NYHA functional Class I-II symptoms, and a small clot burden **(B)** Fibrinolytic therapy may be considered as a first-line therapy for patients with a thrombosed left-sided prosthetic valve, NYHA functional Class III-IV symptoms, and a small clot burden if surgery is high risk or not available **(B)** Fibrinolytic therapy may be considered for patients with an obstructed, thrombosed left-sided prosthetic valve who have NYHA functional Class II-IV symptoms and a large clot burden if emergency surgery is high risk or not available **(C)** Intravenous UFH as an alternative to fibrinolytic therapy may be considered for patients with a thrombosed valve who are in NYHA functional Class I-II and have a small clot burden **(C)**	

ACC/AHA = American College of Cardiology/American Heart Association; NYHA = New York Heart Association; UFH = unfractionated heparin.

TABLE 62G–13 ACC/AHA Guidelines for Patient Follow-up after Prosthetic Valve Implantation

Class	Indication	Level of Evidence
General Patient Follow-up		
Class I (indicated)	For patients with prosthetic heart valves, a history, physical examination, and appropriate tests should be performed at the first postoperative outpatient evaluation, 2 to 4 wk after hospital discharge. This should include a transthoracic Doppler echocardiogram if a baseline echocardiogram was not obtained before hospital discharge.	C
	For patients with prosthetic heart valves, routine follow-up visits should be conducted annually, with earlier reevaluations (with echocardiography) if there is a change in clinical status.	C
Class IIb (weak supporting evidence)	Patients with bioprosthetic valves may be considered for annual echocardiograms after the first 5 yr in the absence of a change in clinical status.	C
Class III (not indicated)	Routine annual echocardiograms are not indicated in the absence of a change in clinical status in patients with mechanical heart valves or during the first 5 yr after valve replacement with a bioprosthetic valve.	C
Follow-up of the Patient with Complications		
Class I (indicated)	Patients with LV systolic dysfunction after valve surgery should receive standard medical therapy for systolic heart failure. This therapy should be continued even if there is improvement of LV dysfunction.	B

ACC/AHA = American College of Cardiology/American Heart Association; LV = left ventricular.

TABLE 62G–14 ACC/AHA Guidelines for the Evaluation and Treatment of Coronary Artery Disease in Patients with Valvular Heart Disease

Indication	Class I (Indicated)	Class IIa (Strong Supportive Evidence)	Class IIb (Weak Supportive Evidence)	Class III (Not Indicated)
Diagnosis of CAD	Coronary angiography is indicated before valve surgery (including infective endocarditis) or mitral balloon commissurotomy in patients with chest pain, other objective evidence of ischemia, decreased LV systolic function, history of CAD, or coronary risk factors (including age). Patients undergoing mitral balloon valvotomy need not undergo coronary angiography solely on the basis of coronary risk factors **(C)** Coronary angiography is indicated in patients with apparently mild to moderate valvular heart disease but with progressive angina (Canadian Heart Association functional Class II or greater), objective evidence of ischemia, decreased LV systolic function, or overt congestive heart failure **(C)** Coronary angiography should be performed before valve surgery in men aged 35 years or older, premenopausal women aged 35 years or older who have coronary risk factors, and postmenopausal women **(C)**	Surgery without coronary angiography is reasonable for patients having emergency valve surgery for acute valve regurgitation, aortic root disease, or infective endocarditis **(C)**	Coronary angiography may be considered for patients undergoing catheterization to confirm the severity of valve lesions before valve surgery without pre-existing evidence of CAD, multiple coronary risk factors, or advanced age **(C)**	Coronary angiography is not indicated in young patients undergoing nonemergency valve surgery when no further hemodynamic assessment by catheterization is deemed necessary and there are no coronary risk factors, no history of CAD, and no evidence of ischemia **(C)** Patients should not undergo coronary angiography before valve surgery if they are severely hemodynamically unstable **(C)**
Treating CAD during aortic valve replacement	Patients undergoing AVR with significant stenoses (≥70% reduction in luminal diameter) in major coronary arteries should be treated with bypass grafting **(C)**	In patients undergoing AVR and coronary bypass grafting, use of the left internal thoracic artery is reasonable for bypass of stenoses of the left anterior descending coronary artery ≥50% to 70% **(C)** For patients undergoing AVR with moderate stenosis (50% to 70% reduction in luminal diameter), it is reasonable to perform coronary bypass grafting in major coronary arteries **(C)**		
Aortic valve replacement in patients undergoing CABG	AVR is indicated in patients undergoing CABG who have severe AS who meet the criteria for valve replacement **(C)**	AVR is reasonable in patients undergoing CABG who have moderate AS (mean gradient 30 to 50 mm Hg or Doppler velocity 3 to 4 m/sec) **(B)**	AVR may be considered in patients undergoing CABG who have mild AS (mean gradient <30 mm Hg or Doppler velocity <3 m/sec) when there is evidence, such as moderate to severe valve calcification, that progression may be rapid **(C)**	

ACC/AHA = American College of Cardiology/American Hospital Association; AS = aortic stenosis; AVR = aortic valve replacement; CABG = coronary artery bypass grafting; CAD = coronary artery disease; LV = left ventricular.

The guidelines support the practice of bypassing all significant coronary artery stenoses when possible in patients undergoing aortic valve replacement.

References

1. Bonow RO, Carabello B, De Leon Jr. AC, et al: ACC/AHA guidelines for the management of patients with valvular heart disease: A report of the American College of Cardiology/American Heart Association Task Force on Practice Guidelines (Committee on Management of Patients with Valvular Heart Disease). J Am Coll Cardiol 32:1486, 1998.
2. Bonow RO, Carabello BA, Chatterjee K, et al: ACC/AHA 2006 guidelines for the management of patients with valvular heart disease: A report of the American College of Cardiology/American Heart Association Task Force on Practice Guidelines (writing committee to revise the 1998 guidelines for the management of patients with valvular heart disease) developed in collaboration with the Society of Cardiovascular Anesthesiologists and endorsed by the Society for Cardiovascular Angiography and Interventions and the Society of Thoracic Surgeons. J Am Coll Cardiol 48:e1, 2006.
3. Cheitlin MD, Armstrong WF, Aurigemma GP, et al: ACC/AHA/ASE 2003 guideline update for the clinical application of echocardiography: A report of the American College of Cardiology/American Heart Association Task Force on Practice Guidelines (ACC/AHA/ASE Committee to Update the 1997 Guidelines for the Clinical Application of Echocardiography). J Am Coll Cardiol 42:954, 2003.
4. Bonow RO, Cheitlin MD, Crawford MH, et al: 36th Bethesda Conference: Recommendations for determining eligibility for competition in athletes with cardiovascular abnormalities. Task Force 3: Valvular heart disease. J Am Coll Cardiol 45:1334, 2005.
5. Maron BJ, Araujo CG, Thompson PD, et al: Recommendations for preparticipation screening and the assessment of cardiovascular disease in masters athletes: An advisory for healthcare professionals from the working groups of the World Heart Federation, the International Federation of Sports Medicine, and the American Heart Association Committee on Exercise, Cardiac Rehabilitation, and Prevention. Circulation 103:327, 2001.
6. Bonow RO, Bennett S, Casey DE Jr, et al: ACC/AHA clinical performance measures for adults with chronic heart failure: A report of the American College of Cardiology/American Heart Association Task Force on Performance Measures (writing committee to develop heart failure clinical performance measures) endorsed by the Heart Failure Society of America. J Am Coll Cardiol 46:1144, 2005.
7. Feldman T, Wasserman HS, Herrmann HC, et al: Percutaneous mitral valve repair using the edge-to-edge technique: Six-month results of the EVEREST Phase I Clinical Trial. J Am Coll Cardiol 46:2134, 2005.
8. Khambadkone S, Coats L, Taylor A, et al: Percutaneous pulmonary valve implantation in humans: Results in 59 consecutive patients. Circulation 112:1189, 2005.
9. Cribier A, Eltchaninoff H, Tron C, et al: Early experience with percutaneous transcatheter implantation of heart valve prosthesis for the treatment of end-stage inoperable patients with calcific aortic stenosis. J Am Coll Cardiol 43:698, 2004.

CHAPTER 63

Epidemiology, 1713
Groups of Patients, 1713

Etiological
Microorganisms, 1716

Pathogenesis, 1718

Pathophysiology, 1719

Clinical Features, 1720

Diagnosis, 1721
Laboratory Tests, 1722
Imaging, 1722

Treatment, 1722
Antimicrobial Therapy for Specific
    Organisms, 1723
Surgical Treatment of Intracardiac
    Complications, 1727
Treatment of Extracardiac
    Complications, 1729
Response to Therapy, 1730

Prevention, 1731

Future Perspectives, 1732

References, 1732

Guidelines, 1734

Infective Endocarditis

Adolf W. Karchmer

The characteristic lesion of infective endocarditis (IE), the vegetation, is a variably sized amorphous mass of platelets and fibrin with abundant enmeshed microorganisms and moderate inflammatory cells. Infection involves heart valves most commonly but also occurs at the site of a septal defect, on chordae tendineae, or on mural endocardium. Infections of arteriovenous shunts, arterioarterial shunts (patent ductus arteriosus), or coarctation of the aorta are clinically and pathologically similar to IE. Many species of bacteria cause IE; nevertheless, streptococci, staphylococci, enterococci, and fastidious gram-negative coccobacilli cause the majority of cases of IE.

IE is often called acute or subacute. Acute IE is caused typically, although not exclusively, by *Staphylococcus aureus.* It presents with marked toxicity and progresses over days to several weeks to valvular destruction and metastatic infection. Subacute IE, usually caused by viridans streptococci, enterococci, coagulase-negative staphylococci, or gram-negative coccobacilli, evolves over weeks to months with only modest toxicity and rarely causes metastatic infection.

EPIDEMIOLOGY

The incidence of IE remained relatively stable from 1950 through 2000 at about 3.6 to 7.0 cases per 100,000 patient-years.[1,2] In selected areas the incidence may be increased because of the concentration of populations at uniquely high risk of infection, specifically intravenous drug users. For example, from 1988 to 1990, 11.6 episodes per 100,000 population were reported from metropolitan Philadelphia (Delaware Valley) with injection drug abuse accounting for approximately half of the cases. The stable incidence is illustrated in Olmsted County, Minnesota, where from 1970 to 2000 the 5-year interval IE incidence ranged from 5.0 to 7.0 per 100,000 person-years, and in France the IE incidence in 1991 and 1999 was 3.1 and 2.6 per 100,000 population, respectively.[2,3] Risk factors in industrialized countries have shifted, however, from chronic rheumatic and congenital heart disease to intravenous drug use, degenerative valve disease in the elderly, intracardiac devices, health care–associated infection, and hemodialysis. Endocarditis usually occurred more frequently in men than in women, with a 2:1 ratio. The median age of patients has gradually increased from 30 to 40 years of age in the early antibiotic era to 47 to 69 years recently. The age-specific incidence of endocarditis increases from 5 cases per 100,000 person-years among persons younger than 50 years of age to 15 to 30 cases per 100,000 person-years in the sixth through eighth decades of life.[1,3] From 50 to 75 percent of patients with native valve endocarditis (NVE) have predisposing valve conditions. The nature of the predisposing conditions and, in part, the microbiology of IE correlates with the age of patients (Table 63-1). Recent case series from large tertiary care referral centers have not only illustrated the previously noted shift in risk factors but also concomitant changes in microbiology, in particular that *Staphylococcus aureus* exceeds streptococci as a causative agent.[4,5] In contrast, population-based series, particularly if not dominated by cases among drug abusers, illustrate the continued importance of rheumatic and congenital valvular disease as predispositions and the predominance of streptococci as causal agents.[2,3,6] Where NVE among adults is not skewed dramatically by IV drug abuse and nosocomial infection, the microbiology is as shown in Table 63-1.

Groups of Patients

CHILDREN. In the Netherlands, IE was noted in 1.7 and 1.2 per 100,000 male and female children younger than 10 years, respectively. IE has been noted with increasing frequency among neonates. It often involves the tricuspid valve of structurally normal hearts and arises as a consequence of infected intravascular catheters or cardiac surgery. The vast majority of children with IE occurring after the neonatal period have identifiable structural cardiac abnormalities (see Table 63-1). Congenital heart abnormalities are present in 75 to 90 percent of cases. In many cases IE occurs at the site of surgical repair and reflects the persistent risk for infection after complex reconstructive surgery. Neither secundum atrial septal defects nor patent ductus arteriosus and pulmonic stenosis after repair are associated with IE. Mitral valve prolapse in association with a regurgitant murmur predisposes to IE in children. The clinical features and echocardiographic findings of IE in children are similar to those noted among adults with NVE or prosthetic valve endocarditis (PVE), respectively.

ADULTS. *Mitral valve prolapse* (MVP), a prominent predisposing structural cardiac abnormality in adults, accounts for 7 to 30 percent of NVE not related to drug abuse or nosocomial infection. The frequency of MVP in IE is not entirely a direct reflection of relative risk but rather a function of the frequency of the lesion in the general population This increased risk of endocarditis is largely confined to patients with prolapse, thickened valve leaflets (>5 mm), and mitral regurgitation murmur, especially among men and patients older than 45 years (see Chap. 62). Among patients with MVP and a systolic murmur, the incidence of IE is 52 per 100,000 person-years, compared with a rate of 4.6 per 100,000 person-years among those with prolapse and no murmur or among the general population. The microbiology and morbidity of IE engrafted on MVP is similar to that of NVE that is not associated with drug abuse.

Rheumatic heart disease as a predisposing cardiac lesion for IE has become less prevalent in industrialized nations. In patients with rheumatic heart disease, endocarditis occurs most frequently on the mitral valve followed by the aortic valve.

Congenital heart disease is the substrate for IE in 10 to 20 percent of younger adults and 8 percent of older adults. Among adults, the common predisposing lesions are patent ductus arteriosus, ventricular septal defect, and bicuspid aortic valve, the latter particularly found among older men (>60 years).

Infection with *human immunodeficiency virus* (HIV), unless associated with IV drug abuse, is not a significant risk factor for IE. Among HIV-infected persons who are not IV drug abusers, organisms typical of NVE and those that are uniquely associated with bacteremia in patients with AIDS, such as *Bartonella* spp., *Salmonella* spp. and *Streptococcus pneumoniae*, cause IE. Notably, 40 percent of cases were nosocomial.[7] In HIV-infected IV drug abusers, endocarditis is frequent and the risk and mortality are related to progressive immunodeficiency, inversely to CD4 counts <400 cells/mm^3.[8]

INTRAVENOUS DRUG ABUSERS. The risk for IE among IV drug abusers, 2 to 5 percent per patient-year, is several-fold greater than that for patients with rheumatic heart disease or prosthetic valves. From 65 to 80 percent of cases of IE in this population occur in men who typically range in age from 27 to 37 years. IE is located on the tricuspid valve in 46 to 78 percent, mitral valve in 24 to 32 percent, and aortic valve in 8 to 19 percent; as many as 16 percent of patients have infection at multiple sites. The valves were normal before infection in 75 to 93 percent of patients. IV drug abuse is a risk factor for recurrent NVE.

MICROBIOLOGY. *S. aureus* causes more than 50 percent of IE occurring in IV drug abusers overall and 60 to 70 percent of infections involving the tricuspid valve (Table 63-2). The well-established predilection for *S. aureus* to infect normal heart valves is noted in addicts. Although the phenomenon of *S. aureus* infection of normal tricuspid valves is not unique to addicts, the high frequency is characteristic. Streptococci and enterococci infect previously abnormal mitral or aortic valves in addicts. Infection of right and left heart valves by *Pseudomonas aeruginosa* and other gram-negative bacilli and left heart valves by fungi occurs with increased frequency among drug abusers. Unusual organisms related to injection of contaminated materials cause endocarditis in these patients, e.g., *Corynebacterium* species, *Lactobacillus*, *Bacillus cereus*, and nonpathogenic *Neisseria* species. Polymicrobial endocarditis accounts for 3 to 5 percent of cases of IE.

The clinical manifestations of IE in IV drug abusers depend on the valves involved and, to a lesser degree, on the infecting organism. Pleuritic chest pain, shortness of breath, cough, and hemoptysis occur with tricuspid valve

CH 63

TABLE 63–1	Predisposing Conditions and Microbiology of Native Valve Endocarditis			
Conditions and Microbiology	**Children (%)**		**Adults (%)**	
	Neonates	*2 mo-15 yr*	*15-60 yr*	*>60 yr*
Predisposing Conditions				
RHD		2-10	25-30	8
CHD	28	75-90*	10-20	2
MVP		5-15	10-30	10
DHD			Rare	30
Parenteral drug abuse			15-35	10
Other			10-15	10
None	72†	2-5	25-45	25-40
Microbiology				
Streptococci	15-20	40-50	45-65‡	30-45‡
Enterococci		4	5-8	15
S. aureus	40-50	25	30-40‡	25-30‡
Coagulase-negative staphylococci	10	5	3-5	5-8
GNB	10	5	4-8	5
Fungi	10	1	1	Rare
Polymicrobial	4		1	Rare
Other			1	2
Culture negative	4	0-15	3-10	5

*50% of cases follow surgery and may involve implanted devices and foreign material.

†Often tricuspid valve IE.

‡In recent large series from tertiary centers, the referral bias combined with health care–associated IE and prevalent IV drug abuse result in a reversal in the relative frequency of IE caused by *S. aureus* and streptococci (see text).

CHD = congenital heart disease; DHD = degenerative heart disease; GNB = gram-negative bacteria—frequently *Haemophilus* species, *Actinobacillus actinomycetemcomitans*, *Cardiobacterium hominis*; MVP = mitral valve prolapse; RHD = rheumatic heart disease.

TABLE 63–2	Microbiology of Endocarditis Associated with Intravenous Drug Abuse			
	Number of Cases (%) of Endocarditis in Drug Addicts*			
Organisms	*Right-Sided N = 346*	*Left-Sided N = 204*	*Total N = 675*	*Spain (1977-1993)† N = 1529*
Streptococci‡	17 (5)	31 (15)	80 (12)	131 (8.5)
Enterococci	7 (2)	49 (24)	59 (9)	21 (1)
Staphylococcus aureus	267 (77)	47 (23)	396 (57)	1138 (74)
Coagulase-negative staphylococci	—	—		44 (3)
Gram-negative bacilli§	7 (5)	26 (13)	45 (7)	23 (1.5)
Fungi (predominantly *Candida* species)	—	25 (12)	26 (4)	18 (1)
Polymicrobia/miscellaneous	28 (8)	20 (10)	49 (7)	48 (3)
Culture negative	10 (3)	6 (3)	20 (3)	106 (7)

*Ten patients with right- and left-sided infective endocarditis are counted twice.

†Data from Miro JM, del Rio A, Mestres CA: Infective endocarditis in intravenous drug abusers and HIV-1 infected patients. Infect Dis Clin North Am 16:273-95, 2002.

‡Includes viridans streptococci, *Streptococcus bovis*, other non–group A groupable streptococci, *Abiotrophia* species (nutritionally variant streptococci).

§*Pseudomonas aeruginosa*, *Serratia marcescens*, and Enterobacteriaceae.

endocarditis, particularly when caused by *S. aureus.* In 65 to 75 percent of patients, chest x-rays reveal abnormalities related to septic pulmonary emboli. Murmurs of tricuspid regurgitation are noted in less than one half of these patients. Infection of the aortic or mitral valve in addicts clinically resembles IE seen in patients who are not drug abusers. HIV infection has been noted in 27 to 73 percent of IV drug abusers with IE (see Chap. 67).

PROSTHETIC VALVE ENDOCARDITIS. Epidemiological studies suggest that prosthetic valve endocarditis (PVE) constitutes 10 to 30 percent of all cases of IE in developed countries.[3,4,6,9] In metropolitan Philadelphia, 0.94 cases of IE per 100,000 population involved prosthetic valves. In patients undergoing valve surgery between 1965 and 1995, the cumulative incidence of PVE estimated actuarially ranged from 1.4 to 3.1 percent at 12 months and 3.0 to 5.7 percent at 5 years.[10] The frequency is greatest during the initial 6 months after valve surgery (particularly during the initial 5 to 6 weeks) and thereafter declines to a lower but stable rate (0.2 to 0.35 percent per year).[10]

PVE has been called "early" when symptoms begin within 60 days of valve surgery and "late" with onset thereafter. These terms were established to distinguish PVE that arose early as a complication of valve surgery from later infection that was likely to be community acquired. In fact, many cases with onset between 60 days and 1 year after surgery relate to the surgical admission despite their delayed presentation or are related to health care. Specific risk factors for PVE, other than a history of IE, have not been clearly defined. During the initial months after valve implantation, mechanical prostheses are at greater risk of infection than bioprosthetic valves but after 12 months, the risk of infection of bioprostheses exceeds that of mechanical valves. By 5 years after valve surgery, the rates of PVE for the two valve types are comparable.[10]

MICROBIOLOGY. The microbiology of PVE, when considered by time of onset, reflects in part the presumed nosocomial, health care–associated, or community acquisition of infection (Table 63-3). Coagulase-negative staphylococci, primarily *Staphylococcus epidermidis,* are a prominent cause of early PVE. *S. aureus,* gram-negative bacilli, enterococci, and fungi (particularly *Candida* species) are also common causes of PVE during this period. Early PVE caused by *Legionella* species, atypical mycobacteria, mycoplasma, and fungi other than *Candida* has been reported. The microbiology of late PVE resembles that of community-acquired NVE; streptococci, *S. aureus,* enterococci, and coagulase-negative staphylococci are the major causes. Nosocomial and health care–associated late PVE has increased recently.[11]

Pathology. In contrast to the largely leaflet-confined pathology of NVE, infection on bioprostheses during the year after implantation or on mechanical prostheses commonly extends beyond the valve ring into the annulus and periannular tissue causing dehiscence of the prosthesis with hemodynamically significant paravalvular regurgitation and conduction disturbances. Bulky vegetations can interfere with valve function at the mitral site and cause valve stenosis (Fig. 63-1).[12]

Among 85 patients with mechanical valve PVE in whom the site of infection was examined at surgery or autopsy, annulus invasion was noted in 42 percent, myocardial abscess in 14 percent, valve obstruction in 4 percent, and pericarditis in 2 percent.[10,12] Among 85 patients with bioprosthetic PVE, 29 of 49 (59 percent) with infection within a year after surgery had invasive disease—in contrast to only 9 of 36 patients (25 percent) with infection occurring

TABLE 63–3	Microbiology of Prosthetic Valve Endocarditis 1970-2003	
	Number of Cases (%)* with Time of Onset After Valve Surgery	
Organisms	**Early (N = 218)** *<12 mo*	**Late (N = 272)** *>12 mo*
Streptococci[†]	5 (2)	77 (28)
Pneumococci	—	—
Enterococci	20 (9)	36 (13)
Staphylococcus aureus	42 (19)	45 (17)
Coagulase-negative staphylococci	72 (33)	31 (11)
Fastidious gram-negative coccobacilli (HACEK group)[‡]	—	11 (4)
Gram-negative bacilli	34 (16)	17 (6)
Fungi, *Candida* species	16 (7)	5 (2)
Polymicrobial/miscellaneous	6 (3)	15 (6)
Diphtheroids	10 (5)	7 (3)
Coxiella burnetii	—	5 (2)
Culture negative	13 (6)	23 (8)

*Data from Karchner AW, Longworth DL: Infections of intracardiac devices. Infect Dis Clin North Am 16:477-505, 2002; Rivas P, Alonso J, Moya J, et al: The impact of hospital-acquired infections on the microbial etiology and prognosis of late-onset prosthetic valve endocarditis. Chest 128:764-771, 2005.

[†]Includes viridans streptococci, *Streptococcus bovis,* other non-group A groupable streptococci, *Abiotrophia* species (nutritionally variant streptococci).

[‡]Includes *Hemophilus* species, *Actinobacillus actinomycetemcomitans, Cardiobacterium hominis, Eikenella* species, and *Kingella* species.

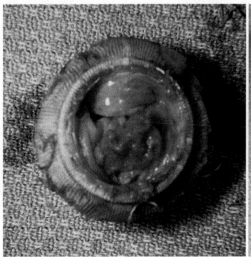 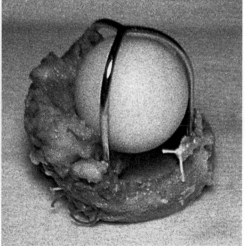

A   B

FIGURE 63–1 A, A large vegetation caused by *Candida albicans* partially occludes the orifice of a bioprosthetic valve removed from the mitral position. **B,** A Starr-Edwards prosthesis removed from the aortic position, where this large vegetation related to *Aspergillus* infection partially obstructed the outflow tract but also allowed regurgitation by preventing valve closure. *(**A,** Reproduced from Karchmer AW: Infections of prosthetic heart valves. In Korzeniowski OM [ed]: Cardiovascular Infection, vol X, Atlas of Infectious Diseases. Philadelphia, Churchill Livingstone, 1998, p 5.7.)*

more than 1 year postoperatively. In surgically treated bioprosthetic IE, invasion was confirmed in 15 of 19 cases (79 percent) with onset in the initial 12 months after surgery, but in only 22 of 71 bioprostheses (31 percent) when infection began more than 12 months after surgery.[10] Aortic site and clinical onset within a year of valve surgery correlate with an increased risk of invasive infection. Infected prosthetic valves can be distinguished from uninfected valves microscopically. Histological examination of infected mechanical and bioprosthetic valves reveals a neutrophil-rich inflammatory infiltrate with neovascularization and possibly microorganisms, whereas the inflammatory infiltrate in vegetations or thrombi adherent to uninfected valves is composed primarily of macrophages and lymphocytes.

Signs and symptoms in patients developing PVE within 60 days of cardiac surgery may be obscured by surgery or other postoperative complications. Peripheral signs of endocarditis (5 to 14 percent) and central nervous system emboli (10 percent) occur less frequently in these patients than in those with PVE occurring later after surgery. Among patients with later onset PVE, congestive heart failure (CHF) occurs in 40 percent, cerebrovascular complications in 26 to 28 percent, and peripheral signs in 15 to 28 percent.[10,12] Among patients with PVE treated since 1980, in-hospital mortality overall ranges from 14 to 41 percent and that for early and late infection from 30 to 46 and 19 to 34 percent, respectively.[9,11] Mortality for *S. aureus* PVE regardless of time of onset remains high, 36 to 47 percent.[13-15]

HEALTH CARE–ASSOCIATED ENDOCARDITIS. Health care–associated endocarditis includes true nosocomial IE as well as IE arising in the community after a recent hospitalization or as a direct consequence of long-term indwelling devices, such as central venous lines, tunneled lines, and hemodialysis catheters. Health care–associated endocarditis, unrelated to concurrent cardiac surgery, makes up 5 to 29 percent of all cases of IE in various series and may involve normal or abnormal native valves, including the tricuspid, transvenous pacemakers and defibrillators, and prosthetic valves.[6,10,11] Hemodialysis is independently associated with *S. aureus* IE.[4,16]

The onset of health care–associated IE is usually acute, and although a changing murmur may be heard, other classic signs of endocarditis are infrequent. Mortality rates among these patients, many of whom are elderly and have serious underlying diseases, are high (27 to 38 percent).[6]

MICROBIOLOGY. Gram-positive cocci are the predominant cause of health care–associated IE with occasional cases caused by Candida species and various gram-negative bacilli.[6,11] Among 128 episodes from four series, *S. aureus* caused 57 episodes, coagulase-negative staphylococci 19, enterococci 21, streptococci 10, *Candida* species 8, and gram-negative bacilli 7; 6 cases were culture negative.

Catheter-associated *S. aureus* bacteremia occurs with sufficient frequency to be the predominant predisposing factor for health care–associated IE.[16] Transesophageal echocardiography (TEE) is recommended to exclude IE in patients with catheter-related *S. aureus* bacteremia (see Chap. 14). Patients with *S. aureus* catheter-related bacteremia who have abnormal heart valves, prosthetic valves, or persisting fever or bacteremia for 3 to 4 days after catheter removal and initiation of therapy are at high risk for IE and should be treated for presumed IE.

ETIOLOGICAL MICROORGANISMS

VIRIDANS STREPTOCOCCI. These streptococci, which cause 30 to 65 percent of NVE cases unrelated to drug abuse and health care, are normal inhabitants of the oropharynx, characteristically produce alpha hemolysis when grown on sheep blood agar, and are usually nontypable using the Lancefield system.[2,6] Using earlier taxonomy, the non-beta hemolytic streptococci causing NVE were distributed as follows: *Streptococcus mitior* (31 percent of cases), *Streptococcus sanguis* (24 percent), *Streptococcus bovis* (27 percent), *Streptococcus mutans* (7 percent), *Streptococcus milleri* (now called *Streptococcus anginosus* group and includes *Streptococcus intermedius, anginosus,* and *constellatus*) (4 percent), *Streptococcus faecalis* (now *Enterococcus faecalis*) (7 percent), and *Streptococcus salivarius* and other species (2 percent). Nutritional variant organisms that require media supplemented with either pyridoxal hydrochloride or L-cysteine for growth, previously speciated as *Streptococcus adjacens* or *Streptococcus defectivus,* cause 5 percent of cases of streptococcal NVE. These organisms have been reclassified as *Granulicatella* species and *Abiotrophia defectiva* species, respectively. *Gemella morbillorum,* previously called *Streptococcus morbillorum,* share some characteristics with nutritionally variant organisms and should be treated with similar antibiotic therapy.[17]

The viridans streptococci had been, in general, highly susceptible to penicillin (minimum inhibitory concentration [MIC] < 0.1 µg/ml for 83 percent). Recently a larger percent of these have penicillin MICs >0.1 µg/ml. The streptococci are killed in a synergistic manner by penicillin plus gentamicin.

***STREPTOCOCCUS BOVIS* AND OTHER STREPTOCOCCI.** *S. bovis,* part of the gastrointestinal tract normal flora, cause 20 to 40 percent of the episodes of streptococcal NVE.[3] Although superficially resembling the enterococci, the distinction is important because *S. bovis* are highly penicillin susceptible, in contrast to the relative penicillin resistance of enterococci. *S. bovis* type I endocarditis is frequently associated with coexistent polyps or malignancy in the colon; accordingly, colonoscopy is warranted in these patients.

Group A streptococci, which can infect normal valves, cause rare episodes of endocarditis. Among IV drug abusers, group A streptococci have caused tricuspid valve IE similar to that noted with *S. aureus.* Group B organisms, *Streptococcus agalactiae,* are part of the normal flora of the mouth, genital tract, and gastrointestinal tract. Group B streptococci infect normal and abnormal valves and cause a morbid NVE syndrome with a high incidence of systemic emboli and septic musculoskeletal complications (arthritis, discitis, osteomyelitis).[18] The *S. anginosus* group are highly pyogenic organisms that cause destructive extracardiac infections and IE with intracardiac complications. Beta-hemolytic (group A, B, C, and G) streptococcal IE often occurs in the absence of valvular disease and has an acute onset and frequent intracardiac or extracardiac complications. IE caused by beta hemolytic streptococci and the *S. anginosus* group commonly requires surgical treatment.[18,19]

STREPTOCOCCUS PNEUMONIAE. Although pneumococcal bacteremia occurs frequently, *S. pneumoniae* accounts for only 1 to 3 percent of NVE cases.[20] Pneumococcal IE frequently involves a normal aortic valve and progresses rapidly with valve destruction, myocardial abscess formation, and acute CHF. The diagnosis of IE is often delayed until intracardiac complications or systemic emboli are evident. The clinical presentation, complications, and outcome of endocarditis caused by penicillin-susceptible and penicillin-resistant *S. pneumoniae* are similar. Almost half of the patients require cardiac surgery because of valve dysfunction, CHF, or persisting fever. Mortality (35 percent) is related to left-sided heart failure and not to the penicillin susceptibility of the infecting strain.[20]

ENTEROCOCCI. *E. faecalis* and *Enterococcus faecium* cause 85 and 10 percent of cases of enterococcal IE, respectively. Enterococci, which are part of the normal gastrointestinal flora and cause genitourinary tract infection, account for 5 to 15 percent of cases of both

NVE and PVE (see Tables 63-2 and 63-3).[2,4,6,12,21] Disease typically occurs with equal frequency in older men (often from a urinary tract portal of entry) and women, and 15 percent of cases are nosocomial.[21] Enterococci infect either normal or abnormal valves and prosthetic valves and occur with acute or subacute onset. Mortality rates are comparable to those noted with viridans streptococcal IE.

Enterococci are resistant to cephalosporins, semisynthetic penicillinase-resistant penicillins (oxacillin and nafcillin), and therapeutic concentrations of aminoglycosides. Most enterococci have been inhibited by modest concentrations of the cell wall–active antibiotics: penicillin, ampicillin, vancomycin, and teicoplanin (not licensed in the United States). Bactericidal antienterococcal activity can be achieved by combining an inhibitory cell wall–active agent and streptomycin or gentamicin. This bactericidal activity, called *synergy*, is essential for optimal treatment of enterococcal IE. Strains of enterococci that are resistant to penicillin and ampicillin, resistant to vancomycin, or highly resistant to streptomycin and gentamicin have been identified as causes of IE. These resistant strains of enterococci may be unresponsive to standard antienterococcal regimens and defy development of synergistic bactericidal therapy.[22] The antibiotic susceptibility of any enterococcus causing IE must be thoroughly evaluated if optimal therapy is to be assured.

STAPHYLOCOCCI. The coagulase-positive staphylococci are a single species: *S. aureus.* Of the 13 species of coagulase-negative staphylococci that colonize humans, *S. epidermidis* has emerged as an important pathogen in the setting of implanted devices and health care–associated infection.

S. aureus. This organism is a major cause of IE in all population groups (see Tables 63-1, 63-2, and 63-3). As a result of the increasing importance of health care–associated infection and IV drug use in causing IE, *S. aureus* is the most common cause of IE noted in two large international series from tertiary care centers.[4,23] *S. aureus* IE is characterized by a highly toxic febrile illness, frequent focal metastatic infection, a 30 to 50 percent rate of CHF, and central nervous system complications.[4,16,23] A cerebrospinal fluid polymorphonuclear pleocytosis, with or without *S. aureus* cultured from the cerebrospinal fluid, is common. Heart murmurs are often initially absent but are ultimately heard in 75 to 85 percent as a consequence of intracardiac damage. The mortality rate in non-addicts with left-sided *S. aureus* endocarditis ranges from 16 to 65 percent overall and is increased with age, with significant underlying diseases, or when IE is complicated by a major neurological event, perivalvular abscess and valve dysfunction, or CHF.[4,16,23] Among addicts, left-sided *S. aureus* IE resembles that in non-addicts. With *S. aureus* IE limited to the tricuspid valve (see Fig. 14-68), systemic complications are rare and mortality rates are only 2 to 4 percent, although occasional patients suffer overwhelming septic pulmonary emboli, pyopneumothorax, and severe respiratory insufficiency.

Coagulase-Negative Staphylococci. These organisms, specifically *S. epidermidis,* are a major cause of PVE, particularly during the initial year after valve surgery, an important cause of nosocomial IE, and the cause of 3 to 8 percent of NVE, usually in the setting of prior valve abnormalities (see Tables 63-1 and 63-2).[24] Non-epidermidis species cause NVE that is not associated with health care. Coagulase negative staphylococcal NVE is often complicated and fatal.[24] *Staphylococcus lugdunensis,* a community-acquired, antibiotic-susceptible coagulase-negative species, causes valve damage and frequently requires surgical intervention.

GRAM-NEGATIVE BACTERIA. The HACEK organisms (*Haemophilus parainfluenzae, Hemophilus aphrophilus, Actinobacillus actinomycetemcomitans, Cardiobacterium hominis, Eikenella corrodens,* and *Kingella kingae*), which are part of the upper respiratory tract and oropharyngeal flora, infect abnormal cardiac valves, causing subacute NVE, and cause PVE that occurs a year or more after valve surgery. Although fastidious and slow growing, HACEK organisms are usually detected in blood cultures within 5 days of incubation; occasionally more prolonged incubation is required. HACEK NVE has been associated with large vegetations and a high incidence of systemic emboli.

P. aeruginosa is the gram-negative bacillus that most commonly causes endocarditis. The Enterobacteriaceae, despite causing frequent episodes of bacteremia, are implicated in only sporadic cases of IE. Mortality rates for gram-negative bacillus IE are high (50 percent).

Neisseria gonorrhoeae, a rare cause of endocarditis today, infects the aortic valve of young patients and causes valve destruction and intracardiac abscesses. Although this organism is generally susceptible to ceftriaxone, antibiotic resistance is widespread among *N. gonorrhoeae;* accordingly, treatment must be based on the susceptibility of the implicated isolate. Other *Neisseria* species (nongonococcal, nonmeningococcal) cause rare episodes of IE, usually in the setting of preexisting valvulopathy.

OTHER ORGANISMS. *Corynebacterium* species, called *diphtheroids,* although often contaminants in blood cultures, cannot be ignored when isolated from multiple blood cultures. They are an important cause of PVE and a surprisingly common cause of endocarditis involving abnormal valves.[12] *Listeria monocytogenes,* a small gram-positive rod, causes occasional cases of IE involving abnormal left heart valves and prosthetic devices. *Tropheryma whippelii,* the cause of Whipple disease, has caused a cryptic afebrile form of IE with associated arthralgias but without diarrhea as well as valvular disease as part of typical Whipple disease. The diagnosis has been established by identification of the organism on excised valves using periodic acid–Schiff stain or by polymerase chain reaction (PCR). IE caused by *T. whippelii* often does not fulfill the Duke criteria for diagnosis (Table 63-4); thus, detection requires a high index of suspicion.

The rickettsia *C. burnetii,* an uncommon cause of IE in the United States, is a prominent cause of IE in other parts of the world. After acute infection by *C. burnetii* (Q fever), persons with abnormal mitral or aortic valves, particularly those with prosthetic valves, may develop insidious subacute IE. Patients with acute Q fever and echocardiogram-confirmed valvulopathy should receive prolonged antibiotic treatment with doxycycline plus hydroxychloroquine to prevent IE.[25] IE commonly manifests with low-grade fever, fatigue, weight loss, and CHF. Hepatosplenomegaly, digital clubbing, and an immune complex vasculitis–induced purpuric rash are not uncommon. Vegetations are small, have smooth surfaces, and are not uniformly visible on echocardiogram. The diagnosis is typically based on high immunoglobulin G antibody titers to phase I *C. burnetii* antigens plus immunoglobulin A antibody or on demonstration of the organism in excised cardiac valves by immunohistological or Gimenez staining or by PCR testing.

Bartonella quintana and *Bartonella henselae,* which together may cause 3 percent of NVE, can be isolated from blood cultures by prolonged incubation and special techniques. In the absence of special culturing efforts, PCR detection of genetic material in excised vegetations, or serological testing, many cases would have been "culture negative." *B. henselae,* which causes cat-scratch disease and, in the HIV-infected population, bacillary angiomatosis and hepatic peliosis, causes IE in patients with prior valve injury and cat exposure. *B. quintana,* the agent of trench fever, causes IE on normal valves largely in homeless people who are exposed to infected body lice. *Bartonella* IE arises insidiously; diagnosis is often delayed, and CHF and systemic emboli frequently complicate infection. Treatment commonly requires valve surgery.[26] On the basis of serological testing, *Chlamydia* species have been suggested as the cause of frequent episodes of IE. Because of the extensive serological cross-reaction between *Chlamydia* and *Bartonella,* many of these episodes have actually been *Bartonella* IE.

FUNGI. *Candida albicans,* nonalbicans *Candida* species, *Histoplasma,* and *Aspergillus* species are the most common of the many fungal organisms identified as causing IE. Unusual so-called emerging fungi and molds account for 25 percent of cases. Among 269 cases of fungal IE described between 1965 and 1995, 25 percent were nosocomial. Risk factors include previous valve surgery, antibiotic use, injection drug abuse, intravascular catheters, surgery other than cardiac,

TABLE 63–4 | Diagnosis of Infective Endocarditis (Modified Duke Criteria)

Definite Infective Endocarditis
Pathological criteria
   Microorganisms: demonstrated by culture or histology in a vegetation, *or* in a vegetation that has embolized, *or* in an intracardiac abscess, *or*
   Pathological lesions: vegetation or intracardiac abscess present, confirmed by histology showing active endocarditis
Clinical criteria, using specific definitions listed below
   Two major criteria, *or*
   One major and three minor criteria, *or*
   Five minor criteria

Possible Infective Endocarditis
One major criterion and one minor criterion or three minor criteria

Rejected
Firm alternative diagnosis for manifestations of endocarditis, *or*
Sustained resolution of manifestations of endocarditis, with antibiotic therapy for 4 days or less, *or*
No pathological evidence of infective endocarditis at surgery or autopsy, after antibiotic therapy for 4 days or less

Criteria for Diagnosis of Infective Endocarditis
Major Criteria
Positive blood culture
   Typical microorganism for infective endocarditis from two separate blood cultures
      Viridans streptococci, *Streptococcus bovis*, HACEK group *or*
      Staphylococcus aureus or community-acquired enterococci in the absence of a primary focus, *or*
   Persistently positive blood culture, defined as recovery of a microorganism consistent with infective endocarditis from:
      Blood cultures (≥2) drawn more than 12 hr apart, *or*
      All of three or a majority of four or more separate blood cultures, with first and last drawn at least 1 hr apart
   Single positive blood culture for *Coxiella burnetii* or antiphase I IgG antibody titer >1:800
Evidence of endocardial involvement
   Positive echocardiogram (TEE advised for PVE or complicated infective endocarditis)
      Oscillating intracardiac mass, on valve or supporting structures, *or* in the path of regurgitant jets, *or* on
         implanted material, in the absence of an alternative anatomical explanation, *or*
      Abscess, *or*
      New partial dehiscence of prosthetic valve, *or*
   New valvular regurgitation (increase or change in preexisting murmur not sufficient)

Minor Criteria
Predisposition: predisposing heart condition *or* intravenous drug use
Fever ≥38.0°C (100.4°F)
Vascular phenomena: major arterial emboli, septic pulmonary infarcts, mycotic aneurysm, intracranial hemorrhage, conjunctival hemorrhages,
   Janeway lesions
Immunological phenomena: glomerulonephritis, Osler nodes, Roth spots, rheumatoid factor
Microbiological evidence: positive blood culture but not meeting major criterion as noted previously* *or* serologic evidence of active infection with
   organism consistent with infective endocarditis

*Excluding single positive cultures for coagulase-negative staphylococci and organisms that do not cause endocarditis commonly.
IgG = immunoglobulin G; PVE = prosthetic valve endocarditis; TEE = transesophageal echocardiography.
Adapted from Durack DT, Lukes AS, Bright DK: New criteria for diagnosis of infective endocarditis: Utilization of specific echocardiographic findings. Am J Med 96:200, 1994; modified per Li JS, Sexton DJ, Mick N, et al: Proposed modifications to the Duke criteria for the diagnosis of infective endocarditis. Clin Infect Dis 30:633, 2000.

CH 63

and immunocompromised state. The frequency of the last three risk factors has increased, and virtually all fungal IE patients have two or more risk factors. Fever, murmurs, embolization including major limb artery occlusion, neurological abnormalities, and CHF are common. Blood cultures are positive commonly when IE is caused by *Candida* species but rarely when caused by mycelial organisms. Culture and histological examination of vegetations and peripheral emboli, when possible, yield a microbiological diagnosis in 75 to 95 percent of cases.

PATHOGENESIS

The interactions between the human host and selected microorganisms that culminate in IE involve the vascular endothelium, hemostatic mechanisms, the host immune system, gross anatomical abnormalities in the heart, surface properties of microorganisms, enzyme and toxin production by microorganisms, and peripheral events that initiate bacteremia. Each component is in itself complex, influenced by many factors. Occasionally these interactions result in a pathogenetic sequence wherein microorganisms gain access to the bloodstream, rapidly adhere to valve surfaces, become persistent at the site of adherence, proliferate to cause local damage and vegetation growth, and ultimately disseminate hematogenously with or without emboli. Studies have begun

to elucidate the pathogenesis of IE caused by viridans streptococci and *S. aureus*.[1,27] The rarity of endocarditis in spite of frequent bacteremia indicates that the intact endothelium is relatively resistant to infection. It is hypothesized that platelet-fibrin deposition occurs spontaneously on abnormal valves and at sites of cardiac endothelium injury or inflammation and that these deposits, called nonbacterial thrombotic endocarditis (NBTE), are the sites at which microorganisms adhere during bacteremia to initiate IE.[1,27]

DEVELOPMENT OF NONBACTERIAL THROMBOTIC ENDOCARDITIS. Two major mechanisms appear pivotal in the formation of NBTE: endothelial injury and a hypercoagulable state. NBTE, thought to be a result of hypercoagulability, has been found in 1.3 percent of patients at autopsy and is more common with increasing age and in patients with malignancy, disseminated intravascular coagulation, uremia, burns, systemic lupus erythematosus, valvular heart disease, and intracardiac catheters. NBTE is found at the valve closure contact line on the atrial surfaces of the mitral and tricuspid valves and on the ventricular surfaces of the aortic and pulmonic valves, the sites of infected vegetations in patients with IE.

Three hemodynamic circumstances may injure the endothelium, initiating NBTE: (1) a high-velocity jet striking endothelium; (2) flow from a high- to a low-pressure chamber;

and (3) flow across a narrow orifice at high velocity. During bacteremia, blood flow through a narrowed orifice deposits bacteria maximally at the low-pressure sink immediately beyond an orifice as a consequence of the Venturi effect or at the site where a jet stream strikes a surface. These are the same sites where NBTE forms as a result of endothelial injury or hypercoagulability. The superimposition of NBTE formation and preferential deposition of bacteria helps to explain the distribution of infected vegetations.

CONVERSION OF NONBACTERIAL THROMBOTIC ENDOCARDITIS TO INFECTIVE ENDOCARDITIS. Bacteremia is the event that converts NBTE to IE. The frequency and magnitude of bacteremia associated with daily activities and health care procedures appear related to specific mucosal surfaces and skin, the density of colonizing bacteria, the disease state of the surface, and the extent of the local trauma. Bacteremia rates are highest for events that traumatize the oral mucosa, particularly the gingiva, and progressively decrease with procedures involving the genitourinary tract and the gastrointestinal tract. An infected surface is associated with an increased risk of bacteremia. For viable circulating microorganisms to reach NBTE, they must be resistant to the complement-mediated bactericidal activity of serum.

The adherence of microorganisms to the NBTE or to apparently intact valve endothelium is a pivotal early event in the development of IE. Bacterial surface molecules (adhesins) mediate adherence to NBTE that has formed on exposed host extracellular matrix molecules or on valve endothelium. Collectively, these adhesins are known as microbial surface components recognizing adhesive matrix molecules (MSCRAMMs). Streptococci that produce surface polysaccharides called glucans or dextran cause endocarditis more frequently than strains that do not produce dextran. Surface dextran mediates the adherence of streptococci to platelet fibrin lattices and injured valves and facilitates the development of endocarditis in experimental models.[1,27] Dextran production, however, is not universal among the major microbial causes of IE; thus, other mechanisms of adherence are likely. For example, Fim A protein of *Streptococcus parasanguis*, which belongs to a family of oral mucosal adhesins in viridans streptococci, facilitates adherence to fibrin and development of experimental endocarditis.[27]

Fibronectin, an important factor in the pathogenesis of IE, has been identified in lesions on heart valves and is produced by endothelial cells, platelets, and fibroblasts in response to vascular injury; a soluble form binds with fibrinogen and fibrin to exposed subendothelial collagen. Receptors for fibronectin, MSCRAMMs, are present on the surface of *S. aureus*; viridans streptococci; group A, C, and G streptococci; enterococci; *S. pneumoniae*; and *C. albicans*. Fibronectin has numerous binding domains and thus can bind simultaneously to fibrin, collagen, cells, and microorganisms and facilitate adherence of bacteria to the valve at the site of injury or NBTE. Fibronectin-binding proteins A and B in *S. aureus* are critical in the induction of experimental endocarditis. Clumping factor (or fibrinogen-binding surface protein) of *S. aureus* also mediates the binding of these organisms to platelet fibrin thrombi and to aortic valves in models of endocarditis.[1,27] The glycocalyx or slime on the surface of *S. epidermidis* does not appear to function as an adhesin but may render organisms more virulent by enhancing their ability to avoid eradication by host defenses.

The mechanism by which virulent organisms colonize and infect intact valvular endothelium is less clearly understood. In elderly people, degenerative valve sclerosis may be associated with local inflammation, that in turn may promote endothelial cells to express integrins that bind fibronectin and other extracellular matrix molecules. Particulate material injected during IV drug abuse might stimulate similar endothelial events. These endothelial changes could promote *S. aureus* adherence through MSCRAMMs to apparently normal valves.[1,27] Adherent *S. aureus* trigger their own internalization by intact endothelial cells. Multiplication of the organism intracellularly results in cell death, which in turn disrupts the endothelial surface and initiates formation of platelet-fibrin deposits and additional sites for bacterial adherence and subsequently IE.

After adherence to NBTE or the endothelium, bacteria must persist and multiply if IE is to develop. Resistance of viridans streptococci and *S. aureus* to platelet antimicrobial proteins is associated with increased ability to cause experimental endocarditis.[1,27] Persistence and multiplication result in a complex dynamic process during which the infected vegetation increases in size by platelet-fibrin aggregation, microorganisms multiply and are shed into the blood, and vegetation fragments embolize. Staphylococcal and streptococcal surface proteins bind to platelets and promote aggregation and growth of the vegetation. Organisms that bind and aggregate platelets are more virulent in experimental models.[27] In addition, both streptococci and staphylococci increase local procoagulant activity by inducing fibrin-adherent monocytes to elaborate tissue factor (a tissue thromboplastin that binds to activated factor VII to initiate clotting).[27] Also, *S. aureus* can induce tissue factor production by endothelial cells, which would facilitate endocarditis development on normal valves.[27] Multiple replications of this cycle from adherence to multiplication and platelet-fibrin deposition result in clinical IE.

PATHOPHYSIOLOGY

Aside from the constitutional symptoms of infection, which are probably mediated by cytokines, the clinical manifestations of IE result from (1) the local destructive effects of intracardiac infection, (2) the embolization of bland or septic fragments of vegetations to distant sites resulting in infarction or infection, (3) the hematogenous seeding of remote sites during continuous bacteremia, and (4) an antibody response to the infecting organism with subsequent tissue injury caused by deposition of preformed immune complexes or antibody-complement interaction with antigens deposited in tissues.

The intracardiac consequences of IE range from an infected vegetation with no attendant tissue damage to infection that destroys valves and adjacent structures. Distortion or perforation of valve leaflets, rupture of chordae tendineae, and perforations or fistulas between major vessels and cardiac chambers or between chambers themselves may result in CHF that is progressive (Fig. 63-2). Infection may extend into paravalvular tissue and result in abscesses and persistent fever related to antibiotic-unresponsive infection, disruption of the conduction system with electrocardiographic conduction abnormalities and clinically relevant arrhythmias, or purulent pericarditis. Large vegetations, particularly at the mitral valve, can result in functional valvular stenosis and hemodynamic deterioration.[12] In general, intracardiac complications involving the aortic valve evolve more rapidly than those associated with the mitral valve; nevertheless, the progression is highly variable and unpredictable in individual patients.

Clinically apparent emboli occur in 11 to 43 percent of patients.[28] Pathological evidence of emboli at autopsy is more frequent (45 to 65 percent). Pulmonary emboli, which are often septic, occur in 66 to 75 percent of IV drug abusers with tricuspid valve IE. IE caused by virulent organisms, particularly *S. aureus,* beta-hemolytic streptococci, or other pyogenic organisms is complicated more frequently by met-

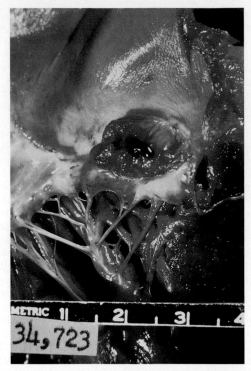

FIGURE 63–2 A normal valve with a large, bulky vegetation caused by *Staphylococcus aureus* infection. Clot is present centrally in the vegetation, obscuring a valve fenestration.

TABLE 63–5		Clinical Features of Infective Endocarditis	
Symptoms	Percent of Patients	Signs	Percent of Patients
Fever	80-85	Fever	80-90
Chills	42-75	Murmur	80-85
Sweats	25	Changing/new murmur	10-40
Anorexia	25-55	Neurological abnormalities[†]	30-40
Weight loss	25-35	Embolic event	20-40
Malaise	25-40	Splenomegaly	15-50
Dyspnea	20-40	Clubbing	10-20
Cough	25	Peripheral manifestations	
Stroke	13-20	Osler nodes	7-10
Headache	15-40	Splinter hemorrhage	5-15
Nausea/vomiting	15-20	Petechiae	10-40
Myalgia/arthralgia	15-30	Janeway lesion	6-10
Chest pain*	8-35	Retinal lesion/Roth spots	4-10
Abdominal pain	5-15		
Back pain	7-10		
Confusion	10-20		

*More common in intravenous drug abusers with right-sided infective endocarditis.
[†]Central nervous system.

astatic infection, often with local signs and symptoms or persistent fever during therapy, than IE due to avirulent bacteria (e.g., viridans streptococci).[16] Metastatic infection assumes particular importance when the required therapy is more than the antibiotics indicated for IE (e.g., when abscesses require drainage or meningitis requires antibiotics penetrating into the cerebrospinal fluid).

CLINICAL FEATURES

The interval between the presumed initiating bacteremia and the onset of symptoms of IE is estimated to be less than 2 weeks in more than 80 percent of patients with NVE. Interestingly, in some patients with intraoperative or perioperative infection of prosthetic valves, the incubation period may be prolonged (5 or more months).[12]

Fever is almost universal (Table 63-5). However, it may be absent or minimal in elderly persons or in those with CHF, severe debility, or chronic renal failure and occasionally in patients with NVE caused by coagulase-negative staphylococci. *Heart murmurs* are usually emblematic of the lesion predisposing to IE. Murmurs are commonly not audible in patients with tricuspid valve IE. The new or changing regurgitant murmurs indicative of valve damage are relatively infrequent in subacute NVE and are more prevalent in acute IE and PVE (e.g. that due to *S. aureus*). They are frequently harbingers of CHF. *Enlargement of the spleen* is more common in subacute IE of long duration.

The classic peripheral manifestations of IE are encountered less frequently today and are virtually absent in IE restricted to the tricuspid valve.[28] *Petechiae*, the most common of these manifestations, are found on the palpebral conjunctiva, the buccal and palatal mucosa, and the extremities. They are not specific for endocarditis even on the conjunctiva. *Splinter* or *subungual hemorrhages* are dark red, linear, or occasionally flame-shaped streaks in the proximal nail bed. Distal lesions at the nail tip are probably

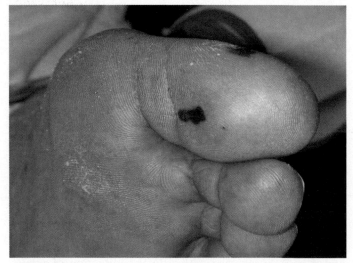

FIGURE 63–3 Digit infarcts in a patient with infective endocarditis due to *Staphylococcus aureus*. (Courtesy of Alan J. Lesse, M.D.)

caused by trauma. *Osler nodes* are small, tender subcutaneous nodules in the pulp of the digits, or occasionally more proximal, that persist for hours to several days. *Janeway lesions* are small erythematous or hemorrhagic macular nontender lesions on the palms and soles and are the consequence of septic embolic events. Embolic infarcts in the digits (Fig. 63-3) are common in left-sided *S. aureus* IE. *Roth spots*, oval retinal hemorrhages with pale centers, are infrequent findings in IE. Neither these nor Osler nodes are pathognomonic for IE.

Musculoskeletal symptoms, unrelated to focal infection, are relatively common in patients with IE. These include arthralgias and myalgias, occasional true arthritis with nondiagnostic but inflammatory synovial fluid findings, and prominent back pain without demonstrable infection of vertebrae, disc space, epidural space, or sacroiliac joint. In patients with arthritis or back pain, focal infection must be excluded because additional therapy may be required.

Symptomatic systemic emboli are relatively common and frequently antedate or coincide with the diagnosis of IE; the incidence decreases promptly during administration of effective antibiotic therapy. Embolic events are infrequent after 2 weeks of therapy. Findings vary but the risks of emboli generally increase with large vegetations (>10 mm), mitral vegetations, *S. aureus* IE, and increasing vegetation size during therapy.[4,29] Embolic stroke syndromes, predominantly involving the middle cerebral artery territory, occur in 15 to 20 percent of patients with NVE and PVE.[12] Coronary artery emboli are common findings at autopsy but rarely result in transmural infarction. Emboli to the extremities may produce pain and overt ischemia, and emboli to mesenteric arteries may cause abdominal pain, ileus, and guaiac-positive stools.

Neurological symptoms and signs are caused most commonly by embolic strokes, are more frequent when IE is caused by *S. aureus*, and are associated with increased mortality rates.[30] Intracranial hemorrhage, which occurs in 5 percent of patients, results from rupture of a mycotic aneurysm, rupture of an artery related to septic arteritis at the site of embolic occlusion, or hemorrhage into an infarct. Cerebritis with microabscesses complicates IE caused by invasive pathogens such as *S. aureus*, but large brain abscesses are rare. Purulent meningitis complicates some episodes of IE caused by *S. aureus* or *S. pneumoniae*, but more typically the cerebrospinal fluid, if abnormal, has an aseptic profile. Other neurological manifestations include severe headache (a potential clue to a mycotic aneurysm), seizures, and encephalopathy.

Congestive heart failure primarily results from valve destruction or distortion or rupture of chordae tendineae. Intracardiac fistulas, myocarditis, or coronary artery embolization may occasionally contribute to the genesis of CHF, as obviously can underlying cardiac disease.

Renal insufficiency as a result of immune complex–mediated glomerulonephritis occurs in less than 15 percent of patients with IE. Azotemia as a result of this process may develop or progress during initial therapy but usually improves with continued administration of effective antibiotic therapy. Focal glomerulonephritis and embolic renal infarcts cause hematuria but rarely result in azotemia. Impaired hemodynamics or antimicrobial toxicities (interstitial nephritis or aminoglycoside toxicity) are the most common cause of renal dysfunction in patients with IE.

DIAGNOSIS

The symptoms and signs of endocarditis are often constitutional and, when localized, often result from a remote complication rather than reflect the intracardiac infection itself (see Table 63-5). Consequently, to avoid overlooking the diagnosis of IE, a high index of suspicion must be maintained. The diagnosis must be investigated when patients with fever present with one or more of the cardinal elements of IE: a predisposing cardiac lesion or behavior pattern, bacteremia, embolic phenomenon, and evidence of an active endocardial process. Among patients with a predisposition to IE, unexplained weight loss, malaise, azotemia, and anemia should prompt consideration of IE even in the absence of fever. Among patients with prosthetic heart

valves, the presence of fever or new prosthesis dysfunction at any time warrants considering this diagnosis. Even when the illness seems typical of endocarditis, the definitive diagnosis requires positive blood cultures or positive cultures (or histology or PCR recovery of the DNA of a microorganism) from the vegetation or an embolus. There are many culture-negative mimics of IE: atrial myxoma, acute rheumatic fever, systemic lupus erythematosus or other collagen-vascular disease, marantic endocarditis, the antiphospholipid syndrome, carcinoid syndrome, renal cell carcinoma with increased cardiac output, and thrombotic thrombocytopenic purpura.

The modified Duke criteria provide a schema that facilitates evaluating patients for endocarditis (see Table 63-4).[31] Clinical and laboratory data, including echocardiography, should be collected in a manner that allows one to assess the presence or absence of the listed major and minor criteria. Finding evidence of two major or one major plus three minor or five minor criteria establishes a clinical diagnosis of "definite endocarditis," whereas finding one major plus one minor or three minor criteria indicates "possible endocarditis." When used judiciously over the entire evaluation (i.e., not limited to initial findings), these criteria are sensitive and specific for the diagnosis of IE.[31] Erroneous rejection of the diagnosis of endocarditis is unlikely. When these diagnostic criteria are used to guide therapy, patients who are categorized with possible endocarditis should be treated as if they have IE. Requiring at least one major plus one minor criterion or three minor criteria to designate possible endocarditis reduces the potential for overdiagnosis (failure to reject the diagnosis).[31] Nevertheless, because the echocardiogram cannot fully distinguish healed vegetations and other valvular masses from actively infected vegetations, these guidelines are vulnerable to misidentifying patients as having culture-negative IE when vegetations that complicate marasmus, malignancy, cryptic collagen-vascular disease, the antiphospholipid antibody syndrome, or previously treated IE are detected. To use bacteremia caused by coagulase-negative staphylococci or diphtheroids (organisms that may cause IE but more often contaminate blood cultures) to support the diagnosis of endocarditis, blood cultures must be persistently positive or the organisms recovered in several sporadically positive cultures must be proved to represent a single clone.[31]

ECHOCARDIOGRAPHY. Inclusion of echocardiographic evidence of endocardial infection in these criteria recognizes the high sensitivity of two-dimensional echocardiography with color Doppler, especially if biplane or multiplanar TEE and transthoracic echocardiography (TTE) are combined (see Chap. 14), and the relative infrequency of false-positive studies when experienced operators use specific definitions for vegetations.[32] TEE provides improved resolution and allows visualization of smaller vegetations compared with TTE (see Fig. 14-67). The sensitivity of TTE for the detection of vegetations in patients with NVE is approximately 65 percent, whereas that of TEE in these patients is 85 to 95 percent. The likelihood of a false negative study can be reduced to 5 to 10 percent if TEE is repeated.[33] TEE is the preferred approach in patients in whom TTE is technically suboptimal and is the procedure of choice for imaging the pulmonic valve and patients with suspected PVE.[32] Among patients with PVE, the diagnostic sensitivity of TTE is 15 to 35 percent. In contrast, the sensitivity of TEE for detecting signs of PVE ranges from 82 to 96 percent with mechanical or bioprosthetic devices in the aortic or mitral position. Thus, the highly sensitive TEE helps to preclude the diagnosis of IE when the clinical suspicion is low; when the clinical suspicion is high, even these studies cannot exclude the diagnosis or need for treatment.[32] When initial TEE is negative and the clinical suspicion of IE remains, repeating TEE in 7 to 10 days is advocated.[17]

The American Heart Association recommends echocardiography evaluation in all patients with suspected IE.[17] Echocardiography should not be used as a screening test for IE in unselected patients with positive blood cultures or in evaluating patients with fevers of unknown origin when the clinical probability of IE is low.[32] A decision analysis evaluation of echocardiography for diagnosis of NVE in patients with bacteremia suggests that, assuming the diagnostic enhancement of TEE over TTE is 15 percent, the most cost-effective strategy (yielding optional quality-adjusted life-years) is as follows: (1) if prior probability of IE is less than 2 percent, treat for bacteremia without echocardiography; (2) if prior probability is 2 to 4 percent, use TTE; and (3) if prior probability is 5 to 45 percent, use TEE initially in lieu of TTE. If the prior probability of IE is greater than 45 percent, therapy for IE without

CH 63

Infective Endocarditis

echocardiography is cost-effective, although imaging is preferred to evaluate for complications and other risks. For an approach to using echocardiography advocated by the American Heart Association, see Figure 63-4.

Studies suggest that among patients with a high prior probability of NVE, data derived from a TEE rarely alters independent decisions to treat for endocarditis based on the clinical presentation and TTE. Exceptions to this, when TEE provides pivotal information, include when TTE is technically inadequate, when PVE is sought, and when there is *S. aureus* or enterococcal bacteremia. In patients with clinically uncomplicated catheter-associated *S. aureus* bacteremia, where the risk of IE ranges from 6 to 23 percent, using TEE to seek vegetations and determine the duration of antibiotic therapy (4 to 6 weeks versus 2 weeks—i.e., treatment for IE or not) is more cost effective and less morbid than empirical selection of either treatment duration.

Despite the sensitivity of TEE in detecting vegetations in patients with proven IE, echocardiography does not itself provide a definite diagnosis. Vegetations and valve dysfunction may be demonstrated, but determination of causality requires clinical or direct anatomical and microbiological confirmation. In addition to noninfected vegetations, thickened valves, ruptured chordae or valves, valve calcification, and nodules may be mistaken for infected vegetations, indicating the specificity limitations of isolated echocardiography.

ESTABLISHING THE MICROBIAL CAUSE. A microbial cause of IE is established by recovering the infecting agent from the blood or by identifying it in vegetations or embolic material. In detecting the continuous bacteremia of IE, there is no advantage to obtaining blood cultures in relation to fever or from arterial blood. In patients who have not received prior antibiotics and who will ultimately have blood culture–positive IE, it is likely that 95 to 100 percent of all cultures obtained will be positive and that one of the first two cultures will be positive in at least 95 percent of patients. Prior antibiotic therapy is a major cause of blood culture–negative IE, particularly when the causative microorganism is highly antibiotic susceptible. After subtherapeutic antibiotic exposure, the time required for reversion to positive cultures is directly related to the duration of antimicrobial therapy and the susceptibility of the causative agent; days to a week or more may be required.

OBTAINING BLOOD CULTURES. Three separate sets of blood cultures, each from a separate venipuncture, obtained over 24 hours, are recommended to evaluate patients with suspected endocarditis.[32] Each set should include a bottle containing an aerobic medium and one containing thioglycollate broth (anaerobic medium); at least 10 ml of blood should be placed into each bottle.[34] If a clinically stable patient has received an antimicrobial agent during the past several weeks, it is prudent to delay therapy so that repeated cultures can be obtained on successive days without further confounding by antibiotics.[34] If endocarditis caused by fungi or unusual bacteria (*Legionella* species or *Bartonella* species) is suspected, the laboratory should be consulted for guidance regarding optimal culture techniques. Serological tests can be used to make the presumptive diagnosis of endocarditis caused by *Brucella* species, *Legionella* species, *Bartonella* species, *C. burnetii*, or *Chlamydia* species. Using special techniques, including PCR and antigen detection, these agents and others that are difficult to recover in blood culture can be identified in blood or vegetations.[32,35,36]

In evaluating positive blood cultures, sustained bacteremia, which is typical of IE, should be distinguished from transient bacteremia. When several blood cultures obtained over 24 hours or more are positive, the diagnosis of IE must be considered. The identity of the organism is also helpful in determining the intensity with which the diagnosis is entertained. Organisms can be divided into those that commonly cause IE, those that rarely cause IE, and the intermediate-behaving organisms, such as enterococci and *S. aureus*, which, when in the blood, may or may not indicate IE. Finally, the presence or absence of alternative sources for the bacteremia aids in the assessment of bacteremia.

Laboratory Tests

Anemia, with normochromic normocytic red blood cell indices, a low serum iron level, and low serum iron-binding capacity, is found in 70 to 90 percent of patients. Anemia worsens with increased duration of illness and thus in acute IE may be absent. In subacute IE, the white blood cell count is usually normal; in contrast, a leukocytosis with increased segmented granulocytes is common in acute IE. Thrombo-

cytopenia occurs only rarely. The *erythrocyte sedimentation rate* (ESR) is elevated (average approximately 55 mm/hr) in almost all patients with IE; the exceptions are those with CHF, renal failure, or disseminated intravascular coagulation. Other tests often indicate immune stimulation or inflammation: circulating immune complexes, rheumatoid factor, quantitative immune globulin determinations, cryoglobulins, and C-reactive protein. Although the results of these tests parallel disease activity, the tests are costly and not efficient ways to diagnose IE or monitor response to therapy. Circulating immune complexes are detectable and complement is depressed in patients with diffuse immune complex glomerulonephritis. The *urinalysis* is often abnormal, even when renal function remains normal. Proteinuria and microscopic hematuria are noted in 50 percent of patients.

Imaging

ECHOCARDIOGRAPHY. Echocardiography (see also Chap. 14) may identify patients at high risk for complications or with a need for surgery and provide information central to the management of IE. Valve dysfunction, obstructing vegetations, or evidence of decompensated CHF can be visualized and quantitated by echocardiogram with Doppler. Some degree of regurgitation by Doppler is almost universal early in the course of NVE and PVE and does not necessarily predict progressive hemodynamic deterioration. Extension of infection beyond the valve leaflet results in abscesses in the annulus or adjacent structures, mycotic aneurysms of the sinus of Valsalva or mitral valve, intracardiac fistulas, and purulent pericarditis. Myocardial abscesses are more readily detected by TEE than TTE in patients with NVE or PVE (see Fig. 14-69). The sensitivity and specificity for abscess detection are 28 percent and 98 percent for TTE, compared with 87 percent and 95 percent for TEE. TEE is also more sensitive and accurate than TTE for recognizing subaortic invasive disease and valve perforations. Progressive CHF, new electrocardiographic conduction changes, changes in heart murmurs, and evidence of pericarditis warrant prompt evaluation by TEE to facilitate decisions regarding care. To facilitate long-term care, valve morphology and function, vegetation size, and ventricular function should be determined by TTE at the conclusion of treatment.

MAGNETIC RESONANCE AND COMPUTED TOMOGRAPHIC IMAGING. These techniques have identified paravalvular extension of infection, aortic root aneurysms, and fistulas; however, their utility relative to echocardiography has not been established.

SCINTIGRAPHY. Efforts to identify vegetations and intracardiac abscess in patients with IE and in animal models have used scintigraphy with gallium-67 citrate, indium-111-labeled granulocytes, and indium-111-labeled platelets. These efforts have not been sufficiently sensitive or anatomically localizing to be useful clinically.

TREATMENT

Two major objectives must be achieved to treat IE effectively. The infecting microorganism in the vegetation must be eradicated. Failure to accomplish this results in relapse of infection. Also, invasive, destructive intracardiac and focal extracardiac complications of infection must be resolved if morbidity and mortality are to be minimized. The second objective often exceeds the capacity of effective antimicrobial therapy and requires cardiac or other surgical intervention.

Bacteria in vegetations multiply to population densities approaching 10^9 to 10^{10} organisms per gram of tissue, become metabolically dormant, and are difficult to eradicate. Clinical experience and animal model experiments suggest that optimal therapy requires bactericidal antibiotics or antibiotic combinations rather than bacteriostatic agents. To reach effective antibiotic concentrations in avascular vegetations by passive diffusion, high serum concentrations must be achieved. Parenteral antimicrobial therapy is used whenever feasible to achieve suitable serum antibiotic concentrations and to avoid the potentially erratic absorption of orally administered therapy. Treatment is continued for prolonged periods to ensure eradication of dormant microorganisms.

In selecting antimicrobial therapy for patients with IE, one must consider the MIC and the ability of potential agents to kill the causative organism. The MIC is the lowest concentration that inhibits growth, and the minimum bactericidal concentration (MBC) is the lowest concentration that decreases a standard inoculum of organisms 99.9 percent during 24 hours. For the vast majority of streptococci and staphylococci, the MIC and MBC of penicillins, cephalosporins, or vancomycin are the same or differ by only a factor of 2 to 4. Organisms for which the MBC for these antibiotics is 10-fold or greater than the MIC are occasionally encountered. This phenomenon has been termed *tolerance*. Most of the tolerant strains are simply killed more slowly than nontolerant strains, and with prolonged incubation (48 hours) their MICs and MBCs are similar. Enterococci exhibit what superficially appears to be tolerance when tested against penicillins and vancomycin; however, these organisms are, in fact, not killed by these agents but are merely inhibited even after longer incubation times. Enterococci can be killed by the combined activity of selected penicillins or vancomycin and an aminoglycoside. This enhanced antibiotic activity of the combination against enterococci, if of sufficient magnitude, is called *synergy* or a *synergistic bactericidal* effect. A similar effect can be seen with these combinations against streptococci and staphylococci.

A synergistic bactericidal effect is required for optimal therapy of enterococcal endocarditis and has been used to achieve more effective therapy or effective short-course therapy of IE caused by other organisms. Tolerance in streptococci or staphylococci has not been correlated with decreased cure rates or delayed responses to treatment with penicillins, cephalosporins, or vancomycin and is not an indication for combination therapy. In fact, regimens are designed using the MICs of these organisms.[17]

The regimens recommended for the treatment of IE caused by specific organisms are designed to provide concentrations of antibiotics in serum and deep in vegetations that exceed the organism's MIC throughout most of the interval between doses. Although antibiotic concentrations in vegetations of patients with IE have been measured infrequently, the success of the recommended regimens suggests that this goal has been achieved. Accordingly, for optimal therapy, it is important that the recommended regimens be followed carefully.

Antimicrobial Therapy for Specific Organisms

The antimicrobial therapy for endocarditis should eradicate the causative agent while causing little or no toxicity. Therapy requires specific susceptibility data for the causative organism. Antibiotic modifications may be needed to accommodate end-organ dysfunction, allergies, or anticipated toxicities. In anticipation of the possible need to modify therapy, the organism causing endocarditis should be saved until successful therapy has been completed. With the exception of staphylococcal endocarditis, the antimicrobial regimens recommended for the treatment of NVE and PVE are similar, although more prolonged treatment is often advised for PVE.[10,12,17]

PENICILLIN-SUSCEPTIBLE VIRIDANS STREPTOCOCCI OR *STREPTOCOCCUS BOVIS*. Multiple regimens provide highly effective, comparable therapy for patients with uncomplicated NVE caused by penicillin-susceptible streptococci and *S. bovis* (Table 63-6). The 4-week regimens yield bacteriological cure rates of 98 percent. The synergistic combination of penicillin or ceftriaxone plus gentamicin for 2 weeks is as effective in selected cases as treatment with the 4-week regimens.[17,37] The short course combination regimens are recommended for patients who have uncom-

TABLE 63–6	Treatment for Native Valve Endocarditis Caused by Penicillin-Susceptible Viridans Streptococci and *Streptococcus bovis* (Minimum Inhibitory Concentration <0.1 μg/ml)*	
Antibiotic	**Dosage and Route†**	**Duration (wk)**
Aqueous penicillin G	12-18 million units/24 hr IV either continuously or every 4 hr in six equally divided doses	4
or		
Ceftriaxone	2 gm once daily IV or IM	4
Aqueous penicillin G	12-18 million units/24 hr IV either continuously or every 4 hr in six equally divided doses	2
or		
Ceftriaxone	2 gm once daily IV or IM	2
plus		
Gentamicin	3 mg/kg/day IM or IV as a single daily dose or divided in equal doses every 8 hr	2
Vancomycin	30 mg/kg/24 hr IV in two equally divided doses, not to exceed 2 gm/24 hr unless serum levels are monitored	4

*For nutritionally variant organisms (*Granulicatella* species, *G. morbillorum*, *Abiotrophia defectiva*), see Table 63-8.

†Dosages given are for patients with normal renal function. Vancomycin and gentamicin doses must be reduced for treatment of patients with renal dysfunction. Vancomycin and gentamicin doses are calculated using ideal body weight (men = 50 kg + 2.3 kg per inch over 5 feet; women = 45.5 kg + 2.3 kg per inch over 5 feet). Vancomycin doses are adjusted to yield 1-hour postinfusion serum concentration of 30-45 μg/ml and trough of 15 μg/ml. Gentamicin administered every 8 hr should be adjusted to achieve a 1-hr peak concentration of 3 to 3.5 μg/ml and a trough of <1.0 μg/ml. To achieve these parameters in patients with renal dysfunction may require lengthening of the dose-to-dose interval.

Modified from Baddour LM, Wilson WR, Bayer AS, et al: Infective endocarditis: Diagnosis, antimicrobial therapy, and management of complications. Circulation 111:3167-84, 2005.

plicated NVE and who are not at increased risk for aminoglycoside toxicity. Patients with endocarditis caused by nutritionally variant organisms (*Granulicatella* species, or *Abiotrophia defectiva*), *G. morbillorum,* endocarditis involving a prosthetic valve or endocarditis complicated by a mycotic aneurysm, myocardial abscess, perivalvular infection, or an extracardiac focus of infection should not be treated with a short-course regimen.

From 2 to 8 percent of viridans streptococci and *S. bovis* causing endocarditis are highly resistant to streptomycin (MIC >2000 μg/ml) and are not killed synergistically by penicillin plus streptomycin but are killed synergistically by penicillin plus gentamicin. Consequently, gentamicin is recommended for use in the short-course combination regimen. Ceftriaxone 2 gm once daily plus either gentamicin (3 mg/kg) or netilmicin (4 mg/kg) given as a single daily dose for 14 days has effectively treated endocarditis caused by penicillin-susceptible streptococci. The nutritionally variant organisms are generally more resistant to penicillin than viridans streptococci; thus IE caused by these organisms is treated with regimens recommended for enterococcal endocarditis (see Table 63-8); however, outcome remains unsatisfactory.

For the treatment of streptococcal endocarditis in patients with a history of immediate allergic reactions (urticarial or anaphylactic reactions) to a penicillin or cephalosporin antibiotic, vancomycin is recommended (see Table 63-6). Patients with other forms of penicillin allergy (delayed maculopapular skin rash) may be treated cautiously with the ceftriaxone regimens (see Table 63-6). For patients with

PVE caused by penicillin-susceptible streptococci, treatment with 6 weeks of penicillin is recommended, with or without gentamicin 3 mg/kg/day in three divided doses given during the initial 2 weeks.[10,12,17]

RELATIVELY PENICILLIN-RESISTANT STREPTOCOCCI. Treatment with 4 weeks of high-dose parenteral penicillin or ceftriaxone plus an aminoglycoside (primarily gentamicin for the reasons noted previously) during the initial 2 weeks is recommended for endocarditis caused by streptococci with MICs for penicillin between 0.2 and 0.5 μg/ml (Table 63-7). Patients who cannot tolerate penicillin because of immediate hypersensitivity reactions can be treated with vancomycin alone. For those with nonimmediate penicillin hypersensitivity, effective treatment can be accomplished either with vancomycin alone or with the ceftriaxone-gentamicin regimen (see Table 63-6). NVE caused by streptococci that are "fully" resistant to penicillin (MIC >0.5 μg/ml) or PVE caused by relatively or fully penicillin-resistant organisms should be treated for 6 weeks with penicillin or ceftriaxone plus gentamicin (doses per Table 63-7) or vancomycin alone.[17]

***STREPTOCOCCUS PYOGENES, STREPTOCOCCUS PNEUMONIAE,* AND GROUP B, C, AND G STREPTOCOCCI.** Endocarditis caused by these streptococci has been either refractory to antibiotic therapy or associated with extensive valvular damage. Penicillin G in a dose of 3 million units IV every 4 hours for 4 weeks is recommended for the treatment of group A streptococcal endocarditis. Ceftriaxone or vancomycin, depending upon the degree of penicillin allergy, in doses noted in Table 63-7 are treatment alternatives.

IE caused by group G, C, or B streptococci is more difficult to treat than that caused by penicillin-susceptible viridans streptococci. Consequently, the addition of gentamicin to the first 2 weeks of a 4-week regimen using high doses of penicillin is often advocated (see Table 63-7).[19] Early cardiac surgery to correct intracardiac complications is needed in almost one half of these cases and may improve outcome.[18,19]

In selecting treatment for pneumococcal IE, both antibiotic resistance in the infecting strain and coexisting meningitis are important considerations.[20] The treatment of IE caused by penicillin-susceptible pneumococci (MIC ≤0.1 μg/ml) with or without concomitant meningitis is penicillin G 4 million units IV every 4 hours, ceftriaxone 2 gm IV every 12 hours, or cefotaxime 4 gm IV every 6 hours. In the absence of meningitis, these regimens are effective for IE caused by pneumococci that are relatively penicillin resistant (MIC 0.1 to 1.0 μg/ml). If IE, including that caused by relatively penicillin-resistant isolates when complicated by meningitis, is caused by a penicillin-resistant (MIC = 2.0 μg/ml) or cefotaxime-resistant (MIC = 2.0 μg/ml) pneumococcus, therapy with ceftriaxone 2 gm IV every 12 hours or cefotaxime 4 gm IV every 6 hours plus vancomycin 15 mg/kg IV every 12 hours is preferred. CHF rather than penicillin resistance is associated with mortal-

ity; thus intervention early with cardiac surgery is essential for an optimal outcome.[20]

ENTEROCOCCI. Optimal therapy for enterococcal endocarditis requires synergistic bactericidal interaction of an antimicrobial targeted against the bacterial cell wall (penicillin, ampicillin, or vancomycin) and an aminoglycoside that is able to exert a lethal effect (streptomycin or gentamicin). High-level resistance, defined as the inability of high concentrations of streptomycin (1000 or 2000 μg/ml) or gentamicin (500 to 2000 μg/ml) to inhibit the growth of an enterococcus, predicts the agent's inability to exert this lethal effect and to participate in the bactericidal synergistic interaction. Similarly, resistance to the cell wall targeted agents indicates their inability to contribute to synergistic killing. The standard regimens recommended for the treatment of enterococcal endocarditis (Table 63-8) are designed to achieve bactericidal synergy and result in cure rates of approximately 85 percent, compared with 40 percent with single-agent, nonbactericidal treatment. Isolates with high-level gentamicin resistance are not routinely high level streptomycin-resistant. In the absence of high-level resistance to streptomycin in a causative strain, streptomycin, 7.5 mg/kg intramuscularly (IM) or IV every 12 hours to achieve a 1 hour peak serum concentration of approximately 20 to 35 μg/ml and a trough of < 10 μg/ml, can be substituted for gentamicin in the standard regimens. The streptomycin dose must be reduced if renal function is decreased. The vancomycin-aminoglycoside regimen (see Table 63-8) is recommended only for patients allergic to penicillin. Desensitization to penicillin may be desirable when preexisting renal dysfunction favors avoiding the potentially more nephrotoxic vancomycin-aminoglycoside combination. Therapy is administered for 4 to 6 weeks, with the longer course used to treat patients with PVE or IE that was symp-

TABLE 63-7	Treatment for Native Valve Endocarditis Caused by Strains of Viridans Streptococci and *Streptococcus bovis* Relatively Resistant to Penicillin G (Minimum Inhibitory Concentration >0.1 μg/ml and <0.5 μg/ml)	
Antibiotic	**Dosage and Route***	**Duration (wk)**
Aqueous penicillin G	24 million units/24 hr IV either continuously or every 4 hr in six equally divided doses	4
or Ceftriaxone *plus*	2 gm once daily IV or IM	
Gentamicin	3 mg/kg/day IM or IV as a single daily dose or divided in equal doses every 8 hr	2
Vancomycin	30 mg/kg/24 hr IV in two equally divided doses, not to exceed 2 gm/24 hr unless serum levels are monitored	4

*Dosages are for patients with normal renal function; see Table 63-6 footnote.
Modified from Baddour LM, Wilson WR, Bayer AS, et al: Infective endocarditis: Diagnosis, antimicrobial therapy, and management of complications. Circulation 111:3167-84, 2005.

TABLE 63-8	Standard Therapy for Endocarditis Caused by Enterococci*	
Antibiotic	**Dosage and Route†**	**Duration (wk)**
Aqueous penicillin G	18-30 million units/24 hr IV given continuously or every 4 hr in six equally divided doses	4-6
plus Gentamicin	1 mg/kg IM or IV every 8 hr	4-6
Ampicillin	12 gm/24 hr IV given continuously or every 4 hr in six equally divided doses	4-6
plus Gentamicin	1 mg/kg IM or IV every 8 hr	6
Vancomycin‡	30 mg/kg/24 hr IV in two equally divided doses not to exceed 2 gm/24 hr unless serum levels are monitored	6
plus Gentamicin	1 mg/kg IM or IV every 8 hr	6

*All enterococci causing endocarditis must be tested for antimicrobial susceptibility to select optimal therapy. These regimens are for treatment of endocarditis caused by enterococci that are susceptible to penicillin, ampicillin, or vancomycin and not highly resistant to gentamicin. These may also be used for treatment of endocarditis caused by penicillin-resistant (minimum inhibitory concentration >0.5) viridans streptococci and nutritionally variant organisms or enterococcal prosthetic valve endocarditis.
†Dosages are for patients with normal renal function. See Table 63-6, footnote.
‡For patients allergic to penicillin/ampicillin. Alternatively, desensitize to penicillin. For enterococcal IE, cephalosporins are not alternatives to penicillin/ampicillin in penicillin-allergic patients.
Modified Baddour LM, Wilson WR, Bayer AS, et al: Infective endocarditis: Diagnosis, antimicrobial therapy, and management of complications. Circulation 111:3167-84, 2005.

tomatic for more than 3 months or is complicated. Careful monitoring of patients clinically, and of serum creatinine and aminoglycoside levels is required to prevent nephrotoxicity and ototoxicity.

Favorable outcomes with regimens using foreshortened courses of aminoglycosides suggest that the aminoglycoside component of combination therapy can be abbreviated if toxicity becomes significant. Of 93 patients treated for enterococcal IE (66 with NVE, 27 with PVE), 75 (81 percent) were cured, 15 (16 percent) died, and 3 (3 percent) relapsed.[38] Cure was achieved with a median duration of cell wall–active antimicrobial therapy and aminoglycoside therapy of 42 and 15 days, respectively. In 39 of the patients who were cured, aminoglycosides were administered for 21 days or less. Experimental data and very limited clinical data suggest that double beta-lactam antibiotic therapy may be bactericidal and provide a non-nephrotoxic alternative treatment: for *E. faecalis,* ceftriaxone or cefotaxime plus ampicillin, or for *E. faecium* imipenem plus ampicillin.[17,37]

Enterococci causing endocarditis must be tested for high-level resistance to both streptomycin and gentamicin and susceptibility to penicillin, ampicillin, and vancomycin (Table 63-9). High-level resistance to gentamicin predicts resistance to all other aminoglycosides except streptomycin. Using these data, an attempt should be made to design a regimen containing a cell wall active agent to which the isolate is susceptible plus gentamicin or streptomycin depending on the absence of high-level resistance. If a bactericidal synergistic regimen is not feasible, an alternative treatment plus possible surgery should be considered (see Table 63-9).[17,22]

STAPHYLOCOCCI

ANTIBIOTIC RESISTANCE. In excess of 90 percent of *S. aureus* and coagulase-negative staphylococci, whether acquired in the hospital or community, produce beta-lactamase and thus are resistant to penicillin, ampicillin, and the ureidopenicillins. Penicillin-resistant *S. aureus* can be further subdivided into isolates that are either methicillin susceptible, i.e., susceptible to penicillinase-resistant beta-lactam antibiotics (nafcillin, oxacillin, cloxacillin, and cefazolin) or methicillin-resistant, i.e., resistant to all beta-lactam antibiotics but susceptible, with rare exceptions, to vancomycin, teicoplanin (not approved for use in the United States), and daptomycin. Previously, the majority of *S. aureus* infections were caused by methicillin-susceptible isolates. Methicillin-resistant *S. aureus* (MRSA) primarily infected patients who were hospitalized, residents of extended care facilities, or in selected other populations such as IV drug abusers and hemodialysis-dependent persons. Multidrug resistant MRSA infections have increased in these populations accounting for 30 to 60 percent of *S. aureus* infections and have spread into the community.[39]

Additionally, a new genetically distinct MRSA has become widespread in the community and is extending into health care institutions as well.[40,41] In two large multinational series of *S. aureus* IE, 15 percent (1979 to 1999) and 27 percent (2000 to 2003) of cases were caused by MRSA.[4,23] Currently, empirical therapy for suspected *S. aureus* IE should be effective against MRSA. Coagulase-negative staphylococci causing community-acquired infections are frequently methicillin susceptible, whereas those causing nosocomial infections, including IE, are commonly methicillin resistant. Methicillin-resistant coagulase-negative staphylococci may not always phenotypically express this resistance (a property called *heteroresistance*). Consequently, special testing may be required to detect this resistance. Most methicillin-resistant strains remain susceptible to vancomycin, teicoplanin, and daptomycin. *S. aureus* and coagulase-negative staphylococci with reduced susceptibility (and occasionally overt resistance) to vancomycin, teicoplanin, and daptomycin have emerged as pathogens.[16,42] Among staphylococci killed by beta-lactam antibiotics or vancomycin, the bactericidal effects of these agents can be enhanced by aminoglycosides.[37] Combinations of semisynthetic penicillinase–resistant penicillins or vancomycin with rifampin do not result in predictable bactericidal synergism; nevertheless, rifampin has unique activity against staphylococcal infections that involve foreign material and is included in regimens for staphylococcal PVE.[12,43] Staphylococcal infections involving prosthetic heart valves are treated differently from NVE caused by the same species (Table 63-10).[10,12,17,43]

STAPHYLOCOCCAL NATIVE VALVE ENDOCARDITIS. The semisynthetic penicillinase–resistant penicillins are the cornerstones of the treatment of endocarditis caused by methicillin-susceptible staphylococci. When patients have a nonimmediate penicillin allergy, a first-generation cephalosporin can be used. The synergistic interaction of beta-lactam antibiotics with an aminoglycoside has not increased the cure rates for staphylococcal endocarditis; however, treatment with these combinations has modestly accelerated the eradication of staphylococci in vegetations and in the blood.[37,43] To achieve this potential benefit, gentamicin may be added to beta-lactam antibiotic therapy for *S. aureus* IE during the initial 3 to 5 days of treatment.[17,37,43] Even this abbreviated aminoglycoside therapy may be associated with renal dysfunction; nephrotoxicity will be exacerbated by more prolonged administration of gentamicin.[37,42] The role for combination therapy is less well defined in NVE caused by coagulase-negative staphylococci; pooled data suggest improved cure rates with combination therapy.

In IV drug addicts, methicillin-susceptible *S. aureus* endocarditis that is uncomplicated and limited to the right heart valves has been effectively treated with 2 weeks of semisynthetic penicillinase-resistant penicillin (but not vancomycin) given alone or in combination with an aminoglycoside (doses as noted in Table 63-10). Patients with right-sided *S. aureus* who develop peripheral signs suggesting left-sided infection are not candidates for abbreviated therapy. Vancomycin or daptomycin (6 mg/kg once daily) for 4 weeks is recommended when right-sided IE is caused by MRSA.[17,42]

Left-sided NVE caused by methicillin-resistant staphylococci requires treatment with vancomycin (see Table 63-10). Trimethoprim-sulfamethoxazole treatment of IE caused by *S. aureus* susceptible to this antimicrobial has been only moderately successful. Methicillin-resistant staphylococci are usually susceptible to linezolid and daptomycin; however, experience using either agent for treatment of left-sided endocarditis caused by MRSA is limited.[42] Teicoplanin (not

TABLE 63–9	Strategy for Selecting Therapy for Enterococcal Endocarditis Caused by Strains Resistant to Components of the Standard Regimen

I. Ideal therapy includes a cell wall–active agent plus an effective aminoglycoside to achieve bactericidal synergy (see text)

II. Cell wall–active antimicrobial
  A. Determine MIC for ampicillin and vancomycin; test for beta-lactamase production (nitrocefin test)
  B. If ampicillin and vancomycin susceptible, use ampicillin
  C. If ampicillin resistant (MIC ≥ 16 µg/ml) and vancomycin susceptible, use vancomycin
  D. If beta-lactamase produced, use vancomycin or consider ampicillin-sulbactam
  E. If ampicillin resistant and resistant to vancomycin (MIC >8 µg/ml) and teicoplanin* (MIC ≥ 8 µg/ml), see IV C, D[†]

III. Aminoglycoside to be used with cell wall–active antimicrobial
  A. If no high-level resistance to streptomycin (MIC <1000 or 2000 µg/ml) or gentamicin (MIC <500-2000 µg/ml), use gentamicin or streptomycin
  B. If high-level resistance to gentamicin (MIC >500-2000 µg/ml), test streptomycin; if no high-level resistance to streptomycin, use streptomycin (See IV B)
  C. If high-level resistance to gentamicin and streptomycin, omit aminoglycoside therapy; use prolonged therapy (8-12 wk) with cell wall–active antimicrobial if the organism is susceptible (see II A-E) or alternative therapy (see IV C, D, E)[†]

IV. Alternative regimens and approaches (use with consultative assistance of infectious disease specialist)
  A. Single-drug therapy (see III C) and possible surgical intervention
  B. Consider ampicillin, vancomycin (or teicoplanin), streptomycin based on absence of high-level resistance
  C. Consider quinupristin/dalfopristin therapy for infective endocarditis caused by susceptible *Enterococcus faecium* and surgical intervention
  D. Consider linezolid therapy with or without surgical intervention
  E. Daptomycin active in vitro against vancomycin-resistant enterococci but little clinical data for this treatment

*Not approved by the Food and Drug Administration for use in the United States; may be available by compassionate-use protocol.

[†]See Stevens MP, Edmond MB: Endocarditis due to vancomycin-resistant enterococci: Case report and review of the literature. Clin Infect Dis 41:1134-42, 2005.

MIC = minimum inhibitory concentration.

CH 63

Infective Endocarditis

TABLE 63–10	Treatment for Staphylococcal Endocarditis in the Absence of Prosthetic Material	
Antibiotic	**Dosage and Route***	**Duration**
Methicillin-Susceptible Staphylococci[†]		
Nafcillin or oxacillin	2 gm IV every 4 hr	4-6 wk
With optional addition of gentamicin	1 mg/kg IM or IV every 8 hr	3-5 d
Cefazolin	2 gm IV every 8 hr	4-6 wk
With optional addition of gentamicin	1 mg/kg IM or IV every 8 hr	3-5 d
Vancomycin[‡]	30 mg/kg/24 hr IV in two equally divided doses, not to exceed 2 gm/24 hr unless serum levels are monitored	4-6 wk
Methicillin-Resistant Staphylococci		
Vancomycin	30 mg/kg/24 hr IV in two equally divided doses, not to exceed 2 gm/24 hr unless serum levels are monitored	4-6 wk

*Dosages are for patients with normal renal function. See Table 63-6, footnote.
[†]For treatment of endocarditis caused by penicillin-susceptible staphylococci (minimum inhibitory concentration ≤0.1 μg/ml), aqueous penicillin G (18-24 million units/24 hr) can be used for 4-6 wk instead of nafcillin or oxacillin.
[‡]Cefazolin, or vancomycin may be used in selected penicillin-allergic patients contingent on degree of allergic response.
Modified from Baddour LM, Wilson WR, Bayer AS, et al: Infective endocarditis: Diagnosis, antimicrobial therapy, and management of complications. Circulation 111:3167-84, 2005.

CH 63

available in the United States) is a possible alternative. Teicoplanin is initiated at a dose of 6 mg/kg twice daily for 3 to 4 days until a trough serum concentration of 20 to 30 μg/ml is achieved; thereafter, 10 mg/kg is administered daily to maintain this trough concentration. Teicoplanin doses must be adjusted if renal function is decreased. Combining gentamicin with vancomycin to enhance activity against MRSA is associated with nephrotoxicity and is not recommended.[17] The addition of rifampin to vancomycin for treatment of methicillin-resistant *S. aureus* NVE has not been beneficial.

STAPHYLOCOCCAL PROSTHETIC VALVE ENDOCARDITIS. *S. aureus* and coagulase-negative staphylococcal PVE should be treated with three antibiotics in combination (Table 63-11).[12,17,43] Rifampin provides unique antistaphylococcal activity when infection involves foreign bodies. However, rifampin-resistant staphylococci rapidly emerge when rifampin is used alone or in combination with only vancomycin or a beta-lactam antibiotic to treat staphylococcal PVE.[10,12] Consequently, staphylococcal PVE is treated with two antimicrobials plus rifampin.[10,12,17,43] I prefer to delay rifampin therapy until treatment with two effective antistaphylococcal agents has been administered for 48 hours.

For PVE caused by methicillin-resistant staphylococci, treatment is initiated with vancomycin plus gentamicin, with rifampin added if the organism is susceptible to gentamicin. If the organism is resistant to gentamicin, an alternative antibiotic to which the organism is susceptible should be sought. This could be another aminoglycoside or a quinolone.[12] If the organism is resistant to these, trimethoprim/sulfamethoxazole or linezolid could be considered. For treatment of PVE caused by methicillin-susceptible staphylococci, a semisynthetic penicillinase–resistant penicillin should be substituted for vancomycin in the combination regimen (see Table 63-11). Because heteroresistance may confound detection of methicillin-resistance in coagulase-negative staphylococci, these organisms should be considered methicillin resistant, particularly when PVE occurs during the initial postoperative year, until susceptibility is conclusively established.

TABLE 63–11	Treatment of Staphylococcal Endocarditis in the Presence of a Prosthetic Valve or Other Prosthetic Material	
Antibiotic	**Dosage and Route***	**Duration (wk)**
Regimen for Methicillin-Resistant Staphylococci		
Vancomycin	30 mg/kg/24 hr IV in two equally divided doses, not to exceed 2 gm/24 hr unless serum levels are monitored	≥6
plus		
Rifampin *and*	300 mg PO every 8 hr	≥6
gentamicin[†]	1.0 mg/kg IM or IV every 8 hr	2
Regimen for Methicillin-Susceptible Staphylococci		
Nafcillin or oxacillin[‡]	2 gm IV every 4 hr	≥6
plus		
Rifampin *and*	300 mg PO every 8 hr	≥6
gentamicin[†]	1.0 mg/kg IM or IV every 8 hr	2

*Dosages are for patients with normal renal function. See Table 63-6, footnote.
[†]Use during initial 2 wk of treatment. If strain is gentamicin resistant, see text for alternatives.
[‡]Cefazolin 2 gm IV every 8 hr can be used in lieu of these agents in patients with nonimmediate-type penicillin allergy. Vancomycin is used with immediate-type allergy.
Modified from Baddour LM, Wilson WR, Bayer AS, et al: Infective endocarditis: Diagnosis, antimicrobial therapy, and management of complications. Circulation 111:3167-84, 2005.

TABLE 63–12	Treatment for Endocarditis Caused by HACEK Microorganisms*	
Antibiotic	**Dosage and Route[†]**	**Duration (wk)**
Ceftriaxone[‡]	2 gm once daily IV or IM	4
Ampicillin/Sulbactam	12 gm/24 hr IV given every 4 hr in six equally divided doses	4

*HACEK microorganisms are *Hemophilus* species, *Actinobacillus actinomycetemcomitans*, *Cardiobacterium hominis*, *Eikenella corrodens*, and *Kingella* species.
[†]Dosages are for those with normal renal function. See Table 63-6, footnote.
[‡]Cefotaxime or another third- or fourth-generation cephalosporin in comparable doses may be substituted for ceftriaxone. See text for treatment of patients unable to take beta-lactam antibiotics.
Modified from Baddour LM, Wilson WR, Bayer AS, et al: Infective endocarditis: Diagnosis, antimicrobial therapy, and management of complications. Circulation 111:3167-84, 2005.

Coagulase-negative staphylococcal PVE that occurs within the initial year after valve placement is often complicated by perivalvular extension of infection, and valve replacement surgery is required for cure.[12] Similarly, patients with *S. aureus* PVE frequently have intracardiac complications; their outcome is improved if early surgical intervention is combined with appropriate combination antimicrobial therapy.[9,13-15]

HAEMOPHILUS SPECIES, ACTINOBACILLUS ACTINOMYCETEMCOMITANS, CARDIOBACTERIUM HOMINIS, EIKENELLA CORRODENS, AND KINGELLA SPECIES (HACEK ORGANISMS). HACEK organisms, previously universally susceptible to ampicillin, may produce beta-lactamase resulting in ampicillin resistance. Given the marked susceptibility of both beta-lactamase–producing and non-beta-lactamase–producing HACEK to third- or fourth-generation cephalosporins, ceftriaxone or a comparable third-generation cephalosporin is recommended for treatment of NVE or PVE caused by these organisms (Table 63-12).[17] Although clinical data are limited, treatment with a fluoroquinolone has been recommended for patients who cannot tolerate a beta-lactam antibiotic.[17]

OTHER PATHOGENS. Recommendations for therapy of IE caused by unusual organisms are contained in the American Heart Association Scientific Statement.[17] Amphotericin desoxycholate or a less toxic liposomal amphotericin formulation, at full doses, often combined with 5-fluorocytosine, is recommended for treatment of *Candida* endocarditis. Prolonged medical treatment with fluconazole has been effective in occasional patients with *Candida* NVE and PVE who do not have intracardiac complications. Nevertheless, surgical intervention shortly after beginning amphotericin treatment remains the standard treatment for *Candida* endocarditis. Sporadic cases of Candida NVE and PVE have been successfully treated with caspofungin, a fungicidal echinocandin agent.[44] Prolonged or indefinite oral azole therapy has been advocated for patients treated either medically or surgically.[17]

Many corynebacteria (diphtheroids) causing IE remain susceptible to penicillin, vancomycin, and aminoglycosides. Strains susceptible to aminoglycosides are killed synergistically by penicillin in combination with an aminoglycoside. *Corynebacterium jeikeium*, although often resistant to penicillin and aminoglycosides, is killed by vancomycin. NVE or PVE caused by *Corynebacterium* species can be treated with the combination of penicillin plus an aminoglycoside or vancomycin, contingent on the susceptibilities of the causative strain.

Susceptibility of Enterobacteriaceae (*Escherichia coli, Klebsiella, Enterobacter, Serratia, Salmonella,* and *Proteus* species) to cephalosporins, ureidopenicillins, and carbapenems has become unpredictable. IE caused by these organisms is treated with high doses of a highly active beta-lactam plus full doses of an aminoglycoside (i.e., gentamicin 1.7 mg/kg every 8 hours).[17] If susceptible, the preferred treatment for *P. aeruginosa* IE is tobramycin (8 mg/kg/day IV once daily with peak and trough serum concentrations of 15 to 20 µg/ml and <2 µg/ml, respectively) plus piperacillin, ceftazidime, or cefipime.[17]

C. burnetii IE is difficult to eradicate. Prolonged therapy (at least 4 years) using doxycycline (100 mg twice daily) or another tetracycline combined with a quinolone has been advocated. Treatment with doxycycline combined with hydroxychloroquine for 18 to 48 months (mean 31 months, median 26 months) may be more effective than longer courses of doxycycline plus a quinolone.[45] Surgery is important in effective treatment.

CULTURE-NEGATIVE ENDOCARDITIS. Special studies must be performed to diagnose IE caused by fastidious bacteria and other organisms and to detect noninfectious mimics of IE (marantic endocarditis, atrial myxoma, antiphospholipid antibody syndrome, acute rheumatic fever, hypernephroma, carcinoid syndrome, and so on). Clinical and epidemiological clues, such as acute versus subacute presentation, a partial response to prior antibiotics, or the presence and duration of prosthetic valve, are important information in designing therapy. Recommended therapy for patients with suspected NVE who received confounding antibiotic therapy is either ampicillin-sulbactam plus gentamicin (3 mg/kg/day) or vancomycin plus gentamicin and ciprofloxacin, and for those with suspected PVE it is vancomycin plus gentamicin, cefepime and rifampin.[17] For patients with suspected IE in whom negative cultures are not confounded by prior antibiotics, fastidious organisms must be considered. *Bartonella* species (in the United States) and *C. burnetii* may be the most common of these causes. Suspected *Bartonella* IE is treated with 6 weeks of ceftriaxone plus gentamicin (1 mg/kg every 8 hours for at least 2 weeks) with an additional 6 weeks of doxycycline (100 mg IV or PO every 12 hours) if diagnostic studies are confirmatory (see Diagnosis).[26,46] Surgical intervention should be considered for those who do not fully respond to empirical antimicrobial therapy. If surgical intervention is undertaken, a detailed microbiological and pathological examination of excised material must be performed to establish an etiological diagnosis (see Diagnosis).

TIMING THE INITIATION OF ANTIMICROBIAL THERAPY. Cost-containment pressures frequently result in initiation of antimicrobial therapy for suspected endocarditis immediately after blood cultures have been obtained. This practice is appropriate for patients with acute IE that is highly destructive and rapidly progressive and for those presenting with hemodynamic decompensation requiring urgent surgical intervention. Precipitous initiation of therapy in hemodynamically stable patients with suspected subacute endocarditis does not prevent early complications and may, by compromising subsequent blood cultures, obscure the etiological diagnosis. In the latter patients, particularly in those who have received antibiotics recently, delaying antibiotic therapy briefly pending the results of the initial blood cultures is prudent. If these cultures are not immediately positive, this delay provides an important opportunity to obtain additional blood cultures without the confounding effect of empirical treatment.

MONITORING THERAPY FOR ENDOCARDITIS. Patients must be carefully monitored during therapy and for several months thereafter. Failure of antimicrobial therapy, myocardial or metastatic abscess, emboli, hypersensitivity to antimicrobial agents, and other complications of therapy (catheter-related infection, thrombophlebitis) or intercurrent illness may be manifested by persistent or recurrent fever. Adverse reactions occur in 33 percent of patients treated for IE with beta-lactam antimicrobials. These include fever, rash, neutropenia and hepatic and renal toxicity. The serum concentration of vancomycin or aminoglycosides should be measured periodically. This allows dose adjustment to ensure optimal therapy and to avoid adverse events. Renal function should be monitored in patients receiving these two antimicrobials, and the complete blood count monitored in patients receiving high-dose beta-lactam antibiotics or vancomycin. Repeated blood cultures should be obtained during the initial days of therapy or if fever persists or recurs to determine whether the bacteremia has been controlled and to detect relapse or new infections.

OUTPATIENT ANTIMICROBIAL THERAPY. Technical advances allowing safe administration of complex antimicrobial regimens combined with well-developed home care systems that provide supplies and monitor outpatient treatment make it feasible to treat patients with endocarditis on an outpatient basis. Doing so can significantly reduce the cost of therapy. However, only patients who have responded to initial therapy and are free of fever, who are not experiencing threatening complications, who will be compliant with therapy, and who have a home situation that is physically suitable should be considered for outpatient treatment. Because most threatening complications of IE occur during the initial 2 weeks of therapy, some clinicians have suggested that treatment during this period be administered in the inpatient setting or an outpatient setting that provides daily physician oversight. Patients treated at home must be apprised of potential complications, instructed to seek advice promptly when encountering unexpected or untoward clinical events, and have regular physician supervision and laboratory monitoring. Outpatient therapy must not result in compromises leading to suboptimal treatment.

Surgical Treatment of Intracardiac Complications

Cardiac surgical intervention has an increasingly important role in the treatment of infection that is unresponsive to antibiotics as well as the intracardiac complications of endocarditis. Retrospective data suggest that mortality is unacceptably high when these aspects of IE are treated with antibiotics alone, whereas mortality is reduced when treatment combines antibiotics and surgical intervention.[47,48] The indications for cardiac surgery evolve from these experiences (Table 63-13).

CONGESTIVE HEART FAILURE. Medical therapy of NVE that is complicated by moderate to severe (New York Heart Association [NYHA] Class III and IV) CHF related to new or worsening valvular dysfunction results in mortality rates of 50 to 90 percent. Survival rates for a similar group of patients treated with antibiotics and cardiac surgery are

TABLE 63–13	Cardiac Surgery in Patients with Infective Endocarditis

Indications
Moderate to severe congestive heart failure caused by valve dysfunction
Unstable prosthesis, prosthesis orifice obstructed
Uncontrolled infection despite optimal antimicrobial therapy
Unavailable effective antimicrobial therapy: endocarditis caused by fungi, *Brucellae, Pseudomonas aeruginosa* (aortic or mitral valves)
Staphylococcus aureus PVE with an intracardiac complication
Relapse of PVE after optimal therapy
Fistula to pericardial sac

Relative Indications*
Perivalvular extension of infection, intracardiac fistula, myocardial abscess with persistent fever
Poorly responsive *S. aureus* NVE (aortic or mitral valves)
Relapse of NVE after optimal antimicrobial therapy
Culture-negative NVE or PVE with persistent fever (≥10 d)
Large (>10 mm diameter) hypermobile vegetation (with or without prior arterial embolus)†
Endocarditis caused by highly antibiotic-resistant enterococci

*Surgery commonly required for optimal outcome.
†See text regarding the decision for surgical intervention.
NVE = native valve endocarditis; PVE = prosthetic valve endocarditis.

60 to 80 percent.[47] In an analysis controlled for bias against operating on severely ill patients with NVE, surgery on those with moderate to severe CHF was associated with a significantly improved 6-month survival when compared to medical treatment.[48] Survival rates among surgically treated patients with PVE complicated by valvular dysfunction and CHF are 45 to 85 percent; in contrast, few patients with these complications are alive at 6 months when treated with antibiotics alone.[10,12] Patients with aortic valve dysfunction not only account for the majority of surgically treated patients but also require surgery on a more urgent basis when CHF supervenes. Severe mitral valve insufficiency, nevertheless, results in inexorable CHF and ultimately requires surgical intervention. Echocardiography indicating significant valvular regurgitation during the initial week of endocarditis treatment does not reliably predict the patients who require valve replacement during active endocarditis. Alternatively, despite the absence of significant valvular regurgitation on early echocardiography, marked CHF may still develop. Thus, decisions about surgical intervention should be based on careful serial monitoring. On occasion, very large vegetations on the mitral valve, particularly a mitral valve prosthesis, result in significant obstruction and require surgery.[12]

UNSTABLE PROSTHESES. Dehiscence of an infected prosthetic valve is a manifestation of paravalvular infection and often results in hemodynamically significant valvular dysfunction. Surgical intervention is recommended for PVE patients with these complications.[12] The risk of invasive infection is increased among patients with onset of PVE within the year after valve implantation and those with infection of aortic valve prostheses. Endocarditis in these patients is often caused by invasive antimicrobial-resistant organisms; consequently, the benefit of combined medical-surgical therapy is enhanced. Patients who appear clinically stable but who have overtly unstable and hypermobile prostheses, a finding indicative of dehiscence in excess of 40 percent of the circumference, are likely to experience progressive valve instability and warrant urgent surgery. Occasional patients with PVE caused by noninvasive, highly antibiotic-susceptible organisms, (e.g., streptococci), despite a favorable clinical course, experience minor valve dehiscence without prosthesis instability or hemodynamic deterioration. Surgical treatment of these patients can be deferred unless clear indications arise.

UNCONTROLLED INFECTION OR UNAVAILABLE EFFECTIVE ANTIMICROBIAL THERAPY. Surgical intervention has improved the outcome of IE when maximal antibiotic therapy fails to eradicate infection. Surgical intervention is recommended for fungal PVE or NVE, particularly with intracardiac complications. Endocarditis caused by some gram-negative bacilli (e.g., *P. aeruginosa, Burkholderia cepacia, Brucella* species) may not be eradicated by maximal tolerable antibiotic therapy and may require surgical excision of the infected tissue to achieve cure.[32] Surgical intervention is recommended when enterococcal endocarditis caused by a strain resistant to synergistic bactericidal therapy does not respond to initial therapy or relapses. Perivalvular invasive infection is in some instances a form of ineradicable infection. Relapse of PVE after optimal antimicrobial therapy reflects invasive disease or the difficulty in eradicating infection involving foreign devices and merits surgical intervention.[12] In contrast, patients with uncomplicated NVE who relapse, unless infected with a highly resistant microorganism, are often treated again with intensified, prolonged antimicrobial therapy.

S. AUREUS PROSTHETIC VALVE ENDOCARDITIS. Crude mortality rates for *S. aureus* PVE treated medically range from 48 to 73 percent as contrasted to 28 to 48 percent for treatment with antibiotics plus surgery.[9,14,15] Management strategy is undoubtedly distorted by selection bias—the most ill patients often being denied surgery. Among 33 cases of *S. aureus* PVE, analyzed in a multivariate model to adjust for confounding variables, the presence of intracardiac complications was associated with a 13.7-fold increased risk of death, and surgical intervention during active disease was accompanied by a 20-fold reduction in mortality.[13] Data suggest that early surgical treatment can improve outcome of patients with *S. aureus* PVE and intracardiac complications.[9,13,14] Some patients less than 50 years old, with an American Society of Anesthesiologist score of III, and neither intracardiac nor central nervous system complications, may do well with medical therapy.[15]

PERIVALVULAR INVASIVE INFECTION. Perivalvular abscess or intracardiac fistula formation occurs in 10 to 14 percent of patients with NVE and 45 to 60 percent of those with PVE.[12] Persistent, otherwise unexplained fever despite appropriate antimicrobial therapy or pericarditis in patients with aortic valve endocarditis suggests infection extending beyond the valve leaflet. New-onset and persistent electrocardiographic conduction abnormalities, although not a sensitive indicator of perivalvular infection (28 to 53 percent), are relatively specific (85 to 90 percent). TEE is superior to TTE for detecting invasive infection in patients with NVE and PVE. Doppler and color flow Doppler or contrast two-dimensional echocardiography optimally defines fistulas. Abscesses suspected but not detected by initial and repeated TEE may be detected by cardiac magnetic resonance, including magnetic resonance angiography. Cardiac catheterization adds little to these imaging studies and is not recommended unless coronary angiography is needed.

Cardiac surgery should be considered to débride abscesses, allowing eradication of uncontrolled infection and to reconstruct cardiac structures, restoring hemodynamics and alleviating CHF. Sporadic patients with small, structurally insignificant abscesses in which the cavity is open to the circulatory stream have been treated medically; close serial monitoring is mandatory.[17]

LEFT-SIDED S. AUREUS ENDOCARDITIS. Because this infection is difficult to control, highly destructive, and associated with high mortality (25 to 47 percent), some investigators have suggested that these patients should be considered for surgical treatment when the response to antimicrobial therapy is not prompt and complete. Patients with *S. aureus* left-sided NVE and vegetations that are visible by TTE (versus requiring TEE) are at increased risk for arterial emboli and death and thus should be considered for surgery. IV drug abusers with *S. aureus* endocarditis limited to the tricuspid or pulmonary valves often experience prolonged fever during antimicrobial therapy; nevertheless, the vast majority respond to antimicrobial therapy and do not require surgery.

UNRESPONSIVE CULTURE-NEGATIVE ENDOCARDITIS. Patients who have culture-negative endocarditis and do not respond to empirical antimicrobial therapy, particularly those with PVE, should be considered for surgical intervention. If endocarditis is not marantic, persistent fever likely represents either unrecognized perivalvular infection or ineffective antimicrobial therapy. Causative organisms can be seen, cultured, or detected by molecular techniques in vegetation specimens in 40 to 70 percent of these patients.[35,36] Thus surgery may help clarify the etiology as well as facilitate treatment.

LARGE VEGETATIONS (>10 MM) AND THE PREVENTION OF SYSTEMIC EMBOLI. In pooled data and meta-analysis, systemic embolization was increased in patients with vegetations greater than 10 mm versus those with smaller or undetectable vegetations (33 to 37 percent versus 19 percent). Additionally, mitral valve location increases the risk of an embolic event.[29,49] Although a relation may exist between vegetation characteristics—including size, mobility, and extent (number of leaflets involved)—and embolic complications, the implications for surgical intervention are not clear. Nevertheless, some researchers have concluded that vegetation characteristics alone might warrant surgery to prevent arterial emboli. This recommendation can be questioned, as can the recommendation for valve surgery after two major arterial emboli.[32]

In deciding to intervene with cardiac surgery to prevent arterial emboli, many factors must be considered carefully. The rate of systemic or cerebral emboli in patients with NVE and PVE decreases during the course of effective antibiotic therapy.[29] Also, it is not clear that valve replacement reduces the frequency of systemic emboli. The morbidity and mortality caused by cerebral and coronary emboli, the major events to be prevented, must be compared with the immediate and long-term risks of valve replacement or, if feasible, vegetectomy and valve repair. Adverse surgical outcomes include perioperative mortality, recrudescent endocarditis on the prosthesis, thromboembolic complications, and valve dysfunction requiring repeat surgery. Additionally, the hazards of warfarin anticoagulation and late-onset PVE must be considered. The sum of the clinical findings, risk of embolization, and other surgically correctable intracardiac complications may be sufficient to justify surgery in spite of these immediate and remote hazards. However, only on rare occasions is vegetation size alone or a prior systemic embolus a sufficient independent indication for surgical intervention.[29,32]

Repair of Intracardiac Defects

TECHNIQUES. New surgical techniques to address severe tissue destruction in NVE and PVE have been developed. Although these are beyond the scope of this discussion, examples include valve composite graft replacement of the aortic root, use of sewing skirts attached to the prostheses, and homograft replacement of the aortic valve and root with coronary artery reimplantation. Repair of the mitral valve in patients with acute or healed endocarditis may avoid the need for insertion of prosthetic materials and the associated hazards. Although tricuspid valvulectomy without valve replacement has been advocated for treatment of uncontrolled tricuspid valve infection in IV drug abusers at high risk for recidivism and recurrent endocarditis, the likelihood of refractory right-sided CHF after valvulectomy makes tricuspid valve repair preferable. Cardiac transplantation has been used to salvage an occasional patient with refractory destructive endocarditis.

TIMING OF SURGICAL INTERVENTION. When endocarditis is complicated by valvular regurgitation and significant CHF, surgical intervention before the development of severe intractable hemodynamic dysfunction is recommended, regardless of the duration of antimicrobial therapy.[17,47,48,50] Postoperative mortality correlates with the severity of preoperative hemodynamic dysfunction; consequently, this approach is justified.[17] In patients who have valvular dysfunction and in whom infection is controlled and cardiac function is compensated, surgery may be delayed until antimicrobial therapy has been completed. If infection is not controlled or if function is not compensated, surgery should be performed promptly.

More specific recommendations for timing of surgery have been presented.[47] Strong clinical evidence suggests emergent (same day) surgery for acute aortic regurgitation

with mitral valve preclosure, sinus of Valsalva rupture into the right heart, and fistula to the pericardial sac; urgent (1 to 2 days) surgery for valve obstruction, unstable prosthesis, acute aortic or mitral regurgitation with CHF (NYHA Class III to IV), septal perforation, perivalvular extension of infection, and no effective antimicrobial therapy; and early elective surgery for progressive paravalvular regurgitation, valve dysfunction and persistent fever, and fungal IE.

It may be desirable to delay surgical intervention to avoid worsening of neurological status or death in patients who have sustained recent neurological injury. Among patients who have had a nonhemorrhagic embolic stroke, exacerbation of cerebral dysfunction occurs during cardiac surgery in 44 percent of cases when the interval between the stroke and surgery is 7 days or less; in 17 percent when the interval is 8 to 14 days; and in 10 percent or less when more than 2 weeks has elapsed. After hemorrhagic intracerebral events, the risk for neurological worsening or death with cardiac surgery persists at 20 percent even after 1 month.[51] Thus, when the response of IE to antimicrobial therapy and hemodynamic status permit, delaying cardiac surgery for 2 to 3 weeks after a significant embolic infarct and at least a month after intracerebral hemorrhage (with prior repair of a mycotic aneurysm) has been recommended.[51] Alternatively, in patients at immediate risk of death in the absence of cardiac surgery, operation during the early days after cerebral infarction has been advocated as life saving in spite of potential neurological risk.

DURATION OF ANTIMICROBIAL THERAPY AFTER SURGICAL INTERVENTION. Inflammatory changes and bacteria visible with Gram stain have been found in vegetations removed from patients who had successfully completed standard recommended antibiotic therapy for IE—29 of 53 (55 percent) still taking antibiotics; 7 of 15 (47 percent) without antibiotics for less than a month; and 4 of 18 (22 percent) without antibiotics for 1 to 6 months. Cultures of these vegetations yielded bacteria in 5, 0, and 1 instances, respectively.[52] If vegetation cultures are negative, neither visible bacteria nor PCR detection of bacterial DNA indicates that antimicrobial therapy has failed or that a full course of antibiotic therapy is needed postoperatively.[52-54] The duration of antimicrobial therapy after surgery depends on the length of preoperative therapy, the antibiotic susceptibility of the causative organism, the presence of paravalvular invasive infection, and the culture status of the vegetation. In general, for uncomplicated NVE caused by relatively antibiotic-responsive organisms with negative cultures of operative specimens, the duration of preoperative plus postoperative therapy should at least equal a full course of recommended therapy with perhaps 2 weeks or less of therapy postoperatively.[53] For patients with prostheses sewn into a débrided abscess cavity or with positive intraoperative cultures, a full course of therapy should be given postoperatively.[17] Patients with PVE should receive a full course of antimicrobial therapy postoperatively when the causative organism is seen or cultured in resected material.[12]

Treatment of Extracardiac Complications

SPLENIC ABSCESS. Three to 5 percent of patients with IE develop a splenic abscess.[50] Although splenic defects can be identified by ultrasonography and computed tomography, these tests in isolation usually cannot reliably discriminate between abscess and the far more common infarct. Persistent fever and progressive enlargement of the lesion during antimicrobial therapy suggest that it is an abscess, which can be confirmed by percutaneous needle aspiration. Successful therapy of splenic abscesses requires drainage percutaneously or a splenectomy.[17,32] If possible, abscesses in the spleen should be treated effectively before valve replacement surgery; alternatively, splenectomy should be performed as soon thereafter as surgical risks permit.[32]

CH 63

Infective Endocarditis

MYCOTIC ANEURYSMS AND SEPTIC ARTERITIS. From 2 to 10 percent of patients with IE have mycotic aneurysms, and half of these involve cerebral vessels. Cerebral mycotic aneurysms occur at the branch points in cerebral vessels and are generally located distally over the cerebral cortex, particularly in branches of the middle cerebral artery. Aneurysms arise either from occlusion of vessels by septic emboli with secondary arteritis and vessel wall destruction or from injury caused by bacteremia seeding the vessel wall through the vasa vasorum. *S. aureus* is commonly implicated in the former mechanism and viridans streptococci in the latter. Devastating intracranial hemorrhage is the initial clinical event in many patients with mycotic aneurysms. Focal deficits from embolic events, persistent focal headache, unexplained neurological deterioration, or cerebrospinal fluid with erythrocytes and xanthochromia may be premonitory. Cerebral angiography is required to evaluate patients with suspected small aneurysms or intracerebral hemorrhage. Magnetic resonance or spiral computed tomographic angiography, each of which has a 90 to 95 percent sensitivity for aneurysms >5 mm, has been recommended for patients experiencing premonitory symptoms, especially if cardiac surgery or anticoagulant therapy is planned.[32] Rupture or leakage may occur at any point before or during early antibiotic therapy, or rarely later. Mortality is 80 percent with aneurysm rupture.

Unruptured mycotic aneurysms should be followed during antimicrobial therapy. Half of these may resolve.[32] If feasible anatomically, aneurysms that have ruptured should be repaired.[55] Surgery should be considered for a single aneurysm that enlarges during or after antimicrobial therapy. Anticoagulant therapy should be avoided in patients with a persisting mycotic aneurysm. Aneurysms occasionally rupture after completion of standard antimicrobial therapy; however, there is no accurate estimation of risk for late rupture. Prevailing opinion favors the resection of single aneurysms that persist after therapy whenever possible without serious neurological injury.[55] The potential existence of occult aneurysms in patients without neurological symptoms or in those who have had a nondiagnostic angiographic evaluation is not considered a contraindication to anticoagulant therapy after completion of antimicrobial therapy.

Extracranial mycotic aneurysms should be managed as outlined for cerebral aneurysms. Those that leak, that are expanding during therapy, or that persist after therapy should be repaired. Particular attention should be given to aneurysms that involve intraabdominal arteries, rupture of which could result in life-threatening hemorrhage.[32]

ANTICOAGULANT THERAPY. Patients with PVE involving devices that would usually warrant maintenance anticoagulation are continued on careful anticoagulant therapy with either warfarin or heparin.[12] Some investigators advise that anticoagulant therapy be withdrawn from patients with *S. aureus* PVE during the initial 2 weeks of treatment.[17] In the absence of an accepted indication, anticoagulation is not initiated as prophylaxis against IE-related thromboembolism in patients with PVE involving devices that do not usually require this therapy. Anticoagulant therapy in patients with NVE is limited to patients for whom there is a clear indication and for whom there is not a known increased risk for intracranial hemorrhage. If central nervous system complications occur in patients who have IE and who are receiving anticoagulant therapy, anticoagulation should be reversed immediately.[12] In a randomized blinded trial, aspirin, 325 mg daily, did not reduce the risk of emboli and was likely associated with increased bleeding.[56]

Response to Therapy

Within a week after initiation of effective antimicrobial therapy, almost 70 percent of patients with NVE or PVE are afebrile and 90 percent have defervesced by the end of the second week of treatment.[12] Fever during therapy persists longer in patients with *S. aureus, P. aeruginosa,* or culture-negative IE as well as IE characterized by microvascular phenomena and major embolic complications. Persistence or recurrence of fever more than 10 days after initiation of antibiotic therapy identifies patients with increased mortality rates and with complications of infection or therapy.[12]

Patients with prolonged or recurrent fever should be evaluated for intracardiac complications, focal extracardiac septic complications, intercurrent nosocomial infections, recurrent pulmonary emboli (patients with right-sided IE), drug-associated fever, additional underlying illnesses, and, if appropriate, in-hospital substance abuse. Blood cultures should be repeated and the antimicrobial susceptibility of the causative organism should be reevaluated. Fever attributed to the antimicrobial therapy may warrant revision of treatment if a suitable alternative is available. In the absence of effective alternative therapy, treatment can be continued despite drug fever if there is no significant end-organ toxicity. Many clinical and laboratory features of IE are slow to resolve despite effective antimicrobial therapy. The increased ESR and anemia may not correct until after therapy has been completed.

Mortality rates for large series of patients with NVE treated since 1980 ranged from 13 to 20 percent.[3,5,6,23] Death from IE has been associated with increased age (>65 to 70 years old), underlying diseases, infection involving the aortic valve, development of CHF, nosocomial origin, *S. aureus* infection, renal failure, and central nervous system complications.[5,6,30] Early surgical treatment of CHF due to valve dysfunction has decreased the mortality associated with CHF. As a result, neurological events and septic complications, e.g., uncontrolled infection and myocardial abscess, have accounted for a larger proportion of deaths in recent series.

Mortality rates among patients with IE caused by viridans streptococci, enterococci, and *S. bovis* have ranged from 4 to 16 percent. Mortality rates are higher for left-sided NVE caused by other organisms: *S. aureus*, 25 to 47 percent; nonviridans streptococci (groups B, C, and G), 13 to 50 percent;[19] *C. burnetii*, 5 to 37 percent; *P. aeruginosa*, Enterobacteriaceae, and fungi, greater than 50 percent.

When adjusted for bias introduced by denying surgery to severely ill patients, surgical intervention, versus medical treatment for the described surgical indications is associated with significant reduction in mortality at 6 months (16 versus 33 percent).[48,50]

Outcome for patients with PVE, as contrasted with NVE, has been less favorable. Before 1980, mortality rates for PVE with onset less than 60 days after surgery and PVE with later onset averaged 70 and 45 percent, respectively. With the recognition that PVE outcome would benefit from surgical intervention, mortality rates have decreased to 14 to 36 percent.[9,11,12] Among patients with PVE treated surgically, survival rates at 4 to 6 years ranged from 50 to 82 percent. Long-term survival was adversely affected by the presence of moderate or severe CHF at discharge. Survival rates are not related to time of onset after cardiac surgery.

Among patients with NVE (non-addicts) discharged after medical or medical-surgical therapy, survival was 71 to 88 percent at 5 years and 61 to 81 percent at 10 years.[50,52] Among patients treated surgically for NVE, survival at 5 years ranged from 70 to 80 percent.

RELAPSE AND RECURRENCE. Relapse of IE usually occurs within 2 months of discontinuing antibiotic treatment. Patients who have NVE caused by penicillin-susceptible viridans streptococci and who receive a recommended course of therapy experience less than 2 percent relapse. From 8 to 20 percent of patients with enterococcal IE relapse after standard therapy. Patients with IE caused by *S. aureus,* Enterobacteriaceae, or fungi are more likely to experience overt failure of therapy rather than relapse; nevertheless, 4 percent of patients with *S. aureus* IE suffer relapse. Relapse of fungal endocarditis at long intervals after treatment has been reported. Relapse occurs in 10 percent of patients with PVE overall and in 6 to 15 percent of those treated surgically.

Among non-addicts with an initial episode of NVE or PVE, 4.5 to 7 percent experience one or more additional episodes.[52] Recurrent IE episodes share the clinical and microbiological features and response to therapy noted in primary episodes. IV drug abuse is now the most common predisposing factor for recurrent IE.

PREVENTION

The American Heart Association has recently issued new and dramatically restricted recommendations for the chemoprophylaxis for IE.[57] These recommendations reflect an evaluation of data documenting procedure-related bacteremia; the antibiotic susceptibility of procedure-related bacteremic organisms that cause endocarditis most commonly; the results of prophylaxis studies in animal models of endocarditis; population-based studies of endocarditis and the prevalence of valvulopathy at risk for endocarditis; the association of excess morbidity with specific forms of endocarditis; and retrospective and prospective studies of endocarditis prophylaxis. The committee recommends prophylactic antibiotics be used in conjunction with dental/oral procedures only in those patients with underlying cardiac conditions at the highest risk for a severe morbid outcome as a consequence of endocarditis. The recommendations are acknowledged to be "less well established by evidence" and to represent the consensus opinion of experts. The committee's reasoning is summarized below.

GENERAL METHODS. The incidence of IE can be significantly reduced by total surgical correction of some congenital lesions, such as patent ductus arteriosus, ventricular septal defect, and pulmonary stenosis. Maintaining good oral hygiene, which decreases the frequency of bacteremia that accompanies daily activities, is an important preventive measure. Oral hygiene and dental health should be addressed before prosthetic valves are placed electively. Some activities or procedures likely to induce bacteremia should be avoided. Oral irrigating devices are not recommended. The use of central intravascular catheters and urinary catheters should be minimized. Infections associated with bacteremia must be treated promptly and, if possible, eradicated before the involved tissues are incised or manipulated.

CHEMOPROPHYLAXIS. Transient bacteremia occurs commonly after manipulation of the teeth and periodontal tissues and various dental procedures. Additionally, transient bacteremia frequently develops during routine daily activities involving the oral cavity: brushing and flossing teeth, using water irrigation devices, and chewing. Considering the relative infrequency of dental visits or oral surgery, the cumulative exposure of cardiac structures to bacteremia is dramatically greater from routine daily activities than from dental procedures. It has been estimated that brushing teeth twice daily for a year results in 154,000 times greater bacteremia exposure than extraction of a single tooth, the dental procedure that induces the greatest risk of bacteremia.[58] Thus, the risk of seeding cardiac structures is far greater from routine daily activities than from dental manipulations. Furthermore, the ability of antibiotics or topical antiseptics to prevent or reduce bacteremia precipitated by dental procedures is not established and is impaired even further by the gradual increase in the frequency of resistance of viridans streptococci to antibiotics previously advocated for prophylaxis: penicillin, amoxicillin, cephalexin, clarithromycin, erythromycin, azithromycin, and clindamycin.

The causal association of dental manipulations with endocarditis is not established, and, in fact, the often implied association may result from biased observations. Population-based studies in the Netherlands concluded that dental procedures caused at best only a small fraction of IE cases and that prophylaxis, even if totally effective, would prevent only a small number of cases. Strom and associates did not find premorbid dental procedures increased in patients with endocarditis when compared with uninfected controls.[59] In France, the estimate of IE related to unprotected procedures in patients with predisposing cardiac lesions was 1 episode per 46,000 procedures (1 per 10,700 and 1 per 54,300, with prosthetic and native valve predispositions, respectively).[60] Others have estimated the risk to be 10-fold lower. Thus, a huge prophylaxis effort may be required to prevent one case of IE.

The committee recognized the absence of data documenting that antibiotic prophylaxis prevents endocarditis as a result of procedure-induced bacteremia; however, it could not exclude that a small number of IE cases could be prevented by antibiotic prophylaxis. Nevertheless, in weighing the benefits, potential adverse events, and cost associated with antibiotic prophylaxis, the committee considered that prophylaxis was not warranted based upon a lifetime increased risk of IE related to cardiac disease, but rather that prophylaxis should be restricted to those patients whose cardiac abnormality places them at the highest risk for a morbid outcome from IE (Table 63-14). Notably, prophylaxis is no longer recommended for patients with mitral valve prolapse or for cardiac conditions other than those noted (see Table 63-14).

The new guidelines advise prophylaxis be used in the high-risk group before any dental procedures that involve gingival tissue, the periapical region of a tooth, or perforate oral mucosa. Procedures not warranting prophylaxis include routine intraoral anesthetic injection through uninfected tissue, taking dental radiographs, placement or adjustment of removable prosthodontic or orthodontic brackets or appliances, shedding of deciduous teeth, or bleeding due to lip or oral mucosa trauma.[57] The regimens recommended are single-dose modifications of those previously advocated (Table 63-15). These same regimens are considered appropriate for at-risk patients (see Table 63-14) who will undergo incision or biopsy of the respiratory mucosa such as tonsillectomy, adenoidectomy, or bronchoscopy.

The causal relationship between gastrointestinal and genitourinary tract procedures and IE is less well defined than that for dental procedures. Consequently, antibiotics are not recommended to prevent endocarditis when at-risk patients undergo these procedures.[57] When at-risk patients (see Table 63-14) with established gastrointestinal or genitourinary tract infection are to receive antibiotic therapy or are to receive antibiotics to prevent wound infections or procedure-induced sepsis, it is reasonable to include an agent active against enterococci. Eradication of genitourinary tract infection, especially that caused by enterococci, before manipulation is advised. Similarly, in at-risk patients undergoing surgery on infected skin or musculoskeletal tissue, antibiotic therapy should include an agent active

TABLE 63–14	Cardiac Conditions Associated with the Highest Risk of Adverse Outcome from Endocarditis for Which Prophylaxis with Dental Procedures Is Recommended

Prosthetic cardiac valve
Previous infective endocarditis
Congenital heart disease
   Unrepaired cyanotic congenital heart disease, including those with palliative shunts and conduits
   Completely repaired congenital heart disease with prosthetic material or device either by surgery or catheter intervention during the first 6 months after the procedure*
   Repaired congenital heart disease with residual defects at the site or adjacent to the site of a prosthetic patch or prosthetic device (which inhibit endothelialization)
Cardiac transplantation recipients who develop cardiac valvulopathy

*Prophylaxis is recommended because endothelialization of prosthetic material occurs within 6 months after the procedure.
Adapted from Wilson W, Taubert KA, Gewitz M, et al: Prevention of infective endocarditis: Recommendations of the American Heart Association. Circulation, 2007.

TABLE 63–15 Regimens for Prophylaxis Against Endocarditis: Use with Dental, Oral, and Upper Respiratory Tract Procedures

Setting	Regimen Administered 30-60 Min before Procedure*
Standard regimen[†]	Amoxicillin 2.0 gm PO
Amoxicillin/penicillin-allergic patients	Cephalixin 2 gm PO[†] *or* Azithromycin or clarithromycin 500 mg PO *or* Clindamycin 600 mg PO
Patients unable to take oral medications	Ampicillin 2.0 gm IM or IV *or* Cefazolin or ceftriaxone 1 gm IV[†]
Ampicillin/amoxicillin/penicillin-allergic patients unable to take oral medications	Clindamycin 300 mg IV 30 min before procedure, then 150 mg 6 hr after initial dose

*Dosages for adults. Initial pediatric dosages are as follows: Ampicillin or amoxicillin, 50 mg/kg; clindamycin, 20 mg/kg; azithromycin or clarithromycin, 15 mg/kg.
[†]Cephalosporins are not used in patients with history of anaphylaxis, angioedema, or urticaria associated with penicillin, ampicillin, or cephalosporins.
Adapted from Wilson W, Taubert KA, Gewitz M, et al: Prevention of infective endocarditis: Recommendations of the American Heart Association. Circulation, 2007.

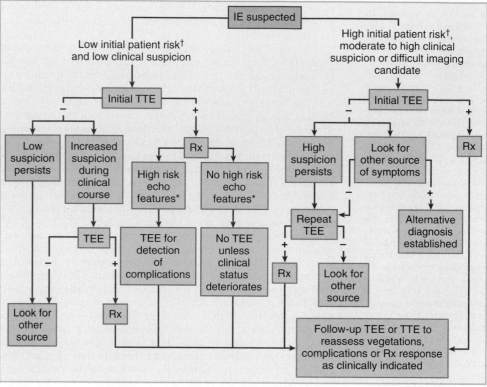

FIGURE 63–4 Schematic approach to the diagnostic use of echocardiography. High-risk echocardiographic features include large vegetations, valve insufficiency, suggestion of perivalvular extension, or ventricular dysfunction. Patients with high initial risk include those with prosthetic heart valves, complex congenital heart disease, prior IE, new murmur, and heart failure. Rx indicates initiation of antibiotic therapy for IE. IE = infective endocarditis; TEE = transesophageal echocardiography; TTE = transthoracic echocardiography. (*Reproduced from Bayer AS, Bolger AF, Taubert KA, et al: Diagnosis and management of infective endocarditis and its complications. Circulation 98:2936-48, 1998.*)

against anticipated or documented *S. aureus* (including methicillin-resistant strains) and beta-hemolytic streptococci.

Patients with cardiac lesions (see Table 63-14) should be given written material about their predisposing lesion and the recommended antibiotic prophylaxis.

FUTURE PERSPECTIVES

The continued significant mortality and morbidity associated with IE stimulate ongoing efforts to improve diag-
nostic, preventive, and therapeutic strategies. Molecular detection of nonviable, nonculturable, and even routine causative organisms are likely and will provide more rapid, efficient, and sensitive diagnostic tests. The increasing prominence of *S. aureus* as a cause of IE and its increasing resistance to antibiotics have stimulated efforts to develop staphylococcal vaccines. If proved to be efficacious, a vaccine could protect patients at continuous high risk for *S. aureus* IE (e.g., patients with chronic health care exposure (hemodialysis) and implanted cardiac devices). New antibiotics are under development for treatment of resistant gram-positive bacteria, including MRSA. Groups of investigators are collaborating to develop large prospectively collected endocarditis case data bases. Using sophisticated analytic techniques, these investigators will address therapeutic questions that are not amenable to randomized clinical trails. They may even be able to mount large randomized-blinded trials to assess therapy for selected forms of IE. The forthcoming information will allow evidenced-based decision-making for difficult areas of treatment, such as surgical indications and treatment of unusual causes of IE.

REFERENCES

Epidemiology

1. Moreillon P, Que YA: Infective endocarditis. Lancet 363:139-49, 2004.
2. Tleyjch IM, Steckelberg JM, Murad HS, et al: Temporal trends in infective endocarditis: A population-based study in Olmsted County, Minnesota. JAMA 293:3022-8, 2005.
3. Hoen B, Alla F, Selton-Suty C, et al: Changing profile of infective endocarditis: Results of a 1-year survey in France. JAMA 288:75-81, 2002.
4. Fowler VG, Jr., Miro JM, Hoen B, et al: Staphylococcus aureus endocarditis: A consequence of medical progress. JAMA 293:3012-21, 2005.

5. Chu VH, Cabell CH, Benjamin DK, Jr., et al: Early predictors of in-hospital death in infective endocarditis. Circulation 109:1745-9, 2004.

6. Martin-Davila P, Fortun J, Navas E, et al: Nosocomial endocarditis in a tertiary hospital: An increasing trend in native valve cases. Chest 128:772-9, 2005.

7. Miro JM, del Rio A, Mestres CA: Infective endocarditis in intravenous drug abusers and HIV-1 infected patients. Infect Dis Clin North Am 16:273-95, 2002.

8. Wilson LE, Thomas DL, Astemborski J, et al: Prospective study of infective endocarditis among injection drug users. J Infect Dis 185:1761-6, 2002.

9. Habib G, Tribouilloy C, Thuny F, et al: Prosthetic valve endocarditis: Who needs surgery? A multicentre study of 104 cases. Heart 91:954-9, 2005.

10. Karchmer AW, Longworth DL: Infections of intracardiac devices. Infect Dis Clin North Am 16:477-505, 2002.

11. Rivas P, Alonso J, Moya J, et al: The impact of hospital-acquired infections on the microbial etiology and prognosis of late-onset prosthetic valve endocarditis. Chest 128:764-71, 2005.

12. Karchmer AW: Infections of prosthetic heart valves. In Waldvogel F, Bisno AL (eds): Infections Associated with Indwelling Medical Devices, 3rd ed. Washington, DC: American Society for Microbiology; 2000, pp 145-72.

13. John MVD, Hibberd PL, Karchmer AW, et al: *Staphylococcus aureus* prosthetic valve endocarditis: Optimal management and risk factors for death. Clin Infect Dis 26:1302-9, 1998.

14. Chirouze C, Cabell CH, Fowler VG, Jr., et al: Prognostic factors in 61 cases of *Staphylococcus aureus* prosthetic valve infective endocarditis from the International Collaboration on Endocarditis merged database. Clin Infect Dis 38:1323-7, 2004.

15. Sohail MR, Martin KR, Wilson WR, et al: Medical versus surgical management of *Staphylococcus aureus* prosthetic valve endocarditis. Am J Med 119:147-54, 2006.

16. Petti CA, Fowler VG, Jr. *Staphylococcus aureus* bacteremia and endocarditis. Infect Dis Clin North Am 16:413-35, 2002.

Etiologic Microorganisms

17. Baddour LM, Wilson WR, Bayer AS, et al: Infective Endocarditis: Diagnosis, antimicrobial therapy, and management of complications. Circulation 111:3167-84, 2005.

18. Sambola A, Miro JM, Tornos MP, et al: *Streptococcus agalactiae* infective endocarditis: Analysis of 30 cases and review of the literature, 1962-1998. Clin Infect Dis 34:1576-84, 2002.

19. Lefort A, Lortholary O, Casassus P, et al: Comparison between adult endocarditis due to beta-hemolytic streptococci (serogroups A, B, C, and G) and *Streptococcus milleri:* A multi-center study in France. Arch Intern Med 162:2450-6, 2002.

20. Martinez E, Miro JM, Almirante B, et al: Effect of penicillin resistance of *Streptococcus pneumoniae* on the presentation, prognosis, and treatment of pneumococcal endocarditis in adults. Clin Infect Dis 35:130-9, 2002.

21. McDonald JR, Olaison L, Anderson DJ, et al: Enterococcal endocarditis: 107 Cases from the international collaboration on endocarditis merged database. Am J Med 118:759-66, 2005.

22. Stevens MP, Edmond MB: Endocarditis due to vancomycin-resistant enterococci: Case report and review of the literature. Clin Infect Dis 41:1134-42, 2005.

23. Miro JM, Anguera I, Cabell CH, et al: *Staphylococcus aureus* native valve infective endocarditis: Report of 566 episodes from the International Collaboration on Endocarditis merged database. Clin Infect Dis 41:507-14, 2005.

24. Chu VH, Cabell CH, Abrutyn E, et al: Native valve endocarditis due to coagulase-negative staphylococci: Report of 99 episodes from the International Collaboration on Endocarditis merged database. Clin Infect Dis 39:1527-30, 2004.

25. Fenollar F, Thuny F, Xeridat B, Lepidi H, Raoult D. Endocarditis after acute Q fever in patients with previously undiagnosed valvulopathies. Clin Infect Dis 42:818-21, 2006.

26. Raoult D, Fournier PE, Vandenesch F, et al: Outcome and treatment of *Bartonella* endocarditis. Arch Intern Med 163:226-30, 2003.

Pathogenesis, Clinical Features, and Diagnosis

27. Moreillon P, Que YA, Bayer AS: Pathogenesis of streptococcal and staphylococcal endocarditis. Infect Dis Clin North Am 16:297-318, 2002.

28. Crawford MH, Durack DT: Clinical presentation of infective endocarditis. Cardiol Clin 21:159-66, 2003.

29. Vilacosta I, Graupner C, San Roman JA, et al: Risk of embolization after institution of antibiotic therapy for infective endocarditis. J Am Coll Cardiol 39:1489-95, 2002.

30. Hasbun R, Vikram HR, Barakat LA, et al: Complicated left-sided native valve endocarditis in adults: Risk classification for mortality. JAMA 289:1933-40, 2003.

31. Li JS, Sexton DJ, Mick N, et al: Proposed modifications to the Duke criteria for the diagnosis of infective endocarditis. Clin Infect Dis 30:633-8, 2000.

32. Bayer AS, Bolger AF, Taubert KA, et al: Diagnosis and management of infective endocarditis and its complications. Circulation 98:2936-48, 1998.

33. Baddour LM, Wilson WR, Bayer AS, et al: Diagnosis, antimicrobial therapy, and management of complications. A statement for healthcare professionals from the Committee on Rheumatic Fever, Endocarditis, and Kawasaki Disease, Council on Cardiovascular Disease in the Young, and the Councils on Clinical Cardiology, Stroke, and Cardiovascular Surgery and Anesthesia, American Heart Association. Circulation 111:e394-e433, 2005

34. Towns ML, Reller LB: Diagnostic methods current best practices and guidelines for isolation of bacteria and fungi in infective endocarditis. Infect Dis Clin North Am 16:363-76, 2002.

35. Lisby G, Gutschik E, Durack DT: Molecular methods for diagnosis of infective endocarditis. Infect Dis Clin North Am 16:393-412, 2002.

36. Grijalva M, Horvath R, Dendis M, et al: Molecular diagnosis of culture negative infective endocarditis: Clinical validation in a group of surgically treated patients. Heart 89:263-8, 2003.

Treatment

37. Le T, Bayer AS: Combination antibiotic therapy for infective endocarditis. Clin Infect Dis 36:615-21, 2003.

38. Olaison L, Schadewitz K: The Swedish Society for Infectious Diseases Quality Assurance Study Group for Endocarditis. Enterococcal endocarditis in Sweden, 1995-1999: Can shorter therapy with aminoglycosides be used? Clin Infect Dis 34:159-66, 2002.

39. National Nosocomial Infections Surveillance System. National Nosocomial Infections Surveillance (NNIS) system report, data summary from January 1992 through June 2003, issued August 2003. Am J Infect Contr 31:481-98, 2003.

40. Fridkin SK, Hageman JC, Morrison M, et al: Methicillin-resistant *Staphylococcus aureus* disease in three communities. N Engl J Med 352:1436-1444, 2005.

41. Seybold U, Kourbatova EV, Johnson JG, et al: Emergence of community-associated methicillin-resistant *Staphylococcus aureus* USA300 genotype as a major cause of health care-associated blood stream infections. Clin Infect Dis 42:647-56, 2006.

42. Fowler VG, Jr., Boucher HW, Corey GR, et al: Daptomycin versus standard therapy for bacteremia and endocarditis caused by *Staphylococcus aureus.* N Engl J Med 355:653-65, 2006.

43. Drinkovic D, Morris AJ, Pottumarthy S, et al: Bacteriological outcome of combination versus single-agent treatment for staphylococcal endocarditis. J Antimicrob Chemother 52:820-5, 2003.

44. Lye DCB, Hughes A, O'Brien D, Athan E: *Candida glabrata* prosthetic valve endocarditis treated successfully with fluconazole plus capsofungin without surgery: A case report and literature review. Eur J Clin Microbiol Infect Dis 24:753-5, 2005.

45. Raoult D, Houpikian P, Tissot Dupont H, et al: Treatment of Q fever endocarditis: Comparison of two regimens containing doxycycline and ofloxacin or hydroxychloroquine. Arch Intern Med 159:167-73, 1999.

46. Rolain JM, Brouqui P, Koehler JE, et al: Recommendations for treatment of human infections causes by *Bartonella* species. Antimicrob Agents Chemother 48:1921-33, 2004.

47. Olaison L, Pettersson G: Current best practices and guidelines: Indications for surgical intervention in infective endocarditis. Infect Dis Clin North Am 16:453-75, 2002.

48. Vikram HR, Buenconsejo J, Hasbun R, Quagliarello VJ: Impact of valve surgery on 6-month mortality in adults with complicated, left-sided native valve endocarditis: A propensity analysis. JAMA 290:3207-14, 2003.

49. Mangoni ED, Adinolfi LE, Tripodi MF, et al: Risk factors for "major" embolic events in hospitalized patients with infective endocarditis. Am Heart J 146:311-6, 2003.

50. Netzer ROM, Altwegg SC, Zollinger E, et al: Infective endocarditis: Determinants of long term outcome. Heart 88:61-6, 2002.

51. Eishi K, Kawazoe K, Kuriyama Y, et al: Surgical management of infective endocarditis associated with cerebral complications: Multicenter retrospective study in Japan. J Thorac Cardiovasc Surg 110:1745-55, 1995.

52. Morris AJ, Drinkovic D, Pottumarthy S, et al: Gram stain, culture, and histopathological examination findings for heart valves removed because of infective endocarditis. Clin Infect Dis 36:697-704, 2003.

53. Morris AJ, Drinkovic D, Pottumarthy S, et al: Bacteriological outcome after valve surgery for active infective endocarditis: Implications for duration of treatment after surgery. Clin Infect Dis 41:187-194, 2005.

54. Rovery C, Greub G, Lepidi H, et al: PCR detection of bacteria on cardiac valves of patients with treated bacterial endocarditis. J Clin Micro 43:163-7, 2005.

55. Phuong LK, Link M, Wijdicks E: Management of intracranial infections aneurisms: A series of 16 cases. Neurosurgery 51:1145-52, 2002.

56. Chan KL, Dumesnil JG, Cujec B, et al: A randomized trial of aspirin on the risk of embolic events in patients with infective endocarditis. J Am Coll Cardiol 42:775-80, 2003.

Prevention

57. Wilson W, Taubert KA, Gewitz M, et al: Prevention of infective endocarditis—recommendations by the American Heart Association. A guideline from the American Heart Association Rheumatic Fever, Endocarditis, Kawasaki Disease Committee, Council on Cardiovascular Disease in the Young and the Council on Clinical Cardiology, Council on Cardiovascular Surgery and Anesthesia and the Quality of Care and Outcomes Research Interdisciplinary Working Group. Circulation, 2007 (in press).

58. Roberts GJ: Dentists are innocent! "Everyday" bacteremia is the real culprit: A review and assessment of the evidence that dental surgical procedures are a principal cause of bacterial endocarditis in children. Pediatr Cardiol 20:217-325, 1999.

59. Strom BL, Abrutyn E, Berlin EA, et al: Dental and cardiac risk factors for infective endocarditis: A population-based, case-control study. Ann Intern Med 129:761-769, 1998.

60. Duval X, Alla F, Hoen B, et al: Estimated risk of endocarditis in adults with predisposing cardiac conditions undergoing dental procedures with or without antibiotic prophylaxis. Clin Infect Dis 42:e102-e107, 2006.

Infective Endocarditis

The American Heart Association guidelines have been evolving for the last 50 years, with the most recent key updates on recommendations for antibiotic prophylaxis published in 1997[1] and 2007,[2] with a scientific statement with recommendations for diagnosis and management of this condition in 1998.[3] Other guidelines with recommendations relevant to this condition include American College of Cardiology/ American Heart Association (ACC/AHA) guidelines for management of valvular heart disease published in 2006[4] and guidelines for use of echocardiography published in 1997.[5]

PREVENTION

The 2007 AHA guidelines represent a marked departure from prior recommendations, and greatly reduce the patient population for which prophylactic antibiotics are recommended. These new guidelines note that prior recommendations were based upon research showing that antimicrobial prophylaxis is effective for prevention of experimental infective endocarditis in animal models. However, these guidelines acknowledge the lack of evidence that antimicrobial prophylaxis is effective in humans for prevention of endocarditis after dental, gastrointestinal, or genitourinary procedures. The expert committee also considered the complexity of prior guidelines, which required stratification of patients and procedures on their risk for infective endocarditis.

The 2007 guidelines committee concluded that only an extremely small number of cases of infective endocarditis might be prevented by antibiotic prophylaxis for dental procedures even if such prophylaxis was 100% effective. Accordingly, the revised guidelines recommend infective endocarditis prophylaxis for dental procedures only for patients with underlying cardiac conditions associated with the highest risk of adverse outcomes from infective endocarditis (Table 63G-1). For patients with these conditions, antibiotic prophylaxis is recommended for dental procedures that involve manipulation of gingival tissue or the periapical region of teeth or perforation of the oral mucosa. The guidelines recommend a single dose of amoxicillin or ampicillin as the preferred prophylactic agent for individuals who do not have a history of type I hypersensitive reactions to a penicillin. For individuals who are allergic to penicillins or amoxicillin, alternative recommendations include first-generation oral cephalosporins, clindamycin, azithromycin, or clarithromycin.

Antibiotic administration is not recommended for patients undergoing genitourinary or gastrointestinal tract procedures solely for the purpose of preventing endocarditis. This recommendation is in contrast with previous guidelines that recommended endocarditis antibiotic prophylaxis before some procedures and not others. Antibiotic prophylaxis for bronchoscopy is not recommended unless the procedure involves incision of the respiratory tract mucosa.

CH 63

TABLE 63G–1	Cardiac Conditions and Dental Procedures for Which Antibiotic Prophylaxis Is Recommended

Cardiac Conditions Associated with the Highest Risk of Adverse Outcome from Endocarditis for Which Prophylaxis with Dental Procedures Is Recommended

Prosthetic cardiac valve

Previous infective endocarditis

Congenital heart disease (CHD)

    Unrepaired cyanotic CHD, including those with palliative shunts and conduits

    Completely repaired CHD with prosthetic material or device either by surgery or catheter intervention during the first 6 months after the procedure*

    Repaired CHD with residual defects at the site or adjacent to the site of a prosthetic patch or prosthetic device (which inhibit endothelialization)

    Except for the conditions listed above, antibiotic prophylaxis is no longer recommended for any other form of CHD

Cardiac transplantation recipients who develop cardiac valvulopathy

Dental Procedures for which Endocarditis Prophylaxis is Recommended for High Risk Patients (see above)

All dental procedures and events that involve manipulation of gingival tissue or the periapical region of teeth or perforation of the oral mucosa **except** the following:

- Routine anesthetic injections through noninfected tissue
- Taking dental radiographs
- Placement of removable prosthodontic or orthodontic appliances
- Adjustment of orthodontic appliances
- Placement of orthodontic brackets
- Shedding of deciduous teeth and bleeding from trauma to the lips or oral mucosa

*Prophylaxis is recommended because endothelialization of prosthetic material occurs within 6 months of the procedure.

From Wilson W, Taubert KA, Gewitz M, et al: Prevention of infective endocarditis. Recommendations by the American Heart Association. Circulation 2007 (in press).

INDICATIONS FOR ECHOCARDIOGRAPHY

Echocardiography is strongly supported in virtually all patients with suspected or known infective endocarditis, but the 1997 ACC/AHA guidelines on echocardiography[4] do not recommend transesophageal echocardiography (TEE) as the initial test of choice in the diagnosis of native valve endocarditis (Table 63G-2). The guidelines urge use of TEE when specific questions are not adequately addressed by an initial

TABLE 63G–2 ACC/AHA Guidelines for Evaluation and Treatment of Endocarditis

Indication	Class I	Class IIa	Class IIb	Class III
Echocardiography in infective endocarditis: native valves	1. Detection and characterization of valvular lesions, their hemodynamic severity, and/or ventricular compensation* 2. Detection of vegetations and characterization of lesions in patients with congenital heart disease in whom infective endocarditis is suspected 3. Detection of associated abnormalities (e.g., abscesses, shunts)* 4. Reevaluation studies in complex endocarditis (e.g., virulent organism, severe hemodynamic lesion, aortic valve involvement, persistent fever or bacteremia, clinical change, or symptomatic deterioration) 5. Evaluation of patients with high clinical suspicion of culture-negative endocarditis*	1. Evaluation of bacteremia without a known source* 2. Risk stratification in established endocarditis*	1. Routine reevaluation in uncomplicated endocarditis during antibiotic therapy	1. Evaluation of fever and nonpathological murmur without evidence of bacteremia
Echocardiography in infective endocarditis: prosthetic valves	1. Detection and characterization of valvular lesions, their hemodynamic severity, and/or ventricular compensation* 2. Detection of associated abnormalities (e.g., abscesses, shunts)* 3. Reevaluation in complex endocarditis (e.g., virulent organism, severe hemodynamic lesion, aortic valve involvement, persistent fever or bacteremia, clinical change, or symptomatic deterioration) 4. Evaluation of suspected endocarditis and negative cultures* 5. Evaluation of bacteremia without a known source*	1. Evaluation of persistent fever without evidence of bacteremia or new murmur*	1. Routine reevaluation in uncomplicated endocarditis during antibiotic therapy*	1. Evaluation of transient fever without evidence of bacteremia or new murmur

Continues

CH 63

Infective Endocarditis

TABLE 63G–2 ACC/AHA Guidelines for Evaluation and Treatment of Endocarditis—cont'd

Indication	Class I	Class IIa	Class IIb	Class III
Surgery for native valve endocarditis (criteria also apply to repaired mitral and aortic allograft or autograft valves)	1. Acute AR or MR with heart failure 2. Acute AR with tachycardia and early closure of the mitral valve 3. Fungal endocarditis 4. Evidence of annular or aortic abscess, sinus or aortic true or false aneurysm 5. Evidence of valve dysfunction and persistent infection after a prolonged period (7 to 10 d) of appropriate antibiotic therapy, as indicated by presence of fever, leukocytosis, and bacteremia, provided there are no noncardiac causes for infection	1. Recurrent emboli after appropriate antibiotic therapy 2. Infection with gram-negative organisms or organisms with a poor response to antibiotics in patients with evidence of valve dysfunction	1. Mobile vegetations >10 mm	1. Early infections of the mitral valve that can probably be repaired 2. Persistent pyrexia and leukocytosis with negative blood cultures
Surgery for prosthetic valve endocarditis (criteria exclude repaired mitral and aortic allograft or autograft valves)	1. Early prosthetic valve endocarditis (first 2 mo or less after surgery) 2. Heart failure with prosthetic valve dysfunction 3. Fungal endocarditis 4. Staphylococcal endocarditis not responding to antibiotic therapy 5. Evidence of paravalvular leak, annular or aortic abscess, sinus or aortic true or false aneurysm, fistula formation, or new-onset conduction disturbances 6. Infection with gram-negative organisms or organisms with a poor response to antibiotics	1. Persistent bacteremia after a prolonged course (7 to 10 d) of appropriate antibiotic therapy without noncardiac causes for bacteremia 2. Recurrent peripheral embolus despite therapy	1. Vegetation of any size on or near the prosthesis	

*Transesophageal echocardiography may provide incremental value in addition to information obtained by transthoracic imaging.

ACC/AHA = American College of Cardiology/American Heart Association; AR = aortic regurgitation; MR = mitral regurgitation; MVP = mitral valve prolapse.

From Bonow RO, Carabello B, Chatterjee K, et al: ACC/AHA 2006 guidelines for the management of patients with valvular heart disease: Executive summary: A report of the American College of Cardiology/American Heart Association Task Force on Practice Guidelines (Committee on Management of Patients with Valvular Heart Disease). Circulation 114:450, 2006.

transthoracic echocardiography (TTE) evaluation, such as if the TTE is of poor quality, if the TTE is negative despite a high clinical suspicion of endocarditis, if a prosthetic valve is involved, and if there is a high suspicion such as in a patient with staphylococcal bacteremia or in an elderly patient with valvular abnormalities that make diagnosis by TTE difficult.

Diagnosis of prosthetic valve endocarditis with TTE is more difficult than diagnosis of endocarditis of native valves. Thus, the ACC/AHA guidelines suggest a lower threshold for performance of TEE in patients with prosthetic valves and suspected endocarditis (see Table 63G-2).

SURGERY FOR ACTIVE ENDOCARDITIS

The ACC/AHA guidelines for valvular heart disease support performance of surgery for patients with life-threatening congestive heart failure or cardiogenic shock related to active endocarditis. Indications for surgery for patients with stable endocarditis are considered less clear (see Table 63G-2).

References

1. Dajani AS, Taubert KA, Wilson W, et al: Prevention of bacterial endocarditis: Recommendations by the American Heart Association. Circulation 96:363, 1997.
2. Wilson W, Taubert KA, Gewitz M, et al. Prevention of infective endocarditis. Recommendations by the American Heart Association. Circulation 2007 (in press).
3. Bayer AS, Bolger AF, Taubert KA, et al: Diagnosis and management of infective endocarditis and its complications. Circulation 98:2936, 1998.
4. Bonow RO, Carabello B, Chatterjee K, et al: ACC/AHA 2006 guidelines for the management of patients with valvular heart disease: Executive summary: A report of the American College of Cardiology/American Heart Association Task Force on Practice Guidelines (Committee on Management of Patients with Valvular Heart Disease). Circulation 114:450, 2006.
5. Cheitlin MD, Alpert JS, Armstrong WF, et al: ACC/AHA guidelines for the clinical application of echocardiography: A report of the American College of Cardiology/American Heart Association Task Force on Practice Guidelines (Committee on Clinical Application of Echocardiography). Circulation 95:1686, 1997.

CHAPTER 64

Dilated Cardiomyopathy, 1739
Specific Cardiomyopathies with a
  Dilated Phenotype, 1743
Alcoholic Cardiomyopathy, 1744

Restrictive and Infiltrative
Cardiomyopathy, 1749

Amyloidosis, 1751

Inherited and Acquired
Infiltrative Disorders Causing
Restrictive
Cardiomyopathy, 1753
Fabry Disease, 1754
Gaucher Disease, 1754
Hemochromatosis, 1754
Glycogen Storage Disease, 1755
Inflammatory Causes of Infiltrative
  Cardiomyopathy, 1755
Endomyocardial Disease, 1756
Löffler Endocarditis: The Hyper-
  eosinophilic Syndrome, 1756
Endomyocardial Fibrosis, 1757
Endocardial Fibroelastosis, 1758

Neoplastic Infiltrative
Cardiomyopathy—Carcinoid
Heart Disease, 1758

Arrhythmogenic Right
Ventricular
Dysplasia/Cardiomyopathy, 1759

Summary and Future
Perspectives, 1760

References, 1760

The Dilated, Restrictive, and Infiltrative Cardiomyopathies

Joshua M. Hare

Cardiomyopathies are diseases of heart muscle that result from a myriad of insults such as genetic defects, cardiac myocyte injury, or infiltration of myocardial tissues. Thus, cardiomyopathies result from insults to both cellular elements of the heart, notably the cardiac myocyte, and processes that are external to cells such as deposition of abnormal substances into the extracellular matrix. Cardiomyopathies are traditionally defined on the basis of structural and functional phenotypes (Table 64-1), notably dilated (characterized primarily by an enlarged ventricular chamber and reduced cardiac performance),[1] hypertrophic (characterized primarily by thickened, hypertrophic ventricular walls and enhanced cardiac performance), and restrictive (characterized primarily by thickened, stiff ventricular walls that impede diastolic filling of the ventricle; cardiac systolic performance is typically close to normal).[2] A fourth, and more recently appreciated, structural and functional phenotype is a cardiomyopathy that primarily involves the right ventricle—arrhythmogenic right ventricular dysplasia/cardiomyopathy. The dilated cardiomyopathy phenotype is often viewed as a "final common pathway" of numerous types of cardiac injuries and is the most common cardiomyopathic phenotype.[3]

The use of the term *cardiomyopathy* was previously reserved for primary diseases of the heart, not including processes affecting valvular structures, coronary vasculature, or pericardium. Because of the recognition of the final common pathway phenomenon, the use of the term cardiomyopathy to denote specific cardiomyopathies such as ischemic cardiomyopathy[4] or valvular cardiomyopathy has entered into common use (see Table 64-1). There is biological support for this because there is substantial (but clearly not complete[5]) overlap in the altered signaling pathways and compensatory mechanisms in the failing heart, regardless of underlying etiology.[3]

SPECIFIC CAUSES. Classifying the causes of cardiomyopathy continues to be a challenge, and a satisfactory and uniformly agreed upon classification system remains in evolution.[6-8] Classification schemes are plagued by the fact that as the causal basis of heart muscle disease becomes increasingly understood, it is also appreciated that for a given etiology there may be a spectrum of phenotypes that can overlap or evolve. For example, both myocarditis and amyloidosis can have a spectrum of phenotypes ranging from restrictive to dilated. Recently, a new classification of cardiomyopathies that incorporates molecular insights was proposed by an American Heart Association Scientific Statement panel.[6] This classification divides cardiomyopathy into primary and secondary causes (see Table 64-1; Tables 64-2 and 64-3), in a manner similar to traditional classification schemes, but added important subcharacterization of the primary cardiomyopathies into genetic, mixed, and acquired groups (Fig. 64-1). From the clinical perspective, where the objective is to diagnose and deliver effective therapy that may be etiology specific, there is

major overlap with the concept of an acquired primary cardiomyopathy and a secondary cardiomyopathy. An important new addition to the genetic subgroup is that of ion channel disorders, which often are not accompanied by structural heart disease but clearly can be considered a primary disorder of the heart (see Chap. 9 for further discussion). Ischemic heart disease can also lead to a cardiomyopathy, and is discussed in Chapters 25, 50, and 54. The hypertrophic cardiomyopathies are discussed in Chapters 8 and 65.

Operationally, disagreement regarding classifying cardiomyopathies does not necessarily impede patient management. Rather the disagreement reinforces the key principle in patient evaluation—there are many primary, secondary, and systemic disorders that manifest with cardiac dysfunction and/or congestive heart failure. Accordingly, the patient with an abnormality in cardiac structure or function requires comprehensive evaluation for a broad array of disorders. The main goal of this approach is to identify disorders that cause reversible cardiac dysfunction, capable of significant improvement with treatment of the underlying etiology of the heart failure.[9,10] Thus, a key principle for managing the cardiomyopathy patient is an exhaustive evaluation to determine the underlying etiological diagnosis. Throughout this chapter the issue of reversibility will be addressed (see also Chap. 22). In contrast to the principle that the underlying etiological basis of cardiomyopathy is broad, is the therapeutic concept that therapies for heart failure are somewhat similar. A common approach of addressing patient's volume status and use of neurohormonal blockade is appropriate management regardless of etiology (see Chap. 25). Only now are specific etiology-based therapies entering into clinical testing.

DILATED CARDIOMYOPATHY

The hallmarks of dilated cardiomyopathy (DCM), the most common cardiomyopathy, are enlargement of one or both of the ventricles and systolic dysfunction (Figs. 64-2

TABLE 64–1 | Classification of the Cardiomyopathies

Disorder	Description
Dilated cardiomyopathy	Dilation and impaired contraction of the left or both ventricles
	Caused by familial-genetic, viral, and/or immune, alcoholic-toxic, or unknown factors or is associated with recognized cardiovascular disease
Hypertrophic cardiomyopathy	Left and/or right ventricular hypertrophy, often asymmetrical, which usually involves the interventricular septum
	Mutations in sarcoplasmic proteins cause the disease in many patients
Restrictive cardiomyopathy	Restricted filling and reduced diastolic size of either or both ventricles with normal or near-normal systolic function
	Is idiopathic or associated with other disease (e.g., amyloidosis, endomyocardial disease)
Arrhythmogenic right ventricular cardiomyopathy	Progressive fibrofatty replacement of the right, and to some degree left, ventricular myocardium
	Familial disease is common
Unclassified cardiomyopathy	Diseases that do not fit readily into any category
	Examples include systolic dysfunction with minimal dilation, mitochondrial disease, and fibroelastosis
Specific Cardiomyopathies	
Ischemic cardiomyopathy	Arises as dilated cardiomyopathy with depressed ventricular function not explained by the extent of coronary artery obstructions or ischemic damage
Valvular cardiomyopathy	Arises as ventricular dysfunction that is out of proportion to the abnormal loading conditions produced by the valvular stenosis and/or regurgitation.
Hypertensive cardiomyopathy	Arises with left ventricular hypertrophy with features of cardiac failure related to systolic or diastolic dysfunction
Inflammatory cardiomyopathy	Cardiac dysfunction as a consequence of myocarditis
Metabolic cardiomyopathy	Includes a wide variety of causes, including endocrine abnormalities, glycogen storage disease, deficiencies (such as hypokalemia), and nutritional disorders
General systemic disease	Includes connective tissue disorders and infiltrative diseases such as sarcoidosis and leukemia
Muscular dystrophies	Includes Duchenne, Becker-type, and myotonic dystrophies
Neuromuscular disorders	Includes Friedreich ataxia, Noonan syndrome, and lentiginosis
Sensitivity and toxic reactions	Includes reactions to alcohol, catecholamines, anthracyclines, irradiation, and others
Peripartum cardiomyopathy	First becomes manifest in the peripartum period, but it is probably a heterogeneous group

Derived from Richardson P, McKenna W, Bristow M, et al: Report of the 1995 World Health Organization/International Society and Federation of Cardiology Task Force on the Definition and Classification of Cardiomyopathies. Circulation 93:841, 1996. Copyright 1996, American Heart Association.

CH 64

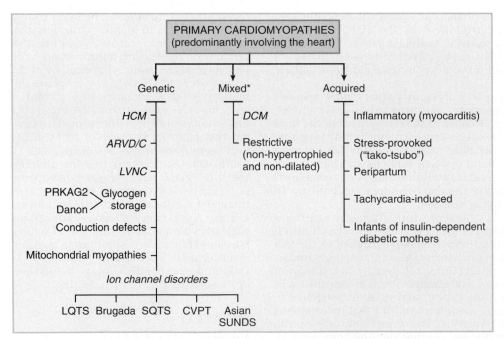

FIGURE 64–1 Primary and specific cardiomyopathies that primarily manifest with cardiac involvement. HCM = hypertrophic cardiomyopathy; DCM = dilated cardiomyopathy; ARVD/C = arrhythmogenic right ventricular dysplasia/cardiomyopathy; LVNC = left-ventricular noncompaction; PRKAG2 = gene encoding the γ-2-regulatory subunit of the AMP-activated protein kinase; LQTS = long-QT syndrome; SQTS = short-QT syndrome; CVPT = catecholaminergic polymorphic ventricular tachycardia; SUNDS = sudden unexplained nocturnal death syndrome. (*From Maron BJ, et al: Circulation 2006;113:1807-1816, copyright 2006, The American Heart Association.*)

and 64-3). It is not uncommon for chamber enlargement to precede signs and symptoms of congestive heart failure. Recent classification revision attempts recognize that chamber dilation is part of the spectrum of genetic and environmental disorders affecting the heart; thus a patient presenting with DCM may have a broad array of cardiac or systemic conditions (see Table 64-2). Nevertheless, DCM is an important and frequent clinical presentation. In 50 percent or more of patients with a DCM, an etiological basis will not be identified, in which case the patient is referred to as having an *idiopathic* DCM.[1,9]

NATURAL HISTORY. The natural history of DCM remains incompletely understood. This is because this diagnosis clearly contains a variety of etiologies and patients have highly variable presentations. Patient presentations can range from asymptomatic left ventricular dysfunction to mild, moderate, or severe congestive heart failure. Different

TABLE 64–2	The Etiologic Basis of Primary and Secondary Cardiomyopathy in a Large Referral Population.*	
Diagnosis		**Number (%)**
Idiopathic cardiomyopathy		616 (50)
Myocarditis		111 (9)
Ischemic heart disease		91 (7)
Cardiomyopathy due to infiltrative myocardial disease		59 (5)
Amyloidosis		36
Sarcoidosis		14
Hemochromatosis		9
Peripartum cardiomyopathy		51 (4)
Cardiomyopathy due to hypertension		49 (4)
Cardiomyopathy due to infection with the human immunodeficiency virus		45 (4)
Cardiomyopathy due to connective-tissue disease		39 (3)
Scleroderma		12
Systemic lupus erythematosus		9
Marfan syndrome		3
Polyarteritis nodosum		3
Dermatomyositis or polymyositis		3
Nonspecific connective-tissue disease		3
Ankylosing spondylitis		2
Rheumatoid arthritis		1
Relapsing polychondritis		1
Wegener granulomatosis		1
Mixed connective-tissue disease		1
Cardiomyopathy due to substance abuse		37 (3)
Chronic alcohol abuse		28
Cocaine abuse		9
Cardiomyopathy due to doxorubicin therapy		15 (1)
Cardiomyopathy due to other causes		117 (10)
Restrictive cardiomyopathy		28
Familial cardiomyopathy		25
Valvular heart disease		19
Endocrine dysfunction		
Thyroid disease		7
Carcinoid		2
Pheochromocytoma		1
Acromegaly		1
Neuromuscular disease		4
Neoplastic heart disease		6
Congenital heart disease		4
Complication of coronary-artery bypass surgery		4
Radiation		3
Critical illness		3
Endomyocardial fibroelastosis		1
Thrombotic thrombocytopenic purpura		1
Rheumatic carditis		1
Drug therapy (not including doxorubicin)		
Leukotrienes		2
Lithium		1
Prednisone		1
Total		1230 (100)

*Final Diagnoses in 1230 Patients with Initially Unexplained Cardiomyopathy.
From Felker GM, Thompson RE, Hare JM, et al: Underlying causes and long-term survival in patients with initially unexplained cardiomyopathy. N Engl J Med 342:1077, 2000. Copyright 2000, Massachusetts Medical Society.

studies report wide-ranging estimates of annual mortality that are between 10 and 50 percent.[11] Traditionally, it is held that symptomatic heart failure is invariably progressive. However, several factors suggest that this concept should be reexamined. First, there has been an impact of therapy on the natural history of patients. Whereas the one-year mortality in the placebo arm was approximately 50 percent in the Cooperative North Scandinavian Enalapril Survival Study (CONSENSUS) conducted in the 1980s, similar patients experienced ~20 percent annual mortality in the Carvedilol Prospective Randomized Cumulative Survival (COPERNICUS) conducted in the 1990s (see Chap. 25). There is also growing awareness that treatment with pharmacological therapies that antagonize the neurohormonal system can lead to myocardial recovery or "reverse left ventricular remodeling" in some patients with DCM (see Chap. 22). Finally, it is reported that between 25 and 33 percent of patients presenting with new-onset DCM experience meaningful cardiac recovery.[12]

PROGNOSIS. The prognosis of DCM may be much more variable than previously appreciated.[11] Several features of the clinical presentation may be valuable in predicting patient outcome (Table 64-4). In addition, the underlying etiology of the cardiomyopathy clearly has a substantial impact on the natural history, thus warranting an exhaustive search for causes (Fig. 64-4). Some cardiomyopathies have excellent long-term survival, whereas others, particularly amyloidosis and human immunodeficiency virus (HIV)-related disease, carry grave prognoses.[9]

In terms of idiopathic DCM, the natural history may not be inextricably progressive, and patients may experience variable courses. In some cases, patients may enter into periods of stability during which symptoms completely stabilize; such periods can last years or even decades. Associated but not clearly linked with periods of stability is reverse remodeling, a phenomenon appreciated only in the last decade (see Chap.22). Reverse remodeling may be spontaneous or in response to pharmacological or device therapy. Alternatively, it is clear that some patients may experience sudden deterioration after a period of stability or never experience a quiescent time.[13] It is also critical to appreciate that certain patients may have severe and life-threatening hemodynamic embarrassment at initial presentation. For these patients a diagnostic evaluation including an endomyocardial biopsy should be rapidly performed; these patients are critically ill and frequently require inotropic or mechanical support as a life-saving therapy.

The determinants of the natural history are not entirely clear but several studies suggest that biomarkers or panels of laboratory values may have prognostic value.[11] As discussed subsequently, there is growing appreciation for the genetic component of DCM, and it is likely that inherited predisposition plays a major role in the natural history of this disorder.

Pathology

MACROSCOPIC EXAMINATION. Gross inspection of the heart demonstrates four chamber enlargement (see Fig. 64-3). Most often the ventricular walls are increased in thickness consistent with the myocyte hypertrophy that accompanies this disorder. Increasing chamber thickness is attributed to a compensatory mechanism aimed at reducing wall stress and is thus thought to play a beneficial role, averting further chamber remodeling.[3] The valvular structures themselves are normal, although chamber enlargement frequently leads to a dilation of the valvular orifice. Intracavitary thrombi are often noted and are preferentially located in the ventricular apices. The coronary circulation is most commonly normal, although the presence of nonocclusive epicardial disease can raise a diagnostic conundrum wherein the degree of cardiomyopathy is "out of proportion to the underlying coronary artery disease." A definition for ischemic cardiomyopathy has been arbitrarily set at a requirement for a greater than 70 percent stenosis in a major epicardial coronary artery, although pathological studies have reported greater degrees of disease.[4] Preferential involvement of the right ventricle should suggest the

CH 64

The Dilated, Restrictive, and Infiltrative Cardiomyopathies

TABLE 64–3	Functional Classification of the Cardiomyopathies		
Dilated		**Restrictive**	**Hypertrophic**
Symptoms			
Congestive heart failure, particularly left sided		Dyspnea, fatigue	Dyspnea, angina pectoris
Fatigue and weakness		Right-sided congestive heart failure	Fatigue, syncope, palpitations
Systemic or pulmonary emboli		Signs and symptoms of systemic disease, e.g., amyloidosis, iron storage disease	
Physical Examination			
Moderate to severe cardiomegaly; S_3, S_4		Mild to moderate cardiomegaly; S_3 or S_4	Mild cardiomegaly
Atrioventricular valve regurgitation, especially mitral		Atrioventricular valve regurgitation; inspiratory increase in venous pressure (Kussmaul sign)	Apical systolic thrill and heave; brisk carotid upstroke
			S_4 common
			Systolic murmur that increases with Valsalva maneuver
Chest Roentgenogram			
Moderate to marked cardiac enlargement, especially left ventricular		Mild cardiac enlargement	Mild to moderate cardiac enlargement
Pulmonary venous hypertension		Pulmonary venous hypertension	Left atrial enlargement
Electrocardiogram			
Sinus tachycardia		Low voltage	Left ventricular hypertrophy
Atrial and ventricular arrhythmias		Intraventricular conduction defects	ST segment and T wave abnormalities
ST segment and T wave abnormalities		Atrioventricular conduction defects	Abnormal Q waves
Intraventricular conduction defects			Atrial and ventricular arrhythmias
Echocardiogram			
Left ventricular dilation and dysfunction		Increased left ventricular wall thickness and mass	Asymmetrical septal hypertrophy (ASH)
Abnormal diastolic mitral valve motion secondary to abnormal compliance and filling pressures		Small or normal-sized left ventricular cavity	Narrow left ventricular outflow tract
		Normal systolic function	Systolic anterior motion (SAM) of the mitral valve
		Pericardial effusion	Small or normal-sized left ventricle
Radionuclide Studies			
Left ventricular dilation and dysfunction (RVG)		Infiltration of myocardium (^{201}Tl)	Small- or normal-sized left ventricle (RVG)
		Small- or normal-sized left ventricle (RVG)	Vigorous systolic function (RVG)
		Normal systolic function (RVG)	Asymmetrical septal hypertrophy (RVG or ^{201}Tl)
Cardiac Catheterization			
Left ventricular enlargement and dysfunction		Diminished left ventricular compliance	Diminished left ventricular compliance
Mitral and/or tricuspid regurgitation		"Square root sign" in ventricular pressure recordings	Mitral regurgitation
Elevated left- and often right-sided filling pressures		Preserved systolic function	Vigorous systolic function
Diminished cardiac output		Elevated left- and right-sided filling pressures	Dynamic left ventricular outflow gradient

RVG = radionuclide ventriculogram; ^{201}Tl = thallium-201.

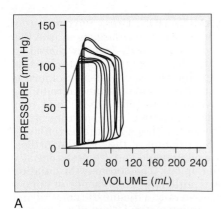
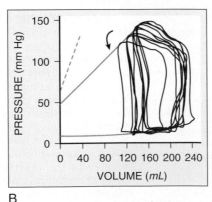

A B

FIGURE 64–2 The dilated cardiomyopathy phenotype. Pressure volume loops depict the features of dilated cardiomyopathy. The slope of the end-systolic pressure volume relation (ESPVR, arrow) is an excellent load-independent index of myocardial contractility. Compared with the normal heart (left, **A**), the dilated cardiomyopathy heart is enlarged, and has depressed contractility and diastolic dysfunction. Dashed line in **B** represents normal ESPVR. LV = left ventricular. *(From Hare JM: Etiologic Basis of Congestive Heart Failure. In Colucci WS [ed]: Atlas of Heart Failure. 4th ed. Copyright 2005, Current Medicine LLC.)*

diagnoses of arrhythmogenic right ventricular dysplasia/cardiomyopathy (ARVD/C) or cor pulmonale (secondary to pulmonary hypertension)

HISTOLOGICAL EXAMINATION. Histological evaluation of the myocardium reveals varying degrees of myocyte hypertrophy and interstitial fibrosis (see Fig. 64-3).[4] Fibrosis most often affects the left ventricular subendocardium or throughout the myocardium in interstitial or perivascular patterns. A finding of replacement fibrosis, an island of fibrotic tissue, often signifies a small area of tissue necrosis and suggests an ischemic etiology. It has been difficult to identify characteristic immunological or infectious findings; however, progress is being made in this regard, particularly with regard to viral persistence within the heart (see later). Scattered cells considered to be lymphocytes are a frequent observation and may lead to a diagnosis of borderline myocarditis. This does not appear to affect prognosis.[14]

Etiology

DCM accounts for approximately 25 percent of the cases of congestive heart failure in the United States.[15] The majority of the additional cases are due to specific cardiomyopathies, most notably ischemic or hypertensive cardiomyopathies,[16] or nonsystolic heart failure.[17] The DCM phenotype can manifest from specific systemic diseases or primary acquired processes, and intensive diagnostic evaluations in referral centers can reveal a specific associated cause of cardiomyopathy in ~50 percent of patients; the remaining 50 percent are assigned the diagnosis of exclusion, idiopathic DCM.[9,10] It is increasingly being appreciated that many of the so-called cases of idiopathic DCM result from underlying genetic abnormalities or previous environmental insults that are difficult to detect at the time of clinical presentation.[8] With the advent of sophisticated molecular and imaging technologies in clinical medicine, it is likely that in the future an increasing number of the idiopathic cases will have a specific diagnosis assigned.

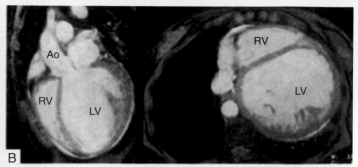

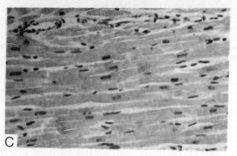
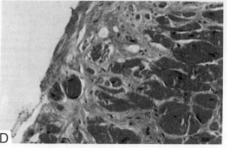

FIGURE 64–3 Dilated cardiomyopathy. Gross and microscopic appearance. Affected hearts exhibit four-chamber enlargement as shown by gross cardiac specimen **(A)** and with cardiac magnetic resonance imaging **(B)**. Cardiac myocytes are hypertrophied **(D)** with variable size and enlarged nuclei compared with normally aligned myocytes **(C)**. In addition there is significant interstitial deposition of fibrotic tissue **(D)**. Ao = aorta; LV = left ventricle; RV = right ventricle. *(From Hare JM: Etiologic Basis of Congestive Heart Failure. In Colucci WS [ed]: Atlas of Heart Failure. 4th ed. Copyright 2005, Current Medicine LLC.)*

Specific Cardiomyopathies with a Dilated Phenotype

Clinically there are a host of important causes of secondary DCM that include alcohol and cocaine abuse (see Chap. 68), HIV infection (see Chap. 67), metabolic abnormalities, as well as the cardiotoxicity of anticancer drugs—most notably doxorubicin and newly introduced drugs that inhibit tyrosine kinases (e.g., herceptin and imitinab) (see Chap.85) (see Table 64-1). The following four specific disorders are particularly important to recognize in that correct diagnosis has a major impact on patient management and chance for recovery.

STRESS ("TAKO-TSUBO" OR "BROKEN HEART SYNDROME").[18] An acute cardiomyopathy can be provoked by a stressful or emotional situation (see Chap. 25). This cardiomyopathy is most common among middle-aged women, appears to be related to catecholamine release, and in most cases is fully reversible with supportive care (Fig. 64-5). Electrocardiogram (ECG) findings of myocardial infarction in the presence of left ventricular dysfunction and absence of epicardial coronary stenoses should prompt the diagnosis. Endomyocardial biopsy is of value to exclude myocarditis, which can also mimic acute myocardial infarction, and demonstrates contraction band necrosis.

PERIPARTUM CARDIOMYOPATHY. Peripartum cardiomyopathy[19-21] is defined as a cardiomyopathy manifesting between the last month of pregnancy and 6 months postpartum. The etiology is unclear, but inflammatory factors are highly implicated and some studies reveal a high incidence of lymphocytic inflammation. Peripartum cardiomyopathy is common in Africa but also manifests in the developed world; it has an excellent long-term natural history if patients survive the initial period (see Fig. 64-4),

TABLE 64–4	Factors Associated with an Adverse Outcome in Dilated Cardiomyopathy		
Clinical	**Noninvasive**	**Invasive**
NYHA Class III/IV	Low LV ejection fraction	High LV filling pressures
Increasing age	Marked LV dilation	
Low exercise peak oxygen consumption	Low LV mass	
Marked intraventricular conduction delay	Moderate mitral regurgitation	
Complex ventricular arrhythmias	Abnormal diastolic function	
Abnormal signal-averaged ECG	Abnormal contractile reserve	
Evidence of excessive sympathetic stimulation	Right ventricular dilation or dysfunction	
Protodiastolic gallop (S_3)		
Elevated serum BNP		
Elevated uric acid		
Decreased serum sodium		

BNP = brain natriuretic peptide, ECG = electrocardiogram; LV = left ventricular; NYHA = New York Heart Association.

during which time hemodynamic compromise may be severe.[19] It is important to differentiate peripartum cardiomyopathy from a chronic cardiomyopathy exacerbated by the volume load occurring during pregnancy.[20] Women who recover are at increased risk of recurrences with subsequent pregnancies—women with full recovery are more likely to tolerate a subsequent pregnancy than are those with residual left ventricular dysfunction.[21]

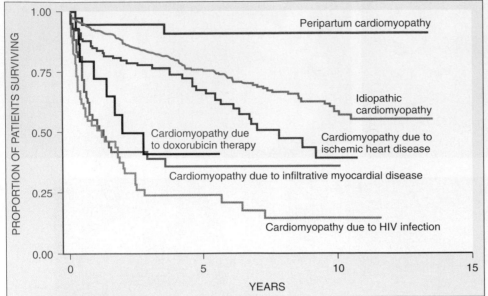

CH 64

FIGURE 64–4 Variable survival in patients with dilated cardiomyopathy depending on underlying etiological basis. HIV = human immunodeficiency virus. *(From Felker GM, et al: N Engl J Med 342:1077-1084, 2000. Copyright 2000, Massachusetts Medical Society.)*

TACHYCARDIA-INDUCED CARDIOMYOPATHY. Patients may develop a DCM with congestive heart failure in the face of recurrent or persistent tachycardias. The most common association is with atrial fibrillation or supraventricular tachycardia (SVT). There is a high rate of full recovery with control of the arrhythmia.[22] This cardiomyopathy is notable for the degree to which it resembles idiopathic DCM phenotypically, yet is characterized by a remarkable degree of recovery in left ventricular function once the arrhythmia is controlled. Patients presenting with an atrial or supraventricular arrhythmia should undergo definitive therapy to control heart rate and to restore normal sinus rhythm. Additionally, patients should be treated with standard neurohormonal blocking agents and carefully monitored with echocardiography in the weeks to months following presentation for signs of recovery.

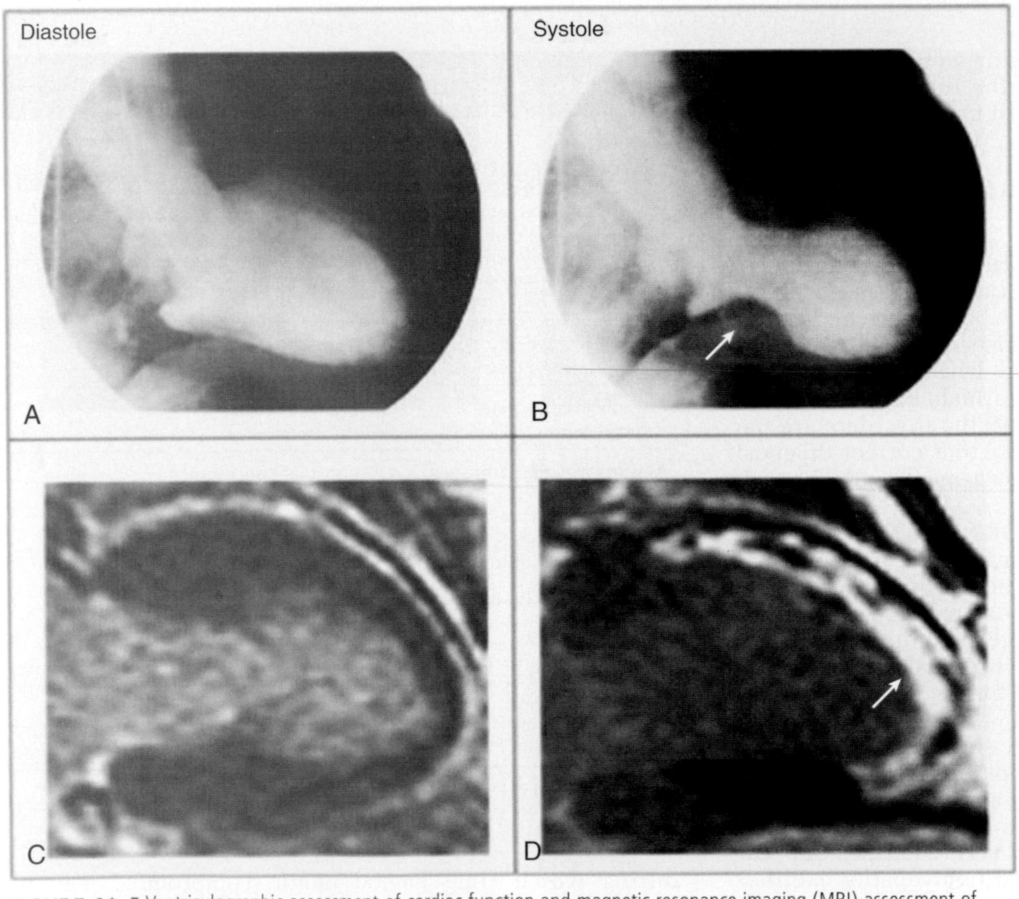

Alcoholic Cardiomyopathy

Alcoholic cardiomyopathy is a common cause of DCM and the most common secondary cardiomyopathy. Phenotypically and clinically, it closely resembles idiopathic DCM (see also Chap. 68). The disorder is linked to ongoing excessive alcohol consumption and appears to be both dose-related and responsive to cessation of alcohol exposure. Alcohol exposure also increases risk for comorbidities that can contribute to cardiovascular disease, such as hypertension, stroke, arrhythmias, and sudden death.

There is strong epidemiological evidence that the effects of alcohol are dose-related in susceptible hosts, and that moderate alcohol consumption has cardioprotective effects (see Chap. 25). The mechanisms for the deleterious effects of alcohol include (1) direct toxicity of alcohol or its metabolites; (2) nutritional deficiency common in alcoholics such as thiamine deficiency, which causes beriberi heart disease (see Chap. 44); and (3) rarely, toxicity of specific additives to the alcoholic beverage (e.g.

FIGURE 64–5 Ventriculographic assessment of cardiac function and magnetic resonance imaging (MRI) assessment of myocardial viability at admission in a patient with stress cardiomyopathy. Contrast-enhanced ventriculography during diastole, in **A,** and systole, in **B,** demonstrate apical and midventricular akinesis, with relative sparing of the base of the heart (arrow). **C,** MRI in the long-axis view reveals that the akinetic regions seen on ventriculography are dark and hypoenhanced, consistent with the presence of viable myocardium. **D,** presented for purposes of comparison, shows hyperenhancement (arrow), indicative of necrosis and decreased viability, after an acute anterior myocardial infarction. *(From Wittstein IS, Thiemann DR, Lima JA, et al: Neurohumoral features of myocardial stunning due to sudden emotional stress. N Engl J Med 352:539, 2005. Copyright 2005, Massachusetts Medical Society.)*

cobalt cardiomyopathy associated with certain beers).[23] Cardiomyopathy caused by beer containing cobalt sulfate was described in the 1960s. Recognition led to removal of the cobalt from beer, and no further cases have been appreciated.

The mechanisms of alcohol-induced left ventricular dysfunction are incompletely understood. Experimental studies show that alcohol and its metabolite acetaldehyde can disrupt cardiac calcium cycling, mitochondrial respiration, myocardial synthesis of proteins and lipid, signal transduction, and myocardial redox state.[24-26] There is also evidence to support a direct toxic effect of alcohol on both cardiac and skeletal myocytes, which may in turn increase the rate of cellular apoptosis.[27] Some, but not all, studies have suggested that electrolyte disturbances may contribute to alcohol toxicity. There are clearly host factors involved in alcohol-related myotoxicity because all alcoholics do not develop cardiomyopathy. Genetic factors play a role as evidenced by studies showing that individuals with the angiotensin-converting enzyme DD genotype have an increased risk of developing alcoholic cardiomyopathy.[28]

PATHOLOGY. Gross and histological evaluation of the heart reveals nonspecific findings that are essentially indistinguishable from those of idiopathic DCM, with interstitial fibrosis, myocyte dropout, variable degrees of myocyte hypertrophy and evidence of small-vessel coronary artery disease. Ultrastructural evaluation with electron microscopy demonstrates enlarged and disorganized mitochondria and glycogen-containing vacuoles.

Clinical Manifestations

The typical presentation of alcoholic cardiomyopathy is in the fourth to sixth decades of life with a male predilection. Affected individuals have a history of extensive consumption of any variety of alcoholic beverage including hard alcohol, beer, or wine, most often for periods exceeding 10 years. Affected females appear to have a lower cumulative dose exposure than do males, although experimental results suggest that females may have protective factors.[29] Malnutrition is implicated as a causal factor,[30] but the syndrome is seen in all socioeconomic strata, and a careful alcohol consumption history is warranted in all subjects presenting with cardiomyopathy. Mild reductions in cardiac performance manifest in chronic alcoholics before symptoms appear. In the symptomatic phase, abnormalities in both systolic and diastolic function characterize ventricular function. In terms of hepatic disease, it is unusual for cardiomyopathy and cirrhosis to coexist, although cirrhotic patients often have asymptomatic ventricular dysfunction. The onset of symptoms ranges from progressive exercise limitation to acute fulminant heart failure in the setting of biventricular dilatation and hypokinesis. Not infrequently, the initial finding is paroxysmal atrial fibrillation. Patients present with symptoms that include fatigue, dyspnea, orthopnea, and paroxysmal nocturnal dyspnea. Palpitations accompany SVTs, especially atrial fibrillation, and syncope often results from ventricular (and possibly supraventricular) arrhythmias. Atypical chest pain may be present but typical angina pectoris should prompt an evaluation for coronary artery disease and aortic stenosis.

PHYSICAL EXAMINATION. Findings on physical examination closely resemble those of idiopathic DCM. The pulse pressure may be narrow with elevated diastolic pressure caused by systemic vasoconstriction. Displaced apical impulse, protodiastolic and presystolic gallop sounds are frequently present, and an apical murmur of mitral regurgitation is common. Fluid retention marked by elevated jugular venous pressure and peripheral edema are typical. A finding more common in alcoholic cardiomyopathy is associated skeletal muscle myopathy, often affecting the shoulder and pelvic girdle; the extent of skeletal muscle abnormalities is proportionate to those of the heart.

LABORATORY EXAMINATION. Cardiomegaly is frequently detected on chest roentgenogram along with pulmonary congestion, pulmonary venous hypertension, and pleural effusions. ECG abnormalities are often present and may precede the development of symptoms. A frequent presentation is that of the "holiday heart syndrome" characterized by palpitations, chest discomfort, or syncope after binge drinking episodes. These episodes are caused by atrial fibrillation, atrial flutter, or frequent premature ventricular contractions. Alcohol may precipitate these arrhythmias in nonalcoholics as well, possibly linked to hypokalemia. SVTs occur frequently in individuals with overt alcoholic cardiomyopathy, and sudden cardiac death caused by ventricular fibrillation is also not uncommon. Additional ECG abnormalities include atrioventricular conduction delay, most often first-degree heart block, bundle branch block, left ventricular hypertrophy, poor precordial R wave progression, and repolarization abnormalities. QT interval prolongation is common. Alcohol cessation may, within a period of days, lead to resolution of ST segment and T wave abnormalities. Hemodynamic, echocardiographic, and nuclear imaging findings are essentially indistinguishable from those observed in the DCM patient.

MANAGEMENT. The cornerstone of successfully treating the patient with alcoholic cardiomyopathy is cessation of alcohol consumption, which can have significant benefits in improving symptoms of heart failure. Ongoing alcohol consumption clearly worsens prognosis. In addition, a regimen of neurohormonal blockers should be prescribed. It is also reasonable, particularly in the setting of decompensated heart failure, to administer thiamine in the event that malnutrition may play a role in the presentation. Anticoagulation should only be considered in the presence of a clear-cut and pressing indication because of the increased risk of trauma, catastrophic bleeding, and supratherapeutic anticoagulation caused by hepatic dysfunction.

Etiological Basis for Idiopathic Dilated Cardiomyopathy

Rapidly advancing knowledge in four areas is shedding light on pathophysiological mechanisms that may contribute to DCM and may, in turn, lead to new therapeutic approaches. These areas include (1) familial and genetic factors,[31] (2) inflammatory and infectious factors—particularly viral infection,[32] (3) cytotoxicity, and (4) cell loss and abnormalities in endogenous repair mechanisms.[33]

GENETIC AND FAMILIAL FACTORS

Studies of the genetics of DCM offer major insights into the etiology of the disease. Two general lines of evidence initially suggested a genetic component to DCM. Familial studies indicated that in excess of 20 percent of patients with DCM had other family members with the condition, and conversely certain inherited conditions, particularly muscular dystrophies, had cardiomyopathy as a component.[31,34] There are now abundant gene linkage studies with multiple genes identified; autosomal dominant and recessive, as well as X-linked modes of inheritance, exist (see Chap. 8).[7,31]

Most of the genes encode for structural elements of the cell, notably members of the dystrophin-associated glycoprotein complex, or components of the sarcomeric contractile machinery (Table 64-5). A particularly interesting and novel mutation is described in the gene encoding phospholamban.[35] This mutation implicates abnormalities in the excitation-contraction cascade as a cause of cardiomyopathy and supports attempts to treat cardiomyopathy with other elements of the calcium cycling machinery (i.e., deliv-

TABLE 64–5 | **List of Molecular Defects in Familial Dilated Cardiomyopathy (FDC)**

Gene	Protein	Function
Autosomal Dominant FDC Phenotype		
ACTC	Cardiac action	sarcomeric protein; muscle contraction
DES	Desmin	dystrophin-associated glycoprotein complex; transduces contractile forces
SGCD	δ-Sarcoglycan	dystrophin-associated glycoprotein complex; transduces contractile forces
MYH7	β-Myosin heavy chain	sarcomeric protein; muscle contraction
TNNT2	Cardiac troponin T	sarcomeric protein; muscle contraction
TPM1	α-Tropomyosin	sarcomeric protein; muscle contraction
TTN	Titin	sarcomere structure/extensible scaffold for other proteins
VCL	Metavinculin	sarcomere structure; intercalated discs
MYBPC	Myosin-binding protein C	sarcomeric protein; muscle contraction
MLP/CSRP3	Muscle LIM protein	sacromere stretch; sensor/Z discs
ACTN2	α-Actinin-2	sarcomere structure; anchor for myofibrillar actin
PLN	Phospholamban	sarcoplasmic reticulum Ca^{2+} regulator; inhibits SERCA2 pump
ZASP/LBD3	Cypher/LIM binding domain 3	cytoskeletal assembley; involved in targeting and clustering of membrane proteins
MYH6	α-Myosin heavy chain	sarcomeric protein; muscle contraction
ABCC	SUR2A	regulatory subunit of Kir6.2, an inwardly rectifying cardiac K_{ATP} channel
LMNA	Lamin A/C	inner leaflet, nuclear membrane protein; confers stability to nuclear membrane; gene expression
X-linked FDC		
DMD	Dystrophin	primary component of dystrophin-associated glycoprotein complex; transduces contractile force
TAZ/G4.5	Tafazzin	unknown
Recessive FDC		
TNN13	cardiac troponin I	sarcomeric protein, muscle contraction

Derived from Burkett EL, Hershberger RE: Clinical and genetic issues in familial dilated cardiomyopathy. J Am Coll Cardiol 45:969, 2005. Copyright 2005, American College of Cardiology.

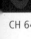

CH 64

ery of the gene encoding for the sarcoplasmic reticulum calcium pump [SERCA]).[36]

The fact that genetic abnormalities play a role offers insights into the phenotype in general. Clearly, genetic predisposition may be a central factor in the development of primary and secondary DCMs. Genetic defects may be primary causes of DCM, or they may act as predisposing factors in the setting of an environmental stressor–host-environment interaction. Primary examples of the latter are viral infections and hypertension, wherein exposure may lead to DCM only in subpopulations of exposed individuals. Genetic predisposition may be of fundamental importance in the variable natural history of DCM and may contribute to responsiveness to therapy.[37]

INFLAMMATORY AND INFECTIOUS MYOCARDITIS.

The diagnosis and management of infectious myocarditis is discussed in Chapter 66 and is reviewed here only briefly. Myocarditis may result from viral (or other pathogen) infection, autoimmune disease, or a combination (autoimmune reaction stimulated by a viral infection).[38] It is also increasingly possible that genetic factors increase the risk of developing cardiac disease following viral infection.

It has long been postulated that viral infection in susceptible hosts may be a proximate cause of cardiomyopathy and may serve as a precursor to the development of DCM. This hypothesis has been difficult to prove because of challenges in confirming viral infection in affected individuals coupled with the fact that common viruses are implicated in viral cardiomyopathy leading to concerns of a high false-positive rate when viruses are detected in patients with heart failure. Lymphocytic myocarditis with or without myocyte necrosis has been considered the hallmark diagnostic finding necessary for a diagnosis, and criteria established for the histological evaluation are termed the *Dallas criteria*.[38] The link between myocarditis and viral heart disease is problematic because true inflammatory myocarditis can occur in the absence of an infectious agent (see later). As discussed in Chapter 66 the application of the polymerase chain reaction (PCR) to detect viral particles in myocardial samples taken from patients with DCM has provided important insights into the role played by viruses in heart muscle disease.

Two general mechanisms for postviral cardiac injury have been invoked: autoimmune reactions or direct tissue injury resulting from viral infection of the heart (see Chap. 66). Both of these mechanisms are incompletely proved and remain controversial. The presence or absence of inflammation on endomyocardial biopsy, which varies greatly from study to study, is used to substantiate immunological injury. However, other studies have suggested different criteria (e.g., complement or immunoglobulins). The postviral hypothesis has increasing support, and viral material has been detected on the basis of elevated viral titers, presence of viral genomic material using PCR, and detection of viral particles.

AUTOIMMUNITY

Studies support abnormalities of humoral and cellular immunity in DCM. Two general theories are proposed for an autoimmune cause of DCM (1) viral components incorporate into the cardiac myocyte membrane, stimulating an antigenic response, or (2) anti-heart antibodies are generated as a result of myocardial damage as opposed to being the proximate cause. Certain specific human leukocyte antigen (HLA) class II antigens (particularly DR4) are associated with DCM. Additionally, numerous circulating antimyocardial antibodies have been measured in DCM patients that react with a variety of antigens, including the myosin heavy chain, the beta adrenoceptor, the muscarinic receptor, sarcolemmal sodium-potassium adenosine triphosphatase, laminin, and mitochondrial proteins. Whether anti-inflammatory therapies have efficacy in treating DCM has been difficult to prove; corticosteroid trials have been neutral, but there are ongoing attempts to test the value of immunoabsorption strategies.

CYTOTOXICITY AND DERANGED INTRACELLULAR SIGNALING

The direct action of various circulating factors is implicated in the pathophysiology of myocyte dysfunction. For example, tumor necrosis factor and endothelin levels are elevated in

DCM. The exact role of these factors remains incompletely understood and therapies to antagonize their effects have not been definitively established.

An additional molecular mechanism gaining increased experimental and clinical support is that of nitroso-redox imbalance—an intracellular phenomenon characterized by dysregulation of nitric oxide production coupled with increased production of reactive oxygen species.[39] This imbalance is described in experimental animal models and in humans with DCM and causes cellular dysfunction and possibly cytotoxicity.[40] Although not definitively proved, one mechanism postulated to explain the response of DCM patients to hydralazine-isosorbide dinitrate is a restoration of nitroso-redox balance (see Chap.25).

INJURY, CELL LOSS, AND ENDOGENOUS REPAIR

A variety of other causes related to damage to cellular constituents of the heart are proposed as etiological factors. Although none are accepted as the absolute cause, the variety of mechanisms highlights the notion of a final common pathway, with various insults converging on a set of mechanisms that all result in a common phenotypic response to injury. Many of the mechanisms such as endocrine disturbances or toxic exposures derive from the existence of specific examples of secondary cardiomyopathies. The appearance of DCM in only a small fraction of subjects with a common disorder is supportive of the idea that specific host (gene)-environment interactions lead to the cardiac manifestations of the exposure.

Ischemia due to hyperreactivity or spasm of the microvasculature may contribute to diffuse myocyte necrosis and replacement fibrosis. The classic disorder in which this is manifest is scleroderma heart disease. Increased myocyte apoptosis is described in DCM and ARVD/C, leading to the suggestion that augmented cell loss may contribute to the development of left ventricular remodeling in DCM processes. Although there are an increasing number of experimental studies supporting cardiac recovery when antiapoptotic agents are administered in animal models,[41] the exact role of apoptosis in these conditions is not known. Further, the role of cell loss in DCM has become more interesting in light of recent accumulating data supporting the idea that endogenous cardiac stem cells repopulate cardiac myocytes throughout life, thereby serving a homeostatic balancing mechanism for ongoing cell loss and cell replacement following tissue injury (see Chap. 29). Indeed, studies already support the idea of cardiac stem cell senescence contributing to the development of human cardiomyopathy.[33] Thus, depletion or dysfunction of endogenous cells with capacity to divide and differentiate in cardiac cellular constituents may be a central pathophysiological contributor to cardiomyopathic processes.[33]

Clinical Evaluation of the Dilated Cardiomyopathies

HISTORY

DCM affects individuals of all ages, including neonates and children.[42,43] In adults, the incidence of DCM is estimated to be between 5 and 8 per 100,000 persons per year. DCM is most frequent in middle age and affects men to a greater degree than women. Although, the incidence of ischemic cardiomyopathy is higher than DCM, these two diagnoses account for an equal number of heart transplantations performed.

The clinical presentation of patients with heart failure is discussed in Chapter 23. In the case of DCM the clinical presentation of patients can vary substantially. In some patients, symptoms develop very gradually and diagnosis can result from the detection of cardiomegaly on routine chest roentgenogram. Patients presenting with clear-cut symptoms of congestive heart failure report the development of progressive symptoms for periods varying from weeks to months. Intercurrent illnesses frequently precipitate congestive heart failure in individuals with DCM. A significant minority of patients with DCM present with aggressive, life-threatening congestive heart failure (fulminant heart failure) that can require the most intensive forms of mechanical intervention.[14] The causes of the fulminant presentation vary from idiopathic cardiomyopathy to fulminant lymphocytic myocarditis to giant cell myocarditis (see Chap. 66).[14,44] The determinants of these various forms of clinical presentation are poorly understood.

EVALUATION FOR SECONDARY CARDIOMYOPATHIES. An initial history must focus on identifying etiological factors (see Tables 64-1 and 64-2). A past or associated history of rheumatological, endocrine, or infectious diseases or of previous neoplasia should be sought. In patients with a history of cancer, treatment with anthracyclines, tyrosine kinase inhibitors, or irradiation are particularly relevant. The family history can often reveal heritable forms of cardiomyopathy. Patients should be questioned regarding the consumption of alcohol, tobacco, and illicit drugs. Travel history can reveal exposure to geographically related infectious pathogens.

The most typical symptoms are those of congestive heart failure and include dyspnea, fatigue and volume gain. A minority of patients report chest pain, which can signify epicardial coronary disease, subendocardial disease, or pulmonary embolism. A report of abdominal discomfort or anorexia is frequent in late stages of the disease and suggests hepatomegaly or bowel edema, respectively.

Common late complications include thromboembolic events, which may be systemic, originating from dislodgment of left atrial and ventricular intracardiac or pulmonary thrombi from the lower extremity venous system.

Physical Examination

The physical examination for patients with heart failure is discussed in Chapters 11 and 23. Particular attention should be paid in the physical examination toward excluding findings of valvular heart disease. S_3 and S_4 gallops are invariably present in DCM. The S_3 must be differentiated from a pericardial knock or an opening snap of mitral stenosis, both of which are higher pitched sounds than the S_3. Patients with fulminant heart failure of new onset will frequently be tachycardic and will develop a gallop rhythm in which S_3 and S_4 fuse. Attention should be paid to differentiating right-sided gallops and murmurs so as to consider the possibility of right-sided involvement.

NONINVASIVE EVALUATION

The diagnostic evaluation of patients with heart failure is discussed in Chapter 23. For patients presenting with DCM, the initial evaluation should focus on identifying reversible and secondary causes. Even though the presentation of the patient with a dilated ventricle and heart failure may be fairly uniform, a wide array of specific and secondary cardiomyopathies may cause a clinical presentation of a DCM. The first step in the diagnostic evaluation involves screening biochemical testing, including serum electrolytes, phosphorus, calcium, and markers of renal function (serum creatinine and urea).[9] Endocrine function should be screened, notably thyroid function (hyper- and hypothyroidism) and possibly urinary evaluation of catecholamine levels to exclude pheochromocytoma. To screen for rheumatological conditions, an antinuclear antibody (ANA) and erythrocyte sedimentation rate (ESR) should be obtained. When suspected, rarer causes of cardiomyopathy can be excluded with blood testing. For example, lyme titers can be a useful screen for lyme carditis. Iron studies may assist in evaluating hemochromatosis and HIV testing is valuable.

The use of biomarkers, such as troponin, to assess myocardial necrosis, and the use of circulating brain natriuretic peptide (BNP or pro-BNP) levels may serve as useful adjunctive strategies to help determine patient diagnosis and/or prognosis (see Chap. 23). Further, there is increasing support for the use of serum uric acid levels as a prognostic marker.[11] A chest roentgenogram offers supporting evidence for the diagnosis and in some cases is the initial mode of detection. Cardiomegaly may be appreciated, as may evidence of pulmonary vascular redistribution. Rarely interstitial and alveolar edema are present on initial presentation. With advancing heart failure, pleural effusions are present and dilated azygos veins and superior vena cava indicate right-sided volume overload.

ELECTROCARDIOGRAPHY. There are no specific electrocardiographic findings signifying DCM. Sinus tachycardia is often present in proportion to the degree of heart failure. Typical changes in the QRS complex include poor R wave progression, intraventricular conduction delays, and left bundle branch block. A wide QRS complex portends a worse prognosis and has now emerged as a clinical indicator of responsiveness to cardiac resynchronization therapy (see Chaps. 25 and 34). Patients with substantial left ventricular fibrosis may exhibit anterior Q waves even in the absence of a discrete scar or epicardial coronary artery obstructions. A broad array of abnormalities may manifest, such as nonspecific ST segment and T wave abnormalities as well as P wave alterations, notably left atrial abnormality. Nonsustained ventricular tachycardia is extremely common on 24-hour ambulatory monitoring, and represents a predictor of all-cause mortality. Persistent supraventricular or ventricular tachyarrhythmias represent an important etiological factor for ventricular dysfunction,[22] and restoration of sinus rhythm or heart rate control may lead to recovery of ventricular function. Control of atrial fibrillation is also important because of atrial transport issues contributing to cardiac output. Additionally atrial fibrillation should prompt consideration of tachycardia-induced cardiomyopathy.

ECHOCARDIOGRAPHY. Echocardiography is a cornerstone in the evaluation and management of patients with DCM (see also Chap. 23). Two-dimensional echocardiography is a highly useful and readily available technique to assess ventricular size and performance and to exclude associated valvular or pericardial abnormalities. Doppler echocardiography permits the evaluation of valvular regurgitation or stenosis and the quantification of cardiac output. Doppler detection of restrictive filling patterns may indicate disease of greater severity. Pericardial effusion may be present. Performing echocardiography during dobutamine stimulation may identify occult coronary artery disease by provoking regional wall motion abnormalities differentiating these patients from those with idiopathic DCM. Moreover, significant contractile reserve during dobutamine infusion represents a positive prognostic finding.

RADIONUCLIDE IMAGING. Nuclear imaging protocols for *myocardial perfusion stress imaging* may be useful to exclude an ischemic cause of dilated heart failure. *Radionuclide ventriculography* also provides evidence of cardiac structure and function, showing increased chamber volumes at end-diastole and end-systole; provides quantification of reduced ejection fraction in either of both ventricles; and can elucidate the regional nature of wall motion abnormalities (see Chap.16); not always necessary, this technique can be of particular value if echocardiography is technically suboptimal.

CARDIAC MAGNETIC RESONANCE IMAGING (MRI) AND MULTIDETECTOR COMPUTED TOMOGRAPHY. Cardiac MRI and multidetector computed tomography are relatively new imaging modalities that are likely to become increasingly useful to evaluate patients with cardiomyopathies (see Chap. 17).[45,46] Specific cardiomyopathic disorders in which MRI has proved particularly valuable include ARVD/C,[47] endocardial fibroelastosis, myocarditis,[48] amyloidosis,[49] and sarcoidosis. MRI evaluation is also emerging as a critical tool to understand DCM pathophysiology and may contribute to identifying patients at particular risk for complications such as sudden cardiac death (e.g., within DCM subsets—those with or without areas of replacement fibrosis that may predispose to electrical instability and sudden cardiac death.)[50] Cardiac MRI is also emerging as an important tool in the delineation of infiltrative and inflammatory cardiomyopathies.

INVASIVE EVALUATION INCLUDING ENDOMYOCARDIAL BIOPSY. *Catheterization*—the exclusion of epicardial coronary disease is essential in the management of the patient presenting with DCM. Because DCM and heart failure increase the false-positive and false-negative rates of noninvasive nuclear assessment for myocardial ischemia, performance of *coronary angiography* is often necessary to exclude epicardial coronary obstructive disease.[4] It is increasingly relevant to obtain hemodynamic assessments in individuals presenting with acute or worsening heart failure. Use of these diagnostic tests is currently nonuniform.[51] Catheterization usually reveals elevated left ventricular end-diastolic and pulmonary artery wedge pressures. Pulmonary arterial hypertension may be of variable degrees—ranging from mild to severe. The right ventricle is frequently involved and enlarged, hemodynamically manifesting with increased right ventricular end-diastolic, right atrial, and central venous pressures.

Left ventriculography demonstrates varying degrees of ventricular dilation and diffuse chamber hypokinesis. There may be a degree of regionality to the decreased function resembling ischemic heart disease, although a diffuse pattern is frequently present. Filling defects may be present because of left ventricular thrombi, and mild mitral regurgitation is not unusual. It is not always possible to distinguish between left ventricular dilation due to severe mitral regurgitation associated with primary mitral valve disease and DCM with secondary mitral regurgitation.

Coronary arteriography is particularly important to exclude coronary obstructive disease. In patients with DCM, the arterial circulation is typically normal although vasodilator function may be abnormal.

BIOPSY. The role of endomyocardial biopsy to evaluate the myocardium histologically remains highly controversial in the evaluation of the patient presenting with structural heart disease and/or symptoms of heart failure.[10,52,53] This procedure, which is routine in the management of heart transplant recipients, allows the acquisition of small pieces of myocardium using a flexible bioptome. Currently available bioptomes are advanced transvenously, most commonly using a right internal jugular venous approach, to the right ventricular septum. If required, the left ventricular septum may be sampled using a transarterial approach. This procedure is currently performed with either fluoroscopic or echocardiographic guidance. Although not reported in the literature, the widespread use of disposable bioptomes, which have replaced reusable Stanford-Caves devices, has led to a reduction of complications—particularly right ventricle perforation.

Perhaps the most compelling reason in favor of routine biopsy is the detection of a few relatively rare diseases in which accurate diagnosis yields a life-threatening disease with specific management.[14,54] For example, lymphocytic and giant cell myocarditis must be detected early in the course of the presentation for patients to survive and can only be separated from each other by histological evaluation. Biopsy is also an established method for grading the severity of anthracycline cardiomyopathy and has potential similar value for cardiac amyloidosis. A biopsy that is negative for inflammation is also valuable in patients with rapidly progressive severe decompensated heart failure, insofar as it may prompt advancing to aggressive mechanical support earlier in the patient's clinical course. However, the widespread use of the myocardial biopsy is no longer routinely recommended. Ultimately, the determination of whether to perform the procedure remains a balance between exposing a patient to a low-yield procedure in the entire population versus the life-saving potential in a relatively fewer number of patients. In patients with fulminant heart failure, particularly those with new-onset cardiomyopathy, the risk-benefit assessment is more clearly in favor of performing a biopsy to more rationally allocate patients for emergent heart transplantation listing or for insertion of a mechanical assist device. Patients who have fulminant lymphocytic myocarditis have excellent long-term prognosis following short-term hemodynamic support; those with giant cell myocarditis should be aggressively immunosuppressed or listed for heart transplantation; and those with idiopathic cardiomyopathy (suggested by the absence of myocardial inflammation on biopsy) should be aggressively supported and converted to conventional therapy once stabilized. Not infrequently, the endomyocardial biopsy reveals an unsuspected cause of cardiomyopathy.

Management

PHARMACOLOGICAL AND DEVICE THERAPY

Whereas the concept of specific etiology-based therapies represents an ongoing quest for patients with DCM, the general treatment for these patients should follow the practice guidelines for all patients with heart failure (see Guidelines: Management of Heart Failure[55] and Chaps. 25 and 34). Indeed, treatment with neurohormonal antagonists to prevent disease progression and the use of diuretics to maintain the volume balance are the therapeutic cornerstones for the management of patients with DCM.[55] Similarly, the use of prophylactic implantable cardiac defibrillators and biventricular pacemakers are indicated in appropriate patients with nonischemic and ischemic DCM (see Chapter 34).[55]

SURGERY

The surgical management for patients with heart failure is discussed in Chapter 27. Patients with valvular heart disease, coronary artery disease, pericardial disease, or congenital heart defects should have these conditions corrected surgically, when appropriate. Other specific operations geared toward the cardiomyopathic heart include approaches motivated by the concept of restoring chamber geometry or interventions to provide mechanical support. Approaches to achieving reverse remodeling surgically include left ventricular reconstruction or implantation of external restraint devices (see Chap. 27). Left ventricular assist devices provide aggressive mechanical support to patients with advanced decompensated heart failure (see Chap. 28).

EMERGING SPECIFIC THERAPIES. Only recently are specific etiology-based therapies being evaluated. These include agents to eradicate persistent viral infections and immunomodulatory agents (see Chaps. 29 and 66). Stem cells for cardiac regeneration are in clinical trials (see Chap. 29).

RESTRICTIVE AND INFILTRATIVE CARDIOMYOPATHY

Relative to the dilated and hypertrophic cardiomyopathies, restrictive cardiomyopathy occurs with lower frequency in the developed world. Specific forms of restrictive cardiomyopathy, such as endomyocardial disease (Table 64-6) are important causes of morbidity and mortality common in specific geographical locales, especially in underdeveloped countries.[56,57] The pathophysiological feature that defines restrictive cardiomyopathy is the increase in stiffness of the ventricular walls, which causes heart failure because of impaired diastolic filling of the ventricle (see also Chaps. 22 and 26).[16] In early stages of the syndrome, systolic function may be normal, although deterioration in systolic function is usually observed as the disease progresses.[2]

Restrictive cardiomyopathy must be distinguished from constrictive pericarditis, which is also characterized by normal or nearly normal systolic function but abnormal ventricular filling (see Chap. 70).[2] Differentiation of these two conditions represents a classic diagnostic challenge and is one of significant clinical importance because pericardial constriction may be treated successfully with pericardiectomy.

Approximately 50 percent of cases of restrictive cardiomyopathy result from specific clinical disorders, whereas the remainder represent an idiopathic process (Fig. 64-6). The most common specific cause of restrictive cardiomyopathy is infiltration caused by amyloidosis—there are both acquired and genetic causes of amyloid.[2] Although there are other specific pathological presentations associated with restrictive cardiomyopathy, their precise etiology often remains obscure. Like dilated cardiomyopathy, there are inflammatory and genetic factors important in the etiology of restrictive cardiomyopathy. The identification of specific infiltrative processes may have prognostic and therapeutic implications (Fig. 64-7).[9] The abnormal diastolic properties of the ventricle are attributable to myocardial fibrosis, infiltration, or scarring of the endomyocardial surface. Myocyte hypertrophy is common, particularly in idiopathic restrictive cardiomyopathy (see Fig. 64-6).

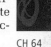

TABLE 64–6	Classification of Types of Restrictive Cardiomyopathy According to Cause

Myocardial
Noninfiltrative
Idiopathic cardiomyopathy*
Familial cardiomyopathy
Hypertrophic cardiomyopathy
Scleroderma
Pseudoxanthoma elasticum
Diabetic cardiomyopathy

Infiltrative
Amyloidosis*
Sarcoidosis*
Gaucher disease
Hurler disease
Fatty infiltration

Storage Disease
Hemochromatosis
Fabry disease
Glycogen storage disease

Endomyocardial
Endomyocardial fibrosis*
Hypereosinophilic syndrome
Carcinoid heart disease
Metastatic cancers
Radiation*
Toxic effects of anthracycline*
Drugs causing fibrous endocarditis (serotonin, methysergide, ergotamine, mercurial agents, busulfan)

*These conditions are more likely than the others to be encountered in clinical practice.

From Kushwaha S, Fallon JT, Fuster V: Restrictive cardiomyopathy. N Engl J Med 336:267, 1997. Copyright 1997, Massachusetts Medical Society.

CARDIAC CATHETERIZATION AND ENDOMYOCARDIAL BIOPSY

A classic diagnostic challenge is to differentiate restrictive cardiomyopathy from constrictive pericarditis, which manifests with similar clinical and hemodynamic features. Cardiac catheterization is a key step in this evaluation (see also Chap. 70). Whereas there is equalization of diastolic pressures in constrictive pericarditis (pressures differ by no more than 5 mm Hg), they may vary to a greater extent in restrictive cardiomyopathy. Pulmonary hypertension is worse in restrictive cardiomyopathy, with systolic pulmonary pressures often exceeding 50 mm Hg. In constrictive pericarditis, the plateau of right ventricular diastolic pressure is usually at least one third of peak systolic pressure; in restrictive cardiomyopathy this is most often lower.

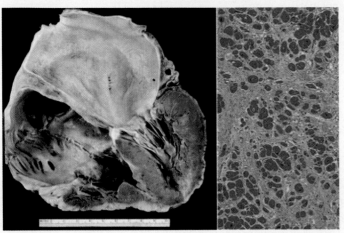

FIGURE 64–6 Pathology of idiopathic restrictive cardiomyopathy in a 63-year-old woman. **Left,** Gross cardiac specimen, shown in four-chamber format, demonstrating prominent biatrial enlargement, with normal-sized ventricles. **Right,** Light microscopy showing marked interstitial fibrosis (light pink areas). Hematoxylin and eosin; magnification ×120. *(From Ammash NM, Seward JB, Bailey KR, et al: Clinical profile and outcome of idiopathic restrictive cardiomyopathy. Circulation 101:2490, 2000. Copyright The American Heart Association.)*

Hemodynamically both conditions have a rapid early diastolic pressure decline followed by a rapid rise and plateau in early diastole, the so-called *square root sign*. The atrial pressure tracing manifests either a classic square root pattern or an M or W waveform when the *x* descent is also rapid. Both *a* and *v* waves are prominent and frequently have the same amplitude. Right- and left-sided atrial filling pressures are elevated, although in the case of restrictive cardiomyopathy the LV filling pressure typically is 5 mm Hg, or more, greater than the right ventricular diastolic pressure. This difference may be accentuated by Valsalva maneuver, exercise, or a fluid challenge.

Endomyocardial biopsy can also be valuable in the evaluation of these patients to exclude an infiltrative process or cardiomyopathic-appearing myocytes. A normal-appearing biopsy supports the diagnosis of a pericardial process. Surgical exploration is needed far less often, given the availability of biopsy and imaging technology (see later).

Prognosis

Restrictive cardiomyopathy carries a variable prognosis dependent on etiology (see Fig. 64-7). Most often, especially in the case of amyloidosis, it is invariably progressive with an accelerated mortality.[58,59] There is no specific therapy for the idiopathic form of restrictive cardiomyopathy, but intensive fluid and supportive management is required to maintain a patient with a reasonable quality of life. There are ongoing aggressive attempts to devise therapies for secondary forms of restrictive cardiomyopathy tailored to the etiology: (e.g., iron removal in hemochromatosis or enzyme replacement therapy in Fabry disease).

CLINICAL MANIFESTATIONS. Patients with restrictive cardiomyopathy frequently present with exercise intolerance that results from an impaired ability to augment cardiac output during increasing heart rate because of the restriction of diastolic filling. Other notable symptoms are weakness, dyspnea, and edema, and exertional chest pain is reported by some but not all patients. With advancing disease, profound edema occurs that includes peripheral edema, hepatomegaly, ascites, and anasarca. These patients represent the most difficult volume management because of the balance between volume status and hypotension that can result during diuresis because of reduced preload filling of the ventricles. Physical examination is notable for an elevated jugular venous pulse, often with the Kussmaul sign, and a rising jugular pressure during inspiration (because of the restriction to filling). Both S_3 and S_4 gallops are common and the apical pulse is palpable (in contrast to constrictive pericarditis). Patients with restrictive cardiomyopathy are highly prone to developing atrial fibrillation.[2]

LABORATORY STUDIES. Computed tomography and MRI are valuable for differentiating constrictive and restrictive disease. A thickened pericardium supports the diagnosis of pericardial constriction. Other ancillary tests also may be helpful. For example, chest roentgenography may detect pericardial calcification. The ECG may disclose atrial fibrillation. Echocardiography should be routinely performed in patients suspected of restrictive cardiomyopathy or constriction, and may reveal biatrial dilation and increasing wall thickness associated with myocardial infiltration, as well as alterations in the appearance of the

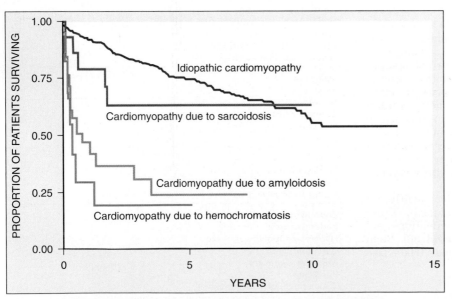

FIGURE 64–7 Adjusted Kaplan-Meier estimates of survival among patients with infiltrative cardiomyopathies. Survival of patients with idiopathic cardiomyopathy is shown for comparison. *(From Felker GM, Thompson RE, Hare JM, et al: Underlying causes and long-term survival in patients with initially unexplained cardiomyopathy. N Engl J Med 342:1077, 2000. Copyright 2000, Massachusetts Medical Society.)*

myocardium (e.g., speckling). Doppler echocardiography supplemented with tissue Doppler reveals evidence of myocardial relaxation with increased early left ventricular filling velocity, decreased atrial filling velocity, and decreased isovolumetric relaxation time. The latter findings are additionally useful for the discrimination from constrictive disease.[2,60] Recently BNP levels were proposed as a test to discriminate between restrictive cardiomyopathy and constrictive disease, with concentrations approximately five times greater in the former compared with the latter.[61]

AMYLOIDOSIS

ETIOLOGY AND TYPES. Amyloidosis is a unique disease process that results from tissue deposition of proteins that have a unique secondary structure (twisted beta-pleated sheet fibrils) (Fig. 64-8). Amyloid may be found in almost any organ but does not produce clinically evident disease unless tissue infiltration is extensive. Several classification systems have been used to characterize the different clinical presentations of amyloidosis. *Primary amyloidosis* results from the deposition of portions of immunoglobulin light chain (designated as AL) within tissues. In the vast majority of cases, the excess production of this protein results from a monoclonal expansion of plasma cells

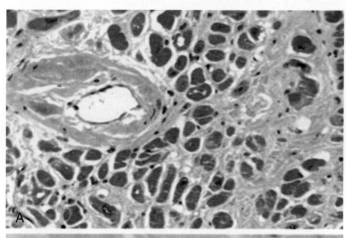

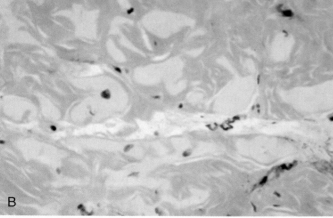

FIGURE 64–8 Histological phenotype of cardiac amyloidosis. **A,** Endomyocardial biopsy specimen, stained with hematoxylin and eosin, from a patient with cardiac amyloidosis. The amyloid stains light pinkish red and is seen as an amorphous material that separates the darker-staining myocytes. **B,** Staining of the tissue from the same patient using sulfated Alcian blue. The amyloid stains turquoise green and the myocytes stain yellow, characteristic of amyloid. *(From Falk RH: Diagnosis and management of the cardiac amyloidoses. Circulation 112:2047, 2005. Copyright, The American Heart Association.)*

in the setting of multiple myeloma. Rarely, a patient with a plasma cell dyscrasia may develop restrictive cardiomyopathy due to deposition of light chains in a nonamyloid manner. Importantly, the latter form of disease may be reversible. Historically, primary amyloidosis occurred from other chronic untreated inflammatory conditions. *Secondary amyloidosis* (also known as *reactive systemic amyloidosis*) results from the excess production of a nonimmunoglobulin protein known as AA.

FAMILIAL AMYLOIDOSIS. In the past decade, there has been growing recognition that various familial diseases can lead to amyloid deposition in the heart. An autosomal dominant form results from the deposition of a variant form of prealbumin serum carrier termed *transthyretin*. Multiple (>80) point mutations in the transthyretin gene are associated with amyloidosis. Transthyretin amyloidosis usually produces one of three different clinical scenarios—nephropathy, neuropathy, or cardiomyopathy. Isolated cardiomyopathy occurring with older age, associated with the Ile 122 variant, is more common in individuals of African-American descent.[62] Given that transthyretin is produced hepatically, liver transplantation may be contemplated in affected individuals who are detected early.

SENILE SYSTEMIC AMYLOIDOSIS. This form of amyloidosis results from amyloid deposition of proteins that are either like atrial natriuretic peptide or transthyretin.[63] This form of amyloidosis is increasing in incidence as the population ages. Although it affects individuals of older age, the prognosis is better than that of AL disease.[63] Deposition of amyloid in the atria and pulmonary vessels is often found at autopsy in octogenarians and may be a risk factor for atrial fibrillation.

Cardiac Amyloidosis

Cardiac amyloidosis is an invariably progressive infiltrative cardiomyopathy that carries a grave prognosis.[58] Cardiac involvement may be present in up to one third of patients with primary amyloidosis resulting from plasma cell dyscrasias. When the heart is studied pathologically, AL protein deposits are present invariably at necropsy even if clinically silent in life. Myocardial infiltration tends to be less with secondary amyloidosis, in which the AA protein deposits tend to be smaller and more perivascular in location, where they are less likely to produce myocardial dysfunction.

Approximately one quarter of patients with transthyretin-induced (familial) amyloidosis experience clinically significant cardiac involvement that is often marked by involvement of the conduction system. Neurological and/or renal involvement may also predominate in this form of amyloidosis. Patients will typically present with clinical symptoms after the age of 35. In one half of the cases involving deposition of transthyretin, the mode of death is cardiac, either from heart failure or sudden cardiac death. In senile amyloidosis, deposits vary from isolated atrial involvement to extensive ventricular infiltration causing severe restrictive cardiomyopathy. Cardiac amyloidosis is observed more frequently in men than in women and is rare before the age of 40.

PATHOLOGY. The term *amyloidosis* was coined by Virchow and means "starch-like." The heart infiltrated with amyloid appears tan and waxy and is rubbery in consistency. The atria are also significantly enlarged (see Fig. 64-8). Histologically, amyloid deposits can be detected with Congo red or Sirius red staining and are present between cardiac myocytes.[16,58] Amyloidosis may cause focal thickening of the cardiac valves but infrequently leads to valvular dysfunction. In addition, amyloid may deposit within the media and adventitia of intramural coronary arteries and may cause impairment in coronary perfusion.

CLINICAL MANIFESTATIONS

There are four overlapping cardiovascular syndromes that may occur with cardiovascular involvement of amyloidosis, including restrictive cardiomyopathy, systolic heart failure, orthostatic hypotension, and presentation with conduction system disease.

RESTRICTIVE CARDIOMYOPATHY. Amyloid infiltration and circulating immunoglobulins produce classic restrictive physiology leading to increased diastolic chamber stiffness with a resultant impairment of left ventricular filling. The impairment of chamber filling leads to fluid retention and peripheral edema, hepatomegaly, and elevated jugular venous pressure. Hemodynamic measurements reveal the classic dip and plateau square root sign. One feature differentiating amyloidosis from constrictive pericarditis is the rate of early diastolic filling, which is accelerated in pericardial disease but is diminished in amyloidosis.

SYSTOLIC HEART FAILURE. Although systolic function may be normal early in the disease, it frequently deteriorates late in the disease as the degree of amyloid deposition increases. Deposition of amyloid in the atrium can also lead to atrial arrest, even though the sinus node is fully functional. The loss of atrial transport function may contribute to worsening heart failure, particularly in the face of restrictive cardiac physiology. Patients may also exhibit angina pectoris, although epicardial coronary arteries are normal angiographically. This form of the disease is usually relentlessly progressive.

ORTHOSTATIC HYPOTENSION. Approximately 10 percent of affected individuals will exhibit orthostasis caused by amyloid infiltration of the autonomic nervous system, blood vessels, or both.[64] Infiltration of the heart and adrenal glands may contribute to the pathogenesis of this variant. Renal failure resulting in the nephrotic syndrome and volume retention can worsen the postural hypotension. Patients with amyloidosis frequently experience frank syncope often associated with emotional or physical stress.[65] Syncope during exertion represents an extremely poor prognosis, with demise likely within 3 months.

CONDUCTION SYSTEM DISEASE. Abnormal propagation of cardiac electrical signals is the least common form of amyloidosis and may result in arrhythmias and conduction disturbances. Sudden cardiac death, caused by malignant arrhythmias or conduction block, is an important mode of death. Episodes of syncope may herald more severe events such as sudden cardiac death.

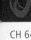

CH 64

PHYSICAL EXAMINATION. Most commonly, patients with cardiac amyloidosis present with signs of congestive heart failure. The jugular venous pulse is elevated, often massively, and there are signs of systemic edema with hepatomegaly, ascites, and edema. On auscultation apical systolic murmurs due to mitral regurgitation and S_3 gallops are frequently present, although the S_4 is typically absent when there is atrial infiltration with amyloid that leads to impaired atrial contraction. The blood pressure is normal to reduced, and the pulse pressure may be quite narrow, consistent with low cardiac output.

NONINVASIVE TESTING. Cardiomegaly is present on chest roentgenography in patients with systolic dysfunction but not in those with restrictive presentations. Pulmonary congestion will be detected if heart failure is present. The electrocardiogram most often reveals low QRS voltage, and bundle branch block and abnormal axis are also common. A pattern of old anterior myocardial infarction may be simulated by diminutive or absent R waves in the right precordial leads, or by inferior Q waves. Amyloid infiltration of the atrium predisposes to atrial fibrillation, and ventricular arrhythmias are also common. Signal-averaged electrocardiography has proved valuable in predicting increased risk for sudden cardiac death. Atrioventricular conduction defects are common, are particularly prominent in familial amyloidosis with polyneuropathy, and may portend a poor prognosis. Electrophysiological testing is usually necessary to detect significant intrahisian block. Sinus node dysfunction is also common and the ECG may show sick sinus syndrome.

ECHOCARDIOGRAPHY. Echocardiograpahy is quite valuable and reveals increased ventricular wall thickness with small intracavitary chambers, enlarged atria, and a thickened interatrial septum. As noted, systolic function is normal early in the course of the disease but progressive left ventricular dysfunction ensues with advancing amyloid deposition. The walls of the ventricles often reveal a distinctive appearance with a sparkling and granular texture, most likely resulting from the amyloid deposition itself. The cardiac valves may have a thickened appearance but typically have normal excursion. Pericardial effusions may be present but do not advance to tamponade. Patterns of chamber hypertrophy are, on occasion, regional, leading to a pattern reminiscent of hypertrophic cardiomyopathy. The echocardiographic appearance of thickened left ventricular walls associated with low voltage on ECG is valuable for differentiation from pericardial disease. Both Doppler echocardiography and radionuclide ventriculography are valuable to evaluate diastolic dysfunction, the degree of which offers prognostic information.

RADIONUCLIDE AND MRI CARDIAC IMAGING. Technetium-99m pyrophosphate scintigraphy, and other agents that bind to calcium may be valuable for amyloid detection. This tool is frequently strongly positive when amyloidosis is extensive and correlates with the degree of cardiac infiltration; however, false-negative results may occur. Both MRI and indium-labeled antimyosin antibody imaging are useful for the detection of cardiac amyloid involvement. Cardiac MRI has a very high sensitivity for the detection of cardiac amyloid, and may also be valuable in measuring the extent of amyloid deposition in the heart, which may be of significant prognostic importance.[49] There are specialized agents which may detect sympathetic denervation in patients with cardiac amyloidosis.

Diagnosis

In the past, systemic amyloidosis was frequently diagnosed at autopsy. However, the increasing awareness and the availability of endomyocardial biopsy now allows for ante-mortem diagnosis in the majority of patients (see Fig. 64-8). Biopsy of alternative tissue locations, such as the abdominal fat pad, the rectum, gingiva, bone marrow, liver, or kidney, is also useful for the detection of systemic amyloidosis. For the diagnosis of cardiac amyloidosis, endomyocardial biopsy performed by an experienced operator is safe and definitive and allows evaluation of the extent of tissue infiltration, which may offer prognostic information.[59] Tissue may be examined by immunohistochemistry to identify specific amyloid proteins, which is increasingly important for targeted therapy. Measurement of circulating serum proteins may also be diagnostically valuable. The importance of seeking the identity of the specific amyloidogenic protein is underscored by a study showing that unsuspected hereditary amyloidosis was detected in nearly 10 percent of patients initially thought to have primary (AL) amyloidosis.

Management

Patients with cardiac amyloidosis have few treatment options, although there are ongoing attempts to modify the severe natural history of this disorder (Fig. 64-9).[66,67] Approaches for patients with AL amyloidosis involve chemotherapy with alkylating agents alone or in combination with autologous bone marrow stem cell transplantation.[68] Heart transplantation with concomitant autologous bone marrow transplants has been reported with variable degrees of success with a 39 percent 4-year survival in one study and 30 percent 5-year survival in another, although amyloid is likely to recur in the transplanted heart.[69] Nevertheless, survival rates may exceed those if the patient is left untreated. Moreover, combination bone-marrow and cardiac transplantation may offer better survival rates in the future. For patients with transthyretin amyloid, liver transplantation may remove the source of the abnormal amyloidogenic protein.[70] No form of therapy is effective in the senile form

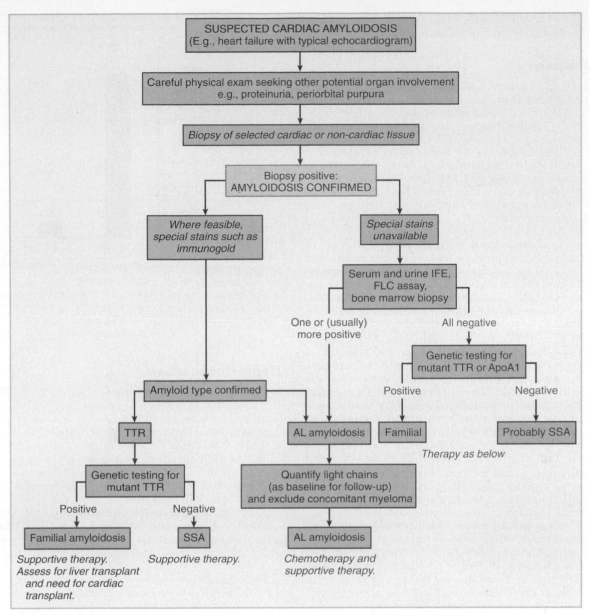

FIGURE 64–9 Flow diagram outlining the evaluation of a patient with suspected cardiac amyloidosis. Clinical evaluation may reveal clues that strengthen the likelihood of amyloidosis, but a tissue diagnosis is mandatory. Although special staining of the biopsy may confirm the type of amyloid, further workup of amyloid (AL) is required to exclude myeloma and to quantify free-light chains. If the biopsy stains positive for transthyretin, further testing is needed to determine whether this is a wild-type or mutant transthyretin. ApoA1 = Apoprotein type A1; IFE = immunofixation electrophoresis; FLC = free-light-chain; SSA = senile systemic amyloidosis; TTR = transthyretin. *(From Falk RH: Diagnosis and management of the cardiac amyloidoses. Circulation 112:2047, 2005. Copyright, The American Heart Association.)*

of amyloidosis, although the clinical course is more benign than in primary amyloidosis.

In terms of conventional cardiac medications, the use of digitalis glycosides requires additional vigilance because patients with cardiac amyloidosis have increased sensitivity to digitalis preparations. In spite of this, digitalis glycosides are sometimes useful for successfully controlling the ventricular rate in atrial fibrillation. Calcium-channel antagonists also require caution because their negative inotropic effect has the potential to exacerbate heart failure. Pacemakers are frequently indicated for conduction system disturbances, and implantable cardioverter-defibrillators (ICDs) should be considered for appropriate patients. Perhaps the mainstay of symptom relief in volume overloaded patients is the judicious use of diuretics, which requires very careful titration, in combination with rigorous fluid restriction. Vasodilator agents may also afford symptom relief and enhance diuresis but must be used cautiously

to avoid systemic hypotension. Anticoagulation should be considered in the case of atrial standstill or atrial fibrillation.

INHERITED AND ACQUIRED INFILTRATIVE DISORDERS CAUSING RESTRICTIVE CARDIOMYOPATHY

The heritable metabolic disorders resulting from the myocardial accumulation or infiltration of abnormal metabolic products represent an important cause of restrictive cardiomyopathy. These disorders produce classic restrictive cardiomyopathy with diastolic impairment and variable degrees of systolic dysfunction. The heritable metabolic disorders include Fabry disease, Gaucher disease, the glycogenoses, and the mucopolysaccharidoses. Early diagnosis is increasingly important because of the availability, in some cases, of effective enzyme replacement therapy.

Fabry Disease

Fabry disease, also referred to as *angiokeratoma corporis diffusum universale*, is an X-linked recessive disorder that results in deficiency of alpha-galactosidase A, a lysosomal enzyme, and the resultant accumulation of glycosphingolipids (most notably globotriaosylceramide) in lysosomes.[71] The major clinical features result from the accumulation of glycolipid substrate in the endothelium. More than 160 different mutations are described that have varying impact, ranging from absence of alpha-galactosidase activity to an attenuated level of activity of this enzyme. Patients with absent alpha-galactosidase activity exhibit widespread systemic manifestations with prominent kidney and cutaneous manifestations, whereas those with an attenuated level of enzyme activity have atypical variants of Fabry disease that may cause isolated myocardial disease. Histological evaluation of the heart demonstrates diffuse involvement of the myocardium, vascular endothelium, conduction system, and valves—most notably the mitral valve (see Fig. 64-e1 on website).

CARDIAC FINDINGS. Patients with Fabry disease often experience angina pectoris and myocardial infarction caused by the accumulation of lipid species in the coronary endothelium, although epicardial coronary arteries are angiographically normal. The ventricular walls are thickened and have mildly diminished diastolic compliance with normal systolic function. Mild mitral regurgitation may be present. Diastolic abnormalities detected by Doppler echocardiography may be one of the earlier manifestations preceding cardiac hypertrophy. Males almost always present with symptomatic cardiovascular involvement, whereas female carriers may be completely asymptomatic or have only minimal symptoms.[72] Other common features of the disorder include systemic hypertension, congestive heart failure, and mitral valve prolapse. Echocardiography demonstrates increased ventricular wall thickness, which may mimic hypertrophic cardiomyopathy.[71] Whereas echocardiography may not be sufficient to do so, cardiac MRI may be able to differentiate Fabry disease from other infiltrative processes such as amyloidosis (see Fig. 64-e2 on website).[72] The surface ECG may reveal a short PR interval, atrioventricular block, and ST segment and T wave abnormalities. The endomyocardial biopsy and low plasma alpha-galactosidase A activity offer a definitive diagnosis, which has therapeutic implications because enzyme replacement therapy for Fabry disease is safe and effective.[73] Administration of recombinant alpha-galactosidase A can ameliorate the stores of globotriaosylceramide from the heart and other tissues, leading to symptomatic, clinical, and echocardiographic improvement (Fig. 64-10).[72,73]

Gaucher Disease

Gaucher disease results from a heritable deficiency of beta-glucosidase, which leads to an accumulation of cerebrosides in diffuse organs including spleen, liver, bone marrow, lymph nodes, brain, and heart. Cardiac disease manifests as a stiffened ventricle caused by reduced chamber compliance, leading to impaired cardiac performance. Other manifestations include left ventricular failure and enlargement, hemorrhagic pericardial effusion, and sclerotic, calcified left-sided valves. Gaucher disease is responsive to enzyme replacement therapy, or in more extreme cases, hepatic transplantation; both therapies contribute to reducing tissue infiltration by cerebrosides and can lead to varying degrees of clinical improvement.[74]

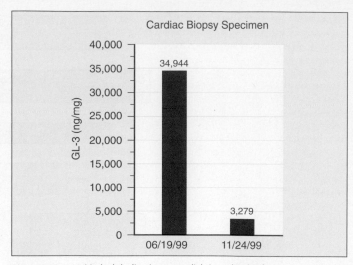

FIGURE 64–10 Marked decline in myocardial tissue levels of globotriaosylceramide (GL-3) in a patient with Fabry disease who was treated with enzyme replacement therapy. *(From Waldek S: PR interval and the response to enzyme-replacement therapy for Fabry's disease. N Engl J Med 348:1186, 2003. Copyright 2003, Massachusetts Medical Society.)*

Hemochromatosis

Hemochromatosis results from excessive deposition of iron in a variety of parenchymal tissues, notably the heart, liver, gonads, and pancreas. The classic pentad is a symptom complex of heart failure, cirrhosis, impotence, diabetes, and arthritis. The most frequent form of hemochromatosis is inherited as an autosomal recessive disorder (see Chap. 10) that arises from a mutation in the *HFE* gene, which codes for a transmembrane protein that is responsible for regulating iron uptake in the intestine and liver. Hemochromatosis may also arise from ineffective erythropoiesis secondary to a defect in hemoglobin synthesis, as well as from chronic liver disease, or may be acquired as a result of chronic and excessive oral or parenteral intake of iron (or blood transfusions).[75]

Iron deposition in the heart is almost always accompanied by varying degrees of infiltration of the liver, spleen, pancreas, and bone marrow, although the degrees of different organ system involvement may not parallel each other. Cardiac involvement produces a mixed pattern of systolic and diastolic dysfunction that is often accompanied by arrhythmias. The severity of hemochromatosis is less and age of onset is later in women because of the menstrual loss of iron. Cardiac toxicity results directly from the free iron moiety in addition to adverse effects of tissue infiltration. Death results most frequently from cirrhosis and hepatocellular carcinoma, whereas cardiac mortality accounts for an additional one third of the mortality and is particularly important in the group of male patients who present at relatively younger ages.

PATHOLOGY. Grossly the hearts are dilated and ventricular walls are thickened. Iron deposits locate preferentially in the myocyte sarcoplasmic reticulum, more frequently in ventricular versus atrial cardiomyocytes. Frequently, the conduction system is involved and loss of myocytes with fibrosis is often present. The degree of iron deposition correlates with the extent of myocardial dysfunction.

CLINICAL MANIFESTATIONS. Symptoms at presentation vary widely, and some patients are asymptomatic although evidence exists for myocardial involvement. Echocardiography reveals increased left ventricular wall thickness, ventricular dilation, and ventricular dysfunction.

Both computed tomography and MRI are useful to detect early subclinical myocardial involvement at a time when therapy is most effective.[76] ECG manifestations occur with advancing cardiac involvement and include ST segment and T wave abnormalities, and supraventricular arrhythmias.

Clinical and echocardiographic features usually are diagnostic, and endomyocardial biopsy is confirmatory but because of false negativity cannot definitively rule out the diagnosis. Evaluation of iron metabolism may aid in the diagnosis. Plasma iron levels are elevated, total iron-binding capacity is low or normal, and serum ferritin, urinary iron, liver iron, and especially saturation of transferrin are markedly elevated. Management should include repeated phlebotomies and/or treatment with chelating agents such as desferrioxamine. For advanced disease, cardiac transplantation carries acceptable 5- and 10-year survival rates.[77]

Glycogen Storage Disease

Patients with type II, III, IV, and V glycogen storage diseases may have cardiac involvement. However, survival to adulthood is rare with the exception of patients with type III disease (glycogen debranching enzyme deficiency). The most typical cardiac involvement is left ventricular hypertrophy, with electrocardiographic and echocardiographic findings, often with the absence of symptoms. A subset of patients may present with overt cardiac dysfunction, arrhythmias, and presentation of a DCM.

Inflammatory Causes of Infiltrative Cardiomyopathy

Sarcoidosis

Sarcoidosis is a systemic inflammatory condition characterized by the formation of noncaseating granulomas, most commonly involving the lungs, reticuloendothelial system, and skin. Sarcoid has been reported to involve essentially all tissues including the heart, which is recognized in 20 to 30 percent of autopsies of affected patients. Cardiac impairment may also arise secondary to pulmonary sarcoidosis, in which case extensive pulmonary fibrosis leads to advancing right-sided heart failure. The main clinical manifestations of sarcoid heart disease result from infiltration of the conduction system and myocardium, producing heart block, malignant arrhythmias, heart failure, and sudden cardiac death. Patients with cardiac sarcoidosis may also present with a restrictive cardiomyopathy caused by increased ventricular chamber stiffness.[44,54]

PATHOLOGY. Noncaseating granulomas surrounded by multinucleated giant cells are the diagnostic feature of the disorder and are found in multiple organs. In the heart they infiltrate the myocardium and lead to the formation of fibrotic scars. The condition must be separated from two other inflammatory conditions of the heart—chronic active myocarditis and giant cell myocarditis (see Chap. 66). Giant cell myocarditis, which is characterized by diffuse giant cell inflammation in the absence of discrete granulomas, has a much more fulminant course than cardiac sarcoid (Fig. 64-11). In sarcoidosis, the granulomas may involve discrete areas of the ventricular walls in a patchy fashion, increasing the likeli-

hood of a false-negative endomyocardial biopsy result. Granulomas are most commonly observed in the interventricular septum and left ventricular free wall, and patients with conduction system disease typically have involvement of the basal portion of the interventricular septum. Left ventricular aneurysm formation may occur with extensive transmural free wall involvement. In terms of the coronary anatomy, the large conductance vessels are usually spared, but small coronary artery branches may be involved.

CLINICAL MANIFESTATIONS. The clinical manifestations result from infiltration of the conduction system and myocardium. The most devastating presentation is that of sudden death due to malignant ventricular arrhythmia. Patients may also present with heart block, congestive heart failure, and syncope. Both atrial and ventricular arrhythmias are common.[78] Patients may be asymptomatic despite significant cardiac involvement. Heart failure may result from direct myocardial involvement or cor pulmonale due to extensive pulmonary fibrosis. Survival may range from months to years, with the presence of a positive endomyocardial biopsy heralding a grave outcome. Excellent long-term outcome may be achieved with aggressive immunosuppression. Isolated cardiac sarcoid has been reported.

The initial detection of cardiac sarcoidosis often results from the presence of bilateral hilar lymphadenopathy on chest roentgenogram in individuals with clinical or ECG findings suggesting myocardial disease. Endomyocardial biopsy should be performed if available due to the importance of positive findings, but it has a high false-negative rate.[79] Multiple imaging modalities assist in assessing diagnosis and prognosis. Echocardiography may demonstrate either global or regional left ventricular dysfunction and rarely may reveal aneurysm formation. Echocardiography is also valuable to evaluate right ventricular hypertrophy and to estimate pulmonary artery systolic pressures. Cardiac MRI is emerging as a highly sensitive and specific test.[80] Other modalities include myocardial nuclear imaging with thallium-201 or technetium-99m, which can reveal segmental perfusion defects due to granulomatous inflammation, and (^{18}F)-fluorodeoxyglucose positron emission tomography, which can reveal focal uptake consistent with sarcoid. Uptake of technetium pyrophosphate, gallium, or labeled antimyosin antibody may also contribute to making the diagnosis.

The *physical examination* may show evidence of extracardiac sarcoid or may be totally normal. An apical systolic murmur due to mitral regurgitation is frequently present, often arising from cardiac chamber dilation as opposed to direct papillary muscle infiltration. Murmurs of tricuspid regurgitation, pulmonic regurgitation, and right-sided third heart sounds suggest pulmonary hypertension and cor pulmonale. Both S$_3$ and S$_4$ are frequently appreciated.

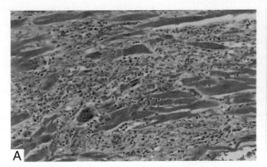
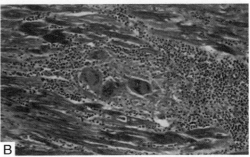

FIGURE 64–11 Sarcoid versus giant cell myocarditis. Giant cell myocarditis (**A**) is characterized by lymphocytic infiltration, myocyte necrosis, and giant cells. Sarcoidosis (**B**) is characterized by the presence of true noncaseating granulomas. *(From Hare JM: Etiologic basis of congestive heart failure. In Colucci WS [ed]: Atlas of Heart Failure. 4th ed. Copyright 2005, Current Medicine LLC.)*

Electrocardiography typically demonstrates nonspecific findings suggestive of myocardial involvement, with T wave abnormalities commonly present. The ECG is highly valuable to assess the degree of conduction system involvement in terms of intraventricular delays and atrioventricular block (see Fig. 64-e3 on website). Q waves may be present indicating severe and extensive myocardial replacement and fibrosis. Typical findings on echocardiography include left-ventricular dilation with global or regional hypokinesis, right-sided enlargement and hypertrophy, possible left ventricular aneurysm formation, and not infrequently, pericardial effusion. Occasionally, increased echogenicity suggests an infiltrative process.

MANAGEMENT. Sarcoidosis is generally treated with immunosuppression. Conduction disturbance, arrhythmias, and myocardial dysfunction may all respond to corticosteroids. Steroids effectively halt the progression of inflammation, and some studies suggest that therapy may offer improved survival. Other drugs that may be of benefit in sarcoidosis include hydroxychloroquine, methotrexate, and cyclophosphamide. It is important to distinguish cardiac sarcoidosis from giant cell myocarditis, a much more aggressive disorder that requires intensive immunosuppression and frequently mechanical support or heart transplantation (see Chap. 66). Whereas antiarrhythmic therapy is often ineffective for controlling malignant arrhythmias, ICD therapy is appropriate for patients at risk for sudden cardiac death. Implantation of a permanent pacemaker is often required in the case of conduction system disease. Heart or heart-lung transplantation should be considered in the case of intractable heart failure, although recurrence of sarcoid may occur in the grafted organ.

Endomyocardial Disease

Definition and Pathogenesis

A common form of restrictive cardiomyopathy found in a geographical location close to the equator is known as endomyocardial disease (EMD). EMD is common in equatorial Africa, and manifests less frequently in South America, Asia, and nontropical countries, including the United States. Two variants are described that, despite similar phenotypes, are likely unique processes, both manifesting as aggressive endocardial scarring obliterating the ventricular apices and subvalvular regions. Endomyocardial fibrosis or Davies disease is the first variant and occurs primarily in tropical regions, and the second, Löffler endocarditis parietalis fibroplastica, or the hypereosinophilic syndrome, is encountered in more temperate zones. Although the pathological appearance of these two disorders is similar, there are sufficient differences between the two disorders, suggesting that they indeed are two distinct entities. Löffler endocarditis is more aggressive and rapidly progresses, affects mainly males, and is associated with hypereosinophilia, thromboemboli, and systemic arteritis; endomyocardial fibrosis occurs in a younger distribution, affects young children, and is only variably associated with eosinophilia.

DIFFERENCES BETWEEN LÖFFLER ENDOCARDITIS AND ENDOMYOCARDIAL FIBROSIS

Overlap between Löffler endocarditis and endomyocardial fibrosis is suggested by the observation that both diseases are attributable to the direct toxic effects of eosinophils in the myocardium. It is suggested that hypereosinophilia (regardless of cause) produces the first phase of EMD, which is characterized by necrosis, intense myocarditis, and arteritis (i.e., Löffler endocarditis). This phase lasts for a period of months and is then followed by a thrombotic stage a year following the initial presentation, in which nonspecific thickening of the myocardium with a layer of thrombus replaces the inflammatory portion of myocardium. In the late phase, final healing is achieved by the formation of fibrosis, at which point the clinical features of endomyocar-

dial fibrosis are present. Most of the support for this three-stage pathophysiology, namely necrotic, thrombotic, and fibrotic, comes from autopsy studies. Nonetheless, definitive evidence that each patient passes sequentially through these stages is lacking.

ROLE OF EOSINOPHILS

The mechanisms by which eosinophils participate in the development of cardiac disease remains incompletely understood. These cells have the capacity to directly infiltrate tissues or release factors that may exert toxicity. The observation that patients with Löffler endocarditis have degranulated eosinophils in their peripheral blood supports the idea that these granules contain cardiotoxic substances, capable of causing the necrotic phase of EMD, which leads to the thrombotic and fibrotic phases once the eosinophilia resolves. It is conceivable that this effect may occur only in temperate zones of the world, as the link between eosinophilia and endomyocardial fibrosis is less clear (although parasitic diseases have increased incidence), suggesting that in tropical countries endomyocardial fibrosis may result from a different mechanism. Factors implicated include elevated cerium levels and hypomagnesemia.

Löffler Endocarditis: The Hypereosinophilic Syndrome

In temperate climates, EMD is closely associated with significant hypereosinophilia, which can have several different etiologies. Hypereosinophilia associated with Löffler endocarditis usually is characterized by eosinophil counts exceeding 1500 per mm^3 for at least 6 months. Most patients with this degree of hypereosinophilia will have cardiac involvement. The eosinophilia may be secondary to leukemia, reactive disorders such as parasite infection, allergies, granulomatous syndromes, hypersensitivity, or neoplastic disorders. In addition, patients with Churg-Strauss syndrome, characterized by asthma or allergic rhinitis and a necrotizing vasculitis often have cardiac involvement.[81]

PATHOLOGY. The hypereosinophilic syndrome involves several organ systems beyond the heart, including the lungs, brain, and bone marrow. Both chambers of the heart are involved and manifest with endocardial thickening of the inflow regions and ventricular apices. Histologically there are variable degrees of eosinophilic myocarditis of the myocardium and subendocardium, thrombosis and inflammation of small intramural coronary vessels, mural thrombosis containing eosinophils, and endocardial fibrotic thickening several millimeters thick.

CLINICAL MANIFESTATIONS. Patients with hypereosinophilic syndrome exhibit weight loss, fever, cough, rash, and congestive heart failure. Early in the course of cardiac involvement, patients may be asymptomatic, but with progression in excess of 50 percent, patients will have overt congestive heart failure and/or cardiomegaly. Murmurs of mitral regurgitation are common. Systemic emboli occur frequently—resulting in neurological and renal sequelae. Death results from heart failure associated with renal, hepatic, or pulmonary involvement.

LABORATORY EXAMINATION. *Chest roentgenography* may demonstrate an enlarged cardiac silhouette accompanied by evidence of pulmonary congestion or, less frequently pulmonary infiltrates. Changes on the *electrocardiogram* are nonspecific and include ST segment and T wave abnormalities. Atrial fibrillation and conduction defects, most notably right bundle branch block, are often noted. The *echocardiogram* often shows regional thickening of the posterobasal portion of the left ventricular wall, with substantial impairment in the motion of the posterior leaflet of the mitral valve. The apex may be obliterated by thrombus. The atria are often dilated, and there is Doppler ultrasound evidence of atrioventricular regurgitation. As is typical for restrictive cardiomyopathy, systolic function is often normal. Hemodynamic measurements support a restrictive cardiomyopathic appearance with abnormal diastolic filling, secondary to the dense endocardial scarring and reduced size of the ventricular cavity from the organized thrombus. Regurgitation through atrioventricular valves results from involvement of their respective supporting structures. *Cardiac catheterization* reveals markedly elevated ventricular filling pressures, and there may be evidence of tricuspid or mitral regurgitation. A characteristic feature on *angiocardiography* is largely preserved systolic function with obliteration of the apex of the ventricles. *Endomyocardial biopsy* can provide diagnostic confirmation, but is not always positive.

MANAGEMENT. There is a role for both medical and surgical therapy in improving quality and quantity of life in patients with Löffler endocarditis. There is evidence that both corticosteroids and cytotoxic drugs such as hydroxyurea may have an important favorable effect on survival. In refractory patients, treatment with interferon may offer a valuable adjunctive therapy. Routine supportive cardiac therapy with diuretics, neurohormonal blockade, and anticoagulation as indicated is appropriate for management of these patients. Surgical therapy consisting of endocardiectomy and valve replacement or repair appears to provide significant symptomatic palliation once the fibrotic stage of the disease manifests.

Endomyocardial Fibrosis

Endomyocardial fibrosis is a disorder found typically in tropical and subtropical Africa, notably in Uganda and Nigeria, and as such is a major cause of morbidity and mortality, accounting for 25 percent of cases of congestive heart failure and death in equatorial Africa.[82,83] The disease is increasingly recognized in other tropical and subtropical regions within 15 degrees of the equator including India, Brazil, Colombia, and Sri Lanka.[57] Importantly, it is also recognized in the Middle East, particularly Saudi Arabia.[83] Cardiac dysfunction occurs because of fibrous lesions that affect the inflow of the right and/or left ventricles and that may also involve the atrioventricular valves, thereby producing regurgitant lesions. Endomyocardial fibrosis has increased incidence among the Rwanda tribe of Uganda and in individuals of low socioeconomic status.[56] It affects both sexes equally, is most common in children[82] and young adults, but has been described in individuals into the sixth decade of life. Although most cases occur in black individuals, there are occasional presentations in white subjects residing in temperate climates. There are rare reports of endomyocardial fibrosis in individuals who have not resided in tropical areas.

PATHOLOGY. Endomyocardial fibrosis affects both the right and left ventricles in approximately 50 percent of patients, purely the left in 40 percent, and the right ventricle alone in the remaining 10 percent.[57,83] The typical gross appearance is that of a normal to slightly enlarged heart. The right atrium may be dilated in proportion to the severity of right ventricular involvement. There is often a pericardial effusion, which may be large. The right-sided heart border may be indented due to apical scarring. The hallmark feature of the disorder is fibrotic obliteration of the apex of the affected ventricle(s) (Fig. 64-12). The fibrosis involves the papillary muscles and chordae tendineae leading to atrioventricular valve distortion and regurgitation. In the left ventricle, the fibrosis extends from the apex to the posterior mitral valve leaflet, usually sparing the anterior mitral leaflet and the ventricular outflow tract. Endocardial calcific deposits can be present involving diffuse areas of the ventricle. The fibrotic tissue often creates a nidus for thrombus formation, which can be extensive. Atrial thrombi also occur. The process usually does not involve the epicardium and the coronary artery obstruction is distinctly uncommon.

HISTOLOGICAL FINDINGS. Endomyocardial fibrosis is clearly apparent histologically, presenting as a thick layer of collagen overlaying loosely arranged connective tissue.[83] In addition, there are fibrous and granular septations extending into the underlying myocardial tissue. Myocyte hypertrophy is common.[57] Whereas cellular infiltration is uncommon, interstitial edema is frequently present. Fibroelastosis that is found in the ventricular outflow tracts beneath the semilunar valves often represents a secondary process caused by local trauma. Examination of intramural coronary arteries may show involvement with medial degeneration, the deposition of fibrin, and fibrosis.

CLINICAL MANIFESTATIONS. The symptomatic status of patients at presentation relates to which ventricles are involved. Pulmonary congestion signals left-sided involvement, whereas predominantly right-sided disease may mimic restrictive cardiomyopathy and/or constrictive pericarditis. Atrioventricular valve regurgitation is common. The disease may be heralded by an acute febrile illness or may be simply insidious. Endomyocardial fibrosis is a relentless and progressive process, although the time course of decline may vary considerably, with some patients appearing to have periods of stability. Modes of death include progressive heart failure, infection, infarction, sudden cardiac death, and complications of surgery. Atrial fibrillation and ascites are reported to be a poor prognostic indicators.[84,85]

RIGHT VENTRICULAR ENDOMYOCARDIAL FIBROSIS. In pure or predominant right ventricular involvement, the right ventricular

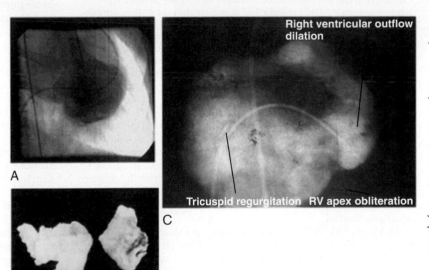

FIGURE 64–12 Right- and left-sided endomyocardial fibrosis (EMF). **A,** Left-sided EMF is characterized by apical obliteration, patchy filling defects, and severe mitral regurgitation. **B,** The management of EMF often requires surgical excision of the endocardial fibrosis. Depicted are pieces of excised endocardial fibrosis. **C,** Right ventricular (RV) angiogram of a patient with RV EMF showing right ventricular outflow tract dilation, RV apex obliteration, and tricuspid regurgitation. (*A and B* from Joshi R, Abraham S, Kumar AS: New approach for complete endocardiectomy in left ventricular endomyocardial fibrosis. J Thorac Cardiovasc Surg 125:40, 2003; *C,* from Seth S, Thatai D, Sharma S, et al: Clinico-pathological evaluation of restrictive cardiomyopathy (endomyocardial fibrosis and idiopathic restrictive cardiomyopathy) in India. Eur J Heart Fail 6:723, 2004.)

apex is characterized by fibrous obliteration, which may extend to involve the supporting structures of the tricuspid valve, with ensuing tricuspid regurgitation. Patients exhibit an elevated jugular venous pressure, a prominent v wave with rapid *y* descent, and a right-sided S₃ gallop. There is prominent hepatomegaly with a pulsatile liver, ascites, splenomegaly, and peripheral edema, but pulmonary congestion is typically absent because of the lack of left-sided involvement. In this regard, pulmonary artery and pulmonary capillary wedge pressures are normal. A large pericardial effusion is often present. The right atrium may be enormously dilated. The *electrocardiogram* often has findings consistent with right-sided enlargement, especially a qR pattern in lead V_1, and supraventricular arrhythmias are common. The *chest roentgenogram* often demonstrates obvious right atrial prominence, a pericardial effusion, and calcification in the walls of the right and, less frequently, the left ventricle. *Echocardiography* demonstrates thickening of the right ventricle with obliteration of the apex, a dilated atrium, hyperechoic endocardial surfaces, and abnormal septal motion in patients with tricuspid regurgitation. On *angiography,* the right ventricular apex is typically not visualized because of fibrous obliteration; tricuspid regurgitation, right atrial enlargement, and filling defects in the right atrium caused by thrombi may be present.

LEFT VENTRICULAR ENDOMYOCARDIAL FIBROSIS. In cases of predominant *left-sided* disease, fibrosis involves the ventricular apex and often the chordae tendineae or the posterior mitral valve leaflet producing mitral regurgitation. The associated murmur may be late systolic, characteristic of a papillary muscle dysfunction murmur, or may be pansystolic. Findings of pulmonary hypertension may be prominent, and an S₃ protodiastolic gallop is frequently present. The *electrocardiogram* usually shows ST segment and T wave abnormalities, low-voltage QRS complexes if a pericardial effusion is present, or left ventricular hypertrophy. Left atrial abnormality is often noted. As with right-sided involvement, atrial fibrillation is often present and portends a poor prognosis. *Echocardiography* reveals increased endocardial echoreflectivity preserved systolic function, apical obliteration, an enlarged atrium, pericardial effusion of varying size, and Doppler ultrasound evidence of mitral regurgitation. Pulmonary hypertension is typically observed during *cardiac catheterization,* as well as left atrial hypertension and a reduced cardiac index. *Left ventriculography* shows mitral regurgitation, and ventricular filling defects caused by intracavitary thrombi may be present. Coronary *arteriography* usually excludes obstructive epicardial vessel stenoses.

BIVENTRICULAR ENDOMYOCARDIAL FIBROSIS. Biventricular endomyocardial fibrosis is more common then either isolated right- or left-sided disease. The typical clinical presentation of EMF resembles right ventricular EMF; however, a murmur of mitral regurgitation is indicative of left-sided involvement. Unless left ventricular involvement is extensive, severe pulmonary hypertension is absent and the right-sided findings are the predominant mode of presentation. Approximately 15 percent of patients will experience systemic embolization and only 2 percent will have infective endocarditis.

DIAGNOSIS. Detection of endomyocardial fibrosis in individuals from the appropriate geographical area requires typical clinical and laboratory findings as well as angiography. Eosinophilia is variably present and may result from parasitic infection.[56] Endomyocardial biopsy is diagnostic, but false-positives can occur because of the patchy nature of the disease. Insofar as myocardial biopsy may be complicated by systemic emboli, left-sided myocardial biopsy is contraindicated.

MANAGEMENT. The medical management of endomyocardial fibrosis remains challenging. One third to one half of patients with advanced disease die within 2-years, whereas those who are less symptomatic fare better. The development of atrial fibrillation is a poor prognostic indicator, although symptomatic relief can be achieved with rate control.[84] Heart failure is difficult to control, and diuretics are effective only in early stages of disease, losing efficacy with advanced ascites. Once EMF progresses to severe endocardial fibrosis, surgical resection with atrioventricular valve replacement on affected sides is the treatment of choice.[86] Surgical therapy consisting of endocardiectomy and valve replacement or repair usually results in hemodynamic improvement with reductions in ventricular filling pressures, increased cardiac output, and normalized angio-

graphic appearance (see Fig. 64-12). Operative mortality is quite high, between 15 and 25 percent, and may be lower if valve replacement is not necessary.[87] Fibrosis may recur, although there are case reports of excellent long-term survival.[88]

Endocardial Fibroelastosis

Endocardial fibroelastosis (EFE) is a disorder of fetuses and infants of unclear etiology, that is characterized by deposition of collagen and elastin leading to ventricular hypertrophy and diffuse endocardial thickening.[89] Although the cause is incompletely understood, there have been reports of associations with viral infections (especially mumps), metabolic disorders, autoimmune disease, and congenital left-sided obstructive lesions. Like DCM, EFE usually progresses to severe congestive heart failure and subsequent death. The echocardiographic finding of a highly reflective endocardial surface of the ventricular myocardium suggests EFE.[89]

NEOPLASTIC INFILTRATIVE CARDIOMYOPATHY—CARCINOID HEART DISEASE

The carcinoid syndrome results from the metastasis of carcinoid tumors from the gut to the heart.[90] The symptoms include marked cutaneous flushing, diarrhea, bronchoconstriction, and endocardial plaques composed of a unique type of fibrous tissue. The symptom complex is caused in large part by the release of serotonin and other circulating substances secreted by the tumor. Essentially all patients experience diarrhea and flushing, 50 percent have cardiac lesions detected echocardiographically, and about 25 percent of the patients have severe right-sided involvement.

Carcinoid tumors originate largely from the gut, with 60 to 90 percent being found in the small bowel and appendix, and the remainder arising from other regions of the gastrointestinal tract or the bronchi. Carcinoid tumors arising in the ileum pose the greatest risk of metastasis, most likely affecting regional lymph nodes and the liver. The carcinoid tumors arising in the liver affect the heart. The severity of the cardiac lesions is related to the circulating concentrations of serotonin and 5-hydroxyindoleacetic acid (its primary metabolite), which are produced primarily by the carcinoid tumors in the liver. The observation that the right side of the heart is preferentially affected in the carcinoid syndrome reflects inactivation of the circulating toxic substances in the lung; the 5 to 10 percent of individuals presenting with left-sided lesions are likely to have right-to-left shunts or tumor involvement of the lungs.

PATHOLOGY. The characteristic lesions are fibrous plaques involving locations "downstream" of the tricuspid and pulmonic valves, the endocardium, and the intima of the venae cavae, pulmonary artery, and coronary sinus. Both stenotic and regurgitant valvular lesions result from fibrotic distortion originating in the plaques.[90] The plaque material appears as a layer of fibrous tissue composed of smooth muscle cells, collagen, and mucopolysaccharides overlying the endocardium, and in some cases extending into the underlying regions. Interestingly, identical pathology results from exposure to the anorectic drugs fenfluramine and dexfenfluramine. Occasionally there is actual metastasis of the tumor to one or both of the ventricles.

CLINICAL MANIFESTATIONS. Cardiac murmurs indicating right-sided valve involvement are widely appreciated. A systolic murmur of tricuspid regurgitation along the left sternal border is almost always present and pulmonic

CH 64

valve murmurs of either stenosis or regurgitation may also be present. The *chest roentgenogram* may be either normal or may show cardiac enlargement and pleural effusions or nodules. The pulmonary artery trunk is most often not enlarged, and poststenotic dilation is also absent, differentiating pulmonic involvement from congenital pulmonic stenosis. Although there are no specific changes on the *electrocardiogram* diagnostic of carcinoid heart disease, it is not uncommon to encounter right atrial enlargement without other findings of right ventricular hypertrophy, nonspecific ST segment, and T wave abnormalities and sinus tachycardia. Patients with advanced disease are likely to have low QRS voltage. *Echocardiography* often reveals tricuspid or pulmonary valve thickening, and enlargement of the right atrium and ventricle; a minority of patients may have a small pericardial effusion. *Cardiac MRI* may offer additional value in evaluating the right side of the heart that may be difficult to image with echocardiography.[91]

MANAGEMENT. For mild congestive heart failure, standard therapy with diuretics and neurohormonal antagonists is appropriate. Both somatostatin analogues and chemotherapy can lead to improved symptoms and possibly enhanced survival, but neither is effective at ameliorating progressive cardiac disease in patients with carcinoid syndrome. A key element of management is relief of stenotic lesions of the tricuspid and pulmonary valves. This may be achieved with either *balloon valvuloplasty* or surgery, both of which can achieve symptomatic relief. Operative mortality is traditionally high, but it has improved significantly in experienced centers.[90]

ARRHYTHMOGENIC RIGHT VENTRICULAR DYSPLASIA/ CARDIOMYOPATHY

Arrhythmogenic right ventricular dysplasia/cardiomyopathy (ARVD/C), first described in 1977 by Fontaine and coworkers, is a genetic form of cardiomyopathy characterized prototypically by fibrofatty infiltration of the right ventricle (Figs. 64-13 and 64-14). ARVD/C accounts for 20 percent of cases of sudden cardiac death, and, importantly, among young athletes dying suddenly, the prevalence of this condition is higher.[92,93]

PRESENTING SYMPTOMS AND NATURAL HISTORY. Patients typically present between the teenage years to the forties, with only 10 percent falling outside of this age range. The natural history of the disorder is characterized by four phases—a concealed phase in which

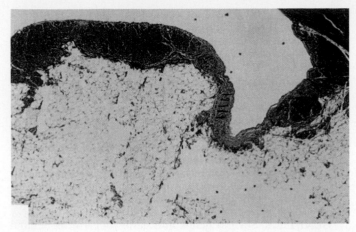

FIGURE 64–13 Arrhythmogenic right ventricular dysplasia/cardiomyopathy (ARVD/C). Histological appearance of ARVD/C showing fibrosis, adipose infiltration, and myocardial thinning. *(From Hare JM. Etiologic basis of congestive heart failure. In Colucci WS [ed]: Atlas of Heart Failure. 4th ed. Copyright 2005, Current Medicine LLC.)*

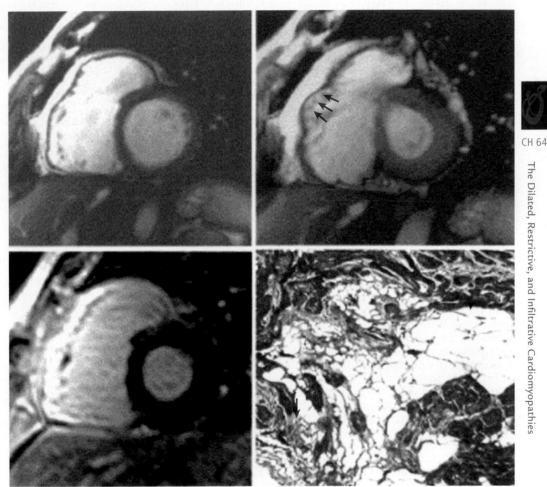

FIGURE 64–14 Arrhythmogenic right ventricular dysplasia/cardiomyopathy (ARVD/C). The **top left and right panels** represent the end-diastolic and end-systolic frames of a short-axis cine magnetic resonance image (MRI) showing an area of dyskinesia on right ventricular (RV) free wall characterizing a focal ventricular aneurysm (arrows). The **bottom left panel** displays the delayed-enhanced MRI with increased signal intensity within the RV myocardium (arrows), at the location of RV aneurysms. The **bottom right panel** shows the corresponding endomyocardial biopsy. Trichrome stain of the right ventricle at high magnification shows marked replacement of the ventricular muscle by adipose tissue. The adipose tissue cells (arrowhead) are irregular in size and infiltrate the ventricular muscle. There is also abundant replacement fibrosis (arrow). There is no evidence of inflammation. *(From Tandri H: JACC 45:98-103, 2005. Copyright 2005, American College of Cardiology.)*

CH 64

The Dilated, Restrictive, and Infiltrative Cardiomyopathies

patients are asymptomatic, a phase characterized by an overt clinical manifestation of an electrical system disturbance, progression to signs and symptoms of right ventricular failure, and finally frank biventricular congestive heart failure. Accordingly, presenting symptoms range from palpitations to syncope, and sudden cardiac death. A majority of patients who subsequently experience sudden cardiac death have a history of syncope, which thus represents an important prognostic event.[93] Progression to heart failure occurs in the minority of patients, but is the predominant mode of death in individuals who are protected from sudden cardiac death by ICD implantation.

PATHOLOGY. Characteristically, a heart affected with ARVD/C heart exhibits fatty or fibrofatty replacement of the myocardium predominantly affecting the right ventricle. Rarely the process extends to the left ventricles.

GENETICS. Several genes and gene loci are associated with ARVD/C, and both autosomal dominant and recessive modes of inheritance are described. Implicated genes include desmoplakin, junctional plakoglobin (JUP), the cardiac ryanodine receptor plakophilin-2 (PKP2), and transforming growth factor-β3. JUP mutations are causally implicated in Naxos disease, a syndrome characterized by ARVD/C, wooly hair, and palmoplantar ketoderma. Individuals with mutations in PKP2 present at younger ages and are more likely to have malignant arrhythmias.[92] This finding suggests the prognostic importance of genetic testing for ARVD/C.

DIAGNOSIS. A task force has set diagnostic criteria to aid in the study and characterization of ARVD/C. The diagnostic criteria involve features obtained from imaging, ECG, signal-averaged ECG and histological criteria, as well as a positive family history and a history of arrhythmias. Early diagnosis of ARVD/C remains challenging. Whereas endomyocardial biopsy may offer valuable diagnostic information, cardiac MRI is emerging as a more definitive diagnostic tool.[47] The main limitation of endomyocardial biopsy is a high false-negative rate because of sampling error and the fact that the right ventricle septum may lack the characteristic histological changes. Tandri and colleagues have reported that characterization of the ventricular wall morphology with delayed enhancement gadolinium MRI correlated well with histological findings as well as with inducibility of ventricular tachycardia during electrophysiological testing.[47]

MANAGEMENT. Patients diagnosed with ARVD/C should receive an ICD. Antiarrhythmic therapy is appropriate prior to ICD insertion and in some cases after, in patients who have recurrent ICD firings. Use of an ICD can have an enormous clinical impact in reducing the major cause of mortality in affected individuals. It is also recommended that patients receive neurohormonal blockade with angiotensin-converting enzyme inhibitors and β-adrenoreceptor antagonists. In individuals progressing to overt heart failure, management involves the same principles for the treatment of other forms of cardiomyopathy. Consideration of heart transplantation is indicated for patients with overt biventricular failure.

SUMMARY AND FUTURE PERSPECTIVES

Our current understanding of cardiomyopathic processes are still fairly rudimentary as evidenced by the large percentage of patients who are assigned as having idiopathic disease. New strides are being made with respect to genetics and cellular biology (stem cells) that are revealing important insights into the etiology, natural history, and potentially the management of dilated, restrictive, and right ventricular cardiomyopathy. The strong genetic basis of several cardio-

myopathic disorders coupled with new high throughput technologies will allow for the possibility of widespread genetic testing of affected individuals and their family members. Genetic testing will also facilitate understanding of which patients have a genetic cause of their disease as opposed to a genetic predisposition to an environmental insult. In addition to genetics, measurement of expressed genes (transcriptomics) and proteins (proteomics) has the potential to aid in understanding etiology, prognosis, and individualized responses to therapy (personalized medicine). A key example of the latter is the attempt to identify patients with a viral cause of cardiomyopathy and treat those patients with appropriate antiviral therapy. The most recent new advance with significant future implications is the observation that the body, including the bone marrow and the heart, possesses reservoirs of endogenous stem cells—the discovery of these cells offers new insights into the causes of cardiomyopathy and may, in the future, provide a new therapeutic avenue.

REFERENCES

Dilated Cardiomyopathy

1. Dec GW, Fuster V: Idiopathic dilated cardiomyopathy. N Engl J Med 331:1564-1575, 1994.
2. Ammash NM, Seward JB, Bailey KR, et al: Clinical profile and outcome of idiopathic restrictive cardiomyopathy. Circulation 101:2490-2496, 2000.
3. Mann DL, Bristow MR: Mechanisms and models in heart failure: The biomechanical model and beyond. Circulation 111:2837-2849, 2005.
4. Hare JM, Walford GD, Hruban RH, et al: Ischemic Cardiomyopathy—endomyocardial biopsy and ventriculographic evaluation of patients with congestive-heart-failure, dilated cardiomyopathy and coronary-artery disease. J Am Coll Cardiol 20:1318-1325, 1992.
5. Kittleson MM, Minhas KM, Irizarry RA, et al: Gene expression analysis of ischemic and nonischemic cardiomyopathy: Shared and distinct genes in the development of heart failure. Physiol Genomics 21:299-307, 2005.
6. Maron BJ, Towbin JA, Thiene G, et al: Contemporary definitions and classification of the cardiomyopathies—An American Heart Association Scientific Statement from the Council on Clinical Cardiology, Heart Failure and Transplantation Committee; Quality of Care and Outcomes Research and Functional Genomics and Translational Biology Interdisciplinary Working Groups; and Council on Epidemiology and Prevention. Circulation 113:1807-1816, 2006.
7. Towbin JA, Bowles NE: The failing heart. Nature 415:227-233, 2002.
8. Thiene G, Corrado D, Basso C: Cardiomyopathies: is it time for a molecular classification? Eur Heart J 25:1772-1775, 2004.
9. Felker GM, Thompson RE, Hare JM, et al: Underlying causes and long-term survival in patients with initially unexplained cardiomyopathy. N Engl J Med 342:1077-1084, 2000.
10. Ardehali H, Qasim A, Cappola T, et al: Endomyocardial biopsy plays a role in diagnosing patients with unexplained cardiomyopathy. Am Heart J 147:919-923, 2004.
11. Levy WC, Mozaffarian D, Linker DT, et al: The Seattle heart failure model—Prediction of survival in heart failure. Circulation 113:1424-1433, 2006.
12. McNamara DM, Holubkov R, Starling RC, et al: Controlled trial of intravenous immune globulin in recent-onset dilated cardiomyopathy. Circulation 103:2254-2259, 2001.
13. Teuteberg JJ, Lewis EF, Nohria A, et al: Characteristics of patients who die with heart failure and a low ejection fraction in the new millennium. J Cardiac Fail 12:47-53, 2006.
14. McCarthy RE, Boehmer JP, Hruban RH, et al: Long-term outcome of fulminant myocarditis as compared with acute (nonfulminant) myocarditis. N Engl J Med 342:690-695, 2000.
15. Braunwald E, Bristow MR: Congestive heart failure: Fifty years of progress. Circulation 102:14-23, 2000.
16. Hare JM: The etiologic basis of congestive heart failure. In Colucci WS, (ed): Atlas of Heart Failure. Philadelphia, Current Medicine LLC, 2005, pp 34-58.
17. Owan TE, Hodge DO, Herges RM, et al: Trends in prevalence and outcome of heart failure with preserved ejection fraction. N Engl J Med 355:251-259, 2006.
18. Wittstein IS, Thiemann DR, Lima JAC, et al: Neurohumoral features of myocardial stunning due to sudden emotional stress. N Engl J Med 352:539-548, 2005.
19. Felker GM, Jaeger CJ, Klodas E, et al: Myocarditis and long-term survival in peripartum cardiomyopathy. Am Heart J 140:785-790, 2000.
20. Elkayam U, Akhter MW, Singh H, et al: Pregnancy-associated cardiomyopathy—Clinical characteristics and a comparison between early and late presentation. Circulation 111:2050-2055, 2005.
21. Elkayam U, Tummala PP, Rao K, et al: Maternal and fetal outcomes of subsequent pregnancies in women with peripartum cardiomyopathy. N Engl J Med 344:1567-1571, 2001.
22. Redfield MM, Kay GN, Jenkins LS, et al: Tachycardia-related cardiomyopathy: A common cause of ventricular dysfunction in patients with atrial fibrillation referred for atrioventricular ablation. Mayo Clinic Proc 75:790-795, 2000.

CH 64

23. Clyne N, Hofman-Bang C, Haga Y, et al: Chronic cobalt exposure affects antioxidants and ATP production in rat myocardium. Scand J Clin Lab Invest 61:609-614, 2001.

24. Vary TC, Deiter G: Long-term alcohol administration inhibits synthesis of both myofibrillar and sarcoplasmic proteins in heart. Metab Clin Exp 54:212-219, 2005.

25. Aistrup GL, Kelly JE, Piano MR, et al: Biphasic changes in cardiac excitation-contraction coupling early in chronic alcohol exposure. Am J Physiol Heart Circ Physiol 291:H1047-H1057, 2006.

26. Fatjo F, Fernandez-Sola J, Lluis M, et al: Myocardial antioxidant status in chronic alcoholism. Alcoholism Clin Exp Res 29:864-870, 2005.

27. Fernandez-Sola J, Fatjo F, Sacanella E, et al: Evidence of apoptosis in alcoholic cardiomyopathy. Hum Pathol 37:1100-1110, 2006.

28. Fernandez-Sola J, Nicolas JM, Oriola J, et al: Angiotensin-converting enzyme gene polymorphism is associated with vulnerability to alcoholic cardiomyopathy. Ann Int Med 137:321-326, 2002.

29. Vary TC, Leese JM, Kimball SR: Gender modulates the response to chronic alcohol intoxication in heart. FASEB J 19:A1596, 2005.

30. Nicolas JM, Garcia G, Fatjo F, et al: Influence of nutritional status on alcoholic myopathy. Am J Clin Nutr 78:326-333, 2003.

31. Burkett EL, Hershberger RE: Clinical and genetic issues in familial dilated cardiomyopathy. J Am Coll Cardiol 45:969-981, 2005.

32. Poller W, Kuhl U, Tschoepe C, et al: Genome-environment interactions in the molecular pathogenesis of dilated cardiomyopathy. J Mol Med 83:579-586, 2005.

33. Chimenti C, Kajstura J, Torella D, et al: Senescence and death of primitive cells and myocytes lead to premature cardiac aging and heart failure. Circ Res 93:604-613, 2003.

34. Lee DS, Pencina MJ, Benjamin EJ, et al: Association of parental heart failure with risk of heart failure in offspring. N Engl J Med 355:138-147, 2006.

35. Schmitt JP, Kamisago M, Asahi M, et al: Dilated cardiomyopathy and heart failure caused by a mutation in phospholamban. Science 299:1410-1413, 2003.

36. Sakata S, Lebeche D, Sakata Y, et al: Mechanical and metabolic rescue in a type II diabetes model of cardiomyopathy by targeted gene transfer. Mol Ther 13:987-996, 2006.

37. McNamara DM, Tam SW, Sabolinski ML, et al: Aldosterone synthase promoter polymorphism modulates outcome in black patients with heart failure: Results from the A-HeFT trial. J Am Coll Cardiol 48:1277-1282, 2006.

38. Baughman KL: Diagnosis of myocarditis—Death of Dallas criteria. Circulation 113:593-595, 2006.

39. Hare JM: Nitroso-redox balance in the cardiovascular system. N Engl J Med 351:2112-2114, 2004.

40. Damy T, Ratajczak P, Shah AM, et al: Increased neuronal nitric oxide synthase-derived NO production in the failing human heart. Lancet 363:1365-1367, 2004.

41. Wencker D, Chandra M, Nguyen K, et al: A mechanistic role for cardiac myocyte apoptosis in heart failure. J Clin Invest 111:1497-1504, 2003.

42. Lipshultz SE, Sleeper LA, Towbin JA, et al: The incidence of pediatric cardiomyopathy in two regions of the United States. N Engl J Med 348:1647-1655, 2003.

43. Cox GF, Sleeper LA, Lowe AM, et al: Factors associated with establishing a causal diagnosis for children with cardiomyopathy. Pediatrics 118:1519-1531, 2006.

44. Cooper LT, Berry GJ, Shabetai R: Idiopathic giant-cell myocarditis—Natural history and treatment. N Engl J Med 336:1860-1866, 1997.

45. Bomma CS, Prakasa K, Dalal D, et al: Multi-detector computer tomography in evaluation of arrhythmogenic right ventricular dysplasia. J Am Coll Cardiol 45:282A-283A, 2005.

46. Vogel-Claussen J, Rochitte CE, Wu KC, et al: Delayed enhancement MR imaging: Utility in myocardial assessment. Radiographics 26:795-U168, 2006.

47. Tandri H, Saranathan M, Rodriguez ER, et al: Noninvasive detection of myocardial fibrosis in arrhythmogenic right ventricular cardiomyopathy using delayed-enhancement magnetic resonance imaging. J Am Coll Cardiol 45:98-103, 2005.

48. Mahrholdt H, Goedecke C, Wagner A, et al: Cardiovascular magnetic resonance assessment of human myocarditis—A comparison to histology and molecular pathology. Circulation 109:1250-1258, 2004.

49. Maceira AM, Joshi J, Prasad SK, et al: Cardiovascular magnetic resonance in cardiac amyloidosis. Circulation 111:186-193, 2005.

50. Nazarian S, Bluemke DA, Lardo AC, et al: Magnetic resonance assessment of the substrate for inducible ventricular tachycardia in nonischemic cardiomyopathy. Circulation 112:2821-2825, 2005.

51. Kurtz CE, Gerber Y, Weston SA, et al: Use of ejection fraction tests and coronary angiography in patients with heart failure. Mayo Clin Proc 81:906-913, 2006.

52. Ardehali H, Kasper EK, Baughman KL. Diagnostic approach to the patient with cardiomyopathy: Whom to biopsy. Am Heart J 149:7-12, 2005.

53. Mills RM, Lauer MS: Endomyocardial biopsy: A procedure in search of an indication. Am Heart J 147:759-760, 2004.

54. Okura Y, Dec GW, Hare JM, et al: A clinical and histopathologic comparison of cardiac sarcoidosis and idiopathic giant cell myocarditis. J Am Coll Cardiol 41:322-328, 2003.

55. Hunt SA, Abraham WT, Chin MH, et al: ACC/AHA 2005 Guideline Update for the Diagnosis and Management of Chronic Heart Failure in the Adult. Circulation 112:E154-E235, 2005.

Restrictive and Infiltrative Cardiomyopathy

56. Rutakingirwa M, Ziegler JL, Newton R, et al: Poverty and eosinophilia are risk factors for endomyocardial fibrosis (EMF) in Uganda. Trop Med Internat Health 4:229-235, 1999.

57. Seth S, Thatai D, Sharma S, et al: Clinico-pathological evaluation of restrictive cardiomyopathy (endomyocardial fibrosis and idiopathic restrictive cardiomyopathy) in India. Euro J Heart Fail 6:723-729, 2004.

58. Falk RH: Diagnosis and management of the cardiac amyloidoses. Circulation 112:2047-2060, 2005.

59. Rahman JE, Helou EF, Gelzer-Bell R, et al: Noninvasive diagnosis of biopsy-proven cardiac amyloidosis. J Am Coll Cardiol 43:410-415, 2004.

60. Ha JW, Ommen SR, Tajik AJ, et al: Differentiation of constrictive pericarditis from restrictive cardiomyopathy using mitral annular velocity by tissue Doppler echocardiography. Am J Cardiol 94:316-319, 2004.

61. Leya FS, Arab D, Joyal D, et al: The efficacy of brain natriuretic peptide levels in differentiating constrictive pericarditis from restrictive cardiomyopathy. J Am Coll Cardiol 45:1900-1902, 2005.

Amyloidosis

62. Jacobson DR, Pastore RD, Yaghoubian R, et al: Variant-sequence transthyretin (isoleucine 122) in late-onset cardiac amyloidosis in black Americans. N Engl J Med 336:466-473, 1997.

63. Ng B, Connors LH, Davidoff R, et al: Senile systemic amyloidosis presenting with heart failure—A comparison with light chain-associated amyloidosis. Arch Int Med 165:1425-1429, 2005.

64. Bernardi L, Passino C, Porta C, et al: Widespread cardiovascular autonomic dysfunction in primary amyloidosis: Does spontaneous hyperventilation have a compensatory role against postural hypotension? Heart 88:615-621, 2002.

65. Chamarthi B, Dubrey SW, Cha K, et al: Features and prognosis of exertional syncope in light-chain associated AL cardiac amyloidosis. Am J Cardiol 80:1242, 1997.

66. Parikh S, de Lemos JA: Current therapeutic strategies in cardiac amyloidosis. Curr Treat Options Cardiovasc Med 7:443-448, 2005.

67. Campbell P, Murdock C: Cardiac amyloidosis—sustained clinical and free light chain response to low dose thalidomide and corticosteroids. Int Med J 36:137-U22, 2006.

68. Seldin DC, Anderson JJ, Sanchorawala V, et al: Improvement in quality of life of patients with AL amyloidosis treated with high-dose melphalan and autologous stem cell transplantation. Blood 104:1888-1893, 2004.

69. Alloni A, Pellegrini C, Ragni T, et al: Heart transplantation in patients with amyloidosis: Single-center experience. Transplant Proc 36:643-644, 2004.

Inherited and Acquired Infiltrative Disorders

70. Delahaye N, Rouzet F, Sarda L, et al: Impact of liver transplantation on cardiac autonomic denervation in familial amyloid polyneuropathy. Medicine 85:229-238, 2006.

71. Pieroni M, Chimenti C, de Cobelli F, et al: Fabry's disease cardiomyopathy—Echocardiographic detection of endomyocardial glycosphingolipid compartmentalization. J Am Coll Cardiol 47:1663-1671, 2006.

72. Glass RBJ, Astrin KH, Norton KI, et al: Fabry disease: Renal sonographic and magnetic resonance imaging findings in affected males and carrier females with the classic and cardiac variant phenotypes. J Comput Assist Tomogr 28:158-168, 2004.

73. Eng CM, Guffon N, Wilcox WR, et al: Safety and efficacy of recombinant human alpha-galactosidase: A replacement therapy in Fabry's disease. N Engl J Med 345:9-16, 2001.

74. Connock M, Burls A, Frew E, et al: The clinical effectiveness and cost-effectiveness of enzyme replacement therapy for Gaucher's disease: A systematic review. Health Technol Assess 10:1, 2006.

75. Hoffbrand AV: Diagnosing myocardial iron overload. Eur Heart J 22:2140-2141, 2001.

76. Ptaszek LM, Price ET, Hu MY, et al: Early diagnosis of hemochromatosis-related cardiomyopathy with magnetic resonance imaging. J Cardiovasc Magnet Res 7:689-692, 2005.

77. Caines AE, Kpodonu J, Massad MG, et al: Cardiac transplantation in patients with iron overload cardiomyopathy. J Heart Lung Transplant 24:486-488, 2005.

78. Koplan BA, Soejima K, Baughman K, et al: Refractory ventricular tachycardia secondary to cardiac sarcoid: Electrophysiologic characteristics, mapping, and ablation. Heart Rhythm 3:924-929, 2006.

79. Ardehali H, Howard DL, Hariri A, et al: A positive endomyocardial biopsy result for sarcoid is associated with poor prognosis in patients with initially unexplained cardiomyopathy. Am Heart J 150:459-463, 2005.

80. Smedema JP, Snoep G, van Kroonenburgh MPG, et al: Evaluation of the accuracy of gadolinium-enhanced cardiovascular magnetic resonance in the diagnosis of cardiac sarcoidosis. J Am Coll Cardiol 45:1683-1690, 2005.

81. Pela G, Tirabassi G, Pattoneri P, et al: Cardiac involvement in the Churg-Strauss syndrome. Am J Cardiol 97:1519-1524, 2006.

82. Marijon E, Ou P: What do we know about endomyocardial fibrosis in children of Africa? Pediatr Cardiol 27:523-524, 2006.

83. Hassan WM, Fawzy ME, Al Helaly S, et al: Pitfalls in diagnosis and clinical, echocardiographic, and hemodynamic findings in endomyocardial fibrosis—A 25-year experience. Chest 128:3985-3992, 2005.

84. Barretto ACP, Mady C, Nussbacher A, et al: Atrial fibrillation in endomyocardial fibrosis is a marker of worse prognosis. Int J Cardiol 67:19-25, 1998.

85. Barretto ACP, Mady C, Oliveira SA, et al: Clinical meaning of ascites in patients with endomyocardial fibrosis. Arq Bras Cardiol 78:196-199, 2002.

86. Joshi R, Abraham S, Kumar AS: New approach for complete endocardiectomy in left ventricular endomyocardial fibrosis. J Thorac Cardiovasc Surg 125:40-42, 2003.

87. Moraes F, Lapa C, Hazin S, et al: Surgery for endomyocardial fibrosis revisited. Eur J Cardiothorac Surg 15:309-312, 1999.

88. Cherian SM, Jagannath BR, Nayar S, et al: Successful reoperation after 17 years in a case of endomyocardial fibrosis. Ann Thorac Surg 82:1115-1117, 2006.

89. Pedra SRFF, Smallhorn JF, Ryan G, et al: Fetal cardiomyopathies—Pathogenic mechanisms, hemodynamic findings, and clinical outcome. Circulation 106:585-591, 2002.

The Dilated, Restrictive, and Infiltrative Cardiomyopathies

90. Moller JE, Pellikka PA, Bernheim AM, et al: Prognosis of carcinoid heart disease—Analysis of 200 cases over two decades. Circulation 112:3320-3327, 2005.

91. Bastarrika G, Cao MG, Cano D, et al: Magnetic resonance imaging diagnosis of carcinoid heart disease. J Comput Assist Tomog 29:756-759, 2005.

92. Dalal D, Molin LH, Piccini J, et al: Clinical features of arrhythmogenic right ventricular dysplasia/cardiomyopathy associated with mutations in plakophilin-2. Circulation 113:1641-1649, 2006.

93. Dalal D, Nasir K, Bomma C, et al: Arrhythmogenic right ventricular dysplasia—A United States experience. Circulation 112:3823-3832, 2005.

CH 64

CHAPTER 65

Hypertrophic Cardiomyopathy

Barry J. Maron

Definition, Prevalence, and Nomenclature, 1763

Genetic Basis, 1763

Morphology, 1764
Left Ventricular Hypertrophy, 1764
Mitral Valve, 1765
Histopathology, 1765

Pathophysiology, 1766
Left Ventricular Outflow
  Obstruction, 1766
Myocardial Ischemia, 1767
Diastolic Dysfunction, 1767

**Family Screening
Strategies, 1767**

Clinical Features, 1767
Physical Examination Findings, 1767
Symptoms, 1767
Electrocardiographic Findings, 1768
Influence of Gender and Race, 1768

Athletes, 1768
Athlete's Heart and Hypertrophic
  Cardiomyopathy, 1768
Preparticipation Screening, 1768

Clinical Course, 1768
Natural History, 1768
Heart Failure, 1769
Risk Stratification and Sudden
  Cardiac Death, 1769

Management, 1770
Prevention of Sudden Death, 1770
Medical Treatment, 1770
Nonmedical Treatment, 1772
Other Management Issues, 1773

Future Directions, 1773

References, 1773

Hypertrophic cardiomyopathy (HCM), the most common of the genetic cardiovascular diseases, is caused by a multitude of mutations in genes encoding proteins of the cardiac sarcomere.[1-3] HCM is characterized by heterogeneous clinical expression, unique pathophysiology, and a diverse clinical course, including sudden cardiac death (SCD) in the young.[1,3,4] In addition, HCM may be responsible for heart failure–related disability at virtually any age.[5] Since the modern description of HCM almost 50 years ago, our understanding of the complexity and clinical spectrum of this disease has evolved dramatically. This chapter represents a contemporary summary of HCM with respect to diagnosis, natural history, and management.

DEFINITION, PREVALENCE, AND NOMENCLATURE

HCM is characterized by a thickened but nondilated left ventricle in the absence of another cardiac or systemic condition capable of producing the magnitude of hypertrophy evident (e.g., aortic valve stenosis, systemic hypertension, and some expressions of athlete's heart).[1-3] Several epidemiological studies have reported the prevalence of the HCM phenotype as about 0.2 percent in the general population (e.g., 1:500), inferring that there are 500,000 people with this disease in the United States.[1] This occurrence is far greater than previously thought and, given the uncommon presence of patients with HCM in general cardiology practice, suggests that most affected individuals may remain undiagnosed. HCM is a global disease, with most interest and reporting of cases from the United States and Canada, Western Europe, Israel, and Asia (Japan and China).[6]

Teare published the first modern report of this disease in 1958, in which he described "asymmetrical hypertrophy of the heart" as responsible for the sudden cardiac death of a small number of young people. Subsequently, the disease acquired a confusing array of names, all presumably describing the same clinical entity, and most have emphasized left ventricular (LV) outflow obstruction, a highly visible feature of the disease.[1,5] Thus, such names as idiopathic hypertrophic subaortic stenosis, hypertrophic obstructive cardiomyopathy, and muscular subaortic stenosis (as well as their acronyms, IHSS, HOCM, and MSS) were once widely used.[1,2] However, obstruction to LV outflow is not invariable (although common), and many patients have the nonobstructive form.[7] Hence, the preferred and generally accepted name for this condition is hypertrophic cardiomyopathy (HCM).[1,2]

GENETIC BASIS (see Chap. 10)

HCM is transmitted as a mendelian trait with an autosomal dominant pattern of inheritance.[1-3,8-11] Molecular studies, conducted intensively over more than a decade, have provided access to definitive laboratory-based diagnosis by detecting pathological disease-causing mutations (even without obvious clinical evidence of the disease), affording important insights into the broad clinical expression of HCM and genetic counseling, as well as promoting recognition of greater numbers of patients.

Eleven mutated sarcomeric genes are presently associated with HCM, most commonly beta-myosin heavy chain (the first identified) and myosin-binding protein C.[8-11] The other nine genes appear to account for far fewer cases and include troponin T and I, alpha-tropomyosin, regulatory and essential myosin light chains, titin, alpha-actin, alpha-myosin heavy chain, and muscle LIM protein (MLP). This intergenetic diversity is compounded by considerable intragenetic heterogeneity, with a number of different mutations identified in each gene (total, more than 400 individual mutations; www.cardiogenomics.med.harvard.edu). Characteristic diversity of the HCM phenotype (even within closely related family members) is likely attributable to the disease-causing mutations, as well as to the influence of modifier genes and environmental factors.[8] Neither the number of HCM genes nor disease-causing mutations is known and many others undoubtedly remain to be identified.

In addition, nonsarcomeric protein mutations in two genes involved in cardiac metabolism (e.g., gamma-2 regulatory subunit of the adenosine monophosphate [AMP]–activated protein kinase, *PRKAG2*, and lysosome-associated membrane protein 2, *LAMP-2*, Danon disease) are responsible for primary cardiac glycogen storage cardiomyopathies in older children and young adults, with a clinical presentation mimicking or indistinguishable from sarcomeric HCM and often associated with ventricular preexcitation.[12] A number of other diseases occurring largely in infants and children up to 4 years of age are associated with prominent thickening of the LV wall, which may resemble or mimic typical HCM caused by sarcomere protein mutations.[2] These cardiomyopathies most frequently include Noonan syndrome, an autosomal dominant cardiofacial condition associated with a variety of other cardiac defects (most commonly, dysplastic pulmonary valve stenosis and atrial septal defect) caused by mutations in *PTPN11*, a gene encoding the nonreceptor protein tyrosine phosphatase SHP-2 genes.[2]

MORPHOLOGY

Left Ventricular Hypertrophy

At necropsy, hearts from patients with HCM are usually increased in weight, often more than 500 gm. Because the LV cavity is characteristically small or normal in size, the greater LV mass is almost entirely the result of increased wall thickness[1-3] (Figs. 65-1 and 65-2). LV hypertrophy is both the gross anatomical marker and a major determinant of many important clinical features of the disease.

Clinical diagnosis of HCM is usually made with two-dimensional echocardiographic imaging.[1] Cardiac magnetic resonance imaging (CMR) has an expanding role in the noninvasive diagnosis of HCM by virtue of its high-resolution tomographic imaging capability.[13] CMR is complementary to echocardiography by clarifying technically ambiguous LV wall thicknesses or visualizing areas of segmental hypertrophy (specifically, in the anterolateral free wall; Fig. 65-3) or by delineating LV apical pathology, including hypertrophy and aneurysm formation, often not identifiable with echocardiography.[13]

Echocardiographic studies in large numbers of patients have defined the morphological features of the HCM phenotype, particularly its diversity with respect to the distribution and magnitude of LV wall thickening[1,3] (see Fig. 65-1). Even closely related relatives, with the same genetic substrate, usually show dissimilar phenotypes, with the exception of identical twins, in whom LV hypertrophy is morphologically identical.[13]

Asymmetrical patterns of hypertrophy are characteristic of this disease, in which one (or more) regions of the LV wall are of greater thickness than other areas, frequently with sharp transitions between contiguous segments. However, there is no single or "classic" morphologic form in HCM; virtually all possible patterns of LV hypertrophy have been reported, including genetically affected individuals with normal LV wall thicknesses.[3] Hypertrophy may frequently be diffuse and involve portions of both the ventricular septum and LV free wall, including some patients with the most marked hypertrophy observed in any cardiac disease, with wall thicknesses ranging up to 60 mm (see Fig. 65-1). Although such marked hypertrophy corresponds to the generally held perception of HCM as a condition characterized by substantial and diffuse hypertrophy, the disease phenotype in a considerable proportion of patients

CH 65

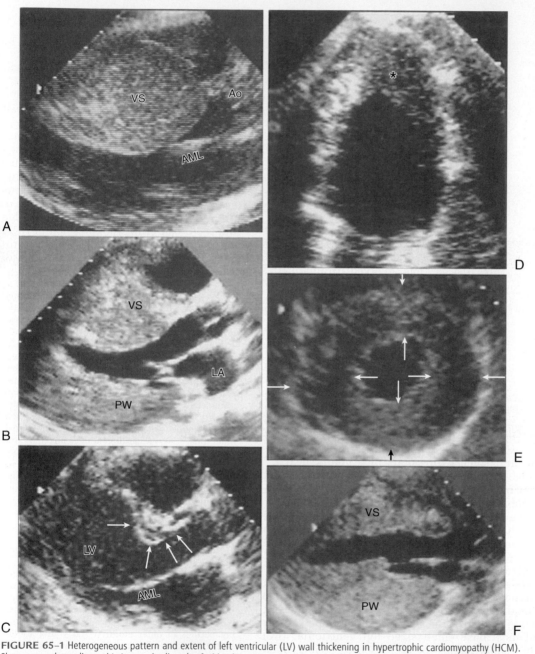

FIGURE 65–1 Heterogeneous pattern and extent of left ventricular (LV) wall thickening in hypertrophic cardiomyopathy (HCM). Shown are echocardiographic images in diastole. **A,** Massive asymmetrical hypertrophy of ventricular septum (VS) with thickness more than 50 mm. **B,** Septal hypertrophy with distal portion considerably thicker than proximal region. **C,** Hypertrophy confined to proximal septum just below aortic valve (arrows). **D,** Hypertrophy localized to left ventricular apex (asterisk)—that is, apical HCM. **E,** Relatively mild hypertrophy in concentric (symmetrical) pattern showing similar or identical thicknesses within each segment (paired arrows). **F,** Inverted pattern with posterior free wall (PW) thicker (40 mm) than anterior VS. Calibration marks = 1 cm. Ao = aorta; AML = anterior mitral leaflet; LA = left atrium. *(From Maron BJ, Casey SA, Poliac LC: Hypertrophic cardiomyopathy: A systematic review. JAMA 287:1308, 2002. With permission of the American Medical Association.)*

(40 percent) paradoxically shows relatively mild and localized hypertrophy of the LV wall, often confined to the basal anterior septum, but occasionally to the posterior (inferior) septum, anterolateral or posterior free wall, or apex. Segmental wall thickening confined to the most distal portion of LV chamber (apical HCM), is a morphological form often associated with a "spade" deformity of the left ventricle and marked T wave negativity on the electrocardiogram (ECG[14]; see Fig. 65-1). Consequently, it is possible for overall LV mass to be normal (or nearnormal) in many HCM patients when wall thickening is localized to only a small portion of the chamber.

LV hypertrophy commonly develops dynamically after a period of prolonged latency. Typically, the HCM phenotype may be incomplete until adolescence, when patients often show spontaneous and striking increases in wall thickness (i.e., average 100 percent change) and more widespread distribution of hypertrophy associated with accelerated growth and maturation. These structural changes, which may also occur later in midlife, are part of genetically predetermined remodeling and are not usually related to the development of symptoms or arrhythmic events. In genetically affected individuals, electrocardiographic abnormalities or subclinical diastolic dysfunction identified by Doppler tissue imaging may precede evidence of LV hypertrophy on the echocardiogram.[15] At present, there is no conclusive evidence that the right ventricle is often substantially involved in the cardiomyopathic process.

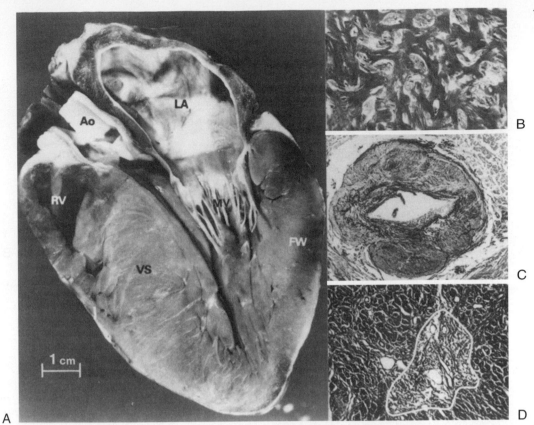

FIGURE 65–2 Morphological components of disease process in hypertrophic cardiomyopathy (HCM). **A,** Heart sectioned in cross-sectional long-axis plane. Left ventricular (LV) wall thickening is asymmetrical, confined primarily to the ventricular septum (VS), which bulges prominently into the small LV outflow tract. **B,** Septal myocardium shows greatly disorganized architecture with adjacent hypertrophied cardiac muscle cells arranged perpendicularly and obliquely. **C,** Intramural coronary artery with thickened wall, caused primarily by medial hypertrophy, and narrowed lumen. **D,** Area of replacement fibrosis in septum adjacent to abnormal intramural coronary artery. FW = left ventricular free wall; Ao = aorta; LA = left atrium; RV = right ventricle. (*From Maron BJ: Hypertrophic cardiomyopathy. Lancet 350:127, 1997. With permission.*)

Mitral Valve

Structural abnormalities of the mitral valve apparatus, including diverse alterations in valvular size and shape, are evident in two thirds of patients studied at necropsy or surgery and represent primary morphological features of HCM.[1,3] The mitral valve may be up to twice normal size because of elongation of both leaflets or segmental enlargement of either the anterior leaflet or the midportion of the posterior leaflet. An important subset of patients may have anomalous insertion of anterolateral papillary muscle directly into the anterior mitral leaflet, causing muscular midcavity obstruction.[1,3]

Histopathology

Cardiac muscle cells (myocytes) in the ventricular septum and LV free wall show increased transverse diameter and bizarre shapes, often maintaining intercellular connections with several adjacent cells.[1,3] Many myocytes (and myofibrils) are arranged in chaotic disorganized patterns, at oblique and perpendicular angles (see Fig. 65-2). Areas of disorganized cardiac muscle cells are evident in 95 percent of patients dying of HCM, usually occupying substantial portions of hypertrophied as well as nonhypertrophied LV myocardium, including 33 percent of the ventricular septum and 25 percent of the free wall.[1,3] Marked cellular disorganization present in infants with HCM suggests that this architectural abnormality may be present from birth.

Abnormal intramural coronary arteries with wall thickening (caused by increased intimal and medial components) and narrowed lumen are present in 80 percent of patients at necropsy, most frequently within or in close proximity to areas of replacement fibrosis[1,3] (see Fig. 65-2). This microvascular small vessel disease is responsible for clinically silent myocardial ischemia, myocyte death, and repair in the form of replacement scars, which may be transmural (see Fig. 65-2). In addition, volume of the interstitial (matrix) collagen compartment, constituting the structural LV framework, is greatly expanded. Matrix components (e.g., perimysial coils, pericellular weaves, struts) are increased in number, morphologically abnormal, and arranged in disorganized patterns.

It is likely that the disorganized architectural pattern and replacement scarring characteristic of LV myocardium in patients with HCM impair transmission of electrophysiological impulses and predispose to disordered patterns and increased dispersion of electrical depolarization and repolarization. This could serve as an electrically unstable

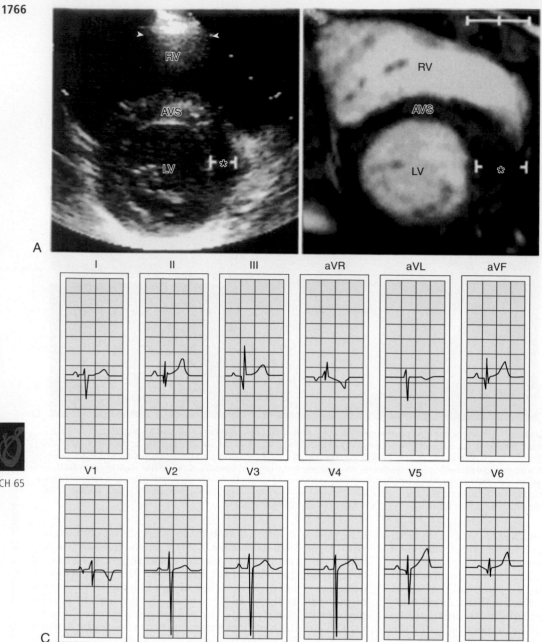

FIGURE 65–3 Diagnostic images from a 13-year-old identical twin with nonobstructive hypertrophic cardiomyopathy (HCM). Two-dimensional echocardiogram **(A)** and comparative cardiac magnetic resonance (CMR) **(B)** images in short-axis at end-diastole and 12-lead electrocardiogram (ECG) **(C)**. **A,** Normal echocardiographic thickness of all left ventricular (LV) wall segments, including anterolateral free wall (asterisk). **B,** CMR shows segmental hypertrophy confined to anterolateral LV free wall (20 mm) and small portion of contiguous anterior septum, not identified by echocardiography (asterisk). **C,** Abnormal ECG with Q waves in leads II, III, AVF, and V$_6$, deep S waves in right precordial leads, and diminished left precordial R waves. Calibration marks = 1 cm. RV = right ventricle; AVS = anterior ventricular septum. *(From Rickers C, Wilke NM, Jerosch-Herold M, et al: Utility of cardiac magnetic resonance imaging in the diagnosis of hypertrophic cardiomyopathy. Circulation 112:855, 2005. With permission of the American Heart Association.)*

CH 65

obstruction to specific risk for sudden cardiac death, usually in patients without significant heart failure symptoms, is weak.[5]

Subaortic obstruction in HCM represents true mechanical impedance to outflow, producing markedly increased intraventricular pressures, which may be detrimental to LV function, probably by increasing myocardial wall stress and oxygen demand.[1,5,16] In the vast majority of patients, obstruction is produced by systolic anterior motion (SAM) of the mitral valve and midsystolic contact with the ventricular septum. Characteristic of SAM, particularly in young patients, is abrupt anterior motion of the mitral valve, in which the elongated leaflets move toward the ventricular septum with a sharp-angled 90-degree bend. Magnitude of the outflow gradient can be reliably estimated with continuous-wave Doppler and is directly related to the duration of mitral valve–septum contact.

SAM is generated by (1) LV ejection producing a high-velocity jet, which streams through a narrowed outflow tract, pulling the mitral leaflets toward the septum (i.e., Venturi phenomenon) and/ or by (2) a drag effect—that is, hydrodynamic pushing force of flow directly on the leaflets. Mitral regurgitation, as a consequence of SAM, is posteriorly directed and is usually only mild to moderate in degree.[1] Severe mitral regurgitation in an HCM patient raises the possibility of an intrinsic mitral valve abnormality, such as myxomatous degeneration with mitral valve prolapse.

Subaortic gradients and systolic ejection murmurs in HCM are often dynamic, showing spontaneous variability.[1] Also, outflow gradient may be reduced or abolished by interventions that decrease myocardial contractility (e.g., beta-adrenergic blocking drugs) or increased ventricular volume or arterial pressure (e.g., squatting, isometric handgrip, phenylephrine). Alternatively, gradients can be augmented by circumstances in which arterial pressure or ventricular volume is reduced (e.g., Valsalva maneuver, nitroglycerin or amyl nitrite, blood loss or dehydration), or with increased contractility, such as premature ventricular contractions,

substrate and nidus for reentry ventricular tachyarrhythmias and sudden death.

PATHOPHYSIOLOGY

Left Ventricular Outflow Obstruction

Long-standing LV outflow tract obstruction under basal conditions (gradient, ≥30 mm Hg) is a determinant of HCM-related progressive heart failure symptoms and cardiovascular death[5,16] (Fig. 65-4). The relationship of

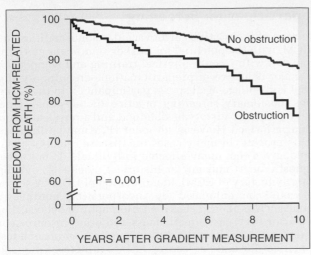

FIGURE 65–4 Left ventricular outflow tract obstruction. Probability of progression to severe heart failure (NYHA Class III or IV), or death from heart failure or stroke, in patients with LV outflow obstruction exceeds that in patients without obstruction (relative risk, 4.4; *P* < 0.001). Patients already in Class III or IV at study entry were excluded. HCM = hypertrophic cardiomyopathy. *(From Maron MS, Olivotto I, Betocchi S, et al: Effect of left ventricular outflow tract obstruction on clinical outcome in hypertrophic cardiomyopathy. N Engl J Med 348:295, 2003. With permission of the Massachusetts Medical Society.)*

isoproterenol, standing, or exercise. Consuming a heavy meal or a small amount of alcohol can also transiently increase the subaortic gradient.

A large proportion of HCM patients without SAM or outflow obstruction at rest may nevertheless generate outflow gradients with physiological exercise, whether or not symptoms are present.[7] Fully 70 percent of an unselected hospital-based HCM cohort have the propensity to develop an outflow gradient ≥30 mm Hg (and ≥50 mm Hg in the majority), either at rest or with exercise; only 30 percent of HCM patients have the true nonobstructive form.[7] Assessment of subaortic gradients with exercise echocardiography has an important role in the evaluation of those HCM patients without obstruction at rest.

Myocardial Ischemia

Regional myocardial ischemia, in the absence of coronary artery disease, commonly occurs in HCM as demonstrated by a dipyridamole stress ECG, atrial pacing, reversible exercise-induced thallium-201 perfusion defects, replacement fibrosis at autopsy, CMR delayed enhancement, and reduced myocardial blood flow in response to dipyridamole with positron emission tomography.[1] Potential mechanisms by which myocardial ischemia leads to replacement fibrosis include abnormalities of the microvasculature and inadequate capillary density with respect to greatly increased LV mass.

Diastolic Dysfunction

Abnormalities in LV relaxation and filling can be identified in about 80 percent of HCM patients, and presumably contribute to or are responsible for heart failure symptoms of exertional dyspnea, although not consistently related to the severity of LV hypertrophy.[1] The rapid filling phase is significantly prolonged and associated with decreased rate and volume of LV filling. In addition, there is usually (in sinus rhythm) a compensatory increase in the contribution of atrial systole to overall filling. Reduced ventricular compliance in HCM probably results largely from those factors

determining the passive elastic properties of the LV chamber, such as hypertrophy, replacement scarring, and interstitial fibrosis, as well as the disorganized cellular architecture. Difficulty in clinically measuring diastolic function represents an obstacle to defining its precise pathophysiological role in HCM patients; diastolic dysfunction is presumed to be the basic mechanism by which heart failure occurs in patients with nonobstructive HCM.

FAMILY SCREENING STRATEGIES

In clinical practice, prospective screening of family members for HCM usually takes place without access to DNA analysis and is performed primarily with two-dimensional echocardiography and 12-lead ECG, as well as history taking and physical examination. Recommended screening strategy calls for such evaluations on a 12- to 18-month basis, usually beginning by age 12.[17] If these studies do not show evidence of LV hypertrophy by the time full growth is achieved (18 to 21 years), it had been customary to conclude that a HCM-causing mutation is probably absent.

However, recognition that morphological conversions to the HCM phenotype can uncommonly occur later in adulthood has altered the practice of family screening and genetic counseling.[17] Consequently, because it is no longer possible to offer unequivocal reassurance that a normal echocardiogram obtained at maturity defines a genetically unaffected relative, it may be prudent to pursue the disease-causing mutation by genetic testing or extend clinical surveillance into adulthood at about 5-year intervals for adult phenotype–negative family members.[17]

CLINICAL FEATURES

Physical Examination Findings

Physical examination findings in patients with HCM are variable and related in large measure to the hemodynamic state. In patients with obstruction to LV outflow, a double or triple LV apical impulse may be palpable, reflecting the outward systolic thrust caused by ventricular contraction, a presystolic accentuated atrial contraction, and expansion of early diastolic filling.

Initial clinical suspicion of HCM is frequently triggered by recognition of a heart murmur on examination. Patients with obstruction have a medium-pitch systolic ejection murmur along the lower left sternal border and at the apex, which varies in intensity with the magnitude of the subaortic gradient, either at rest (supine or standing), with the Valsalva maneuver, or during and immediately following exercise. Most patients with loud murmurs of at least grade 3/6 have outflow gradients exceeding 30 mm Hg. The apical murmur may be holosystolic and characteristic of coexistent mitral regurgitation. Associated with LV outflow obstruction, arterial pulses are unusually sharp and rise rapidly, with a distinct bisferiens contour. Carotid pulse recordings are bifid, with a shortened upstroke time and prolonged systolic ejection. Conversely, physical findings in patients without outflow obstruction may be subtle; the systolic murmur is characteristically soft, although a forceful LV apical impulse may arouse suspicion of HCM.

Symptoms

Symptoms of heart failure in the presence of preserved LV function may become evident at any age, from young children to the elderly, consisting of exertional limitation caused by dyspnea and/or fatigue, and occasionally orthopnea or paroxysmal nocturnal dyspnea.[1,3] Such functional disability may be accompanied by chest pain, typical or atypical of midsternal angina pectoris, likely resulting from abnormalities of LV microvasculature and ischemia. Patients may also experience impaired consciousness with syncope (or near-syncope) or lightheadedness and palpitations caused by various mechanisms, including arrhythmias. The severity and nature of symptoms may be similar in patients with or without obstruction to LV outflow.[1]

Electrocardiographic Findings

The 12-lead ECG is abnormal in 90 to 95 percent of probands with HCM and in 75 percent of asymptomatic relatives.[1,3] ECGs show a wide variety of abnormal patterns, some of which may be distinctly bizarre, including increased voltages consistent with LV hypertrophy, ST-T changes including marked T wave inversion in the lateral precordial leads, left atrial enlargement, deep and narrow Q waves, and diminished R waves in the lateral precordial leads.[18] However, no particular electrocardiographic pattern is characteristic or predictive of future events. Normal ECGs are most common in asymptomatic family members, but do not provide reliable prognostic information regarding outcome. Increased voltages (tall R waves or deep S waves) are only weakly correlated with the magnitude of LV hypertrophy evident on echocardiogram and do not differentiate between obstructive and nonobstructive forms of the disease.[18]

Influence of Gender and Race

Transmitted as an autosomal dominant trait, HCM occurs with equal frequency in men and women.[8] However, women are underdiagnosed and achieve clinical recognition much less frequently, with more pronounced symptoms, and at older ages than men.[19] Furthermore, women show a higher risk for progression to advanced heart failure or death often associated with outflow obstruction; men and women do not differ regarding risk for sudden death or overall mortality.[19] Although HCM has been documented in many races,[1,6,14,20] it appears to be clinically underrecognized in African Americans. Most competitive athletes who die suddenly of HCM are previously undiagnosed African Americans.[20] Apical hypertrophy, as part of the broad HCM disease spectrum, is more common in but not limited to Japanese patients.[14]

ATHLETES

Athlete's Heart and Hypertrophic Cardiomyopathy

Long-term athletic training can produce physiologically increased LV diastolic cavity dimension, wall thickness, and calculated mass, known as "athlete's heart."[21] Absolute increases in wall thicknesses are usually modest, but may be more substantial in some trained individuals participating in the rowing and cycling sports. A diagnostic dilemma may arise in distinguishing clinically benign physiological hypertrophy as a consequence of athletic training from pathological conditions, such as HCM. Clinical parameters which support the diagnosis of HCM in trained athletes in the gray zone of overlap between the two conditions, with maximum LV wall thicknesses of 13 to 14 mm, include a disease-causing sarcomeric protein mutation identified by genetic testing, recognition of HCM in a relative, a transmitral Doppler waveform consistent with altered LV relaxation and filling, and LV end-diastolic cavity dimension less than 45 mm.[21] Parameters favoring physiological hypertrophy include regression of wall thickness following a short (4- to 6-week) period of deconditioning or enlarged LV cavity, greater than 55 mm.[21]

Preparticipation Screening

Detection of preexisting cardiovascular abnormalities such as HCM, with the potential for SCD or significant morbidity associated with intense physical training and competition, is a major objective of preparticipation screening for high school and college-aged sports participants.[21] In the United States, customary screening practice dictates that a personal and family history be obtained and a physical examination performed. However, although HCM may be diagnosed by this process, in many cases the disease remains unsuspected, given that many affected individuals do not have a diagnostic heart murmur or historical clues (e.g., syncope or family history of HCM). Identification of HCM by screening would be enhanced by incorporating noninvasive testing, such as 12-lead electrocardiography or echocardiography. However, cost-effectiveness and other resource considerations probably make routine application of such tests impractical for mass screening of U.S. athletes. Frequency of borderline and false-positive test results (and the uncertainty that accompanies such circumstances), as well as the possibility that the HCM phenotype may not always be detectable with echocardiography prior to age 16, represent additional limitations to high school screening.

CLINICAL COURSE

Natural History

HCM is a unique cardiovascular disease with the potential for clinical presentation during any phase of life, from infancy to old age (birth to >90 years).[1-3] Patients at the extremes of this age range appear to have the same genetic defects and basic disease process, although not necessarily the same natural history, as other patients.[1,9-11] Over the last decade, greater clarity and understanding have emerged regarding the overall clinical course of HCM. In community-based patient populations, uncontaminated by tertiary center referral bias (and more representative of the true disease state) overall HCM-related mortality rates of about 1 percent/year have been reported (Fig. 65-5), although somewhat higher in children (i.e., 2 percent/year).[1,3] Annual mortality rates of 3 to 6 percent derived from highly selected cohorts at major referral centers (incorporating substantial patient referral bias) were skewed toward high-risk patients and are no longer relevant to the contemporary patient population.[1,3]

The clinical course is typically variable, and patients may remain stable over long periods of time, with up to 25 percent of a hospital-based HCM cohort achieving normal life expectancy with little or no disability, and without the necessity for major therapeutic interventions.[1,3] HCM in adults (particularly older than 50) does not add to overall total mortality beyond that expected for the general population, underscoring that many patients deserve reassurance regarding their prognosis (see Fig. 65-5).[1,3,7,18]

However, subgroups at higher risk for important disease complications and premature death reside within a HCM patient population. Many patients proceed along specific adverse pathways, punctuated by clinical events that ultimately dictate treatment strategies[1,3-5,16,22-25] (Fig. 65-6): (1) premature sudden and unexpected death, most commonly in adolescents and young adults; (2) progressive symptoms of heart failure with exertional dyspnea and functional limitation (often accompanied by chest pain) in the presence of preserved LV systolic function; (3) advanced heart failure (end-stage phase) characterized by systolic dysfunction and LV remodeling; and (4) complications attributable to atrial fibrillation (AF), such as embolic stroke and heart

CH 65

failure. However, predicting clinical course and outcome for individual patients with HCM is encumbered by its markedly diverse disease expression and the long period of potential risk for young patients.[1,2]

Heart Failure

Whereas some degree of heart failure is frequent in HCM, progression to severe functional limitation (i.e., New York Heart Association [NYHA] Class III or IV) is uncommon, occurring in 10 to 15 percent of the overall patient population.[1,3,5,16,22,26-28] Principal determinants of progressive heart failure, with preserved LV systolic function, appear to be LV outflow obstruction and AF or, in some cases, diastolic dysfunction. Marked increase in left atrial size (transverse dimension $\geq$50 mm)[26] and microvascular dysfunction evident by positron-emission tomography[27] have also been reported to predict long-term outcome and heart failure death. In contrast to the risk for sudden death in HCM, which bears a linear relationship to increasing magnitude of LV hypertrophy, greater LV wall thickness is not associated with the likelihood of developing severe heart failure.[28] Cardiac events are unusual in the first decade of life, and HCM is a rare cause of severe heart failure in infants or very young children; such a clinical presentation is an unfavorable prognostic sign.[1,3]

About 3 percent of HCM patients manifest the end stage of HCM characterized by systolic dysfunction, with an ejection fraction of less than 50 percent, in which progressive heart failure (and often AF) are associated with heterogeneous patterns of LV remodeling, most commonly wall thinning and/or cavity dilation.[22] The clinical course is unpredictable, but the frequency of progression to refractory heart failure, heart transplantation, and sudden death is substantial (11 percent/year). The most reliable risk marker for evolution to the end stage is a family history of the end stage.[22]

Risk Stratification and Sudden Cardiac Death

SCD in HCM may occur at a wide range of ages, but most commonly during adolescence and young adulthood, less than 30 to 35 years of age.[1,3,4] Events are arrhythmia-based, caused by primary ventricular tachycardia (VT) or ventricular fibrillation (VF), with a predilection for the early morning hours.[1,3] SCD is often the initial clinical manifestation in asymptomatic individuals, many of whom had not been diagnosed during life. While most patients who die suddenly do so associated with sedentary or modest physical activity, an important proportion of such events is associated with vigorous exertion.[4]

HCM is the most common cause of SCD in young people, including competitive athletes[1,3,4] (Fig. 65-7). This observation is the basis for the standard and prudent recommendation to disqualify young athletes with HCM from intense competitive sports to reduce their risk for sudden death, under the guidelines of Bethesda Conference 36.[29] At present, the greatest risk for sudden death appears to be associated with one of the following clinical markers[1,3,23-25,30,31] (Fig. 65-8): (1) for secondary prevention, prior cardiac arrest or sustained ventricular tachycardia; and for primary prevention—(2) family history of one or more premature HCM-related deaths, particularly if sudden and multiple; (3)

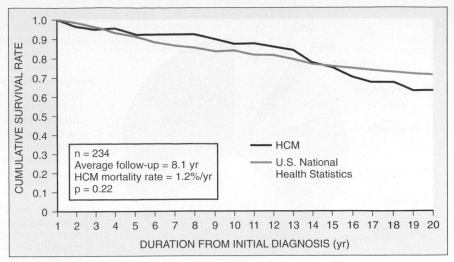

FIGURE 65–5 Cumulative survival in a community-based adult hypertrophic cardiomyopathy (HCM) population. Total mortality in 234 HCM patients (1 percent/year) does not differ significantly from that expected in the general U.S. population after adjustment for age, gender, and race. (From Maron BJ, Casey SA, Poliac LC, et al: Clinical course of hypertrophic cardiomyopathy in a regional United States cohort. JAMA 281:650, 1999. With permission of the American Medical Association.)

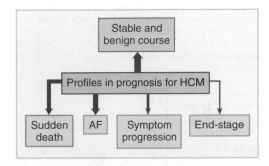

FIGURE 65–6 Principal pathways of disease progression in hypertrophic cardiomyopathy (HCM). Widths of respective arrows approximate the frequency of occurrence in an HCM population. AF = atrial fibrillation. (From Maron BJ, McKenna WJ, Danielson GK, et al: American College of Cardiology/European Society of Cardiology Clinical Expert Consensus Document on Hypertrophic Cardiomyopathy. J Am Coll Cardiol 42:1687, 2003. With permission of the American College of Cardiology.)

CH 65

syncope, especially in the young and related to exertion; (4) hypotensive or attenuated blood pressure response to exercise; (5) multiple, repetitive (or prolonged) nonsustained ventricular tachycardia on serial ambulatory (Holter) monitoring; and (6) massive LV hypertrophy (wall thickness, $\geq$30 mm), most relevant to young patients. In contrast, mild degrees of LV hypertrophy are generally associated with lower or negligible risk for SCD or disease progression.[23]

Other high-risk subgroups have also emerged within the heterogeneous HCM disease spectrum, including the following: LV apical aneurysm associated with regional myocardial scarring and monomorphic ventricular tachycardia; end-stage phase with systolic dysfunction; and, in some patients, following percutaneous alcohol septal ablation with transmural infarction.[22,32-34] Although the subaortic gradient ($\geq$30 mm Hg at rest) is a determinant of progressive heart failure and death, the specific relationship to SCD is weak and insufficient to regard obstruction as a primary HCM risk marker.[5]

Elderly patients are not usually targeted for risk stratification, given that HCM-related SCD is uncommon in this age group and survival to advanced age (without overt disease manifestations) itself generally declares lower risk

Hypertrophic Cardiomyopathy

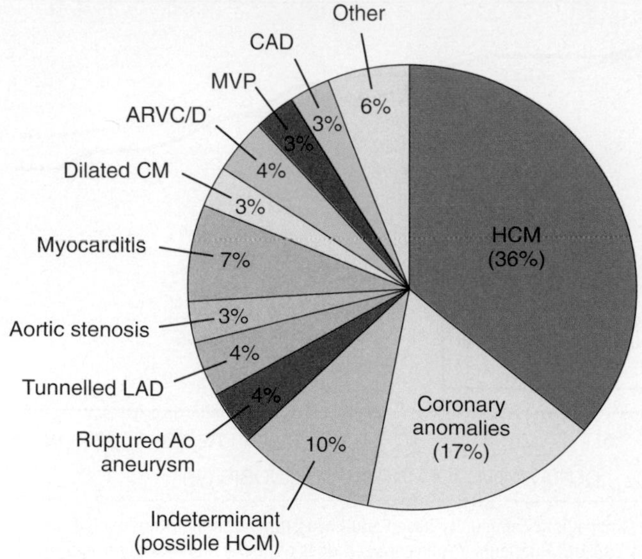

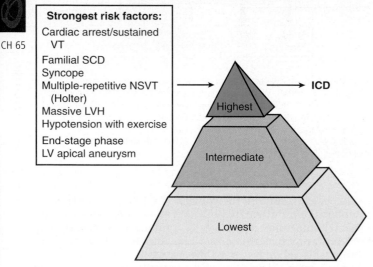

FIGURE 65–7 Causes of sudden cardiac death in young competitive athletes, with hypertrophic cardiomyopathy (HCM) being the most common. Ao = aorta; LAD = left anterior descending coronary artery; CM = cardiomyopathy; ARVC/D = arrhythmogenic right ventricular cardiomyopathy/dysplasia; MVP = mitral valve prolapse; CAD = coronary artery disease. *(From Maron BJ, Thompson PD, Puffer JC, et al: Cardiovascular preparticipation screening of competitive athletes. A statement for health professionals from the Sudden Death Committee [clinical cardiology] and Congenital Cardiac Defects Committee [cardiovascular disease in the young], American Heart Association. Circulation 94:850, 1996. With permission of the American Heart Association.)*

Strongest risk factors:

Cardiac arrest/sustained VT

Familial SCD

Syncope

Multiple-repetitive NSVT (Holter)

Massive LVH

Hypotension with exercise

End-stage phase

LV apical aneurysm

ICD

Highest

Intermediate

Lowest

FIGURE 65–8 Clinical parameters that identify high-risk status for sudden cardiac death (SCD) in hypertrophic cardiomyopathy (HCM). One or more of the risk factors justifies consideration for an implantable cardioverter-defibrillator (ICD) in the context of primary or secondary prevention. LV = left ventricular; LVH = left ventricular hypertrophy; NSVT = nonsustained ventricular tachycardia; VT = ventricular tachycardia. *(From Maron BJ, Estes NAM III, Maron MS, et al: Primary prevention of sudden death as a novel treatment strategy in hypertrophic cardiomyopathy. Circulation 107:2872, 2003. With permission of the American Heart Association.)*

status. It is also acknowledged that the current risk stratification algorithm is probably incomplete, and some HCM patients without any of the accepted primary prevention risk factors may be at risk for SCD.

It has been proposed that certain mutations responsible for HCM could represent prognostic markers conveying a favorable or adverse outcome, including the risk for SCD

(see Chap. 10).[8] For example, early genotype-phenotype studies identified certain beta-myosin heavy chain and troponin T mutations to be associated with a higher frequency of premature death compared with other mutations, such as those involving myosin-binding protein C or alpha-tropomyosin. More recently, the prognostic significance of disease-causing mutations in HCM for risk stratification and decision-making in the clinical management of individual patients has been questioned.[35] The prognosis attached to adult gene carriers without LV hypertrophy appears to be benign. There is no evidence to justify routinely precluding such individuals from most activities or employment opportunities.

Although the intramuscular course of the proximal left anterior descending coronary artery segment (i.e., myocardial bridging, tunneled coronary artery) has been proposed as a risk factor for SCD, its significance in HCM remains unresolved.[36] In addition, there is little or no role for conventional laboratory electrophysiological testing with programmed ventricular stimulation to segregate high- from low-risk patients. Such arrhythmias provoked in the laboratory are generally regarded as nonspecific electrophysiological responses to multiple ventricular extrastimuli, and are highly dependent on the level of aggression in the protocol.[1,3] The vulnerable electrophysiological substrate for reentrant arrhythmias in HCM has also been investigated by an extrastimulus-based method that assesses paced electrogram fractionation, which reflects asynchronous delayed activation and the disrupted myocardial architecture in this disease.[37]

MANAGEMENT

Prevention of Sudden Death

The implantable cardioverter-defibrillator (ICD) has proven effective and reliable in patients with HCM by aborting potentially lethal ventricular tachyarrhythmias, both for secondary prevention with implantation after cardiac arrest (11 percent/year), or as primary (prophylactic) prevention in the presence of one or more risk factors (4 percent/year).[38] Patients judged to be at high risk for sudden death based on traditional risk factor analysis deserve consideration for the prevention of SCD with the ICD.[31,38]

Prophylactic, empirical pharmacological treatment with amiodarone (or beta blockers or verapamil) for asymptomatic high-risk patients to reduce SCD risk is now an obsolete strategy, abandoned largely because of lack of evidence for efficacy and the emergence of the ICD as an effective preventive therapy.[1] Furthermore, antiarrhythmic treatment with amiodarone is probably unrealistic, given the likelihood of important side effects over the long risk period involved with young patients.[1,38] For primary prevention patients the number of risk factors is unrelated to the likelihood that an appropriate device intervention will interrupt VT or VF. A substantial proportion of patients with prophylactic ICDs experiencing such life-saving therapy (35 percent) have only one risk marker.[38] Noteworthy in HCM is the extended time period that may elapse between the clinical decision to implant an ICD and the moment at which the device terminates a highly unpredictable ventricular tachyarrhythmia. In HCM, there appears to be virtually no risk for catastrophe associated with the implantation procedure itself.[38]

Medical Treatment (Fig. 65-9)

HEART FAILURE. HCM patients manifest heart failure symptoms within one of two clinical profiles, largely requiring different therapeutic strategies. The more usual circumstance is characterized by exertional dyspnea and fatigue, indicative of elevated pulmonary venous pressures, in the presence of normal or hyperdynamic systolic function. Such symptoms are related to diastolic dysfunction, outflow tract obstruction or microvascular myocardial ischemia, or combinations of these pathophysiological variables. Response of heart failure symptoms to medical treatment is highly variable and is often empirically tailored to the requirements of individual patients. Since the mid-1960s, various beta-adrenergic receptor blocking drugs have been used extensively to relieve and control symptoms of heart failure in patients with obstructive or nonobstructive HCM.[1] Long-acting preparations of propranolol, atenolol, metoprolol, or nadolol are now commonly used. Beta blockers improve symptoms by slowing heart rate and reducing the force of LV contraction, thus augmenting ventricular filling and relaxation, and by decreasing myocardial oxygen consumption. By inhibiting sympathetic stimulation of the heart, beta blockers have the potential to blunt the outflow gradient triggered under physiologic exercise conditions.

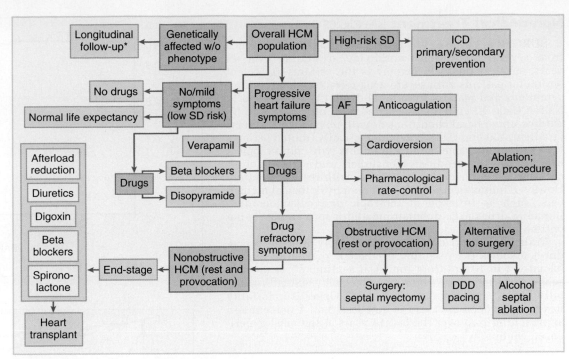

FIGURE 65–9 Clinical presentation and treatment strategies for patient subgroups within the broad hypertrophic cardiomyopathy (HCM) clinical spectrum. *No specific treatment or intervention indicated, except under exceptional circumstances. AF = atrial fibrillation; DDD = dual-chamber; ICD = implanted cardioverter-defibrillator; SD = sudden death. *(From Maron BJ, McKenna WJ, Danielson GK, et al: American College of Cardiology/European Society of Cardiology Clinical Expert Consensus Document on Hypertrophic Cardiomyopathy. J Am Coll Cardiol 42:1687, 2003. With permission of the American College of Cardiology.)*

Verapamil improves symptoms and exercise capacity, largely in patients without marked obstruction to LV outflow, because of its beneficial effect on ventricular relaxation and filling.[1] However, some patients with both greatly elevated pulmonary venous pressures and marked obstruction may be susceptible to pulmonary edema and sudden death while taking verapamil. Disopyramide may be initiated as a third option (in combination with a beta blocker) to ameliorate symptoms, when other drugs fail to achieve control, and does not appear to be proarrhythmic in HCM.[39] Diuretic agents can be administered judiciously, either alone or in conjunction with beta blockers or verapamil, to reduce pulmonary congestion, LV filling pressures, and symptoms.

In HCM, medical treatment is usually initiated with beta blockers or verapamil, although either drug may be administered first. There is no evidence that combining these drugs is advantageous, and together they may excessively lower heart rate and/or blood pressure.

Therapeutic strategies for patients with end-stage LV systolic dysfunction are similar to those employed for congestive heart failure in other cardiac diseases and may include the administration of beta blockers, angiotensin-converting enzyme (ACE) inhibitors or angiotensin receptor blockers, and diuretics, or possibly digoxin, spironolactone, as well as warfarin.[22] The end stage represents a risk factor for SCD and a potential indication for a prophylactic ICD as a bridge to heart transplantation.[22]

Plasma brain natriuretic peptide (BNP) levels are independently related to the magnitude of heart failure symptoms in HCM.[40] However, the BNP level has limited clinical value as a biomarker for heart failure in this disease because of substantial overlap among patients with different symptom levels, as well as confounding variables such as increased LV wall thickness and age.

ATRIAL FIBRILLATION. The most common sustained arrhythmia in HCM is AF, which frequently accounts for unexpected hospital admissions and lost productivity, and often requires aggressive therapeutic intervention.[1,3] Paroxysmal episodes or chronic AF occurs in 20 percent of HCM patients, increasing in incidence with age, and linked to enlargement of the left atrium.[41] AF is reasonably well-tolerated by about one third of patients and has not proved to be an independent determinant of SCD in this disease.[41] Of note, AF is associated with embolic stroke (incidence, 1 percent/year; prevalence, 6 percent), progressive heart failure, disability, and sometimes death, particularly when associated with outflow obstruction at rest or with arrhythmia onset at younger than 50 years of age.[41]

Paroxysmal AF may occasionally be responsible for acute clinical decompensation, requiring emergent electrical or pharmacological cardioversion. Although data in HCM patients are limited, amiodarone is considered most effective in reducing AF recurrences. With chronic AF, beta blockers and verapamil will usually control heart rate; atrioventricular (AV) node ablation and permanent ventricular pacing are rarely required. Because of the potential for clot formation and embolization, anticoagulant therapy with warfarin is indicated in AF patients. Because only one or two paroxysms of AF have been associated with risk for systemic thromboembolism in HCM, the threshold for initiation of anticoagulant therapy is low.[1,41] However, such clinical decisions should be tailored to individual patients after considering obligatory life-style modifications, risk of hemorrhagic complications, and expectations for compliance. Some success in treating refractory AF complicating HCM has been reported in a small number of patients with the surgical maze procedure and by catheter ablation with pulmonary vein isolation.[42]

SURGERY. Based on the uniformly excellent experience from several institutions worldwide, extending over 45 years, surgical septal myectomy is the primary treatment option for patients with severe drug-refractory heart failure symptoms and marked functional disability (equivalent to NYHA Class III and IV), associated with obstruction to LV outflow under basal conditions or with physiologic exercise (gradient, ≥50 mm Hg).[43-45] Symptomatically limited patients with only provocable outflow gradients (with physiological exercise) are also candidates for surgery and achieve a clinical benefit similar to that of patients with rest obstruction. However, inducing gradients with nonphysiological maneuvers, such as infusion of inotropic and catecholamine-inducing drugs (e.g., dobutamine and isoproterenol) is not optimal practice.

Transaortic ventricular septal myectomy (Morrow procedure) involves the resection of a small portion of muscle (usually 2 to 10 gm) from the basal septum.[1,3,43] Some surgeons perform a more aggressive myectomy, extending distally in the septum for about 7 cm.[44,45] Operative mortality has steadily decreased and is now less than 1 percent and approaching zero over the last 12 years at the most experienced centers.[45]

The primary objective of surgical septal myectomy is reduction in heart failure symptoms and improved quality of life by relieving outflow obstruction. Indeed, 95 percent of patients undergoing myectomy experience permanent abolition or substantial reduction in the basal outflow gradient, without compromise in global LV function.[43-45] Long-term follow-up studies have reported relief of symptoms in 85 percent of patients over periods up to 25 years, with a 10-year postoperative survival of 83 percent.[43,44] There is no evidence that myectomy predisposes patients to the end-stage phase with systolic dysfunction and LV remodeling. Extensive experience with septal myectomy has substantiated that obstructive HCM represents a mechanical and surgically reversible form of heart failure.

In addition, there is evidence that myectomy beneficially alters the clinical course of HCM. Operated patients achieve long-term survival equivalent to that expected in the general population and superior to nonoperated HCM patients with outflow obstruction, as well as reduction in SCD risk[44] (Fig. 65-10). Surgical myectomy is not recommended for asymptomatic (or mildly symptomatic) patients, nor is there conclusive evidence that prophylactic surgical relief of obstruction conveys a long-term clinical benefit in quality of life and survival. However, as a matter of practice, symptomatic young children with obstructive HCM have customarily undergone septal myectomy at levels of functional limitation less than NYHA Class III.

Occasionally, patients demonstrate outflow obstruction from a mechanism other than SAM, in which anomalous papillary muscle insertion directly into the anterior mitral leaflet (without interposition of chordae tendineae) produces muscular midventricular obstruction.[1,3] Distally extended myectomy is the preferred strategy for relief of muscular obstruction resulting from this congenital malformation of the mitral apparatus.[44,45]

DUAL-CHAMBER PACING. Fifteen years ago, permanent dual-chamber pacing was promoted as an alternative to myectomy for obstructive HCM patients with severe refractory symptoms. However, several randomized studies demonstrated that subjectively perceived symptomatic benefit from pacing is not accompanied by objective evidence of improved exercise capacity and appears mainly to represent a placebo effect.[1,3] Although reduction in subaortic gradient may occur in some patients with pacing, this benefit is usually modest and inconsistent, particularly compared with that achieved by myectomy.[1] Although selected older patients (over 65 years) may benefit from pacing, the role for this treatment modality in HCM has become particularly limited.[1,3]

ALCOHOL SEPTAL ABLATION. The recently introduced modality of percutaneous alcohol septal ablation has

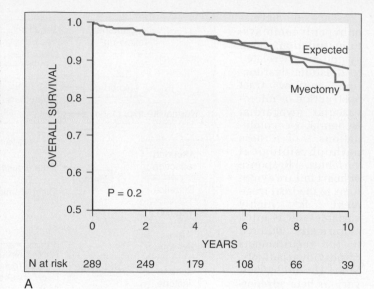

A

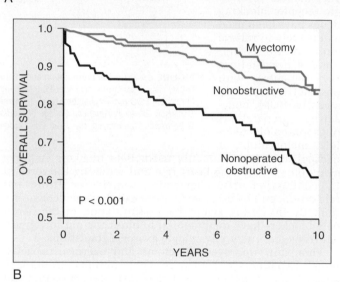

B

FIGURE 65–10 Long-term survival following surgical septal myectomy. **A,** Survival free from all-cause mortality after myectomy for obstructive hypertrophic cardiomyopathy (HCM) (*N* = 289) compared with age- and gender-matched U.S. population. **B,** Survival free from all-cause mortality in three HCM patient subgroups—surgical myectomy (*n* = 289), nonoperated with obstruction (*n* = 228), and nonobstructive (*n* = 820). Overall log rank and myectomy versus nonoperated obstructive HCM, *P* < 0.001. *(From Ommen SR, Maron BJ, Olivotto I, et al: Long-term effects of surgical septal myectomy on survival in patients with obstructive hypertrophic cardiomyopathy. J Am Coll Cardiol 46:470, 2005. With permission of the American College of Cardiology.)*

experienced rapidly increasing popularity.[33,46-50] With this procedure, 1 to 3 ml of 96 to 98 percent alcohol is introduced into a major septal perforator coronary artery to create necrosis and permanent myocardial infarction in the proximal septum. This scarring leads to progressive thinning and restricted excursion of the ventricular septum, outflow tract enlargement, and ultimately to reduction of subaortic obstruction and mitral regurgitation, thereby mimicking the LV remodeling that results from surgical myectomy.[33,46-50]

Alcohol ablation may substantially reduce LV outflow tract gradient and heart failure symptoms in many patients, although follow-up is necessarily short (average, 2 to 3 years) compared with myectomy (up to 45 years).[46-50] Nonrandomized comparative data analyses have shown gradient reduction produced by alcohol ablation to be similar although somewhat less consistent and complete than with myec-

CH 65

tomy[33,46,50]; about 20 percent of patients may require repeated alcohol ablations because of an unsatisfactory hemodynamic and symptomatic result following the first procedure.[45]

Because percutaneous septal ablation has been perceived to be less invasive and more accessible than surgical myectomy, its penetration into cardiological practice has been so extensive as to raise the possibility that the threshold for ablation has been lowered (with respect to severity of symptoms and obstruction).[1,33] Indeed, an American College of Cardiology/European Society of Cardiology expert consensus panel[1] has recommended surgical septal myectomy as the primary management option for patients with severe refractory symptoms and marked outflow obstruction. Alcohol ablation is regarded as an alternative treatment strategy for selected patients—that is, those of particularly advanced age, with significant comorbidity and increased operative risk, without access to expert surgical centers, or strongly adverse to surgical intervention.[1]

However, long-term issues remain unresolved, most prominently the clinical significance of the alcohol-induced transmural scar (occupying about 10 percent of the LV wall), which represents a potentially unstable arrhythmogenic substrate that could raise the risk for SCD in some patients.[32,34,45,49] Reported procedural mortality for alcohol septal ablation at experienced centers (2 percent) is slightly higher than for surgery at HCM referral institutions.[45] For several practical reasons, it is unlikely that a randomized myectomy versus ablation trial will be carried out to resolve these issues.

Other Management Issues

PREGNANCY. There is no evidence that HCM patients are at increased risk during pregnancy and delivery. Maternal mortality is particularly rare and confined to the very small subset of women with high-risk clinical profiles.[51] Such patients should be afforded specialized, preventive obstetrical care. Otherwise, most HCM patients can undergo normal vaginal delivery, without necessity for cesarean section, but with the possible exception of those with marked outflow obstruction.

BACTERIAL ENDOCARDITIS. This is an uncommon complication of HCM (prevalence, less than 1 percent) and virtually confined to patients with the obstructive form. Vegetations most commonly involve the anterior mitral leaflet or septal endocardium at the site of mitral valve–septum contact. For bacterial endocarditis prevention, standard antimicrobial prophylaxis according to American Heart Association recommendations is indicated prior to dental or surgical procedures.

FUTURE DIRECTIONS

The last decade has witnessed substantial understanding of the diagnosis, clinical profile, natural history, and management of HCM. Future clinical directions will include the development of more precise risk stratification strategies to identify those patients at unacceptably high risk for sudden death more accurately and deserving of consideration for implantable defibrillator therapy. Also, there will be a continuing effort to define the most appropriate role for alcohol septal ablation as an alternative to surgical septal myectomy in the management of severely symptomatic drug-refractory patients with outflow obstruction. Finally, the identification of other disease-causing mutations responsible for HCM will enhance the sensitivity of DNA-based laboratory diagnosis.

REFERENCES

Definition and Prevalence

1. Maron BJ, McKenna WJ, Danielson GK, et al: American College of Cardiology/European Society of Cardiology Clinical Expert Consensus Document on Hypertrophic Cardiomyopathy. J Am Coll Cardiol 42:1687, 2003.

2. Maron BJ, Towbin JA, Thiene G, et al: Contemporary definitions and classification of the cardiomyopathies. An American Heart Association Scientific Statement. Circulation 113:1807, 2006.

3. Maron BJ: Hypertrophic cardiomyopathy: A systematic review. JAMA 287:1308, 2002.

4. Maron BJ: Sudden death in young athletes. N Engl J Med 349:1064, 2003.

5. Maron MS, Olivotto I, Betocchi S, et al: Effect of left ventricular outflow tract obstruction on clinical outcome in hypertrophic cardiomyopathy. N Engl J Med 348:295, 2003.

6. Zou Y, Song L, Wang Z, et al: Prevalence of idiopathic hypertrophic cardiomyopathy in China: A population-based echocardiographic analysis of 8080 adults. Am J Med 116:14, 2004.

7. Maron MS, Olivotto I, Zenovich AG, et al: Hypertrophic cardiomyopathy is predominantly a disease of left ventricular outflow tract obstruction; Circulation 114:216, 2006.

Genetics and Pathophysiology

8. Seidman JG, Seidman CE: The genetic basis for cardiomyopathy: From mutation identification to mechanistic paradigms. Cell 104:557, 2001.

9. Niimura H, Patton KK, McKenna WJ, et al: Sarcomere protein gene mutations in hypertrophic cardiomyopathy of the elderly. Circulation 105:446, 2002.

10. Richard P, Charron P, Carrier L, et al: Hypertrophic cardiomyopathy. Distribution of disease genes, spectrum of mutations, and implications for a molecular diagnosis strategy. Circulation 107:2227, 2003.

11. Arad M, Penas-Lado M, Monserrat L, et al: Gene mutations in apical hypertrophic cardiomyopathy. Circulation 112:2805, 2005.

12. Arad M, Maron BJ, Gorham JM, et al: Glycogen storage diseases presenting as hypertrophic cardiomyopathy. N Engl J Med 352:362, 2005.

13. Rickers C, Wilke NM, Jerosch-Herold M, et al: Utility of cardiac magnetic resonance imaging in the diagnosis of hypertrophic cardiomyopathy. Circulation 112:855, 2005.

14. Kitaoka H, Doi Y, Casey SA, et al: Comparison of prevalence of apical hypertrophic cardiomyopathy in Japan and the United States. Am J Cardiol 92:1183, 2003.

15. Ho CY, Sweitzer NK, McDonough B, et al: Assessment of diastolic function with Doppler tissue imaging to predict genotype in preclinical hypertrophic cardiomyopathy. Circulation 105:2992, 2002.

16. Kofflard MJ, ten Cate FJ, van der Lee C, van Domburg RT: Hypertrophic cardiomyopathy in a large community-based population: Clinical outcome and identification of risk factors for sudden cardiac death and clinical deterioration. J Am Coll Cardiol 41:987, 2003.

17. Maron BJ, Seidman JG, Seidman CE: Proposal for contemporary screening strategies in families with hypertrophic cardiomyopathy. J Am Coll Cardiol 44:2125-2132, 2004.

18. Montgomery JV, Harris KM, Casey SA, et al: Relation of electrocardiographic patterns to phenotypic expression and clinical outcome in hypertrophic cardiomyopathy. Am J Cardiol 96:270, 2005.

19. Olivotto I, Maron MS, Adabag AS, et al: Gender-related differences in the clinical presentation and outcome of hypertrophic cardiomyopathy. J Am Coll Cardiol 46:480, 2005.

20. Maron BJ, Carney KP, Lever HM, et al: Relationship of race to sudden cardiac death in competitive athletes with hypertrophic cardiomyopathy. J Am Coll Cardiol 41:974, 2003.

21. Maron BJ, Pelliccia A: The heart of trained athletes: Cardiac remodeling and the risks of sports including sudden death. Circulation 114;1633, 2006.

22. Harris KM, Spirito P, Maron MS, et al: Prevalence, clinical profile and significance of left ventricular remodeling in the end-stage phase of hypertrophic cardiomyopathy. Circulation 114;216, 2006.

23. Spirito P, Bellone P, Harris KM, et al: Magnitude of left ventricular hypertrophy predicts the risk of sudden death in hypertrophic cardiomyopathy. N Engl J Med 342:1778, 2000.

24. Monserrat L, Elliott PM, Gimeno JR, et al: Nonsustained ventricular tachycardia in hypertrophic cardiomyopathy: An independent marker of sudden death risk in young patients. J Am Coll Cardiol 42:873, 2003.

25. Elliott PM, Gimeno B, Mahon NG, et al: Relation between severity of left ventricular hypertrophy and prognosis in patients with hypertrophic cardiomyopathy. Lancet 357:420, 2001.

26. Nistri S, Olivotto I, Betocchi S, et al: Prognostic significance of left atrial size in patients with hypertrophic cardiomyopathy (from the Italian Registry for Hypertrophic Cardiomyopathy). Am J Cardiol 98:960, 2006.

27. Cecchi F, Olivotto I, Gistri R, et al: Coronary microvascular dysfunction and prognosis in hypertrophic cardiomyopathy. N Engl J Med 349:1027, 2003.

28. Maron MS, Zenovich AG, Casey SA, et al: Significance and relationship between magnitude of left ventricular hypertrophy and heart failure symptoms in hypertrophic cardiomyopathy. Am J Cardiol 95:1329, 2005.

29. Maron BJ, Zipes DP: Introduction: Eligibility recommendations for competitive athletes with cardiovascular abnormalities—general considerations. J Am Coll Cardiol 45:1318, 2005.

30. Adabag AS, Casey SA, Kuskowski MA, et al: Spectrum and prognostic significance of arrhythmias on ambulatory Holter electrocardiogram in hypertrophic cardiomyopathy. J Am Coll Cardiol 45:697, 2005.

31. Maron BJ, Estes NAM III, Maron MS, et al: Primary prevention of sudden death as a novel treatment strategy in hypertrophic cardiomyopathy. Circulation 107:2872, 2003.

32. Boltwood CM Jr, Chien W, Ports T: Ventricular tachycardia complicating alcohol septal ablation. N Engl J Med 351:1914, 2004.

CH 65

33. Kimmelstiel CD, Maron BJ: Role of percutaneous septal ablation in hypertrophic obstructive cardiomyopathy. Circulation 109:452, 2004.

34. Simon RD, Crawford FA 3rd, Spencer WH 3rd, Gold MR: Sustained ventricular tachycardia following alcohol septal ablation for hypertrophic cardiomyopathy. PACE 28:1354, 2005.

35. Ackerman MJ, Van Driest SL, Ommen SR, et al: Prevalence and age dependence of malignant mutations in the beta-myosin heavy chain and troponin T genes in hypertrophic cardiomyopathy: a comprehensive outpatient perspective. J Am Coll Cardiol 39:2042, 2002.

36. Sorajja P, Ommen SR, Nishimura RA, et al: Myocardial bridging in adult patients with hypertrophic cardiomyopathy. J Am Coll Cardiol 42:889, 2003.

37. Saumarez RC, Chojnowska L, Derksen R, et al: Sudden death in noncoronary heart disease is associated with delayed paced ventricular activation. Circulation 107:2595, 2003.

Management

38. Maron BJ, Shen W-K, Link MS, et al: Efficacy of implantable cardioverter-defibrillators for the prevention of sudden death in patients with hypertrophic cardiomyopathy. N Engl J Med 342:365, 2000.

39. Sherrid MV, Barac I, McKenna WJ, et al: Multicenter study of the efficacy and safety of disopyramide in obstructive hypertrophic cardiomyopathy. J Am Coll Cardiol 45:1251, 2005.

40. Maron BJ, Tholakanahalli VN, Casey SA, et al: Usefulness of B-type natriuretic peptide assay in the assessment of symptomatic state in hypertrophic cardiomyopathy. Circulation 109:984, 2004.

41. Olivotto I, Cecchi F, Casey SA, et al: Impact of atrial fibrillation on the clinical course of hypertrophic cardiomyopathy. Circulation 104:2517, 2001.

42. Kilicaslan F, Verma A, Saad E, et al: Efficacy of catheter ablation of atrial fibrillation in patients with hypertrophic obstructive cardiomyopathy. Heart Rhythm 3:275, 2006.

43. Woo A, Williams WG, Choi R, et al: Clinical and echocardiographic determinants of long-term survival following surgical myectomy in obstructive hypertrophic cardiomyopathy. Circulation 111:2033, 2005.

44. Ommen SR, Maron BJ, Olivotto I, et al: Long-term effects of surgical septal myectomy on survival in patients with obstructive hypertrophic cardiomyopathy. J Am Coll Cardiol 46:470, 2005.

45. Maron BJ, Dearani JA, Ommen SR, et al: The case for surgery in obstructive hypertrophic cardiomyopathy. J Am Coll Cardiol 44:2044, 2004.

46. Firoozi S, Elliott PM, Sharma S, et al: Septal myotomy-myectomy and transcoronary septal alcohol ablation in hypertrophic obstructive cardiomyopathy. A comparison of clinical, haemodynamic and exercise outcomes. Eur Heart J 23:1617, 2002.

47. Kuhn H, Seggewiss H, Geitzen FH, et al: Catheter-based therapy for hypertrophic obstructive cardiomyopathy. First in-hospital outcome analysis of the German TASH Registry. Z Cardiol 93:23, 2004.

48. Faber L, Seggewiss H, Welge D, et al: Echo-guided percutaneous septal ablation for symptomatic hypertrophic obstructive cardiomyopathy: 7 years of experience. Eur J Echocardiogr 5:347, 2004.

49. Valeti US, Nishimura RA, Holmes DR, et al: Comparison of surgical septal myectomy and alcohol septal ablation by cardiac magnetic resonance imaging in patients with hypertrophic obstructive cardiomyopathy. J Am Coll Cardiol 49:350, 2007.

50. Qin JX, Shiota T, Lever HM, et al: Outcome of patients with hypertrophic obstructive cardiomyopathy after percutaneous transluminal septal myocardial ablation and septal myectomy surgery. J Am Coll Cardiol 38:1994, 2001.

51. Autore C, Conte MR, Pinccininno M, et al: Risk associated with pregnancy in hypertrophic cardiomyopathy. J Am Coll Cardiol 40:1864, 2002.

CHAPTER 66

Myocarditis

Peter P. Liu and Heinz-Peter Schultheiss

Definition and Incidence, 1775
Myocarditis, 1775
Dilated Cardiomyopathy, 1775

Epidemiology, 1776

Specific Etiological Agents, 1776
Viruses, 1776
Bacteria, 1778
Protozoal Infections, 1779
Metazoal Myocardial Diseases, 1780
Hypersensitivity Reactions—Vaccines and Drugs, 1780
Physical Agents, 1781

Pathophysiology, 1781
Viral Entry, 1781
Immune Activation and Viral Persistence, 1782
Innate Immunity, 1782
Acquired Immunity, 1783
Cardiac Remodeling, 1784

Clinical Presentation, 1784
Acute Myocarditis, 1784
Fulminant Myocarditis, 1784
Giant Cell Myocarditis, 1784
Chronic Active Myocarditis, 1784

Diagnostic Approaches, 1785
Clinical Symptoms, 1785
Laboratory Testing, 1785
Cardiac Magnetic Resonance Imaging, 1786
Myocardial Biopsy, 1787

Prognosis, 1787

Therapeutic Approaches, 1788
Supportive Therapy, 1788
Immunosuppression, 1789
Interferon, 1789
Intravenous Immunoglobulin, 1790
Immune Adsorption Therapy, 1790
Immune Modulation, 1790
Hemodynamic Support, 1790
Vaccination, 1791

Future Perspectives, 1791

References, 1791

Myocarditis is defined as "inflammation of the heart muscle." The most common causes today are infectious agents such as viruses or parasites or autoimmune conditions. True cases of viral myocarditis are likely more common than currently diagnosed, largely because of its protean manifestations and reliance on myocardial biopsies for pathological confirmation. The availability of new diagnostic modalities such as cardiac magnetic resonance (CMR) imaging will help to increase the appropriate identification of suspected cases. New molecular tools to identify viral genome from cardiac tissues also help in defining the appropriate etiology.

The pathogenesis of myocarditis is a classic paradigm of cardiac injury, followed by immunological response from the host as cardiac inflammation. The relative incidence of viral etiologies is continuously evolving as new diagnostic tools based on molecular epidemiology become available. Just as important, if the host immune response is overwhelming or inappropriate, the inflammation may destroy the heart tissue acutely or lingers and produces cardiac remodeling leading to dilated cardiomyopathy, heart failure, or death. For the appropriate diagnosis of myocarditis, a heightened clinical suspicion is required. Composite diagnostic criteria are also evolving. Fortunately for the majority of patients, clinical myocarditis is often self-limited if proper support and follow-up are available. A general rule of thumb for the prognosis of viral myocarditis is that one third will recover, one third will remain with some degree of cardiac dysfunction, and the final one third will deteriorate and require intensive therapy including transplantation. Because of the high incidence of ultimate recovery, aggressive therapy including ventricular assist is indicated for patients with severe hemodynamic compromise. With the evolution of new understanding of pathophysiology and new therapies for this condition, the outlook for myocarditis is continuing to improve.

classic myocarditis refers to inflammation of the heart muscle as a result of exposure to either discrete external antigens such as viruses, bacteria, parasites, and drugs or internal triggers such as autoimmune activation against self-antigens.[1] The classic Dallas criteria for the pathological diagnosis of myocarditis require the presence of inflammatory cells simultaneously with evidence of myocyte necrosis on the same microscopic section when examining a myocardial biopsy. Borderline myocarditis is characterized by inflammatory cell infiltrate without myocardial necrosis (Fig. 66-1).[2] However, the Dallas criteria have been criticized for being overly restrictive and not easily reproducible. A broader definition including the presence of viral genome or molecular markers of immune activation has since evolved, but consensus has not yet been achieved on these additional measures.[3]

Not surprisingly, then, the precise incidence of myocarditis is difficult to ascertain, depending on inclusion and diagnostic criteria applied. One estimate has been about 8 to 10 per 100,000 of the population. However, because of failure to make the appropriate diagnosis or failure to detect subclinical cases, many deaths caused by myocarditis may go unrecognized. Therefore the prevalence of myocarditis among unselected autopsy series is as high as 1 to 5 per 100. Recent pathological series examining young adults who had suffered sudden deaths suggested an even higher incidence of myocarditis ($\approx$8.6 percent).[4] When patients with only idiopathic dilated cardiomyopathy are considered, myocarditis accounts for 10 to 40 percent of the cases overall.[5] This suggests that clinical myocarditis is not clinically suspected in a large number of cases, leading to deaths or severe heart failure.

DEFINITION AND INCIDENCE

Myocarditis

Myocarditis broadly refers to inflammation of the heart muscle. Inflammation can be found after any form of injury to the heart including ischemic damage, me-chanical trauma, and genetic cardiomyopathies. However,

Dilated Cardiomyopathy

(see also Chap. 64)

Dilated cardiomyopathy refers to disorders of the heart muscle associated with an increased internal diameter of the left ventricular (LV) chamber. This generally

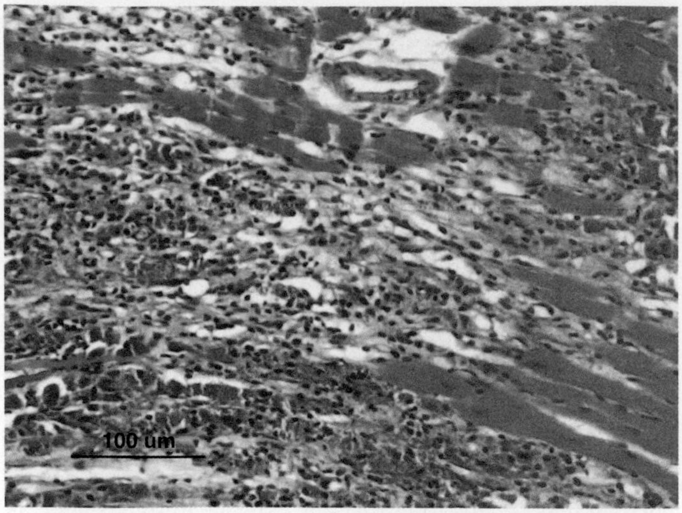

FIGURE 66–1 Myocardial biopsy section under high power. This section is diagnostic of myocarditis by the Dallas criteria. The Dallas criteria require the presence of a lymphocyte-rich inflammatory infiltrate associated with myocyte degeneration or necrosis in the same view (hematoxylin and eosin stain). However, the Dallas criteria is viewed as overly conservative, in view of the patchy nature of the inflammatory foci, and less than ideal reproducibility.

includes cardiac dysfunction *not* associated with overt ischemic heart disease. About one third of dilated cardiomyopathy can be attributed to single gene mutations involving cytoskeletal defects such as actin, dystrophin complex, plakoglobin, or laminin. Myocarditis may also be an antecedent event leading to dilated cardiomyopathy with ventricular dilation as a consequence of inflammation-induced myocyte loss and interstitial fibrosis.

Viruses such as Coxsackie virus can also elaborate proteases that directly modify the cytoskeleton components such as the dystrophin complex in the heart, leading to ventricular dilation.[6] Dilated cardiomyopathy is associated with relatively poor prognosis and is one of the commonest indications for cardiac transplantation worldwide.

EPIDEMIOLOGY

Myocarditis has been more often a diagnosis of exclusion, rather than a specific diagnosis. However, the incidence of myocarditis is increasing, with the advent of newer molecular diagnostic techniques in place of the absolute requirement of inflammatory cell infiltrates on myocardial biopsy. For example, a recent biopsy series from Schultheiss and colleagues in Germany demonstrated that a significant proportion of patients presenting with classical myocarditis showed only the presence of viral genome on myocardial biopsy, rather than classic inflammatory cell infiltrates required by the Dallas criteria.[7,8] Their series of 245 patients with dilated cardiomyopathy demonstrated a viral positivity using polymerase chain reaction (PCR) technique in 67 percent of patients, and surprisingly none of these biopsies had inflammatory infiltrates in the myocardium that would have qualified for the Dallas criteria of myocarditis.[7,8]

Meanwhile, the increasing prevalence of human immunodeficiency virus (HIV) infection with the improved survival of patients with acquired immunodeficiency syndrome (AIDS) introduced the new condition of HIV-associated myocarditis (see also Chap. 67). The latter condition is associated with poor prognosis and is likely related to both the HIV infection and multiple comorbidities in these patients.[9]

Changing Etiology and Divergent Geographical Distribution

The etiological agents accounting for myocarditis has changed not only temporally, but also geographically around the globe. Previously the commonest etiological agents globally have been enteroviruses, with Coxsackie viruses predominating. However, more recent series have indicated that the traditional dominance of Coxsackie viruses has been replaced by a broader spectrum of viral etiologies including adenoviruses, parvoviruses, and cytomegaloviruses. A distinct viral profile is also evolving in different regions of the globe.

In Europe Kuhl and Schultheiss' recent series of biopsies from 245 patients with dilated cardiomyopathy found that 51.4 percent of the biopsies tested positively for parvovirus B19, 21.6 percent for human herpesvirus-6, 9.4 percent for enterovirus, and 1.6 percent for adenovirus.[7] Interestingly, 27.3 percent had evidence of multiple infections.

In contrast, Bowles and Towbin[10] analyzed biopsies from 624 patients with PCR and found overall viral positivity was 38 percent (or 239/624). On analysis, 22.8 percent tested positive for adenovirus and 13.6 percent tested positive for enterovirus. Only 1 percent tested positive for parvovirus. This group of patients was younger, resided mainly in North America, and certainly showed a distinct viral etiological profile (Fig. 66-2). Meanwhile, in Japan the incidence of hepatitis C virus (HCV) infection in the heart, particularly related to a hypertrophic cardiomyopathy, dominated the etiological profile. Both HCV antibodies and genome have been detected in the serum and myocardial biopsies of patients with myocarditis.[11]

Globally, a common cause of dilated cardiomyopathy in the third world is still Chagas disease, an inflammatory myocarditis caused by the parasite *Trypanosoma cruzii*. Therefore there are major regional differences in the etiological profile of myocarditis, showing the footprints of genetic and environmental interaction. Some of these differences may be caused by differences in the prevalence of these viruses in the local population, but others may be caused by differences of definition and inclusion criteria.

SPECIFIC ETIOLOGICAL AGENTS

Myocarditis most commonly results from an external inflammatory trigger such as a virus, inducing a host immune response that may range from minimally transient response to fulminant, overwhelming inflammation. Characterization of the etiological triggers has benefited significantly from molecular tools such as PCR amplification or in situ hybridization to detect external agents such as viral genome. These techniques have shown that the viral genome may persist in the myocardium for variable periods of time, with or without the accompaniment of an inflammatory cell infiltrate.

Recent series of molecular analysis in patients with suspected myocarditis have confirmed that indeed viruses are the most common etiological agents associated with the condition (Table 66-1). Meta-analysis of PCR studies in patients who had heart biopsies with clinically suspected myocarditis or cardiomyopathy demonstrated an odds ratio of 3.8 for viral presence when compared with control patients. The persistence of viral genome in the myocardium is also associated with progressive ventricular dysfunction and worse outcome during follow-up.[12]

Viruses

Enteroviruses Including Coxsackie Viruses

The most common etiological agent for viral myocarditis has traditionally been the enteroviruses, single-stranded

RNA viruses that include the Coxsackie virus and echoviruses. Because Coxsackie viruses have also infected susceptible strains of mice, they are also the model system on which the current understanding of pathophysiology of viral myocarditis in humans is based.

Current evidence suggests that Coxsackie viruses enter the host gastrointestinal or respiratory system using the coxsackie-adenoviral receptor (CAR) for cell entry. The latter is a junctional protein important for cell–cell communication and is critical for internalization of the virus.[13,14] CAR localization is particularly concentrated in the cardiovascular, immune, and neurological systems. Utilization of the CAR receptor for viral entry also triggers the host immune activation through its associated receptor tyrosine kinases, leading to the subsequent inflammatory response. The virus is usually cleared from the host by the immune system in 1 to 2 weeks; however, in some instances, the virus genome can persist in the host myocardium for 6 months or longer, constituting a nidus for chronic inflammatory response and a known risk factor for worse prognosis.

More recent series of myocarditic patients have demonstrated a decrease in the prevalence of enteroviruses as etiological agents, particularly in Western Europe. This could be related to the development of herd immunity after a period of prolonged exposure, leading to a temporary decrease in the prevalence of infections in the community.

Adenovirus

Adenovirus is a deoxyribonucleic acid (DNA) virus that commonly infects the human mucosal surface, particularly in the pediatric population. Adenoviruses also use the CAR (shared with Coxsackie virus) and integrin receptor to gain entry into cells. Adenoviral infections can be much more virulent than Coxsackie viruses and can cause extensive cell deaths without comparable inflammatory response. The immunological profile associated with adenovirus is different from that found with enterovirus, with markedly decreased CD2, CD3, and cD45RO T-lymphocyte counts in those with the adenoviral genome present in the myocardium.[15]

Parvovirus

A new entry in the epidemiology of myocarditis is the parvovirus B19 family of viruses. Parvoviruses are single-stranded DNA viruses that cause common childhood infections such as the fever and exanthem seen in "fifth disease."[16] However, in a recent biopsy series from Europe, parvovirus B19 genome has been found in more than 51 percent of the patients with dilated cardiomyopathy.[7] Questions have been raised about whether this is mere association, contamination, or truly causal. Cases of myocarditis or

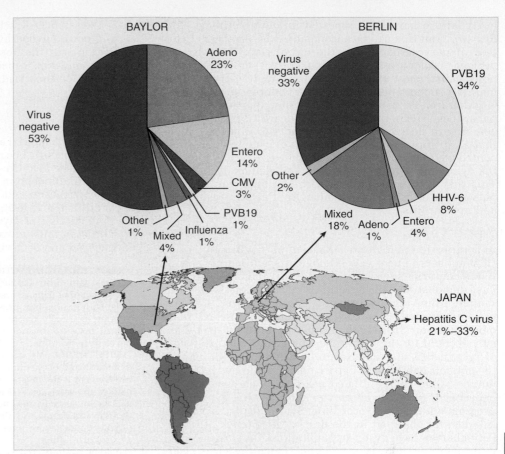

FIGURE 66–2 The viral etiological profiles differ in different parts of the world. European biopsy series (from Berlin, $N = 245$) show the dominance of parvovirus B19 (PVB19), herpesvirus (HHV), and enteroviruses (Entero).[7] On the other hand, North American biopsy series (from Baylor, $N = 624$) showed dominance of adenovirus (Adeno), enterovirus, and very few parvoviruses.[10] Japanese series, on the other hand ($N = 61$), show a dominance of hepatitis C virus, partly caused by the high prevalence of hepatitis C infection in the population.[69] CMV = cytomegalovirus; mixed = two or more different viral genomes detected in the same biopsy.

TABLE 66–1	Etiological Agents Causing Myocarditis
Viral (Most Common) Adenovirus Coxsackie virus/Enterovirus Cytomegalovirus Parvovirus B19 Hepatitis C virus Influenza Human immunodeficiency virus Herpes virus Epstein-Barr virus Mixed infections **Bacterial** Mycobacterial species *Chlamydia pneumoniae* Streptococcal species *Mycoplasma pneumoniae* *Treponema pallidum* **Fungal** Aspergillus Candida Coccidioides Cryptococcus Histoplasma **Protozoal** *Trypanosoma cruzi*	**Parasitic** Schistosomiasis Larva migrans **Toxins** Anthracyclines Cocaine **Hypersensitivity** Clozapine Sulfonamides Cephalosporins Penicillins Tricyclic antidepressants **Autoimmune Activation** Smallpox vaccination Giant cell myocarditis Churg-Strauss syndrome Sjögren syndrome Inflammatory bowel disease Celiac disease Sarcoidosis Systemic lupus erythematosus Takayasu arteritis Wegener granulomatosis

heart failure have been reported following clinical "fifth disease," and this can be accompanied by persistent detection of parvovirus B19 in the circulation. Patients with parvovirus myocarditis are frequently symptomatic with nonspecific chest pain, and interestingly parvovirus is mainly resident and trophic in the endothelial cells of the vasculature. Persistent viral infection, particularly with parvovirus B19, in patients with myocarditis has been associated with decreased flow-mediated vasodilation.[17] Endothelial dysfunction from the parvovirus infection may contribute to local inflammation and vasospasm, producing the symptoms of chest pain and ventricular dysfunction. This may also be consistent with the high prevalence of parvovirus infection in patients with diastolic dysfunction and myocarditis.[8]

Hepatitis C Virus

In contrast to the high prevalence of parvovirus in Europe, HCV appears to be a new etiological agent mainly seen in Asian countries such as Japan.[11] Myocardial biopsy samples have demonstrated the hepatitis C viral genome, with serum samples showing confirmatory antibody rise in those patients affected. Hepatitis C infection is also overall much more prevalent in Asia than other parts of the world and may account for the higher detection rates. The phenotype of myocarditis also appears to be different, with many of the patients exhibiting a hypertrophic cardiomyopathy phenotype rather than a dilated heart. This may suggest that hepatitis C directly alters the growth and hypertrophy program within the myocardium. Symptomatic myocarditis is generally observed in the first to third week of illness. Patients may have dyspnea, palpitations, and anginal chest pain; fatalities have been reported. Once the virus clears, the heart has been reported to return to normal function and morphology.

Human Immunodeficiency Virus

With improved survival in patients with HIV infections, the presence of ventricular dysfunction and associated myocarditis is also increasing in prevalence (see also Chap. 67). From histological analysis of postmortem cases infected with HIV, 14 of 21 patients (67 percent) had criteria for myocarditis, and this increased to 83 percent in another study concentrating on high-risk patients. In asymptomatic patients with HIV infection the annual incidence of progression to dilated cardiomyopathy has been estimated at 15.9 cases per 1000 individuals.[9] Often it is impossible to determine the precise cause of the ventricular dysfunction in a given patient because it may be attributable to the HIV infection itself, immunological dysregulation, side effects of antiretroviral treatment, opportunistic coinfection or comorbid conditions, or a combination of any of these factors.

Influenza

During epidemics, 5 to 10 percent of infected patients may experience cardiac symptoms. The presence of preexisting cardiovascular disease greatly increases the risk of morbidity and mortality.[18] Cardiac involvement typically occurs within 4 days to 2 weeks of the onset of the illness. Death may be associated with massive hemorrhagic pulmonary edema caused by viral or bacterial involvement of the lungs.

Mixed Viral Infections

Another interesting new finding is the presence of mixed or multiple etiological agents from a single myocardial biopsy using multiplexed molecular detection tools. It appears that multiple viruses can enhance each others' virulence in a given host by cooperating as coinfections. This may occur for both Coxsackie viruses and adenoviruses because they share the same CAR, which can be upregulated in the presence of cardiomyopathy.[19] Conversely, this may also be an indication that the host's immune system is incapable of clearing multiple types of viruses because of a genetic defect, which then leads to worse ventricular function and outcome.[12]

Bacteria

Virtually any bacterial agent can cause myocardial dysfunction. This occurs because of activation of inflammatory mediators (see also Chap. 22) through specific interactions with toll-like receptors 2 and 4, bacterial invasion, microabscess formation, and toxins elaborated by the pathogen. Other clinical manifestations of the infection mask or delay the appreciation of myocardial involvement. Accordingly, the clinician must always be alert for cardiac involvement during systemic bacterial infections.

CLOSTRIDIAL INFECTION. Cardiac involvement is common in patients with clostridial infections with multiple organ involvement. The myocardial damage results from the toxin elaborated by the bacteria, with gas bubbles present in the myocardium. An inflammatory infiltrate is usually absent. *Clostridium perfringens* may cause myocardial abscess formation with myocardial perforation and resultant purulent pericarditis.

DIPHTHERIA. Myocardial involvement is a serious complication of diphtheria and occurs in up to one half of cases. Indeed, myocardial involvement is the most common cause of death in this infection and half of the fatal cases demonstrate cardiac involvement.[20] Cardiac damage is caused by the liberation of a toxin that inhibits protein synthesis by interfering with the transfer of amino acids from soluble RNA to polypeptide chains under construction. The toxin appears to have a particular affinity for the cardiac conducting system. Antitoxin should be administered as rapidly as possible. Antibiotic therapy is of less urgency. The development of complete atrioventricular block is an ominous complication, and mortality is high despite insertion of a transvenous pacemaker.

STREPTOCOCCAL INFECTION. The most commonly detected cardiac finding after beta-hemolytic streptococcal infection is acute rheumatic fever. Involvement of the heart by the streptococcus may produce a myocarditis that is distinct from acute rheumatic carditis. It is characterized by an interstitial infiltrate composed of mononuclear cells with occasional polymorphonuclear leukocytes, and the infiltrate may be focal or diffuse. Electrocardiographic abnormalities including prolongation of the PR and QT intervals occur frequently. Rarely this may result in sudden death, conduction disturbances, and arrhythmias.

TUBERCULOSIS. Involvement of the myocardium by *Mycobacterium tuberculosis* (not tuberculous pericarditis) is rare. Tuberculous involvement of the myocardium occurs by means of hematogenous or lymphatic spread or directly from contiguous structures and may cause nodular, miliary, or diffuse infiltrative disease.[21] On occasion, it may lead to arrhythmias including atrial fibrillation and ventricular tachycardia, complete atrioventricular block, heart failure, LV aneurysms, and sudden death.

WHIPPLE DISEASE Although overt involvement is rare, intestinal lipodystrophy, or Whipple disease, is not uncommonly associated with cardiac involvement. Periodic acid–Schiff–positive macrophages can be found in the myocardium, pericardium, coronary arteries, and heart valves of patients with this disorder. Electron microscopy has demonstrated rod-shaped structures in the myocardium similar to those found in the small intestine, representing the causative agent of the disease, *Tropheryma whippelii*, a gram-negative bacilli related to the actinomycetes.[22] An associated inflammatory infiltrate and foci of fibrosis may be present. The valvular fibrosis may be severe enough to result in aortic regurgitation and mitral stenosis. Although usually asymptomatic, nonspecific electrocardiographic changes are most common; systolic murmurs, pericarditis, complete heart block, and even overt congestive heart failure may occur. Antibiotic therapy appears to be effective in treating the basic disease, but relapses can occur, often more than 2 years after initial diagnosis.

Spirochetal Infections—Lyme Carditis

Lyme disease is caused by a tickborne spirochete (*Borrelia burgdorferi*). It usually begins during the summer months with a characteristic rash (erythema chronicum migrans), followed by acute neurological, joint, or cardiac involvement, and usually little long-term sequelae.[23] About 10 percent of patients with Lyme disease develop evidence of transient cardiac involvement, the most common manifestation being variable degrees of atrioventricular block. Syncope caused by complete heart block is frequent with cardiac involvement because often there is an associated depression of ventricular escape rhythms. Diffuse ST segment and T wave abnormalities are transient and usually asymptomatic. A positive gallium scan is compatible with cardiac involvement, and the demonstration of spirochetes in myocardial biopsies of patients with Lyme carditis suggests a direct cardiac effect. Patients with second-degree or complete heart block should be hospitalized and undergo continuous electrocardiographic monitoring. Temporary transvenous pacing may be required for a week or longer in patients with high-grade block. Although the efficacy of antibiotics is not established, clinicians routinely use antibiotics in patients with Lyme carditis. Intravenous antibiotics are suggested, although oral antibiotics can be used when there is only mild cardiac involvement. It is thought that treating the early manifestations of the disease will prevent development of late complications.

Protozoal Infections

Chagas Disease

Chagas disease is still one of the commonest causes of dilated cardiomyopathy worldwide. The World Health Organization estimates that there are 18 million infected cases worldwide and that 5 million people will develop symptomatic disease.[24] The causative organism is the protozoa *Trypanosome cruzii*, spread by arthropods as the vector in endemic regions in the world, most notably in South America (Fig. 66-3). Organs other than the heart may also be involved. The parasite incites an intense acquired T-lymphocyte–mediated inflammatory response in the host, akin to viral myocarditis, leading to extensive scarring and remodeling of the myocardium, resulting in Chagastic cardiomyopathy. Treatment is most effective during the acute phase of the

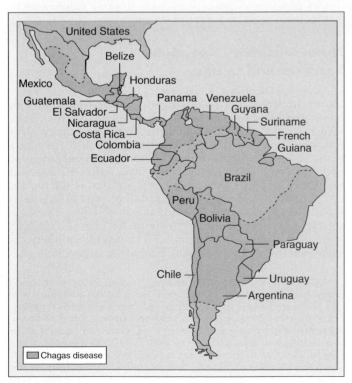

FIGURE 66–3 Distribution of Chagas disease in the Americas. *(Modified from Acquatella H: Chagas' disease. In Abelmann WH, Braunwald E (eds): Atlas of Heart Disease. Cardiomyopathies, Myocarditis, and Pericardial Disease. Philadelphia, Current Medicine, 1995, pp 8.1-8.18.)*

disease. Ultimately, prevention through public health measures will be most cost effective.

The natural history of Chagas disease is characterized by three phases: acute, latent, and chronic. During the acute phase, the disease is transmitted to humans (usually younger than 20 years of age) through the bite of a reduviid bug (subfamily Triatominae), which harbors the parasite in its gastrointestinal tract. Acute trypanosomiasis occurs after inoculation by the protozoa and is symptomatic in only 10 percent of the patients, yet this phase can also be fatal in 10 percent of patients.[25] Pathological examination during the acute phase often reveals parasites in the cardiac fibers with a marked cellular infiltrate, particularly around cardiac cells that have ruptured and released the parasites. Involvement may extend into the endocardium, resulting in thrombus formation, and into the epicardium, resulting in pericardial effusion. The pathogenesis of the myocardial lesions of acute Chagas disease appears to relate in large part to immune lysis by antibody and cell-mediated immunity directed against antigens released from *T. cruzi*–infected cells.

Clinical manifestations of acute trypanosomiasis include fever, muscle pains, sweating, hepatosplenomegaly, myocarditis with congestive heart failure, pericardial effusion, and, occasionally, meningoencephalitis. Most patients recover, even though young children most frequently develop clinical acute disease and can be seriously ill.

Latent trypanosomiasis follows the acute stage and is generally asymptomatic. Electrocardiographic changes often appear during the latent stage and are a marker for the eventual clinical heart failure and increased mortality. A progressive cardiomyopathy may develop in about 30 percent of the infected patients. In the advanced chronic stage of the disease, cardiac dilation typically involves all the cardiac chambers, although right-sided enlargement may predominate.[26] Pathological examination reveals lesions of the cardiac nerves, compatible with parasympathetic denervation. Cardiac enlargement with hypertrophy of all cardiac chambers also occurs. In more than half of patients the ventricular apex is thin and bulging, resembling an aneurysm. Thrombus formation is frequent and may fill much of the apex and, at times, the right atrium.

Clinical manifestations include anginal chest pain, heart failure (predominantly right-sided), conducting system disease, and sudden death. On examination, tricuspid regurgitation is often present. The S2 is widely split, often with an accentuated pulmonic component, reflecting the combined effects of right bundle branch block and pulmonary hypertension. Autonomic dysfunction is common. Deaths result from pump failure or sudden arrhythmias. The chest radiograph often demonstrates severe cardiomegaly, with or without pulmonary venous hypertension. The serum aldolase level is usually elevated. Right bundle branch block, left anterior hemiblock, atrial fibrillation, and ventricular premature depolarizations are the most common electrocardiographic findings in patients with chronic Chagas disease. Many patients have clinically silent conduction abnormalities that can be demonstrated on electrophysiology. In chronic Chagas disease, multifocal ventricular premature depolarizations are common, particularly after exercise, and bouts of ventricular tachycardia can occur. Ventricular arrhythmias are particularly common during and after exercise. Atrial arrhythmias including atrial fibrillation (often with a slow ventricular response) can also occur. Thromboembolic phenomena are a frequent complication, occurring in more than 50 percent of the patients. The echocardiographic findings in advanced cases are distinctive, with LV posterior wall hypokinesis and relatively preserved interventricular septal motion, frequently with an apical aneurysm.

Clinical predictors of outcome in Chagas heart disease were recently examined in 424 Brazilian patients.[27] Six major independent predictors of outcome were identified: (1) New York Heart Association functional Class III or IV, (2) cardiomegaly, (3) segmental or global wall motion abnormality on echocardiography, (4) nonsustained VT on Holter, (5) low QRS voltage on electrocardiogram (ECG), and (6) male sex. When each factor was assigned a point score of 5, 5, 5, 3, 3, 2, and 2, respectively, the authors developed a risk-scoring system to classify patients as high risk (12 to 20 points), intermediate risk (7 to 11 points), and low risk (0 to 6 points). The 10-year mortality rates for low-risk, intermediate-risk, and high-risk patients of the study group were 10, 44, and 84 percent, respectively. The scoring system was validated against a separate database of 1053 patients with Chagas disease.

In terms of serodiagnosis, the complement-fixation test (Machado-Guerreiro test) is most useful in diagnosis; it has high sensitivity and specificity for the identification of chronic Chagas disease. Also used in diagnosis are the indirect immunofluorescent antibody test, the enzyme-linked immunosorbent assay, and the hemagglutination test. Perhaps the most widely used test in endemic areas is the detection of parasites in the blood of patients with chronic Chagas disease (which occurs in up to 50 percent of cases) by means of xenodiagnosis. The patient is bitten by reduviid bugs bred in the laboratory; the subsequent identification of parasites in the intestine of the insect is proof of infection in the human host.

In terms of treatment, patients with Chagas disease may respond to beta blockade, and some evidence indicates that captopril, early in the course of disease, may alleviate disease in animal models. Major efforts are aimed at interrupting transmission of the parasite to humans; such vector control methods have been generally successful. They may prevent not only the initial infection but also reinfection that may play a role in determining the severity of the resulting cardiomyopathy. Amiodarone appears to be effective in controlling the ventricular arrhythmias frequently seen in patients with Chagas disease, although its impact on survival is uncertain. Implantable cardioverter defibrillators are indicated for patients with life-threatening arrhythmias, but this is not a financially viable option for the vast majority of patients. Anticoagulation may be of some benefit in preventing recurrent thromboembolic episodes. Antiparasitic agents such as nifurtimox, benznidazole, and itraconazole are effective in reducing parasitemia and are useful in acute disease. In chronic disease, encouraging data suggest that benznidazole may slow the disease progression and increase the rate of negative seroconversion.[28] However, this was a nonrandomized open trial, supporting the need for a future randomized trial. A promising future approach is vaccination, although an effective vaccine is not yet available.

CH 66

METAZOAL MYOCARDIAL DISEASES

ECHINOCOCCUS (HYDATID CYST). Echinococcus is endemic in many sheep-raising areas of the world, particularly Argentina, New Zealand, Greece, North Africa, and Iceland; however, cardiac involvement in patients with hydatid disease is uncommon (<2 percent). The usual host of *Echinococcus granulosus* is the dog, but humans may serve as intermediate hosts if they accidentally ingest ova from contaminated dog feces. When cardiac involvement is present, the cysts are usually intramyocardial in the interventricular septum or LV free wall. A myocardial cyst can degenerate and calcify, develop daughter cysts, or rupture. Rupture of the cyst is the most dreaded complication; rupture into the pericardium can result in acute pericarditis, which may progress to chronic constrictive pericarditis. Rupture into the cardiac chambers can result in systemic or pulmonary emboli. Rapidly progressive pulmonary hypertension can occur with rupture of right-sided cysts, with subsequent embolization of hundreds of scolices into the pulmonary circulation. The liberation of hydatid fluid into the circulation can produce profound, fatal circulatory collapse caused by an anaphylactic reaction to the protein constituents of the fluid. Estimates indicate that only 10 percent of patients with cardiac hydatid cysts have clinical symptoms. The ECG may reflect the location of the cyst. Chest pain is usually caused by rupture of the cyst into the pericardial space with resultant pericarditis. Large cystic masses sometimes produce right-sided obstruction. The chest radiograph may show an abnormal cardiac silhouette or a calcified lobular mass adjacent to the left ventricle. Two-dimensional echocardiography, computed tomography, or magnetic resonance imaging may aid in the detection and localization of heart cysts. Eosinophilia, when present, is a useful adjunctive finding. The Casoni skin test, or serological evaluation for echinococcus, has a limited role in cardiac diagnosis. In terms of therapy, despite the availability of effective drugs such as mebendazole and albendazole, surgical excision is generally recommended, even for asymptomatic patients. This is because of the significant risk of rupture of the cyst and its attendant serious and sometimes fatal consequences.

TRICHINOSIS. Infestation with *Trichinella spiralis* is common, but clinically detectable cardiac involvement occurs in only a minority of patients. Symptomatic involvement is uncommon and may be responsible for the fatalities. Less frequently, death is caused by pulmonary embolism secondary to venous thrombosis or neurological complications. Although the parasite can invade the heart, it does not usually encyst there, and it is rare to find larvae or larval fragments in the myocardium. The heart may be dilated and flabby, and a pericardial effusion may be present. A prominent focal infiltrate composed of lymphocytes and eosinophils can be found, with occasional microthrombi in the intramural arterioles. Areas of muscle degeneration and necrosis are present. The clinical myocarditis in trichinosis is usually mild and goes unnoticed, but in occasional cases it is manifested by heart failure and chest pain, usually appearing around the third week of the disease. Electrocardiographic abnormalities are detected in approximately 10 percent of patients with trichinosis and parallel the time course of clinical cardiac involvement, initially appearing in the second or third week and usually resolving by the seventh week of the illness. The most common electrocardiographic abnormalities are repolarization abnormalities and ventricular premature complexes. The diagnosis is usually based on the demonstration of a positive indirect immunofluorescent antibody test in a patient with the clinical features of trichinosis. Eosinophilia, when present, is a supportive finding. The skin test is usually but not invariably positive. Treatment is with anthelmintics and corticosteroids; dramatic improvement in cardiac function has been reported after their use.

Hypersensitivity Reactions—Vaccines and Drugs

Multiple medications have been implicated in contributing to hypersensitivity myocarditis. The condition may be accompanied by constitutional symptoms such as fever, skin rash, peripheral eosinophilia, and sinus tachycardia following ingestions of a particular drug that may be new to the patient's regimen or that has been previously ingested and exposed to for a long time. Myocardial biopsy may reveal eosinophilic or lymphocytic infiltrates during the acute phase. Eosinophilic necrotizing myocarditis may rapidly deteriorate into hemodynamic collapse. However, the latter scenario is a rare exception because the majority of cases will recover fully on withdrawal of the offending agent, and rarely are there any hemodynamic sequelae.

SMALLPOX VACCINATION. Although smallpox has been eradicated from the world, its re-emergence as a potential bioterror threat has prompted a recent series of repeat vaccinations by the U.S. Department of Defense. Widespread smallpox vaccination in late 2002 by the Department of Defense was followed unexpectedly by an increase in the incidence of myocarditis temporally coupled to the vaccination. The incidence of myopericarditis has been estimated to be around 7.8 cases per 100,000 vaccinations. One case of eosinophilic-lymphocytic myocarditis has been proven by biopsy.[29] Fortunately, this latter case responded well to high-dose steroids. This complication from the existing vaccine preparation may preclude that the vaccine be given widely to the population unless the risk of bioterror vastly exceeds the corresponding risk of myocarditis.

CLOZAPINE. An exception to the general safety of psychotropic drugs for the heart is clozapine, currently indicated for resistant schizophrenia.[30] To date, 15 cases of myocarditis and 8 cases of cardiomyopathy have been recorded in patients who have been prescribed this drug. Five of the myocarditis cases have died, all within 3 weeks of initiating therapy. This suggests a rapid-onset hypersensitivity myocarditis, and patients should be monitored closely during the initiation phase of the therapy.

TRICYCLICS. Although sinus tachycardia, postural hypotension, disturbances in rhythm, abnormalities of atrioventricular conduction, and even sudden death can be seen in patients taking tricyclic antidepressants, particularly in cases of overdose, important depression of LV function usually does not occur, even in patients with preexisting heart disease. Clinicians have expressed concern over using tricyclic antidepressants in patients with prior myocardial infarction and/or preexisting ventricular arrhythmias because these agents have a class I antiarrhythmic effect, prolong the QT interval, and might be proarrhythmic in these settings. The selective serotonin reuptake inhibitors are remarkably free of cardiovascular toxicity and do not appear to depress ventricular function. More frequently, they produce side effects by interacting with the metabolism of drugs mediated through the cytochrome-P450 enzyme system.

PHENOTHIAZINES. The phenothiazines are associated with a variety of cardiac disturbances including electrocardiographic changes, atrial and ventricular arrhythmias, and sudden death. Postural hypotension can also be seen. The cardiac effects are largely dose dependent. But electrocardiographic abnormalities can be observed even at low doses, such as lengthening of the QT interval and T wave changes.

Physical Agents

A wide variety of substances other than infectious agents can act on the heart and damage the myocardium. In some cases the damage is acute, transient, and associated with evidence of an inflammatory myocardial infiltrate with myocyte necrosis (e.g., with the arsenicals and lithium). Other agents that damage the myocardium can lead to chronic changes with resulting histological evidence of fibrosis and a clinical picture of a dilated or restrictive cardiomyopathy. Numerous chemicals and drugs (both industrial and therapeutic) can lead to cardiac damage and dysfunction. Several physical agents (e.g., radiation and excessive heat) can also contribute directly to myocardial damage.

RADIATION. The cardiac effects of radiation therapy are discussed in Chapter 85. Briefly, radiation therapy can lead to a variety of cardiac complications that arise long after the completion of radiation therapy including pericarditis with effusion, tamponade, or constriction; coronary artery fibrosis and myocardial infarction; valvular abnormalities; myocardial fibrosis; and conduction disturbances. Although radiation probably results in some degree of tissue damage in all patients, clinically significant cardiac involvement occurs in the minority of patients, usually long after the radiation treatment has ended. Radiation-induced cardiac damage is related to the cumulative dose of the radiation and the mass of heart irradiated. The late cardiac damage that may follow irradiation appears to result from a long-lasting injury of the capillary endothelial cells, which leads to cell death, capillary rupture, and microthrombi. Because of this damage to the microvasculature, ischemia results and is followed by myocardial fibrosis. In addition to microvascular damage, the major epicardial coronary arteries can become narrowed, especially at the ostia.

Occasionally a patient will develop acute cardiac complications after radiation therapy. Typically this may manifest as acute pericarditis. A mild, transient, asymptomatic depression of LV function is sometimes seen early after radiation therapy. The more common clinical expressions of radiation heart disease occur months or years after the exposure. The pericardium is the most common site of clinical involvement, with findings of chronic pericardial effusion or pericardial constriction (see Chap. 85). Myocardial damage occurs less frequently and is characterized by myocardial fibrosis with or without endocardial fibrosis or fibroelastosis. Left and/or right ventricular dysfunction at rest or with exercise appears to be a common, albeit usually asymptomatic, finding 5 to 20 years after radiation therapy. Often there is a latent period of a decade or more between the radiation exposure and

the development of ventricular dysfunction or valvular deformity. Electrocardiographic abnormalities, heart block, accelerated atherosclerosis, and a variety of arrhythmias may be seen months or years after therapeutic radiation, although ultimate clinical significance is unclear.

HEAT STROKE. Heat stroke results from failure of the thermoregulatory center following exposure to high ambient temperature. It is manifested principally by hyperpyrexia, renal insufficiency, disseminated intravascular coagulation, and central nervous system dysfunction. However, electrocardiographic abnormalities appear to be common in heat stroke; pulmonary edema and transient right and/or left ventricular dysfunction may occur, along with hypotension and circulatory collapse. Pathological changes include dilation of the right side of the heart, particularly the right atrium. Hemorrhages of the subendocardium and the subepicardium are frequently seen at necropsy and often involve the interventricular septum and posterior wall of the left ventricle. Histological findings include degeneration and necrosis of muscle fibers, as well as interstitial edema. Sinus tachycardia is invariably present, whereas atrial and ventricular arrhythmias are usually absent. Transient prolongation of the QT interval may be seen along with ST segment and T wave abnormalities. It can take up to several months for these repolarization abnormalities to resolve. Serum enzyme levels can be elevated and may reflect myocardial damage, at least in part, although concomitant rhabdomyolysis is often present.

HYPOTHERMIA. Low temperature can also result in myocardial damage. Cardiac dilation can occur, with epicardial petechiae and subendocardial hemorrhages. Microinfarcts are found in the ventricular myocardium, presumably related to abnormalities in the microcirculation. The lesions are not caused by the low temperature per se but appear to be the result of the circulatory collapse, hemoconcentration, capillary slugging, and depressed cellular metabolism that accompany hypothermia. Clinical manifestations of hypothermia include sinus bradycardia, conduction disturbances, atrial (and occasionally ventricular) fibrillation, hypotension, a fall in cardiac output, reversible myocardial depression, and a characteristic deflection of the terminal portion of the QRS pattern (Osborn wave). Treatment includes core warming (often utilizing extracorporeal blood warming), cardiopulmonary resuscitation, and management of pulmonary, hematological, and renal complications. Notwithstanding its potential cardiac risks, mild therapeutic hypothermia appears to improve neurological outcome after cardiac arrest and is a currently accepted practice.

PATHOPHYSIOLOGY

Current understanding of the pathogenesis of viral myocarditis is derived mostly from enteroviral models of myocarditis in the mouse, and the principles have been generalized to other types of myocarditis.[1,31] The disease represents a delicate interaction between the virus and the host. Myocarditis can be considered to have three phases in its pathophysiology. The first is the viral phase, followed by immunological response phase (including innate and acquired immunity components), followed by cardiac remodeling phase (Fig. 66-4).

Viral Entry

Viral myocarditis is initiated by the introduction of a virus of pathogenic strain (e.g., an enterovirus such as coxsackie virus CVB3), which invades the susceptible host through a portal of entry via a virus internalizing receptor on the cell surface. The virus ultimately reaches the myocardium through hematogenous or lymphangitic spread. For the coxsackievirus and many others, the virus is initially processed in the lymphoid organs such as the spleen, where the virus will proliferate in immune cells themselves including macrophages and T and B lymphocytes. It is paradoxically through the host immune activation that the viruses reach the actual target organs (heart and pancreas in the cases of CVB3). Once the virus reaches the myocyte, it will again use its specific receptor or receptor-complex for target cell entry. For the Coxsackie virus, this includes the CAR[13,19,32]

CH 66

Myocarditis

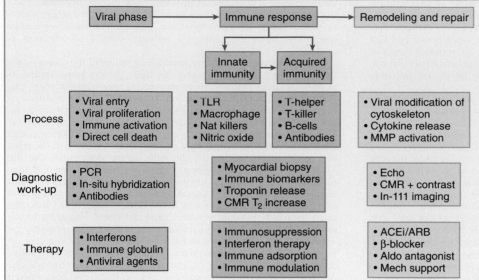

FIGURE 66–4 Conceptual framework of the three pathophysiological stages leading to chronic myocarditis including viral phase, immune response phase and remodeling, and repair phase. The immune response can be subdivided into innate and acquired immune response, with significant collaboration between the two processes. Both the viral and immune processes contribute to the cell deaths, cardiac remodeling, and inflammatory response by the host. The therapeutic efficacy, unfortunately, has not been as well documented because of heterogeneity of the population, high rates of spontaneous improvement, and small sample size of the studies. ACEi = angiotensin-converting enzyme inhibitors; Aldo = aldosterone; ARB = angiotensin receptor blocker; CMR = cardiac magnetic resonance; Mech = mechanical; MMP = matrix metalloproteinases; Nat = natural; PCR = polymerase chain reaction; TLR = toll-like receptors.

and the attachment and virulence determining co-receptor, decay accelerating factor (DAF), or CD55 (Fig. 66-5).[33,34]

Enteroviruses use the CAR complex, hence the high frequency of coxsackie and adenovirus infection in myocarditis. CAR is a member of the immunoglobulin superfamily and is a tight junction protein particularly present in the heart, brain, and gut.[14,34] Through the activation of this receptor complex, the negative strand RNA of the Coxsackie virus will enter the cell and is reverse-transcribed into a positive strand to act as a template for subsequent viral RNA duplication. The polycistronic RNA encodes a large polyprotein that contains its own cleavage enzyme and important viral capsid subunits VP1-VP4. Exuberant viral replication in a susceptible host lacking suitable immunity defenses can cause acute myocardial damage and early death of the host.

Entry of the virus through the receptor also activates its signaling system including tyrosine kinase $p56^{lck}$, Fyn, and Abl. Activation of these signals modifies the host cell cytoskeleton to permit more viral entry. At the same time, these signals also mediate the activation of T cells, which are critically dependent on $p56^{lck}$ and Fyn. Interestingly, the presence of heart tissue damage and inflammation upregulate the CAR and increase the susceptibility of the host to Coxsackie virus infection.[19]

Immune Activation and Viral Persistence

Although viral entry triggers the immune activation, the immune system has a dual role. On one hand, it is activated to eliminate as many virus-infected cells as possible to control in the infection. On the other hand, the response needs to be modulated by negative controls; otherwise there will be excessive tissue damage from an inflammatory response with organ dysfunction. The virus has an elaborate system in place to escape host immunological surveillance including molecular mimicry, proliferation in immunocytes, and upregulation of its own receptors, and it

can persist in the myocyte for months to years.

Viral persistence can expose the host to persistent antigenic trigger and chronic immune activation, as well as potentially chronic myocarditis. Persistence of the viral genome, such as Coxsackie virus in the myocyte, has been directly linked to the development of dilated cardiomyopathy through cytoskeleton remodeling. Knowlton and colleagues[6,35] have identified that the enteroviral protease 2A can directly cleave the dystrophin-sarcoglycan complex located at the myocyte-extracellular matrix junction. This can directly lead to myocyte remodeling and subsequent cardiac dilation.

Innate Immunity

The earliest responses of the host to the presence of foreign genome sequences are members of the innate immune system. Innate immunity is an evolutionarily ancient host protective system that provides early warnings for the cells to deal with an adverse external environment. The commonest pathways for innate immunity to be triggered by the foreign virus are the ubiquitous toll-like receptors (TLRs), which are an expanding family of cell surface receptors that recognized general molecular patterns without the high specificity conferred by acquired immune players such as T and B cells. For example, TLR-3, which recognizes double-stranded RNA, and TLR-4, which is the receptor for bacterial lipopolysaccharide (LPS), are present in abundance in the myocardium. The presence of foreign genetic material can be detected by the TLRs, leading to signaling activation that ultimately leads to activation of transcription factors such as NF-κB, with subsequent cytokine production, and interferon regulatory factors (IRFs) leading to interferon production (see Fig. 66-5). The activation of TLRs signals through adaptors and kinases such as MyD88 and IRAKs.

In murine models of myocarditis, many components of innate immunity are upregulated immediately on viral exposure including MyD88 and IRAK4,[31,36] leading to NF-κB activation. Excessive NF-κB activation and cytokine release is detrimental to the host, and reductions of cytokines such as tumor necrosis factor (TNF) or decoy for NF-κB can improve the outcomes of myocarditis.[37] Interestingly, the activation of NF-κB appears to be modulated by the interferon production pathways including interferon regulator factors (IRFs) such as IRF-3.[36] Downregulation of MyD88 and in turn NF-κB and activation of acquired immunity is accompanied by the upregulation of type I interferons (interferons alpha and beta). Interferon is critical for host protection and survival, and its absence leads to excessive viral proliferation and direct cardiac damage.[38] Type I interferon thus may have an ideal dual role of controlling viral proliferation, as well as downregulation of acquired immune pathways of T-cell activation and clonal expansion. Besides the positive regulators of host defense responses outlined earlier, there are also systems of negative modulators that will counteract the excessive cytokine activation. One system is the intracellular suppressors of cytokine signaling (SOCS) system that negatively regulate innate immune response.[39] The SOCS system particularly downregulates cytokine signals going through the gp130 receptor on the myocytes. Normal signals through the gp130 receptor serve to stabilize the dystrophin complex and confer protection for the host. This appears to be an SOCS-3 dependent phenomenon, as cardiac restricted overexpression of SOCS-3 in a transgenic model led to gp130 instability and worse outcome.

Acquired Immunity

Acquired immunity refers to the ability of the immune system to recognize and respond specifically to a single viral or tissue antigen, through T and B cells that recognize specific peptide sequences. This system is triggered by the recognition of a precise "foreign" molecular pattern by the variable region of the T-cell receptor. The T cell is then stimulated to clonally expand to attack the source of "antigen," which could be from the viral coat protein, or sometimes from parts of the myocardium (such as myosin), which may resemble the pattern of the virus (molecular mimicry), triggering autoimmunity. However, this process is dependent on co-stimulation from inflammatory signals, often linked to innate immunity signaling activated earlier in the injury process.

The result of acquired immune activation is the production of T killer cells that can directly attack the virus and virally infected cells. The activation of T cells also leads to B-cell activation and the production of specific antibodies to neutralize the antigen. This results in subacute and chronic inflammation observed in myocarditis and contributes to the subsequent myocyte necrosis, fibrosis, and remodeling. The critical contributory role of the signals through the acquired immune pathways has been examined in mouse models of myocarditis. A common downstream signaling pathway from the T-cell receptor is the tyrosine kinase p56^{lck}. Interestingly, p56^{lck} is the same tyrosine kinase signal attached to the CAR-DAF receptor complex for viral entry. When p56^{lck} is genetically removed from the mouse by transgenic knockout techniques, the mouse is no longer susceptible to the inflammation seen in typical myocarditis, and the mortality is almost completely eliminated.[40] T cells, when present, will attempt to seek out the infected cells and destroy them using mechanisms such as cytokine-mediated signaling[41] or perforin-mediated cell deaths. This confirms that the T-cell receptor activation sequence ultimately leads to the detrimental phenotype of the disease and supports the concept that decreasing inflammation from acquired immunity, while finding ways to control the virus through innate immunity, will lead to the most beneficial outcomes of the disease.

To understand why certain individuals develop overwhelming myocarditis after exposure to the virus and rapidly die from the disease, whereas others do not even show inflammation, we have been methodically mapping the major determinants of the host immune system using

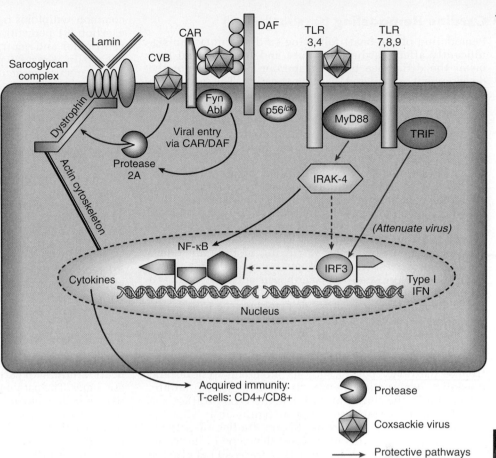

FIGURE 66–5 The pathogenesis of viral myocarditis, such as that caused by Coxsackie virus. The virus enters the cell membrane through internalization receptors of coxsackie-adenovirus receptor (CAR). The latter can in turn trigger receptor–associated kinases such as p56^{lck}, Fyn, and Abl, to alter host myocyte cytoskeleton to facilitate viral entry. Viruses such as the Coxsackie virus can directly produce enzymes such as protease 2A that can dissemble the important cytoskeletal components such as dystrophin-sarcoglycan complex, leading to myocyte remodeling and destruction. Engagement of the receptor also activates tyrosine kinases, which are important also for T-cell clonal expansion and linking between the innate and the acquired immune system. The virus also activates the innate immunity by engaging toll-like receptors (TLRs), through adaptors such as MyD88, and TRIF. Activation and translocation of NF-κB on one hand will produce cytokines and trigger-acquired immunity such as CD4/CD8 T-cell mobilization. On the other hand, this can be attenuated by the activation of IRF-3 and type I interferon (IFN) production. The latter may be protective through multiple mechanisms including attenuation of the virus. CVB = Coxsackie B virus; DAF = decay accelerating factor; IRAK = interleukin receptor associated kinase, a signaling protein in innate immune pathway; IRF = interferon regulatory factor.

molecular targeting strategies in knockout mice. Earlier work identified that components of innate immunity, such as interferon and IRF-3, are critical for host survival, yet T-cell signaling and activation is injurious to the host. Through CD4$^-$/CD8$^-$ knockout mice, we have established that both CD4 and CD8 T cells contribute to the host autoimmune inflammatory disease, accompanied by a shift of cytokine profile from Th1 to Th2 response.[42] More recently, we have identified that p56^{lck} triggers downstream extracellular signal-regulated kinase activation in the host target cell and appears to be critical for the determinant of host susceptibility.[41] To validate these observations, we have also investigated the function of the associated tyrosine phosphatase CD45 linked in function to the p56^{lck} kinase and confirmed that CD45$^{-/-}$ animals are also resistant to viral myocarditis.[43] After careful dissection, it was apparent that CD45 is an important src, as well as JAK/STAT phosphatase, and virally triggered CD45 activation shuts down interferon production. Interferon levels are markedly increased once CD45 is removed, and the host is indeed rescued through this dual protective process.

Cardiac Remodeling (see also Chap. 22)

Remodeling of the heart following cardiac injury can significantly affect cardiac structure and function and may mean the difference between appropriate healing or the development of dilated cardiomyopathy. The virus can directly enter the endothelial cells and myocytes and, through intracellular interactions with the host protein synthetic and signaling pathways, lead to direct cell death or hypertrophy. The virus can also modify the myocyte cytoskeleton, as mentioned earlier, and lead to dilated cardiomyopathy.

The inflammatory process outlined earlier from both innate and acquired immunity can lead to cytokine release, activation of matrix metalloproteinases that digest the interstitial collagen and elastin framework of the heart. Indeed, the matrix metalloproteinases of the collagenase and elastase families can lead to cardiac remodeling and dysfunction and contribute to the worsening of inflammation.[44] More recently, the family of matrix metalloproteinases including urokinase-type plasminogen activator has been found to contribute to cardiac dilatation and inflammation.[45] In addition, activation of cytokines such as transforming growth factor-beta (TGF-β) can lead to activation of the SMAD signaling cascade and lead to production of profibrotic factors leading to pathological fibrosis. The final result can lead to the development of dilated or hypertrophic cardiomyopathy, with its attendant systolic and diastolic dysfunction, and progressive heart failure. Interestingly, the ability to modulate the viral proliferation or inflammatory response can also significantly alter the outcomes in terms of fibrosis. Recent studies in patients receiving interferon therapy suggest that type I interferons may be able to modulate not only the viral load but also the fibrotic outcomes in the matrix of the affected hearts.[46]

CH 66

CLINICAL PRESENTATION

Myocarditis has a wide-ranging clinical presentation, which contributes to the difficulties in diagnosis and classification. The clinical presentation can range from asymptomatic electrocardiographic or echocardiographic abnormalities to symptoms of cardiac dysfunction, arrhythmias or heart failure to hemodynamic collapse. Transient electrocardiographic or echographic abnormalities have been observed frequently during community viral outbreaks or influenza epidemics, but most patients remain asymptomatic from a cardiac point of view and have little long-term sequelae. Myocarditis typically has a bimodal distribution in terms of age in the population, with the acute presentation more commonly seen in young children and teenagers. In contrast, the presenting symptoms are more subtle and insidious, often with dilated cardiomyopathy and heart failure in the older adult population. Felker and colleagues[47] have observed earlier in consecutive cases of new-onset dilated cardiomyopathy in adults that 9 to 16 percent have classic myocarditis on biopsy by the Dallas criteria.[47] The difference in presentation is likely related to the maturity of the immune system—the young tend to have an exuberant response to the initial exposure of a provocative antigen. On the other hand, the older individual would have developed a greater degree of tolerance and shown chronic inflammatory response only to the chronic presence of a foreign antigen or a dysregulated immune system, which predisposes to autoimmunity.

Acute Myocarditis

Classically, patients with myocarditis present with nonspecific symptoms related to the heart. In a recent series of 245 patients with clinically suspected myocarditis, the most common symptoms include fatigue (82 percent); dyspnea on exertion (81 percent); arrhythmias (55 percent, both supraventricular and ventricular); palpitations (49 percent); and chest pain at rest (26 percent).[7] The latter can be difficult to distinguish from acute ischemic syndromes because they result in release of troponin, ST segment elevation on ECG, and segmental wall motion abnormalities on echocardiogram. Therefore, the symptoms can be quite nonspecific, although some symptoms indicate cardiac involvement. Viral prodrome of fever, chills, myalgias, constitutional symptoms occur between 20 and 80 percent of the cases, can be readily missed by the patient, and thus cannot be relied upon for diagnosis.

Many cases of myocarditis present with de novo onset of heart failure, particularly when the patient is middle-aged or older. When the health care team fails to identify other causes of heart failure, viral myocarditis along with idiopathic dilated cardiomyopathy become the diagnosis of exclusion. To distinguish myocarditis from idiopathic dilated cardiomyopathy, almost one third of the cases of viral myocarditis will recover to normal cardiac function with appropriate supportive therapy, which is less frequent in genetic dilated cardiomyopathy.

Fulminant Myocarditis

Less frequently, the patient may present with dramatic acute heart failure with cardiogenic shock in the absence of other etiologies. The patient is usually toxic in appearance, accompanied by low blood pressure and cardiac output, and often requires high-dose vasopressor support or even a ventricular assist device (VAD). In one series, 14 of 147 (10.2 percent) patients with clinical myocarditis presented in a fulminant fashion, with the triad of hemodynamic compromise, rapid onset of symptoms (usually within 2 weeks), and fever.[48] The patients have on echocardiography characteristically severe global ventricular dysfunction but minimally dilated left ventricles. Pathology on endomyocardial biopsy shows multiple foci of inflammation and necrosis but does not match the clinical phenotypic severity. Much of this is likely related to high levels of cytokine production by the host, leading to significant reversible cardiac depression. On follow-up, 93 percent of the original cohorts were alive and transplant-free 11 years following initial biopsy, compared with only 45 percent in those with more classic forms of acute myocarditis. This underscores the importance of supporting patients with myocarditis as aggressively as possible to maximize chances of recovery.

Giant Cell Myocarditis

Giant cell myocarditis is another subclass of myocarditis in which the patient develops heart failure and follows a progressive, relentless, downhill course, and biopsy confirms the presence of giant cells and active inflammation on the histological sections. The Giant Cell Myocarditis Study observed that 75 percent of the patients presented with significant heart failure symptoms on first encounter. Other symptoms may include arrhythmias or heart block. Unfortunately, patients with giant cell myocarditis often have an aggressive downhill course, with extremely poor prognosis and a median survival of less than 6 months. Some may temporarily respond to an aggressive immunosuppressive regimen. Most patients will require cardiac transplantation if they qualify for the local listing criteria as candidates (see also Chap. 27).

Chronic Active Myocarditis

This group represents the vast majority of older adult patients with myocarditis, and the onset is often insidious and difficult to pinpoint. The patient presents with symptoms compatible with moderate ventricular dysfunction such as fatigue and dyspnea. Myocardial biopsy pathology may show active myocarditis, but more frequently it is only borderline or generalized chronic myopathic changes with fibrosis and myocyte drop-out. Some may progress to diastolic dysfunction with excessive fibrosis, thus resembling restrictive cardiomyopathy.

DIAGNOSTIC APPROACHES

The diagnosis of myocarditis has traditionally required a histological diagnosis according to the classic Dallas criteria to secure the diagnosis.[2] However, because of its low sensitivity caused by the patchy nature of the inflammatory infiltrates in the myocardium, as well as the reluctance of clinicians to perform an invasive diagnostic procedure, myocarditis is severely underdiagnosed. Because the incidence of the disease is likely much higher than appreciated, a high level of clinical suspicion, together with a hybrid of clinical and laboratory criteria, and new imaging modalities may help to secure the diagnosis without necessarily resorting to biopsy in all cases.

With the advent of a number of new diagnostic strategies for myocarditis, one may now *strongly suspect myocarditis* if two of the following criteria are present, and the diagnosis would be *highly probable as myocarditis* if there are three or more criteria present: (1) compatible clinical symptoms; (2) evidence of cardiac structural/functional defect or myocardial damage *in the absence* of active regional coronary ischemia; (3) regional delayed contrast enhancement or increased T_2 signal on CMR imaging; and (4) presence of inflammatory cell infiltrate or positive viral genome signals on myocardial biopsy or pathology (Table 66-2). Of course, myocardial biopsy still provides the most specific diagnosis for myocarditis.

For example, myocarditis as a diagnosis should be suspected when a young patient presents with unexplained symptoms of heart failure or chest pain, but the coronary arteries are found to be normal on angiography. When young patients such as this individual present with minimal risk factors for coronary disease present with acute chest pain or ischemic electrocardiographic abnormalities, 32 percent will turn out to have biopsy evidence of acute myocarditis according to the Dallas criteria.[9] An even higher proportion will also be viral genome–positive on molecular analysis. A major limitation to the accurate diagnosis of myocarditis is the lack of highly sensitive and specific tools that are noninvasive and widely applicable. The commonly discussed modalities and their reported sensitivities and specificities are outlined in Table 66-3.

Clinical Symptoms

The clinical symptoms of myocarditis are not specific and depend heavily on the mode of presentation as outlined earlier. Younger patients most often complain of chest pain and fatigue. Patients with cardiac dysfunction may present with new-onset heart failure, dyspnea, or fatigue. Some patients are have symptoms of supraventricular or ventricular arrhythmias including palpitations, presyncope, and syncope. In most severe cases, such as those with fulminant myocarditis, patients may present with cardiogenic shock and intractable arrhythmias. Some patients may present with constitutional symptoms such as fever and viral prodrome. However, these are infrequent and unreliable for diagnosis.

Laboratory Testing

Severe myocarditis will lead to myocardial damage secondary to the presence of inflammatory cell infiltrates and cyto-

TABLE 66–2	Expanded Criteria for Diagnosis of Myocarditis

Suspicious for myocarditis = 2 positive categories

Compatible with myocarditis = 3 positive categories

High probability of being myocarditis = all 4 categories positive
(Any matching feature in category = positive for category)

Category I: Clinical Symptoms
Clinical heart failure
Fever
Viral prodrome
Fatigue
Dyspnea on exertion
Chest pain
Palpitations
Presyncope or syncope

Category II: Evidence of Cardiac Structural/Functional Perturbation *in the Absence* of Regional Coronary Ischemia
Echocardiography evidence
Regional wall motion abnormalities
Cardiac dilation
Regional cardiac hypertrophy
Troponin release
High sensitivity (>0.1 ng/ml)
Positive indium-111 antimyosin scintigraphy
and
Normal coronary angiography *or*
Absence of reversible ischemia by coronary distribution on perfusion scan

Category III: Cardiac Magnetic Resonance Imaging
Increased myocardial T_2 signal on inversion recovery sequence
Delayed contrast enhancement following gadolinium-DTPA infusion

Category IV: Myocardial Biopsy—Pathological or Molecular Analysis
Pathology findings compatible with Dallas criteria
Presence of viral genome by polymerase chain reaction or in situ hybridization

TABLE 66–3	Comparison of Efficacy of Various Diagnostic Modalities for Myocarditis

Diagnostic Modality	Sensitivity Range	Specificity Range
ECG changes (e.g., AV block, Q, ST changes)	47%	?
Troponin (lower threshold of >0.1 mg/ml)	34%-53%	89%-94%
CK-MB	6%	?
Antibodies to virus or myosin	25%-32%	40%
Indium-111 antimyosin scintigraphy	85%-91%	34%-53%
Echocardiography (ventricular dysfunction)	69%	?
Cardiac magnetic resonance imaging	86%	95%
Myocardial biopsy (Dallas criteria of pathology)	35%-50%	78%-89%
Myocardial biopsy (viral genome by PCR)	38%-65%	80%-100%

? = indeterminant or poor; AV = atrioventricular; CK-MB = cytosine kinase isoenzyme; ECG = electrocardiogram; PCR = polymerase chain reaction.

kine activation, as well as some contribution directly from virus-mediated cell deaths. These processes can severely depress cardiac function and produce evidence of cardiac damage. This can be detected as leakage of *cardiac enzymes* such as creatine kinase (CK) or troponin when the damage is severe or chronic (see Table 66-2). However, in most cases the leakage of enzymes is relatively minor, and standard laboratory testing for CK or its isoform CK-MB is too insensitive (overall sensitivity for myocarditis is only 8 percent). Enzyme biomarkers such as troponin are more useful when high-sensitivity thresholds are used. For example, when a serum troponin T threshold of greater than 0.1 ng/ml as a cutoff is used, the sensitivity can be increased from 34 to 53 percent without compromising specificity. Similar findings have been noted for troponin I. Other biomarkers such as cytokines, complement, or antiviral or antiheart antibodies are either too insensitive or inadequately standardized to make them generally useful clinically.

The cardiac damage can also manifest as electrocardiographic *abnormalities* that range from T wave inversions to frank ST segment elevation and bundle branch block, depending on the region and extent of inflammatory damage. The series by Kuhl and colleagues noted that arrhythmias including both supraventricular and ventricular arrhythmias may be present in 55 percent of the patients.[12]

Imaging techniques such as *2-D echocardiography* are useful as an initial diagnostic evaluation of the patient to detect the regional ventricular dysfunction that often accompanies the condition. Parameters of ventricular remodeling including chamber dilation, regional hypertrophy, and regional wall motion abnormalities are often seen with myocarditis, but these changes may be indistinguishable from those of myocardial ischemia or infarction at the outset. The absence of matching regional coronary disease and evidence of rapid recovery of ventricular dysfunction during follow-up are general clues to the diagnosis of myocarditis. Retrospective analysis of echocardiograms from 42 patients with biopsy-proven myocarditis identified ventricular dysfunction in 69 percent of the patients, but the presence of cardiac dilatation is much more variable. Newer techniques such as tissue characterization and tissue Doppler imaging may permit better diagnostic accuracy in the future. Additional validation studies will be necessary to determine their ultimate clinical role. However, echocardiography is certainly useful as a follow-up imaging modality to monitor natural history of the patient's ventricular function or response to treatment. 2-D echocardiography may also help to distinguish fulminant from more classical forms of myocarditis, with the former showing less diastolic dimensional increase but increased septal thickness and the latter showing a much greater degree of ventricular dilatation.

Indium-111 labeled *antimyosin antibody imaging* can potentially identify myocytes that have lost cell membrane integrity, permitting binding of antibody to the intracellular myosin through immunological or viral damage. Indium-111 antibody imaging has shown in a series of patients with suspected myocarditis to have good sensitivity (83 percent) but lower specificity (53 percent). The combination of a positive antimyosin scan with nonventricular dilation predicts a high frequency of positive myocardial biopsy and may be used as a set of noninvasive first-stage diagnostic work-up.

Cardiac Magnetic Resonance
Imaging (see also Chap. 17)

A new approach to the diagnosis of myocarditis is CMR imaging. CMR imaging is attractive for the detection of myocarditis because of its ability to characterize tissue according to water content and changes in contrast kinetics. CMR also allows visualization of the entire myocardium and is thus well suited to detect the local patchy nature of the myocarditic lesions.[49] The local inflammatory process in myocarditis leads to cytokine release and mobilization of inflammatory cells to the infected foci. This in turn produces local changes in membrane permeability, tissue edema, and ultimately tissue fibrosis. These changes directly affect the T_2 relaxation parameters of the tissues, which depend on water content. Furthermore, extracellular contrast agents such as gadolinium DTPA will also distribute and clear differently in inflamed or scarred tissue when compared with normal tissue, leading to changes in T_1 relaxation and thus contrast changes or delayed enhancement on T_1-weighted images (Fig. 66-6).

Evaluation of the relative accuracy of CMR in the detection of myocarditis has demonstrated the relative merit of using a T_2-weighted imaging strategy such as inversion recovery sequence. This approach of detecting myocarditic lesions showed a sensitivity of 84 percent and specificity of 74 percent on the basis of biopsy or natural history evidence of myocarditis.[50] The addition of T_2-weighted imaging to the more commonly used gadolinium-DTPA–based extracellular T_1 altering contrast agent and the inclusion of local delayed enhancement further increased the diagnostic accuracy to more than 90 percent by collation of all of the current studies.[49] The delayed contrast enhancement phenomena is often associated with the recent cardiac necrosis or a healing of the myocardium following myocardial infarction, but in the setting of myocarditis can also be used to further increase the sensitivity and specificity of diagnosis. The mechanism is not clear but may be related to the deposition of local collagen bundles during the healing process that can also temporarily bind the gadolinium-DTPA to delay its clearance.

The ability to localize areas of tissue signature abnormality together with regional wall motion abnormality visualized on the CMR has permitted contrast-enhanced CMR to also guide subsequent myocardial biopsy. Mahrholt and colleagues[51] used this CMR-guided cardiac biopsy in 32 patients with suspected myocarditis. Biopsy in these abnormal regions showed remarkable positive and negative predictive values of 71 and 100 percent, respectively.[51] Interestingly, CMR suggested that the lateral wall actually may be the most common location for lesion development, and not the septum, from which most of the biopsy samples have been taken previously.

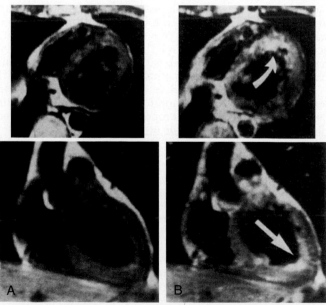

FIGURE 66–6 A, Precontrast T_1-weighted transaxial **(top)** and coronal **(bottom)** magnetic resonance images through the left ventricle in a patient with myocarditis. **B,** Postcontrast magnetic resonance images at the same levels after contrast injection. Note enhancement of the myocardial signal in the septum and apical region (arrows). *(From Matsouka H, Hamada M, Honda T, et al: Evaluation of acute myocarditis and pericarditis by Gd-DTPA enhanced magnetic resonance imaging. Eur Heart J 15:283, 1994.)*

Because of the relatively noninvasive nature of CMR, this imaging technique could also be repeated to follow the patient's natural history of the condition and monitor response to therapy.

Myocardial Biopsy

Histological Evaluation

The Dallas criteria for the diagnosis of myocarditis represented the first attempt to standardize the pathological definition of myocarditis. The Dallas criteria require an inflammatory infiltrate and associated myocyte necrosis or damage not characteristic of an ischemic event. Borderline myocarditis requires a less intense inflammatory infiltrate and no light microscopic evidence of myocyte destruction. Despite its insensitivity for detecting myocarditis, it remains the gold standard for making the unequivocal diagnosis.

The reasons for the insensitivity of Dallas criteria are many, and some of them are outlined here. Because of the patchy nature of the myocarditic lesions in the myocardium, standard myocardial biopsy of sampling myocardial tissue of approximately 30 mg in mass is a "hit and miss" phenomenon. Chow and McManus[52] first demonstrated this insensitivity by biopsying postmortem hearts from patients with myocarditis. They demonstrated that with a single endomyocardial biopsy, histological myocarditis could be demonstrated in only 25 percent of cases. Even with five random biopsies, the correct diagnosis of myocarditis by the classic Dallas criteria could be reached in only about two thirds of subjects. This is further compounded by a recent magnetic resonance imaging study showing that the earliest myocardial inflammatory abnormalities in myocarditis were located commonly in the lateral wall of the left ventricle, a site difficult to reach with standard bioptome.[51] Therefore, there is considerable built-in sampling error and insensitivity with the standard diagnosis of myocarditis using endomyocardial biopsies. To compound the situation further, there are also variations in the interpretation of histological samples by expert pathologists experienced in reading cardiac biopsies. For example, of the 111 patients recruited in the original National Institutes of Health (NIH) Myocarditis Treatment Trial diagnosed with myocarditis by heart biopsy, only 64% had that diagnosis confirmed by the expert pathology panel during consensus reading of the same biopsy samples later in time.[53]

The current American College of Cardiology/American Heart Association (ACC/AHA) guidelines for the treatment of heart failure consider endomyocardial biopsy as a class IIb recommendation.[54] Myocardial biopsy is generally reserved for patients with rapidly progressive cardiomyopathy refractory to conventional therapeutic management or an unexplained cardiomyopathy that is associated with progressive conduction system disease or life-threatening ventricular arrhythmias. It should also be considered when cardiovascular signs or symptoms develop in a patient with a systemic disease known to cause LV dysfunction. It is not routinely indicated in patients with all suspected myocarditis.

RISKS OF ENDOMYOCARDIAL BIOPSY

Studies suggest that the complication rate of myocardial biopsy in patients with dilated cardiomyopathy is approximately 2 to 5 percent. Approximately half of these complications are related to venous access, and the remainder to the biopsy procedure itself. Complications related to venous access include inadvertent arterial puncture, pneumothorax, vasovagal reaction, or bleeding after sheath removal. The use of ultrasonographically guided techniques to identify the internal jugular vein and/or guide in vein cannulation improves the success rate and decreases the complication rate and access time. Complications associated with the procedure include arrhythmias, cardiac conduction abnormalities, and cardiac perforation, which can lead to pericardial tamponade and, rarely, death. Patients with perforation report pain, which otherwise should not be experienced during the procedure. These patients may deteriorate rapidly because of the rapid accumulation of blood in the pericardial space and underlying LV dysfunction. The rapid accumulation of blood in the pericardial space can form a clot acutely, which may interfere with percutaneous pericardial evacuation of blood. Patients who cannot be immediately resuscitated by percutaneous pericardiocentesis should have open chest evacuation of the hematoma. This requires coordination with cardiovascular surgery and preparation in the laboratory for the occurrence of these rare, but expected, complications. The complication rate with biopsies via the femoral vein is at least equivalent to that experienced with a jugular venous procedure. Performance of LV biopsies shares similar perforation complication rates, despite the greater wall thickness of the left ventricle.

Molecular Evaluation

Although the traditional Dallas criteria based on standard pathological analysis of myocardial biopsies have limitations, advances in molecular techniques for detecting the viral genome and inflammatory activation within the same biopsy have expanded our ability to detect viral myocarditis significantly, delineate the potential viral etiology, and improve the sensitivity of the biopsy as a diagnostic technique.

Molecular detection techniques for viral genome such as in situ hybridization seeking the presence of viral genetic signatures in a pathological sample or multiplexed PCR amplification of the RNA from the biopsy itself have increased the sensitivity of detecting virus signatures in the heart. These techniques have demonstrated that viral ribonucleic acid can be significantly associated with symptoms and prognosis. However, the surprise was that the presence of viral genome is entirely independent of the presence or absence of inflammatory cells on the same biopsy. Thus a tissue sample can be Dallas criteria–positive only, molecularly positive only, both, or neither. This underscores that myocarditis is truly a disease of the molecular trigger by the virus or the immunological response by the host—either alone will be able to produce the disease syndrome.

Additional analysis of immunological activation on the biopsy tissues may also provide information. The tissues can be analyzed for inflammatory cell infiltration subtypes, or signal activation, such as cytokine and complement signals. The tissues can also be analyzed for the upregulation of major histocompatibility (MHC) antigens. Although the sensitivity of specificity of MHC antigen upregulation has been shown to be 80 and 85 percent, respectively, from studies of small sample size, this has not been replicated in larger series. Nevertheless, MHC expression has been used to guide therapy of patients with myocarditis and inflammatory cardiomyopathy in one study evaluating immunosuppressive therapy.[55]

PROGNOSIS

Patients with acute myocarditis and mild cardiac involvement generally will recover in the majority of cases without long-term sequelae. However, patients with more advanced cardiac dysfunction accompanying myocarditis may have a more varied outlook. Of these, at least one third of the patients will have residual ventricular dysfunction, about 25 percent may progress to transplantation or death and the remainder will recover to normal ventricular function.[47]

Specific subgroups of patients with myocarditis have significantly differential outcome. Patients with fulminant myocarditis have an excellent long-term prognosis, with one series documenting transplant-free survival of 93 percent in 11 years.[48] In contrast, patients with giant cell myocarditis have an extremely poor prognosis, with median survival of less than 6 months, and most will require transplantation to avoid succumbing to the disease (Fig. 66-7). On the other hand, patients with chronic active myocarditis with dilated cardiomyopathy, as those recruited into the NIH Myocarditis Treatment Trial, still have a relatively poor prognosis. These patients all had the diagnosis of myocarditis based on the Dallas biopsy criteria and showed a mortality of 20 percent at 1 year and 56 percent at 4.3 years, with many cases of chronic heart failure despite optimal medical management (Fig. 66-8).[53]

Several studies have attempted to identify clinical variables that can predict adverse outcomes in viral myocarditis. Although many of these variables cannot be replicated from study to study, several factors do appear to predict death or transplantation including presentation with syncope, bundle branch block on ECG, or an ejection frac-

tion of less than 40 percent. On the other hand, 2-D echocardiographic evidence of a small left atrial and LV size were predictive of myocardial recovery from a small study of 15 patients. Although general pathological features of myocyte necrosis or inflammatory cell infiltration on the biopsy almost never predict prognosis, the resolution of myocarditis on follow-up biopsy or absence of Azan-Mallory staining of cardiac myocytes (a marker of cellular edema and/or myocytolysis) do appear to herald functional ventricular recovery.[56]

Why and colleagues[57] reported that among 120 patients with dilated cardiomyopathy, the group (34 percent) that was positive for enteroviral minus strand ribonucleic acid had a significantly worse outcome over 2 years (68 versus 92 percent, $p = 0.02$), when compared with those who were enteroviral genome negative.[57] More recently, Kuhl[12] also demonstrated that viral genome persistence on myocardial biopsy predicted more rapid deterioration of ventricular function during follow-up. Interestingly, molecular markers of cell apoptosis may turn out to be a good prognostic marker. Fuse and colleagues[36] from Japan found that serum levels of soluble Fas and Fas ligand were significantly higher in patients with fatal myocarditis compared with survivors. Sheppard[58] more recently examined the patients who participated in the Intervention in Myocarditis and Acute Cardiomyopathy (IMAC II) trial. Patients with myocardial expression of Fas ligand or tumor necrosis factor receptor 1 (TNFR1) showed minimal recovery, which again suggests that excessive apoptosis is a poor prognosticator in patients with acute myocarditis. Because of the diversity of outcomes in patients with myocarditis and the general lack of dramatic response to treatment, meticulous follow-up of patients to determine their natural history is important. This will also help to determine the need for continuation or additional therapy and ongoing risk determination.

THERAPEUTIC APPROACHES

Supportive Therapy

The first-line therapy for all patients with myocarditis and heart failure is supportive care (see also Chap. 25). A small proportion of patients will require hemodynamic support that ranges from vasopressors (see Chap. 24) to intraaortic balloon pump to VADs (see Chap. 28) (Fig. 66-9). These patients should be treated as any patient with clinical heart failure including initial diuretics to remove excessive volume overload if present. Patients may also benefit from intravenous vasodilators such as nitroglycerin or nesiritide in appropriate doses with appropriate monitoring to improve cardiac output and lower filling pressures (see Chap. 24). The patient should then be initiated on recommended therapy for heart failure, such as angiotensin modulators (angiotensin-converting enzyme [ACE] inhibitors or angiotensin receptor blockers) and beta blockers, as soon as they are clinically stable and able to tolerate these medications (see Chap. 25). The patient should follow the current ACC/AHA/ESC/CCS guidelines for heart failure care.[54,59]

Although there is usually an urgent discussion of whether immunosuppressive therapies should be used for patients with myocarditis, what is not well recognized is the fact that the traditional heart failure therapies may already have a significant antiinflammatory effect. ACE inhibitors together with beta blockers represent the cornerstones of modern heart failure therapy. It has been previously well documented that angiotensin is a potent proinflammatory and prooxidative agent. ACE inhibitors have been shown to decrease the expression of adhesion molecules on the surface of the endothelium. ACE inhibitors also have general anti-inflammatory properties in terms of attenuating inflam-

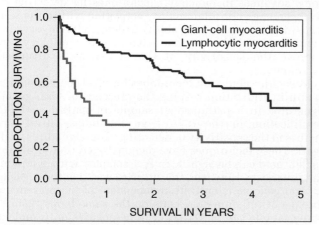

FIGURE 66–7 Prognosis in patients with giant cell myocarditis. Patients with giant cell myocarditis have much worse survival when compared with lymphocytic myocarditis, particularly in the acute phase soon after presentation.

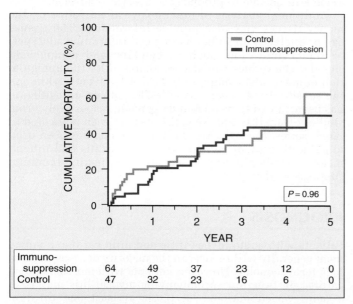

FIGURE 66–8 The cumulative mortality data from the National Institutes of Health–sponsored Myocarditis Treatment Trial. The mortality curve confirms the general poor prognosis of patients with myocarditis who unfortunately did not demonstrate that the immunosuppressive treatment (red line) conferred any mortality benefit over standard medical therapy (control, blue line). Overall, 20 percent of the patients were dead in 1 year, and 54 percent died during 4.3 years of follow-up. A temporary improvement in the immunosuppressive arm was not sustained. (*Modified from Mason JW, O'Connell JB, Herskowitz A, et al: A clinical trial of immunosuppressive therapy for myocarditis. The Myocarditis Treatment Trial Investigators. N Engl J Med 333:269, 1995.*)

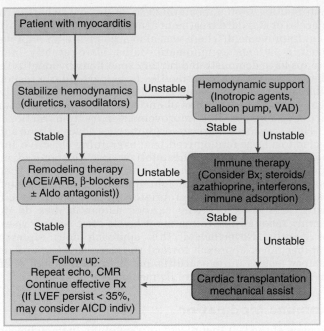

FIGURE 66–9 Treatment algorithms for patients with myocarditis, depending on hemodynamic stability and response to general supportive and remodeling treatment regimen at each step. All patients should have aggressive support and appropriate follow-up. Immunotherapy at the present time is still mainly to support those have failed to spontaneously improve. ACEi = angiotensin-converting enzyme inhibitors; AICD = automatic implantable cardioverter-defibrillator; Aldo = aldosterone; ARB = angiotensin receptor blockers; Bx = biopsy; indiv = based on individual assessment of risk versus benefit; VAD = ventricular assist device.

matory cell mobilization and cytokine release. The effects of ACE inhibitors observed to date in heart failure and atherosclerosis are consistent with its effect on inflammation. Although beta blockers have traditionally been associated mainly with blockade of the adrenergic system, more recently there has been appreciation that they may also affect inflammatory cytokine signaling. In a canine model of heart failure, the effective use of beta blockade in this setting can significantly reduce cytokine gene expression in the myocardium. This is accompanied by improvement in ventricular function and reverses remodeling of the left ventricle.

Immunosuppression

Because inflammatory cell infiltrates have consistently been found on the myocardial biopsies or autopsies of patients who have myocarditis, the general belief has been that immunosuppression should be beneficial for myocarditis. However, this is an unproven hypothesis, as current understanding of inflammation suggests that the immune response can be as much protective as harmful and that broad immunosuppressive regimens may produce as much harm as benefit. To date, there is no shortage of small trials evaluating a variety of immunosuppressive regimens. However, all of them are fraught with significant limitations including (1) the high degree of spontaneous improvement in the control and treatment arms, (2) the small sample size with a heterogeneous collection of recruited patients, (3) the patchy nature of myocardial biopsy detection of myocarditis, and (4) the lack of relationship between pathological abnormalities and clinical prognosis.

The first systematic approach to evaluate immune modulatory therapy in heart disease is the NIH-sponsored Myocarditis Treatment Trial (see Fig. 66-8). In this trial, patients with biopsy-proven myocarditis according to the Dallas criteria were randomized to receive either conventional therapy including ACE inhibitors and standard anti–heart failure regimen or the addition of immunosuppressive therapy. The immunosuppressive therapy regimen consisted of steroids, azathioprine, or cyclosporine. The results showed that that there was a significant improvement in ejection fraction in both arms of the randomized trial, such that at the end of follow-up period at 4.3 years, there was no significant difference between the two arms.[53] The overall outcome of patients with myocarditis and dilated cardiomyopathy is still poor in the trial. Predictors of improvement included high initial LV ejection fraction (LVEF), less intensive conventional therapy, and short duration of symptoms. When examining the survival in more detail, there was a trend for improvement in the immunosuppressed arm while the treatment was actively being administered. However, because the immunosuppression was given for only 6 months and was discontinued thereafter, the effect was not sustained. In retrospect, during the time conducting the Myocarditis Treatment Trial, the clinical approach was focused on overly simplified notion of immune activation in myocarditis and heart failure. The immunosuppressive regimen used was nonspecific for the innate or acquired arms of immunity. In addition, there was no delineation of the viral etiology in the trial itself. Finally, the patients in the trial were at various stages of development of cardiomyopathy and the sample size was not adequate in retrospect to detect a transient albeit potentially important benefit over the short term.[1] A recent series from Italy examined 112 patients with active biopsy-proven myocarditis caused by failure of conventional therapy, of whom 41 were treated with prednisone and azathioprine. The responders to the immunosuppressive regimen were 90 percent positive for cardiac autoantibodies, and no evidence of persisting viral genome existed.[60] This suggested that predictors of response to immunosuppression may evolve.

On the basis of the results of the foregoing studies, immunosuppression should not be routinely considered for patients with myocarditis. However, patients with giant cell myocarditis, myocarditis caused by autoimmune or hypersensitivity reactions, or patients with severe hemodynamic compromise and deteriorating conditions may benefit from a trial of immunosuppressive therapy in the hope of stabilizing hemodynamic condition of the patient. The best responders may be those with an active autoimmune response without persisting viral genome. Clinicians must be aware that this will unlikely influence the ultimate mortality of the patient but may improve the short-term natural history.

Interferon

Type I interferons (interferons alpha and beta) exert antiviral activity by virtue of their ability to phosphorylate interferon-stimulated genes (ISGs) in the host innate immune system. These ISGs together can lead to degradation of foreign viral RNA, and the small GTPase Mx (a component of the ISG) can interfere with the accumulation of viral RNA and coat protein. Interferon beta has been shown to be most effective in animal models of viral myocarditis, and we have demonstrated recently that interferon beta knockout animals (IFN-$\beta^{-/-}$) have a higher viral titer, increased inflammatory cell infiltrate, increased mortality, and worse cardiac function.[38]

To determine if this strategy can be applied to patients, Kuhl and colleagues[46] have evaluated 22 patients with dilated cardiomyopathy and biopsy evidence of viral persistence. The patients were treated with subcutaneous interferon beta for 24 weeks. The interferon treatment eliminated the viral genome from all patients, and ventricular function improved in 15 of 22 patients. The mean LVEF improved from 44.6 to 53.1 percent ($p < 0.001$). Overall, the patients also improved in clinical status. These encouraging phase II results have paved the way for an ongoing worldwide phase III trial of interferon β in patients with dilated cardiomyopathy. Preliminary data in the phase III trial suggested that there is a significant improvement in both symptoms and ventricular function when compared with standard heart failure therapy. If this is replicated, it will be a significant advancement for the treatment of myocarditis.

Intravenous Immunoglobulin

Many causes of acute-onset dilated cardiomyopathy including peripartum cardiomyopathy likely represent an autoimmune inflammatory process in the myocardium that is triggered by a transient viral infection. Instead of anticytokine therapy or active immune suppression, a possible strategy is to infuse passive immunization through the infusion of immune globulins. In cases of pediatric heart failure, particularly myocarditis, uncontrolled studies suggested a potential benefit with intravenous immunoglobulins.

Retrospective analysis suggests that of patients with peripartum cardiomyopathy (many of whom also had concurrent myocarditis), those who received intravenous immunoglobulin appear to have better ventricular function during follow-up.[61] To test this hypothesis more thoroughly and prospectively in adults, McNamara and Feldman[62] conducted a randomized, double-blinded trial involving 62 patients with acute heart failure and randomized the patients with 2 g/kg of intravenous immunoglobulin or placebo. They followed the patients for changes in LVEF from the baseline to 6 months and 12 months (IMAC II trial).[62] Overall, there was impressive improvement of LVEF from 25 to 41 percent at 6 months and to 42 percent at 12 months; however, the improvement was identical in both the intravenous immunoglobulin treatment arm, as well as the placebo arm. The transplant-free survival was 92 percent at 1 year. In the IMAC trial, the patients spontaneously improved LVEF significantly with or without immunoglobulin treatment. The rapid improvement in LV ejection fraction in the control precluded any possibility of demonstrating a treatment effect. In retrospect the evaluation of this agent in a more advanced chronic cardiomyopathy population with evidence of inflammation in the heart may have produced a more definitive result. Accordingly, at present there is no primary indication for immunoglobulins in myocarditis, except perhaps in the pediatric population and those refractory to immunosuppressive therapy.

Immune Adsorption Therapy

A physical approach to remove potential cardiac depressant factors is immune adsorption therapy through the plasmapheresis of peripheral blood. Suggestions have been made that in addition to cytokines, circulating antibodies may target against specific components of the myocyte under stress, such as the beta adrenergic receptor, the adenosine triphosphate carrier, or even the myosin molecule, leading to eventual cell dysfunction and cell death. Various strategies have been developed to capture these cardiodepressant factors or antibodies using immune adsorption columns.

In one earlier randomized trial using immune adsorption therapy, 34 patients were randomized to standard therapy or immune adsorption therapy aimed to remove antibodies against the beta adrenergic receptor.[63] After 1 year of treatment, the treated group demonstrated a change of LV ejec-

tion fraction from a mean of 22 to 38 percent, whereas the placebo or standard treatment arm did not show any significant improvement. There was also accompanying improvement in patients' symptomatic status. More recently, other groups have demonstrated further specificity by identifying the IgG-3 subclass of antibodies to be particularly responsible for cardiac depression.[64,65] Patients who had effective removal of the IgG-3 class of antibodies are those who particularly demonstrated improvement in ejection fraction.

However, these innovative approaches have not been subjected to a large randomized trial examining objective endpoints such as deaths or hospitalization with standardized immunoadsorption columns or treatment protocols. There is also no mechanistic insight into the treatment benefit caused by the lack of appropriate animal models. Specifically, it is not clear why cardiac autoantibodies do not simply rebound to pretreatment levels after several weeks or months. Nevertheless, this approach does represent another novel approach toward the removal of proinflammatory factors in myocarditis and heart failure and offers the opportunity to explore its mechanism of benefit.

Immune Modulation

In view of the fact that direct anti-cytokine therapy has not been successful, alternative strategies have been sought to abrogate cytokine effects through indirect strategies. A novel technique in which autologous whole blood is irradiated with ultraviolet radiation and reinjected back into the patient intramuscularly has been shown to decrease markers of inflammation. The mechanisms related to this therapy are not clear, but it is thought that the irradiation triggers apoptosis in the white blood cells in the blood and in turn induces tolerance or anergy in activated immune cell clones in the host. A preliminary study involving 75 heart failure patients in functional class III or IV were randomized to receive either immune modulation therapy or placebo on top of standard therapy for 6 months.[66] At the end of the follow-up period, there was no difference in the primary endpoint of the 6-minute walk test, but surprisingly there was a significant reduction in the risk of death ($p = 0.022$) and hospitalization ($p = 0.008$) in the immune modulation group. There was also a suggestion of improved quality of life in the treated patients. This has resulted in a large follow-up mortality/morbidity trial involving more than 2400 patients (ACCLAIM), which concluded in late 2006. As noted in Chapter 29, preliminary results indicated that the overall trial did not reach the primary endpoint of reduction in mortality or hospitalization. However, there appears to be significant risk reduction in patients with class II symptoms who have not reached the stages of advanced heart failure. The mechanisms accounting for this interesting finding are yet to be elucidated but do offer additional support to the concept that modulating the immunological response in some patients with ventricular dysfunction can significantly modify the outcome.

Hemodynamic Support (see also Chap. 28)

Although there has been no universally applicable specific therapy for patients with myocarditis, general supportive measures, even for those patients with hemodynamic compromise, have been effective because a significant portion of patients recover spontaneously. Patients with myocarditis presenting with profound hemodynamic compromise secondary to fulminant myocarditis or cardiogenic shock can be supported effectively with support devices ranging from intraaortic balloon pumps to full VADs. Indeed, many cases of spontaneous recovery following VAD support

CH 66

without the need for transplantation, or so-called "bridge to recovery," are in patients with the primary diagnosis of myocarditis. For example, Simon and colleagues[67] reported from a single-center series of 154 patients receiving VAD therapy, of whom 10 had successful recovery without transplantation.[67] The majority of cases were nonischemic cardiomyopathy including myocarditis in three patients and peripartum cardiomyopathy in four patients.

Vaccination

If viruses continue as the most common etiology for myocarditis and dilated cardiomyopathy, one may consider in the future the possibility of targeted vaccination. Patients who may be genetically susceptible to myocarditis may receive vaccination against the commonest causative agents and thus obviate the risk of developing the disease altogether. One example is the disappearance of endocardial fibroelastosis causing dilated cardiomyopathy in children associated with the mumps vaccination program.[68] If vaccination is effective, this could lead to an effective prevention program of myocarditis and dilated cardiomyopathy, with attendant reduction in cost and improvement in morbidity and mortality.

FUTURE PERSPECTIVES

Myocarditis serves as an excellent model to study host injury and repair. The outcome is critically dependent on the virulence of the causative agent, the ability of the host immune system to mount an appropriate response, and the ability of the host to repair the injury effectively and efficiently. Future determination of the genetic risk factors leading to the phenotype of myocarditis and its potential interactions with the environment, as well as the ability to predict who will or will not recover, will be beneficial in identifying those at particular high risk for developing long-term sequelae.

Meanwhile, the diagnostic techniques are evolving to identify novel blood-based biomarkers reflecting cardiac inflammation through microarray and proteomic analysis of tissues of laboratory models, as well as patient samples. The goal in the near future is to develop a blood-based diagnostic tool or panel with sufficient sensitivity and specificity to obviate the need for myocardial biopsies. The combination of blood samples of biomarkers together with imaging techniques such as CMR imaging may help to properly diagnose and stage the disease and avoid the current problem of severe underdiagnosis caused by dependence on Dallas criteria by biopsy.

With the understanding of new pathophysiological mechanisms, new therapies are also being developed and evaluated in clinical trials. Ongoing interferon and immune-modifying strategies may become more refined as data determining their relative efficacies compared with traditional therapies become available. This may help to develop more evidence-based guidelines for treatment of these ill patients. In addition, the increased refinement of ventricular assist strategies to support patients and ultimately wean them from support without necessary transplantation represents another unique opportunity to improve the outcomes for the patients presenting with dramatic hemodynamic collapse. One long-term goal would be to identify individuals at risk for myocarditis and evaluate the opportunity and cost-effectiveness of developing a combination vaccine to prevent the development of disease in these individuals despite exposure to the causative agents.

REFERENCES

Incidence and Epidemiology

1. Liu P, Mason J: Advances in the understanding of myocarditis. Circulation 104:1076, 2001.
2. Aretz HT, Billingham ME, Edwards WD, et al: Myocarditis, a histopathologic definition and classification. Am J Cardiovasc Pathol 1:3, 1987.
3. Baughman KL: Diagnosis of myocarditis: Death of Dallas criteria. Circulation 113:593, 2006.
4. Fabre A, Sheppard MN: Sudden adult death syndrome and other non-ischaemic causes of sudden cardiac death. Heart 92:316, 2006.
5. Nugent AW, Daubeney PE, Chondros P, et al: The epidemiology of childhood cardiomyopathy in Australia. N Engl J Med 348:1639, 2003.
6. Xiong D, Yajima T, Lim BK, et al: Inducible cardiac restricted expression of enteroviral protease 2A is sufficient to induce dilated cardiomyopathy. Circulation 115:94, 2007.
7. Kuhl U, Pauschinger M, Noutsias M, et al: High prevalence of viral genomes and multiple viral infections in the myocardium of adults with "idiopathic" left ventricular dysfunction. Circulation 111:887, 2005.
8. Tschope C, Bock CT, Kasner M, et al: High prevalence of cardiac parvovirus B19 infection in patients with isolated left ventricular diastolic dysfunction. Circulation 111:879, 2005.
9. Magnani JW, Dec GW: Myocarditis: Current trends in diagnosis and treatment. Circulation 113:876, 2006.
10. Bowles NE, Ni J, Kearney DL, et al: Detection of viruses in myocardial tissues by polymerase chain reaction. Evidence of adenovirus as a common cause of myocarditis in children and adults. J Am Coll Cardiol 42:466, 2003.
11. Matsumori A: Hepatitis C virus infection and cardiomyopathies. Circ Res 96:144, 2005.

Etiologic Agents

12. Kuhl U, Pauschinger M, Seeberg B, et al: Viral persistence in the myocardium is associated with progressive cardiac dysfunction. Circulation 112:1965, 2005.
13. Martino T, Petric M, Weingartl H, et al: The coxsackie-adenovirus receptor (CAR) is used by reference strains and clinical isolates representing all 6 serotypes of coxsackievirus group B, and by swine vesicular disease virus. J Virology 271:99, 2000.
14. Coyne CB, Bergelson JM: Virus-induced Abl and Fyn kinase signals permit coxsackievirus entry through epithelial tight junctions. Cell 124:119, 2006.
15. Pauschinger M, Bowles NE, Fuentes-Garcia FJ, et al: Detection of adenoviral genome in the myocardium of adult patients with idiopathic left ventricular dysfunction. Circulation 99:1348-1354, 1999.
16. Young NS, Brown KE: Parvovirus B19. N Engl J Med 350:586, 2004.
17. Vallbracht KB, Schwimmbeck PL, Kuhl U, et al: Endothelium-dependent flow-mediated vasodilation of systemic arteries is impaired in patients with myocardial virus persistence. Circulation 110:2938, 2004.
18. Craver RD, Sorrells K, Gohd R: Myocarditis with influenza B infection. Pediatr Infect Dis J 16:629, 1997.
19. Noutsias M, Fechner H, de Jonge H, et al: Human coxsackie-adenovirus receptor is colocalized with integrins alpha(v)beta(3) and alpha(v)beta(5) on the cardiomyocyte sarcolemma and upregulated in dilated cardiomyopathy: Implications for cardiotropic viral infections. Circulation 104:275, 2001.
20. Kneen R, Nguyen MD, Solomon T, et al: Clinical features and predictors of diphtheritic cardiomyopathy in Vietnamese children. Clin Infect Dis 39:1591, 2004.
21. Afzal A, Keohane M, Keeley E, et al: Myocarditis and pericarditis with tamponade associated with disseminated tuberculosis. Can J Cardiol 16:519, 2000.
22. Silvestry FE, Kim B, Pollack BJ, et al: Cardiac Whipple disease: Identification of Whipple bacillus by electron microscopy of a patient before death. Ann Intern Med 126:214, 1997.
23. Nowakowski J, Nadelman RB, Sell R, et al: Long-term follow-up of patients with culture-confirmed Lyme disease. Am J Med 115:91, 2003.
24. Barrett MP, Burchmore RJ, Stich A, et al: The trypanosomiasis. Lancet 362:1469, 2003.
25. Hagar J, Rahimtoola S: Chagas' heart disease. Curr Prob Cardiol 20:825, 1995.
26. Hagar JM, Rahimtoola SH: Chagas' heart disease in the United States. N Engl J Med 325:763, 1991.
27. Rassi A Jr, Rassi A, Little WC, et al: Development and validation of a risk score for predicting death in Chagas' heart disease. N Engl J Med 355:799, 2006.
28. Viotti R, Vigliano C, Lococo B, et al: Long-term cardiac outcomes of treating chronic Chagas disease with benznidazole versus no treatment: A nonrandomized trial. Ann Intern Med 144:724, 2006.
29. Murphy JG, Wright RS, Bruce GK, et al: Eosinophilic-lymphocytic myocarditis after smallpox vaccination. Lancet 362:1378, 2003.
30. Killian JG, Kerr K, Lawrence C, Celermajer DS: Myocarditis and cardiomyopathy associated with clozapine. Lancet 354:1841, 1999.

Pathophysiology

31. Ayach B, Fuse K, Martino T, Liu P: Dissecting mechanisms of innate and acquired immunity in myocarditis. Curr Opin Cardiol 18:175, 2003.
32. Bergelson JM, Cunningham JA, Droguett G, et al: Isolation of a common receptor for Coxsackie B viruses and adenoviruses 2 and 5. Science 275:1320, 1997.
33. Martino TA, Petric M, Brown M, et al: Cardiovirulent coxsackieviruses and the decay-accelerating factor (CD55) receptor. Virology 244:302, 1998.

CH 66

Myocarditis

34. Liu PP, Opavsky MA: Viral myocarditis: Receptors that bridge that immune with the cardiovascular systems. Circ Res 86:253, 2000.

35. Badorff C, Lee GH, Lamphear BJ, et al: Enteroviral protease 2A cleaves dystrophin: Evidence of cytoskeletal disruption in an acquired cardiomyopathy. Nat Med 5:320, 1999.

36. Fuse K, Chan G, Liu Y, et al: Myeloid differentiation factor-88 plays a crucial role in the pathogenesis of coxsackievirus B3 induced myocarditis, and influences type I interferon production. Circulation 112:2276, 2005.

37. Liu PP, Le J, Nian M: NF-kB Decoy: Targeting the heart of inflammatory heart disease. Circ Res 89:850, 2001.

38. Deonarain R, Cerullo D, Fuse K, et al: Protective role for interferon-beta in coxsackievirus B3 infection. Circulation 110:3540, 2004.

39. Yajima T, Yasukawa H, Jeon ES, et al: Innate defense mechanism against virus infection within the cardiac myocyte requiring gp130-STAT3 signaling. Circulation 114:2364, 2006.

40. Liu P, Aitken K, Kong YY, et al: Essential role for the tyrosine kinase p56lck in coxsackievirus B3 mediated heart disease. Nature Med 6:429, 2000.

41. Opavsky MA, Martino T, Rabinovitch M, et al: Enhanced ERK-1/2 activation in mice susceptible to coxsackievirus-induced myocarditis. J Clin Invest 109:1561, 2002.

42. Opavsky MA, Penninger J, Aitken K, et al: Susceptibility to myocarditis is dependent on the response of αβ T lymphocytes to coxsackieviral infection. Circ Res 85:551, 1999.

43. Irie-Sasaki J, Sasaki T, Matsumoto W, et al: CD45 is a JAK phosphatase and negatively regulates cytokine receptor signaling. Nature 409:349, 2001.

44. Lee JK, Zaidi SHE, Liu P, et al: A serine elastase inhibitor reduces inflammation and fibrosis and preserves cardiac function following experimental murine myocarditis. Nature Med 4:1383, 1998.

45. Heymans S, Pauschinger M, De Palma A, et al: Inhibition of urokinase-type plasminogen activator or matrix metalloproteinases prevents cardiac injury and dysfunction during viral myocarditis. Circulation 114:565, 2006.

Clinical Presentation and Diagnosis

46. Kuhl U, Pauschinger M, Schwimmbeck PL, et al: Interferon-beta treatment eliminates cardiotropic viruses and improves left ventricular function in patients with myocardial persistence of viral genomes and left ventricular dysfunction. Circulation 107:2793, 2003.

47. Felker GM, Thompson RE, Hare JM, et al: Underlying causes and long-term survival in patients with initially unexplained cardiomyopathy. N Engl J Med 342:1077, 2000.

48. McCarthy RE, Boehmer JP, Hruban RH, et al: Long-term outcome of fulminant myocarditis as compared with acute (nonfulminant) myocarditis. N Engl J Med 342:690, 2000.

49. Liu PP, Yan AT: Cardiovascular magnetic resonance for the diagnosis of acute myocarditis: Prospects for detecting myocardial inflammation. J Am Coll Cardiol 45:1823, 2005.

50. Abdel-Aty H, Boye P, Zagrosek A, et al: Diagnostic performance of cardiovascular magnetic resonance in patients with suspected acute myocarditis: comparison of different approaches. J Am Coll Cardiol 45:1815, 2005.

51. Mahrholdt H, Goedecke C, Wagner A, et al: Cardiovascular magnetic resonance assessment of human myocarditis: A comparison to histology and molecular pathology. Circulation 109:1250, 2004.

52. Chow LH, Radio SJ, Sears TD, McManus BM: Insensitivity of right ventricular endomyocardial biopsy in the diagnosis of myocarditis. J Am Coll Cardiol 14:915, 1989.

53. Mason JW, O'Connell JB, Herskowitz A, et al; Investigators MTT: A clinical trial of immunosuppressive therapy for myocarditis. N Engl J Med 333:269, 1995.

54. Hunt SA, Abraham WT, Chin MH, et al: ACC/AHA 2005 Guideline Update for the Diagnosis and Management of Chronic Heart Failure in the Adult: A report of the American College of Cardiology/American Heart Association Task Force on Practice Guidelines (Writing Committee to Update the 2001 Guidelines for the Evaluation and Management of Heart Failure). Circulation 112:1825, 2005.

55. Wojnicz R, Nowalany-Kozielska E, Wojciechowska C, et al: Randomized, placebo-controlled study for immunosuppressive treatment of inflammatory dilated cardiomyopathy: two-year follow-up results. Circulation 104:39, 2001.

56. Mann DL: Determinants of myocardial recovery in myocarditis has the time come for molecular fingerprinting? J Am Coll Cardiol 46:1043, 2005.

57. Why HJ, Meany BT, Richardson PJ, et al: Clinical and prognostic significance of detection of enteroviral RNA in the myocardium of patients with myocarditis or dilated cardiomyopathy. Circulation 89:2582, 1994.

58. Sheppard R, Bedi M, Kubota T, et al: Myocardial expression of fas and recovery of left ventricular function in patients with recent-onset cardiomyopathy. J Am Coll Cardiol 46:1036, 2005.

59. Arnold JM, Liu P, Demers C, et al: Canadian Cardiovascular Society consensus conference recommendations on heart failure 2006: Diagnosis and management. Can J Cardiol 22:23, 2006.

60. Frustaci A, Chimenti C, Calabrese F, et al: Immunosuppressive therapy for active lymphocytic myocarditis: Virological and immunologic profile of responders versus nonresponders. Circulation 107:857, 2003.

61. Bozkurt B, Villaneuva FS, Holubkov R, et al: Intravenous immune globulin in the therapy of peripartum cardiomyopathy. J Am Coll Cardiol 34:177, 1999.

62. McNamara DM, Holubkov R, Starling RC, et al: Controlled trial of intravenous immune globulin in recent-onset dilated cardiomyopathy. Circulation 103:2254, 2001.

63. Muller J, Wallukat G, Dandel M, et al: Immunoglobulin adsorption in patients with idiopathic dilated cardiomyopathy. Circulation 101:385, 2000.

64. Staudt A, Bohm M, Knebel F, et al: Potential role of autoantibodies belonging to the immunoglobulin G-3 subclass in cardiac dysfunction among patients with dilated cardiomyopathy. Circulation 106:2448, 2002.

65. Staudt A, Schaper F, Stangl V, et al: Immunohistological changes in dilated cardiomyopathy induced by immunoadsorption therapy and subsequent immunoglobulin substitution. Circulation 103:2681, 2001.

66. Torre-Amione G, Sestier F, Radovancevic B, Young J: Effects of a novel immune modulation therapy in patients with advanced chronic heart failure: Results of a randomized, controlled, phase II trial. J Am Coll Cardiol 44:1181, 2004.

67. Simon MA, Kormos RL, Murali S, et al: Myocardial recovery using ventricular assist devices: prevalence, clinical characteristics, and outcomes. Circulation 112:I32, 2005.

68. Ni J, Bowles NE, Kim YH, et al: Viral infection of the myocardium in endocardial fibroelastosis. Molecular evidence for the role of mumps virus as an etiologic agent. Circulation 95:133, 1997.

69. Matsumori A, Yutani C, Ikeda Y, et al: Hepatitis C virus from the hearts of patients with myocarditis and cardiomyopathy. Lab Invest 80:1137, 2000.

CHAPTER 67

Background, 1793

Left Ventricular
Dysfunction, 1793
Left Ventricular Systolic
Dysfunction, 1793
Left Ventricular Diastolic
Dysfunction, 1797

Pericardial Effusion, 1797

Infective Endocarditis, 1798

Nonbacterial Thrombotic
Endocarditis, 1799

Cardiovascular Malignancy, 1799

Isolated Right Ventricular
Disease, 1799

Pulmonary Hypertension, 1799
Vasculitis, 1800

Accelerated
Atherosclerosis, 1800

Autonomic Dysfunction, 1800

Long QT Interval, 1800

Complications of Therapy
for HIV, 1801
Major Adult Complications, 1801
Perinatal Transmission and Vertically
Transmitted HIV Infection, 1802
Monitoring Recommendations, 1803

Future Perspectives, 1803

References, 1804

Cardiovascular Abnormalities in HIV-Infected Individuals

Stacy D. Fisher and Steven E. Lipshultz

BACKGROUND

Infection with the human immunodeficiency virus (HIV) is one of the leading causes of acquired heart disease and specifically of symptomatic heart failure (Table 67-1). Cardiac complications of HIV infection tend to occur late in the disease or are associated with related therapies and are therefore becoming more prevalent as therapy and longevity improve.[1-6] Complicated drug therapies for HIV infection have sustained life but may increase cardiovascular risk and accelerate atherosclerotic disease.[1,7]

Some 38.6 million adults and children were living with HIV infection at the end of 2005. In the United States, approximately 10 percent of those infected are older than age 50. Between 2001 and 2005, the number of people on antiretroviral therapy in low- and middle-income countries increased from 240,000 to approximately 1.3 million. Nevertheless, only one in five people worldwide who need antiretroviral therapy have access to it.[8] The 2- to 5-year incidence of symptomatic heart failure ranges from 4 to 28 percent,[1,9] suggesting a prevalence of symptomatic HIV-related heart failure of between 4 and 5 million cases worldwide. Among HIV-infected children, up to 10 years of age, 25 percent die with chronic cardiac disease[10] and 28 percent experience serious cardiac events after an AIDS-defining illness.[10,11] Antiretroviral therapy clearly increases survival. Early in the epidemic, HIV infections were chiefly found in homosexual men; currently, however, most new cases occur in injection drug users and heterosexual partners of infected persons. New infection rates have plateaued, and minority groups remain overrepresented.[8]

A range of cardiac abnormalities (see Table 67-1) associated with HIV infection has been suggested by autopsy studies; the conditions, in order of frequency, are pericardial effusion, lymphocytic interstitial myocarditis, dilated cardiomyopathy (frequently with myocarditis), infective endocarditis, and malignancy (myocardial Kaposi sarcoma and B-cell immunoblastic lymphoma).[11] Even more prevalent are drug effects and interactions, which directly challenge the cardiovascular system.

LEFT VENTRICULAR DYSFUNCTION

Left Ventricular Systolic Dysfunction

CLINICAL PRESENTATION. In HIV-infected patients, concurrent pulmonary infections, pulmonary hypertension, anemia, portal hypertension, malnutrition, or malignancy can alter or confuse the characteristic signs that define heart failure in other populations. Thus, patients with left ventricular systolic dysfunction can be asymptomatic or can present with New York Heart Association Class III or IV heart failure.

Echocardiography (see Chap. 14) is useful for assessing left ventricular systolic function in this population and, in addition to diagnosing left ventricular dysfunction, often reveals either low to normal wall thickness or left ventricular hypertrophy and a dilated left ventricle.[5,12] Echocardiography should be performed in any patient at elevated cardiovascular risk, with any clinical manifestations of cardiovascular disease, or with unexplained or persistent pulmonary symptoms or viral coinfections at baseline and every 1 to 2 years thereafter, or as clinically indicated.[5,11]

An electrocardiogram (ECG) (see Chap. 12) can reveal nonspecific conduction defects or repolarization changes. The chest radiograph has low sensitivity and specificity for congestive heart failure in patients with HIV infection.[13] In small studies of HIV-infected patients and large populations of patients without HIV infection, brain natriuretic peptide levels have been inversely correlated with left ventricular ejection fraction and can be useful in the differential diagnosis of congestive cardiomyopathy in HIV-infected patients.[14]

Patients with encephalopathy are more likely to die of congestive heart failure than those without encephalopathy (hazard ratio, 3.4).[15] HIV persists in reservoir cells in the myocardium and the cerebral cortex, even after antiretroviral therapy. These cells seem to be important in the development and progression of cardiomyopathy and encephalopathy. Reservoir cells may hold HIV on their surfaces for extended periods and cause progressive tissue damage by chronic release of cytotoxic cytokines.

INCIDENCE. A 4-year observational study of 296 patients with a spectrum of HIV-related disease before highly active antiretroviral therapy (HAART) found 44 (15 percent) with dilated cardiomyopathy (fractional shortening less than 28 percent, with global left ventricular hypokinesis), 13 (4 percent) with isolated right ventricular dysfunction (right ventricle larger than left ventricle on standard two-dimensional views), and 12 (4 percent) with borderline left ventricular dysfunction (left ventricular end-systolic diameter larger than 58 mm but fractional shortening more than 28 percent, or global dysfunction reported by one or two but not all three observers) (Fig. 67-1).[1] Dilated cardiomyopathy was strongly associated with a CD4 count of less than 100 cells/ml.[5]

Left ventricular dysfunction is a common consequence of HIV infection in children. In a study of 205 children infected with HIV by maternal-fetal transmission (enrolled at a median age of 22 months; observed with echocardiography every 4 to 6 months and with electrocardiography, Holter monitoring, and chest radiography every year), the prevalence of decreased left ventricular function (fractional shortening less than 28 percent) was 5.7 percent. The 2-year cumulative incidence was 15.3 percent.[5] The cumulative incidence of symptomatic congestive heart failure, use of cardiac medications, or both, was 10 percent over 2 years.[16]

PATHOGENESIS. A wide variety of possible causative agents has been postulated in HIV-related cardiomyopathy (see Table 67-1), including myocardial infection with HIV itself, opportunistic infections, viral infections, autoimmune response to viral infection, cardiotoxicity or direct mitochondrial injury from therapeutic or illicit drugs, nutritional deficiencies, and cytokine overexpression.

TABLE 67-1	Summary of HIV-Associated Cardiovascular Diseases			
Disease Type	**Possible Causes**	**Incidence/Prevalence**	**Diagnosis**	**Treatment**
Dilated cardiomyopathy	Drug-related: cocaine, AZT, IL-2, doxorubicin, interferon Infectious: HIV, *Toxoplasma*, coxsackievirus group B, EBV, CMV, adenovirus Metabolic or endocrine: selenium or carnitine deficiency, anemia, hypo-calcemia, hypophosphatemia, hyponatremia, hypokalemia, hypo-albuminemia, hypo-thyroidism, growth hormone deficiency, adrenal insufficiency, hyper-insulinemia, hemochromatosis, pheochromocytoma, sarcoidosis, amyloidosis Cytokines: TNF-α, nitric oxide, TGF-β, endothelin-I, interleukins Immunodeficiency: CD4 < 100 cells/mm³ Autoimmune	Up to 8% of asymptomatic patients Up to 25% of autopsy cases Systolic > diastolic	Chest radiographic findings: non-specific conduction abnormalities, PVCs, PACs Echocardiographic findings: low-normal LV wall thickness, increased LV mass, dilated LV, systolic LV dysfunction Possible laboratory studies: troponin T, brain natriuretic peptide level, CD4 count, viral load, viral PCR, *Toxoplasma* serology, thyroid-stimulating hormone, cortisol, carnitine, selenium, serum ACE, vanillylmandelic acid, amyloid, urine analysis, stress testing, myocardial biopsy, cardiac catheterization	Diuretics, digoxin, ACE inhibitors, beta blockers ***Adjunctive treatment in HIV patients:*** treatment of infection; nutritional replacement; IVIG; intensify antiretroviral therapy ***Follow-up:*** serial echocardiography
Pericardial	Bacteria: *Staphylococcus, Streptococcus, Proteus, Klebsiella, Enterococcus, Listeria, Nocardia, Mycobacterium* Viral pathogens: HIV, HSV, CMV, adenovirus, echovirus Other pathogens: *Cryptococcus, Toxoplasma, Histoplasma* Malignancy: Kaposi sarcoma, lymphoma, capillary leak, wasting, malnutrition Hypothyroidism Immunodeficiency Uremia	11%/year, spontaneous resolution in 42% of affected patients; ~30% increase in 6-month mortality	Pericardial rub on examination Echocardiography Fluid analysis for Gram stain and culture, cytology ECG: low voltage, PR depression Associated pleural and peritoneal fluid analysis Pericardial biopsy	Treat the cause ***Follow-up:*** serial echocardiography; intensify antiretroviral therapy; pericardiocentesis or window
Infective endocarditis	Autoimmune Bacteria: *Staphylococcus aureus* or *S. epidermidis, Salmonella, Streptococcus, Haemophilus para-influenzae, Pseudallescheria boydii,* HACEK Fungal: *Aspergillus fumigatus, Candida, Cryptococcus neoformans*	6% increased incidence in IVDA, regardless of HIV status	Blood cultures; echocardiography	IV antibiotics, valve replacements
Nonbacterial thrombotic endocarditis	Valvular damage, vitamin C deficiency, malnutrition, wasting, DIC, hypercoagulable state, prolonged acquired immunodeficiency	Rare but clinically relevant emboli in 42% of cases	Echocardiography	Anticoagulation, treat vasculitis or underlying illness
Malignancy	Kaposi sarcoma, non–Hodgkin lymphoma, leiomyosarcoma, low CD4 count, prolonged immunodeficiency, HHV-8, EBV	Approximately 1% incidence, usually metastatic in HIV-positive patients	Echocardiography, biopsy	Chemotherapy possible
Right ventricular and pulmonary disease	Recurrent pulmonary infections, pulmonary arteritis, microvascular pulmonary emboli		ECG, echocardiog-raphy, right heart catheterization	Diuretics, treat underlying lung infection or disease, anticoagulation

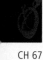

CH 67

TABLE 67–1	Summary of HIV-Associated Cardiovascular Diseases—cont'd			
Disease Type	**Possible Causes**	**Incidence/Prevalence**	**Diagnosis**	**Treatment**
Primary pulmonary hypertension	Plexogenic pulmonary arteriopathy	0.5%	ECG, echocardiog-raphy, right heart catheterization	Anticoagulation, vasodilators, prostacyclin analogues
Vasculitis	Drug therapy with antibiotics and antivirals	Increasing incidence	Clinical diagnosis	Systemic corticosteroids, withdrawal of drug
Accelerated atherosclerosis	Protease inhibitors, atherogenesis with virus-infected macrophages, chronic inflammation, glucose intolerance, dyslipidemia	Up to 8% prevalence	Stress testing, echocardiography, lipid profile, CT angiography, calcium scoring	Minimize risk factors
Autonomic dysfunction	CNS disease, drug therapy, prolonged immunodeficiency, malnutrition	Increased in patients with CNS disease	Tilt-table test, Holter monitoring	Procedural precautions
Arrhythmias	Drug therapy, pentamidine, autonomic dysfunction, acidosis, electrolyte abnormalities		ECG: long QT, Holter monitoring, exercise stress testing	Discontinue drug, procedural precautions
Lipodystrophy	Drug therapy: protease inhibitors		Echocardiography, lipid profile, cardiac catheterization, coronary calcium score	Lipid therapy (beware of drug interactions), aerobic exercise, altered antiretroviral therapy, cosmetic surgery, fat implantation

ACE = angiotensin-converting enzyme; AZT = azidothymidine; CMV = cytomegalovirus; CNS = central nervous system; DIC = disseminated intravascular coagulation; EBV = Epstein-Barr virus; ECG = electrocardiogram; HHV = human herpesvirus; HIV = human immunodeficiency virus; HSV = herpes simplex virus; HTN = hypertension; IL-2 = interleukin-2; IVDA = intravenous drug abuse; IVIG = intravenous immunoglobulin; LV = left ventricular; PAC = premature atrial complex; PCR = polymerase chain reaction; PVC = premature ventricular complex; TGF = transforming growth factor; TNF = tumor necrosis factor.

Myocarditis is perhaps the best-studied of the possible causes. Dilated cardiomyopathy can be related to a direct action of HIV on the myocardial tissue or to proteolytic enzymes or cytokine mediators induced by HIV alone or in conjunction with co-infecting viruses.[16-18] *Toxoplasma gondii,* coxsackievirus group B, Epstein-Barr virus, cytomegalovirus, adenovirus, and HIV in myocytes have been found in biopsy specimens.

Autopsy and biopsy results have revealed only scant and patchy inflammatory cell infiltrates in the myocardium.[11,17] HIV can clearly infect myocardial interstitial cells but not the cardiac myocyte. Increased numbers of infected interstitial cells have been found in patients with confirmed myocarditis, in which proteolytic enzymes or increased levels of tumor necrosis factor-alpha (TNF-α) or interleukin may injure the myocytes. Increased levels of TNF-α, inducible nitric oxide synthase, and interleukin-6 in affected patients and experimental models have been reported.[17]

Notably, HIV-related cardiomyopathy is often not associated with any specific opportunistic infection, and approximately 40 percent of patients have not experienced any opportunistic infection before the onset of cardiac symptoms.[11]

CYTOKINE ALTERATIONS. HIV infection increases the production of TNF-α, which alters intracellular calcium homeostasis and increases nitric oxide production, transforming growth factor-beta, and endothelin-1 upregulation.[15] High levels of nitric oxide induced experimentally had a negative inotropic effect and were cytotoxic to myocytes.

In one study, HIV-infected individuals with dilated cardiomyopathy were much more likely to have myocarditis and had a broader spectrum of viral infections than HIV-negative patients with idiopathic dilated cardiomyopathy. Also, levels of TNF-α and induced nitric oxide synthase were higher in myocytes from the HIV-infected patients with dilated cardiomyopathy (particularly those with viral coinfections), and these levels varied inversely with the CD4 count. Immunodeficiency may favor the selection of those viral variants with increased pathogenicity or enhance the cardiovirulence of viral strains.[15,17]

NUTRITIONAL DEFICIENCIES. Nutritional deficiencies are common in HIV infection, particularly in those with late-stage disease. Poor absorption and diarrhea both lead to electrolyte imbalances and deficiencies in elemental nutrients. Deficiencies of trace elements have been associated with cardiomyopathy. For example, selenium deficiency increases the virulence of coxsackievirus to cardiac tissue.[11] Selenium replacement reverses cardiomyopathy and restores left ventricular function in nutritionally depleted patients. Levels of vitamin B_{12}, carnitine, and growth and thyroid hormones can also be altered in HIV disease; all have been associated with left ventricular dysfunction.

PATHOGENESIS IN CHILDREN. In children with vertically transmitted HIV infection, two mechanisms of pathogenesis have been described. One is dilation of the left ventricle with a reduction in the ratio of thickness to end-systolic dimension of the ventricle. The other is concentric hypertrophy of the muscle; with dilation, the ratio of thickness to end-systolic dimension remains normal or is increased.[5]

COURSE OF DISEASE. Patients with asymptomatic left ventricular dysfunction (fractional shortening less than 28 percent, with global left ventricular hypokinesis) may have transient disease by echocardiographic criteria. In one serial echocardiographic study, three of six patients with abnormal fractional shortening had normal readings after a mean of 9 months. The three patients with persistently depressed left ventricular function died within 1 year of baseline.[11]

PROGNOSIS. Mortality in HIV-infected patients with cardiomyopathy is increased, independently of CD4 count, age, sex, and HIV risk group. The median survival to AIDS-related death was 101 days in patients with left ventricular dysfunction and 472 days in patients with a normal heart at a similar stage of infection before HAART therapy (see Fig. 67-1).[1,11] Isolated right ventricular dysfunction or borderline left ventricular dysfunction did not place patients at risk.

CH 67

Cardiovascular Abnormalities in HIV-Infected Individuals

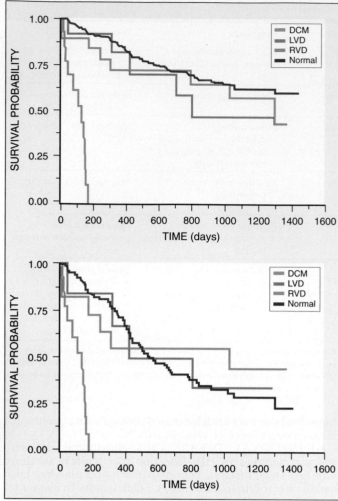

FIGURE 67–1 Top, Survival curves for 296 HIV-infected patients with structurally normal hearts, dilated cardiomyopathy (DCM), left ventricular dysfunction (LVD), or right ventricular dysfunction (RVD). **Bottom,** Time to death related to AIDS in 81 patients with CD4+ cell counts less than 20 × 10^6 cells/L. *(From Currie PF, Jacob AJ, Foreman AR, et al: Heart muscle disease related to HIV infection: Prognostic implications. Br Med J 309:1605, 1994.)*

In the Pediatric Pulmonary and Cardiovascular Complications of Vertically Transmitted HIV Infection (P2C2 HIV) study of children with vertically transmitted HIV infection (median age, 2.1 years), 5-year cumulative survival was 64 percent.[10] Mortality was higher in children with baseline measurements showing depressed left ventricular fractional shortening or increased left ventricular dimension, thickness, mass, wall stress, heart rate, or blood pressure. Decreased left ventricular fractional shortening and increased wall thickness also predicted survival after adjustment for age, height, CD4 count, HIV RNA copy number, clinical center, and encephalopathy.[3,10]

Fractional shortening was abnormal for up to 3 years before death, whereas wall thickness identified a population at risk only 18 to 24 months before death. Thus, in children, fractional shortening may be a useful long-term predictor and wall thickness may be a useful short-term predictor of mortality.[19]

Postmortem cardiomegaly was associated with echocardiographic evidence of increased left ventricular mass and documented chronically increased heart rate before death but not with anemia, encephalopathy, or HIV viral load.[12] In HIV-infected children, mild persistent depression of left ventricular (LV) function and elevated LV mass were associated with higher all-cause mortality.[19]

Rapid-onset congestive heart failure has a grim prognosis in HIV-infected adults and children, with more than 50 percent of patients dying from primary cardiac failure within 12 months of presentation.[10,11] Chronic-onset heart failure may respond better to medical therapy in these patients.

THERAPY. Therapy for dilated cardiomyopathy associated with HIV infection is generally similar to therapy for nonischemic cardiomyopathy and includes diuretics, digoxin, beta blockers, aldosterone antagonists, and angiotensin-converting enzyme inhibitors, as tolerated. No studies have investigated the efficacy of specific cardiac therapeutic regimens other than intravenous immunoglobulin.[2]

Opportunistic or other infections should be sought aggressively and treated to improve or resolve the cardiomyopathy. Right ventricular biopsy may be useful for identifying infectious causes of failure and for suggesting targeted therapy.[11,13] However, right ventricular biopsy is probably underused.

After medical therapy is begun, serial echocardiographic studies should be performed at 4-month intervals (Fig. 67-2).[13] Monitoring recommendations for testing and timing of follow-up are based on studies relating impairment of fractional shortening to a worse prognosis. If function continues to worsen or the clinical course deteriorates, a biopsy should be considered. Patients with congestive heart failure who have not responded to 2 weeks of medical therapy may benefit from cardiac catheterization and endomyocardial biopsy, which may reveal lymphocytic infiltrates suggesting myocarditis or treatable opportunistic infections (by special stains), permitting aggressive therapy of an underlying pathogen. Tissue should be evaluated for the presence of abnormal mitochondria that could suggest benefit from an antiretroviral drug holiday. Angiography should be performed selectively if there are risk factors for atherosclerotic disease or suggestive clinical symptoms.[13]

Intravenous immunoglobulins have had some success in treating acute congestive cardiomyopathy and nonspecific myocarditis in patients who are not infected with HIV. Immunoglobulin therapy is beneficial in Kawasaki disease, an immunologically mediated illness with cardiac dysfunction resembling that seen with HIV disease. Monthly immunoglobulin infusions in HIV-infected children have minimized left ventricular dysfunction, increased left ventricular wall thickness, and reduced peak left ventricular wall stress (Fig. 67-3), suggesting that impaired myocardial growth and left ventricular dysfunction can be immunologically mediated.[2]

The apparent efficacy of immunoglobulin therapy may be the result of immunoglobulins removing cardiac autoantibodies or dampening the secretion or effects of cytokines and cellular growth factors. Immunomodulatory therapy may be helpful in special circumstances or in children with declining left ventricular function.

Patients should be evaluated for nutritional status, and any with deficiencies should receive supplements. Supplementation with selenium, carnitine, multivitamins, or all three can be helpful, especially in anorexic patients or those with wasting or diarrhea syndromes.

Heart transplantation has been reported in one HIV-infected man believed to have anthracycline-related cardiomyopathy. At 24 months of follow-up, his course was complicated by more frequent and higher grade episodes of rejection than average, but otherwise it was relatively uneventful and productive.[20] Liver and kidney transplantation in this population has also now been reported with greater frequency and generally acceptable outcomes. Transplantation therapy is not currently widely available but is an area of active consideration and discussion.

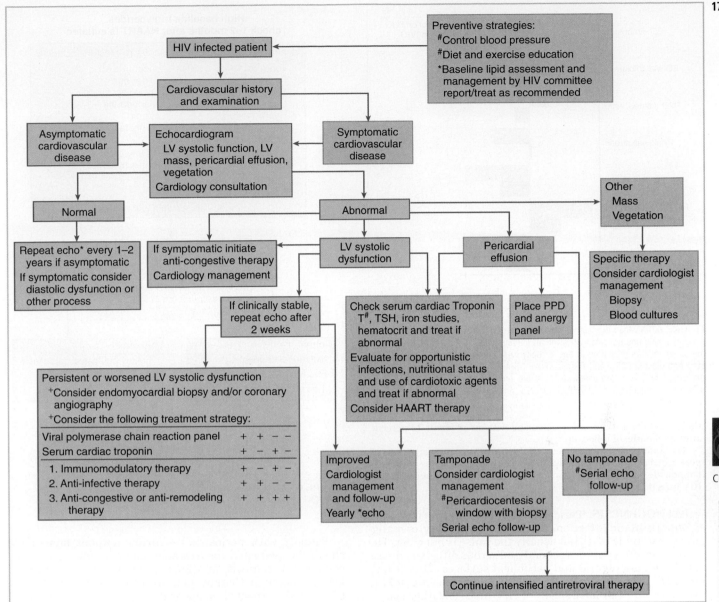

FIGURE 67–2 Cardiac dysfunction in HIV-infected patients. *Evidence-based. #Non-HIV standard of care data. +Thought for future research. HAART = highly active antiretroviral therapy; LV = left ventricular; PPD = purified protein derivative; TSH = thyroid-stimulating hormone. *(From Dolin R, Masur H, Saag MS [eds]: AIDS Therapy. 2nd ed. New York, Churchill Livingstone, 2003, p 817.)*

ANIMAL MODELS. Chronic pathogenic simian immunodeficiency virus (SIV) infection in rhesus macaques has resulted in marked depression of left ventricular ejection fraction and extensive coronary arteriopathy suggestive of a cell-mediated immune response.[21] Notably, 9 of 15 chronically infected macaques who died of SIV had myocardial pathology with lymphocytic myocarditis, and 9 had coronary arteriopathy (6 alone and 3 in combination with myocarditis). Coronary arteriopathy was associated with evidence of vessel occlusion and recanalization, with associated areas of myocardial necrosis in 4 animals. Two animals had marasmic endocarditis, and one had a left ventricular mural thrombus. Animals with cardiac pathology were emaciated to a greater extent than those with SIV and similar periods of infection who did not experience cardiac pathology.

Transgenic mouse models with cardiac pathological changes have been used in research studies. This may help evaluate the impact of environmental factors, therapeutic or illicit drugs, or drug combinations in the cause and therapy of HIV-associated myocarditis.[22]

Left Ventricular Diastolic Dysfunction

Clinical and echocardiographic findings have suggested that diastolic dysfunction is relatively common in long-term survivors of HIV infection. Left ventricular diastolic dysfunction may precede systolic dysfunction.[7,16,19]

PERICARDIAL EFFUSION (see Chap. 70)

CLINICAL PRESENTATION. HIV-infected patients with pericardial effusions generally have a lower CD4 count than those without effusions, marking more advanced disease.[7,19] Effusions are generally small and asymptomatic.

INCIDENCE. Asymptomatic pericardial effusions are common in HIV-infected patients. The 5-year Prospective Evaluation of Cardiac Involvement in AIDS (PRECIA) study found that 16 of 231 patients (59 patients with asymptomatic HIV, 62 with AIDS-related complex, and 74 with AIDS) had pericardial effusions.[23] Three had an effusion on enrollment, and 13 experienced effusions during follow-up (12 had AIDS). Pericardial effusions were small (maximum pericardial space less than 10 mm at end diastole) in 13 and asymptomatic in 14 patients. The incidence of pericardial effusion in those with AIDS was 11 percent/year. The prevalence of effusion in AIDS patients rises over

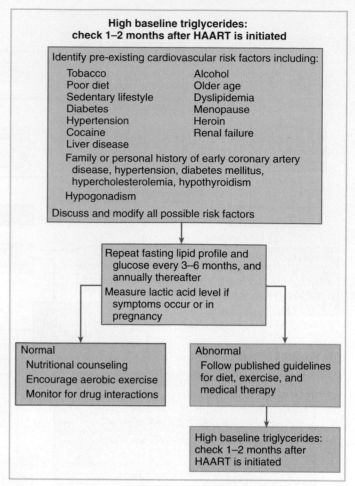

FIGURE 67–3 Mean echocardiographically measured cardiac dimensions in patients taking and not taking intravenous immunoglobulin (IVIG). All measurements are presented as age- or body surface area–adjusted Z scores. ED = end-diastolic; ES = end-systolic. *(From Lipshultz SE, Orav EJ, Sanders SP, et al: Immunoglobulins and left ventricular structure and function in pediatric HIV infection. Circulation 92:2220, 1995. © 1995, American Heart Association.)*

FIGURE 67–4 Cardiovascular considerations when initiating highly active antiretroviral therapy (HAART).

time, reaching a mean in asymptomatic patients of about 22 percent after 25 months of follow-up.[23]

HIV infection should be suspected whenever young patients have pericardial effusion or tamponade. In a retrospective series of cardiac tamponade cases in a city hospital, 13 of 37 patients (35 percent) had HIV infection.[11]

PATHOGENESIS. Pericardial effusion may be related to an opportunistic infection, metabolic abnormality, or malignancy (see Table 67-1), but usually the cause is not clear. The effusion is often part of a generalized serous effusive process also involving pleural and peritoneal surfaces. This "capillary leak" syndrome may be related to enhanced cytokine production in the later stages of HIV disease. Other causes can include uremia from HIV-associated nephropathy and drug nephrotoxicity. Fibrinous pericarditis with or without effusion has also been well described, constituting 9 percent of cardiac lesions found in AIDS patients in one autopsy series.[23]

COURSE OF DISEASE AND PROGNOSIS. Effusion markedly increases mortality. For example, in the PRECIA study, it nearly tripled the risk of death among AIDS patients.[23] Also, 2 of 16 patients with effusions experienced pericardial tamponade. Pericardial effusion may, however, resolve spontaneously in up to 42 percent of patients.[11,18]

MONITORING AND THERAPY. Screening echocardiography is recommended for HIV-infected individuals, regardless of the stage of disease.[13] All HIV-infected patients with evidence of heart failure, Kaposi sarcoma, tuberculosis, or other pulmonary infections should undergo baseline echocardiography and electrocardiographic testing.[13] Patients should undergo pericardiocentesis if they have pericardial effusion and clinical signs of tamponade (e.g., elevated jugular venous pressure, dyspnea, hypotension, persistent tachycardia, pulsus paradoxus) or echocardiographic signs of tamponade (e.g., continuous-wave Doppler evidence of respiratory variation in valvular inflow, septal bounce, right ventricular diastolic collapse, a large effusion).

Patients with pericardial effusion without tamponade should be evaluated for treatable opportunistic infections, such as tuberculosis, and for malignancy. HAART should be considered if therapy has not already been instituted (Fig. 67-4). Repeated echocardiography is recommended after 1 month, or sooner if clinical symptoms direct (see Fig. 67-2).

INFECTIVE ENDOCARDITIS (see Chap. 63)

Injection drug users are at greater risk than the general population for infective endocarditis, chiefly of right-sided heart valves. Surprisingly, HIV-infected patients may not have a higher incidence of endocarditis than people with similar risk behaviors.[7]

Because the autoimmune response to bacterial endocarditis is often largely responsible for the valvular destruction associated with endocarditis, the course of the disease in HIV-infected patients may vary. For example, HIV-infected patients have a higher risk of salmonella endocarditis than immunocompetent patients because they are more likely to be exposed to salmonella bacteremia during salmonella infection. However, they respond better to antibiotic therapy and may be less likely to sustain valvular damage because of their impaired immune response.[11,18,24]

Common organisms associated with endocarditis in HIV-infected patients include *Staphylococcus aureus* and *Salmonella* species. Fungal endocarditis with organisms such as *Aspergillus fumigatus, Candida* species, and *Cryptococ-*

cus neoformans are more common in intravenous drug users with HIV than in those without it and again may be responsive to therapy (see Table 67-1).[11]

Fulminant courses of infective endocarditis with high mortality can occur in late-stage AIDS patients with poor nutritional status and severely compromised immune systems, but several patients have been successfully treated with antibiotic therapy. Operative indications in HIV-infected patients with endocarditis include hemodynamic instability, failure to sterilize blood cultures after appropriate intravenous antibiotics, and severe valvular destruction in patients with a reasonable life expectancy after recovery from surgery.

NONBACTERIAL THROMBOTIC ENDOCARDITIS

Nonbacterial thrombotic endocarditis (or marantic endocarditis) involves large, friable, sterile vegetations that form on the cardiac valves. These lesions have been associated with disseminated intravascular coagulation and systemic embolization. Lesions are rarely diagnosed ante mortem; among patients who do receive the diagnosis, clinically relevant emboli occur in a high percentage of cases.[11] In the early HIV epidemic, several case series suggested a high incidence of this uncommon disorder; however, few cases have since been reported, and almost none have been found in prospective series. Marantic endocarditis should be suspected in any patient with systemic embolization, but should be considered rare in AIDS patients.

Treatment of nonbacterial thrombotic endocarditis should focus on reducing the underlying disease causing coagulation abnormalities, valvular endothelial damage, or both. An anticoagulation risk-benefit assessment must be made on an individual basis.

CARDIOVASCULAR MALIGNANCY (see Chap. 69)

Malignancy affects many AIDS patients, generally in the later stages of disease. Cardiac malignancy is usually metastatic disease.

Kaposi sarcoma (angiosarcoma) is associated with human herpesvirus 8 and affects up to 35 percent of AIDS patients, particularly homosexuals, with an incidence inversely related to the CD4 count. Autopsy studies have found that 28 percent of HIV-infected patients with widespread Kaposi sarcoma have cardiac involvement but this is rarely described as a primary cardiac tumor.[3] Kaposi sarcoma has not been found invading the coronary arteries but is often an endothelial cell neoplasm with a predilection in the heart for subpericardial fat around the coronary arteries.[3]

Kaposi sarcoma involving the heart is generally an incidental finding at autopsy and rarely causes cardiac symptoms. Specific symptoms can be related to pericardial effusion associated with the epicardial location of the tumor. Pericardial fluid in patients with cardiac Kaposi sarcoma is typically serosanguineous, without malignant cells or infection.[3]

Kaposi sarcoma is difficult to treat, although most affected patients die from opportunistic infections related to the advanced stage of immunodeficiency rather than from the malignancy. Protease inhibitors have significantly decreased the incidence of Kaposi sarcoma from its reported incidence in the pre-HAART era.[25]

Primary cardiac malignancy associated with HIV infection is generally caused by cardiac lymphoma. Non–Hodgkin lymphomas are 25 to 60 times more common in HIV-infected individuals. They are the first manifestation of AIDS in up to 4 percent of new cases.[3] Patients with primary cardiac lymphoma can present with dyspnea, right-sided heart failure, biventricular failure, chest pain, or arrhythmias. Cardiac lymphoma is associated with rapid progression to cardiac tamponade, symptoms of congestive heart failure, myocardial infarction, tachyarrhythmias, conduction abnormalities, or superior vena cava syndrome. Pericardial fluid typically reveals malignant cells but can be histologically normal. Systemic multiagent chemotherapy with and without concomitant radiation or surgery has been beneficial in some patients but overall the prognosis is poor.[3] HAART has not substantially affected the incidence of HIV-related non–Hodgkin lymphomas.

Leiomyosarcoma, associated with Epstein-Barr virus, is a rare malignant tumor of smooth muscle origin with an increased incidence in children with AIDS. Leiomyosarcomas are largely noncardiac and often involve the arterial wall.[3] An intracardiac mass in late-stage HIV infection is associated with a uniformly poor prognosis.

ISOLATED RIGHT VENTRICULAR DISEASE

Isolated right ventricular hypertrophy, with or without right ventricular dilation, is relatively uncommon in HIV-infected individuals and is generally related to pulmonary disease that increases pulmonary vascular resistance. Possible causes include multiple bronchopulmonary infections, pulmonary arteritis from the immunological effects of HIV disease, or microvascular pulmonary emboli caused by thrombus or contaminants in injected drugs. In two patients with severe right ventricular dysfunction, in the absence of pulmonary disease or left ventricular dysfunction, right ventricular function returned to normal with antiviral therapy and decreased viral load.[26]

PULMONARY HYPERTENSION (see Chap. 73)

Primary pulmonary hypertension has been described in a disproportionate number of HIV-infected individuals, primarily in case reports. Primary pulmonary hypertension has been estimated to occur in about 0.5 percent of hospitalized AIDS patients.[4,7] In one series of patients with pulmonary hypertension associated with right ventricular hypertrophy and failure, clinical findings included dyspnea on exertion, hypoxemia, restrictive lung disease with decreased diffusing lung capacity for carbon monoxide, and right ventricular hypertrophy on the electrocardiogram (ECG).[4] Histological analysis has often revealed plexogenic pulmonary arteriopathy characterized by remodeling of the pulmonary vasculature, with intimal fibrosis and replacement of normal endothelial structure. All these patients had clear lung fields on examination and chest radiography and normal perfusion scans.

Pulmonary hypertension is often explained by lung infections, venous thromboembolism (see Chap. 72), or left ventricular dysfunction. Pulmonary hypertension found on screening echocardiography or right heart catheterization warrants further examination for treatable pulmonary infections.

Primary pulmonary hypertension has been reported in HIV-infected patients without a history of thromboembolic disease, intravenous drug use, or pulmonary infections associated with HIV.[4] One autopsy and one biopsy specimen revealed precapillary muscular pulmonary artery and arteriole medial hypertrophy, fibroelastosis, and eccentric intimal fibrosis, without direct viral infection of pulmonary artery cells. These findings suggests mediator release from infected cells elsewhere. Primary pulmonary hypertension has also been found in hemophiliacs receiving lyophilized factor VIII, intravenous drug users, and patients with left ventricular dysfunction, obscuring any relationship with HIV.[4] It may be that HIV causes endothelial damage and mediator-related vasoconstriction of the pulmonary arteries.

The CD4 count has been independently associated with survival, and pulmonary hypertension was the direct cause of death in 72 percent of those affected. Survival rates at 1, 2, and 3 years were 73, 60, and 47 percent, respectively. Survival rates in New York Heart Association functional Class III or IV patients at the time of diagnosis were 60, 45, and 28 percent.[27]

Therapy includes anticoagulation (on the basis of individual risk-benefit analysis), vasodilator agents as tolerated, and endothelin antagonists.[28] Safe and effective therapy has been reported using treprostinil (a subcutaneous prostacyclin analogue)[29] and epoprostenol in combination with antiretroviral agents.

Vasculitis (see Chap. 84)

Most types of vasculitis have been reported in HIV-infected patients. Vasculitis should be suspected in patients with fever of unknown origin, unexplained multisystem disease, unexplained arthritis or myositis, glomerulonephritis, peripheral neuropathy (especially mononeuritis multiplex), or unexplained gastrointestinal, cardiac, or central nervous system ischemia. Immunomodulatory therapy, chiefly with systemic corticosteroid therapy, has been successful.

ACCELERATED ATHEROSCLEROSIS (see Chap. 38)

Accelerated atherosclerosis has been observed in young HIV-infected adults and children without traditional coronary risk factors.[30,31] Pronounced coronary lesions were dis-

covered at autopsy in several HIV-positive patients 23 to 32 years of age who died unexpectedly. Cytomegalovirus was present in two of eight patients, and hepatitis B virus was found in two of eight patients. None had evidence of cocaine use.

Premature cerebrovascular disease is common in AIDS patients. The prevalence of stroke in AIDS patients was estimated to be 8 percent on review of autopsy records between 1983 and 1987. Of the patients with stroke, 4 of 13 had evidence of cerebral emboli and the embolus had a clear cardiac source in 3 of those 4. After percutaneous coronary interventions (see Chap. 55), restenosis may be higher than in other populations.[32]

Protease inhibitor therapy markedly alters lipid metabolism and can be associated with premature atherosclerotic disease. Chronic inflammatory states have also been associated with premature atherosclerotic vascular disease. Atherosclerotic disease in the HIV-infected patient is believed to have multifactorial causes and is prone to plaque rupture, possibly related to the host environment (Figs. 67-5 and 67-6).[37]

Protease inhibitor therapy, and specifically HAART overall, however, have clearly improved morbidity and mortality, with no short-term evidence of increased cardiovascular mortality.[33] Lipodystrophy, including fat redistribution with increased truncal obesity, temporal wasting, increased triglyceride levels, elevated small dense low-density lipoprotein levels, and glucose intolerance, should be recognized and treated because of an elevated 10-year cardiovascular risk.[7,31] Risk stratification based on traditional risk factors plus diet, alcohol intake, physical exercise, hypertriglyceridemia, cocaine use, heroin use, thyroid disease, renal disease, and hypogonadism should be considered for long-term cardiac preventive care (see Fig. 67-4).[13,31,33]

Fat redistribution is seen in 42 percent of children after more than 5 years of antiretroviral therapy.[30] Routine physical and laboratory assessment should be part of routine follow-up to balance cardiovascular risk and necessary HIV therapies. Diet and exercise modification are recommended to reduce cardiovascular risk.

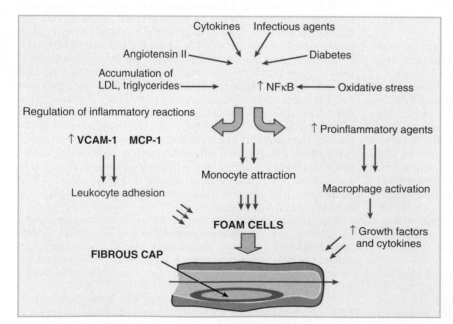

FIGURE 67–5 Foam cells and fibrous cap formation. LDL = low-density lipoprotein; NF-κB = nuclear factor kappa B; VCAM-1 = vascular cell adhesion molecule-1. *(From Fisher SD, Miller TL, Lipshultz SE: Impact of HIV and highly active antiretroviral therapy on leukocyte adhesion molecules, arterial inflammation, dyslipidemia, and atherosclerosis. Atherosclerosis 185:1, 2006.)*

AUTONOMIC DYSFUNCTION (see Chap. 89)

Early clinical signs of autonomic dysfunction in HIV-infected patients include syncope and presyncope, diminished sweating, diarrhea, bladder dysfunction, and impotence. In one study, heart rate variability, Valsalva ratio, cold pressor testing, and hemodynamic responses to isometric exercise, tilt-table testing, and standing have shown that autonomic dysfunction occurs in patients with HIV and is pronounced in AIDS patients. AIDS patients undergoing HAART are relatively protected. Patients with HIV-associated nervous system disease have the greatest abnormalities in autonomic function (Fig. 67-7).[34]

LONG QT INTERVAL (see Chaps. 32 and 35)

HIV infection is associated with QT prolongation and torsades de pointes ventricular tachycardia; the incidence increases with progression to AIDS.[35] Hepatitis C is independently associated with increased QT duration, and co-infection with HIV nearly doubles the risk of clinically important QT prolongation (i.e., QTc values of 470 milliseconds or longer). The risk of QT prolongation was 16 percent with HIV alone and 30 percent with both HIV and hepatitis C infections.[36]

COMPLICATIONS OF THERAPY FOR HIV

Major Adult Complications

Potent antiretroviral medications and HAART, which generally combines three or more agents and usually includes a protease inhibitor, have clearly increased the life span and quality of life of HIV-infected patients.[9] However, protease inhibitors, particularly when used in combination therapy or in HAART, are associated with lipodystrophy, fat wasting and redistribution, metabolic abnormalities, hyperlipidemia, insulin resistance, and increased atherosclerotic risk (see Fig. 67-4). HIV-infected patients treated with protease inhibitors have reported substantial decreases in total body fat with peripheral lipodystrophy (fat wasting of the face, limbs, and buttocks) and relative conservation or enhancement of central adiposity (truncal obesity, breast enlargement, and "buffalo hump") compared with patients who have not received protease inhibitors. Lipid alterations associated with protease inhibitors include higher triglyceride, total cholesterol, insulin, lipoprotein(a), and C-peptide levels and lower high-density lipoprotein levels, all contributing to an atherogenic profile.[31]

Lipid abnormalities vary with different protease inhibitors. Ritonavir has the most adverse effects on lipids, with a mean increase in total cholesterol of 2.0 mmol/liter and a mean increase in triglycerides of 1.83 mmol/liter. More modest increases of total cholesterol without marked triglyceride increases are found in patients taking indinavir and nelfinavir. Combination with saquinavir does not elevate the total cholesterol further. Protease inhibitor therapy increases lipoprotein(a) by 48 percent in patients with elevated pretreatment values (higher than 20 mg/dl).[37] In some cases, switching protease inhibitors may reverse elevations in triglyceride levels and in abnormal fat deposition. Low-level aerobic exercise may also help reverse lipid abnormalities.[7,38]

Zidovudine or azidothymidine (AZT) has been implicated in skeletal muscle myopathies. In culture, AZT causes a dose-dependent destruction of human myotubes. Human cultured cardiac muscle cells treated with AZT develop mitochondrial abnormalities, and non-nucleoside reverse transcriptase inhibitors in general have been associated with altered mitochondrial DNA replication.[39] However, cardiac myopathies have not been evident in clinical data. Rarely, patients with left ventricular dysfunction have improved with cessation of AZT therapy.

Intravenous pentamidine, used to treat *Pneumocystis jiroveci* (formerly known as *P. carinii*) pneumonia in patients intolerant of trimethoprim-sulfamethoxazole, has been associated with cases of torsades de pointes and refractory ventricular tachycardia.[11,39] Pentamidine should be reserved for patients whose QTc interval is 48 milliseconds or longer. A number of medication reactions and interactions have occurred during the treatment of HIV infection and are a

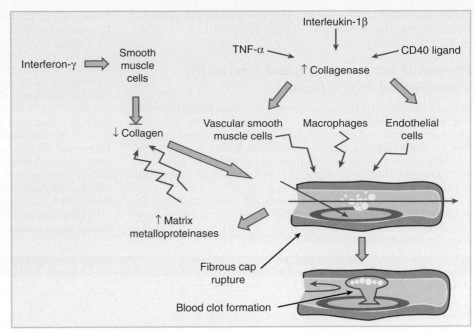

FIGURE 67–6 Rupture of fibrous cap and blood clot formation. (See also Chap. 38.) *(From Fisher SD, Miller TL, Lipshultz SE: Impact of HIV and highly active antiretroviral therapy on leukocyte adhesion molecules, arterial inflammation, dyslipidemia, and atherosclerosis. Atherosclerosis 185:11, 2006.)*

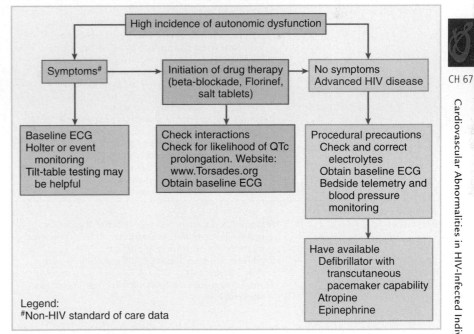

FIGURE 67–7 Evaluation and management of dysautonomia. ECG = electrocardiography. *(Modified from Dolin R, Masur H, Saag MG [ed]:. AIDS Therapy. 2nd ed. New York, Churchill Livingstone, 2003, p 817.)*

1802 major cause of cardiac emergencies in HIV-infected patients. Common cardiac drug interactions are outlined in Table 67-2.

Perinatal Transmission and Vertically Transmitted HIV Infection

Most children with HIV are infected in the perinatal period, but HIV transmission can be minimized if mothers are given antiretroviral therapy in the second and third trimesters or short courses before parturition.[40] The incidence of vertical transmission can be limited to less than 2 percent with current therapies, some including up to 6 months of neonatal AZT.

Rates of congenital cardiovascular malformations in cohorts of HIV-uninfected and HIV-infected children born to HIV-infected mothers range from 5.6 to 8.9 percent. These rates are 5 to 10 times higher than those reported in population-based epidemiological studies but are not higher than in normal populations similarly screened.[11]

In the same cohorts, serial echocardiograms obtained at 4- to 6-month intervals have shown subclinical cardiac abnormalities to be common, persistent, and often progressive.[5] Some have dilated cardiomyopathy (left ventricular contractility 2 standard deviations, SDs, or more below the normal mean and left ventricular end-diastolic dimension 2 SDs or more above the mean) and some have mildly increased cardiac mass for height and weight. Depressed left ventricular function correlated with immune dysfunction at baseline but not longitudinally, suggesting that the CD4 cell count may not be a useful surrogate marker of HIV-associated left ventricular dysfunction. The development of encephalopathy is highly correlated with a decline in fractional shortening.

CH 67

TABLE 67–2	Cardiovascular Actions and Interactions of Drugs Commonly Used in HIV Therapy*	
Class	**Cardiac Drug Interactions**	**Cardiac Side Effects**
Antiretrovirals		
Nucleoside reverse transcriptase inhibitors	Zidovudine and dipyridamole	Rare: lactic acidosis, hypotension, accelerated risk with cardiopulmonary bypass Zidovudine: skeletal muscle myopathy, myocarditis
Nonnucleoside reverse transcriptase inhibitors	Calcium channel blockers, warfarin, beta blockers, nifedipine, quinidine, steroids, theophylline Delavirdine—can cause serious toxic effects if given with antiarrhythmics and calcium channel blockers	
Protease inhibitors	Metabolized by cytochrome P-450, interact with other drugs metabolized through this pathway, such as selected antimicrobials, antidepressants and antihistamines, cisapride, HMG CoA reductase inhibitors (e.g., lovastatin, simvastatin), sildenafil Potentially dangerous interactions that require close monitoring or dose adjustment; can occur with amiodarone, disopyramide, flecainide, lidocaine, mexiletine, propafenone, quinidine Ritonavir—most potent cytochrome activator (CYP3A) and P-glycoprotein inhibitor; most likely to interact Indinavir, amprenavir, nelfinavir—moderate Saquinavir—lowest probability to interact Calcium channel blockers, prednisone, quinine, beta blockers (1.5- to 3-fold increase) Decrease theophylline concentrations	Implicated in premature atherosclerosis, dyslipidemia, insulin resistance, diabetes mellitus, fat wasting and redistribution
Antiinfectives		
Antibiotics	Rifampin: reduces therapeutic effect of digoxin by inducing intestinal P-glycoprotein, reduces protease inhibitor concentration and effect Erythromycin: cytochrome P-450 metabolism and drug interactions Trimethoprim-sulfamethoxazole (Bactrim): increases warfarin effects	Erythromycin: orthostatic hypotension, ventricular tachycardia, bradycardia, torsades de pointes (with drug interactions) Clarithromycin: QT prolongation and torsades de pointes Trimethoprim-sulfamethoxazole: orthostatic hypotension, anaphylaxis, QT prolongation, torsades de pointes, hypokalemia Sparfloxacin (fluoroquinolones): QT prolongation
Antifungal agents	Amphotericin B: digoxin toxicity Ketoconazole or itraconazole: cytochrome P-450 metabolism and drug interactions—increases levels of sildenafil, warfarin, HMG CoA reductase inhibitors, nifedipine, digoxin	Amphotericin B: hypertension, arrhythmia, renal failure, hypokalemia, thrombophlebitis, bradycardia, angioedema, dilated cardiomyopathy; liposomal formulations still have potential for electrolyte imbalance and QT prolongation Ketoconazole, fluconazole, itraconazole: QT prolongation and torsades de pointes
Antiviral agents	Ganciclovir: zidovudine	Foscarnet: reversible cardiac failure, electrolyte abnormalities Ganciclovir: ventricular tachycardia, hypotension
Antiparasitic		Pentamidine: hypotension, QT prolongation, arrhythmias (torsades de pointes), ventricular tachycardia, hyperglycemia, hypoglycemia, sudden death; these effects enhanced by hypomagnesemia and hypokalemia

TABLE 67–2 | **Cardiovascular Actions and Interactions of Drugs Commonly Used in HIV Therapy*—cont'd**

Class	Cardiac Drug Interactions	Cardiac Side Effects
Chemotherapeutic Agents	Vincristine, doxorubicin: decrease digoxin level	Vincristine: arrhythmia, myocardial infarction, cardiomyopathy, autonomic neuropathy Recombinant human interferon-alpha: hypertension, hypotension, tachycardia, acute coronary events, dilated cardiomyopathy, arrhythmias, sudden death, atrioventricular block, peripheral vasodilation Contraindicated in patients with unstable angina or recent myocardial infarction Interleukin-2: hypotension, arrhythmia, sudden death, myocardial infarction, dilated cardiomyopathy, capillary leak, thyroid alterations Anthracyclines (doxorubicin, daunorubicin, mitoxantrone): myocarditis, cardiomyopathy Liposomal anthracyclines: as above for doxorubicin; also, vasculitis
Other Systemic corticosteroids	Corticosteroids: decrease salicylate levels, increase gastric ulceration in combination with salicylates	Corticosteroids: ventricular hypertrophy, cardiomyopathy, hyperglycemia
Pentoxifylline		Pentoxifylline: decreased triglyceride levels, arrhythmias, chest pain Megestrol acetate: edema, thrombophlebitis, hyperglycemia
Megestrol acetate (Megace)		Epoetin alfa (erythropoietin): hypertension, ventricular dysfunction
Methadone		Prolonged QT interval
Amphetamines		Increased heart rate and blood pressure

HMG CoA = 3-hydroxy-3-methylglutaryl coenzyme A.

In children with vertically transmitted HIV-1 infection, disease can progress rapidly or slowly.[10,23] Rapid progressors have higher heart rates, higher respiratory rates, and lower fractional shortening on serial examinations than nonrapid progressors and HIV-uninfected children who are similarly screened. Rapid progressors have higher 5-year cumulative mortality, higher HIV-1 viral loads, and lower CD8+ (cytotoxic) T-cell counts than nonrapid progressors. Knowing the patterns of disease allows more aggressive therapy to be initiated earlier in rapid progressors.

Monitoring Recommendations

Routine, systematic, cardiac evaluation, including a comprehensive history and thorough cardiac examination, is essential for the care of HIV-infected adults and children. The history should include traditional risk factors, environmental exposures, and therapeutic and illicit drug use. Routine blood pressure monitoring is important because HIV-infected individuals have been reported to experience hypertension at a younger age and more frequently than in the general population.[11,13,18]

Routine electrocardiography and Holter monitoring are not warranted unless patients have symptoms such as palpitations, syncope, stroke, or dysautonomia. These tests can also be useful for baseline and monitoring before, during, and after therapies, such as pentamidine, methadone, or antibiotics that may prolong the QT interval.[13,18]

Asymptomatic cardiac disease related to HIV can be fatal, and cardiac symptoms are often disguised by secondary effects of HIV infection, so systematic echocardiographic monitoring is warranted. We recommend an echocardiogram at the time of HIV diagnosis and every 1 to 2 years thereafter (see Fig. 67-2). Symptomatic patients with HIV infection without cardiovascular abnormalities should have

annual echocardiographic follow-up. Echocardiography should also be considered in patients with unexplained or persistent pulmonary symptoms and in those with viral coinfection at risk for myocarditis.[13]

An international consensus panel has recommended slightly less aggressive echocardiographic monitoring, with a baseline, for any patient at high risk or with any clinical manifestation of cardiovascular disease, and serial studies should be repeated every 1 to 2 years or as clinically indicated.[41] Patients with cardiac symptoms should have a formal cardiac assessment, including baseline echocardiography, electrocardiography, and Holter monitoring, and should begin directed therapy.[13] Brain natriuretic peptide levels may be helpful in diagnosing ventricular dysfunction.

In patients with left ventricular dysfunction, serum troponin assays are indicated. Serum troponin level elevations warrant consideration of cardiac catheterization and endomyocardial biopsy. Myocarditis proved by biopsy indicates consideration of therapy with intravenous immunoglobulin.[2] Cytomegalovirus inclusions on the biopsy specimen support the use of antiviral therapy, and abnormal mitochondria should encourage consideration of a drug holiday from zidovudine. Echocardiography should be repeated after 2 weeks of therapy to allow a more aggressive approach if left ventricular dysfunction persists or worsens and to encourage continued therapy if improvement has occurred.[13]

FUTURE PERSPECTIVES

As longevity improves in HIV-infected patients, cardiovascular disease will predominate as a cause of mortality and will surface as a vital area of research. Research may translate to other populations if HIV can be used as a model of chronic immunosuppression in a large population. Understanding genetic predispositions to QT prolongation may guide therapy, and understanding the causes of cardiomyopathy may benefit diverse research efforts, such as the effects of cytokine, mitochondrial, and neurohormonal pathways. Observations of increased mortality related to LV mass and very mild LV dysfunction may enhance diagnostic testing in at-risk populations affected by other poorly understood cardiomyopathies.

REFERENCES

Classics

1. Currie PF, Jacob AJ, Foreman AR, et al: Heart muscle disease related to HIV infection: Prognostic implications. BMJ 309:1605, 1994.
2. Lipshultz SE, Orav EJ, Sanders SP, Colan SD: Immunoglobulins and left ventricular structure and function in pediatric HIV infection. Circulation 92:2220, 1995.
3. Jenson HB, Pollock BH: Cardiac cancers in HIV-infected patients. *In* Lipshultz SE (ed): Cardiology in AIDS. New York, Chapman & Hall, 1998.
4. Saidi A, Bricker JT: Pulmonary hypertension in patients infected with HIV. *In* Lipshultz SE (ed): Cardiology in AIDS. New York, Chapman & Hall, 1998, pp 255-263.
5. Lipshultz SE, Easley KA, Orav EJ, et al: Cardiac dysfunction and mortality in HIV-infected children: The Prospective P2C2 HIV Multicenter Study. Pediatric Pulmonary and Cardiac Complications of Vertically Transmitted HIV Infection (P2C2 HIV) Study Group. Circulation 102:1542, 2000.
6. Felker GM, Thompson RE, Hare JM, et al: Underlying causes and long-term survival in patients with initially unexplained cardiomyopathy. N Engl J Med 342:1077, 2000.

Background

7. Morse CG, Kovacs JA: Metabolic and skeletal complications of HIV infection: The price of success. JAMA 296:844, 2006.
8. UNAIDS: 2006 Report on the Global AIDS Epidemic (http://www.unaids.org).
9. Bozzette S, Ake CF, Tam HK, et al: Cardiovascular and cerebrovascular events in patients treated for human immunodeficiency virus infection. N Engl J Med 348:702, 2003.
10. Al-Attar I, Orav EJ, Exil V, et al: Predictors of cardiac morbidity and related mortality in children with acquired immunodeficiency syndrome. J Am Coll Cardiol 41:1598, 2003.
11. Fisher SD, Lipshultz SE: Cardiac disease. *In* Dolin R, Masur H, Saag MS (eds): AIDS Therapy. 2nd ed. New York, Churchill Livingstone, 2003, pp 814-826.

Left Ventricular Systolic and Diastolic Dysfunction

12. Kearney DL, Perez-Atayde AR, Easley KA, et al: Postmortem cardiomegaly and echocardiographic measurements of left ventricular size and function in children infected with the human immunodeficiency virus. The Prospective P(2)C(2) HIV Multicenter Study. Cardiovasc Pathol 12:140, 2003.
13. Lipshultz SE, Fisher SD, Lai WW, Miller TL: Cardiovascular risk factors, monitoring, and therapy for HIV-infected patients. AIDS 17:S96, 2003.
14. Carrillo-Jimenez R, Treadwell TL, Goldfine H, et al: Brain natriuretic peptide and HIV-related cardiomyopathy. AIDS Read 12:501, 2002.
15. Fisher SD, Bowles NE, Towbin JA, Lipshultz SE: Mediators in HIV-associated cardiovascular disease: A focus on cytokines and genes. AIDS 17:S29, 2003.
16. Starc TJ, Lipshultz SE, Easley KA, et al: Incidence of cardiac abnormalities in children with human immunodeficiency virus infection: The prospective P2C2 HIV study. J Pediatr 141:327, 2002.
17. Currie PF, Boon NA: Immunopathogenesis of HIV-related heart muscle disease: Current perspectives. AIDS 17:S21, 2003.
18. Sudano I, Spieker LE, Noll G, et al: Cardiovascular disease in HIV infection. Am Heart J 151:1147, 2006.
19. Fisher SD, Easley KA, Orav EJ, et al: Mild dilated cardiomyopathy and increased left ventricular mass predict mortality: The prospective P2C2 HIV Multicenter Study. Am Heart J 150:439, 2005.
20. Calabrese LH, Albrecht M, Young J, et al: Successful cardiac transplantation in an HIV-1-infected patient with advanced disease. N Engl J Med 348:2323, 2003.

Animal Models

21. Shannon RP, Simon MA, Mathier MA, et al: Dilated cardiomyopathy associated with simian AIDS in nonhuman primates. Circulation 101:185, 2000.
22. Lewis W: Use of the transgenic mouse in models of AIDS cardiomyopathy. AIDS 17:S36, 2003.

Pericardial Effusion

23. Harmon WG, Dadlani GH, Fisher SD, Lipshultz SE: Myocardial and pericardial disease in HIV. Curr Treat Options Cardiovasc Med 4:497, 2002.

Infective Endocarditis

24. Martin-Davila P, Navas E, Fortun J, et al: Analysis of mortality and risk factors associated with native valve endocarditis in drug users: The importance of vegetation size. Am Heart J 150:1099, 2005.

Cardiovascular Malignancy

25. Bruno R, Sacchi P, Filice G: Overview on the incidence and the characteristics of HIV-related opportunistic infections and neoplasms of the heart: Impact of highly active antiretroviral therapy. AIDS 17:S83, 2003.

Right Ventricular Dysfunction and Pulmonary Hypertension

26. Rangasetty UC, Rahman AM, Hussain N: Reversible right ventricular dysfunction in patients with HIV infection. South Med J 99:197, 2006.
27. Nunes H, Humbert M, Sitbon O, et al: Prognostic factors for survival in human immunodeficiency virus-associated pulmonary arterial hypertension. Am J Respir Crit Care Med 167:1433, 2003.
28. Sitbon O, Gressin V, Speich R, et al: Bosentan for the treatment of human immunodeficiency virus-associated pulmonary arterial hypertension. Am J Respir Crit Care Med 170:1212, 2004.
29. Cea-Calvo L, Escribano Subias P, Tello De Menesses R, et al: [Treatment of HIV-associated pulmonary hypertension with treprostinil.] Rev Esp Cardiol 56:421, 2003.

Accelerated Atherosclerosis

30. Ene L, Goetghebuer T, Hainaut M, et al: Prevalence of lipodystrophy in HIV-infected children: A cross-sectional study. Eur J Pediatr 166:13, 2007.
31. Grinspoon S, Carr A: Cardiovascular risk and body-fat abnormalities in HIV-infected adults. N Engl J Med 352:48, 2005.
32. Boccara F, Teiger E, Cohen A, et al: Percutaneous coronary intervention in HIV-infected patients: Immediate results and long term prognosis. Heart 92:543, 2006.
33. Hadigan C, Meigs JB, Wilson PW, et al: Prediction of coronary heart disease risk in HIV-infected patients with fat redistribution. Clin Infect Dis 36:909, 2003.

Autonomic Dysfunction

34. Correia D, Rodrigues De Resende LA, Molina RJ, et al: Power spectral analysis of heart rate variability in HIV-infected and AIDS patients. Pacing Clin Electrophysiol 29:53, 2006.

Long QT Intervals

35. Sani MU, Okeahialam BN: QTc interval prolongation in patients with HIV and AIDS. J Natl Med Assoc 97:1657, 2005.
36. Nordin C, Kohli A, Beca S, et al: Importance of hepatitis C coinfection in the development of QT prolongation in HIV-infected patients. J Electrocardiol 39:199, 2006.

Complications of Therapy for HIV

37. Fisher SD, Miller TL, Lipshultz SE: Impact of HIV and highly active antiretroviral therapy on leukocyte adhesion molecules, arterial inflammation, dyslipidemia, and atherosclerosis. Atherosclerosis 185:1, 2006.
38. Nanavati KA, Fisher SD, Miller TL, Lipshultz SE: HIV-related cardiovascular disease and drug interactions. Am J Cardiovasc Drugs 4:315, 2004.
39. Zareba KM, Miller TL, Lipshultz SE: Cardiovascular disease and toxicities related to HIV infection and its therapies. Expert Opin Drug Saf 4:1017, 2005.

Perinatal Transmission and Vertically Transmitted HIV Infection

40. Manavi K: A review on infection with human immunodeficiency virus. Best Pract Res Clin Obstet Gynaecol 20:923, 2006.
41. Volberding PA, Murphy RL, Barbaro G, et al: The Pavia consensus statement. AIDS 17:S170, 2003.

CH 67

CHAPTER 68

Toxins and the Heart

Richard A. Lange and L. David Hillis

Introduction, 1805

Ethanol, 1805
Effects of Ethanol on Cardiac Myocyte
Structure and Function, 1805
Effects of Ethanol on Organ
Function, 1805
Ethanol and Systemic Arterial
Hypertension, 1806
Ethanol and Lipid Metabolism, 1806
Coronary Artery Disease, 1806
Arrhythmias, 1807
Sudden Death, 1808

Cocaine, 1808
Pharmacology and Mechanisms of
Action, 1808
Cocaine-Related Myocardial Ischemia
and Infarction, 1808
Cocaethylene, 1810
Cocaine-Induced Myocardial
Dysfunction, 1810
Arrhythmias, 1811
Endocarditis, 1811
Aortic Dissection, 1811

Amphetamines, 1811

Catecholamines, 1811

Inhalants, 1812

Antiretroviral Agents (Protease
Inhibitors), 1812

Ergotamine and Serotonin
Agonists, 1812

Appetite Suppressants, 1812

Pergolide (Permax), 1812

Chemotherapeutic Agents, 1812

Environmental Exposures, 1813
Cobalt, 1813
Lead, 1813
Mercury, 1813
Antimony, 1813
Arsenic, 1814
Carbon Monoxide, 1814
Thallium, 1814

References, 1814

INTRODUCTION

Many toxins, some of which are used by a substantial fraction of the population, may affect the heart adversely. As a result, it is important to understand the myriad of ways in which these substances may influence the cardiovascular system. This chapter focuses on commonly prescribed pharmacologic agents, as well as frequently used illicit drugs including cocaine and amphetamines. Chapter 85 discusses the toxicities of various chemotherapeutic agents in greater detail.

ETHANOL

Some two thirds of Americans occasionally consume ethanol, and approximately 10 percent are considered to be heavy consumers. Although the ingestion of a moderate amount of ethanol (usually defined as three to nine drinks per week) appears to be associated with a reduced risk of cardiovascular disease, the consumption of excessive amounts has the opposite effect. When ingested in substantial amounts, ethanol may cause ventricular systolic and/or diastolic dysfunction, systemic arterial hypertension, angina pectoris, arrhythmias, and even sudden cardiac death.

Effects of Ethanol on Cardiac Myocyte Structure and Function

Ethanol may cause myocardial damage via several mechanisms (Table 68-1).[1] First, ethanol and its metabolites, acetaldehyde and acetate, may exert a direct toxic effect on the myocardium. Second, deficiencies of certain vitamins (e.g., thiamine), minerals (e.g., selenium), or electrolytes (e.g., magnesium, phosphorus, or potassium) that sometimes occur in heavy ethanol consumers may adversely affect myocardial function. Third, certain substances that are sometimes added to alcoholic beverages, such as lead (often found in "moonshine" alcohol) or cobalt, may be toxic to the myocardium.

Ethanol impairs excitation-contraction, mitochondrial oxidative phosphorylation, and cardiac contractility by adversely affecting the function of the sarcolemmal membrane, the sarcoplasmic reticulum, mitochondria, and contractile proteins. Electron microscopic studies of the hearts of experimental animals in close temporal proximity to heavy ethanol ingestion demonstrate dilated sarcoplasmic reticula and swollen mitochondria, with fragmented cristae and glycogen-filled vacuoles. With sustained exposure to ethanol, myofibrillar degeneration and replacement fibrosis appear. In addition to the effects of ethanol on the myocardial contractile apparatus, acute or chronic consumption may adversely influence myofibrillar protein synthesis. Microscopically, the hearts of chronic heavy consumers of ethanol manifest an increased accumulation of collagen in the extracellular matrix, as well as increased intermolecular cross-links.

Effects of Ethanol on Organ Function

Chronic heavy ethanol ingestion may induce left ventricular diastolic and/or systolic dysfunction. Diastolic dysfunction, which is caused, at least in part, by interstitial fibrosis of the myocardium, is often demonstrable in heavy consumers of ethanol even in the absence of symptoms or obvious signs. About half of asymptomatic chronic alcoholics have echocardiographic evidence of left ventricular hypertrophy with preserved systolic performance. By Doppler echocardiography, the left ventricular relaxation time is often prolonged, the peak early diastolic velocity is reduced, and the acceleration of early diastolic flow is slowed—all manifestations of left ventricular diastolic dysfunction. Abnormal increases in left ventricular filling pressure during volume or pressure loading may be observed.

Ethanol may induce asymptomatic left ventricular systolic dysfunction even when it is ingested by healthy individuals in relatively small quantities, as occurs in subjects who are considered "social" drinkers. As many as 30 percent of asymptomatic chronic alcoholics have echocardiographic evidence of left ventricular systolic dysfunction. With continued heavy ethanol ingestion, these subjects often develop symptoms and signs of congestive heart failure, which is due to a dilated cardiomyopathy. In fact, ethanol abuse is the leading cause of nonischemic dilated cardiomyopathy in industrialized countries, accounting for approximately half of those who are diagnosed with this entity. The likelihood of developing an ethanol-induced dilated cardiomyopathy correlates with the amount of ethanol that

TABLE 68–1	Mechanisms of Ethanol-Induced Myocardial Injury

Direct Toxic Effects
Uncoupling of the excitation/contraction system
Reduced calcium sequestration in sarcoplasmic reticulum
Inhibition of sarcolemmal ATP-dependent Na^+/K^+ pump
Reduction in mitochondrial respiratory ratio
Altered substrate utilization
Increased interstitial/extracellular protein synthesis

Toxic Effect of Metabolites
Acetaldehyde
Ethyl esters

Nutritional or Trace Metal Deficiencies
Thiamine
Selenium

Electrolyte Disturbances
Hypomagnesemia
Hypokalemia
Hypophosphatemia

Toxic Additives
Cobalt
Lead

is consumed in a lifetime. Most men who develop an ethanol-induced dilated cardiomyopathy have consumed more than 80 gm of ethanol (i.e., 1 liter of wine, 8 standard-sized beers, or one-half pint of hard liquor) per day for at least 5 years. Women appear to be even more susceptible to ethanol's cardiotoxic effects in that they may develop a dilated cardiomyopathy following the consumption of a smaller amount of ethanol per day and per lifetime when compared with their male counterparts.

With abstinence from ethanol, left ventricular systolic and diastolic function often improve; the earlier in the course of ethanol consumption that abstinence is initiated, the more pronounced the benefit. Even subjects with markedly symptomatic ethanol-induced dilated cardiomyopathy may manifest a substantial improvement in left ventricular systolic function and symptoms of heart failure with complete abstinence or a dramatic reduction in ethanol consumption. Although most of this improvement occurs in the first 6 months of abstinence, it often continues for as long as 2 years of observation.

Although many heavy ethanol consumers develop a dilated cardiomyopathy, others do not, thereby suggesting individual variability in susceptibility to ethanol's cardiotoxic effects. In this regard, some studies have suggested that genetic polymorphisms in the angiotensin-converting enzyme (ACE) gene may play a role in the development of ethanol-induced dilated cardiomyopathy. Subjects who are homozygous for the deletion polymorphism of the ACE gene (so-called *DD*) have increased plasma and cardiac levels of ACE. In the absence of ethanol consumption, these homozygotes are at increased risk of developing left ventricular hypertrophy and idiopathic dilated cardiomyopathy. Similarly, alcoholics who are homozygous for this deletion polymorphism are more likely to develop a dilated cardiomyopathy than alcoholic subjects without it.[2]

Ethanol and Systemic Arterial Hypertension (see Chaps. 40 and 41)

Experts estimate that ethanol is of etiologic importance in up to 11 percent of men with hypertension. Individuals who consume more than 2 drinks daily are 1.5 to 2 times more likely to have hypertension when compared with age- and gender-matched nondrinkers.[3] This effect is dose related

and is most prominent when the daily ethanol intake exceeds 5 drinks (i.e., 30 gm of ethanol).[4] "Social" ethanol consumption is associated with a modest rise in systolic arterial pressure, whereas heavy consumption may lead to a substantial increase. Although the mechanism by which ethanol induces a rise in systemic arterial pressure is poorly understood, previous studies have demonstrated that ethanol consumption increases plasma levels of catecholamines, renin, and aldosterone, each of which may cause systemic arterial vasoconstriction. In individuals with ethanol-induced hypertension, abstinence is often followed by a normalization of systemic arterial pressure.

Ethanol and Lipid Metabolism

Ethanol consumption inhibits the oxidation of free fatty acids by the liver, which stimulates hepatic triglyceride synthesis and the secretion of very low-density lipoprotein cholesterol. Most commonly, therefore, ethanol consumption causes hypertriglyceridemia. In addition, it may cause an increase in the serum concentrations of total cholesterol and low-density lipoprotein (LDL). Regular ethanol consumption increases the serum concentration of high-density lipoprotein (HDL) cholesterol. Subjects with hyperlipidemia should be encouraged to limit their ethanol intake.[5]

Coronary Artery Disease

(see also Chaps. 39 and 45)

Heavy ethanol use is associated with an increased incidence of atherosclerotic coronary artery disease and resultant cardiovascular morbidity and mortality. This increase may result, at least in part, from the increased likelihood that heavy ethanol consumers compared with nondrinkers have systemic arterial hypertension, an increased left ventricular muscle mass (with concomitant diastolic and/or systolic dysfunction), and hypertriglyceridemia. In addition, heavy ethanol drinkers often smoke cigarettes. In contradistinction, mild to moderate ethanol intake (two to seven drinks per week) appears to be associated with a decreased risk of cardiovascular morbidity and mortality in both men and women. This reduced risk of cardiovascular morbidity and mortality among consumers of moderate amounts of ethanol—when compared with nondrinkers or heavy consumers—is supported by numerous retrospectively and prospectively conducted studies. The French were noted to have a reduced incidence of coronary artery disease when compared with inhabitants of other countries with similar dietary habits (the so-called *French paradox*). Although this diminished incidence initially was attributed to the antioxidant and hemostatic properties of red wine, similar findings subsequently were reported in mild to moderate consumers of other alcoholic beverages and in other study populations.[6] Several prospectively performed cohort studies have demonstrated that drinkers of moderate amounts of ethanol are 40 to 70 percent less likely to manifest coronary artery disease or ischemic stroke when compared with nondrinkers or heavy consumers.[6] Some studies have suggested that the consumption of all alcoholic beverages exerts such an effect, whereas others have reported that this so-called *cardioprotection* is strongest with the consumption of wine.[7] The mechanism(s) by which the consumption of moderate amounts of ethanol reduces cardiovascular risk appear to be multifactorial, in that moderate consumption exerts several beneficial effects including (a) an increase in the serum concentrations of HDL cholesterol and apolipoprotein A-I, (b) inhibition of platelet aggregation, (c) a decreased serum fibrinogen concentration, (d) increased antioxidant activity (from the phenolic compounds and flavonoids contained in red wine), and (e) improved fibrinolysis (resulting from increased concentrations of endogenous tissue plasminogen activator and a concomitant decrease in endogenous plasminogen activator inhibitor activity) (Fig. 68-1).[5]

Some studies have suggested that the cardioprotective effects of moderate ethanol intake are manifest only in those with increased risk for coronary artery disease (i.e., those older than 50 to 60 years of age, men with an LDL cholesterol concentration >200 mg/dl, and women with multiple risk factors for atherosclerosis). Other studies have demonstrated that light to moderate ethanol consumption is associated with similar risk reductions in coronary artery disease among diabetic and nondiabetic men and women (Fig. 68-2).[8,9]

In subjects without known cardiac disease, the decrease in cardiovascular mortality that is associated with moderate ethanol intake results largely from a reduction in the incidence of sudden death (Fig. 68-3). Of the more than 21,000 men in the Physicians Health Study, those who consumed two to four or five to six drinks per week had a significantly reduced risk of sudden death (relative risks, 0.40 and 0.21, respectively) when compared with those who rarely or never drank. In contrast, heavy ethanol consumption (i.e., six or more drinks per day) or binge drinking was associated with an increased risk of sudden death.

In survivors of myocardial infarction (MI), moderate ethanol consumption appears to reduce subsequent mortality.[10] In the setting of an acute MI, the recent ingestion of ethanol does not appear to reduce infarct size or the propensity for the subsequent appearance of an arrhythmia or heart failure.

Arrhythmias

Ethanol consumption is associated with a variety of atrial and ventricular arrhythmias, most commonly (a) atrial or ventricular premature beats, (b) supraventricular tachycardia, (c) atrial flutter, (d) atrial fibrillation, (e) ventricular tachycardia, or (f) ventricular fibrillation. The most common ethanol-induced arrhythmia is atrial fibrillation. Ethanol is of etiologic importance in about one third of subjects with new-onset atrial fibrillation; in those younger than 65 years of age, it may be responsible for as many as two thirds of subjects. Most episodes occur after binge drinking, usually on weekends or holidays—hence the term "holiday heart." Electrophysiological testing in humans without cardiac disease has shown that ethanol enhances the vulnerability to the induction of atrial flutter and fibrillation. The treatment of these ethanol-induced arrhythmias is abstinence.

Ethanol may be arrhythmogenic via several mechanisms. In many ethanol consumers, concomitant factors may predispose to arrhythmias including cigarette smoking, electrolyte disturbances, metabolic abnormalities, hypertension, or sleep apnea. Acute ethanol ingestion induces a diuresis, which is accompanied by the concomitant urinary loss of sodium, potassium, and magnesium. The presence of myocardial interstitial fibrosis, ventricular hypertrophy, cardiomyopathy, and autonomic dysfunction also may enhance the likelihood of dysrhythmias.

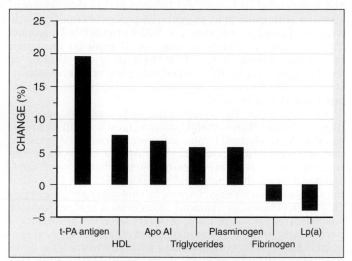

FIGURE 68–1 Percentage change in various serologic variables caused by the ingestion of 30 gm of ethanol daily.[5] The ingestion of ethanol, 30 gm daily, for 1 to 9 weeks was associated with increased serum concentrations of tissue type plasminogen activator (t-PA) antigen, high-density lipoprotein (HDL) cholesterol, apolipoprotein A1 (Apo A1), serum triglycerides, and serum plasminogen, as well as decreased concentrations of serum fibrinogen and lipoprotein(a) [Lp(a)]. The reduced risk of cardiovascular events seen in subjects who consume moderate amounts of ethanol may be caused, at least in part, by these beneficial changes in serologic variables.

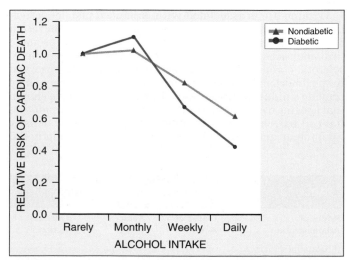

FIGURE 68–2 Ethanol consumption and relative risk of cardiac death according to diabetic status, with data from the Physicians Health Study.[8,9] Light to moderate alcohol consumption is associated with similar risk reductions in cardiac death among diabetic and nondiabetic men.

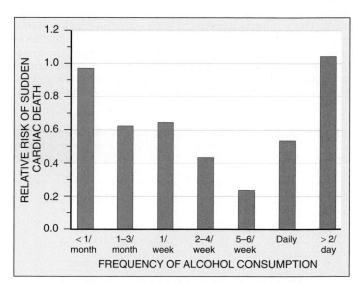

FIGURE 68–3 Ethanol consumption and the risk of sudden cardiac death among U.S. male physicians. In comparison to those who had less than 1 drink per month (far left bar), those who consumed small or moderate amounts of ethanol (middle bars) had a reduced risk of sudden cardiac death. In contrast, those who consumed at least two drinks per day (far right bar) had an increased risk

Sudden Death

Heavy ethanol consumption is associated with an increased incidence of sudden death independent of the presence of coronary artery disease. The incidence of ethanol-induced sudden death increases with age and the amount of ethanol that is ingested. For example, the daily ingestion of more than 80 gm of ethanol is associated with a 3-fold increased incidence of mortality when compared with a daily consumption of a lesser amount.

COCAINE

Cocaine is currently the most commonly used illicit drug among subjects seeking care in hospital emergency departments, and it is the most frequent cause of drug-related deaths reported by medical examiners in the United States.[11] Its widespread use is attributable to (a) its ease of administration, (b) the ready availability of relatively pure drug, (c) its relatively low cost, and (d) the misperception that its recreational use is safe. As cocaine abuse has increased in frequency, the number of cocaine-related cardiovascular complications including angina pectoris, MI, cardiomyopathy, and sudden death has increased (Table 68-2).

Pharmacology and Mechanisms of Action

Cocaine (benzoylmethylecgonine) is an alkaloid extracted from the leaf of the *Erythroxylon coca* bush, which grows primarily in South America. It is available in two forms: the hydrochloride salt and the "freebase." Cocaine *hydrochloride* is prepared by dissolving the alkaloid in hydrochloric acid to form a water-soluble powder or granule, which can be taken orally, intravenously, or intranasally (so-called "chewing," "mainlining," or "snorting," respectively). The *freebase* form is manufactured by processing the cocaine with ammonia or sodium bicarbonate (baking soda). Unlike the hydrochloride form, "freebase" cocaine is heat stable so that it can be smoked. It is known as "crack" because of the popping sound that it makes when heated.

Cocaine hydrochloride is well absorbed through all mucous membranes; therefore users may achieve a high blood concentration with intranasal, sublingual, vaginal, or rectal administration. The route of administration determines the rapidity of onset and duration of action (Table 68-3). The euphoria associated with smoking crack cocaine occurs within seconds and is short lived. Crack cocaine is considered the most potent and addictive form of the drug. Cocaine is metabolized by serum and liver cholinesterases to water-soluble metabolites (primarily benzoylecgonine and ecgonine methyl ester), which are excreted in the urine.

TABLE 68–2	Cardiovascular Complications of Cocaine Use
Myocardial ischemia	
Angina pectoris	
Myocardial infarction	
Sudden death	
Arrhythmias	
Pulmonary edema	
Myocarditis	
Endocarditis	
Aortic dissection	

Because cocaine's serum half-life is only 45 to 90 minutes, it is detectable in blood or urine only for several hours after its use. However, its metabolites persist in blood or urine for 24 to 36 hours after its administration.

When applied locally, cocaine acts as an anesthetic by virtue of its inhibition of membrane permeability to sodium during depolarization, thereby blocking the initiation and transmission of electrical signals. When given systemically, it blocks the presynaptic reuptake of norepinephrine and dopamine, thereby producing an excess of these neurotransmitters at the site of the postsynaptic receptor (Fig. 68-4). In short, cocaine acts as a powerful sympathomimetic agent.

Cocaine-Related Myocardial Ischemia and Infarction

Since 1982, numerous reports have associated cocaine use and myocardial ischemia and infarction.[11] In one survey of 10,085 adults, aged 18 to 45 years, 25 percent of nonfatal MIs were attributed to cocaine use.[12] Cocaine-related myocardial ischemia or infarction may result from (a) increased myocardial oxygen demand in the setting of a limited or fixed oxygen supply; (b) marked coronary arterial vasoconstriction; and (c) enhanced platelet aggregation and thrombus formation (Fig. 68-5).

By virtue of its sympathomimetic effects, cocaine increases the three major determinants of myocardial oxygen demand: heart rate, left ventricular wall tension, and left ventricular contractility. At the same time, the ingestion of even small amounts of the drug causes vasoconstriction of the epicardial coronary arteries (so-called *inappropriate vasoconstriction*), in that myocardial oxygen supply decreases as demand increases. Cocaine induces vasoconstriction in normal coronary arteries but exerts a particularly marked vasoconstrictive effect in diseased segments. As a result, cocaine users with atherosclerotic coronary artery disease probably have an especially high risk for an ischemic event after cocaine use. Cocaine-induced coronary arterial vasoconstriction results primarily from the stimulation of coronary arterial alpha-adrenergic receptors because it is reversed by phentolamine (an alpha-adrenergic antagonist) and exacerbated by propranolol (a beta-adrenergic antagonist). In addition, cocaine causes increased endothelial production of endothelin (a potent vasoconstrictor) and decreased production of nitric oxide (a potent vasodilator), which also may promote vasoconstriction.

Cocaine use is associated with enhanced platelet activation and aggregability, as well as an increased concentration of plasminogen activator inhibitor, which may promote thrombus accumulation. The presence of premature atherosclerotic coronary artery disease, which has been observed in postmortem studies of long-term cocaine users, may provide a nidus for thrombosis. In vitro studies have shown that cocaine causes structural abnormalities in the endothelial-cell barrier, increasing its permeability to low-density lipoprotein and enhancing the expression of endothelial

TABLE 68–3	Pharmacokinetics of Cocaine According to the Route of Administration		
Route of Administration	Onset of Action	Peak Effect	Duration of Action
Inhalation (smoking)	3-5 sec	1-3 min	5-15 min
Intravenous	10-60 sec	3-5 min	20-60 min
Intranasal or other mucosal	1-5 min	15-20 min	60-90 min

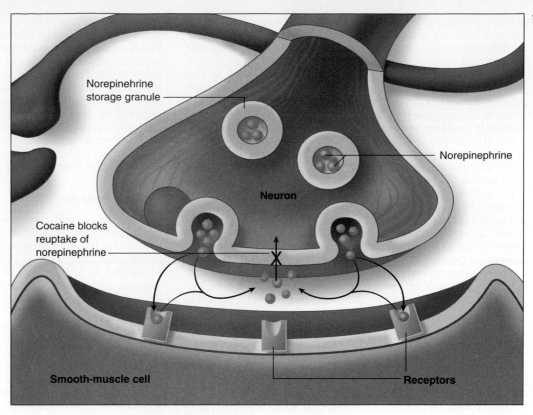

FIGURE 68–4 The mechanism by which cocaine alters sympathetic tone. Cocaine blocks the reuptake of norepinephrine by the preganglionic neuron (X), resulting in excess amounts of this neurotransmitter at receptor sites at the postganglionic site.

Norepinehrine storage granule

Norepinephrine

Neuron

Cocaine blocks reuptake of norepinephrine

Smooth-muscle cell

Receptors

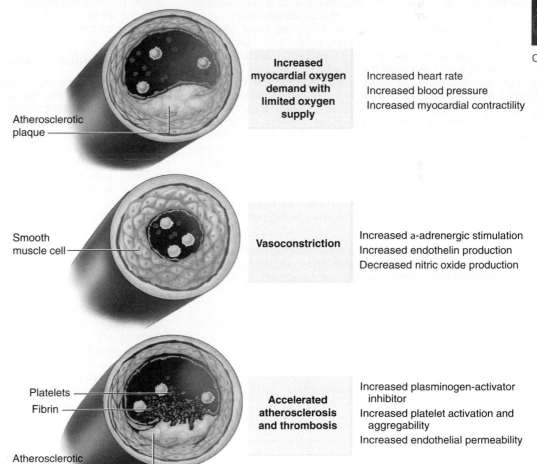

FIGURE 68–5 Mechanisms by which cocaine may induce myocardial ischemia or infarction. Cocaine may induce myocardial ischemia or infarction by increasing the determinants of myocardial oxygen demand in the setting of limited oxygen supply **(top),** causing intense coronary arterial vasoconstriction **(middle),** or inducing accelerated atherosclerosis and thrombosis **(bottom).**

Atherosclerotic plaque

Increased myocardial oxygen demand with limited oxygen supply

Increased heart rate
Increased blood pressure
Increased myocardial contractility

Smooth muscle cell

Vasoconstriction

Increased a-adrenergic stimulation
Increased endothelin production
Decreased nitric oxide production

Platelets
Fibrin

Accelerated atherosclerosis and thrombosis

Increased plasminogen-activator inhibitor
Increased platelet activation and aggregability
Increased endothelial permeability

Atherosclerotic plaque

adhesion molecules (thereby favoring leukocyte migration), all of which are associated with atherogenesis.

Chest pain is the most common cardiovascular complaint of patients seeking medical assistance following cocaine use. Approximately 6 percent of those who come to the emergency department with cocaine-associated chest pain have enzymatic evidence of myocardial necrosis. Most subjects with cocaine-related MI are young, nonwhite, male cigarette smokers without other risk factors for atherosclerosis who have a history of repeated cocaine use (Table 68-4). Similar to cocaine, cigarette smoking induces coronary arterial vasoconstriction through an alpha-adrenergic mechanism. The deleterious effects of cocaine on myocardial oxygen supply and demand are exacerbated substantially by concomitant cigarette smoking. Following concomitant cocaine use and smoking, heart rate and systemic arterial pressure increase markedly, and coronary arterial vasoconstriction is more intense than with either alone.

In subjects who are considered otherwise to be at low risk for MI, the risk of infarction is increased 24-fold during the 60 minutes after cocaine use. The occurrence of MI after cocaine use appears to be unrelated to the amount ingested, its route of administration, and the frequency of its use: Cocaine-related infarction has been reported with doses ranging from 200 to 2000 mg, after ingestion by all routes, and in habitual and first-time users. About half the patients with cocaine-related MI have no angiographic evidence of atherosclerotic coronary artery disease. Therefore when subjects with no or few risk factors for atherosclerosis, particularly those who are young or have a history of substance abuse, present with acute MI, urine and blood samples should be analyzed for cocaine and its metabolites.

Cardiovascular complications resulting from cocaine-related MI are relatively uncommon, with ventricular arrhythmias occurring in 4 to 17 percent, congestive heart failure in 5 to 7 percent, and death in less than 2 percent. This low incidence of complications is caused, at least in part, by the young age and absence of extensive multivessel coronary artery disease of most patients with cocaine-related infarction. If complications develop, most occur within 12 hours of presentation to the hospital.[13] Following hospital discharge, continued cocaine use and recurrent chest pain are common. Occasionally a patient has recurrent nonfatal or fatal MI.

Most subjects with cocaine-related myocardial ischemia or infarction have chest pain within an hour of cocaine use, when the blood cocaine concentration is highest. However, an occasional individual notes the onset of symptoms several hours after the administration of the drug, when the blood cocaine concentration is low or even undetectable. With cocaine ingestion, the diameter of the coronary arteries decreases as the drug concentration increases. Then, as the drug concentration declines, the vasoconstriction resolves. Thereafter, as the concentrations of cocaine's major metabolites (benzoylecgonine and ecgonine methyl ester) rise, "delayed" (i.e., recurrent) coronary arterial vasoconstriction occurs, thereby providing an explanation of why myocardial ischemia or infarction has been reported to occur several hours after drug use.

Cocaethylene

In individuals who use cocaine in temporal proximity to the ingestion of ethanol, hepatic transesterification leads to the production of a unique metabolite, cocaethylene. Cocaethylene is often detected postmortem in subjects who are presumed to have died of cocaine and ethanol toxicity. Similar to cocaine, cocaethylene blocks the reuptake of dopamine at the synaptic cleft, thereby possibly potentiating the systemic toxic effects of cocaine. In experimental animals, in fact, cocaethylene is more lethal than cocaine. In humans the combination of cocaine and ethanol causes a substantial increase in myocardial oxygen demand. The concomitant use of cocaine and ethanol is associated with a higher incidence of disability and death than either agent alone. Individuals presumably dying of a combined cocaine-ethanol overdose have much lower blood cocaine concentrations than those presumably dying of a cocaine overdose alone, thereby suggesting an additive or synergistic effect of ethanol on the catastrophic cardiovascular events that are induced by cocaine.

Cocaine-Induced Myocardial Dysfunction

Long-term cocaine abuse has been associated with left ventricular hypertrophy, as well as left ventricular diastolic and/or systolic dysfunction. Several reports have described dilated cardiomyopathy in long-term cocaine abusers, and others have described profound but reversible myocardial depression after binge cocaine use. Approximately 7 percent of long-term chronic users without cardiac symptoms have radionuclide ventriculographic evidence of left ventricular systolic dysfunction.

Cocaine may adversely affect left ventricular systolic function by several mechanisms. First, as noted previously, cocaine may induce myocardial ischemia or infarction. Second, the profound repetitive sympathetic stimulation induced by cocaine is similar to that observed in patients with pheochromocytoma; either may induce a cardiomyopathy and characteristic microscopic changes of subendocardial contraction band necrosis. Third, the concomitant administration of adulterants or infectious agents may cause myocarditis, which has been seen on occasion in intravenous cocaine users studied post mortem. Fourth, studies in experimental animals have shown that cocaine alters cytokine production in the endothelium and in circulating leukocytes, induces the transcription of genes responsible for changes in the composition of myocardial collagen and myosin, and induces myocyte apoptosis.

Aside from the effects of long-term cocaine use on myocardial performance, it may cause an acute deterioration of left ventricular systolic and/or diastolic function. In some subjects, this deterioration results from metabolic and/or acid-base disturbances that accompany cocaine intoxication, whereas in others it may be caused by a direct toxic effect of the drug. The intracoronary infusion of cocaine (in an amount sufficient to produce a concentration in coronary

TABLE 68–4	Characteristics of Patients with Cocaine-Induced Myocardial Infarction (MI)
Dose of Cocaine	
5-6 lines (150 mg) to as much as 2 gm	
Serum concentration, 0.01-1.02 mg/liter	
Frequency of Use	
Reported in chronic, recreational, and first-time users	
Route of Administration	
Occurs with all routes of administration	
75% of reported MIs occurred after intranasal use	
Age	
Mean, 34 (range, 17-71) yr	
20% younger than 25 yr	
Gender	
80-90% male	
Timing	
Often within minutes of cocaine use	
Reported as late as 5-15 hr after use	

sinus blood similar in magnitude to the peripheral blood concentration found in abusers presumably dying of cocaine intoxication) exerts a deleterious effect on left ventricular systolic and diastolic function. It seems feasible that cocaine or its metabolites alter the manner in which myocytes handle calcium.

Arrhythmias

Cardiac dysrhythmias may occur with cocaine (Table 68-5), but the precise arrhythmogenic potential of the drug is poorly defined. In many instances, the dysrhythmias ascribed to cocaine occur in the setting of profound hemodynamic or metabolic derangements, such as hypotension, hypoxemia, seizures, or MI. Nonetheless, because of cocaine's sodium-channel–blocking properties and its ability to enhance sympathetic activation, it is considered a likely cause of cardiac arrhythmias.[14] The development of lethal arrhythmias with cocaine use may require an underlying substrate of abnormal myocardium. Studies in experimental animals have shown that cocaine precipitates ventricular arrhythmias only in the presence of myocardial ischemia or infarction. In humans, life-threatening arrhythmias and sudden death in association with cocaine use occur most often in those with myocardial ischemia or infarction or in those with nonischemic myocellular damage. Long-term cocaine use is associated with increased left ventricular mass and wall thickness, which is known to be a risk factor for ventricular dysrhythmias. In some cocaine users, such an increased mass may provide the substrate for arrhythmias.

Cocaine may affect the generation and conduction of cardiac impulses by several mechanisms. First, its sympathomimetic properties may increase ventricular irritability and lower the threshold for fibrillation. Second, it inhibits action potential generation and conduction (i.e., it prolongs the QRS and QT intervals) as a result of its sodium-channel–blocking effects. In so doing, it acts in a manner similar to that of a class I antiarrhythmic agent. Accordingly, torsades de pointes has been observed following cocaine use. Third, cocaine increases the intracellular calcium concentration, which may result in afterdepolarizations and triggered ventricular arrhythmias. Fourth, it reduces vagal activity, thereby potentiating its sympathomimetic effects.

Endocarditis

Although the intravenous administration of any illicit drug is associated with an increased risk of bacterial endocardi-

TABLE 68–5	Cardiac Dysrhythmias and Conduction Disturbances Reported with Cocaine Use
Sinus tachycardia	
Sinus bradycardia	
Supraventricular tachycardia	
Bundle branch block	
Complete heart block	
Accelerated idioventricular rhythm	
Ventricular tachycardia	
Ventricular fibrillation	
Asystole	
Torsades de pointes	
Brugada pattern (right bundle branch block with ST segment elevation in leads V_1, V_2, and V_3)	

tis, the intravenous use of cocaine appears to be accompanied by a greater risk of endocarditis than the intravenous administration of other drugs. The reason for this enhanced risk of endocarditis in intravenous cocaine users is unknown, but several hypotheses have been proposed. The increase in heart rate and systemic arterial pressure that accompanies cocaine use may induce valvular injury that predisposes to bacterial invasion. Cocaine's immunosuppressive effects may increase the risk of infection. The manner in which cocaine is manufactured, as well as the adulterants that are often present in it, may increase the risk of endocarditis. In contradistinction to the endocarditis that is associated with other drugs, the endocarditis of cocaine users more often involves the left-sided cardiac valves.

Aortic Dissection

Aortic dissection or rupture has been temporally related to cocaine use; therefore it should be considered as a possible cause of chest pain in cocaine users. In one study of 38 patients with acute aortic dissection, 14 (37 percent) were related to cocaine use, with an average interval from cocaine use to the onset of symptoms of 12 (range, 0 to 24) hours.[15] Dissection probably results from a cocaine-induced increase in systemic arterial pressure. In addition to aortic rupture, the cocaine-related rupture of mycotic and intracerebral aneurysms has been reported.

AMPHETAMINES

Amphetamines were previously prescribed for the treatment of obesity, attention deficit disorder, and narcolepsy; at present, their use is strictly limited. The most frequently abused amphetamines are dextroamphetamine, methcathinone, methamphetamine, methylphenidate, ephedrine, propylhexedrine, phenmetrazine, and 3,4-methylene-dioxymethamphetamine (MDMA, also known as *ecstasy*). *Ice* is a freebase form of methamphetamine that can be inhaled, smoked, or injected. Because amphetamines are sympathomimetic agents, their use has been associated with systemic arterial hypertension, MI, myocardial damage consistent with catecholamine excess, and lethal arrhythmias.[16,17] Similar to cocaine, amphetamines may induce intense coronary arterial vasoconstriction with or without thrombus formation.[18] Finally, subjects with dilated cardiomyopathy following repetitive amphetamine use have been described.

CATECHOLAMINES

Catecholamines, administered exogenously or secreted by a neuroendocrine tumor (e.g., pheochromocytoma or neuroblastoma), may produce acute myocarditis (with focal myocardial necrosis and inflammation), cardiomyopathy, tachycardia, and arrhythmias. Similar abnormalities have been described with the excessive use of beta-adrenergic agonist inhalants and methylxanthines in patients with severe pulmonary disease. The secretion of large amounts of endogenous catecholamines, as may occur in subjects with subarachnoid hemorrhage or intense stress, has been associated with the appearance of transient left ventricular apical dyskinesis and anterior electrocardiographic T wave inversions. This entity, known as *takotsubo* or *stress cardiomyopathy,* is more likely to occur in women than men. It resolves spontaneously when catecholamine secretion abates.[19,20]

Several mechanisms may be responsible for the acute and chronic myocardial damage associated with catecholamines. They may exert a direct toxic effect on the myocardium through changes in autonomic tone, enhanced lipid mobility, calcium overload, free radical production, or increased sarcolemmal permeability. Alternatively, myocardial damage may be secondary to a sustained increase in myocardial oxygen demands and/or decrease in myocardial oxygen supply (the latter due to catecholamine-induced coronary arterial vasoconstriction or platelet aggregation).

INHALANTS

The inhalants may be classified as organic solvents, organic nitrites (such as amyl nitrite or amyl butyl), and nitrous oxide. The organic solvents include toluene (airplane glue), Freon, kerosene, gasoline, carbon tetrachloride, acrylic paint sprays, shoe polish, degreasers, nail polish remover, typewriter correction fluid, adhesives, and lighter fluid. These solvents are most often inhaled by children or young adolescents. Acute or chronic inhalant use occasionally has been reported to induce cardiac abnormalities, most commonly dysrhythmias; rarely, inhalant use has been associated with myocarditis, MI, and sudden death. The inhalation of Freon, for example, can sensitize the myocardium to catecholamines; in these individuals, fatal arrhythmias have been reported to occur when the user is startled during inhalation.

ANTIRETROVIRAL AGENTS (PROTEASE INHIBITORS) (see also Chap. 67)

Subjects treated with HIV protease inhibitors have been observed to have severe hypertriglyceridemia (serum triglycerides >1000 mg/dl) and marked elevations in lipoprotein(a).[21] Not surprisingly, therefore, patients who are maintained on these agents have an increased risk of atherosclerosis.[22] Dilated cardiomyopathy in association with HIV antiretroviral therapy has been reported.[23-25] In mice, zidovudine produces a cardiomyopathy, with pathologic changes demonstrable in the mitochondria, and similar ultrastructural mitochondrial changes have been observed in myocardial biopsy specimens from HIV-infected patients treated with this agent.[25] In one individual, zidovudine's discontinuation resulted in a reversal of cardiac dysfunction.

ERGOTAMINE AND SEROTONIN AGONISTS

Two medications used to treat subjects with migraine headaches, ergotamine and sumatriptan, have been associated with acute MI. Ergotamine causes vasoconstriction of intercerebral and extracranial arteries; rarely, its use has been associated with coronary arterial vasospasm and acute MI. Its vasoconstrictor effects are exaggerated by concomitant caffeine ingestion or beta-adrenergic blocker use. Sumatriptan, a selective 5-hydroxytryptamine agonist, also exerts its therapeutic effects by inducing cerebral arterial vasoconstriction. Several reports have been made of patients in whom coronary vasospasm and acute MI occurred following the administration of therapeutic doses of sumatriptan, some of which were complicated by ventricular tachycardia/fibrillation and sudden cardiac death.

APPETITE SUPPRESSANTS (see Chap. 62)

Exposure to the appetite suppressants fenfluramine or dexfenfluramine, alone or in combination with phenter-

mine, has been implicated in the pathogenesis of certain valvular abnormalities. Fenfluramine (Pondimin), a sympathomimetic amine, promotes the release of serotonin and blocks its neuronal uptake; dexfenfluramine (Redux) is the dextroisomer of fenfluramine. Phentermine (Adipex, Fastin, Ionamin) is a noradrenergic central nervous system stimulant.

The association of appetite suppressant use and valvular abnormalities was first described in 1997, when subjects receiving the combination of fenfluramine and phentermine were noted to have unusual valvular morphology and resultant regurgitation of both left- and right-sided heart valves. All had aortic and/or mitral regurgitation, and half had tricuspid regurgitation.[26] Echocardiographic and histopathological findings resembled those described in patients with carcinoid or ergotamine-induced valvular heart disease. Grossly, the aortic and mitral valve leaflets and chordae tendineae were thickened and had a glistening white appearance. Histologically, leaflet architecture was intact; a plaque-like encasement of the leaflets and chordal structures was noted; and proliferative myofibroblasts surrounded by an abundant extracellular matrix were observed. As a result of these observations, the manufacturer withdrew fenfluramine and dexfenfluramine from the market. Because no valvular abnormalities have been associated with the use of phentermine alone, it is still available.

The risk of valvular heart disease associated with exposure to fenfluramine or dexfenfluramine, alone or in combination with phentermine, has been addressed in several studies, with the prevalence of valvular regurgitation varying from less than 1 percent to as much as 26 percent.[27,28] This apparent wide-ranging risk is attributable to differences in study type, patient populations, varying definitions of regurgitation, and differing durations of treatment with these agents. The prevalence of "significant" valvular regurgitation appears to be related directly to the duration of exposure to the anorectic agents. In most subjects, the valvular abnormalities stabilize or improve after the agents are discontinued.[29]

Currently, it is recommended that all persons exposed to fenfluramine or dexfenfluramine for any period of time, alone or in combination with other agents, should undergo a thorough cardiovascular assessment to determine the presence or absence of cardiopulmonary symptoms or signs. Those with symptoms or signs suggestive of valvular disease (e.g., dyspnea or a new murmur) should undergo echocardiographic evaluation.

PERGOLIDE (PERMAX)

Pergolide is a dopamine receptor agonist that is used in the treatment of subjects with Parkinson disease. During pergolide treatment, a small number of individuals have developed cardiac valvulopathy.[30] In some of them, the symptoms or signs of valvulopathy improved with discontinuation of the drug, whereas others necessitated valve replacement surgery. Pathologically, the excised valves appeared similar morphologically and microscopically to the valvulopathy associated with the carcinoid syndrome or the use of ergot alkaloids.

CHEMOTHERAPEUTIC AGENTS
(see also Chap. 85)

Several chemotherapeutic agents may adversely affect cardiac function. Certain of these substances have been reported to induce hypertension, acute cardiomyopathy, myocardial ischemia or infarction, dysrhythmias, and/or sudden death (Table 68-6).[31,32] Among the agents that cause cardiotoxicity, the anthracyclines are known to induce acute myocarditis and longstanding cardiomyopathy. Trastuzumab, a recently approved antibody directed against the human epidermal growth factor receptor-2 (HER2 receptor), improves survival in patients with metastatic breast cancer. In a minority of subjects, it causes a decrease in left ventricular ejection fraction, which is especially likely to occur if it is administered in conjunction with paclitaxel or anthracyclines. In contrast to anthracycline cardiotoxicity, however, the cardiotoxicity associated with trastuzumab is not cumulative or dose dependent, and cardiac function often returns to normal after it is discontinued. As a result, its repeat administration once cardiac function has normalized is acceptable.

Up to 29 percent of patients who receive paclitaxel as a chemotherapeutic agent develop transient asymptomatic bradycardia. More substantial cardiac disturbances including atrioventricular block, left bundle branch block, ventricular tachycardia, or myocardial ischemia occur in up to 5 percent of subjects. When paclitaxel is given in combination with doxorubicin, the risk of cardiotoxicity may be higher: Some reports have suggested that heart failure developed in up to 20 percent of patients treated with this combination. Finally, 5-fluorouracil may cause myocardial ischemia or infarction by inducing coronary vasospasm.

ENVIRONMENTAL EXPOSURES

Cobalt

In the mid-1960s, an acute and fulminant form of dilated cardiomyopathy was described in heavy beer drinkers. It was suggested that the cobalt chloride, which was added to the beer as a foam stabilizer, was the causative agent; therefore its addition was discontinued. Subsequently, this acute and severe form of cardiomyopathy disappeared. More recently, several reports of dilated cardiomyopathy after occupational exposure to cobalt have appeared; in these individuals, high concentrations of cobalt were demonstrated in endomyocardial biopsy specimens.

Lead

Patients with lead poisoning typically have complaints that are referable to the gastrointestinal and central nervous systems. On occasion, subjects with lead poisoning have electrocardiographic abnormalities, atrioventricular conduction defects, and overt congestive heart failure; rarely, myocardial involvement may contribute to or be the principal cause of death.

Mercury

Occupational exposure to metallic mercuric vapors may cause systemic arterial hypertension and myocardial failure. Although some studies have suggested that a high mercury content of fish may counteract the beneficial effects of its ω-3 fatty acids, thereby increasing the risk of atherosclerotic cardiovascular disease,[33] more recent assessments have not supported an association between total mercury exposure and the risk of coronary artery disease.[34]

Antimony

Various antimony compounds previously have been used in the treatment of patients with schistosomiasis. Their use is

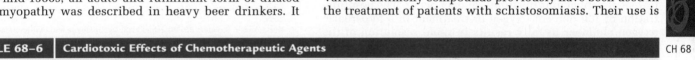

TABLE 68–6	Cardiotoxic Effects of Chemotherapeutic Agents	
Agent	**Short-Term Toxicity**	**Long-Term Toxicity**
Doxorubicin	Arrhythmias, pericarditis-myocarditis syndrome, MI, SCD	Cardiomyopathy/CHF
Mitoxantrone	CHF, ↓LVEF, MI, electrocardiographic changes, arrhythmias	
Cyclophosphamide	Hemorrhagic cardiac necrosis, reversible systolic dysfunction, electrocardiographic changes, CHF	
Ifosfamide	Electrocardiographic changes, CHF, arrhythmias	
Cisplatin	Myocardial ischemia, Raynaud phenomenon, electrocardiographic changes	
Fluorouracil	MI, AP, cardiogenic shock, SCD, dilated cardiomyopathy	
Trastuzumab	Ventricular dysfunction, CHF	Cardiomyopathy
Paclitaxel	SCD, bradyarrhythmias, myocardial dysfunction, CHF, MI	
Amsacrine	Ventricular arrhythmia, electrocardiographic changes	Cardiomyopathy
Cytarabine	CHF, pericarditis, arrhythmias	
Interferon-α-2a	Exacerbates underlying cardiac disease, hypotension, arrhythmias	Cardiomyopathy
Interleukin-2	Myocardial injury/myopericarditis, ventricular arrhythmias, hypotension, SCD	Dilated cardiomyopathy
Mitomycin	CHF	CHF
Vincristine	MI, hypotension, cardiovascular autonomic neuropathy	
Vinblastine	MI, Raynaud phenomenon	
Busulfan	Endocardial fibrosis, pulmonary fibrosis, pulmonary hypertension, cardiac tamponade	
Tretinoin	Pleural-pericardial effusions, MI	
Pentostatin	AP, MI, arrhythmias	CHF
Etoposide	MI, electrocardiographic changes	
Teniposide	Arrhythmias	

AP = angina pectoris; CHF = congestive heart failure; LVEF = left ventricular ejection fraction; MI = myocardial infarction; SCD = sudden cardiac death.

often associated with electrocardiographic abnormalities including prolongation of the QT interval and T wave flattening or inversion. Rarely, chest pain, bradycardia, hypotension, ventricular arrhythmias, and sudden death have been reported.

Arsenic

Arsenic exposure typically occurs from pesticide poisoning. Its cardiac manifestations include pericardial effusion, myocarditis, and various electrocardiographic abnormalities including QT interval prolongation with T wave inversion.

Carbon Monoxide

Carbon monoxide has a higher affinity for hemoglobin than does oxygen; as a result, elevated blood concentrations of carbon monoxide lead to reduced tissue oxygen delivery. Although central nervous system symptoms are the predominant manifestations of carbon monoxide poisoning, cardiac toxicity may occur because of myocardial hypoxia or a direct toxic effect of the gas on myocardial mitochondria. Such cardiac involvement may appear promptly after carbon monoxide exposure or may be delayed for several days. Sinus tachycardia and various arrhythmias including ventricular extrasystoles and atrial fibrillation are common; bradycardia and atrioventricular block may occur in more severe cases. Angina pectoris or MI may be precipitated by carbon monoxide exposure in patients with or without underlying coronary artery disease. Electrocardiographic ST segment and T wave abnormalities occur commonly, and transient ventricular dysfunction may occur. The administration of 100 percent oxygen or treatment in a hyperbaric oxygen chamber usually results in rapid resolution of the cardiac abnormalities.

CH 68

Thallium

Thallium salts are toxic when inhaled, ingested, or absorbed through the skin. Gastrointestinal and neurologic symptoms of poisoning occur within 12 to 24 hours of a single toxic dose (more than 1 gm in adults). Several weeks after acute exposure, individuals are predisposed to cardiac arrhythmias and sudden death.

REFERENCES

Ethanol

1. Lucas DL, Brown RA, Wassef M, Giles TD: Alcohol and the cardiovascular system: Research challenges and opportunities. J Am Coll Cardiol 45:1916, 2005.
2. Fernandez-Sola J, Nicolas JM, Oriola J, et al: Angiotensin-converting enzyme gene polymorphism is associated with vulnerability to alcoholic cardiomyopathy. Ann Intern Med 137:321, 2002.
3. Klatsky AL: Alcohol and cardiovascular disease—more than one paradox to consider. Alcohol and hypertension: Does it matter? Yes. J Cardiovasc Risk 10:21, 2003.
4. Thadhani R, Camargo CA Jr, Stampfer MJ, et al: Prospective study of moderate alcohol consumption and risk of hypertension in young women. Arch Intern Med 162:569, 2002.
5. Rimm EB, Williams P, Fosher K, et al: Moderate alcohol intake and lower risk of coronary heart disease: Meta-analysis of effects on lipids and haemostatic factors. BMJ 319:1523, 1999.
6. Mukamal KJ, Conigrave KM, Mittleman MA, et al: Roles of drinking pattern and type of alcohol consumed in coronary heart disease in men. N Engl J Med 348:109, 2003.
7. Gronbaek M, Becker U, Johansen D, et al: Type of alcohol consumed and mortality from all causes, coronary heart disease, and cancer. Ann Intern Med 133:411, 2000.
8. Koppes LL, Dekker JM, Hendriks HF, et al: Meta-analysis of the relationship between alcohol consumption and coronary heart disease and mortality in type 2 diabetic patients. Diabetologia 49:648, 2006.
9. Ajani UA, Gaziano JM, Lotufo PA, et al: Alcohol consumption and risk of coronary heart disease by diabetes status. Circulation 102:500, 2000.
10. Mukamal KJ, Maclure M, Muller JE, et al: Prior alcohol consumption and mortality following acute myocardial infarction. JAMA 285:1965, 2001.

Cocaine

11. Lange RA, Hillis LD: Cardiovascular complications of cocaine use. N Engl J Med 345:351, 2001.
12. Qureshi AI, Suri MF, Guterman LR, et al: Cocaine use and the likelihood of nonfatal myocardial infarction and stroke: Data from the Third National Health and Nutrition Examination Survey. Circulation 103:502, 2001.
13. Weber JE, Shofer FS, Larkin GL, et al: Validation of a brief observation period for patients with cocaine-associated chest pain. N Engl J Med 348:510, 2003.
14. Bauman JL, DiDomenico RJ: Cocaine-induced channelopathies: Emerging evidence on the multiple mechanisms of sudden death. J Cardiovasc Pharmacol Ther 7:195, 2002.
15. Hsue PY, Salinas CL, Bolger AF, et al: Acute aortic dissection related to crack cocaine. Circulation 105:1592, 2002.

Amphetamines/Methamphetamines

16. Jacobs W: Fatal amphetamine-associated cardiotoxicity and its medicolegal implications. Am J Forens Med Pathol 27:156, 2006.
17. Lai TI, Hwang JJ, Fang CC, Chen WJ: Methylene 3,4 dioxymethamphetamine-induced acute myocardial infarction. Ann Emerg Med 42:759, 2003.
18. Costa GM, Pizzi C, Bresciani B, et al: Acute myocardial infarction caused by amphetamines: A case report and review of the literature. Ital Heart J 2:478, 2001.

Catecholamines

19. Wittstein IS, Thiemann DR, Lima JA, et al: Neurohumoral features of myocardial stunning due to sudden emotional stress. N Engl J Med 352:539, 2005.
20. Akashi YJ, Nakazawa K, Sakakibara M, et al: Reversible left ventricular dysfunction "takotsubo" cardiomyopathy related to catecholamine cardiotoxicity. J Electrocardiol 35:351, 2002.

Antiretroviral Agents (Protease Inhibitors)

21. Steinhart CR, Emon MF: Risks of cardiovascular disease in patients receiving antiretroviral therapy for HIV infection: Implications for treatment. AIDS Read 14:86, 2004.
22. Kulasekaram R, Peters BS, Wiersbicki AS: Dyslipidemia and cardiovascular risk in HIV infection. Curr Med Res Opin 21:1717, 2005.
23. Sudano I, Spieker LE, Noll G, et al: Cardiovascular disease in HIV infection. Am Heart J 151:1147, 2006.
24. Zareba KM, Lavigne JE, Lipshultz SE: Cardiovascular effects of HAART in infants and children of HIV-infected mothers. Cardiovasc Toxicol 4:271, 2004.
25. Lewis W: Mitochondrial DNA replication, nucleoside reverse-transcriptase inhibitors, and AIDS cardiomyopathy. Prog Cardiovasc Dis 45:305, 2003.

Appetite Suppressants

26. Connolly HM, Crary JL, McGoon MD, et al: Valvular heart disease associated with fenfluramine-phentermine. N Engl J Med 337:581, 1997.
27. Mast ST, Gersing KR, Anstrom KJ, et al: Association between selective serotonin-reuptake inhibitor therapy and heart valve regurgitation. Am J Cardiol 87:989, 2001.
28. Sachdev M, Miller WC, Ryan T, Jollis JG: Effect of fenfluramin-derivative diet pills on cardiac valves: A meta-analysis of observational studies. Am Heart J 144:1065, 2002.
29. Weissman NJ, Panza JA, Tighe JF, et al: Natural history of valvular regurgitation 1 year after discontinuation of dexfenfluramine therapy. A randomized, double-blind, placebo-controlled trial. Ann Intern Med 134:267, 2001.

Pergolide

30. Waller EA, Kaplan J, Heckman MG: Valvular heart disease in patients taking pergolide. Mayo Clin Proc 80:1016, 2005.

Chemotherapeutic Agents

31. Simbre AV, Duffy SA, Dadlani GH, et al: Cardiotoxicity of cancer chemotherapy: Implications for children. Pediatr Drugs 7:187, 2005.
32. Yeh ET: Cardiotoxicity induced by chemotherapy and antibody therapy. Ann Rev Med 57:485, 2006.

Environmental Exposures

33. Guallar E, Sanz-Gallardo MI, van't Veer P, et al: Mercury, fish oils, and the risk of myocardial infarction. N Engl J Med 347:1747, 2002.
34. Yoshizawa K, Rimm EB, Morris JS, et al: Mercury and the risk of coronary heart disease in men. N Engl J Med 347:1755, 2002.

CHAPTER 69

Primary Tumors of the Heart

Bruce McManus and Cheng-Han Lee

Clinical Presentation, 1815
Systemic Manifestations, 1815
Embolic Phenomena, 1816
Cardiac Manifestations, 1816
Metastatic Diseases, 1817

Benign Tumors, 1817
Myxomas, 1817
Rhabdomyomas, 1822
Fibromas and Hamartomas, 1823
Hemangiomas and
    Lymphangiomas, 1823

Malignant Tumors, 1824
Angiosarcomas, 1824
Rhabdomyosarcomas, 1825
Leiomyosarcomas, 1825
Other Sarcomas, 1825

Management of Primary Cardiac
Tumors, 1826

References, 1827

Primary tumors of the heart are rare across all age groups, with a reported prevalence of 0.001 to 0.03 percent in autopsy series.[1] Secondary involvement of the heart by extracardiac tumors is 20 to 40 times more common than by primary cardiac tumors.[1-3] The first premortem diagnosis of a primary cardiac tumor, a cardiac myxoma, was made by Goldberg in 1952. Since then, many more primary cardiac tumors have been reported in the literature.[1] Despite rarity, there are multiple recognized histologic types of primary cardiac tumors. Excluding tumors that are primarily based in the pericardium like mesotheliomas and teratomas (see Chap. 70), the overwhelming majority of primary cardiac tumors are mesenchymal tumors that display the full spectrum of differentiation as do those seen in the soft tissue. About 75 percent of all primary cardiac tumors are regarded as benign neoplasms, with cardiac myxoma accounting for at least half of them. However, the oncologic designation of benignity understates the potentially devastating effect any benign primary cardiac tumor may impose on the patient. By virtue of their anatomic locations, primary cardiac tumors are capable of producing a myriad of cardiac, embolic, and systemic symptomatologies, sometimes with fatal consequences. Of the remaining 25 percent of primary cardiac tumors that are considered to be malignant neoplasms, the majority are sarcomas, with lymphomas being the next most common. Because many symptoms of malignant primary cardiac tumors occur relatively late in the disease course, findings of locally infiltrative or systemically widespread disease at initial presentation are not uncommon.

The diagnosis of primary cardiac tumors is frequently challenging. The symptoms associated with most primary cardiac tumors are nonspecific, and they often mimic far more commonly encountered disease entities. Further, many tumors present with mild and vague symptoms such that most routine work-ups will fail to identify the underlying abnormality. This elusiveness often results in a delay in the diagnosis of disease. Fortunately, the more widespread use of noninvasive and relatively sensitive imaging modalities such as cardiac echocardiography, computed tomography (CT), cardiac magnetic resonance (CMR), and positron emission tomography (see Chaps. 14, 16, 17, and 18) should facilitate the identification of cardiac lesions. However, the consideration of primary cardiac tumor in the differential diagnosis combined with a high index of suspicion is also paramount in arriving at the correct diagnosis. In addition to the diagnostic challenges, the management of some primary cardiac tumors is also not straightforward even when the histologic diagnosis has been made. Many benign primary cardiac tumors are now found incidentally in asymptomatic individuals. Therefore the treatment decision requires a thorough analysis of the potential benefits and harms of the surgery versus conservative management. Because of our limited experience with the natural clinical course of many primary cardiac tumors, this treatment decision may be difficult to reach.

CLINICAL PRESENTATION

Primary cardiac tumors are great masqueraders of many commonly encountered cardiac and systemic diseases. Depending on the location, size, mobility, friability, and histologic type of the lesions, cardiac tumors can produce a variety of symptoms and clinical findings. The types of clinical manifestations that are produced by primary cardiac tumors overall can be divided into four general mechanistic categories—systemic manifestations, embolic manifestations, cardiac manifestations, and phenomena secondary to metastatic diseases. Systemic manifestations refer to the constitutional symptoms and paraneoplastic syndromes that can be associated with some primary cardiac tumors. Embolic manifestations refer to the phenomenon of pulmonary and systemic embolism caused by tumor emboli themselves and/or tumor-associated thromboemboli. Cardiac manifestations encompass a multitude of abnormalities that include mechanical interference with myocardial function/valvular function/coronary blood flow, conduction disturbances, and pericardial fluid accumulation. Metastatic diseases are features of malignant primary cardiac tumors, and a plethora of clinical manifestations are possible depending on the site of tumor metastases.

Systemic Manifestations

Primary cardiac tumors, whether benign or malignant, are capable of producing a multitude of systemic symptoms that can add to the challenge of reaching the proper diagnosis. Patients with primary cardiac tumors may experience constitutional symptoms of fever, chills, fatigue, malaise, and weight loss. In addition, these symptoms mimic those of several connective tissue diseases and vasculitides such as myalgia, arthralgia, muscle weakness, and Raynaud phenomenon.[4,5] Routine laboratory tests may reveal evidence of leukocytosis, polycythemia, anemia, thrombocytosis, thrombocytopenia, hypergammaglobulinemia, and increased erythrocyte sedimentation rate. These systemic manifestations are believed to be produced by secretory products released by the tumor and/or by tumor necrosis. Among the benign primary cardiac tumors, cardiac myxomas are the most notorious for causing systemic symptoms, and an elevated serum interleukin-6 (IL-6) frequently found in these patients is believed to mediate such symptoms.[6,7] Malignant primary cardiac tumors, similar to their counterparts from extracardiac sites, are also frequently associated with constitutional findings.

Embolic Phenomena

Primary cardiac tumors can cause systemic and/or pulmonary embolism by way of tumor emboli or thromboemboli that are released from or formed on the surface of the tumor, respectively. The propensity of cardiac tumors to cause embolic phenomena depends largely on the predominant origin of the tumor (intramural or intracavitary), the type of the tumor, and the friability of the intraluminal tumor surface.[8] Among the benign primary cardiac neoplasms, cardiac myxomas are most frequently associated with embolic findings, especially when the tumor possesses a villous surface.[8] Other benign primary cardiac neoplasms that are known to produce emboli include papillary fibroelastomas and hemangiomas/lymphangiomas.[9-11] Embolism related to malignant primary cardiac tumors is not uncommon because many malignant tumors have a friable and sometimes necrotic luminal surface. However, systemic/pulmonary metastases from the malignant tumor must be excluded because they can produce similar manifestations. Primary cardiac tumors can embolize to almost any organ, resulting in ischemia, infarction, and even delayed aneurysm formation in the organs or the body sites involved.[1,5,12,13] Embolism can sometimes occur concurrently in multiple organs and/or body sites. Systemic emboli are typically caused by a left-sided tumor, although right-sided tumors can also result in systemic emboli if there is concurrent right-to-left shunting through a patent foramen ovale. The brain is the most common site of involvement for systemic emboli produced by primary cardiac tumors, and the involvement of both hemispheres and multiple regions is seen more than 40 percent of the time.[12] The multifocal nature of cerebral involvement should therefore prompt a search for embolic origin with echocardiography and carotid Doppler ultrasound in these instances. Cerebral embolism most commonly results in a transient ischemic attack or an ischemic stroke, but intracranial hemorrhage may occur as well. Depending on the region of the brain involved, patients may experience a variety of psychiatric and neurologic disturbances that range in severity from mild vertigo to seizure and even a comatose state. Delayed aneurysm formation presumably at the site of previous cerebral tumor emboli represents another dreadful complication of the disease.[13] In addition to the brain, the tumor emboli or tumor-associated thromboemboli can occur in almost any organ or tissue. This includes tumor emboli to a coronary artery that can result in clinical findings of myocardial infarction that can further conceal the underlying abnormality. Careful examination of embolectomy specimens is therefore important because it may reveal evidence of tumor emboli. In contrast to systemic emboli, pulmonary embolization is typically caused by a right-sided tumor, although in rare instances emboli from a left-sided tumor located proximal to the site of a left-to-right intracardiac shunt can also result in pulmonary embolism. Consideration should be given to the possible presence of a primary cardiac tumor in patients presenting with findings of pulmonary embolism when no identifiable source of emboli surfaces after conventional assessment.

Cardiac Manifestations

The cardiac manifestations of primary cardiac tumors can result from direct mechanical interference with myocardial/valvular function, interruption of coronary blood flow, interference with electrophysiological conduction, and stimulation of pericardial fluid accumulation. The propensity for various cardiac manifestations depends primarily on the location of the tumor (pericardial, intramural, or intracavitary); the chamber involved; the size; and the infiltrative nature. Pericardial tumors are not addressed in this chapter because they are dealt with elsewhere (see Chap. 70).

Primary cardiac tumors that are completely or predominantly intramural or myocardial in location are typically asymptomatic, especially if the sizes are small. Large intramural tumors that are located within or pressing on major cardiac conduction pathways may, however, cause a wide variety of arrhythmias including complete heart block or asystole in more severe cases.[4] In addition, large intramural tumors may also compress the cardiac cavities, obstruct the ventricular outflow tract, or contribute to insufficiency of the mitral valve.

In contrast to intramural tumors, primary cardiac tumors with a significant intracavitary component tend to cause more symptoms for patients. Further, intracavitary tumors that are pedunculated and mobile can be especially problematic because of their tendency to interfere with valvular and myocardial function. The precise cardiac manifestations depend also on the locale of a tumor in the heart. For left atrial tumors, intracavitary lesions that are pedunculated and mobile can interfere with the mitral valve and produce clinical findings typical of mitral regurgitation that include fatigue, dyspnea, orthopnea, paroxysmal nocturnal dyspnea, cough, hemoptysis, chest pain, pulmonary edema, and peripheral edema. However, the presence of findings atypical for mitral regurgitation such as the aforementioned systemic and constitutional symptoms should prompt further investigation. These symptoms can be sudden in onset, intermittent, and positional. Physical examination may reveal signs of pulmonary congestion with an S3 and loud and widely split S1, the presence of a holosystolic murmur most prominent at the apex with radiation to the axilla, the presence of a diastolic murmur from turbulent blood flow through the mitral orifice, and the presence of a tumor "plop." Such tumor "plop" is thought to result from the tumor striking the endocardial wall or the abrupt halt of tumor excursions. It occurs later than an opening snap but earlier than an S3. For intracavitary tumors located in the right atrium, findings of right heart failure that include fatigue, peripheral edema, ascites, hepatosplenomegaly, and elevated jugular venous pressure (JVP) with prominent a-wave are the most common cardiac presentations.

Because of the right atrial location, the diagnosis is often delayed with an average time interval from presentation to the correct diagnosis of 3 years. Patients frequently present with rapidly progressive right heart failure and also new-onset heart murmurs because of mechanical interference with the tricuspid valve by the tumor. In patients with a patent foramen ovale, the build-up of right atrial pressure can produce right-to-left intracardiac shunting and result in systemic hypoxia, cyanosis, clubbing, and polycythemia. Occasionally, patients may also present with superior vena cava (SVC) syndrome caused by a large right atrial tumor. Physical examination may reveal findings of peripheral edema, hepatosplenomegaly, ascites, elevated JVP with prominent a-wave and steep y descent, and an early diastolic murmur or holosystolic murmur that exhibits significant respiratory or positional variation.

Right ventricular tumors with a significant intracavitary component may obstruct the filling or the outflow of the right ventricle and as such can produce right-sided congestive heart failure that includes dyspnea, peripheral edema, ascites, and hepatosplenomegaly. Precordial auscultation may reveal a systolic ejection murmur at the left sternal border, an S3, and a delayed P2. An elevated JVP and Kussmaul sign may also be present. These findings may vary significantly depending on the position of the patient. Lastly, left ventricular tumors with a significant intracavitary component can obstruct the left ventricular outflow tract and produce findings of left-sided heart failure and syncope, as well as atypical chest pain from obstruction of a coronary artery either by direct tumor involvement or tumor emboli. Physical examination may reveal evidence of pulmonary edema, low blood pressure, and systolic murmurs that mimic the findings of aortic or subaortic stenosis. The murmurs and blood pressure may display considerable positional variation. In the case of malignant primary cardiac tumors such as angiosarcomas and primary cardiac lymphomas, malignant hemorrhagic pericardial effusion may be present. Life-threatening cardiac tamponade and cardiac rupture leading to sudden death may also occur.[14-16]

Metastatic Diseases

Truly metastatic diseases are by definition features of malignant primary cardiac tumors. Most malignant primary cardiac tumors are detected at a late stage with systemic dissemination present. In some cases, symptoms secondary to the metastatic disease may represent the initial clinical manifestation of the malignant primary cardiac tumor.[17] Common sites of metastases for most primary cardiac sarcomas like angiosarcomas and rhabdomyosarcomas include lung, brain, and bone,[14,18,19] although metastases to the liver, lymph node, adrenal gland, spleen, and skin have also been reported.

DIAGNOSTIC APPROACH

Primary cardiac tumors are among the most challenging disease entities to diagnose because of their rarity and their highly variable and usually nonspecific clinical presentations. Therefore it is understandable that clinicians who first encounter a patient with a primary cardiac tumor generally attribute the findings to other, more commonly encountered disease entities and proceed to work up the patient accordingly. Thus the key to proper and timely diagnosis of a primary cardiac tumor lies not necessarily in its immediate diagnostic recognition, but rather in the consideration of primary cardiac tumor in the differential diagnosis. In addition, clinicians need to maintain a high index of suspicion for rare entities like primary cardiac tumors, especially when there are atypical features present. A thorough clinical evaluation including a complete history and physical examination coupled with appropriate laboratory tests are necessary because pertinent information may be present to help support a possible diagnosis of primary cardiac tumor (Table 69-1) or secondary cardiac tumor. When the diagnosis of cardiac tumor is considered in the differential diagnosis, the most ideal initial method of evaluation is echocardiography (see Chap. 14), either transthoracic or transesophageal depending on the clinical circumstances. The sensitivities of transthoracic and transesophageal echocardiography for detecting a cardiac mass are 93 and 97 percent, respectively.[20] If and when a cardiac lesion is identified, chest CT with contrast enhancement and CMR with contrast are superior modalities for characterizing the lesions and delineating the extent of tumor involvement (see Chaps. 17 and 18). They can also help to exclude the possibility of a tumor that originates from adjacent mediastinal structures. Features suggestive of malignant cardiac tumors include presence of a large broad-based lesion occupying most of the affected cardiac chamber, hilar lymphadenopathy, extensive pericardial involvement, and hemorrhagic pericardial effusions. However, the diagnosis of a cardiac tumor, whether benign or malignant, cannot be made with imaging studies alone, and histologic evaluation is necessary for definitive diagnosis. Depending on the clinical settings, tissue diagnosis may be made with less invasive methods such as cytologic evaluation of pericardial/pleural fluids, echo-guided percutaneous cardiac biopsy, or echo-guided transvenous cardiac biopsy.[14,21,22] However, a negative biopsy obtained through these less invasive methods does not rule out a diagnosis of malignancy because the false-negative rate of these methods can be significant. Therefore more invasive methods of tumor biopsy through mediastinoscopy or even thoracotomy may be necessary in order to obtain a definitive diagnosis. In the scenarios in which the presence of a malignant cardiac tumor is confirmed through tissue diagnosis or strongly suspected on the basis of clinical and imaging findings, a full metastatic

work-up should be performed if clinically feasible. Of note is that the great majority of malignant cardiac tumors represent local or distant metastases by an extracardiac tumor, and most malignant primary cardiac tumors are diagnosed at an advanced stage with distant metastases already present. Therefore a thorough physical examination and a complete series of imaging may help locate probable extracardiac origin of the primary tumor or identify potential metastatic lesions from the primary cardiac tumor. This information will help in the disease staging and prognostication, as well as the planning of a treatment course.

BENIGN TUMORS

Myxomas

Myxoma is the most common type of primary cardiac tumor, accounting for 30 to 50 percent of all primary tumors of the heart.[1] It has an annual incidence of 0.5 per million population and most commonly presents in adults 30 to 50 years of age, although it can occur in nearly all age groups ranging from 1 to 83 years.[7] Sixty-five percent of cardiac myxomas occur in women, and 4.5 to 10 percent of cardiac myxomas are familial.[7] Although there was debate in the past about whether cardiac myxoma was, indeed, a neoplastic entity or an organized thrombus, recent gene expression and immunohistochemical studies have shown that cardiac myxoma is a neoplasm with tumor cells arising most likely from multipotent mesenchymal cells.[23-29] Other features suggestive of its being a neoplastic process include its ability to recur, its occurrence in multiple sites, and occurrence in families. Despite several documented reports of metastases to various anatomic sites, the typical cardiac myxoma is regarded as a benign neoplasm in a conventional sense and the reported metastases most likely represent tumor growth from embolic tumor fragments that are deposited along the arterial circulation in different remote sites.

The pathogenesis of cardiac myxoma is poorly understood, especially for those that occur sporadically. Recent studies have, however, shed more light on the pathogenesis of familial cases of cardiac myxomas. Carney syndrome accounts for the majority of familial cases of cardiac myxoma and for 7 percent of all cardiac myxomas.[24] Carney syndrome or complex is an autosomal dominant syndrome characterized by myxoma formation in cardiac and several extracardiac locations, spotty skin pigmentation, endocrine hyperactivity and other tumors such as testicular Sertoli cell tumor, psammomatous melanotic schwannoma, pituitary adenoma, and thyroid tumors.[24] The cardiac myxomas occurring in the setting of Carney syndrome and sporadic cases are histologically indistinguishable. However, cardiac myxomas associated with Carney syndrome show no age or gender predilection, can be single or multiple, can occur in any intracardiac location, and tend to recur with a rate of 20 percent despite adequate surgical excision. In contrast, sporadic cases of cardiac myxoma tend to occur in women of middle age and as isolated lesions in the left atrial aspect of interatrial septum. Sporadic cases have a lower recurrence rate (≈3 percent) than those mentioned previously. Etiologically, mutations in PRKAR1A, a regulatory subunit 1A of cAMP-dependent protein kinase A (PKA) and in MYH8, a non-PKA phosphorylated perinatal myosin isoform, are believed to be responsible for cardiac myxoma formation in most individuals with Carney syndrome. The precise mechanism of tumorigenesis involving these mutations in the formation of myxomas is unknown. However, there may be a role for genetic testing for these mutations in asymptomatic kindreds of individuals with myxomas to guide further investigation and management.[30]

Clinically, patients with symptomatic cardiac myxoma can have a variety of nonspecific findings depending on the size, location, and mobility of the myxoma. However, the

TABLE 69-1 Characteristic Clinicopathologic Features of Primary Cardiac Tumors

Primary Cardiac Tumors	Epidemiologic Features	Common Clinical Presentations	Clinical Association	Common Locations	Pathologic Features
Myxomas	30-50 yr, F > M, 5-10% familial	Cardiac mechanical and rhythm disturbances, embolic symptoms, systemic symptoms	5-10% associated with Carney syndrome/complex	Left atrium (83%), right atrium (13%), subendocardial	Pedunculated solitary tumor (>90%) with a stalk attached to subendothelial base
Lipomas	All ages, M = F	Cardiac mechanical and rhythm disturbances	None	Subendocardial and subepicardial tumor, no chamber predilection	
Lipomatous hypertrophy	70 yr, obese patient, M > F	Cardiac rhythm disturbances	None	Atrial septum	Significant thickening of the atrial septum
Papillary fibroelastomas	Elderly	Embolic symptoms		80-90% on valvular endocardium, aortic valve most common	1 cm lesion with delicate papillary fronds, single in 91%
Rhabdomyomas	80% < 1 yr, 50% familial	Cardiac mechanical and rhythm disturbances	50% associated with tuberous sclerosis	Ventricles > atria	Multiple small (<1 mm) lesions found in most tuberous sclerosis–associated cases and in 50% of sporadic cases
Fibromas	90% in children, M = F	Cardiac mechanical and rhythm disturbances	A small subset associated with Gorlin syndrome	Interventricular septum and left ventricular free wall in >90%	Solitary intramural tumor (5-cm average size)
Hemangiomas/Lymphangiomas	All ages	Cardiac mechanical and rhythm disturbances, embolic symptoms	Occasional association with extracardiac hemangiomas in the gastrointestinal tract and on the face, Kasabach-Merritt syndrome	Ventricles > atria	Multiple tumors in 30%
Angiosarcomas	30-50 yr, M > F	Cardiac mechanical and rhythm disturbances, embolic symptoms, systemic/constitutional symptoms, metastatic disease		90% in right atrium	Intramural mass with protrusion into the cavity, infiltrative, frequent involvement of pericardium
Rhabdomyosarcomas	Children and young adults, M > F	Cardiac mechanical and rhythm disturbances, systemic/constitutional symptoms, metastatic disease	Hypereosinophilia	No chamber predilection	Multiple lesions seen in 60%, infiltrative
Leiomyosarcomas	30-40, M = F	Cardiac mechanical and rhythm disturbances, systemic/constitutional symptoms, metastatic disease		70-80% in left atrium, may involve pulmonary trunk	Solitary lesion in 70%, infiltrative
Lymphomas	62-67 yr, can affect all ages, M > F	Cardiac mechanical and rhythm disturbances, embolic symptoms, systemic/constitutional symptoms	HIV infection, immunocompromised state, posttransplantation	Right side of the heart in 69-72%	Single lesion in 66% and multiple lesions in 34%, may cause pericardial effusion

majority of the patients will present with at least one of the classic triad of obstructive cardiac, embolic, and constitutional/systemic signs.[1,5] The obstructive cardiac findings including dizziness, dyspnea, cough, pulmonary edema, and congestive heart failure are the result of mechanical interference with the mitral valve by the tumor and account for the most common presenting findings in the triad. Tumor embolism is another common basis for clinical presentation and can affect the systemic and/or pulmonary circulation depending on the location of the tumor and the patency of the foramen ovale. Cardiac myxoma is the most common primary cardiac tumor to produce tumor emboli, and it has been reported to embolize to virtually any organ or tissue. Constitutional and nonembolic systemic findings secondary to cardiac myxoma include several nonspecific symptoms such as fever, weight loss, fatigue, myalgia, arthralgia, muscle weakness, and Raynaud syndrome.[5,6,31] These nonspecific symptoms often create the most confusion and difficulty in the diagnosis because they may mimic immunologic diseases. They are believed to be related to IL-6 release by the cardiac myxoma tumor cells. A significant subset (approximately two thirds) of patients with cardiac myxoma have abnormal electrocardiograms (ECGs), commonly showing evidence of left atrial enlargement, although a variety of abnormalities can be seen.[5,8,32] However, atrial arrhythmias or conduction disturbances are rare. On chest radiograph, about one third of patients have normal findings. Evidence of elevated left atrial pressure such as left atrial enlargement, vascular redistribution, prominent pulmonary trunk, and pulmonary edema is found in 53 percent of patients with left atrial myxoma.[4] Cardiomegaly is seen in 37 and 50 percent of left and right atrial myxomas, respectively. Intracardiac tumor calcification is a rare finding in left atrial myxomas but is found in 56 percent of patients with right atrial myxoma. The typical imaging modalities used for diagnostic and preoperative assessment purposes include CT, CMR, and echocardiography. Most cardiac myxomas appear as spherical or ovoid masses with lobular contour on CT and MRI scans.[4] Two thirds of myxomas are heterogeneous, whereas one third appear homogeneous on CT (see Chap. 18).

Contrast-enhanced CT reveals that most myxomas have an overall attenuation lower than that of myocardium, few such tumors have equivalent attenuation, but in no instance have the tumors showed higher attenuation. CMR shows heterogeneous signal intensity in 90 percent of cardiac myxomas, with the T1-weighted images showing isointense signal in 79 percent and hyperintense signal in 14 percent of the cases (see Chap. 17). Cine gradient-echo CMR is a new modality that appears to be superior to other imaging modalities in the assessment of cardiac tumors because it allows for better visualization of the size, location, and point of attachment of the tumor.[4] Echocardiography is the most commonly used modality for diagnostic purposes, and transesophageal echocardiography is the recommended method for initial assessment of suspected cardiac lesions.[3]

Cardiac myxoma most commonly occurs in the left atrium (Fig. 69-1). A recent meta-analysis showed that 83 percent of cardiac myxomas occur in the left atrium (see Fig. 14-103), 12.7 percent occur in the right atrium, and 1.3 percent of cardiac myxomas are biatrial.[7] Occurrence in the ventricles is uncommon, with only 1.7 and 0.6 percent of cardiac myxomas occurring in the left ventricle and the right ventricle, respectively.[1] The majority (>90 percent) of cardiac myxomas are solitary, although multiple synchronous cardiac myxomas can occur, especially in the setting of Carney syndrome. Cardiac myxomas are generally pedunculated tumors with a fibrovascular stalk attaching to the subendothelial base. The usual site of attachment is the interatrial septum in the region of the fossa ovalis (see Fig. 18-27).[5,33] Rarely, cardiac myxoma can involve heart valves directly. Most cardiac myxomas have sizes ranging from 4 to 8 cm in diameter, although they can reach a size of 16 cm.[4,5,8] The mean weight is 37 gm, with a range of 15 to 180 gm. Approximately half of the cardiac myxomas have a smooth compact surface, whereas the remaining half have a villous surface. Evidence suggests that myxomas with villous surface are more likely to embolize.[8] On cross-section, cardiac myxomas have a gelatinous appearance, although foci of hemorrhage, calcification (Fig. 69-2), ossification (see Fig. 18-27), and cystic change can also be present.[4] Histologically, cardiac myxoma contains sparsely distributed uniform spindle- and stellate-shaped cells within an extensive myxoid stroma. Though generally hypocellular, the degree of cellularity can vary from tumor to tumor. Tumor spindle- and stellate-shaped cells typically possess round/oval nuclei, with indistinct nucleoli and indistinct cell borders. Binucleate or multinucleate cells may be seen. Mitotic figures are rarely present. The myxoid stroma is composed of acid mucopolysaccharides that are hyaluronidase sensitive. The stroma typically contains prominent thin-walled vessels. Necrosis, calcification, and Gamna bodies (calcified elastic fibers) can be seen in a small subset of cardiac myxomas.[4,5] Smooth muscle cells and fibroblasts are occasionally present in the stroma.[29] A mixed inflammatory infiltrate is commonly seen. Although infrequently seen, cardiac myxomas may contain epithelial/glandular, hematopoietic, chondroid, and thymic elements.[29,34,35] Experts suspect that these heterotopic elements represent a form of choristoma. Even more rarely, malignant transformation of these heterotopic elements can occur, giving rise to various malignancies.[34] Histochemically, both the stroma and the tumor cells stain positive with PAS, whereas only the stroma shows positive staining with Alcian blue. Immunohistochemically, the stromal tumor cells show vimentin positivity and variable S-100 and NSE positivity, but never keratin positivity.[29] When embolic myxoma is suspected in embolectomy specimens, calretinin and IL-6 may be useful in differentiating between embolic myxoma and myxoid thrombus.[8,36]

The treatment for symptomatic cardiac myxoma is prompt surgical resection of the tumor with the patients placed on cardiopulmonary bypass.[37] Complete excision is the goal, although it may not be plausible in all instances.[38] Immediate postoperative mortality in most series ranges from 0 to 7.5 percent.[5,33,39] Other common postoperative complications include arrhythmias, which may require long-term medication.[33] Recurrence occurs in about 3 percent of tumors, although the rate is higher with familial cardiac myxomas and can occur anywhere from 3 months up to 14 years postoperatively.[5,23-25] Recurrences can be local or in extracardiac locations such as the brain, lung, skeletal muscle, bone, kidney, gastrointestinal tract, skin, and other soft tissue sites. Recurrence of myxoma in the brain, which likely represents growth of the embolized tumor fragments, can be difficult to manage, but chemotherapy is not recommended because embolic myxomas do not truly represent metastatic diseases.[40] A particularly rare but potentially life-threatening complication is the development of cerebral aneurysm secondary to embolic tumor fragments.[13] Long-term follow-up of such patients with cardiac myxoma is highly recommended.

LIPOMAS AND LIPOMATOUS HYPERTROPHY OF THE ATRIAL SEPTUM

Benign lipomatous tumor is the second most common primary neoplasm of the heart and can be divided into two major groups primarily on the basis of the degree of encapsulation—lipoma and lipomatous hypertrophy of the atrial septum. Cardiac lipomas can occur sporadi-

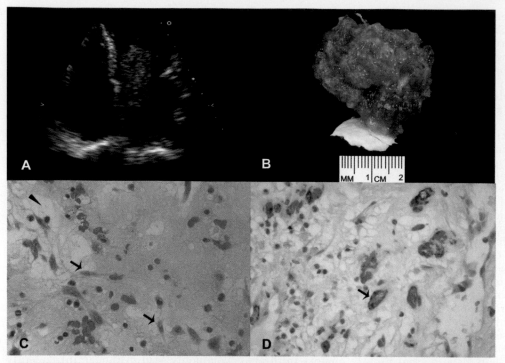

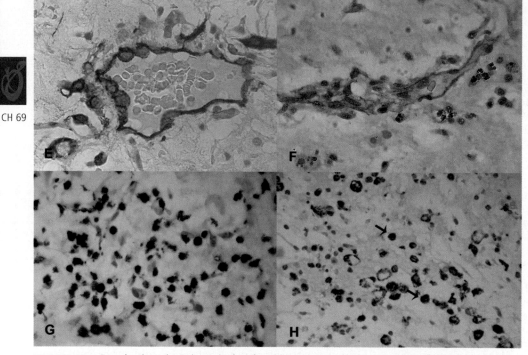

FIGURE 69–1 Four-chamber echocardiograph of a left atrial myxoma in a 71-year-old woman, showing a mass on the left side of the heart (A) projecting from the atrial septum through the mitral valve into the left ventricle. B, Gross photograph of the left atrial myxoma that was surgically excised from the same woman. Grossly, the tumor is a pedunculated, variegated mass with a friable, gelatinous texture. C, Hematoxylin and eosin staining of the loose, proteoglycan-rich tumor (×200). The tumor is highly vascular; with vessels containing red blood cells admixed with lipidic cells present in a network throughout the tumor matrix (arrow). Immunohistochemical staining for vessels was positive for alpha smooth muscle actin, CD 34, and CD 31 (D, E, and F, respectively; ×400). Staining for leukocyte common antigen is positive for mononuclear cells (G; ×400). Staining for CD 68 shows several macrophages (H; ×400), some of which are hemosiderin laden, reflecting previous hemorrhage, a common occurrence in myxomas.

tricular surfaces.[1] They originate most commonly in the subepicardial and subendocardial locations (see Fig. 17-15), though intramyocardial lesions have also been reported. Subendocardial lipomas with prominent intracavitary component can interfere with mechanical function of the heart, resulting in symptoms of heart failure.[43] Subepicardial tumors are usually asymptomatic, but large lesions may cause compression of the heart and produce pericardial effusion.[1] Intramyocardial lipoma may interfere with electrical conduction in the heart and cause arrhythmias. Diagnostically, even though transesophageal echocardiography can be used to assess the location, size, and mobility of these cardiac lesions, it may not be possible to accurately determine the tissue type because typical cardiac lipomas have a nonspecific appearance on ultrasound.[41,44] CT scan can provide better tissue characterization because cardiac lipomas display a low attenuation signal similar to subcutaneous or mediastinal fat (see Chap. 18).[41] Grossly, cardiac lipomas usually occur as single well-encapsulated masses, though multiple lesions can occur, especially in patients with tuberous sclerosis.[41] Size typically ranges from 1 to 8 cm in diameter. Similar to lipomas found in other sites, cardiac lipoma is histopathologically composed of mature fat cells with occasional fibrous connective tissue (fibrolipoma) and vacuolated brown fat (hibernoma-like). Areas of degeneration and extensive radiographically apparent calcification may be present.[45] The treatment for symptomatic cardiac lipomas is surgical resection, and the postoperative prognosis is excellent.[1,43]

In contrast to lipoma, lipomatous hypertrophy of the atrial septum (LHAS) (Fig. 69-3), also known as *massive fatty deposits of the atrial septum*, is a nonencapsulated excessive accumulation of fat in the atrial septum at the level of fossa ovalis that is greater than 2 cm in thickness and typically occurs in elderly, obese, male patients. A recent study revealed that this disease as diagnosed by CT scan may have an incidence as high as 2.2 percent, which is considerably higher than previously estimated.[44] The mean age of diagnosis in most series is about 70 years and tends to occur in obese patients.[44] The etiology of lipomatous hypertrophy of the atrial septum is unknown, and there is controversy regarding whether the condition truly represents a neoplasm in most instances.[1,44,46] Its apparent association with advanced age and obesity has led to the suggestion that it may represent a metabolic process. However, the

cally at all ages with equal frequency in both sexes.[41] Although lipomas from other body sites such as skin frequently show cytogenetic abnormalities involving chromosome 12 in q15,[42] the molecular and genetic basis of cardiac lipomas is not elucidated. Clinically, most cardiac lipomas are asymptomatic and typically present as incidental findings. However, the tumor can produce a variety of symptoms depending on its size and location. Cardiac lipomas can occur at any atrial and ven-

observed occurrence in nonobese patients suggests otherwise.[1] Clinically, the great majority of lipomatous hypertrophy of the atrial septum does not cause any symptoms. Occasionally, it can result in a variety of rhythm disturbances and even sudden death.[41] In rare instances in which the tumor protrudes into the right atrium and the superior vena cava, patients can present with symptoms secondary to blood flow obstruction.[47] CT and CMR are the most desirable modalities for the

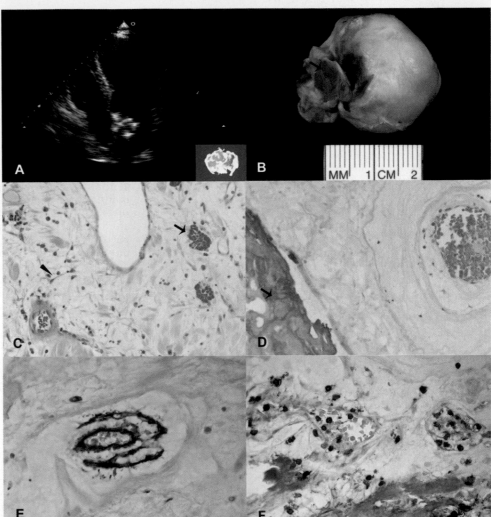

FIGURE 69–2 **A,** Four-chamber echocardiographic view of the heart with a mass in the left atrium of the heart. **A, Inset,** Ex vivo radiograph of the calcified myxoma with dense areas of calcifications that correspond to echo densities seen. **B,** Gross photograph of a surgically excised, partially calcified left atrial myxoma from a 77-year-old man with a cream-yellow glistening surface (arrow—cut surface of the atrial septum that attached to a short myxomal stalk. Of note is the neighboring focal hemorrhage.) **C,** Hematoxylin and eosin staining (×200) of the tumor after decalcification showing hemosiderin-laden macrophages (arrow) and lipidic cells (arrowhead). **D,** The arrow shows "watermark" postdecalcification (×200). **E,** Immunohistochemical staining for endothelial cells was positive for CD 34 (×400). **F,** Staining with leukocyte common antigen is positive for mononuclear cells (×400).

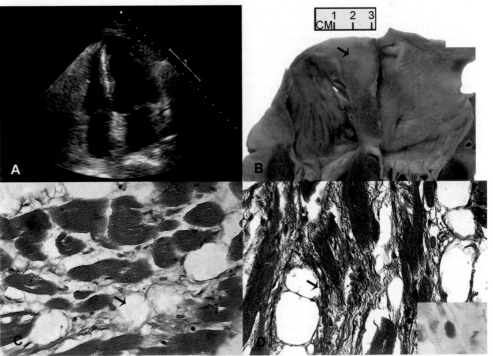

FIGURE 69–3 **A,** Four-chamber echocardiograph of the heart from a 72-year-old woman with lipomatous hypertrophy of the atrial septum. (Image courtesy of Dr. Kenneth Gin, University of British Columbia, Division of Cardiology.) Lipomatous hypertrophy of the atrial septum in a heart from a 62-year-old man. **B,** The atrial septum superior to the fossa ovale was measured to have a thickness greater than 3 cm (arrow). **C,** Hematoxylin and eosin staining shows myocardium among mature and immature adipocytes and scant inflammatory cells (×400). **D,** Movat pentachrome staining (×400) shows myocytes in red and associated excess collagen in yellow (arrow). **D, Inset,** Chloracetate esterase staining shows the presence of mast cells (×400).

diagnosis of lipomatous hypertrophy of the interatrial septum because they are superior to echocardiography in differentiating between fat and connective tissue. On imaging, the atrial septum is thickened to up to 7 cm, whereas normally it is less than 1 cm.[44,48] Accumulation of the fat beneath the atrial septal endocardium may bulge into the right atrium. Histologically, lipomatous hypertrophy of the atrial septum contains an infiltrating mixture of mature fat and vacuolated adipose cells resembling brown fat with enlarged cardiac myocytes. There is a focal excess of fibrous tissue. No mitotic activity is observed in the face cells in contrast to liposarcoma.[1] Occasional mononuclear cells are present, and mast cells are also not uncommon in association with the adipose cells. LHAS with symptomatic arrhythmias can be managed medically, whereas surgical excision should be restricted to the rare cases in which the disease causes symptomatic hemodynamic obstruction.[44,49]

PAPILLARY TUMORS OF THE HEART VALVES

Papillary fibroelastoma is the third most common primary cardiac tumor with an incidence of up to 0.33 percent in autopsy series.[50] It is believed to be an acquired lesion with a slow growth rate that is distinct from Lambl excrescences.[11,51] Little is known about the etiology of this disease, and experts debate whether it represents a reactive, hamartomatous, or neoplastic process.[1] Clinically, most patients with papillary fibroelastoma are asymptomatic. However, a review of the literature shows that nearly half of patients can be symptomatic.[50] Common presenting symptoms include transient ischemic attacks, stroke, angina, myocardial infarction, and dyspnea with cerebral embolic symptoms present in more than half of the symptomatic patients.[50] Rarely, patients present with subacute bacterial endocarditis–like findings, and pulmonary embolism and sudden death have also been reported. In contrast to other cardiac neoplasms like cardiac myxoma, the embolic material from papillary fibroelastoma is believed to be fibrin or thrombus originating from the tumor surface because fragments of tumor have only rarely been found in the vessels involved.[52] Transesophageal echocardiography is the recommended imaging modality for the diagnosis and characterization of papillary fibroelastoma (see Fig. 14-105), with a sensitivity and specificity of 89 and 88 percent, respectively, for lesions measuring 2 cm or greater.[53] A papillary fibroelastoma generally appears as a round, oval or irregular lesion that is well demarcated and homogeneous on echocardiography. Even though papillary fibroelastoma can be found anywhere in the heart, 80 to 90 percent are found on the valvular endocardium.[53] The aortic valve is the most common site of origin for papillary fibroelastoma (37 to 45 percent), although it can also originate on the mitral, tricuspid, or pulmonary valves and less commonly on the left atrial and left ventricular endocardium.[50,53-55] The lesions are single in 91 percent of the cases,[53] though multiple papillary fibroelastomas from different sites can be found in a small subset of patients.[56,57] The average size of a reported papillary fibroelastoma is about 1 cm in diameter, and it can range from 0.2 to 4.6 cm. Grossly, the papillary fibroelastoma has often been compared with the sea anemone because of the numerous and delicate papillary fronds. The tumor is soft; white to tan; and often friable with adherent thrombus, which likely represents the source of the emboli. Forty-four percent of papillary fibroelastomas have a 1- to 3-mm stalk, and this mobile type of papillary fibroelastoma appears more likely to give rise to embolism.[50,53,58] Papillary fibroelastoma has a distinct histologic appearance with the narrow, elongated, avascular papillary fronds. The surface is covered by a single layer of endothelial cells frequently with attached fibrin thrombi, and the matrix of the papillary fronds consists of variable amounts of mucopolysaccharides, collagen, elastic fibers, and rare spindle cells resembling smooth muscle cells or fibroblasts. The treatment for papillary fibroelastoma is surgical excision with either reconstitution or, less commonly, replacement of the valve.[50,58] In prospective studies involving 45 patients with suspected papillary fibroelastomas based on transesophageal echocardiography, 6.6 percent of the patients went on to develop embolic-type symptoms in a 1-year follow-up period.[53] However, the risk of papillary fibroelastoma–related complication must be weighed against the risk of surgery from patient to patient. Asymptomatic patients with small, left-sided, nonmobile-type papillary fibroelastomas can be cautiously observed, whereas patients with larger (1 cm or greater) and/or mobile-type papillary fibroelastomas should be considered for excision.[50,53,58] In terms of the use of systemic anticoagulation to prevent the embolic complications of papillary fibroelastoma, no data are currently available to support its use. The prognosis for patients with surgically respectable papillary fibroelastoma is excellent, and there is no reported case of recurrence to date.[53]

Rhabdomyomas

Cardiac rhabdomyomas are the most frequently encountered primary cardiac tumor in infants and children. Nearly 80 percent of the reported cases of cardiac rhabdomyomas occur in patients younger than the age of 1,[26] and increasing number of cases are being recognized due to the routine use of prenatal ultrasound. However, rare cases of cardiac rhabdomyomas occurring in adults have been encountered and these adult-type cardiac rhabdomyomas do show some phenotypic differences from the more typically encountered fetal-type rhabdomyomas.[59] Etiologically, the fetal-type cardiac rhabdomyomas are congenital lesions that appear to behave more consistently in manner with a hamartoma than a neoplasm with their complete lack of mitotic activity and their tendency to degenerate and atrophy spontaneously. Because about half of the patients presenting with cardiac rhabdomyomas have tuberous sclerosis, it is speculated that mutation of TSC1 and TSC2 genes may be responsible for the formation of this hamartoma.[60]

Alternatively, some researchers have suggested that cardiac rhabdomyomas represent a form of diffuse glycogen storage disease, but the focal nature of the lesion and the lack of extracardiac involvement would suggest otherwise.[1] Clinically, the fetal-type rhabdomyomas can result in stillbirth or early postnatal death if the tumor causes significant hemodynamic impairment. Obstruction may occur to either the right ventricular or left ventricular outflow tract if the tumor has a prominent intracavitary component, and significant cardiac murmurs can be found in these instances. Although also found in some cases of fetal-type rhabdomyoma, arrhythmias represent the most common presentation for adult-type rhabdomyomas.[59,61] However, for both fetal-type and adult-type rhabdomyomas, patients may be asymptomatic if the lesions are small. The diagnosis of fetal-type rhabdomyoma is usually made on prenatal ultrasound or postnatal echocardiography. The presence of a family history of tuberous sclerosis and multifocality of the lesion would suggest a diagnosis of tuberous sclerosis–associated cardiac rhabdomyoma.[62] Grossly, cardiac rhabdomyoma arises more commonly in the ventricles, although up to 30 percent of cases can involve either atrium.[1,63] Cases associated with tuberous sclerosis typically occur as multiple, less than 1-mm lesions, although multiple lesions are also seen in 50 percent of the sporadic cases.[1] The lesion typically appears as a yellow-gray, firm, circumscribed lobulated mass, and the size of the tumor can range from less than 1 mm to 9 cm. Histologically, cardiac rhabdomyoma is a well-demarcated lesion composed of enlarged cells with clear cytoplasm and occasional "spider cells."[1] The cytoplasm is rich in glycogen, as confirmed by the PAS stain. The lesional cells also stain positively for myoglobin, desmin, actin, and vimentin. In contrast to the fetal type rhabdomyoma, adult-type cardiac rhabdomyoma resembles the extracardiac rhabdomyoma found in the head and neck region of adults histologically and shows higher cellularity with focal presence of tightly packed small cells and inconspicuous vacuolated spider cells.[59,61] As with fetal-type rhabdomyoma, mitotic activity should be absent in adult-type rhabdomyoma. Therapeutically, because most cardiac rhabdomyomas show spontaneous regression before age 6, conservative clinical observation is the mainstay of management in up to 80 percent of cases.[1] In symptomatic cases showing significant outflow tract obstruction or arrhythmias, surgical excision with removal of the culprit portion of the lesion is sufficient. No recurrence has been documented to date for cardiac rhabdomyomas, and the prognosis of this disease is excellent.

CH 69

Fibromas and Hamartomas

Cardiac fibroma is the second most common primary cardiac neoplasm in infants and children after rhabdomyoma.[1] About 90 percent of the reported cases occur in children, although fibromas can present in any age group ranging from a few days of age to 83 years. Some cases of cardiac fibroma have also been diagnosed prenatally by ultrasound.[64] There is no sex predilection, and the majority of cases appear to be nonfamilial.[1] The exact nature of cardiac fibroma is unknown, and it is unclear whether it represents a hamartoma or a true neoplasm. The majority of cardiac fibromas behave like hamartomas with no tendency to recur or grow aggressively.[1] However, some cardiac fibromas behave as benign neoplasms with the ability to recur but never metastasize. Although most cardiac fibromas appear to occur sporadically, some appear to develop as part of the Gorlin syndrome (nevoid basal cell carcinoma syndrome).[65]

Clinically, congestive heart failure, heart murmurs, arrhythmias, and syncope are the more common presenting findings in patients with cardiac fibroma.[1] Less common presenting findings include sudden death and atypical chest pain. However, up to one third of patients with cardiac fibroma can remain asymptomatic. The ECG can show a number of abnormalities including evidence of left ventricular hypertrophy, right ventricular hypertrophy, bundle branch block, and A-V block, as well as ventricular tachycardia.[66] Chest radiography may reveal cardiomegaly with or without focal bulge, and calcification is visible in 15 percent of cases. Because of its tendency to occur in children, cardiac fibroma must be considered in the differential diagnosis for children with unexplained CHF, arrhythmias, cardiomegaly, murmur, and pericardial effusion. On echocardiography, cardiac fibroma usually appears as a solitary homogeneous echogenic lesion (see Fig. 14-104).[64] For preoperative assessment, CT and CMR are more desirable for evaluating the resectability of the lesion. Grossly, cardiac fibromas typically appear as solitary, rounded, intramural masses with a fibrous, whorled cut surface.[1] The mass can be grossly circumscribed or infiltrative with a pushing margin. The average size of the tumor is 5 cm, although lesions up to 10 cm in size have been reported.[1] The usual location of the tumor is in the ventricular septum or the left ventricular free wall with occurrence in the right ventricle or the atria seen in less than 10 percent of cases. Histologically, cardiac fibroma shows a proliferation of monomorphic fibroblasts with little or no cellular atypia. The degree of cellularity decreases with age, whereas the amount of collagen deposition increases with age.[1]

Mitotic activity is usually absent but can be present in infants that are only a few months old.[1] A variable amount of elastic fibers and lymphocytic and histiocytic infiltrates may exist. Immunohistochemical examination may demonstrate some degree of smooth muscle actin positivity, but staining for desmin, CD-34, and S-100 should be negative.[67] The differential diagnosis, especially in the more cellular cases, includes low-grade fibrosarcoma and inflammatory myofibroblastic tumors. Because of the potential for cardiac fibroma to cause arrhythmias and occasionally recur, complete surgical resection in symptomatic cases is recommended. The postoperative prognosis is typically good, although some surgical attempts in infants younger than 4 months of age have resulted in death.[1] If complete resection is not feasible, palliative partial resection may be considered. Periodic echocardiography may be necessary to monitor for recurrence of the tumor. For large, unresectable tumors, cardiac transplantation may be considered if symptoms such as arrhythmias persist.

Hemangiomas and Lymphangiomas

Primary benign vascular tumors of the heart include hemangiomas, lymphangiomas, and hemangioendotheliomas. Lymphangiomas and hemangioendotheliomas are extremely rare with only a few reported cases in the literature.[1] In comparison, cardiac hemangioma is more frequently seen and accounts for less than 2 percent of primary cardiac neoplasms.[9] Hemangioma can occur in any age group ranging from a few months to the seventh decade of life.[1] Cardiac hemangiomas are considered to be benign neoplasms with potential for recurrence, but the etiology is not defined. Patients with cardiac hemangioma may remain asymptomatic. In symptomatic patients, the clinical presentation of cardiac hemangioma is variable. Depending on the nature and location of the tumor, patients can present with arrhythmias[1,10]; congestive heart failure[1,10]; pericardial effusion; ventricular outflow tract obstruction; pseudoangina[10]; cerebral embolism[9,10]; and, in more extreme cases, sudden death. In some instances, giant cardiac hemangioma can result in Kasabach-Merritt syndrome characterized by thrombosis, consumptive thrombocytopenia, and coagulopathy. Cardiac hemangioma can occasionally be associated with hemangioma in extracardiac sites such as the gastrointestinal tract and on the skin or face. Echocardiography is a sensitive, noninvasive method for detecting the tumor, with cardiac hemangioma appearing typically as a hyperechoic lesion.[3] Coronary angiography can sometimes demonstrate blood supply to the tumor, with the presence of "tumor blush."[3,10] On chest CT, cardiac hemangioma is characterized by heterogeneous signal with intense enhancement in most cases after contrast material administration.[3,68] On CMR, cardiac hemangiomas appear as masses with intermediate signal intensity on T1-weighted images and hypointense signal on T2-weighted images (see Chap. 17), and there may be rapid enhancement during contrast infusion.[69] Grossly, cardiac hemangiomas can range from less than 1 cm to 8 cm in size and can occur as intracavitary, intramural, or epicardial/pericardial lesions. They can occur in any chamber, although occurrences in the ventricles are more frequent than in the atria. Multiple tumors are seen in about 30 percent of cases.[70] Although usually well demarcated, some cardiac hemangiomas can have an infiltrative border, which makes complete surgical resection difficult.[1] Histologically, the appearance of cardiac hemangiomas is similar to hemangiomas arising in other sites. Three main histological subtypes exist: (1) the cavernous hemangioma, which is composed of multiple thin- or thick-walled dilated vessels; (2) the capillary hemangioma, which is composed of lobules of endothelial cells forming small, capillary-like vessels; and (3) arteriovenous hemangioma, which is composed of dysplastic thick-walled arterioles, venous-like vessels, and capillaries. The cavernous type of cardiac hemangioma tends to not show a rapid signal enhancement with contrast administration on imaging because of the slow blood flow.[3] In contrast to angiosarcoma, necrosis, marked nuclear atypia, and mitotic activity are not seen in hemangioma. In symptomatic patients, radical resection of the tumor is recommended because of the potential for recurrence, especially if the resection is incomplete.[10] The postoperative prognosis is excellent in resectable cases.[70] Because cardiac hemangiomas may regress spontaneously, conservative management may be considered in asymptomatic patients, particularly if complex and potentially hazardous excision is required.[3] However, in all cases, periodic echocardiography is recommended to examine for recurrence or tumor growth.

Approximately one fourth of all cardiac tumors are considered malignant, and about one half to three quarters of all malignant primary cardiac tumors are sarcomas with primary cardiac lymphomas being the next most common group.[1,71] Of note is that metastatic tumors to the heart are 20 to 40 times more common. Most common malignancies that involve the heart or pericardium include lung and breast cancer. However, Hodgkin's disease; non-Hodgkin's lymphomas; malignant melanoma; numerous primary gastrointestinal malignancy; and various types of sarcomas arising from extracardiac locations can also secondarily involve the heart. Therefore it is important, as well as logical, to consider the possibility that a cardiac lesion confirmed histologically to be a sarcoma may actually be a metastasis from a sarcoma located in another anatomic location. A thorough clinical examination combined with a series of imaging studies should help to rule out this possibility. The more common malignant primary tumors of the heart (excluding malignant mesothelioma that arise from the pericardium) include angiosarcomas, leiomyosarcomas, rhabdomyosarcomas, malignant fibrous histiocytomas, undifferentiated sarcomas, fibrosarcomas, and malignant lymphomas. Other rarely encountered primary cardiac sarcomas include liposarcomas, synovial sarcomas, and malignant peripheral nerve sheath tumors. In general the individual histologic subtypes of primary cardiac sarcomas do not appear to influence the outcome as significantly as the histologic grade of the sarcomas, which is evaluated on the basis of a combination of mitotic activity, amount of necrosis, and degree of cellular differentiation. Sarcomas showing high mitotic activity (>5 mitotic figures/10 high-power fields), extensive tumor necrosis, and poor cellular differentiation have a worse prognosis than sarcomas without these features.[1] The presence of metastases also confers a poorer prognosis. In terms of imaging studies, nearly all sarcomas occurring in the heart are aggressive tumors that show a highly infiltrative pattern of growth. They often appear on CT or CMR as large, heterogeneous, broad-based masses that frequently occupy most of the affected cardiac chambers.[3] The tumors may also show evidence of extension into other cardiac chambers and the pericardium, and there may also be associated pericardial effusions and hilar lymphadenopathy.

Angiosarcomas

Primary cardiac angiosarcoma is the most common primary cardiac sarcoma in adults, accounting for 30 to 37 percent of the cases.[1,2,72] Other malignant vascular tumors such as Kaposi sarcoma and malignant epithelioid hemangioendothelioma are even rarer by comparison. Cardiac angiosarcomas typically occur in adults 30 to 50 years old but can occur in almost any age group from 2 to 80 years. A slight male predilection exists.[2,18] With the exception of a single report of familial occurrence of cardiac angiosarcomas, all others appear to occur sporadically.[73] Little is known about the oncogenesis of angiosarcoma. Complex cytogenetic changes and mutations in *p53* have been identified in some angiosarcomas.[73,74] Clinically, patients with primary cardiac angiosarcomas typically present with advanced disease, with 66 to 89 percent of patients already demonstrating evidence of metastatic disease at initial presentation.[2] Initial findings may include dyspnea, chest pain, heart murmur, constitutional symptoms, arrhythmias, superior vena cava syndrome, and evidence of congestive heart failure.[1,2,14,75,76] Because of the propensity of cardiac angiosarcoma to involve pericardium, pericardial effusion and cardiac tamponade may also be the presentation.[14,15,71] Less commonly, symptoms related to the metastatic disease such as strokelike neurologic symptoms secondary to cerebral metastases are the initial presentation in patients with cardiac angiosarcoma.[2,77] The ECG may reveal nonspecific ST changes, arrhythmias, and atrioventricular (AV) block. The chest radiograph may show nonspecific changes like cardiomegaly, widened mediastinum, hilar lymphadenopathy, and pleural effusion.[72] Transesophageal echocardiography is the initial imaging modality of choice[14,72] for detection of the lesion, but echocardiography has limited ability to demonstrate tumor infiltration and cannot depict mediastinal and extracardiac involvement. CT and CMR are therefore required[72] for a better characterization of the tumor growth and involvement (Fig. 69-4). Angiosarcomas typically appear as low-attenuation, invasive, irregular nodular masses showing heterogeneous enhancement with contrast on CT and heterogeneous mass on CMR (see Fig. 17-16). They fre-

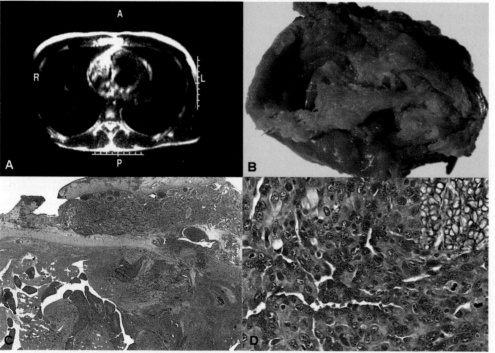

FIGURE 69–4 Cardiac magnetic resonance (CMR) imaging of the heart of a 20-year-old man with an angiosarcoma in the right atrium (**A**). CMR confirmed findings from a transesophageal echocardiogram that showed a 3 × 3 × 3.5-cm intraarterial mass with extension toward the inferior vena cava. **B,** Angiosarcoma tumor resected from the right atrium of a 20-year-old man. This tumor was surgically resected from the superior vena cava down to the annulus of the tricuspid valve. The surgical resection specimen shows a tan-red, multilobulated tumor mass. Section of angiosarcoma (hematoxylin and eosin, **C** and **D** (**D**, ×400). **D, Inset,** A brightly positive staining for CD31 in tumor cells. (**A** and **C,** *Courtesy of Drs. Gerald Berry and Kizhake Kurian, Department of Pathology, Stanford University, Calif., and Department of Cardiovascular Medicine, UFSHC at Jacksonville, Fla., respectively.* **B** and **D,** *From Kurian KC, Weisshaar D, Parekh H, et al: Primary cardiac angiosarcoma: Case report and review of the literature. Cardiovasc Pathol 15:110, 2006.*)

quently show extensive pericardial involvement and hemorrhagic pericardial effusions.[3] For histologic diagnosis, invasive methods like transvenous echo-guided cardiac biopsy may provide diagnostic material, but a negative biopsy result does not rule out the possibility of angiosarcoma.[14,21] Alternatively, biopsy of the metastatic lesion in a more accessible location or cytology examination on pericardiocentesis fluid may also assist in the diagnosis.[14] Grossly, angiosarcomas typically appear as large, multilobular, dark brown intramural masses that may protrude into or replace most of the atrial cavity.[1] About 90 percent of angiosarcomas arise in the right atrium, and this is thought to contribute to the late onset of symptoms. Involvement of adjacent structures such as the tricuspid valve, pulmonary valve, and vena cava, as well as extension into the pericardium, may occur. Histologically, cardiac angiosarcomas usually exhibit evidence of endothelial differentiation with formation of vascular channels and/or papillary structures.[1] In contrast to benign vascular lesions, the lining cells are atypical and form irregular anastomosing sinusoid structures, and mitotic activity is also present. In some cases the tumor is composed primarily of anaplastic or spindle cells with little evidence of endothelial derivation, and the identification of poorly formed vascular channels or intracytoplasmic vacuole containing red blood cells can aid in the diagnosis. Immunohistochemical study can be used to further support evidence of endothelial differentiation by demonstrating CD31, CD34, and vWF positive immunophenotype in the tumor cells.[78] Novel lymphatic endothelial markers including D2-40 and LYVE-1 can further identify tumors showing more lymphatic endothelial differentiation than vascular endothelial differentiation.[79-81] Cardiac angiosarcomas are aggressive-behaving neoplasms that are associated with a poor prognosis and mean survival of 9 to 10 months.[76] This is partially because of the late detection of the disease—most patients present with advanced-stage disease. Common sites of metastases include lung, liver, brain, and bone, although metastases to lymph nodes, adrenal glands, spleen, and skin have also been reported.[14,18] Even though no consistent, effective treatment has been identified for cardiac angiosarcoma to date,[76] a multidisciplinary approach to the treatment of cardiac angiosarcoma is advocated.[15,18] Such an integrated approach includes a combination of surgery, irradiation, adjuvant/neoadjuvant chemotherapy, and immunotherapy using interleukin-12 (IL-12). The aim of the surgery is still complete tumor resection.[82] Neoadjuvant chemotherapy may be administered to reduce the tumor mass and facilitate surgical excision.[83] The use of heart transplantation remains controversial in this setting.[2] For patients with advanced-stage unresectable disease, palliative treatment including the use of metallic stents for SVC syndrome and for severe right ventricular outflow tract obstruction may help to improve the patients' short-term quality of life.[2,83]

Rhabdomyosarcomas

Cardiac rhabdomyosarcomas are the most common primary sarcoma of the heart in children. The average age of disease presentation is in the second decade of life, but it can also occur in young adults. A slight male predominance, especially in the pediatric population, exists.[1] Because of its rarity, the etiology of primary cardiac rhabdomyosarcomas remains elusive. Findings of congestive heart failure, arrhythmias, cardiac murmurs, and constitutional symptoms are common presentations of the disease.[1] Occasional cases are also associated with hypereosinophilia, hypertrophic osteoarthropathy, and polyarthritis.[84,85] Nonspecific ECG and chest radiography findings are often present. As with other cardiac sarcomas, transthoracic and transesophageal echocardiography are reasonable imaging modalities in the initial work-up of the patient suspected to have a cardiac lesion.[19,85] Chest CT or CMR are necessary for better delineation of the nature, origin, and extent of the lesion, especially if a malignant lesion is suspected.[19,85] Although echo-guided transvenous cardiac biopsy may be attempted for tissue diagnosis, a negative result cannot be relied on because there is a high rate of false negatives. In contrast to angiosarcomas, cardiac rhabdomyosarcomas show no predilection for a specific cavity, and multiple lesions are frequently present (60 percent).[19,85] The histologic features of cardiac rhabdomyosarcomas are similar to their extracardiac counterparts. The embryonal type and pleomorphic type of rhabdomyosarcomas are more commonly seen as primary tumors in the heart, whereas the alveolar type of rhabdomyosarcomas is typically found as a metastatic disease to the heart.[1] Cardiac rhabdomyosarcomas are aggressive neoplasms with a tendency to produce local and distant metastases, most commonly to the lung and lymph nodes, although spread to various other organs has also been documented previously.[19] Cardiac rhabdomyosarcomas have a dismal prognosis, and survival is usually less than 1 year. Tumors demonstrating a high mitotic activity, extensive tumor necrosis, lack of cellular differentiation, and extensive myocardial and pericardial extension are associated with the worst prognosis.[1,85] The primary aim of treatment is complete surgical resection, but the highly infiltrative nature of tumor often precludes such a possibility. Further, the tumor has a poor response to radiation and chemotherapy.[86] In selected cases, heart transplant may be considered if no obvious distant metastases are present.[85]

Leiomyosarcomas

Leiomyosarcomas are malignant mesenchymal tumors that demonstrate histologic and immunophenotypic evidence of smooth muscle differentiation. The mean age of presentation is in the fourth decade, and there is no apparent sex predilection.[1] The exact oncogenesis of leiomyosarcomas is not known. The common clinical presentations include dyspnea, pericardial effusions, chest pain, atrial arrhythmias, and congestive heart failure.[1,87,88] Approximately 70 to 80 percent of leiomyosarcomas arise from the left atrium, and they tend to extend into the pulmonary trunk.[87] The tumor is typically solitary but can be multiple in 30 percent of patients.[1,88] Echocardiography can help to identify the cardiac lesion, and contrast-enhanced CT or CMR can help to further characterize the nature and extent of tumor growth.[88,89] Histologically, typical leiomyosarcomas show intersecting fascicles of spindle cells with blunt ended nuclei and well-defined eosinophilic cytoplasm with longitudinal striations. Some leiomyosarcomas contain a large number of highly atypical pleomorphic cells. Immunohistochemical demonstration of smooth muscle differentiation in the form of smooth muscle actin and desmin positivity is required to confirm the diagnosis of leiomyosarcoma, especially for pleomorphic tumors.

Cardiac leiomyosarcomas are rapidly growing tumors with a high rate of local recurrence and distant metastases, and the prognosis is poor with a mean survival of 6 months after diagnosis.[87] Because of the tendency of leiomyosarcomas to recur, cardiac transplantation is not a realistic option. Effective treatment of this progressively lethal disease is unknown. Palliative surgery may be considered in severely symptomatic patients to improve their quality of life.

Other Sarcomas

Besides rhabdomyosarcomas, other nonvascular sarcomas include malignant fibrous histiocytomas, undifferentiated sarcomas, osteosarcomas, fibrosarcomas, myxosarcomas, synovial sarcomas, and malignant peripheral nerve sheath tumors.[1] With the exception of malignant fibrous histiocytomas, the remaining types of sarcomas occur extremely rarely as primary tumors of the heart. The majority of these sarcomas arise in the left atrium, and they can produce symptoms and signs of chest pain, congestive heart failure, valvular insufficiency, arrhythmias, and systemic embolism.[1,3] Constitutional symptoms and those secondary to tumor metastases are also frequently encountered. As with angiosarcomas, rhabdomyosarcomas, and leiomyosarcomas, the other primary cardiac sarcomas are all highly aggressive tumors that show little or no response to chemotherapy and radiation therapy. Complete surgical excision is often attempted in resectable cases, but local recurrences and metastatic disease are common even after apparently complete surgical excision. The mean survival is typically less than 1 year for the different histologic types of primary cardiac sarcomas,[3] and palliative surgery may help to improve patients' quality of life.

LYMPHOMAS

Primary cardiac lymphomas are rare neoplasms that account for 1.3 to 2 percent of all primary cardiac tumors.[16,22] They can arise both in immunocompetent and immunocompromised individuals with occurrences in immunocompromised individuals being more common.[90] In recent years there have been increasing reports of primary cardiac lymphomas, particularly in association with HIV infections. In the scenarios of solid organ transplantation, posttransplantation lymphoproliferative disease (PTLD) is another setting in which primary cardiac lymphoma can occur,[91] in this case caused by chronic immunosuppression and Epstein-Barr virus infection. Lymphomas associated with HIV and PTLD usually have extracardiac involvement at presentation, and isolated cardiac involvement is rare. The average patient age at diagnosis of primary cardiac lymphomas is 62 to 67 years with a range of 13 to 90 years,[16,22] and there is a slight male predominance. The common clinical presentations of primary cardiac lymphomas include chest pain, congestive heart failure, pericardial effusion, palpitation, and arrhythmias.[16,22,90] Constitutional symptoms may be present in a subset of patients.[22] Less common presentations of primary cardiac lymphomas are cardiac tamponade, pulmonary and systemic embolism,[92,93] superior vena cava syndrome, and sudden death.[16] Routine chemistry shows elevation of lactate dehydrogenase in 16 to 23 percent of patients and elevation in sedimentation rate in 20 percent.[16] ECG findings are nonspecific and not uncommonly reveal evidence of AV block and supraventricular arrhythmias.[22,94,95] Chest radiograph is typically not helpful, but echocardiography, especially transesophageal, is excellent for initial visualization of such cardiac lesions. CT and CMR are superior at delineating the infiltrative nature of the tumor (see Fig. 18-28), and CMR has the highest sensitivity for detecting primary cardiac lymphomas.[22] However, the CT and CMR signals of primary cardiac lymphomas are not specific, and histopathologic diagnosis is required for definitive diagnosis. Cytology of pericardial effusion has proved to be diagnostic in 60 percent of cases.[22] Transesophageal, echo-guided, transvenous biopsy and percutaneous intracardiac biopsy may provide diagnostic tissue samples. However, if all else fails, biopsy performed through mediastinoscopy or thoracotomy may be necessary in some cases for diagnosis. Grossly, primary cardiac lymphomas involve the right side of the heart in 69 to 72 percent of the cases.[16,22] It appears as a single lesion in 66 percent and multiple lesions in 34 percent of the cases.[16] Pericardial effusion is present in 49 percent of the cases and, in some cases, only the pericardial effusion may be evident. Primary cardiac lymphomas range from 3 to 12 cm in size with a mean of 7 cm.[16] Histologically, about 80 percent of primary cardiac lymphomas found in immunocompetent individuals are of the diffuse large cell B-cell lymphoma type, though cases of small cell lymphomas, Burkitt lymphomas, and T-cell lymphomas have also been reported.[16] In immunocompromised patients, small noncleaved or immunoblastic lymphomas are more commonly seen. Flow cytometry and immunohistochemistry can aid in the diagnosis and determination of specific subtypes of cardiac lymphomas. Therapeutically, primary cardiac lymphomas are similar to any aggressive lymphomas arising from other sites in that they are all sensitive to chemotherapy treatment. Early implementation of anthracycline-based chemotherapy with or without radiation therapy has become the main-

stay of treatment for primary cardiac lymphomas,[22] and radical surgical excision is generally discouraged.[97] More recently, the use of Rituximab, a monoclonal antibody targeted against CD20, in combination with conventional chemotherapy, has shown some promise in improving patient survival.[98,99] Overall, because of the aggressive nature of most primary cardiac lymphomas, the current prognosis of primary cardiac lymphoma remains relatively poor regardless of the treatment given, and about 60 percent of patients die of the disease within 2 months after the initial diagnosis.[16] In contrast, the prognosis of patients with primary cardiac PTLD is better and a trial of reduced immunosuppression is the recommended initial approach in all cases.[37]

MANAGEMENT OF PRIMARY CARDIAC TUMORS

Management of primary cardiac tumors is discussed briefly and in detail in earlier sections.[37] Because of the rarity of primary cardiac neoplasms, no prospective randomized controlled trials have been performed to date. The treatment of benign primary cardiac tumors is mostly surgical, and the urgency of surgical intervention depends primarily on the symptomatology of the patient and the type of tumor, although consideration should also be given to the general medical status of the patient. For most benign cardiac tumors, no clinical data will allow clinicians to prospectively assess the annual risks of the patient for tumor-related complications. This can sometimes create therapeutic dilemmas, especially if the patient is a poor surgical candidate and minimally symptomatic. For cardiac myxomas, prompt complete surgical excision after diagnosis, regardless of whether the patient is currently symptomatic, is strongly recommended because of the risk of significant morbidity or mortality from tumor embolism and/or severe hemodynamic compromise. Similarly, because of the risk of embolism, prompt surgical excision is also recommended for patients with papillary fibroelastomas if they are large (1 cm or greater) and/or of the mobile type, although conservative management for patients with small, left-sided, and nonmobile-type papillary fibroelastoma may also be considered.[50,53,58] In contrast, surgical intervention for patients with cardiac lipomas or LHAS should be restricted to those with significant hemodynamic dysfunction.[37] For patients with cardiac fibromas or hemangiomas/lymphangiomas, complete surgical resection in symptomatic cases is recommended because of the potential for tumor recurrence if the resection is incomplete. Surgery is generally curative for benign primary cardiac tumors like myxomas, and the prognosis of the surgically resectable tumors is generally excellent.

The treatment of malignant primary cardiac tumors like sarcomas and lymphomas is guided primarily by experiences derived from the treatment of their extracardiac pathologic counterparts. For primary cardiac sarcomas, surgery is the mainstay of therapy and offers the only chance for curative therapy, although it is usually limited by early metastases and local spread or recurrence. Most operations are palliative and are performed to relieve cardiac compression or hemodynamic obstruction with partial resection and/or placement of stents.[37] Neoadjuvant chemotherapy may be administered to reduce the tumor mass and facilitate surgical excision in some cases.[83] For cardiac angiosarcomas, an integrated approach that includes a combination of surgery, irradiation, adjuvant/neoadjuvant chemotherapy, and immunotherapy using IL-12 is currently advocated for clinically suitable candidates. For other primary cardiac sarcomas, chemotherapy is the treatment of first choice for sarcomas that are unresectable or that present with extracardiac metastases, and combinations of several agents are more effective than single-agent therapy. Radiation therapy may play an adjunct role in these cases. Despite the use of these conventional systemic therapies, the mean survival of most primary cardiac sarcomas is typically less than 1 year regardless of the histologic types[3] and palliative surgery may offer the only mean to improve patients' quality of life.

As reviewed in detail earlier,[37] primary cardiac lymphomas are generally sensitive to systemic chemotherapy. Prompt implementation of conventional chemotherapy with or without radiation therapy has become the mainstay of treatment for primary cardiac lymphomas,[22] and radical surgical excision is generally discouraged.[97] The use of Rituximab may also be considered in some cases.[98,99] For PTLD, early diagnosis is essential to its successful management and a trial of reduced immunosuppression is the recommended initial approach in all cases.

FUTURE OUTLOOK

The diagnosis and the treatment of primary cardiac tumors can be an unexpected challenge for clinicians and surgeons because of their rarity and the lack of clearly defined guidelines in their management. For the initial evaluation of a suspected cardiac mass, echocardiography will likely remain the preferred modality in the years and perhaps decades to come. Although CT and CMR are superior to echocardiography at identifying and characterizing cardiac lesions, emerging imaging modalities such as combined positron-emission tomography and CT (PET-CT) with the use of novel radiopharmaceutical agents may eventually prove to be more sensitive and specific for diagnosing and characterizing the lesions.[100,101] Furthermore, although not yet demonstrated, it is highly probable that PET-CT will become a more valuable tool for detecting recurrent primary cardiac tumors and/or metastases of primary cardiac tumors.[100]

With the more widespread use of various imaging modalities and the aging population, it is conceivable that more cases of primary cardiac tumors, especially of benign varieties, will be uncovered incidentally in patients who are not experiencing any clinical symptoms. The management of these patients may become a clinical dilemma, especially for the tumor types for which the conventional treatment is radical tumor excision. Therefore it is crucial for us to gain a better appreciation for the natural history of many of these benign primary cardiac tumors when they present as small, asymptomatic lesions. For instance, understanding the annual risk of embolism for small papillary fibroelastomas or small, nonpedunculated myxomas with smooth surfaces will allow proper assessment of the risks and benefits of surgical intervention. Given the rarity of these diseases, an international consortium/network may be required to accumulate the treatment and follow-up data of patients with primary cardiac tumors. Such a source of information will undoubtedly provide valuable data for the clinicians and patients in determining the most appropriate management plan. A similar collective effort is also necessary for primary cardiac sarcomas. Despite our best intentions and effort thus far, primary cardiac sarcomas are in the vast majority of cases incurable diseases with dismal prognoses.

Studies using high-throughput gene array technology to examine gene expression level or copy number changes in tumors may be a reasonable initial step for identifying genes of interest in the different subtypes of primary cardiac sarcomas.[102] Again, an international network or tumor registry can assist in collecting tissues from surgical specimens of patients undergoing curative or palliative surgical excision for their primary cardiac sarcomas. Furthermore, because of our lack of understanding of primary cardiac sarcomas and sarcomas in general, the classification of sarcomas is in a constant state of evolution.[103] One of the more noteworthy changes stems from our recognition that many sarcomas once considered to be malignant fibrous histiocytomas (MFHs) in the past actually represent poorly differentiated types of other sarcomas like leiomyosarcomas and myxofibrosarcomas.[104] A new term, *undifferentiated pleomorphic sarcoma*, has now replaced MFH, reflecting the fact that this tumor truly lacks evidence of specific mesenchymal differentiation.

Acknowledgments

The authors are deeply indebted to Ms. Lise Matzke for her incredible assistance with all aspects of this chapter. We also appreciate the generosity and expertise of Dr. Gerald J. Berry—Stanford University, Stanford, Calif.; Dr. Kizhake C. Kurian—University of Florida Health Science Center, Jacksonville; Dr. Glenn Taylor—The Hospital for Sick Children, Toronto; Dr. Kenneth Gin—Vancouver General Hospital, Vancouver, B.C.; and Dr. Suzanne Chan—British Columbia Children's Hospital, Vancouver. Without their contributions, this work would not have been possible.

REFERENCES

1. Burke A, Virmani R: Fascicle 16, 3rd series: Tumors of the heart and the great vessels. *In:* Atlas of Tumor Pathology. Washington, DC, Armed Forces Institute of Pathology, 1996.
2. Best AK, Dobson RL, Ahmad AR: Best cases from the AFIP: Cardiac angiosarcoma. Radiographics 23:S141, 2003.
3. Grebenc ML, Rosado de Christenson ML, Burke AP, et al: Primary cardiac and pericardial neoplasms: Radiologic-pathologic correlation. Radiographics 20:1073, 2000; quiz 1110, 1112.

Clinical Presentation

4. Grebenc ML, Rosado-de-Christenson ML, Green CE, et al: Cardiac myxoma: Imaging features in 83 patients. Radiographics 22:673, 2002.
5. Pinede L, Duhaut P, Loire R: Clinical presentation of left atrial cardiac myxoma. A series of 112 consecutive cases. Medicine (Baltimore) 80:159, 2001.
6. Mendoza CE, Rosado MF, Bernal L: The role of interleukin-6 in cases of cardiac myxoma. Clinical features, immunologic abnormalities, and a possible role in recurrence. Tex Heart Inst J 28:3, 2001.
7. Kuon E, Kreplin M, Weiss W, Dahm JB: The challenge presented by right atrial myxoma. Herz 29:702, 2004.
8. Acebo E, Val-Bernal JF, Gomez-Roman JJ, Revuelta JM: Clinicopathologic study and DNA analysis of 37 cardiac myxomas: A 28-year experience. Chest 123:1379, 2003.
9. Kocak H, Ozyazicioglu A, Gundogdu C, Sevimli S: Cardiac hemangioma complicated with cerebral and coronary embolization. Heart Vessels 20:296, 2005.
10. Kipfer B, Englberger L, Stauffer E, Carrel T: Rare presentation of cardiac hemangiomas. Ann Thorac Surg 70:977, 2000.
11. Fox E, Brunson C, Campbell W, Aru G: Cardiac papillary fibroelastoma presents as an acute embolic stroke in a 35-year-old African American male. Am J Med Sci 331:91, 2006.
12. Ekinci EI, Donnan GA: Neurological manifestations of cardiac myxoma: A review of the literature and report of cases. Intern Med J 34:243, 2004.
13. Sabolek M, Bachus-Banaschak K, Bachus R, et al: Multiple cerebral aneurysms as delayed complication of left cardiac myxoma: A case report and review. Acta Neurol Scand 111:345, 2005.
14. Brandt RR, Arnold R, Bohle RM, et al: Cardiac angiosarcoma: Case report and review of the literature. Z Kardiol 94:824, 2005.
15. Sakaguchi M, Minato N, Katayama Y, Nakashima A: Cardiac angiosarcoma with right atrial perforation and cardiac tamponade. Ann Thorac Cardiovasc Surg 12:145, 2006.
16. Chalabreysse L, Berger F, Loire R, et al: Primary cardiac lymphoma in immunocompetent patients: A report of three cases and review of the literature. Virchows Arch 441:456, 2002.
17. Pomper GJ, Gianani R, Johnston RJ, Rizeq MN: Cardiac angiosarcoma: An unusual presentation with cutaneous metastases. Arch Pathol Lab Med 122:273, 1998.
18. Sinatra R, Brancaccio G, di Gioia CR, et al: Integrated approach for cardiac angiosarcoma. Int J Cardiol 88:301, 2003.
19. Villacampa VM, Villarreal M, Ros LH, et al: Cardiac rhabdomyosarcoma: Diagnosis by MR imaging. Eur Radiol 9:634, 1999.

Diagnostic Approach

20. Meng Q, Lai H, Lima J, et al: Echocardiographic and pathologic characteristics of primary cardiac tumors: A study of 149 cases. Int J Cardiol 84:69, 2002.
21. Nitta R, Sakomura Y, Tanimoto K, et al: Primary cardiac angiosarcoma of the right atrium undiagnosed by transvenous endocardial tumor biopsy. Intern Med 37:1023, 1998.
22. Anghel G, Zoli V, Petti N, et al: Primary cardiac lymphoma: Report of two cases occurring in immunocompetent subjects. Leuk Lymphoma 45:781, 2004.

Benign Tumors

23. Terracciano LM, Mhawech P, Suess K, et al: Calretinin as a marker for cardiac myxoma. Diagnostic and histogenetic considerations. Am J Clin Pathol 114:754, 2000.
24. Wilkes D, Charitakis K, Basson CT: Inherited disposition to cardiac myxoma development. Nat Rev Cancer 6:157, 2006.
25. Orlandi A, Ciucci A, Ferlosio A, et al: Cardiac myxoma cells exhibit embryonic endocardial stem cell features. J Pathol 209:231, 2006.
26. Amano J, Kono T, Wada Y, et al: Cardiac myxoma: Its origin and tumor characteristics. Ann Thorac Cardiovasc Surg 9:215, 2003.
27. Kodama H, Hirotani T, Suzuki Y, et al: Cardiomyogenic differentiation in cardiac myxoma expressing lineage-specific transcription factors. Am J Pathol 161:381, 2002.
28. Kono T, Koide N, Hama Y, et al: Expression of vascular endothelial growth factor and angiogenesis in cardiac myxoma: A study of fifteen patients. J Thorac Cardiovasc Surg 119:101, 2000.
29. Pucci A, Gagliardotto P, Zanini C, et al: Histopathologic and clinical characterization of cardiac myxoma: Review of 53 cases from a single institution. Am Heart J 140:134, 2000.

30. Aspres N, Bleasel NR, Stapleton KM: Genetic testing of the family with a Carney-complex member leads to successful early removal of an asymptomatic atrial myxoma in the mother of the patient. Australas J Dermatol 44:121, 2003.

31. Mochizuki Y, Okamura Y, Iida H, et al: Interleukin-6 and "complex" cardiac myxoma. Ann Thorac Surg 66:931, 1998.

32. Komiya N, Isomoto S, Hayano M, et al: The influence of tumor size on the electrocardiographic changes in patients with left atrial myxoma. J Electrocardiol 35:53, 2002.

33. Ipek G, Erentug V, Bozbuga N, et al: Surgical management of cardiac myxoma. J Card Surg 20:300, 2005.

34. Miller DV, Tazelaar HD, Handy JR, et al: Thymoma arising within cardiac myxoma. Am J Surg Pathol 29:1208, 2005.

35. Pucci A, Bartoloni G, Tessitore E, et al: Cytokeratin profile and neuroendocrine cells in the glandular component of cardiac myxoma. Virchow Arch 443:618, 2003.

36. Val-Bernal JF, Acebo E, Gomez-Roman JJ, Garijo MF: Anticipated diagnosis of left atrial myxoma following histological investigation of limb embolectomy specimens: A report of two cases. Pathol Int 53:489, 2003.

37. Rosenberg FM, Chan A, Lichtenstein SV, McManus BM: Cardiac neoplasms. Curr Treat Options Cardiovasc Med 1:243, 1999.

38. Bjessmo S, Ivert T: Cardiac myxoma: 40 years' experience in 63 patients. Ann Thorac Surg 63:697, 1997.

39. Selkane C, Amahzoune B, Chavanis N, et al: Changing management of cardiac myxoma based on a series of 40 cases with long-term follow-up. Ann Thorac Surg 76:1935, 2003.

40. Altundag MB, Ertas G, Ucer AR, et al: Brain metastasis of cardiac myxoma: Case report and review of the literature. J Neurooncol 75:181, 2005.

41. Salanitri JC, Pereles FS: Cardiac lipoma and lipomatous hypertrophy of the interatrial septum: Cardiac magnetic resonance imaging findings. J Comput Assist Tomogr 28:852, 2004.

42. Mitelman F: Catalog of chromosome aberrations in cancer (version 1). New York: Wiley-Liss, 1998.

43. Akram K, Hill C, Neelagaru N, Parker M: A left ventricular lipoma presenting as heart failure in a septuagenarian: A first case report. Int J Cardiol 114:386, 2007.

44. Heyer CM, Kagel T, Lemburg SP, et al: Lipomatous hypertrophy of the interatrial septum: A prospective study of incidence, imaging findings, and clinical symptoms. Chest 124:2068, 2003.

45. Nova M, Stoiner I: A rationale for a stone on the heart—subepicardial lipoma. Cardiovasc Pathol 15:176, 2006.

46. Meaney JF, Kazerooni EA, Jamadar DA, Korobkin M: CT appearance of lipomatous hypertrophy of the interatrial septum. Am J Roentgenol 168:1081, 1997.

47. Christiansen S, Stypmann J, Baba HA, et al: Surgical management of extensive lipomatous hypertrophy of the right atrium. Cardiovasc Surg 8:88, 2000.

48. Roberts WC: Primary and secondary neoplasms of the heart. Am J Cardiol 80:671, 1997.

49. Nadra I, Dawson D, Schmitz SA, et al: Lipomatous hypertrophy of the interatrial septum: A commonly misdiagnosed mass often leading to unnecessary cardiac surgery. Heart 90:e66, 2004.

50. Howard RA, Aldea GS, Shapira OM, et al: Papillary fibroelastoma: Increasing recognition of a surgical disease. Ann Thorac Surg 68:1881, 1999.

51. Sumino S, Paterson HS: No regrowth after incomplete papillary fibroelastoma excision. Ann Thorac Surg 79:e3, 2005.

52. Roberts WC: Papillary fibroelastomas of the heart. Am J Cardiol 80:973, 1997.

53. Sun JP, Asher CR, Yang XS, et al: Clinical and echocardiographic characteristics of papillary fibroelastomas: A retrospective and prospective study in 162 patients. Circulation 103:2687, 2001.

54. Saad RS, Galvis CO, Bshara W, et al: Pulmonary valve papillary fibroelastoma. A case report and review of the literature. Arch Pathol Lab Med 125:933, 2001.

55. Georghiou GP, Erez E, Vidne BA, et al: Tricuspid valve papillary fibroelastoma: An unusual cause of intermittent dyspnea. Eur J Cardiothorac Surg 23:429, 2003.

56. Davoli G, Bizzarri F, Enrico T, et al: Double papillary fibroelastoma of the aortic valve. Tex Heart Inst J 31:448, 2004.

57. Eslami-Varzaneh F, Brun EA, Sears-Rogan P: An unusual case of multiple papillary fibroelastoma, review of literature. Cardiovasc Pathol 12:170, 2003.

58. Nawaz MZ, Lander AR, Schussler JM, et al: Tumor excision versus valve replacement for papillary fibroelastoma involving the mitral valve. Am J Cardiol 97:759, 2006.

59. Burke AP, Gatto-Weis C, Griego JE, et al: Adult cellular rhabdomyoma of the heart: A report of 3 cases. Hum Pathol 33:1092, 2002.

60. Vaughan CJ, Veugelers M, Basson CT: Tumors and the heart: Molecular genetic advances. Curr Opin Cardiol 16:195, 2001.

61. Krasuski RA, Hesselson AB, Landolfo KP, et al: Cardiac rhabdomyoma in an adult patient presenting with ventricular arrhythmia. Chest 118:1217, 2000.

62. Gamzu R, Achiron R, Hegesh J, et al: Evaluating the risk of tuberous sclerosis in cases with prenatal diagnosis of cardiac rhabdomyoma. Prenat Diagn 22:1044, 2002.

63. Chen X, Hoda SA, Edgar MA: Cardiac rhabdomyoma. Arch Pathol Lab Med 126:1559, 2002.

64. Kim TH, Kim YM, Han YM, et al: Perinatal sonographic diagnosis of cardiac fibroma with MR imaging correlation. Am J Roentgenol 178:727, 2002.

65. Bossert T, Walther T, Vondrys D, et al: Cardiac fibroma as an inherited manifestation of nevoid basal-cell carcinoma syndrome. Tex Heart Inst J 33:88, 2006.

66. Wong JA, Fishbein MC: Cardiac fibroma resulting in fatal ventricular arrhythmia. Circulation 101:E168, 2000.

67. de Montpreville VT, Serraf A, Aznag H, et al: Fibroma and inflammatory myofibroblastic tumor of the heart. Ann Diagn Pathol 5:335, 2001.

68. Oshima H, Hara M, Kono T, et al: Cardiac hemangioma of the left atrial appendage: CT and MR findings. J Thorac Imaging 18:204, 2003.

69. Moniotte S, Geva T, Perez A, et al: Images in cardiovascular medicine. Cardiac hemangioma. Circulation 112:e103, 2005.

70. Kojima S, Sumiyoshi M, Suwa S, et al: Cardiac hemangioma: A report of two cases and review of the literature. Heart Vessels 18:153, 2003.

Malignant Tumors

71. Farah HH, Jacob M, Aragam J: Images in cardiology: A case of cardiac angiosarcoma presenting as pericardial tamponade. Heart 86:665, 2001.

72. Deetjen AG, Conradi G, Mollman S, et al: Cardiac angiosarcoma diagnosed and characterized by cardiac magnetic resonance imaging. Cardiol Rev 14:101, 2006.

73. Casha AR, Davidson LA, Roberts P, et al: Familial angiosarcoma of the heart. J Thorac Cardiovasc Surg 124:392, 2002.

74. Zu Y, Perle MA, Yan Z, et al: Chromosomal abnormalities and p53 gene mutation in a cardiac angiosarcoma. Appl Immunohistochem Mol Morphol 9:24, 2001.

75. Amonkar GP, Deshpande JR: Cardiac angiosarcoma. Cardiovasc Pathol 15:57, 2006.

76. Kurian KC, Weisshaar D, Parekh H, et al: Primary cardiac angiosarcoma: Case report and review of the literature. Cardiovasc Pathol 15:110, 2006.

77. Liassides C, Katsamaga M, Deretzi G, et al: Cerebral metastasis from heart angiosarcoma presenting as multiple hematomas. J Neuroimaging 14:71, 2004.

78. Weiss SW, Enzinger GJ: Enzinger and Weiss's Soft Tissue Tumors. 4th ed. St. Louis, Mosby–Harcourt Brace, 2001.

79. Arai E, Kuramochi A, Tsuchida T, et al: Usefulness of D2-40 immunohistochemistry for differentiation between kaposiform hemangioendothelioma and tufted angioma. J Cutan Pathol 33:492, 2006.

80. Kahn HJ, Bailey D, Marks A: Monoclonal antibody D2-40, a new marker of lymphatic endothelium, reacts with Kaposi's sarcoma and a subset of angiosarcomas. Mod Pathol 15:434, 2002.

81. Xu H, Edwards JR, Espinosa AR, et al: Expression of a lymphatic endothelial cell marker in benign and malignant vascular tumors. Hum Pathol 35:857, 2004.

82. Hoffmeier A, Scheld HH, Tjan TD, et al: Ex situ resection of primary cardiac tumors. Thorac Cardiovasc Surg 51:99, 2003.

83. Totaro M, Miraldi F, Ghiribelli C, et al: Cardiac angiosarcoma arising from pulmonary artery: Endovascular treatment. Ann Thorac Surg 78:1468, 2004.

84. Lo Re V III, Fox KR, Ferrari VA, et al: Hypereosinophilia associated with cardiac rhabdomyosarcoma. Am J Hematol 74:64, 2003.

85. Grandmougin D, Fayad G, Decoene C, et al: Total orthotopic heart transplantation for primary cardiac rhabdomyosarcoma: Factors influencing long-term survival. Ann Thorac Surg 71:1438, 2001.

86. Aksoylar S, Kansoy S, Bakiler AR, et al: Primary cardiac rhabdomyosarcoma. Med Pediatr Oncol 38:146, 2002.

87. Ishikawa K, Takanashi S, Mihara W, et al: Surgical treatment for primary cardiac leiomyosarcoma causing right ventricular outflow obstruction. Circ J 69:121, 2005.

88. Clarke NR, Mohiaddin RH, Westaby S, Banning AP: Multifocal cardiac leiomyosarcoma. Diagnosis and surveillance by transoesophageal echocardiography and contrast enhanced cardiovascular magnetic resonance. Postgrad Med J 78:492, 2002.

89. Ogimoto A, Hamada M, Ohtsuka T, et al: Rapid progression of primary cardiac leiomyosarcoma with obstruction of the left ventricular outflow tract and mitral stenosis. Intern Med 42:827, 2003.

90. Rockwell L, Hetzel P, Freeman JK, Fereshetian A: Cardiac involvement in malignancies. Case 3. Primary cardiac lymphoma. J Clin Oncol 22:2744, 2004.

91. Nart D, Nalbantgil S, Yaqdi T, et al: Primary cardiac lymphoma in a heart transplant recipient. Transplant Proc 37:1362, 2005.

92. Binder J, Pfleger S, Schwarz S: Images in cardiovascular medicine. Right atrial primary cardiac lymphoma presenting with stroke. Circulation 110:e451, 2004.

93. Quigley MM, Schwartzman E, Boswell PD, et al: A unique atrial primary cardiac lymphoma mimicking myxoma presenting with embolic stroke: A case report. Blood 101:4708, 2003.

94. Engelen MA, Juergens KU, Breithardt G, Eckardt L: Interatrial conduction delay and atrioventricular block due to primary cardiac lymphoma. J Cardiovasc Electrophysiol 16:926, 2005.

95. Fujisaki J, Tanaka T, Kato J, et al: Primary cardiac lymphoma presenting clinically as restrictive cardiomyopathy. Circ J 69:249, 2005.

96. Giunta R, Cravero RG, Granata G, et al: Primary cardiac T-cell lymphoma. Ann Hematol 83:450, 2004.

97. Rolla G, Bertero MT, Pastena G, et al: Primary lymphoma of the heart. A case report and review of the literature. Leuk Res 26:117, 2002.

98. Dawson MA, Mariani J, Taylor A, et al: The successful treatment of primary cardiac lymphoma with a dose-dense schedule of rituximab plus CHOP. Ann Oncol 17:176, 2006.

99. Nakagawa Y, Ikeda U, Hirose M, et al: Successful treatment of primary cardiac lymphoma with monoclonal CD20 antibody (rituximab). Circ J 68:172, 2004.

Future Outlook

100. Messa C, Di Muzio N, Picchio M, et al: PET/CT and radiotherapy. Q J Nucl Med Mol Imaging 50:4, 2006.

101. von Schulthess GK, Steinert HC, Hany TF: Integrated PET/CT: Current applications and future directions. Radiology 238:405, 2006.

102. Nielsen TO, West RB, Linn SC, et al: Molecular characterization of soft tissue tumors: A gene expression study. Lancet 359:1301, 2002.

103. Fletcher CD: The evolving classification of soft tissue tumors: An update based on the new WHO classification. Histopathology 48:3, 2006.

104. Fletcher CD, Gustafson P, Rydholm A, et al: Clinicopathologic re-evaluation of 100 malignant fibrous histiocytomas: Prognostic relevance of subclassification. J Clin Oncol 19:3045, 2001.

CHAPTER 70

Anatomy and Physiology of the
Pericardium, 1829

The Passive Role of the Normal
Pericardium in Heart Disease, 1830

Acute Pericarditis, 1830
Etiology, Epidemiology, and
Pathophysiology, 1830
History and Differential Diagnosis, 1831
Physical Examination, 1832
Laboratory Testing, 1832
Natural History and Management, 1833
Relapsing and Recurrent
Pericarditis, 1834

Pericardial Effusion and
Tamponade, 1834
Etiology, 1834
Pathophysiology and
Hemodynamics, 1834
Clinical Presentation, 1836
Laboratory Testing, 1837
Management of Pericardial Effusion and
Tamponade, 1838

Constrictive Pericarditis, 1842
Etiology, 1842
Pathophysiology, 1842
Clinical Presentation, 1843
Physical Examination, 1843
Laboratory Testing, 1843
Differentiating Constrictive Pericarditis
from Restrictive
Cardiomyopathy, 1845
Management, 1846

Effusive-Constrictive
Pericarditis, 1846

Specific Causes of Pericardial
Disease, 1846
Viral Pericarditis, 1846
Bacterial Pericarditis, 1847
Pericardial Disease and Human
Immunodeficiency Virus, 1847
Tuberculous Pericarditis, 1848
Fungal Pericarditis, 1848
Uremic Pericarditis and Dialysis-
Associated Pericardial Disease, 1849
Early Post–Myocardial Infarction Pericarditis
and Dressler Syndrome, 1849
Postpericardiotomy and Postcardiac
Injury Pericarditis, 1850
Radiation-Induced Pericarditis, 1850
Metastatic Pericardial Disease, 1850
Primary Pericardial Tumors, 1851
Autoimmune and Drug-Induced
Pericardial Disease, 1851
Drug-Induced Pericarditis, 1851
Hemopericardium, 1851
Thyroid-Associated Pericardial
Disease, 1852
Pericardial Disease in Pregnancy, 1852
Congenital Anomalies of the
Pericardium, 1852

References, 1852

Pericardial Diseases

Martin M. LeWinter

ANATOMY AND PHYSIOLOGY OF THE PERICARDIUM

The pericardium is composed of two layers,[6] the *visceral* pericardium, a membrane composed of a single layer of mesothelial cells adherent to the epicardial surface of the heart, and the fibrous *parietal* layer, which is about 2 mm thick in normal humans and surrounds most of the heart. The parietal pericardium is largely acellular and contains both collagen and elastin fibers. Collagen is the major structural component and appears as wavy bundles at low levels of stretch. With further stretch the bundles straighten, resulting in increased stiffness of the tissue. The visceral pericardium reflects back near the origins of the great vessels, becoming continuous with and forming the inner layer of the parietal pericardium. The pericardial space or sac is contained within these two layers and normally contains up to 50 ml of serous fluid. The reflection of the visceral pericardium is a few centimeters proximal to the junctions of the caval vessels with the right atrium; thus portions of these vessels lie within the pericardial sac (Fig. 70-1). Posterior to the left atrium, the reflection occurs at the oblique sinus of the pericardium. The left atrium is largely extrapericardial. The parietal pericardium has ligamentous attachments to the diaphragm, sternum, and other structures in the anterior mediastinum. These ensure that the heart occupies a relatively fixed position within the thoracic cavity regardless of respiration and body position. The only noncardiovascular macrostructures associated with the pericardium are the phrenic nerves, which are enveloped by the parietal pericardium.

Although pericardiectomy does not result in obvious negative consequences, the normal pericardium does have functions.[1,4] As noted earlier, it maintains the position of the heart relatively constant. It may also function as a barrier to infection and provides lubrication between visceral and parietal layers. The pericardium is well innervated with mechanoreceptors and chemoreceptors and phrenic afferents.[7] The normal roles of these receptors are incompletely understood, but they probably participate in reflexes arising from the pericardium and/or epicardium (e.g., the Bezold-Jarisch reflex), as well as transmission of pericardial pain. The pericardium also secretes prostaglandins and related substances that may modulate neural traffic and coronary tone by effects on coronary receptors.[8]

The best-characterized mechanical function of the normal pericardium is its *restraining* effect on cardiac volume.[1,4] This reflects the mechanical properties of the pericardial tissue.[4] The parietal pericardium has a tensile strength similar to rubber. At low applied stresses similar to those at physiological or subphysiological cardiac volumes, it is elastic (Fig. 70-2, top), meaning that small forces result in large amounts of stretch. As stretch increases, the tissue fairly abruptly becomes stiff and resistant to further stretch. The point on the pericardial stress-strain relation (see Fig. 70-2, top) where this transition occurs probably corresponds to stresses present around the upper range of physiologic cardiac volumes and is likely related to straightening of collagen bundles.

The *pressure-volume relation* of the pericardial sac parallels the properties of the isolated tissue[1,4] (Fig. 70-2, bottom, left curve); a relatively flat, compliant segment transitions relatively abruptly to a noncompliant segment, with the transition in the range of the upper limit of normal total cardiac volume. Thus the pericardial sac has a relatively small reserve volume. When exceeded, the pressure within the sac operating on the surface of the heart increases rapidly and is transmitted to the inside of the cardiac chambers. The shape of the pericardial pressure-volume relation accounts for the fact that once a critical level of effusion is reached, relatively small amounts of additional fluid cause large increases in intrapericardial pressure and have marked effects on cardiac function. Conversely, removal of small amounts of fluid in patients with cardiac tamponade can result in striking improvement.

The shape of the pericardial pressure-volume relation suggests that it can normally restrain cardiac volume (i.e., the force it exerts on the surface of the heart can significantly limit filling, with a component of *intracavitary* filling pressure representing transmission of the pericardial pressure). This has been examined by using flattened balloons specially designed to measure contact pressures between surfaces.[1,4] These studies demonstrate a substantial pericardial contact pressure, especially when the upper limit of normal cardiac volume is exceeded. The contact pressure is proportionally more important for the right heart, whose filling pressures are normally lower than the left heart. In some studies, pericardial pressure was found to be virtually identical to right heart filling pressure, whereas in others

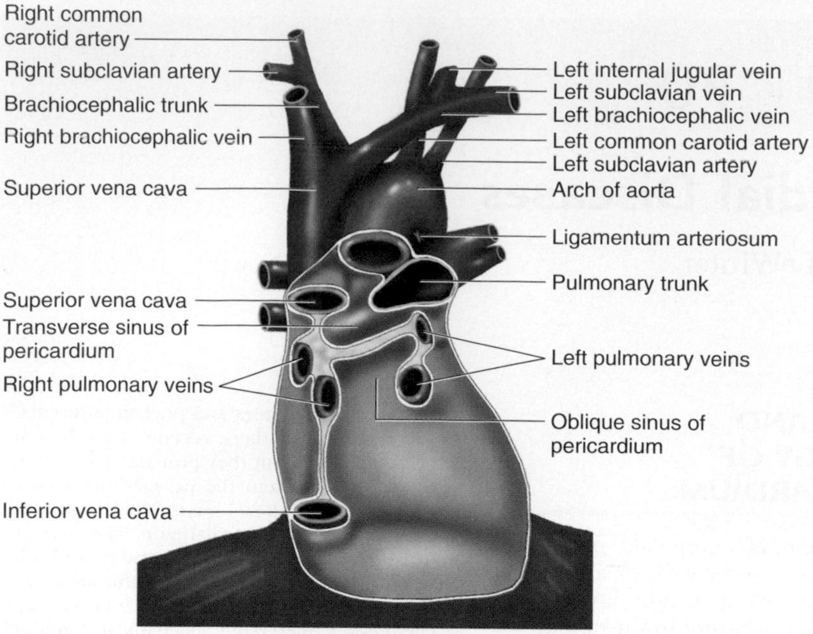

Right common carotid artery

Right subclavian artery

Brachiocephalic trunk

Right brachiocephalic vein

Superior vena cava

Superior vena cava

Transverse sinus of pericardium

Right pulmonary veins

Inferior vena cava

Left internal jugular vein
Left subclavian vein
Left brachiocephalic vein
Left common carotid artery
Left subclavian artery
Arch of aorta

Ligamentum arteriosum

Pulmonary trunk

Left pulmonary veins

Oblique sinus of pericardium

FIGURE 70–1 The pericardial reflections near the origins of the great vessels shown after removal of the heart. Note that portions of the caval vessels are within the pericardial space. *(From Johnson D [ed]: The pericardium. In Standring S, et al (eds): Gray's Anatomy, St. Louis, Mosby, 2005, pp 995-996.)*

it was not as high but once again quite significant in relation to the right heart pressure.[4]

Pericardial contact pressure has also been estimated by quantifying the change in the right and left heart diastolic pressure-volume relation before and after pericardiectomy.[1,4] A decrease in pressure at a given volume is the effective pericardial pressure at that volume. Studies in canine hearts using this approach indicate negligible pericardial restraint at low normal filling volumes, with contact pressures in the 2 to 4 mm Hg range at the upper end of the normal range. With additional filling, contact pressure rapidly increases. At left-sided filling pressure (≈25 mm Hg), estimated contact pressure is approximately 10 mm Hg, accounting for most of the *right heart* pressure at this level of filling. Thus the normal pericardium can *acutely* restrain cardiac volume and influences intra cavitary filling pressure. Moreover, patients with normal preoperative cardiac volumes undergoing pericardiotomy in conjunction with heart surgery develop mild postoperative increases in cardiac mass and volume (similar to volume overload), consistent with relief of underlying, normally occurring restraint to filling by the pericardium.[9]

The normal pericardium also contributes to diastolic interaction,[1,4] the transmission of intracavitary filling pressure to adjoining chambers. Thus, for example, a portion of right ventricular (RV) diastolic pressure is transmitted to the left ventricle across the interventricular septum and contributes to left ventricular (LV) diastolic pressure. Because its presence increases RV intracavitary pressure, the normal pericardium amplifies diastolic interaction. Thus as cardiac volume increases above the physiological range, the pericardium contributes increasingly to intracavitary filling pressures, directly because of the external contact pressure and indirectly because of increased diastolic interaction.

THE PASSIVE ROLE OF THE NORMAL PERICARDIUM IN HEART DISEASE

When the cardiac chambers dilate rapidly, the restraining effect of the pericardium and its contribution to diastolic interaction can become markedly augmented, resulting in a hemodynamic picture resembling both cardiac tamponade and constrictive pericarditis. The most common example is acute RV myocardial infarction (MI),[10] usually in conjunction with inferior LV MI. Here, the right heart dilates markedly and rapidly such that total heart volume exceeds the

pericardial reserve volume. As a result of increased pericardial constraint and augmented diastolic interaction, left- and right-sided filling pressures equilibrate at elevated levels and a paradoxical pulse and inspiratory increase in systemic venous pressure (Kussmaul sign) may be observed. Other conditions where similar effects are seen include acute pulmonary embolus and subacute mitral regurgitation.[1,4]

Chronic cardiac dilation (e.g., caused by dilated cardiomyopathy or regurgitant valvular disease) can result in cardiac volumes well in excess of the normal pericardial reserve volume. Despite this, exaggerated restraining effects are not ordinarily encountered. This implies that the pericardium undergoes chronic adaptation to accommodate marked increases in cardiac volume. In experimental chronic volume overload, the pericardial pressure-volume relation shifts to the right and its slope decreases (see Fig. 70-2, bottom, right curve); in other words, it becomes more compliant in association with increased pericardial area and mass and a decreased effect on the LV diastolic pressure-volume relation.[1,4] Thus apparent growth of pericardial tissue occurs in response to chronic stretch. Presumably, a similar effect occurs with large, slowly accumulating pericardial effusions, which typically do not cause tamponade.

ACUTE PERICARDITIS

Etiology, Epidemiology, and Pathophysiology

Table 70-1 is a partial list of diseases that can involve the pericardium. Acute pericarditis, defined as symptoms and/or signs resulting from pericardial inflammation of no more than 1 to 2 weeks' duration, can occur in a wide variety of these diseases (denoted by asterisks), but the majority of cases are idiopathic.[11-13] The term *idiopathic* is used to denote acute pericarditis for which no specific etiology can be found by routine diagnostic testing as outlined later. Most cases of acute idiopathic pericarditis are presumed to be viral in etiology, but testing for specific viruses is not routinely done because of cost and the fact that this knowledge rarely alters management.

The incidence of acute pericarditis is difficult to quantify because there are undoubtedly many undiagnosed cases. At autopsy, the frequency is approximately 1 percent.[11,14] Pericarditis is relatively common in patients presenting to the emergency department, accounting for up to 5 percent of those with nonischemic chest pain[14] and approximately 1 percent of cases with electrocardiographic ST elevation.[15] The fraction of all acute cases accounted for by *idiopathic* pericarditis is also uncertain and is influenced by population demographics and regional and seasonal variation in viral infections. However, 80 to 90 percent seems a reasonable estimate.[11-14] This percentage is lower in patients with pericarditis who require hospitalization and higher in young, previously healthy patients. Tuberculous pericarditis is included in Table 70-1 as a cause of acute pericarditis, but it usually presents with more chronic symptoms. Bacterial pericarditis is also included because it can present with signs and symptoms of acute pericardial inflammation, but these patients are usually critically ill and other components of their illness including pericardial effusions, sepsis, and pneumonias typically dominate the picture. Pericardi-

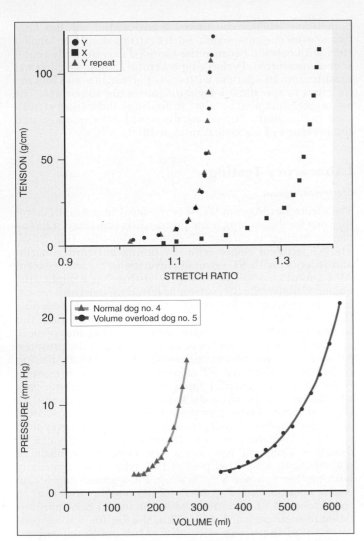

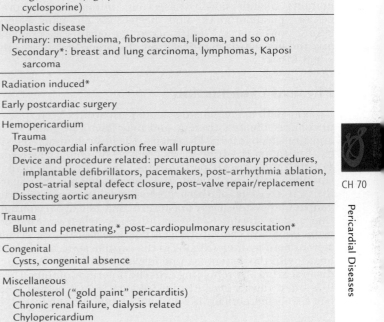

FIGURE 70–2 Top, Relationship between stretch and tension in vitro in normal human pericardial tissue. The tissue has been stretched in two, mutually orthogonal directions (X, Y). Note relatively abrupt transition from relatively flat to steep, inelastic relationship. In addition, the tissue is anisotropic, i.e., the relation between tension and stretch depends on the direction of stretch. **Bottom,** pressure-volume relationship of the normal canine pericardium **(left)** and after four weeks of cardiac dilation due to volume overload **(right).** Note the relatively abrupt transition to a steep relationship in normal pericardium and marked shift to the right and flattening after chronic volume overload. *(Top, From Lee M-C, Fung YC, Shabetai R, LeWinter MM: Biaxial mechanical properties of the human pericardium and canine comparisons. Am J Physiol 22:H75, 1987; **Bottom,** From Freeman G, LeWinter M: Pericardial adaptations during chronic cardiac dilation in dogs. Circ Res 54:294, 1984.)*

TABLE 70–1	Categories of Pericardial Disease and Selected Specific Etiologies

Idiopathic*

Infectious
 Viral* (echovirus, coxsackievirus, adenovirus, cytomegalovirus, hepatitis B, infectious mononucleosis, HIV/AIDs)
 Bacterial* (*Pneumococcus, Staphylococcus, Streptococcus,* mycoplasma, Lyme disease, *Haemophilus influenzae, Neisseria meningitidis,* and others)
 Mycobacteria* *(Mycobacterium tuberculosis, Mycobacterium avium-intracellulare)*
 Fungal (histoplasmosis, coccidiomycosis)
 Protozoal

Immune-inflammatory
 Connective tissue disease* (systemic lupus erythematosus, rheumatoid arthritis, scleroderma, mixed)
 Arteritis (polyarteritis nodosa, temporal arteritis)
 Inflammatory bowel disease
 Early post–myocardial infarction
 Late post–myocardial infarction (Dressler syndrome),* late postcardiotomy/thoracotomy,* late posttrauma*
 Drug induced* (e.g., procainamide, hydralazine, isoniazid, cyclosporine)

Neoplastic disease
 Primary: mesothelioma, fibrosarcoma, lipoma, and so on
 Secondary*: breast and lung carcinoma, lymphomas, Kaposi sarcoma

Radiation induced*

Early postcardiac surgery

Hemopericardium
 Trauma
 Post–myocardial infarction free wall rupture
 Device and procedure related: percutaneous coronary procedures, implantable defibrillators, pacemakers, post-arrhythmia ablation, post-atrial septal defect closure, post-valve repair/replacement
 Dissecting aortic aneurysm

Trauma
 Blunt and penetrating,* post–cardiopulmonary resuscitation*

Congenital
 Cysts, congenital absence

Miscellaneous
 Cholesterol ("gold paint" pericarditis)
 Chronic renal failure, dialysis related
 Chylopericardium
 Hypothyroidism and hyperthyroidism
 Amyloidosis
 Aortic dissection

*Etiologies that can present as acute pericarditis.
HIV/AIDS = human immunodeficiency virus/acquired immunodeficiency syndrome.

CH 70

Pericardial Diseases

tis occurring 24 to 72 hours after transmural MI caused by local inflammation and the delayed pericarditis of Dressler syndrome were once common (see Chap. 50). Their incidence has declined since the advent of thrombolytics and mechanical revascularization. With these exceptions, the distribution of etiologic diagnoses for acute pericarditis has changed little over time. This contrasts with pericardial effusion and constriction, whose epidemiology has changed considerably.

The pathophysiology of *uncomplicated* acute pericarditis is straightforward (i.e., symptoms and signs result from inflammation of pericardial tissue). A minority of cases are complicated, as discussed later. Some cases are associated with myocarditis.[11-14] Coexistent myocarditis is usually manifest solely by release of biomarkers such as creatine kinase and troponin I (see Chap. 66).[16,17] Occasionally,

however, significant myocardial dysfunction occurs in conjunction with clinically manifest pericarditis.

History and Differential Diagnosis

Acute pericarditis almost always presents with chest pain.[11,12] A few cases are diagnosed during evaluation of associated symptoms such as dyspnea or fever or incidentally in conjunction with noncardiac manifestations of systemic diseases such as rheumatoid arthritis or systemic lupus erythematosus (SLE). The pain of pericarditis can be severe. It is variable in quality but often sharp and almost always pleuritic. It usually does not have the viselike, constricting, or oppressive features of ischemic discomfort. Pericardial pain typically has a relatively rapid onset and sometimes begins remarkably abruptly. It is most commonly substernal, but can also be centered in the left anterior chest or epigastrium. Left arm radiation is not unusual. The most characteristic radiation is the trapezius ridge, which is highly specific for pericarditis. Pericardial pain is almost always relieved by sitting forward and worsened by lying down. Associated symptoms can include dyspnea, cough, and occasionally hiccoughs. An antecedent history of fever and/or symptoms suggesting a viral syndrome are common. It is important to carefully review the past medical history for clues to specific etiological diagnoses. A history of cancer or an autoimmune disorder, high fevers with shaking chills, skin rash, or weight loss should alert the physician to specific diseases that can cause pericarditis.

The differential diagnosis of chest pain is extensive (see Chaps. 11 and 49). Diagnoses most easily confused with pericarditis include pneumonia or pneumonitis with pleurisy (which may coexist with pericarditis), pulmonary embolus/infarction, costochondritis, and gastroesophageal reflux disease. Acute pericarditis is usually relatively easily distinguished from myocardial ischemia/infarction on clinical and other grounds, but coronary angiography is occasionally required to resolve this issue. Other considerations include aortic dissection, intraabdominal processes, pneumothorax, and herpes zoster pain before skin lesions appear. Finally, acute pericarditis is occasionally the presenting manifestation of a preceding, clinically silent MI.

Physical Examination

Patients with *uncomplicated* acute pericarditis often appear uncomfortable and anxious and may have low-grade fever and sinus tachycardia. Otherwise, the only abnormal physical finding is the friction rub caused by contact between visceral and parietal pericardium. The classic rub is distinctive, easily recognized, and pathognomonic of pericarditis. It consists of three components corresponding to ventricular systole, early diastolic filling, and atrial contraction and is similar to the sound made when walking on crunchy snow. The rub is usually loudest at the lower left sternal border, often extends to the cardiac apex, and is best heard with the patient leaning forward. It is often dynamic, disappearing and returning over short periods of time. Thus it is often rewarding to listen frequently to a patient who has suspected pericarditis without an audible rub initially.

Sometimes what is considered a pericardial rub has only two or even one component. Such findings should be labeled rubs with caution because the sound(s) may actually represent a murmur(s). Performing a careful, complete physical examination in a patient with acute pericarditis and looking for clues to specific etiologic diagnoses are important. The examiner must also be alert to findings indicating significant pericardial effusion, as discussed subsequently, and the presence of coexistent myocarditis.

Laboratory Testing

Electrocardiogram

The electrocardiogram (ECG) is the most important laboratory test for diagnosing acute pericarditis (see Chap. 12). The classic finding is diffuse ST segment elevation (Fig. 70-3). The ST segment vector typically points leftward, anterior and inferior, with ST segment elevation in all leads except AVR and often V1. Thus the term "diffuse" is a slight misnomer. Usually, the ST segment is coved upward and resembles the current of injury of acute, transmural ischemia. However, the distinction between acute pericarditis and transmural ischemia is usually not difficult because of more extensive lead involvement in pericarditis and the presence of much more prominent reciprocal ST segment depression in ischemia. However, ST elevation in pericarditis sometimes involves a smaller number of leads, in which case the distinction is more difficult. In other cases the ST segment more closely resembles early repolarization. Here again, pericarditis usually involves more leads than typical early repolarization. As with the rub, ECG changes can be dynamic. Frequent recordings can yield a diagnosis in patients with suspected pericarditis who present initially with neither rub nor ST elevation. PR segment depression is also common (see Fig. 70-3). PR depression can occur in the absence of ST elevation and be the initial ECG manifestation of acute pericarditis.[11,12] Thus the finding is diagnostically useful in patients with neither rub nor ST elevation.

ECG abnormalities other than ST elevation and PR depression are unusual in patients presenting soon after the onset of symptoms of acute pericarditis. Subsequent ECG changes are quite variable.[11] In some, the ECG reverts to normal over days or weeks. In others, the elevated ST segment passes through the isoelectric point and progresses to ST segment depression and T wave inversions in leads with upright QRS complexes. The latter changes can persist for weeks and months. They have no known significance in patients who have otherwise recovered. In patients presenting late after the onset of symptoms, these ECG changes can be difficult to distinguish from myocardial ischemia.

ECG abnormalities other than the above should be considered carefully because they suggest diagnoses other than idiopathic pericarditis and/or the presence of complications. As examples, AV block may indicate Lyme disease, pathological Q waves can signify a previous silent MI with pericardial

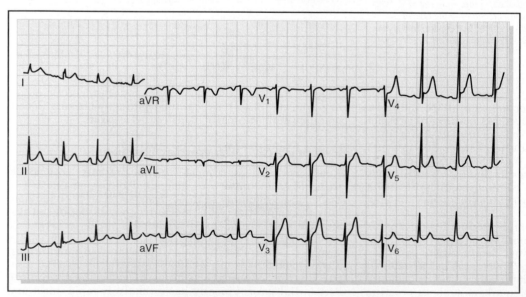

FIGURE 70–3 ECG in acute pericarditis. Both diffuse ST segment elevation and PR segment depression exist.

pain as its first manifestation, and low voltage or electrical alternans point toward significant effusion.

Hemogram

Modest elevations of the white blood cell count, typically 11,000 to 13,000 ml³ with a mild lymphocytosis, are common in acute idiopathic pericarditis. Higher counts are an alert for the presence of other etiologies, as is anemia. The erythrocyte sedimentation rate (ESR) should be no more than modestly elevated in acute idiopathic pericarditis. Unusually high values may be a clue to etiologies such as autoimmune diseases or tuberculosis.

Cardiac Enzymes and Troponin Measurements

Surprisingly large numbers of patients with a diagnosis of acute pericarditis without other evidence of myocarditis (see Chap. 66) or MI (see Chap. 50) have elevated creatine kinase MB fraction and/or troponin I values.[16,17] This suggests a significant incidence of concomitant, otherwise silent myocarditis. Pericarditis patients with elevated biomarkers of myocardial injury almost always have ST segment elevation. Another concern in patients with elevated biomarkers is silent MI presenting with subsequent pericarditis. Post-MI pericarditis usually (but not always) occurs after MIs with transmural ECG changes. Lastly, some patients have modest elevations of troponin I without creatine kinase changes.[16,17] It has been suggested that this is caused by adjacent epicardial inflammation rather than a true myocarditis.

Chest Radiograph (see Chap. 15)

The chest radiograph is usually normal in uncomplicated acute idiopathic pericarditis. Occasionally, small pulmonary infiltrates or pleural effusions are present, presumably because of viral or possibly mycoplasma infections. Other than this, pulmonary parenchymal or other abnormalities suggest diagnoses other than idiopathic pericarditis. Thus bacterial pericarditis often occurs in conjunction with severe pneumonia. Tuberculous pericarditis can occur with or without associated pulmonary infiltrates. Mass lesions and enlarged lymph nodes suggestive of neoplastic disease also have great significance. Pulmonary vascular congestion may signal coexistent, severe myocarditis. Small to even moderate effusions may not cause an abnormal cardiac silhouette; thus even modest enlargement is a cause for concern that a significant effusion is present.

Echocardiography (see Chap. 14)

The echocardiogram is normal in most patients with acute idiopathic pericarditis. The main reason for its performance is to exclude an otherwise silent effusion. No modern data delineate the incidence of effusions in such patients. Most do not have effusions, but small ones are fairly common and not a cause for concern. Moderate or larger effusions are unusual and may signal a diagnosis other than idiopathic pericarditis. Echocardiography is also useful in delineating whether associated myocarditis is severe enough to alter ventricular function, as well as in detection of MI.

Natural History and Management

Recently, the European Society of Cardiology published guidelines for the diagnosis and management of pericardial diseases.[13] Although these are useful, there have been virtually no randomized clinical trials devoted to the diagnosis or management of pericardial disease. Therefore it is important to keep in mind that controlled data to support the following recommendations for management of acute pericarditis, as well as other pericardial diseases, are limited.

TABLE 70–2	Initial Approach to the Patient with Definite or Suspected Acute Pericarditis

1. If diagnosis is suspected but not certain, listen frequently for pericardial rub and obtain frequent ECGs to look for diagnostic findings.

2. If diagnosis suspected or certain, obtain the following tests to determine if a specific etiologic diagnosis is likely or significant associated conditions and/or complications are present:
   — Chest radiograph
   — Hemogram
   — Echocardiogram
   — Creatine kinase with MB fraction, troponin I
   — Echocardiogram
   — Consider serum ANA if patient is young female

3. If diagnosis is certain, initiate therapy with a NSAID.

ANA = anti-nuclear antibody; NSAID = nonsteroidal antiinflammatory drug.

Initial management should be focused on screening for specific etiologies that would alter management, detection of effusion and other echocardiographic abnormalities, alleviation of symptoms, and appropriate treatment if a specific etiology is discovered. Initially, we recommend obtaining the laboratory data discussed earlier (i.e., ECG, hemogram, chest radiograph, creatine kinase and troponin I, and echocardiography). In young women, it is not unreasonable to test for SLE. Table 70-2 summarizes our recommendations for initial assessment and treatment of patients with definite or suspected acute pericarditis.

Acute idiopathic pericarditis is a self-limited disease without significant complications or recurrence in 70 to 90 percent of patients.[11-14,18] If laboratory data support the clinical diagnosis, symptomatic treatment with nonsteroidal antiinflammatory drugs (NSAIDs) should be initiated.[11-14] Because of its excellent safety profile, we prefer ibuprofen (600 to 800 mg po three times daily) with discontinuation if pain is no longer present after 2 weeks. Many patients have gratifying responses to the first dose or two of an NSAID, and most respond fully and need no additional treatment. Reliable patients with no more than small effusions who respond well to NSAIDs need not be admitted to a hospital.[19] Patients who do not respond well initially, have larger effusions, or suspicion of an etiology other than idiopathic pericarditis should be hospitalized for additional observation, diagnostic testing, and treatment as needed.

Patients who respond slowly or inadequately to NSAIDs may require supplementary narcotic analgesics to allow time for a full response and/or a brief course of colchicine or prednisone. Colchicine is administered as a 2 to 3 mg oral loading dose followed by 1 mg daily for 10 to 14 days.[20,21] Prednisone 60 mg by mouth is administered daily for 2 days with tapering to zero over a week. We prefer colchicine because there is some evidence that corticosteroids may encourage relapses.[14,22] In any case, it is unusual to not achieve a satisfactory response to this regimen. Colchicine has also been suggested as an alternative to NSAIDs for initial treatment.[20,21]

Complications of acute pericarditis include effusion, tamponade, and constrictive pericarditis. How many patients with acute pericarditis have moderate or larger effusions is unknown, but it is almost certainly less than 5 percent. As discussed earlier, a significant effusion increases the chance that a specific etiology will be identified. Management of effusion is discussed later. The chance of developing constrictive pericarditis following a bout of acute pericarditis is also unknown, but is undoubtedly extremely low. Strictly speaking, myocarditis is not a complication of pericarditis but an associated condition.

Relapsing and Recurrent Pericarditis

Perhaps 15 to 30 percent of patients with acute, apparently idiopathic pericarditis who respond satisfactorily to treatment as outlined earlier suffer a relapse after completion of initial therapy.[1,11-14] A minority develop recurrent bouts of pericardial pain, which can be chronic and debilitating. Recurrent pain is not necessarily associated with objective signs of pericardial inflammation. Some patients with what is initially thought to be idiopathic pericarditis manifest evidence of a specific etiology as they develop recurrences. Accordingly, a repeat evaluation for specific causes, especially autoimmune disorders, is appropriate. A pericardial biopsy to look for a specific etiology in patients with recurrent pain *without effusion* is rarely indicated because it is unlikely that a diagnosis will actually result or the information obtained will alter management.

Treatment of recurrent pain is empirical. For an initial relapse, a second 2-week course of a NSAID is often effective. A course of colchicine may be at least as effective.[20] For bouts of recurrent pericardial pain beyond an initial relapse, we favor colchicine prophylaxis.[20] Substantial experience has accumulated using chronic colchicine as prophylaxis for recurrent pericardial pain including that caused by idiopathic pericarditis and other etiologies (postthoracotomy, SLE). This experience strongly suggests that colchicine is at least as effective as corticosteroid therapy and has a much more favorable side effect profile. As earlier, the usual dose is a 2- to 3-mg oral load followed by 1 mg by mouth daily. Initiation of prophylactic therapy does not preclude simultaneous use of NSAIDs or corticosteroids, although as discussed earlier, colchicine alone is often effective for acute episodes. The most common difficulty in using colchicine is nausea and/or diarrhea, which results in dose reduction or termination in 10 to 15 percent of patients.

CH 70

Patients with recurrent pericardial pain despite NSAIDs and colchicine (or who cannot tolerate colchicine) are a challenging management problem. One option is a short course of prednisone as outlined earlier whenever symptoms first appear. Maintenance corticosteroid therapy should be avoided if at all possible. Nonsteroidal immunosuppressive therapy with drugs such as azathioprine and cyclophosphamide is another alternative, but published experience is extremely limited.[23] Low-dose maintenance therapy with these drugs may reduce the need for intermittent or maintenance corticosteroids and do so with fewer side effects. A recent report[24] suggests that intermittent administration of human immunoglobulins may be effective. Pericardiectomy has occasionally been employed for recurrent pericarditis, but appears to be effective in only a small minority of patients.[11-14]

PERICARDIAL EFFUSION AND TAMPONADE

Etiology

Idiopathic pericarditis and any infection, neoplasm, autoimmune, or inflammatory process (including postradiation and drug induced) that can cause pericarditis can cause an effusion (see Table 70-1).[13,14,25,26] Effusions are common early after cardiac surgery, but it is unusual for them to cause tamponade and they almost always resolve within several weeks. A lengthy list of miscellaneous, noninflammatory diseases can cause effusion (see Table 70-1). Patients with severe circulatory congestion may have small to moderate transudative effusions. Bleeding into the pericardial sac occurs after blunt and penetrating trauma (see Chap. 71),

following post-MI rupture of the free wall of the left ventricle, as a complication of percutaneous cardiac procedures and device implantation, and rarely after entrance of a sharp object (e.g., needles) into the cardiovascular system. Retrograde bleeding is an important cause of death because of aortic dissection (see Chap. 56). Lastly, patients are occasionally encountered with large, silent pericardial effusions and no evidence of pericarditis.[27] Effusions in these patients are generally stable, but there is a significant incidence of tamponade over time.

Of diseases that can cause effusion, those with a high incidence of progression to tamponade are bacterial (including mycobacteria), fungal, and human immunodeficiency virus (HIV)-associated infections (see Chap. 67) and neoplastic involvement. Although large effusions caused by acute idiopathic pericarditis are unusual, because of its high frequency this form of pericarditis accounts for a significant percentage of tamponade cases. Approximately 20 percent of large, symptomatic effusions without an obvious cause based on routine diagnostic examination constitute the initial presentation of a previously unrecognized cancer.[28] Details of pericardial effusion pertinent to specific disease entities are discussed later in this chapter.

Pathophysiology and Hemodynamics

Formation of an effusion is a component of the response to inflammation when there is an inflammatory and/or infectious process affecting the pericardium. The latter is also likely the case with pericardial tumor implants (see Chap. 69). Lymphomas occasionally cause effusion in association with enlarged mediastinal lymph nodes[1] by obstructing pericardial lymph drainage. The pathophysiology of effusions in situations with no obvious inflammation (e.g., uremia) is poorly understood.

Cardiac tamponade is characterized by a continuum from an effusion causing minimally detectable effects to full-blown circulatory collapse. Clinically, the most critical point occurs when an effusion reduces the volume of the cardiac chambers such that cardiac output begins to decline. Determinants of the hemodynamic consequences of pericardial effusion are the level of pressure in the pericardial sac and the ability of the heart to compensate for elevated pressure. The pressure depends on the amount of fluid and the pericardial pressure-volume relation. As discussed earlier, the pericardium normally has little reserve volume. As a result, relatively modest amounts of rapidly accumulating fluid can have major effects on cardiac function. Large, slowly accumulating effusions are often well tolerated, presumably because of chronic changes in the pericardial pressure-volume relation described earlier. The compensatory response to a significant pericardial effusion includes increased adrenergic stimulation and parasympathetic withdrawal, which cause tachycardia and increased contractility.[1,29] Patients who cannot mount a normal adrenergic response (e.g., those receiving beta-adrenergic blocking drugs) are more susceptible to the effects of a pericardial effusion. In the terminal stages of tamponade, a depressor reflex with paradoxical bradycardia may supervene.

The hemodynamic consequences of pericardial effusion have fascinated physiologists and physicians for years.[1,2,25,26,29] Non–steady-state responses to an abrupt increase in pericardial pressure provide insights into the mechanisms of these hemodynamic derangements. Figure 70-4 shows an experiment in a dog in which aortic and pulmonary arterial flow (stroke volume) were measured beat to beat before and after a large amount of fluid was rapidly introduced into the pericardial sac over one to two cardiac cycles,[2] indicated by the arrow. This causes an immediate decrease in pulmonary arterial stroke volume but no change in aortic stroke volume. Two beats later aortic stroke volume decreases, and eventually a new steady state is achieved with equivalent decreases

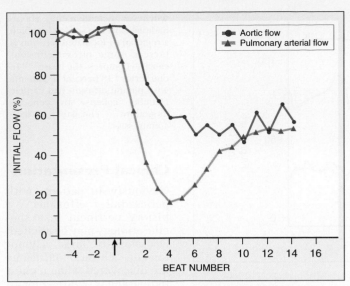

FIGURE 70-4 Beat-to-beat changes in pulmonary arterial and aortic stroke volume (as percentage of control) following abrupt production of cardiac tamponade (at arrow). Pulmonary arterial stroke volume decreases immediately, but there is a brief lag before aortic stroke volume decreases. Pulmonary arterial stroke volume is lower than aortic stroke volume until a new steady state is reached. *(From American Heart Association from Ditchey R, Engler R, LeWinter M, et al: The role of the right heart in acute cardiac tamponade in dogs. Circ Res 48:701, 1981.)*

TABLE 70-3	Hemodynamics in Cardiac Tamponade and Constrictive Pericarditis	
	Tamponade	**Constriction**
Paradoxical pulse	Usually present	Present in $\approx^1/_3$
Equal left/right filling pressures	Present	Present
Systemic venous wave morphology	Absent *y* descent	Prominent *y* descent (M or W shape)
Inspiratory change in systemic venous pressure	Decrease (normal)	Increase or no change (Kussmaul sign)
"Square root" sign in ventricular pressure	Absent	Present

in aortic and pulmonary arterial stroke volume. During the time required to achieve a new steady state, pulmonary stroke volume is less than aortic stroke volume. The transient inequality in left and right heart output results in net transfer of blood out of the pulmonary and into the systemic circulation and may explain the decrease in pulmonary vascularity on chest radiograph in tamponade. In parallel studies[1] right heart volume was shown to decrease more than left heart volume in response to a given increase in pericardial pressure. These results indicate that high pericardial pressure exerts its effect mainly by impeding right heart filling, with much of the effect on the left heart caused by secondary underfilling. In studies employing regional tamponade,[30] the importance of right heart compression was confirmed. These observations also provide a mechanism for the observations that atrial and ventricular diastolic collapse in tamponade are usually confined to the right heart.

As fluid accumulates in the pericardial sac, left- and right-sided atrial and ventricular diastolic pressures rise and in severe tamponade equalize at a pressure similar to that in the pericardial sac, typically 15 to 20 mm Hg (Fig. 70-5). Equalization is closest during inspiration. Thus the pressure in the pericardial sac dictates the intracavitary filling pressure, and the *transmural* filling pressures of the cardiac chambers are low. Correspondingly, cardiac volumes progressively decline. The small end-diastolic ventricular volume (decreased preload) mainly accounts for the small stroke volume. Because of compensatory increases in contractility, end-systolic volume also decreases, but not enough to normalize stroke volume (hence the importance of tachycardia in maintaining cardiac output). Because transmural right heart filling pressure is normally lower than left heart filling pressure (upper limit of mean right atrial pressure $\approx$7 mm Hg, mean left atrial pressure $\approx$12 mm Hg), as fluid accumulates, filling pressure increases more rapidly in the right than the left heart until equalization is achieved.

In addition to elevated and equal intracavitary filling pressures, markedly reduced transmural filling pressures, and small cardiac volumes, two other hemodynamic abnormalities are characteristic of tamponade. One is loss of the *y* descent of the right atrial or systemic venous pressure (see Fig. 70-5). The *x* and *y* descents of the venous pressure waveform correspond to periods when flow is increasing. Loss of the *y* descent has been explained on the basis of the concept that total heart volume is fixed in severe tamponade.[1,25,26,29] Thus blood can enter the heart only when blood is simultaneously leaving. The right atrial *y* descent begins when the tricuspid valve opens (i.e., when blood is not leaving the heart). Thus no blood can enter the heart, and the *y* descent is lost. In contrast, the *x* descent occurs during ventricular ejection. Because blood is leaving the heart, venous inflow can increase and the *x* descent is retained. Loss of the *y* descent can be

difficult to discern at the bedside but is easily appreciated in recordings of systemic venous or right atrial pressure and provides a useful clue to the presence of significant tamponade.

The second characteristic hemodynamic finding is the paradoxical pulse (Fig. 70-6), an abnormally large decline in systemic arterial pressure during inspiration (usually defined as a >10 mm Hg drop in systolic pressure). Other causes of *pulsus paradoxus* include constrictive pericarditis, pulmonary embolus, and pulmonary disease with large variation in intrathoracic pressure. In severe tamponade the arterial pulse is impalpable during inspiration. The mechanism of the paradoxical pulse is multifactorial, but respiratory changes in systemic venous return are certainly important.[1,5,25,26,29] In tamponade, in contrast to constrictive pericarditis, the normal inspiratory *increase* in systemic venous return is retained. Therefore the normal *decline* in systemic venous pressure on inspiration is present (Kussmaul sign is *absent*). The increase in right heart filling occurs, once again, under conditions in which total heart volume is fixed and left heart volume markedly reduced to start. The interventricular septum shifts to the left in exaggerated fashion on inspiration, encroaching on the left ventricle such that its stroke volume and pressure generation are abnormally reduced (see Fig. 70-6). Although the inspiratory increase in right heart volume (preload) causes an increase in RV stroke volume, this requires several cardiac cycles to increase LV filling and stroke volume and counteract the septal shift. Other factors that may contribute to the paradoxical pulse include increased afterload caused by transmission of negative intrathoracic pressure to the aorta and traction on the pericardium caused by the descent of the diaphragm, which increases pericardial pressure. Associated with these complex mechanisms are the striking findings that left and right heart pressure and stroke volume variations are exaggerated and 180 degrees out of phase (see Fig. 70-6). Table 70-3 lists the major hemodynamic findings of tamponade in comparison with constrictive pericarditis.

When preexisting elevations in diastolic pressures and/or volume exist, tamponade can occur without a paradoxical pulse.[1,25,26,29] Examples are patients with LV dysfunction, aortic regurgitation, and atrial septal defect. In patients with retrograde bleeding into the pericardial sac because of aortic dissection, tamponade may occur without a paradoxical pulse because of aortic valve disruption and regurgitation.

Although left- and right-sided filling pressures are usually 15 to 20 mm Hg in severe tamponade, tamponade can occur at lower levels of filling pressure, a phenomenon termed *low pressure tamponade*.[1,25,29] Low pressure tamponade occurs when there is a decrease in blood volume in the setting of a preexisting effusion that would not otherwise be significant. Under these conditions, a modestly elevated pericardial pressure can lower transmural filling pressure to levels where stroke volume is compromised. Because the venous pressure is only modestly elevated or even normal, the diagnosis may not be suspected. Low pressure tamponade is observed during hemodialysis, where it is signaled by hypotension during a dialysis run, in patients with blood loss and dehydration, and when diuretics are administered to patients with effusions.

Pericardial effusions can be loculated or localized, resulting in regional tamponade as sometimes encountered after cardiac surgery.[25,29,31] Regional tamponade may cause atypical hemodynamic abnormalities that can simulate heart failure (i.e., reduced cardiac output with unilateral filling pressure elevation). However, reports of hemodynamics in regional tamponade are scarce and it is difficult to generalize about this entity. Regional tamponade should be suspected

CH 70

Pericardial Diseases

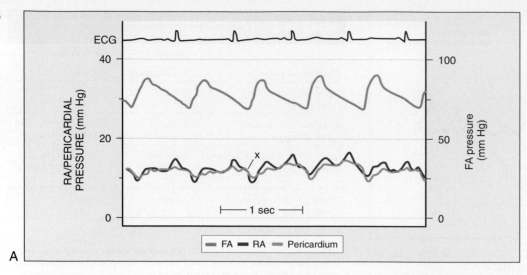

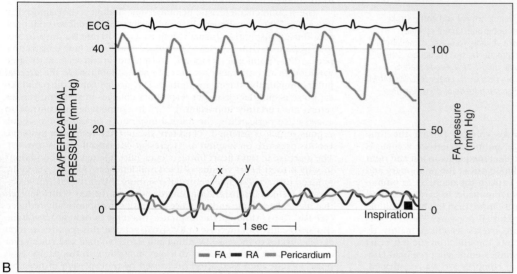

FIGURE 70–5 Femoral arterial (FA), right atrial (RA), and pericardial pressure before **(A)** and after **(B)** pericardiocentesis in a patient with cardiac tamponade. Both RA and pericardial pressure are about 15 mm Hg before pericardiocentesis. In this case there was a negligible paradoxical pulse. Note presence of *x* descent but absence of *y* descent before pericardiocentesis. Pericardiocentesis results in marked increase in FA pressure and marked decrease in RA pressure. During inspiration, pericardial pressure becomes negative, there is clear separation between RA and pericardial pressure, and *y* descent is now evident and prominent, suggesting the possibility of an effusive-constrictive picture. *(Modified from Lorell BH, Grossman W: Profiles in constrictive pericarditis, restrictive cardiomyopathy and cardiac tamponade. In Baim DS, Grossman W [eds]: Grossman's Cardiac Catheterization, Angiography, and Intervention. Philadelphia, Lippincott Williams & Wilkins, 2000, p 840.)*

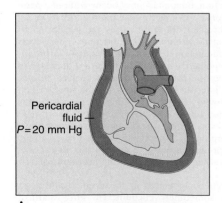

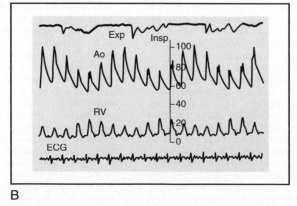

FIGURE 70–6 A, Schematic illustration of leftward septal shift with encroachment of left ventricular volume during inspiration in cardiac tamponade. **B,** Respiration marker and aortic and right ventricular pressure tracings in cardiac tamponade. A paradoxical pulse and marked, 180-degree, out-of-phase respiratory variation exists in right- and left-sided pressures. *(From Shabetai R: The Pericardium. New York, Grune & Stratton, 1981, p 266.)*

whenever hemodynamic abnormalities exist in a setting in which a regional or loculated effusion is present. Large pleural effusions can also compress the heart.[32,33] In one series[32] 18 percent of patients with pleural effusion had cardiac chamber collapse by echocardiography, consistent with compression.

Clinical Presentation

Obviously, in patients with pericardial effusions a history pertinent to a specific etiology may be elicited. Occasionally, large, asymptomatic chronic effusions are discovered when a chest radiograph is obtained for an unrelated reason.[27] As discussed earlier, specific etiologies are usually not found in these cases. Many patients with effusions also have pericardial pain. However, effusions do not by themselves cause symptoms unless tamponade is present. Patients with tamponade may complain of true dyspnea, the mechanism of which is uncertain because no pulmonary congestion occurs. This is difficult to distinguish from tachypnea reflecting shock and respiratory alkalosis. Other symptoms reflect the extent to which the cardiac output is reduced. Pericardial pain and/or a nonspecific sense of discomfort often dominate the clinical picture. In our experience, patients with tamponade almost always are more comfortable sitting forward.

A careful, complete physical examination of patients with pericardial effusion may provide clues to a specific etiology. In pericardial effusion without tamponade, the cardiovascular examination is normal except that if the effusion is large, the cardiac impulse may be difficult or impossible to palpate and the heart sounds muffled. Tubular breath sounds may be heard in the left axilla or left base because of bronchial compression. *Beck's triad* of hypotension, muffled heart sounds, and elevated jugular venous pressure remains a useful clue to the presence of severe tampon-

CH 70

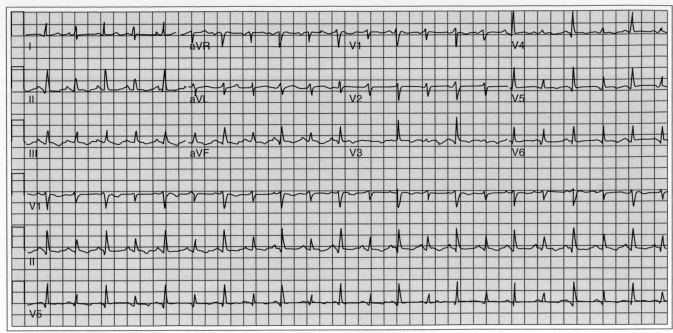

FIGURE 70–7 ECG in cardiac tamponade showing electrical alternans. *(From Lau TK, Civitello AB, Hernandez A, Coulter SA: Cardiac tamponade and electrical alternans. Tex Heart Inst J 48:67, 2002. Copyright 2002 Texas Heart Institute.)*

ade. Patients with tamponade are almost always uncomfortable, with signs reflecting varying degrees of reduced cardiac output and shock including tachypnea; diaphoresis; cool extremities; peripheral cyanosis; depressed sensorium; and, rarely, yawning.[34] Hypotension is usually present, although in early stages compensatory mechanisms maintain the blood pressure. A paradoxical pulse is the rule, but it is important to be alert to those situations in which it may not be present. The paradoxical pulse is quantified by cuff sphygmomanometry by noting the difference between the pressure at which Korotkoff sounds first appear and that at which they are present with each heart beat. In severe tamponade, the inspiratory decrease in arterial pressure is palpable and most obvious in arteries that are distant from the heart. Tachycardia is the rule unless heart rate–lowering drugs have been administered, conduction system disease coexists, or a preterminal bradycardic reflex has supervened. The jugular venous pressure is markedly elevated except in low-pressure tamponade, and the y descent is absent (see Fig. 70-5), although once again the latter can be difficult to appreciate at the bedside. The normal decrease in venous pressure on inspiration is retained. Examination of the heart usually, but not invariably, reveals a reduced or absent cardiac impulse, and, of course, a friction rub may also be present. Tamponade can be confused with anything that causes hypotension, shock, and elevated jugular venous pressure including myocardial failure, right heart failure caused by pulmonary embolus or other causes of pulmonary hypertension, and RV MI.

Laboratory Testing

Electrocardiogram

The ECG abnormalities characteristic of pericardial effusion and tamponade are reduced voltage and electrical alternans (Fig. 70-7).[1,29] Reduced voltage is nonspecific and can be caused by several other conditions including emphysema, infiltrative myocardial disease, and pneumothorax. Electrical alternans is specific but relatively insensitive for large effusions. It is caused by anterior-posterior swinging

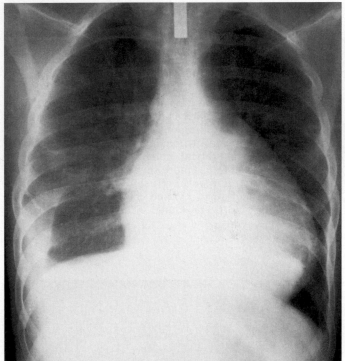

FIGURE 70–8 Anteroposterior chest radiograph in a patient with a large pericardial effusion (see text). *(From Kabbani SS, LeWinter M: Cardiac constriction and restriction. In Crawford MH, DiMarco JP [eds]: Cardiology. St. Louis, Mosby, 2001, pp 5, 15.5.)*

of the heart with each heartbeat. When pericarditis coexists, the usual ECG findings may be present.

Chest Radiograph (see Chap. 15)

The cardiac silhouette remains normal until pericardial effusions are at least moderate in size. With moderate and larger effusions, the anteroposterior cardiac silhouette assumes a rounded, flasklike appearance (Fig. 70-8). Lateral views may reveal the pericardial fat pad sign, a linear lucency between the chest wall and the anterior surface of the heart representing separation of parietal pericardial fat from epicardium. The lungs characteristically appear oligemic.

Echocardiography (see Chap. 14)

Because of convenience and ease of application, M-mode and two-dimensional Doppler echocardiography remain the standard noninvasive diagnostic methods for detection of pericardial effusion and assessment of tamponade. A pericardial effusion appears as a lucent separation between parietal and visceral pericardium (Fig. 70-9). With a true effusion, separation is present for the entire cardiac cycle. Small effusions are first evident over the posterobasal left ventricle. As the fluid increases, it spreads anteriorly, laterally, and behind the left atrium, where its limit is demarcated by the visceral pericardial reflection. Ultimately, the separation becomes circumferential. Ordinarily, tamponade does not occur without a circumferential effusion and the diagnosis should be viewed with skepticism if this is not the case. However, effusions can be regional and/or loculated and, as discussed earlier, cause regional tamponade. Computed tomography (CT) and magnetic resonance (MR) are more precise than echocardiography for imaging the pericardium itself. However, frondlike or shaggy-appearing structures in the pericardial space detected by echocardiography suggest clots and/or chronic inflammatory or neoplastic pericardial processes.

As discussed earlier, tamponade is best considered as a spectrum of severity of cardiac compression. Several findings indicate that tamponade is severe enough to cause at least some degree of hemodynamic compromise. Early diastolic collapse of the right ventricle (Fig. 70-10) and collapse of the right atrium (which occurs during *ventricular* diastole) (Fig. 70-11) are sensitive and specific signs that appear relatively early during tamponade.[3,25,26,29] Both occur when the pericardial pressure transiently exceeds the intracavitary pressure. Right atrial collapse is considered more sensitive, and RV collapse more specific for tamponade.[26] As noted earlier, a large *pleural* effusion can also cause right-sided chamber collapse. LV and left atrial collapse have been reported with regional effusions after cardiac

surgery[3,25,26] but are unusual. The cardiac chambers are small in tamponade and, as discussed earlier, in extreme cases the heart swings anteroposteriorly within the effusion. Distention of the caval vessels that does not diminish with inspiration is also a useful sign.

Reflecting the hemodynamic abnormalities discussed earlier, Doppler velocity recordings demonstrate exaggerated respiratory variation in right- and left-sided venous and valvular flow, with marked inspiratory increases on the right and decreases on the left[25,26,29] (Fig. 70-12). As a result of reduced systemic venous inflow during early diastole with loss of the y descent, most caval and pulmonary venous inflow occurs during ventricular systole. These flow patterns were found to have a sensitivity of 75 percent and a specificity of 91 percent for diagnosing tamponade.[35] The *absence* of chamber collapse is especially useful in excluding tamponade in patients with effusions, but its presence is less well correlated with tamponade than abnormal venous flow patterns. Newer techniques such as tissue Doppler do not yet have a well-defined, additive role in cardiac tamponade. In most cases of pericardial effusion, transthoracic echocardiography provides sufficient diagnostic information to make informed management decisions. Although transesophageal studies provide better-quality images, they are often impractical in sick patients. However, the transesophageal approach can easily be employed in intubated patients.

Other Imaging Modalities

Pericardial effusion causes damping or abolition of cardiac pulsation. Accordingly, fluoroscopy is useful in the cardiac catheterization laboratory for detection of acute, procedural-related effusions.

Computed tomography (CT) (see Chap. 18) and magnetic resonance imaging (MRI) (see Chap. 17) are useful adjuncts to echocardiography in the characterization of effusion and tamponade.[36,37] Neither is ordinarily required and/or advisable in sick patients who require prompt management and treatment decisions. They have an important ancillary role in situations in which hemodynamics are atypical and the presence and severity of tamponade is less certain, and they are invaluable when echocardiography is technically inadequate. Both CT and MRI provide more detailed quantitation and regional/spatial localization than echocardiography and are especially useful for loculated and regional effusions. Pericardial thickness can be measured with both, allowing indirect assessment of the severity and chronicity of inflammation. Clues to the nature of pericardial fluid can be gained from CT attenuation coefficients. Attenuation similar to water suggests transudative, greater than water malignant, bloody or purulent, and less than water chylous effusion. MRI can be used to make similar distinctions. Real-time CT or MR cine displays provide similar information as echocardiography for assessment of tamponade (e.g., septal shifting and chamber collapse), and both are invaluable when other pathology in the chest is suspected in association with or as a cause of pericardial effusion.

Management of Pericardial Effusion and Tamponade

Management of pericardial effusion is dictated first and foremost by whether tamponade is present or has a high chance of developing in the near term.[25,26,29] Situations

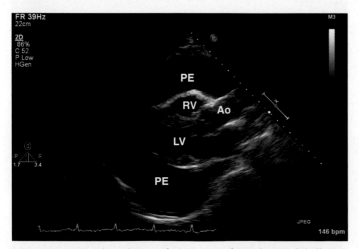

FIGURE 70–9 2D echocardiogram of a large, circumferential pericardial effusion. (*From Kabbani SS, LeWinter M: Cardiac constriction and restriction. In Crawford MH, DiMarco JP [eds]: Cardiology. St. Louis, Mosby, 2001, pp 5, 15.5.*)

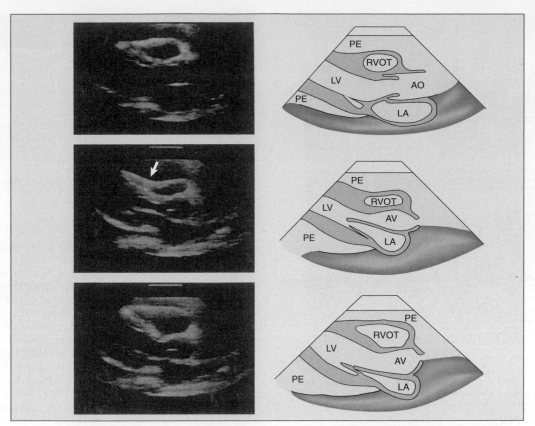

FIGURE 70–10 2D echocardiogram illustrating diastolic collapse or indentation of the right ventricle in cardiac tamponade. **Top,** Systole. **Middle,** Early diastole with indentation indicated by arrow. **Bottom,** Late diastole with return of normal configuration. PE, pericardial effusion; RVOT, right ventricular outflow tract; LV, left ventricle; LA, left atrium; AV, aortic valve. *(From Weyman AE: Principles and Practice of Echocardiography. Philadelphia, Lea & Febiger, 1994, p 1119.)*

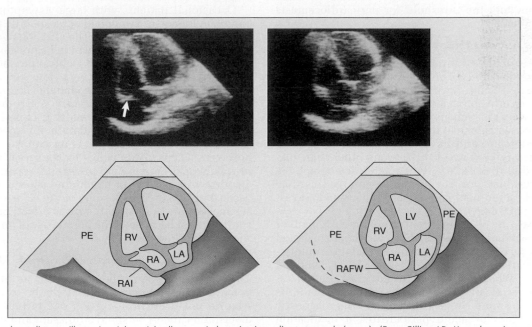

FIGURE 70–11 2D echocardiogram illustrating right atrial collapse or indentation in cardiac tamponade (arrow). *(From Gilliam LD: Hemodynamic compression of the right atrium: A new echocardiographic sign of cardiac tamponade. Circulation 68:294, 1983.)*

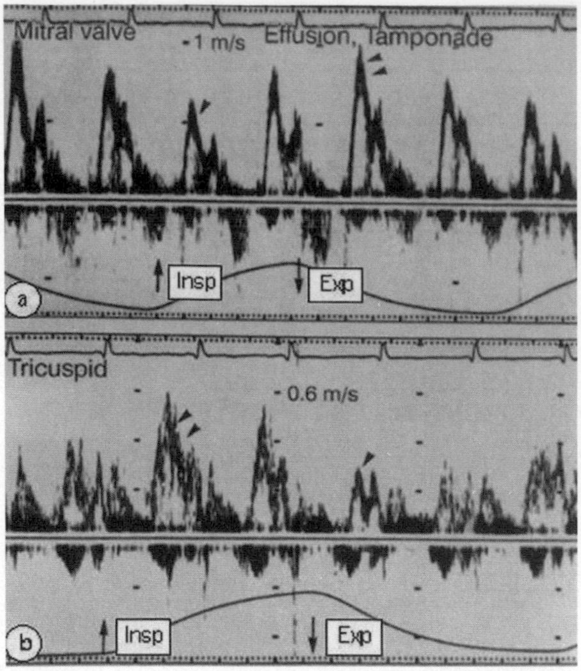

CH 70

FIGURE 70–12 Transmitral and tricuspid Doppler velocity recordings in cardiac tamponade showing marked, 180 degrees out of phase respiratory variations. *(From Oh JK, Hatle LK, Mulvagh SL, Tajik AJ: Transient constrictive pericarditis: Diagnosis by two-dimensional Doppler echocardiography. Mayo Clin Proc 68:1158, 1993.)*

TABLE 70–4	Initial Approach to the Patient with a Pericardial Effusion

1. Determine if tamponade is present or threatened on the basis of history, physical examination, and echocardiogram.

2. If tamponade is not present or threatened, follow these guidelines:
   — If etiology is not apparent, consider diagnostic tests as for acute pericarditis.
   — If effusion is large, consider course of a NSAID or corticosteroid and, if no response, consider closed pericardiocentesis.

3. If tamponade is present or threatened, follow this guideline:
   — Urgent or emergent closed pericardiocentesis or careful monitoring if trial of medical treatment to reduce effusion is considered appropriate.

where tamponade should be considered a near-term threat include suspected bacterial or tuberculous pericarditis, bleeding into the pericardial space, and any situation in which there is a moderate to large effusion that is not thought to be chronic and/or is increasing in size. When tamponade is present or threatened, clinical decision requires urgency and the threshold for pericardiocentesis should be low (Table 70-4).

Effusions Without Actual or Threatened Tamponade

In the absence of actual or threatened tamponade, management can be more leisurely. This cohort of patients includes several categories. Some have acute pericarditis with a small to moderate effusion detected as part of routine evaluation. Others undergo echocardiography because of the presence of diseases known to involve the pericardium. The rest are asymptomatic and have effusions detected when diagnostic tests are performed for reasons other than suspected pericardial disease (e.g., when echocardiography is performed to evaluate an unexpectedly enlarged cardiac silhouette on chest radiograph or CT or MR is used to investigate thoracic pathology).

In many cases of effusion when tamponade is neither present nor threatened, a cause will be evident or suggested on the basis of the history (e.g., known neoplastic or autoimmune disease, radiation therapy) and/or previously obtained diagnostic tests. When a diagnosis is not clear, an assessment of specific etiologies of pericardial disease should be undertaken. This should in general include the diagnostic tests recommended for acute pericarditis, a medication review, and anything else dictated by the clinical picture. Thus skin testing for tuberculosis and screening for neoplastic and autoimmune diseases and infections (e.g., Lyme disease) and hypothyroidism should be considered. At the same time, careful judgment should be exercised in the selection of tests. Thus a patient with severe heart failure and circulatory congestion with a small, asymptomatic effusion does not need extensive testing. In contrast, patients

with evidence of a systemic disease deserve careful attention. Serial titers of antibodies to viruses are usually not helpful in these cases because the results may be nonspecific or negative despite a viral etiology. However, situations occasionally arise in which evidence of a viral etiology, if present, is helpful in clarifying diagnostic dilemmas, providing reassurance, and avoiding unnecessary diagnostic testing and/or treatments. In these situations it may be useful to save serum obtained at presentation, should there be a need to measure viral titers at a later date.

In most of these patients, pericardiocentesis (closed or open with biopsy) need only be undertaken for diagnostic purposes and is usually not required. As discussed earlier, in many cases a diagnosis will either be obvious when the effusion is first noted or become evident as part of initial investigations. Moreover, in this setting analysis of pericardial fluid *alone* in general has a low yield for providing a specific diagnosis.[25,26,38,39] In occasional situations where pericardiocentesis is necessary for diagnostic purposes, consideration should be given to open drainage with biopsy.

Occasional patients with large, asymptomatic effusions and no evidence of tamponade or a specific etiology constitute a special category.[27,38,39] The effusions are by definition chronic because tamponade would be present if this was not the case. They are in general stable, and specific etiologies usually do not emerge over time. However, a minority progress to tamponade in an unpredictable fashion. After closed pericardiocentesis, the effusions typically do not reaccumulate.[27,38,39] Thus there is a rationale for closed pericardiocentesis following routine evaluation for specific etiologies, as outlined earlier. This decision can be individualized, however, because little is lost by conservative management in reliable patients. Before undertaking pericardiocentesis, a course of a NSAID or colchicine should be considered[40] because this will shrink some of the effusions. A course of corticosteroids may have the same effect, but this remains controversial because of the possibility of an increased likelihood of recurrence.

Effusions with Actual or Threatened Tamponade

These patients should be considered as having a true or potential medical emergency. With the exception of those who do not want prolongation of life (mainly those with metastatic cancer), hospital admission and careful hemodynamic and echocardiographic monitoring are mandatory. Most patients require pericardiocentesis to treat or prevent tamponade. Treatment should be carefully individualized, and thoughtful clinical judgment is critical. Thus, for example, patients with acute, apparently idiopathic pericarditis who have no more than mild tamponade can be treated with a course of a NSAID and/or colchicine and monitored in the hope that their effusions will shrink rapidly. Patients with autoimmune diseases can be treated in the same way and/or with a course of corticosteroids. Patients with *possible* bacterial infections or bleeding into the pericardial sac *whose effusions are no more than moderate in size* may in some cases be suitable for initial conservative management and careful monitoring because the risk of closed pericardiocentesis is increased with smaller effusions.

Hemodynamic monitoring with a pulmonary artery balloon catheter is often useful, especially in those with threatened or mild tamponade in whom a decision is made to defer pericardiocentesis. Monitoring is also helpful *after* pericardiocentesis to assess reaccumulation and the presence of underlying constrictive disease (see Fig. 70-5), as discussed subsequently. However, insertion of a pulmonary artery catheter should not be allowed to delay definitive therapy in critically ill patients.

For most patients in this category, management should be directed toward urgent or emergent pericardiocentesis. Once actual or threatened tamponade is diagnosed, intravenous hydration should be instituted, especially in patients who mistakenly receive diuretics because of an incorrect diagnosis of heart failure. In patients with tamponade who are critically ill, intravenous positive inotropes (dobutamine, dopamine) can be employed but are of limited efficacy. Hydration and positive inotropes are temporizing measures and should not be allowed to substitute for or delay pericardiocentesis.

In the vast majority of circumstances, closed pericardiocentesis is the initial treatment of choice. Before proceeding it is important to be confident that there is indeed an effusion large enough to cause tamponade, especially if hemodynamics are atypical. Loculated effusions, as well as effusions containing clots or fibrinous material, are also of concern because the risk and difficulty of closed pericardiocentesis are increased. In these situations, if removal of pericardial fluid is thought to be necessary, an open approach should be considered for safety and to obtain pericardial tissue and create a window.

The most commonly employed approach to closed pericardiocentesis is subxiphoid needle insertion performed under echocardiographic guidance to minimize the risk of puncture of the myocardium and assess completeness of fluid removal.[41] Once the needle has entered the pericardial space, a modest amount of fluid should be removed (perhaps 50 to 150 ml) in an effort to produce some degree of hemodynamic improvement. Then a guidewire should be inserted, and the needle replaced with a pigtail catheter. The catheter can be manipulated with continuing echocardiographic guidance to maximize the amount of fluid removed. In a large series from the Mayo Clinic,[41] the procedural success rate was 97 percent and the complication rate was 4.7 percent (major, 1.2 percent; minor, 3.5 percent). The procedure should be performed in the cardiac catheterization laboratory with experienced personnel in attendance, unless the patient is too ill to be moved. If echocardiographic guidance is unavailable, the needle should be directed toward the right shoulder and then replaced with a catheter for subsequent fluid removal. Fluoroscopy-guided drainage is an alternative when echocardiography cannot be used.

If a pulmonary artery catheter has been inserted into the right heart, pulmonary capillary wedge and systemic arterial pressures and cardiac output should be monitored before, during, and after the procedure. Ideally, pericardial fluid pressure should also be measured. As discussed earlier, removal of relatively small amounts of fluid can result in substantial hemodynamic improvement. Hemodynamic monitoring before and after pericardiocentesis is useful for several reasons. Initial measurements confirm and document the severity of tamponade. Assessment after completion establishes a baseline to assess reaccumulation. As discussed later, some patients presenting with tamponade have a coexisting component of constriction (i.e., effusive-constrictive pericarditis),[42] which is difficult to detect when an effusion dominates the picture. Filling pressures that remain elevated after pericardiocentesis and the appearance of venous waveforms typical of constriction (rapid x and y descents) indicate coexistent constriction.

Following pericardiocentesis, repeat echocardiography and in many cases continued hemodynamic monitoring are useful to assess fluid reaccumulation. The duration of monitoring is a matter of judgment, but typically pulmonary artery catheter pressures are measured for about 24 hours and a follow-up echocardiogram is performed immediately before its removal. If hemodynamic changes indicating reaccumulation appear, echocardiography should be performed sooner. The intrapericardial catheter should be left in place for several days to allow continued fluid removal, which minimizes recurrences[13,25,26] and assists delivery of intrapericardial drugs if indicated.

Open pericardiocentesis is occasionally preferred for the initial removal of pericardial fluid. Loculated effusions and/or effusions that are borderline in size are drained more safely in the operating room. Recurring effusions, especially those causing tamponade, are often initially drained using a closed approach because of logistical considerations. However, open pericardiocentesis with biopsy and establishment of a pericardial window are preferred for most recurrences that are severe enough to cause tamponade. Creation of a window reliably eliminates future episodes of tamponade and provides pericardial tissue to assist in diagnosis. The surgeon should inspect the pericardium carefully and obtain multiple biopsies. Percutaneous balloon and tube pericardiostomy techniques have also been used for drainage.[43,44] These methods appear to be safe and effective for producing pericardial windows, but at present are available in only a few centers.

Analysis of Pericardial Fluid

Previous information about the composition of normal pericardial fluid was obtained in small numbers of subjects. Ben-Horin and colleagues[45] recently reassessed this in a larger group undergoing heart surgery with no evidence of pericardial disease. The fluid has the features of a plasma ultrafiltrate. However, lactate dehydrogenase levels were 2.4 times that of serum and mean protein levels were 0.6 times that of serum. Lymphocytes were the predominant cell type.

Although analysis of pericardial fluid does not usually have a high yield in identifying the etiology of pericardial disease, careful analysis can be rewarding. *Assuming a diagnosis is not known before fluid removal*, routine pericardial fluid measurements should include specific gravity, white blood cell count and differential, hematocrit, and protein content.[13,25,26,45] Although most effusions are exudates, detection of a transudate reduces the diagnostic possibilities considerably. Blood in pericardial fluid is nonspecific. Moreover, pericardial blood usually undergoes rapid fibrinolysis. Chylous effusions can occur after traumatic or surgical injury to the thoracic duct or obstruction by a neoplastic process. Occasionally they are idiopathic. Cholesterol rich ("gold paint") effusions occur in severe hypothyroidism.

Pericardial fluid should be routinely stained and cultured for detection of bacteria, including tuberculosis, and fungi. As much fluid as possible should be submitted for detection of malignant cells because there is a reasonably high yield for diagnosis of malignancy in patients with pericardial involvement. In tuberculous pericardial disease, several tests other than culture of fluid and examination of biopsy specimens are useful.[13,25,26,46-48] These include adenosine deaminase (ADA), interferon-gamma, and polymerase chain reaction (PCR), as discussed in more detail later. Unless some other cause is evident, we believe that a relatively rapid test for tuberculosis (ADA, PCR) should be routine because of the general difficulty of diagnosing tuberculous pericarditis and the delays involved in making a diagnosis by culture. There may be a role for routine measurement of selected tumor markers as a general screen for malignant effusion and an adjunct to direct detection of malignant cells.[13]

Pericardioscopy and Percutaneous Biopsy

Some experts advocate the routine use of pericardioscopic-guided biopsy in patients with pericardial effusion who do not have an etiologic diagnosis. Seferovic and colleagues[49] compared the diagnostic yield of percutaneous, fluoroscopy-guided parietal pericardial biopsy (3 to 6 samples) to targeted, pericardioscopic-guided biopsy with either limited (3 to 6 samples) or extended sampling (18 to 20 samples). Tissue was examined by routine histology. Pericardioscopic biopsy was found to have a higher sampling efficiency than fluoroscopic guidance and a much higher diagnostic yield. Extended sampling performed best, leading to a new diagnosis in 41 percent and a specific etiology in 53 percent of cases, which is comparable to open biopsy. The technique was especially useful in detecting malignant involvement, and few complications occurred. However, pericardioscopy is technically challenging, few individuals have significant experience, and the number of institutions at which it is available is limited. Moreover, in earlier reports major complications were occasionally encountered.[49] Most importantly, it is not clear that its use will significantly improve long-term outcomes in patients with pericardial disease. Accordingly, we believe that routine pericardioscopic biopsy is not yet warranted.

CONSTRICTIVE PERICARDITIS

Etiology

Constrictive pericarditis is the end stage of an inflammatory process involving the pericardium. Virtually any inflamma-

TABLE 70–5	Causes of Constrictive Pericarditis
Idiopathic	
Irradiation	
Postsurgical	
Infectious	
Neoplastic	
Autoimmune (connective tissue) disorders	
Uremia	
Posttrauma	
Sarcoid	
Methysergide therapy	
Implantable defibrillator patches	

tory process listed in Table 70-1 can cause constriction. In the developed world the cause is most commonly idiopathic, postsurgical, or radiation injury[14,25,26] (Table 70-5). Tuberculosis was the most common cause of constrictive pericarditis in the developed world before development of effective drug therapy. It remains important in developing countries. Although constriction can follow an initial insult by as little as several months, it usually takes years to develop. The end result is dense fibrosis, often calcification, and adhesions of the parietal and visceral pericardium. Usually scarring is more or less symmetrical and impedes filling of all heart chambers. In a subset of patients the process develops relatively rapidly and is reversible. This variant is seen most commonly following cardiac surgery.[50] The clinical presentation is usually dominated by signs and symptoms of right-heart failure.

Pathophysiology

The pathophysiological consequence of pericardial scarring is markedly restricted filling of the heart.[25,26] This results in elevation and equilibration of filling pressures in all chambers and the systemic and pulmonary veins. In early diastole the ventricles fill abnormally rapidly because of markedly elevated atrial pressures and accentuated early diastolic ventricular suction, the latter related to small end-systolic volumes. During early to mid-diastole, ventricular filling abruptly ceases when intracardiac volume reaches the limit set by the stiff pericardium. As a result, almost all ventricular filling occurs early in diastole. Systemic venous congestion results in hepatic congestion, peripheral edema, ascites, and sometimes anasarca and cardiac cirrhosis. Reduced cardiac output is a consequence of impaired ventricular filling and causes fatigue, muscle wasting, and weight loss. In "pure" constriction, contractile function is preserved, although ejection fraction can be reduced as a consequence of reduced preload. The myocardium is occasionally involved in the chronic inflammation and fibrosis, leading to true contractile dysfunction that can at times be quite severe. The latter predicts a poor response to pericardiectomy.

Failure of transmission of intrathoracic pressure changes during respiration to the cardiac chambers is an important contributor to the pathophysiology of constrictive pericarditis (Fig. 70-13). These changes continue to be transmitted to the pulmonary circulation. Thus on inspiration the drop in intrathoracic pressure (and therefore pulmonary venous pressure) is not transmitted to the left heart.[5,25,26] Consequently, on inspiration the small pulmonary vein to left atrial pressure gradient that normally drives left heart filling is reduced, resulting in decreased left atrial and transmitral inflow. The inspiratory decrease in LV filling allows an increase in RV filling and an interventricular septal shift to the left. The opposite sequence occurs with expiration.

High systemic venous pressure and reduced cardiac output result in compensatory retention of sodium and water by the kidneys. Inhibition of atrial natriuretic peptide also contributes to renal sodium retention and further exacerbates increases in systemic venous and left-sided filling pressures.[51]

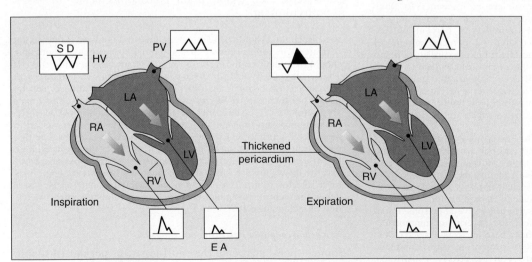

FIGURE 70–13 Schematic representation of transvalvular and central venous flow velocities in constrictive pericarditis. During inspiration the decrease in left ventricular filling results in a leftward septal shift, allowing augmented flow into the right ventricle. The opposite occurs during expiration. EA = mitral inflow; HV = hepatic vein; LA = left atrium; LV = left ventricle; PV = pulmonary venous flow; RA = right atrium; RV = right ventricle.

Clinical Presentation

The usual presentation consists of signs and symptoms of predominantly right heart failure. At a relatively early stage these signs and symptoms include lower extremity edema, vague abdominal complaints, and some degree of passive hepatic congestion. As the disease becomes more severe, hepatic congestion worsens and can progress to ascites and/or anasarca, as well as jaundice caused by cardiac cirrhosis. Signs and symptoms ascribable to elevated pulmonary venous pressures such as exertional dyspnea, cough, and orthopnea may also appear with progressive disease. Atrial fibrillation and tricuspid regurgitation, which further exacerbate venous pressure elevation, may also appear at this stage. In the end stage of constrictive pericarditis, the effects of a chronically low cardiac output are prominent including severe fatigue, muscle wasting, and cachexia. Less common symptoms include recurrent pleural effusions and syncope. Constrictive pericarditis can be mistaken for any cause of right heart failure, as well as end-stage primary liver disease. Of course, venous pressure is not elevated in the latter circumstance.

Physical Examination

Physical findings include markedly elevated jugular venous pressure with a prominent, rapidly collapsing *y* descent. This, combined with a normally prominent *x* descent, results in an M- or W-shaped venous pressure contour. At the bedside, this is best appreciated as two prominent descents with each cardiac cycle. In patients in atrial fibrillation the *x* descent is lost, leaving only the prominent *y* descent. The latter is difficult to distinguish from tricuspid regurgitation, which, as noted earlier, may itself occur as a consequence of constrictive pericarditis. *Kussmaul sign,* an inspiratory increase in systemic venous pressure, is usually present,[1,25,26] or the venous pressure may simply fail to decrease on inspiration. Kussmaul sign reflects loss of the normal increase in right heart venous return on inspiration, even though tricuspid flow increases. These characteristic abnormalities of the venous waveform contrast markedly with those in tamponade. A paradoxical pulse occurs in perhaps one third of patients with constrictive pericarditis and is especially common when there is an effusive-constrictive picture (see later). It is best explained by the aforementioned lack of transmission of decreased intrathoracic pressure to the left heart chambers. Table 70-3 is a comparison of hemodynamic findings in cardiac tamponade and constrictive pericarditis.

In cases with extensive calcification and adhesion of the heart to adjacent structures, the position of the cardiac point of maximal impulse may fail to change with changes in body position. However, the most notable cardiac finding is the pericardial knock, an early diastolic sound best heard at the left sternal border and/or the cardiac apex. It occurs slightly earlier and has a higher acoustic frequency content than a third heart sound. The knock corresponds to the early, abrupt cessation of ventricular filling. Widening of second heart sound splitting may also be present. As noted, significant numbers of patients have secondary tricuspid regurgitation with its characteristic systolic murmur.

Abdominal examination reveals hepatomegaly, often with palpable venous pulsations, with or without ascites. Other signs of chronic hepatic congestion include jaundice, spider angiomata, and palmar erythema. Lower extremity edema is usually present, and anasarca occurs in some cases. As noted earlier, with end-stage constriction, muscle wasting, cachexia, and massive ascites and edema of the scrotum and lower extremities may appear.

Laboratory Testing

Electrocardiogram

No specific ECG findings exist. Nonspecific T wave abnormalities are often observed, as well as reduced voltage. Left atrial abnormality may also be present. Atrial fibrillation is present in significant numbers of patients.

Chest Radiograph (see Chap. 15)

The cardiac silhouette can be enlarged secondary to a coexisting pericardial effusion. Pericardial calcification is seen in a minority of patients and should raise the suspicion of tuberculous pericarditis (Fig. 70-14), but calcification per se is not diagnostic of constrictive physiology. The lateral chest film is useful to detect pericardial calcification along the right heart border and in the atrioventricular groove. Isolated calcification of the LV apex or posterior wall suggests ventricular aneurysm rather than pericardial calcification. Pleural effusions are occasionally noted and can be a presenting sign of constrictive pericarditis. When left heart filling pressures are markedly elevated, pulmonary vascular congestion and redistribution can be present.

Echocardiogram (see Chap. 14)

M-mode and two-dimensional echocardiography findings include pericardial thickening, abrupt displacement of the interventricular septum during early diastole (septal "bounce"),[5,13,25,26] and signs of systemic venous congestion such as dilation of hepatic veins and distention of the inferior vena cava with blunted respiratory fluctuation. Premature pulmonic valve opening as a result of elevated RV early diastolic pressure may also be observed. Exaggerated septal shifting during respiration is often present.

Lack of transmission of intrathoracic pressure to the cardiac chambers and resulting mitral and tricuspid inflow patterns in constrictive pericarditis have been discussed earlier. In accordance with these patterns, Doppler flow velocity measurements reveal exaggerated respiratory variation in both mitral inflow velocity and tricuspid-mitral inflow differences, with the latter 180 degrees out of phase (see Fig. 70-13). Although there is some overlap with cardiac tamponade, these inflow

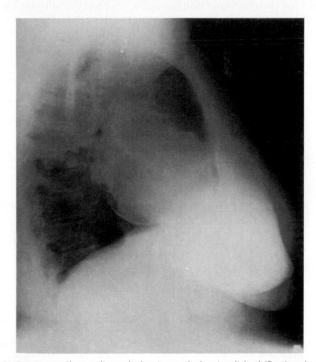

FIGURE 70-14 Chest radiograph showing marked pericardial calcifications in a patient with constrictive pericarditis.

patterns have good sensitivity and specificity for constrictive pericarditis and also help distinguish restrictive cardiomyopathy from constrictive pericarditis.[5,13,25,26] Typically, patients with constriction demonstrate greater than or equal to a 25 percent increase in mitral E velocity during expiration compared with inspiration and increased diastolic flow reversal with expiration in the hepatic veins. Mitral E wave deceleration time is usually, but not always, less than 160 ms. These Doppler findings have excellent sensitivity and specificity for diagnosing constrictive pericarditis. However, a subset of patients (up to 20 percent) with constriction do not exhibit typical respiratory changes, most likely because of markedly increased left atrial pressure or possibly a mixed constrictive-restrictive pattern caused by myocardial involvement by the constrictive process. In patients without typical respiratory mitral-tricuspid flow velocity findings, examination after maneuvers that decrease preload (head-up tilt, sitting) can unmask characteristic respiratory variation in mitral E velocity.[25,26] *Tissue Doppler* examination reveals increased E′ velocity of the mitral annulus, as well as septal abnormalities corresponding to the "bounce."[52-54] Tissue Doppler appears to be at least as sensitive as conventional echocardiography-Doppler for diagnosing constriction.

Similar patterns of respiratory variation in mitral inflow velocity can be observed in chronic obstructive lung disease, RV infarction, pulmonary embolism, and pleural effusion. These conditions have other clinical and echocardiographic features that differentiate them from constrictive pericarditis. Superior vena caval flow velocities are helpful in distinguishing constrictive pericarditis from chronic obstructive pulmonary disease. Patients with pulmonary disease display a marked increase in inspiratory superior vena caval systolic forward flow velocity, which is not seen in constriction.

Transesophageal echocardiography can be used as a valuable adjunct in assessing constrictive pericarditis. It is superior to transthoracic echocardiography for measuring pericardial thickness and has an excellent correlation with CT for this purpose.[55] Moreover, when mitral inflow velocities by transthoracic echocardiography are technically inadequate or equivocal, measurement of pulmonary venous Doppler velocities using the transesophageal approach demonstrates pronounced respiratory variation, larger than that observed across the mitral valve.[56]

Cardiac Catheterization and Angiography (see Chap. 19)

Cardiac catheterization in patients with suspected constrictive pericarditis provides documentation of the hemodynamics of constrictive physiology and assists in discriminating between constrictive pericarditis and restrictive cardiomyopathy.[1,13,25] Although there is limited need for contrast ventriculography, coronary angiography is used to detect occult coronary artery disease in those being considered for pericardiectomy. In addition, on rare occasions external pinching or compression of the coronary arteries or outflow tract regions by the constricting pericardium is detected.

Right and left heart pressures should be recorded simultaneously at equisensitive gains. Right atrial, RV diastolic, pulmonary capillary wedge, and pre-a wave LV diastolic pressure are elevated and equal, or nearly so, at approximately 20 mm Hg. Differences of more than 3 to 5 mm Hg between left and right heart filling pressures are rarely encountered. The right atrial pressure tracing shows a preserved *x* descent, a prominent *y* descent, and roughly equal a and v wave height, with the resultant M or W shape configuration. Both RV and LV pressures reveal an early, marked diastolic dip followed by a plateau ("dip and plateau" or "square root" sign) (Fig. 70-15). Pulmonary artery and RV systolic pressures are usually modestly elevated, in the 35 to 45 mm Hg range. Pulmonary hypertension is not a feature of constrictive pericarditis and is indicative of coexisting cardiac or pulmonary disease. Hypovolemia (e.g., secondary to diuretic therapy) can mask typical hemodynamic findings. Rapid volume challenge of 1000 ml of normal saline over 6 to 8 minutes may reveal the hemodynamic features of constrictive pericarditis.[57] Stroke volume is almost always reduced, but resting cardiac output can be preserved because of tachycardia. Depression of stroke volume is primarily related to reduced diastolic filling. In the absence of extensive coexisting myocardial involvement, LV ejection fraction is normal or slightly reduced.

Computed Tomography and Magnetic Resonance Imaging

CT (see Chapter 18) provides detailed images of the pericardium and is especially helpful in detecting even minute amounts of pericardial calcification (Fig. 70-16).[36,37] Its major disadvantage is the frequent need for iodinated contrast medium administration to best display findings of pericardial pathology. The thickness of the normal pericardium measured by CT is less than 2 mm. MRI[36,37] (see Chapter 17) provides a detailed and comprehensive examination of the pericardium without the need for iodinated contrast or ionizing radiation. It is somewhat less sensitive for detecting calcification than CT. The "normal" pericardium visualized by MRI has been reported to be up to 4 mm in thickness. This measurement most likely reflects the entire pericardial "complex," with physiological fluid representing a significant component of the measured thickness.

Demonstration of a thickened pericardium with or without calcification indicates acute and/or chronic pericarditis. If there is clinical evidence of impaired diastolic filling, pericardial thickening, especially if calcification is

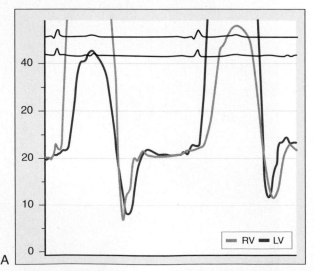

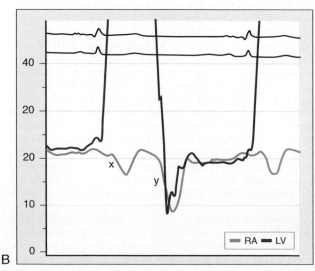

FIGURE 70–15 Pressure recordings in a patient with constrictive pericarditis. **A,** Simultaneous right ventricular (RV) and left ventricular (LV) pressure tracings with equalization of diastolic pressure, as well as "dip and plateau" morphology. **B,** Simultaneous right atrial (RA) and LV pressure with equalization of RA and LV diastolic pressure. The y descent is prominent. (*From Vaitkus PT, Cooper KA, Shuman WP, Hardin NJ: Images in cardiovascular medicine: Constrictive pericarditis. Circulation 93:834, 1996.*)

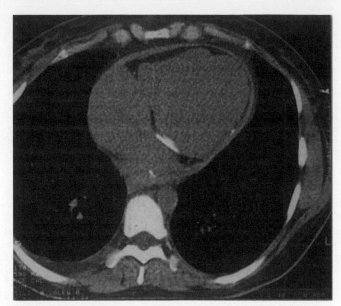

FIGURE 70–16 CT scan showing increased pericardial thickness and mild calcification in a patient with constrictive pericarditis.

TABLE 70–6	Hemodynamic and Echocardiographic Features of Constrictive Pericarditis Compared with Restrictive Cardiomyopathy	
	Constriction	**Restriction**
Prominent *y* descent in venous pressure	Present	Variable
Paradoxical pulse	≈$^1/_3$ cases	Absent
Pericardial knock	Present	Absent
Equal right-left side filling pressures	Present	Left at least 3-5 mm Hg > right
Filling pressures >25 mm Hg	Rare	Common
Pulmonary artery Systolic pressure >60 mm Hg	No	Common
"Square root" sign	Present	Variable
Respiratory variation in left-right pressures/flows	Exaggerated	Normal
Ventricular wall thickness	Normal	Usually increased
Atrial size	Possible LA enlargement	Biatrial enlargement
Septal "bounce"	Present	Absent
Tissue Doppler E′ velocity	Increased	Reduced
Pericardial thickness	Increased	Normal

present, is virtually diagnostic of constriction. Absence of pericardial thickening argues against the diagnosis of constriction but does not rule it out. The pericardium can be globally or focally thickened. Localized compression of the heart caused by focal thickening is reported and occurs much more commonly on the right than the left side. In patients being considered for pericardiectomy, detailed descriptions of the location and severity of thickening and calcification aid the surgeon with respect to both risk stratification and planning of surgery. Additional findings include distorted ventricular contours, hepatic venous congestion, ascites, pleural effusions, and occasionally pericardial effusion. Cine acquisition (MRI or CT) shows abnormal motion of the interventricular septum in early diastole. Finally, enhanced uptake of gadolinium appears useful for detection of pericardial inflammation.[58]

A cohort of patients with well-documented constriction yet no pericardial thickening at all based on measurements in pathological specimens, despite histologic evidence of chronic inflammation and calcification, has been reported. These patients constituted 18 percent of all those with constrictive pericarditis in a large Mayo Clinic series.[59] Almost all had normal pericardial thickness by CT. Calcification and distorted ventricular contours occurred in a majority, providing clues to the diagnosis despite normal thickness.

Differentiating Constrictive Pericarditis from Restrictive Cardiomyopathy

Because treatment is radically different, distinguishing constrictive pericarditis from restrictive cardiomyopathy is extremely important (Table 70-6). Their presentation and course overlap in many respects. An unequivocal pericardial knock points to constriction, but prominent third heart sounds in restrictive disease can confuse bedside differentiation. ECG and chest radiographic findings are mostly nonspecific. However, a calcified pericardium indicates constrictive pericarditis, whereas a low-voltage QRS suggests amyloidosis. Some useful echocardiographic distinctions can be made. Patients with restrictive cardiomyopathy usually have thick-walled ventricles caused by infiltrative processes such as amyloidosis. Marked biatrial enlargement

is also common in restriction. In constriction the most distinctive finding is the septal "bounce." As discussed earlier, the pericardium is usually thickened in constriction, but this may be difficult to assess with transthoracic echocardiography. As noted, transesophageal echocardiographic measurements of pericardial thickness correlate well with CT measurements,[55] although they are limited by their narrow field of view.

Doppler measurements are also useful in differentiating constrictive from restrictive physiology.[5,25,26,56] Enhanced respiratory variation in mitral inflow velocity (>25 percent) is seen in constriction, whereas in restriction mitral inflow velocity varies by less than 10 percent (see Fig. 70-13). In restriction, pulmonary venous systolic flow is markedly blunted and diastolic flow is increased. This is not observed in constriction. Hepatic veins demonstrate enhanced expiratory flow reversal with constriction, in contrast to increased inspiratory flow reversal in restriction. Tissue Doppler echocardiography and color M-mode flow propagation are complementary to mitral Doppler respiratory variation in distinguishing constriction from restrictive cardiomyopathy. Higher E′ values at the mitral annulus in constriction versus restrictive cardiomyopathy are reported to have a higher sensitivity for making the distinction than do mitral inflow parameters.[52,53]

Hemodynamic differentiation between constrictive pericarditis and restrictive cardiomyopathy in the cardiac catheterization laboratory can be difficult. However, careful attention to the hemodynamic profile usually makes the distinction (see Table 70-6). In both conditions, RV and LV diastolic pressures are markedly elevated. In restrictive cardiomyopathy, diastolic pressure in the left ventricle is usually higher than in the right ventricle by at least 3 to 5 mm Hg, whereas in constrictive pericarditis left- and right-sided diastolic pressures typically track closely and rarely differ by more than 3 to 5 mm Hg. Pulmonary hypertension is common with restrictive cardiomyopathy but rare in constrictive pericarditis. The absolute level of atrial or ventricular diastolic pressure elevation is also sometimes useful in distinguishing the two conditions, with extremely high pressures (>25 mm Hg) much more common in restrictive cardiomyopathy.[25,26]

CT and MRI, because of their superior ability to provide detailed assessment of pericardial thickness and calcification, are useful in differentiating constriction from restriction.[36,37] Patients in whom constriction is occasionally present with normal pericardial thickness have been discussed earlier. Detection of pericardial calcification or distorted ventricular contours is helpful in making the correct diagnosis in these patients. Endomyocardial biopsy (or abdominal fat pad biopsy in amyloidosis) is often helpful in documenting the etiology of restrictive cardiomyopathy. However, normal biopsy findings do not exclude it. In a small series brain natriuretic peptide levels differed markedly, being elevated in restrictive cardiomyopathy and normal in constriction.

Availability of the multiple diagnostic techniques discussed earlier has made it rare to have to resort to exploratory thoracotomy to distinguish constriction from restriction. In difficult cases it is important to obtain as much diagnostic information as possible.

Management

Constrictive pericarditis is a progressive disease. With the exception of patients with transient constrictive pericarditis, surgical pericardiectomy is the only definitive treatment. Transient constriction should be suspected in patients presenting relatively earlier after cardiac surgery or with relatively rapid development of symptoms. Such patients can be monitored for several months to look for spontaneous improvement. They may respond to a course of corticosteroids, and there is little to lose by managing them in this way. Patients with major comorbidities and/or severe debilitation are sometimes considered to be at too high risk to undergo pericardiectomy. Otherwise, surgery should not be delayed once the diagnosis is made. Medical management with diuretics and salt restriction is useful for relief of fluid overload and edema, but patients ultimately become refractory. Because sinus tachycardia is a compensatory mechanism, beta-adrenergic blockers and calcium antagonists that slow the heart rate should be avoided. In patients with atrial fibrillation and a rapid ventricular response, digoxin is recommended as initial treatment to slow the ventricular rate before resorting to beta blockers or calcium antagonists. In general, the rate should not be allowed to drop below 80 to 90 beats/min.

Pericardiectomy can be performed through either a median sternotomy or a left fifth interspace thoracotomy and involves radical excision of as much of the parietal pericardium as possible.[13] The visceral pericardium is then inspected. Resection should be considered if it is involved in the disease process. Most surgeons initially attempt to perform the operation without cardiopulmonary bypass. The latter should be available as back-up and is frequently required to assist access to the lateral and diaphragmatic surfaces of the LV and allow safe removal of a maximal amount of pericardial tissue. Ultrasonic or laser debridement[13,60] is useful as an adjunct to conventional surgical débridement or as the sole technique in high-risk patients with extensive, calcified adhesions between pericardium and epicardium.

Hemodynamic and symptomatic improvement is achieved in some patients immediately after operation. In others symptomatic improvement may be delayed for weeks to months. From 70 to 80 percent of patients remain free from adverse cardiovascular outcomes at 5 years, and 40 to 50 percent at 10 years after pericardiectomy.[61] Long-term results are worst in patients with radiation-induced disease, impaired renal function, relatively high pulmonary artery systolic pressure,

reduced LV ejection fraction, low serum sodium, and advanced age.[61,62] In an echocardiographic analysis, LV diastolic function returned to normal in 40 percent of patients early and 57 percent late after pericardiectomy.[63] Persistence of abnormal diastolic filling was correlated with postoperative symptomatic status. Delayed or inadequate responses to pericardiectomy have been attributed to long-standing disease with myocardial atrophy or fibrosis, incomplete pericardial resection, and the development of recurrent cardiac compression by mediastinal inflammation and fibrosis. Lack of improvement after pericardiectomy may also be caused by inadequate resection of visceral pericardium. Worsening of tricuspid regurgitation can also cause hemodynamic deterioration after pericardiectomy.

Pericardiectomy has a 5 to 15 percent perioperative mortality in patients with constrictive pericarditis. In the Cleveland Clinic series,[61] 63 percent of patients were alive after a median follow-up period of 6.9 years, but long-term results have been quite variable. Early mortality results primarily from low cardiac output, often in debilitated patients with prolonged cardiopulmonary bypass and difficult pericardial dissections. Sepsis, uncontrolled hemorrhage, and renal and respiratory insufficiency also contribute to early mortality.[61,62] The highest mortality occurs in patients with class III/IV preoperative symptoms, supporting our recommendation of early pericardiectomy.

EFFUSIVE-CONSTRICTIVE PERICARDITIS

A number of patients with pericardial disease present with a syndrome combining elements of effusion/tamponade and constriction. They often have a subacute course initially. An inflammatory effusion may dominate the picture early, with constrictive findings more prominent later. As noted previously, these patients are often identified when hemodynamics fail to normalize following pericardiocentesis. Sagrista-Sauleda and colleagues[42] defined effusive-constrictive pericarditis in this setting as a failure of the right atrial pressure to decline by at least 50 percent to a level below 10 mm Hg when the pericardial pressure was reduced to near 0 mm Hg by pericardiocentesis. In their series of patients at a referral center, 8 percent of those requiring pericardiocentesis met these criteria. Etiologies are diverse, but the most common are idiopathic, malignancy, radiation, and tuberculosis. Physical, hemodynamic, and echocardiographic findings are often mixtures of those associated with effusion and constriction and may vary with time as the syndrome progresses. Diagnosis may require acquisition of pericardial fluid and biopsies if the etiology is not obvious and tamponade does not mandate pericardiocentesis. Being cautious in the performance of closed pericardiocentesis in these patients is important if they do not have large effusions. Management is tailored to the specific etiology, if known. A common thread for these patients is that they often ultimately require pericardiectomy.

SPECIFIC CAUSES OF PERICARDIAL DISEASE

Viral Pericarditis

Etiology and Pathophysiology

Viral pericarditis is the most common form of pericardial infection.[13,14,64] It is caused by either direct damage resulting from viral replication or immune responses. Numerous viruses have been implicated (HIV is discussed separately later). Echo and Coxsackie viruses are the most common, and they track seasonal patterns of infection. Cytomegalovirus has a predilection for immunocompromised patients.

Other than identification of specific viral particles, the most definitive way to diagnose viral pericarditis is detection of DNA by PCR or in situ hybridization in pericardial fluid or tissue. As discussed earlier, this is rarely necessary for management.

Clinical Features and Management

These have been discussed earlier in conjunction with the syndrome of acute pericarditis. In patients with chronic, confirmed viral pericarditis, several immune-mediated treatments are under investigation,[13] but none have been shown to be effective to date.

Bacterial Pericarditis

Etiology and Pathophysiology

Bacterial pericarditis is usually characterized by a purulent effusion. A wide variety of organisms can be causative.[13,14,65,66] Direct extension from pneumonia or empyema accounts for a majority of cases. The most common agents are staphylococci, pneumococci, and streptococci. Hematogenous spread during bacteremia and contiguous spread after thoracic surgery or trauma are also important mechanisms. Hospital-acquired, penicillin-resistant staphylococcal pericarditis following thoracic surgery has been increasing. Anaerobic organisms are also increasing in frequency. Concomitant infection in the mediastinum, head, or neck is commonly associated with anaerobes.[66]

Bacterial pericarditis can also result from rupture of perivalvular abscesses into the pericardial space (see Chap. 63). Rarely, pericardial invasion spreads along facial planes from the oral cavity, particularly periodontal and peritonsillar abscesses. The pericardium can become infected in the course of meningococcal sepsis with or without concurrent meningitis. In contrast to the usual purulent fluid, Neisseria can evoke a sterile effusion accompanied by systemic reactions such as arthritis, pleuritis, and ophthalmitis. This does not require antibiotic therapy and responds to antiinflammatory drugs.

Clinical Features

The clinical presentation of bacterial pericarditis is usually high-grade fever with shaking chills and tachycardia, but these may be absent in debilitated patients. Patients may complain of dyspnea and chest pain. A pericardial friction rub is present in the majority. Bacterial pericarditis can take a fulminant course with rapid development of tamponade and may be unsuspected because associated illnesses such as severe pneumonia or mediastinitis following thoracic surgery dominate the clinical picture. Laboratory findings include leukocytosis with marked left shift. Pericardial fluid shows polymorphonuclear leukocytosis, low glucose, high protein, and elevated lactate dehydrogenase levels. Frank pus is occasionally drained. The chest radiograph shows widening of the cardiac silhouette if the effusion is large. With gas-producing organisms a lucent air fluid interface may be observed. The ECG shows typical ST segment and T wave changes of acute pericarditis, along with low voltage if there is a large effusion. Echocardiography almost always demonstrates a significant pericardial effusion with or without adhesions. Cardiac tamponade is common and can be confused with septic shock.

Management

Suspected or proven bacterial pericarditis should be considered a medical emergency, and prompt closed pericardiocentesis or surgical drainage performed.[13,14,65] We recommend at least 3 to 4 days of subsequent catheter drainage. The actual length is dependent on the volume and nature (i.e.,

purulence) of the fluid. Fluid should be Gram stained and cultured for aerobic and anaerobic bacteria with appropriate antibiotic sensitivity testing. Fungal and tuberculosis staining and cultures should also be performed. Blood, sputum, urine, and recent surgical wounds should all be cultured. Broad-spectrum antibiotics should be started promptly and then modified according to culture results. Anaerobic coverage is critical when pericarditis associated with head and neck infections is suspected.

Purulent pericardial effusions are likely to recur. Thus surgical drainage with construction of a window is often necessary. In patients with thick, purulent effusions and dense adhesions, extensive pericardiectomy may be required to achieve adequate drainage and prevent the development of constrictive pericarditis. Early surgical drainage may also help prevent late constriction. Intrapericardial streptokinase has been administered to selected patients with purulent and/or loculated effusions and may obviate the need for a window.[67] The prognosis of bacterial pericarditis is generally poor,[14,65,68] with survival in the range of 30 percent even in modern series.

Pericardial Disease and Human Immunodeficiency Virus (see Chap. 67)

Etiology and Pathophysiology

A wide variety of pericardial diseases have been reported in patients infected with the human immunodeficiency virus (HIV). An estimated 20 percent of HIV patients have pericardial involvement at some time. Pericardial disease is the most common cardiac manifestation of HIV, and the most common abnormality is an effusion.[69-71] Most are small; asymptomatic; and, in the developed world, idiopathic. Effusions may also be part of a generalized sero-effusive process involving pleural and peritoneal surfaces. This "capillary leak" syndrome is likely related to enhanced cytokine expression in the later stages of HIV disease. Moderate to large effusions are more frequent with more advanced stages of infection. Congestive heart failure, Kaposi sarcoma, tuberculosis, and other pulmonary infections are independently associated with moderate to large effusions, but most remain idiopathic. In some cases the HIV virus itself appears to be the etiology. Tuberculosis is the most common etiology of pericardial effusion in African HIV patients, in whom the disease is particularly aggressive.[72] Other less frequent forms of pericardial disease include involvement by various neoplasms, classic acute pericarditis, and myopericarditis. Constrictive pericarditis is rare. When present it is usually secondary to *Mycobacterium tuberculosis*.[69]

Clinical Features

Symptomatic patients with pericardial disease usually present with dyspnea or chest pain secondary to pericardial inflammation and/or a large effusion. Large, symptomatic effusions are often caused by infection or neoplasm. The most common infectious agents identified in symptomatic effusions are *M. tuberculosis* and *Mycobacterium avium-intracellulare*. However, a wide variety of organisms, often unusual, have been implicated including *Cryptococcus neoformans*, cytomegalovirus, and *Mycobacterium kansasii*. Lymphomas and Kaposi sarcoma are the most common neoplasms associated with effusion (see Chap. 69).

Management

Asymptomatic patients with small to moderate pericardial effusions do not require treatment. Most are idiopathic and usually remain asymptomatic or resolve spontaneously. Symptomatic, large effusions should be drained, and an identifiable cause sought. Even though they are often small and asymptomatic, pericardial effusion in HIV disease usually occurs in the context of or heralds the onset of full-blown acquired immune deficiency syndrome and is strongly associated with a shortened survival independent of CD4 count.[73] Six-month mortality for patients with pericardial effusion is ninefold greater than those without an effusion.[73] The impact of highly active antiretroviral therapy on HIV-related pericardial disease has not yet been described.

Tuberculous Pericarditis

Etiology and Pathophysiology

The incidence of pericardial tuberculosis has decreased markedly in the developed world in parallel with decreased pulmonary tuberculosis. Among patients with pulmonary tuberculosis, 1 to 8 percent develop pericardial involvement.[13,74] In a modern series of acute to subacute pericardial disease, tuberculosis was diagnosed in only 4 percent overall and in 7 percent of patients who developed cardiac tamponade. Similarly, tuberculosis was diagnosed in only 1 of 135 patients with constrictive pericarditis in a Mayo Clinic series. However, pericardial tuberculosis remains a major problem in immunocompromised hosts and the third world, especially Africa.[74] As discussed earlier, tuberculous pericarditis is by far the most common cause of pericardial disease in African HIV patients. Evidence of pericardial involvement in HIV patients in African countries where tuberculosis and HIV are endemic is usually sufficient to prompt antituberculous therapy.[74] Pericardial involvement by tuberculosis is usually secondary to retrograde spread from peribronchial, peritracheal, or mediastinal lymph nodes or hematogenous spread from the primary focus. Less commonly, the pericardium is involved by the breakdown and contiguous spread of a necrotic lesion in the lung.

Clinical Features

The clinical presentation of tuberculous pericarditis is usually subacute to chronic, with fever, malaise, and dyspnea in association with a pericardial effusion. Cough, night sweats, orthopnea, weight loss, and ankle edema are also common. The most frequent findings are radiographic cardiomegaly, pericardial rub, fever, and tachycardia. Findings related to large effusions, paradoxical pulse, hepatomegaly, increased venous pressure, pleural effusion, and distant heart sounds are common, as is severe hemodynamic compromise. Many patients are classified as having a subacute, effusive-constrictive syndrome, and a number develop late constrictive pericarditis despite antituberculous treatment.[42,74] Clinical evidence of pulmonary tuberculosis may be absent or subtle, one of the chief reasons the diagnosis is sometimes unsuspected.

Diagnosing tuberculous pericardial disease has been notoriously difficult.[1,13,47,64] A definitive diagnosis is made by isolating the organism from pericardial fluid or biopsy. However, the yield for isolation from pericardial fluid is low. In a series of 41 patients with subacute tuberculous pericarditis, *M. tuberculosis* grew in only 4 of 13 cultures of pericardial fluid.[75] The probability of making a diagnosis is increased if both pericardial fluid and biopsy specimens are examined early in the effusive stage of the disease. Thus there is a definite role for pericardial biopsy. Pericardial tissue reveals either granulomas or organisms in 80 to 90 percent of cases. The optimal diagnostic work-up (as well as management) of suspected tuberculous pericarditis includes a pericardial window with fluid and tissue sent for culture and histopathological examination. The presence of granulomas without bacilli in biopsy tissue is helpful but not diagnostic of tuberculous pericarditis because granulomas can be found in rheumatoid and sarcoid pericardial disease. A positive tuberculin skin test increases suspicion, but a negative test does not exclude the diagnosis, especially in immunocompromised hosts. A positive skin test is also less helpful in populations with a high endemic incidence of tuberculosis.

Measurement of adenosine deaminase (ADA), an enzyme produced by white blood cells in pericardial fluid, was the first modern test to markedly improve the accuracy and speed of diagnosis of tuberculous pericarditis.[13,47,74,75] ADA greater than 40 units/liter in pericardial fluid has a sensitivity and specificity greater than 90 percent. Increased interferon-gamma in pericardial fluid is an additional marker. Combined with ADA it provides even greater diagnostic accuracy. Most recently, PCR to detect *M. tuberculosis* DNA has been used and can be performed in minute amounts of pericardial fluid. Use of one or more of these modern tests should be routine whenever tuberculous pericarditis is suspected.

Management

The goals of therapy are to treat symptoms, as well as tamponade if present, and prevent the progression to constriction. Multidrug antimycobacterial treatment is mandatory and has greatly decreased mortality. The role of corticosteroids and the issue of open surgical drainage versus closed pericardiocentesis have been debated for some time. The largest study to address these issues was performed in South Africa and reported in 1988.[76] After initial evaluation, patients were randomly allocated to open biopsy and complete surgical drainage of fluid or percutaneous pericardiocentesis as needed. Patients were further randomized to receive or not receive prednisolone. All patients were treated with isoniazid, streptomycin, rifampin, and pyrazinamide. The outcomes suggested that patients who undergo open drainage are less likely to require repeat pericardiocentesis, and there was a trend in the open drainage group toward reduced development of constriction. Corticosteroids did not influence the risk of death or progression to constriction but did speed the resolution of symptoms and decrease reaccumulation of fluid. Subsequent meta-analyses[13] tend to support these conclusions, but individual studies have been inconclusive and there are no modern, appropriately powered, controlled trials of corticosteroid use. No studies have addressed the use of corticosteroids in HIV-positive patients with tuberculous pericarditis, in whom outcomes could well be different. If corticosteroids are administered, high doses (1 to 2 mg/kg/day with tapering over 6 to 8 weeks) are recommended[13] because rifampicin induces their hepatic metabolism. Because data are inconclusive, selection of closed versus open drainage and corticosteroid are based on clinical judgment. Finally, there is no rationale for the use of corticosteroids once established constriction is present.

FUNGAL PERICARDITIS

Etiology and Pathophysiology

Fungal infections can rarely cause pericarditis. They are mainly caused by locally endemic organisms such as *Histoplasma* or *Coccidioides* or opportunistic fungi such as *Candida* and *Aspergillus*.[13,64] Other fungi reported to cause pericardial disease include *Blastomyces*, *Cryptococcus*, and *Pneumocystis carinii*. Histoplasmosis is the most common. It is endemic in Ohio, the Mississippi River Valley, and the Western Appalachians; is acquired by inhalation; and can infect otherwise healthy patients living in endemic areas. Coccidiomycosis is endemic in the Southwest. The organism is acquired by inhalation of chlamydospores.[77] Immunocompromised patients and those taking corticosteroids or broad-spectrum antibiotics and drug addicts are at increased risk for opportunistic fungal pericarditis.

Clinical Features and Management

Pericardial histoplasmosis usually occurs in a previously healthy young patient and is thought to represent an inflammatory process in response to infection of adjacent mediastinal lymph nodes.[13,64] Accordingly, isolation of organisms from pericardial fluid is unusual. The fluid is serous, xanthochromic, or hemorrhagic. The disease usually begins with respiratory symptoms followed by pericardial pain. Effusion leading to tamponade occurs in almost half the cases. The diagnosis must be considered in endemic zones and is aided by rising complement fixation titers. Providing effusions are drained as needed; pericardial involvement eventually resolves with or without anti-inflammatory drugs. Antifungal agents are indicated only for disseminated histoplasmosis.

Coccidiomycosis pericarditis occurs as a complication of progressive, disseminated infection.[13,64,77] Patients are chronically ill and debilitated. Pericardial involvement does not occur in the self-limited influenza-like form of the infection. Physical findings suggestive of cardiac compression may be the first clues to the diagnosis. Treatment is directed at the disseminated infection with intravenous amphotericin B. Pericardiocentesis is of course indicated when tamponade occurs.

Pericarditis caused by opportunistic fungi such as *Candida* and *Aspergillus* usually occurs in patients who are immunosuppressed or receiving broad-spectrum antibiotics, as well as patients recovering from open heart surgery.[13,64] Pericardial involvement usually occurs in the setting of disseminated fungal infection. The prognosis is poor, and the diagnosis is often made at autopsy.

Uremic Pericarditis and Dialysis-Associated Pericardial Disease (see Chap. 88)

Etiology and Pathophysiology

The incidence of classic uremic pericarditis has decreased markedly since the introduction of widespread dialysis. Its pathophysiology has never been fully elucidated, but it is correlated with blood levels of blood urea nitrogen (BUN) and creatinine. Toxic metabolites, hypercalcemia, hyperuricemia, hemorrhagic, viral, and autoimmune mechanisms have all been proposed as etiological factors.[1,13,78] The acute or subacute phase is characterized by shaggy, hemorrhagic, fibrinous exudates on both parietal and visceral surfaces with minimal inflammatory cellular reaction. Subacute or chronic constriction may develop with organization of the effusion and formation of thick adhesions within the pericardial space. Large, gradually accumulating effusions are typical.

Dialysis-associated pericardial disease is now much more common than classic uremic pericarditis.[13,78] It is characterized by de novo appearance of pericardial disease in patients undergoing chronic dialysis, despite the fact that BUN and creatinine are normal or only mildly elevated. Its mechanism(s) and relation to classic uremic pericarditis are unclear. Small pericardial effusions are often caused by volume overload.

Clinical Features

In modern populations of dialysis patients, the clinical presentation is sometimes that of acute pericarditis with chest pain, fever, leukocytosis, and pericardial friction rub. Small, asymptomatic effusions are common. Alternatively, patients can present with a pericardial effusion causing hypotension during or after ultrafiltration (low-pressure tamponade). Although conventional cardiac tamponade with acute or subacute hemodynamic compromise can occur, the extremely large, asymptomatic effusions typical of classic uremic pericarditis are unusual today.

The ECG is usually not markedly affected and reflects a high incidence of associated abnormalities (LV hypertrophy, previous MI, electrolyte abnormalities). The chest radiograph may demonstrate cardiac enlargement related to myocardial dysfunction, volume overload, or pericardial effusion. Because asymptomatic effusions of small to moderate size are common, the presence of typical pericardial pain and/or a friction rub is necessary for the diagnosis of pericarditis.

Management

The management of classic uremic pericarditis is intensive hemodialysis and drainage in patients with effusions causing hemodynamic compromise.[1,13,64,78] Patients with symptomatic pericarditis almost always respond to intensi-

fication of dialysis. Heparin should be used cautiously during hemodialysis because of the possibility of causing hemorrhagic pericarditis with tamponade. Pericardial effusions without hemodynamic compromise usually resolve after several weeks of intensive hemodialysis.

Treatment of pericardial disease appearing de novo in patients on chronic dialysis is empirical.[13,64,78] Tamponade obviously requires drainage. In our experience, intensifying dialysis is variably beneficial, presumably because these patients are already receiving most of its benefits. Use of NSAIDs for pericardial pain is reasonable, but corticosteroids are probably ineffective. Experience with colchicine is scarce. A pericardial window may be required and is usually the most effective approach in patients with recurring effusions. For patients requiring drainage, instillation of a nonabsorbable corticosteroid in the pericardial space has been beneficial in small series of patients.

Early Post–Myocardial Infarction Pericarditis and Dressler Syndrome (see Chap. 50)

Etiology and Pathophysiology

Early post-MI pericarditis occurs during the first 1 to 3 days and no more than a week after the index event.[1,13] It is caused by transmural necrosis with inflammation affecting the adjacent visceral and parietal pericardium. Pericardial involvement is correlated with infarct size. Autopsy studies indicate that approximately 40 percent of patients with large, Q-wave MIs have pericardial inflammation. Thrombolysis and mechanical revascularization appear to have reduced the incidence of this form of pericarditis by at least 50 percent. The earlier revascularization is initiated, the lower the incidence of pericarditis.

Late pericarditis is characterized by pleuropericardial involvement with pericardial and/or pleural effusions.[1,13,64] The syndrome was initially described by Dressler and had an estimated incidence of 3 to 4 percent of MI patients. Its incidence appears to have also markedly diminished since the onset of reperfusion therapy. Dressler syndrome is believed to have an autoimmune etiology caused by sensitization to myocardial cells at the time of MI. Antimyocardial antibodies have been demonstrated. As noted earlier, Dressler syndrome is a polyserositis. In contrast to early post-MI pericarditis, inflammation is diffuse and not localized to the myocardial injury site.

Clinical Features

Most commonly, early post-MI pericarditis is asymptomatic and identified by auscultation of a rub, usually within 1 to 3 days after presentation. Rubs in this setting are notoriously evanescent. Many are monophasic (usually systolic) and can be confused with murmurs of mitral regurgitation or ventricular septal defect. Acute post-MI pericarditis virtually never causes tamponade by itself. However, tamponade occurs in association with LV free wall rupture. Because of its association with large MIs, early post-MI pericarditis should alert the clinician to this possibility, especially if an effusion is present. Symptomatic patients develop pleuritic chest pain within the above time frame. Distinguishing pericardial pain from recurrent ischemic discomfort is important. Ordinarily, this is not difficult on clinical grounds. However, the typical ECG changes of acute pericarditis are uncommon post-MI. Pericardial inflammation is localized to the infarcted area; hence ECG changes usually involve subtle re-elevation of the ST segment in originally involved leads. An atypical T-wave evolution consisting of persistent upright T waves or early normalization of inverted

T waves has also been described and appears to be highly sensitive for early post-MI pericarditis.

Dressler syndrome occurs as early as 1 week to a few months after acute MI. Symptoms include fever and pleuritic chest pain. The physical examination may reveal pleural and/or pericardial friction rubs. The chest radiograph may show a pleural effusion and/or enlargement of the cardiac silhouette, and the ECG often demonstrates ST elevation and T wave changes typical of acute pericarditis. Although pericardial effusions are common, tamponade is unusual.

Management

Although associated with large, transmural MIs, early post-MI pericarditis per se is almost invariably a benign process that does not appear to *independently* affect in-hospital mortality. Treatment is entirely symptomatic. Augmentation of the usual low-dose aspirin administered to MI patients (650 mg three to four times per day for 2 to 5 days) or acetaminophen is usually effective.[13,64] Corticosteroids and perhaps some non-aspirin NSAIDs interfere with conversion of an MI into a scar, resulting in greater wall thinning and a higher incidence of post-MI rupture.[13,26] Thus these drugs should be avoided. Because significant hemopericardium is extremely rare with early post-MI pericarditis and there is no evidence that heparin increases its risk, heparin administration need not be modified because of its presence. Virtually no cases of hemopericardium in patients with early post-MI pericarditis receiving anti-platelet regimens for percutaneous coronary interventions have been reported. Nonetheless, it seems prudent to administer these regimens with caution when pericarditis is present.

Although Dressler syndrome is a self-limited disorder, admission to hospital for observation and monitoring should be considered if there is a substantial pericardial effusion or, as is often the case, other conditions (e.g., pulmonary infarction) are also being considered. Aspirin or other NSAIDs are effective for symptomatic relief.[13,64] Colchicine is also likely effective. A short course of prednisone, 40 to 60 mg per day with a 7- to 10-day taper, can be used in patients not responding to the previously described treatment or for recurrent symptoms.

POSTPERICARDIOTOMY AND POSTCARDIAC INJURY PERICARDITIS (see Chap. 71)

Blunt or penetrating injury of the chest and heart with myocardial contusion can cause associated acute pericarditis (see Chap. 65). Pericarditis is rarely of clinical significance compared with other effects of the trauma. However, pericarditis can develop days to months following cardiac surgery, thoracotomy, or chest trauma. The pathogenesis of this syndrome is thought to involve production of antiheart antibodies in response to myocardial injury.[13] A systemic inflammatory response occurs and is characterized by low-grade fever, mild leukocytosis, and pleuropericardial inflammation with associated chest discomfort. The chest radiograph typically shows pleural effusions. A few patients demonstrate pulmonary infiltrates. The ECG reveals changes consistent with acute pericarditis in about 50 percent of cases. The echocardiogram usually shows a small to moderate pericardial effusion, but tamponade is rare. NSAIDs are first-line treatment, with an excellent response usually occurring within 48 hours of initiation. Colchicine is also likely effective. Treatment should be maintained for 2 to 3 weeks. Corticosteroid therapy is reserved for patients with unresponsive, severe, or recurrent symptoms.

RADIATION-INDUCED PERICARDITIS

Mediastinal and thoracic radiation is standard treatment for a variety of thoracic neoplasms. Hodgkin disease, non-Hodgkin lymphoma, and breast carcinoma are the most common neoplasms associated with radiation pericarditis (see Chaps. 63 and 83). Factors that influence pericardial injury include total dose delivered, the amount of cardiac silhouette exposed, the nature of the radiation source, and the duration and fractionation of therapy. The incidence of clinically evident pericarditis in conjunction with modern techniques of radiation delivery is approximately 2 percent.[13,64] However, the incidence can be as high as 20 percent when the entire pericardium is exposed.

Radiation pericarditis takes one of two forms: an acute illness with chest pain and fever or a delayed form of pericardial injury that can occur years after treatment. Self-limited, asymptomatic effusions are common soon after radiation, but tamponade is unusual. Late manifestations of radiation injury occur from about a year to up to 20 years after exposure. Patients can present with symptomatic pericarditis and effusion with or without cardiac compression or circulatory congestion caused by constrictive pericarditis. Effusions can evolve into constriction (i.e., an effusive-constrictive syndrome).

Radiation-induced pericarditis and effusion can be confused with malignant effusions. Malignant effusions are usually associated with other evidence of disease recurrence and metastases. Hypothyroidism induced by mediastinal radiation can also contribute to pericardial effusion. Pericardiocentesis with fluid analysis for malignant cells and thyroid function tests differentiate radiation-induced effusion from other etiologies. Large, symptomatic pericardial effusions may be drained either percutaneously or surgically. Recurrent pericardial effusions are usually best treated surgically with either a window or pericardiectomy. Pericardiectomy is the treatment of choice for patients with constrictive physiology. However, perioperative mortality in this group of patients is higher than with idiopathic constrictive pericarditis.

METASTATIC PERICARDIAL DISEASE (see Chap. 69)

Pericardial tumor implants are the usual cause of effusion in patients with known malignancies, although, as noted earlier, obstruction of lymphatic drainage by enlarged mediastinal nodes is occasionally observed.[1,13,28,64,79] Malignancy is a leading cause of cardiac tamponade in developed countries. Lung carcinoma is the most common, accounting for approximately 40 percent of malignant effusions, with breast carcinoma and lymphomas responsible for about another 40 percent. Gastrointestinal carcinoma, melanoma, and sarcomas are less common. With the advent of HIV disease, the incidence of Kaposi sarcoma and lymphomatous involvement of the pericardium have increased markedly.

Pericardial tumor implants can cause pericardial pain. However, the dominant feature is usually an effusion. Effusive-constrictive patterns are common. An asymptomatic, incidentally discovered pericardial effusion can be the presenting sign of pericardial involvement in patients with malignancies. However, most patients present with symptomatic effusions and/or tamponade. The ECG is variable but usually shows nonspecific T-wave abnormalities with low-voltage QRS. ST segment elevation is somewhat unusual but can occur. In addition to echocardiography, CT and MR imaging are useful in evaluating the extent of metastatic disease to the pericardium and adjacent structures.

In most cancer patients with effusions, it is important that metastatic involvement of the pericardium be confirmed by identification of malignant cells and/or tumor markers in pericardial fluid. This is because of occasional patients who have obstructed lymphatic drainage causing effusion, the possibility of confusion with radiation induced-disease, and the fact that other forms of pericardial disease can occur in patients who have cancer. However, there are many exceptions in which clinical judgment dictates that pericardial fluid need not be obtained, especially when effusions are not large and specific treatment (e.g., instillation of drugs in the pericardial space) is not being contemplated.

Evaluating the life expectancy of patients is essential before performing pericardiocentesis and choosing treatment modalities. In terminally ill patients, drainage of effusions should be performed only to relieve symptoms. However, patients with better prognoses deserve a more aggressive approach, which can be gratifying in a surprisingly large number. In many cases a single drainage will provide prolonged relief, as well as providing fluid for analysis. For this reason, this should be the initial step in most patients, with several days of drainage and careful attention to detection of reaccumulation. For recurrences and perhaps in some cases of a first effusion, intrapericardial instillation of tetracycline or chemotherapeutic agents has a reasonable record of success.[13] Cisplatin appears to be effective in treating pericardial involvement by lung adenocarcinoma.[80] Thiotepa[81] has a good record with a variety of malignancies. External beam radiation therapy is an option in patients with radiation sensitive tumors. A pericardial window or even complete surgical pericardiectomy should be considered in patients with recurrent effusions not responding to the previously mentioned measures who continue to have a good prognosis otherwise.[82]

PRIMARY PERICARDIAL TUMORS

A number of primary pericardial neoplasms have been reported. All are exceedingly rare. They include malignant mesotheliomas, fibrosarcomas, lymphangiomas, hemangiomas, teratomas, neurofibromas, and lipomas.[13,83] Because of their rarity, it is difficult to generalize about their clinical presentation and course. In general, they are locally invasive and/or compress cardiac structures or are detected from an abnormal cardiac silhouette on chest radiograph. Mesotheliomas and fibrosarcomas are lethal.[84] Others such as lipomas are benign. CT and MR imaging are helpful in delineating the anatomy of these tumors, but surgery is usually required for diagnosis and treatment.

AUTOIMMUNE AND DRUG-INDUCED
PERICARDIAL DISEASE (see Chap. 84)

Pericardial involvement can occur in virtually any autoimmune disease, but the bulk of clinically recognized cases occur in rheumatoid arthritis, SLE, and progressive systemic sclerosis (scleroderma).[13,64] In addition, many drugs have been reported to cause pericarditis as part of an autoimmune process. Maisch and colleagues[85] coined the general term *autoreactive pericarditis* when an autoimmune mechanism is thought to be involved as the cause of pericarditis. Assignment to this group is not dependent on establishing a specific diagnosis (e.g., SLE) but rather on an extensive evaluation including analysis of pericardial fluid that is designed to systematically exclude nonautoimmune etiologies. In a selected cohort, 32 percent of patients with pericardial effusion were found to have autoreactive pericarditis. Maisch and colleagues[85] advocate treatment of these patients with intrapericardial instillation of triamcinolone. However, theirs was not a controlled study, follow-up was relatively short, and a significant number of patients suffered transient Cushing syndrome. Thus the overall effectiveness of this approach is at present uncertain.

RHEUMATOID ARTHRITIS

Pericardial involvement is common in rheumatoid arthritis (see Chap. 84).[1,13,64] Older autopsy studies revealed pericardial inflammation in about 50 percent of patients. However, no contemporary pathological or clinical studies address the incidence of pericardial involvement. Clinically evident pericardial involvement is reported in up to 25 percent of rheumatoid arthritis patients. Patients can present with chest pain, fever, and dyspnea because of acute pericarditis, which usually occurs in conjunction with exacerbation of the underlying disease. Asymptomatic pericardial effusion or cardiac tamponade can also be presenting manifestations. Pericardial fluid is characterized by low glucose; neutrophilic leukocytosis; elevated titers of rheumatoid factor; low complement levels; and, rarely, high cholesterol concentration. Constrictive pericarditis also can occur as the result of long-standing pericardial inflammation. In patients with joint exacerbations, management of associated acute pericarditis or asymptomatic effusion is first and foremost the same as that employed to treat the exacerbation. Pericardial manifestations seem to respond well to high-dose aspirin or NSAIDs. Pericardial effusions causing cardiac tamponade should be drained both to treat tamponade and establish with confidence that there is no other etiology (e.g., infection) in patients who may be receiving immunosuppressive drugs. In general, the response to treatment of underlying disease exacerbations is too slow and uncertain to advocate a period of watchful waiting in the hope that large effusions will shrink. Recurrent tamponade or large effusions are good indications for a pericardial window. Therapy with colchicine has also been shown to be effective for recurrences.[13]

SYSTEMIC LUPUS ERYTHEMATOSUS

Pericarditis is the most common cardiovascular manifestation of SLE.[13,64] Acute pericarditis can be the first manifestation of the disease.[86] Approximately 40 percent of patients with SLE develop pericarditis at some time, usually in conjunction with an overall flare and involvement of other serosal surfaces. Typical patients present with pleuritic chest pain and low-grade fever.[87] Large effusions can occur but are unusual.[87] The ECG often shows typical findings of acute pericarditis. The chest radiograph may show enlargement of the cardiac silhouette if pericardial effusion is present, along with pleural effusions and often parenchymal infiltrates. Pericardial effusions have high protein and low glucose contents and a white blood cell count below 10,000/ml³. As with rheumatoid arthritis, it is important to exclude purulent, fungal, or tuberculous pericarditis because many patients are treated

with immunosuppressants. Most patients respond to corticosteroids and/or immunosuppressive therapy used to treat disease flares. Hemodynamic compromise secondary to cardiac tamponade is estimated to occur in up to 10 percent of patients with SLE.[86] Accordingly, we recommend hospitalization to monitor for hemodynamic complications until clinical stability is achieved. Closed drainage combined with corticosteroids is reported to have a good outcome in these patients.[13,86]

PROGRESSIVE SYSTEMIC SCLEROSIS (SCLERODERMA)

In progressive systemic sclerosis, approximately 10 percent of patients have acute pericarditis cases with chest pain and pericardial rub.[13,64] Pericardial involvement is found at autopsy in approximately 50 percent of patients. Pericardial effusion is detected by echocardiography in up to 40 percent. Most are small and asymptomatic, but occasionally large effusions occur. Late constrictive pericarditis has been described. Treatment of acute pericarditis in scleroderma patients is often unrewarding, with an unpredictable response to aspirin and NSAIDs. Although there is no published experience, colchicine should be considered. It is important to perform right heart catheterization in patients presenting with dyspnea or right heart failure to evaluate pulmonary vascular disease, which is relatively common and can be confused with pericardial involvement.

DRUG-INDUCED PERICARDITIS

The great majority of cases of drug-induced pericardial disease occur as a component of drug-induced SLE syndromes.[13] No recent studies of the epidemiology or cause of drug-induced SLE have been done, and the list of offending agents is long. Therefore it is difficult to generalize about current trends. Isoniazid and hydralazine are probably the most common current offenders. Large effusions, tamponade, and even constriction have been reported but are rare in drug-induced SLE pericarditis. In addition to drug cessation, management is dictated by the specific elements of the SLE syndrome present, as well as usual efforts aimed at detection and treatment of effusions. In rare cases, drug-induced pericarditis caused by agents such as penicillin and cromolyn have involved apparent eosinophilic hypersensitivity reactions without a SLE picture.

HEMOPERICARDIUM

Any form of chest trauma can cause hemopericardium (see Chap. 71).[13,64] Post-MI free wall rupture with hemopericardium occurs within several days of transmural MI and is discussed in Chapter 50. Hemopericardium caused by retrograde bleeding into the pericardial sac is an important complication and frequent cause of death in type I dissecting aortic aneurysm (see Chap. 56). These patients may also have the combination of acute volume overload caused by disruption of the aortic valve and tamponade without a paradoxical pulse.

Puncture of atrial or ventricular walls can occur during mitral valvuloplasty and is signaled by abrupt chest pain.[13,64] Tamponade commonly ensues and can occur rapidly or with a delayed course. It is usually managed with percutaneous drainage.

Tamponade is a rare but important complication of percutaneous coronary intervention (PCI)[88,89] (see Chap. 52). The incidence ranges from 0.1 to 0.6 percent and may have increased in the decade of the 1990s in relation to aggressive treatment of complex lesions with atherectomy and debulking devices and stiff and/or hydrophilic guidewires. With more modern equipment and experience, the incidence may be decreasing or at least stabilizing. Cardiac tamponade during PCI is almost always a result of coronary perforation. The clinical presentation is usually abrupt or rapidly progressive cardiac decompensation and severe hypotension, although occasionally it can be delayed and more insidious. The diagnosis of perforation is usually made by the angiographic appearance of extravasation of dye from the coronary circulation into the pericardial space. Loss of cardiac pulsation on fluoroscopy indicates that a significant pericardial effusion is present. Management of tamponade requires sealing the coronary perforation, pericardiocentesis, and reversal of anticoagulation.[13,88,89] If the perforation cannot be managed percutaneously, emergency surgery is indicated.

Pericardial effusion and tamponade can also occur as a complication of catheter-based arrhythmia procedures, especially atrial fibrillation ablations. The incidence is difficult to estimate, but in a recent series it was 1 percent for pulmonary vein isolation and 6 percent for linear ablation procedures.[90] Reduction of energy appears to reduce the incidence. Management is similar to that for coronary perforations.

THYROID-ASSOCIATED PERICARDIAL DISEASE (see Chap. 81)

Patients with severe hypothyroidism develop pericardial effusions in perhaps 25 to 35 percent of cases.[13,91] These can become quite large but rarely, if ever, cause tamponade. Classically, they have high concentrations of cholesterol. The effusions gradually resolve with thyroid replacement. Rarely, effusion can occur in hyperthyroidism.[92]

PERICARDIAL DISEASE IN PREGNANCY (see Chap. 77)

Small, clinically insignificant pericardial effusions are observed in approximately 40 percent of healthy pregnant women.[13,93] No evidence indicates that pregnancy per se influences the incidence, cause, or course of pericardial disease, and it is generally managed no differently than in nonpregnant patients. However, colchicine is contraindicated and pericardiocentesis should be performed only for effusions causing tamponade and/or if a treatable infectious etiology is suspected. Early during pregnancy, fluoroscopically guided pericardiocentesis should be avoided.

CONGENITAL ANOMALIES OF THE PERICARDIUM

Pericardial Cysts

Pericardial cysts are rare, benign congenital malformations.[13,83] They are usually fluid filled, located at the right costophrenic angle, and identified as an incidental finding on a chest radiograph. The diagnosis is usually confirmed by echocardiography. Management is conservative.

Congenital Absence of the Pericardium

Congenital absence of the pericardium is rare. Usually part or all of the left side of the parietal pericardium is absent, but partial absence of the right side has also been reported.[13,94] Partial absence of the left pericardium is often associated with other cardiac anomalies including atrial septal defect, bicuspid aortic valve, or pulmonary malformations. It is often symptomatic and may even allow herniation of portions of the heart through the defect and/or torsion of the great vessels, with potentially life-threatening hemodynamic consequences. Recurrent pulmonary infections are occasionally seen. Patients can present with chest pain, syncope, or even sudden death. The ECG typically reveals an incomplete right bundle branch block. Absence of all or most of the left pericardium results in a characteristic chest radiograph with a leftward shift of the cardiac silhouette, elongated left heart border, and radiolucent bands between the aortic knob and the main pulmonary artery and between the left diaphragm and the base of the heart. Echocardiography reveals paradoxical septal motion and RV enlargement. CT or MR imaging can be employed to establish a definitive diagnosis and elaborate the details of the defect. Pericardiectomy should ordinarily be advised to ameliorate symptoms and prevent herniation.

REFERENCES

Classics

1. Shabetai R: The Pericardium. New York, Grune & Stratton, 1981.
2. Ditchey R, Engler R, LeWinter M, et al: The role of the right heart in acute cardiac tamponade in dogs. Circ Res 48:701, 1981.
3. Singh S, Wann LS, Schuchard GH, et al: Right ventricular and right atrial collapse in patients with cardiac tamponade—a combined echocardiographic and hemodynamic study. Circulation 70:966, 1984.
4. LeWinter MM, Myhre EESP, Slinker BK: Influence of the pericardium and ventricular interaction on diastolic function. In Gaasch WH, LeWinter MM (eds): Heart Failure and Left Ventricular Diastolic Function. Philadelphia, Lea & Febiger, 1993, pp 103-117.
5. Hatle LK, Appleton CP, Popp RL: Differentiation of constrictive pericarditis and restrictive cardiomyopathy by Doppler echocardiography. Circulation 79:357,1989.

Anatomy and Physiology of the Pericardium

6. Johnson D (ed): The pericardium. In Standring S, et al (eds): Gray's Anatomy. St. Louis, Elsevier, 2005, pp 995-996.
7. Kostreva DR, Pontus SP: Pericardial mechanoreceptors with phrenic afferents. Am J Physiol 264:H1836, 1993.
8. Miyazaki T, Pride HP, Zipes DP: Prostaglandins in the pericardial fluid modulate neural regulation of cardiac electrophysiological properties. Circ Res 66:163, 1990.
9. Tischler M, Cooper K, LeWinter MM: Increased left ventricular volume and mass following coronary bypass surgery. A role for relief of pericardial constraint? Circulation 87:1921, 1993.

The Passive Role of the Normal Pericardium in Heart Disease

10. O'Rourke RA, Dell'Italia LJ: Diagnosis and management of right ventricular myocardial infarction. Curr Probl Cardiol 29:6, 2004.

Acute Pericarditis

11. Spodick DH: Acute pericarditis: current concepts and practice. JAMA 289:1150, 2003.
12. Lange RA, Hillis LD: Clinical practice. Acute pericarditis. N Engl J Med 351:2195, 2004.
13. Maisch B, Seferovic PM, Ristic AD, et al: Guidelines on the diagnosis and management of pericardial diseases executive summary; the Task Force on the Diagnosis and Management of Pericardial Diseases of the European Society of Cardiology. Eur Heart J 25:587, 2004.
14. Troughton RW, Asher CR, Klein AL: Pericarditis. Lancet 363:717, 2004.
15. Brady WJ, Perron AD, Martin ML, et al: Cause of ST-segment abnormality in ED chest pain patients. Am J Emerg Med 19:25, 2001.
16. Brandt RR, Filzmaier K, Hanrath P: Circulating cardiac troponin I in acute pericarditis. Am J Cardiol 87:1326, 2001.
17. Imazio M, Demichelis B, Cecchi E, et al: Cardiac troponin I in acute pericarditis. J Am Coll Cardiol 42:2144, 2003.
18. Imazio M, Demichelis B, Parrini I, et al: Management, risk factors, and outcomes in recurrent pericarditis. Am J Cardiol 96:736, 2005.
19. Imazio M, Demichelis B, Parrini I, et al: Day-hospital treatment of acute pericarditis: A management program for outpatient therapy. J Am Coll Cardiol 43:1042, 2004.
20. Imazio M, Bobbio M, Cecchi E, et al: Colchicine as first-choice therapy for recurrent pericarditis: Results of the CORE (COlchicine for REcurrent pericarditis) trial. Arch Intern Med 165:1987, 2005.
21. Imazio M, Bobbio M, Cecchi E, et al: Colchicine in addition to conventional therapy for acute pericarditis: Results of the COlchicine for acute PEricarditis (COPE) trial. Circulation 112:2012, 2005.
22. Artom G, Koren-Morag N, Spodick DH, et al: Pretreatment with corticosteroids attenuates the efficacy of colchicine in preventing recurrent pericarditis: A multicentre all-case analysis. Eur Heart J 26:723, 2005.
23. Marcolongo R, Russo R, Laveder F, et al: Immunosuppressive therapy prevents recurrent pericarditis. J Am Coll Cardiol 26:1276, 1995.
24. Peterlana D, Puccetti A, Simeoni S, et al: Efficacy of intravenous immunoglobulin in chronic idiopathic pericarditis: Report of four cases. Clin Rheumatol 24:18, 2005.

Pericardial Effusion and Tamponade

25. Hoit BD: Management of effusive and constrictive pericardial heart disease. Circulation 105:2939, 2002.
26. Little WC, Freeman GL: Pericardial disease. Circulation 113:1622, 2006.
27. Goland S, Caspi A, Malnick S, et al: Idiopathic chronic pericardial effusion. N Engl J Med 342:1449, 2000.
28. Ben-Horin S, Bank I, Guetta V, Livneh A: Large symptomatic pericardial effusion as the presentation of unrecognized cancer: A study in 173 consecutive patients undergoing pericardiocentesis. Medicine (Baltimore) 85:49, 2006.
29. Spodick DM: Acute cardiac tamponade. N Engl J Med 349:684, 2003.
30. Fowler NO, Gabel M: Regional cardiac tamponade: A hemodynamic study. J Am Coll Cardiol 10:164, 1987.
31. Kuvin JT, Harati NA, Pandian NG, et al: Postoperative cardiac tamponade in the modern surgical era. Ann Thorac Surg 74:1148, 2002.
32. Sadaniantz A, Anastacio R, Verma V, Aprahamian N: The incidence of diastolic right atrial collapse in patients with pleural effusion in the absence of pericardial effusion. Echocardiography 20:211, 2003.
33. Kopterides P, Lignos M, Papanikolaou S, et al: Pleural effusion causing cardiac tamponade: Report of two cases and review of the literature. Heart Lung 35:66, 2006.
34. Krantz MJ, Lee JK, Spodick DH: Repetitive yawning associated with cardiac tamponade. Am J Cardiol 94:701, 2004.
35. Merce J, Sagrista-Sauleda J, Permanyer-Miralda G, et al: Correlation between clinical and Doppler echocardiographic findings in patients with moderate and large pericardial effusion: Implications for the diagnosis of cardiac tamponade. Am Heart J 138:759, 1999.
36. Wang ZJ, Reddy GP, Gotway MB, et al: CT and MR imaging of pericardial disease. Radiographics 23:S167-80, 2003.
37. Oyama N, Oyama N, Komuro K, et al: Computed tomography and magnetic resonance imaging of the pericardium: Anatomy and pathology. Magn Res Med Sci 3:145, 2004.
38. Merce J, Sagrista-Sauleda J, Permanyer-Miralda G, et al: Should pericardial drainage be performed routinely in patients who have a large pericardial effusion without tamponade? Am J Med 105:106, 1998.
39. Tsang TS, Barnes ME, Gersh BJ, et al: Outcomes of clinically significant idiopathic pericardial effusion requiring intervention. Am J Cardiol 91:704, 2003.
40. Adler Y, Finkelstein Y, Guindo J, et al: Colchicine treatment for recurrent pericarditis: A decade of experience. Circulation 97:2183, 1998.
41. Tsang TS, Enriquez-Sarano M, Freeman WK, et al: 1127 consecutive therapeutic echocardiographically guided pericardiocentesis: Clinical profile, practice patterns, and outcomes spanning 21 years. Mayo Clin Proc 77:429, 2002.
42. Sagrista-Sauleda J, Angel J, Sanchez A, et al: Effusive-constrictive pericarditis. N Engl J Med 350:469, 2004.
43. Wang HJ, Hsu KL, Chiang FT, et al: Technical and prognostic outcomes of double-balloon pericardiotomy for large malignancy-related pericardial effusions. Chest 122:893, 2002.
44. Del Barrio LG, Morales JH, Delgado C, et al: Percutaneous balloon window for patients with symptomatic pericardial effusion. Cardiovasc Intervent Radiol 25:360, 2002.

45. Ben-Horin S, Shinfeld A, Kachel E, et al: The composition of normal pericardial fluid and its implications for diagnosing pericardial effusions. Am J Med 118:636, 2005.
46. Burgess LJ, Reuter H, Carstens ME, et al: The use of adenosine deaminase and interferon-gamma as diagnostic tools for tuberculous pericarditis. Chest 122:900, 2002.
47. Permanyer-Miralda G: Acute pericardial disease: approach to the aetiologic diagnosis. Heart 90:252, 2004.
48. Mayosi BM, Burgess LJ, Doubell AF: Tuberculous pericarditis. Circulation 112:3608, 2005.
49. Seferovic PM, Ristic AD, Maksimovic R, et al: Diagnostic value of pericardial biopsy: Improvement with extensive sampling enabled by pericardioscopy. Circulation 107:978, 2003.

Constrictive Pericarditis

50. Haley JH, Tajik AJ, Danielson GK, et al: Transient constrictive pericarditis: Causes and natural history. J Am Coll Cardiol 43:271, 2004.
51. Leya FS, Arab D, Joyal D, et al: The efficacy of brain natriuretic peptide levels in differentiating constrictive pericarditis from restrictive cardiomyopathy. J Am Coll Cardiol 45:1900, 2005.
52. Rajagopalan N, Garcia MJ, Rodriguez L, et al: Comparison of new Doppler echocardiographic methods to differentiate constrictive pericardial heart disease and restrictive cardiomyopathy. Am J Cardiol 87:86, 2001.
53. Ha JW, Ommen SR, Tajik AJ, et al: Differentiation of constrictive pericarditis from restrictive cardiomyopathy using mitral annular velocity by tissue Doppler echocardiography. Am J Cardiol 94:316, 2004.
54. Sengupta PP, Mohan JC, Mehta V, et al: Doppler tissue imaging improves assessment of abnormal interventricular septal and posterior wall motion in constrictive pericarditis. J Am Soc Echocardiogr 18:226, 2005.
55. Izumi C, Iga K, Sekiguchi K, et al: Usefulness of the transgastric view by transesophageal echocardiography in evaluating thickened pericardium in patients with constrictive pericarditis. J Am Soc Echocardiog 15:1004, 2002.
56. Tabata T, Kabbani S, Murray RD, et al: Differences in the respiratory variation between pulmonary venous and mitral inflow Doppler velocities in patients with constrictive pericarditis with and without atrial fibrillation. J Am Coll Cardiol 37:1936, 2001.
57. Abdalla IA, Murray RD, Lee JC, et al: Does rapid volume loading during transesophageal echocardiography differentiate constrictive pericarditis from restrictive cardiomyopathy? Echocardiography 19:125, 2002.
58. Taylor AM, Dymarkowski S, Verbeken EK, Bogaert J: Detection of pericardial inflammation with late-enhancement cardiac magnetic resonance imaging: initial results. Eur Radiol 16:569, 2006.
59. Talreja DR, Edwards WD, Danielson GK, et al: Constrictive pericarditis in 26 patients with histologically normal pericardial thickness. Circulation 108:1852, 2003.
60. Hirai S, Hamanaka Y, Mitsui N, et al: Surgical treatment of chronic constrictive pericarditis using an ultrasonic scalpel. Ann Thorac Cardiovasc Surg 11:204, 2005.
61. Ling LH, Oh JK, Schaff HV, et al: Constrictive pericarditis in the modern era: Evolving clinical spectrum and impact on outcome after pericardiectomy. Circulation 100:1380, 1999.
62. Bertog SC, Thambidorai SK, Parakh K, et al: Constrictive pericarditis: Etiology and cause-specific survival after pericardiectomy. J Am Coll Cardiol 43:1445, 2004.
63. Trotter MC, Chung KC, Ochsner JL, McFadden PM: Pericardiectomy for pericardial constriction. Am Surg 62:304, 1996.

Specific Causes of Pericardial Disease

64. Maisch B, Ristic AD: Practical aspects of the management of pericardial disease. Heart 89:1096, 2003.
65. Sagrista-Sauleda J, Barrabes JA, Permanyer-Miralda G, Soler-Soler J: Purulent pericarditis; review of a 20-year experience in a general hospital. J Am Coll Cardiol 22:1661, 1993.
66. Brook I: Pericarditis due to anaerobic bacteria. Cardiology 97:55, 2002.
67. Tomkowski WZ, Gralec R, Kuca P, et al: Effectiveness of intrapericardial administration of streptokinase in purulent pericarditis. Herz 29:802, 2004.

68. Keersmaekers T, Elshot SR, Sergeant PT: Primary bacterial pericarditis. Acta Cardiol 57:387, 2002.
69. Silva-Cardoso J, Moura B, Martins L, et al: Pericardial involvement in Human Immunodeficiency Virus infection. Chest 115:418, 1999.
70. Barbaro G: Pathogenesis of HIV-associated cardiovascular disease. Adv Cardiol 40:49, 2003.
71. Gowda RM, Khan IA, Mehta NJ, et al: Cardiac tamponade in patients with human immunodeficiency virus disease. Angiology 54:469, 2003.
72. Ntsekhe M, Hakim J: Impact of human immunodeficiency virus infection on cardiovascular disease in Africa. Circulation 112:3602, 2005.
73. Heidenreich P, Eisenberg M, Keel L, et al: Pericardial effusion in AIDS: Incidence and survival. Circulation 92:3229, 1995.
74. Mayosi BM, Burgess LJ, Doubell AF: Tuberculous pericarditis. Circulation 112:3608, 2005.
75. Barbara W, Trautner O, Rabih O: Tuberculous pericarditis: Optimal diagnosis and management. Clin Infectious Dis 33:954, 2001.
76. Strang JI, Kakaza HHS, Gibson DG, et al: Controlled clinical trial of complete open surgical drainage and of prednisolone in treatment of tuberculous pericardial effusion in Transkei. Lancet 2:759, 1988.
77. Arsura EL, Bobba RK, Reddy CM: Coccidioidal pericarditis. Int J Infect Dis 10:86, 2006.
78. Alpert MA, Ravenscraft MD: Pericardial involvement in end-stage renal disease. Am J Med Sci 325:228, 2003.
79. Imazio M, Demichelis B, Parrini I, et al: Relation of acute pericardial disease to malignancy. Am J Cardiol 95:1393, 2005.
80. Bischiniotis TS, Lafaras CT, Platogiannis DN, et al: Intrapericardial cisplatin administration after pericardiocentesis in patients with lung adenocarcinoma and malignant cardiac tamponade. Hellenic J Cardiol 46:324, 2005.
81. Martinoni A, Cipolla CM, Cardinale D, et al: Long-term results of intrapericardial chemotherapeutic treatment of malignant pericardial effusions with thiotepa. Chest 126:1412, 2004.
82. Frankel KM: Treating malignancy-related effusions. Chest 123:1775, 2003.
83. Duwe BV, Sterman DH, Musani AI: Tumors of the mediastinum. Chest 128:2893, 2005.
84. Eren NT, Akar AR: Primary pericardial mesothelioma. Curr Treat Option Oncol 5:369, 2002.
85. Maisch B, Ristic AD, Pankuweit S: Intrapericardial treatment of autoreactive pericardial effusion with triamcinolone; the way to avoid side effects of systemic corticosteroid therapy. Eur Heart J 23:1503, 2002.
86. Kahl LE: The spectrum of pericardial tamponade in systemic lupus erythematosus. Arthritis Rheum 35:1343, 1992.
87. Weich HS, Burgess LJ, Reuter H: Large pericardial effusions due to systemic lupus erythematosus: A report of eight cases. Lupus 14:450, 2005.
88. Fasseas P, Orford JL, Panetta CJ, et al: Incidence, correlates, management, and clinical outcome of coronary perforation: Analysis of 16,298 procedures. Am Heart J 147:140, 2004.
89. Witzke CF, Martin-Herrero F, Clarke SC, et al: The changing pattern of coronary perforation during percutaneous coronary intervention in the new device era. J Invasive Cardiol 16:257, 2004.
90. Hsu LF, Jais P, Hocini M, et al: Incidence and prevention of cardiac tamponade complicating ablation for atrial fibrillation. Pacing Clin Electrophysiol 28(Suppl 1): S106, 2005.
91. Kabadi UM, Kumar SP: Pericardial effusion in primary hypothyroidism. Am Heart J 120:1393, 1990.
92. Nakata A, Komiya R, Ieki Y, et al: A patient with Graves' disease accompanied by bloody pericardial effusion. Intern Med 44:1064, 2005.
93. Ristic AD, Seferovic PM, Ljubic A, et al: Pericardial disease in pregnancy. Herz 28:209,2003.
94. Nasser WK, Helman C, Tavel ME, et al: Congenital absence of the left pericardium. Clinical, electrocardiographic, radiograph, hemodynamic, and angiographic findings in six cases. Circulation 41:469, 1970.

CH 70

Pericardial Diseases

CHAPTER 71

Incidence, 1855

Etiology and Patterns of Cardiac
Trauma, 1855
Penetrating Cardiac Trauma, 1855
Blunt Cardiac Trauma, 1855
Iatrogenic Cardiac Injury, 1856
Intracardiac Foreign Bodies/
    Missiles, 1856
Metabolic
    Cardiac Injury/Burns, 1856
Electrical Injury, 1857

Clinical Presentation and
Pathophysiology, 1857
Penetrating Cardiac Trauma, 1857
Blunt Cardiac Trauma, 1857
Pericardial Trauma, 1858

Evaluation, 1858
Prehospital/Emergency
    Department, 1858
FAST/Ultrasonography/
    Echocardiography, 1858
Subxiphoid Pericardial Window/
    Pericardiocentesis, 1858

Evaluation of Blunt Cardiac
Injury, 1859
Electrocardiography, 1859
Cardiac Enzymes, 1859
Echocardiography, 1859

Treatment, 1859
Prehospital/Emergency
    Department, 1859
Definitive Treatment, 1859
Results, 1860
Complications, 1860
Follow-up, 1860

References, 1862

Traumatic Heart Disease

Matthew J. Wall, Jr., Danny Chu, and Kenneth L. Mattox

INCIDENCE

Trauma is the fourth leading cause of death in the United States, particularly in persons younger than 40 years of age. Thoracic trauma is responsible for 25 percent of the deaths from vehicular accidents. The actual incidence of cardiac injury is unknown because of the diverse causes and classifications. Cardiac injury may account for 10 percent of deaths from gunshot wounds.[1] Penetrating cardiac trauma is a highly lethal injury, with relatively few victims surviving long enough to reach the hospital. In a series of 1198 patients with penetrating cardiac injuries in South Africa, only 6 percent of patients reached the hospital with any signs of life.[2] With improvements in organized emergency medical transport systems, up to 45 percent of those who sustain significant heart injury may reach the emergency department.

Blunt cardiac injuries have been reported less frequently than penetrating injuries.[1,3,4] However, 10 to 70 percent of motor vehicle fatalities may have been the result of blunt cardiac rupture.

ETIOLOGY AND PATTERNS OF CARDIAC TRAUMA

Traumatic heart disease is categorized on the basis of the mechanism of injury (Table 71-1).

Penetrating Cardiac Trauma

Penetrating trauma is the most common cause of significant cardiac injury seen in the hospital setting, with the predominant etiology being from guns and knives.[5-7] Other mechanisms such as shotguns, ice picks, and fence post impalement have also been reported.

The location of injury to the heart often correlates with the location of injury on the chest wall. Because of anterior location, the anatomical chambers at greatest risk for injury are the right and left ventricles. A review of 711 patients with penetrating cardiac trauma reported 54 percent sustained stab wounds and 42 percent had gunshot wounds. The right ventricle was injured in 40 percent of the cases, the left ventricle in 40 percent, the right atrium in 24 percent, and the left atrium in 3 percent. One third of cardiac injuries involved multiple cardiac structures.[6] Significant intracardiac injuries involved the coronary arteries ($n = 39$), valvular apparatus (mitral) ($n = 2$), intracardiac fistulas (i.e., ventricular septal defects [VSDs]) ($n = 14$), and unusual injuries ($n = 10$). Only 2 percent of patients surviving the initial injury and undergoing an operation required reoperation for a residual defect, and the majority of these repairs were performed on a semielective basis.[6]

Blunt Cardiac Trauma

Nonpenetrating or *blunt cardiac trauma* has replaced the term "cardiac contusion" and describes injury ranging from minor bruises of the myocardium to cardiac rupture. It can be caused by direct energy transfer to the heart or compression of the heart between the sternum and the vertebral column at the time of the accident. It can even include cardiac contusion and cardiac rupture during external cardiac massage as part of cardiopulmonary resuscitation (CPR). Within this spectrum, blunt cardiac injuries can manifest as free septal rupture, free wall rupture, coronary artery thrombosis, cardiac failure, complex and simple dysrhythmias, and/or rupture of chordae tendineae or papillary muscles.[3] The incidence can be as high as three fourths of the patients with severe bodily trauma. Mechanisms include motor vehicle accidents, vehicular-pedestrian accidents, falls, crush injuries, blasts, assaults, CPR, and recreational events. Such injury is often associated with sternal or rib fractures. In one report a fatal cardiac dysrhythmia occurred when the sternum was struck by a baseball,[8] which may be a form of commotio cordis.[9]

Cardiac rupture carries a significant risk of mortality. The biomechanics of cardiac rupture include direct transmission of increased intrathoracic pressure to the chambers of the heart; hydraulic effect from a large force applied to the abdominal or extremity veins, causing force to be transmitted to the right atrium; decelerating force between fixed and mobile areas, which explains atriocaval tears; myocardial contusion, necrosis, and delayed rupture; and penetration from a broken rib or fractured sternum.[1,10]

Blunt rupture of the cardiac septum occurs most frequently in late diastole or early systole near the apex of the heart. Multiple ruptures and disruption of the conduction system have been reported.[4] From autopsy data, blunt cardiac trauma with ventricular rupture most often

TABLE 71–1	Etiology of Traumatic Heart Diseases

I. Penetrating
  A. Stab wounds—knives, swords, ice picks, fence posts, wire, sports
  B. Gunshot wounds—handguns, rifles, nail guns, lawnmower projectiles
  C. Shotgun wounds—Close range versus distant

II. Nonpenetrating (blunt)
  A. Motor vehicle accident
    1. Seat belt
    2. Air bag
  B. Vehicular-pedestrian accident
  C. Falls from height
  D. Crushing—industrial accident
  E. Blasts—explosives, grenades
  F. Assault (aggravated)
  G. Sternal or rib fractures
  H. Recreational—sporting events, rodeo, baseball

III. Iatrogenic
  A. Catheter induced
  B. Pericardiocentesis induced

IV. Metabolic
  A. Traumatic response to injury
  B. "Stunning"
  C. Systemic inflammatory response syndrome

V. Others
  A. Burn
  B. Electrical
  C. Factitious—needles, foreign bodies
  D. Embolic—missiles

involves the left ventricle, followed by the right ventricle, and, least often, the left atrium. Ventricular septal defect (VSD) can occur, with the most common tear involving both the membranous and the muscular portions of the septum. Injury to only the membranous portion of the septum is the least common blunt VSD. Traumatic rupture of the thoracic aorta is associated with lethal cardiac rupture in almost 25 percent of cases.[11] Blunt pericardial rupture results from pericardial tears secondary to increased intraabdominal pressure or lateral decelerative forces. Tears can occur on the left side, most often parallel to the phrenic nerve; to the right of the pleuropericardium; to the diaphragmatic surface of the pericardium; and finally to the mediastinum. Cardiac herniation with cardiac dysfunction can occur in conjunction with these tears. The heart can be displaced into either pleural cavity or even into the peritoneum. In the instance of right pericardial rupture, the heart can become torsed, leading to the surprising discovery of an "empty" pericardial cavity at resuscitative left anterolateral thoracotomy. With a left-sided cardiac herniation through a pericardial tear, a distending heart prevents the heart from returning to the pericardium and the term *strangulated heart* has been applied. Venous filling is impaired, and unless the cardiac herniation is reduced, hypotension and cardiac arrest can occur.[12]

Iatrogenic Cardiac Injury

Iatrogenic cardiac injury can occur with central venous line insertion, cardiac catheterization procedures, and pericardiocentesis. Cardiac injuries caused by central venous lines usually occur with placement from either the left subclavian or the left internal jugular vein.[13] Perforation causing tamponade has also been reported with a right internal jugular introducer sheath for transjugular intrahepatic portocaval shunts. Vigorous insertion of left-sided central lines,

especially during dilation of the line tract, can lead to cardiac perforations. Even appropriate technique carries a discrete rate of iatrogenic injury secondary to central venous catheterization. Common sites of cardiac injury include the superior vena caval–atrial junction and the superior vena cava–innominate junction. These small perforations often lead to a compensated cardiac tamponade. Drainage by pericardiocentesis is often unsuccessful, and evacuation via subxiphoid pericardial window or full median sternotomy is sometimes required. Once access to the pericardial space is gained, the site of injury has often sealed and may be difficult to find.

Complications from coronary catheterization including perforation of the coronary arteries, cardiac perforation, and aortic dissection can be catastrophic and require emergency surgical intervention. The incidence of coronary perforation with balloon angioplasty is estimated to be 0.1 to 0.2 percent, but with advanced interventional techniques (e.g., rotablation, directional atherectomy, coronary artery stenting, and laser ablation), the incidence may be as high as 3 percent.[14]

Other potential iatrogenic causes of cardiac injury include external and internal cardiac massage, right ventricular injury during pericardiocentesis, and intracardiac injections.[15]

Intracardiac Foreign Bodies/Missiles

Intrapericardial and intracardiac foreign bodies can cause complications of acute suppurative pericarditis, chronic constrictive pericarditis, foreign body reaction, and hemopericardium.[16] Intrapericardial foreign bodies that have been reported to result in complications include bullets, hand grenades, shrapnel, knitting needles, and hypodermic needles. Needles and similar foreign bodies have been noted after deliberate insertion by patients, usually those with psychiatric diagnoses. A report by LeMaire and colleagues[16] advocated removal of those intrapericardial foreign bodies that are greater than 1 cm in size, that are contaminated, or that produce symptoms.

Intracardiac missiles are foreign bodies that are embedded in the myocardium, retained in the trabeculations of the endocardial surface, or free in a cardiac chamber. These are the result of direct penetrating thoracic injury or injury to a peripheral venous structure with embolization to the heart. Location and other conditions determine the type of complications that can occur and the treatment required. Observation might be considered when the missile is right sided, embedded completely in the wall, contained within a fibrous covering, not contaminated, and producing no symptoms. Right-sided missiles can embolize to the lung, at which point they can be removed if large. In rare cases they can embolize "paradoxically" through a patent foramen ovale or atrial septal defect.[17] Left-sided missiles can manifest as systemic embolization shortly after the initial injury. Diagnosis is pursued with radiographs in two projections, fluoroscopy, echocardiography, or angiography. Treatment of retained missiles is individualized. Removal is recommended for missiles that are left sided, larger than 1 to 2 cm, rough in shape, or that produce symptoms.[17] Although a direct approach, either with or without cardiopulmonary bypass, has been advocated in the past, a large percentage of right-sided foreign bodies can now be removed by interventional radiologists.

Metabolic Cardiac Injury/Burns

Metabolic cardiac injury refers to cardiac dysfunction in response to traumatic injury and may be associated with injuries caused by burns, electrical injury, sepsis, the systemic inflammatory response syndrome, and multisystem trauma.[18-20] The exact mechanism responsible for this dysfunction is unclear, but responses to trauma can induce a release of cytokines that may have a direct effect on the myocardium. Endotoxin; tumor necrosis factor-alpha; tumor necrosis factor-beta; interleukin-1; interleukin-6; interleukin-10; catecholamines (epinephrine, norepinephrine); cell-adhesion molecules; and nitric oxide are all possible responsible mediators.[21-23]

Metabolic cardiac injury can manifest clinically as conduction disturbances or decreased contractility leading to decreased output. Myocardial depression can occur in response to the mediator storm and can alter calcium utilization and depression of the myocyte responsiveness to beta-adrenergic stimulation.[24-25] Myocytes have altered calcium utilization in patients with injuries from burns. The activation of constitutive nitric oxide synthase can modulate cardiac responsiveness to cholinergic and adrenergic stimulation, and production of inducible nitric oxide synthase can depress myocyte contractile responsiveness to beta-adrenergic agonists. The myocardial depressive effects appear to be reversible.[20]

Treatment of metabolic cardiac injury has been supportive, with correction of the initiating insults, but some practitioners have attempted to address the involved mediators using intravenous milrinone, corticosteroids, arginine, granulocyte-macrophage colony-stimulating factor, and glutamate.[24-26] Use of an intraaortic counterpulsation balloon pump can be considered to treat such myocardial depression, but controlled series do not exist to test this hypothesis.

Cardiac complications in the early postburn period are a major cause of death. The initial cardiovascular effect of burn injury is attributable to the profound reduction in cardiac output that can occur within minutes of the injury. The overall cardiac response has been described as an ebb and flow pattern, with the initial ebb phase lasting between 1 and 3 days marked by hypovolemia and myocardial depression and the flow phase characterized by a prolonged period of increased metabolic demand with increased cardiac output and peripheral blood flow. The reduction in cardiac output observed in the initial period of burn injury is the result of a dramatic and rapid decrease in intravascular volume and of direct myocardial depression. Hypovolemia results from the capillary leak caused by endothelial injury and may be mediated by platelet-activating factor, complement, cytokines, arachidonic acid, or oxygen free radicals. Myocardial depression manifested by a decrease in myocardial contractility and abnormalities in ventricular compliance becomes apparent with a total body surface area burn of 20 to 25 percent. Myocardial-depressant factor, tumor necrosis factor, vasopressin, oxygen free radicals, and interleukins may be responsible for the depression.[27-29]

Electrical Injury

Cardiac complications are a common cause of death after electrical injury. An estimated 1100 to 1300 deaths occur annually in the United States from electrical injury (including lightning strikes). The cardiac complications after electrical injury include immediate cardiac arrest; acute myocardial necrosis with or without ventricular failure; pseudoinfarction; myocardial ischemia; dysrhythmias; conduction abnormalities; acute hypertension with peripheral vasospasm; and asymptomatic, nonspecific abnormalities evident on an electrocardiogram (ECG). Damage from electrical injury is due to direct effects on the excitable tissues, heat generated from the electrical current, and accompanying associated injuries (e.g., falls, explosions, fires).[30]

CLINICAL PRESENTATION AND PATHOPHYSIOLOGY

Penetrating Cardiac Trauma

Wounds involving the anatomical area, which includes the epigastrium and precordium within 3 cm of the sternum, carry a high incidence of cardiac injury. Stab wounds present a more predictable path of injury than gunshot wounds. Patients with cardiac injury can present with a clinical spectrum from full cardiac arrest with no vital signs to asymptomatic with normal vital signs. Up to 80 percent of stab wounds that injure the heart eventually manifest tamponade. The weapon injures the pericardium and heart, but as the weapon is removed, the pericardium seals and may not allow blood to escape. Rapid bleeding into the pericardium favors clotting rather than defibrination.[1] As pericardial fluid accumulates, a decrease in ventricular filling occurs, leading to a decrease in stroke volume. A compensatory rise in catecholamines leads to tachycardia and increased right heart filling pressures. The limits of distensibility are reached as the pericardium is filled with blood, and the septum shifts toward the left side, further compromising left ventricular function. If this cycle persists, ventricular function can continue to deteriorate, leading to irreversible shock. As little as 60 to 100 ml of blood in the pericardial sac can produce the clinical picture of tamponade.[1]

The rate of accumulation depends on the location of the wound. Because it has a thicker wall, wounds to the right ventricle seal themselves more readily than wounds to the right atrium. Patients with injuries to the coronary arteries present with rapid onset of tamponade combined with cardiac ischemia. With injuries to the left ventricle, the decompensated state can worsen, leading to cardiac arrest. The right side of the heart can compensate for injuries, and rapid deterioration may not occur. Patients with this sort of injury can benefit from early diagnosis and immediate intervention.

The classic findings of Beck's triad (muffled heart sounds, hypotension, and distended neck veins) are seen in only 10 percent of trauma patients. Pulsus paradoxus (a substantial fall in systolic blood pressure during inspiration) and Kussmaul's sign (increase in jugular venous distention on inspiration) may be present but are not reliable signs.[31] A valuable and reproducible sign of pericardial tamponade is a narrowing of the pulse pressure. An elevation of the central venous pressure often accompanies rapid and cyclic hyperresuscitation with crystalloid solutions, but in such instances a widening of the pulse pressure occurs.

In contrast to stab wounds, gunshot wounds to the heart are more frequently associated with hemorrhage than with tamponade. Twenty percent of gunshot wounds to the heart manifest as tamponade. With firearms, the kinetic energy is greater and the wounds to the heart and pericardium are frequently larger. Thus these patients present in arrest and exsanguination into a pleural cavity more often.[31]

Blunt Cardiac Trauma

As in penetrating cardiac trauma, clinically severe blunt cardiac trauma (e.g., cardiac rupture) manifests as either tamponade or as hemorrhage, depending on the status of the pericardium. If the pericardium is intact, tamponade develops; if it is not intact, extrapericardial bleeding occurs and hypovolemic shock ensues. Tamponade is sometimes combined with hypovolemia, thus complicating the clinical presentation.

Blunt cardiac injury can be divided into clinically significant and clinically insignificant injuries. Clinically significant injuries include cardiac rupture (ventricular or atrial), septal rupture, valvular dysfunction, coronary thrombosis, and caval avulsion. These injuries manifest as tamponade, hemorrhage, or severe cardiac dysfunction. Septal rupture and valvular dysfunction (leaflet tear, papillary muscle, or chordal rupture) can initially appear without symptoms but later demonstrate the delayed sequela of heart failure.[1]

Blunt cardiac injury can also appear as a dysrhythmia, most commonly premature ventricular contractions, the precise mechanism of which is unknown. Ventricular tachycardia can occur and degenerate into ventricular fibrillation. Supraventricular tachyarrhythmias can also occur. These symptoms commonly occur within the first 24 to 48 hours after injury.

Pericardial Trauma

Small isolated tears in the pericardium (see Chap. 70) can lead to cardiac herniation. This is a rare complication of pericardial rupture and depends on the size of the pericardial tear. If large enough, cardiac herniation can occur, leading to acute cardiac dysfunction.[1,12] Traumatic pericardial rupture is rare. Most patients with pericardial rupture do not survive transport to the hospital due to other significant associated injuries. The overall mortality of those who are treated at trauma centers with such injury remains as high as 64 percent.[32] Motor vehicle accident is the most common etiology of pericardial rupture. Sixty percent of pericardial ruptures occur along the left pleuropericardial surface.[32] An overwhelming majority of these cases are diagnosed either intraoperatively or on autopsy.[12] The clinical presentation of pericardial rupture can mimic that of pericardial tamponade with associated cardiac electrical-mechanical dissociation due to cardiac herniation and impaired venous return. When the heart returns to its normal position in the pericardial sac, venous return becomes normal again. Positional hypotension is the hallmark of cardiac herniation due to pericardial rupture,[12] whereas pericardial tamponade is associated with persistent hypotension until the pericardium is decompressed. Therefore a high index of suspicion must be present when evaluating polytrauma patients with unexplained positional hypotension.

CH 71

EVALUATION

Prehospital/Emergency Department

The evaluation of suspected heart injury differs, depending on whether the presenting patient is clinically stable or in extremis. The diagnosis of heart injury requires a high index of suspicion. On initial presentation to the emergency center, airway, breathing, and circulation (ABCs) under the Advanced Trauma Life Support protocol are evaluated and established.[33] Two large-bore intravenous catheters are inserted, and blood is typed and cross-matched. The patient undergoes focused abdominal sonogram for trauma (FAST)[34] and is examined for the Beck triad of muffled heart sounds, hypotension, and distended neck veins, as well as for pulsus paradoxus and Kussmaul sign. These findings suggest cardiac injury but are present in only 10 percent of patients with cardiac tamponade. If the FAST demonstrates pericardial fluid in an unstable patient (systemic blood pressure <90 mm Hg), transfer to the operating room for definitive repair or damage control is recommended.

Patients in extremis require immediate surgical intervention and often require emergency thoracotomy for resuscitation. The clear indications for emergency department

thoracotomy by surgical personnel include the following[35,36]:

1. Salvageable postinjury cardiac arrest (e.g., patients who have witnessed cardiac arrest with high likelihood of intrathoracic injury, particularly penetrating cardiac wounds)
2. Severe postinjury hypotension (i.e., systolic blood pressure <60 mm Hg) due to cardiac tamponade, air embolism, or thoracic hemorrhage

If, after resuscitative thoracotomy, vital signs are regained, the patient is transferred to the operating room for definitive repair. The patient with confirmed pericardial fluid by FAST, with normal vital signs (systemic blood pressure >90 mm Hg), may undergo a thorough evaluation to identify associated injuries. If other injuries are excluded, then open exploration may be required to exclude cardiac injury. In the absence of known causes of pericardial fluid (e.g., malignant pericardial effusion), a missed cardiac injury can lead to delayed bleeding, deterioration, or death.

Chest radiography is nonspecific, but it can identify hemothorax or pneumothorax and demonstrate an enlarged cardiac silhouette suggesting pericardial fluid. Other possibly indicated examinations include ultrasonography, central venous pressure measurements, subxiphoid pericardial window, thoracoscopy, and laparoscopy.

FAST/Ultrasonography/Echocardiography

Surgeons are increasingly performing ultrasonography (see Chap. 14) for thoracic trauma, paralleling the use of ultrasonography for blunt abdominal trauma. The FAST examination evaluates four anatomic windows for the presence of intraabdominal or pericardial fluid.[34,37] Ultrasonography in this setting is not intended to reach the precision of studies performed in the radiology suite but is merely intended to determine the presence of abnormal fluid collections, which aids in surgical decision making.[38] Ultrasonography is safe, portable, and expeditious and can be repeated as indicated. If performed by a trained surgeon, the FAST examination has a sensitivity of nearly 100 percent and a specificity of 97.3 percent.[37] As the use of FAST evolves, the most universally agreed indication is evaluation for pericardial fluid.

To evaluate more subtle findings of blunt cardiac injury, such as wall motion, valvular, or septal abnormalities in the stable patient, transthoracic echocardiography or transesophageal echocardiography (TEE) can be used.

Subxiphoid Pericardial Window/ Pericardiocentesis

Subxiphoid pericardial window has been performed both in the emergency department and in the operating room with the patient under either general or local anesthesia. Via a subxiphoid vertical incision, a small hole is made in the pericardium to determine the presence of blood. In a prospective study, Meyer and coworkers[39] compared the subxiphoid pericardial window with echocardiography in cases of penetrating heart injury and reported that the sensitivity and specificity of subxiphoid pericardial window were 100 percent and 92 percent, respectively, compared with 56 percent and 93 percent with echocardiography. They suggested that the difference in sensitivity may have been due to the presence of hemothorax, which can be confused with pericardial blood, or due to the fact that the blood had drained into the pleura.[39]

The disadvantage of a subxiphoid pericardial window is that it is an invasive procedure, and if a major injury is found, a second thoracic incision is required for definitive repair. Although there has been significant controversy in the past with regard to the indication for subxiphoid pericardial window, recent enthusiasm for ultrasonographic evaluation has almost eliminated the role of subxiphoid pericardial window in the evaluation of cardiac trauma.[40]

Pericardiocentesis has had significant historical support, especially when the majority of penetrating cardiac wounds were produced by ice picks and the (surviving) patients arrived several hours and/or days after injury. In such instances there was a natural triage of the more severe cardiac injuries and the intrapericardial blood had become defibrinated and was easy to remove. Currently, many trauma surgeons discourage pericardiocentesis for acute trauma. In general, pericardiocentesis has historically been used as a diagnostic or therapeutic maneuver to drain non-clotting pericardial fluid. In the setting of trauma, cardiac tamponade is acute and caused by hemorrhage. Clot forms quickly and is not amenable to needle drainage. Recurrence of tamponade with subsequent increase in mortality, as well as a significant incidence of false-negative results and potential for iatrogenic injury, makes pericardiocentesis a far less than optimal diagnostic tool.[15]

Indications for its use may apply in the case of iatrogenic injury caused by cardiac catheterization, at which time immediate decompression of the tamponade may be life saving, or in the trauma setting when a surgeon is not available.

EVALUATION OF BLUNT CARDIAC INJURY

Electrocardiography

In cases of blunt cardiac injury, conduction disturbances are common. Thus a screening 12-lead ECG (see Chap. 12) can be helpful for evaluation. Sinus tachycardia is the most common rhythm disturbance seen. Other possible disturbances include T wave and ST segment changes, sinus bradycardia, first-degree atrioventricular block, right bundle branch block, right bundle branch block with hemiblock, third-degree block, atrial fibrillation, premature ventricular contractions, ventricular tachycardia, and ventricular fibrillation.

Cardiac Enzymes

Much has been written previously about the use of cardiac enzyme determinations in evaluating blunt cardiac injury. However, no correlation among serum assays (e.g., creatine phosphokinase myocardial band, cardiac troponin T, cardiac troponin I) and identification and prognosis of injury has been demonstrated with blunt cardiac injury.[41-43] Therefore cardiac enzyme assays should not be performed unless one is evaluating concomitant coronary artery disease.[43]

Echocardiography

Transthoracic echocardiography (see Chap. 14) has limited use in evaluating blunt cardiac trauma because most patients also have significant chest wall injury, thus rendering the test suboptimal. Its major use is in diagnosing intrapericardial blood inferring other injuries. In stable patients, TEE is a more sensitive test in evaluating blunt cardiac injury. Cardiac septal defects and valvular insufficiency are readily diagnosed with TEE. Ventricular dysfunction can often mimic cardiac tamponade in its clinical presentation. Echocardiography is particularly useful in older patients with preexisting ventricular dysfunction. However, most blunt

TREATMENT

Prehospital/Emergency Department

Only a small subset of patients with significant cardiac injury ever reaches the emergency department, and expeditious transport to an appropriate facility is essential to survival. Transport times of less than 5 minutes and successful endotracheal intubation are positive factors for survival.[45]

Definitive Treatment

Penetrating Injury

Definitive treatment involves surgical exposure through an anterior thoracotomy or median sternotomy. The mainstays of treatment are relief of tamponade and hemorrhagic control. Concomitantly, correction of acidosis and hypothermia and reestablishment of effective coronary perfusion are pursued by appropriate resuscitation.

Exposure of the heart is accomplished via a left anterolateral thoracotomy (Fig. 71-1), which allows access to the pericardium and heart and exposure for aortic cross-clamping if necessary. This incision can be extended across the sternum to gain access to the right side of the chest and for better exposure of the right atrium or right ventricle. Manual access to the right hemithorax from the left side of the chest can be achieved through the anterior mediastinum by blunt dissection. This maneuver allows rapid evaluation of the right side of the chest for major injuries without transecting the sternum. Once the left pleural space is entered, the lung is retracted to expose the descending thoracic aorta for cross-clamping. The amount of blood present in the left chest indicates whether one is dealing with hemorrhage or tamponade. The pericardial sac anterior to the phrenopericardial vessels and phrenic nerve is opened, injuries are rapidly identified, and repair is performed.

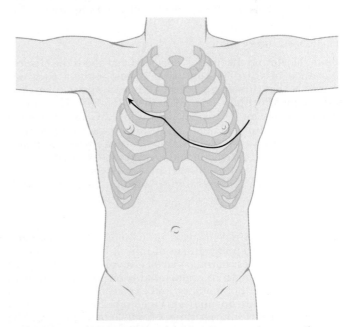

FIGURE 71–1 Left anterior thoracotomy (extension across the sternum if required). See text. (*Redrawn from Baylor College of Medicine, 2005.*)

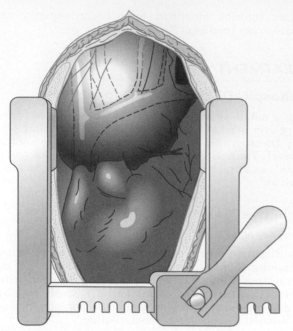

FIGURE 71–2 Median sternotomy (extension to the neck has been performed to address an injury of the great vessels). See text. *(Redrawn from Baylor College of Medicine, 2005.)*

In selected cases, particularly stab wounds to the precordium, median sternotomy (Fig. 71-2) can be used. This incision allows excellent exposure to the anterior structures of the heart, but difficulty with access to the posterior mediastinal structures and descending thoracic aorta for cross-clamping may be encountered.

Cardiorrhaphy should be performed by experienced surgeons. Poor technique can result in enlargement of the lacerations or injury to the coronary arteries. If the initial treating physician is uncomfortable with the suturing technique, digital pressure can be applied until a more experienced surgeon arrives. Other techniques that have been described include the use of a Foley balloon catheter and a skin stapler (Fig. 71-3). Injuries adjacent to coronary arteries can be managed by placing the sutures deep to the artery (Fig. 71-4). Mechanical support is not often required in the acute setting.[7]

Blunt Cardiac Injury

Much debate and discussion has occurred about the clinical relevance of "cardiac contusion." Most trauma surgeons conclude that this diagnosis should be eliminated because it does not affect how one treats these injuries. Thus a normotensive patient with a normal initial ECG and suspected blunt cardiac injury is managed in observation units, with no expected clinical significance. Patients with an abnormal ECG are admitted for monitoring and treated accordingly. Patients who present in cardiogenic shock are evaluated for a structural injury, which is then repaired.[46]

Results

Factors determining survival in patients with traumatic cardiac injury are mechanism of injury, location of injury, associated injuries, coronary artery involvement, presence of tamponade, length of prehospital transport, requirement for resuscitative thoracotomy, and experience of the trauma team. The overall hospital survival rate for patients with penetrating heart injuries ranges from 30 to 90 percent. The survival rate for patients with stab wounds is 70 to 80 percent, whereas survival after gunshot wounds is between 30 and 40 percent.[31] Cardiac rupture has a worse prognosis than penetrating injuries to the heart, with a survival rate of approximately 20 percent.

Complications

Primary injury-related cardiac complications include coronary artery injury; valvular apparatus injury (annulus, papillary muscles, and chordae tendineae); intracardiac fistulas; arrhythmias; and delayed tamponade. These delayed sequelae have been reported to have a broad incidence (4 to 56 percent), depending on the definition of complication.

Coronary artery injury is a rare complication, occurring in 5 to 9 percent of patients with cardiac injuries, with a 69 percent mortality rate.[6] A coronary artery injury is most often controlled by simple ligation, but bypass grafting using a saphenous vein may be required for proximal left anterior descending injuries (with total cardiopulmonary bypass).[6] With a resurrection of the old concept of coronary artery bypass grafting without cardiopulmonary bypass (off-pump bypass), this technique can theoretically be used for cases of these injuries in the highly unlikely event that the patient is hemodynamically stable.

Valvular apparatus dysfunction is rare (0.2 to 9 percent) and can occur with both blunt and penetrating trauma.[3,6] The aortic valve is most frequently injured, followed by the mitral and tricuspid valves, though many victims of aortic valve injuries die at the scene. Often these injuries are identified after the initial cardiorrhaphy and resuscitation have been performed. Timing of repair depends on the patient's condition. If severe cardiac dysfunction exists at the time of the initial operation, immediate valve repair or replacement may be required; otherwise, delayed repair is more commonly advised.[6]

Intracardiac fistulas include VSDs, atrial septal defects, and atrioventricular fistulas, with an incidence of 1.9 percent among cardiac injuries. Management depends on symptoms and degree of cardiac dysfunction, with only a minority of these patients requiring repair.[6] These injuries are often identified after primary repair is accomplished, and they can be repaired after the patient has recovered from the original and associated injuries. Cardiac catheterization and detailed echocardiography should be accomplished before repair so that specific anatomical sites of injury and incision planning can be accomplished.

Dysrhythmias can occur as a result of blunt injury, ischemia, or electrolyte abnormalities and are addressed according to the injury (Table 71-2).

Delayed pericardial tamponade is rare. It has been reported to occur as early as 1 hour after initial operation and as long as 76 days after the injury.[47]

Follow-up

Secondary sequelae in survivors of cardiac trauma include valvular abnormalities and intracardiac fistulas.[6,39,48] These abnormalities can be identified intraoperatively by gross palpation of a thrill[6] or with the use of TEE. TEE may not be feasible, however, in the acutely injured patient. Early postoperative clinical examination and ECG findings are unreliable.[6,48] Thus echocardiography is recommended during the initial hospitalization to identify occult injury and establish a baseline study. Because the incidence of late sequelae can be as high as 56 percent, follow-up echocardiography 3 to 4 weeks after injury has been recommended.[39,48]

In summary, the approach to the patient follows a well-defined plan. Patients with penetrating trauma arriving alive at a trauma center can have hemopericardium diagnosed by echocardiography/FAST. Urgent operation per-

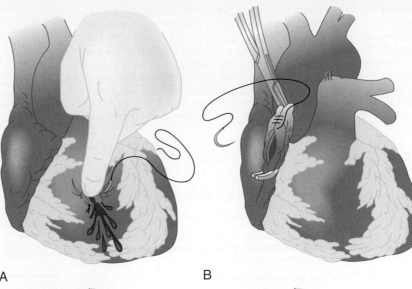

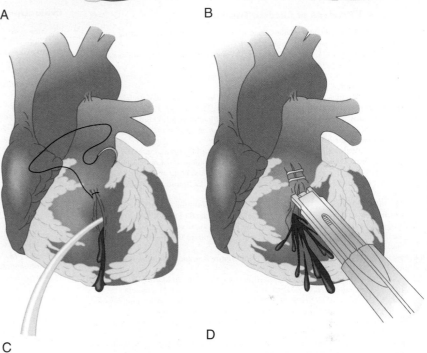

FIGURE 71–3 Temporary techniques to control bleeding. **A,** Finger occlusion. **B,** Partial occluding clamp. **C,** Foley balloon catheter. **D,** Skin staples. *(Redrawn from Baylor College of Medicine, 2005.)*

A

B

C

D

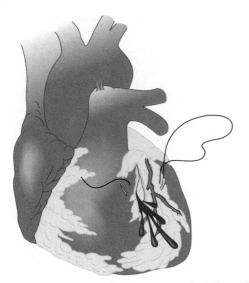

FIGURE 71–4 Injuries adjacent to coronary arteries can be addressed by placing sutures deep, avoiding injury to the artery. *(Redrawn from Baylor College of Medicine, 2005.)*

TABLE 71–2	Dysrhythmias Associated with Cardiac Injury
Penetrating Cardiac Injury	
Sinus tachycardia	
ST segment changes associated with ischemia	
Supraventricular tachycardia	
Ventricular tachycardia/fibrillation	
Blunt Cardiac Injury	
Sinus tachycardia	
ST segment, T wave abnormalities	
Atrioventricular blocks, bradycardia	
Ventricular tachycardia/fibrillation	
Electrical Injury	
Sinus tachycardia	
ST segment, T wave abnormalities	
Bundle branch blocks	
Axis deviation	
Prolonged QT	
Paroxysmal supraventricular tachycardia	
Atrial fibrillation	
Ventricular tachycardia, fibrillation (alternating current)	
Asystole (lightning strike)	

1862 formed in the trauma resuscitation area or the operating room can result in survival. Blunt cardiac trauma can produce either minor ECG changes or frank rupture of the septum, free wall, or cardiac valves. Associated injuries are not uncommon. Stable patients can undergo evaluation in a cardiac evaluation unit, but unstable patients require rapid imaging and urgent operation. Late sequelae of fistula, coronary occlusion, and heart failure are rare and are most often detected by echocardiography within the first year after injury.

REFERENCES

Incidence

1. Ivatury RR: Injury to the heart. *In* Moore EE, Feliciano DV, Mattox KL (eds): Trauma. 5th ed. New York, McGraw-Hill, 2004.
2. Campbell NC, Thomsen SR, Murkart DJ, et al: Review of 1198 cases of penetrating cardiac trauma. Br J Surg 84:1737, 1997.
3. Lin JC, Ott RA: Acute traumatic mitral valve insufficiency. J Trauma 47:165, 1999.
4. Schaffer RB, Berdat PA, Seiler C, Carrel TP: Isolated rupture of the ventricular septum after blunt chest trauma. Ann Thorac Surg 67:853, 1999.

Etiology and Patterns of Cardiac Trauma

5. Asensio JA, Berne JD, Demetriades D, et al: One hundred five penetrating cardiac injuries: A 2-year prospective evaluation. J Trauma 44:1073, 1998.
6. Wall MJ Jr, Mattox KL, Chen CD, Baldwin JC: Acute management of complex cardiac injuries. J Trauma 42:905, 1997.
7. Asensio JA, Soto SN, Forno W, et al: Penetrating cardiac injuries: A complex challenge. Injury 32:533, 2001.
8. Amerongen RV, Rosen M, Winnik G, Horwitz J: Ventricular fibrillation following blunt chest trauma from a baseball. Pediatr Emerg Care 13:107, 1997.
9. Maron BJ, Link MS, Wang PJ, et al: Clinical profile of commotio cordis: An underappreciated cause of sudden death in young during sports and other activities. J Cardiovasc Electrophysiol 10:114, 1999.
10. Bakaeen FG, Wall MJ Jr, Mattox KL: Successful repair of an avulsion of the superior vena cava from the right atrium inflicted by blunt trauma. J Trauma 59:1486, 2005.
11. Howanitz EP, Buckley D, Galbraith TA, et al: Combined blunt traumatic rupture of the heart and aorta: Two case reports and review of the literature. J Trauma 30:506, 1990.
12. Wall MJ Jr, Mattox KL, Wolf DA: The cardiac pendulum—blunt rupture of the pericardium with strangulation of the heart. J Trauma 59:136, 2005.
13. Baumgartner FJ, Rayhanabad J, Bongard FS, et al: Central venous injuries of the subclavian-jugular and innominate-caval confluences. Tex Heart Inst J 26:177, 1999.
14. Medizinische Klinik IV: Perforation und Ruptur Koronaryarterien. Herz 23:311, 1998.
15. Ivatury RR, Simon RJ, Rohman M: Cardiac complications. *In* Mattox KL (ed): Complications of Trauma. New York, Churchill Livingstone, 1994, pp 409-428.
16. LeMaire SA, Wall MJ Jr, Mattox KL: Needle embolus causing cardiac puncture and chronic constrictive pericarditis. Ann Thorac Surg 65:1786, 1998.
17. Symbas PN, Symbas PJ: Missiles in the cardiovascular system. Surg Clin North Am 7:343, 1997.
18. Huang YS, Yang ZC, Tan BG, et al: Pathogenesis of early cardiac myocyte damage after sear burns. J Trauma 46:428, 1999.
19. Kirkpatrick AW, Chun R, Brown R, Simons RK: Hypothermia and the trauma patient. Can J Surg 42:333, 1999.
20. Sharkey SW, Shear W, Hodges M, Herzog CA: Reversible myocardial contraction abnormalities in patients with an acute non-cardiac illness. Chest 114:98, 1998.
21. Kumar A, Thota V, Dee L, et al: TNF-alpha and IL-1 are regulators for depression of in vitro myocardial cell contractility induced by serum from humans with septic shock. J Exp Med 183:949, 1996.
22. Meldrum DR, Shenkar R, Sheridan BC, et al: Hemorrhage activates myocardial NF-kappa and increases TNF-alpha in the heart. J Mol Cell Cardiol 29:2849, 1997.

23. Horton JW, Lin C, Maass D: Burn trauma and tumor necrosis factor alpha alter calcium handling by cardiomyocytes. Shock 10:270, 1998.
24. Horton JW, White J, Maass D, Sanders B: Arginine in burn injury improves cardiac performance and prevents bacterial translocation. J Appl Physiol 84:695, 1998.
25. Heinz G, Geppert A, Delle Karth G, et al: IV milrinone for cardiac output increase and maintenance: Comparison in nonhyperdynamic SIRS/sepsis and congestive heart failure. Intensive Care Med 25:620, 1999.
26. Flohe S, Borgermann J, Dominquez FE, et al: Influence of granulocyte-macrophage colony-stimulating factor (GM-CSF) on whole blood endotoxin responsiveness following trauma, cardiopulmonary bypass, and severe sepsis. Shock 12:17, 1999.
27. Maass DL, White J, Horton JW: IL-1beta and IL-6 act synergistically with TNF-alpha to alter cardiac contractile function after burn trauma. Shock 18:360, 2002.
28. Horton JW: Oxygen free radicals contribute to postburn cardiac cell membrane dysfunction. J Surg Res 61:97, 1996.
29. Horton JW: Cellular basis for burn-mediated cardiac dysfunction in adult rabbits. Am J Physiol 271:H2615, 1996.
30. Lee RC: Injury by electrical forces: pathophysiology, manifestations, and therapy. Curr Probl Surg 34:677, 1997.

Clinical Presentation and Pathophysiology

31. Brown J, Grover FL: Trauma to the heart. Chest Surg Clin North Am 7:325, 1997.
32. Galindo Gallego M, Lopez-Cambra MJ, Fernandez-Acenero MJ, et al: Traumatic rupture of the pericardium. Case report and literature review. J Cardiovasc Surg (Torino) 37:187, 1996.

Evaluation

33. American College of Surgeons, Committee on Trauma: Advanced Trauma Life Support. Chicago, American College of Surgeons, 1997.
34. Rozycki GS, Feliciano DV, Schmidt JA, et al: The role of surgeon performed ultrasound in patients with possible cardiac wounds. Ann Surg 223:737, 1996.
35. Biffl WD, Moore EE, Johnson JL: Emergency department thoracotomy. *In* Moore EE, Feliciano DV, Mattox KL (eds): Trauma. 5th ed. New York, McGraw-Hill, 2004.
36. Working Group, Ad Hoc Subcommittee on Outcomes, American College of Surgeons-Committee on Trauma Practice Management Guidelines for Emergency Department Thoracotomy. J Am Coll Surg 193:303, 2001.
37. Rozycki GS, Schmidt JA, Oschner MG, et al: The role of surgeon-performed ultrasound in patients with possible penetrating wounds: A prospective multicenter study. J Trauma 45:190, 1998.
38. Mattox KL, Wall MJ Jr: Newer diagnostic measures and emergency management. Chest Surg Clin North Am 7:214, 1997.
39. Meyer DM, Jessen ME, Grayburn PA: Use of echocardiography to detect occult cardiac injury after penetrating thoracic trauma: A prospective study. J Trauma 39:902, 1995.
40. Feliciano DV, Rozycki GS: Advances in the diagnosis and treatment of thoracic trauma. Surg Clin North Am 79:1417, 1999.
41. Adams JE III, Davila-Roman VG, Bessey PQ, et al: Improved detection of cardiac contusion with cardiac troponin I. Am Heart J 131:308, 1996.
42. Ferjani M, Droc G, Dreux S, et al: Circulating cardiac troponin T in myocardial contusion. Chest 111:427, 1997.
43. Bertinchant JP, Polge A, Mohty D, et al: Evaluation of incidence, clinical significance and prognostic value of circulating cardiac troponin I and T elevation in hemodynamically stable patients with suspected myocardial contusion after blunt chest trauma. J Trauma 48:924, 2000.
44. Karalis DG, Victor MF, Davis GA, et al: The role of echocardiography in blunt chest trauma: A transthoracic and transesophageal echocardiographic study. J Trauma 36:53, 1994.

Treatment

45. Durham LA, Richardson R, Wall MJ, et al: Emergency center thoracotomy: Impact of prehospital resuscitation. J Trauma 32:779, 1992.
46. Mattox KL, Flint LM, Carrico CJ, et al: Blunt cardiac injury (formerly termed "myocardial contusion") (editorial). J Trauma 31:653, 1991.
47. Aaland MO, Sherman RT: Delayed pericardial tamponade in penetrating chest trauma: Case report. J Trauma 31:1563, 1991.
48. Mattox KL, Limacher MC, Feliciano DV, et al: Cardiac evaluation following heart injury. J Trauma 25:758, 1985.

CH 71

CHAPTER 72

Pulmonary Embolism

Samuel Z. Goldhaber

Epidemiology, 1863

Pathophysiology, 1864
Hypercoagulable States, 1864
Relationship Between Deep Venous
   Thrombosis and Pulmonary
   Embolism, 1864

Diagnosis, 1865

Management, 1870
Risk Stratification, 1870
Anticoagulation, 1871

Prevention, 1878

Future Perspectives, 1879

References, 1879

Pulmonary embolism (PE) and deep venous thrombosis (DVT) afflict millions of individuals worldwide and account for several hundred thousand deaths annually in the United States. Few health care providers realize that the case fatality rate for PE, approximately 15 percent, exceeds the mortality rate for acute myocardial infarction. During the past 5 years, a remarkable transition started in North America. The lay public began to become aware of the magnitude of disability from venous thromboembolism (VTE), which encompasses PE and DVT.

The same features of VTE that fascinate the public have kept clinical scientists spellbound by this illness. VTE is a common problem yet often difficult to diagnose. It strikes a wide range of individuals, from teenagers to nonagenarians. Its onset is usually unpredictable, and the likelihood of recurrence after completing a time-limited course of anticoagulation remains uncertain. Though most individuals survive, VTE impairs quality of life by increasing susceptibility to chronic thromboembolic pulmonary hypertension and chronic venous insufficiency. It also exerts a psychological toll on patients who wonder whether they will suffer a recurrent event, whether it will affect their family members, and whether it will lower their quality of life and shorten their lifespan.

Chest CT scanning has for the most part replaced lung scanning as the principal diagnostic test for PE. Coupled with clinical likelihood assessment, the diagnosis of PE has become much more straightforward and far less murky than in the past, when nondiagnostic lung scans required either invasive pulmonary angiography or empirical diagnostic decision-making regarding the presence or absence of PE.

For PE management, risk stratification is of paramount importance. High-risk patients may benefit from thrombolysis or embolectomy in addition to anticoagulation. Accurate prognostication relies on clinical assessment of general appearance, heart rate, blood pressure, and respiratory rate, as well as novel factors such as elevation of cardiac biomarkers, right ventricular hypokinesis judged by echocardiogram, and right ventricular enlargement detected by chest CT scan. Clinicians have learned to use these prognostic indicators to predict adverse outcomes rapidly and accurately, even if patients appear clinically stable.

The selection of immediately active parenteral anticoagulant drugs has expanded beyond unfractionated heparin (UFH). Low-molecular-weight heparins (LMWH) and fondaparinux provide convenient once or twice daily weight-based dosing as an alternative to a continuous intravenous infusion of UFH dosed by adjusting the activated partial thromboplastin time (aPTT). These alternatives to unfractionated heparin also minimize the possibility of developing heparin-induced thrombocytopenia. Meanwhile, immediately effective oral anticoagulants given in fixed dose are being developed to replace warfarin. These new oral agents include anti-Xa agents, direct thrombin inhibitors, and even oral heparin. None requires dose adjustment or laboratory coagulation monitoring (see also Chap. 82).

Finally, a major challenge remains: preventing VTE by implementing evidence-based pharmacological or mechanical measures. Hospitalized surgical patients routinely receive prophylaxis. However, multiple surveys and audits reveal that many hospitalized general medical and medical subspecialty patients do not receive guideline-mandated preventive measures against VTE. Strategies to improve implementation of prophylaxis include enhanced education, performance-based incentives, and electronic alerts to the responsible physician.

EPIDEMIOLOGY

The death rate from PE increases with age and is higher in African-American than in white patients.[1] The incidence of VTE has also risen, primarily because of an increase in the diagnosis of DVT. The incidence is similar among men and women.[2] About half the cases of VTE are idiopathic and occur without antecedent trauma, surgery, immobilization, or diagnosis of cancer.[3] Several gene polymorphisms associate independently with an increased risk of VTE apart from those with widely known prothrombotic effects, such as factor V Leiden. These include polymorphisms in ADRB2, an inflammatory mediator, and LPL, an enzyme with a key role in lipid metabolism.[4] The biggest recent breakthrough in epidemiology is discovering an association between arterial atherosclerosis and VTE. Arterial events are more common in patients with VTE.[5] This finding is of special relevance to cardiologists and other arterial vascular medicine specialists.

The previous uncertainty about the clinical relevance of asymptomatic proximal DVT no longer exists. Asymptomatic proximal leg DVT has a high associated mortality rate among patients hospitalized with medical illnesses. The 90-day mortality rate in hospitalized medical patients was 14 percent for those with asymptomatic proximal leg DVT at day 21, compared with a 1.9 percent 90-day mortality rate for those with no DVT at day 21.[6] This finding underscores the appropriateness of targeting asymptomatic proximal leg DVT as an endpoint in clinical trials of thromboprophylaxis.

Table 72-1 lists major acquired risk factors for PE. An especially problematic risk factor is obesity, which has become pandemic in the United States. Obesity doubles or triples the likelihood of VTE.[7] As patients survive longer with cancer, the frequency of VTE is increasing because cancer patients have twice the incidence of VTE as noncancer patients. This increased

TABLE 72–1	Major Acquired Risk Factors for Venous Thromboembolism
Advancing age	
Arterial disease including carotid and coronary disease	
Obesity	
Cigarette smoking	
Chronic obstructive pulmonary disease	
Personal or family history of venous thromboembolism	
Recent surgery, trauma, or immobility including stroke	
Acute infection	
Long-haul air travel	
Cancer	
Pregnancy, oral contraceptive pills, or hormone replacement therapy	
Pacemaker, implantable cardiac defibrillator leads, or indwelling central venous catheters	

TABLE 72–2	Major Thrombophilias Associated with Venous Thromboembolism
Inherited	
Factor V Leiden resulting in activated protein C resistance	
Prothrombin gene mutation 20210	
Antithrombin III deficiency	
Protein C deficiency	
Protein S deficiency	
Acquired	
Antiphospholipid antibody syndrome	
Hyperhomocysteinemia	

CH 72

risk of VTE accompanies not only adenocarcinomas of the pancreas, stomach, lung, esophagus, prostate, and colon, but also threatens patients with "liquid tumors" such as myeloproliferative disease, lymphoma, and leukemia.[8] The VTE incidence is highest among patients initially diagnosed with metastatic disease.[9] Less well-known acquired risk factors include acute infection[10] and chronic obstructive pulmonary disease.[11] The epidemiology of PE is also a women's health issue. Pregnancy, hormonal contraception,[12] and postmenopausal hormonal therapy[13] each contribute to increased risk.

Perhaps the most frequently discussed acquired risk factor is long-haul air travel. The risk of fatal PE in this setting is less than 1 in 1 million.[14] However, when death occurs, it is dramatic and especially tragic because the victim is often an otherwise healthy young person. It appears that among some individuals, there is activation of the coagulation system during air travel.[15] The reason for hypercoagulability remains uncertain. However, the mechanism does not appear to be caused by hypobaric hypoxia.[16]

Hospitalized patients with medical illnesses such as pneumonia or congestive heart failure have a high risk of developing VTE. The stasis and immobilization associated with postoperative venous thrombosis may paradoxically increase after hospital discharge because, with short hospital lengths of stay, patients may be too weak and debilitated at home to ambulate after surgery. Vigilance is required to ensure that appropriate patients receive extended VTE prophylaxis at the time of hospital discharge.

Independent risk factors for VTE also include nursing home confinement, cancer, and cancer chemotherapy, in addition to diabetes mellitus.[17] In a prospective registry of 5451 patients with ultrasonographically confirmed DVT, the five most common comorbidities were hypertension, surgery within 3 months, immobility within 30 days, cancer, and obesity.[18]

Upper extremity DVT is an increasingly important clinical entity because of more frequent placement of pacemakers and internal cardiac defibrillators, as well as more frequent use of chronic indwelling catheters for chemotherapy and nutrition. Patients with upper extremity DVT are at risk for PE, superior vena caval syndrome, and loss of vascular access.[19]

PATHOPHYSIOLOGY

Hypercoagulable States

In 1856 Rudolf Virchow postulated a triad of factors that predispose to intravascular coagulation: (1) local trauma to the vessel wall, (2) hypercoagulability, and (3) stasis. Classically, the pathogenesis of PE has been dichotomized as caused by either "inherited" (primary) or acquired (secondary) risk factors. It appears likely, however, that a combination of thrombophilia (Table 72-2) and acquired risk factors often precipitates overt thrombosis.

PRIMARY HYPERCOAGULABLE STATES. Normally, a specified amount of activated protein C (aPC) can be added to plasma to prolong the aPTT. Patients with "aPC resistance" have a blunted aPTT prolongation and a predisposition to developing PE and DVT. The phenotype of aPC resistance is associated with a single point mutation, designated factor V Leiden, in the factor V gene. Factor V Leiden triples the risk of developing VTE. This genetic mutation is also a risk factor for recurrent pregnancy loss, possibly caused by placental vein thrombosis. Use of oral contraceptives by patients with factor V Leiden increases the risk of VTE by at least 10-fold.

A single-point mutation in the 3′ untranslated region of the prothrombin gene (G-to-A transition at nucleotide position 20210) is associated with increased levels of prothrombin. In the Physicians' Health Study, the prevalence of the prothrombin gene mutation was 3.9 percent, and this mutation doubled the risk of venous thrombosis.

One of the most serious thrombophilic disorders is the antiphospholipid antibody syndrome, which is acquired, not inherited. Patients with this syndrome have increased risk of recurrent arterial or venous thrombosis or pregnancy loss.[20]

A careful family history remains the most rapid and cost-effective method of identifying a predisposition to venous thrombosis. Investigation with blood tests can be misleading. For example, consumption coagulopathy caused by venous thrombosis may be misdiagnosed as deficiency of antithrombin III, protein C, or protein S. Heparin administration can depress antithrombin III levels. Use of warfarin ordinarily causes a mild deficiency of protein C or S. Both oral contraceptives and pregnancy depress protein S levels.

Relationship Between Deep Venous Thrombosis and Pulmonary Embolism

When venous thrombi detach from their sites of formation, they flow through the venous system toward the vena cava. They pass through the right atrium and right ventricle, then enter the pulmonary arterial circulation. An extremely large embolus may lodge at the bifurcation of the pulmonary artery, forming a saddle embolus (Fig. 72-1, top). More com-

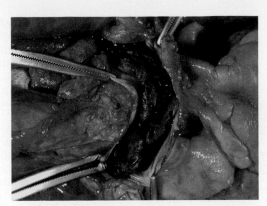

FIGURE 72-1 This 41-year-old woman with poorly controlled hypertension suffered an intracerebral hemorrhage, complicated six days later by acute pulmonary embolism. Emergency catheter embolectomy was unsuccessful, and she suffered cardiac arrest. At autopsy, a large saddle embolus extended from the root of the pulmonary artery into the left and right lungs.

monly, a major pulmonary vessel is occluded (see Fig. 72-1, bottom). Many patients with large PEs do not have ultrasonographic evidence of DVT, probably because the clot has already embolized to the lungs.

RIGHT VENTRICULAR DYSFUNCTION. The extent of pulmonary vascular obstruction and the presence of underlying cardiopulmonary disease are probably the most important factors determining whether right ventricular dysfunction ensues.[21] As obstruction increases, pulmonary artery pressure rises. Further increases in pulmonary vascular resistance and pulmonary hypertension are caused by secretion of vasoconstricting compounds such as serotonin, reflex pulmonary artery vasoconstriction, and hypoxemia. The overloaded right ventricle[22] releases cardiac biomarkers including pro-brain natriuretic peptide, brain natriuretic peptide, and troponin, all of which predict an increased likelihood of an adverse clinical outcome.[23]

VENTRICULAR INTERDEPENDENCY. The sudden rise in pulmonary artery pressure reflects an abrupt increase in right ventricular afterload, with consequent elevation of right ventricular wall tension followed by right ventricular dilation and dysfunction (Fig. 72-2). As the right ventricle dilates, the interventricular septum shifts toward the left, with resultant underfilling and decreased left ventricular diastolic distensibility. With underfilling of the left ventricle, systemic cardiac output and systolic arterial pressure both decline, potentially impairing coronary perfusion and producing myocardial ischemia. Elevated right ventricular wall tension following massive PE[24] reduces right coronary flow, increases right ventricular myocardial oxygen demand, and causes ischemia. Perpetuation of this cycle can lead to right ventricular infarction, circulatory collapse, and death.

Summary of Pathophysiology

PE can have the following pathophysiological effects: (1) increased pulmonary vascular resistance caused by vascular obstruction, neurohumoral agents, or pulmonary artery baroreceptors; (2) impaired gas exchange caused by increased alveolar dead space from vascular obstruction and hypoxemia from alveolar hypoventilation, low ventilation-perfusion units, and right-to-left shunting, as well as impaired carbon monoxide transfer caused by loss of gas-exchange surface; (3) alveolar hyperventilation caused by reflex stimulation of irritant receptors; (4) increased airway resistance due to bronchoconstriction; and (5) decreased pulmonary compliance due to lung edema, lung hemorrhage, and loss of surfactant.[25]

DIAGNOSIS

Diagnosis of PE is more difficult than treatment or prevention. Fortunately, noninvasive diagnostic approaches have become increasingly reliable. The greatest challenges are to remember to consider the possible diagnosis of PE and realize that it can masquerade as many other illnesses. It can also occur concomitantly with other illnesses, thereby confounding the diagnostic work-up. The most useful approach is the clinical assessment of likelihood, based on presenting symptoms and signs, in conjunction with judicious diagnostic testing. When PE is not highly suspected, a normal plasma D-dimer enzyme-linked immunosorbent assay (ELISA) usually suffices to rule out this condition. When PE is highly suspected, especially with an elevated D-dimer ELISA, chest CT scanning is the best imaging test. Of note is that acute respiratory failure caused by other illnesses such as asthma or pneumonia may mimic PE.

A French group studied 1529 consecutive outpatients suspected of PE in 117 emergency departments by assessing the appropriateness of diagnostic management.[26] When PE was diagnosed, appropriate criteria were used in 92 percent of patients. In contrast, when PE was excluded, *inappropriate* criteria were used in 57 percent of patients. Of 506 patients receiving *inappropriate* diagnostic management that led to exclusion of PE, 39 had recurrent events within the following 3 months (7.7 percent). Of these 39 patients, 29 suffered unexplained sudden death. In contrast, of those 418 patients excluded using *appropriate* diagnostic management, only 5 (1.2 percent) had recurrent events in the follow-up period. Two factors predisposed to inappropriate diagnostic management: (1) lack of a written diagnostic algorithm and (2) failure to use clinical probability scoring of each patient. The two most common errors were (1) ruling out PE on the basis of a normal venous ultrasound of the legs and (2) not doing additional testing after finding an abnormally elevated D-dimer test.

Another problem is that patients often delay seeking medical attention.[27] In a study of 1152 patients with confirmed DVT or PE at 70 North American medical centers, 21 percent of DVT patients received diagnoses more than 1 week after symptom onset. Among PE patients, 17 percent were diagnosed more than 1 week after symptom onset.

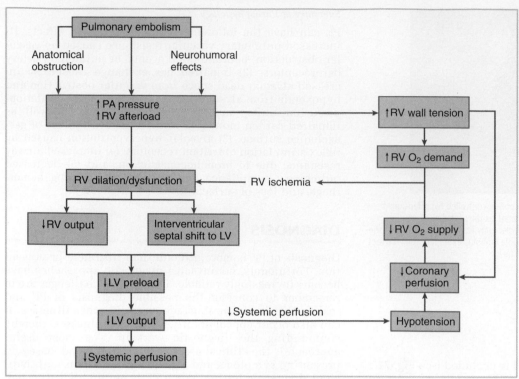

FIGURE 72–2 Pathophysiology of right ventricular dysfunction. LV = left ventricular; PA = pulmonary artery; RV = right ventricular.

TABLE 72–3	Most Common Symptoms or Signs of Pulmonary Embolism

Symptoms
Otherwise unexplained dyspnea
Chest pain, either pleuritic or "atypical"

Signs
Tachypnea
Tachycardia
Low-grade fever
Tricuspid regurgitation murmur
Accentuated P2

CLINICAL PRESENTATION. Clinical suspicion of PE is of paramount importance in guiding diagnostic testing. Clinical *gestalt* and clinical experience are helpful, but the incremental gain in diagnostic accuracy is small when comparing attending physicians with interns.[28]

Dyspnea is the most frequent symptom, and tachypnea is the most frequent sign of PE (Table 72-3). In general, severe dyspnea, syncope, or cyanosis portends a major life-threatening PE, which is often devoid of chest pain. Paradoxically, severe pleuritic pain often signifies that the embolism is small and located in the distal pulmonary arterial system, near the pleural lining.

PE should be suspected in hypotensive patients when (1) there is evidence of venous thrombosis or predisposing factors for it and (2) there is clinical evidence of acute cor pulmonale (acute right ventricular failure) such as distended neck veins, a right-sided S_3 gallop, a right ventricular heave, tachycardia, or tachypnea, especially if (3) there are echocardiographic findings of right ventricular dilation and hypokinesis or electrocardiographic evidence of acute cor pulmonale manifested by a new S1Q3T3 pattern, new incomplete right bundle branch block, or right ventricular ischemia (Fig. 72-3).

A reliable clinical decision scoring system[29] can stratify patients into high clinical probability or non–high clinical probability of PE with a rapid seven-question bedside assessment (Table 72-4). This approach was validated in a large Dutch study in which almost half of the patients could be categorized as "PE unlikely." In this low-risk group, only about 5 percent of patients were subsequently diagnosed with PE.[30]

DIFFERENTIAL DIAGNOSIS. The differential diagnosis of PE is broad and covers a spectrum from life-threatening disease such as acute myocardial infarction to innocuous anxiety states (Table 72-5). Some patients have concomitant PE and other illnesses. For example, if pneumonia or heart failure does not respond to appropriate therapy, the possibility of coexisting PE should be considered. Idiopathic pulmonary hypertension may present with sudden exacerbations that mimic acute PE.

Clinical Syndromes of Pulmonary Embolism

Classification of acute PE into three syndromes (Table 72-6) can assist prognostication and decisions regarding clinical management. Massive PE occurs rarely in most hospitals. In contrast, submassive PE and small to moderate PE occur with about equal frequency.

MASSIVE PULMONARY EMBOLISM. Patients with massive PE are susceptible to cardiogenic shock and multisystem organ failure. Renal insufficiency, hepatic dysfunction, and altered mentation are common findings. They usually have thrombosis affecting at least half of the pulmonary arterial vasculature. Clot is typically present bilaterally. Dyspnea is usually the most noticeable symptom; chest pain is unusual; transient cyanosis is common; and systemic arterial hypotension requiring pressor support is frequent. Excessive fluid boluses may worsen right heart failure and render therapy more difficult.

MODERATE TO LARGE ("SUBMASSIVE") PULMONARY EMBOLISM. These patients frequently present with right ventricular hypokinesis, as well as elevations in troponin, pro-BNP, or BNP, but they maintain normal systemic arterial pressure. Usually, one third or more of the pulmonary artery vasculature is obstructed. If there is no prior history of cardiopulmonary disease, they may appear clinically well, but this initial impression is often misleading. They are at risk for recurrent (and possibly fatal) PE, even with adequate anticoagulation. Most survive, but they may require escalation of therapy with pressor support or mechanical ventilation. Therefore, especially if right ventricular dysfunction persists, one should consider using

TABLE 72–11	Diagnostic Tests for Suspected Pulmonary Embolism
Test	**Comments**
Oxygen saturation	Nonspecific but can raise suspicion if there is a sudden, otherwise unexplained decrement.
D-dimer	An excellent "rule out" test if normal, especially if accompanied by non–high clinical suspicion (see Table 72-4).
Electrocardiogram	May be normal, especially in younger, previously healthy individuals. May provide alternative diagnosis such as myocardial infarction or pericarditis.
Lung scanning	Usually does not definitively diagnose or exclude PE. Being replaced by chest CT except for patients with (1) anaphylaxis to contrast agent, (2) renal insufficiency, or (3) pregnancy.
Chest CT	The most accurate diagnostic imaging test for PE (see Table 72-9). May be problematic if CT result and clinical decision rule score (see Table 72-4) are discordant.
Pulmonary angiography	Invasive, costly, uncomfortable. Has ceded to chest CT its designation as "diagnostic gold standard."
Echocardiography	Best used as a prognostic test in patients with established PE, rather than as a diagnostic test (see Table 72-10). Many patients with large PE will have normal echocardiograms.
Venous ultrasonography	Excellent for diagnosing acute symptomatic proximal DVT, but a negative test does not rule out PE because a recent leg DVT may have embolized completely. Calf vein imaging is operator dependent.
Magnetic resonance imaging	Reliable only for imaging large, proximal pulmonary arteries

TABLE 72–12	Clinical Predictors of Increased Mortality
Systolic blood pressure less than or equal to 100 mm Hg	
Age older than 70 years	
Heart rate higher than 100 beats/min	
Congestive heart failure	
Chronic lung disease	
Cancer	

TABLE 72–13	Cardiac Biomarkers and Imaging Predictors of Increased Mortality
Elevated troponin I or troponin T	
Elevated BNP or pro-BNP	
Right ventricular hypokinesis on echocardiogram	
Right ventricular enlargement on chest CT	

BNP = brain natriuretic peptide; CT = computed tomography.

likelihood of an adverse outcome, principally because these PE patients have suffered right ventricular microinfarction.[51] Elevations of pro-BNP[52] and BNP[53] indicate myocardial stretch caused by right ventricular pressure overload. These patients also have an increased risk of a complicated hospital course, with a higher likelihood of recurrent PE, respiratory failure requiring mechanical ventilation, hypotension requiring vasopressors, and death.

The standard imaging test for risk stratification is echocardiography. Right ventricular hypokinesis is an independent risk factor for a poor prognosis.[54] The combination of right ventricular hypokinesis and elevated cardiac biomarkers identifies the highest-risk group of PE patients.[55,56]

The newest approach to risk stratification involves further analysis of the cardiac images obtained on the chest CT scan used to diagnosis acute PE. Right ventricular enlargement is defined as a right ventricular diameter that is 90 percent or greater than the size of the left ventricular diameter. On multivariable analysis, right ventricular enlargement emerges as an independent risk factor for death and nonfatal clinical complications.[57,58]

Anticoagulation (see Chap. 82)

UNFRACTIONATED HEPARIN. Unfractionated heparin (UFH) is a highly sulfated glycosaminoglycan that is partially purified most commonly from porcine intestinal mucosa. Its molecular weight ranges from 3000 to 30,000 and averages 15,000. Heparin acts primarily by binding to antithrombin III (AT III), a protein that inhibits the coagulation factors thrombin (factor IIa), Xa, IXa, XIa, and XIIa. Heparin subsequently promotes a conformational change in AT III that accelerates its activity approximately 100- to 1000-fold. This prevents additional thrombus formation and permits endogenous fibrinolytic mechanisms to lyse clot that has already formed. Heparin does *not* directly dissolve thrombus that already exists. The efficacy of heparin is limited because clot-bound thrombin is protected from heparin-antithrombin III inhibition. Furthermore, heparin resistance can occur because UFH binds to plasma proteins.

An activated partial thromboplastin time (aPTT) at least one and one-half times greater than the control value should provide a minimum therapeutic level of UFH. Commonly, the therapeutic range is 60 to 80 seconds. However, there are many different PTT reagent kits and virtually no stan-

support with mechanical ventilation or pressors while the PE is managed with aggressive medical, interventional angiographic, or surgical therapy (Fig. 72-6). The three key components for risk stratification are (1) clinical evaluation; (2) cardiac biomarkers such as troponin, pro-BNP, and BNP; and (3) assessment of right ventricular size and function.

Clinical evaluation is straightforward if the patient looks and feels perfectly well. The International Cooperative Pulmonary Embolism Registry[48] identified 6 major clinical predictors of increased mortality within 30 days (Table 72-12).[49] Clinical assessment should be supplemented by cardiac biomarkers and imaging predictors of increased mortality (Table 72-13).

The practitioner should assess right ventricular dysfunction on physical examination by seeking distended jugular veins, a systolic murmur of tricuspid regurgitation, or an accentuated P2. Obese necks may make jugular vein assessment difficult. Noisy emergency departments can obscure the subtle auscultatory findings of right ventricular dysfunction. The ECG may show features that predict an adverse clinical outcome. These include right bundle branch block, Q waves in leads III and AVF, low voltage, atrial arrhythmias, and ST segment elevation or depression in leads V4-V6.[50]

Measurement of cardiac biomarkers has provided a major step forward in risk assessment of patients with acute PE. Elevation of cardiac troponins I or T portends an increased

CH 72

Pulmonary Embolism

dardization of aPTT levels. The dose response to intravenous UFH is highly variable. Even when a therapeutic aPTT is achieved, subsequent measurements are usually not within the desired therapeutic range.

Heparin is the cornerstone of treatment for acute PE. Before starting heparin, evaluate potential risk factors for bleeding, such as a prior history of bleeding with anticoagulation, thrombocytopenia, vitamin K deficiency, increasing age, underlying diseases, and concomitant drug therapy. The most frequently overlooked portion of the physical examination is a rectal examination for occult blood. Withhold heparin in patients with active major bleeding, and consider nonpharmacological treatment with insertion of an inferior vena caval filter.

Initiate UFH as soon as acute PE is suspected, unless a severe bleeding problem such as active gastrointestinal bleeding is detected. Begin with a bolus of 5000 to 10,000 units of intravenous UFH, followed by a continuous intravenous infusion based on weight. Most patients require at least 30,000 units/24 hour. Many nomograms such as that of Raschke[59] assist in adjusting the dose of continuous intravenous UFH, with guidelines provided by the patient's weight and aPTT (Table 72-14). Although there is a trend toward the use of LMWH for patients who present with acute PE, the shorter half-life of UFH is advantageous if there is a possibility that the patient will require insertion of an inferior vena caval filter, thrombolysis, or embolectomy. The option of high-dose subcutaneous UFH is often overlooked. Subcutaneous UFH can be effectively and safely administered either by adjusting the dose according to the PTT[60] or by administering a fixed dose of UFH adjusted according to weight.[61]

LOW-MOLECULAR-WEIGHT HEPARIN. LMWH consists of fragments of UFH that exhibit less binding to plasma proteins and endothelial cells than UFH. Therefore LMWH has greater bioavailability, more predictable dose response, and a longer half-life than UFH.[62] These features permit weight-based LMWH dosing, without laboratory tests for dose adjustment in most instances. Consequently, LMWHs have revolutionized the management of DVT and converted the treatment from a mandatory minimum 5-day hospitalization to either an overnight stay or outpatient strategy for most patients (Table 72-15). Success of this approach requires a reliable administrative and clinical infrastructure to ensure meticulous follow-up.

A large randomized trial in patients with acute DVT showed that subcutaneously administered LMWH is at least as effective and safe as a continuous infusion of intravenous UFH.[63] A meta-analysis of randomized

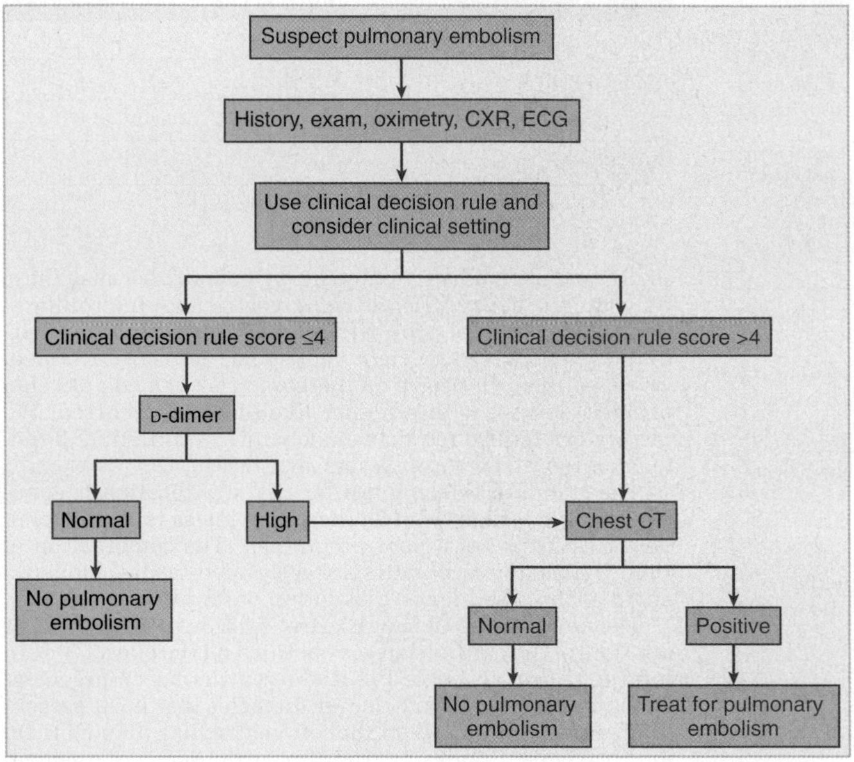

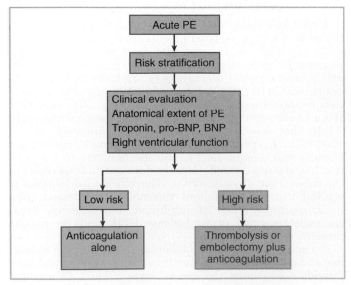

FIGURE 72–5 Integrated diagnostic approach. CT = computed tomography; ELISA = enzyme-linked immunosorbent assay; PA-Gram = pulmonary arteriogram.

FIGURE 72–6 Management strategy for acute pulmonary embolism (PE), based on risk stratification. BNP = brain natriuretic peptide.

TABLE 72–14	Intravenous Unfractionated Heparin "Raschke Nomogram"
Variable	**Action**
Initial heparin bolus	80 U/kg bolus, then 18 U/kg/hr
aPTT <35 seconds (<1.2 × control)	80 U/kg bolus, then increase by 4 U/kg/hr
aPTT 35 to 45 seconds (1.2 to 1.5 × control)	40 U/kg bolus, then increase by 2 U/kg/hr
aPTT 46 to 70 seconds (1.5 to 2.3 × control	No change
aPTT 71 to 90 seconds (2.3 to 3 × control)	Decrease infusion rate by 2 U/kg/hr
aPTT >90 seconds (>3 × control)	Hold infusion 1 hr, then decrease infusion rate by 3 U/kg/hr

aPTT = activated partial thromboplastin time.
From Raschke RA, Reilly BR, Guidry JR, et al: The weight-based heparin dosing nomogram compared with a "standard care" nomogram: A randomized controlled trial. Ann Intern Med 119:874, 1993.

TABLE 72–15	Low-Molecular-Weight Heparins			
Name	Status	Molecular Weight (Daltons)	Anti-Xa/ anti-IIa ratio	Treatment Dose
Enoxaparin	FDA approved for DVT treatment	4800	3.9	1 mg/kg twice daily (approved as an inpatient or outpatient dose), or 1.5 mg/kg once daily (inpatient dose only)
Dalteparin	FDA approved, but not for DVT treatment	5000	2.2	100 U/kg twice daily, or 200 U/kg once daily
Nadroparin	Not available in the United States	4500	3.5	4100 U twice daily for patients weighing <50 kg, 6150 U twice daily for 50-70 kg, and 9200 U twice daily for >70 kg
Reviparin	Not available in the United States	3900	3.3	3500 U twice daily for patients weighing 35-45 kg, 4200 U twice daily for 46-60 kg and 6300 U twice daily for >60 kg
Tinzaparin	FDA approved for DVT treatment	4500	1.5	175 U/Kg once daily

DVT = deep venous thrombosis; FDA = Food and Drug Administration.

trials comparing 3674 patients with acute DVT receiving LMWH versus UFH demonstrated that LMWH reduced the mortality rate over 3 to 6 months of follow-up by 29 percent. The major bleeding complication rate was reduced by 43 percent. LMWH was highly cost effective compared with UFH for DVT management.

The U.S. Food and Drug Administration (FDA) has approved outpatient treatment of DVT *without PE* using enoxaparin 1 mg/kg every 12 hours for a minimum of 5 days. Warfarin is usually begun on the first evening of therapy, and enoxaparin is continued until a stable and therapeutic international normalized ratio (INR) of 2 to 3 is achieved. The dose of enoxaparin must be decreased in patients with renal insufficiency because LMWH is primarily renally excreted. The FDA approved the same enoxaparin dosing regimen for inpatient treatment of DVT *with or without PE,* as well as an alternative dosing regimen of 1.5 mg/kg once daily.

The FDA has *not* approved LMWH for treatment of patients presenting primarily with symptomatic PE. Nevertheless, LMWH is being used "off label" with increasing frequency for this indication. An individual patient data meta-analysis has shown that the efficacy and safety of enoxaparin for DVT treatment is not modified by the presence of symptomatic PE.[64] A meta-analysis of 1951 acute PE patients from 12 randomized controlled trials compared LMWH with UFH.[65] No statistically significant difference was found between the two treatment strategies, but there was a trend toward fewer recurrences and fewer major bleeding complications with LMWH.

LMWH has also been used off label as monotherapy without warfarin. In a trial of 672 patients with VTE and cancer, those randomized to dalteparin 200 U/kg once daily for 6 months had a much lower recurrence rate than patients receiving UFH: 8.8 percent versus 17.4 percent.[66] In a randomized controlled trial of 60 PE patients, extended 3-month treatment with enoxaparin as monotherapy for symptomatic acute PE appeared feasible and shortened the duration of hospitalization compared with patients receiving standard treatment.[67] In a subsequent 3-month PE trial of 40 patients, enoxaparin monotherapy was compared with enoxaparin as a bridge to warfarin. The study population encompassed a broad range of risk—30 percent had elevated troponin levels; 28 percent had moderate or severe right ventricular dysfunction on echocardiography; and 25 percent received thrombolysis. No difference occurred between the LMWH and UFH patients with respect to efficacy or safety outcomes.[68]

LMWH is usually dosed according to weight. However, if a quantitative assay is desired, an anti-Xa level can be obtained. Whether anti-Xa levels can be used reliably to improve efficacy and safety remains controversial. No broad-based consensus exists regarding therapeutic and toxic levels. A therapeutic level is estimated to be between 0.5 and 1 unit/ml. The peak level is reached 3 to 6 hours after subcutaneous injection. The plasma anti-Xa level may be useful in five situations: (1) UFH anticoagulation with baseline elevated aPTT caused by a lupus anticoagulant or anticardiolipin antibodies, (2) LMWH dosing in obese patients, (3) LMWH dosing in patients with renal dysfunction, (4) pregnancy,[69] and (5) determining the origin of an unexpected bleeding or clotting problem in patients receiving what appeared to be appropriate anticoagulant dosing.

FONDAPARINUX. Fondaparinux is an anticoagulant pentasaccharide that specifically inhibits activated Factor X. By selectively binding

TABLE 72–16	Fondaparinux Dosing for Patients with Acute Pulmonary Embolism or DVT		
Patient weight	<50 kg	50-100 kg	>100 kg
Daily dose of fondaparinux*	5 mg	7.5 mg	10 mg

*Assumes normal renal function.

to ATIII, fondaparinux potentiates (about 300 times) the neutralization of Factor Xa by ATIII. Fondaparinux does not inactivate thrombin (activated Factor II) and has no known effect on platelet function. Its predictable and sustained pharmacokinetic properties allow for a fixed-dose, once-daily subcutaneous injection, without the need for coagulation laboratory monitoring or dose adjustment. Fondaparinux does not cross-react with heparin-induced antibodies, and there is no documented case of fondaparinux-induced thrombocytopenia. No specific antidote for fondaparinux-associated bleeding exists.

The FDA has approved fondaparinux for initial treatment of acute PE and acute DVT as a bridge to oral anticoagulation with warfarin. The subcutaneous dosing regimen to treat VTE is straightforward (Table 72-16). The dose for prophylaxis is a fixed low dose of 2.5 mg once daily, regardless of body weight. However, fondaparinux elimination is prolonged in patients with renal impairment because the major route of elimination is urinary excretion of unchanged drug.

A randomized controlled trial of 2213 acute PE patients compared subcutaneous fondaparinux administered in a fixed dose once daily without coagulation monitoring versus intravenous UFH adjusted according to the aPTT.[70] Each regimen was given as a bridge to oral anticoagulation. In this largest ever anticoagulation trial of acute PE patients, there was no statistically significant difference between the two groups with respect to recurrent events or major bleeding. However, there was a trend toward fewer recurrences with fondaparinux (3.8 percent) compared with UFH (5 percent). A randomized controlled trial of 2205 acute DVT patients compared fondaparinux once daily versus enoxaparin 1 mg/kg twice daily.[71] Each drug was given as a bridge to oral anticoagulation. No difference between the two anticoagulation regimens occurred with respect to recurrent events or major bleeding.

WARFARIN. Warfarin is a vitamin K antagonist that prevents gamma carboxylation activation of coagulation factors II, VII, IX, and X. The full anticoagulant effect of warfarin may not be apparent for 5 days, even if the prothrombin time, used to monitor warfarin's effect, becomes elevated more rapidly. Elevation in the prothrombin time, used to adjust the dose of warfarin, may initially reflect depletion of coagulation factor VII, which has a short half-life of about 6 hours, whereas factor II has a long half-life of about 5 days. The prothrombin time should be standardized and reported according to the INR, not the prothrombin time ratio or the prothrombin time expressed in seconds. For VTE patients, the usual target INR range is between 2 and 3.

Warfarin is a difficult drug to dose and monitor. Warfarin is dosed by an "educated guess" coupled with trial and error. Considerable controversy exists over the optimal initial warfarin dose and whether it should be 5 mg or 10 mg. One open-label, randomized trial compared 2 warfarin initiation nomograms (5 mg versus 10 mg) in 50 patients with acute VTE.[72] All participants received fondaparinux for at least 5 days as a "bridge" to warfarin. The primary endpoint was defined as the number of days necessary to achieve 2 consecutive INR values greater than 1.9. The median time to 2 consecutive INRs was 5 days in both groups (p = 0.69), whether or not the initial dose was 5 or 10 mg, using the appropriate nomograms for following dose adjustment. These encouraging results should provide clinicians with increased warfarin dosing options, specifically two different reliable and effective nomograms for patients presenting with acute VTE.

WARFARIN PHARMACOGENOMICS. A wide variation in dose-response and frequent bleeding complications characterize the initiation of warfarin therapy. Genetic determinants of warfarin dose-response have recently been identified. Therefore a comprehensive pharmacogenetics approach to warfarin therapy has the potential to improve the safety and effectiveness of warfarin initiation.[73] Maintenance warfarin dosing can be estimated from demographic, clinical, and pharmacogenetic factors.[74]

Some patients have an extremely low warfarin dose requirement of 1.5 mg or less in the absence of liver dysfunction, drug interaction, or concomitant disease. They usually possess CYP2C9 variant alleles associated with impaired hydroxylation of S-warfarin.[75] If their warfarin pharmacogenetic profile is not known when warfarin is initiated, these individuals have a potentially high risk of bleeding complications.[76] Screening for CYP2C9 variants, with rapid turnaround of the results, may allow clinicians to develop individualized dosing protocols to reduce the risk of excessive anticoagulation.

Recently, vitamin K receptor gene haplotypes that can help stratify patients into low-, intermediate-, or high-dose warfarin groups have been discovered. Variants in the gene encoding vitamin K epoxide reductase complex 1 (VKORC1) explain about 25 percent of the variance in warfarin dosage.[77] Genetic profiles from CYP2C9 and VKORC1 can be combined to improve categorization of individual warfarin dose requirements.[78]

WARFARIN OVERLAP WITH HEPARIN. If warfarin is initiated as monotherapy without UFH, LMWH, or fondaparinux, a paradoxical exacerbation of hypercoagulability may occur, increasing the likelihood of recurrent thrombosis. Warfarin monotherapy decreases the levels of two endogenous anticoagulants, proteins C and S, thus increasing thrombogenic potential. By overlapping warfarin for at least 5 days with an immediately effective parenteral anticoagulant, the procoagulant effect of unopposed warfarin can be counteracted.

MONITORING WARFARIN. Monitoring warfarin requires walking a tightrope. Excessive dosing predisposes to bleeding complications. Subtherapeutic dosing makes patients vulnerable to recurrent VTE. All patients taking warfarin should wear a medical alert bracelet or necklace. This allows emergency medical personnel to reverse warfarin quickly if major trauma causes catastrophic bleeding.

Warfarin is plagued by multiple drug-drug and drug-food interactions. Most antibiotics increase the INR, but some, like rifampin, lower the INR. Even benign-sounding drugs such as acetaminophen increase the INR in a dose-dependent manner. The warfarin dose should be reduced when managing debilitated or elderly patients. On the other hand, green leafy vegetables have vitamin K and lower the INR. Avid green vegetable eaters usually require higher than average doses of warfarin. Concomitant medications with antiplatelet effects may increase the bleeding risk without increasing the INR. These include fish oil supplements, vitamin E, and alcohol.

Centralized anticoagulation clinics, staffed by nurses or pharmacists, have eased the administrative burden of prescribing warfarin and have assisted in safer and more effective anticoagulation. In an observational cohort study of 6645 patients receiving warfarin, 3323 were managed by a centralized clinical pharmacy anticoagulation service.[79] Personal physicians managed the control group of 3322 patients. Those managed by the anticoagulation service were 39 percent less likely to suffer an anticoagulation therapy-related complication. Improved outcome was mediated largely through improved maintenance of warfarin within the targeted INR range. Patients managed by the centralized service had therapeutic INRs for 63.5 percent of the study period compared with the control group, in whom INRs were therapeutic for 55.2 percent of time.

A systematic review and metaregression found that the setting for anticoagulation management is crucial in determining its success.[80] This report encompassed 50,208 patients from 67 studies. Patients managed by anticoagulation clinics or clinical trials remained in the therapeutic INR range 66 percent of the time. However, patients managed by community practices were therapeutic for only 57 percent of the study period.

"Point-of-care" devices provide the INR result in 2 minutes by use of a drop of whole blood obtained from a fingertip puncture. Appropriately selected patients can be taught to obtain their own INRs and to self-manage their warfarin dosing at home. A randomized trial of 737 patients compared self-management with conventional management.[81] No difference occurred between the two groups with respect to frequency of maintaining the target INR value. However, major anticoagulation-related complications, mostly thromboembolic, were more frequent in the conventionally managed patients compared with the self-managed patients: 7.3 versus 2.2 percent.

A systematic review and meta-analysis studied self-monitoring and self-adjusting of oral anticoagulation among 3049 patients in 14 trials.[82] Compared with conventional management, self-monitoring of INR was associated with a 55 percent reduction in thromboembolic events and a 39 percent reduction in all-cause mortality. A 35 percent decrease occurred in major hemorrhage. Those patients capable of both self-monitoring and self-adjusting therapy had fewer thromboembolic events (73 percent less) and 63 percent lower mortality compared with those who undertook self-monitoring alone.

COMPLICATIONS OF ANTICOAGULATION. The most important adverse effect of anticoagulation is hemorrhage. Major bleeding during anticoagulation may unmask a previously silent lesion such as bladder or colon cancer. Resumption of anticoagulation at a lower dose or implementing alternative therapy depends on the severity of the bleeding, the risk of recurrent thromboembolism, and the extent to which bleeding may have resulted from excessive anticoagulation.

To manage bleeding caused by heparin, cessation of UFH or LMWH will usually suffice. However, the anticoagulation effect will persist longer with LMWH than with UFH. With life-threatening or intracranial hemorrhage, protamine sulfate can be administered at the time heparin is discontinued. Protamine, a strongly basic protein, immediately reverses anticoagulant activity by forming a stable complex with the acidic heparin. However, protamine only partially inhibits the anticoagulant activity of LMWH. The dose is approximately 1 mg/100 units of heparin, administered slowly (e.g., 50 mg over 10 to 30 minutes). Protamine sulfate may cause allergic reactions, particularly in diabetic patients who have had prior exposure to protamine after using neutral protamine Hagedorn (NPH) insulin.

Heparin-induced thrombocytopenia is now recognized as a serious, pervasive, and perhaps increasingly frequent immune system-mediated complication. It is about 10 times more common with UFH than with LMWH.[83] IgG antibodies bind to a heparin-platelet factor 4 complex and activate platelets, causing release of prothrombotic microparticles, platelet consumption, and thrombocytopenia.[84] The microparticles promote excessive thrombin generation, which can result in paradoxical thrombosis. The thrombosis is usually extensive DVT or PE but can be manifested as myocardial infarction, stroke, or unusual arterial thrombosis such as mesenteric arterial thrombosis. One should suspect heparin-induced thrombocytopenia when the platelet count decreases to less than 100,000 or to less than 50 percent of baseline. Typically, heparin-induced thrombocytopenia occurs after 5 to 10 days of heparin exposure. UFH or LMWH should be immediately discontinued, and platelets should not be transfused. A direct thrombin inhibitor[85] such as argatroban, bivalirudin, or lepirudin should be used. The clinician should document heparin-induced thrombocytopenia in the patient's medical record[86] and instruct him or her to carry a special wallet card with details of the diagnosis and nadir platelet count.[87]

With warfarin, the risk of bleeding increases as the INR increases. Among a cohort of 979 outpatients with a first episode of INR greater than 5, 0.96 percent developed major hemorrhage.[88] In a meta-analysis of 33 studies with 4374 patient-years of oral anticoagulation, the rate of intracranial bleeding was 1.15 per 100 patient-years.[89] Paradoxically, for patients who develop warfarin-associated intracerebral hemorrhage, the INR is often less than 3 at the time of diagnosis. Nevertheless, mortality from intracerebral hemorrhage increases as the INR level rises.[90] One review of warfarin-associated hemorrhage documented only a brief warning period during which a slightly elevated INR predicted an imminent bleeding event.[91] Therefore the dose of warfarin should be adjusted downward when an "intranormal rise" in the INR occurs, such as an increase from 2.2 to 2.8 in patients whose target INR range is 2 to 3.

Life-threatening bleeding caused by warfarin has traditionally required immediate treatment with enough cryoprecipitate or fresh frozen plasma to normalize the INR and achieve immediate hemostasis. Recombinant human factor VIIa concentrate provides safe and rapid reversal of warfarin-induced excessive anticoagulation and appears to be a more reliable approach to warfarin reversal.[92] Recombinant VIIa was beneficial in a randomized placebo-controlled trial of patients with acute intracerebral hemorrhage not associated with warfarin.[93] Treatment within 4 hours limited the expansion of brain hematoma, reduced mortality, and improved functional outcome, with a small increase in the frequency of thromboembolic events.

Prior to "reversing" an elevated INR, it is useful to ensure that the abnormal laboratory value is "real" and not artifactual. An INR specimen that is not assayed promptly after blood collection can be spuriously high. In addition, "point of care" machines generally have higher INRs than central laboratories for patients who are intensively anticoagulated with warfarin. Point of care machine readings are often unreliable when the INR value exceeds 4. These abnormally high INR results should generally be verified with standard central laboratory instrumentation before adjusting the warfarin dose downward.[94]

Some patients with an INR less than 9 but without overt bleeding simply require interruption of warfarin therapy until the INR drifts down to the therapeutic range. To treat minor bleeding or a confirmed INR that exceeds 9 without any bleeding, the traditional approach is prescription of vitamin K 10 mg subcutaneously. This strategy usually reverses the effects of warfarin within 12 hours but makes patients relatively refractory to warfarin for up to 2 weeks. Merely withholding one or two doses of warfarin and administering 2.5 mg of oral vitamin K is a reliable and safe method for rapidly correcting an elevated INR in the absence of serious bleeding. A meta-analysis of 21 studies comparing oral and subcutaneous vitamin K had counterintuitive findings. Oral vitamin K was superior to subcutaneous vitamin K for reversal of excessively elevated INRs.[95]

NOVEL ANTICOAGULANTS. Multiple new anticoagulants in development may offer more convenient, safer, and possibly more effective anticoagulation than warfarin. Most of these drugs under development are administered in fixed doses without obligatory laboratory coagulation testing or dose adjustment. They have few drug-drug or drug-food interactions. The most common targets are thrombin and factor Xa.[96] Oral heparin is also being developed. Direct factor Xa inhibitors include rivaroxaban and apixaban. An oral direct thrombin inhibitor in phase III trials is dabigatran. Another oral direct thrombin inhibitor, ximelagatran, never received approval from the FDA because of liver toxicity.[97]

OPTIMAL DURATION OF ANTICOAGULATION. Management is more straightforward for provoked rather than unprovoked VTE (Table 72-17). For patients with first-time PE or proximal leg DVT provoked by surgery, trauma, oral contraceptives, pregnancy, or hormone replacement, the optimal duration of anticoagulation is 6 months with a target INR between 2 and 3. For patients with a first-time isolated calf or upper extremity DVT, with any of the same provoking factors, the optimal duration of anticoagulation is 3 months, with a target INR between 2 and 3. For a second VTE with the same provoking factors, most clinicians double the duration of anticoagulation. The American College of Chest Physicians (ACCP), however, recommends indefinite duration anticoagulation for these patients.[98] For a third VTE, a broad and strong consensus supports lifelong anticoagulation.

For patients with cancer and a first episode of DVT, there is disagreement concerning the optimal type of anticoagulant and the optimal duration of therapy. Many clinicians administer warfarin, even though the ACCP and the 2006 National Comprehensive Cancer Network Guidelines (http://www.nccn.org) recommend LMWH as monotherapy without warfarin. The FDA has not approved LMWH in this setting, although the Canadian equivalent to the FDA has approved LMWH for monotherapy in cancer patients. Many clinicians also administer a fixed 6 months of anticoagulation for cancer patients with VTE, even though the ACCP recommends indefinite duration anticoagulation in this clinical setting.

More than half of patients with PE have persistent imaging defects on lung scan or chest CT 6 months after the initial event.[99] Further resolution of thrombi appears to reach a plateau phase, but persistent defects rarely cause clinical problems. Therefore I do not recommend routine follow-up imaging in patients with PE who have received an uncomplicated course of 6 months of anticoagulation.

The most important risk factors for recurrence after discontinuing anticoagulation are (1) unprovoked or idiopathic VTE, (2) prior VTE, and (3) male gender. Patients with a first symptomatic PE have a higher risk of recurrent VTE than those with a first DVT. PE patients also have higher risk of symptomatic PE when they suffer a recurrent event.[100] For unknown reasons, the risk of VTE recurrence is much higher in men than in women after stopping anticoagulant treatment. In a meta-analysis of 15 studies enrolling 5416 individuals, men had a 50 percent higher rate of recurrence.[101] The lower risk of recurrence in women persisted even after adjusting for hormone replacement therapy or pregnancy. Low HDL cholesterol levels also predispose to an increased risk of recurrent VTE.[101a]

The presence of a thrombophilic disorder is considered much less important now than even a few years ago in determining the risk of recurrence and the need for indefinite duration anticoagulation. The Leiden University

TABLE 72–17	Optimal Duration of Anticoagulation
Clinical Setting	**Recommendation**
First provoked PE/proximal leg DVT	6 mo
First provoked upper extremity DVT or isolated calf DVT	3 mo
Second provoked VTE	12 mo or indefinite duration
Third VTE	Indefinite duration
Cancer	6 mo or indefinite duration
Unprovoked VTE	Consider indefinite duration

DVT = deep vein thrombosis; PE = pulmonary embolism; VTE = venous thromboembolism.

Medical Center followed 474 VTE patients for an average of 7.3 years.[102] All patients underwent extensive thrombophilia testing. Clinical factors appeared more important than laboratory abnormalities in predicting recurrence.

Patients with VTE outside the setting of surgery, trauma, cancer, oral contraceptives, pregnancy, or hormone replacement therapy are classified as having unprovoked or idiopathic VTE. This includes patients with VTE in the setting of long-haul air travel. A series of randomized trials using extended-duration; low-intensity warfarin anticoagulation (target INR between 1.5 and 2)[103]; standard intensity anticoagulation[104]; or the experimental oral direct thrombin inhibitor, ximelegatran[105]; as well as a meta-analysis[106] have demonstrated fewer recurrent events with indefinite duration rather than time-limited anticoagulation. Despite prolonged courses of anticoagulation, there does not appear to be a significant increase in major hemorrhage. However, no long-term cohort studies exist to demonstrate that 5, 10, or 20 years of anticoagulation are beneficial for these VTE patients. This causes unease among patients and their physicians. In theory, based on the available evidence from randomized trials, a 30-year-old patient with an idiopathic isolated calf DVT is a candidate for lifelong anticoagulation. The ACCP softly suggests "that patients with first-episode idiopathic DVT be considered for indefinite anticoagulation therapy." At Brigham and Women's Hospital, we recommend 6 months of full-intensity anticoagulation (INR 2 to 3), followed by indefinite-duration, low-intensity anticoagulation (INR 1.5 to 2) for all suitable patients with idiopathic VTE.

The question arises whether anticoagulant treatment can be tailored with biomarkers to optimize the duration of anticoagulation.[107] Persistent abnormally elevated D-dimer levels after withdrawal of anticoagulation may reflect an ongoing hypercoagulable state. In the placebo group of the PREVENT Trial, patients with unprovoked VTE received only 6 months of anticoagulation. D-dimer was measured 7 weeks after discontinuing warfarin.[108] The subsequent recurrence rate was 12 percent per year in those with elevated D-dimer levels compared with 5.6 percent per year in those with normal levels. Thus D-dimer might be useful to prognosticate recurrence after an initial 6 months of anticoagulation. Another approach in patients with idiopathic VTE involves measuring peak thrombin generation after discontinuation of anticoagulation.[109] Those patients with low levels of thrombin generation had low rates of recurrence.

INFERIOR VENA CAVAL FILTERS. The two major indications for placement of an inferior vena caval (IVC) filter are: (1) major hemorrhage that precludes anticoagulation and (2) recurrent PE despite well-documented anticoagulation. Eight-year follow-up of a randomized controlled trial of filters shows that filters reduce the risk of PE, increase the risk of DVT, and have no long-term impact on survival.[110] Nevertheless, insertion of filters has markedly increased, with a 25-fold rise in use in the United States over the past two decades.[111] In a prospective DVT registry of 5451 patients at 183 U.S. sites, 14 percent underwent insertion of filters.[112] Some patients have a temporary contraindication to anticoagulation. Under these circumstances, placement of a nonpermanent, retrievable filter may be appropriate. Retrievable filters can be left in place for weeks to months or can remain permanently, if necessary, because of a trapped large clot or a persistent contraindication to anticoagulation.[113] In a cohort of 220 patients receiving retrievable filters, the complication rate was 11.8 percent; retrieval was attempted in only 25 percent of the cohort with a success rate of 93 percent.[113a]

FIBRINOLYSIS. The FDA has approved alteplase for massive PE. The dose is 100 mg as a continuous infusion over 2 hours, without concomitant heparin. Guidelines for heparin before and after alteplase are provided in Table

72-18. The ACCP advises: "For most patients with PE, we recommend clinicians **not** use thrombolytic therapy. . . . For patients who are hemodynamically unstable, we suggest use of thrombolytic therapy."

When successfully utilized, thrombolysis will (1) reverse right-sided heart failure by physical dissolution of anatomically obstructing pulmonary arterial thrombus, thereby reducing right ventricular pressure overload; (2) prevent the continued release of serotonin and other neurohumoral factors that can worsen pulmonary hypertension; and (3) dissolve thrombus in the pelvic or deep leg veins, thereby decreasing the likelihood of recurrent PE. Theoretically, thrombolysis may also improve capillary blood flow and decrease the likelihood of developing chronic thromboembolic pulmonary hypertension.

MAPPET-3, the largest randomized trial of thrombolytic therapy versus heparin alone, studied patients with submassive PE who had the combination of normal blood pressure and right ventricular dysfunction.[114] Tissue plasminogen activator, compared with placebo, halved the frequency of escalation of therapy—defined as the need for pressors, mechanical ventilation, cardiopulmonary resuscitation, or open-label thrombolysis—and did not increase major bleeding. Open-label thrombolysis was the major endpoint that drove MAPPET-3 in favor of tissue plasminogen activator. Because the decision to use open-label thrombolysis after the initial randomization treatment was subjective, the trial has been criticized, and its findings have not been widely accepted.

A meta-analysis of 748 patients in 11 prior randomized thrombolysis trials found that in the subset of trials that included major PE, the mortality rate was halved and the major bleeding rate doubled among thrombolysis-treated subjects.[115] Thrombolysis will be tested in submassive PE patients in an ambitious 85-center, 12-country European trial that is scheduled to begin in 2007 and plans to enroll about 1100 patients over a 3-year period. The endpoints will be objective and will include death, resuscitation from cardiac arrest, mechanical ventilation, and prolonged use of vasopressors. The objective is to reduce the rate of death or cardiovascular collapse from 14 percent to 7 percent. If successful, this new trial will be larger than all previous placebo-controlled trials combined.

The potential benefits of thrombolysis must be weighed against the risk of hemorrhage. Clinical trials tend to underestimate the frequency of adverse drug reactions because high-risk patients are often excluded. Those patients who

TABLE 72–18	Use of Heparin Before and After Thrombolysis

1. Discontinue the continuous infusion of intravenous UFH as soon as the decision has been made to administer thrombolysis.

2. Proceed to order thrombolysis. Use the U.S. Food and Drug Administration–approved regimen of alteplase 100 mg as a continuous infusion over 2 hours.

3. Do not delay the thrombolysis infusion by obtaining an activated partial thromboplastin time (aPTT).

4. Infuse thrombolysis as soon as it becomes available.

5. At the conclusion of the 2-hr infusion, obtain a STAT aPTT.

6. If the aPTT is <80 sec (which is almost always the case), resume UFH as a continuous infusion without a bolus.

7. If the aPTT exceeds 80 sec, hold off from resuming heparin for 4 hr and repeat the aPTT. At this time, the aPTT has virtually always declined to <80 sec. If this is the case, resume continuous infusion intravenous UFH without a bolus.

STAT = immediately; UFH = unfractionated heparin.

are enrolled receive extremely close monitoring. In the International Cooperative Pulmonary Embolism Registry, with 2454 patients enrolled from 52 hospitals in 7 countries, the intracerebral hemorrhage rate was 3 percent among those patients treated with thrombolysis. Increasing age is a major independent risk factor for hemorrhagic complications after PE thrombolysis. In a German multicenter PE registry of 428 women and 291 men, thrombolysis was associated with a 79 percent reduction in 30-day mortality in men, but no statistically significant reduction in women.[116] Women had a 27 percent rate of major bleeding compared with 15 percent in men.

At Brigham and Women's Hospital, we tend to prescribe thrombolysis to patients with submassive PE who have moderate or severe right ventricular enlargement on chest CT or right ventricular dysfunction on echocardiogram. We are especially likely to use thrombolysis when patients have elevation in cardiac biomarkers, as well as right ventricular hypokinesis. Despite more than two decades of experience with thrombolysis for acute PE, review of our alteplase-treated patients revealed a major bleeding rate of 19 percent.[117]

Unlike patients receiving myocardial infarction thrombolysis, patients with PE have a wide "window" for effective use of thrombolysis. Specifically, patients who receive thrombolysis up to 14 days after new symptoms or signs maintain an effective response, probably because of the bronchial collateral circulation. Therefore patients should be considered potentially eligible for thrombolysis if they present with new symptoms or signs within 2 weeks.

DEEP VENOUS THROMBOSIS INTERVENTIONS. Indications for DVT thrombolysis remain controversial because no convincing reduction in leg ulceration or recurrent DVT has yet been demonstrated. Pooling results from previous trials of anatomically large DVT suggest a reduction in post-thrombotic syndrome.[118] Common indications for thrombolysis include extensive iliofemoral or upper extremity venous thrombosis. Totally occlusive venous thrombosis usually does not improve if the agent is infused through a peripheral vein. Therefore DVT thrombolysis is almost always administered locally through a catheter. This intervention is frequently combined with catheter-directed suction embolectomy, venous angioplasty, and venous stenting.

CATHETER EMBOLECTOMY. Interventional catheterization techniques for massive PE include mechanical fragmentation of thrombus with a standard pulmonary artery catheter, clot pulverization with a rotating basket catheter, percutaneous rheolytic thrombectomy, and pigtail rotational catheter embolectomy. Another approach is simultaneous mechanical clot fragmentation and pharmacological thrombolysis. Catheter embolectomy occasionally results in extraction of massive pulmonary arterial thrombus. More often, multiple tiny clot fragments are suctioned through the catheter, with modest angiographic improvement, resulting nevertheless in rapid restoration of normal blood pressure with a decrease in hypoxemia. Catheter techniques have been limited by poor maneuverability, mechanical hemolysis, macroembolization, and microembolization. A new percutaneous thrombectomy catheter is under development and shows promise.[119] It aspirates, macerates, and removes pulmonary artery thrombus. In animal models of massive PE, it has rapidly reversed cardiogenic shock without device-related complications (Fig. 72-7). Another novel approach is temporary pulmonary stent placement as emergency treatment of acute PE.[120] The stent is made from woven Nitinol and has a distal blunt end and proximal crimped end. In an animal model of massive PE, there was marked improvement in pulmonary angiograms, coupled with reductions in tachycardia and pulmonary hypertension, and improved mean arterial pressure.

SURGICAL EMBOLECTOMY. Emergency surgical embolectomy with cardiopulmonary bypass has reemerged as an effective strategy for managing patients with massive PE and systemic arterial hypotension or submassive PE with right ventricular dysfunction[121] in whom contraindications preclude thrombolysis (Fig. 72-8). This operation is also suited for acute PE patients who require surgical excision of a right atrial thrombus or closure of a patent foramen ovale. Surgical embolectomy can also rescue patients refractory to thrombolysis.[122] The results of embolectomy will be optimized if patients are referred before the onset of cardiogenic shock. In one study, 47 patients underwent surgical embolectomy in a 4-year period, with a 96 percent survival rate.[123] We perform the procedure off bypass, with normothermia, without aortic cross-clamping or cardioplegic or fibrillatory arrest. Avoiding blind instrumentation of the fragile pulmonary arteries is imperative. Extraction is limited to directly visible clot, which can be accomplished through the segmental pulmonary arteries.

EMOTIONAL SUPPORT. Patients find PE to be emotionally draining. They and their families require constant reassurance that most patients have good outcomes once the diagnosis has been established. They must learn to cope with PE-related issues such as genetic predisposition, potential long-term disability, changes in lifestyle related to anticoagulation, and the possibility of suffering a recurrent event. By discussing the implications of PE with patients and their families, we can allay the emotional burden. A Pulmonary Embolism Support Group for patients can fill this need. Our group meets at the hospital once every 3 weeks in the evening. Although these sessions have an educational component, the major emphasis is on discussing the anxieties and day-to-day difficulties that occur in the aftermath of PE.

MASSIVE PULMONARY EMBOLISM. Hospitals should establish written protocols and rehearse interdisciplinary management for patients with massive PE. The policies and procedures to treat massive PE should become as firmly established and enforced as those for acute ST segment elevation myocardial infarction. Some management tips are presented in Table 72-19. Rapid integration of historical information, physical findings, and laboratory data along with an integrated team approach among cardiologists, emergency department physicians, radiologists, and cardiac surgeons is crucial to maximize success. Immediate patient referral to hospitals specializing in massive PE should be considered. In a series of 108 patients who presented with

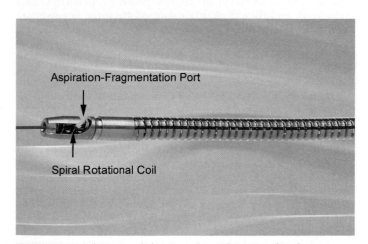

FIGURE 72–7 Pulmonary embolectomy catheter. The Aspirex thrombectomy device is an 11-French over-the-wire catheter for the treatment of patients with massive pulmonary embolism. This device aspirates, macerates, and removes thrombus through an L-shaped aspiration-fragmentation port by high-speed rotation of a spiral coil.

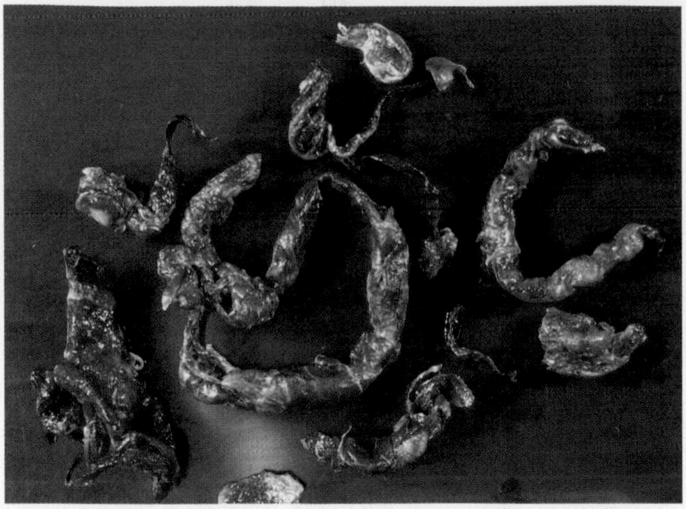

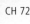

FIGURE 72–8 This 72-year-old woman presented with presyncope, hypotension, and hypoxia. She was diagnosed with massive pulmonary embolism by chest computed tomography scan and underwent emergency pulmonary embolectomy.

TABLE 72–19	Massive Pulmonary Embolism

Bolus high-dose intravenous unfractionated heparin as soon as massive pulmonary embolism is suspected.

Begin continuous infusion unfractionated heparin to achieve a target activated partial thromboplastin time of at least 80 sec.

Try volume resuscitation with no more than 500-1000 ml of fluid.

Excessive volume resuscitation will worsen right ventricular failure.

Have a low threshold for administration of vasopressors and inotropes.

Decide whether thrombolysis can be safely administered, without a high risk of major hemorrhage.

If thrombolysis is too risky, consider placement of an inferior vena caval filter, catheter embolectomy, or surgical embolectomy.

Do not use a combination of thrombolysis and vena caval filter insertion. The prongs of the filter insert into the caval wall. Concomitant thrombolysis predisposes to caval wall hemorrhage.

Consider immediate referral to a tertiary care hospital specializing in massive pulmonary embolism.

CH 72

massive PE and hypotension, a counterintuitive observation was that thrombolysis did not reduce mortality or recurrent PE. Vena caval filter insertion did prevent recurrence and markedly lowered mortality.[124]

POSTTHROMBOTIC SYNDROME AND CHRONIC VENOUS INSUFFICIENCY. Dysfunction of the valves of the deep venous system is most often a consequence of damage from prior DVT. Obstruction of the deep veins may limit the outflow of blood, causing increased venous pressure with muscle contraction. Abnormal hemody-namics in the large veins of the leg are transmitted into the microcirculation. The eventual result is venous microangiopathy.[125]

Many patients with VTE are plagued with chronic lower leg swelling and calf discomfort that can become problematic years after the initial event. Physical findings may include varicose veins, abnormal pigmentation of the medial malleolus, and venous ulceration. The economic impact is high because of time lost from work and the expense of medical diagnosis and treatment. Chronic venous disease is associated with a reduced quality of life, especially in relation to increased pain, decreased physical function, and decreased mobility.[126] A mainstay of therapy is vascular compression stockings, below knee, 30 to 40 mm Hg. Compression stockings improve venous hemodynamics, reduce edema, and minimize skin discoloration. By alleviating calf discomfort, stockings improve the quality of life. Risk factors for developing postthrombotic syndrome include proximal (rather than calf) DVT, male gender, and high D-dimer levels after completing a course of anticoagulation.[127] Patients with postthrombotic syndrome also have an increased risk of recurrent VTE.

CHRONIC THROMBOEMBOLIC PULMONARY HYPER-TENSION. Chronic thromboembolic pulmonary hypertension occurs much more frequently after acute PE than had been classically believed. The old teaching was that chronic thromboembolic pulmonary hypertension had a prevalence of 1 in 500 or 1 in 1000 cases of acute PE. New data indicate the frequency is between 1 and 4 percent.[128,129] Although acute PE is the initiating event, pulmonary vascular remodeling may cause severe pulmonary hypertension out of proportion to the pulmonary vascular obliteration observed on pulmonary angiography.[130] To complicate matters further, there may be an overlap between chronic thromboembolic pulmonary hypertension and idiopathic pulmonary artery

hypertension, which is characterized by in situ pulmonary artery thrombosis.[131]

Primary therapy is pulmonary thromboendarterectomy, which, if successful, can reduce and at times even cure pulmonary hypertension.[132,132a] The operation involves a median sternotomy, institution of cardiopulmonary bypass, and deep hypothermia with circulatory arrest periods. Incisions are made in both pulmonary arteries into the lower-lobe branches. Pulmonary thromboendarterectomy removes organized thrombus by establishing an endarterectomy plane in all involved vessels. At the University of California at San Diego, almost 2000 patients debilitated by chronic pulmonary hypertension caused by PE have undergone pulmonary thromboendarterectomy with good results and at an acceptable risk. When surgery is not feasible, balloon pulmonary angioplasty can be considered. This procedure is associated with functional improvement and improved exercise tolerance.[133]

PREVENTION

PE is difficult to diagnose, expensive to treat, and occasionally lethal despite therapy. Therefore preventive measures are of paramount importance. Fortunately, numerous prophylaxis options are available (Table 72-20). North American[134] and European[135] consensus conferences have provided detailed guidelines with various mechanical measures and pharmacological agents. Often multiple options are available for each category of risk. The specific prophylaxis modality chosen within a risk group is less important than adhering to the standard that all hospitalized patients will receive preventive measures appropriate to their risk level. The concept of prophylaxis is gaining increased acceptance, partly because of the medicolegal liability of physicians who omit prophylaxis among hospitalized patients with risk factors for venous thrombosis. Computer-generated alerts to physicians whose hospitalized patients are not receiving prophylaxis can reduce the frequency of symptomatic PE and DVT.[136]

Routine use of VTE prophylaxis is more reliably established among surgeons than among medical physicians.[136a] Perhaps this is because VTE prophylaxis was first tested in a large-scale international multicenter surgical trial in 1975.[137] The 4121 mostly general surgical patients were randomized to receive heparin 5000 units three times daily for 1 week or no heparin prophylaxis. The first heparin injection was administered 2 hours before the skin incision. The difference in outcome was dramatic in the two groups: 16 controls and 2 heparin group patients died of massive, autopsy-confirmed PE. The fatal hemorrhage rate was virtually identical: five controls and four heparin group patients. Though cost effective,[138] VTE prophylaxis is ordered less frequently among hospitalized medical than hospitalized surgical patients.[139] In a Canadian audit of 1894 medical admissions, 90 percent should have received VTE prophylaxis.[140] Some form of prophylaxis was administered to 23 percent of all patients, but only 16 percent received appropriate evidence-based prophylaxis. Patients with cancer had a 60 percent lower chance of receiving prophylaxis than other medical patients.

MECHANICAL MEASURES. Mechanical measures consist of graduated compression stockings and intermittent pneumatic compression devices, which enhance endogenous fibrinolysis and increase venous blood flow. These measures can be used in combination. Mechanical measures are especially worthwhile among patients who have an absolute contraindication to anticoagulation. A meta-analysis of intermittent pneumatic compression devices was undertaken in 2270 postoperative patients from 15 studies. In comparison to no prophylaxis, intermittent pneumatic compression devices reduced the risk of DVT by 60 percent.[141] Intermittent pneumatic compression combined with pharmacological prophylaxis can achieve an extremely low DVT rate in the postoperative setting.[142]

PHARMACOLOGICAL AGENTS. Pharmacological prophylaxis options include UFH, LMWH, fondaparinux, and warfarin. The American College of Chest Physicians does not consider aspirin to confer meaningful prophylaxis against VTE. For prophylaxis in the setting of total hip replacement or hip fracture, the clinician should extend prophylaxis for 4 weeks. For cancer surgery patients, enoxaparin for 4 weeks postoperatively is superior to enoxaparin for 1 week.[143]

PROPHYLAXIS STRATEGIES IN MEDICAL PATIENTS. Hospitalized medical patients are at risk for DVT and PE. The risk is greatest in intensive care units, but it persists among less critically ill patients with diagnoses that include congestive heart failure, respiratory failure, pneumonia, or other serious infection. These venous thromboses can often be prevented with low, fixed, prophylactic doses of LMWH, such as enoxaparin 40 mg once daily,[144] dalteparin 5000 units once daily,[145] or fondaparinux 2.5 mg once daily.[146] Nevertheless, in the DVT FREE Registry of 5451 DVT patients, 2295 of the 3894 patients (59%) who did not receive prophylaxis were medical patients.

FUTURE PERSPECTIVES

Routine preventive measures have previously been an option that physicians could choose to use or ignore. However, a cultural and regulatory shift has begun. The National Quality Forum, the Joint Commission on Accreditation of Hospitals, and the Leapfrog Group are calling for mandatory preventive measures. The public is starting to advocate for prevention as well. These efforts will accelerate with the release of the U.S. Surgeon General's 2007 "Call to Action" on DVT. This initiative will provide the public with educational materials on VTE prevention and treatment that are specifically targeted for a lay audience. The Office of the Surgeon General will provide medical professionals with updates on VTE epidemiology, diagnosis, management, and prophylaxis. The North American Thrombosis Forum, a nonprofit organization, has been established to enhance education of health care professionals and the public on issues related to VTE (www.NATFonline.org).

CH 72

Pulmonary Embolism

TABLE 72–20	Regimens for Venous Thromboembolism Prevention
Condition	**Prophylaxis**
Hospitalization with medical illness	Unfractionated heparin 5000 units SC TID **or** Enoxaparin 40 mg SC QD **or** Dalteparin 5000 units SC QD **or** Fondaparinux 2.5 mg SC QD (in patients with a heparin allergy such as heparin-induced thrombocytopenia) **or** Graduated compression stockings/intermittent pneumatic compression for patients with contraindications to anticoagulation Consider combination pharmacological and mechanical prophylaxis for high-risk patients Consider surveillance lower extremity ultrasonography for intensive care unit patients
General surgery	Unfractionated heparin 5000 units SC BID or TID **or** Enoxaparin 40 mg SC QD **or** Dalteparin 2500 or 5000 units SC QD
Major orthopedic surgery	Warfarin (target INR 2 to 3) **or** Enoxaparin 30 mg SC BID **or** Enoxaparin 40 mg SC QD **or** Dalteparin 2500 or 5000 units SC QD **or** Fondaparinux 2.5 mg SC QD
Neurosurgery	Unfractionated heparin 5000 units SC BID **or** Enoxaparin 40 mg SC QD **and** Graduated compression stockings/intermittent pneumatic compression Consider surveillance lower extremity ultrasonography
Oncologic surgery	Enoxaparin 40 mg SC QD
Thoracic surgery	Unfractionated heparin 5000 units SC TID **and** Graduated compression stockings/intermittent pneumatic compression

BID = twice daily; INR = international normalized ratio; QD = daily; SC = subcutaneous; TID = three times daily.

REFERENCES

Epidemiology

1. Stein PD, Kayali F, Olson RE: Estimated case fatality rate of pulmonary embolism, 1979 to 1998. Am J Cardiol 93:1197, 2004.
2. Stein PD, Beemath A, Olson RE: Trends in the incidence of pulmonary embolism and deep vein thrombosis in hospitalized patients. Am J Cardiol 95:1525, 2005.
3. Cushman M, Tsai AW, White RH, et al: Deep vein thrombosis and pulmonary embolism in two cohorts: The longitudinal investigation of thromboembolism etiology. Am J Med 117:19, 2004.
4. Zee RY, Cook NR, Cheng S, et al: Polymorphism in the beta2-adrenergic receptor and lipoprotein lipase genes as risk determinants for idiopathic venous thromboembolism: A multilocus, population-based, prospective genetic analysis. Circulation 113:2193, 2006.
5. Bova C, Marchiori A, Noto A, et al: Incidence of arterial cardiovascular events in patients with idiopathic venous thromboembolism: A retrospective cohort study. Thromb Haemost 96:132, 2006.
6. Vaitkus PT, Leizorovicz A, Cohen AT, et al: Mortality rates and risk factors for asymptomatic deep vein thrombosis in medical patients. Thromb Haemost 93:76, 2005.
7. Stein PD, Beemath A, Olson RE: Obesity as a risk factor in venous thromboembolism. Am J Med 118:978, 2005.
8. Stein PD, Beemath A, Meyers FA, et al: Incidence of venous thromboembolism in patients hospitalized with cancer. Am J Med 119:60, 2006.
9. Chew HK, Wun T, Harvey D, et al: Incidence of venous thromboembolism and its effect on survival among patients with common cancers. Arch Intern Med 166:458, 2006.
10. Smeeth L, Cook C, Thomas S, et al: Risk of deep vein thrombosis and pulmonary embolism after acute infection in a community setting. Lancet 367:1075, 2006.
11. Tillie-Leblond I, Marquette CH, Perez T, et al: Pulmonary embolism in patients with unexplained exacerbation of chronic obstructive pulmonary disease: Prevalence and risk factors. Ann Intern Med 144:390, 2006.
12. David PS, Boatwright EA, Tozer BS, et al: Hormonal contraception update. Mayo Clin Proc 81:949, 2006.
13. Curb JD, Prentice RL, Bray PF, et al: Venous thrombosis and conjugated equine estrogen in women without a uterus. Arch Intern Med 166:772, 2006.
14. Parkin L, Bell ML, Herbison GP, et al: Air travel and fatal pulmonary embolism. Thromb Haemost 95:807, 2006.
15. Schreijer AJ, Cannegieter SC, Meijers JC, et al: Activation of coagulation system during air travel: A crossover study. Lancet 367:832, 2006.
16. Toff WD, Jones CI, Ford I, et al: Effect of hypobaric hypoxia, simulating conditions during long-haul air travel, on coagulation, fibrinolysis, platelet function, and endothelial activation. JAMA 295:2251, 2006.
17. Heit JA: The epidemiology of venous thromboembolism in the community: Implications for prevention and management. J Thromb Thrombolysis 21:23, 2006.
18. Goldhaber SZ, Tapson VF: A prospective registry of 5451 patients with ultrasound-confirmed deep vein thrombosis. Am J Cardiol 93:259, 2004.
19. Joffe HV, Kucher N, Tapson VF, Goldhaber SZ: Upper-extremity deep vein thrombosis: A prospective registry of 592 patients. Circulation 110:1605, 2004.

20. Lim W, Crowther MA, Eikelboom JW: Management of antiphospholipid antibody syndrome: A systematic review. JAMA 295:1050, 2006.
21. Konstantinides S: Pulmonary embolism: Impact of right ventricular dysfunction. Curr Opin Cardiol 20:496, 2005.
22. Piazza G, Goldhaber SZ: The acutely decompensated right ventricle: Pathways for diagnosis and management. Chest 128:1836, 2005.
23. Kucher N, Printzen G, Goldhaber SZ: Prognostic role of brain natriuretic peptide in acute pulmonary embolism. Circulation 107:2545, 2003.
24. Kucher N, Goldhaber SZ: Management of massive pulmonary embolism. Circulation 112:e28, 2005.
25. Goldhaber SZ, Elliott CE: Acute pulmonary embolism: Part I. Epidemiology, pathophysiology, and diagnosis. Circulation 108:2726, 2003.

Diagnosis

26. Roy PM, Meyer G, Vielle B, Le Gall C, et al, for the EMDEPU Study Group: Appropriateness of diagnostic management and outcomes of suspected pulmonary embolism. Ann Intern Med 144:157, 2006.
27. Elliott CG, Goldhaber SZ, Jensen RL: Delays in diagnosis of deep vein thrombosis and pulmonary embolism. Chest 128:3372, 2005.
28. Kabrhel C, Camargo CA Jr, Goldhaber SZ: Clinical gestalt and the diagnosis of pulmonary embolism: does experience matter? Chest 127:1627, 2005.
29. Wells PS, Ginsberg JS, Anderson DR, et al: Use of a clinical model for safe management of patients with suspected pulmonary embolism. Ann Intern Med 129:997, 1998.
30. van Belle A, Buller HR, Huisman MV, et al: Effectiveness of managing suspected pulmonary embolism using an algorithm combining clinical probability, D-dimer testing, and computed tomography. JAMA 295:172, 2006.
31. Khairy P, O'Donnell CP, Landzberg MJ: Transcatheter closure versus medical therapy of patent foramen ovale and presumed paradoxical thromboemboli: A systematic review. Ann Intern Med 139:753, 2003.
32. Meissner I, Khandheria BK, Heit JA, et al: Patent foramen ovale: innocent or guilty? Evidence from a prospective population-based study. J Am Coll Cardiol 47:440, 2006.
33. Dunn KL, Wolf JP, Dorfman DM, et al: Normal D-dimer levels in emergency department patients suspected of acute pulmonary embolism. J Am Coll Cardiol 40:1475, 2002.
34. Stein PD, Hull RD, Patel KC, et al: D-dimer for the exclusion of acute venous thrombosis and pulmonary embolism: A systematic review. Ann Intern Med 140:589, 2004.
35. Kearon C, Ginsberg JS, Douketis J, et al: An evaluation of D-dimer in the diagnosis of pulmonary embolism: A randomized trial. Ann Intern Med 144:812, 2006.
36. Punukollu G, Gowda RM, Vasavada BC, Khan IA: Role of electrocardiography in identifying right ventricular dysfunction in acute pulmonary embolism. Am J Cardiol 96:450, 2005.
37. Stein PD, Kayali F, Olson RE: Trends in the use of diagnostic imaging in patients hospitalized with acute pulmonary embolism. Am J Cardiol 93:1316, 2004.
38. Goldhaber SZ: Multislice computed tomography for pulmonary embolism—a technological marvel. N Engl J Med 352:1812, 2005.
39. Schoepf UJ, Goldhaber SZ, Costello P: Spiral computed tomography for acute pulmonary embolism. Circulation 109:2160, 2004.
40. Moores LK, Jackson WL Jr, Shorr AF, Jackson JL: Meta-analysis: Outcomes in patients with suspected pulmonary embolism managed with computed tomographic pulmonary angiography. Ann Intern Med 141:866, 2004.
41. Quiroz R, Kucher N, Zou KH, et al: Clinical validity of a negative computed tomography scan in patients with suspected pulmonary embolism: A systematic review. JAMA 293:2012, 2005.
42. Perrier A, Roy PM, Sanchez O, et al: Multidetector-row computed tomography in suspected pulmonary embolism. N Engl J Med 352:1760, 2005.
43. Stein PD, Fowler SE, Goodman LR, et al: Multidetector computed tomography for acute pulmonary embolism. N Engl J Med 354:2317, 2006.
44. Perrier A, Bounameaux H: Accuracy or outcome in suspected pulmonary embolism. N Engl J Med 354:2383, 2006.
45. The PIOPED Investigators: Value of the ventilation/perfusion scan in acute pulmonary embolism. Results of the prospective investigation of pulmonary embolism diagnosis (PIOPED). JAMA 263:2753, 1990.
46. Blum A, Bellou A, Guillemin F, et al: Performance of magnetic resonance angiography in suspected acute pulmonary embolism. Thromb Haemost 93:503, 2005.
47. Stevens SM, Elliott CG, Chan KJ, et al: Withholding anticoagulation after a negative result on duplex ultrasonography for suspected symptomatic deep venous thrombosis. Ann Intern Med 140:985, 2004.

Management

48. Goldhaber SZ, Visani L, De Rosa M: Acute pulmonary embolism: Clinical outcomes in the International Cooperative Pulmonary Embolism Registry (ICOPER). Lancet 353:1386, 1999.
49. Kucher N, Rossi E, De Rosa M, Goldhaber SZ: Prognostic role of echocardiography among patients with acute pulmonary embolism and a systolic arterial pressure of 90 mm Hg or higher. Arch Intern Med 165:1777, 2005.
50. Geibel A, Zehender M, Kasper W, et al: Prognostic value of the ECG on admission in patients with acute major pulmonary embolism. Eur Respir J 25:843, 2005.
51. Konstantinides S, Geibel A, Olschewski M, et al: Importance of cardiac troponins I and T in risk stratification of patients with acute pulmonary embolism. Circulation 106:1263, 2002.
52. Binder L, Pieske B, Olschewski M, et al: N-terminal pro-brain natriuretic peptide or troponin testing followed by echocardiography for risk stratification of acute pulmonary embolism. Circulation 112:1573, 2005.
53. Sohne M, Ten Wolde M, Boomsma F, et al: Brain natriuretic peptide in hemodynamically stable acute pulmonary embolism. J Thromb Haemost 4:552, 2006.
54. Goldhaber SZ: Echocardiography in the management of pulmonary embolism. Ann Intern Med 136:691, 2002.
55. Giannitsis E, Katus HA: Risk stratification in pulmonary embolism based on biomarkers and echocardiography. Circulation 112:1520, 2005.
56. Scridon T, Scridon C, Skali H, et al: Prognostic significance of troponin elevation and right ventricular enlargement in acute pulmonary embolism. Am J Cardiol 96:303, 2005.
57. Quiroz R, Kucher N, Schoepf UJ, et al: Right ventricular enlargement on chest computed tomography: prognostic role in acute pulmonary embolism. Circulation 109:2401, 2004.
58. Schoepf UJ, Kucher N, Kipfmueller F, et al: Right ventricular enlargement on chest computed tomography: A predictor of early death in acute pulmonary embolism. Circulation 110:3276, 2004.
59. Raschke RA, Reilly BR, Guidry JR, et al: The weight-based heparin dosing nomogram compared with a "standard care" nomogram: A randomized controlled trial. Ann Intern Med 119:874, 1993.
60. Writing Committee for the Galilei Investigators: Subcutaneous adjusted-dose unfractionated heparin vs fixed-dose low-molecular-weight heparin in the initial treatment of venous thromboembolism. Arch Intern Med 164:1077, 2004.
61. Kearon C, Ginsberg JS, Julian JA, et al: Comparison of fixed-dose weight-adjusted unfractionated heparin and low-molecular-weight heparin for acute treatment of venous thromboembolism. JAMA 296:935, 2006.
62. Becattini C, Agnelli G, Emmerich J, et al: Initial treatment of venous thromboembolism. Thromb Haemost 96:242, 2006.
63. Merli G, Spiro TE, Olsson CG, et al: Subcutaneous enoxaparin once or twice daily compared with intravenous unfractionated heparin for treatment of venous thromboembolic disease. Ann Intern Med 134:191, 2001.
64. Mismetti P, Quenet S, Levine M, et al: Enoxaparin in the treatment of deep vein thrombosis with or without pulmonary embolism: An individual patient data meta-analysis. Chest 128:2203, 2005.
65. Quinlan DJ, McQuillan A, Eikelboom JW: Low-molecular-weight heparin compared with intravenous unfractionated heparin for treatment of pulmonary embolism: A meta-analysis of randomized, controlled trials. Ann Intern Med 140:175, 2004.
66. Lee AYY, Levine MN, Baker RI, et al: Low-molecular-weight heparin versus a coumarin for the prevention of recurrent venous thromboembolism in patients with cancer. N Engl J Med 349:146, 2003.
67. Beckman JA, Dunn K, Sasahara AA, Goldhaber SZ: Enoxaparin monotherapy without oral anticoagulation to treat acute symptomatic pulmonary embolism. Thromb Haemost 89:953, 2003.
68. Kucher N, Quiroz R, McKean S, et al: Extended enoxaparin monotherapy for acute symptomatic pulmonary embolism. Vasc Med 10:251, 2005.
69. Seshadri N, Goldahber SZ, Elkavam U, et al: The clinical challenge of bridging anticoagulation with low-molecular-weight heparin in patients with mechanical prosthetic heart valves: An evidence-based comparative review focusing on anticoagulation options in pregnant and nonpregnant patients. Am Heart J 150:27, 2005.
70. The Matisse Investigators: Subcutaneous fondaparinux versus intravenous unfractionated heparin in the initial treatment of pulmonary embolism. N Engl J Med 349:1695, 2003.
71. Buller HR, Davidson BL, Decousus H, et al: Fondaparinux or enoxaparin for the initial treatment of symptomatic deep venous thrombosis: A randomized trial. Ann Intern Med 140:867, 2004.
72. Quiroz R, Gerhard-Herman M, Kosowsky JM, et al: Comparison of a single end point to determine optimal initial warfarin dosing (5 mg versus 10 mg) for venous thromboembolism. Am J Cardiol 98:535, 2006.
73. Voora D, McLeod HL, Eby C, Gage BF: The pharmacogenomics of coumarin therapy. Pharmacogenomics 6:503, 2005.
74. Gage BF, Eby C, Milligan PE, et al: Use of pharmacogenetics and clinical factors to predict the maintenance dose of warfarin. Thromb Haemost 91:87, 2004.
75. Joffe HV, Xu R, Johnson FB, et al: Warfarin dosing and cytochrome P450 2C9 polymorphisms. Thromb Haemost 91:1123, 2004.
76. Higashi MK, Veenstra DL, Kondo LM, et al: Association between CYP2C9 genetic variants and anticoagulation-related outcomes during warfarin therapy. JAMA 287:1690, 2002.
77. Rieder MJ, Reiner AP, Gage BF, et al: Effect of VKORC1 haplotypes on transcriptional regulation and warfarin dose. N Engl J Med 352:2285, 2005.
78. Vecsler M, Loebstein R, Almog S, et al: Combined genetic profiles of components and regulators of the vitamin K-dependent gamma-carboxylation system affect individual sensitivity to warfarin. Thromb Haemost 95:205, 2006.
79. Witt DM, Sadler MA, Shanahan RL, et al: Effect of a centralized clinical pharmacy anticoagulation service on the outcomes of anticoagulation therapy. Chest 127:1515, 2005.
80. van Walraven C, Jennings A, Oake N, et al: Effect of study setting on anticoagulation control: A systematic review and metaregression. Chest 129:1155, 2006.
81. Menendez-Jandula B, Souto JC, Oliver A, et al: Comparing self-management of oral anticoagulant therapy with clinic management: A randomized trial. Ann Intern Med 142:1, 2005.
82. Heneghan C, Alonso-Coello P, Garcia-Alamino JM, et al: Self-monitoring of oral anticoagulation: A systematic review and meta-analysis. Lancet 367:404, 2006.
83. Martel N, Lee J, Wells PS: Risk for heparin-induced thrombocytopenia with unfractionated and low-molecular-weight heparin thromboprophylaxis: A meta-analysis. Blood 106:2710, 2005.

CH 72

84. Jang IK, Hursting MJ: When heparins promote thrombosis: Review of heparin-induced thrombocytopenia. Circulation 111:2671, 2005.

85. Di Nisio M, Middeldorp S, Buller HR: Direct thrombin inhibitors. N Engl J Med 353:1028, 2005.

86. Arepally GM, Ortel TL: Heparin-induced thrombocytopenia. N Engl J Med 355:809, 2006.

87. Baroletti SA, Goldhaber SZ: Heparin-induced thrombocytopenia. Circulation 114: e355, 2006.

88. Garcia DA, Regan S, Crowther M, Hylek EM: The risk of hemorrhage among patients with warfarin-associated coagulopathy. J Am Coll Cardiol 47:804, 2006.

89. Linkins LA, Choi PT, Douketis JD: Clinical impact of bleeding in patients taking oral anticoagulant therapy for venous thromboembolism: A meta-analysis. Ann Intern Med 139:893, 2003.

90. Rosand J, Eckman MH, Knudsen KA, et al: The effect of warfarin and intensity of anticoagulation on outcome of intracerebral hemorrhage. Arch Intern Med 164:880, 2004.

91. Kucher N, Connolly S, Beckman JA, et al: International normalized ratio increase before warfarin-associated hemorrhage: brief and subtle. Arch Intern Med 164:2176, 2004.

92. Deveras RA, Kessler CM: Reversal of warfarin-induced excessive anticoagulation with recombinant human factor VIIa concentrate. Ann Intern Med 137:884, 2002.

93. Mayer SA, Brun NC, Begtrup K, et al: Recombinant activated factor VII for acute intracerebral hemorrhage. N Engl J Med 352:777, 2005.

94. Dorfman DM, Goonan EM, Boutilier MK, et al: Point-of-care (POC) versus central laboratory instrumentation for monitoring oral anticoagulation. Vasc Med 10:23, 2005.

95. Dezee KJ, Shimeall WT, Douglas KM, et al: Treatment of excessive anticoagulation with phytonadione (vitamin K): A meta-analysis. Arch Intern Med 166:391, 2006.

96. Weitz JI: Emerging anticoagulants for the treatment of venous thromboembolism. Thromb Haemost 96:274, 2006.

97. Arora N, Goldhaber SZ: Anticoagulants and transaminase elevation. Circulation 113:e698, 2006.

98. Buller HR, Agnelli G, Hull RD, et al: Antithrombotic therapy for venous thromboembolic disease: The seventh ACCP conference on antithrombotic and thrombolytic therapy. Chest 126:401S, 2004.

99. Nijkeuter M, Hovens MM, Davidson BL, Huisman MV: Resolution of thromboemboli in patients with acute pulmonary embolism: A systematic review. Chest 129:192, 2006.

100. Eichinger S, Weltermann A, Minar E, et al: Symptomatic pulmonary embolism and the risk of recurrent venous thromboembolism. Arch Intern Med 164:92, 2004.

101. McRae S, Tran H, Schulman S, et al: Effect of patient's sex on risk of recurrent venous thromboembolism: A meta analysis. Lancet 368:371, 2006.

101a. Eichinger S, Pechenik N, Hron G, et al: High-density lipoprotein and the risk of recurrent venous thromboembolism. Circulation 115:1609, 2007.

102. Christiansen SC, Cannegieter SC, Koster T, et al: Thrombophilia, clinical factors, and recurrent venous thrombotic events. JAMA 293:2352, 2005.

103. Ridker PM, Goldhaber SZ, Danielson E, et al: Long-term, low-intensity warfarin therapy for the prevention of recurrent venous thromboembolism. N Engl J Med 348:1425, 2003.

104. Kearon C, Ginsberg JS, Kovacs MJ, et al: Comparison of low-intensity warfarin therapy with conventional-intensity warfarin therapy for long-term prevention of recurrent venous thromboembolism. N Engl J Med 349:631, 2003.

105. Schulman S, Wahlander K, Lundstrom T, et al: Secondary prevention of venous thromboembolism with the oral direct thrombin inhibitor ximelagatran. N Engl J Med 349:1713, 2003.

106. Ost D, Tepper J, Mihara H, et al: Duration of anticoagulation following venous thromboembolism: A meta-analysis. JAMA 294:706, 2005.

107. Kamphisen PW: Can anticoagulant treatment be tailored with biomarkers in patients with venous thromboembolism? J Thromb Haemost 4:1206, 2006.

108. Shrivastava S, Ridker PM, Glynn RJ, et al: D-dimer, factor VIII coagulant activity, low-intensity warfarin and the risk of recurrent venous thromboembolism. J Thromb Haemost 4:1208, 2006.

109. Hron G, Kollars M, Binder BR, et al: Identification of patients at low risk for recurrent venous thromboembolism by measuring thrombin generation. JAMA 296:397, 2006.

110. Eight-year follow-up of patients with permanent vena cava filters in the prevention of pulmonary embolism: The PREPIC (Prevention du Risque d'Embolie Pulmonaire par Interruption Cave) randomized study. Circulation 112:416, 2005.

111. Stein PD, Kayali F, Olson RE: Twenty-one-year trends in the use of inferior vena cava filters. Arch Intern Med 164:1541, 2004.

112. Jaff MR, Goldhaber SZ, Tapson VF: High utilization rate of vena cava filters in deep vein thrombosis. Thromb Haemost 93:1117, 2005.

113. Stein PD, Alnas M, Skaf E, et al: Outcome and complications of retrievable inferior vena cava filters. Am J Cardiol 94:1090, 2004.

113a. Mismetti P, Rivron-Guillot K, Quenet S, et al: A prospective long-term study of 220 patients, with a retrievable vena cava filter for secondary prevention of venous thromboembolism. Chest 131:223, 2007.

114. Konstantinides S, Geibel A, Heusel G, et al: Heparin plus alteplase compared with heparin alone in patients with submassive pulmonary embolism. N Engl J Med 347:1143, 2002.

115. Wan S, Quinlan DJ, Agnelli G, Eikelboom JW: Thrombolysis compared with heparin for the initial treatment of pulmonary embolism: A meta-analysis of the randomized controlled trials. Circulation 110:744, 2004.

116. Geibel A, Olschewski M, Zehender M, et al: Possible gender-related differences in the risk-to-benefit ratio of thrombolysis for acute submassive pulmonary embolism. Am J Cardiol 99:103, 2007.

117. Fiumara K, Kucher N, Fanikos J, Goldhaber SZ: Predictors of major hemorrhage following fibrinolysis for acute pulmonary embolism. Am J Cardiol 97:127, 2006.

118. Emmerich J, Meyer G, Decousus H, Agnelli G: Role of fibrinolysis and interventional therapy for acute venous thromboembolism. Thromb Haemost 96:251, 2006.

119. Kucher N, Windecker S, Banz Y, et al: Percutaneous catheter thrombectomy device for acute pulmonary embolism: In vitro and in vivo testing. Radiology 236:852, 2005.

120. Schmitz-Rode T, Verma R, Pfeffer JG, et al: Temporary pulmonary stent placement as emergency treatment of pulmonary embolism. J Am Col Cardiol 48:812, 2006.

121. Sukhija R, Aronow WS, Lee J, et al: Association of right ventricular dysfunction with in-hospital mortality in patients with acute pulmonary embolism and reduction in mortality in patients with right ventricular dysfunction by pulmonary embolectomy. Am J Cardiol 95:695, 2005.

122. Meneveau N, Seronde MF, Blonde MC, et al: Management of unsuccessful thrombolysis in acute massive pulmonary embolism. Chest 129:1043, 2006.

123. Leacche M, Unic D, Goldhaber SZ, et al: Modern surgical treatment of massive pulmonary embolism: Results in 47 consecutive patients after rapid diagnosis and aggressive surgical approach. J Thorac Cardiovasc Surg 129:1018, 2005.

124. Kucher N, Rossi E, De Rosa M, Goldhaber SZ: Massive pulmonary embolism. Circulation 113:577, 2006.

125. Eberhardt RT, Raffetto JD: Chronic venous insufficiency. Circulation 111:2398, 2005.

126. Bergan JJ, Schmid-Schonbein GW, Coleridge Smith PD, et al: Chronic venous disease. N Engl J Med 355:488, 2006.

127. Stain M, Schonauer V, Minar E, et al: The post-thrombotic syndrome: Risk factors and impact on the course of thrombotic disease. J Thromb Haemost 3:2671, 2005.

128. Pengo V, Lensing AW, Prins MH, et al: Incidence of chronic thromboembolic pulmonary hypertension after pulmonary embolism. N Engl J Med 350:2257, 2004.

129. Becattini C, Agnelli G, Pesavento R, et al: Incidence of chronic thromboembolic pulmonary hypertension after a first episode of pulmonary embolism. Chest 130:172, 2006.

130. Hoeper MM, Mayer E, Simonneau G, Rubin LJ: Chronic thromboembolic pulmonary hypertension. Circulation 113:2011, 2006.

131. Farber HW, Loscalzo J: Pulmonary arterial hypertension. N Engl J Med 351:1655, 2004.

132. Jamieson SW, Kapelanski DP, Sakakibara N, et al: Pulmonary endarterectomy: Experience and lessons learned in 1500 cases. Ann Thorac Surg 76:1457, 2003; discussion 1462.

132a. Rubens FD, Bourke M, Hynes M, et al: Surgery for chronic thromboembolic pulmonary hypertension—Inclusive experience from a national referral center. Ann Thorac Surg 83:1075, 2007.

133. Feinstein JA, Goldhaber SZ, Lock JE, et al: Balloon pulmonary angioplasty for treatment of chronic thromboembolic pulmonary hypertension. Circulation 103:10, 2001.

Prevention

134. Geerts WH, Pineo GF, Heit JA, et al: Prevention of venous thromboembolism. Chest 126:338S, 2004.

135. Nicolaides AN, Fareed J, Kakkar AK, et al: Prevention and treatment of venous thromboembolism: International consensus statement (guidelines according to scientific evidence). Int Angiol 25:101, 2006.

136. Kucher N, Koo S, Quiroz R, et al: Electronic alerts to prevent venous thromboembolism among hospitalized patients. N Engl J Med 352:969, 2005.

136a. Zurawska U, Parasuraman S, Goldhaber SZ: Prevention of pulmonary embolism in gneral surgery patients. Circulation 115:e302, 2007.

137. International Multicentre Trial: Prevention of fatal postoperative pulmonary embolism by low doses of heparin. Lancet 2:45, 1975.

138. Avorn J, Winkelmayer WC: Comparing the costs, risks, and benefits of competing strategies for the primary prevention of venous thromboembolism. Circulation 110: IV25, 2004.

139. Goldhaber SZ, Turpie AGG: Prevention of venous thromboembolism among hospitalized medical patients. Circulation 111:e1, 2005.

140. Kahn SR, Panju A, Geerts W, et al: Multicenter evaluation of the use of venous thromboembolism prophylaxis in acutely ill medical patients in Canada. Thromb Res 119:145, epub2006.

141. Urbankova J, Quiroz R, Kucher N, Goldhaber SZ: Intermittent pneumatic compression and deep vein thrombosis prevention. A meta-analysis in postoperative patients. Thromb Haemost 94:1181, 2005.

142. Turpie AGG, Bauer KA, Caprini JA: Fondaparinux combined with intermittent pneumatic compression (IPC) versus IPC alone in the prevention of venous thromboembolism after major abdominal surgery: The randomized APOLLO study. Session Type: Oral Session. Blood 106L, Abstract # 270, 2005.

143. Bergqvist D, Agnelli G, Cohen AT, et al: Duration of prophylaxis against venous thromboembolism with enoxaparin after surgery for cancer. N Engl J Med 346:975, 2002.

144. Samama MM, Cohen AT, Darmon JY, et al: A comparison of enoxaparin with placebo for the prevention of venous thromboembolism in acutely ill medical patients. Prophylaxis in Medical Patients with Enoxaparin Study Group. N Engl J Med 341:793, 1999.

145. Leizorovicz A, Cohen AT, Turpie AG, et al: Randomized, placebo-controlled trial of dalteparin for the prevention of venous thromboembolism in acutely ill medical patients. Circulation 110:874, 2004.

146. Cohen AT, Davidson BL, Gallus AS, et al: Efficacy and safety of fondaparinux for the prevention of venous thromboembolism in older acute medical patients: Randomised placebo controlled trial. BMJ 332:325, 2006.

pulmonary vascular resistance. Prostaglandins I_2 (PGI_2) and E_1 (PGE_1) are active pulmonary vasodilators, whereas $PGF_{2\alpha}$ and PGA_2 are pulmonary vasoconstrictors. Counterregulatory actions have been ascribed to prostacyclin (PGI_2) and thromboxane within the pulmonary circulation. Prostacyclin functions through cell-surface G protein–coupled receptors linked to different signaling pathways.

Pulmonary endothelial cells have an abundance of prostacyclin synthase, whereas platelets are replete with thromboxane synthase. Both convert the cyclic endoperoxide precursors PGG_2 and PGH_2 into specific bioactive eicosanoids. Prostacyclin is a powerful vasodilator and inhibitor of platelet aggregation through activation of cyclic adenosine monophosphate (cAMP). Its metabolic half-life in the bloodstream is less than one circulation time, with its metabolite 6-ketoprostaglandin $F_{1\alpha}$ having little biological activity.

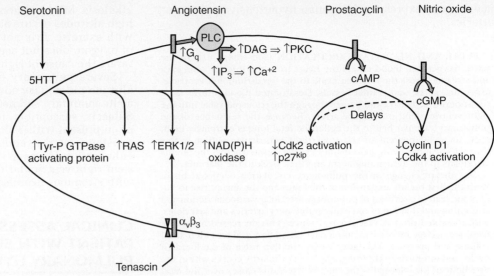

FIGURE 73–1 Growth factor signaling pathways in pulmonary vascular smooth muscle cells. Mechanisms involved in smooth muscle growth involve serotonin, angiotensin II, prostacyclin, nitric oxide, the matrix protein tenascin, and $\alpha_v\beta_3$ integrin signaling. These stimulatory signals, despite triggering different pathways of intracellular signaling, all result in smooth muscle cell growth. Tyr-P GTPase = tyrosine P guanosine triphosphatase; IP_3 = inositol 1,4,5-triphosphate; RAS = renal artery stenosis; PLC = phospholipase C; DAG = diacylglycerol; PKC = protein kinase C; cAMP = cyclic adenosine monophosphate; cGMP = cyclic guanosine monophosphate; NAD(P)H = nicotinamide adenine dinucleotide phosphate (reduced). *(From Tuder RM, Zaiman AL: Prostacyclin analogs as the brakes for pulmonary artery smooth muscle cell proliferation. Am J Respir Cell Mol Biol 26:171, 2002.)*

Release of prostacyclin by endothelial cells causes relaxation of the underlying vascular smooth muscle and prevents platelet aggregation within the bloodstream. Thromboxane is synthesized in platelets and macrophages. It also has a short half-life. Thromboxane is a potent agonist for platelet aggregation and vasoconstriction, and it may function as a growth factor for smooth muscle cells by acting via protein kinase C–linked pathways.

NITRIC OXIDE. The biological action of nitric oxide (NO) is similar to that of prostacyclin in the way in which it relaxes vascular smooth muscle.[3] It differs, however, in that its effects are mediated by rising levels of cyclic guanosine monophosphate (cGMP). Endothelial NO synthase is found in the vascular endothelium of the normal pulmonary vasculature, where it is responsible for generating NO to regulate vascular tone. Release of NO occurs in response to a multitude of physiological stimuli, which include thrombin, bradykinin, and shear stress. In addition to its direct hemodynamic effects, NO inhibits platelet activation and confers an important antithrombotic property on the endothelial surface. NO also inhibits the growth of vascular smooth muscle cells and is probably involved in vascular remodeling in response to injury. NO is also important in the signal transduction of angiogenesis, in that VEGF receptor activation results in increased NO production.

ENDOTHELIN. Endothelin (ET) is a potent mitogenic and vasoconstrictor peptide that also plays a role in the regulation of pulmonary vascular tone. ET-1 is the predominant isoform of endothelin in the cardiovascular system, generated through the cleavage of pre-pro ET-1 to big ET-1 and then to ET-1. ET-1 is found in endothelial cells and released toward the vascular smooth muscle cell, consistent with a paracrine role, but it is also produced by smooth muscle cells and cardiomyocytes. ET-1 has vasoconstrictive and mitogenic effects, stimulates the production of growth factors such as VEGF and basic fibroblast growth factor, and potentiates the effects of transforming growth factor-beta (TGF-β) and platelet-derived growth factor. ET-1 biosynthesis is regulated by physiochemical factors such as blood

flow, pulsatile stretch, hypoxia, and thrombin. Endogenous inhibitors of ET-1 synthesis include nitric oxide and prostacyclin.

ET-1 exerts its major vascular effects through activation of two distinct G protein–coupled ET_A and ET_B receptors. ET_A receptors are found in the medial smooth muscle layers of the blood vessels and atrial and ventricular myocardium. When stimulated, ET_A receptors induce vasoconstriction and cellular proliferation by increasing intracellular calcium. ET_B receptors are localized on endothelial cells and to some extent on smooth muscle cells and macrophages. The activation of ET_B receptors stimulates the release of nitric oxide and prostacyclin and prevents apoptosis. Normally, there is a balance between production and clearance, which is mediated by the ET_B receptor such that circulating endothelin is at a low level.

SEROTONIN. Serotonin is an important constituent of platelet-dense granules and is released on activation. Serotonin is a vasoconstrictor that promotes smooth muscle cell hypertrophy and hyperplasia. Normal endothelial cells respond to serotonin by enhancing the release of NO, thereby leading to vascular smooth muscle relaxation and vasodilation. In the setting of endothelial dysfunction, serotonin is unable to stimulate NO release and increases vascular smooth muscle tone, thereby leading to vasoconstriction. In addition, serotonin can act as a growth factor, contributing to medial hypertrophy and promoting vascular remodeling.

ANGIOTENSIN II. This peptide is generated in the lung by means of enzymatic conversion of angiotensin I, a potent pulmonary vasoconstrictor. Angiotensin II stimulates cell proliferation, extracellular matrix protein synthesis, and smooth muscle cell migration. In chronically hypoxic rats, the development of pulmonary hypertension and right ventricular hypertrophy is associated with a significant increase in membrane-bound right ventricular angiotensin-converting enzyme (ACE) activity. ACE protein and mRNA expression are focally increased in rat pulmonary arteries with medial hypertrophy from chronic hypoxia. There is also increased ACE immunoreactivity at sites of increased matrix gene expression in human hypertensive pulmonary arteries.

FETAL AND NEONATAL CIRCULATION (see Chap. 61). In the fetus, oxygenated blood enters the heart from the inferior vena cava and streams across the foramen ovale to the left atrium, left ventricle, ascending aorta, and cranial vessels. Desaturated blood returns from the superior vena cava and passes through the tricuspid valve into the right ventricle and pulmonary artery. Because the resistance of the pulmonary vascular bed in the collapsed fetal lung is extremely high, only 10 to 30 percent of the total right ventricular output passes through the lungs, with the remainder being shunted across the ductus arteriosus to the descending aorta and then back to the placenta.

An abrupt change in the pulmonary circulation occurs at birth. With the first breath, expansion of the lungs and the abrupt rise in Po_2 of blood lead to a reversal of pulmonary arteriolar vasoconstriction and stretching and dilation of muscular pulmonary arteries and arterioles, with a marked drop in vascular resistance. This decreased resistance facilitates a large increase in pulmonary blood flow and raises left atrial volume and pressure. The latter closes the flap valve of the foramen ovale, and interatrial right-to-left shunting ordinarily ceases within the first hour of life. Normally, the ductus arteriosus closes over the next 10 hours as a result of contraction of the thick smooth muscle bundles within its wall in response to rising arterial oxygen tension and a change in the prostaglandin milieu. Following the initial dramatic fall in pulmonary vascular resistance at birth, a continuous decline occurs over the first few months of life, associated with thinning of the media of muscular pulmonary arteries and arterioles until the normal adult pattern is achieved.

AGING. In older adults, the main pulmonary artery becomes mildly dilated, and shallow atheromas may develop in the elastic pulmonary arteries. Mild medial thickening and eccentric intimal fibrosis may occur in the muscular pulmonary arteries; the capillaries become slightly thicker and the veins are frequently involved by intimal hyalinization, with mild luminal narrowing. Pulmonary artery pressure and pulmonary vascular resistance increase with advanced age, similar to increases that occur in systemic vascular resistance. Changes in the pulmonary arteries are also affected by reduced compliance of left ventricular filling with age that is passively reflected back on the pulmonary vascular bed.

Exercise

With moderate exercise, a large increase in pulmonary blood flow is normally accompanied by only a small increase in pulmonary artery pressure. Exercise results in an increase in left atrial pressure that is progressive with exercise intensity and accounts for most of the increase in observed pulmonary arterial pressure. This marked effect of downstream pressure on upstream pressure is unique to the lung circulation inasmuch as systemic arterial pressure during exercise is independent of right atrial pressure. Because of the high vascular compliance in the normal lung microcirculation, an increase in left atrial pressure that results from the increased flow will act to distend the small vessels, contributing to the fall in pulmonary vascular resistance during exercise. Microcirculatory distention increases the surface area for diffusion and slows passage of red blood cells through the lung, which facilitates oxygen transfer.

Altitude

Life at high altitudes is associated with pulmonary hypertension of variable severity, reflecting the range of susceptibilities of different persons to the pulmonary vasoconstrictive effect of chronic hypoxia. Altitude decreases the inspired partial pressure of oxygen (Po_2) because of a decrease in barometric pressure. At sea level, Po_2 is on average 150 mm Hg. At high altitudes (3000 to 5500 m), Po_2 decreases to 80 to 100 mm Hg and, at extreme altitudes (5500 to 8840 m), Po_2 decreases to 40 to 80 mm Hg. Corresponding alveolar Po_2 (PAo_2) and arterial Po_2 (Pao_2) depend on the hypoxic ventilatory response and associated respiratory alkalosis. Mild pulmonary hypertension in adults living at high altitudes occurs at rest and may increase substantially with exercise. It is not immediately reversed by breathing of oxygen, does not seem to limit exercise capacity, and is rarely the cause of right ventricular failure.

Severe pulmonary hypertension may occur with high-altitude pulmonary edema, infantile or adult forms of subacute mountain sickness, and chronic mountain sickness.[4] Subjects susceptible to high-altitude pulmonary edema often present with a slight increase in pulmonary vascular resistance at rest and exercise at sea level and with an enhanced pulmonary vascular reactivity to hypoxia. Transient right ventricular dysfunction has also been described with strenuous exercise at high altitude.

CLINICAL ASSESSMENT OF THE PATIENT WITH SUSPECTED PULMONARY HYPERTENSION

History

A careful and detailed history of the patient with suspected pulmonary hypertension is often revealing.[5] Because the earliest abnormalities in patients with pulmonary hypertension are manifest with exercise, it is typical that presenting symptoms are effort-related. Because pulmonary hypertension can have an insidious onset, patients commonly experience dyspnea with effort that they attribute either to aging or to weight gain. With the onset of right ventricular failure, lower extremity edema from venous congestion is characteristic. Angina is also a common symptom, generally representing more advanced disease. It likely represents reduced coronary blood flow to a markedly hypertrophied right ventricle and has the typical qualities of angina from coronary artery disease. As the cardiac output becomes fixed and eventually falls, patients may have episodes of syncope or near-syncope. Syncope occurs because of exercise-induced right ventricular failure, whereby the heart rate becomes the only mechanism available to increase cardiac output, which has limited effectiveness. Patients with pulmonary hypertension related to left ventricular diastolic dysfunction will characteristically have orthopnea and paroxysmal nocturnal dyspnea. Patients with underlying lung disease may also report episodes of coughing. Hemoptysis is relatively uncommon in patients with pulmonary hypertension and may be associated with underlying thromboembolism and pulmonary infarction. Some patients with advanced mitral stenosis also present with hemoptysis.

Physical Examination

Cardiovascular findings consistent with pulmonary hypertension and right ventricular pressure overload include a large a wave in the jugular venous pulse, a low-volume carotid arterial pulse with a normal upstroke, a left parasternal (right ventricular) heave, a systolic pulsation produced by a dilated, tense pulmonary artery in the second left interspace, an ejection click and flow murmur in the same area, a closely split second heart sound with a loud pulmonic component, and a fourth heart sound of right ventricular origin. Late in the course, signs of right ventricular failure (e.g., hepatomegaly, peripheral edema, and ascites) may be present. Patients with severe pulmonary hypertension may also have prominent v waves in the jugular venous pulse as a result of tricuspid regurgitation, a third heart sound of right ventricular origin, a high-pitched early diastolic murmur of pulmonic regurgitation, and a holosystolic murmur of tricuspid regurgitation. Tricuspid regurgitation is a reflection of right ventricular dilation. Cyanosis is a late finding and usually attributable to a markedly reduced cardiac output, with systemic vasoconstriction and ventilation-perfusion mismatch in the lung. Uncommonly, the left laryngeal nerve becomes paralyzed as a consequence of compression by a dilated pulmonary artery (Ortner syndrome).

CONCOMITANT DISEASE. Patients whose pulmonary hypertension is associated with another condition will also have clinical features of that disease. For example, patients with scleroderma typically report Raynaud's phenomenon, dysphagia, sclerodactyly, and nonspecific arthritic symptoms. Patients with portal hypertension usually give a history of underlying chronic liver disease and may present with ascites that can be from the liver disease, right heart failure, or both. Many patients with congenital heart disease have a known history, but atrial septal defects in adults are frequently missed and patients may have symptoms manifest only later in life. These patients often have marked cyanosis that worsens with exercise. Patients with pulmonary venous hypertension, or pulmonary hypertension associated with lung disease, can also have extreme levels of hypoxemia. In patients with chronic obstructive pulmonary disease (COPD), the clinical signs are often obscured by hyperinflation of the chest. The jugular venous pressure may also be difficult to assess in patients with COPD because of large swings in intrathoracic pressure.

Diagnostic Tests

A number of tests are available for the assessment of pulmonary arterial hypertension (PAH).[6]

LABORATORY TESTS. The results of these studies (Table 73-2) are usually normal in patients with pulmonary hypertension. If chronic arterial oxygen desaturation exists, polycythemia should be present. A number of investigators have reported hypercoagulable states, abnormal platelet function, defects in fibrinolysis, and other abnormalities of coagulation in patients with PAH. Abnormal liver function test results can indicate right ventricular failure, with resultant systemic venous hypertension.

Brain natriuretic peptide (BNP) levels are elevated in patients with pulmonary hypertension and correlate positively with the pulmonary artery pressure. BNP is secreted predominantly from cardiac ventricles through a constitutive pathway and is affected by the degree of myocardial stretch, damage, and ischemia in the ventricle.

Uric acid levels are elevated in patients with pulmonary hypertension and correlate with hemodynamics. Although the mechanism is uncertain, it may relate both to overproduction and impaired uric acid excretion caused by the low cardiac output and tissue hypoxia.

There is an increased incidence of thyroid disease in patients with PAH,[7] which can mimic the symptoms of right ventricular (RV) failure. Consequently, it is advised that thyroid function tests be monitored serially in all patients.

CHEST RADIOGRAPHY (see Chap. 15). Radiographic examination of the chest in patients with pulmonary hypertension shows enlargement of the main pulmonary artery and its major branches, with marked tapering of peripheral arteries. The right ventricle and atrium may also be enlarged. Dilation of the right ventricle gives the heart a globular appearance, but right ventricular hypertrophy or dilation is not easily discernible on a plain chest radiograph. Encroachment of the retrosternal air space on the lateral film may be a helpful sign to confirm that the enlarged silhouette is a result of right ventricular dilation. The lung fields should be clear, and often appear darkened from the relative oligemia caused by a low cardiac output.

ELECTROCARDIOGRAPHY (see Chap. 12). The detection of right ventricular hypertrophy on the electrocardiogram is highly specific but has a low sensitivity. The electrocardiogram in patients with PAH usually exhibits right atrial and right ventricular enlargement. T wave inversion, representing the repolarization abnormalities associated with right ventricular hypertrophy (RVH) are usually seen in the anterior precordial leads and may be mistaken for anteroseptal ischemia. These electrocardiographic abnormalities are usually less pronounced in patients with COPD than in patients with other forms of pulmonary hypertension because of the relatively modest degree of pulmonary hypertension that occurs and because of the effects of hyperinflation.

ECHOCARDIOGRAPHY (see Chap. 14). Echocardiography usually demonstrates enlargement of the right atrium and ventricle, normal or small left ventricular dimensions, and a thickened interventricular septum.[8] Abnormal septal motion as a result of the right ventricular pressure overload is characteristic. Detection of right ventricular hypertrophy by echocardiography is limited by its ability to differentiate the right ventricular wall from its surrounding structures. Moreover, correlations between the thickness of the right ventricular wall and the right ventricular mass are poor, even when measured at autopsy. Right ventricular dysfunction is difficult to quantitate echocardiographically, but the position and curvature of the intraventricular septum provide an indication of right ventricular afterload.[6] Echocardiographic findings that portend a poor prognosis include pericardial effusion and a markedly diminished left ventricular cavity.

Doppler echocardiographic estimates of right ventricular systolic pressures can be obtained by measuring the velocity of the tricuspid regurgitant jet and using the Bernoulli formula (see Chap. 14). Although Doppler measurements correlate with right ventricular systolic pressure, they are relatively imprecise (±20 mm Hg) and are not a substitute for catheterization if a correct measurement of pulmonary pressure is needed.[9] Doppler echocardiography has also demonstrated that left ventricular diastolic dysfunction develops from the pulmonary hypertensive state, with marked dependence on atrial contraction for ventricular filling.

RADIONUCLIDE VENTRICULOGRAPHY (see Chap. 16). Radionuclide ventriculography can provide useful information regarding right ventricular function, provided that adequate separation of the cardiac chambers can be accomplished. Because radioactive counts are proportional to volume, variations in the geometric configuration of the ventricles are less important. Although pulmonary artery pressure cannot be estimated with this technique, there is an inverse relationship between pulmonary artery pressure and right ventricular ejection fraction.

TABLE 73–2	Clues for Interpretation of Diagnostic Tests for Pulmonary Hypertension
Test	**Notable Findings**
Chest x-ray	Enlargement of central pulmonary arteries reflects level of PA pressure and duration.
Electrocardiography	Right axis deviation and precordial T wave abnormalities are early signs.
Pulmonary function tests	Elevated pulmonary artery pressure causes restrictive physiology.
Perfusion lung scan	Nonsegmental perfusion abnormalities can occur from severe pulmonary vascular disease.
Chest computed tomography scan	Minor interstitial changes may reflect diffuse disease; mosaic perfusion pattern indicates thromboembolism and/or left heart failure.
Echocardiography	Right ventricular enlargement will parallel the severity of the pulmonary hypertension.
Contrast echocardiography	Minor right to left shunting rarely produces hypoxemia.
Doppler echocardiography	This is too unreliable for following serial measurements to monitor therapy.
Exercise testing	This is very helpful to assess the efficacy of therapy. Severe exercise-induced hypoxemia should cause consideration of a right-to-left shunt.

PULMONARY FUNCTION TESTS. Although pulmonary function in patients with PAH is often completely normal, reductions in lung volumes of 20 percent are common, making the differentiation from interstitial lung disease on the basis of PFTs difficult. A significant obstructive pattern is not characteristic and suggests obstructive airways disease. In patients with PAH, the diffusing capacity for carbon monoxide (DLCO) is reduced to approximately 60 to 80 percent of predicted; there is no clear correlation between severity of the disease and the DLCO. The presence of arterial hypoxemia is caused by ventilation-perfusion mismatch and/or reduced mixed venous oxygen saturations resulting from low cardiac output. The degree of arterial hypoxemia is often slight to moderate. A severe reduction of Pao_2 and Sao_2 can be caused by right-to-left intracardiac or extracardiac shunts and/or intrapulmonary shunts. Consequently, Pao_2 and Sao_2 may vary markedly among patients with different constellations of associated abnormalities. Patients with pulmonary venous hypertension often have severe hypoxemia for reasons that are unclear.

Approximately 20 percent of patients with systemic sclerosis have an isolated reduction in DLCO, which, when severe (less than 55 percent of predicted), can be associated with the development of PAH. In patients with limited systemic sclerosis, a fall in DLCO in the presence of normal lung volumes often precedes the onset of PAH.

LUNG SCINTIGRAPHY. A perfusion lung scan is an important test in making the correct diagnosis of pulmonary hypertension. Patients with PAH may reveal a relatively normal perfusion pattern or diffuse, patchy, perfusion abnormalities. A perfusion lung scan will reliably distinguish patients with PAH from those who have pulmonary hypertension secondary to chronic pulmonary thromboembolism (Fig. 73-2).

COMPUTED TOMOGRAPHY (see Chap. 18). Chest computed tomography (CT) scans are very helpful in the assessment of patients with pulmonary hypertension. Spiral chest CT scans have been used successfully in diagnosing chronic thromboembolic pulmonary hypertension. In addition to visualization of thrombi in the pulmonary vasculature with contrast enhancement, a mosaic pattern of variable attenuation compatible with irregular pulmonary perfusion can be determined on the nonenhanced CT scan. Marked variation in the size of segmental vessels is also a specific feature of chronic thromboembolic disease. The sensitivity and specificity of spiral CT scanning to diagnose pulmonary embolism are highly variable, and related in large part to the sophistication of the scanner. In some patients, it may be necessary to perform perfusion lung scanning along with spiral CT scanning to make a correct diagnosis.

High-resolution CT is the best test by which to diagnose interstitial lung disease. It has a high degree of specificity, but its sensitivity is low. However, patients with PAH without coexisting lung disease should have normal lung parenchyma. Thus, although CT tends to underrepresent the extent of the disease, the presence of any interstitial abnormality would suggest that interstitial lung disease is underlying the pulmonary hypertension. A high-resolution CT scan of the chest is also an accurate means of detecting emphysema, and may demonstrate emphysema in patients with little or no abnormality detected by pulmonary function tests

PULMONARY ANGIOGRAPHY. Pulmonary angiography establishes the correct diagnosis in patients with pulmonary hypertension in whom a perfusion lung scan suggests segmental or lobar defects. Although pulmonary angiography carries an increased risk in patients with pulmonary hypertension, it can be performed safely if adequate precautions are taken. Maintenance of adequate oxygenation by the administration of supplemental oxygen and the avoidance of vasovagal reactions, and rapid treatment of those that occur with intravenous atropine, should reduce the associated risk in this patient group. Continuous arterial pressure monitoring is advised, and nonionic contrast agents appear to be better tolerated.

EXERCISE TESTING (see Chap. 13). The use of a symptom-limited exercise test can be very helpful in the evaluation of patients with pulmonary hypertension. The 6-minute walk test is commonly used in clinical trials as an endpoint for efficacy of therapy in patients with pulmonary hypertension.[10] It has been correlated with workload, heart rate, oxygen saturation, and dyspnea response. Its drawbacks include the fact that anthropometric factors such as gait speed, age, weight, muscle mass, and length of stride can affect the test results. Treadmill testing has also been used and compares with the 6-minute walk test in reflecting drug efficacy. The Naughton protocol uses a treadmill with increases in work of 1 metabolic equivalent (MET) increments at 2-minute stages to allow patients with very limited exercise tolerance to perform.

Cardiopulmonary exercise testing using an upright bicycle and measurements of gas exchange has the potential to grade the severity of exercise limitation in patients with pulmonary hypertension noninvasively.[11] The breathlessness of patients with pulmonary hypertension during exercise can be related to the relative hypoperfusion of their lungs, which causes an increase in dead space ventilation manifest by a hyperbolic increase in minute ventilation.[12] This can be exacerbated by lactic acidosis and hypoxemia as a result of their inability to increase cardiac output with exercise. Thus, dyspnea with pulmonary hypertension is attributable to worsening ventilation-perfusion mismatching, lactic acidosis, and arterial hypoxemia.

CARDIAC CATHETERIZATION (see Chap. 19). In addition to confirming the diagnosis and allowing the exclusion of other causes, cardiac catheterization also establishes the severity of disease and allows an assessment of prognosis. By definition, patients with PAH should have a low or normal pulmonary capillary wedge pressure. Because this is a critical measurement in distinguishing a patient with PAH from one with pulmonary venous hypertension, several quality measures must be established in the catheterization laboratory to ensure that correct values are obtained. The transducers must be carefully adjusted to reflect the height of the midchest of every patient. Pressures should never be determined by the digital readout from the laboratory's computer, because these measurements represent an average of several heartbeats and ignore respiratory influences. In addition, the electronically integrated mean pressure can differ greatly from the actual wedge pressure. Instead, measurements of all pressures are properly made at end-expiration to avoid incorporating negative intrathoracic pressures. When a reproducible wedge pres-

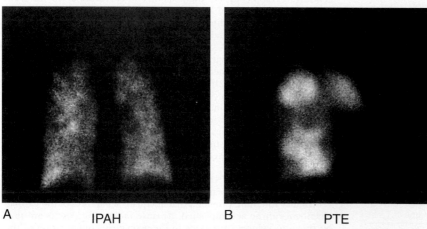

FIGURE 73–2 Perfusion lung scans in patients with pulmonary hypertension. **A,** Patient with idiopathic pulmonary hypertension (IPAH). **B,** Patient with pulmonary thromboembolism causing pulmonary hypertension (PTE). Both perfusion scans are abnormal. The scan from the patient with IPAH shows a mottled distribution in a nonsegmental, nonanatomical manner. The scan from the patient with PTE reveals lobar, segmental, and subsegmental defects highly suggestive of an anatomical obstruction to pulmonary blood flow.

sure cannot be obtained, direct measurement of left ventricular end-diastolic pressure is advised. If the wedge pressure is increased, it should be correlated with left ventricular end-diastolic pressure and not attributed to a falsely elevated reading. It has been shown that left ventricular diastolic compliance becomes impaired in patients with PAH and parallels the severity of the disease; thus, pulmonary capillary wedge pressure tends to rise slightly in the late stages of PAH, although it rarely exceeds 16 mm Hg.

It can be extremely difficult to pass a catheter into the pulmonary artery in patients with pulmonary hypertension because of the tricuspid regurgitation, dilated right atrium and ventricle, and low cardiac output. A specific flow-directed thermodilution balloon catheter has been developed for patients with pulmonary hypertension (American Edwards Laboratories, Irvine, CA); it has an extra port for the placement of a 0.28-inch guidewire to provide better stiffness to the catheter. The risk associated with cardiac catheterization in patients with pulmonary hypertension is extremely low in experienced hands, but deaths have been reported.

TESTING WITH VASODILATORS. Several vasodilators are of value in the assessment of pulmonary vasoreactivity in patients with PAH (Table 73-3).[13] Adenosine is an intermediate product in the metabolism of adenosine triphosphate that has potent vasodilator properties through its action on specific vascular receptors. It is believed to stimulate the endothelial cell and vascular smooth muscle receptors of the A_2 type, which induce vascular smooth muscle relaxation by increasing cyclic adenosine monophosphate. In patients with PAH, adenosine has been shown to be a potent vasodilator and predictive of the chronic effects of intravenous prostacyclin as well as the calcium channel blockers. Adenosine has an extremely short half-life (less than 5 seconds), which provides a safety net by its rapid dissolution should any adverse side effects occur. It is administered intravenously as an infusion in doses of 50 µg/kg/min and titrated upward every 2 minutes until uncomfortable symptoms develop (e.g., chest tightness or dyspnea).

Epoprostenol has been used as an acute test of vasoreactivity in patients with PAH. Like adenosine, its short half-life allows use of the drug to be discontinued if any acute adverse effects result. Also similar to adenosine, it is administered incrementally, at 2 ng/kg/min, and increased every 15 to 30 minutes until systemic effects such as headache, flushing, or nausea occur, which limits the acute dose titration. Favorable acute effects from epoprostenol are predictive of a favorable response to calcium channel blockers.

Adenosine and epoprostenol possess potent inotropic properties, in addition to their ability to vasodilate the pulmonary vascular bed. When using these drugs for the acute testing of patients, one needs to pay particular attention to changes in cardiac output that occur in association with the changes in pulmonary arterial pressure. An increase in cardiac output with no change in pulmonary arterial pressure will result in a reduction in calculated pulmonary vascular resistance, and may be erroneously interpreted as a vasodilator response.

Nitric oxide is also a useful drug to test pulmonary vasoreactivity. Because it binds very rapidly to hemoglobin with high affinity and is thereby inactivated, inhalation of NO gas results in selective pulmonary vascular effects without influencing the systemic circulation. Inhalation of NO by patients with PAH has been shown to produce a reduction in pulmonary vascular resistance acutely, similar to that achieved with intravenous adenosine, and also to predict the effectiveness of calcium channel blockers. NO differs importantly from adenosine and epoprostenol in that it has little effect on cardiac output. It is usually given via facemask at 20 to 40 ppm.

It must be emphasized that hemodynamic assessment of the entire circulatory system is essential when determining the influence of drugs in these patients. Small changes in pulmonary artery pressure are usually caused by variability rather than direct drug influence. Changes in pulmonary vascular resistance cannot be directly measured but are computed by the change in pulmonary pressure and cardiac output simultaneously. Because thermodilution cardiac output, the method that is most commonly used in these patients, can be associated with large errors in reproducibility, particular care should be taken in the methodology of thermodilution used in these patients. In addition, when an underlying right-to-left shunt exists, the Fick determination of cardiac output is required.

Changes in pulmonary capillary wedge pressure can have important influences on the determination of pulmonary vascular resistance. A rising capillary wedge pressure secondary to increased cardiac output may be the first sign of impending left ventricular failure and an adverse effect of a drug, whereas the calculated pulmonary vascular resistance may become lower and suggest a beneficial effect. Right atrial pressure also reflects the filling characteristics

TABLE 73-3	Hemodynamic Assessment of Vasodilators in Pulmonary Hypertension	
Parameter Measured	**Desired Acute Changes**	**Comments**
Mean pulmonary artery pressure (PAP)	>10-mm Hg decrease; ideally, mean PAP below 30 mm Hg	Must not be associated significant fall in systemic blood pressure
Pulmonary vascular resistance (PVR)	>33% decrease; ideally, PVR below 6 units	Cardiac output unchanged or increased
Pulmonary capillary wedge pressure	No change	Increase in wedge pressure suggests pulmonary venoocclusive disease or coexisting left ventricular dysfunction
Cardiac output	Increase	Increase should be from increased stroke volume rather than increased heart rate
Heart rate	No significant change	Chronic increased heart rate will result in RV failure; watch for bradycardia if using high doses of diltiazem
Systemic arterial oxygen saturation	Increase if reduced on room air, little change if normal	Decrease in systemic arterial oxygen saturation suggests lung disease or right-to-left shunt; prohibits chronic use
Pulmonary artery (mixed venous) oxygen saturation	Increase	Should parallel increase in cardiac output and improved tissue oxygenation

of the right ventricle. A right atrial pressure increase in the face of rising cardiac output suggests right ventricular diastolic dysfunction. The resting heart rate is a physiological parameter of marked importance in patients with congestive heart failure, and treatments that cause an increased heart rate are likely to yield deleterious long-term results. Finally, the systemic arterial oxygen content should be evaluated in patients with pulmonary hypertension. Effective vasodilator drugs can result in vasodilation of blood vessels supplying poorly ventilated areas of the lung and can worsen hypoxemia. This effect is particularly noticeable in patients with underlying chronic lung disease.

CLASSIFICATION OF PULMONARY HYPERTENSION

Pulmonary hypertension, in its simplest sense, refers to any elevation in the pulmonary arterial pressure above normal. The presence of pulmonary hypertension may reflect a serious underlying pulmonary vascular disease, which can be progressive and fatal, or simply an obligatory passive elevation in the pulmonary artery pressure in response to elevated pressures in the left heart. Consequently, an accurate diagnosis of the cause of pulmonary hypertension in a patient is essential to establish an effective treatment plan. In addition, therapies that may be beneficial for patients with some types of pulmonary hypertension may be harmful for patients with other types.

The diagnosis of pulmonary hypertension relies on establishing an elevation in pulmonary artery pressure above normal. Published norms have come from cardiac catheterizations performed in young subjects at rest without any evidence of cardiopulmonary disease. The upper limit of normal for pulmonary artery mean pressure is 19 mm Hg. However, this assumes that there are no abnormalities in downstream pressures of the left atrium or left ventricle, or an increased cardiac output. That is why a patient can have pulmonary hypertension from the standpoint of an elevated pulmonary artery pressure, but normal pulmonary vascular resistance. Parameters for normal pulmonary arterial systolic pressure derived by echocardiographic Doppler studies have been published that suggest that the upper limit of normal of pulmonary arterial systolic pressure in the general population may be higher than previously appreciated. The Centers for Disease Control and Prevention has surveyed the number of hospitalizations of persons with pulmonary hypertension in the United States from 1980 to 2002.[14] They found that there was a dramatic increase since 1990, with 260,000 hospitalizations and 15,668 deaths reported annually since 2000.

There are patients whose resting hemodynamics are normal but in whom marked elevations in pulmonary pressure occur with exercise. It has been presumed that this represents an early stage of pulmonary vascular disease. However, because patients may have a hypertensive response to exercise with respect to the systemic vasculature, a similar type of response may also occur in the pulmonary vasculature. The diagnosis of exercise-induced pulmonary hypertension by echocardiographic Doppler studies is particularly unreliable because of inherent errors in the Doppler estimates of pulmonary artery pressure.

In 1998, a new classification for pulmonary hypertension was developed at the World Symposium on Pulmonary Hypertension, cosponsored by the World Health Organization. This classification catalogued clinical conditions based on common pathobiological features to serve as a guide in the clinical assessment and treatment of these patients.

CH 73

TABLE 73–4	Revised Clinical Classification of Pulmonary Hypertension*

Pulmonary arterial hypertension (PAH)
  Idiopathic (IPAH)
  Familial (FPAH)
  Associated with (APAH)
    Collagen vascular disease
    Congenital systemic-to-pulmonary shunts
    Portal hypertension
    Human immunodeficiency virus (HIV) infection
    Drugs and toxins
    Other (thyroid disorders, glycogen storage disease, Gaucher disease, hereditary hemorrhagic telangiectasia, hemoglobinopathies, myeloproliferative disorders, splenectomy)
  Associated with significant venous or capillary involvement
    Pulmonary venoocclusive disease (PVOD)
    Pulmonary capillary hemangiomatosis (PCH)
  Persistent pulmonary hypertension of the newborn

Pulmonary hypertension with left heart disease
  Left-sided arterial or ventricular heart disease
  Left-sided valvular heart disease

Pulmonary hypertension associated with lung disease and/or hypoxemia
  Chronic obstructive pulmonary disease
  Interstitial lung disease
  Sleep-disordered breathing
  Alveolar hypoventilation disorders
  Chronic exposure to high altitude
  Developmental abnormalities

Pulmonary hypertension caused by chronic thrombotic and/or embolic disease
  Thromboembolic obstruction of proximal pulmonary arteries
  Thromboembolic obstruction of distal pulmonary arteries
  Nonthrombotic pulmonary embolism (tumor, parasites, foreign material)

Miscellaneous
  Sarcoidosis, histiocytosis X, lymphangiomatosis, compression of pulmonary vessels (adenopathy, tumor, fibrosing mediastinitis)

*Venice, 2003.
From Simmoneau G, Galie N, Rubin LJ, et al: Clinical classification of pulmonary hypertension. J Am Coll Cardiol 43:5S, 2004.

Modifications to this classification have been proposed (Table 73-4). In addition, a functional classification patterned after the New York Heart Association functional classification for heart disease has been developed to allow comparisons of patients with respect to the clinical severity of the disease process (Table 73-5).

PAH refers to pulmonary vascular disease affecting the arterioles, resulting in an elevation in pressure and vascular resistance. Although idiopathic PAH (formerly referred to as primary pulmonary hypertension or PPH), is relatively rare, with an estimated incidence of 1 to 2 per million in the population, severe PAH associated with other conditions is considerably more common The most common cause is associated with connective tissue disease states, primarily scleroderma, including the CREST syndrome (calcinosis cutis, Raynaud's phenomenon, esophageal dysfunction, sclerodactyly, and telangiectasia), and mixed connective tissue disease. PAH is also relatively common in patients with congenital heart defects, especially those with ventricular septal defects or a patent ductus arteriosus. Other comorbid conditions include cirrhosis with portal hypertension and human immunodeficiency virus (HIV) infection.

TABLE 73–5	WHO Functional Classification of Pulmonary Hypertension

Class I—Patients with pulmonary hypertension but without resulting limitation of physical activity. Ordinary physical activity does not cause undue dyspnea or fatigue, chest pain, or syncope.

Class II—Patients with pulmonary hypertension resulting in slight limitation of physical activity. They are comfortable at rest. Ordinary physical activity causes undue dyspnea or fatigue, chest pain, or syncope.

Class III—Patients with pulmonary hypertension resulting in marked limitation of physical activity. They are comfortable at rest. Less than ordinary activity causes undue dyspnea or fatigue, chest pain, or syncope.

Class IV—Patients with pulmonary hypertension with inability to carry out any physical activity without symptoms. These patients manifest signs of right heart failure. Dyspnea and/or fatigue may even be present at rest. Discomfort is increased by any physical activity.

TYPES OF PULMONARY HYPERTENSION

Idiopathic Pulmonary Arterial Hypertension

Idiopathic pulmonary arterial hypertension (IPAH) is the diagnosis given to patients with pulmonary hypertension of unexplained cause. Although the name of the disease stems from its distinction from pulmonary hypertension secondary to known cardiac or pulmonary causes, IPAH should not be considered as only pulmonary hypertension for which no cause can be found. The clinical features, usual age of onset, progression of the disease, and autopsy findings make IPAH a distinct clinical entity and distinguish it from other forms of pulmonary hypertension, even though its diagnosis requires careful exclusion of secondary causes.

Pathological Features

Morphological abnormalities in each cell line of the pulmonary vasculature have been described in cases of IPAH.[15] The endothelium in particular displays marked heterogeneity in the pulmonary vascular bed. Although endothelial dysfunction has been clearly described in cases of PAH, discordance between phenotype and function has been noted. It is not known at what stage during the evolution of PAH endothelial cell proliferation occurs. It has been proposed, however, that a somatic mutation rather than nonselective cell proliferation in response to injury accounts for the growth advantage of endothelial cells in patients with IPAH. Heterogeneity in the smooth muscle and fibroblast populations also contributes to discordance between phenotype and function. Interconversion between cell types (fibroblast to smooth muscle cell or endothelium to smooth muscle cell), in addition to neovascularization, may occur.

Smooth muscle cell hypertrophy and increased connective tissue and extracellular matrix are found in the large muscular and elastic arteries. In the subendothelial layer, increased thickness may be the result of recruitment and/or proliferation of smooth muscle–like cells. It is possible that precursor smooth muscle cells are in a continuous layer in the subendothelial layer along the entire pulmonary artery. These cells are similar to the pericytes responsible for the appearance of muscle in normally nonmuscular arteries and that contribute to intimal thickening in larger arteries. Alterations in the extracellular matrix secondary to proteolytic enzymes also play a role in the pathology of PAH. Matrix-degrading enzymes can release mitogenically active growth factors that stimulate smooth muscle cell proliferation. In addition, elastase and matrix metalloproteinases

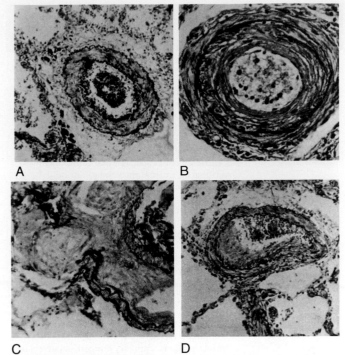

FIGURE 73–3 Photomicrographs of pulmonary arterial histological lesions seen in cases of clinically unexplained pulmonary hypertension. All slides were stained with Verhoeff–van Gieson stain. **A,** Medical hypertrophy (original magnification, ×100). **B,** Concentric laminar intimal fibrosis, seen most often in association with plexiform lesions (original magnification, ×200). **C,** Plexiform lesion demonstrating obstruction in the arterial lumen, aneurysmal dilation, and proliferation of anastomosing vascular channels (original magnification, ×200). **D,** Eccentric intimal fibrosis, often seen in association with organized microthrombi but also present in many patients with plexiform lesions (original magnification, ×100). *(From Palevsky HI, Schloo BL, Pietra GG, et al: Primary pulmonary hypertension: Vascular structure, morphometry and responsiveness to vasodilator agents. Circulation 80:1207, 1989.)*

contribute to the upregulation of proliferation. Degradation of elastin has also been shown to stimulate upregulation of the glycoprotein fibronectin, which in turn stimulates smooth muscle cell migration.

HYPERTENSIVE PULMONARY ARTERIOPATHY. The most common vascular changes in PAH can best be characterized as a hypertensive pulmonary arteriopathy, which is present in 85 percent of cases (Table 73-6). These changes involve medial hypertrophy of the arteries and arterioles, often in conjunction with other vascular changes. Isolated medial hypertrophy is uncommon and, when present, it has been assumed to represent an early stage of the disease. The intimal proliferation may appear as concentric laminar intimal fibrosis, eccentric intimal fibrosis, or concentric nonlaminar intimal fibrosis. The frequency of these findings differs from case to case and within regions of the same lung in the same patient. In addition, plexiform and dilation lesions, as well as a necrotizing arteritis, may be seen throughout the lungs. The fundamental nature of the plexiform lesion remains a mystery. Morphologically, it represents a mass of disorganized vessels with proliferating endothelial cells, smooth muscle cells, myofibroblasts, and macrophages. Several studies have demonstrated the involvement of growth factors that have been implicated in angiogenesis. Whether the plexiform lesion represents impaired proliferation or angiogenesis remains unclear (Fig. 73-3).

THROMBOTIC PULMONARY ARTERIOPATHY. The other major pattern of vascular changes in PAH is that of a thrombotic pulmonary arteriopathy. Typical features

TABLE 73–6	Histopathological Classification of Hypertensive Pulmonary Vascular Disease
Classification	**Characteristic Histopathological Features**
Arteriopathy	
Isolated medial hypertrophy*	Medial hypertrophy: increase of medial muscle in muscular arteries, muscularization of nonmuscularized arterioles; no appreciable intimal or luminal obstructive lesions; no plexiform lesions
Plexogenic pulmonary	Plexiform and dilation lesions; medial hypertrophy; eccentric or concentric laminar and nonlaminar arteriopathy, intimal thickening; fibrinoid necrosis, arteritis, and thrombotic lesions
Thrombotic pulmonary	Thrombi (fresh, organizing, or organized and colander lesions); eccentric and concentric nonlaminar arteriopathy, intimal thickening, varying degrees of medial hypertrophy; no plexiform lesions
Isolated pulmonary arteritis	Active or healed arteritis, limited to pulmonary arteries; varying degrees of medial hypertrophy, intimal fibrosis, and thrombotic lesions; no plexiform lesions; no systemic arteritis
Venopathy	
Pulmonary venoocclusive disease	Eccentric intimal fibrosis and recanalized thrombi within diseased pulmonary veins and venules; arterialized veins, capillary congestion, alveolar edema and siderophages, dilated lymphatics, pleural and septal edema, and arterial medial hypertrophy; intimal thickening and thrombotic lesions
Microangiopathy	
Pulmonary capillary	Infiltrating thin-walled blood vessels throughout pulmonary parenchyma, hemangiomatosis pleura, bronchi, and walls of pulmonary veins and arteries; medial hypertrophy and intimal thickening of muscular pulmonary arteries and arterioles

*Medial hypertrophy includes muscularization of arterioles.
From Pietra GG: Pathology of primary pulmonary hypertension. *In* Rubin LJ, Rich S (eds): Primary Pulmonary Hypertension. New York, Marcel Dekker, 1997, pp 19-61. Courtesy of Marcel Dekker, Inc.

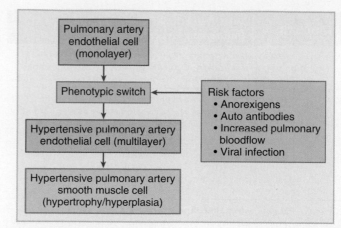

FIGURE 73–4 Proposed pathway leading to pulmonary hypertensive endothelial and smooth muscle cell changes. It is believed that endothelial cells undergo a phenotypic switch as a result of exposure to a number of identified risk factors, which results in the emergence of an apoptosis-resistant cell line. This hypertensive endothelial cell signals a change in the smooth muscle cells that promotes proliferation and vasoconstriction.

include medial hypertrophy of the arteries and arterioles, with both eccentric and concentric nonlaminar intimal fibrosis. The presence of colander lesions, which represent recanalized thrombi, is also typical. These lesions are believed to arise as a result of primary in situ thrombosis of the small vascular arteries and not from recurrent pulmonary embolism.

Many patients will have characteristics of both patterns of arteriopathy of varying degrees. This would suggest that the vascular changes from PAH occur across a spectrum, and are likely influenced by genetic and environmental factors.

Causative Factors

By definition, the precise cause of IPAH is unknown, but it probably represents the clinical expression of PAH as the final common pathway from multiple biological abnormalities within the pulmonary circulation.[16-19] As understanding of vascular biology has improved, many studies indicate abnormalities in pulmonary endothelial cell function as causing or contributing to the development of pulmonary hypertension in humans (Fig. 73-4). It is now understood that the endothelial cell regulates pulmonary smooth muscle cell tone. Dysfunction of the counterregulatory systems within the pulmonary vascular bed seems to be common in cases of pulmonary hypertension. The normal pulmonary vascular endothelial cell maintains the vascular smooth muscle in a state of relaxation. The finding of increased pulmonary vascular reactivity and vasoconstriction in patients with IPAH suggests that a marked vasoconstrictive tendency underlies the development of IPAH in predisposed individuals, possibly as a result of inappropriate smooth muscle hypertrophy.

An equally important causative feature of IPAH is the widespread development of in situ thrombosis of the small pulmonary arteries, with intraluminal thrombin deposition.[20] Abnormalities in platelet activation and function and biochemical features of a procoagulant environment within the pulmonary vasculature support a role of thrombosis in disease initiation in some patients. Interactions between growth factors, platelets, and the vessel wall suggest that thrombin may play a fundamental role in many of the pathobiological processes described in patients with PPH and in disease progression. A prothrombotic state can arise as a consequence of impaired fibrinolysis, enhanced coagulation, or increased platelet activation. Platelet activation not only promotes thrombosis, but also leads to the release of granules that contain mitogenic agents and vasoconstrictive substances (Fig. 73-5).

DYSFUNCTIONAL ENDOTHELIUM. The dysfunctional pulmonary hypertensive endothelial cell phenotype is characterized by uncontrolled proliferation, increased production of vasoconstrictor mediators such as endothelin, expression of 5-lipooxygenase, and decreased synthesis of prostacyclin.[21] In patients with IPAH, expression of prostacyclin synthase is reduced in pulmonary arteries ranging from 1 mm to less than 100 μm in diameter, which suggests that the reduction in prostacyclin synthesis in otherwise morphologically normal to minimally remodeled vessels may play a role in the early stages of pathogenesis. Alternatively, endothelial cells of pulmonary small arteries may become dysfunctional as the disease progresses and pulmonary artery pressure progressively rises. Loss of expression of prostacyclin synthase is one of the phenotypic alterations present in pulmonary endothelial cells in cases of severe pulmonary hypertension.

Reduced expression of the endothelial isoform of NO synthase has been demonstrated in the pulmonary vasculature and correlates inversely with the extent and severity of morphological lesions. Endothelial nitric oxide synthase (eNOS) is increased in plexiform lesions, however, and may be part of a compensatory process. Endothelin may also play a role in the elevated pulmonary vascular tone. Because it has a long half-life, subtle disturbances in production or release could lead to sustained vasoconstriction. It appears that regardless of whether abnormal endothelial function is the underlying cause of IPAH, progression of the disease is invariably accompanied by worsening of endothelial function, which itself can promote disease progression.

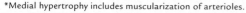

CH 73

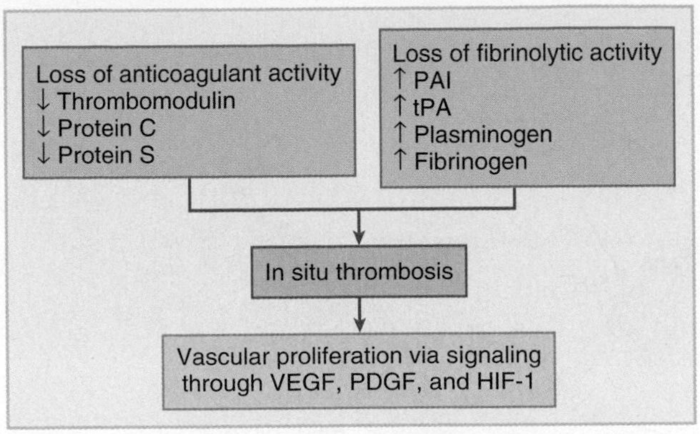

FIGURE 73–5 Proposed mechanisms of thrombosis-induced pulmonary vascular growth. The loss of normal anticoagulant activity by a reduction in circulating anticoagulants, and a loss in normal fibrinolytic activity by an increase in local procoagulants, produces in situ thrombosis of the pulmonary arterioles, which have an underlying abnormal endothelial cell surface. Histologically, this will most often appear as eccentric intimal pads in the arteriolar vessels. The result is vascular proliferation via specific growth factor signaling pathways that can initiate or sustain pulmonary vascular disease. PAI-1 = plasminogen activator inhibitor–1; tPA = tissue plasminogen activator; VEGF = vascular endothelial growth factor; PDGF = platelet-derived growth factor; HIF-1 = hypoxia inducible factor-1.

A striking feature of the pulmonary vasculature in patients with IPAH is intimal proliferation and, in some vessels, it causes virtually complete vascular occlusion. Several growth factors have been implicated in the development of this type of vascular pathology, including basic fibroblast growth factor from the endothelium[22] and platelet-derived growth factor (PDGF) from platelets. Enhanced growth factor release, activation, and intracellular signaling may lead to smooth muscle cell proliferation and migration, as well as extracellular matrix synthesis. Even advanced lesions show evidence of in situ activity of ongoing synthesis of connective tissue proteins such as elastin, collagen, and fibronectin.

LOCAL HEMODYNAMICS. Several studies have suggested that local hemodynamics can influence pulmonary vascular remodeling. A classic example is the pulmonary hypertension that occurs in congenital systemic-to-pulmonary shunts. It is believed that endothelial cells can release mediators that induce vascular smooth muscle cell growth in response to changes in pulmonary blood flow or pressure. Experimental data suggest that medial hypertrophy can be converted to a neointimal pattern when pulmonary vascular injury is coupled with increased pulmonary blood flow. These neointimal lesions are composed of smooth muscle cells that are immunoreactive to antialpha smooth muscle actin antibody. It is now accepted that hemodynamic shear stress acts through the endothelium to regulate vessel tone and the chronic restructuring of blood vessels.

Endothelial denudation also results in platelet adherence to exposed tissue collagen, with release of platelet-derived smooth muscle mitogens that also have vasoconstrictor properties. This process in turn leads to an inflammatory response and thrombosis, thereby narrowing the lumen of pulmonary vessels. In a person who is susceptible, whether on a genetic or an acquired basis, intense vasoconstriction may lead to fibrinoid necrosis of the arteriolar wall and the development of plexiform lesions. Ultimately, the vessels are reduced in number, and the residua of these destroyed vessels can be seen histologically as "ghost vessels." Destruction of large numbers of pulmonary arterioles reduces the cross-sectional area of the pulmonary vascular bed, thereby producing a permanent increase in pulmonary vascular resistance and fixed pulmonary hypertension. The latter in turn damages other blood vessels and initiates a vicious cycle, with progressively rising pulmonary arterial pressure.

Increased shear stress in the pulmonary microvasculature makes the endothelial cells more vulnerable to apoptosis. One theory has proposed that this might also allow for the emergence of an apoptosis-resistant cell line, which localizes proliferative vascular remodeling. This theory is attractive because it accounts for many of the pathobiological phenomena described in IPAH, including the intense intimal proliferation that leads to obliteration of the arteriolar lumen and resorption of the distal vasculature. It might also explain the seemingly opposite response of the pulmonary vasculature in IPAH in the early stages (heralded by reversible vasoconstriction) as opposed to the later stages (heralded by absence of vasoconstriction and accompanied by intense vascular proliferation).

ION CHANNELS. Potassium channels are found throughout the pulmonary vascular bed. They consist of voltage-dependent and calcium-dependent potassium channels (see Chap. 31). The role of these channels has been studied primarily in the presence of acute hypoxia in animals. It is believed that potassium channels modulate adult pulmonary vascular tone. It is probable that calcium channels also serve a regulatory role in modulating vascular tone, particularly the L-type calcium channel. Inhibition of the voltage-regulated potassium channel by hypoxia or drugs can produce vasoconstriction and has been described in pulmonary artery smooth muscle cells harvested from patients with IPAH.[23] It has been suggested that defects in the potassium channel of pulmonary resistance smooth muscle cells are involved in the initiation or progression of pulmonary hypertension. A genetic defect related to potassium channels in the lungs of patients with IPAH that leads to vasoconstriction may be one mechanism for the development of IPAH in some patients.

SEROTONIN. Elevated plasma levels of serotonin and reduced platelet serotonin concentration have been described in IPAH patients. One series has reported increased serotonin levels in patients with pulmonary hypertension associated with the use of fenfluramine and with connective tissue disease. Of interest is that after six of these patients underwent heart-lung transplantation, they had persistently elevated concentrations of plasma serotonin and decreased platelet serotonin concentrations, suggesting that the abnormality in platelet serotonin handling was a primary process in the evolution of their pulmonary hypertension. Mutations in the serotonin transporter and 5-hydroxytryptamine 2B (5-HT$_{2B}$) receptor have now been reported in patients with IPAH (Fig. 73-6).[24,25]

ELASTOLYTIC ENZYMES. High elastin turnover and neosynthesis of elastin have been attributed to degradation of elastin from the increased activity of serine elastase. A cause-and-effect relationship between elastase and pulmonary vascular disease was demonstrated when elastase inhibitors were shown to be effective in attenuating the development and retarding the progression of pulmonary hypertension in monocrotaline-injected hypoxic rats. Progression of pulmonary hypertension may involve a series of switches in smooth muscle cell phenotype and proliferation to account for medial hypertrophy and smooth muscle cell migration, resulting in neointimal formation. Structural and functional alterations in the endothelial cell could result in loss of barrier function and allow leakage into the subendothelium of a serum factor normally excluded from this region. Enzymes released from precursor or mature smooth muscle cells activate growth factors normally stored in the extracellular matrix, such as basic fibroblast growth factor and TGF-β, which are known to induce smooth muscle cell hypertrophy and proliferation and increase connective tissue protein synthesis. In muscular arteries, release of growth factors would result in hypertrophy of the vessel wall.

OTHER VASCULAR PROTEINS. Increased plasma levels of adrenomedullin occur in PAH and hypoxic pulmonary hypertension.[26] Increased levels of mRNA for adrenomedullin and its receptor suggest that it is part of a compensatory mechanism for maintaining normal pulmonary blood flow. Vasoactive intestinal peptide decreases pulmonary artery pressure and pulmonary vascular resistance and inhibits platelet activation and smooth muscle cell proliferation. Increased levels have been reported in PAH.[27]

Genetics

An important concept in the development of PAH is that the disease develops in patients with an underlying genetic predisposition following exposure to specific stimuli, which serve as triggers. Predisposition to the development of pulmonary hypertension has been noted by the marked heterogeneity in responses of the pulmonary vasculature in various disease states. Examples include the considerable variability among individuals to vasoconstrictive stimuli such as hypoxia or acidosis, which can produce marked pulmonary hypertension in one person and be essentially without effect in another.[28] The pulmonary arterial pressure response to hypoxia is particularly high in individuals with blood group A. This variability in responsiveness of the pulmonary vascular bed undoubtedly accounts for the fact that pulmonary edema develops in only a minority of individuals on exposure to high altitude. Also, the severity of

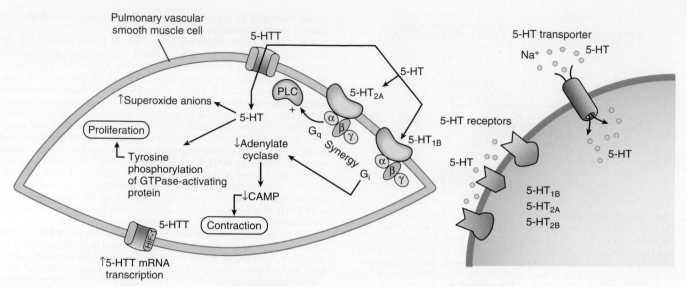

FIGURE 73-6 Serotonin receptors and transporter in pulmonary artery smooth muscle cells. Serotonin and its plasmic membrane transporter play a central role in the pathogenesis of pulmonary arterial smooth muscle cell proliferation in pulmonary arterial hypertension (PAH). Serotonin levels are increased, and pulmonary smooth muscle cells have heightened proliferation, which has been attributed to the overexpression of the serotonin transporter. 5-HT = 5-hydroxytryptamine; 5-HTT = 5-hydroxytryptamine transporter; CAMP = cyclic adenosine monophosphate; GTPase = guanosine triphosphatase. *(From Humbert M, Morrell NW, Archer SL, et al: Cellular and molecular pathobiology of pulmonary arterial hypertension. J Am Coll Cardiol 43:13S, 2004.)*

pulmonary hypertension and level of pulmonary vascular resistance vary considerably among individuals with congenital heart disease and comparably sized ventricular septal defects. Presumably, a genetic basis underlies these differences in pulmonary vascular reactivity, just as there appears to be a genetic basis for the increased reactivity of the systemic vascular bed in essential systemic hypertension.

FAMILIAL PULMONARY ARTERIAL HYPERTENSION. Idiopathic PAH has been diagnosed in families worldwide. The prevalence of familial PAH (FPAH) is uncertain, but it occurs in at least 6 percent of cases, and the incidence is likely higher.[29] Many unique features are associated with the transmission and development of FPAH. The age of onset is variable and the low penetrance of the gene confers only about a 20 percent likelihood of development of the disease. Many individuals in families with PAH inherit the gene and have progeny in whom PAH never develops. The observation that fewer males are born in PAH families than in the population at large suggests that the PAH gene might influence fertilization or cause male fetal wastage. Patients with FPAH have a similar female-to-male ratio, age of onset, and natural history of the disease as those with IPAH.

Documentation of FPAH can be difficult, because remote common ancestry occurs in patients with PAH, and skip generations caused by incomplete penetrance or by variable expression can mimic sporadic disease. Vertical transmission has been demonstrated in as many as five generations in one family and is indicative of a single autosomal dominant gene for PAH. Genetic anticipation has been described in FPAH since the early reports

Bone Morphogenetic Protein Receptor Type 2 Gene. Using linkage analysis, the locus designated PPH-1 on chromosome 2q33 led to the discovery of the *PPH-1* gene. *PPH-1* is the Human Genome Organization–approved designation DGB:1381541.[30-33] The bone morphogenetic protein receptor type 2 gene (*BMPR-2*) codes for a receptor member of the TGF-β family (Fig. 73-7). *BMPR-2* modulates vascular cell growth by activating the intracellular pathways of Smad and LIM kinase. Normally, this gene produces proteins 2,4 and 7, which signal through heterodimeric complexes of

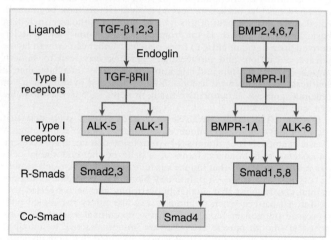

FIGURE 73–7 Transforming growth factor-beta (TGF-β) signaling pathway. The pathways involved in pulmonary arterial hypertension (PAH) are shown. TGF-β receptor type 2 (R2), and bone morphogenic protein (BMP) R2 are present on most cell surfaces as homodimers or heterooligomers. With ligand binding, the type 2 receptor phosphorylates the type 1 receptor in its juxtamembrane domain. The activated type 1 receptor then phosphorylates a receptor-regulated Smad (R-Smad); thus, the type 1 receptors determine the specificity of the signal. Smads 1, 5, and 8 are specific for the BMP signaling pathway and the ALK-1 pathway. Once activated by phosphorylation, the R-Smads interact with the common mediator Smad 4 to form hetero-oligomers that are translocated to the nucleus. ALK = activin receptor kinase.

BMPR types 2 and 1A receptors to suppress vascular smooth cell growth. The mutations ascribed to the locus interrupt the BMP-mediated signaling pathway, resulting in a predisposition to proliferation rather than apoptosis of cells within small pulmonary arteries. These molecular studies have suggested that the target cells within the pulmonary arterial wall are sensitive to *BMPR-2* gene dosage and that the TGF-β pathway mediated through *BMPR-2* is critical for the maintenance and/or normal response to injury of the pulmonary vasculature. It is clear, however, that additional factors, either environmental or genetic, are required in the pathogenesis of the disease. Recent data have supported the hypothesis that the predominant molecular mechanism underlying PAH is haploinsufficiency for *BMPR-2*. How defects in *BMPR-2* contribute to endothelial cell proliferation, smooth muscle cell hypertrophy, and fibroblast deposition in patients with PAH remains unclear. It is interesting to note that about one in four cases of IPAH actually have germline mutations in the gene encoding the *BMPR-2* receptor. Patients with both hereditary hemorrhagic telangiectasia and IPAH have been described and found to have mutations of the *ALK1* gene, also within the TGF-β superfamily.

Other Genetic Factors. Other factors that have been associated with PAH would support the concept that polymorphisms in several other genes could contribute to the development of PAH. Willers and associates and Machado and colleagues have demonstrated that there is overexpression of serotonin transporter (5-hydroxytryptamine transporter, 5-HTT) in pulmonary arteries and platelets from all the patients with PAH they studied, and that increased activity of 5-HTT is responsible for the associated smooth muscle hyperplasia.[34,35] In addition, they recently demonstrated that 5-HTT expression is elevated in cultured pulmonary artery smooth muscle cells from patients with PAH and that proliferation was also increased and related to 5-HTT expression and 5-HTT activity. 5-HTT is encoded by a single gene on chromosome 17q11.2, and a variant in the

upstream promotor region of the *5-HTT* gene has been described. This polymorphism, with long (L) and short (S) forms, affects 5-HTT expression and function, with the L allele inducing a greater rate of *5-HTT* gene transcription than the S allele. This L-allelic variant was found to be present in homozygous form in 65 percent of PPH patients but only in 27 percent of control subjects. *5-HTT* gene polymorphism could also contribute to interindividual differences in hypoxia-induced 5-HTT expression and potentially affect susceptibility to hypoxic PAH.

Defects in a common vascular signaling pathway involving angiopoetin-1 have also been described.[36] Increased signaling has been noted which causes phosphorylation of the endothelial-specific TIE-2 receptor. This reduces the level of the BMPR-1A receptor which is necessary for normal BMPR-2 signaling. Du and colleagues[36] have suggested that this pathway is nonspecific, in that it is involved in all forms of PAH (Fig. 73-8).

Clinical Features

NATURAL HISTORY AND SYMPTOMS. The most extensive study on the natural history of IPAH was reported from the National Institutes of Health (NIH) Registry on Primary Pulmonary Hypertension from 1981 to 1987. The study included the long-term follow-up of 194 patients in whom IPAH was diagnosed by established clinical and

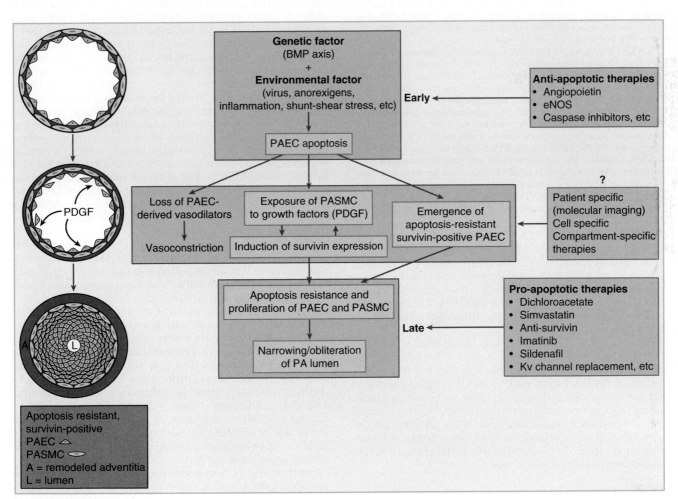

FIGURE 73-8 Apoptosis-based theory for the development of pulmonary arterial hypertension (PAH) and its therapeutic implications. Early PAH is characterized by increased apoptosis in the endothelial layer, whereas late PAH is characterized by suppressed apoptosis and increased proliferation in the intima and media. Patients in early stages of PAH may benefit more from antiapoptotic approaches, whereas patients presenting in late stages will benefit from proapoptotic strategies. BMP = bone morphogenetic protein; PA = pulmonary artery; PAEC = pulmonary artery endothelial cell; PASMC = pulmonary artery smooth muscle cell; PDGF = platelet-derived growth factor; eNOS = endothelial nitric oxide synthase. (*From Michelakis ED: Spatio-temporal diversity of apoptosis within the vascular wall in pulmonary arterial hypertension. Circ Res 98:172, 2006.*)

hemodynamic criteria. Sixty-three percent of the patients were female, and the mean age was 36 ± 15 years (range, 1 to 81 years) at the time of diagnosis. The mean interval from the onset of symptoms to diagnosis was 2 years, and the most common initial symptoms were dyspnea (80 percent), fatigue (19 percent), syncope or near-syncope (13 percent), and Raynaud phenomenon (10 percent). No ethnic differentiation was observed, with 12.3 percent of patients being black and 2.3 percent being Hispanic.

HEMODYNAMICS. Univariate analysis from the NIH Registry has pointed to the mean right atrial pressure, mean pulmonary artery pressure, and cardiac index, as well as the DLCO, as being significantly related to mortality. The New York Heart Association (NYHA) functional classification was also strongly related to survival.

Right ventricular failure from pulmonary hypertension is a result of chronic pressure overload and associated volume overload, with the development of tricuspid regurgitation. However, animal and clinical studies have suggested that right ventricular ischemia is an important factor. The mechanism of right ventricular failure in patients with pulmonary hypertension is complex. The chronic pressure overload that induces right ventricular hypertrophy and reduced contractility has been shown to cause a reduction in coronary blood flow to the right ventricular myocardium, which can produce right ventricular ischemia, both acutely and chronically. Such right ventricular dysfunction appears to be a result of a reduction in right ventricular coronary artery driving pressure. In animals, acute right ventricular failure secondary to right ventricular hypertension was overcome by increasing central aortic pressure, which resulted in an increase in right ventricular coronary driving pressure. Others have also reported that a moderate increase in aortic pressure is accompanied by a large increase in right ventricular myocardial perfusion when the autonomic nervous system is blocked with an alpha blocker.

LEFT VENTRICULAR FUNCTION. On occasion, patients with pulmonary hypertension have a reduced left ventricular ejection fraction and even regional wall motion abnormalities of the left ventricle. In the past, these findings had been attributed to mechanisms related to interventricular dependence, which suggests that in some way a dysfunctional right ventricle can lead to a dysfunctional left ventricle. Clearly, the shared interventricular septum can affect the function of both ventricles. More recently, extrinsic compression of the left main coronary artery by the pulmonary artery in patients with chronic pulmonary hypertension has been described and may be associated with classic angina-like symptoms. It is advisable to look for extrinsic compression of the left main coronary artery with coronary angiography in patients with long-standing pulmonary hypertension who have abnormal left ventricular function.

CLINICAL COURSE. The clinical course of patients with IPAH can be highly variable. However, with the onset of overt right ventricular failure manifested by worsening symptoms and systemic venous congestion, patient survival is generally limited to approximately 6 months. Understanding the clinical course of patients with IPAH is important, especially when considering major interventional therapy such as organ transplantation.[37,38]

The most common cause of death in patients with IPAH in the NIH Registry was progressive right-sided heart failure (47 percent). Sudden cardiac death was limited to patients who were in NYHA functional Class IV, suggesting that it is a manifestation of end-stage disease rather than a phenomenon that occurs early or unpredictably in the clinical course of the disease. The remainder of the patients died of other medical complications, such as pneumonia or bleeding, which suggests that patients with IPAH do not tolerate coexistent medical conditions well.

Management

LIFESTYLE CHANGES

The diagnosis of IPAH does not necessarily imply total disability for the patient. However, physical activity can be associated with elevated pulmonary artery pressure inasmuch as marked hemodynamic changes have been docu-

mented to occur early in the onset of increased physical activity. For that reason, graded exercise activities, such as bike riding or swimming, in which patients can gradually increase their workload and easily limit the extent of their work, are thought to be safer than isometric activities. Isometric activities such as lifting weights or stair climbing can be associated with syncopal events and should be limited or avoided.

PREGNANCY ISSUES

The subject of pregnancy should also be discussed with women of childbearing age. The physiological changes that occur in pregnancy can potentially activate the disease and result in death of the mother and/or the child. In addition to the increased circulating blood volume and oxygen consumption that will increase right ventricular work, circulating procoagulant factors and the risk of pulmonary embolism from deep vein thrombosis and amniotic fluid are serious concerns. Syncope and cardiac arrest have also been reported to occur during active labor and delivery, and a syndrome of postpartum circulatory collapse has been described. For these reasons, surgical sterilization should be given strong consideration by women with IPAH or their husbands, and pregnancy should be strongly discouraged.

MEDICAL THERAPIES

Medical therapies have been developed that are targeted at reversing the severity of pulmonary hypertension via many different pathways (Fig. 73-9).[39,40] However, these patients suffer from right heart failure and thus measures that have been shown to be effective in heart failure are often used.

DIGOXIN. Animal studies in right ventricular systolic overload have shown that prior administration of digoxin helps prevent the reduction in contractility of the right ventricle. Clinically, it has been shown that digoxin can exert a favorable hemodynamic effect when given acutely to patients with right ventricular failure from pulmonary hypertension. An increase in resting cardiac output of approximately 10 percent was noted, which is similar to observations made in patients with left ventricular systolic failure. In addition, it was also observed that digoxin causes a significant reduction in circulating norepinephrine, which was markedly increased. Digitalis toxicity in patients with pulmonary hypertension and normal renal function is uncommon.

DIURETICS. These drugs appear to be of marked benefit in symptom relief of patients with IPAH. Their traditional role has been limited to patients manifesting right ventricular failure and systemic venous congestion. However, patients with advanced IPAH can have increased left ventricular filling pressures that contribute to the symptoms of dyspnea and orthopnea, which can be relieved with diuretics. Diuretics may also serve to reduce right ventricular wall stress in patients with concomitant tricuspid regurgitation and volume overload. The fear that diuretics will induce systemic hypotension is unfounded, because the main factor limiting cardiac output is pulmonary vascular resistance and not pulmonary blood volume. Patients with severe venous congestion may require high doses of loop diuretics or the use of combined diuretics. In these cases, electrolyte levels need to be carefully monitored to avoid hyponatremia and hypokalemia.

In humans, elevated plasma aldosterone concentrations are associated with endothelial dysfunction, left ventricular hypertrophy, and cardiac death. Spironolactone has been demonstrated to enhance the beneficial effect of ACE inhibition on mortality in patients with congestive heart failure (see Chap. 25). Given the similarities between left and right heart failure on activation of the renin-angiotensin-aldosterone system, it seems reasonable to use aldosterone antagonists in patients with pulmonary hypertension.

SUPPLEMENTAL OXYGEN.
Hypoxic pulmonary vasoconstriction can contribute to pulmonary vascular disease in patients with alveolar hypoxia from parenchymal lung disease. Supplemental low-flow oxygen alleviates arterial hypoxemia and attenuates the pulmonary hypertension in patients with these disorders. Although most patients with IPAH do not exhibit resting hypoxemia, those who experience arterial oxygen desaturation with activity may benefit from ambulatory supplemental oxygen, because increased oxygen extraction develops in the face of fixed oxygen delivery. Patients with severe right-sided heart failure and resting hypoxemia resulting from markedly increased oxygen extraction at rest should be treated with continuous oxygen therapy to maintain their arterial oxygen saturation above 90 percent. Patients with hypoxemia caused by a right-to-left shunt via a patent foramen ovale do not improve their level of oxygenation to an appreciable degree with supplemental oxygen.

ANTICOAGULANTS. Oral anticoagulant therapy is widely recommended for patients with PAH, although its clinical efficacy as a therapy is difficult to prove. A retrospective review of patients with PPH monitored over a 15-year period at the Mayo Clinic has suggested that patients who received warfarin had improved survival over those who did not. The influence of warfarin therapy has been investigated in patients with IPAH who failed to respond to high doses of calcium channel blockers. Significant improvement in survival was observed in patients who received anticoagulation, with a 1-year survival rate of 91 percent and a 3-year survival rate of 47 percent, as compared with 1- and 3-year rates of 62 and 31 percent, respectively, in patients who did not receive anticoagulants. The current recommendation is to use warfarin in relatively low doses, as has been recommended for prophylaxis of venous thromboembolism, with the international normalized ratio (INR) maintained at 2.0 to 3.0 times that of controls.

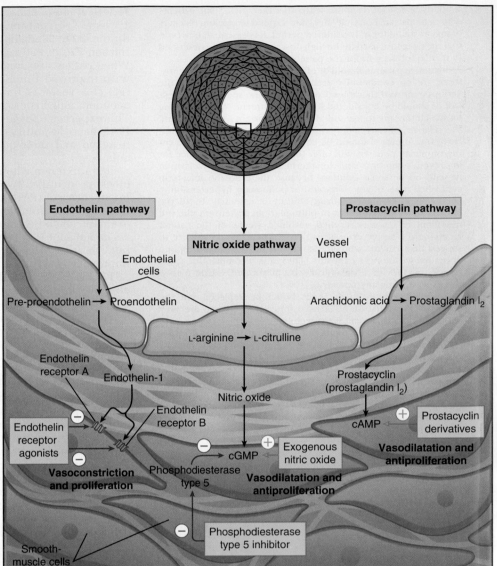

FIGURE 73–9 Targets for current therapies in pulmonary arterial hypertension (PAH). Three pathways involved in the pathogenesis of PAH are shown. These pathways correspond to important therapeutic targets and illustrate how currently approved therapies might work in PAH at the cellular level. Vasoconstriction and cellular proliferation are the dominant processes. There is currently no way of knowing which pathway(s) might be important in any given patient. Although the use of therapies in combination has appeal, there are little data currently indicating that this approach is efficacious. (*From Humbert M, Sitbon O, Simonneau G: Treatment of pulmonary arterial hypertension. N Engl J Med 351:1425, 2004.*)

Principles of Drug Treatment of Pulmonary Arterial Hypertension

- Establish a correct diagnosis. The symptoms of pulmonary hypertension attributable to PAH can be indistinguishable from pulmonary hypertension of other causes. However, the treatments vary markedly. In addition, treatments that may be helpful in PAH can often be harmful and even dangerous in other conditions. For these reasons, it is absolutely essential that a correct diagnosis of the cause be made in every case. Lack of an obvious history should not be relied on as adequate, because patients with congenital heart disease may never have been told of a heart murmur, and patients with chronic thromboembolic pulmonary hypertension often have no antecedent history of pulmonary embolism. Given the poor survival of pulmonary hypertension of any cause, every patient should undergo thorough testing, including cardiac catheterization, prior to initiating therapy.

- Obtain baseline assessments of the disease. To determine whether the treatments of PAH are effective, it is important to evaluate the patient's response objectively. Regardless of which test or tests are used (e.g., exercise testing, catheterization), an adequate baseline assessment of the patient's disease must be obtained to monitor the patient's response to therapy.

- Test vasoreactivity. Because of the dramatic effect that calcium blockers have on improving survival in patients who are vasoreactive, patients should be tested at the time of diagnosis so that potentially reactive patients are not missed.

- Reactive patients should undergo a trial of calcium channel blockers. Calcium blockers are the drugs of choice in those patients who demonstrate vasoreactivity at the time of testing. There is no evidence to suggest that these patients would have a similarly beneficial response with other therapies. Some patients who demonstrate reactivity may not respond to calcium blockers or may respond for only a limited period. It is essential, however, that the drugs are used in the high doses that have been described to realize full benefit for the patient (see earlier).

- Nonreactive patients should be offered other therapies. Currently, there are no comparative trials regarding the efficacy of the various approved therapies. Consequently, no specific treatment can or should be considered first-line treatment. When deciding on which therapy to use initially, it is important to keep in mind the relative efficacy, safety, and cost of the various therapies. However, foremost should be consideration of which treatment the physician believes will offer the patient the best chance for improved symptoms and long-term survival. This will often depend on personal opinion, because there are no long-term controlled trials of any therapies for pulmonary hypertension.
- Follow-up assessment of drug efficacy is essential. In all the clinical trials for treatment of pulmonary hypertension, the full treatment effect was reached within 4 weeks of the patient receiving the active drug at full dose. There is no evidence to suggest that patients who do not respond initially might respond over time with longer exposure. Thus, it is recommended that a repeat measure of drug efficacy be performed within 6 to 8 weeks of starting any new drug treatment.
- Treatments that are ineffective should be replaced. All the approved therapies for PAH have inherent risks and are very expensive. If a treatment is deemed ineffective by an assessment of efficacy, a different treatment should be substituted rather than added. Patients who clinically fail all treatments should be considered for lung transplantation (see later).
- Benefits and risks of combination therapies are largely unknown. The use of these treatments in combination is becoming popular. However, the only randomized controlled trial of combination therapy demonstrating efficacy has been the addition of oral sildenafil to stable patients with PAH on intravenous epoprostenol (currently unpublished). Other combination trials are underway.
- Repeated measures of efficacy should be adhered to. Evidence has suggested that these therapies may lose efficacy over time. Thus, even in patients in whom it has been shown that drug therapy has been helpful initially, serial assessments of drug efficacy should be performed indefinitely to check for loss of efficacy over time.

VASODILATOR THERAPY

Because of early reports showing a reduction in pulmonary artery pressure following the acute administration of vaso-dilators, it has been presumed that vasodilators are the mainstay of treatment in patients with IPAH. This presumption is not supported by the published literature. Vasodilators are effective in a subset of patients with IPAH, but many complexities regarding vasodilator administration make their use in these patients difficult. The final common cellular pathway by which vasodilators work is through a reduction of intracellular calcium in the vascular smooth muscle cell. The same mechanism is also attributable to cellular growth inhibition. Indeed, most vasodilators have been shown to possess growth inhibitory properties of smooth muscle cells in culture. It is likely that the chronic effects of these agents in patients with pulmonary hypertension represent both mechanisms.

CALCIUM CHANNEL BLOCKERS. Of the vasodilators prescribed for patients with IPAH, calcium channel blockers appear to have the widest use. Early studies using conventional doses have failed to demonstrate a chronic sustained benefit. Moreover, calcium channel blockers have properties that could worsen the underlying pulmonary hypertension, including negative inotropic effects on right ventricular function and reflex sympathetic stimulation, which may increase the resting heart rate. It has been reported that 10 to 20 percent of patients with IPAH who are challenged with very high doses of calcium channel blockers may manifest a dramatic reduction in pulmonary artery pressure and pulmonary vascular resistance, which, on

serial catheterization, has been maintained for more than 15 years.[41] It appears essential that high doses (e.g., amlodipine, 20 to 30 mg/day; nifedipine, 180 to 240 mg/day; diltiazem, 720 to 960 mg/day) be used to realize full benefit. When patients respond favorably, quality of life is restored with improved functional class, and survival (94 percent rate at 5 years) is improved when compared with nonresponders and historical control subjects (36 percent rate). This experience suggests that a select subset of patients with IPAH have the ability to have their pulmonary hypertension reversed and their quality of life and length of survival enhanced.

It is unknown whether the response to calcium channel blockers identifies two subsets of patients with IPAH, different stages of IPAH, or a combination of both. However, it is essential to point out that patients who do not exhibit a dramatic hemodynamic response to calcium channel blockers do not appear to benefit from their long-term administration. Patients who do respond will show marked clinical improvement within the first few months.

PROSTACYCLINS. Prostacyclins have been found to be effective in the therapy of pulmonary arterial hypertension.[42] Continuous intravenous infusion of *epoprostenol* has been shown in randomized clinical trials to improve quality of life and symptoms related to IPAH, exercise tolerance, hemodynamics, and short-term survival. The long-term effects of epoprostenol in IPAH include its vasodilator and antithrombotic effects, but its effects may also be importantly related to its ability to normalize cardiac output. Patients may have a reduction in pulmonary vascular resistance of more than 50 percent, even if no acute hemodynamic effects are noted. Epoprostenol is administered through a central venous catheter that is surgically implanted and delivered by an ambulatory infusion system. The delivery system is complex and requires patients to learn the techniques of sterile drug preparation, operation of the pump, and care of the intravenous catheter. Most serious complications that have occurred with epoprostenol therapy have been attributable to the delivery system and include catheter-related infections and temporary interruption of the infusion because of pump malfunction. Anecdotal reports of rebound pulmonary hypertension occurring in patients in whom the infusion was interrupted suggest that great care must be taken to ensure that the infusion is never stopped.

Side effects related to epoprostenol include flushing, headache, nausea, diarrhea, and a unique type of jaw discomfort that occurs with eating. In most patients, these symptoms are minimal and well tolerated. Chronic foot pain and a poorly defined gastropathy with prolonged use develop in some patients. To date, epoprostenol has been given to patients with PAH for more than 15 years with favorable effectiveness. In some patients (NYHA Class IV) who are critically ill, it serves as a bridge to lung transplantation by stabilizing the patient to a more favorable preoperative state. Patients who are less critically ill may do so well with epoprostenol therapy that the need to consider transplantation may be delayed, perhaps indefinitely.

The optimal dose of epoprostenol has never been determined, but doses between 25 and 40 ng/kg/min are typical. A high cardiac output state has been reported in a series of patients with IPAH receiving chronic epoprostenol therapy and is consistent with the drug having positive inotropic effects. Whether the effect is a direct one on the myocardium or indirect via neurohormonal activation has not been determined. Although most patients with IPAH have reduced cardiac output on initial examination, the development of a chronic high-output state could have long-term detrimental effects on underlying cardiac function. The follow-up assessment of patients receiving intravenous epoprostenol is variable among medical centers, but it does appear important to determine the cardiac output response to therapy periodically to optimize dosing.

The experience with epoprostenol in patients with IPAH for more than 10 years has been reported by two large centers (Fig. 73-10).[43,44] Survival rates longer than 5 years were markedly improved compared with survival in historical control subjects and the natural history predicted by the NIH Registry. Predictors of survival included NYHA functional class, exercise tolerance, and acute vasodilator responsiveness. Both studies provided important data for identifying patients who would do well over the long term, versus those in whom transplantation should be considered.

Treprostinil is a stable prostacyclin analogue that has pharmacological actions similar to those of epoprostenol, but differs in that it is chemically stable at room temperature and neutral pH and has a longer half-life (4 hours). Its pharmacological properties allow it to be administered through continuous subcutaneous infusion, thus eliminating the need for a central venous catheter and refrigeration during administrations. Infusion site pain is common. In a large randomized clinical trial in patients with pulmonary arterial hypertension, treprostinil was effective in increasing distance walked in 6 minutes, symptoms of dyspnea associated with exercise, and hemodynamics.[45] Treprostinil has also been approved for intravenous administration, and uncontrolled clinical trials have shown comparable efficacy to epoprostenol on exercise testing and hemodynamics.[46] The optimal dose of treprostinil has never been determined, but doses of 50 to 80 ng/kg/min are typical. Because there is no difference in bioavailability between the subcutaneous and intravenous routes, patients can be easily transitioned from one route of administration to the other without the need for adjusting the dosage.

A key element of the long-term efficacy of the parenteral prostacyclins appears to be related to the strategy of upward dose titration of the drug over time. It is important to increase the dose to tolerated side effects in patients who remain symptomatic, because there is a direct relationship to the dose of drug and improvement in exercise testing and hemodynamics. Once an optimal dose has been achieved, the dose is kept constant thereafter. Patients who deteriorate after a long period of stability usually do not respond to further dose increases.

Iloprost, an analogue of prostacyclin, has been approved for use via inhalation. In randomized clinical trials, inhaled iloprost was shown to have an acute effect on hemodynamics similar to those of inhaled nitric oxide. When iloprost was given chronically, patients reported an improvement in exercise, manifested by a postinhalation 6-minute walk test, and in hemodynamics.[47] Because of the short half-life of iloprost, however, it requires frequent (up to 12/day) inhalations. Iloprost is given by 2.5- or 5.0-μg ampules via dedicated nebulizer.

Beraprost is an orally active prostacyclin analogue that has been evaluated in randomized double-blind placebo-controlled multicenter trials in patients with PAH. In one large European trial (the ALPHABET study), beraprost improved exercise capacity and symptoms over a 12-week period but had no significant effect on cardiopulmonary hemodynamics or functional class. A similar trial conducted in the United States, however, showed similar efficacy at 12 weeks, only to document the loss of effectiveness over 1 year.[48] This is the only trial to follow patients for a period of 1 year and underscores how initial improvements with therapies in these patients might not be sustained for longer periods. At present, beraprost is only approved for use in Japan.

ENDOTHELIN RECEPTOR BLOCKERS. *Bosentan* is a nonselective endothelin receptor blocker that is approved as a treatment of pulmonary arterial hypertension.[49,50] In a large randomized clinical trial, bosentan showed a significant improvement in 6-minute walk distance after 16 weeks as compared with placebo.[51] It also was shown to lengthen the composite endpoint of time to clinical worsening, which included death, lung transplantation, hospitalization for pulmonary hypertension, lack of improvement, or worsening leading to discontinuation in the need for epoprostenol therapy. Importantly, there was a dose-dependent increase in hepatic transaminase levels noted from the medication, with significant elevations in 14 percent of the patients randomized to the higher dosage (250 mg twice daily). The approved dosage of bosentan is 125 mg twice daily.

CH 73

Pulmonary Hypertension

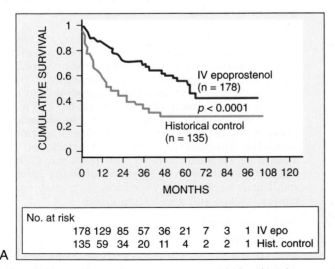
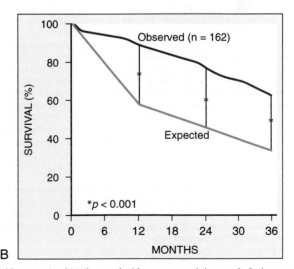

FIGURE 73–10 Kaplan-Meier survival estimates in patients with idiopathic pulmonary arterial hypertension (IPAH) treated with epoprostenol therapy. **A,** Patient survival is compared with patients with IPAH matched for New York Heart Association functional class and who never received epoprostenol therapy. **B,** Patient survival compared with untreated patients with IPAH from the NIH Registry survival prediction equation. The observed survival with epoprostenol therapy from both studies was remarkably similar and considerably better than what would have been expected. (*A* from Sitbon O, Humbert M, Nunes H, et al: Long-term intravenous epoprostenol infusion in primary pulmonary hypertension. J Am Coll Cardiol 40:780, 2002; *B* from McLaughlin V, Shillington A, Rich S: Survival in primary pulmonary hypertension. The impact of epoprostenol therapy. Circulation 106:1477, 2002.)

PHOSPHODIESTERASE TYPE 5 INHIBITORS. *Sildenafil* is a phosphodiesterase type 5 (PDE5) inhibitor initially approved to treat erectile dysfunction, and more recently PAH. PDE5 inhibitors produce pulmonary vasodilation by promoting an enhanced and sustained level of cGMP, an identical effect to that of inhaled NO.[52] When tested as a single oral agent, sildenafil has been shown to be a selective pulmonary vasodilator with equal efficacy to that of inhaled NO in lowering pulmonary artery pressure and pulmonary vascular resistance. Sildenafil has a preferential effect on the pulmonary circulation because of the high expression of this isoform in the lung. A large, randomized, clinical trial demonstrated that sildenafil caused significant improvements in 6-minute walk distance and hemodynamics in patients with PAH.[53] The recommended dosage is 20 mg three times daily, but dosages as high as 80 mg three times daily have been used safely.

Invasive Techniques

ATRIAL SEPTOSTOMY. The rationale for the creation of an atrial septostomy in patients with PAH is based on experimental and clinical observations suggesting that an intraatrial defect allowing right-to-left shunting in the setting of severe pulmonary hypertension might be of benefit.[54] Although countless patients have undergone this procedure worldwide, it should still be considered investigational. Indications for the procedure include recurrent syncope and/or right ventricular failure, despite maximum medical therapy, as a bridge to transplantation if deterioration occurs in the face of maximum medical therapy, or when no other option exists. Because the disease process in PAH appears to be unaffected by the procedure, the long-term effects of atrial septostomy must be considered palliative.

The rate of procedure-related mortality with atrial septostomy in patients with PAH is high, and thus the procedure should be attempted only in institutions with an established record for the treatment of advanced pulmonary hypertension and experience in performing atrial septostomy with a low rate of morbidity. It should not be performed in a patient with impending death and severe right ventricular failure or a patient receiving maximum cardiorespiratory support. Predictors of procedure-related failure or death have been identified and include a mean right atrial pressure higher than 20 mm Hg, a pulmonary vascular resistance index higher than 55 units/m², or a predicted 1-year survival rate of less than 40 percent.

The mechanisms responsible for the beneficial effects of atrial septostomy remain unclear. Possibilities include increased oxygen delivery at rest and/or with exercise, reduced right ventricular end-diastolic pressure or wall stress, improvement in right ventricular function as by the Frank-Starling curve, or relief of ischemia.

HEART-LUNG AND LUNG TRANSPLANTATION (see Chap. 27). Heart-lung transplantation has been performed successfully in patients with PAH since 1981.[55] Because these patients have pulmonary vascular disease and severe right ventricular dysfunction, it was originally believed that heart-lung transplantation was the only transplantation option. Widespread application of heart-lung transplantation, however, has been limited by the number of centers with expertise to perform the procedure, the scarcity of suitable donor organs, and the very long waiting times required for patients with end-stage right-sided heart failure. Consequently, bilateral or double-lung transplantation and single-lung transplantation have been performed successfully in patients with PAH. Hemodynamic studies have shown an immediate reduction in pulmonary artery pressure and pulmonary vascular resistance associated with improvement in right ventricular function.

The ages of recipients of heart-lung and lung transplants for pulmonary hypertension have ranged from 2 months to 61 years. The operative mortality rate ranges between 16 and 29 percent and is somewhat higher for recipients of a single-lung transplant. The 1-year survival rate is between 70 and 75 percent, the 2-year survival rate is between 55 and 60 percent, and the 5-year survival rate is between 40 and 45 percent. Transplantation should be reserved for patients with pulmonary hypertension who have progressed in spite of optimal medical management. It is generally accepted that patients should be considered for transplantation when they have WHO functional class III or IV disease in spite of therapy with a parenteral prostacyclin. Recent changes in the prioritization of lung transplant recipients, however, are making it increasingly difficult for these patients to become trans-

planted. Although their postoperative mortality is higher than patients with lung disease, their long-term survival is comparable. The major long-term complications in patients who survive the operation are the high incidence of bronchiolitis obliterans in the transplanted lungs, acute organ rejection, and opportunistic infection.[56]

Pulmonary Arterial Hypertension Associated with Congenital Heart Disease (see Chap. 61)

Pulmonary hypertension can develop in adults with an atrial septal defect. It is presumed that chronically increased pulmonary blood flow may have effects on pulmonary endothelium through mechanical means that cause perturbations in the integrity of the vascular wall and lead to the development of pulmonary vascular disease. Increased pulmonary blood flow from hyperthyroidism and beriberi have been reported to be associated with the development of unexplained pulmonary hypertension, which suggests that high pulmonary blood flow, rather than mere coincidence, is the basis for the development of pulmonary hypertension in patients with pretricuspid shunts, such as atrial septal defect or anomalous pulmonary venous drainage.

If a congenital cardiovascular defect causes pulmonary hypertension from the time of birth, the small muscular arteries of the fetal lung may undergo delayed or only partial involution, with subsequent persistently high levels of pulmonary vascular resistance. This is especially true in lesions in which a left-to-right shunt enters the right ventricle or pulmonary artery directly (i.e., a posttricuspid valve shunt, such as ventricular septal defect or patent ductus arteriosus). These patients experience a higher incidence of severe and irreversible pulmonary vascular damage than those in whom the shunt is proximal to the tricuspid valve (pretricuspid shunts, as in atrial septal defect and partial anomalous pulmonary venous drainage).

Pathology

The extent of reversibility of pulmonary vascular obstructive disease in the presence of congenital heart disease varies. From an anatomical point of view, reversible conditions are those in which the decreased pulmonary arteriolar cross-sectional area is the result of medial hypertrophy and vasoconstriction; irreversibility is associated with the presence of necrotizing arteritis and plexiform lesions in these small vessels.

The classification by Heath and Edwards of six grades of structural change was developed to characterize the severity of the pulmonary vascular disease and to predict reversibility that would allow surgical correction. The vascular changes that occur in pulmonary hypertension associated with congenital heart disease, however, are identical to those seen in IPAH. Early changes are characterized by hypertrophy of the media and intimal proliferation of small, muscular, pulmonary arteries and arterioles. Advanced disease is characterized by the presence of concentric laminar fibrosis with obliteration of many arterioles and small arteries, complex plexiform, angiomatous, and cavernous lesions, and necrotizing arteritis.

Clinical Considerations

EISENMENGER SYNDROME. This refers to any anomalous circulatory communication that leads to obliterative pulmonary vascular disease, including pretricuspid and posttricuspid shunts. The long-term prognosis of patients with Eisenmenger syndrome appears to be better than that of patients with other conditions associated with pulmonary hypertension. Survival of patients with Eisenmenger syndrome has been reported to be 80 percent at 10 years, 77 percent at 15 years, and 42 percent at 25 years. Survival is typically related to mean right atrial pressure and pulmonary vascular resistance.

When pulmonary vascular resistance has increased so that the patient shunts right to left, surgical closure of the anomalous circulatory communication will be associated with a prohibitive immediate risk and, if the patient survives, will usually fail to relieve pulmonary hypertension. Surgery may in fact hasten death in survivors who had either balanced shunts or predominant right-to-left shunts, because closure of the right-to-left communication merely increases the load on an already overburdened right ventricle. Structural changes in the pulmonary vascular bed are evident in pulmonary arteriograms, which reveal dilated central pulmonary arteries and narrowing of the peripheral branches.

Treatment

Intravenous epoprostenol therapy has been shown to improve exercise tolerance, quality of life, and hemodynamics in patients with congenital heart disease, irrespective of the severity or duration of the condition. It is effective in patients who have had previous surgical repair of their defect and in those who have not. No increased incidence of systemic side effects has been noted in patients who have a persistent right-to-left shunt. In patients who have bidirectional shunts, the use of epoprostenol may be a therapeutic strategy to enable a patient who is considered inoperable to become eligible for surgery at a later date. Treprostinil has also been used effectively in patients with congenital heart disease.

A useful assessment for these patients is exercise testing with pulse oximetry. Patients with little or no pulmonary vascular disease should continue to shunt left to right during exercise, and thus their pulse oximetry should be normal throughout. Patients with bidirectional shunting may have normal resting pulse oximetry but typically it will fall during exercise, reflecting shunt reversal. The magnitude of the fall may be helpful in deciding how to intervene. Patients with advanced pulmonary vascular disease will have hypoxemia at rest, which should worsen significantly with any level of exercise activity.

Pulmonary Arterial Hypertension Associated with Connective Tissue Diseases (see Chap. 84)

Scleroderma, including the CREST syndrome, is the most common cause of pulmonary hypertension in connective tissue disease states.[57] Scleroderma is associated with pulmonary hypertension in as many as one third of patients and with CREST syndrome in as many as 50 percent. The high incidence suggests that periodic screening with echocardiography in these patients may be reasonable. Although pulmonary hypertension may occur as a result of entrapment and obstruction of the pulmonary microvasculature by interstitial inflammation or fibrosis, patients initially seen with severe pulmonary hypertension usually have a pulmonary vasculature with histological features that resemble those of PAH. Patients with systemic lupus erythematosus also have pulmonary hypertension, although less commonly than patients with scleroderma. Mixed connective tissue disease is a less common form of connective tissue disease, but pulmonary hypertension may occur in as many as two thirds of these patients. Pulmonary hypertension has also been described in patients with polymyositis, dermatomyositis, and rheumatoid arthritis.

Because connective tissue diseases may have an insidious onset and slowly progressive course, early recognition

of the symptoms of pulmonary hypertension may be difficult. Although easy fatigability may be a feature of the connective tissue disease, it may also be an initial symptom of pulmonary hypertension. Dyspnea is still the most common initial symptom and should not be attributed to advancing age. Syncope, presyncope, or peripheral edema represents advanced pulmonary hypertension and right-sided heart failure. Physical findings of an elevated jugular venous pressure and an increased pulmonic component of the second heart sound, along with a right ventricular fourth heart sound, are typical features of pulmonary hypertension and warrant an evaluation for pulmonary hypertension. A murmur of tricuspid regurgitation generally reflects more advanced disease. Arterial hypoxemia is characteristic and should also prompt an evaluation of possible pulmonary hypertension in these patients. Most of these patients will have some coexisting interstitial lung disease, which may not be apparent on chest CT scanning or from pulmonary function tests. A reduced DLCO on pulmonary function tests, however, has been shown to be highly predictive of the presence of pulmonary vascular disease.

The prognosis of patients with connective tissue disease in whom pulmonary hypertension develops is poor. Conventional therapy with digitalis, diuretics, and anticoagulation has been recommended to provide a survival benefit similar to the practice in PAH. Because hypoxemia is so common, patients should be tested with pulse oximetry during exercise, and supplemental oxygen used whenever indicated., All the clinical trials involving PAH have included patients with mixed connective tissue disease, and all the approved therapies apply to the connective tissue diseases. The principles of drug selection and management for IPAH apply equally to patients with connective tissue disease, although their long-term efficacy is lower.

Pulmonary Arterial Hypertension Associated with Portal Hypertension

Pulmonary abnormalities have been commonly associated with the development of hepatic cirrhosis and portal hypertension and include hypoxemia and intrapulmonary shunting, portal-pulmonary shunting, impaired hypoxic pulmonary vasoconstriction, and pulmonary hypertension. Although the relative risk associated with the development of pulmonary hypertension in patients with portal hypertension is unknown, a large postmortem study from the Johns Hopkins Hospital has shown that the prevalence of unexplained or pulmonary hypertension in patients with cirrhosis is 5.6 times higher than that of IPAH alone. A modest increase in pulmonary artery systolic pressure is not unusual in patients with cirrhosis and portal hypertension. The increase in pulmonary artery pressure is usually passive and relates to the increase in cardiac output and/or blood volume and is associated with near-normal pulmonary vascular resistance. Published studies have indicated a strong association between portal hypertension and pulmonary hypertension, regardless of whether liver disease is present. Although the mechanisms are uncertain, several possibilities are consistent. Portal hypertension itself induces numerous modifications in the vascular media that may trigger a cascade of intracellular signals and/or cause activation or repression of various genes in endothelial and smooth muscle cells. Increased levels of several vasoactive mediators, cytokines, and growth factors have been demonstrated in patients with portal hypertension, including serotonin and interleukin-1. Other angiogenic factors such as hepatocyte growth factor or vascular endothelial growth factor may be involved in pulmonary artery remodeling.

Patients in whom PAH develops in association with cirrhosis appear to be similar to patients without cirrhosis, with the sole exception that they tend to have higher cardiac output and consequently lower calculated systemic and pulmonary vascular resistance, which is characteristic of the cirrhotic state. Treatment of portal pulmonary hypertension generally follows the guidelines developed for treating patients with PAH. Although severe pulmonary hypertension is considered a contraindication to liver transplantation because of the risk of irreversible right-sided heart failure, successful liver transplantation has been reported in patients with very mild pulmonary hypertension treated successfully with intravenous epoprostenol.

Pulmonary Arterial Hypertension Associated with Human Immunodeficiency Virus Infection (see Chap. 67)

Although well documented, it remains unclear how HIV infection results in an increased incidence of PAH in HIV-infected patients. A direct pathogenic role of HIV seems unlikely, inasmuch as no viral constituents have been detected in the vascular endothelium of these patients. On the other hand, reports of pulmonary arteriopathy with intimal proliferation in monkeys experimentally infected with the simian immunodeficiency virus and in a murine model of acquired immunodeficiency syndrome have suggested a pathogenetic link between infection with an immunodeficiency virus and the development of PAH, possibly mediated by release of inflammatory mediators or by autoimmune mechanisms. A large case-control study of HIV-associated PAH conducted in the Swiss HIV Cohort Study reported the cumulative incidence to be 0.6 percent in the entire HIV-infected population. PAH was diagnosed in patients in all stages of HIV infection and without an obvious relationship to immune deficiency, because it was unrelated to the CD4 cell counts. The clinical and hemodynamic features of these patients were similar to those of patients with PAH.

Pulmonary Arterial Hypertension Related to Anorexigens

Several anorexigens have been demonstrated to cause pulmonary hypertension in humans. The first observation was made in 1967, when an epidemic of PAH was associated with the use of aminorex in Europe coincident with its introduction in the general population. The mechanism by which aminorex causes pulmonary hypertension remains uncertain, but it has similarities to both adrenaline and ephedrine in its chemical structure. The clinical features of pulmonary hypertension were identical to those attributed to PAH.

The association between the use of fenfluramine appetite suppressants and the development of PAH was established in the International Primary Pulmonary Hypertension Study (IPPHS), a case-control study conducted in Europe in 1992 to 1994. Ultimately, the marked increase in the number of cases of PAH and cardiac valvulopathy ascribed to the use of fenfluramine drugs in the United States led to their withdrawal in 1997. In most patients, the development of pulmonary hypertension was progressive, despite withdrawal of the appetite suppressants.[58] In addition, many of the patients did not develop clinical symptoms of PAH for at least 5 years after their last ingestion. Although the drugs mainly identified in the IPPHS were the fenfluramines, anorexigens such as amphetamines were also implicated.

The mechanism by which the fenfluramines and aminorex produce pulmonary hypertension has been investigated. Experimental studies have demonstrated that these drugs can cause pulmonary vasoconstriction by inhibiting voltage-gated potassium channels in the smooth muscle cells of resistance level pulmonary arteries. Although the degree of pulmonary vasoconstriction noted was small, it increased dramatically when NO synthase was inhibited. One study compared NO production in patients with PAH and patients with pulmonary hypertension associated with the use of anorexigens. It appears that the latter group had a deficiency in basal NO production when compared with patients with PAH, which suggests that NO may be a compensatory product of the pulmonary arterial endothelium that increases in pulmonary hypertension to counteract the effects of chronic vasoconstriction.

Pulmonary Hypertension Related to Sickle Cell Disease

Cardiopulmonary complications are common in sickle cell disease. The cause of pulmonary hypertension, which has been reported in 20 to 32 percent of sickle cell disease patients, is multifactorial, with contributing factors including hemolysis, impaired nitric oxide bioavailability, chronic hypoxemia, high cardiac output, thromboembolism, and parenchymal and vascular injury caused by sequestration of sickle erythrocytes, chronic liver disease, and asplenia.[59]

In a series of 195 consecutive patients with sickle cell disease screened with echocardiography, pulmonary hypertension, defined as a tricuspid regurgitant jet higher than 2.5 m/sec by Doppler echocardiography, was diagnosed in 32 percent. Most had mild pulmonary hypertension, with only 9 percent of patients having a tricuspid regurgitant velocity higher than 3.0 m/sec. A self-reported history of cardiovascular or renal complications, increased systolic blood pressure, high lactate dehydrogenase levels, high alkaline phosphatase levels, and low transferrin levels were all significant independent correlates of pulmonary hypertension. Notably, only 18 patients in this series underwent a right heart catheterization. These patients had a mean pulmonary artery pressure of 35 mm Hg, pulmonary capillary wedge pressure of 17 mm Hg, and cardiac output of 10.2 liters/min. In this series, tricuspid regurgitant velocity of higher than 2.5 m/sec was strongly associated with an increased risk of death during the median follow-up period of 18 months. Whether the pulmonary hypertension itself truly reduces survival, or is simply a marker of more advanced sickle cell disease, remains unclear.

In general, the hemodynamic profile of most patients with pulmonary hypertension in the setting of sickle cell disease is distinct from those with IPAH and is characterized by a more modest elevation in pulmonary artery pressure, an elevation in left heart filling pressures, and invariably a markedly elevated cardiac output. It is likely that left-sided heart disease, or pulmonary venous hypertension, is a contributing factor in most patients. Intensification of sickle cell disease therapy, such as with hydroxyurea or exchange transfusions, should be the mainstay of ttreatment. There have been no controlled trials demonstrating benefit from pulmonary vasodilator therapy. Patients with sickle cell disease can also have an increased risk of thromboembolism, and pulmonary thromboendarterectomy may be indicated in certain cases.

Persistent Pulmonary Hypertension of the Newborn

Three forms of persistent pulmonary hypertension of the newborn have been described. In the hypertrophic type, the muscular tissue of the pulmonary arteries is hypertrophied and extends peripherally to the acini. Medial hypertrophy causes narrowing of the arteries, an increase in pulmonary pressure, and a reduction in pulmonary blood flow. It is believed to be the result of sustained fetal hypertension from chronic vasoconstriction caused by chronic fetal distress. In the hypoplastic type, the lungs, including the pulmonary arteries, are underdeveloped, usually as the result of a congenital diaphragmatic hernia or prolonged leakage of amniotic fluid. The cross-sectional area of the pulmonary vascular bed is inadequate for normal neonatal pulmonary blood flow. In the reactive type, lung histology is presumably normal but vasoconstriction causes pulmonary hypertension. High levels of vasoconstrictive mediators such as thromboxane, norepinephrine, and leukotrienes may be responsible and may result from streptococcal infection or acute asphyxia at birth.

Although persistent pulmonary hypertension of the newborn can vary in severity, severe cases are usually life-threatening. It is usually associated with severe hypoxemia and the need for mechanical ventilation. Echocardiographic findings of severe pulmonary hypertension and right-to-left shunting at the level of the ductus arteriosus or foramen ovale are common. Inhaled nitric oxide has provided encouraging results through improvement in oxygenation in these patients. Intravenous epoprostenol has also been used and may even have additive effects to those of inhaled NO. Alveolar capillary dysplasia is a very rare cause of persistent pulmonary hypertension of the newborn and is characterized by a developmental abnormality in the pulmonary vasculature. The antemortem diagnosis can be made only with open-lung biopsy. Despite aggressive treatment with NO, epoprostenol, and even extracorporeal membrane oxygenation, survival in the setting of alveolar capillary dysplasia is rare.

Pulmonary Venoocclusive Disease

Pulmonary venoocclusive disease is a rare form of PAH.[60] The histopathological diagnosis is based on the presence of obstructive eccentric fibrous intimal pads in the pulmonary veins and venules. Arterialization of the pulmonary veins is often present and is associated with alveolar capillary congestion. Other changes of chronic pulmonary hypertension, such as medial hypertrophy and muscularization of the arterioles with eccentric intimal fibrosis, may also be seen. The pulmonary venous obstruction explains the increased pulmonary capillary wedge pressure described in patients in the late stages of the disease and the increase in basilar bronchovascular markings noted on the chest radiograph. These clinical findings, along with a perfusion lung scan showing diffuse, patchy nonsegmental abnormalities, are suggestive of the diagnosis on a clinical basis. The chest CT scan may be helpful, revealing smooth interlobular septal thickening, ground-glass opacities, and a mosaic attention pattern. The treatment of pulmonary venoocclusive disease is unsatisfactory. Anecdotal reports of success with calcium blockers or epoprostenol have been tempered by reports of these treatments producing fulminant pulmonary edema. Any therapy needs particularly close supervision, and early referral of the patient for lung transplantation should be considered.

Pulmonary Capillary Hemangiomatosis

Pulmonary capillary hemangiomatosis was first described in 1978 as a very rare cause of pulmonary hypertension. Because of the few reports

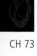

CH 73

in the medical literature, it is hard to characterize this abnormality.[61] The typical chest radiographic appearance is a diffuse bilateral reticular nodular pattern associated with enlarged central pulmonary arteries. Ventilation-perfusion scans are often abnormal and may show matched or unmatched defects. The most characteristic finding on high-resolution CT scan is diffuse bilateral thickening of the interlobular septa and small centrilobular, poorly circumscribed, nodular opacities. Diffuse ground-glass opacities have also been described. Histological findings often include irregular small nodular foci of thin-walled capillary-sized vessels that diffusely invade the lung parenchyma, bronchiolar walls, and adventitia of large vessels. These nodular lesions are often associated with alveolar hemorrhage. Changes of hypertensive arteriopathy manifest by intimal fibrosis and medial hypertrophy are also common. Most patients appear to be young adults and present with dyspnea and/or hemoptysis. It is difficult to distinguish pulmonary capillary hemangiomatosis from IPAH clinically. A hereditary form with probable autosomal recessive transmission has been reported.

The clinical course of patients with this condition is usually one of progressive deterioration leading to severe pulmonary hypertension, right-sided heart failure, and death. Intravenous epoprostenol has been used, but it has been reported with the associated development of severe pulmonary edema. The only definitive treatment for these patients is bilateral lung transplantation.

Pulmonary Venous Hypertension

Pathophysiology

Increased resistance to pulmonary venous drainage is a mechanism common to several conditions of diverse causes in which pulmonary hypertension occurs. Altered resistance to pulmonary venous drainage may be the result of diseases affecting the left ventricle or pericardium or mitral or aortic valves, or of rare entities such as cor triatriatum and left atrial myxoma.

The severity of pulmonary hypertension depends, in part, on the performance of the right ventricle. In response to an acute stress such as pulmonary embolism, the normal right ventricle of an adult living at sea level can achieve systolic pulmonary pressures of 45 to 50 mm Hg, above which right ventricular failure supervenes. Systolic pressures exceeding these levels can be generated only by a hypertrophied right ventricle. If right ventricular infarction or ischemia has occurred or if the right and left ventricles are both affected by a myopathic process, right ventricular failure occurs at lower pulmonary artery pressure and severe elevations in pulmonary artery pressure may not develop, despite an increase in pulmonary vascular resistance.

In the presence of a normal right ventricle, an increase in left atrial pressure initially results in a fall in both pulmonary vascular resistance and the pressure gradient across the lungs. These reductions may reflect distention of a population of compliant small vessels, recruitment of additional vascular channels, or both. With further increases in left atrial pressure, pulmonary arterial pressure rises along with pulmonary venous pressure, so that at a constant pulmonary blood flow, the pressure gradient between the pulmonary artery and veins and pulmonary vascular resistance remains constant. When pulmonary venous pressure approaches or exceeds 25 mm Hg on a chronic basis, a disproportionate elevation in pulmonary artery pressure occurs, so that the pressure gradient between the pulmonary artery and veins rises while pulmonary blood flow remains constant or falls. This is indicative of an elevation in pulmonary vascular resistance that is caused, in part, by pulmonary vasoconstriction. Such patients may have some of the pathological features of IPAH (see later), and it may be this subgroup that benefits from therapy directed at pulmonary hypertension.

PULMONARY ARTERIAL VASOCONSTRICTION. Considerable variability in pulmonary arterial vasoconstriction

occurs in response to pulmonary venous hypertension. Marked reactive pulmonary hypertension with pulmonary artery systolic pressures in excess of 80 mm Hg occurs in somewhat less than one third of patients whose pulmonary venous pressures are elevated more than 25 mm Hg. The fact that severe reactive pulmonary hypertension develops in fewer than one third of patients with severe mitral stenosis suggests a broad spectrum of pulmonary vascular reactivity to chronic increases in pulmonary venous pressure. Although less well characterized, chronic elevation of pulmonary venous pressures as a result of other disorders, such as left ventricular diastolic dysfunction, also results in a disproportionate elevation in pulmonary artery pressures in a subset of patients.

The mechanisms involved in elevating pulmonary vascular resistance are unclear. In addition to hypertrophy of the media of the vasculature, a neural component may be present. An elevation in pulmonary venous pressure may also narrow or close airways, which may diminish ventilation and lead to hypoxia and vasoconstriction, and interstitial pulmonary edema secondary to pulmonary venous hypertension may encroach on the vascular lumen. Some patients may also have a genetic predisposition, allowing the chronically elevated pulmonary venous pressures to serve as a trigger for the development of structural changes similar to those found in IPAH.

Pathology

Structural changes in the pulmonary vascular bed develop in association with chronic pulmonary venous hypertension, irrespective of its origin. At the ultrastructural level, these changes include swelling of pulmonary capillary endothelial cells, thickening of their basal lamina, and wide separation of groups of connective tissue fibrils, indicative of interstitial edema. With persistence of the edema, reticular and elastic fibrils proliferate and the alveolar capillaries become embedded in dense connective tissue. The permeability of interendothelial junctions depends on pulmonary capillary pressure, with leakage of large molecules (40,000 to 60,000 Da) occurring at capillary pressures in excess of approximately 30 mm Hg.

Light microscopic examination of the lungs of patients with pulmonary venous hypertension shows distention of pulmonary capillaries, thickening and rupture of the basement membranes of endothelial cells, and transudation of erythrocytes through these ruptured membranes into the alveolar spaces, which contain fragments of disintegrating erythrocytes. Pulmonary hemosiderosis is commonly observed and may progress to extensive fibrosis. In the late stages of pulmonary venous hypertension, areas of hemorrhage may be scattered throughout the lungs, edema fluid and coagulum may collect in the alveolar spaces, and widespread organization and fibrosis of pulmonary alveoli may be present. Occasionally, particularly in patients with chronic pulmonary venous hypertension caused by mitral valve disease, the alveolar spaces become ossified. Pulmonary lymphatics may become markedly distended and give the appearance of lymphangiectasis, particularly when pulmonary venous pressure chronically exceeds 30 mm Hg. Structural alterations in the small pulmonary arteries, arterioles, and venules include medial hypertrophy, intimal fibrosis and, rarely, necrotizing arteritis.

Causative Factors

Pulmonary hypertension secondary to elevation of the pulmonary venous pressure occurs in left ventricular dysfunction (see Chaps. 25 and 26), mitral and aortic valve disease (see Chap. 62), cardiomyopathy (see Chaps. 64 and 65), cor triatriatum (see Chap. 61), and pericardial disease (see Chap. 70).

Pulmonary hypertension is a common and well-recognized complication of left ventricular systolic dysfunction. Right ventricular dysfunction and pulmonary hypertension are independent predictors of survival in patients with left ventricular systolic dysfunction.[62] Patients with a high pulmonary artery pressure on right heart catheterization and a low right ventricular ejection fraction have a sevenfold higher risk of death compared with heart failure patients with a normal pulmonary artery pressure and right ventricular ejection fraction. Treatment of pulmonary systolic venous hypertension as a result of left ventricular systolic dysfunction should include traditional therapy for the underlying disease. Both epoprostenol and endothelin receptor antagonists have been studied in these patients and have been demonstrated to increase mortality or have no benefit, respectively.

Pulmonary venous hypertension related to left ventricular diastolic dysfunction is less appreciated than that related to systolic dysfunction, and is more commonly mistaken for IPAH (see Chap. 26). The prevalence of pulmonary hypertension in patients with diastolic dysfunction is not well characterized. Patients tend to be older than IPAH patients and not infrequently have other conditions that may contribute to pulmonary hypertension, including obesity and obstructive sleep apnea. Historical factors that favor the diagnosis of pulmonary venous hypertension as opposed to IPAH include symptoms of paroxysmal nocturnal dyspnea and orthopnea and a history of systemic hypertension and diabetes. Atrial fibrillation is uncommon in IPAH and its presence should increase the suspicion for pulmonary venous hypertension. Absence of right axis deviation on the electrocardiogram is common in those with pulmonary venous hypertension. Left atrial enlargement on the echocardiogram also suggests pulmonary venous rather than PAH. Although echocardiographic techniques for the assessment of left ventricular diastolic function are advancing, right heart catheterization is required to document left heart filling pressures in those thought to have IPAH. If an ideal wedge pressure tracing cannot be obtained, a direct measurement of left ventricular end diastolic pressure with a pigtail catheter should be made. To make the diagnosis of PAH, the pulmonary capillary wedge pressure or left ventricular end-diastolic pressure must be 15 mm Hg. Left heart filling pressures higher than this establish the diagnosis of pulmonary venous hypertension. In certain cases, such as in a patient in whom the index of suspicion for diastolic dysfunction is high, a fluid challenge at the time of right heart catheterization may further clarify the diagnosis. The reduction in diastolic filling time that occurs with an increased heart rate during exercise may further increase left heart filling pressures and, as a result, pulmonary artery pressures.

Treatment

Treatment of left ventricular diastolic dysfunction is difficult and has been reviewed.[63] In patients with pulmonary venous hypertension caused by left ventricular diastolic dysfunction, we recommend aggressive blood pressure control, usually with a target blood pressure of less than 110/60 mm Hg, and optimal fluid management. Comorbid diseases such as obesity, diabetes, and obstructive sleep apnea must be addressed. ACE inhibitors and nitrates, over time, may allow for left ventricular remodeling. Atrial fibrillation is not well tolerated in such patients and every attempt should be made to maintain sinus rhythm. No trials of PAH-specific therapies have been performed to date in patients with pulmonary venous hypertension as a result of left ventricular diastolic dysfunction, and these drugs must be used with extreme caution in this population. PAH-specific

therapies may increase pulmonary blood flow to a noncompliant left ventricle and result in pulmonary edema.

Pulmonary hypertension as a result of mitral stenosis has been well characterized, and tends to resolve with time after effective treatment of the mitral stenosis (see Chap. 62). Pulmonary hypertension occurs occasionally in the setting of severe aortic stenosis, and portends a poor prognosis.[64] Although severe pulmonary hypertension was an independent predictor of perioperative mortality in this study, aortic valve replacement was associated with a reduction in pulmonary artery pressures and improvement in New York Heart Association functional class. The prognosis of those with pulmonary hypertension and severe aortic stenosis who did not undergo surgery was poor, with a 20 percent survival after a median of 436 days.

Pulmonary Arterial Hypertension Associated with Disorders of the Respiratory System

Diseases of the lung parenchyma are a common cause of pulmonary hypertension. The pathogenic mechanisms that can lead to pulmonary hypertension in this setting are shown in Table 73-7.

Chronic Obstructive Pulmonary Disease

Chronic obstructive pulmonary disease is the fourth leading cause of death in the United States, affecting more than 16 million people. The incidence, morbidity rate, and mortality rate of COPD vary widely among countries and are rising. The variation is possibly related to differences in exposure to risk factors, as well as to differences in individual susceptibility.

Chronic obstructive pulmonary disease is a heterogeneous group of diseases that share a common feature—the airways are narrowed, which results in an inability to exhale completely. Although there are numerous disorders that fall under the heading of COPD, the two largest components are emphysema and chronic bronchitis. Although

TABLE 73–7	Potential Pathogenic Mechanisms Leading to Pulmonary Arterial Hypertension and Cor Pulmonale	
Mechanisms	**Example(s)**
Primary	
Anatomical decrease in cross-sectional area (vessel destruction; encroachment on lumen by hypertrophy) of the pulmonary resistance vessels	Interstitial fibrosis and granuloma
Vasoconstriction of pulmonary resistance vessels	Hypoxia and acidosis
Contributory	
Large increments in pulmonary blood flow	Exercise
Increased pressures on the left side of the heart and pulmonary veins	Left ventricular failure or pulmonary venoocclusive disease
Increased viscosity of the blood	Secondary polycythemia or chronic hypoxia
Unproved	
Compression of pulmonary resistance vessels by raised alveolar pressures in their vicinity	Asthmatic bronchitis
Bronchial arterial-pulmonary arterial anastomoses	Expanded bronchial circulation

From Fishman AP: Pulmonary hypertension and cor pulmonale. *In* Fishman AP: Pulmonary Diseases and Disorders. 2nd ed. New York, McGraw-Hill, 1988, p 1001.

CH 73

clear-cut distinctions between these components can often be made, there is considerable overlap as to the dominant abnormality in the individual patient, in whom features of both may be manifest. Chronic bronchitis is a condition associated with excessive tracheal bronchial mucus production sufficient to cause cough with expectoration for at least 3 months of the year for more than 2 consecutive years. Emphysema is defined as the permanent abnormal distention of the air spaces distal to the terminal bronchi, with destruction of the alveolar septa. In lungs from patients with COPD studied postmortem, the major site of air flow obstruction has been shown to be in the small airways.

Definitions of COPD have been prepared by expert panels of the American Thoracic Society, the European Respiratory Society, the British Thoracic Society, and the Global Initiative for Chronic Obstructive Lung Disease (GOLD). Despite some subtle differences, all four expert panels made essentially the same key points:

1. Irreversible air flow obstruction is a cardinal feature of COPD.
2. Although limited reversibility of airflow obstruction in response to bronchodilator drugs is common, absence of such reversibility does not preclude bronchodilator treatment.
3. Neither asthma with complete reversibility nor chronic airflow obstruction caused by other diagnosable conditions such as cystic fibrosis, obliterative bronchiolitis, or panbronchiolitis is included in the definition of COPD.
4. Tobacco smoking is the major, but not the only, risk factor for COPD.
5. The cause of irreversible airflow obstruction in patients with COPD is the presence in the lungs of bronchiolitis or small airway disease and emphysema, which are present to a variable mix among patients.

Of all these definitions, the GOLD definition has gained widespread acceptance because of its simplicity and emphasis on spirometry as the standard for the diagnosis of airflow obstruction.

RISK FACTORS. Cigarette smoking is the most commonly identified correlate with COPD and accounts for 80 to 90 percent of the risk of developing COPD. It has been estimated that 15 percent of one pack/day smokers and 25 percent of two pack/day smokers develop COPD during their lifetime. Other potential environmental causes include air pollution, occupational exposures, and infection. It is likely that there are important interactions between environmental factors and a genetic predisposition to COPD. Individuals who are homozygous for alpha$_1$-antitrypsin deficiency develop severe emphysema in the third and fourth decades of life. Dusty occupational environments are well-established risks but probably not major factors in North America.

PATHOGENESIS. A chronic inflammatory process is involved in COPD that differs from that seen in asthma, with different inflammatory cells, mediators, inflammatory effects, and responses to treatment. Most inflammation in cases of COPD occurs in the peripheral airways (bronchioles) and lung parenchyma. The progression of COPD is strongly associated with an increase in the volume of tissue in the wall and with the accumulation of inflammatory mucous exudates in the lumen of the small airways.[65] There is increased destruction of lung parenchyma and an increased number of macrophages and T lymphocytes, which are predominantly CD8+ (cytotoxic) T cells.[65] Importantly, eosinophils are not as prominent as they are in asthma, except during an exacerbation. Other inflammatory mediators that are elevated in patients with COPD include leukotriene B$_4$, which is chemotactic for neutrophils, tumor necrosis factor-alpha (TNF-α), and interleukin-8. Macrophages also appear to play an important role, because the cells are 5 to 10 times more numerous, activated, and localized to the sites of damage, and have the capability to produce the pathological changes of COPD. Macrophages also appear to be activated by cigarette smoke and other irritants to release neutrophil-chemotactic factors, such as leukotriene B$_4$ and interleukin-8. Neutrophils and macrophages also release multiple proteinases that break down connective tissue in the lung parenchyma, resulting in emphysema, and stimulate mucus secretion (Fig. 73-11). In addition to inflammation, an imbalance of proteinases and antiproteinases in the lungs and oxidative stress are also important in the pathogenesis of COPD.[76]

SYSTEMIC EFFECTS OF COPD. These include increased circulating concentrations of interleukin-6 and of acute-phase proteins such as C-reactive protein. Weight loss in patients with COPD has been associated with increased circulating levels of TNF-α and soluble TNF

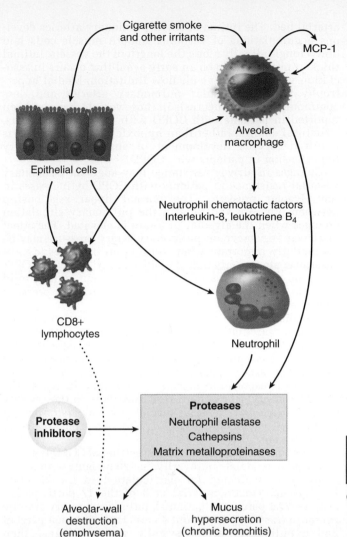

FIGURE 73–11 Inflammatory mechanisms in chronic obstructive pulmonary disease. Cigarette smoke and other irritants activate macrophages and airway epithelial cells in the respiratory tract, which release neutrophil chemotactic factors, including interleukin-8 and leukotriene B$_4$. Neutrophils and macrophages then release proteases that break down connective tissue in the lung parenchyma, resulting in emphysema, and also stimulate mucus hypersecretion. Proteases are normally counteracted by protease inhibitors, including alpha$_1$-antitrypsin, secretory leukoprotease inhibitor, and tissue inhibitors of matrix metalloproteinases. Cytotoxic T cells (CD8+ lymphocytes) may also be involved in the inflammatory cascade. MCP-1 denotes monocyte chemotactic protein 1, which is released by and affects macrophages. (*From Barnes PJ: Chronic obstructive pulmonary disease. N Engl J Med 343:269, 2000.*)

receptors and with increased release of TNF-α from circulating cells. The subsequent elevation of circulating levels of leptin may lead to weight loss and skeletal muscle wasting in COPD patients. The low-grade systemic inflammation present in patients with moderate to severe airflow obstruction is thought to play a role in the increased cardiovascular risk for COPD patients.[66]

PULMONARY HYPERTENSION IN COPD. Most commonly, pulmonary hypertension in COPD patients has multiple causative factors, including pulmonary vasoconstriction caused by alveolar hypoxia, acidemia, and hypercarbia, the compression of pulmonary vessels by the high lung volume, the loss of small vessels in the vascular bed in regions of the emphysema and lung destruction, and increased cardiac output and blood viscosity from polycythemia secondary to hypoxia (see Table 73-7). Of these, hypoxia is the most important factor and is associated with pathological changes that occur characteristically in the peripheral pulmonary arterial bed. The intima of small pulmonary arteries develops accumulations of vascular smooth muscle cells laid down longitudinally along the length of the vessels. Intimal thickening appears to be an early event that occurs in association with progressive air flow limitation. Medial hypertrophy in the muscular pulmonary arteries and, less commonly, fibrinoid necrosis in these vessels, has also been reported in patients with COPD with chronic PAH. Thus, structural change, rather than hypoxic vasoconstriction, is required for the development of sustained pulmonary hypertension in patients with COPD.

Changes in airway resistance may augment pulmonary vascular resistance in patients with COPD by increases in the alveolar pressure. The normal linear relationship between pressure and flow in the pulmonary circulation changes when the alveolar pressure is elevated. The effect of airway resistance on pulmonary artery pressure may be particularly important when ventilation increases (e.g., in cases of acute exacerbation of COPD). In patients with COPD, even the small increases in flow that occur during mild exercise may increase pulmonary artery pressure significantly.

Alveolar hypoxia is a potent arterial constrictor in the pulmonary circulation that reduces perfusion with respect to ventilation in an attempt to restore Pao_2. In patients with COPD, there is a positive correlation between the $Paco_2$ and pulmonary artery pressure. Polycythemia, which may develop in response to chronic hypoxemia, increases the blood viscosity, which may also contribute to the severity of PAH. Pulmonary arterial thrombosis may also occur in patients with COPD and may be a result of peripheral airway inflammation.

Pulmonary hypertension in the setting of COPD is generally mild to moderate in severity. In 120 patients with severe emphysema evaluated for participation in the National Emphysema Treatment Trial at 3 of the 17 participating centers (77.5 percent of patients), pulmonary artery systolic pressure was between 30 and 45 mm Hg.[67] Thirteen percent had a pulmonary artery systolic pressure higher than 45 mm Hg and the mean pulmonary artery pressure was higher than 35 mm Hg in only 5 percent of patients.

More recently, the cardiopulmonary hemodynamics of a retrospective series of 998 patients with COPD has been published.[68] Twenty-seven patients had severe pulmonary hypertension, defined as a mean pulmonary artery pressure higher than 40 mm Hg. Interestingly, 16 of these 27 had another possible cause of pulmonary hypertension, such as anorexigen exposure, connective tissue disease, thromboembolic disease, or left ventricular disease. In only 11 patients, or 1.1 percent, was COPD the only potential cause of the pulmonary hypertension. The median mean pulmonary artery pressure in these 11 patients was 48 mm Hg. They had an unusual pattern of cardiopulmonary abnormalities with mild to moderate airway obstruction, severe hypoxemia, hypocapnia, and a very low diffusing capacity for carbon monoxide. In a similar series, among 215 patients with severe COPD who underwent right heart catheterization to evaluate candidacy for lung transplantation or lung volume reduction surgery, pulmonary hypertension, defined as a mean pulmonary artery pressure higher than 25 mm Hg, was present in 50.2 percent of patients.[69] The pulmonary hypertension was characterized as moderate (mean pulmonary artery pressure, 35 to 45 mm Hg) in 9.8 percent and severe (mean pulmonary artery pressure, higher than 45 mm Hg) in 3.7 percent. A cluster analysis identified a subgroup of atypical patients characterized by moderate impairment of pulmonary mechanics with moderate to severe pulmonary hypertension and severe hypoxemia. These observations have suggested that a different biological mechanism results in changes in the pulmonary vascular bed in susceptible patients and that severe pulmonary hypertension occurs in the presence of lung disease, rather than as a result of the lung disease. For example, a genetic predisposition to pulmonary hypertension in COPD patients as a result of a 5-HTT polymorphism has been described, which may predispose to more severe pulmonary hypertension in hypoxemic patients with COPD.[70]

In the vast majority of COPD patients, pulmonary hypertension is mild, and treatment should be directed at the underlying COPD. Patients who present with severe pulmonary hypertension should be evaluated for another disease process responsible for the high pulmonary arterial pressures before it is attributed to the COPD. Specific treatment of pulmonary hypertension in the setting of COPD has not been adequately studied.

EVALUATION OF THE PATIENT WITH CHRONIC OBSTRUCTIVE PULMONARY DISEASE

The diagnosis of COPD should be considered in patients with chronic cough, sputum production, dyspnea, or history of exposure to risk factors for the disease. Key indicators for considering a diagnosis of COPD are listed in Table 73-8. Although an important part of patient care, the physical examination is relatively insensitive for diagnosing pulmonary hypertension and COPD. Clinical signs are often obscured by hyperinflation of the chest. Spirometry is the gold standard by which to diagnose and categorize COPD. Spirometry should measure the maximal volume of air forcibly exhaled from the point of maximal inhalation (forced vital capacity, FVC) and the volume of air exhaled during the first second of this maneuver (forced expiratory volume in 1 second, FEV_1). The ratio of these two components (FEV_1/FVC) should then be calculated. Patients with COPD typically show a decrease in both FEV_1 and FVC. An FEV_1/FVC ratio of less than 70 percent and a postbronchodilator FEV_1 of less than 80 percent of predicted confirms the presence of airflow limitation that is not fully reversible. However, even patients who do not demonstrate

CH 73

TABLE 73–8	Key Indicators for Considering a Diagnosis of Chronic Obstructive Pulmonary Disease (COPD)*
Stage	**Characteristics**
Chronic cough	Present intermittently or every day Often present throughout the day; seldom only nocturnal
Chronic sputum production	Any pattern of chronic sputum production may indicate COPD
Dyspnea that is	Progressive (worsens over time) Persistent (present every day) Described by the patients as "increased effort to breathe," "heaviness," "air hunger," or "gasping" Worse on exercise Worse during respiratory infections
History of exposure to risk factors, especially	Tobacco smoke Occupational dusts and chemicals Smoke from home cooking and heating fuels

*Consider COPD and perform spirometry if any of these indicators are present. These indicators are not diagnostic by themselves, but the presence of multiple key indicators increases the probability of a diagnosis of COPD. Spirometry is needed to establish a diagnosis of COPD.

Modified from Pauwels RA, Buist AS, Calverley PM, et al: Global strategy for the diagnosis, management, and prevention of chronic obstructive pulmonary disease. Am J Respir Crit Care Med 163:1256, 2001.

reversibility with a short-acting bronchodilator can benefit symptomatically from long-term bronchodilator treatment.

ECHOCARDIOGRAPHY. Although echocardiography is an invaluable tool in the evaluation of most forms of pulmonary hypertension, its usefulness is more limited in cases of COPD because hyperinflation of the lungs and marked respiratory variations in intrathoracic pressures often result in suboptimal images. In one study, Doppler echocardiography was used to estimate systolic pulmonary artery pressure in a cohort of 374 lung transplantation candidates.[9] Of these patients, 68 percent had obstructive lung disease, 28 percent had interstitial lung disease, and 4 percent had pulmonary vascular disease. The prevalence of pulmonary hypertension was 18 percent among the COPD population, 59 percent among those with interstitial lung disease, and 100 percent among those with pulmonary vascular disease. Estimation of the systolic pulmonary artery pressure was possible in only 44 percent of the patients. Although the correlation between systolic pulmonary artery pressure estimated by echocardiography and that measured at the time of cardiac catheterization was good, 52 percent of the pressure measurements were found to be inaccurate, defined as a more than 10-mm Hg difference compared with the measured pressure at the time of cardiac catheterization. Furthermore, 48 percent of patients were misclassified as having pulmonary hypertension by echocardiography. Sensitivity, specificity, and positive and negative predictive values of systolic pulmonary artery pressure estimation by echocardiography for the diagnosis of pulmonary hypertension were 85, 55, 52, and 87 percent, respectively. Although the right ventricle was adequately visualized in nearly all the patients, detection of right ventricular abnormalities did not enhance the poor positive predictive value of the Doppler echocardiogram. Given the inaccuracy of the echocardiogram in patients with pulmonary disease, an elevated estimated systolic pulmonary artery pressure obtained by echocardiography must be interpreted with caution, because approximately half of the time it will represent a false-positive finding.

PROGNOSIS AND PREDICTORS OF SURVIVAL

Chronic obstructive pulmonary disease is usually a progressive disease, and a patient's lung function can be expected to deteriorate over time, even with the best available care. Although pulmonary hypertension progresses slowly in patients with COPD, its presence confers a poor prognosis. Survival was significantly less in the COPD patients with severe pulmonary hypertension described by Chaouat and colleagues compared with COPD patients with or without mild to moderate pulmonary hypertension (Fig. 73-12).[68]

A study with a 10-year follow-up was conducted on a cohort of 870 patients with severe COPD. Among 609 patients with severe emphysema randomized to the medical therapy arm of the National Emphysema Treatment Trial, the following variables were predictive of survival in a multivariate analysis: increasing age, oxygen uptake, lower total lung capacity, higher residual volume, lower maximal cardiopulmonary exercise testing workload, greater proportion of emphysema in the lower lung zone versus the upper lung zone, lower upper–to–lower lung perfusion ratio, and modified BODE (*b*ody mass index, airflow *o*bstruction, *d*yspnea, *e*xercise capacity).[71] Once endotracheal intubation is necessary, the prognosis is usually poor and the survival after 1 year is usually lower than 40 percent. Pulmonary embolism is a common cause of death, with the frequency estimated to be approximately 11 percent. Among patients with COPD

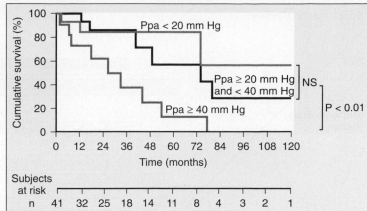

FIGURE 73–12 Survival of patients with chronic obstructive pulmonary disease (COPD) and no other detectable cause of pulmonary hypertension. The probability of survival of each group according to the pulmonary artery pressure (Ppa) was estimated using the Kaplan-Meier method and compared using the log-rank test. Eleven patients with a Ppa of 40 mm Hg or greater, 16 patients with Ppa of less than 40 mm Hg and 20 mm Hg or greater, and 14 patients with Ppa less than 20 mm Hg were at risk at baseline. NS = not significant. (*From Chaouat A, Bugnet AS, Kadaoui N, et al: Severe pulmonary hypertension and chronic obstructive pulmonary disease. Am J Respir Crit Care Med 172:192, 2005.*)

in the intensive care unit, pulmonary embolism was the most frequent cause of death, at 40.6 percent.

MANAGEMENT

The overall approach to the management of stable COPD should revolve around a stepwise increase in treatment, depending on the severity of the disease. Disease severity is determined by the severity of symptoms and air flow limitation as well as other factors, including the frequency and severity of exacerbations, complications, respiratory failure, and comorbid factors, including cardiovascular disease and sleep-related disorders, in addition to the general health status of the patient. Patient education is paramount to the effective treatment of COPD. Treatment of COPD has been well summarized in two reviews (Fig. 73-13).[72,73]

SMOKING CESSATION. The importance of smoking cessation cannot be overemphasized. The most comprehensive of the guidelines prepared on smoking cessation is "Treating Tobacco Use and Dependence," an evidence-based guideline sponsored by the U.S. Department of Health and Human Services. The guideline and the meta-analysis on which it is based are available on line.[74]

PULMONARY REHABILITATION. The goals of pulmonary rehabilitation in COPD patients are to reduce symptoms, improve quality of life, and increase physical and emotional participation in daily activities. Although a large study of 200 patients with disabling COPD demonstrated no difference in hospital admission among the patients randomized to receive rehabilitation versus the control patients, the rehabilitation group showed greater improvements in walking ability and general and disease-specific health status. Pulmonary rehabilitation should be considered for patients with COPD who have dyspnea or other respiratory symptoms, reduced exercise tolerance, a restriction in activities because of their disease, or impaired health status.[75]

PHARMACOLOGICAL TREATMENT. Pharmacological therapy is used to prevent and control symptoms, reduce the frequency and severity of exacerbations, improve health status, and improve exercise tolerance. Although none of these medications has been demonstrated to modify the long-term decline in lung function, this should not preclude the use of these therapies to control symptoms.

CH 73

Pulmonary Hypertension

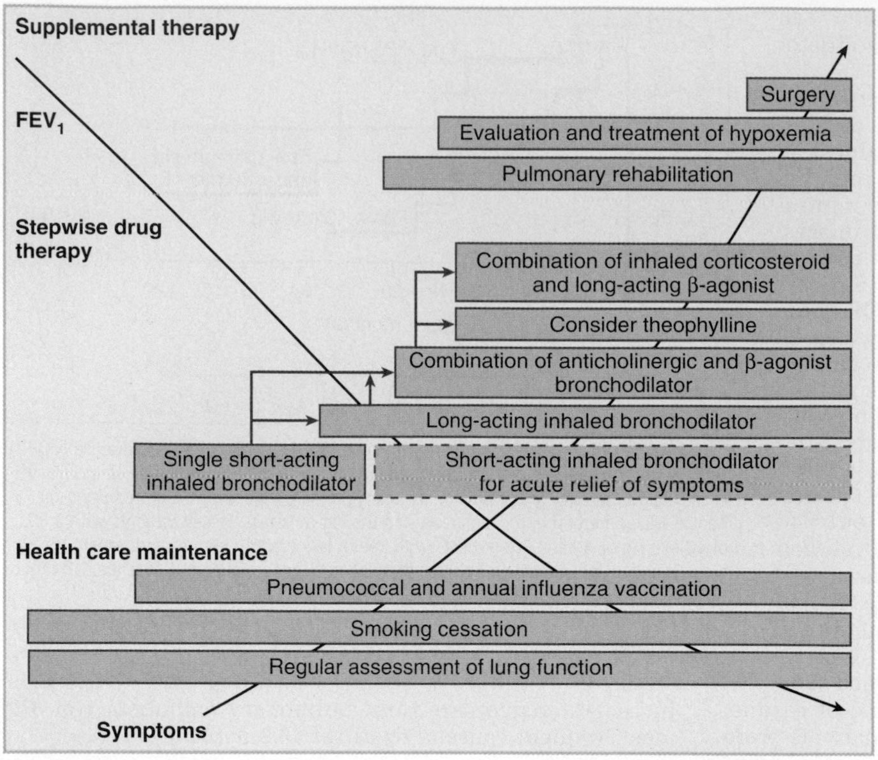

FIGURE 73–13 Algorithm for the treatment of chronic obstructive pulmonary disease. FEV_1 = forced expiratory volume in 1 second. (From Sutherland ER, Cherniack RM: Management of chronic obstructive pulmonary disease. N Engl J Med 350:2692, 2004.)

Bronchodilators and Corticosteroids. Bronchodilators are central to the management of COPD and can be used on an as-needed basis for relief of persistent or worsening symptoms or on a regular basis to help prevent and reduce symptoms. The choice of a beta$_2$ agonist, anticholinergic agent, theophylline, or combination therapy depends on the availability and individual response in terms of symptom relief and side effects. Glucocorticoids act at multiple points in the inflammatory cascade, although their effects in COPD are more modest as compared with bronchial asthma.

Other Pharmacological Treatments. The use of vasodilators has been disappointing in the treatment of COPD patients, even those with pulmonary hypertension. No agent other than oxygen has been shown convincingly to vasodilate the pulmonary circulation in patients with COPD. Because of the potential for worsening ventilation-perfusion mismatch, vasodilators may worsen hypoxemia. Evidence regarding the use of digoxin in COPD patients is insufficient to make recommendations, although short-term intravenous digoxin has improved cardiac output and reduced circulating norepinephrine levels in patients with right ventricular dysfunction caused by PPH. Influenza and pneumococcal vaccines are recommended for prophylaxis.

OXYGEN. Hypoxemia is a common finding in patients with advanced COPD and is easily corrected with low-flow supplemental O_2. In key clinical trials, long-term O_2 therapy clearly improved the survival of hypoxemic patients with COPD. The therapeutic goal is to maintain the Sao$_2$ higher than 90 percent during rest, sleep, and exertion.

NONINVASIVE VENTILATION. Noninvasive positive-pressure ventilation has been reported to improve gas exchange, sleep efficiency, quality of life, and functional status in patients with restrictive lung disease and chronic respiratory failure; however, its usefulness in patients with COPD is not as well established. Uncontrolled studies have demonstrated that noninvasive positive-pressure ventila-

tion used at home may improve oxygenation and reduce hospital admissions in patients with severe COPD and hypercapnia and improve long-term survival, although large controlled clinical trials are now needed. The combination of noninvasive positive-pressure ventilation and long-term O_2 therapy may be more effective but, again, large trials are needed before this approach can be recommended.

LUNG VOLUME REDUCTION SURGERY. Volume reduction surgery, which was originally described by Brantigan, has been advocated in selected patients with advanced emphysema. The surgical technique involves removing 20 to 30 percent of the volume of each lung by means of sternotomy, sequential thoracotomy, or thoracoscopy to reduce the severe hyperinflation commonly seen in patients with severe COPD. A randomized trial comparing the results of lung volume reduction surgery with medical therapy for severe emphysema has been reported.[76] A total of 1218 patients with severe emphysema who underwent pulmonary rehabilitation were randomly assigned to undergo lung volume reduction surgery or to receive continued medical therapy. An interim analysis determined that patients with a FEV$_1$ less than 20 percent of that predicted and either homogeneous distribution of emphysema on CT scan or carbon monoxide diffusing capacity that was 20 percent or less of that predicted were at high risk for death after lung volume reduction surgery, with a low probability of functional benefit. Such patients were subsequently excluded from entry into the trial. Overall, there was a death rate of 0.11/person-year in both treatment groups, although it was determined that certain subgroups might benefit. Among patients with predominantly upper lobe emphysema and low exercise capacity, the mortality rate was lower in the surgery group than in the medical therapy group. Among patients with non–upper lobe emphysema and high exercise capacity, the mortality rate was higher in the surgery group than in the medical therapy group.

Exercise Capacity. Despite the lack of survival advantage, exercise capacity improved by more than 10 W in 28, 22, and 15 percent of patients in the surgery group after 6, 12, and 24 months, respectively, as compared with 4, 5, and 3 percent of patients in the medical therapy group. Patients in the surgery group were also significantly more likely to have improvements in 6-minute walk distance, percentage of predicted value for FEV$_1$, general and health-related quality of life, and degree of dyspnea. Thus, patients with predominantly upper lobe emphysema and a low maximal workload have a lower mortality rate and a greater probability of improvement in exercise capacity with lung volume reduction surgery, and should be considered for the procedure. In contrast, patients with predominantly non–upper lobe emphysema and high maximal workload had a higher mortality rate and little functional improvement, regardless of treatment received. These symptomatic improvements after lung volume reduction surgery appear to wane with time, and long-term data from the large National Emphysema Treatment Trial may be enlightening. Lung volume reduction is a palliative procedure that does not halt, but only slows, the rate of functional decline for COPD. The disease will still progress, and symptoms will likely worsen.

LUNG TRANSPLANTATION. COPD is the most common indication for lung transplantation worldwide. Lung transplantation is a viable treatment option in patients with advanced pulmonary parenchymal or pulmonary vascular disease who have exhausted medical management. Both single-lung transplantation and bilateral lung transplantation result in significant improvement in postoperative lung function, exercise capacity, and quality of life. The choice of the procedure needs to be individualized. In general, single-lung transplantation is used for emphysema because of the scarcity of organ donors, lower perioperative morbidity and mortality rates, and comparable improvement in exercise capacity compared with bilateral lung transplantation. However, postoperative spirometry findings, single breath-diffusing capacity, and arterial oxygen tension are all significantly higher in bilateral lung transplantation compared with single-lung transplantation, which may benefit young patients with emphysema because the higher pulmonary reserve will offset any decline in lung function caused by infection or rejection. In most centers, bilateral lung transplantation is reserved for patients with suppurative lung disease or pulmonary vascular disease. The 1- and 5-year survival rates for single and bilateral lung transplantation for emphysema are approximately 80 and 40 percent, respectively.

Interstitial Lung Diseases

Interstitial lung diseases represent various conditions that involve the alveolar walls, perialveolar tissue, and other contiguous supporting structures. Pulmonary hypertension occurs in patients with interstitial lung diseases and is often associated with obliteration of the pulmonary vascular bed by lung destruction and fibrosis. The mechanism for pulmonary hypertension may be related to hypoxemia, a loss of effective pulmonary vasculature from lung destruction, and/or by indirectly triggering a pulmonary vasculopathy. Interstitial lung disease may be caused by environmental inhalant exposures, such as to asbestos, drugs, and chemotherapeutic agents, radiation, and recurring aspiration pneumonias. A large number of patients have interstitial lung disease of unknown origin, the most common being idiopathic pulmonary fibrosis and interstitial lung disease associated with connective tissue disease.

ADULT CYSTIC FIBROSIS. Cystic fibrosis is the most common lethal genetic disease in whites and occurs in approximately 1 of every 2000 live births. As the disease progresses, patients develop disabling lung disease and eventually respiratory failure, pulmonary hypertension, and cor pulmonale. The pathophysiology of pulmonary hypertension in cystic fibrosis is believed to be related to progressive destruction of the lung parenchyma and the pulmonary vasculature and to pulmonary vasoconstriction secondary to hypoxemia. The development of pulmonary hypertension in patients with cystic fibrosis carries a grave prognosis. The mean survival time from onset has been reported to be as short as 8 months. Typically, patients have severe hypoxemia, which may be a result of and a causative factor in the disease.

One study has evaluated patients with cystic fibrosis and pulmonary hypertension in depth.[110] Right ventricular hypertrophy appears to be a precursor of right ventricular failure and an indicator of the onset of pulmonary hypertension. The severity of the pulmonary hypertension appeared to correlate significantly with declining pulmonary function, as well as with the degree of oxygen desaturation with exercise. In this study, patients who developed pulmonary hypertension had a much worse prognosis (average survival, 15 months) compared with those without pulmonary hypertension (average survival, 33 months). Once lung function is severely limited (FEV$_1$ less than 40 percent of predicted), the prevalence of pulmonary hypertension may be as high as 40 percent. Because hypoxemia is universally found, supplemental oxygen is considered to be the mainstay of treatment in this group.

Sleep-Disordered Breathing and Pulmonary Hypertension (see Chap. 74)

Observational studies have demonstrated a wide variation in the incidence of pulmonary hypertension as a complication of sleep apnea, with a wide range of severity. The number affected was found to range from 17 to 52.6 percent, although these studies had variable entry criteria and some included patients with coexistent COPD.[77] The diagnosis of pulmonary hypertension in obstructive sleep apnea patients is also clouded by the coexistence of systemic hypertension,

obesity, and diastolic dysfunction. Successful treatment with continuous positive airway pressure improves pulmonary hemodynamics in patients with obstructive sleep apnea,[78] supporting the relationship between these two disease entities. Acute pulmonary hemodynamic changes during obstructive apneas have been well defined; however, the extent to which these translate into persistent daytime pulmonary hypertension remains less certain.

Alveolar Hypoventilation Disorders

Alveolar hypoventilation disorders are characterized by hypoxemia and mechanical disorders of the ventilatory system which, in concert, may cause pulmonary hypertension.

CHEST WALL DISORDERS. Thoracovertebral deformities that can result in restrictive pulmonary syndromes, chronic alveolar hypoventilation, and pulmonary hypertension include idiopathic kyphoscoliosis, spinal tuberculosis, congenital spinal developmental abnormalities, spinal cord injury and other childhood myelopathies, ankylosing spondylitis, or other congenital and acquired muscular skeletal conditions, such as pectus excavatum. Pulmonary hypertension frequently occurs in patients with thoracovertibular deformities. Pulmonary hypertension is related to the reduction of the vascular bed because of hypoventilation and hypoxia. Usually, symptoms are slowly progressive. Hypoxemia can be seen from ventilation-perfusion mismatch or underlying atelectasis. In patients with advanced disease, intermittent positive-pressure breathing and noninvasive ventilation have been used successfully, as well as supplemental oxygen in patients who are hypoxemic.

NEUROMUSCULAR DISEASE. The development of right-sided heart failure is an unusual manifestation of respiratory failure solely caused by respiratory muscle weakness. It usually develops in response to hypoxic and hypercapnic stimuli in patients with chronic forms of these disorders. Weakness of the respiratory muscles can be caused by generalized muscle disease, such as myopathic infiltrating diseases or muscular dystrophy (see Chap. 87) or, more commonly, by such neurological disorders as a cord lesion at or below the third cervical vertebra, amyotrophic lateral sclerosis, myasthenia gravis, poliomyelitis, and Guillain-Barré syndrome. The diagnosis of respiratory muscle weakness is confirmed by the finding of a restrictive ventilatory defect and a marked impairment of maximal respiratory pressures. Nocturnal ventilatory support, with positive or negative pressure, has become established as effective therapy in appropriate cases, and its beneficial effects are well recognized.

DIAPHRAGMATIC PARALYSIS. Bilateral diaphragmatic paralysis is an uncommon and rarely recognized cause of pulmonary hypertension. Diaphragmatic paralysis is a result of phrenic nerve injury, which can be traumatic or secondary to an underlying motor neuron disease. It may occur after cardiac surgery, as a manifestation of Lyme disease, after radiation therapy, or as a manifestation of other neurological disorders. When an affected patient is upright, ventilation may be normal or almost so, but when the patient is supine, gas exchange deteriorates. The diagnosis may be suspected in a patient with supine breathlessness, disturbed sleep pattern, paradoxical motion of the abdomen on inspiration, and low vital capacity in the upright position.

Patients with nontraumatic bilateral diaphragmatic paralysis may go unrecognized until they present with respiratory failure or pulmonary hypertension. The diagnosis can be suspected when the vital capacity is reduced by more than 40 percent of that predicted and paradoxical motion of the hemidiaphragms is noted by fluoroscopy. Patients can also have unilateral paralysis of the diaphragm, which is more common but is associated with fewer symptoms and physiological abnormalities. The treatment should always be directed toward correcting the underlying chronic neuromuscular disease, if present, and addressing nocturnal hypoventilation with noninvasive ventilatory techniques. Intermittent positive airway pressure is an effective therapy.

Pulmonary Hypertension Caused by Chronic Thrombotic or Embolic Obstruction of the Pulmonary Arteries (see Chap. 72)

Chronic thromboembolic pulmonary hypertension is an underdiagnosed disorder, and the true prevalence is still unclear. Pulmonary embolism, either as a single episode or as recurrent events, is thought to be the initiating process, followed by progressive vascular remodeling. However, more than half of patients with chronic thromboembolic pulmonary hypertension may not have a history of clinically overt pulmonary embolism.[79] Whereas the incidence was originally believed to be approximately 0.1 to 0.5 percent of patients who survive an acute pulmonary embolus, more recent data have suggested a higher incidence. In a prospective study of 223 patients who presented with an acute pulmonary embolism followed for a median of 94 months, the incidence of symptomatic chronic thromboembolic pulmonary hypertension was 3.1 percent at 1 year and 3.8 percent at 2 years.[80] Risk factors for the development of chronic thromboembolic pulmonary hypertension were previous episodes of acute pulmonary embolism, larger perfusion defects, and a younger age. The natural history of chronic thromboembolic pulmonary hypertension is poor and is related to the severity of the pulmonary hypertension.

Rather than having inherent fibrinolytic resolution of the thromboembolism with restoration of vascular patency, the thromboemboli in these patients fail to resolve adequately. They undergo organization and incomplete recanalization and become incorporated into the vascular wall. Commonly, they are in the subsegmental, segmental, and lobar vessels, although it is believed that chronic thromboembolism tends to propagate in a retrograde manner, leading to slowly progressive vascular obstruction. The development of a pulmonary hypertensive arteriopathy, similar to that seen in patients with other forms of pulmonary hypertension, has been documented in nonobstructive lung regions as well as in vessels distal to partially or completely occluded proximal pulmonary arteries. These small vessel changes therefore appear to be a significant contributor to the hemodynamic progression seen in many patients.

An identifiable hypercoagulable state is found in only a minority of patients. The lupus anticoagulant is present in 10 to 20 percent of patients with chronic thromboembolic pulmonary hypertension, whereas inherited deficiencies of protein C, protein S, and antithrombin III as a group can be identified in up to 5 percent of this population. Other risk factors for the development of chronic thromboembolic pulmonary hypertension have been identified, including chronic inflammatory disorders, myeloproliferative syndromes, the presence of a ventriculoatrial shunt, and splenectomy.[81]

Patient Evaluation

Chronic thromboembolic pulmonary hypertension involving the proximal pulmonary arteries is a well-characterized entity. The slowly progressive nature of the course of chronic thromboembolic pulmonary hypertension allows right ventricular hypertrophy to ensue, which compensates for the increased pulmonary vascular resistance. However, because of progressive thrombosis or vascular changes in the "uninvolved" vascular bed, the pulmonary hypertension becomes progressive and the patient manifests the clinical symptoms of dyspnea,

fatigue, hypoxemia, and right-sided heart failure. Patients may present with progressive dyspnea on exertion and/or signs of right heart failure after a single or recurrent episode of overt pulmonary embolism. Some patients experience a reprieve between the acute event and the clinical signs of chronic thromboembolic pulmonary hypertension, which may last from a few months to many years.

The findings on clinical examination of patients with chronic thromboembolic pulmonary hypertension are similar to those of other patients with pulmonary hypertension, with the exception of the following features. These patients tend to have lower cardiac outputs than patients with IPAH, which is often reflected in the reduced carotid arterial pulse volume. In addition, on occasion, bruits can be heard over areas of the lung that represent vessels with partial occlusions, but they must be carefully listened for. It is important to make the diagnostic distinction between patients with chronic thromboembolic pulmonary hypertension and those with other forms of pulmonary hypertension, because the treatments are so different. For the former group, a potentially curative therapy through thromboendarterectomy is available, whereas for the latter group effective pharmacological regimens are now evolving.

PERFUSION LUNG SCAN. The perfusion lung scan is usually adequate to identify patients with this disorder and is an important reason why lung scans are recommended for all patients who present with pulmonary hypertension (see Fig. 73-2). However, the lung scan typically underestimates the severity of the central pulmonary arterial obstruction. Therefore, patients who present with one or more mismatched segmental or larger defects should undergo pulmonary angiography. This continues to be the gold standard for defining the pulmonary vascular anatomy and is performed to determine whether chronic thromboembolic obstruction is present, to determine its location and surgical accessibility, and to rule out other diagnostic possibilities. Maturation and organization of clot results in vessel retraction and partial recanalization, resulting in several angiographic patterns suggestive of chronic thromboembolic disease—pouch defect, pulmonary webs or bands, intimal irregularities, abrupt narrowing of major pulmonary vessels, and obstruction of main, lobar, or segmental pulmonary arteries, frequently at their point of origin. Bronchial artery collaterals may be present. Because chronic thromboembolic pulmonary hypertension is usually bilateral, the presence of unilateral central pulmonary artery obstruction should prompt consideration of other diagnoses, such as pulmonary vascular tumors or extravascular compression from a lung carcinoma, hilar or mediastinal adenopathy, or mediastinal fibrosis. Pulmonary angiography can be performed safely in these patients if careful attention is given to the hemodynamic state. Nonionic contrast medium has been demonstrated to cause no major hemodynamic effects, even in patients with severe chronic thromboembolic pulmonary hypertension, and is preferred. Hypotension and/or bradycardia should be immediately treated with atropine.

COMPUTED TOMOGRAPHY (see Chap. 18). CT scanning can be a great aid in diagnosing chronic thromboembolic pulmonary hypertension (Fig. 73-14). Using high-resolution nonenhanced CT, areas of increased attenuation that do not obscure the vessels and that have a ground-glass appearance have been characterized as a mosaic pattern corresponding to hypoperfusion of the lung. Although this pattern is consistent with chronic thromboembolic pulmonary hypertension, it may also be seen in patients with cystic fibrosis, those with bronchiectasis, and lung transplant recipients, but it is virtually never seen in patients with IPAH. The contrast-enhanced CT features suggestive of chronic thromboembolic pulmonary hypertension include evidence of organized thrombus lining the pulmonary vessels in an eccentric or concentric fashion, enlargement of the right ventricle and central pulmonary arteries, variation in size of segmental arteries (relatively smaller in the affected segments compared with uninvolved segments), bronchial artery collaterals, and parenchymal changes to pulmonary infarcts. Marked variation in the size of the segmental vessels is more specific for chronic thromboembolic pulmonary hypertension and is believed to represent involvement of the segmental vessels caused by thromboemboli. It has been reported that these findings might also be mimicked in patients with fibrosing mediastinitis.

CARDIAC CATHETERIZATION. Patients with chronic thromboembolic pulmonary hypertension tend to have higher right atrial pressures and lower cardiac outputs than comparable patients with IPAH for the same level of pulmonary artery pressure. Because this is a disease that generally is progressive, the hemodynamic indications for surgical intervention are an elevation of pulmonary artery pressure and pulmonary vascular resistance for a period of more than 3 months, despite adequate anticoagulation.

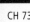

CH 73

cular resistance and perioperative mortality. It is also important to assess the comorbid conditions preoperatively. Although severe left ventricular dysfunction is the only absolute contraindication to pulmonary thromboendarterectomy, advanced age, severe right ventricular dysfunction, and other significant comorbid illnesses increase the perioperative morbidity and mortality risks. Right ventricular dysfunction is not considered a contraindication to surgery, because right ventricular function has been noted to improve once the obstruction of the pulmonary blood flow has been removed. It is a true endarterectomy, requiring establishment of a dissection plane at the level of the media. The procedure is performed on cardiopulmonary bypass and usually requires periods of complete circulatory arrest to allow for a bloodless field and define an adequate endarterectomy plane.

An operative classification of thromboembolic disease has been established and may be useful in terms of prognostication.[82] Among 202 patients who underwent pulmonary thromboendarterectomy, intraoperative classification of thromboembolism was defined as follows: type 1 (37.6 percent), thrombus in the main lobar pulmonary arteries; type 2 (40 percent), intimal thickening and fibrosis proximal to the segmental arteries; type 3 (18.8 percent), disease within distal segmental arteries only; and type 4 (3.4 percent), distal arteriolar vasculopathy without visible thromboembolic disease. Although all four patient groups were similar with respect to age, preoperative pulmonary artery pressures, and pulmonary vascular resistance, patients with proximal thromboembolic disease (groups 1 and 2) had a significantly greater improvement in pulmonary artery systolic pressure and pulmonary vascular resistance. There was also a greater increase in postoperative cardiac index and decrease in right ventricular systolic pressure in these patients as compared with those who had disease in the segmental or distal branches (groups 3 and 4). Although in previous series the operative mortality rate has been reported to be fairly high, the 1-month survival rates in patients who fell into groups 1 and 2 were 98.7 and 97.5 percent, respectively, whereas the 1-month survival rates in patients in groups 3 and 4 were 86.8 and 85.7 percent, respectively.

POSTOPERATIVE MANAGEMENT. Postoperative management can be extremely challenging. Patients in whom a large volume of central thrombus is removed, associated with backbleeding from the distal vascular segments and an immediate fall in the pulmonary artery pressure, usually have an extremely good postoperative course and long-term follow-up. Patients in whom small amounts of thrombus can be removed, in whom the thrombus becomes fragmented at the time of thromboendarterectomy, or in whom there is no distal backbleeding from the segment where the thrombus was removed usually have a difficult postoperative course. In addition, lack of a significant fall in pulmonary artery pressure and an increase in cardiac output portends a difficult postoperative recovery. These patients may need mechanical ventilation and inotropic support for days to weeks during periods of slow recovery. Much of their mortality risk appears to be related to severe right ventricular dysfunction, which actually initially worsens during the surgical procedure. Reperfusion injury, manifest by profound hypoxemia and pulmonary infiltrates corresponding to the segments where thrombus was removed, occurs in approximately 15 to 20 percent of patients and can be extensive. The only effective management of this complication is sustained assisted ventilation and oxygen supplementation. Attempts to reverse this with corticosteroids or other agents have not been successful. Other complications include atrial fibrillation, pneumonia, delirium, pneumothorax, pancreatitis, *Clostridium difficile* infection, colitis, and gastroin-

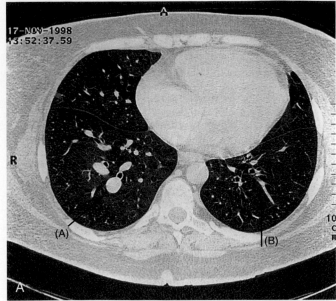

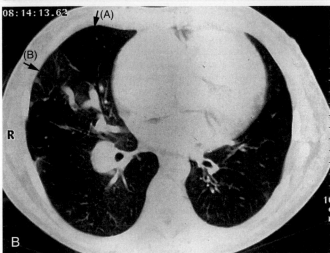

FIGURE 73–14 Chest computed tomography scans in a patient with chronic thromboembolic pulmonary hypertension. **A,** Helical scan with contrast medium enhancement of the pulmonary vasculature shows a marked disparity in vessel size between the involved vessels (A), which are enlarged from thrombus, and the uninvolved vessels (B). **B,** Non–contrast-enhanced high-resolution scan illustrates a marked mosaic pattern manifest by differences in density of regions of the lung parenchyma reflecting the perfused areas (B) and the nonperfused areas (A), also consistent with underlying thromboembolic disease.

Treatment

Pulmonary thromboendarterectomy is considered in patients who are symptomatic and have evidence of hemodynamic or ventilatory impairment at rest or with exercise. Operability is determined by the location and extent of proximal thromboemboli. Thrombi must involve the main, lobar, or proximal segmental arteries. It is important to evaluate whether the amount of surgically accessible thrombus is compatible with a degree of hemodynamic impairment. Failure to reduce the pulmonary vascular resistance with endarterectomy significantly, usually a result of the small vessel arteriopathy that may accompany this disease, is associated with a higher perioperative mortality rate and worse long-term outcome.

Patients undergoing surgery usually have a preoperative pulmonary vascular resistance more than 4 Wood units, and typically in the range of 10 to 12 Wood units. There is a close relationship between preoperative pulmonary vas-

testinal bleeding. Those survivors who have a good result, with a significant reduction in postoperative pulmonary vascular resistance at 48 hours, can expect to realize an improvement in functional class and exercise tolerance. Life-long anticoagulation with a goal INR ratio of 2.5 to 3.5 is indicated postoperatively.

Idiopathic Pulmonary Arterial Hypertension Versus Chronic Thromboembolic Pulmonary Hypertension

There are patients whose clinical presentation and evaluation findings are virtually identical to those of patients with IPAH but who on autopsy have widespread thrombotic lesions throughout their pulmonary vasculature. It is unclear whether they represent IPAH with an excessive tendency toward thrombosis or chronic thromboembolic pulmonary hypertension with persistent thromboemboli only at the arteriolar level. Often, the lung scan will show a perfusion pattern characterized by a diffuse mottled abnormality. Because of the poor outcomes after surgery of patients with very distal thromboembolic disease, medical management has been attempted. Small, open-label, uncontrolled trials have suggested a benefit of the oral prostacyclin analogue beraprost sodium, the phosphodiesterase inhibitor sildenafil, and the endothelin receptor antagonist bosentan in patients with nonoperable chronic thromboembolic pulmonary hypertension.[83-85]

Pulmonary Hypertension Caused by Disorders Directly Affecting the Pulmonary Vasculature

Schistosomiasis

Although schistosomiasis is extremely rare in North America, hundreds of millions of people are affected worldwide, particularly in developing countries. The development of pulmonary hypertension almost always occurs in the setting of hepatosplenic disease and portal hypertension. Clinical features appear when ova embolize to the lungs, where they induce formation of delayed hypersensitivity granulomas. In addition, deposition of fibrous tissue causes narrowing, thickening, and occlusion of the pulmonary arterioles. Histologically, focal changes related directly to the presence of schistosome ova may be located in the alveolar tissue or in the pulmonary arteries, and plexiform or angiomatoid lesions may be found. Fibrosis surrounds most focal lesions. The clinical symptoms and radiographic findings in these patients who develop pulmonary hypertension are not distinctive. In developing countries, this condition can be confused with primary pulmonary hypertension.

The diagnosis of schistosomiasis-induced pulmonary hypertension is confirmed by finding the parasite ova in the urine or stools of persons with symptoms. However, the insidious onset of pulmonary vascular disease years after infection makes finding these parasite ova difficult. Active infections are treated with praziquantel, which kills the adult worms and stops further destruction of tissue by ova deposition. Reversal of pathological lesions in the lungs after therapy has not been documented.

Sarcoidosis

Sarcoidosis is a multisystemic granulomatous disease of unknown origin characterized by an enhanced cellular immune response at the sites of involvement. Although any organ can be involved, sarcoidosis most commonly affects the lungs and intrathoracic lymph nodes. The clinical manifestation and natural history of sarcoidosis vary greatly, but the lung is involved in more than 90 percent of patients. The most common presenting symptoms are cough and shortness of breath, which is of a progressive nature. As the disease progresses in the lung parenchyma, extensive interstitial fibrosis is the result. In addition, obstructive airway disease, fibrocystic disease, bronchiectasis, endobronchial granulomas, and lobar atelectasis are common consequences of lung involvement.

Cardiac involvement from sarcoidosis appears to be more common than previously thought and may be present in up to one third of cases. Consequently, patients presenting with dyspnea should undergo a thorough cardiac evaluation for the possibility of cardiac involvement. Noncaseating granulomas may infiltrate the myocardium and leave fibrotic scars and, if enough of the myocardium is involved, patients will develop clinical features of a restrictive cardiomyopathy (see Chap. 64). Patients with cardiac involvement from sarcoidosis also present with varying degrees of heart block, arrhythmias, and/or clinical features of biventricular diastolic heart failure. Sudden death can be a common manifestation of cardiac sarcoid, and it is one of the most feared sequelae. The prognosis of patients with cardiac involvement from sarcoidosis is variable but can be poor. Usually, a trial of corticosteroids is given in the hope that it will alter the natural history of the disease.

The echocardiogram often demonstrates diffuse or regional wall motion abnormalities in patients with cardiac involvement. It is not uncommon, however, to find the features of pulmonary hypertension. Pulmonary hypertension detected by Doppler echocardiography techniques may be the result of restrictive cardiomyopathy from sarcoid and needs to be clearly distinguished from pulmonary hypertension caused by direct pulmonary vascular involvement, because the clinical management of these two conditions differs dramatically.

Pulmonary hypertension is most commonly the result of chronic severe fibrocystic sarcoidosis. Patients have chronic progressive dyspnea with effort, a chest radiograph demonstrating severe diffuse interstitial fibrotic lung disease, and pulmonary function test results that reflect severe restrictive physiology and hypoxemia. In these cases, the resulting pulmonary hypertension is usually mild to moderate and typical of patients presenting with restrictive lung disease of any cause.

MANAGEMENT. Management is generally focused on reversing any acute exacerbations of the lung disease and giving supplemental oxygen, when indicated. Some patients with sarcoidosis, however, have mild to moderate restrictive lung disease with severe pulmonary hypertension, presumed to be caused by granulomatous vasculitis of the pulmonary vessels. It is critically important in the cardiopulmonary evaluation of the patient presenting with underlying sarcoidosis and dyspnea to distinguish whether the symptoms are from chronic interstitial lung disease, restrictive cardiomyopathy, or pulmonary vascular disease. Although the traditional treatment of these patients has been unsatisfactory, it has been demonstrated that some patients have a very favorable response to intravenous epoprostenol therapy. Although interstitial lung involvement from sarcoidosis can result in mild pulmonary hypertension, a subset of patients present with severe pulmonary hypertension believed to be caused by direct pulmonary vascular involvement. It appears that, as with other secondary causes, these patients are predisposed to the development of pulmonary vascular disease triggered in some way by the sarcoid disease process. Although the use of intravenous epoprostenol chronically may reverse the right-sided heart failure and dramatically improve these patients' pulmonary hemodynamics, it will have no impact on any underlying fibrotic lung disease and/or hypoxemia, which still may render the patients symptomatic and dyspneic.

FUTURE PERSPECTIVES

It has become apparent that the clinical manifestation of pulmonary hypertension is a final common pathway of diverse abnormalities in the pulmonary circulation to a number of disease states. Animal models of pulmonary hypertension have illustrated how changes in specific molecular pathways can produce pulmonary hypertension, and how blocking these pathways can lead to reversal of advanced disease. Clinical experience has also shown that reversing what had once been considered end-stage pathological changes is possible. As the molecular pathways involved in pulmonary hypertension are becoming elucidated and understood, drugs that block these pathways will hold promise as future treatments. Therapies targeted to block specific tyrosine kinase pathways are clinically available and have great potential. Although the presence of redundant pathways and multiple abnormalities will make clinical progress more challenging, clinical trials using growth factor inhibitors are already in the planning stages.[86]

REFERENCES

1. Kasper M: Phenotypic characterization of pulmonary arteries in normal and diseased lung. Chest 128:547S, 2005.
2. Weir EK, Lopez-Barneo J, Buckler KJ, Archer SL: Acute oxygen-sensing mechanisms. N Engl J Med 353:2042, 2005.
3. Ichinose F, Roberts JD Jr, Zapol WM: Inhaled nitric oxide: A selective pulmonary vasodilator: Current uses and therapeutic potential. Circulation 109:3106, 2004.
4. Voelkel N: High-altitude pulmonary edema. N Engl J Med 346:1606, 2002.

Clinical Assessment of the Patient with Pulmonary Hypertension

5. McGoon M, Gutterman D, Steen V, et al: Screening, early detection, and diagnosis of pulmonary arterial hypertension: ACCP evidence-based clinical practice guidelines. Chest 126:14S, 2004.
6. Barst RJ, McGoon M, Torbicki A, et al: Diagnosis and differential assessment of pulmonary arterial hypertension. J Am Coll Cardiol 43:40S, 2004.
7. Chu JW, Kao PN, Faul JL, Doyle RL: High prevalence of autoimmune thyroid disease in pulmonary arterial hypertension. Chest 122:1668, 2002.
8. Raymond R, Hinderliter A, Willis P, et al: Echocardiographic predictors of adverse outcomes in primary pulmonary hypertension. J Am Coll Cardiol 39:1214, 2002.
9. Arcasoy SM, Christie JD, Ferrari VA, et al: Echocardiographic assessment of pulmonary hypertension in patients with advanced lung disease. Am J Respir Crit Care Med 167:735, 2003.
10. Enright PL, McBurnie MA, Bittner V, et al: The 6-minute walk test: A quick measure of functional status in elderly adults. Chest 123:387, 2003.
11. Oudiz RJ, Barst RJ, Hansen JE, et al: Cardiopulmonary exercise testing and six-minute walk correlations in pulmonary arterial hypertension. Am J Cardiol 97:123, 2006.
12. Sun X-G, Hansen J, Oudiz R, Wasserman K: Pulmonary function in primary pulmonary hypertension. J Am Coll Cardiol 41:1028, 2003.
13. Badesch DB, Abman SH, Ahearn GS, et al: Medical therapy for pulmonary arterial hypertension: ACCP evidence-based clinical practice guidelines. Chest 126:35S, 2004.
14. Hyduk A, Croft J, Ayala C, et al: Pulmonary hypertension surveillance—United States, 1980-2002. MMRWR Surveill Summ 54:1, 2005.

Idiopathic Pulmonary Arterial Hypertension

15. Pietra GG, Capron F, Stewart S, et al: Pathologic assessment of vasculopathies in pulmonary hypertension. J Am Coll Cardiol 43:25S, 2004.
16. Farber HW, Loscalzo J: Pulmonary arterial hypertension. N Engl J Med 351:1655, 2004.
17. Runo JR, Loyd JE: Primary pulmonary hypertension. Lancet 361:1533, 2003.
18. Humbert M, Morrell NW, Archer SL, et al: Cellular and molecular pathobiology of pulmonary arterial hypertension. J Am Coll Cardiol 43:13S, 2004.
19. Eddahibi S, Morrell N, d'Ortho MP, et al: Pathobiology of pulmonary arterial hypertension. Eur Respir J 20:1559, 2002.
20. Gorlach A, BelAiba RS, Hess J, Kietzmann T: Thrombin activates the p21-activated kinase in pulmonary artery smooth muscle cells. Role in tissue factor expression. Thromb Haemost 93:1168, 2005.
21. Budhiraja R, Tuder RM, Hassoun PM: Endothelial dysfunction in pulmonary hypertension. Circulation 109:159, 2004.
22. Benisty JI, McLaughlin VV, Landzberg MJ, et al: Elevated basic fibroblast growth factor levels in patients with pulmonary arterial hypertension. Chest 126:1255, 2004.
23. Mandegar M, Yuan JX-J: Role of K+ channels in pulmonary hypertension. Vasc Pharmacol 38:25, 2002.
24. Marcos E, Fadel E, Sanchez O, et al: Serotonin-induced smooth muscle hyperplasia in various forms of human pulmonary hypertension. Circ Res 94:1263, 2004.

25. Eddahibi S, Raffestin B, Hamon M, Adnot S: Is the serotonin transporter involved in the pathogenesis of pulmonary hypertension? J Lab Clin Med 139:194, 2002.
26. Nagaya N, Kyotani S, Uematsu M, et al: Effects of adrenomedullin inhalation on hemodynamics and exercise capacity in patients with idiopathic pulmonary arterial hypertension. Circulation 109:351, 2004.
27. Petkov V, Mosgoeller W, Ziesche R, et al: Vasoactive intestinal peptide as a new drug for treatment of primary pulmonary hypertension. J Clin Invest 111:1339, 2003.
28. Elliott CG, Glissmeyer EW, Havlena GT, et al: Relationship of BMRP2 mutations and vasoreactivity in pulmonary arterial hypertension. Circulation 113:2509, 2006.
29. Newman JH, Trembath RC, Morse JA, et al: Genetic basis of pulmonary arterial hypertension. J Am Coll Cardiol 43:33S, 2004.
30. Richter A, Yeager ME, Zaiman A, et al: Impaired transforming growth factor-beta signaling in idiopathic pulmonary arterial hypertension. Am J Respir Crit Care Med 170:1340, 2004.
31. Zhang S, Fantozzi I, Tigno DD, et al: Bone morphogenetic proteins induce apoptosis in human pulmonary vascular smooth muscle cells. Am J Physiol Lung Cell Mol Physiol 285:L740, 2003.
32. Teichert-Kuliszewska K, Kutryk MJ, Kuliszewski MA, et al: Bone morphogenetic protein receptor-2 signaling promotes pulmonary arterial endothelial cell survival: Implications for loss-of-function mutations in the pathogenesis of pulmonary hypertension. Circ Res 98:209, 2006.
33. Wong WK, Knowles JA, Morse JH: Bone morphogenetic protein receptor type II C-terminus interacts with c-Src: Implication for a role in pulmonary arterial hypertension. Am J Respir Cell Mol Biol 33:438, 2005.
34. Willers ED, Newman JH, Loyd JE, et al: Serotonin transporter polymorphisms in familial and idiopathic pulmonary arterial hypertension. Am J Respir Crit Care Med 173:798, 2006.
35. Machado RD, Koehler R, Glissmeyer E, et al: Genetic association of the serotonin transporter in pulmonary arterial hypertension. Am J Respir Crit Care Med 173:793, 2006.
36. Du L, Sullivan C, Chu D, et al: Signaling molecules in nonfamilial pulmonary hypertension. N Engl J Med 348:500, 2003.
37. McLaughlin VV, Presberg KW, Doyle RL, et al: Prognosis of pulmonary arterial hypertension: ACCP evidence-based clinical practice guidelines. Chest 126:78S, 2004.
38. Wensel R, Opitz C, Anker S, et al: Assessment of survival in patients with primary pulmonary hypertension. Circulation 106:319, 2002.
39. Humbert M, Sitbon O, Simonneau G: Treatment of pulmonary arterial hypertension. N Engl J Med 351:1425, 2004.
40. Galie N, Manes A, Branzi A: Emerging medical therapies for pulmonary arterial hypertension. Prog Cardiovasc Disease 45:213, 2002.
41. Sitbon O, Humbert M, Jais X, et al: Long-term response to calcium channel blockers in idiopathic pulmonary arterial hypertension. Circulation 111:3105, 2005.
42. Badesch DB, McLaughlin VV, Delcroix M, et al: Prostanoid therapy of pulmonary arterial hypertension. J Am Coll Cardiol 43:56S, 2004.
43. Sitbon O, Humbert M, Nunes H, et al: Long-term intravenous epoprostenol infusion in primary pulmonary hypertension. J Am Coll Cardiol 40:780, 2002.
44. McLaughlin V, Shillington A, Rich S: Survival in primary pulmonary hypertension. The impact of epoprostenol therapy. Circulation 106:1477, 2002.
45. Simonneau G, Barst RJ, Galie N, et al: Continuous subcutaneous infusion of treprostinil, a prostacyclin analogue, in patients with pulmonary arterial hypertension: A double-blind, randomized, placebo-controlled trial. Am J Respir Crit Care Med 165:800, 2002.
46. Tapson VF, Gomberg-Maitland M, McLaughlin VV, et al: Safety and efficacy of IV treprostinil for pulmonary arterial Hypertension: A prospective, multicenter, open-label, 12-week trial. Chest 129:683, 2006.
47. Olschewski H, Simonneau G, Galie N, et al: Inhaled iloprost for severe pulmonary hypertension. N Engl J Med 347:322, 2002.
48. Barst RJ, McGoon M, McLaughlin V, et al: Beraprost therapy for pulmonary arterial hypertension. J Am Coll Cardiol 41:2119, 2003.
49. Rich S, McLaughlin VV: Endothelin receptor blockers in cardiovascular disease. Circulation 108:2184, 2003,.
50. Channick RN, Sitbon O, Barst RJ, et al: Endothelin receptor antagonists in pulmonary arterial hypertension. J Am Coll Cardiol 43:62S, 2004.
51. Rubin L, Badesch D, Barst R, et al: Bosentan therapy for pulmonary arterial hypertension. N Engl J Med 346:896, 2002.
52. Wharton J, Strange JW, Moller GM, et al: Antiproliferative effects of phosphodiesterase type 5 inhibition in human pulmonary artery cells. Am J Respir Crit Care Med 172:105, 2005.
53. Galie N, Ghofrani HA, Torbicki A, et al: Sildenafil citrate therapy for pulmonary arterial hypertension. N Engl J Med 353:2148, 2005.
54. Kleptko W, Mayer E, Sandoval J, et al: Interventional and surgical modalities of treatment for pulmonary arterial hypertension. J Am Coll Cardiol 43:73S, 2004.
55. Doyle RL, McCrory D, Channick RN, et al: Surgical treatments/interventions for pulmonary arterial hypertension. Chest 126:63S, 2004.
56. Hertz M, Taylor D, Trulock E, et al: The registry of the international society for heart and lung transplantation: Nineteenth official report—2002. J Heart Lung Transplant 21:950, 2002.
57. Schachna L, Wigley FM, Chang B, et al: Age and risk of pulmonary arterial hypertension in scleroderma. Chest 124:2098, 2003.

Pulmonary Hypertension with Associated Conditions

58. Rich S, Shillington A, McLaughlin V: Comparison of survival in patients with pulmonary hypertension associated with fenfluramine to patients with primary pulmonary hypertension. Am J Cardiol 92:1366, 2003.
59. Gladwin MT, Sachdev V, Jison ML, et al: Pulmonary hypertension as a risk factor for death in patients with sickle cell disease. N Engl J Med 350:886, 2004.

CH 73

Pulmonary Hypertension

60. Runo J, Vnencak-Jones C, Prince M, et al: Pulmonary veno-occlusive disease caused by an inherited mutation in bone morphogenetic protein receptor II. Am J Respir Crit Care Med 167:889, 2003.

61. Almagro P, Julia J, Sanjaume M, et al: Pulmonary capillary hemagiomatosis associated with primary pulmonary hypertension. Medicine 81:417, 2002.

62. Ghio S, Gavazzi A, Capana C, et al: Independent and additive prognostic value of right ventricular function and pulmonary artery pressure in patients with chronic heart failure. J Am Coll Cardiol 37:183, 2005.

63. Aurigemma GP, Gaasch WH: Diastolic heart failure. N Engl J Med 351:1097, 2004.

64. Malouf JF, Enriquez Sarano M, Pellikka PA, et al: Severe pulmonary hypertension in patients with severe aortic valve stenosis: Clinical profile and prognositc implications. J Am Coll Cardiol 40:789, 2002.

65. Hogg JC, Chu F, Utokaparch S, et al: The nature of small-airway obstruction in chronic obstructive pulmonary disease. N Engl J Med 350:2645, 2004.

66. Sin DD, Man SF: Why are patients with chronic obstructive pulmonary disease at increased risk of cardiovascular diseases? The potential role of systemic inflammation in chronic obstructive pulmonary disease. Circulation 107:1514, 2003.

67. Scharf SM, Iqbal M, Keller C, et al: Hemodynamic characterization of patients with severe emphysema. Am J Respir Crit Care Med 166:314, 2002.

68. Chaouat A, Bugnet AS, Kadaoui N, et al: Severe pulmonary hypertension and chronic obstructive pulmonary disease. Am J Respir Crit Care Med 172:189, 2005.

69. Thabut G, Dauriat G, Stern JB, et al: Pulmonary hemodynamics in advanced COPD candidates for lung volume reduction surgery or lung transplantation. Chest 127:1531, 2005.

70. Eddahibi S, Chaouat A, Morrell N, et al: Polymorphism of the serotonin transporter gene and pulmonary hypertension in chronic obstructive pulmonary disease. Circulation 108:1839, 2003.

71. Martinez FJ, Foster G, Curtis JL, et al: Predictors of mortality in patients with emphysema and severe airflow obstruction. Am J Respir Crit Care Med 173:1326, 2006.

72. Sutherland ER, Cherniach RM: Management of chronic obstructive pulmonary disease. N Engl J Med 350:2689, 2004.

73. Celli BR, MacNee W; ATS/ERS Task Force: Standards for diagnosis and treatment of patients with COPD a summary of the ATS/ERS position paper. Eur Respir J 23:932, 2004.

74. U.S. Department of Health and Human Services, Office of the Surgeon General: Tobacco Cessation Guideline (http://www.surgeongeneral.gov/tobacco/default.htm), 2006.

75. Troosters T, Casaburi R, Gosselink R, et al: Pulmonary rehabilitation in chronic obstructive pulmonary disease. Am J Respir Crit Care Med 172:19, 2005.

76. National Emphysema Treatment Trial Research Group: A randomized trial comparing lung-volume-reduction surgery with medical therapy for severe emphysema. N Engl J Med 348:2059, 2003.

77. Atwood CW, McCrory D, Garcia JGN, et al: Pulmonary artery hypertension and sleep-disorder breathing: ACCP evidence-based clinical practice guidelines. Chest 126(Suppl):72S, 2004.

78. Sajkov D, Wang T, Saunders NA, et al: Continuous positive airway pressure treatment improves pulmonary hemodynamics in patients with obstructive sleep apnea. Am J Resp Crit Care Med 165:152, 2002.

79. Lang IM: Chronic thromboembolic pulmonary hypertension—not so rare after all. N Engl J Med 350:2236, 2004.

80. Pengo V, Lensing AWA, Prins MH, et al: Incidence of chronic thromboembolic pulmonary hypertension after pulmonary embolism. N Engl J Med 350:2257, 2004.

81. Boderman D, Jakowitsch J, Adlbrecht C, et al: Medical conditions increasing the risk of chronic thromboembolic pulmonary hypertension. Thromb Haemost 93:512, 2005.

82. Thistlethwaite PA, Mo M, Madani MM, et al: Operative classification of thromboembolic disease determines outcome after pulmonary endarterectomy. J Thorac Cardiovasc Surg 124:1203, 2002.

83. Ono F, Nagaya N, Okumura H, et al: Effect of orally active prostacyclin analogue on survival in patients with chronic thromboembolic pulmonary hypertension without major vessel obstruction. Chest 123:1583, 2003.

84. Ghofrani HA, Schermuly RT, Rose F, et al: Sildenafil for long-term treatment of nonoperable chronic thromboembolic pulmonary hypertension. Am J Respir Crit Care Med 167:1139, 2003.

85. Hoeper MM, Kramm T, Wilkens H, et al: Bosentan therapy for inoperable chronic thromboembolic pulmonary hypertension. Chest 128:2363, 2005.

86. Schermuly RT, Dony E, Ghofrani HA, et al: Reversal of experimental pulmonary hypertension by PDGF inhibition. J Clin Invest 115:2811, 2005.

CH 73

CHAPTER 74

Normal Sleep Physiology, 1915

Sleep Disorders, 1915
Obstructive Sleep Apnea, 1915
Central Sleep Apnea (Cheyne-Stokes Respirations), 1917

Screening and Diagnosis of Sleep Disorders, 1918
History and Examination, 1918
Screening Tools for Obstructive Sleep Apnea, 1919
Polysomnography, 1919

Sleep Apnea Therapy, 1919
Obstructive Sleep Apnea, 1919
Central Sleep Apnea, 1920

References, 1921

Sleep Apnea and Cardiovascular Disease

Apoor S. Gami and Virend K. Somers

NORMAL SLEEP PHYSIOLOGY

Sleep, which usually comprises up to one third of our lifetime, is a complex and dynamic physiological process.[1] Rapid eye movement (REM) sleep comprises about 25 percent of a night of sleep. It is a tonic state punctuated by periods of phasic activity, during which autonomic and cardiac functions are erratic. Thermoregulation is absent, sympathetic neural drive increases, heart rate increases and its variability decreases, and blood pressure increases. Non–rapid eye movement (NREM) sleep comprises about 75 percent of a night of sleep and is subdivided into four stages. During NREM sleep, in contrast to REM sleep, autonomic and cardiac regulation is stable. Sympathetic neural activity decreases and parasympathetic tone predominates, which decreases the arterial baroreceptor set point, heart rate, blood pressure, cardiac output, and systemic vascular resistance. Because of the predominance of parasympathetic neural tone, it is not unusual for healthy individuals to have sinus bradycardia, marked sinus arrhythmia, sinus pauses, or first-degree and type I second-degree atrioventricular block during sleep. Thus, the majority of sleep is quiescent in regard to cardiac function, with the exception being the dynamic changes of phasic REM sleep.

SLEEP DISORDERS

Various sleep disorders can interrupt normal sleep physiology. The two principal disorders with a recognized impact on cardiovascular function and disease are obstructive sleep apnea (OSA) and central sleep apnea (CSA).

Obstructive Sleep Apnea

Definition and Physiology

OSA is a sleep-related breathing disorder. Its principal feature is upper airway occlusion, which causes partial or complete cessation of airflow. This causes hypoxia and strenuous ventilatory efforts, followed by a transient arousal to a lighter stage of sleep and restoration of airway patency and airflow. The sequence of events can recur hundreds of times nightly. In symptomatic individuals, the condition is called the obstructive sleep apnea syndrome, or the obstructive sleep apnea–hypopnea syndrome.

An obstructive apnea is defined as the absence of air flow for at least 10 seconds in the presence of active ventilatory efforts, which are reflected by thoracoabdominal movements. An obstructive hypopnea is defined as a more than 50% decrease in thoracoabdominal movements for at least 10 seconds associated with a more than 4% decrease in oxygen saturation. The apnea-hypopnea index (AHI) is the average number of apneic and hypopneic events per hour of sleep, and it is the most common metric to describe the severity of OSA. OSA is present when the AHI is 5 or more and is considered severe when the AHI is 30 or more; however, these are essentially arbitrary thresholds created by expert consensus. In the context of cardiovascular disease and risk assessment, low AHI thresholds are reasonable because, as discussed later, clinically important cardiovascular outcomes are associated with an AHI as low as (and even lower than) 5.[2]

The mechanisms of OSA relate to the structure and function of the pharyngeal musculature and the state of the central nervous system during sleep.[3] The patency of the upper airway is determined by pharyngeal dilator and abductor muscle tone competing against negative transmural pharyngeal pressures during inspiration. The supine position makes airway collapse more likely because of the posterior displacement of the tongue, soft palate, and mandible. People with micrognathia, retrognathia, tonsillar hypertrophy, macroglossia,

and acromegaly are especially predisposed to OSA. Also, changes in central nervous system activity during sleep, particularly in REM sleep, decrease diaphragmatic activity (i.e., ventilatory drive) and pharyngeal muscle tone, which destabilizes the airway and favors airway collapse. Sedative-hypnotic medications or alcohol may compound these effects and increase the risk of obstructive apneas and hypopneas. Apneas terminate because of transient arousals to a lighter sleep stage, which are demonstrable with electroencephalographic recordings, but may not result in subjective awakening or awareness. Peripheral and central chemoreceptors, which are activated by the hypoxemia and hypercapnia of apnea, elicit postapneic hyperventilation, also contributing to electroencephalographic arousals.

Pathophysiological Mechanisms Linking Obstructive Sleep Apnea to Cardiovascular Disease

Individuals with OSA demonstrate an increased sensitivity of the peripheral chemoreceptors, which results in an increased ventilatory response to hypoxemia during sleep and wakefulness.[2] Activation of the chemoreceptors also stimulates sympathetic traffic to skeletal vasculature, which results in peripheral vasoconstriction. During apneas, as hypoxemia worsens, peripheral sympathetic activity markedly increases and blood pressure acutely rises.[2] Severe oxygen desaturations may be associated with ventricular ectopy. In some individuals, peripheral sympathetic over-activity may be accompanied by cardiac parasympathetic activity, which results in peripheral vasoconstriction and bradycardia (i.e., the homeostatic "diving reflex" that simultaneously decreases myocardial oxygen demand and increases cerebral and cardiac perfusion).[2] Even during daytime wakefulness, individuals with OSA have persistently heightened sympathetic activity, partly because of tonic chemoreflex activation.

These mechanisms may manifest clinically by the lack of the usual dip in nocturnal blood pressure, drug-resistant hypertension (see Chaps. 40 and 41), automatic tachycardias driven by sympathetic activity, and profound nocturnal bradycardias caused by cardiac vagal activity. Common nocturnal arrhythmias, such as marked sinus arrhythmia and second-degree atrioventricular block (Mobitz type I), are exacerbated, and higher degree conduction abnormalities, such as long sinus pauses and advanced atrioventricular block, may occur transiently (see Chaps. 32 and 35). The chronically elevated sympathetic activity results in increased resting heart rates, decreased heart rate variability, and increased blood pressure variability. In conjunction with structural heart disease or heart failure, this may have prognostic implications. The common occurrence of baroreflex dysfunction in patients with hypertension and heart failure may offset the protective effects of the baroreflex on chemoreflex-mediated sympathetic driven pressure surges.

The inspiratory efforts against a collapsed airway during an obstructive apnea generate marked negative intrathoracic pressures, which themselves cause acute cardiac structural and hemodynamic effects.[2,4] Whereas normal inspiratory pressures are about −8 cm H_2O, individuals with OSA can generate intrathoracic pressures of −30 cm H_2O or lower. This increases venous return to the right heart, produces ventricular interdependence, decreases left ventricular compliance and filling, and results in decreased cardiac output. Coupled with heightened peripheral sympathetic activity, these changes can directly increase cardiac afterload and detrimentally affect left ventricular systolic function. Acute diastolic dysfunction and increases in left atrial transmural pressure also occur, which may cause acute atrial or pulmonary vein stretch. This is evidenced by increases in atrial natriuretic peptide levels and the common symptom of nocturia in individuals with OSA. These changes, in association with oscillations in sympathetic and parasympathetic tone, may promote the initiation of atrial fibrillation during sleep.[5] The intrathoracic pressure fluctuations may cause chronic diastolic dysfunction and left atrial enlargement, associated with OSA independently of obesity and hypertension.

OSA also results in the production of important neurohumoral mediators of cardiac and vascular disease.[6] Individuals with OSA have increased production of the potent vasoconstrictor endothelin and impaired endothelial function, which affect vasomotion. OSA has also been associated with systemic inflammation, reflected by increases in C-reactive protein and serum amyloid A levels, which may advance atherosclerosis and is associated with increased cardiovascular risk. Perhaps through its effects on sympathetic activity or because of sleep deprivation, OSA may increase insulin resistance, which promotes cardiovascular risk via multiple pathways.[7] Lastly, OSA is associated with increased levels of leptin, a hormone secreted by fat cells that is also associated with cardiovascular events.[6]

Obstructive Sleep Apnea and Cardiovascular Disease Associations and Outcomes

The true prevalence of OSA in the population is unknown, because most people with OSA have not undergone polysomnography and remain undiagnosed. Population-based studies have estimated that 1 in 5 middle-aged Western adults with a body-mass index (BMI) of 25 to 28 kg/m² have OSA, and 1 in 20 are symptomatic, with the OSA syndrome.[8] OSA is strongly associated with obesity, and there is a direct relationship between BMI and the AHI index.[9] OSA is present in over 40 percent of those with a BMI of 30, and it is especially common in individuals with a BMI of 40. OSA is associated with multiple metabolic abnormalities, including abdominal obesity, diabetes, and dyslipidemia, and is highly prevalent in patients with the metabolic syndrome.[7] Given its putative roles in predisposing to and exacerbating insulin resistance, which is thought to be the underlying pathophysiology of the metabolic syndrome,

OSA could conceivably play a role in the development of the syndrome in some individuals.

OSA is highly prevalent in patients with cardiovascular disease (Table 74-1). It has been estimated to be present in up to half of patients with hypertension,[10] half of patients with acute stroke,[11] half of patients with atrial fibrillation requiring cardioversion,[12] one third of patients with lone atrial fibrillation,[13] one third of patients with coronary artery disease,[2] and one tenth to one third of patients with heart failure.[2] Many of these cardiovascular disease associations may occur because of the comorbidities of OSA—namely, obesity and its metabolic consequences—which together increase the risk of organic heart disease. However, large cohort observational studies have suggested that OSA itself may lead to incident cardiovascular disease. This was first demonstrated in a study of systemic hypertension,[10] in which it was demonstrated that in 709 normotensive people, the AHI correlated independently and directly with the development of hypertension over a period of 4 years. Even individuals with a "normal" AHI (0.1 to 4.9) had a 42 percent greater risk of incident hypertension compared with individuals with an AHI of 0.[10] OSA may also be a risk factor for new-onset atrial fibrillation. In 3542 people followed for an average of about 5 years after diagnostic polysomnography, nonelderly adults (younger than 65 years old) with OSA (AHI = 5) were more likely than those without OSA to have incident atrial fibrillation (Fig. 74-1). The severity of nocturnal oxygen desaturation was associated with the magnitude of this risk independently of other atrial fibrillation risk factors, including obesity, hypertension, and heart failure.[14] Reliable evidence also exists for the direct effects of OSA on left ventricular systolic function. Interventional studies of continuous positive airway pressure (CPAP), which can effectively abolish obstructive apneas and hypopneas (see later), have shown that it acutely and chronically increases the left ventricular ejection fraction by an average of about 8%.[15] OSA also may increase the risk of stroke, myocardial infarction, and death. In 1022 older adults followed for an average of about 3.5 years after diagnostic polysomnography, OSA (AHI = 5) was independently associated with a doubling of the risk of incident stroke or death.[16] In another 1651 men followed for an average of about 10 years, those with untreated severe OSA (AHI = 30) had a nearly threefold risk of death from stroke or myocardial infarction, and a more than threefold risk of coronary revascularization or nonfatal myocardial infarction or stroke, independently of important comorbidities, compared with healthy men (Fig. 74-2).[17] Finally, the unique nocturnal pathophysiology of OSA may be associated with an increased risk of nocturnal cardiac events. A retrospective study of 112 individuals who had undergone polysomnography and then had sudden cardiac death found that those with OSA had a peak in sudden cardiac death during the sleeping hours, which contrasted with the nadir of sudden cardiac death during this

TABLE 74–1	Estimated Prevalence of Obstructive Sleep Apnea in Patients with Cardiovascular Diseases
Cardiovascular Disease	**Prevalence (%)**
Hypertension	50
Coronary artery disease	33
Heart failure with systolic dysfunction	30-40
Acute stroke	50
Atrial fibrillation requiring cardioversion	50
Lone atrial fibrillation	33

period in those without OSA and in the general population (Fig. 74-3).[18] Currently, however, available evidence does not definitely implicate OSA as an independent cause of cardiovascular events. Figure 74-4 summarizes the pathophysiology of OSA, its possible intermediate cardiovascular disease mechanisms, and its cardiovascular disease associations and risks.

Central Sleep Apnea (Cheyne-Stokes Respirations)

Definition and Physiology

CSA refers to multiple forms of periodic breathing, in which ventilation waxes and wanes, gradually alternating between hyperpnea and apnea. CSA may occur in infants and in people traveling to high altitudes. CSA, in the form of Cheyne-Stokes respirations, is also associated with heart failure (see Chaps. 22 to 24).

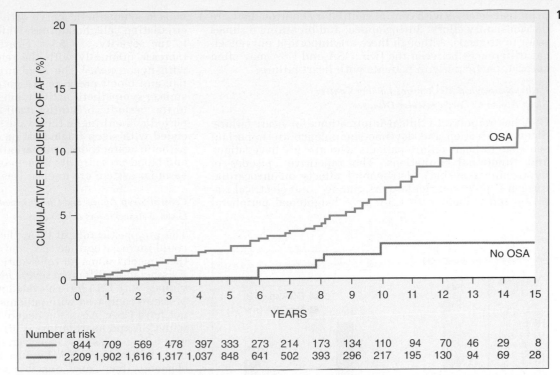

FIGURE 74-1 The cumulative frequency of new-onset atrial fibrillation in 3542 adults younger than 65 years old, followed for an average 4.6 years after diagnostic polysomnography. Individuals with OSA (obstructive sleep apnea) are shown with the blue line, and individuals without OSA are shown by the orange line. AF = atrial fibrillation. *(Modified from Gami AS, Hodge DO, Herges RM, et al: Obstructive sleep apnea, obesity, and the risk of incident atrial fibrillation. J Am Coll Cardiol 49:565, 2007.)*

CSA, like OSA, is considered a sleep-related breathing disorder, even though its characteristic ventilatory patterns may also present subtly during wakefulness. Its principal defect is an instability of ventilatory control, which results in oscillations in the arterial partial pressure of carbon dioxide ($PaCO_2$) above and below the apneic threshold, producing periodic hyperpnea and apnea.[19] Ventilation is controlled by feedback loops that integrate information from multiple sources (e.g., central and peripheral chemoreceptors, intrapulmonary receptors, ventilatory muscle afferents) to limit fluctuations in $PaCO_2$ and the arterial partial pressure of oxygen (PaO_2). Control of ventilation becomes uns when a phase delay exists between the inputs (chemosensors) and responses (ventilatory muscles) in these feedback loops, and also when the gain of these feedback loops is increased so that small inputs produce exaggerated responses.[19]

Patients with heart failure have ventilatory instability and CSA because of their heightened chemosensitivity to $PaCO_2$ (high loop gain) and long circulation time (phase delay). Increased chemosensitivity chronically decreases $PaCO_2$ closer to the apneic threshold. Also, stimulation of pulmonary irritant mechanoreceptors by increased left ventricular filling pressures and pulmonary edema causes hyperventilation beyond what is necessary to normalize the $PaCO_2$.[19] This hyperpnea leads to hypocapnia beyond the apneic threshold, and the central efferents to the ventilatory muscles become suppressed, resulting in apnea. In heart failure, this may be exacerbated by the prolonged lung to periphery circulation time, which is inversely proportional to cardiac output. During apnea, declining PaO_2 and rising $PaCO_2$ ultimately initiate breathing, which may or may not be followed by an arousal. Arousals directly lead to hyperpnea and promote the periodic breathing of CSA, because the same PCO_2 that was present during sleep is relatively hypercapnic for the awake state.

It is important to note the fundamental physiological differences between OSA and CSA. In OSA, the principal defect is with pharyngeal muscle structure and function, ventilatory efforts continue during apnea, and arousals lead to airway patency and resumed breathing. In CSA, the

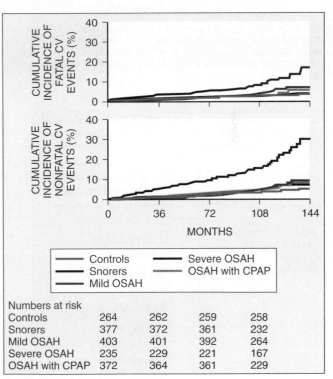

FIGURE 74-2 Cumulative frequency of fatal **(top)** and nonfatal **(bottom)** cardiovascular events in 1651 men followed for an average of 10.1 years. CPAP = continuous positive airway pressure; CVS = cardiovascular or stroke; OSAH = obstructive sleep apnea-hypopnea syndrome. *(Modified from Marin JM, Carrizo SJ, Vicente E, et al: Long-term cardiovascular outcomes in men with obstructive sleep apnoea-hypopnoea with or without treatment with continuous positive airway pressure: An observational study. Lancet 365:1046, 2005.)*

principal defect is with central ventilatory control, there are no ventilatory efforts during apnea, and breathing resumes prior to arousals. Although there are important physiological differences between the two, OSA and CSA may often coexist, particularly in patients with heart failure.

Pathophysiological Mechanisms Linking Central Sleep Apnea to Cardiovascular Disease

CSA has important clinical implications for heart failure. Sleep deprivation and daytime somnolence are important sequelae in heart failure patients who already have fatigue and functional limitations. The repetitive episodes of hypoxemia may have detrimental effects on myocardial oxygen supply, ventricular performance, and electrical stability. Individuals with CSA have heightened peripheral muscle sympathetic nerve activity and elevated levels of circulating catecholamines, which may be directly related to the severity of CSA.[20] Heart rate and blood pressure increase gradually with the rate of ventilation and peak with hyperpnea.[20] The mechanisms of the elevated heart rate and blood pressure are not directly related to hypoxemia or sympathetic activity, but instead are directly related to the periodic breathing itself and even manifest during periodic breathing in the awake state. Whereas CSA is associated with sleep fragmentation, cyclical hypoxemia, sympathetic overactivity, and periodicity of increased heart rate and blood pressure, its direct consequences for the cardiovascular system are unclear (see later).

Central Sleep Apnea and Cardiovascular Disease Associations and Outcomes

The prognostic role of CSA, the mechanisms by which it could increase cardiac risk, and the usefulness of targeting these mechanisms for intervention have been debated. CSA is associated with more severe forms of heart failure.[20] Individuals with CSA have elevated pulmonary capillary wedge pressure compared with patients with heart failure who do not have CSA. Also, the degree of hypocapnia in patients with CSA and heart failure is directly related to left ventricular filling pressures. However, not all patients with severe heart failure have CSA, because the key pathophysiological elements that cause unstable ventilatory control are not always present. The prevalence of CSA in patients with heart failure has been estimated at 30 to 40 percent.[21] Some small prospective studies assessing its prognostic value have shown that the risk of cardiac transplantation and death are directly related to the severity of CSA, represented by the central apnea-hypopnea index.[22] It is possible this is partly because of its associated increase in sympathetic activity, which is a known prognostic factor in heart failure. Also, patients with heart failure and CSA are more likely to have premature ventricular contractions, which may reflect ventricular electrical instability and a heightened risk of sudden cardiac death. However, large prospective systematic analyses of the relationship of CSA with significant heart failure outcomes or sudden cardiac death are lacking.[22]

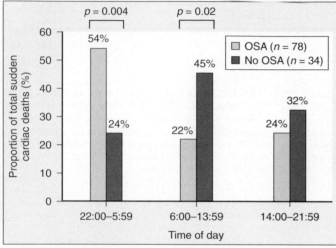

FIGURE 74–3 The day-night pattern of sudden cardiac death in individuals with and without polysomnogram-confirmed obstructive sleep apnea (OSA). *(Modified from Gami AS, Howard DE, Olson EJ, et al: Day-night pattern of sudden death in obstructive sleep apnea. N Engl J Med 352:1206, 2005. © 2005 Massachusetts Medical Society.)*

SCREENING AND DIAGNOSIS OF SLEEP DISORDERS

History and Examination

After snoring, which is ubiquitous in people with OSA, the most common symptom of OSA is excessive daytime sleepiness. The latter is defined as falling asleep during daytime activities, such as reading, conversing, eating, or driving. Another related but distinct symptom is tiredness on waking from sleep. An important symptom of OSA is witnessed nocturnal apnea, which is usually reported by the bed partner of the patient. Other symptoms may include nightly gasping or choking episodes, nighttime or morning headaches, morning dry mouth or sore throat, gastroesophageal acid reflux, and nocturia. Cognitive and memory difficulties, as well as psychological and behavioral changes, may be associated with severe OSA.[1]

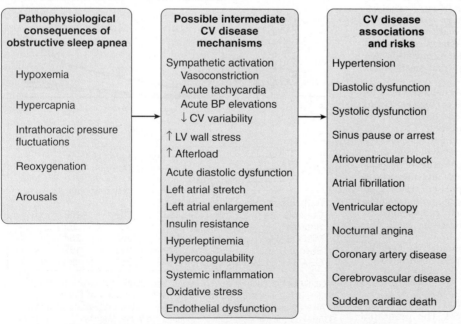

FIGURE 74–4 The pathophysiology of obstructive sleep apnea (OSA) may acutely and chronically elicit multiple intermediate cardiovascular disease mechanisms, which may promote the association of OSA with a number of cardiovascular conditions and diseases.

The physical examination in people with OSA may be normal, but it is usually notable for an overweight or obese body habitus. However, about 40 percent of obese people do not have OSA (and about 30 percent of people with OSA are not obese).[9] Increased neck circumference, particularly when more than 17 inches, is more specific than the body-mass index for predicting OSA. Certain cranial features, such as a low soft palate, narrow oropharynx, large uvula, micrognathia, and retrognathia, also predispose to OSA.[9]

Symptoms of CSA are not very specific, particularly in those with symptomatic heart failure. Snoring may not be present in individuals with CSA. Observations of the characteristic crescendo-decrescendo ventilatory pattern by a patient's bed partner may be helpful, but may be difficult for them to identify. The physical examination is not specific for CSA beyond the findings of heart failure, although CSA is more common in male or lean heart failure patients.

Screening Tools for Obstructive Sleep Apnea

Even an expert's subjective prediction of OSA based on a patient's history and physical alone has a diagnostic accuracy of only about 50 percent. Multiple prediction models have been developed by researchers to assess the likelihood of OSA. Most agree that age, body-mass index, neck circumference, hypertension, loud and habitual snoring, and witnessed apneas are the most sensitive and specific characteristics of OSA.[23] The Multiple Sleep Latency Test and the Maintenance of Wakefulness Test are both laboratory-based studies that require dedicated resources and time to quantify a patient's degree of somnolence objectively. The Epworth Sleepiness Scale is a simple questionnaire with a 24-point score that provides a standardized approach to determine and compare individuals' sense of sleepiness, which otherwise may be difficult to characterize precisely. The score seems to reasonably correlate with the severity of OSA. The Berlin Questionnaire is a risk stratification tool for OSA that incorporates body-mass index, history of hypertension, and multiple questions about daytime sleepiness, snoring frequency and severity, and falling asleep while driving. It has been validated in a primary care practice population, and later was shown to be accurate in a cardiology clinic population.[12] The predictive accuracy of any model is determined by the prevalence of OSA in the population in which it is applied. In patients with cardiovascular disease, in whom the prevalence of OSA is high, it is especially important to use variables with a high specificity for OSA, such as neck circumference and witnessed apneas. Overnight pulse oximetry has been used to screen for OSA; however, there are several limitations to its use and more research is necessary to identify its appropriate role.[24]

Polysomnography

Polysomnography is the current gold standard test for the diagnosis of sleep-disordered breathing, including OSA and CSA.[1] Traditionally, this is performed during a full night and, if indicated, is repeated on another night to apply and titrate continuous positive airway pressure (CPAP) therapy. Split-night studies, in which the diagnostic study occurs during the first half of the night and CPAP titration occurs during the second half of the night, are increasingly used as a more cost-effective diagnostic-therapeutic strategy. Polysomnography consists of continuous measurement during sleep of the electroencephalogram, oculogram, submental and tibial electromyogram, electrocardiogram, naso-

oral air flow, peripheral oxygen saturation, and excursions of the thoracic and abdominal walls. Together, these provide comprehensive information regarding sleep efficiency, sleep architecture, arousals and their causes, disordered breathing events, oscillations in oxygen saturation, and cardiac arrhythmias during specific sleep stages or events. Major limitations to obtaining polysomnography in the large population of patients with cardiovascular disease who probably have OSA or CSA are the cost (about $2000) and access to sleep centers. In fact, it has been estimated that over 60 percent of U.S. adults with OSA are undiagnosed. In response to this, the development and prospective evaluation of portable sleep monitoring devices have been instituted.[24] Ongoing discussions continue among expert organizations regarding the appropriate characteristics of the ideal screening and diagnostic modalities for sleep apnea.

SLEEP APNEA THERAPY

Obstructive Sleep Apnea

Positive Airway Pressure Therapy

Positive airway pressure (PAP) therapy effectively splints open the airway, preventing its collapse and resultant apneas. It is applied via naso-oral masks, nasal masks, or nasal pillows. The machine sits on a bedside table, and current models have a memory card to record time of use for assessing compliance. Continuous PAP is the principal therapy used. Autotitrating PAP machines and bilevel PAP machines are sometimes used for patients who do not tolerate standard continuous PAP.

A number of potential drawbacks of PAP therapy create obstacles to widespread acceptance by individual patients. These include claustrophobia, rhinitis or nasal congestion, nose bleeds, abrasions of the bridge of the nose, and air leaks because of poor fit of the device. Usually, these can be managed with conscientious attention to the patient's specific needs and regular follow-up. Noncompliant patients often are unaware of the alternative devices and adjunctive measures that recently have become available, and that may help mitigate these common side effects and complications.

Multiple cardiovascular benefits have been demonstrated with effective PAP therapy in individuals with OSA.[25] Nocturnal hypoxemia is relieved and sympathetic activity decreases, not only during sleep but also in daytime normoxic wakefulness. Similarly, PAP can promote significant decreases in blood pressure during sleep and daytime, particularly in patients with uncontrolled daytime hypertension. PAP therapy is effective in relieving symptoms in some OSA patients with nocturnal myocardial ischemia or angina. In patients with heart failure and OSA, PAP causes direct improvements in left ventricular systolic function and, over several months of therapy, leads to increased left ventricular ejection fraction and improved functional status.[15] Long-term observational studies have suggested that OSA patients who use PAP are at decreased risk of major adverse cardiovascular events, such as myocardial infarction, coronary revascularization, stroke, and death.[17] Large randomized controlled trials assessing the effects of PAP on long-term cardiovascular outcomes have not been reported and it is unknown whether PAP will reduce cardiovascular events or death.[25] Current indications for CPAP therapy in patients with OSA are listed in Table 74-2.

Other Therapies

Treatment of obesity via life style modification is effective in attenuating or curing OSA.[26] Pharmacological therapy for OSA is ineffective.[27] Mechanical devices other than PAP

TABLE 74–2	Indications for Continuous Positive Airway Pressure (CPAP) for Obstructive Sleep Apnea Treatment

Adults for whom surgery is a likely alternative to CPAP, with either
1. An apnea-hypopnea index ≥ 15

or

2. An apnea-hypopnea index ≥ 5 in a patient with symptoms (e.g., excessive daytime sleepiness, impaired cognition, mood disorders, insomnia), hypertension, ischemic heart disease, or history of stroke

Based on the Centers for Medicare and Medicaid Services, U.S. Department of Health and Human Services: Medicare Coverage Database, National Coverage, Continuous Positive Airway Pressure (CPAP) Therapy For Obstructive Sleep Apnea (OSA) (http://www.cms.hhs.gov/mcd).

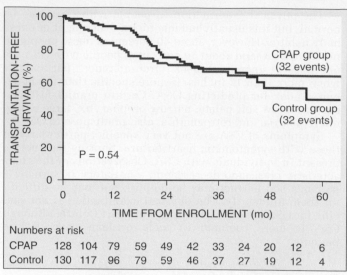

FIGURE 74–5 Survival free of cardiac transplantation in 258 patients with New York Heart Association Class II to IV heart failure symptoms and central sleep apnea, who were randomized to continuous positive airway pressure (CPAP) therapy or no CPAP and followed for an average of 2 years. *(Modified from Bradley TD, Logan AG, Kimoff RJ, et al: Continuous positive airway pressure for central sleep apnea and heart failure. N Engl J Med 353:2025, 2005. © 2005 Massachusetts Medical Society.)*

include oral appliances that maintain an anterior position of the tongue or the entire mandible.[28] These may be efficacious in patients with OSA that is mild or exclusive to the supine position. For patients with positional (supine) OSA, wearing a well-fitting shirt with a tennis ball sewn tightly to the midback should maintain a nonsupine sleep position, although there are insufficient data to prove its efficacy.

Surgical options exist for the treatment of OSA.[29] Bariatric surgery incidentally cures OSA in most morbidly obese patients; however, OSA returns if weight is regained. A number of surgeries that modify the oropharynx should be considered second-line therapies to weight loss and PAP. These are options for patients with specific craniofacial characteristics amenable to each specific approach. These include tonsillectomy, adenoidectomy, nasal septal surgery, uvulopalatopharyngoplasty, the Le Fort type 1 osteotomy, and mandibular-hyoid advancement. Tonsillectomy is more effective in children or thin adults. Tracheostomy, which was the first treatment ever effectively applied for OSA, is completely successful in abolishing obstructive apneas, but should be reserved for patients with the motivation and support to maintain the apparatus.

Central Sleep Apnea

Positive Airway Pressure Therapy

The rationale for using positive pressure ventilation in patients with CSA is based not on treating CSA per se, but rather on treating heart failure. The same hemodynamic benefits of continuous PAP therapy shown in OSA patients have been reported in patients with heart failure and CSA— namely, decreased sympathetic activity, decreased ventricular afterload, and increased left ventricular ejection fraction.[30] Concomitant with these changes, the severity of CSA decreases. In the largest controlled trial performed to clarify the potential benefits of continuous PAP in this population, 258 patients with New York Heart Association Class II to IV heart failure and CSA were randomized to effective therapy with continuous PAP or no therapy and followed for 2 years.[31] The trial was stopped early. Improvements occurred in a number of intermediate variables, such as the apnea-hypopnea index, circulating catecholamine concentrations, nocturnal oxygen saturations, left ventricular ejection fraction, and 6-minute walk distance. However, no survival benefit was observed (Fig. 74-5).

Adaptive pressure support servoventilation, another form of PAP, has been shown in short-term controlled trials to improve CSA, daytime somnolence, neurohormonal activity, and ventricular wall stress, as reflected by B-type natriuretic peptide concentrations; however, no changes in left ventricular systolic function were observed, and long-term outcome studies have not been reported.[22]

Other Therapies

Low-flow oxygen supplementation may abolish CSA in some patients.[22] Two randomized placebo-controlled trials in heart failure patients have shown that nocturnal administration of low-flow oxygen by nasal cannula immediately improved the apnea-hypopnea index, oxygen saturations, and sleep architecture and that 1 week of nocturnal oxygen supplementation improves functional capacity. A controlled study of 24 patients with heart failure has shown that implantation of a biventricular permanent pacemaker improves indices of CSA (both the apnea-hypopnea index and minimum nocturnal oxygen saturation) and sleep quality after about 4 months.[32]

Small studies have shown improvements in CSA with the administration of theophylline; however, there are no large long-term studies assessing the safety of theophylline, a methylxanthine, in heart failure patients.[22] Another experimental intervention successful in directly abolishing CSA is the inhalation of a gas mixture that has a carbon dioxide tension as little as 1 to 3 mm Hg higher than ambient air. This resets the resting hypocapnic state of heart failure further from the apneic threshold.[22] The safety of delivering CO_2-enriched air to heart failure patients has not been assessed, and this is not applied clinically.

It remains unknown whether it is beneficial to abolish CSA in heart failure patients. Whether CSA is a marker of the severity of the underlying heart disease rather than a mediator of risk and whether it is a worthwhile target for intervention to improve cardiovascular prognosis remain to be determined. Generally, therapies that improve heart failure (e.g., angiotensin-converting enzyme inhibitors, biventricular pacing) also improve CSA. Pending further studies, treatment directed specifically at CSA, such as oxygen or CPAP, should probably be reserved for patients with severe daytime somnolence or symptoms attributable to nocturnal hypoxemia (angina or significant arrhythmias). Otherwise, optimization of heart failure management should remain the principal goal.

REFERENCES

Obstructive Sleep Apnea

1. Kryger MH, Roth T, Dement WC (eds): Principles and Practice of Sleep Medicine. 4th ed. Philadelphia, Elsevier/Saunders, 2005.
2. Shamsuzzaman AS, Gersh BJ, Somers VK: Obstructive sleep apnea: Implications for cardiac and vascular disease. JAMA 290:1906, 2003.
3. Ryan CM, Bradley TD: Pathogenesis of obstructive sleep apnea. J Appl Physiol 99:2440, 2005.
4. Shivalkar B, Van de Heyning C, Kerremans M, et al: Obstructive sleep apnea syndrome: More insights on structural and functional cardiac alterations, and the effects of treatment with continuous positive airway pressure. J Am Coll Cardiol 47:1433, 2006.
5. Gami AS, Friedman PA, Chung MK, et al: Therapy insight: Interactions between atrial fibrillation and obstructive sleep apnea. Nat Clin Pract Cardiovasc Med 2:145, 2005.
6. Wolk R, Gami AS, Garcia-Touchard A, Somers VK: Sleep and cardiovascular disease. Curr Probl Cardiol 30:625, 2005.
7. Svatikova A, Wolk R, Gami AS, et al: Interactions between obstructive sleep apnea and the metabolic syndrome. Curr Diab Rep 5:53, 2005.
8. Young T, Peppard PE, Gottlieb DJ: Epidemiology of obstructive sleep apnea: A population health perspective. Am J Respir Crit Care Med 165:1217, 2002.
9. Gami AS, Caples SM, Somers VK: Obesity and obstructive sleep apnea. Endocrinol Metab Clin North Am 32:869, 2003.
10. Narkiewicz K, Wolf J, Lopez-Jimenez F, Somers VK: Obstructive sleep apnea and hypertension. Curr Cardiol Rep 7:435, 2005.
11. Brown DL: Sleep disorders and stroke. Semin Neurol 26:117, 2006.
12. Gami AS, Pressman G, Caples SM, et al: Association of atrial fibrillation and obstructive sleep apnea. Circulation 110:364, 2004.
13. Porthan KM, Melin JH, Kupila JT, et al: Prevalence of sleep apnea syndrome in lone atrial fibrillation: A case-control study. Chest 125:879, 2004.
14. Gami AS, Hodge DO, Herges RM, et al: Obstructive sleep apnea, obesity, and the risk of incident atrial fibrillation. J Am Coll Cardiol 49:565, 2007.
15. Kaneko Y, Floras JS, Usui K, et al: Cardiovascular effects of continuous positive airway pressure in patients with heart failure and obstructive sleep apnea. N Engl J Med 348:1233, 2003.
16. Yaggi HK, Concato J, Kernan WN, et al: Obstructive sleep apnea as a risk factor for stroke and death. N Engl J Med 353:2034, 2005.
17. Marin JM, Carrizo SJ, Vicente E, Agusti AG: Long-term cardiovascular outcomes in men with obstructive sleep apnoea-hypopnoea with or without treatment with continuous positive airway pressure: An observational study. Lancet 365:1046, 2005.
18. Gami AS, Howard DE, Olson EJ, Somers VK: Day-night pattern of sudden death in obstructive sleep apnea. N Engl J Med 352:1206, 2005.

Central Sleep Apnea

19. White DP: Pathogenesis of obstructive and central sleep apnea. Am J Respir Crit Care Med 172:1363, 2005.
20. Lanfranchi PA, Somers VK: Sleep-disordered breathing in heart failure: Characteristics and implications. Respir Physiol Neurobiol 136:153, 2003.
21. Oldenburg O, Lamp B, Faber L, et al: Sleep-disordered breathing in patients with symptomatic heart failure. A contemporary study of prevalence in and characteristics of 700 patients. Eur J Heart Fail 2006 Oct 5 (Epub ahead of print).
22. Pepin JL, Chouri-Pontarollo N, Tamisier R, Levy P: Cheyne-Stokes respiration with central sleep apnoea in chronic heart failure: Proposals for a diagnostic and therapeutic strategy. Sleep Med Rev 10:33, 2006.

Screening and Diagnosis of Sleep Disorders

23. Young T, Shahar E, Nieto FJ, et al: Predictors of sleep-disordered breathing in community-dwelling adults: The Sleep Heart Health Study. Arch Intern Med 162:893, 2002.
24. Littner MR: Portable monitoring in the diagnosis of the obstructive sleep apnea syndrome. Semin Respir Crit Care Med 26:56, 2005.

Sleep Apnea Therapy

25. Giles TL, Lasserson TJ, Smith BJ, et al: Continuous positive airways pressure for obstructive sleep apnoea in adults. Cochrane Database Syst Rev (1):CD001106, 2006.
26. Veasey SC, Guilleminault C, Strohl KP, et al: Medical therapy for obstructive sleep apnea: A review by the Medical Therapy for Obstructive Sleep Apnea Task Force of the Standards of Practice Committee of the American Academy of Sleep Medicine. Sleep 29:1036, 2006.
27. Smith I, Lasserson TJ, Wright J: Drug therapy for obstructive sleep apnoea in adults. Cochrane Database Syst Rev (2):CD003002, 2006.
28. Ng A, Gotsopoulos H, Darendeliler AM, Cistulli PA: Oral appliance therapy for obstructive sleep apnea. Treat Respir Med 4:409, 2005.
29. Sundaram S, Bridgman SA, Lim J, Lasserson TJ: Surgery for obstructive sleep apnoea. Cochrane Database Syst Rev (2):CD001004, 2005.
30. Javaheri S: Central sleep apnea in congestive heart failure: Prevalence, mechanisms, impact, and therapeutic options. Semin Respir Crit Care Med 26:44, 2005.
31. Bradley TD, Logan AG, Kimoff RJ, et al: Continuous positive airway pressure for central sleep apnea and heart failure. N Engl J Med 353:2025, 2005.
32. Sinha AM, Skobel EC, Breithardt OA, et al: Cardiac resynchronization therapy improves central sleep apnea and Cheyne-Stokes respiration in patients with chronic heart failure. J Am Coll Cardiol 44:68, 2004.

CH 74

Sleep Apnea and Cardiovascular Disease

PART IX

Cardiovascular Disease in Special Populations

CHAPTER 75

Demographics/Epidemiology, 1923

Pathophysiology, 1924

Medication Therapy, 1926
Chronic Medication
  Administration, 1926

Vascular Disease, 1931
Hypertension, 1931
Coronary Artery Disease, 1934
Carotid Artery Disease/Stroke, 1940
Peripheral Artery Disease, 1942

Heart Failure, 1943

Arrhythmias, 1946
Sinus Node Dysfunction, 1946
Atrioventricular Conduction
  Disease, 1946
Atrial Arrhythmias, 1946
Ventricular Arrhythmias, 1947

Valvular Disease, 1947
Aortic Valve Disease, 1947
Aortic Regurgitation, 1949
Mitral Annular Calcification, 1949
Mitral Stenosis, 1949
Mitral Regurgitation, 1949

Future Directions, 1949

References, 1949

Cardiovascular Disease in the Elderly

Janice B. Schwartz and Douglas P. Zipes

DEMOGRAPHICS/EPIDEMIOLOGY[1]

The proportion of people aged 65 years and older in the United States is projected to increase from 12.4 percent (35 million) of the population in 2000 to 19.6 percent in 2030 (71 million) and 82 million in 2050. The number of people older than 80 years of age is projected to double from 9.3 million in 2000 to 19.5 million in 2030 and more than triple by 2050. Women represented 59 percent of persons older than 65 years of age in 2000 and are estimated to comprise 56 percent of the older population in 2030 (Fig. 75-1). If current projections hold, increases in the percentage of racial minorities will occur. From 2000 to 2030, the proportion of persons older than 65 years of age who are members of racial minority groups (e.g., African American, American Indian-Alaska Native, Asian-Pacific Islander) is expected to increase from 11.3 to 16.5 percent, and the proportion of Hispanics is expected to increase from 5.6 to 10.9 percent. Almost half of people older than 65 years of age in the United States in 2000 had after-tax incomes at the poverty level (41 percent of 65- to 74-year-olds and 56 percent of those older than 75 years of age), and this trend is likely to continue.[2] Global trends are similar, with the worldwide population older than 65 years of age projected to increase to 973 million or 12 percent in 2030 and make up about 20 percent of the population in 2050. Increases will be greatest in undeveloped nations. Estimates are for twice as many women as men older than 80 years and three times as many women as men older than 90 years.

Cardiovascular disease is the most frequent diagnosis in elderly people and is the leading cause of death in both men and women older than 65 years of age. Hypertension occurs in one half to two thirds of people older than 65 years of age, and heart failure (HF) is the most frequent hospital discharge diagnosis among older Americans. The profile of these common cardiovascular diseases differs in older patients from that in younger patients. Systolic, but not diastolic, blood pressure increases with aging, resulting in increased pulse pressure. Systolic hypertension becomes a stronger predictor of cardiovascular events, especially in women. Heart failure with preserved systolic function becomes more common at older ages and is more common in women. Coronary artery disease (CAD) is more likely to involve multiple vessels and left main artery disease and is equally likely in women as in men older than 65 years of age. Equal numbers of older men and women present with acute myocardial infarction (MI) until age 80, after which more women present. More than 80 percent of all deaths attributable to cardiovascular disease occur in people older than 65 years with approximately 60 percent of deaths in patients older than 75 years.

Importantly, cardiovascular disease in older people is not seen in isolation. Eighty percent of older Americans have at least one chronic medical condition, and half have at least two. Arthritis affects about 60 percent of persons older than 65 years, and diabetes affects about 20 percent (Fig. 75-2). Ear, nose, and throat problems, vision disorders, and orthopedic problems are also common. As U.S. adults live longer, the prevalence and incidence of dementia that impairs memory, decision-making capability, orientation to physical surroundings, and language also increase. The prevalence of Alzheimer's disease is estimated at 10 percent in community-dwelling Caucasians older than 65 years and higher in African-American and Hispanic populations. By age 80, approximately 40 percent of people may be affected.[3] One third of Medicare beneficiaries with Alzheimer's disease have CAD, one quarter have had a stroke, and 22 percent have diabetes.[4]

The high morbidity and mortality from cardiovascular disease in the elderly warrant aggressive approaches to prevention and treatment that have been shown to be effective in older patients. Compelling data demonstrate reduced morbidity and mortality rates for the treatment of hypertension, heart failure, atrial fibrillation, acute coronary syndromes, CAD, stroke, diabetes, and lipid abnormalities in older patients 60 to 74 years of age, although

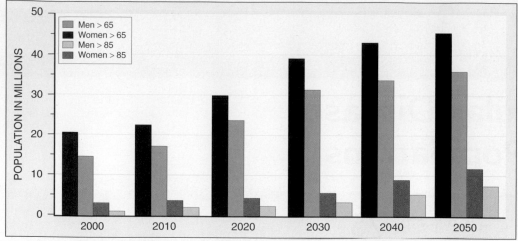

FIGURE 75–1 U.S. population estimates projected from 2000 until 2050. Dark pink bars represent numbers of women older than 65 years. Dark blue bars represent men older than 65 years. Light pink bars represent numbers of women older than 85 years. Light blue bars represent numbers of men older than 85 years in millions of people. (*From the U.S. Census Bureau.*)

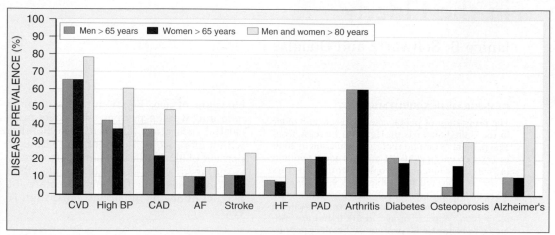

FIGURE 75–2 Prevalence of cardiovascular and other common chronic medical illnesses in older persons in the United States. Data are percentages. Blue bars represent data for men older than 65 years, pink bars represent women older than 65 years, and yellow bars represent men and women older than 80 years. AF = atrial fibrillation; CAD = coronary artery disease; CVD = cardiovascular disease; HF = heart failure; BP = hypertension (all forms); PAD = peripheral artery disease.

data on minorities and women are limited. Few trials of cardiovascular therapies have enrolled significant numbers of men or women older than 75 years of age, elderly patients with multisystem disease, or elderly patients with cognitive impairment, and none have addressed cardiovascular therapies in the nursing home population. When clinical trials enroll older patients, participants may differ markedly from the majority of older patients. The projected increase in numbers of older people from previously understudied and undertreated groups presents both medical and economic challenges for cardiovascular disease treatment.

PATHOPHYSIOLOGY

Neither a universal definition of "elderly" nor an accurate biomarker for aging exists. Although physiological changes associated with aging do not appear at a specific age and do not proceed at the same pace in all individuals, most definitions of elderly are based on chronological age. The World Health Organization uses 60 years of age to define "elderly," whereas most U.S. classifications use the age of 65 years. Gerontologists subclassify older age groups into *young old* (60-74 years), *old old* (75-85 years), and *very old* (older than 85 years of age). Clinicians often separate older patients into two subgroups—those 65 to 80 years of age and those older than 80 years of age—to highlight the frailty, reduced capacity (physical and mental), and presence of multiple disorders that are more common after 80 years of age.

Hallmarks of cardiovascular aging in humans[5-7] include progressive increases in systolic blood pressure, pulse pressure (Fig. 75-3), pulse wave velocity, left ventricular (LV) mass, and increased incidence of CAD and atrial fibrillation. Reproducible age-related decreases are seen in rates of early LV diastolic filling, maximal heart rates (Fig. 75-4), maximal cardiac output (see Fig. 75-4), maximum aerobic capacity or maximal oxygen consumption (VO_{2max}), exercise-induced augmentation of ejection fraction, reflex responses of heart rate, heart rate variability, and vasodilation in response to beta-adrenergic stimuli or endothelial-mediated vasodilator compounds (Fig. 75-5).

Cellular, enzymatic, and molecular alterations in the arterial vessel wall include migration of activated vascular smooth muscle cells into the intima, with increased matrix production caused by altered activity of matrix metalloproteinases, angiotensin II, transforming growth factor-beta, intercellular cell adhesion molecules, and production of collagen and collagen cross-linking. Loss of elastic fibers, increases in fibronectin, and calcification also occur. These processes lead to arterial dilatation and increased intimal thickness resulting in increased vascular stiffness. Increased arterial stiffness is manifested by increases in pulse-wave velocity away from the heart and increased and earlier pulse wave reflections back toward the heart (often estimated as the aortic augmentation index). In both animal and human models of aging, endothelial cell production of nitric oxide (NO) decreases with age, endothelial cell mass decreases and is associated with increased cell senescence and apoptosis and increased NO consumption caused by age-dependent increases in vascular superoxide anion production. These changes contribute to reduced endothelial cell NO-mediated vasodilatory responses of the peripheral and coronary vasculature. Vascular responses to beta-adrenergic agonists and alpha-adrenergic blockade are also reduced with aging. In contrast, responses to non–endothelial-derived compounds such as nitrates or nitroprusside are preserved with aging but may vary by vascular bed or be altered by diseases such as hypertension or diabetes.

Changes in the extracellular matrix of the myocardium parallel those in the vasculature with increased collagen, increased fibril diameter and collagen cross-linking, an increase in the ratio of type I to type III collagen, decreased elastin content, and increased fibronectin. A shift in the balance between matrix metalloproteinases and tissue inhibitors of matrix metalloproteinases that favors increased production of extracellular matrix may also occur. Fibroblast proliferation is induced by growth factors, in particular angiotensin-transforming growth factors, tumor necrosis factor-alpha, and platelet-derived growth factor. These changes are accompanied by cell loss and altered cellular function.[8,9] In the atria, decreased sinus node cells and extracellular matrix changes contribute to sinus node dysfunction and atrial fibrillation. Collagen, elastic tissue, and calcification changes in or near the central fibrous body and the atrioventricular (AV) node or proximal

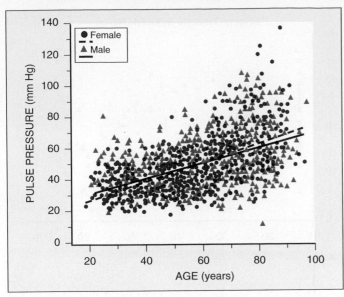

FIGURE 75–3 Pulse pressure (systolic minus diastolic pressure) with aging in apparently healthy subjects enrolled in the Baltimore Longitudinal Study of Aging. *(Reprinted from Pearson JD, Morrell CH, Brant LJ, et al: J Gerontol Med Sci 53: M177-M183, 1997).*

bundle branches contribute to conduction abnormalities and annular valvular calcification. In the ventricle, collagen deposition and extracellular matrix changes contribute to loss of cells, hypertrophy of myocytes with changes in myosin subforms, and altered myocardial calcium handling.[10] Changes in myocardial calcium handling include reduced or delayed inactivation of L-type transmembrane calcium current, decreased and delayed intracellular ionized calcium uptake by cardiac myocyte sarcoplasmic reticulum (in part caused by reduced calcium adenosine triphosphatase [SERCA2] activity), and reduced and delayed outwardly directed potassium rectifier current activation. The result is prolongation of the membrane action potential and inward calcium current with prolongation of both contraction and relaxation.[8,10,11]

Age-related changes are also seen in the intravascular environment. Increases in fibrinogen, coagulation factors V, VIII, IX, and XIIa, and von Willebrand factor are seen without countering increases in anticoagulant factors. Platelet phospholipid content is altered and platelet activity is increased with increased binding of platelet-derived growth factor to the arterial wall in older individuals compared with younger individuals. Increased levels of plasminogen activator inhibitor (PAI-1) are seen with aging, especially during stress, resulting in impaired fibrinolysis. Circulating prothrombotic inflammatory cytokines, especially interleukin-6, also increase with age and may play a role in the pathogenesis of acute coronary syndromes. Adipose cells associated with obesity are also sources of PAI-1 and inflammatory cytokines. All these changes also potentiate development of atherosclerosis.[8,12,13]

Consistent changes in the autonomic nervous system accompany aging and influence cardiovascular function. For the beta-adrenergic system, age-related changes include decreased receptor numbers, altered G protein coupling, and altered G protein–mediated signal transduction. Age-related decreases in alpha-adrenergic platelet receptors and decreased alpha-adrenergic–mediated arterial vasoreactivity of forearm blood vessels occur, whereas alpha-adrenergic–mediated changes in human hand veins appear to be preserved. Dopaminergic receptor content and dopaminergic transporters decrease, and cardiac contractile responses to dopaminergic stimulation may be blunted with aging. Decreased sensitivity and responses to parasympathetic stimulation are seen in cardiac and vascular tissues, whereas increased central nervous system (CNS) effects are frequently seen in aging models.[5,6,8,14-17] The combined age-related autonomic changes lead to decreased baroreflex function and responses to physiological stressors with increased sensitivity to parasympathetic stimulation of the CNS.

Several unifying hypotheses for age-related changes throughout the body have been proposed and include cumulative oxidative damage, inflammatory responses to cellular stress or infection, and programmed cell death. Some of the age-related cardiovascular changes can be partially, if not totally, reversed. Exercise improves endothelial function, measures of arterial stiffness, and baroreceptor function in older

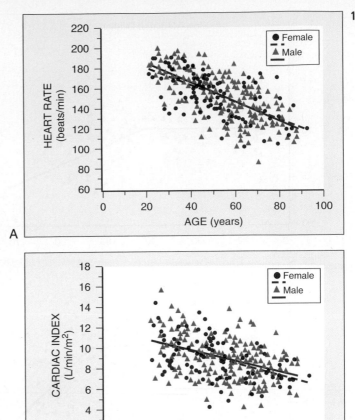

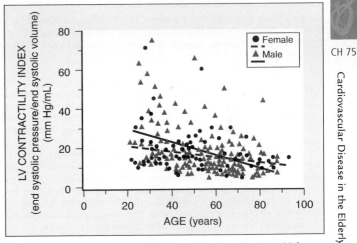

FIGURE 75–4 Maximum exercise heart rate **(A)**, cardiac index **(B)**, and left ventricular (LV) contractility index **(C)** in men and women in the Baltimore Longitudinal Study of Aging who had been prescreened to exclude clinical and occult cardiovascular disease. *(Reprinted from Fleg JL, O'Connor FC, Gerstenblith G, et al: Impact of age on the cardiovascular response to dynamic upright exercise in healthy men and women. J Appl Physiol 78:890-900, 1995.)*

people. Caloric restriction slows aging and age-related cardiac changes, as well as increasing maximal lifespan in several small animal models. In humans, caloric restriction decreases weight, blood pressure, and risk factors for atherosclerosis and has improved indices of diastolic function in cross-sectional studies.[18-21] Pharmacological approaches with antiinflammatory and antioxidant vitamin administration or omega-3 free fatty acids for either primary or secondary prevention have not been successful in humans, although dietary antioxidant intake has been associated with slowing of age-related changes in the vasculature and medications such as angiotensin-converting enzyme

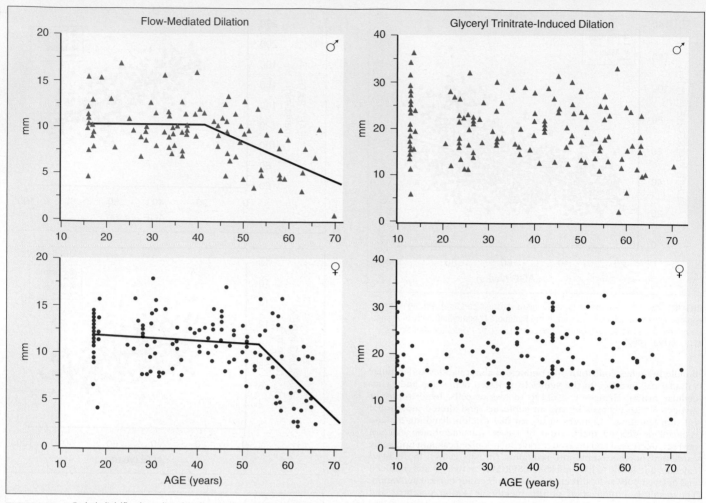

FIGURE 75-5 Endothelial (flow)-mediated and nonendothelial (glyceryl trinitrate)-induced arterial dilation in apparently healthy men and women. Age-associated declines are seen in flow-mediated dilation but not in glyceryl trinitrate–induced dilation. Age-related changes occur earlier in men compared with women. *(Reprinted from Celermajer DS, Sorensen KE, Spiegelhalter DJ, et al: J Am Coll Cardiol 24:471-476, 1994.)*

(ACE) inhibitors, aldosterone antagonists, or beta blockers may influence the vascular and cardiac remodeling associated with hypertension, atherosclerosis, or heart failure.[22-29] Agents that directly target advanced glycation endproducts, collagen cross-linking, and inflammation are being evaluated.[30]

Age-related changes create a cardiovascular system faced with increased pulsatile load and one that is less able to increase output in response to stress. Age-related changes also limit maximal capacity and decrease reserve capacity, contributing to lower thresholds for symptoms in the presence of cardiovascular diseases that become more common with increasing age. Table 75-1 summarizes age-related cardiovascular changes contrasted with cardiovascular disease.

MEDICATION THERAPY: MODIFICATIONS FOR THE OLDER PATIENT

The vast majority of therapeutic interventions for the elderly are pharmacological, making appropriate drug selection and modification of dosing regimens for the older patient important.

LOADING DOSES OF MEDICATIONS (see Chap. 6). On average, body size decreases with aging and body composition changes, resulting in decreased total body water, intravascular volume, and muscle mass. Age-related changes are continuous but most pronounced after 75 to 80 years of age. Women tend to weigh less and have smaller body and intra-

vascular volumes and muscle mass than men at all ages. Higher serum concentrations of medications are found in older patients, and especially older women, if initial doses are the same as in younger patients. Weight adjustment for loading doses of the cardiovascular drugs digoxin, lidocaine, and other type I antiarrhythmic drugs; type III antiarrhythmic drugs; aminoglycoside antibiotics; chemotherapy regimens; and unfractionated heparin are standard. When fibrinolytic drugs have been administered without weight-based dosage adjustments, increased risk of intracranial hemorrhage results with older age, smaller body weight, and female sex (in addition to hypertension and prior cerebrovascular disease).[31,32] Increased risk of bleeding in older patients is also seen after administration of "standard doses" of low-molecular-weight heparins in combination with other lytic agents. In contrast, increased risk of intracranial bleeding in older patients is not seen in trials using weight-based dosing.[33]

Routine dosage/weight adjustments should be made in loading doses of medications, especially those with low therapeutic-to-toxicity ratios resulting in doses that are usually lower in older patients, especially older women.

Chronic Medication Administration

RENAL CLEARANCE (see Chap. 88). Renal function is gaining more recognition as a prognostic indicator for outcomes of patients with cardiovascular disease and cardiovascular interventions.[34-36] Renal

TABLE 75–1	Differentiation Between Age-Associated Changes and Cardiovascular Disease in Older People	
Organ	**Age-Associated Changes**	**Cardiovascular Disease**
Vasculature	Increased intimal thickness Arterial stiffening Increased pulse pressure Increased pulse wave velocity Early central wave reflections Decreased endothelial-mediated vasodilation	Systolic hypertension Coronary artery obstruction Peripheral artery obstruction Carotid artery obstruction
Atria	Increased left atrial size Atrial premature complexes	Atrial fibrillation
Sinus node	Decreased maximal heart rate Decreased heart rate variability	Sinus node dysfunction, sick sinus
Atrioventricular node	Increased conduction time	Type II block, third-degree block
Valves	Sclerosis, calcification	Stenosis, regurgitation
Ventricle	Increased left ventricular wall tension Prolonged myocardial contraction Prolonged early diastolic filling rate Decreased maximal cardiac output Right bundle branch block Ventricular premature complexes	Left ventricular hypertrophy Heart failure (with or without preserved systolic function) Ventricular tachycardia, fibrillation

TABLE 75–2	Estimated Glomerular Filtration Rate (eGFR) by Age, Sex, and Race														
	Cr = 1					**Cr = 1.2**					**Cr = 1.5**				
Age (yr)	*45*	*55*	*65*	*75*	*85*	*45*	*55*	*65*	*75*	*85*	*45*	*55*	*65*	*75*	*85*
Caucasian men	86*	82	80	77	75	70	67	65	63	61	_54_	_52_	_50_	_48_	_47_
Caucasian women	64	61	_59_	_57_	_56_	_52_	_50_	_48_	_47_	_45_	_40_	_38_	_37_	_36_	_35_
African American men	104	100	97	94	91	84	81	78	76	74	65	63	61	_59_	_57_
African American women	77	74	72	70	68	63	60	_58_	_56_	_55_	_48_	_46_	_45_	_44_	_43_

*Data are average eGFR/1.73 m² for serum creatinine of 1 mg/dl (Cr = 1), 1.2 mg/dl (Cr = 1.2), and 1.5 mg/dl (Cr = 1.5) for Caucasian and African American men and women. Underscores indicate eGFR <60 ml/min/1.73 m² classified as moderate decreases in GFR or stage 3 chronic renal disease (ICD-9-CM code 585.3).

From Manjunath G, Sarnak M, Levey A: Prediction equations to estimate glomerular filtration rate: An update. Curr Opin Nephrol Hypertens 10:785-792, 2001 and Levey A, Bosch J, Lewis J, et al: A more accurate method to estimate glomerular filtration rate from serum creatinine: A new prediction equation. Ann Intern Med 130:461-470, 1999.

clearance by all routes (glomerular filtration, renal tubular reabsorption and secretion) decreases with age and is lower in women compared with men at all ages. Considerable intersubject variability exists, but a general estimate is a 10 percent decline in glomerular filtration per decade with 15 to 25 percent lower rates in women compared with men. One of the earliest algorithms to estimate creatinine clearance includes age, sex, weight, and serum creatinine (mg/dl) concentrations as variables:

$$\text{Creatinine clearance} = (140 - \text{age [yr]} \times \text{weight [kg]})/$$
$$(\text{creatinine}^{\dagger} \times 72) \text{ multiplied by } 0.85 \text{ for women}^{37}$$

and highlights that significant decreases in renal elimination can be present in older patients in the presence of normal serum creatinine measurements. With elevations of serum creatinine, severe renal impairment is likely to be present. A more recently validated algorithm that incorporates creatinine, age, race, and sex as variables nonlinearly is reported to estimate glomerular filtration rate (eGFR) in the elderly and obese.[38,39]

$$\text{Glomerular filtration rate} = 186.3^{*} \times (\text{creatinine}^{\dagger})^{-1.154} \times$$
$$(\text{age})^{-0.203} \times 1.212 \text{ (if African American)} \times 0.742 \text{ (if female)}$$

---

*Use 175 if a standardited serum creatinine assay is used.
†mg/dl; for SI units (μmol/l), divide creatinine by 88.4.

eGFR is expressed as ml per minute per 1.73 m². Adjustments for body surface area yielding eGFR in ml/min are necessary for appropriate adjustment in medication doses for patients who are very large or very small. Importantly, the clinician should recognize that renal clearance estimation algorithms predict Caucasian women older than the age of 60 to have stage 3 decreased renal function or moderate renal failure (Table 75-2) (see National Kidney Foundation criteria and online creatinine clearance and eGFR calculator at http://www.kidney.org). Failure to adjust dosages of renally cleared narrow therapeutic index medications such as thrombolytic agents, low-molecular-weight heparin, and glycoprotein (GP) IIb/IIIa inhibitors has resulted in increased bleeding and intracerebral hemorrhages in clinical trials and routine clinical practice.[40-43] Risk of bleeding increases with age, and excess dosing is associated with increased risk of bleeding in women and men. Bleeding risk attributable to dosing is reported to be much higher in women and may account for up to 25 percent of excess bleeding risk in women treated with GP IIb/IIIa inhibitors.[41] Routine estimation of glomerular filtration (or creatinine clearance) for risk assessment before contrast administration, procedures, surgery, or administration of renally cleared medications can guide efforts to reduce adverse effects and provides an opportunity for quality improvement.

Limitations of current algorithms to estimate either GFR or creatinine clearance include lack of accuracy during hemodynamic instability or acute renal damage and derivation from populations without significant numbers of older or minority patients. Cystatin is being evaluated as a marker of renal clearance that reflects changes in renal function more rapidly and may reflect age-related changes without sex differences.[44-46]

HEPATIC (AND INTESTINAL) CLEARANCE. Most studies show decreases in oxidative drug metabolism/clearance by the cytochrome P450 (CYP) system with aging, suggesting that lower amounts of drug per unit time (or day) should be given to older patients compared with younger patients. Cardiovascular drugs showing such age-related changes in hepatic clearance include alpha blockers (doxazosin, prazosin, terazosin); some beta blockers (metoprolol, propranolol, timolol); calcium channel blockers (dihydropyridines, diltiazem, verapamil); several 3-hydroxy-3-methylglutaryl coenzyme A (HMG CoA) reductase inhibitors (atorvastatin, fluvastatin); and the benzodiazepines (midazolam). Variability in age-related changes is marked, however, and the effects of disease states, gender, race, and medication interactions are usually greater than those of age in patient populations.[47-49] CYP drug clearance is usually faster in men compared with women, even after correction for weight, suggesting that women should get lower dosages per unit time and weight than men. The exceptions are CYP 3A substrates such as atorvastatin, midazolam, nifedipine, and verapamil (see Chap. 6 on CYP pathways of metabolism), which are cleared faster in women. Additional information on sex-specific medication adjustments has been recently reviewed.[50,51]

Genetic variation in drug metabolism exists, and allelic variants for most of the CYP enzymes have been described that can affect drug clearance and responses. The CYP2D6 enzyme is polymorphic and can produce distinct phenotypes of ultra-rapid, rapid, slow, and ultra-slow drug clearance (see Chap. 6), but clinical dosing has not yet been based on pharmacogenetic analyses. One fairly consistent cardiovascular example of the impact of pharmacogenetic variants is that of warfarin and variant haplotypes of its metabolizing enzyme, CYP2C9, which are associated with lower initial warfarin requirements and increased bleeding with standard initial dosages in Caucasians.[52] When present, variants in the vitamin K epoxide reductase complex may play a greater role. Overanticoagulation during chronic warfarin therapy, however, is more closely associated with environmental factors. The risk of marked Q-T prolongation during exposure to drugs with Q-T prolonging properties may be altered by underlying genetic factors of both channel pharmacology and drug metabolism.[53] Age effects are additive to genetically determined differences in the pharmacokinetics of drugs metabolized by CYP2D6 and CYP2C9/19. Further information can be found at the NIH-sponsored Pharmacogenetics Research Network website (www.pharmgkb.org) or the Human Cytochrome P450 Allele Nomenclature Committee website (www.imm.ki.se/CYPalleles/).[54]

Drugs metabolized by the conjugative reactions of glucuronidation (morphine, diazepam), sulfation (methyldopa), or acetylation (procainamide) do not appear to be affected by aging in general but show disease-related effects, may show frailty-related decreases, and show consistently lower clearance in women compared with men.

A growing body of knowledge suggests that the overall clinical pharmacological profile in an individual may reflect the presence, expression, and activity of multiple drug metabolizing and/or transporting proteins, as well as drug receptors that vary among ethnic groups and are also modulated by environmental factors. The multitude of factors that show variation may explain the relative paucity of data demonstrating the impact of pharmacogenomics (see Chap. 6) on cardiovascular therapeutics.

ELIMINATION HALF-LIVES. In general, elimination half-lives of drugs increase with age, so the time between dosage adjustments needs to be increased in older patients before the full effect of a given dose can be assessed. Conversely, increased time is necessary for complete drug elimination from the body and dissipation of the effects of a drug.

Age-related changes in protein binding of drugs are not usually found. Changes in free drug concentrations caused by drugs competing for binding sites can occur, although these changes are predicted to be transitory. Clinically significant examples involve warfarin and changes in anticoagulation when additional drugs are added to therapy. For example, markedly increased prolongation of coagulation times can occur when amiodarone is added to warfarin therapy (see Chap. 33). Drug interactions must be considered whenever an agent is added to warfarin therapy. Table 75-3 summarizes general guidelines for drug dosing in older patients.

ADVERSE DRUG EVENTS AND DRUG INTERACTIONS. Adverse drug events are estimated to affect

TABLE 75–3	Guidelines for Medication Prescribing in Older Patients
In general, loading doses should be reduced—weight (or body surface area) can be used to estimate loading dose requirements; doses in women are usually less than in men.
Use estimates of glomerular filtration to guide dosing of renally cleared medications and contrast administration; reduce doses of metabolically or hepatically cleared drugs.
Time between dosage adjustments and evaluation of dosing changes should be longer in older patients than younger patients.
Routine use of strategies to avoid drug interactions is essential—incorporating reference materials, a team approach, and quality improvement initiatives are effective strategies.
Knowledge of effects of noncardiac medications is necessary.
Assessment of adherence and attention to factors contributing to nonadherence should be part of the prescribing process.
Physicians must be familiar with the patient's source of prescription medication coverage including Medicare D legislation and provide patient education and assistance with obtaining critical medications.
Multidisciplinary approaches to monitoring medication therapy may increase successful outcomes of medication therapy.

millions of people per year and account for up to 5 percent of hospital admissions.[55] Cardiovascular medications such as digoxin, warfarin, diuretics, and calcium channel blockers are among those most frequently cited as responsible for "preventable" adverse drug events in community-dwelling elderly and hospitalized elderly patients.[56,57] The odds ratio of severe adverse drug events with cardiovascular medications has been reported to be 2.4 times that of other medications in hospitalized patients.[58] In ambulatory primary care settings for adult patients, selective serotonin reuptake inhibitors (SSRIs), beta blockers, ACE inhibitors, and nonsteroidal antiinflammatory drugs (NSAIDs) are identified in adverse drug events.[59] In nursing home patients, drugs associated with adverse drug events are more frequently antibiotics, anticoagulants and antiplatelet drugs, atypical and typical antipsychotic drugs, antidepressants, antiseizure medications, or opioids.[60] Adverse drug effects may present with "atypical" symptoms such as mental status changes and impaired cognition in the older patient.

The strongest risk factor for adverse drug-related events is the number of drugs prescribed, independent of age. Chronic administration of four drugs is associated with a risk of adverse effects of 50 to 60 percent; administration of 8 to 9 drugs increases the risk to almost 100 percent (Fig. 75-6). Although the goal is to prescribe as few drugs as possible in the elderly, the presence of multiple diseases and multidrug regimens for common cardiovascular diseases often results in polypharmacy. A recent national survey of noninstitutionalized people older than 65 years of age found that more than 40 percent used 5 or more different medications each week, whereas 12 percent used 10 or more different medications per week.[61] American College of Cardiology/American Heart Association (ACC/AHA) guidelines for the pharmacological treatment of patients after uncomplicated myocardial infarction and for the management of chronic heart failure recommend use of more than three drugs. Current regimens for treatment of the common disorders of diabetes and osteoporosis in the elderly similarly include two to four drugs. Strategies that minimize the chance of drug interactions and adverse drug effects are thus essential.

PHARMACOKINETIC INTER-ACTIONS. Pharmacokinetic interactions that alter the concentration of concomitantly administered medications are more likely if drugs that are metabolized by or inhibit the same pathway are coadministered. Tables in Chapter 6 list examples of cardiovascular drugs by metabolic pathway with examples of inducers and inhibitors and interactions. The most potent inhibitors of the CYP oxidative enzymes are amiodarone (all CYP isoforms); the azole antifungal drugs itraconazole and ketoconazole (CYP3A); and protease inhibitors (CYP3A), followed by erythromycin (CYP3A) and terfenadine (CYP3A).[62] Oral hypoglycemic agents are commonly prescribed drugs in the elderly, and coadministration of sulfonamide antibiotics with sulfonylureas can lead to hypoglycemia, in part because of CYP2C9 inhibition. Some drugs are administered as "prodrugs" and metabolized to active agents (cardiovascular examples include many ACE inhibitors and clopidogrel). Inhibition of the antiplatelet effects of clopidogrel by coadministration of atorvastatin that decreases clopidogrel activation (CYP3A) has been reported.[63]

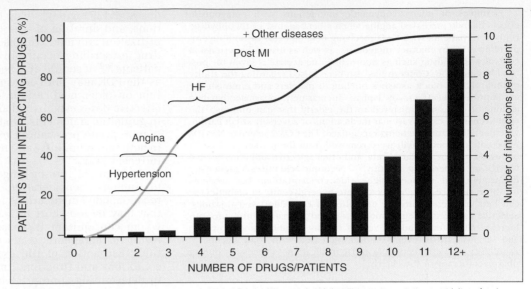

FIGURE 75–6 The relationship between the number of drugs consumed and drug interactions. Current guidelines for the pharmacological management of patients with heart failure (HF) or myocardial infarction (post MI) place them at high risk for drug interactions. *(Reprinted from Schwartz JB: Clinical Pharmacology, ACCSAP V, 2003, American College of Cardiology, Bethesda, Md, as modified from Nolan L and O'Malley K: Age Aging 1989; Denham, Br Med Bull, 1990.)*

Inducibility of enzyme activity can lower concentrations of medications and lead to ineffective therapy. The antituberculous drug rifampin is the most potent inducer of CYP1A and CYP3A. With mandatory screening of nursing home residents for tuberculosis, treatment with rifampin may be initiated. Coadministered dosages of drugs cleared by CYP1A and CYP3A may need to be increased during rifampin administration and decreased on discontinuation of rifampin. The clinical importance of this interaction was recognized with markedly decreased cyclosporine levels during rifampin coadministration; recently, reduced clopidogrel inhibition of platelet aggregation by atorvastatin has been reported following rifampin administration.[63] Other clinically relevant CYP inducers include carbamazepine (all CYPs); dexamethasone and phenytoin (CYP2C); caffeine, cigarette smoke, lansoprazole, and omeprazole (CYP1A); St. John's wort (CYP3A); and troglitazone.[62] Diet-drug and herb-drug interactions also occur.[64,65]

Despite the predictability of some of these interactions, many hospital admissions of elderly patients for drug toxicity involve administration of drugs known to interact.[66] Because of the multiplicity of potential interactions and release of new medications and discovery of new interactions, use of pharmacy or computerized and online tools that provide comprehensive up-to-date information and guidelines for avoiding drug interactions is highly recommended. Available tools include the *Physicians' Desk Reference* (PDR—traditional, pocket, or online versions), PDR handbook of drug interactions (traditional, computer version, or hand-held computer version available free of charge at www.PDR.net), the Medical Letter and Medical Letter Drug Interactions Program (computer-based), and Epocrates for the hand-held computer (available free of charge at www.epocrates.com), or online pharmacology texts or databases (e.g., www.fda.gov/cder, drug reactions section; www.druginteractions.org; http://medicine.iupui.edu/flockhart). Many individual hospitals, health care systems, and pharmacies provide internal reference sources. Specialized clinics, use of specific algorithms, and computer-based dosage programs to monitor oral anticoagulant therapy in outpatients have been shown to reduce bleeding-related complications.[67]

Other approaches that have been shown to reduce adverse drug reactions in older patients include involvement of pharmacy-trained individuals to assess the appropriateness of doses and medication counseling using multidisciplinary care team members. A major limitation to the success of all of these approaches is the frequent lack of complete and readily accessible information on medication consumption and disease state information, especially in the older patient with multiple diseases and physicians. Integrated medical record and pharmacy information, interactive databases, and computerized physician order entry with clinical decision support have been recommended to reduce adverse drug events and improve medication therapy. Importantly, use of such systems has achieved these goals.[68,69] Such systems, however, are not yet widely implemented. In contrast, mandated drug utilization review efforts appear ineffective.[70]

ADVERSE PHARMACODYNAMIC EFFECTS. Age-related changes in cardiovascular physiology and dynamics affect pharmacodynamics (see Table 75-1). Greater age-related CNS sensitivity to parasympathetic stimulation may explain the increased frequency of adverse effects such as urinary retention, constipation and fecal impaction, and worsened cognition in older patients who receive drugs with anticholinergic properties. Gastrointestinal transit time is generally increased in the elderly, and constipation is a frequent complaint of hospitalized elderly, less active elderly, and institutionalized elderly. Drug-induced constipation and bowel obstruction can occur in older patients receiving bile acid sequestrants, anticholinergic medications, opiates, and verapamil.

Pharmacodynamic drug interactions are more likely to occur between drugs acting on the same system. A classic example of additive effects that can produce hypotension and postural hypotension in the elderly is the coadministration of direct vasodilators or nitrates combined with alpha blockers, beta blockers, calcium channel blockers, ACE inhibitors, angiotensin receptor blockers (ARBs), diuretics, sildenafil, or tricyclic antidepressants. Other examples are bradycardia with combinations of amiodarone, beta-adrenergic blocking drugs, digoxin, diltiazem, or verapamil; and bleeding caused by increased inhibition of platelet and clotting factors with combinations of aspirin, NSAIDs (including some cyclo-oxygenase [COX]-2 selective inhibitors), warfarin, and/or clopidogrel. Increased potassium concentrations caused by combined administration of ACE inhibitors, ARBs, aldosterone and renin antagonists, and potassium-sparing diuretics in older patients are cited as causes of serious adverse drug reactions (ADRs) that are preventable.[60,71] Combinations of NSAIDs including selective COX-2 inhibitors with ACE inhibitors can also decrease potassium excretion with resultant hyperkalemia or can cause a decrease in renal function in the older patient. Combinations of drugs that produce Q-T interval prolongation can result in torsades de pointes arrhythmias (see Chap. 35). Importantly, noncardiac drugs such as antibiotics (azithromycin, clarithromycin, erythromycin, gatifloxacin, gemfloxacin, moxifloxacin), antidepressants (amitriptyline, fluoxetine, lithium, venlafaxine), antipsychotics (haloperidol, risperidone), tamoxifen, or vardenafil, which may be used in the elderly and generally produce only moderate increases in the Q-T interval, may have additive effects with cardiovascular drugs such as the class IA, IC, and III antiarrhythmic drugs isradipine, nicardipine, and ranolazine (see Chap. 33; online updated lists of medications that prolong the Q-T are available at www.Qtdrugs.org).

CH 75

Cardiovascular Disease in the Elderly

Examples of pharmacodynamic interactions with antagonistic effects include increased angina when a beta agonist or theophylline is given to patients with CAD receiving beta blockers or nondihydropyridine calcium channel antagonists, as well as loss of hypertension control when a drug such as fludrocortisone acetate is given for postural hypotension. Concern has also been raised regarding the ability of ibuprofen to block aspirin's binding to platelets and diminish the cardioprotective effects of aspirin. Increasingly, pharmacodynamic actions of drugs administered to the elderly that can diminish the effectiveness of cardiovascular medications or adversely affect cardiovascular risk factors are being recognized. The COX-2 selective NSAIDs rofecoxib and valdecoxib were removed from the market because of increased cardiovascular events, and other selective and nonselective NSAIDs are undergoing scrutiny.[72,73] Nicotinic acid raises high-density lipoprotein and reduces triglyceride concentrations but worsens insulin resistance and can exacerbate hyperglycemia in diabetics, as can beta blockers (with the exception of carvedilol) and thiazides. Selective estrogen receptor modulators and aromatase inhibitors can increase cholesterol and the risk of venous thromboembolic events, and serious cardiac events appear increased with some agents.[74,75] Familiarity with effects of noncardiac medications is necessary during pharmacotherapy of the elderly.

INAPPROPRIATE PRESCRIBING IN THE ELDERLY.
Lists of medications considered "inappropriate" for routine use in the elderly because of adverse effects or lack of efficacy have been compiled.[76-78] The updated 2003 Beers criteria[78] can be accessed online at http://archinte.ama-assn.org/cgi/reprint/163/22/2716.pdf. Long-acting benzodiazepines, sedative and hypnotic agents, long-acting oral hypoglycemic agents, selected analgesics and NSAIDs, first-generation antihistamines, antiemetics, and gastrointestinal antispasmodics are usually considered "inappropriate" in the elderly. Although most cardiovascular medications are not considered "inappropriate" for use in the older patient, amiodarone, clonidine, disopyramide, doxazosin, ethacrynic acid, guanethidine, and guanadrel have been classified as generally inappropriate in the elderly. More recent definitions of "inappropriate drug use" include failure to consider drug-disease interactions and failure to adjust drug dosages for age-related changes (i.e., digoxin at doses >0.125 mg/day), drug duplication, drug-drug interactions, and duration of use. Using these criteria, most drug utilization review studies conclude that inappropriate drug prescribing occurs in a significant fraction of older patients.[60,79] It should also be recognized that resources such as the PDR may not contain geriatric prescribing information on older medications or present data on minimally effective doses established after drug marketing approval or in guideline statements. Disturbingly, analyses suggest that inappropriate prescribing of medications to older patients in both the community and nursing homes has not decreased in recent years.[79-81]

Appropriate prescribing of medications is evolving to include consideration of discontinuing guideline-recommended medications in patients with life expectancy that may be too short to achieve long-term benefits, or in whom concomitant diseases such as end-stage dementia result in therapeutic goals related primarily to quality of life.[82] Estimation of life expectancy from both comorbid conditions and functional measures is gaining acceptance in determining appropriateness for screening for diseases, preventive strategies, and therapeutic decision-making for older adults.[83-85] Recent models that estimate life expectancy use data likely to be available during routine clinical care or at the time of hospital discharge[84,86] and are simpler than those from earlier cardiovascular studies. Table 75-4 presents one model developed from a large and diverse sample of community-dwelling elderly in the United States. It demonstrates the importance of noncardiac factors that often are not considered during cardiac care but that contribute significantly to overall mortality in the elderly. A logical approach to choosing appropriate medications, as well as other therapies, would incorporate consideration of remaining life expectancy, time until benefit, treatment targets, and goals of care for the individual older patient.

ADHERENCE. Medication adherence is commonly thought to be lower in older patients compared with younger patients. In one report, hospitalization for decompensated

TABLE 75–4 Estimation of 4-Year Mortality in the Elderly Using Medical and Functional Information

		Points
Age (yr)	60-64	1
	65-69	2
	70-74	3
	75-79	4
	80-84	5
	>85	7
Male sex		2
Diabetes mellitus		1
Cancer		2
Lung disease		2
Heart failure		2
BMI < 25		1
Current smoker		2
Assistance needed for		
Bathing		2
Managing finances		2
Difficulty		
Walking several blocks		2
Pushing/pulling heavy objects		1

Score	4-Year Mortality (%)
0	0-1
1	1
2	1.5
3	3.5
4	5
5	5-8
6	9
7	12-15
8	19-20
9	20-24
10	27-28
11	43-45
12	44-48
13	54-59
≥14	64-67

BMI = body mass index.

Modified from Lee S, Lindquist K, Segal M, Covinsky K: Development and validation of a prognostic index for 4-year mortality in older adults. JAMA 295:801, 2006.

congestive heart failure was attributed to medication non-compliance in 42 percent of elderly patients.[87] Contributing factors include the cost of medications, difficulty with understanding directions because of small print of written directions, hearing impairment, impaired memory, inadequate instructions, complex dosing regimens, difficulties with packaging materials, or insufficient patient or family or caregiver education on medication use. Of these, the most limiting are thought to be the cost of medications, poor patient education regarding medications, and cognitive impairment in elderly patients, especially those living alone. In a study of Medicare beneficiaries with CAD, use of HMG CoA reductase inhibitors was directly related to drug payment coverage.[88]

Of note is that physicians routinely overestimate patient adherence with medications.[89,90] Assessment of adherence should be part of care, and issues related to potential contributors to medication nonadherence should be addressed by prescribing health care professionals. Unfortunately, there are few trials of interventions to improve medication adherence with resources usually available in clinical settings.[91] Strategies to overcome these obstacles include programs for low-income seniors, visual or memory aids, medication-dispensing tools, use of geriatric-friendly packaging, assessment of cognitive status and patient understanding, and inclusion of caregivers or family members in discussions regarding medications.

MEDICARE D. January 1, 2006 marked the beginning of prescription-drug coverage under the Medicare Prescription Drug and Modernization Act of 2003 in the United States. The Medicare D legislation created a complex plan involving government-contracted private industry coverage requiring individual enrollment. Elements common to all plans are deductibles of $250 per year and partial payment of annual drug costs up to the estimated average annual drug expenditure for seniors of $2250 per year and then a gap in payment until costs exceed $3600 for all but low-income seniors (i.e., patients "dually eligible" for Medicaid and Medicare and those with incomes of 100 to 150 percent poverty levels). A multitude of plans are offered in regions that vary in benefits, copays, covered formulary medications, and tiers of medications with differing levels of copays within formularies. Implementation has been described as chaotic, and physicians and pharmacists have had the task of educating a significant number of patients and families. The potential for improving medication access, adherence, and therapy exists, but the impact of the program is yet to be determined. Many plans rely on utilization-management techniques, making it key that physicians are involved to initiate processes or appeal for continuation of nonformulary critical medications (termed *exceptions*), for medications during changes of plans or to monitor chronically ill patients forced to switch to therapeutic alternatives. Patterns of problems with plan denials or coverage appeals can be reported to the Physician Regulatory Issues Team at the Center for Medicare Services. Specific medications excluded from coverage by the law include those "inappropriate" for use in the elderly (such as barbiturates and benzodiazepines, see earlier) but also include over-the-counter medications, vitamins, and products for symptomatic relief of colds or cough and medications not used for "medically accepted" indications. Individual plans may choose to provide some of these products such as nonsedative antihistamines and over-the-counter proton pump inhibitors. The program is evolving, and updated information for physicians and patients is available on Internet sites including www.Medicare.gov, www.MedicareToday.org, www.HLC.org, www.cms.hhs.gov, www.ama-assn.org, www.acponline.org, and www.accesstobenefits.org, and by calling 800-633-4227.

Hypertension (see Chaps. 40 and 41)

PREVALENCE AND INCIDENCE. Diastolic (>90 mm Hg) and/or systolic (>140 mm Hg) hypertension occurs in half to two thirds of people older than 65 years and in 75 percent of people older than 80 years.[92] The prevalence varies by race (or genetics) and is slightly higher in African Americans and Hispanics compared with non-Hispanic whites.[93] The profile of hypertension is altered by aging. Systolic hypertension becomes more prevalent with aging, whereas diastolic blood pressure is relatively constant from 50 to 80 years of age, with average diastolic pressures higher in men than women from ages 50 to 80 years. Systolic blood pressure rises with aging in both men and women but rises more steeply in women. Systolic blood pressure is lower in women compared with men until about age 50 (average age of menopause) but rises to levels equal to those of men by age 65 years. "Isolated" systolic hypertension, without elevation of diastolic blood pressure, is present in about 8 percent of sexagenarians and more than 25 percent of the population older than 80 years of age. A large percentage of people are unaware that they have hypertension, and hypertension is not controlled in many older patients, especially older women and those older than 80 years of age.

TREATMENT. Relative risks for cardiovascular events associated with increasing blood pressure do not decline with older age, and absolute risk increases markedly in older patients, emphasizing the need for treatment of hypertension in the elderly.[92] Randomized clinical trials in elderly patients over the past three decades have unequivocally demonstrated that treatment of diastolic and/or systolic hypertension in the elderly confers cardiovascular benefits (Table 75-5). All but one of these studies utilized thiazide diuretics, beta blockers, and/or calcium channel blockers and did not enroll patients older than 80 years of age. Several randomized trials have compared antihypertensive agents (diuretics to a calcium channel blocker or an ACE inhibitor) in exclusively older populations, but a clear distinction in relative benefits has not emerged.[94-96] Recent large, randomized mortality trials that compare single or combination hypertensive regimens that include ACE inhibitors or ARBs have enrolled elderly patients within study populations and have analyzed cardiovascular outcomes, as well as surrogate endpoints (see Chaps. 40 and 41).[97] The overall conclusions are that there is cardiovascular benefit for treatment of systolic or diastolic blood pressure in the elderly; that combination drug regimens including a diuretic are usually required to approach blood pressure targets; and that different combinations of pharmacological agents may have advantages based on the patients' concomitant diseases, genetics, or risk factors. Meta-analyses have suggested greater stroke benefit with dihydropyridine calcium channel blockers and that ACE inhibitors are associated with cardiac benefit, primarily in men.[98,99] Only one trial of treatment for systolic hypertension in the elderly has reported reduced rates of dementia with treatment.[100] In the elderly patient with uncomplicated hypertension (especially systolic), agents that decrease pulse pressure may be preferable to agents that further widen pulse pressure. The emphasis should be on diagnosis and treatment of hypertension that requires combination regimens in older patients rather than the choice of initial individual therapeutic agents.

In addition to recommendations based on concomitant cardiovascular diseases recognized in hypertension treatment guidelines (Table 75-6),[97,101] other conditions in the elderly warrant consideration to optimize effects; minimize adverse effects, cost, and the number of medications; and increase adherence. Arthritis is second in prevalence to cardiovascular disease in the elderly, and NSAIDs are among the most frequently consumed drugs (prescription and over-the-counter) in older people. In addition to the potential for adverse renal effects and/or hyperkalemia when given

						Risk Reduction			
Trial	N	Age (yr)	Type		Drug(s)	Stroke	CAD	HF	All CVD
HDFP (1)	2374	60-69	D		Chlor + Res or Meth	44%	15%	NR	16%
Australian (2)	582	60-69	D		Chlor (+)	33%	18%	NR	31%
EWPHE (3)	840	>60	D (+ S)		HCTZ + TR (+)	36%	20%	22%	29%
Coope (4)	884	60-79	D (+ S)		Beta (ATEN) (+)	42%	−3%	32%	24%
STOP-HTN (5)	1627	70-84	D (+ S) HCTZ + Am or Beta			47%	13%	51%	40%
MRC (6)	4396	65-74	D(+ S)		HCTZ + Am or Beta	25%	19%	NR	17%
SHEP (7)	4736	≥60	S		Chlor	33%	27%	55%	32%
Syst-Eur (8)	4695	≥60	S		CCB (NITR)	42%	26%	36%	31%
STONE (9)	1632	60-79	S		CCB (NIF)	57%	6%	68%	60%
Syst-China (10)	2394	≥60	S		CCB (NITR)	38%	33%	38%	37%
SCOPE (11)	4973	70-89	S +/or D		ARB (CAND)	24%	NR	NR	11% (NS)

TABLE 75–5 | Trials of Blood Pressure Reduction in the Elderly

All CVD = all cardiovascular disease composite endpoint; Am = amiloride; ARB = angiotensin receptor blocker; ATEN = atenolol; Beta = beta-blocker; CAD = coronary artery disease; CAND = candesartan; CCB = calcium channel blocker; Chlor = chlorthalidone; D = diastolic; HCTZ = hydrochlorothiazide; HF = heart failure; N = number of subjects; NIF = nifedipine; NITR = nitrendipine; NR = not reported; NS = not statistically significant; Res = reserpine; S = systolic; TR = triamterene; Type = type of hypertension.

From randomized trials of pharmacologic blood pressure reduction in the elderly: (1) HDFP: Five-year findings of the hypertension detection and follow up program: I. Reduction in mortality of persons with high blood pressure, including mild hypertension. JAMA 242:2562-2571, 1979. Five-year findings of the hypertension detection and follow-up program: II. Mortality by race-sex and age. Hypertension detection and follow-up program cooperative. JAMA 242:2572-2577, 1979. (2) Management Committee. Med J Aust 77:398-402, 1981. (3) Amery A, Birkenhäger W, Brixko P, et al: Mortality and morbidity results from the European Working Party on High Blood Pressure in the Elderly trial. Lancet i:1349-1354, 1985. (4) Coope J, Warrender TS: Randomised trial of treatment of hypertension in elderly patients in primary care. BMJ 293:1145-1151, 1986. (5) Dahlöf B, Lindholm LH, Hansson L, et al: Morbidity and mortality in the Swedish Trial in Old Patients with Hypertension (STOP-hypertension). Lancet 338:1281-1285, 1991. (6) MRC Working Party. Medical Research Council trial of treatment of hypertension in older adults: Principal results. BMJ 304:405-412, 1992. (7) Medical research council trial of treatment of hypertension in older adults: Principal results. MRC Working Party. Br Med J 304:405-412, 1992. (8) SHEP Cooperative Research Group. Prevention of stroke by antihypertensive drug treatment in older persons with isolated systolic hypertension: Final results of the Systolic Hypertension in the Elderly Program (SHEP). JAMA 265:3255-3264, 1991. (9) Staessen JA, Fagard R, Thijs LT, et al: Randomised double-blind comparison of placebo and active treatment for older patients with isolated systolic hypertension. Lancet 350:757-764, 1997. (10) Gong L, Zwang W, Zhu Y: Shanghai trial of nifedipine in the elderly. Seventh European Meeting on Hypertension, June 9-12, 1995, Milan, Italy. (11) Liu L, Wang JG, Gong L, et al; Systolic Hypertension in China (Syst-China) Collaborative Group: Comparison of active treatment and placebo for older patients with isolated systolic hypertension. J Hypertens 16:1823-1829, 1998. (11) Lithell H, Hansson L, Skoog I, et al; Study on Cognition and Prognosis in the Elderly (SCOPE): Principal results of a randomized double-blind intervention trial. J Hypertens 21:875-886, 2003.

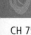

CH 75

in combination with ACE inhibitors, ARBs, or aldosterone antagonists, loss of blood pressure control and HF have been precipitated by nonselective NSAIDs, as well as COX-2 selective NSAIDs. Age-related bone loss accelerates in older men and women and is the major contributing cause of osteoporosis. Osteoporosis, in turn, is a major risk factor for fractures in older people, with the lifetime risk of osteoporotic fracture in Americans estimated at 40 percent for women and 13 percent for men. Thiazide administration has been associated with higher bone mineral density and a reduction in risk of hip fractures in epidemiological studies and preservation of bone mineral density compared with placebo in older adults, suggesting a noncardiac treatment benefit in older patients. Older patients for whom thiazide diuretics may not be a good choice include patients with urinary frequency problems—stress incontinence, urinary frequency and/or incontinence caused by prostatic hypertrophy, overactive bladders, and patients needing assistance with toileting. Drugs that do not increase urinary frequency may have higher adherence in these patients.

Table 75-6 presents suggested antihypertensive regimens in older patients on the basis of the presence of hypertension *and* concomitant diseases. Additional data on frequent geriatric problems and medications to use or avoid are available at www.geriatricsatyourfingertips.com.

ADDITIONAL CONSIDERATIONS IN THE OLDER PATIENT WITH HYPERTENSION. Both the Seventh Report of the Joint National Committee on Prevention, Detection, Evaluation, and Treatment of High Blood Pressure (JNC 7)[97] and the European Guidelines for the Management of Arterial Hypertension[101] recommend lower initial drug dosages and slower medication titration in older patients, as well as the need to monitor for postural hypotension.

A decrease in standing systolic blood pressure is estimated to be present in 15 percent of 70- to 74-year-old community-dwelling men or women and in up to 30 percent of patients with systolic hypertension. Postural hypotension of greater than 20 mm Hg or 20 percent of systolic pressure is a risk factor for falls and fractures that carries significant morbidity and mortality.[102] Antihypertensive medications add to the risk of postural hypotension, as do many anti-parkinson agents, antipsychotic agents, or tricyclic antidepressant drugs. The frailest and oldest of the elderly may reside in long-term care facilities. Approximately 30 to 70 percent of these patients are hypertensive, and 30 percent have postural hypotension. Diuretic therapy appears to be effective in controlling systolic blood pressure in these patients and may also decrease postural hypotension. Postural blood pressure changes should be assessed (after >5 minutes supine, immediately after standing, and 2 minutes after standing) in older patients, and volume depletion avoided.

Postprandial declines in both systolic and diastolic blood pressure occur in hospitalized, institutionalized, and community-dwelling elderly. The greatest decline occurs about 1 hour after eating, with blood pressure returning to fasting levels 3 to 4 hours after eating. Vasoactive medications with rapid absorption and peaks should not be administered with meals.

Table 75-7 summarizes the approach to hypertension in older patients.

CURRENT CONTROVERSIES

- *Target blood pressures for systolic blood pressure in the very old.* Achieving a target systolic blood pressure of less than 140 mm Hg was not accomplished in the majority of older patients in trials of systolic hypertension. Meta-analyses of randomized trial data have concluded that there are cardiovascular morbidity

TABLE 75–6	Considerations for Pharmacological Therapy of Older Patients with Hypertension and Other Disorders	
Hypertension +	Efficacy Considerations	Toxicity/Adverse Effect Considerations
Arthritis	—	ACE, ARB, aldosterone antagonist interactions with NSAIDs
Atrial fibrillation	Beta blocker,* calcium channel blocker (non-DHP),* amiodarone	Interactions with warfarin
Atrioventricular block	—	Beta blockers, non-DHP calcium channel blockers
Carotid disease/stroke	Calcium channel blocker,* ACEI†	
Constipation	—	Verapamil
Coronary artery disease	Beta blocker,*† calcium channel blocker*†	Nitrates and postural hypotension
Dementia	Clonidine‡	
Depression	—	SSRIs and hyponatremia
Diabetes	ACE,*† ARB,*† calcium channel blocker (non-DHP),† beta blocker†	Chlorpropamide and hyponatremia
Gout		Diuretics
Heart failure	ACE,*† ARB*† + loop diuretic,*† ± beta blocker*† ± aldosterone antagonist*†§	Calcium channel blockers (possible) ACE, ARB, aldosterone antagonist and hyperkalemia
Hyponatremia	—	Diuretic (especially with SSRI)
Incontinence	—	Diuretic
Myocardial infarction	Beta blocker,*† ± ACE,*† ± aldosterone antagonist†	ACE, ARB, aldosterone antagonist and hyperkalemia
Osteoporosis	—	Thiazides and bone loss
Peripheral artery disease	Calcium channel blocker (DHP)*	Beta blocker (if severe)
Postural hypotension	Thiazide¶	Alpha blocker, calcium channel blocker (DHP)
Prostatic hypertrophy	Alpha blocker*	
Renal failure	ACE,*† ARB,*† ACE + ARB; loop diuretic*	Aldosterone antagonists
Ventricular arrhythmias	Beta blocker*	Thiazide, loop diuretics, and hypokalemia

*Recommendations for first-line therapy from the European Society of Cardiology guidelines for the management of arterial hypertension.[101]
†Recommendations for second-line agents usually added to thiazide diuretics from The Seventh Report of the Joint National Committee on Prevention, Detection, Evaluation, and Treatment of High Blood Pressure.[97]
‡Only available transdermal formulation for patients unable to swallow or who refuse oral medications.
§Systolic heart failure only.
¶Nursing home patients.
ACEI = angiotensin-converting enzyme inhibitor; ARB = angiotensin receptor blocking inhibitor; DHP = dihydropyridine; NSAIDs = nonsteroidal antiinflammatory drugs; SSRIs = selective serotonin reuptake inhibitors.

benefits without mortality benefit for treatment of hypertension in patients older than 80 years but have also reported a slightly higher overall risk of death in treated hypertensives older than 80 years of age compared with reduced deaths in patients 60 to 80 years of age. Preliminary results from an ongoing large trial of hypertension treatment in patients older than 80 years of age also suggest that stroke reduction may be balanced by excess cardiovascular mortality.[103]

- *Differences in central versus peripheral blood pressure.* Effects of blood pressure-lowering agents on derived central aortic pressure may differ despite similar effects on brachial blood pressure. This observation provides a plausible explanation for differential benefit of agents such as calcium channel blockers in the elderly, but the clinical outcomes of central versus peripheral blood pressure-lowering needs further evaluation.
- *Lifestyle modifications.* Smaller trials have shown weight loss and sodium restriction to be effective in older patients from 65 to 75 years of age. Manipulation of dietary calcium can also reverse some of the age-related changes in blood pressure. Increased activity can lower blood pressure and improve function in elderly patients without many of the potential adverse effects of medications, yet lifestyle modification attempts are markedly underutilized and are without validated regimens for older patients.
- Impact of blood pressure treatment on development of dementia. Trials or substudies of ongoing trials will address this question.[103]

TABLE 75–7	Approach to Hypertension in Older Patients

Systolic and diastolic hypertension should be treated; current recommendations are based on brachial artery measurements:
- Diastolic target is <90 mm Hg
- Systolic target is <140 mm Hg (individualization is necessary for patients older than 80 years of age)

The focus should be on achieving blood pressure control, not initial therapy

Multiple medications are usually required in older patients, and combinations should be based on concomitant diseases

Drug dosing regimens should be adjusted for age- and disease-related changes in drug metabolism and potential drug-drug interactions

Patients should be monitored for adverse effects and drug interactions, especially:
- Postural hypotension and postprandial hypotension
- Hypovolemia with diuretics
- Hyperkalemia with angiotensin-converting enzyme, angiotensin receptor blocker, or aldosterone antagonists

Coronary Artery Disease (see Chaps. 45 to 50)

PREVALENCE AND INCIDENCE. Both the prevalence and severity of atherosclerotic CAD increase with age in men and women. Autopsy studies show that more than half of people older than the age of 60 years have significant CAD with increasing prevalence of left main or triple-vessel CAD with older age. Using electrocardiogram (ECG) evidence of MI, abnormal echocardiogram, carotid intimal thickness, or abnormal ankle-brachial index as measures of subclinical vascular disease in community-dwelling elderly in the Cardiovascular Health Study, abnormalities were detected in 22 percent of women and 33 percent of men aged 65 to 70 years and 43 percent of women and 45 percent of men older than age 85 years.[104-106] The lifetime risk of developing symptomatic CAD is estimated as 1 in 3 for men and 1 in 4 for women with onset of symptoms about 10 years earlier in men compared with women, and with hypertension, diabetes, and lipid abnormalities influencing individual risk.[107]

By 80 years of age, similar frequencies of symptomatic CAD of about 20 to 30 percent are seen in men and women. Because of the increasing proportion of women at older ages, however, population studies show more absolute numbers of women with angina compared with men in the community, with these women less likely to receive evidence-based therapy for stable angina, aggressive therapy for acute coronary syndromes, or diagnostic evaluations.[108-111]

Diagnosis

ESTIMATION OF RISK. Risk factors and tools such as those developed from the Framingham study in younger populations may be less accurate in the very old.[112] Elevated blood pressure confers risk, but its predictive value is less in older patients with cardiovascular disease or HF. Total cholesterol and low-density lipoprotein cholesterol (LDL-c) decline in predictive power in the elderly, and these and individual lipoproteins may not predict cardiovascular disease or death risk in older women.[113-115] Data exclusively from older patients suggest that high-density lipoprotein cholesterol (HDL-c) should be considered in risk assessment. Increased pulse pressure and measures of arterial stiffness also assume importance in risk assessment in older people. Predictive models that incorporate traditional risk factors (e.g., smoking, blood pressure, selected lipid levels, diabetes) and age-specific markers such as pulse pressure or arterial stiffness with further adjustment for sex may provide the best current estimates of cardiovascular risk in older people without known CAD.[116-118]

The Cardiovascular Health Study, a large population-based prospective study of community-dwelling adults older than age 65, has found the strongest predictors of death caused by an acute cardiac event to be a history of cardiac disease, myocardial infarction, or HF.[119] Diabetes was also associated with an increased risk of fatality, whereas other traditional risk factors such as hypertension, cholesterol levels, and body mass index were not. A diagnosis of stable angina has similarly been shown to identify increased risk for coronary events and mortality in older and younger patients.[120] Newer noncardiac markers such as cystatin-C may predict both cardiac and noncardiac death.[121]

HISTORY. Anginal symptoms are more likely to be absent and ischemia is more likely to be silent in older patients compared with young patients. Symptoms are likely to be termed "atypical" in older patients because the description differs from the classic description of substernal pressure with exertion. Symptoms may be described primarily as dyspnea, shoulder or back pain, weakness, fatigue (in women), or epigastric discomfort and may be precipitated by concurrent illnesses. Some older patients describe symptoms with effort, but others may not because of limited physical exertion or altered manifestations of pain caused by concomitant diabetes or possible age-related changes. Symptoms in these patients may occur at rest or during mental artress. Memory impairment may also limit the accuracy of the history. Lack of symptoms during evidence of myocardial ischemia on ECG (silent ischemia) has been reported in 20 to 50 percent of patients 65 years or older.

TESTING FOR ISCHEMIA (see Chap. 49). The high prevalence of resting ST-T wave abnormalities on ECG in older people results in a modest age-associated reduction in specificity of exercise electrocardiography. Treadmill exercise testing can provide prognostic information in patients able to exercise sufficiently and can also provide information regarding functional capacity and exercise tolerance. Exercise results can be enhanced by the use of modified protocols beginning with low-intensity exercise. ACC/AHA Guidelines on Exercise Testing estimate a slightly higher sensitivity (84 percent) and lower specificity (70 percent) in patients older than 75 years than in younger patients (see www.acc.org or www.americanheart.org). Echocardiography and nuclear testing can be used to overcome some of the limitations of ECG interpretation. In older patients unable to exercise, pharmacological agents such as dipyridamole or adenosine can be used with nuclear scintigraphy to assess myocardial perfusion at rest and after vasodilation, or agents such as dobutamine can be combined with echocardiography or other imaging techniques to assess ventricular function at rest and during increased myocardial demand.

The Screening for Heart Attack Prevention and Education (SHAPE) Task Force has proposed new practice guidelines that call for noninvasive screening with imaging (computed tomography [CT] for measurement of coronary artery calcification score [CACS] and B-mode ultrasound for measurement of carotid and carotid plaque) of all asymptomatic men 45 to 75 years of age and asymptomatic women 55 to 75 years of age (except those defined as very low risk).[122] The SHAPE authors recognize that application of the universal screening paradigm may not be cost effective in persons aged 75 years and older and that it would be more reasonable to treat these individuals as high risk. The value of such screening for asymptomatic CAD in the elderly is not known. What is known, however, is that the presence of coronary calcifications is high and neither the presence nor degree of coronary calcification has correlated with coronary flow decrease in the older population. Data are especially limited for women.[123,124] The high prevalence of hypertension, diabetes, obesity, and inactivity in the elderly including those aged 65 to 75 years would suggest that increased efforts in improving diet and activity levels, smoking cessation, treatment of hypertension and diabetes, and optimizing renal function would be of greater benefit on overall morbidity and mortality than screening with vascular imaging studies in the asymptomatic elderly.

Treatment

MEDICAL

Therapeutic goals and management goals that have been established for chronic stable angina are targeted at symptom relief with nitrates, beta blockers, calcium antagonists, and partial free fatty acid inhibitors or risk reduction and slowing the progression of disease with lifestyle modifications, lipid-lowering agents, and aspirin (see Chap. 54). Secondary prevention efforts are targeted at interventions conferring benefit within the anticipated lifespan of the patient.[125] Those with immediate benefits such as lifestyle changes of smoking cessation, increased activity, and weight control have a stronger likelihood of benefit. Aspirin benefits in men are established, whereas benefits in women, especially older women, are not as clear. Review of administrative databases report that only a fraction (19 percent) of community-dwelling elderly with either cardiovascular disease or diabetes receive lipid-lowering therapy with statins.[111,126,127] Increased use of cholesterol-lowering agents has been suggested as an area for quality of care improvement efforts.

Benefit from lipid-lowering regimens may not occur until after several years of treatment, with most data coming from secondary prevention trials of HMG CoA reductase inhibitors (Table 75-8). The Heart Protection Study (HPS) enrolled significant numbers of women and those older than age 73 with CAD and concomitant disease. The HPS demonstrated decreased total mortality in prespecified subgroups of women, patients older than 75 years of age, diabetics, and patients without elevated LDL cholesterol levels. The PROspective Study of Pravastatin in the Elderly at Risk (PROSPER) studied equal numbers of men and women aged 70 to 82 years who either had CHD or were at risk for cardiac events. A significant reduction in the primary composite endpoint of CHD death, nonfatal MI, and stroke, as well as in the secondary endpoint of CHD death plus nonfatal MI after 3 years of treatment, was reported. Prespecified subgroup analyses showed benefit for secondary prevention but not primary prevention, and in men but not women. Risk reduction was related to HDL-c but not LDL-c or apolipoprotein (apo) B. The incidence of rhabdomyolysis is low with

HMG CoA reductase inhibitors in randomized controlled trials. A higher incidence of statin-induced rhabdomyolysis has been observed when statins are used outside clinical trials.[128] Identified risk factors for statin-induced myopathy are older age (older than 80 years of age, and in women more than men), smaller body frame and frailty, multisystem disease (including chronic renal insufficiency, especially because of diabetes), the perioperative period, coadministration of certain medications (fibrates, nicotinic acid, cyclosporine, azole antifungals, macrolide antibiotics, erythromycin, clarithromycin, nefazodone, verapamil, amiodarone), hypothyroidism, and alcohol abuse. With higher doses, the incidence of myopathy also increases. An observational study of 7924 French patients, of whom 30 percent were older than age 65 years, receiving "high-dosage" statin therapy (atorvastatin 40 or 80 mg/day, fluvastatin 80 mg/day, pravastatin 40 mg/day, or simvastatin 40 or 80 mg/day) for at least 3 months found 10.5 percent of patients had muscular symptoms, with the incidence of muscle pain related to activity levels. Muscular pain required analgesics in 39

TABLE 75-8 | Major Trials of Lipid-Lowering Therapy with Elderly Participants

	Patients	N	% > 65(n) (% women, n)	Drug (Dose)	Major Results
Secondary Prevention					
Scandinavian Simvastatin Survival (4S) Trial (1,2)	CAD	4,444	23% (1021) (19%, 827)	Simvastatin (20-40 mg/d)	Reduced all-cause and CAD mortality, CAD events, coronary revascularization, and stroke
Cholesterol and Recurrent Events (CARE) Trial (3,4)	Post MI	4,159	31% (1283) (14%, 576)	Pravastatin (40 mg/d)	Reduced CAD mortality, death or events, coronary revascularization, and stroke
Long-term Intervention with Pravastatin in Ischemic Disease (LIPID) Study (5)	Post MI or unstable angina	9,014	39% (3514) (17%, 1516)	Pravastatin (40 mg/d)	Reduced all-cause mortality, CAD death or events, coronary revascularization, and stroke
Veterans Affairs Cooperative Studies Program High-Density Lipoprotein Cholesterol Intervention Trial (VA-HIT) (6)	CAD + high cholesterol and low HDL	2,531	76%* (1936) (0, 0)	Gemfibrozil (1200 mg/d)	Reduced death from cardiovascular causes, no difference in coronary revascularization rates
Heart Protection Study (HPS) (7)	CAD + other vascular disease, diabetes or hypertension	>20,000	28%† (5806) (33%, 5082)	Simvastatin (40 mg/d)	Reduced all cause mortality, reduced cardiovascular events, reduced coronary revascularizations, and reduced stroke
Pravastatin in elderly individuals at risk The PRO spective study of (PROSPER) (8)	CVD or high risk	5,804	100% (5804) (52%, 3000)	Pravastatin (40 mg/d)	Reduced composite endpoint of CHD death, nonfatal MI, and stroke; as well as CHD death plus nonfatal MI
Primary Prevention					
Antihypertensive and Lipid-Lowering Treatment to Prevent Heart Attack Trial (ALLHAT-LLT) (9)	Hypertension + one additional CVD risk factor	10,355	55%‡ (5707) (49%, 5051) 60% minorities	Pravastatin (40 mg/d) + anti-HTN	No significant reductions in total mortality, CHD or stroke with pravastatin versus usual care
Anglo-Scandinavian Cardiac Outcomes Trial—Lipid Lowering Arm (ASCOT-LLA) (10)	Hypertension + 3 additional CVD risk factors	10,305	64% (6570) (19%, 1942)	Atorvastatin (10 mg/d) + anti-HTN	Reduced cardiovascular deaths and nonfatal MI (no significant reduction in total mortality)

*Age older than 60.

†Age older than 70 years.

‡Age older than 65 years.

anti-HTN = antihypertensive medication; CAD = coronary artery disease; CHD = coronary heart disease; CVD = cardiovascular disease; HDL = high-density lipoprotein; MI = myocardial infarction.

From (1) Randomised trial of cholesterol lowering in 4444 patients with coronary heart disease: The Scandinavian Simvastatin Survival Study (4S). Lancet 344:1383-1389, 1994. (2) Miettinen T, Pyorala K, Olsson A, et al: Cholesterol-lowering therapy in women and elderly patients with myocardial infarction or angina pectoris. Findings from the Scandinavian Simvastatin Survival Study (4S). Circulation 96:4211-4218, 1997. (3) Sacks F, Pfeffer M, Moye L, et al: The effect of pravastatin on coronary events after myocardial infarction in patients with average cholesterol levels. Cholesterol and Recurrent Events Trial Investigators. N Engl J Med 335:1001-1009, 1996. (4) Lewis S, Moye L, Sacks F, et al: Effect of pravastatin on cardiovascular events in older patients with myocardial infarction and cholesterol levels in the average range. Results of the Cholesterol and Recurrent Events (CARE) Trial. Ann Intern Med 129:681-689, 1998. (5) The Long-Term Intervention with Pravastatin in Ischaemic Disease (LIPID) Study Group: Prevention of cardiovascular events and death with pravastatin in patients with coronary heart disease and a broad range of initial cholesterol levels. N Engl J Med 339:1349-1357, 1998. (6) Rubins H, Robins S, Collins D, et al; Veterans Affairs High-Density Lipoprotein Cholesterol Intervention Trial Study Group: Gemfibrozil for the secondary prevention of coronary heart disease in men with low levels of high-density lipoprotein cholesterol. N Engl J Med 341:410-418, 1999. (7) Heart Protection Study Collaborative Group: MRC/BHF Heart Protection Study of cholesterol lowering with simvastatin in 20,536 high-risk individuals: A randomised placebo-controlled trial. Lancet 360:7-22, 2002. (8) Shepherd J, Blauw G, Murphy M, et al: Pravastatin in elderly individuals at risk of vascular disease (PROSPER): A randomized controlled trial. Lancet 360:1623-1630, 2002. (9) ALLHAT Officers and Coordinators for the ALLHAT Collaborative Research Group: Major outcomes in moderately hypercholesterolemic, hypertensive patients randomized to pravastatin vs. usual care: The Antihypertensive and Lipid Lowering Treatment to Prevent Heart Attack Trial (ALLHAT-LLT). JAMA 288:2998-3007, 2002. (10) Sever P, Dahlof B, Poulter N, et al; ASCOT Investigators: Prevention of coronary and stroke events with atorvastatin in hypertensive patients who have average or lower-than-average cholesterol concentrations, in the Anglo-Scandinavian Cardiac Outcomes Trial—Lipid Lowering Arm (ASCOT-LLA): A multicentre randomised controlled trial. Lancet 361:1149-1158, 2003. For a comprehensive list that includes ongoing studies of statin trials, see Gotto AM: The benefits of statin therapy—what questions remain. Clin Cardiol 28:499-503, 2005.

CH 75

Cardiovascular Disease in the Elderly

percent, 38 percent reported inability to perform moderate exertion during daily activities, and 4 percent were either confined to bed or unable to work.[129] Although higher doses of statins for 6 years have been shown to decrease the number of CHD events in white male CAD patients (mean age of 61 years at study entry), risk of death from all causes was not reduced.[130] No outcome data on aggressive lipid lowering in CAD patients older than age 65, or for older women with CAD, are available.

Symptoms of myopathy may be difficult to differentiate from other types of musculoskeletal disorders or pain in the older patient or may not be recognized because of cognitive impairment. The most common complaints may also be nonspecific or described as "flulike," and fatigue may be nearly as common as muscle pain. In older patients the smallest effective dose should be used. Signs and symptoms should be monitored, and there should be a low threshold for laboratory tests. Muscle strength testing may be helpful in evaluating symptoms in older patients including simple assessments of ability to rise from a chair or climb stairs. Aggressive lipid lowering should be reserved for selected younger elderly patients with longer life expectancy and should be accompanied by monitoring for adverse effects.

STATINS FOR PRIMARY PREVENTION. The elderly have not been the target of most primary prevention trials of lipid lowering. Of the two early large primary prevention trials of lipid lowering with HMG CoA reductase inhibitors, one only enrolled men up to age 64 and the other had an upper age cutoff of 73 years of age.[131,132] The Antihypertensive and Lipid-Lowering Treatment to Prevent Heart Attack Trial (ALLHAT) compared unblinded treatment of hypertension plus lipid-lowering therapy with "usual care" in hypertensives with at least one additional CHD risk factor (see Table 75-8). Half of the participants were older than age 65 years (*n* = 5707), and 60 percent were minorities. No benefit of statin therapy (over blood pressure treatment effects) was found in any subgroup, with cholesterol reduction in the treated group smaller than in prior placebo-controlled statin trials. The Lipid Lowering Arm of the Anglo-Scandinavian Cardiac Outcomes Trial (ASCOT-LLA) tested the effects of lipid lowering in hypertensive patients up to age 79 years without increased lipids but with at least three additional CHD risk factors (see Table 75-8). ASCOT-LLA was stopped after 3.3 years because of a significant reduction in the composite cardiovascular endpoint of fatal and nonfatal cardiac events without significant differences in all-cause mortality. Prespecified subgroups of women, diabetics, patients with metabolic syndrome, nonobese, and those with prior vascular diseases did not show CHD benefit.

CURRENT CONTROVERSIES: LIPID-LOWERING STRATEGIES IN THE ELDERLY

- Primary prevention with statin administration, especially in women.
- CHD and mortality risk-related to lipid subfractions-HDL-c versus LDL-c versus apo B
- Benefit of secondary prevention with statins on total mortality or CHD mortality in women or minorities
- HDL-c as a treatment target
- Optimal targets (and doses) for lipid lowering
- Frequency of statin-induced myalgias/myopathy in older patients
- Extent of underutilization of statins in clinical practice
- Benefits of lipid lowering on cerebrovascular disease

SPECIAL CONSIDERATIONS WITH PHARMACOLOGICAL TREATMENT OF THE ELDERLY CAD PATIENT. (See also "Medication Therapy—Modifications for the Older Patient" earlier). Marked vasodilation caused by rapid absorption or higher peak effects of isosorbide dinitrates can exacerbate postural hypotension, so agents with smooth concentration versus time profiles such as mononitrates or transdermal formulations may be preferred for daily administration, although cost may be prohibitive. Beta blockers have not been shown to increase the occurrence of depression in randomized trials, but beta blockers that are not lipophilic (e.g., atenolol, nadolol) may produce fewer CNS effects. Calcium channel blockers, especially the dihydropyridines, can produce pedal edema more frequently in the older

patient. Shorter-acting formulations can produce or exacerbate postural hypotension and should be avoided. Verapamil can exacerbate constipation, especially in the inactive elderly. Both beta blockers and nondihydropyridine calcium channel blockers should be avoided in the presence of sick sinus node disease. In older women, hormone replacement therapy is not indicated for either primary prevention of CHD or treatment of CHD. Adverse effects of dizziness, constipation, nausea, asthenia, headache dyspepsia and abdominal pain with the newer piperazine derivative ranolazine are more common in elderly patients, and women may have less exercise benefit with ranolazine compared with men.

REVASCULARIZATION

There is increased experience with both percutaneous coronary intervention (PCI) and coronary artery bypass grafting (CABG) in older patients (see Chap. 55). Half of all PCI and CABG procedures are performed in patients older than 65 years of age, with one third of coronary artery revascularization procedures performed in patients older than 70 years of age, and increasing numbers of women are undergoing revascularization. Randomized trials of revascularization have demonstrated efficacy and successful outcomes in patients, usually with limited numbers of older patients (Table 75-9). The Bypass Angioplasty Revascularization Investigation (BARI) trial of patients with multivessel disease included 109 patients older than the age of 75 years. Patients aged 65 to 80 had higher early morbidity and mortality after CABG compared with PCI but greater angina relief and fewer repeat procedures after CABG. Stroke was more common after CABG than after PCI (1.7 versus 0.2 percent), and HF and pulmonary edema were more common after PCI (4.0 versus 1.3 percent). The 5-year survival rate was more than 80 percent for both procedures (86 percent after CABG and 81.4 percent after PCI) in these highly selected patients, with women and minorities underrepresented.

Information about the outcomes of elderly patients following revascularization as part of "routine" clinical care is emerging from clinical and administrative databases (Fig. 75-7). These patients tend to be older, have more multivessel disease and comorbid conditions than those in randomized studies, have lower long-term survival rates, and have complication rates that are higher than reported in randomized trials. Early CABG mortality rates increase from less than 2 percent in patients younger than 60 years of age to between 6 and 8 percent in patients older than age 75 years with rates approaching 10 percent in patients older than age 80. Elderly women are at highest risk, in part because of comorbid conditions. In a single site series of CABG patients with ejection fractions less than 35 percent, early-operative mortality was higher in older patients and 5-year survival was less than 30 percent for patients 75 years of age and older.[133] For patients older than the age of 90 years, operative mortality has been reported as 11.8 percent from the Society of Thoracic Surgeons Database. Renal function, usually estimated by algorithms that include age and sex in addition to creatinine, has emerged as an important predictor of morbidity and mortality after CABG.[35,133]

PCI AND PCI VERSUS CABG. Registry data suggest in-hospital mortality risk of PCI of less than 1 percent in patients younger than 60 years of age that increases to about 4 percent in patients older than 75 years and is greater than 5 percent in patients older than 80 years of age (see Fig. 75-7). The Northern New England Cardiovascular Disease Study Group reported preliminary nonrandomized data from nearly 1700 patients older than the age of 80 treated for two- or three-vessel disease (excluding left main) that found better in-hospital mortality and short-term survival for PCI versus CABG (in-hospital mortality 3 percent versus 6 percent, respectively.)[134] For those surviving past 6 months, survival was better for patients who underwent CABG. PCI data were from bare metal stent implants, and CABG data were from on-pump procedures in more than 85 percent.

Nonfatal complications with procedures also increase with age. PCI is associated with a slightly less than 1 percent risk of permanent stroke or coma, and CABG is associated with a 3 to 6 percent incidence of permanent stroke or coma in patients older than 75 years of age. In the

Trial Name	Enrollment Yr	Treatment Comparisons	Number Enrolled	Age Inclusion	Number enrolled ≥75 yr of Age
CASS	1970s	CABG versus medical	780	Age ≤65 yr	0
VA	1970s	CABG versus medical	686	None	0
European	1970s	CABG versus medical	767	Age <65 yr	0
RITA	1980s-1990s	CABG versus PCI	1011	None	22
EAST	1980s-1990	CABG versus PCI	392	None	36
GABI	1986-1991	CABG versus PCI	359	Age <75 yr	0
CABRI	1980s-1990s	CABG versus PCI	1054	Age ≤75 yr	0
BARI	Late 1980s-1990s	CABG versus PCI	1829	Age <80 yr	109
ERACI	1980s	CABG versus PCI	127	Age <76 yr	N/A (few)
ACME	Late 1980s	PCI versus medical	328	N/A (mean = 60 yr)	N/A
ARTS	1997-1998	PCI + stent versus CABG	1205	Age ≤83 yr	70*
TIME	1996-2000	PCI or CABG versus medical	282	>75 yr	282
Senior-PAMI	>2000	Thrombolysis versus PCI	483	>70 yr	N/A

TABLE 75–9 | Representation of Elderly Patients with Coronary Artery Disease in Trials of Revascularization

ACME = Angioplasty Compared to Medicine Study (VA study); ARTS = Arterial Revascularization Therapy Study Trial; BARI = Bypass Angioplasty Revascularization Investigation; CABG = coronary artery bypass grafting; CABRI = Coronary Artery versus Bypass Revascularization Investigation; CASS = Coronary Artery Surgery Study; EAST = Emory Angioplasty versus Surgery Trial; ERACI = Argentine Randomized Trial of Percutaneous Transluminal Coronary Angioplasty versus Coronary Artery Bypass Surgery in Multivessel Disease; European = European Coronary Surgery Study; GABI = German Angioplasty versus Bypass Surgery Trial; N/A = not available; PCI = percutaneous coronary intervention; RITA = Randomized Intervention Treatment of Angina; Senior PAMI = Senior Primary Angioplasty in Myocardial Infarction Trial; TIME = Trial of Invasive versus Medical Therapy in Elderly patients; VA = VA Cooperative Study of Coronary Artery Bypass for Stable Angina.

*Personal communication.

immediate postoperative period, longer durations of ventilatory support, greater need for inotropic support and intraaortic balloon placement, and greater incidence of atrial fibrillation, bleeding, delirium, renal failure, perioperative infarction, and infection are seen in older patients compared with younger patients. *N*-acetylcysteine has been reported to prevent contrast-induced nephropathy from PCI. The highest rates of complications are usually seen in older women and in patients undergoing emergency procedures.

In addition to the increased immediate mortality and morbidity associated with revascularization in older patients, the duration of disability and rehabilitation after procedures is usually longer in the older person. The risk of postoperative cognitive impairment in older patients detected with neuropsychological testing has been estimated as 25 to 50 percent after CABG.[135-137] Smaller randomized trials have reported both improved cognitive outcomes and no difference in outcomes with use of off-pump versus on-pump CABG. Reports of lack of differences in quality of life between the two approaches in the first year after surgery have been more consistent in younger than older patients. Meta-analyses suggest that early outcomes may be improved in elderly patients with off-pump compared with on-pump CABG.[138]

Preoperative considerations in the older patients should address cognition and the potential need for in-home assistance or extended care hospitalization after surgery. Postoperative considerations should also include evaluation for depression (see later).

One study compared invasive (PCI or CABG) versus optimized medical therapy in CAD patients older than 75 years with angina refractory to standard therapy (TIME) (see Table 75-9). Although the initial analysis at 6 months reported an advantage for revascularization, the advantage was no longer present at 1 year. Revascularization presented an early risk of death and complications whereas optimized medical therapy carried a chance of later events (hospitalization and revascularization) without a clear advantage of either strategy. This study enrolled significant numbers of patients older than 75 years and enrolled significant numbers of women (40 percent).

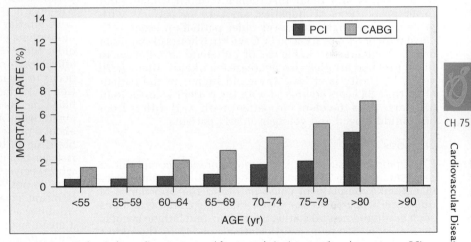

FIGURE 75–7 In-hospital mortality rates reported for revascularization procedures by age group. PCI = percutaneous intervention of all types, CABG = coronary artery bypass graft surgery. *(From the National Cardiovascular Revascularization Network as reported by Alexander K, Anstrom K, Muhlbaier L, et al: Outcomes of cardiac surgery in patients ≥80 years: Results from the National Cardiovascular Network. JACC 35:731-738, 2000 (www.sgcard.org); Batchelor W, Anstrom K, Muhlbaier L, et al: Contemporary outcome trends in the elderly undergoing percutaneous coronary interventions: Results in 7472 octogenarians. JACC 36:723-730, 2000; and from the Society of Thoracic Surgeons Database, Bridges C, Edwards F, Peterson E, et al: Cardiac surgery in nonagenarian and centenarians. JACS 197:347-356, 2003. Data were not available for PCI in patients older than 90 years of age.)*

SPECIAL CONSIDERATIONS IN THE OLDER PATIENT UNDERGOING REVASCULARIZATION. ACC/AHA Coronary Artery Bypass Surgery and PCI Guidelines conclude that age alone should not be used as the sole criterion when considering revascularization procedures (see www.acc.org or www. americanheart.org). Individualized prognostic information based on multiple clinical factors and respect for patient preference in the decision-making process has a clear role. The possibility of disability or prolonged hospitalization after interventions must be considered and accurately conveyed to the patient. Short- and long-term benefits should be considered in the context of anticipated life span and quality of life of the patient. Death, recurrent angina, or MI may not be viewed as carrying the same negative impact as a disabling stroke to many older patients. For the patient unable to make decisions, involvement of family members or agents is key to choices reflecting the prior wishes of the patient.

CURRENT ISSUES IN REVASCULARIZATION OF THE ELDERLY

- Modifiable risk factors for revascularization mortality and morbidity in older patients
  - Role of N-acetylcysteine in preventing contrast-induced nephropathy with PCI
  - Target for glucose control periprocedurally
  - Age-adjusted PCI and CABG protocol regimens
- Prevention of cognitive decline after CABG
- Benefits of on- versus off-pump surgery, especially in women
- Comparisons between medical therapy and revascularization
- Appropriate selection criteria for specific therapies for octogenarians and nonagenarians

Acute Coronary Syndromes (see Chaps. 50 to 53)

About 60 percent of hospital admissions for acute myocardial infarction (AMI) are in people older than 65 years, and approximately 85 percent of deaths caused by AMI occur in this group. With increasing age, the gender composition of patients presenting with AMI changes from predominantly men presenting in middle age, to an equal number of men and women presenting between the ages of 75 and 84, to the majority of patients with AMI being women older than 80 years of age. Mortality rates are usually higher in older women than in older men with AMI, as are adverse outcomes with thrombolytics, fibrinolytics, and glycoprotein (GP) IIb/IIIa inhibitors. As age increases past 65 years, there are more patients with functional limitation, HF, prior coronary disease, and renal insufficiency; more women; and lower proportions of diabetics, smokers, or patients with prior revascularization. Fewer older patients present with chest pain or ST elevation on ECG within 6 hours of symptom onset. Angiographic evidence of collateral circulation to infarct-related arteries also decreases markedly after age 70 years. Mortality is at least threefold higher in the patient older than 85 years compared with the patient younger than 65 years. Thus the older old patient with AMI differs from both middle-aged and younger elderly patients.

DIAGNOSIS

Chest pain or discomfort is the most common complaint in patients up to age 75 years, but after age 80 years a minority of patients complain of chest pain and the prevalence of diaphoresis decreases (see Chap. 49). Nonspecific symptoms such as altered mental status, confusion, and fatigue become increasingly common manifestations of MI in the oldest patients. Older patients may also present with sudden pulmonary edema or neurological symptoms such as syncope or stroke. The ECG is also more likely to be nondiagnostic without ST-segment elevation but with baseline abnormalities of ventricular hypertrophy or intraventricular conduction or pacing (see Chap. 12). The combination of nonspecific symptoms and nondiagnostic ECG findings leads to delays in diagnosis and implementation of therapy and highlights the importance of rapid laboratory testing for circulating markers of myocardial damage such as the troponins.

TREATMENT

REPERFUSION

Thrombolysis (see Chap. 51). Randomized clinical trials of the effects of thrombolysis enrolled few patients older than 75 to 80 years of age, and those enrolled represented a younger, healthier subset of the elderly in the community. For patients up to the age of 75 years, most trials show that fibrinolytic, antiplatelet, and antithrombin therapy is associated with a survival advantage compared with placebo that may be similar to or less than that seen in younger

patients.[139] Complication rates of minor and major bleeding and transfusion rates are higher in older patients compared with younger patients with all agents, especially with improper dosing of antiplatelet and antithrombin agents. Population-based studies have suggested that community-dwelling elderly patients older than age 75 years treated with thrombolytics have an increased risk of intracranial hemorrhage (ICH) that approximates 1.4 percent,[140] and some subgroups may not have an overall benefit from use of thrombolytics.[141,142] Those with high risk for ICH include patients older than 75 years, women, African Americans, small size (<65 kg in women and <80 kg in men), prior stroke, and systolic blood pressure >160 mm Hg. Fibrin-specific agents such as tissue plasminogen activator are also associated with increased stroke risk caused by ICH in the older than 75- to 80-year age group. Most agents are administered in combination with low-molecular-weight heparins, and dosage adjustments for weight and estimated glomerular filtration may decrease risks of bleeding. Even with dose adjustments, however, the risk of bleeding appears increased in older patients.[143] Cardiac rupture risk with thrombolysis is also increased in patients older than 70 years of age and in women, with an incidence of 0.5 to 2 percent. The risk of cardiac rupture does not appear to be related to the intensity of anticoagulation.

Antithrombotic Agents. Trial data show aspirin reduces mortality in patients older than 70 years and is recommended for routine administration to older patients with AMI,[144] although older patients have been less likely to receive aspirin than younger patients in routine clinical practice. The addition of clopidogrel to aspirin after non–ST-elevation MI reduces major event rates by 20 percent, with similar absolute reductions in patients younger and older than 65 years, without significant data on patients older than 75 years.[145] Newer GP IIb/IIIa inhibitors appear efficacious in older patients, although net benefit may not occur in patients over age 75 years when given in combination with half-doses of thrombolytics. In clinical trials, bleeding risk including intracranial hemorrhage is increased about twofold with GP IIb/IIIa inhibitors, with the risk being about 2 percent. Registry data estimate the increased risk of bleeding to be similar, with an estimated twofold greater risk for bleeding (or 2 percent) in patients undergoing PCI who receive GP IIb/IIIa inhibitors compared with patients who do not.[146] A review of the U.S. Food and Drug Administration adverse event reports in the presence of GP IIb/IIIa inhibitor administration found the deaths in patients with a mean age of 69 to be associated with excessive bleeding, with intracranial bleeding as the most common site of fatal bleeds.[147]

Antiplatelet and antithrombin agents have narrow therapeutic windows with dosing recommendations based on weight and renal function. Prospective observational analyses have shown that more than 40 percent of patients with acute coronary syndromes receiving unfractionated heparin, low-molecular-weight heparin, or GP IIb/IIIa inhibitors receive at least one dose in excess of guidelines.[40] Factors associated with excess dosing were older age, female sex, renal insufficiency, low body weight, diabetes mellitus, and congestive HF. Bleeding increased relative to the degree of excess dose and to the number of agents administered in excess. Mortality was higher and length of hospital stay was longer in patients administered excess dosing. Women had twofold higher rates of major bleeding than men and were three times more likely to receive excess GP IIb/IIIa doses than men. Approximately 25 percent of the bleeding risk was attributable to excess dosing in women versus 4.4 percent in men.[41] A randomized, controlled clinical trial for treatment of acute MI with PCI with eptifibatide administration has also reported increased bleeding resulting from lack of dose adjustment for reduced renal function.[43] These data highlight the need for adjustment of dosing of antithrombin and antiplatelet agents for estimated renal clearance (see Table 75-2).

Invasive Strategies. Results from several studies and database reviews have suggested that primary angioplasty in experienced centers is associated with improved outcomes compared with thrombolytic strategies in elderly patients with ST-elevation acute MI (see Chap. 52).[139] Even when mortality is reduced with primary PCI compared with thrombolytic therapy, in-hospital mortality of patients older than the age of 75 years is estimated to be fivefold higher (5 percent) than patients younger than 75 years, and 1-year mortality is 7-fold greater (11 percent). Advantages of PCI over thrombolytics in acute coronary syndromes of younger individuals may not be apparent unless patients can undergo revascularization within 90 minutes of presentation. Achieving this may be less likely in older patients with delays in diagnosis and/or transport to experienced centers. Acute procedural success rates are also somewhat lower than in younger MI populations and are associated with increased bleeding at the access site, as well as increased transfusion requirements. PCI procedures are also associated with an increased risk for contrast-mediated renal dysfunction in older patients.

The potential benefits of PCI compared with those of fibrinolysis in older patients with acute MI were directly compared in the Senior PAMI (Primary Angioplasty in Myocardial Infarction) study. The study was stopped early because of low recruitment, but preliminary reports found primary PCI to be superior to thrombolytic therapy from ages 65 to 79 with no advantage of primary PCI over thrombolysis in those older than 80 years of age.[148] Death rates were 16 to 19 percent in patients older than 80 years of age. The only subset of older patients with MI that have long-term survival advantages with early revascularization compared with medical stabilization in clinical trials is the subset with cardiogenic shock caused by LV failure.[149]

ADDITIONAL PHARMACOLOGICAL AGENTS

Beta Blockers. Beta blocker administration is recommended for all patients with AMI regardless of age in the absence of contraindications. Age-related dosage adjustments are appropriate.

Angiotensin-Converting Enzyme Inhibitors. In the presence of LV systolic dysfunction or anterior wall MI, ACE inhibitors are recommended within the first 24 hours of onset of AMI. ACE inhibitors are recommended after 24 hours for all other MI patients, especially those with reduced LV ejection and prior MI. As with other agents in the elderly, smaller initial doses and slower titration are indicated, as is close monitoring of renal function.

GUIDELINES AND CLINICAL PRACTICE OF ACUTE CORONARY SYNDROME CARE IN THE ELDERLY. In an analysis of community practice outcomes as part of the Can Rapid Risk Stratification of Unstable Angina Patients Suppress Adverse Outcomes With Early Implementation of the ACC/AHA Guidelines (CRUSADE), the use of five recommended therapies, including early use of aspirin, beta blockers, heparin, GP IIb/IIIa inhibitors and cardiac catheterization, were evaluated.[150] The risk of in-hospital mortality declined as a function of the number of guideline-recommended therapies given in patients aged 75 years and older, with greater benefit with use of guideline-recommended therapies in older compared with younger patients. The guidelines recommend special attention to altered dosing and sensitivity of older patients and the need for close observation for adverse effects of intensive medical and interventional management in elderly subgroups with acute coronary syndromes.

Post-Myocardial Infarction

MEDICATIONS

Recommendations for administration of aspirin, beta blockers, ACE inhibitors or ARBs, and lipid lowering drugs for the post-MI patient are based on clinical trial data showing benefit in populations that have included elderly patients.

Data suggest that these agents are underutilized in older patients, especially women and minorities. Analyses of care delivery to Medicare recipients estimate that 24 percent of eligible patients 65 years of age or older are not prescribed aspirin at the time of discharge following acute MI, and 50 percent are not prescribed a beta blocker.[151] Patients older than 75 years of age are even less likely to receive these therapies than patients 65 to 74 years of age. In contrast, calcium antagonist drugs may be more frequently prescribed in the older post-MI patient than younger post-MI patients. Routine administration of antiarrhythmic agents after MI (with the exception of beta blockers) has no role (see Chap. 33).

ANTIDEPRESSANTS. Depression is considered relatively common in the elderly, affecting 10 percent of community-dwelling older people (see Chap. 86). The prevalence of depression in patients after MI is estimated at 20 to 30 percent for major depression and up to 50 percent for potentially significant symptoms of depression.[152] Studies have shown associations between depression and low perceived social support and increased cardiac morbidity and mortality in post-MI patients[153] and in patients undergoing CABG.[154] Individual trials of counseling interventions in patients with depression have not shown cardiac benefit, whereas meta-analyses suggest benefit.[155] Trials have addressed the efficacy and safety of SSRI antidepressant therapy in patients with depression after acute coronary syndromes or myocardial infarction. The results suggest benefits of SSRI use on either cardiac events and mortality (perhaps because of antiplatelet properties) or quality of life and overall function, especially in patients with a prior history of depression.

General recommendations for all older patients with chronic medical diseases include screening for depression. Initial screening can take the form of a simple two-question test followed by additional evaluation for patients with answers suggesting the presence of depression. Alternatively, the nine-item Patient Health self-report questionnaire screening instrument can be used in literate patients, or the geriatric depression screen for older patients can be administered.[156] Increasing evaluation and use of SSRIs (citalopram, escitalopram, fluoxetine, fluvoxamine, paroxetine, and sertraline) and mixed-mechanism antidepressants (bupropion, venlafaxine, duloxetine, nefazodone, trazodone, and mirtazapine) has led to recognition of side effects, as well as efficacy. Of particular importance to the cardiologist is hyponatremia with SSRIs and that antiplatelet effects of SSRIs can increase the risk of bleeding when used in combination with warfarin, low-molecular-weight heparin, or aspirin or in patients with hereditary platelet defects.[157] The first-generation SSRI fluoxetine has been associated with an increased risk of syncope in elderly patients.

MODIFICATIONS IN THERAPY FOR OLDER POST-MI PATIENTS. Analyses of older post-MI patients who were prescribed beta blockers showed a greater risk of rehospitalization with HF if given high doses compared with low doses.[158] Higher use of beta blockers in the post-MI regimen of older patients might possibly be reached if recommendations were for lower and better-tolerated doses of these drugs.

HORMONE REPLACEMENT THERAPY. Randomized trials comparing administration of hormone replacement therapy in the form of combined estrogen and progesterone or estrogen alone have shown overall lack of cardiovascular morbidity or mortality benefit and potential harm for both secondary and primary prevention in postmenopausal women. Selective estrogen modulators have also been evaluated. Similar to estrogen, raloxifene lowered LDL cholesterol and increased HDL cholesterol but did not decrease coronary event rates in a placebo-controlled trial (Raloxifene Use for the Heart (RUTH)) in 10,101 postmenopausal women who had CHD or multiple risk factors for CHD.[159] Stroke rates and thromboembolism rates were increased with raloxifene. A comparison of raloxifene to tamoxifen for prevention of breast cancer in women at high risk for breast cancer found equivalent efficacy in invasive breast cancer reduction, equivalent risks for ischemic disease and stroke, and a lower risk of thromboembolic events with raloxifene.[160] Estrogen, estrogen plus progesterone, raloxifene, and tamoxifen cannot be recommended for cardiovascular disease prevention or treatment.

CH 75

Cardiovascular Disease in the Elderly

The feasibility and improvement with intensive exercise interventions have been shown for both the frailest elderly residing in the community as well as in the nursing home. The recent Cardiac Rehabilitation in Advanced Age (CR-AGE) trial compared hospital-based cardiac rehabilitation with home-based cardiac rehabilitation in cognitively intact patients from ages 46 to 86 with recent MI.[161] Similar improvement in total work capacity and health-related quality of life was seen with home-based rehabilitation compared with hospital-based rehabilitation in all age groups without improvement in the control group. The improvement, however, was somewhat smaller in the group older than age 75. Benefits decreased over time after hospital rehabilitation but were maintained with home cardiac rehabilitation. Complications were similar across groups, whereas costs were lower in the home rehabilitation group.

Table 75-10 summarizes the approach to the older patient with CAD.

Carotid Artery Disease/Stroke

PREVALENCE/INCIDENCE

Stroke is the third leading cause of death and is the most common cause of disability in the United States (see Chap. 58). The risk of stroke increases with age and doubles for each decade after age 55 years. Framingham data estimate the 10-year probability of stroke at 11 percent in men age 65 and 7 percent for women age 65. At age 80, the probability increases to 22 and 24 percent for men and women, respectively. After age 85 years, women are at greater risk than men. Carotid stenosis is responsible for approximately 25 percent of strokes, and atrial fibrillation for approximately 15 percent. Although transient ischemic attacks (TIAs) signal a high short-term risk of stroke, 70 percent of strokes are first events leading to increasing emphasis on primary prevention. Nonmodifiable risk factors for stroke include age, sex (men > women), race/ethnicity (African Americans > Caucasians), and a family history of stroke. Modifiable risk factors for noncardioembolic ischemic stroke or TIA in the elderly are hypertension, smoking and passive smoking, hyperlipidemia, lack of physical activity, inadequate treatment of atrial fibrillation, carotid artery disease, and HF. Diabetes confers additional risk. Sleep apnea has recently been identi-

fied as a potentially modifiable risk factor, as has estrogen administration to postmenopausal women (see Chap. 74).

Diagnosis

The diagnosis of TIA is made following a spell of neurological impairment lasting less than 24 hours that is produced by ischemia in a discrete vascular territory in the brain. The diagnosis is usually based on clinical history alone. Neurological deficits will not be present unless there has been prior stroke or disease. Diagnosis of significant carotid disease is usually made in the presence of a stenosis greater than 70 to 80 percent defined by noninvasive imaging with Doppler ultrasound, magnetic resonance angiography, or less frequently with CT angiography (see Chaps. 14, 17, and 18). Carotid bruits may or may not be present, and carotid disease may be asymptomatic. A lopsided face, weak arm, and garbled speech are the most common warning signs of stroke. The Face, Arm, Speech, Time (FAST) mnemonic can help identify patients with a potential stroke. Rapid triage to neuroimaging for diagnosis and selection of appropriate therapy is advised. The Brain Attack Coalition advocates establishment of both primary stroke centers and comprehensive stroke centers to care for patients with complex stroke types, severe deficits, or multiorgan disease.[162]

Treatment

ACUTE STROKE MANAGEMENT[163]

Brain imaging is required to guide the selection of acute interventions. CT is used most commonly with magnetic resonance imaging as an alternative. Blood pressure management in the setting of acute stroke remains controversial with aggressive reduction in pressure not generally recommended. When hypertension is treated, intravenous agents are recommended for initial therapy (labetalol or nicardipidine for systolic or mixed hypertension with diastolic pressures <140 mm Hg; nitroprusside for diastolic pressures >140 mm Hg). Blood pressure control should precede thrombolytic therapy. Pharmacological thrombolysis with recombinant tissue plasminogen activator (rt-PA) is recommended for selected patients with ischemic stroke with a measurable neurological deficit (see Chap. 58) in whom it can be administered within 3 hours of stroke onset. Most contraindications relate to potential bleeding caused by trauma, surgery, MI, active bleeding, anticoagulation, low platelets, prior intracranial hemorrhage or suggestion of subarachnoid hemorrhage, uncontrolled hypertension, and the presence of a major deficit. The subtypes of ischemic stroke are not thought to influence responses to rtPA. No age-specific recommendations for rtPA have been made, but delays in diagnosis are more likely in the elderly. Symptomatic hemorrhagic transformation of the infarction after rtPA administration occurs in slightly more than 5.2 percent of patients and can be reduced by proper patient selection. Orolingual angioedema occurs in about 5 percent and is more common in patients taking ACE inhibitors and those with ischemia in the frontal cortex and insula. The role of intraarterial thrombolysis alone or in combination with intravenous thrombolysis is undergoing evaluation. Data support administration of aspirin within 48 hours of acute stroke for most patients but do not support early anticoagulation with unfractionated or low-molecular-weight heparin or use of other antiplatelet agents. The 2005 stroke guidelines conclude that none of the methods of mechanical thrombolysis have been adequately tested to allow recommendations.[163] The poststroke management should include early initiation of rehabilitation therapy, a swallow screening testing for dysphagia, an active secondary stroke prevention program, and proactive prevention of venous thrombi. Evaluation for depression and medical

TABLE 75–10	Approach to the Older Patient with Coronary Artery Disease (CAD)

Morbidity and mortality from CAD and CAD treated medically or with revascularization increases with age, especially in patients older than age 75, after which there are no clear advantages of one method of treatment of CAD over another.

Clinically recognized CAD or heart failure confer the greatest risk for cardiac death and warrant aggressive secondary prevention strategies.

For acute coronary syndromes the following apply:
For patients 65-79 yr of age presenting to a hospital where direct PCI can be performed rapidly by experienced operators, PCI may have an advantage over thrombolysis.
For patients older than age 80, reperfusion therapy with thrombolytic agents initiated rapidly after presentation (in the absence of contraindications) is the first choice.

Decisions regarding medical therapy versus revascularization or for PCI versus CABG should be based on the role of CAD in the context of the individual older patient's overall health, lifestyle, projected life span, and preferences.

Anticipated procedural complication rates should reflect the age and health status of the patient, not complication rates from series of younger patients:
Recovery times will be prolonged from all procedures.
Depression should be evaluated.

CABG = coronary artery bypass graft; PCI = percutaneous coronary intervention.

therapy for depression or emotional lability is also strongly recommended.[164]

PREVENTION

Secondary and primary prevention is targeted at modifiable risk factors. Evidence-based recommendations are for antiplatelet therapy in patients with prior stroke, TIA, or myocardial infarction and anticoagulation in high-risk patients such as those with stroke on aspirin or with atrial fibrillation (see Chap. 35). Carotid artery interventions should be considered for patients with severe lesions or symptomatic disease.[165] Clinical trials with limited numbers of elderly and very elderly have also demonstrated that LDL cholesterol reduction with statins reduces the risk of stroke in patients with cardiovascular disease (CVD) or major CVD risk factors.[166] A trial of aggressive lipid lowering for prevention of stroke in patients with a mean age of 63 years had preliminary findings of reduced stroke rate without a difference between groups in all-cause mortality at 5 years but with more hemorrhagic strokes with aggressive lipid lowering.[167] The benefit of LDL-c reduction on prevention of stroke is less clear in the elderly, and aggressive lipid lowering has not been investigated. Smoking cessation and avoidance of second-hand smoke, weight control, limited alcohol intake, and increased activity are part of a preventive strategy. Primary prevention with low-dose aspirin is recommended for women at high risk, as is avoidance of estrogen therapy.

MEDICATIONS

ANTIPLATELET DRUGS

Aspirin reduces the long-term risk of stroke, as well as cardiovascular events, after stroke or TIA and is considered standard therapy after a stroke regardless of patient age. The beneficial role of other agents such as the thienopyridine drugs ticlopidine and clopidogrel that inhibit platelet aggregation by blocking platelet adenosine diphosphate receptors is less clear. Ticlopidine-induced hematological side effects have limited its clinical use. Clopidogrel has substantially lower rates of hematological side effects compared with ticlopidine but is considerably more expensive than aspirin. Secondary prevention trials with clopidogrel that enrolled stroke patients found reductions in composite endpoints that included stroke, but the effect was not as great as the reduction in peripheral artery disease events. Combined aspirin and clopidogrel have failed to show additive benefit in two large clinical trials but markedly increase moderate and major bleeding. The combination is not recommended.[168,169] Combined aspirin and extended-release dipyridamole have been reported to prevent more strokes than placebo or ASA or dipyridamole but are associated with greater gastrointestinal intolerance, headache, cost, and drug discontinuation.[170] A comparison of warfarin and aspirin did not find significant differences in the prevention of recurrent ischemic stroke or death or occurrence of serious adverse events.[171]

In most reports, bleeding complications with antiplatelet drugs are more frequent in older compared with younger patients. No dose-response relationship was observed for the protective effects of aspirin from 50 to 1000 mg/day, whereas larger doses increased the risk of gastrointestinal bleeding. Although the minimally effective dose for aspirin has not been determined, lower doses are recommended for the older patient, in particular.

ANTICOAGULANT DRUGS

Antithrombotic prophylaxis should be individualized on the basis of the estimated risk for stroke during aspirin therapy and the risk for bleeding during anticoagulation with warfarin. For older patients at moderate and higher risk for stroke, anticoagulation with warfarin is appropriate, unless contraindicated. The target INR is 2-3. Both initial and maintenance warfarin doses are usually lower in older adults compared with middle-aged patients, with initiation of warfarin at the estimated maintenance dosage of warfarin (usually 2-5 mg daily in the elderly) recommended, followed by frequent monitoring (see www.americangeriatrics.org and www.warfarindosing.org). See Table 75-11 for a summary of the approach to anticoagulation in the older patient.

SURGICAL AND ENDOVASCULAR APPROACHES

Several clinical trials have demonstrated that carotid endarterectomy (CEA) in symptomatic patients with 70 to 99 percent internal carotid artery (ICA) stenosis who have had a stroke or TIA attributable to the stenosis is safe and effective in reducing the risk of ipsilateral carotid ischemia.[165] Surgery has performed better compared with medical treatment in preventing disabling ipsilateral stroke (Fig. 75-8).[172] Benefit is less certain in patients with stenosis of 50 to 69 percent. Benefit is greatest in those with more severe stenosis, those older than age 75, in men, and in those with recent stroke. Revascularization is not recommended for patients with lesions of less than 50 percent. In asymptomatic patients with carotid stenoses, revascularization carries a risk and is less likely to benefit the patient. To achieve a net beneficial effect of CEA versus medical therapy alone, the combined mortality and morbidity rate should be less than 3 percent for asymptomatic patients and less than 7 percent for symptomatic patients. Increased risk of perioperative stroke or death is seen with surgery for completed stroke (versus TIA), female sex, age older than 75 years, systolic blood pressure greater than 180 mm Hg, and a history of peripheral vascular disease. Intracranial vascular disease and bilateral carotid disease also increase the risk of stroke or death.

Data on carotid angioplasty and stenting (CAS) for symptomatic and asymptomatic patients have emerged, but data comparing CEA with CAS are limited. A recent Cochrane review of randomized trials comparing endovascular therapy with surgical endarterectomy showed no difference at 1 year in the rate of stroke or death, with a lower rate of minor complications for endovascular therapy.[173] Preliminary results from ongoing trials suggest an overall disadvantage of stenting compared with CEA and that older patients, especially those older than 70-80 years of age, have the highest periprocedural rates of stroke and death, even with distal protection devices. Risk of stroke or death within 30 days of carotid stenting has been reported as between 1 and 2 percent for patients up to 69 years of age, 5.3 percent for patients 70 to 79 years of age, and 12.1 percent for patients older than 80 years of age. It is recommended that the requirement for a less than 3 percent

TABLE 75–11	Approach to Anticoagulation in Older Patients
Obtain complete medication and nutraceutical intake data to anticipate warfarin requirements, interactions, contraindications, and necessary adjustment	
Educate patient, family, and/or caregivers on diet, alcohol effects, drug interactions, and need for monitoring and communication	
Initiate at low doses—often at 2 mg, not to exceed 5 mg	
Monitor closely and titrate slowly; consider use of the following: Anticoagulation clinics Finger-stick self-testing programs (patient, family, or caregiver)	
Consider warfarin effects of all medication, supplement, and diet changes	
Use preventive measures for osteoporosis	

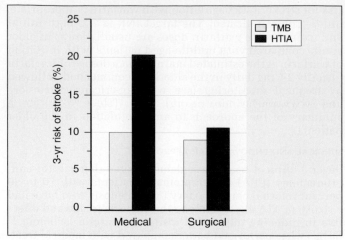

FIGURE 75–8 Three-year risk of ipsilateral stroke in patients with at least 50 percent stenosis and transient monocular blindness (TMB) or hemispheric transient ischemic attack (HTIA) in the North American Symptomatic Carotid Endarterectomy Trial (NASCET). *(From Benevente O, Eliasziw M, Streifler J, et al: Prognosis after transient monocular blindness associated with carotid artery stenosis. N Engl J Med 345:1084-1090, 2000.)*

TABLE 75–12	Approach to the Older Patient with Stroke

Prevention is key
 Treat hypertension, diabetes, smoking, physical inactivity, elevated lipids, obesity, and sleep apnea and limit alcohol intake
 Anticoagulate patients with atrial fibrillation (in the absence of contraindications)

Acute stroke treatment
 Evaluate rapidly—use neuroimaging for diagnosis and to guide therapy
 Aspirin within 48 hr
 Recombinant tissue plasminogen activator (rt-PA) within 3 hr in selected patients
 Anticoagulation is not recommended
 Initiate rehabilitation early
 Routinely evaluate and treat for depression

Secondary prevention
 Aspirin (at lower doses), clopidogrel, or aspirin plus extended release dipyridamole
 Aspirin + clopidogrel is not recommended
 Consider warfarin for patients with strokes while receiving aspirin

Carotid revascularization
 Symptomatic patients with 70-99% ICA stenosis without other risk(s) for short-term mortality
 Selected patients with high-risk lesions by operators with low mortality rates
 Carotid endarterectomy is the standard
 Oldest patients have the worst results with transvascular carotid interventions

ICA = internal carotid artery.

complication rate be required for carotid stenting, as well as CEA for asymptomatic lesions. Currently, CAS is considered an alternative to carotid endarterectomy in patients who are known to have a higher operative complication rate because of medical conditions or technical contraindications to surgery (e.g., previous neck surgeries or radiation), restenosis after endarterectomy, or intracranial lesions in patients that have failed medical therapy, and when procedural risks do not exceed acceptable limits defined for CEA.[165,173]

Table 75-12 summarizes the general approach to the older patient with stroke.

CURRENT CONTROVERSIES
- Time window for effectiveness of thrombolytic therapy in acute stroke
- Optimal endovascular techniques for carotid disease
- Role of endovascular procedures versus surgical procedures

Peripheral Artery Disease

Prevalence and Incidence

Peripheral artery disease is the clinical term used to denote stenotic, occlusive, and aneurysmal disease of the aorta and its branch arteries, exclusive of the coronary arteries. Lower extremity peripheral arterial disease (PAD) is common among older men and women (see Chap. 57). The frequency of intermittent claudication increases with age from 0 to 6 percent in people aged 45 to 54 years to about 9 percent of patients aged 65 to 74 years. Patients with known atherosclerotic coronary, carotid, or renal artery disease are likely to have concomitant lower extremity PAD. At ages up to 69 years, risk factors are age plus diabetes, smoking, dyslipidemia, hypertension, or hyperhomocysteinemia. Some experts consider elevations of C-reactive protein a risk factor. After age 70, age alone is a risk factor for lower extremity PAD, which is equally prevalent in older men and women. When an ankle brachial index of 0.9 is used to identify lower extremity PAD, significant PAD is diagnosed in 17 to 20 percent of men and 21 percent of women older than 55 years of age, with somewhat higher rates in African Americans compared with Caucasians. Individuals with PAD have approximately equal relative risk of death from cardiovascular causes as patients with coronary or cerebrovascular disease. Community-based studies have demonstrated the prevalence of PAD, but physician unawareness has limited use of risk factor–modifying therapies.[174]

Diagnosis

Intermittent claudication is the earliest and most frequent presenting symptom in about one third of patients with PAD. More than half of patients with abnormal ankle brachial index measurements indicating peripheral arterial disease have "atypical" leg discomfort. About 20 percent of patients with PAD are asymptomatic. As disease severity progresses, patients may describe fewer symptoms related to PAD as they avoid activities that precipitate symptoms. Screening for peripheral arterial disease with the ankle-brachial index (ABI) is recommended in all patients older than 70 years of age; patients 50 to 69 years of age who smoke or have diabetes; patients younger than 50 years with diabetes and one other atherosclerosis risk factor; patients with leg symptoms with exertion; abnormal results on vascular examinations of the leg; and patients with coronary, carotid, or renal arterial disease.[175] In patients with symptoms of intermittent claudication and normal ABI at rest, measurement of the ABI after exercise is recommended. In patients with functional impairment, insufficient response to therapies (see later) and lack of other diseases that would limit activity, pulse volume recording, duplex ultrasound imaging, computed tomographic angiography, or magnetic resonance angiography may assist in evaluating further therapeutic options. Invasive digital subtraction angiography usually precedes endovascular interventions. Signs of acute limb ischemia include pain, paralysis, paresthesias, pulselessness, and pallor. The new appearance of any of these symptoms warrants evaluation.

Treatment (see ACC/AHA Practice Guidelines and Hankey et al[176])

Initial therapy for PAD should be directed at smoking cessation, formal/supervised exercise training programs (recently approved for reimbursement), and weight loss in overweight patients to improve symptoms and walking impairment. A trial of pharmacological therapy with cilostazol should be considered in patients with lower extremity PAD and intermittent claudication who do not have HF. Pentoxifylline is a second-line alternative therapy that can be used in patients with HF. To reduce overall mortality risk and slow progression of disease, diabetes, elevated lipid levels, and other cardiovascular risk factors such as hypertension should be treated. Antiplatelet therapy with aspirin or clopidogrel will not improve claudication but may reduce the risk of cardiovascular events, slow progression of disease, and improve results of revascularization procedures. A role for ACE inhibitors even in the absence of hypertension (as defined by older definitions) has been suggested.[176] Benefits of arginine, L-carnitine, and ginkgo biloba are less clear.

Decreased sensation because of age, cognitive impairment, neuropathy, diabetes, increased risk of cutaneous damage from minor trauma with age, and decreased vision increase the chance of missing early signs of critical limb ischemia in older patients. The patient with PAD and/or caregiver should be educated on limb hygiene, frequent examination, and early reporting of lesions, and health care professionals must inspect limbs as a routine part of clinical care.

Revascularization can be performed using endovascular or surgical techniques for individuals with unacceptable responses to pharmacological or life-style modifications, limiting disability, or critical limb ischemia that threatens limb viability. Interventional procedures have been most successful for disease of the iliac arteries. Guidelines to standardize nomenclature and treatment by lesion recommendations for percutaneous and surgical revascularization strategies have been published by both surgical and medical organizations. Guidelines address choices between surgical- and catheter-based approaches, as well as methods of catheter-based approaches that are rapidly evolving and undergoing evaluation.[177] Decisions should be based on symptoms, responses to therapies, comorbid conditions, quality of life, and recognition of higher morbidity and longer surgical recovery times in older patients, as well as the morbidity and mortality results of the operator. No age restrictions to therapeutic approaches exist. Table 75-13 presents the general approach to the older patient with lower extremity PAD. Disease of the aorta is discussed in Chapter 56.

CURRENT CONTROVERSIES

- Best screening tool for PAD in the elderly
- Optimal pharmacological therapies and endovascular techniques
- Role of endovascular procedures versus surgical procedures

TABLE 75–13	Approach to the Older Patient with Peripheral Artery Disease (PAD)
Treatment of cardiovascular risk factors, aspirin, and supervised walking-based exercise programs are first-line therapy.
Medications can improve symptoms (cilostazol > clopidogrel > pentoxifylline; cilostazol should not be used in patients with heart failure).
Estrogen and progesterone should be avoided in women with PAD.
Revascularization options include PCI for iliac disease, but long-term efficacy requires surgical approaches at the femoropopliteal and infrapopliteal level.
Surgical morbidity and mortality increase with age, and postoperative recovery times can be prolonged. All are highest in the setting of surgery for critical ischemia or limb salvage.

PCI = percutaneous coronary intervention.

HEART FAILURE (see Chaps. 22 to 24)

Prevalence and Incidence

HF has become primarily a disorder of the elderly. HF contributes to at least 20 percent of hospital admissions of patients older than 65 years of age with approximately three quarters of HF hospitalizations occurring in patients older than 65 years and more than 85 percent of HF deaths occurring in patients older than 65 years of age. HF was reported as one of their medical conditions by 0.1 percent of people 18 to 39 years old, by approximately 4 percent of people 65 to 74 years old, and by about 6 percent of people 75 to 105 years old in a recent national health interview survey.[178] In the Cardiovascular Health Study of independent community-dwelling subjects 66 to 103 years old ($n = 4842$), HF defined by physician report and medical record review developed at a rate of 19.3/1000 patient years. The incidence increased from 10.6/1000 person-years in participants 65 to 69 years of age at the initial evaluation to 42.5/1000 person-years in those older than 80 years of age (Fig. 75-9). Asymptomatic LV systolic dysfunction is estimated to occur in another 3 to 5 percent of the community with higher prevalence at older ages. The incidence and prevalence of HF is higher in men than women at all ages, and HF is more likely to result from CAD in men than women. However, because more women are alive at older ages, there are more older women than older men presenting for care for HF and the cause is less likely to be ischemic. HF of any type is associated with a reduction in life span, as well as decreased quality of life and recurrent hospitalizations. Although HF treatments are improving, average 5-year mortality for HF patients with systolic dysfunction is approximately 50 percent and is at least 25 percent for HF patients with preserved systolic function (normal ejection fraction). Prognosis is worse in patients older than 65 years of age (Fig. 75-10). In community-based cohorts, overall survival after onset of HF has improved over the past two decades, but there has been less improvement among women and elderly patients with HF.[179,180]

Age-Related Changes in Ventricular Function (see Chap. 21)

In contrast to middle-aged patients with HF, factors other than LV systolic function contribute to HF in the elderly population. Signs and symptoms of HF in older patients often occur in the presence of preserved LV function evaluated as ejection fraction. This clinical presentation has been referred to as HF with normal ejection fraction or diastolic HF. Diastolic HF may be seen in 40 to 80 percent of older patients with HF and is almost twice as frequent in women as men. The pathophysiology is primarily attributed to LV diastolic dysfunction (a leftward and upward shifted end-diastolic pressure-volume relationship), in which LV diastolic chamber size is normal or reduced despite elevated filling pressures resulting in decreased stroke volume and cardiac output. A history of hypertension is often present, and increased circulating blood volume is present in a subset.[181] Endocardial biopsies from HF patients without CAD showed structural and functional differences in cardiomyocytes from patients with diastolic HF compared to cardiomyocytes from patients with abnormal systolic ejection fraction.[182] Myocytes from patients with diastolic HF had increased diameter and higher myofibrillar density and developed greater passive force and had greater calcium sensitivity. Myocardial collagen volume fraction was equally elevated. Although HF with preserved systolic function has a slightly better short-term prognosis than HF with abnormal function, there is a fourfold higher mortality risk compared with subjects free of HF.

CH 75

Cardiovascular Disease in the Elderly

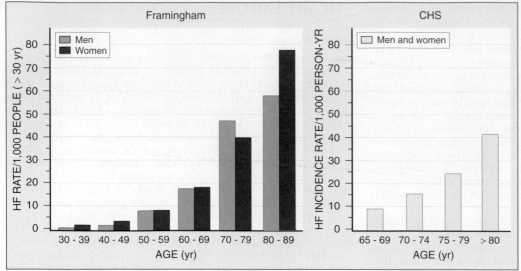

FIGURE 75–9 Prevalence and incidence rates of heart failure (HF) with aging in longitudinal studies. Prevalence rates of HF by age for men and women in the Framingham Study are shown in the left panel, and incidence rates of congestive heart failure by age, gender, and race from the Cardiovascular Health Study (CHS) are shown in the right panel. *(Framingham data are from Ho KK, Pinsky J, Kannel W, Levy D: The epidemiology of heart failure: Framingham Study. JACC 22(Suppl A):6A-13A, 1993, and CHS data are from Gottdiener J, Arnold A, Aurigemma G, et al: Predictors of congestive heart failure in the elderly: the Cardiovascular Health Study. JACC 35:1628-1637, 2000.)*

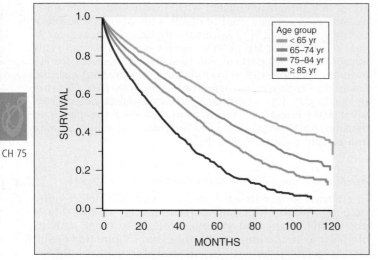

FIGURE 75–10 Age-stratified mortality (adjusted for gender and race) for patients with a diagnosis of heart failure in the Resource Utilization Among Congestive Heart Failure (REACH) study of 29,686 health care recipients during the years 1989-1999. *(Reprinted with permission from McCullough P, Philbin E, Spertus J, et al: Confirmation of a heart failure epidemic: findings from the Resource Utilization Among Congestive Heart Failure (REACH) Study. JACC 39:60-69, 2002.)*

Diagnosis

Exercise intolerance is the primary symptom in chronic HF of either systolic (see Chap. 25) or diastolic (see Chap. 26) cause. Dyspnea and fatigue are prominent symptoms in patients with HF, but fatigue also accompanies many chronic illnesses such as pulmonary disease, thyroid abnormality, anemia, or depression. Complaints of shortness of breath, orthopnea or development of nocturnal cough, or paroxysmal nocturnal dyspnea suggest the presence of HF. Despite the prevalence of HF documented in the elderly, less than half of patients with moderate or severe diastolic or systolic dysfunction as measured by Doppler echocardiography had recognized HF in a recent community-based study.[183] Poten-

tial explanations for unrecognized HF in the older patient include the nonspecificity of complaints of fatigue, ascribing symptoms to aging or comorbid conditions, reduction in activities to avoid symptoms, and memory impairment leading to poor historical information. In addition, physical examination may not be as definitive as in younger individuals. Peripheral edema can occur because of age-related changes in venous tone, decreased skin turgor, or prolonged sedentary states. Evaluation of volume status based on neck veins may also be difficult in the older patient. Rales and a third heart sound may only be present during episodes of acute decompensation, and differentiation of HF from pneumonia may be difficult in older patients less likely to present with temperature elevations. With diastolic HF, fourth heart sounds may be present but third heart sounds are seldom present. Chest radiography will show pulmonary congestion during acute exacerbations and for some time following an episode; cardiomegaly will be present in systolic HF but may or may not be present in HF with preserved ejection fraction. Because of the difficulties with diagnosing HF in the older patient by physician examination or by conventional radiography, use of echocardiography and serum markers of HF take on greater diagnostic importance. Measurement of natriuetic peptides such as B-type natriuretic peptide (BNP) or N-terminus (NT) pro-BNP can improve diagnostic accuracy in patients with dyspnea presenting for acute care, and may be helpful in evaluating older patients with dyspnea and nonspecific symptoms or multiple comorbidities. Levels of natriuretic peptides increase with age and renal decline and are higher in women, so interpretation in older patients requires consideration of these factors.[184] For NT pro-BNP, cutoffs for HF diagnosis are age-specific with almost four-fold higher cutoff value for patients over age 75 years compared to those less than 75 years of age. For BNP, a twofold higher cutoff value has been suggested for patients with eGFR less than 60 ml/min/1.73 M2 (the eGFR for most Caucasian women older than 65 years of age, as explained earlier).

Treatment

Most data from randomized, double-blind studies of therapy for HF are from studies of younger middle-aged men with systolic dysfunction resulting from ischemic CAD and few major medical comorbidities. Guidelines for the management of patients with chronic HF have been published by several organizations and are available at www.acc.org, www.americanheart.org, or www.onlinejcf.com. The elderly HF population differs markedly from patients who have been enrolled in large trials of systolic HF treatment, and limited trial data are available to guide treatment of the older patient with HF and preserved or normal ejection fraction. Conceptually, strategies that have demonstrated benefit for systolic HF may benefit patients with HF with preserved ejection fraction. Because the direct applicability of clinical trial findings and HF treatment guidelines to the majority of older HF patients, especially women and those residing in long-term care facilities, is unknown, it is important to consider care in the context of the individual patient and his or her goals, comorbid conditions, and estimated life expectancy.

HEART FAILURE WITH DECREASED SYSTOLIC FUNCTION (SYSTOLIC HEART FAILURE)

Pharmacological therapy is targeted at control of systolic and diastolic hypertension (see earlier), use of diuretics to control pulmonary congestion, and pulmonary edema and control of ventricular response rate in patients with atrial fibrillation. Most systolic HF trials have tested therapies on a background of digitalis and diuretic administration. The role of digoxin has been addressed in the DIG trial with analyses suggesting a morbidity and hospitalization benefit for most HF patients, with possible mortality benefit in patients with digoxin concentrations between 0.5 and 0.9 ng/ml.[185] Efficacy with the addition of ACE inhibitors and ARBs has been demonstrated in trials that have included elderly patients, and additional efficacy has been shown for diabetes, which is present in at least 10 percent of the older population.[186] Caution and close monitoring are necessary with use of ACE inhibitors in the elderly, especially when given at "full doses" used in studies of younger patients. Beta blockers are usually considered next and can be instituted at low doses during periods of clinical stability. At least one trial of a vasodilating beta blocker in elderly patients with HF with decreased (and preserved) ejection fractions has reported reduced combined endpoints of all-cause death and/or hospitalization for HF, with nonsignificant differences in all-cause death.[187,188] Direct vasodilators may have less of a role in older patients with increased likelihood of orthostatic hypotension. Studies of aldosterone antagonists and selective aldosterone blockers have enrolled limited numbers of older patients, especially minorities or women. Benefit may be seen with these drugs used at lower doses in patients with severe HF, but age-related decreases in renal function increase the risk for hyperkalemia. Data for natriuretic peptides in older patients are also lacking. Sex differences in HF etiology and prognosis have been suggested, but there are no sex specific recommendations to date.

NONPHARMACOLOGICAL STRATEGIES. Dietary sodium restriction is advised, and moderate physical activity should be encouraged if feasible. Cardiac resynchronization therapy can decrease hospitalizations and reduce mortality in selected patients with symptomatic systolic HF and prolonged cardiac repolarization or QRS intervals on the ECG. Biventricular pacing and defibrillator trials have not included significant numbers of elderly patients. Guidelines, as well as clinical judgment, dictate that such therapies be considered on an individual basis and, when estimated longevity from all causes is long enough to confer benefit (see Chap. 34). Revascularization therapies are considered in the setting of ischemia (see Chaps. 27 and 28). The few highly selected patients older than age 65 years who have received cardiac transplantation appear to have survival times similar to those of younger patients with slightly more morbidity and mortality because of the surgical procedure but lower rates of rejection compared with younger patients.

Heart Failure with Preserved Left Ventricular Ejection Fraction (Diastolic Heart Failure)

Management is based on control of physiological factors (blood pressure, heart rate, blood volume, and myocardial ischemia) that are known to exert important effects on ventricular relaxation and the treatment of diseases known to cause diastolic HF. Diuretics are advised for therapy of diastolic HF in the ACC/AHA Guidelines for Evaluation and Management of Heart Failure and the Heart Failure Society Guidelines. Circulating blood volume is a major determinant of ventricular filling pressure, and the use of diuretics may improve breathlessness in patients with diastolic HF (as well as those with systolic HF). Digoxin was reported to yield symptomatic improvement and decreased hospitalizations (without mortality benefit) in the DIG study in patients with diastolic and systolic HF. In more recent analyses of the smaller subset of patients with normal ejection fractions enrolled in the DIG study, no benefit of digoxin was detected in patients with mild to moderate HF that were in normal sinus rhythm and receiving diuretics and ACE inhibitors.[189] The risk-benefit ratio of digoxin in women with HF has also been questioned. Small studies of HF in the elderly with preserved LV function suggest that ACE inhibitors or ARBs may improve functional class, exercise duration, ejection fraction, diastolic filling, and LV hypertrophy. In the only large trial to date of ARBs for diastolic HF in the elderly, morbidity was reduced but primary endpoints for mortality reduction were not achieved.[190] As noted earlier, a vasodilating beta blocker has been shown to improve morbidity in older patients with diastolic and systolic HF.[187,188] Although calcium channel antagonists can improve measures of diastolic function during short-term use, definitive data on outcomes with chronic administration for diastolic HF are not available. Data are also lacking on nitrates, but some clinicians find them helpful in reducing orthopnea if given at bedtime. Finally, spironolactone and other aldosterone antagonists have not been tested in patients with diastolic HF.

ADDITIONAL CONSIDERATIONS FOR THE OLDER PATIENT WITH HEART FAILURE. Elderly patients with HF have the highest rehospitalization rate of all adult patient groups. Education and involvement of the patient, family members, and/or caregivers is key to the management of older patients with HF. Recognition of warning signs of worsening failure, understanding of medication regimens, diet adjustments, and the role of regular moderate physical activity should be emphasized. Reliance cannot be on classical symptoms of HF. Weight should be measured daily with a mechanism for rapid communication of information and timely adjustment of diuretic dosages in order to prevent exacerbations of HF. Multidisciplinary team approaches with patient contacts between office visits and more frequent contact during the transitional period after hospital discharge can be highly beneficial and reduce rehospitalization rates.[191,192] Use of primary care preventive strategies such as influenza vaccination can also reduce hospitalizations for HF in older people.[193]

For very old patients or those with progressive symptoms of severe HF, goals of improving symptoms and quality of life and preventing acute exacerbations and hospitalization rather than prolongation of life become the emphasis. Palliative care programs may have special expertise in the management of symptoms such as dyspnea with opiates and in providing support for family and caregivers, as well as the patient with advanced HF (Table 75-14).[194]

CURRENT CONTROVERSIES/ISSUES in HF in the elderly include the following:
- BP target for older patients with HF
- Optimal treatment for diastolic HF
- Impact of exercise training on mortality
- Optimal use of case management teams for HF in the elderly
- Role of nutrition
- Role of renal dysfunction, anemia, and/or treatment with erythropoietin on outcomes
- Role of ultrafiltration
- Role of devices in patients older than 75 to 80 years of age or older patients with significant comorbid conditions
- Role of cross-link breaking agents to reduce ventricular stiffening

CH 75

Cardiovascular Disease in the Elderly

TABLE 75-14	Approach to the Older Patient with Heart Failure (HF)

Symptoms may be nonspecific in the older patient—suspect HF.
   Consider HF diagnosis in patients with fatigue, dyspnea, exercise intolerance, or low activity.

Diagnosis may be assisted by use of echocardiography or serum markers of HF.

HF may be present in the older patient with preserved systolic function (ejection fraction), especially older women.

Aggressive treatment of hypertension or diabetes when present may improve HF outcomes.

Treat symptoms with a goal of improving quality of life and morbidity:
   Control blood pressure-systolic and diastolic.
   Treat ischemia.
   Control atrial fibrillation rate.
   Promote physical activity.
   Adjust medications for age and disease-related changes in kinetics and dynamics.

Educate and involve patients, family members, or caregivers in management of HF:
   Monitor weight.
   Consider use of multidisciplinary team approaches.

ARRHYTHMIAS

PATHOPHYSIOLOGY AND AGE-RELATED ECG CHANGES

Cell loss and collagen infiltration occur in the area of the sinus node, throughout the atria, the central fibrous body, and cytoskeleton of the heart with increasing age. Changes are most marked in the area of the sinus node with destruction of up to 90 percent of cells by age 75 years. The correlation between pathology and sinus node function, however, is poor and sinus node function is preserved in most elderly patients, although sinoatrial conduction is decreased. Collagen infiltration and fibrosis is of lesser magnitude in the area of the AV node and more marked in the left and right bundle branches. Conduction times through the atrioventricular (AV) node increase with aging with the site of delay above the His bundle. Despite age-related collagen infiltration, His-Purkinje conduction times are not usually increased by aging alone.

Resting heart rate is not altered by age but maximal heart rate (see Fig. 75-4), and beat-to-beat variability in heart rate decrease with age because of decreases in sinus node responses to beta-adrenergic and parasympathetic stimulation (see Chap. 89). On the surface ECG, the P-R interval increases and the R, S, and T wave amplitude decrease. The QRS axis shifts leftward. This shift may reflect increased LV mass or interstitial fibrosis of the anterior fascicular radiation. Right bundle branch block is found in 3 percent of healthy people older than 85 years, up to 20 percent of centenarians, and in 8 to 10 percent of older patients with heart disease but is not associated with cardiac morbidity or mortality. The presence of left bundle branch block increases with age and is more likely to be associated with cardiovascular disease. Similarly, nonspecific intraventricular conduction delays become more frequent with increasing age and are usually related to underlying myocardial disease. Repolarization times throughout the myocardium increase with age, and surface ECG Q-T intervals increase.

Atrial ectopy has been found on ECG recordings in 10 percent of community-dwelling elderly without known cardiac disease and up to 80 percent during 24-hour ambulatory ECG recordings. Brief episodes of atrial tachyarrhythmias are seen on 24-hr ambulatory ECGs in up to 50 percent of community-dwelling elderly. Premature ventricular complexes also increase in prevalence and frequency with age. Ventricular ectopic beats are seen on ECG in 6 to 11 percent of elderly patients without known cardiovascular disease and in up to 76 percent on 24-hour ambulatory ECG recordings. In the absence of cardiac disease, these age-related findings have not been associated with subsequent cardiovascular events (see Table 75-1).

Sinus Node Dysfunction

Bradycardia caused by sinus node dysfunction and/or AV conduction disease is more common as age increases. The mean age of patients undergoing permanent pacemaker implantation is approximately 74 years, with 70 percent of new pacemaker recipients being older than the age of 70 years. In the United States, 85 percent of pacemaker implantations are in patients older than the age of 65 years, with up to 30 percent implanted in patients older than 80 years. The most common indication is for sinus node dysfunction,

Atrioventricular Conduction Disease

First-degree AV block is diagnosed in 6 to 10 percent of healthy elderly. Higher degree AV block is less common. Transient type II AV block occurs in 0.4 to 0.8 percent of 24-hour ambulatory ECGs of community-dwelling elderly and transient third-degree AV block in less than 0.2 percent. These arrhythmias usually represent advanced conduction system disease, requiring pacemaker implantation (see Chap. 35). Acquired AV block is the second most important indication for permanent pacemaker implantation.

Prior and recent studies[195-197] have compared outcomes with single-chamber versus dual-chamber pacing devices in older patients with sinus node dysfunction or AV node disease (see Chap. 34). The overall conclusion is that dual-chamber pacing does not provide a significant 2- to 6-year survival advantage or benefit with respect to cardiovascular death or stroke, For some patients, quality of life or HF symptoms may be improved or atrial fibrillation may be less common with atrial based pacing, but procedural complication rates and reoperation rates before discharge are higher with dual-chamber pacemaker implantation.[198,199]

CURRENT CONTROVERSIES

- Optimal pacing mode for individual patients with sinus and AV node disease
- Role of resynchronization therapy in the elderly

Atrial Arrhythmias

Atrial fibrillation (AF, see Chap. 35) is seen on 24-hour ambulatory recordings in 10 percent of community-dwelling older patients. The incidence of AF doubles with each decade beginning at age 60, so that by ages 80 to 89 years the incidence of AF is estimated to be 8 to 10 percent. The median age of patients with AF in the United States is 75 years, with approximately 70 percent of AF patients between the ages of 65 and 85 years. Age-adjusted prevalence of AF is higher in men, but the overall number of men and women of all ages with AF is about equal, with higher numbers of women with AF at 75 years of age and older. AF in the population is projected to have a 2.5-fold increase in prevalence over the next 50 years.[200] Hospitalizations for AF have already increased.

In population-based studies,[201] 10 to 12 percent of patients with a history of AF report no history of cardiopulmonary disease, whereas only 4 percent of patients with permanent AF in the clinical practice setting have AF without cardiopulmonary disease (lone AF). Hypertension, ischemic heart disease, HF, valvular disease, and diabetes are the most common conditions associated with AF. Thyroid disease should also be considered in the older patient.

TREATMENT (See ACC/AHA/ESC Guidelines). AF is rarely an isolated condition in the older patient. The risks for stroke associated with AF combined with the high prevalence of other stroke risk factors mandates a focus on antithrombotic therapy (anticoagulation), management of associated conditions, and rate control to improve symptoms.

Randomized studies have found no significant difference in long-term outcome between rate control or rhythm control, and it is the unusual older patient who requires

CH 75

rhythm control to provide symptom relief.[202] Patients should be anticoagulated with warfarin in the absence of contraindications (see Table 75-11). The target INR is 2 to 2.5 in older patients in whom close monitoring of INRs can be performed. Low, fixed warfarin doses of 1 mg are not efficacious. Patients older than age 75 may require less than half the dose of middle-aged patients for equivalent anticoagulation. Warfarin dosing guidelines for the elderly recommend initiation of warfarin at the estimated maintenance dosage of warfarin, 2 to 5 mg daily (see www.americangeriatrics.org and www.warfarindosing.org). Drug interaction information should be consulted whenever warfarin is being initiated or a drug is added to or deleted from a patient's medication regimen.

Chronic warfarin administration may contribute to osteoporosis. Vitamin K plays a role in bone metabolism, and oral anticoagulation with warfarin antagonizes vitamin K. In analyses of women receiving chronic oral anticoagulation compared with nonanticoagulated cohorts, increased risk of osteoporosis and higher rates of vertebral and rib fractures were associated with oral anticoagulation for more than 12 months.[203] Measures to prevent osteoporosis should accompany long-term anticoagulation with warfarin (calcium and vitamin D in most; bisphosphonates and calcitonin, if needed). See Table 75-15 for a summary of the approach to the older patient with AF.

CURRENT CONTROVERSIES

- Optimal rate control
- Estimating bleeding risk
- Indications for rhythm control in older patients

Ventricular Arrhythmias

Treatment of PVCs with most type I antiarrhythmic agents has been either of no benefit or has decreased survival. If patients have symptoms, administration of a beta blocker may be helpful. Sustained ventricular tachycardia and ventricular fibrillation require treatment in patients of any age (see Chap. 35 and ACC/AHA/ESC Guidelines).

VALVULAR DISEASE (see also Chap. 62)

PATHOPHYSIOLOGY AND AGE-RELATED CHANGES. Age-related changes in the fibromuscular skeleton of the heart include myxomatous degeneration and collagen infiltration termed *sclerosis*. Sclerosis of the aortic valve is present in up to 30 percent of the elderly, with the prevalence of sclerosis detected on echocardiography increasing as age increased from 65 years to more than 85 years in the Cardiovascular Health Study. Further age-related changes include calcification of the aortic valve leaflets, aortic annulus, base of the semilunar cusps, and the mitral annulus. Aortic valve calcium detected by electron beam computed tomography increases over time,[204] with progression from valvular sclerosis to stenosis with a transvalvular pressure gradient in a significant percentage of patients[205] (Table 75-16). Aortic sclerosis appears to parallel atherosclerotic progression in other vessels. This may explain the increased risk of MI and death from cardiovascular causes in patients with aortic sclerosis without evidence of stenosis.[206] Risk factors identified for progression include hypertension; hyperlipidemia; smoking; end-stage renal disease; congenital bicuspid valves; and, in some series, diabetes, shorter stature, and male sex. In older patients, fibrosis and valve calcification is now the most common cause of valvular stenoses, especially at the aortic position. Ischemic or hypertensive disease has become the most common cause of valvular regurgitation, especially at the mitral valve. Similarly, pulmonary and tricuspid regurgitation in the elderly are usually secondary to pulmonary hypertension and dilation of the right ventricle resulting from LV ischemia, HF, or pulmonary disease. Less common etiologies of mild to moderate mitral or aortic regurgitation are ruptured chordae, endocarditis, trauma, aortic dissection, or rheumatic heart disease.

Infective endocarditis is seen in about equal frequency in younger and older patients but is more likely to be associated with nosocomial infections with the use of intravascular catheters or other devices, the presence of prosthetic implants, pacemaker leads, atheromas, or mitral annular calcification in older patients. Polymicrobial infections are uncommon in the elderly, and the most frequent pathogens are group D streptococci and enterococcus, *Staphylococcus epidermidis*, and *Streptococcus viridans* (see Chap. 63).

Treatment for symptomatic valvular disease relies on surgical approaches. Surgery in older patients between 70 and 80 years of age is increasingly common, but experience with those older than 90 years of age is limited and carries a high surgical mortality rate.

Aortic Valve Disease

AORTIC STENOSIS

The prevalence of aortic stenosis in patients older than 65 years is estimated at 2 percent for severe stenosis, 5 percent for moderate stenosis, and 9 percent for mild stenosis. Aortic stenosis in more than 90 percent of older patients involves calcification of the aortic annulus and semilunar cusps of trileaflet valves without commissural fusion. The pathophysiological consequences of aortic stenosis are independent of cause and include LV hypertrophy, elevated LV diastolic pressures, and decreased stroke volume in patients of all ages. For any given

CH 75

Cardiovascular Disease in the Elderly

TABLE 75-15	Approach to the Older Patient with Atrial Fibrillation (AF)
AF is frequent in the elderly and confers a risk of stroke.	
Routine examinations or ECG evaluations should be targeted toward detection of AF.	
Thyroid disease and medical conditions should be controlled.	
Anticoagulation is the chief weapon against stroke. Both greater potential benefit and risk for fatal intracranial bleeding are present at ages older than 75 yr, especially in women. Careful attention to anticoagulation monitoring is necessary. Aspirin does not usually provide stroke risk reduction in older patients but has similar overall bleeding complication rates as warfarin.	
Rate control produces equivalent benefits with lower costs and morbidity than attempts at rhythm control. Useful agents in the elderly include digoxin (rest control), beta blockers, nondihydropyridine calcium channel blockers, and amiodarone with dose adjustments for age, weight, and diseases.	

TABLE 75-16 · Prevalence of Aortic Valve Abnormalities Detected by Echocardiography in the Cross-sectional Cardiovascular Health Study of 5201 Medicare Subjects over 65 Years of Age*

| | Aortic Valve Abnormality | | | |
	None	*Sclerosis*	*Stenosis*	*Valve Replacement*
All subjects	3736 (72%)	1329 (26%)	88 (2%)	23 (0.4%)
Women	2249 (76%)	641 (22%)	43 (1.5%)	12 (0.4%)
Men	1487 (67%)	688 (31%)	45 (2%)	11 (0.5%)
65-74 y old	2684 (78%)	697 (20%)	43 (1.3%)	16 (0.5%)
Women	1654 (82%)	344 (17%)	20 (1.0%)	9 (0.4%)
Men	1030 (73%)	353 (25%)	23 (1.6%)	7 (0.5%)
75-84 y old	962 (62%)	542 (35%)	37 (2.4%)	7 (0.5%)
Women	546 (66%)	259 (31%)	22 (2.7%)	3 (0.4%)
Men	416 (58%)	283 (39%)	15 (2.1%)	4 (0.6%)
85+ y old	90 (48%)	90 (48%)	8 (4%)	0 (0%)
Women	49 (56%)	38 (43%)	1 (1%)	0
Men	41 (41%)	52 (52%)	7 (7%)	0

Data are expressed as number (%) of subjects.
*Reproduced from Stewart BF, Siscovick D, Lind BK, et al with permission. J Am Coll Cardiol. 29(3):630-634, 1997.

degree of aortic stenosis, LV hypertrophy and decreased LV compliance are greater in patients older than age 65 compared with younger patients. Approximately 50 percent of patients with severe aortic stenosis will have significant CAD, further influencing LV function, symptoms, and morbidity.

DIAGNOSIS. Symptoms can be exertional angina, syncope, or HF and may be precipitated by atrial arrhythmias such as atrial fibrillation. Symptoms may be absent in inactive older patients or may not be elicited from patients with memory impairment. Physical findings of calcific aortic valve stenosis in older patients differ from those seen with rheumatic aortic stenosis and do not accurately reflect the degree of stenosis. The age-related arterial changes of decreased compliance and increased stiffness mask carotid artery findings associated with rheumatic aortic stenosis in younger individuals (see Chap. 83). The carotid artery upstroke and peak may appear normal, and carotid amplitude may be unaltered or increased even in the presence of severe calcific stenosis. The presence of decreased carotid upstroke and volume (in the absence of carotid disease) usually indicates severe stenosis. Aortic sclerosis and aortic stenosis both produce systolic ejection murmurs. The volume of the murmur depends on flow, as well as the pressure gradient, and does not reflect the severity of stenosis. It may be absent in low-output states reflecting severe aortic valve obstruction. The murmur may be high pitched and musical as opposed to harsh and of low frequency. The loudness of the second heart sound may be preserved. Hypertension is common in the elderly, making LV hypertrophy on ECG or ventricular enlargement on chest radiograph similarly of little diagnostic help. Thus, Doppler echocardiography has become the clinical standard for diagnosis of aortic stenosis in the elderly. In the setting of low cardiac output, maneuvers (vasodilators, inotropes) to increase output may be helpful in quantifying stenosis. Catheterization is less commonly used to make the diagnosis, but coronary angiography is usually performed to evaluate CAD in older patients before surgical interventions.

MANAGEMENT. Management of the older patient with aortic stenosis (Table 75-17) is similar to that of younger patients with recognition of the increased likelihood of concomitant coronary disease and diseases of other organs (see Chap. 62 and ACC/AHA Guidelines). Antibiotic prophylaxis should be used to prevent bacterial endocarditis. Risk factors should be treated. Although current concepts suggest a relationship between cholesterol concentrations and calcification of valves, as well as cardiac vessels, that would support aggressive lipid lowering in patients with calcific aortic sclerosis and stenosis, intensive lipid-lowering therapy did not slow the progression of calcific aortic stenosis or induce its regression in a small, randomized, double-blind, placebo-controlled trial.[204,207-209]

Surgical morbidity and mortality relate to the severity and duration of aortic stenosis, degree of LV hypertrophy, presence or absence of HF or CAD, concomitant diseases (especially renal), and urgency and complexity of the procedure. Combined valve replacement and CABG are associated with higher perioperative morbidity and mortality than isolated valve replacement. Estimates of average operative mortality for older patients who have undergone valve replacement with or without CABG as part of clinical care have been reported as 6 percent for high-volume surgery centers and 13 percent in low-volume surgery centers.[210] Perioperative renal failure, pulmonary insufficiency, stroke, late cognitive impairment, and late death rates are higher than in younger individuals. Postoperative hospitalization and rehabilitation times are usually longer in older patients. Appropriate selection of patients includes assessment of the burden of disease in addition to that of valve disease, anticipated lifespan independent of valve disease, and symptom status. Surgical risk assessment tools may be helpful but have not been specifically developed for older patients (see www.sts.org and www.euroscore.org).[211] The frailer the patient and the more comorbidities, the more likely that perioperative mortality will outweigh the benefit.

Biological tissue valves are frequently implanted in elderly patients on the basis of a number of factors including shorter anticipated life expectancy, longer bioprosthesis durability with older age, and avoidance of chronic anticoagulation. Estimated structural failure rates of current bioprosthetic valves are about 1 percent per patient year in patients older than 65 years of age, and mechanical valves should be considered for younger old patients or those with longer estimated life spans. Aortic balloon valvotomy is not considered an acceptable alternative to surgery. Observed mortality rates for patients after aortic valvuloplasty are similar to that in patients with severe symptomatic aortic stenosis that do not undergo surgery. When aortic balloon valvuloplasty is used in symptomatic patients who are not surgical candidates, hemodynamics and symptoms improve initially, but there is a high (>10 percent) procedural morbidity and mortality, with rapid restenosis and recurrence of symptoms within months in most series. Valvotomy may serve as a bridge to valve surgery in hemodynamically unstable patients (cardiogenic shock), patients undergoing emergent noncardiac surgery, and in patients with severe comorbidities who are too ill to undergo cardiac surgery.[212]

Asymptomatic older patients with aortic stenosis and their families should be educated on signs and symptoms related to aortic stenosis and followed regularly for development of symptoms. Clinicians can monitor the rate of hemodynamic progression by changes in aortic jet velocity and aortic valve area on Doppler echocardiography. Sudden death in asymptomatic patients with aortic stenosis occurs, but the frequency in prospective studies using echocardiography is estimated at less than 1 percent, much lower than previous estimates of 3 to 5 percent in retrospective studies. Operative mortality in older patients exceeds either of these rates. Thus asymptomatic older patients with severe AS are not usually recommended for surgical interventions.

CURRENT CONTROVERSIES

- Underlying mechanisms responsible for age-related valvular sclerosis and calcification
- Role of lipid-lowering therapy in prevention of or slowing of aortic valve sclerosis/calcification
- Management/frequency of monitoring of asymptomatic older patients with AS
- Use of anticoagulation with biologic valves during the first 3 months after surgery

TABLE 75–17	Approach to the Older Patient with Suspected Valvular Disease
Physical examination cannot reliably assess the severity of valvular lesions in most older patients.	

Doppler echocardiography is the clinical standard for diagnosis and evaluation of the severity of valve lesions.
    Differentiates sclerosis from stenosis
    Can assist in monitoring progression of stenosis
    Quantitates regurgitation
    Assesses calcification of valves and supporting structures	

Age is a predictor of worse outcomes for the natural history of valvular lesions, as well as surgical approaches.	
Surgery is definitive therapy for valvular lesions with age, coronary artery disease, additional diseases, projected lifespan, and desired lifestyle as factors in evaluating surgical options.	

Aortic Regurgitation

The prevalence of aortic regurgitation also increases with age. Mild aortic regurgitation was detected by Doppler echocardiography in 13 percent of patients older than 80 years and moderate or severe regurgitation in 16 percent in a recent series.[213] Causes of aortic regurgitation in the older patient include primary valvular disease (myxomatous or infective) or aortic root disease and dilation secondary to hypertension or dissection. Significant aortic regurgitation in older patients is usually seen in combination with aortic stenosis. When infective aortic regurgitation occurs in the elderly, the clinical manifestations may be insidious and nonspecific and symptoms fewer than in younger patients with endocarditis. CNS symptoms are common and may predict a less favorable clinical outcome. Patients who have acute HF and pulmonary congestion as the manifestation of aortic valve endocarditis have a mortality rate of 50 to 80 percent. Age is a predictor of worse outcome for the natural history of aortic regurgitation. The life span of older patients with chronic severe aortic regurgitation who do not undergo valve replacement has been estimated at 2 years after onset of HF in earlier observational studies.

Aortic regurgitation can be diagnosed by presence of the classic diastolic murmur on physical examination. The finding of a widened pulse pressure usually associated with aortic regurgitation in younger patients is of limited diagnostic value in the older patient because age-related changes in the vasculature usually produce a widened pulse pressure in older people. Doppler echocardiography is the usual method of quantitation of the regurgitation and assessment of ventricular function. Patients older than 75 years are more likely to develop symptoms or LV dysfunction at earlier stages of LV dilation, have more persistent ventricular dysfunction and HF symptoms after surgery, and worse postoperative survival rates than younger patients.

Mitral Annular Calcification

Mitral annular calcification is a chronic degenerative process that is age-related and is seen more commonly in women compared with men and in people older than 70 years of age. An increased prevalence of mitral annular calcification is seen in patients with systemic hypertension, increased mitral valve stress, mitral valve prolapse, raised LV systolic pressure, aortic valve stenosis, chronic renal failure, secondary hyperparathyroidism, atrial fibrillation, and aortic atherosclerosis. As with aortic calcific processes, mitral annular calcification is associated with risk factors for the development of coronary atherosclerosis and may reflect generalized atherosclerosis. Mitral annular calcification may produce mitral stenosis, mitral regurgitation, infective endocarditis, atrial arrhythmias, or heart block. It is an independent risk factor for systemic embolism and stroke, with the risk of stroke directly related to the degree of mitral annular calcification.

Mitral Stenosis

Increasing numbers of older patients now present with symptomatic mitral stenosis. Symptoms are the same as in the younger patient and include exertional dyspnea, orthopnea, paroxysmal nocturnal dyspnea, and pulmonary edema or right HF. Physical findings of calcific mitral stenosis differ from those of rheumatic mitral stenosis, and neither a loud first heart sound nor an opening snap is usually heard. The characteristic diastolic rumbling murmur is usually present. Quantification of stenosis is usually accomplished by Doppler echocardiography. Older patients are more likely to have heavy calcification and fibrosis of the valve leaflets and subvalvular fusion, making them less likely to benefit from percutaneous valvotomy than younger patients. The success rate of valvotomy in older patients is less than 50 percent, with procedural mortality rates of 3 percent and higher complication rates than in younger patients. Long-term clinical improvement is also lower, and mortality is higher. Highly selected older patients may be candidates for percutaneous approaches, but surgical valve replacement remains the standard.

Mitral Regurgitation

Myxomatous degeneration and ischemic papillary muscle dysfunction or rupture caused by CAD and myocardial infarction as causes of mitral regurgitation in the older patient are increasing. Rheumatic mitral disease is declining, and endocarditis etiology is unchanged. Mitral regurgitation may also be seen in the setting of LV dilation because of HF.

Acute MR presents with HF and pulmonary edema, but this may also be the initial presentation for medical care of the older patient with chronic MR. Chronic MR may be asymptomatic, especially in the sedentary patient. In symptomatic patients, initial complaints are usually easy fatigability and decreasing exercise tolerance caused by low forward cardiac output, followed by dyspnea on exertion, orthopnea, paroxysmal nocturnal dyspnea, and dyspnea at rest as the left ventricle function fails. Right HF may also occur. Findings on examination are not altered by age, and a holosystolic murmur is usually present along with displacement of the LV apical impulse and third heart sound or early diastolic flow rumble. Comprehensive 2-D transthoracic echocardiography with Doppler is recommended to evaluate LV size and function, RV and left atrial size, pulmonary artery pressure, and severity of mitral regurgitation. Transesophageal echocardiography is used when transthoracic echocardiography is suboptimal. Medical treatment of chronic MR is age independent and includes afterload reduction, diuretics as needed for HF, management of AF, and antibiotic prophylaxis. When symptoms cannot be controlled, surgical options are based on valvular anatomy, LV function, and the extent of comorbid diseases. Mitral valve repair is preferred to mitral valve replacement, when possible, in the older patient. Transesophageal echocardiography is recommended in the evaluation of surgical candidates to assess feasibility and guide repair. Cardiac catheterization is used when there is a discrepancy between symptoms and noninvasive findings and to evaluate CAD. Older age is a risk factor for hospital mortality with isolated mitral valve surgery. Elderly patients with MR have less successful surgical outcomes than older patients with aortic stenosis. The average operative mortality for MV replacement in the elderly exceeds 14 percent in the United States and is more than 20 percent in low-volume surgery centers.[210] Risks are reduced somewhat if mitral repair rather than mitral valve replacement is performed but increased with the need for combined CABG surgery for CAD that is often present in older patients. Series reporting mitral valve repair results (alone and with CABG) estimate early death rates in patients older than age 70 of 9 percent.[214] Survival after combined mitral valve replacement and CABG at 5 years may be as low as 50 percent.

ADDITIONAL CONSIDERATIONS IN THE ELDERLY. Drug-induced valve disease is uncommon, but there are case reports of fibroproliferative lesions producing valvular insufficiency or regurgitation in older patients on chronic treatment with the anti-Parkinson disease dopamine receptor agonist pergolide.[215]

FUTURE DIRECTIONS

Increasing emphasis is being placed on preventive strategies for CVD in older patients and improving the quality of care using current therapies that were not designed for the elderly. A major limitation is the lack of understanding of the mechanisms underlying many age-related cardiovascular changes or diseases. Increased investigation at both the basic level and clinical level is necessary to identify therapies that will benefit older patients on the basis of both the pathophysiology of age-related CV disease and the frequent presence of comorbid diseases. Caring for patients near the end of their lives is different than caring for patients with longer life expectancies. Research and training will be necessary to achieve coordinated care for the older patient, and both medical and social factors must be considered to provide optimal care.

Demographics/Epidemiology

1. Centers for Disease Control and Prevention: MMWR Series on Public Health and Aging. MMWR 52:101-106, 2003.
2. U.S. Census Bureau: Income 2001 (http://www.census.gov/hhes/income). Accessed July 15, 2003.
3. Clark C, Karlawish J: Alzheimer disease: Current concepts and emerging diagnostic and therapeutic strategies. Ann Intern Med 138:400-410, 2003.
4. National Academy on an Aging Society: Alzheimer's Disease and Dementia. A Growing Challenge. Washington, DC, National Academy on an Aging Society, 2000.

Pathophysiology

5. Lakatta E, Levy D: Arterial and cardiac aging: Major shareholders in cardiovascular disease enterprises: Part II: The aging heart in health: Links to heart disease. Circulation 107:346-354, 2003.
6. Lakatta E, Levy D: Arterial and cardiac aging: major shareholders in cardiovascular disease enterprises: Part I: Aging arteries a "set up" for vascular disease. Circulation 107:139-146, 2003.
7. Kass D: Age-related changes in ventricular-arterial coupling: Pathophysiologic implications. Heart Fail Rev 7:51-62, 2002.
8. Lakatta E: Arterial and cardiac aging: Major shareholders in cardiovascular disease enterprises: Part III: Cellular and molecular clues to heart and arterial aging. Circulation 107:490-497, 2003.
9. Anversa P, Nadal-Ginard B: Myocyte renewal and ventricular remodelling. Nature 415:240-243, 2002.
10. Lakatta E, Sollott S: Perspectives on mammalian cardiovascular aging: Humans to molecules. Comp Biochem Physiol A Mol Integr Physiol 132:699-721, 2002.
11. Zhou Y, Lakatta E, Xiao R: Age-associated alterations in calcium current and its modulation in cardiac myocytes. Drugs Aging 13:159-171, 1998.
12. Wilkerson W, Sane D: Aging and thrombosis. Semin Thromb Hemost 28:555-568, 2002.
13. Willerson J: Systemic and local inflammation in patients with unstable atherosclerotic plaques. Prog Cardiovasc Dis 44:469-478, 2002.
14. Seals D, Esler M: Human ageing and the sympathoadrenal system. J Physiol 528:407-417, 2000.
15. Rehman H, Masson E: Neuroendocrinology of ageing. Age Ageing 30:279-287, 2001.
16. Kaasinen V, Rinne J: Functional imaging studies of dopamine system and cognition in normal aging and Parkinson's disease. Neurosci Biobehav Rev 26:785-793, 2002.
17. Hess P, Fleg J, Mirza Z, et al: Effects of normal aging on left ventricular lusitropic, inotropic, and chronotropic responses to dobutamine. J Am Coll Cardiol 47:1440-1447, 2006.
18. Walford R, Mock D, Verdery R, MacCallum T: Calorie restriction in biosphere 2: Alterations in physiologic, hematologic, hormonal, and biochemical parameters in humans restricted for a 2-year period. J Gerontol A Biol Sci Med Sci 57:B211-224, 2002.
19. Fontana L, Meyer T, Klein S, Holloszy J: Long-term calorie restriction is highly effective in reducing the risk for atherosclerosis in humans. Proc Natl Acad Sci U S A 101:6659-6663, 2004.
20. Heilbronn L, de Jonge L, Frisard M, et al: Pennington CALERIE Team: Effect of 6-month calorie restriction on biomarkers of longevity, metabolic adaptation, and oxidative stress in overweight individuals. JAMA 295:1539-1548, 2006.
21. Meyer TE, Kovacs SJ, Ehsani AA, et al: Long-term caloric restriction ameliorates the decline in diastolic function in humans. J Am Coll Cardiol 47:398-402, 2006.
22. Eidelman R, Hollar D, Hebert P, et al: Randomized trials of vitamin E in the treatment and prevention of cardiovascular disease. Arch Intern Med 164:1552-1556, 2004.
23. Bonaa K, Njolstad I, Ueland P, et al: NORVIT Trial Investigators: Homocysteine lowering and cardiovascular events after acute myocardial infarction. N Engl J Med 354:1578-1588, 2006.
24. Hooper L, Thompson R, Harrison R, et al: Risks and benefits of omega 3 fats for mortality, cardiovascular disease, and cancer: Systematic review. BMJ 332:752-760, 2006.
25. The Heart Outcomes Prevention Evaluation (HOPE) Investigators: Homocysteine lowering with folic acid and B vitamins in vascular disease. N Engl J Med 354:1567-1577, 2006.
26. Gale C, Ashurst H, Powers H, Martyn C: Antioxidant vitamin status and carotid atherosclerosis in the elderly. Am J Clin Nutr 74:402-408, 2001.
27. Miquel J: Can antioxidant diet supplementation protect against age-related mitochondrial damage? Ann N Y Acad Sci 959:508-516, 2002.
28. Remme W: Aldosterone and myocardial infarction—are aldosterone antagonists needed to prevent remodelling or does ACE inhibition suffice? Cardiovasc Drugs Ther 15:297-298, 2001.
29. Hansson L: ACE inhibition and left ventricular remodelling. Eur Heart J 18:1203-1204, 1997.
30. Zieman S, Kass D: Advanced glycation endproduct crosslinking in the cardiovascular system: Potential therapeutic target for cardiovascular disease. Drugs 64:459-470, 2004.

Medication Therapy

31. Gurwitz J, Gore J, Goldberg R, et al: Risk for intracranial hemorrhage after tissue plasminogen activator treatment for acute myocardial infarction. Participants in the National Registry of Myocardial Infarction 2. Ann Intern Med 129:597-604, 1998.
32. Van de Werf F, Barron H, Armstrong P, et al: Incidence and predictors of bleeding events after fibrinolytic therapy with fibrin-specific agents. Eur Heart J 22:2253-2261, 2001.
33. Van de Werf F: ASSENT-3: Implications for future trial design and clinical practice. Eur Heart J 23:911-912, 2002.
34. Shlipak MG, Fried LF, Cushman M, et al: Cardiovascular mortality risk in chronic kidney disease. Comparison of traditional and novel risk factors. JAMA 293:1737-1745, 2005.
35. Cooper W, O'Brien S, Thourani V, et al: Impact of renal dysfunction on outcomes of coronary artery bypass surgery: Results from the Society of Thoracic Surgeons' National Adult Cardiac Database. Circulation 113:1056-1062, 2006.
36. Barrett B, Parfrey P: Preventing nephropathy induced by contrast medium. N Engl J Med 354:379-386, 2006.
37. Cockcroft DW, Gault MH: Prediction of creatinine clearance from serum creatinine. Nephron 16:31-41, 1976.
38. Manjunath G, Sarnak M, Levey A: Prediction equations to estimate glomerular filtration rate: An update. Curr Opin Nephrol Hypertens 10:785-792, 2001.
39. Stevens L, Coresh J, Greene T, Levey A: Assessing kidney function—measured and estimated glomerular filtration rate. N Engl J Med 354:2473-2483, 2006.
40. Alexander K, Chen A, Roe M, et al: CRUSADE Investigators. Excess dosing of antiplatelet and antithrombin agents in the treatment of non-ST-segment elevation acute coronary syndromes. JAMA 294:3108-3116, 2005.
41. Alexander K, Chen A, Newby L, et al: CRUSADE Investigators: Sex differences in major bleeding with glycoprotein IIb/IIIa inhibitors: Results from CRUSADE. Circulation 114:1380-1387, 2006.
42. Lansky A, Pietras C, Costa R, et al: Gender differences in outcomes after primary angioplasty versus primary stenting with and without abciximab for acute myocardial infarction: Results of the Controlled Abciximab and Device Investigation to Lower Late Angioplasty Complications (CADILLAC) trial. Circulation 111:1611-1618, 2005.
43. Kirtane A, Piazza G, Murphy S, et al: TIMI Study Group: Correlates of bleeding events among moderate- to high-risk patients undergoing percutaneous coronary intervention and treated with eptifibatide. Observations from the PROTECT-TIMI-30 Trial. J Am Coll Cardiol 47:2374-2379, 2006.
44. Ognibene A, Mannucci E, Caldini A, et al: Cystatin C reference values and aging. Clin Biochem 2006 Apr 21:Epub ahead of print.
45. Wasen E, Isoaho R, Mattila K, et al: Estimation of glomerular filtration rate in the elderly: A comparison of creatinine-based formulae with serum cystatin C. J Intern Med 256:70-78, 2004.
46. Grubb A, Bjork J, Lindstrom V, et al: A cystatin-C based formula without anthropometric variables estimates glomerular filtration rate better than creatinine clearance using the Cockcroft-Gault formula. Scand J Clin Lab Invest 65:153-162, 2005.
47. Kang D, Verotta D, Krecic-Shepard ME, et al: Population analyses of sustained release verapamil in patients: Age, race, and sex effects. Clin Pharmacol Ther 73:31-40, 2003.
48. Kang D, Verotta D, Schwartz J: Population analyses of amlodipine in patients living in the community and nursing homes. Clin Pharmacol Ther 79:114-124, 2006.
49. Schwartz J: Erythromycin breath test results in elderly, very elderly, and frail elderly persons. Clin Pharmacol Ther 79:440-448, 2006.
50. Schwartz J: Gender-specific implications for cardiovascular medication use in the elderly: optimizing therapy for older women. Cardiol Rev 11:275-298, 2003.
51. Schwartz J: The influence of sex on pharmacokinetics. Clin Pharmacokin 42:4-10, 2003.
52. Humphries S, Hingorani A: Pharmacogenetics: Progress, pitfalls and clinical potential for coronary heart disease. Vascul Pharmacol 44:119-125, 2006.
53. Roden D: Proarrhythmia as a pharmacogenomic entity: A critical review and formulation of a unifying hypothesis. Cardiovasc Res 67:419-425, 2005.
54. Sim S, Ingelman-Sundberg M: The human cytochrome P450 Allele Nomenclature Committee Web site: Submission criteria, procedures, and objectives. Methods Mol Biol 320:183-191, 2006.
55. Committee: To err is human: Building a safer health system. In Kohn LT, Donaldson M (eds): Washington, DC, National Academy of Sciences, 2000 (http://books.nap.edu/catalog.php?record_id=9728; accessed 4/12/07).
56. Onder GPC, Landi F, Cesari M, et al: Adverse drug reactions as cause of hospital admission: Results from the Italian Group of Pharmacoepidemiology in the Elderly (GIFA). JAGS 50:1962-1968, 2002.
57. Gurwitz JH, Harrold LR, Rothschild J, et al: Incidence and preventability of adverse drug events among older persons in the ambulatory setting. JAMA 289:1107-1116, 2003.
58. Bates D, Miller E, Cullen D, et al: ADE Prevention Study Group: Patient risk factors for adverse drug events in hospitalized patients. Arch Intern Med 159:2553-2560, 1999.
59. Gandhi TK, Borus J, Seger AC, et al: Adverse drug events in ambulatory care. N Engl J Med 348:1556-1564, 2003.
60. Gurwitz J, Field T, Judge J, et al: The incidence of adverse drug events in two large academic long-term care facilities. Am J Med 118:251-258, 2005.
61. Kaufman DKJ, Rosenberg L, Anderson TE, Mitchell AA: Recent patterns of medication use in the ambulatory adult population of the United States. The Slone Survey. JAMA 287:337-344, 2002.
62. Flockhart D: Clinically relevant CYP inducers and inhibitors (http://medicine.iupui.edu/flockhart/clinlist.htm). Accessed May 16, 2006.
63. Lau WC, Waskell LA, Watkins PB, et al: Atorvastatin reduces the ability of clopidogrel to inhibit platelet aggregation: A new drug-drug interaction. Circulation 107:32-37, 2003.

CH 75

64. De Smet P: Herbal remedies. N Engl J Med 347:2046-2056, 2002.

65. Ioannides C: Pharmacokinetic interactions between herbal remedies and medicinal drugs. Xenobiotica 32:451-478, 2002.

66. Juurlink DN, Kopp A, Laupacis A, Redelmeier DA: Drug-drug interactions among elderly patients hospitalized for drug toxicity. JAMA 289:1652-1658, 2003.

67. Schulman S: Care of patients receiving long-term anticoagulant therapy. N Engl J Med 349:675-683, 2003.

68. Perlin JB, Roswell RH: The Veterans Health Administration: Quality, value, accountability, and information as transforming strategies for patient-centered care. Am J Manag Care 10:828-836, 2004.

69. Kuperman G, Bigson R: Computer physician order entry: benefits, costs, and issues. Ann Intern Med 139:31-39, 2003.

70. Briesacher B, Limcangco R, Simoni-Wastila L, et al: Evaluation of nationally mandated drug use reviews to improve patient safety in nursing homes: A natural experiment. J Am Geriatr Soc 53:991-996, 2005.

71. Juurlink D, Mamdani M, Kopp A, et al: Drug-drug interactions among elderly patients hospitalized for drug toxicity. JAMA 289:1652-1658, 2003.

72. Drazen J: Cox-2 inhibitors—a lesson in unexpected problems. N Engl J Med 352:1131-1132, 2005.

73. Psaty B, Furberg C: Cox-2 inhibitors—lessons in drug safety. N Engl J Med 352:1133-1135, 2005.

74. Smith I, Dowsett M: Aromatase inhibitors in breast cancer. N Engl J Med 348:231-242, 2003.

75. A comparison of letrozole and tamoxifen in postmenopausal women with early breast cancer. The Breast International Group (BIG) 1-98 Collaborative Group. N Engl J Med 353:2747-2757, 2005.

76. Beers M: Explicit criteria for determining potentially inappropriate medication by the elderly. Arch Intern Med 157:1531-1536, 1997.

77. Hanlon JT, Boult C, Artz MB, et al: Use of inappropriate prescription drugs by older people. JAGS 50:26-34, 2002.

78. Fick D, Cooper J, Wade W, et al: Updating the Beers Criteria for potentially inappropriate medication use in older adults. Arch Intern Med 163:2716-2724, 2003.

79. Simon S, Chan K, Soumerai S, et al: Potentially inappropriate medication use by elderly persons in U.S. Health Maintenance Organizations, 2000-2001. J Am Geriatr Soc 53:227-232, 2005.

80. Rochon P, Lane C, Bronskill S, et al: Potentially inappropriate prescribing in Canada relative to the US. Drugs Aging 21:939-947, 2004.

81. Curtis L, Ostbye T, Sendersky V, et al: Inappropriate prescribing for elderly Americans in a large outpatient population. Arch Intern Med 164:1621-1625, 2004.

82. Holmes H, Hayley D, Alexander G, Sachs G: Reconsidering medication appropriateness for patients late in life. Arch Intern Med 166:605-609, 2006.

83. Walter L, Covinsky K: Cancer screening in elderly patients: A framework for individualized decision making. JAMA 285:2750-2756, 2001.

84. Lee S, Lindquist K, Segal M, Covinsky K: Development and validation of a prognostic index for 4-year mortality in older adults. JAMA 295:801-808, 2006.

85. O'Connor P: Adding value to evidence-based clinical guidelines. JAMA 294:741-743, 2005.

86. Walter L, Brand R, Counsell S, et al: Development and validation of a prognostic index for 1-year mortality in older adults after hospitalization. JAMA 285:2987-2994, 2001.

87. Michalsen A, Konig G, Thimme W: Preventable causative factors leading to hospital admission with decompensated heart failure. Heart 80:437-441, 1998.

88. Federman A, Adams A, Ross-Degnan D, et al: Supplemental insurance and use of effective cardiovascular drugs among elderly Medicare beneficiaries with coronary heart disease. JAMA 286:1732-1739, 2001.

89. Barat I, Andreasen F, Damsgaard E: Drug therapy in the elderly: What doctors believe and patients actually do. Br J Clin Pharmacol 51:615-622, 2001.

90. Piette J, Heisler M, Wagner T: Cost-related medication underuse. Do patients with chronic illnesses tell their doctors? Arch Intern Med 164:1749-1755, 2004.

91. McDonald HPGA, Haynes RB: Interventions to enhance patient adherence to medication prescriptions. Scientific Review. JAMA 288:2868-2879, 2002.

Vascular Disease

92. LLoyd-Jones D, Evans J, Levy D: Hypertension in adults across the age spectrum. Current outcomes and control in the community. JAMA 294:466-472, 2005.

93. Hajjar I, Kotchen T: Trends in prevalence, awareness, treatment, and control of hypertension in the United States, 1988-2000. JAMA 290:199-206, 2003.

94. Wing LM, Reid CM, Ryan P, et al: Second Australian National Blood Pressure Study Group. A comparison of outcomes with angiotensin-converting enzyme inhibitors and diuretics for hypertension in the elderly. N Engl J Med 348:583-592, 2003.

95. Randomized double-blind comparison of a calcium antagonist and a diuretic in elderly hypertensives. National Intervention Cooperative Study in Elderly Hypertensives Study Group. Hypertension 34:1129-1133, 1999.

96. Malacco E, Mancia G, Rappelli A, et al: Treatment of isolated systolic hypertension: The SHELL study results. Blood Press 12:160-167, 2003.

97. Chobanian AV, Bakris GL, Black HR, et al: National High Blood Pressure Education Program Coordinating Committee. The Seventh Report of the Joint National Committee on Prevention, Detection, Evaluation, and Treatment of High Blood Pressure. The JNC 7 Report. JAMA 289:2560-2572, 2003.

98. Angeli F, Verdecchia P, Reboldi G, et al: Calcium channel blockade to prevent stroke in hypertension: A meta-analysis of 13 studies with 103,793 subjects. Am J Hypertens 17:817-822, 2004.

99. Verdecchia P, Reboldi G, Angeli F, et al: Angiotensin-converting enzyme inhibitors and calcium channel blockers for coronary heart disease and stroke prevention. Hypertension 46:386-392, 2005.

100. Forette F, Seux ML, Staessen JA, et al: Syst-Eur Investigators: The prevention of dementia with antihypertensive treatment. Arch Intern Med 162:2046-2052, 2002.

101. Guidelines Committee: 2003 European Society of Hypertension—European Society of Cardiology guidelines for the management of arterial hypertension. J Hypertens 21:1011-1053, 2003 (http://www.eshonline.org/documents 2003_guidelines.pdf).

102. Tinetti M: Preventing falls in elderly persons. N Engl J Med 348:42-49, 2003.

103. Bulpitt C, Beckett N, Cooke J, et al: Hypertension in the Very Elderly Trial Working Group: Results of the pilot study for the Hypertension in the Very Elderly Trial. J Hypertens 12:2409-2417, 2003.

Coronary Artery Disease

104. Kuller L, Fisher L, McClelland R, et al: Differences in prevalence of and risk factors for subclinical vascular disease among black and white participants in the Cardiovascular Health Study. Arterioscler Thromb Vasc Biol 18:283-293, 1998.

105. Newman AB, Shemanski L, Manolio TA, et al: Ankle-arm index as a predictor of cardiovascular disease and mortality in the Cardiovascular Health Study. Arterioscler Thromb Vasc Biol 19:538-545, 1999.

106. Kuller L, Borhani N, Furberg C, et al: Prevalence of subclinical atherosclerosis and cardiovascular disease and association with risk factors in the Cardiovascular Health Study. Am J Epidemiol 139:1164-1179, 1994.

107. Wilson P, D'Agostino R, Levy D, et al: Prediction of coronary heart disease using risk factor categories. Circulation 97:1837-1847, 1998.

108. Daly C, Clemens F, Sendon JLL, et al: Gender differences in the management and clinical outcome of stable angina. Circulation 113:490-498, 2006.

109. Vaccarino V, Rathore S, Wenger N, et al: National Registry of Myocardial Infarction Investigators: Sex and racial differences in the management of acute myocardial infarction, 1994 through 2002. N Engl J Med 353:671-682, 2005.

110. Anand S, Xie C, Mehta SR, et al: CURE Investigators. Differences in the management and prognosis of women and men who suffer from acute coronary syndromes. J Am Coll Cardiol 46:1845-1851, 2005.

111. Blomkalns A, Chen A, Hochman J, et al: CRUSADE Investigators. Gender disparities in the diagnosis and treatment of non-ST-segment elevation acute coronary syndromes: Large-scale observations from the CRUSADE (Can Rapid Risk Stratification of Unstable Angina Patients Suppress Adverse Outcomes with Early Implementation of the American College of Cardiology/American Heart Association Guidelines) National Quality Improvement Initiative. J Am Coll Cardiol 45:832-837, 2005.

112. Kannel W, D'Agostino R, Sullivan L, Wilson P: Concept and usefulness of cardiovascular risk profiles. Am Heart J 148:16-26, 2004.

113. Ariyo A, Thach C, Tracy R: Cardiovascular Health Study Investigators: Lp(a) lipoprotein, vascular disease, and mortality in the elderly. N Engl J Med 349:2108-2115, 2003.

114. Psaty B, Anderson M, Kronmal R, et al: The association between lipid levels and the risks of incident myocardial infarction, stroke, and total mortality: The Cardiovascular Health Study. J Am Geriatr Soc 52:1639-1647, 2004.

115. Stork S, Feelders R, van den Beld A, et al: Prediction of mortality risk in the elderly. Am J Med 119:519-525, 2006.

116. Sesso H, Stampfer M, Rosner B, et al: Systolic and diastolic blood pressure, pulse pressure, and mean arterial pressure as predictors of cardiovascular disease risk in men. Hypertension 36:801-807, 2000.

117. Mattace-Raso F, van der Cammen T, Hofman A, et al: Arterial stiffness and risk of coronary heart disease and stroke. The Rotterdam Study. Circulation 113:657-663, 2006.

118. Hansen T, Staessen J, Torp-Pederson C, et al: Prognostic value of aortic pulse wave velocity as index of arterial stiffness in the general population. Circulation 113:664-670, 2006.

119. Pearte C, Furberg C, O'Meara E, et al: Characteristics and baseline clinical predictors of future fatal versus nonfatal coronary heart disease events in older adults. The Cardiovascular Health Study. Circulation 113:2177-2185, 2006.

120. Hemingway H, McCallum A, Shipley M, et al: Incidence and prognostic implications of stable angina pectoris among women and men. JAMA 295:1404-1411, 2006.

121. Shlipak M, Sarnak M, Katz R, et al: Cystatin C and the risk of death and cardiovascular events among elderly persons. N Engl J Med 352:2049-2060, 2005.

122. Naghavi M, Falk E, Hecht H, et al: SHAPE Task Force: From vulnerable plaque to vulnerable patient—Part III: Executive summary of the Screening for Heart Attack Prevention and Education (SHAPE) Task Force report. Am J Cardiol 98(Suppl):2H-15H, 2006.

123. Mieres J, Shaw L, Arai A, et al: Role of noninvasive testing in the clinical evaluation of women with suspected coronary artery disease: Consensus statement from the Cardiac Imaging Committee, Council on Clinical Cardiology, and the Cardiovascular Imaging and Intervention Committee, Council on Cardiovascular Radiology and Intervention, American Heart Association. Circulation 111:682-696, 2005.

124. Redberg R: Coronary artery calcium: Should we rely on this surrogate marker? Circulation 113:336-337, 2006.

125. Williams M, Fleg J, Ades P, et al: Secondary prevention of coronary heart disease in the elderly (with emphasis on patients >75 years of age). An American Heart Association Scientific Statement from the Council on Clinical Cardiology Subcommittee on Exercise, Cardiac Rehabilitation, and Prevention. Circulation 105:1735-1743, 2002.

126. Ko D, Mamdani M, Alter D: Lipid-lowering therapy with statins in high-risk elderly patients: The treatment-risk paradox. JAMA 291:1864-1870, 2004.

127. Avezum A, Makdisse M, Spencer F, et al: GRACE Investigators: Impact of age on management and outcome of acute coronary syndrome: Observations from the Global Registry of Acute Coronary Events (GRACE). Am Heart J 149:67-73, 2005.

128. Antons K, Williams C, Baker S, Phillips P: Clinical perspectives of statin-induced rhabdomyolysis. Am J Med 119:400-409, 2006.

129. Bruckert E, Hayem G, Dejager S, et al: Mild to moderate muscular symptoms with high-dosage statin therapy in hyperlipidemic patients—the PRIMO Study. Cardiovasc Drugs Ther 19:403-414, 2005.

130. LaRosa J, Grundy S, Waters D, et al: Treating to New Targets (TNT) Investigators. Intensive lipid lowering with atorvastatin in patients with stable coronary disease. N Engl J Med 352:1425-1435, 2005.

131. Downs J, Clearfield M, Weis S, et al: Primary prevention of acute coronary events with lovastatin in men and women with average cholesterol levels. Results of AFCAPS/TexCAPS. JAMA 279:1615-1622, 1998.

132. Shepherd J, Cobbe S, Ford I, et al: Prevention of coronary heart disease with pravastatin in men with hypercholesterolemia. N Engl J Med 333:1301-1307, 1995.

133. Hillis GS, Zehr K, Williams A, et al: Outcome of patients with low ejection fraction undergoing coronary artery bypass grafting. Renal function and mortality after 3.8 years. Circulation 114(Suppl):I-414-419, 2006.

134. Dacey L, Likosky D, Ryan T, et al: Northern New England Cardiovascular Disease Study Group. Long-term survival following CABG surgery vs. PCI in 1693 octogenarians with multivessel coronary disease. The Society of Thoracic Surgeons Annual Meeting, Chicago, 2006.

135. Newman MF, Kirchner J, Phillips-Bute B, et al: Neurological Outcome Research Group and the Cardiothoracic Anesthesiology Research Endeavors Investigators. Longitudinal assessment of neurocognitive function after coronary-artery bypass surgery. N Engl J Med 344:395-402, 2001.

136. Jensen B, Hughes P, Rasmussen L, et al: Cognitive outcomes in elderly high-risk patients after off-pump versus conventional coronary artery bypass grafting: A randomized trial. Circulation 113:2790-2795, 2006.

137. Silbert B, Scott D, Evered L, et al: A comparison of the effect of high and low dose fentanyl on the incidence of postoperative cognitive dysfunction after coronary artery bypass surgery in the elderly. Anesthesiology 104:1137-1145, 2006.

138. Panesar S, Athanasious T, Nair S, et al: Early outcomes in the elderly: A meta-analysis of 4921 patients undergoing coronary artery bypass grafting—comparison between off-pump and on-pump techniques. Heart 12:1808, 2006.

139. Mehta R, Granger C, Alexander K, et al: Reperfusion strategies for acute myocardial infarction in the elderly. State of the art paper. J Am Coll Cardiol 45:471-478, 2005.

140. Brass LM, Lichtman JH, Wang Y, et al: Intracranial hemorrhage associated with thrombolytic therapy for elderly patients with acute myocardial infarction: Results from the Cooperative Cardiovascular Project. Stroke 31:1802-1811, 2000.

141. Berger A, Radford M, Wang Y, et al: Thrombolytic therapy in older patients. J Am Coll Cardiol 36:366-374, 2000.

142. Thiemann D, Coresh J, Schulman S, et al: Lack of benefit for intravenous thrombolysis in patients with myocardial infarction who are older than 75 years. Circulation 101:2239-2246, 2000.

143. Yusuf S, Mehta SR, Chrolavicius S, et al: Comparison of fondaparinux and enoxaparin in acute coronary syndromes. The Fifth Organization to Assess Strategies in Acute Ischemic Syndromes Investigators. N Engl J Med 354:1464-1476, 2006.

144. Antiplatelet Trialists' Collaboration: Collaborative meta-analysis of randomised trials of antiplatelet therapy for prevention of death, myocardial infarction and stroke in high risk patients. BMJ 324:71-86, 2002.

145. Sabatine M, Cannon C, Gibson C, et al: CLARITY-TIMI 28 Investigators: Addition of clopidogrel to aspirin and fibrinolytic therapy for myocardial infarction with ST-segment elevation. N Engl J Med 352:1179-1189, 2005.

146. Horwitz P, Berlin J, Sauer W, et al: Registry Committee of the Society for Cardiac Angiography Interventions. Bleeding risk of platelet glycoprotein IIb/IIIa receptor antagonists in broad-based practice (results from the Society for Cardiac Angiography and Interventions Registry). Am J Cardiol 91:803-806, 2003.

147. Brown D: Deaths associated with platelet glycoprotein IIb/IIIa inhibitor treatment. Heart 89:535-537, 2003.

148. Sixon S, Grines C, O'Neill W: The year in interventional cardiology. J Am Coll Cardiol 47:1689-1706, 2006.

149. Hochman J, Sleeper L, Webb J, et al: SHOCK Investigators. Early revascularization and long-term survival in cardiogenic shock complicating acute myocardial infarction. JAMA 295:2511-2515, 2006.

150. Alexander K, Roe M, Kulkarni S, et al: Evolution of cardiovascular care for elderly patients with non-ST-segment elevation acute coronary syndromes. Results from CRUSADE. J Am Coll Cardiol 46:1490-1495, 2005.

151. Berwen D, Galusha D, Lewis J, et al: National and state trends in quality of care for acute myocardial infarction between 1994-1995 and 1998-1999. Arch Intern Med 163:1430-1439, 2003.

152. Thombs B, Bass E, Ford D, et al: Prevalence of depression in survivors of acute myocardial infarction. J Gen Intern Med 21:30-38, 2006.

153. Bush D, Ziegelstein R, Tayback M, et al: Even minimal symptoms of depression increase mortality risk after acute myocardial infarction. Am J Cardiol 88:337-341, 2001.

154. Connerney I, Shapiro P, McLaughlin J, et al: Relation between depression after coronary artery bypass surgery and 12-month outcome: A prospective study. Lancet 358:1766-1771, 2001.

155. Dusseldorp E, van Elderen T, Maes S, et al: A meta-analysis of psychoeducational programs for coronary heart disease patients. Health Psychol 18:506-519, 1999.

156. Whooley M: Depression and cardiovascular disease. JAMA 296:2874-2881, 2006.

157. Serebruany VL: Selective serotonin reuptake inhibitors and increased bleeding risk: Are we missing something? Am J Med 119:113-116, 2006.

158. Rochon P, Tu J, Anderson G, et al: Rate of heart failure and 1-year survival for older people receiving low-dose beta-blocker therapy after myocardial infarction. Lancet 356:639-644, 2000.

159. Barrett-Connor E, Mosca L, Collins P, et al: Raloxifene Use for The Heart (RUTH) Trial Investigators. Effects of Raloxifene on Cardiovascular Events and Breast Cancer in Postmenopausal Women. N Engl J Med 355:125, 2006.

160. Vogel V, Costantino J, Wickerham D, et al: National Surgical Adjuvant Breast and Bowel Project (NSABP). Effects of tamoxifen vs raloxifene on the risk of developing invasive breast cancer and other disease outcomes: The NSABP Study of Tamoxifen and Raloxifene (STAR) P-2 trial. JAMA 295:2727-2741, 2006.

161. Marchionni N, Fattirolli F, Fumagalli S, et al: Improved exercise tolerance and quality of life with cardiac rehabilitation of older patients after myocardial infarction. Results of a randomized, controlled trial. Circulation 107:2201-2206, 2003.

162. Alberts M, Latchaw R, Selman W, et al: Brain Attack Coalition: Recommendations for comprehensive stroke centers. A consensus statement from the Brain Attack Coalition. Stroke 36:1597-1618, 2005.

163. Adams H, Adams R, Del Zoppo G, Goldstein L: Guidelines for the early management of patients with ischemic stroke. 2005 Guidelines Update. A scientific statement from the Stroke Council of the American Heart Association/American Stroke Association. Stroke 36:916-921, 2005.

164. Bates B, Choi J, Duncan P, et al: Veterans Affairs/Department of Defense clinical practice guideline for the management of adult stroke rehabilitation care. Executive summary. Circulation 36:2049-2056, 2005.

165. Sacco R, Adams R, Alberts M, et al: Guidelines for prevention of stroke in patients with ischemic stroke or transient ischemic attack. A statement for healthcare professionals from the American Heart Association/American Stroke Association Council on Stroke: Co-sponsored by the Council on Cardiovascular Radiology and Intervention: The American Academy of Neurology affirms the value of this guideline. Circulation 113:e409-e449, 2006.

166. Baigent C, Keech A, Kearnery P, et al: Cholesterol Treatment Trialists' (CTT) Collaborators. Efficacy and safety of cholesterol-lowering treatment: Prospective meta-analysis of data from 90,056 participants in 14 randomized trials. Lancet 366:1267-1278, 2005.

167. The SPARCL Investigators: The Stroke Prevention by Aggressive Reduction in cholesterol Levels (SPARCL) study. Cerebrovasc Dis 21(Suppl 4):1, 2006.

168. Diener H, Bogousslavsky J, Brass L, et al: Aspirin and clopidogrel compared with clopidogrel alone after recent ischaemic stroke or transient ischaemic attack in high-risk patients (MATCH): Randomised, double-blind placebo-controlled trial. Lancet 364:331-337, 2004.

169. Bhatt D, Fox K, Hacke W, et al: CHARISMA Investigators. Clopidogrel and aspirin versus aspirin alone for the prevention of atherothrombotic events. N Engl J Med 354:1706-1717, 2006.

170. Diener H, Cunha L, Forbes C, et al: European Stroke Prevention Study-2: Dipyridamole and acetylsalicylic acid in the secondary prevention of stroke. J Neurol Sci 143:1-13, 1996.

171. Mohr J, Thompson J, Lazar R, et al: A comparison of warfarin and aspirin for the prevention of recurrent ischemic stroke. N Engl J Med 345:1444-1451, 2001.

172. Barnett H, Meldrum H, Eliasziw M: North American Symptomatic Carotid Endarterectomy Trial (NASCET) collaborators. The appropriate use of carotid endarterectomy. CMAJ 166:1169-1179, 2002.

173. Coward L, Featherstone R, Brown M: Safety and efficacy of endovascular treatment of carotid artery stenosis compared with carotid endarterectomy: A Cochrane systematic review of the randomized evidence. Stroke 36:905-911, 2005.

Peripheral Artery Disease

174. Hirsch AT, Criqui MH, Treat-Jacobson D, et al: The PARTNERS program: A national survey of peripheral arterial disease detection, awareness, and treatment. JAMA 286:1317-1324, 2001.

175. Hirsh A, Haskal Z, Hertzer N, et al: ACC/AHA 2005 Practice Guidelines for the management of patients with peripheral arterial disease (lower extremity, renal, mesenteric, and abdominal aortic): Executive Summary: A collaborative report from the American Association for Vascular Surgery/Society for Vascular Surgery, Society for Cardiovascular Angiography and Interventions, Society for Vascular Medicine and Biology, Society of Interventional Radiology, and the ACC/AHA Task Force on Practice Guidelines (Writing Committee to Develop Guidelines for the Management of Patients with Peripheral Arterial Disease). Circulation 113:1474-1547, 2006.

176. Hankey G, Norman P, Eikelboom J: Medical treatment of peripheral artery disease. JAMA 295:547-553, 2006.

177. Singh K, Patel M, Zidar J, Kandzari D: Peripheral arterial disease: An overview of endovascular therapies and contemporary treatment strategies. Rev Cardiovasc Med 7:55-68, 2006.

Heart Failure

178. Ni H: Prevalence of self-reported heart failure among US adults: Results from the 1999 National Health Interview Survey. Am Heart J 146:1-4, 2003.

179. Roger VL, Weston S, Redfield M, et al: Trends in heart failure incidence and survival in a community-based population. JAMA 292:344-350, 2004.

180. Barker W, Mullooly J, Getchell W: Changing incidence and survival for heart failure in a well-defined older population, 1970-1974 and 1990-1994. Circulation 113:799-805, 2006.

181. Maurer M, King D, Rumbarger E, et al: Left heart failure with a normal ejection fraction: identification of different pathophysiologic mechanisms. J Card Failure 11:177-187, 2005.

182. van Heerebeek L, Borbely A, Niessen H, et al: Myocardial structure and function differ in systolic and diastolic heart failure. Circulation 113:1966-1973, 2006.

183. Redfield M, Jacobsen S, Burnett J, et al: Burden of systolic and diastolic ventricular dysfunction in the community. Appreciating the scope of the heart failure epidemic. JAMA 289:194-202, 2003.

CH 75

184. Silver M, Yancy C, McCullough P, et al: BNP Consensus Panel 2004: A clinical approach for the diagnostic, prognostic, screening, treatment monitoring, and therapeutic roles of natriuretic peptides in cardiovascular diseases. CHF 10(Suppl 3):1-30, 2004.

185. Ahmed A, Rich M, Love T, et al: Digoxin and reduction in mortality and hospitalization in heart failure: A comprehensive post hoc analysis of the DIG trial. Eur Heart J 27:178-186, 2006.

186. Turnbull F, Neal B, Algert C, et al: Blood Pressure Lowering Treatment Trialists' Collaboration: Effects of different blood pressure-lowering regimens on major cardiovascular events in individuals with and without diabetes mellitus: Results of prospectively designed overviews of randomized trials. Arch Intern Med 165:1410-1419, 2005.

187. Flather M, Shibata M, Coats A, et al: Randomized trial to determine the effect of nebivolol on mortality and cardiovascular admission in elderly patients with heart failure (SENIORS). Eur Heart J 26:215-225, 2005.

188. Ghio S, Magrini G, Serio A, et al: SENIORS Investigators: Effects of nebivolol in elderly heart failure patients with or without systolic left ventricular dysfunction: Results of the SENIORS echocardiographic substudy. Eur Heart J 27:562-568, 2006.

189. Ahmed A, Rich M, Fleg J, et al: Effects of digoxin on morbidity and mortality in diastolic heart failure: The ancillary digitalis investigation group trial. Circulation 114:397-403, 2006.

190. Yusuf S, Pfeffer M, Swedberg K, et al: Effects of candesartan in patients with chronic heart failure and preserved left-ventricular ejection fraction: The CHARM-Preserved trial. Lancet 362:777-781, 2003.

191. Rich M, Beckham V, Wittenberg C, et al: A multidisciplinary intervention to prevent the readmission of elderly patients with congestive heart failure. N Engl J Med 333:1190-1195, 1995.

192. Naylor M, Brooten D, Campbell R, et al: Transitional care of older adults hospitalized with heart failure: A randomized controlled trial. J Am Geriatr Soc 52:672-684, 2004.

193. Nichol K, Nordin J, Mullooly J, et al: Influenza vaccination and reduction in hospitalizations for cardiac disease and stroke among the elderly. N Engl J Med 348:1322-1332, 2003.

194. Pantilat S, Steimle A: Palliative care for patients with heart failure. JAMA 291:2476-2482, 2004.

Arrhythmias

195. Lamas G, Lee K, Sweeney M, et al: Mode selection trial in sinus-node dysfunction. Ventricular pacing or dual-chamber pacing for sinus-node dysfunction. N Engl J Med 346:1854-1862, 2002.

196. Kerr C, Connolly S, Abdollah H, et al: Canadian Trial of Physiological Pacing: Effects of physiological pacing during long-term follow-up. Circulation 109:357-362, 2004.

197. Toff W, Camm A, Skehan J: United Kingdom Pacing and Cardiovascular Events Trial Investigators. Single-chamber versus dual-chamber pacing for high-grade atrioventricular block. N Engl J Med 353:145-155, 2005.

198. Healey J, Toff W, Lamas G, et al: Cardiovascular outcomes with atrial-based pacing compared with ventricular pacing: Meta-analysis of randomized trials, using individual patient data. Circulation 114:11-17, 2006.

199. Martinez C, Tzur A, Hrachian H, et al: Pacemakers and defibrillators: Recent and ongoing studies that impact the elderly. Am J Ger Cardiol 15:82-87, 2006.

200. Tsang T, Petty G, Barnes M, et al: The prevalence of atrial fibrillation in incident stroke cases and matched population controls in Rochester, Minnesota. Changes over three decades. J Am Coll Cardiol 42:93-100, 2003.

201. Nieuwlatt R, Capucci A, Camm A, et al: European Heart Survey Investigators: Atrial fibrillation management: A prospective survey in ESC member countries: The Euro Heart Survey on Atrial Fibrillation. Eur Heart J 26:2422-2432, 2005.

202. de Denus S, Sanoski C, Carlsson J, et al: Rate vs. rhythm control in patients with atrial fibrillation: A meta-analysis. Arch Intern Med 165:258-262, 2005.

203. Caraballo P, Heit J, Atkinson E, et al: Long-term use of oral anticoagulants and the risk of fracture. Arch Intern Med 159:1750-1756, 1999.

Valvular Disease

204. Shavelle D, Takasu J, Budoff M, et al: HMG CoA reductase inhibitor (statin) and aortic valve calcium. Lancet 359:1125-1126, 2002.

205. Faggiano P, Antonini-Canterin F, Erlicher A, et al: Progression of aortic valve sclerosis to aortic stenosis. Am J Cardiol 91:99-101, 2003.

206. Otto C, Lind B, Kitzman D, et al: Association of aortic-valve sclerosis with cardiovascular mortality and morbidity in the elderly. N Engl J Med 341:142-147, 1999.

207. Peltier M, Trojette F, Enriquez-Sarano M, et al: Relation between cardiovascular risk factors and nonrheumatic severe calcific aortic stenosis among patients with a three-cuspid aortic valve. Am J Cardiol 91:97-99, 2003.

208. Bellamy M, Pellikka P, Klarich K, et al: Association of cholesterol levels, hydroxymethylglutaryl coenzyme-a reductase inhibitor treatment, and progression of aortic stenosis in the community. JACC 40:1723-1730, 2002.

209. Cowell S, Newby D, Prescott R, et al: Scottish Aortic Stenosis and LIpid Lowering Trial, Impact on Regression (SALTIRE) Investigators. A randomized trial of intensive lipid-lowering therapy in calcific aortic stenosis. N Engl J Med 352:2389-2397, 2005.

210. Goodney P, O'Connor G, Wennberg D, Birkmeyer J: Do hospitals with low mortality rates in coronary artery bypass also perform well in valve replacement? Ann Thorac Surg 76:1131-1136, 2003.

211. Ambler G, Omar R, Royston P, et al: Generic, simple risk stratification model for heart valve surgery. Circulation 112:224-231, 2005.

212. Kauterman K, Michaels A, Ports T: Is there any indication for aortic valvuloplasty in the elderly? Am J Geriatr Cardiol 12:190-196, 2003.

213. Aronow W, Ahn C, Kronzon I: Comparison of echocardiographic abnormalities in African-American, Hispanic, and white men and women aged >60 years. Am J Cardiol 87:1131-1133, 2001.

214. Lee R, Sundt TI, Moon M, et al: Mitral valve repair in the elderly: Operative risk for patients over 70 years of age is acceptable. J Cardiovasc Surg 44:157-161, 2003.

215. Flowers C, Racoosin J, Lu S, Beitz J: The US Food and Drug Administration's registry of patients with pergolide-associated valvular heart disease. Mayo Clin Proc 78:730-731, 2003.

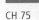

CHAPTER 76

Cardiovascular Disease in Women

L. Kristin Newby and Pamela S. Douglas

Background, 1955

Scope of the Problem, 1955

Coronary Artery Disease Risk
Factors and Risk Factor
Modification, 1956
Unmodifiable Risk Factors, 1956
Potentially Modifiable Risk
    Factors, 1956
Life Style Risk Factors, 1957
Global Assessment of Risk Factors for
    Coronary Heart Disease, 1957

Presentation with Acute
Coronary Disease, 1957
Imaging for Diagnosis and
    Prognosis, 1958
Evidence-Based Therapy in
    Women, 1958
ACC/AHA STEMI and UA/NSTEMI
    ACS Guidelines, 1961
Invasive Management and
    Revascularization, 1961
Glycoprotein IIb/IIIa Inhibitors, 1962
Bleeding with Antithrombotic
    Therapy, 1962
Sex Differences in Treatment, 1962
Cardiac Rehabilitation, 1963

Heart Failure, 1963

Peripheral Arterial
Disease, 1964

Future Perspective, 1964

References, 1964

BACKGROUND

Throughout history, differences between men and women in health and in illness have fascinated researchers and clinicians alike. The Institute of Medicine's Committee on Understanding the Biology of Sex and Gender Differences defined *sex* as "the classification of living things, generally as male or female according to their reproductive organs and functions assigned by the chromosomal complement."[1] *Gender*, on the other hand, was defined as "a person's self-representation as male or female or how that person is responded to by social institutions on the basis of the individual's gender presentation." Women (XX) and men (XY) differ in their genetic complement by but a single chromosome out of the 46 that define the human species. However, the influence of this single chromosomal difference affects both the expression of disease and the psychosocial and behavioral characteristics and work environments of individuals, which may protect from or enhance susceptibility to cardiovascular disease. In this discussion of cardiovascular disease in women, both of these definitions come into play to explain differences in the occurrence, presentation with, or course of cardiovascular disease, and in some cases treatment and response to therapy.

SCOPE OF THE PROBLEM

Cardiovascular disease is the leading cause of death among women, regardless of race or ethnicity, accounting for nearly 500,000 deaths in the United States each year and causing the deaths of 1 in 3 women; this amounts to more deaths from heart disease than from stroke, lung cancer, chronic obstructive lung disease, and breast cancer combined.[2] About half of these deaths result from coronary heart disease. Despite these sobering statistics and estimates that a 40-year-old woman has a lifetime risk of cardiovascular disease of 32 percent,[3] and although awareness of cardiovascular disease as the leading cause of death has increased, still only about 55 percent of women identify cardiovascular disease as their greatest health risk.[4] Although mortality from heart disease has declined gradually among men since 1979 (by 30 to 50 percent), mortality from heart disease in women has increased during that same period.[2] For coronary heart disease in specific, mortality rates have fallen for both men and women over this time period, but much more rapidly in men than women.[2] A greater proportion of women (52 percent) than men (42 percent) with myocardial infarction die of sudden cardiac death before reaching the hospital, and two thirds of women who suffer a myocardial infarction never completely recover.[2,5] Since the late 1970s, hospital discharges from heart failure among women, a consequence of predominantly ischemic and hypertensive heart disease, have also increased at a markedly faster rate than among men.[2] Thus, understanding even subtle differences between men and women in development or progression of cardiovascular disease, use of proven therapies, and response to therapy is paramount.

Experts in industrialized societies have long recognized that the first presentation with coronary heart disease occurs approximately 10 years later among women than men, most commonly after menopause. The worldwide INTERHEART Study, a large cohort study of more than 52,000 individuals with myocardial infarction, first demonstrated that this approximate 8- to 10-year difference in age of onset among men compared with women holds widely around the world, across various socioeconomic, climatic, and cultural environments.[6] Although coronary artery disease in general manifests earlier in less well-developed countries, the approximate 8- to 10-year age gap in time of onset between men and women is universal (Table 76-1). Despite this delay in onset, mortality from coronary heart disease is increasing more rapidly among women than men in both the developed and developing world.[7] Further, younger, premenopausal women, not older women, carried a mortality excess compared with similarly aged men presenting with myocardial infarction in the National Registry of Myocardial Infarction (NRMI).[8]

Experts have widely speculated that this age difference reflects premenopausal protection from development of atherosclerotic coronary disease afforded by circulating estrogen, which is markedly reduced at menopause. However, despite this plausible biological explanation for the difference between the sexes in age of first onset of coronary disease, replacement of estrogen after menopause has been shown not to be effective in preventing clinical cardiovascular events.[9-12] For a summary of hormonal influence on atherosclerotic vascular disease and the spectrum of observational and clinical trials research on postmenopausal hormone therapy, the reader can consult an excellent review by Ouyang and colleagues.[13]

TABLE 76–1	Comparison of Age of First Myocardial Infarction among Women and Men across Geographic Region	
Region	Median Age Women	Median Age Men
Western Europe	68 (59-76)	61 (53-70)
Central/Eastern Europe	68 (59-74)	59 (50-68)
North America	64 (52-75)	58 (49-68)
South America/Mexico	65 (56-73)	59 (50-68)
Australia/New Zealand	66 (59-74)	58 (50-67)
Middle East	57 (50-65)	50 (44-57)
Africa	56 (49-65)	52 (46-61)
South Asia	60 (50-66)	52 (45-60)
China/Hong Kong	67 (62-72)	60 (50-68)
Southeast Asia/Japan	63 (56-68)	55 (47-64)

Modified from Yusuf S, Hawken S, Ounpuu S, et al: Effect of potentially modifiable risk factors associated with myocardial infarction in 52 countries (the INTERHEART study): Case-control study. Lancet 364:937, 2004.

CORONARY ARTERY DISEASE RISK FACTORS AND RISK FACTOR MODIFICATION

The classic risk factors for coronary atherosclerosis are commonly divided into those that are potentially modifiable to mitigate risk (diabetes, hypertension, hyperlipidemia, cigarette smoking, obesity, and sedentary life style) and those that are not modifiable (age and family history). With a few exceptions, these factors have similar influence on cardiovascular risk across the sexes.

Unmodifiable Risk Factors

Age

Age is one of the most powerful risk factors for development of cardiovascular disease and accompanying clinical events. Although the prevalence of cardiovascular disease with increasing age varies modestly according to sex (prior to the fifth decade of life, prevalence in men is greater than in women, but in the sixth decade, prevalence equalizes and in subsequent decades becomes greater in women), the magnitude of the association of age with clinical cardiovascular events is similar among men and women.[2]

Family History

Family history of coronary heart disease is a second unmodifiable risk factor. It is well established that coronary heart disease and death from cardiovascular disease have a hereditary component.[14,15] In a minority of families, the predilection for coronary disease is monogenic, with transmission occurring in a mendelian pattern (see also Chap. 8). An example is a family recently identified to have a mutation in the *MEF2A* gene.[16] In contrast, the majority of coronary artery disease is complex, likely reflecting contribution of multiple genes, with variations in several genes, each contributing modestly to a predisposition to atherosclerosis and atherothrombotic clinical events.

Whether sex differences exist in the frequency of genetic polymorphisms that influence the occurrence of cardiovascular events remains an open question. However, the statistical association of gene variants with coronary disease differs in men and women, suggesting that different pathways may operate in the manifestation of cardiovascular

disease between the sexes.[17] Two of 112 polymorphisms in 71 candidate genes were associated with myocardial infarction in women: stromelysin-1, a member of the matrix metalloproteinase family of enzymes that are believed to be involved in plaque rupture (relative risk [RR] of 4.7 [99 percent confidence interval (CI) 2.0 to 12.2]) and, much less strongly, plasminogen activator inhibitor-1 (PAI-1). In contrast, in men, two different genes were associated with myocardial infarction: the gap junction protein, connexon 37 (RR 1.7, 95 percent CI 1.1 to 1.6), and p22 (phox), a component of the NAD(P)H redox system (RR 0.7, 95 percent CI 0.6 to 0.9). This apparent sex-related difference in the association of genetic polymorphisms with clinical disease phenotypes may be less related to the presence or absence of the genetic mutation itself in men and women than to the influences of sex on variation in the expression of various genes or the downstream responses to the gene's products.

Evidence indicates that variations in sex hormones and their levels between men and women or other differences related to the presence or absence of Y chromosome genes including, but not limited to, those that regulate cellular function could influence these observed associations. Indeed, ex vivo male macrophages responded to androgens with upregulation of 27 atherosclerosis-associated genes resulting in increased foam cell formation and enhanced lysosomal low-density lipoprotein (LDL) cholesterol degradation, whereas ex vivo female cells did not show a response in any of the 588 genes tested.[18] Such differences may help to explain observed differences in the pathophysiology of atherosclerosis including plaque composition (more cellular and fibrous tissue in women),[19] endothelial function (estrogen-induced coronary vasodilation), and hemostasis (higher fibrinogen and factor VII levels in women).[20-22] Further, the underlying inciting pathophysiology of atherothrombotic coronary events varies in women and men and may be influenced by both genetics and sex-based differences including the effects of estrogen that influence gene expression and protein production or activity. For example, women are twice as likely to have plaque erosion (37 percent in women versus 18 percent in men), and men more frequently have plaque rupture as the underlying inciting event (82 percent in men versus 63 percent in women).[23] With the continued evolution of ribonucleic acid (RNA) microarray technology and proteomics capabilities, it will become increasingly feasible to determine expression patterns of tens of thousands of genes and the presence and relative abundance of their protein products simultaneously. Although only limited work has explored sex differences in gene expression or proteomics, further work in this area may provide important insights into development, diagnosis, and tailored treatment of cardiovascular disease in women and men.

Potentially Modifiable Risk Factors

Hypertension

Hypertension is an increasingly common risk factor among the U.S. population, with 65 million affected individuals in National Health and Nutrition Examination (NHANE) surveys from 1999 to 2000.[24] Overall, more than 35 million women had hypertension, a 15 percent higher prevalence than that in men. The prevalence of hypertension increased with age in both sexes, but from 45 to 54 years of age the escalation was greater among women than men, the difference in prevalence reaching statistical significance at age 75 and beyond. In subjects younger than 35 years of age, hypertension was significantly more prevalent among men than women.

In a meta-analysis of 61 prospective studies of hypertension involving more than 1 million previously healthy adults between the ages of 49 and 89, the association with ischemic heart disease risk was only slightly stronger in women than in men.[25] In this study the slope of the association between ischemic heart disease mortality and blood pressure was fairly constant, arguing against a "threshold" systolic pressure below which disease risk is not further reduced. An analysis of men and women in the Framingham Heart Study supports this position by showing that the gradient of cardiovascular risk extended to high normal and normal blood pressures in both sexes.[26]

Unfortunately, women remain one of the populations most likely to be undertreated when they have an established diagnosis of hypertension, and even more concerning, little progress has been made in improving rates of treatment and control over the past decade. Whereas treatment and control rates in men increased by an absolute 9.8 and 15.3 percent, respectively, between the NHANE surveys spanning 1988-1994 and a follow-up survey from 1999 to 2000, the treatment and control rates in women were essentially unchanged (increases of only 1.9 and 0.5 percent, respectively).[27]

Diabetes and the Metabolic Syndrome (see Chap. 43)

The prevalence of diabetes in the United States is escalating rapidly. Between 2000 and 2001, the prevalence of diabetes rose by 8.2 percent, and in 2003, women older than 20 years of age comprised slightly more than half (10.1 million) of the 20.1 million patients with diabetes.[2] Of these women, 7.1 million had a physician diagnosis of diabetes, but 3 million had undiagnosed diabetes. Further, of the 14.7 million people in the United States with prediabetes, defined as impaired glucose tolerance or a fasting blood glucose of 110 to less than 126 mg/dl, women accounted for 6.1 million.[2] Cardiovascular disease is twice as common among women with diabetes as those without, they are four times as likely to be hospitalized, and women have a higher risk for most clinical events than men.[2]

Metabolic syndrome relates closely to insulin resistance and comprises a constellation of at least three of the following risk factors: abdominal obesity, an atherogenic lipid profile (excessive triglycerides and/or inadequate high-density lipoprotein [HDL] cholesterol), blood pressure of 130/85 mm Hg or higher, and a fasting glucose concentration of 110 mg/dl or greater. At any given LDL cholesterol level, metabolic syndrome increases the risk for coronary heart disease. Because of this, the National Cholesterol Education Program (NCEP) Adult Treatment Panel III considers metabolic syndrome a secondary target of risk-reduction therapy.[28] After adjustment for age, metabolic syndrome appears to be highly prevalent in both sexes, with little difference in rates between women and men.[29]

Hyperlipidemia (see Chap. 42)

More than half of women in the United States have a total cholesterol greater than 200 mg/dl, and 36 percent have LDL greater than 130 mg/dl, incidences similar to the general population.[2] However, more favorably, whereas 22.6 percent of Americans overall have an HDL less than 40 mg/dl, only 12.6 percent of women are in this range,[2] leading to the establishment of a higher cut point of greater than 50 mg/dl for the normal level in women. The relative risk for coronary disease events associated with elevation of various lipid variables was determined in a nested case-control study from the Nurses Health Study. Among 32,826 healthy women who provided blood samples at baseline, the multivariable adjusted relative risks (adjusted for high-sensitivity C-reactive protein [hsCRP], homocysteine, and other traditional cardiac risk factors) for the highest quintiles of lipid variables were: apolipoprotein B (apo B) (RR = 4.1 [2 to 8.3], low levels of HDL (RR 2.6 [1.4 to 5]), LDL (RR 3.1 [1.7 to 5.8]), and triglycerides (RR 1.9 [1 to 3.9]).[30] Adverse changes in lipid profiles accompany menopause.[31] Perimenopausal triglyceride levels are the most erratic but followed roughly the same pattern of increase as total and LDL cholesterol, which increase on average by an absolute 10 percent from levels 6 months premenopause. Menopause influences HDL cholesterol less dramatically. HDL declines gradually in the 2 years preceding menopause and then levels after menopause. The postmenopausal increase in cardiovascular disease risk may result partly from these lipid alterations.

The 1988-1994 NHANE surveys showed that serum cholesterol concentrations in U.S. adults were on a downward trend. However, lipid profiles changed little between the 1988-1994 and 1999-2000 NHANE surveys. In the follow-up survey, the prevalence of hypercholesterolemia was similar for men and women, and of all adults with high total cholesterol, only 35 percent were aware of their diagnosis and rates were similar among men and women. Only 10.2 percent of dyslipidemic women were under treatment compared with 12 percent overall, and among treated women, only 3.7 percent achieved a total cholesterol concentration of 5.2 mmol/liter compared with 5.4 percent overall.[32] As with hypertension, these findings highlight the need for a stronger commitment to prevention, treatment, and control of hypercholesterolemia, with enhanced focus on women.

Life Style Risk Factors

In 2003, 61.6 percent of American women were overweight, defined as a body mass index (BMI) greater than 25 kg/m²; 29 percent did not engage in leisure-time physical activity; and 18.5 percent were smokers.[2] Further, the prevalence of obesity (BMI > 30 kg/m²) in women has increased gradually but markedly from 12.2 percent in 1991 to 20.8 percent in 2001.[33]

Global Assessment of Risk Factors for Coronary Heart Disease (see Chap. 39)

Primary findings of the large case-control INTERHEART Study provide some of the best data to date on the relationship of clinical parameters with the risk of ischemic heart disease worldwide, including patterns of association of myocardial infarction risk among women compared with men.[6] Overall, after adjustment, nine risk factors accounted for 90.4 percent of the population attributable risk (PAR) for myocardial infarction (94 percent of the PAR among women and 90 percent among men). The risk factors were (1) apo B/apo A-I ratio; (2) cigarette smoking; (3) hypertension; (4) diabetes; (5) abdominal obesity; (6) psychosocial factors (an index based on combining parameter estimates for depression, stress at work or home, financial stress, one or more life events, locus of control scores); (7) fruit and vegetable intake; (8) exercise; and (9) alcohol intake.

Although the strength of association of most risk factors with myocardial infarction was similar among women and men, the INTERHEART Study confirmed a markedly stronger association of diabetes with myocardial infarction among women compared with men (Fig. 76-1).[6] Psychosocial factors also tended to associate more strongly with increased risk among women, though the difference was less in magnitude. In addition, healthy life-style choices including regular exercise and modest alcohol consumption provided stronger protection among women than men, and there was a tendency for fruit and vegetable intake to be more favorable among women. Although further work is necessary to define the underpinnings of these observations, they nonetheless have important implications for counseling and management of women to prevent cardiovascular events.

PRESENTATION WITH ACUTE CORONARY DISEASE

A number of symptoms are commonly associated with myocardial infarction in both sexes including chest pain, pressure or squeezing; pain radiating to the neck, shoulder, back, arms, or jaw; palpitations; dyspnea; heartburn, nausea, vomiting, or abdominal pain; diaphoresis; and dizziness. Women may experience milder symptoms or describe them somewhat differently and may more frequently experience

Risk factor	Sex	Control (%)	Case (%)	Odds ratio (99% CI)	PAR (99% CI)
Current smoking	F	9.3	20.1	2.86 (2.36–3.48)	15.8% (12.9–19.3)
	M	33.0	53.1	3.05 (2.78–3.33)	44.0% (40.9–47.2)
Diabetes	F	7.9	25.5	4.26 (3.51–5.18)	19.1% (16.8–21.7)
	M	7.4	16.2	2.67 (2.36–3.02)	10.1% (8.9–11.4)
Hypertension	F	28.3	53.0	2.95 (2.57–3.39)	35.8% (32.1–39.6)
	M	19.7	34.6	2.32 (2.12–2.53)	19.5% (17.7–21.5)
Abdominal obesity	F	33.3	45.6	2.26 (1.90–2.68)	35.9% (28.9–43.6)
	M	33.3	46.5	2.24 (2.03–2.47)	32.1% (28.0–36.5)
Psychosocial index	F	-	-	3.49 (2.41–5.04)	40.0% (28.6–52.6)
	M	-	-	2.58 (2.11–3.14)	25.3% (18.2–34.0)
Fruits/veg	F	50.3	39.4	0.58 (0.48–0.71)	17.8% (12.9–24.1)
	M	39.6	34.7	0.74 (0.66–0.83)	10.3% (6.9–15.2)
Exercise	F	16.5	9.3	0.48 (0.39–0.59)	37.3% (26.1–50.0)
	M	20.3	15.8	0.77 (0.69–0.85)	22.9% (16.9–30.2)
Alcohol	F	11.2	6.3	0.41 (0.32–0.53)	46.9% (34.3–60.0)
	M	29.1	29.6	0.88 (0.81–0.96)	10.5% (6.1–17.5)
ApoB/ApoA1 ratio	F	14.1	27.0	4.42 (3.43–5.70)	52.1% (44.0–60.2)
	M	21.9	35.5	3.76 (3.23–4.38)	53.8% (48.3–59.2)

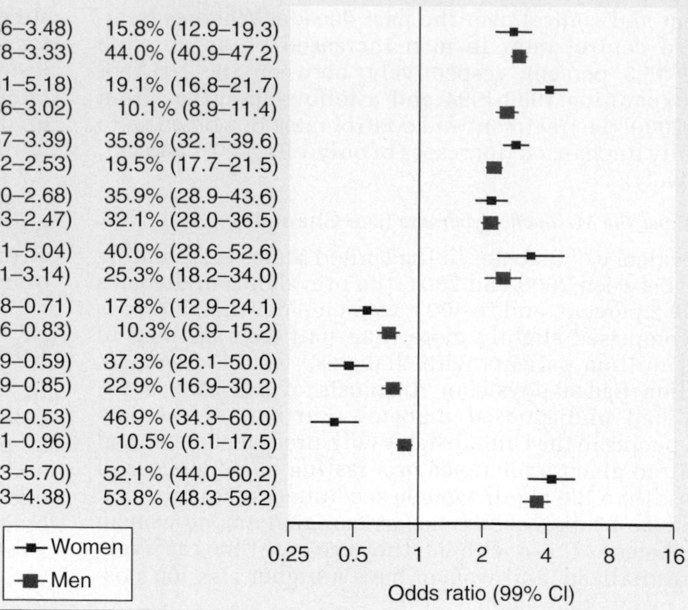

Women
Men

Odds ratio (99% CI)

FIGURE 76–1 Relative risks associated with various cardiac risk factors among men (M) and women (F) in the INTERHEART Study. PAR = population attributable risk. *(From Yusuf S, Hawken S, Ounpuu S, et al: Effect of potentially modifiable risk factors associated with myocardial infarction in 52 countries [the INTERHEART study]: Case-control study. Lancet 364:937, 2004.)*

CH 76

nonspecific prodromal symptoms such as fatigue.[34] A study of 127 men and 90 women by Milner and colleagues[35] showed that among patients who presented to the emergency department with symptoms of coronary disease other than chest pain, there were several sex-related differences in symptoms. Dyspnea, nausea/vomiting, indigestion, fatigue, sweating, and arm or shoulder pain as presenting symptoms in the absence of chest pain were all more frequent among women than men. However, the Myocardial Infarction Triage and Intervention investigators demonstrated that chest pain was present in almost all women (99.6 percent) and men (99 percent) who experienced a documented acute myocardial infarction.[36] In addition to symptom differences, women with myocardial infarction have more comorbidities including hypertension and present later in the course of symptoms and more frequently with high-risk clinical findings of heart failure and tachycardia.[37]

Women (4 million visits/year) are hospitalized more frequently for evaluation of chest pain than men (2.4 million visits/year),[2] but it has been well documented that women who present with chest pain or even more clearly with acute coronary syndromes (ACS) are more likely than men to have a noncardiac etiology and less severe obstructive coronary lesions or other nonatherosclerotic etiologies such as vasospasm.[38] Recent data from the National Institutes of Health (NIH)–sponsored Women's Ischemia Syndrome Evaluation study confirm a marked discordance between observed rates of coronary artery disease and the predicted probability of coronary disease (Fig. 76-2).[5] This discordance was pervasive across age groups, and angina was classified as typical or atypical.

Imaging for Diagnosis and Prognosis

Compounding observations of differences in presentation and the discordance between predicted probability of disease and actual disease, there is a paucity of data regarding the best diagnostic strategy for assessing women with chest pain to establish or exclude a diagnosis of coronary

artery disease. Thus recommendations for use of stress testing in women often derive from studies performed predominantly in men. Further, accuracy in the clinical setting is often confounded by use of tests among women with low pretest probability, yielding multiple false-positive tests. However, in one small study, the results of exercise stress testing according to the Duke Treadmill score appeared at least as good for both diagnosis and prognosis in women as in men, with a higher negative predictive value in women.[39]

In general, recommendations for stress testing with imaging parallel those in men.[40] In a consensus statement from the American Heart Association (AHA) on imaging in women, Mieres and colleagues[41] summarized the available data on diagnostic stress testing and derived an algorithm to guide the use of exercise testing with or without cardiac imaging in women with chest pain. Figure 76-3 demonstrates the algorithm for use in intermediate- or high-risk women with atypical or typical chest pain symptoms. In general, imaging in symptomatic women is recommended for those at intermediate or high risk for coronary artery disease.[41] Both stress echocardiographic and stress gated myocardial single-photon emission computed tomographic (SPECT) nuclear imaging appear to perform similarly in women for diagnosis,[42] and both were given similar recommendations for stress testing in women in the AHA position statement.[41] Importantly, available evidence suggests that the prognostic utility of either form of imaging with stress testing is similar (Fig. 76-4) and describes a gradient of risk that is similar in men and women.[42]

Evidence-Based Therapy in Women

Women in Clinical Research

Randomized clinical trials with adequate power to demonstrate clinically meaningful differences between treatments, interventions, or management strategies should guide their use in practice. Assessing treatment effect within a subgroup is usually underpowered and fraught with the likelihood of type I error as a result of multiple comparisons. That said, consistency of findings across subgroups provides reassurance that the trial results are generalizable. Using observational studies to assess treatment benefits and risks is complex and subject to multiple recognized and unrecognized biases, which may lead to erroneous conclusions. The story of hormone replacement therapy for primary and secondary prevention of cardiovascular events is an excellent example in that multiple observational studies had shown dramatic reductions in coronary heart disease death or myocardial infarction among users of hormone replacement therapy. However, a series of large randomized clinical trials later demonstrated that not only did hormone replacement therapy fail to reduce coronary heart disease events, in some cases events actually increased among those randomly assigned to receive hormone therapy compared with those assigned to placebo treatment.[9-12]

Unfortunately, in a systematic review surveying the literature for all randomized clinical trials in myocardial infarction from 1966 to 2000, Lee and colleagues[43] demonstrated that there was a marked discordance between the representation of women among myocardial infarction patients and their representation in clinical trials (Fig. 76-5). Even most recently, whereas women sustained 45 percent of all myocardial infarctions, they represented only 27 percent of patients enrolled in randomized clinical trials of treatments for acute myocardial infarction. Thus recruitment of women in proportion to their representation among patients with the cardiovascular disease of interest is paramount to support the extension of the results of clinical trials to women.

Practice Guidelines to Codify Treatment Recommendations

In general, American College of Cardiology (ACC)/AHA Guidelines for management of ST-segment elevation and non-ST-segment elevation myocardial infarction, as well as chronic coronary disease, are silent or neutral on treatment by

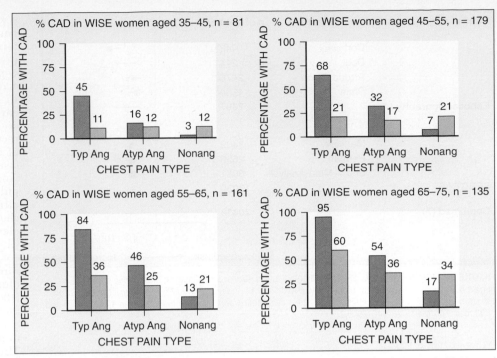

FIGURE 76–2 Observed rates of coronary artery disease (CAD) at angiography (yellow bars) compared with Diamond probability of CAD (purple bars). Atyp Ang = atypical angina; Nonang = nonanginal pain; Typ Ang = typical angina. *(From Shaw LJ, Bairey Merz, Pepine CJ, et al: Insights from the NHLBI-sponsored Women's Ischemia Syndrome Evaluation [WISE] Study. Part I: Gender differences in traditional and novel risk factors, symptom evaluation, and gender-optimized diagnostic strategies. J Am Coll Cardiol 47:4S, 2006.)*

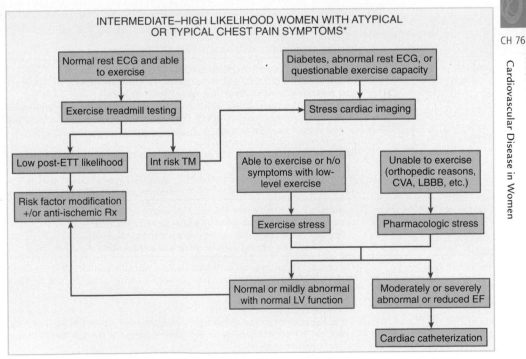

FIGURE 76–3 Algorithm for stress testing in women with moderate to high risk of coronary artery disease and presenting with typical or atypical symptoms. CVA = cerebrovascular accident; ECG = electrocardiogram; EF = ejection fraction; ETT = exercise treadmill test; h/o = history of; LBBB = left bundle branch block; LV = left ventricular; TM = treadmill. *(From Mieres JH, Shaw LJ, Arai A, et al: Role of noninvasive testing in the clinical evaluation of women with suspected coronary artery disease: Consensus statement from the Cardiac Imaging Committee, Council of Clinical Cardiology, and the Cardiovascular Imaging and Intervention Committee, Council on Cardiovascular Radiology and Intervention, American Heart Association. Circulation 111:682, 2005.)*

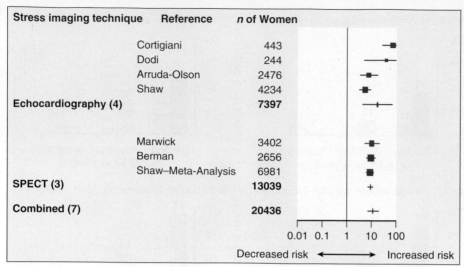

Stress imaging technique	Reference	*n* of Women
	Cortigiani	443
	Dodi	244
	Arruda-Olson	2476
	Shaw	4234
Echocardiography (4)		**7397**
	Marwick	3402
	Berman	2656
	Shaw–Meta-Analysis	6981
SPECT (3)		**13039**
Combined (7)		**20436**

0.01 0.1 1 10 100

Decreased risk ← → Increased risk

FIGURE 76–4 Prognostic utility of echocardiographic and nuclear stress imaging among women. SPECT = single-photon emission computed tomography. *(From Shaw LJ, Vasey C, Sawada S, et al: Impact of gender on risk stratification by exercise and dobutamine stress echocardiography: Long-term mortality in 4234 women and 6898 men. Eur Heart J 26:447, 2005.)*

sex.[38,44-46] In addition to these "gender-neutral" guidelines, the AHA maintains a broadly endorsed set of prevention guidelines specifically for women (Table 76-2).[47] To take into account the lower numbers of women in most randomized clinical trials of cardiovascular prevention strategies and medications, in addition to ranking recommendations by class and strength of evidence, these guidelines added a score that addresses generalizability to women. Since these guidelines were published, three major randomized clinical trials have been published that shed further light on the class I and class III recommendations (see also Chaps. 39 and 45).

The Women's Health Study (WHS) randomized 39,876 healthy women older than 45 years to low-dose aspirin (100 mg on alternate days) or placebo and followed them for 10 years for first occurrence of death, nonfatal myocardial infarction, or nonfatal stroke.[48] This trial provides important insights into the use of aspirin for primary prevention in women. Although the overall

TABLE 76–2	Recommendations from the Women's Evidence-Based Prevention Guidelines
Clinical Area	**Recommendations**
Class I Recommendations	
Life Style Interventions	Smoking cessation; avoid second-hand smoke
	30 min of moderate-intensity physical activity on most (preferably all) days of the week
	Cardiac rehabilitation/risk reduction program post-MI, post–coronary intervention, and if chronic angina
	Overall healthy eating pattern; limit saturated fat to <10% of calories, cholesterol to <300 mg/d, limit trans fatty acids
	Weight maintenance/reduction to BMI 18.5-24.9 kg/m²
Major Risk Factor Interventions	Encourage optimal BP < 120/80 through life style approaches
	Pharmacotherapy if BP > 140/90 or lower if end-organ damage or diabetes
	Use thiazide diuretics unless absolute contraindication
	Optimal lipid targets: LDL < 100 mg/dl, HDL > 50 mg/dl, triglycerides <150 mg/dl, non-HDL cholesterol <130 mg/dl
	In high-risk women or elevated LDL, reduce intake of saturated fat to <7% of calories and cholesterol to <200 mg/day and reduce trans fatty acids
	Drug therapy for lipid abnormalities:
	High risk—initiate if LDL ≥ 100 mg/dl; statin therapy if high risk and LDL < 100 mg/dl; niacin or fibrate if HDL is low or non-HDL cholesterol high
	Intermediate risk—initiate if LDL ≥ 130 mg/dl; niacin or fibrate if HDL is low or non-HDL cholesterol high
	Life style and pharmacotherapy to achieve near normal (<7%) HbA1c in women with diabetes
Preventive Drug Regimens	Aspirin in high-risk women (75-162 mg daily) or clopidogrel if aspirin allergic or intolerant
	Beta blockers indefinitely post-MI unless contraindicated
	ACE inhibitors in high-risk women unless contraindicated
	ARBs in high-risk women with heart failure or EF < 40%
Atrial Fibrillation/ Stroke Prevention	For chronic or paroxysmal atrial fibrillation, warfarin to INR 2.0-3.0 unless low risk
	Aspirin (325 mg daily) if contraindication to warfarin or at low risk for stroke (<1%/yr)
Class III Recommendations	
	Hormone therapy:
	Do not start or continue estrogen + progestin for primary or secondary prevention
	Do not initiate or continue other forms of hormone therapy for prevention of cardiovascular disease pending results of ongoing trials
	Antioxidants:
	Do not use antioxidant supplements for cardiovascular disease prevention
	Aspirin:
	Routine use of aspirin in low-risk women is not recommended

ACE = angiotensin-converting enzyme; ARB = angiotensin receptor blocker; BMI = body mass index; BP = blood pressure; EF = ejection fraction; HbA1c = hemoglobin A1c; HDL = high-density lipoprotein; INR = international normalized ratio; LDL = low-density lipoprotein; MI = myocardial infarction.
Modified from Mosca L, Appel LJ, Benjamin E, et al: Evidence-based guidelines for cardiovascular disease prevention in women. J Am Coll Cardiol 43:900, 2004.

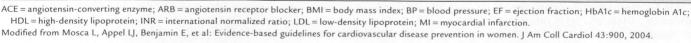

study showed a nonsignificant 9 percent reduction in the primary composite endpoint (RR 0.91 [95 percent CI 0.80 to 1.03]), when the individual endpoints were examined, there was heterogeneity of effect. There was no effect of aspirin on the rate of nonfatal myocardial infarction (RR 1.02 [95 percent CI 0.84 to 1.25]) or cardiovascular death (RR 0.95 [0.74 to 1.22]). However, aspirin reduced stroke risk by 17 percent overall (RR 0.83 [95 percent CI 0.69 to 0.99]), and ischemic stroke by 24 percent (RR 0.76 [95 percent CI 0.63 to 0.93]). Hemorrhagic stroke increased nonsignificantly (RR 1.24 [95 percent CI 0.82 to 1.87]), but gastrointestinal bleeding requiring transfusion was significantly increased (RR 1.40 [95 percent CI 1.07 to 1.83]). Of note, this study revealed significant age × treatment interactions for the effect of aspirin on the primary composite endpoint and the individual endpoint of nonfatal myocardial infarction. Whereas the benefit of aspirin in reducing ischemic stroke was consistent across all age groups, only in those older than 65 years did aspirin significantly reduce the risk of nonfatal myocardial infarction (RR 0.66 [95 percent CI 0.44 to 0.97]). Thus consideration of the use of aspirin in primary prevention requires a careful assessment of multiple potential risks and benefits of treatment before prescription in an individual woman.

The recently completed Pravastatin or Atorvastatin Evaluation and Infection Trial–Thrombolysis in Myocardial Infarction 22 trial demonstrated the safety and effectiveness of more aggressive lipid-lowering therapy with statins.[49] In this study an intensive regimen of 80 mg of atorvastatin reduced LDL cholesterol by 51 percent to a median of 62 mg/dl compared with a reduction of 22 percent to a median of 95 mg/dl in the pravastatin 40 mg arm. This greater reduction of LDL cholesterol translated into a 16 percent reduction in the hazard for death or major cardiac events at a mean follow-up of 2 years. No difference occurred in the safety or efficacy profile among women and men. Thus evidence now exists for even more aggressive lowering of LDL cholesterol in secondary prevention than reflected in current guideline recommendations.

The results of the Women's Health Initiative estrogen-only trial provide additional support for the class III recommendation for use of hormone replacement therapy to prevent first coronary disease event.[12] In this trial, 10,739 postmenopausal women without a uterus were randomized to placebo or 0.625 mg of oral conjugated equine estrogens daily. The trial was stopped early by its Data and Safety Monitoring Board in February 2004. At that point, there was no significant benefit of conjugated equine estrogens on the primary composite endpoint of death or nonfatal myocardial infarction (RR 0.91 [0.75 to 1.12]), but the incidence of stroke (RR 1.39 [95 percent CI 1.10 to 1.77]) and pulmonary embolus (RR 1.34 [0.87 to 2.06]) increased in the estrogen arm. Thus it appears that like estrogen + progesterone, no cardiovascular benefit and potential harm result from postmenopausal administration of conjugated equine estrogens. Because of these and similar results of other studies of hormone replacement therapy, the U.S. Food and Drug Administration has placed a black box warning on the labeling of all estrogen-containing compounds.

ACC/AHA STEMI and UA/NSTEMI ACS Guidelines

The ST-segment elevation myocardial infarction (STEMI) guidelines are silent on sex-specific recommendations, providing completely sex- and gender-neutral treatment

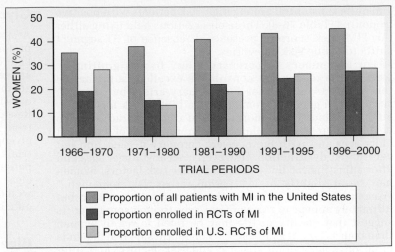

FIGURE 76–5 Underrepresentation of women in clinical trials of acute myocardial infarction (MI) relative to their representation among all patients with acute MI. RCTs = randomized clinical trials. *(From Lee PY, Alexander KP, Hammill BG, et al: Representation of elderly persons and women in published randomized trials of acute coronary syndromes. JAMA 286:708, 2001.)*

recommendations.[44] The unstable angina/non-ST-segment elevation myocardial infarction (UA/NSTEMI) guidelines provide the following class I summary recommendation regarding treatment of women: "Women with UA/NSTEMI should be managed in a manner similar to men. Specifically, women, like men with UA/NSTEMI, should receive aspirin and clopidogrel. Indications for noninvasive and invasive testing are similar in women and men. (*Level of Evidence: B*)."[38] However, the literature suggests that subtle differences exist between the sexes and have relevance to the care of individual patients (see later discussion).

Invasive Management and Revascularization

A recent meta-analysis of trials of percutaneous coronary intervention (PCI) confirmed that women more frequently suffer vascular complications of their procedures compared with men.[50] In addition, many studies in predominantly elective PCI demonstrate a tendency to higher in-hospital mortality among women than men. However, late mortality was similar between the sexes. Findings were similar for the use of primary PCI to treat acute myocardial infarction, showing higher in-hospital, but similar late, mortality.

Three randomized clinical trials of early invasive strategies for management of NSTEMI showed conflicting results with regard to treatment benefit in women. Whereas the Fragmin and Fast Revascularization during Instability in Coronary (FRISC) II, Randomised Intervention Trial of unstable Angina 3 (RITA 3), and Treat Angina with Aggrastat and determine Cost of Therapy with Invasive or Conservative Strategy–Thrombolysis in Myocardial Infarction 18 (TACTICS-TIMI 18) trials showed treatment benefit among men, the FRISC II trial showed that women did worse with the early invasive strategy. The RITA 3 trial showed that results were neutral among women, but the TACTICS-TIMI 18 trial showed that women appeared to benefit from the early invasive strategy.[51-53] Although differences in the frequency of use of bypass surgery and the early hazard discussed by Lansky may have contributed to these observations, Glasser and colleagues[51] demonstrated a critical principle of the relationship of risk-to-treatment benefit that may be even more salient in explaining the results of these trials.[51] For low-risk patients (as evidenced by normal troponins) treatment effect becomes neutral, whereas it is modest overall

1962 and quite substantial among high-risk patients with positive troponins (Table 76-3). These observations held using either the TIMI risk score or presence or absence of ST-segment shifts to define risk categories.

For a summary of coronary artery bypass grafting in women, the reader can consult the excellent summary in the ACC/AHA guidelines for coronary artery bypass graft surgery.[54] In general, women have a higher risk for perioperative morbidity and mortality, but in many studies much of this difference is explained by presentation of women at older ages and with more severe coronary disease and left ventricular dysfunction. However, even at younger ages and after adjusting for body size and other risk factors, women may be at slightly higher perioperative risk than men.[55] Women have more postoperative depression than men but ultimately appear to recover similarly, though some reports suggest that quality of life may be rated lower in women than men as far out as 1 year.[56-58] Long-term survival depends more on concomitant disease and risk factors, and after adjustment it is similar in women and men. Thus the guidelines recommend: "Coronary bypass surgery should therefore not be delayed or denied to women who have the appropriate indications for revascularization."[52]

TABLE 76–3	Benefit of an Early Invasive Strategy by Sex and Risk Stratum in TACTICS-TIMI 18*	
6-Mo Endpoints (OR)	**Women**	**Men**
Death	0.94 (0.37-2.44)	0.75 (0.36-1.56)
Death or myocardial infarction	0.45 (0.24-0.88)	0.68 (0.43-1.05)
Death, myocardial infarction, or rehospitalization		
Overall	0.72 (0.47-1.11)	0.64 (0.47-0.88)
Troponin positive	0.56 (0.32-0.97)	0.53 (0.35-0.79)
Troponin negative	1.46 (0.78-2.72)	1.02 (0.64-1.62)

*Data shown are adjusted odds ratio (OR) with 95% confidence interval in parentheses.

From Glasser R, Herrmann HC, Murphy SA, et al: Benefit of an early invasive management strategy in women with acute coronary syndromes. JAMA 288:3124, 2002.

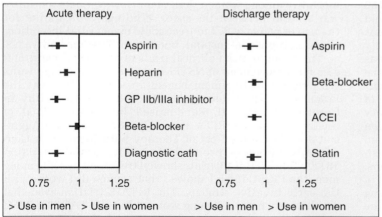

FIGURE 76–6 Use of guidelines-recommended therapies among women compared with men in the CRUSADE registry. ACEI = angiotensin converting enzyme inhibitor; cath = cardiac catheterization; Gp IIb/IIIa = glycoprotein IIB/IIIA. (From Blomkalns AL, Chen AY, Hochman JS, et al; CRUSADE Investigators: Gender disparities in the diagnosis and treatment of non-ST-segment elevation acute coronary syndromes: Large-scale observations from the CRUSADE [Can Rapid Risk Stratification of Unstable Angina Patients Suppress Adverse Outcomes with Early Implementation of the American College of Cardiology/American Heart Association Guidelines] National Quality Improvement Initiative. J Am Coll Cardiol 45:832, 2005.)

Glycoprotein IIb/IIIa Inhibitors

A similar picture emerges with the small molecule glycoprotein IIb/IIIa inhibitors, with initial studies indicating heterogeneity of treatment effect by sex. Although men appeared to benefit from eptifibatide treatment, women had an increased rate of death or myocardial infarction at 30 days in the Platelet Glycoprotein IIb/IIIa in Unstable Angina: Receptor Suppression Using Integrilin Therapy (PURSUIT) trial.[59] A subsequent meta-analysis of all small molecule glycoprotein IIb/IIIa inhibitor (eptifibatide or tirofiban) trials revealed similar results in aggregate.[60] However, once patients were stratified by risk using troponin results, it was clear that the treatment benefit extended to both men and women at high risk for adverse outcomes and that adverse outcomes occurred mostly in low-risk individuals.

Bleeding with Antithrombotic Therapy

The differential treatment effects observed among women and men with the small molecule glycoprotein IIb/IIIa inhibitors and the relationship with risk for ischemic complications may be partly explained by the counterbalancing higher risk for complications of therapy, particularly bleeding. In a recent analysis from the Can Rapid risk stratification of Unstable angina patients Suppress ADverse outcomes with Early implementation of the ACC/AHA Guidelines (CRUSADE) registry, of patients receiving antithrombotic therapy with unfractionated heparin, enoxaparin, and/or a small molecule glycoprotein IIb/IIIa inhibitor, 42 percent received at least 1 initial dose outside of recommended dosing ranges.[61] Such overdosing was associated with increased likelihood of bleeding that increased with the number of agents that were overdosed. Women were significantly more likely to be overdosed than men, in part because of advanced age and associated renal impairment, as well as lower body weight. Several studies have now shown that bleeding and the use of blood transfusions are associated with increased ischemic outcomes among patients with ACS[62-64]; thus treating women at lower risk for adverse ischemic outcomes exposes them to both inherent bleeding risks of treatment and those associated with inappropriate dosing, to which they are more prone, that may offset or exceed any benefit of therapy. Careful attention, particularly to adjustments in dosing for body weight and estimated creatinine clearance, is critically important to ensure safe use of these therapies.

Sex Differences in Treatment

Despite abundant data in aggregate to support the use of existing evidence-based therapy similarly among women as men and sex- and gender-neutral practice guidelines for their use, undertreatment of women relative to men persists. In a recent analysis from the CRUSADE registry of patients with non-ST-segment elevation ACS, use of all therapies for acute management and discharge management were suboptimal, but after adjustment for confounders, use of guidelines-recommended therapies was lower in men than women for all agents except beta blockers in the acute setting (Fig. 76-6).[65] Among more than 345,000 patients with ST-segment elevation myocardial infarction, the NRMI-1 investigators similarly observed lower rates of use of aspirin, beta blockers, and heparin among women compared with men and later administration of fibrinolytic therapy among women.[66] Equally important, women appear to have greater risk than men for nonadherence to long-term use of evidence-based medications in secondary pre-

CH 76

vention, particularly aspirin, statins, and angiotensin-converting enzyme (ACE) inhibitors.[67] Although the cause of these disparities in treatment and adherence is likely multifactorial, concerted efforts to correct them will be necessary in order for women to achieve the full potential of available therapies.

One important component of the strategy to improve adherence to cardiovascular disease guidelines appears to lie in both women's awareness of disease risk and physicians' awareness of guidelines and ability to correctly assess and assign risk level. Although the number of women who recognize cardiovascular disease as the leading cause of death among women has increased to 55 percent in a recent survey, in that same survey only 48 percent of women correctly identified the optimal blood pressure level, 37 percent for HDL, 21 percent for LDL, and 31 percent for blood sugar.[68] However, when present, individual awareness that one's level was not healthy did prompt initiation of steps to lower risk.

In a related study, 500 randomly selected physicians were surveyed about their awareness of and adherence to cardiovascular prevention guidelines.[69] Surprisingly, fewer than 1 in 5 physicians knew that more women than men die each year from cardiovascular disease. Using case studies, the investigators evaluated physicians' assessment of a patient's risk. Regardless of specialty, assignment of risk was strongly associated with the recommendation for lifestyle or treatment interventions, but importantly from these case studies, more women at calculated intermediate risk were perceived by physicians as being at low risk than occurred for intermediate-risk men. Thus improved physician assessment of risk may play an important role in reducing undertreatment relative to guidelines recommendations.

Use of standardized treatment algorithms and participation in quality improvement programs may improve overall adherence to treatment guidelines and lessen sex-related undertreatment. The ACC's Guidelines Applied in Practice (GAP) discharge tool is one such strategy that appears to be effective in increasing use of guidelines-recommended therapies at discharge in both men and women.[70] Importantly, initial results suggest that use of the tool may be associated with lower mortality among women at 1 year.

Cardiac Rehabilitation (see also Chap. 46)

In a 2004 systematic review and meta-analysis of randomized controlled trials of exercised-based cardiac rehabilitation after myocardial infarction that represented 48 trials since 1970, 21 included only men, 26 included both men and women, and 20 percent of all participants were women.[71] In aggregate, these trials showed a 20 percent reduction in total mortality and a 26 percent reduction in cardiac mortality among patients randomized to exercise-based cardiac rehabilitation compared with controls receiving usual care. Improvements in lipid levels and blood pressure and greater rates of smoking cessation were also found. Detailed analyses of men and women were not performed, but conclusions were general regarding the benefits of exercise-based cardiac rehabilitation postmyocardial infarction. In keeping with these findings, the ACC/AHA guidelines for the management of patients with ST-segment elevation myocardial infarction provide a class I recommendation for "cardiac rehabilitation/secondary prevention programs, when available . . . for patients with STEMI, particularly those with multiple modifiable risk factors and/or those moderate- to high-risk patients in whom supervised exercise training is warranted. (*Level of Evidence: C*)."[44] The guidelines for management of patients with non–ST-segment elevation ACS recommend such programs

specifically for individuals who smoke.[38] Despite these recommendations, women are less likely than men to participate in cardiac rehabilitation after acute myocardial infarction.[72]

HEART FAILURE (see Chaps. 25 and 26)

In 2003 there were 550,000 incident cases of heart failure in the United States with an absolute population prevalence that was similar in women (2.6 million individuals) and men (2.4 million individuals).[2] However, women account for 61 percent of heart failure deaths, heart failure more frequently complicates acute myocardial infarction in women (46 percent of cases) than men (22 percent), and survival after diagnosis has increased more in men than women over the past two decades.[2] Women also account for more hospital discharges for heart failure each year than men, a gap that has widened since 1979 (Fig. 76-7).[2]

The underlying pathophysiology of heart failure also appears to be different in women and men. In the Medicare population, patients with heart failure and preserved systolic function are 80 percent women.[73] Alcoholic cardiomyopathy occurs less frequently in women than men; however, this may be because of the lower prevalence of alcoholism among women because alcohol may in fact be more toxic to the myocardium in women, with a lower total dose required to produce cardiomyopathy.[74] In a study of 105,388 patients admitted with acute decompensated heart failure, women accounted for 52 percent of cases but, compared with men, more frequently had preserved left ventricular function (51 versus 28 percent).[75] In this study, men and women had similar length of stay and adjusted in-hospital mortality. Diuretic therapy was used similarly, but women received vasoactive agents less frequently and although both sexes were undertreated with evidence-based oral therapies for heart failure, women were less likely than men to receive them. Additional data from the Acute Decompensated Heart Failure National Registry (ADHERE) indicate that approximately half of patients admitted for management of heart failure have preserved systolic function and that these patients are more frequently women.[76] Recent reports from both the Mayo Clinic and the province of Ontario, Canada reflect these findings of female prevalence among patients with heart failure with preserved left ventricular function.[77,78] Further, these reports show an increasing prevalence of heart failure with preserved left ventricular function and indicate that its prognosis, which is similar to that of

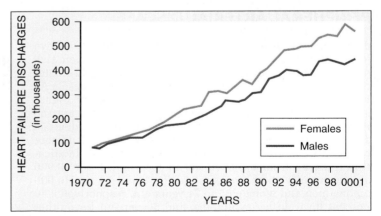

FIGURE 76–7 Trends in hospital discharges for heart failure since 1979 by sex. (*From Thom T, Hasse N, Rosamond W, et al: Heart disease and stroke statistics—2006 update: A report from the American Heart Association Statistics Committee and Stroke Statistics Subcommittee. Circulation 113:e85, 2006.*)

heart failure with systolic dysfunction, has remained essentially unchanged for more than a decade.

Because most evidence for management of heart failure arises from trials in which left ventricular systolic dysfunction predominated or was a critical inclusion criterion and in which men predominated, it is challenging to assess the utility of these therapies in women, particularly when preserved systolic function is much more prominent among women with heart failure. In the absence of such data, the current ACC/AHA heart failure guidelines recommend as a class I recommendation: "Groups of patients including (a) high-risk ethnic minorities (e.g., blacks), (b) groups underrepresented in clinical trials, and (c) any groups believed to be underserved should, in the absence of specific evidence to direct otherwise, have clinical screening and therapy in a manner identical to that applied to the broader population. (*Level of Evidence: B*)."[79] In women, caution should be given to digoxin dosing, especially among elderly women with diminished renal function, and recognition of different side effect profiles, such as increased frequency of cough with ACE inhibitors, may be important.[79]

Implantable cardioverter-defibrillator (ICD) device implantation and cardiac resynchronization therapy are increasingly important components of management of patients with heart failure and ischemic heart disease with left ventricular systolic dysfunction. The utility of and indication for ICD implantation and cardiac resynchronization therapy are reviewed in Chaps. 25 and 34. Further, the reader is referred to an excellent recent review on this topic by Goldberger and Lampert.[80] Although multiple studies have provided evidence for use of these therapies, none of the studies, alone or in aggregate, have enrolled sufficient patients to allow meaningful conclusions regarding utility in women compared with men. Therefore guidelines are broadly inclusive and recommend use of ICD therapy for secondary prevention in all patients with "otherwise good clinical function and prognosis, for whom prolongation of survival is a goal."[79]

Transplantation as treatment for heart failure is used less frequently among women than men. This is in part because of the older age of women with heart failure and differences in women's desires for transplantation.[81] According to AHA statistics, in the United States in 2004, 72.4 percent of transplant patients were men.[2] Among transplanted patients, 1-year survival rates were only slightly less among women (84.6 percent) compared with men (86.4 percent). This gap widened slightly at 3 years (76.1 percent versus 78.9 percent, respectively, in women and men) and at 5 years (68.5 versus 72.2 percent).

PERIPHERAL ARTERIAL DISEASE

Approximately 8 million Americans are believed to have lower extremity peripheral arterial disease, and their risk of death from cardiovascular disease is nearly sixfold greater than individuals without peripheral arterial disease.[2] As with coronary disease, the prevalence is slightly higher among men than women.[82] Smoking and diabetes are the most potent risk factors for peripheral arterial disease. According to a recent summary by the AHA, only 10 percent of patients overall complain of classic intermittent claudication (ranging from 6 per 10,000 in men and 3 per 10,000 among women 30 to 44 years old to 61 and 54 per 10,000 among men and women 65 to 74 years old, respectively); 40 percent have no leg symptoms, and 50 percent have other atypical symptoms.[2] Particularly in elderly women, up to 66 percent may have no symptoms. For an in-depth summary of the epidemiology, diagnosis, and management of peripheral arterial disease, the reader can consult the 2005 publi-

cation of the AHA/ACC practice guidelines for this disease state.[83] In general, recommendations for diagnosis and management are sex/gender neutral (see also Chap. 57).

The population prevalence of renal artery stenosis is not well established but in older adults has been determined in one study at 8.4 percent and was more common among men (9.1 percent) than women (5.5 percent).[84] Ninety percent of lesions are caused by atherosclerosis, but fibromuscular dysplasia is a particularly prevalent pathophysiology in young women with hypertension and renal artery stenosis.[83] Guidelines for diagnosis and treatment are similar in women and men.

Mesenteric arterial disease predominates in women; approximately two thirds of acute presentations are in elderly women (median age 70 years old), and 70 percent of chronic intestinal ischemia occurs in women.[83] Without treatment, acute intestinal ischemia is nearly always fatal. Surgical treatment to remove ischemic bowel and revascularize is given a class I, level of evidence B, recommendation in the guidelines for management of peripheral arterial disease.[83] Despite surgical treatment, mortality remains in the 70 percent range. Percutaneous revascularization and surgical revascularization are recommended in the appropriate settings.[83] Abdominal aortic aneurysms caused by atherosclerotic disease are more prevalent among men than women and are more prevalent in both sexes among older individuals and smokers.[83] Treatment recommendations are sex/gender neutral.

FUTURE PERSPECTIVE

Cardiovascular disease is common among women, and as the population ages, the number of women living with coronary disease and its sequelae, such as heart failure, will only increase. In general, although underrepresentation of women in clinical trials persists, existing treatments appear to be equally effective in both women and men. Despite increasing awareness among physicians and women about cardiovascular disease risk, women are more likely to be undertreated, and for some therapies are more susceptible to complications from treatment. Increased attention to careful selection of therapies for use according to risk and careful monitoring of dosing will be imperative to modulate the balance of benefit and risk in women. The growth in our understanding of genetic susceptibility to cardiovascular disease and rapid advances in genomic, proteomic, and metabolomic techniques promise to elucidate further the underpinnings of differences in disease pathophysiology among men and women that may ultimately lead to new therapies and personalized, perhaps sex-specific, application of new or existing therapies in the coming years.

REFERENCES

General and Risk Factors in Women

1. Wizemann TM, Pardue ML (eds): Institute of Medicine Committee on Understanding the Biology of Sex and Gender Differences. Exploring the Biological Contributions to Human Health. Does Sex Matter? Washington, DC, National Academy Press, 2001.
2. Thom T, Hasse N, Rosamond W, et al: Heart disease and stroke statistics—2006 update: A report from the American Heart Association Statistics Committee and Stroke Statistics Subcommittee. Circulation 113:e85, 2006.
3. Lloyd-Jones DM, Larson MG, Beiser A, Levy D: Lifetime risk of developing coronary heart disease. Lancet 353:89, 1999.
4. Mosca L, Mochari H, Christian A, et al: National study of women's awareness, preventive action, and barriers to cardiovascular health. Circulation 113:525, 2006.
5. Shaw LJ, Bairey Merz CN, Pepine CJ, et al: Insights from the NHLBI-sponsored Women's Ischemia Syndrome Evaluation (WISE) Study. Part I: Gender differences in traditional and novel risk factors, symptom evaluation, and gender-optimized diagnostic strategies. J Am Coll Cardiol 47:4S, 2006.

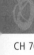

6. Yusuf S, Hawken S, Ounpuu S, et al: Effect of potentially modifiable risk factors associated with myocardial infarction in 52 countries (the INTERHEART study): Case-control study. Lancet 364:937, 2004.

7. Yusuf S, Reddy S, Ôunpuu S, Anand S: Global burden of cardiovascular diseases: Part I: General considerations, the epidemiologic transition, risk factors, and impact of urbanization. Circulation 104:2746, 2001.

8. Vaccarino V, Parsons L, Every NR, et al: Sex-based differences in early mortality after myocardial infarction. National Registry of Myocardial Infarction 2 Participants. N Engl J Med 341:217, 1999.

Hormone Therapy

9. Hulley S, Grady D, Bush T, et al; Heart and Estrogen/Progestin Replacement Study (HERS) Research Group: Randomized trial of estrogen plus progestin for secondary prevention of coronary heart disease in postmenopausal women. JAMA 280:605, 1998.

10. Grady D, Herrington D, Bittner V, et al; HERS Research Group: Cardiovascular disease outcomes during 6.8 years of hormone therapy: Heart and Estrogen/Progestin Replacement Study follow-up (HERS II). JAMA 288:49, 2002. Erratum in: JAMA 288:1064, 2002.

11. Manson JE, Hsia J, Johnson KC, et al; Women's Health Initiative Investigators: Estrogen plus progestin and the risk of coronary heart disease. N Engl J Med 349:523, 2003.

12. Anderson GL, Limacher M, Assaf AR, et al; Women's Health Initiative Steering Committee: Effects of conjugated equine estrogen in postmenopausal women with hysterectomy: The Women's Health Initiative randomized controlled trial. JAMA 291:1701, 2004.

13. Ouyang P, Michos ED, Karas RH: Hormone replacement therapy and the cardiovascular system: Lessons learned and unanswered questions. J Am Coll Cardiol 47:1741, 2006.

Genetics

14. Zdravkovic S, Wienke A, Pedersen NL, et al: Heritability of death from coronary heart disease: A 36-year follow-up of 20 966 Swedish twins. J Intern Med 252:247, 2002.

15. Murabito JM, Pencina MJ, Nam BH, et al: Sibling cardiovascular disease as a risk factor for cardiovascular disease in middle-aged adults. JAMA 294:3117, 2005.

16. Wang L, Fan C, Topol SE, et al: Mutation of MEF2A in an inherited disorder with features of coronary artery disease. Science 302:1578, 2003.

17. Yamada Y, Izawa H, Ichihara S, et al: Prediction of the risk of myocardial infarction from polymorphisms in candidate genes. N Engl J Med 347:1916, 2002.

Mechanisms of CAD in Women

18. Ng MKC, Quinn CM, McCrohon JA, et al: Androgens up-regulate atherosclerosis-related genes in macrophages from males but not females: Molecular insights into gender differences in atherosclerosis. J Am Coll Cardiol 42:1306, 2003.

19. Burke AP, Farb A, Malcom GT, et al: Effect of risk factors on the mechanism of acute thrombosis and sudden coronary death in women. Circulation 97:2110, 1998.

20. English JL, Jacobs LO, Green G, et al: Effect of the menstrual cycle on endothelium dependent vasodilation of the brachial artery in normal young women. Am J Cardiol 82:256, 1998.

21. Sader MA, McCredie RJ, Griffiths KA, et al: Oestradiol improves arterial endothelial function in healthy men receiving testosterone. Clin Endocrinol (Oxf) 54:175, 2001.

22. Weksler B: Hemostasis and thrombosis. In Douglas PS (ed): Cardiovascular Health and Disease in Women. 2nd ed. Philadelphia, WB Saunders, 2002, pp 157-177.

23. Arbustini E, Dal Bello B, Morbini P, et al: Plaque erosion is a major substrate for coronary thrombosis in acute myocardial infarction. Heart 82:269, 1999.

Specific Risk Factors in Women

24. Fields LE, Burt VL, Cutler JA, et al: The burden of adult hypertension in the United States 1999 to 2000: A rising tide. Hypertension 44:398, 2004.

25. Lewington S, Clarke R, Qizilbash N, et al; Prospective Studies Collaboration: Age-specific relevance of usual blood pressure to vascular mortality: A meta-analysis of individual data for one million adults in 61 prospective studies. Lancet 360:1903, 2002.

26. Vasan RS, Larson MG, Leip EP, et al: Impact of high-normal blood pressure on the risk of cardiovascular disease. N Engl J Med 345:1291, 2001.

27. Hajjar I, Kotchen TA: Trends in prevalence, awareness, treatment, and control of hypertension in the United States, 1988-2000. JAMA 290:199, 2003.

28. Expert Panel on Detection, Evaluation, and Treatment of High Blood Cholesterol in Adults: Executive Summary of the Third Report of the National Cholesterol Education Program (NCEP) Expert Panel on Detection, Evaluation, and Treatment of High Blood Cholesterol in Adults (Adult Treatment Panel III). JAMA 285:2486, 2001.

29. Ford ES, Giles WH, Dietz WH: Prevalence of the metabolic syndrome among US adults: Findings from the third National Health and Nutrition Examination Survey. JAMA 287:356, 2002.

30. Shai I, Rimm EB, Hankinson SE, et al: Multivariate assessment of lipid parameters as predictors of coronary heart disease among postmenopausal women: Potential implications for clinical guidelines. Circulation 110:2824, 2004.

31. Jensen J, Nilas L, Christiansen C: Influence of menopause on serum lipids and lipoproteins. Maturitas 12:321, 1990.

32. Ford ES, Mokdad AH, Giles WH, Mensah GA: Serum total cholesterol concentrations and awareness, treatment, and control of hypercholesterolemia among US adults: Findings from the National Health and Nutrition Examination Survey, 1999 to 2000. Circulation 107:2185, 2003.

33. Mokdad AH, Ford ES, Bowman BA, et al: Prevalence of obesity, diabetes, and obesity-related health risk factors, 2001. JAMA 289:76, 2003.

34. Kyker KA, Limacher MC: Gender differences in presentation and symptoms of coronary artery disease. Curr Womens Health Rep 2:115, 2002.

35. Milner KA, Funk M, Richards S, et al: Gender differences in symptom presentation associated with coronary heart disease. Am J Cardiol 84:396, 1999.

36. Kudenchuk PJ, Maynard C, Martin JS, et al; MITI Project Investigators: Comparison of presentation, treatment, and outcome of acute myocardial infarction in men versus women (The Myocardial Infarction Triage and Intervention Registry). Am J Cardiol 78:9, 1996.

37. McGuire DK, Newby LK, Biswas MS, Hochman JS: The elderly, women, and patients with diabetes mellitus. In Theroux P (ed): Acute Coronary Syndromes: A Companion to Braunwald's Heart Disease. Philadelphia, Elsevier Science, 2003, pp 553-573.

38. Braunwald E, Antman EM, Beasley JW, et al: ACC/AHA guidelines update for the management of patients with unstable angina and non-ST-segment elevation myocardial infarction. A report of the American College of Cardiology/American Heart Association Task Force on Practice Guidelines (Committee on the Management of Patients with Unstable Angina), 2002 (http://www.acc.org/clinical/guidelines/unstable/unstable.pdf). Accessed June 30, 2006.

39. Alexander KP, Shaw LJ, DeLong ER, et al: Value of exercise treadmill testing in women. J Am Coll Cardiol 32:1657, 1998.

40. Gibbons RJ, Balady GJ, Bricker JT, et al: ACC/AHA Guidelines update for exercise testing. A report of the American College of Cardiology/American Heart Association Task Force on Practice Guidelines (Committee on Exercise Testing), 2002 (www.acc.org/clinical/guidelines/exercise/dirIndex.htm). Accessed July 16, 2006.

41. Mieres JH, Shaw LJ, Arai A, et al: Role of noninvasive testing in the clinical evaluation of women with suspected coronary artery disease: Consensus statement from the Cardiac Imaging Committee, Council of Clinical Cardiology, and the Cardiovascular Imaging and Intervention Committee, Council on Cardiovascular Radiology and Intervention, American Heart Association. Circulation 111:682, 2005.

42. Shaw LJ, Vasey C, Sawada S, et al: Impact of gender on risk stratification by exercise and dobutamine stress echocardiography: Long-term mortality in 4234 women and 6898 men. Eur Heart J 26:447, 2005.

43. Lee PY, Alexander KP, Hammill BG, et al: Representation of elderly persons and women in published randomized trials of acute coronary syndromes. JAMA 286:708, 2001.

Evidence Base for Cardiovascular Therapy in Women

44. Antman EM, Anbe DT, Armstrong PW, et al: ACC/AHA guidelines for the management of patients with ST-elevation myocardial infarction. A report of the American College of Cardiology/American Heart Association Task Force on Practice Guidelines (Committee to Revise the 1999 Guidelines for the Management of Patients with Acute Myocardial Infarction. Circulation 110:e82, 2004.

45. Smith SC Jr, Allen J, Blair SN, et al: AHA/ACC guidelines for secondary prevention for patients with coronary and other atherosclerotic vascular disease: 2006 update. J Am Coll Cardiol 47:2130, 2006.

46. Gibbons RJ, Abrams J, Chatterjee K, et al: ACC/AHA guidelines update for the management of patients with chronic stable angina-summary article. A report of the American College of Cardiology/American Heart Association Task Force on Practice Guidelines (Committee on the Management of Patients with Chronic Stable Angina). Circulation 107:149, 2003.

47. Mosca L, Appel LJ, Benjamin E, et al: Evidence-based guidelines for cardiovascular disease prevention in women. J Am Coll Cardiol 43:900, 2004.

48. Ridker PM, Cook NR, Lee I-M, et al: A randomized trial of low-dose aspirin in the primary prevention of cardiovascular disease in women. N Engl J Med 352:1293, 2005.

49. Cannon CP, Braunwald E, McCabe CH, et al; Pravastatin or Atorvastatin Evaluation and Infection Therapy–Thrombolysis in Myocardial Infarction 22 Investigators. Intensive versus moderate lipid lowering with statins after acute coronary syndromes. N Engl J Med 350:1495, 2004. Erratum in N Engl J Med 354:778, 2006.

50. Lansky AJ, Hochman JS, Ward PA, et al: Percutaneous coronary intervention and adjunctive pharmacotherapy in women: A statement for healthcare professionals from the American Heart Association. Circulation 111:940, 2005.

51. Glasser R, Herrmann HC, Murphy SA, et al: Benefit of an early invasive management strategy in women with acute coronary syndromes. JAMA 288:3124, 2002.

52. Lagerqvist B, Safstrom K, Stahle E, et al; FRISC II Study Group Investigators: Is early invasive treatment of unstable coronary artery disease equally effective for both women and men? FRISC II Study Group Investigators. J Am Coll Cardiol 38:41, 2001.

53. Clayton TC, Pocock SJ, Henderson RA, et al: Do men benefit more than women from an interventional strategy in patients with unstable angina or non-ST-elevation myocardial infarction? The impact of gender in the RITA 3 trial. Eur Heart J 25:1641, 2004.

54. Eagle KA, Guyton RA, Davidoff R, et al: ACC/AHA guideline update for coronary artery bypass graft surgery. A report of the American College of Cardiology/American Heart Association Task Force on Practice Guidelines (Committee to Update the 1999 Guidelines for Coronary Artery Bypass Graft Surgery), 2004. (http://www.acc.org/clinical/guidelines/cabg/cabg.pdf). Accessed July 12, 2006.

55. Vaccarino V, Abramson JL, Veledar E, Weintraub WS: Sex differences in hospital mortality after coronary artery bypass surgery: Evidence for a higher mortality in younger women. Circulation 105:1176, 2002.

56. Vaccarino V, Lin ZQ, Kasl SV, et al: Sex differences in health status after coronary artery bypass surgery. Circulation 108:2642, 2003.

57. Keresztes PA, Merritt SL, Holm K, et al: The coronary artery bypass experience: Gender differences. Heart Lung 32:308, 2003.

58. LeGrande MR, Elliott PC, Murphy BM, et al: Health related quality of life trajectories and predictors following coronary artery bypass surgery. Health and Quality of Life Outcomes 4:49, 2006.

59. The PURSUIT Trial Investigators: Inhibition of platelet glycoprotein IIb/IIIa with eptifibatide in patients with acute coronary syndromes. Platelet Glycoprotein IIb/IIIa in Unstable Angina: Receptor Suppression Using Integrilin Therapy. N Engl J Med 339:436, 1998.

60. Boersma E, Harrington RA, Moliterno DJ, et al: Platelet glycoprotein IIb/IIIa inhibitors in acute coronary syndromes: A meta-analysis of all major randomised clinical trials. Lancet 359:189, 2002. Erratum in: Lancet 359:2120, 2002.

61. Alexander KP, Chen AY, Roe MT, et al; CRUSADE Investigators: Excess dosing of antiplatelet and antithrombin agents in the treatment of non-ST-segment elevation acute coronary syndromes. JAMA 295:628, 2006.

62. Rao SV, Jollis JG, Harrington RA, et al: Relationship of blood transfusion and clinical outcomes in patients with acute coronary syndromes. JAMA 292:1555, 2004.

63. Rao SV, O'Grady K, Pieper KS, et al: Impact of bleeding severity on clinical outcomes among patients with acute coronary syndromes. Am J Cardiol 96:1200, 2005.

64. Yusuf S, Mehta SR, Chrolavicius S, et al; Fifth Organization to Assess Strategies in Acute Ischemic Syndromes Investigators. Comparison of fondaparinux and enoxaparin in acute coronary syndromes. N Engl J Med 354:1464, 2006.

65. Blomkalns AL, Chen AY, Hochman JS, et al; CRUSADE Investigators: Gender disparities in the diagnosis and treatment of non-ST-segment elevation acute coronary syndromes: Large-scale observations from the CRUSADE (Can Rapid Risk Stratification of Unstable Angina Patients Suppress Adverse Outcomes with Early Implementation of the American College of Cardiology/American Heart Association Guidelines) National Quality Improvement Initiative. J Am Coll Cardiol 45:832, 2005.

66. Vaccarino V, Rathore SS, Wenger NK, et al; National Registry of Myocardial Infarction Investigators: Sex and racial differences in the management of acute myocardial infarction, 1994 through 2002. N Engl J Med 353:671, 2005.

67. Newby LK, Allen LaPointe NM, Chen AY, et al: Long-term adherence to evidence-based secondary prevention therapies in coronary artery disease. Circulation 113:203, 2006.

68. Mosca L, Mochari H, Christian A, et al: National study of women's awareness, preventive action, and barriers to cardiovascular health. Circulation 113:525, 2006.

69. Mosca L, Linfante AH, Benjamin EJ, et al: National study of physician awareness and adherence to cardiovascular disease prevention guidelines. Circulation 111:499, 2005.

70. Jani SM, Montoye C, Mehta R, et al: Sex differences in the application of evidence-based therapies for the treatment of acute myocardial infarction. Arch Int Med 166:1164, 2006.

71. Taylor RS, Brown A, Ebrahim S, et al: Exercise-based rehabilitation for patients with coronary heart disease: Systematic review and meta-analysis of randomized controlled trials. Am J Med 116:682, 2004.

72. Witt BJ, Jacobsen SJ, Weston SA, et al: Cardiac rehabilitation after myocardial infarction in the community. J Am Coll Cardiol 44:988, 2004.

Heart Failure in Women

73. Masoudi FA, Havranek EP, Smith G, et al: Gender, age, and heart failure with preserved left ventricular systolic function. J Am Coll Cardiol 41:217, 2003.

74. Fernandez-Sola J, Nicolas-Arfelis JM: Gender differences in alcoholic cardiomyopathy. J Gend Specif Med 5:41, 2002.

75. Galvao M, Kalman J, DeMarco T, et al: Gender differences in in-hospital management and outcomes in patients with decompensated heart failure: Analysis from the Acute Decompensated Heart Failure National Registry (ADHERE). J Card Fail 12:100, 2006.

76. Yancy CW, Lopatin M, Stevenson LW, et al; ADHERE Scientific Advisory Committee and Investigators: Clinical presentation, management, and in-hospital outcomes of patients admitted with acute decompensated heart failure with preserved systolic function: A report from the Acute Decompensated Heart Failure National Registry (ADHERE) Database. J Am Coll Cardiol 47:76, 2006. Erratum in J Am Coll Cardiol 47:1502, 2006.

77. Owan TE, Hodge DO, Herges RM, et al: Trends in prevalence and outcome of heart failure with preserved ejection fraction. N Engl J Med 355:251, 2006.

78. Bhatia RS, Tu JV, Lee DS, et al: Outcome of heart failure with preserved ejection fraction in a population-based study. N Engl J Med 355:260, 2006.

79. Hunt SA, Abraham WT, Chin MH, et al: ACC/AHA Guideline update for the diagnosis and management of chronic heart failure in the adult. A report of the American College of Cardiology/American Heart Association Task Force on Practice Guidelines (Writing Committee to Update the 2001 Guidelines for the Evaluation and Management of Heart Failure), 2005 (http://www.acc.org/clinical/guidelines/failure//index.pdf). Accessed June 25, 2006.

80. Goldberger Z, Lampert R: Implantable cardioverter-defibrillators: Expanding indication and technologies. JAMA 295:809, 2006.

81. Aaronson KD, Schwartz JS, Goin JE, et al: Sex differences in patient acceptance of cardiac transplant candidacy. Circulation 91:2753, 1995.

PAD in Women

82. Criqui MH: Peripheral arterial disease—epidemiological aspects. Vasc Med 6(Suppl):3, 2001.

83. Hirsch AT, Haskal ZJ, Hertzer NR, et al: ACC/AHA 2005 guidelines for the management of patients with peripheral arterial disease (lower extremity, renal, mesenteric, and abdominal aortic): A collaborative report from the American Association for Vascular Surgery/Society for Vascular Surgery, Society for Cardiovascular Angiography and Interventions, Society for Vascular Medicine and Biology, Society of Interventional Radiology, and the ACC/AHA Task Force on Practice Guidelines (Writing Committee to Develop Guidelines for the Management of Patients with Peripheral Arterial Disease), 2005. (http://www.acc.org/clinical/guidelines/pad/index.pdf). Accessed July 16, 2006.

84. Hansen KJ, Edwards MS, Craven TE, et al: Prevalence of renovascular disease in the elderly: A population-based study. J Vasc Surg 36:443, 2002.

CHAPTER 77

Pregnancy and Heart Disease

Carole A. Warnes

Hemodynamic Changes, 1967
During Pregnancy, 1967
During Labor and Delivery, 1968

Evaluation, 1968
Physical Examination, 1968
Imaging, 1969

**Management During
Pregnancy, 1969**
Medical Therapy, 1969
Surgical Management, 1969
High-Risk Pregnancies, 1969

Cardiovascular Diseases, 1970
Congenital Heart Disease, 1970
Pulmonary Hypertension, 1971
Rheumatic and Acquired Valvular
    Heart Disease, 1972
Connective Tissue Disorders, 1974
Cardiomyopathies, 1974
Coronary Artery Disease, 1975
Hypertension, 1975
Arrhythmias, 1975

**Cardiovascular Drug
Therapy, 1976**

Contraception, 1977
Oral Contraceptives, 1977
Tubal Sterilization, 1977

Future Perspectives, 1978

References, 1978

Guidelines, 1979

Approximately 2 percent of pregnancies involve maternal cardiovascular disease and, as such, this poses an increased risk to both mother and fetus. Most women with cardiovascular disease can experience pregnancy with proper care, but a careful prepregnancy evaluation is mandatory. Sometimes, cardiac disease may manifest for the first time in pregnancy, because the hemodynamic changes may compromise a limited cardiac reserve. Conversely, the symptoms and signs of a normal pregnancy may mimic the presence of cardiac disease. Lightheadedness, dizziness, shortness of breath, peripheral edema, and even syncope often occur in the course of a normal pregnancy and, for the unwary physician, cardiac disease may be suspected. An understanding of the normal cardiac examination of a pregnant patient is therefore important. For those physicians counseling patients with cardiac disease about the potential risks of a pregnancy, a comprehensive knowledge of the underlying defect, as well as of the hemodynamic changes that pregnancy will impose, is imperative.

With the declining incidence of rheumatic heart disease in Western countries, most maternal cardiac disease is now congenital in origin. Other cardiovascular problems seen include cardiomyopathies, both dilated and hypertrophic, and valvular disease, such as bicuspid aortic valve and mitral valve prolapse. Less common problems include pulmonary hypertension and, rarely, coronary artery disease. Prepregnancy counseling is important to give prospective mothers appropriate information about the advisability of pregnancy and discuss the risks to her and the fetus. Such patients should be seen in a high-risk pregnancy unit and have a clinical examination, electrocardiogram, and chest x-ray. An echocardiogram facilitates a detailed evaluation of myocardial function, valvular disease, and pulmonary pressures. For patients with congenital heart disease, their perception of normal activity may be skewed, and an exercise test is helpful in delineating their true functional aerobic capacity. In general, patients who cannot achieve more than 70 percent of their predicted functional aerobic capacity are unlikely to tolerate a pregnancy safely. During this visit, it is important to take a careful family history to assess whether there is any congenital heart disease in the family. Genetic counseling may also be considered, if necessary. A careful discussion of the maternal and fetal risks should be made at the time of prepregnancy counseling and, if the mother is going to pursue a pregnancy, a strategy should be outlined regarding the frequency of follow-up by the cardiologist, and a plan should be put in place for labor and delivery.[1]

A multicenter Canadian study has suggested that maternal cardiac risk may be predicted by the use of a risk index.[2] Four predictors of maternal cardiac events are as follows: (1) prior cardiac event (e.g., heart failure, transient ischemic attack, or stroke before pregnancy) or arrhythmia; (2) baseline New York Heart Association (NYHA) class higher than Class II or cyanosis; (3) left heart obstruction (mitral valve area smaller than 2 cm^2, aortic valve area less than 1.5 cm^2, or peak left ventricular outflow tract gradient more than 30 mm Hg by echocardiography); and (4) reduced systemic ventricular systolic function (ejection fraction less than 40 percent). Each of 599 pregnancies was assigned 1 point when each predictor was present. No pregnancy received more than 3 points. The estimated risk of a cardiac event in pregnancies with 0, 1, and more than 1 point was 5, 27, and 75 percent, respectively. It was concluded that those with a low cardiac risk of 0 could safely be delivered in a community hospital, but those at intermediate or high cardiac risk (risk score of 1 or more) should be delivered at a regional center.

During pregnancy, a multidisciplinary team approach is recommended, with close collaboration with the obstetrician, so that the mode, timing, and location of delivery can be planned.[3] The management should be tailored to the specific needs of the patient. During pregnancy, fetal growth is monitored by the obstetric team and, for the woman with congenital heart disease, a fetal cardiac echocardiogram is offered at about 22 to 26 weeks of pregnancy to determine whether the baby has a congenital cardiac anomaly.

HEMODYNAMIC CHANGES

During Pregnancy

The hemodynamic changes are profound and begin early in the first trimester. The plasma volume begins to increase in the sixth week of pregnancy and, by the second trimester, approaches 50 percent above baseline (Fig. 77-1). The plasma volume then tends to plateau until delivery. This increased plasma volume is followed by a slightly lesser rise in red cell mass, which results in the relative anemia of pregnancy. The heart rate begins to increase to about 20 percent above baseline to facilitate the increase in cardiac output (Fig. 77-2). Uterine blood flow increases with placental growth, and there is a fall in peripheral resistance. This decreased peripheral resistance may result in a slight fall in blood pressure, which also begins in the first trimester. The venous pressure in the lower extremities rises, which is why approximately 80 percent of healthy pregnant women develop pedal edema. The adaptive changes of a normal pregnancy result in an increase in cardiac output, which also begins in the first trimester and, by the end of the second trimester, approaches 30 to 50 percent above baseline.

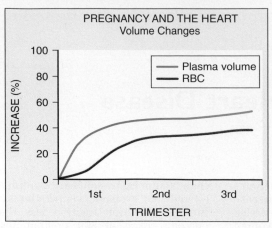

FIGURE 77–1 Plasma volume and red blood cell (RBC) increase during the three trimesters of pregnancy. The plasma volume increases to approximately 50 percent above baseline by the second trimester and then virtually plateaus until delivery.

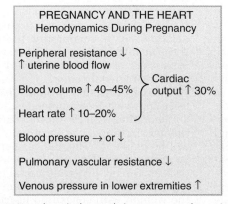

FIGURE 77–2 Hemodynamic changes during pregnancy relate to increased cardiac output and a fall in peripheral resistance. Blood pressure in most patients remains the same or falls slightly. Venous pressure in the legs increases, causing pedal edema in many patients.

CH 77

These hemodynamic changes may cause problems for the mother with cardiac disease. The added volume load may obviously compromise a patient who has impaired ventricular function and limited cardiac reserve. Stenotic valvular lesions (e.g., aortic stenosis) are less well tolerated than regurgitant lesions, because the decrease in peripheral resistance exaggerates the gradient across the aortic valve. Similarly, the tachycardia of pregnancy reduces the time for diastolic filling in a patient with mitral stenosis, with resultant increase in left atrial pressure. In a similar fashion, the tachycardia of pregnancy reduces the time for diastolic filling in a patient with mitral stenosis, with resultant increase in left atrial pressure. In contrast, with a lesion such as mitral regurgitation, the afterload reduction helps offset the volume load on the left ventricle that gestation imposes.

During Labor and Delivery

The hemodynamic changes during labor and delivery are abrupt. With each uterine contraction, up to 500 ml of blood is released into the circulation, prompting a rapid increase in cardiac output and blood pressure. The cardiac output is often 50 percent above baseline during the second stage of labor and may be even higher at the time of delivery. During a normal vaginal delivery, approximately 400 ml of blood is lost. In contrast, with a cesarean section, about 800 ml of blood is often lost and, as such, may pose a more significant hemodynamic burden to the parturient. Following delivery of the baby, there is an

abrupt increase in venous return, in part because of autotransfusion from the uterus but also because the baby no longer compresses the inferior vena cava. In addition, there continues to be autotransfusion of blood in the 24 to 72 hours after delivery, and this is when pulmonary edema may occur.

All these abrupt changes mandate that for the high-risk patient with cardiac disease, a multidisciplinary approach during labor and delivery is essential. The cardiologist and obstetrician should work with the anesthesiologist to determine the safest mode of delivery.

For most patients with cardiac disease, a vaginal delivery is feasible and preferable and a cesarean section is only indicated for obstetric reasons. Exceptions to this include the patient who is anticoagulated with warfarin, because the baby is also anticoagulated and vaginal delivery carries an increased risk to the fetus of intracranial hemorrhage. Cesarean section may also be considered in patients who have a dilated unstable aorta (e.g., Marfan syndrome), severe pulmonary hypertension, or a severe obstructive lesion, such as aortic stenosis. High-risk patients should be delivered in a center where expertise is available to monitor the hemodynamic changes of labor and delivery, and intervene when necessary. If vaginal delivery is elected, fetal and maternal electrocardiographic monitoring should be performed. Delivery can be accomplished with the mother in the left lateral position so that the fetus does not compress the inferior vena cava, thereby maintaining venous return. The second stage should be assisted, if necessary (e.g., forceps or vacuum extraction), to avoid a long labor. Blood and volume loss should be replaced promptly. For those patients with tenuous hemodynamics, Swan-Ganz catheterization before active labor facilitates optimization of the hemodynamics and should be continued for at least 24 hours after delivery, when pulmonary edema commonly occurs.

Although there is no consensus regarding the administration of antibiotic prophylaxis at the time of delivery for patients with lesions vulnerable to infective endocarditis, many institutions routinely give antibiotics because of the documented bacteremia. This can occur even during an uncomplicated delivery.[4]

EVALUATION

Physical Examination (see Chap. 11)

Because of the altered hemodynamics during pregnancy, the physical examination of a healthy pregnant woman changes and may mimic the presence of cardiac disease. The heart rate increases and the pulse volume is often bounding. By the middle of the second trimester, the jugular venous pressure may be elevated, with brisk descents, because of the volume overload and reduced peripheral resistance. The apical impulse is more prominent and, on auscultation, the first sound may appear loud. Commonly, there is an ejection systolic murmur at the left sternal edge, never more than grade 3/6 in intensity, which relates to increased flow through the left or right ventricular outflow tract. A third sound is very common. There should be no diastolic murmur. The second sound may also appear accentuated, and these combined auscultatory features may raise the suspicion of an atrial septal defect and/or pulmonary hypertension. Continuous murmurs may also be heard, either from a cervical venous hum or a mammary souffle. Peripheral edema is common as pregnancy advances. If there is any concern that the physical examination suggests cardiac disease, transthoracic echocardiogram should be performed. This facilitates the evaluation of ventricular size and function, valvular heart disease, any potential shunts (e.g., atrial septal defect, ventricular septal defect), and a noninvasive assessment of pulmonary artery pressure.

Imaging (see Chaps. 14 to 18)

CHEST RADIOGRAPHY. A chest x-ray is not obtained routinely in any pregnant patient because of concern about radiation to the fetus but should be considered in any patient when there are concerns about her cardiac status and new onset of dyspnea or failure. The chest x-ray in a normal healthy patient may show slight prominence of the pulmonary artery and, as pregnancy advances, elevation of the diaphragm may suggest an increase in the cardiothoracic ratio.

TRANSTHORACIC ECHOCARDIOGRAPHY. This is the cornerstone of cardiac evaluation in pregnancy and facilitates differentiation of the features of cardiac pathology from those of a normal pregnancy. It is used most frequently to determine the presence or absence of normal ventricular function, assess the status of native and prosthetic valve disease and, by using the tricuspid regurgitant velocity, assess pulmonary artery pressure. For those patients with congenital heart disease, a detailed assessment of any shunt and complex anatomy may be made.

During pregnancy, because of the increased cardiac output, the velocities across the left and right ventricular outflow tracts increase, which may mimic an increase in outflow tract gradient. Careful examination of the two-dimensional anatomical appearances will help differentiate this from a true valvular abnormality, and calculation of valve area will be helpful. Similarly, because of the increased stroke volume, any valvular regurgitation will appear to be accentuated. Serial echocardiograms may be particularly useful in a patient with a mechanical valve prosthesis who is vulnerable to thrombosis during pregnancy. The valve area calculation, in addition to pressure half-time determination, may be more helpful than a simple measurement of valve gradient; this may appear to be increased as pregnancy advances because the circulation becomes more hyperkinetic and cardiac output increases.

In patients with impaired ventricular function, particularly those with cardiomyopathy, echocardiography plays the most important role in assessing left ventricular function. In a normal pregnancy, the left ventricular end-diastolic measurement is increased and there may be similar increases in right ventricular size, as well as the volumes of both atria. Measurement of ejection fraction is determined by changes in preload and afterload and, in the supine position, preload may be reduced because the fetus may compress the inferior vena cava. Some studies have suggested that the ejection fraction increases in normal patients during pregnancy, but not all reports agree with this view.

TRANSESOPHAGEAL ECHOCARDIOGRAPHY. Transesophageal echocardiography is seldom performed during pregnancy but may be necessary to provide more detailed imaging of valvular pathology, presence or absence of a shunt, or presence or absence of a thrombus. In addition, it may be useful to determine the presence or absence of endocarditis to facilitate the detection of a valvular vegetation or perivalvular abscess. Transesophageal echocardiography can be performed safely, although careful monitoring of maternal oxygen saturation is necessary if midazolam is used for sedation. Antibiotic prophylaxis is unnecessary.

FETAL ECHOCARDIOGRAPHY. Fetal echocardiography has been a major advance in the last 20 years and excellent imaging of the fetal heart can usually be obtained by 20 weeks' gestation. The four-chamber view may be obtained in most pregnancies and should demonstrate two atrioventricular valves, the crux of the heart, and whether two ventricles of equal size are present. The patent foramen ovale should also be demonstrated. Typically, the heart should be smaller than one third of the size of the fetal thorax.

MANAGEMENT DURING PREGNANCY

Medical Therapy

Patients who are otherwise healthy may require little or no specific treatment other than the usual obstetric recommendations and monitoring. Patients who are NYHA Class I or II may need to limit strenuous exercise and get adequate rest, supplementation of iron and vitamins to minimize the anemia of pregnancy, a low-salt diet if there is concern about ventricular dysfunction, and regular cardiac and obstetric evaluations, the frequency of which must be individualized. Patients who are NYHA Class III or IV may need hospital admission for bed rest and close monitoring and may require early delivery if there is maternal hemodynamic compromise.

Surgical Management

Cardiac surgery is seldom necessary during pregnancy and should be avoided whenever possible. There is a higher risk of fetal malformation and loss if cardiopulmonary bypass is performed in the first trimester; if performed in the last trimester, there is a higher likelihood of precipitating premature labor. The "optimal time" appears to be between 20 and 28 weeks of gestation and the fetal outcome may be improved by using normothermic rather than hypothermic extracorporeal circulation, higher pump flows, higher pressures (mean blood pressure of 60 mm Hg), and as short a bypass time as possible.[5] Obstetric monitoring of the fetus during the procedure is recommended so that fetal bradycardia may be dealt with promptly and uterine contractions may be controlled. Despite these interventions, the current risk of fetal loss is still at least 10 percent, and is probably higher when the cardiac surgery is emergent. Maternal functional class is an important predictive factor for maternal death. A multidisciplinary approach is preferable to optimize the outcome for both mother and baby.

High-Risk Pregnancies

In some situations, the maternal risk of pregnancy is very high and the patient should be counseled to avoid pregnancy, and sometimes even consider termination of pregnancy if it occurs (Table 77-1). No data exist regarding the precise level of pulmonary hypertension that poses a major threat to the mother but in my experience, systolic pulmonary artery pressures higher than 60 to 70 percent of the systemic pressure are likely to be associated with maternal compromise; in these circumstances, pregnancy is best avoided. Women who have a left ventricular ejection fraction less than 40 percent from any cause are not likely to withstand the volume load that pregnancy imposes and should be advised not to get pregnant. Because pregnancy is associated with a decrease in peripheral resistance, symptomatic patients with significant stenotic cardiac lesions (see Table 77-1) are likely to deteriorate during a pregnancy. Patients with a dilated aortic root more than 40 mm are vulnerable to progressive aortic dilation, dissection, and rupture during pregnancy, particularly those patients with Marfan syndrome. This occurs not only because of the increased stroke volume, but probably also because the gestational hormonal changes may be additive to the underlying histological abnormality in the aortic media. Estrogen inhibits collagen and elastin synthesis in the aorta and

TABLE 77–1	High-Risk Pregnancies
Pulmonary hypertension	
Dilated cardiomyopathy, ejection fraction < 40 percent	

Symptomatic obstructive lesions:
   Aortic stenosis
   Mitral stenosis
   Pulmonary stenosis
   Coarctation of the aorta	

Marfan syndrome with aortic root > 40 mm	
Cyanotic lesions	
Mechanical prosthetic valves	

progesterone has been shown to accelerate the deposition of noncollagenous proteins in the aortas of rats.[6]

CARDIOVASCULAR DISEASES

Congenital Heart Disease (see Chap. 61)

Most maternal cardiac disease in Western societies is now congenital in origin. This relates to the enormous advances in congenital cardiac surgery over the last 50 years, so that most babies born with congenital heart disease, even with complex lesions, now survive to adulthood. Some patients will present for the first time in pregnancy with symptoms and learn that they have congenital heart disease. Other patients with repaired defects may encounter cardiac problems during pregnancy. All patients, whether or not they have had cardiac repair, should have a detailed evaluation and appropriate counseling before pregnancy is considered.[7]

ATRIAL SEPTAL DEFECT. Secundum atrial septal defect is one of the most common congenital heart defects. Patients with even a large secundum atrial septal defect (ASD) usually tolerate pregnancy without complication unless there is coexistent pulmonary hypertension or atrial fibrillation. The volume load on the right ventricle is usually well tolerated. Meticulous attention should be paid to the maternal leg veins, particularly during peridelivery, because deep venous thrombosis could precipitate a paradoxical embolus and stroke. Elective closure of an atrial septal defect by device or operative repair is preferable before pregnancy is contemplated.

VENTRICULAR SEPTAL DEFECT. Patients with small defects usually tolerate pregnancy without difficulty. In the setting of a large ventricular septal defect and pulmonary hypertension, patients should be counseled not to proceed with a pregnancy (see later discussion of Eisenmenger syndrome).

PATENT DUCTUS ARTERIOSUS. Small ducts with normal or near-normal pressures usually cause no hemodynamic perturbations during pregnancy. In the setting of a large shunt, the added volume load of pregnancy might precipitate left ventricular failure. Those with pulmonary hypertension should be counseled not to have a pregnancy.

AORTIC STENOSIS. Aortic stenosis in women of childbearing age usually occurs secondary to a bicuspid aortic valve. A detailed two-dimensional anatomical and Doppler echocardiographic assessment of the valve function should be performed before pregnancy is contemplated. In addition, there should be a careful examination of the entire thoracic aorta, because bicuspid aortic valve is associated with an aortopathy and, even with a functionally normal valve, an aortic dilation or ascending aortic aneurysm may

be present. Pregnancy is usually considered contraindicated if the aortic dimension is larger than 4.5 cm.

Mild aortic stenosis is usually well tolerated, provided the patient has a normal exercise capacity and no symptoms.[8] Moderate stenosis is sometimes well tolerated, but the patient needs to be evaluated carefully prepregnancy. In the absence of symptoms, with a normal exercise test without ST-T wave changes, pregnancy with a compliant patient who is carefully managed is likely to be successful. Those with severe aortic stenosis (valve area smaller than 1 cm^2) or a mean gradient greater than 50 mm Hg should be counseled not to have a pregnancy. The decrease in peripheral resistance during pregnancy will exaggerate the aortic gradient and may precipitate symptoms. Patients may respond to bed rest and the administration of beta blockers, but an early delivery may be necessary. The risk to the mother of continuing the pregnancy versus delivering a baby early by cesarean section needs to be balanced. Labor and delivery can be particularly problematic in such patients because of the abrupt hemodynamic changes, particularly the abrupt fall in afterload when the baby is delivered. Blood loss at the time of parturition can also precipitate maternal collapse. Epidural analgesia needs to be carefully and slowly administered, and spinal block should be avoided because of the potential for hypotension. Delivery may be facilitated by central venous pressure monitoring or the use of a Swan-Ganz catheter to maintain optimum hemodynamics. This should be continued for at least 24 hours after delivery.

Several small reports have reviewed percutaneous aortic balloon valvuloplasty during pregnancy; this can be accomplished provided the valve anatomy is favorable and the procedure is performed by an experienced interventionalist.[9] Radiation exposure of the fetus can be minimized by lead screening of the mother's abdomen and pelvis. It should be performed in centers with extensive experience and surgical back-up and, if performed after 26 weeks of pregnancy, should have obstetric standby in case of premature labor.

PULMONARY STENOSIS. Pulmonary stenosis is usually well tolerated during pregnancy, particularly if the right ventricular pressure is less than 70 percent of systemic pressure and sinus rhythm is maintained. If necessary, balloon pulmonary valvuloplasty can be performed, with shielding of the fetus from radiation.

CYANOTIC HEART DISEASE. Cyanosis poses risks for both mother and fetus.[10] The decrease in peripheral resistance that accompanies pregnancy augments the right-to-left shunt and may exaggerate the maternal cyanosis. Because of the erythrocytosis that accompanies cyanosis and the propensity to thrombosis, women who develop venous thrombosis are at risk of paradoxical embolus and stroke. Maternal hypoxia imposes a pronounced handicap to fetal growth and survival. Presbitero and colleagues[11] have evaluated 44 women with 96 pregnancies (excluding patients with Eisenmenger syndrome) and confirmed earlier studies that the degree of maternal cyanosis has a profound impact on fetal outcome. When the maternal oxygen saturation is less than 85 percent, the fetal outcome is poor, with only 2 in 17 pregnancies (12 percent) resulting in live-born infants (Table 77-2). Conversely, when the maternal oxygen saturation is 90 percent or higher, 92 percent of the pregnancies result in a live birth. Maternal cardiovascular complications occurred in 14 patients (32 percent). Eight patients had heart failure, and bacterial endocarditis occurred in 2 patients, both with palliated tetralogy of Fallot. Two patients had thrombotic complications, one pulmonary and one cerebral.

In addition to the degree of maternal cyanosis, right ventricular function must be assessed prepregnancy by echocardiography or magnetic resonance imaging (MRI). The

TABLE 77–2	Fetal Outcome in Cyanotic Congenital Heart Disease and Its Relationship to Maternal Cyanosis		
Parameter	No. of Pregnancies	No. of Live Births	Percentage Born Alive
Hemoglobin, gm/dl*			
≤16	28	20	71
17-19	40	18	45
≥20	26	2	8
Arterial oxygen saturation (%)†			
≤85	17	2	12
85-89	22	10	45
≥90	13	12	92

*Hemoglobin concentration unknown in two pregnancies.
†Arterial oxygen saturation unknown in 44 pregnancies.
From Presbitero P, Somerville J. Stone S, et al: Pregnancy in cyanotic congenital heart disease. Outcome of mother and fetus. Circulation 89:2673, 1994.

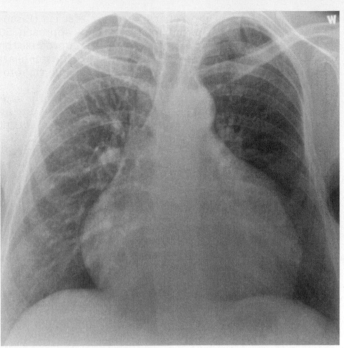

FIGURE 77–3 Chest radiograph of a 40-year-old woman with late repair of tetralogy of Fallot who presented in the first 4 weeks of pregnancy. She did not know she was pregnant at the time of the radiograph. She had severe pulmonary regurgitation and severe tricuspid regurgitation, with brief episodes of nonsustained supraventricular tachycardia. Despite the right atrial and right ventricular enlargement, pregnancy was accomplished successfully with an early delivery, and she subsequently had pulmonary valve replacement and tricuspid annuloplasty with good result. Had she presented before pregnancy, she would have been counseled to have surgery before pregnancy was undertaken.

type of maternal cardiac lesion present will also affect the propensity of the baby to inherit congenital cardiac disease. For those women with conotruncal abnormalities (tetralogy or pulmonary atresia), screening for 22q11 deletion is recommended, because this has autosomal dominant transmission, and the offspring have a 50 percent chance of inheriting the genetic defect.[12]

TETRALOGY OF FALLOT. Most women of childbearing age with tetralogy of Fallot will have had prior surgical repair and, as such, should be free of cyanosis. An occasional patient will be seen in adulthood who has not had prior surgery or may have been palliated with a surgically created shunt (e.g., Blalock-Taussig). In these cases, pregnancy may pose a risk depending on the degree of cyanosis, as noted earlier. The fall in peripheral resistance augments the right-to-left shunt through the ventricular septal defect, causing worsening cyanosis, and this poses a risk for mother and fetus.

For those patients with prior definitive surgical repair, a careful assessment of any hemodynamic residua and sequelae should be undertaken before giving advice about the safety of a pregnancy. The clinical and echocardiographic evaluation should focus on the presence of lesions, such as residual pulmonary regurgitation, which is common after repair, and associated right ventricular dysfunction and tricuspid regurgitation (Fig. 77-3). The volume load of pregnancy may not be well tolerated in these circumstances,[13,14] and superimposed atrial and even ventricular arrhythmias may add to the hemodynamic stresses. Additional volume lesions such as ventricular septal defects and aortic regurgitation should be evaluated, as well as residual right ventricular outflow tract obstruction. For those women with a good surgical repair, good exercise capacity, and minimal residua, pregnancy may be well tolerated, provided that they are properly managed.[14,15] Genetic counseling should be offered during prepregnancy counseling to look for 22q11 deletion. If there is no parental chromosomal abnormality and no family history of other congenital cardiac disease, the risk of the fetus having a congenital cardiac anomaly is approximately 5 to 6 percent, similar to the risk of inheritance of many congenital cardiac lesions.

EBSTEIN ANOMALY. The safety of a pregnancy in these patients depends on right ventricular size and function, degree of tricuspid regurgitation, and presence or absence of an atrial communication. The latter is present in approximately 50 percent of patients and, if the patient is cyanotic at rest, the risk of pregnancy increases considerably. An atrial communication poses the added potential risk of a stroke from a paradoxical embolus, and meticulous atten-

tion should be paid to the mother's leg veins for the possibility of deep venous thrombosis. Atrial arrhythmias may not be well tolerated in pregnancy with this anomaly and both atrial fibrillation and reentry tachycardia are common. Accessory bypass tracts causing preexcitation may precipitate rapid tachycardias, which add to the burden of a poorly functioning right ventricle.

CONGENITALLY CORRECTED TRANSPOSITION (L-TRANSPOSITION). Patients with this anomaly have atrioventricular discordance and ventriculoarterial discordance; thus, the systemic ventricle is the morphological right ventricle. Patients may have a successful pregnancy as long as the ejection fraction of the systemic ventricle is preserved and there are no significant associated anomalies. The most common of these is systemic atrioventricular valve (tricuspid) regurgitation, which contributes to systemic ventricular dysfunction. Other lesions such as ventricular septal defect, pulmonary stenosis, and complete heart block may coexist and may compromise the ability to have a successful pregnancy.

Pulmonary Hypertension

Pulmonary hypertension, regardless of the cause, carries a high mortality when associated with pregnancy.[16] Causes include thromboembolic disease, anorexic drugs, valvular heart disease, and primary pulmonary hypertension. The most common cause in childbearing years, however, is secondary to a shunt in the setting of congenital heart disease (e.g., ventricular septal defect, patent ductus arteriosus, or atrial septal defect). When the pulmonary hypertension exceeds approximately 60 percent of systemic levels, pregnancy is more likely to be associated with complications. In the setting of severe pulmonary vascular disease (Eisenmenger syndrome), maternal mortality may approach 50 percent. The volume load of pregnancy may compromise the poorly functioning right ventricle and precipitate heart failure. The fall in peripheral resistance augments right-to-left shunting and may precipitate more cyanosis.

The time around labor and delivery is particularly dangerous and the highest incidence of maternal death is during parturition and the puerperium. There may be an abrupt decrease in afterload as the baby is delivered and hypovolemia from blood loss can cause hypoxia, syncope, and sudden death. Vagal responses to pain may also be life-threatening. Death may also occur from pulmonary embolism or in situ pulmonary infarction. In the largest retrospective review, Gleicher and associates[17] reported 44 documented cases of Eisenmenger syndrome with 70 pregnancies. Of these patients, 52 percent died in connection with a pregnancy and 34 percent of vaginal deliveries resulted in maternal death. Three of four cesarean sections also resulted in maternal death; however, the numbers were small and it is likely that those patients represented a higher risk cohort, because they were the most hemodynamically unstable. Only 25.6 percent of pregnancies reached term, and more than half of the deliveries were premature. Perinatal mortality was 28.3 percent and was significantly associated with prematurity. Current recommendations are still that termination of pregnancy is the safer option although, in patients with pulmonary hypertension, this too may be a more complex procedure and cardiac anesthesia is probably helpful in this regard. Low-dose subcutaneous heparin may be administered during bed rest, but there is no evidence that it improves maternal survival. The mode of delivery needs to be discussed carefully. If the vaginal route is selected, it should be performed in an intensive care unit. Epidural analgesia must be cautiously administered to minimize peripheral vasodilation. A prolonged second stage should be avoided. Meticulous attention should be paid to the peripheral venous system and a thromboguard or compression pump may help prevent peripheral venous thrombosis. Cesarean section delivery is probably preferable,[18] with cardiac anesthesia. In-hospital monitoring should be continued for at least 2 weeks after delivery.

No studies have suggested a more favorable outcome with the use of pulmonary vasodilators, although case reports have suggested a more successful maternal outcome. Nitric oxide can be administered via nasal canula or face mask, and successful pregnancy has also been reported with intravenous epoprostenol. Sildenafil has also been used but, with all these agents, maternal death may still occur days or weeks after delivery.[19]

In summary, the mortality for patients with severe pulmonary hypertension and pregnancy is prohibitively high. Appropriate advice regarding contraception should be given to all patients. Estrogen-containing contraceptives are contraindicated in this setting.

Rheumatic and Acquired Valvular Heart Disease (see Chap. 83)

Because of the declining incidence of rheumatic heart disease in Western countries, rheumatic heart disease is infrequent in North America but remains very prevalent in developing countries. The most common problem encountered is mitral stenosis, which tends to worsen during pregnancy because of the increase in cardiac output coupled with the increase in heart rate; this shortens the diastolic filling time and exaggerates the mitral valve gradient. Any decrease in stroke volume causes a further reflex tachycardia, all of which contribute to an elevated left atrial pressure. The onset of atrial fibrillation may precipitate acute pulmonary edema. A study of Canadian women has reported no maternal death, but 35 percent of pregnancies were associated with cardiac complications.[20] Patients should have a careful echocardiographic evaluation of their mitral valve gradient, valve area, and pulmonary pressures before proceeding with a pregnancy. An exercise echocardiogram may also be helpful in delineating the hemodynamic response to effort in terms of mitral gradient and the presence or absence of pulmonary hypertension.

The cornerstone of therapy for the symptomatic patient is beta blockade.[21] This slows the heart rate, prolongs the diastolic filling time, and can result in marked improvement in symptoms. Bed rest may also be helpful to slow the heart rate and minimize cardiac demands.[22] The judicious use of diuretics is appropriate if there is pulmonary edema. Anticoagulants should probably be given if the patient is on bed rest and should certainly be administered in the setting of atrial fibrillation. In unusual circumstances, when the mother is refractory to medical therapy, balloon valvuloplasty may be performed if the valve anatomy is favorable and there is no concomitant mitral regurgitation.[23,24] Rarer still, surgical valvotomy may be performed, with the caveats described earlier.

Mitral and aortic regurgitation are fairly well tolerated in pregnancy, provided the regurgitation is no more than moderate, the mother is symptom-free prior to pregnancy, and ventricular function is well preserved. Closer monitoring during pregnancy is usually warranted, however, particularly for those with mitral regurgitation, because the left ventricle tends to dilate as pregnancy progresses and this may exacerbate the degree of mitral regurgitation. Early delivery may be necessary if there is maternal hemodynamic compromise.

Prosthetic Valves

Pregnancy for the woman with a prosthetic valve poses risks for mother and baby and has been called a "double jeopardy" situation. The choice of a prosthetic valve for the woman of childbearing age involves a detailed discussion of the relative risks so that she can make an informed decision about whether to select a tissue or mechanical prosthesis. Tissue valves are less thrombogenic than mechanical valves and therefore are generally less problematic in pregnancy, because they do not routinely involve the use of warfarin. The disadvantage is their tendency to degenerate after an average of 10 years, necessitating a reoperation, with its attendant risks and potential mortality. Mechanical prostheses, in contrast, have a greater longevity but require anticoagulation and, whichever anticoagulant strategy is chosen during pregnancy, there is a higher chance of fetal loss, placental hemorrhage, and prosthetic valve thrombosis. Thus, each type of valve has a risk-benefit ratio; the choices are reviewed here.

Tissue Prostheses

The most common types of tissue valves used currently are porcine or pericardial valves. For patients in sinus rhythm, they confer the advantage that warfarin is not required, although many patients take a daily baby aspirin (81 mg). These valves are all vulnerable to structural degeneration and calcification, which occurs more rapidly in younger patients. In addition, mitral prostheses tend to degenerate faster than those in the aortic position. There is some evidence that pregnancy may accelerate valve degeneration and, in some retrospective series, a second valve replacement was necessary in approximately one third of patients within 2 years of delivery.[25] This is not universally accepted, however, and other large series have shown no difference in structural valve degeneration in young women who had a pregnancy versus those who did not. Nonetheless, all tissue valves will degenerate, necessitating a second operation with an operative risk that is usually higher than the first. In some series, the mortality of a second valve replacement may be as high as 6 percent, and it must be recognized that if death occurs after the mother has had a successful pregnancy, the young child is left without a mother.[26] Thus, at the time of counseling women of childbearing age about valve choice the surgical results from the individual's institution should be reviewed. These may vary considerably, based on both surgical volume and expertise.

Homografts pose similar problems of structural deterioration and reoperation. The Ross operation, in which an autograft pulmonary valve is placed in the aortic position and a tissue prosthesis (usually porcine) is implanted in the pulmonary position, is associated with good outcomes during pregnancy when the hemodynamics are good. Nonetheless, the Ross procedure essentially exchanges one valvular problem for two, and ultimately the tissue pulmonary prosthesis must be replaced, as well as the aortic prosthesis.

Mechanical Prostheses and Anticoagulant Treatment

The management of pregnancy when the mother has a mechanical valve prosthesis is controversial and no universal consensus exists. There is no perfect strategy and each modality is associated with some hazard for the mother and/or the fetus. Before any approach is adopted, it is crucial to explain the risks to the patient. During pregnancy, maternal blood is highly thrombogenic, because there is an increased concentration of clotting factors and increased platelet adhesiveness, combined with decreased fibrinolysis. These changes in clotting parameters make the risk of valve thrombosis and thromboembolism significant.

UNFRACTIONATED HEPARIN. Unfractionated heparin is a large molecule that does not cross the placenta and does not cause developmental abnormalities in the fetus. Laboratory control of activated partial thromboplastin time (APTT) is difficult, however, in part because of the variation in response to standard doses and the wide variation in the reagents used to monitor doses. The APTT ratio should be maintained at a level of at least 2, which corresponds to an antifactor Xa (anti-Xa) level of more than 0.55 unit/ml in approximately 90 percent of patients.[27] Unfractionated heparin has been used subcutaneously and intravenously and is often begun in the first trimester, as soon as pregnancy is diagnosed, to minimize fetal exposure to warfarin at the critical time of fetal embryogenesis. It is usually continued until week 13 or 14 of pregnancy, when fetal embryogenesis is almost complete, and then warfarin is substituted. Some physicians continue heparin throughout pregnancy to avoid any fetal exposure to warfarin, but unfractionated heparin has been shown to be a poor anticoagulant in pregnancy. One large retrospective European study comparing different anticoagulation strategies has shown that most maternal complications (e.g., valve thrombosis, stroke, death) occur while mothers are taking heparin.[28] Most complications occur with mechanical mitral tilting disc prostheses, and this observation has been supported by many other studies, particularly with older generation prostheses.[29] One meta-analysis by Chan and colleagues[30] has shown that using heparin early in the first trimester virtually eliminates the risk of fetal embryopathy but at the expense of maternal valve thrombosis, which occurred with a frequency of 9 percent. If unfractionated heparin is the selected treatment strategy, the midinterval APTT should be at least twice that of the control or an anti-Xa level of 0.35 to 0.7 unit/ml should be maintained.[27]

LOW-MOLECULAR-WEIGHT HEPARIN. Low-molecular-weight heparin is an attractive alternative to unfractionated heparin because of its ease of use and superior bioavailability. Deaths have been reported with its use, however, usually associated with maternal valve thrombosis. The American College of Chest Physicians has suggested that it may be used and the anticoagulant effect carefully monitored by measuring the anti-Xa level. It is recommended that it be administered subcutaneously every 12 hours and the dose adjusted, so that a 4-hour postinjection anti-Xa level is maintained at approximately 1.0 to 1.2 unit/ml, perhaps measured weekly.[27] The addition of low-dose aspirin, 75 to 162 mg/day, has also been recommended. There are no large prospective trials to confirm the usefulness of low-molecular-weight heparin in this setting, however, and reported studies are confined to small groups. Certainly, dosing based on weight alone has been shown to be inadequate to maintain most pregnant women in the therapeutic range as measured by anti-Xa activity,[31] and the pharmacokinetics change throughout pregnancy.[32] One retrospective study has reviewed published series between 1989 and 2004.[33] There were 74 women with 81 pregnancies, most of whom had mitral prostheses. Thromboemboli occurred in 10 of 81 pregnancies (12 percent) and all these patients had mitral prostheses. In 60 pregnancies, low-molecular-weight heparin was used throughout and, in 21 pregnancies, was used only in the first trimester and again at term. In 51 pregnancies, anti-Xa levels were monitored and, in 30 pregnancies, a fixed dose was used. All 10 patients with thromboemboli were on heparin throughout pregnancy and 9 of them were on a fixed-dose regimen. This underscores the need for meticulous monitoring of anti-Xa levels, and Oran and associates[33] have recommended that the 4- to 6-hour postinjection level be maintained at 1 IU/ml. Thus, the use of low-molecular-weight heparin remains controversial, with no large prospective series and no evidence-based data to support which levels of anti-Xa should be maintained. It should be discontinued at least 24 hours before delivery if epidural analgesia is to be used, because it has a prolonged effect and there is risk of spinal hematoma. Unfractionated heparin can be substituted peridelivery because it can be started and stopped abruptly. With all strategies, anticoagulants should be resumed as soon as possible after delivery.

WARFARIN. Fetal exposure to warfarin in the first trimester may be associated with fetal embryopathy. In its mildest form, this may be only bony stippling (chondrodysplasia punctata), but in its most severe form it may be manifested as nasal hypoplasia, optic atrophy, and mental retardation. The reported fetal risk of embryopathy varies widely, but probably averages 6 percent. This risk is reduced by initiating heparin before 6 weeks of pregnancy, but the disadvantage is an increased risk of maternal valve thrombosis. Warfarin also appears to increase the risk of fetal loss and spontaneous abortion.

The risk of fetal embryopathy may be dose-related, and a study by Vitale and colleagues[34] has suggested that the risk is very low if the maternal warfarin dose is 5 mg or less. Thus, the anticoagulant approach for the woman with a mechanical valve needs to be individualized. For the woman with an older generation or tilting disc mitral prosthesis, particularly if she is in atrial fibrillation, the safer approach may be to treat her with warfarin for the first 34 to 35 weeks of pregnancy, particularly if her dose is less than 5 mg/day. This must be fully discussed with the patient before she gets pregnant, not only for the medicolegal implications, but so that all the risks and benefits are understood. For those patients at lesser risk, heparin therapy (with the provisos noted earlier) may be selected as soon as pregnancy is diagnosed, warfarin substituted at 13 to 14 weeks, and heparin restarted at approximately 35 weeks in anticipation of delivery.

The most common connective tissue disorder is the Marfan syndrome, which is a disorder of fibrillin and is inherited in an autosomal dominant inheritance pattern. Preconception counseling is essential to advise prospective parents about the risks of transmission to the offspring and the risks of cardiovascular complications for the mother. A careful clinical and echocardiographic cardiovascular evaluation should be performed. This would usually include MRI or computed tomography (CT) assessment of the entire aorta to look for aortic dilation or dissection. Pregnancy is usually contraindicated if the ascending aorta is larger than 40 mm in diameter, although the exact dimension is still a matter of debate. One recent study has suggested that pregnancy is relatively safe up to a diameter of 45 mm.[35] Associated cardiovascular problems also need to be evaluated, including the presence or absence of aortic regurgitation and mitral valve prolapse with associated regurgitation. Many patients are on long-term treatment with beta-adrenergic blockers to slow the progression of aortic regurgitation. These should be continued during pregnancy if there is any aortic dilation. Periodic echocardiographic surveillance every 6 to 8 weeks is recommended to monitor the mother's aortic root size, with the interval dependent on the initial echocardiographic findings. Any chest pain should be promptly evaluated to rule out dissection. During labor and delivery, pushing should be avoided, with an assisted second stage if necessary.

A prospective study of 45 pregnancies in 21 women with Marfan syndrome by Rossiter and colleagues[36] has shown that most patients had little or no change in aortic root diameter during pregnancy, but two patients had aortic dissection; one with an aortic root diameter of 42 mm had rapid aortic dilation to 52 mm by the third trimester and 68 mm at 2 months' postpartum. These results underscore that women with Marfan syndrome must be advised that pregnancy is not uniformly safe, and aortic dilation may be unpredictable, although much more likely to occur when the aortic root is larger than 40 mm.

Cardiomyopathies (see Chaps. 64 and 65)

Dilated Cardiomyopathy

Patients with idiopathic dilated cardiomyopathy are usually counseled not to have a pregnancy if the ejection fraction is lower than 40 percent. Because angiotensin-converting enzyme (ACE) inhibitors are contraindicated in pregnancy, ventricular function must be assessed without this drug. Careful echocardiographic evaluation should be performed before pregnancy. Exercise testing may also be helpful, because women with ejection fractions of 40 to 50 percent may not tolerate pregnancy well if they have a poor functional aerobic capacity. Symptomatic patients who proceed with a pregnancy may need hydralazine for afterload reduction, bed rest, and low-dose diuretics for heart failure. Early delivery may also be necessary.

Peripartum Cardiomyopathy

Peripartum cardiomyopathy (PPCM) is a dilated cardiomyopathy, documented with echocardiographic left ventricular dysfunction occurring in the last month of pregnancy or within 5 months of delivery.[37] Patients with a prior history of myocardial disease are excluded from this definition, although this makes the diagnosis challenging in many women who have had neither a chest X-ray nor an echocardiogram to confirm that they had previously normal ventricular function. This makes the actual incidence unknown, but it is probably approximately 1 in 3000. Risk factors include multiparity, being black, older maternal age, and preeclampsia. In a recent retrospective study of 123 women with PPCM,[38] a history of hypertension was obtained in 43 percent of patients, and twin pregnancies were reported in 13 percent. Consistent with earlier studies, most patients (75 percent) presented in the first month postpartum, perhaps suggesting an autoimmune cause rather than the pregnancy exacerbating a preexisting cardiomyopathy. This theory is supported by the documentation of autoantibodies in some cases.

The treatment of PPCM is the same as for other forms of congestive heart failure, except that ACE inhibitors and angiotensin receptor blocking agents (ARBs) are contraindicated in pregnancy. Hydralazine, beta blockers, and digoxin have all been used and are safe, and diuretics may decrease preload and improve symptoms.[39] Intracardiac thrombus and embolism are common, and consideration should be given to anticoagulation with unfractionated heparin in those with an ejection fraction lower than 35 percent.[40] Early fetal delivery may be necessary in women needing hospitalization for heart failure. Myocarditis is a causative factor in some cases, with a reported incidence between 8.8 and 78 percent. The role of endomyocardial biopsy is controversial, but probably should be considered and performed by those with considerable experience. Immunosuppressive treatment should be given to those with proven myocarditis.

Normalization of ventricular function occurs in about 50 percent of patients and appears more likely if the ejection fraction is more than 30 percent at the time of diagnosis.[38] Most physicians counsel against a second pregnancy, even if the ventricular function does return to normal, because PPCM will recur in approximately 30 percent of cases. This may result in significant clinical deterioration and even death.[41,42]

Hypertrophic Cardiomyopathy

A wide spectrum of anatomical and hemodynamic abnormalities exists in hypertrophic cardiomyopathy, including left ventricular outflow tract obstruction, mitral regurgitation, arrhythmias, and diastolic dysfunction. Some patients are asymptomatic with minimal hemodynamic disturbance; others are profoundly limited, with marked hemodynamic perturbations. A careful personal history, review of family history, electrocardiography, exercise test, and transthoracic echocardiography should precede counseling about the advisability of a pregnancy. The prospective parents should be informed about the autosomal dominant inheritance pattern, which has variable penetrance. Currently, over 200 genetic mutations have been identified, and genetic counseling and family screening are appropriate before pregnancy is contemplated.

Most women with hypertrophic cardiomyopathy tolerate pregnancy well. The decrease in afterload that might exacerbate the outflow gradient is largely offset by the maternal increase in plasma volume. Medications such as beta blockers, which alleviate the outflow tract obstruction, may be continued throughout pregnancy, but the dose may need to be increased. Patients who have significant symptoms before pregnancy (usually related to severe left ventricular outflow tract obstruction) may not do well and become hemodynamically unstable. Common symptoms include palpitation, angina, and breathlessness. In a retrospective study of 127 women with 271 pregnancies, 36 women (28.3 percent) reported cardiac symptoms but 90 percent were symptomatic before pregnancy.[43] Heart failure occurred postnatally in two women but there were no maternal deaths. Arrhythmia-related deaths in pregnancy have been reported, however.[44] Low-dose diuretics may be helpful to treat heart failure in pregnancy, but care must be taken not to volume-deplete the patient and exacerbate the left ventricular outflow gradient. Meticulous attention to hemodynamics should be made at the time of delivery. Epidural anesthesia and spinal block should be avoided in case of hypotension, and blood loss should be promptly replaced. The Valsalva maneuver should be avoided and the second stage should be facilitated as necessary. Cesarean section is indicated for obstetric reasons only.

Coronary Artery Disease (see Chaps. 50 to 54)

Coronary artery disease is uncommon in women of child-bearing age but may occur, particularly in the setting of diabetes and tobacco abuse. Acute myocardial infarction is rare and, when it occurs, pregnancy increases the maternal risk three- to fourfold. The most common cause is coronary artery dissection, and the most common site is in the left anterior descending coronary artery.[45] The treatment should be urgent coronary angiography, with a consideration of percutaneous coronary intervention and stenting.[21] The vulnerability to coronary artery dissection during pregnancy may relate to the presence of hypertension and also to the changes in elastin and collagen synthesis incurred by the hormonal changes of pregnancy.

A recent United States population-based study[46] has reported 44 deaths related to acute myocardial infarction, for a case fatality rate of 5.1 percent. The odds of acute myocardial infarction were 30-fold higher for women age 40 years and older than for women younger than 20 years. The odds were more than fivefold higher for black women age 35 years and older. Thrombus may also occur without atherosclerotic disease and atherosclerosis with or without intracoronary thrombus is found in some cases, presumably related to the clotting diathesis that occurs during pregnancy.

Hypertension (see Chaps. 40 and 41)

Hypertension in pregnancy is an important cause of maternal morbidity and mortality. The different types of hypertension seen in pregnancy are defined in Table 77-3. Gestational hypertension is distinguished from preeclampsia by the lack of proteinuria. About 50 percent of patients will develop preeclampsia, however, so close monitoring is warranted.[47] It develops in approximately 25 percent of patients with chronic hypertension. Preeclampsia is a much more worrisome development and tends to occur more commonly in primiparous women and those with twin pregnancies. They do not usually develop frank hypertension until the second half of gestation. The cause is not entirely clear but may relate to endothelial dysfunction causing abnormal remodeling of the placental spiral arteries.[48] Hypertension is just one feature of the diffuse endothelial dysfunction, which is associated with vasospasm, reduced end-organ perfusion, and activation of the coagulation cascade.[21]

Although antihypertensive medications are effective in treating chronic hypertension that has worsened during pregnancy, they are not effective in preventing preeclampsia. When preeclampsia develops, bed rest is usually initiated, with salt restriction and close monitoring, and magnesium sulfate is often administered in an effort to prevent eclamptic seizures and prolong the pregnancy, thereby facilitating fetal maturity. Urgent delivery is usually necessary, however, following which the blood pressure usually normalizes rapidly.

The treatment of other types of hypertension in pregnancy involves bed rest, salt restriction, and antihypertensive medications. Beta blockers, particularly labetalol (see "Cardiovascular Drug Therapy" and Table 77-4), have been used with good effect, although there is a long safety record

TABLE 77–3	Classification of Hypertension in Pregnancy[41]
Classification	**Features**
Chronic hypertension	Hypertension (blood pressure, [BP] ≥ 140 mmHg systolic or ≥ 90 mm Hg diastolic) present before pregnancy or diagnosedbefore 20th week of gestation
Gestational hypertension	New hypertension with BP of 140/90 mm Hg on two separate occasions, without proteinuria, arising de novo after 20th week of pregnancy; BP normalizes by 12 weeks postpartum
Preeclampsia superimposed on chronic hypertension	Increased BP above patient's baseline, change in proteinuria, or evidence of end-organ dysfunction
Preeclampsia-eclampsia	Proteinuria (>0.3 gm over 24 hours or 2+/4+ in two urine samples) in addition to new hypertension; edema no longer included in this diagnosis because of poor specificity; when proteinuria is absent, disease suspected with increased BP associated with headache, blurred vision, abdominal pain, low platelet count, or abnormal liver enzyme levels

From Gifford RW, August PA, Cunningham G, et al: Report of the National High Blood Pressure Education Program Working Group on High Blood Pressure in Pregnancy. Am J Obstet Gynecol 183:S1, 2000.

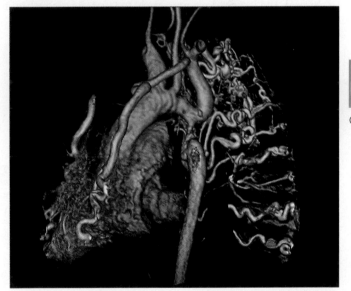

FIGURE 77–4 Magnetic resonance imaging scan of a 34-year-old with severe coarctation of the aorta (near interruption), with multiple and very large collateral vessels. She had had two prior pregnancies with preeclampsia and the coarctation had gone unnoticed.

with methyldopa, which has no adverse effect on mother or baby.

Coarctation of the aorta needs to be considered (Fig. 77-4).

Arrhythmias (see Chaps. 32 to 35)

Because of the physiological changes of pregnancy, the heart may be more vulnerable to arrhythmias during this time. Potential contributing factors include the increase in preload causing more myocardial irritability, increased heart rate, which may affect the refractory period, fluid and electrolyte shifts, and changes in catecholamine levels. Worsening arrhythmias is not a consistent feature, however, and many women with a past history of tachycardia may not notice any change in the frequency of symptoms, and some even improve. The presenting symptom complex may be difficult to separate from the normal symptoms of pregnancy, including a sensation of fast heartbeat and skipped beats, which most commonly are supraventricular ectopics. The general approach should include taking a careful history, looking for any precipitating causes, and ruling out any concomitant medical problems (e.g., thyroid disease) by performing appropriate laboratory tests, such as complete blood count, electrolyte level measurement, and thyroid function determination. The clinical examination may help define whether the arrhythmia occurs in the setting of a normal heart or whether there is any underlying organic heart disease. If there is any doubt after the clinical examination, a transthoracic echocardiogram should be obtained. If the mother has no underlying cardiac disease, pharmacological treatment should be administered if she is symptomatic or if the arrhythmia poses a risk to the mother or baby. In general, supraventricular and ventricular ectopic beats require no therapy. If there is underlying organic disease, the precipitating cause should be treated, if possible and, if this does not resolve, the arrhythmia medical therapy should be initiated.

The most common arrhythmia is atrial reentry tachycardia. Treatment of this type of arrhythmia is generally the same as for nonpregnant women, but with added concern about the effects of medications on the fetus (see Table 77-4). In general, the lowest dose necessary to treat the arrhythmia should be administered, and there should be a periodic evaluation of whether it is necessary to continue treatment. Atrial fibrillation is usually an indication that there is underlying structural heart disease. If the arrhythmia is unresponsive to medical therapy, electrical cardioversion may be performed and is not usually harmful to the fetus. Some have recommended that during elective cardioversion, fetal monitoring should be performed in case transient fetal bradycardia is present.

Premature ventricular complexes are common during pregnancy and usually require no treatment. Ventricular tachycardia is rare but may be a consequence of ischemic heart disease or cardiomyopathy. The treatment depends on the rate of tachycardia and the hemodynamic status of the mother. The choices of medications are listed in Table 77-4; electrical cardioversion should be performed if there is hemodynamic compromise.

CARDIOVASCULAR DRUG THERAPY
(see Chap. 6)

When administration of cardiovascular drugs is being contemplated during pregnancy, the U.S. Food and Drug Administration (FDA) classification of these drugs must be considered. The reader is referred to more detailed information in this regard. Category X drugs are those for which fetal abnormalities have been demonstrated in animal or human studies, and the drug is contraindicated (e.g., warfarin). Almost all cardiovascular drugs are classified as category C, which means that animal studies have revealed adverse fetal effects, but there are no controlled data in women. A medication should only be given if the benefits outweigh the potential risk to the fetus. Important principles to be considered when using cardiovascular medications for pregnant women include the use of drugs with the longest safety record, using the lowest dose and shortest duration necessary and generally avoiding a multidrug regimen, if possible. All these issues need to be reviewed carefully with the prospective mother at the time of prepregnancy counseling. A list of cardiovascular medications that might be considered in pregnancy is given in Table 77-4.

ASPIRIN. This crosses the placenta, and concern exists about its effect on fetal prostaglandins, which might cause

TABLE 77–4	Cardiovascular Drugs in Pregnancy
Drug	**Potential Fetal Side Effects**
Amiodarone	Goiter, hypothyroidism and hyperthyroidism, IUGR
Angiotensin-converting enzyme inhibitor	Contraindicated; IUGR, oligohydramnios, renal failure, abnormal bone ossification; FDA class X
Aspirin	Baby aspirin not harmful
Beta blocker	Relatively safe; IUGR, neonatal bradycardia, hypoglycemia
Calcium channel blocker	Relatively safe; few studies; concern regarding uterine tone at time of delivery
Digoxin	Safe; no adverse effects
Flecainide	Relatively safe; limited data; used to treat fetal arrhythmias
Hydralazine	Safe; no major adverse effects
Lasix	Safe; caution regarding maternal hypovolemia and reduced placental blood flow
Lidocaine	Safe; high doses may cause neonatal central nervous system depression
Methyldopa	Safe; considered by some to be drug of choice for hypertension in pregnancy
Procainamide	Relatively safe; limited data; has been used to treat fetal arrhythmias, no major fetal side effects
Propafenone	Limited data
Quinidine	Relatively safe; rarely associated with neonatal thrombocytopenia; minimal oxytocic effect
Warfarin	Fetal embryopathy; placental and fetal hemorrhage; central nervous system abnormalities; FDA class X

IUGR = intrauterine growth retardation.

closure of the fetal ductus arteriosus. Baby aspirin (81 mg), however, has been used safely in pregnancy without premature closure of the fetal duct. It may be useful adjunctive therapy when the mother has a mechanical valve prosthesis and can help prevent valve thrombosis.

AMIODARONE. Amiodarone and its iodine component cross the placenta and may cause neonatal goiter. The risks and benefits of its use, however, need to be balanced; if it has proved effective in controlling serious maternal arrhythmias, it may be safer for the mother to continue its use during pregnancy.

ANGIOTENSIN-CONVERTING ENZYME INHIBITORS. These are contraindicated in pregnancy, because they are associated with abnormal renal development in the fetus as well as oligohydramnios and intrauterine growth retardation.

BETA-ADRENERGIC RECEPTOR BLOCKERS. These have been used extensively during pregnancy for treatment of arrhythmias, hypertrophic cardiomyopathy, and hypertension. They cross the placenta but are not teratogenic. Concern exists, however, particularly regarding fetal growth, because they have been demonstrated to cause fetal growth retardation. They may also be associated with neonatal bradycardia and hypoglycemia. More concern exists with regard to atenolol than some of the other beta-blocking agents. From a practical perspective, however, although the risk-benefit ratio needs to be considered, beta blockers have been used safely during pregnancy, although it is recommended that fetal growth be monitored more carefully.

CALCIUM CHANNEL BLOCKERS. These have been used to treat both arrhythmias and hypertension. There are limited data regarding their use. Most experience probably exists with verapamil, and no major adverse fetal effects have been recorded. Diltiazem and nifedipine have also been used, but studies are limited.

DIGOXIN. This has been used during pregnancy for many decades and, whereas it does cross the placenta, no adverse effects with its use have been reported.

DIURETICS. These agents, most commonly furosemide, may be used to treat congestive heart failure during pregnancy and sometimes are used for the treatment of hypertension. Aggressive use of diuretics, however, may cause reduction in placental blood flow and have a detrimental effect on fetal growth.

WARFARIN. This is usually contraindicated in the first trimester of pregnancy, because it crosses the placenta and may cause fetal embryopathy. As noted earlier (see "Mechanical Prostheses and Anticoagulant Treatment"), however, there may be some high-risk situations in which the mother and physician determine that the safer approach is to continue warfarin therapy, particularly when the maternal dose is 5 mg or lower. Concern exists in the third trimester about labor and delivery, because the immature fetal liver does not metabolize warfarin as rapidly as the mother's liver. After discontinuation of warfarin, reversal of anticoagulation occurs more rapidly in the mother, whereas reversal of anticoagulation in the fetus may take up to 1 week because of the immature fetal liver. Vaginal delivery when the fetus is anticoagulated is contraindicated because of the risk of fetal hemorrhage. Therefore, switching to an alternative anticoagulant such as heparin must be done well before labor is anticipated.

CONTRACEPTION

For women with cardiac disease, appropriate contraceptive advice should be given before they become sexually active. This is particularly true for those with congenital heart disease who, like other adolescents without heart disease, often become sexually active in their early teens; For some, pregnancy may pose a high risk of morbidity and even mortality. Patients need to be given detailed advice about various contraceptive methods and their effectiveness, and each patient should understand the relative risks and benefits of each modality. The approach should be individualized, also bearing in mind the patient's likely compliance

BARRIER CONTRACEPTION. Male and female condoms help protect against sexually transmitted disease but must be used correctly and require some dexterity. Even when used appropriately, they have a recognized failure rate of approximately 15 pregnancies/100 woman-years of use. The decision to use a barrier method, therefore, depends on how critical it is for the woman to avoid pregnancy and on compliance and the ability to use a condom correctly.

INTRAUTERINE DEVICES. Intrauterine devices (IUDs) may be used in parous women, with failure rates of approximately 3 pregnancies/100 woman-years. Complications include infection and arrhythmia at the time of insertion. A vasovagal response occurring in a patient with idiopathic pulmonary arterial hypertension or secondary pulmonary hypertension, such as Eisenmenger syndrome, could be life-threatening, and many physicians therefore avoid using an IUD in such patients. More recently developed IUDs are more effective in preventing pregnancy than earlier devices, particularly those that are loaded with progesterone, which suppresses endometrial activity and thickens cervical mucus. Antibiotic prophylaxis should be used around the time of insertion.

Oral Contraceptives

Combination estrogen-progesterone oral preparations are very effective, with an extremely low failure rate and, for this reason, coupled with ease of use, are widely taken. For the woman with heart disease, however, concern exists because of increased risk of venous thromboembolism, atherosclerosis, hyperlipidemia, hypertension, and ischemic heart disease, particularly for those who are older than 40 years and for those who smoke. In addition, patients with congenital heart disease who have cyanosis, atrial fibrillation or flutter, mechanical prosthetic heart valves, or a Fontan circulation probably should avoid estrogen-containing preparations. Those with impaired ventricular function from any cause (probably an ejection fraction less than 40 percent) or with a history of any prior thromboembolic event should avoid warfarin.

Progesterone-only contraceptives are less reliable than combined preparations, with failure rates of 2 to 5 pregnancies/100 woman-years. They require that the woman take the pill at the same time every day for optimum efficacy, and this requires considerable motivation on the part of the patient. There is a paucity of data about adverse effects of progesterone agents on the cardiovascular system, but probably these are safe for most women with heart disease.

DEPOT PROGESTERONE. Injectable progesterone, given three times monthly, is effective and is an attractive alternative for patients who may have problems with compliance with oral medications. Some patients find fluid retention and irregular menstruation to be problematic, but otherwise cardiovascular contraindications are the same as those for progesterone.

Tubal Sterilization

This may be performed laparoscopically or via a laparotomy. For patients who have tenuous cardiac hemodynamics, there may be some risk of cardiac instability, and cardiac anesthesia may be preferable. This is particularly important, for example, in patients with primary or secondary pulmonary hypertension when general anesthesia may be hazardous and insufflation of the abdomen may elevate the diaphragm and contribute to unstable cardiorespiratory function. More recently, tubal sterilization has been accomplished with the use of an intrafallopian plug, which is inserted endoscopically.

FUTURE PERSPECTIVES

Appropriate pregnancy counseling for women with cardiac disease is problematic. Few physicians have expertise or training to manage such patients, particularly those women with congenital heart disease. Few if any evidence-based guidelines are available, and most published data involve isolated case reports or small cohort studies. Many questions remain unanswered. Although successful pregnancy is possible in many women with heart disease, does the volume load cause subtle long-term deterioration in ventricular dysfunction in those with limited cardiac reserve?[49] What is the ideal management strategy for women with mechanical valve prostheses? These continued uncertainties emphasize the need for the institution of multicenter research initiatives to answer prospectively the many questions that remain.

REFERENCES

General

1. Connolly H, Warnes C: Pregnancy and contraception. *In* Gatzoulis MA, Webb GD, Daubeney PE (eds): Diagnosis and Management of Adult Congenital Heart Disease. Edinburgh, Churchill Livingstone, 2003, pp 135-177.
2. Siu SC, Sermer M, Colman JM, et al: Prospective multicenter study of pregnancy outcomes in women with heart disease. Circulation 104:515, 2001.
3. Thorne SA: Pregnancy in heart disease. Heart 90:450, 2004.
4. Elkayam U, Bitar F: Valvular heart disease and pregnancy. Part I: Native valves. J Am Coll Cardiol 46:223, 2005.
5. Arnoni RT, Arnoni AS, Bonini RC, et al: Risk factors associated with cardiac surgery during pregnancy. Ann Thorac Surg 76:1605, 2003.
6. Wolinsky H: Effects of estrogen and progestogen treatment on the response of the aorta of male rats to hypertension: Morphological and chemical studies. Circ Res 30:341, 1972.
7. Stout K: Pregnancy in women with congenital heart disease: the importance of evaluation and counselling. Heart 91:713, 2005.

Congenital Heart Disease

8. Silversides CK, Colman JM, Sermer M, et al: Early- and intermediate-term outcomes of pregnancy with congenital aortic stenosis. Am J Cardiol 91:1386, 2003.
9. Myerson SG, Mitchell AR, Ormerod OJ, et al: What is the role of balloon dilation for severe aortic stenosis during pregnancy? J Heart Valve Dis 14:147, 2005.
10. Warnes CA: Cyanotic congenital heart disease. *In* Oakley C, Warnes CA (eds): Heart Disease in Pregnancy. 2nd ed. BMJ Books, 2007, pp 43-58.
11. Presbitero P, Somerville J, Stone S, et al: Pregnancy in cyanotic congenital heart disease. Outcome of mother and fetus. Circulation 89:2673, 1994.
12. Beauchesne LM, Warnes CA, Connolly HM, et al: Prevalence and clinical manifestations of 22q11.2 microdeletion in adults with selected conotruncal anomalies. J Am Coll Cardiol 45:595, 2005.
13. Khairy P, Ouyang DW, Fernandes SM, et al: Pregnancy outcomes in women with congenital heart disease. Circulation 113:517, 2006.
14. Meijer JM, Pieper PG, Drenthen W, et al: Pregnancy, fertility, and recurrence risk in corrected tetralogy of Fallot. Heart 91:801, 2005.
15. Veldtman GR, Connolly HM, Grogan M, et al: Outcomes of pregnancy in women with tetralogy of Fallot. J Am Coll Cardiol 44:174, 2004.
16. Warnes CA: Pregnancy and pulmonary hypertension. Int J Cardiol 97(Suppl 1):11, 2004.
17. Gleicher N, Midwall J, Hochberger D, et al: Eisenmenger's syndrome and pregnancy. Obstet Gynecol Surv 34:721, 1979.
18. Bonnin M, Mercier FJ, Sitbon O, et al: Severe pulmonary hypertension during pregnancy: mode of delivery and anesthetic management of 15 consecutive cases. Anesthesiology 102:1133; discussion, 1135A, 2005.
19. Lacassie HJ, Germain AM, Valdes G, et al: Management of Eisenmenger syndrome in pregnancy with sildenafil and L-arginine. Obstet Gynecol 103:1118, 2004.

Rheumatic and Acquired Valvular Heart Disease

20. Silversides CK, Colman JM, Sermer M, et al: Cardiac risk in pregnant women with rheumatic mitral stenosis. Am J Cardiol 91:1382, 2003.
21. The Task Force on the Management of Cardiovascular Diseases During Pregnancy of the European Society of Cardiology: Expert consensus document on management of cardiovascular diseases during pregnancy. Eur Heart J 24:761, 2003.
22. Reimold SC, Rutherford JD: Clinical practice. Valvular heart disease in pregnancy. N Engl J Med 349:52, 2003.
23. Routray SN, Mishra TK, Swain S, et al: Balloon mitral valvuloplasty during pregnancy. Int J Gynaecol Obstet 85:18, 2004.
24. Aggarwal N, Suri V, Goyal A, et al: Closed mitral valvotomy in pregnancy and labor. Int J Gynaecol Obstet 88:118, 2005.
25. Jamieson WR, Miller DC, Akins CW, et al: Pregnancy and bioprostheses: Influence on structural valve deterioration. Ann Thorac Surg 60(Suppl 2):S282, 1995.
26. Hung L, Rahimtoola SH: Prosthetic heart valves and pregnancy. Circulation 107:1240, 2003.
27. Bates SM, Greer IA, Hirsh J, et al: Use of antithrombotic agents during pregnancy: The Seventh ACCP Conference on Antithrombotic and Thrombolytic Therapy. Chest 126:627S, 2004.
28. Sbarouni E, Oakley CM: Outcome of pregnancy in women with valve prostheses. Br Heart J 71:196, 1994.
29. Elkayam U, Bitar F: Valvular heart disease and pregnancy. Part II: Prosthetic valves. J Am Coll Cardiol 46:403, 2005.
30. Chan WS, Anand S, Ginsberg JS: Anticoagulation of pregnant women with mechanical heart valves: A systematic review of the literature. Arch Intern Med 160:191, 2000.
31. Barbour LA, Oja JL, Schultz LK: A prospective trial that demonstrates that dalteparin requirements increase in pregnancy to maintain therapeutic levels of anticoagulation. Am J Obstet Gynecol 191:1024, 2004.
32. Sephton V, Farquharson RG, Topping J, et al: A longitudinal study of maternal dose response to low-molecular-weight heparin in pregnancy. Obstet Gynecol 101:1307, 2003.
33. Oran B, Lee-Parritz A, Ansell J: Low-molecular-weight heparin for the prophylaxis of thromboembolism in women with prosthetic mechanical heart valves during pregnancy. Thromb Haemost 92:747, 2004.
34. Vitale N, De Feo M, De Santo LS, et al: Dose-dependent fetal complications of warfarin in pregnant women with mechanical heart valves. J Am Coll Cardiol 33:1637, 1999.

Connective Tissue Disorders

35. Meijboom LJ, Vos FE, Timmermans J, et al: Pregnancy and aortic root growth in the Marfan syndrome: A prospective study. Eur Heart J 26:914-920, 2005.
36. Rossiter JP, Repke JT, Morales AJ, et al: A prospective longitudinal evaluation of pregnancy in the Marfan syndrome. Am J Obstet Gynecol 173:1599, 1995.

Cardiomyopathies

37. Pearson GD, Veille JC, Rahimtoola S, et al: Peripartum cardiomyopathy: National Heart, Lung, and Blood Institute and Office of Rare Diseases (National Institutes of Health) workshop recommendations and review. JAMA 283:1183, 2000.
38. Elkayam U, Akhter MW, Singh H, et al: Pregnancy-associated cardiomyopathy: Clinical characteristics and a comparison between early and late presentation. Circulation 111:2050, 2005.
39. Sliwa K, Fett J, Elkayam U: Peripartum cardiomyopathy. Lancet 368:687, 2006.
40. Phillips SD, Warnes WC: Peripartum cardiomyopathy: Current therapeutic perspectives. Curr Treat Options Cardiovasc Med 6:481, 2004.
41. Elkayam U, Tummala PP, Rao K, et al: Maternal and fetal outcomes of subsequent pregnancies in women with peripartum cardiomyopathy. N Engl J Med 344:1567, 2001.
42. Sliwa K, Forster O, Zhanje F, et al: Outcome of subsequent pregnancy in patients with documented peripartum cardiomyopathy. Am J Cardiol 93:1441, 2004.
43. Thaman R, Varnava A, Hamid MS, et al: Pregnancy related complications in women with hypertrophic cardiomyopathy. Heart 89:752, 2003.
44. Autore C, Conte MR, Piccininno M, et al: Risk associated with pregnancy in hypertrophic cardiomyopathy. J Am Coll Cardiol 40:1864, 2002.

Coronary Artery Disease

45. Maeder M, Ammann P, Angehrn W, et al: Idiopathic spontaneous coronary artery dissection: Incidence, diagnosis and treatment. Int J Cardiol 101:363, 2005.
46. James AH, Jamison MG, Biswas MS, et al.: Acute myocardial infarction in pregnancy: A United States population-based study. Circulation 113:1564, 2006.

Hypertension, Arrhythmias

47. Barton JR, O'Brien J M, Bergauer NK, et al: Mild gestational hypertension remote from term: Progression and outcome. Am J Obstet Gynecol 184:979, 2001.
48. Lain KY, Roberts JM: Contemporary concepts of the pathogenesis and management of preeclampsia. JAMA 287:3183, 2002.
49. Guedes A, Mercier LA, Leduc L, et al: Impact of pregnancy on the systemic right ventricle after a Mustard operation for transposition of the great arteries. J Am Coll Cardiol 44:433, 2004.

CH 77

Pregnancy and Heart Disease

Recommendations for the management of heart disease in pregnancy appear in various American College of Cardiology/American Heart Association (ACC/AHA) guidelines. These include guidelines on valvular heart disease,[1] atrial fibrillation,[2] supraventricular tachycardias,[3] and stroke,[4] as well as the 2003 scientific statement on warfarin therapy.[5] Of note, the European Society of Cardiology has published a comprehensive consensus paper on the management of cardiovascular disease during pregnancy.[6]

ATRIAL FIBRILLATION

Atrial fibrillation (AF) is rare during pregnancy and is usually associated with another underlying cause, such as mitral stenosis, congenital heart disease, or hyperthyroidism. Diagnosis and treatment of the underlying condition causing the dysrhythmia are of utmost importance. Antithrombotic therapy is recommended for all pregnant women with atrial fibrillation. The type of therapy should be chosen with regard to the stage of pregnancy (Table 77G-1).[2] Ventricular rate should be controlled with digoxin or a nondihydropyridine calcium channel antagonist to control the rate of ventricular response. Direct-current cardioversion can be performed without fetal damage in women who become hemodynamically unstable because of AF. Administration of quinidine or procainamide is a reasonable approach for cardioversion in pregnant women with AF who are hemodynamically stable.

VALVULAR DISEASE

Many women with valvular heart disease can be successfully managed throughout pregnancy, labor, and delivery with conservative medical measures. Symptomatic or severe valvular lesions should be addressed and rectified before conception and pregnancy whenever possible.[1] Drugs should be avoided when possible.

Mitral Stenosis. Pregnant women with mild to moderate mitral stenosis can almost always be managed with judicious use of diuretics and beta blockade. A cardioselective beta blocker may prevent deleterious effects of epinephrine blockade on myometrial tissue. Women with severe mitral stenosis should be considered for percutaneous balloon mitral valvotomy before conception, if possible. Percutaneous balloon valvotomy is a reasonable option for women who develop severe symptoms during pregnancy.

Mitral Regurgitation. Mitral regurgitation can usually be managed medically with diuretics and vasodilator therapy. If surgery is required, repair is always preferred.

Aortic Stenosis. Pregnant women with mild obstruction and normal left ventricular systolic function can be managed conservatively throughout pregnancy. Those with moderate to severe obstruction or symptoms should be advised to delay conception until aortic stenosis can be corrected. Women with severe aortic stenosis who develop symptoms may require percutaneous aortic balloon valvotomy or surgery before labor and delivery.

Aortic Regurgitation. Isolated aortic regurgitation can usually be managed with diuretics and vasodilator therapy when needed. Surgery during pregnancy should be contemplated only for control of refractory symptoms.

Endocarditis Prophylaxis. The guidelines do not recommend routine antibiotic prophylaxis in patients with valvular heart disease undergoing uncomplicated vaginal delivery or cesarean section unless infection is suspected. For high-risk patients, such as those with prosthetic heart valves or a prior history of endocarditis, antibiotics are considered optional.

SUPRAVENTRICULAR TACHYCARDIAS

Premature atrial beats, which are commonly observed during pregnancy, are generally benign and well tolerated. In patients with mild symptoms and structurally normal hearts, no treatment other than reassurance should be provided. Given that all commonly used antiarrhythmic drugs cross the placental barrier to some extent, antiarrhythmic drug therapy should be used only if symptoms are intolerable or if the tachycardia causes hemodynamic compromise (Table 77G-2).[3] Catheter ablation should be recommended for women with symptomatic tachyarrhythmias before they contemplate pregnancy. Because of the potential problem of recurring tachyarrhythmias during pregnancy, the policy of withdrawing antiarrhythmic drugs and resuming them later can be recommended only as an alternative in selected cases. Catheter ablation is the procedure of choice for drug-refractory, poorly tolerated supraventricular tachycardia (SVT). If needed, it should be performed in the second trimester.

STROKE

Pregnancy increases the risk for stroke and complicates the selection of acute and preventive treatments. Guidelines for acute treatment have not yet been established. Recommendations for stroke prevention in pregnant women made by the American Heart Association and American Stroke Association[4] focus on anticoagulation and antiplatelet strategies (Table 77G-3), which are similar to those for management of valvular heart disease during pregnancy.

HYPERTROPHIC CARDIOMYOPATHY

Women with hypertrophic cardiomyopathy are generally not at increased risk during pregnancy and undergo normal vaginal delivery without the necessity for cesarean section.[7] Morbidity and mortality appear to be confined principally to women with high-risk clinical profiles, who should receive specialized preventive obstetrical care during pregnancy.

ANTICOAGULATION

The 2006 ACC/AHA guidelines on valvular heart disease offer complex recommendations for the management of anticoagulation in pregnant patients with mechanical prosthetic heart valves (Table 77G-4). These guidelines reflect high complication rates in pregnant women managed with subcutaneous heparin and support the use of intravenous heparin during the first trimester. After the 36th week of pregnancy, transition from warfarin to heparin is recommended in anticipation of labor.

The AHA's 2003 Scientific Statement on anticoagulation[5] notes a dilemma for physicians managing anticoagulation for pregnant patients. Three options are available:

1. Heparin or low-molecular-weight heparin throughout pregnancy
2. Warfarin throughout pregnancy, changing to heparin or low-molecular-weight heparin at 38 weeks' gestation with planned labor induction at about 40 weeks
3. Heparin or low-molecular-weight heparin in the first trimester of pregnancy, switching to warfarin in the second trimester, continuing it until about 38 weeks' gestation, and then changing to heparin or low-molecular-weight heparin at 38 weeks with planned labor induction at about 40 weeks

These strategies are complicated by the fact that low-molecular-weight heparin is not approved by the U.S. Food and Drug

TABLE 77G-1 ACC/AHA Recommendations for Management of Atrial Fibrillation (AF) During Pregnancy

Class	Indication	Level of Evidence
Class I (indicated)	Control the rate of ventricular response with digoxin, a beta blocker, or a calcium channel antagonist.	C
	Perform electrical cardioversion in patients who become hemodynamically unstable because of the dysrhythmia.	C
	Administer antithrombotic therapy (anticoagulant or aspirin) throughout pregnancy to all patients with AF (except those with lone AF).	C
Class IIb (weak supportive evidence)	Attempt pharmacological cardioversion by administration of quinidine, procainamide, or sotalol in hemodynamically stable patients who develop AF during pregnancy.	C
	Administer heparin to patients with risk factors for thromboembolism during the first trimester and last month of pregnancy. Unfractionated heparin may be administered either by continuous intravenous infusion in a dose sufficient to prolong the activated partial thromboplastin time to 1.5 to 2 times the control (reference) value or by intermittent subcutaneous injection in a dose of 10,000 to 20,000 units every 12 h, adjusted to prolong the midinterval (6 h after injection) activated partial thromboplastin time to 1.5 times control. Limited data are available to support the subcutaneous administration of low molecular-weight heparin for this indication.	C
	Administer an oral anticoagulant during the second trimester to patients at high thromboembolic risk.	C

ACC = American College of Cardiology; AHA = American Heart Association.

TABLE 77G-2 ACC/AHA Recommendations for Treatment Strategies for Supraventricular Tachycardias During Pregnancy

Indication	Class I (Indicated) [Level of Evidence]	Class IIa (Strong Supportive Evidence) [Level of Evidence]	Class IIb (Weak Supportive Evidence) [Level of Evidence]	Class III (Not Indicated) [Level of Evidence]
Acute conversion of PSVT	Vagal maneuver [C] Adenosine [C] DC cardioversion [C]	Metoprolol,* propranolol* [C]	Verapamil [C]	
Prophylactic therapy	Digoxin [C]	Propranolol* [B]	Quinidine, propafenone,† verapamil [C]	Atenolol‡ [B]
	Metoprolol*	Sotalol,* flecainide† [C]	Procainamide [B] Catheter ablation [C]	Amiodarone [C]

*Beta-blocking agents should not be taken in the first trimester, if possible.
†Consider AV node–blocking agents in conjunction with flecainide and propafenone for certain tachycardias.
‡Atenolol is categorized in class C (drug classification for use during pregnancy) by legal authorities in some European countries.
ACC/AHA = American College of Cardiology/American Heart Association; AV = atrioventricular; DC = direct current; PSVT = paroxysmal supraventricular tachycardia.

CH 77

TABLE 77G-3 AHA/ASA Recommendations for Stroke Prevention During Pregnancy

Class	Indication	Level of Evidence
Class IIb (weak supportive evidence)	For pregnant women with ischemic stroke or TIA and high-risk thromboembolic conditions, such as known coagulopathy or mechanical heart valves, the following options may be considered: adjusted-dose UFH throughout pregnancy, e.g., a subcutaneous dose every 12 hr with activated partial thromboplastin time monitoring; adjusted-dose LMWH with factor Xa monitoring throughout pregnancy; or UFH or LMWH until week 13, followed by warfarin until the middle of the third trimester, when UFH or LMWH is then reinstituted until delivery.	C
	Pregnant women with lower risk conditions may be considered for treatment with UFH or LMWH in the first trimester, followed by low-dose aspirin for the remainder of the pregnancy	C

AHA/ASA = American Heart Association/American Stroke Association; LMWH = low-molecular-weight heparin; TIA = transient ischemic attack; UFH = unfractionated heparin.

Class	Indication	Level of Evidence
TABLE 77G–4	**AHA Recommendations for Anticoagulation Regimens in Pregnant Patients with Mechanical Prosthetic Valves**	
Class I (indicated)	Continuous therapeutic anticoagulation with frequent monitoring.	B
	If warfarin discontinued between wk 6 and 12 of gestation, replace with continuous intravenous UFH, dose-adjusted UFH, or dose-adjusted subcutaneous LMWH.	C
	Up to 36 wk of gestation, the therapeutic choice of continuous intravenous or dose-adjusted subcutaneous UFH, dose-adjusted LMWH, or warfarin should be discussed fully.	C
	If dose-adjusted LMWH is used, the LMWH should be administered twice daily subcutaneously to maintain the anti-Xa level between 0.7 and 1.2 units/ml 4 h after administration.	C
	If dose-adjusted UFH is used, the aPTT should be at least twice control.	C
	If warfarin is used, the INR goal should be 3.0 (range, 2.5 to 3.5).	C
	Warfarin should be discontinued starting 2 to 3 wk before planned delivery and continuous intravenous UFH given instead.	C
Class IIa (strong supportive evidence)	It is reasonable to avoid warfarin between wk 6 and 12 of gestation because of the high risk of fetal defects.	C
	It is reasonable to resume UFH 4 to 6 h after delivery and begin oral warfarin in the absence of significant bleeding.	C
	It is reasonable to give low-dose aspirin (75 to 100 mg/d) in the second and third trimesters of pregnancy in addition to anticoagulation with warfarin or heparin.	C
Class III (not indicated)	LMWH should not be administered unless anti-Xa levels are monitored 4 to 6 h after administration.	C
	Dipyridamole should not be used instead of aspirin as an alternative antiplatelet agent because of its harmful effects on the fetus.	B

AHA = American Heart Association; aPTT = activated partial thromboplastin time; INR = international normalized ratio; LMWH = low-molecular-weight heparin; UFH = unfractionated heparin.

Administration (FDA) for use in any patient with a mechanical prosthetic heart valve, and the FDA has issued an advisory warning against the use of enoxaparin (Lovenox) in pregnant women with mechanical prosthetic heart valves. The guidelines note that some data indicate that low-molecular-weight heparin appears to be safe in nonpregnant patients with mechanical heart valves, but the expert panel could not recommend its use directly, given the status of FDA-approved indications.

References

1. Bonow RO, Carabello BA, Kanu C, et al: ACC/AHA 2006 guidelines for the management of patients with valvular heart disease: A report of the American College of Cardiology/American Heart Association Task Force on Practice Guidelines (writing committee to revise the 1998 Guidelines for the Management of Patients With Valvular Heart Disease): Developed in collaboration with the Society of Cardiovascular Anesthesiologists: Endorsed by the Society for Cardiovascular Angiography and Interventions and the Society of Thoracic Surgeons. Circulation 114:e84, 2006.
2. Fuster V, Ryden LE, Cannom DS, et al: ACC/AHA/ESC 2006 Guidelines for the Management of Patients With Atrial Fibrillation—Executive Summary. A Report of the American College of Cardiology/American Heart Association Task Force on Practice Guidelines and the European Society of Cardiology Committee for Practice Guidelines (Writing Committee to Revise the 2001 Guidelines for the Management of Patients With Atrial Fibrillation). Circulation 114:257, 2006.
3. Blomstrom-Lundqvist C, Scheinman MM, Aliot EM, et al: ACC/AHA/ESC guidelines for the management of patients with supraventricular arrhythmias—executive summary. A report of the American College of Cardiology/American Heart Association Task Force on Practice Guidelines and the European Society of Cardiology Committee for Practice Guidelines (Writing Committee to Develop Guidelines for the Management of Patients With Supraventricular Arrhythmias) developed in collaboration with NASPE-Heart Rhythm Society. J Am Coll Cardiol 42:1493, 2003.
4. Adams H, Adams R, Del Zoppo G, et al: Guidelines for the early management of patients with ischemic stroke: 2005 guidelines update. A scientific statement from the Stroke Council of the American Heart Association/American Stroke Association. Stroke 36:916, 2005.
5. Hirsh J, Fuster V, Ansell J, et al: American Heart Association/American College of Cardiology Foundation guide to warfarin therapy. J Am Coll Cardiol 41:1633, 2003.
6. Oakley C, Child A, Jung B, et al: Expert consensus document on management of cardiovascular diseases during pregnancy. Eur Heart J 24:761, 2003.
7. Maron BJ, McKenna WJ, Danielson GK, et al: American College of Cardiology/European Society of Cardiology clinical expert consensus document on hypertrophic cardiomyopathy. A report of the American College of Cardiology Foundation Task Force on Clinical Expert Consensus Documents and the European Society of Cardiology Committee for Practice Guidelines. J Am Coll Cardiol 42:1687, 2003.

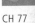

CH 77

Pregnancy and Heart Disease

CHAPTER 78

Introduction, 1983

Physical Activity, Exercise, and
Sports—Definitions, 1983

Benefits of Exercise, 1984

Risks of Exercise, 1985

Exercise Prescription for Health
and Fitness, 1986

Screening, 1986
Medical Office Setting, 1986
Health and Fitness Facilities, 1988
Athletes, 1988

Exercise and Sports in Persons
with Cardiovascular
Disease, 1988
Coronary Artery Disease, 1988
Hypertension, 1989
Valvular Heart Disease, 1989
Cardiomyopathy, 1989
Arrhythmias, 1989
Congenital Heart Disease, 1989

Future Perspectives, 1990

References, 1990

Exercise and Sports Cardiology

Gary J. Balady and Philip A. Ades

INTRODUCTION

Thousands of years ago the ancient Greeks recognized the importance of exercise and sport, but an interesting paradox now exists. A large volume of evidence from epidemiological observational studies, cohort studies, randomized controlled trials, and basic research, primarily conducted during the past 30 years, provides unequivocal evidence that exercise and physical activity confer health. The publication of the 1996 Surgeon General's report on physical activity and health[1] was a seminal event that moved the promotion of physical activity to the top of America's national public health agenda. Physical inactivity is now recognized as an independent risk factor for the development of cardiovascular disease.[2] Nonetheless, only a small proportion of Americans engage in sufficient physical activity. The Centers for Disease Control and Prevention indicates that approximately 25 to 45 percent of adult Americans participate in recommended levels of physical activity, and 25 percent report no regular leisure-time physical activity whatsoever.[3] Although the world benefits from advancements in technology that lead to increased productivity and improved quality of life, the price is paid, in part, by the generation of a sedentary society that spends much of its time in cars, at computer stations, and in front of televisions and video screens.

While medical professionals, public health leaders, and community leaders continue their unprecedented efforts to promote increased physical activity through a variety of venues that range from casual walks to participation in organized sports, health care providers need to support these efforts for their patients. Health care providers should do so in the context of optimizing the benefits of participation while minimizing the small but potential associated risks. This chapter presents these issues with an overview of the classifications of exercise and sports; scientific data regarding the benefits of exercise and mechanisms by which these benefits occur; the risks of exercise; the exercise prescription; and screening and recommendations for participation in exercise and athletic competition with a particular emphasis on persons with specific cardiovascular conditions.

PHYSICAL ACTIVITY, EXERCISE, AND SPORTS—DEFINITIONS

To understand the many issues surrounding exercise and sports and subsequently make important activity-related clinical decisions, a review of standard definitions[1] is essential. *Physical activity* refers to any activity in which skeletal muscle contraction and relaxation results in bodily movement and requires energy. The *intensity* of physical activity can be described in terms of the energy required per unit of time for the performance of the activity. This energy requirement can be quantified in absolute terms by measuring the oxygen uptake during the activity, using respiratory gas analysis. It can also be estimated using standard regression equations, as a multiple of resting energy expenditure (metabolic equivalent [MET]), with one MET defined as the oxygen requirement in the resting, awake individual (3.5 ml/kg of body weight/min).

The intensity of a physical activity can also be defined in relative terms by expressing it as a proportion of the individual's maximal capacity (e.g., the percentage of maximal oxygen uptake, or the percentage of maximum heart rate). Alternatively, activity intensity can be expressed as a measure of the force of muscle contraction required (in pounds or kilograms). When defining the amount of physical activity or exercise, an important interrelationship exists between the total dose of activity and the intensity at which the activity is performed. *Dose* refers to the total amount of energy expended in physical activity expressed in terms of kilocalories or METhours, whereas intensity reflects the rate of energy expenditure during such activity.

Exercise or *exercise training* is planned physical activity that is performed with the goal of improving or preserving physical fitness. *Physical fitness* is a set of attributes that enables an individual to perform physical activity. Physical fitness is best assessed by directly measuring peak or maximum oxygen uptake during a graded exercise test. Although this is not always practical, it is more commonly estimated from the peak MET level attained, or reporting the peak work rate (e.g., speed and grade of a treadmill, watts on a stationary cycle) during graded exercise tests.[1]

Although most types of exercise involve both endurance and resistance training, one training type usually predominates (see Table 78-1). The physiological responses to exercise depend on the type of exercise performed. *Endurance exercise* (also referred to as *aerobic, dynamic,* or *isotonic exercise*) consists of activity involving high-repetition movements against low resistance. Regular endurance exercise is also referred to as *endurance training* because it usually leads to an improved functional capacity, thereby enabling the individual to exercise for a longer duration or at a higher work rate. *Resistance exercise* involves low-repetition movements against high resistance, in which muscle tension develops predominantly without much muscle shortening. Regular resistance training leads to increased strength and is also referred to as *power or strength training*. Figure 78-1 demonstrates the classification of several types of sports as related to the peak static and dynamic components achieved during competition.[5] The classification does not take into account differences in environment (altitude, temperature, air quality) in which the sport is performed. Each of these can influence the physiological responses during sports activity as well.

Finally, a distinction must be made between competitive and recreational sports, as the physiological and emotional demands during training and performance are perceived to be quite different.[6] *Competitive athletes* participate in an organized sport that places a high premium on athletic excellence and achievement and requires systematic training and regular competition. These athletes characteristically extend themselves to high levels of effort for long periods of time, often doing so regardless of other considerations. *Recreational athletes* engage in activities that do not require regular systematic training or the pursuit of excellence and do so on either a regular or inconsistent basis. Hence they do not have the same pressure to excel as do the competitive athletes.

BENEFITS OF EXERCISE (see Chap. 46)

Physical activity is associated with lower all-cause mortality rates in healthy individuals,[2,6,7] individuals with chronic diseases,[8] diabetic persons,[9] and the elderly.[10] Although studies on men and women demonstrate that remote activity performed decades earlier without subsequent maintenance appears to have no long-term benefit, the risk for all-cause mortality decreases among inactive men and women who subsequently become more physically active.[2] Physical fitness can be more readily measured than physical activity. A consistent and graded relationship has been demonstrated between peak exercise capacity attained during exercise testing and subsequent mortality in both men[11] and women.[6] Regular exercise training in patients with coronary artery disease[12] and in patients with heart failure[13] has demonstrated a reduction in mortality and cardiovascular events in separate meta-analyses, although this has not been conclusively demonstrated in single cohort studies.

The specific mechanisms by which physical activity reduces mortality and cardiovascular events are likely multifactorial, and extend beyond a reduction in cardiovascular risk factors, because beneficial effects have been shown on thrombosis, endothelial function, inflammation, and autonomic tone. The magnitude of blood pressure reduction attained with exercise is modest and in mildly hypertensive persons yields an effect that is similar to pharmacological monotherapy.[14] Physical activity and exercise induce several important and beneficial effects on glucose metabolism including increased insulin sensitivity, decreased hepatic glucose production, preferential use of glucose over fatty acids by exercising muscle, and reduced obesity.[15] In addition, regular exercise may prevent the onset of diabetes mellitus.[16] A widely known fact is that overweight and obesity are associated with significant increases in cardiovascular morbidity and mortality.[17] Exercise training appears to be an important component of weight loss programs, although most randomized controlled trials show only modest reductions in weight. Studies suggest that exercise is necessary to maintain weight loss and prevent weight regain after diet-induced weight loss.[18] The effects of exercise on lipid profiles demonstrate the greatest benefit on triglycerides, modest changes in high-density lipoprotein (HDL), and little to no change in low-density lipoprotein (LDL) levels.[2] However, some data suggest that exercise training reduces the concentration of atherogenic, small, dense LDL particles.[19] A recent

CH 78

		A. Low (<40% max O₂)	B. Moderate (40–70% max O₂)	C. High (>70% max O₂)
Increasing static component	III. High (>50% MVC)	Bobsledding/luge,*† field events (throwing), gymnastics,*† martial arts,* sailing, sport climbing, water skiing,*† weight lifting,*† windsurfing*†	Body building,*† downhill skiing,*† skateboarding,*† snowboarding,*† wrestling*	Boxing,* canoeing/kayaking, cycling,*† decathlon, rowing, speed-skating,*† triathlon*†
	II. Moderate (20–50% MVC)	Archery, auto racing,*† diving,*† equestrian,*† motorcycling*†	American football,* field events (jumping), figure skating,* rodeoing,*† rugby,* running (sprint), surfing,*† synchronized swimming†	Basketball,* ice hockey,* cross-country skiing (skating technique), lacrosse,* running (middle distance), swimming, team handball
	I. Low (<20% MVC)	Billiards, bowling, cricket, curling, golf, riflery	Baseball/softball,* fencing, table tennis, volleyball	Badminton, cross-country skiing (classic technique), field hockey,* orienteering, race walking, racquetball/squash, running (long distance), soccer,* tennis

Increasing dynamic component →

FIGURE 78–1 Classification of sports. This classification is based on peak static and dynamic components achieved during competition. The increasing dynamic component is related to the estimated percent of maximal oxygen uptake (max O₂) achieved and results in an increasing cardiac output. The increasing static component is related to the estimated percent of maximal voluntary contraction (MVC) attained and results in an increasing blood pressure. The lowest total cardiovascular demands are shown in green and the highest in red. Blue, yellow, and purple depict low moderate, moderate, and high moderate total cardiovascular demands. * = danger of bodily collision; † = increased risk if syncope occurs. *(From Mitchell JH, Haskell W, Snell P, Van Camp SP: Task Force 8: Classification of sports. J Am Coll Cardiol 45:1364, 2005, with permission from the American College of Cardiology Foundation.)*

study of monozygotic twins shows a strong genetic component to HDL levels that can be slightly but favorably modified by vigorous activity.[20]

Further evidence suggests that exercise training has beneficial effects on the fibrinolytic system, and many studies report an inverse relationship between physical activity or fitness and inflammatory markers.[21] Chronic exercise training appears to have an important and favorable influence on endothelial function in both peripheral[22] and coronary arteries.[23] Improved endothelial vasodilator function may result, in part, from increased nitric oxide production and a net reduction in oxidative stress,[25] as well as an increase in endothelial progenitor cells.[26] Such improvements may contribute to a reduction in adverse cardiovascular events.[27] Finally, exercise training appears to modulate favorably the balance between sympathetic and parasympathetic tone, an effect associated with improvements in survival.[28]

Changes in the muscular, cardiovascular, and neurohumoral systems that result from exercise training improve functional capacity and strength. These changes are referred to as the *training effect* and enable an individual to exercise to higher peak work rates with lower heart rates at each submaximal level of exercise. A decline in maximal exercise capacity is associated with aging, and a longitudinal study demonstrates that this is more marked with each successive decade of life.[29] Although regular exercise may attenuate this loss of exercise capacity at any age, it does not appear to prevent the progressively greater decline with advancing age.[29]

TABLE 78–1	Cardiovascular Causes of Sudden Death in Young Athletes	
Cause		**Percent of All Causes**
Hypertrophic cardiomyopathy		26.4
Coronary-artery anomalies		13.7
Left ventricular hypertrophy of indeterminate causation*		7.5
Myocarditis		5.2
Ruptured aortic aneurysm (Marfan syndrome)		3.1
Arrhythmogenic right ventricular cardiomyopathy		2.8
Tunneled (bridged) coronary artery		2.8
Aortic-valve stenosis		2.6
Atherosclerotic coronary artery disease		2.6
Dilated cardiomyopathy		2.3
Myxomatous mitral-valve degeneration		2.3

*Findings suggestive but not diagnostic of hypertrophic cardiomyopathy.

Modified from Maron BJ: Sudden death in young athletes. N Engl J Med 349:1064, 2003.

RISKS OF EXERCISE

Although exercise has many benefits, the risks during exercise and sports activities are low. Most hazards involve the cardiovascular and musculoskeletal systems. These differ relative to the participant's age, gender, physical fitness, underlying cardiovascular and medical conditions, and the activity or sport in which the individual is engaged. Accordingly, the cardiovascular risk-benefit ratio should be assessed for each individual for any given activity. Age exerts a major influence on cardiovascular risk during exercise. Exercise-related death in persons older than the age of 35 years usually results from atherosclerotic coronary artery disease, whereas genetic or congenital cardiac malformations predominate in younger individuals.[4] Among high school and college athletes, the sports-related, nontraumatic, sudden death rate per year is estimated to be 1 in 133,333 male athletes and 1 in 769,230 female athletes.[30] A prospective series of somewhat older Italian athletes (mean age 26 years) who had undergone a national preparticipation screening program reports the rate of sudden death to be 2.3 per 100,000 athletes/year, with a rate in men that is more than twice that of women.[31] The cardiovascular causes of sudden death in young athletes are shown in Table 78-1. The reported rates of exertionally related sudden death among middle-aged persons vary, in part, because of the methods of data collection and reporting, the type of activity involved, and the population studied. Prospectively collected data on men[32] and women[33] demonstrate that the risk of sudden death during moderate to vigorous exertion is quite low. Among middle-aged men without known cardiovascular disease in the Physicians' Health Study, the absolute risk during any episode of vigorous exertion was 1 per 1.51 million *episodes* of exertion.[32] The absolute risk reported among middle-aged women of the Nurses' Health Study during moderate to vigorous exertion was 1 per 36.5 million *hours* of exertion.[33] In addition, evidence indicates that heavy exertion may trigger an acute myocardial infarction; however, even less precise estimates are available for this occurrence in the general population. Importantly, these studies[32,33] and others clearly demonstrate that the risk of an adverse event is transiently increased during the period of exertion, particularly among sedentary persons with occult or known coronary artery disease when performing an unaccustomed, vigorous physical activity. Conversely, the overall risk is significantly lower among those who engage in habitual moderate to vigorous physical activity and exercise.

Traumatic and musculoskeletal injuries during exercise and sports activities constitute an important and sometimes disabling risk of participation but are beyond the scope of this chapter. However, blunt, nonpenetrating chest blows may trigger ventricular fibrillation and sudden cardiac death. This condition is known as *commotio cordis* and appears responsible for about 20 percent of sudden deaths in young athletes in the United States.[4,34] It most commonly occurs in baseball, ice hockey, football, lacrosse, and martial arts and is often the result of direct bodily contact from the ball or puck, or between players. Methods for prevention of this devastating and often fatal event are discussed in detail earlier (see Chap. 36).[34]

Although the risks of each sport vary, long-distance marathon road racing deserves special mention. Marathoning in the United Stated has become widely popular, particularly among middle-aged individuals. Among the 314 marathons that took place in 2005, there were 382,000 finishing times recorded. Approximately 82 percent of men and women marathoners are 35 years old or older, and 3 percent of men and 1 percent of women are 60 years old or older.[35] A recent report demonstrates that the risk of sudden cardiac death during marathon road racing is approximately 1.1 per 100,000 race participants and that this risk appears to be decreasing relative to prior estimates, while the likelihood of survival is increasing. The authors attribute this improved survival to the greater availability of automated cardiac defibrillators at these events.[36] The risk of marathon racing among persons with recognized or occult cardiovascular disease is not known, but it would be expected to be greater. Although it is widely known that marathon racing can lead to metabolic derangements, hyponatremia due to overhydration has recently been recognized as an important and preventable risk.[37] Several studies have demonstrated structural and biochemical evidence of transient myocardial injury, as well as systolic and diastolic dysfunction in both the right and left ventricles. Some of these abnormalities may persist up to 1 month after the race[38]; however, the clinical significance of these findings is uncertain.

EXERCISE PRESCRIPTION FOR HEALTH AND FITNESS

Consensus papers and guidelines from the American Heart Association,[2,39] the American College of Sports Medicine,[40] the Institute of Medicine,[41] and the U.S. Surgeon General[1] all recommend that *adults exercise for 30 to 60 minutes at moderate-intensity levels (e.g., brisk walking) on most, if not all, days of the week with the goal of achieving weekly energy expenditure of at least 1000 kcal.* This is considered the most basic exercise prescription. It is simple, effective, and based on scientific evidence. This physical activity can be accomplished in a single daily session or during multiple shorter intervals throughout the day. If exercise is of low-intensity (e.g., slow walking), it should be performed more frequently and for longer duration.

Numerous exercise-training studies have evaluated the frequency, intensity, and duration of the training sessions required to achieve physical fitness and muscular strength (Table 78-2). Improvements in peak oxygen uptake of 15 to 30 percent are usually achieved for sedentary individuals using the regimen as outlined for endurance training. Intermittent activity at comparable exercise intensity and total duration can confer fitness benefits similar to those of continuous activity.[2] Details regarding the exercise prescription are provided elsewhere.[39,40] Chapter 46 presents in detail the prescription for exercise training in persons with known cardiovascular disease. Issues regarding exercise and sports participation in persons with specific cardiovascular conditions are discussed later. All cardiac patients who are poised to begin an exercise training program should have an exer- cise test that should be repeated annually or at any time the patient's condition warrants. Exercise intensity can be ascertained by an exercise test using the heart rate reserve method and the peak heart rate from the exercise test (see Table 78-2). If angina or ischemic ST-segment depression occurs during the exercise test, the training heart rate should be a minimum of 10 beats/min below the heart rate at which the abnormality occurs.

SCREENING (see Chap. 65)

Concerted efforts to promote physical activity and exercise aim to increase levels of regular physical activity throughout the U.S. population including the nearly one fourth of adult Americans who have some form of cardiovascular disease. Although the benefits of exercise generally outweigh the risks, adequate screening and evaluation are important to identify and counsel persons with underlying cardiovascular disease in order to minimize those risks before they begin exercising at *vigorous* levels (≥60 percent heart rate reserve or ≥77 percent peak heart rate) (see Table 78-2). Yet screening should not constitute an impediment to the widespread implementation of physical activity.

Screening can take place in many different settings and venues: during office visits with the health care provider[39,40,42]; at health and fitness centers on enrollment or periodic guest use[43]; using self-screening tools made available by the American Heart Association (AHA) and other organizations; and during preseason physical examinations for young athletes who want to engage in a particular sport.[44,45] If underlying cardiovascular disease is suspected or detected by any of these evaluations, appropriate medical referral for further assessment is necessary.

Medical Office Setting

Details regarding medical screening are provided elsewhere.[39,40,42] Abnormalities in any of the key elements of the history and physical examination as shown in Table 78-3 should prompt further evaluation and testing. Using the AHA risk classification scheme (Table 78-4), health care providers can assess whether *vigorous* exercise training can be permitted and what level of supervision and monitoring, if any, are necessary. Exercise testing is important in the

TABLE 78–2	Exercise Prescription for Endurance and Resistance Training
Endurance Training	
Frequency: 3-5 d/wk⁻¹	**Modality:** Aerobics, Arm ergometry, Cross-country ski machines, Combined arm/leg cycle, Elliptical machines, Jogging/running, Rowing, Stairclimber, Swimming, Walking
Intensity: 55-90% maximum HR or 40-85% maximum VO₂ or HRR	
Duration: 20-60 min	
Resistance Training	
Frequency: 2-3 d/wk⁻¹	**All Major Muscle Groups** *Arms/shoulders:* Biceps curl, Triceps extension, Overhead press, Lateral raises, *Chest/back:* Bench press, Lateral pull down/pull-ups, Bent-over/Seated row, *Legs:* Leg extensions, curls, press, Adductor/abductor
Intensity: 1-3 sets of 8-15 RM for each muscle group	

Modalities listed above are not all inclusive.

HR = heart rate; maximum HR = 220 minus age, or peak HR on exercise test; HRR = heart rate reserve = (peak-resting HR) × % (plus resting HR); RM = maximum number of times a load can be lifted before fatigue; VO₂ = measured oxygen uptake.

Modified from Whaley MH (ed): American College of Sports Medicine Guidelines for Exercise Testing and Prescription. 7th ed. New York, Lippincott Williams & Wilkins, 2006.

TABLE 78-3	American Heart Association Consensus Panel Recommendations for Preparticipation Athletic Screening
Family History	
1. Premature sudden cardiac death	
2. Heart disease in surviving relatives younger than 50 years old	
Personal History	
3. Heart murmur	
4. Systemic hypertension	
5. Fatigue	
6. Syncope/near-syncope	
7. Excessive/unexplained exertional dyspnea	
8. Exertional chest pain	
Physical Examination	
9. Heart murmur (supine/standing)	
10. Femoral arterial pulses (to exclude coarctation of aorta)	
11. Stigmata of Marfan syndrome	
12. Brachial blood pressure measurement (sitting)	

From Maron BJ, Douglas PS, Graham TP, et al: Task Force 1: Preparticipation screening and diagnosis of cardiovascular disease in athletes. J Am Coll Cardiol 45:1322, 2005, with permission from the American College of Cardiology Foundation.

TABLE 78–4 | American Heart Association Risk Classification for Exercise Training

Class A: Apparently Healthy Individuals

This classification includes the following:

(A1) Children, adolescents, men younger than 45 yr, and women younger than 55 yr who have no symptoms or known presence of heart disease or major coronary risk factors

(A2) Men 45 years old or older and women 55 years old or older who have no symptoms or known presence of heart disease and with fewer than 2 major cardiovascular risk factors

(A3) Men 45 years old or older and women 55 years old or older who have no symptoms or known presence of heart disease and with 2 or more major cardiovascular risk factors

Activity guidelines: No restrictions other than basic guidelines

Supervision required: None

ECG and blood pressure monitoring: Not required

Note: Persons classified as Class A2 and particularly Class A3 should undergo a medical examination and possibly a medically supervised exercise test before engaging in vigorous exercise.

Class B: Presence of Known, Stable Cardiovascular Disease with Low Risk for Complications with Vigorous Exercise, but Slightly Greater Than for Apparently Healthy Individuals

This classification includes individuals with any of the following diagnoses:

1. CAD (angina, myocardial infarction, coronary revascularization, abnormal exercise test, and abnormal coronary angiograms) whose condition is stable and who have the clinical characteristics outlined below
2. Valvular heart disease—excluding severe valvular stenosis or regurgitation with the clinical characteristics as outlined below
3. Congenital heart disease—risk stratification for patients with congenital heart disease should be guided by the 26th Bethesda Conference recommendations (36th Bethesda Conference report)
4. Cardiomyopathy—ejection fraction ≤ 30%; includes stable patients with heart failure with clinical characteristics as outlined below; not hypertrophic cardiomyopathy or recent myocarditis
5. Exercise test abnormalities that do not meet any of the high risk criteria outlined in class C below

Clinical Characteristics: (Must Include All of the Following)

1. New York Heart Association (NYHA) Class I or II
2. Exercise capacity ≥ 6 METs
3. No evidence of "congestive" heart failure
4. No evidence of myocardial ischemia or angina at rest nor on the exercise test at or below 6 METs
5. Appropriate rise in systolic blood pressure during exercise
6. Absence of sustained or nonsustained ventricular tachycardia at rest or with exercise
7. Ability to satisfactorily self-monitor intensity of activity

Activity guidelines: Activity should be individualized with exercise prescription provided by qualified individuals and approved by primary health care provider.

Supervision required: Medical supervision during initial prescription session is beneficial. Supervision is provided by appropriate, trained, nonmedical personnel for other exercise sessions until the individual understands how to monitor his or her activity.

Medical personnel should be trained and certified in Advanced Cardiac Life Support (ACLS).

Nonmedical personnel should be trained and certified in Basic Life Support (which includes cardiopulmonary resuscitation).

ECG and blood pressure monitoring: Useful during the early prescription phase of training, usually 6 to 12 sessions.

Class C: Those at Moderate to High Risk for Cardiac Complications During Exercise and/or Unable to Self-Regulate Activity or Understand Recommended Activity Level

This classification includes individuals with any of the following diagnoses:

1. CAD with the clinical characteristics outlined below
2. Valvular heart disease—excluding severe valvular stenosis or regurgitation with the clinical characteristics as outlined below
3. Congenital heart disease—risk stratification for patients with congenital heart disease should be guided by the 36th Bethesda Conference recommendations (36th Bethesda Conference report)
4. Cardiomyopathy—ejection fraction < 30%; includes stable patients with heart failure with clinical characteristics as outlined below; not hypertrophic cardiomyopathy or recent myocarditis
5. Complex ventricular arrhythmias not well controlled

Clinical Characteristics (Any of the Following)

1. NYHA Class III or IV
2. Exercise test results
   - Exercise capacity < 6 METs
   - Angina or ischemic ST depression at a workload <6 METs
   - Fall in systolic blood pressure below resting levels during exercise
   - Nonsustained ventricular tachycardia with exercise
3. Previous episode of primary cardiac arrest (i.e., cardiac arrest that did not occur in the presence of an acute myocardial infarction or during a cardiac procedure)
4. A medical problem that the physician believes may be life threatening

Activity guidelines: Activity should be individualized with exercise prescription provided by qualified individuals and approved by primary health care provider.

Supervision: Medical supervision should exist during all exercise sessions until safety is established.

ECG and blood pressure monitoring: Continuous monitoring during exercise sessions is recommended until safety is established, which is usually 12 sessions or more.

Note: Class C patients who have successfully completed a series of supervised exercise sessions may be reclassified to Class B providing that the safety of exercise at the prescribed intensity is satisfactorily established by appropriate medical personnel, and that the patient has demonstrated the ability to self-monitor.

Class D: Unstable Disease with Activity Restriction: Exercise for Conditioning Purposes Is Not Recommended

This classification includes individuals with any of the following conditions:

1. Unstable ischemia
2. Severe and symptomatic valvular stenosis or regurgitation
3. Congenital heart disease—criteria for risk that would prohibit exercise conditioning in patients with congenital heart disease should be guided by the 36th Bethesda Conference recommendations (36th Bethesda Conference report)
4. Heart failure that is not compensated
5. Uncontrolled arrhythmias
6. Other medical conditions that could be aggravated by exercise

Activity guidelines: No activity is recommended for conditioning purposes. Attention should be directed to treating the subject and restoring patient to Class C or better. Daily activities must be prescribed on the basis of individual assessment by the subject's personal physician.

CAD = coronary artery disease; ECG = electrocardiogram; MET = metabolic equivalent test.

Reprinted from Fletcher GF, Balady GJ, Amsterdam EA, et al: Exercise standards for testing and training: A statement for health professionals from the American Heart Association. Circulation 104:1694, 2001, with permission from the American Heart Association.

risk stratification process for individuals deemed to be at greater risk of having underlying heart disease, particularly coronary artery disease, or individuals with diabetes. It also allows the establishment of appropriate and specific safety precautions, target exercise training heart rate, and initial levels of exercise training work rates.

Health and Fitness Facilities

The AHA recommends that all facilities offering exercise equipment or services should conduct cardiovascular screening of all new members and/or prospective users.[43] Details regarding such screening are presented elsewhere.[43] The use of simple screening tools, such as the Physical Activity Readiness Questionnaire (PAR-Q),[40] are recommended with appropriate medical evaluation and follow-up as indicated.

Athletes

Screening of competitive athletes prior to participation in organized sports is a particularly challenging issue and is discussed in detail earlier (see also Chap. 9).[4,46,47] Approximately 10 to 15 million athletes live in the United States. Although sudden cardiac death among these athletes is uncommon, it is nonetheless a tragic and potentially avoidable event. The risk for sudden death during exercise in young persons is much lower than among middle-aged adults because so few young persons have advanced coronary artery disease and because congenital and genetic cardiovascular problems that cause sudden cardiac death (see Table 78-1) are so rare. The estimated prevalence of these conditions in the young athletic population is 0.2 percent.[47] Mass screening of athletes can be particularly difficult because individuals with these life-threatening conditions generally lack symptoms and have unrevealing physical examinations. In addition, the evaluation can be confounded by the normal physiological changes in autonomic tone and in cardiac size and structure that occur with prolonged and intense training, a condition known as the *athlete's heart*.[44] The electrocardiogram, which can appear abnormal in about 40 percent of elite athletes, reflects these changes and may demonstrate increased cardiac mass, chamber dimensions, and wall thickness. Methods to distinguish the normal athletic heart from the hypertrophic cardiomyopathy are discussed earlier (see Chap. 65).

Because no screening test or procedure will yield 100 percent sensitivity and specificity for the detection of a life-threatening cardiovascular abnormality or guarantee a zero-risk outcome, what can be done to enhance their detection and reduce the occurrence of adverse events? The AHA does not recommend routine electrocardiography or echocardiography in the initial mass screening evaluation of young athletes because of their diagnostic and cost limitations when applied to this population.[45,47] However, these tests may be an important part of subsequent evaluations in the medical office setting, as clinically indicated. Importantly, those responsible for screening evaluations and supervision of athletes should become familiar with the most common causes of sudden death in athletes (see Table 78-1). This will heighten their awareness of the signs and symptoms of associated cardiac conditions during the initial assessment and at any time during athletic participation. The initial medical history and physical should include all of the key elements as defined by the AHA (see Table 78-3). Abnormal findings should prompt appropriate medical referral and further cardiovascular testing, as indicated. Finally, athletes and coaches should be advised that if the athlete develops chest discomfort, syncope or presyncope, excessive dyspnea, palpitations, or other unusual symptoms during training or competition, he or she should report to medical personnel for an appropriate evaluation.

EXERCISE AND SPORTS IN PERSONS WITH CARDIOVASCULAR DISEASE

The presence of structural heart disease once signified the imposition of a sedentary lifestyle and a near total avoidance of physical activity and competitive sports. Yet compelling evidence now exists that regular exercise reduces cardiovascular events and cardiovascular mortality in individuals with known coronary heart disease (CHD).[12] Furthermore, in the setting of other cardiovascular conditions such as arterial hypertension, valvular heart disease, and chronic heart failure, regular exercise results in an increased functional capacity, an improved quality of life, and improved cardiovascular risk factors.[13,43] Thus after careful evaluation, most individuals with structural heart disease can safely participate in prescribed physical activity. Participation in competitive sports for individuals with structural heart disease depends on the type and severity of heart disease present, the type and intensity of the sport being pursued, and the level of risk or harm that could occur from participation.[46] The 36th Bethesda Conference report presents details regarding recommendations for participation.[49] Participation in competitive sports is a beneficial activity and should be precluded only after a full cardiovascular examination and a knowledgeable assessment of potential harm from participation. Experts also recognize, however, that individuals participating in competitive sports cannot always properly judge the significance of cardiac-related symptoms or if it is prudent to terminate physical exertion in the heat of competition.

Coronary Artery Disease

A large body of scientific evidence, developed since the 1970s primarily in cardiac rehabilitation programs, has shown that regular exercise reduces total and cardiovascular mortality in individuals with recently diagnosed CHD (see Chap. 46).[12] However, a relative paucity of data exists in competitive athletes with established CHD regarding the risk of athletic participation. The risk of competitive athletics is likely increased to some degree in all patients with established CHD, and the risk of exercise-related events parallels the extent of disease, the presence of left ventricular (LV) dysfunction, inducible ischemia, and electrical instability along with the intensity of the competitive sport and intensity of effort.[50] Athletes with CHD diagnosed by any method should have their LV function assessed and should undergo maximal exercise testing to assess exercise capacity, the presence of angina or inducible ischemia, and the presence of exercise-induced arrhythmias. In general, two levels of risk can be defined on the basis of testing[50]:

1. *Mildly increased risk* is predicted by the presence of preserved LV function at rest, a normal exercise tolerance for age, an absence of exercise-induced ischemia or complex ventricular arrhythmias, an absence of hemodynamically significant coronary stenosis, and/or having undergone successful coronary revascularization.
2. *Substantially increased risk* is identified by the presence of any of the following: impaired LV systolic function at rest (ejection fraction < 50 percent), evidence of exercise-induced myocardial ischemia or complex ventricular arrhythmias, or hemodynamically significant stenosis of a major coronary artery to a degree of 50 percent or more luminal narrowing if coronary angiography was performed. The 36th Bethesda Conference recommendations

CH 78

for participation in competitive sport suggest that athletes in the mildly increased risk group can participate in low dynamic and low/moderate static competitive sports such as golf, bowling, diving, or motorcycling but not in more strenuous competitive sports such as cycling, running, or basketball (see Fig. 78-1).[50] Athletes in the substantially increased risk category should generally be restricted to only the lowest intensity competitive sports. These athletes should be reminded about the nature of prodromal symptoms and instructed to cease sports activity promptly should such symptoms appear.

Hypertension

Arterial hypertension is the most common cardiovascular condition observed in competitive athletes. It has long been recognized that individuals with systemic hypertension benefit from regular physical activity as it reduces blood pressure,[14] protects against stroke,[51] and protects against obesity-induced hypertension.[52] The presence of stage I hypertension in the absence of target organ damage, including left ventricular hypertrophy (LVH) on echocardiography, should not limit eligibility for any competitive sport, given adequate control of blood pressure with medication or lifestyle therapies. Athletes with more severe hypertension (stage II), even without target organ damage such as LVH, should be restricted particularly from high static sports until blood pressure is controlled by either lifestyle modification or drug therapy.[52] Hypertension per se has not been incriminated as a cause of sudden cardiac death in young competitive athletes, thus treatment aims to prevent the occurrence of target organ damage and long-term sequelae such as stroke or myocardial infarction.

Valvular Heart Disease (see Chap. 62)

In general, patients with left-sided valvular regurgitation or stenosis that is mild in severity and who are asymptomatic with exercise testing, without other contraindications, can participate in regular physical activity and essentially all competitive sports. Most patients with significant mitral stenosis are sufficiently symptomatic that participation in competitive sports is not an issue. Patients with atrial fibrillation on anticoagulants should not participate in sports with a risk for bodily contact. Individuals with mild to moderate mitral regurgitation who are in sinus rhythm with normal LV size and function and normal pulmonary artery pressures can participate in all competitive sports.[53] Patients with significant mitral regurgitation should be followed longitudinally with serial echocardiograms for changes in LV ejection fraction and end-systolic volume.[53] Individuals with severe mitral regurgitation and definite LV enlargement, pulmonary hypertension, or LV systolic dysfunction should not participate in any competitive sports.

Aortic stenosis can cause sudden death in young competitive athletes.[4] Importantly, most, but not all, episodes of exertional sudden death have occurred in individuals with severe aortic stenosis. The progressive nature of aortic stenosis mandates longitudinal follow-up with serial echocardiography. Although athletes with mild aortic stenosis (valve area > 1.5 cm^2) can participate in exercise and competitive sports, individuals with asymptomatic, moderate aortic stenosis should engage in only lower-intensity sports and/or competition limited to sports with only a moderate or less component of static or dynamic effort (see Fig. 78-1). Individuals with severe aortic stenosis or moderate stenosis with symptoms should not engage in any competitive sports and should also limit the intensity of regular exercise. Finally, the risk of exercise and competitive sports in patients with aortic insufficiency depends both on its severity and on the clinical setting. For example, in the setting of a dilated proximal aorta, even with only mild regurgitation, only low-intensity exercise or sports can be recommended.[53] On the other hand, in the case of mild or moderate aortic insufficiency with normal or only mildly increased end-diastolic volumes and a normal aorta, athletes can participate in all competitive sports. Finally, patients with severe aortic insufficiency and LV diastolic diameters of greater than 67 mm or mild-to-moderate insufficiency with symptoms should not participate in any competitive sports.

Cardiomyopathy

Hypertrophic cardiomyopathy (see Chap. 65), myocarditis, and arrhythmogenic right ventricular dysplasia are known antecedents to sudden cardiac death in young athletes,[4] and thus present contraindications to intense exercise and most competitive sports, with the possible exception of those of low intensity.[54] On the other hand, patients with stable NYHA Class II to III chronic heart failure caused by ischemic cardiomyopathy or idiopathic dilated cardiomyopathy appear to be able to participate safely in supervised cardiac rehabilitation training programs with transition to home programs without a substantially increased risk of cardiac death.[13] These programs have demonstrated clinical benefits including an increased exercise capacity, an improved quality of life, and a possible survival benefit.[13] The symptoms of individuals with Class II to III chronic heart failure and systolic LV dysfunction generally limit high-intensity competitive sports.

Arrhythmias

A complaint of syncope or of palpitations occurring during physical exertion or sports participation requires full evaluation. In particular, structural heart disease must be ruled out and the cause of these symptoms must be determined. These evaluations should include, but not be limited to, echocardiography, an electrocardiogram, exercise stress testing, and ambulatory monitoring. In the presence of structural heart disease, individuals with ventricular or supraventricular tachyarrhythmias should generally be excluded from intensive exercise or sports competition until definitive therapy can be accomplished.[55] Depending on the severity of the structural heart disease, in some cases, if arrhythmias are controlled with medications or ablation, exercise and competition can be reconsidered. However, the presence of an intracardiac defibrillator to prevent sudden cardiac death has not been deemed to be an adequately tested therapy in a setting where sudden cardiac death might otherwise be brought on by exercise.[54] Sinus bradycardia, sinus pause, and sinus arrest of less than 3 seconds are common in endurance-trained athletes and generally require no further evaluation or preclusion of exercise. When vasovagal syncope is diagnosed, despite its favorable prognosis, athletes with this condition should not participate in sports such as automobile racing or downhill ski racing, in which even a momentary loss of consciousness could be hazardous. For more extensive detail relating to the risk of specific arrhythmias, see the 36th Bethesda Conference report.[55]

Congenital Heart Disease

The most common congenital heart diseases that have been associated with untoward events during sports competition are hypertrophic cardiomyopathy (see Chap. 65), coronary artery anomalies, Marfan syndrome, and congenital aortic valve stenosis.[56] Other congenital lesions that are frequently

CH 78

Exercise and Sports Cardiology

associated with elevated pulmonary resistance must also be considered. Hypertrophic cardiomyopathy is the most common underlying cause of sudden cardiac death during sports participation in young athletes and is therefore considered a disqualifying diagnosis for sports competition and intensive exercise (see Chap. 65).[4] Congenital coronary anomalies of wrong sinus origin in which a coronary artery passes between great arteries are the second most common cause of sudden death in young athletes.[4] As such, this diagnosis should result in exclusion from all participation in sports. Participation can be reconsidered after successful surgical correction in an athlete without ischemia or arrhythmias during maximal exercise testing. Coronary anomalies should be considered in athletes with exertional syncope, chest pain, or symptomatic ventricular arrhythmias and can be diagnosed by echocardiography, CT scanning, magnetic resonance imaging, or coronary arteriography.

Marfan syndrome is an autosomal dominant disorder of connective tissue with an estimated prevalence of 1 in 5000 to 10,000 individuals. Cardiac manifestations include progressive dilatation of the aortic root or descending aorta, which predisposes to dissection and rupture, and mitral valve prolapse with associated mitral regurgitation. The risk for aortic rupture is usually linked to dilatation of the proximal aorta to greater than 50 mm, although even lesser levels of dilation increase risk. Athletes with aortic root dilations of greater than 40 mm, moderate or worse mitral regurgitation, or a family history of dissection or sudden death in a Marfan relative can participate in only low-intensity competitive sports (see Fig. 78-1). Weightlifting has been specifically linked with aortic dissection in athletes with cystic medial necrosis and should be considered relatively contraindicated in Marfan syndrome.[57]

Finally, a variety of congenital heart lesions linked to pulmonary hypertension present a risk during exercise and competitive sports.[56] In general, in the absence of other contraindications, if the pulmonary artery systolic pressure is less than 30 mm Hg, athletes can participate in all sports. If, however, the pulmonary systolic pressure exceeds 30 mm Hg in the presence of an uncorrected intracardiac shunt, a full evaluation and individual exercise prescription is required for athletic participation. Patients with cyanotic congenital heart disease are generally too symptomatic to participate in intense exercise or competitive sports, although from a medical point of view they should be precluded from participation. Variants of tetralogy of Fallot, atrial septal defects, ventricular septal defects, and Ebstein anomaly all require full evaluation before an individualized decision regarding athletic participation can be made. The final decision should take into account the severity of the lesion, the pulmonary pressure at rest and during exercise, and the intensity of the sport being considered. In cases of mild or fully corrected lesions with normal pulmonary pressures, full participation can be considered. Details of these and other congenital conditions can be reviewed in the proceedings of the 36th Bethesda Conference report.[56]

FUTURE PERSPECTIVES

As our society becomes more sedentary and the resulting adverse health consequences like obesity and diabetes increase, major and sustained efforts at physical activity promotion are necessary. Although a broad approach requires a concerted and multifaceted effort involving health policymakers, schools, work sites, insurers, media and others, health care providers have a primary responsibility toward the individual. Medical education of physicians, nurses, and other health care providers must incorporate training in physical activity and exercise counseling, as well as screening for exercise and sports-related risk. Health care providers must routinely evaluate the activity status of their patients and promote the adoption of a physically active lifestyle. Accordingly, health care providers must be familiar with the physiological demands of exercise and specific sports such that they may appropriately evaluate and mitigate risk while not unduly proscribing participation.

Many of the recommendations made regarding screening and counseling individuals about their participation in exercise and sports are based on expert consensus. Because of the wide range and varied nature of the physiological demands of sports and associated training, as well as the great variation in the presence and severity of underlying cardiovascular disease and comorbidities of prospective participants, it is unlikely that there will ever be adequate scientific data to precisely define individual risk. However, the continued generation of carefully collected outcome data regarding adverse event rates during specific sports-related activities, as well as the underlying cause of those events, can fill many gaps in the available information and help to further refine risk assessment. In the meantime, available guidelines must be promulgated and implemented by the medical community and those involved with athletic screening and training. Standardization of medical screening forms to contain key elements of the history and physical examination (see Table 78-3) and algorithms that outline steps for further evaluation should be established for athletic screening at all levels of competition from school to professional athletics. Finally, all those involved with directly supervising exercise and sports-related activities in any venue must be facile with the prompt recognition of an adverse event, alerting of emergency medical systems, provision of cardiopulmonary resuscitation, and use of the automated external defibrillator (AED), where available. The AHA and the 36th Bethesda Conference report[58] have outlined recommendations regarding the availability of AEDs at health and fitness facilities, sports arenas, and other venues of competitive athletic programs.

REFERENCES

Background on Physical Activity and Cardiovascular Disease

1. U.S. Department of Health and Human Services: Physical activity and health: A report of the surgeon general. Atlanta, Centers for Disease Control and Prevention, 1996.
2. Thompson PD, Buchner D, Pina IL, et al: Exercise and physical activity in the prevention and treatment of atherosclerotic cardiovascular disease: A statement from the Council on Clinical Cardiology (Subcommittee on Exercise, Rehabilitation, and Prevention) and the Council on Nutrition, Physical Activity, and Metabolism (Subcommittee on Physical Activity). Circulation 107:3109, 2003.
3. Centers for Disease Control and Prevention: Physical activity trends—United States, 2000-2001. MMWR 53:764, 2003.
4. Maron BJ: Sudden death in young athletes. N Engl J Med 349:1064, 2003.
5. Mitchell JH, Haskell W, Snell P, Van Camp SP: Task Force 8: Classification of sports. J Am Coll Cardiol 45:1364, 2005.
6. Gulati M, Pandey DK, Arnsdorf MF, et al: Exercise capacity and the risk of death in women—The St. James Women Take Heart Project. Circulation 108:1554, 2003.
7. Paffenbarger RS, Hyde RT, Wing A, et al: Physical activity, all-cause mortality, and longevity of college alumni. N Engl J Med 314:605, 1986.
8. Martinson BC, O'Connor PJ, Pronk NP: Physical inactivity and short-term all-cause mortality in adults with chronic disease. Arch Intern Med 161:1173, 2001.
9. Tanasescu M, Leitzmann MF, Rimm EB, et al: Physical activity in relation to cardiovascular disease and total mortality among men with type 2 diabetes. Circulation 107:2435, 2003.
10. Landi F, Cesari M, Lattanzio F, et al: Physical activity and mortality in frail, community-living, elderly patients. J Gerontol A Biol Sci Med Sci 59:833, 2004.

Cardiovascular Benefits of Physical Activity

11. Myers J, Prakash M, Froelicher V, et al: Exercise capacity and mortality among men referred for exercise testing. N Engl J Med 346:793, 2002.
12. Taylor RS, Brown A, Ebrahim S, et al: Exercise-based rehabilitation for patients with coronary heart disease: Systematic review and meta-analysis of randomized controlled trials. Am J Med 116:682, 2004.

13. Piepoli MF, Davos C, Francis DP, Coats AJ: ExTraMATCH Collaborative. Exercise training meta-analysis of trials in patients with chronic heart failure (ExTraMATCH). BMJ 328:189, 2004.

14. Whelton SP, Chin A, Xin X, et al: Effect of aerobic exercise on blood pressure: A meta-analysis of randomized, controlled trials. Ann Intern Med 136:493, 2002.

15. Sigal RJ, Kenney GP, Wasserman DH, et al: Physical activity/exercise and type 2 diabetes: A consensus statement from the American Diabetes Association. Diabetes Care 29:1433, 2006.

16. Knowler WC, Barrett-Connor E, Fowler SE, et al: Reduction in the incidence of type 2 diabetes with lifestyle intervention or metformin. N Engl J Med 346:393, 2002.

17. Klein S, Burke LE, Bray GA, et al: Clinical implications of obesity with specific focus on cardiovascular disease. A statement for professionals from the American Heart Association Council on Nutrition, Physical Activity, and Metabolism. Circulation 110:2952, 2004.

18. Saris WH, Blair SN, van Baak MA, et al: How much physical activity is enough to prevent unhealthy weight gain? Outcome of the IASO 1st Stock Conference and consensus statement. Obes Rev 4:101, 2003.

19. Kraus WE, Houmard JA, Duscha BD, et al: Effects of the amount and intensity of exercise on plasma lipoproteins. N Engl J Med 347:1483, 2002.

20. Williams PT, Blanche PJ, Krauss RM: Behavioral versus genetic correlates of lipoproteins and adiposity in identical twins discordant for exercise. Circulation 112:350, 2005.

21. Kasapis C, Thompson PD: The effects of physical activity on C-reactive protein and inflammatory markers: A systematic review. J Am Coll Cardiol 45:1563, 2005.

22. Linke A, Schoene N, Gielen S, et al: Endothelial dysfunction in patients with chronic heart failure: Systemic effects of lower-limb exercise training. J Am Coll Cardiol 37:392, 2001.

23. Hambrecht R, Wolf A, Geilen S, et al: Effect of exercise on coronary endothelial function in patients with coronary artery disease. N Engl J Med 342:454, 2000.

24. Hambrecht R, Adams V, Erbs S, et al: Regular physical activity improves endothelial function in patients with coronary artery disease by increasing phosphorylation of endothelial nitric oxide synthase. Circulation 107:3152, 2003.

25. Adams V, Linke A, Krankel N, et al: Impact of regular physical activity on the NAD(P)H kinase and angiotensin receptor system in patients with coronary artery disease. Circulation 111:555, 2005.

26. Steiner S, Neissner A, Ziegler S, et al: Endurance training increases the number of endothelial progenitor cells in patients with cardiovascular risk and coronary disease. Atherosclerosis 181:305, 2005.

27. Halcox JP, Schenki WH, Zalos G, et al: Prognostic value of coronary vascular endothelial dysfunction. Circulation 106:653, 2002.

28. Adamson PB, Smith AL, Abraham WT, et al: Continuous autonomic assessment in patients with symptomatic heart failure: Prognostic value of heart rate variability measured by implanted cardiac resynchronization device. Circulation 110:2389, 2004.

29. Fleg JL, Morrell CH, Bos AG, et al: Accelerated longitudinal decline of aerobic capacity in healthy older adults. Circulation 112:674, 2005.

Cardiovascular Disease and Athletes

30. VanCamp SP, Bloor CM, Muelle FU, et al: Non-traumatic sports deaths in high school and college athletes. Med Sci Sports Exerc 27:641, 1995.

31. Gorrado D, Hasso C, Rizzoli G, et al: Does sports activity enhance the risk of sudden death in adolescents and young adults? J Am Coll Cardiol 42:1959, 2003.

32. Albert CM, Mittleman MA, Chae CU, et al: Triggering of sudden death from cardiac causes by vigorous exertion. N Engl J Med 343:1355, 2000.

33. Whang W, Manson JE, Hu FB, et al: Physical exertion, exercise, and sudden cardiac death in women. JAMA 295:1399, 2006.

34. Maron BJ, Estes NAM, Link MA: Task Force 11: Commotio Cordis Task Force 8: Classification of sports. J Am Coll Cardiol 45:1371, 2005.

35. Marathonguide.com Staff: USA Marathoning: 2005 Overview. (http://www.marathonguide.com/features/Articles/2005RecapOverview.cfm). Accessed August 4, 2006.

36. Roberts WO, Maron BJ: Evidence for decreasing occurrence of sudden cardiac death associated with the marathon. J Am Coll Cardiol 46:1373, 2005.

37. Almond CSD, Shin AY, Fortescue EB, et al: Hyponatremia among runners in the Boston Marathon. N Engl J Med 352:1550, 2005.

38. Neilan TG, Yoerer DM, Douglas PS, et al: Persistent and reversible cardiac dysfunction among amateur marathon runners. Eur Heart J 27:1079, 2006.

39. Fletcher GF, Balady GJ, Amsterdam EA, et al: Exercise standards for testing and training: A statement for health professionals from the American Heart Association. Circulation 104:1694, 2001.

40. Whaley MH (ed): American College of Sports Medicine Guidelines for Exercise Testing and Prescription. 7th ed. New York, Lippincott Williams & Wilkins, 2006.

41. Brooks GA, Butte NF, Rand WM, et al: Chronicle of the Institute of Medicine physical activity recommendation: How a physical activity recommendation came to be among dietary recommendations. Am J Clin Nutr 79(Suppl):921S, 2004.

42. Maron B, Arujo C, Thompson P, Fletcher G, et al: Recommendations for preparticipation screening and the assessment of cardiovascular disease in master athletes. Circulation 103:327, 2001.

43. Balady GJ, Chaitman B, Driscoll D, et al: American Heart Association/American College of Sports Medicine Joint Scientific Statement: Recommendations for Cardiovascular Screening, Staffing, and Emergency Policies at Health/Fitness Facilities. Circulation 97:2283,1998.

44. Maron BJ, Douglas PS, Graham TP, et al: Task force 1: Preparticipation screening and diagnosis of cardiovascular disease in athletes. J Am Coll Cardiol 45:1322, 2005.

45. Maron BJ, Thompson PS, Puffer JC, et al: Cardiovascular preparticipation screening of competitive athletes. Circulation 94:850, 1996.

Physical Activity and Sports in Patients with Cardiovascular Disease

46. Maron BJ, Zipes DP: Introduction: Eligibility recommendations for competitive athletes with cardiovascular abnormalities—general considerations. J Am Coll Cardiol 45:1318, 2005.

47. Maron BJ, Chaitman BR, Ackerman MJ, et al: Recommendations for physical activity and recreational sports participation for young patients with genetic cardiovascular diseases. Circulation 109:2807, 2004.

48. Ades PA: Cardiac rehabilitation and the secondary prevention of coronary heart disease. N Engl J Med 345:892, 2001.

49. 36th Bethesda Conference: Eligibility recommendations for competitive athletes with cardiovascular abnormalities. J Am Coll Cardiol 45:1313, 2005.

50. Thompson PD, Balady GJ, Chaitman BR, et al: Task Force 6: Coronary artery disease. J Am Coll Cardiol 4:1348, 2005.

51. Lee CD, Folsom AR, Blair SN: Physical activity and stroke risk: A meta-analysis. Stroke 34:2475, 2003.

52. Kaplan NM, Gidding SS, Pickering TG, et al: Task Force 5: Systemic hypertension. J Am Coll Cardiol 45:1346, 2005.

53. Bonow RO, Cheitlin MD, Crawford MH, et al: Task Force 3: Valvular heart disease. J Am Coll Cardiol 45:1334, 2005.

54. Maron BJ, Ackerman MJ, Nishimura RA, et al: Task Force 4: HCM and other cardiomyopathies, mitral valve prolapse, myocarditis, and Marfan syndrome. J Am Coll Cardiol 45:1340, 2005.

55. Zipes DP, Ackerman MJ, Estes NA III, et al: Task Force 7: Arrhythmias. J Am Coll Cardiol 45:1354, 2005.

56. Graham TP Jr, Driscoll DJ, Gersony WM, et al: Task Force 2: Congenital heart disease. J Am Coll Cardiol 45:1326, 2005.

57. Elefteriades JA, Hatzaras I, Tranquilli MA, et al: Weight lifting and rupture of silent aortic aneurysms. JAMA 290:2803, 2003.

58. Myerberg RJ, Estes NAM, Fontaine JM, et al: Task Force 10: Automated external defibrillators. Task Force 8: Classification of sports. J Am Coll Cardiol 45:1369, 2005.

CHAPTER 79

Medical Management of the Patient Undergoing Cardiac Surgery

Richard J. Gray and Dhun H. Sethna

Organization of the
Program, 1993

Preoperative Risk
Analysis, 1993
Advanced Age/Gender, 1993
Ethnicity/Race, 1994
Reoperation, 1994
Baseline Laboratory Values, 1994
Preoperative Drug Therapy, 1994

Preoperative Medical
Conditions, 1995
Pregnancy, 1995
Renal Dysfunction, 1995
Atrial Fibrillation, 1996
Pulmonary Disease, 1996
Neurological Disease, 1996
Hepatic Cirrhosis, 1996
Connective Tissue Disease, 1996
Human Immunodeficiency Virus
   Type-1, 1996
Hematology/Oncology, 1996

Preoperative Risk
Calculation, 1996

The "Normal" Postoperative
Convalescence, 1998
Cardiovascular Convalescence, 1998
Pulmonary Convalescence, 1998
Neurological Convalescence, 1998
Postoperative Chest Pain, 1999
Postoperative Drug Therapy, 1999
Hospital Course, 2000

Postoperative Morbidity, 2000
Cardiovascular Morbidity, 2000
Postoperative Pulmonary
   Morbidity, 2004
Postoperative Bleeding, 2004
Postoperative Renal
   Dysfunction, 2005
Postoperative Neurological
   Morbidity, 2006
Postoperative Gastrointestinal
   Morbidity, 2008
Postoperative Infection, 2008
Postoperative Endocrine
   Abnormalities, 2009

References, 2009

ORGANIZATION OF THE PROGRAM

The way in which a surgical program is organized is as important to its success as any other single factor. The most successful programs, defined by low surgical mortality and morbidity, are generally characterized by larger surgical volume (and large per surgeon volume) and are organized tightly around surgical leadership, with a limited role for referring physicians, cardiologists, and consultants unless they are a regular and direct part of the surgical service. Very large and successful programs often have a single or small number of separate surgical practice groups. The minimization of variation through standardized protocols, recognized widely in medical literature, is critical in a cardiac surgical program for improving patient satisfaction and improving quality by decreasing confusion over patient management approaches. Quality assurance is a must in any program; given the scope of the usual team, inclusion of nursing and other physician members (anesthesia, cardiology, critical care, and others) is important, with time spent reviewing data on surgical outcomes. Significant adverse events should be examined by the leader of the quality initiative to determine if a case presentation should be made in the context of peer review.

There is much demand for data on outcomes, both voluntary and required, and some are publicly reported. The Society of Cardiac Surgeons (STS) is the most widely used and reported data base. The Leapfrog Group, a consortium of some of the largest employers and health care purchasers in the United States, recognizes and rewards leaps in quality and patient value through proprietary quality scores that assess hospitals with cardiac surgery programs regarding their participation in the STS and the rankings of risk-adjusted outcomes to national averages. The Joint Commission on Accreditation of Healthcare Organizations (JCAHO) surveys use cardiac surgical data in the credentialing process. There are commercial quality-reporting organizations, such as Health Grades, which use MedPar (Medicare) data sets in developing scores or rankings of cardiac surgical programs. There is also a public reporting of these data by the U.S. Department of Health and Human Services in a program called "Hospital Compare." The biggest development is the mandatory public reporting of cardiac surgical data in several states (eleven states in all at present) involving either isolated coronary artery bypass surgery (CABG) or a wider scope of operations. Although probably leading to better quality of care,[1] it has not been without controversy, with allegations of case selection designed to enhance results and out-referrals of complex cases.[2]

PREOPERATIVE RISK ANALYSIS

Advanced Age/Gender

More than 60 percent of octogenarian patients have at least one nonfatal postoperative complication.[3] Besides twice the risk of death from a cardiac intervention, they show markedly higher risk of prolonged ventilation time, reoperation for bleeding, and pneumonia leading to hospital stays that are, on average, 2 days longer than their younger counterparts.[4] Outcomes are worse after valve surgery in the elderly with a high 17 percent hospital mortality.[5] More perioperative complications occur in patients older than 75 years who have low body mass indices (BMI < 23).[6] Off-pump surgery using only arterial conduits confers an operative survival benefit leading to an enhanced long-term quality of life.[7,8] With improving techniques and greater attention to detail, select nonagenarians can also undergo CABG with a 95 percent 30-day survival; the only statistically significant risk factor for death is emergency surgery.[9] However, complications can be expected in 67 percent of patients, resulting in prolonged average ICU stay (12 days; median, 5 days), and longer average hospital stay (17.5 days; median, 11 days).

In retrospective cohort studies of large data bases involving 15,000 to 54,425 patients undergoing CABG, early mortality was found to be significantly higher in women after adjustment for confounding factors, including low body surface area (BSA).[10,11] On the other hand, a survey conducted between 1992 and 2002 of 3760 consecutive patients who underwent isolated CABG showed no differences in in-hospital mortality or 5-year survival between men and women.[12] Malignant ventricular arrhythmias, calcified aorta, and preoperative renal failure are poor prognostic signs in women. The benefit of open heart surgery at 2-year follow-up is equivalent in both genders in terms of quality of life as assessed by the 36-item short form health survey questionnaire (SF36), although women show lower baseline scores.[13]

Ethnicity/Race

In a survey conducted in 2004, 44 percent of cardiovascular surgeons thought that, among patients with cardiac risk factors, black patients were not as likely as white patients to receive cardiac diagnostic tests and procedures.[14] Thirteen percent agreed that cardiac care disparities occur "often" or "somewhat often" based on patients' race/ethnicity, independent of their insurance and education (see Chap. 2). But only 3 percent said that disparities were likely to occur in their own clinical setting. However, in one follow-up study after CABG, African-American patients experienced twice the mortality at 5 years compared to their white counterparts, despite similar medical insurance coverage.

CASE VOLUME

As a discriminator of quality of care and mortality, the use of hospital volumes of cardiac surgery, which may combine the experience of a wide range of individual surgeons, has been said to be "only slightly better than a coin flip."[15] A retrospective cohort of 948,093 Medicare patients undergoing CABG with cardiopulmonary bypass (CPB) in 870 U.S. hospitals from 1996 to 2001 showed considerable variation in adjusted mortality within the low-volume group (1 to 17 percent) as well as within the high-volume group (2 to 11 percent) so that the volume criterion alone was a poor discriminator of mortality (c statistic = 0.51). Of the 660 low-volume hospitals, 253 (38 percent) had risk-adjusted mortality rates that were similar to or lower than the overall risk-adjusted mortality of some of the high-volume hospitals.

Volume statistics of individual surgeons seem to be a better quality criterion. In a study of first time isolated CABG operations, patients treated by low-volume surgeons (1 to 50 cases annually) had significantly higher mortality rates than those treated by medium-volume surgeons (51 to 100 cases annually; 7.0 versus 3.8 percent), high-volume surgeons (101 to 150 cases annually; 7.0 versus 2.7 percent), or very-high-volume surgeons (>151 cases annually; 7.0 versus 3.2 percent).[16] The adjusted odds ratio of hospital in-patient deaths declined with increasing surgeon volume, with the odds of in-patient death for those patients treated by low-volume surgeons being 1.52 times those of medium-volume surgeons, 1.89 times those of high-volume surgeons, and 2.04 times those of very-high-volume surgeons. Hospital volume and surgeon volume effects on CABG outcomes are probably interdependent.[17]

SURGICAL TECHNIQUE

Conventional sternotomy with CPB is still the standard in most institutions (see Chap. 54). Alternative approaches should be used as tools within a decision-making algorithm driven by patient-related factors of coronary anatomy and comorbidity, and the surgeon's own experience. Off-pump beating-heart CABG has the possibility to eliminate intraoperative global myocardial ischemia and to be an acceptable surgical option for patients after acute myocardial infarction (MI); it is associated with lower postoperative mortality and morbidity. Minimally invasive direct CABG (MIDCAB), conducted through a left thoracotomy, is limited to patients with amenable coronary anatomy. Port-access CABG requires CPB with cardiac arrest but avoids sternotomy. Off-pump CABG (OPCAB) may be considered using a median sternotomy or with MIDCAB procedures. Meta-analysis indicates that OPCAB appears to be as good as, or superior to, on-pump CABG in terms of reduced length of hospital stay, operative morbidity, and operative mortality, including decreased need for intraaortic balloon pump placement, rate of postoperative renal failure, and hemorrhage-related reexploration, especially in high risk patients (see Chap. 54).[18-20]

More studies are required before firm conclusions can be drawn concerning the effect of OPCAB on midterm mortality, angina recurrence, and repeat intervention. After risk adjustment, patients with critical left main stem stenosis or those with diffuse coronary disease requiring endarterectomy can undergo OPCAB safely, with results comparable with on-pump CABG. Anatomical factors against OPCAB

include target vessel size less than 1.25 mm, calcification, intramyocardial location of target vessels, and multiple stenoses. The risk of reduced graft patency also needs to be considered when choosing OPCAB as a tailored strategy in selected patients. Given that OPCAB can be performed safely, patients in the moderate or high risk range, i.e., elderly with multiple comorbidities, or emergency patients operated within the first 48 hours of acute MI, could preferentially be treated using OPCAB. Experienced OPCAB surgeons have a low risk of acute conversion to CPB. Acutely converted patients have a moderately increased risk of in-hospital death and serious complications that are difficult to quantify because conversion is infrequent and unpredictable.

Reoperation

In many centers, hospital mortality for reoperative CABG is approaching that of primary CABG.[21] Aggressive risk-factor reduction (see Chap. 45) and extensive arterial coronary revascularization at primary CABG should result in fewer coronary reoperations.[22] In a study of elective redo-CABG patients, minimal tissue dissection and target vessel revascularization without CPB did not add significant benefit with regard to perioperative morbidity and mortality.

Baseline Laboratory Values

Elevated preprocedural systemic markers of inflammation have been associated with adverse clinical outcomes after CABG. Higher preoperative white blood cell count has been independently associated with higher perioperative myocardial necrosis (MB CK release) and 1-year mortality.[23] The risk for perioperative cerebrovascular accident (CVA) is also increased starting at preoperative white cell count of 9×10^9/L and rising at higher ranges.[24] The white cell count has a significant impact on CVA and neuropsychological outcomes.[25] However, reducing the perioperative inflammatory response with leukocyte filtration does not seem to be efficacious in improving short-term outcomes.[26] Preoperative C-reactive protein (CRP) greater than 1.0 mg/dl carries a higher risk of overall postoperative death, cardiac death, low cardiac output syndrome, and any cerebrovascular complication, with reduced overall long-term survival.[27,28] Patients with high baseline CRP levels are at higher risk of having postoperative atrial fibrillation (AF) following on-pump and off-pump surgery.[29] Low basal free T_3 concentration has been shown to reliably predict the occurrence of postoperative AF in CABG patients.[30] Serum troponin (cTnI) levels measured within 24 hours before elective CABG further identifies a subgroup of patients with higher risk for perioperative MI, low cardiac output syndrome, and high in-hospital mortality.[31] Preoperative cTnI measurement before emergency CABG is a powerful and independent determinant of in-hospital mortality and major adverse cardiac events in acute coronary syndromes (see Chap. 53).[32]

Preoperative Drug Therapy

Preoperative aspirin taken within 5 days preceding CABG is associated with significantly lower in-hospital mortality without increased risk of reoperation for bleeding or need for blood transfusion.[33] In patients who have had OPCAB, it does not increase bleeding-related complications, mortality rate, or other morbidities.[34]

The risk versus benefit of preoperative administration of clopidogrel remains unresolved. Based on multivariable models, preoperative clopidogrel is an independent risk factor for increased transfusion requirements and prolonged ICU and hospital length of stay.[35] Among in-hospital referral patients, preoperative clopidogrel administered within 5 days before CABG increases early mortality and morbidity, and the risk of death is greatest when the drug is given within 48 hours of surgery.[36] It is recommended that surgery in patients on clopidogrel should be performed using standard heparinization and antifibrinolytic strategies; platelets transfused before chest closure have a beneficial effect on hemostasis.[37] Aprotinin reduces bleeding and transfusion requirements of packed red blood cells, platelets, and total blood units in patients on clopidogrel who need urgent or elective CABG.[38,39] Preoperative use of clopidogrel has also been shown not to be associated with increased major or life-threatening bleeding or need for surgical reexploration, or higher risk of blood and blood product transfusion after CABG.[40] A post hoc analysis of the CURE trial reported that patients who underwent early CABG after non-ST elevation acute coronary syndrome showed significant improvement in cardiovascular outcomes with preoperative clopidogrel therapy, with no significant increase in life-threatening postoperative bleeding.[41]

Preoperative enoxaparin given less than 12 hours before CABG is associated with lower postoperative hemoglobin values and higher rates of transfusion when compared to preoperative continuous unfractionated heparin administration.[42] Intraoperative heparin resistance may also be increased, requiring more heparin to maintain the desired activated clotting time, leading to higher heparin concentrations and lower antithrombin values compared with control patients.[43]

Preoperative statin therapy confers a protective benefit on postoperative outcomes because the odds of experiencing early mortality and morbidity are significantly less in the statin-pretreated patients (see Chaps. 42 and 45).[44,45] In one study, statins were associated with reduced primary combined endpoint, death, and MI after surgery—regardless of inflammatory markers, with additional protection observed in patients with positive troponin T levels.[46] Treatment with atorvastatin 40 mg/day, initiated 7 days before surgery, significantly reduces the incidence of postoperative AF after elective cardiac surgery with CPB and shortens hospital stay.[47]

PREOPERATIVE MEDICAL CONDITIONS

Pregnancy

Cardiac surgery during pregnancy is associated with increased maternal (8.6 percent) and fetal (18.6 percent) mortality rates.[48] Poor functional class has been associated with a higher risk of maternal death, as is the use of vasoactive drugs, age, type of surgery, and reoperation. Maternal age more than 35 years, functional class, reoperation, emergency surgery, type of myocardial protection, and anoxic time can have adverse effects on fetal survival.

CARDIOVASCULAR RISK FACTORS (also see Chap. 39)

CIGARETTE SMOKING. Smoking is a strong risk factor for the development of postoperative respiratory complications, which are twice as common in smokers (29.5 percent) as nonsmokers (13.6 percent) and ex-smokers (14.7 percent).[49] Patients who have stopped smoking for more than six months have complication rates similar to those who have never smoked. Even smoking cessation for more than 2 months can significantly reduce the rate of respiratory complications (57.1 versus 14.5 percent).

OBESITY. Despite the perception that obesity increases the risk of in-hospital and early (1 year) mortality and morbidity in CABG operations, the clinical outcomes of these patients are not so different from other patients when proper attention is given to detail.[50-52] However, long-term survival may be reduced, and higher rates of AF, bleeding, reoperation, renal, and gastrointestinal complications may occur.[53] In particular, BMI > 40 leads to significantly more complications, including a higher incidence of postoperative sternal wound infections, prolonged ventilation, and longer hospital stay.

DIABETES. The outcome in patients after cardiac surgery using CPB is negatively influenced by the presence of diabetes (see Chap. 60), with insulin-dependent type II diabetics showing a significantly higher rate of major postoperative complications including acute renal failure, deep sternal wound infection, and prolonged postoperative stay when compared to nondiabetics and those not taking insulin.[54,55] Although there may not be a higher risk of in-hospital mortality, longevity has been shown to be significantly reduced over a 5-year follow-up period. In-hospital resource utilization may be expected to be higher in diabetics: each 50 mg/dl blood glucose increase has been shown to be associated with longer postoperative days, higher hospitalization charges by $2824, and increased hospitalization cost by $1769.[56] OPCAB in diabetic patients can significantly reduce postoperative morbidity and length of stay compared with coronary operation on CPB.[57] The absence of diabetes-related target organ damage, specifically renal failure or peripheral vascular disease, is associated with long-term survival after CABG that is similar to or only slightly less than that in patients without diabetes.[58] Diabetes does not affect the early postoperative and midterm results, including 1-year graft patency, in patients with multivessel disease undergoing total arterial vascularization and OPCAB. The metabolic syndrome is associated with faster degeneration of bioprosthetic valves.[59]

PERIPHERAL VASCULAR DISEASE. Patients with peripheral vascular disease (see Chap. 57) undergoing CABG have better intermediate survival out to 3 years than similar patients undergoing PCI.[60] Off-pump CABG is safe in such patients with acceptable results and a reduced incidence of postoperative stroke.[61] However, they are at higher risk for limb ischemia, leg wound healing and infection, especially after intraaortic balloon counterpulsation therapy. About 10 percent of patients scheduled for CABG have associated unsuspected abdominal aortic aneurysm (see Chap. 56); whether this justifies routine preoperative echocardiographic screening remains undetermined.[62] When calcification of the ascending aorta is detected on chest x-ray, computed tomography (CT) evaluation should be considered to map out the locations of calcium. Alternatively, intraoperative epiaortic ultrasound may be useful to avoid vascular disruption or stroke during cannulation or proximal anastomoses of bypass grafts. The most severe aortic calcification known as "porcelain aorta" may require OPCAB or an alternative approach to cannulation or proximal grafting.

Renal Dysfunction (see Chap. 88)

Because coronary artery disease remains the most frequent cause of death in patients with end-stage renal disease, it is inevitable that a substantial percentage of patients with varying severities of renal dysfunction need surgical revascularization. Risk stratification is superior using estimated or measured glomerular filtration rate (GFR) rather than serum creatinine, as the association with adverse outcomes is stronger with estimated creatinine clearance than with serum creatinine level.[63] Cystatin C, a cystine protease inhibitor, has proved to be a simple and more sensitive measure of overall renal function than serum creatinine and can be used with serum creatinine in the routine assessment of renoprotective strategies.[64]

Preoperative serum creatinine between 1.47 and 2.25 mg/dl is an important predictor of worse in-hospital mortality, morbidity, and midterm survival after CABG.[65] Mild elevation of preoperative creatinine level (1.3 to 2.0 mg/dl) can significantly increase the probability of perioperative mortality, low cardiac output, hemodialysis and prolonged hospital stay.[66] Total mortality in patients with lower GFRc (GFRc < 71.1 ml·min^{-1}·1.73 m^{-2}) is significantly increased.[67] Nondialysis-dependent patients with renal dysfunction undergoing CABG experience higher in-hospital mortality, stroke, and atrial arrhythmia, with need for prolonged ventilation and longer postoperative stay.[68] Midterm (5 year) survival is also significantly reduced. Dialysis dependence is an additional major risk that may be reduced with OPCAB.[69] Patients who have undergone kidney transplantation show better survival than those on dialysis.[70] In one study from a single institution, preoperative renal insufficiency, mitral valve disease, and left ventricular (LV) dysfunction were associated with adverse early outcomes.[71]

Patients with serum creatinine >2.0 mg/dl or dialysis dependence who have had an acute or recent MI undergo CABG with an 8 to 10 percent hospital mortality, and a higher risk of pulmonary complications and AF.[72]

Atrial Fibrillation

Preexisting AF in patients undergoing CABG is not associated with increased in-hospital mortality or major morbidity; however, it is a risk factor for reduced 5-year survival (see Chap. 35).[73] In one study, median survival in propensity-matched patients with AF was 8.7 years versus 14 years for those without it.[74] Spontaneous cardioversion to sinus rhythm during surgery is transient in the majority of patients and is not associated with midterm survival benefit. Notwithstanding, if patients in AF require surgical revascularization, it is appropriate to consider performing a concomitant surgical ablation procedure.

Pulmonary Disease

Preoperative chronic obstructive pulmonary disease (COPD), defined as those undergoing active therapy or having a $FEV_1 < 75$ percent of predicted, leads to a higher mortality (7 percent) and higher incidence (50 percent) of postoperative respiratory complications, especially pneumonia, requiring prolonged ICU and hospital stay.[75] The subgroup of elderly patients (>75 years) with COPD who are on steroids have prohibitive postoperative mortality.

Neurological Disease

Preoperative stroke carries a higher risk of developing postoperative neurological complications. An accepted rule of thumb is to wait 2 or 3 months after a stroke before placing a patient on CPB. Patients with remote CVA, even though they may have completely recovered, often exhibit signs of reactivation whereby some or all of the previous symptoms reappear, albeit in a milder form. Although the prognosis for recovery is good, several weeks are sometimes needed.

Carotid artery occlusive disease occurs in 1.5 to 6 percent of patients with coronary artery disease and may be associated with postoperative stroke. Although mandatory preoperative screening with bilateral duplex ultrasound of all patients is still done in some institutions, limiting this process to patients older than 65 years, those with a carotid bruit, or those with suspected or established cerebrovascular disease can reduce the screening load by nearly 40 percent with negligible impact on surgical management or neurological outcomes.[76] In those cases in which critical, symptomatic carotid artery stenosis coexists at the time of scheduled CABG, a combined or staged CABG and carotid endarterectomy procedure can be done with excellent results. It still remains unclear whether a combined or staged technique shows superior outcomes over the other.

Patients with advanced Parkinsonism require considerable nursing care after cardiac surgery, and their inability to generate a good cough effort requires aggressive respiratory care. ICU and hospital stay may be prolonged, and discharge to an extended care facility is often necessary. Abnormal peripheral vascular tone secondary to autonomic dysfunction, manifested in its extreme form as the Shy-Drager syndrome, can cause hemodynamic problems in the perioperative period. Although there is no absolute score from the Mini-Mental Status Examination that provides a cutoff for declaring a patient inoperable, the indications for surgery in patients with Alzheimer disease who are severely disoriented, confused, and incapable of independent living should be strongly considered on an individual basis with a view against operation. Preoperative depression is an independent risk factor for postoperative mortality.[77]

Hepatic Cirrhosis

Liver disease may be associated with complex multifactorial coagulopathies. Cardiac operation can be performed safely in patients with mild or moderately advanced hepatic cirrhosis with a 6 percent early mortality. Complication rates can be high at 39 percent for Pugh Class A patients, and 80 percent in Pugh Class B and C based on one study,[78] but rates may be lower for OPCAB in such patients.[79]

Connective Tissue Disease

CABG appears to be safe in patients with connective tissue diseases (see Chap. 84) (rheumatoid arthritis and systemic lupus) with acceptable early results.[80] Wound complications may be a problem, and the use of steroids or other immunomodulating agents is associated with increased postoperative complications. Chronic steroid therapy in general does not increase mortality or overall morbidity but it may be associated with a greater chance of developing atrial arrhythmias or of requiring prolonged ventilation.[81]

Human Immunodeficiency Virus Type-1

Although the incidence of active infectious endocarditis in patients with immunodeficiency virus type-1 (HIV-1) has been reduced, noninfectious valvular disease and coronary artery disease are on the rise in such patients (see Chap. 67). Those patients requiring cardiac surgery show a high (22 percent) overall mortality with 58 percent actuarial 15-year survival, and no blunting of the CD4 response induced by antiretrovirals.[82] The late causes of death are usually not AIDS-related.

Hematology/Oncology

Whether cardiac surgery is justifiable in patients with malignant tumors is determined by the long-term outcome of the treated malignancy. One study showed that fatal progression of the tumor can occur if the time interval between the occurrence of the malignancy and cardiac surgery is short.[83] Cardiac operations can be performed with acceptable mortality (4.1 percent) in patients with hematological malignancies but with significant morbidity rates (50 percent), most often bleeding and infection.[84]

Antiphospholipid syndrome (APS) is a rare coagulation disorder associated with recurrent arterial and venous thrombotic events (see Chap. 82). Patients with APS undergoing cardiac surgery belong to a high-risk subgroup, and some patients with unexplained perioperative thromboembolic complications, such as graft occlusion, may turn out to have an undiagnosed APS.[85] Patients with glucose-6-phosphate dehydrogenase deficiency who are undergoing cardiac surgery may have a more complicated course with a longer ventilation time, more hypoxia, increased hemolysis, and a need for more blood transfusion.[86] Because this difference may be caused by subnormal free radical deactivation, strategies that minimize bypass in general and free radicals specifically may be beneficial. Patients with glycoprotein IIIa allele $Pl^{A1/A2}$ genetic polymorphism (Pl^{A1} homozygotes) who undergo CABG show increased postoperative bleeding that is further accentuated by preoperative aspirin therapy.[87]

PREOPERATIVE RISK CALCULATION

Intra-institutional and inter-institutional benchmarking requires scoring systems with reliability (calibration) and stability over the complete spectrum of periprocedural risk. Three mortality measures have traditionally been used to estimate perioperative outcomes: in-hospital, 30-day, and procedural (either in-hospital or 30-day) mortality. In the same patient population, the in-hospital mortality is generally the lowest rate, whereas the procedural mortality rate is usually the highest.[88] Additionally, because complications occur more frequently than death, risk-adjusted major morbidity may differentially impact quality of care and enhance a surgical team's ability to assess their quality. A further limitation of standard risk models is that risk associated with some preoperative variables can change significantly over time after surgery, and assessments that assume constant risk during the postoperative follow-up period may substantially overestimate or underestimate risk.[89] Diabetes adds little incremental risk immediately after surgery, but the risk increases steadily and doubles at 9.5 years after surgery (see Chap. 60). Age, chronic obstructive pulmonary disease, and urgent or emergent status also show risk-changing by 50 to 60 percent over a decade. Avoidance of CPB does not confer significant clinical advantages in all high-risk coronary patients; instead, there are particular subsets of patients for whom beating heart surgery can be particularly indicated, and others for whom on-pump revascularization seems a better solution (see Chap. 54).[90] Off-pump surgery improves in-hospital outcome only in the subset of patients at highest risk. Off-pump patients have more early and late cardiac complications, whereas patients operated on-pump exhibit a higher incidence of postoperative systemic organ dysfunction. Adaptation of the operation to the individual patient is probably the best way to improve outcomes.

Over the decades, a host of risk models have been proposed for the estimation of in-hospital mortality in patients undergoing cardiac surgery, such as the Bernstein-Parsonnet model, the New York State model, and the Northern New England model. Two successful and widely used models are the EuroSCORE additive model which also comes in a full logistical version, and the Society of Thoracic Surgeons (STS) model. In the latter instance, using the STS database, models have been developed for postoperative mortality and composite endpoint, and for postoperative morbidity including stroke, renal failure, reoperation, prolonged ventilation, and sternal infection.[91] When different models (Parsonnet score, EuroSCORE, ACC/AHA score and three UK Bayes models [old, new complex, and new simple]) were used in a study for comparing inter-institutional 30-day mortality, only two of the scores were found to be useful in comparing institutions.[92] All six systems in this study performed moderately well at ranking patients, suggesting that individual risk models may be useful for patient management. The study concluded that more results are needed from other institutions to confirm that the models are suitable for institutional risk-adjusted comparisons.

THE EUROSCORE

The EuroSCORE (Table 79-1) is the most rigorously evaluated scoring system in modern cardiac surgery. It has been used not only for estimating perioperative mortality risk but also for assessing 3-month mortality, length of stay, and specific postoperative complications such as renal failure, sepsis and/or endocarditis, and respiratory failure in the whole context of cardiac surgery, and to predict ICU cost and ICU stay of more than 2 days after open heart surgery.[93,94]

The validity of the EuroSCORE has been assessed by several individual centers within and outside Europe. It has a significantly better discriminatory power to predict 30-day mortality than the STS risk algorithm for patients undergoing CABG.[95] The additive EuroSCORE gives excellent discrimination that is as good as the logistic version of the model, but it greatly underestimates risk in high-risk patients when compared to the logistic version.[96] Internationally, the evidence is highly suggestive that the additive version generally overestimates mortality at lower scores (EuroSCORE 6) and underestimates mortality at higher values (EuroSCORE >13).[97] The additive model is also less precise and exhibits a predictive distortion, which should be accounted for, particularly when employing it at the individual patient level.[98] The logistic EuroSCORE is more accurate at predicting mortality in simultaneous CABG and valve surgery as the additive EuroSCORE signifi-

TABLE 79–1	The Additive EuroSCORE	
Risk Factor	**Definition**	**Score**
Patient-Related Factors		
Age	Per 5 years or part thereof (>60 yr)	1
Sex	Female	1
Chronic pulmonary disease	Long-term use of bronchodilators or steroids for lung disease	1
Extracardiac arteriopathy	Any one or more of the following: claudication, carotid occlusion or >50% stenosis, previous or planned intervention on the abdominal aorta, limb arteries, or carotid arteries	2
Neurological dysfunction	Disease severely affecting ambulation or day-to-day functioning	2
Previous cardiac surgery	Requiring opening of the pericardium	3
Serum creatinine	>200 mmol/liter preoperatively	2
Active endocarditis	Patient still receiving antibiotic treatment for endocarditis at the time of surgery	3
Critical preoperative state	Any one or more of the following: ventricular tachycardia or fibrillation or aborted sudden death, preoperative cardiac massage, preoperative ventilation before arrival in the operating room, preoperative inotropic support, intraaortic balloon counterpulsation, or preoperative acute renal failure (anuria or oliguria <10 ml/hr)	3
Cardiac-Related Factors		
Unstable angina	Rest angina requiring IV nitrates until arrival in the operating room	2
LV dysfunction	Moderate or LVEF 0.30-0.50	1
	Poor or LVEF<0.30	3
Recent myocardial infarct	<90 days	2
Pulmonary hypertension	Systolic PA pressure >60 mm Hg	2
Operation-Related Factors		
Emergency	Carried out on referral before the beginning of the next working day	2
Other than isolated CABG	Major cardiac procedure other than or in addition to CABG	2
Surgery on thoracic aorta	For disorder of ascending, arch, or descending aorta	3
Postinfarct septal rupture		4

EuroSCORE	Patients	Died (%)	Observed	Expected
0-2 (low risk)	4,529	36 (0.8)	(0.56-1.10)	(1.27-1.29)
3-5 (medium risk)	5,977	182 (3.0)	(2.62-3.51)	(2.90-2.94)
6 plus (high risk)	4,293	480 (11.2)	(10.25-12.16)	(10.93-11.54)
Total	14,799	698 (4.7)	(4.37-5.06)	(4.72-4.95)

CABG=coronary artery bypass grafting; IV=intravenous; LV=left ventricular; LVEF=left ventricular ejection fraction; PA=pulmonary artery.
Adapted from Nashef SA, Rogues F, Michel P, et al: European system for cardiac operative risk evaluation (EuroSCORE). Eur J Cardiothorac Surg 16:9-13, 1999.

cantly underpredicts in this high-risk group.[99] The logistic version should be used to predict mortality when possible. If this is not feasible, a modified additive score could be employed at the bedside.

For valvular heart disease, the EuroSCORE has been used to predict not only in-hospital mortality for which it was originally designed, but also long-term mortality in the whole context of heart valve surgery (see Chap. 62).[100] The Northern New England (NNE) risk model and the Providence Health System Cardiovascular Study Group (PHS) risk model are additional commonly applied algorithms for valvular heart disease. Both allow similar assessment of prevalence and mortality, and a new unified model has been proposed.[101] A scoring system using blood tests and clinical risk factors to determine thromboembolic risk after heart valve replacement has been described, and may be used to guide prosthesis choice and antithrombotic management.[102]

THE "NORMAL" POSTOPERATIVE CONVALESCENCE

The usual postoperative course is influenced by changes in physiology as a result of anesthesia, surgical trauma, and CPB, which make these patients unique from other hospitalized medical and surgical patients. The use of CPB can be associated with a systemic inflammatory response syndrome (SIRS) which has been reviewed in detail.[103] This "whole body inflammation" response can lead to a "postpump syndrome" which is clinically expressed as fever, leukocytosis, abnormal coagulation, hypoxemia (from neutrophil aggregation and lysis in pulmonary vasculature), increased pulmonary capillary permeability, renal dysfunction, and cognitive dysfunction.

Constipation is a nearly universal complaint as is diminished appetite, even profound anorexia. In some instances, constipation is accompanied by a distorted sense of taste (dysgeusia). Zinc sulfate (20 mg orally every 8 hours) may be helpful despite normal zinc levels. When persisting for more than 48 hours, regardless of the cause, consideration of alternative forms of alimentation (nasogastric feeding or even peripheral or central intravenous) are warranted, especially in the elderly. Urinary retention is fairly common early postoperatively in men as a result of prostatic hypertrophy and is aggravated by bed rest, overdistention of the bladder, and diuretic use. Prolonged use of an indwelling Foley catheter can also contribute to urinary retention from diminished bladder tone and prostatic edema.

Cardiovascular Convalescence

Sinus tachycardia of 100 to 120 beats/min may occur a few hours after surgery without apparent cause and should lead to assessment of adequacy of blood volume, low cardiac output syndrome, pericardial effusion or tamponade, infection (even without fever), and occult hyperthyroidism. A prominent pericardial friction rub is expected while the pericardial chest tubes are still in place. Orthostatic hypotension can be recurring and problematic in some patients, persisting for up to 2 weeks or so after surgery. It may be associated with persistent sinus tachycardia with the heart rate relatively fixed at 100 to 120 beats/min. Investigation of intravascular volume status, liberalization of salt intake, and reevaluation of antihypertensive medications or diuretics that may have been ordered, are indicated. Tightly fitting veno-occlusive stockings are occasionally helpful, as well as instructions to the patient about slowly arising from lying or sitting positions.

Pulmonary Convalescence

Most patients are still intubated when arriving in the ICU from the operating room but should be suitable for extubation within 12 hours; recent practice is to extubate patients ideally within 4 to 6 hours after operation. Such rapid weaning or "fast tracking" should be encouraged in elective, hemodynamically stable patients with adequate gas exchange who have no evidence of heart failure, excessive bleeding, or neurological complications. In one study, the 30-day mortality rate for "fast tracked" patients was 0.34 percent, mean intensive care time was 5 hours 52 minutes, mean time to extubation was 3 hours 10 minutes, mean readmission rate to intensive care was 0.34 percent and mean hospital stay from day of operation (inclusive) was 5.65 days.[104] This process increased throughput by 14.6 percent (compared to standard practices), allowing intensive care beds to be used by more than one patient each day leading to significant cost savings by reducing the nursing ratio per patient. Immediate extubation after OPCAB appears to reduce the incidence of postoperative AF independent of comorbidities. Periextubation tachycardia should be controlled with intravenous esmolol.

Atelectasis is common; the usual suspects include general anesthesia, manual compression of the lung during operation, one lung ventilation during minimally invasive surgery, apnea during CPB, and postoperative poor coughing or deep inspirations, gastric distention, interstitial lung water, and pleural effusions. Systematic literature reviews and a randomized study have failed to show that routine, prophylactic use of incentive spirometry, continuous positive airway pressure (CPAP), or physical therapy lower pulmonary morbidity in the usual patient, reflecting the low morbidity of most cases of postoperative atelectasis.[105,106] However, preoperative inspiratory muscle training in high-risk patients may reduce the incidence of postoperative pulmonary complications.[107] Pleural effusions develop in 40 to 50 percent of patients after CABG and usually resolve spontaneously within 2 to 6 weeks with no specific therapy or, at most, gentle diuresis. Effusions occurring 2 to 3 weeks after surgery may represent a postpericardiotomy syndrome that occurs in 10 to 40 percent of patients; they, too, resolve spontaneously over a few months.

Neurological Convalescence

Ulnar and median nerve injury has been described after CABG in 1.9 to 18 percent of patients as a result of a fractured first rib after sternotomy, stretch or compression injury of the brachial plexus from sternal retraction, awkward arm positioning, or needle trauma at internal jugular puncture.[108] In one small study, fracture of the first rib or of the costotransverse articulation as diagnosed by radionuclide bone scan was described in 15 percent of patients. Ulnar involvement follows the typical pattern of sensory distribution, generally numbness of the small finger and the medial portion of the ring finger in the affected limb. Median neuropathy results in motor weakness of the muscles of the hand and forearm, typically noted when the patient is unable to grasp a cup or eating cutlery. Resolution occurs in even the most serious cases, usually by 2 to 3 months. Numbness or tingling related to the leg incision wound has been reported in 61 percent of patients, of whom 37 percent improve within 3 months. However, up to 41 percent may have persistent numbness beyond 2 years. Incisional leg pain has been reported by 46 percent of patients, of whom 77 percent show improvement by 3 months and only 10 percent experience pain persisting beyond 2 years.

Neurological dysfunction may occur because of surgical trauma or ischemic neuropathy after the radial artery is removed as a conduit for CABG. In a consecutive series of 50 patients, the incidence of any neurological symptoms was 32 percent in the early postoperative period.[109] There were no major neurological hand complications in the presence of adequate collateral arterial blood supply. All reported

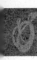

CH 79

neurological complaints were associated with sensory conduction deceleration of no clinical significance in EMG investigations of median nerve sensory-motor and ulnar nerve motor conduction. Pre- and postoperative radial nerve motor and sensory conduction records were statistically similar. The technique of radial artery harvesting does not seem to influence outcomes.

Visual symptoms are common and often consist of poor visual acuity, blurring, or scotoma. Many patients will describe prominent "floaters" that they had not experienced previously; others report seeing various spots and stripes. Because spontaneous recovery may take up to 6 months, it is ill-advised to change eyeglasses during this time in all but the most severely affected patients.

POSTOPERATIVE LABORATORY VALUES

Hematocrit levels are usually in the low 30s; even though the root cause of the usual postoperative anemia is related to hemodilution and blood loss, there may be features of anemia of "chronic disease." Platelet count <100,000 is common but thrombocytopenia much below 50,000 should be investigated. Mild metabolic acidosis with serum bicarbonate levels of 18 to 26 mEq/L and pH of 7.3 or above may occur and usually resolve with rewarming and improvement in cardiac output. Potassium levels can change rapidly, and need regular and frequent surveillance and a replacement protocol. Calcium levels may often be depressed to 7.0 mg/dl or less due to hemodilution; this rarely requires treatment—but more profound lowering, especially in the presence of hypotension, should be treated. Phosphate levels should be routinely measured immediately after surgery and appropriate therapy instituted because significant hypophosphatemia is common (34.3 percent) and may be associated with considerable morbidity, including prolonged ventilation, increased cardioactive drug requirements, and a prolonged hospital stay.[110] Cardiopulmonary bypass is associated with increases in catecholamine and cortisol levels exacerbates hyperglycemia; these changes are induced to a lesser degree by off-pump surgery. A high peak serum glucose level during CPB is an independent risk factor for death and morbidity in diabetic patients and nondiabetic patients.[111] An insulin nomogram or protocol is needed at least briefly to avoid diabetic ketoacidosis in diabetic patients and to improve leukocyte chemotaxis. Serum cTnI levels measured 24 hours after cardiac surgery predict short-, medium-, and long-term mortality, and remain independently predictive when adjusted for all other potentially confounding variables.[112] CABG is associated with a marked reduction in serum homocysteine and folate levels in the early postoperative period.[113] This reduction is, at least in part, independent of hemodilution and may be caused by an altered homocysteine turnover because of an increased consumption of glutathione during and soon after CABG.

PERIOPERATIVE ELECTROCARDIOGRAPHIC CHANGES

Hemiblocks are the most common postoperative anomaly and are generally transient—many are gone within 48 hours and the majority by hospital discharge. There is dispute about the long-term significance, with some believing that they do not worsen prognosis. Conversely, left bundle branch block as well as nonspecific interventricular conduction delay, both seen less often, are associated with a worse long-term prognosis and in the authors' experience, are associated with a significant risk of cardiac death in the first year after surgery.[114] The appearance of new Q waves should raise the concern of an MI, but unmasking of previously evident Q waves of a remote inferior wall MI has been reported, as well as disappearance of anterior Q waves. The older literature suggested that myocardial revascularization had revitalized a hibernating region that had remained viable yet had ischemia severe enough to prevent electrocardiographic depolarization.

PERIOPERATIVE CHEST X-RAY

The early postoperative chest x-ray often has a "wet" appearance with pulmonary venous upward redistribution despite normal or even low cardiac filling pressure, most likely caused by the reported decrease in colloid osmotic pressure and increase in pulmonary extravascular water. Radiographic atelectasis (commonly affecting the left lower lobe) or pleural effusion, or both, are seen in 63 percent of patients. The incidence is higher by CT scanning. Air may occasionally be seen in the pericardium as well as within the abdominal cavity via diaphragmatic eventration, and is usually benign except when it appears later or in the presence of ongoing abdominal disease.

Postoperative Chest Pain

Persistent need for parenteral narcotic medication should lead to a reevaluation to rule out fracture of the sternum or ribs, costochondral subluxation, or mediastinal wound problems such as dehiscence, instability, or infection. Pain associated with thoracotomy is more severe than with median sternotomy because it involves incising muscles. The pain of leg incisions can be more intense than the pain of a well-stabilized sternotomy. Lingering nonanginal chronic postoperative pain occurred in more than 20 percent of patients in one report. When patients with and without chronic postoperative pain were compared, the former group had significantly higher levels of anxiety and depression, and they perceived their health-related quality of life as more compromised.[115]

Good alternatives to opiates include naproxen, which may result in increased chest tube drainage but no apparent increase in other complications.[116] COX-2 inhibitors such as etodolac and diclofenac may produce better postoperative pain relief with less side effects than opiates, albeit with a short-lasting impairment of renal function.[117] Patient-controlled analgesia (PCA) and intrathecal morphine may be selectively used. Sternal wire removal should be offered to patients with anterior chest wall pain persisting late after sternotomy, when other serious postoperative complications have been excluded.

Ischemic pain may simulate preoperative symptoms but may be different following surgery. A beneficial response to nitroglycerin should be rapid and consistent with the expected time course. Suspicious pain should trigger an ECG and cardiac biomarker assessment for graft closure. For those with less certain ECG findings, atrial pacing (using the surgically implanted temporary pacing wires) for 90-second intervals at heart rates of 70, 90, 110, 130, and 150 beats per minute can be useful and can be combined with thallium-201 scintigraphy. Because early graft closure is usually thrombotic in nature, intravenous heparin is often added cautiously to avoid pericardial hemorrhage. With objective evidence of ECG changes or biomarker elevation, a strategic approach should be outlined by both the cardiologist and the cardiac surgeon. Knowledge about the downstream condition of coronary vessels and anastomotic site may greatly aid in understanding of the likelihood and potential consequences of specific graft closure. Coronary angiography or cardiac CT angiography, if it is to be performed, must be predicated on a reasonable certainty that an important graft is in jeopardy and on the expectation that a secondary attempt at revascularization is likely to succeed.

Postoperative Drug Therapy

Early postoperative use of enoxaparin and unfractionated heparin is associated with a significant increase in reexploration for postoperative bleeding, often at a significantly delayed time period after the initial surgery.[118] It has been suggested that the antiplatelet effect of aspirin may be impaired after CPB, but not after CABG without CPB. Hence, increased platelet turnover after CPB seems to contribute to aspirin resistance because an increased number of platelets might be competent to form thromboxane within the dosing intervals. Clopidogrel (75 mg/day for 5 days) may not inhibit platelet aggregation in the first 5 postoperative days and, therefore, should not be used as a sole antiplatelet agent early after CABG.[119] OPCAB patients can safely receive clopidogrel in the early postoperative period without increased risk for mediastinal hemorrhage when it is started 4 hours postoperatively, if the chest tube output is <100 ml/hour for 4 hours, and then daily.[120] Clopidogrel therapy was independently associated with decreased symptom recurrence and adverse cardiac events following OPCAB. Extending clopidogrel use beyond 30 days did not have a significant effect on defined endpoints.[121] Calcium channel blockers may be associated with significantly reduced mortality after cardiac surgery, including CABG.[122]

Hospital Course

Fast-track anesthesia has allowed early (<24 hours) transfer out of the ICU. Virtually all patients are suitable for fast track recovery. Patients with advanced age, high APACHE score, and reexploration are likely to have prolonged ICU stays (>3 days) with higher ICU mortality when renal, respiratory, or heart failure is present.[123] Readmission to the ICU after fast-track anesthesia, although uncommon at 3.3 percent, is associated with a longer second ICU stay and significant mortality.[124] Forty-three percent of ICU readmissions occur within 24 hours of discharge, and are commonly the result of pulmonary problems (47 percent), usually difficulty in clearing secretions, or arrhythmias (20 percent).

Although length of hospital stay will vary with the surgical procedure and many other factors, hospital discharge on the third to fifth postoperative day should be the goal for the patient having a straightforward CABG or valve procedure using CPB. Earlier discharge is possible in OPCAB patients—in one study, 55.8 percent of patients were discharged on the day after OPCAB with no deaths, but they had a high readmission rate of 12.7 percent.[125] Early discharge was unusual in patients with diabetes, renal failure, or recent infarction. Previous bypass, obesity, acute MI, and hypertension were associated with readmission. Discharge medications should include aspirin (81 to 325 mg), other antithrombotic drugs as dictated by a valve procedure or prior drug-eluting coronary stent, statins for those with coronary artery disease, an oral analgesic such as acetaminophen (Tylenol) with codeine, a stool softener, a beta blocker, and short-term use of any special agents used for arrhythmia management.

POSTOPERATIVE MORBIDITY

Cardiovascular Morbidity

Hypotension and Low Cardiac Output

Preoperative ventricular dysfunction is the most important determinant of postoperative low output. Additional determinants of low cardiac output include poor myocardial preservation with a long CPB pump run resulting in myocardial edema, loss of high-energy phosphates, and accumulation of oxygen-free radicals; surgical technical mishap; and perioperative MI. Distinction between intrinsic cardiac dysfunction and pericardial tamponade is essential and can present challenges not seen in nonsurgical patients. Although equalized right atrial (RA) and pulmonary capillary wedge (PCW) pressures may be the presenting situation in the surgical patient when both are low (8 to 10 mm Hg), clots can form in the pericardium resulting in nonuniform cavity compression. A common area for such clots is around the right atrium at the site of venous cannulation. This can result, for instance, in compression of the right atrium with cervical vein distention with low cardiac filling pressures.[126] Selective restriction of left atrial filling has also been observed associated with high right-sided filling pressures and low left atrial pressures. With intravenous fluid administration, PCW pressure should increase out of proportion to RA pressure (eventually exceeding the RA pressure by 5 mm Hg) in the absence of tamponade. The exception will be the patient with single chamber (right atrial) compression by pericardial clot or even a lower PCW pressure caused by clot in the region of the left atrium. Transthoracic or transesophageal bedside echo are useful to confirm normal LV contraction and the presence of pericardial blood. Technetium-tagged RBC nuclear studies with delayed imaging have proved useful in difficult cases.[127] Many surgeons simply prefer taking the patient back for exploration if tamponade is suspected but cannot be confirmed.

Hemodynamic monitoring is essential in the management of postoperative low output syndromes; however, there are pitfalls, some unique to the cardiac surgical patient. The correlation of PCW pressure or pulmonary artery diastolic pressure with LV end-diastolic pressure has been questioned in the early hours after surgery due to altered ventricular compliance from hypothermia and myocardial edema and elevated pulmonary vascular resistance. Pulmonary ventilation using positive end-expiratory pressure (PEEP) in excess of the left atrial pressure will also invalidate this relationship. Directly measured diastolic systemic or pulmonary pressures can be falsely low because of underdamping of monitoring systems. PCW pressures can appear spuriously low because of overwedging of the balloon device. Thermodilution output calculations can be inaccurate in the setting of severe tricuspid regurgitation. For these reasons, overall clinical assessment of the patient and the trend of hemodynamic performance are more important than any single measurement.

Management of hypotension or low output syndrome starts with ensuring adequate oxygenation and hematocrit and a check for acidosis. Then filling pressures should be optimized with intravenous volume to raise PCW pressure to 18 to 20 mm Hg, but this may need to be higher if there is LV hypertrophy or other cause of LV diastolic stiffness. There may be a blunted elevation of filling pressures with fluid administration in the vasodilated patient caused by sedation, fever, rewarming, or other factors. The heart rate may need to be adjusted with atrial or atrial-ventricular (AV) sequential pacing to a maximum of 90 to 100 beats/min. AV synchrony is vital to maintaining cardiac function at this time.

VASOACTIVE DRUGS. If low output or hypotension persists, vasoactive drugs are needed and should be chosen based on the framework shown in Table 79-2. Commonly used vasoactive agents, their mode of action, and dosages are discussed elsewhere in this text. Dopamine is a first choice; dobutamine, with predominantly beta$_1$ adrenergic stimulation with mild and competing alpha$_1$ and beta$_2$ adrenergic effects, results in less effect on vascular tone or heart rate. Dobutamine is indicated to improve myocardial contractility with less tendency for increases in LV filling pressures or systemic vascular resistance (SVR) than dopamine and with less tachycardia or arrhythmias. Because it does not act to release norepinephrine from endogenous stores (unlike dopamine), it may be useful when endogenous stores of norepinephrine are depleted, as in chronic heart failure. The myocardial inotropic effects of both are blunted with effective chronic beta-blockade. Early postoperative increases in myocardial oxygen consumption with these agents are accompanied by larger increases in coronary blood flow and no change in lactate release, indicating that ischemia is not present despite an increase in cardiac work.[128]

TABLE 79–2	Hemodynamic Manipulation			
BP	**PCWP**	**CO**	**SVR**	**Treatment**
↓	↑N	↓	↑	Inotrope
↓	N	N↑	↓	Alpha agent
↑	↑	↓	↑	Vasodilator

BP=blood pressure; CO=cardiac output; PCWP=pulmonary capillary wedge pressure; SVR=systemic vascular resistance.

Epinephrine, indicated to increase cardiac output and to raise blood pressure, is generally reserved for unresponsiveness to dopamine or dobutamine. There is significant renal vascular constriction with epinephrine, and beneficial increases in cardiac performance may be overshadowed by tachycardia and increased myocardial oxygen consumption resulting in myocardial ischemia if there is incomplete revascularization or residual ischemia.

Norepinephrine is indicated to raise blood pressure with little effect on heart rate or tachyarrhythmias. Its use is limited by increases in myocardial work and decreases in vital organ perfusion, especially the kidneys. It can also be used in conjunction with other agents, such as phentolamine (a weak alpha blocker and direct vascular smooth muscle relaxant) or dopamine to blunt the intense alpha constricting effects, resulting in increases in blood pressure and vascular resistance with no change in heart rate, cardiac output, or filling pressures, and with less renal vascular constriction.

Isoproterenol leads to major increases in contractility with an even greater increase in heart rate and tendency toward arrhythmias, with some reduction in SVR. There is a significant increase in myocardial oxygen demand and tendency for shunting of systemic blood flow away from splanchnic and renal sites. The beta$_2$ effects result in lower pulmonary vascular resistance and bronchodilation. The clinical indications for use are limited to its dromotropic benefits in improving AV conduction or increasing automaticity in cases of torsades or asystolic arrest, and to its significant inotropic effects in situations in which tachycardia is less of a problem as in heart transplantation. It is sometimes used for isolated right ventricular failure because it lowers right ventricular afterload.

Phenylephrine is a pure vasocontricting agent, useful for treating severe systemic vasodilation (vasoplegia), which occurs infrequently as a reaction to large doses of protamine given to reverse heparin, or as a result of the systemic inflammatory response to CPB. Another indication is in patients receiving chronic treatment with angiotensin-converting enzyme inhibitors, who may exhibit this hemodynamic picture during attempted weaning from CPB; a novel approach to preventing vasoplegia in these patients is the infusion of phenylephrine in the dosage of 0.03 μg/min during CPB. Phenylephrine is also the pressor agent of choice in treating hypotension unresponsive to fluid administration in patients with hypertrophic cardiomyopathy and severe LV outflow obstruction (see Chap. 65).

The "inodilators" amrinone and milrinone improve cardiac output by a reduction in vascular resistance and some increase in inotropy with little increase in heart rate. They have effects similar to dobutamine but with less increase in heart rate. Because of their unique mechanism of action, they can be used in addition to catecholamines such as dobutamine or alone in the case of catecholamine resistance. As second-line drugs, use is limited to resistance, continued hypotension, or tachycardia with catecholamines, alone or in conjunction with a pressor. They have special value in treating right ventricular failure as well. Unlike virtually all other vasoactive drugs, their relatively long duration of action must be kept in mind (>3 hours for amrinone; >2 hours for milrinone) during weaning to fully appreciate intrinsic cardiac performance.

A few other agents deserve mention, including calcium chloride which, given in the dose of 0.5 to 1.0 gm intravenously, will produce a modest and short-lived increase in blood pressure and SVR. Nesiritide, a recombinant B-type natriuretic peptide with vasodilating and natriuretic properties, has been used to improve cardiac output and natriuresis in severe chronic symptomatic heart failure with persistently elevated preload and afterload with limited preload response to diuretics.[129] It has been used successfully in early postoperative patients with severe LV dysfunction and persistently elevated SVR, especially in the presence of renal impairment where its renal arteriolar dilation is beneficial.[130]

RIGHT VENTRICULAR FAILURE. Acute right ventricular decompensation can lead to LV failure with catastrophic results. As with LV dysfunction, checking for oxygen saturation, optimizing heart rate and maintaining AV synchrony, correcting acidosis, and optimizing preload, afterload, and intrinsic ventricular performance are all important. Maintaining ventilator settings to avoid high-peak inspiratory pressures will help reduce pulmonary vascular resistance. However, there are certain caveats. In the surgical patient, unlike the medical patient with right ventricular infarction, fluid administration can be useful to improve right ven-

tricular function, but the limits of RA pressure elevation are less forgiving and can lead to rapid deterioration of LV function. Because the right-sided cardiac chambers are very capacious, significant volume increase may occur with only modest increases in RA pressure, resulting in leftward shift of the intraventricular septum, thereby encroaching on LV filling. Inotropic agents that improve ventricular function but reduce pulmonary artery pressures are important, so dobutamine would be preferred over dopamine and epinephrine would be preferred over norepinephrine.

Phosphodiesterase inhibitors may play a useful role, depending on systemic pressure. They generally improve ventricular contractility and reduce pulmonary artery pressures and also may have positive lusitropic effects on diastolic relaxation. However, they may also lower blood pressure, which as a rule is the limiting factor in managing severe right-sided failure. This usually requires a combination of agents with careful titration of each. Prostaglandin E$_1$ given in smaller doses will have a selective effect on pulmonary vascular resistance with little systemic effects.[131]

The selective infusion of different drugs into the right side (intravenous vasodilator/inotrope) and left side (inotrope/constrictor into the left atrium), although attractive, has not been successful in the authors' experience because of the dominantly systemic effect of these agents, especially in the presence of poor cardiac function. Exceptions would be various inhaled agents such as nitric oxide which, because of its unique route of administration and short half-life, results in a decrease in pulmonary resistance with little effect on SVR and systemic blood pressure. Unfortunately, it is very expensive, is complicated to use, and must be properly mixed with oxygen to avoid toxicity. Epoprostenol (prostacyclin, prostaglandin I$_2$) is a very short-acting, selective pulmonary vasodilator that, when inhaled, will lower pulmonary afterload with little effect on systemic pressure.[132] Iloprost, another prostacyclin analogue, lowers pulmonary vascular resistance for up to 2 hours with little effect on systemic pressures when given via aerosol.[133]

MECHANICAL CIRCULATORY SUPPORT. Intraaortic balloon counterpulsation can be placed preoperatively to stabilize the patient with high-risk ischemic heart disease, including those with recurring ischemia with precarious coronary anatomy, severe LV dysfunction, or mechanical complications of MI, such as ventricular septal rupture or acute mitral regurgitation. The postoperative indication is persistent low output or hypotension, despite safely tolerated dosages of inotropic drugs. As cardiac function improves in anticipation of balloon removal, drug support should be reduced and maintained at low levels.

Other devices can be used short term when maximal medical therapy and intraaortic balloon counterpulsation are not sufficient, including extracorporeal membrane oxygenation (ECMO) and ventricular assist devices (see Chap. 27).

Postoperative Hypertension

Defined by a mean arterial pressure of 105 mm Hg, an increase of 20 mm Hg over baseline,[134] or systolic pressure over 140 mm Hg, postoperative hypertension is a common occurrence after most cardiac operations. It is especially common and severe following valve surgery, particularly after relief of aortic stenosis. Patients who were hypertensive preoperatively and those on beta blockers preoperatively are also more prone to exhibit postoperative hypertension. Because it usually manifests early (within 1 to 2 hours), the risk is that of arterial anastomosis disruption and mediastinal bleeding, myocardial ischemia caused by excessive afterload and, if severe, the risk of stroke. Integrity of saphenous vein or internal thoracic arterial grafts may also be compromised.

Elevated serum catecholamines have been implicated as an etiological factor, along with elevation of renin, angiotensin, vasopressin, and sympathetic activity. Although it is epinephrine levels that are most profoundly elevated in the first several hours after surgery, the norepinephrine levels remain elevated for several days. Further evidence of the central role played by norepinephrine is the observation that patients with postoperative hypertension have norepinephrine levels that are consistently elevated at two- to sevenfold the upper limits of normal, whereas epinephrine levels are normal in some and only modestly elevated in others.

The hemodynamic picture is often that of normal or slightly reduced cardiac output and significant elevation of SVR. Consequently a vasodilator, most commonly nitroprusside, is used extensively for treatment. A potential concern is that of excessive reduction of diastolic pressure leading to decreased coronary blood flow and myocardial ischemia. As a result, nitroglycerin is also used in this situation. Postoperative hypertension can also be seen in the setting of hyperdynamic cardiovascular function with sinus tachycardia, normal or elevated cardiac output, and normal or slightly elevated SVR. Esmolol or labetalol given as a continuous infusion are common choices in this setting.

Perioperative Myocardial Infarction

Acute ischemic injury of the myocardium is caused primarily by the limitations of myocardial protection during the procedure. Because coronary blood flow is absent during aortic cross-clamping for surgery utilizing CABG, success depends directly on the ability to reduce myocardial oxygen requirements to a negligible level. The STS data base reports the national incidence of perioperative MI for 2005 to be 1.1 percent, based on the diagnostic criteria of CK-MB (or CK) at least five times the upper limits of normal at <24 hours postoperatively and if >24 hours, one of the following: evolutionary ST segment elevation; new Q waves in two or more contiguous leads or new left bundle branch block; or CK-MB (or CK) at least three times the upper limits of normal. The clinical risk factors appear to be older age and longer pump time as well as elevated LV end-diastolic pressure, unstable angina, and left main coronary disease.

The patient with perioperative MI usually emerges from the surgery with new Q waves that persist. "Pseudo" Q waves mimicking inferior wall infarction may occur as a result of a marked left axis shift. The occurrence of perioperative MI seems to have an adverse impact on survival acutely, but there is disagreement about any impact on long-term survival, with some reporting reduced survival and others showing impact related only to enzyme level.[135]

The mechanism of MI occurring days or weeks after the procedure is often bypass graft closure. The pattern of enzyme release, climbing to a peak a few hours after surgery, rather than the more common immediate tapering, suggests a mechanism other than the expected enzyme release from inadequate myocardial preservation and other operative events. In one report, cTnI cutoff levels of 13 ng/ml identified patients at higher risk of hospital death (9.5 versus 0.7 percent) and were the only independent predictor, but had no influence on mortality at 2 years' follow-up. In the case of CK-MB, a cut-off of >40 ng/ml was associated with higher perioperative mortality, but at 1 year this association no longer persisted. OPCAB appears to be associated with less release of cardiac enzymes but with no influence on survival at 1 year.

Postcardiotomy Syndrome

Controversy still exists regarding the etiology of the postcardiotomy syndrome. Anti-heart antibodies, present in high titers in virtually all cases, have implicated an autoimmune response.[136] Triggers for this are thought to be hemopericardium, traumatic pericarditis, or denatured myocardium. Engle and coworkers found frequent coprevalence of high titers of anti-heart antibodies in all patients with postpericardiotomy syndrome as well as a fourfold increase in antibody to adenovirus or Coxsackie B_1 to B_6 virus in 70 percent of affected patients, leading to the speculation that this is an immunological reaction triggered by acute or latent virus infection. A distinctive seasonal (spring, summer) occurrence pattern and the presence of high titers of viruses known to produce pericarditis also suggest that this is viral related. The incidence seems to be less in adults than in children and is age dependent. Signs and symptoms range from a low-grade fever, with or without white blood cell count elevation, to a profound illness with pericardial and pleuritic pain, myalgias, and lassitude with fever up to 104°F. A pericardial friction rub and often a pleural rub along with effusions are common. Elevated white cell count with a leftward shift and elevated sedimentation rate are also seen commonly. Table 79-3 shows the relative frequency of typical symptoms and physical findings in a group of 45 such patients.[137] Chest x-ray findings of cardiomegaly or pleural effusion are useful, but nonspecific. The ECG, if demonstrating diffuse ST segment elevation, may be helpful but T wave changes alone are not specific, and the ECG can be entirely normal. The echocardiographic finding of a small pericardial effusion is also not specific.

The time of appearance can be as early as 1 week after surgery, but most cases appear 2 to 3 weeks after surgery, and can appear for up to 2 months. The most serious consequences are pericardial constriction, bypass graft closure, and tamponade. Tamponade itself is uncommon. The pericardial fluid is serosanguineous, and moderate or even large effusions detected by echocardiography can usually be managed conservatively—as long as the patient remains compensated without signs of tamponade.

Therapy with oral prednisone 70 to 80 mg/day with tapering over 10 to 14 days is indicated. In the early phase of the presentation, inpatient treatment is appropriate unless the symptoms and involvement are very mild. Specifically, the systolic pressure should be above 100 mm Hg; the pulse pressure above 30 mm Hg; and the heart rate no higher than 110 beats/min. The patient should be examined frequently for evidence of increasing pulsus paradoxus or decreased urine output. Pericardial drainage is indicated when these parameters suggest tamponade (see Chap. 70) although, as noted earlier, tamponade is uncommon. Pericardiocentesis poses special risks in patients with anteriorly placed coronary grafts. The fluid can be loculated, and catheter drainage should not be attempted unless there is echocardiographic evidence of fluid anteriorly or around the cardiac apex. For these reasons pericardiocentesis should be done in the operating room or in an ICU setting, using echocardiographic guidance and only by experienced individuals. Special care is needed in skin preparation to avoid bacterial contamination. The recurrence of fluid accumulation occurs with a reported incidence of 13 percent in a pediatric population to as high as 50 percent in adults in one report. A significant rate of early bypass graft occlusion occurring as a consequence of postpericardiotomy syndrome has been reported with and without constriction, and, along with the goal of symptomatic relief, is a reason for aggressive medical therapy.

TABLE 79-3	Typical Signs and Symptoms in Postpericardiotomy Syndrome Patients*	
Sign or Symptom	No. of Patients	Incidence, %
Fever	45	100
Increased incisional pain	43	95
Pericardial or pleural rub	43	95
Malaise and weakness	31	69
Increased white blood cell count	38	84
Increased erythrocyte sedimentation rate	36	80
Pericardial or pleural fluid	30	67
Asymptomatic	2	4

*Modified from Urschel HC, Razzuk MA, Gardner M: Coronary artery bypass occlusion secondary to postcardiotomy syndrome. Ann Thorac Surg 22:528, 1976.

Constrictive Pericarditis

Constrictive pericarditis following open heart surgery may appear as early as 2 weeks or as late as several years after the procedure, the majority appearing between 3 and 12 months postoperatively.[138] The presentation is similar to that caused by other causes of constriction (see Chap. 70), where the hallmarks are distended neck veins, peripheral edema, ascites, and hepatosplenomegaly. Echocardiography is valuable in making the diagnosis (see Chap. 14), and definitive diagnosis using cardiac CT has also been reported (see Chap. 18).[139] When constriction is suspected but cannot be confirmed by equalized diastolic pressures, rapid intravenous volume infusion may illustrate the true hemodynamic features. Most patients will require surgery, consisting of either localized or radical pericardiectomy, and the surgical results are generally favorable. Patients presenting within 2 months of surgery warrant a trial of medical therapy consisting of diuretics and steroids because of the high likelihood of a more inflammatory component with less fibrosis. The mechanisms proposed for constriction include postpericardiotomy syndrome, the use of povidone-iodine pericardial irrigation, and the late effects of hemopericardium.[140]

Perioperative Arrhythmias

SUPRAVENTRICULAR TACHYARRHYTHMIAS. The incidence of atrial tachyarrhythmias after CABG is at least 30 percent, and is higher in valve-related procedures. AF is the most common arrhythmia, with an incidence of 20 to 40 percent, usually occurring between postoperative day 3 and 5. Hemodynamic compromise, systemic embolism, and anticoagulation-related complications, including pericardial tamponade, may complicate the management of such patients. Independent predictors of AF include advanced age, history of AF, diabetes, duration of CPB and cross-clamp time, inadequate protection of the atria during cross-clamping, postoperative elevation of both epinephrine and norepinephrine, and high-dose postoperative nonsteroidal antiinflammatory drug use. Meta analysis of 14 studies (16,505 patients) has shown a slightly lower incidence of AF (19 percent) with off-pump CABG than CABG with CPB (24 percent), including the elderly. Similar arrhythmias also occur in patients having noncardiac thoracic surgical procedures, but at reduced frequency.

No preventive strategies have been successful in eliminating the problem of postoperative AF, and the most successful approaches reduce the incidence by about one half. Sotalol has been shown to be effective in prevention, but is a negative inotropic agent and can cause QT prolongation with polymorphic ventricular tachycardia including torsades de pointes. Amiodarone is effective when started preoperatively,[141] intraoperatively[142] or postoperatively.[143] Biatrial pacing has also shown efficacy when applied for the first 3 days postoperatively.

Treatment of AF or atrial flutter begins with control of the heart rate (see Chap. 35); both metoprolol and esmolol are available intravenously and have the advantage of rapid onset of action and 50 percent likelihood of conversion to sinus rhythm. Diltiazem affects rate control and cardioversion to a lesser extent, but may be associated with hypotension, which can be avoided to some degree by pretreatment with intravenous calcium chloride, 1 gm intravenously. There is the possibility of complete AV block when combining intravenous beta blockers and calcium antagonists, so that pacing wires should be in place and connected to a pacing device. In one study of 640 consecutive CABG patients, amiodarone and early electrical cardioversion was more effective than non-amiodarone therapies for restoring sinus rhythm. Digoxin is not a first-line agent for prophy-

laxis, but can be given intravenously in low daily doses to supplement beta blocker effects. Other approaches to acute pharmacological conversion proven useful include: procainamide, propafenone, ibutilide, and dofetilide. The latter two agents are useful when negative inotropism is not tolerated or if bronchospasm is an issue with beta blocking agents. Both prolong the QT interval and exhibit proarrhythmic properties and should be stopped as soon as cardioversion takes place. Patients with new AF after CABG, converted to normal sinus rhythm before hospital discharge, have a benign course. Antiarrhythmic therapy as short as 1 week may be appropriate in these patients.

Low-energy cardioversion using biatrial epicardial wires implanted during surgery is effective and safe in conscious patients. Overdrive atrial pacing is very effective using temporary epicardial atrial pacing wires placed at surgery if the underlying rhythm is atrial flutter or paroxysmal atrial tachycardia. When the type of rhythm is not clear, an atrial electrogram can be extremely helpful. Bipolar electrograms can be recorded by attaching one epicardial lead to each of the two arm leads of the ECG patient cable using an alligator clip. By recording standard lead I on the lead selector, a bipolar atrial electrogram is recorded. A unipolar recording can be performed by attaching the atrial lead to the precordial patient monitoring lead. If there is any sign of organized regular depolarization of the left atrium, a trial of overdrive pacing is indicated. Starting at a pacing rate of just under the atrial flutter rate with maximal stimulus output, the pacing rate is slowly increased by 10-beat increments until atrial entrainment occurs. Failure to correct the rhythm can be caused by a number of factors, including a broken pacemaker wire or loss of contact with the epicardial surface. If only one such wire is broken, unipolar pacing is possible using the remaining functioning wire as a negative pole and an electrode patch close to the wire as the other electrode. The threshold for capture may rise above the level of output of commercially available pacing units (which is usually 20 ma), in which case repeat attempts after dosing with an antiarrhythmic agent may be successful. Occasionally atrial pacing will convert atrial flutter to fibrillation. Because the ventricular response rate is often slower and more responsive to negative chronotropic agents, this is usually a preferred rhythm. Rapid atrial pacing that is unable to convert to sinus rhythm may induce a level of higher grade AV blockade, resulting in a more controlled ventricular response rate despite persistent flutter. Heparin anticoagulation should be considered for the patient who has not converted in 24 hours and earlier if there is a history of atrial tachyarrhythmias prior to surgery. Cardioversion is reserved for patients exhibiting acute hemodynamic instability. It is desirable to have an anesthesiologist performing the sedation if possible. For elective cardioversion, anteriorposterior paddles are preferred with the posterior paddle placed at the lower tip of the scapula.

VENTRICULAR ARRHYTHMIAS. Ventricular ectopy including nonsustained ventricular tachycardia requiring at least a short course of therapy has been reported in up to 50 percent of patients, with high occurrence between postoperative days 3 and 5. Possible mechanisms include the previously mentioned elevation of circulating catecholamines, clinical or subclinical myocardial necrosis, and electrolyte abnormalities. Reports on the clinical meaning of ventricular ectopy are conflicting; one study showing that even a single ventricular ectopic beat on a resting ECG predicts a poor outcome after bypass, and a more recent study showed no difference in survival based on the presence or absence of complex ventricular ectopy on ambulatory monitoring in a post-bypass population carefully selected for normal preoperative ventricular function. Until more definitive data are available, it is prudent to individualize therapy based on known or suspected risk factors such as LV function and the patient's medical history (see Chap. 35).

An initial approach is to use atrial pacing which will often reduce the ectopy, without resorting to drugs. The decision to use procainamide to suppress simple ventricular ectopy is a common choice. For nonsustained ventricular tachycardia, magnesium and amiodarone are commonly used. For sustained ventricular tachycardia, overdrive pacing, cardioversion or intravenous amiodarone are used.[144]

CONDUCTION DEFECTS. Complete AV block, like lesser degrees of AV block, can be caused by incomplete washout of cardioplegia solution, antiarrhythmic drugs, or their toxicity. When it occurs as a specific result of the surgical procedure, it most often follows aortic valve replacement and may be transient. If caused by trauma or surgical manipulation in the area of the AV node or bundle of His, it may be temporary but often lasts several days. Surgical transection of the node during aortic valve replacement is a well-known complication and leads to permanent AV blockade.

Varying degrees of AV block are more common after aortic valve replacement than other types of cardiovascular surgery. Because of the proximity of the main bundle of His, a "danger zone" exists in the region of the noncoronary cusp and its adjacent portion of the right coronary artery above the junction of the membranous and muscular septum. Calcium débridement or suture placement in this zone was more likely to produce complete heart block.[145] Improvement in preoperative complete heart block may occur in up to 29 percent of patients after successful aortic valve replacement and can occur for up to 18 months after surgery. Elimination of medications that may potentially contribute to AV block is indicated, and the need for pacing is dependent on the adequacy of heart rate and escape mechanism. Factors weighing against recovery and the potential need for a permanent pacemaker include a heavily calcified AV node or aortic valve ring with extension into the septum, appearance of AV block hours or days after surgery, and to a lesser extent, a significant preoperative conduction defect. In the absence of excessive calcification, optimism is warranted, and it may be realistic to wait for up to 10 days for recovery before implanting a permanent pacemaker.

Surgically placed epicardial pacemaker wires are commonly used and can be life saving. Paired placement on the right atrium and right ventricle enhances diagnostic capability and allows for pacing of all modes of bradycardia and for overdrive pacing. Until used, the wires are kept in a clean, dry, electrically isolated dressing. Removal is usually planned for the day before hospital discharge and is accomplished using gentle, steady traction. Resistance can be overcome by placing the wires on a small amount of gentle traction. For patients receiving warfarin anticoagulation, the INR should be allowed to drift down close to normal (INR 1.5). The patient should be at bed rest for 2 hours after removal. On rare occasions, when removal is not possible; the wire is retracted as far out as possible and cut close to the skin. Leaving a retained wire behind is definitely not desirable because chronic or recurring sinus tract drainage can result.

Postoperative Pulmonary Morbidity

Pulmonary complications after cardiac surgery have been reviewed in detail by Weissman.[146] In a large, multicenter administrative data base of 51,351 patients who underwent CABG, the incidence of adult respiratory distress syndrome/pulmonary edema was 4.9 percent, pneumonia 0.8 percent, and other respiratory complications 3.0 percent.[147] Clinical observations suggest a 7.5 percent incidence of pulmonary morbidity, with an associated 21 percent mortality, in

cardiac surgery patients with use of CPB. Heart failure is a major cause of postoperative pulmonary morbidity, and preoperative LV systolic dysfunction has a greater correlation with postoperative respiratory failure than reduced preoperative pulmonary function. Observational and randomized studies, and one propensity analysis study from the STS data base, suggest that the incidence of pulmonary complications is lower in patients receiving OPCAB. Small studies of patients undergoing mini-sternotomy or anterior thoracotomy have not convincingly shown reductions in respiratory complications.

Data from the STS data base indicate that 6.0 percent of patients undergoing CABG using median sternotomy require mechanical ventilation for more than 48 hours, with higher incidence of 2 week hospital stay (6 percent) and higher mortality (11.3 percent) than patients undergoing off-pump surgery, including patients with COPD.[148] Factors that predispose to prolonged ventilation include low albumin, low cardiac output state, persistent postoperative bleeding, neurological complications, acute renal failure, bloodstream infections, and intraabdominal complications. Postoperative AF may lead to hemodynamic instability requiring reintubation.

PNEUMONIA

Pneumonia has been reported in 2 to 22 percent of cardiac surgery patients, and may be associated with up to 27 percent mortality. Clinical presentation occurs, on average, 4 days after surgery and ranges from fever with productive cough to acute respiratory failure requiring prolonged ventilation. Silent aspiration leading to pneumonia occurs commonly in the elderly, especially those with neurological or cognitive impairment. Other reported predisposing factors include use of H_2-receptor blockers (which increase colonization of gastric fluid with gram-negative organisms, which are then microaspirated) or broad spectrum antibiotics, presence of nasogastric tube (which facilitates microaspiration), reintubation, prolonged mechanical ventilation, and transfusion of four or more units of blood products. Diagnosis is difficult because of frequent concomitant atelectasis and pleural effusions and, hence, a high index of suspicion is warranted. Gram-negative organisms are the most common, but gram-positive bacteria appearing in the sputum before surgery are often the culprits in pneumonia occurring within 3 days of CABG. Resistant strains are emerging. Ventilator-associated pneumonia (VAP) occurs in 8 percent of patients after cardiac surgery, rising to 9 to 21 percent in those with respiratory failure, and 44 percent when intubation is longer than 7 days. It has been suggested that the risk of pneumonia increases by 1 percent with each day of mechanical ventilation. Mortality of VAP can be as high as 75 percent because of associated multiorgan failure.

ACUTE RESPIRATORY DISTRESS SYNDROME

Acute respiratory distress syndrome (ARDS) is characterized by the presence of bilateral interstitial infiltrates on chest x-ray, a pulmonary capillary wedge pressure of less than 18 mm Hg, and the presence of arterial hypoxemia leading to PaO_2/FiO_2 ratio less than 200. It occurs in less than 2 percent of patients undergoing CPB, but is associated with mortality up to 80 percent because of associated multiorgan failure. It remains unclear whether off-pump or minimally invasive procedures reduce the occurrence of ARDS. The etiology of ARDS is multifactorial and includes pulmonary endothelial trauma caused by the whole body inflammation on CPB, cessation of ventilation during CPB, translocation of enteric endotoxins secondary to intestinal hypoperfusion and ischemia, reperfusion injury, hypothermia, with contributions from untoward reactions to protamine and transfusion products. Management is aimed at general multiorgan supportive care. Prevention of ventilator-associated pulmonary mechanotrauma through the use of small tidal volumes (6 ml/kg) has been shown to reduce mortality by 25 percent; the associated permissive hypercapnea is not detrimental.[149] The use of heparin-coated circuits, hollow fiber membrane oxygenators, or high-dose steroids to modulate the systemic inflammatory response has not been shown consistently to improve outcomes.

Postoperative Bleeding

Coagulopathy is common after CPB and is related to reductions in coagulation factors, fibrinolysis, inadequate reversal of heparinization, excessive protamine administration, other perioperative drugs, and defective platelet formation. It has been suggested that CPB-induced platelet aggregation may not be caused by factors released from the tubing or its coating but may be initiated by short bouts of high shear stress, and its continuation is critically dependent on adenosine diphosphate.[150] Patients undergoing off-pump surgery show protection against activation of coagulation and fibrinolysis and against endothelial injury only during the intraoperative period; this is followed by the development of a prothrombotic pattern comparable to that of patients undergoing on-pump surgery lasting at least as late as 30 days after surgery.[151] Hemodilution with low intraoperative hematocrit levels (<19 percent) has been shown not to contribute to postoperative bleeding.[152] In contrast to standard coagulation testing (prothrombin time, fibrinogen level, D-dimer, and platelet count), platelet function as assessed by thrombelastography and whole blood aggregometry may predict both bleeding and thrombosis after off-pump CABG.[153]

Pharmacological approaches and perioperative use of antithrombotic drugs (see Chap. 82) to reduce blood loss and transfusions in the perioperative period have been reviewed.[154,155] Lysine analogues such as epsilon aminocaproic acid (Amicar) or tranexamic acid are inexpensive and effectively reduce chest tube drainage and transfusion requirements after CPB. Serine protease inhibitors such as high-dose aprotinin are expensive and, in addition, reduce the inflammatory response associated with CPB. Meta-analysis shows no significant difference in efficacy between the two classes. The specific use of aprotinin after cardiac surgery has been reviewed.[156] Aprotinin offers both hemostatic and antithrombotic benefits through its antifibrinolytic effects, by inhibiting contact activation, reducing platelet dysfunction, and attenuating the inflammatory response to CPB. It is not associated with a change in mortality, MI, or renal failure risk, but is associated with a reduced risk of stroke and a trend toward reduced incidence of AF.[157] In a retrospective study of 1524 cardiac surgery patients at high risk for postoperative stroke, the administration of full-dose aprotinin but not half-dose aprotinin was associated with a lower incidence of stroke.[158] It has been proposed that the higher level of kallikrein inhibition obtained with full dosing may be required for end-organ protection. The drug reduces perioperative bleeding during off pump CABG.[159] Desmopressin acetate (DDAVP) causes a 2- to 20-fold increase in plasma levels of factor VIII and von Willebrand factor and releases tissue plasminogen activator (tPA) and prostacyclin from vascular endothelium. The drug may be useful in mild to moderate forms of hemophilia or von Willebrand disease, in uremic patients with platelet dysfunction, and in certain forms of postoperative platelet dysfunction based on specific testing. Recombinant activated factor VII (rFVIIa) as rescue therapy in severe, uncontrollable, nonsurgical, postoperative hemorrhage after cardiac surgery is efficacious and safe, and it is not associated with adverse neurological or cardiovascular effects.[160]

Risk factors for reexploration for bleeding after CABG include advanced age, smaller body mass index, nonelective cases, and five or more distal anastomoses. Preoperative aspirin and heparin are risk factors for the on-pump CABG group. Patients needing reexploration are at higher risk of complications if the time to reexploration is prolonged.[161] Chest reexploration in ICU for bleeding or tamponade after heart surgery can be a safe alternative to return to the operating room.[162]

Judicious use of packed red blood cells is warranted as perioperative packed red blood cell transfusion carries the potential for exposure to a variety of cellular and humoral antigens, disease transmission, and immunomodulation.

Reduced transfusion is associated with reduced risk-adjusted 1-year survival after CABG, with the largest proportion of deaths occurring within 30 days.[163,164] In a group of cardiac surgery patients, the risk of pneumonia increased by 5 percent per unit of red blood cells or platelets received, with higher risk for each day that the blood was stored. However, recent observations suggest that the administration of blood per se may not lead to increased postoperative infection.[165] Point-of-care coagulation monitoring using thrombelastography has been shown to reduce postoperative transfusion requirements. Preoperative erythropoietin administered over weeks is associated with higher postoperative hemoglobin concentrations with modest reductions in transfusion requirements.[166] Alternatively, intraoperative autologous heparinized blood removal before CPB in hemodynamically stable patients and retransfused after CPB, intraoperative cell salvage, and autotransfusion of washed salvaged red blood cells also reduces need for transfusion. The volume remaining in the oxygenator and tubing set should be returned without cell processing or hemofiltration. Using the hard shell cardiotomy reservoir from the heart-lung machine, autotransfusion of the shed mediastinal blood can be continued hourly up to 18 hours after operation. Using these methods, homologous red cell transfusion may be avoided in up to 98.6 percent of patients. However, cardiotomy suction and autotransfusion of mediastinal shed blood may contribute to the perioperative inflammatory response.[167] Closed circuit extracorporeal circulation (CCECC) for CABG is associated with a significant reduction of red blood cell damage and activation of coagulation cascades similar to off-pump surgery when compared with conventional CPB; in contrast, fibrinolysis markers and IL-6 were markedly increased in CCECC postoperatively.[168] A substantially lower need for postoperative blood transfusions and a comparable hemorrhage-related reexploration rate suggests that OPCAB may avoid the morbidity and mortality associated with excessive postoperative blood loss.[169] There is a tendency toward less activation of coagulation and fibrinolysis in low-risk patients during elective OPCAB when compared with on-pump surgery.[170]

Postoperative Renal Dysfunction

The development of acute renal failure following cardiac surgery (see Chap. 88) is an uncommon but devastating complication with high morbidity and up to 42 percent 30-day mortality.[171] Significant risk factors for death are complex procedures, gastrointestinal complications, long cross-clamp time (>88 minutes), reexploration, and advanced age (>75 years). Additional independent factors contributing to the poor postoperative outcome and cardiac instability associated with acute renal failure are elevated preoperative creatinine, postoperative pulmonary edema, sepsis, multiple organ failure, hypotension, and preoperative renal failure.[172] Although CPB is considered to be an important contributor to renal injury, OPCAB improves only early mortality; long-term survival has been shown to be better in those revascularized on-pump, possibly because of more complete revascularization with CPB.

Patients with normal preoperative renal function can develop unexpected postoperative acute renal failure requiring dialysis when they undergo urgent or emergent surgery or experience intraoperative technical complications. Such patients usually have longer CPB and cross-clamp times.[173] Patients with preoperative renal dysfunction commonly experience worsening of renal function even when the perioperative course is uncomplicated, and often require dialysis in hospital or after discharge. Although in-hospital mortality may be relatively low, midterm mortality is increased compared to those who do not require dialysis. Those with large increases in postoperative creatinine (>50 percent) have higher 90-day mortality after CABG compared with patients with lower creatinine increases.[174]

Patients with elevated preoperative serum creatinine may be transfused with Hartmann solution preoperatively (30 to 50 ml/hour for 8 to 12 hours). Intraoperative mannitol (25 gm) or dopamine infusion at 3.0 to 4.5 µg/kg/min are often given; furosemide (20 to 100 mg) or hemofiltration should be considered during CPB. Fenoldopam mesylate (0.08 µg/kg/min) infusion starting at the induction of anesthesia and continued for at least the next 24 hours may reduce the risk of acute renal failure in high-risk patients.[175] Maintaining high mean perfusion pressure (around 80 mm Hg), reducing pump time, and optimizing hemodynamics with pharmacological or mechanical support are also beneficial. Infection control and renal protection should be stressed. Early and aggressive use of continuous venovenous hemofiltration postoperatively in patients with volume overload and high serum creatinine is associated with better than expected survival.

Postoperative Neurological Morbidity

Cognitive Dysfunction

Cognitive dysfunction after cardiac surgery has been reviewed.[176] It is a common short-term (33 to 83 percent) and long-term (20 to 60 percent) development, and may resolve after days to weeks or may remain as a permanent disorder, especially in terms of memory impairment. However, small studies indicate that prospective longitudinal neuropsychological performance of patients with CABG may be no different from that of comparable nonsurgical control subjects with coronary artery disease at 3 months or 1 year after baseline examination.[177] This suggests that the generally reported cognitive decline during the early postoperative period after CABG may be transient and reversible. Baseline impairment before surgery in patients with coronary artery disease may also be higher than generally suspected. Pathological findings point to a complex etiology involving the interplay of anesthesia effects, systemic inflammation, cerebral microemboli, and cerebral hypoperfusion. Long-term cognitive function and magnetic resonance imaging (MRI) evidence of brain injury are similar after off-pump and on-pump CABG. Off-pump surgery does not appear to consistently offer immunity from adverse neurocognitive outcomes, suggesting that the clinical decline may not be specific to the use of CPB, but may also occur in patients with similar risk factors for cardiovascular and cerebrovascular disease.

Cognitive dysfunction is clinically expressed as impairment of memory, concentration, language comprehension, and social integration, and is usually evaluated with a battery of neuropsychological tests assessing the cognitive domains of attention, language, verbal and visual memory, visual construction, executive function, and psychomotor and motor speed. The clinical syndrome occurs more commonly in the elderly and those with low educational status, limited social support, diabetes, and severe noncoronary atherosclerotic disease.[178] Women appear more likely to suffer injury to brain areas subserving visuospatial processing. Intraoperative hemodynamic instability, hypoxia, elevated preoperative creatinine, poor preoperative LV function, medications, and postoperative infections have been described as additional risk factors. A higher incidence of the apolipoprotein e 4 (APO e 4) in these patients has suggested a genetic susceptibility. Reduced preoperative endotoxin immunity has been proposed as a predictor of postoperative cognitive dysfunction in the elderly; a significant positive association between serum concentrations of S100B protein and neuropsychological function has been reported. The success of neuroprotective therapeutic interventions, including high-dose steroids, has been limited. Preoperative cerebral MRI may be used to predict the risk for cognitive dysfunction after CABG.

Stroke

Stroke and encephalopathy after cardiac surgery has been reviewed in detail.[179] Stroke after cardiac surgery is defined as any new permanent (manifest stroke) or temporary neurological deficit or deterioration (transient ischemic attack or prolonged reversible ischemic neurological deficit) and is confirmed by CT or MRI whenever possible. Brain MRI with diffusion-weighted imaging (DWI) is the most sensitive and accurate neurological imaging technique, and is preferred over conventional MRI (T2 and Flair) because it can reveal significantly more lesions, especially in a "watershed" distribution.[180] Stroke patients with hypoperfused brain tissue may be identified by comparing the mismatch between DWI and perfusion-weighted imaging. If DWI is not feasible, then head CT should be obtained.

The development of major stroke following CABG has been reported to be 1.5 to 5 percent in prospective studies and about 0.8 to 3.2 percent in retrospective analysis. When neurological or psychometric analyses are performed before and after the operation, the occurrence of cerebral damage has varied from 15 to 40 percent. When more sensitive biochemical markers of brain cell damage are used, there is evidence of neurological abnormality in more than 60 percent of patients. Clinically silent infarction may be far more frequent and could contribute to long-term cognitive dysfunction in patients after cardiac procedures. Serial measurement of serum S-100B protein in the initial 12 hours after CPB has been used to predict early postoperative brain injury.[181] Preoperative assessment of white matter disease by cerebral MRI imaging may also help predict the patient's risk of developing cerebral injury.[182] Use of a risk prediction model for stroke indicates that most strokes occur among patients at low or medium preoperative risk, suggesting that many of these strokes may be preventable.[183]

Most strokes develop within the first 2 days after surgery, and are up to two times more common in combined cardiac procedures or technically challenging operations.[184] Multivariable analysis has identified 10 variables that were independent predictors of stroke: history of cerebrovascular disease, peripheral vascular disease, diabetes, hypertension, previous cardiac surgery, preoperative infection, urgent operation, CPB time more than 2 hours, need for intraoperative hemofiltration, and high transfusion requirement. The temperature at which CPB is performed is not a significant factor. Stroke risk may be reduced but not eliminated with OPCAB versus conventional CABG.[184]

Perioperative stroke confers significant mortality and morbidity. The 30-day mortality for stroke patients can be 10 times greater than that of those who do not suffer stroke.[186] The greatest risk of death is noted within the first year after surgery.[187] Five-year survival is lower among patients who had major functional limitations before discharge, among those who had hypoperfusion strokes, and among patients who were discharged to locations other than home or rehabilitation facilities. Patients with ascending aortic atherosclerosis, older age (70 years), preoperative unstable angina, chronic obstructive pulmonary disease, and carotid artery disease are at risk for late postoperative stroke (new strokes during 5-year follow-up) after CABG.[188] Approximately 20 percent of patients with valve prostheses have a late embolic stroke within 15 years after valve replacement.[189] Some risk factors, such as smoking, mitral mechanical prostheses, aortic tilting-disc valves, and mitral valve surgery in the setting of LV dysfunction, are potentially modifiable.

Encephalopathy

Encephalopathy defined as diffuse brain injury occurs in 8 to 32 percent of patients depending on its manifestation, which can range from coma to confusion, agitation, and combativeness. Like stroke, it is associated with high mortality and prolonged length of hospital stay, with additional convalescence often required in a nursing home or assisted living facility. Psychotic symptoms are independently associated with prolonged ICU length of stay, multiorgan failure or shock, cardiac arrest, and higher in-hospital death after surgery.[190] Important risk factors are advanced age, carotid bruits, hypertension, diabetes, or a previous history of stroke. Perioperative hypothermia (<33°C), hypoxemia, low hematocrit, renal failure, increased serum sodium levels, infection, and stroke can be independent precipitating factors. Prompt diagnostic and therapeutic intervention aimed at the underlying problem may improve outcomes. Postoperative delirium is common after cardiac operations, and the increased use of beating-heart surgery without CPB may lead to a lower occurrence of this complication.

REDUCING RISK OF POSTOPERATIVE STROKE AND ENCEPHALOPATHY

Evidence is accumulating that patients who get perioperative encephalopathy and stroke have more preexisting cerebrovascular disease than was recognized earlier—as evidenced by routine preoperative MRI scans.[191] The main perioperative causes of neurological dysfunction are microemboli caused by air, blood cell aggregates, calcium, or aortic atheroma associated with the pump oxygenator, the potential risk of air embolization during aortic cannulation, atheroembolism from the ascending aorta, and clots from the left ventricle. There is an independent, direct association between degree of hemodilution during CPB and risk of perioperative stroke, with each percent decrease in hematocrit being associated with a 10 percent increase in the odds of suffering perioperative stroke.[192] CT studies of the head suggest that a main mechanism of brain injury is cerebral embolization rather than cerebral hypoperfusion. Studies have also demonstrated a higher incidence of perioperative stroke (5 percent) in patients with abnormal preoperative regional cerebral perfusion, which is associated with older age, current tobacco use, and diabetes mellitus.[193] The role of atheroembolism as a recognized complication of cardiac surgery has been reviewed by Djaiani.[194] The incidence of postoperative stroke increases with increased levels of aortic manipulation.[195] OPCAB reduces stroke rates by minimizing aortic manipulation. AF after CABG has also been shown to be associated with the development of embolic postoperative stroke, usually occurring late (>7 days) after operation.[196]

Although macroembolization is less common during modern cardiac surgery, microembolization remains a problem despite attention to routine precautions such as arterial filtration, reservoir filtration, filtration within the pump oxygenator, venting the aorta and—in the case of a diseased aorta—using femoral cannulation, retrograde cardioplegia through the coronary sinus, bilateral internal thoracic arteries, and insertion of proximal anastomoses on the carotid or innominate arteries. Transesophageal echocardiography, epiaortic scanning, and transcranial Doppler studies have documented embolic showers to the head during aortic cross clamping and unclamping. Superior neurological outcomes are achieved by using intraaortic filters to capture particulate debris and avoiding partial aortic clamping during OPCAB (no touch technique). In one study of 700 consecutive patients, the incidence of stroke was significantly lower in the no-touch group.[197] Logistic regression has identified partial aortic clamping as the only independent predictor of stroke, influencing this risk 28-fold. Pulsatile flow, despite modest improvements in cerebral perfusion, does not seem to offer benefits in the incidence of stroke. Maintaining high mean arterial pressure (80 to 100 mm Hg) on CPB does lead to fewer strokes than lower mean pressure (50 to 60 mm Hg). Magnesium administration is safe and improves short-term postoperative neurological function after cardiac surgery, particularly in preserving short-term memory and cortical control over brainstem functions.[198]

Neuropathy

Phrenic nerve injury is a function of pericardial slush use and surgical dissection of the internal thoracic artery. When no topical ice slush is used, an elevated left hemidiaphragm, manifest as the diaphragm being two or more intercostal spaces higher than the opposite side, occurs in 2.5 percent of cases. This incidence is increased to 26 percent when topical ice slush is used, and is further raised to 39 percent when the left internal thoracic artery is dissected. The right phrenic nerve is at risk of injury in 4 percent of patients during high mobilization of the right internal thoracic artery.[199] Phrenic nerve injury can be prevented if the pericardiophrenic branch of the internal thoracic artery is preserved. The hemidiaphragm remains elevated in 80 percent of patients at the end of 1 month, and 22 percent at the end of 1 year. Spontaneous recovery may be anticipated in two-thirds of patients in whom the injury is identified postoperatively. High right internal thoracic artery harvesting should be used with caution in patients with preoperative pulmonary dysfunction in whom phrenic nerve injury would be poorly tolerated. Bilateral diaphragmatic paralysis has a prolonged time course of recovery.

Vocal cord palsy after adult cardiac surgery has been comprehensively reviewed.[200] The cumulative incidence is 1.1 percent (33 in 2980 patients). It may also be caused by injury of the recurrent laryngeal nerves by surgical dissection or nonsurgical mechanisms such as tracheal intubation and central venous catheterization. Other reported surgical mechanisms of injury are harvesting of internal thoracic artery and topical cold cardioprotection. Bilateral nerve palsy has been lethal on at least one occasion.

The risk of perioperative optic neuropathy associated with cardiac surgery in which CPB is used is low (roughly 0.1 percent) but the outcomes can be devastating.[201] Factors that lead to the condition remain unknown, although the presence of systemic vascular disease and both an absolute and relative drop in hemoglobin during the perioperative period seem to be important. Because this condition often causes profound permanent visual loss, it has been recommended that patients, particularly those with systemic vascular disease, be made aware of this potential complication when cardiac surgery with CPB is planned. In one study of neurological complications after CABG, 17 percent had evidence of retinal infarction. Half were asymptomatic; others complained of visual disturbances such as reading difficulty or haziness in the peripheral vision. Despite the presence of definite pathological changes, recovery of visual acuity can be expected. Cortical blindness can occur and may be missed during brief daily hospital visits with patients. One should be alerted when the patient appears to stare through rather than focus on the objects of intended vision. When asked, the patient is unable to read or comprehend the content, often turning the reading material in various directions to help clarify confusion. Despite profound dysfunction, patients may not spontaneously mention such symptoms and occasionally may flatly deny their presence (Anton syndrome).[202] CT or diffusion-weighted MRI may be useful in differentiating retinal from cortical causes of visual disturbances. The prognosis for symptomatic improvement is good, but detectable visual abnormalities often remain.

Neuropsychiatric Changes

Depression is common after surgery, especially in patients with the tendency preoperatively. It can start in the first week, worsens for 2 to 3 weeks, and usually resolves by 6 weeks. Clinically significant depression such as that which interferes with daily activity and postoperative recovery, not showing signs of improvement by 4 to 6 weeks, should be formally evaluated and treated, especially if present prior to surgery. Severe psychotic symptoms are seen in 2.1 percent of postoperative patients.[203] Higher age, renal failure, dyspnea, heart failure, and LV hypertrophy are independent preoperative predisposing factors. Perioperative hypothermia (<33°C), hypoxemia, low hematocrit, renal failure, hypernatremia, infection, and stroke are independent precipitating factors. Psychotic symptoms have been shown to be independently associated with a prolonged length of stay in the intensive care unit, multiorgan failure or shock, cardiopulmonary resuscitation, and in-hospital death after surgery.

Postoperative Gastrointestinal Morbidity

Abdominal organ morbidity after cardiac surgery has been thoughtfully reviewed by Hessel.[204] In his analysis of 37 reports between 1976 and 2004 covering more than 172,000 operations, the incidence of GI complications averaged about 1.2 percent (range 0.2 to 5.5 percent) and was associated with a high 33 percent average mortality (range: 13 to 87 percent) accounting for nearly 15 percent of all cardiac surgery deaths. In the STS data base for 1997 (*www.sts.org/doc/* 2986), the incidence was 2.8 percent in 206,143 reported cases, which was about the same frequency as reoperation for bleeding, renal failure, and stroke, and nearly two to three times more frequent than sternal infection, perioperative MI, acute respiratory failure, dialysis, and multiorgan failure. Gastrointestinal bleeding was the most common; mesenteric ischemia, pancreatitis, and cholecystitis were next in frequency; paralytic ileus, perforated peptic ulcer, hepatic failure, diverticular disease, pseudo-obstruction of the colon, small-bowel obstruction, and multiorgan failure were less common. Intestinal infarction was invariably fatal, and high mortalities, averaging 70 percent, were associated with intestinal ischemia (which is usually of the nonocclusive type) and hepatic failure.

Damage to gastrointestinal organs can occur from hypoperfusion caused by vasoconstriction on CPB, atheroembolism, or perioperative hemodynamic instability leading to reduced mucosal blood flow with mucosal ischemia characterized by low mucosal pH. The systemic inflammatory response syndrome (SIRS) from endotoxemia, which can be initiated by splanchnic ischemia, has also been proposed as a mechanism. Complement activation on CPB, release of leukotriene B4 and tumor necrosis factor, and plasmin formation result in damage to endothelial and mucosal cells and extracellular matrix, as well as capillary leakage and microthrombi.

Identifying patients at higher risk for gastrointestinal morbidity and optimizing their perioperative hemodynamic management is the cornerstone for lowering this complication. Prolonged postoperative mechanical ventilation longer than 24 hours is a risk factor; others include advanced age, low ejection fraction, perioperative inotropic or mechanical support, transfusions, arrhythmias, history of renal dysfunction, reoperation, emergency surgery, and poor NYHA functional classification. Splanchnic blood flow may be improved with preoperative volume loading (1.5 ml/kg/hr of crystalloid or up to 600 ml of 6 percent hetastarch), phosphodiesterase inhibitors (milrinone), and selective gut decontamination (oral polymyxin, tobramycin, and amphotericin preoperatively for 3 days). Vasopressors should be avoided; the benefits of dopamine and dobutamine remain uncertain. The conduct of CPB may be of value: high flows, minimized circuits with low prime volumes, pulsatile flow,

maintaining hematocrit >25, minimizing atheroembolization, and perioperative administration of aspirin have been shown to contribute to reduced gastrointestinal morbidity. Early diagnosis of bowel ischemia is difficult, although very high lactate levels, persistent metabolic acidosis, leukocytosis, and ileus may be clues. An aggressive approach including early utilization of colonoscopy, peritoneal lavage, and early interventional angiography with dilation or papaverine infusion and, occasionally, surgical intervention, may be life saving.

Postoperative Infection

Obesity is the single most important risk factor for postoperative sternal dehiscence, with or without infection, after any type of cardiac operation.[205] Prophylactic sternal reinforcement seems to prevent this complication by preventing nonunion or malunion which can subsequently lead to deep sternal wound infections and mediastinitis. The current standard for sternotomy closure remains the method of wire-cerclage. Application of rigid plate fixation for sternal osteotomies affords greater stability of the sternum.[206] The application of collagen-gentamicin (260 mg gentamicin) sponges within the sternotomy before wound closure has been suggested to reduce the risk for postoperative sternal wound infections with no adverse effects on renal function.[207] Bilateral internal thoracic artery harvesting has carried a higher risk of sternal infection; skeletonization of both internal thoracic arteries, in contrast to harvesting in a pedicled fashion, significantly reduces this risk.[208] There is no difference in the incidence of sternal dehiscence, superficial or deep sternal infection among diabetic patients receiving a single internal thoracic artery or double skeletonized internal thoracic arteries.[209] Tracheostomy after median sternotomy is occasionally associated with a higher risk of deep sternal wound infection, and may be associated with significant mortality up to 55 percent.[210]

Prophylactic antibiotics, usually cefazolin, are traditionally given at induction and a second dose before wound closure with *Staphylococcus aureus* as the indicator microorganism. It has been shown that conventional doses do not provide targeted antimicrobial cefazolin plasma levels during the entire surgical procedure when CPB time exceeds 120 minutes.[211] Patients with shorter bypass times and those undergoing profound hypothermic circulatory arrest are better protected, but the generally used protocol of prophylaxis is not optimal for all patients.

Wound complications are common, with an incidence of about 32 percent after traditional saphenous vein harvesting, and with 65 percent of the patients requiring antibiotics. Radial artery infections secondary to catheterization for blood pressure monitoring are rare (0.2 percent) but potentially serious complications.[212] Strict, systematic changing of arterial lines on a timely basis is warranted. A high suspicion index, aggressive surgical treatment of bacterial arteritis, and appropriate intravenous antibiotics are critical. Early surgical intervention is necessary in cases of infected radial artery pseudoaneurysms.

Postoperative sternal wound complications after cardiac surgical procedures are classified as uninfected dehiscence (El Oakley class 1), superficial infections (El Oakley class 2A), and deep sternal wound infections (El Oakley class 2B). Deep sternal wound infection is a serious and expensive complication with a mortality rate of 15 to 20 percent despite current treatment methods. An algorithm for the management of poststernotomy complications has been proposed.[213] First-line therapy for postoperative mediastinitis is closed-drainage aspiration with Redon catheters. Preservation of the sternum should be the principal aim of surgical treatment of deep sternal wound infection. Early diagnosis, aggressive surgical débridement, and the use of vacuum-assisted systems lead to good long-term results with sternum preservation, complete healing, and nearly normal quality of life. Vacuum techniques are superior to the conventional technique of open packing and allow earlier freedom from mediastinal microbiological cultures and earlier wiring, resulting in shorter hospital stays and improved long-term survival.[214,215] Sternal resection and musculocutaneous or omental flap is a therapeutic option in extreme circumstances, and leads to safe, effective control of the infection with acceptable results in terms of pain control and quality of life.[216] However, flap coverage without osseous closure makes subsequent reoperation difficult.

Recurrence rates of sternal infections remain high at nearly 20 percent. In one study, severe recurrent staphylococcal mediastinitis was treated with either granulated sugar wound dressing or with wound débridement, v-shape sternectomy and associated muscle flap surgery. Complete cure was achieved earlier using this approach with lower hospital mortality and shorter hospital stays.[217] Conservative management with the sugar dressing method was most effective in the sickest patients (such as those requiring hemodialysis, tracheostomy, inotropic support), with no further recurrences.

Postoperative Endocrine Abnormalities

Tight glucose control, defined as glucose less than 130 mg/dl for more than 50 percent of measurements, is mandatory after cardiac surgery and requires a standard protocol and metrics to track protocol performance.[218] Reduced postoperative infections, especially mediastinitis, are experienced in diabetic patients and even in nondiabetic patients when intensive insulin therapy is used to keep blood glucose below 110 mg/dl.[219] High-dose insulin treatment (short-acting insulin 1 IU/kg/hr with 30 percent glucose 1.5 ml/kg/hr administered separately) with emphasis on strict control of blood glucose level is associated with lower blood glucose levels, better postoperative myocardial contractile function with less need for inotropic support, and lower lactate levels.[220]

Diabetes insipidus after CABG has been ascribed to altered left atrial non-osmoreceptor function that provokes altered antidiuretic hormone activity during the period of asystole on CPB.[221] The euthyroid sick syndrome (nonthyroid illness syndrome) in CABG patients is considered to be a nonspecific response to stress.[222] Reduction in serum total triiodothyronine (T_3) and free T_3 levels are associated with substantially elevated reversed T_3 levels, with values of thyroid-stimulating hormone, thyroxine, and free thyroxine remaining within normal limits. It has been proposed that intravenous T_3 may have a potential role in the management of postoperative low cardiac output states (see Chap. 81).

REFERENCES

1. Hannan EL, O'Donnell JF, Kilburn H Jr., et al: Investigation of the relationship between volume and mortality for surgical procedures performed in New York state hospitals. JAMA 262:503, 1989.
2. Zinman D: Heart surgeons rated: State reveals patient mortality records. Newsday, Nassau and Suffolk Ed. December 18:3, 1991.

Preoperative Risk Assessment

3. Weissman C: Pulmonary complications after cardiac surgery. Semin Cardiothorac Vasc Anesth 8:185, 2004.
4. Scott D, Barnett LS, Halpin AM, et al: Postoperative complications among octogenarians after cardiovascular surgery. Ann Thorac Surg 76:726, 2003.
5. Edwards MB, Taylor KM: Outcomes in nonagenarians after heart valve replacement operation. Ann Thorac Surg 75:830, 2003.
6. Maurer MS, Luchsinger JA, Wellner R, et al: The effect of body mass index on complications of cardiac surgery in the oldest old. J Am Geriatr Soc 50:988, 2002.
7. Paul A, Kurlansky DB, Williams EA, et al: Arterial grafting results in reduced operative mortality and enhanced long-term quality of life in octogenarians. Ann Thorac Surg 76:418, 2003.
8. Matsuura K, Kobayashi J, Tagusari O, et al: Off-pump coronary artery bypass grafting using only arterial grafts in elderly patients. Ann Thorac Surg 80:144, 2005.
9. Bacchetta MD, Ko W, Girardi LN, et al: Outcomes of cardiac surgery in nonagenarians: A 10-year experience. Ann Thorac Surg 75:1215, 2003.
10. Guru V, Fremes SE, Tu JV, et al: Time-related mortality for women after coronary artery bypass graft surgery: A population-based study. J Thorac Cardiovasc Surg 127:1158, 2004.
11. Blankstein R, Ward RP, Arnsdorf M, et al: Female gender is an independent predictor of operative mortality after coronary artery bypass graft surgery. Circulation 112 (suppl I):I-323, 2005.
12. Ioannis K, Toumpoulis CE, Anagnostopoulos SK, et al: Assessment of independent predictors for long-term mortality between women and men after coronary artery bypass grafting: Are women different from men? J Thorac Cardiovasc Surg 131:343, 2006.
13. Falcoz PE, Chocron S, Laluc F, et al: Gender analysis after elective open heart surgery: A two-year comparative study of quality of life. Ann Thorac Surg 81:1637, 2006.
14. Stephanie L, Taylor AF, Arvind K, et al: Racial and ethnic disparities in care: The perspectives of cardiovascular surgeons. Ann Thorac Surg 81:531, 2006.
15. Karl F, Welke MJ, Barnett MS, et al: Limitations of hospital volume as a measure of quality of care for coronary artery bypass graft surgery. Ann Thorac Surg 80:2114, 2005.
16. Hsyien-Chia W, Chao-Hsiun T, Herng-Ching L, et al: Association between surgeon and hospital volume in coronary artery bypass graft surgery outcomes: A population-based study. Ann Thorac Surg 81:835, 2006.
17. Anoar Z, Thomas A, Schwann CJ, et al: Is Hospital procedure volume a reliable marker of quality for coronary artery bypass surgery? A comparison of risk and propensity adjusted operative and midterm outcomes. Ann Thorac Surg 79:1961, 2005.

18. Geert JMG, van der Heijden HM, Nathoe EWL, et al: Meta-analysis on the effect of off-pump coronary bypass surgery. Eur J Cardiothorac Surg 26:81-84, 2004.
19. Wijeysunder DN, Beattie WS, Djaiani G, et al: Off-pump coronary artery surgery for reducing mortality and morbidity: Meta-analysis of randomized and observational studies. J Am Coll Cardiol 46(5):872-882, 2005.
20. Parolari A, Alamanni F, Polvani G, et al: Meta-analysis of randomized trials comparing off-pump with on-pump coronary artery bypass graft patency. Ann Thorac Surg 80: 2121, 2005.
21. Joseph F, Sabik EH III, Blackstone PL, et al: Is reoperation still a risk factor in coronary artery bypass surgery? Ann Thorac Surg 80:1719, 2005.
22. Joseph F, Sabik EH III, Blackstone A, et al: Influence of patient characteristics and arterial grafts on freedom from coronary reoperation. J Thorac Cardiovasc Surg 131:90, 2006.
23. Newall N, Grayson AD, Oo AY, et al: Preoperative white blood cell count is independently associated with higher perioperative cardiac enzyme release and increased 1-year mortality after coronary artery bypass grafting. Ann Thorac Surg 81:583, 2006.
24. Albert AA, Beller CJ, Walter JA, et al: Preoperative high leukocyte count: A novel risk factor for stroke after cardiac surgery. Ann Thorac Surg 75:1550, 2003.
25. Newall N, Grayson AD, Oo AY, et al: Relationship between white cell count, neuropsychologic outcome, and microemboli in 161 patients undergoing coronary artery bypass surgery. J Thorac Cardiovasc Surg 131:1358, 2006.
26. Robert F, Salamonsen JA, Anderson M, et al: Total leukocyte control for elective coronary bypass surgery does not improve short-term outcome. Ann Thorac Surg 79:2032, 2005.
27. Biancari F, Lahtinen J, Lepojärvi S, et al: Preoperative C-reactive protein and outcome after coronary artery bypass surgery. Ann Thorac Surg 76:2007, 2003.
28. Kangasniemi OP, Biancari F, Luukkonen F, et al: Preoperative C-reactive protein is predictive of long-term outcome after coronary artery bypass surgery. Eur J Cardiothorac Surg 29:983, 2006.
29. Lo B, Fijnheer R, Nierich AP, et al: C-Reactive protein is a risk indicator for atrial fibrillation after myocardial revascularization. Ann Thorac Surg 79:1530, 2005.
30. Cerillo AG, Bevilacqua S, Storti S, et al: Free triiodothyronine: A novel predictor of postoperative atrial fibrillation. Eur J Cardiothorac Surg 24:487, 2003.
31. Thielmann M, Massoudy P, Neuhäuser M, et al: Risk stratification with cardiac troponin I in patients undergoing elective coronary artery bypass surgery. Eur J Cardiothorac Surg 27:861, 2005.
32. Thielmann M, Massoudy P, Neuhauser M, et al: Prognostic value of preoperative cardiac troponin I in patients undergoing emergency coronary artery bypass surgery with non ST-elevation or ST-elevation acute coronary syndromes. Circulation 114 (suppl I):I-448, 2006.
33. Bybee KA, Powell BD, Valeti U, et al: Preoperative aspirin therapy is associated with improved postoperative outcomes in patients undergoing coronary artery bypass grafting. Circulation 112 (suppl I):I-286, 2005.
34. Arun K, Srinivasan AD, Grayson D, et al: Effect of preoperative aspirin use in off-pump coronary artery bypass operations. Ann Thorac Surg 76:41, 2003.
35. Michael E, Halkos JH, Levy EC, et al: Early experience with activated recombinant factor VII for intractable hemorrhage after cardiovascular surgery. Ann Thorac Surg 79:1303, 2005.
36. Ascione R, Ghosh A, Rogers CA, et al: In-hospital patients exposed to clopidogrel before coronary artery bypass graft surgery: A word of caution. Ann Thorac Surg 79:1210, 2005.
37. Englberger L, Faeh B, Berdat P, et al: Impact of clopidogrel in coronary artery bypass grafting. Eur J Cardiothorac Surg 26:96, 2004.
38. Lindvall G, Sartipy I, van der Linden J: Aprotinin reduces bleeding and blood product use in patients treated with clopidogrel before coronary artery bypass grafting. Ann Thorac Surg 80:922, 2005.
39. Van der Linden J, Lindvall G, Sartipy U: Aprotinin decreases postoperative bleeding and number of transfusions in patients on clopidogrel undergoing coronary artery bypass graft surgery. Circulation 112 (suppl I):I-276, 2005.
40. Karabulut H, Toraman F, Evrenkaya S, et al: Clopidogrel does not increase bleeding and allogenic blood transfusion in coronary artery surgery. Eur J Cardiothorac Surg 25:419, 2004.
41. Fox KA, Mehta SR, Peters R, et al: Benefits and risks of the combination of clopidogrel and aspirin in patients undergoing surgical revascularization for non-ST-elevation acute coronary syndrome: The Clopidogrel in Unstable angina to prevent Recurrent ischemic Events (CURE) Trial. Circulation 110:1202, 2004.
42. Edward H, Kincaid ML, Monroe DL, et al: Effects of preoperative enoxaparin versus unfractionated heparin on bleeding indices in patients undergoing coronary artery bypass grafting. Ann Thorac Surg 76:124, 2003.
43. Pleym H, Videm V, Wahba A, et al: Heparin resistance and increased platelet activation in coronary surgery patients treated with enoxaparin preoperatively. Eur J Cardiothorac Surg 29:933, 2006.
44. Leslie L, Clark JS, Ikonomidis FA, et al: Preoperative statin treatment is associated with reduced postoperative mortality and morbidity in patients undergoing cardiac surgery: An 8-year retrospective cohort study. J Thorac Cardiovasc Surg 131:679, 2006.
45. Pan W, Pintar T, Anton J, et al: Statins are associated with a reduced incidence of perioperative mortality after coronary artery bypass graft surgery. Circulation 110 (suppl II):II-45, 2004.
46. Pascual A, Arribas JM, Tornel PL, et al: Preoperative statin therapy and troponin t predict early complications of coronary artery surgery. Ann Thorac Surg 81:78-83, 2006.
47. Patti G, Chello M, Candura M, et al: Randomized trial of atorvastatin for reduction of postoperative atrial fibrillation in patients undergoing cardiac surgery. Circulation 114:1455, 2006.

48. Arnoni RT, Arnoni AS, Bonini RCA, et al: Risk factors associated with cardiac surgery during pregnancy. Ann Thorac Surg 76:1605, 2003.

49. Ngaage DL, Martins E, Orkell E, et al: The impaction of the duration of mechanical ventilation on the respiratory outcome in smokers undergoing cardiac surgery. Cardiovasc Surg 10:345, 2002.

50. Lindhout AH, Wouters CW, Noyez L: Influence of obesity on in-hospital and early mortality and morbidity after myocardial revascularization. Eur J Cardiothorac Surg 26:535, 2004.

51. Christopher H, Wigfield JD, Lindsey AM, et al: Is extreme obesity a risk factor for cardiac surgery? Eur J Cardiothorac Surg 29:434, 2006.

52. Orhan G, Biçer Y, Aka SA, et al: Coronary artery bypass graft operations can be performed safely in obese patients. Eur J Cardiothorac Surg 25:212, 2004.

53. Habib RH, Zacharias A, Schwann TA, et al: Effects of obesity and small body size on operative and long-term outcomes of coronary artery bypass surgery: A propensity-matched analysis. Ann Thorac Surg 79:1976, 2005.

54. Nicola L, Giuseppe N, Mario G, et al: Coronary artery bypass grafting in type II diabetic patients: A comparison between insulin-dependent and non-insulin-dependent patients at short- and mid-term follow-up. Ann Thorac Surg 76:1149, 2003.

55. Kubal C, Srinivasan AK, Grayson AD, et al: Effect of risk-adjusted diabetes on mortality and morbidity after coronary artery bypass surgery. Ann Thorac Surg 79:1570, 2005.

56. Carlos A, Estrada JA, Young L, et al: Outcomes and perioperative hyperglycemia in patients with or without diabetes mellitus undergoing coronary artery bypass grafting. Ann Thorac Surg 75:1392, 2003.

57. Srinivasan AK, Grayson AD, Fabri BM: On-pump versus off-pump coronary artery bypass grafting in diabetic patients: A propensity score analysis. Ann Thorac Surg 78:1604, 2004.

58. Leavitt BJ, Sheppard L, Maloney C, et al: Effect of diabetes and associated conditions on long-term survival after coronary artery bypass graft surgery. Circulation 110 (suppl II):II-41, 2004.

59. Briand M, Pibarot P, Despres JP, et al: Metabolic syndrome is associated with faster degeneration of bioprosthetic valves. Circulation 114 (suppl I):I-512, 2006.

60. Daniel J, O'Rourke HB, Quinton WP, et al: Survival in patients with peripheral vascular disease after percutaneous coronary intervention and coronary artery bypass graft surgery. Ann Thorac Surg 78:466, 2004.

61. Shishir K, Ghassan M, Antony D, et al: Coronary surgery in patients with peripheral vascular disease: Effect of avoiding CPB. Ann Thorac Surg 77:1245, 2004.

62. Monney P, Hayoz D, Tinguely F, et al: High prevalence of unsuspected abdominal aortic aneurysms in patients hospitalised for surgical coronary revascularisation. Eur J Cardiothorac Surg 25:65, 2004.

63. Noyez L, Plesiewicz I, Verheugt FW: Estimated creatinine clearance instead of plasma creatinine level as prognostic test for postoperative renal function in patients undergoing coronary artery bypass surgery. Eur J Cardiothorac Surg 29:461, 2006.

64. Abu-Omar Y, Mussa S, Naik MJ, et al: Evaluation of cystatin C as a marker of renal injury following on-pump and off-pump coronary surgery. Eur J Cardiothorac Surg 27:893, 2005.

65. Zakeri R, Freemantle N, Barnett V, et al: Relation between mild renal dysfunction and outcomes after coronary artery bypass grafting. Circulation 112 (suppl I):I-270, 2005.

66. Antunes PE, Prieto D, Ferrão de Oliveira J, et al: Renal dysfunction after myocardial revascularization. Eur J Cardiothorac Surg 25:597, 2004.

67. van de Wal RMA, van Brussel BL, Voors AA, et al: Mild preoperative renal dysfunction as a predictor of long-term clinical outcome after coronary bypass surgery. J Thorac Cardiovasc Surg 129:330, 2005.

68. Mohan P, Devbhandari AJ, Duncan AD, et al: Effect of risk-adjusted, non-dialysis-dependent renal dysfunction on mortality and morbidity following coronary artery bypass surgery: A multi-centre study. Eur J Cardiothorac Surg 29:964, 2006.

69. Beckermann J, Van Camp J, Li S, et al: On-pump versus off-pump coronary surgery outcomes in patients requiring dialysis: Perspectives from a single center and the United States experience. J Thorac Cardiovasc Surg 131:1261, 2006.

70. Massad MD, Kpodonu J, Lee J, et al: Outcome of coronary artery bypass operations in patients with renal insufficiency with and without renal transplantation. Chest 128:855, 2005.

71. Zhang L, Garcia JM, Hill PC, et al: Cardiac surgery in renal transplant recipients: Experience from Washington Hospital Center. Ann Thorac Surg 81:1379, 2006.

72. Trachiotis GD, Hanumara D, McKenna L, et al: Surgical revascularization after acute myocardial infarction in patients with end-stage renal disease. Eur J Cardiothorac Surg 26:671, 2004.

73. Rogers CA, Angelini GD, Culliford LA, et al: Coronary surgery in patients with preexisting chronic atrial fibrillation: Early and midterm clinical outcome. Ann Thorac Surg 81:1676, 2006.

74. Quader MA, McCarthy PM, Gillinov AM, et al: Does preoperative atrial fibrillation reduce survival after coronary artery bypass grafting? Ann Thorac Surg 77:1514, 2004.

75. Canver CC, Nichols RD, Kronke GM: Influence of age-specific lung function on survival after coronary bypass. Ann Thorac Surg 66:144, 1998.

76. Durand DJ, Perler BA, Roseborough GS, et al: Mandatory versus selective preoperative carotid screening: A retrospective analysis. Ann Thorac Surg 78:159, 2004.

77. Ho PM, Masoudi FA, Spertus JA, et al: Depression predicts mortality following cardiac valve surgery. Ann Thorac Surg 79:1255, 2005.

78. Lin CH, Lin FY, Wang SS, et al: Cardiac surgery in patients with liver cirrhosis. Ann Thorac Surg 79:1551, 2005.

79. Hayashida N, Shoujima T, Teshima H, et al: Clinical outcome after cardiac operations in patients with cirrhosis. Ann Thorac Surg 77:500, 2004.

80. Birdas TJ, Landis JT, Haybron D, et al: Outcomes of coronary artery bypass grafting in patients with connective tissue diseases. Ann Thorac Surg 79:1610, 2005.

81. Pai KR, Ramnarine IR, Grayson AD, et al: The effect of chronic steroid therapy on outcomes following cardiac surgery: A propensity-matched analysis. Eur J Cardiothorac Surg 28:138, 2005.

82. Mestres CA, Chuquiure JE, Claramonte X, et al: Long-term results after cardiac surgery in patients infected with the human immunodeficiency virus type-1 (HIV-1). Eur J Cardiothorac Surg 23:1007, 2003.

83. Mistiaen WP, Van Cauwelaert P, Muylaert P, et al: Effect of prior malignancy on survival after cardiac surgery. Ann Thorac Surg 77:1593, 2004.

84. Fecher AM, Birdas TJ, Haybron D, et al: Cardiac operations in patients with hematologic malignancies. Eur J Cardiothorac Surg 25:537, 2004.

85. Massoudy P, Cetin SM, Thielmann M, et al: Antiphospholipid syndrome in cardiac surgery—An underestimated coagulation disorder? Eur J Cardiothorac Surg 28:133, 2005.

86. Gerrah R, Shargal Y, Elami A: Impaired oxygenation and increased hemolysis after cardiopulmonary bypass in patients with glucose-6-phosphate dehydrogenase deficiency. Ann Thorac Surg 76:523, 2003.

87. Morawski W, Sanak M, Cisowski M, et al: Prediction of the excessive perioperative bleeding in patients undergoing coronary artery bypass grafting: Role of aspirin and platelet glycoprotein IIIa polymorphism. J Thorac Cardiovasc Surg 130:791, 2005.

Preoperative Risk Calculation

88. Donald S, Likosky WC, Nugent RA, et al: Comparison of three measurements of cardiac surgery mortality for the Northern New England Cardiovascular Disease Study Group. Ann Thorac Surg 81:1393, 2006.

89. Gao D, Grunwald GK, Rumsfeld JS, et al: Time-varying risk factors for long-term mortality after coronary artery bypass graft surgery. Ann Thorac Surg 81:793, 2006.

90. Gaudino M, Glieca F, Alessandrini F, et al: High risk coronary artery bypass patient: Incidence, surgical strategies, and results. Ann Thorac Surg 77:574, 2004.

91. Laurie A, Shroyer W, Coombs LP, et al: The society of thoracic surgeons: 30-Day operative mortality and morbidity risk models. Ann Thorac Surg 75:1856, 2003.

92. Asimakopoulos G, Al-Ruzzeh S, Ambler G, et al: An evaluation of existing risk stratification models as a tool for comparison of surgical performances for coronary artery bypass grafting between institutions. Eur J Cardiothorac Surg 23:935, 2003.

93. Nilsson J, Algotsson L, Höglund P, et al: EuroSCORE predicts intensive care unit stay and costs of open heart surgery. Ann Thorac Surg 78:1528, 2004.

94. Toumpoulis IK, Anagnostopoulos CE, Swistel DG, et al: Does EuroSCORE predict length of stay and specific postoperative complications after cardiac surgery? Eur J Cardiothorac Surg 27:128, 2005.

95. Nilsson J, Algotsson L, Höglund P, et al: Early mortality in coronary bypass surgery: The EuroSCORE versus The Society of Thoracic Surgeons risk algorithm. Ann Thorac Surg 77:1235, 2004.

96. Jin R, Grunkemeier GL: Additive vs. logistic risk models for cardiac surgery mortality. Eur J Cardiothorac Surg 28:240, 2005.

97. Gogbashian A, Sedrakyan A, Treasure T: EuroSCORE: A systematic review of international performance. Eur J Cardiothorac Surg 25:695, 2004.

98. Zingone B, Pappalardo A, Dreas L: Logistic versus additive EuroSCORE. A comparative assessment of the two models in an independent population sample. Eur J Cardiothorac Surg 26:1134, 2004.

99. Karthik S, Srinivasan AK, Grayson AD, et al: Limitations of additive EuroSCORE for measuring risk stratified mortality in combined coronary and valve surgery. Eur J Cardiothorac Surg 26:318, 2004.

100. Toumpoulis IK, Anagnostopoulos CE, Toumpoulis SK, et al: EuroSCORE predicts long-term mortality after heart valve surgery. Ann Thorac Surg 79:1902, 2005.

101. Jin R, Grunkemeier GL, Starr AS, et al: Validation and refinement of mortality risk models for heart valve surgery. Ann Thorac Surg 80:471, 2005.

102. Butchart EG, Ionescu A, Payne N, et al: A new scoring system to determine thromboembolic risk after heart valve replacement. Circulation 108 (suppl II):II-68, 2003.

Normal Postoperative Convalescence

103. Laffey JG, Boylan JF, Cheng DCH: The systemic inflammatory response to cardiac surgery. Anesthesiology 97:215, 2002.

104. Flynn M, Reddy S, Shepherd W, et al: Fast-tracking revisited: Routine cardiac surgical patients need minimal intensive care. Eur J Cardiothorac Surg 25:116, 2004.

105. Johnson D, Kelm C, Thomson D, et al: The effect of physical therapy on respiratory complications following cardiac valve surgery. Chest 109:638, 1996.

106. Pasquina P, Tramer MR, Walder B: Prophylactic respiratory physiotherapy after cardiac surgery: Systematic review. BMJ 327:1379, 2003.

107. Hulzebos EHJ, Helder PJM, Favie NJ, et al: Preoperative intensive inspiratory muscle training to prevent postoperative pulmonary complications in high risk patients undergoing CABG surgery. JAMA 296:1851-1857, 2006.

108. Breuer AC, Furlan AJ, Hansen MR, et al: Neurologic complications of open heart surgery. Clevel Clin Q 48:205-206, 1981.

109. Ikizler M, Ozkan S, Dernek S, et al: Does radial artery harvesting for coronary revascularization cause neurological injury in the forearm and hand? Eur J Cardiothorac Surg 28:420, 2005.

110. Cohen J, Kogan A, Sahar G, et al: Hypophosphatemia following open heart surgery: Incidence and consequences. Eur J Cardiothorac Surg 26:306, 2004.

CH 79

111. Doenst T, Wijeysundera D, Karkouti K, et al: Hyperglycemia during CPB is an independent risk factor for mortality in patients undergoing cardiac surgery. J Thorac Cardiovasc Surg 130:1144, 2005.

112. Croal BL, Hillis GL, Gibson PH, et al: Relationship between postoperative cardiac troponin I levels and outcome of cardiac surgery. Circulation 114:1468, 2006.

113. Storti S, Cerillo AG, Rizza A, et al: Coronary artery bypass grafting surgery is associated with a marked reduction in serum homocysteine and folate levels in the early postoperative period. Eur J Cardiothorac Surg 26:682, 2004.

114. Bateman TM, Weiss MH, Czer LSC, et al: Fascicular conduction distutbances and ischemic heart disease: Adverse prognosis despite coronary revascularization. J Am Coll Cardiol 5:632, 1985.

115. Taillefer MC, Carrier M, Bélisle S, et al: Prevalence, characteristics, and predictors of chronic nonanginal postoperative pain after a cardiac operation: A cross-sectional study. J Thorac Cardiovasc Surg 131:1274, 2006.

116. Bainbridge D, Cheng DC, Martin JE, et al: NSAID—analgesia, pain control and morbidity in cardiothoracic surgery. Can J Anesth 53:46, 2006.

117. Immer FF, Immer-Bansi AS, Trachsel N, et al: Pain treatment with a COX-2 inhibitor after coronary artery bypass operation: A randomized trial. Ann Thorac Surg 75:490, 2003.

118. Jones HU, Muhlestein JB, Jones KW, et al: Early postoperative use of unfractionated heparin or enoxaparin is associated with increased surgical re-exploration for bleeding. Ann Thorac Surg 80:518, 2005.

119. Lim E, Cornelissen J, Routledge T, et al: Clopidogrel did not inhibit platelet function early after coronary bypass surgery: A prospective randomized trial. J Thorac Cardiovasc Surg 128:432, 2004.

120. Halkos ME, Cooper WA, Petersen R, et al: Early administration of clopidogrel is safe after off-pump coronary artery bypass surgery. Ann Thorac Surg 81:815, 2006.

121. Gurbuz AT, Zia A, Vuran AC, et al: Postoperative clopidogrel improves mid-term outcome after off-pump coronary artery bypass graft surgery: A prospective study. Eur J Cardiothorac Surg 29:190, 2006.

122. Wijeysundera DN, Beattie WS, Rao V, et al: Calcium antagonists are associated with reduced mortality after cardiac surgery: A propensity analysis. Thorac Cardiovasc Surg 127:755, 2004.

123. Hein OV, Birnbaum J, Wernecke K, et al: Prolonged intensive care unit stay in cardiac surgery: Risk factors and long-term-survival. Ann Thorac Surg 81:880, 2006.

124. Kogan A, Cohen J, Raanani E, et al: Readmission to the intensive care unit after "fast-track" cardiac surgery: Risk factors and outcomes. Ann Thorac Surg 76:503, 2003.

125. Baisden CE, Bolton JWR, Riggs MW: Readmission and mortality in patients discharged the day after off-pump coronary bypass surgery. Ann Thorac Surg 75:68, 2003.

Postoperative Cardiovascular Morbidity

126. Batmen T, Gray R, Chaux A, et al: Right atrial tamponade caused by hematoma complicating coronary artery bypass graft surgery: Clinical hemodynamic and scintigraphic correlates. J Thorac Cardiovasc Surg 84:413, 1982.

127. Bateman TM, Czer L, Kass RM, et al: Cardiac causes of shock early after open heart surgery: Etiologic classification by radionuclide ventriculography. Circulation 71:1153, 1985.

128. Sethna DH, Gray R, Moffitt EA, et al: Dobutamine and cardiac oxygen balance in patients following myocardial revascularization. Anesth Analg 61:917, 1982.

129. Gordon G, Rastegar H, Khabbaz K, et al: Perioperative use of nesiritide in adult cardiac surgery. Anesth Analg 98:SCA1, 2004.

130. Moazamin N, Damiano RJ, Bailey MS, et al: Nesiritide (BNP) in the management of postoperative cardiac patients. Ann Thorac Surg 75:1974, 2003.

131. Camara ML, Aris A, Alvarez J, et al: Hemodynamic effects of prostaglandin E and isoproterenol early after cardiac operations for mitral stenosis. J Thorac Cardiovasc Surg 103:1177, 1992.

132. De Wet CJ, Affleck DG, Jacobsohn E, et al: Inhaled prostacyclin is safe, effective and affordable in patients with pulmonary hypertension, right heart dysfunction, and refractory hypoxemia after cardiothoracic surgery. J Thorac Cardiovasc Surg 127:1058, 2004.

133. Rex S, Busch T, Vettelschoss M, et al: Intraoperative management of severe pulmonary hypertension during cardiac surgery with inhaled iloprost. Anesthesiology 99:745, 2003.

134. Gray R, Bateman TB, Czer LSC, et al: Use of esmolol in hypertension after cardiac surgery. Am J Cardiol 56:49F, 1985.

135. Gray R, Matloff JM, Conklin CM, et al: Perioperative myocardial infarction: Late clinical course after coronary artery bypass surgery. Circulation 66:1185, 1982.

136. Engle MA, McCabe JC, Ebert PA, et al: The postpericardiotomy syndrome and antiheart antibodies. Circulation 49:401, 1974.

137. Urschel HC, Razzuk MA, Gardner M: Coronary artery bypass occlusion secondary to postcardiotomy syndrome. Ann Thorac Surg 22:528, 1976.

138. Ng SH, Dorosti K, Sheldon WC: Constrictive pericarditis following cardiac surgery—Cleveland Clinic experience: Report of 12 cases and review. Cleve Clin Q 51:39, 1983.

139. Bateman TM, Gray R, Whiting JS, et al: Cine-computed tomographic evaluation of aorto-coronary bypass graft patency. J Am Coll Cardiol 8:693, 1986.

140. Kutcher MA, King SB, Alimurung BN, et al: Constrictive pericarditis as a complication of cardiac surgery: Recognition of an entity. Am J Cardiol 50:742, 1982.

141. Daoud EG, Strickberger SA, Man KC, et al: Preoperative oral amiodarone as prophylaxis against atrial fibrillation after heart surgery. N Engl J Med 337:1785, 1997.

142. White CM, Giri S, Tsikouris JP, et al: A comparison of two individual amiodarone regimens to placebo in open heart surgery patients. Ann Thorac Surg 74:69, 2002.

143. Yazigi A, Rahbani P, Zied HA, et al: Postoperative oral amiodarone as prophylaxis against atrial fibrillation after coronary artery surgery. J Cardiothorac Vasc Anesth 16:603, 2002.

144. Pinto RP, Romerill DB, Nasser WK, et al: Prognosis of patients with frequent premature ventricular complexes and nonsustained ventricular tachycardia after coronary artery bypass surgery. Clin Cardiol 19:321, 1996.

145. Gray R, Bateman TM, Czer LSC, et al: Esmolol: A new ultrashort-acting beta-adrenergic blocking agent for rapid control of heart rate in postoperative supraventricular tachyarrhythmias. J Am Coll Cardiol 5:1451, 1985.

Postoperative Pulmonary Morbidity

146. Weissman C: Pulmonary complications after cardiac surgery. Sem Cardiothorac Vasc Anesth 8:185, 2004.

147. Mack MJ, Brown PP, Kugelmass AD, et al: Current status and outcomes of coronary revascularization 1999-2002: 148,000 Surgical and percutaneous procedures. Ann Thorac Surg 77:761, 2004.

148. Shroyer ALW, Coombs LP, Peterson ED, et al: The Society of Thoracic Surgeons. 30-Day operative mortality and morbidity risk models. Ann Thorac Surg 75:1856, 2003.

149. The Acute Respiratory Syndrome Network: Ventilation with lower tidal volumes as compared with traditional tidal volumes for acute lung injury and the acute respiratory distress syndrome. N Engl J Med 342:1301, 2000.

Postoperative Bleeding

150. Borgdorff P, Tangelder GJ: Pump-induced platelet aggregation with subsequent hypotension: Its mechanism and prevention with clopidogrel. J Thorac Cardiovasc Surg 131:813, 2006.

151. Parolari A, Mussoni L, Frigerio M, et al: Increased prothrombotic state lasting as long as one month after on-pump and off-pump coronary surgery. Thorac Cardiovasc Surg 130:303, 2005.

152. Dial S, Delabays E, Albert M, et al: Hemodilution and surgical hemostasis contribute significantly to transfusion requirements in patients undergoing coronary artery bypass. Thorac Cardiovasc Surg 130:654, 2005.

153. Poston R, Gu J, Manchio J, et al: Platelet function tests predict bleeding and thrombotic events after off-pump coronary bypass grafting. Eur J Cardiothorac Surg 27:584, 2005.

154. Ozier Y, Schlumberger S: Pharmacological approaches to reducing blood loss and transfusions in the surgical patient. Can J Anesth 53(6 suppl):S21, 2006.

155. Vincentelli A, Jude B, Belisle S: Antithrombotic therapy in cardiac surgery. Can J Anesth 53(6 suppl):S89, 2006.

156. Mangano DT, Tudor IC, Dietzel C: The risk associated with aprotinin in cardiac surgery. N Engl J Med 354:353, 2006.

157. Sedrakyan A, Treasure T, Elefteriades JA: Effect of aprotinin on clinical outcomes in coronary artery bypass graft surgery: A systematic review and meta-analysis of randomized clinical trials. J Thorac Cardiovasc Surg 128:442, 2004.

158. Frumento RJ, O'Malley CM, Bennett-Guerrero E, et al: Stroke after cardiac surgery: A retrospective analysis of the effect of aprotinin dosing regimens. Ann Thorac Surg 75:479, 2003.

159. Poston RS, White C, Gu J, et al: Aprotinin shows both hemostatic and antithrombotic effects during off-pump coronary artery bypass grafting. Ann Thorac Surg 81:104, 2006.

160. Bishop CV, Renwick WEP, Hogan C, et al: Recombinant activated factor VII: Treating postoperative hemorrhage in cardiac surgery. Ann Thorac Surg 81:875, 2006.

161. Karthik S, Grayson AD, McCarron EE, et al: Reexploration for bleeding after coronary artery bypass surgery: Risk factors, outcomes, and the effect of time delay. Ann Thorac Surg 78:527, 2004.

162. Charalambous CP, Zipitis CS, Keenan DJ, et al: Chest reexploration in the intensive care unit after cardiac surgery: A safe alternative to returning to the operating theater. Ann Thorac Surg 81:191, 2006.

163. Kuduvalli M, Oo AY, Newall N, et al: Effect of perioperative red blood cell transfusion on 30-day and 1-year mortality following coronary artery bypass surgery. Eur J Cardiothorac Surg 27:592, 2005.

164. Koch CG, Li L, Duncan AI, et al: Transfusion in coronary artery bypass grafting is associated with reduced long-term survival. Ann Thorac Surg 81:1650, 2006.

165. Ali ZA, Lim E, Motalleb-Zadeh R, et al: Allogenic blood transfusion does not predispose to infection after cardiac surgery. Ann Thorac Surg 78:1542, 2004.

166. Murphy GJ, Rogers CS, Lansdowne WB, et al: Safety, efficacy, and cost of intraoperative cell salvage and autotransfusion after off-pump coronary artery bypass surgery: A randomized trial. Thorac Cardiovasc Surg 130:20, 2005.

167. Westerberg M, Bengtsson A, Jeppsson A: Coronary surgery without cardiotomy suction and autotransfusion reduces the postoperative systemic inflammatory response. Ann Thorac Surg 78:54, 2004.

168. Wippermann J, Albes JM, Hartrump M, et al: Comparison of minimally invasive closed circuit extracorporeal circulation with conventional cardiopulmonary bypass and with off-pump technique in CABG patients: Selected parameters of coagulation and inflammatory system. Eur J Cardiothorac Surg 28:127, 2005.

169. Frankel TL, Stamou SC, Lowery RC, et al: Risk factors for hemorrhage-related reexploration and blood transfusion after conventional versus coronary revascularization without CPB. Eur J Cardiothorac Surg 27:494, 2005.

170. Vedin J, Antovic A, Ericsson A, et al: Hemostasis in off-pump compared to on-pump coronary artery bypass grafting: A prospective, randomized study. Ann Thorac Surg 80:586, 2005.

Postoperative Renal Dysfunction

171. Luckraz H, Gravenor MB, George R, et al: Long and short-term outcomes in patients requiring continuous renal replacement therapy post CPB. Eur J Cardiothorac Surg 27:906, 2005.

Medical Management of the Patient Undergoing Cardiac Surgery

172. Elahi MM, Lim MY, Joseph RN, et al: Early hemofiltration improves survival in post-cardiotomy patients with acute renal failure. Eur J Cardiothorac Surg 26:1027, 2004.

173. Gaudino M, Luciani N, Giungi S, et al: Different profiles of patients who require dialysis after cardiac surgery. Ann Thorac Surg 79:825, 2005.

174. Brown JR, Cochran RP, Dacey LJ, et al: Preoperative increases in serum creatinine are predictive of increased 90-day mortality after coronary artery bypass grafting. Circulation 114 (suppl. I):I-409, 2006.

175. Ranucci M, Soro G, Barzaghi N, et al: Fenoldopam prophylaxis of postoperative acute renal failure in high-risk cardiac surgery patients. Ann Thorac Surg 78:1332, 2004.

Postoperative Neurologic Morbidity

176. Gao L, Taha R, Gauvin D, et al: Postoperative cognitive dysfunction after cardiac surgery. Chest 128:3664, 2005.

177. Selnes OA, Grega MA, Borowicz LM Jr, et al: Cognitive changes with coronary artery disease: A prospective study of coronary artery bypass graft patients and nonsurgical controls. Ann Thorac Surg 75:1377, 2003.

178. Ho PM, Arciniegas DB, Grigsby J, et al: Predictors of cognitive decline following coronary artery bypass graft surgery. Ann Thorac Surg 77:597, 2004.

179. McKhann GM, Grega MA, Borowicz LM Jr, et al: Stroke and encephalopathy after cardiac surgery: An update. Stroke 37:562, 2006.

180. Wityk RJ, Goldsborough MA, Hillis A, et al: Diffusion—and perfusion weighted brain magnetic resonance imaging in patients with neurologic complications after cardiac surgery. Arch Neurol 58:571, 2001.

181. Ueno T, Iguro Y, Yamamoto H, et al: Serial measurement of serum S-100B protein as a marker of cerebral damage after cardiac surgery. Ann Thorac Surg 75:1892, 2003.

182. Andréll P, Jensen C, Norrsell H, et al: White matter disease in magnetic resonance imaging predicts cerebral complications after coronary artery bypass grafting. Ann Thorac Surg 79:74, 2005.

183. Likosky DS, Leavitt BJ, Marrin CAS, et al: Intra- and postoperative predictors of stroke after coronary artery bypass grafting. Ann Thorac Surg 76:428, 2003.

184. Bucerius J, Gummert JF, Borger MA, et al: Stroke after cardiac surgery: A risk factor analysis of 16,184 consecutive adult patients. Ann Thorac Surg 75:472, 2003.

186. Baker RA, Hallsworth LJ, Knight JL: Stroke after coronary artery bypass grafting. Ann Thorac Surg 80:1746, 2005.

187. Dacey LJ, Likosky DS, Leavitt BJ, et al: Perioperative stroke and long-term survival after coronary artery bypass graft surgery. Ann Thorac Surg 79:532, 2005.

188. Schachner T, Zimmer A, Nagele G, et al: Risk factors for late stroke after coronary artery bypass grafting. J Thorac Cardiovasc Surg 130:485, 2005.

189. Ruel M, Masters RG, Rubens FD, et al: Late incidence and determinants of stroke after aortic and mitral valve replacement. Ann Thorac Surg 78:77, 2004.

190. Giltay EJ, Huijskes R, Kho KH, et al: Psychotic symptoms in patients undergoing coronary artery bypass grafting and heart valve operation. Eur J Cardiothorac Surg 30:140, 2006.

191. Goto T, Baba T, Honma K, et al: Magnetic resonance imaging and postoperative neurologic dysfunction in the elderly patients undergoing coronary artery bypass surgery. Ann Thorac Surg 72:137, 2001.

192. Karkouti K, Djaiani G, Borger MA, et al: Low hematocrit during cpb is associated with increased risk of perioperative stroke in cardiac surgery. Ann Thorac Surg 80:1381, 2005.

193. Moraca R, Lin E, Holmes JH IV, et al: Impaired baseline regional cerebral perfusion in patients referred for coronary artery bypass. J Thorac Cardiovasc Surg 131:540, 2006.

194. Djaiani GN: Aortic arch atheroma: stroke reduction in cardiac surgical patients. Sem Cardiothorac Vasc Anesth 10:143, 2006.

195. Kapetanakis EI, Stamou SC, Dullum MKC, et al: The impact of aortic manipulation on neurologic outcomes after coronary artery bypass surgery: A risk-adjusted study. Ann Thorac Surg 78:1564, 2004.

196. Lahtinen J, Biancari F, Salmela E, et al: Postoperative atrial fibrillation is a major cause of stroke after on-pump coronary artery bypass surgery. Ann Thorac Surg 77:1241, 2004.

197. Lev-Ran O, Braunstein R, Sharony R, et al: No-touch aorta off-pump coronary surgery: The effect on stroke. J Thorac Cardiovasc Surg 129:307, 2005.

198. Bhudia SK, Cosgrove DM, Naugle RI, et al: Magnesium as a neuroprotectant in cardiac surgery: A randomized clinical trial. J Thorac Cardiovasc Surg 131:853, 2006.

199. Deng Y, Byth K, Paterson HS: Phrenic nerve injury associated with high free right internal thoracic artery harvesting. Ann Thorac Surg 76:459, 2003.

200. Dimarakis I, Protopapas AD: Vocal cord palsy as a complication of adult cardiac surgery: Surgical correlations and analysis. Eur J Cardiothorac Surg 26:773, 2004.

201. Kalyani SD, Miller NR, Dong LM, et al: Incidence of and risk factors for perioperative optic neuropathy after cardiac surgery. Ann Thorac Surg 78:34, 2004.

202. Meyendorf R: In Becker R (ed): Psychopathological and Neurological Dysfunctions following Open Heart Surgery. Berlin, New York, Springer Verlag, 1982, pp 16-31.

203. Giltay EJ, Huijskes R, Kho KH, et al: Psychotic symptoms in patients undergoing coronary artery bypass grafting and heart valve operation. Eur J Cardiothorac Surg 30:140, 2006.

Postoperative Gastrointestinal Morbidity, Infection and Endocrine Abnormalities

204. Hessel EA II: Abdominal organ injury after cardiac surgery. Sem Cardiothorac Vasc Anesth 8:243, 2004.

205. Molina JE, Lew RS, Hyland KJ: Postoperative sternal dehiscence in obese patients: Incidence and prevention. Ann Thorac Surg 78:912, 2004.

206. Song DH, Lohman RF, Renucci JD, et al: Primary sternal plating in high-risk patients prevents mediastinitis. Eur J Cardiothorac Surg 26:367, 2004.

207. Friberg O, Svedjeholm R, Söderquist B, et al: Local gentamicin reduces sternal wound infections after cardiac surgery: A randomized controlled trial. Ann Thorac Surg 79:153, 2005.

208. De Paulis R, de Notaris S, Scaffa R, et al: The effect of bilateral internal thoracic artery harvesting on superficial and deep sternal infection: The role of skeletonization. J Thorac Cardiovasc Surg 129:536, 2005.

209. Momin AU, Deshpande R, Potts J, et al: Incidence of sternal infection in diabetic patients undergoing bilateral internal thoracic artery grafting. Ann Thorac Surg 80:1765, 2005.

210. Force SD, Miller DL, Petersen R, et al: Incidence of deep sternal wound infections after tracheostomy in cardiac surgery patients. Ann Thorac Surg 80:618, 2005.

211. Caffarelli AD, Holden JP, Baron EJ, et al: Plasma cefazolin levels during cardiovascular surgery: Effects of CPB and profound hypothermic circulatory arrest. J Thorac Cardiovasc Surg 131:1338, 2006.

212. El-Hamamsy I, Dürrleman N, Stevens LM, et al: Incidence and outcome of radial artery infections following cardiac surgery. Ann Thorac Surg 76:801, 2003.

213. Doyle AJ, Large SR, Murphy F: Sternal wound dehiscence after internal mammary artery harvesting. Logical management. Part 2. Interact Cardiovasc Thorac Surg 4:511, 2005.

214. Fuchs U, Zittermann A, Stuettgen B, et al: Clinical outcome of patients with deep sternal wound infection managed by vacuum-assisted closure compared to conventional therapy with open packing: A retrospective analysis. Ann Thorac Surg 79:526, 2005.

215. Sjogren J, Nilsson J, Gustafsson R, et al: The impact of vacuum-assisted closure on long-term survival after post-sternotomy mediastinitis. Ann Thorac Surg 80:1270, 2005.

216. Immer FF, Durrer M, Mühlemann KS, et al: Deep sternal wound infection after cardiac surgery: Modality of treatment and outcome. Ann Thorac Surg 80:957, 2005.

217. De Feo M, De Santo LS, Romano G, et al: Treatment of recurrent staphylococcal mediastinitis: Still a controversial issue. Ann Thorac Surg 75:538, 2003.

218. Carr JM, Sellke FW, Fey M, et al: Implementing tight glucose control after coronary artery bypass surgery. Ann Thorac Surg 80:902, 2005.

219. Van den Berghe G, Wouters P, Weekers F, et al: Intensive insulin therapy in the critically ill patient. N Engl J Med 345:1359, 2001.

220. Koskenkari JK, Kaukoranta PK, Kiviluoma KT, et al: Metabolic and hemodynamic effects of high-dose insulin treatment in aortic valve and coronary surgery. Ann Thorac Surg 80:511, 2005.

221. Kuan P, Messenger JC, Ellestad MH: Transient central diabetes insipidus after aortocoronary bypass operations. Am J Cardiol 52:1181-1183, 1983.

222. Cerillo AG, Sabatino L, Bevilacqua S, et al: Nonthyroidal illness syndrome in off-pump coronary artery bypass grafting. Ann Thorac Surg 75:82, 2003.

CHAPTER **80**

Introduction, 2013

Assessment of Risk, 2013
Ischemic Heart Disease, 2013
Hypertension, 2014
Heart Failure, 2014

Valvular Heart Disease, 2015

Congenital Heart Disease
in Adults, 2015

Arrhythmias, 2016

Decision to Undergo Diagnostic
Testing, 2016

Tests to Improve Identification
and Definition of Cardiovascular
Disease, 2018

Overview of Anesthesia Used in
Cardiac Patients Undergoing
Noncardiac Surgery, 2020
Spinal and Epidural Anesthesia, 2021
Monitored Anesthesia Care, 2021
Intraoperative Hemodynamics and
    Myocardial Ischemia, 2021

Postoperative
Management, 2021
Overview of Postoperative Response
    to Surgery, 2021
Postoperative Intensive Care, 2021
Postoperative Pain
    Management, 2022

Surveillance and Implications
of Perioperative Cardiac
Complications, 2022

Strategies to Reduce Cardiac Risk
of Noncardiac Surgery, 2022
Surgical Revascularization, 2022
Pharmacological Interventions, 2024
Nonpharmacological
    Interventions, 2026

References, 2027

Guidelines, 2028

Anesthesia and Noncardiac Surgery in Patients with Heart Disease

Lee A. Fleisher and Kim A. Eagle

INTRODUCTION

Cardiovascular morbidity and mortality represent a significant risk in the patient with known, or risk factors for, cardiovascular disease undergoing noncardiac surgery. The costs of perioperative myocardial injury add substantially to the total health care expenditures, with an average increased length of stay of 6.8 days for patients with perioperative myocardial ischemic injury. The implications of perioperative cardiovascular complications not only affect the immediate period but may also influence outcome over the subsequent 1 to 2 years. Over the past three decades there has been a steady progression of knowledge beginning with identification of those at greatest risk to recent randomized trials to identify strategies to reduce perioperative cardiovascular complications. To disseminate best practices, guidelines have been developed to provide information for management of high-risk patients. This chapter attempts to distill this information, incorporating the available guidelines while acknowledging that these guidelines are constantly evolving with new information available.

ASSESSMENT OF RISK

The identification of perioperative cardiac risk has been an area of active study for three decades, and much of the work has focused on the development of clinical risk indices. The most recent index was developed in a study of 4315 patients aged 50 years or older undergoing elective major noncardiac procedures in a tertiary-care teaching hospital. Six independent predictors of complications were identified and included in a Revised Cardiac Risk Index (RCRI): high-risk type of surgery, history of ischemic heart disease, history of congestive heart failure, history of cerebrovascular disease, preoperative treatment with insulin, and preoperative serum creatinine greater than 2.0 mg/dl, with increasing cardiac complication rates noted with increasing number of risk factors.[1] The RCRI has become the standard tool in the literature for assessing the prior probability of perioperative cardiac risk in a given individual and serves to direct the decision to perform cardiovascular testing and implement perioperative management protocols. RCRI is discussed throughout the rest of the chapter.

Ischemic Heart Disease

A patient may be evaluated by numerous care systems before noncardiac surgery. The patient may be seen by a primary caregiver or a cardiologist.

However, many patients are only evaluated by the surgeon or anesthesiologist immediately before surgery. The stress of noncardiac surgery may raise heart rate (HR) preoperatively, which has been associated with a high incidence of symptomatic and asymptomatic myocardial ischemia. Therefore the preoperative clinical evaluation of the patient may identify stable or unstable coronary artery disease (CAD). Patients with acute coronary syndromes such as unstable angina or decompensated heart failure of ischemic origin have a high risk of developing further decompensation, myocardial necrosis, and death during the perioperative period. Such patients clearly warrant further evaluation and medical stabilization. If the noncardiac surgery is truly emergent, there are several case series using intra-aortic balloon bump counterpulsation as a means of providing short-term myocardial protection beyond maximal medical therapy.

If the patient does not have unstable symptoms, then the identification of known or symptomatic stable CAD or risk factors for CAD can guide the need for further diagnostic evaluation or changes in perioperative management. In determining the extent of the preoperative evaluation, it must be remembered that testing should not be performed unless the results will affect perioperative management. These management changes include cancellation of surgery for prohibitive risk compared with benefit, delay of surgery for further medical management, coronary interventions before noncardiac surgery, use of an intensive care unit, and changes in monitoring. As discussed later, the potential benefit of preoperative coronary revascularization has been questioned and there may be less of a need for extensive testing.

The patient with stable angina represents a continuum from mild angina with extreme exertion to dyspnea with angina after walking up a few stairs. The patient who only manifests angina after strenuous exercise often does not demonstrate signs of left ventricular dysfunction and generally can be stabilized with adequate medical therapy, particularly treatment with beta-blocking agents. In contrast, a patient with dyspnea on mild exertion would be at high risk for developing perioperative ventricular dysfunction, myocardial ischemia, and possible myocardial infarction (MI). Such patients have a high probability of having extensive CAD, and additional monitoring or cardiovascular testing should be contemplated, depending on the surgical procedure, institutional factors, and prior evaluation.

Traditionally, coronary risk assessment for noncardiac surgery in patients with a prior MI was based on the time interval between the MI and surgery. Multiple studies demonstrated an increased incidence of reinfarction after noncardiac surgery if the prior MI was within 6 months of the operation. With improvements in perioperative care, this time interval has become shortened.[2] However, the relative importance of the intervening time interval is less relevant in the current era of thrombolytics, angioplasty, and routine coronary risk stratification after an acute MI. Although some patients with a recent MI may continue to have myocardium at risk for subsequent ischemia and infarction, most patients in the United States will have had their critical coronary stenosis evaluated and revascularized or will be on maximal medical therapy. The American Heart Association/American College of Cardiology Task Force on Perioperative Evaluation of the Cardiac Patient Undergoing Noncardiac Surgery has suggested that the highest-risk cohort is a patient within 6 weeks of his or her MI, a time period during which plaque and myocardial healing occur. After that period, risk stratification is based on the presentation of disease (i.e., those with active ischemia being at highest risk).[3,4]

Hypertension

In the 1970s a series of case studies that were presented changed the prevailing thought that antihypertensive agents should be discontinued before surgery. The reports suggested that poorly controlled hypertension was associated with untoward hemodynamic responses and that antihypertensive agents should be continued perioperatively. However, several large prospective studies did not establish mild-to-moderate hypertension as an independent predictor of postoperative cardiac complications such as cardiac death, postoperative MI, heart failure, or arrhythmias. Therefore much of the approach to the patient with hypertension relies on management strategies from the nonsurgical literature.

A hypertensive crisis in the postoperative period, defined as a diastolic blood pressure (BP) greater than 120 mm Hg and clinical evidence of impending or actual end organ damage, poses a definite risk of MI and cerebrovascular accident. Diagnostic criteria include papilledema or other evidence of increased intracranial pressure, myocardial ischemia, or acute renal failure. Several precipitants of hypertensive crises have been identified including preeclampsia or eclampsia, pheochromocytomas, abrupt clonidine withdrawal before surgery, the use of chronic monoamine oxidase inhibitors with or without sympathomimetic drugs in combination, and inadvertent discontinuation of antihypertensive therapy.

Chronic hypertension may indirectly predispose patients to perioperative myocardial ischemia because CAD is more prevalent in these patients. Even in the absence of CAD, patients with chronic hypertension may have episodes of myocardial ischemia, perhaps due to impaired coronary vasodilator reserve and autoregulation such that higher arterial pressures are required to maintain adequate perfusion of vital organs. Because of vascular stiffness, hypertensive patients are also predisposed to hypotension and hence lower filling pressures. Thus hypertensive patients with

known peripheral and coronary vascular disease must have preoperative BP levels monitored and controlled.

The Study of Perioperative Ischemia Research Group, in which patients had continuous perioperative electrocardiogram monitoring, showed that a history of hypertension was one of five independent predictors of postoperative ischemia and one of three independent predictors of increased postoperative mortality. Patients with a history of hypertension had almost twice the risk of developing postoperative myocardial ischemia and almost four times the risk of postoperative death than did patients without hypertension in the first 48 hours postoperatively.

Thus whether patients with mild-to-moderate hypertension should be considered at greater than average risk of perioperative myocardial ischemia remains uncertain because of often conflicting reports from the past 20 years. Surgery generally need not be postponed or canceled in the otherwise uncomplicated patient with mild-to-moderate hypertension.[3] Antihypertensive medications should be continued perioperatively,[5] and BP should be maintained near preoperative levels to reduce the risk of myocardial ischemia. In patients with more severe hypertension, such as diastolic BP greater than 110 mm Hg, the potential benefits of delaying surgery in order to optimize antihypertensive medications should be weighed against the risk of delaying the surgical procedure. With rapid-acting intravenous agents, BP can usually be controlled within a matter of several hours. Weksler and colleagues[6] studied 989 chronically treated hypertensive patients who presented for noncardiac surgery with diastolic BP between 110 and 130 mm Hg and who had no previous MI, unstable or severe angina pectoris, renal failure, pregnancy-induced hypertension, left ventricular hypertrophy, previous coronary revascularization, aortic stenosis, preoperative dysrhythmias, conduction defects, or stroke. The control group had their surgery postponed and remained in the hospital for BP control, and the study patients received 10 mg of nifedipine intranasally delivered. No statistically significant differences in postoperative complications were observed, suggesting that this subset of patients without significant cardiovascular comorbidities can proceed with surgery despite elevated BP the day of surgery.

Isolated systolic hypertension (systolic BP > 160 mm Hg and diastolic BP < 90 mm Hg) has been identified as a risk factor for cardiovascular complications in the general population, and successful treatment reduces the future risk of stroke. However, only one study has directly assessed the relationship between cardiovascular disease and preoperative isolated systolic hypertension. In a multicenter study of patients undergoing coronary artery bypass grafting (CABG), the presence of isolated systolic hypertension has been associated with a 30 percent increased incidence of cardiovascular complications compared with normotensive individuals.[7] Because it is unknown if these findings can be generalized to the noncardiac surgery and whether treatment will affect outcome, definition of the best approach will require further study. Treatment of systolic hypertension in the elderly is particularly challenging because the diastolic pressures are often low and unusually sensitive to hypovolemia.

Heart Failure

Heart failure associates in virtually all studies with perioperative cardiac morbidity after noncardiac surgery. Goldman and colleagues identified a third heart sound or signs of heart failure as portending the highest perioperative risks.[8] For patients who present for noncardiac surgery with signs or symptoms of heart failure, its underpinnings require characterization before major noncardiac surgery. The pre-

CH 80

operative evaluation should aim to identify the underlying coronary, myocardial, and/or valvular heart disease and assess the severity of systolic and diastolic dysfunction. Treatment of decompensated hypertrophic cardiomyopathy is different than dilated cardiomyopathy, and thus the preoperative evaluation can influence perioperative management. In particular, this assessment may influence perioperative fluid and vasopressor management. Ischemic cardiomyopathy is of greatest concern because the patient has a substantial risk for developing further ischemia leading to myocardial necrosis and potentially a downward spiral. In such patients, a pulmonary artery catheter or transesophageal echocardiography may be helpful.

Obstructed hypertrophic cardiomyopathy was formerly regarded as a high-risk condition associated with high perioperative morbidity. A retrospective review of perioperative care in 35 patients, however, suggested that the risk of general anesthesia and major noncardiac surgery is low in such patients. However, this study did suggest that spinal anesthesia may be relatively contraindicated in view of the sensitivity of cardiac output to preload in this condition. Haering and colleagues[9] studied 77 patients with asymmetrical septal hypertrophy who were retrospectively identified from a large database. Forty percent of patients had one or more adverse perioperative cardiac events including one patient who had an MI and ventricular tachycardia that required emergent cardioversion. The majority of the events were perioperative congestive heart failure. No perioperative deaths occurred. Unlike the original cohort of patients, the type of anesthesia was not an independent risk factor. Important independent risk factors for adverse outcome (as seen generally) included major surgery and increasing duration of surgery.

VALVULAR HEART DISEASE

The presence of aortic stenosis places the patient at increased risk, with those with critical stenosis associated with the highest risk of cardiac decompensation in patients undergoing elective noncardiac surgery. Kertai[10] has reported a substantially higher rate of perioperative complications in patients with severe aortic stenosis compared with patients with moderate aortic stenosis (31 percent [5/16] versus 11 percent [10/92]). The presence of any of the classic triad of angina, syncope, and heart failure in a patient with aortic stenosis should alert the clinician to the need for further evaluation and potential interventions, usually valve replacement. However, many patients with severe or critical aortic stenosis may be asymptomatic. Preoperative patients with aortic systolic murmurs warrant a careful history and physical examination and often further evaluation. Importantly, several recent case series of patients with critical aortic stenosis demonstrate that, when necessary, noncardiac surgery can be performed with acceptable risk.[11,12] For the most part, these cases have included patients with few or no symptoms but a valve area less than 0.05 cm^2. Alternatively, aortic valvuloplasty represents an option for occasional patients. Although the long-term outcome of patients who undergo aortic balloon valvuloplasty is generally poor primarily because of restenosis, this procedure may be used for temporary benefit surrounding noncardiac surgery in patients who cannot undergo valve replacement in the short term. The considerable procedure-related morbidity and mortality risk must be carefully considered before recommending this strategy as a means to try to lower the risk of noncardiac surgery.

Mitral valve disease tends to cause less risk of perioperative complications than aortic stenosis. However, occult mitral stenosis from rheumatic heart disease is still encountered on occasion and can lead to severe left heart failure in the presence of tachycardia and/or volume loading. In contrast to aortic valvuloplasty, mitral valve balloon valvuloplasty often yields reasonable short- and long-term benefit, especially in younger patients with predominant mitral stenosis but without severe mitral valve leaflet thickening or significant subvalvular fibrosis and calcification.

In the perioperative patient with a functioning prosthetic heart valve, the major issues are antibiotic prophylaxis and anticoagulation. All patients with prosthetic valves who undergo procedures that can cause transient bacteremia should be prophylaxed.[13] In patients with prosthetic valves, the risk of increased bleeding during a procedure while receiving antithrombotic therapy must be weighed against the increased risk of a thromboembolism caused by stopping the therapy. The common practice for patients undergoing noncardiac surgery with a mechanical prosthetic valve in place is for the cessation of oral anticoagulants 3 days before surgery. This allows the international normalized ratio to fall to less than 1.5 times normal. The oral anticoagulants can then be resumed on postoperative day 1. Using a similar protocol, Katholi and colleagues[14] had no perioperative episodes of thromboembolism or hemorrhage in 25 patients. An alternative approach in patients at high risk for thromboembolism is the conversion to heparin during the perioperative period. The heparin can then be discontinued 4 to 6 hours before surgery and resumed shortly thereafter. Many current prosthetic valves have a lower risk of valve thrombosis than the older ball-in-cage valves, for instance, so the risk of heparin may outweigh the benefit in the perioperative setting. According to the American Heart Association/American College of Cardiology Guidelines, heparin can usually be reserved for those who have had a recent thrombosis or embolus (arbitrarily within 1 year), those with demonstrated thrombotic problems when previously off therapy, those with the Björk-Shiley valve, and those with more than three risk factors (atrial fibrillation, previous thromboembolism, hypercoagulable condition, and mechanical prosthesis).[15] A lower threshold for recommending heparin should be considered in patients with mechanical valves in the mitral position, in whom a single risk factor would be sufficient evidence of high risk. Subcutaneous low-molecular-weight heparin offers an alternative outpatient approach.[16] Having a discussion between the surgeon and cardiologist regarding the optimal perioperative management is critical.

CONGENITAL HEART DISEASE IN ADULTS

Congenital heart disease afflicts 500,000 to 1 million adults in the United States alone. The nature of both the underlying anatomy and any anatomic correction affect the perioperative plan and incidence of complications, which include infection, bleeding, hypoxemia, hypotension, and paradoxical embolization. A major concern in the patient with congenital heart disease is the presence of pulmonary hypertension and Eisenmenger syndrome. It has traditionally been thought that regional anesthesia should be avoided in these patients because of the potential for sympathetic blockade and worsening of the right to left shunt. However, a review of the published literature incorporating 103 cases found that overall perioperative mortality was 14 percent; patients receiving regional anesthesia had a mortality of 5 percent, whereas those receiving general anesthesia had a mortality of 18 percent.[17] The authors concluded that most deaths probably occurred as a result of the surgical procedure and disease and not anesthesia. Although perioperative and peripartum mortalities were high, many anesthetic agents and techniques had been used with success. Patients with congenital heart disease are at risk for infective endocarditis and should receive antibiotic prophylaxis. A recent review discusses the anesthetic management of these patients in detail.[18]

ARRHYTHMIAS (see Chaps. 33 and 35)

Cardiac arrhythmias are common in the perioperative period, particularly in the elderly or patients undergoing thoracic surgery. Predisposing factors include prior arrhythmias, underlying heart disease, hypertension, perioperative pain (e.g., hip fractures), severe anxiety, and other situations that heighten adrenergic tone. A prospective study of 4181 patients who were 50 years of age or older demonstrated supraventricular arrhythmia in 2 percent of patients during and 6.1 percent after surgery. Perioperative atrial fibrillation raises several concerns including an incidence of stroke.[19] Therefore early treatment to restore sinus rhythm or control the ventricular response and initiate anticoagulation is indicated. Amar and colleagues[20] evaluated the prophylactic value of intravenous diltiazem in a randomized, placebo-controlled trial in high-risk thoracic surgery and reported that prophylactic diltiazem reduced the incidence of clinically significant atrial arrhythmias. Balser and colleagues[21] studied 64 cases of postoperative supraventricular tachyarrhythmia. After adenosine administration, patients who remained in supraventricular tachyarrhythmia were prospectively randomized to receive either intravenous diltiazem or intravenous esmolol for ventricular rate control and reported that intravenous esmolol produced a more rapid (2-hour) conversion to sinus rhythm than did intravenous diltiazem. The literature has recently been reviewed, and an algorithm for treatment produced (Fig. 80-1).[19]

Although ventricular arrhythmias were originally identified as a risk factor for perioperative morbidity, more recent studies have not confirmed this finding. O'Kelly studied a consecutive sample of 230 male patients with known CAD or at high risk of CAD who were undergoing major noncardiac surgical procedures. Preoperative arrhythmias were associated with the occurrence of intraoperative and postoperative arrhythmias. However, nonfatal MI and cardiac death were not significantly more frequent in those with prior perioperative arrhythmias. Amar and colleagues[22] studied 412 patients undergoing major thoracic surgery and determined that the incidence of nonsustained ventricular tachycardia was 15 percent but was not associated with poor outcome. Despite this finding, the presence of an arrhythmia in the preoperative setting should provoke a search for underlying cardiopulmonary disease, ongoing myocardial ischemia or infarction, drug toxicity, or metabolic derangements.

Conduction abnormalities can increase perioperative risk and may require the placement of a temporary or permanent pacemaker. On the other hand, patients with intraventricular conduction delays, even in the presence of a left or right bundle branch block, and no history of advanced heart block or symptoms rarely progress to complete heart block perioperatively. Since transthoracic pacing units have become available, the need for temporary transvenous pacemakers has decreased.

DECISION TO UNDERGO DIAGNOSTIC TESTING

The American College of Cardiology/American Heart Association Guidelines on Perioperative Cardiovascular Evaluation for Noncardiac Surgery have proposed an algorithm based on expert opinion, which will likely be updated in the next revision of the Guidelines to reflect recent randomized trials.[4,5] The current algorithm uses a step-wise Bayesian strategy that relies on assessment of clinical markers, prior coronary evaluation and treatment, functional capacity, and surgery-specific risk as outlined later. Successful use of the algorithm requires an appreciation for different levels of risk attributable to certain clinical circumstances, levels of functional capacity, and types of surgery.

Multiple studies have attempted to identify clinical risk markers for perioperative cardiovascular morbidity and mortality. As described earlier, patients with unstable coronary syndromes and severe valvular disease have active cardiac conditions. Patients with known stable CAD have intermediate risk. Other clinical risk factors in the RCRI make up the remainder of the intermediate risk predictors (history of congestive heart failure, history of cerebrovascular disease, preoperative treatment with insulin, and preoperative serum creatinine >2.0 mg/dl).[23] Cardiovascular disease has clinical risk markers, each associated with variable levels of perioperative risk, which have been classified as "low-risk factors." The classification of perioperative clinical risk

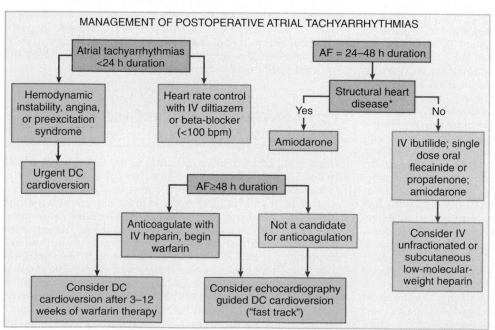

FIGURE 80–1 Proposed algorithm for the treatment of postoperative atrial tachyarrhythmias. AF = atrial fibrillation/flutter; DC = direct current; bpm = beats/min. * Structural heart disease is defined as the presence of one of the following: left ventricular hypertrophy with wall thickness >1.4 cm, mitral valve disease, coronary artery disease, or heart failure. (*Reproduced with permission from Amar D: Perioperative atrial tachyarrhythmias. Anesthesiology 97:1618, 2002.*)

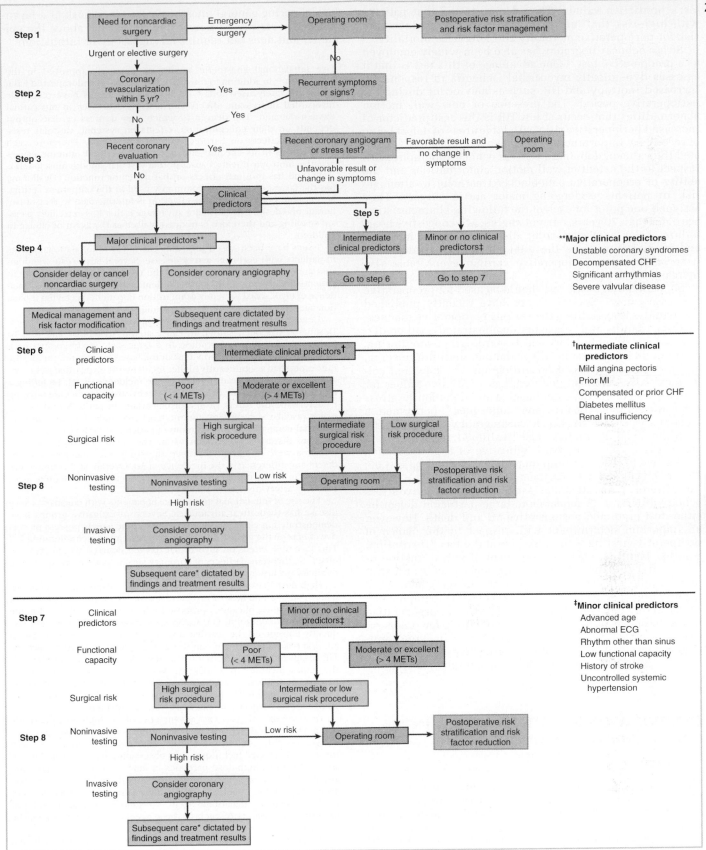

FIGURE 80–2 The American College of Cardiology/American Heart Association (ACC/AHA) Task Force on Perioperative Evaluation of Cardiac Patients Undergoing Noncardiac Surgery has proposed an algorithm for decisions regarding the need for further evaluation. This represents one of multiple algorithms proposed in the literature. The algorithm is based on expert opinion and incorporates six steps. First, the clinician must evaluate the urgency of the surgery and the appropriateness of a formal preoperative assessment. Next, the clinician must determine whether the patient has had a previous revascularization procedure or coronary evaluation. Those patients with unstable coronary syndromes should be identified, and appropriate treatment should be instituted. The decision to have further testing depends on the interaction of the clinical risk factors, surgery-specific risk, and functional capacity. (Reproduced with permission from the ACC/AHA Guidelines for Perioperative Cardiovascular Evaluation for Noncardiac Surgery Update. Reproduced with permission from Eagle KA, Berger PB, Calkins H, et al: ACC/AHA guideline update for perioperative cardiovascular evaluation for noncardiac surgery—executive summary: A report of the ACC/AHA Task Force on Practice Guidelines *(Committee to Update the 1996 Guidelines on Perioperative Cardiovascular Evaluation for Noncardiac Surgery). J Am Coll Cardiol 39:542, 2002.)*

test's predictive value.[32] They demonstrated that patients with high-risk thallium scans had particularly increased risk for perioperative morbidity and long-term mortality.

Stress echocardiography has also been widely employed as a preoperative test.[33] One advantage of this test is that it assesses dynamically myocardial ischemia in response to increased inotropy and HR, such as may occur during the perioperative period. The presence of new wall motion abnormalities that occur at low HR is the best predictor of increased perioperative risk, with large areas of defect being of secondary importance.[33] Boersma and colleagues[34] evaluated the value of dobutamine stress echocardiography with respect to the extent of wall motion abnormalities and the ability of preoperative beta-blocker treatment to attenuate risk in patients undergoing major aortic surgery. They assigned one point for each of the following characteristics: age older than 70 years, current angina, MI, congestive heart failure, prior cerebrovascular disease, diabetes mellitus, and renal failure.[34] As the total number of clinical risk factors increases, perioperative cardiac event rates also increase.

So, which diagnostic test should be used for preoperative risk assessment? Several groups have recently published meta-analyses examining the various preoperative diagnostic tests. Mantha and colleagues demonstrated good predictive values of ambulatory electrocardiogram monitoring, radionuclide angiography, dipyridamole thallium imaging, and dobutamine stress echocardiography.[35] Shaw and colleagues[36] also demonstrated excellent predictive values for both dipyridamole thallium imaging and dobutamine stress echocardiography. Beattie and colleagues[37] performed a meta-analysis of 25 stress echocardiography studies and 50 thallium imaging studies. The likelihood ratio for stress echocardiography was more indicative of a postoperative cardiac event than thallium imaging (likelihood ratio, 4.09; 95 percent CI, 3.21 to 6.56 versus 1.83; 1.59 to 2.10; $p = 0.001$). The difference was attributable to fewer false-negative stress echocardiograms. A moderate-to-large perfusion defect by either test predicted postoperative MI and death. However, an important determinant with respect to the choice of preoperative testing is the expertise at the local institution. Another factor is whether assessment of valve function or myocardial thickness is of interest, where echocardiography may be preferred. Stress nuclear imaging may have slightly higher sensitivity, but stress echocardiography may be less likely to be falsely positive. The role in preoperative risk assessment of newer imaging modalities for preoperative assessment using magnetic resonance imaging, multislice computed tomography imaging, coronary calcium scores, and positron emission tomography is rapidly evolving.

OVERVIEW OF ANESTHESIA USED IN CARDIAC PATIENTS UNDERGOING NONCARDIAC SURGERY

Three classes of anesthetics exist: general, regional, and local/sedation or monitored anesthesia care (MAC). General anesthesia can best be defined as a state including unconsciousness, amnesia, analgesia, immobility, and attenuation of autonomic responses to noxious stimulation. General anesthesia can be achieved with inhalational agents, intravenous agents, or a combination (frequently termed a *balanced technique*). Additionally, general anesthesia can be achieved with or without an endotracheal tube. Laryngoscopy and intubation were traditionally thought to be the time of greatest stress and risk for myocardial ischemia, but extubation may be a time of greater risk. Alternative methods

for delivering general anesthesia are via a mask or a laryngeal mask airway—a newer device that fits above the epiglottis and does not require laryngoscopy or intubation.

Five inhalational anesthetic agents are currently approved in the United States in addition to nitrous oxide, although enflurane and halothane are rarely used today. All inhalational agents have reversible myocardial depressant effects and lead to decreases in myocardial oxygen demand. The degree to which they depress cardiac output depends on their concentration, effects on systemic vascular resistance, and effects on baroreceptor responsiveness. Therefore each agent differs in its specific effects on HR and BP. Isoflurane causes negative inotropic effects, causes potent vascular smooth muscle relaxation, and has minimal effects on baroreceptor function. Desflurane has the fastest onset and is commonly used in the outpatient setting. Sevoflurane's onset and offset of action is intermediate to that of isoflurane and desflurane. Its major advantage is that it is extremely pleasant smelling and therefore is frequently used as the agent of choice in children.

Issues have been raised regarding the safety of inhalational agents in patients with coronary artery disease. Several large-scale, randomized and nonrandomized studies of the use of inhalational agents in patients undergoing CABG have not demonstrated any increased incidence of myocardial ischemia or infarction in patients receiving inhalation agents versus narcotic-based techniques.

Concerns regarding the safety of desflurane have also been raised. Desflurane has been shown to cause airway irritability and lead to tachycardia in volunteer studies. In a large-scale study comparing a narcotic-based anesthetic to a desflurane-based anesthetic, the desflurane group had a significantly higher incidence of myocardial ischemia, although there was no difference in the incidence of MI. Including a narcotic with desflurane can avoid this tachycardia. Studies are ongoing to determine the safety profile of desflurane in patients undergoing major vascular surgery. Sevoflurane has been studied in one randomized trial compared with isoflurane in patients at high risk for cardiovascular disease. No differences in the incidence of myocardial ischemia were observed; however, the study was underpowered to detect any difference in the incidence of MI. Overall, at this time there appears to be no one best inhalation anesthetic for the patient with coronary artery disease.

The use of inhalational anesthetics in patients with coronary artery disease has theoretical advantages. Several investigative groups have demonstrated in vitro and in animals that these agents possess protective effects on the myocardium similar to ischemic preconditioning.[38,39] This favorable effect on myocardial oxygen demand would serve to offset the theoretical effects of coronary steal in patients with chronic coronary occlusion.

High-dose narcotic techniques offer the advantage of hemodynamic stability and lack of myocardial depression. In the early 1980s, Lowenstein and colleagues proposed a high-dose narcotic technique for patients undergoing CABG. Narcotic-based anesthetics were frequently considered the "cardiac anesthesia" and advocated for use in all high-risk patients including those undergoing noncardiac surgery. The disadvantage of these traditional high-dose narcotic techniques is the requirement for postoperative ventilation. An ultra-short-acting narcotic (remifentanil) was introduced into clinical practice, obviating the need for prolonged ventilation. It has been used in patients undergoing cardiac surgery and can assist early extubation.

Despite the theoretical advantages of a high-dose narcotic technique, several large-scale trials in patients undergoing CABG showed no difference in survival or major morbidity compared with the inhalation-based technique. This observation has in part led to the abandonment of high-dose narcotics in much of cardiac surgery and an emphasis on early extubation. Most anesthesiologists use a "balanced" technique. This involves the administration of lower doses of narcotics with an inhalational agent. This allows the anesthesiologist to derive the benefits of each of these agents, while minimizing the side effects.

An alternative mode of delivering general anesthesia is with the intravenous agent propofol. Propofol is an alkyl phenol that can be used for both induction and maintenance of general anesthesia. It can result in profound hypotension due to reduced arterial tone with no change in HR. The major advantage of propofol is its rapid clearance with few residual effects on awakening; however, it is expensive, so its current use tends to be limited to operations of brief duration. Despite its hemodynamics effects, it has been used extensively to assist early extubation after coronary artery bypass surgery. Current evidence indicates that there is no one best general anesthetic technique for patients with coronary artery disease undergoing noncardiac surgery and has led to the abandonment of the concept of a "cardiac anesthetic."

SPINAL AND EPIDURAL ANESTHESIA

Regional anesthesia includes the techniques of spinal and epidural, as well as peripheral, nerve blocks. Each technique has its advantages and risks. Peripheral techniques, such as brachial plexus or Bier blocks, offer the advantage of causing minimal or no hemodynamic effects. In contrast, spinal or epidural techniques can produce sympathetic blockade, which can reduce BP and slow HR. Spinal anesthesia and lumbar or low thoracic epidural anesthesia can also evoke reflex sympathetic activation above the blockade, which might lead to myocardial ischemia.

The primary clinical difference between epidural and spinal anesthesia is the ability to provide continuous anesthesia or analgesia via placement of an epidural catheter as opposed to a single dose in spinal anesthesia, although some clinicians will place a catheter in the intrathecal space. Although the speed of onset depends on the local anesthetic agent used, spinal anesthesia and its associated autonomic effects occur sooner than the same agent administered epidurally. Because a catheter is usually left in place for epidural anesthesia, it can be more easily titrated. Epidural catheters can also be used postoperatively to provide analgesia.

A great deal of research has compared regional versus general anesthesia for patients with coronary artery disease, particularly in patients undergoing infrainguinal bypass surgery. In one meta-analysis, overall mortality was reduced by about one third in patients allocated to neuraxial blockade, although the findings were controversial because most of the benefit was observed in older studies.[40] Reductions in MI and renal failure also occurred.

MONITORED ANESTHESIA CARE

MAC encompasses local anesthesia administered by the surgeon both with or without sedation. In a large-scale cohort study, MAC was associated with increased 30-day mortality in a univariate analysis compared with general anesthesia, although it did not remain significant in multivariate analysis once patient comorbidity was taken into account.[41] The major issue with MAC is the ability to adequately block the stress response because inadequate analgesia associated with tachycardia may be worse than the potential hemodynamic effects of general or regional anesthesia. Since the introduction of the newer short-acting intravenous agents, essentially general anesthesia can now be administered without an endotracheal tube. This can allow the anesthesiologist to provide intense anesthesia for short or peripheral procedures without the potential effects of endotracheal intubation and extubation and therefore blurs the distinction between general anesthesia and MAC. Using an analysis of closed insurance claims, Domino and colleagues[42] demonstrated a high incidence of respiratory complications with MAC.

Intraoperative Hemodynamics and Myocardial Ischemia

Over the past two decades numerous studies have explored the relationship between hemodynamics and perioperative ischemia and MI. Tachycardia is the strongest predictor of perioperative ischemia. Although traditionally an HR greater than 100 beats/min defines tachycardia, slower HRs may result in myocardial ischemia. As described later, control of HR using beta blockers does decrease the incidence of myocardial ischemia and infarction.[42-46] Poldermans and colleagues[31] demonstrated that control of HR lowers the incidence of perioperative MI, with the greatest benefit if HR is controlled to less than 70 beats/min. Although concern about beta blockers causing intraoperative hypotension in patients with CAD has been raised, no evidence supports such a contention. In CABG, the vast majority of episodes of intraoperative ischemia do not correlate with hemodynamic changes.[47] In the absence of tachycardia, hypotension has not been shown to be associated with myocardial ischemia.

POSTOPERATIVE MANAGEMENT

Overview of Postoperative Response to Surgery

To determine the best approach to preoperative testing, it is important to understand the pathophysiology of perioperative cardiac events. A full discussion of the pathophysiology of perioperative MI has been published.[48] All surgical procedures cause a stress response, although the extent of the response depends on the extent of the surgery and the use of anesthetics and analgesics to reduce the response. The stress response can lead to increases in HR and BP, which can precipitate episodes of myocardial ischemia in areas distal to coronary artery stenoses. Prolonged myocardial ischemia (either prolonged individual episodes or cumulative duration of shorter episodes) can cause myocardial necrosis and perioperative MI and death.[49] Identification of patients with a high risk of coronary artery stenoses, through either history or cardiovascular testing, can lead to implementation of strategies to reduce morbidity from supply/demand mismatches.[50] As described earlier, beta-blocking agents can reduce the increased demand, whereas coronary revascularization may improve supply-related issues in patients with critical stenoses.

A major mechanism of MIs in the nonoperative setting is plaque rupture of a noncritical coronary stenosis with subsequent coronary thrombosis (see Chaps. 38 and 50). Because the perioperative period is marked by tachycardia and a hypercoagulable state, plaque disruption and thrombosis may occur quite commonly. Because the nidus for the thrombosis is a noncritical stenosis, preoperative cardiac evaluation may fail to identify such a patient before surgery, although control of HR may decrease the propensity of the plaque to rupture. The areas distal to the noncritical stenosis would not be expected to have collateral coronary flow, and therefore any acute thrombosis may have a greater detrimental effect than it would in a previously severely narrowed vessel. In the absence of fixed coronary narrowing elsewhere, preoperative cardiovascular testing will clearly not identify these patients. Contrariwise, if the postoperative MI is due to prolonged increase in myocardial oxygen demand in patients with one or more critical fixed stenosis, then one would expect that preoperative testing would identify such patients.

Evidence from several autopsy and postinfarction angiography studies after surgery supports both mechanisms. Ellis and colleagues[51] demonstrated that one third of all patients sustained events in areas distal to noncritical stenoses. Dawood and colleagues[52] demonstrated that fatal perioperative MI occurs predominantly in patients with multivessel coronary disease, especially left main and three-vessel disease; however, the severity of preexisting underlying stenosis did not predict the resulting infarct territory. This analysis suggested that fatal events occurred primarily in patients with advanced fixed stenoses, but that the infarct may result from plaque rupture in a mild or only moderately stenotic segment of diseased vessel.

Postoperative Intensive Care

Over the past several years, provision of intensive care by intensivists has become a patient safety goal. Pronovost and colleagues[53] performed a systematic review of the literature on physician staffing patterns and clinical outcomes in critically ill patients. They grouped intensive care unit (ICU) physician staffing into low-intensity (no intensivist or elective intensivist consultation) or high-intensity (mandatory intensivist consultation or closed ICU [all care directed by intensivist]) groups. High-intensity staffing was associated with lower hospital mortality in 16 of 17 studies (94 percent) and with a pooled estimate of the relative risk for hospital mortality of 0.71 (95 percent CI, 0.62 to 0.82). High-intensity staffing was associated with a lower ICU mortality in 14 of 15 studies (93 percent) and with a pooled estimate of the relative risk for ICU mortality of 0.61 (95 percent CI, 0.50 to 0.75). High-intensity staffing reduced hospital length of stay (LOS) in 10 of 13 studies and reduced ICU LOS in 14 of 18 studies without case-mix adjustment. High-intensity staffing was associated with reduced hospital LOS in two of four studies and ICU LOS in both studies that adjusted for case mix. No study found increased LOS with high-intensity staffing after case-mix adjustment. High-intensity versus low-intensity ICU physician staffing is associated with reduced hospital and ICU mortality and hospital and ICU LOS.

Postoperative Pain Management

Postoperative analgesia may reduce perioperative cardiac morbidity.[54] Because postoperative tachycardia and catecholamine surges probably promote myocardial ischemia and/or coronary plaque rupture, and because postoperative pain can produce tachycardia and increased catecholamines, effective postoperative analgesia may reduce cardiac complications. Additionally, postoperative analgesia may reduce the hypercoagulable state. Epidural anesthesia may reduce platelet aggregability compared with general anesthesia. Whether this related to the intraoperative or postoperative management is unclear. In an analysis of Medicare claims data, the use of epidural analgesia (as determined by billing codes for postoperative epidural pain management) was associated with decreased risk of death at 7 days.[55] Future research will focus on how best to deliver postoperative analgesia to maximize the potential benefits in reducing complications.

SURVEILLANCE AND IMPLICATIONS OF PERIOPERATIVE CARDIAC COMPLICATIONS

The optimal and most cost-effective strategy for monitoring high-risk patients for major morbidity after noncardiac surgery is unknown. Myocardial ischemia and infarctions that occur postoperatively are usually silent, most likely due to the confounding effects of analgesics and postoperative surgical pain. Creatine kinase (CK)-MB is also less specific for myocardial necrosis postoperatively because this marker can rise during aortic surgery and after mesenteric ischemia. Further confounding the issue is the observation that most perioperative MIs do not cause ST segment elevation, and nonspecific ST-T wave changes are common after surgery with or without MI. Therefore the diagnosis of a perioperative MI is particularly difficult using these traditional tests.

The approach to detection of perioperative MI has recently evolved with the use of troponin T and I. Adams and colleagues studied 108 patients undergoing high-risk surgery and obtained measures of CK-MB, total CK, cardiac troponin I, daily electrocardiograms, and pre-operative and postoperative echocardiograms.[56] Troponin I had a specificity of 99 percent, whereas CK-MB had a specificity of 81 percent. Lee and colleagues[57] measured CK-MB and troponin T levels in 1175 patients undergoing noncardiac surgery and created receiver-operating characteristic curves. They found that troponin T had a similar performance for diagnosing perioperative MI but significantly better correlation for major cardiac complications developing after an acute MI. Metzler and colleagues[58] examined the sensitivity of troponin assay at variable cut-off levels—a value of greater than 0.6 ng/ml demonstrated a positive predictive value of 87.5 percent and a negative predictive value of 98 percent. Manach and colleagues studied 1152 consecutive patients who underwent abdominal infrarenal aortic surgery and identified four patterns of cardiac troponin I (cTn-I) release after surgery.[59] One group did not have any abnormal levels, whereas a second group had only mild elevations of cTn-I. Interestingly, the two groups demonstrated elevations of cTn-I consistent with a periopera-tive myocardial infarction (PMI). One demonstrated acute (<24 hour) and early elevations of cTn-I above threshold, and the other demonstrated prolonged low levels of cTn-I release, followed by a delayed (>24 hour) elevation of cTnI. The authors suggest that these two different patterns represent two distinct pathophysiologies: acute coronary occlusion for early morbidity and prolonged myocardial ischemia for late events.

Traditionally, perioperative MIs were associated with a 30 to 50 percent short-term mortality. However, recent series have reported a fatality rate of perioperative MIs at less than 20 percent.[49] This improvement may result from more reliable detection of small, nonfatal MIs. A shift in the timing of a perioperative MI is also apparent. Studies from the 1980s suggested a peak incidence of the second and third postoperative days. Badner and colleagues,[60] using troponin I as a marker for MI, suggested that the immediate and first postoperative days showed the highest incidence, as confirmed in other studies. Again, it is likely that this change relates to more robust surveillance methods, not a fundamental shift in how or when myocardial ischemia or infarct occur.

Increasing evidence associates a perioperative MI or biomarker elevation with worse long-term outcome. Lopez-Jimenez and colleagues[61] found that abnormal troponin T levels were associated with an increased incidence of cardiovascular complications within 6 months of surgery. Kim and colleagues[62] studied perioperative tropo-nin I levels in 229 patients having aortic or infrainguinal vascular surgery or lower extremity amputation.[62] Twenty-eight patients (12 percent) had postoperative troponin I levels greater than 1.5 ng/ml, which was associated with a 6-fold increased risk of 6-month mortality and a 27-fold increased risk of MI. Furthermore, they observed a relationship between troponin I concentration and mortality. Landesberg and colleagues[63] demonstrated that postoperative CK-MB and troponin, even at low cutoff levels, are independent and complementary predictors of long-term mortality after major vascular surgery.

STRATEGIES TO REDUCE CARDIAC RISK OF NONCARDIAC SURGERY

Surgical Revascularization

Coronary revascularization has been suggested as a means of reducing perioperative risk surrounding noncardiac surgery. Previous retrospective evidence indicates that prior successful preoperative revascularization may decrease postoperative cardiac risk twofold to fourfold in patients undergoing elective vascular surgery. The strongest evidence comes from the Coronary Artery Surgery Study (CASS) Registry, which enrolled patients from 1978 to 1981. The operative mortality for patients with CABG before noncardiac surgery was 0.9 percent but was significantly higher (2.4 percent) in patients without prior CABG. However, there was a 1.4 percent mortality rate associated with the CABG procedure itself. Eagle and colleagues[64] reported a long-term analysis of patients entered into CASS and assigned to medical or surgical therapy for coronary artery disease for more than 10 years who subsequently underwent 3368 noncardiac operations in the years following assignment of coronary treatment. Intermediate-risk surgery such as abdominal, thoracic, or carotid endarterectomy was associated with a combined morbidity and mortality of 1 to 5 percent with a small but significant improvement in outcome in patients who had undergone prior revascularization. The most significant improvement in outcome was in patients undergoing major vascular surgery such as abdominal or lower extremity revascularization. However, this observational study did not randomize patients and was undertaken in the 1970s and 1980s before significant advances in medical, surgical, and percutaneous coronary strategies.[64] Landesberg and colleagues[65] reported retrospectively reviewed long-term outcome in 578 major vascular procedures. By multivariate analysis, age, type of vascular surgery, presence of diabetes, previous MI, and moderate-severe ischemia on preoperative perfusion imaging independently predicted mortality, and preoperative coronary revascularization predicted improved survival. Long-term survival after major vascular surgery significantly improved if patients with moderate to severe ischemia on preoperative perfusion imaging underwent selective coronary revascularization.

Several cohort studies have examined the benefit of percutaneous coronary intervention (PCI) before noncardiac surgery. Posner and colleagues used an administrative data set of patients who underwent PCI and noncardiac surgery in Washington State.[66] They matched patients with coronary disease undergoing noncardiac surgery with and without prior PCI and looked at cardiac complications. In this nonrandomized design, they noted a significantly lower rate of 30-day cardiac complications in patients who underwent PCI at least 90 days before the noncardiac surgery. Importantly, PCI within 90 days of noncardiac surgery did not improve outcome. Although the explanation for these results is unknown, they may support the notion that PCI performed "to get the patient through surgery" may not improve perioperative outcome because cardiac complications may not occur in patients with stable and/or asymptomatic coronary stenosis and PCI may actually destabilize coronary plaques that become manifest in the days or weeks after noncardiac surgery. Moreover, the advent of drug-eluting stents that involve prolonged antiplatelet therapy may promote operative bleeding complications or increase subacute stent thrombosis if antiplatelet treatment stops perioperatively.

Several randomized trials now address the value of both CABG and PCI in a subset of patients. McFalls and colleagues[67] reported the results of a multicenter randomized trial in the Veterans Administration Health System in which patients with documented CAD on coronary angiography, excluding those with left main disease or severely depressed ejection fraction (<20 percent), were randomized before elective major vascular surgery to CABG (59 percent) or PCI (41 percent) versus routine medical therapy. At 2.7 years after randomization, mortality in the revascularization group was not significantly different (22 percent) compared with the no-revascularization group (23 percent). Within 30 days after the vascular operation, a postoperative MI, defined by elevated troponin levels, occurred in 12 percent of the revascularization group and 14 percent of the no-revascularization group ($p = 0.37$). The authors suggested that coronary revascularization is not indicated in patients with stable CAD and further support the lack of efficacy of PCI or CABG for single- or double-vessel disease before noncardiac surgery. In a reanalysis of the data, the completeness of the revascularization affects the rate of perioperative MI with CABG being more effective than PCI.[68] As described earlier, Poldermans and colleagues[31] randomized patients at intermediate risk to testing and interventions or no testing and demonstrated no difference in 30-day cardiac events. Given the results of the older cohort series, further research is necessary to define the value of prophylactic coronary artery revascularization in the highest-risk patients.

One issue in interpreting the results is that length of time between the coronary revascularization and noncardiac surgery most likely affects its protective effect and potential risks. Back and colleagues[69] studied 425 consecutive patients undergoing 481 elective major vascular operations at an academic VA Medical Center. Coronary revascularization was classified as recent (CABG, <1 year; percutaneous transluminal coronary angioplasty [PTCA], <6 months) in 35 cases (7 percent), prior (1 year ≤ CABG < 5 years, 6 months ≤ PTCA < 2 years) in 45 cases (9 percent), and remote (CABG, ≥5 years; PTCA, ≥2 years) in 48 cases (10 percent). Outcomes in patients with previous PTCAs were similar to those after CABG ($p = 0.7$). Significant differences in adverse cardiac events and mortality were found between patients with CABG done within 5 years or PTCA within 2 years (6.3 and 1.3 percent, respectively), individuals with remote revascularization (10.4 and 6.3 percent, respectively), and nonrevascularized patients stratified at high risk (13.3 and 3.3 percent, respectively) or intermediate/low (2.8 and 0.9 percent, respectively) risk. The authors concluded that previous coronary revascularization (CABG, >5 years; PTCA, >2 years) may provide only modest protection against adverse cardiac events and mortality following major arterial reconstruction.

PCI using coronary stenting poses several special issues. Kaluza and colleagues[70] reported the outcome in 40 patients who underwent prophylactic coronary stent placement less than 6 weeks before major noncardiac surgery requiring a general anesthesia. They reported 7 MIs, 11 major bleeding episodes, and 8 deaths. All deaths and MIs, as well as 8 of 11 bleeding episodes, occurred in patients subjected to surgery fewer than 14 days after stenting. Four patients expired after undergoing surgery 1 day after stenting. Wilson and colleagues[71] reported on 207 patients who underwent noncardiac surgery within 2 months of stent placement. A total of 8 patients died or suffered an MI, and all 8 were among the 168 patients undergoing surgery 6 weeks after stent placement. Vincenzi and colleagues[72] studied 103 patients and reported that the risk of a perioperative cardiac event was 2.11-fold greater in patients with recent stents (<35 days before surgery) as compared with PCI more than 90 days before surgery.[72] The importance of delaying surgery was reported despite the fact that the authors either continued antiplatelet drug therapy or only briefly interrupted it; heparin was administered to all patients. Leibowitz and colleagues[73] studied a total of 216 consecutive patients who had a PCI within 3 months of noncardiac surgery (112 PTCA and 94 stent).[73] A total of 26 patients (12 percent) died, 13 in the stent group (14 percent) and 13 in the PTCA group (11 percent), a nonsignificant difference. The incidence of acute MI and death within 6 months did not differ significantly (7 and 14 percent in the stent group and 6 and 11 percent in the PTCA group, respectively). Significantly more events occurred in the 2 groups when noncardiac surgery was performed within 2 weeks of percutaneous coronary intervention. On the basis of the accumulating data, elective noncardiac surgery after PCI, with or without stent placement, should be delayed for 4 to 6 weeks.

Drug eluting stents may represent an even greater problem during the perioperative period on the basis of a series of recent analyses in the nonoperative setting and several perioperative case reports. Data is emerging that suggest that the risk of thrombosis continues for at least 1 year after insertion.[74,75] Nasser and colleagues described two patients with in-stent thrombosis occurring 4 and 21 months after implantation of sirolimus-eluting stents.[76] A science advisory from the American Heart Association, American College of Cardiology, Society for Cardiovascular Angiography and Interventions, American College of Surgeons, and American Dental Association was published in 2007 that stresses the importance of 12 months of dual antiplatelet therapy after placement of a drug-eluting stent.[77] It also recommends postponing elective surgery for 1 year, and, if surgery cannot be deferred, considering the continuation of aspirin during the perioperative period in high-risk patients with drug-eluting stents.

Beta-Blocking Agents

Beta blockers are the best-studied medical treatment, and guidelines for their use in the perioperative period have been published recently. Mangano and colleagues[43] administered atenolol or placebo beginning the morning of surgery and continuing for 7 days postoperatively in a cohort of 200 patients with known coronary disease or risk factors for CAD undergoing high-risk noncardiac surgery. They demonstrated a marked reduction in the incidence of perioperative myocardial ischemia, although no differences in the rates of perioperative MI. Importantly, survival improved markedly at 6 months in the atenolol group and continued for at least 2 years. The authors speculated that the lower incidence of myocardial ischemia was the result of less plaque destabilization, with a resultant reduction in subsequent MI or death in the 6 months after noncardiac surgery. Issues of randomization and uneven distribution of risk factors and treatment at baseline and on discharge with beta blockers may, at least in part, account for the findings. However, Poldermans and colleagues[46] studied the perioperative use of bisoprolol versus routine care in elective major vascular surgery in the Dutch Echocardiographic Cardiac Risk Evaluation Applying Stress Echo (DECREASE) trial. This medication was started at least 7 days preoperatively, titrated to achieve a resting HR less than 60 beats per minute, and continued postoperatively for 30 days. Of note, the study was confined to patients with at least one clinical marker of cardiac risk (prior MI, diabetes, angina pectoris, heart failure, age older than 70 years, or poor functional status), and evidence of inducible myocardial ischemia on a preoperative dobutamine stress echocardiogram. Patients with extensive regional wall abnormalities (large zones of myocardial ischemia) were excluded. Bisoprolol reduced perioperative MI or cardiac death by nearly 80 percent in this high-risk population. Because of the selection criteria, the efficacy of bisoprolol in the highest-risk group, those who would be considered for coronary revascularization or modification or cancellation of the surgical procedure, cannot be determined from this trial. However, the event rate in the placebo group (nearly 40 percent) suggests that all but the highest-risk patients were enrolled in the trial.

Boersma and colleagues[34] re-evaluated the value of dobutamine stress echocardiography with respect to the extent of wall motion abnormalities and use of beta blockers during surgery for the entire cohort of patients screened for the DECREASE trial. They assigned one point for each of the following characteristics: age older than 70 years, current angina, MI, congestive heart failure, prior cerebrovascular event, diabetes mellitus, and renal failure. As the total number of clinical risk factors increased, perioperative cardiac event rates also increased (Fig. 80-3). When the risk of death or MI was stratified by perioperative beta-blocker usage, there was no significant improvement in those without any of the prior risk factors. In those with a risk factor score between 1 and 3, which represented more than half of all patients, the rate of cardiac events fell from 3 to 0.9 percent by effective beta blockade. Most importantly, in those with fewer than 3 risk factors, comprising 70 percent of the population, beta-blocker therapy was effective in reducing cardiac events in those with new wall motion abnormalities in 1 to 4 segments (33 versus 2.8 percent), having a smaller effect in those without new wall motion abnormalities (5.8 versus 2 percent). Beta blockers were not protective in those patients with new wall motion abnormalities in greater than five segments. This group with risk factors and extensive wall motion abnormalities on preoperative stress echo may be the group to consider for prophylactic coronary revascularization.

Brady and colleagues[78] randomized 103 patients without previous MI who had infrarenal vascular surgery to oral metoprolol or placebo from admission until 7 days after surgery. Perioperative beta blockade with metoprolol did not seem to reduce 30-day cardiovascular events, but it was underpowered to do so. The study did show that metoprolol reduced the time from surgery to discharge. Lindenauer and colleagues[79] retrospectively reviewed the records of 782,969 patients and determined who received beta-blocker treatment during the first 2 hospital days. The relationship between perioperative beta-blocker treatment and the risk of death varied directly with cardiac risk; among the 580,665 patients with a revised cardiac risk index score of 0 or 1, treatment was associated with no benefit and possible harm, whereas among the patients with a revised cardiac risk index score of 2, 3, or 4 or more, the adjusted odds ratios for death in the hospital were 0.88

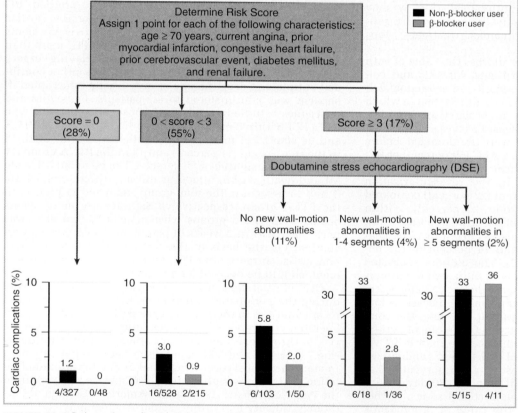

FIGURE 80–3 Perioperative cardiac risk and death in different populations of patients enrolled in the Dutch Echocardiographic Cardiac Risk Evaluation Applying Stress Echo trial. Risk is defined according to clinical risk and use of beta blockers both as part of the randomized and nonrandomized cohorts of individuals. Patients with risk factors and a positive stress test demonstrating one to four areas of regional wall motion abnormality on dobutamine stress echocardiography were randomized to perioperative bisoprolol titrated preoperatively to a heart rate less than 60 beats/min versus standard care. For all other patients who were not randomized but were on preoperative beta blockers, the medication was switched to bisoprolol targeted to a heart rate less than 60 beats per minute. *(Reproduced with permission from Boersma E, Poldermans D, Bax JJ, et al: Predictors of cardiac events after major vascular surgery: Role of clinical characteristics, dobutamine echocardiography, and beta-blocker therapy. JAMA 285:1865, 2001.)*

CH 80

(95 percent CI, 0.80 to 0.98), 0.71 (95 percent CI, 0.63 to 0.80), and 0.58 (95 percent CI, 0.50 to 0.67), respectively.

A study of 497 vascular surgery patients randomized to a fixed dose of metoprolol versus placebo demonstrated no difference in perioperative outcome.[80] A trial of metoprolol in diabetic patients without known coronary disease undergoing a diverse group of surgical procedures was unable to demonstrate any difference in perioperative outcomes.[81]

The current Focused Update to the ACC/AHA Guidelines on perioperative beta blockade advocate that perioperative beta-blockade is a class I indication for certain patient populations. It should be used in patients previously on beta blockers and those with a positive stress test undergoing major vascular surgery.[82] The use of these agents in those without active CAD or undergoing less invasive procedures is advocated as a class IIa recommendation. On the basis of recent studies, beta blockers may not be effective unless the HR is well controlled and may not be effective in lower-risk patients (Table 80-4).

Several pragmatic considerations pertain to the use of perioperative beta blockers in those currently not taking these agents. Several authors have recently demonstrated that the majority of patients presenting for noncardiac surgery, and even for vascular surgery, have not been started on beta blockers. One concern of anesthesiologists is related to the acute administration of beta-blocking agents on the morning of surgery. The combined effect of acute HR decrease coupled with the induction of anesthesia in a patient who had previously been beta blocker naïve has anecdotally been associated with marked bradycardia and hypotension. Treatment of these events may lead to wide swings in HR and BP and less HR control than desired. Thus the approach to the use of beta blockers depends on the preoperative status, type of surgery, cardiac risk factors, and any results of cardiac stress testing. Ideally, the beta-blocker therapy should be initiated more than 7 days in advance similar to the protocol by Poldermans, and longer-acting agents such as atenolol or bisoprolol should be used. Analyzing a large database, Redelmeier demonstrated improved perioperative survival in patients administered atenolol compared with metoprolol.[83] If the patient is undergoing nonvascular surgery or vascular surgery and has indications for beta-blocker therapy independent of surgery but is not currently taking beta blockers, then initiation of beta blockers several days preoperatively by the internist, cardiologist, or other primary care provider would be appropriate to ensure a stable beta-blocker level on the day of surgery. If several days of beta-blocker therapy cannot be achieved,

the potential risks of new-onset beta-blocker therapy during induction of either general, epidural, or spinal anesthesia may outweigh the benefits of beginning drug therapy the morning of surgery. Because the study by Mangano did not demonstrate any difference in in-hospital outcome and the approach of Raby and colleagues demonstrated similar efficacy with respect to perioperative ischemia, we suggest inducing general anesthesia or providing regional anesthesia before starting beta-blocker therapy.[44] If the induction is associated with tachycardia, then administration of esmolol would be appropriate. After adequate anesthesia and analgesia are achieved, then HR should be controlled and maintained below 70 beats/min. Feringa and colleagues[84] demonstrated that higher doses of beta blockers and tight HR control are associated with reduced perioperative myocardial ischemia and troponin T release and improved long-term outcome in vascular surgery patients.

Alpha$_2$-Agonists

Several randomized trials have evaluated the value of prophylactic alpha$_2$-agonists as a means of reducing perioperative cardiac morbidity. Wallace and colleagues[85] evaluated alpha$_2$-agonists compared with placebo in high-risk patients undergoing noncardiac surgery. They reported similar results to those of Mangano and colleagues and demonstrated marked improvement in 2 years' survival in the alpha$_2$-agonist group. Licker and colleagues[27] have reported on a cardioprotection protocol involving preoperative alpha$_2$-agonist administration and intraoperative and postoperative beta-blocker administration compared with historical controls that did not use preoperative testing or this pharmacological protocol.[27] They reported markedly improved perioperative and long-term survival and reduced perioperative troponin levels in the more contemporary group employing the cardio-protection protocol. A meta-analysis of published studies demonstrated that perioperative clonidine reduced cardiac ischemic episodes in patients with known, or at risk of, coronary arterial disease without increasing the incidence of bradycardia, although the studies were underpowered to evaluate the efficacy for reduction of perioperative cardiac morbidity.[86]

Nitroglycerin

Only two randomized trials have evaluated the potential protective effect of prophylactic nitroglycerin in reducing perioperative cardiac complications after noncardiac surgery. In a small study by Coriat and colleagues in patients

CH 80

TABLE 80–4	Recommendations for Perioperative Beta-Blocker Therapy Based on Published Randomized Clinical Trials		
	Low Cardiac Patient Risk	**Intermediate Cardiac Patient Risk**	**CHD or High Cardiac Patient Risk**
Vascular Surgery	Class IIb Level of Evidence: C	Class IIb Level of Evidence: C	*Patients found to have myocardial ischemia on preoperative testing* Class I Level of Evidence: B* Class IIa Level of Evidence: B†
High-/Intermediate-Risk Surgery	‡	Class IIb Level of Evidence: C	Class IIa Level of Evidence: B
Low-Risk Surgery	‡	‡	‡

*Applies to patients found to have coronary ischemia on preoperative testing.

†Applies to patients found to have coronary heart disease.

‡Indicates insufficient data. See text for further discussion.

CHD = coronary heart disease.

Reproduced with permission from Fleisher L, Beckman J, Brown K, et al: ACC/AHA 2006 Guideline Update on Perioperative Cardiovascular Evaluation for Noncardiac Surgery: Focused Update on Perioperative Beta-Blocker Therapy. A Report of the American College of Cardiology/American Heart Association Task Force on Practice Guidelines (Writing Committee to Update the 2002 Guidelines on Perioperative Cardiovascular Evaluation for Noncardiac Surgery). Circulation 113:2662, 2006.

undergoing carotid endarterectomy, high-dose (1 µg/kg/min) nitroglycerin was more effective than lower-dose (0.5 mcg/kg/min) nitroglycerin in reducing the incidence of myocardial ischemia, but MI did not occur in either group.[87] Importantly, the anesthetic used in this study was an oxygen/pancuronium/fentanyl method and therefore inhalational agents were not administered. Dodds studied nitroglycerin versus placebo using a balanced anesthetic technique and reported no difference in the rates of myocardial ischemia or infarction.[88] Taken together, the evidence suggests that prophylactic nitroglycerin does not reduce the incidence of perioperative cardiac morbidity, although neither trial was powered to detect a modest benefit of nitroglycerin. Because prophylactic nitroglycerin has considerable hemodynamic effects and is not known to prevent MI or cardiac death, it would seem prudent to avoid the prophylactic use of nitroglycerin, although there are clear indications for its use as treatment once myocardial ischemia develops.

Statin Therapy

In addition to their cholesterol-lowering properties, statins have anti-inflammatory and plaque-stabilizing properties. Given the potential mechanisms of perioperative MIs, statins could have theoretical benefits. Poldermans and colleagues[89] performed a case-controlled study of 2816 patients who underwent major vascular surgery from 1991 to 2000. Statin therapy was significantly less common in patients experiencing a postoperative MI compared with controls (8 versus 25 percent; $p < 0.001$). The adjusted odds ratio for perioperative mortality among statin users as compared with nonusers was 0.22 (95 percent CI; 0.10 to 0.47). Lindenauer and colleagues[90] used administrative data to study a cohort of 780,591 patients; 77,082 patients (9.9 percent) received lipid-lowering therapy perioperatively, and 23,100 (2.96 percent) died during the hospitalization.[91] Using multivariate modeling and propensity matching, the number needed to treat to prevent a postoperative death was 85 (95 percent CI; 77 to 98) and varied from 186 among patients at lowest risk to 30 among those with a revised cardiac risk index score of 4 or more. Durazzo and colleagues[91] randomized 100 patients to receive 20 mg atorvastatin or placebo once a day for 45 days.[92] The incidence of cardiac events was more than three times higher with placebo (26 percent) compared with atorvastatin (8 percent; $p = 0.031$). Patients given atorvastatin exhibited a significant decrease in the rate of cardiac events, compared with the placebo group, within 6 months after vascular surgery ($p = 0.018$). The accumulating evidence suggests that statin therapy should continue during the perioperative period, and consideration should be given for starting statin therapy in high-risk patients, particularly those with established atherosclerosis, because one could argue that the patient should have been on a statin already.

Nonpharmacological Interventions

Temperature

Frank and colleagues completed a randomized trial of regional versus general anesthesia for lower extremity vascular bypass procedures and noted an association between hypothermia (temperature < 35°C) and myocardial ischemia.[92] They subsequently performed a randomized trial in 300 high-risk patients undergoing a diverse group of intermediate- and high-risk procedures and randomized patients to maintenance of normothermia or routine care. They observed a significantly reduced incidence of perioperative cardiac morbidity and mortality within 24 hours of surgery in the group that was kept normothermic.

Electrocardiographic, Hemodynamic, and Echocardiographic Monitoring

Multiple studies have demonstrated the predictive value correlating perioperative ST-segment changes and major cardiac events, as described earlier. Furthermore, the duration, either cumulative or continuous, of perioperative ST changes strongly predicts poor outcomes. Therefore ST-segment monitoring has become a standard during the intraoperative and intensive care unit periods for high-risk patients. However, patients at low to moderate risk may also develop ST segment changes. These changes may not reflect true myocardial ischemia, as suggested in a recent series.[93]

The period of greatest risk of a postoperative cardiac event may be the time when the patient is on the ward and unmonitored. Many of the monitoring companies have developed ST segment telemetry monitors, but they have not been tested to any large degree in the perioperative period. This issue of whether early treatment of prolonged ST segment changes will lead to improved outcome remains unresolved. Until such studies are completed, the efficacy of such monitors remains debatable.

A great deal of controversy surrounds the value of pulmonary artery catheterization for noncardiac surgery. Several small, randomized trials did not demonstrate a significant reduction in major cardiac morbidity and mortality in patients undergoing aortic surgery. A large-scale cohort study performed by Polanczyk and colleagues,[94] in which patients who had pulmonary catheters placed were matched to those who did not, using a propensity score also failed to demonstrate any significant benefit. In fact, they observed an increased incidence of congestive heart failure and untoward noncardiac outcomes in the pulmonary artery catheter group. More recently, a total of 1994 patients were randomized to goal-directed therapy guided by a pulmonary catheter with standard care without the use of a pulmonary catheter for patients undergoing urgent or elective major surgery.[95] No difference in survival occurred, but there was a higher rate of pulmonary embolism in the catheter group compared with the standard care group. Therefore current evidence does not support the routine use of pulmonary artery catheterization for high-risk patients undergoing major noncardiac surgery. Further work will be required to understand if these results can be generalized to the high-risk vascular surgical population and to determine the benefits of the pulmonary artery catheters in specific clinical situations.

Transesophageal echocardiography (TEE) represents another means of assessing intraoperative cardiac function. It is an extremely sensitive, noninvasive tool to monitor intraoperative wall motion abnormalities and fluid status. In patients undergoing aortic cross clamping, TEE proved to have a significantly better sensitivity for detecting intraoperative ischemia than electrocardiographic monitoring. For noncardiac surgery, a study of TEE, 2-lead electrocardiography, and 12-lead electrocardiography demonstrated minimal additive value of TEE over 2-lead electrocardiography.[96] Although TEE for routine monitoring of intraoperative ischemia in noncardiac surgery may have minimal additive value over ST segment recording for predicting patients who will sustain perioperative morbidity, TEE monitoring may be valuable to guide treatment in patients with unstable hemodynamics in whom filling status and/or myocardial function are uncertain.

Transfusion Threshold

A great deal of controversy surrounds the optimal hemoglobin level at which to transfuse high-risk noncardiac surgical patients. No randomized trials have evaluated the optimal transfusion threshold, although there is a great deal of anecdotal evidence. Several small cohort studies have shown that hematocrits in the 27 to 29 percent range represent the point below which incidence of myocardial ischemia and potentially MI increases.[97,98] A large-scale trial of transfusion triggers in the ICU did not document increased morbidity and mortality with a transfusion threshold of a hemoglobin less than 7 gm/dl, but there were trends toward increased morbidity in the subset of patients with ischemic heart disease. The evidence suggests that patients with known ischemic heart disease that has not been revascularized should be maintained perioperatively with a hemoglobin greater than 9 gm/dl.

REFERENCES

Preoperative Risk Stratification

1. Reddy PR, Vaitkus PT: Risks of noncardiac surgery after coronary stenting. Am J Cardiol 95:755, 2005.
2. Rivers SP, Scher LA, Gupta SK, Weith FJ: Safety of peripheral vascular surgery after recent acute myocardial infarction. J Vasc Surg 11:70, 1990.
3. Eagle KA, Brundage BH, Chaitman BR, et al: Guidelines for perioperative cardiovascular evaluation for noncardiac surgery. Report of the American College of Cardiology/American Heart Association Task Force on Practice Guidelines (Committee on Perioperative Cardiovascular Evaluation for Noncardiac Surgery). J Am Coll Cardiol 27:910, 1996.
4. Eagle KA, Berger PB, Calkins H, et al: ACC/AHA guideline update for perioperative cardiovascular evaluation for noncardiac surgery—executive summary: a Report of the American College of Cardiology/American Heart Association Task Force on Practice Guidelines (Committee to Update the 1996 Guidelines on Perioperative Cardiovascular Evaluation for Noncardiac Surgery). J Am Coll Cardiol 39:542, 2002.
5. Eagle K, Brundage B, Chaitman B, et al: Guidelines for perioperative cardiovascular evaluation of the noncardiac surgery. A report of the American Heart Association/American College of Cardiology Task Force on Assessment of Diagnostic and Therapeutic Cardiovascular Procedures. Circulation 93:1278, 1996.
6. Weksler N, Klein M, Szendro G, et al: The dilemma of immediate preoperative hypertension: To treat and operate, or to postpone surgery? J Clin Anesth 15:179, 2003.
7. Aronson S, Boisvert D, Lapp W: Isolated systolic hypertension is associated with adverse outcomes from coronary artery bypass grafting surgery. Anesth Analg 94:1079, 2002.
8. Goldman L, Caldera DL, Nussbaum SR, et al: Multifactorial index of cardiac risk in noncardiac surgical procedures. N Engl J Med 297:845, 1977.
9. Haering JM, Comunale ME, Parker RA, et al: Cardiac risk of noncardiac surgery in patients with asymmetric septal hypertrophy. Anesthesiology 85:254, 1996.
10. Kertai MD, Bountioukos M, Boersma E, et al: Aortic stenosis: an underestimated risk factor for perioperative complications in patients undergoing noncardiac surgery. Am J Med 116:8, 2004.
11. Torsher LC, Shub C, Rettke SR, Brown DL: Risk of patients with severe aortic stenosis undergoing noncardiac surgery. Am J Cardiol 81:448, 1998.
12. Zahid M, Sonel AF, Saba S, Good CB: Perioperative risk of noncardiac surgery associated with aortic stenosis. Am J Cardiol 96:436, 2005.

Management of the Perioperative Cardiac Patient

13. Dajani A, Taubert K, Wilson W, et al: Prevention of bacterial endocarditis. Recommendations by the American Heart Association. JAMA 277:1794, 1997.
14. Katholi RE, Nolan SP, McGuire LB: The management of anticoagulation during noncardiac operations in patients with prosthetic heart valves. A prospective study. Am Heart J 96:163, 1978.
15. Bonow RO, Carabello B, de Leon AC Jr, et al: Guidelines for the management of patients with valvular heart disease: Executive summary. A report of the American College of Cardiology/American Heart Association Task Force on Practice Guidelines (Committee on Management of Patients with Valvular Heart Disease). Circulation 98:1949, 1998.
16. Ezekowitz MD: Anticoagulation management of valve replacement patients. J Heart Valve Dis 11(Suppl):S56, 2002.
17. Martin JT, Tautz TJ, Antognini JF: Safety of regional anesthesia in Eisenmenger's syndrome. Reg Anesth Pain Med 27:509, 2002.
18. Galli KK, Myers LB, Nicolson SC: Anesthesia for adult patients with congenital heart disease undergoing noncardiac surgery. Int Anesthesiol Clin 39:43, 2001.
19. Amar D: Perioperative atrial tachyarrhythmias. Anesthesiology 97:1618, 2002.
20. Amar D, Roistacher N, Rusch VW, et al: Effects of diltiazem prophylaxis on the incidence and clinical outcome of atrial arrhythmias after thoracic surgery. J Thorac Cardiovasc Surg 120:790, 2000.
21. Balser JR, Martinez EA, Winters BD, et al: Beta-adrenergic blockade accelerates conversion of postoperative supraventricular tachyarrhythmias. Anesthesiology 89:1052, 1998.
22. Amar D, Zhang H, Roistacher N: The incidence and outcome of ventricular arrhythmias after noncardiac thoracic surgery. Anesth Analg 95:537, 2002.
23. Lee TH, Marcantonio ER, Mangione CM, et al: Derivation and prospective validation of a simple index for prediction of cardiac risk of major noncardiac surgery. Circulation 100:1043, 1999.

24. Reilly DF, McNeely MJ, Doerner D, et al: Self-reported exercise tolerance and the risk of serious perioperative complications. Arch Intern Med 159:2185, 1999.
25. Bartels C, Bechtel J, Hossmann V, Horsch S: Cardiac risk stratification for high-risk vascular surgery. Circulation 95:2473, 1997.
26. Froehlich JB, Karavite D, Russman PL, et al: American College of Cardiology/American Heart Association preoperative assessment guidelines reduce resource utilization before aortic surgery. J Vasc Surg 36:758, 2002.
27. Licker M, Khatchatourian G, Schweizer A, et al: The impact of a cardioprotective protocol on the incidence of cardiac complications after aortic abdominal surgery. Anesth Analg 95:1525, 2002.
28. Almanaseer Y, Mukherjee D, Kline-Rogers EM, et al: Implementation of the ACC/AHA guidelines for preoperative cardiac risk assessment in a general medicine preoperative clinic: improving efficiency and preserving outcomes. Cardiology 103:24, 2005.
29. Legner VJ, Doerner D, McCormick WC, Reilly DF: Clinician agreement with perioperative cardiovascular evaluation guidelines and clinical outcomes. Am J Cardiol 97:118, 2006.
30. Falcone RA, Nass C, Jermyn R, et al: The value of preoperative pharmacologic stress testing before vascular surgery using ACC/AHA guidelines: A prospective, randomized trial. J Cardiothorac Vasc Anesth 17:694, 2003.
31. Poldermans D, Bax JJ, Schouten O, et al: Should major vascular surgery be delayed because of preoperative cardiac testing in intermediate-risk patients receiving beta-blocker therapy with tight heart rate control? J Am Coll Cardiol 48:964, 2006.
32. Fleisher LA, Rosenbaum SH, Nelson AH, et al: Preoperative dipyridamole thallium imaging and Holter monitoring as a predictor of perioperative cardiac events and long term outcome. Anesthesiology 83:906, 1995.
33. Poldermans D, Arnese M, Fioretti PM, et al: Improved cardiac risk stratification in major vascular surgery with dobutamine-atropine stress echocardiography. J Am Coll Cardiol 26:648, 1995.
34. Boersma E, Poldermans D, Bax JJ, et al: Predictors of cardiac events after major vascular surgery: Role of clinical characteristics, dobutamine echocardiography, and beta-blocker therapy. JAMA 285:1865, 2001.
35. Mantha S, Roizen MF, Barnard J, et al: Relative effectiveness of four preoperative tests for predicting adverse cardiac outcomes after vascular surgery: A meta-analysis. Anesth Analg 79:422, 1994.
36. Shaw LJ, Eagle KA, Gersh BJ, Miller DD: Meta-analysis of intravenous dipyridamole-thallium-201 imaging (1985 to 1994) and dobutamine echocardiography (1991 to 1994) for risk stratification before vascular surgery [see comments]. J Am Coll Cardiol 27:787, 1996.
37. Beattie WS, Abdelnaem E, Wijeysundera DN, Buckley DN: A meta-analytic comparison of preoperative stress echocardiography and nuclear scintigraphy imaging. Anesth Analg 102:8, 2006.

Cardiovascular Effects of Anesthetic Agents

38. Toller WG, Kersten JR, Pagel PS, et al: Sevoflurane reduces myocardial infarct size and decreases the time threshold for ischemic preconditioning in dogs. Anesthesiology 91:1437, 1999.
39. Chen Q, Camara AK, An J, et al: Sevoflurane preconditioning before moderate hypothermic ischemia protects against cytosolic [Ca(2+)] loading and myocardial damage in part via mitochondrial K(ATP) channels. Anesthesiology 97:912, 2002.
40. Rodgers A, Walker N, Schug S, et al: Reduction of postoperative mortality and morbidity with epidural or spinal anaesthesia: Results from overview of randomised trials. BMJ 321:1493, 2000.
41. Cohen M, Duncan PG, Tate RB: Does anesthesia contribute to operative mortality? JAMA 260:2859, 1988.
42. Bhananker SM, Posner KL, Cheney FW, et al: Injury and liability associated with monitored anesthesia care: A closed claims analysis. Anesthesiology 104:228, 2006.

Perioperative Use of Beta-Adrenergic Blocking Agents

43. Mangano DT, Layug EL, Wallace A, Tateo I: Effect of atenolol on mortality and cardiovascular morbidity after noncardiac surgery. Multicenter Study of Perioperative Ischemia Research Group. N Engl J Med 335:1713, 1996.
44. Raby KE, Brull SJ, Timimi F, et al: The effect of heart rate control on myocardial ischemia among high-risk patients after vascular surgery [see comments]. Anesth Analg 88:477, 1999.
45. Wallace A, Layug B, Tateo I, et al: Prophylactic atenolol reduces postoperative myocardial ischemia. McSPI Research Group [see comments]. Anesthesiology 88:7, 1998.
46. Poldermans D, Boersma E, Bax JJ, et al: The effect of bisoprolol on perioperative mortality and myocardial infarction in high-risk patients undergoing vascular surgery. Dutch Echocardiographic Cardiac Risk Evaluation Applying Stress Echocardiography Study Group [see comments]. N Engl J Med 341:1789, 1999.

Assessment of Perioperative Infarction and Ischemia

47. Leung JM, O'Kelly BF, Mangano DT, et al: Relationship of regional wall motion abnormalities to hemodynamic indices of myocardial oxygen supply and demand in patients undergoing CABG surgery. Anesthesiology 73:802, 1990.
48. Landesberg G: The pathophysiology of perioperative myocardial infarction: Facts and perspectives. J Cardiothorac Vasc Anesth 17:90, 2003.
49. Landesberg G, Luria MH, Cotev S, et al: Importance of long-duration postoperative ST-segment depression in cardiac morbidity after vascular surgery. Lancet 341:715, 1993.
50. Fleisher LA, Eagle KA: Clinical practice. Lowering cardiac risk in noncardiac surgery. N Engl J Med 345:1677, 2001.

2028

51. Ellis SG, Hertzer NR, Young JR, Brener S: Angiographic correlates of cardiac death and myocardial infarction complicating major nonthoracic vascular surgery. Am J Cardiol 77:1126, 1996.

52. Dawood MM, Gutpa DK, Southern J, et al: Pathology of fatal perioperative myocardial infarction: Implications regarding pathophysiology and prevention. Int J Cardiol 57:37, 1996.

53. Pronovost PJ, Angus DC, Dorman T, et al: Physician staffing patterns and clinical outcomes in critically ill patients: A systematic review. JAMA 288:2151, 2002.

54. Kehlet H, Holte K: Effect of postoperative analgesia on surgical outcome. Br J Anaesth 87:62, 2001.

55. Wu CL, Hurley RW, Anderson GF, et al: Effect of postoperative epidural analgesia on morbidity and mortality following surgery in Medicare patients. Reg Anesth Pain Med 29:525, discussion 15, 2004.

56. Adams JE, Sicard GA, Allen BT, et al: Diagnosis of perioperative myocardial infarction with measurement of cardiac troponin I. N Engl J Med 330:670, 1994.

57. Lee TH, Thomas EJ, Ludwig LE, et al: Troponin T as a marker for myocardial ischemia in patients undergoing major noncardiac surgery. Am J Cardiol 77:1031, 1996.

58. Metzler H, Gries M, Rehak P, et al: Perioperative myocardial cell injury: The role of troponins. Br J Anaesth 78:386, 1997.

59. Le Manach Y, Perel A, Coriat P, et al: Early and delayed myocardial infarction after abdominal aortic surgery. Anesthesiology 102:885, 2005.

60. Badner NH, Knill RL, Brown JE, et al: Myocardial infarction after noncardiac surgery. Anesthesiology 88:572, 1998.

61. Lopez-Jimenez F, Goldman L, Sacks DB, et al: Prognostic value of cardiac troponin T after noncardiac surgery: 6-month follow-up data. J Am Coll Cardiol 29:1241, 1997.

62. Kim LJ, Martinez EA, Faraday N, et al: Cardiac troponin I predicts short-term mortality in vascular surgery patients. Circulation 106:2366, 2002.

63. Landesberg G, Shatz V, Akopnik I, et al: Association of cardiac troponin, CK-MB, and postoperative myocardial ischemia with long-term survival after major vascular surgery. J Am Coll Cardiol 42:1547, 2003.

Preoperative Coronary Revascularization

64. Eagle KA, Rihal CS, Mickel MC, et al: Cardiac risk of noncardiac surgery: Influence of coronary disease and type of surgery in 3368 operations. CASS Investigators and University of Michigan Heart Care Program. Coronary Artery Surgery Study. Circulation 96:1882, 1997.

65. Landesberg G, Mosseri M, Wolf YG, et al: Preoperative thallium scanning, selective coronary revascularization, and long-term survival after major vascular surgery. Circulation 108:177, 2003.

66. Posner KL, Van Norman GA, Chan V: Adverse cardiac outcomes after noncardiac surgery in patients with prior percutaneous transluminal coronary angioplasty. Anesth Analg 89:553, 1999.

67. McFalls EO, Ward HB, Moritz TE, et al: Coronary-artery revascularization before elective major vascular surgery. N Engl J Med 351:2795, 2004.

68. Ward HB, Kelly RF, Thottapurathu L, et al: Coronary artery bypass grafting is superior to percutaneous coronary intervention in prevention of perioperative myocardial infarctions during subsequent vascular surgery. Ann Thorac Surg 82:795, discussion 1, 2006.

69. Back MR, Stordahl N, Cuthbertson D, et al: Limitations in the cardiac risk reduction provided by coronary revascularization prior to elective vascular surgery. J Vasc Surg 36:526, 2002.

70. Kaluza GL, Joseph J, Lee JR, et al: Catastrophic outcomes of noncardiac surgery soon after coronary stenting. J Am Coll Cardiol 35:1288, 2000.

71. Wilson SH, Fasseas P, Orford JL, et al: Clinical outcome of patients undergoing noncardiac surgery in the two months following coronary stenting. J Am Coll Cardiol 42:234, 2003.

72. Vicenzi MN, Meislitzer T, Heitzinger B, et al: Coronary artery stenting and noncardiac surgery—a prospective outcome study. Br J Anaesth 96:686, 2006.

73. Leibowitz D, Cohen M, Planer D, et al: Comparison of cardiovascular risk of noncardiac surgery following coronary angioplasty with versus without stenting. Am J Cardiol 97:1188, 2006.

74. Moreno R, Fernandez C, Calvo L, et al: Meta-analysis comparing the effect of drug-eluting versus bare metal stents on risk of acute myocardial infarction during follow-up. Am J Cardiol 99:621, 2007.

75. Pfisterer M, Brunner-La Rocca HP, Buser PT, et al: Late clinical events after clopidogrel discontinuation may limit the benefit of drug-eluting stents: An observational study of drug-eluting versus bare-metal stents. J Am Coll Cardiol 48:2584, 2006.

76. Nasser M, Kapeliovich M, Markiewicz W: Late thrombosis of sirolimus-eluting stents following noncardiac surgery. Catheter Cardiovasc Interv 65:516, 2005.

77. Grines CL, Bonow RO, Casey DE Jr, et al: Prevention of premature discontinuation of dual antiplatelet therapy in patients with coronary artery stents: A science advisory from the American Heart Association, American College of Cardiology, Society for Cardiovascular Angiography and Interventions, American College of Surgeons, and American Dental Association, with representation from the American College of Physicians. J Am Coll Cardiol 49:734, 2007.

Medical Management of Perioperative Ischemia

78. Brady AR, Gibbs JS, Greenhalgh RM, et al: Perioperative beta-blockade (POBBLE) for patients undergoing infrarenal vascular surgery: Results of a randomized double-blind controlled trial. J Vasc Surg 41:602, 2005.

79. Lindenauer PK, Pekow P, Wang K, et al: Perioperative beta-blocker therapy and mortality after major noncardiac surgery. N Engl J Med 353:349, 2005.

80. Yang H, Raymer K, Butler R, et al: Metoprolol after vascular surgery (MaVS). Can J Anesth 51:A7, 2004.

81. Juul AB, Wetterslev J, Gluud C, et al: Effect of perioperative beta blockade in patients with diabetes undergoing major non-cardiac surgery: Randomised placebo controlled, blinded multicentre trial. BMJ 332:1482, 2006.

82. Fleisher L, Beckman J, Brown K, et al: ACC/AHA 2006 Guideline Update on Perioperative Cardiovascular Evaluation for Noncardiac Surgery: Focused Update on Perioperative Beta-Blocker Therapy. A Report of the American College of Cardiology/American Heart Association Task Force on Practice Guidelines (Writing Committee to Update the 2002 Guidelines on Perioperative Cardiovascular Evaluation for Noncardiac Surgery), 2006.

83. Redelmeier D, Scales D, Kopp A: Beta blockers for elective surgery in elderly patients: Population based, retrospective cohort study. BMJ 331:932, 2005.

84. Feringa HH, Bax JJ, Boersma E, et al: High-dose beta-blockers and tight heart rate control reduce myocardial ischemia and troponin T release in vascular surgery patients. Circulation 114:I344, 2006.

85. Wallace AW, Galindez D, Salahieh A, et al: Effect of clonidine on cardiovascular morbidity and mortality after noncardiac surgery. Anesthesiology 101:284, 2004.

86. Nishina K, Mikawa K, Uesugi T, et al: Efficacy of clonidine for prevention of perioperative myocardial ischemia: A critical appraisal and meta-analysis of the literature. Anesthesiology 96:323, 2002.

87. Coriat P: Intravenous nitroglycerin dosage to prevent intraoperative myocardial ischemia during noncardiac surgery. Anesthesiology 64:409, 1986.

88. Dodds TM, Stone JG, Coromilas J, et al: Prophylactic nitroglycerin infusion during noncardiac surgery does not reduce perioperative ischemia. Anesth Analg 76:705, 1993.

89. Poldermans D, Bax JJ, Kertai MD, et al: Statins are associated with a reduced incidence of perioperative mortality in patients undergoing major noncardiac vascular surgery. Circulation 107:1848, 2003.

90. Lindenauer PK, Pekow P, Wang K, et al: Lipid-lowering therapy and in-hospital mortality following major noncardiac surgery. JAMA 291:2092, 2004.

91. Durazzo AE, Machado FS, Ikeoka DT, et al: Reduction in cardiovascular events after vascular surgery with atorvastatin: A randomized trial. J Vasc Surg 39:967, 2004.

92. Frank SM, Fleisher LA, Breslow MJ, et al: Perioperative maintenance of normothermia reduces the incidence of morbid cardiac events. A randomized clinical trial. JAMA 277:1127, 1997.

93. Fleisher LA, Zielski MM, Schulman SP: Perioperative ST-segment depression is rare and may not indicate myocardial ischemia in moderate-risk patients undergoing noncardiac surgery. J Cardiothorac Vasc Anesth 11:155, 1997.

Perioperative Monitoring of the Cardiac Patient

94. Polanczyk CA, Rohde LE, Goldman L, et al: Right heart catheterization and cardiac complications in patients undergoing noncardiac surgery: An observational study. JAMA 286:309, 2001.

95. Sandham JD, Hull RD, Brant RF, et al: A randomized, controlled trial of the use of pulmonary-artery catheters in high-risk surgical patients. N Engl J Med 348:5, 2003.

96. Eisenberg MJ, London MJ, Leung JM, et al: Monitoring for myocardial ischemia during noncardiac surgery. A technology assessment of transesophageal echocardiography and 12-lead electrocardiography. The Study of Perioperative Ischemia Research Group. JAMA 268:210, 1992.

97. Hogue CW Jr, Goodnough LT, Monk TG: Perioperative myocardial ischemic episodes are related to hematocrit level in patients undergoing radical prostatectomy. Transfusion 38:924, 1998.

98. Nelson AH, Fleisher LA, Rosenbaum SH: Relationship between postoperative anemia and cardiac morbidity in high-risk vascular patients in the intensive care unit. Crit Care Med 21:860, 1993.

CH 80

GUIDELINES *Thomas H. Lee*

Reducing Cardiac Risk with Noncardiac Surgery

Guidelines on the assessment and management of perioperative cardiovascular risk for patients undergoing noncardiac surgery were published by an American College of Cardiology/American Heart Association (ACC/AHA) task force in 1996 and updated in 2002.[1] Guidelines were also published by the American College of Physicians (ACP) in 1997,[2] but these guidelines preceded more recent research that has shifted the focus of management from noninvasive risk stratification to risk reduction through strategies such as the use of perioperative beta blockade. The latest update from the ACC/AHA in 2006 focuses on perioperative beta blocker therapy.[3]

Both the ACC/AHA and ACP guidelines emphasize the importance of a directed history and physical examination, including assessment of patient functional capacity. Clinicians are urged to give attention to noncardiac comorbid conditions as well as cardiac issues. The

ACC/AHA guidelines note but do not endorse any single risk prediction decision aid; instead, these guidelines recommend a stepwise algorithm to identify patients most appropriate for noninvasive testing for further risk stratification (see Fig. 80-2).

The ACC/AHA guidelines also offer a simple alternative approach for clinicians to decide whether noninvasive cardiac testing is needed (Fig. 80G-1). The guidelines recommend noninvasive testing if any two of these three factors are present:

Intermediate clinical predictors are present (Canadian class 1 or 2 angina, prior myocardial infarction based on history or pathological Q waves, compensated or prior heart failure, or diabetes)

Poor functional capacity (less than 4 METs [metabolic equivalents])

High-risk surgical procedure (e.g., emergency major operation, aortic repair or peripheral vascular surgery, prolonged surgical procedure with large fluid shifts or blood loss)

ACC/AHA recommendations for the use of tests in patients undergoing noncardiac surgery are summarized in Table 80G-1. The routine 12-lead electrocardiogram (ECG) is supported for use in patients with high or intermediate clinical risk factors, including diabetes, or recent chest pain. The guidelines recommend restraint in the use of ECGs in asymptomatic patients undergoing low-risk procedures. Routine use of echocardiography to assess left ventricular function is discouraged unless patients have heart failure or dyspnea of unknown cause. Similarly, routine use of exercise or pharmacological stress testing in asymptomatic patients without evidence of coronary artery disease is considered a Class III indication (not supported by evidence).

The recommendations for use of coronary angiography (see Table 80G-1) reflect the goal of improving the patient's long-term cardiovas-

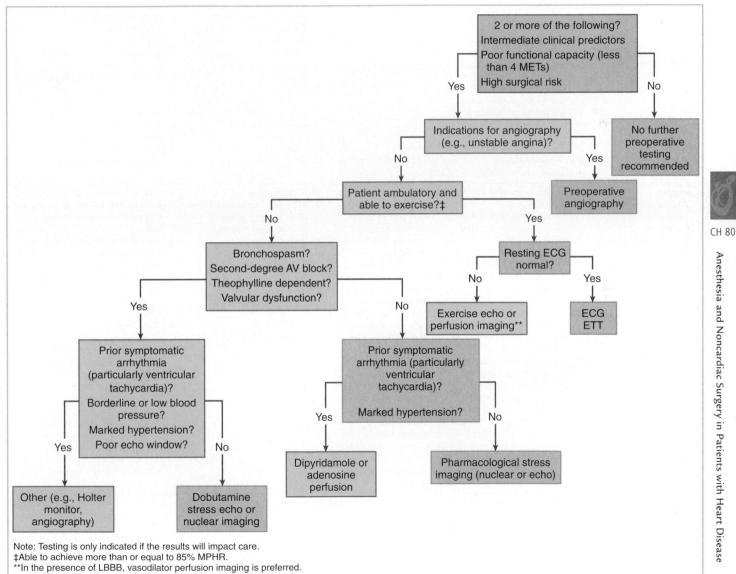

Note: Testing is only indicated if the results will impact care.
‡Able to achieve more than or equal to 85% MPHR.
**In the presence of LBBB, vasodilator perfusion imaging is preferred.

FIGURE 80G-1 Supplemental preoperative evaluation. AV = atrioventricular; ECG = electrocardiogram; ETT = exercise tolerance test; LBBB = left bundle branch block; MET = metabolic equivalent. (From Eagle KA, Berger PB, Calkins H, et al; American College of Cardiology; American Heart Association: ACC/AHA guideline update for perioperative cardiovascular evaluation for noncardiac surgery—executive summary. A report of the American College of Cardiology/American Heart Association Task Force on Practice Guidelines [Committee to Update the 1996 Guidelines on Perioperative Cardiovascular Evaluation for Noncardiac Surgery]. J Am Coll Cardiol 39:542, 2002.)

CH 80

Anesthesia and Noncardiac Surgery in Patients with Heart Disease

TABLE 80G–1 American College of Cardiology/American Heart Association Recommendations for Use of Ancillary Tests in Patients Undergoing Noncardiac Surgery

Indication	Class I (Indicated)	Class IIa (Good Supportive Evidence)	Class IIb (Weak Supportive Evidence)	Class III (Not Indicated)
Preoperative 12-lead rest ECG	1. Recent episode of chest pain or ischemic equivalent in clinically intermediate- or high-risk patients scheduled for an intermediate- or high-risk operative procedure	1. Asymptomatic persons with diabetes mellitus	1. Patients with prior coronary revascularization 2. Asymptomatic man older than 45 yr or woman older than 55 yr with two or more atherosclerotic risk factors 3. Prior hospital admission for cardiac causes	1. As a routine test in asymptomatic subjects undergoing low-risk operative procedures
Preoperative noninvasive evaluation of left ventricular function	1. Patients with current or poorly controlled heart failure	1. Patients with prior heart failure and patients with dyspnea of unknown origin		1. As a routine test of left ventricular function in patients without prior heart failure
Exercise or pharmacological stress testing	1. Diagnosis of adult patients with intermediate pretest probability of CAD 2. Prognostic assessment of patients undergoing initial evaluation for suspected or proven CAD; evaluation of subjects with significant change in clinical status 3. Demonstration of proof of myocardial ischemia before coronary revascularization 4. Evaluation of adequacy of medical therapy 5. Prognostic assessment after an acute coronary syndrome (if recent evaluation unavailable)	1. Evaluation of exercise capacity when subjective assessment is unreliable	1. Diagnosis of CAD patients with high or low pretest probability; those with resting ST depression less than 1 mm, those undergoing digitalis therapy, and those with ECG criteria for left ventricular hypertrophy 2. Detection of restenosis in high-risk asymptomatic subjects within the initial months after PCI	1. For *exercise* stress testing, diagnosis of patients with resting ECG abnormalities that preclude adequate assessment (e.g., preexcitation syndrome, electronically paced ventricular rhythm, resting ST depression greater than 1 mm, or left bundle branch block) 2. Severe comorbidity likely to limit life expectancy or candidacy for revascularization 3. Routine screening of asymptomatic men or women without evidence of CAD 4. Investigation of isolated ectopic beats in young patients
Coronary angiography in perioperative evaluation before (or after) noncardiac surgery	Patients with suspected or known CAD: 1. Evidence for high risk of adverse outcome based on noninvasive test results 2. Angina unresponsive to adequate medical therapy 3. Unstable angina, particularly when facing intermediate-risk* or high-risk* noncardiac surgery 4. Equivocal noninvasive test results in patients at high clinical risk† undergoing high-risk* surgery	1. Multiple markers of intermediate clinical risk† and planned vascular surgery (noninvasive testing should be considered first) 2. Moderate to large region of ischemia on noninvasive testing but without high-risk features and without lower LVEF 3. Nondiagnostic noninvasive test results in patients of intermediate clinical risk† undergoing high-risk* noncardiac surgery 4. Urgent noncardiac surgery while convalescing from acute MI	1. Perioperative MI 2. Medically stabilized Class III or IV angina and planned low-risk or minor* surgery	1. Low-risk* noncardiac surgery with known CAD and no high-risk results on noninvasive testing 2. Asymptomatic after coronary revascularization with excellent exercise capacity (≥7 METs) 3. Mild stable angina with good left ventricular function and no high-risk noninvasive test results 4. Noncandidate for coronary revascularization because of concomitant medical illness, severe left ventricular dysfunction (e.g., LVEF < 0.20), or refusal to consider revascularization 5. Candidate for liver, lung, or renal transplantation older than 40 yr as part of evaluation for transplantation, unless noninvasive testing reveals high risk for adverse outcome

*Cardiac risk according to type of noncardiac surgery. High risk—emergent major operations, aortic and major vascular surgery, peripheral vascular surgery, anticipated prolonged surgical procedure associated with large fluid shifts and blood loss; intermediate risk—carotid endarterectomy, major head and neck surgery, intraperitoneal and intrathoracic surgery, orthopedic surgery, or prostate surgery; low risk—endoscopic procedure, superficial procedure, cataract surgery, breast surgery.

†Cardiac risk according to clinical predictors of perioperative death, MI, or HF. High clinical risk—unstable angina, acute or recent MI with evidence of important residual ischemic risk, decompensated HF, high degree of atrioventricular block, symptomatic ventricular arrhythmias with known structural heart disease, severe symptomatic valvular heart disease, or patient with multiple intermediate-risk markers such as prior MI, HF, and diabetes; intermediate clinical risk—Canadian Cardiovascular Society class I or II angina, prior MI by history or ECG, compensated or prior HF, diabetes mellitus, renal insufficiency.

CAD = coronary artery disease; ECG = electrocardiogram; HF = heart failure; LVEF = left ventricular ejection fraction; MET = metabolic equivalent; MI = myocardial infarction; PCI = percutaneous coronary intervention.

From Eagle KA, Berger PB, Calkins H, et al: ACC/AHA guideline update for perioperative cardiovascular evaluation for noncardiac surgery—executive summary: A report of the American College of Cardiology/American Heart Association Task Force on Practice Guidelines (Committee to Update the 1996 Guidelines on Perioperative Cardiovascular Evaluation for Noncardiac Surgery). J Am Coll Cardiol 39:542, 2002.

TABLE 80G–2	American College of Cardiology/American Heart Association (ACC/AHA) 2006 Guidelines on the Use of Perioperative Beta Blocker Therapy for Noncardiac Surgery			

Class I (Indicated) [Level of Evidence]	Class IIa (Good Supportive Evidence) [Level of Evidence]	Class IIB (Weak Supportive Evidence) [Level of Evidence]	Class III (Not Indicated) [Level of Evidence]
Continue beta blocker therapy in patients undergoing surgery who are receiving a beta blocker to treat angina, symptomatic arrhythmias, hypertension, or other ACC/AHA Class I guideline indications. [C]	Consider a beta blocker for patients undergoing vascular surgery in whom preoperative assessment identifies coronary heart disease. [B]	Possibly consider a beta blocker for patients undergoing intermediate- or high-risk procedures, including vascular surgery, in whom preoperative assessment identifies intermediate cardiac risk as defined by the presence of a single clinical risk factor.* [C]	Do not institute beta blocker therapy in patients undergoing surgery who have one or more absolute contraindications to beta blockade. [C]
Institute beta blockade for patients undergoing vascular surgery at high cardiac risk because of the finding of ischemia on preoperative testing. [B]	Consider a beta blocker for patients in whom preoperative assessment for vascular surgery identifies high cardiac risk as defined by the presence of multiple clinical risk factors.* Consider a beta blocker for patients in whom preoperative assessment identifies coronary heart disease or high cardiac risk as defined by the presence of multiple clinical risk factors* and who are undergoing vintermediate- or high-risk procedures.	Possibly consider a beta blocker in patients undergoing vascular surgery with low cardiac risk who are not currently on a beta blocker. [C]	

*From Eagle KA, Berger PB, Calkins H, et al; American College of Cardiology; American Heart Association: ACC/AHA guideline update for perioperative cardiovascular evaluation for noncardiac surgery—executive summary. A report of the American College of Cardiology/American Heart Association Task Force on Practice Guidelines [Committee to Update the 1996 Guidelines on Perioperative Cardiovascular Evaluation for Noncardiac Surgery]. J Am Coll Cardiol 39:542, 2002.

TABLE 80G–3	American College of Cardiology/American Heart Association Recommendations for Use of Interventions in Patients Undergoing Noncardiac Surgery			

Indication	Class I (Indicated)	Class IIa (Good Supportive Evidence)	Class IIb (Weak Supportive Evidence)	Class III (Not Indicated)
Perioperative beta blockers Other perioperative medical therapy	See Table 80G-2.		Alpha₂ agonists: perioperative control of hypertension, or known CAD or major risk factors for CAD	Alpha₂ agonists: contraindication to alpha₂ agonists
Intraoperative nitroglycerin	High-risk patients previously taking nitroglycerin who have active signs of myocardial ischemia without hypotension	As a prophylactic agent for high-risk patients to prevent myocardial ischemia and cardiac morbidity, particularly in those who have required nitrate therapy to control angina		Patients with signs of hypovolemia or hypotension
Intraoperative use of pulmonary artery catheters		Patients at risk for major hemodynamic disturbances most easily detected by a pulmonary artery catheter who are undergoing a procedure that is likely to cause these hemodynamic changes (e.g., suprarenal aortic aneurysm repair in a patient with angina) in a setting with experience in interpreting the results	Either the patient's condition or the surgical procedure (but not both) places the patient at risk for hemodynamic disturbances (e.g., supraceliac aortic aneurysm repair in a patient with a negative stress test).	No risk of hemodynamic disturbances
Perioperative ST segment monitoring		When available, proper use of computerized ST segment analysis in patients with known CAD or undergoing vascular surgery may provide increased sensitivity to detect myocardial ischemia during the perioperative period and may identify patients who would benefit from further postoperative and long-term interventions	Patients with single or multiple risk factors for CAD.	Patients at low risk for CAD

CAD = coronary artery disease.

From Eagle KA, Berger PB, Calkins H, et al; American College of Cardiology; American Heart Association: ACC/AHA guideline update for perioperative cardiovascular evaluation for noncardiac surgery—executive summary. A report of the American College of Cardiology/American Heart Association Task Force on Practice Guidelines [Committee to Update the 1996 Guidelines on Perioperative Cardiovascular Evaluation for Noncardiac Surgery]. J Am Coll Cardiol 39:542, 2002.

CH 80

Anesthesia and Noncardiac Surgery in Patients with Heart Disease

cular prognosis and of minimizing the chances of the patient having an acute complication during the planned procedure. In general, the same indications that are used to determine whether a nonsurgical patient warrants coronary angiography should be used in the preoperative setting, but the threshold for performing angiography should decrease if the patient is to undergo a higher risk surgical procedure.

RISK REDUCTION INTERVENTIONS

The guidelines emphasize that "It is almost never appropriate to recommend coronary bypass surgery or other invasive interventions such as coronary angioplasty in an effort to reduce the risk of noncardiac surgery when they would not otherwise be indicated." Thus, most of the attention of the guidelines is given to medical therapies and monitoring interventions for higher risk patients.

The 2006 update focuses on the perioperative use of beta blockers mainly because the Physicians Consortium for Performance Improvement and the Surgical Care Improvement Project identified perioperative beta blockade as a quality measure. In this update, beta blockers receive support for use in various patient subgroups. The guidelines strongly support their use in patients with coronary heart disease or at high cardiac risk who are undergoing vascular surgery, as well as for those who are taking a beta blocker to treat angina, hypertension, or symptomatic arrhythmias or other ACC/AHA Class I guideline recommendations. The guidelines are somewhat less supportive of their use in other populations (Table 80G-2), for whom the ideal target populations, doses, and routes of beta blocker administration have yet to be delineated. Practical considerations such as how, when, and how long to continue perioperative beta blocker therapy also remain uncertain.

Evidence for the perioperative use of alpha$_2$-agonists was considered less convincing. Intraoperative nitroglycerin is supported for patients with acute ischemic syndromes who must undergo noncardiac procedures on an urgent basis. The guidelines warn that prophylactic use of nitroglycerin must take into account the anesthetic plan and patient's hemodynamics and must recognize the risk of vasodilation and hypovolemia during anesthesia and surgery. The ACC/AHA task force did not find sufficient evidence to balance risks and benefits

of intraaortic balloon counterpulsation for patients with myocardial ischemic syndromes or routine use of transesophageal echocardiography.

The guidelines acknowledge data (primarily from observational studies) questioning the value of pulmonary artery catheterization for patients undergoing noncardiac surgery, but note that this procedure might provide valuable information in patients at highest risk for and from hemodynamic shifts with major procedures (Table 80G-3). These recommendations preceded a large randomized controlled trial that did not find benefit from pulmonary artery catheterization in elderly high-risk surgical patients.[4] There was some support for use of ST segment monitoring to detect perioperative ischemia, but the guidelines acknowledge that no studies have shown that this intervention improves outcome when therapy is based on the resulting data.

Perioperative surveillance for acute coronary syndromes using routine ECGs and cardiac serum biomarkers is considered unnecessary in clinically low-risk patients undergoing low-risk operative procedures. In patients with high or intermediate clinical risk who have known or suspected coronary artery disease and who are undergoing high- or intermediate-risk surgical procedures, the guidelines recommend performance of ECGs at baseline, immediately after the surgical procedure, and daily on the first 2 days after surgery. For detection of myocardial injury, cardiac troponin measurements 24 hours postoperatively and on day 4 or hospital discharge (whichever comes first) are recommended.

References

1. Eagle KA, Berger PB, Calkins H, et al: ACC/AHA guideline update for perioperative cardiovascular evaluation for noncardiac surgery—executive summary: A report of the American College of Cardiology/American Heart Association Task Force on Practice Guidelines (Committee to Update the 1996 Guidelines on Perioperative Cardiovascular Evaluation for Noncardiac Surgery). J Am Coll Cardiol 39:542, 2002.
2. Guidelines for assessing and managing the perioperative risk from coronary artery disease associated with major noncardiac surgery. American College of Physicians. Ann Intern Med 127:309, 1997.
3. Fleisher LA, Beckman JA, Brown KA, et al: ACC/AHA 2006 guideline update on perioperative cardiovascular evaluation for noncardiac surgery: Focused update on perioperative beta-blocker therapy. J Am Coll Cardiol 47:2343, 2006.
4. Sandham JD, Hull RD, Brant RF, et al: A randomized, controlled trial of the use of pulmonary-artery catheters in high-risk surgical patients. N Engl J Med 348:5, 2003.

PART X

Cardiovascular Disease and Disorders of Other Organs

Pituitary Gland, 2033
Growth Hormone, 2033
Cardiovascular Manifestations of
    Acromegaly, 2034
Adrenal Corticotropic Hormone and
    Cortisol, 2035
Cushing Disease, 2035
Hyperaldosteronism, 2036
Addison Disease, 2037

Parathyroid Disease, 2037

Thyroid Gland, 2038
Hemodynamic Alterations in Thyroid
    Disease, 2040
Hyperthyroidism, 2040
Hypothyroidism, 2042
Amiodarone and Thyroid
    Function, 2044

Pheochromocytoma, 2045

Future Perspectives, 2046

References, 2046

CHAPTER 81

Endocrine Disorders and Cardiovascular Disease

Irwin Klein

Medical science has few areas in which basic science investigation links more closely to clinical observations and therapy than in cardiovascular endocrinology. As our understanding of the cellular and molecular effects of various hormones evolves, we can better understand the clinical manifestations that arise from both excess hormone secretion and glandular failure leading to hormone deficiency states. More than 200 years ago Caleb Hillier Parry, an English physician, described a woman with goiter and palpitations whose "each systole shook the whole thorax." He was the first to suggest the notion that there was a connection between diseases of the heart and enlargement of the thyroid gland. The cardiovascular abnormalities associated with pathologic changes of endocrine glands were recognized before the identification of the specific hormones produced by these glands. This chapter reviews the spectrum of cardiac disease states that arise from changes in specific endocrine function. This approach allows us to explore the cellular mechanisms by which various hormones can alter the cardiovascular system through actions on the cardiac myocyte, vascular smooth muscle cells, and other target cells and tissues.

PITUITARY GLAND

The pituitary gland consists of two distinct anatomical portions. The anterior or adenohypophysis contains six different cell types, five of which produce polypeptide or glycoprotein hormones, and the sixth is classically referred to as nonsecretory chromophobic cells. Of these cell types, the somatotrophic cells, which secrete human growth hormone (hGH), and the corticotropic cells, which produce adrenocorticotropic hormone (ACTH), can contribute to cardiac disease. The posterior pituitary or neurohypophysis is the anatomical location for the nerve terminals that secrete vasopressin (antidiuretic hormone) or oxytocin.

Growth Hormone

In adults, excessive growth hormone secretion before the fusion of bony epiphysis leads to gigantism, whereas increased secretion of hGH after maturation of the long bones leads to acromegaly. The growth-promoting factor obtained from extracts of the pituitary gland was first identified by Evans and Long in the early 1920s. Almost 50 years later the protein sequence and structure of hGH was first identified, and its role as one member of a family of growth-promoting (somatic) factors emerged.

Growth hormone exerts its cellular effects through two major pathways. The first is by hormone binding to specific growth hormone receptors on target cells. These receptors have been identified in heart, skeletal muscle, fat, liver, and kidney and in many additional cell types throughout fetal development.[1] The second growth-promoting effect of hGH results from stimulation of synthesis of the insulin-like growth factor type 1 (IGF-1). This protein is produced primarily in liver, but other cell types can produce IGF-1 under the influence of hGH.

Shortly after the identification of the IGF family, it was proposed that most actions of growth hormone were mediated through this second messenger. Clinical disease activity of patients with growth hormone excess (acromegaly) correlates better with serum levels of IGF-1 than with hGH. The ability to promote glucose uptake and cellular protein synthesis gave rise to the term *insulin-like*. IGF-1 binds to its cognate IGF-1 receptor localized on virtually all cell types. Transgenic experiments have demonstrated that the presence of IGF-1 receptors on cell types is closely linked to the ability of those cells to divide. Ingenious studies in which the IGF-1 receptor was overexpressed in cardiac myocytes reportedly produced an increased myocyte number, mitotic rate, and the ability of postdifferentiated myocytes to replicate. The harnessing of this action holds potential benefit for genetic manipulation and repair of the diseased myocardium.

Infusion of either hGH or IGF-1 acutely changes cardiovascular hemodynamics. The acute increases in cardiac contractility and cardiac output may be caused, at least in part, by a decrease in systemic vascular resistance and cardiac afterload.[2] Short-term administration of both hGH and IGF-1 does not increase blood pressure, implying that the increase in cardiac output is indeed a result of changes in systemic vascular resistance.[3,4]

Cardiovascular Manifestations of Acromegaly

Acromegaly is a relatively uncommon condition (approximately 900 new cases each year in the United States). Acromegaly and pituitary-dependent human gigantism are associated with markedly increased morbidity and mortality primarily from cardiovascular disease. Untreated acromegaly, identified by its characteristic clinical signs and symptoms and by increased hGH secretion, markedly shortens life expectancy with less than 20 percent of patients surviving beyond 60 years. Multiple studies implicate increased neoplasia arising from the gastrointestinal tract, colon polyps, colon cancer, and pulmonary disease in this increased mortality.[5] However, the cardiovascular and cerebrovascular changes including hypertension, cardiomegaly, congestive heart failure, and cerebral vascular accidents continue to serve as the major events that limit survival.[6] Cardiovascular involvement in acromegaly is a chronic insidious process that was first recognized by Pierre Marie in 1886.

The cardiovascular and hemodynamic effects of acromegaly vary considerably depending on age, severity of disease, and disease duration.[7] Patients diagnosed with less than 5 years of disease activity had no significant change in systolic or diastolic blood pressure, but echocardiographic determination of left ventricular mass index increased almost 35 percent and cardiac index increased 24 percent.[8] Measures of systolic function including stroke index increased significantly, and systemic vascular resistance rose by 20 percent. Left ventricular diastolic function was normal.[6,7] These studies stand in contrast to the reports that longer duration of acromegaly produces left ventricular dysfunction and cardiomyopathy. In untreated acromegaly, global left ventricular diastolic dysfunction accompanies cardiac hypertrophy. Regional myocardial systolic strain abnormalities identified by Doppler imaging reversed with treatment.[9]

Known cardiac disease risk factors including hypertension, insulin resistance, diabetes mellitus, and hyperlipidemia frequently occur in patients with acromegaly. Although initial reports suggest that impairment of cardiac function in longstanding acromegaly was caused by accelerated atherosclerosis, a postmortem study revealed significant coronary artery disease in only 11 percent of patients dying from disease-related causes. Angiography demonstrates the presence of either normal or dilated coronary arteries in most cases. Nuclear stress testing is positive in less than 25 percent of patients and overall allows us to conclude that atherosclerosis and ischemic heart disease are unlikely to account for the marked degrees of biventricular cardiac hypertrophy, cardiac failure, and cardiovascular mortality. A rather specific functional and histological myocyte change appears to arise in the setting of prolonged excess serum levels of hGH and IGF-1.[8] Up to two thirds of acromegalic patients have echocardiographic criteria for left ventricular hypertrophy (LVH).[6,7] The right ventricle also increases in mass in acromegaly, indicating a more generalized process beyond systemic hypertension.[9] Asymmetrical septal hypertrophy, initially thought to be common in patients with acromegaly, is an unusual finding. Acromegaly increases the prevalence of both aortic and mitral valve disease, which persists despite disease cure.[10] In patients with uncontrolled acromegaly, progressive mitral valve regurgitation and left ventricular strain occur.[11] Acromegalic patients may present with dilatation of the aortic root, and defects of the cardiac conduction system have been reported.[7,12]

Histological evaluation of acromegalic cardiac tissue reveals an increase in myocyte size (hypertrophy) without an increase in cell number. Acromegaly produces interstitial fibrosis and infiltration of a variety of inflammatory cells including mononuclear cells consistent with myocarditis.[6] The absence of cell necrosis in the presence of an inflammatory reaction has raised the question of whether part of these histological findings can be accounted for by IGF-1–promoted programmed cell death (apoptosis).

Functional changes accompany pathological involvement of the heart in acromegaly.[8,9] Although approximately 10 percent of newly diagnosed patients have signs and symptoms of cardiac compromise, this percentage increases markedly with disease duration.[11-13] Some studies report a low incidence of overt left ventricular failure, suggesting that supervening factors including hypertension, type 2 diabetes, and hyperlipidemia are necessary to impair function. In acromegaly, LVH and congestive heart failure can occur in longstanding disease without hypertension, indicating that high levels of growth hormone and/or IGF-1 can produce cardiac myopathic changes per se.[12] Importantly, successful therapy reverses many, if not all, of these findings.[14,15]

Electrocardiogram (ECG) abnormalities including left axis deviation, septal Q-waves, ST-T wave depression, abnormal QT dispersion, and conduction system defects occur in up to 50 percent of acromegalic patients. A variety of dysrhythmias including atrial and ventricular ectopic beats, sick sinus syndrome, as well as supraventricular and ventricular tachycardias can occur.[6] The finding of a fourfold increase in complex ventricular arrhythmias and late potentials observed in a signal average ECG, thought to be predictors of ventricular irritability, were also more common in active acromegaly when compared with treated patients.[12] In contrast, exercise stress testing with ECG monitoring did not show inducible rhythm disturbances or evidence of ischemia, suggesting that left ventricular rhythm disturbances did not relate to any underlying ischemia.

Secondary hypertension associated with acromegaly occurs in 20 to 40 percent of patients.[5-7] Given the overall high prevalence rate of hypertension in the adult population and the insidious onset of acromegaly, determining whether hypertension is secondary or merely coincidental is difficult. The improvement with therapy, however, suggests that they are related.[15] Although epidemiological studies of survival in acromegaly initially suggested that hypertension was not an independent risk factor for mortality, in a survey of patients dying of the disease it was demonstrated that mean blood pressures were higher than in those who survived.[5] The mechanism underlying hypertension in acromegaly is not clearly understood. Newly diagnosed patients with short-duration disease had systolic and diastolic blood pressures no different from age- and sex-matched controls, whereas cardiac index was significantly increased. It does appear that in longstanding acromegalic patients, the arterial intimal thickness is increased and these changes respond to hGH lowering.[2,6]

Growth hormone administration promotes sodium retention and volume expansion and appears to have a potent antinatriuretic effect independent of any effect on aldosterone.[3,16] Studies of the renin-angiotensin-aldosterone system show a failure to optimally inhibit renin release by volume expansion. Patients with acromegaly have a paradoxical increase in blood pressure to angiotensin II inhibitors. The role of hyperinsulinemia in the hypertension of acromegaly has been questioned. Increased serum insulin can contribute to urinary sodium retention, impairment of endothelial-dependent vasodilation, and increased sympathetic activity.

DIAGNOSIS

In 99 percent of cases, acromegaly arises from benign adenomas of the anterior pituitary gland.[5,15] At the time of diagnosis the majority of these neoplasms are classified as macroadenomas (>10 mm) and patients have clinical evidence of disease for more than 10 years. The diagnosis can be confirmed by demonstrating a serum growth hormone greater than 5 ng/dl and a serum IGF-1 level greater than 300 μIU/ml measured 1 hour after a 100 gm glucose load. In the majority of patients fasting growth hormone levels are greater than 10 ng/ml. Tumor localization can be established by magnetic resonance imaging dedicated to the pituitary gland. Rarely, growth hormone–releasing hormone (GH-RH) can be secreted, causing diffuse hyperplasia of the pituitary. The existence of such changes must lead to the consideration of a neoplastic lesion residing in other parts (ectopic) of the endocrine system.

THERAPY

Transsphenoidal surgery with resection of the adenoma is the procedure of choice for initial management. If hGH and/or IGF-1 remain elevated, radiotherapy in older patients or dopamine or somatostatin receptor agonists in younger patients can be used to restore serum growth hormone and IGF-1 levels to normal. Octreotide acetate is a pharmacological analogue to somatostatin and is effective in the vast majority of patients to lower hGH to less than 5 ng/ml. It may be primary therapy to both lower IGF-1 levels and shrink tumor size in selected cases.[15,17] The cardiovascular complications of acromegaly including hypertension, LVH and left ventricular dysfunction improve with treatment, and survival is significantly better in patients achieving disease remission.[7,11] A recently approved growth hormone receptor antagonist, pegvisomant, can normalize IGF-1 levels in long-term therapy and may play a role in somatostatin-resistant patients.[14,15]

Adrenal Corticotropic Hormone and Cortisol

The adrenal corticotropic cells in the anterior pituitary synthesize a large protein (pro-opiomelanocortin), which is then processed within the corticotropic cell into a family of smaller proteins that include alpha-melanocyte stimulating hormone, beta-endorphin, and ACTH. ACTH in turn binds to specific cells within the adrenal gland. The adrenal gland anatomically consists of two major segments: the cortex and the medulla. The cortex zona glomerulosa produces aldosterone, and the zona fasciculata produces primarily cortisol and some androgenic steroids. The zona reticularis also produces cortisol and androgens. ACTH regulates synthesis of cortisol in the zona fasciculata and reticularis. The zona glomerulosa shows a much lesser degree of ACTH responsiveness and responds primarily to angiotensin II by increased aldosterone secretion.

Cushing Disease

Excess cortisol secretion and its attendant clinical disease states can arise either from excess pituitary release of ACTH (Cushing disease) or through the adenomatous or rarely malignant neoplastic process arising in the adrenal gland itself (Cushing syndrome). Well-characterized conditions of both adrenal glucocorticoid, as well as mineralocorticoid excess, appear to result from the excessively high levels of

(ectopic) ACTH produced by small cell carcinoma of the lung, carcinoid tumors, pancreatic islet cell tumors, medullary thyroid cancer, and other adenocarcinomas and hematologic malignancies.

Cortisol, a member of the glucocorticoid family of steroid hormones, binds to monomeric receptors located within the cytoplasm of many cell types (Fig. 81-1). The unliganded glucocorticoid receptors are bound to heat shock protein complexes. After binding cortisol, the receptors dissociate from these complexes, homodimerize or occasionally heterodimerize, translocate to the nucleus, and function as transcription factors. A variety of cardiac genes contain glucocorticoid response elements in their promoter region that confer glucocorticoid responsiveness.[18] These genes include those that encode the voltage-gated potassium channel, as well as protein kinases, which serve to phosphorylate and regulate voltage-gated sodium channels. This expression may be chamber specific and play a role in the developing fetal heart.[19]

The cardiac effects of glucocorticoid excess in Cushing disease rise from both the direct effects of glucocorticoids on the heart as well as from the effects of glucocorticoids on the liver, skeletal muscle, and fat tissue.[18-20] Accelerated atherosclerosis can result from abnormal glucose metabolism with hyperglycemia and hyperinsulinemia, hypertension, and altered clotting and platelet function. The mechanism for cortisol-mediated hypertension is multifactorial. Studies have shown that, in contrast to aldosterone-induced hypertension, the central administration of glucocorticoids lowers blood pressure. Thus cortisol-mediated hypertension appears not to result from activation of the mineralocorticoid receptor. In addition, antagonism of glucocorticoid effects via its cytosolic receptor can block cortisol-induced elevations of glucose and insulin but not those related to blood pressure.[21,22] Interestingly, one study suggested that inhibition of sodium retention, is also insufficient to block the cortisol-mediated rise in blood pressure pointing to the changes in vascular reactivity, systemic vascular resistance, and nitric oxide–mediated vasodilatation as candidates for the hypertensive effect.[18]

The rise in serum glucose and the development of insulin resistance may give rise to activation of proinflammatory cytokines such as tumor necrosis factor-alpha and interleukin-6 (IL-6), which may underlie the accelerated atherosclerosis of insulin resistance found in other endocrine disease states.[21] Thus while acting classically as an antiinflammatory hormone, cortisol excess can promote inflammation and accelerate atherosclerosis by producing insulin resistance, changes in corticosteroid binding protein, and regulation of a variety of pro-inflammatory cytokines. The centripetal obesity characteristic of glucocorticoid excess resembles that seen in the insulin resistance syndromes.[21] Excess androgen production resulting from increased ACTH stimulation of the adrenal cortex may also accelerate atherosclerosis in both men and women.

The increased cardiovascular morbidity and mortality of Cushing syndrome can in large part be explained by cerebrovascular disease, peripheral vascular disease, coronary artery disease with myocardial infarction, and chronic congestive heart failure.[20,22] All expected changes in the setting of accelerated atherosclerosis result from hypertension and hyperlipidemia.[23] Studies of left ventricular structure and function have shown hypertrophy and impaired contractility in 40 percent of patients.[24] Cushing syndrome can present as dilated cardiomyopathy.[25] In addition, the marked muscle weakness resulting from corticosteroid-induced skeletal myopathy contributes to impaired exercise tolerance.

Patients with Cushing disease can exhibit a variety of ECG changes. The duration of the P-R interval appears to correlate directly with adrenal cortisol production rates. The mechanism underlying this may relate to either the expression or the regulation of the voltage-gated sodium channel (SCN5A). Changes in ECGs, specifically P-R and QT intervals, may also arise as a result of the direct (nongenomic) effects of glucocorticoids on the voltage-gated potassium channel (Kv1.5) in a variety of excitable tissues.[18,20]

A particular complex of cardiac and adrenal lesions, referred to as Carney complex, combines Cushing syndrome, cardiac myxoma, and a variety of pigmented dermal lesions

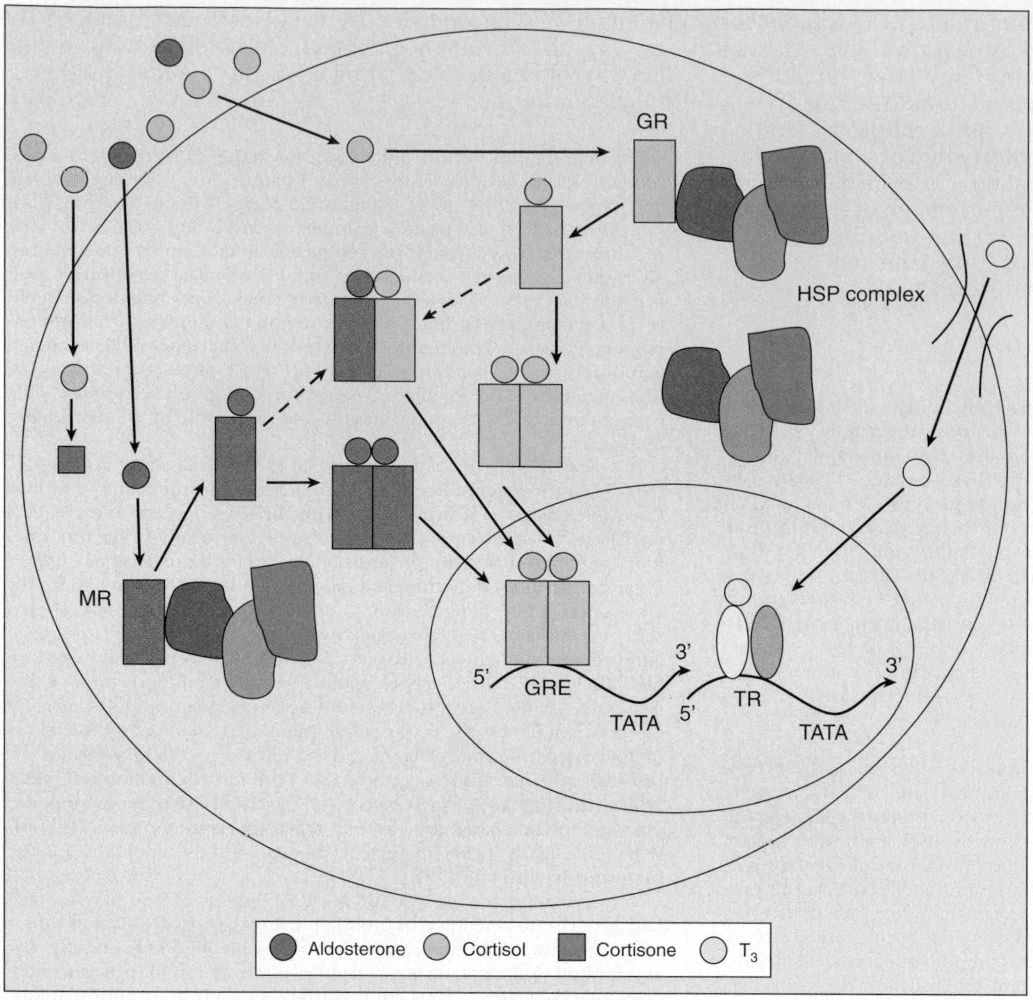

FIGURE 81–1 Scheme of a generalized nuclear hormone receptor mechanism of action. The mineralocorticoid receptor (MR) has similar affinities for aldosterone and cortisol. Circulating levels of cortisol are 100 to 1000 times greater than that of aldosterone. In MR-responsive cells, the enzyme 11 beta-hydroxysteroid dehydrogenase metabolizes cortisol to cortisone, thereby allowing aldosterone to bind to MR. MR and the glucocorticoid receptor (GR) are cytoplasmic receptors that, after binding ligand, translocate to the nucleus and bind to glucocorticoid response elements (GREs) in the promoter regions of responsive genes. Triiodothyronine (T_3) enters the cell by facilitated diffusion and binds to thyroid hormone receptors (TRs), which are bound to thyroid hormone response elements (TREs) in the promoter regions of T_3-responsive genes. HSP = heat shock protein. *(Courtesy of Dr. S. Danzi.)*

clinical signs and symptoms of Cushing syndrome. In nonsurgical patients, the adrenal enzyme inhibitor ketoconazole can reverse excess cortisol production. Even mild or subclinical degrees of Cushing syndrome (adrenal "incidentaloma") appear to increase the risk for cardiovascular disease.[27]

Hyperaldosteronism

Aldosterone production by the zona glomerulosa is under the control of the renin angiotensin system.[28,29] Renin secretion responds primarily to changes in intravascular volume. Aldosterone synthesis and secretion is primarily regulated by angiotensin II, which binds to the angiotensin II type I receptor on the cells of the zona glomerulosa.[28,29]

The mechanism of action of aldosterone on target tissues resembles that reported for glucocorticoids (see Fig. 81-1).[30] Aldosterone is taken up into cells and binds to the mineralocorticoid receptor, which then translocates to the nucleus and promotes the expression of aldosterone-responsive genes.[28] In addition to kidney cells, where mineralocorticoid receptors control sodium transport, in vitro studies have demonstrated these receptors in rat cardiac myocytes. These receptors respond to mineralocorticoid stimulation with an increase in protein synthesis.[30,31] Whether these changes correspond to any relevant in vivo cardiac effects is unclear, but aldosterone may augment the development of cardiac hypertrophy in hypertension. Genetically engineered mice with an inactive mineralocorticoid receptor gene show classic features of mineralocorticoid deficiency and require sodium supplementation to survive. The aldosterone antagonists spironolactone and eplerenone compete for receptor binding in the cytosol (see Fig. 81-1). Recent studies have defined a role for the drugs in the treatment of left ventricular dysfunction, heart failure, and hypertension.[32,33]

Although the major cause of increased serum aldosterone is in the physiological response to the activation of the renin angiotensin system, there are well-recognized aldosterone-producing benign adrenal adenomas (Conn syndrome). Primary hyperaldosteronism augments sodium retention, causes hypertension, increases renal loss of magnesium and potassium, decreases arterial compliance with a rise in systemic vascular resistance and resulting vascular damage, and alters the sympathetic and parasympathetic neural regulation. Many of the changes in the heart and cardiovascular system in hyperaldosteronism result from the associated hypertension.[33] The degree of LVH, however, exceeds that expected from the hypertension alone, perhaps

(not café-au-lait).[26] This monogenic autosomal dominant trait maps to the Q2 region of chromosome 17. Myxomas most commonly occur in the left atrium but occur throughout the heart, occur at young ages, and be multicentric.

DIAGNOSIS

Diagnosis of Cushing disease and syndrome require demonstration of increased cortisol production as reflected by an elevated 24-hour, urinary-free cortisol. ACTH measurements to determine whether the disease is pituitary, adrenal, or ectopically based and anatomical localization with magnetic resonance imaging of the suspected lesions confirms the laboratory tests.

TREATMENT

The treatment of excess cortisol production depends on the underlying mechanisms. In Cushing disease, transsphenoidal hypophysectomy can partially or completely reverse the increased ACTH production of the anterior pituitary. Cushing syndrome requires surgical removal of one (adrenal adenoma, adrenal carcinoma) or both (multiple nodular) adrenal glands. Immediately after surgery it is necessary to replace both cortisol and mineralocorticoid (fludrocortisone) to prevent adrenal insufficiency. Treatment of the ectopic ACTH syndrome requires identification and treatment of the neoplastic process. Patients treated with exogenous steroids for more than 1 month often develop

because of the increase in volume, as well as pressure load resulting from increased aldosterone action.[33] The hyperaldosterone-mediated hypokalemia and much of the associated hypertension respond to the surgical removal of a unilateral (or occasionally bilateral) benign adrenal adenoma(s).[34]

Addison Disease

Long before recognition that the glands situated just above the upper pole of each kidney (suprarenal) synthesize and secrete glucocorticoids and mineralocorticoids, Thomas Addison described the association of atrophy with loss of function of these structures with marked changes in the cardiovascular system. The hypovolemia, hypotension, and acute cardiovascular collapse resulting from renal sodium wasting, hyperkalemia, and loss of vascular tone are the hallmarks of acute Addisonian crisis, one of the most severe endocrine emergencies. Adrenal insufficiency most commonly arises from bilateral loss of adrenal function on an autoimmune basis; as a result of infection, hemorrhage, or metastatic malignancy; or in selected cases of inborn errors of steroid hormone metabolism.[35] In contrast, secondary adrenal insufficiency, which results from pituitary-dependent loss of ACTH secretion, leads to a fall in glucocorticoid production, whereas mineralocorticoid production including aldosterone remains at relatively normal levels. Recent studies have addressed the issue of relative hypothalamic-pituitary-adrenal insufficiency in acutely ill patients.[36] Although the actual existence of such an entity and diagnostic criteria for establishing this occurrence remains to be validated, it has reopened the question of the need for stress dose cortisol treatment of critical illness.

Addison disease can occur at any age. The noncardiac symptoms including increased pigmentation, abdominal pain with nausea and vomiting, and weight loss can be chronic, whereas the tachycardia, hypotension, and electrolyte abnormalities herald impending cardiovascular collapse and crisis.[35] Blood pressure measurements uniformly show low diastolic pressure (<60 mm Hg) with significant orthostatic changes reflecting volume loss. Laboratory findings of hyponatremia and hyperkalemia indicate loss of aldosterone production (renin levels are high). The hyperkalemia can alter the ECG, producing low amplitude P waves and peaked T waves.[36] Newly diagnosed, untreated patients with Addison disease have reduced left ventricular, end-systolic, and end-diastolic dimensions compared with controls. Cardiac atrophy is an unusual condition. It is seen in malnutrition caused by anorexia, in astronauts after prolonged space flight, in populations with sodium-deficient diets, and characteristically with Addison disease (tear drop heart) (Fig. 81-2). This atrophy reflects a response to decreases in cardiac workload because restoration of normal plasma volume with both mineralocorticoid and glucocorticoid replacement increases ventricular mass.[37]

DIAGNOSIS

Acute adrenal insufficiency will characteristically occur in the setting of an acute stress, infection, or trauma in a patient with chronic autoimmune adrenal insufficiency or in children with congenital abnormalities of cortisol metabolism. It can also occur from bilateral adrenal hemorrhage in patients with severe systemic infection or diffuse intravascular coagulation.[35] Secondary adrenal insufficiency can occur in the setting of hypopituitarism, which in most situations is chronic; however, acute changes caused by pituitary hemorrhage (apoplexy) or pituitary inflammation (lymphocytic hypophysitis) can occur. Patients treated with long-term suppressive doses of corticosteroids (>10 mg of prednisone for more than 1 month) can develop acute adrenal insufficiency should such treatment be precipitously stopped.

The diagnosis is established when, in the morning or during severe stress, cortisol levels are low (<8 μg/dl) and fail to rise above 20 μg/dl 30 minutes after an intravenous (IV) injection of 0.25 mg of cosyntropin. The diagnosis in the setting of acute illness caused by a variety of causes may be more difficult, and a low (<10 μg/dl) morning serum level of cortisol may suffice to suggest impaired control of secretion.[36]

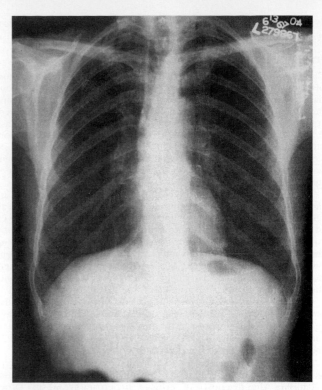

FIGURE 81–2 Routine chest radiograph of a patient with Addison disease related to tuberculosis. In addition to the small cardiac silhouette, there are calcified lymph nodes in the hilum of the right lung. *(Courtesy of Dr. J. B. Naidich.)*

TREATMENT

Management of acute Addisonian crisis needs to address three major issues. The first is adequate hydrocortisone replacement, 100 mg given as an initial IV bolus and then 100 mg every 8 hours for the first 24 hours, tapering the dose for the next 72 to 96 hours. The second is the restoration of intravascular fluid deficit using large volumes of normal saline with 5 percent dextrose. Last is the need to identify and treat any underlying precipitating cause including infection, acute cardiac or cerebral ischemia, or intraabdominal emergency. Chronic treatment is with oral corticosteroid and mineralocorticoid (fludrocortisone 0.1 mg/day) replacement.[37]

PARATHYROID DISEASE

Diseases of the parathyroid glands can produce cardiovascular disease and alter cardiac function by two mechanisms. The first is through changes in the secretion of parathyroid hormone, a protein hormone, which exerts effects on the heart, vascular smooth muscle cells, and endothelial cells.[38] Second is by way of changes in serum calcium. Serum ionized calcium regulates the synthesis and secretion of parathyroid hormone (PTH) by an exquisitely sensitive negative feedback mechanism.

PTH can bind to its receptor and alter the spontaneous beating rate of neonatal cardiac myocytes by an increase in intracellular cyclic adenosine monophosphate (cAMP). PTH can also alter calcium influx and cardiac contractility in adult cardiac myocytes. In vascular smooth muscle cells this causes vasodilation. In addition to PTH, a structurally related parathyroid hormone–related peptide (PTHrP) is synthesized and secreted in a variety of tissues including cardiac myocytes. Interestingly, PTHrP can bind to the PTH receptor on cardiac cells and stimulate cAMP accumulation and contractile activity and regulate L-type calcium currents. Thus the direct effects of increased serum levels of PTHrP on the heart and systemic vasculature can accom-

CH 81

Endocrine Disorders and Cardiovascular Disease

pany a variety of paraneoplastic syndromes characterized by hypercalcemia.[38]

HYPERPARATHYROIDISM

Classical primary hyperparathyroidism producing hypercalcemia most often arises as a result of the adenomatous enlargement of one of four parathyroid glands. The cardiovascular actions of hypercalcemia include an increase in cardiac contractility, a shortening of the ventricular action potential duration primarily through changes in phase 2, and blunting of the T-wave and changes in the ST segment occasionally suggesting cardiac ischemia.[39] The Q-T interval is shortened, occasionally accompanied by decreases in the PR interval as well. Treatment with digitalis glycosides appears to increase sensitivity of the heart to hypercalcemia.

Hypercalcemia has been linked to pathological changes in the heart including the myocardial interstitium, the conducting system, and calcific deposits in the valve cusps and annuli. Although initially observed in fairly longstanding and severe hypercalcemia, so-called *metastatic calcifications* can also occur in secondary parathyroid disease arising from chronic renal failure in which the serum calcium-phosphorus product constant is exceeded. Whereas left ventricular systolic function is maintained in primary hyperparathyroidism, severe or chronic disease may impair diastolic function.[40]

Presumably as a result of the direct effect of calcium on vascular smooth muscle tone, patients with primary hyperparathyroidism have increased arterial pressure. PTH acts as a direct vasodilator and increased dietary calcium can decrease arterial pressure, so complex mechanisms link PTH to blood pressure.[39,40]

A simultaneous increase in serum immunoreactive PTH (best represented by the intact PTH assay) with an elevation of serum calcium establishes the diagnosis of primary hyperparathyroidism. Other causes include hypercalcemia of malignancy with an increased level of PTHrP or arising from direct bony metastasis, or a neoplastic (lymphoma) or nonneoplastic (sarcoidosis) diseases leading to an increase in synthesis and release of 1,25-dihydroxyvitamin D_3. Treatment of hyperparathyroidism is the surgical removal of the parathyroid adenoma.

HYPOCALCEMIA

Low serum levels of total and ionized calcium directly alter myocyte function. Hypocalcemia prolongs phase 2 of the action potential duration and the Q-T interval. Severe hypocalcemia can impair cardiac contractility and gives rise to a diffuse musculoskeletal syndrome including tetany and rhabdomyolysis. Primary hypoparathyroidism is a rare disease that can be seen after surgical removal of the parathyroid

glands, in the setting of polyglandular dysfunction syndromes, as the result of glandular agenesis (Di George) syndrome, and in the rare but heritable disorder pseudohypoparathyroidism.

The most common cause of a low serum calcium is chronic renal failure and high PTH levels. In such patients it appears that the effects of chronically high levels of PTH (secondary hyperparathyroidism) on the heart and cardiovascular system predominate.[38] The ability of PTH to stimulate G protein–coupled receptors may impair myocyte contractility and contribute to the LVH commonly observed in patients with chronic renal failure.[38] Systemic vascular resistance is often low, potentially reflecting the vasodilatory action of PTH.

THYROID GLAND

The thyroid gland and the heart share a close relationship arising in embryology. In ontogeny the thyroid and heart anlage migrate together. The close physiological relationship is affirmed by predictable changes in cardiovascular function across the entire range of thyroid disease states. In fact, cardiovascular manifestations are some of the most common and characteristic findings of hyperthyroidism.[41] To approach the diagnosis and management of thyroid hormone–mediated cardiac disease states, it is important to understand the cellular mechanisms of thyroid hormone on the heart and vascular smooth muscle cells.[42]

CELLULAR MECHANISMS OF THYROID HORMONE ACTION ON THE HEART

Under the regulation of thyroid stimulating hormone (thyrotropin, TSH), the thyroid gland has the unique property of concentrating serum iodide and through a series of enzymatic steps synthesizes predominantly tetraiodothyronine (T_4 85 percent) and a smaller percentage of triiodothyronine (T_3 15 percent) (Fig. 81-3).[43] The major source of T_3 synthesis is by conversion by 5′ monodeiodination primarily in the liver and to a lesser degree in the kidney.[44] A variety of studies have confirmed T_3 as the active form of thyroid hormone that accounts for the vast majority of biological effects including stimulation of tissue thermogenesis, alterations in the expression of various cellular protein, and actions on the heart and vascular smooth muscle cells.[41,45] Serum-free T_3 in turn is taken up by a process of facilitated diffusion within cells, where it appears to pass without additional protein binding to the cell nucleus (Fig. 81-4). Most data indicate that the cardiac myocyte cannot metabolize T_4 to T_3. Therefore despite the presence of the relevant enzymes, all of the observed nuclear actions and changes in gene expression result from changes in blood levels of T_3. The cardiac myocyte expresses both the alpha and beta isoforms of the thyroid hormone receptors (TRs), which arise from two separate genes. These genes give rise to splice variants TRalpha$_1$ and TRalpha$_2$, of which only the former binds thyroid hormone, as well as TRbeta$_1$, TRbeta$_2$, and TRbeta$_3$.[45] As reported for the steroid and retinoic acid family of receptor proteins, the TRs act by binding as either homodimers or heterodimers to the thyroid hormone response elements (TREs) in a promoter region of specific genes.[45] Binding to the promoter regions can either activate or repress gene expression.[46]

Thyroid hormone transcriptionally regulates many cardiac proteins (Table 81-1). They include structural and regulatory proteins, as well as a variety of cardiac membrane ion channels and cell surface receptors, thus providing a molecular mechanism

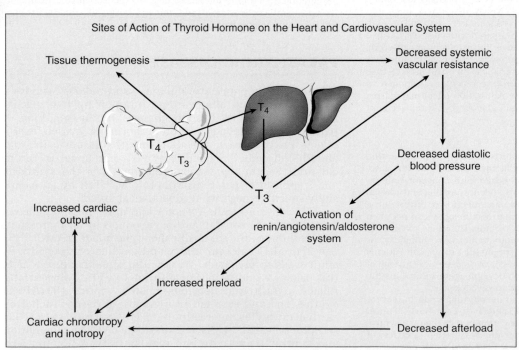

FIGURE 81–3 Schematic representation of thyroid hormone metabolism and the effects of triiodothyronine (T_3) on the heart and systemic vasculature. T_4 = tetraiodothyronine.

to explain many of the diverse effects of thyroid hormone on the heart. The first reported and the best studied to date has been the myosin heavy chain isoforms alpha and beta) The human ventricle expresses primarily beta myosin, and there appear to be few, if any, alterations in isoform expression accompanying thyroid disease states. Changes in myosin heavy chain isoform expression occur in the human atria in a variety of disease states including congestive heart failure, and whether these changes are thyroid hormone mediated remains to be determined.[47]

The sarcoplasmic reticulum calcium-activated ATPase is an important ion pump that determines the magnitude of myocyte calcium cycling (see also Chap. 21). The reuptake of calcium into the sarcoplasmic reticulum early in diastole in part determines the rate at which the left ventricle relaxes (isovolumetric relaxation time, IVRT).[41] The activity of SERCA2 in turn is regulated by the polymeric protein phospholamban with its ability to inhibit SERCA activity further modified by

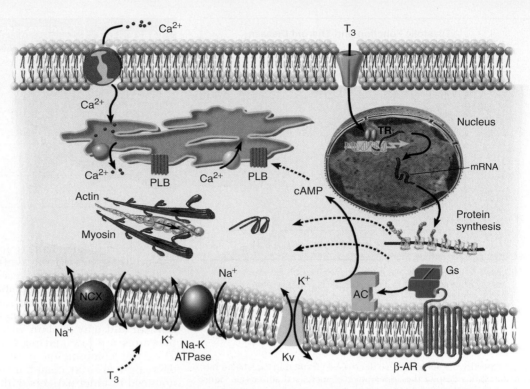

FIGURE 81–4 Triiodothyronine (T_3) enters the cell and binds to nuclear T_3 receptors. The complex then binds to thyroid hormone response elements and regulates transcription of specific genes. Nonnuclear T_3 actions on ion channels for sodium (Na^+), potassium (K^+), and calcium (Ca^{2+}) ions are indicated. AC = adenylyl cyclase; ATPase = adenosine triphosphatase; β-AR = beta adrenergic receptor; cAMP = cyclic adenosine monophosphate; Gs = guanine nucleotide binding protein subunit; Kv = voltage-gated potassium channel; mRNA = messenger RNA; NCX = sodium channel; PLB = phospholamban; TR = T_3 receptor protein.

the level of phosphorylation of the individual phospholamban monomers.[48] Inotropic agents that enhance cardiac contractility through increases in myocyte cAMP do so by stimulating the phosphorylation of phospholamban. Thyroid hormone inhibits the expression of phospholamban and increases phospholamban phosphorylation.[49] Genetically engineered animals deficient in phospholamban do not further increase cardiac contractility after exposure to excess thyroid hormone.[48] These data indicate that thyroid hormone exerts most of its direct effects on cardiac contractility by regulating calcium cycling through the SERCA-phospholamban system both transcriptionally and posttranscriptionally. This molecular mechanism can explain why diastolic function varies inversely across the entire spectrum of thyroid disease states including even mild, subclinical hypothyroidism (Fig. 81-5).[41,50,51] In addition, beta-adrenergic blockade of the heart in hyperthyroidism does not decrease the rapid diastolic relaxation, further dissociating the thyroid hormone from the adrenergic effects of thyrotoxicosis.[41]

Changes in other myocyte genes including Na^+/K^+ ATPase account for the increase in basal oxygen consumption of the experimental hyperthyroid heart and explain the decrease in digitalis sensitivity of hyperthyroid patients. A variety of studies have shown that thyroid hormone can regulate the genetic expression of its own nuclear receptors within the cardiac myocyte (see Table 81-1).

In addition to the well-characterized nuclear effects of thyroid hormone, a growing body of cardiac responses to thyroid hormone appear to be mediated through nongenomic mechanisms[52] as suggested by their relatively rapid onset of action (faster than can be accounted for by changes in gene expression and protein synthesis) and failure to be affected by inhibitors of gene transcription. The significance of these diverse actions remains to be established but may explain the ability of acute T_3 treatment to alter cardiovascular hemodynamics. They may alter the functional properties of membrane ion channels and pumps including the sodium channel and the inward rectifying potassium current (I_k).

THYROID FUNCTION TESTING

A number of sensitive and specific laboratory tests can establish a diagnosis of thyroid disease with a high degree of precision. Serum TSH is the most widely used and most sensitive measure for the diag-

TABLE 81–1	Thyroid Hormone Regulation of Cardiac Gene Expression	
Positively Regulated	**Negatively Regulated**
Alpha-myosin heavy chain	Beta-myosin heavy chain
Sarcoplasmic reticulum Ca²⁺-ATPase	Phospholamban
Na⁺, K⁺-ATPase	Na⁺/Ca²⁺ exchanger
Voltage-gated potassium channels (Kv1.5, Kv4.2, Kv4.3)	Thyroid hormone receptor alpha1
Atrial and brain natriuretic peptide	Adenylyl cyclase (AC) types V, VI
Malic enzyme	Guanine nucleotide–binding protein G_i
Beta-adrenergic receptor	
Guanine nucleotide–binding protein G_s	
Adenine nucleotide transporter 1	

ATPase = adenosine triphosphatase.

nosis of both hypothyroidism and hyperthyroidism.[53] Serum TSH levels uniformly increase (>5 µIU/ml) in patients with primary hypothyroidism, and conversely, because of the normal feedback of excess levels of T_4 (and T_3) on the pituitary synthesis and secretion of TSH, the levels are low (<0.04 to 0.01 µIU/ml) in hyperthyroidism. Measures of free T_4 can be useful when coexistent hepatic, nutritional, or genetic disease may alter thyroxine-binding globulin content. Autoimmune thyroid disease (Hashimoto and Graves) can be further diagnosed by the use of serologic measures of antithyroid antibodies, most specifically antithyroid peroxidase (anti-TPO) or antithyroglobulin antibodies.

THYROID HORMONE–CATECHOLAMINE INTERACTION

Early observations of the heart in hyperthyroidism emphasize the similarity to that of hyperadrenergic states and moreover propose enhanced sensitivity to catecholamines in this setting. This postulate forms the basis for the test described by Goetsch in 1918 in which hyperthyroidism could be diagnosed by demonstrating a marked cardioacceleration and blood pressure response to small, subcutaneous doses of epineph-

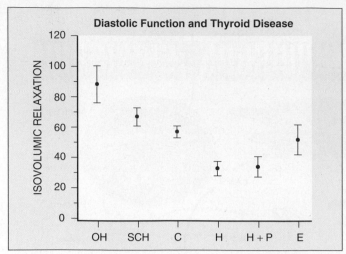

FIGURE 81-5 Diastolic function as measured by the isovolumic relaxation time varies over the entire range of thyroid disease including overt hypothyroidism (OH), subclinical hypothyroidism (SCH), control (C), hyperthyroidism (H), hyperthyroidism after beta-adrenergic blockade (H + P), and hyperthyroidism after treatment to restore normal thyroid function studies (E).

TABLE 81-2	Cardiovascular Changes with Thyroid Disease		
Parameter	Normal	Hyperthyroid	Hypothyroid
Systemic vascular resistance (dyne-cm · sec ^{5})	1500-1700	700-1200	2100-2700
Heart rate (beats/min)	72-84	88-130	60-80
Cardiac output (liter/min)	5.8	>7.0	<4.5
Blood volume (% of normal)	100	105.5	84.5

rine. Hyperthyroid subjects have decreased circulating catecholamine concentrations despite the appearance of increased adrenergic signs and symptoms. Increased beta$_1$ adrenergic receptors on cardiac myocytes observed in experimental hyperthyroidism provide a mechanism for enhanced catecholamine sensitivity. A recent carefully controlled study of subhuman primates, however, found no increase in sensitivity of the heart or cardiovascular system to catecholamines in experimental hyperthyroidism.[54] Accompanying the increased levels of beta$_1$-adrenergic receptors and guanosine triphosphate binding proteins, thyroid hormone decreases the expression of cardiac-specific (V, VI) adenylyl cyclase catalytic subunit isoforms and thereby maintains cellular response to beta-adrenergic agonists within normal limits.[55]

Hemodynamic Alterations in Thyroid Disease

Changes in myocardial contractility and cardiovascular hemodynamics occur across the entire spectrum of thyroid disease (Table 81-2; also see Fig. 81.5).[41] Multiple studies including those in experimental animals, as well as invasive and noninvasive measurements in patients, indicate that triiodothyronine regulates cardiac inotropy and chronotropy through a variety of both direct and indirect mechanisms.[41,56-59] Figure 81-3 represents the integrated schema by which T$_3$ acts on tissues throughout the body to increase tissue thermogenesis. Direct effects on vascular smooth muscle cells decrease systemic vascular resistance of the arterioles of the peripheral circulation.[56,59] A decrease in mean arterial pressure and activation of the renin-angiotensin-aldosterone system occurs, as does an increase in renal sodium reabsorption. The increase in plasma volume coupled with an increase in erythropoietin leads to an increase in blood volume and a rise in cardiac preload.[58] Thus a combination of lower systemic vascular resistance (by as much as 50 percent), coupled with increases in venous return and preload, increases cardiac output. Cardiac output may more than double in hyperthyroidism and conversely may decrease by as much as 30 to 40 percent in hypothyroidism. Recent studies using positron emission tomography (PET) measurements of acetate metabolism have demonstrated that the marked increase in cardiac output in hyperthyroidism is accomplished with no change in energy efficiency.[60]

Triiodothyronine appears to reduce systemic vascular resistance by both direct effects on vascular smooth muscle

cells and through changes in the vascular endothelium potentially involving the synthesis and secretion of nitric oxide.[56] T$_3$ can produce a vasodilatory effect within hours after administration to patients undergoing coronary artery bypass grafting, as well as patients with chronic congestive heart failure.[47,59] Arterial compliance also falls in hyperthyroidism and may explain why mean arterial and diastolic pressures are low and peak systolic pressures increase.[57] Thus the combination of increased cardiac output and decreased arterial compliance, which may be more pronounced in older patients with some degree of arterial vascular disease, leads to systolic hypertension in up to 30 percent of patients.[57] In hypothyroidism, systemic vascular resistance may increase as much as 30 percent. Mean arterial pressure rises with up to 20 percent of patients having significant diastolic hypertension.[57] Even mild hypothyroidism may decrease endothelial-derived relaxing factors.[61] The diastolic hypertension of hypothyroidism is frequently associated with a low renin level and a decrease in hepatic synthesis of renin substrate. This leads to a characteristically low level of salt sensitivity, again reinforcing the importance of an increase in systemic vascular resistance underlying the mechanism for diastolic hypertension.[62]

Hyperthyroidism

Cardiovascular symptoms are an integral and often the predominant clinical presentation of patients with hyperthyroidism (Table 81-3). Palpitations resulting from both an increase in the rate and force of cardiac contractility are present in the majority of patients. The increase in heart rate results from both an increase in sympathetic tone and a decrease in parasympathetic stimulation. Heart rates >90 beats per minute both at rest and during sleep commonly occur, the normal diurnal variation in heart rate is blunted and the increase during exercise is exaggerated. Many hyperthyroid patients experience exercise intolerance and exertional dyspnea, due in part to weakness in skeletal and respiratory muscle.[41,63] In the setting of a low vascular resistance and increased preload, cardiac functional reserve is compromised and cannot further rise to accommodate the demands of submaximal or maximal exercise.[63]

A subset of thyrotoxic patients can experience angina-like chest pain. In older patients with known or suspected coronary artery disease, the increase in cardiac work associated with the increase in cardiac output and cardiac contractility of hyperthyroidism can produce myocardial ischemia, which can respond to beta-adrenergic blocking agents or the restoration of a euthyroid state. In rare patients, usually younger women, there is a syndrome of chest pain at rest associated with ischemic ECG changes. Cardiac catheterization has demonstrated that the majority of these patients have angiographically normal coronary arteries;

TABLE 81–3	Cardiovascular Symptoms of Hyperthyroidism
Palpitations	Angina-like chest pain
Exercise intolerance	Peripheral edema
Dyspnea	Congestive heart failure

however, coronary vasospasm has been reported similar to that found in variant angina. Myocardial infarction rarely develops, and these patients appear to respond to calcium channel blockers or to nitroglycerin.

Recent reports have shown that hyperthyroidism is associated with a significant degree of pulmonary hypertension (pulmonary artery systolic pressure >75 mm Hg), which was reversible after treatment of the Graves disease. This observation implies that although systemic vascular resistance is decreased with thyrotoxicosis, peripheral vascular resistance is not. Perhaps all patients with unexplained pulmonary hypertension should be evaluated for thyroid disease with measurement of serum TSH.[57,64]

Atrial Fibrillation

The most common rhythm disturbance in patients with hyperthyroidism is sinus tachycardia.[43] Its clinical impact, however, is overshadowed by patients with atrial fibrillation resulting from thyrotoxicosis. The prevalence of atrial fibrillation and the less common forms of supraventricular tachycardia in this disease ranges from 2 to 20 percent.[65,66] When compared with a control population with normal thyroid function and a prevalence of atrial fibrillation of 2.3 percent, the prevalence of atrial fibrillation in overt hyperthyroidism was 13.8 percent.[66] In a study of more than 13,000 hyperthyroid patients, the prevalence rate for atrial fibrillation was less than 2 percent, perhaps because of earlier recognition and disease treatment. When that same group of patients was analyzed for age distribution, it was seen that there was a stepwise increase in prevalence in each decade peaking at approximately 15 percent in patients older than 70 years.[65] This latter study confirms essentially all reports that atrial fibrillation caused by hyperthyroidism is more common with advancing age. In a study of unselected patients presenting with atrial fibrillation, less than 1 percent were caused by overt hyperthyroidism. Thus the yield of abnormal thyroid function testing including a low serum TSH appears to be low in patients with new-onset atrial fibrillation. However, the ability to restore thyrotoxic patients to a euthyroid state and sinus rhythm justifies TSH testing in most patients with the recent onset of otherwise unexplained atrial fibrillation or other supraventricular arrhythmias.

Treatment of atrial fibrillation in the setting of hyperthyroidism includes beta-adrenergic blockade using one of a variety of beta₁ selective or nonselective agents to control the ventricular response. This symptomatic measure can be accomplished rapidly, whereas the treatments leading to restoration of the euthyroid state require more time. Digitalis has been used to control the ventricular response in hyperthyroidism-associated atrial fibrillation, but because of the increased rate of digitalis clearance and decreased sensitivity of the drug action resulting from high cellular levels of Na^+/K^+ ATPase and lastly with decreased parasympathetic tone, patients usually require higher doses of this medication. Anticoagulation in patients with hyperthyroidism and atrial fibrillation is controversial.[41,67] The potential for systemic or cerebral embolization must be weighed against the risk of bleeding and complications related to this therapy. Whether hyperthyroid patients are at increased risk for systemic embolization per se is not totally resolved.[68] In a retrospective study of patients with hyperthyroidism, it was age rather than the presence of atrial fibrillation that was the main risk factor for embolization. Retrospective analysis of large series

of patients did not demonstrate a prevalence of thromboembolic events greater than the reported risk of major bleeding from warfarin treatment.[67] Thus in younger patients with hyperthyroidism and atrial fibrillation in the absence of other heart disease, hypertension, or other independent risk factors for embolization, the benefits of anticoagulation have not been proven and might be outweighed by the risk. Aspirin provides an alternative for lowering risk for embolic events in young people and can be used safely.[43]

Successful treatment of hyperthyroidism with either radioiodine or antithyroid drugs and restoration of normal serum levels of T_4 and T_3 are associated with reversion to sinus rhythm in two thirds of patients within 2 to 3 months.[65] In older patients or in the setting of atrial fibrillation of longer duration, the rate of reversion to sinus rhythm is lower and therefore electrical or pharmacological cardioversion should be attempted, but only after the patient has been rendered euthyroid. The majority of patients (90 percent) can be restored to sinus rhythm either by electrical cardioversion or pharmacological measures, and many will remain in sinus rhythm for periods up to 5 years or more. In a regimen that added disopyramide 300 mg per day for 3 months after successful cardioversion, patients were more likely to remain in sinus rhythm than those not treated.[67,68]

HEART FAILURE

The cardiovascular alterations in hyperthyroidism include increased resting cardiac output and enhanced cardiac contractility (Fig. 81-6; also see Table 81-2). Nevertheless, a minority of patients present with symptoms including dyspnea on exertion, orthopnea, and paroxysmal nocturnal dyspnea, as well as signs demonstrating peripheral edema, neck vein distention, and an S_3 indicative of heart failure (see Table 81-3). This complex of findings coupled with a failure to increase the LV ejection fraction with exercise has suggested the possibility of a hyperthyroid cardiomyopathy. The term often used in this setting—*high output failure*—is not appropriate because although resting cardiac output is as much as two to three times normal, the exercise intolerance does not appear to be a result of cardiac failure but rather of skeletal muscle weakness.[41,63] High output states, however, can increase renal sodium reabsorption, expand plasma volume, and cause development of peripheral edema, pleural effusions, and venous hypertension. Interestingly, whereas systemic vascular resistance falls with hyperthyroidism, the pulmonary vascular bed is not similarly affected and, as a result of the increase in output to the pulmonary circulation, there is an increase in pulmonary artery pressures.[57,64] This results in a rise in mean venous pressure, neck vein distention, hepatic congestion, and peripheral edema of the type associated with primary pulmonary hypertension or right heart failure.[41,57,64]

Patients with longstanding hyperthyroidism and marked sinus tachycardia or atrial fibrillation can develop low cardiac output, impaired cardiac contractility with a low ejection fraction, an S_3 and pulmonary congestion, all consistent with congestive heart failure.[41] Review of such cases suggests that impairment in left ventricular function results from prolonged high heart rate and the development of rate-related heart failure. When the left ventricle becomes dilated, mitral regurgitation may also develop. Recognition of this entity is important because treatments aimed at slowing heart rate or controlling the ventricular response in atrial fibrillation appear to improve left ventricular function even before initiation of antithyroid therapy.[41] Because these patients are critically ill they should be managed in an intensive care unit setting. Some patients with hyperthyroidism (similar to the overall congestive heart failure population) do not tolerate initiation of beta-adrenergic blocking drugs in full doses, and treatment can be started with lower doses of short-acting beta-blocking drugs in conjunction with classic forms of treatment of acute congestive heart failure including diuresis.

The increase in rate-pressure product and oxygen consumption that results from hyperthyroidism can impair cardiac function in older patients with known or suspected ischemic, hypertensive, or valvular heart disease. It is important to recognize promptly hyperthyroidism in older patients as they are at higher risk of cardiovascular and cerebral vascular events both before[69] and subsequent to treatment.[70]

TREATMENT

Treatment of patients with thyrotoxic cardiac disease should include a beta-adrenergic antagonist to lower the heart rate to 10 or 15 percent above normal. This will cause the tachycardia-mediated component of ventricular dysfunction to improve, whereas the direct inotropic effects of thyroid hormone will persist (see Fig. 81-4).[41] The rapid onset of action and the improvement in many of the signs and symptoms of

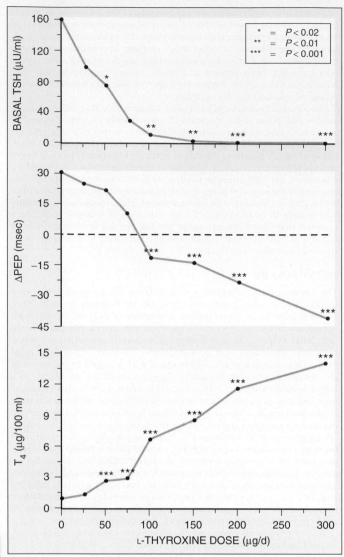

FIGURE 81–6 Response to stepwise L-thyroxine sodium treatment of hypothyroid patients as assessed by serum thyrotropin (TSH), serum tetraiodothyronine (T_4), and the improvement in left ventricular contractility as measured noninvasively by the change in the preejection period (PEP). *(From Crowley WF Jr, Ridgway EC, Bough EW, et al: Noninvasive evaluation of cardiac function in hypothyroidism. Response to gradual thyroxine replacement. N Engl J Med 296:1, 1977.)*

hyperthyroidism indicate that most patients with overt symptoms should receive beta-blocking agents. Definitive therapy can then be accomplished safely with iodine-131 alone or in combination with an antithyroid drug.

Hypothyroidism

In contrast to the dramatic clinical signs and symptoms of hyperthyroidism, the cardiovascular findings of hypothyroidism are more subtle.[71] Mild degrees of bradycardia, diastolic hypertension, a narrow pulse pressure and a relatively quiet precordium, and decreased intensity of the apical impulse are characteristic. Hemodynamic changes of hypothyroidism are diametrically opposite to that of hyperthyroidism (see Table 81-2) and explain many of the physical findings. Despite the decrease in cardiac output and contractility of the hypothyroid myocardium, recent studies of myocardial metabolism by PET scan have shown energy inefficiency of the hypothyroid myocardium. The oxygen cost of work increases primarily as a result of the increase

in afterload.[72] Treatment of hypothyroid patients with the restoration of a euthyroid state resolves these changes in parallel with a return of systemic vascular resistance to lower levels.[71,72]

Hypothyroidism also produces increases in total and low-density lipoprotein (LDL) cholesterol in proportion to the rise in serum TSH.[73] Although thyroid hormone can alter cholesterol metabolism through multiple mechanisms including a decrease in biliary excretion, it appears that changes in LDL metabolism caused by decreases in LDL receptor number are a primary mechanism.[74,75]

Serum creatine kinase is elevated by anywhere from 50 percent to 10-fold in up to 30 percent of patients with hypothyroidism. Analysis of isoform specificity indicates that greater than 96 percent is MM consistent with a skeletal muscle origin of increased enzyme release.[74] In contrast to the half-life of creatine kinase after acute myocardial infarction (12 hours), the half-life in hypothyroidism after initiation of standard oral thyroid hormone replacement is approximately 10 to 14 days. Pericardial effusions can occur consistent with observation that patients with hypothyroidism have an increase in volume of distribution of albumin and a decrease in lymphatic clearance function. Occasionally the pericardial effusions are quite large, causing the appearance of cardiomegaly on chest radiograph. Although rare, tamponade with hemodynamic compromise can occur. Echocardiography demonstrates small to moderate effusions in up to 30 percent of overtly hypothyroid patients, which resolve over a period of weeks to months after initiation of thyroid hormone replacement.[71]

As a result of changes in ion channel expression, the ECG in hypothyroidism is characterized by sinus bradycardia, low voltage, and prolongation of the action potential duration and the QT interval. The latter in turn predisposes the patients to ventricular arrhythmias, and cases of patients with acquired torsades de pointes that have improved or completely resolved with thyroid hormone replacement have been reported.[41]

As a result of increases in risk factors including hypercholesterolemia, hypertension, and elevated levels of homocysteine, patients with hypothyroidism may have increased risk for atherosclerosis and coronary and systemic vascular disease.[73-75] Recent studies have shown increases in abdominal aortic atherosclerosis in elderly women patients with even mild hypothyroidism.[76] Whether patients with hypothyroidism have an increase in coronary artery disease is an important clinical issue. Recent findings suggest increased cardiovascular morbidity and mortality with untreated subclinical hypothyroidism.[77] Noninvasive studies including thallium scanning have demonstrated abnormalities in perfusion suggestive of myocardial ischemia, but these defects appear to resolve with thyroid hormone treatment.

In patients younger than 50 years of age with no history of heart disease, it is possible to initiate full replacement doses of L-thyroxine (100 μg to 150 μg per day) without concern for untoward cardiac effects. In patients older than age 50 with known or suspected coronary artery disease, the issue is more complicated. In patients with known coronary artery disease and a coexistent diagnosis of hypothyroidism, three major issues need to be addressed.

The first is whether coronary artery revascularization is required before initiating thyroid hormone replacement. If patients are not candidates for percutaneous intervention, coronary artery bypass grafting can be accomplished in patients with unstable angina, left main coronary artery disease, or three-vessel disease with impaired left ventricular function, even in the setting of overt hypothyroidism. Rarely a patient has sufficiently profound hypothyroidism to prolong bleeding times and partial thromboplastin times, requiring preoperative supplementation of clotting factors. Thyroid hormone replacement can be delayed until the postoperative period, when it can be administered in full dose either parenterally or orally.[41]

The second is in patients with known stable cardiac disease in whom cardiac revascularization is not clinically indicated. Treatment of such patients should begin with low doses (12.5 μg) of L-thyroxine and increased stepwise (12.5-25 μg) every 6 to 8 weeks until serum TSH is normal. Thyroid hormone replacement in this setting and its ability to lower systemic vascular resistance and lower afterload, as

TABLE 81–4	Muscle Disease Syndromes: Clinical Characterization
Statin-Induced	**Hypothyroid-Related**
Myopathy—any associated disease	**Myalgia**—nonspecific muscle symptoms, cramping, especially nocturnal, variable CK level
Myalgia—muscle aches/weakness without CK elevation	**Myopathy**—impaired endurance usually with CK elevation; pseudomyotonia
Myositis—symptoms plus elevated CK	**Hoffmann syndrome**—impaired function; pseudohypertrophy, often marked CK elevations
Rhabdomyolysis—symptoms plus markedly elevated CK levels	

CK = creatine kinase.

well as improve myocardial efficiency, can actually decrease clinical signs of myocardial ischemia. Beta-adrenergic blocking agents are an ideal concomitant therapy to control heart rate.

Third is the group of patients who, although potentially at risk for coronary artery disease, exhibit no clinical signs or symptoms. In this group thyroid hormone replacement can be started at low doses generally in the range of 25 to 50 µg per day and increased 25 µg every 6 to 8 weeks until serum TSH is normal. Should signs or symptoms of ischemic heart disease develop, the same recommendations apply as to patients with known underlying heart disease.

In all patients, thyroid hormone replacement should continue until serum TSH is normal and the patients are clinically euthyroid. The concept that these patients benefit from maintenance of "mild hypothyroidism" is not supported by the known effects of thyroid hormone on the heart and cardiovascular system.[41,71,72] Thyroid hormone replacement should be accomplished by purified preparations of levothyroxine sodium. Preparations containing T_4 with T_3 (thyroid extract) or the existing purified preparations of T_3 do not offer benefit. The short half-life of T_3 and the inability to maintain serum levels within normal range in patients so treated can add to cardiac risk.[78] An interesting issue is whether some patients with statin-induced myopathy have underlying thyroid disease as a contributing factor. The myopathy/myalgia symptoms of both conditions are similar (Table 81-4), and thyroid function testing with TSH should be part of the evaluation of these patients.[74]

DIAGNOSIS

Hashimoto disease, postradioiodine therapy for Graves disease, and iodine deficiency (in parts of the world where that remains a public health problem) are the leading causes of hypothyroidism and produce diagnostic elevation in serum TSH.[53] Thus the finding of an elevated TSH is sufficient to establish the diagnosis and form the basis for treatment. In routine practice additional testing with a serum T_4 and T_3 resin uptake is confirmatory. The prevalence of hypothyroidism is estimated at 3 to 4 percent for overt disease and 7 to 10 percent for the milder forms of disease. Thus TSH screening can be advised for all adults and particularly in patients with hypertension, hypercholesterolemia, hypertriglyceridemia, coronary or peripheral vascular disease, and unexplained pericardial or pleural effusions and for a variety of musculoskeletal syndromes or statin-associated myopathy.[43,79]

TREATMENT

The response to treatment of hypothyroidism is predictable, especially from a cardiovascular perspective. Stepwise thyroid hormone replacement using levothyroxine sodium (Levoxyl, Synthroid) incrementally decreases serum TSH, serum cholesterol, and serum creatine kinase and improves left ventricular performance. Full replacement is accomplished when serum TSH is normal.[53] In the rare condition of myxedema coma, which is characterized by patients with severe and longstanding hypothyroidism who develop hypothermia, altered mental status, hypotension, bradycardia, and hypoventilation, the need for thyroid hormone replacement is more emergent and treatment can be accomplished with either 100 µg a day of T4 or 25 to 50 µg a day of T_3 administered intravenously. These patients often require intensive care unit monitoring with volume repletion, gentle warming, and ven-

tilatory support in the face of CO_2 retention. Administration of hydrocortisone (100 mg q8h) should be undertaken until results of serum cortisol testing are obtained. When treated in this manner, hemodynamics including systemic vascular resistance, cardiac output, and heart rate improve within 24 to 48 hours.

SUBCLINICAL THYROID DISEASE

In contrast to overt symptomatic thyroid disease, subclinical thyroid disease implies the absence of classic hyperthyroid or hypothyroid related symptoms in patients with thyroid dysfunction. The definition has been further refined to include the demonstration of an abnormal TSH level in the face of normal serum levels of total T_4, free T_4, total T_3 and free T_3.[53,80] With the advent of widespread TSH screening, the magnitude of subclinical thyroid disease may exceed that of overt disease by threefold to fourfold.[75]

SUBCLINICAL HYPOTHYROIDISM

Subclinical hypothyroidism defined as a TSH above the upper range of the reference population (usually >5 µIU/ml) is seen in up to 9 percent of unselected populations, and clearly prevalence increases with advancing age.[75] In contrast to younger patients in whom there is a strong female predilection, in older populations, this difference is lost. Subclinical hypothyroidism alters lipid metabolism, atherosclerosis, cardiac contractility, and systemic vascular resistance. Cholesterol levels rise in parallel with increments in TSH elevations starting at 5 µIU/liter. A large study of women in Rotterdam showed that atherosclerosis and myocardial infarction increased with odds ratios of 1.7 and 2.3 in subclinical hypothyroid women, respectively. Interestingly, the presence of antithyroid antibodies as a measure of autoimmune thyroid disease indicated heightened risk.[76] Restoration of serum TSH to normal after thyroid hormone replacement improved lipid levels, lowered systemic vascular resistance, and improved cardiac contractility.[81] Patients with subclinical hypothyroidism have prolonged isovolumic relaxation times, whereas systolic contractile function does not change (see Fig. 81-6). Replacement with L-thyroxine sodium at a mean dose of 68 µg per day (range 50 to 100 µg per day) restored isovolumic relaxation times to normal and when compared with the same patients before therapy, systemic vascular resistance declined and systolic function significantly improved.[82] A variety of studies have indicated that the changes in systemic vascular resistance result from alterations in endothelium-dependent vasodilation.[50,61] Taken together, it seems appropriate to recommend thyroid hormone replacement for all patients with subclinical hypothyroidism from a cardiovascular perspective. The lack of untoward cardiac effects observed when serum TSH levels normalize indicate that the potential benefits far outweigh the risks of treatment.[41,50,73,80]

SUBCLINICAL HYPERTHYROIDISM

Subclinical hyperthyroidism is diagnosed when serum TSH is low (<0.1 µIU/ml) and both T_4 and T_3 are normal.[53] The significance of subclinical hyperthyroidism was conclusively established from a study of atrial fibrillation in patients 60 years of age or older in the Framingham cohort.[83] Prevalence of atrial fibrillation after 10 years was 28 percent in the subclinical hyperthyroid patient population compared with 11 percent in patients with normal thyroid function with a relative risk of 3.1 (Fig. 81-7). A large U.S. study of patients 65 years or older confirmed and extended this result.[84] A population-based study of more than 1000 individuals with subclinical hyperthyroidism not receiving L-thyroxine therapy or antithyroid medication demonstrated that a TSH level of less than 0.5 was associated with twofold increased mortality with relative risk of 2.3 to 3.3 from all causes, which in turn was largely accounted for by increases in cardiovascular mortality.[84]

Although the cardiovascular changes are well established, the management of patients with subclinical hyperthyroidism is controversial. Therapy can be individualized with regard to three specific groups. The first group includes patients receiving thyroid hormone replacement for hypothyroidism in whom the low TSH is believed to be the result of excess medication and reduction of the dose is indicated.[84] The second group includes patients with a prior diagnosis of thyroid cancer currently receiving L-thyroxine for the express purpose of TSH suppression. In younger patients beta-adrenergic blocking agents can reverse many, if not all, of the cardiovascular manifestations including heart rate control, LVH, and atrial ectopy. In older patients the degree of TSH suppression can be relaxed by lowering the T_4 dosage.[86]

The third group includes those patients in whom subclinical hyperthyroidism results from endogenous thyroid gland overactivity includ-

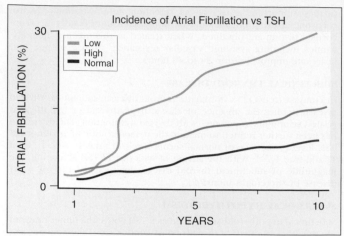

FIGURE 81–7 Atrial fibrillation in subclinical hyperthyroidism. Low thyrotropin (thyroid-stimulating hormone, TSH) designates patients who have serum TSH less than 0.1 µIU/ml. *(Modified from Sawin CT: Subclinical hyperthyroidism and atrial fibrillation. Thyroid 12:501, 2002.)*

ing Graves disease or nodular goiter. In this category younger patients appear to have little or no untoward effects, whereas older patients are potentially at risk from atrial fibrillation. In patients older than the age of 60 years, antithyroid therapy (methimazole 5 to 10 mg per day) can produce improvement, and in patients who do respond consideration should be given to the use of radioiodine for definitive treatment.[41]

Amiodarone and Thyroid Function

Amiodarone is an iodine-rich, antiarrhythmic agent effective in the treatment of both ventricular and atrial tachyarrhythmias. It is currently used extensively in patients with a variety of cardiac diseases. As a result of the 30 percent by weight iodine content, this drug commonly causes abnormalities in thyroid function testing in patients treated for either short or long periods of time.[87] The finding that dronedarone, a noniodinated benzofuran antiarrhythmic, does not alter thyroid function is reinforced by this concept.[88] Similar to other iodinated drugs, amiodarone inhibits the 5′ monodeiodination of T_4 both in the liver and in the pituitary.[44] Inhibition of T_4 metabolism in the liver decreases serum T_3 and increases serum T_4, while serum TSH levels initially remain normal. With more chronic treatment and as the total iodide content of the body rises, there is a potential for inhibition of T_4 synthesis and release from the thyroid gland, producing a rise in TSH. In patients with underlying goiter, autoimmune thyroid disease, or enzymatic defects in thyroid hormone biosynthesis, and in some patients without any risk factors there is a progression to overt chemical and clinical hypothyroidism with a marked rise in serum TSH.[87] The overall prevalence of hypothyroidism in amiodarone-treated patients is reported to be between 15 and 20 percent. Importantly, the symptoms of hypothyroidism in this setting can be quite subtle, and significant hypothyroidism can occur even in their absence.[71]

Thyroid function should be measured every 3 months in all patients receiving amiodarone. The effect on thyroid function does not depend on dose and can occur anytime after initiating treatment, and because of the high lipid solubility and long half-life of the drug, for periods up to a year after discontinuing therapy.[87]

Less common but perhaps more challenging is the development of amiodarone-induced thyrotoxicosis. Although initially not observed in the iodine-replete American population, the experience from Italy suggested that it occurred with a prevalence as high as 10 percent.[87] The onset was often sudden and could occur shortly after drug initiation, during chronic treatment, or up to 1 year after stopping therapy. Although the pathogenesis is multifactorial, early studies distinguished two forms of amiodarone-induced thyrotoxicosis. Type I occurs primarily in patients with preexisting thyroid disease and most commonly in iodine-deficient areas. These patients may rarely have an increase in 24-hour radioiodine uptake measures and frequently some measures of thyroid autoimmunity including antithyroid antibodies. Color flow Doppler sonography of the thyroid gland has a "characteristic" appearance consistent with other forms of autoimmune thyroid disease. In contrast, type II disease was identified as a form of thyroiditis presumably mediated by a variety of proinflammatory cytokines including IL-6.[89] This is primarily a destructive process causing release of preformed thyroid hormone, which may continue for periods of weeks and months and is most often associated with a low to absent radioiodine uptake. Further experience has shown that these two types have substantial overlap for many of the distinguishing parameters.

Because of the increased thyroidal and total body iodine content, use of iodine-131 is almost always ineffective.[41] Similarly, treatment with antithyroid drugs has marginal effectiveness. Corticosteroids (prednisone 20 to 40 mg per day) have been recommended and proven to be of benefit perhaps with increased utility in patients with type II disease in whom serum levels of IL-6 are high.[87] Alternatively, corticosteroids can be instituted in all patients because, when effective, the response usually occurs within 1 to 2 weeks of initiating treatment. In patients unresponsive to glucocorticoids with evidence of hyperthyroidism including weight loss, tachycardia, palpitations, worsening angina, or other untoward cardiac effects, treatment with antithyroid therapy (Tapazole 10 to 30 mg/day) and potassium perchlorate (if available) is variably effective.[89] Treatment can cause significant side effects including bone marrow toxicity from the potassium perchlorate. A recent report confirms that total thyroidectomy can be performed safely and is an effective means of rapidly reversing the hyperthyroidism. Preoperative treatment with beta-adrenergic blocking drugs is indicated, and there have been no reported cases of resulting thyroid storm.[90]

An important issue is whether amiodarone-mediated thyroid dysfunction should mandate discontinuation of the drug. There is no evidence that stopping the amiodarone hastens the resolution of the chemical hyperthyroidism. Because certain patients require amiodarone therapy to manage arrhythmias, and because the duration of drug retention in the body in lipid-soluble stores is in excess of 6 months, it seems prudent to continue amiodarone therapy while making separate management plans to deal with the thyroid dysfunction.

CHANGES IN THYROID HORMONE METABOLISM THAT ACCOMPANY CARDIAC DISEASE

In addition to the changes in thyroid function, which can result from classic thyroid disease, there are primary alterations in serum total and free T_3 and occasionally serum T_4 that accompany a variety of acute and chronic illnesses including sepsis, starvation, and cardiac disease (see Fig. 81-3).[91] In the absence of thyroid gland abnormality, changes in serum T_3 levels result from alterations in thyroid hormone metabolism. These cases have been referred to as "nonthyroidal illness." The mechanism for this decrease in serum T_3 is multifactorial and in part related to a decrease in 5′ monodeiodination in the liver.[41,44]

Population-based study of patients with cardiac disease has shown that a low serum T_3 level strongly predicts all-cause and cardiovascular mortality.[92,93] Following uncomplicated acute myocardial infarction, serum T_3 levels fall by about 20 percent and reach a nadir after approximately 96 hours. Experimental myocardial infarction in animal models produces a similar decrease in serum T_3, and replacement of T_3 levels to normal has been reported to increase left ventricular contractile function.[47]

Both children and adults undergoing cardiac surgery with cardiopulmonary bypass demonstrate a predictable fall in serum T_3 in the perioperative period.[94] Although treatment strategies using acute administration of intravenous T_3 to adults after coronary artery bypass grafting have shown an improvement in cardiac output and a fall in systemic vascular resistance, there was no alteration in overall mortality. When the prevalence of atrial fibrillation was studied in this group of patients, however, it was shown to be decreased by as much as 50 percent when compared with age-matched controls.[95] Pediatric cardiac patients, especially those undergoing surgery in the neonatal period, demonstrate an even greater decline in serum T_3 that can last for longer periods of time. The low postoperative T_3 level identifies patients at increased risk for morbidity and mortality.[96] A recent prospective randomized study has shown that especially in neonates, the degree of therapeutic intervention and the need for postoperative inotropic agents is decreased by the administration of T_3 in doses sufficient to restore serum T_3 levels to normal.[97]

In patients with chronic congestive heart failure the fall in serum T_3 is proportional to the severity of heart failure as assessed by New York Heart Association classification.[47,93] Up to 30 percent of patients with heart failure have a low serum T_3, which occurs both in patients treated with amiodarone and those who are not. In view of the deleterious effects of hypothyroidism on the myocardium, T_3 replacement may be of benefit. Human studies using a novel form of T_3 that is capable of restoring serum T_3 levels to normal and avoiding the peaks and valleys of drug levels currently associated with existing drug preparations will be required to answer this question.

Pheochromocytoma

Pheochromocytomas are primarily benign tumors arising from neuroectodermal chromaffin cells primarily within the adrenal medulla and abdomen, but they may arise anywhere within plexi of sympathetic adrenergic nerves. Although the prevalence is probably less than 1 per 2000 cases of diastolic hypertension, the importance of pheochromocytoma derives from the dramatic mode in which symptoms can present. Various autopsy studies have shown that in 75 percent of patients the diagnosis was not clinically suspected, and in more than half it was believed to be a factor contributing to mortality.[98]

Most pheochromocytomas are 1 cm or greater in size, the vast majority arise as a unilateral adrenal lesion, and extraadrenal tumors are more common in children.[99] Although most tumors are sporadic, approximately 10 percent are familial and the latter are more often bilateral or occur in an extraadrenal location. When pheochromocytoma coexists with medullary thyroid carcinoma or occasionally with hyperparathyroidism, it is a designated *multiple endocrine neoplasia* (MEN) *syndrome type II.* These patients have a mutation in the RET proto-oncogene. In patients with MEN2B, pheochromocytomas coexist with medullary thyroid cancer and mucosal neuromas frequently seen on the lips and tongue. In patients with neurofibromatosis, pheochromocytoma may be present in up to 1 percent of patients, and in the von Hippel-Lindau disease, pheochromocytoma develops in association with cerebellar or retino-angiomas.

Pheochromocytoma presents clinically with headache, palpitations, excessive sweating, tremulousness, chest pain, weight loss, and a variety of other constitutional complaints. Hypertension may be episodic but is most commonly constant and is paradoxically associated with orthostatic hypotension on arising in the morning. The paroxysmal attacks and classic symptoms result from episodic excess catecholamine secretion.[98]

The first onset of hypertension caused by pheochromocytoma can be at the time of elective surgical intervention for an unrelated condition. As a result of norepinephrine release with an increase in systemic vascular resistance, cardiac output is minimally, if at all, increased despite increases in heart rate. The ECG can show LVH, as well as the presence of inverted T waves suggesting left ventricular strain. Although ventricular and atrial ectopy and episodes of supraventricular tachycardia can occur, there is little to distinguish the LVH from that of essential hypertension.[98]

Reports of impaired left ventricular function and cardiomyopathy have been made in patients with pheochromocytoma. The mechanism underlying this is complex and includes increased left ventricular work and LVH from associated hypertension, potential adverse effects of excess catecholamines on myocyte structure and contractility, and changes in coronary arteries including thickening of the media, presumably potentially impairing blood flow to the myocardium. Histologic evidence of myocarditis is present postmortem in patients with previously diagnosed or undiagnosed disease.[98] The possibility of catecholamine-stimulated tachycardia in turn mediating left ventricular dysfunction should be addressed because treatments designed to slow the heart rate may improve left ventricular function.

Release of catecholamines from pheochromocytomas involves diffusion out of chromaffin cells, as well as release of storage vessels accounting for the demonstration of chromogranin A in the circulation. The primary catecholamine released is norepinephrine, but increases in epinephrine can also be measured. Demonstration of elevated serum dopamine implies the possibility of malignant transformation, which in turn suggests that the tumor may arise in an extra-adrenal site. Rarely pheochromocytoma can arise within the heart, presumably from chromaffin cells, which are part of the adrenergic autonomic paraganglia.[100]

DIAGNOSIS

Diagnosis is established by demonstrating an increase in norepinephrine or epinephrine or its metabolites either in serum or blood. Quantitative 24-hour urinary metanephrines are the most reliable screening procedures, and plasma catecholamines, when obtained under proper conditions, are also fairly sensitive.[100,101] A variety of provocative tests have been used to increase plasma catecholamines in patients with episodic disease. In contrast, the clonidine-suppression test is safe and will suppress plasma norepinephrine by more than 50 percent in essential hypertensive patients but not in those with pheochromocytoma.[99] Imaging modalities include magnetic resonance imaging, which has a high degree of specificity, and computed tomographic scan, which has a high degree of sensitivity because adrenal lesions are of sufficient size to be detected. Further studies with isotopic precursors of catecholamine biosynthesis including ^{131}I-metaiodobenzylguanidine (MIBG) are useful for confirming that anatomic lesions are producing catecholamines.[101]

TREATMENT

Definitive treatment of pheochromocytoma requires removal of the lesion. Accurate preoperative localization has reduced operative mortality and eliminates the need for exploratory laparotomy. Endoscopic procedures are now standard.[102] Preoperative pharmacological management includes 7 to 14 days of alpha-adrenergic blockade usually with prazosin or phenoxybenzamine. Beta-adrenergic blocker therapy is considered contraindicated before establishing sufficient alpha blockade. If supraventricular arrhythmias or unremitting tachycardia is present, beta$_1$-selective agents such as atenolol are preferred.[101] Operative intervention requires constant blood pressure monitoring, and the use of intravenous phentolamine, or sodium nitroprusside may be required to treat episodic hypertension.[98,102] Postoperative management includes the use of large volumes of crystalloid-containing fluids to maintain blood volume and prevent hypotension. Glucose may be necessary to replace depleted liver glycogen stores. Success of surgery can be determined both by effective blood pressure and symptomatic improvement but also with measurement of urinary catecholamines at 4 weeks after the procedure. In patients who are not candidates for surgical treatment, metyrosine can decrease catecholamine synthesis and improve the majority of cardiovascular signs and symptoms.[102]

The recognition that a variety of naturally occurring hormones have such profound effects on the heart and cardiovascular system suggests that these actions can be captured to treat a variety of cardiovascular diseases. The ability of thyroid hormone to lower cholesterol, enhance cardiac contractility (especially diastolic function) via novel transcription-based mechanisms, and at the same time lower systemic vascular resistance provides a platform on which novel therapies can be devised. Similarly, the ability of vasoactive intestinal peptide to lower pulmonary artery pressure opens the possibility of treating patients with pulmonary hypertension arising from many different causes.

REFERENCES

(For references to the older literature, please consult the 7th edition of *Braunwald's Heart Disease*, Chapter 79).

Acromegaly

1. Lu C, Schwartzbauer G, Sperling MA, et al: Demonstration of direct effects of growth hormone on neonatal cardiomyocytes. J Biol Chem 276:22892, 2001.
2. Napoli R, Guardasole V, Angelini V, et al: Acute effects of growth hormone on vascular function in human subjects. J Clin Endocrinol Metab 88:2817, 2003.
3. Colao A, Vitale G, Pivonello R, et al: The heart: An end-organ of GH action. Eur J Endocrinol 151(Suppl):S93, 2004.
4. Brevetti G, Marzullo P, Silvestro A, et al: Early vascular alterations in acromegaly. J Clin Endocrinol Metab 87:3174, 2002.
5. Mestron A, Webb SM, Astorga R, et al: Epidemiology, clinical characteristics, outcome, morbidity and mortality in acromegaly based on the Spanish Acromegaly Registry (Registro Espanol de Acromegalia, REA). Eur J Endocrinol 151:439, 2004.
6. Clayton RN: Cardiovascular function in acromegaly. Endocr Rev 24:272, 2003.
7. Bruch C, Herrmann B, Schmermund A, et al: Impact of disease activity on left ventricular performance in patients with acromegaly. Am Heart J 144:538, 2002.
8. Colao A, Spinelli L, Cuocolo A, et al: Cardiovascular consequences of early-onset growth hormone excess. J Clin Endocrinol Metab 87:3097, 2002.
9. Di Bello V, Bogazzi F, Di Cori A, et al: Myocardial systolic strain abnormalities in patients with acromegaly: A prospective color Doppler imaging study. J Endocrinol Invest 29:544, 2006.
10. Colao A, Spinelli L, Marzullo P, et al: High prevalence of cardiac valve disease in acromegaly: An observational, analytical, case-control study. J Clin Endocrinol Metab 88:3196, 2003.
11. van der Klaauw AA, Bax JJ, Roelfsema F, et al: Uncontrolled acromegaly is associated with progressive mitral valvular regurgitation. Grow Horm IGF Res 16:101, 2006.
12. Herrmann BL, Bruch C, Saller B, et al: Acromegaly: Evidence for a direct relation between disease activity and cardiac dysfunction in patients without ventricular hypertrophy. Clin Endocrinol (Oxf) 56:595, 2002.
13. Damjanovics SS, Neskovic AN, Petakov MS, et al: High output heart failure in patients with newly diagnosed acromegaly. Am J Med 112:610, 2002.
14. Trainer PJ, Drake WM, Katznelson L, et al: Treatment of acromegaly with the growth hormone-receptor antagonist pegvisomant. N Engl J Med 342:1171, 2000.
15. Clemmons DR, Chihara K, Freda PU, et al: Optimizing control of acromegaly: Integrating a growth hormone receptor antagonist into the treatment algorithm. J Clin Endocrinol Metab 88:4759, 2003.
16. Fazio S, Cittadini A, Biondi B, et al: Cardiovascular effects of short-term growth hormone hypersecretion. J Clin Endocrinol Metab 85:179, 2000.
17. Colao A, Pivonello R, Auriemma RS, et al: Predictors of tumor shrinkage after primary therapy with somatostatin analogues in acromegaly: A prospective study in 99 patients. J Clin Endocrinol Metab 91:2112, 2006.

Adrenal Cortex

18. Whitworth JA, Mangos GJ, Kelly JJ: Cushing, cortisol, and cardiovascular disease. Hypertension 36:912, 2000.
19. Wintour EM: Cortisol as a growth hormone for the fetal heart. Endocrinology 147:3641, 2006.
20. Colao A, Pivonello R, Spiezia S, et al: Persistence of increased cardiovascular risk in patients with Cushing's disease after five years of successful cure. J Clin Endocrinol Metab 84:2664, 1999.
21. Fernandez-Real J, Ricard W: Insulin resistance and chronic cardiovascular inflammatory syndrome. Endocr Rev 24:278, 2003.
22. Suzuki T, Shibata H, Ando T, et al: Risk factors associated with persistent postoperative hypertension in Cushing's syndrome. Endocr Res 26:791, 2000.
23. Faggiano A, Pivonello R, Spiezia S, et al: Cardiovascular risk factors and common carotid artery caliber and stiffness in patients with Cushing's disease during active disease and 1 year after disease remission. J Clin Endocrinol Metab 88:2527, 2003.
24. Muiesan ML, Lupia M, Salvetti M, et al: Left ventricular structural and functional characteristics in Cushing's syndrome. J Am Coll Cardiol 41:2275, 2003.
25. Marazuela M, Aguilar-Torres R, Benedicto A, et al: Dilated cardiomyopathy as a presenting feature of Cushing's syndrome. Int J Cardiol 88:331, 2003.

26. Bertherat J: Carney complex (CNC). Orphanet J Rare Dis 6:21, 2006.
27. Ambrosi B, Sartorio A, Pizzocaro A, et al: Evaluation of haemostatic and fibrinolytic markers in patients with Cushing's syndrome and in patients with adrenal incidentaloma. Exp Clin Endocrinol Diabetes 108:294, 2000.
28. Mortensen RM, Williams GH: Aldosterone action. In DeGroot L, Jameson L (eds): Endocrinology. Philadelphia, Saunders, 2001, p 1783.
29. Carey RM, Siragy HM: Newly recognized components of the renin-angiotensin system: Potential roles in cardiovascular and renal regulation. Endocr Rev 24:261, 2003.
30. Young MJ, Funder JW: Mineralocorticoid receptors and pathophysiological roles for aldosterone in the cardiovascular system. J Hypertens 20:1465, 2002.
31. White PC: Aldosterone: Direct effects on and production by the heart. J Clin Endocrinol Metab 88:2376, 2003.
32. Szucs TD, Holm MV, Schwenkglenks M, et al: Cost-effectiveness of eplerenone in patients with left ventricular dysfunction after myocardial infarction—an analysis of the Ephesus Study from a Swiss perspective. Cardiovasc Drugs Ther 20:193, 2006.
33. Matsumura K, Fujii K, Oniki H, et al: Role of aldosterone in left ventricular hypertrophy in hypertension. Am J Hypertens 19:13, 2006.
34. Dolmatch B, Nesbitt S, Vongpatanasin W: Primary hyperaldosteronism: Effect of adrenal vein sampling on surgical outcome. Arch Surg 141:497, 2006.
35. Espinosa G, Santos E, Cervera R, et al: Adrenal involvement in the antiphospholipid syndrome: Clinical and immunologic characteristics of 86 patients. Medicine (Baltimore) 82:106, 2003.
36. Cooper MS, Stewart PM: Corticosteroid insufficiency in acutely ill patients. N Engl J Med 348:727, 2003.
37. Fallo F, Betterle C, Budano S, et al: Regression of cardiac abnormalities after replacement therapy in Addison's disease. Eur J Endocrinol 140:425, 1999.

Parathyroid Disease

38. Schluter K, Piper HM: Cardiovascular actions of parathyroid hormone and parathyroid hormone-related peptide. Cardiovasc Res 37:34, 1998.
39. Stefenelli T, Abela C, Frank H, et al: Cardiac abnormalities in patients with primary hyperparathyroidism: Implications for follow-up. J Clin Endocrinol Metab 82:106, 1997.
40. Andersson P, Rydberg E, Willenheimer R: Primary hyperparathyroidism and heart disease—a review. Eur Heart J 25:1776, 2004.

Thyroid Disease

41. Klein I, Ojamaa K: Thyroid hormone and the cardiovascular system. N Engl J Med 344:501, 2001.
42. Dillmann WH: Cellular action of thyroid hormone on the heart. Thyroid 12:447, 2002.
43. Klein I, Danzi S: The cardiovascular system in thyrotoxicosis. In Braverman LE, Utiger RD, (eds): Werner & Ingbar's The Thyroid: A fundamental and Clinical Text. 9th ed. Philadelphia, Lippincott Williams & Wilkins, 2005, p 559.
44. Koenig RJ: Regulation of type 1 iodothyronine deiodinase in health and disease. Thyroid 15:835, 2005.
45. Harvey CB, Williams GR: Mechanism of thyroid hormone action. Thyroid 12:441, 2002.
46. Danzi S, Klein I: Thyroid hormone-regulated cardiac gene expression and cardiovascular disease. Thyroid 12:467, 2002.
47. Ojamaa K, Ascheim D, Hryniewic K, et al: Thyroid hormone therapy of cardiovascular disease. Cardiovasc Rev Rep 23:20, 2002.
48. Carr AN, Kranias EG: Thyroid hormone regulation of calcium cycling proteins. Thyroid 12:453, 2002.
49. Ojamaa K, Kenessey A, Klein I: Thyroid hormone regulation of phospholamban phosphorylation in the rat heart. Endocrinology 141:2139, 2000.
50. Biondi B, Klein I: Hypothyroidism as a risk factor for hypothyroidism. Endocrine 24:1, 2004.
51. Virtanen VK, Saha HH, Groundstroem KW, et al: Thyroid hormone substitution therapy rapidly enhances left-ventricular diastolic function in hypothyroid patients. Cardiology 96:59, 2001.
52. Davis PJ, Davis FB: Nongenomic actions of thyroid hormone on the heart. Thyroid 12:459, 2002.
53. Demers LM, Spencer CA: Laboratory medicine practice guidelines, laboratory support for the diagnosis and monitoring of thyroid disease. Thyroid 13:3, 2003.
54. Hoit BD, Khoury SF, Shao Y, et al: Effects of thyroid hormone on cardiac beta-adrenergic responsiveness in conscious baboons. Circulation 96:592, 1997.
55. Ojamaa K, Klein I, Sabet A, et al: Changes in adenylyl cyclase isoforms as a mechanism for thyroid hormone modulation of cardiac beta-adrenergic receptor responsiveness. Metabolism 49:275, 2000.
56. Park KW, Kai HB, Ojamaa K, et al: The direct vasomotor effect of thyroid hormones on rat skeletal muscle resistance arteries. Anesth Analg 85:734, 1997.
57. Danzi S, Klein I: Thyroid hormone and blood pressure regulation. Curr Hypertens Rep 5:513, 2003.
58. Biondi B, Palmieri EA, Lombardi G, et al: Effects of thyroid hormone on cardiac function: The relative importance of heart rate, loading conditions, and myocardial contractility in the regulation of cardiac performance in human hyperthyroidism. J Clin Endocrinol Metab 87:968, 2002.
59. Schmidt B, Martin N, Georgens AC, et al: Nongenomic cardiovascular effects of triiodothyronine in euthyroid male volunteers. J Clin Endocrinol Metab 87:1681, 2002.
60. Bengel FM, Lehnert J, Ibrahim T, et al: Cardiac oxidative metabolism, function, and metabolic performance in mild hyperthyroidism: A noninvasive study using positron emission tomography and magnetic resonance imaging. Thyroid 13:471, 2003.

61. Taddei S, Caraccio N, Virdis A, et al: Impaired endothelium-dependent vasodilatation in subclinical hypothyroidism: Beneficial effect of levothyroxine therapy. J Clin Endocrinol Metab 88:3731, 2003.

62. Marcisz C, Jonderko G, Kucharz EJ: Influence of short-time application of a low sodium diet on blood pressure in patients with hyperthyroidism or hypothyroidism during therapy. Am J Hypertens 14:995, 2001.

63. Kahaly GJ, Kampmann C, Mohr-Kahaly S: Cardiovascular hemodynamics and exercise tolerance in thyroid disease. Thyroid 12:473, 2002.

64. Virani SS, Mendoza CE, Ferreira AC, et al: Graves disease and pulmonary hypertension. Tex Heart Inst J 30:314, 2003.

65. Shimizu T, Koide S, Noh JY, et al: Hyperthyroidism and the management of atrial fibrillation. Thyroid 12:489, 2002.

66. Auer J, Scheibner P, Mische T, et al: Subclinical hyperthyroidism as a risk factor for atrial fibrillation. Am Heart J 142:838, 2001.

67. Nakazawa H, Lythall DA, Noh J, et al: Is there a place for the late cardioversion of atrial fibrillation? A long-term follow-up study of patients with post-thyrotoxic atrial fibrillation. Eur Heart J 21:327, 2000.

68. Fuster V, Ryden LE, Asinger RW, et al: ACC/AHA/ESC Guidelines for the management of patients with atrial fibrillation. J Am Coll Cardiol 38:1266, 2001.

69. Franklyn JA, Maisonneuve P, Sheppard MC, et al: Mortality after the treatment of hyperthyroidism with radioactive iodine. N Engl J Med 338:712, 1998.

70. Flynn RW, MacDonald TM, Jung RT, et al: Some cardiovascular diseases occur with increased frequency in patients treated for hyperthyroidism or hypothyroidism. J Clin Endocrinol Metab 91:2159, 2006.

71. Klein I: The cardiovascular system in hypothyroidism. In Braverman LE, Utiger RD (eds): Werner & Ingbar's The Thyroid: A Fundamental and Clinical Text. 9th ed. Philadelphia, Lippincott Williams & Wilkins, 2005, p 774.

72. Bengel FM, Nekolla SC, Ibrahim T, et al: Effect of thyroid hormones on cardiac function, geometry, and oxidative metabolism assessed noninvasively by positron emission tomography and magnetic resonance imaging. J Clin Endocrinol Metab 85:1822, 2000.

73. Cappola AR, Ladenson PW: Hypothyroidism and atherosclerosis. J Clin Endocrinol Metab 88:2438, 2003.

74. Rush J, Danzi S, Klein I: Role of thyroid disease in the development of statin-induced myopathy. Endocrinologist 16:279, 2006.

75. Canaris GJ, Manowitz NR, Mayor G, et al: The Colorado thyroid disease prevalence study. Arch Intern Med 160:526, 2000.

76. Hak AE, Pols HAP, Visser TJ, et al: Subclinical hypothyroidism is an independent risk factor for atherosclerosis and myocardial infarction in elderly women: The Rotterdam Study. Ann Intern Med 132:270, 2000.

77. Walsh JP, Bremner AP, Bulsara MK, et al: Subclinical thyroid dysfunction as a risk factor for cardiovascular disease. Arch Intern Med 165:2467, 2005.

78. Brokhin M, Klein I: Low T3 syndrome in a patient with acute myocarditis. Clin Cornerstone 2(Suppl):28, 2005.

79. Thompson PD, Clarkson P, Karas RH: Statin-induced myopathy. JAMA 289:1681, 2003.

80. Rodondi N, Aujesky D, Vittinghoff E, et al: Subclinical hypothyroidism and the risk of coronary heart disease. Am J Med 119:541, 2006.

81. Monzani F, Di Bello V, Caraccio N, et al: Effect of levothyroxine on cardiac function and structure in subclinical hypothyroidism: A double blind, placebo-controlled dtudy. J Clin Endocrinol Metab 86:1110, 2001.

82. Biondi B, Fazio S, Palmieri EA, et al: Left ventricular diastolic dysfunction in patients with subclinical hypothyroidism. J Clin Endocrinol Metab 84:2064, 1999.

83. Sawin CT: Subclinical hyperthyroidism and atrial fibrillation. Thyroid 12:501, 2002.

84. Cappola AR, Fried LP, Arnold AM, et al: Thyroid status, cardiovascular risk, and mortality in older adults. JAMA 295:1033, 2006.

85. Parle, JV, Maisonneuve P, Sheppard MC, et al: Prediction of all-cause and cardiovascular mortality in elderly people from one low serum thyrotropin result: A 10-year cohort study. Lancet 358:861, 2001.

86. Burmeister LA, Flores A: Subclinical thyrotoxicosis and the heart. Thyroid 12:495, 2002.

Amiodarone

87. Martino E, Bartalena L, Bogazzi F, et al: The effects of amiodarone on the thyroid. Endocr Rev 22:240, 2001.

88. Kathofer S, Thomas D, Karle CA: The novel antiarrhythmic drug dronedarone: comparison with amiodarone. Cardiovasc Drug Rev 23:217,2005.

89. Bogazzi F, Bartalena L, Cosci C, et al: Treatment of type II amiodarone-induced thyrotoxicosis by either iopanoic acid or glucocorticoids: A prospective, randomized study. J Clin Endocrinol Metab 88:1999, 2003.

90. Williams M, Lo Gerfo P: Thyroidectomy using local anesthesia in critically ill patients with amiodarone-induced thyrotoxicosis: A review and description of the technique. Thyroid 12:523, 2002.

Changes in Thyroid Hormone Metabolism in Cardiac Disease

91. DeGroot LJ: Dangerous dogmas in medicine: The nonthyroidal illness syndrome. J Clin Endocrinol Metab 84:151, 1999.

92. Iervasi G, Pingitore A, Landi P, et al: Low-T3 syndrome: A strong prognostic predictor of death in patients with heart disease. Circulation 107:708, 2003.

93. Pingitore A, Landi P, Taddei MC, et al: Triiodothyronine levels for risk stratification of patients with chronic heart failure. Am J Med 118:132, 2005.

94. Portman MA, Fearneyhough C, Ning W, et al: Triiodothyronine repletion in infants during cardiopulmonary bypass for congenital heart disease. J Thorac Cardiovasc Surg 120:604, 2000.

95. Klemperer JD, Klein I, Ojamaa K, et al: Triiodothyronine therapy lowers the incidence of atrial fibrillation after cardiac operations. Ann Thorac Surg 61:1323, 1996.

96. Mainwaring RD, Capparelli E, Schell K, et al: Pharmacokinetic evaluation of triiodothyronine supplementation in children after modified Fontan procedure. Circulation 101:1423, 2000.

97. Chowdhury D, Parnell V, Ojamaa, K, et al: Usefulness of triiodothyronine (T3) treatment after surgery for complex congenital heart disease in infants and children. Am J Cardiol 84:1107, 1999.

Pheochromocytoma

98. Bravo EL: Pheochromocytoma. Cardiol Rev 10:44, 2002.

99. Manger WM, Gifford RW: Pheochromocytoma. J Clin Hypertens (Greenwich) 4:62, 2002.

100. Lenders JW, Pacak K, Eisenhofer G: New advances in the biochemical diagnosis of pheochromocytoma: Moving beyond catecholamines. Ann N Y Acad Sci 970:29, 2002.

101. Schiff RL, Welsh GA: Perioperative evaluation and management of the patient with endocrine dysfunction. Med Clin North Am 87:175, 2003.

102. Eigelberger MS, Duh QY: Pheochromocytoma. Curr Treat Options Oncol 2:321, 2001.

103. Danzi S, Klein I: Potential uses of T3 in the treatment of human disease. Clin Cornerstone 2(Suppl):9, 2005.

CH 81

Endocrine Disorders and Cardiovascular Disease

CHAPTER 82

Basic Mechanisms of Hemostasis and Thrombosis, 2049
Vascular Endothelium, 2049
Coagulation, 2050
Anticoagulant (Antithrombotic) Mechanisms, 2052
Platelets, 2054
Central Role of Thrombin, 2056

Thrombophilic Disorders, 2056
Inherited Thrombophilia, 2056
Acquired Thrombophilia, 2060

Antithrombotic Drugs, 2062
Heparin and Related Drugs, 2062
　Low-Molecular-Weight
　　Heparins, 2063
　Other Glycosaminoglycan-Derived
　　Drugs, 2065
Warfarin, 2065
Thrombin Inhibitors and Other
　Specific Coagulation
　Inhibitors, 2066
Thrombolytic (Fibrinolytic)
　Drugs, 2067
Antiplatelet Agents, 2068

References, 2075

Hemostasis, Thrombosis, Fibrinolysis, and Cardiovascular Disease

Barbara A. Konkle, Daniel Simon, and Andrew I. Schafer

BASIC MECHANISMS OF HEMOSTASIS AND THROMBOSIS

The human hemostatic system has evolved as a remarkably orchestrated scheme of linked activities designed to preserve the integrity of blood circulation. Hemostasis is regulated to promote blood fluidity under normal circumstances. It is also prepared to clot blood with speed and precision to arrest blood flow and prevent exsanguination whenever and wherever the integrity of the circulation is disrupted. Finally, hemostasis can restore blood flow and perfusion on subsequent healing of a damaged vessel. The major components of the hemostatic system are (1) the vessel wall itself, (2) plasma proteins (the coagulation and fibrinolytic factors), and (3) platelets. These constituents function virtually inseparably (Fig. 82-1). Although they are discussed in this chapter individually, it is important to recognize the interdependence of the actions of the vessel wall, plasma clotting factors, and platelets.

Vascular Endothelium (see Chap. 38)

Endothelial cells arise from hemangioblasts, which collect in blood islands, the precursors of blood vessels, in the yolk sac of the developing embryo.[1] Hemangioblasts differentiate into both primitive endothelial cells (angioblasts) and hematopoietic cells.[2] The endothelial cell progenitors that arise from hemangioblasts have the capacity to form new blood vessels (a process termed *vasculogenesis*) under the influence of vascular endothelial growth factors (VEGFs) and their tyrosine kinase receptors, as well as other tyrosine kinase receptors and their ligands. Endothelial cell precursors may actually circulate in adult human blood, and their numbers may increase as they participate in neovascularization (angiogenesis), vascular healing, and remodeling in response to ischemia, injury, tumor growth, and other pathological processes.[3] Thus, circulating endothelial cells, currently measured by various methods, may be a biomarker of vascular disease.[4] Endothelial cell progenitors enter the adult circulation from bone marrow–derived angioblasts, as well by shedding from the vessel wall.

A monolayer of endothelial cells lines the intimal surface of the entire circulatory tree, thereby representing the only stationary cell type that components of blood ever contact under normal circumstances. The endothelial surface of the adult human is enormous; it is composed of about 1 to 6×10^{13} cells, weighs approximately 1 kg, and covers a surface area equivalent to about six tennis courts. Yet, as recently as the first half of the 20th century, endothelial cells were viewed simply as barriers of blood flow, acting "merely in a negative manner," "similarly to a layer of paraffin or oil." Today, we recognize that endothelium is a dynamic organ with complex metabolic capabilities, including the ability to control vascular permeability, the flow of biologically active molecules and nutrients, cell-cell and cell-matrix interactions within the vessel wall, blood flow and vascular tone, interactions of blood cells, the inflammatory response, and angiogenesis.[5]

Endothelium is also an ideal regulator of hemostasis.[6] It is endowed with a remarkable repertoire of activities that permit it to transform rapidly from a potent antithrombotic to a prothrombotic surface wherever the need arises. Indeed, attempts to reproduce these properties in clinical settings, such as cardiovascular prostheses, extracorporeal circuits, and bypass grafts by pharmacological or even gene transfer methods, have proven challenging.

Normal quiescent endothelium constitutively displays a potent antithrombotic (thromboresistant) surface to blood (Fig. 82-2). It expresses anticoagulant, profibrinolytic, and platelet inhibitory properties. Whenever endothelium is activated or perturbed, however, it can quickly become a prothrombotic surface that actually promotes coagulation, inhibits fibrinolysis, and activates platelets. These are not entirely uniform phenomena, however. Throughout the circulatory tree, even within a single organ, there is marked heterogeneity in the phenotype of endothelial cells.[7] With respect to hemostasis, for example, endothelial cells from different tissues are heterogeneous in their expression of the various antithrombotic and prothrombotic mediators. Vascular bed–specific phenotypic characteristics of endothelium may account for the distinctively focal nature of thrombosis in the face of systemic abnormalities of hemostasis.[7] This endothelial heterogeneity results from genetic and environmental factors. Exposure to different microenvironmental stimuli, in-cluding variable hemodynamic forces, extracellular matrix composition, and cellular and humoral mediators, contributes significantly to the heterogeneity of endothelial phenotypes that develops throughout the circulation.

The specific antithrombotic and prothrombotic properties of endothelial cells noted in Figure 82-2 are described in more detail in the following sections. The hemostatic conversion of the vessel wall is trig-

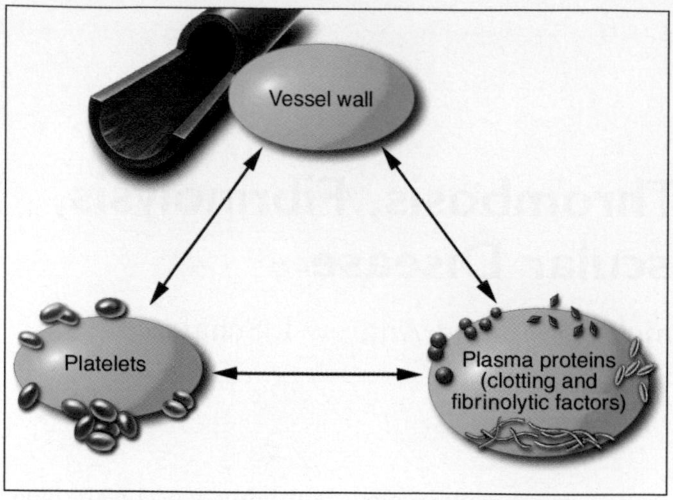

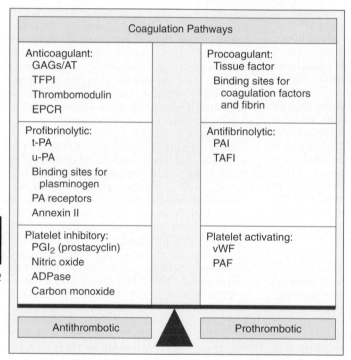

FIGURE 82–1 Interactions between the major components of the hemostatic system—the vessel wall, plasma proteins (clotting and fibrinolytic factors), and platelets.

Coagulation Pathways

Anticoagulant: GAGs/AT TFPI Thrombomodulin EPCR	Procoagulant: Tissue factor Binding sites for coagulation factors and fibrin
Profibrinolytic: t-PA u-PA Binding sites for plasminogen PA receptors Annexin II	Antifibrinolytic: PAI TAFI
Platelet inhibitory: PGI$_2$ (prostacyclin) Nitric oxide ADPase Carbon monoxide	Platelet activating: vWF PAF
Antithrombotic	Prothrombotic

FIGURE 82–2 Balance of antithrombotic and prothrombotic properties of vascular endothelium. In general, antithrombotic properties dominate in quiescent endothelium under normal physiological conditions. In contrast, prothrombotic properties are expressed whenever endothelium is perturbed or activated. AT = antithrombin; EPCR = endothelial cell protein C receptor; GAGs = glycosaminoglycans; PAF = platelet-activating factor; PAI = plasminogen activator inhibitor; TAFI = thrombin-activatable fibrinolysis inhibitor; TFPI = tissue factor pathway inhibitor; t-PA = tissue-type plasminogen activator; u-PA = urokinase-type plasminogen activator; vWF = von Willebrand factor. *(Modified from Rosendaal FR: Venous thrombosis: A multicausal disease. Lancet 353:1167, 1999.)*

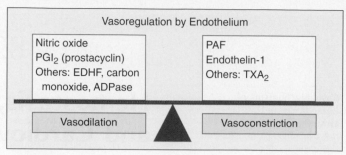

FIGURE 82–3 Regulation of vascular tone by the balance of endothelium-derived vasodilators and vasoconstrictors. ADPase = adenosine diphosphatase; EDHF = endothelium-derived hyperpolarizing factor; PAF = platelet-activating factor; TXA$_2$ = thromboxane A$_2$.

dino nitrogen atoms of L-arginine by the action of a group of enzymes known as nitric oxide synthases (NOSs). The major isoform of NOS present in endothelial cells, eNOS, is constitutively active and is further activated by stimuli that increase intracellular calcium, including several receptor-dependent agonists (e.g., thrombin) and hemodynamic forces (shear stress and cyclic stretch).[8] NO acts as a potent vasodilator as well as an inhibitor of platelet adhesion and platelet aggregation by stimulating soluble guanylate cyclase and thereby elevating intracellular levels of cyclic guanosine monophosphate in vascular smooth muscle cells and platelets. Vascular cell–derived carbon monoxide (CO), a product of heme degradation by heme oxygenase, may exert similar actions on vascular function.[9] Prostaglandin I$_2$ (PGI$_2$, prostacyclin) is a major endothelium-derived oxygenation product of arachidonic acid, synthesized by the sequential actions of cyclooxygenase (COX) and prostacyclin synthase.[10] Prostacyclin, like NO, is both a vasodilator and inhibitor of platelet aggregation (but not adhesion), exerting these actions by stimulating adenylate cyclase and thereby elevating intracellular cyclic adenosine monophosphate (cAMP) levels in target vascular smooth muscle and platelets. Endothelium-derived hyperpolarizing factors[5] (EDHF), which include epoxyeicosatrienoic acids,[11] hydrogen peroxide[12] and potassium ions, are also vasodilators elaborated by endothelial cells. Endothelial ecto-adenosine diphosphatase (ADPase), or CD39,[13] is a membrane-associated platelet inhibitor but may also indirectly promote vasodilation by generating adenosine. These vasodilator properties of endothelium are counterbalanced by endothelium-derived vasoconstrictors, including platelet-activating factor, endothelin-1, and thromboxane A$_2$ (TXA$_2$).[14]

In many cases, endothelium-derived vasodilators are also platelet inhibitors and, conversely, endothelium-derived vasoconstrictors can also be platelet activators. The net effect of vasodilation and inhibition of platelet function is to promote blood fluidity, whereas the net effect of vasoconstriction and platelet activation is to promote hemostasis. Thus, blood fluidity and hemostasis can be exquisitely regulated by the balance of antithrombotic-prothrombotic and vasodilatory-vasoconstrictor properties of endothelial cells, which are often coordinately modulated by their relative states of quiescence and activation (see Figs. 82-2 and 82-3).[6] Endothelial vasodilator dysfunction may predict cardiovascular events. It can be assessed by in vivo endothelial vasomotor testing in the peripheral or coronary circulations or by measurement of circulating markers of endothelial dysfunction.[15]

Coagulation

Plasma coagulation proteins (clotting factors) normally circulate in plasma in their biologically inactive zymogen (or

gered by mechanical damage or by perturbation and activation of the vascular cells by factors such as cytokines, endotoxin, hypoxia, and hemodynamic forces.

Similarly, as illustrated in Figure 82-3, a delicate balance exists in regard to the capability of endothelial cells to modulate vascular tone. An important physiological vasodilator released by endothelial cells is nitric oxide (NO), a simple diatomic gas synthesized from the terminal guani-

proenzyme) forms. When mechanical injury or inflammatory and other systemic stimuli alter the thromboresistant nature of the vascular system, the coagulation system is activated. If the physiological antithrombotic defenses can be overwhelmed, the result will be the formation of hemostatic thrombi composed of platelets and fibrin. In cases in which activation of the coagulation system is triggered by focal vascular injury, the occlusive hemostatic thrombus will be precisely localized at and limited to the site of damage.

The sequence of coagulation protein reactions that culminate in the formation of fibrin was originally described as a waterfall or cascade (Fig. 82-4). The coagulation cascade is a highly coordinated and regulated series of linked enzymatic reactions that involves the sequential activation of plasma zymogens to serine proteases. Each protease then catalyzes the subsequent zymogen-protease transition by cleavage of peptide bonds. This sequence constitutes a biochemical amplifier in which a small initiating stimulus rapidly generates high levels of the end product, fibrin. Our understanding of the coagulation cascade has undergone refinement with the recognition that it actually involves a series of linked enzymatic multiprotein complexes, each consisting of a serine protease, one or more cofactor proteins, divalent cations, and a cellular surface (e.g.,

platelet membranes), which favor assembly of these components.[16,17]

Two pathways of blood coagulation exist, the so-called extrinsic or tissue factor pathway and the so-called intrinsic or contact activation pathway. These two pathways of activation of the coagulation cascade converge to form a common pathway, which leads to the generation of the pivotal coagulation enzyme thrombin. Thrombin not only catalyzes the conversion of fibrinogen to fibrin but also serves an important role in sustaining the cascade by feedback activation of coagulation factors at several strategic sites (see Fig. 82-4).

EXTRINSIC (TISSUE FACTOR) PATHWAY. The extrinsic pathway, also referred to as the tissue factor pathway, probably initiates coagulation in vivo. The immediate trigger is the injury-induced expression of the integral membrane glycoprotein tissue factor on the surfaces of activated endothelial cells and blood cells (particularly leukocytes), cells that normally do not express tissue factor activity on their surfaces.[17,18] Alternatively, vascular damage can expose blood to tissue factor expressed on the surfaces of or deposited in the extracellular space endothelial or smooth muscle cells or macrophages (see Chap. 38). The serine protease factor VIIa (activated factor VII) circulates in blood at trace levels but possesses very poor enzymatic activity in its free form. Exposure of blood to cell surface tissue factor activates coagulation by binding this free factor VIIa. The tissue factor–factor VIIa complex then acts as a bimolecular enzyme to autocatalyze the conversion of factor VII to VIIa rapidly, thereby generating more tissue factor–factor VIIa complexes and amplifying this initial hemostatic response.[19] Factor Xa and thrombin can also induce factor VII activation (see Fig. 82-4); in fact, these two enzymes may be kinetically preferred over the tissue factor–factor VIIa complex as physiological activators of factor VII.

The final reaction in the extrinsic pathway is the activation of factor X to factor Xa. This step can be catalyzed directly by the tissue factor–factor VIIa bimolecular enzyme complex. Alternatively, the complex can indirectly activate factor X by initially converting factor IX to factor IXa (providing communication between the extrinsic and intrinsic pathways of coagulation), which then activates factor X. This indirect route of factor X activation is probably favored kinetically.

INTRINSIC (CONTACT ACTIVATION) PATHWAY. This pathway of coagulation is triggered by the autoactivation of factor XII to its active serine protease form (factor XIIa) on negatively charged surfaces, optimally in the presence of two other contact activation proteins, prekallikrein and high-molecular-weight kininogen.[20] A physiological negatively charged surface for contact activation of factor XII and the intrinsic pathway of coagulation has not been identified. However, this pathway is important for in vitro activation of coagulation, and knowledge of this pathway is necessary for interpretation of coagulation laboratory testing. In this pathway, factor XIIa converts the zymogen factor XI to its corresponding serine protease, factor XIa. Factor XIa, in turn, can then activate factor IX to IXa. In the final step in the intrinsic pathway, the plasma zymogen factor X undergoes activation to factor Xa by factor IXa, a reaction that requires the activated form of the plasma cofactor, factor VIIIa. Factor VIIIa is generated by thrombin-induced limited proteolysis of factor VIII.

The most compelling support that coagulation is not initiated by the intrinsic pathway derives from the clinical observation that individuals with inherited deficiencies of any of the contact activation factors (e.g., factor XII, prekallikrein, high-molecular-weight kininogen) do not have a bleeding tendency. In fact, these proteins may play important roles in other physiological systems, such as vasoregu-

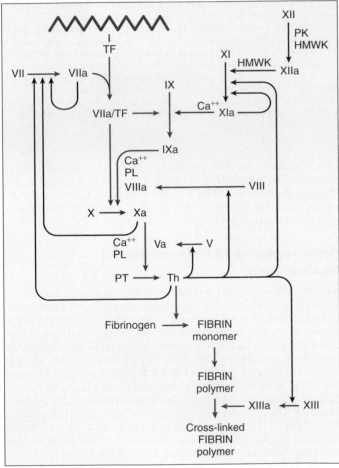

FIGURE 82–4 The coagulation cascade. This scheme emphasizes understanding of the importance of the tissue factor pathway in initiating clotting in vivo, the interactions between pathways, and the pivotal role of thrombin in sustaining the cascade by feedback activation of coagulation factors. HMWK = high-molecular-weight kininogen; PL = phospholipid; PT = prothrombin; TF = tissue factor; PK = prekallikrein; Th = thrombin. *(Modified from Schafer AI: The primary and secondary hypercoagulable states. In Schafer AI [ed]: Molecular Mechanisms of Hypercoagulable States. Austin, TX, Landes Bioscience, 1997, pp 1-48.)*

lation and the inflammatory response, and as antithrombotic and profibrinolytic agents.[20] In contrast, those with deficiencies of factors XI, IX, or VIII have clinical bleeding tendencies, and therefore these proteins in the intrinsic pathway appear to play important roles in hemostasis. The participation of factor XI in hemostasis therefore probably does not depend on its activation by factor XIIa but rather on its positive feedback activation by thrombin. Thus, this positive feedback loop (see Fig. 82-4) would permit factor XIa to function in the propagation and amplification, rather than in the initiation, of the coagulation cascade.

COMMON PATHWAY. Factor Xa, which can be formed through the actions of either the tissue factor–factor VIIa complex or factor IXa (with factor VIIIa as a cofactor), initiates the common pathway of coagulation by converting the inactive plasma zymogen prothrombin to thrombin, the pivotal protease of the coagulation system. The essential cofactor for this reaction is factor Va, which like the homologous factor VIIIa, is produced by thrombin-induced limited proteolysis of factor V. As noted earlier and further described later, thrombin is a multifunctional enzyme, but its major role in the common pathway is to convert soluble plasma fibrinogen to an insoluble fibrin matrix.[21] Fibrin polymerization involves an orderly process of intermolecular associations. Thrombin also activates factor XIII (fibrin-stabilizing factor) to factor XIIIa, a transglutaminase that covalently cross-links and thereby stabilizes the fibrin clot.

The coagulation cascade that culminates in fibrin formation would occur extremely inefficiently and slowly in fluid phase plasma. However, the assembly of these clotting factors on activated cell membrane surfaces greatly accelerates their reaction rates and also serves to localize blood clotting to sites of vascular injury.[17,22] In addition, proteases in the coagulation factor complexes assembled on cell surfaces are sequestered from inactivation by their physiological antithrombotic regulators (described later), further enhancing the efficiency of membrane-dependent reactions. The critical cell membrane components on which these coagulation reactions proceed are acidic phospholipids. These phospholipid species are not normally exposed on resting cell membrane surfaces. However, when vascular injury or inflammatory stimuli activate platelets, monocytes, or endothelial cells, the procoagulant head groups of the membrane anionic phospholipids translocate to the surfaces of these cells or are shed as part of microparticles, making them available to support and promote the plasma coagulation reactions.[23]

PHOSPHOLIPID-ASSOCIATED ENZYME COMPLEXES. Major membrane phospholipid-associated enzyme complexes in the coagulation cascade include the Xase (or "tenase") and prothrombinase complexes (Fig. 82-5). Each complex consists of a serine protease enzyme, its zymogen substrate, and its cofactor assembled in association with each other on the membrane surface. The extrinsic Xase complex consists of the tissue factor–factor VIIa enzyme complex and its zymogen substrates, factors IX and X. The intrinsic Xase complex consists of factor IXa as the enzyme, factor X as its substrate, and factor VIIIa as the cofactor. The prothrombinase complex consists of factor Xa as the enzyme, prothrombin (factor II) as its substrate, and factor Va as the cofactor. Factor IXa generated by the extrinsic Xase complex becomes the enzyme of the intrinsic Xase complex. Factor Xa, generated by the extrinsic Xase or intrinsic Xase complex, becomes the enzyme of the prothrombinase complex. These successive reaction complexes of coagulation most likely occur by diffusion of products along the same cell membrane surface.

The final enzyme product, thrombin serves multiple purposes. A major terminating reaction, also shown in Figure

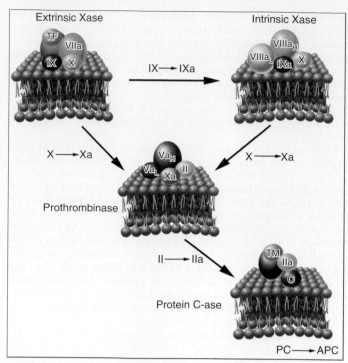

FIGURE 82–5 Schematic representation of the phospholipid membrane–associated enzyme complexes of coagulation. Each vitamin K–dependent serine protease (factors VIIA, IXA, and Xa and alpha-thrombin [IIa]) is shown in association with its cofactor protein (tissue factor [TF], factors VIIIa and VA, and thrombomodulin [TM]) and zymogen substrate(s) (factors IX and X, prothrombin [II] and protein C [C]) on the membrane surface. The cofactor proteins, factor VIIIa and factor VA, are characterized by a two-domain structure and consist of heavy (H) and light (L) chains that are bridged together by Ca²⁺ ions. Both domains are required for cofactor-membrane association and cofactor-protease binding. *(Modified from Jenny NS, Mann KG: Coagulation cascade: An overview. In Loscalzo J, Schafer AI [eds]: Thrombosis and Hemorrhage. 2nd ed. Baltimore, Williams & Wilkins, 1998, pp 3-27.)*

82-5, involves membrane assembly of the protein C-ase complex, in which free thrombin (factor IIa) binds to the integral membrane protein, thrombomodulin, which serves as the site for activation of protein C, a major antithrombotic protein discussed later.

Anticoagulant (Antithrombotic) Mechanisms

Several physiological antithrombotic mechanisms act in concert to prevent clotting under normal circumstances. Optimal activity of each of the anticoagulant systems depends on the integrity of vascular endothelium. Thus, these physiological mechanisms preserve blood fluidity in the intact circulation and also limit blood clotting to specific focal sites of vascular injury. Endogenous inhibitors of platelets include endothelial PGI₂, nitric oxide, ADPase, and carbon monoxide (see Fig. 82-2). Other anticoagulant systems can also limit fibrin, including antithrombin, the protein C–protein S–thrombomodulin system and tissue factor pathway inhibitor (TFPI). The fibrin that forms despite these anticoagulant defenses can then undergo degradation by the fibrinolytic system (Fig. 82-6).

ANTITHROMBIN. Antithrombin (or antithrombin III) is the major plasma protease inhibitor of thrombin and the other clotting factors. It is a single-chain glycoprotein that is synthesized primarily in the liver and belongs to the serine protease inhibitor (serpin) family of proteins.[24] Antithrombin neutralizes thrombin and other activated coagulation factors by forming a complex between the active site of

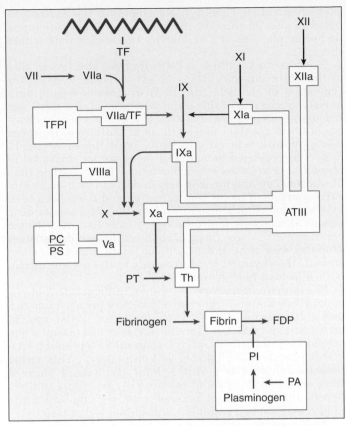

FIGURE 82-6 Sites of action of the four major physiological antithrombotic pathways—antithrombin (AT); protein C/protein S (PC/PS); tissue factor pathway inhibitor (TFPI); and the fibrinolytic system, consisting of plasminogen, plasminogen activator (PA), and plasmin (PI). *(From Schafer AI: The primary and secondary hypercoagulable states.* In *Schafer AI [ed]: Molecular Mechanisms of Hypercoagulable States. Austin, TX, Landes Bioscience, 1997, pp 1-48.)*

the enzyme and the reactive center (Arg393 and Ser394) of antithrombin. The rate of formation of these inactivating complexes increases by a factor of several thousand in the presence of heparin. Heparin and heparan sulfate proteoglycans are actually present as endogenous components of the vessel wall. Thus, antithrombin inactivation of thrombin and other activated clotting factors probably occurs physiologically on vascular surfaces. Inherited quantitative or qualitative deficiencies of antithrombin lead to a lifelong predisposition to venous thromboembolism.[25]

PROTEIN Z. Protein Z–dependent protease inhibitor (ZPI) is a heparin-independent inhibitor of factor Xa.[26] Protein Z is a vitamin K–dependent protein that circulates in plasma in a complex with ZPI. Inhibition of factor Xa by ZPI, a member of the serpin superfamily of proteinase inhibitors, is enhanced 1000-fold by protein Z. Low levels of protein Z appear not to be an independent risk factor for thrombosis, but enhance the thrombotic risk in patients with additional thrombophilias, most notably factor V Leiden.[27] A nonsense polymorphism in ZPI has been recently found to increase the risk of venous thrombosis.[28]

PROTEIN C–PROTEIN S–THROMBOMODULIN. Protein C is another plasma glycoprotein synthesized by the liver, which becomes an anticoagulant when it is activated by thrombin through cleavage of an Arg169-Leu170 bond in its heavy chain.[29] The thrombin-induced activation of protein C occurs physiologically on thrombomodulin, a transmembrane proteoglycan binding site for thrombin on endothelial cell surfaces.[30] Thrombomodulin thus serves an antithrombotic function by binding and thereby removing thrombin from the circulation and also by promoting the generation

of active protein C, active as an anticoagulant. The binding of protein C to its receptor on endothelial cells (endothelial cell protein C receptor) allows its concentration in proximity to the thrombin-thrombomodulin complex, therefore enhancing its efficiency of activation. Activated protein C acts as an anticoagulant by cleaving multiple bonds and thereby destroying the membrane-bound activated forms of coagulation factors V (Va) and VIII (VIIIa). A cofactor, protein S, accelerates this reaction. Like protein C, protein S is a glycoprotein that undergoes vitamin K–dependent post-translational carboxylations to form gamma-carboxyglutamic acid (Gla) residues. Protein S acts as a cofactor by increasing the affinity of activated protein C for phospholipids in the formation of the membrane-bound protein C-ase complex (see Fig. 82-5). Quantitative or qualitative deficiencies of protein C or protein S, or resistance to the action of activated protein C by a specific mutation at its target cleavage site in factor Va (factor V Leiden), lead to hypercoagulable states.[25]

TISSUE FACTOR PATHWAY INHIBITOR. TFPI is a plasma protease inhibitor that regulates the tissue factor–induced extrinsic pathway of coagulation.[31] Unlike other coagulation inhibitors, which are members of the serpin family, TFPI is a multivalent Kunitz-type serine protease inhibitor. This structure permits TFPI to exert dual inhibitory actions against both tissue factor–factor VIIa (mediated by its Kunitz-1 domain binding to factor VIIa; see Fig. 82-6) as well as factor Xa (mediated by its Kunitz-2 binding to factor Xa). TFPI circulates bound to lipoproteins. Heparin can release TFPI from endothelial cells, where it is bound to glycosaminoglycans, and from platelets.[32] Impairment of TFPI activity and antibodies to TFPI have been demonstrated in patients with antiphospholipid antibody syndrome.[33] Lipoprotein(a), Lp(a), can bind and inactivate TFPI, a novel mechanism by which Lp(a) may promote thrombosis. Low levels of TFPI constitute a risk factor for venous thrombosis; association with oral contraceptive use might contribute to the thrombotic tendency in this setting.[35]

FIBRINOLYTIC SYSTEM. Any thrombin that escapes inhibition by the physiological anticoagulant systems described earlier is available to convert fibrinogen to fibrin. In response, the endogenous fibrinolytic system is then activated to dispose of intravascular fibrin and thereby maintain or reestablish the patency of the circulation. Just as thrombin is the key protease enzyme of the coagulation system, plasmin is the major protease enzyme of the fibrinolytic system, acting to digest fibrin to fibrin degradation products (Fig. 82-7).

Plasminogen, the inactive zymogen form of plasmin, is synthesized primarily in the liver and circulates in plasma in high (micromolar) concentrations. It is a single-chain glycoprotein, which has significant sequence homology with apolipoprotein(a). Elevated plasma levels of Lp(a) are associated with atherosclerotic cardiovascular risk.[36] Indeed, one possible atherogenic mechanism for Lp(a) might be to inhibit fibrinolysis by competing with plasminogen for plasmin generation.

Plasminogen Activators. Plasminogen activators cleave the Arg560-Val561 bond of plasminogen to generate the active enzyme plasmin, a two-chain molecule that derives its heavy chain (or A chain) from the amino-terminal region and its light chain (or B chain) from the carboxy terminal region of plasminogen. The enzyme-active site of plasmin resides in the B chain, whereas the A chain contains lysine-binding sites. The lysine-binding sites of plasmin (and plasminogen) permit it to bind to fibrin, so that physiological fibrinolysis is fibrin-specific.[37] The serine protease plasmin has actions beyond fibrinolysis; plasmin also plays important roles in embryogenesis, tissue remodeling, wound healing, angiogenesis, and cell migration.[37]

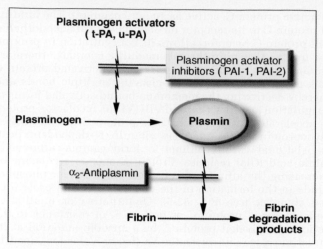

FIGURE 82–7 Schema of the fibrinolytic system and its control. PAI-1, -2 = plasminogen activator inhibitors 1, 2; t-PA = tissue-type plasminogen activator; u-PA = urokinase-type plasminogen activator.

The major physiological plasminogen activators that convert plasminogen to plasmin are tissue-type plasminogen activator (t-PA) and urokinase-type plasminogen activator (u-PA).[37] Endothelial cells release both these serine proteases into plasma in trace concentrations. Plasmin can convert t-PA from its single-chain form to a two-chain molecule, in which the heavy and light chains are disulfide-bonded. Both the single-chain and double-chain forms of t-PA are catalytically active to convert plasminogen to plasmin. In contrast, single-chain u-PA (scu-PA) has little enzyme activity and must be converted to its disulfide-bonded, two-chain active form by hydrolysis of a Lys158-Ile159 bond. t-PA and u-PA are released from endothelial cells by various humoral factors (e.g., growth factors, hormones, cytokines), as well as hemodynamic forces, but many of these stimuli also induce the release of plasminogen activator inhibitors.

Both plasminogen (through its lysine-binding sites) and t-PA possess specific affinity for fibrin and thereby bind selectively to clots. The assembly of a ternary complex, consisting of fibrin, plasminogen, and t-PA, promotes the localized interaction between plasminogen and t-PA and thereby greatly accelerates the rate of plasminogen activation to plasmin. Moreover, partial degradation of fibrin by plasmin exposes new plasminogen and t-PA binding sites in carboxy terminus lysine residues of fibrin fragments to enhance these reactions further. This sequence creates a highly efficient mechanism to generate plasmin focally on the fibrin clot, which then becomes plasmin's substrate for digestion to fibrin degradation products. Thus, the fibrin surface itself importantly regulates its own degradation by providing binding sites for fibrinolytic proteins.

In addition to its interactions with fibrin, components of the fibrinolytic system are also efficiently assembled on cell surfaces, similar to the coagulation system, to localize and kinetically optimize the generation of plasmin.[37,38] Specific binding sites for plasminogen and t-PA identified with annexin II reside on the surfaces of endothelial cells and other cell surfaces to catalyze plasminogen activation. u-PA receptors (u-PAR) also localize on endothelial cells and other cell types.

The capacity of endothelial cells to synthesize and release plasminogen activators and then to bind these and other components of the fibrinolytic system provides a powerful paracrine mechanism to concentrate and activate fibrinolysis in proximity to intravascular thrombi contiguous to sites of endothelial damage. Receptors for the fibrinolytic proteins also localize on the surfaces of other cell types, including platelets and leukocytes that accumulate within thrombi.[37]

Plasmin cleaves fibrin at different rates at different sites of the fibrin molecule. This orderly process leads to the generation of characteristic fibrin fragments during fibrinolysis. At the end of this sequential proteolysis, the D and E domains of fibrin are liberated. The sites of plasmin cleavage of fibrin are the same as those in fibrinogen. However, when plasmin acts on covalently cross-linked fibrin, D-dimers are released; hence, D-dimers can be measured in plasma as a relatively specific test of fibrin (rather than fibrinogen) degradation. D-dimer assays can be used as sensitive markers of blood clot formation and some have been validated for clinical use to exclude the diagnosis of deep venous thrombosis and pulmonary embolism in selected populations[39,40] (see Chap. 72). Fibrin(ogen) degradation products may have potent anticoagulant and antiplatelet actions, thereby further contributing to the net antithrombotic effects of fibrinolysis.

Fibrinolytic Inhibitors. As shown in Figure 82-7, physiological regulation of fibrinolysis occurs primarily at two levels: (1) plasminogen activator inhibitors (PAIs), specifically PAI-1 and PAI-2, inhibit the physiological plasminogen activators; and (2) alpha$_2$-antiplasmin inhibits plasmin. PAI-1 is the primary inhibitor of t-PA in plasma.[37] This serine protease inhibitor is a single-chain glycoprotein derived from endothelial cells and other cell types. PAI-1 inhibits t-PA by the formation of a complex between the active site of t-PA and the bait residues (Arg346-Met347) of PAI-1.

Alpha$_2$-antiplasmin is a single-chain glycoprotein serpin synthesized predominantly by the liver. It is the main inhibitor of plasmin in human plasma, forming a 1:1 stoichiometric complex with plasmin that inactivates the enzyme.[41] Alpha$_2$-macroglobulin also inhibits plasmin, but at a much slower rate than alpha$_2$-antiplasmin; therefore, alpha$_2$-macroglobulin has questionable importance in the physiological regulation of fibrinolysis.

Further regulation of fibrinolysis occurs by a unique feedback mechanism of thrombin generation via the thrombin-activatable fibrinolysis inhibitor (TAFI).[42] Thrombin activates TAFI, a reaction that is increased more than 1000-fold in the presence of endothelial cell thrombomodulin. Thus, thrombomodulin on the endothelial cell creates a direct molecular link between the coagulation and fibrinolytic systems—it converts thrombin to an antifibrinolytic enzyme by directing it to TAFI activation.[42] TAFI suppresses fibrinolysis through the removal of carboxy terminal lysine residues on fibrin monomers, eliminating plasminogen and t-PA binding sites that normally serve to augment t-PA–mediated conversion of plasminogen to plasmin. Elevated TAFI levels and TAFI polymorphisms may be a mild risk factor for venous thrombosis, and may increase the risk of venous thromboembolism (VTE) recurrence in patients with high factor VIII, IX, or XI levels.[42] A clear relationship with coronary artery disease has not been established.[45]

Platelets

Platelets are fragments released into blood from bone marrow megakaryocytes, a process that is regulated primarily by the hormone thrombopoietin, and circulate with an average life span of 7 to 10 days.[46] These cell fragments have no nuclei and therefore possess minimal capacity to synthesize new protein. The antithrombotic properties of intact vascular endothelium include potent platelet inhibitors (Fig. 82-8A; see Fig. 82-2). These inhibitors include PGI$_2$, NO, and CO, labile molecules released by endothelial cells that act locally as autacoids, and ADPase, an ectonu-

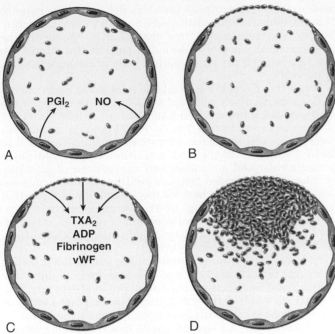

FIGURE 82–8 Sequence of events in platelet activation. **A,** Under normal conditions, a monolayer of endothelial cells lines the intimal surface of the circulatory tree, releasing platelet inhibitory mediators such as PGI₂ (prostacyclin) and nitric oxide (NO). **B,** At a site of vascular injury (depicted from 11 to 1 o'clock), endothelium is lost and platelets undergo "adhesion" (platelet–vessel wall interactions) to subendothelial structures that are now exposed (e.g., collagen). **C,** Adherent platelets are activated and release granule constituents (e.g., ADP, fibrinogen, von Willebrand factor [vWF]) and thromboxane A₂ (TXA₂). D, Substances released from activated platelets recruit additional platelets from the circulation to the site of injury and mediate the process of platelet "aggregation" (platelet-platelet interactions), resulting in the formation of an occlusive platelet plug. ADP = adenosine diphosphate.

cleotidase of endothelial membranes that breaks down platelet-activating ADP.

ADHESION. Vascular intimal injury impairs the antiplatelet properties of endothelium locally and exposes previously cryptic, thrombogenic, subendothelial substances (e.g., collagen) to flowing blood. Circulating platelets recognize sites of vascular disruption and adhere to the site of injury (see Fig. 82-8B). Adhesion results in the formation of a monolayer of platelets on the denuded vascular intimal surface. Platelet adhesion (i.e., platelet–vessel wall interaction) is mediated primarily by von Willebrand factor (vWF), a protein that assembles into a multimeric molecular mass that ranges from about 550 to more than 10,000 kDa, one of the largest soluble proteins in plasma.[47] vWF is synthesized by endothelial cells and megakaryocytes, where it is stored in Weibel-Palade bodies and alpha granules, respectively, before its regulated secretion. Released vWF is present in plasma and in the extracellular matrix of the subendothelial vessel wall, to which the platelets are anchored. The large vWF multimers serve as the primary molecular glue to attach platelets to a damaged vessel wall with sufficient strength to withstand the high levels of shear stress that would tend to detach them with the flow of blood. The receptor for vWF on the platelet surface, glycoprotein (GP) Ib, is part of the platelet membrane GP Ib–IX–V complex.[48] Higher levels of shear stress on the arterial side of the circulation promote the interaction between vWF and platelet membrane GP Ib.[48] Platelet adhesion is also facilitated by direct binding to subendothelial collagen by means of specific platelet membrane collagen receptors, including alpha₂-beta₁ integrin (also known as GP Ia/IIa) and the

immunoglobulin (Ig) superfamily member GP VI.[49] Under conditions of high shear stress in small arteries, GP Ib and GP VI act in concert to tether platelets rapidly to the exposed extracellular matrix of the injured vessel wall through their respective ligands, vWF and collagen.[50] Subsequently, the generation of intracellular signals from GP Ib and GP VI leads to platelet activation (see next paragraph) and activation of integrins to reinforce the initial adhesion process.

ACTIVATION. Adherent platelets then become activated (see Fig. 82-8C). Platelet activation results from the combined actions of several agonists that bind to their respective membrane receptors on adherent platelets, mobilize intracellular calcium, and transmit platelet-activating intracellular signals.[51] These platelet stimuli include humoral mediators in plasma (e.g., epinephrine, thrombin), mediators released from activated cells (e.g., ADP, serotonin), and vessel wall extracellular matrix constituents that come in contact with adherent platelets (e.g., collagen, vWF). Several of these stimuli can synergistically activate platelets and may also act in concert with shear forces that platelets encounter simultaneously. Activated platelets undergo the release reaction, during which they secrete prepackaged constituents of their cytoplasmic granules—ADP, adenosine triphosphate, and serotonin from the dense granules; soluble adhesive proteins (fibrinogen, vWF, thrombospondin, fibronectin), growth factors (including platelet-derived growth factor, transforming growth factor [TGF]-alpha and TGF-beta), and procoagulants (platelet factor 4, factor V) from the alpha granules. Simultaneously, activated platelets synthesize de novo and release the potent platelet activator and vasoconstrictor TXA₂. TXA₂ is the major cyclooxygenase product of arachidonic acid metabolism in platelets. As described later in the section on antiplatelet agents, aspirin inhibits cyclooxygenase and thereby blocks TXA₂ synthesis in platelets.[52]

AGGREGATION. The products of the platelet release reaction, including secreted granule constituents and TXA₂, mediate the final phase of platelet activation, the process of aggregation (see Fig. 82-8D).[51] During platelet aggregation (platelet-platelet interaction), additional platelets are recruited from the circulation to the site of vascular injury, leading to the formation of an occlusive platelet thrombus. As discussed earlier, the platelet plug is anchored and stabilized by the fibrin mesh that develops simultaneously as the product of the coagulation cascade. At lower shear levels (e.g., in the venous circulation), the molecular glue that mediates aggregation is fibrinogen, which can be derived either from plasma or from the alpha-granule releasate of activated platelets. At higher shear levels (e.g., in arteries), vWF itself, which is also the ligand that mediates platelet adhesion, can substitute for fibrinogen as the ligand of aggregation. Fibrinogen or vWF binds to specific platelet membrane receptors that are located in the GP IIb/IIIa (or alpha_IIb-beta₃) integrin complex.

The GP IIb/IIIa complex is the most abundant receptor on the platelet surface. Its alpha subunit (GP IIb, or alpha_IIb) is expressed specifically on platelets, but its beta₃ subunit (GP IIIa) is shared by other integrins, including receptors on vascular cells. Ligand-binding GP IIb/IIIa complexes are not normally exposed in their active forms on the surfaces of quiescent circulating platelets. However, platelet activation converts GP IIb/IIIa into competent receptors by means of specific signal transduction pathways,[53] enabling GP IIb/IIIa to bind fibrinogen and vWF. Recognition of fibrinogen and other ligands by the active GP IIb/IIIa complex involves the Arg-Gly-Asp (RGD) tripeptide sequence (located at positions 95-97 and 572-574 of each of the two A-alpha chains of fibrinogen). When two activated platelets with functional GP IIb/IIIa each bind the same fibrinogen molecule, fibrinogen can form a bridge between the two platelets (Fig. 82-9).

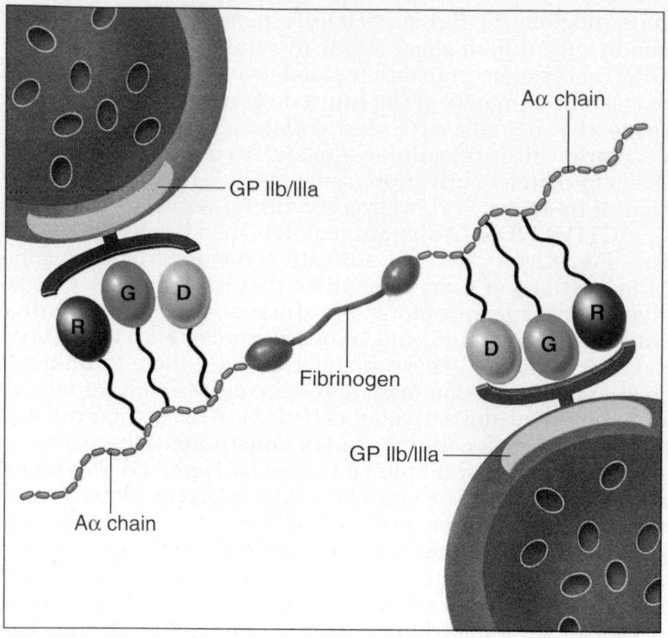

FIGURE 82–9 Linkage of two activated platelets by fibrinogen, which binds to its receptors in the platelet glycoprotein (Gp) IIb/IIIa complex by means of tripeptide RGD (arginine–glycine–aspartic acid) sequences located on the α chains of dimeric fibrinogen. The high density of GP IIb/IIIa complexes on the surfaces of activated platelets permits the rapid formation of a network of fibrinogen bridges, leading to platelet aggregation at the site of vascular injury. (In regions of high shear stress, such as in diseased coronary arteries, von Willebrand factor may replace fibrinogen as the primary aggregating ligand. Like fibrinogen, the von Willebrand factor molecule has RGD sequences that mediate this process.) The result of platelet aggregation is the formation of an occlusive platelet thrombus. (*From Schafer AI: Antiplatelet therapy with glycoprotein IIb/IIIa receptor inhibitors and other novel agents. Tex Heart Inst J 24:90, 1997.*)

Thus, multivalent adhesive proteins like fibrinogen link activated GP IIb/IIIa complexes on adjacent platelets. Because the surface of each platelet has about 50,000 GP IIb/IIIa fibrinogen binding sites, numerous activated platelets recruited to the site of vascular injury can rapidly form an occlusive aggregate by means of a dense network of intercellular fibrinogen bridges.[54] In addition to its RGD sequences, the gamma chains of fibrinogen also contain a 12–amino acid residue (dodecapeptide HHLGGAKQAGDV) that can also bind to the platelet GP IIb/IIIa receptor. These events of ligand binding to activated platelet membrane GP IIb/IIIa receptors, which mediate the process of platelet aggregation, have served as targets for antiplatelet therapy with GP IIb/IIIa antagonists.[55]

Following ligand binding to activated integrins on platelet surfaces, downstream intraplatelet signaling events are initiated, referred to as "outside-in" signaling.[53,54] This process leads to full platelet spreading, irreversible aggregation, and clot retraction. Clot retraction depends on the interaction of platelet GP IIb/IIIa with extracellular fibrin and with intracellular actin-myosin filaments. These events bring platelets into closer contact with each other, creating a protected environment in the gaps between aggregated platelets, preventing the escape of platelet activators from within the gaps, and thereby promoting the continued growth and stability of the hemostatic plug.[56]

Central Role of Thrombin

Thrombin plays a pivotal role in coordinating, integrating, and regulating hemostasis. Depending on the circumstances, it can promote or prevent blood clotting. This multifaceted effect of thrombin has been referred to as the "thrombin paradox."[57,58] At least three variables determine the balance of prothrombotic and antithrombotic activities of thrombin: (1) the concentration of free thrombin in blood; (2) the presence or absence of endothelial cells at thrombin's site of action; and (3) the physiological state of the endothelium (if present).

When free thrombin is available in blood at high concentrations, particularly at a site of vascular injury where the antithrombotic influence of endothelium is lost, thrombin potently induces clotting (Fig. 82-10). This enzyme catalyzes several coagulation factor activation reactions that lead to fibrin formation, factor XIII activation to promote fibrin cross-linking, and activation and aggregation of platelets. Membranes of activated platelets facilitate thrombin generation by providing a surface for the assembly of coagulation factors and cofactors (Fig. 82-11; described earlier). Conversely, thrombin is a potent activator of platelets, stimulating the availability of additional activated platelet surface for further thrombin generation.

At lower concentrations of thrombin and in the presence of intact, nonactivated or noninflamed endothelium, the antithrombotic effects of thrombin predominate (see Fig. 82-10). Low levels of thrombin stimulate increased levels of the endogenous circulating anticoagulant, activated protein C.[57] Accordingly, a J-shaped curve describes the relationship between the thrombotic potential of blood and free thrombin concentration (Fig. 82-12).[58] Furthermore, in the presence of normal endothelial cells in the intact circulation (see Fig. 82-10), endothelial thrombomodulin removes free thrombin from blood and low concentrations of thrombin stimulate t-PA release and the release of antiplatelet PGI_2 and NO from endothelial cells. Inflammation results in decreased endothelial thrombomodulin expression, diminishing its antithrombotic effect.[59] Thus, thrombin plays a central role in modulating the state of blood coagulability, depending on its free concentration in blood and the presence or absence of intact nonactivated endothelial cells at its site of action.

THROMBOPHILIC DISORDERS

Pathological arterial or venous thromboembolism results from a complex interplay of inherited and acquired risk factors. The major risk factor for arterial thrombosis in adults is atherosclerosis (see Chap. 38). This section will focus on inherited and acquired risk factors for venous or both venous and arterial thrombosis, as shown in Table 82-1. An individual's likelihood of suffering a venous thromboembolic event over his or her lifetime results from a combination of risk factors (Fig. 82-13). Many, and possibly most, individuals with venous thromboembolism have one or more underlying genetic disorder(s) that predispose them to thrombosis throughout life (inherited hypercoagulable states or thrombophilias). Actual clinical episodes of venous thromboembolism would be expected to be precipitated by overt or subclinical acquired thrombogenic triggers. Although an individual's risk at any given time cannot currently be defined completely, research studies are moving toward that goal.

Inherited Thrombophilia

FACTOR V LEIDEN. Factor V (FV) Leiden is the most common inherited thrombophilia, with a prevalence in whites of approximately 5 percent and as high as 20 to 40 percent in patients with VTE, depending on selection criteria.[60] Factor V Leiden results from a single mutation (G1691A) in the factor V gene, which results in replacements of arginine at amino acid 506 with a glutamine. This site is one of three activated protein C (APC) cleavage sites in factor V, at which APC, with free protein S as a cofactor, inactivates factor V and thus inhibits blood clot formation (see Fig. 82-6). Individuals heterozygous for this mutation have an approximately three- to eightfold increased risk of VTE and those who are homozygous have an approximately 50- to 80-fold increased risk of VTE. Interestingly, it appears to be a stronger risk factor for deep venous thrombosis (DVT) than for pulmonary embolism. Some have speculated that a more adherent clot is formed in these individuals, which is therefore less likely to embolize. Although the mutation is most common in white patients, and rare in those from sub-Saharan Africa and Asia, its prevalence in the United States in African Americans is approximately 1 percent and in Asian Americans 0.5 percent, which is as or more common than protein C, protein S, or antithrombin (AT) deficiency (Table 82-2).[61,62]

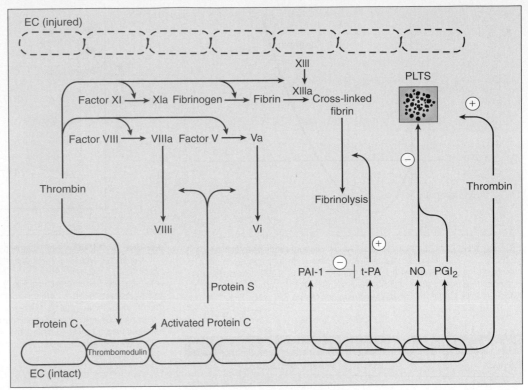

FIGURE 82–10 Central role of thrombin in modulating the state of blood coagulability, depending on the presence or absence of intact endothelial cells (EC) at its site of action. In the presence of intact EC (lower part of figure), free thrombin is removed from the circulation by EC thrombomodulin, and the antithrombotic effects of thrombin predominate—activation of protein C, release of tissue-type plasminogen activator (t-PA), and release of platelet inhibitory nitric oxide (NO) and prostaglandin I_2 (PGI₂) by intact EC. In the absence of intact EC (upper part of figure), free thrombin is available in blood at higher concentrations and its prothrombotic effects predominate—activation of coagulation factors, fibrin formation and cross-linking, and activation of platelets (PLTS). PAI-1 = plasminogen activator inhibitor-1.

Factor V (FV) Leiden does not appear to be an obvious general risk factor for myocardial infarction (MI) or ischemic stroke. This has been supported by large cohort studies, including the Physician's Health Study, the Cardiovascular Health Study, and the Copenhagen City Heart Study. A meta-analysis evaluated 18 studies, including 4623 patients with MI (7.4 percent with FV Leiden) and 12,856 controls (7.4 percent with FV Leiden).[63] In certain subsets of patients, particularly those with concomitant cardiac risk factor, those younger than 55 years, and women, hereditary thrombophilias such as factor V Leiden may confer a higher risk of arterial thrombosis.[64] One study found a statistically significant increased risk of early MI in women who smoked cigarettes, but not in women who did not smoke.[65] Other studies have not confirmed this finding. The risk of ischemic stroke is also not increased in adults with FV Leiden but may be in children.[64] Stroke risk may also increase in women with the FV Leiden mutation who take oral contraceptives.[66]

Women with the FV Leiden mutation have an enhanced risk of thrombosis with hormone therapy, including oral contraceptives (OCPs) and postmenopausal hormone replacement (HRT).[67] The risk of VTE with OCP use in women heterozygous for the mutation is increased 20- to 50-fold, compared with three- to fivefold in women without thrombophilia. A higher risk is seen in women using third-generation versus second-generation OCPs because of different relative protective effects of the progestins.[68] Because young women have a low underlying risk of DVT (approximately 1 in 10,000/year), the number of women who will actually suffer a DVT, even when risk is increased significantly, is low in this age group. The risk of VTE in women receiving HRT is increased 13- to 14-fold versus two- to fourfold in women without FV Leiden or other identified underlying thrombophilia. Hormone-induced VTE in thrombophilic women occurs earlier after initiation of therapy than in women without an identified thrombophilia.

The FV Leiden mutation accounts almost exclusively for the inherited form of the laboratory phenomenon of APC resistance. Rare cases of other factor V mutations affecting APC cleavage have been reported. APC resistance was first described as impairment of APC-mediated

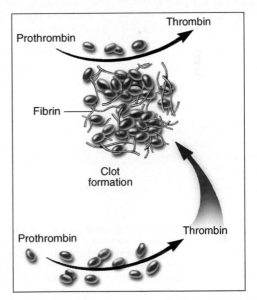

FIGURE 82–11 Reciprocal interaction between thrombin generation and platelet activation. The oval objects represent platelets. Membranes of activated platelets facilitate thrombin generation by providing a surface for assembly of coagulation factors. Conversely, thrombin is a potent activator of platelets, thus acting to promote and amplify activation of the coagulation system. This reciprocal interaction results in the accelerated and tightly focused formation of a hemostatic plug composed of platelets and fibrin. *(From Schafer AI: The primary and secondary hypercoagulable states. In Schafer AI [ed]: Molecular Mechanisms of Hypercoagulable States. Austin, TX, Landes Bioscience, 1997, pp 1-48.)*

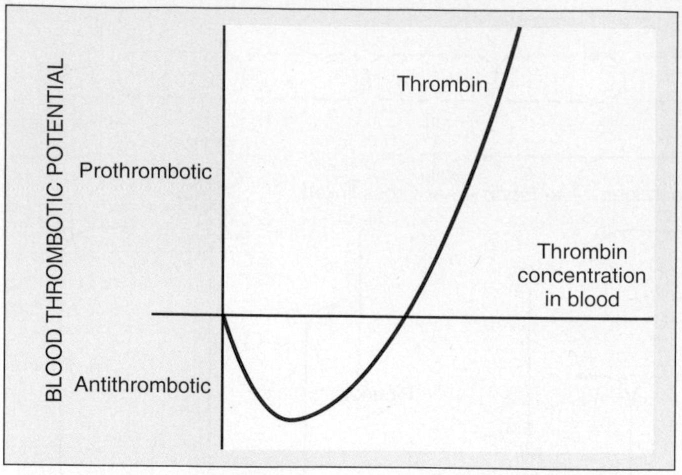

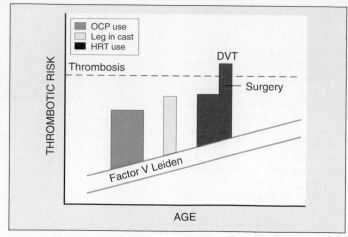

FIGURE 82–12 The thrombin paradox. At low concentrations of thrombin, protein C is activated and elevated activated protein C exhibits antithrombotic activity. At increasingly higher levels of thrombin, the procoagulant properties of thrombin become dominant and prothrombotic potential is markedly increased. *(Modified from Griffin JH: The thrombin paradox. Nature 378:337, 1995.)*

FIGURE 82–13 Thrombotic risk over time. Shown schematically is an individual's thrombotic risk over time. An underlying factor V Leiden mutation provides a theoretically constant increased risk. Thrombotic risk increases with age; intermittently, oral contraceptive (OCP), hormone replacement (HRT) use, or other events increase that risk further. At some point, the cumulative risk may increase to the threshold for thrombosis and result in deep venous thrombosis (DVT). (**Note:** The magnitude and duration of risk portrayed in the figure are meant for example only and may not precisely reflect the relative risk determined by clinical study.) *(Modified from Rosendaal FR: Venous thrombosis: A multicausal disease. Lancet 353:1167, 1999.)*

TABLE 82–1	Risk Factors for Thrombosis
Venous	**Venous and Arterial**
Inherited	Inherited
Factor V Leiden	Homocysteinuria
Prothrombin *G20210A*	Dysfibrinogenemia
Antithrombin deficiency	
Protein C deficiency	Mixed—hyperhomocysteinemia
Protein S deficiency	
Elevated factor VIII activity	
Acquired	Acquired
Age	Malignancy
Previous thrombosis	Antiphospholipid antibody
Immobilization	syndrome
Major surgery	Hormone therapy (oral
Pregnancy and puerperium	contraceptives and
Hospitalization	hormone replacement
Activated protein C resistance,	therapy)
nongenetic	Polycythemia vera
	Essential thrombocythemia
	Paroxysmal nocturnal
	hemoglobinuria
Unknown*	
Elevated factor VII, IX, XI, von	
Willebrand factor	
Elevated levels of thrombin-	
activatable fibrinolysis inhibitor	
Low levels of tissue factor	
pathway inhibitor	

*Unknown whether risk factor is inherited or acquired.

prolongation of the activated partial thromboplastin time (aPTT) in the plasma of selected thrombophilic patients.[69] This abnormality, in the absence of FV Leiden, has been associated with an increased risk of thrombosis, but the testing cannot be well standardized and the clinical usefulness of this finding is unclear. APC resistance is acquired in many conditions, including hormone therapy, pregnancy, and antiphospholipid antibody syndrome, but its role in the pathogenesis of thrombosis in these conditions has not been defined. Many laboratories use a factor V–specific APC resistance test that is highly sensitive and specific for the factor V Leiden mutation. Only other factor V mutations affecting APC cleavage and, rarely, lupus anticoagulants, have been reported to produce false-positive results in this assay.

PROTHROMBIN GENE MUTATION. A polymorphism in the 3′ untranslated region of the prothrombin (PT) gene (*G20210A*) is associated with a two- to threefold increased risk of VTE.[25] This mutation is found predominantly in whites (1 to 6 percent), is uncommon in African Americans (0.2 percent) and is rare in other racial groups.[70] Although this mutation is not in the coding region of the prothrombin gene, it appears to result in increased prothrombin levels. Overall, studies have not shown a greater risk of VTE recurrence in those heterozygous for the factor V Leiden or PT *G20210A* mutation. Thus, these states alone do not modify general recommendations for duration of anticoagulation following a single episode of VTE.[60]

Like factor V Leiden, PT *G20210A* is associated with an increased risk of venous, but generally not arterial, thrombosis. Because PT *G20210A* is such a mild risk factor, thrombosis usually occurs in the setting of additional risk factors, genetic or acquired. The risk of VTE increases in patients heterozygous for both the factor V Leiden and PT *G20210A* mutations above that for either mutation alone. Because both variants are common in white populations, homozygous and compound heterozygous states are encountered.

Hormone therapy further increases the thrombotic risk in patients with PT *G20210A*. The VTE risk in those heterozygous for this mutation who use OCPs increases 16-fold.[71] In addition, a markedly increased risk of cerebral venous thrombosis, a rare clinical event, has occurred in women using OCPs who are heterozygous for this mutation.[72]

ANTITHROMBIN DEFICIENCY. AT deficiency was the first described inherited risk factor for thrombosis.[24,25] Inherited AT deficiency can be the result of a quantitative (type 1) or qualitative (type II) abnormality, the latter manifest by decreased function, with a normal protein level. Complete AT deficiency has not been described and is likely incompatible with life. Patients with inherited type 1 deficiency carry the highest risk of thrombosis; their probability of thrombosis, based on small cohort studies, is up to 85 percent by the age of 50. Population studies do not support such a high risk. The discrepancy is likely seen because of a number of factors, including issues with testing, acquired AT deficiency not carrying the same risk of thrombosis, and possible additional unrecognized genetic defects in the most affected families. In AT-deficient individuals who

Group	Factor V Leiden	Prothrombin *G20210A*	↓ Protein C*	↓ Protein S*	↓ AT*
White Americans	3-7	1-3			
African Americans	~1	0-0.2	0.2-0.5	0.1-1	0.02-0.04
Hispanic Americans	~2	†			
Asian Americans	~0.05	†			
Native Americans	~1	†			

TABLE 82–2 | Ethnic Distribution of Inherited Thrombophilia in the United States (Prevalence, %)

*The prevalence of protein C, protein S, or antithrombin deficiency is not known to vary by ethnic origin of the population tested.
†Unknown.

present with thrombosis, anticoagulation measures are usually continued indefinitely. Although rare cases of arterial thrombosis have been reported, AT deficiency is predominantly a risk for VTE. Venous thrombosis at unusual sites, including the portal and mesenteric veins, has been reported.

PROTEINS C AND S DEFICIENCIES. As described earlier, free protein S serves as a cofactor for activated protein C in the inactivation of factors V and VIII (see Fig. 82-6). Homozygous deficiency of protein C or S presents in infancy as purpura fulminans. The risk of thrombosis in individuals heterozygous for these mutations is unclear, because reports vary, but is probably increased approximately 10-fold.[25,73] Interestingly, chronic venous abnormalities have been noted with increased frequency in protein C–deficient individuals without a prior history of thrombosis, suggesting that the risk of thrombosis with familial protein C deficiency may be underestimated.[74] There appears to be significant variability among affected families, which may result from additional inherited factors. Factor V Leiden can contribute to increased thrombotic risk in families with protein C or protein S deficiency. Because FV Leiden is so common, at least in white populations, a combination of these defects can occur, and the combined effect may be enhanced by a double hit of the same anticoagulant pathway. Whereas rare cases of arterial thrombosis, particularly for protein S deficiency, have been reported, deficiencies of these are predominantly, if not exclusively, risk factors for VTE.

Acquired deficiencies not clearly associated with a thrombotic risk and difficulties in laboratory testing make their diagnosis challenging.[73] Ideally, an inherited deficiency is confirmed in family members. Proteins C and S are affected by vitamin K deficiency, warfarin ingestion, and liver disease, all of which tend to reduce their levels. Mildly decreased protein C levels can be an early marker of liver disease.

Functional protein S assays are used as initial testing for protein S deficiency in many laboratories.[73] This test has a significant false-positive rate and should not be used alone to diagnose protein S deficiency without further testing or family studies. Acquired protein S deficiency, particularly a low free protein S level, occurs in a number of settings, including pregnancy, inflammatory states, and hormone use. Whereas a decreased level of free protein S with a normal total protein S level is frequently an acquired condition, individuals with inherited deficiency may have a similar picture (type III deficiency or type I in older individuals), making the distinction difficult. A diagnosis of protein S deficiency should be made with caution in individuals taking medications or with conditions known to affect protein S levels.

HOMOCYSTEINE. Homocysteine is a sulfhydryl amino acid formed from the demethylation of dietary methionine (Fig. 82-14).[75] Homocysteine may be remethylated to methionine by donation of a methyl group from methyltetrahydrofolate (MTHF) in a reaction catalyzed by methionine synthase using vitamin B_{12} as an essential cofactor, or from betaine. MTHF is derived from the reduction of 5,10-methylene tetrahydrofolate in a reaction catalyzed by MTHF

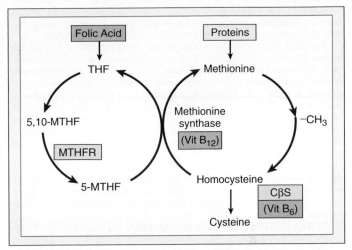

FIGURE 82–14 Homocysteine metabolism. Metabolism of homocysteine can occur through remethylation to methionine, a reaction that requires the enzyme methionine synthase and the cofactor, vitamin B_{12}, or through transsulfuration to cysteine via initial condensation with serine to form cystathionine, in a reaction catalyzed by cystathionine-β-synthase (CβS) followed by hydrolysis by the enzyme γ-cystathionase to cysteine and alpha-ketobutyrate. Both steps in the transsulfuration pathway require vitamin B_6 as a cofactor. In the liver, remethylation also occurs with betaine as the methyl donor (not shown). Methyltetrahydrofolate is derived from the reduction of 5,10-methylene tetrahydrofolate in a reaction catalyzed by methylene tetrahydrofolate reductase (MTHFR). Enzymes in which mutations occur that may increase thrombotic risk are depicted in blue. Vitamins, supplementation with which is used for therapy, are depicted in red. MTHF = methylene tetrahydrofolate; THF = tetrahydrofolate.

reductase (MTHFR). Homocysteine can also condense with serine to form cystathionine, a reaction catalyzed by cystathionine β-synthase (CβS). Vitamin B_6 is an essential cofactor in this reaction.

Patients with severe deficiencies in the enzymes methionine synthase, MTHFR, and, particularly, CβS can have marked elevations in plasma homocysteine (hyperhomocysteinemia) and suffer from premature atherosclerosis and arterial and venous thrombosis.[75] Homocysteinuria, almost exclusively caused by homozygous CβS deficiency, is rare, with a frequency in the general population of 1/250,000, and is manifest by mental retardation, ectopic lenses, and skeletal abnormalities, as well as premature atherosclerosis and thrombosis. Approximately 25 percent of affected individuals will suffer a vascular occlusive event by age 16 and approximately 50 percent will do so by age 29. In a review of reported cases, 51 percent were VTE, 32 percent cerebrovascular accidents (CVAs), 11 percent peripheral vascular disease (PVD), and 4 percent MIs. Pathogenic effects of markedly elevated homocysteine levels are supported by in vitro studies and include induction of smooth muscle proliferation, accelerated oxidation of low-density lipoprotein (LDL) cholesterol, direct endothelial toxicity, impairment of endothelium-derived nitric oxide, decreased synthesis of heparan sulfate proteoglycan, and induction of proinflammatory changes, including increased tissue factor synthesis, decreased cell surface expression of thrombomodulin, and increased expression of vascular adhesion molecule-1.[75]

The strong association of markedly elevated homocysteine levels with atherosclerotic and thrombotic disease has prompted the evaluation of the effects of less marked elevations of homocysteine[95] (see Chaps. 39 and 45). Mild (16 to 24 μmol/liter) or moderate (25 to 100 μmol/liter) hyperhomocysteinemia usually results from mutations in MTHFR and/or acquired dietary deficiencies of vitamin B_{12}, folic acid, or vitamin B_6, which are cofactors in homocysteine metabolism. Prospective studies have not found the relationship of hyperhomocysteinemia to atherosclerotic vascular disease to be as strong, and a meta-analysis of prospective studies has suggested at best a weak association.[75,76]

In assessing VTE risk, several meta-analyses have found only a modest association in individuals with elevated fasting homocysteine levels.[77] Although MTHFR mutations that can result in higher plasma homocysteine levels are common, fasting plasma homocysteine levels, and not the presence of specific mutations, correlate with increased thrombotic risk.[78] Many small studies evaluating thrombophilic factors have reported that elevated homocysteine levels further increase the risk of thrombosis in those with other causes of thrombophilia.[79]

Elevated plasma homocysteine levels usually respond to vitamin supplementation, particularly folic acid. However, two recent studies have found no decrease in cardiovascular events in high-risk patients treated over 5 years or in patients with myocardial infarction treated over 40 months with folic acid, vitamin B_6, and vitamin B_{12} compared with placebo.[80,81] Vitamin treatment was associated with substantial reductions in plasma homocysteine levels but not with significant reduction in clinical endpoints. In a third prospective trial, neither of two dosage regimens of triple-vitamin therapy resulted in significant improvement in secondary stroke prevention, despite dose-dependent reductions in homocysteine levels.[82] The lack of clinical benefit of vitamin therapy in patients with vascular disease suggests that the homocysteine hypothesis is incorrect or that vitamin therapy may have other, potentially adverse effects that offset its homocysteine-lowering benefit.

OTHER INHERITED THROMBOPHILIAS. Increased levels of procoagulants may augment risk of thrombosis. The strongest association is with elevated factor VIII levels.[83] Persistently elevated FVIII levels, remote from acute events, can be inherited and, in that setting, can increase the risk of VTE fivefold (individuals with FVIII higher than 150 units/dl versus those with FVIII lower than 100 units/dL). As a risk factor for thrombosis, FVIII levels are independent of vWF levels. Elevated vWF levels were found to be a risk factor for VTE independent of FVIII levels in one study, but not in another.[83] Elevated factor VIII levels may increase the risk of VTE recurrence, with the highest levels imparting the greatest risk. One study found a 37 percent likelihood of recurrence at 2 years in individuals with FVIII levels above the 90th percentile of the normal range.[84]

Elevated fibrinogen levels are associated with an increased risk of atherothrombotic disease, but not VTE (see Chap. 39). However, this likely reflects an inflammatory response, and inherited factors resulting in increased fibrinogen levels do not clearly associate with an increased risk of thrombosis.[85] Also, lowering fibrinogen levels has not been shown to decrease risk. Increased prothrombin (factor II) levels not caused by the prothrombin *G20210A* mutation have been associated with an increased risk of thrombosis, similar to that seen in individuals with the PT *G20210A* mutation.[71] Elevated factor IX, XI, or VII levels may be weakly associated with an increased risk of VTE.[85] Other than for FVIII, there is no evidence that levels of these factors should alter management of VTE at this time. In the future, multiple levels may be assessed in a multifactorial approach to thrombotic risk. Until such an approach is validated by clinical studies, testing these factors as part of a routine thrombophilia evaluation cannot be recommended.

Inherited heparin cofactor II deficiency is currently not considered to be a significant risk factor for thrombosis. Routine testing of patients with thromboembolic disease for heparin cofactor II deficiency is not recommended. Qualitative abnormalities of fibrinogen (dysfibrinogenemias) are not usually associated with clinical manifestations, although both mild bleeding symptoms and venous or arterial thrombosis have been reported. These are inherited in an autosomal dominant fashion. Because thrombosis-related dysfibrinogenemia is so rare, its inclusion in a thrombophilia evaluation is not routine.[86] Low levels of TFPI are associated with an increased risk of venous thrombosis.[87] Plasminogen deficiency, previously proposed as a thrombophilic condition, has not been substantiated in studies of deficient families.

Acquired Thrombophilia

Most cases of VTE are, at least in part, caused by acquired conditions (see Chap. 72). Age itself is a strong risk factor for VTE, with the underlying risk in octogenarians (baseline risk of approximately 1 in 100/year) being 100-fold that of young children (baseline risk of approximately 1 in 100,000/year).[88] Thrombotic risk in acquired situations as assessed in the Leiden Thrombophilia Study is shown in Table 82-3.

Immobilization, surgery, and bed rest are all well-documented risk factors for thrombosis. Hospitalization and nursing home residence was found to account for almost 60 percent of new VTE cases occurring in a community setting.[89] Criteria for risk stratification of patients hospitalized and/or having surgery have been developed and guide the use of prophylactic anticoagulation in those settings.[90] Prolonged air travel has received significant publicity as a risk factor for VTE. Studies have suggested a two- to threefold increased risk of VTE, with a greater risk after longer flights (more than 5000 miles or 8 hours).[91] In a recent study, air travel was found to result in activation of the clotting system measured by thrombin-antithrombin complexes, which was not found in those with similar immobilization or in controls.[92] The effect was greatest in women with the FV Leiden mutation who were taking combined OCPs.[92]

Malignancy associates strongly with thrombosis and should always be considered in adults who present with venous thrombosis, particularly if it is idiopathic in those with no family history of thrombosis. Evaluation of these individuals beyond age-appropriate recommended cancer screening has not been shown to prolong survival, although decision analysis based on the SOMIT trial, a randomized

TABLE 82–3	Thrombosis Risk in Acquired Situations: Data from the Leiden Thrombophilia Study			
Risk Factor	Patients, N = 474 (n, %)	Controls, N = 474 (n, %)	Odds Ratio	95% Confidence Interval
Surgery	85 (18)	17 (3.6)	5.9	3.4-10.1
Hospitalization	59 (12)	6 (1.3)	11.1	4.7-25.9
Immobilization	17 (3.6)	2 (0.4)	8.9	2.0-38.2
Pregnancy	8 (5.0)	2 (1.3)	4.2	0.9-19.9
Puerperium	13 (8.2)	1 (0.6)	14.1	1.8-10.9
Oral contraceptives	109 (70)	65 (38)	3.8	2.4-6.0

From the Leiden Thrombophilia Study, a population based case-control study. Cases were unselected consecutive patients aged 18-70 yr, with a first objectively diagnosed deep vein thrombosis. Controls were acquaintances of cases or spouses of (other) cases. Controls were matched for age and genders and subjects with active malignancies were excluded. Time window for surgery, hospitalization (without surgery), and immobilization (not in the hospital, immobilized >13 days) was 1 yr preceding the index date. For puerperium, it was delivery 30 days or less before the index date, and for pregnancy and oral contraceptives it was at the index date. Data on pregnancy, puerperium, and oral contraceptive use refer to women of childbearing age only.

Modified from Bauer KA, Rosendaal FR, Heit JA: Hypercoagulability: Too many tests, too much conflicting data. Hematology 353-368, 2002.

trial of extensive screening versus routine medical examination in patients with idiopathic VTE, found it beneficial to perform abdominal-pelvic computed tomography (CT) scans with or without mammography and/or sputum cytology. Many individuals presenting with thrombosis and diagnosed with malignancy have abnormalities on physical examination or routine laboratory or radiological studies. Those with myeloproliferative disorders, notably polycythemia vera and essential thrombocythemia (ET), have an increased risk of venous and arterial thrombosis, and therefore a complete blood count should be part of a thrombophilia evaluation.

HORMONE THERAPY AND PREGNANCY. Hormone therapy carries an increased risk of VTE and this risk may be increased significantly in thrombophilic women, as discussed earlier. Second-generation OCPs and hormone replacement therapy increase the risk of thrombosis two- to fourfold.[67] Because middle-aged women have an underlying risk of VTE approximately 10-fold greater than that of young women, they are more likely to experience thrombosis when placed on hormonal therapy. Third-generation OCPs, which contain less estrogen and a different progestin, are associated with a twofold increased risk of VTE compared with second-generation products. The contraceptive patch appears to result in an increased risk of thrombosis, possibly greater than seen with oral preparations. OCP use is associated with an increased risk of peripheral arterial disease[94] and a modest increase in myocardial infarction.[95] The pathogenesis of hormone-induced thrombosis is not clear. Estrogens have many different effects on the coagulation system, including increases in procoagulant factors, reductions in free protein S and antithrombin levels, and acquired protein C resistance. Hormone-induced increases in fibrinolytic activity do not counterbalance this procoagulant effect.[67]

Pregnancy is associated with a four- to fivefold increase in VTE, with the greatest risk period occurring in the first 6 weeks postpartum[96] (see Chap. 77). The rate of VTE is higher in women who are older than 35 years, African American, or have underlying medical conditions or complications of pregnancy.[97] Most DVTs are in the left leg and thrombosis of the left iliac system is not uncommon. The risk of VTE increases further in thrombophilic women,[98] but prophylactic antepartum anticoagulation is not indicated in women without a prior history of VTE, unless a more severe underlying thrombophilia is present, such as AT deficiency, homozygous factor V Leiden, or combined defects. Low-molecular-weight heparin (LMWH) has become the treatment of choice for VTE during pregnancy because there is evidence that it does not cross the placenta and, compared with unfractionated heparin (UFH), has a more predictable dose response, longer plasma half-life, less risk of heparin-induced thrombocytopenia, and probably a lower risk of heparin-induced osteoporosis.[99]

ANTIPHOSPHOLIPID ANTIBODY SYNDROME (APS). APS is defined by a characteristic constellation of clinical and laboratory abnormalities, including an increased risk of thrombosis. Clinical findings may include unexplained venous or arterial thrombosis, pregnancy morbidity, including repeated miscarriages or fetal growth retardation, and neurological manifestations. Rare patients with APS present with life-threatening multiple organ involvement, referred to as catastrophic APS.[101] This syndrome is characterized by rapid-onset thrombosis with multiple organ dysfunction, disseminated small vessel thrombosis, and evidence of systemic inflammatory response syndrome with acute respiratory distress syndrome (ARDS).

APS is associated with persistent antibodies to certain phospholipid-binding proteins. These antibodies, and particularly antibodies to the phospholipid cardiolipin (anticardiolipin antibodies, ACAs), can be induced by infections or drugs, but in those settings they are not clearly associated with thrombosis. True APS likely results from an autoimmune reaction, either not associated with a defined autoimmune disorder, designated primary APS, or associated with an autoimmune disease, such as systemic lupus erythematosus (SLE), designated secondary APS.

The antibodies found in individuals with this syndrome are actually directed against phospholipid-binding proteins, not against phospholipid itself. Actually, most positive ACA reactions require beta$_2$-glycoprotein 1 (β_2GP1) in the assay, which is an abundant protein in bovine and human plasma. Antibodies against other phospholipid-binding proteins, most notably against prothrombin, but also protein C, protein S, annexin V, and TFPI, may also be found in this syndrome. The role of these autoantibodies in the pathogenesis of APS has not been elucidated. Two mechanisms have been proposed whereby antiphospholipid antibodies promote thrombosis: (1) interfering with phospholipid-dependent anticoagulant pathways, including APC and TFPI functions; and (2) binding to vascular and blood cell surfaces and inducing cell activation.[102]

Patients with APS may have antibodies that react only in an immunoassay, as described earlier, or that interfere with phospholipid-dependent tests (termed *lupus anticoagulants*), or both. The presence of persistent antibodies to β_2GP1 appear to be better predictors of thrombosis than antibodies to prothrombin, but testing for anti-β_2GP1 antibodies has not clearly been shown to improve the diagnosis of APS over the use of ACA determinations alone. Antiprothrombin antibodies do not prevent conversion of prothrombin to thrombin, but may result in prothrombin deficiency, which rarely associates with bleeding, in contrast to the more characteristic thrombotic tendency of APS.

A number of laboratory tests are used to diagnosis lupus anticoagulants (LAs).[100,102,103] Many of these tests have been developed to detect LAs by modifications that make them more sensitive to interactions of the antibody with the phospholipid component of the assay. The aPTT may be prolonged, depending on the strength of the LAs and the aPTT reagent used. A widely used test, which when positive probably correlates best with an increased risk of thrombosis, is the dilute Russell's viper venom test (dRVVT). Prolongation of the dRVVT will correct when mixed with normal plasma if the prolongation is caused by factor deficiency, which could be inherited secondary to liver disease, vitamin K deficiency, or warfarin therapy. Heparin will function as an inhibitor and the test will not correct when mixed with normal plasma, resulting in a false positive test. Many dRVVT assay procedures absorb out heparin, eliminating this problem; however, positive values in a patient on heparin should be repeated when the patient is off heparin at a later date to confirm the finding. Laboratory confirmation of a lupus anticoagulant requires prolongation of a phospholipid-dependent test that does not correct with mixing, but does correct with the addition of the correct phospholipid, usually a phospholipid assembled into a structure denoted as hexagonal phase or platelet membranes (platelet neutralization procedure).

Arterial and/or venous thrombosis recurrence rates in patients with true APS have been reported to be as high as 70 percent, making this an indication for long-term anticoagulation. Patients with SLE or rheumatoid arthritis with persistently positive ACAs or LAs have a higher rate of venous and arterial thrombosis than those without these laboratory findings. Findings from two randomized trials have supported an international normalized ratio (INR) target of 2 to 3 in patients with APS and arterial or venous thrombosis.[104,105] However, both trials excluded patients with prior recurrence on warfarin. Aspirin appears to be as effective as moderate-intensity warfarin for preventing recurrent stroke in patients with prior stroke and a single positive test result for antiphospholipid antibody.[106] There is a subset of patients who will develop recurrent arterial or venous thrombosis, even at higher levels of anticoagulation, who require alternative prophylactic approaches.[107]

ANTITHROMBOTIC DRUGS

Heparin and Related Drugs

Because its onset of action is practically immediate when administered parenterally, heparin is the anticoagulant of choice when rapid anticoagulation is required. Commercial preparations of unfractionated heparin consist of a heterogeneous mixture of glycosaminoglycans, with molecular weights ranging from 3000 to 30,000.[108] However, only about one third of the molecules in these products are active as anticoagulants. Heparin exerts its anticoagulant effect by interacting with antithrombin (Fig. 82-15). A specific pentasaccharide sequence in heparin accounts for its ability to bind with high affinity to lysine sites on antithrombin. In the absence of heparin, antithrombin binds to and neutralizes thrombin and other activated clotting factors (see earlier) slowly; however, heparin-bound antithrombin undergoes a conformational change that dramatically accelerates its ability to bind to and neutralize these factors. In these reactions, arginine reactive centers in antithrombin bind to the enzyme-active site serines of thrombin and other serine protease coagulation factors, thereby inhibiting their activities. Heparin then dissociates from these complexes and can be reused to bind to other antithrombin molecules. Heparin thus acts as a true catalyst in accelerating the neutralization of thrombin and other activated clotting factors by antithrombin.[108] Fibrin-bound thrombin is relatively protected from inactivation by the heparin-antithrombin complex.

Heparin is poorly absorbed from the gastrointestinal tract and therefore is administered parenterally. The complex pharmacokinetics of unfractionated heparin is a result of its nonspecific binding to many plasma proteins (including some acute-phase reactants) and to vascular and blood cells. Provided that the doses used are adequate, the efficacy and safety of heparin are comparable when administered by continuous intravenous infusion or by subcutaneous injection.[108] Intermittent intravenous injections of heparin are associated with more bleeding complications than continuous intravenous infusion.

UNFRACTIONATED HEPARIN MONITORING. Because of unfractionated heparin's often unpredictable pharmacokinetics and its narrow therapeutic range, therapy with this agent requires laboratory monitoring for proper dosing.[108] This is performed conventionally with the activated partial thromboplastin time (aPTT), a test sensitive to the inhibitory effects of heparin on thrombin, factor Xa, and factor IXa. For the treatment of acute coronary syndromes, weight-based dosing is recommended, because this approach results in more prompt anticoagulation without an increased risk of bleeding compared with other approaches.[109] Treatment for ST elevation myocardial infarction (STEMI) is initiated with a bolus of 60 units/kg (maximum, 4000 units) followed by an initial infusion of 12 units/kg/hr (maximum 1000 units/hr), adjusted to maintain the aPTT at 1.5 to 2.0 times control (approximately 50 to 70 seconds); for unstable angina and non-ST elevation myocardial infarction (NSTEMI), an initial bolus of 60 to 70 units/kg (maximum, 5000 units) followed by a 12- to 15-units/kg/hr infusion is recommended (see Chaps. 51 and 53). For DVT or pulmonary embolism, treatment is initiated with an 80-units/kg bolus, followed by 18 units/kg/hr, with a target aPTT that has been standardized in the laboratory to reflect heparin levels measured by anti-Xa levels of 0.3 to 0.7 unit/ml (see Chap. 72).

The aPTT is sensitive over a heparin range of 0.1 to 1.0 unit/ml. Because the aPTT becomes immeasurably prolonged at heparin concentrations of more than 1.0 unit/ml, this test is unsuitable for monitoring heparin dosage during percutaneous coronary interventions (angioplasty and stenting) and during cardiac bypass surgery, in which patients require higher levels of anticoagulation with heparin (see Chaps. 52 and 55). In these procedures, heparin can be monitored by the activated clotting time (ACT) because this test provides a graded response to heparin concentrations in the range of 1 to 5 units/ml. Hemochron (ITC, Edison, NJ) and HemoTec (Medtronic Inc, Parker, Co) devices are commonly used to measure the ACT and the Hemochron ACT values generally exceed those of the HemoTec ACT by up to 30 percent, although considerable variability exists. Several studies have retrospectively related ACT values to clinical outcomes after PCI. A retrospective analysis of data from 5216 patients receiving heparin during PCI has suggested that ischemic complications at 7 days are 34 percent lower with a Hemochron ACT in the range of 350 to 375 seconds than they were with an ACT between 171 and 295 seconds.[110] Although ischemic complications were reduced at higher levels of ACT, this was at the cost of progressively increased bleeding, from 8.6 percent at ACTs shorter than 350 seconds to 12.4 percent at ACTs of 350 to 375 seconds. A substantial increase in bleeding events was observed when ACT values exceeded 400 seconds.[110] For percutaneous intervention (PCI), heparin is given in doses of 70 to 100 IU/kg and a target ACT between 250 and 350 seconds is advocated in the absence of adjunctive GP IIb/IIIa inhibition; in contrast, a target ACT of 200 to 250 seconds is advocated when heparin (bolus dose of unfractionated heparin [UFH], 40 to 70 IU/kg) is given in conjunction with a GP IIb/

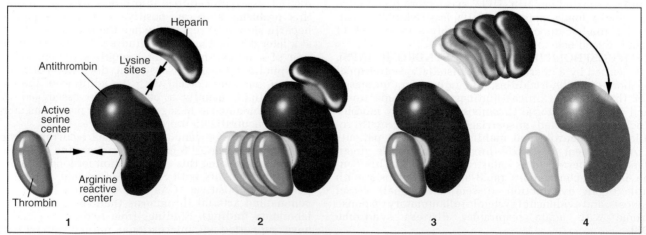

FIGURE 82–15 Mechanism of heparin action. See text for explanation. (*Modified from Rosenberg RD: Hemorrhagic disorders: I. Protein interactions in the clotting mechanism.* In *Beck WS [ed]: Hematology. 5th ed. Cambridge, MIT Press, 1991, pp 507-542.*)

IIIa inhibitor. Removal of the femoral sheath should be delayed until the ACT is between 150 and 180 seconds. Routine use of intravenous heparin after PCI is no longer used because several randomized studies have shown that prolonged heparin infusions do not reduce ischemic complications and are associated with a higher rate of bleeding at the catheter insertion site.

Low-dose subcutaneous unfractionated heparin has also been used to prevent (rather than treat) venous thromboembolism in high-risk patients. Doses of 5000 units every 8 or 12 hours generally do not prolong the aPTT and therefore do not require monitoring in this setting.

LOW-MOLECULAR-WEIGHT (LMWH) HEPARINS.

Low-molecular-weight heparins (see Chap. 51) are manufactured from standard, unfractionated heparin by chemical or enzymatic depolymerization that yields fragments about one third the size of unfractionated heparin.[132,133] Inhibition of thrombin requires that heparin bind to both antithrombin and thrombin, thereby forming a ternary complex (Fig. 82-16). This requires that heparin contain at least 18 saccharide residues, including the high-affinity pentasaccharide sequence that binds to antithrombin. In contrast, inhibition of factor Xa requires that heparin bind only to antithrombin; hence, only the pentasaccharide sequence of heparin is needed. Most heparin chains in LMWH preparations have fewer than 18 saccharide units and therefore are of insufficient length to bind to both antithrombin and thrombin, but can catalyze the inhibition of factor Xa by antithrombin, provided that they contain the essential pentasaccharide sequence. Thus, the effects of LMWH in the coagulation cascade are restricted to relatively selective inactivation of factor Xa, whereas standard (unfractionated) heparin has equivalent inhibitory activity against factor Xa and thrombin.

Low-molecular-weight heparin has theoretical advantages over standard heparin.[111] First, unlike unfractionated heparin, it can inhibit platelet-bound factor Xa. Second,

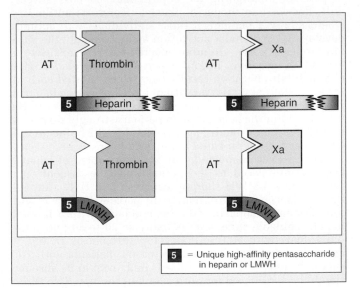

FIGURE 82–16 Mechanisms of inhibitory action of unfractionated heparin (heparin) and low-molecular-weight heparin (LMWH) on thrombin and factor Xa. Both unfractionated heparin and LMWH bind to antithrombin (AT) through a high-affinity pentasaccharide sequence (5) that both types of heparin contain. Inhibition of thrombin (left side of figure) requires formation of a ternary complex of heparin with antithrombin and thrombin. Unfractionated heparins have sufficient length (18 saccharide residues or more, including the pentasaccharide sequence) to accomplish this, but LMWHs do not. In contrast, inhibition of factor Xa (right side of figure) requires that heparin bind only to antithrombin, which unfractionated heparin and LMWH can catalyze equally effectively through their common pentasaccharide sequences. Thus, LMWH (but not unfractionated heparin) inactivates factor Xa selectively relative to thrombin.

LMWH binds less readily to plasma proteins (including acute-phase reactants) and vascular and blood cells, and LMWH is more resistant to neutralization by platelet factor 4; this results in a longer plasma half-life, more predictable bioavailability, and more favorable pharmacokinetics than standard heparin. Third, LMWH has less pronounced effects on platelet function and vascular integrity. The longer plasma half-life and more predictable anticoagulant response of LMWH preparations allow their administration as fixed-dose, once-daily, or twice-daily subcutaneous injections, without the need for laboratory monitoring.

The convenience of use of LMWH has been extended to outpatient management of patients with uncomplicated acute venous thromboembolism, a situation that previously required continuous intravenous heparin infusion in the hospital (see Chap. 72). Although several LMWH preparations have been approved for use in North America and Europe, they are prepared by different depolymerization methods and have somewhat different molecular compositions, pharmacological properties, and anticoagulant profiles. Therefore, caution may need to be exercised in the interchangeability of these LMWH products.[112,113]

Although enoxaparin has demonstrated advantages over unfractionated heparin in low to moderate risk patients with acute coronary syndromes treated conservatively, enoxaparin therapy was no better than unfractionated heparin in patients with unstable angina or NSTEMI at high risk for ischemic cardiac complications managed with an early invasive approach based on the results of the SYNERGY (Superior Yield of the New Strategy of Enoxaparin, Revascularization and Glycoprotein IIb/IIIa Inhibitors) trial.[114] Furthermore, more bleeding was observed with enoxaparin, with a statistically significant increase in TIMI (thrombolysis in myocardial infarction) major bleeding (9.1 versus 7.6 percent; $P = 0.008$).

COMPLICATIONS OF HEPARIN AND LMWH.

The major complication of heparin is bleeding. Early studies have suggested that treatment with LMWH causes significantly less bleeding than with unfractionated heparin; however, data from more recent and larger studies do not show as great a difference in bleeding risks between the two preparations (see Chap. 51). Factors that predispose to increased bleeding risk include advanced age, serious concurrent illness, heavy consumption of alcohol, concomitant use of aspirin, and renal failure.[115] LMWHs are cleared by renal excretion and should be used with caution in patients with renal insufficiency. In the TIMI 11A trial, a multicenter dose-ranging trial to evaluate the safety of enoxaparin in the treatment of patients with non-ST segment elevation acute coronary syndrome, patients with a creatine clearance of less than 40 ml/min had higher trough and peak anti-Xa activity and were more likely to have major hemorrhagic events than subjects with normal renal function.[116]

Because of the relatively short half-life of unfractionated heparin, simple discontinuation is usually adequate to control bleeding complications. Protamine sulfate can be used in emergency situations with serious bleeding. Protamine, a strongly basic protein, almost instantaneously neutralizes heparin, which is highly negatively charged. Protamine is effective in neutralizing the antithrombin activity of LMWH but does not completely reverse its antifactor Xa activity.

Two distinct types of thrombocytopenia are associated with heparin therapy.[117] The more common form, which may occur in up to 15 percent of patients receiving therapeutic doses of heparin, is a benign and self-limited side effect. This dose-dependent, non—immune-mediated type of thrombocytopenia rarely causes severe reductions in the platelet count or clinical complications and usually does not require discontinuation of heparin. In contrast, the immune form of heparin-induced thrombocytopenia (HIT) can, paradoxically, cause serious limb- and life-threatening arterial as well as venous thrombosis (heparin-induced thrombocytopenia with thrombosis, HITT). The mechanism in these cases is the interaction of antibody (usually IgG) with a complex of heparin and platelet factor 4 on the surfaces of platelets from which platelet factor 4 is released on activation (Fig. 82-17A).[117] This complex results in the activation of platelets and monocytes through their FcRγIIa

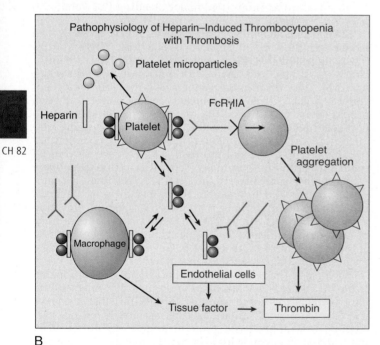

A

B

FIGURE 82–17 A, Pathophysiology of heparin-induced thrombocytopenia. With platelet activation, platelet factor 4 (PF4) is released from the platelet alpha granule and binds the surface of the activated platelet. PF4, a very basic protein, can complex with circulating negatively charged heparin, forming an antigenic complex. **B,** Pathophysiology of heparin-induced thrombocytopenia with thrombosis. PF4/heparin antibodies can activate coagulation by a number of mechanisms, including (1) activation of platelets via the platelet FCRγIIa receptor, resulting in platelet microparticle formation and the provision of a phospholipid surface for coagulation, and (2) activation of endothelial cells and monocytes, resulting in tissue factor expression, initiation of coagulation, and ultimately thrombin formation, which results in amplification of coagulation and further platelet activation. *(Courtesy of D. Cines, University of Pennsylvania, Philadelphia.)*

receptors or on the surface of endothelial cells, where released platelet factor 4 also binds (see Fig. 82-17B).[118]

In HIT, patients develop absolute or relative (greater than 50 percent drop in platelet count) thrombocytopenia in a reproducible and diagnostic manner.[119] Thrombocytopenia begins at least 4 days after the initiation of heparin and rarely occurs more than 14 days after this point. The exceptions are patients who received heparin within the recent past, usually within the past 3 months, and have circulating antiheparin–platelet factor 4 antibodies. In those individuals, reexposure to heparin can abruptly decrease platelet count, and systemic reactions can occur. However, except in this situation, prior exposure to heparin does not alter the time course of HIT. The decline in platelet count in HIT is usually moderate, with a typical nadir of 50,000 to 60,000/mm[3]. However, HIT can cause severe thrombocytopenia even in the absence of thrombosis and, conversely, heparin-induced thrombosis can actually occur with a normal platelet count. Immune-mediated HIT is not heparin dose–dependent and can develop with low-dose heparin or even with heparin flushes or the use of heparin-bonded catheters. Delayed-onset HIT has been described, a clinical scenario in which patients present a few weeks after heparin exposure with thrombosis and strongly positive testing for HIT, with or without thrombosis.[120,121] The pathogenesis of this variant is unclear but may result from ongoing antigenic stimulation, possibly from complexes bound to the vascular wall.

No single definitive laboratory test can ascertain the diagnosis of HIT, and HIT remains a clinical diagnosis supported by laboratory testing.[117,122] Laboratory testing for HIT can involve functional assays in which the heparin-induced activation of platelets in vitro is tested by aggregation, serotonin release, or platelet activation markers. Alternatively, enzyme immunoassays of antibody–heparin–platelet factor 4 complexes can be used to test for HIT. The latter have a high sensitivity but low specificity for HIT. Up to 70 percent of patients undergoing cardiopulmonary bypass surgery will develop antiheparin–platelet factor 4 antibodies, whereas only 2 percent of those individuals will actually develop HIT.[122] Platelet activation assays, notably the serotonin release assay, are more specific but less sensitive. In general, a negative immunoassay result excludes HIT, although false-negative results have been reported early in the presentation, while the patient is still receiving heparin, presumably because of antigen excess. Therefore, if the initial test finding is negative in patients strongly suspected of HIT, treatment modifications should still be made and laboratory testing repeated a few days later.

When HIT is suspected, any source or route of heparin being administered to the patient must be discontinued immediately. LMWH therapy can result in HIT, although the incidence is approximately 10 percent that seen with unfractionated heparin. HIT is associated with a marked hypercoagulable state, and as many as 30 to 50 percent of individuals with HIT will develop thrombosis in the 30 days after diagnosis.[117] For this reason, patients with HIT should be assessed for thrombosis and, even in its absence, should be considered for anticoagulant therapy. Two direct thrombin inhibitors have been studied and shown to have efficacy as anticoagulants in this setting—recombinant hirudin (lepirudin) and argatroban, a small-molecule synthetic antithrombin.[122] Results from a retrospective observational analysis in 181 patients have suggested that the previously recommended dose of lepirudin in patients with HIT is too high and that the use of a reduced dose may be safer with regard to bleeding, without compromising antithrombotic efficacy.[123] LMWHs should not be substituted for heparin because they have strong cross reactivity with HIT sera.

The pentasaccharide fondaparinux (see later) may have a role in treatment of HIT. By size, it may have altered binding to platelet factor 4 (PF4) and provide less antigenic stimulus. Antiheparin PF4 antibodies were found in patients treated with fondaparinux, but none reacted with PF4-fondaparinux and none of the 2726 patients treated prophylactically for orthopedic surgery developed HIT.[124]

Other side effects of heparin include cumulative dose-dependent osteoporosis, skin necrosis, alopecia, hypersensitivity reactions, and hypoaldosteronism.[125] Heparin is the anticoagulant of choice during pregnancy; unlike warfarin, it does not cross the placenta and is not teratogenic. However, warfarin may be needed in women with mechanical heart valves who are at high risk of thromboembolism, at least in the periods of low risk of teratogenicity, because of the increased effectiveness of warfarin in this setting (see Chap. 77).[126]

OTHER GLYCOSAMINOGLYCAN-DERIVED DRUGS. Heparan sulfate, dermatan sulfate, and proteoglycans are endogenous heparin-like molecules with antithrombotic activity.[127] Several of these endogenous glycosaminoglycans have been developed as clinical anticoagulants. Danaparoid (Orgaran), a mixture of low-molecular-weight anticoagulant glycosaminoglycans, predominantly heparan sulfate (84 percent) plus dermatan sulfate (12 percent), was removed from the U.S. market.[128] Heparins that can be absorbed orally are under development and some have entered clinical trials, although their efficacy has yet to be documented.

Fondaparinux, a chemically synthesized methoxyl derivative of the naturally occurring antithrombin-binding pentasaccharide, selectively catalyzes the inactivation of factor Xa by antithrombin without inhibiting thrombin (see Fig. 82-15). Once-daily treatment with fondaparinux (2.5 mg subcutaneously) initiated in the early postoperative period is as or more effective than a LMWH preparation in preventing venous thromboembolism after hip or knee surgery and when given to medical patients and patients undergoing abdominal surgery who are at high risk of thrombosis, without increasing the risk of bleeding. In therapeutic doses (5 mg for less than 50 kg, 7.5 mg for 50 to 100 kg, and 10 mg for more than 100 kg), fondaparinux is as effective as unfractionated heparin for symptomatic pulmonary embolism and deep vein thrombosis, respectively.[129] Emerging clinical trial data from over 40,000 patients have supported the use of fondaparinux as an anticoagulant in acute coronary syndromes. In patients presenting with unstable angina and non-ST segment elevation myocardial infarction, the results of the OASIS-5 (Fifth Organization to Assess Strategies in Acute Ischemic Syndromes) study have recently shown that fondaparinux (2.5 mg daily) is similar to enoxaparin (1 mg/kg twice daily) in reducing the risk of ischemic events, but substantially reduce major bleeding and improve long-term mortality compared with enoxaparin.[130] In ST-segment elevation myocardial infarction (OASIS-6), fondaparinux compared with unfractionated heparin was found to reduce mortality and reinfarction significantly without increasing bleeding or strokes.[131]

Fondaparinux is administered by subcutaneous injection, and its elimination half-life of 17 to 21 hours allows once-daily dosing. There is no known antidote for reversal of the anticoagulant effect of fondaparinux. Even with a low bleeding risk, its long half-life may become an issue in the clinical management of patients receiving this drug. It is also difficult to monitor the anticoagulant effects of fondaparinux, which likely contributed to the increased risk of thrombotic complications in patients undergoing primary PCI in OASIS-6.[131] Additional synthetic pentasaccharides for anticoagulation are under clinical study, including the drug idraparinux, which has a longer half-life than fondaparinux.

Warfarin

Warfarin (Coumadin) is the most frequently used oral anticoagulant. Oral anticoagulants, which are derivatives of coumarins, exert their anticoagulant actions as vitamin K antagonists.[132,133] The reduced form of vitamin K, vitamin KH_2, is normally required as a cofactor for the gamma-carboxylation of glutamic acid residues in coagulation factors II (prothrombin), VII, IX, and X (Fig. 82-18). This posttranslational modification is necessary to allow the coagulation factors to bind to and form calcium-dependent complexes on cellular phospholipid surfaces. Coumarins block the reductase enzymes required to recycle vitamin K epoxide to vitamin KH_2 after the gamma-carboxylation reaction, thereby depleting the active vitamin K cofactor.

Warfarin is rapidly and almost completely absorbed from the gastrointestinal tract and circulates bound to albumin with a mean plasma half-life of approximately 40 hours.[133] Metabolism is affected by inherited allelic variants of P450 CYP2C9, which catalyzes the conversion of S-warfarin to its inactive metabolite. Subjects homozygous for the least active alleles are more likely to require a low warfarin dose and to experience warfarin-related bleeding complications.[134] Polymorphisms in the vitamin K epoxide reductase (VKOR) gene also influence anticoagulant response. Genetic testing for CYP2C9 and VKOR polymorphisms to improve individual warfarin dosing is under study (see Chap. 72).

Numerous drugs alter the anticoagulant response to warfarin by pharmacokinetic or pharmacodynamic interac-

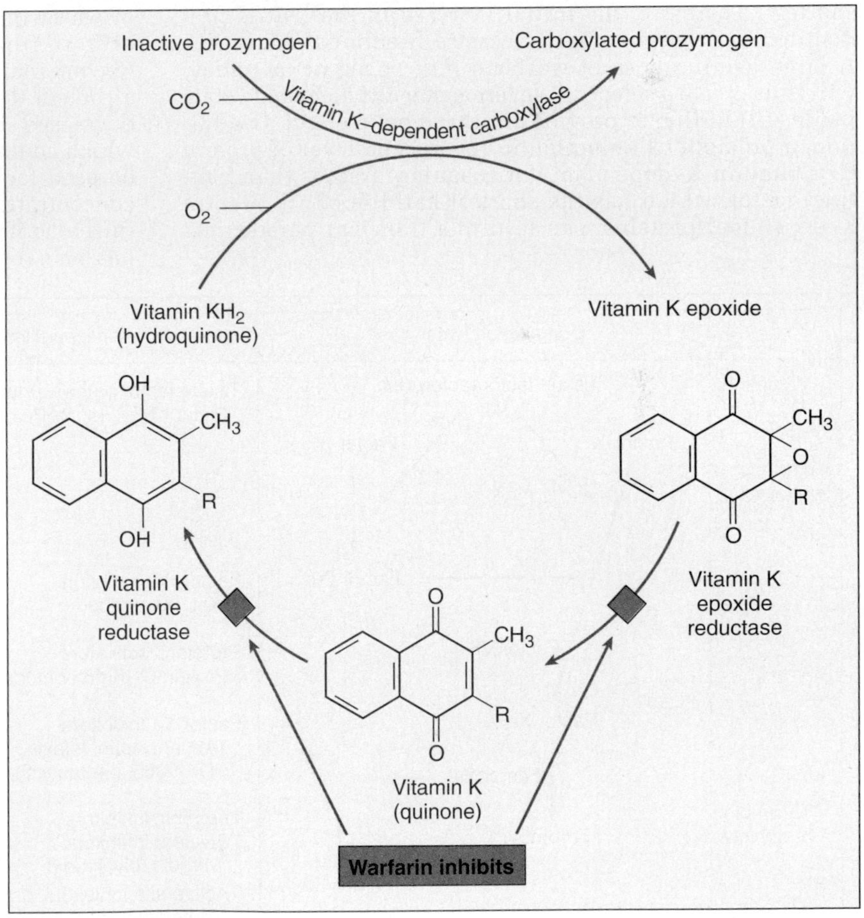

FIGURE 82–18 Vitamin K cycle and its inhibition by warfarin. Warfarin inhibits vitamin K epoxide reductase and vitamin K quinone reductase and consequently blocks the conversion of vitamin K epoxide to vitamin KH_2. Vitamin KH_2 is a cofactor for the carboxylation of inactive proenzymes (factors II, VII, IX, and X) to their active forms. *(From Furie B, Furie BC: Molecular basis of vitamin K-dependent gamma-carboxylation. Blood 75:1753, 1990.)*

tions.[133] Drugs such as phenylbutazone, erythromycin, fluconazole, cimetidine, amiodarone, clofibrate, isoniazid, and propranolol increase warfarin levels, whereas drugs such as cholestyramine, barbiturates, rifampin, and sucralfate decrease warfarin levels. Similarly, dietary variations in vitamin K alter warfarin's anticoagulant effects; high vitamin K intake in the diet (including nutritional supplements and vitamin preparations) reduces the anticoagulant response to warfarin. Conversely, liver disease, malabsorption, and hypermetabolic states enhance the anticoagulant effect of warfarin.

MONITORING. Oral anticoagulant therapy requires laboratory monitoring with the prothrombin time. To standardize prothrombin time reporting, the INR is used to correct for differences in the thromboplastin reagents used by different laboratories. The optimal therapeutic range of warfarin for the prevention of venous thromboembolism and systemic embolism from atrial fibrillation and tissue heart valves targets an INR of 2.0 to 3.0. Higher intensity anticoagulation (INR, 2.5 to 3.5) is required in patients with mechanical prosthetic heart valves.

Loading doses of warfarin should not be used in initiating oral anticoagulation. Although warfarin has a rapid onset of action, its optimal antithrombotic effect requires several days. The activity of all four vitamin K-dependent clotting factors must be inhibited to achieve clinically effective anticoagulation. The effects of warfarin require depletion of circulating clotting factors that are already gamma-carboxylated and hence biologically active when warfarin is started. The vitamin K–dependent clotting factors have different half-lives, with factor VII having the shortest. Therefore, the initial increase in the INR is predominantly because of a decrease in functional factor VII. A large loading dose of warfarin (i.e., 10 mg or more/day) will thus create a selective, severe factor VII deficiency state while still failing to provide antithrombotic effect. In addition, a precipitous reduction in the plasma level of protein C, a vitamin K–dependent anticoagulant (rather than clotting) factor, which has the shortest half-life of all vitamin K–dependent proteins, can lead to a transient paradoxical hypercoagulable state during the first 36 hours of warfarin therapy (see later).[133] Therefore, the initial dose of warfarin should approximate the chronic maintenance dose that is anticipated, generally in the range of 4 to 6 mg/day in most adults.

COMPLICATIONS. Skin necrosis, a very rare complication that occurs within the first few days of starting warfarin therapy, tends to occur in patients with underlying inherited protein C or protein S deficiency. As noted earlier, it is likely related to the initial precipitous decrease in protein C levels, especially in individuals who may already have a congenitally low level of protein C. This leads to a transient prothrombotic imbalance, particularly with the use of large loading doses of warfarin.

As with heparin, bleeding complications are the most frequent adverse effects of warfarin. For an individual patient, the cumulative risk of bleeding complications relates directly to the intensity and duration of anticoagulant therapy. Major bleeding on warfarin occurs at a rate of 5 to 7 percent/year.[135] When the INR exceeds the therapeutic range, discontinuing or reducing the dose of warfarin is usually sufficient; stopping warfarin generally normalizes the INR within about 3 days. If more rapid reversal of warfarin effect is required because of extreme elevations of the INR or clinical bleeding, vitamin K can be administered orally or parenterally. Vitamin K given orally has been shown to be superior to that given by subcutaneous injection, because the latter is ineffective in some patients.[136] However, particularly when vitamin K is given at higher doses, a transient resistance to reanticoagulation with warfarin may be subsequently encountered. Emergency reversal of warfarin effect can be rapidly achieved by the infusion of fresh frozen plasma (usually starting with 2 to 4 units). Recombinant factor VIIa (rFVIIa) will reduce the INR,[137] although this needs to be correlated in clinical study with decreased bleeding. Prothrombin complex concentrates, which contain coagulation factors II, VII, IX and X, can also be used for emergency reversal.[138] Products with balanced concentrations of these factors are currently not available in the United States. Clinical efficacy with these products has been reported although, as for rFVIIa, larger prospective trials are needed to determine the efficacy and safety of these drugs in this setting. Algorithms for the management of elevated INR with or without bleeding have been proposed.[139]

Thrombin Inhibitors and Other Specific Coagulation Inhibitors

Newly developed anticoagulants specifically target inactivation of thrombin, factor Xa, factor IXa, and the factor VIIa–tissue factor complex, as well as inactivation of factors VIIIa and Va by enhancement of the protein C anticoagulant pathway (Fig. 82-19).[140] Except for the direct thrombin inhibitors, most of these agents still await evaluation in phase 3 trials.

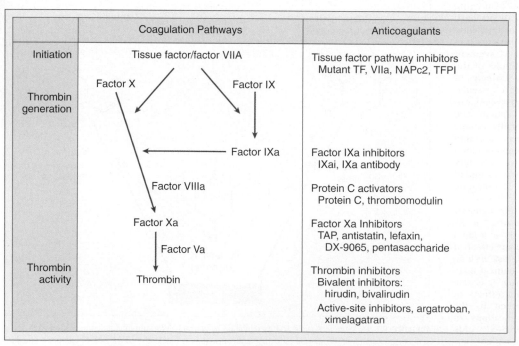

FIGURE 82–19 Activation and inhibitors of coagulation. New anticoagulants act by inhibiting the tissue factor pathway (initiation), thrombin generation, and thrombin activity. Ximelagatran is the product of the active thrombin inhibitor melagatran. *(Modified from Hirsh J, Weitz JI: New antithrombotic agents. Lancet 353:1431, 1999.)*

THROMBIN INHIBITORS. Direct thrombin inhibitors inactivate both free (fluid phase) thrombin and fibrin-bound thrombin. In this respect, these agents differ from heparin and its low-molecular-weight derivatives, which require complex formation with antithrombin and thus are weak inhibitors of clot-bound thrombin.[140,141]

The thrombin molecule has distinct functional domains. The active site of thrombin is the catalytic site that possesses serine protease activity. "Exosite 1" of thrombin serves to dock substrates in the proper orientation and is the binding site for fibrin(ogen). Direct thrombin inhibitors interact with one or both of these sites. Hirudin and bivalirudin are more specific for thrombin than active site inhibitors because they are bivalent, binding to thrombin at both the active site and exosite 1. In contrast, low-molecular-weight thrombin inhibitors such as argatroban and efegatran bind only to the active site of thrombin. Because the active site of thrombin resembles that of other serine proteases, these active site inhibitors are less selective for thrombin than the bivalent inhibitors.

Hirudin, the prototype of the direct thrombin inhibitors, is a 65–amino acid polypeptide originally isolated from the saliva of *Hirudo medicinalis*, the medicinal leech. Hirudin is now produced by recombinant DNA technology (lepirudin). It binds tightly to thrombin, forming a slowly reversible 1:1 stoichiometric complex. In this complex, the amino terminus of hirudin binds to the active site and its carboxy terminal binds to exosite 1 of thrombin.

Bivalirudin (Angiomax) is a synthetic 20–amino acid polypeptide composed of a peptide sequence (D-Phe-Pro-Arg-Pro) directed at the active site of thrombin and linked to a dodecapeptide analogue of the exosite 1-binding carboxy terminal of hirudin. Thus, like hirudin, bivalirudin interacts bivalently with both the active site and exosite 1 of thrombin, forming a 1:1 stoichiometric complex. However, once bound, thrombin cleaves the Arg-Pro bond and thereby removes the active site–binding part of bivalirudin, leaving only a low-affinity, weaker inhibitory interaction with thrombin. Consequently, the potent thrombin inhibitory effect of bivalirudin is short-lived, conferring a potential safety advantage. Although the anticoagulant effect of bivalirudin dissipates quickly because of its short half-life of 25 minutes, there is no rapid reversal agent available. In patients with severe impairment of renal function, the half-life may be increased significantly. Following PCI with bivalirudin, sheath removal should be delayed for 2 hours for patients with normal renal function, and up to 8 hours for patients on dialysis.

Several low-molecular-weight direct thrombin inhibitors have been developed. These less specific agents target only the active site of thrombin. Argatroban is the prototype of the noncovalent class of these active site inhibitors, which also includes napsagatran, inogatran, and melagatran.

Direct thrombin inhibitors have theoretical advantages over unfractionated heparin—activity against fibrin-bound thrombin, less nonspecific protein binding, direct action without a cofactor, absence of known inhibitors, and less platelet binding. These benefits ultimately result in more effective and reliable thrombin inhibition, less platelet activation, less thrombocytopenia, and a more predictable pharmacokinetic profile, obviating the need to measure ACTs.

Clinical trials with bivalirudin, including REPLACE-2 (Randomized Evaluation in PCI Linking Angiomax to Reduced Clinical Events-2)[142] and ACUITY (Acute Catheterization and Urgent Intervention Triage Strategy),[143] have explored the efficacy and safety of bivalirudin alone compared with combination therapy with unfractionated heparin and glycoprotein IIb/IIIa inhibitors in patients undergoing PCI (REPLACE-2) or presenting with unstable angina–non-ST segment elevation myocardial infarction (ACUITY). These trials have proposed a new paradigm for evaluating the net clinical benefit of antithrombotic strategies by combining efficacy (major adverse cardiovascular events, including death, myocardial infarction, and urgent revascularization) and safety (major and minor bleeding) parameters as the primary clinical trial endpoint. This combined efficacy–safety endpoint has evolved from the growing appreciation that bleeding is a powerful independent predictor of mortality. Indeed, in a pooled analysis of more than 34,000 patients enrolled in acute coronary syndrome trials, a major bleeding event raises the risk of death by a factor of five, underscoring the clinical impact of bleeding.[144] Although the precise mechanism linking

bleeding and mortality is uncertain, the link between bleeding and mortality is largely temporal (i.e., most deaths occur soon after the acute event), consistent across a range of patient subgroups, and related to severity (mortality rises with severity of the bleeding complication). The findings of REPLACE-2[142] and ACUITY[143] have indicated that bivalirudin monotherapy is noninferior to unfractionated heparin and GP IIb/IIIa when the combined efficacy and safety endpoint is evaluated (see Chap. 55). Combination efficacy and safety endpoints and noninferiority design are controversial.[145]

Orally administered direct thrombin inhibitors have been developed and one, ximelagatran, completed phase 3 clinical trials but was withdrawn from further development because of serious liver injury observed in studies of venous thromboembolism prophylaxis and treatment. Additional oral direct thrombin inhibitors that may evade hepatotoxicity are in clinical development.

OTHER SPECIFIC COAGULATION INHIBITORS. Human platelets express dual thrombin receptors, protease-activated receptor 1 (PAR1) and PAR4. PAR1 and PAR4 antagonists are under development to prevent arterial thrombosis.[146] Inhibitors of factor Xa (see Fig. 82-19) include tick anticoagulant peptide (TAP), antistatin, and lefaxin.[140] The latter two are extracts of the salivary glands of two species of leeches. All are potent and specific factor Xa inhibitors that are available in recombinant forms. DX-9065 is a synthetic, low-molecular-weight, reversible factor Xa inhibitor that has oral bioavailability. Experimental agents that inhibit factor IXa include a monoclonal antibody and active site-blocked factor IXa.[140] Specific inhibitors of the tissue factor pathway under study include the following: a soluble mutant form of tissue factor that has decreased cofactor function for factor VIIa–induced activation of factor X, active site-blocked factor VIIa (VIIai), which competes with factor VII for tissue factor binding; NAPc2, a small, nematode-derived anticoagulant protein that binds to factor X and inhibits factor VIIa within the factor VII/tissue factor complex[147]; and recombinant TFPI.[140] Protein C activators that have been studied as therapeutic anticoagulants include plasma, recombinant forms of protein C, and recombinant soluble thrombomodulin. Recombinant human activated protein C, or drotrecogin alfa (activated), has antithrombotic, antiinflammatory, and profibrinolytic properties. A randomized, double-blind, placebo-controlled trial has shown that this agent significantly reduces mortality in patients with severe sepsis, although with an increased risk of bleeding.[148]

Thrombolytic (Fibrinolytic) Drugs

The common mechanism of action of currently available thrombolytic (fibrinolytic) agents, including streptokinase, urokinase, and alteplase (recombinant tissue-type plasminogen activator [rt-PA]), involves the conversion of the inactive plasma zymogen, plasminogen, to the active fibrinolytic enzyme, plasmin (see Fig. 82-7; also see Chap. 51).[149] Plasmin has relatively weak substrate specificity and can degrade not only fibrin but also any protein that has an arginyl-lysyl bond, including fibrinogen. Indiscriminate plasmin lysis of both fibrin and fibrinogen can produce a systemic state of fibrin(ogen)olysis (or a systemic lytic state), with potential serious systemic bleeding, so attempts have been made to develop thrombolytic agents that generate plasmin preferentially at the fibrin surface in a preformed thrombus (fibrin-specific agents). Plasmin associated with fibrin is protected from rapid inhibition by alpha₂-antiplasmin (see earlier) and can thereby effectively degrade the fibrin of a clot.

Streptokinase and urokinase induce a systemic lytic state, with extensive systemic activation of the fibrinolytic system, deplete alpha₂-antiplasmin, and degrade circulating fibrinogen. In contrast, the physiological plasminogen activators t-PA and scu-PA activate plasminogen preferentially at the fibrin surface. The promise of a marked reduction in the risk of hemorrhage with second-generation fibrin-specific agents has not been fulfilled in large clinical trials, however. This may be caused by the inability of plasmin to discriminate between fibrin in pathological thrombi, which is the desired target, and fibrin in physiological hemostatic plugs, the lysis of which will induce bleeding.

STREPTOKINASE. Streptokinase is isolated from hemolytic streptococci and produced from bacterial cultures. The mechanism of activation of plasminogen by streptokinase is unique among plasminogen activators in that streptokinase itself possesses no enzymatic activity.[149] Streptokinase forms a complex with plasminogen, and it is the streptokinase-plasminogen complex that actually possesses enzymatic activity toward plasminogen. The streptokinase-plasminogen complexes are thereby converted to streptokinase-plasmin complexes, and the enzyme-active sites in the streptokinase-plasmin complexes are the same as those in plasmin. The streptokinase-plasmin(ogen) complexes activate circulating and fibrin-bound plasminogen relatively indiscriminately, producing a systemic lytic state.

Because of its bacterial source, streptokinase is antigenic. Most individuals have preexisting antibodies resulting from previous streptococcal infection. The administration of streptokinase stimulates the rapid formation of high titers of neutralizing antistreptokinase antibodies, which suffice to neutralize standard doses of streptokinase. Although antibody titers may return to near-baseline levels as early as 2 years after a single dose, once streptokinase has been used, subsequent thrombolytic treatment should be with an immunologically unrelated agent because of the uncertain efficacy of repeated treatment. Streptokinase causes transient hypotension in many patients and significant allergic reactions in some, including a serum sickness–type syndrome, fever, rash, and bronchospasm.

UROKINASE. Urokinase, or two-chain urokinase-type plasminogen activator (tcu-PA), is a trypsin-like serine protease composed of two polypeptide chains linked by a disulfide bridge.[149] Urokinase is produced from cultures of human fetal kidney cells. It directly activates plasminogen to plasmin, leading to relatively nonspecific degradation of fibrin, fibrinogen, and other plasma proteins, depletion of circulating alpha$_2$-antiplasmin, and a systemic lytic state. Urokinase is not antigenic and does not cause allergic reactions.

TISSUE-TYPE PLASMINOGEN ACTIVATOR. Tissue-type plasminogen activator is a naturally occurring molecule released from vascular endothelial cells. For therapeutic thrombolysis, it is produced commercially by recombinant DNA technology (rt-PA; alteplase) and, as a second-generation agent, is relatively fibrin-specific.[149]

Tissue-type plasminogen activator, a single-chain serine protease, activates plasminogen directly. Fibrin significantly enhances the efficiency of plasminogen activation by t-PA. The basis for the relative fibrin specificity of t-PA action has been described earlier in the section on the fibrinolytic system.

Tissue-type plasminogen activator is converted by plasmin to a disulfide-linked two-chain form. Alteplase consists mainly of the single-chain form of t-PA. Both the single-chain and two-chain forms of t-PA are cleared from plasma according to a two-compartment model, with initial half-lives of 3 to 6 minutes and terminal half-lives of 40 to 50 minutes. The currently preferred dosage regimen of fibrin-selective alteplase for coronary thrombolysis consists of weight-adjusted, accelerated (front-loaded) administration (see Chap. 51). The front-loaded administration of alteplase achieves a mean steady-state plasma concentration during the initial 30 minutes that is 45 percent higher than that achieved with standard infusion, although it does not alter the plasma half-life.

VARIANTS OF PLASMINOGEN ACTIVATORS. Some thrombolytic agents have been engineered to alter the pharmacokinetic and functional properties of currently used drugs favorably. They were designed to have prolonged half-lives, improve enzymatic efficiency, enhance local concentrations in the clot by altered binding to fibrin and stimulation by fibrin, and confer resistance to plasma protease inhibitors.[149]

Variants of u-PA have been developed and evaluated in clinical studies.[149] Saruplase is a nonglycosylated, single-chain recombinant u-PA. Clinical trials have demonstrated similar efficacy of this drug to other thrombolytics but, in some studies, increased bleeding complications occurred. M23 is a single-chain molecule composed of the kringle and protease domains of saruplase and the carboxy terminal fragment of the direct thrombin inhibitor hirudin, providing both fibrinolytic and antithrombotic activity.

A number of t-PA mutants have been developed. These can be classified according to those in which amino acid substitutions have been made (monteplase, tenecteplase) and those with deletion mutants (reteplase, lanoteplase, pamiteplase). In monteplase, there is a cysteine to serine substitution at position 84, resulting in an increased half-life of the drug compared with native t-PA. Tenecteplase contains amino acid substitutions at three sites: threonine at position 103 is replaced by asparagine; asparagine at position 117 is replaced by glutamine; and four amino acids—lysine, histidine, arginine, and arginine—are

replaced by alanine-alanine-alanine-alanine at positions 296 through 299. Tenecteplase is characterized by a prolonged half-life, increased fibrin specificity, and increased resistance to inhibition by PAI-1.[150]

Reteplase (r-PA) is a single-chain nonglycosylated deletion variant of t-PA, containing only the kringle-2 and serine protease domains. This deletion mutant has a prolonged half-life and therefore can be administered by bolus injection. Another third-generation drug is lanoteplase (n-PA), which retains kringle-1, kringle-2, and protease domains and also has a glutamine substituted for asparagine at position 117. It has an even longer half-life (37 minutes) and can be administered by single-bolus, weight-adjusted injection.[150] Pamiteplase is a modified t-PA with deletion of the kringle-1 domain and a point substitution of glutamine for arginine at position 274. These modifications make the drug resistant to plasmin-mediated cleavage.

The t-PA of saliva from the vampire bat *Desmodus rotundus* (bat-PA) has potent and relatively fibrin-specific thrombolytic properties.[187,190] Different molecular forms of bat-PA have been purified, characterized, cloned, and expressed. These are being evaluated in preclinical ex vivo and animal studies.

Antiplatelet Agents

The sequence of events involved in the process of platelet activation is described in detail in the previous section on platelets (Fig. 82-20; see Fig. 82-8). Inhibition of platelet function can target any one of these activation steps.[151] Platelet blockade would be expected to be most effective if it is directed at the initial (adhesion; see Fig. 82-20A) or final (aggregation; see Fig. 82-20D) points in the sequence. Antiplatelet agents targeted at any one of the intermediate events should be less potent, because platelet adhesion is followed by the binding of several specific agonists to their respective receptors and the activation of several simultaneous intracellular pathways (e.g., ADP release, TXA$_2$ synthesis) that act in concert to induce the final step of platelet aggregation. Therefore, pharmacological interruption of only one of these intermediate steps (e.g., with aspirin, clopidogrel) may permit platelet activation through alternative uninhibited pathways. Therapeutic approaches to inhibit platelet adhesion have yet to be translated into clinical practice. In contrast, considerable clinical evidence has now validated powerful therapeutic strategies to block the final step of platelet aggregation mediated by the interaction of fibrinogen (or vWF) with its receptor platelet GP IIb/IIIa (see Fig. 82-20D).

ASPIRIN. Aspirin (acetylsalicylic acid), known for more than 50 years to have antithrombotic efficacy, has stood the test of time as an effective, inexpensive, and relatively safe drug for the prevention of various thrombotic and vascular disorders, particularly in the arterial circulation, where platelets are the predominant participants in the thrombotic process.[151,152] However, there are several clinical settings in which aspirin fails to provide full (or even partial) antithrombotic benefit.[153,154]

Aspirin is readily absorbed from the stomach and upper small intestine and is then hydrolyzed to release free acetyl groups. This moiety acetylates serine residues at position 529 of cyclooxygenase (COX; prostaglandin–G/H synthase), which leads to irreversible inactivation of the enzyme (Fig. 82-21). Aspirin and other nonsteroidal anti-inflammatory drugs (NSAIDs) inhibit COX enzymes, which exist in at least two isoforms, COX-1 and COX-2. Aspirin and older agents in this class are nonselective inhibitors of COX-1 and COX-2; newer selective inhibitors of COX-2 are termed *coxibs*.[155] Inactive acetylated COX cannot function to catalyze the oxygenation of arachidonic acid to prostaglandin G$_2$, blocking the formation of TXA$_2$, a potent mediator of platelet aggregation and vasoconstrictor. Because anucleate platelets essentially are unable to synthesize new, nonacetylated COX, aspirin blocks the function of platelets exposed to it for their remaining lifetime (normally, 7 to 10 days) in the circulation. This accounts for the lengthy therapeutic effect of aspirin, despite its plasma half-life of only 20 minutes.

Aspirin inhibits platelet TXA$_2$ production and ex vivo aggregation rapidly, with maximal effects achieved within 15 to 30 minutes of oral administration of a dose as low as 81 mg. A single oral dose of 100 mg of aspirin almost completely suppresses platelet TXA$_2$ synthesis in normal individuals and patients with cardiovascular disease. Daily administration of only 30 to 50 mg of aspirin exerts a cumulative effect and similarly results in almost complete inhibition of platelet TXA$_2$ production within 7 to 10 days. These aspirin effects on platelet TXA$_2$ formation generally correlate well with inhibition of ex vivo platelet aggregability and prolongation of the skin bleeding time. Although platelet function remains impaired for 4 to 7 days after a single dose of aspirin, reflecting the life span of irreversibly inhibited platelets, the prolonged bleeding time generally returns to normal within 24 to 48 hours of aspirin ingestion. This discrepancy results from the release from bone marrow into the circulation of a sufficient cohort of uninhibited platelets after the elimination of aspirin from blood to restore normal in vivo hemostasis (bleeding time), even before complete normalization of ex vivo platelet function.

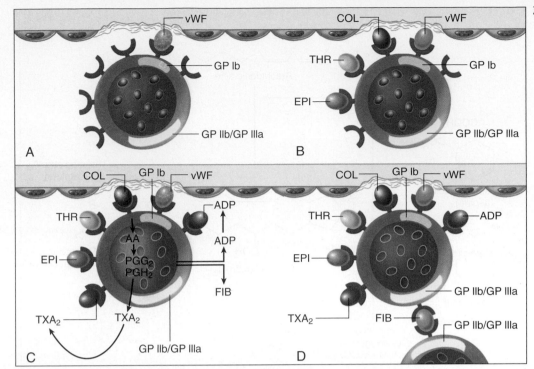

FIGURE 82–20 Sequence of events in platelet activation, with potential targets for antiplatelet therapy. **A,** Platelet adhesion to the injured vascular intimal surface is mediated by von Willebrand factor (vWF) binding to its receptor on platelet membrane glycoprotein (GP) IIb. **B,** Adherent platelets are also anchored to the damaged vessel wall by binding of subendothelial collagen (COL) to its platelet surface COL receptors. Other platelet stimuli in blood, including thrombin (THR) and epinephrine (EPI), bind to their respective receptors. **C,** In response to these different stimuli, adherent platelets are activated and release thromboxane A$_2$ (TXA$_2$) and adenosine diphosphate (ADP), which bind to their own respective platelet receptors and amplify the activation process. **D,** Platelet aggregation is mediated by fibrinogen (FIB) binding to its receptors on adjoining platelets, forming fibrinogen bridges. The FIB receptor is formed by the complexing of GP IIb/IIIa in the membrane of activated platelets. AA = arachidonic acid; PGG$_2$ and PGH$_2$ = labile prostaglandin endoperoxides. *(Modified from Schafer AI: Antiplatelet therapy with glycoprotein IIb/IIIa receptor inhibitors and other novel agents. Tex Heart Inst J 24:90, 1997.)*

Aspirin also inhibits COX in vascular endothelial cells, leading to suppression of platelet inhibitory and vasodilatory endothelium-derived PGI$_2$; this would be expected to offset the antiplatelet effects of aspirin. Attempts to design platelet selective aspirin regimens have not been translated into clinical feasibility. Nevertheless, ample evidence supports the predominantly antithrombotic effects of aspirin in vivo, possibly because of mechanisms in addition to platelet TXA$_2$ inhibition.

NONASPIRIN NSAIDs. Nonaspirin NSAIDs similarly inhibit COX. Unlike aspirin, however, these other NSAIDs inhibit the enzyme reversibly, and therefore their durations of TXA$_2$ and platelet inhibitory action depend on the clearance of the drugs from the circulation.[151] There is considerable variability in the extent and duration of the effects of various NSAIDs on ex vivo platelet aggregation and bleeding time prolongation. Nonaspirin NSAIDs reversibly inhibit COX by preventing its arachidonic acid substrate from gaining access to the active site of the enzyme.

COX-1, the constitutive isoform of COX, is present in platelets and produces TXA$_2$. Aspirin and the traditional NSAIDs are nonselective inhibitors of both COX-1 and COX-2.[155] The newer COX-2–specific inhibitors were designed to maximize the antiinflammatory effects mediated by the COX-2 isoform while minimizing the common side effects (e.g., bleeding, gastric toxicity) attributed to the COX-1 isoform. Therefore, the antiplatelet potency of the new COX-2 inhibitors is several orders of magnitude lower than that of aspirin and standard NSAIDs, and generally cannot be assumed to afford antithrombotic protection. In fact, COX-2 inhibitors appear to increase cardiovascular risk. Meta-analysis of randomized trials that included a comparison of a selective COX-2 inhibitor versus placebo or a selective COX-2 inhibitor versus a traditional NSAID of at least 4 weeks' duration have shown that randomization to a selective COX-2 is associated with a 42 percent relative increase in the incidence of serious vascular events (relative risk, 1.42; 95 percent confidence interval, 1.13 to 1.78; $P = 0.003$), with

no significant heterogeneity among the different selective COX-2 inhibitors.[256] Although the precise mechanism(s) for this adverse affect is unknown, concerns have been raised about the cardiovascular safety of these agents because of their inhibition of COX-2–dependent PGI$_2$ production (Fig. 82-22).[155]

Interaction of NSAIDs with COX may prevent acetylation of the enzyme by aspirin. This suggests that the concomitant administration of nonselective NSAIDs (e.g., ibuprofen), but not COX-2–selective NSAIDs, may actually antagonize the effects of aspirin on COX by competitive interaction and consequently blunt aspirin's antiplatelet efficacy.[157] The mechanism of this pharmacodynamic interaction is competition between aspirin and NSAIDs for a common docking site within the COX channel, which aspirin binds to in platelets before irreversible acetylation of Ser529.[158]

OTHER THROMBOXANE INHIBITORS. Triflusal (4-trifluoromethyl derivative of salicylate) and its active metabolite (3-hydroxy-4-trifluoromethylbenzoic acid) inhibit COX, but also block phosphodiesterase and nitric oxide release. Triflusal may be associated with a lower risk of hemorrhagic complications compared with aspirin.[158] Figure 82-20C illustrates other opportunities to interrupt platelet TXA$_2$ synthesis and/or action in addition to COX blockade. The reduced incidence of atherosclerotic cardiovascular disease in Greenland Eskimos has been attributed, at least in part, to their diets rich in fish oils, which contain omega-3 polyunsaturated fatty acids. A major omega-3 fatty acid in fish oils is eicosapentaenoic acid, which incorporates into phospholipids of cell membranes and competes with arachidonic acid as a substrate for COX. The product of eicosapentaenoic acid oxygenation is TXA$_3$, an eicosanoid devoid of the potent platelet-activating and vasoconstrictor actions of arachidonic acid–derived TXA$_2$. Large and often unpalatable dosages (more than 10 gm eicosapentaenoic acid daily) of medicinal fish oils are required to simulate changes in platelet membrane fatty acid content attained with Eskimo diets and thereby produce antiplatelet actions.

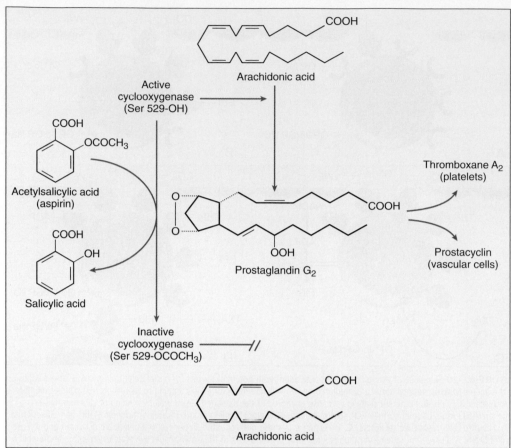

FIGURE 82–21 Aspirin (acetylsalicylic acid) inhibition of cyclooxygenase (prostaglandin-G/H synthase). Aspirin acetylates serine at position 529 of cyclooxygenase, rendering the enzyme inactive. Acetylated cyclooxygenase does not function to catalyze the oxygenation of arachidonic acid to prostaglandin G₂. Aspirin thereby blocks the formation of thromboxane A₂ (in platelets) and prostacyclin (in vascular cells). *(From Loscalzo J, Schafer AI: Anticoagulants, antiplatelet agents, and fibrinolytics. In Loscalzo J, Creager MA, Dzau MV [eds]: Vascular Medicine: A Textbook of Vascular Biology and Diseases. Philadelphia, Lippincott Williams & Wilkins, 1996.)*

CLOPIDOGREL AND OTHER ADP RECEPTOR ANTAGONISTS. Clopidogrel (Plavix) is a thienopyridine derivative. The thienopyridine derivatives selectively and irreversibly inhibit the P2Y12 ADP receptor, which participates importantly in platelet activation and aggregation.[151,160] As ADP receptor blockers, these drugs inhibit ADP-induced platelet aggregation (see Fig. 82-20C) and, when given in combination with aspirin, thienopyridines inhibit platelet aggregation to a greater extent than either agent alone.[151]

Presumably because it must be converted to an active form in vivo, clopidogrel has a relatively slow onset of antiplatelet action. With repeated daily dosages of 75 mg of clopidogrel, partial inhibition of platelet aggregation occurs from the second day of treatment and reaches steady-state inhibition after 4 to 7 days. Using a larger loading dose of clopidogrel (300 to 900 mg) results in more rapid onset (2 to 6 hours) of platelet inhibition[160] Pretreatment with clopidogrel prior to PCI improves 30-day outcomes compared with those not pretreated.[160,161] To achieve the pretreatment benefit of early clopidogrel, patients should be treated more than 12 to 15 hours prior to PCI.[162] Use of a 600-mg clopidogrel loading dose may allow the pretreatment period to be reduced to as short as 2 hours prior to PCI[163] and does not appear to increase the risk of bleeding.[164]

The antiplatelet activity of clopidogrel generally persists for 4 to 8 days after discontinuation of the drug, reflecting the circulating lifetime of platelets and consistent with an irreversible antiplatelet effect, as is the case with aspirin. However, the time course of functional recovery after the discontinuation of clopidogrel is highly variable, raising some concerns regarding the routine 5-day waiting period used before proceeding to coronary artery bypass graft surgery in patients receiving clopidogrel without platelet function testing.

Broad indications now exist for the use of thienopyridine derivatives as antiplatelet agents in PCI[165] and acute coronary syndromes.[166] Thienopyridine use was propelled by landmark studies demonstrating dramatic, nearly fivefold reductions in acute and subacute stent thrombosis when aspirin was used in combination with a thienopyridine post-PCI compared with combinations of aspirin, warfarin, and dipyridamole.[167] Although dual antiplatelet therapy is the standard of care for PCI and acute coronary syndromes, recent trials have established boundaries of benefit (see Chap. 55). Oral anticoagulation has proven superior to clopidogrel plus aspirin for the prevention of events in patients with atrial fibrillation at high risk of stroke.[168] Clopidogrel plus aspirin was also not significantly more effective than aspirin alone in reducing the rate of myocardial infarction, stroke, or death from cardiovascular causes in a broad population of patients at high risk for atherothrombotic events.[169]

Four randomized clinical trials have directly compared ticlopidine in combination with ASA after stenting. Meta-analysis has demonstrated that clopidogrel is associated with a significant reduction in the incidence of major adverse cardiac events (odds ratio [OR], 0.50; $P = 0.001$) and mortality (OR, 0.43; $P = 0.001$) compared with ticlopidine.[170] Use of ticlopidine has been virtually abandoned in the United States because of its increased risk of neutropenia, which occurs in up to 1 percent of patients and is usually reversible with discontinuation of the drug.[151] The risk of this adverse effect is much lower (about 0.1 percent) with clopidogrel. In addition, thrombotic thrombocytopenic purpura, a serious and sometimes fatal disorder, is a rare complication of therapy with both ticlopidine and clopidogrel. Thrombotic thrombocytopenic purpura typically occurs within 2 to 8 weeks of initiation of the thienopyridine and has been noted in 0.02 percent of patients receiving ticlopidine after coronary stenting.[171] Other side effects, including gastrointestinal symptoms, pruritus, urticaria, and bleeding, also appear to occur less often with clopidogrel than with ticlopidine.

New P2Y12 receptor antagonists are under development. Prasugrel (CS-747, LY640315), a novel potent thienopyridine P2Y12 receptor antagonist, may achieve higher levels of inhibition of ADP-induced platelet aggregation than currently approved doses of clopidogrel and is currently being evaluated in a phase 3 clinical trial against clopidogrel.

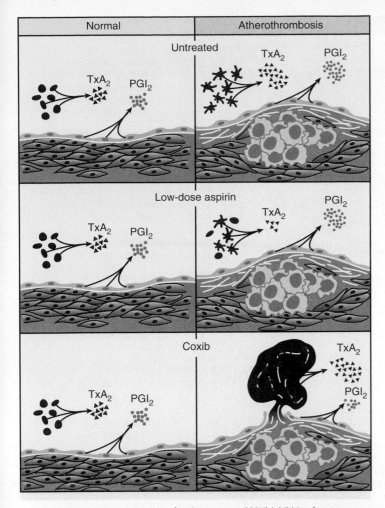

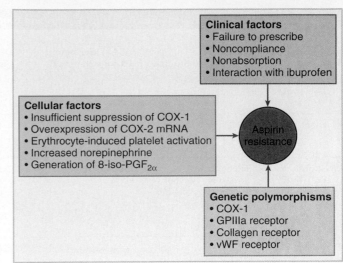

FIGURE 82–23 Possible mechanisms of apparent aspirin resistance. COX = cyclooxygenase; GP = glycoprotein; vWF = von Willebrand factor. *(From Bhatt DL: Aspirin resistance. More than just a laboratory curiosity. J Am Coll Cardiol 32:1127, 2004.)*

FIGURE 82–22 Consequences of cyclooxygenase (COX) inhibition for prostacyclin and thromboxane A_2 production in normal and atherosclerotic arteries. Endothelial cells are shown as a source of prostacyclin (PGI_2) and platelets as a source of thromboxane A_2 (TxA_2) under untreated conditions **(top row)** or treated with low-dose aspirin **(middle row)** or a coxib **(bottom row)** in the normal **(left panel)** and atherosclerotic artery **(right panel)** for comparison. COX-1 is the only isoenzyme expressed in platelets; endothelial cells express both COX-1 and COX-2. In the normal artery, the balance between PGI_2 and TxA_2 production favors PGI_2 and inhibition of platelet-dependent thrombus formation. In the atherosclerotic artery, both PGI_2 and TxA_2 production is increased, in part because of increased platelet activation with compensatory PGI_2 formation via both COX-1 and COX-2 in endothelial cells; the net effect is an imbalance favoring TxA_2 production and platelet-dependent thrombus formation. Low-dose aspirin selectively impairs COX-1–mediated TxA_2 production in platelets, restoring the next antithrombotic balance. Coxib use suppresses COX-2–dependent PGI_2 production in endothelial cells, which has only a marginal effect on the net antithrombotic balance because of the importance of COX-1 as a source of PGI_2 in the normal state. In the setting of atherosclerosis, however, COX-2 plays a greater role as a source of PGI_2 and more TxA_2 is produced; thus, inhibiting COX-2 has a more profound effect on prostanoid balance, favoring TxA_2 production and promoting platelet-dependent thrombosis. *(From Antman EM, DeMets D, Loscalzo J: Cyclooxygenase inhibition and cardiovascular risk. Circulation 112:759, 2005.)*

There are also two reversible P2Y12 inhibitors, AZD6140 and cangrelor. AZD6140 is the first oral, reversible ADP receptor antagonist. Doses of AZD6140, 100 and 200 mg twice daily, were well tolerated and were superior to clopidogrel, 75 mg daily, as determined by ex vivo platelet inhibition studies.[172] Initial experience with intravenous cangrelor, a rapid, reversible, and ultra-short-acting inhibitor of platelet aggregation via competitive binding to the ADP P2Y12 platelet receptor, suggests an acceptable risk of bleeding and adverse cardiac events in PCI, with less prolongation of bleeding time than that observed with GP IIb/IIIa receptor antagonists.[173] Both agents are being evaluated clinically in PCI and acute coronary syndrome trials.

Antiplatelet Drug Resistance

Variability in the response to antiplatelet drugs has been recognized for decades. Antiplatelet drug resistance, or nonresponsiveness, refers to the clinical observation of the inability of the antiplatelet agent to prevent thrombotic vascular events or the laboratory phenomenon of reduced effect(s) of the antiplatelet agent on one or more tests of platelet function. The mechanisms of aspirin and clopidogrel resistance, or nonresponsiveness, are incompletely defined. In the case of aspirin, a number of cellular, clinical, and genetic factors likely contribute to the aspirin resistance that occurs in 5 to 40 percent of patients (Fig. 82-23).[153] Clopidogrel nonresponsiveness or hyporesponsiveness occurs in up to 30 percent of patients.[153] The metabolic activity of hepatic P-450 3A4 is largely responsible for converting clopidogrel to its active thiol metabolite, which binds to and inhibits the P2Y12 ADP receptor. Increasing the clopidogrel dose or hepatic P-450 3A4 activity enhances the platelet inhibitory response of clopidogrel.[174] For both drugs, the important contribution of patient noncompliance cannot be underestimated.

Prospective studies linking laboratory measures of antiplatelet drug resistance to adverse clinical outcomes have been reported (Table 82-4). The largest outcome study reported to date is a nested case-control study of 976 aspirin-treated patients with documented or at high-risk of cardiovascular disease from the Heart Protection Outcomes Evaluation data base.[175] Aspirin responsiveness was categorized into quartiles by urinary 11-dehydrothromboxane B_2 levels, a marker of in vivo thromboxane generation. After 5 years of follow-up, patients in the highest quartile had a 1.8-fold (95 percent confidence interval [CI] 1.2 to 2.7; $P = 0.009$) increased risk of the composite of MI, stroke, or cardiovascular death compared with those in the lowest quartile. The risks of MI (OR, 2.0; 95 percent CI, 1.2 to 2.7; $P = 0.006$) or cardiovascular death (OR, 3.50; 95 percent CI, 1.7 to 7.4; $P < 0.001$) both increased significantly. Aspirin nonresponsiveness also appears to be a marker of adverse outcomes in patients undergoing elective PCI and treated with aspirin at 80 to 300 mg daily for at least 7 days.[176] Using an aggregation-based point of care assay, 29 (19.2 percent) of the 151 enrolled patients were found to be aspirin-resistant. Despite clopidogrel pretreatment with a loading dose of 300 mg at least 12 hours prior to the intervention and procedural anticoagulation with unfractionated heparin, aspirin-resistant patients had a 2.9-fold increased risk of myocardial necrosis as determined by creatine kinase-MB elevation compared with aspirin-sensitive patients.

TABLE 82–4 | **Prospective Studies Relating Aspirin and Clopidogrel Resistance to Adverse Clinical Events**

Study	Population Studied	ASA/Clopidogrel Dosage (mg/day)	Definition of ASA or Clopidogrel Resistance	Prevalence of ASA or Clopidogrel Resistance	Adverse Clinical Events
Grotemeyer et al, 1993*	Stroke patients (N = 180)	ASA, 1500	Platelet reactivity index >1.25	ASA, 33%	~10-fold increased risk of vascular death, MI, or stroke at 2 yr
Mueller, 1997†	PAD patients (N = 100)	ASA, 100	≥20% reduction in platelet function using CWBA	ASA, ~60%	87% increased risk of reocclusion at angioplasty site at 1 yr
Eikelboom et al, 2002[175]	Patients with CAD, stroke, PAD, or DM plus one or more CV risk factor(s) (N = 976)	Not specified	Quartiles of urinary 11-dehydro-thromboxane B_2 levels	Not specified	1.8-fold increased risk of cardiovascular death, MI, or stroke at 5 yr
Gum et al, 2003‡	Patients with stable CV disease (N = 326)	ASA, 325	≥70% ADP-induced and ≥20% AA-induced optical platelet aggregation	ASA, 5.2%	~Fourfold increased risk of death, MI, or stroke at 1.8 yr
Chen et al, 2004[176]	Patients undergoing elective PCI (N = 151)	ASA, 80-300	ARU ≥ 550 in point of care platelet aggregation assay	ASA, 19.2%	2.9-fold increased risk of CK-MB elevation after PCI
Matetzky et al, 2004[177]	Patients with primary PCI for STEMI (N = 60)	ASA, 300 mg initially, then 200 mg daily; clopidogrel 300 mg loading dose and 75 mg daily	Clopidogrel response by quartiles	Lowest quartile (<20% inhibition to ADP)	Major adverse cardiovascular events—quartile I = 40%; quartile II = 6.7%; quartiles III and IV = 0%
Lev et al, 2006[177]	Patients undergoing PCI (N = 150)	ASA, 81-325 mg daily; clopidogrel, 300 mg loading dose and 75 mg daily	ASA—(1) 0.5 mg/ml arachidonic acid–induced aggregation ≥ 20%; (2) 5 μmol/liter ADP-induced platelet aggregation ≥70%; and (3) ARU ≥ 550 by VerifyNow ASA test; clopidogrel—baseline minus posttreatment aggregation ≤10% in response to both 5 and 20 μmol/liter ADP	ASA, 12.4% Clopidogrel, 24% Dual resistance, 6%	CPK-MB elevation; ASA-resistant versus ASA-sensitive, 38.9% versus 18.3%; clopidogrel-resistant versus clopidogrel-sensitive, 32.4% versus 17.3%; dual-resistant versus sensitive, 44.4% versus 15.8%

*Grotemeyer KH, Scharafinski HW, Husstedt IW: Two-year follow-up of aspirin responder and aspirin non responder. A pilot-study including 180 post-stroke patients. Thromb Res 71:397, 1993.

†Mueller MR, Salat A, Stangl P, et al: Variable platelet response to low-dose ASA and the risk of limb deterioration in patients submitted to peripheral arterial angioplasty. Thromb Haemost 78:1003, 1997.

‡Gum PA, Kottke-Marchant K, Welsh PA, et al: A prospective, blinded determination of the natural history of aspirin resistance among stable patients with cardiovascular disease. J Am Coll Cardiol 41:961, 2003.

AA = arachidonic acid; ADP = adenosine diphosphate; ARU = aspirin reaction unit; ASA = aspirin; CK = creatine kinase; CV = cardiovascular; CWBA = corrected whole blood aggregometry; DM = diabetes mellitus; MI = myocardial infarction; PAD = peripheral arterial disease; PCI = percutaneous coronary intervention; STEMI = ST elevation myocardial infarction.

Prospective trials relating clopidogrel responsiveness to clinical outcome are more limited in number than aspirin resistance studies. Clopidogrel responsiveness and clinical outcomes were evaluated in patients with STEMI undergoing primary PCI.[177] Patients received clopidogrel 300 mg on completion of PCI and 75 mg daily for 3 months and were stratified into quartiles according to the percentage reduction of ADP (5 mol/liter)-induced platelet aggregation at day 6 compared with baseline. Patients in the first quartile were defined as clopidogrel-resistant. At 6-month follow-up, clopidogrel-resistant patients developed recurrent ischemic cardiovascular events (40 percent) at a significantly higher rate than patients with intermediate (6.7 percent) or high (0 percent) levels of platelet inhibition. Resistance to both aspirin and clopidogrel was evaluated in elective PCI patients.[178] Using criteria based on light transmission aggregometry or point of care assay, the incidence of aspirin and clopidogrel resistance was 12.7 and 24 percent, respectively; dual resistance was observed in 6.0 percent of patients. There was a significant increase in the incidence of creatine kinase-MB elevation in aspirin-resistant patients, when compared with aspirin-sensitive patients, and trends for more frequent creatine kinase-MB elevation were noted in dual drug-resistant and clopidogrel-resistant patients compared with dual drug-sensitive and clopidogrel-sensitive patients, respectively.

Numerous studies have documented interindividual variability in platelet inhibitory responsiveness to oral antiplatelet drugs. A growing body of evidence has demonstrated that hyporesponsiveness or nonresponsiveness to antiplatelet drugs in the laboratory (i.e., resistance) is associated with adverse clinical events in diverse populations of patients with atherosclerotic disease in stable and unstable phases as well as in the post–percutaneous coronary and post–peripheral intervention settings. However, there are major limitations of the currently available data. The number of patients studied in all these reports is small, and the study designs are not adequate for controlling confounding variables. The definition of antiplatelet resistance is not uniform. In studies of aspirin, dosage varied and treatment compliance was not verified. Widespread clinical application of antiplatelet resistance will require additional studies on larger populations that define antiplatelet resistance in a standardized manner, using assays with consistency and reproducibility that correlate measurements with clinical outcomes and that provide strategies for modifying antiplatelet regimens to improve outcome (e.g., increasing dose of antiplatelet agent, adding or substituting a second antiplatelet agent).

PHOSPHODIESTERASE INHIBITORS

Dipyridamole. The mechanism of antiplatelet action of dipyridamole is unclear. Although this drug can stimulate PGI_2 synthesis, potentiate the platelet inhibitory effects of PGI_2, raise platelet cAMP levels by inhibiting phosphodiesterase, and block uptake of adenosine into vascular and blood cells, these potential antiplatelet actions generally do not occur at therapeutically achievable drug concentrations.[151] Unlike aspirin, dipyridamole does not prolong the bleeding time or inhibit ex vivo platelet aggregation at therapeutic doses. Numerous clinical trials have failed to demonstrate the antithrombotic efficacy of dipyridamole when it is used alone in any clinical setting. However, it may enhance the effect of warfarin in preventing systemic embolization from mechanical heart valve prostheses and add to the beneficial effect of aspirin in preventing the progression of peripheral occlusive arterial disease or, when used in a sustained-release preparation, may be useful in the secondary prevention of ischemic stroke.[179,180]

Cilostazol. Cilostazol is a quinolone derivative that is a potent inhibitor of platelet phosphodiesterase-3 and has vasodilatory effects. It may be beneficial in the treatment of intermittent claudication caused by peripheral vascular disease, an indication for which it has been approved by the U.S. Food and Drug Administration.[151] A 6-month course of cilostazol reduced angiographic restenosis (36 percent relative risk reduction) after bare metal stenting.[181] Aspirin plus cilostazol may be used as an alternative to aspirin plus a thienopyridine in patients who are intolerant to ticlopidine and clopidogrel.[182]

GLYCOPROTEIN IIb/IIIa ANTAGONISTS (see Chaps. 51 and 55).

Regardless of the stimulus for their activation, platelet activation depends on their membrane binding sites for fibrinogen and vWF in the GP IIb/IIIa complex (see Fig. 82-20D). This mechanism provides the rationale for pharmacological intervention directed against the platelet GP IIb/IIIa complex. The role of the platelet GP IIb/IIIa complex in platelet activation is discussed in more detail earlier (in the section on platelets). Because GP IIb/IIIa antagonists do not block TXA_2 production by activated platelets, concomitant use of aspirin may enhance their antithrombotic efficacy.

Platelet GP IIb/IIIa antagonists generally belong to one of the following classes: (1) monoclonal antibody against GP IIb/IIIa; (2) peptide (peptidomimetic) antagonists, many of which contain the RGD sequence that can compete with fibrinogen for its GP IIb/IIIa binding site; and (3) nonpeptide (nonpeptide-mimetic) antagonists of GP IIb/IIIa. Three intravenous drugs currently available for percutaneous coronary intervention or acute coronary syndromes represent the prototypes for these groups: abciximab (c7E3 Fab, ReoPro), a monoclonal antibody; eptifibatide (Integrilin), a peptide antagonist; and tirofiban (Aggrastat), a nonpeptide mimetic (see Chaps. 51 and 52).[151]

Abciximab is a humanized Fab fragment engineered from murine monoclonal antibody 7E3 directed against GP IIb/IIIa. Unlike the small-molecule agents, abciximab interacts with the GP IIb/IIIa receptor at sites distinct from the ligand-binding RGD sequence site, and exerts its inhibitory

effect noncompetitively.[183] The antibody has unusual pharmacokinetics, with most of the drug cleared from plasma within 26 minutes, but much slower clearance from the body, with a functional half-life up to 7 days. Because of the high affinity of abciximab for GP IIb/IIIa, the number of abciximab molecules bound to platelets is considerably higher than the free plasma pool of the drug for the duration of treatment. Platelet-associated abciximab can be detected for more than 14 days after the infusion is stopped.[184] With an average period of platelet circulation of approximately 7 days, it appears that abciximab molecules can freely dissociate and reassociate with GP IIb/IIIa as the turnover of platelets in the circulation continues, thus prolonging the biological half-life of the drug.

Abciximab binds to and inhibits not only GP IIb/IIIa, but also cross-reacts with alpha$_v$-beta$_3$ and the leukocyte integrin Mac-1.[185] Cross-reactivity with $G_p\alpha_v\beta_3$ has raised the possibility that abciximab may favorably modulate intimal hyperplasia and restenosis, because smooth muscle cells express alpha$_v$-beta$_3$ basally, and at higher levels postvascular injury. However, clinical studies have not consistently demonstrated the clinical significance of abciximab's reactivity with structures other than GP IIb/IIIa.

The design of the cyclic heptapeptide eptifibatide is based on barbourin, a 73–amino acid peptide isolated from the venom of the Southeastern pygmy rattlesnake, *Sistrurus miliaris barbouri*.[191] With the recommended double-bolus (180-µg/kg bolus followed 10 minutes later by 180-µg/kg second bolus) and infusion (2 µg/kg/min) regimen, peak plasma levels are established shortly after the bolus doses, and slightly lower concentrations are subsequently maintained throughout the infusion period; plasma concentration decreases rapidly after the infusion is discontinued. Eptifibatide has an elimination half-life of 2.5 hours, with most of the drug eliminated through renal mechanisms.[186] A lower infusion dose (1 µg/kg/min) of eptifibatide is recommended in patients with creatinine clearance less than 50 ml/min. Substantial recovery of platelet aggregation is apparent within 4 hours of discontinuation of infusion.[186]

Tirofiban, a peptidometic inhibitor, occupies the binding pocket on GP IIb/IIIa and thereby competitively inhibits platelet aggregation mediated by fibrinogen or vWF.[151] The stoichiometry of both tirofiban and eptifibatide is more than 100 molecules of drug per GP IIb/IIIa needed to achieve full platelet inhibition. This compares with a stoichiometry of 1.5 molecules of abciximab for each receptor.[187] Like eptifibatide, substantial recovery of platelet aggregation is apparent within 4 hours of completion of infusion.[186]

The clinical experience with oral GP IIb/IIIa antagonists (e.g., sibrafiban, orbofiban, xemilofiban) has been disappointing. There have been six phase 3 trials conducted with oral GP IIb/IIIa inhibitors, all with no improvement in outcome. Meta-analysis of these trials has demonstrated an increased bleeding risk and increased mortality in patients treated with oral GP IIb/IIIa inhibitors.[188] The lack of clinical benefit for these agents as compared with the established efficacy with intravenous inhibitors may result in part from inadequate in vivo platelet GP IIb/IIIa blockade. Oral GP IIb/IIIa antagonists may also cause paradoxical platelet activation. Ligand-mimetic GP IIb/IIIa blockers can have intrinsic platelet-activating properties or can stimulate outside-in signal transduction, leading to paradoxical platelet aggregation. These ligand-mimetic properties of GP IIb/IIIa antagonists may also cause thrombocytopenia (see later).[189]

Pharmacodynamics and Optimal Dosing with GP IIb/IIIa Inhibitors. Both preclinical and clinical pharmacodynamic studies have set the range of greater than 80 percent inhibition of platelet aggregation by light transmission aggregometry as the target for clinically effective antiplatelet activity. The level of platelet inhibition varies between the three GP IIb/IIIa inhibitors following the recommended bolus and infusions.[190] In general, the bolus and infusion regimen of abciximab and the double-bolus and infusion regimen of eptifibatide

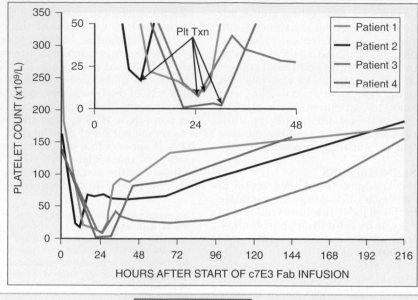

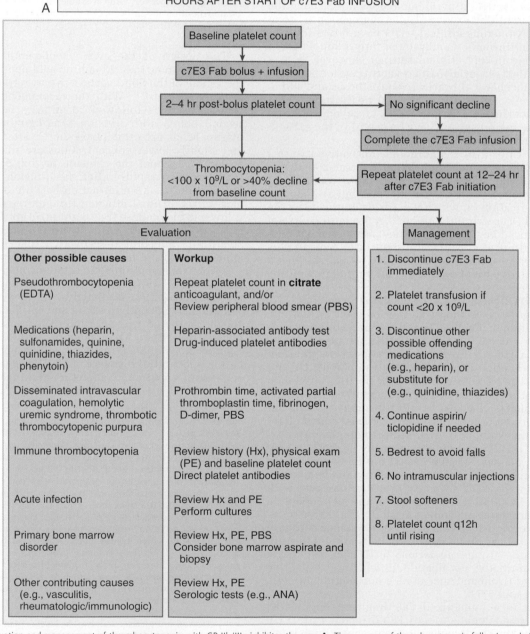

CH 82

FIGURE 82–24 Evaluation and management of thrombocytopenia with GP IIb/IIIa inhibitor therapy. **A,** Time course of thrombocytopenia following administration of abciximab. Platelet counts before and during therapy and after recovery in four patients who developed acute profound thrombocytopenia after receiving c7E3 Fab bolus plus infusion. **Inset,** Platelet counts during the first 48 hours and first platelet transfusion (Plt Txn) given. **B,** Platelet-monitoring algorithm, thrombocytopenia workup, and treatment strategies for patients receiving abciximab or other glycoprotein (GP) IIb/IIIa antagonist. ANA = antinuclear antibody; EDTA = ethylenediaminetetraacetic acid. *(From Berkowitz SD, Harrington RA, Rund MM, Tcheng JE: Acute profound thrombocytopenia after c7E3 Fab (abciximab) therapy. Circulation 95:809, 1997.)*

cause rapid and profound inhibition of platelet function. Several studies have documented that the FDA-approved bolus and infusion regimen for tirofiban achieves suboptimal levels of platelet inhibition for up to 4 to 6 hours, which probably accounted for the inferior clinical results in the PCI setting.[187] The degree of platelet inhibition appears central to the efficacy of GP IIb/IIIa inhibitors. Achieving more than 95 percent platelet inhibition 10 minutes after the bolus in patients undergoing PCI was associated with a 55 percent reduction in major adverse cardiac events compared with those patients with less than 95 percent platelet inhibition.[190]

Facilitated PCI with Thrombolytic Therapy and GP IIb/IIIa in Combination (see Chaps. 51 and 52). Effective and rapid reperfusion of the infarct-related coronary artery is the critical goal in the treatment of acute myocardial infarction. The optimal pharmacological strategy for bridging between admission and performance of PCI in a patient with acute myocardial infarction has not been defined. Although several drugs or combinations of drugs may meet the requirements for effective facilitated PCI, comparative evidence and clinical efficacy regarding the optimal regimen is lacking. Several studies have been performed to assess the safety and efficacy of combination therapy using half-dose thrombolytic therapy and various GP IIb/IIIa inhibitors pre-PCI to improve baseline angiographic patency of the infarct-related artery. Each of these trials has demonstrated improved early patency of the infarct-related artery compared with full-dose thrombolytic therapy alone. However, this benefit may be at the expense of increased major bleeding.[191] Improvement of hard clinical endpoints using this combination has yet to be shown and one study[192] of reteplase plus abciximab versus abciximab alone has demonstrated no significant difference in final infarct size using technetium-99m sestamibi.

Complications. Bleeding complications with currently approved intravenous platelet GP IIb/IIIa antagonists have primarily involved vascular access puncture sites in patients undergoing percutaneous intervention. Reduction and weight adjustment in adjunctive heparin dosing in patients undergoing coronary interventions have reduced the incidence of these bleeding problems. No increase in intracerebral hemorrhage has been observed with the GP IIb/IIIa antagonists.

GP IIb/IIIa Antagonists and Thrombocytopenia. In a meta-analysis of eight clinical trials, abciximab increased the incidence of mild thrombocytopenia (defined as a platelet count ranging from 50,000 to 90,000 or 100,000/mm^3) compared with the placebo group (4.2 versus 2.0 percent; $P < 0.001$; OR, 2.13).[193] Eptifibatide or tirofiban with heparin did not increase mild thrombocytopenia compared with placebo with heparin (OR, 0.99). Patients receiving abciximab with heparin also had more than twice the frequency of severe thrombocytopenia (platelet count ranging from 20,000 to 50,000/mm^3) than those receiving placebo with heparin (1.0 versus 0.4 percent; $P = 0.01$; OR, 2.48). Eptifibatide or tirofiban with heparin did not cause a significant excess of severe thrombocytopenia compared with placebo with heparin. Acute coronary syndrome trials tend to report a higher incidence of thrombocytopenia compared with PCI trials, possibly because longer heparin infusions may produce heparin-induced thrombocytopenia.[193]

Profound thrombocytopenia (platelet count less than 20,000/mm^3) occurs in 0.1 to 0.5 percent of patients treated with intravenous agents, and the incidence appears to be slightly higher with abciximab. An algorithm for evaluation of these patients has been proposed (Fig. 82-24).[194] Pseudothrombocytopenia caused by platelet clumping and HIT must be ruled out in these patients. True thrombocytopenia requires the immediate cessation of GP IIb/IIIa therapy. In most cases, the platelet count usually returns to normal within 48 to 72 hours. Regardless of cause, thrombocytopenia in patients undergoing PCI is associated with more ischemic events, bleeding complications, and transfusions.[195]

The mechanism(s) of thrombocytopenia is unknown. A precipitous decrease in platelet count may occur within 1 to 2 hours of initial exposure, or there may be a significant

decline several days after initiation of therapy. Readministration of abciximab, but not the small-molecule inhibitors (eptifibatide and tirofiban), is associated with a slightly increased risk of recurrent thrombocytopenia.[196]

REFERENCES

Basic Mechanisms of Hemostasis and Thrombosis

1. Park C, Ma YD, Choi K: Evidence for the hemangioblast. Exp Hematol 33:965, 2005.
2. Jaffredo T, Nottingham W, Liddiard K, et al: From hemangioblast to hematopoietic stem cell: An endothelial connection? Exp Hematol 33:1029, 2005.
3. Sata M: Role of circulating vascular progenitors in angiogenesis, vascular healing, and pulmonary hypertension: Lessons from animal models. Arterioscler Thromb Vasc Biol 26:1008, 2006.
4. Blann AD, Woywodt A, Bertolini F, et al: Circulating endothelial cells. Biomarker of vascular disease. Thromb Haemost 93:228, 2005.
5. Moncada S, Higgs EA (eds): The Vascular Endothelium. New York, Springer, 2006.
6. Schafer AI: Vascular endothelium: In defense of blood fluidity. J Clin Invest 99:1143, 1997.
7. Aird WC: Endothelial cell heterogeneity and atherosclerosis. Curr Atheroscler Rep 8:69, 2006.
8. Searles CD: Transcriptional and posttranslational regulation of endothelial nitric oxide synthase expression. Am J Physiol Cell Physiol 291:C803, 2006.
9. Durante W, Schafer AI: Carbon monoxide and vascular cell function. Int J Mol Med 2:255, 1998.
10. Smyth EM, FitzGerald GA: Human prostacyclin receptor. Vitam Horm 65:149, 2002.
11. Fleming I, Busse R: Endothelium-derived epoxyeicosatrienoic acids and vascular function. Hypertension 47:629, 2006.
12. Shimokawa H, Morikawa K: Hydrogen peroxide is an endothelium-derived hyperpolarizing factor in animals and humans. J Mol Cell Cardiol 39:725, 2005.
13. Marcus AJ, Broekman MJ, Drosopoulos JH, et al: Role of CD39 (NTPDase-1) in the thromboregulation, cerebroprotection, and cardioprotection. Sem Thromb Hemost 31:234, 2005.
14. Busse R, Fleming I: Regulation of endothelium-derived vasoactive autacoid production by hemodynamic forces. Trends Pharmacol Sci 24:24, 2003.
15. Lerman A, Zeiher AM: Endothelial function. Cardiac events. Circulation 111:363, 2005.
16. Hoffman MM, Monroe DM: Rethinking the coagulation cascade. Curr Hematol Rep. 4:391, 2005.
17. Mann KG, Butenas S, Brummel K: The dynamics of thrombin formation. Arteriosler Thromb Vasc Biol 23:17, 2003.
18. Versteeg HH, Ruf W: Emerging insights in tissue factor-dependent signaling events. Semin Thromb Hemost 32:24, 2006.
19. Mackman N: Role of tissue factor in hemostasis and thrombosis. Blood Cells MolDis 36:104, 2006.
20. Kitchens CS: The contact system. Arch Pathol Lab Med 126:1382, 2002.
21. Mosesson MW: Fibrinogen structure and fibrin clot assembly. Semin Thromb Hemost 24:169, 1998.
22. Roberts HR, Hoffman M, Monroe DM: A cell-based model of thrombin generation. Semin Thromb Hemost 32(Suppl 1):32, 2006.
23. Lopez JA, Del Conde I, Shrimpton CN: Receptors, rafts, and microvesicles in thrombosis and inflammation. J Thromb Haemost 3:1737, 2005.
24. Quinsey NS, Greedy AL, Bottomley SP, et al: Antithrombin: In control of coagulation. Int J Biochem Cell Biol 36:386, 2004.
25. Crowther MA, Kelton JG: Congenital thrombophilic states associated with venous thrombosis: A qualitative overview and proposed classification system. Ann Intern Med 138:128, 2003.
26. Broze GJ Jr: Protein Z-dependent regulation of coagulation. Thromb Haemost 86:8, 2001.
27. Martinelli I, Razzari C, Biguzzi E, et al: Low levels of protein Z and the risk of venous thromboembolism. J Thromb Haemost 3:2817, 2005.
28. Corral J, Gonzalez-Conejero R, Soria JM, et al: A nonsense polymorphism in the protein Z-dependent protease inhibitor increases the risk for venous thrombosis. Blood 108:177, 2006.
29. Simmonds RE, Rance J, Lane DA: Regulation of coagulation. In Loscalzo J, Schafer AI (eds): Thrombosis and Hemorrhage. 3rd ed. Philadelphia, Lippincott Williams & Wilkins, 2003, pp 35-61.
30. Li YH, Shi GY, Wu HL: The role of thrombomodulin in atherosclerosis: From bench to bedside. Cardiovasc Hematol Agents Med Chem 4:183, 2006.
31. Lwaleed BA, Brass PS: Tissue factor pathway inhibitor: structure, biology and involvement in disease. J Pathol 208:327, 2006.
32. Tobu M, Ma Q, Iqbal O, et al: Comparative tissue factor pathway inhibitor release potential of heparins. Clin Appl Thromb Hemost 11:37, 2005.
33. Forastiero RR, Martinuzzo ME, Broze Jr GJ: High titers of autoantibodies to tissue factor pathway inhibitor are associated with the antiphospholipid syndrome. J Thromb Haemost 1:718, 2003.
34. Caplice NM, Panetta C, Peterson TE, et al: Lipoprotein(a) binds and inactivates tissue factor pathway inhibitor: a novel link between lipoproteins and thrombosis. Blood 98:2980, 2001.
35. Dahm A, Rosendaal FR, Anderson TO, Sandset PM: Tissue factor pathway inhibitor anticoagulant activity: Risk for venous thrombosis and effect of hormonal state. Br J Haematol 132:333, 2006.

36. Berglund L, Ramakrishnana R: Lipoprotein(a): An elusive cardiovascular risk factor. Arterioscler Thromb Vasc Biol 24:2219, 2004.

37. Castellino FJ, Ploplis VA: Structure and function of the plasminogen/plasmin system. Thrombo Haemost 93:647, 2005.

38. Miles LA, Hawley SB, Baik N, et al: Plasminogen receptors: The sine qua non of the cell surface plasminogen activation. Front Biosci 10:1754, 2005.

39. Hull RD. Diagnosing pulmonary embolism with improved certainty and simplicity. JAMA 295:213, 2006.

40. Kearon C, Ginsberg JS, Douketis J, et al; Canadian Pulmonary Embolism Diagnosis Study (CANPEDS) Group: An evaluation of D-dimer in the diagnosis of pulmonary embolism: A randomized trial. Ann Intern Med 144:812, 2006.

41. Vaughan DE, Declerck PJ: Regulation of fibrinolysis. In Loscalzo J, Schafer AI (eds): Thrombosis and Hemorrhage, 3rd ed. Philadelphia, Lippincott Williams & Wilkins, 2003, pp 105-119.

42. Nesheim M: Thrombin and fibronolysis. Chest 124(3 Suppl):335, 2003.

43. Verdu J, Marco P, Benlloch S, et al: Thrombin activatable fibrinolysis inhibitor (TAFI) polymorphisms and plasma TAFI levels measured with an ELISA insensitive to isoforms in patients with venous thromboembolic disease (VTD). Thromb Haemost 95:585, 2006.

44. Eichinger S, Schonauer V, Weltermann A, et al: Thrombin-activatable fibrinolysis inhibitor and the risk for recurrent venous thromboembolism. Blood 103:3773, 2004.

45. Mornage PE, Tregouet DA, Frere C, et al; PRIME Study Group: TAFI gene haplotypes, TAFI plasma levels and future risk of coronary heart disease: The PRIME Study. J Thromb Haemost 3:1503, 2005.

46. Kaushansky K: The molecular mechanisms that control thrombopoiesis. J Clin Invest 115:3339, 2005.

47. Mendolicchio GL, Ruggeri ZM: New perspectives on von Willebrand factor functions in hemostasis and thrombosis. Semin Hematol 42:5, 2005.

48. Berndt MC, Shen Y, Dopheide SM, et al: The vascular biology of the glycoprotein Ib-IX-V complex. Thromb Haemost 86:178, 2001.

49. Furie B, Furie BC: Thrombus formation in vivo. J Clin Invest 115:3355, 2005.

50. Nieswandt B, Watson SP: Platelet-collagen interactions: Is GP VI the central receptor? Blood 102:449, 2003.

51. Jurk K, Kehrel BE: Platelets: Physiology and biochemistry. Semin Thromb Haemost 31:381, 2005.

52. Yu Y, Cheng Y, Fan J, et al: Differential impact of prostaglandin H synthase 1 knockdown on platelets and parturition. J Clin Invest 115:986, 2005.

53. Shattil SJ, Newman PJ: Integrins: Dynamic scaffolds for adhesion and signaling in platelets. Blood 104:1606, 2004.

54. Bennett JS: Structure and function of the platelet integrin $\alpha_{IIb}\beta_3$. J Clin Invest 115:3363, 2005.

55. Vorcheimer DA, Becker R: Platelets in atherosclerosis. Mayo Clin Proc 81:59, 2006.

56. Brass LF, Zhu L, Stalker TJ: Minding the gaps to promote thrombus growth and stability. J Clin Invest 115:3385, 2005.

57. Davie EW, Kulman JD: An overview of the structure and function of thrombin. Semin Thromb Hemost 32(Suppl 1):3, 2006.

58. Griffin JH: The thrombin paradox. Nature 378:337, 1995.

59. Esmon CT: Inflammation and the activated protein C anticoagulant pathway. Semin Thromb Hemost 32(Suppl 1):49, 2006.

Thrombophilic Disorders

60. Bauer KA: Management of thrombophilia. J Thromb Haemost 1:1429, 2003.

61. Itakura H: Racial disparities in resk factors for thrombosis. Curr Opin Hematol 12:364, 2005.

62. Dowling NF, Austin H, Dilley A, et al: The epidemiology of venous thromboembolism in Caucasians and African-Americans: The GATE study. J Thromb Haemost 1:80, 2003.

63. Juul K, Tybjaerg-Hansen A, Steffensen R, et al: Factor V Leiden: The Copenhagen city heart study and 2 meta-analyses. Blood 100:3, 2002.

64. Feinbloom D, Bauer KA: Assessment of hemostatic risk factors in predicting arterial thrombotic events. Arterioscler Thromb Vasc Biol 25:2043, 2005.

65. Rosendaal FR, Siscovick DS, Schwartz SM, et al: Factor V Leiden (resistance to activated protein C) increases the risk of myocardial infarction in young women. Blood 89:2817, 1997.

66. Slooter AJ, Rosendaal FR, Tanis BC, et al: Prothrombotic conditions, oral contraceptives, and the risk of ischemic stroke. J Thromb Haemost 3:1213, 2005.

67. Stein S, Konkle BA: Thrombotic risk of oral contraceptives, postmenopausal hormone replacement, and selective estrogen receptor modulators (SERMs). In Kitchens CS, Alving BM, Kessler CM (eds): Consultative Hemostasis and Thrombosis. Philadelphia, WB Saunders, 2002, pp 427-436.

68. Alhenc-Gelas M, Plu-Bureau G, Guillonneau S, et al: Impact of progestagens on activated protein C (APC) resistance among users of oral contraceptives. J Thromb Haemost 2:1594, 2004.

69. Dahlback B: The discovery of activated protein C resistance. J Thromb Haemost 1:3, 2003.

70. Dilley A, Austin H, Hooper WC, et al: Prevalence of the prothrombin 20210 G-to-A variant in blacks: Infants, patients with venous thrombosis, patients with myocardial infarction, and control subjects. J Lab Clin Med 132:452, 1998.

71. Legnani C, Cosmi B, Valdre L, et al: Venous thromboembolism, oral contraceptives and high prothrombin levels. J Thromb Haemost 1:112, 2002.

72. Martinelli I, Sacchi E, Landi G, et al: High risk of cerebral-vein thrombosis in carriers of a prothrombin-gene mutation and in users of oral contraceptives. N Engl J Med 338:1793, 1998.

73. Goodwin AJ, Rosendaal FR, Kottke-Marchant K, Bovill EG: A review of the technical, diagnostic, and epidemiologic considerations for protein S assays. Arch Pathol Lab Med 126:1349, 2002.

74. Emmerich J, Vossen CY, Callas PW, et al: Chronic venous abnormalities in symptomatic and asymptomatic protein C deficiency. J Thromb Haemost 3:1428, 2005.

75. Undas A, Brozek J, Szczeklik A: Homocysteine and thrombosis: From basic science to clinical evidence. Thromb Haemost 94:907, 2005.

76. Mangoni AA, Jackson SH: Homocysteine and cardiovascular disease: Current evidence and future prospects. Am J Med 112:556, 2002.

77. den Heijer M, Lewington S, Clarke R: Homocysteine, MTHFR and risk of venous thrombosis: A meta-analysis of published epidemiological studies. J Thromb Haemost 3:292, 2005.

78. Ray JG, Shmorgun D, Chan WS: Common C677T polymorphism of the methylene-tetrahydrofolate reductase gene and the risk of venous thromboembolism: Meta-analysis of 31 studies. Pathophys Haemost Thromb 32:51, 2002.

79. Keijzer MBAJ, den Heijer M, Blom HJ, et al: Interaction between hyperhomocysteinemia, mutated methylenetetrahydrofolatereductase (MTHFR) and inherited thrombophilic factor in recurrent venous thrombosis. Thromb Haemost 88:723, 2002.

80. The Heart Outcomes Prevention Evaluation (HOPE) 2 Investigators: Homocysteine lowering with folic acid and B vitamins in vascular disease. N Engl J Med 354:1567, 2006.

81. Bonaa KH, Njolstad I, Ueland PM, et al; NORVIT Trial Investigators: Homocysteine lowering and cardiovascular events after acute myocardial infarction. N Engl J Med 354:1578, 2006.

82. Toole JF, Malinow MR, Chambless LE, et al: Lowering homocysteine in patients with ischemic stroke to prevent recurrent stroke, myocardial infarction, and death: The Vitamin Intervention for Stroke Prevention (VISP) randomized controlled trial. JAMA 291:565, 2004.

83. Martinelli I: von Willebrand factor and factor VIII as risk factors for arterial and venous thrombosis. Semin Hematol 42:49, 2005.

84. Kyrle PA, Minar E, Hirschl M, et al: High plasma levels of factor VIII and the risk of recurrent venous thromboembolism. N Engl J Med 343:457, 2000.

85. Tsai AW, Cushman M, Rosamond WD, et al: Coagulation factors, inflammation markers, and venous thromboembolism: The longitudinal investigation of thromboembolism cause (LITE). Am J Med 113:636, 2002.

86. Haynes T: Dysfibrinogenemia and thrombosis. Arch Pathol Lab Med 126:1387, 2002.

87. Dahm A, Rosendaal FR, Andersen TO, Sandset PM: Tissue factor pathway inhibitor anticoagulant activity: Risk for venous thrombosis and effect of hormonal state. Br J Haematol 132:333, 2006.

88. Bauer KA, Rosendaal FR, Heit JA: Hypercoagulability: Too many tests, too much conflicting data. Hematology 353-368, 2002.

89. Heit JA: Venous thromboembolism: Disease burden, outcomes and risk factors. J Thromb Haemost 3:1611, 2005.

90. Geerts WH, Pineo GF, Heit JA, et al: Prevention of venous thromboembolism: The seventh ACCP conference on antithrombotic and thrombolytic therapy. Chest 126:338S, 2004.

91. Aryal KR, Al-Khaffaf H: Venous thromboembolic complications following air travel: What's the quantitative risk? A literature review. Eur J Vasc Endovasc Surg 31:187, 2006.

92. Schreijer AJM, Cannegieter SC, Meijers JCM, et al: Activation of coagulation system during air travel: A crossover study. Lancet 367:832, 2006.

93. Di Nisio M, Otten HM, Piccioli A, et al: Decision analysis for cancer screening in idiopathic venous thromboembolism. J Thromb Haemost 3:2391, 2005.

94. van den Bosch MAAJ, Kemmeren JM, Tanis BC, et al: The RATIO study: Oral contraceptives and the risk of peripheral arterial disease in young women. J Thromb Haemost 1:439, 2003.

95. Baillargeon JP, McClish DK, Essah PA, Nestler JE: Association between the current use of low-dose oral contraceptives and cardiovascular aterial disease: A meta-analysis. J Clin Endocrinol Metab 90:3863, 2005.

96. Heit J, Kobbervig C, James A, et al: Trends in the incidence of deep vein thrombosis and pulmonary embolism during pregnancy or the puerperium: A 30-year population-based study. Ann Intern Med 143:697, 2005.

97. James AH, Jamison MG, Brancazio LR, Myers ER: Venous thromboembolism during pregnancy and the postpartum period: Incidence, risk factors, and mortality. Am J Obstet Gynecol 194:1311, 2006.

98. Robertson L, Wu O, Langhorne P, et al; The Thrombosis: Risk and Economic Assessment of Thrombophilia Screening (TREATS) Study: Thrombophilia in pregnancy: A systematic review. Br J Haematol 132:171, 2006.

99. Bates SM, Greer IA, Hirsh J, Ginsberg JS: Use of antithrombotic agents during pregnancy: The seventh ACCP conference on antithrombotic and thrombolytic therapy. Chest 126:627S, 2004.

100. Miyakis S, Lockshin MD, Atsumi T, et al: International consensus statement on an update of the classification criteria for definite antiphospholipid syndrome (APS). J Thromb Haemost 4:295, 2006.

101. Vora SK, Asherson RA, Erkan D: Catastrophic antiphospholipid syndrome. J Intens Care Med 21:144, 2006.

102. de Groot PG, Derksen RH: Pathophysiology of the antiphospholipid syndrome. J Thromb Haemost 3:1854, 2005.

103. Ortel TL: The antiphospholipid syndrome: What are we really measuring? How do we measure it? And how do we treat it? J Thromb Thrombolysis 21:79, 2006.

104. Crowther MA, Ginsberg JS, Julian J, et al: A comparison of two intensities of warfarin for the prevention of recurrent thrombosis in patients with the antiphospholipid antibody syndrome. N Engl J Med 349:1133, 2003.

105. Finazzi G, Marchioli R, Brancaccio V, et al: A randomized clinical trial of high-intensity warfarin versus. conventional antithrombotic therapy for the prevention of recurrent thrombosis in patients with the antiphospholipid syndrome (WAPS). J Thromb Haemost 3:848, 2005.

106. Levine SR, Brey RL, Tilley BC, et al: Antiphospholipid antibodies and subsequent thrombo-occlusive events in patients with ischemic stroke. JAMA 291:576, 2001.

107. Lim W, Crowther MA, Eikelbloom JW: Management of antiphospholipid antibody syndrome: A systematic review. JAMA 295:1050, 2006.

Antithrombotic Drugs

108. Hirsh J, Raschke R: Heparin and low-molecular-weight heparin. Chest (Suppl) 26:188S, 2004.

109. Antman EM, Anbe DT, Armstrong PW, et al: ACC/AHA guidelines for the management of patients with ST-elevation myocardial infarction—executive summary. J Am Coll Cardiol 44:671, 2004.

110. Chew DP, Bhatt DL, Lincoff AM, et al: Defining the optimal activated clotting time during percutaneous coronary intervention: Aggregate results from 6 randomized trials. Circulation 103:961, 2001.

111. Notescu EA, Shapiro NL, Chevalier A, Amin AN: A pharmacologic overview of current and emerging anticoagulants. Cleve Clin J Med 72:S14, 2005.

112. Nenci GG: Low molecular weight heparins: Are they interchangeable? No. J Thromb Haemost 1:12, 2003.

113. Prandoni P: Low molecular weight heparins: Are they interchangable? Yes. J Thromb Haemost 1:10, 2003.

114. Ferguson JJ, Califf M, Antman EM, et al: Enoxaparin vs. unfractionated heparin in high-risk patients with non-ST-segment elevation acute coronary syndromes managed with an intended early invasive strategy: Primary results of the SYNERGY randomized trial. JAMA 292:45, 2004.

115. Ginsberg JS: Pharmacology of heparin-related compounds and coumarin derivatives. In Loscalzo J, Schafer AI (eds): Thrombosis and Hemorrhage. 3rd ed. Philadelphia, Lippincott Williams & Wilkins, 2003, pp 937-948.

116. Becker RC, Spencer FA, Gibson M, et al: Influence of patient characteristics and renal function on factor Xa inhibition pharmacokinetics and pharmacodynamics after enoxaparin administration in non-ST-segment elevation acute coronary syndromes. Am Heart J 143:753, 2002.

117. Arepally GM, Ortel TL: Heparin-induced thrombocytopenia. N Engl J Med 355:809, 2006.

118. Poncz M: Mechanistic basis of heparin-induced thrombocytopenia. Semin Thorac Cardiovasc Surg 17:73, 2005.

119. Warkentin TE, Kelton JG: Temporal aspects of heparin-induced thrombocytopenia. N Engl J Med 344:1286, 2001.

120. Warkentin TE, Kelton JG: Delayed-onset heparin-induced thrombocytopenia and thrombosis. Ann Intern Med 135:502, 2001.

121. Warkentin TE, Bernstein RA: Delayed-onset HIT and cerebral thrombosis after a single administration of unfractionated heparin. N Engl J Med 348:1067, 2003.

122. Greinacher A, Warkentin TE: Recognition, treatment, and prevention of heparin-induced thrombocytopenia: Review and update. Thromb Res 188:165, 2006.

123. Tardy B, Lecompte T, Boelhen F, et al: Predictive factors for thrombosis and major bleeding in an observational study in 181 patients with heparin-induced thrombocytopenia treated with lepirudin. Blood 108:1492, 2006.

124. Warkenten TE, Cook RJ, Marder VJ, et al: Anti-platelet factor 4/heparin antibodies in orthopedic surgery patients receiving antithrombotic prophylaxis with fondaparinux or enoxaparin. Blood 106:3791, 2005.

125. Warkentin TE: Nonhemorrhagic complications of antithrombotic therapy. In Spandorfer J, Konkle B, Merli G (eds): Management and Prevention of Thrombosis IN Primary Care. New York, Oxford University Press, 2001, pp 202-220.

126. Ginsberg J, Chan WS, Bates S, Kaatz S: Anticoagulation of pregnant women with mechanical heart valves. Arch Intern Med 163:694, 2003.

127. Freedman JE, Loscalzo J: New antithrombotic strategies. In Loscalzo J, Schafer AI (eds): Thrombosis and Hemorrhage. 3rd ed. Philadelphia, Lippincott Williams & Wilkins, 2003, pp 978-995.

128. Ibbotson T, Perry CM: Danaparoid: A review of its use in thromboembolic and coagulation disorders. Drugs 62:2283, 2002.

129. Bauersachs RM: Fondaparinux: An update on new study results. Eur J Clin Invest 35(Suppl 1):27, 2005.

130. Yusuf S, Mehta SR, Chrolauicius S, et al: Comparison of fondaparinux and enoxaparin in acute coronary syndromes. N Engl J Med 354:1425, 2006.

131. Yusuf S, Mehta SR, Chrolavicius S, et al: Effects of fondaparinux on mortality and reinfarction in patients with acute ST-segment elevation myocardial infarction: The OASIS-6 randomized trial. JAMA 295:1519, 2006.

132. Keller C, Matzdorff AC, Kemkes-Matthes B: Pharmacology of warfarin and clinical implications. Semin Thromb Hemost 25:13, 1999.

133. Ansell J, Hirsh J, Doller L, et al: The pharmacology and management of the vitamin K antagonists. Chest 126(Suppl):204S, 2004.

134. Kamali F, Dirmohamed M: The future prospects of pharmacogenetics in oral antecoagulation therapy. Br J Clin Pharmacol 61:746, 2006.

135. Schafer AI: Warfarin for venous thromboembolism—walking the dosing tightrope. N Engl J Med 348:1478, 2003.

136. Crowther MA, Douketis JD, Schnurr T, et al: Oral vitamin K lowers the international normalized ratio more rapidly than subcutaneous vitamin K in the treatment of warfarin-associated coagulopathy: A randomized, controlled trial. Ann Intern Med 137:251, 2002.

137. Deveras RAE, Kessler CM: Reversal of warfarin-induced excessive anticoagulation with recombinant human factor VIIa concentrate. Ann Intern Med 137:884, 2002.

138. Hanley JP: Warfarin reversal. J Clin Pathol 57:1132, 2004.

139. Heit JA: Mapping out the future in venous thromboembolism and acute coronary syndromes. Semin Thromb Hemost 28:33, 2002.

140. Bates SM, Wertz JI: The status of new anticoagulants. Am Heart J 134:3, 2006.

141. Kaplan KL, Francis CW: Direct thrombin inhibitors. Semin Hematol 39:187, 2002.

142. Lincoff AM, Bittl JA, Harrington RA, et al: Bivalirudin and provisional glycoprotein IIb/IIIa blockade compared with heparin and planned flycoprotein IIb/IIIa blockade during percutaneous coronary intervention: REPLACE-2 randomized trial. JAMA 289:853, 2003.

143. Stone GW, Bertrand M, Colombo A, et al: Acute catheterization and urgent intervention triage strategy (ACUITY) trial: Study design and rationale. Am Heart J 148:764, 2004.

144. Eikellboom JW, Mehta SR, Anand SS, et al: Adverse impact of bleeding on prognosis in patients with acute coronary syndromes. Circulation 114:774, 2006.

145. Antman EM: Should bivalirudin replace heparin during percutaneous coronary interventions? JAMA 289:903, 2003.

146. Wu CC, Teng CM: Comparison of the effects of PAR1 antagonists, PAR4 antagonists, and their combination on thrombin-induced human platelet activation. Eur J Pharmacol 546:142, 2006.

147. AH, Peters RJ, Bijsterveld NR, et al: Recombinant nematode anticoagulant protein CZ, an inhibitor of the tissue factor/factor VIIa complex, in patients undergoing elective coronary angioplasty. J Am Coll Cardiol 41:2147, 2003.

148. Bernard GR, Vincent J-L, Laterre P-F, et al: Efficacy and safety of recombinant human activated protein C for severe sepsis. N Engl J Med 344:699, 2001.

149. Leopold JA, Loscalzo J: Pharmacology of thrombolytic agents. In Loscalzo J, Schafer AI (eds): Thrombosis and Hemorrhage. 3rd ed. Philadelphia, Lippincott Williams & Wilkins, 2003, pp 949-977.

150. Al-Shwafi KA, de Meester A, Pirenne B, Col JJ: Comparative fibrinolytic activity of front-loaded alteplase and the single-bolus mutants tenecteplase and lanoteplase during treatment of acute myocardial infarction. Am Heart J 145:217, 2003.

151. Roth GJ: Antiplatelet therapy. In Colman RW, Marder VG, Clowes AW, et al (eds). Hemostasis and Thromboses. 5th ed. Philadelphia, Lippincott Williams & Wilkins, 2006, pp 1725-1738.

152. Mehta P: Aspirin in the prophylaxis of coronary artery disease. Curr Opin Cardiol 17:552, 2002.

153. Gurbel TA, Tantry US: Aspirin and clopidogrel resistance: Consideration and management. J Intervent Cardiol 19:439, 2006.

154. Schafer AI: Genetic and acquired determinants of individual variability of response to antiplatelet drugs. Circulation 108:910, 2003.

155. Antman EM, DeMets D, Loscalzo J: Cyclooxygenase inhibition and cardiovascular risk. Circulation 112:759, 2005.

156. Kearney PM, Baigent C, Godwin J, et al: Do selective cyclo-oxygenase-2 inhibitors and traditional non-steroidal anti-inflammatory drugs increase the risk of athero-thromboses? Meta-analysis of randomized trials. BMJ 332:1302, 2006.

157. FitzGerald GA, Patrono C: The coxibs, elective inhibitors of cyclooxygenase-2. N Engl J Med 345:433, 2001.

158. Catella-Lawson F, Reilly MP, Kapoor SC, et al: Cyclooxygenase inhibitors and the antiplatelet effects of aspirin. N Engl J Med 345:1809, 2001.

159. Matias-Guiu J, Ferro JM, Alverez-Sabin J, et al: Comparison of triflusal and aspirin for prevention of vascular events in patients after cerebral infarction: the TACIP Study: A randomized, double-blind, multicenter trial. Stroke 34:840, 2003.

160. Phillips DR, Conley PB, Sinha U, Andre P: Therapeutic approaches in arterial thromboses. J Thromb Haemost 3:1577, 2005.

161. Steinhubl SR, Berger PB, Mann JT 3rd, et al: Early and sustained dual oral antiplatelet therapy following percutaneous coronary intervention: A randomized controlled trial. JAMA 288:2411, 2002.

162. Steinhubl SR, Berger PB, Brennan DM, Topol EJ, CREDO Investigators: Optimal timing for the initiation of pre-treatment with 300 mg clopidogrel before percutaneous coronary intervention. J Am Coll Cardiol 47:939, 2006.

163. Kastrati A, von Beckerath N, Joost A, et al: Loading with 600 mg clopidogrel in patients with coronary artery disease with and without chronic clopidogrel therapy. Circulation 110:1916, 2004.

164. Patti G, Colonna G, Pasceri V, et al: Randomized trial of high loading dose of clopidogrel for reduction of periprocedural myocardial infarction in patients undergoing coronary intervention: Results from the ARMYDA-2 (Antiplatelet therapy for Reduction of MYocardial Damage during Angioplasty) study. Circulation 111:2099, 2005.

165. Smith SC Jr., Feldman TE, Hirshfeld JW Jr, et al: ACC/AHA SCAI 2005 guideline update for percutaneous coronary intervention—summary article: A report of the American College of Cardiology/American Heart Association Task Force on Practice Guidelines. Catheter Cardiovasc Interv 67:87, 2006.

166. Braunwald E, Antman EM, Beasley JW, et al: ACC/AHA guildline update for the management of patients with unstable angina and non-ST-segment elevationmyocardial infarction—2002: Summary article: A report of the American College of Cardiology/American Heart Association Task Force on Practice Guidelines (Committee on the Management of Patients with Unstable Angina). Circulation 106:1893, 2002.

167. Leon MB, Baum DS, Popma JJ, et al: A clinical trial comparing three antithrombotic drug regimens after coronary-artery stenting. N Engl J Med 339:1665, 1998.

168. ACTIVE Writing Group on behalf of the ACTIVE Investigators; Connnolly S, Pogue J, Hart R, et al: Clopidogrel plus aspirin versus oral anticoagulation for atrial fibrillation in the Atrial fibrillation Clopidogrel Trial with Irbesartan for prevention of Vascular Events (ACTIVE W): A randomized controlled trial. Lancet 367:1903, 2006.

169. Bhatt DL: Can clopidogrel and aspirn lower mortality in patients with acute myocardial infarction? Nat Clin Pract Cardiovasc Med 3:520, 2006.

170. Bhatt DL, Bertrand ME, Berger PB, et al: Meta-analysis of randomized and registry comparisons of ticlopidine after stenting. J Am Coll Cardiol 39:9, 2002.

171. Bennett CL, Connors JM, Carwile JM, et al: Thrombotic thrombocytopenic purpura associated with clopidogrel. N Engl J Med 342:1773, 2000.

172. Husted S, Emanuelsson H, Heptinstall S, et al: Pharmacodynamics, pharmacokinetics, and safety of the oral reversible P2Y12 antagonist AZD6140 with aspirin in patients with atherosclerosis: A double-blind comparison to clopidogrel with aspirin. Eur Heart J 27:1038, 2006.

173. Greenbaum AB, Grines CL, Bittl JA, et al: Initial experience with an intravenous P2Y12 platelet receptor antagonist in patients undergoing percutaneous coronary

CH 82

Hemostasis, Thrombosis, Fibrinolysis, and Cardiovascular Disease intervention: Results from a 2-part, phase II, multicenter, randomized, placebo- and active-controlled trial. Am Heart J 151:689.e1, 2006.

174. Lau WC, Gurbel PA, Watkins PB, et al: Contribution of hepatic cytochrome P450 3A4 metabolic activity to the phenomenon of clopidogrel resistance. Circulation 109:166, 2004.

175. Eikelboom JW, Hirsh J, Weitz JI, et al: Aspirin-resistant thromboxane biosynthesis and the risk of myocardial infarction, stroke, or cardiovascular death in patients at high risk for cardiovascular events. Circulation 105:1650, 2002.

176. Chen WH, Lee PY, Ng W, et al: Aspirin resistance is associated with a high incidence of myonecrosis after non-urgent percutaneous coronary intervention despite clopidogrel pretreatment. J Am Coll Cardiol 43:1122, 2004.

177. Matetzky S, Shenkman B, Guetta V, et al: Clopidogrel resistance is associated with increased risk of recurrent atherothrombotic events in patients with acute myocardial infarction. Circulation 109:3171, 2004.

178. Lev EI, Patel RT, Maresh KJ, et al: Aspirin and clopidogrel drug response in patients undergoing percutaneous coronary intervention: The role of dual drug resistance. J Am Coll Cardiol 47:27, 2006.

179. Halkes PH: Acetylsalicylic acid and dipyridamole offer better secondary protection than acetylsalicylic acid only following transient ischaemic attack or cerebral infarction of aterial origin; the European/Australasian Stroke Prevention in Reversible Ischaemic Trial (ESPRIT). Ned Tijdshr Geneeskd 150:1832, 2006.

180. De Schryver EL, Algra A, van Gijn J: Dipyridamole for preventing stroke and other vascular events in patients with vascular disease. Cochrane Database System Rev (1):CD001820, 2003.

181. Douglas JS Jr, Holmes DR Jr, Kereiakes DJ, et al: Coronary stent restenosis in patients treated with cilostazol. Circulation 112:2826, 2005.

182. Ge J, Han Y, Jiang H, et al; RACTS Trial Investigators. RACTS: A prospective randomized Antiplatelet trial of cilostazol versus ticlopidine in patients undergoing coronary stenting: Long-term clinical and angiographic outcome. J Cardiovasc Pharmacol 46:162, 2005.

183. Plow EF, Cierniewski CS, Xiao Z et al: Alpha IIb beta3 and its antagonism at the new millennium. Thromb Haemost 86:34, 2001.

184. Mascelli MA, Lance ET, Damaraju L, et al: Pharmacodynamic profile of short-term abciximab treatment demonstrated prolonged platelet inhibition with gradual recovery from GP IIb/IIIa receptor blockade. Circulation 97:1680, 1998.

185. Coller BS. Potential non-glycoprotein IIb/IIIa effects of abciximab. Am Heart J 138(1 Pt 2):S1-S5, 1999.

186. Simon DI, Xu H, Ortlepp S, et al: 7E3 monoclonal antibody directed against the platelet glycoprotein IIb/IIIa cross-reacts with the leukocyte integrin Mac-1 and blocks adhesion to fibrinogen and ICAM-1. Arterioscler Thromb Vasc Biol 17:528, 1997.

187. Kleiman NS: GP IIb/IIIa antagonists. Clinical experience and potential uses in cardiology. Drugs R D 1:361, 1999.

188. Newby LK, Califf RM, White HD, et al: The failure of orally administred glycoprotein IIb/IIIa inhibitors to prevent recurrent cardiac events. Am J Med 112:647, 2002.

189. Peter K, Bode C: Procoagulant activities of glycoprotein IIb/IIIa receptor blockers. In Sasahara AA, Loscalzo J (eds): New Therapeutic Agents in Thrombosis and Thrombolysis. 2nd ed. New York, Marcel Dekker, 2003, pp 401-411.

190. Steinhubl SR: Antiplatelet agents in cardiology: The choice of therapy. Ann Thorac Surg 70(Suppl 2):S3, 2000.

191. Giugliano RP, Roe MT, Harrington RA, et al; INTEGRITI Investigators: Combination reperfusion therapy with eptifibatide and reduced-dose tenecteplase for ST-elevation myocardial infarction: Results of the integrilin and tenecteplase in acute myocardial infarction (INTEGRITI) Phase II Angiographic Trial. J Am Coll Cardiol 41:1251, 2003.

192. Kastrati A, Mehilli J. Schlotterbeck K, et al; Bavarian Reperfusion Alternatives Evaluation (BRAVE) Study Investigators: Early administration of reteplase plus abciximab versus. abciximab alone in patients with acute myocardial infarction referred for percutaneous coronary intervention: a randomized controlled trial. JAMA 291:947, 2004.

193. Dasgupta H, Blankenship JC, Wood GC, et al: Thrombocytopenia complicating treatment with intravenous glycoprotein IIb/IIIa receptor inhibitors: A pooled analysis. Am Heart J 140:206, 2000.

194. Berkowitz SD, Harrington RA, Rund MM, Tcheng JE: Acute profound thrombocytopenia after C7E3 Fab (abciximab) therapy. Circulation 95:809, 1997.

195. Merlini PA, Rossi M, Menozzi A, et al: Thrombocytopenia caused by abciximab or tirofiban and its association with clinical outcome in patients undergoing coronary stenting. Circulation 109:2203, 2004.

196. Tcheng JE, Kereiakes DJ, Lincoff AM, et al: Abciximab readministration: Results of the ReoPro Readministration Registry. Circulation 104:870, 2001.

CHAPTER 83

Rheumatic Fever

B. Soma Raju and Zoltan G. Turi

Epidemiology, 2079
Decline in Rheumatic Fever, 2079

Evaluation, 2081
Diagnosis, 2081
    Physical Examination, 2082
    Echocardiography, 2083
Laboratory Findings, 2084

Treatment, 2085
Therapeutic Modalities, 2085

Future Directions, 2086

Classic Reading, 2086

References, 2086

Rheumatic fever (RF) is an autoimmune disorder that remains incompletely characterized in regard to its basic elements—cause, pathophysiology, diagnosis, and treatment—despite evidence of its existence dating to at least the 1600s, when Sydenham described several of its classic features. Although there have been substantial advances in immunological studies, a number of issues confound accurate diagnosis of the disease—hence, major modifications or review of the Jones criteria have occurred four times in the past six decades (Fig. 83-1). The classic understanding that the disease is a postsuppurative streptococcal pharyngitis cascade, leading variably to arthritis, chorea, dermal manifestations and, most importantly, carditis, has withstood challenge. Immunological studies have confirmed the presence of epitopes on the bacterial surface that mimic cardiac myosin, as well as antigens found in valve, skin, joint, and brain tissue, and account for the immunological cross-reactive attack characteristic of RF. Because no single diagnostic tool or laboratory test exists, RF is diagnosed on the basis of a composite of clinical criteria, without firm consensus on sensitivity, specificity, or accuracy.

The sequelae of carditis account for most of the morbidity and virtually all the mortality associated with RF. As a cause of heart disease in adults, RF has declined dramatically in industrialized nations, albeit with episodic outbreaks, and is generally declining in developing countries as well. Rheumatic heart disease (RHD) once accounted for nearly half the admissions for heart disease around the world and remains common in developing nations, but accounts for less than 1 percent of cardiac admissions in industrialized states. The primary consequences of RF, rheumatic mitral and aortic valve disease in adults, are declining worldwide, even in developing countries where the disease remains prevalent. The diagnostic and treatment algorithms are still largely based on descriptive series and expert opinion panels, with relatively few randomized controlled trials comparing treatment modalities. Because failure to diagnose RF results in lack of secondary prophylaxis to prevent RHD, increasing attention is being focused on improving sensitivity of diagnosis in areas where the disease is endemic.

EPIDEMIOLOGY

After human immunodeficiency virus (HIV), tuberculosis, and malaria, group A streptococcus has a global mortality range comparable to that of the pathogens causing hepatitis, measles, and *Haemophilus* influenza.[1] *Streptococcus pyogenes* is responsible for a spectrum of disease, ranging from pharyngitis to glomerulonephritis, necrotizing fasciitis. and toxic shock syndrome. However, suppurative pharyngitis is the only well-established prequel to acute RF. It was estimated in 2005 that approximately 15.6 million people had RF or RHD, with sub-Saharan Africa and South Central Asia accounting for the majority of cases.[1]

Given the causal association between group A beta-hemolytic streptococci (GABHS) and RF, their epidemiology also appears to be linked. Whereas most pharyngitis (80 percent) is viral in cause, GABHS is isolated in up to 75 percent of cases from children with symptoms of severe bacterial pharyngitis. Antistreptolysin O (ASLO) titers more than 200 Todd units occur in up to 50 percent of asymptomatic children in the prime age group for RF, 6 to 15 years, reflecting in part the frequent occurrence (estimated to be once yearly) of pharyngitis in this age group, approximately 15 to 20 percent of which is caused by GABHS.[2] RF in children younger than age 5 years is uncommon. Recurrence occurs most commonly in adolescents and young adults, and is rare beyond age 34.[3] Data from the early antibiotic era have suggested that from 0.3 to 3 percent of those with untreated GABHS pharyngitis develop acute RF. There is no clear gender, race, or geographic predisposition to the development of RF, although certain end-organ manifestations, such as postpubertal chorea and the development of mitral stenosis, are more common in females. GABHS is present in 10 to 30 percent of asymptomatic individuals in the prime RF age groups in the United States, and higher in many countries. A history of pharyngitis has been reported for most cases of acute RF in most series, but only in 30 percent of cases in a more recent outbreak in the United States. The carrier state, defined by absence of clinical history or rise in antibody titers, is not associated with occurrence of acute RF.

Decline in Rheumatic Fever

The decline in incidence of RF began prior to the modern antibiotic era, and accelerated with the introduction of penicillin. The possible explanations for the preantibiotic era decline include improvement in environmental factors, decrease in rheumatogenicity of streptococcal strains, and improved specificity in diagnosis, likely influenced by the introduction of the Jones criteria, prior to which children with minor manifestations such as isolated arthralgias were frequently assigned a diagnosis of RF. The fact that mortality from acute carditis also decreased in the preantibiotic era suggests that the virulence of rheumatogenic strains has decreased as well. Figure 83-2 demonstrates the decreasing mortality associated with RF in the United States, along with milestones in its diagnosis and management.

The incidence of RF in industrialized states is now estimated as less than 1/100,000 people, whereas rates higher than 100 per 100,000 people continue to be seen in endemic areas. Both the diagnosis and treatment of RF involve special

2080 considerations in poorer nations, where RHD remains the main cause of acquired heart disease, especially in the first three decades of life. Socioeconomic, epidemiologic, cultural, and other factors influence applicability of some of the standard algorithms for diagnosis and management in

these countries. The prevalence of RHD follows a similar pattern as RF. WHO statistics described 39.5 percent of New England cardiac admissions as related to RHD in 1928 and 23.5 percent in 1951. By the 1990s, RHD accounted for less than 0.5 percent of primary discharge diagnoses in the United States. In contrast, rates comparable to those of the 1950s have been sustained in the poorest nations, as well as in isolated subpopulations such as Australian aborigines. Crowding, including rampant population growth, inadequate medical facilities, lack of antibiotics for initial therapy of pharyngitis and for secondary prevention after RF, and lack of medical personnel have sustained the prevalence of RF and RHD. Nevertheless, there is a general trend in most developing nations toward declining frequency of the disease,[4] in part because of better availability of basic health care, associated in many cases with over-the-counter dispensing of antibiotics.

The outbreaks of RF in the United States in the 1980s prompted intensive investigation of the disease in an industrialized nation. RF occurred in areas without the classic risk factors attributed to susceptible populations and appears to have been triggered by the reappearance of rheumatogenic strains of *S. pyogenes.*

PATHOBIOLOGY

The elements of the classic triad of agent, host, and environment all play major roles in the pathogenesis of RF. The agent responsible, GABHS, has more than 100 subtypes defined by M-protein surface molecules. Specific M-protein subtypes appear to be rheumatogenic, typically mucoid, strains that adhere well to pharyngeal tissue. The antiphagocytic properties of M protein allow persistence of bacteria in tissues for up to 2 weeks, until specific antibodies are created. M-protein, *N*-acetylglucosamine, and several other epitopes mimic myocardium (myosin and tropomyosin), heart valves (laminin), synovia (vimentin), skin (keratin), and subthalamic and caudate nuclei in the brain (lysogangliosides). Superantigenic activity triggered by M-protein fragments as well as streptococcal toxins have also been implicated in B-cell– and T-cell–mediated autoimmune reactivity. T cells activated against myosin and bacterial epitopes react to valve tissue with as yet incompletely defined host factors that may enhance the inflammatory response in heart valves.[5] Considerable heterogeneity exists in the epitopes associated with RF in different geographic areas, as well as in the genes that encode for M proteins—the chromosomal emm sequence types that have been associated with GABHS pharyngitis and RF. Other properties of GABHS, such as production of serum opacity factor, differentiate strains associated with RF from those associated with glomerulonephritis. Patients who develop RF appear to manifest a hyperimmune response to GABHS, and the level of the immune response appears to correlate with the severity of RF manifestations. The decline in incidence of RF has paralleled the decrease in rheumatogenic M-protein strains isolated from the throats of children with pharyngitis during the past for decades.[6] whereas conversely, the reappearance of RF in the United States has been associated with an increase in mucoid strains known to be rheumatogenic.[7]

The risk of developing RF is associated with the extent of the immune response to the pharyngitis, genetic susceptibility, and prior history of RF. The highest rate of RF after untreated GABHS pharyngitis appears to be in those who have had previous RF, as high as 50 percent, compared to the 3 percent or lower rate in patients without prior RF, providing a strong mandate for long-term secondary prophylaxis antibiotic therapy. The evidence that hosts are genetically predisposed to developing RF is significant, with

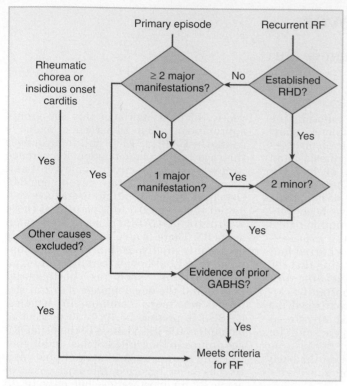

FIGURE 83–1 Algorithm for diagnosis of acute rheumatic fever (RF), incorporating the 1992 revision of the Jones criteria and the World Health Organization (WHO) expert consultation report (2002-2003).[2] The WHO modifications incorporated in the flowchart are more sensitive and less specific than those incorporated in the American Heart Association criteria. GABHS = group A beta-hemolytic streptococci; RHD = rheumatic heart disease.

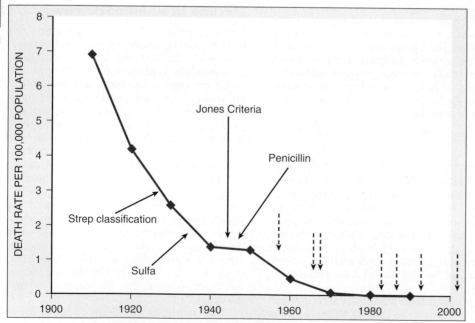

FIGURE 83–2 Decline in mortality from rheumatic fever in the United States during the 20th century. Note that the decline began well before the availability of penicillin. Dashed arrows mark the multiple modifications or revisions of the Jones Criteria or WHO expert opinion reviews and recommendations. *(Modified from Gordis L: The virtual disappearance of rheumatic fever in the United States: Lessons in the rise and fall of disease. T. Duckett Jones memorial lecture. Circulation 72:1155, 1985.)*

CH 83

varying human leukocyte antigen (HLA) class II alleles, as well as various other genetic markers, being identified in populations known to be susceptible. The expression of a B-cell alloantigen, D8/17, appears to be both sensitive and specific in some endemic areas for screening patients with RF, as well as patients with prior RF and first-degree relatives; the antibody binds to M protein and to human cardiac tissue.[8] As with HLA class II allele typing, this finding is not consistent across populations with RHD.

Finally, environmental elements correlate strongly with development of RF. Where epidemic pharyngitis has been documented, such as in military barracks prior to antibiotic availability, approximately 3 percent developed RF. With the element of overcrowding removed, during the same period, the RF rate was approximately 1/10th as common. It has been hypothesized that this is caused by the increased virulence of strains associated with rapid transmission across multiple hosts.

PATHOLOGY

In patients dying of rheumatic carditis, autopsy findings have demonstrated verrucous vegetations on the valve leaflets, along with extensive inflammation and edema. In the exudative phase, during the first few weeks after the onset of RF, fibrinoid degeneration of collagen is noted. Inflammation is seen in left ventricular endocardium, with lymphocytic, macrophage and, in a minority of cases, plasma cell, polymorphonuclear leukocyte, eosinophil, and mast cell infiltration. In the proliferative phase, from 1 to 6 months after the onset of RF, Aschoff bodies, granulomatous lesions pathognomonic for rheumatic carditis, are seen, and can be found in valve tissue as well as endocardium, myocardium, and pericardium. Although Aschoff bodies can be demonstrated as early as the second week of onset of RF, they may be present chronically without evidence of ongoing carditis. Rheumatic arthritis is manifest by edema, lymphocytic and polymorphonuclear infiltration, and fibrinoid lesions that resolve. In patients with chorea, inflammatory changes have been noted in the cerebral cortex, cerebellum, and basal ganglia.

EVALUATION

Diagnosis

Acute RF (ARF) occurs after GABHS pharyngitis, and probably not after other infections caused by *S. pyogenes*. The postsuppurative pharyngitis phase is frequently followed by migratory polyarthritis and carditis, the most common manifestations of ARF, typically within the first 2 to 3 weeks after infection, in contrast with Sydenham chorea, which is less frequent and occurs 1 to 6 months later. The cutaneous manifestations, erythema marginatum, and subcutaneous nodules are far less common, typically do not occur in isolation, appear within the first few weeks in the case of the former, and after 1 month or more for the latter.

Jones Criteria

Prior to the introduction of the Jones criteria in 1944, RF diagnosis was based on a wide and inconsistent range of symptoms, including minor arthralgias, fevers, and abdominal pain, resulting in substantial overdiagnosis. Because RF was the major cause of mortality in children and adolescents, there was a substantial need for accurate diagnosis to assess disease incidence, patient management algorithms, and efficacy of treatment. Thus, specificity was emphasized and has remained the prevailing focus of multiple revisions. It should be noted that the Jones criteria generally, and the revisions specifically, have been based more on expert consensus than on clinical trials. The major criteria—carditis, polyarthritis, chorea, erythema marginatum and subcutaneous nodules—have been unchanged since the first modification in 1956. Minor criteria include the clinical findings of arthralgia and fever and laboratory findings of elevated acute-phase reactants. Evidence of a prior group A streptococcal infection, either positive throat culture or streptococcal antigen test, or elevated or rising streptococcal antibody titer has been incorporated since 1965 as an *essential* criterion for the diagnosis of ARF. Although neither evidence of GABHS presence in the pharynx nor elevated or rising antibody titers is specific for an acute attack of GABHS pharyngitis, the requirement adds to the overall specificity of the Jones criteria. The more recent modifications have sought increased specificity by emphasizing arthritis over arthralgia and by eliminating various elements from the minor criteria, such as epistaxis, abdominal and precordial pain, pulmonary findings, prolonged PR interval, anemia, and elevated white counts, all of which are nonspecific for acute RF. The original revisions emphasized evidence of prior RF, because in that susceptible group the possibility of recurrence is much more likely. With the 1992 revision, emphasis has shifted to the use of the guidelines to diagnose an *initial* attack of RF. The 2004 WHO report (see Fig. 83-1) addressed the issue of recurrent RF, in particular for patients with established RHD, and suggested algorithms for increasing the overall sensitivity of the diagnosis.[2] Whereas two major or one major and two minor manifestations plus evidence of preceding GABHS infection are required for a primary episode of RF or recurrent RF without established RHD, in the setting of RHD, two minor criteria are deemed to be sufficient to make the diagnosis with reasonable specificity if there is evidence of recent streptococcal infection. The 1992 Jones criteria listed two exceptions to the requirement that evidence for antecedent GABHS infection be established—chorea and low-grade carditis. Because of the long latency period before symptoms of chorea occur, laboratory evidence may be absent, as it may be in the chronic low-grade carditis that follows many cases of RF.

The tradeoff in sensitivity for specificity warns against the use of a single finding, such as fever, monoarthritis, arthralgia, or elevation of the erythrocyte sedimentation rate (ESR) or C-reactive protein (CRP) level to make the diagnosis of RF.[9,10] However, in countries where the disease is prevalent, laboratory data may not be available, and clinical findings such as monoarthritis or polyarthralgias may be used in a diagnosis of "probable rheumatic fever" in vulnerable age groups where a number of minor manifestations are present, in particular if there is evidence of antecedent GABHS infection. Some of these patients will subsequently manifest evidence of having had RF. The importance of such a controversial "probable" category is the suspicion raised for possible subsequent development of carditis, with the benefits of serial follow-up examinations and, in particular, the administration of chronic secondary antibiotic prophylaxis. The most recent guidelines continue to be questioned in developing countries, where patient presentation may be too late for some elements of the Jones criteria to be observed or where over-the-counter treatment with antiinflammatory or antibiotic agents may obscure elements of the criteria. Both the Jones and WHO criteria are deemed too insensitive by some practitioners caring for patients in endemic areas; they are concerned about inadequate secondary prophylaxis in patients who do not meet these criteria but who have a high incidence of subsequent RHD.

A number of clinical conditions mimic acute RF (Table 83-1). In addition, forme frustes of arthritis and chorea, both associated with GABHS infections, have been described (see later). Special considerations apply if a first attack of RF occurs in adulthood. In this setting, arthritis dominates, with a lower incidence of carditis; the other major manifestations are rare. Although the Jones criteria can be met, they become less specific, and other causes need to be excluded.

TABLE 83–1	Differential Diagnosis of Rheumatic Arthritis, Carditis, and Chorea

Polyarthritis
Infectious
  Staphylococcus, gonococcus
  Endocarditis
  Lyme disease
  Mycobacterial, fungal
  Viral
Reactive
  Poststreptococcal
  Enteric infection
  Reiter syndrome
  Inflammatory bowel
Connective tissue disease
  Rheumatoid arthritis
  Systemic lupus
  Systemic vasculitis
Miscellaneous
  Gout
  Leukemia, lymphoma
  Sarcoidosis
  Cancer
  Familial Mediterranean fever
  Henoch-Schönlein purpura
  Mucocutaneous disorders
  "Growth pains" in children
  Serum sickness

Carditis
Murmur
  Physiological murmur
  Mitral valve prolapse
  Bicuspid aortic valve
  Anemia
  Straight back syndrome

Congenital heart disease
  Ventricular septal defect
  Subvalvular aortic stenosis
  Primum atrial septal defect
Viral myocarditis
Endocarditis
Pericarditis

Chorea
Familial chorea—Huntington
Hormone-induced
  Oral contraceptives
  Pregnancy
Drug-induced
  Anticonvulsants
  Antidepressants
  Metoclopramide
Connective tissue
  Systemic lupus
  Periarteritis
Lyme disease
Wilson disease
Atypical seizures
Hyperthyroidism
Hypoparathyroidism
Tourette syndrome
PANDAs

PANDAS = **p**ediatric **a**utoimmune **n**europsychiatric **d**isorders **a**ssociated with streptococcal infection.

Modified from Pinals RS: Polyarthritis and fever. N Engl J Med 330:769, 1994; Kothari SS: Active rheumatic carditis. *In* Narula J, Virman R, Srinath Reddy K, Tandon R (eds): Rheumatic Fever. Washington, DC, American Registry of Pathology, Armed Forces Institute of Pathology, 1999, p 265; and Swedo SE: Sydenham's chorea: a model for childhood autoimmune neuropsychiatric disorders. JAMA 272:1788, 1994.

CH 83

Carditis

Rheumatic carditis is associated with virtually all the major sequelae of RF, including mortality. Approximately 40 to 60 percent of RF episodes result in RHD.[1] Carditis typically manifests as valvulitis, detected by the presence of mitral regurgitation (MR) or, less commonly, aortic regurgitation on auscultation. It can be responsible for acute and chronic myocardial dysfunction and acute, although not chronic, pericardial disease. An important consideration is that neither myocarditis nor pericarditis can be expected to occur in the absence of valvulitis and, if evidence of valvular involvement is not present, alternate nonrheumatic causes must be considered.

PHYSICAL EXAMINATION

There are a number of hallmarks of acute carditis noted on physical examination of a patient with an initial episode of RF. There may be a prominent left ventricular (LV) impulse secondary to cardiac enlargement but not as localized as with chronic MR. Because of recent onset, there is usually at most only mild LV dilation. Sinus tachycardia is common, but atrial fibrillation is rare. The first heart sound may vary from normal to diminished intensity, either because of MR, prolonged PR interval, or both. The second heart sound is normally or widely or variably split, depending on the degree of the MR. The pulmonary component of the second sound is accentuated with the presence of pulmonary hypertension caused by severe MR. Although classically the aortic second sound is diminished in chronic aortic insufficiency, in acute RF it is usually normal, even with significant aortic regurgitation, because mobility of the aortic valve is not affected early. A third heart sound is common, and cannot be used as a marker for severity of MR, because children frequently have an S_3 heart sound without associated pathology. The soft, blowing, pansystolic murmur of MR is a hallmark of carditis in RF. The murmur is best heard at the apex and selectively conducted to the axilla and back; the latter suggests severe MR. A nonpansystolic murmur may occur when MR is mild, although it retains its high-frequency, soft, blowing character, which distinguishes it from the physiological murmurs seen in children. The apical diastolic murmur of Carey Coombs is often related to the severity of MR, but is also associated with flow disturbances caused by mitral valve deformity secondary to valvulitis, in addition to the increased flow in diastole. The murmur is typically middiastolic as opposed to the late diastolic accentuation seen with mitral stenosis. The aortic valve is involved in a minority of cases (up to 40 percent) and is associated with an early diastolic murmur of aortic regurgitation best heard along the base and left sternal border. Aortic insufficiency in the absence of MR is uncommon. A murmur of functional tricuspid regurgitation may occur in the setting of severe heart failure, pulmonary hypertension, and right ventricular dilation, with associated neck vein distention and other hallmarks of tricuspid insufficiency.

The severity of left ventricular dysfunction, even in the acute setting, appears to correlate with the extent of valvulitis rather than with any myocardial injury. Rheumatic myocarditis, in the setting of preserved LV function, is not associated with the troponin level elevation seen in viral myocarditides.[11] Both echocardiographic data and postmortem pathology findings are consistent with severe heart failure in acute RF, being secondary to altered myocardial mechanics caused by MR rather than secondary to myocarditis. Traditionally, the diagnosis has been made on the basis of auscultation of mitral or, less commonly, aortic insufficiency in the setting of heart failure, with cardiomegaly in the most severe cases. Severe MR is most commonly associated with the worst prognosis—acute and sometimes refractory and fatal heart failure. This subgroup is most likely to develop significant chronic RHD, with an incidence as high as 90 percent. There is a linear relationship between the severity of MR during the first episode of RF and subsequent RHD.

Because the valvulitis can be transient, repeated auscultation is appropriate. Whereas acute carditis may result in fulminant pulmonary edema, in a significant percentage of patients the carditis is subclinical, setting the stage for scarring of the mitral or aortic valve apparatus with manifestations occurring years or decades later. Rheumatic tricuspid disease is uncommon, and pulmonic valve disease rare. Although left ventricular dysfunction secondary to chronic valvulitis is thought to account for the majority of myocardial dysfunction seen, there is a characteristic regional wall motion abnormality seen in patients, primarily in the inferobasal segment of the heart adjacent to the mitral valve. The valvulitis typically involves the leaflets, but extends into the submitral apparatus in a significant percentage of cases. In the setting of LV dysfunction or pericarditis without valvular involvement, the consensus is that the pathology is unlikely to be secondary to RF. Because pericarditis alone is not diagnostic of rheumatic carditis, detection of an associated valvular lesion is important. Pericardial involvement is usually associated with significant valvulitis and may result in an effusion, but large effusions, chronic constriction, or tamponade are rare. Tachycardia and various arrhythmias are nonspecific findings. The use of endomyocardial biopsy for the diagnosis of rheumatic carditis has been explored but has not provided sufficient additional diagnostic information to warrant its use. The use of radionuclide tracers for the detection of inflammation has also not been of additional diagnostic benefit.

Recurrent carditis occurs with very high frequency in subsequent episodes of RF. Pericarditis, new cardiac murmurs, and increase in cardiac silhouette size have been the traditional basis for a diagnosis of recurrent or "mimetic" carditis. Patients with prior rheumatic carditis are predisposed to bacterial endocarditis and the greater exposure to infection in the population already susceptible to RF, because of crowding and nonhygienic conditions, makes excluding endocarditis in patients with fever and heart murmurs especially important, particularly when other major Jones criteria are absent.

ECHOCARDIOGRAPHY

Several studies have used echocardiography as a more sensitive tool than auscultation to detect valve pathology. Primarily mitral but occasional aortic insufficiency has been diagnosed in a minority of putative RF patients in whom characteristic murmurs were not heard, although this finding has not been uniform. Because echocardiographic-Doppler findings in the absence of auscultatable murmurs are not specific for rheumatic valvulitis, the use of echocardiography alone to justify a diagnosis of carditis for this major Jones criterion is a subject of controversy. Despite the development of criteria to differentiate pathological from functional regurgitation, including posterior direction of the mitral jet, holosystolic flow, significant turbulence in the MR jet, and MR seen in orthogonal planes, in general the inclusion of patients with "silent carditis" or "echocarditis" has been thought to result in overdiagnosis. MR in particular is seen in other febrile illnesses. Longitudinal studies of patients with carditis by echoardiography but not physical examination may shed light on the long-term implications of "silent carditis."

There is considerable inconsistency in the literature regarding the echocardiographic findings characteristic of acute rheumatic carditis. Mitral insufficiency is the most common finding, associated subsequently (but not acutely) with restricted leaflet motion rather than prolapse and with ventricular but not annular dilation. When chordal rupture occurs, however, both flail leaflets and prolapse *are* seen. Nodular lesions are seen in a significant minority (25 percent). Although it has been suggested that echocardiography may be helpful in settings such as concomitant pericarditis, in which auscultation may be difficult, MR is usually moderate or severe when pericarditis is secondary to RF and the murmur is detectable, despite a friction rub, which is frequently intermittent. Echocardiography *is* useful for confirming the findings on auscultation, excluding nonrheumatic causes (e.g., physiological murmurs or congenital heart disease), and sequential follow-up of valvular insufficiency, cardiac chamber size, pulmonary hypertension, valve thickening, and left ventricular systolic function (see Chaps 14 and 62).

Arthritis

Polyarthritis is the most frequent manifestation of RF, occurring in up to 75 percent of patients with acute symptoms. It is typically very painful, migratory, and limited to the major joints of the arms and legs. It is the earliest manifestation after streptococcal pharyngitis, occurring within 2 to 3 weeks after onset of RF, and may be the only clinically apparent manifestation in one third to half of patients. The arthritis is self-limited, with symptoms and findings varying from minor arthralgias to severe arthritis with erythema, warmth, and swelling. Joint aspiration may reveal moderate leukocytosis. A common characteristic is tenderness out of proportion to other findings. During the migratory phase, multiple joints can be involved in different phases of inception and resolution. Inflammation in individual joints lasts 1 to 2 weeks and the polyarthritis as a whole resolves in 1 month or less. Chronic sequelae and disability do not appear to occur, with the rare exception of Jaccoud arthropathy, an unusual periarticular fibrosis that is not specific for RF. The arthritis phase frequently overlaps with the onset of carditis, and the two manifestations appear to be inversely related in severity—patients with severe arthritis appear to have less severe manifestations of carditis, and vice versa. Considerable debate has taken place over the differing patterns of joint manifestations in industrialized and developing countries, and whether arthralgias or single-joint arthritis should be made a major criterion in areas where the diagnosis may otherwise be missed, largely because of late presentation. In general, because it resolves completely, the long-term importance of the arthritis of RF is that it draws attention to the presence of carditis that might otherwise be missed in asymptomatic individuals.

A number of conditions resemble the migratory polyarthritis of RF (see Table 83-1). In general, failure of symptoms to respond to salicylates suggests nonrheumatic arthritis. In contrast, if salicylates are given early in the course, they may blunt the full appearance of the syndrome, resulting in monoarthritis. Other forms of infectious arthritis, including Lyme disease, other autoimmune disorders, and acute leukemia can present with polyarthritis, ironically including a serum sickness syndrome induced by penicillin. Bacterial endocarditis with joint involvement is especially important to consider. One syndrome, poststreptococcal reactive arthritis, occurs early after streptococcal pharyngitis without other manifestations of RF, may affect the small joints of the upper extremities, is much less responsive to salicylates, and lasts for a longer period. These patients should be monitored for the development of RHD and secondary prophylaxis is recommended (Fig. 83-3). Arthritis in the absence of an elevated ASLO titer is unlikely to be related to RF.

Chorea

Sydenham chorea manifests as involuntary, irregular movements, fibrillatory muscle movements of the tongue, characteristic spooning with external rotation of the hands, and abolition of the movements with sleep. This major component of the Jones criteria is a uniquely delayed manifestation of ARF, with a wide range in reported incidence between 5 and 35 percent, a latency period of 1 to 7 months, and choreiform manifestations that may last for months, occasionally years. Importantly, there is a substantial risk of subsequent RHD in these patients, found in one study to be more than 50 percent.[3] Although this particular type of chorea is the classic neurological manifestation of RF, attention has focused on various other neurological and psychological manifestations of the disease, including short- and long-term emotional lability, obsessive-compulsive behavior, and other central nervous manifestations such as seizures and chronic migraine. This too appears to be immunologically mediated, with evidence of antibodies to brain tissue.[12] Whereas Sydenham chorea does not result in residual neurological deficits per se, psychiatric disturbances occur in a small but significant number of patients in the decades following the chorea. Recurrences are common. Because of the late manifestation of chorea, laboratory evidence of prior streptococcal infection is far less common than with carditis or arthritis. Thus, consideration of the differential diagnosis is particularly relevant. This includes seizures, connective tissue disorders, other types of chorea, and toxic reactions to various drugs, including oral contraceptives. Like arthritis, chorea can be a manifestation of Lyme disease. A syndrome of *p*ediatric *a*utoimmune *n*europsychiatric *d*isorders *a*ssociated with *s*treptococcal infections (PANDAS), like poststreptococcal reactive arthritis, has a temporal relationship to GABHS infection, but is not associated with other features of RF.[13] Immunological cross-reactivity between basal ganglia and GABHS epitopes has been hypothesized as the mechanism.

Cutaneous Manifestations

Both major cutaneous criteria of RF typically occur in single-digit percentage rates. Subcutaneous nodules typically occur in patients with moderate to severe rheumatic carditis and, like other noncardiac manifestations, resolve completely. They occur several weeks after the onset of cardiac findings, consist of firm nodules found over major joints and bony prominences, and are asymptomatic, sometimes evanescent, typi-

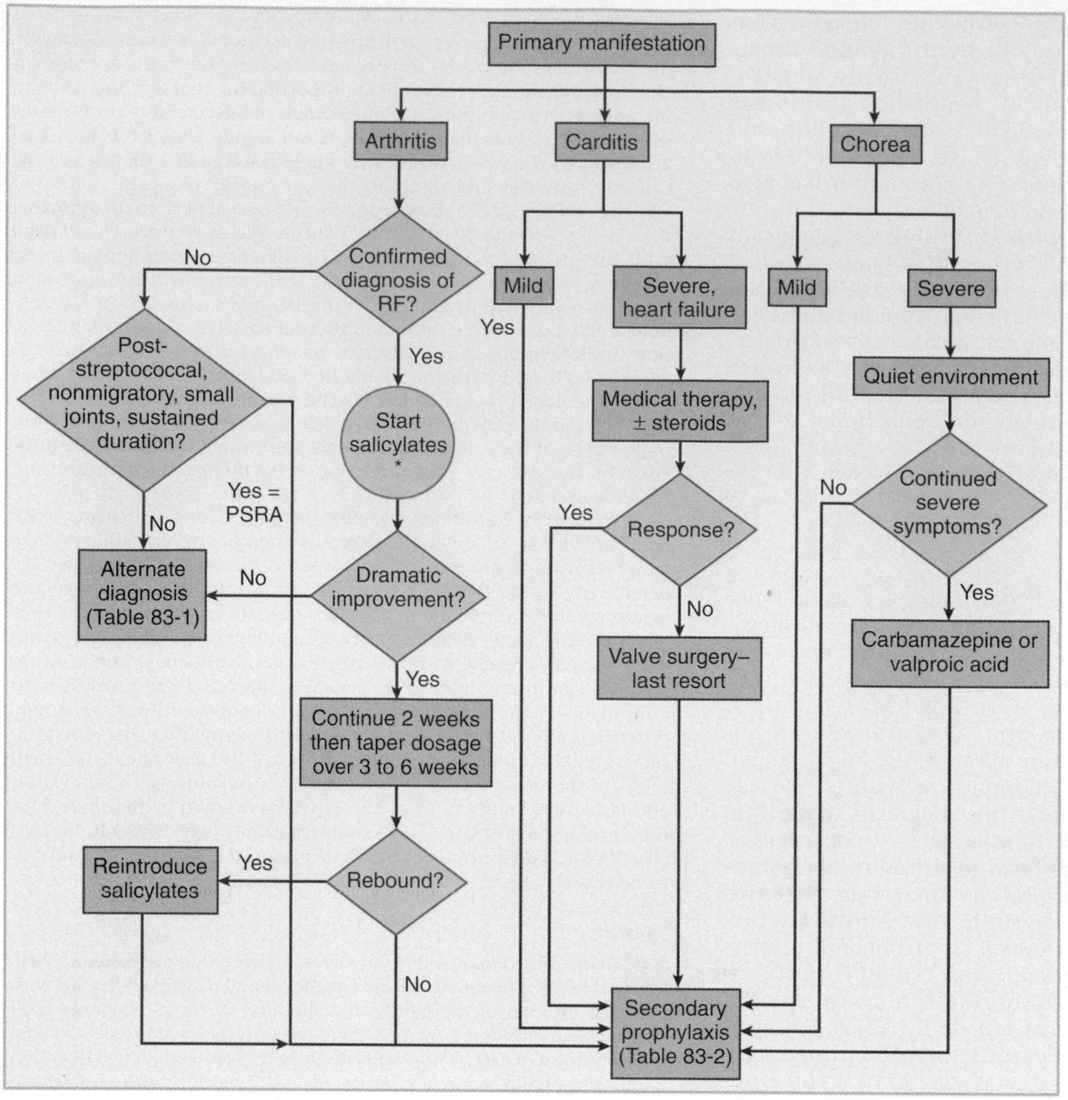

FIGURE 83–3 Algorithm for management of rheumatic fever (RF) and its primary manifestations. *Salicylates are also indicated for fever and arthralgia, but there is no evidence of effectiveness for carditis or chorea. PSRA = poststreptococcal reactive arthritis. *(Modified from Thatai D, Turi ZG: Current guidelines for the treatment of patients with rheumatic fever. Drug 57:545, 1999.)*

cally resolving within weeks to 1 or 2 months. They are not diagnostic of RF and can be seen with other autoimmune disorders. Similarly, erythema marginatum typically occurs in conjunction with carditis, although with a milder course and, unlike subcutaneous nodules, may last for months or years. It tends to occur over the trunk or proximal extremities, early in the course of RF. Erythema marginatum is also not specific for RF and occurs with sepsis and drug reactions, among other settings. It also resembles the cutaneous findings seen in juvenile rheumatoid arthritis and Lyme disease.

Laboratory Findings

Both ESR and CRP are significantly elevated in RF, and may remain so for months. They are reliable markers for the severity of the autoimmune response and inflammatory activity associated with arthritis and carditis, and their time course generally correlates with activity of the disease, although some masking may be induced by anti-inflammatory agents. Because of the late onset of chorea, the acute-phase reactants, like the anti-GABHS titers, are frequently no longer elevated. CRP levels, unlike ESR, are not influenced by comorbidities such as anemia and congestive heart failure.

The electrocardiographic findings of RF include sinus arrhythmias, with tachycardia related to fever, pericarditis,

or myocarditis. However, bradycardia occurs in a significant minority of cases. Conduction disturbances have been described in 30 percent or more of patients, typically first-degree AV block, but including small numbers with second- or third-degree block. AV block is not specific for valvular involvement or for rheumatic carditis. When associated with RF, heart block is secondary to inflammation of periatrioventricular nodal tissues, with possibly increased vagal tone as well; pathological studies have demonstrated lesions in or around the His bundle. The presence of conduction abnormalities does not correlate with prognosis or predict subsequent valvular manifestations. The QT interval is frequently prolonged, although not necessarily beyond normal limits, and rare episodes of torsades de pointes as well as sudden death have been reported.

Demonstration of antecedent streptococcal infection by throat culture or streptococcal antigen testing, with elevated or rising streptococcal antibody titers, adds considerably to the specificity standards of the Jones criteria. The presence of a positive throat culture alone is of limited value, because many individuals are carriers, whereas a negative culture may be secondary to elimination of GABHS from the pharynx by immune response prior to patient presentation or to antibiotic already administered. As with RF, accurate diagnosis of GABHS pharyngitis can be difficult, especially if laboratory facilities are limited. A clinical spectrum that suggests bacterial infection, including lymphadenopathy, fever, severe throat symptoms, and tonsillar-pharyngeal swelling or exudate in the absence of viral upper respiratory symptoms makes the diagnosis relatively specific. Because 20 percent or more of pharyngitis is secondary to GABHS, and because GABHS is present in a significant number of patients in a carrier state, the decision to treat with antibiotics is ultimately based on the clinical manifestations of pharyngitis and perceived risk, including the age of the patient and prevalence of RF in the community. Rapid streptococcal antigen tests are generally specific but have lower sensitivity. Baseline antibody levels exhibit substantial age and geographic variability, with high levels during the peak ages of vulnerability to RF. In contrast, *rising* streptococcal antibody titers, including antistreptolysin O, anti-deoxyribonuclease B, antihyaluronidase, and streptozyme are more specific, although they are affected by non-GABHS infections. The time course of antibody level increase is within 1 month of onset of streptococcal pharyngitis and plateaus for 3 to 6 months, following which a decline is seen, with levels elevated from the patient's baseline that typically last 1 year or less.

TREATMENT

The sine qua non of treatment is acute antimicrobial therapy to remove GABHS from the pharynx and continuous antibiotics for secondary prevention. Effective antibiotic treatment acutely (starting less than 10 days after the onset of pharyngitis) almost completely eliminates risk of the disease. Once the RF is manifest, the treatment algorithm varies, depending on manifestations of major criteria (see Fig. 83-3). The course of RF covers a spectrum from mild, which resolves without treatment, to severe and recurrent, with consequent end-stage heart disease. Long-term monitoring for carditis and RHD is generally warranted, even if symptoms resolve early. The first line of symptomatic therapy has traditionally been antiinflammatory agents, ranging from salicylates to steroids. However, evidence has suggested that the natural course of the disease itself is not influenced by antiinflammatory therapy. Evidence for bed rest is from the preantibiotic era, and many practitioners now treat RF patients on an outpatient basis, except for those presenting with carditis, for whom bed rest, at a minimum during the symptomatic stage, is empirically applied.

Prevention Strategies

Primary Prevention. Effective eradication of GABHS from the pharynx defines the role of primary prevention of RF. Patients with apparent bacterial pharyngitis and positive test results for GABHS should be treated as early as possible in the suppurative phase. The differential diagnosis, in addition to viral infection, includes non-GABHS and gonococcal pharyngitis. Penicillin is uniformly effective for GABHS if the drug is taken orally for a full 10-day course, or benzathine penicillin is injected, because penicillin-resistant GABHS has not been demonstrated. The particular advantage of benzathine penicillin G is that it avoids compliance issues. The alternatives for penicillin-allergic patients, as well as for oral therapy, are outlined in Table 83-2.

Secondary Prevention. The method of choice for preventing RF recurrence is continuous administration of benzathine penicillin every 4 weeks. Because of low or nondetectable penicillin levels during the fourth week after injection, higher frequency (every 3 weeks) has been recommended in endemic areas or for patients at high risk, although evidence for improved prophylaxis has not been compelling. Patients with documented RF should have continuous secondary prevention instituted as soon as the primary GABHS treatment regimen has been completed. Parenteral therapy is preferable, largely because of better compliance than with a twice-daily oral regimen; the latter should be reserved primarily for patients deemed to be at low risk for recurrent RF. A number of recommendations regarding the duration of therapy have been made, with the important variables being patient age, known RHD, time since last episode of RF, number of episodes of RF, family history of RF or RHD, occupational exposure (e.g., teachers), and environmental factors, such as living in endemic areas.[2] For the duration of the antimicrobial therapy, the minimum recommendations are 5 years or until age 18 (whichever is longer) in the absence of carditis, 10 years or until age 25 (whichever is longer) for patients with mild or apparently healed carditis, and life-long for patients with moderate or severe carditis. Confounding factors have been reluctance of rural practitioners to administer parenteral antibiotics for fear of allergic reactions and, for similar reasons, regulations prohibiting parenteral administration in hospitals in some developing countries. The actual risk of anaphylaxis, estimated to be 0.2 percent, is less in children under age 12. Because benzathine penicillin injection is the most effective method of delivery, it is essential that only truly penicillin-allergic patients be given alternative antibiotic regimens.

Therapeutic Modalities

Carditis

Salicylates and nonsteroidals have no specific role in rheumatic carditis, with the exception of treatment of concomitant pericarditis. It has generally been accepted that acute carditis benefits from aggressive antiinflammatory therapy with steroids. There is no evidence base to support this in the modern era; a meta-analysis of eight randomized controlled trials has failed to demonstrate superiority of steroids, immunoglobulins, or salicylates over placebo in the progression of RHD.[14] Nevertheless, in the setting of severe, potentially life-threatening heart failure, steroid administration is widespread but empirical; randomized trials using modern diagnostic tools to assess the effect on cardiac func-

TABLE 83–2	Antibiotic Therapy for Acute Rheumatic Fever (RF) and Long-Term Prophylaxis			
Initial Treatment of Group A Beta-Hemolytic Streptococcal Pharyngitis (Adult Dosages)				
Antibiotic	*Dose*	*Frequency*	*Duration*	*Comments*
Benzathine penicillin G	1.2 million units IM	One time	Acutely only	↓ Compliance issues ↑ Pain
Penicillin V	500 mg Po	b.i.d.	10 days	
Amoxicillin	500 mg Po	t.i.d.	10 days	
Cephalosporins or erythromycin	Varies by drug	Varies by drug	10 days	Erythromycin if penicillin-allergic*
Secondary Prophylaxis Regimen for Patients with Documented RF (Adult Dosages)[†]				
Antibiotic	*Dose*	*Frequency*	*Comments*	
Benzathine penicillin G	1.2 million units IM	q3-4 wk	↓ Compliance issues ↑ Pain	
Penicillin V	250 mg Po	b.i.d.		
Erythromycin	250 mg Po	b.i.d.	Alternative for penicillin-allergic patients*	
Sulfonamides	1 gm Po	Daily	Alternative for penicillin-allergic patients	

*Some areas have a high rate of macrolide-resistant group A streptococci.
†Duration of therapy ranges from 5 years to life-long (see text). For patients with poststreptococcal reactive arthritis, recommended duration is 1 year in nonendemic areas, 5 years where RF is prevalent if no evidence of carditis appears.
Modified from Rheumatic fever and rheumatic heart disease. World Health Organ Tech Rep Ser 923:1, 2004.

tion are required to address the issue. Treatment of cardiac manifestations otherwise follows established guidelines, including management of congestive heart failure and severe valvular regurgitation (see Chaps. 25 and 62). Unless valvular regurgitation and severe congestive heart failure are refractory to drug therapy, valve surgery is avoided for acute RF patients. Surgical morbidity and mortality have been significant and failed repair leading to valve replacement frequent, although postoperative ventricular function generally improves significantly, consistent with regurgitation rather than myocardial dysfunction being the primary mechanism leading to heart failure.

The natural course of the disease without secondary prophylaxis was extensively studied in the preantibiotic era in RHD hospitals where patients were treated for late manifestations of the disease, virtually all cardiac. Patients with recurrent episodes of carditis developed severe mitral and aortic valve disease and end-stage congestive heart failure, often with severe pulmonary hypertension, right heart failure and, occasionally, end-stage liver disease secondary to passive congestion.

Arthritis

Salicylates are the first line of therapy for migratory polyarthritis because of their highly effective analgesic, antiinflammatory, and antipyretic properties. Nonsteroidal antiinflammatory drugs are effective alternative therapy. Aspirin (100 mg/kg/day in four or more divided doses) is both therapeutic and diagnostic; failure of the pain to resolve within 24 hours suggests alternative causes of arthritis. Although salicylate levels can be followed (15 to 30 mg/dl is the therapeutic range), these data are usually not available in endemic areas; instead, patients are monitored for tinnitus and gastrointestinal toxicity. Early administration of salicylates or nonsteroidal agents does have the potential to mask the evolving clinical picture (e.g., arthritis when medication is given for arthralgias). Steroids are typically not used, because they offer no therapeutic advantage and may mask the presence of other illnesses causing the arthritis, such as lupus, or exacerbate other causes, such as infectious arthritis.

Chorea

Traditional modalities of treatment have included sedation and empirical use of antiseizure or antipsychotic medications. In addition, several recent small series,[15-17] one a randomized controlled trial, have studied corticosteroids, along with plasmapheresis and intravenous immunoglobulins, for the possibility that the severity and time course of symptoms could be altered. However, the evidence base is not conclusive, the interventions potentially toxic and, pending larger studies, a conservative approach to a largely self-limited disorder seems most appropriate. For patients with refractory symptoms, modest evidence has suggested some efficacy for carbamazepine or valproic acid.

FUTURE DIRECTIONS

A universal streptococcal vaccine has been elusive, partly because of the number and variability of antigenic stimulants, making the use of a vaccine identifying specific epitopes ineffective.[18] A simple and inexpensive screening test for identifying patients and populations genetically susceptible to RF has not been developed, nor is there a readily available, universally applicable, and inexpensive screening test for GABHS antibodies. With the 1992 Jones criteria modifications, the pendulum has swung toward ensuring specificity at the cost of sensitivity. Given the relatively modest cost of secondary prophylaxis and the prohibitive costs associated with RHD in developing countries where RF remains endemic, systematic longitudinal studies of more sensitive diagnostic algorithms using various technologies will be important. Too few treatment modalities for RF have undergone rigorous trials, resulting in a relatively weak evidence base for current or proposed management algorithms. Although initial episodes of RF appear to be declining with better health care delivery in some developing nations, public health efforts to prevent recurrences have the potential to decrease the global health care burden of RF substantially. Competition for limited health care resources, with a growing prevalence of ischemic heart disease in developing countries, has limited the financing of potentially highly cost-effective preventive health care programs.

CLASSIC READING

Guidelines for the diagnosis of rheumatic fever. Jones Criteria, 1992 update. Special Writing Group of the Committee on Rheumatic Fever, Endocarditis, and Kawasaki Disease of the Council on Cardiovascular Disease in the Young of the American Heart Association. JAMA 268:2069, 1992.

Krishna Kumar R, Rammohan R, Narula J, Kaplan EL: Epidemiology of streptococcal pharyngitis, rheumatic fever and rheumatic heart disease. In Narula J, Virman R, Srinath Reddy K, Tandon R (eds): Rheumatic Fever. Washington, DC, American Registry of Pathology, Armed Forces Institute of Pathology, 1999, pp 41-68.

REFERENCES

1. Carapetis JR, Steer AC, Mulholland EK, Weber M: The global burden of group A streptococcal diseases. Lancet Infect Dis 5:685, 2005.
2. Rheumatic fever and rheumatic heart disease. World Health Organ Tech Rep Ser 923:1, 2004.
3. Carapetis JR, McDonald M, Wilson NJ: Acute rheumatic fever. Lancet 366:155, 2005.
4. Jose VJ, Gomathi M: Declining prevalence of rheumatic heart disease in rural school-children in India: 2001-2002. Indian Heart J 55:158, 2003.
5. Guilherme L, Kalil J, Cunningham M: Molecular mimicry in the autoimmune pathogenesis of rheumatic heart disease. Autoimmunity 39:31, 2006.
6. Shulman ST, Stollerman G, Beall B, et al: Temporal changes in streptococcal M protein types and the near-disappearance of acute rheumatic fever in the United States. Clin Infect Dis 42:441, 2006.
7. Veasy LG, Tani LY, Daly JA, et al: Temporal association of the appearance of mucoid strains of Streptococcus pyogenes with a continuing high incidence of rheumatic fever in Utah. Pediatrics 113:e168, 2004.
8. Harrington Z, Visvanathan K, Skinner NA, et al: B-cell antigen D8/17 is a marker of rheumatic fever susceptibility in Aboriginal Australians and can be tested in remote settings. Med J Aust 184:507, 2006.
9. Carapetis JR, Currie BJ: Rheumatic fever in a high-incidence population: The importance of monoarthritis and low grade fever. Arch Dis Child 85:223, 2001.
10. Ferrieri P: Proceedings of the Jones Criteria workshop. Circulation 106:2521, 2002.
11. Kamblock J, Payot L, Iung B, et al: Does rheumatic myocarditis really exists? Systematic study with echocardiography and cardiac troponin I blood levels. Eur Heart J 24:855, 2003.
12. Kirvan CA, Swedo SE, Kurahara D, et al: Streptococcal mimicry and antibody-mediated cell signaling in the pathogenesis of Sydenham's chorea. Autoimmunity 39:21, 2006.
13. Snider LA, Swedo SE: PANDAS: Current status and directions for research. Mol Psychiatry 9:900, 2004.
14. Cilliers AM, Manyemba J, Saloojee H: Anti-inflammatory treatment for carditis in acute rheumatic fever. Cochrane Database Syst Rev (2):CD003176, 2003.
15. Genel F, Arslanoglu S, Uran N, et al: Sydenham's chorea: Clinical findings and comparison of the efficacies of sodium valproate and carbamazepine regimens. Brain Dev 24:73, 2002.
16. Garvey MA, Snider LA, Leitman SF, et al: Treatment of Sydenham's chorea with intravenous immunoglobulin, plasma exchange, or prednisone. J Child Neurol 20:424, 2005.
17. Paz JA, Silva CA, Marques-Dias MJ: Randomized double-blind study with prednisone in Sydenham's chorea. Pediatr Neurol 34:264, 2006.
18. Shet A, Kaplan E: Addressing the burden of group A streptococcal disease in India. Indian J Pediatr 71:41, 2004.

CHAPTER 84

Rheumatic Diseases and the Cardiovascular System

Brian F. Mandell and Gary S. Hoffman

General Principles, 2087

Vasculitis, 2087
Approach to Proving the Diagnosis of Vasculitis, 2087
Forms of Vasculitis Relevant to Cardiologists and Cardiovascular Surgeons, 2087

Vasculitis of Small or Medium-Sized Vessels That May Affect the Cardiovascular System, 2093
Churg-Strauss Syndrome, 2093
Polyarteritis Nodosa, 2093

Systemic Rheumatological Disorders, 2094
Rheumatoid Arthritis, 2094
HLA-B27–Associated Spondyloarthropathies, 2096
Systemic Lupus Erythematosus, 2096
Antiphospholipid Antibody Syndrome, 2098
Scleroderma, 2099
Polymyositis and Dermatomyositis, 2100
Sarcoidosis, 2101

References, 2102

GENERAL PRINCIPLES

Systemic rheumatological conditions often involve the cardiovascular system. Patients may first come to medical attention because of constitutional symptoms, muscle or joint pain, fever, regional or visceral ischemia, or organ failure. Rheumatological events that affect the heart and vessels range from being inapparent to catastrophic. The cardiovascular specialist may be the first to recognize that cardiovascular disease may have a primary immunological basis. Examples include patients with vasculitis, who may present with claudication, aortic aneurysms, and ischemic heart disease (Takayasu or giant cell arteritis), and patients with systemic lupus erythematosus who develop acute or chronic pericarditis or valvular abnormalities. This chapter will review the vasculitides and rheumatological conditions that may cause conditions encountered by the cardiovascular specialist.

VASCULITIS

Discrimination between the various forms of vasculitis begins with the concept of primary (i.e., primary process is immune dysregulation, without a known trigger) versus secondary (i.e., the cause [hepatitis, bacterial endocarditis] or associated disease [rheumatoid arthritis or systemic lupus] is known and inflammation–immune-mediated injury requires treatment or removal of the causative agent or underlying disease). Not knowing which group a patient fits in could lead to inappropriate use of immunosuppressive therapy, which may have adverse or lethal consequences. Examples of secondary vasculitides include vasculitis secondary to sepsis, particularly endocarditis, drug toxicity, and poisonings, malignancies, cardiac myxomas, and multifocal emboli from large-vessel aneurysms (Table 84-1). Each can mimic vasculitis or cause multifocal ischemia or infarction, with accompanying vasculitis. The greatest certainty in the diagnosis of primary vasculitis is in the setting of classic clinical and laboratory patterns—for example, a 70-year-old woman with new-onset severe headache, temporal region pain, hip and shoulder girdle stiffness, visual aberration (amaurosis or blindness), and a high erythrocyte sedimentation rate (ESR). This picture would be so compatible with giant cell arteritis as not to require biopsy evidence of the diagnosis. Unfortunately, many patients with vasculitis do not present with such recognizable features. Instead, one may have to depend on combinations of less typical clues. A patient with ischemic digits, active urinary sediment, and peripheral neuropathy is likely to have vasculitis, especially if the previously noted secondary causes of vasculitis and its mimics have already been ruled out. The presence of a purpuric rash, particularly if it is palpable (Fig. 84-1), furthers the probability of this diagnosis, which can be confirmed by a simple skin biopsy. Such features occurring in the setting of an established autoimmune disease (e.g., rheumatoid arthritis, systemic lupus erythematosus [SLE], Sjögren syndrome, or relapsing polychondritis) enhance the likelihood of vasculitis being present. The physician must still distinguish primary from secondary causes.

Approach to Proving the Diagnosis of Vasculitis

Definitive proof of the diagnosis depends on visualizing vasculitic lesions in affected tissue. The greatest success in achieving a tissue diagnosis comes from biopsy of abnormal or symptomatic sites. In patients with proven vasculitis, the yield from biopsies of clinically normal sites is considerably less than 20 percent. Therefore, a biopsy of apparently normal tissue is not recommended. Biopsies of abnormal organs provide diagnostically useful information in over 65 percent of cases. Biopsies of involved viscera have less than 100 percent yields because needle organ-penetrating biopsies often do not directly visualize the affected tissue and uniform involvement of vessels in affected viscera is uncommon.

A biopsy may not be practical in certain circumstances, such as systemic illness with symptoms of visceral ischemia, carotidynia, or findings of unequal pulses or blood pressures. Because biopsy of large vessels is usually impractical, angiography may be helpful. In this setting, vascular stenoses and/or aneurysms that cannot be explained on the basis of atherosclerosis may provide sufficient circumstantial evidence to proceed with treatment for primary systemic vasculitis.

Forms of Vasculitis Relevant to Cardiologists and Cardiovascular Surgeons

Takayasu Arteritis

Takayasu arteritis (TA) is an idiopathic large-vessel vasculitis of young adults that affects the aorta and its major branches.

EPIDEMIOLOGY. Women are affected about 10 times more often than men. The median age at onset is 25 years. Although TA is best known to occur in Asia, the distribution of the disease is worldwide and has been reported in all races and ethnicities. The incidence of TA is estimated to occur in 2.6 in 1,000,000 persons in the United States and 1.26 in 1,000,000 in northern Europe.[1] Autopsy series from Japan have noted a higher incidence, with 1 in every 3000 autopsies having features of TA.[2]

PATHOGENESIS. Although the cause of TA is unknown, studies of acute lesions reveal mononuclear cell infiltrates that appear to have accessed the vessel wall through the vasa vasorum and subsequently migrate to the macroluminal intima. These cells are predominantly macrophages, T, gamma-delta, cytotoxic, and natural killer lymphocytes. There is also a small admixture of B lymphocytes. The presence of various cytokines, including interleukin-6 (IL-6) and tumor necrosis factor (TNF) in these granulomatous lesions has suggested various therapeutic approaches using biological agents.[3]

CLINICAL FEATURES. In TA, arterial stenoses occur three to four times more often than aneurysms. Claudication (more than 60 percent upper versus approximately 30 percent lower extremities) is the most common complaint and bruits (approximately 80 percent), blood pressure, and pulse asymmetries (60 to 80 percent) are the most common findings. Aneurysms are most common and clinically most significant in the aortic root, where they can lead to valvular regurgitation (approximately 20 percent) (Fig. 84-2A, left; see Fig. 84-2B). Hypertension is most often caused by renal artery stenosis, but can also be associated with suprarenal aortic stenosis or a chronically damaged, rigid aorta. Cardiac, renal, and central nervous system (CNS) vascular diseases

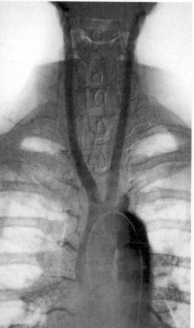

FIGURE 84–1 Palpable purpura. Vascular inflammation at the level of capillaries and venules leads to exudation of formed elements and the color and texture of lesions noted in these patients. The person on the right is a young woman with Henoch-Schönlein vasculitis or purpura (HSP). The elderly man on the left has a similar lesion. However, in this case it was associated with hepatitis C, acquired in the course of transfusions for heart surgery. Hepatitis C virus (HCV) infection led to cryoglobulinemia and secondary vasculitis. The treatment for each patient is different. The one with HSP, who does not have extracutaneous disease, only requires reassurance and monitoring for her usually self-limiting problem, whereas the patient with HCV and vasculitis requires antiviral therapy.

TABLE 84–1	Diseases That Can Mimic Primary Systemic Vasculitis
Sepsis, especially endocarditis	
Drug toxicity, poisoning 　Cocaine 　Amphetamines 　Ephedra 　Phenylpropanolamine	
Coagulopathy 　Anticardiolipin antibody syndrome 　Disseminated intravascular coagulation	
Malignancy (solid organ or "liquid" tumors)	
Cardiac myxoma	
Multifocal emboli from large-vessel aneurysms (cholesterol, mycotic)	
Ehlers-Danlos syndrome (vascular ectatic type)	
Fibromuscular dysplasia	

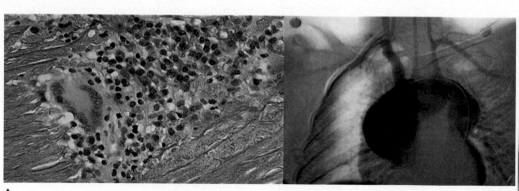

A

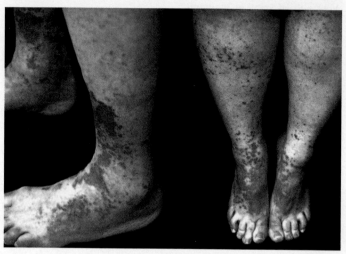

B

FIGURE 84–2 Takayasu disease. **A,** Takayasu arteritis. Granulomatous inflammation and medial destruction **(left panel)** has led to marked aortic root dilation **(right panel)** in a 17-year-old female high school student who developed symptoms of congestive heart failure and exertional angina. She also had diffuse narrowing of the left common carotid artery and irregular dilation of the innominate artery. **B,** Occlusion of both subclavian arteries has led to leg pressures being the only reliable measure of central aortic pressure.

are the principal causes of severe morbidity and mortality. Estimates of mortality range from a low of approximately 3 percent at 5 years[4] to approximately 35 percent at 5 years follow-up.[1,4]

Symptoms of large-vessel abnormalities or the finding of hypertension, especially in young patients, necessitate examination of extremity pulses and blood pressures for asymmetry and a search for bruits. Increasing extremity or visceral ischemia, malaise, myalgias, arthralgias, night sweats, and fever may indicate active disease. When such symptoms occur in the setting of an elevated ESR, active disease is assumed to be present. However,, many patients may not have any constitutional or new vascular symptoms, and as many as 50 percent may have normal ESRs and still experience progressive disease.[1,4] The following findings indicate that active TA can occur in this setting:

1. New vascular abnormalities on sequential angiographic studies in patients who were thought to be in remission
2. Presence of inflammatory changes in bypass biopsy specimens from patients in whom surgery was performed because of critical flow abnormalities in the setting of clinically quiescent disease[1,4]

Until we can judge the degree of disease activity in TA better, outcomes will be compromised. Studies using refinements in magnetic resonance imaging (MRI)[5] and positron emission tomography (PET) techniques may enable the clinician to detect qualitative abnormalities in the vessel wall that imply inflammatory change. Definitive prospective studies that clearly define the operating characteristics of PET have not been done. However, preliminary data about its usefulness have been encouraging. Sequential fluorodeoxyglucose PET studies may become useful to determine response to therapy.[6]

The cardiac sequelae of TA result more often from aortic regurgitation and inadequately treated hypertension than from arteritis affecting the coronary vessels.[1,4] Indirect evidence from echocardiography studies has also suggested that left ventricular systolic dysfunction may be caused by myocarditis in about 18 percent of patients.[7] When coronary artery vasculitis is detected (less than 5 percent), it is most frequent in the ostial regions. However, more distal involvement has also been reported and both types of lesions may occur in the same patient. These observations underscore the importance of considering vasculitis in the differential diagnosis of young patients with ischemic symptoms.

DIFFERENTIAL DIAGNOSIS. Certain congenital diseases cause abnormalities of tissue matrix and aortic regurgitation (e.g., Marfan syndrome, Ehlers-Danlos syndrome). However, these conditions are not associated with stenotic lesions in large vessels, which is the most common feature of TA. Inborn genetic errors that affect matrix structure are also not associated with systemic symptoms, abnormal acute-phase reactants, anemia, or thrombocytosis, which may be present with large-vessel vasculitis. The young female predominance of TA distinguishes it from patients with typical atherosclerosis, a disease much more likely to affect the lower extremity large vessels than the arms and the abdominal aorta than the aortic root. Infectious causes of large-vessel aneurysms (e.g., bacterial, syphilitic, mycobacterial, fungal) must be considered in both genders and all age groups, but are *not* usually associated with vascular stenoses affecting the arch vessels. Certain autoimmune diseases may be complicated by large-vessel vasculitis, but they are readily discerned by their associated characteristics (e.g., systemic lupus, Cogan syndrome, Behçet disease, spondyloarthropathies) and unique age preferences (e.g., Kawasaki disease and giant cell arteritis of the elderly). Sarcoidosis can closely mimic TA. Making the correct diagnosis depends on other characteristic features of sarcoidosis being present (e.g., proliferative synovitis, skin lesions, Bell palsy, hilar adenopathy). There are no specific diagnostic tests for TA. The diagnosis is based on clinical features in conjunction with vascular imaging abnormalities. In patients who undergo vascular surgery, histopathological abnormalities may further support the diagnosis.

TREATMENT. Although almost all patients with TA improve when treated with high doses of corticosteroid (CS) (e.g., prednisone, 1 mg/kg/day), relapses are common with tapering of CS therapy. CS-resistant or relapsing patients may respond to the addition to daily therapy of cyclophosphamide (approximately 2 mg/kg) or weekly therapy with methotrexate (approximately 20 mg).[1,4,8] About 40 percent of patients who are treated with a cytotoxic agent and CS will achieve remission but, over time, about half these patients will also relapse, leading to the need for chronic immunosuppressive therapy in many patients.[1,4] Such unsatisfactory results have led to ongoing studies that seek to take advantage of new insights into pathogenesis. Preliminary studies have demonstrated that treatment designed to block TNF may dramatically improve most patients (14 of 15) with TA who have relapsed during tapering of steroid therapy.[9]

A discussion of pharmacological therapy for TA only addresses one important aspect of care. Other important issues include treatment of the anatomical effects of vascular lesions. Patients with TA may have signs of clinical deterioration caused by fixed critical stenoses or aneurysms. Hypertension affects approximately 40 to 90 percent of patients.[1,4] In Asia, India, and Mexico, TA is one of the most common causes of hypertension in the adolescent and young adult population. One of the most common errors in clinical management relates to the physician not knowing whether blood pressure recordings in an extremity are representative of aortic root pressure. Because over 90 percent of patients have stenotic lesions and the most common site of stenosis is the subclavian and innominate arteries, blood pressure in one or both arms may underestimate pressure in the aorta. Elevated aortic root pressure, when unrecognized and untreated, enhances the risks of hypertensive complications. This potential dilemma can best be appreciated when angiographic procedures include intravascular pressure recordings, which should always be included in patients with stenoses and possible gradients. The importance of knowing the distribution and severity of all vascular lesions cannot be overemphasized. In the setting of renal insufficiency, the potential of contrast agents to cause further renal impairment may limit exploring the extent of all potential vascular lesions. However, if no contraindications are present, patients should have the entire aorta and its primary branches included in vascular imaging studies. MR angiography lacks the ability to measure intravascular pressures. If the clinical examination does not suggest that lesions affecting extremity-recorded blood pressures are present and extremity pressures are equal, a MR study may be sufficient to delineate other vascular lesions without resorting to catheter-guided angiography.

Whenever feasible, anatomical correction of clinically significant lesions should be considered, especially in the setting of renal artery stenosis and hypertension. In about 20 percent of patients, aortic root involvement may lead to valvular insufficiency, angina, and congestive heart failure (see Fig. 84-2).[1,4] Severe or progressive changes may require aortic surgery, with or without valve replacement. Because subclavian and carotid stenoses are among the most common lesions in TA, severe symptomatic stenoses of these vessels should be preferably treated by grafts that have originated from the aortic root and not from an arch vessel to another arch vessel. The latter may be followed by loss of the graft because of new stenosis in an initially spared subclavian or carotid artery. Conversely, a graft from the ascending aorta is a safer conduit long term because the ascending aorta in TA essentially never becomes stenotic. Mesenteric and celiac artery stenoses are usually asymptomatic and only rarely require surgery. Angioplasty and intravascular stents have met with restenosis far more often than bypass, which is preferred whenever feasible.[1,4] It is always preferable to operate on patients who are in remission; however, judgment of disease activity in TA may be difficult. Consequently, *all* bypass surgeries should include vascular biopsy specimens for histopathological evaluation. Findings from surgical specimens should guide the need for postoperative immunosuppressive treatment.

The care of patients with TA requires a team approach that includes clinicians familiar with the proper use of immunosuppressive therapies, vascular imaging or intervention specialists and, in the setting of critical stenoses or aneurysms, cardiovascular physicians and surgeons. For most patients, medical and surgical therapies provide important palliation.

Giant Cell Arteritis of the Elderly

Giant cell arteritis (GCA) and Takayasu arteritis are the principal diseases associated with sterile granulomatous inflammation of large and medium-sized vessels.

EPIDEMIOLOGY. In the United States, GCA affects approximately 18/100,000 population who are older than 50 years of age (mean, 74 years). Although not understood, it is particularly interesting that the incidence of GCA is much greater in northern latitudes. For example, in Iceland and Denmark, the incidence is 27 and 21/100,000, respectively, in the age group older than 50 years. Although females predominate in frequency of being affected (2 to 3:1), this is not as striking as in TA (6 to 10:1). The demographic characteristics of GCA are the same as for patients with polymyalgia rheumatica (PMR), and in fact 30 to 50 percent of patients with GCA may concurrently have features of PMR.[10]

PATHOGENESIS. Although the cause of GCA remains unknown, the inflammatory lesion begins in the adventitia. The vasa vasorum are the conduit for the mononuclear cells (dendritic cells, macrophages, and Th1-type lymphocytes) that mediate vascular injury. Dendritic cells participate in the process by presenting to lymphocytes the putative antigen that is believed to "drive" GCA. This is supported by the finding of clonality of approximately 4 percent of T lymphocytes in the vessel wall. Clonality is not found in peripheral blood lymphocytes, thus further enhancing the likelihood that a responsible antigen is presented in the adventitia or media. Vascular lesions are initially rich in proinflammatory cytokines such as IL-1, IL-6, TNF, and interferon-gamma (IFN-γ). Intermediate lesions harbor mediators of matrix destruction (e.g., metalloproteinases, reactive oxygen and nitrogen species). In later stages, growth factors such as platelet-derived growth factor (PDGF) and fibroblast growth factor (FGF) participate in stimulating myointimal proliferation, leading to vessel stenosis.

CLINICAL FEATURES. The most characteristic features of GCA are new onset of atypical and often severe headaches, scalp and temporal artery tenderness, acute visual loss, polymyalgia rheumatica, and pain in the muscles of mastication (Table 84-2). Concurrence of such abnormalities with an increase in the ESR supports a clinical diagnosis of GCA and treatment should be started, even without proof of diagnosis from a temporal artery biopsy. The diagnosis is doubtful if dramatic improvement does not occur within 24 to 72 hours. The yield of positive temporal artery biopsies in patients clinically diagnosed with GCA is about 50 to 80 percent, depending on the pretest probability of GCA. Patients with a high ESR, who had presented to an ophthalmologist with symptoms of new-onset atypical headache

and visual loss, are more likely to have a positive biopsy than patients cared for by their generalist who present with symptoms of vague limb girdle pain, headache, and malaise.

GCA may produce clinically apparent aortitis in at least 15 percent of cases and involve the primary branches of the aorta, especially the subclavian arteries, in a similar number of individuals.[10,11] Postmortem studies have suggested that large-vessel involvement is far more common than clinically appreciated. Consequently, some patients with GCA may present with features that resemble those of TA. Among the elderly with inflammatory large-vessel disease, the same considerations and precautions must be applied in GCA as in patients with TA—the need to identify an extremity that provides a reliable blood pressure equivalent to aortic root pressure, follow-up to include careful observation for new bruits, pulse and blood pressure asymmetry, and the possible development of aortic aneurysms. Studies have demonstrated that patients with GCA were more than 17 times more likely than age-matched controls to have thoracic aortic aneurysms and about 2.5 times more likely than age-matched controls to have abdominal aortic aneurysms.[11] Half of patients with thoracic aortic aneurysms died as a result of those lesions. Because aneurysms were found in the course of routine care or at postmortem, these may be conservative estimates. The finding of large-vessel disease, including aortic aneurysms, in elderly persons with GCA should not merely be assumed to be secondary to atheromatous disease. It is not surprising that about half of all patients with GCA have objective features of cardiac disease. However, it appears that myocardial infarction caused by GCA is rare or rarely appreciated because histopathological findings in coronary arteries are infrequently sought in the group of patients whose mean age is 74 years.

DIFFERENTIAL DIAGNOSIS. Mimics of GCA include other vasculitides that may cause musculoskeletal pain, headache, visual aberrations, fever, and malaise. Although these include Wegener granulomatosis, Churg-Strauss vasculitis, microscopic polyangiitis, and others, it is relatively simple to rule these out based on more characteristic features of those illnesses being present (e.g., upper and/or lower airway disease and features of small-vessel vasculitis). Rarely, the GCA phenotype may be part of a paraneoplastic process. If polymyalgia rheumatica is the most compelling symptom of GCA, the differential then also includes polymyositis and proximal-onset rheumatoid arthritis. No precise serological test exists for GCA. Diagnosis is based on a clinically compatible presentation, concurrent highly abnormal acute-phase reactants (more than 80 percent of cases), a positive temporal artery biopsy (50 to 80 percent of cases) or angiographic abnormalities of large vessels (Fig. 84-3) compatible with GCA.

TREATMENT. CS treatment continues to be the most effective therapy for GCA. Prednisone (approximately 0.7 to 1 mg/kg/day) will reduce symptoms within 1 to 2 days and often eliminate symptoms within 1 week. About 2 to 4 weeks after clinical and laboratory parameters, particularly the ESR, have normalized, tapering of CS can begin. Unfortunately, the ESR does not always normalize, even with disease control, so it should not be relied on as the only measure of disease activity. Occasional patients may either not achieve complete remission or not be able to be tapered off CS. Cytotoxic and other immunosuppressive agents, including anti-TNF monoclonal antibodies, have not proved efficacious in controlled comparative trials.[12,13] Two more recent studies have demonstrated that the use of low-dose aspirin reduces cranial ischemic events (blindness and stroke) three- to fourfold compared with patients who have not received such therapy. In the absence of contraindications, low-dose aspirin should be provided for all patients with GCA.[14,15]

Idiopathic Aortitis

Aortitis is a recognized feature of TA and GCA. It may also occur in diseases such as Behçet disease, Cogan syndrome, and in children as a complication of Kawasaki disease. Occasionally, it is an unanticipated finding in patients undergoing surgery for aortic valve regurgitation, aneurysm

TABLE 84–2	Clinical Profile of Giant Cell Arteritis
Abnormality	**Frequency (%)**
Atypical headache	60-90
Tender temporal artery	40-70
Systemic symptoms not attributable to other diseases	20-50
Fever	20-50
Polymyalgia rheumatica	30-50
Acute visual abnormalities	12-40
Transient ischemic attack or stroke	5-10

Claudication
  "Jaw"
  Extremities
	
	30-70
	5-15

Aortic aneurysm	15-20
Dramatic response to CS	~100
Positive temporal artery biopsy	~50-80

CS=corticosteroids.

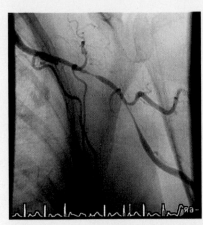

FIGURE 84-3 Giant cell arteritis. Takayasu-like lesions involving the subclavian and axillary arteries in a case of giant cell arteritis are shown.

resection, or coarctation.[16] Little is known about the frequency and clinical characteristics of idiopathic aortitis. (Aortitis in the context of retroperitoneal fibrosis is a separate topic that will not be discussed in this chapter.)

EPIDEMIOLOGY. A 20-year review of pathological specimens from consecutive aortic surgeries at the Cleveland Clinic Foundation has revealed that 52 of 1204 specimens (4.3 percent) were classified as idiopathic aortitis. Sixty-seven percent of patients with idiopathic aortitis were women.[16]

PATHOGENESIS. Unless the patient with idiopathic aortitis had a past history of GCA or TA, the mechanisms of disease have remained unexplored.

CLINICAL FEATURES. In our series, 96 percent of cases with idiopathic aortitis had findings limited to the thoracic aorta. These data are similar to those from large postmortem series in which aortas have been examined in spite of the absence of overt aortic disease during life. In 96 percent of our cases, symptoms of systemic illness had not been present at the time of surgery. In 69 percent of cases, idiopathic aortitis was not related to a current or past history of systemic disease. However, in 31 percent (16 of 52), aortitis was associated with a past history of GCA, TA, systemic lupus, Wegener granulomatosis, and various other disorders. Thus, a past history of these illnesses and reporting them presumably being in remission becomes suspect in the setting of a newly recognized thoracic root aneurysm.

DIFFERENTIAL DIAGNOSIS. Patients with idiopathic aortitis vary in age from childhood to the very elderly. Consequently, differential diagnostic considerations might include Kawasaki disease, TA, GCA, systemic lupus, sarcoidosis, Cogan syndrome, Behçet disease, spondyloarthropathies, rheumatoid arthritis, rheumatic fever, and aortitis caused by infectious agents (e.g., TB, syphilis, mycoses, and bacteria). Symptoms or findings of these diseases may immediately allow prioritization of diagnostic choices. However, some processes may be clinically silent and diagnosis may be aided by ancillary laboratory studies (e.g., rapid plasma reagin [RPR], antinuclear antibody [ANA]), skin tests (e.g., purified protein derivative [PPD]), cultures, and special stains of surgical specimens. Because idiopathic aortitis is a syndrome that requires ruling out all causes of aortitis that may have specific therapies (e.g., antibiotics), no diagnostic tests for this entity exist, apart from histopathological assays.

TREATMENT. In our experience with 36 patients, followed for a mean period of 42 months and analyzed retrospectively, new aneurysms were identified in 6 of 25 patients not treated with CS and none of 11 patients treated with CS. Although this observation would suggest that such therapy is indicated in this setting, there were marked variations of dose and duration of therapy that led to uncertainty about CS efficacy. Because only 17 percent of all patients subsequently developed new aneurysms over 3.5 years, we do not believe that all such patients require medical treatment.[16] These observations suggest that inflammatory disease may be isolated to the aortic root in most patients. To justify treatment, one would have to prove the existence of ongoing inflammatory disease. We approach this by routine history and physical, laboratory evaluation (complete blood count [CBC], ESR, C-reactive protein [CRP]), and imaging studies (MRI or MR angiography of the entire aorta and its primary branches). Because new lesions may

occur over time, patients with idiopathic aortitis identified at the time of surgery should be periodically evaluated for recurrence. If disease definitely recurs, treatment should be pursued as recommended for TA and GCA. Although proof of the effectiveness of this approach is lacking, it can be defended based on the similarities of these conditions and demonstrated efficacy in GCA and TA.

Kawasaki Disease

Kawasaki disease (KD) is an acute febrile systemic illness of childhood. It is the principal cause of acquired heart disease in children in Japan and the United States.

EPIDEMIOLOGY. KD occurs primarily in children younger than 4 or 5 years old. Peak incidence is in children younger than 2 years old. Boys are affected 1.5 times more often than girls. KD almost never occurs beyond the age of 8 years (mean age in Japan is 12 months and in the United States 2.8 years). Although all racial groups can be affected, Asian children have the highest incidence of KD (50 to 200/100,000 children younger than 5 years of age versus 6-15/100,000 in the U.S.). Asian Americans have a higher incidence of KD than African Americans, in whom the incidence exceeds that of white Americans.[17] Although siblings of patients with KD are infrequently affected, KD does affect siblings more often than the general age-matched population (2.1 versus 0.19 percent). When siblings are affected, symptoms often occur shortly after their family member had become ill. This raises questions about an infectious cause in the setting of an immunological predisposition.[17-20]

PATHOGENESIS. Fever, rash, conjunctivitis, adenopathy, and geographic clustering suggest an infectious cause. However, no agent has yet been identified. The following are possible causes:

1. An undiscovered pathogen is responsible for KD.
2. A known infectious agent plays a role in triggering an abnormal immune response, but the pathogen itself is cleared.
3. A pathogen triggers disease by molecular mimicry to normal host antigens.
4. A sequence of stochastic events leads to clinically apparent disease, but by the time the patient presents, the most critical early features of pathogenesis have disappeared.

The essential absence of disease in neonates invites speculation about protection from maternal antibodies, although the rarity of KD in adults suggests protection may occur through acquired immunity.[19,20]

The acute phase of illness is characterized by widespread evidence of immunoinflammatory activation. This includes high levels of acute-phase reactants, leukocytosis with a left shift, lymphocytosis with a predominance of polyclonal B cells, and thrombocytosis that frequently reaches 1,000,000/mm^3. Blood T lymphocytes, including CD4$^+$ and CD8$^+$cells, increase in number and show signs of activation. In spite of these observations, children with acute KD are often anergic, indicating T-cell dysfunction. Increased blood levels of a broad range of cytokines and soluble forms of endothelial cell adhesion molecules indicate widespread immune activation. Cytokine-mediated endothelial cell activation and cytotoxic factors to endothelial cells may play an important early role in pathogenesis. Pathology specimens reveal vasculitis with endothelial cell edema, necrosis, desquamation, and a changing profile of leukocytes in the vessel wall, first being neutrophils and later macrophages and T lymphocytes. After months, the inflammatory infiltrate diminishes and, as it fades, myointimal proliferation may produce stenoses or wall weakening may lead to aneurysm formation. In either case, the stage is set for subsequent thrombosis.[19,20]

CLINICAL FEATURES. The most prominent features are included in the case definition guidelines of the Centers for

TABLE 84–3 | **Definition of Kawasaki Syndrome**

Fever ≥5 days, without other explanation, plus at least four of the following:
1. Bilateral conjunctival injection
2. Mucous membrane changes—injected or fissured lips; injected pharynx or "strawberry" tongue.
3. Extremity abnormality—erythema of palms, soles, edema of hands, feet, or generalized or peripheral desquamation (hands, feet).
4. Rash (polymorphous)
5. Cervical lymphadenopathy (usually a single node >1.5 cm)

Associated manifestations
  Irritability
  Sterile pyuria, meatitis
  Perineal erythema and desquamation
  Arthralgias, arthritis
  Abdominal pain, diarrhea
  Aseptic meningitis
  Hepatitis
  Obstructive jaundice
  Hydrops of gallbladder
  Uveitis
  Sensorineural hearing loss
  Cardiovascular changes

80% cases <4 years old; rare, >8 years old
CDC=Centers for Disease Control and Prevention.
Modified from Barron K: Kawasaki disease: Etiology, pathogenesis and treatment. Cleve Clin J Med 69(Suppl 2):69, 2002.

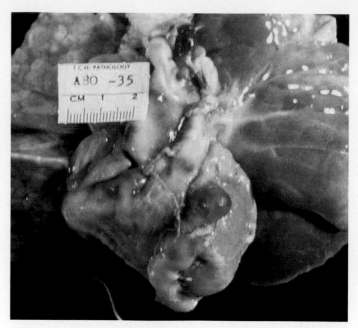

FIGURE 84–4 Giant coronary artery aneurysms caused by Kawasaki disease. Note the bulbous protrusion from the left anterior descending coronary artery. (*Courtesy of Dr. Karyl Barron.*)

Disease Prevention and Control (Table 84-3). These guidelines lack any specific serological diagnostic test. The illness is usually self-limiting, within 4 to 8 weeks, and mortality is 2 percent.

Cardiac abnormalities include pericardial effusions (approximately 30 percent), myocarditis, mitral regurgitation (approximately 30 percent), aortitis and aortic regurgitation (infrequent), congestive heart failure, and atrial and ventricular arrhythmias.[19,20] Electrocardiographic findings include decreased R wave voltage, ST segment depression, and T wave flattening or inversion. Slowed conduction may be seen with prolonged PR or QT prolongation. In untreated patients or patients treated with aspirin alone, coronary artery aneurysms occur in about 20 to 25 percent of cases within 2 weeks and are associated with a mortality rate of approximately 2 percent. Early diagnosis and treatment with aspirin and intravenous immune globulin (IVIG) have reduced the death rate to well below 1 percent and the prevalence of coronary artery aneurysms to approximately 5 percent. Deaths usually result from acute coronary artery thrombosis in aneurysms that form following vasculitis. Noninvasive techniques disclose coronary artery aneurysms in approximately 20 percent of patients, compared with 60 percent shown by angiography. Aneurysms usually appear 1 to 4 weeks after onset of fever. New aneurysms seldom form after 6 weeks. Aneurysms are more common in the proximal than distal coronary arteries. Although larger ("giant") aneurysms (larger than 8 mm) (Fig. 84-4) are among the most likely to later thrombose and occlude, leading to infarction and even sudden death, endothelial abnormalities and intimal proliferation in smaller lesions (smaller than 4 mm) may lead to cardiac ischemia as well. About half of all small aneurysms will undergo angiographic regression within 1 to 2 years. Giant aneurysms rarely regress. The vascular remodeling process in injured vessels includes fibromuscular proliferation that can lead to stenoses. Myocardial infarction may result from thrombus formation in aneurysms or severe stenoses, and occurs most commonly in the first year after illness, but less often in young adults.[17,19,20]

Data from postmortem studies have also demonstrated vasculitis of the aorta, celiac, carotid, subclavian, and pulmonary arteries. Rare case reports of gut vasculitis in KD exist. Gastrointestinal (GI) morbidity may depend more on small-vessel than large-vessel disease.

DIFFERENTIAL DIAGNOSIS. Given the resemblance of KD to infectious diseases, competing diagnoses include bacterial, spirochetal (e.g., leptospirosis), rickettsial (e.g., Rocky Mountain spotted fever), and viral illnesses. Drug reactions, poisonings (e.g., mercury), juvenile rheumatoid arthritis, systemic lupus, other vasculitides, and malignancies, especially lymphomas and leukemias, may also share aspects of KD.

TREATMENT. Before the use of high dosages of aspirin and IVIG, coronary artery aneurysms were relatively common. However, such treatment appears to have reduced the incidence of aneurysms to approximately 5 percent.[17,19] The current standard of care consists of 2 gm/kg of IVIG as a single infusion. Treatment provided within the first 10 days of illness shows efficacy most convincingly. Aspirin (80 to 100 mg/kg/day until the patient is afebrile) has both anti-inflammatory and anti-thrombotic effects. After fever subsides, the dose of aspirin is reduced (3 to 5 mg/kg/day) to achieve primarily antiplatelet effects. This treatment should continue until the platelet count and other inflammatory markers return to normal (about 8 weeks). Long-term low-dose aspirin is recommended for children with echocardiogram-demonstrated aneurysms, although controlled studies have not proved the efficacy of such therapy. A small subset of KD patients is resistant to conventional therapy. They constitute a group that is most prone to aneurysm formation and long-term disease sequelae. The use of corticosteroids in this group and other patients remains controversial. The reported increased frequency of coronary artery aneurysms in an early report of CS-treated patients has not been seen by others.[19]

Recommendations for long-term follow-up by the American Heart Association include consideration of anticoagulation therapy in children with multiple giant aneurysms and known obstructive lesions, and evaluation by stress testing during adolescence. Severe coronary artery lesions have been treated by bypass, but if disease is widespread and bypass not possible, transplantation should be considered.[19]

Coronary artery bypass procedures have been reserved for patients with severe obstructive lesions, such as those involving the main left coronary artery (LCA) or at least two of three major coronary arteries. Internal thoracic artery grafts have appeared to fare better than saphenous vein grafts. Data on percutaneous interventions, including those using drug-eluting stents, are limited.

VASCULITIS OF SMALL OR MEDIUM-SIZED VESSELS THAT MAY AFFECT THE CARDIOVASCULAR SYSTEM

Churg-Strauss Syndrome

Churg-Strauss syndrome (CSS; allergic angiitis and granulomatosis) is a very rare syndrome that typically includes a history of asthma, eosinophilia, pulmonary infiltrates, upper airway inflammation, and a variable frequency of renal, neurological, cutaneous, and cardiac involvement. Histopathological observations from involved lesions reveal eosinophilic granulomatous infiltrates and vasculitis.

EPIDEMIOLOGY. The most generous estimates of annual incidence of CSS are 2.4 cases/1,000,000 persons annually. Those affected may be children or adults, with the peak age group being 35 to 50 years old. Significant gender bias does not exist.[21,22]

PATHOGENESIS. The cause of CSS remains unknown. Nonetheless, authorities have recommended withdrawal of any newly introduced drugs or treatments (e.g., desensitization), and avoidance to new environmental stimuli (e.g., farm, workplace, if relevant to the medical history). A role for leukotriene antagonists, as used in the treatment of asthma, in precipitating CSS is the subject of controversy. Most would agree that if such an agent were introduced just before emergence of CSS, it should be discontinued.

Whether antineutrophil cytoplasmic antibodies (ANCAs) play a role in CSS is uncertain. ANCAs occur in only 40 percent or fewer cases, suggesting that if they play a role, it is not an essential one. Nonetheless, two prospective studies have suggested that the presence of ANCA may influence disease expression. In both studies, in ANCA-positive patients, renal disease was more common and cardiac disease was less common.[21,22] Most often, the immunofluorescent pattern for ANCA in CSS is perinuclear (P pattern) but, in a minority of cases, it can be cytoplasmic (C pattern). The specific antigen targeted by ANCA is usually myeloperoxidase (MPO), but in some cases it will be proteinase 3 (PR-3) and the corresponding immunofluorescent pattern will be C.

The granulomatous nature of CSS lesions suggests an involvement of Th1 lymphocytes and macrophages, although ANCA, if relevant, and eosinophils, argue for a role of Th2-biased lymphocytes. The latter are a source of IL-5, which increases eosinophil production and release from the bone marrow.

CLINICAL FEATURES. By definition, the diagnosis requires a past or present history of asthma. Nonetheless, rare cases have been recognized with only a history of allergies and allergic rhinitis. Systemic symptoms are present in 70 to 100 percent of cases from different series. Chest imaging reveals infiltrates, usually multifocal, in 30 to 75 percent. Much less often, pulmonary nodules may be seen, as in Wegener granulomatosis (WG); however, in CSS, nodules are very unlikely to cavitate, a finding that is common in WG. Cardiac disease in CSS is the most common cause of death. It is reported in 15 to 55 percent of cases and may include pericarditis, myocarditis, and coronary arteritis. Congestive heart failure occurs in 15 to 30 percent of cases. Mesenteric ischemia (approximately 5 percent) contributes significantly to morbidity and mortality. It may be manifest by frank blood per rectum, melena, or bowel perforation. Many more patients have abdominal pain (30 to 60 percent) for which the ultimate cause is suspected to be CSS. The small intestine and colon are the sites more often affected. Peripheral neurological abnormalities (sensory and/or motor) affect over two thirds of patients. Although these features are not life-threatening, they can be a source of profound morbidity. Musculoskeletal symptoms and rashes may be seen in approximately half of all patients and renal disease (glomerulonephritis) is seen in at least a third.

DIFFERENTIAL DIAGNOSIS. CSS may be confused with WG. Patients who suffer from WG do not have an unusually high frequency of allergies, asthma, and striking eosinophilia, but in some patients with WG, eosinophils can be approximately 10 percent of the total white blood cell count. In WG, the most common ANCA pattern is C and antibody is usually directed to proteinase 3 (70 to 80 percent of ANCA-positive cases). Pulmonary nodules may cavitate in WG, an event that would be very rare in CSS.

Other considerations in the differential are parasitic infections, especially helminths (e.g., larvae and adults of hookworm, ascaris, trichinella, strongyloides, filaria, flukes) that may produce chronic eosinophilia by stimulating IL-5 in affected organs. Because helminths may migrate through the lungs, infiltrates and bronchospasm may result, producing a picture of eosinophilic pneumonia and asthma. Idiopathic hypereosinophilic syndrome (HES) is a diagnosis to be considered only after all other causes of eosinophilia have been ruled out. In some cases, it is part of a leukoproliferative syndrome and may be associated with splenomegaly, cytogenetic abnormalities, myelofibrosis, myelodysplasia, anemia, and abnormal red blood cell forms. When such findings are not present, the absence of vasculitis and asthma distinguishes HES from CSS. HES is of particular interest to cardiologists because of the risks of cardiac fibrosis, ventricular apical necrosis, and intraventricular thrombus formation. Emboli from the ventricles may lead to pulmonary infarction or systemic circulatory events, including stroke and peripheral occlusive lesions. Myocarditis and cardiac fibrosis may lead to a restrictive cardiomyopathy.

TREATMENT. Corticosteroids (most often prednisone, 1 mg/kg/day orally) usually produce dramatic improvement. In patients with critical organ system involvement (heart, brain, kidneys, gut) it may be prudent to provide pulse IV therapy (1 gm/day of methylprednisolone) for 1 to 3 days. Although recommended, this regimen has never been the subject of controlled clinical trials. Patients who are critically ill should also receive a second agent (most often, cyclophosphamide [CP]). CP is used daily in a dose of 2 mg/kg, assuming normal renal function. In the presence of renal impairment, the dose must be proportionately reduced to avoid severe bone marrow suppression. Long-term CP therapy carries many risks. Although once the standard of care, CP is now used to induce remission and then, after 3 to 6 months, if remission continues, even though CSs are being tapered, CP is switched to maintenance therapy with daily azathioprine or weekly methotrexate.

Polyarteritis Nodosa

Polyarteritis nodosa (PAN) is a nongranulomatous disease of only medium-sized arteries. The older PAN literature has been a source of confusion. Those series included patients with both PAN and microscopic polyangiitis (MPA), a disease that can have features of PAN but is defined by the presence of small-vessel vasculitis (capillaries, venules, and arterioles). Today, cases of nongranulomatous vasculitis with glomerulonephritis (renal capillaritis) and pulmonary infiltrates (alveolitis or capillaritis) would be considered MPA. and not PAN. The Chapel Hill Consensus Conference (CHCC) on Nomenclature set forth these guidelines. The guidelines also stress that PAN and MPA are not immune complex mediated and are not secondary forms of vasculitis, as might be caused by infections, hepatitis virus, or systemic lupus and other rheumatological diseases.

EPIDEMIOLOGY. Because not all authors strictly adhere to the CHCC guidelines, it is difficult to know the incidence of PAN. Even liberal application of these guidelines indicates that PAN is a rare disease, with an annual incidence of less than 1/100,000. Some authors include vasculitis caused by hepatitis, mediated by immune complexes and cryoglobulins, in this figure. Men and women are equally affected. PAN may affect people of any age, but the incidence peaks between 40 and 60 years of age.

PATHOGENESIS. When one properly excludes cases associated with hepatitis, the cause of medium-sized vessel vasculitis compatible with PAN is unknown. The histopa-

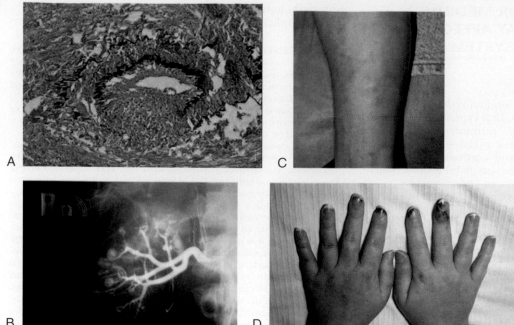

FIGURE 84–5 Polyarteritis nodosa (PAN). In PAN, the likelihood of having adequate collateral circulation to maintain tissue viability following vasoocclusion is less than that seen in other vasculitides. **A,** Section of a muscular artery showing destruction of the internal elastic lamina (from 5 to 8 o'clock), as well as intimal thickening and stenosis. Although aneurysms may be visually more striking on angiography, vascular occlusive lesions **(B)** may contribute to high-renin hypertension and renal failure. **C,** Palpable subcutaneous nodules on the patient's forearms that were painful. **D,** Infarcts on the fingers caused by severe digital artery involvement.

tiology of lesions varies and often evolves in time, at first having a predominance of neutrophils and later mononuclear cells. Granulomas and increased numbers of eosinophils *are not* present. Necrotizing changes may follow, with weakening of the vessel wall and aneurysm formation or myointimal proliferation, causing stenosis and occlusion.

CLINICAL FEATURES. Systemic symptoms are present in at least 50 percent of all patients in different series. Any organ system can be involved. However, if one adheres to CHCC guidelines, several features should not be included because they reflect microvascular (capillary-venule) disease—palpable purpura, pulmonary infiltrates, or hemorrhage and glomerulonephritis. In contrast, these may be findings in MPA.

PAN would more typically include deep skin inflammatory changes that may produce painful nodules (similar to erythema nodosum) or progress to infarction and gangrene (30 to 50 percent), neuropathy (especially mononeuritis multiplex, 20 to 50 percent), renal infarction and insufficiency (approximately 10 to 30 percent), hypertension (approximately 30 percent), segmental pulmonary infarctions (less than 40 percent), and cardiac disease (10 to 30 percent; congestive failure, angina, infarction, pericarditis). Although musculoskeletal symptoms occur in over 50 percent of all PAN patients, they are not a helpful differential diagnostic feature. As noted for CSS, markers of poor prognosis include ischemia or infarction of critical organs (brain, gut, kidneys, and heart). Although clinically apparent heart disease may only affect less than one third of cases, postmortem examination may reveal medium-sized vessel vasculitis or consequences of hypertension (left ventricular hypertrophy, congestive heart failure) in up to 75 percent.[21]

DIFFERENTIAL DIAGNOSIS. The discussion of epidemiology and classification (see earlier) has addressed this issue. However, it is important to reemphasize that certain infections may cause inflammation of medium-sized vessels. All patients with clinical findings that resemble PAN should be tested for hepatitis B and C. A PAN-like presentation is most often associated with hepatitis B virus (HBV) and cryoglobulinemia, whereas an MPA-like presentation occurs more frequently in association with HCV infection and cryoglobulinemia. Rarely, infection with human immunodeficiency virus (HIV) may present in this fashion. In immunocompromised hosts, cytomegalovirus (CMV) should also be sought as a possible cause of small and medium-sized vessel disease. The PAN-MPA–like spectrum obligates a search for bacterial and fungal infections as causes of endocarditis or endovascular vegetations. Use and abuse of vasoactive drugs (e.g., cocaine, amphetamines, ephedrine) should also be considered (see Chap. 68). A subsequent section of this chapter discusses sarcoidosis with vasculitis, another disease that can affect vessels of any size. PAN is not associated with ANCA. No serological diagnostic tests exist for PAN; the diagnosis depends on biopsy or angiographic proof of medium-sized vessel inflammation (Fig. 84-5).

TREATMENT. The guidelines for treatment are the same as those for CSS. Not all patients with PAN require the addition of a cytotoxic agent (cyclophosphamide, methotrexate, or azathioprine). However, in the setting of critical organ disease, one should not hesitate to use these agents.

Other primary vasculitides such as hypersensitivity vasculitis, Henoch-Schönlein purpura, and WG may all have cardiac consequences. However, because vasculitis-mediated heart disease is infrequent in these disorders, they will not be addressed further here. The principles of treatment are similar to those noted for CSS and PAN, with the exception that WG therapy always requires the addition of a cytotoxic agent. Although primary cardiac involvement from vasculitis is not common in WG, preliminary reports have suggested that atherosclerosis may occur in an accelerated fashion in these patients compared with controls that are matched for age, gender, and conventional risk factors.[23,24] This story is similar to the one that has emerged for SLE and rheumatoid arthritis (see later). The association of chronic inflammatory disease and increased cardiovascular risk would suggest that patients with these conditions be evaluated by experts in preventive cardiology so that an aggressive approach may be implemented to reverse treatable cofactors for accelerated atherosclerosis. Whether accelerated atherosclerosis is of equal concern in large-vessel vasculitis is suspect, but unproven.

SYSTEMIC RHEUMATOLOGICAL DISORDERS

Rheumatoid Arthritis

Rheumatoid arthritis (RA) is the most common form of chronic inflammatory polyarthritis. Rheumatoid factor (RF) is present in approximately 70 percent of patients. Its presence does not confirm the diagnosis of RA; it is frequently detected in other diseases. including chronic viral hepatitis and bacterial endocarditis. A newer test, anticyclic citrullinated peptide, adds specificity to serological diagnosis of the patient with a compatible clinical syndrome; it is not detected in RF-positive patients with hepatitis C and arthritis. Systemic complications of RA include pericarditis, pleuritis, vasculitis, compressive neuropathies, interstitial lung disease, atherosclerotic cardiovascular disease, and Sjögren and Felty syndromes. There is also a slightly increased prevalence of lymphoma, which is important to remember when estimating the risk of drug-induced lymphoproliferative disease in patients with RA.

EPIDEMIOLOGY. RA affects approximately 1 to 3 percent of the population. The disease affects patients of all ages, but is most frequently diagnosed in women (more than 2:1) during their third to fifth decades of life. Patients with a positive circulating rheumatoid factor or human leukocyte antigen (HLA)–DR4 are more likely to have severe erosive joint disease and extraarticular manifestations.

PATHOGENESIS. The cause of RA is unknown. There is a genetic predisposition, but this is seemingly polygenic. There may be an infectious trigger, but no agent has been proved to cause disease. An abnormal and persistent T-cell response triggers macrophage activation. Tumor necrosis factor, interleukin-1, and other cytokines sustain the chronic inflammatory response, which includes angiogenesis, proliferation of synovial tissue, and bone remodeling.

CLINICAL FEATURES. RA is a chronic symmetrical polyarthritis that affects small and large joints, especially the metacarpophalangeal joints and wrists, although sparing the lumbar and thoracic spines and distal interphalangeal joints. Characteristic radiographic damage to the joints occurs in most patients, and may be detected early in the course of the disease with MRI.

RA affects the pericardium in approximately 40 percent of patients, as indicated by echocardiographic and necropsy studies (see Chap. 70). Chronic, asymptomatic effusive pericardial disease is more common than acute pericarditis.[25] However, the frequency of symptomatic pericardial disease in outpatients with RA has been estimated as less than 0.5 percent in a series of 41 selected patients with severe RA. Asymptomatic pericardial abnormalities were commonly observed on echocardiography in the era before current aggressive approaches to treatment of the disease. Patients with rheumatoid pericardial disease are generally older and have longstanding RA. The electrocardiogram (ECG) is usually normal in patients with chronic pericardial disease, but may show characteristic changes in acute pericarditis. Coexistent small pleural effusions are common and may reflect rheumatoid serositis or hemodynamic effects of the pericarditis. Pericardial calcification can occur, mimicking tuberculous pericarditis, but this is uncommon.

Limited data have been published on the nature of pericardial fluid in RA. Fluid is frequently blood-tinged, with leukocyte counts ranging from scant to more than 30,000/mm³, generally with a neutrophil predominance. The glucose level in the pericardial fluid may be low when compared with serum glucose levels, similar to markedly depressed glucose levels reported in rheumatoid pleural effusions. The presence of rheumatoid factor in the fluid does not confirm the diagnosis of RA pericarditis. Constrictive pericarditis can occur and must be distinguished from restrictive cardiomyopathy, which is a rare complication of secondary amyloidosis in patients with longstanding RA.

Treatment of clinical pericarditis includes the use of nonsteroidal antiinflammatory drugs (NSAIDs), intensified systemic immunosuppressive therapy, pericardial steroid injections, or pericardiocentesis if hemodynamic compromise occurs. If systemic therapy is ineffective or already at an intense level, patients with recurrent pericardial effusions may require a pericardial window. Constriction should be surgically treated. The current use of aggressive medical therapy early in the course of rheumatoid disease may decrease the frequency of extraarticular complications of RA, including pericardial involvement.

RA does not usually cause clinically significant myocarditis, but congestive heart failure probably occurs with increased prevalence. Secondary amyloidosis is rare in rheumatoid disease, but can cause cardiomyopathy and

atrioventricular block. Tachyarrhythmias can occur as a result of rheumatoid pericarditis. Focal cardiac involvement with rheumatoid nodules has been well described and has been associated with conduction block. All levels of block have been described and, once established, may not respond to antiinflammatory or immunosuppressive therapies. Concerns have been raised regarding an increased risk of death and hospitalization in patients with severe congestive heart failure (CHF) but no RA who received high-dose infliximab (an anti-TNF agent)[25] in a clinical trial. This complication has not been observed with standard dosing of etanercept, an alternative anti-TNF agent.

Autopsy studies have indicated frequent involvement of the cardiac valves and aorta, but these rarely have clinical significance. Slowly progressive granulomatous valvulitis may be difficult, if not impossible, to distinguish from disease unrelated to RA. A rapidly progressive aortic valvulitis, advancing to the need for valve replacement caused by regurgitation over less than 5 years, has been described. Rheumatoid aortitis, with involvement of the aortic valve, has been reported, but aortitis is not frequently recognized antemortem. RA does not cause primary pulmonary hypertension (PHtn). However, secondary hypertension may result from rheumatoid lung disease.

Patients with RA have a decreased life expectancy. The leading cause of death is cardiovascular disease,[26] with a relative risk of at least 2 compared with age-matched normal controls. Potential risk factors for coronary artery disease (CAD) in patients with RA include the chronic systemic inflammatory state, generation of proatherosclerotic high-density lipoprotein (HDL forms), use of selective or nonselective NSAIDs, underusage of aspirin, and use of corticosteroids, which may accelerate atherosclerosis. The relative contributions of these factors to the acceleration of CAD, coronary events, and increased prevalence of CHF are not clear. Significant ischemic disease may be clinically silent because of the relative inactivity of patients with severe RA. Special consideration should be given to the patient with RA about to undergo major noncardiac surgery. Although currently unsupported by adequate evidence, it is reasonable to consider longstanding RA as an intermediate risk factor in assessing preoperative risk, similar to patients with renal insufficiency in the American Heart Association (AHA) guidelines. Coronary arteritis is a rarely reported complication of RA.

DIFFERENTIAL DIAGNOSIS. Rheumatoid arthritis, in the absence of characteristic radiographic erosive changes, remains a diagnosis of exclusion. Other conditions that can cause a symmetrical small and large joint polyarthritis include chronic hepatitis B and C, SLE, several vasculitides, including PAN and WG, and crystal-induced arthropathies. Early or acute RA can also be confused with bacterial endocarditis and other infections, such as parvovirus or rubella. Lyme disease (*Borrelia* infection), which can cause cardiac conduction disease, produces an oligoarticular large joint arthritis that does not mimic RA.

TREATMENT. Current treatment regimens for the treatment of RA emphasize aggressive disease-modifying therapy as soon as the diagnosis is made. Combination therapy with agents such as methotrexate, sulfasalazine, leflunomide, hydroxychloroquine, and low-dose prednisone is frequently used. Nonsteroidal antiinflammatory drugs are no longer the mainstay of therapy, especially because of the following: (1) they have not been shown to alter the course of RA; (2) they are associated with an increased risk of GI bleeding; and (3) chronic use of cyclooxygenase-1 or -2 inhibitors has been linked to adverse cardiovascular outcomes. Antagonists of TNF are extremely effective agents, although cost and the unknown long-term effects of therapy are of concern in their use. The increased use of effective therapy may be associated with a decreased incidence of extraarticular complications of RA. Notable is the concern over increased cardiac morbidity and mortality with the use of infliximab in some patients with severe RA.[27] The data do not clearly preclude the use of these agents in patients with mild and controlled CHF, but increased vigilance is warranted. Given the increased prevalence of CAD in patients with RA, even in the absence of typical risk factors, aggressive attention to lifestyle, blood pressure control, and low-density lipoprotein (LDL) levels seems prudent.

HLA-B27–Associated Spondyloarthropathies

The RF-negative spondyloarthropathies include ankylosing spondylitis, psoriatic arthritis, inflammatory bowel disease–associated arthritis, and postinfectious reactive arthritis.

EPIDEMIOLOGY. The vast majority of white patients with ankylosing spondylitis and many patients with other spondyloarthropathies have the HLA-B27 gene; however, most individuals who carry this gene do not have spondyloarthritis. Patients with spondyloarthropathy share several features that distinguish them from rheumatoid arthritis. Although females do suffer from these disorders, ankylosing spondylitis and reactive arthritis are male-dominant diseases. The spondyloarthropathies are less common than RA.

PATHOGENESIS. The spondyloarthropathies have been historically grouped together because of shared clinical characteristics and the disproportionate presence of the B27 antigen. Recent studies with transgenic rats expressing the human B27 antigen have shown that these animals, when raised in a non–germ-free environment, exhibit inflammation of skin, spine, and other tissues similar to that seen in human patients. This strongly supports the role that B27 plays in the pathogenesis of the inflammation. The presence of the B27 gene may permit an abnormal immune response to gut or mucosal bacterial antigens, which are cross-reactive with tissue antigens present in joints, skin, and other tissues. The abnormal response includes breaking of tolerance to specific self-antigens and the perpetuation of localized inflammation. This theory has not been confirmed, and the antigens have not been reproducibly delineated. Because not all patients with spondyloarthropathies have the B27 antigen, either there are alternative pathogenic mechanisms or the current ability to define the HLA-B locus at a molecular rather than serological level limits our full understanding of its pathogenetic role.

CLINICAL FEATURES. Unlike rheumatoid arthritis, the entire spine, not just the cervical region, may be involved. Sacroiliac joint involvement is frequent, and may be the only musculoskeletal manifestation. Large peripheral joints are commonly involved but, unlike in RA, involvement tends to be asymmetrical. There frequently is inflammation of the tendons, ligaments, or joint capsules at the point of attachment to bone (enthesis; thus, the term *enthesitis*). Diffuse tendon sheath involvement may produce "sausage" digits. In the United States, 90 percent of white patients with ankylosing spondylitis and approximately 60 percent of patients with inflammatory bowel disease–related spondylitis have the HLA-B27 gene. The carriage rate of HLA-B27 in healthy U.S. whites is approximately 10 percent. It is much lower in African Americans and Asians. Presence of the gene predisposes to anterior uveitis and perhaps cardiac conduction disease and proximal aortitis. Thus, patients with psoriatic arthritis, enteropathic arthritis, and reactive arthritis, as well as ankylosing spondylitis, are predisposed to these complications. Patients may express extraskeletal B27-associated complications without overt rheumatic disease. Most importantly, determining the presence of the HLA-B27 gene is *not* a diagnostic test.

Pericarditis, although reported, is not characteristic of the spondyloarthropathies. CAD does not occur at an increased rate (but has not been well studied), and coronary arteritis is not expected. Diastolic dysfunction has been reported[28] in patients who have HLA-B27 but is rarely of clinical significance. Cardiac conduction disease has been well described in patients with ankylosing spondylitis and other B27-associated disorders. Up to one third of patients with ankylosing spondylitis develop conduction disease. Atrioventricular conduction block may initially be intermittent, but tends to progress. Conduction disease is more common in male patients, and as many as 20 percent of males with permanent pacemakers carry the HLA-B27 gene. Conduction disease may be the only abnormality associated with the HLA-B27 gene. Electrophysiological studies have indicated that the level of block is usually at the AV node and is not fascicular.[28] Atrial fibrillation may occur more commonly than expected in patients with the HLA-B27 gene.

Aortic root disease has been reported in up to 100 percent of ankylosing spondylitis patients who also had aortic valve involvement in an autopsy series.[29] Characteristic findings have included thickening of the aortic root with subsequent dilation. Aortic cusp nodularity with proximal thickening comprises the subaortic bump, which was found in 74 percent of 44 selected patients with ankylosing spondylitis[30] using transesophageal echocardiography. In this study, aortic regurgitation developed in 50 percent of patients, and 20 percent of patients developed congestive heart failure, underwent valve replacement, had a stroke, or died as compared with only 3 percent of age- and gender-matched volunteers. The aortic lesions progressed in 24 percent of patients and resolved in an additional 20 percent of patients over approximately a 2-year follow-up. The severity of aortic root disease was associated with the patient's age and duration of spondylitis. Dilation and stiffening of the aortic root may contribute to the aortic regurgitation. Hence, the regurgitant murmur, as in syphilitic aortitis, may be best heard along the right sternal border. However, an electrocardiographic and transthoracic echocardiographic study of 100 Swiss men with ankylosing spondylitis of more than 15 years' duration showed no significant increase in valvular or conduction disease.[30] Given the relatively small number of patients with spondylitis studied, and the fact that patients studied at autopsy represent a limited subset, routine echocardiographic screening for aortitis is prob-ably not warranted. Careful physical examination for the development of aortic regurgitation seems a reasonable approach.

DIFFERENTIAL DIAGNOSIS. The B27-associated spondyloarthropathies are characterized by inflammation of the spine, with morning stiffness of the involved areas. Unlike RA, the peripheral arthritis is usually asymmetrical, with frequent involvement of large joints. The specific spondyloarthropathies are clinically distinguished by their associated extraarticular features (e.g., psoriasis, balanitis, urethritis, oral and/or genital ulcers). Cardiac involvement seems linked more to the presence of the HLA-B27 gene than to any specific rheumatic disorder.

TREATMENT. For years, the spondyloarthropathies have been treated symptomatically, with marginal success, with NSAIDs and physical therapy. Modification of the disease course has not been well documented from such therapy. The disease-modifying drugs used successfully in patients with RA (methotrexate, sulfasalazine) have minimal efficacy in relieving the symptoms and findings of spinal inflammation, although they are variably successful in treating peripheral arthritis. The B27 extraarticular manifestations are treated, as needed, with corticosteroids (uveitis) or surgery (aortic regurgitation, aortitis). The anti-TNF agents (etanercept, infliximab, adalimumab) have demonstrated clinical efficacy in treating the symptoms of spondylitis; whether they will be beneficial for treating or preventing cardiovascular manifestations is currently unknown. As noted earlier, the use of these agents in patients with significant CHF requires vigilance.

Systemic Lupus Erythematosus

SLE is a systemic autoimmune disease characterized by the presence of immune complexes, autoantibodies, and ANAs in the setting of a constellation of clinical features, which may include serositis, arthritis, glomerulonephritis, CNS dysfunction, hemolytic anemia, thrombocytopenia, and leukopenia. Antiphospholipid antibodies (APLA) are present in more than 20 percent of lupus patients and may predispose the individual patient to arterial and venous thrombosis, pulmonary hypertension, or miscarriage (see Chap. 82).

EPIDEMIOLOGY. SLE is more common in women and can occur at any age. Both idiopathic and drug-induced lupus have cardiac manifestations. Reversible drug-induced lupus is well recognized following treatment with various cardiac medications, including procainamide, quinidine, and hydralazine.

PATHOGENESIS. Over 95 percent of patients with SLE have ANAs; however, the presence of even high titers of ANA is *not* diagnostic of SLE. Anti–double-stranded DNA is more specific for SLE but is present in only 50 to 70 percent of patients with idiopathic SLE, often in those with glomerulonephritis. SLE is an autoantibody and immune complex disorder, with immunoglobulin and complement deposition in involved organs, including the heart. The view of SLE as only an immune complex disorder is an oversimplification. Evidence to support this concept includes the following: (1) removal of complexes by apheresis does not dramatically alter the course of the disease; (2) immune deposits can be found in tissue (skin, heart) without resultant inflammation; (3) antibodies may have immunological consequences without being in the form of circulating complexes with antigen; and (4) T-cell hyperreactivity and loss of T-cell tolerance are acknowledged components of SLE. Some lupus animal models have been associated with retroviral infections, but there are no consistently demonstrable viral agents in humans with SLE. Twin studies have suggested an important role for genetic factors.

CLINICAL FEATURES. Pericarditis is the most commonly recognized cardiac problem in SLE.[31] Imaging and autopsy series have demonstrated pericardial involvement in more than 60 percent of patients, although clinically significant pericarditis occurs in less than 30 percent. Unexplained chest pain is common in patients with SLE, but is more likely caused by manifestations other than pericarditis. Pericarditis may occur as the initial manifestation of SLE, appear at any point during the disease course, or occur as a complication of chronic renal disease. Pericardial fluid has generally demonstrated a neutrophil predominance, elevated protein level, and low or normal glucose level. Complement levels in pericardial fluid tend to be low, but this is not a characteristic unique to SLE. The fluid is indistinguishable from that obtained from patients with bacterial pericarditis, and infection must therefore be excluded. Pericardial tamponade may rarely occur at any point in the course of SLE, including the initial presentation. When effusions occur in the setting of chronic renal failure, it is difficult to distinguish uremic from lupus pericarditis. Pericarditis, as well as tamponade, can occur with drug-induced lupus. Constrictive pericarditis, presumably as a sequela of lupus pericarditis, can occur.

Coronary arteritis, resulting in ischemic syndromes, rarely occurs in patients with SLE. The distinction between CAD and coronary arteritis may require sequential angiographic studies, with documentation of more rapid change in luminal images than is usually seen with CAD. Despite the young age of many patients with lupus, atherosclerosis remains the most common cause of ischemic cardiac disease and the most common cause of death in patients with chronic illness. Young patients with SLE may experience a myocardial infarction as the initial manifestation of their coronary artery disease. Middle-aged women with lupus are more than 50 times likely to have a myocardial infarction[32]

than are age- and gender-matched controls without SLE. The prevalence of subclinical CAD is high as determined by scintigraphy, electron beam computed tomography, and autopsy studies. Risk factors for accelerated atherosclerosis include disease duration, period of time treated with corticosteroids, postmenopausal status and hypercholesterolemia. Recently, proatherosclerotic forms of HDL have been described in patients with SLE.[33] An aggressive approach to the management of recognized risk factors for CAD should be implemented in all patients with SLE, especially because lupus-associated independent risk factors have not been fully defined.

Additional causes of acute coronary syndromes in SLE include thrombosis, often related to the presence of APLA (see earlier), and embolism from nonbacterial vegetative endocarditis (Libman-Sacks). The presence of APLA may predispose to thrombosis and has been associated in some echocardiographic studies with valve thickening and nonbacterial endocarditis. Antiendothelial cell antibodies may accelerate atherogenesis. The presence of APLA independently predicted coronary artery disease in a subset analysis of the Helsinki heart study. Treatment of ischemic disease in patients with SLE is similar to those patients with routine atherosclerotic disease, but an extremely aggressive approach to reducing known risk factors is warranted. The rare patient with coronary arteritis should be treated with high-dose corticosteroids, and those patients with thrombotic disease related to APLA should receive long-term anticoagulation. Aspirin is probably *not* sufficient as an anticoagulant; although controlled therapeutic trial evidence is lacking in patients with CAD. Thrombocytopenia is common in patients with APLA, and may complicate therapeutic decisions.

Myocardial dysfunction in lupus is usually multifactorial and may result from immunological injury, ischemia, valvular disease, or coexistent problems such as hypertension. Acute myocarditis is infrequent, but can be the initial presentation of SLE. Patients with peripheral skeletal myositis are reportedly at increased risk for myocarditis. Measurement of troponin I may be of value in documenting cardiac involvement, but the MB fraction of creatine kinase (CK)-MB may be significantly elevated in the presence of skeletal myositis, even in the absence of myocarditis. Noninvasive studies have demonstrated abnormal systolic and diastolic function in patients with active SLE. These changes often reverse with control of disease activity. Acute or chronic congestive heart failure caused by SLE, in the absence of other confounding factors, is not common. Endomyocardial biopsy of the patient with cardiomyopathy and suspected lupus may not provide a specific diagnosis of lupus. The biopsy generally reveals patches of myocardial fibrosis, sparse interstitial mononuclear cell infiltrates, and occasional myocyte necrosis with immune complex deposition, even in areas devoid of inflammatory changes. If unexplained acute LV failure occurs in patients with active SLE, a trial of corticosteroid therapy is warranted.

Tachyarrhythmias can occur in patients with SLE secondary to pericarditis. Sinus tachycardia may be the earliest manifestation of myocarditis. A gallium scan may be abnormal in lupus myocarditis, but this has not been adequately validated. Abnormal heart rate variability may be caused by autonomic dysfunction or occult myocarditis. Abnormal myocardial single-photon emission computed tomography (SPECT) scans have been noted, even in some patients with a normal resting echocardiogram.[34] Unexplained sinus tachycardia, which resolves with treatment of SLE, can occur in the presence of active lupus, even when evidence of cardiac dysfunction is absent. Occult pulmonary embolism should be considered as a cause of tachycardia in patients with SLE, especially in the presence of APLAs.

Conduction disease is not expected in SLE, but babies born to mothers with SLE and some other systemic autoimmune disease have an increased incidence of congenital complete AV block. The pathogenic mechanism is the transmission of maternal anti-Ro and anti-La antibodies in utero, causing myocardial inflammation and fibrosis of the conduction system.[35] The risk for developing complete AV block in infants born to mothers carrying this antibody is low. However, women with systemic autoimmune diseases known to be associated with this antibody should be screened for its presence prior to pregnancy. If present, the fetus should be followed throughout pregnancy with ultrasound studies to detect fetal conduction abnormality or hydrops. AV block usually appears after the first trimester of pregnancy, and is almost always irreversible. If recognized early, dexamethasone *may* be successful in reversing fetal myocarditis in utero. Data to support this intervention are limited. Pacemaker placement is frequently necessary in the infant and may be required shortly after delivery.

Valvular pathology in SLE is common. Recognized 50 years ago as noninfectious vegetations (Libman-Sacks endocarditis), transesophageal studies have shown valvular abnormalities in over 50 percent of patients with SLE.[36] Valvular thickening is the most common echocardiographic finding, followed by vegetations and valvular insufficiency. The vegetations generally localize on the atrial side of the mitral valve and the arterial side of the aortic valve and are usually nonmobile. Over time, the lesions may resolve or worsen; fibrosis may cause retraction of the valve, causing regurgitation. Less commonly, the vegetations on the valve may occlude the orifice, causing stenosis. Valvulitis (Fig. 84-6), with valve fenestrations and rapidly progressing dysfunction, can occur. The nonbacterial vegetations rarely embolize and cause stroke syndromes. Several studies have demonstrated an increased prevalence of cardiac valve dysfunction in the presence of APLA, with or without SLE. Because vegetations may occur in APLA-negative patients with SLE, multiple mechanisms may affect heart valves in lupus patients. Because of the high prevalence of valvular abnormalities in patients with SLE, it has been suggested that all patients with SLE receive antibiotic prophylaxis for endocarditis. Adequate studies do not exist to allow objective evaluation of this proposal. There are reports of mitral and aortic valve replacement in patients with SLE.[37] Valve repair has also been described.[38] Recurrence of valve disease, particularly thrombosis, may affect prosthetic valves.

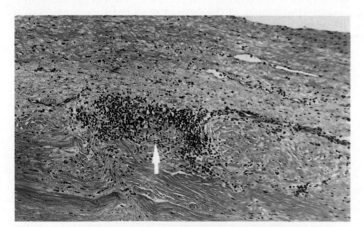

FIGURE 84–6 Valvulitis in systemic lupus erythematosus (SLE). Patients with SLE can develop valve dysfunction caused by bland vegetations (Libman-Sacks endocarditis), valve-associated thrombosis, and rarely true valvulitis. This photomicrograph illustrates aortic valve valvulitis that was discovered at the time of surgery for aortitis and aortic insufficiency (×400). The white arrow indicates a cluster of infiltrating leukocytes.

Based on Doppler echocardiography, pulmonary artery hypertension is common in SLE.[39] Clinically significant pulmonary hypertension is less common. Causes of the development of pulmonary hypertension include thromboembolic disease associated with APLAs, intimal proliferation of the pulmonary artery and, very rarely, arteritis of the pulmonary vessels. Successful heart-lung transplantation has been reported in a patient with SLE and progressive pulmonary hypertension. Aortitis with associated valvular insufficiency can rarely occur in SLE.[40]

DIFFERENTIAL DIAGNOSIS. Among the most common features of SLE are antinuclear antibodies (more than 95 percent), arthralgias and arthritis (60 to 90 percent), constitutional symptoms (50 to 75 percent), rash (50 to 80 percent), Raynaud vasospasm (30 to 60 percent), and glomerulonephritis (30 to 75 percent). Characteristic features that enhance diagnostic likelihood include butterfly rash, sun-sensitive skin eruptions, discoid skin lesions, hemocytopenias (especially thrombocytopenia and leukopenia), antibodies to double-stranded DNA and Sm (anti-Smith), hypocomplementemia, and characteristic findings on biopsies of involved sites. Diseases that can be confused with SLE include dermatomyositis, infections, particularly endocarditis, lymphomas, thrombotic thrombocytopenic purpura, immune thrombocytopenic purpura, Still disease, and sarcoidosis. The pattern of cardiac involvement in SLE is not uniquely diagnostic.

TREATMENT. There is no single treatment for SLE. The specific manifestations are managed on an individual basis. Life-threatening organ involvement is controlled by high-dose corticosteroids, often with the addition of cyclophosphamide, azathioprine, or mycophenolate. Patients with mild pericarditis without threat of hemodynamic compromise are generally treated with a short course of NSAID therapy, unless there is a contraindication, such as renal insufficiency. Corticosteroids are used for more severe disease. If prompt response to steroid therapy does not occur, large sterile pericardial effusions, particularly those accompanied by fever and/or hemodynamic compromise, are best treated with drainage and, if recurrent, consideration of a pericardial window. Arteritis and myocarditis are treated with high-dose corticosteroids, with or without adjunctive cyclophosphamide or azathioprine. Corticosteroid therapy may be tried for acute valvulitis; the indications for surgery are the same as for other causes of valvular dysfunction.

Antiphospholipid Antibody Syndrome

Antiphospholipid antibody syndrome (APLAS) (see Chap. 82) is defined as the presence of either APLA or a lupus anticoagulant *and* a history of otherwise unexplained recurrent venous or arterial thrombosis, or frequent second or third trimester miscarriages. Mild thrombocytopenia, hemolytic anemia, and livedo reticularis are commonly present. APLAs are common (10 to 30 percent) in SLE, although not all these patients will exhibit the clinical syndrome. Low to moderate levels of APLA can also accompany a number of infectious and other autoimmune diseases, usually without clinical consequence. In the absence of an underlying systemic disease, APLAS is termed *primary*. The presence of APLA or a lupus anticoagulant, in the absence of sequelae, does not routinely warrant therapy.

EPIDEMIOLOGY. The true prevalence of the antiphospholipid antibody syndrome is unknown. The demonstration of a lupus anticoagulant or antiphospholipid antibody does not define the clinical syndrome, which requires a coincident clinical thrombotic or embolic event(s).

PATHOGENESIS. See Chapter 82.

CLINICAL FEATURES. Venous thromboembolic disease is the most common manifestation and most often occurs in the legs and lungs. Arterial thrombosis often leads to stroke, but can occur in a wide range of locations. Primary APLAS is not associated with pericarditis, myocarditis, or conduction disease. Cardiac manifestations include thrombotic CAD, intracardiac thrombi, and nonbacterial endocarditis.[41] Heart valve abnormalities occur in approximately 30 percent of patients with primary APLAS and include leaflet thickening, thrombotic masses extending from the valve ring or leaflets, or vegetations. The mitral valve is affected more frequently than the aortic valve and regurgitation is far more common than stenosis (Fig. 84-7). Most valvular involvement is clinically silent. The first manifestation of valvular involvement with APLAS may be a thromboembolic event, such as stroke. The incidence of superimposed

bacterial endocarditis is not known. Treatment of clinically significant valvular or intracardiac masses is high-dose anticoagulation with heparin and then chronic warfarin,[42] with or without the addition of aspirin. Management of heparin dosing, in the setting of a lupus anticoagulant, which prolongs the baseline prothrombin time (PTT), may require consultation with the coagulation laboratory[43] and use of special assays. Vegetations may resolve with anticoagulation therapy over several months,[44] but may also resolve spontaneously. Patients with APLA are at risk for myocardial infarction (MI) and reocclusion following coronary intervention or bypass grafting. Aggressive prophylactic anticoagulation should be used perioperatively in patients with APLA and previous thrombosis. Pulmonary hypertension can occur in patients with APLA secondary to chronic thromboembolic disease. APLA may promote pulmonary artery intimal proliferation.

DIFFERENTIAL DIAGNOSIS. The differential diagnosis of APLAS includes SLE, thrombocytopenic purpura (TTP), idiopathic thrombocytopenic purpura (ITP), and frequently occult neoplasia. SLE can involve the heart, as discussed earlier. TTP can cause coronary ischemia, but not valvular disease; occult neoplasia has been associated with nonbacterial thrombotic endocarditis.

TREATMENT. The primary therapy of APLAS is anticoagulation, generally to a level similar to what is used for patients with prosthetic valves. Preliminary studies have suggested that aspirin is reasonable treatment for arterial disease and a prospective trial has indicated that an international normalized ratio (INR) around 2.0 to 2.5 is sufficient (older retrospective studies had suggested a target INR of 3.0) for venous thrombosis. Monitoring of the anticoagulation level can be difficult in the presence of a prolonged PTT, but use of weight-based algorithms or low-molecular-weight heparin while waiting for a full warfarin effect makes this easier. There are no long-term controlled studies on the effect of chronic anticoagulation and valve disease. Valve replacement can be successfully accomplished in these patients; the indications for surgery are the same as for other patients. The considerations for the type of valve may be influenced by the need for lifelong anticoagulation in these patients, independent of the valve replacement.

Scleroderma

Scleroderma (progressive systemic sclerosis, CREST syndrome) and its variants are characterized by microvascular occlusive disease with vasospasm and intimal proliferation in conjunction with various patterns of cutaneous and parenchymal fibrosis. Although early lesions are inflammatory, the most obvious clinical manifestations result from enhanced fibrosis.

EPIDEMIOLOGY. Scleroderma, particularly progressive systemic sclerosis (PSS), is a rare disease. An increased prevalence occurs in certain populations, such as the Choctaw Native Americans. The average age of onset is between 45 and 65 years. Children are infrequently affected. Among younger individuals, there is a female bias (approximately 7:1 versus 3:1 for entire scleroderma cohorts).

PATHOGENESIS. The cause of scleroderma is unknown. An increased frequency of autoimmune disorders and autoantibodies in relatives of patients suggests the importance of genetic factors. Nonetheless, scleroderma extremely rarely affects both members of twin pairs, indicating that if inheritance plays a role, it is complex, almost certainly polygenic, and perhaps influenced by environmental factors. The latter view is supported by the association of scleroderma-like conditions with exposures to "tainted" oils (rapeseed oil) and drugs (certain preparations of L-tryptophan).

The earliest lesions are mononuclear infiltrates, primarily T lymphocytes, surrounding small arteries. Endothelial injury and vascular leak probably accounts for the edema seen in the early stages of scleroderma in some patients.

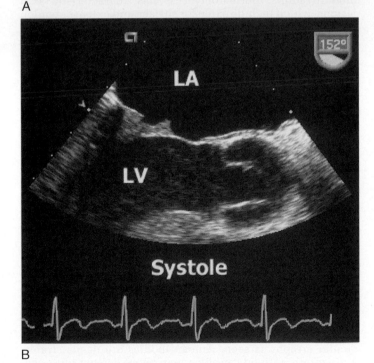

FIGURE 84–7 A, B, Transesophageal echocardiogram demonstrating large sterile vegetations in a 41-year-old male with a previous history of deep venous thrombosis, symptoms of dyspnea on exertion, and a holosystolic apical murmur. A transthoracic echocardiogram demonstrated severe mitral regurgitation. The presence of opposing lesions on both the anterior (right) and posterior (left) leaflets of the mitral valve, also known as "kissing" vegetations, is characteristic of the anticardiolipin antibody syndrome. *(Courtesy of Dr. Mario Garcia, Cleveland Clinic, Cleveland, OH.)*

Immunocyte and endothelial cell activation yields release of cytokines (e.g., transforming growth factor-beta [TGF-β], PDGF, IL-4); this is linked to an increase in fibroblast production of extracellular matrix, especially types I and III collagen and glycosaminoglycans. Over 90 percent of patients are ANA-positive in both PSS and the more limited CREST (*c*alcinosis, *R*aynaud phenomenon, *e*sophageal dysmotility, *s*clerodactyly, *t*elangiectasia) variant. This observation demonstrates a likely role for both T- and B-cell dysregulation.

CLINICAL FEATURES. Raynaud phenomenon usually precedes skin "hardening" and occurs in more than 90 percent of patients, again supporting the initial and critical role of vascular dysfunction. Common features among patients with limited (CREST) or generalized PSS are arthralgias (more than 90 percent), proximal weakness (more than 60 percent), esophageal dysmotility (more than 80 percent), telangiectasias (90 percent with CREST, approximately 60 percent with generalized disease) and pulmonary fibrosis (35 percent of CREST, 70 percent generalized). Renal crisis[45] is 20-fold more common in generalized disease than in CREST (20 versus 1 percent). Calcinosis may occur in both subtypes, but is twice as common in the CREST variant (40 versus 20 percent). Generalized PSS is distinguished by proximal cutaneous fibrosis. Thus, the term *limited* is not meant to indicate the absence of risk of visceral disease, but only refers to the distribution of skin lesions. The pattern of visceral involvement differs somewhat between CREST and PSS.

Pericardial involvement is common in PSS, and includes fibrinous pericarditis in up to 70 percent of patients at autopsy.[46] Echocardiography demonstrates small pericardial effusions in less than 40 percent of patients. Acute pericarditis syndromes, including significant effusions, also occur.[45] The presence of moderate or large pericardial effusions is an independent risk factor for mortality. Pericarditis with effusions may require corticosteroid therapy, but there is concern over the risk of inducing scleroderma renal crisis with the use of corticosteroids.

Necropsy and endomyocardial biopsies demonstrate the presence of patchy fibrosis, occasionally with contraction band necrosis. These findings may result from intermittent intense ischemia produced by microvascular occlusion, perhaps caused by vasospasm. The epicardial coronary arteries are generally angiographically normal. However, approximately 80 percent of PSS and 65 percent of CREST patients have fixed perfusion defects on scintigraphic imaging. Myocardial infarctions have been documented in PSS patients who have angiographically normal coronary arteries. Ventricular conduction abnormalities are common and, along with a septal pseudoinfarct pattern, correlate with reduced myocardial function with exercise. Electrical abnormalities can be found throughout the conduction system, and ventricular ectopy is present in more than 60 percent of patients. Patients with scleroderma, especially those with a history of palpitations or syncope, are prone to sudden death. The risk of sudden death is further increased in patients with coexistent skeletal myositis. Primary valvular disease is not common. Renal crisis[47] may be associated with minimal or extreme hypertension, rapidly rising creatinine level, microangiopathy, thrombocytopenia, and left ventricular failure. Treatment is with angiotensin-converting enzyme (ACE) inhibitors, not corticosteroids. The goal is rapid control of the blood pressure in the low-normal range.

Pulmonary hypertension occurs in both limited scleroderma and PSS, and is a major clinical problem. It may be caused by intrinsic pulmonary artery disease or may be secondary to interstitial fibrosis.[48] Patients with CREST, as well as PSS, should undergo periodic echocardiography to screen for asymptomatic pulmonary hypertension.

DIFFERENTIAL DIAGNOSIS. Initially, prior to skin hardening (sclerodactyly), SLE, RA, or severe primary Raynaud disease can be confused with early scleroderma. Buerger disease does not lead to thick tight skin and is more often seen in male smokers, but can cause Raynaud's phenomenon and digital necrosis (see Chap. 57). Cryoglobulinemia and its primary causes (hepatitis, malignancy, other systemic autoimmune diseases) should be excluded in patients presenting with principally vascular symptoms and ischemic lesions. Eosinophilic fasciitis, carcinoid syndrome, and several paraneoplastic syndromes can rarely also cause some diagnostic confusion. In time, the emergence of features typical of scleroderma enables clarification of diagnosis.

TREATMENT. At present, there is no proven effective treatment to limit the underlying mechanisms responsible for progression of PSS. A controlled trial has suggested that cyclophosphamide may slow pulmonary progression in some patients. Treatment of Raynaud vasospasm is symptomatic. Gastric reflux is often severe, and can be improved by avoiding food and liquid intake before reclining, not assuming a fully horizontal position (wedged pillows for beds or raising head of bed), and by aggressive antacid regimens with proton pump inhibitors. Renal crisis usually responds to aggressive control of blood pressure; ACE inhibitors are the initial agents of choice. A few complications (e.g., myositis, alveolitis, pericarditis) may respond to corticosteroids, but steroid use increases the risk for renal crisis. Conduction disease and arrhythmias are treated as they would be in the absence of PSS. Pulmonary hypertension may respond to vasodilator therapy with endothelin antagonists or prostanoids.

Polymyositis and Dermatomyositis

Myositis with resultant weakness of proximal more than distal skeletal muscles characterizes polymyositis (PM) and dermatomyositis. The creatinine kinase (CK) level is usually elevated. Respiratory muscles can be clinically involved. Both conditions can be associated with fever and interstitial lung disease. Other visceral organ involvement is uncommon in adults. Dermatomyositis has characteristic skin lesions, which include extensor surface and extensor tendon erythema, Gottron papules overlying knuckles, elbows, and knees, edema of the eyelids, and a photosensitive diffuse papular eruption with scaling. Dermatomyositis, in a minority of older patients, may be a paraneoplastic syndrome.

EPIDEMIOLOGY. The incidence of inflammatory myositis is about 2 to 10 new cases/1,000,000 population annually. People in all races and ethnicity groups may develop PM or dermatomyositis. An overall predilection favors females, 2.5:1. However, in children, there is less gender bias (1:1) and, when myositis coexists with other autoimmune diseases (e.g., SLE, scleroderma—"overlap syndromes"), gender bias is enhanced (10:1 females). When myositis coexists with malignancy in the adult population (mean age, 60), it is not gender-biased. Inflammatory myositis can affect patients of all ages. Juvenile dermatomyositis has no association with malignancy. However, it may be associated with visceral arteritis, which can cause bowel ischemia.

PATHOGENESIS. The cause of these disorders is unknown. Involved muscles are infiltrated with lymphocytes, and the lymphocyte subsets and histopathological pattern of inflammation differ between the two disorders. Polymyositis is characterized by endomysial mononuclear cell infiltration, although in dermatomyositis there is a greater amount of perivascular inflammation, and perifascicular atrophy is seen. Autoantibodies are demonstrable, and certain antibody profiles may be associated with specific clinical patterns of presentation of PM and response to therapy; currently, however, these autoantibodies cannot be used to dictate reliably therapeutic decisions. The increased frequency of other autoimmune diseases in relatives, as in scleroderma and lupus, suggests at least some genetic component in pathogenesis.

CLINICAL FEATURES. Both diseases affect skeletal muscle, but can also affect the heart. Pericarditis is not common, but can occur when polymyositis occurs as part of an overlap syndrome with other autoimmune diseases, such as SLE or PSS. Coronary arteritis and ischemic CAD are rarely part of these overlap syndromes. Localized or generalized myocardial dysfunction is common by echocardiographic assessment, but infrequently causes clinical failure. The cardiomyopathy may be steroid-responsive. Corticosteroid myopathy, a complication of treatment that can mimic PM, although with a normal CK, generally affects skeletal but not respiratory or cardiac muscle. PM and dermatomyositis frequently affect the conduction system. In an electrocardiographic study of 77 patients, 23 percent had conduction block,[49] which can occur in the absence of cardiomyopathy, usually in the absence of symptoms. Pulmonary hypertension can occur, but is usually secondary to interstitial lung disease. Acute alveolitis can at times mimic acute CHF. Acute dysphagia caused by muscle dysfunction can predispose to aspiration.

DIFFERENTIAL DIAGNOSIS. PM causes a chronically elevated CK level and/or proximal weakness. Statin therapy can cause myopathy, and occasionally an elevated CK level, and thus can mimic PM. Myalgias are more common than in PM, and weakness less common. Other drugs can also induce elevations in the CK level, and drug-induced myopathy should always be considered before proceeding with diagnostic tests for PM (e.g., electromyography, biopsy). Hypothyroidism can mimic PM and is easily ruled out by appropriate laboratory studies. Inclusion body myositis causes an elevated CK level, but usually is more indolent than PM and frequently also involves the distal muscles. The distinction is important, because it is less responsive to therapy. Polymyalgia rheumatica is not associated with an increase in muscle enzyme levels or weakness and may be associated with giant cell arteritis. Dermatomyositis is recognized by one of several characteristic rashes, although SLE can closely mimic dermatomyositis in some patients.

TREATMENT. There are no controlled trials to guide treatment decisions. Nonetheless, initial therapy of inflammatory myositis when an underlying malignancy is not identified includes high doses of daily oral corticosteroids. In severe disease—that is, in the setting of proximal dysphagia or myocarditis—a "pulse" regimen of several grams of methylprednisolone is often prescribed. Many clinicians frequently use a second agent (e.g., methotrexate, azathioprine, cyclosporine, tacrolimus) along with corticosteroids from the outset or if the patient demonstrates a chronic requirement for high-dose corticosteroid therapy. Long-term immunosuppressive therapy is frequently required. Refractory cases may respond to the addition of monthly high-dose IVIG therapy.

Sarcoidosis

Sarcoidosis is a granulomatous inflammatory disease of unknown cause that primarily affects the lung parenchyma, but can cause significant adenopathy, arthropathy, myositis, fever, renal, liver, skin, eye, and cardiac disease.

EPIDEMIOLOGY. Sarcoidosis can affect men and women of all ages. The peak incidence is in the second to fourth decades. Very few cases are diagnosed in childhood. The prevalence varies with the degree of vigilance applied to screening and susceptibility of populations. Consequently, in Sweden, the prevalence is 64/100,000, although in the United States it has variably been reported as 10 to 40/100,000. The manifestations of the disease are seemingly different in different populations. Scandinavians seem more predisposed to acute sarcoid (Löfgren syndrome). There appears to be a preponderance of cases with cardiac involvement reported from Japan. African Americans and Hispanics are more prone to severe multisystem disease.

PATHOGENESIS. The cause of sarcoidosis is unknown. A multicenter U.S. study of sarcoidosis has found limited evidence to support an environmental or occupational exposure cause for sarcoidosis. In contrast, studies have linked infectious agents, including mycobacterial and propionibacterial organisms, with sarcoidosis. Evidence of polyclonal B-cell activation in the blood and several reports of transmission of sarcoidosis to recipients of organs donated by patients with sarcoidosis have also supported the presence of a transmissible agent, despite the general successful use of immunosuppressive therapy. Analysis of tissue involved with sarcoidosis reveals that T-helper lymphocytes drive the granulomatous inflammatory response. There is evidence for a genetic predisposition to sarcoidosis, including familial clustering and shared HLA haplotypes in different populations.

CLINICAL PRESENTATION. Pericarditis has been frequently described and necropsy studies have documented cardiac involvement in 27 percent of patients, but clinically significant pericarditis is uncommon. The granulomatous infiltrative disease of the myocardium is often asymptomatic, but can cause arrhythmias, conduction disease and, rarely, otherwise unexplained congestive heart failure (see Chap. 66). Granulomatous infiltration may be patchy, with a predilection toward involvement of the left ventricle, particularly the upper septal area. This distribution influences the likelihood of obtaining a diagnostic right-sided endomyocardial biopsy. Use of gallium imaging may be helpful in determining the need for and duration of immunosuppressive therapy, but this approach has not been proved in any formal trial. Sarcoid-dilated cardiomyopathy may be difficult to distinguish from idiopathic cardiomyopathy or occasionally from giant cell myocarditis. Conduction disease is more common than pump dysfunction in patients with sarcoidosis.[50] Biopsy may help distinguish sarcoidosis from idiopathic or giant cell myocarditis, but the diagnostic yield of endomyocardial biopsy is low.[51] Active sarcoidosis is generally believed to be steroid-responsive. However, myocardial involvement with sarcoid can result in large patches of fibrotic scar that may be arrhythmogenic but no longer respond to steroids. Scar is often significantly underestimated by imaging studies and biopsy.

Pulmonary artery hypertension and cor pulmonale can occur in sarcoidosis, generally as a result of pulmonary fibrosis. Systemic vasculitis is an uncommon complication of sarcoidosis. Its prevalence remains unknown. Sarcoid vasculitis can affect small- to large-caliber vessels, including the aorta. The latter presentation can be easily confused with Takayasu arteritis (Fig. 84-8). African American patients appear predisposed to developing large vessel involvement.

DIFFERENTIAL DIAGNOSIS. Clinically, there are many mimics of systemic sarcoidosis, including chronic viral hepatitis, granulomatous hepatitis, SLE, Still disease, lymphoma, HIV infection, fungal infections, and Sjögren syndrome. When tissue specimens are available, special stain and culture assays should be performed to seek fungal and mycobacterial infection. The ACE level should *not* be relied on as a diagnostic test. Cardiac sarcoidosis is usually diagnosed by the presence of otherwise unexplained cardiomyopathy or conduction disease in the presence of documented pulmonary or hepatic sarcoidosis. Despite inherent sampling errors, myocardial biopsy is desirable when reasonable. Cardiac MRI is a useful diagnostic test.

TREATMENT. Although corticosteroid therapy may be palliative for all forms of sarcoidosis, including vasculitis, relapses of the disease are common and may preclude total withdrawal of treatment. Myocardial involvement is generally treated with long-term therapy, and frequently steroid-sparing therapies such as methotrexate are empirically added. Morbidity from disease and treatment is common. There are no controlled trials of therapeutic interventions in cardiac sarcoid, and specifically there is no evidence to guide the duration of therapy. The serum ACE level is an imperfect guide to therapy. Malignant ventricular arrhythmias may result from scarring and may not respond to antiinflammatory therapies.

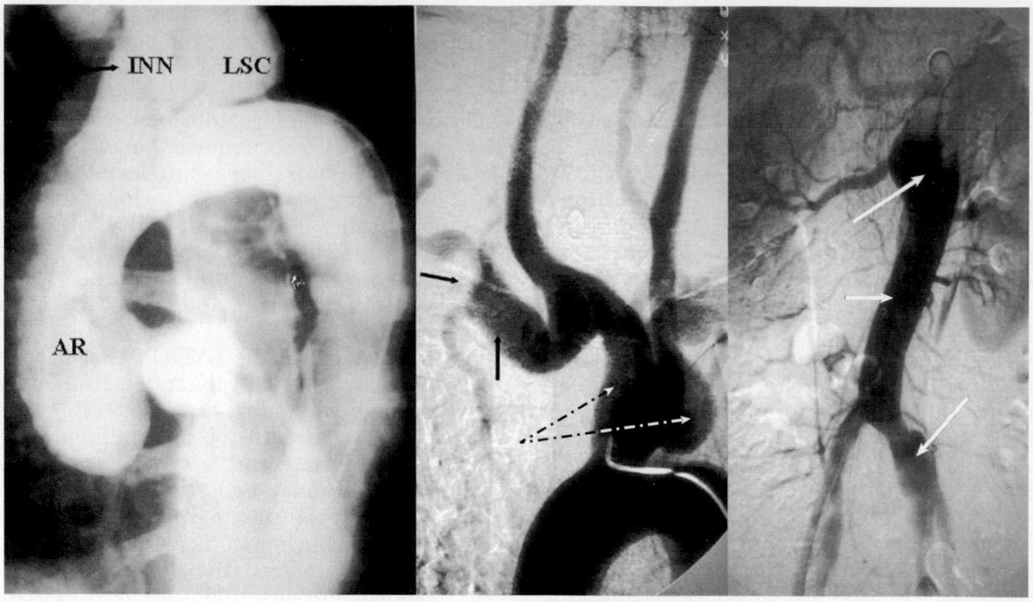

FIGURE 84-8 Sarcoid vasculitis shown in this aortogram from a 20-year-old African-American man who presented with chronic polyarthritis, uveitis, Bell palsy, and upper extremity claudication. The angiogram shows aneurysmal dilation of the innominate and proximal subclavian arteries (dotted arrows), the entire aortic root (AR) **(left panel)**, occlusion of both subclavian vessels (arrows) associated with arm claudication **(middle panel)**, and stenosis of the iliac vessels **(right panel)**. Note how sarcoid vasculitis can mimic Takayasu arteritis (TA). However, TA is associated with stenoses three to four times more often than aneurysms. Therefore, this angiographic picture should raise the differential diagnosis of TA. INN = innominate artery; LSC = left subclavian artery.

REFERENCES

Takayasu Arteritis

1. Kerr GS, Hallahan CW, Giordano J, et al: Takayasu's arteritis. Ann Intern Med 120:919, 1994.
2. Hashimoto Y, Tanaka M, Hata A, et al: Four years follow-up study in patients with Takayasu arteritis and severe aortic regurgitation; assessment by echocardiography. Int J Cardiol 54(Suppl):173-176, 1997.
3. Seko Y, Sato O, Takagi A, et al: Restricted usage of T-cell receptor V alpha-V beta genes in infiltrating cells in aotic tissue of patients with Takayasu's arteritis. Circulation 93:1788-1790, 1996.
4. Maksimowicz-McKinnon K, Clark TM, Hoffman GS: Takayasu's arteritis: Limitations of therapy and guarded prognosis in an American cohort. Arthritis Rheum 56:1000-1009, 2007.
5. Tso E, Flamm SD, White RD, et al: Takayasu's arteritis: Utility of magnetic resonance imaging in diagnosis and treatment. Arthritis Rheum 46:1634-1642, 2002.
6. Webb M, Chambers A, Al-Nahhas A, et al: The role of F-FDG PET in characterizing disease activity in Takayasu arteritis. Eur J Nucl Med Mol Imaging 31:627-634, 2004.
7. Pfizenmaier DH, Al Atawi FO, Castillo K, et al: Predictor of left ventricular dysfunction in patients with Takayasu's arteritis or giant cell aortitis. Clin Exp Rheumatol 22(Suppl 36):S41-45), 2004.
8. Hoffman GS, Leavitt RY, Kerr GS, et al: Treatment of Takayasu's with methotrexate. Arthritis Rheum 37:578-582, 1994.
9. Hoffman GS, Merkel PA, Brasington RD, et al: Anti-tumor necrosis factor therapy in patients with difficult to treat Takayasu arteritis. Arthritis Rheum 50:2296-2304, 2004.

Giant Cell Arteritis

10. Weyand CM, Goronzy JJ: Medium and large vessel vasculitis. N Engl J Med 349:160, 2003.
11. Evans JM, O'Fallon WM, Hunder GG: Increased incidence of aortic aneurysm and dissection in giant cell (temporal) arteritis. Ann Intern Med 122:502-507, 1995.
12. Hoffman GS, Cid MC, Rendt KE, et al: Infliximab-GCA Study Group: Prednisone and infliximab for giant cell arteritis: A randomized, double-blind, placebo-controlled, multicenter study of efficacy and safety. Ann Intern Med (in press).
13. Hoffman GS, Cid MC, Hellmann DB, et al: A multicenter, randomized, double-blind, placebo-controlled trial of adjuvant methotrexate treatment for giant cell arteritis. Arthritis Rheum 46:1309-1318, 2002.
14. Nesher GN, Berkun Y, Mates M, et al: Low-dose aspirin and prevention of cranial ischemic complications in GCA. Arthritis Rheum 50:1332-1337, 2004.
15. Lee MS, Smith SD, Galor A, Hoffman GS: Antiplatelet and anticoagulant therapy in patients with giant cell arteritis. Arthritis Rheum 54:3306-3309, 2006.

Idiopathic Aortitis

16. Rojo-Leyva F, Ratliff N, Cosgrove DM, Hoffman GS: Study of 52 patients with idiopathic aortitis from a cohort of 1,204 surgical cases. Arthritis Rheum 43:901-907, 2000.

Kawasaki Disease

17. Newburger JW, Takahashi M, Gerber MA, et al: Diagnosis, treatment, and long-term management of Kawasaki disease: A statement for health professionals from the Committee on Rheumatic Fever, Endocarditis and Kawasaki Disease, Council on Cardiovascular Disease in the Young, American Heart Association. Circulation 110:2747-2471, 2004.
18. Davis RL, Waller PL, Mueller BA, et al: Kawasaki syndrome in Washington state: Race-specific incidence rates and residential proximity to water. Arch Pediatr Adolesc Med 149:66-69, 1995.
19. Barron K: Kawasaki disease: Etiology, pathogenesis and treatment. Cleve Clin J Med 69(Suppl 2):69-78, 2002.
20. Barron KS: Kawasaki disease. In Hoffman GS, Weyand CM (eds): Inflammatory Disease of Blood Vessels. New York, Marcel Dekker, 2002, pp 305-319.

Churg-Strauss Syndrome, Polyarteritis Nodosa

21. Sable-Fourtassou R, Cohen P, Mahr A, et al: Antineutrophil cytoplasmic antibodies and the Churg Strauss syndrome. Ann Intern Med 143:632-638, 2005.
22. Sinico RA, Di Toma L, Maggiore U, et al: Prevalence and clinical significance of antineutrophil cytoplasmic antibodies in Churg Strauss syndrome. Arthritis Rheum 52:2926-2935, 2005.

Rheumatoid Arthritis

23. Raza K, Thambyrajah J, Townsend JN, et al: Suppression of inflammation in primary systemic vasculitis restores vascular endothelial function: Lessons for atherosclerotic disease? Circulation 102:1470-1472, 2000.
24. deLeeuw K, Sanders J-S, Stegeman C, et al: Accelerated atherosclerosis in patients with Wegener's granulomatosis. Ann Rheum Dis 64:753-759, 2005.
25. Kitas G, Banks MJ, Bacon PB: Cardiac involvement in rheumatoid disease. Clin Med 1:18-21, 2001.
26. Solomon DH, Karlson EW, Rimm EB, et al: Cardiovascular morbidity and mortality in women diagnosed with rheumatoid arthritis. Circulation 11:1307-1307, 2003.
27. Sarzi-Puttini P, Atzeni F, Shoenfeld Y, Ferraccioli G : TNF-α, rheumatoid arthritis, and heart failure: A rheumatological dilemma. Autoimmunity Rev 4:153-161, 2005.

HLA-B27–Associated Spondyloarthropathies

28. Bergfeldt L: HLA-B27–associated cardiac disease. Ann Intern Med 127:621-629, 1997.
29. Roldan CA, Chavez J, Wiest PW, et al: Aortic root disease associated with ankylosing spondylitis. J Am Coll Cardiol 32:1397-1404, 1998.
30. Brunner F, Kunz A, Weber U, Kissling R: Ankylosing spondylitis and heart abnormalities: Do cardiac conduction disorders, valve regurgitation and diastolic dysfunction occur more often in male patients with diagnosed ankylosing spondylitis for over 15 years than in the normal population? Clin Rheumatol 25:24-29, 2005.

Systemic Lupus Erythematosus

31. Moder KG, Miller TD, Tazelaar HD: Cardiac involvement in systemic lupus erythematosus. Mayo Clin Proc 74:275-284, 1999.

32. Manzi S, Meilahn EN, Rairie JE, et al: Age-specific incidence rates of myocardial infarction and angina in women with systemic lupus erythematosus: Comparison with the Framingham study. Am J Epidemiol 145:408-415, 1997.

33. McMahon M, Grossman J, FitzGerald J, et al: Proinflammatory high-density lipoprotein as a biomarker for atherosclerosis in patients with systemic lupus erythematosus and rheumatoid arthritis. Arthritis Rheum 54:2541-2549, 2006.

34. Laganà B, Schillaci O, Tubani L, et al: Lupus carditis: Evaluation with technetium-99m MIBI myocardial SPECT and heart rate variability. Angiology 50:143-148, 1999.

35. Finkelstein Y, Adler Y, Harel L, et al: Anti-Ro (SSA) and anti-La (SSB) antibodies and complete congenital heart block. Ann Intern Med 148:204-208, 1997.

36. Roldan CA, Shively BK, Crawford MH: An echocardiographic study of valvular heart disease associated with systemic lupus erythematosus. N Engl J Med 335:1424-1430, 1996.

37. Fluture A, Chaudhari S, Frishman WH: Valvular heart disease and systemic lupus erythematosus: Therapeutic implications. Heart Dis 5(5):349-353, 2003.

38. Perez-Villa F, Font J, Azqueta M, et al: Severe valvular regurgitation and antiphospholipid antibodies in systemic lupus erythematosus: A prospective, long-term follow-up study. Arthritis Rheum 53:460-467, 2005.

39. Johnson SR, Gladman DD, Urowitz MB, et al: Pulmonary hypertension in systemic lupus. Lupus 13:506-509, 2004.

40. Ohara N, Myiata T, Kurata A, et al: Ten years' experience of aortic aneurysm associated with systemic lupus erythematosus. Eur J Vasc Endovasc Surg 19:288-293, 2000.

Antiphospholipid Antibody Syndrome

41. Hojnik M, George J, Ziporen L, Shoenfeld Y: Heart valve involvement (Libman-Sacks endocarditis) in the antiphospholipid syndrome. Circulation 92:1579-1587, 1996.

42. Lim W, Crowther MA, Eikelboom JW: Management of antiphospholipid antibody syndrome: A systematic review. JAMA 295:1050-1057, 2006.

43. Bartholomew J: Dosing of heparin in the presence of a lupus anticoagulant. J Clin Rheumatol 4:307-311, 1998.

44. Agirbasli MA, Hansen DE, Byrde BF: Resolution of vegetations with anticoagulation after myocardial infarction in primary antiphospholipid syndrome. Echocardiography 10:877-880, 1997.

Scleroderma

45. Rhew EY, Barr WG: Scleroderma renal crisis: New insights and developments. Curr Rheumatol Rep 6:129-136, 2004.

46. Byers RJ, Marshall DAS, Freemont AJ: Pericardial involvement in systemic sclerosis. Ann Rheum Dis 45:393-394, 1997.

47. Steen V: The heart in systemic sclerosis. Curr Rheumatol Rep 6:137-140, 2004.

48. Chang B, Schachna L, White B, et al: Natural history of mild-moderate pulmonary hypertension and the risk factors for severe pulmonary hypertension in scleroderma. J Rheumatol 33:269-274, 2006.

Polymyositis and Dermatomyositis

49. Stern R, Godblold J, Chess Q, Kagen L: ECG abnormalities in polymyositis. Arch Intern Med 144:2185-2188, 1984.

Sarcoidosis

50. Doughan AR, Williams BR: Cardiac sarcoidosis. Heart 92:282-288, 2006.

51. Uemura A, Morimoto SI, Hiramissu S, et al: Histological diagnostic rate of cardiac sarcoidosis: Evaluation of endomyocardial biopsies. Am Heart J 138:299-302, 1999.

CH 84

Rheumatic Diseases and the Cardiovascular System

Direct Complications of
Neoplasia, 2105
Cardiac Tumors, 2105
Pericardial Involvement, 2105
Superior Vena Cava
    Obstruction, 2106
Valvular Heart Disease, 2108
Ischemic Heart Disease, 2108
Arrhythmias, 2108

Indirect Cardiovascular
Complications of
Neoplasia, 2108
Hyperviscosity, 2108

Cardiovascular Complications of
Cancer Therapeutic Agents, 2108
Traditional Chemotherapeutic
    Agents, 2108
Targeted Therapeutics, 2111
Complications of Radiation
    Therapy, 2115

Management of Heart Failure
Induced by Cancer Therapeutic
Agents, 2116

Future Perspectives, 2116

References, 2116

CHAPTER 85

The Cancer Patient and Cardiovascular Disease

Thomas Force

Patients with cancer frequently develop complications in the cardiovascular system. These complications can occur as a result of locally invasive disease or distant spread. Pericardial effusions with tamponade and superior vena cava syndrome are relatively common manifestations of advanced cancers. The cardiovascular system can also be affected by indirect complications, most notably hyperviscosity syndromes, resulting from myeloproliferative disorders or leukemias. Finally, several of the therapies used to treat cancer, including radiation, traditional chemotherapeutics, and so-called targeted therapeutics, that are aimed at factors that are causal or that promote cancer growth and metastasis, can also be toxic to the heart and cardiovascular system. Because cardiovascular disease and cancer are common diseases, and share common risk factors, they often coexist in patients. It has become increasingly clear that optimal care of oncology patients by cardiologists and oncologists requires an understanding of both disciplines.

DIRECT COMPLICATIONS OF NEOPLASIA

Cardiac Tumors

Primary tumors of the heart are uncommon and are usually benign (see Chap. 69). Briefly, the classes of primary tumors that involve the heart include myxomas (which account for 25 to 50 percent of all primary cardiac tumors), papillary fibroelastomas (10 percent), rhabdomyomas (of which approximately 50 percent occur in association with tuberous sclerosis), lipomas, and hemangiomas (5 to 10 percent).[1] Malignant tumors are usually sarcomas (angiosarcoma being most common) or lymphomas, although primary lymphomas of the heart occur much less frequently than secondary involvement.

In contrast, direct extension of tumors, hematogenous spread, and retrograde lymphatic extension to the heart are common.[2] Based on autopsy studies, involvement of the heart or pericardium occurs in 10 to 12 percent of all patients with malignancies. Tumors most likely to involve the heart are primary lung tumors (36 percent of all patients with cardiac involvement). The grouping of lymphoma, leukemia, and Kaposi sarcoma accounts for 20 percent, breast cancer for 7 percent, and esophageal cancer for 6 percent. Most of these involve the heart by direct extension or regional lymphatic invasion. Metastases to the myocardium are much less common and are often caused by hematogenous spread of melanomas or lymphomas. From 46 to 71 percent of patients with melanoma have metastases to the myocardium and/ or pericardium. Although a relatively rare cancer, mesotheliomas commonly invade the pericardium (74 percent of patients) or myocardium (25 percent of patients). Patients with myocardial metastases of any origin often present with sudden onset of arrhythmia or, more rarely, conduction abnormalities.

Pericardial Involvement

PERICARDIAL EFFUSION. The differential diagnosis of a pericardial effusion (see Chap. 70) in a patient with a known malignancy includes malignant effusion, radiation-induced or drug-induced pericarditis, idiopathic pericarditis, infectious (including tuberculosis, fungal, or bacterial), or iatrogenic, secondary to procedures. In one series, approximately 40 percent of patients with cancer and a pericardial effusion were found to have either radiation-induced (10 percent) or idiopathic (32 percent) effusions,[2] although other series have reported even higher rates.[3] Drug-induced pericarditis is typically seen after high-dose anthracycline or cyclophosphamide therapy (see later, "Cardiovascular Complications of Cancer Therapeutic Agents").

CARDIAC TAMPONADE. Approximately one third of patients with pericardial involvement will present with impaired cardiac function, and cardiac compression can progress to tamponade, demanding immediate drainage. Patients' symptoms include chest pain, fever, dyspnea, cough, and peripheral edema. Tamponade without two or more signs of an inflammatory process (typical pain, friction rub, fever, diffuse ST segment elevation) is more likely to be malignant (2.9-fold increase in risk).[3] On examination, heart sounds may be distant, and jugular venous distention and pulsus paradoxus, often with a narrow pulse pressure, are present. The Kussmaul sign, which is a paradoxical rise in the jugular venous pulse with inspiration, can also be seen but is not specific for tamponade and is also seen in constrictive pericarditis, restrictive cardiomyopathy, and right ventricular infarction. In some cases, the electrocardiogram (ECG) may show low voltage and, rarely, electrical alternans. The chest x-ray often shows an enlarged cardiac silhouette. Echocardiography demonstrates the effusion, which is usually large, although it does not have to be if the fluid has accumulated quickly. The diagnosis of tamponade physiology is based on diastolic inversion (or collapse) of the right ventricular free wall on echocardiography. Right atrial compression may also be seen. However, tamponade can occur with loculated effusions and, in these cases, typical echocardiographic signs may be absent.

The acute treatment of tamponade includes careful fluid replacement as a temporizing measure if the patient is believed to be volume-depleted and hemodynamics are compromised.[3] Echocardiography-guided pericardiocentesis is required. Fluid should be sent for a full battery of diagnostic tests because, as noted, the cause is commonly noncancerous, even in patients with known cancer. If the effusion is malignant, cytological examination of the pericardial fluid is positive in approximately 85 percent of patients.

Although no randomized clinical trials of various strategies have been done, the risk of recurrence of the effusion appears to be reduced by extended catheter drainage (3 ± 2 days; 11.5 percent recurrence) as opposed to simple pericardiocentesis (36 percent recurrence).[4,5] Recurrence of pericardial effusion can often be treated with repeat pericardiocentesis with extended catheter drainage. Some have used intrapericardial instillation of chemotherapeutic agents or sclerosing agents (e.g., thiotepa, tetracycline), but it is not clear that this approach is more effective than extended catheter drainage. Occasionally, percutaneous balloon pericardiotomy or pericardiectomy may be required, but patients with malignant effusions have such a poor prognosis (median survival of 135 days in one series of 275 patients),[4] invasive procedures should be avoided, if possible. Therapy is directed at the underlying tumor.

CONSTRICTIVE PERICARDITIS. Constrictive or effusive-constrictive pericarditis is a late complication of chest irradiation that may be becoming more common because of the longer survival of patients with breast cancer and Hodgkin's disease who typically receive chest irradiation. In a retrospective study of 635 patients with Hodgkin's disease, 44 patients developed delayed pericarditis, and

pericardiectomy was required in 12.[6] This study included patients who had received mantle irradiation with and without subcarinal block, and rates are lower when blocking is used. The median range for time between radiation therapy and pericardiectomy is 7 to 13 years.[7] In a series of 163 patients undergoing pericardiectomy for constrictive pericarditis of various causes, prior irradiation significantly adversely affected both perioperative mortality (21.4 versus 2.7 percent for postradiation versus idiopathic constrictive pericarditis) and long-term survival.[3,7] Reasons for this include mediastinal fibrosis from the radiation, which limits the amount of pericardium that can be removed, increasing the risk of residual constriction. In addition, a restrictive myopathy that can follow chest irradiation and can accompany constrictive pericarditis adds significant additional morbidity and mortality. Patients may have underlying myocardial fibrosis and should be evaluated for this prior to considering pericardiectomy because excluding these patients reduces perioperative mortality.[3]

Superior Vena Cava Obstruction

Superior vena cava syndrome (SVCS) occurs when obstruction of the thin-walled superior vena cava (SVC) interrupts venous return of blood to the right atrium from the head, upper extremities, and thorax. The SVC is encircled by lymph nodes that drain from the right thoracic cavity and the lower left thorax (Fig. 85-1). SVCS often manifests with slowly progressive symptoms worsening over weeks and recruitment of collateral circulation via several venous systems, including the azygos and internal mammary. When symptoms occur abruptly, SVCS can constitute a medical emergency.[8]

SYMPTOMS. Obstruction of the SVC can be caused by malignant or benign disease. Clinically, patients report the progressive development of shortness of breath (60 percent), facial swelling (50 percent), cough (24 percent), arm swelling (18 percent), chest pain (15 percent), and dysphagia (9 percent) as well as distorted vision, hoarseness, nausea, headache, and syncope. Physical findings include venous distention over the neck (66 percent) and chest wall (54 percent), facial edema (46 percent), plethora (19 percent), and cyanosis (19 percent). Symptoms may be exacerbated by lying in a supine position or bending forward. Patients with this syndrome may develop life-threatening complications, such as laryngeal or cerebral edema.

CAUSATIVE FACTORS. Seventy-five to 85 percent of cases of SVCS result from neoplasia (Table 85-1), with lung cancer accounting for most cases.[8] Of patients with lung cancer, 2 to 5 percent develop SVCS. However, 10 to 20 percent of patients with small cell lung cancer (SCLC), which constitutes only 20 percent of lung cancers, develop SVCS, accounting for almost 40

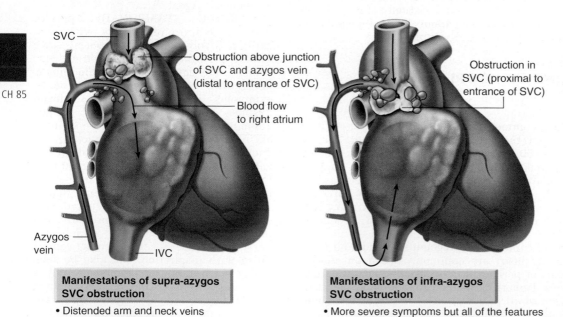

Manifestations of supra-azygos SVC obstruction

- Distended arm and neck veins
- Edema of neck, face, and arms
- Congested mucous membranes (mouth)
- Dilated, tortuous vessels on upper chest and back

Manifestations of infra-azygos SVC obstruction

- More severe symptoms but all of the features for obstruction distal to entrance of SVC
- Dilation of collateral vessels on anterior and posterior abdominal wall with downward blood flow into IVC, then back to heart

A   B

FIGURE 85–1 Anatomy of superior vena cava (SVC) syndrome. Lymph nodes may obstruct blood return above the entrance of the azygos vein **(A)**, resulting in edema of the face, neck, and arms and distended veins in the neck and arms and over the upper chest. Obstruction below the return of the azygos vein **(B)** results in retrograde flow through the azygos via collateral veins to the inferior vena cava (IVC), resulting in all the symptoms and signs in **A** plus dilation of the veins over the abdomen as well. *(Modified from Skarin AT [ed]: Atlas of Diagnostic Oncology. 3rd ed. Philadelphia, Elsevier Science, 2003.)*

TABLE 85–1	Malignancies Associated with Superior Vena Cava Syndrome (SVCS) in Adults*	
Neoplastic Diagnosis	**Percentage of SVCS**	**Disease-Associated SVCS (%)**
Lung cancer, stage 3B or 4	48-81	
Small-cell lung cancer		15-45
Squamous cell cancer		20-25
Adenocarcinoma		5-25
Large-cell carcinoma		4-30
Lymphoma	2-21	
Diffuse large-cell lymphoma		64
Lymphoblastic lymphoma		33
Breast cancer	11	

*Includes lung cancer, lymphomas, and metastases from other solid tumors; 75% to 85% of patients with SVCS have neoplastic disease.

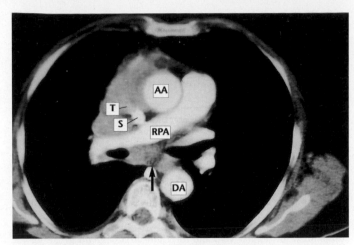

FIGURE 85–2 Superior vena cava syndrome in a case of diffuse large-cell lymphoma. This computed tomography image with intravenous contrast at the level of the right pulmonary artery (RPA) shows a tumor (T) infiltrating into the area of the superior vena cava (S), which is narrowed. Tumor is also present in the subcarinal space (arrow). AA = ascending aorta; DA = descending aorta. *(From Skarin AT [ed]: Atlas of Diagnostic Oncology. 3rd ed. Philadelphia, Elsevier Science, 2003.)*

TABLE 85–2	Yields of Various Procedures for Diagnosis in Patients with Superior Vena Cava Syndrome
Procedure	**% Diagnostic**
Thoracotomy	98
Mediastinoscopy	90
Thoracentesis	71
Lymph node biopsy	67
Bronchoscopy	52
Sputum cytology	49

percent of patients with SVCS and lung cancer. Of patients with lung cancer–associated SVCS, 80 percent have right-sided primary lesions.

Lymphoma is the second most common cause of neoplasia-associated SVCS, comprising 2 to 21 percent of SVCS patients. Diffuse large cell lymphoma is the most common (64 percent), followed by lymphoblastic lymphoma (33 percent). Similar to patients with lung cancer, only 1 to 5 percent of patients with lymphoma develop SVCS (21 percent of lymphoblastic lymphomas and 7 percent of diffuse large cell lymphomas). Of patients with primary mediastinal B-cell lymphoma with sclerosis, 57 percent developed SVCS. Although Hodgkin lymphoma often involves the mediastinum, SVCS rarely develops. Thymoma and germ cell tumors are other primary mediastinal malignancies that occasionally cause SVCS. The most common metastatic disease that causes SVCS is breast cancer, accounting for 11 percent of SVCS cases.

DIFFERENTIAL DIAGNOSIS. Benign causes of SVC obstruction not associated with neoplasia result from mediastinal fibrosis caused by radiotherapy or histoplasmosis, tuberculosis, collagen-vascular disease, arteriovenous shunts, or SVC thrombosis as a complication of central venous catheters, pacemaker leads, peritoneovenous shunts, Swan-Ganz catheters, or hyperalimentation catheters. Pacemakers and implantable cardioverter defibrillators result in up to 30 percent of local venous thrombosis, in some cases associated with infection; however, SVC obstruction is uncommon and relates to acute or previous lead infection or retention of a severed lead.[9] Other benign causes include granulomas, congenital anomalies, and mediastinal fibrosis from histoplasmosis.

DIAGNOSTIC PROCEDURES. In a patient with characteristic symptoms of SVC obstruction, physical evaluation is usually informative and raises a high level of suspicion. In patients with SVCS caused by neoplasia, 60 percent lack a prior history of cancer. A mass is generally present on the chest radiograph, with superior mediastinal widening and often pleural effusions. Computed tomography (CT) provides critical additional information (Fig. 85-2). Contrast-enhanced CT can document the presence of obstruction and establish the level, extent, and therapeutic options by mapping collateral and patent vasculature to aid interventional access and document any pulmonary emboli. Increased use of imaging in patients with cancer has identified many asymptomatic patients with impending SVC obstruction, allowing early radiation therapy to prevent or delay obstruction. The CT scan can illustrate the strategic relationship of growing tumor masses or the development of nonocclusive, early intraluminal thrombus. Magnetic resonance imaging (MRI) can also perform this role effectively.

The causes of SVCS include intraluminal, mural, and extraluminal obstruction. Intraluminal causes include bland and neoplastic thrombus as well as direct tumor extension. Bland thrombus is usually associated with intravenous lines or infected pacemaker leads, although it is an uncommon cause of complete occlusion. A paraneoplastic bland thrombus can also occur, and tumor vascularization can be used to differentiate a bland from a neoplastic thrombus. Mural causes include strictures resulting from radiation therapy. Extraluminal causes are usually direct compression by bronchogenic tumors or malignant lymphadenopathy and represent the most common causes detected by imaging.

Because the underlying cause will guide any therapeutic recommendations, obtaining tissue samples to define the cause is essential (Table 85-2). Sputum cytology can establish the diagnosis in almost half of patients. Biopsy of enlarged lymph nodes, when present, is frequently a relatively noninvasive method to obtain reliable tissue diagnosis. Thoracentesis can establish the diagnosis of malignancy in 70 percent of patients with pleural effusions. A diagnosis is made in most of the remaining cases with bronchoscopy, including brushing, washing, and biopsy samples. A marrow biopsy may be diagnostic of lymphoma or SCLC. If the diagnosis remains obscure, percutaneous transthoracic CT-guided fine-needle biopsy is a safe and effective method of diagnosis. When other methods have been unsuccessful, mediastinoscopy has a high diagnostic yield but a somewhat higher risk of complications (5 percent).

MANAGEMENT (see Chap. 59). During medical evaluation and before institution of specific therapy, oxygen is administered to reduce the cardiac output and venous pressure; head elevation, diuretics, and a low-salt diet are used to reduce edema. Dehydration increases the risk of further thrombosis, however. In patients with SVCS caused by malignant tumors, radiotherapy and chemotherapy are the most common first-line treatment options. Steroids can, in some cases, decrease inflammation or tumor-associated obstruction, but may obscure the diagnosis of lymphoma.

Increasingly, endovascular stenting is proving to provide more rapid and longer lasting relief of the obstruction.[10] Despite the historical concern that invasive diagnostic procedures in the setting of increased intrathoracic venous pressure would result in severe bleeding and complications of anesthesia, complication rates in experienced centers have proved acceptably low. Stent insertion has a high percentage of technical success, with rapid relief of symptoms. Adjuvant radiation therapy and chemotherapy can be used. Anticoagulation has not been proven to provide benefit in patients with neoplasia-associated SVCS and may interfere with diagnostic biopsies and interventions. Surgical treatment involves the insertion of a bypass graft between the left innominate or jugular vein and the right atrial appendage, using an autologous or Dacron graft. However, this operation is very invasive and difficult. Therefore, it should be avoided if possible and, if necessary, performed only in patients with a relatively long life expectancy. In the chronic situation devoid of vascular interventions, patients may develop a network of chest wall and azygos-hemiazygos collateral vessels that effectively restore venous return to the right heart.

Oncological treatment of SVCS focuses on determining as rapidly as possible the histological type of the primary lesion so that curative therapy for lymphomas, germ cell tumors, and even SCLC, can be instituted, or so that palliation for advanced non–SCLCs and other metastatic solid tumors can be provided (see Table 85-2). The prognosis of patients who present with SVCS depends greatly on the prognosis of the underlying neoplasm. Combination chemotherapy with or without radiation therapy relieves SVCS symptoms within 1 to 2 weeks in patients with newly diagnosed SCLC and lymphoma.

Valvular Heart Disease

Cardiac valves can be involved directly by primary or metastatic tumor, by bacterial or candidal infections, with nonbacterial thrombotic endocarditis, by trauma from semipermanent catheters inserted to facilitate treatment, and as a late effect of radiation therapy (see later, "Complications of Radiation Therapy").

Nonbacterial thrombotic endocarditis can be seen in autoimmune disorders and can also complicate the course of various malignancies, most commonly adenocarcinomas from the gastrointestinal tract and lung.[11] Morbidity and mortality mainly result from systemic embolism. In one study, 200 nonselected ambulatory patients with solid tumors evaluated for evidence of thromboembolic events and for plasma D-dimer levels were compared with a control group of 100 consecutive patients without overt heart disease referred to echocardiography for the detection of an occult arterial embolic source. Of 38 cancer patients with cardiac valvular vegetations from the group of 200, the valves affected were mitral (19), aortic (18), and tricuspid (1). Primary lesions were lymphoma (10), lung (9), and pancreatic (3). Thromboembolism to extremities was diagnosed in 4 patients, cerebrovascular accidents were diagnosed in 2, and 4 patients had silent segmental left ventricular wall motion abnormalities on echocardiography. Nine of 38 patients (24 percent) with vegetations developed thromboembolism, as compared with 13 of 162 patients without vegetations (8 percent; $P = 0.013$). D-Dimer levels were increased in 19 of 21 patients (90 percent) with thromboembolism and in 76 of 149 patients without (51 percent; $P = 0.001$).[11] Treatment of cancer-related nonbacterial thrombotic endocarditis remains difficult.

Ischemic Heart Disease

Given the similar risk factors for certain cancers and coronary artery disease (CAD), especially smoking, particulate matter air pollution, and age, patients will commonly have both diseases. Furthermore, as discussed in detail later, several cancer therapies can be toxic to the cardiovascular system, including the coronary arteries, producing unstable angina or myocardial infarction (MI). Depending on the type and level of aggressiveness of the chosen cancer therapeutic approach, and the risk factor profile of the patient, it is reasonable to consider a baseline evaluation for the presence and severity of CAD prior to initiation of the therapy, even in the absence of symptoms or objective signs of disease. Although there are no firm guidelines that address this issue, patients who will receive agents known to induce unstable angina or MI (see later) should probably undergo stress and imaging studies to screen for CAD prior to treatment.

Arrhythmias

Arrhythmias in cancer patients are caused most commonly by coexisting abnormalities rather than by the cancer itself. Thus, although arrhythmia-inducing metastases to the myocardium or pericardium certainly occur, more commonly arrhythmias will be caused by hypoxemia (as a result of extensive carcinomas of the lung, metastases to the lung, or pulmonary infection), electrolyte imbalances, cardiotoxic radiation and cancer therapeutics, or comorbidities, such as chronic obstructive pulmonary disease. Resuscitation of patients with end-stage cancer is often attempted but the chance of survival is low. In one series, 0 of 171 patients in whom cardiac arrest was anticipated because of worsening metabolic status survived to discharge. In contrast, 22 percent survived in whom the arrest was not anticipated.[12] These findings highlight the need for careful attention to end-of-life decisions with end-stage patients, thereby avoiding painful and costly interventions that are usually futile.

INDIRECT CARDIOVASCULAR COMPLICATIONS OF NEOPLASIA

Hyperviscosity

Hyperviscosity can result from a number of causes, including erythrocytosis (from polycythemia vera), thrombocytosis, which can be reactive or secondary to a myeloproliferative disorder (essential thrombocytosis), leukocytosis, occasionally seen in acute leukemias, and an increase in plasma protein levels (seen with multiple myeloma and Waldenström macroglobulinemia). For further information on the cardiovascular complications of hyperviscosity and its treatment, see Chapter 85 Online Supplement on the website.

CARDIOVASCULAR COMPLICATIONS OF CANCER THERAPEUTIC AGENTS

Drug development in cancer therapeutics has changed more dramatically in the last decade than in any other era. In this section, the cardiovascular toxicity of traditional chemotherapeutic agents and of the newer targeted therapeutic agents are discussed. (see also Chap. 68.)

Traditional Chemotherapeutic Agents

Anthracyclines

The anthracyclines currently approved in the United States, doxorubicin (Adriamycin), daunorubicin (Cerubidine), epirubicin (Ellence), and idarubicin (Idamycin PFS), are key components of many chemotherapeutic regimens, having demonstrated efficacy in lymphomas and many solid tumors, including breast and small cell lung cancer.[13] This class of agents is clearly the most cardiotoxic to date, acutely producing arrhythmias, left ventricular (LV) dysfunction, and pericarditis, and chronically producing LV dysfunction and heart failure (HF) (Table 85-3). The toxicity is strongly dose-related. Initial retrospective analyses have suggested that the incidence of HF is 2.2 percent overall and 7.5 percent in patients receiving a cumulative dose of 550 mg/m². However, more recent studies have suggested that the incidence is higher than this.[14] The incidence rises significantly for cumulative doses above 400 to 450 mg/m² for doxorubicin. Consequently, for most tumors, oncologists typically limit the dose to 450 to 500 mg/m².[13] If patients develop anthracycline cardiomyopathy, it is often within the first year of completing therapy, with a median of 5 to 9 months. However, the cardiomyopathy may be progressive over years.[15]

Risk factors for cardiotoxicity, in addition to doses above 450 mg/m², include advanced age, history of cardiac disease, and prior mediastinal irradiation (Fig. 85-3). Predictors of cardiotoxicity based on assessment of LV function include a baseline LV ejection fraction (EF) less than 50 percent or a decline in LVEF of more than 10 percent on treatment to a level less than 50 percent. Diastolic dysfunction may be the first abnormality noted.[16] Children may be particularly susceptible to anthracycline cardiotoxicity and, in one series, 5 percent developed HF at 15 years of follow-up and the incidence increased to 10 percent for cumulative doses

Parameter	Frequency	Comments
Left Ventricular Dysfunction–Heart Failure		
Anthracyclines		
Doxorubicin (and others)	+++	Highly dose-dependent; risk factors include age (old and young), prior mediastinal XRT, history of heart disease, decreased ejection fraction (EF), drop in EF on drug therapy, female gender (for children), and other agents (especially trastuzumab); risk decreased by liposomal encapsulation or dexrazoxane.
Mitoxantrone	++	Derivative with somewhat lower risk; efficacy questionable; used in patients with multiple sclerosis at lower doses
Alkylating agents		
Cyclophosphamide, ifosfamide	+	Primarily seen with high dose "conditioning" regimens; risk factors are prior mediastinal XRT or anthracycline drug therapy, and imatinib or pentostatin (?); also can have myocarditis, pericarditis, myocardial necrosis
Mitomycin	+	Risk increased with high doses, anthracyclines, or XRT
Taxanes		
Paclitaxel	++	Seen with concurrent anthracycline therapy; caused by retarded metabolism of anthracycline' largely preventable with dosing regimen; not seen with docetaxel; trastuzumab increases risk of heart failure (HF)
Targeted therapeutics		
Trastuzumab	++	Relatively uncommon as single agent; increased risk with anthracyclines, paclitaxel, cyclophosphamide
Imatinib, dasatinib	++	Frequency not clear but probably <5%; can be severe; can also cause severe fluid retention with peripheral edema, pleural and pericardial effusion not secondary to left ventricular (LV) dysfunction
Sunitinib	+++	LV dysfunction common
Bevacizumab	++	HF can be seen in setting of severe hypertension, which occurs in 10-25% of patients, depending on dose; anthracyclines may increase HF risk
ATRA	++	With retinoic acid syndrome (see text)
Ischemic Syndromes		
5-Fluorouracil (5-FU), capecitabine	++	Acute coronary syndromes (ACS); patients with CAD at increased risk; recurs with rechallenge; vasospasm likely mechanism
Cisplatin, carboplatin	++	ACS caused by vasospasm and/or vascular injury; hypertension common
Interferon-α	+	Risk of ischemia increased in patients with CAD; hypertension common
Bevacizumab	++	Arterial thrombotic events in 8.5% of patients >65 yr
Vinca alkaloids	+	~1% risk of cardiac events; ischemia possibly caused by coronary spasm
Sorafenib	++	2.5% risk of ACS in preapproval trials
Hypertension		
Cisplatin	++++	
Bevacizumab	++++	
Sunitinib	++++	
Hypotension		
Rituximab	++	Infusion reactions
Alemtuzumab	+++	Infusion reactions
Interleukin (IL)-2, denileukin	++++	Capillary leak syndrome
Interferon-α	+++	Within first few hours after treatment
ATRA	++	In setting of retinoic acid syndrome
Arrhythmias		
Paclitaxel	+	Bradyarrhythmias; ventricular tachycardia rare
Thalidomide	++	Bradyarrhythmias
Arsenic trioxide	++++	Prolonged QT; rarely, torsades de pointes
Rituximab	++	Occur during or shortly after infusion

ATRA = all-*trans*-retinoic acid; XRT = radiation therapy.
Relative frequency of the cardiotoxicity is scored as follows: + = <1%; ++ = 1-5%; +++ = 6-10%; ++++ = >10%.
Modified from Yeh ET, Tong AT, Lenihan DJ, et al: Cardiovascular complications of cancer therapy: Diagnosis, pathogenesis, and management. Circulation 109:3122, 2004.

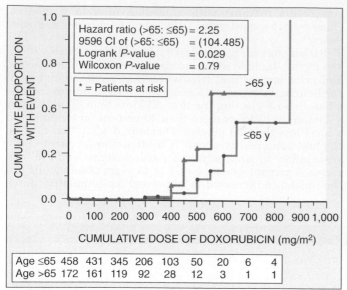

Age ≤65	458	431	345	206	103	50	20	6	4
Age >65	172	161	119	92	28	12	3	1	1

FIGURE 85-3 Risk of doxorubicin-associated congestive heart failure by patient age. This graphically depicts the cumulative doxorubicin dose at the onset of doxorubicin-associated congestive heart failure in 630 patients according to patient age older or younger than 65 years (y). *(Redrawn from Swain SM, Whaley FS, Ewer MS: Congestive heart failure in patients treated with doxorubicin: A retrospective analysis of three trials. Cancer 97:2869, 2003.)*

of 550 mg/m^2.[17] In addition to dose and mediastinal irradiation, age at diagnosis and female gender are predictors for adverse outcomes in children. Unlike in adults, HF may appear years after treatment has been stopped and may be progressive.[18]

Endomyocardial biopsy is the most sensitive method to detect anthracycline cardiotoxicity, with typical findings being cytosolic vacuolization, lysis of myofibrils, and cellular swelling, findings more typical of a necrotic form of cell death. However, abnormalities on electron microscopy have not been shown to correlate highly with risk of development of HF and are often present in patients at cumulative doses well below those associated with an increased risk of HF. Given the technical nature of the procedure and inherent risks, this is not a practical way to detect or follow patients with anthracycline cardiotoxicity, and serial determination of LV function, although insensitive, is the currently accepted method.

The cellular mechanisms leading to anthracycline cardiotoxicity remain unclear but are believed, in part, to involve oxidant stress leading to iron oxidation and generation of free radicals that damage cell and organelle membranes via peroxidation of lipids.[19] Other contributing factors include activation of calpains, proteases that degrade structural proteins in the cardiomyocyte, including titin. The oxidized iron hypothesis has led to the use of dexrazoxane (Zinecard), a chelator of intracellular iron. Although the compound does reduce the incidence of cardiotoxicity, concerns were raised in one trial that it might also reduce efficacy of the anthracycline.[20] This was not seen in a later meta-analysis, however, and the drug is now approved in the United States. American Society of Clinical Oncology recommendations have suggested that the use of dexrazoxane be limited to patients who have received more than 300 mg/m^2 of doxorubicin or the equivalent.[21]

Other strategies have been used to limit anthracycline cardiotoxicity, including the use of epirubicin, a stereoisomer of doxorubicin. This agent has less cardiotoxicity than doxorubicin at comparable doses, and 900 to 1000 mg/m^2 of epirubicin produces cardiotoxicity comparable to 450 to 500 mg/m^2 of doxorubicin. However, efficacy of the two agents is comparable at equivalent doses.[13] The agent is used much more in Europe than the United States at this time. Other strategies include encapsulating doxorubicin within liposomes (Myocet, approved in Europe), with or without adding a polyethylene glycol coat (Doxil). The liposome encapsulation is believed to reduce delivery of the drug

to the heart, and polyethylene glycol increases the half-life and delivery to the tumor. It appears that either strategy does reduce cardiotoxicity, as assessed by clinical criteria or assessment of LV function, and although concerns were raised in one study over possible reduced tumor response rate for the Myocet preparation, this does not appear to be the case.[22] Mitoxantrone (Novantrone), an anthracycline derivative that is also used in the treatment of patients with multiple sclerosis, can also cause cardiac dysfunction.[16]

Patients should have a baseline determination of LV function prior to initiating anthracycline therapy, and should be monitored periodically after that, especially when the cumulative dose rises above 300 to 350 mg/m^2 for doxorubicin or above the comparable doses for the other anthracyclines. It is important to note that history and physical examination alone will miss a substantial number of patients with significant deterioration in LV function. Use of the criteria noted earlier concerning risk factors, baseline LV function, and deterioration of LV function, in combination with dosage consideration, can be used to risk-stratify patients for the development of HF. Routine use of troponin measurements is not highly predictive except in patients receiving high-dose chemotherapy (for treatment of aggressive malignancies). In those patients, an elevated troponin I level predicted those going on to develop LV dysfunction with high sensitivity, albeit low predictive accuracy. A negative troponin I strongly predicted patients whose LV function would not deteriorate.[23] A recent report has suggested that prophylactic angiotensin-converting enzyme (ACE) inhibitor therapy in patients with elevated troponin I levels can prevent progression to HF.[24]

Early studies of anthracycline cardiotoxicity have suggested a more than 40 percent mortality with digoxin- or diuretic-based therapy but, with more modern approaches to the management of patients with HF, the prognosis is much better.[15] In one study in children that used prophylactic enalapril, there was significantly less deterioration in LV function at 3 years of follow-up.[25] Unfortunately, in other studies, it appears that the beneficial effect of ACE inhibition in children may not be long-lasting.[18]

Taxanes

The taxanes, paclitaxel (Taxol) and docetaxel (Taxotere), disrupt microtubular networks as their mechanism of antitumor activity and are effective in breast cancer. Used alone, they have relatively little cardiotoxicity. In one large study, cardiac toxicity occurred in 14 percent of patients, but 76 percent of these events were asymptomatic bradycardia. Heart block can also occur. However, when paclitaxel is combined with doxorubicin, cardiotoxicity is increased, and 18 percent of patients developed HF in one trial. This was found to be secondary to retardation of metabolism of the doxorubicin. When paclitaxel was administered 30 minutes after doxorubicin and the doxorubicin dose was kept to 360 mg/m^2, the decline in ejection fraction was greater than that with the combination of doxorubicin plus cyclophosphamide, although the rates of HF were low and not statistically different between the groups.[26] Docetaxel does not retard metabolism of doxorubicin and also does not lead to an increase in HF. Similarly, epirubicin plus a taxane does not increase HF.

Alkylating Agents and Antimetabolites

These classes of agents generally have low incidences of cardiotoxicity. Cyclophosphamide (Cytoxan) is relatively well-tolerated when used at conventional doses but, in patients receiving conditioning regimens prior to autologous stem cell transplantation, which use high-dose cyclophosphamide, acute cardiotoxicity can occur.[27] As opposed to the total cumulative dosage for anthracyclines, dosage of an individual course of treatment is more predictive for cyclophosphamide. Risk factors include prior anthracycline therapy or mediastinal radiation, and possibly prior imatinib therapy.[16,28] Clinically, patients may present with HF, myocarditis, or pericarditis. In one series of 17 consecutive patients receiving induction therapy, none of whom developed HF, LV dilation by MRI was evident from the onset.[27] Mechanisms underlying the toxicity are believed to be injury of both endothelial cells and myocytes, and a picture of hemorrhagic myocardial necrosis can emerge. Those who survive the acute phase typically do not have residual LV dysfunction. High-dose ifosfamide (Ifex) induces HF in 17 percent of patients.

Cisplatin (Platinol)-based regimens are the cornerstone of therapy for testicular germ cell cancer, the most common malignancy in men aged 20 to 40 years, with 80 percent of those with disseminated nonseminoma achieving long-term survival.[29] Thus, in addition to short-term toxicity, long-term toxicity is a concern in this group. Cisplatin is notable for causing hypertension, which is sometimes severe. Acute chest pain syndromes, including MI, have also been reported, possibly related to coronary spasm. Because cisplatin is often used in combination with bleomycin, an agent that can induce Raynaud's phenomenon in approximately one third of patients, long-term vascular toxicity is particularly a concern.[30] Indeed, after a median 10-year follow-up of patients treated with platinum-based regimens (cisplatin or carboplatin [Paraplatin]) versus radiation therapy, 6.7 percent of patients after chemotherapy and 10 percent of patients after irradiation suffered a cardiac event, for a relative risk of 2.4- to 2.8-fold compared with patients treated with surgery only.[30] Changes in the ratio of carotid intima-media thickness were detected as early as 10 weeks following a course of cisplatin-based chemotherapy.[29] The morbidity data have led to calls for more conservative approaches to patients at low risk for cancer recurrence.[30]

5-Fluorouracil (5-FU; Adrucil) is used in the treatment of many solid tumors and regimens based on this agent are the mainstay of treatment for colorectal cancer. 5-FU can cause acute ischemic syndromes ranging from angina to MI, and this can occur in patients without CAD (approximately 1 percent of patients), although it is more common in patients with preexisting disease (4 to 5 percent). Overall, rates range from 0.55 to 8 percent,[31] although more sensitive methods of detecting possible subclinical ischemia (ambulatory electrocardiographic monitoring) find much higher rates. Discontinuing treatment and standard antianginal therapies usually lead to resolution of symptoms, but ischemia often recurs if therapy is reinitiated. An alternative agent, capecitabine (Xeloda), which is often used in combination with oxaliplatin (Eloxatin) in colorectal and breast cancer, is metabolized to 5-FU, preferentially in tumor cells, suggesting that it may have less cardiotoxicity. However, one retrospective review (that excluded patients with "significant" cardiac disease) has found an incidence of 6.5 percent major cardiac events for the combination, including angina (4.6 percent), MI, ventricular tachycardia (VT), and sudden death.[31] Vasospasm is believed to be the mechanism triggering ischemia, although thromboembolic events are also increased. It is not clear at this point whether prophylactic nitrates prevent ischemic events. Capecitabine monotherapy appears to have a lower incidence of cardiac toxicity compared with 5-FU monotherapy.[31]

Other Chemotherapeutic Agents

TAMOXIFEN. Tamoxifen (Nolvadex) is widely used in the treatment of breast cancer. Based largely on experimental data, it had been proposed to have cardioprotective effects. However, in a large 13,388 patient trial, in women both with and without coronary artery disease, tamoxifen

therapy did not reduce or increase the incidence of fatal MI, nonfatal MI, unstable angina, or severe angina.[32] Concerns have been raised, however, that stroke risk might be increased somewhat.[33]

PROTEASOME INHIBITORS. Bortezomib (Velcade) is an inhibitor of the proteasome system responsible for degrading improperly folded proteins and proteins that are no longer needed in the cell (e.g., some proteins driving early phases of cellular proliferation need to be destroyed for later phases of the cell cycle to go forward).[34] The drug is approved for use in patients with multiple myeloma, a B-cell malignancy with overgrowth of monotypic plasma cells in the bone marrow. The concept behind its use is that malignant cells have altered proteins regulating the cell cycle, leading to more rapid cell division and increased accumulation of damaged proteins as a result. Therefore, the continued health of the malignant cell, as opposed to normal cells, may be more dependent on degradation of the damaged proteins. In support of this concept, proteasome inhibitors are more toxic to proliferating malignant cells in culture than normal cells.[35] Targets include activation of endoplasmic reticulum stress pathways leading to activation of proapoptotic factors (c-Jun N-terminal kinase [JNK]), and inactivation of survival factors, such as nuclear factor kappa B (NF-κB).[34] There are limited data at present on the cardiotoxicity of bortezomib, but cardiomyocytes have an active proteasome system, raising concerns that inhibiting the proteasome may be cardiotoxic. However, in the phase III trials of the drug, HF was reported in 5 percent of patients but was reported in 4 percent of patients in the dexamethasone arm of the trial (www.mlnm.com/products/velcade/full_prescrib_velcade.pdf; Millennium Pharmaceuticals, Inc., 2006).

ADDITIONAL AGENTS. A discussion of the cardiotoxicity of additional agents, including cytokines (IL-2, aldesleukin [Proleukin] and denileukin diftitox) and interferons, histone deacetylase (HDAC) inhibitors (Trichostatin A and suberoylanilide hydroxamic acid), topoisomerase inhibitors (etoposide and teniposide), purine analogues (pentostatin and cladribine), all-*trans*-retinoic acid (ATRA), arsenic trioxide, and thalidomide and lenalidomide, can be found in the Chapter 85 Online Supplement on the website.

Targeted Therapeutics

The treatment of a number of malignancies has changed radically over the past few years with the advent of so-called targeted therapies. As opposed to traditional chemotherapeutics, which target basic cellular processes present in most cells, these therapies target factors that are specifically dysregulated in cancerous cells. It was hoped that this approach would reduce toxicities typical of standard chemotherapeutics (e.g., alopecia, gastrointestinal [GI] toxicity, myelotoxicity), and at the same time be more effective at treating the cancer. In some situations this has been the case, but concerns about cardiotoxicity have surfaced for some agents.[36]

Prior to a discussion of the agents and their toxicities, it is essential to understand these agents and how they work, and also something about the theories behind their development. The vast majority of the targeted cancer therapeutics inhibit the activity of tyrosine kinases (Table 85-4).[37] Tyrosine kinases (TKs) attach phosphate groups to tyrosine residues of other proteins, thereby changing the activity, subcellular localization, or rate of degradation of the protein. In the normal cell, these wild-type (i.e., normal) tyrosine kinases play many roles in regulating basic cellular functions. However, in leukemias and cancers, the gene encoding the causal (or contributory) TK is amplified (leading to overexpression) or mutated, leading to a constitutively acti-

TABLE 85–4 | **Tyrosine Kinase Targets in Malignant Hematological Disorders and Solid Tumors**

Tyrosine Kinase	Activating Mechanisms	Cancer	Therapy*	Cardiotoxicity?†
Hematological Disorders				
ABL	Transloc	CML, ALL, AML	I/D/N	Y
ARG	Transloc	AML	I/D/N	Y
ALK	Transloc	ALCL		
FGFR1	Transloc	aCML	PD0173074	?
FGFR3	Transloc; mut	MM	PD0173074	?
FLT3	Duplic; mut	AML	Lestaurtinib	?
			Su/So	Y
c-FMS	Mut	MDS/AML		
NTRK3	Transloc	AML		
PDGFRα	Del; transloc	HES/SM	I/Su	Y
PDGFRβ	Transloc	CMML; AML	I/D/Su	Y
JAK2	Mut; transloc	PCV/ET/IMF		
c-KIT	Mut; overexp	AML/SM	I/D/Su/So	Y
SYK	Transloc	MDS		
Solid Tumors				
ALK	Transloc	IMT		
EGFR	Overexp; mut; del	NSCLC; ovarian; SCCHN; RCC; C-R	G/E/Cetux	N
HER2	Overexp; mut	Breast; lung	Tras	Y
			Lapatinib	N
EGFR3	Overexp	Clear cell sarcoma		
c-KIT	Mut; del; dup	GIST; SCLC; sarcoma	I/D/Su/So	Y
c-MET	Overexp; mut; fusion	SCLC; gastric; melanoma; renal		
NTRK1	Transloc	PTC		
PDGFRα	Overexp; mut; del	Glioblastoma; GIST; osteosarcoma	I/Su/So	Y
RET	Mut	MEN-2A/B	Su	Y
VEGFR-1/-2	Overexp; VEGF	NSCLC; breast Renal; C-R; prostate	Su/Beva/So	Y

*Prediction of therapeutic efficacy in some cases is based on preclinical studies or on in vitro data showing inhibition of the tyrosine kinase.

†For many of these kinases, cardiotoxicity occurs but rates are not known as yet.

The following abbreviations are used in the table: Tyrosine kinases: ABL=Abelson tyrosine kinase; ARG=Abl-related gene (ABL2); ALK=anaplastic lymphoma kinase; FGFR=fibroblast growth factor receptor; FLT3=Fms-like tyrosine kinase 3; NTRK=neurotrophin receptor kinase; PDGFR=platelet-derived growth factor receptor; JAK (Janus kinase); c-KIT=stem cell factor receptor; SYK=spleen tyrosine kinase; EGFR=epidermal growth factor receptor; HER2=human EGFR-2; c-MET=hepatocyte growth factor receptor; RET=ret proto-oncogene. Activating mechanisms: Transloc=chromosomal translocations producing fusion proteins with the tyrosine kinase; Mut=activating point mutations in the kinase; Duplic=duplications; Del=deletions; Overexp=overexpression of the kinase. Cancers: CML=chronic myeloid leukemia; ALL=acute lymphoblastic leukemia; AML=acute myeloid leukemia; ALCL=anaplastic large-cell lymphoma; MM=multiple myeloma; MDS=myelodysplastic syndrome; HES=hypereosinophilic syndrome; SM=systemic mastocytosis; CMML=chronic myelomonocytic leukemia; PCV=polycythemia vera; ET=essential thrombocytosis; IMF=idiopathic myelofibrosis; IMT=inflammatory myofibroblastic tumor; NSCLC=non–small cell lung cancer; SCCHN=squamous cell carcinoma of head and neck; RCC=renal cell carcinoma; C-R=colorectal cancer; GIST=gastrointestinal stromal tumor; SCLC=small cell lung cancer; PTC=papillary thyroid cancer; MEN=multiple endocrine neoplasia. Targeted therapeutics: I=imatinib (Gleevec); D=dasatinib (Sprycel); N=nilotinib; Su=sunitinib (Sutent); G=gefitinib (Iressa); E=erlotinib (Tarceva); Cetux=cetuximab (Erbitux); Tras=trastuzumab (Herceptin); Beva=bevacizumab (Avastin); So=sorafenib (Nexavar); Va=vatalinib.

Modified from Krause DS, Van Etten RA: Tyrosine kinases as targets for cancer therapy. N Engl J Med 353:172, 2005.

CH 85

vated state that drives proliferation of the cancerous clonal cells and/or blocks their normal death (see Table 85-4).[37] Inhibiting these kinases could then retard cell proliferation and/or induce cell death. Cardiotoxicity arises when the normal kinase, present in cardiomyocytes, which is also inhibited by the agent, plays a central role in maintenance of cardiomyocyte homeostasis. In some cases, cardiotoxicity of these drugs may be predictable, but usually it is not. This is because the targeted kinase was not known to provide a maintenance function, or because of off-target effects (i.e., inhibition of TKs other than those the drug was designed to target). Most tyrosine kinase inhibitors (TKIs) compete with ATP for binding to a pocket in the kinase that is moderately well conserved across many TKs.[38] There are approximately 500 protein kinases in the human genome, of which approximately 90 are TKs.[39] Most companies test their TKIs against no more than 40 to 50 kinases. Thus, there may be several additional TKs that are inhibited and many additional serine or threonine kinases (the other major family) that are inhibited, and these will generally not be known to the oncologist or cardiologist caring for the patient. Therefore, if known targets of a drug play no role in cardiomyocyte homeostasis, but patients present with HF after initiation of therapy, the possibilities of off-target effects accounting for toxicity versus HF from other causes must be considered.

Drugs and Their Targets

Because numerous drugs are approved or in development for each molecular target, rather than organizing this section by drug, it is organized by molecular target (see Table 85-4). Then, as new agents are released, they will be able to be viewed in relation to their target(s), allowing some ability to predict possible adverse outcomes (see Table 85-4). The role of the mutant gene product in the pathogenesis of the cancer, and the role of the normal gene product in the heart and vasculature, if known, will be discussed so that cardiotoxicity can be better understood. Where there are no data on cardiotoxicity, theoretical concerns will be raised.

The first molecularly targeted therapies, trastuzumab (Herceptin) and imatinib (Gleevec), illustrate the two general classes of these agents—humanized monoclonal antibodies targeting growth factor receptors on the surface of the cancer cell (trastuzumab), and small-molecule inhibitors of receptors or of intracellular pathways regulating growth of the cancer cells (imatinib). All generic names for monoclonal antibodies end in "-mab" and all small-molecule inhibitors end in "-nib."

HER2 RECEPTOR AND TRASTUZUMAB

The growth factor receptor, Her2 (human epidermal growth factor receptor-2), is amplified in 15 to 30 percent of breast cancers and Her2-positive cancers carry a worse prognosis.[40] This amplification, and the resulting overexpression (up to 100-fold) and activation of Her2, both enhances cell cycle progression (and thus proliferation) and inhibits apoptosis of the cancer cells. Trastuzumab is a humanized monoclonal antibody that binds to and inhibits the activity of the Her2 receptor.[41] Treatment of patients with trastuzumab improves survival in patients with metastatic disease and, when used in the adjuvant setting postsurgery, reduces recurrences of the cancer.[41-43]

Traztusumab is very well-tolerated as far as side effect profile. However, it can induce HF in a percentage of patients. The original trials with trastuzumab indicated that 3 to 7 percent of patients developed left ventricular dysfunction and this incidence was increased to 27 percent by concomitant use of doxorubicin (with 16 percent being New York Heart Association [NYHA] Class III or IV).[44] This is in comparison to rates of 8 percent total and 3 percent NYHA Class III or IV HF with anthracyclines plus cyclophosphamide. When trastuzumab was used with paclitaxel, 13 percent of patients developed cardiotoxicity versus only 1 percent with paclitaxel alone.

More recently, trastuzumab cardiotoxicity has been analyzed in three key trials in breast cancer patients that assessed efficacy of the agent in the adjuvant setting.[42,43] In one trial,[42] patients who underwent surgery plus adjuvant or neoadjuvant chemotherapy and/or radiotherapy, were randomized to received herceptin or simply observation. Patients were excluded if after chemotherapy or irradiation they (1) received more than 360 mg/m² of doxorubicin or 720 mg/m² of epirubicin, (2) received prior mediastinal radiation, or (3) had an EF less than 55 percent. In addition, patients were excluded for a history of HF, CAD with prior Q wave MI, angina requiring medication, uncontrolled hypertension, valvular disease, or "unstable arrhythmias."[42] At 1 year of follow-up, 7.1 percent of patients in the trastuzumab arm versus 2.2 percent in the observation arm had significant declines in LVEF, and 1.7 percent in the trastuzumab arm versus 0 percent in the observation arm developed symptomatic HF. These figures therefore represent short-term risks for trastuzumab in otherwise healthy patients with no cardiac morbidities and normal LV function who had received moderate doses of adjuvant chemotherapy and no mediastinal radiation.

The other two studies,[43] which also excluded patients with a cardiac history and low EF or a decline in EF on doxorubicin-cyclophosphamide therapy, examined patients treated with more aggressive regimens—doxorubicin plus cyclophosphamide followed by (1) placebo versus paclitaxel versus paclitaxel plus trastuzumab, followed by (2) placebo versus trastuzumab. Follow-up was for a mean of 27 months. Of note, 6.7 percent of patients were prohibited from entering the trastuzumab phase of the trial because of an LVEF below the limit of normal following doxorubicin-cyclophosphamide. In this trial, 8.7 percent of patients in the trastuzumab arms versus 1.6 percent in the no-trastuzumab arm developed symptomatic HF. Furthermore, 2.2 to 4.1 percent developed severe HF on trastuzumab versus 0.2 to 0.8 percent on placebo. Significant declines in EF were roughly twice as likely, occurring in 18 to 34 percent of patients on trastuzumab versus 8 to 17 percent on placebo. The lower rates in these later three trials,[42,43] compared with earlier studies,[41,44] reflect not only enrolling more highly selected patients, but also administering doxorubicin and trastuzumab sequentially rather than concurrently. Even given the lower rates, overall approximately 20 percent of patients were withdrawn from this trial for cardiac reasons.[45] The more recent trials largely enrolled node-positive patients.[41,44] However, it is possible that clinical practice will move toward treating node-negative patients, for whom the prognostic significance of Her2 positivity is only modest.[46] It will be important to analyze risk-benefit in node-negative patients, in whom even the relatively low rates of HF may outweigh benefits.[46]

MECHANISMS OF TOXICITY. That trastuzumab was cardiotoxic is not altogether surprising because mice in which the Her2 gene (designated ErbB2 in mice) was knocked out, developed a spontaneous dilated cardiomyopathy.[47] Thus the ErbB2 receptor, at least in mice, appears to serve a "maintenance" function in cardiomyocytes. Furthermore,

cardiomyocytes isolated from the knockout hearts were more susceptible to anthracycline toxicity, consistent with the concept that inhibition of Her2 in patients may have amplified the severity of doxorubicin toxicity by preventing repair. Consistent with this, neuregulin, the endogenous ligand for Her2, can decrease anthracycline cardiotoxicity.[19] Cellular mechanisms of the toxicity of ErbB2 inhibition may include activation of the intrinsic-mitochondrial proapoptotic pathway by downregulating antiapoptotic BclxL and upregulating BclxS, leading to mitochondrial dysfunction and cell death.[48]

NATURAL HISTORY OF TRASTUZUMAB TOXICITY. Debate continues over the degree to which herceptin cardiotoxicity is reversible. Clearly, ultrastructural abnormalities on biopsy appear to be minimal, and patients respond well to standard HF regimens.[49] Some can continue on treatment without recurrence of HF. In follow-up in one of the adjuvant trials, of 27 patients with herceptin-induced HF (herceptin given after anthracycline plus cyclophosphamide, with or without paclitaxel), only 1 patient was persistently symptomatic.[45] Furthermore, overall LV function at more than 6 months of follow-up improved for the group versus on-treatment values. However, LV function remained depressed compared with baseline in 17 of 24 patients. Longer term follow-up is required to evaluate this issue fully.

Many additional agents targeting Her2 are in development, including some TKIs. Although previous experience with trastuzumab raises concerns, and LV function must be watched, one of these TKIs, lapatinib, that targets both the epidermal growth factor receptor (EGFR) and Her2, have shown surprisingly little cardiotoxicity in early trials. The reason for this is not clear and must be confirmed in larger studies, but may reflect the underlying differences in mechanisms of action of mAbs versus TKIs, including complement-dependent cell lysis and antibody-dependent cell-mediated cytotoxicity that is triggered by mAbs but not TKIs.

BCR-ABL AND IMATINIB

The first targeted small-molecule inhibitor to be used successfully in malignancies was imatinib.[50] This agent inhibits the activity of the fusion protein, Bcr-Abl, which arises from the chromosomal translocation that creates the Philadelphia chromosome, and is the causal factor in approximately 90 percent of cases of chronic myeloid leukemia (CML) and some cases of B-cell acute lymphoblastic leukemia (ALL).[37] This translocation creates a constitutively active protein kinase that drives proliferation and inhibits apoptosis in bone marrow stem cells, leading to the leukemias. Imatinib has revolutionized the treatment of CML, and now 90 percent of patients are alive 5 years after diagnosis with a disease that was uniformly fatal prior to the development of imatinib.[50]

Recently, imatinib was reported to cause HF.[51] In contrast to trastuzumab, the cardiotoxicity of imatinib was surprising because c-Abl, the wild-type kinase expressed in all cells, including cardiomyocytes, that is also inhibited by imatinib, was not known to play a role in maintenance of cardiomyocyte viability. In cardiomyocytes, inhibition of c-Abl led to activation of stress responses, culminating in marked mitochondrial dysfunction and cell death (Fig. 85-4).[51] The incidence of LV dysfunction with imatinib is not known because assessment of LV function was not included in any of the trials with this agent. However, significant peripheral edema and dyspnea were reported in the trials, and one small study has suggested that screening brain natriuretic peptide (BNP) levels could help differentiate edema and dyspnea caused by LV dysfunction from that due to other causes.[52] Trials with a new more potent Bcr-Abl (and

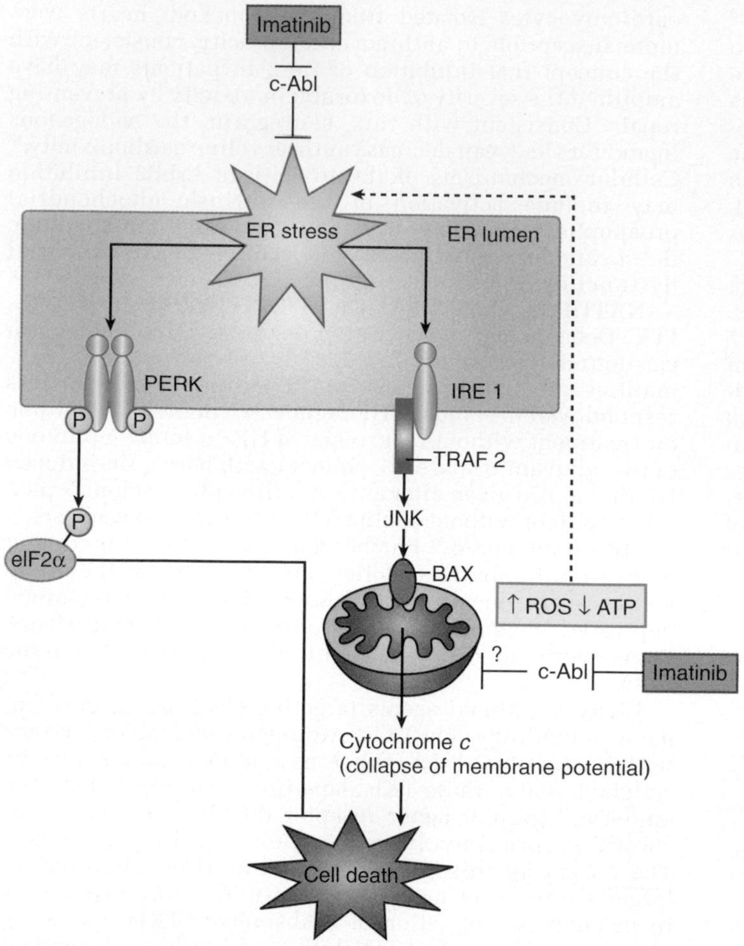

FIGURE 85-4 Targeted tyrosine kinase inhibition can lead to cellular apoptosis. Under stress, cell will activate the endoplasmic reticulum (ER) stress response (also called the unfolded protein response), which is initially protective (e.g., phosphorylation of eIF2α by PERK [PKR-like ER kinase] blocks general protein translation, thereby limiting ATP consumption). If the stress is prolonged, however, it can lead to IRE1 (integral membrane protein of the endoplasmic reticulum)–TRAF2 (tumor necrosis factor receptor associated factor 2)–mediated c-Jun N-terminal kinase (JNK) signaling, which leads to translocation of BAX to the mitochondrial membrane. The result is cytochrome c release and collapse of the mitochondrial membrane potential. The nonreceptor tyrosine kinase c-Abl may act to suppress the ER stress response indirectly by preventing mitochondrial collapse, or directly through an as yet unidentified mechanism. Anticancer drugs that target tyrosine kinases (e.g., imatinib mesylate) may promote apoptosis and heart damage by inhibiting c-Abl, thereby leading to a sustained ER stress response. ROS = reactive oxygen species. *(Redrawn from Mann DL: Targeted cancer therapeutics: The heartbreak of success. Nat Med 12:881, 2006.)*

c-Abl) inhibitor, dasatinib (Sprycel),[53] that also inhibits Bcr-Abl mutants that have become resistant to imatinib caused by additional mutations in the kinase domain, reported a 4 percent incidence of HF and, in half these patients, HF was grade 3 or 4 in severity (NCI grading of severity, in which grade 3 equates to symptomatic HF with an EF of 20 to 40 percent; www.sprycell.com/pdf/pi.pdf; Bristol-Myers Squibb Company, 2006). The median duration of treatment in this trial was only 6 months. However, patients need to be on treatment for life because CML recurs when the drug is stopped. Patients could only be enrolled in this trial if they had normal cardiac function, again highlighting the fact that patients in clinical trials may not reflect the patient population as a whole that will be receiving the drug. Other agents of this group will be released soon, including nilotinib (which also prolongs the QT interval by 15 to 30 msec)[54] and, until rates of cardiotoxicity are known, patients treated with these agents should be monitored.

EPIDERMAL GROWTH FACTOR RECEPTOR ANTAGONISTS

EGFR antagonists are in fairly widespread use for a number of solid tumors, although their efficacy has been generally modest. These agents are either monoclonal antibodies (e.g., cetuximab [Erbitux], panitumumab) or small-molecule inhibitors (gefitinib [Iressa] or erlotinib [Tarceva]). In contrast to inhibition of Her2, cardiotoxicity with EGFR inhibitors seems to be very rare. Thus, other causes of HF should be aggressively sought in patients on these agents presenting with HF.

VASCULAR ENDOTHELIAL GROWTH FACTOR AND VASCULAR ENDOTHELIAL GROWTH FACTOR RECEPTOR ANTAGONISTS

There is great interest in drug development for agents targeting the vascular supply of tumors. Because vascular endothelial cell growth factor (VEGF) and two of its receptors, VEGF-R1 and VEGF-R2, are key regulators of angiogenesis and are overexpressed in many solid tumors, they represent prime candidates.[55] The monoclonal antibody bevacizumab (Avastin) targets VEGF-A and, when combined with chemotherapy, enhanced survival in metastatic colorectal cancer and metastatic, nonsquamous, non-SCLC,[55,56] leading some to suggest that "antivascular" therapies may soon be incorporated into many regimens for solid tumors.[57] Hypertension is relatively common with bevacizumab. It is dose-related and can reach grade 3 or 4 severity in 8 to 18 percent of patients (www.gene.com/products/information/oncology/avastin/insert.jsp; Genentech, Inc., 2006). Proteinuria was also increased in some trials. Based on a meta-analysis of five trials, concerns have also been raised over the approximately twofold increase in arterial (but not venous) thromboembolic events. In this analysis, age and prior thromboembolic events were risk factors. In patients older than 65 years, 8.5 percent developed arterial thromboembolic events versus 2.9 percent for the chemotherapy-alone arm. Stroke risk was increased approximately fourfold (1.9 versus 0.5 percent). Theoretical concerns about the use of these agents in patients with CAD have also been advanced, based on the potential reduction in collateral vessel formation. Finally, HF is relatively uncommon with bevacizumab monotherapy (approximately 2 percent), but rises to approximately 4 percent when patients have received prior anthracyclines or irradiation, and to 14 percent with concurrent anthracycline therapy.

Approved agents targetins VEGF-Rs include sunitinib (Sutent) and sorafenib (Nexavar), and vatalinib is in development. However, hypertension is common with these agents as well. Furthermore, sunitinib and sorafenib are part of a recent trend toward targeting multiple kinases involved in cancer progression. Although this makes sense for treating cancers, multitargeted TKIs raise additional concerns about cardiotoxicity. In one trial, sorafenib was associated with acute coronary syndromes in 2.9 percent of patients (compared with 0.4 percent in the placebo arm; www.univgraph.com/bayer/inserts/nexavar.pdf; Bayer Pharmaceuticals, Inc., 2006). It is now clear that sunitinib is associated with LV dysfunction and CHF. In one study, 10% of patients had significant treatment-emergent decreases in LVEF.[58] Patients with cardiac events in the year prior were excluded from participation. Until more data are available, a baseline evaluation of LV function is recommended for all patients going on sunitinib. Patients on therapy, especially those with cardiac disease, should be followed closely.

The same approach should apply to patients on sorafenib and, possibly, vatalinib.

Several drugs, including imatinib and sunitinib, inhibit c-Kit, the receptor for stem cell factor that is overexpressed or mutated in several leukemias. c-Kit is also expressed on the surface of some hematopoietic stem and progenitor cells capable of adopting endothelial cell fates. Indeed, mice deleted for c-kit undergo LV dilation and have greater deteriorations in LV function following experimental MI, suggesting a key role for c-Kit–positive cells in postinfarct repair.[59] These studies are cause for some concern for the chronic inhibition of c-Kit.

JANUS KINASE/SIGNAL TRANSDUCER AND ACTIVATOR OF TRANSCRIPTION ANTAGONISTS

An activating point mutation in the nonreceptor TK Janus kinase-2 (JAK2) is present in most patients with polycythemia vera and in some with idiopathic myelofibrosis with myeloid metaplasia.[37] Mutant JAK2 appears to act, at least in part, by activating a transcription factor, signal transducer and activator of transcription 3 (STAT3) in the leukemic cells. However, STAT3 also plays critical roles in maintaining capillary density in the heart based on studies with a mouse deleted for the *stat3* gene.[60] STAT3 appears to be particularly important as the animals age. Mechanisms include direct regulation of VEGF expression, induction of pro-angiogenic cytokines, and suppression of antiangiogenic gene programs in the heart. Of note, the STAT3 knockout mouse is also more susceptible to doxorubicin-induced cardiotoxicity.[60] These findings suggest that a careful examination of cardiotoxicity of JAK2 inhibitors that are currently in development is in order.

VASCULAR DISRUPTING AGENTS

Another class of agents, the so-called vascular disrupting agents (VDAs), target endothelial cells. A phase I trial of one such agent, ZD6126, which targets the tubulin network of the endothelial cell, was complicated by pulmonary thromboembolism, asymptomatic creatine kinase (CK)-MB release, and declines in LVEF.[57] Thus, results of additional clinical trials of this and other vascular disrupting agents, which appear to target normal as well as tumor vasculature, will be of interest for determining their potential for vascular toxicity.

OTHER MONOCLONAL ANTIBODIES

In addition to the toxicities specific to the receptors that are inhibited (see earlier), monoclonal antibodies, including cetuximab, which is a chimeric immunoglobulin G1 (IgG1) monoclonal antibody that binds to EGFR with high specificity and with a higher affinity than epidermal growth factors, and two antibodies used in lymphocytic leukemias or lymphomas, alemtuzumab (Campath, targeting the lymphoid antigen, CD52), and rituximab (Rituxan, targeting CD20), commonly induce infusion-related reactions (flu-like symptoms) that can occasionally be severe, leading to hypotension, bronchospasm, skin rashes, urticaria, or angioedema.[61] Care is supportive and is usually effective.

MODULATORS OF APOPTOSIS

Although no agents in this category have yet been approved, this is an area of great interest to the pharmaceutical industry. The concept that modulation of apoptotic factors could be accomplished in vivo, and could produce significant effects, has been largely studied in animal models of acute ischemic injury (stroke and MI). In these models, in which inhibition of caspases has been achieved by small peptide inhibitors, there was reduced injury.[62,63] One small-molecule, nonpeptide inhibitor, IDN6556 (Pfizer, Inc.), was

in Phase II clinical trials. However, for cancer, the general concept would be to enhance rather than inhibit apoptosis. A number of strategies are being pursued, including small molecules that lead to activation of caspase 3, an executioner caspase critical to apoptosis, and small molecules that are inhibitors of prosurvival pathways.[62] Another area of interest is inhibition of the IAP (inhibitor of apoptosis) family. IAPs are overexpressed in some cancers and these cells are relatively resistant to apoptosis. Strikingly, virus-mediated gene transfer of IAPs to the brain has been shown to reduce ischemic injury in stroke models.[62] Thus, strategies for cancer therapeutics targeting apoptotic pathways are often diametrically opposed to strategies for cardiovascular therapeutics.[64] Therefore, development of agents targeting apoptotic pathways in cancer will be of concern for potential cardiovascular toxicity.

Complications of Radiation Therapy

Radiation of the chest can lead to abnormalities of the pericardium, myocardium, valves, and coronary arteries.[6] Patients with Hodgkin disease who receive direct mediastinal irradiation are at particular risk of developing cardiovascular complications. In one detailed study of 48 Hodgkin disease patients 6 to 28 years postirradiation, findings suggestive of right ventricular conduction delay (R-SR' in right precordial leads) were identified in 60 percent of patients. Multiple abnormalities were found on echocardiography including valve abnormalities (43 percent, with aortic and mitral regurgitation of at least mild severity in 19 and 21 percent, respectively.[65] The rate of valvular abnormalities was higher in this study than in an earlier study,[66] in which 24 percent of patients were found to have left-sided regurgitant lesions, probably caused by the lower number of patients in the earlier study receiving 30 Gy or more of radiation, believed to be the threshold dose below which regurgitant lesions are rare.[65] The long-term consequences of this are not clear, but some patients in the high-dose irradiation study were followed for 25 years (mean, 16.5 years), and no patients required valve replacement.[65]

More strikingly, patients postirradiation demonstrated a complex of decreased LV mass, decreased chamber size, and decreased wall thickness and, in 22 percent of patients, this was associated with significantly impaired diastolic filling, suggesting a restrictive cardiomyopathy. Although reduced LV systolic function was detected, it was less common (10 percent) and not severe. Thus, modern approaches to mediastinal irradiation do not appear to lead to important reductions in systolic function, but cardiotoxicity, manifest as diastolic dysfunction, may be a significant problem. Supporting the functional importance of these abnormalities, 30 percent of patients had peak O_2 consumption of less than 20 ml/kg/m², values that are graded as severely reduced in typical HF populations.[65]

Adults are at risk of irradiation-induced cardiac damage even if they have not received direct mediastinal irradiation. For example, a large meta-analysis of 40 randomized trials of patients with breast cancer has shown that irradiation leads to decreased breast cancer deaths, but the overall survival was not changed, with the difference being caused by an excess of cardiovascular deaths in the irradiated patients.[67] In contrast, other studies have demonstrated improved overall survival in radiotherapy-treated patients.[68,69] It is believed that the difference between the latter two studies and the meta-analysis, which included studies from many years before, is probably the result of improved technologies and use of strategies designed to avoid irradiation of the heart and great vessels. This is not to say that there is no risk. For example, the development of CAD appears to be both dose- and volume-related.[70] Although the relative risk (RR) of high-dose and -volume irradiation for MI was only 1.3 (not significant), the RR of death from ischemic heart disease was 2.5, and the RR for any cardiovascular disease was 2.0. Differences became apparent as early as 4 to 5 years posttreatment and continued to increase over 10 to 12 years.[70] The lack of an increase in death from MI with an overall increase in CAD death suggests that small-vessel and microvascular disease may be critical. Patients with preexisting CAD are particularly susceptible to radiation-induced vascular injury. However, patients with no known CAD and no risk factors for CAD also present with disease.

Patients can present with the full spectrum of abnormalities, including angina, MI, HF, and sudden death. Management of patients is similar to that of typical patients with CAD except that mediastinal fibrosis can significantly complicate coronary artery bypass graft surgery. In addition to symptomatic CAD, in one report of 12 breast cancer patients who were asymptomatic from a cardiac standpoint 1 year postirradiation, 50 percent developed evidence of significant flow-limiting disease based on a new defect on perfusion imaging.[71] Other manifestations, including pericarditis, pericardial effusion, and constrictive pericarditis, were discussed earlier. Their incidence appears to be decreasing with modern approaches.[16]

MANAGEMENT OF HEART FAILURE INDUCED BY CANCER THERAPEUTIC AGENTS

At present, the guidelines of the Heart Failure Society of America and the American Heart Association/American College of Cardiology (AHA/ACC) do not contain specific recommendations for treatment of patients with what is presumed to be cancer therapeutic agent–induced HF. However, it is probably most reasonable at this time to approach the patient as one would any patient with newly diagnosed HF, as discussed in Chapter 25. In this regard, it is critical to exclude other potential causes for HF (see Table 25-2) before assuming that chemotherapy has caused the HF. Several of the agents discussed above, including trastuzumab, imatinib, and sunitinib, appear to have some degree of reversibility of LV dysfunction with aggressive treatment with ACE inhibitors and beta blockers. In many cases, patients need to continue on the cancer treatment, and a number of anecdotal case reports have suggested that patients whose LV dysfunction largely resolves after withdrawal of the agent and institution of a HF regimen may be safely rechallenged with the agent, although continuing the HF regimen. Clearly, however, at this point there is insufficient evidence to conclude whether this approach is generally safe, so no clear recommendations can be made, and any rechallenge should be undertaken with great caution.

FUTURE PERSPECTIVES

Many more targets exist for drug development for leukemias and solid tumors (see Table 85-3). Although effective inhibitors for these targets are not yet available, given the intense interest in this area by the pharmaceutical industry, they will likely become available at some point. Clinicians will be faced with a host of novel therapeutics (some of the multitargeted TKI group) and the prospect of trying to predict which will have adverse effects on the cardiovascular system. It will be important to take note of the targets of each new inhibitor and, if adverse effects on the cardiovas-

cular system of inhibiting one of these targets are known, based on studies with earlier agents, the new agent should be assumed to be cardiotoxic until proven otherwise. The keys for the future will be to develop better strategies to identify targets to avoid, thereby limiting cardiotoxicity. When the target cannot be avoided (i.e., when it is causal), the goal will be to develop prophylactic therapies to prevent or minimize cardiotoxicity in high-risk patients. When that fails, we need to develop effective approaches to the management of patients with cardiotoxicity so that progression of HF can be prevented and patients can continue on what is often life-saving treatment. In this endeavor, oncologists and cardiologists must collaborate.

REFERENCES

Complications of Neoplasia

1. Luna A, Ribes R, Caro P, et al: Evaluation of cardiac tumors with magnetic resonance imaging. Eur Radiol 15:1446, 2005.
2. Chiles C, Woodard PK, Gutierrez FR, Link KM: Metastatic involvement of the heart and pericardium: CT and MRI imaging. RadioGraphics 21:439-449, 2001.
3. Maisch B, Seferovic PM, Ristic AD, et al: Guidelines on the diagnosis and management of pericardial diseases. Eur Heart J 25:587-610, 2004.
4. Tsang TS, Seward JB, Barnes ME, et al: Outcomes of primary and secondary treatment of pericardial effusion in patients with malignancy. Mayo Clin Proc 75:248-253, 2000.
5. Tsang TS, Barnes DJ, Gersh BJ: Outcomes of clinically significant idiopathic pericardial effusion requiring intervention. Am J Cardiol 91:704-707, 2002.
6. Lee PJ, Mallik R: Cardiovascular effects of radiation therapy. Cardiol Rev 13:80-86, 2005.
7. Bertog SC, Thambidorai SK, Prarakh K, et al: Constrictive pericarditis: Etiology and cause-specific survival after pericardiectomy. J Am Coll Cardiol 43:1445-1452, 2004.
8. Wudel LJ, Nesbitt JC: Superior vena cava syndrome. Curr Treat Options Oncol 2:77, 2001.
9. Teo N, Sabharwal T, Rowland E, et al: Treatment of superior vena cava obstruction secondary to pacemaker wires with balloon venoplasty and insertion of metallic stents. Eur Heart J 23:1465, 2002.
10. Rowell NP, Gleeson FV: Steroids, radiotherapy, chemotherapy and stents for superior vena cava obstruction in carcinoma of the bronchus: A systematic review. Clin Oncol 14:338-351, 2002.
11. Edoute Y, Haim N, Rinkevich D, et al: Cardiac valvular vegetations in cancer patients: A prospective echocardiographic study of 200 patients. Am J Med 102:252-258, 1997.
12. Ewer MS, Kish SK, Martin CG, et al: Characteristics of cardiac arrest in cancer patients as a precitor of survival after cardiopulmonary resuscitation. Cancer 92:1905-1912, 2001.

Cardiovascular Complications of Cancer Therapeutic Agents

13. Ng R, Better N, Green MD: Anticancer agents and cardiotoxicity. Semin Oncol 33:2-14, 2006.
14. Swain SM, Whaley FS, Ewer MS: Congestive heart failure in patients treated with doxorubicin: A retrospective analysis of three trials. Cancer 97:2869-2879, 2003.
15. Jensen BV, Skoversusgaard T, Nielsen SL: Functional monitoring of anthracycline cardiotoxicity: A prospective, blinded, long-term observational study of outcome in 120 patients. Ann Oncol 13:699-709, 2002.
16. Yeh ET, Tong AT, Lenihan DJ, et al: Cardiovascular complications of cancer therapy: Diagnosis, pathogenesis, and management. Circulation 109:3122-3131, 2004.
17. Kremer LC, van Dalen EC, Offringa M, et al: Anthracycline-induced clinical heart failure in a cohort of 607 children: Long-term follow-up study. J Clin Oncol 19:191-196, 2001.
18. Lipshultz SE, Lipsitz SR, Sallan SE, et al: Chronic progressive cardiac dysfunction years after doxorubicin therapy for childhood acute lymphoblastic leukemia. J Clin Oncol 23:2629-2636, 2005.
19. Peng X, Chen B, Lim CC, Sawyer DB: The cardiotoxicity of anthracycline chemotherapeutics. Mol Intervent 5:163-171, 2005.
20. Swain SM, Whaley FS, Gerber MC, et al: Cardioprotection with dexrazoxane for doxorubicin-containing therapy in advanced breast cancer. J Clin Oncol 15:1318-1332, 1997.
21. Schuchter LM, Hensley ML, Meropol NJ, Winer EP: 2002 update of recommendations for the use of chemotherapy and radiotherapy protectants. J Clin Oncol 20:2895-2903, 2002.
22. Ewer MS, Martin FJ, Henderson C, et al: Cardiac safety of liposomal anthracyclines. Semin Oncol 31:161-181, 2004.
23. Cardinale D, Sandri MT, Colombo A, et al: Prognostic value of troponin I in cardiac risk stratification of cancer patients undergoing high-dose chemotherapy. Circulation 109:2749-2754, 2004.
24. Cardinale D, Colombo A, Sandri MT, et al: Prevention of high-dose chemotherapy-induced cardiotoxicity in high-risk patients by angiotensin-converting enzyme inhibition. Circulation 114:2474-2481, 2006.
25. Silber JH, Cnaan A, Clark BJ, et al: . Enalapril to prevent cardiac function decline in long-term survivors of pediatric cancer exposed to anthracyclines. J Clin Oncol 22:820-828, 2004.

26. Biganzoli L, Cufer T, Bruning P, et al: Doxorubicin-paclitaxel: A safe regimen in terms of cardiac toxicity in metastatic breast carcinoma patients. Results from a European Organization for Research and Treatment of Cancer multicenter trial. Cancer 97:40-45, 2003.

27. Kuittinen T, Husso-Saastamoinen M, Sipola P, et al: Very acute cardiac toxicity during BEAC chemotherapy in non-Hodgkin's lymphoma patients undergoing autologous stem cell transplantation. Bone Marrow Transplant 36:1077-1082, 2005.

28. Sohn SK, Kim JG, Kim DH, Lee KB: Cardiac morbidity in advanced chronic myelogenous leukaemia patients treated by successive allogeneic stem cell transplantation with busulphan/cyclophosphamide conditioning after imatinib mesylate administration. Br J Haematol 121:469-472, 2003.

29. Nuver J, Smit AJ, van der Meer J, et al: Acute chemotherapy-induced cardiovascular changes in patients with testicular cancer. J Clin Oncol 23:9130-9137, 2005.

30. Huddart RA, Norman A, Shahidi M, et al: Cardiovascular disease as a long-term complication of treatment for testicular cancer. J Clin Oncol 21:1513-1523, 2003.

31. Ng M, Cunningham D, Norman ARL The frequency and pattern of cardiotoxicity observed with capecitabine used in conjunction with oxaliplatin in patients treated for advanced colorectal cancer (CRC). Eur J Cancer 41:1542-1546, 2005.

32. Reis SE, Costantino JP, Wickerham DL, van der Meer J: Cardiovascular effects of tamoxifen in women with and without heart disease: Breast cancer prevention trial. National Surgical Adjuvant Breast and Bowel Project Breast Cancer Prevention Trial Investigators. J Natl Cancer Inst 93:16-21, 2001.

33. Chlebowski RT, Anderson GL, Geller M, Col N: Coronary heart disease and stroke with aromatase inhibitor, tamoxifen, and menopausal hormone therapy use. Clin Breast Cancer 6:S58-S64, 2006.

34. Chauhan D, Hideshima T, Mitsiades C, et al: Proteasome inhibitor therapy in multiple myeloma. Mol Cancer Ther 4:686-692, 2005.

35. Chauhan D, Hideshima T, Anderson KC: Proteasome inhibition in multiple myeloma: Therapeutic implication. Annu Rev Pharmacol Toxicol 45:465-476, 2005.

36. Force T, Krause D, Van Etten RA: Molecular mechanism of cardiotoxicity of tyrosine kinase inhibition. Nat Rev Cancer, 2007 (in press).

37. Krause DS, Van Etten RA: Tyrosine kinases as targets for cancer therapy. N Engl J Med 353:172-187, 2005.

38. Force T, Kuida K, Namchuk M, et al: Inhibitors of protein kinase signaling pathways: Emerging therapies for cardiovascular disease. Circulation 109:1196-1205, 2004.

39. Manning G, Whyte DB, Martinez R, et al: The protein kinase complement of the human genome. Science 298:1912-1934, 2002.

40. Burstein HJ: The distinctive nature of HER2-positive breast cancers. N Engl J Med 353:1652-1654, 2005.

41. Slamon DJ, Leyland-Jones B, Shak S, et al: Use of chemotherapy plus a monoclonal antibody against HER2 for metastatic breast cancer that overexpresses HER2. N Engl J Med 344:783-792, 2001.

42. Piccart-Gebhart MJ, Procter M, Leyland-Jones B, et al: Trastuzumab after adjuvant chemotherapy in HER2-positive breast cancer. N Engl J Med 353:1659-1672, 2005.

43. Romond EH, Perez EA, Bryant J, et al: Trastuzumab plus adjuvant chemotherapy for operable HER2-positive breast cancer. N Engl J Med 353:1673-1684, 2005.

44. Seidman A, Hudis C, Pierri MK, et al: Cardiac dysfunction in the trastuzumab clinical trials experience. J Clin Oncol 20:1215-1221, 2002.

45. Tan-Chiu E, Yothers G, Romond E, et al: Assessment of cardiac dysfunction in a randomized trial comparing doxorubicin and cyclophosphamide followed by paclitaxel, with or without trastuzumab as adjuvant therapy in node-positive, human epidermal growth factor receptor 2-overexpressing breast cancer: NSABP B-31. J Clin Oncol 23:7811-7819, 2005.

46. Levine MN: Trastuzumab cardiac side effects: Only time will tell. J Clin Oncol 23:7775-7776, 2005.

47. Crone SA, Zhao YY, Fan L, et al: ErbB2 is essential in the prevention of dilated cardiomyopathy. Nat Med 8:459-465, 2002.

48. Grazette L, Boecker W, Matsui T, et al: Inhibition of ErbB2 causes mitochondrial dysfunction in cardiomyocytes: Implications for herceptin-induced cardiomyopathy. J Am Coll Cardiol 44:2231-2238, 2004.

49. Ewer MS, Vooletich MT, Durand JB, et al: Reversibility of trastuzumab-related cardiotoxicity: New insights based on clinical course and response to medical treatment. J Clin Oncol 23:7820-7826, 2005.

50. Deininger M, Buchdunger E, Druker BJ: The development of imatinib as a therapeutic agent for chronic myeloid leukemia. Blood 105:2640-2653, 2005.

51. Kerkela R, Grazette L, Yacobi R, et al: Cardiotoxicity of the cancer therapeutic agent imatinib mesylate. Nat Med 12:908-916, 2006.

52. Park YH, Park HJ, Kim BS, et al: BNP as a marker of the heart failure in the treatment of imatinib mesylate. Cancer Lett ePub:Jan 4, 2006, 2006.

53. Talpaz M, Shah NP, Kantarjian H, et al: Dasatinib in imatinib-resistant Philadelphia chromosome–positive leukemias. N Engl J Med 354:2531-2541, 2006.

54. Kantarjian H, Giles F, Wunderle L, et al: Nilotinib in imatinib-resistant CML and Philadelphia chromosome–positive ALL. N Engl J Med 354:2542-2551, 2006.

55. Morabito A, De ME, Di MM, et al: Tyrosine kinase inhibitors of vascular endothelial growth factor receptors in clinical trials: Current status and future directions. Oncologist 11:753-764, 2006.

56. Dy GK, Adjei AA: Angiogenesis inhibitors in lung cancer: A promise fulfilled. Clin Lung Cancer 7(Suppl 4):S145-S149, 2006.

57. van Heeckeren WJ, Bhakta S, Ortiz J, et al: Promise of new vascular-disrupting agents balanced with cardiac toxicity: Is it time for oncologists to get to know their cardiologists? J Clin Oncol 24:1485-1488, 2006.

58. Motzer RJ, Hutson TE, Tomczak P, et al: Sunitinib versus interferon alpha in metastatic renal-cell carcinoma. E Engl J Med 365:115, 2007.

59. Ayach BB, Yoshimitsu M, Dawood F, et al: Stem cell factor receptor induces progenitor and natural killer cell-mediated cardiac survival and repair after myocardial infarction. Proc Nat Acad Sci U S A 103:2304-2309, 2006.

60. Hilfiker-Kleiner D, Limbourg A, Drexler H: STAT3-mediated activation of myocardial capillary growth. Trends Cardiovasc Med 15:152-157, 2005.

61. Osterborg A, Karlsson C, Lundin J, et al: Strategies in the management of alemtuzumab-related side effects. Semin Oncol 33:S29-S35, 2006.

62. Lavrik IN, Golks A, Krammer PH: Caspases: Pharmacological manipulation of cell death. J Clin Invest 115:2665-2672, 2005.

63. Reed JC: Apoptosis-based therapies. Nat Rev Drug Disc 1:111-121, 2002.

64. Foo RS, Mani K, Kitsis RN: Death begets failure in the heart. J Clin Invest 115:565-571, 2005.

65. Adams MJ, Lipsitz SR, Colan SD, et al: Cardiovascular status in long-term survivors of Hodgkin's disease treated with chest radiotherapy. J Clin Oncol 22:3139-3148, 2004.

66. Lund MB, Ihlen H, Voss BM, et al: Increased risk of heart valve regurgitation after mediastinal radiation for Hodgkin's disease: An echocardiographic study. Heart 75:591-595, 1996.

67. Early Breast Cancer Trialists' Collaborative Group: Favourable and unfavourable effects on long-term survival of radiotherapy for early breast cancer: An overview of the randomised trials. Lancet 355:1757-1770, 2000.

68. Overgaard M, Hansen PS, Overgaard J, et al: Postoperative radiotherapy in high-risk premenopausal women with breast cancer who receive adjuvant chemotherapy. Danish Breast Cancer Cooperative Group 82b Trial. N Engl J Med 337:949-955, 1997.

69. Overgaard M, Jensen MB, Overgaard J, et al: Postoperative radiotherapy in high-risk postmenopausal breast-cancer patients given adjuvant tamoxifen: Danish Breast Cancer Cooperative Group DBCG 82c randomised trial. Lancet 353:1641-1648, 1999.

70. Gyenes G, Rutqvist LE, Liedberg A, Fornander T: Long-term cardiac morbidity and mortality in a randomized trial of pre- and postoperative radiation therapy versus surgery alone in primary breast Cancer Radiother Oncol 48:185-190, 1998.

71. Gyenes G, Fornander T, Carlens P, et al: Detection of radiation-induced myocardial damage by technetium-99m sestamibi scintigraphy. Eur J Nucl Med 24:286-292, 1997.

CHAPTER **86**

Psychiatric and Behavioral
Aspects of Coronary Heart
Disease, 2119
From Type A Behavior to Type D
    Personality, 2119
Depression and Anxiety, 2119
Psychosocial Factors, 2121
Acute Mental Stress, 2121
Sudden Emotion, 2122

**Arrhythmias and Sudden
Cardiac Death, 2122**

**Psychiatric and Behavioral
Aspects of Hypertension and
Heart Failure, 2123**
Hypertension, 2123
Heart Failure, 2124

**Cardiac Symptoms: Chest Pain
and Palpitations, 2125**
Chest Pain, 2125
Palpitations, 2125
Delay and Denial of Cardiac
    Symptoms, 2125

**Psychiatric Care of the Cardiac
Patient, 2126**
Acute Care of the Hospitalized
    Patient, 2126
Convalescence and Recovery after
    Hospitalization, 2127
Cardiac Rehabilitation
    Programs, 2128

**Psychopharmacology in the
Cardiac Patient, 2128**
Cardiovascular Aspects of
    Psychotropic Agents, 2128
Psychiatric Side Effects of
    Cardiovascular Drugs, 2132
Interactions of Psychotropic and
    Cardiac Drugs, 2132

Future Perspectives, 2133

References, 2133

Psychiatric and Behavioral Aspects of Cardiovascular Disease

Lawson R. Wulsin and Arthur J. Barsky

Daily life offers ample empirical evidence of an intimate relationship between the psyche and the heart. Intense emotions such as anxiety, anger, elation, and sexual arousal are accompanied by predictable increases in heart rate and blood pressure. Our everyday speech is filled with cardiac metaphors—the heart "races" with excitement, "pounds" in eager anticipation, "stands still" in dread, and "aches" with grief. Many cultures have regarded the heart as the seat of emotion, the origin of love, the source of courage, or the abode of the soul. Generous people have "big hearts," and stingy people are "heartless." When you met your first love, your heart "skipped a beat," and you were "broken hearted" when you parted ways. We attend funerals with a "heavy heart" and offer our "heartfelt" condolences. The interaction of heart and psyche works both ways. Emotions and stressful experiences affect the heart directly through the autonomic nervous system, as well as indirectly via neuroendocrine pathways. And conversely, pathologic cardiac activity and function trigger distress and contribute to psychopathology, such as depressive syndromes following myocardial infarctions (MIs) or strokes.

PSYCHIATRIC AND BEHAVIORAL ASPECTS OF CORONARY HEART DISEASE

From Type A Behavior to Type D Personality

Clinicians have long observed that many patients with coronary heart disease (CHD) seem to be compulsive, driven overachievers who are unable to relax and are quick to feel angry and frustrated when things do not proceed as planned. These observations were reinforced in the 1960s by Friedman and Rosenman, who advanced the concept of type A behavior. Type A behavior is suffused with a sense of ambition, time urgency, and anger and hostility; type A people are excessively competitive and aggressive, with an extreme drive for achievement—impatient people leading fast-paced lives in continual and strenuous pursuit of a goal. In contrast, type B people are relaxed, unhurried, less aggressive, and do not get as upset when thwarted. Large-scale, prospective studies in the 1970s and 1980s conducted on initially healthy individuals showed that those with type A behavior pattern, compared with type B individuals, had a significantly elevated rate of developing CHD and MI at 5- to 8.5-year follow-up and had more extensive CHD at the time of angiography. Although some subsequent studies replicated these

findings, a number failed to support the association.[1]

These contradictory findings led to a search for a specific component of type A behavior that might be more closely associated with CHD. This work suggested that anger and/or suppressed anger are the pathogenic components of type A personality. Anger, hostility, antagonistic interactions, cynicism, and mistrust have now been associated in long-term, prospective studies with the incidence of CHD, coronary events, and total mortality. Some studies, however, have failed to find an association between anger and CHD, and in general it appears that hostility and anger may predispose more to the initial cardiac event than adversely influencing the course of already established CHD. To what degree hostility's effect may be mediated through its effect on other risk factors such as lack of social support, smoking, obesity, and alcohol use is unclear. The combination of both anger and low social support may be particularly hazardous. Possible associations among anger and race, socioeconomic status, and gender also represent potential confounds. Although more research is necessary, it does appear that anger and hostility play some role in the development of CHD.

More recently, Denollet and colleagues[2] have examined the effect on CHD outcomes of "type D personality," a set of traits that combine a pattern of anxious and depressive feelings with a tendency toward social inhibition and isolation. Denollet has shown in several controlled studies that people who score high on the 14-item type D questionnaire have higher early mortality rates from CHD disease. Denollet argues that what damages the cardiovascular system is not just depressed mood or feeling bad, but feeling bad alone over many years.[2]

Depression and Anxiety

DEPRESSION. Depression is prevalent in CHD patients but is consistently underdiagnosed by their cardiologists and primary care physicians. Clinically significant depressive symptoms are found in

40 to 65 percent of patients following a MI, and major depressive disorder is found in 15 to 25 percent of such patients.[3] In one study, 31.5 percent of patients with MI experienced major depression while in the hospital or in the year following discharge. The prevalence of depression is also elevated in patients with stable CHD who have not had a recent MI and in patients who have undergone coronary artery bypass grafting (CABG). Depression is often chronic: Three fourths of the patients with major depression 2 weeks after a MI remain depressed 3 months later. Although most subjects in these studies have been men, the risk of depression in women with CHD is twice as high as that of men.[4]

Depression is important in itself because of the considerable suffering it imposes. In addition, depression exacerbates and amplifies cardiac symptoms. Depressed CHD patients have more severe cardiac symptoms than nondepressed CHD patients, even after controlling for the severity of cardiac disease: They have more angina during exercise treadmill testing, terminate the treadmill test sooner, and have more persistent angina following MI. Depression adversely affects compliance with medical therapy, and it is detrimental to cardiac rehabilitation. Depression also predicts a slower resumption of activities, poorer social readjustment, a lower likelihood of returning to work, and poorer quality of life following MI.[5,6] Depression both worsens the prognosis of established CHD and constitutes a risk factor for the development of CHD in healthy individuals; that is, it confers an increased risk of cardiac mortality in both those with and without CHD at baseline.[7] In patients with documented CHD, depression predicts future cardiac events and is associated with significantly elevated rates of cardiac mortality (primarily as a result of sudden cardiac death [SCD]). Following MI, depression increases the risk of reinfarction, cardiac arrest, and death, after adjusting for CHD severity.[8] This risk is elevated for women as well as men, and is not limited to major depressive disorder but also includes milder depressive symptoms. Thus there is a continuous, linear relationship between the severity of depression and the risk of subsequent cardiac events.[9] Major depressive disorder at the time of cardiac catheterization is a significant predictor of subsequent MI, angioplasty, CABG, and death in patients with evidence of CHD, and this effect is independent of disease severity, ejection fraction, and smoking. Depression before undergoing CABG surgery is an independent predictor of rehospitalization, continued surgical pain, and failure to resume previous activity.[10]

For longer follow-up periods, from 5 to 15 years, the relative risk of recurrent MI or cardiac mortality associated with depression is between 1.5 and 6, after controlling for disease severity, smoking, diabetes, and age in multivariate analyses.[9] The degree of risk associated with depression is as great as that associated with traditional risk factors (e.g., cholesterol, smoking, hypertension) and is largely independent of them. In some studies, however, the association between depression and postmyocardial reinfarction is no longer significant when adjusted for all other predictors of cardiac mortality and for possible confounds (e.g., fatigue) that are common to both CHD and depression. Much of the increased cardiac mortality associated with depression appears to be attributable to SCD caused by arrhythmias. This suggests that the effect of depression may be more arrhythmogenic than atherogenic. An interaction effect may exist, in which the co-occurrence of depression with ventricular arrhythmias constitutes a particularly ominous prognostic factor.[11]

Depression as a Risk Factor. Depression also appears to be a risk factor for the development of CHD in healthy individuals, though the evidence here is somewhat less conclusive. In prospective studies of initially healthy community residents without a history of CHD, depression has been associated with an adjusted relative risk between 1.5 and 2 for the subsequent development of CHD, MI, and cardiac death over 6- to 40-year periods in men and in women, and this risk is largely independent of the more traditional risk factors.[12] A dose-response relationship seems to exist such that the more severely depressed the patient is, the greater the risk of developing CHD.

In *summary*, clinical depression predicts poor outcomes for patients with established CHD and is a risk factor for the development of CHD in healthy individuals. It is associated with increased morbidity, mortality, disability, and impaired quality of life. Both major depressive disorder and less severe depressive symptoms contribute to CHD risk. The degree of risk associated with major depression is comparable to that associated with other, established CHD risk factors and is largely independent of them.

Behavioral Mechanisms. Depressed individuals take poorer care of themselves; are less physically active; pay less attention to diet; drink more alcohol; smoke more and have worse quitting rates; have less motivation and energy to exercise regularly; and may be less likely to seek medical care. Depression is associated with poorer adherence to the medical regimen and to cardiac risk factor modification and rehabilitation, and depressed patients are more likely to drop out of exercise programs. For reasons that remain unclear, patients with a range of psychiatric disorders including depression undergo revascularization procedures (percutaneous transluminal coronary angioplasty and CABG) less frequently than those without psychiatric disorders, even after adjusting for disease severity.[13]

Pathophysiological Mechanisms. Several pathophysiological mechanisms may link depression and CHD. First, depression results in autonomic arousal and hypothalamic-adrenocortical and sympathoadrenal hyperactivity. Depressed patients show hyperactivity of the hypothalamic-pituitary-adrenocortical axis and hypercortisolemia, and corticosteroids have atherogenic effects including the induction of high blood pressure and increases in cholesterol and free fatty acids, as well as possible effects on arterial endothelial function.[14] In addition, there is hypersecretion of norepinephrine in depression, and plasma catecholamines stimulate heart rate, blood pressure, and myocardial oxygen consumption. Catecholamines are also proarrhythmic, and an increased incidence of ventricular tachyarrhythmias has been found in depressed patients. (This observation is compatible with the finding that SCD accounts for a large share of the excess cardiac mortality found in depressed CHD patients.)[9,11]

Second, depressed cardiac patients exhibit diminished heart rate variability, resulting from a relative increase in sympathetic tone and/or a relative decrease in parasympathetic tone, which increases the risk of fatal arrhythmias. Third, depression may be accompanied by changes in platelet aggregability. Serotonin plays a major role in depression, and it is also known to influence thrombogenesis and enhance platelet activation and responsiveness to other thrombogenic agents. Serotonin reuptake inhibitor antidepressants appear to normalize this platelet hyperactivity seen in depression.

ANXIETY. Like depression, chronically high levels of anxiety, panic disorder, and phobic anxiety contribute to the risk for the onset and progression of CHD.[15,16] In the former instance, several prospective studies of initially healthy men and women reveal that those who are highly anxious at the outset are more likely to subsequently develop arteriosclerotic plaques, carotid artery intimal thickening, nonfatal MI, and cardiac death. In the Framingham Heart Study high levels of tension predicted increased risk for new CHD and anxiety predicted increased risk for mortality from all causes.[17] One large prospective study found that high levels of phobic anxiety are associated with an increased risk of fatal CHD, particularly from SCD.[15] Anxiety may also worsen the course of established CHD. Thus high levels of anxiety following MI appear to confer a 2.5-fold to 5-fold increased risk of recurrent ischemia, reinfarction, ventricular fibrillation, and SCD. Whether anxiety is more closely related to arrhythmias and SCD than to arteriosclerosis and infarction remains unclear.

Possible mechanisms explaining these associations include sympathetic nervous system upregulation with increased catecholamine production and decreased vagal activity, microvascular angina, and idiopathic cardiomyopathy.

Psychosocial Factors

Psychosocial, cultural, and environmental factors increase the risk of CHD, either independently or in combination. These include social isolation and lack of social support, life stresses (such as job strain), and sociodemographic characteristics. These psychosocial risk factors tend to be associated with each other and often co-occur. For example, job strain and socioeconomic position may be inversely correlated, and depression is associated with social isolation. Furthermore, these psychosocial factors tend to be associated with unhealthy lifestyle behaviors. For example, life stress may be correlated with smoking, increased alcohol consumption, and body weight, and people with fewer social supports are less likely to stop smoking or adhere to the medical regimen.

SOCIAL ISOLATION, LACK OF SOCIAL SUPPORT, AND SOCIAL DISRUPTION. Population-based, cross-sectional surveys reveal that social integration (e.g., being married, having regular contact with friends, and belonging to organizations) is associated with lower levels of CHD. Conversely, social isolation and low social support (living alone, having few friends or family members, and not belonging to organizations, clubs, or churches) is associated with an increased incidence of CHD and a poorer outcome following first diagnosis of CHD.[18] As a predictor of mortality 1 year after MI, low social support is equivalent to such traditional risk factors as hypertension, smoking, and elevated cholesterol. In a recent prospective study of 430 CHD patients, those with fewer than four people in their social network had a 2.4 times greater risk of cardiac mortality after adjusting for differences in age, disease severity, psychological distress, smoking, and income.[19] Social support and depression seem to interact, such that high levels of social support blunt the impact of depression on cardiac mortality.[20]

Animal studies also suggest a protective role for social support against atherogenesis. When research personnel fondle laboratory rabbits placed on an atherogenic diet, the development of coronary atherosclerosis is retarded. Crowding and social disruption of animal colonies, as well as isolation of individual laboratory animals, increase the rates of atherogenesis.

Several mediating mechanisms have been proposed to explain this relationship between social integration and CHD. First, concerned and supportive others may encourage healthy behaviors and adherence to the medical regimen and provide motivation for altering unhealthy behavioral risk factors; conversely, loneliness may foster unhealthy behaviors such as smoking and drinking. Second, social support, by providing comfort, encouragement, and consolation, may attenuate and buffer the individual's emotional and/or physiological response to environmental stress. Finally, significant others can provide practical assistance that mitigates the impact of stressful life events (e.g., lending money, doing errands, providing transportation).

LIFE STRESS AND JOB STRAIN. The relationship between life stress and CHD has long been of interest. Animal work is provocative in this regard. In studies ranging from mice to primates, stressful experimental paradigms that increase aggression and fear and that disturb stable social hierarchies and decrease social affiliation are associated with atherosclerosis. Thus dominant male monkeys fed an atherogenic diet develop coronary atherosclerosis at a higher rate when repeatedly moved from one social group to another rather than when left in a single, stable group.

In humans, two different forms of stress have received particular attention: major life events that tax one's abilities to adapt (e.g., getting divorced, moving, encountering financial difficulties, being involved in a lawsuit) and minor, recurrent irritants and frustrations. Some studies of individuals undergoing major, stressful life events have found an association with the incidence of MI, the development of CHD, or cardiac mortality, but other prospective studies have not. At present, the evidence remains inconclusive.

When turning to recurrent daily stresses, job strain and work-related pressures have received considerable attention. *Job strain* is defined as the combination of high demands with little autonomy or control over one's working conditions, routine, or schedule. Job strain has been associated with an increased risk of CHD in previously healthy people,[21] but its impact on the progress of already established CHD is less clear. Cross-sectional studies in the United States and Europe disclose that both men and women workers with high job strain have a higher prevalence of CHD and higher incidence of MI than do those with low job strain. Longitudinal studies also provide some support for this hypothesis.[22] In a longitudinal study of 812 Finnish employees over a 25-year period, those with high demands from and low levels of control over work conditions had more than double the risk for cardiovascular disease mortality.[21] Marital stress has been found to exert a negative prognostic influence on CHD in women and may be even more important than job stress for women.[23]

SOCIODEMOGRAPHIC CHARACTERISTICS. Lower socioeconomic status (whether assessed by education, occupation, or income) prospectively predisposes healthy people to an increased risk of CHD and CHD patients to a poorer prognosis. The decline in cardiovascular disease mortality over the past 30 years in the United States has been more pronounced among those of higher socioeconomic status, and the reasons for this are not clear. Because beneficial health habits (including not smoking and weight control) tend to be associated with socioeconomic status, they may play a role. Poorer nutrition and difficulty obtaining medical care may contribute, and hostility and depression may be weakly inversely correlated with social position. Stressful life events, greater job strain, lack of social support, and diminished sense of self-control may mediate the relationship between socioeconomic status and CHD. In addition, complex racial and ethnic differences in cardiovascular disease remain poorly understood. Because race and ethnicity tend to be confounded with differences in socioeconomic position, it has been difficult to isolate their effects.

Acute Mental Stress

Acute mental stress has negative cardiovascular consequences. Cardiovascular mortality rises in the month following the death of a loved one, and the incidence of cardiac events rises immediately after natural disasters and among civilians subjected to military attack. The direct cardiovascular effects of acute mental stress have been observed during daily life and with laboratory paradigms of experimental stress. Experimental stress (induced, e.g., by public speaking or accomplishing difficult intellectual tasks under time pressure or in frustrating circumstances) reliably increases heart rate, blood pressure, and myocardial oxygen demands. The effect of acute mental stress on the heart already damaged by preexisting CHD has been studied with relatively sensitive measures of myocardial ischemia such as regional myocardial perfusion and wall motion abnormalities. However, the frequency of mental stress–induced ischemia varies widely, with reports of such stress precipitating myocardial ischemia in 20 to 70 percent of CHD patients.[24]

Mental stress–induced ischemia occurs at lower heart rates and at lower levels of myocardial work than does exercise-induced ischemia, suggesting that decreases in myocardial perfusion may play a role in mental stress–induced ischemia. In a laboratory study of 58 patients with CHD and three levels of LV function (normal, mild-to-moderate ejection fractions of 30 to 50 percent, and severe ejection fractions of <30 percent), ischemia was induced more frequently (50 percent) with mental stress in those with severe LV dysfunction compared with 9 percent of those with normal LV function. Mental stress ischemia may be most important clinically in CHD patients with LV dysfunction.[25]

Mental stress–induced ischemia is more likely to be "silent," or asymptomatic, than is ischemia induced by exercise. In one study, 83 percent of mental stress–induced ischemic episodes were asymptomatic. Approximately one third of CHD patients without exercise-induced ischemia experience mental stress–induced ischemia, suggesting that the two forms of stress induce ischemia by different but related sets of mechanisms.[24]

When CHD patients are monitored during daily life, mental challenges unaccompanied by strenuous physical exertion are frequently associated with transient myocardial ischemia. Such ischemia has been observed, for example, while driving and during public speaking. Although most ischemic episodes during daily life do not appear to be precipitated by psychological or mental stress, a sizable minority (perhaps as many as one fourth) are.

CHD patients who exhibit mental stress–induced ischemia appear to be at increased risk of subsequent fatal and nonfatal cardiac events.[26] This relationship persists after other risk factors (including age, left ventricular function, and prior MI) have been taken into account.

Acute stress may promote ischemic heart disease in a number of ways. First, stress increases myocardial oxygen demands as a result of its hemodynamic effects. Second, vasospasm may reduce coronary blood flow, especially in more severely diseased vessels. Third, the stress response increases circulating cortisol and catecholamines, which activate platelets and promote platelet aggregation and which increase cholesterol and decrease high-density lipoproteins. The net result of these actions is to increase cardiac demand while at the same time decreasing coronary blood supply and to promote plaque rupture and thrombus formation.

Sudden Emotion (see Chap. 64)

The work on anger, depression, and anxiety discussed earlier deals with the long-term consequences and sequelae of enduring, persistent emotions. A body of work also exists on the immediate and acute effects of sudden, intense, negative emotion. Because much of this work focuses on arrhythmias and SCD, it is reviewed in the next section. However, mental activities leading to intense anger or frustration and, to a lesser degree, to anxiety and sadness can trigger myocardial ischemia.[27] The relative risk for MI in the 1 to 2 hours following an episode in which the patients report feeling angry is between 2.3 and 9.[28] Because these intense,

negative emotional states involve sympathetic arousal, they may act by triggering coronary vasospasm, rupture of atherosclerotic plaques, and increased platelet aggregation. Anger and hostility in particular have been associated with increased platelet adhesion.[29] Hostility is also associated with decreased parasympathetic arousal during ambulatory monitoring. When anger is experimentally induced, patients scoring higher on hostility scales exhibit greater sympathetic nervous system–mediated cardiovascular responses than those who are less hostile.[30]

ARRHYTHMIAS AND SUDDEN CARDIAC DEATH (see Chaps. 32, 33, and 35)

Increasing evidence links mentally stressful and emotionally powerful events with lethal arrhythmias and SCD. Intense, overwhelming emotions such as fear and anger have been associated with both benign and lethal arrhythmias including ventricular premature complexes, ventricular tachycardia, and ventricular fibrillation. This effect is most evident in hearts that are already diseased, ischemic, or electrically unstable. At least three lines of investigation into the arrhythmogenic potential of stress and intense emotion exist: retrospective case series of psychological distress immediately preceding lethal arrhythmias or SCD; psychophysiological experiments demonstrating that arrhythmias immediately follow sudden, intense emotion or acute stress; and investigations of the neural control of cardiac rate and rhythm.

OBSERVATIONAL STUDIES. Experts have long suspected that acutely stressful events and sudden, intense emotion can precipitate fatal arrhythmias and SCD, and many anecdotal cases of SCD immediately following severe psychological stress and intense emotional arousal have been reported. Careful psychiatric interviews of patients hospitalized after ventricular tachycardia or ventricular fibrillation revealed that 21 percent had undergone a major emotional disturbance or psychological trigger in the preceding 24 hours. These included interpersonal conflicts, bereavement, public humiliation, marital separation, and business losses. Studies like these suffer from retrospective bias and selective recall, inadequate or absent control groups, and sampling bias. When taken together, however, they nonetheless suggest that acute stress (perhaps in conjunction with other factors such as preexisting CHD) has the power on occasion to precipitate lethal arrhythmias and contribute to SCD.

STRESS AND ARRHYTHMIAS. Other research has probed the link between emotionally provocative daily stresses and arrhythmias. Healthy subjects manifest ventricular ectopy during driving, public speaking, and stressful interviews. Among cardiac patients undergoing ambulatory monitoring, daily life stresses are associated with ectopy. Experimentally induced psychological stress has been shown to lower the ventricular vulnerable period and the threshold for ventricular fibrillation and to increase the frequency of ventricular ectopic beats in patients with preexisting ventricular arrhythmias. Thus it is clear that stressful experiences and events can produce rhythm changes in both normal subjects and CHD patients. The clinical importance of this remains to be established, but the combination of severe, acute mental distress and a myocardium made vulnerable by preexisting disease can result in lethal arrhythmias and SCD.

The link between stress and arrhythmias has been explored in experimental animal work. When dogs are subjected to aversive restraint and electric shock, there is a 49 to 66 percent decrease in the repetitive extrasystole threshold. If a coronary artery occlusion is first produced experimentally, then the same stressful paradigm induces spontaneous ventricular fibrillation. Similarly, when pigs with a coronary artery occlusion are placed in a stressful environment, there is a high incidence of spontaneous ventricular fibrillation.

Some psychiatric disorders, particularly anxiety and depressive disorders, may predispose to SCD. The empirical evidence, however, remains scanty. In one study, psychiatric distress after MI predicted ventricular arrhythmias in the year following the infarct, although subsequent work failed to confirm these findings. Depressed patients with CHD have an increased incidence of significant ventricular arrhythmias.[31] Post-MI depression in particular has been linked to SCD, and much of its negative influence on cardiac mortality in patients with CHD is mediated through SCD. However, a number of methodological problems make this work difficult to interpret, and on balance the evidence at this time must be considered equivocal.

Sociocultural and sociodemographic factors may also play a role in SCD. The inverse relationship between socioeconomic status and cardiac mortality in general is especially robust for SCD, although this may well be confounded by an association between social position and access to emergency medical care. Other work has disclosed that cardiac mortality is significantly higher immediately after, as compared with immediately before, an important religious holiday. In addition, there are well-recognized, culture-specific syndromes in which sudden death follows highly ritualized events with a powerful, culture-specific significance, such as "voodoo death."

NEURAL INFLUENCES ON RATE AND RHYTHM. A number of pathways mediate the neural control of heart rate and rhythm. First, activation of the hypothalamic-adrenomedullary axis increases myocardial irritability and decreases the threshold for inducing ventricular fibrillation. Second, direct sympathetic innervation of the heart exerts a proarrhythmic effect, increasing ventricular ectopy and lowering the threshold for inducing ventricular arrhythmias, especially in the heart with preexisting ischemic damage or electrical instability. Animal work provides evidence of cortical and brain stem influence over cardiac rhythm: Pathways run from the frontal cortex and hypothalamus to the brain stem nuclei controlling cardiovascular function. Thus stimulation of the lateral and posterior hypothalamus lowers the ventricular fibrillation threshold, and blockade of these corticofrontal pathways raise it. In humans, electrocardiographic changes in rhythm and/or repolarization are seen in patients suffering cerebrovascular accidents involving the cortex. Finally, extreme stress and acute psychological trauma can cause myocardial necrosis. In animal models, large quantities of catecholamines, either exogenously administered or stress induced, can result in myofibrillar degeneration and myocardial necrosis. On pathological examination, widespread calcification is found, the result of peroxidation of myocardial lipid membranes and blockage of the calcium-channel pump. This same lesion has also been reported in humans who died suddenly at the peak of extreme psychic stress and trauma.

Implantable cardioverter-defibrillators are increasingly used in the treatment of potentially lethal arrhythmias (see Chap. 34). Although these devices are medically efficacious and generally meet with a high degree of patient acceptance, in a substantial minority of patients (probably between 25 and 50 percent) the implantation of the device results in significant emotional distress (anxiety, depression, anger, withdrawal).[32]

PSYCHIATRIC AND BEHAVIORAL ASPECTS OF HYPERTENSION AND HEART FAILURE

Hypertension (see Chaps. 40 and 41)

Stress, conditioned learning, and autonomic arousal all can elevate blood pressure. Stimulation of brain sites with connections to the sympathetic nervous system have a pressor effect, and many of these sites are in turn connected with higher centers involved in the perception of the environment. However, the transient elevations of blood pressure seen in stressful and provocative situations may be unrelated to the persistent, sustained elevation that constitutes the disease of hypertension.

STRESS AND BLOOD PRESSURE. Stressful environments and challenging or aversive situations transiently increase the blood pressure of both normotensive and hypertensive individuals. This has been demonstrated in field studies using ambulatory monitoring of blood pressure during daily life and in laboratory studies assessing blood pressure reactivity to a discrete stimulus or specific experimental stressor. Some individuals exhibit greater cardiovascular reactivity than others, consistently responding to psychological stressors with greater increases in blood pressure and heart rate, more vasoconstriction and catecholamine secretion, and a more prolonged recovery phase. These individual differences in cardiovascular reactivity emerge early in life and are thought to be stable and enduring. Such hyperreactivity to stress has long been believed to predispose the individual to the eventual development of hypertension (and atherosclerosis), but the empirical evidence remains inconclusive. Several large epidemiological surveys of initially normotensive individuals have found that exaggerated blood pressure responses to psychological and physical stress predict the subsequent development of essential hypertension on long-term follow-up.[33] However, a number of questions remain about the hypothesis that an exaggerated stress response predisposes individuals to hypertension: Cardiovascular reactivity may vary over time; it may vary within the same individual depending on the nature of the stress; and it is not yet clear that transient blood pressure increases in response to such stressors are the precursors of pathological, sustained hypertension.

In surveys examining the relationship between naturally occurring stress and blood pressure, stress has been associated with the onset or worsening of essential hypertension. Job strain in particular has been associated with an elevated prevalence and incidence of hypertension in men (this is less clear in women), and the blood pressures of people in more stressful occupations tend to be higher than those in less stressful jobs. However, it appears that such chronic stress requires the co-occurrence of other etiological factors (e.g., genetic endowment, dietary factors, psychological characteristics) to cause sustained hypertension. This situation may be analogous to that emerging from animal work: Repeated exposure to stress can lead to sustained hypertension in animals that are predisposed to hypertension by genetic endowment or salt ingestion, but not in healthy animals free of such predisposing factors.

PSYCHOLOGICAL STATES. Anger and anxiety are accompanied by increases in peripheral vascular resistance and blood pressure, and anger has long been thought to contribute to the development of essential hypertension. Hostile individuals respond to provocation, conflict, and disagreement with larger increases in blood pressure than people who are less hostile, and there have been reports of higher levels of anger and suppressed anger among hypertensive patients. In a recent prospective study of 3308 citizens age 18 to 30 at enrollment, hostility was significantly associated with a dose-response increase in the 15-year risk for hypertension, independent of standard hypertension risk factors.[34] Other studies, however, have failed to detect an association between anger or aggression and hypertension. A recent meta-analysis of 15 studies of the relationship between anger and blood pressure concluded that the evidence supports "a modest role of self-reported trait anger and anger expression in blood pressure levels."[35] The relationship between anger and hypertension may be stronger in some minority groups than in nonminorities. In sum, the evidence linking anger and hypertension remains equivocal. Recent work has focused on the more-difficult-to-measure construct of repressed or *suppressed* emotion (particularly anger), and there are reports of an association between emotional inhibition and essential hypertension. Although one meta-analysis concluded that there appears to be an association between suppressed anger and resting blood pressure, overall, this literature must still be considered inconclusive.

Other work has examined the role of anxiety. Some evidence indicates that chronically anxious persons develop greater increases in systolic blood pressure over the ensuing years and may also be at increased risk of developing essential hypertension. A quantitative review of 15 prospective studies with greater than 1-year follow-up concluded that there is at least "moderate support" in the evidence for anxiety's independent contribution to the risk for hypertension.[36] However, although several prospective studies confirmed this association, others have not.[10,37] Finally, the possible etiological role of depression has also been investigated. The prevalence of hypertension is reported to be higher in depressed community residents, depressed medical patients, and depressed psychiatric patients than in nondepressed comparison groups. In one population-based study of 1920 citizens, major depression that began more than a year before baseline predicted a significantly increased risk for incident hypertension.[38] In another recent, large, population-based study, the symptoms of depression and anxiety were significantly associated with the development of hypertension, even after adjusting for sociodemographic characteristics, smoking and alcohol use, and blood pressure at inception.[39]

On the basis of this work, relaxation training, meditation, and blood pressure and heart rate biofeedback have been employed to treat hypertension. Relaxation techniques and meditation apparently decrease blood pressure by lowering total vasoconstrictor tone and peripheral resistance, but it is unclear to what degree the treatment effect persists after the discontinuation of active treatment. Several expert groups and consensus panels have concluded that the benefits of such psychological treatments for hypertension have not yet been conclusively demonstrated.[40] On the other hand, several meta-analyses suggest that they are beneficial.[41] For example, a recent, small, controlled trial of individualized stress management reported statistically significant and clinically meaningful reductions of systolic and diastolic blood pressure at 6-month follow-up.[42] Some of the confusion is because the empirical findings seem to vary depending on the study design, methods, and measurements. Although these behavioral techniques may not be effective when used alone, they may provide some incremental benefit when used to augment conventional antihypertensive therapy, perhaps enabling the physician to lower the doses of antihypertensives. This is important because nonadherence to the antihypertensive medication regimen is common and constitutes a major impediment to effective treatment. Relaxation training, meditation, and biofeedback may be most suitable for those patients who report a subjec-

tive sense of stress in their lives and for those who are attracted to the idea of psychological treatments for medical conditions.[42]

SOCIOCULTURAL FACTORS. Epidemiological and animal studies suggest a relationship between high blood pressure and sociocultural conditions. Individuals in more crowded and stressful living and working environments tend to show increased levels of catecholamines, increased cardiovascular reactivity, and higher blood pressures. Essential hypertension tends to be less prevalent in societies with stronger cultural traditions and more commonly shared value systems, as well as in those that are safer and more stable, than in societies with more disintegration, higher crime rates, and less stable social orders. In societies undergoing transition, conflict, or disintegration, blood pressures tend to rise over time, but many factors (e.g., changes in diet) may be contributing. Animal studies seem to corroborate these findings: Mice subjected to crowding or exposed to repeated threats from cats develop sustained high blood pressure.

Heart Failure (see Chaps. 23-25)

The psychiatric and behavioral aspects of congestive heart failure (CHF) have only recently been subjected to study. CHF patients report high levels of psychological distress and diminished quality of life.[43] It appears that the same sorts of psychosocial factors that affect the course and outcome of CHD also influence CHF. Stress and emotional distress have been linked to the onset and exacerbation of CHF, perhaps by increasing heart rate and blood pressure and/or by provoking myocardial ischemia in patients with preexisting CHD. It has been suggested that left ventricular function is impaired during psychological stress,[25] and stress-induced heart failure has been described. In patients with idiopathic cardiomyopathy, experimental psychological stress (mental arithmetic) has been shown to induce changes in left ventricular diastolic function.

Depression has received particular attention in CHF patients because of its high prevalence in the elderly and because it appears to worsen the medical outcome. Approximately one fourth of patients hospitalized for CHF have major depression.[44] Depression is an independent predictor of hospital admission and of increased medical care utilization in CHF.[45] It may also predict subsequent mortality.[46] Depression may also predispose to the development of CHF; in a prospective study of 2500 elderly community residents who were initially free of heart failure, depression at inception independently increased the risk of developing CHF in women, but not in men, over a 14-year follow-up period.[47] Research in this area is complicated by difficulty in differentiating the symptoms of CHF from those of depressive disorder. The anorexia, fatigue, weakness, and insomnia (resulting from orthopnea and paroxysmal nocturnal dyspnea) accompanying CHF can be confused with the symptoms of depression, and the cardiac cachexia of end-stage CHF may also suggest severe depression. When CHF is severe enough to cause cerebral ischemia, then cognitive dysfunction, confusion, and delirium with psychotic symptoms may result. This may at times be difficult to distinguish from anxiety disorder and panic.

Social support is an important moderator of the clinical course of CHF. Elderly women hospitalized with CHF who were without sources of emotional support had a more than threefold increase in the risk of cardiovascular events in the ensuing year than comparable patients with emotional support.[48] Elderly men without emotional support were not at increased risk. Social isolation was also found to be a significant predictor of mortality in CHF patients over a 2-year follow-up period, while controlling for depression, age, and disease severity.[1,48] A recent review of the literature on the influence of social supports on heart failure outcomes found that of 17 studies, 4 found clear relationships between social support and two outcomes, rehospitalization and mortality.[49] Both the number and quality of studies in this area are modest.

CARDIAC SYMPTOMS: CHEST PAIN AND PALPITATIONS

Chest Pain (see Chaps. 11 and 49)

Chest pain, the classic symptom of CHD, is a nonspecific, insensitive, and unreliable indicator of ischemia. Pain does not bear a fixed, one-to-one relationship to demonstrable pathology; many patients with chest pain have no heart disease, and conversely, ischemia and infarction are often asymptomatic. Approximately one fourth of MIs are silent, and 70 to 80 percent of out-of-hospital, ischemic episodes in CHD patients are asymptomatic. Conversely, no cardiac cause can be found to explain most complaints of chest pain. Even in patients with documented CHD, two thirds of chest pain episodes occur in the absence of ST segment depression indicative of ischemia, and approximately one third of revascularized patients continue to have chest pain. Even among patients undergoing coronary angiography for chest pain, 10 to 30 percent have minimal or no angiographic evidence of CHD.

The absence of demonstrable heart disease does not mean that the patient's chest pain is either inconsequential or self-limited. Follow-up studies of chest pain patients with negative angiography and/or negative exercise stress testing reveal persistent distress and disability and a generally poor response to conventional antiischemic therapy. Although rates of MI and of cardiac morbidity and mortality remain low, these patients continue to exhibit elevated levels of symptoms, disability, and medical care utilization. At least half continue to report recurrent chest pain, the persistent belief that they have serious heart disease, and impaired functioning (at work, socially, and in daily activities) at levels that are comparable to that of patients with CHD.

Psychological, psychiatric, and behavioral factors mediate some of this variance in symptoms among CHD patients. Thus emotional distress is highly correlated with reports of chest pain in both those with and without CHD. Mood and daily activities may account for as much of the variability in ambulatory patients' reports of chest pain as does ST depression indicative of ischemia. Several psychological factors differentiate chest pain patients with and without demonstrable cardiac disease. Generalized psychological distress and body awareness is higher in patients with chest pain and normal coronary arteries than in chest pain patients with CHD. When those with normal angiography or normal stress tests are compared with those with positive tests, the former group is younger, is more likely female, somatizes more, and has more psychological distress and a higher prevalence of diagnosable psychiatric disorder. Patients with medically unexplained chest pain, when compared with chest pain patients with abnormal angiographic findings, have elevated rates of panic disorder (≈35 to 50 percent versus 5 percent) and major depression (≈35 to 40 percent versus 5 to 8 percent). Of course, cardiac and psychiatric disorders are not mutually exclusive and therefore not infrequently co-occur. Thus 5 to 23 percent of patients with angiographic evidence of CHD also have panic disorder. These cases of psychiatric and cardiac comorbidity pose especially difficult diagnostic dilemmas, and it is in these patients that panic disorder is most likely to be overlooked. The chest pain seen in panic disorder is more likely to be atypical in clinical character and to be accompanied by palpitations, dizziness, paresthesias, and multiple other somatic symptoms.

Palpitations (see Chap. 32)

Palpitations are among the most common symptoms encountered in medical practice, reported by 16 percent of primary care patients. Yet this subjective sensation corresponds poorly to demonstrable abnormalities of cardiac rate or rhythm. Most palpitations are not accompanied by arrhythmias, and most arrhythmias are not perceived and reported as palpitations. When patients complaining of palpitations undergo 24-hour, ambulatory ECG monitoring, 39 to 85 percent manifest a rhythm disturbance (most being benign and clinically insignificant). Approximately three fourths of these patients with arrhythmias report at least one palpitation during 24 hours of monitoring, but in less than 15 percent of them are their symptoms coincident with the arrhythmia. Thus accurate symptom reports occur in less than 10 percent of all patients being monitored.

A high proportion of patients with palpitations either have a psychiatric cause for their symptom or no etiology can be established. In a careful survey of 190 patients presenting with palpitations, 31 percent were judged to have a psychiatric basis for their presenting symptom and no etiology could be established in an additional 16 percent. The most common psychiatric cause of palpitations is panic disorder, found in more than one fourth of ambulatory medical patients complaining of palpitations. In one study 31 percent of 229 such patients had panic disorder or panic attacks, and in another study 28 percent of patients complaining of palpitations had lifetime panic disorder and 19 percent had current panic disorder.

Palpitations that have no demonstrable cardiac basis may nonetheless be persistent and disturbing. In an observational 1-year follow-up study, 75 percent of palpitation patients reported recurrent symptoms, 19 percent reported impairment of their work performance, and 37 percent reported impairment in their role functioning at home. In another study, 84 percent of palpitation patients remained symptomatic 6 months after initially presenting and had an elevated rate of medical care utilization.

Panic attacks and arrhythmias may be difficult to distinguish clinically. Both may present as palpitations, shortness of breath, and light-headedness, and both not infrequently occur in those who are young and otherwise healthy. Frank syncope, however, is unusual in panic disorder, and if there have been multiple episodes, panic attacks are more stereotyped and more consistent from episode to episode. Recurrent panic attacks tend to lead to agoraphobia, in which the patient first becomes apprehensive about, and then avoids, being left alone, trapped in large crowds, and journeying far from home. Conversely, to make matters more difficult, the sympathetic arousal that may accompany an arrhythmia (and other acute cardiac events such as pulmonary emboli, acute valvular dysfunction, and myocardial ischemia) may be experienced and reported by the patient as acute anxiety or panic rather than as a cardiac event.

Delay and Denial of Cardiac Symptoms

MI patients commonly rationalize, ignore, or deny their symptoms, so the average interval between the onset of symptoms and arrival in an emergency department is between 3 and 9 hours. Such delay poses a serious problem because a high proportion of MI deaths occur soon after the event, and the newer therapies to preserve myocardial tissue require early intervention (see Chap. 51). Delay is greater in women and in the elderly and (paradoxically) in those with a history of previous MI.[50] A crucial determinant of the extent of delay is the length of time before the MI sufferer informs another person of his or her symptoms; once the patient tells someone else, medical attention is usually obtained promptly.

PSYCHIATRIC CARE OF THE CARDIAC PATIENT

Acute Care of the Hospitalized Patient

ANXIETY. The onset or sudden progression of cardiac disease is terrifying. Pain and physical discomfort, the specter of sudden death or prolonged invalidism, and the knowledge that one has a chronic and potentially lethal disease all are profoundly distressing. The initial reaction is almost always one of anxiety. Fears of premature and sudden death loom, and worries about physical, sexual, social, and occupational incapacity materialize and plague patients. They may become terrified of any physical activity or strong emotion, fearing that these will trigger sudden death. As time passes, anxiety may be replaced with despondency and a heightened sense of physical vulnerability and of one's mortality. The individual may come to feel useless, damaged, or diminished. Patients may believe that their job performance and future livelihood have been irrevocably compromised, that they have become worn out and decrepit, and that they face a meager and empty future. They may feel guilty and blame themselves for falling ill, ascribing their plight to their failure to exercise enough, diet sufficiently, or maintain other "healthy" habits. All of this may presage a clinically significant depressive episode.

Several psychiatric and behavioral problems commonly arise in patients while they are hospitalized for an acute cardiac event. The hospitalization itself (in particular, admission to the coronary care or intensive care unit) can be frightening and stressful. Patients suddenly find themselves in an unfamiliar, alien, and frightening world, surrounded by fearsome machines with blinking lights and beeping alarms, subjected to painful procedures and tests about which they know little and understand less, while their lives seemingly hang in the balance from moment to moment. They are cut off from family, friends, neighbors, and all that is familiar. Sustained sleep is next to impossible, and many are afraid to fall asleep, believing that the heart is in greater jeopardy during sleep. Their worst fears are substantiated if they witness the death or cardiac arrest of another patient.

Hospitalized patients should be kept well informed about what is transpiring, what is being done medically for them, and why. They should be told what to expect before procedures are carried out; the functions of equipment should be explained; and the effects and (especially) side effects of medications should be described in advance. The patient should be reassured that anxiety is a normal and entirely appropriate reaction. Early and frequent family visitation generally helps the patient to feel supported. Anxiolytics are often prescribed because anxiety is not only uncomfortable, but its concomitant sympathetic arousal can be medically dangerous. Benzodiazepines are most commonly used for this purpose and should be prescribed on a regular, round-the-clock (rather than as-needed) basis. In the elderly and in those with compromised liver function, the shorter-acting benzodiazepines (e.g., oxazepam or lorazepam) are preferred because they are cleared primarily by the kidney. The pharmacology of anxiolytics is discussed in the following section.

DELIRIUM AND COGNITIVE IMPAIRMENT. Delirium is frequent in hospitalized cardiac patients, especially following cardiac surgery. The delirious patient is confused, disoriented to time and place, has impaired memory and attention, has delusional ideas, and experiences perceptual disturbances such as illusions or hallucinations. The sleep-wake cycle is disrupted, and the level of consciousness and arousal is disturbed, so the patient may be either stuporous and obtunded or hyperalert and agitated. The onset of delirium may be insidious (e.g., insomnia, mild nocturnal confusion, restlessness) and go unnoticed by the staff, or it may be dramatic and abrupt. The patient begins to misinterpret sensory information (e.g., mistaking a shadow for someone lurking in a corner of his or her room) and becomes suspicious and increasingly frightened. As confusion, fear, and excitement mount, frank paranoia sets in and the patient may become agitated, disruptive, belligerent, and out of control. This is a psychiatric emergency because, in their confusion and frenzy, delirious patients may harm themselves accidentally; fall; or pull out therapeutic lifelines, catheters, and implanted devices. The incidence of delirium after cardiac surgery is between 10 and 30 percent, typically following a lucid interval of 3 to 5 days after surgery. The risk factors for postcardiotomy delirium are advanced age (older than 70 years of age); more extensive aortic atherosclerosis (large atheromas may be liberated by surgical manipulation of the aorta); a prior history of neurological disease, particularly preexisting cerebrovascular disease; a history of pulmonary disease, with the concomitant risks of poorer cerebral oxygenation and more hypoxia; and higher doses of narcotics and sedatives.[51]

Treatment of Delirium. This rests on rapid identification and correction of its underlying cause, medication for behavioral control if necessary, and supportive measures to provide comfort and safety. The etiological search is paramount. This means checking for cerebral hypoperfusion or hypoxia, acid-base disturbance, inadequate hydration, fluid and electrolyte imbalance, renal or hepatic failure, endocrine dysfunction, infection, and nutritional deficiency. Alcohol or drug withdrawal is a frequent cause, and the history must be searched carefully with this possibility in mind. Medications must be carefully reviewed because anticholinergics, narcotics, sedative-hypnotics, and H_2 blockers are common causes of delirium. Common offenders include cimetidine, digoxin, aminophylline, anticonvulsants, and all sedatives and hypnotics.

If the patient is agitated, disruptive, or confused enough to require behavioral control, high-potency antipsychotic drugs can be administered. Haloperidol has been widely used for this purpose and is safe and effective in critically ill patients, whether given orally or parenterally (including intravenously in emergency situations). Mild delirious agitation is treated with 0.5 to 2 mg of haloperidol, and moderate delirium with 5 to 10 mg. The severely delirious patient can be given 10 mg or more of haloperidol. If the agitation persists unabated after 20 to 30 minutes, twice the original dose may be readministered. It has a minimal effect on heart rate, blood pressure, and respiration, and extrapyramidal effects are rare when it is administered intravenously. Parenteral droperidol is sometimes used. If excitement, hyperarousal, and motor agitation are especially prominent, the antipsychotic may be supplemented with a short-acting benzodiazepine such as lorazepam. The newer, "atypical" antipsychotics are increasingly used to treat delirium.[52] They appear to be safe and effective but have not yet been studied definitively. Antipsychotic agents are discussed in the following section.

Supportive measures should be undertaken to calm, orient, and comfort the delirious patient. He or she should be reoriented frequently by the staff, and a clock and calendar should be prominently displayed to aid in this process. It is helpful to preserve as much of a normal day-night cycle as is feasible considering the hospital routine. Family visitation should be encouraged because it is helpful in reassuring and calming the patient and in reducing paranoia. Familiar objects such as family photographs should be prominently displayed and plainly visible. Staff need to continually reintroduce themselves, educate the patient about what they are doing, and repeatedly explain the situation. Physical restraint should be employed whenever necessary to prevent self-harm or harm to the staff.

Longer-term cognitive changes also occur following cardiac surgery. These often involve memory, arithmetic skills, and the sequencing of complex actions. Severity of impairments usually fall short of dementia or "mild cognitive impairment," but they do reduce quality of life and raise costs of care. Proposed mechanisms include surgical-related trauma, microemboli, and mild ischemic changes. Clinicians should monitor cognitive function before and after cardiac surgery.[53] Neurocognitive testing of patients following CABG disclosed cognitive decline in 53 percent at discharge, 36 percent at 6 weeks, and in 24 percent of patients 6 months after discharge.[54] This study lacked a noncardiac surgery comparison group, however.

Convalescence and Recovery after Hospitalization

In the weeks and months after hospital discharge, depression is common. Depression is often self-limited, gradually diminishing as the patient resumes his or her old activities and as the specter of the acute episode and the hospitalization recede into the past. Frank discussion of the patient's concerns and specific information about common myths and fears are helpful. Lingering anxiety may lead patients to avoid activities or situations that they fear will provoke symptoms or even sudden death. Early, progressive mobilization is the best antidote. The patient may be dismayed by the degree of exhaustion resulting from even mild exertion, and although this easy fatigability is actually the result of deconditioning, it is mistakenly interpreted as evidence of permanent cardiac damage. As a result, exercise may be assiduously avoided, further exacerbating the problem.

Patients are often apprehensive about returning to work because of the stress it engenders. Many believe that strong emotions can be lethal and try to protect themselves by assiduously avoiding all situations or activities that arouse strong feelings such as sexual activity or watching sports on television. Sexual activity in particular is diminished, and sexual dysfunction is common in both women and men with cardiac disease. Such concerns should be elicited by the physician and then discussed frankly and openly. Recommendations about proscribed and prescribed activities should be as specific as possible; simply saying "use your judgment" or "do it in moderation" is not helpful. Group meetings in which cardiac patients share common concerns, provide mutual support, obtain educational information, and guide the progressive resumption of activities are helpful.

TREATMENT. If depression lasts more than several weeks and meets diagnostic criteria for major depressive disorder, as happens in one third or more of patients in the year after MI, pharmacotherapy is indicated. If left untreated, depression imposes a serious psychosocial burden, medical rehabilitation and recovery are impeded, and the depression itself is likely to become chronic. Because of this and its negative effect on cardiac outcomes, increasing emphasis is being placed on the prompt detection and treatment of post-MI depression. The Sertraline Antidepressant Heart Attack Randomized Trial (SADHART) was a double-blind, randomized, placebo-controlled trial of a selective serotonin reuptake inhibitor (SSRI) for major depressive disorder in patients hospitalized for MI or unstable angina. At 6-month follow-up, when compared with placebo, the more severely depressed patients who received active drug were less depressed, although the less severely depressed patients did not show a treatment effect. The trial showed that sertraline was safe and effective for the treatment of recurrent major depression in patients with recent MI or unstable angina. A 20 percent reduction in life-threatening cardiac events (including nonfatal MI and death) among those on active drug occurred, but this difference in cardiac outcomes was not statistically significant because of the number of patients in the trial.[55]

Depression is the strongest predictor of quality of life in post-MI patients, and in this study treatment with sertraline was associated with clinically meaningful improvements in quality of life over 6 months for those with recurrent depression.[56] In a case-controlled study of smokers hospitalized for MI, SSRI administration was associated with a lowered risk of recurrent MI, suggesting that treatment of depression may reduce its negative prognostic influence on cardiac outcomes.[57] Thus it remains to be definitively demonstrated that the treatment of depression following MI significantly improves cardiac outcomes. The pharmacotherapy of depression is discussed in the following section.

Interest in psychosocial interventions for depression and/or social isolation has also been high. In one study of 435 post-MI patients, a nursing-based psychosocial intervention reduced 1-year cardiac mortality, and the incidence of recurrent MI was significantly lower at 7-year follow-up. However, two subsequent, large, randomized trials of multimodal interventions delivered by nurses or health visitors failed to improve depression or cardiac outcomes.[58] In the Montreal Heart Attack Readjustment Trial (M-HART), a supportive and educational home nursing intervention was provided to the most psychologically distressed post-MI patients. This rather limited intervention was compared with usual care. At 1-year follow-up, the intervention had no effect on psychological distress and no overall effect on cardiac mortality, although it was actually associated with a *higher* mortality rate among women.[59] However, a subgroup analysis revealed that those patients whose psychological distress improved with treatment had more favorable long-term cardiac outcomes.[60] In the Enhancing Recovery in Coronary Heart Disease (ENRICHD) study, 2500 recent MI patients with depression and/or low social support randomly received either cognitive behavior therapy (and SSRI antidepressants if indicated) or care as usual. Preliminary results suggest that there was no benefit in terms of cardiac outcomes or mortality, and outcomes appear worse for women. At the least, one can safely conclude from these studies that when the psychosocial treatment fails to improve depression (because the patient population is not sufficiently depressed or the treatment is not effective enough), then it does not improve cardiac outcomes. In addition, the study suggests that women may benefit less from these psychosocial interventions in terms of cardiac outcomes than men.

Over the long term, some cardiac patients adopt a persistent coping style that is maladaptive and dysfunctional. They may ignore and deny their illness entirely, maintaining that nothing serious has happened at all. They may refuse to acknowledge any limitations or adhere to a therapeutic regimen and generally overdo things. Alternatively, they may capitulate completely to their illness and retreat into unwarranted invalidism, becoming "cardiac cripples" who are preoccupied with their health, terrified by every benign twinge or cramp, and living a life of psychological invalidism and disability. Each of these profoundly maladaptive coping patterns deserves psychotherapeutic attention.

Cardiac Rehabilitation Programs

(see Chap. 46)

Cardiac rehabilitation programs seek to modify biobehavioral risk factors and retard the progression of the disease. These psychosocial, educational, and behavioral programs include various components. Almost all emphasize a formal program of graduated, progressive, aerobic exercise. Most assist patients in smoking cessation, curtailing alcohol abuse, lowering saturated fat intake, and controlling weight.

Most cardiac rehabilitation programs also include psychosocial interventions.[61] These involve the identification of psychosocial stressors and problems (depression, anxiety, anger, social isolation); individual or group counseling to deal with them; and instruction in stress reduction and stress management. The latter often entails relaxation training, which generally combines elements of progressive muscle relaxation, diaphragmatic breathing, and the use of calming mental imagery.

Evaluating the effectiveness of these heterogeneous psychotherapeutic, psychosocial, and behavioral programs is difficult because they vary so widely in quality, content, design, and intensity. Many intervention trials are flawed by small sample size, high dropout rates, lack of randomization, insufficient long-term follow-up, and inadequate comparison or control groups. In addition, as standard cardiac care improves so substantially, it becomes more difficult to demonstrate the incremental benefit of these programs in terms of hard cardiac endpoints. Nonetheless, there are now a substantial number of intervention trials and several careful meta-analyses assessing the incremental benefit of adding a specific psychosocial component to cardiac rehabilitation programs. These studies generally indicate that, when compared with rehabilitation programs without such components, these programs further reduce psychological distress and anxiety and depressive symptoms and improve coping skills and quality of life.[61] The empirical evidence also suggests that they lead to significantly lower rates of cardiac death and nonfatal, recurrent MI.[62,63] When these psychological interventions have been found ineffective against cardiac endpoints, they have at the same time failed to lower psychosocial distress, depression, and anxiety.[63] The cardiac benefits of psychosocial treatment generally seem less clear for women and perhaps for older patients as well.

PSYCHOPHARMACOLOGY IN THE CARDIAC PATIENT

Cardiovascular Aspects of Psychotropic Agents

Antidepressants (Table 86-1)

SELECTIVE SEROTONIN REUPTAKE INHIBITORS

The SSRIs have superseded the tricyclic antidepressants (TCAs) as the first-line agents for treating the cardiac patient with major depressive disorder. Their efficacy is comparable to that of the older TCAs; they are better tolerated, safer in overdose, and have less pharmacological action on the heart. The data thus far suggest that the SSRIs have minimal cardiovascular effects and a large margin of safety in treating patients with even severe heart disease.[64] The SSRIs have little anticholinergic, antihistaminic, or noradrenergic activity and appear to inhibit platelet aggregation.

In healthy patients the SSRIs have no adverse effects on cardiac contractility or conduction, and there is no evidence of cardiotoxicity in overdose. In cardiac populations they do not appear to cause significant ECG or blood pressure changes, although they can slow heart rate. Only rarely do they produce a clinically significant degree of sinus bradycardia. Because the SSRIs interfere with platelet aggregation, they can increase bleeding time. The SSRIs do have the potential to interact with a number of medications used in cardiac patients. They inhibit hepatic cytochrome P450 isoenzymes,[64] a series of isoenzymes involved in the oxidative metabolism of many drugs. These include lipophilic beta blockers (e.g., metoprolol, propranolol); calcium channel blockers; type IC antiarrhythmics; angiotensin-converting enzyme (ACE) inhibitors; anticonvulsants; antihistamines; benzodiazepines; TCAs; codeine; and warfarin. The SSRIs therefore can raise the blood levels of these other agents when coadministered. Caution should be exercised when giving SSRIs to patients on these medications, and in particular the prothrombin time of patients receiving both warfarin and an SSRI should be monitored closely. Because the SSRIs are highly protein bound, they may displace other protein-bound drugs when coadministered, thereby increasing their bioavailability. This interaction can occur with warfarin and digitoxin, but it does not appear to be clinically significant in magnitude.

Because both depression and MI enhance platelet activation, the period of post-MI depression poses excessive risks for thrombotic events. In a recent controlled analysis of 281 patients with acute coronary syndrome (ACS) with or without depression, patients with combined ACS and depression showed the highest levels of platelet factor 4, beta-thromboglobulin, and platelet/endothelial cell adhesion molecule-1 compared with ACS patients without depression or healthy controls.[65] The use of SSRIs to treat depression in patients with CHD or CHF confers additional antiplatelet effects beyond the effect of aspirin.[66] Consequently, SSRI use may modify the dose or the need for aspirin or other antiplatelet medications.

TRICYCLIC ANTIDEPRESSANTS

TCAs were previously the mainstay of antidepressant pharmacotherapy and remain effective agents that are still widely employed. However, their multiple cardiovascular side effects and their potential lethality in overdose are disadvantages in patients with cardiac disease. TCAs act on adrenergic and serotoninergic neurons in the central nervous system and, in the periphery, have anticholinergic properties. They also have quinidine-like effects and produce alpha-adrenergic receptor blockade. They affect heart rate, rhythm, conduction, contractility, and blood pressure. Accordingly, these agents are not generally used in the presence of rhythm or conduction disturbances, severe CHF, or within 4 to 6 weeks of an MI. Among the TCAs, the tertiary amines (e.g., imipramine and amitriptyline) are associated with more side effects, and the secondary amines (e.g., nortriptyline) have a preferable side effect profile in cardiac patients.

The TCAs are type IA antiarrhythmic agents (see Chap. 33) and accordingly depress cardiac conduction, decrease ventricular irritability, and suppress ectopic activity. They slow atrial and ventricular depolarization; increase the QT, PR, and QRS intervals; and decrease T wave amplitude. In the absence of preexisting conduction abnormalities, this action is unlikely to be clinically significant at therapeutic doses. However, second-degree heart block, sick sinus syndrome, bundle branch block, a prolonged QT interval, and the concurrent administration of antiarrhythmic agents all are considered contraindications to their use. In contrast to this antiarrhythmic effect, the TCAs can on occasion

TABLE 86–1	Antidepressants				
Agent	Starting Doses	Maximum Doses	Side Effects		Cardiovascular Effects
Serotonin Reuptake Inhibitors					
Sertraline	25 mg/d	200 mg/d	Sexual dysfunction, nausea, diarrhea, headache		Benign bradycardia
Fluoxetine	10 mg/d	80 mg/d	Sexual dysfunction, anxiety, agitation, insomnia, somnolence		
Citalopram	20 mg/d	60 mg/d	Sexual dysfunction, nausea		
Escitalopram	10 mg/d	30 mg/d	Sexual dysfunction, nausea, diarrhea		
Paroxetine	10 mg/d	60 mg/d	Sexual dysfunction, headache		
Tricyclics					
Amitriptyline	25 mg h.s.	300 mg/d	Sedation, somnolence Dry mouth Blurry vision, postural hypotension		Increased QT, PR, QRS intervals
Imipramine	25 mg h.s.	300 mg/d	Constipation Urinary retention		Decreased T wave amplitude Tachycardia
Nortriptyline	10 mg/d	150 mg/d	Anxiety, insomnia Weight gain		Arrhythmias Postural hypotension
Desipramine	25 mg/d	300 mg/d			
Psychostimulants					
Methylphenidate	5 mg/d	60 mg/d	Anxiety, agitation Insomnia Anorexia		Tachycardia (mild) Hypertension (mild)
Other Agents					
Bupropion	75 mg/d	450 mg/d	Anorexia, nausea Anxiety, agitation Insomnia Seizures		
Venlafaxine	75 mg/d	300 mg/d	Nausea Headache Sexual dysfunction Anxiety, insomnia Somnolence Dizziness		Hypertension (dose related) Tachycardia (dose related)
Duloxetine	20 mg/d	60 mg/d	Nausea Sexual dysfunction Anxiety, insomnia Somnolence		Headache
Mirtazapine	15 mg q.h.s.	45 mg q.h.s.	Sedation, somnolence Weight gain Dry mouth, anticholinergic effects Dizziness Agranulocytosis (rare)		Tachycardia (mild)

be arrhythmogenic, probably by virtue of their prolongation of the QT interval and/or an increase in myocardial norepinephrine resulting from their peripheral inhibition of norepinephrine reuptake. Although the most common such arrhythmias are atrial and ventricular premature beats, these may give way to more malignant ventricular arrhythmias. These toxic, proarrhythmic effects are seen primarily in overdose and are more likely in those with preexisting CHD, a prolonged QT interval, electrical instability, or a recent MI. The TCAs also elevate heart rate 5 to 20 beats/min as a result of their anticholinergic blockade. Although this does not pose a problem in relatively healthy patients, it may be a consideration in those with heart disease.

TCAs produce postural hypotension in up to 20 percent of patients. In the elderly, in whom orthostatic hypotension can produce cerebral hypoperfusion and lead to falls and fractures, this side effect can be crucial. Blood pressure and pulse should be monitored for signs of orthostasis in patients treated with TCAs, especially when initiating treatment and when adjusting the dose. Elderly patients should be advised to stand up slowly after lying or sitting for prolonged periods. The magnitude of this effect is related to the magnitude of pretreatment orthostatic hypotension, and it is more likely to be clinically significant in patients with CHF, impaired left ventricular function, or volume depletion or who are taking antihypertensive medications. Caution is indicated when treating patients with poor ejection fractions because in animal studies TCAs exert a depressant effect on myocardial contractility, although in humans this effect is evident only at toxic doses and only rarely aggravates CHF.

OTHER ANTIDEPRESSANTS

Bupropion, a non-TCA that acts on both the dopamine and norepinephrine systems, causes less hypotension than the TCAs; does not affect cardiac conduction or contractility; and is safely used in patients with cardiac disease. It does not exacerbate ventricular arrhythmias or conduction block in patients with these conditions. An additional benefit of bupropion in cardiac patients is that it is apparently effective in smoking cessation. An increased incidence of seizures is seen at higher doses, and bupropion may occasionally elevate blood pressure and heart rate, though rarely to a clinically significant degree. Because it inhibits the cytochrome P450 isoenzymes, bupropion can raise the levels of beta blockers and type 1C antiarrhythmics when administered concurrently.

Venlafaxine affects the reuptake of both serotonin and norepinephrine. It appears to have few cardiovascular actions and no effect on the ECG. At higher doses venlafaxine has been associated with an elevation in blood pressure and pulse. Unlike the SSRIs, it does not inhibit cytochrome P450 isoenzymes and is not highly protein bound; it may therefore be useful in patients on cardiac medications.

Duloxetine, the newest serotonin and norepinephrine reuptake inhibitor (SNRI), has not been studied in patients with cardiovascular disease. For now we can only assume that we should manage it as we manage venlafaxine, with one important difference. Unlike venlafaxine, duloxetine does not raise blood pressure at high doses.

Trazodone, a triazolopyridine antidepressant, is often used in low doses as a hypnotic. Cardiovascular complications from trazodone are rare. It has few, if any, antiarrhythmic properties, although it has rarely been associated with heart block and ventricular arrhythmias. Because of its weak alpha-adrenergic blockade, it may also produce orthostatic hypotension. *Nefazodone,* a closely related drug, can also occasionally produce orthostatic hypotension and has significant P450 isoenzyme inhibition. Therefore nefazodone can increase the levels of concurrently administered calcium channel blockers, quinidine, and lidocaine.

Mirtazapine is a tetracyclic antidepressant with a complex mechanism of action. It has not been studied in patients with cardiovascular disease, but in noncardiac

populations it does not affect blood pressure or cardiac conduction. It has no anticholinergic activity, but it may increase heart rate slightly.

Psychostimulants such as dextroamphetamine and methylphenidate are used to treat depression in medically compromised and elderly patients. These agents tend to be used when depression is life threatening, when immediate treatment response is crucial (because they have a rapid onset of action), and in depressions with prominent anergia and apathy. Although there is considerable clinical support for their use, empirical evidence of their sustained efficacy over time is lacking. Serious cardiovascular side effects such as tachycardia, hypertension, and arrhythmias are relatively rare, but caution must be exercised when administering these medications to patients with significant hypertension, tachycardia, or ventricular ectopy, and blood pressure and heart rate should be monitored.

NEUROLEPTICS (Table 86-2). Neuroleptic or antipsychotic drugs are used in the treatment of schizophrenia, organic psychoses, and mood disorders that are refractory or have psychotic features. They are also widely used for agitation, confusion, excitement, and behavioral dyscontrol in geriatric patients. Neuroleptic drugs generally affect cardiac conduction and rhythm and produce hypotension. They have alpha-adrenergic blocking and quinidine-like properties, along with anticholinergic activity. They can produce prolongation of the PR and QT intervals, ST segment depression, T wave changes, ventricular arrhythmias, and heart block. Increasing attention has been devoted to their potential to increase the QT interval, leading in rare instances to torsades de pointes. *Thioridazine* is most frequently implicated in this respect.[67] Although the quinidine-like effects of the neuroleptics are usually negligible, they can become significant in patients already taking type I antiarrhythmics or in those with hypokalemia or clinically significant conduction delays. When administering a low-potency neuroleptic along with an antiarrhythmic, the

TABLE 86–2 | **Neuroleptic (Antipsychotic) Agents**

Agent	Starting Doses	Maximum Doses	Side Effects	Cardiovascular Effects
Haloperidol	0.5 mg/d	40 mg/d	Akathisia Dystonia Parkinsonism Tardive dyskinesia Neuroleptic malignant syndrome Rash Anticholinergic effects	Tachycardia QT interval prolongation Torsades de pointes
Clozapine	12.5 mg q.h.s. or b.i.d.	300 mg t.i.d.	Dizziness Somnolence Weight gain Hypersalivation Seizures Agranulocytosis Anticholinergic effects	Tachycardia Postural hypotension
Olanzapine	2.5-5 mg/d	20 mg/d	Sedation Constipation Weight gain Seizures Akathisia Extrapyramidal symptoms	Postural hypotension (mild) QT interval prolongation
Risperidone	0.25-0.5 mg/d	6 mg/d	Somnolence Fatigue Nausea, diarrhea Weight gain Sexual dysfunction Nasal congestion Extrapyramidal symptoms	Hypotension QT interval prolongation Tachycardia

ECG should be monitored for conduction delays. The lower-potency neuroleptics produce more orthostatic hypotension (by means of alpha-adrenergic blockade) and tachycardia (by means of anticholinergic action), and this is of particular concern in the elderly and in the acute MI patient. Orthostasis is more likely to be a problem when these agents are combined with antihypertensives.

The higher-potency neuroleptic agents, such as *haloperidol* and the piperazine phenothiazines, produce fewer of these effects and are therefore preferred in the presence of significant cardiac disease (especially conduction problems) and after cardiac surgery. Haloperidol in particular has been frequently used with safety and efficacy in severely ill cardiac patients. Oral haloperidol does not significantly affect the ECG, and intravenous haloperidol is used in acute emergencies such as agitated deliria. Administration can on rare occasions result in torsades de pointes and even SCD, and the QT interval should therefore be monitored during aggressive intravenous haloperidol therapy.

Experience with the newer "atypical" antipsychotics in cardiac patients is much more limited but suggests a generally similar profile. *Clozapine* can cause tachycardia and orthostatic hypotension and has significant anticholinergic activity (along with a risk of myelosuppression and agranulocytosis). An infrequent association of clozapine with myocarditis and cardiomyopathy has been reported. This risk is greatest in the first month of therapy. *Olanzapine* produces mild orthostatic hypotension but has little effect on the ECG. *Risperidone* produces hypotension and has a quinidine-like effect, prolonging the QT interval, although this may not be of clinical significance. *Ziprasidone* has been associated with QT prolongation and is not recommended in patients with recent MI, heart failure, QT prolongation, or arrhythmias. Thus it is clear that the new atypical neuroleptics, like the phenothiazines and haloperidol, can prolong QT interval. However, the relationship to torsades de pointes and SCD is less clear because the tendency to prolong the QT interval is not closely associated with the tendency to cause torsades de pointes. Recently, concern with atypical antipsychotics has focused on the incidence of new-onset diabetes and increased glucose levels in patients with pre-existing diabetes, on hyperlipidemia, and on the weight gain seen in patients on these agents.[67]

Mood Stabilizers (Table 86-3)

LITHIUM

Lithium exerts minimal cardiotoxicity at therapeutic doses in most patients and can be used safely in cardiac disease if initiated at a low dose, increased gradually, and monitored carefully. Clinically significant, cardiovascular side effects of lithium are rare; they may include sinus node dysfunction and increases in ventricular irritability. Benign, reversible T wave changes (including inversion and flattening) are common with lithium administration and are not clinically significant. The major toxic effects of lithium are neural (confusion, sedation), and the primary concern in cardiac patients is lithium toxicity resulting from decreased renal clearance or hypovolemia. This is of concern in patients with CHF, and it is exacerbated by their diuretics and restricted sodium intake. Sodium depletion decreases renal clearance of lithium. In the kidney, lithium is filtered out at the glomerulus and then reabsorbed in the proximal tubules. Sodium depletion, such as with diuretics, causes an increased proximal reabsorption of sodium, and lithium is reabsorbed more efficiently at the same time. A given lithium dose thus results in a higher blood level. Lithium may still be administered to the patient on diuretics, but levels must be monitored and dosage may need to be reduced. The elderly also require lower lithium doses because of a decline in the glomerular filtration rate. On rare occasion, lithium may worsen arrhythmias in patients with sinus node dysfunction.

ANTICONVULSANTS

These drugs are increasingly prescribed to stabilize the mood of patients with bipolar disorder (manic-depressive illness). Their use in cardiac patients has not yet been systematically studied. *Carbamazepine* has quinidine-like effects and can aggravate heart block, and it may also exacerbate CHF. Carbamazepine can also produce hyponatremia, and this effect is potentiated by other causes of hyponatremia such as diuretics and CHF.

Valproate, although not yet studied widely in cardiac populations, does not appear to have adverse cardiac effects. It can, however, lower the platelet count, decrease fibrinogen levels, and increase the prothrombin time. *Lamotrigine*

TABLE 86-3	Mood Stabilizers			
Agent	**Starting Doses**	**Maximum Doses**	**Side Effects**	**Cardiovascular Effects**
Lithium	300 mg b.i.d.	2100 mg/d (titrate against serum concentration)	Drowsiness, sedation Confusion Nausea, diarrhea Metallic taste Polyuria/polydipsia Tremor Hypothyroidism	T wave inversion or flattening Sinus node dysfunction Ventricular irritability
Carbamazepine	100 mg b.i.d.	1600 mg/d	Dizziness Drowsiness, sedation Ataxia Diplopia, blurred vision Rash Nausea Leukopenia Hyponatremia	Depressed cardiac conduction
Valproate	250 mg b.i.d.	3500 mg/d	Nausea, vomiting, anorexia Sedation Confusion Weight gain Tremor	

TABLE 86–4	Benzodiazepines	
Agent	Starting Doses	Maximum Doses
Short-Acting Benzodiazepines		
Lorazepam	0.5 mg b.i.d.	6 mg/d
Alprazolam	0.5 mg b.i.d.	8 mg/d
Long-Acting Benzodiazepines		
Diazepam	2-5 mg q.d.	40 mg/d
Chlordiazepoxide	5 mg q.d.	100 mg/d
Clonazepam	0.25 mg/d	6 mg/d

is increasingly used in refractory depression and appears to have no significant cardiac effects nor impact on the cytochrome P450 system. *Topiramate* may have a role in the treatment of mania and anxiety. It is renally excreted, and care must be taken to ensure adequate hydration.

BENZODIAZEPINES (Table 86-4)

Benzodiazepines have anxiolytic, sedative, anticonvulsant, and muscle relaxant properties. Anxiety disorders, especially panic disorder and generalized anxiety disorder, are prevalent in patients with cardiac disease. Panic disorder is treated either with a benzodiazepine with antipanic efficacy (such as clonazepam, lorazepam, or alprazolam) or an antidepressant. Generalized anxiety disorder can also be treated with benzodiazepines, buspirone, or SSRIs. Hospitalized cardiac patients are acutely anxious, and benzodiazepines are widely used in coronary care units. They can decrease respiratory drive in patients with chronic obstructive pulmonary disease and chronic hypercapnia but are free of cardiac side effects and are safe in seriously ill cardiac patients, even in the period immediately after MI.

Benzodiazepines with longer half-lives and/or active metabolites (e.g., diazepam, flurazepam, clonazepam, chlordiazepoxide) accumulate in the body with repeated administration. A steady state is reached slowly, and clearance of the drug after discontinuation is prolonged. Thus the benzodiazepines with shorter half-lives and fewer active metabolites (lorazepam, oxazepam) are generally preferable, particularly in the elderly. Intramuscular absorption of these agents, other than lorazepam and midazolam, is erratic and unpredictable. The most prominent side effects are sedation, fatigue, memory complaints, and psychomotor impairment. In hospitalized patients and in the elderly, these effects can result in frank oversedation or delirium. Patients with preexisting cognitive impairment or organic brain syndromes often react to benzodiazepines with further confusion, increased memory loss, behavioral disinhibition, and belligerence. Ambulatory patients should be cautioned about driving and participating in activities requiring a high degree of alertness.

Psychiatric Side Effects of Cardiovascular Drugs

ANTIHYPERTENSIVES. Many antihypertensive agents have central nervous system side effects. Depression is not uncommon with methyldopa, clonidine, reserpine, and guanethidine. Therefore calcium-channel blockers and ACE inhibitors may be preferable in the hypertensive patient with a history of depression. Abrupt discontinuation of antihypertensive agents can cause anxiety, agitation, and vivid dreams. *Methyldopa* is a relatively common cause of insomnia.

BETA-ADRENERGIC RECEPTOR ANTAGONISTS. A longstanding clinical impression is that beta blockers can cause depression. Although there are reports that patients maintained on these agents have an elevated rate of concurrent antidepressant pharmacotherapy, other studies have failed to find an association between beta blocker use and depression. Some of the confusion may stem from the fact that these agents cause sedation, lethargy, fatigue, and impotence, side effects that may be confused with depression. Depression may be more likely in those with a past history of depressive disorder, with use of the more lipophilic agents (e.g., propranolol, metoprolol), and when using higher doses. Beta blockers also occasionally cause vivid dreams and nightmares; hallucinations; and other psychotic symptoms, particularly in the elderly.

CALCIUM CHANNEL BLOCKERS. In general, calcium channel blockers do not have prominent psychiatric side effects. Isolated cases of depression associated with their administration have been reported, but this effect has not been demonstrated conclusively. Care should be taken when these agents are coadministered with the psychotropic drugs that inhibit the cytochrome P450 system, such as nefazodone and high doses of fluoxetine and paroxetine.

ANGIOTENSIN-CONVERTING ENZYME INHIBITORS. These inhibitors appear to have relatively few central nervous system side effects, although they may, on rare occasion, induce depression.

ANTIARRHYTHMICS. *Lidocaine* is a relatively common cause of anxiety, confusion, disorientation, hallucinations, and central nervous system excitement. Confusion, hallucinations, and delirium have also been reported with high doses of quinidine. Procainamide may cause depression, hallucinations, and other psychotic symptoms.

DIGITALIS. Anxiety, depression, visual illusions (e.g., yellow halos), and confusion may be the first signs of digitalis toxicity, but psychiatric symptoms may emerge at therapeutic levels as well.

DIURETICS. Diuretics can induce cognitive mental status changes by causing electrolyte imbalance (e.g., hyponatremia) or hypovolemia, and a secondary mood disorder may also occur, often characterized by anorexia, lethargy, and weakness.

Interactions of Psychotropic and Cardiac Drugs (Table 86-5)

Because many cardiac and psychotropic agents lower blood pressure, additive hypotensive effects are not uncommon (e.g., between TCAs and antihypertensives). Many psychotropic agents slow conduction and prolong the PR, QRS, and QT intervals, and synergistic effects can occur when they are used in conjunction with antiarrhythmic medications, resulting in heart block or the long-QT syndrome. Extreme caution is required if atypical neuroleptics are administered concomitantly with other drugs that increase the QT interval such as *ketoconazole, quinidine,* and *cisapride.* Several interactions occur between the TCAs and cardiac medications: The TCAs interfere with neuronal reuptake of clonidine and guanethidine and thus antagonize their antihypertensive action. They may potentiate the antihypertensive action of prazosin, and the dry mouth induced by TCAs may hinder the absorption of sublingual nitrates.

SSRIs are bound to plasma proteins and can displace other protein-bound drugs, thereby increasing the level of active drug and resulting in possible toxicity. This is particularly salient with *warfarin* and *digitoxin,* although the clinical significance of these interactions is not yet clear. As noted earlier, diuretics may raise *lithium* levels into the toxic range. This can generally be dealt with by reducing the lithium dose, although during acute diuresis the proper adjustment of lithium is difficult because of the massive shifts in sodium and fluid balance.

TABLE 86–5 | **Interactions of Psychotropic and Cardiac Drugs**

Medication	Effect on Cardiac Agent
Interactions Involving Tricyclic Antidepressants	
Type IA antiarrhythmics	Potentiate delay in cardiac conduction; heart block
Antihypertensives: guanethidine, clonidine, reserpine	Antagonize antihypertensive effect; potentiate orthostatic hypotension
Sublingual nitrates	Oral absorption hindered by dry mouth
Alpha-adrenergic blocking agents	Potentiate antihypertensive effect
Interactions Involving Serotonergic Antidepressants	
Lipophilic beta blockers	Increase blood levels because of decreased hepatic degradation
Calcium channel blockers	Increase blood levels because of decreased hepatic degradation
Type IC antiarrhythmics	Increase blood levels because of decreased hepatic degradation
Angiotensin-converting enzyme inhibitors	Increase blood levels because of decreased hepatic degradation
Warfarin	Increase blood levels because of decreased hepatic degradation
Digitoxin	Increase bioavailability because of displacement from protein-binding sites

Medication	Effect on Psychotropic Agent
Interactions Involving Lithium	
Diuretics that cause sodium loss	Increase blood lithium levels
Calcium channel blockers	Enhance lithium toxicity; bradycardia
Angiotensin-converting enzyme inhibitors	Enhance lithium toxicity
Methyldopa	Enhance lithium toxicity

Medication	Effect on Psychotropic or Cardiac Agent
Interactions Involving Carbamazepine	
Calcium channel blockers	Enhance carbamazepine toxicity
Antiarrhythmics	Potentiate delay in cardiac conduction

Idiosyncratic toxic reactions have been reported, along with bradycardia when lithium is coadministered with the calcium channel blockers *verapamil* and *diltiazem* and lithium toxicity precipitated by the use of ACE inhibitors. *Methyldopa* seems to have a number of interactions with psychotropic agents including possible toxicity when combined with lithium. The metabolic degradation of *carbamazepine* may be inhibited by calcium-channel blockers, thereby increasing the risk of carbamazepine toxicity. Carbamazepine and antiarrhythmics may have additive effects in slowing cardiac conduction.

FUTURE PERSPECTIVES

The critical advances in research and clinical care in the next 10 years will depend on (1) a coherent research strategy to elucidate the mechanisms linking depression and anxiety to cardiovascular disease outcomes and (2) clinical trials of treatments for psychiatric disorders that assess both psychiatric and cardiovascular outcomes. Better definition of high-risk groups, based on psychiatric epidemiology and mechanisms, will lead to more effective treatments that reduce the excessive cardiovascular morbidity and mortality that result from unrecognized and undertreated psychiatric disorders.

REFERENCES

Psychiatric and Behavioral Aspects of Coronary Heart Disease

1. Trigo M, Silva D, Rocha E: Psychosocial risk factors in coronary heart disease: Beyond type A behavior. Revista Portuguesa de Cardiologia 24:261, 2005.
2. Denollet J, Pedersen SS, Vrints CJ, Conraads VM: Usefulness of type D personality in predicting five-year cardiac events above and beyond concurrent symptoms of stress in patients with coronary heart disease. Am J Cardiol 97:970, 2006.
3. Rudisch B, Nemeroff C: Epidemiology of comorbid coronary artery disease and depression. Biol Psychiatry 54:227, 2003.
4. Wulsin LR: Is depression a major risk factor for coronary disease? A systematic review of the epidemiologic evidence. Harv Rev Psychiatry 12:79, 2004.
5. Ruo B, Rumsfeld J, Hlatky M, et al: Depressive symptoms and health-related quality of life: The Heart and Soul Study. JAMA 290:215, 2003.
6. Carney RM, Jaffe AS: Treatment of depression following acute myocardial infarction. JAMA 288:750, 2002.
7. Wulsin L, Singal B: Do depressive symptoms increase the risk for the onset of coronary disease? A systematic quantitative review. Psychosom Med 65:201, 2003.
8. Carney RM, Freedland KE: Depression, mortality, and medical morbidity in patients with coronary heart disease. Biol Psychiatry 54:241, 2003.
9. Lespérance F, Frasure-Smith N, Talajic M, et al: Five-year risk of cardiac mortality in relation to initial severity and one-year changes in depression symptoms after myocardial infarction. Circulation 105:1049, 2002.
10. Burg MM, Benedetto MC, Rosenberg R, et al: Presurgical depression predicts medical morbidity 6 months after coronary artery bypass graft surgery. Psychosom Med 65:111, 2003.
11. Carney R, Freedland K, Miller G, Jaffe A: Depression as a risk factor for cardiac mortality and morbidity: A review of potential mechanisms. J Psychosom Res 53:897, 2002.
12. Rugulies R: Depression as a predictor for coronary heart disease: A review and meta-analysis. Am J Prev Med 23:51, 2002.
13. Druss RG, Bradford DW, Rosenheck RA: Mental disorders and use of cardiovascular procedures after myocardial infarction. JAMA 283:506, 2000.
14. Broadley AJM, Korszun A, Jones CJH, et al: Arterial endothelial function is impaired in treated depression. Heart 88:521, 2002.
15. Albert CM, Chae CU, Rexrode KM, et al: Phobic anxiety and risk of coronary heart disease and sudden cardiac death among women. Circulation 111:480, 2005.
16. Rosengren A, Hawken S, Ounpuu S, et al: Association of psychosocial risk factors with risk of acute myocardial infarction in 11119 cases and 13648 controls from 52 countries (the INTERHEART study): Case-control study. Lancet 364:953, 2004.
17. Eaker ED, Sullivan LM, Kelly-Hayes M, et al: Tension and anxiety and the prediction of the 10-year incidence of coronary heart disease, atrial fibrillation, and total mortality: The Framingham Offspring Study. Psychosom Med 67:692, 2005.
18. Mookadam F, Arthur HM: Social support and its relationship to morbidity and mortality after acute myocardial infarction: systematic overview. Arch Intern Med 164:1514, 2004.
19. Brummett BH, Barefoot JC, Siegler IC, et al: Characteristics of socially isolated patients with coronary artery disease who are at elevated risk for mortality. Psychosom Med 63:267, 2001.
20. Frasure-Smith N, Lespérance F, Gravel G, et al: Social support, depression, and mortality during the first year after myocardial infarction. Circulation 101:1919, 2000.
21. Kivimaki M, Leino-Arjas P, Luukkonen R, et al: Work stress and risk of cardiovascular mortality: Prospective cohort study of industrial employees. BMJ 325:857, 2002.
22. Belkic KL, Landsbergis PA, Schnall PL, Baker D: Is job strain a major source of cardiovascular disease risk? Scand J Work Environ Health 30:85, 2004.
23. Orth-Gomér K, Wamala SP, Horsten M, et al: Marital stress worsens prognosis in women with coronary heart disease. JAMA 284:3008, 2000.
24. Ramachandruni S, Fillingim RB, McGorray SP, et al: Mental stress provokes ischemia in coronary artery disease subjects without exercise- or adenosine-induced ischemia. J Am Coll Cardiol 47:987, 2006.
25. Akinboboye O, Krantz DS, Kop WJ, et al: Comparison of mental stress-induced myocardial ischemia in coronary artery disease patients with versus without left ventricular dysfunction. Am J Cardiol 95:322, 2005.
26. Sheps D, McMahon R, Becker L, et al: Mental-stress induced ischemia and all-cause mortality in patients with coronary artery disease. Circulation 105:1780, 2002.

27. Gullette ECD, Blumenthal JA, Babyak M, et al: Effects of mental stress on myocardial ischemia during daily life. JAMA 277:1521, 1997.

28. Müller J, Hallqvist J, Diderichsen F, et al: Do episodes of anger trigger myocardial infarction? A case-crossover analysis in the Stockholm Heart Epidemiology Program (SHEEP). Psychosom Med 61:842, 1999.

29. Markowitz JH: Hostility is associated with increased platelet activity in coronary heart disease. Psychosom Med 60:586, 1998.

30. Suarez EC, Kuhn CM, Schanberg SM, et al: Neuroendocrine, cardiovascular, and emotional responses of hostile men: The role of interpersonal challenge. Psychosom Med 60:78, 1998.

31. Januzzi JL, Stern TA, Pasternak RC, et al: The influence of anxiety and depression on outcomes of patients with coronary artery disease. Arch Intern Med 160:1913, 2000.

32. Bilge AK, Ozben B, Demircan S, et al: Depression and anxiety status of patients with implantable cardioverter defibrillator and precipitating factors. Pacing Clin Electrophysiol 29:619, 2006.

33. Weidner G, Kohlmann C, Horsten M, et al: Cardiovascular reactivity to mental stress in the Stockholm Female Coronary Risk Study. Psychosom Med 63:917, 2001.

34. Yan LL, Liu K, Matthews KA, et al: Psychosocial factors and risk of hypertension: The Coronary Artery Risk Development in Young Adults (CARDIA) study. JAMA 290:2138, 2003.

Psychiatric and Behavioral Aspects of Hypertension and Heart Failure

35. Schum JL, Jorgensen RS, Verhaeghen P, et al: Trait anger, anger expression, and ambulatory blood pressure: A meta-analytic review. J Behav Med 26:395, 2003.

36. Rutledge T, Hogan B: A quantitative review of prospective evidence linking psychological factors with hypertension development. Psychosom Med 64:758, 2002.

37. Shinn EH, Poston WSC, Kimball KT, et al: Blood pressure and symptoms of depression and anxiety: A prospective study. Am J Hypertens 14:660, 2001.

38. Meyer CM, Armenian HK, Eaton WW, Ford DE: Incident hypertension associated with depression in the Baltimore Epidemiologic Catchment area follow-up study. J Affect Disord 83:127, 2004.

39. Jonas BS, Lando JF: Negative affect as a prospective risk factor for hypertension. Psychosom Med 62:188, 2000.

40. Wexler R, Aukerman G: Nonpharmacologic strategies for managing hypertension. Am Fam Physician 73:1953, 2006.

41. Linden W, Chambers LA: Clinical effectiveness of non-drug therapies for hypertension: A meta-analysis. Ann Behav Med 16:35, 1994.

42. Linden W, Lenz JW, Con AH: Individualized stress management for primary hypertension: A randomized trial. Arch Intern Med 161:1071, 2001.

43. MacMahon K, Lip GYH: Psychological factors in heart failure: A review of the literature. Arch Intern Med 162:509, 2002.

44. Freedland KE, Rich MW, Skala JA, et al: Prevalence of depression in hospitalized patients with congestive heart failure. Psychosom Med 65:119, 2003.

45. Sullivan M, Simon G, Spertus J, et al: Depression-related costs in heart failure care. Arch Intern Med 162:1860, 2002.

46. Rumsfeld JS, Jones PG, Whooley MA, et al: Depression predicts mortality and hospitalization in patients with myocardial infarction complicated by heart failure. Am Heart J 150:961, 2005.

47. Williams SA, Kasl SV, Heiat A, et al: Depression and risk of heart failure among the elderly. Psychosom Med 64:6, 2002.

48. Krumholtz HM, Butler J, Miller J, et al: Prognostic impact of emotional support for elderly patients hospitalized with heart failure. Circulation 97:958, 1998.

49. Luttik M L, Jaarsma T, Moser D, et al: The importance and impact of social support on outcomes in patients with heart failure: An overview of the literature. J Cardiovasc Nurs 20:162, 2005.

50. Ryan CJ, Zerwic JJ: Perceptions of symptoms of myocardial infarction related to health care seeking behaviors in the elderly. J Cardiovasc Nursing 18:184, 2003.

Psychiatric Care of the Cardiac Patient

51. Sockalingam S, Parekh N, Bogoch II, et al: Delirium in the postoperative cardiac patient: A review. J Card Surg 20:560, 2005.

52. Schwartz TL, Masand PS: The role of atypical antipsychotics in the treatment of delirium. Psychosomatics 43:171, 2002.

53. Raja PV, Blumenthal JA, Doraiswamy PM: Cognitive deficits following coronary artery bypass grafting: Prevalence, prognosis, and therapeutic strategies. CNS Spectr 9:763, 2004.

54. Newman MF, Kirchner JL, Phillips-Bute B, et al: Longitudinal assessment of neurocognitive function after coronary-artery bypass surgery. N Engl J Med 344:395, 2001.

55. Glassman A, O'Connor C, Califf R, et al: Sertraline treatment of major depression in patients with acute MI or unstable angina. JAMA 288:701, 2002a.

56. Swenson JR: Quality of life in patients with coronary artery disease and the impact of depression. Curr Psychiatry Rep 6:438, 2004.

57. Sauer WH, Berlin JA, Kimmel SE: Selective serotonin reuptake inhibitors and myocardial infarction. Circulation 104:1894, 2001.

58. Taylor CB, Miller NH, Smith PM, et al: The effect of a home-based, case-managed, multifactorial risk-reduction program on reducing psychological distress in patients with cardiovascular disease. J Cardiopulm Rehabil 17:157, 1997.

59. Frasure-Smith N, Lespérance F, Prince RH, et al: Randomized trial of home-based psychosocial nursing intervention for patients recovering from myocardial infarction. Lancet 350:473, 1997.

60. Cossette S, Frasure-Smith N, Lespérance F: Clinical implications of a reduction in psychological distress on cardiac prognosis in patients participating in a psychosocial intervention program. Psychosom Med 63:257, 2001.

61. Ades PA: Cardiac rehabilitation and secondary prevention of coronary heart disease. N Engl J Med 345:892, 2001.

62. Dusseldorp E, van Elderen T, Maes S, et al: A meta-analysis of psychoeducational programs for coronary heart disease patients. Health Psychol 18:506, 1999.

63. Linden W: Psychological treatments in cardiac rehabilitation: Review of rationales and outcomes. J Psychosom Res 48:443, 2000.

Psychopharmacology in the Cardiac Patient

64. Glassman AH: Clinical management of cardiovascular risks during treatment with psychotropic drugs. J Clin Psychiatry 63(Suppl):12, 2002b.

65. Serebruany VL, Glassman AH, Malinin AI, et al: Enhanced platelet/endothelial activation in depressed patients with acute coronary syndromes: Evidence from recent clinical trials. Blood Coagul Fibrinolysis 14:563, 2003b.

66. Serebruany VL, Glassman AH, Malinin AI, et al: Selective serotonin reuptake inhibitors yield additional antiplatelet protection in patients with congestive heart failure treated with antecedent aspirin. Eur J Heart Fail 5:517, 2003a.

67. Glassman AH: Schizophrenia, antipsychotic drugs, and cardiovascular disease. J Clin Psychiatry 66(Suppl):5, 2005.

CHAPTER 87

Muscular Dystrophies, 2135
Duchenne and Becker Muscular
    Dystrophies, 2135
Myotonic Dystrophies, 2137
Emery-Dreifuss Muscular Dystrophies
    and Associated Disorders, 2142
Limb-Girdle Muscular
    Dystrophies, 2144
Facioscapulohumeral Muscular
    Dystrophy, 2145

Friedreich Ataxia, 2145

Less Common Neuromuscular
Diseases Associated with
Cardiac Manifestations, 2147
Periodic Paralyses, 2147

Acute Cerebrovascular
Disease, 2149

Future Perspectives, 2150

References, 2152

Neurological Disorders and Cardiovascular Disease

William J. Groh and Douglas P. Zipes

Cardiovascular disease that occurs secondary to an underlying neurological disorder is either related to a direct involvement of the heart or caused by induced neurohormonal abnormalities that act on the heart. In several neurological disorders, the cardiovascular manifestations can be responsible for a greater risk of morbidity and mortality than the neurological manifestations. This chapter reviews neurological disorders associated with important cardiovascular sequelae.

MUSCULAR DYSTROPHIES

The muscular dystrophies are a diffuse group of heritable disorders in which direct involvement of cardiac muscle is present to a variable degree. The muscular dystrophies that have been observed to manifest cardiovascular involvement can be classified as follows:
1. Duchenne and Becker muscular dystrophies
2. Myotonic dystrophies
3. Emery-Dreifuss muscular dystrophies and associated disorders
4. Limb-girdle muscular dystrophies
5. Facioscapulohumeral muscular dystrophy

Duchenne and Becker Muscular Dystrophies

GENETICS. Both Duchenne and Becker muscular dystrophy are X-linked recessive disorders in which the genetic locus has been identified as an abnormality in the dystrophin gene. The dystrophin protein and dystrophin-associated glycoproteins provide a structural link between the myocyte cytoskeleton and extracellular matrix functioning to link contractile proteins to the cell membrane.[1] Dystrophin messenger RNA is expressed predominantly in skeletal, cardiac, and smooth muscle with lower levels in brain. Absence of dystrophin can lead to membrane fragility resulting in myofibril necrosis and eventual loss of muscle fibers with fibrotic replacement. Abnormalities in dystrophin and in dystrophin-associated glycoproteins underlie the degeneration of cardiac and skeletal muscle in several inherited myopathies including X-linked dilated cardiomyopathy. Beyond the inherited disorders, the loss of dystrophin plays a role in myocyte failure in other cardiomyopathies including sporadic idiopathic, viral myocarditis, and those associated with coronary artery disease. In Duchenne muscular dystrophy, dystrophin is nearly absent, whereas in Becker muscular dystrophy, dystrophin is present but reduced in size or amount. This leads to the characteristic rapidly progressive skeletal muscle disease in Duchenne and the more benign course in Becker muscular dystrophy. The heart as a muscle is involved in both disorders. Specific dystrophin gene mutations are associated with a higher prevalence of cardiomyopathy.[2]

CLINICAL PRESENTATION. Duchenne muscular dystrophy is the most common inherited neuromuscular disorder with an incidence of 30 per 100,000 live male births. Patients typically become symptomatic before age 5, presenting with skeletal muscle weakness that progresses such that the boy becomes wheelchair-bound before 13 years of age (Fig. 87-1). Death occurs commonly by 25 years of age primarily from respiratory dysfunction and, less commonly, heart failure. Use of ventilatory support has lengthened survival. Becker muscular dystrophy is less common (3 per 100,000 live male births); has a more variable presentation of skeletal muscle weakness (Fig. 87-2); and has a better prognosis, with most patients surviving 40 to 50 years.

In both Duchenne and Becker muscular dystrophy, elevated serum creatine kinase activity is observed, over 10-fold and five-fold normal values, respectively.

CARDIOVASCULAR MANIFESTATIONS. The majority of patients with Duchenne muscular dystrophy develop a cardiomyopathy (see Chap. 64), but symptoms may be masked by severe skeletal muscle weakness. Preclinical cardiac involvement is present in one fourth by age 6, with the onset of clinically apparent cardiomyopathy after age 10 common. Predilection for involvement in the posterobasal and posterolateral left ventricle has been observed (Fig. 87-3). As with the skeletal muscle weakness, cardiac involvement in Becker muscular dystrophy is more variable than in Duchenne muscular dystrophy, ranging from none or subclinical to severe cardiomyopathy requiring transplantation. Cardiac involvement in Becker muscular dystrophy is independent of the severity of skeletal muscle involvement, with some but not all investigators observing increased likelihood of cardiovascular disease in older patients. More than half of patients with subclinical or benign skeletal muscle disease were noted to have cardiac involvement if carefully evaluated. Progression in the severity of cardiac involvement is common. Cardiomyopathy can initially solely involve the right ventricle.

Thoracic deformities and a high diaphragm may alter the cardiovascular examination in Duchenne muscular dystrophy. A reduction in the anterior-posterior chest dimension is commonly responsible for a systolic impulse displaced to the left sternal border, a grade 1-3/6 short midsystolic murmur in the

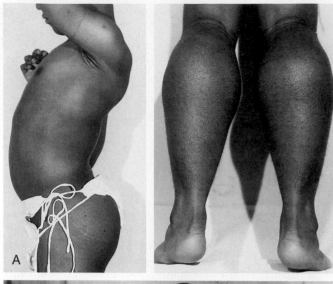

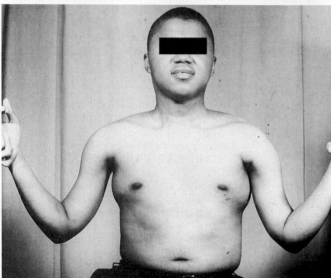

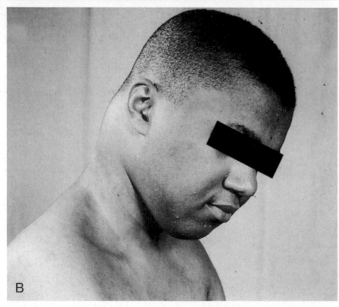

FIGURE 87–1 **A,** Classic X-linked muscular dystrophy. **Left,** Exaggerated lumbar lordosis. **Right,** Calf pseudohypertrophy and shortening of the Achilles tendons. **B,** Seventeen-year-old boy with Duchenne muscular dystrophy. Of note is the striking enlargement (hypertrophy/pseudohypertrophy) of the deltoid and pectoralis major muscles **(upper panel)** and of the trapezius **(lower panel).** In addition, striking enlargement of both calves existed (not shown). (*A and B, Courtesy of Joseph K. Perloff, M.D.*)

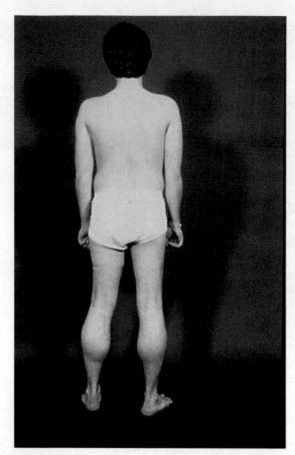

FIGURE 87–2 Becker muscular dystrophy in a 24-year-old male. There is dystrophy of the shoulder girdle and calf pseudohypertrophy. (*Courtesy of Robert M. Pascuzzi, M.D.*)

second left interspace and a loud pulmonary component of the second heart sound. In both Duchenne and Becker muscular dystrophy, mitral regurgitation is commonly observed. The presence of mitral regurgitation is related to posterior papillary muscle dysfunction in Duchenne muscular dystrophy and to mitral annular dilation in Becker muscular dystrophy.

Female carriers of Duchenne and Becker muscular dystrophy are at increased risk of dilation cardiomyopathy.

Electrocardiography (see Chap. 12). In the majority of patients with Duchenne muscular dystrophy, the electrocardiogram (ECG) is abnormal, demonstrating a distinctive pattern of tall R waves and an increased R/S amplitude in V1 and deep narrow Q waves in the left precordial leads related to the characteristic posterolateral left ventricular involvement (Fig. 87-4). In patients with Becker muscular dystrophy, electrocardiographic abnormalities are present in up to 75 percent. The electrocardiographic abnormalities observed include tall R waves and an increased R/S amplitude in V1, similar to that seen in Duchenne muscular dystrophy, but may also show frequent incomplete right bundle branch block. This may be related to early involvement of the right ventricle. In patients with congestive heart failure, left bundle branch block is common.

Arrhythmias (see Chaps. 32-36). In Duchenne muscular dystrophy, persistent or labile sinus tachycardia is the most common arrhythmia recognized. Atrial arrhythmias including atrial fibrillation and atrial flutter occur primarily as a preterminal rhythm. Abnormalities in atrioventricular conduction have been observed, with 10 percent of patients having PR intervals less than 120 ms and an additional 10 percent having prolonged PR intervals. Ventricular arrhythmias occur on monitoring in 30 percent, primarily ventricular premature beats. Complex ventricular arrhythmias have been reported, more commonly in patients with severe skeletal muscle disease. Sudden death occurs in Duchenne muscular dystrophy, typically in patients with end-stage muscular disease. Whether the sudden death is caused by arrhythmias is unclear. Several follow-up studies have shown a correlation between sudden death and the presence of complex ventricular arrhythmias. However, the presence of ventricular arrhythmias was not a predictor for all-cause mortality.[3]

Arrhythmia manifestations in Becker muscular dystrophy typically correspond to the severity of the associated cardiomyopathy. Distal conduction system disease with complete heart block and bundle branch reentry ventricular tachycardia has been observed.

TREATMENT AND PROGNOSIS. Duchenne muscular dystrophy is a progressive disorder with death from a respiratory or cardiac cause. Steroids and steroid derivatives are effective in

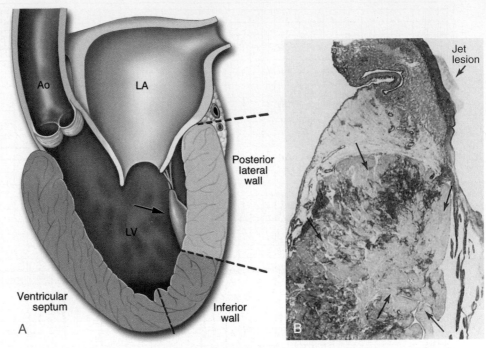

FIGURE 87–3 A, Schematic illustration showing the typical posterobasal myocardial involvement with lateral extension in classic Duchenne muscular dystrophy. The posterolateral papillary muscle is involved (arrow). **B,** Necropsy section showing posterobasal involvement (long arrows) of the left ventricle in a boy with classic Duchenne muscular dystrophy. The posterolateral papillary muscle was involved, resulting in mitral regurgitation and the jet lesion shown at upper right (short arrow). Ao = aorta; LA = left atrium; LV = left ventricle. (*A and B, Courtesy of Joseph K. Perloff, M.D.*)

delaying skeletal muscle disease progression.[4] Gene replacement therapy holds future promise. A primary cardiac etiology for death occurs in one fourth of patients but appears to be playing an increasingly significant role because of delayed mortality from improved respiratory support. An equal distribution of cardiac death from heart failure and sudden death occurs. Yearly imaging for assessment of left ventricular function should be initiated in patients at about 10 years of age. Angiotensin-converting enzyme (ACE) inhibitors and beta blockers can improve left ventricular function in patients treated early.[2,5] Whether these heart failure therapies improve long-term outcomes is unclear.

In patients with Becker muscular dystrophy an improvement in left ventricular function is also observed after treatment with ACE inhibitors and beta blockers.[2] Screening left ventricular imaging should occur as in Duchenne muscular dystrophy. Female carriers of Duchenne and Becker muscular dystrophies do not develop a cardiomyopathy during childhood, and screening can be delayed until later in adolescence. Whether carriers benefit from afterload reduction therapy is unknown, but this would seem reasonable on the basis of shared mechanisms. Once heart failure is established, conventional therapy is indicated. Cardiac transplantation has been reported.

Myotonic Dystrophies

GENETICS

The myotonic dystrophies are autosomal dominant inherited disorders characterized by reflex and percussion myotonia; weakness and atrophy of distal skeletal muscles; and other multisystemic manifestations including endocrine abnormalities, cataracts, cognitive impairment, and cardiac involvement (Fig. 87-5). Two distinct genetic mutations are responsible for the myotonic dystrophies and are reflected in an updated disease classification. In *myotonic dystrophy type 1*, the gene mutation is an amplified and unstable trinucleotide, cytosine-thymine-guanine repeat found on chromosome 19q13.3.

Whereas unaffected patients have 5 to 37 copies of the repeat, patients with myotonic dystrophy have 50 to several thousand repeats. A direct correlation exists between an increasing number of cytosine-thymine-guanine repeats and earlier age of onset and increasing severity of neuromuscular involvement. Cardiac involvement including conduction disease and arrhythmias also correlate with the length of repeat expansion (Fig. 87-6).[6] The cytosine-thymine-guanine repeat typically expands as it is passed from parents to their offspring, giving the characteristic worsening clinical manifestations in subsequent generations, termed *anticipation*.

Myotonic dystrophy type 2, also called proximal myotonic myopathy, has generally less severe skeletal muscle and cardiac involvement than type 1.[7] No congenital presentation or cognitive impairment is apparent in myotonic dystrophy type 2, typically the most severely involved subsets of the type 1 patients. The genetic mutation responsible for myotonic dystrophy type 2 is a large and unstable tetranucleotide repeat expansion, cytosine-cytosine-thymine-guanine, found on chromosome 3q21. Intergenerational contraction of the repeat expansion has been reported, and no apparent relationship exists between the degree of expansion and clinical severity.

Via several molecular mechanisms, an amplified nucleotide repeat expansion on two different chromosomes leads to an analogous clinical syndrome. One mechanism proposed for both myotonic dystrophy types 1 and 2 is the negative effect of the large mutant RNA expansion on nuclear RNA binding proteins.

CLINICAL PRESENTATION. The myotonic dystrophies are the most common inherited neuromuscular disorders in patients presenting as adults. Until recently, studies have not genetically differentiated myotonic dystrophy types 1 and 2, and therefore the clinical characteristics described are likely for a mixed group. Type 1 is significantly more common than type 2 except possibly in certain geographic areas of northern Europe. The global incidence of myotonic dystrophy type 1 has been estimated to be 1 in 8000, although it is higher in certain populations such as French Canadians and lower to nonexistent in other populations such as African blacks. The age at onset of symptoms and diagnosis averages 20 to 25 years. Common early manifestations are

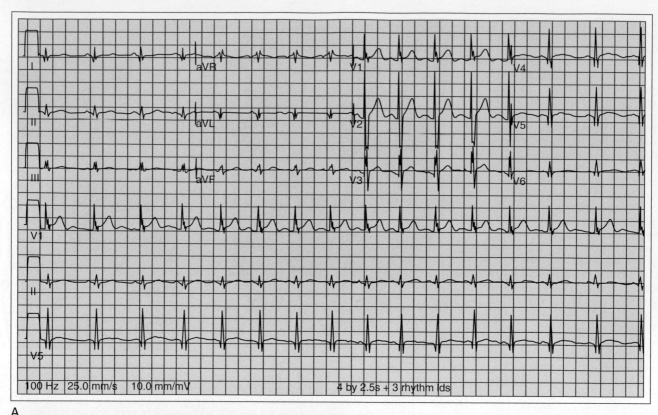

A

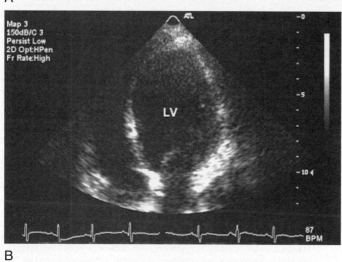

B

FIGURE 87–4 Dilated cardiomyopathy in a 19-year-old male with Duchenne muscular dystrophy. **A,** Electrocardiogram showing a QRS complex that is typical of Duchenne dystrophy with tall R waves in V₁ and deep, narrow Q waves in leads I and aVL. **B,** Two-dimensional echocardiogram (parasternal four chamber) showing a dilated, thinned left ventricle (LV).

weakness in the muscles of the face, neck, and distal extremities. On examination, myotonia (delayed muscle relaxation) can be demonstrated in the grip, thenar muscle group, and tongue (Fig. 87-7). Diagnosis when the patient is asymptomatic is possible using electromyography and genetic testing. In general, cardiac symptoms occur after the onset of skeletal muscle weakness but can be the initial manifestation of the disease.

Myotonic dystrophy type 2 also manifests myotonia, muscle weakness, cataracts, and endocrine abnormalities as in type 1. Age at symptom onset is typically older in myotonic dystrophy type 2.[7]

CARDIOVASCULAR MANIFESTATIONS. Cardiac pathology is commonly seen in myotonic dystrophies primarily involving degeneration (fibrosis and fatty infiltration) of the specialized conduction tissue including the sinus node, atrioventricular node, and His-Purkinje system. Degenerative changes are observed in working atrial and ventricular tissue but rarely progress to a symptomatic dilated cardiomyopathy (Fig. 87-8). Whether there are differences in cardiac pathology between myotonic dystrophy types 1 and 2 is unclear. The primary cardiac manifestations of the myotonic dystrophies are arrhythmias.

Electrocardiography (see Chap. 12). The majority of adult patients with myotonic dystrophy type 1 have electrocardiographic abnormalities. In a large, unselected myotonic population followed in a U.S. neuromuscular clinic setting, 65 percent of patients had an abnormal ECG.[6] Abnormalities included first-degree atrioventricular block in 42 percent, right bundle branch block in 3 percent, left bundle

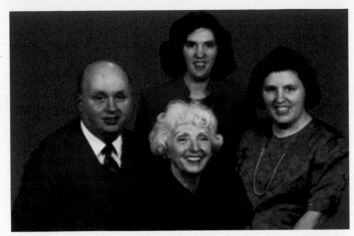

FIGURE 87–5 Myotonic muscular dystrophy in three siblings. The mother **(front)** is unaffected. Premature balding **(left)** and characteristic thin facies **(rear)** are demonstrated.

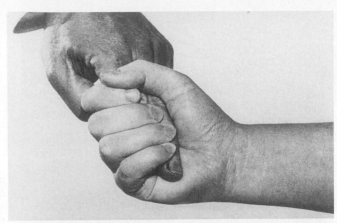

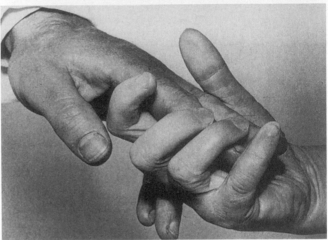

FIGURE 87–7 Grip myotonia in myotonic muscular dystrophy. Inability to release **(bottom)** after exerting grip **(top)**. *(From Engel AG, Franzini-Armstrong C [eds]: Myology: Basic and Clinical. 2nd ed. Vol. II. New York, McGraw-Hill, 1994.)*

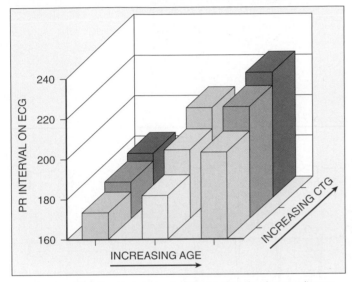

FIGURE 87–6 Relationship between the PR interval on the electrocardiogram (ECG) and age and cytosine-thymine-guanine (CTG) repeat sequence expansion in 342 patients with myotonic dystrophy type 1. A direct relationship between age and CTG repeat sequence expansion and the severity of cardiac conduction disease as quantified by the PR interval exists. The relationship suggests that cardiac involvement in myotonic dystrophy type 1 is a time-dependent degenerative process with rate of progression modulated by the extent of CTG repeat expansion. *(From Groh WJ, Lowe MR, Zipes DP: Severity of cardiac conduction involvement and arrhythmias in myotonic dystrophy type 1 correlates with age and CTG repeat length. J Cardiovasc Electrophysiol 13:444, 2002.)*

branch block in 4 percent, and nonspecific intraventricular conduction delay in 12 percent. Q waves not associated with a known myocardial infarction are common. Electrocardiographic abnormalities progress as the patient ages (Fig. 87-9).

Electrocardiographic abnormalities are less common in myotonic dystrophy type 2, occurring in approximately 20 percent of middle-aged patients.[7]

Echocardiography (see Chap. 14). Left ventricular systolic and diastolic dysfunction, left ventricular hypertrophy, mitral valve prolapse, regional wall motion abnormalities, and left atrial dilation have been reported in myotonic dystrophy type 1 patients with moderate prevalence rates.[8] However, the prevalence of clinical heart failure is significantly lower, estimated at 2 percent. Mild left ven-

tricular hypertrophy and ventricular dilation has been reported in myotonic dystrophy type 2.

Arrhythmias (see Chaps. 32-36). Patients with myotonic dystrophy type 1 demonstrate a wide range of arrhythmias. At cardiac electrophysiological study, the most common abnormality found is a prolonged His-ventricular (HV) interval. Conduction system disease can progress to symptomatic atrioventricular block and necessitate pacemaker implantation. The prevalence of permanent cardiac pacing in patients with myotonic dystrophy type 1 varies widely among studies on the basis of referral patterns and indications used for implantation. Recent pacing guidelines have recognized that asymptomatic conduction abnormalities in neuromuscular diseases such as myotonic dystrophy may warrant special consideration for pacing.[9]

Atrial arrhythmias, primarily atrial fibrillation and atrial flutter, are the most common arrhythmias observed.[6] Ventricular tachycardia can occur. The myotonic dystrophy type 1 patients are at risk of ventricular tachycardia because of reentry in the diseased distal conduction system, as characterized by bundle branch reentry and interfascicular reentry tachycardia (Fig. 87-10). Therapy with right bundle branch or fascicular radiofrequency ablation can be curative.

The incidence of sudden death in patients with myotonic dystrophy type 1 is substantial, and experts believe it is primarily caused by arrhythmias. In a registry of 180 myotonic dystrophy patients from the Netherlands collected from 1950 to 1997, 29 percent of all deaths were classified as sudden presumably because of arrhythmias.[10] This was

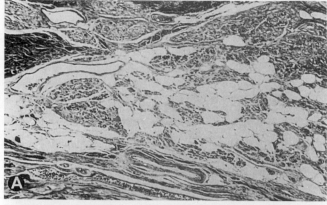
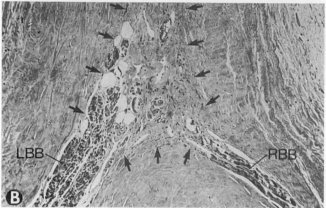

FIGURE 87–8 Histopathology of the atrioventricular bundle in myotonic dystrophy. **A,** Fatty infiltration in a 57-year-old man (Masson trichrome stain, ×90). **B,** Focal replacement fibrosis and atrophy in a 48-year-old woman. Arrows demarcate expected size and shape of the branching atrioventricular bundle (hematoxylin-eosin stain, ×90). LBB = left bundle branch; RBB = right bundle branch. (*A and B, From Nguyen HH, Wolfe JT III, Holmes DR Jr, Edwards WD: Pathology of the cardiac conduction system in myotonic dystrophy: A study of 12 cases. J Am Coll Cardiol 11:662, 1988.*)

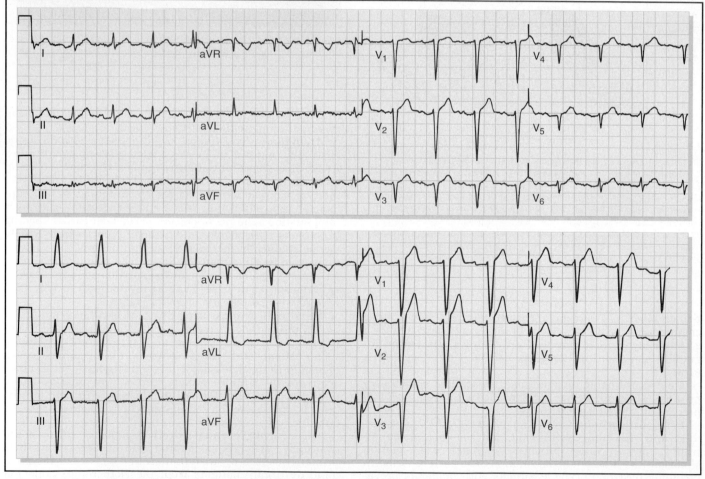

FIGURE 87–9 Electrocardiograms obtained 1 year apart in a 36-year-old man with myotonic dystrophy (the top set is older). Note the abnormal Q waves in the precordial leads. An increasing PR interval and QRS duration are observed, consistent with increasing severity of conduction disease.

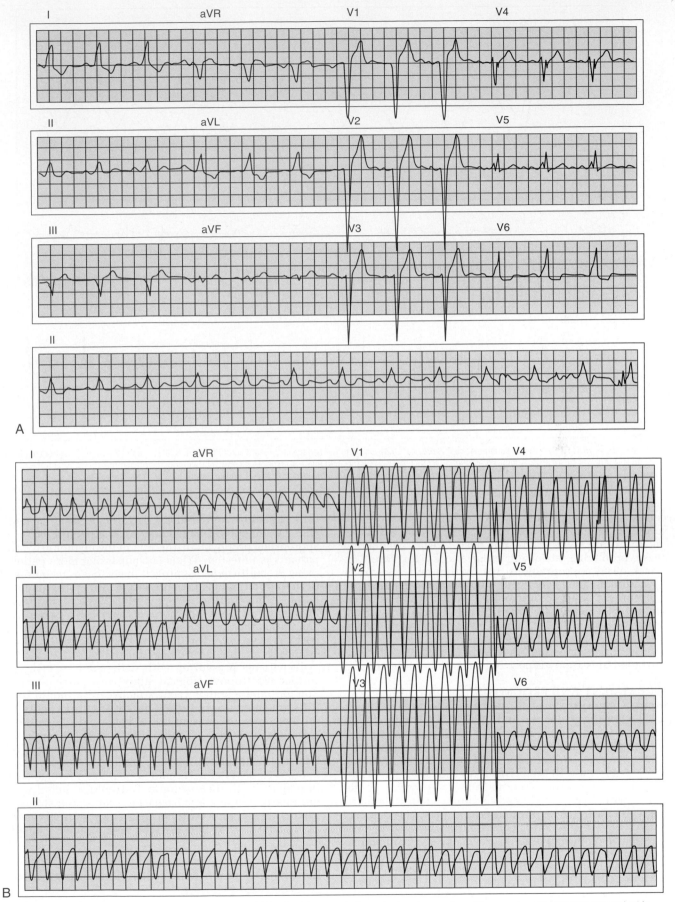

Neurological Disorders and Cardiovascular Disease

FIGURE 87–10 Bundle branch reentry tachycardia in a 34-year-old female with myotonic dystrophy type 1 presenting with a symptomatic (recurrent syncope) wide-complex tachycardia. **A,** Electrocardiogram showing sinus rhythm and a QRS complex with left bundle branch block. **B,** Electrocardiogram showing a rapid monomorphic tachycardia easily inducible at electrophysiological study with left bundle morphology.

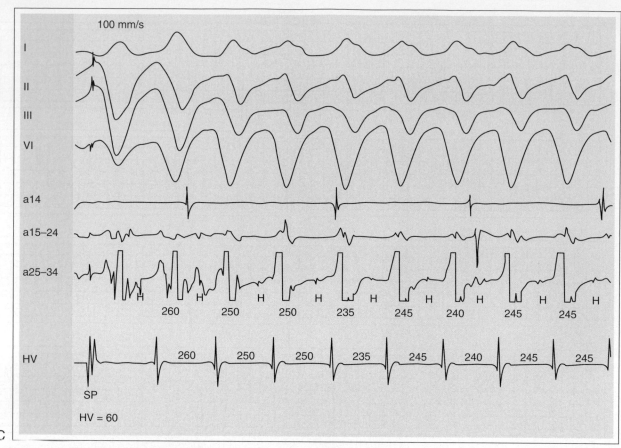

FIGURE 87–10, cont'd C, Recordings during electrophysiological study including the surface electrocardiogram (leads I, II, III, V₁) and intracardiac electrocardiograms. A monomorphic ventricular tachycardia is induced with atrial-ventricular (A-V) dissociation and His-association consistent with bundle branch reentry tachycardia. H = His recording; HRA = high right atrium; HV = RV; RV = right ventricle; a14 = HRA; a15-24 = His proximal; a25-34 = His distal.

secondary only to pneumonia (31 percent) as a cause of death. The mechanisms leading to sudden death in myotonic dystrophy type 1 are not clear. Distal conduction disease producing atrioventricular block can result in the lack of an appropriate escape rhythm and asystole or bradycardia-mediated ventricular fibrillation. Sudden death can occur in myotonic dystrophy type 1 despite previous permanent cardiac pacing, implicating the role of ventricular arrhythmias. Whether a nonarrhythmic cause of sudden death plays a role remains uncertain.

Arrhythmias and sudden death have been reported in myotonic dystrophy type 2 but seem to be rarer than in type 1.[7,11]

TREATMENT AND PROGNOSIS. Because cardiac manifestations can occur in both myotonic dystrophy types 1 and 2, diagnostic evaluation and appropriate therapy should be done for both. As discussed earlier, significant cardiac involvement is more common in myotonic dystrophy type 1 than 2. Cardiac management in patients without myotonic dystrophies is not well established. An echocardiogram can determine if structural abnormalities are present. In the unusual patient with a dilated cardiomyopathy, standard therapy including ACE inhibitors and beta blockers has improved symptoms. Patients presenting with symptoms indicative of arrhythmias such as syncope and palpitations should undergo an evaluation, often including a cardiac electrophysiological study, to determine an etiology. Annual ECGs and 24-hour ambulatory monitoring have been recommended in asymptomatic patients. Significant or progressive electrocardiographic abnormalities despite a lack of symptoms can be an indication for prophylactic pacing or further diagnostic testing. Whether permanent pacemakers protect against sudden death is unclear. Whether implantable cardioverter-defibrillators (ICDs) would be a more appropriate prophylactic therapy in the myotonic dystrophy patients is untested. Trials encompassing more patients by using a multicenter approach have been recommended. Certain families may be more prone to arrhythmia manifestations of myotonic dystrophy. Anesthesia in patients with myotonic dystrophy can increase the risk of atrioventricular block and other arrhythmias. Careful monitoring during the perioperative period with a low threshold for prophylactic temporary pacing is recommended.

In patients presenting with wide complex tachycardia, cardiac electrophysiological study with particular evaluation for bundle branch reentry tachycardia should be done. ICDs are being used in myotonic dystrophy patients.

The course of neuromuscular abnormalities in the myotonic dystrophies is variable. Death from respiratory dysfunction can occur in advanced skeletal muscle disease. Other patients may be only minimally limited by weakness to 60 to 70 years of age. Sudden death can reduce survival in patients with the myotonic dystrophies including those minimally symptomatic from a neuromuscular status. What evaluation and interventions are appropriate and the degree of effectiveness to decrease the risk of sudden death are unclear.

Emery-Dreifuss Muscular Dystrophy and Associated Disorders

GENETICS AND CARDIAC PATHOLOGY. Emery-Dreifuss muscular dystrophy is a rare familial disorder in which skeletal muscle symptoms are often mild but with cardiac involvement that is common and life threatening. The disease is classically inherited in an X-linked recessive fashion, but there is heterogeneity in that families that fit an X-linked dominant, autosomal dominant, and autosomal recessive inheritance pattern have been reported. The gene responsible for the X-linked Emery-Dreifuss muscular dystrophy, *STA,* encodes a nuclear membrane protein termed *emerin.* The lack of emerin in skeletal and cardiac muscle is responsible for the disease phenotype. Mutations in genes found on chromosome 1 encoding two other nuclear membrane proteins, lamins A and C, have been identified as being responsible for a variety of other disorders with a phenotypic expression related to X-linked Emery-Dreifuss muscular dystrophy. The disorders include autosomal dominant and recessive Emery-Dreifuss muscular dystrophy, autosomal dominant dilated cardiomyopathy with conduction disease, autosomal dominant limb-girdle muscular dystrophy with conduction disease, and lipodystrophy with associated cardiac abnormalities.[12]

Nuclear membrane proteins such as emerin and lamins A and C provide structural support for the nucleus and interact with the cell's cytoskeletal proteins. Mutations in the tail regions of lamins A and C are responsible for the majority of cases of autosomal dominant Emery-

Dreifuss muscular dystrophy with a phenotype of both cardiac and skeletal muscle involvement. Mutations in the rod domain of the lamin A/C gene primarily cause isolated cardiac disease including dilated cardiomyopathy, conduction system degeneration, and atrial and ventricular arrhythmias.

CLINICAL PRESENTATION. Emery-Dreifuss muscular dystrophy is characterized by a triad of (1) early contractures of the elbow, Achilles tendon, and posterior cervical muscles; (2) slowly progressing muscle weakness and atrophy primarily in humeroperoneal muscles; and (3) cardiac involvement (Fig. 87-11). The disorder has been labeled "benign X-linked muscular dystrophy" to differentiate the slowly progressive muscular weakness from that of Duchenne muscular dystrophy. A definitive diagnosis can be made in Emery-Dreifuss muscular dystrophy and in carriers using antiemerin antibodies.

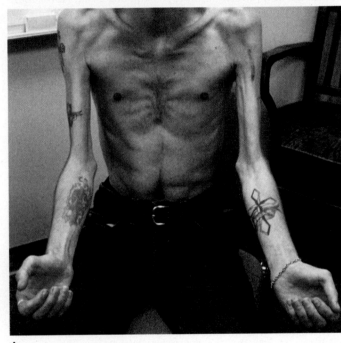

A

FIGURE 87–11 Emery-Dreifuss muscular dystrophy in a 28-year-old male presenting with syncope. **A,** Contractures of the elbow and atrophy in the humeroperoneal muscles. **B,** Electrocardiogram at patient presentation showing atrial fibrillation with slow ventricular rate and a QRS complex with left bundle branch block. *(Courtesy of Robert M. Pascuzzi, M.D.)*

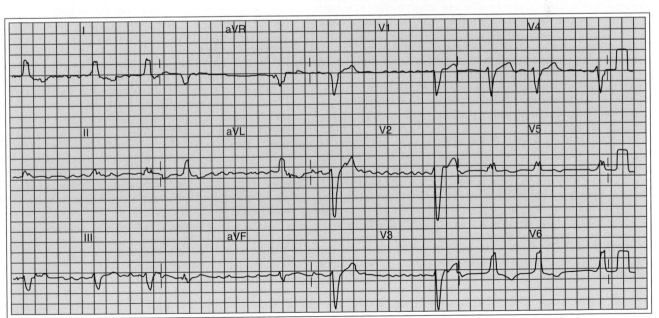

B

In the autosomal dominant and recessive inheritance of Emery-Dreifuss muscular dystrophy, a more variable phenotypic expression and penetrance is typically observed.

A mutation in the lamin A/C gene is also responsible for an autosomal dominantly inherited familial partial lipodystrophy characterized by marked loss of subcutaneous fat, diabetes, hypertriglyceridemia, and cardiac abnormalities.[12]

CARDIOVASCULAR MANIFESTATIONS. Arrhythmias and dilated cardiomyopathy are the major manifestations of cardiac disease in Emery-Dreifuss muscular dystrophy and the associated disorders. In X-linked recessive Emery-Dreifuss muscular dystrophy, abnormalities in impulse generation and conduction are exceedingly frequent. ECGs are generally abnormal by age 20 to 30 years, commonly showing first-degree atrioventricular block. The atria appear to be involved earlier than the ventricles, with atrial fibrillation and atrial flutter or, more classically, permanent atrial standstill and junctional bradycardia observed. Abnormalities in impulse generation or conduction are present in virtually all patients by age 35 to 40 years, and pacing is often required. Ventricular arrhythmias including sustained ventricular tachycardia and ventricular fibrillation have been reported. Invasive cardiac electrophysiological study data are limited in this rare condition.

Mild prolongation of the HV interval, atrial, atrioventricular nodal, and ventricular refractory periods have been observed. Sudden, presumably cardiac, death before age 50 is common. The incidence of sudden death may decrease with prophylactic pacing. Female carriers of X-linked recessive Emery-Dreifuss muscular dystrophy do not develop skeletal muscle disease, but late cardiac disease including conduction abnormalities and sudden death can occur. Although arrhythmia disease is the most common presentation of cardiac involvement in X-linked recessive Emery-Dreifuss muscular dystrophy, a dilated cardiomyopathy can rarely develop. The dilated cardiomyopathy is more common in patients in whom survival has been improved with pacemaker implantation. Both autopsy and endomyocardial biopsies have shown abnormal cardiac fibrosis.

An X-linked dominant Emery-Dreifuss muscular dystrophy with incomplete and age-dependent penetrance has been reported.[13] In the observed families, skeletal muscle involvement was absent or mild and the primary cardiac manifestations were atrial fibrillation, heart block, and sudden death. Women were affected later in life than men.

Patients with disorders caused by lamins A and C mutations typically present at 20 to 40 years of age with cardiac conduction disease, atrial fibrillation, and dilated cardiomyopathy. Skeletal muscle disease is typically subclinical or absent. Progression of a cardiomyopathy to an extent that heart transplantation is required has been observed. Sudden death in those patients with a dilated cardiomyopathy is common. Permanent pacing is often required for symptomatic heart block.

TREATMENT AND PROGNOSIS. Affected patients should be monitored for development of electrocardiographic conduction abnormalities and other arrhythmias. Atrioventricular block can occur with anesthesia. In X-linked recessive Emery-Dreifuss muscular dystrophy, permanent pacing is recommended once conduction disease is evident and can be life-saving. Sudden death even in patients with pacemakers can occur. Prophylactic placement of an ICD has been advocated in patients with disorders caused by lamins A and C mutations if significant electrocardiographic conduction disease is present and pacing is being considered.[14] A referred, nonrandomized patient series in which all participants received ICDs has demonstrated appropriate therapy delivery in a significant proportion.[15]

Whether prophylactic ICDs should be considered only in a certain subgroups of patients or in all patients with Emery-Dreifuss muscular dystrophy and the associated disorders who have significant conduction disease or cardiomyopathy is not clear. History, examination, and cardiac imaging for evaluation of left ventricular function are appropriate in all of the patients with Emery-Dreifuss muscular dystrophy and the associated disorders. Patients with left ventricular dysfunction should benefit from appropriate pharmacological therapy. The patients do appear to benefit from heart transplant. Female carriers of X-linked recessive Emery-Dreifuss muscular dystrophy develop conduction disease, so electrocardiographic monitoring on a routine basis is appropriate.

Limb-Girdle Muscular Dystrophies

GENETICS

The limb-girdle muscular dystrophies constitutes a group of disorders with a limb-pelvic girdle distribution of weakness, but with otherwise heterogeneous inheritance and genetic etiology.[16] Inheritance is most commonly autosomal recessive (limb-girdle muscular dystrophy type 2), but sporadic and autosomal dominant (limb-girdle muscular dystrophy type 1) inheritance is also observed. A genetic-based nomenclature (e.g., 1A, 1B, 2A) was introduced to categorize the increasing number of recognized disorders. The genes involved encode dystrophin-associated glycoproteins, sarcomeric proteins, nuclear membrane proteins, and cellular enzymes.

CLINICAL PRESENTATION. The onset of muscle weakness is variable but usually occurs before 30 years of age. The recessive disorders tend to cause earlier and more severe weakness than the dominant disorders. Creatine kinase levels are typically moderately elevated. Patients commonly present with complaints of difficulty with walking or running secondary to pelvic girdle involvement. As the disease progresses, involvement of the shoulder muscles and then more distal muscles occurs, with sparing of facial involvement. Slow progression to severe disability and death can occur.

CARDIOVASCULAR MANIFESTATIONS. As with many of the features of the limb-girdle muscular dystrophies, heterogeneity is observed in the presence and degree of cardiac involvement.

The limb-girdle muscular dystrophy types 2C to 2F are autosomal recessive disorders caused by mutations in a subunit of the sarcoglycan complex.[17] Patients with sarcoglycanopathies commonly manifest a dilated cardiomyopathy. ECGs show similar abnormalities as in Duchenne and Becker muscular dystrophy including an increased R wave in V1 and lateral Q waves. Using electrocardiographic or echocardiographic evaluations, cardiac abnormalities are detected in up to 80 percent of patients, with a smaller proportion symptomatic. A severe cardiomyopathy including presentation with heart failure in childhood can occur. Sudden death associated with the cardiomyopathy has been reported. Mechanisms by which sarcoglycan abnormalities lead to a dilated cardiomyopathy may include a direct myopathic effect exacerbated by vascular spasm and ischemia increasing cellular dysfunction and death.[18]

Limb-girdle muscular dystrophy type 2I is an autosomal recessive disorder caused by a mutation in the fukutin-related protein gene located on chromosome 19. The mutation is also responsible for a form of congenital muscular dystrophy. The gene abnormality affects glycosylation of a dystrophin-associated glycoprotein. The age at disease onset and severity of skeletal muscle involvement in limb-girdle muscular dystrophy type 2I is variable, with some patients symptomatic in childhood but, more typically, symptoms developing between 20 and 40 years of age. Similar to the sarcoglycanopathies, a high proportion of patients with limb-girdle muscular dystrophy type 2I develop a dilated cardiomyopathy.[19] In a patient series, nearly all patients had evidence of cardiac involvement by age 60. Patients who were heterozygous for a common mutation, C826A, with a different second mutation were affected at a younger age than those homozygous for the C826A mutation. The majority of heterozygous patients had cardiac abnormalities by 20 to 30 years of age. Approximately half of all patients had heart failure symptoms, and some were being considered for cardiac transplantation. In limb-girdle muscular dystrophy type 2I, conduction disease did not occur separately from the structural cardiac involvement.

The autosomal dominant limb-girdle muscular dystrophy type 1B is caused by mutations in the gene encoding lamins A and C, similar to that observed in Emery-Dreifuss muscular dystrophy. Not surprisingly, the clinical phenotype is also similar to Emery-Dreifuss muscular dystrophy with mild skeletal muscle symptoms and more severe cardiac involvement, primarily arrhythmia in nature. Affected patients develop atrioventricular block that often necessitates pacing by early middle age. Sudden death, believed to be cardiac, is common, including in those in whom pacing was previously instituted. A dilated cardiomyopathy can occur.

TREATMENT AND PROGNOSIS. Because of the heterogeneous nature of limb-girdle muscular dystrophy, specific recommendations for routine cardiac evaluation and therapy are based on the genetic classification. Genetic testing can determine those with limb-girdle types 2C-F, 2I, or 1B who are at the highest risk for cardiac involvement. In these patients (and families) cardiac evaluation for arrhythmias and ventricular dysfunction should be done. Patients with dilated cardiomyopathies do appear to respond to standard heart failure therapy.[19] Prophylactic pacing in those with lamins A and C mutations after conduction disease is observed should be considered. The high risk of sudden death despite pacing may point to the ICD as being more appropriate electrical therapy.[14]

Facioscapulohumeral Muscular Dystrophy

GENETICS

Facioscapulohumeral muscular dystrophy is the third most common muscular dystrophy after Duchenne and myotonic, with a prevalence of 1 per 20,000 persons. It is an autosomal dominant disorder in which the genetic locus has been mapped to chromosome 4q35. Genetic heterogeneity has been reported. The diagnosis can be confirmed by a 4q35 *Eco*RI allele size of 38 kilobases or less. This repeat region, termed *D4Z4*, is responsible for binding to a regulatory protein complex that suppresses transcription of adjacent genes.[20] The lack of an appropriate number of D4Z4 repeats results in an overexpression of 4q35 genes and is proposed as the mechanism leading to the facioscapulohumeral muscular dystrophy phenotype. The exact genes that are overexpressed and their protein products are not clear.

CLINICAL PRESENTATION. Muscle weakness tends to follow a slowly progressive but variable course presenting with facial and/or shoulder girdle muscle weakness and progressing to involve the pelvic musculature. Major disability affecting walking eventually occurs in 20 percent of patients.

CARDIOVASCULAR MANIFESTATIONS. Cardiac involvement in facioscapulohumeral muscular dystrophy is reported but does not constitute as significant a problem in prevalence or severity as in other muscular dystrophies. In some series no evidence of cardiac abnormalities was found. Other series have reported a propensity toward arrhythmias, primarily atrial in origin, with atrioventricular conduction abnormalities less common.

TREATMENT AND PROGNOSIS. Because significant clinical cardiac involvement is rare in facioscapulohumeral muscular dystrophy, specific monitoring or treatment recommendations are not well defined. Yearly ECGs have been recommended.

FRIEDREICH ATAXIA

GENETICS

Friedreich ataxia is an autosomal recessive spinocerebellar degenerative disease characterized clinically by ataxia of the limbs and trunk, dysarthria, loss of deep tendon reflexes, sensory abnormalities, skeletal deformities, diabetes mellitus, and cardiac involvement.[21] The disease is linked to chromosome 9, with the gene mutation affecting the encoding of a 210-amino acid protein, frataxin. Frataxin is a mitochondrial protein important in iron homeostasis and respiratory function. Messenger RNA for frataxin is highly expressed in the heart. The mutation responsible for Friedreich ataxia is an amplified trinucleotide (Guanine-Adenine-Adenine [GAA]) repeat found in the first intron of the gene encoding frataxin. Whereas normal patients have fewer than 33 repeats, patients with Friedreich ataxia have 66 to 1500 GAA repeats. In 95 percent of patients both alleles of the gene have the expanded repeat. In 5 percent of patients, a point mutation occurs on one allele in association with an expanded repeat on the other. The GAA repeat disrupts transcription, severely decreasing frataxin synthesis. The decrease in frataxin leads to mitochondrial dysfunction, poor cellular response to oxidative stress, and apoptosis. Endomyocardial biopsies in patients with Friedreich ataxia have shown deficient function in mitochondrial respiratory complex subunits and in aconitase, an iron-sulfur protein involved in iron homeostasis. Abnormal cardiac bioenergetics appear to result from the abnormalities in respiratory function and iron handling.[22] As the GAA triplet size increases, an earlier age of symptom onset, increasing severity of neurological symptoms and worsening left ventricular hypertrophy by echocardiography are observed.[23]

CLINICAL PRESENTATION. The estimated prevalence of Friedreich ataxia is 1 in 50,000. Neurological symptoms usually manifest around puberty and almost always before age 25. Progressive loss of neuromuscular function, with the patient wheelchair bound 10 to 20 years after symptom onset, is the norm. Neurological symptoms precede cardiac symptoms in most but not all cases.

CARDIOVASCULAR MANIFESTATIONS. Friedreich ataxia is commonly associated with a concentric hypertrophic cardiomyopathy (Fig. 87-12). Less commonly, asymmetrical septal hypertrophy is observed. The presence of a left ventricular outflow gradient associated with the septal

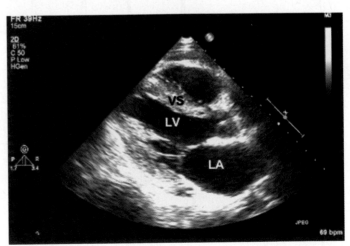

FIGURE 87–12 Hypertrophic cardiomyopathy in a 28-year-old male with Friedreich ataxia. Two-dimensional echocardiogram (parasternal two chamber) showing a thickened ventricular septum (VS) and a dilated left atrium (LA). LV = left ventricle.

hypertrophy has been reported. Presentation with a dilated cardiomyopathy is rarer but can occur (Fig. 87-13). The dilated cardiomyopathy appears to occur as a progressive transition from a hypertrophic cardiomyopathy. The prevalence of hypertrophy varies among studies but does increase in prevalence with a younger age at diagnosis and with increasing GAA trinucleotide repeat length.[23] Up to 95 percent of neurologically symptomatic patients have abnormalities on electrocardiographic and echocardiographic evaluations. Findings are primarily consistent with ventricular hypertrophy. Left ventricular hypertrophy is not always present on ECGs despite echocardiographic evi-

dence. Widespread T-wave inversions are common (Fig. 87-14).

Arrhythmias occur in Friedreich ataxia but are less common than expected considering the high incidence of cardiac involvement. Atrial arrhythmias including atrial fibrillation and flutter are associated with the progression to a dilated cardiomyopathy. Ventricular tachycardia, again in the setting of a dilated cardiomyopathy, has been observed. The hypertrophic cardiomyopathy of Friedreich ataxia is not associated with serious ventricular arrhythmias as observed in the other types of heritable hypertrophic cardiomyopathies. Myocardial fiber disarray is not commonly observed in the hypertrophic cardiomyopathy of Friedreich ataxia. Sudden death has been reported, but a mechanism has not been well characterized.

Endomyocardial biopsies in Friedreich ataxia have demonstrated myocyte hypertrophy and interstitial fibrosis. Histopathological examination has revealed myocyte hypertrophy and degeneration, interstitial fibrosis, active muscle necrosis, bizarre pleomorphic nuclei, and periodic acid–Schiff–positive deposition in both large and small coronary arteries. Degeneration and fibrosis in cardiac nerves and ganglia and the conduction system have also been observed. Deposition of calcium salts and iron has been reported.

TREATMENT AND PROGNOSIS. Idebenone, a free radical scavenger, modestly decreased septal wall thickness and left ventricular

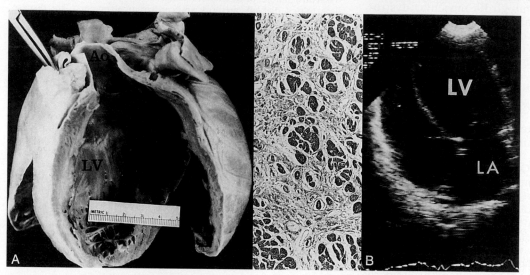

FIGURE 87–13 **A,** Gross and histological specimens from a 17-year-old boy with Friedreich ataxia whose echocardiogram progressed from normal at age 13 years to a minimally dilated, hypocontractile left ventricle (LV) 3 to 4 years later. The gross specimen shows a mildly dilated LV with normal wall thickness; the walls were flabby. The microscopic section from the left ventricular free wall **(middle panel)** shows marked connective tissue replacement. Although specifically sought, small-vessel coronary artery disease was not identified. **B,** Two-dimensional echocardiogram (apical window) showing the mildly dilated, thin-walled LV. LA = left atrium. (*A and B, From Child JS, Perloff JK, Bach PM, et al: Cardiac involvement in Friedreich ataxia. J Am Coll Cardiol 7:1370, 1986.*)

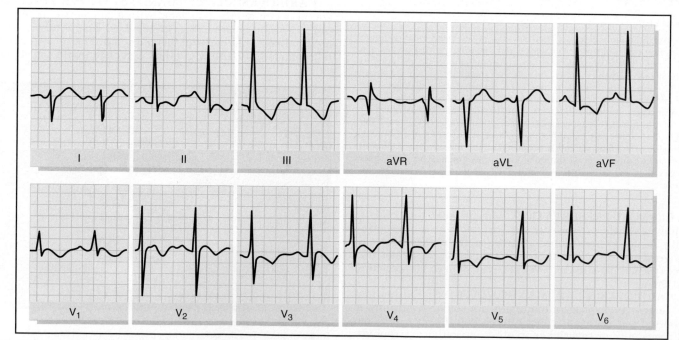

FIGURE 87–14 Electrocardiogram from a 34-year-old man with Friedreich ataxia. Widespread ST and T changes are observed. (*Courtesy of Charles Fisch, M.D., Indiana University School of Medicine, Indianapolis.*)

mass in Friedreich ataxia patients treated in a blinded, placebo-controlled, 1-year trial.[24] Patients with a greater degree of hypertrophy responded best. In another study the majority of patients with depressed left ventricular function showed improvement on serial imaging with idebenone therapy.[25] Whether the modest improvement in cardiac imaging parameters with idebenone therapy also leads to any alteration in the clinical cardiovascular course has not been tested. Idebenone does not appear to improve neurological outcomes.

In the majority of patients with Friedreich ataxia, progressive neurological dysfunction is the norm with death from respiratory failure or infection in the fourth or fifth decades. Cardiac death occurs primarily in those developing a dilated cardiomyopathy. These patients tend to do poorly, with rapid progression to end-stage congestive heart failure.

LESS COMMON NEUROMUSCULAR DISEASES ASSOCIATED WITH CARDIAC MANIFESTATIONS

Periodic Paralyses

GENETICS

The primary periodic paralyses are rare, nondystrophic, autosomal dominant disorders that result from abnormalities in ion channel genes. They can be classified into hypokalemic, hyperkalemic (potassium-sensitive), and normokalemic periodic paralyses with several subclassifications in each.

Hypokalemic periodic paralysis is characterized by episodic attacks of weakness in association with decreased serum potassium levels. Penetrance is complete in males and approximately 50 percent in females. Hypokalemic periodic paralysis has been mapped to chromosome 1q31-32 with subsequent identification of mutations in the alpha$_1$ subunit of the dihydropyridine-sensitive calcium channel. The disease may be genetically heterogeneous, as observed with the identification of a family with hypokalemic periodic paralysis and a mutation in the skeletal muscle sodium channel *(SCN4A)*.[26]

Hyperkalemic periodic paralysis also manifests with episodic weakness but with symptoms worsening with potassium supplementation. Complete penetrance is observed. Potassium levels are usually high but may be normal during an attack. Hyperkalemic periodic paralysis is caused primarily by mutations in the alpha subunit of *SCN4A* found on chromosome 17.[27] Multiple different mutations in this gene have been reported and result in a potassium-sensitive failure of inactivation in the sodium channel. Hyperkalemic periodic paralysis is genetically heterogeneous.

Andersen-Tawil syndrome is a distinct periodic paralysis associated with characteristic dysmorphic physical features, an abnormal QT-U-wave pattern, and ventricular arrhythmias (Fig. 87-15).[28] The periodic paralysis can be hypokalemic, hyperkalemic, or normokalemic. Phenotypic variability and incomplete penetrance is observed. Andersen-Tawil syndrome is linked to chromosome 17q23 with the mutations responsible in the *KCNJ2* gene encoding an inward rectifier potassium protein (Kir2.1) found in the majority of patients.[29] Loss of function in the inward rectifier potassium channel, I_{K1}, results. This affects the terminal repolarization of the cardiac action potential.[30] Some experts have suggested that Andersen-Tawil syndrome be given an alternate long-QT syndrome 7 nomenclature.[31]

CLINICAL PRESENTATION. The primary manifestation of all of the periodic paralyses is episodic weakness. Attacks of weakness tend to be more severe and of longer duration with hypokalemic periodic paralysis than with hyperkalemic periodic paralysis. In all the periodic paralyses, cold, exercise, and rest after exercise can trigger an attack. Ingestion of carbohydrates can trigger an attack in hypokalemic periodic paralysis but may ameliorate an attack in hyperkalemic periodic paralysis.

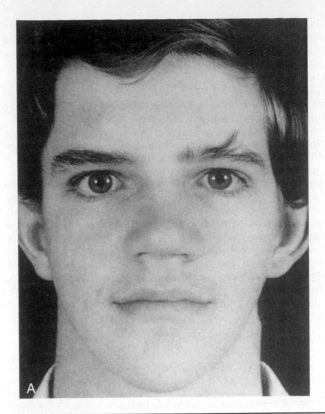

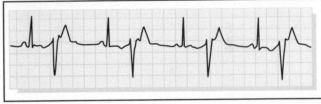

FIGURE 87–15 Andersen-Tawil syndrome in a 22-year-old man. **A,** Characteristic low-set ears and hypoplastic mandible. **B,** Electrocardiographic recording revealing ventricular bigeminy. (***A*** and ***B****, From Tawil R, Ptacek LJ, Pavlakis SG, et al: Andersen's syndrome: Potassium-sensitive periodic paralysis, ventricular ectopy, and dysmorphic features. Ann Neurol 35:326, 1994.)*

CARDIOVASCULAR MANIFESTATIONS. The periodic paralyses are associated with ventricular arrhythmias. Arrhythmias occur primarily in hyperkalemic periodic paralysis and Andersen-Tawil syndrome. Bidirectional ventricular tachycardia has been observed independent of digitalis intoxication. The episodes of bidirectional ventricular tachycardia are independent of attacks of muscle weakness, do not correlate with serum potassium levels, and can convert to sinus rhythm with exercise. Ventricular ectopy is common.

A prolonged QT interval can be observed. In some reports, the prolonged QT interval is episodic and associated with weakness, hypokalemia, or antiarrhythmia therapy. In other cases a prolonged QT can be constant. Andersen-Tawil syndrome is associated with a modest prolongation in the QT interval but more specifically a prolonged and prominent U wave.[30] Ventricular arrhythmias including premature ventricular contractions, ventricular bigeminy, and nonsustained polymorphic ventricular tachycardia, primarily bidirectional tachycardia, are commonly observed in Andersen-Tawil syndrome. Cardiac conduction abnormalities, atypical of long QT syndromes, have been observed in Andersen-Tawil syndrome. Torsades de pointes is observed in Andersen-Tawil syndrome but is less common than in long QT syndromes.

Syncope, cardiac arrest, and sudden death have been reported in the periodic paralyses, most prominently in the Andersen-Tawil syndrome. The factors that portend an increased risk of life-threatening arrhythmias are not clear.

TREATMENT AND PROGNOSIS. The episodes of weakness typically respond to measures that work to normalize potassium levels. Weakness in hyperkalemic periodic paralysis can respond to mexiletine. Weakness in hypokalemic periodic paralysis can respond to acetazolamide. Treatment of electrolytes usually does not improve arrhythmias or, if so, only transiently. Improvement in symptomatic nonsustained ventricular tachycardia associated with a prolonged QT interval has been reported with beta-blocker therapy. Class 1A antiarrhythmic agents can worsen muscle weakness and exacerbate arrhythmias associated with a prolonged QT interval. Bidirectional ventricular tachycardia, not associated with a prolonged QT interval, may not respond to beta-blocker therapy. Amiodarone has been observed to decrease episodes of polymorphic ventricular tachycardia in Andersen-Tawil syndrome. The use of ICDs in patients with Andersen-Tawil syndrome has been described.

MITOCHONDRIAL DISORDERS

GENETICS. The mitochondrial disorders are a heterogeneous group of diseases resulting from abnormalities in mitochondrial DNA and function.[32] The number of distinct disorders is extensive. Mitochondrial DNA is inherited maternally, and most of these disorders are thus transmitted from mother to children of both sexes. Some of the disorders occur sporadically or are inherited in an autosomal fashion. Disease severity can vary among patients and family members because both mutant and normal mitochondrial DNA can be present in tissue in a variable proportion. This is not surprising on the basis of the important metabolic function of mitochondria that these disorders manifest with systemic pathology. Tissue with a high respiratory workload such as brain, skeletal muscle, and cardiac muscle are especially affected.

Mitochondrial disorders, which have cardiac manifestations, present as several clinical phenotypes including chronic progressive external ophthalmoplegia, which includes the Kearns-Sayre syndrome; myoclonus epilepsy with red ragged fibers (MERRF); mitochondrial myopathy, encephalopathy, lactic acidosis and strokelike episodes (MELAS); and Leber hereditary optic neuropathy. Other, more rare mitochondrial point mutation disorders present primarily with cardiac manifestations, typically a hypertrophic or dilated cardiomyopathy.[33] Chronic progressive external ophthalmoplegia is primarily a sporadic disease, whereas the others listed are maternally inherited.

CLINICAL PRESENTATION. *Kearns-Sayre syndrome* is characterized by the clinical triad of progressive external ophthalmoplegia, pigmentary retinopathy, and atrioventricular block. Diabetes, deafness, and ataxia can also be associated. Clinical features of MERRF include myoclonus, seizures, ataxia, dementia, and skeletal muscle weakness. MELAS is the most common of the maternally inherited mitochondrial disorders and is characterized by encephalopathy, subacute strokelike events, migraine-like headaches, recurrent emesis, extremity weakness, and short stature. *Leber hereditary optic neuropathy* manifests as a severe, subacute, painless loss of central vision, predominantly affecting young men.

CARDIOVASCULAR MANIFESTATIONS. In chronic progressive external ophthalmoplegia, most commonly in the Kearns-Sayre syndrome, cardiac involvement manifests primarily as conduction abnormalities.[34] A dilated cardiomyopathy has been reported. In the Kearns-Sayre syndrome, atrioventricular block is common, usually presenting after eye involvement. The HV interval is prolonged, consistent with distal conduction disease. Permanent pacing is often required by age 20. An increased prevalence of electrocardiographic preexcitation has also been reported.

Leber hereditary optic neuropathy can be associated with a short PR interval on the ECG and preexcitation. Supraventricular tachycardia has been reported.

In MERRF and MELAS, cardiac involvement manifesting as hypertrophic (symmetrical or asymmetrical) or dilated cardiomyopathy is observed. Other disorders caused by mitochondrial point mutations can present with a similar cardiac phenotype.[33] Patients can present

with chest pain with electrocardiographic abnormalities and myocardial perfusion defects. Whether the dilated cardiomyopathy represents a progression from the hypertrophic cardiomyopathy or a separate syndrome is not clear. The dilated cardiomyopathy can result in heart failure and death.

Preexcitation has been described with MELAS.

TREATMENT AND PROGNOSIS. In Kearns-Sayre syndrome, the implantation of a pacemaker has been advocated when significant or progressive conduction disease is evident including in asymptomatic patients.[9] The degree of conduction disease that warrants prophylactic pacing is not clear. In Leber hereditary optic neuropathy, a baseline ECG is prudent. In the other mitochondrial disorders, an understanding of the potential for cardiac involvement is necessary. Screening echocardiography has been recommended. Whether other specific screening evaluations are warranted in these disorders is uncertain. Therapy directed at improvement in the respiratory chain defects, for example, with coenzyme Q10, has not been uniformly demonstrated to be of benefit.

SPINAL MUSCULAR ATROPHY

GENETICS AND CLINICAL PRESENTATION. The spinal muscular atrophies are a group of lower motor neuron disorders presenting as progressive, symmetrical, proximal muscular weakness.[35] The disorders are inherited in an autosomal recessive fashion or are sporadic. The spinal muscular atrophies are classified clinically by the age of symptom onset and disease severity. *Type I (Werdnig-Hoffman disease)* has onset during the neonatal period typically with severe limitation of lifespan related to progressive paralysis. *Type II (intermediate form)* and *type III (Kugelberg-Welander disease)* are characterized by later childhood or even adult-onset (type III) and slower progression, typically with survival to adulthood.

The spinal muscular atrophies link to chromosome 5q13. Mutations or deletions in the telomeric *SMN* (survival of motor neuron) gene occur in more than 95 percent of patients. The loss of functional SMN protein results in premature neuronal cell death.[36]

CARDIOVASCULAR MANIFESTATIONS. Cardiac involvement in spinal muscular atrophies includes co-existing complex congenital heart disease, cardiomyopathy, and arrhythmias. Congenital heart disease has been associated with types I and III spinal muscular atrophies. The most common abnormality is atrial septal defect with other abnormalities reported. In spinal muscular atrophy type III, a dilated cardiomyopathy can occur with endomyocardial biopsies demonstrating fibrosis. Progression leading to a fatal outcome has been reported. Arrhythmia abnormalities including atrial standstill, atrial fibrillation, atrial flutter, and atrioventricular block appear to be the most common cardiac manifestation in these diseases. Permanent pacing for atrial standstill and atrioventricular block has been reported.

TREATMENT AND PROGNOSIS. In spinal muscular atrophy type I, severe skeletal muscle involvement with respiratory failure can limit life span to a significant degree such that treatment of associated cardiac abnormalities is often not indicated. In spinal muscular atrophy type III, awareness of the potential for associated cardiac abnormalities is necessary. Permanent pacing may be required. Gene therapy may hold future promise.

DESMIN-RELATED MYOPATHIES

GENETICS AND CLINICAL PRESENTATION. The desmin-related myopathies are a rare group of inherited skeletal muscle dystrophic disorders associated with a cardiomyopathy in more than half of affected patients.[37] Desmin is a cytoskeletal protein that functions as the chief intermediate filament providing support to contracting skeletal and cardiac muscle. A mouse model deficient in desmin develops both a skeletal and cardiac myopathy. The disorder is inherited in an autosomal dominant fashion or is sporadic. Mutations in the desmin gene leading to the inability of the protein to form functioning intermediate filaments are the cause of desmin-related myopathies. Mutations that lead to a cardiomyopathy without an apparent skeletal myopathy have been described.[38]

Patients typically present in their late 20s with distal weakness that progresses proximally. Difficulty with ambulation and, in severe cases, with respiration can occur. Creatine kinase has been observed to be mildly elevated in some patients. Muscle biopsy is diagnostic, showing desmin and other myofibrillar protein deposition with immunostaining.

CARDIOVASCULAR MANIFESTATIONS. The cardiomyopathy associated with the desmin-related myopathies can occur before or after the diagnosis of a skeletal myopathy. The cardiac involvement observed typically consists of conduction system dysfunction before the onset of a dilated or restrictive cardiomyopathy. Syncope with need for pacemaker implantation has been described. Both sudden and heart failure–related deaths can occur. Sudden death can occur despite pacemaker implantation.

TREATMENT AND PROGNOSIS. The desmin-related myopathies should be considered in the differential diagnosis in individuals or families presenting with skeletal and cardiac myopathies. Monitoring for the development of cardiac conduction and structural disease is indicated in affected families. Prophylactic pacemakers or ICDs should be considered in those patients with significant conduction disease, as in other neuromuscular disorders. Heart failure therapy in appropriate patients would seem indicated.

GUILLAIN-BARRÉ SYNDROME

CLINICAL PRESENTATION. The Guillain-Barré syndrome is an acute inflammatory demyelinating neuropathy characterized by peripheral, cranial, and autonomic nerve dysfunction.[39] It is the most common acquired demyelinating neuropathy with an annual incidence of 1 to 2 per 100,000 population. Men are more commonly affected than women. In two thirds of affected patients an acute viral or bacterial illness, typically respiratory or gastrointestinal, precedes the onset of neurological symptoms within 6 weeks. The disorder typically presents with pain, paresthesias, and symmetrical limb weakness that progresses proximally and can involve cranial and respiratory muscles. Approximately one fourth of patients require assisted ventilation.

CARDIOVASCULAR MANIFESTATIONS. Nonambulant patients are at increased risk for deep venous thrombosis and pulmonary emboli. Cardiac involvement in Guillain-Barré syndrome is related to accompanying autonomic nervous system dysfunction that manifests as hypertension, orthostatic hypotension, resting sinus tachycardia, loss of heart rate variability, electrocardiographic ST abnormalities, and both bradycardia and tachycardia. Significant autonomic nervous system dysfunction occurs in about 20 percent of patients with Guillain-Barré syndrome, primarily in severe cases.[39] Microneurographic recordings have shown increased sympathetic outflow during the acute illness that normalizes with recovery.

Life-threatening arrhythmias are common in severe cases of Guillain-Barré syndrome, primarily those requiring assisted ventilation. Arrhythmias observed include asystole, symptomatic bradycardia, rapid atrial fibrillation, and ventricular tachycardia/fibrillation. Deaths caused by arrhythmias occur. Asystole was commonly associated with tracheal suctioning.

TREATMENT AND PROGNOSIS. Supportive care should include deep venous thrombosis prophylaxis in nonambulant patients. Early plasmapheresis or intravenous immunoglobulin can improve recovery. In severely affected patients, especially those requiring assisted ventilation, cardiac rhythm monitoring is mandatory. If serious bradycardia or asystole is observed, temporary or permanent pacing can improve survival. Atropine or isoproterenol during tracheal suctioning can be of benefit. The mortality rate in patients hospitalized with Guillain-Barré syndrome is as high as 15 percent. In patients who recover from Guillain-Barré syndrome, autonomic function also recovers and long-term arrhythmia risk has not been observed.

MYASTHENIA GRAVIS

CLINICAL PRESENTATION. Myasthenia gravis is a disorder of neuromuscular transmission resulting from production of antibody targeted against the nicotinic acetylcholine receptor. The primary symptom, fluctuating weakness, usually begins with the eye and facial muscles and later can involve the large muscles of the limbs. Patients can present at any age, typically at a younger age in women and an older age in men. Myasthenia gravis is usually associated with hyperplasia or a benign or malignant tumor (thymoma) of the thymus gland. The prevalence of myasthenia gravis is 50 to 125 cases per million population.

CARDIOVASCULAR MANIFESTATIONS. A myocarditis can occur in patients with myasthenia gravis, especially in those with thymoma. Up to 16 percent of patients with myasthenia gravis have cardiac manifestations not explained by another etiology. Presentation with arrhythmia symptoms including atrial fibrillation, atrioventricular block, asystole, and unexplained sudden death or heart failure is typical. Autopsy findings are consistent with myocarditis.

TREATMENT AND PROGNOSIS. Myasthenia gravis is treated with anticholinesterase and immunosuppressive agents. Thymectomy is often indicated. Anticholinesterase agents may slow heart rate and cause hypotension. Whether immunosuppressive agents or thymec-

tomy improve associated cardiac disease is unknown. Case reports have described patients developing rapidly progressive and fatal heart failure within weeks after thymoma resection, with histology showing giant cell myocarditis.[40]

EPILEPSY

CARDIOVASCULAR MANIFESTATIONS. Epilepsy is a complex brain disorder characterized by chronic seizures.[41] Patients with epilepsy are at an increased risk of sudden death of unknown cause. Sudden unexpected (unexplained) death in epilepsy (SUDEP) is responsible for 2 to 18 percent of all deaths, with an incidence estimated at 1 per 1000 patient-years.[42] The underlying mechanisms leading to SUDEP are not clear. The majority of witnessed sudden deaths occur at or in proximity to the time of a seizure, with respiratory compromise observed. Severe bradycardia with sinus arrest has been documented to occur in a small number of monitored patients during seizures.[43] Whether the bradycardia has any role in the sudden death observed in epileptic patients is not clear. An undiagnosed primary ventricular arrhythmia disorder such as the long QT syndrome or right ventricular dysplasia can present with symptoms suggestive of epilepsy and thus could be responsible for a small proportion of the sudden deaths.

Risk factors for sudden unexpected death in epilepsy include a higher seizure frequency, a longer duration of epilepsy, and the use of three or more antiepileptic drugs.[44] Epileptic patients with these significant factors can be at as high a risk for sudden death as 1 percent per year.

TREATMENT AND PROGNOSIS. A primary arrhythmia disorder must be considered in the differential diagnosis of epilepsy. Patients with poorly controlled epilepsy should be aggressively evaluated and treated.[42] Nighttime supervision of the epileptic patient may decrease the risk of sudden unexpected death.[45]

ACUTE CEREBROVASCULAR DISEASE (see Chap. 58)

CARDIOVASCULAR MANIFESTATIONS. Acute cerebrovascular diseases including subarachnoid hemorrhage, other stroke syndromes, and head injury can be associated with severe cardiac manifestations.[46] The mechanism by which cardiac abnormalities occur with brain injury appears to be related to autonomic nervous system dysfunction, with both an increased sympathetic and parasympathetic output. Excessive myocardial catecholamine release is primarily responsible for the observed cardiac pathology. Hypothalamic stimulation can reproduce the electrocardiographic changes observed in acute cerebrovascular disease. Electrocardiographic changes associated with hypothalamic stimulation or blood in the subarachnoid space can be diminished with spinal cord transection, stellate ganglion blockade, vagolytics, and adrenergic blockers.

Electrocardiographic abnormalities are observed in approximately 70 percent of patients with subarachnoid hemorrhage.[47] Abnormalities including ST elevation and depression, T wave inversion, and pathologic Q waves are observed. Peaked inverted T waves and a prolonged QT interval can occur in a significant proportion of patients with abnormal ECGs (Fig. 87-16). Hypokalemia can be seen in patients with subarachnoid hemorrhage and can increase the likelihood of QT interval prolongation. Other stroke syndromes are often associated with abnormal ECGs, but whether these are related to the stroke syndrome or to underlying intrinsic cardiac disease is often difficult to discern. A prolonged QT interval is more common in subarachnoid hemorrhage than in other stroke syndromes. Closed head trauma can cause electrocardiographic abnormalities similar to those in subarachnoid hemorrhage including a prolonged QT interval.

Myocardial damage with liberation of myocardial enzymes and subendocardial hemorrhage or fibrosis at autopsy can occur in the setting of acute cerebral disease.[47,48]

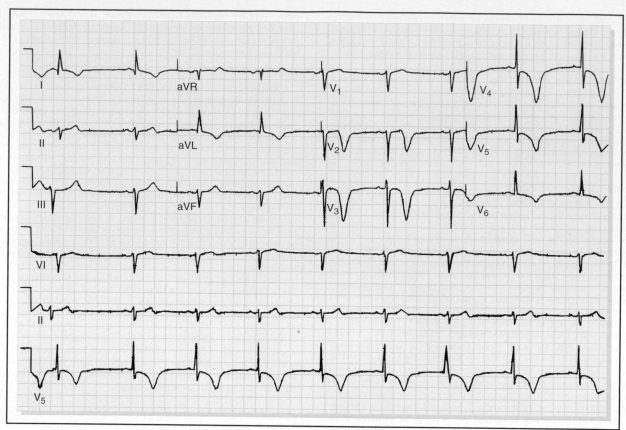

FIGURE 87–16 Electrocardiogram from a patient with cerebral hemorrhage. Deep and symmetrical T wave inversions are observed. *(Courtesy of Charles Fisch, M.D., Indiana University School of Medicine, Indianapolis.)*

Cardiac troponin I level elevation and echocardiographic evidence of left ventricular dysfunction is present in a significant proportion of patients with subarachnoid hemorrhage. Patients with poorer neurological status at admission are more likely to have an increased peak troponin level. Women are at higher risk of myocardial necrosis.

Neurogenic pulmonary edema may accompany the acute neurological insult. The edema can have both a cardiogenic component, related to systemic hypertension, and a noncardiogenic (pulmonary capillary leak) component.

Life-threatening arrhythmias can occur in the setting of acute cerebrovascular disease. Ventricular tachycardia or fibrillation has been observed in patients with subarachnoid hemorrhage and head trauma. A torsades de pointes–type ventricular tachycardia can occur (Fig. 87-17). Often this is observed in the setting of a prolonged QT interval and hypokalemia. Stroke syndromes, other than subarachnoid hemorrhage, appear to be only rarely associated with serious ventricular tachycardias. Atrial arrhythmias including atrial fibrillation and regular supraventricular tachycardia have been observed. Atrial fibrillation is most common in patients presenting with what is believed to be an acute thromboembolic stroke. Separating an effect from the cause can be difficult. Bradycardias including sinoatrial block, sinus arrest, and atrioventricular block occur in up to 10 percent of patients with subarachnoid hemorrhage.

TREATMENT AND PROGNOSIS. Beta-adrenergic blockers appear effective in decreasing myocardial damage and in controlling both supraventricular and ventricular arrhythmias associated with subarachnoid hemorrhage and head trauma. Beta-adrenergic blockers can increase the likelihood of bradycardia and cannot be used in patients with hypotension requiring vasopressors. Life-threatening arrhythmias occur primarily in the first day following the neurological event. Continuous electrocardiographic monitoring during this period is indicated. Careful monitoring of potassium levels, especially in patients with subarachnoid hemorrhage, is warranted. Refractory ventricular arrhythmias have been controlled effectively with stellate ganglion blockade. Electrocardiographic abnormalities reflect unfavorable intracranial factors but do not appear to portend a poor cardiovascular outcome. The magnitude of peak troponin elevation is predictive for adverse patient outcomes including severe disability at hospital discharge and death.[47] Other than the mortality occurring secondary to acute arrhythmias, the observed myocardial necrosis does not appear to play a major factor affecting outcome.

Head injury (blunt trauma or gunshot wound) and cerebrovascular accident are the leading causes of brain death in patients being considered as heart donors. These donors can manifest electrocardiographic abnormalities, hemodynamic instability, and myocardial dysfunction related primarily to adrenergic storm and not to intrinsic cardiac disease. Experimental studies on whether contractile performance recovers with transplantation are still controversial. Optimization of volume status and inotropic support with careful echocardiographic evaluation and possibly left heart catheterization can allow the use of some donor hearts that would have otherwise been rejected.

FUTURE PERSPECTIVES

Increasing understanding of both the mechanisms and clinical presentations of cardiac involvement can occur in neurological diseases. Such knowledge will continue to grow

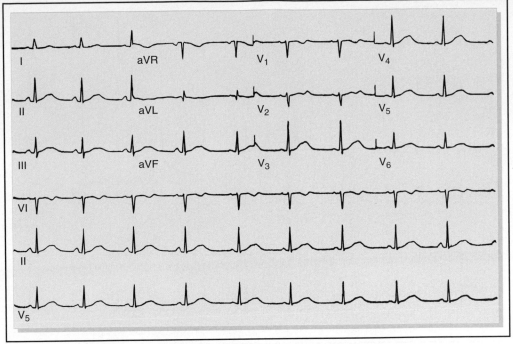

A

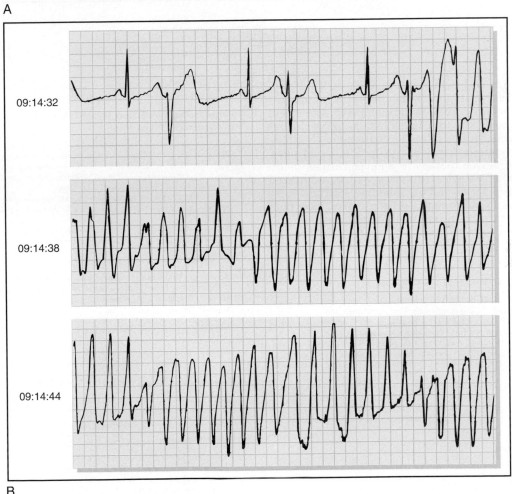

B

FIGURE 87–17 A 49-year-old patient with cerebral hemorrhage. **A,** Electrocardiogram recorded within 3 hours of admission and 4 hours after onset of symptoms. QT interval prolongation is observed. **B,** Electrocardiographic monitoring 6 hours after admission. Ventricular bigeminy precedes the onset of polymorphic ventricular tachycardia. Cardioversion was required. The patient was subsequently treated with a beta-adrenergic blocker without further ventricular tachycardia.

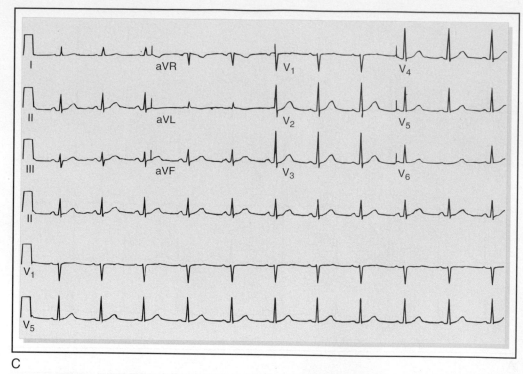

FIGURE 87–17, cont'd C, Electrocardiogram done 2 weeks after admission. The QT interval has normalized.

in the future. As the ability to care for patients with dystrophic muscular diseases improves, the proportion of patients manifesting symptoms related to cardiac involvement will increase. Cardiologists and cardiac electrophysiologists will be more commonly consulted for management of these patients. Controversies regarding appropriate use of pharmacotherapy and device therapy to manage cardiac manifestations in the neurological diseases will be addressed further with patient series and nonrandomized trials. Gene therapy continues to hold much future promise. How both the skeletal and cardiac muscle pathology improves with gene therapy remains to be seen.

REFERENCES

Duchenne and Becker Muscular Dystrophies

1. Lapidos KA, Kakkar R, McNally EM: The dystrophin glycoprotein complex: Signaling strength and integrity for the sarcolemma. Circ Res 94:1023, 2004.
2. Jefferies JL, Eidem BW, Belmont JW, et al: Genetic predictors and remodeling of dilated cardiomyopathy in muscular dystrophy. Circulation 112:2799, 2005.
3. Corrado G, Lissoni A, Beretta S, et al: Prognostic value of electrocardiograms, ventricular late potentials, ventricular arrhythmias, and left ventricular systolic dysfunction in patients with Duchenne muscular dystrophy. Am J Cardiol 89:838, 2002.
4. Chakkalakal JV, Thompson J, Parks RJ, et al: Molecular, cellular, and pharmacological therapies for Duchenne/Becker muscular dystrophies. FASEB 19:880, 2005.
5. Duboc D, Meune C, Lerebours G, et al: Effect of perindopril on the onset and progression of left ventricular dysfunction in Duchenne muscular dystrophy. J Am Coll Cardiol 45:855, 2005.

Myotonic Dystrophies

6. Groh WJ, Lowe MR, Zipes DP: Severity of cardiac conduction involvement and arrhythmias in myotonic dystrophy type 1 correlates with age and CTG repeat length. J Cardiovasc Electrophysiol 13:444, 2002.
7. Day JW, Ricker K, Jacobsen JF, et al: Myotonic dystrophy type 2: molecular, diagnostic and clinical spectrum. Neurology 60:657, 2003.
8. Bhakta D, Lowe MR, Groh WJ: Prevalence of structural cardiac abnormalities in patients with myotonic dystrophy type I. Am Heart J 147:224, 2004.
9. Gregoratos G, Abrams J, Epstein AE, et al: ACC/AHA/NASPE 2002 guideline update for implantation of cardiac pacemakers and antiarrhythmia device. Circulation 106:2145, 2002.
10. de Die-Smulders CE, Howeler CJ, Thijs C, et al: Age and causes of death in adult-onset myotonic dystrophy. Brain 121:1557, 1998.

11. Schoser BG, Ricker K, Schneider-Gold C, et al: Sudden cardiac death in myotonic dystrophy type 2. Neurology 63:2402, 2004.

Emery-Dreifuss Muscular Dystrophies and Associated Disorders

12. van der Kooi AJ, Bonne G, Eymard B, et al: Lamin A/C mutations with lipodystrophy, cardiac abnormalities, and muscular dystrophy. Neurology 59:620, 2002.
13. Sakata K, Shimizu M, Ino H, et al: High incidence of sudden cardiac death with conduction disturbances and atrial cardiomyopathy caused by a nonsense mutation in the STA gene. Circulation 111:3352, 2005.
14. Bushby KM, Beckmann JS: The 105th ENMC sponsored workshop: Pathogenesis in the non-sarcoglycan limb-girdle muscular dystrophies. Neuromusc Disord 13:80, 2003.
15. Meune C, Van Berlo JH, Anselme F, et al: Primary prevention of sudden death in patients with lamin A/C gene mutations. N Engl J Med 354:209, 2006.

Limb-Girdle Muscular Dystrophies

16. Kirschner J, Bonnemann CG: The congenital and limb-girdle muscular dystrophies: Sharpening the focus, blurring the boundaries. Arch Neurol 61:189, 2004.
17. Mathews KD, Moore SA: Limb-girdle muscular dystrophy. Curr Neurol Neurosci Rep 3:78, 2003.
18. Wheeler MT, Allikian MJ, Heydemann A, et al: Smooth muscle cell-extrinsic vascular spasm arises from cardiomyocyte degeneration in sarcoglycan-deficient cardiomyopathy. J Clin Invest 113:668, 2004.
19. Poppe M, Bourke J, Eagle M, et al: Cardiac and respiratory failure in limb-girdle muscular dystrophy 2I. Ann Neurol 56:738, 2004.

Facioscapulohumeral Muscular Dystrophy

20. Gabellini D, Green MR, Tupler R: Inappropriate gene activation in FSHD: A repressor complex binds a chromosomal repeat deleted in dystrophic muscle. Cell 110:339, 2002.

Friedreich Ataxia

21. Lynch DR, Farmer JM, Balcer LJ, et al: Friedreich ataxia: Effects of genetic understanding on clinical evaluation and therapy. Arch Neurol 59:743, 2002.
22. Lodi R, Rajagopalan B, Blamire AM, et al: Cardiac energetics are abnormal in Friedreich ataxia patients in the absence of cardiac dysfunction and hypertrophy: An in vivo 31P magnetic resonance spectroscopy study. Cardiovasc Res 52:111, 2001.
23. Isnard R, Kalotka H, Durr A, et al: Correlation between left ventricular hypertrophy and GAA trinucleotide repeat length in Friedreich's ataxia. Circulation 95:2247, 1997.
24. Mariotti C, Solari A, Torta D, et al: Idebenone treatment in Friedreich patients: One-year-long randomized placebo-controlled trial. Neurology 60:1676, 2003.
25. Hausse AO, Aggoun Y, Bonnet D, et al: Idebenone and reduced cardiac hypertrophy in Friedreich's ataxia. Heart 87:346, 2002.

Less Common Neuromuscular Diseases Associated with Cardiac Manifestations

26. Bulman DE, Scoggan KA, van Oene MD, et al: A novel sodium channel mutation in a family with hypokalemic periodic paralysis. Neurology 53:1932, 1999.

27. Ptacek LJ: Channelopathies: Ion channel disorders of muscle as a paradigm for paroxysmal disorders of the nervous system. Neuromusc Disord 7:250, 1997.

28. Yoon G, Oberoi S, Tristani-Firouzi M, et al: Andersen-Tawil syndrome: Prospective cohort analysis and expansion of the phenotype. Am J Medical Genet 140:312, 2006.

29. Plaster NM, Tawil R, Tristani-Firouzi M, et al: Mutations in Kir2.1 cause the developmental and episodic electrical phenotypes of Andersen's syndrome. Cell 105:511, 2001.

30. Zhang L, Benson DW, Tristani-Firouzi M, et al: Electrocardiographic features in Andersen-Tawil syndrome patients with KCNJ2 mutations: characteristic T-U-wave patterns predict the KCNJ2 genotype. Circulation 111:2720, 2005.

31. Tristani-Firouzi M, Jensen JL, Donaldson MR, et al: Functional and clinical characterization of KCNJ2 mutations associated with LQT7 (Andersen syndrome). J Clin Invest 110:381, 2002.

32. Wallace DC: Mitochondrial defects in cardiomyopathy and neuromuscular disease. Am Heart J 139:S70, 2000.

33. Santorelli FM, Tessa A, D'Amati G, et al: The emerging concept of mitochondrial cardiomyopathies. Am Heart J 141:E1, 2001.

34. Anan R, Nakagawa M, Miyata M, et al: Cardiac involvement in mitochondrial diseases. A study on 17 patients with documented mitochondrial DNA defects. Circulation 91:955, 1995.

35. Iannaccone ST; American Spinal Muscular Atrophy Randomized Trials (AmSMART) Group: Outcome measures for pediatric spinal muscular atrophy. Arch Neurol 59:1445, 2002.

36. Kerr DA, Nery JP, Traystman RJ, et al: Survival motor neuron protein modulates neuron-specific apoptosis. PNAS 97:13312, 2000.

37. Dalakas MC, Park KY, Semino-Mora C, et al: Desmin myopathy, a skeletal myopathy with cardiomyopathy caused by mutations in the desmin gene. N Engl J Med 342:770, 2000.

38. Li D, Tapscoft T, Gonzalez O, et al: Desmin mutation responsible for idiopathic dilated cardiomyopathy. Circulation 100:461, 1999.

39. Hughes RA, Cornblath DR: Guillain-Barré syndrome. Lancet 366:1653, 2005.

40. Joudinaud TM, Fadel E, Thomas-de-Montpreville V, et al: Fatal giant cell myocarditis after thymoma resection in myasthenia gravis. J Thor Cardiovasc Surg 131:494, 2006.

41. Duncan JS, Sander JW, Sisodiya SM, et al: Adult epilepsy. Lancet 367:1087, 2006.

42. Pedley TA, Hauser WA: Sudden death in epilepsy: A wake-up call for management. Lancet 359:1790, 2002.

43. Rugg-Gunn FJ, Simister RJ, Squirrell M, et al: Cardiac arrhythmias in focal epilepsy: A prospective long-term study. Lancet 364:2212, 2004.

44. Walczak TS, Leppik IE, D'Amelio M, et al: Incidence and risk factors in sudden unexpected death in epilepsy: A prospective cohort study. Neurology 56:519, 2001.

Acute Cerebrovascular Disease

45. Langan Y, Nashef L, Sander JW: Case-control study of SUDEP. Neurology 64:1131, 2005.

46. Sakr YL, Ghosn I, Vincent JL: Cardiac manifestations after subarachnoid hemorrhage: A systematic review of the literature. Prog Cardiovasc Dis 45:67, 2002.

47. Naidech AM, Kreiter KT, Janjua N, et al: Cardiac troponin elevation, cardiovascular morbidity, and outcome after subarachnoid hemorrhage. Circulation 112:2851, 2005.

48. Tung P, Kopelnik A, Banki N, et al: Predictors of neurocardiogenic injury after subarachnoid hemorrhage. Stroke 35:548, 2004.

CH 87

Neurological Disorders and Cardiovascular Disease

CHAPTER 88

Cardiorenal Intersection, 2155

Chronic Kidney Disease and Cardiovascular Risk, 2155

Implications of Anemia Caused by Chronic Kidney Disease, 2156

Contrast-Induced Nephropathy, 2158

Prevention of Contrast-Induced Nephropathy, 2159

Acceleration of Vascular Calcification, 2161

Renal Disease and Hypertension, 2162

Diagnosis of Acute Coronary Syndromes in Patients with Chronic Kidney Disease, 2162

Renal Dysfunction as a Prognostic Factor in Acute Coronary Syndromes, 2163

Reasons for Poor Outcomes after Acute Coronary Syndromes in Patients with Renal Dysfunction, 2163

Treatment of Acute Myocardial Infarction in Patients with Renal Dysfunction, 2163

Chronic Kidney Disease Complicating Heart Failure, 2164

Chronic Kidney Disease and Valvular Heart Disease, 2166

Renal Function and Arrhythmias, 2166

Consultative Approach to the Hemodialysis Patient, 2166

Summary, 2168

References, 2169

Interface Between Renal Disease and Cardiovascular Illness

Peter A. McCullough

CARDIORENAL INTERSECTION

The heart and kidney are inextricably linked in terms of hemodynamic and regulatory functions. In a normal 70-kg man, each kidney weighs about 130 to 170 gm and receives blood flow of 400 ml/min per 100 gm, which is approximately 20 to 25 percent of the cardiac output, allowing the needed flow to maintain glomerular filtration by approximately 1 million nephrons (Fig. 88-1). This flow is several times greater per unit weight than the blood flow through most other organs. Although the oxygen extraction is low, the kidneys account for about 8 percent of the total oxygen consumption of the body. The kidney has a central role in electrolyte balance, volume, and blood pressure regulation. Communication between these two organs occurs at multiple levels including the sympathetic nervous system, the renin-angiotensin-aldosterone system (RAAS), antidiuretic hormone, endothelin, and the natriuretic peptides (Fig. 88-2). With the understanding of these systems has come the development of key diagnostic and therapeutic targets in cardiovascular medicine.

The obesity pandemic in developed countries is a central driver of secondary epidemics of type II diabetes mellitus (DM) and hypertension (HTN) often leading to combined chronic kidney disease (CKD) and cardiovascular disease (CVD).[1] Among those with DM for 25 years or more, the prevalence of diabetic nephropathy in type I and type II DM is 57 and 48 percent, respectively.[2] Approximately half of all cases of end-stage renal disease (ESRD) are caused by diabetic nephropathy. With the aging of the general population and cardiovascular care shifting toward the elderly population, an understanding of why decreasing levels of renal function act as a major adverse prognostic factor after a variety of cardiac events is imperative. Considerable evidence shows that CKD accelerates atherosclerosis, myocardial disease, and valvular disease and promotes an array of cardiac arrhythmias leading to sudden death in many cases.[3]

CHRONIC KIDNEY DISEASE AND CARDIOVASCULAR RISK

Chronic kidney disease (CKD) is defined through a range of estimated glomerular filtration rate (eGFR) values by the National Kidney Foundation Kidney Disease Outcomes Quality Initiative (KDOQI).[4] A common definition for CKD stipulates an eGFR of less than 60 ml/min/1.73 m^2 or the presence of kidney damage (Fig. 88-3). Although with normative aging (age 20 to 80), the eGFR declines from about 130 to 60 ml/min/1.73 m^2, a variety of pathobiological processes appear to begin when the eGFR drops below 60 ml/min/1.73 m^2. Most studies of cardiovascular outcomes have found that a critical cut point for the development of contrast-induced nephropathy (CIN), restenosis after percutaneous coronary intervention (PCI), recurrent myocardial infarction (MI), diastolic/systolic heart failure (HF), arrhythmias, and CVD is an eGFR of 60 ml/min/1.73 m^2, which roughly corresponds to a serum creatinine (Cr) greater than 1.5 mg/dl in the general population (Fig. 88-4).[4-8] Because Cr is a crude indicator of renal function and often underestimates renal dysfunction in women and the elderly, calculated measures of eGFR or Cr clearance (CrCl) using the Cockcroft-Gault equation or the Modification of Diet in Renal Disease equation are superior methods for the assessment of renal function.[4] The four-variable Modification of Diet in Renal Disease equation for eGFR is the preferred method because it does not rely on body weight.[4] The equation follows:

$$CrCl = 186.3 \times (\text{serum } Cr^{-1.154}) \times (\text{age}^{-.203})$$

and calculated values are multiplied by .742 for women and by 1.21 for African Americans. A recently approved blood test reflecting renal filtration function is the cystatin C test.[9] Cystatin C is a nonglycosylated, low-molecular-mass (13 kDa) protein produced by all nucleated cells. Its low molecular mass and its high isoelectric point allow it to be freely filtered by the glomerular membrane and 100 percent reabsorbed by the proximal tubule. The serum concentration of cystatin C correlates with eGFR and, in combination with a stable production rate, provides a sensitive marker of renal filtration function. Serum levels of cystatin C are independent of weight and height, muscle mass, age, and sex, making it less variable than

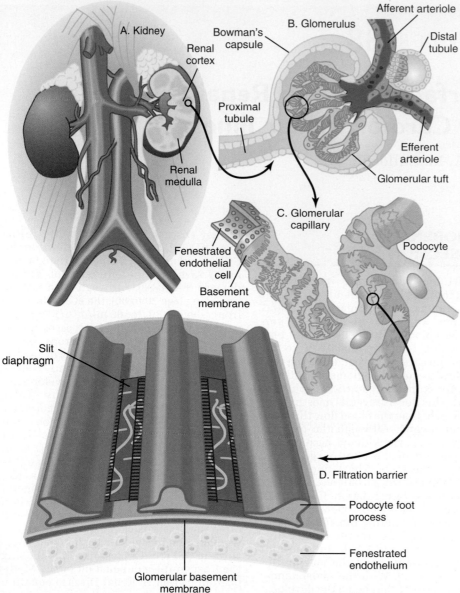

FIGURE 88–1 Normal structure of the glomerular vasculature. Each kidney contains about 1 million glomeruli in the renal cortex **(A). B,** An afferent arteriole entering a Bowman's capsule and branching into several capillaries that form the glomerular tuft; the walls of the capillaries constitute the actual filter. The plasma filtrate (primary urine) is directed to the proximal tubule, whereas the unfiltered blood returns to the circulation through the efferent arteriole. The filtration barrier of the capillary wall contains an innermost fenestrated endothelium, the glomerular basement membrane, and a layer of interdigitating podocyte foot processes **(C). D,** Cross section through the glomerular capillary depicts the fenestrated endothelial layer and the glomerular basement membrane with overlying podocyte foot processes. An ultrathin slit diaphragm spans the filtration slit between the foot processes, slightly above the basement membrane. In order to show the slit diaphragm, the foot processes are drawn smaller than actual scale. *(Modified from Tryggvason K, Patrakka J, Waraiovaara J: Hereditary proteinuria syndromes and mechanisms of proteinuria. N Engl J Med 354:1387-1401, 2006.)*

Cr. Furthermore, measurements can be made and interpreted from a single random sample with reference intervals in women and men being 0.54 and 1.21 mg/liter (median 0.85 mg/liter, range 0.42 to 1.39 mg/liter).

In addition, microalbuminuria at any level of eGFR is considered to represent CKD and has been thought to occur as the result of endothelial dysfunction in glomerular capillaries secondary to the metabolic syndrome, DM, and HTN.[10] The most widely accepted definition of microalbuminuria is a random urine albumin-to-Cr ratio (ACR) of 30 to 300 mg/ gm. An ACR greater than 300 mg/gm is considered gross proteinuria. The random, spot urine ACR is the office test for microalbuminuria recommended as part of the cardiovascular risk assessment done by cardiologists and other

specialists. Microalbuminuria as an independent CVD risk factor for both diabetics and those without DM is covered elsewhere in this text. The Seventh Report of the Joint National Committee on Prevention, Detection, Evaluation, and Treatment of High Blood Pressure (JNC 7) has recognized CKD as an independent cardiovascular risk state.[10] This risk state has a host of vascular and metabolic abnormalities, which are discussed subsequently (Fig. 88-5).[11]

IMPLICATIONS OF ANEMIA CAUSED BY CHRONIC KIDNEY DISEASE

Recognition of the associations among blood hemoglobin (Hb) level, CKD, and CVD is increasing. The most commonly used definition of anemia by the World Health Organization calls for an Hb level less than 13 g/dl in men and less than 12 g/dl in women. Approximately 9 percent of the general adult population meets the definition of anemia at these levels. In general, anemia caused by CKD is present in 20 percent of patients with stable coronary disease and 30 to 60 percent of patients with HF. Hence anemia is a common and easily identifiable potential diagnostic and therapeutic target.[12-13]

Anemia contributes to multiple adverse outcomes, in part because of decreased tissue oxygen delivery and utilization.[13] The cause of anemia in patients with CKD can be multifactorial with a central component being a relative deficiency of erythropoietin-α (EPO), an erythrocyte-stimulating protein (ESP) that is normally produced by renal parenchymal cells in response to blood partial pressure of oxygen. Normal plasma EPO levels range from 10 to 30 IU/ml, but during anemic periods these levels may be elevated up to 100. In patients with CKD and HF, there appears to be a relative EPO deficiency with an inappropriately low EPO level for the measured blood Hb level. This relative deficiency of EPO may not only be related to anemia but may also play a role in impaired vascular repair, thus contributing indirectly to the progression of atherosclerosis. In addition, in the setting of CKD and HF, there are increased levels of tumor necrosis factor-alpha, interleukins 1 and 6, endothelin, matrix metalloproteinases, and other inflammation-related proteins that are produced by the heart itself. These factors can work to directly reduce red blood cell production at the level of the bone marrow and further worsen the anemia. In a recent review, 28 of 29 large prospective studies of HF have found anemia to be an independent predictor of mortality.[14] On average, among those patients with HF, for each 1 g/dl decrement in Hb, there is a 13 percent increase in risk for all-cause mortality.[13] In addition, those patients with anemia and CKD are more likely to progress to ESRD irrespective of their baseline level of renal function. Thus, anemia contributes independently to the progression of CKD.[2] As Hb drops over time, there is a graded increase in HF hospitalizations and death. Conversely, those patients who have had a rise in Hb, whether because of improved nutrition, reduced neurohormonal factors or other unknown factors, enjoy a significant reduction in endpoints over the next several years. This improvement has been associated with a significant reduction in left ventricular mass index, suggesting a favorable change in left ventricular remodeling.[15] The observational data suggest that changes in Hb, either up or down, are associated with clinical consequences. Hence there is a rationale for intervention on the Hb level in order to change the natural history of cardiorenal disease.

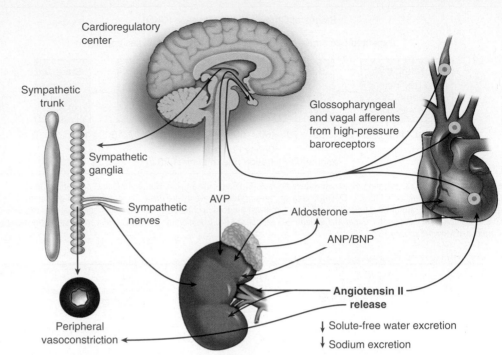

FIGURE 88–2 Major neurohumoral communication systems between the heart and kidney. ANP = A-type natriuretic peptide; AVP = arginine vasopressin; BNP = B-type natriuretic peptide. (*Modified from Schrier RW, Abraham WT: Hormones and hemodynamics in heart failure. N Engl J Med 341:577, 1999.*)

Besides the effect on Hb levels, the pleiotropic effects of ESPs include positive effects on coronary endothelium resulting in an increase in coronary flow reserve. This effect may be mediated through the activation of endothelial nitric oxide synthase via protein kinase B phosphorylation and by preventing endothelial cell apoptosis. These proteins may also have the potential for enhancing myocardial repair in patients with myocardial injury that could minimize the progression of left ventricular dysfunction by recruiting vascular progenitor cells, which can become functional myocardial cells, thereby increasing the contractile function of the injured ventricle. The molecular target for ESPs includes receptors expressed on cardiac myocytes, endothelial cells, and endothelial progenitor cells in addition to hematopoietic stem cells.

Treatment of anemia with exogenous ESPs (EPO and darbepoetin-alpha) in CKD has shown promise in reducing morbidity, particularly that of cardiovascular origin, and in improving survival and quality of life. Darbepoetin-alpha is a genetically engineered form of EPO designed to have a longer half-

Criteria

1. Kidney damage for ≥ 3 months, as defined by structural or functional abnormalities of the kidney, with or without decreased GFR, manifest by *either:*
   - Pathological abnormalities; or
   - Markers of kidney damage, including abnormalities in the composition of the blood or urine, or abnormalities in imaging tests
2. eGFR<60 mL/min/1.73m^2 for ≥ 3 months, with or without kidney damage

Markers of kidney damage	Findings indicating kidney damage
Proteinuria	Albumin-to-creatinine ratio >30 mg/g
Urine sediment abnormalities	Cellular casts, coarse granular casts, fat
Imaging tests	Abnormalities in kidney size Asymmetry in kidney size or function Irregularities in shape (cysts, scars, mass lesions) Stones Hydronephrosis and other abnormalities of the urinary tract Arterial stenosis and other vascular lesions
Abnormalities in blood or urine composition	Nephrotic syndrome Tubular syndromes (renal tubular acidosis, potassium secretory defects, renal glycosuria, renal phosphaturia, Fanconi's syndrome)

FIGURE 88–3 Diagnostic criteria for chronic kidney disease and kidney damage. eGFR = estimated glomerular filtration rate.

life, making once-monthly injections an attractive treatment option.[13] Increasing the Hb level from below 10 g/dl to 12 g/dl has been linked to favorable changes in left ventricular remodeling, improved ejection fraction, improved functional classification, and higher levels of peak oxygen consumption with exercise testing. However, there is a state of equipoise on this issue because treatment with EPO and supplemental iron, which is necessary in approximately 70 percent of cases, has been associated with three problems: (1) increased platelet activ-

ity, thrombin generation, and resultant increased risk of thrombosis; (2) increased endothelin levels, increased asymmetric dimethylarginine, which theoretically reduces nitric oxide availability and results in HTN; and (3) worsened measures of oxidative stress. Two randomized trials in CKD indicate that treatment with ESPs to higher hemoglobin targets resulted in higher CVD events. The Cardiovascular Risk Reduction by Early Anemic Treatment with Epoetin beta in Chronic Kidney Disease Patients (CREATE) Trial randomized 600 patients to

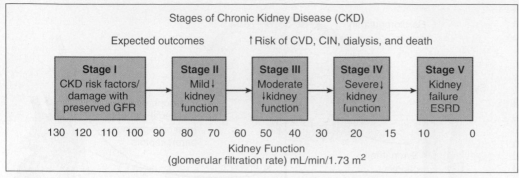

FIGURE 88–4 The classification of chronic kidney disease (CKD) according to the National Kidney Foundation Kidney Disease Outcomes Quality Initiative (KDOQI). Increased rates of adverse events are generally seen below an estimated glomerular filtration rate of 60 ml/min/1.73 m2. CIN = contrast-induced nephropathy; ESRD = end-stage renal disease; GFR = glomerular filtration rate. *(From McCullough PA, Sandberg KR: Epidemiology of contrast-induced nephropathy. Rev Cardiovasc Med 4(Suppl 5):S3-9, 2003.)*

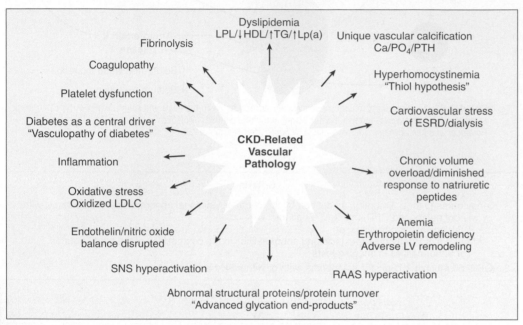

FIGURE 88–5 The pathobiology of the chronic kidney disease (CKD) state and its effects on the cardiovascular system. Ca = calcium; ESRD = end-stage renal disease; HDL = high-density lipoprotein; LDL-C = low-density lipoprotein cholesterol; Lp(a) = lipoprotein (a); LPL = lipoprotein lipase; LV = left ventricle; PO_4 = phosphate; PTH = parathyroid hormone; RAAS = renin-angiotensin-aldosterone system; SNS = sympathetic nervous system; TG = triglyceride. *(Modified from McCullough PA: Why is chronic kidney disease the "spoiler" for cardiovascular outcomes? J Am Coll Cardiol 41;725, 2003.)*

CH 88

CONTRAST-INDUCED NEPHROPATHY

Contrast-induced nephropathy (CIN), a form of acute kidney injury, is most commonly defined as a rise in serum Cr greater than 25 percent or greater than 0.5 mg/dl from baseline after intravascular administration of iodinated contrast (see Chaps. 20 and 55).[19] The frequency of CIN is approximately 13 percent in nondiabetics and 20 percent in diabetics undergoing PCI. It is critical to understand that the risk of CIN is related in a curvilinear fashion to the eGFR (see Fig. 88-6).[20] Fortunately, among patients undergoing PCI, cases of CIN leading to dialysis are rare (0.5 to 2 percent). However, when they occur, they are related to catastrophic outcomes including a 36 percent in-hospital mortality rate and a 2-year survival of only 19 percent.[21] Although not always attributed to CIN, transient rises in Cr are directly related to longer intensive care unit and hospital ward stays (3 and 4 more days, respectively) after bypass surgery.[19] Even transient rises in Cr translate to differences in adjusted long-term outcomes after PCI (Fig. 88-7).[22]

Three core elements in the pathophysiology of CIN are (1) direct toxicity of iodinated contrast material to nephrons, (2) microshowers of atheroemboli to the kidneys, and (3) contrast material– and atheroemboli-induced intrarenal vasoconstriction. Furthermore, as renal function declines, a host of chronic perturbations occur in hemostasis, lipids, endothelial function, protein metabolism, calcium-phosphorus balance, and oxidative stress.[23] Direct toxicity to nephrons with iodinated contrast media appears to be related to the ionicity and osmolality of the contrast media.[24] Microshowers of cholesterol emboli are thought to occur in about 50 percent of percutaneous interventions when a guiding catheter is passed through the aorta.[25] Most of these showers are clinically silent. However, in approximately 1 percent of high-risk cases, an acute cholesterol emboli syndrome can develop, manifested by acute renal failure, mesenteric ischemia, decreased microcirculation to the extremities, and, in some cases, embolic stroke. Because acute kidney injury occurs after coronary artery bypass graft (CABG) surgery with nearly the same risk predictors as in procedures involving contrast media, atheroembolism is considered a common pathogenic feature of both causes of renal failure.[26] Intrarenal vasoconstriction as a pathological vascular response to

treatment with EPO to a target of 13 to 15 versus 10.5 to 11.5 g/dl for 2.5 years and found higher rates of CVD and progression to ESRD in the 13 to 15 g/dl group.[16] The Correction of Hemoglobin and Outcomes in Renal Insufficiency (CHOIR) trial randomized 1432 patients with CKD and treated with EPO to a target of 13.5 versus 11.3 g/dl.[17] The composite endpoint was a combination of mortality and cardiovascular outcomes: stroke, heart attack, and hospitalization caused by congestive heart failure occurred in 125 events in the 13.5 g/dl arm and 97 events in the 11.3 g/dl arm ($p = 0.03$). Thus to have a placebo-controlled trial on this issue is critical because it appears that treatment to higher hemoglobin targets results in worsened CVD outcomes. The ongoing Trial to Reduce Cardiovascular Events with Aranesp Therapy (TREAT), which is a multicenter, double-blind, placebo-controlled randomized trial specifically designed to determine whether patients with CKD (eGFR of 20 to 60 ml/min/1.73 m²), type II DM, and anemia (Hb < 11 g/dl) will experience a reduction in the risk of the composite endpoint of death or cardiovascular morbidity (nonfatal MI, hospitalization for myocardial ischemia, HF, or stroke) when treated with darbepoetin-alpha to raise Hb to 13 g/dl.[18] Until there is clear evidence that the partial correction of anemia has favorable outcomes in CVD, this form of treatment is not recommended for the primary purpose of improving the natural history of CVD.

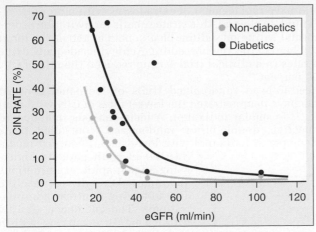

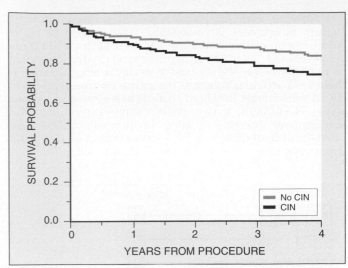

FIGURE 88–6 Rates of contrast-induced nephropathy (CIN) by estimated glomerular filtration rate (eGFR) and diabetic status from the placebo groups of randomized trials. The risk of CIN according to the baseline renal function (eGFR or creatinine clearance in milliliters per minute, as reported) modeled from published data. The fitted function is a drawn quadratic. CIN was defined as serum creatinine increase of 25 percent and/or 0.5 mg/dl. Trials including less than 25 patients were excluded. Risk for CIN according to the baseline renal function is shown separately for patients with (red circles) and without (yellow circles) diabetes on the basis of trials and registries that represent these populations separately. *(Modified from McCullough PA, Adam A, Becker CP, et al: Risk prediction of contrast nephropathy. Am J Cardiol 98:27K-36K, 2006.)*

FIGURE 88–7 Adjusted, long-term outcomes in 7586 patients with and without contrast-induced nephropathy (CIN) after angioplasty; *p* = 0.0001. CIN is defined as a 0.5 mg/dl rise in creatinine after percutaneous coronary intervention. *(Modified from Rihal CS, Textor SC, Grill DE, et al: Incidence and prognostic importance of acute renal failure after percutaneous coronary intervention. Circulation 105:2259, 2002.)*

contrast media and perhaps as an organ response to cholesterol emboli is a final hypoxic-ischemic injury to the kidney in PCI. Hypoxia triggers activation of the renal sympathetic nervous system and results in further reduction in renal blood flow. When these contrast agents are given to animals, there is disagreement about their direct vasoconstrictor or vasodilator effects in the kidney.[27-29] In completely normal human renal blood vessels, contrast agents probably provoke a vasodilation and an osmotic diuresis. However, when there is vascular disease, endothelial dysfunction, and glomerular injury, the contrast agent and the multifactorial insult of renal hypoxia provoke a vasoconstrictive response and mediate ischemic injury (Fig. 88-8). The most important predictor of CIN is underlying renal dysfunction. The "remnant nephron" theory postulates that after sufficient chronic kidney damage has occurred and the eGFR is reduced to less than 60 ml/min/1.73 m², the remaining nephrons must assume the residual filtration load. The residual nephrons also have increased oxygen demands and are more susceptible to ischemic and oxidative injury.[30]

PREVENTION OF CONTRAST-INDUCED NEPHROPATHY

A prevention strategy for CIN should be employed for patients with preexisting CKD (baseline eGFR < 60 ml/min/1.73 m²) and, in particular, those with CKD and DM. The

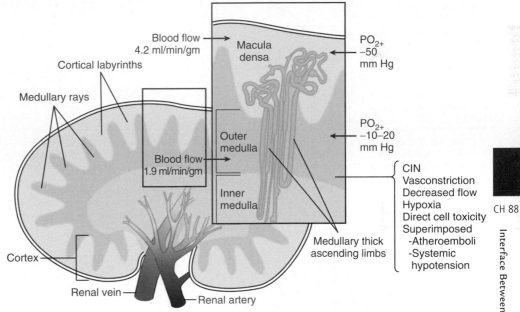

FIGURE 88–8 Pathophysiology of contrast-induced nephropathy (CIN) involves acute ischemia to the outer medulla, the most vulnerable part of the kidney, because of direct cellular toxicity, sustained intrarenal vasoconstriction, and reduction in renal blood flow. This process is worsened by multiple factors including hypoxia, anemia, and systemic hypoperfusion. *(Modified from Brezis M, Rosen S: Hypoxia of the renal medulla-its implications for disease. N Engl J Med 332:674-655, 1995.)*

presence of CKD, DM, and other risk factors including hemodynamic instability, use of intra-aortic balloon counterpulsation, HF, older age, and anemia in the same patient can produce a predicted probability of CIN of more than 50 percent (Fig. 88-9).[31] Thus CIN must be discussed in detail during the informed consent process of high-risk patients before use of intravascular iodinated contrast. The four basic concepts in CIN prevention are (1) hydration and volume expansion; (2) choice and quantity of contrast material; (3) pre-, intra-, and postprocedural end-organ protection with pharmacotherapy; and (4) postprocedural monitoring and expectant care.

Hydration with intravenous normal saline or isotonic sodium bicarbonate is reasonable, starting 3 to 12 hours before the procedure at a rate of 1 to 2 ml/kg/hr.[32-34] In those at risk, at least 300 to 500 ml of intravenous hydration should be received before the contrast material is administered. If there are particular concerns regarding volume overload or HF in individuals in whom clinical assessment of volume status is difficult, a right-heart catheterization may aid management during and after the procedure. The postprocedural hydration target is a urine output of 150 ml/hr. If patients have a diuresis of more than a 150 ml/hr, they should have replacement of extra losses with more intravenous fluid. In general, this strategy calls for hydration orders of normal saline or sodium bicarbonate at 150 ml/hr for at least 6 hours after the procedure. Achieving adequate urine flow rates in a clinical trial setting reduced the rate of CIN by 50 percent.[33]

Head-to-head randomized trials of iodinated contrast agents have demonstrated the lowest rates of CIN with non-ionic, iso-osmolar iodixanol. A meta-analysis included 16 prospective, double-blind, randomized, controlled trials that compared iodixanol with low-osmolar contrast media (LOCM) in adult patients undergoing angiographic examinations and reported Cr values at baseline and following contrast administration.[35] The incidence of CIN (Cr = 0.5 mg/dl) occurring within 72 hours after contrast administration among the iodixanol- and LOCM-treated groups is summarized in Figure 88-10. The pooled data found a reduced risk of CIN with iodixanol (overall odds ratio [OR] = 0.39, 95 percent CI 0.23 to 0.66, $p = 0.0004$). These data are consistent with the hypothesis that iodixanol (290 mOsm/kg) is less nephrotoxic than LOCM agents with osmolalities ranging from 600 to 800 mOsm/kg in the volumes of contrast used in these trials.

Iodixanol was also demonstrated to be less thrombogenic than other contrast agents in the Contrast Media Utilization in High-Risk Percutaneous Transluminal Coronary Angioplasty (COURT) trial, with a 45 percent reduction in major adverse cardiac events compared with ioxaglate meglumine (Hexabrix); hence iodixanol is the contrast agent of choice in patients at high renal risk undergoing PCI.[36] Although it is desirable to limit contrast to the

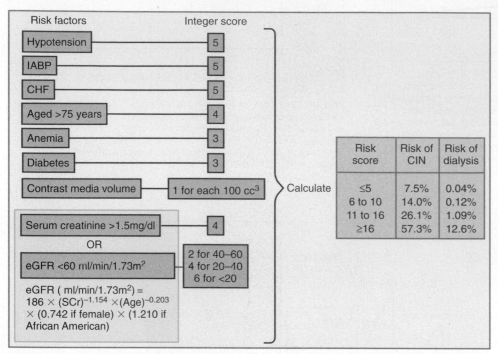

FIGURE 88-9 Risk prediction scheme for the development of contrast-induced nephropathy (CIN) and for serious renal failure requiring dialysis after coronary angiography or percutaneous coronary intervention. Anemia = baseline hematocrit value less than 39 percent for men and less than 36 percent for women. CHF = congestive heart failure functional class III/IV and/or history of pulmonary edema; eGFR = estimated glomerular filtration rate; hypotension = systolic blood pressure less than 80 mm Hg for at least 1 hour requiring inotropic support with medications or intraaortic balloon pump (IABP) within 24 hours periprocedurally. SCr = serum creatinine. *(From Mehran R, Aymong ED, Nikolsky E, et al: A simple risk score for prediction of contrast-induced nephropathy after percutaneous intervention: Development and initial validation. J Am Coll Cardiol 44:1393-1399, 2004.)*

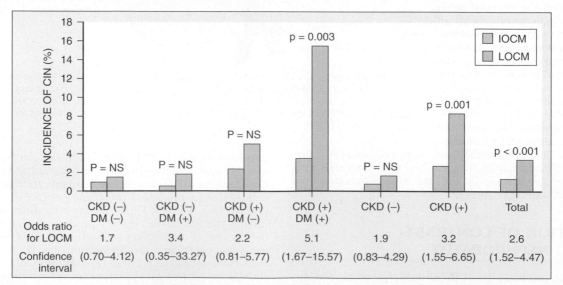

FIGURE 88-10 Incidence of contrast-induced nephropathy (CIN) in patients with or without chronic kidney disease (CKD) or diabetes mellitus (DM) who received iso-osmolar contrast media (IOCM; iodixanol) or low-osmolar contrast media (LOCM) in a meta-analysis of 16 trials. NS = not significant.

smallest volume possible in any setting, there is disagreement about a "safe" contrast limit. The lower the eGFR, the smaller the amount of contrast material necessary to cause CIN. In general, it is desirable to limit the contrast medium to less than 30 ml for a diagnostic and less than 100 ml for an interventional procedure. If staged procedures are planned, it is advantageous to have more than 10 days between the first and second contrast exposures if CIN has occurred with the first procedure.

More than 40 randomized trials have tested various adjunctive strategies in the prevention of CIN.[37] The majority of these trials were small and underpowered, and they did not find the preventive strategy under investigation to be better than placebo. A few lessons have been learned from these trials: (1) diuretics in the form of loop diuretics or mannitol can worsen CIN if there is inadequate volume replacement for the diuresis that follows; (2) low-dose or "renal-dose" dopamine does not provide protection despite its popularity in practice, given the counterbalancing forces of intrarenal vasodilation through the dopamine-1 receptor and the vasoconstricting forces of the dopamine-2, alpha, and beta receptors; and (3) renal toxic agents including nonsteroidal antiinflammatory agents, aminoglycosides, and cyclosporine should not be administered in the periprocedural period. No approved agents for the prevention of CIN are currently available.

A suggested algorithm for risk stratification and prevention of CIN is shown in Figure 88-11. When the eGFR is less than 60 ml/min/1.73 m², then optimal hydration; iodixanol as the contrast agent of choice; and consideration of prophylactic agents including N-acetylcysteine (NAC), statins, aminophylline, ascorbic acid, and prostaglandin E1 can be considered. On the basis of many small, randomized trials, oral or intravenous NAC, a cytoprotective agent against oxidative injury, may be considered effective in the prevention of CIN.[37] A trial of NAC in patients with acute MI undergoing primary angioplasty assigned 354 patients (eGFR ≈ 78 ml/min, ≈15 percent diabetics) to one of three groups: 116 patients were assigned to a standard dose of NAC (a 600 mg intravenous bolus before primary angioplasty and 600 mg orally twice daily for the 48 hours after angioplasty), 119 patients to a double dose of NAC (a 1200 mg intravenous bolus and 1200 mg orally twice daily for the 48 hours after intervention), and 119 patients to placebo.[38] The rates of CIN (>25 percent rise in Cr from baseline) in controls, 17 (15 percent) for standard-dose NAC, and 10 (8 percent) for double-dose NAC; p < 0.001. Overall in-hospital mortality was 13 (11 percent) in the control group, 5 (4 percent) in the standard-dose NAC group, and 3 (3 percent) in the double-dose NAC; p = 0.02. The rates for the composite endpoint of death, acute kidney injury requiring temporary renal-replacement therapy, or the need for mechanical ventilation were 21 (18 percent), 8 (7 percent), and 6 (5 percent) in the three groups, respectively (p = 0.002). Most operators believe that, given the seriousness of CIN, the relative safety of the strategies used, and the evolution of clinical trials shaping our practice, the combination of hydration, use of iodixanol, and use of prophylactic NAC is a reasonable three-pronged approach to

minimize CIN and the risk of acute renal failure requiring dialysis in patients at risk.

Postprocedural monitoring is critical in the current era of short stays and outpatient procedures. In general, high-risk patients in the hospital should have hydration started 12 hours before the procedure and continued at least 6 hours afterward. A serum Cr should be measured 24 hours after the procedure. For outpatients, particularly those with eGFR less than 60 ml/min/1.73 m², either an overnight stay or discharge to home with 48-hour follow-up and Cr measurement is advised. Individuals in whom severe CIN develops have a rise of Cr greater than 0.5 mg/dl in the first 24 hours after the procedure.[39] Thus for those who do not have this degree of Cr elevation and an otherwise uneventful course, discharge to home may be considered. For those with eGFR less than 30 ml/min/1.73 m², the possibility of dialysis should be discussed with the patient and preprocedural nephrology consultation is advised for possible preprocedural and postprocedural hemofiltration and dialysis management.

ACCELERATION OF VASCULAR CALCIFICATION

Atherosclerotic calcification begins as early as the second decade of life, just after fatty streak formation.[40] Coronary artery lesions of young adults have revealed small aggregates of crystalline calcium within the necrotic lipid core of a plaque.[40] Calcium phosphate (hydroxyapatite, $Ca_3[-PO_4]_2-xCa[OH]_2$), which contains 40 percent calcium by weight, precipitates in diseased coronary arteries by a mechanism similar to that found in osteogenesis and remodeling.[41] Hydroxyapatite, the predominant crystalline form in calcium deposits, is formed primarily in vesicles that pinch off from arterial wall cells, within the necrotic core, analogous to the way matrix vesicles pinch off from chondrocytes in developing bone.[41] Coronary artery calcification (CAC) seems to occur exclusively in atherosclerotic arteries and is

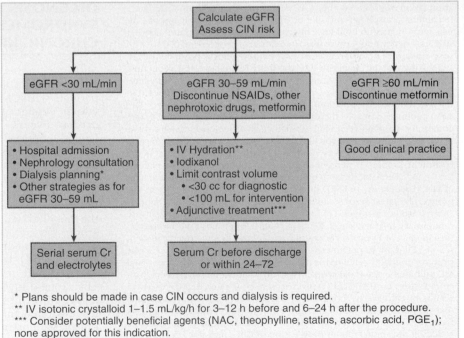

FIGURE 88–11 Algorithm for management of patients receiving iodinated contrast media. CIN = contrast-induced nephropathy; Cr = creatinine; eGFR = estimated glomerular filtration rate; NAC = N-acetylcysteine; NSAIDs = nonsteroidal anti-inflammatory drugs; PGE₁ = prostaglandin E₁. (*Modified from McCullough PA: Rev Cardiovasc Med 7:177-197, 2006.*)

absent in normal vessel walls.[40] Thus the finding of calcification on human imaging studies implies the anatomical presence of atherosclerosis and relates to CAD risk.

When the eGFR falls below 60 ml/min/1.73 m², there is a reduction in the filtration and elimination of phosphorus. Thus subtle degrees of hyperphosphatemia trigger increased release of parathyroid hormone (PTH), causing liberation of calcium stores from bone and potentially accelerating the vascular calcification process.[41] Patients with ESRD have the greatest absolute values and rates of accumulation of CAC.[42] A variety of stimuli can induce vascular smooth muscle cells to assume osteoblast-like functions in vitro including handling of phosphorus, oxidized low-density lipoprotein cholesterol (LDL-C), calcitriol, PTH, and PTH-related peptide. Clinical studies in ESRD suggest that vascular calcification is driven much more by the patient's age, length of time on dialysis, and lipid status.[43] A systematic review of the literature concerning CKD and ESRD ($n = 2919$) found 31 studies that were split on either finding or not finding significance of serum calcium (Ca), serum phosphorus (PO₄), calcium-phosphorus product, PTH, or treatments for calcium-phosphorus (Ca-PO₄) balance including phosphate binders, calcium, and vitamin D analogues in relation to CAC.[43] When taken into consideration, the lipid profiles (primarily reduced high-density lipoprotein cholesterol [HDL-C], elevated triglycerides [TGs], elevated LDL-C, and elevated total cholesterol) were the most predictive factors for CAC in ESRD.

In the Treat to Goal trial, 200 ESRD subjects were randomized to sevelamer (a gastrointestinal phosphate binder with a similar structure to the bile acid–binding resin colesevelam) versus calcium carbonate or calcium acetate and had electron beam computed tomography scans done at baseline and at 52 weeks.[45] Investigators were not blinded to the measures of Ca-PO₄ balance and were allowed to adjust phosphate-binders, dialysate calcium, or use vitamin D analogues. The baseline and final calcium-phosphorus product values were 71 and 48 (difference 23) and 69 and 49 (difference 20) for the sevelamer and calcium groups, respectively. However, there was a large difference in the final LDL-C levels between the sevelamer and the calcium groups, 65 versus 103 mg/dl, respectively; $p < 0.0001$. This is consistent with the known bile-acid sequestrant properties of sevelamer. Accordingly, there was attenuation of progression of CAC with sevelamer with no differences in calcium-phosphorus product or PTH, suggesting the change in CAC was more related to lipid lowering, as has been demonstrated in other studies.[51] Accordingly, there was attenuation of progression of CAC with sevelamer with no differences in calcium-phosphorus product or PTH, suggesting that the change in CAC was more related to LDL-C reduction. This concept has been extended to the Dialysis Clinical Outcomes Revisited (DCOR) trial, the largest outcomes study ever conducted in the hemodialysis population.[52] The 3-year trial involving more than 2100 patients compared the difference in mortality and morbidity outcomes for patients receiving sevelamer hydrochloride versus those using calcium-based phosphate binders. Despite the LDL-C reduction with sevelamer, there was no reduction in mortality between the treatment groups (9 percent relative risk reduction with sevelamer; $p = 0.30$).[46] Thus stabilization of the progression of CAC may be a benefit of LDL-C reduction; in ESRD there were no changes in mortality in this group. The latest results came from the 4D Trial (Deutsche Diabetes Dialyse Studie) in which 1255 type II DM patients with new ESRD were randomized to atorvastatin 20 mg by mouth four times a day or placebo for a median of 4 years.[47] The statin was effective in reducing the median serum LDL-C by 42 percent throughout the study period. However, the primary endpoint—defined as the composite of cardiac death, nonfatal MI, and fatal or nonfatal stroke—was only reduced by 8 percent with atorvastatin; $p = 0.37$. The 4D investigators concluded that the negative results might have been caused by the advanced CVD in the chronic dialysis patients and statin therapy being initiated too late. It appears from the DCOR and 4D trials that LDL-C reduction in ESRD, although reducing the annual rate of progression of CAC, may not affect cardiovascular events or mortality caused by the advanced disease, competing cardiovascular mechanisms for terminal events in ESRD (nonischemic arrhythmias, bradycardia, etc.), and competing noncardiovascular sources of mortality (e.g., sepsis, venous thromboembolism). Thus as of this writing, using CAC as a diagnostic or therapeutic target in patients with CKD or ESRD is not recommended.

RENAL DISEASE AND HYPERTENSION

The kidney is a central regulator of blood pressure and controls intraglomerular pressure through autoregulation. Glomerular injury activates a variety of pathways that increase systemic blood pressure. This effect sets up a vicious circle of more glomerular and tubulointerstitial injury and worsened HTN. A cornerstone of management of combined CKD and CVD is strict blood pressure control (see Fig. 40-14). An optimal blood pressure can be defined as less than 120/80 mm Hg (with systolic blood pressure [SBP] being the more important target), and most patients with CKD and HTN require three or more antihypertensive agents to achieve a goal blood pressure of less than 130/80 mm Hg.[11] Detection and treatment of HTN are outlined elsewhere in this text (see Chaps. 40 and 41). The key life-style issues with CKD and HTN include dietary changes with sodium restriction, weight reduction to a target body mass index less than 25 kg/m², and exercise for 60 minutes per day most days of the week. Pharmacological therapy aims for strict blood pressure control with an agent that antagonizes the RAAS, often in combined action with a thiazide-type diuretic.[48] Dihydropyridine calcium channel blockers alone, because of relative afferent arteriolar dilation, increase intraglomerular pressure and worsen glomerular injury and thus should be avoided as singular agents for blood pressure control. Special diagnostic consideration should be given to the possibility of underlying bilateral renal artery stenosis from the clinical clues of poorly controlled blood pressure on more than three agents, abdominal bruits, smoking history, peripheral arterial disease, and a marked change in serum Cr with administration of angiotensin-converting enzyme inhibitor (ACEI) or angiotensin II receptor blocker (ARB).[49] Although renal artery stenosis accounts for less than 3 percent of ESRD cases, it represents a potentially treatable condition.[50] Diagnostic approaches discussed elsewhere in this text should be considered.

DIAGNOSIS OF ACUTE CORONARY SYNDROMES IN PATIENTS WITH CHRONIC KIDNEY DISEASE

Multiple studies have found that elderly persons and those with DM have higher rates of silent ischemia.[51] Likewise, patients with CKD have shown higher silent ischemia rates, which cluster with serious arrhythmias, HF, and other cardiac events. Hemodialysis patients bear considerable hemodynamic stress three times per week during dialysis sessions. Several studies have demonstrated a relationship between ST segment depression and release of cardiac biomarkers (primarily troponin), before or during dialysis, and poor long-term survival.[52] From a practical perspective, it is important to realize that patients with CKD presenting to the hospital with chest discomfort represent a high-risk group, having a 40 percent cardiac event rate at 30 days.[53] In making the diagnosis of acute MI (AMI) in patients with CKD or ESRD, troponin I is the preferred biomarker based on its kinetic profile in patients with renal impairment.[54] The skeletal myopathy of CKD can elevate creatine kinase, myoglobin, and some troponin T assays, making these tests less desirable. In addition to an elevated biomarker of cardiac injury, supporting evidence of the diagnosis of AMI could be characteristic chest pain, electrocardiographic changes (e.g., ST segment elevation or depression, new Q waves), or the identification of a culprit lesion on angiography. Because of the high event rate and prevalence of CVD among patients with CKD, it is advisable to consider admission to the hospital when the presenting symptom is chest discomfort and the eGFR is less than 60 ml/min/1.73 m² or the patient has ESRD and is receiving dialysis.[55]

RENAL DYSFUNCTION AS A PROGNOSTIC FACTOR IN ACUTE CORONARY SYNDROMES

In the past several decades, considerable advances have been made in the diagnosis and treatment of acute coronary syndromes (ACSs) in the general population. These advances include early paramedic response and defibrillation, coronary care units, and pharmacotherapy including antiplatelet agents, antithrombotics, beta receptor blocking agents, ACEIs, and intravenous thrombolytic agents. Primary angioplasty for ST segment elevation MI (STEMI) has become a well-accepted mode of treatment. These advances, however, have not been tested in patients with CKD or ESRD, primarily because randomized treatment trials generally exclude these patients. Retrospective studies of patients in coronary care units have identified renal dysfunction as the most significant prognostic factor for long-term mortality when adjusting for other clinical factors including age, gender, and comorbidities.[56] In addition, retrospective studies of patients with AMI consistently find renal dysfunction as an independent predictor of death, with a greater impact on mortality than baseline demographics or therapies received.[56] Patients with ESRD have the highest mortality after AMI of any large, chronic disease population (Fig. 88-12).[57]

REASONS FOR POOR OUTCOMES AFTER ACUTE CORONARY SYNDROMES IN PATIENTS WITH RENAL DYSFUNCTION

Four reasons may explain why patients with renal dysfunction have poor cardiovascular outcomes in a variety of settings: (1) excess comorbidities associated with CKD and ESRD, in particular DM and heart failure; (2) therapeutic nihilism; (3) toxicity of therapies; and (4) special biological and pathophysiological factors in renal dysfunction that cause worsened outcomes.[56] In one study by Beattie and coworkers,[6] the comorbidities of patients with STEMI and CKD (mean Cr = 2.7 mg/dl) included older age (mean 70.2 years), DM (38.1 percent), and prior HF (23.2 percent).[6] Those with ESRD had similar rates of comorbidities including age (mean 64.9 years), DM (40.4 percent), and prior HF (31.7 percent). This study found that, among the CKD and ESRD groups, there were lower rates of use of reperfusion therapy (thrombolysis or primary angioplasty) and beta blockers, suggesting some contribution to poor outcomes from underutilization of proven therapies (therapeutic nihilism). Patients with renal dysfunction may present later in their course, have more contraindications, or have other aspects about their presentations that prompt clinicians to use fewer therapies or take a more conservative approach.

Data on the toxicity of treatments for ACSs related to renal dysfunction are often unavailable, primarily because of exclusion of patients with CKD from these trials. The primary defects in thrombosis attributable to uremia are excess thrombin generation and decreased platelet aggregation. Hence patients with CKD and ESRD can have increased rates of coronary thrombotic events and increased bleeding risks at the same time. In patients with renal dysfunction the risks of bleeding increase with aspirin, unfractionated heparin, low-molecular-weight heparin, thrombolytics, glycoprotein IIb/IIIa antagonists, and thienopyridine antiplatelet agents. The reason is primarily that uremia causes platelet dysfunction in a mechanism that is independent of and therefore additive to pharmacologically induced platelet antagonism or antithrombosis.[58] In patients with renal dysfunction, the best measure of bleeding risk is the bleeding time. Unfortunately, the bleeding time is not a practical test for the ACS patient; consequently, clinicians cannot readily assess the a priori bleeding risk for any given CKD or ESRD patient. However, it is unlikely that bleeding complications account for the large differences seen in mortality between CKD and ESRD and those with preserved renal function with AMI.

The final and most important reason why patients with CKD and ESRD have poor outcomes after ACS is the enhanced vascular pathobiology induced by the chronic renal failure state.[56] The processes that contribute to accelerate atherosclerosis include a dyslipidemia characterized by decreased function of lipoprotein lipase, reduced HDL-C, elevated TG, and elevated LDL-C. Elevations in homocysteine and other thiols are present when the eGFR drops below 60 ml/min/1.73 m², enhancing oxidation of LDL-C and progression of atherosclerotic lesions.[23] Renal dysfunction is a highly inflammatory state, associated with higher rates of plaque rupture and incident CVD events. Lastly, chronic hyperactivation of the sympathetic nervous system and an imbalance between endothelin, a powerful vasoconstrictor, and nitric oxide, a local paracrine vasodilator, may worsen HTN and may augment intravascular wall stress that could further contribute to incident CVD events.[23]

TREATMENT OF ACUTE MYOCARDIAL INFARCTION IN PATIENTS WITH RENAL DYSFUNCTION

The clinician must confront the high-risk populations, those with CKD and ESRD, with little evidence on which to base treatment decisions in ACS. Therapies that benefit the general population often yield enhanced benefit in patients with CKD and ESRD. A favorable benefit-to-risk ratio has now been demonstrated for aspirin, beta blockers, ACEI, ARB, aldosterone receptor antagonists, and statins.[59] Therapies that require dose adjustment on the basis of CrCl include low-molecular-weight heparins, bivalirudin, and glycoprotein (GP) IIb/IIIa antagonists (Table 88-1). Given that

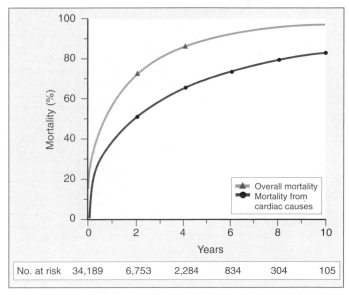

FIGURE 88–12 Cumulative mortality after myocardial infarction in patients with end-stage renal disease from the U.S. Renal Data System. *(Modified from Herzog CA, Ma JZ, Collins AJ: Poor long-term survival after acute myocardial infarction among patients on long-term dialysis. N Engl J Med 339;799, 1998.)*

the major inputs for bleeding risks include older age, low body weight, and renal dysfunction, Table 88-1 also lists agents that are approved in a weight-adjusted dose form and gives the currently recommended dose adjustments for commonly used antiplatelet and antithrombotic agents.[58] It is possible that greater utilization of such therapies, despite the heightened risk for complications, will attenuate the excess mortality reported in the CKD and ESRD populations. No randomized trials of PCI or CABG surgery in patients with CKD or ESRD have occurred. However, in the Bypass Angioplasty Revascularization Investigation (BARI) trial, whether PCI or surgery was used in the management of multivessel coronary disease, CKD and DM were associated with worsened long-term survival (Fig. 88-13).[8] Further research is necessary into the particular pathogenic mechanisms in the renal failure state that promote plaque rupture, accelerate atherosclerosis, lead to ACS complications, and promote the development of HF and arrhythmias.

CHRONIC KIDNEY DISEASE COMPLICATING CONGESTIVE HEART FAILURE (see Chap. 25)

The diagnosis of HF with concomitant renal failure presents a particular challenge. Patients with CKD and, in particular, ESRD have three key mechanical contributors to HF: pressure overload (related to HTN), volume overload, and cardiomyopathy. Approximately 20 percent of patients approaching hemodialysis have a diagnosis of HF.[60] It is unclear how much of this diagnosis can be attributable purely to chronic volume overload from renal failure and how much is caused by impaired systolic or diastolic func-

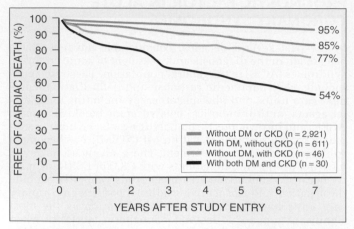

FIGURE 88–13 Freedom from cardiovascular death after angioplasty or bypass surgery in the Bypass Angioplasty Revascularization Investigation (BARI) Trial and Registry, n = 3608. CKD = chronic kidney disease; DM = diabetes mellitus. *(Modified from Szczech LA, Best PJ, Crowley E; Bypass Angioplasty Revascularization Investigation (BARI) Investigators: Outcomes of patients with chronic renal insufficiency in the bypass angioplasty revascularization investigation. Circulation 105:2253, 2002.)*

TABLE 88–1	Recommended Dose Adjustment of Conventional Antithrombotics Used for Acute Coronary Syndromes in Patients with Chronic Kidney Disease and End-Stage Renal Disease			
Agent	**eGFR (ml/min/1.73 m²)** **60-90 ml/min**	**Creatinine Clearance (ml/min)** **30-60 ml/min**	**<30 ml/min**	**Dialysis Dependent**
Aspirin	No adjustment needed	No adjustment needed	No adjustment needed	No adjustment needed
Clopidogrel	No adjustment needed	No adjustment needed	No adjustment needed	No adjustment needed
Ticlopidine	No adjustment needed	No adjustment needed	No adjustment needed	No adjustment needed
Heparin	No guidelines	No guidelines	No guidelines	No guidelines
LMWH	No guidelines	No guidelines	Reduced dose by 30%; factor Xa monitoring advocated	No guidelines
Lepirudin	No guidelines	CrCl 45-60 ml/min or SrCr 1.6-2 mg/dl: Reduce bolus to 0.2 mg/kg IV + decrease infusion rate by 50% (0.075 mg/kg/hr IV) CrCl 30-44 ml/min or SrCr 2.1-3 mg/dl: Reduce bolus to 0.2 mg/kg IV + decrease standard initial infusion rate by 70% (0.045 mg/kg/hr IV)	CrCl 15-29 ml/min or SrCr 3.1-6 mg/dl: Reduce bolus to 0.2 mg/kg IV + decrease infusion rate by 85% (0.0225 mg/kg/hr IV) CrCl <15 ml/min or SrCr >6 mg/dl: Reduce bolus to 0.2 mg/kg IV; No infusion	Reduce the bolus dose to 0.2 mg/kg IV; no infusion
Bivalirudin	No guidelines	Reduce infusion dose by 20%	Reduce infusion dose by 60%	Reduce infusion dose by 90%
Argatroban	No dose adjustment	No dose adjustment	No dose adjustment	
Abciximab	No guidelines Monitoring advocated	No guidelines Monitoring advocated	No guidelines Monitoring advocated	No guidelines Monitoring advocated
Eptifibatide	No guidelines	SrCr 2-4 mg/dl: 135 µg/kg IV bolus + 0.5 µg/kg/min IV infusion	SrCr >4mg/dl Contraindicated	No clinical data In vitro data demonstrate clearance
Tirofiban	No dose adjustment	No dose adjustment	0.2 µg/kg/min IV for 30 min, followed by 0.05 µg/kg/min IV	No clinical data In vitro data demonstrate clearance

CrCl = creatinine clearance; eGFR = estimated glomerular filtration rate; LMWH = low-molecular-weight heparin; SrCr = serum creatinine.
Modified from Sica D: The implications of renal impairment among patients undergoing percutaneous coronary intervention. J Invasive Cardiol 14(Suppl B):30B, 2002.

CH 88

tion. Notably, CKD influences the levels of B-type natriuretic peptide (BNP), a diagnostic blood test for HF. In general, when the eGFR is less than 60 ml/min/1.73 m^2, a higher BNP cut point of 200 pg/ml should be used in the diagnosis of HF.[61] It is now well recognized that CKD (eGFR < 60 ml/min/1.73 m^2), when present in patients with HF, independently predicts poor outcomes.[62] Estimated and actual GFRs clearly can be reduced by decreased renal blood flow related to low cardiac output. However, multiple studies of patients with class II and III HF, in whom a low cardiac output state is not present, have shown decreased survival in a graded fashion related to renal impairment.[62]

The combination of HF and CKD presents a challenge to cardiologists with respect to proven treatment options. ACEI, if tolerated, or ARBs, if ACEI is not tolerated, beta blockers, aldosterone antagonists, and loop diuretics are all acceptable combination therapies.[63] Caveats in the use of ACEI and ARBs are the marked elevation in the serum Cr and acute renal failure that are more likely to occur when the patient is volume depleted or in the presence of occult bilateral renal artery stenosis or equivalent (unilateral renal artery stenosis present in a renal transplant recipient).[64] When initiating therapy to block the RAAS, it is advisable to have the SBP stable and greater than 90 mm Hg, euvolemia, and a drug regimen without concurrent renal toxic agents. The clinician should realize that CKD patients enjoy an improved survival and reduced rates of ESRD on ACEI/ARB agents even though the serum Cr is chronically elevated on these agents because of reductions in intraglomerular pressure. Discontinuation of ACEI/ARB drugs because of moderate, asymptomatic rises in Cr is a common management error. In general, an attempt should be made to use ACEI or ARB in patients down to an eGFR of 15 ml/min/1.73 m^2. Below this level, case reports suggest a high rate of hyperkalemia and the concern of accelerating the course to ESRD and dialysis.

The management of the patient who is already receiving dialysis and in HF requires particular care. In general, proven HF therapies, provided they are tolerated, should be employed along with regular and ad hoc dialysis as needed to control volume overload. In a randomized trial, carvedilol did provide additional benefit in this scenario.[65] In addition, retrospective analysis supports the use of ACEI in patients with ESRD admitted with HF.[66] Lastly, the acute management of decompensated HF in patients with impaired eGFR poses a particularly difficult challenge. In fact, an elevated Cr is the single most common reason for the use of positive inotropes or inodilators in hospitalized patients with HF.[68] No reports of dobutamine leading to long-term favorable outcomes have been reported, and in the short term it increases arrhythmias and mortality. Likewise, milrinone has not been shown to reduce mortality, causes arrhythmias, and must be dose-adjusted when the eGFR drops below 45 ml/min/1.73 m^2 (Table 88-2).[72] Another option is the use of intravenous BNP (nesiritide), which causes primarily venodilation and natriuresis.[69] Completed studies with nesiritide have evaluated the CKD subgroups and found benefit in CKD equal to that in those with preserved renal function, although the overall effect is modestly better than that with intravenous nitroglycerin.[70] Patients with advanced HF have reduced renal blood flow, decreased glomerular filtration rate, enhanced proximal reabsorption of water, and an overall reduced capacity of the nephron to excrete water (Fig. 88-14). Furthermore, reduced effective arterial blood volume is a stimulus for antidiuretic hormone release, which plays a dominant role in worsening water retention (see Fig. 88-14). The clinical signs of this deterioration are an elevation in the serum Cr

TABLE 88-2	Recommended Dose Adjustment of Selected Medical Therapy for Hypertension, Dyslipidemia, Heart Failure, and Arrhythmias in Patients with Chronic Kidney Disease and End-Stage Renal Disease				
		eGFR (ml/min/1.73 m^2) (CrCl ml/min)			
Drug	Elimination Route	90-60	60-30	<30	Dialysis Dependent
Central Adrenergic Blockers					
Clonidine	Renal				↓ Dose 50%
Methyldopa	Renal	q.i.d.	q.i.d.	↓ t.i.d.	↓ b.i.d. or qd
Angiotensin-Converting Enzyme Inhibitors (ACEIs)					
Captopril	Renal				↓ Dose 50%
Enalapril	Hepatic			↓ Dose 25%	↓ Dose 50%
Lisinopril	Renal			↓ Dose 25%	↓ Dose 50%
Ramipril	Renal/GI			↓ Dose 75%	↓ Dose 75%
Benazepril	Renal			↓ Dose 25%	↓ Dose 75%
Inotropic Agents					
Digoxin	Renal/nonrenal		↓ Dose 50%	↓ Dose 50%	↓ Dose 75%; change to q.o.d.
Milrinone	Renal		↓ Dose 25%	↓ Dose 50%	↓ Dose 75%
Antiarrhythmics					
Disopyramide	Renal/hepatic	b.i.d.	b.i.d.	↓ qd	↓ q.o.d.
Flecainide	Renal/hepatic				↓ Dose 25-50%
Mexiletine	Renal/hepatic				↓ Dose 50-75%
Procainamide	Renal/hepatic	q.i.d.	↓ t.i.d.	↓ b.i.d.	↓ b.i.d. or qd
Dofetilide	Renal/nonrenal		↓ Dose 50%	↓ Dose 75%	Contraindicated
Beta Blockers					
Atenolol	Renal			↓ Dose 50%	↓ Dose 75%; ↓ q.o.d.
Sotalol	Renal			↓ Dose 50%	↓ Dose 75%
Others					
Verapamil	Hepatic				↓ Dose 50-75%
Hydralazine		q.i.d.	↓ t.i.d	↓ t.i.d.	↓ b.i.d.
Gemfibrozil	Renal			↓ Dose 50%	↓ Dose 75%
Nicotinic acid	Renal/hepatic			↓ Dose 25%	↓ Dose 25%

CrCl = creatinine clearance; eGFR = estimated glomerular filtration rate; GI = gastrointestinal.

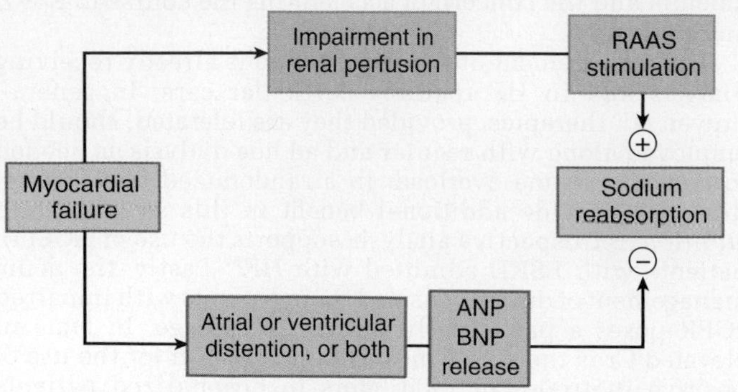

FIGURE 88–14 Pathophysiological processes in combined heart and kidney failure. ANP = A-type natriuretic peptide; BNP = B-type natriuretic peptide; RAAS = renin-angiotensin-aldosterone system. *(From Weber KT: Aldosterone in congestive heart failure. N Engl J Med 345:1689, 2001.)*

and blood urea nitrogen, hyponatremia, volume retention, and excessive thirst. Treatment efforts should be aimed at improving left ventricular systolic function, often in the hospitalized setting, with the intravenous therapies mentioned previously and discussed in detail elsewhere in this text. Small trials utilizing continuous veno-venous ultrafiltration have demonstrated short-term reductions in symptoms, shorter hospital stay, and reductions in rehospitalizations.[71] Until larger trials confirm longer-term benefits in hospitalization and mortality, ultrafiltration can be considered a last-line approach for the patient with refractory cardiorenal failure.

In summary, CKD and HF present a particularly challenging scenario for clinicians and patients. Frequent monitoring and the combined use of renal and cardioprotective strategies are critical. Future research is necessary to confirm anemia correction and ultrafiltration as additional strategies in patients who have cardiorenal syndrome. Dialysis patients, despite having volume reduction with mechanical fluid removal, should have medical therapy with ACEIs or ARBs, beta blockers, and additional agents for blood pressure control if necessary.

CHRONIC KIDNEY DISEASE AND VALVULAR HEART DISEASE

Impaired renal function has been linked to mitral annular calcification and aortic sclerosis. Advanced thickening of the cardiac valves and calcification have been observed in patients with ESRD.[72] Some 80 percent of patients with ESRD have the murmur of aortic sclerosis. Neither of these lesions usually progresses to the point that studies beyond echocardiography are necessary. Bacterial endocarditis may develop in patients with ESRD who have temporary dialysis access catheters.[73] Endocarditis with common pathogens including *Staphylococcus, Streptococcus,* and *Enterococcus,* in the aortic or mitral position, is associated with a mortality rate greater than 50 percent in this setting.[73] It becomes difficult to treat given the continued need for dialysis access and the delay in surgical placement of permanent arteriovenous shunts or fistulas. Unfortunately, surgical mortality associated with valve replacement in ESRD related

to endocarditis is quite high. In the setting of ESRD, when valve surgery is carried out for endocarditis or other causes of valve failure, there has been no difference in survival among those who received tissue or mechanical valve prostheses. Thus tissue valves are a reasonable choice given the complicating issue of chronic anticoagulation and bleeding with dialysis vascular access.

RENAL FUNCTION AND ARRHYTHMIAS

Uremia, hyperkalemia, acidosis, and disorders of calcium-phosphorous balance have all been linked to higher rates of atrial and ventricular arrhythmias.[74] Given a concurrent substrate of left ventricular hypertrophy, left ventricular dilation, HF, and valvular disease, it is not surprising that higher rates of virtually all arrhythmias have been reported in CKD including bradyarrhythmias and heart block.[74] Caveats for practical management include dose adjustment for many antiarrhythmic medications including digoxin, sotalol, and procainamide (see Table 88-2). Of concern, CKD, and ESRD in particular, may cause elevated defibrillation thresholds and failure of implantable cardioverter defibrillators (ICDs).[75] Until this association is better understood, patients receiving ICDs should have frequent surveillance and consideration for noninvasive programmed stimulation for appropriate antitachycardia and defibrillation therapy. Considering the high rates of sudden death in patients with ESRD, clinical trials of prophylactic ICDs in this population are under consideration.

CONSULTATIVE APPROACH TO THE HEMODIALYSIS PATIENT

The prevalence of angiographically significant coronary artery disease (CAD) ranges from 25 percent in young, non-diabetic hemodialysis patients to 85 percent in older ESRD patients with long-standing DM.[76-77] It has been estimated that cardiac death in dialysis patients younger than age 45 is 100 times greater than that in the general population.[77]

The prevalence and severity of CAD among patients with ESRD is daunting in terms of both occurrence and extent of poor outcomes. Medicare beneficiaries with CKD prior to initiation of dialysis are 60 percent more likely to have a billing claim submitted for the diagnosis of CVD and 70 percent more likely to have a claim submitted for "atherosclerotic heart disease."[78] Of those incident to dialysis, a substantial proportion, perhaps the majority, have established CAD. In diabetic renal transplant candidates, 30 percent will have one or more lesions with greater than 75 percent stenosis.[77] When comparing the patients who undergo evaluation for CAD, those with ESRD have substantially more numerous and severe coronary artery lesions, as well as more severe left ventricular dysfunction.[77]

The patient with incipient ESRD who has been placed on dialysis can be considered the highest cardiovascular risk patient in medicine with expected rates of CVD death that are many-fold that expected for a non-ESRD patient, even those with a burden of several cardiovascular risk factors. ESRD is more than a cardiovascular risk equivalent, warranting meticulous efforts to achieve goals mandated by conventional guidelines (Table 88-3).

Despite the use of multiple medications, most published series of ESRD patients from either clinical trials or registries indicate the mean systolic blood pressure is approximately 155 mm Hg. Indeed, 80 percent of ESRD patients have HTN and it is adequately controlled in only 30 percent.[79] Long-term cardiorenal protection involves two

TABLE 88–3	Therapeutic Opportunities to Improve Cardiovascular Care in Patients with End-Stage Renal Disease
Therapeutic Opportunity	**Rationale**
Weight loss/weight maintenance at BMI ≤ 25 kg/m²	Improvement of the dysmetabolic syndrome and diabetes
Low sodium intake	Reduce blood pressure Make blood pressure more responsive to medications Reduce volume retention between dialysis sessions
Aspirin 81 mg p.o. qd or clopidogrel 75 mg p.o. qd if aspirin intolerant	Primary prevention of AMI and stroke
Lipid control (diet, statin, fibrates, niacin, others) —LDL-C < 100 mg/dl —TG < 150 mg/dl —HDL-C > 50 mg/dl	Possible primary prevention of AMI, stroke, and CVD death Possible reduction in progression of CKD
Blood pressure control to target of SBP < 130 mm Hg (optimal <120 mm Hg) —RAAS blocking agents —Beta-blocking agents —Other add-on agents	Primary prevention of AMI, stroke, heart failure, and CVD death Preserve residual urine volume in peritoneal dialysis patients Reduce left ventricular hypertrophy Treatment of subclinical cardiac ischemia
Blood glucose control in diabetes	Reduction in risk of AMI, stroke, and CVD death Reduction in worsened nephropathy/retinopathy
Reduce homocysteine —Folic acid —Vitamin B₆ and B₁₂	Possible reduction in risk of AMI, stroke, and CVD death

AMI = acute myocardial infarction; BMI = body mass index; CVD = cardiovascular disease; HDL-C = high-density lipoprotein cholesterol; LDL-C = low-density lipoprotein cholesterol; RAAS = renin-angiotensin-aldosterone system; TG = triglycerides.
Modified from McCullough PA: Acute coronary syndromes in patients with renal failure. Curr Cardiol Rep 5:266, 2003.

important concepts: blood pressure control to a much lower target of an SBP less than 130 mm Hg and use of an agent that blocks the RAAS such as an ACEI or ARB as the base of therapy. How can an ACEI/ARB be effective in a patient with ESRD, particularly one who is anephric? The RAAS appears to have considerable redundancy and can maintain its function, if not increase its overall level of activity without participation by the kidneys.[80] Hence this hyperactivation of the RAAS is a target for therapy in ESRD because ACEI/ARB have been demonstrated to reduce LVH and possibly improve survival in ESRD.[81] A small trial demonstrated that ramipril was related to preservation of residual urine output in those receiving peritoneal dialysis, which is a consistently favorable management issue in ESRD.[82] A retrospective study found that although only approximately 20 percent of patients with ESRD and CAD receive ACEI, those who were given these agents after CAD events had improved all-cause mortality over the next 5 years.[83] The common difficulty with ACEI/ARB is worsened hyperkalemia in patients with ESRD. As tolerated, the clinician should consider adjusting the dialytic regimen to improve potassium removal from the system. From all sources of evidence to date, patients with ESRD appear to benefit from ACEI/ARB therapy provided the serum potassium and blood pressure can be adequately controlled.

With an ACEI/ARB as a base of therapy, the antihypertensive regimen can be further modified according to blood pressure–lowering efficacy and CAD event reduction. Beta blockers can be used as both antihypertensive and antiischemic agents.[84] In those with HF, beta blockers improve left ventricular ejection fraction and reduce rates of hospitalization, sudden death, and all-cause mortality.[85-86] Large relative risk reductions in all-cause mortality have been reported for patients who receive beta blockers with ESRD after CAD events.[86]

After inclusion of ACEI/ARB and beta blockers in the ESRD blood pressure regimen, the remaining choices should be based on ease of management, compliance, and lack of adverse effects. The goal is to create a blood pressure environment for the cardiovascular system in which the mean

SBP, on 24-hour monitoring, for example, is at least less than 130 mm Hg. Guidelines for non-ESRD patients state that the optimal SBP should be less than 120 mm Hg.[11,48] The difficult task in the ESRD patient is to achieve these goals without having hypotension during dialysis sessions. Given the high rates of severe CAD in ESRD, hypotension during dialysis can worsen clinical and subclinical ischemia recognized as chest discomfort, shortness of breath, ST-segment depression on electrocardiography, and elevations of cardiac troponin on blood testing.[87]

The National Kidney Foundation Guidelines support LDL-C reduction, in most cases with a statin, in patients with ESRD irrespective of the relative risk reductions in CVD events observed to date in clinical trials.[88-89] In addition, agents that reduce TG levels and raise HDL-C including nicotinic acid and fibrates can be used according to the National Cholesterol Education Project Adult Treatment Panel III (NCEP-ATP-III) Guidelines.[90]

In ESRD with DM, blood glucose control to a target glycohemoglobin less than 7 mg/dl can be expected to reduce rates of microvascular (retinopathy) and, to a lesser extent, clinically important atherosclerotic disease elsewhere (e.g., AMI, stroke, CVD death).[91] Likewise, smoking cessation as another basic reduction maneuver is recommended in patients with ESRD.[92] The effect of aspirin on renal endpoints is unknown; however, given its CVD protective effect, it is recommended for adult patients with ESRD.[93] For those who are aspirin-intolerant, general cardiology guidelines recommend the use of clopidogrel, although there are no published studies of clopidogrel on cardiovascular outcomes in ESRD.

Three analyses suggest that patients with ESRD with CAD who receive conservative medical management do fare the worst of all the groups (Fig. 88-15).[93-96] So the first step after stress-imaging, in an ESRD patient with symptomatic CAD, is to make an attempt at angiography and revascularization. Usually multivessel CAD is found, so the next question is what is the optimal approach—multivessel PCI or CABG surgery? It is widely accepted that patients with ESRD undergoing mechanical coronary revascularization procedures are at increased risk for adverse events including death. Dialysis-dependent patients undergoing CABG surgery face a 4.4 times greater risk of in-hospital death, a 3.1 times greater risk of mediastinitis, and a 2.6 times greater risk of stroke compared with those patients undergoing CABG surgery who were not on dialysis.[97] Although newer surgical techniques have been successful in high-risk patients with renal failure, the long-term results, compared with traditional surgical and percutaneous techniques, are not yet known. In general, despite this significant "upfront" risk of surgery, the literature suggests the superiority of CABG surgery compared with percutaneous interventions in patients with ESRD.[94] In single-vessel CAD and multivessel CAD without good bypass targets, recent trends suggest that PCI with stenting is a favorable approach for patients with ESRD (see Fig. 88-15).[94] As drug-eluting stents become more widely used in ESRD, they may make an impact in the high restenosis rates seen in this population and may tip the risk-benefit scale in favor of PCI.[98]

In summary, patients with ESRD have more than coronary artery disease risk equivalent status in their baseline CAD risk assessment. An aggressive approach with medical management for CAD is warranted, even in the case of subclinical CAD. A low threshold for diagnostic testing should be held in ESRD patients (Fig. 88-16). When significant CAD is found, ESRD patients appear to benefit from revascularization compared with conservative medical management and, if clinically reasonable, should be given that opportunity for improved survival and reduction in future cardiac events.

SUMMARY

Recognition has increased over the past decade that patients with CKD have a high risk for CVD. Frequent clinical scenarios in which renal function influences care include CIN, ACS, HF, valvular disease, and arrhythmias. Results from retrospective studies and clinical trial subgroups form the basis of current recommendations, given the lack of prospective randomized trials in CKD and ESRD. Further study of the adverse metabolic milieu of CKD is likely to lead to generalizable diagnostic and therapeutic targets for the future management of renal patients with cardiovascular illness.

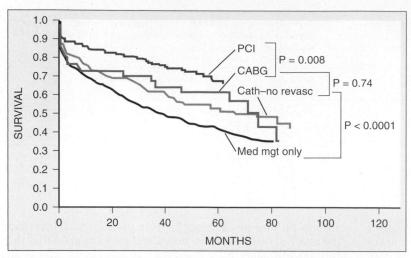

FIGURE 88–15 Long-term survival according to CAD management strategy in patients with creatinine clearance (CRCl) of 60 ml/min or end-stage renal disease (ESRD) on dialysis. CABG = coronary artery bypass graft; Cath—no revasc = catheterization—no revascularization; med mgt = medical management; PCI = percutaneous coronary intervention. *(From Keeley EC, Kadakia R, Soman S, et al: Analysis of long-term survival after revascularization in patients with chronic kidney disease presenting with acute coronary syndromes. Am J Cardiol 92:509-514, 2003.)*

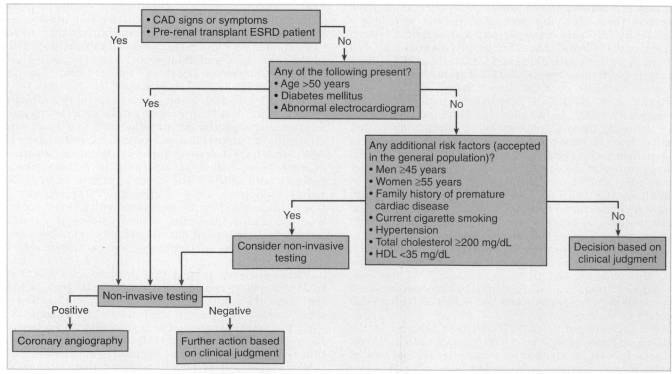

FIGURE 88–16 Approach to the end-stage renal disease (ESRD) patient with coronary artery disease. CAD = coronary artery disease; HDL = high-density lipoprotein. *(Modified from McCullough PA: Evaluation and treatment of coronary artery disease in patients with end-stage renal disease. Kidney Int Suppl 95:s51-58, 2005.)*

REFERENCES

Epidemiology and Outcomes

1. Lewis CE, Jacobs DR Jr, McCreath H, et al: Weight gain continues in the 1990s: 10-year trends in weight and overweight from the CARDIA study. Coronary Artery Risk Development in Young Adults. Am J Epidemiol 151:1172, 2000.
2. Bakris GL, Williams M, Dworkin L, et al: Preserving renal function in adults with hypertension and diabetes: A consensus approach. National Kidney Foundation Hypertension and Diabetes Executive Committees Working Group. Am J Kidney Dis 36:646, 2000.
3. McCullough PA: Cardiorenal risk: An important clinical intersection. Rev Cardiovasc Med 3:71, 2002.
4. National Kidney Foundation: Clinical practice guidelines for chronic kidney disease: Evaluation, classification, and stratification. Am J Kidney Dis 2(Suppl 1):S46, 2002.
5. McCullough PA, Soman SS, Shah SS, et al: Risks associated with renal dysfunction in patients in the coronary care unit. J Am Coll Cardiol 36:679, 2000.
6. Beattie JN, Soman SS, Sandberg KR, et al: Determinants of mortality after myocardial infarction in patients with advanced renal dysfunction. Am J Kidney Dis 37:1191, 2001.
7. Chertow GM, Lazarus JM, Christiansen CL, et al: Preoperative renal risk stratification. Circulation 95:878, 1997.
8. Szczech LA, Best PJ, Crowley E; the Bypass Angioplasty Revascularization Investigation (BARI) Investigators: Outcomes of patients with chronic renal insufficiency in the bypass angioplasty revascularization investigation. Circulation 105:2253, 2002.
9. Filler G, Bokenkamp A, Hofmann W, et al: Cystatin C as a marker of GFR—history, indications, and future research. Clin Biochem 38:1-8, 2005.
10. Sarnak MJ, Levey AS, Schoolwerth AC, et al; American Heart Association Councils on Kidney in Cardiovascular Disease, High Blood Pressure Research, Clinical Cardiology, and Epidemiology and Prevention: Kidney disease as a risk factor for development of cardiovascular disease: A statement from the American Heart Association Councils on Kidney in Cardiovascular Disease, High Blood Pressure Research, Clinical Cardiology, and Epidemiology and Prevention. Circulation 108:2154-2169, 2003.
11. Chobanian AV, Bakris GL, Black HR; the National Heart, Lung, and Blood Institute Joint National Committee on Prevention, Detection, Evaluation, and Treatment of High Blood Pressure; National High Blood Pressure Education Program Coordinating Committee: The Seventh Report of the Joint National Committee on Prevention, Detection, Evaluation, and Treatment of High Blood Pressure: The JNC 7 report. JAMA 289:2560, 2003.

Anemia and Chronic Kidney Disease

12. NKF-DOQI clinical practice guidelines for the treatment of anemia of chronic renal failure. National Kidney Foundation-Dialysis Outcomes Quality Initiative. Am J Kidney Dis 30(Suppl 3):S192-240, 1997.
13. McCullough PA, Lepor NE: The deadly triangle of anemia, renal insufficiency, and cardiovascular disease: Implications for prognosis and treatment. Rev Cardiovasc Med 6:1-10, 2005.
14. Silverberg DS, Wexler D, Iaina A: The role of anemia in the progression of congestive heart failure. Is there a place for erythropoietin and intravenous iron? J Nephrol 17:749-761, 2004.
15. Anand I, McMurray JJ, Whitmore J, et al: Anemia and its relationship to clinical outcome in heart failure. Circulation 110:149-154, 2004.
16. Cardiovascular Risk Reduction by Early Anemic Treatment with Epoetin beta in Chronic Kidney Disease Patients (CREATE) Trial. European Renal Association/European Dialysis and Transplantation Association Annual Scientific Meeting, June 2005.
17. Singh A, Reddan D: Correction of Hemoglobin and Outcomes in Renal Insufficiency (CHOIR) Trial. National Kidney Foundation 2006 Spring Clinical Meeting, April 19-23, 2006, Chicago.
18. Mix TC, Brenner RM, Cooper ME, et al: Rationale—Trial to Reduce Cardiovascular Events with Aranesp Therapy (TREAT): Evolving the management of cardiovascular risk in patients with chronic kidney disease. Am Heart J 149:408-413, 2005.

Percutaneous Coronary Interventions and Contrast-Induced Nephropathy

19. McCullough P: Outcomes of contrast-induced nephropathy: Experience in patients undergoing cardiovascular intervention. Catheter Cardiovasc Interv 67:335-343, 2006.
20. McCullough PA, Manley HJ: Prediction and prevention of contrast nephropathy. J Interv Cardiol 14:547, 2001.
21. Pannu N, Wiebe N, Tonelli M; Alberta Kidney Disease Network: Prophylaxis strategies for contrast-induced nephropathy. JAMA 295:2765-2779, 2006.
22. Rihal CS, Textor SC, Grill DE, el al: Incidence and prognostic importance of acute renal failure after percutaneous coronary intervention. Circulation 105:2259, 2002.
23. Yerkey MW, Kernis SJ, Franklin BA, et al: Renal dysfunction and acceleration of coronary disease. Heart 90:961-966, 2004.
24. Andersen KJ, Christensen EI, Vik H: Effects of iodinated x-ray contrast media on renal epithelial cells in culture. Invest Radiol 29:955, 1994.
25. Keeley EC, Grines CL: Scraping of aortic debris by coronary guiding catheters: A prospective evaluation of 1,000 cases. J Am Coll Cardiol 32:1861, 1998.
26. Wijeysundera DN, Karkouti K, Beattie WS, et al: Improving the identification of patients at risk of postoperative renal failure after cardiac surgery. Anesthesiology 104:65-72, 2006.

27. Denton KM, Shweta A, Anderson WP: Preglomerular and postglomerular resistance responses to different levels of sympathetic activation by hypoxia. J Am Soc Nephrol 13:27, 2002.
28. Uder M, Humke U, Pahl M, et al: Nonionic contrast media iohexol and iomeprol decrease renal arterial tone: Comparative studies on human and porcine isolated vascular segments. Invest Radiol 37:440, 2002.
29. Rauch D, Drescher P, Pereira FJ, et al: Comparison of iodinated contrast media-induced renal vasoconstriction in human, rabbit, dog, and pig arteries. Invest Radiol 32:315, 1997.
30. McCullough PA: Beyond serum creatinine: Defining the patient with renal insufficiency and why? Rev Cardiovasc Med 4(Suppl 1):S2-S6, 2003.
31. Mehran R, Aymong ED, Nikolsky E, Lasic Z, et al: A simple risk score for prediction of contrast-induced nephropathy after percutaneous coronary intervention: Development and initial validation. J Am Coll Cardiol 44:1393-1399, 2004.
32. Mueller C, Buerkle G, Buettner HJ, et al: Prevention of contrast media-associated nephropathy: Randomized comparison of 2 hydration regimens in 1620 patients undergoing coronary angioplasty. Arch Intern Med 162:329, 2002.
33. Stevens MA, McCullough PA, Tobin KJ, et al: A prospective randomized trial of prevention measures in patients at high risk for contrast nephropathy: Results of the P.R.I.N.C.E. Study. Prevention of Radiocontrast Induced Nephropathy Clinical Evaluation. J Am Coll Cardiol 33:403, 1999.
34. Merten GJ, Burgess WP, Gray LV, et al: Prevention of contrast-induced nephropathy with sodium bicarbonate: a randomized controlled trial. JAMA 291:2328-2334, 2004.
35. Stacul F, Bertrand ME, McCullough PA, Brinker J: Contrast-induced nephropathy (CIN) following iso-osmolar (IOCM) versus low-osmolar contrast media (LOCM) in patients undergoing angiography and predicting factors for CIN: A meta-analysis. Eur Congress Radiol B-934, 2004.
36. Davidson CJ, Laskey WK, Hermiller JB, et al: Randomized trial of contrast media utilization in high-risk PTCA: The COURT trial. Circulation 101:2172, 2000.
37. Tepel M, Aspelin P, Lameire N: Contrast-induced nephropathy: a clinical and evidence-based approach. Circulation 113:1799-1806, 2006.
38. Marenzi G, Assanelli E, Marana I, et al: N-acetylcysteine and contrast-induced nephropathy in primary angioplasty. N Engl J Med 354:2773-2782, 2006.
39. Guitterez N, Diaz A, Timmis GC, et al: Determinants of serum creatinine trajectory in acute contrast nephropathy. J Interv Cardiol 15:349-354, 2002.

Accelerated Vascular Calcification

40. Stary HC: The sequence of cell and matrix changes in atherosclerotic lesions of coronary arteries in the first forty years of life. Eur Heart J 11(suppl E):3-19, 1990.
41. Demer LL, Tintut Y, Parhami F: Novel mechanisms in accelerated vascular calcification in renal disease patients. Curr Opin Nephrol Hypertens 11:437-443, 2002.
42. McCullough PA, Soman S: Cardiovascular calcification in patients with chronic renal failure: are we on target with this risk factor? Kidney Int Suppl Sep:S18-24, 2004.
43. McCullough PA, Sandberg KR, Dumler F, Yanez JE: Determinants of coronary vascular calcification in patients with chronic kidney disease and end-stage renal disease: A systematic review. J Nephrol 17:205-215, 2004.
44. McCullough PA: Effect of lipid modification on progression of coronary calcification. J Am Soc Nephrol 16(Suppl 2):S115-119, 2005.
45. Chertow GM, Burke SK, Raggi P; Treat to Goal Working Group: Sevelamer attenuates the progression of coronary and aortic calcification in hemodialysis patients. Kidney Int 62:245-252, 2002.
46. Suki W, Zabaneh R, Cangiano J, et al: The DCOR trial—a prospective, randomized trial assessing the impact on outcomes of sevelamer in dialysis patients. American Society of Nephrology Renal Week 2005; Nov. 8-13, 2005; Philadelphia. Abstract PO745.
47. Wanner C, Krane V, Marz W, et al; German Diabetes and Dialysis Study Investigators: Atorvastatin in patients with type 2 diabetes mellitus undergoing hemodialysis. N Engl J Med 21;353:238-248, 2005. Erratum in: N Engl J Med 353:1640, 2005.

Renal Disease and Hypertension

48. Kidney Disease Outcomes Quality Initiative (K/DOQI): K/DOQI clinical practice guidelines on hypertension and antihypertensive agents in chronic kidney disease. Am J Kidney Dis 43(Suppl 1):S1-290, 2004.
49. Cohen MG, Pascua JA, Garcia-Ben M, et al: A simple prediction rule for significant renal artery stenosis in patients undergoing cardiac catheterization. Am Heart J 150:1204-1211, 2005.
50. Fatica RA, Port FK, Young EW: Incidence trends and mortality in end-stage renal disease attributed to renovascular disease in the United States. Am J Kidney Dis 37:1184, 2001.

Ischemic Heart Diseases in Patients with Impaired Renal Function

51. Conti CR: Silent cardiac ischemia. Curr Opin Cardiol 17:537, 2002.
52. Freda BJ, Tang WH, Van Lente F, et al: Cardiac troponins in renal insufficiency: Review and clinical implications. J Am Coll Cardiol 40:2065-2071, 2002.
53. McCullough PA, Nowak RM, Foreback C, et al: Emergency evaluation of chest pain in patients with advanced kidney disease. Arch Intern Med 162:2464, 2002.
54. McCullough PA, Nowak RM, Foreback C, et al: Performance of multiple cardiac biomarkers measured in the emergency department in patients with chronic kidney disease and chest pain. Acad Emerg Med 9:1389, 2002.
55. McCullough PA: Acute coronary syndromes in patients with renal failure. Curr Cardiol Rep 5:266, 2003.
56. McCullough PA: Why is chronic kidney disease the "spoiler" for cardiovascular outcomes? J Am Coll Cardiol 41:725, 2003.

CH 88

Interface Between Renal Disease and Cardiovascular Illness

57. Herzog CA, Ma JZ, Collins AJ: Poor long-term survival after acute myocardial infarction among patients on long-term dialysis. N Engl J Med 339:799, 1998.

58. Sica D: The implications of renal impairment among patients undergoing percutaneous coronary intervention. J Invasive Cardiol 14(Suppl B):30B, 2002.

59. McCullough PA: Evaluation and treatment of coronary artery disease in patients with end-stage renal disease. Kidney Int Suppl Jun:s51-58, 2005.

Heart Failure in Patients with Kidney Disease

60. Schreiber BD: Congestive heart failure in patients with chronic kidney disease and on dialysis. Am J Med Sci 325:179, 2003.

61. McCullough PA, Duc P, Omland T; BNP Multinational Study Investigators: B-type natriuretic peptide and renal function in the diagnosis of heart failure: An analysis from the breathing not properly multinational study. Am J Kidney Dis 41:571, 2003.

62. Al-Ahmad A, Rand WM, Manjunath G, et al: Reduced kidney function and anemia as risk factors for mortality in patients with left ventricular dysfunction. J Am Coll Cardiol 38:955, 2001.

63. Shlipak MG: Pharmacotherapy for heart failure in patients with renal insufficiency. Ann Intern Med 138:917, 2003.

64. Schoolwerth AC, Sica DA, Ballermann BJ, Wilcox CS; Council on the Kidney in Cardiovascular Disease and the Council for High Blood Pressure Research of the American Heart Association: Renal considerations in angiotensin converting enzyme inhibitor therapy: A statement for healthcare professionals from the Council on the Kidney in Cardiovascular Disease and the Council for High Blood Pressure Research of the American Heart Association. Circulation 104:1985, 2001.

65. Cice G, Ferrara L, D'Andrea A, et al: Carvedilol increases two-year survival in dialysis patients with dilated cardiomyopathy: A prospective, placebo-controlled trial. J Am Coll Cardiol 41:1438, 2003.

66. McCullough PA, Sandberg KR, Yee J, Hudson MP: Mortality benefit of angiotensin-converting enzyme inhibitors after cardiac events in patients with end-stage renal disease. J Renin Angiotensin Aldosterone Syst 3:188, 2002.

67. Smith GL, Vaccarino V, Kosiborod M, et al: Worsening renal function: What is a clinically meaningful change in creatinine during hospitalization with heart failure? J Card Fail 9:13, 2003.

68. Jain P, Massie BM, Gattis WA, et al: Current medical treatment for the exacerbation of chronic heart failure resulting in hospitalization. Am Heart J 145(Suppl):S3, 2003.

69. Keating GM, Goa KL: Nesiritide: A review of its use in acute decompensated heart failure. Drugs 63:47, 2003.

70. Butler J, Emerson C, Peacock WF, et al: The efficacy and safety of B-type natriuretic peptide (nesiritide) in patients with renal insufficiency and acutely decompensated congestive heart failure. Nephrol Dial Transplant 19:391, 2004.

71. Jaski BE, Miller D: Ultrafiltration in decompensated heart failure. Curr Heart Fail Rep Sep;2:148-154, 2005.

Valvular Heart Disease and Arrhythmias in Patients with Kidney Disease

72. Umana E, Ahmed W, Alpert MA: Valvular and perivalvular abnormalities in end-stage renal disease. Am J Med Sci 325:237, 2003.

73. Manian FA: Vascular and cardiac infections in end-stage renal disease. Am J Med Sci 325:243, 2003.

74. Soman SS, Sandberg KR, Borzak S, et al: The independent association of renal dysfunction and arrhythmias in critically ill patients. Chest 122:669, 2002.

75. Wase A, Basit A, Nazir R, et al: Impact of chronic kidney disease upon survival among implantable cardioverter-defibrillator recipients. J Interv Card Electrophysiol 11:199-204, 2004.

Consultative Approach to the Hemodialysis Patient

76. Centers for Disease Control and Prevention (CDC): Incidence of end-stage renal disease among persons with diabetes—United States, 1990-2002. MMWR Morb Mortal Wkly Rep 54:1097-1100, 2005.

77. Reddan DN, Szczech LA, Tuttle RH, et al: Chronic kidney disease, mortality, and treatment strategies among patients with clinically significant coronary artery disease. J Am Soc Nephrol 14:2373-2380, 2004.

78. Szczech LA, Reddan DN, Owen WF, et al: Differential survival following coronary revascularization procedures among patients with renal insufficiency. Kidney Int 60:292-299, 2001.

79. Agarwal R, Nissenson AR, Batlle D, et al: Prevalence, treatment, and control of hypertension in chronic hemodialysis patients in the United States. Am J Med 115:291-297, 2003.

80. Vlahakos DV, Hahalis G, Vassilakos P, et al: Relationship between left ventricular hypertrophy and plasma renin activity in chronic hemodialysis patients. J Am Soc Nephrol 8:1764-1770, 1997.

81. Hampl H, Sternberg C, Berweck S, et al: Regression of left ventricular hypertrophy in hemodialysis patients is possible. Clin Nephrol 58(Suppl 1):S73-96, 2002.

82. Li PK, Chow KM, Wong TY, et al: Effects of an angiotensin-converting enzyme inhibitor on residual renal function in patients receiving peritoneal dialysis. A randomized, controlled study. Ann Intern Med 139:105-112, 2003.

83. McCullough PA: Opportunities for improvement in the cardiovascular care of patients with end-stage renal disease. Adv Chronic Kidney Dis 11:294-303, 2004.

84. Bakris GL: Role for beta-blockers in the management of diabetic kidney disease. Am J Hypertens 16(9 Pt 2):7S-12S, 2003.

85. Cice G, Ferrara L, D'Andrea A, et al: Carvedilol increases two-year survival in dialysis patients with dilated cardiomyopathy: A prospective, placebo-controlled trial. J Am Coll Cardiol 41:1438-1444, 2003.

86. McCullough PA, Sandberg KR, Borzak S, et al: Benefits of aspirin and beta-blockade after myocardial infarction in patients with chronic kidney disease. Am Heart J 144:226-232, 2002.

87. Porter GA, Norton TL, Lindsley J, et al: Relationship between elevated serum troponin values in end-stage renal disease patients and abnormal isotopic cardiac scans following stress. Ren Fail 25:55-65, 2003.

88. Buemi M, Senatore M, Corica F, et al: Statins and progressive renal disease. Med Res Rev 22:76-84, 2002.

89. National Kidney Foundation: K/DOQI clinical practive guidelines for managing dyslipidemias in chronic kidney disease. Executive summary. New York, 2003.

90. Grundy SM, Cleeman JI, Merz CN, et al; National Heart, Lung, and Blood Institute; American College of Cardiology Foundation; American Heart Association: Implications of recent clinical trials for the National Cholesterol Education Program Adult Treatment Panel III guidelines. Circulation 110:227-239, 2004. Review. Erratum in: Circulation 10;110:763, 2004.

91. American Diabetes Association: Standards of medical care for patients with diabetes mellitus. Diabetes Care 26(Suppl 1):S33-50, 2003.

92. Biesenbach G, Zazgornik J: Influence of smoking on the survival rate of diabetic patients requiring hemodialysis. Diabetes Care 19:625-628, 1996.

93. Winchester JF: Therapeutic uses of aspirin in renal diseases. Am J Kidney Dis 28(Suppl 1):S20-23, 1996.

94. Keeley EC, McCullough PA: Coronary revascularization in patients with coronary artery disease and chronic kidney disease. Adv Chronic Kidney Dis 11:254-260, 2004.

95. Reddan DN, Szczech LA, Tuttle RH, et al: Chronic kidney disease, mortality, and treatment strategies among patients with clinically significant coronary artery disease. J Am Soc Nephrol 14:2373-2380, 2003.

96. Keeley EC, Kadakia R, Soman S, et al: Analysis of long-term survival after revascularization in patients with chronic kidney disease presenting with acute coronary syndromes. Am J Cardiol 92:509-514, 2003.

97. Opsahl JA, Husebye DG, Helseth HK, et al: Coronary artery bypass surgery in patients on maintenance dialysis: Long-term survival. Am J Kidney Dis 12:271-274, 1988.

98. McCullough PA, Berman AD: Percutaneous coronary interventions in the high-risk renal patient: Strategies for renal protection and vascular protection. Cardiol Clin 23:299-310, 2005.

CHAPTER 89

Introduction, 2171

Overview of Neural Circulatory Control, 2171
Baroreceptors, 2171
Cardiopulmonary Baroreceptors, 2172
Heart Rate Modulation, 2172
Breathing and the Chemoreflexes, 2172
The Diving Reflex, 2172

Autonomic Testing, 2172
Orthostatics, 2173
Valsalva Maneuver, 2173
Baroreflex Sensitivity, 2173
Heart Rate Variability, 2173
Heart Rate Recovery, 2174
Chemoreflexes, 2174
Tilt-Table Testing, 2174

Autonomic Dysregulation, 2174
Sympathetic Dysautonomias, 2174
Parasympathetic Dysautonomias, 2175

Primary Chronic Autonomic Failure, 2175
Pure Autonomic Failure, 2175
Multiple System Atrophy, 2175
Parkinson Disease with Autonomic Failure, 2175
Diagnosis and Therapy, 2175

Secondary Autonomic Failure, 2176

Autoimmune Autonomic Failure, 2176

Congenital Autonomic Failure, 2176

Orthostatic Intolerance, 2176
Postural Tachycardia Syndrome, 2176
Neurally Mediated Syncope, 2177
Chronic Fatigue Syndrome, 2177
Baroreflex Failure, 2178
Norepinephrine Transporter Deficiency, 2178
Addison Disease, 2178

Variants of Neurocardiogenic Syncope, 2178
Aortic Stenosis, 2178
Renal Failure and Hemodialysis, 2178
Right Coronary Thrombolysis, 2179
Inferior Wall Myocardial Infarction, 2179
Hypertrophic Obstructive Cardiomyopathy, 2179
Blood Phobia, 2179

Disorders of Increased Sympathetic Outflow, 2180
Neurogenic Essential Hypertension, 2180
Panic Disorder, 2180
Congestive Heart Failure, 2181
Obstructive Sleep Apnea, 2182
Pheochromocytoma, 2182
Sleep, 2182
Bed Rest, 2182

Disorders of Increased Parasympathetic Tone, 2182
Sinus Arrhythmia, 2182

References, 2183

Cardiovascular Manifestations of Autonomic Disorders

Suraj Kapa and Virend K. Somers

INTRODUCTION

Cardiovascular function is closely linked and responsive to numerous endogenous and exogenous factors. This interplay is mediated through rapid and often subtle neurohormonal changes. One of the most important mechanisms by which rapid circulatory control is achieved is the autonomic nervous system, which modulates cardiac function through direct effects on the heart and vascular tone in response to intrinsic and extrinsic cues. These include dynamic volume changes, acid-base disturbances, postural changes, and other physiologic and pathologic events. This chapter builds on the review in the earlier edition.[1] Aspects of the NIH Conference on Clinical Disorders of the Autonomic Nervous System are highlighted,[2] and a more comprehensive bibliography is provided.

OVERVIEW OF NEURAL CIRCULATORY CONTROL

The autonomic nervous system may be subdivided into sympathetic, parasympathetic, and enteric components. The principal cardiovascular influences are mediated through the sympathetic and parasympathetic systems. The interplay between these two systems and their relative balance help determine cardiovascular responses under a variety of conditions. These responses usually take the form of changes in blood pressure or heart rate. The physiology by which blood pressure and heart rate react to autonomic cues is important to understanding how disorders of the autonomic nervous system can affect cardiovascular function.

BARORECEPTORS

Autonomic responses, capillary shift mechanisms, hormonal responses, and kidney and fluid balance mechanisms all interact to maintain blood pressure control. Of these, the autonomic nervous system offers the most rapid response system. Neural circulatory regulation occurs via either increased contractility of the heart or vasoconstriction of the arterial or venous circulations in response to information received from baroreceptors. This afferent information is synthesized and integrated, and appropriate responses are generated, in the vasomotor center of the brain (Fig. 89-1).

The reflexes by which blood pressure is maintained are collectively known as the *baroreflex*, which includes arterial baroreceptors (also known as the *high pressure receptors*) and cardiopulmonary receptors (the *low pressure receptors*). Under normal physiologic circumstances, sympathetic activity is inhibited and parasympathetic activity predominates. Arterial baroreceptors, which are the most sensitive, are located in the carotid sinuses, aortic arch, and at the origin of the right subclavian artery. The carotid sinus baroreceptors are innervated by the glossopharyngeal nerve (CN IX), and the aortic arch baroreceptors are innervated by the vagus nerve (CN X). Baroreceptors are stretch-dependent mechanoreceptors that sense changes in pressure, transmitting via afferents to the nucleus tractus solitarius (NTS) in the brain stem. When distended, the baroreceptors are activated and generate action potentials increasing in frequency in correlation to the amount of stretch. Thus spike frequency is used as a surrogate measure of blood pressure at the level of the NTS, with higher frequency correlating with higher blood pressure.

The arterial baroreceptors are tonically active under normal circumstances at mean arterial pressures (MAP) above 70 mm Hg, which is termed the *baroreceptor set point*. With MAPs below the set point, baroreceptors become essentially silent. However, the set point may vary with persistent blood pressure changes, such as in chronic hypertension in which the set point is increased or in chronic hypotension in which it is decreased (see Chap. 40). The set point may vary depending on other endogenous factors and disease states.

Integration of baroreceptor afferent signals is achieved at the level of the NTS. The NTS sends inhibitory fibers to the vasomotor center, which regulates the sympathetic nervous system, and excitatory fibers to vagal nuclei that regulate the parasympathetic system. Activation of the NTS (associated with increased action potential frequency from arterial baroreceptors) stimulates parasympathetic outflow, while an inactive nucleus induces sympathetic activation and parasympathetic inhibition. Sympathetic activation leads to increased cardiac contractility, increased heart rate, venoconstriction, and arterial vasoconstriction, ultimately leading to increased blood pressure via elevation of total peripheral resistance and cardiac output. Parasympathetic activation leads to a decrease in heart rate and a minor decrease in contractility, resulting in a decrease in blood pressure.

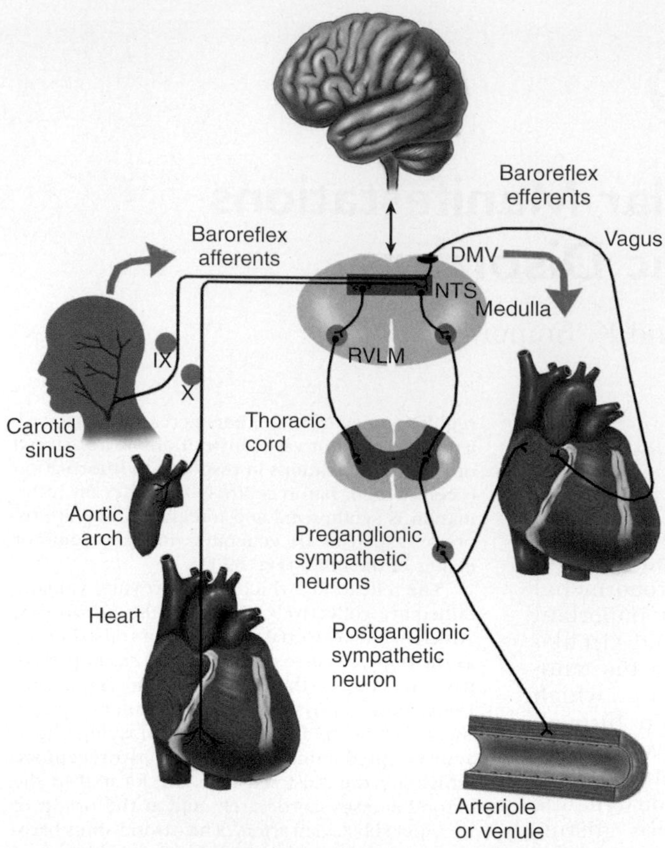

FIGURE 89–1 Autonomic components of the baroreflex.[1] Note that the baroreflex is primarily mediated via the glossopharyngeal and vagus nerves via input from the carotid sinus and aortic arch baroreceptors and cardiac mechanoreceptors. Cortical overlay has an influence on transmission and processing within the baroreflex arc. In turn, the baroreceptor reflex modulates parasympathetic and sympathetic input to the heart and circulation via the vagus nerve and spinal input to preganglionic and postganglionic sympathetic neurons. DMV = dorsal motor nucleus of the vagus; NE = norepinephrine; NTS = nucleus tractus solitarii; RVLM = rostroventrolateral medulla. *(Courtesy of Dr. André Diedrich.)*

Coupling of sympathetic inhibition with parasympathetic activation allows the baroreflex to maximize blood pressure reduction. Conversely, sympathetic activation with parasympathetic inhibition allows for an increase in blood pressure.

CARDIOPULMONARY BARORECEPTORS

Although the arterial baroreceptors are the most sensitive receptors, low-pressure receptors in the heart and venae cavae termed *cardiopulmonary receptors* also play a role in blood pressure modulation. They primarily respond to changes in volume but also to chemical stimuli. They project via vagal afferents to the NTS and via spinal sympathetic afferents to the spinal cord. Stimulation results in vasodilation and inhibition of vasopressin release. Furthermore, a stretch stimulus depresses renal sympathetic nerve activity[3] and has been shown to play a role in modulating renin release, resulting in diuresis and natriuresis,[4] thus regulating whole body fluid volume to maintain blood pressure homeostasis.[1]

HEART RATE MODULATION

Modulation of heart rate is another means by which the autonomic nervous system maintains normal blood pressure and exerts control over the cardiovascular system. Increases in heart rate are achieved through increases in contractile frequency via sympathetic activation. This is in part mediated through the arterial baroreflex. The cardiopulmonary receptors have only limited direct influence on heart rate control.

Under normal circumstances, at rest, the intrinsic sinus nodal rate is 95 to 110 beats/min, but efferent parasympathetic input via the vagus nerve suppresses the sinus nodal rate to 60 to 70 beats/min. During rest, there is little sympathetic efferent input and a low concentration

of catecholamines. This changes with any movement away from the resting state, as with physical exertion, when sympathetic activity increases and parasympathetic activity decreases. On termination of exertion, the recovery of resting heart rate is again largely governed by parasympathetic dominance.

Although cardiac automaticity is intrinsic to pacemaker activity (see Chap. 31), the autonomic nervous system plays a primary role under normal conditions in defining heart rate and rhythm. The parasympathetic influence is achieved via acetylcholine release from the vagus nerve, which increases conductance of potassium across the cell membrane. In addition, acetylcholine inhibits the hyperpolarization-activated pacemaker current. This effect is quickly dispersed because of the high acetylcholinesterase concentration around the sinus node. The sympathetic influence is achieved by release of epinephrine and norepinephrine, which cause cAMP-mediated phosphorylation of membrane proteins and a resultant increase in the inward calcium current, resulting in accelerated slow diastolic depolarization. Also, other endogenous factors, such as nitric oxide, influence channel function and further modulate autonomic control of heart rate.[5]

BREATHING AND THE CHEMOREFLEXES

The chemoreflexes are modulators of sympathetic activation and play an important role in cardiovascular autonomic tone. The chemoreceptors are most simply divided into their central and peripheral components. The peripheral chemoreceptors are located in the carotid bodies and respond to hypoxemia, whereas the central chemoreceptors are in the brainstem and respond mostly to hypercapnia. Hypoxemia or hypercapnia results in hyperventilation and vascular sympathetic activation. Inhibitory influences on the chemoreflex drive are seen with stretch of the pulmonary afferents and with activation of the baroreflex, both of which have a greater influence on peripheral rather than central chemoreflexes.[6]

In numerous clinical conditions there is a substantial role of the chemoreflexes in modulation of neural circulatory control. One is sleep apnea (see Chap. 74), in which the sympathetic vasoconstrictor response to hypoxia is potentiated because of elimination of the inhibitory influence on the chemoreflexes by stretch of the pulmonary afferents.[7] Another is hypertension, in which the ventilatory response to hypoxemia is increased and there is also an increase in sympathetic tone. This may be caused in part by impaired baroreflex sensitivity in hypertensive patients,[8] but also to an increased chemoreflex drive. The increased chemoreflex sensitivity to hypoxemia in obstructive sleep apnea patients can be reversed by use of 100 percent oxygen, with which reductions in heart rate, blood pressure, and sympathetic outflow are seen. Administering 100 percent oxygen to patients with borderline hypertension and to spontaneously hypertensive rats also reduces not only ventilation but also vasoconstrictor tone.

THE DIVING REFLEX (Fig. 89-2)

Under circumstances of prolonged apnea, a unique state of simultaneous increased parasympathetic drive to the heart and increased sympathetic drive to the vasculature occurs. This is seen in diving mammals and sometimes in humans during prolonged submersion in water. In response to hypoxia, the body usually seeks to increase ventilation and blood flow to end organs to maintain tissue oxygenation. However, in response to prolonged hypoxia in the absence of breathing, the body no longer experiences replenishment of oxygen stores and the normal homeostatic mechanisms alter so as to maintain oxygen delivery to organs vital to life, namely the brain and heart. This is achieved by decreasing oxygen delivery to much of the rest of the body via increased sympathetic vasoconstriction. This increased sympathetic outflow, however, does not constrict the cerebral vasculature due to the fact that cerebral vascular tone is under autoregulatory control. Furthermore, myocardial oxygen demand is decreased because of bradycardia caused by an increase in parasympathetic tone. For these reasons it is possible for individuals under exceptional circumstances to survive for prolonged periods of up to 5 minutes or more under anoxic conditions.

AUTONOMIC TESTING

Testing of autonomic function may occur at the bedside or via sophisticated instrumentation and long-term studies. Experimental evidence for an association between lethal arrhythmias and increased sympathetic or reduced vagal activity has spurred development of several quantitative markers of autonomic activity. Generally the two easiest and most economical means of studying the interplay between autonomic and cardiac function are via orthostatics and the Valsalva maneuver, though both are nonspecific. When a patient presents with syncope, a cost-effective means of differentiating a neurocardiogenic cause is with a tilt-table test (see Chaps. 32 and 37). Furthermore, studies of baroreflex sensitivity, heart rate variability, heart rate recovery, and chemoreflexes have been shown to help in direct assessment of autonomic dysfunction. Finally, blood levels of norepinephrine and its metabolites may assist in discriminating between different types of dysautonomias.

Orthostatics

Orthostatic hypotension is defined as a decrease of more than 20 mm Hg in systolic pressure or a decrease of more than 10 mm Hg in diastolic pressure after rising to a standing position from a supine position. Blood pressure and heart rate measurement should be done once symptoms develop or after 3 minutes have passed after rising to the standing position.[2] If the patient is unable to stand, then orthostatics may be done after the patient has risen to a sitting position with feet dangling over the edge of the bed. Orthostatic hypotension is an inability of the cardiopulmonary system to maintain sufficient blood pressure and adequate cerebral perfusion against gravity. Generally, on rising from a supine position, an average person may lose about 700 ml of blood from the thorax. This results in decreased stroke volume, as well as a decreased systolic pressure and increased diastolic pressure. Compensation occurs via an increase in heart rate and slight peripheral vasoconstriction. Individuals intolerant of orthostasis may get venous pooling secondary to decreased muscle and vascular tone and may develop a decreased circulating blood volume in response to standing. When testing orthostatics, it is important to note that a significant decrease in blood pressure without a corresponding rise in heart rate suggests abnormal autonomic innervation to the heart and may represent an underlying neuropathy.

Valsalva Maneuver

The Valsalva maneuver becomes useful in testing patients at the bedside when done in conjunction with continuous electrocardiographic monitoring. During monitoring, the patient will blow continuously into a closed system for 12 seconds at 40 mm Hg and the fastest heart rate during the maneuver is divided by the slowest heart rate immediately afterward. A quotient of less than 1.4 is suggestive of autonomic impairment. However, this is quite nonspecific. For example, patients with congestive heart failure are less able to restrict blood return to the right atrium and do not exhibit the typical hemodynamic response.[1]

Baroreflex Sensitivity

Baroreflex sensitivity is a measure of parasympathetic input to the sinus node. Testing baroreflex control of heart rate involves measuring the reflex increase in R-R interval in

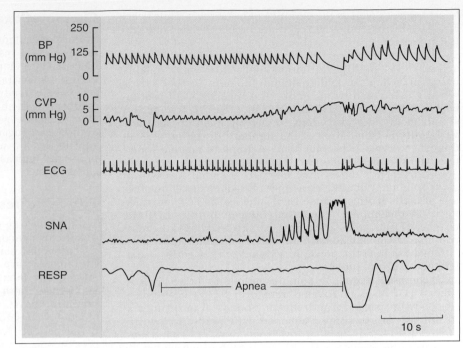

FIGURE 89–2 The diving reflex. Shown are recordings of intra-arterial blood pressure (BP), central venous pressure (CVP), electrocardiogram (ECG), sympathetic nerve activity (SNA), and respiration (RESP) during apnea lasting 30 seconds. SNA is reflected by frequency and amplitude of bursts. Toward the end of the apneic period are noted increases in BP, CVP, and SNA in addition to progressive bradycardia with eventual complete heart block. Furthermore, O_2 saturation fell to 92 percent. With release of apnea, ECG and SNA changes resolve with some temporarily continued elevation in BP. *(From Somers VK, Dyken ME, Mark AL, Abboud FM: Parasympathetic hyperresponsiveness and bradyarrhythmias during apnoea in hypertension. Clin Auton Res 2:171, 1992.)*

response to an increase in blood pressure. The increase in blood pressure has historically been achieved by use of an alpha-adrenergic agonist, most often phenylephrine. Intravenous injection of a bolus of phenylephrine induces a 20 to 30 mm Hg increase in systolic pressure. Generally a linear relationship exists between the increase in the R-R interval and the increase in systolic pressure. The slope is used to quantify the sensitivity of the arterial baroreflex. This is repeated three to five times to obtain an average slope. The slope is typically steep in healthy individuals but decreases with advancing age and flattens even more with severe cardiovascular disease like hypertension or heart failure.

As a measure of autonomic function, baroreflex sensitivity decreases (i.e., shows a flatter slope) with sympathetic dominance and increases (i.e., shows a steeper slope) with parasympathetic dominance. In the search for noninvasive ways to measure baroreflex sensitivity, various devices and maneuvers have been used. The FINAPRES (from finger arterial pressure) device is one such example and has been used in the Autonomic Tone and Reflexes after Myocardial Infarction (ATRAMI) study. Spontaneous increases and decreases in blood pressure, as well as associated RR changes, have been employed to determine the "spontaneous baroreflex." Furthermore, spectral techniques used to analyze the relationship between beat-to-beat oscillations of blood pressure and R-R intervals are being studied as possible alternatives to the more invasive method of phenylephrine infusion.

Heart Rate Variability

Heart rate variability has become a commonly used but difficult-to-interpret means of studying the interplay between the autonomic nervous system and cardiovascular function. The phenomenon being measured in heart rate variability is that of the oscillation in the interval between consecutive heart beats, as well as the variance of heart rates. Thus heart rate variability studies the oscillation of both heart rate and R-R intervals.

The actual measurement of heart rate variability has been achieved via multiple different modalities, most notably using time domain and frequency domain methods. It is usually calculated by analyzing the time series of beat-to-beat intervals from ECG or arterial pressure tracings. A simple example of time domain measurement of heart rate variability is calculation of the standard deviation of beat-to-beat intervals. The time domain graph of a value shows how the signal changes over time. The frequency domain graph, however, shows how much of a signal lies within given frequency bands over a range of frequencies. It involves use of mathematical transforms, such as the Fourier transform, to decompose a function into an infinite or finite number of frequencies. Spectral density analysis is the most common frequency domain method used and involves measurement of how the power of a signal or time series is distributed with frequency.

A common frequency domain method involves application of the discrete Fourier transform to the beat-to-beat interval time series. The frequency bands of most interest in humans are the high frequency (HF) band, the low frequency (LF) band, the very low frequency (VLF) band, and the ultra low frequency (ULF) band, each of which has its own physiologic correlate. The HF band lies between 0.15 and 0.4 Hz and is driven by respiration, appearing to derive mainly from vagal activity. The LF band, which lies between 0.04 and 0.15 Hz, appears to derive from vagal and sympathetic activity and is believed to reflect delay in the baroreceptor loop. The VLF band lies between 0.0033 and 0.04 Hz and has been attributed to physical activity. Finally, the ULF band lies between 0 and 0.0033 Hz and is associated with day/night variation.

Other means of calculating heart rate variability include phase domain measurement and other nonlinear dynamic methods. The information provided by each measuring method, however, is complementary and ought to be taken together to define and understand the characteristics of heart rate variability in a given disorder.

The utility of heart rate variability as a measure of autonomic function and as a predictor of mortality has been suggested by multiple studies. In the 1970s Wolf and colleagues showed a higher risk of postinfarction mortality with reduced heart rate variability, and Ewing and colleagues developed simple bedside tests to use short-term R-R differences as a means of detecting autonomic neuropathy in diabetics. In the late 1980s heart rate variability was shown to be an independent predictor of post–myocardial infarction mortality. More recently, altered heart rate variability has been associated with other pathologic conditions such as hypertension,[9] hemorrhagic shock,[10] and septic shock.[11] Heart rate variability has been accepted via international consensus as an independent predictor of mortality after myocardial infarction and as an early warning sign for diabetic neuropathy.

Heart Rate Recovery

During exercise, heart rate rises, initially secondary to a reduction in vagal tone, and then due to increased sympathetic activity. After exercise, parasympathetic reactivation and reduced sympathetic activity contribute to the recovery of resting heart rate. The rate at which the heart rate returns to baseline, measured over the first minute after exercise, is termed the *heart rate recovery*. A delayed heart rate recovery is a marker of decreased vagal activity, which has been shown to be an independent risk factor for sudden cardiac death.[12]

Chemoreflexes

Studies of chemoreflex function are one way of determining the dominant respiratory response in certain diseases. As discussed previously, the hypercapnic response is mediated mainly by central chemoreceptors, whereas the hypoxemic response is mediated by peripheral chemoreceptors. Thus overcoming the hypoxemic response with administration of 100 percent oxygen and studying the impact on sympathetic outflow can suggest the relative role of oxygenation versus ventilation in mediation of neural control in disease processes such as heart failure, hypertension, or obstructive sleep apnea.

Tilt-Table Testing

Tilt-table testing is often done in patients presenting with a history of syncope. The purpose is to diagnose possible dysautonomic causes of syncope. Patients are strapped to a tilt table and are suspended at angles anywhere from 60 to 90 degrees. Some patients may be given isoproterenol to make them more susceptible to syncope. Symptoms, blood pressure, heart rate, electrocardiographic findings, and blood oxygen saturation are recorded, and the test is stopped if the patient experiences symptoms, such as syncope or presyncope, or after a set period of time has passed.

The test is considered positive if the patient experiences symptoms associated with a blood pressure drop or an arrhythmia. These abnormalities are suggestive of dysfunction of the autonomic system. Normally, blood pressure will compensate via an increase in heart rate and constriction of blood vessels in the legs. In some patients, fainting or syncope could be associated with a precipitous drop in blood pressure (vasodepressor syncope) or pulse rate (cardioinhibitory syncope), or a mixed response, thus requiring continuous monitoring of both.

AUTONOMIC DYSREGULATION

Dysautonomias refer to any dysfunction of the autonomic nervous system, whether central, peripheral, or secondary to other disease processes. In general the most common dysautonomias are those affecting the sympathetic system. However, the parasympathetic system and conditions of increased parasympathetic tone, such as during sleep or with endurance training, are also important to understand because they can have significant implications for cardiovascular health.

Dysautonomias may be categorized in numerous ways. Clinically, the division between severe and mild dysautonomias, characterized by the degree of orthostatic intolerance or heart rate abnormalities, is one means of categorization. However, further consideration can be made as to whether the dysfunction is transient or part of a progressive neurodegenerative disease or whether it is the primary pathophysiology or a complication of another disease state. Generally, dysautonomias will present suddenly, whether as a syncopal episode or acute light-headedness, or as a coincidental finding, as with hypertension during a physical examination or orthostatic intolerance during a hospitalization for some other disease process.

Sympathetic Dysautonomias

The sympathetic dysautonomias are by far the most common and may be characterized by disorders of release, function, or re-uptake of the main sympathetic chemical messenger, norepinephrine. Furthermore, local blood flow and clearance of norepinephrine from the circulation may manifest as a dysautonomia. The sympathetic dysautonomias can be generally divided into two groups—those associated with decreased function, in which orthostasis often occurs, and those associated with increased outflow, in which hypertension and/or tachycardia may be present.

Parasympathetic Dysautonomias

The parasympathetic dysautonomias are most often reflected as increases in parasympathetic tone and manifest as exaggerated responses to normal physiologic conditions. Typically parasympathetic tone predominates at rest in normal humans and is balanced by local and neurohormonal responses. Furthermore, the sympathetic response to elevated parasympathetic function also helps to serve as a counterbalance.

PRIMARY CHRONIC AUTONOMIC FAILURE

Orthostatic intolerance is a key manifestation of neurocirculatory failure. It often serves as the presenting symptom. However, not all orthostatic hypotension is symptomatic of neurocirculatory failure. Most cases of orthostatic hypotension result from blood loss, volume depletion, or a prolonged bedridden state. Only rarely does it result from true autonomic failure.

Chronic autonomic failure is distinguishable from acute-onset autonomic dysfunction syndromes by its progressive nature and prognosis. Generally, chronic autonomic failure may be subdivided into secondary and primary failure, with secondary failure being far more common. In cases of secondary failure, the cause is usually clear and treatment involves therapy for the underlying disorder. However, when autonomic failure dominates the clinical presentation and a clear cause is not apparent, this is termed *primary chronic autonomic failure.*[2]

Primary autonomic failure may be subdivided into three major syndromes—pure autonomic failure, multiple system atrophy, and Parkinson disease. Major overlap among these three syndromes exists, and treatment differs among them.

Pure Autonomic Failure

Pure autonomic failure involves orthostatic hypotension in the absence of symptoms or signs of central neurodegeneration. Thus the dysfunction occurs at the level of peripheral neurons and not in the central nervous system. The functional error lies in available levels of norepinephrine, which are low when supine and rise minimally with standing.[1] Thus orthostatic hypotension and an inadequate chronotropic response to standing and the Valsalva maneuver are evident. No direct effect on longevity occurs in these patients.

Multiple System Atrophy

Multiple system atrophy includes autonomic failure with signs and symptoms of progressive central neurodegeneration. It is generally divided into Parkinsonian, cerebellar, and mixed forms. Patients develop symptoms in the sixth or seventh decade of life, exhibiting sympathetic and parasympathetic dysfunction.[1] Aside from orthostatic hypotension, findings may include impotence,[13] loss of sweating, abnormal pupillary responses, reduced intraocular pressure,[14] sleep apnea,[15] and urinary incontinence. In some patients orthostatic angina, which is actually exacerbated by use of nitroglycerin, may occur. The angina appears to be caused by severe orthostatic hypotension and resultant inadequate coronary perfusion. Furthermore, urine production is greater in these patients during the night, leaving patients more hypovolemic in the morning and further exaggerating symptoms.

Orthostatic changes in this disease may be striking, with as much as a 100 mm Hg fall in systolic pressure on standing and a minimal rise in heart rate. Because of the progressive nature and the chronicity, patients may tolerate this precipitous drop in blood pressure relatively well. The drop is believed to be caused by increased venous compliance rather than changes in arterial resistance, which appears to be increased when the patient is both supine and standing.[1] Furthermore, patients often exhibit hypertension when supine, suggesting an inappropriate level of circulating catecholamines. In fact, plasma levels of catecholamines and their metabolites are preserved, but not appropriately elevated on standing.[16]

Patients may exhibit movement disorders similar to those seen in Parkinson disease. However, this is a distinct entity from Parkinsonism with autonomic failure, or atypical Parkinson disease, which includes cell loss and Lewy body formation in the hypothalamus and central sympathetic and parasympathetic nuclei. Distinction is often made on the basis of response to antiparkinsonian medications, particularly levodopa-carbidopa, but this is not a perfect test in distinguishing between the two.

Lifespan in multiple system atrophy is diminished, and patients live on average 9 years from diagnosis. Movement abnormalities are centrally mediated and do not often respond to pharmacological intervention. Furthermore, respiratory compromise can occur progressively with development of nocturnal stridor that may require continuous positive airway pressure.[1]

Parkinson Disease with Autonomic Failure

This entity is similar in clinical appearance to multiple system atrophy with parkinsonian features. The most common cause is diffuse disease of autonomic centers in the brain. This results in similar autonomic dysfunction to that described previously, affecting organs diffusely.

Diagnosis and Therapy

Distinguishing pure autonomic failure from multiple system atrophy and Parkinson disease with autonomic failure tends to be easier than distinguishing between the latter two. Magnetic resonance imaging of the brain in pure autonomic failure will not reveal any central nervous system abnormalities, whereas in the other two, it will demonstrate central lesions. It has been suggested that levodopa-carbidopa can be used to distinguish patients with Parkinson disease, but this drug can worsen orthostatic hypotension and there have been reports of patients diagnosed with multiple system atrophy showing some improvement with therapy.

Neuroimaging techniques have been used to distinguish the three types of autonomic failure. Cardiac sympathetic nerves take up ^{123}I-metaiodobenzylguanidine (^{123}I-MIBG) and 6-(^{18}F)fluoro-dopamine, which radiolabel vesicles in the sympathetic nerve terminals, thus allowing for visualization of cardiac innervation by scintigraphy scan or single-photon emission computed tomography with use of ^{123}I-MIBG or positron emission tomography with use of 6-(^{18}F)fluoro-dopamine. In patients with multiple system atrophy, intact cardiac sympathetic innervation is noted. However, patients with Parkinson disease or pure autonomic failure show no detectable activity in the myocardium on emission scans, consistent with loss of sympathetic innervation of the heart. Thus even though Parkinson disease with autonomic failure may demonstrate central lesions, there is suggestion of an additional postganglionic lesion in these patients, which is distinct from the isolated preganglionic lesion of multiple system atrophy.[2]

Therapy depends on changes in lifestyle in addition to pharmacologic therapy. Research has shown that ingestion of carbohydrates can lower blood pressure and that a meal before bedtime may be helpful in reducing night-time supine hypertension.[17] This depressor effect can be difficult for patients after meals during the day, so caffeine ingestion or use of somatostatin in the case of severe blood pressure decreases can be used to attenuate the hemodynamic response to food. Furthermore, water intake can help increase blood pressure.[18] Physical maneuvers that cause compression of the lower extremities have also been noted to help patients symptomatically.[1]

Pharmacologically, the two main areas of intervention include volume expansion and pressor administration. Use of fludrocortisone, 0.05 to 0.2 mg twice daily, and adding sodium to the diet can help with volume expansion. The use of pressor agents should be considered in the context of the aforementioned postganglionic versus preganglionic nature of the different diseases. In patients with sympathetic cardiac denervation (i.e., pure autonomic failure or Parkinson disease with autonomic failure), midorine (an alpha-adrenoreceptor agonist) or L-threo-3,4-dihydroxyphenylserine (a norepinephrine precursor converted by parenchymal cells) may be useful. However, patients with multiple system atrophy in whom sympathetic innervation is intact may benefit from use of a sympathomimetic amine or alpha-2-adrenoreceptor blocker. Also, ma-huang or yohimbine may be useful because they induce release of norepinephrine from the sympathetic nerve terminal, but they could cause acute hypertension if used improperly.[1]

SECONDARY AUTONOMIC FAILURE

More commonly, autonomic failure occurs in the context of some other disease process and treatment of the underlying process may or may not relieve the autonomic dysfunction. By far the most common cause of secondary autonomic failure is diabetes (see Chap. 43). Diabetic neuropathy is a well-known, long-term complication and all nerves may be affected, both somatic and autonomic. Cardiovascular complications secondary to dysfunction of autonomic control have been described in patients with and without orthostatic hypotension. Heart rate variability may help in detection of diabetic autonomic neuropathy. Nerve conduction abnormalities may not be the only component of autonomic dysfunction in diabetes. Relationships between vascular stiffness and dysfunction of the baroreflex have also been noted. Furthermore, some studies have suggested that the primary dysfunction may be in defective activation of central parasympathetic pathways, as noted in rat and rabbit models.[19] Thus there appear to be both afferent and efferent, as well as sympathetic and parasympathetic, components to the autonomic dysregulation associated with diabetes. Glucose and blood pressure control may protect against neuropathic and microvascular complications and improve autonomic function.

Other common causes of secondary autonomic failure include renal failure,[20] amyloidosis,[21] paraneoplastic syndromes, and vitamin B$_{12}$ deficiency. If antibodies against components of the autonomic nervous system are present in the absence of clinically apparent neoplasm, further assess-

ment for neoplasm should be made given that clinical improvement can be achieved following treatment.[22] HIV can cause autonomic dysfunction independent of effects on cardiac function,[23] as can heavy metal intoxication, particularly with copper, lead, mercury, or thallium.

AUTOIMMUNE AUTONOMIC FAILURE

Severe autonomic failure may result from autoimmune damage to neurons. Disease progression is variable and ranges from days to years.[24] Due to the variable time of presentation, it may be difficult to separate autoimmune autonomic failure from other types of autonomic dysfunction. In addition to orthostatic hypotension, bowel and bladder dysfunction may occur. Plasma catecholamines are usually low and rise minimally with standing. Some reports have shown utility of intravenous gamma globulin in treatment. One case report has also suggested a role for plasma exchange pheresis in treatment.[25]

In addition to autoimmune autonomic failure, autonomic dysfunction may be seen as a complication in severe cases of Guillain-Barré syndrome. In these patients, treatment is often supportive and orthostatic intolerance may be the only symptom. Furthermore, autonomic function may completely return with general motor function. Orthostatic intolerance may also occur as a sequela of prolonged bed rest in these patients.[1]

CONGENITAL AUTONOMIC FAILURE

The first autonomic disorder associated with a defined genetic abnormality was dopamine beta-hydroxylase deficiency. Dopamine beta-hydroxylase converts dopamine to norepinephrine in vesicles in noradrenergic neurons. Thus this is a disorder of sympathetic noradrenergic function. As a result of the norepinephrine deficiency, patients cannot mount a vasoconstrictor response to upright posture and have marked orthostatic hypotension with a blunted rise in heart rate.[1] Also, they have excess quantities of dopamine, which is released in place of norepinephrine, resulting in increased urinary sodium excretion, ptosis, nasal stuffiness, joint hyperextensibility, and retrograde ejaculation in men.[1] Dihydroxyphenylserine has been used with some benefit to restore norepinephrine levels because these patients have normal levels of dopa decarboxylase.[26]

ORTHOSTATIC INTOLERANCE

Orthostatic intolerance (see Chap. 37) is an entity distinct from orthostatic hypotension and is only occasionally characterized by rapid development of orthostatic hypotension. Generally, symptoms are seen in young women who report visual changes, poor concentration while standing, fatigue while standing, tremor, and oftentimes syncope. Several diseases are associated with orthostatic intolerance. These range from problems of localized excess noradrenergic stimulation to abnormalities of the baroreflex response. However, there is considerable overlap in terms of diagnosis, especially among postural tachycardia syndrome, neurally mediated syncope, and chronic fatigue syndrome, which oftentimes coexist in patients presenting with orthostatic intolerance.

Postural Tachycardia Syndrome

Postural orthostatic tachycardia syndrome is a heterogeneous disorder, characterized primarily by orthostatic symptoms, tachycardia, and the absence of significant hypotension. Postural orthostatic tachycardia syndrome is characterized by decreased responsiveness of the baroreflex arc to hypotension and a decrease in transmission of appropriate sympathetic input to the vasculature. However, sympathetic input to the heart and consequently heart rate *responses* are actually increased. This appears to be caused by orthostatic pooling of blood in splanchnic and dependent circulations on standing, causing activation of the cardiac sympathetic system and resultant tachycardia.[2]

Diagnostic criteria for postural orthostatic tachycardia syndrome are controversial and may be based on several criteria including the following:

- Orthostatic tachycardia greater than 30 beats/min
- Transient systolic blood pressure decrease of greater than 20 mm Hg, with recovery within the first minute of tilt
- Standing plasma norepinephrine greater than 600 pg/ml
- Severe orthostatic symptoms

In these patients there is a reduction in the baroreflex index in the presence of alpha and beta receptor hypersensitivity. In order to fully assess whether the cardiac response is normal or not, blood flow in the middle cerebral artery during a head-up tilt test can be assessed, with abnormally rapid declines being associated with an inadequate sympathetic response.[1]

Neurally Mediated Syncope (Fig. 89-3)

Neurally mediated syncope, also known as *neurocardiogenic syncope,* is characterized by periodic syncopal episodes with normal autonomic function between episodes. Patients frequently have vasovagal-like fainting and a reduction in vascular sympathetic activity during the syncopal episode. Several variants of neurally mediated syncope are discussed later in this chapter.

The mechanisms underlying neurally mediated syncope remain controversial but are presumed to be secondary to decreased venous return to the heart resulting from increased peripheral venous pooling of blood, which results in cardiac hypercontractility. One study has documented the complete disappearance of peroneal sympathetic nerve recordings during syncopal episodes in these patients. The hypercontractile response activates cardiac mechanoreceptors, resulting in a paradoxical reflex bradycardia and decreased systemic vascular resistance despite the already decreased venous return, eliciting the characteristic presyncopal symptoms of weakness, light-headedness, feelings of warmth or cold, and ultimate brief loss of consciousness. This reflex bradycardia and hypotension is similar to that evoked by the Bezold-Jarisch reflex.

Potential cardiac causes of syncope must be considered before this diagnosis of exclusion can be made, and prognosis is benign aside from sequelae of any falls that may occur with a syncopal event. However, even then, diagnosis can be difficult.

Situational syncope must be excluded, as well as phobia syndromes or other organic causes. Tilt-table testing has good specificity but uncertain sensitivity in diagnosis and is not always reproducible. Implantable loop recorders, which store 45 minutes of retrospective electrocardiographic data, may also be used and can be activated by patients after each syncopal event. However, the cost is high and the diagnostic benefit remains undefined.

Typically, treatment in these patients is conservative and involves education, particularly in determining potential predisposing factors and recognizing prodromal symptoms when they occur. Increasing fluid and salt intake may also help in avoiding development of syncope. Pharmacological therapy includes beta-blockers, which presumably work via inhibition of mechanoreceptor activation[27]; fludrocortisone, which expands central fluid volume via retention of sodium; and vasoconstrictors and selective serotonin reuptake inhibitors, which may have a role in regulating sympathetic nervous system activity. Although cardiac pacing addresses the bradycardia, it is incompletely effective because it does not compensate for the vasodepressor component.

Chronic Fatigue Syndrome

Chronic fatigue syndrome is characterized by new, unexplained fatigue that lasts for at least 6 months, is unrelieved by rest, and has no clear cause.[2] The etiology of this syndrome is unclear. Some data have suggested that dysautonomia may be common in patients with chronic fatigue syndrome. On the basis of tilt-table testing, more than 60 percent of patients with chronic fatigue show abnormal blood pressure or heart rate responses, with sudden hypotension or severe bradycardia or tachycardia, along with decreased consciousness.[28] Syncopal episodes in these patients are usually associated with a decrease in sympathetic outflow in the absence of ventricular hypovolemia or hypercontractility.

Chronic fatigue patients have not been shown to benefit from treatment with fludrocortisone and high salt intake, unlike most patients suffering from orthostatic intolerance

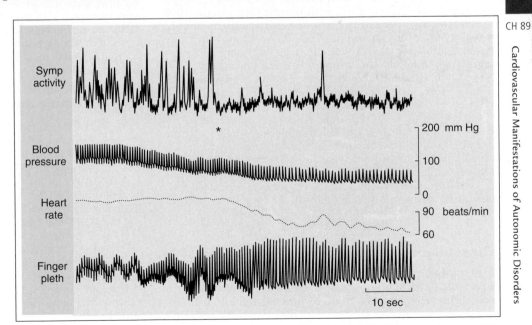

FIGURE 89–3 Recordings of sympathetic nerve activity and blood pressure before and during vasovagal syncope. Note the simultaneous reductions in sympathetic nerve activity, heart rate, and blood pressure that is associated with the episode of syncope (*). Symp = sympathetic; pleth = plethysmography. *(From Wallin BG, Sundlof G: Sympathetic outflow to muscles during vasovagal syncope. J Auton Nerv Syst 6:287, 1982.)*

secondary to sympathetic neurocirculatory failure. Thus it is not clear what the exact mechanism of orthostatic intolerance is in these patients. Alternative treatments may include midorine or beta-adrenoreceptor blockers. Whether relief of any dysautonomic symptoms in these patients may relieve the symptoms of fatigue is unclear.[2] Because these patients are often physically inactive, an exercise conditioning program implemented to improve well-being may help alleviate symptoms.

Baroreflex Failure

Causes of baroreflex failure most often include surgery, radiation therapy,[29] and cerebrovascular accidents.[30] Failure results from damage to afferent neuronal input (via the vagus and glossopharyngeal nerves) or from damage to brain stem nuclei or interneurons.[1] As a result, there is a loss of response to arterial baroreceptor stimulation.

These patients are often seen acutely, presenting with significant pheochromocytoma-like pressor crises associated with palpitations, diaphoresis, and severe headaches. Patients may present after surgical intervention, trauma, or stroke. Blood pressure is labile and may rise to extremely high levels. Some studies have shown that 9 to 30 percent of patients exhibit hypertension consistent with baroreflex failure after carotid endarterectomy.[1] In fact, patients with unilateral involvement may show nearly complete failure as well. The right carotid baroreflex may be more effective than the left carotid, suggesting a difference in clinical outcome depending on which carotid artery is affected.[31]

The clinical presentation may vary over time, and acute episodes during waking hours may mimic a pheochromocytoma, and severe hypotension and bradycardia may occur during sleep. Heart rate and blood pressure change together (concomitant rises or falls in both). Furthermore, there is little or no orthostatic hypotension initially, though it may appear later with prolonged standing. Apneic episodes may occur because of loss of neural afferents from carotid chemoreceptors.[32]

Loss of the baroreflex buffering mechanism results in prolonged and exaggerated responses to a variety of tests, such as the cold pressor test. Plasma and urinary norepinephrine levels may be high, with plasma levels in the 1000 to 3000 pg/ml range. Minor stimuli can result in pressor crises even after successful initial treatment in these patients, and long-term therapy may be necessary. Diagnostically, patients may show a depressor response to a small dose of clonidine but no heart rate response to depressor or pressor infusions, even though heart rate will change with sedation or cortical stimuli.[1]

Initial therapy over the first 72 hours may include nitroprusside and clonidine. Chronically, patients may continue to have labile hypertension and tachycardia alternating with hypotension and bradycardia. This may be effectively treated with clonidine and methyldopa. During periods of excess cortical stimulation (e.g., stress, anxiety), low-dose benzodiazepines and clonidine may help relieve symptoms.[1]

Norepinephrine Transporter Deficiency

In norepinephrine transporter deficiency, there is a deficiency of the membrane norepinephrine transporter. As a result, there is a greater than 98 percent reduction in reuptake of norepinephrine at the sympathetic nerve ending.[33] This results in elevated levels of norepinephrine at the synapse and resultant tachycardia, especially on standing, when norepinephrine delivery is increased despite the already elevated synaptic concentration.

Addison Disease

Adrenal hypofunction, Addison disease, and particularly Addisonian crisis may manifest as a global autonomic dysfunction with particular impact on heart rate and blood pressure. The combined glucocorticoid and mineralocorticoid deficiency may be due to a defect anywhere in the hypothalamic-pituitary-adrenal axis. Glucocorticoid insufficiency contributes to hypotension and may reduce myocardial contractility. In primary Addison's, mineralocorticoid insufficiency disturbs the renin-angiotensin-aldosterone axis and intravascular fluid balance, contributing to the hypotension and tachycardia seen in these patients. The combined effects of glucocorticoid and mineralocorticoid deficiencies lead to decreased intravascular volume with an attenuated cardiac response to stressors, resulting in orthostatic hypotension and eventual circulatory collapse without appropriate treatment. Thus Addison disease can mimic central autonomic dysfunction due to its effects on circulatory control and volume status.

VARIANTS OF NEUROCARDIOGENIC SYNCOPE

Aortic Stenosis (Fig. 89-4)

Exertional syncope is common in aortic stenosis (see Chap. 62) and has often been attributed to carotid sinus hypersensitivity, arrhythmias, or left ventricular failure. The normal compensatory response to exercise involves a rise in blood pressure and heart rate resulting from an increase in cardiac output, peripheral vasoconstriction in inactive muscles, and vasodilation in active muscles. Flamm and colleagues[34] demonstrated that the onset of near-syncope in patients with aortic stenosis was associated with a large reduction in blood pressure and cardiac output to resting levels in the absence of appropriate reflex vasoconstriction. Patients with aortic stenosis and a history of exertional syncope develop paradoxical forearm vasodilation during leg exercise. This muscular vasodilation is presumed to be due to activation of mechanosensitive vagal afferents in response to an outflow obstruction-associated increase in left ventricular end diastolic pressure. The net effect of this process is a reflex vasodilation. However, the vasodilator response is not accompanied by bradycardia, suggesting that the syncopal response to exertion in aortic stenosis is primarily vasodepressor rather than cardioinhibitory in nature.

Renal Failure and Hemodialysis

(Fig. 89-5) (see Chap. 88)

Acute hypotension is a common complication of hemodialysis, though the precise cause is poorly defined. Presumably, the mechanism may be similar to that in hypotension associated with acute hemorrhage, in which there is paradoxical sympathetic withdrawal, vasodilation, and bradycardia. This appears to result from activation of cardiac vagal afferents caused by tachycardia and decreased ventricular filling. Hypotension-prone hemodialysis patients have an initial tachycardia, sympathetic activation, and vasoconstriction, followed by profound hypotension due to paradoxical bradycardia, vasodilation, and sympathetic inhibition. This is different from patients not prone to hypotension who exhibit progressive rises in heart rate and sympathetic activity during dialysis. Furthermore, there is a clear difference in cardiac adaptation to changes in fluid volume, with hypotension-prone patients exhibiting a progressive reduction to near obliteration of left ventricular end-systolic dimensions, whereas there is little change in hypotension-

sion, exhibit a greater incidence of bradycardia and hypotension (>80 percent) than patients with left coronary occlusion (<14 percent) (see Chap. 52). This perceived difference may be caused in part by the preferential distribution of inhibitory cardiac receptors in the inferoposterior wall of the ventricle. Activation of the inhibitory reflex may be caused by either sudden improvement in contractile force of the previously akinetic segment of myocardium, resulting in activation of mechanosensitive vagal afferents, or to the release of free radicals and other metabolic products, resulting in activation of chemosensitive vagal afferents.

Inferior Wall Myocardial Infarction

As stated previously, preferential localization of inhibitory cardiac receptors in the inferoposterior wall of the ventricle is apparent. With infarction, there would be an expected reflex tachycardia; indeed, this is often the case in patients who suffer from an anterior wall infarction. However, patients suffering from an inferior wall infarction may have a relatively increased incidence of bradycardia and hypotension. In fact, during Prinzmetal angina, spasm of vessels supplying the inferior wall more often results in bradycardia when compared with spasm of those vessels supplying the anterior wall, which more often results in tachycardia. This reflex activation of cardiac inhibitory signals also appears to result in inhibition of renal sympathetic activity, further potentiating neurogenic hypotension.

Reflex reduction in cardiac afterload and heart rate may be beneficial in the context of myocardial infarction due to a decrease in myocardial oxygen demand. Thus low-grade activation of the cardiac inhibitory reflex may conceivably contribute to the more favorable prognosis associated with inferior wall myocardial infarction.

Hypertrophic Obstructive Cardiomyopathy

Syncope in hypertrophic obstructive cardiomyopathy (HCM) is associated with a high risk of sudden death (see Chap. 65). In these patients, sudden death has generally been associated with a tendency to develop malignant arrhythmias. However, patients with HCM also demonstrate syncope during sinus rhythm and an abnormal blood pressure response to exercise, suggesting that activation of left ventricular baroreceptors may cause the associated hypotension and hemodynamic collapse. The predisposition to hypotension and bradycardia in these patients appears to result from activation of left ventricular mechanoreceptors. Studies with tilt-table testing in these patients resulted in hypotension in a significant number of patients with a prior history of syncope. Head-up tilt was paired with echocardiography, which revealed reduced cavity sizes and increased fractional shortening with head-up tilt, consistent with conditions that would be favorable to activation of left ventricular mechanoreceptors. This suggests that the cause of syncope in patients with HCM may not just be malignant arrhythmias but may also occur because of inappropriate activation of inhibitory left ventricular mechanoreceptors in response to vigorous ventricular contraction or reduced ventricular cavity size.

Blood Phobia

Many people suffer from blood or injury phobia and experience syncope or presyncope in response to these visual stimuli. Syncope in these patients has been thought to be

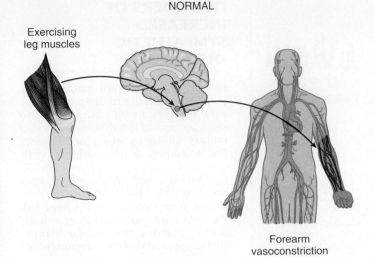

NORMAL

Exercising leg muscles

Forearm vasoconstriction

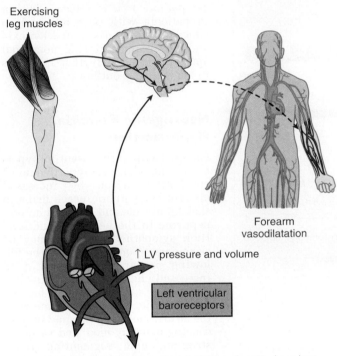

SEVERE AORTIC STENOSIS

Exercising leg muscles

Forearm vasodilatation

↑ LV pressure and volume

Left ventricular baroreceptors

FIGURE 89–4 Syncope in severe aortic stenosis. The schematic shows how afferent impulses from exercising leg muscles relayed to the brain stem normally elicit reflex vasoconstriction in the nonexercising forearm. However, in patients with severe aortic stenosis, increased left ventricular pressure and volume during exercise inhibits and even reverses forearm vasoconstriction by inducing sympathetic withdrawal during exercise. This sympathetic withdrawal has the potential to result in exertional syncope. (*Modified from Mark AL: The Bezold-Jarisch reflex revisited: Clinical implications of inhibitory reflexes originating in the heart. J Am Coll Cardiol 1:90, 1983.*)

resistant patients. This suggests that the mechanism by which hypotension develops in hypotension-prone hemodialysis patients may be via excessive myocardial contraction around an empty chamber, resulting in activation of ventricular mechanoreceptors and resultant cardiac inhibition.

Right Coronary Thrombolysis

Patients with right coronary artery occlusion, following intracoronary thrombolytic therapy and resultant reperfu-

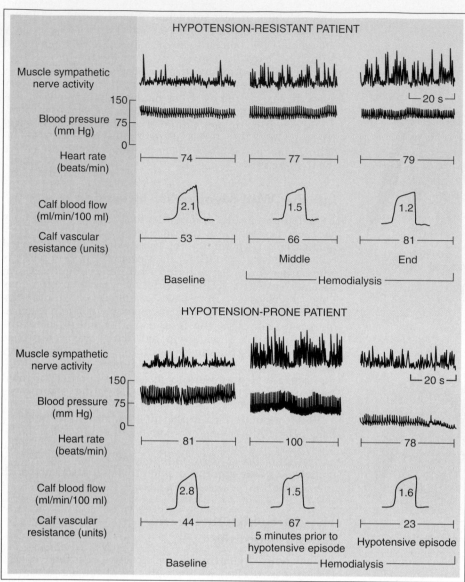

HYPOTENSION-RESISTANT PATIENT

Muscle sympathetic nerve activity

Blood pressure (mm Hg) — 150, 75, 0

Heart rate (beats/min) — 74 — 77 — 79

└ 20 s ┘

Calf blood flow (ml/min/100 ml) — 2.1, 1.5, 1.2

Calf vascular resistance (units) — 53 — 66 — 81

Middle — End

Baseline — Hemodialysis

HYPOTENSION-PRONE PATIENT

Muscle sympathetic nerve activity

Blood pressure (mm Hg) — 150, 75, 0

└ 20 s ┘

Heart rate (beats/min) — 81 — 100 — 78

Calf blood flow (ml/min/100 ml) — 2.8, 1.5, 1.6

Calf vascular resistance (units) — 44 — 67 — 23

5 minutes prior to hypotensive episode — Hypotensive episode

Baseline — Hemodialysis

FIGURE 89–5 Mechanisms of hypotension during hemodialysis. **Top,** Measurements in a patient resistant to dialysis-induced hypotension. **Bottom,** Measurements in a patient prone to hypotension during dialysis. In a hypotension-resistant patient, hemodialysis induces a gradual increase in sympathetic activity and accompanying fall in calf blood flow and increased vascular resistance. This vasoconstriction works in concert with increased heart rate to maintain blood pressure. However, in a hypotension-prone patient, hemodialysis initially induces sympathetic activation that is qualitatively similar to that in the hypotension-resistant patient. However, further hemodialysis causes a marked fall in blood pressure with an associated reduction in sympathetic nerve activity, heart rate, and vascular resistance. This is likely due to activation of ventricular mechanoreceptors due to volume depletion in the setting of tachycardia and increased contractility, resulting in a relative bradycardia and sympathetic inhibition with vasodilation and consequent profound hypotension. *(From Converse RL, Jacobsen TN, Jost CMT, et al: Paradoxical withdrawal of reflex vasoconstriction as a cause of hemodialysis-induced hypotension. J Clin Invest 90:1657, 1992.)*

DISORDERS OF INCREASED SYMPATHETIC OUTFLOW

Increased sympathetic outflow may occur in a number of diseases, either as a primary event contributing to development of the disease or as secondary to the underlying disease. For example, many patients with essential hypertension have chronic sympathetic activation, which may precede the development of sustained hypertension (see Chap. 40). Patients with panic disorder exhibit acute episodes that evoke sympathetic neuronal and adrenomedullary activation, with precipitation of coronary artery spasm. In heart failure patients, chronic elevation in sympathetic tone is noted, as is seen in patients with obstructive sleep apnea, in whom associated hypoxia and hypercapnia during nocturnal apneas may elicit further increases in sympathetic outflow.

Neurogenic Essential Hypertension

Patients with early essential hypertension may have a "hyperdynamic" circulation driven by increased efferent sympathetic nerve firing to skeletal muscle and elevated norepinephrine in the heart and kidneys. High sympathetic outflow may be secondary to one or more of the following: impaired baroreflex gain, increased chemoreflex gain, insulin resistance, and/or genetic factors. Sympathetic activation stimulates the heart, elevating cardiac output, causing neurally mediated vasoconstriction, and augmenting renin secretion and tubular reabsorption of sodium, increasing total body fluid volume.[2] In the long term, secondary end organ and vascular changes may sustain "established" hypertension, even in the absence of overt sympathetic activation and tachycardia.

largely neurogenic and anticipatory in origin because of the high correlation with situational stressors. One recent study suggested that patients suffering from syncope secondary to blood or injury phobia actually have an underlying predisposition toward neurocardiogenic syncope. Patients with a history of blood phobia syncope have been shown to have a higher rate of tilt-induced syncope than controls.[35] These findings suggest that fainting in response to blood or injury may be caused by dysfunction in neural circulatory control and has an associated organic origin. It has been proposed that this dysfunction may secondarily lead to the phobia because of repeated syncopal events.

Panic Disorder

Cardiovascular events during a panic episode may be triggered by increased sympathetic outflow (see Chap. 86). Although the true risk is unknown, it seems that there may be some increased ischemic heart disease in patients with a history of panic disorder. During a panic attack, sympathetic nerve firing increases, as does adrenomedullary secretion of epinephrine.[2] Patients who describe angina pectoris–like symptoms during a panic attack may or may not have electrocardiographic changes consistent with myocardial ischemia. It has been suggested that some patients

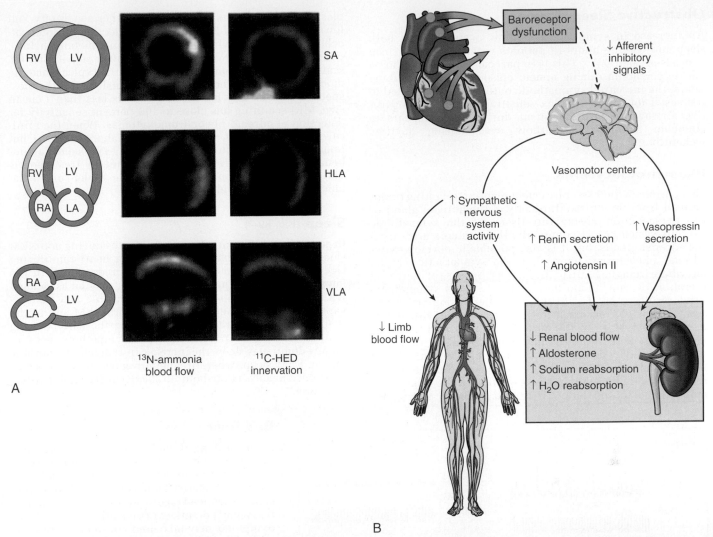

13N-ammonia
blood flow

11C-HED
innervation

A

B

FIGURE 89–6 A, Autonomic denervation of the failing heart. Positron emission tomography images obtained from patients with congestive heart failure (CHF) have demonstrated that there is partial denervation of the left ventricle in these patients. The images above demonstrate the short-axis (SA), horizontal long-axis (HLA), and vertical long-axis (VLA) views of the heart. Ammonia uptake is seen to be relatively homogeneous, which is consistent with intact myocardial perfusion. C-11 hydroxyephedrine (C-HED) uptake marks innervation of the heart and, in patients with heart failure, there is reduced retention that appears to be relatively heterogeneous, suggesting partial denervation of the left ventricle. A known association exists between the extent of denervation and clinical outcome, with higher degrees of denervation associated with increased mortality. Denervation of the heart may affect cardiac and vascular control secondary to defective afferent autonomic input from mechanoreceptors in the left ventricle. **B,** Increased sympathetic activity in CHF. Baroreceptor dysfunction may partly account for the increased sympathetic activity seen in patients with congestive heart failure. Baroreceptor function is impaired in heart failure, in part due to partial sympathetic denervation of the heart. Thus inhibitory input from cardiac mechanoreceptors is decreased despite increased intracardiac volumes. Typically, stimulation of these mechanoreceptors via increased stretch will result in vasodilation and depression of renal sympathetic nerve activity. However, because of partial denervation, there is a lack of appropriate inhibition of the sympathetic nervous system, leading to excess sympathetic activity to the kidney, worsening fluid retention, and to peripheral blood vessels, potentiating vasoconstriction. Thus partial denervation of cardiac mechanoreceptors may result in a neural circulatory profile mimicking that seen in hypovolemia and may, in part, explain the sympathetic activation and fluid retention seen in heart failure. (**A,** From Schwaiger M, Bengal F: Atlas of Heart Diseases: Nuclear Cardiology. Edited by Dilsizian V, Narula J, Braunwald E [series ed.]. Current Medicine, 2006. **B,** Adapted from Nohria A, Cusco J, Creager M: Atlas of Heart Diseases: Heart Failure. Edited by Colucci WS, Braunwald E [series ed.]. Current Medicine, 2004.)

may experience angina-like attacks secondary to coronary artery spasm.

Congestive Heart Failure

(Fig. 89-6) (see Chap. 24)

The failing heart becomes partly sympathetically denervated. Thus historically, adrenergic agonists were used to treat these patients, though this turned out to be more dangerous than helpful. In fact, beta-blocker use in these patients contributed to long-term improvement rather than worsening of heart failure. The reason for this may be partially because although there is low myocardial tissue concentration of norepinephrine, cardiac norepinephrine spillover is increased to levels associated with near-maximal aerobic exercise.[2] Heart failure patients also exhibit baroreflex dysfunction and disrupted heart rate variability. Increased cardiac sympathetic activation, altered baroreflex gain, and blunted heart rate variability have been associated with poorer long-term outcomes. It has been proposed that development of heart failure and increase in sympathetic outflow may occur in conjunction and feed off of one another to further adversely affect cardiac status. While cardiac transplantation may improve some of the autonomic disturbances seen in heart failure, residual autonomic dysfunction may persist.

Obstructive Sleep Apnea

An increase in sympathetic outflow occurs during both sleep and waking hours in patients with obstructive sleep apnea (see Chap. 74).[36] This is in part caused by the hypoxia and hypercapnia during apneic episodes. During waking hours, the increased sympathetic outflow may be related to increased tonic chemoreflex sensitivity. Continuous positive airway pressure treatment during sleep appears to attenuate sympathetic outflow even during daytime wakefulness.

Pheochromocytoma

Pheochromocytoma is a rare catecholamine-secreting tumor derived from the chromaffin cells of the adrenal gland or the paraganglion chromaffin tissue of the sympathetic nervous system. Most commonly, these tumors arise from the adrenal glands, but it is also possible to develop extra-adrenal pheochromocytomas in the sympathetic ganglia anywhere from the brain to the bladder. Because of increased secretion of catecholamines, there is excess sympathetic drive resulting in life-threatening hypertension or cardiac arrhythmias. The excess secretion is associated with lack of normal innervation to the adrenal medulla, and the exact mechanism of secretion is not completely clear, though it may be caused by direct pressure or changes in tumor blood flow. Pheochromocytomas may also be sporadic or familial, with primarily norepinephrine secretion in the former and epinephrine in the latter. Diagnosis requires testing for plasma metanephrine, which has a higher sensitivity and lower specificity, and 24-hour urine collection for total catecholamines, vanillylmandelic acid, and metanephrines, which have a higher specificity and lower sensitivity. CT scanning of the abdomen and pelvis is the typical imaging modality used but is neither the most sensitive nor the most specific, particularly for adrenal tumors less than 1 cm in size. MRI scanning has close to 100 percent sensitivity for detection of adrenal pheochromocytomas. When the clinical suspicion is high due to positive laboratory tests but imaging reveals no source, a scan with ^{131}I-labeled metaiodobenzylguanidine may be useful. Definitive treatment is via surgical resection with appropriate alpha- and beta-blockade preoperatively.

Sleep (Fig. 89-7)

In general, parasympathetic tone increases during non-REM sleep. This is associated with a fall in heart rate during sleep. However, REM sleep, which is predominant in the later hours of sleep, just before waking, may be associated with significant sympathetic activation. This may be relevant to nocturnal angina associated with REM and to the predominance of cardiac events during the early waking hours following sleep. Although parasympathetic activity largely dominates sleep, the increase in sympathetic outflow during REM sleep, when dreams are most likely to occur, may conceivably contribute to tachycardia and cardiac ischemia.

Bed Rest

After prolonged bed rest or after exposure to microgravity, such as in spaceflight, there is a decrease in normal autonomic tone,[37,38] with orthostatic tachycardia and hypotension. Advanced age and vasoactive medications may potentiate orthostatic consequences. Symptoms may take hours to weeks to resolve, with longer periods of bed rest requiring longer periods of time. In some people, compression garments may be useful as interim therapy.[1]

DISORDERS OF INCREASED PARASYMPATHETIC TONE

Increased parasympathetic tone may be associated with a number of physiologic and pathologic conditions including weight loss[39] and spinal cord trauma.[40] Bradyarrhythmias, such as Mobitz type I heart block occurring during sleep, may also be due to abrupt but physiologic increases in parasympathetic tone during REM sleep. Also, the decrease in resting heart rate seen in well-conditioned athletes may be associated with an elevated parasympathetic outflow at rest. However, in general, pathologic disorders of sympathetic outflow are more common than those of parasympathetic tone.

Sinus Arrhythmia

Under normal circumstances the heart is under parasympathetic dominance. Variations from the resting state occur with each breath because of the influence of breathing on the flow of sympathetic and vagal activity to the sinoatrial

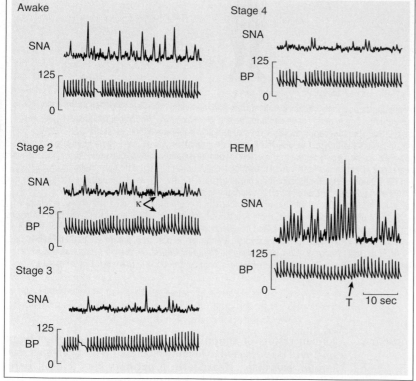

FIGURE 89-7 Recordings of sympathetic activity and mean blood pressure at various stages of sleep. As non-rapid eye movement (REM) sleep deepens, sympathetic nerve activity decreases and blood pressure and variability in blood pressure are gradually reduced. Arousal stimuli elicit increases in sympathetic nerve activity and blood pressure (arrows indicate K-complex on electroencephalogram) in stage 2 sleep. However, during REM sleep, heart rate, blood pressure, and blood pressure variability increase along with an increase in frequency and amplitude of sympathetic nerve activity. The "T" under REM sleep denotes a REM twitch (a momentary period of restoration of muscle tone) and an abrupt inhibition of sympathetic nerve discharge, which is accompanied by an increase in blood pressure. *(From Somers VK, Dyken ME, Mark AL, Abboud F: Sympathetic nerve activity during sleep in normal subjects. N Engl J Med 328:303, 1993.)*

node. With inhalation, vagus nerve activity is inhibited and heart rate begins to increase. With exhalation, this process reverses. This variation of heart rate with breathing is normal and is a sign of cardiac health. Absence of heart rate change with inspiration suggests cardiac disease and disturbed or diseased neural circulatory control.

REFERENCES

Neural Circulatory Control

1. Robertson RH, Robertson D: Cardiovascular manifestations of autonomic disorders. In Zipes DP, Libby P, Bonow R, Braunwald E (eds): Braunwald's Heart Disease: A Textbook of Cardiovascular Disease, 7th edition. Philadelphia, WB Saunders, 2004, pp 2173-2184.
2. Goldstein DS, Robertson D, Esler M, et al: Dysautonomias: Clinical disorders of the autonomic nervous system. Ann Intern Med 137:753, 2002.
3. Ditting T, Hilgers KF, Scrogin KE, et al: Influence of short-term versus long-term cardiopulmonary receptor stimulation on renal and preganglionic adrenal sympathetic nerve activity in rats. Basic Res Cardiol 101:223, 2006.
4. DiBona GF: Physiology in perspective: The wisdom of the body: Neural control of the kidney. Am J Physiol Regul Integr Comp Physiol 289:R633, 2005.
5. Takimoto Y, Aoyama T, Tanaka K, et al: Augmented expression of nitric oxide synthase in the atria parasympathetically decreases heart rate during acute myocardial infarction in rats. Circulation 105:490, 2002.
6. Spicuzza L, Porta C, Bramanti A, et al: Interaction between central-peripheral chemoreflexes and cerebro-cardiovascular control. Clin Auton Res 15:373, 2005.
7. Kara T, Narkiewicz K, Somers VK: Chemoreflexes—physiology and clinical implications. Acta Physiol Scand 177:377, 2003.
8. Lai CJ, Yang CCH, Hsu YY, et al: Enhanced sympathetic outflow and decreased baroreflex sensitivity are associated with intermittent hypoxia-induced systemic hypertension in conscious rats. J Appl Physiol 100:1974, 2006.

Autonomic Testing

9. Schroeder EB, Liao D, Chambless LE, et al: Hypertension, blood pressure, and heart rate variability: The Atherosclerosis Risk in Communities (ARIC) Study. Hypertension 42:1106, 2003.
10. Cooke WH, Convertino VA: Heart rate variability and spontaneous baroreflex sequences: Implications for autonomic monitoring during hemorrhage. J Trauma Inj Infect Crit Care 58:798, 2005.
11. Soriano F, Nogueira A, Cappi S, et al: Heart dysfunction and heart rate variability prognoses in sepsis. Crit Care 8:P75, 2005.
12. Tiukinhoy S: Heart rate profile during exercise as a predictor of sudden death. J Cardiopul Rehab 25:387, 2005.

Autonomic Dysregulation

13. Kirchhof K, Apostolidis AN, Mathias CJ, Fowler CJ: Erectile and urinary dysfunction may be the presenting features in patients with multiple system atrophy: A retrospective study. Int J Impot Res 15:293, 2003.
14. Singleton CD, Robertson D, Byrne DW, Joos KM: Effect of posture on blood and intraocular pressures in multiple system atrophy, pure autonomic failure, and baroreflex failure. Circulation 108:2349, 2003.
15. Yamaguchi M, Arai K, Asahina M, Hattori T: Laryngeal stridor in multiple system atrophy. Eur Neurol 49:154, 2003.
16. Goldstein DS, Holmes C, Sharabi Y, et al: Plasma levels of catechols and metanephrines in neurogenic orthostatic hypotension. Neurology 60:1327, 2003.
17. Colosimo C, Pezzella FR: The symptomatic treatment of multiple system atrophy. Eur J Neurol 9:195, 2002.
18. Shannon JR, Diedrich A, Biaggioni I, et al: Water drinking as a treatment for orthostatic syndromes. Am J Med 112:355, 2002.
19. McDowell T, Hajduczok G, Abboud F, Chapleau M: Baroreflex dysfunction in diabetes mellitus: II. Site of baroreflex impairment in diabetic rabbits. Am J Physiol 266: H244, 2003.
20. Koomans HA, Blankestijn PJ, Joles JA: Sympathetic hyperactivity in chronic renal failure: A wake-up call. J Am Soc Nephrol 15:524, 2004.
21. Ito T, Sakakibara R, Yamamoto T, et al: Urinary dysfunction and autonomic control in amyloid neuropathy. Clin Auton Res 16:66, 2006.
22. Low PA: Autonomic neuropathies. Curr Opin Neurol 15:605, 2002.
23. Brownley KA, Hurwitz BE: Assessment of autonomic and cardiovascular function in HIV disease. Adv Cardiol 40:105, 2003.
24. Klein CM, Vernino S, Lennon VA, et al: The spectrum of autoimmune autonomic neuropathies. Ann Neurol 53:752, 2003.
25. Schroeder C, Vernino S, Birkenfeld AL, et al: Plasma exchange for primary autoimmune autonomic failure. N Engl J Med 353:1585, 2005.
26. Vincent S, Robertson D: The broader view: Catecholamine abnormalities. Clin Auton Res 12(Suppl):I44, 2002.
27. Brignole M: Randomized clinical trials of neurally mediated syncope. J Cardiovasc Electrophysiol 14(Suppl):S64, 2003.
28. Afari N, Buchwald D: Chronic fatigue syndrome: A review. Am J Psychiatry 160:221, 2003.
29. Sharabi Y, Dendi R, Holmes C, Goldstein DS: Baroreflex failure as a late sequela of neck irradiation. Hypertension 42:110, 2003.
30. Semplicini A, Maresca A, Boscolo G, et al: Hypertension in acute ischemic stroke. Arch Intern Med 163:211, 2003.
31. Furlan R, Diedrich A, Rimoldi A, et al: Effects of unilateral and bilateral carotid baroreflex stimulation on cardiac and neural sympathetic discharge oscillatory patterns. Circulation 108:717, 2003.
32. Timmers H: Denervation of carotid baro- and chemo-receptors in humans. J Physiol 553:3, 2003.
33. Schroeder C, Tank J, Boschmann M, et al: Selective norepinephrine reuptake inhibition as a human model of orthostatic intolerance. Circulation 105:347, 2002.
34. Flamm MD, Braniff BA, Kimball R, et al: Mechanism of effort syncope in aortic stenosis. Circulation 36(Suppl):109, 1967.
35. Accurso V, Somers VK: Blood and injury phobia; cause or consequence of fainting? Cardiovasc Rev Rep 23:20, 2003.

Disorders of Increased Sympathetic Outflow

36. Aydin M, Altin R, Ozeren A, et al: Cardiac autonomic activity in obstructive sleep apnea: Time-dependent and spectral analysis of heart rate variability using 24-hour Holter electrocardiograms. Tex Heart Inst J 31:132, 2004.
37. Ertl AC, Diedrich A, Biaggioni I, et al: Human muscle sympathetic nerve activity and plasma noradrenaline kinetics in space. J Physiol 538:321, 2002.
38. Xiao X, Mukkamala R, Sheynberg N, et al: Effects of prolonged bed rest on total peripheral resistance baroreflex. Comp Cardiol 29:53, 2002.

Disorders of Increased Parasympathetic Tone

39. Laaksonen DE, Laitinen T, Schonberg J, et al: Weight loss and weight maintenance, ambulatory blood pressure and cardiac autonomic tone in obese persons with the metabolic syndrome. J Hypertens 21:371, 2003.
40. Gondim FAA, Lopes ACA, Oliveira GR, et al: Cardiovascular control after spinal cord injury. Curr Vasc Pharmacol 2:71, 2004.

The following contributors have indicated that they have a relationship that, in the context of their participation in the writing of a chapter for the Eighth Edition of *Braunwald's Heart Disease,* could be perceived by some people as a real or apparent conflict of interest, but do not consider that it has influenced the writing of their chapter. Codes for the disclosure information (institution[s] and nature of relationship[s]) are provided below.

Relationship Codes

A—Stock options or bond holdings in a for-profit corporation or self-directed pension plan
B—Research grants
C—Employment (full or part-time)
D—Ownership or partnership

E—Consulting fees or other remuneration received by the contributor or immediate family
F—Nonremunerative positions, such as board member, trustee, or public spokesperson

G—Receipt of royalties
H—"Speaker's bureau"

Institution and Company Codes

001—Abbott Labs
002—Accumetrics
003—Acorn Cardiovascular
004—Actelion Pharmaceuticals
005—Active Biotic
006—Adolor
007—AGA Medical
008—Alexion Pharmaceuticals
009—Alnylam
010—Alteon
011—American College of Nutrition
012—American Heart Association
013—Amgen
014—Amorcyte Inc.
015—Anexon
016—Angiodynamics
017—Apotex
018—Arena
019—Armgo Pharma
020—Astellas
021—Astra Zeneca, Inc.
022—Atlas Venture Advisors, Inc.
023—AtheroGenics, Inc.
024—Avanir
025—Aventis
026—Baker Brothers Advisors LLC
027—Barr-Teva Litigation
028—BASS Medical
029—Bayer Italy
030—Bayer Healthcare
031—Beckman-Coulter
032—BGB-New York
033—Biomarin Pharmaceuticals
034—Bioscience Webster
035—Biosite, Inc.
036—BG Medicine
037—Blackwell Publishing
038—Bluhm Cardiovascular Institute
039—BMS
040—BMS-Sanofi

041—Boeringer Ingelheim
042—Boston Scientific Corporation
043—Boston Scientific Inc.
044—Bracco
045—Bristol-Meyers Squibb Company
046—Cardiac Concepts Inc.
047—Cardiac Dimensions
048—CardioDynamics
049—Cardiokine Inc.
050—Cardio DX
051—CardioMems Inc.
052—CDC
053—Centocor
054—CHF Solutions
055—Circulation
056—Cordis Corporation
057—Critical Diagnostics
058—Cryocor
059—Current Protocols in Human Genetics
060—Cytokinetics, Inc.
061—CV Therapeutics, Inc.
062—Dade Behring
063—Daiichi Sankyo
064—Dime
065—Edwards Lifesciences
066—Eisai
067—Eli Lilly and Company
068—Elsevier
069—Emisphere
070—Encysive
071—E Z EM
072—GE Healthcare
073—Genentech
074—Genzyme
075—Geron
076—Gilead Sciences
077—Glaxo Smith Kline
078—GSK
079—Guidant Corporation

080—I3DNL
081—IBM
082—Interleukin Genetics
083—Int'l Life Sciences Health & Environmental Sciences Institute
084—Inverness Medical Inc.
085—ISIS
086—Johnson & Johnson
087—Kowa Research Institute
088—LabCorp
089—Laboratory of Molecular Medicine/HPCGG
090—Lippincott
091—LPath
092—Lung RX
093—Mallinckrodt
094—Medicines Company
095—Medicure
096—Medscape
097—Medtronic, Inc.
098—Merck & Co., Inc.
099—Merck Cardiovascular Scientific
100—Merck/Schering-Plough Corp.
101—MG Medicine
102—Millennium Pharmaceuticals
103—Molecular Insight Pharmaceuticals
104—Myogen
105—National Heart, Lung and Blood Institute
106—NCME
107—Neurological Technologies
108—NIH
109—NIH/Agency for Healthcare Research and Quality
110—Nitromed
111—Northpoint Domain
112—NovaCardia
113—Novartis, Inc.
114—Ortho-Clinical Diagnostics

115—Pfizer, Inc.
116—Philips Medical
117—Physical Logic AG
118—Preventicum
119—Prime
120—Procter and Gamble
121—Protein Design Labs
122—Reliant Pharmaceuticals
123—Regeneron
124—Resmed Foundation
125—Respironics
126—Roche Diagnostics
127—SAB
128—Sanofi-Aventis

129—Sapphire Therapeutics, Inc.
130—Scios, Inc.
131—Servier France
132—Schering
133—Schering Plough Corp.
134—Sciele, Inc.
135—Siemens
136—Siemens Medical Solutions
137—Sigma Tau
138—Stereotaxis
139—St. Jude Medical
140—T2cure
141—Takeda
142—Terumo Heart, Inc.

143—Tethys
144—Thoratec
145—United Therapeutics, Inc.
146—VA
147—Vanderbilt/Genaissance
148—Vascular Biogenics
149—Vasculitis Foundation
150—Ventracor Inc.
151—Vertex
152—Visen Scientific
153—Wyeth
154—Xceed Molecular Scientific
    Advisory Board
155—Xoma

Contributors

Achenbach, Stephan B-132, B-136, E-44, E-45
Antman, Elliot E-67, E-128
Baim, Donald S. C-42
Beckman, Joshua A.
Bettmann, Michael H-16, H-71
Bonow, Robert O. E-65
Braunwald, Eugene B-21, B-30, B-61, B-67, B-98, B-113, B-115, B-128, B-133, E-63, E-115, E-128, E-133
Calkins, Hugh E-97
Carroll, John D. B-166, H-166
Costello, Rebecca C-108, F-11
Creager, Mark A. B-67, B-98, E-5, E-33, E-45, E-74, E-98, E-128, E-137, H-45, H-128
Dilsizian, Vasken A-72, A-103, B-20, B-72, B-103, E-45, E-103, H-20, H-45, H-72, H-93
Dimmeler, Stefanie D-140, E-74, E-79, E-97, E-115, E-140, H-140
Douglas, Pamela S. A-50, A-102, A-111, B-97, E-72, E-77, E-88, E-98, E-99, E-101, E-111, E-152, E-154
Eagle, Kim B-35, B-45, B-115, B-128, E-108, E-115, E-128
Force, Thomas E-113, H-98
Gersh, Bernard J. F-14, F-21, F-43, F-45, F-61, F-113
Goldhaber, Sam B-41, B-66, B-78, B-128, E-39, E-41, E-69, E-128
Goldstein, Larry B. B-7, B-39, B-41, B-52, B-106, B-108, E-86, E-107, E-115

Hoffman, Gary B-108, B-149, E-53, E-73, E-123
Isselbacher, Eric M. H-115
Kaplan, Norman E-113, H-41, H-115, G-90
LeWinter, Martin B-97, B-113, E-97, H-113, H-141
Libby, Peter E-21, E-23, E-41, E-45, E-77, H-21, H-41, H-45, H-77
Lipshultz, Steve B-77, B-113, B-115, B-126, B-155
Mann, Douglas A-97, E-3, E-97, F-19, F-91
Mark, Daniel B-8, B-95, B-97, B-105, B-109, B-115, B-120, E-21, E-25, E-97, E-113, G-68
McLaughlin, Vallerie B-4, B-70, B-92, B-115, B-145, E-4, E-76, H-4, H-76, H-115
McManus, Bruce B-13, B-81, B-113, E-13, E-116
Miller, John B-42, B-97, B-139, E-34, E-42, E-97, E-138, E-139
Morrow, David E-30, E-31, E-57, E-61, E-62, E-73, E-77, E-114, E-126, E-128
Myerburg, Robert E-43, E-79, E-120, E-122, H-43, H-79
Nesto, Richard W. E-78, E-128, H-78, H-128, H-141
Newby, L. Kristin B-12, B-35, B-36, B-40, B-84, B-126, B-133, E-6, E-61, E-86, E-120, E-130, H-40
Olgin, Jeffrey B-58, B-139
Opie, Lionel E-29, G-68

Pennell, Dudley J. B-17, B-97, B-113, B-135, E-97, E-113, E-118, E-135, H-17, H-113
Priori, Silvia B-79, B-97, H-79, H-97
Pyeritz, Reed E. B-74, E-74, H-74
Redfield, Margaret B-10, B-35, B-47, B-79, B-97, B-130, B-139, G-15
Resnic, Frederic S. B-94, B-139, H-139
Ridker, Paul B-1, B-21, B-128, E-1, E-21, E-62, E-85, E-113, E-148
Roden, Dan E-22, E-24, E-26, E-27, E-49, E-61, E-67, E-78, E-79, E-113, E-115, E-128, E-129, E-147, F-97, H-83
Schwartz, Janice E-134
Seidman, Christine F-89, G-59
Seidman, Jonathan C-89, F-89, G-59
Simon, Daniel I. B-2, B-56, B-86, B-133, E-56, E-86, E-128, E-133, H-56, H-67, H-86, H-94, H-128, H-133
Somers, Virend K. B-124, E-46, E-125
Teerlink, John A-60, B-1, B-4, B-45, B-48, B-54, B-60, B-112, B-130, E-1, E-4, E-20, E-28, E-45, E-60, E-75, E-104, E-121, E-153
Warnes, Carole G-37
Yancy, Clyde W. Jr. B-130, E-77, E-97, E-110, E-113, E-130, H-77, H-113
Yoshifumi, Naka E-51, E-142, E-150, H-144
Zeiher, Andreas M. A-140, B-79, B-128, E-79, H-115
Zipes, Douglas P. A-116, B-97, E-97, E-116, E-153

Note: Page numbers followed by f and t indicate figures and tables, respectively.

A

a wave
   abnormal, 129-130, 130f
   in atrial pressure, 451
   in atrial tachycardia, 877
   normal, 128f, 129
Abciximab
   in chronic kidney disease patients,
      2164t
   in diabetes mellitus, 1550
   in myocardial infarction, 1254, 1256
   in percutaneous coronary intervention,
      1307-1308, 1307f, 1310, 1436
   as platelet inhibitor, 2073
   thrombocytopenia from, 2075
   in UA/NSTEMI, 1329
Abdomen
   in heart failure, 563, 591
   in myocardial infarction, 1223-1224
   pain in, in abdominal aortic
      aneurysms, 1459
   physical examination of, 128
Abdominal aorta. See Aorta, abdominal.
Abdominal-jugular reflux. See
      Hepatojugular reflux.
Abetalipoproteinemia, 1079
AbioCor total artificial heart, 692
Abiomed BVS 5000i and AB5000
      ventricular assist devices, 689-690
Ablation therapy. See also Cryoablation.
   in arrhythmias, 803-819
   catheter. See Radiofrequency catheter
      ablation.
   chemical, 819
   septal, in hypertrophic cardiomyopathy,
      1772-1773
Abscess, splenic, in infective
      endocarditis, 1729
Absent pulmonary valve syndrome,
      tetralogy of Fallot with, 1588
Absolute coronary reserve, 1178-1179,
      1180f
Absolute risk, of cardiovascular disease,
      1122, 1122f
Accelerated idioventricular rhythm, 864t-
      865t, 895-896, 896f, 1278
Accelerated-malignant hypertension,
      1045-1046, 1045t, 1046f, 1046t
Acceleration-dependent block,
      electrocardiography in, 172, 172f,
      173f
Accentuated antagonism, 863
Accessory pathways
   atriofascicular, 805
   concealed, 882-884, 882f-883f
      clinical features of, 884
      diagnosis of, 883-884
      electrocardiography in, 172, 172f,
         173f, 882-883, 882f-883f
      management of, 884
   due to preexcitation. See Wolff-
      Parkinson-White syndrome.
   radiofrequency catheter ablation of,
      804-806, 804f-805f

Accessory pathways (Continued)
   schematic representation of, 887f
   septal, 804, 804f, 882
   surgical interruption of, 819f, 820
Accuracy, test, in exercise
      electrocardiography, 206, 206t
ACE. See Angiotensin-converting enzyme
      (ACE).
Acebutotol
   in arrhythmias, 792-793
   pharmacokinetics and pharmacology of,
      1372t
Acetazolamide
   in heart failure, 623
   in periodic paralyses, 2148
N-Acetyl transferase, in drug metabolism
      and elimination, 61t
Acetylcholine
   cardiac effects of, 732-733
   coronary artery spasm from, 488-489
   in coronary blood flow regulation, 1168,
      1170, 1170t
   in Prinzmetal variant angina, 1338
   in sinus node, 728
N-Acetylcysteine (NAC), for prevention of
      contrast-induced nephropathy, 2161
Acetylsalicylic acid. See Aspirin
      (acetylsalicylic acid).
Acidosis
   in coronary blood flow regulation, 1175
   in hypoxic pulmonary vasoconstriction,
      1884
   metabolic, in cardiac arrest, 962
ACIP protocol, for exercise stress testing,
      198
Acorn cardiac support device, 674, 675f
Acquired immunodeficiency syndrome
      (AIDS). See Human
      immunodeficiency virus (HIV)
      infection.
Acromegaly, 2034-2035
Actin
   alpha-cardiac, mutation of, in
      hypertrophic cardiomyopathy, 112t,
      113-114
   structure of, 510, 511f, 512, 515f
Action potential, 737-744
   duration of, in myocardial ischemia,
      204
   inward currents of, 742
   ionic fluxes regulating, 738, 738f
   loss of, in arrhythmogenesis, 745-746,
      746f
   membrane voltages during, 735, 735f,
      735t, 738-739, 738f, 738t, 739f
   phase 0 (upstroke or rapid
      depolarization), 739-740, 739f, 740f,
      742
      fast versus slow channels in, 740, 742
      inward currents in, 742
      mechanism of, 739f, 740, 740f, 742
   phase 1 (early rapid depolarization),
      742-743, 743f
   phase 2 (plateau), 743-744

Action potential (Continued)
   phase 3 (final rapid depolarization), 744
   phase 4 (diastolic depolarization), 744
   phase 4 (resting), 738t, 739
   recording of, 738-739, 738f
Action potential duration (APD)
   alternans, in ventricular fibrillation,
      760, 760f, 761
Activated clotting time, 2062
Activated partial thromboplastin time,
      2062
Activated protein C
   recombinant (drotrecogin alfa), 2067
   resistance to
      factor V Leiden gene mutation and,
         2057-2058
      venous thromboembolism in, 1864
Activities of daily living (ADLs), in
      preoperative risk assessment for
      noncardiac surgery, 2017, 2017t
Acute coronary syndromes, 1210-1211,
      1210f, 1211f. See also Angina
      pectoris; Myocardial infarction.
   chest pain in. See Chest pain, acute.
   in chronic kidney disease
      diagnosis of, 2162-2163
      outcomes of, 2163
      prognosis and, 2163, 2163f
      treatment of, 2163-2164, 2164t
   in elderly persons, 1938-1939
   exercise stress testing in, 209
   as framework for therapeutic strategies,
      1210-1211
   lipid-lowering therapy in, 1088
   long-term risk following,
      pathophysiology of, 1323-1324,
      1324f
   magnetic resonance imaging in, 397
   myocardial perfusion imaging in, 380-
      382, 380f-383f
   natural history of, 1324
   risk stratification in, guidelines for,
      1348t
   spectrum of, 1210, 1210f
   treatment of, economic analysis of,
      36-37
   in women
      cardiac rehabilitation after, 1963
      symptoms of, 1957-1958
      treatment of, 1961-1963, 1962f, 1962t
Acute Decompensated Heart Failure
      National Registry (ADHERE), 586
Acute ischemic stroke. See Stroke, acute
      ischemic.
Acute myocardial infarction. See
      Myocardial infarction.
Acute respiratory distress syndrome,
      postoperative, 2004
Adams-Stokes attacks, in children with
      complete atrioventricular block, 919
Adaptive immunity, in atherogenesis, 993,
      993f
Addison disease, 2037, 2037f, 2178
Adeno-associated viral gene transfer, 81

Adenohypophysis, 2033
Adenoma, aldosterone-producing,
  hypertension in, 1041-1042
Adenosine
  adverse effects of, 800
  in arrhythmias, 799-800
  in atrial flutter, 875
  in atrioventricular nodal reentrant
    tachycardia, 881
  in contraction-relaxation cycle, 526
  in coronary blood flow regulation, 1174,
    1176-1177
  dosage and administration of, 784t,
    799
  electrophysiological characteristics of,
    780t, 781t, 782t, 786t, 799
  indications for, 799-800
  in myocardial infarction, 1264, 1309
  pharmacokinetics of, 784t, 799
  postoperative, 2016
  in pulmonary hypertension, 1889
  for stress myocardial perfusion
    imaging, 364-366, 365f, 366t
  in Wolff-Parkinson-White syndrome,
    892
Adenosine antagonists, in acute heart
  failure, 605
Adenosine deaminase, in tuberculous
  pericarditis, 1848
Adenosine diphosphate (ADP), in
  coronary blood flow regulation, 1175
Adenosine diphosphate (ADP) receptor
  antagonists, in diabetes mellitus,
  1550
Adenosine monophosphate, cyclic (cAMP)
  compartmentalization of, 523
  production of, 522
  protein kinase dependence on, 522-523,
    522f
Adenosine monophosphate–activated
  protein kinase (AMPK), mutation of,
  in glycogen storage cardiomyopathy,
  114
Adenosine triphosphate (ATP), in heart
  failure with normal ejection fraction,
  650
Adenosine triphosphate (ATP) binding
  pocket of myosin filament, 512, 513f,
  515f
Adenosine triphosphate (ATP) potassium
  channel
  in coronary blood flow regulation,
    1174-1175
  mutation of, in dilated cardiomyopathy,
    115t, 116
Adenoviral gene transfer, 80-81
Adenovirus infection, myocarditis in,
  1777
Adenylyl cyclase, 522
Adipose tissue
  biology of, in diabetes mellitus, 1096,
    1096f
  as source of stem/progenitor cells, 699
Adiposity, dyslipidemia and, 1113
Adolescent(s). See also Children.
  cardiac arrest in, primary prevention
    of, 970
  congenital heart disease in. See also
    Congenital heart disease.
    echocardiography in, 1575, 1576f
    management approach to, 1566
Adrenal cortex
  diseases of, 2035-2037
  in myocardial infarction, 1220
Adrenal hyperplasia
  bilateral, hypertension in, 1041-1042
  congenital, hypertension in, 1043

Adrenal medulla, in myocardial
  infarction, 1220
Adrenergic agonists
  in acute heart failure, 601t, 603-604
  alpha, central
    in chronic kidney disease patients,
      2165t
    in hypertension, 1059
  alpha- and beta-, in hypertension, 1061
  beta-, in myocardial infarction,
    1268-1269
Adrenergic inhibitors
  alpha. See Alpha-adrenergic blocking
    agents.
  beta. See Beta blockers.
  in hypertension, 1058-1061, 1059f,
    1059t
  in hypertensive crises, 1066, 1066t
  peripheral. See Peripheral neuronal
    inhibitors.
Adrenergic nerve ending, 1058, 1059f
Adrenergic receptors
  alpha. See Alpha-adrenergic receptors.
  beta. See Beta-adrenergic receptors.
Adrenergic signaling
  alpha, 520f, 521-524, 523f, 524f
  beta, in contraction-relaxation cycle,
    520-524, 520f-524f
Adrenergic system, in heart failure, 542,
  543f
Adrenocorticotropic hormone (ACTH),
  actions of, 2035
Adrenomedullin
  in heart failure, 548-549
  in idiopathic pulmonary arterial
    hypertension, 1893
Adriamycin. See Doxorubicin
  (Adriamycin).
Adult stem cells, 698-699
Adults
  congenital heart disease in
    echocardiography in, 1575
    heart failure in, 1567
    management approach to, 1566
    types of, 1562, 1562t
  polycystic kidney disease in, 94-95
Advance care planning, in end-stage
  heart disease, 719-721, 720t
Advanced glycation end products (AGEs),
  in diabetes mellitus, 1554
Adventitia, of arteries, 988-989, 989f
Aerobic (endurance) exercise, 1983
  in cardiovascular disease, 1153, 1154t
  definition of, 1150t, 1983
  exercise prescription for, 1986t
Affinity chromatography, 78
African Americans
  cardiovascular disease risk factors in,
    23-24
  cardiovascular mortality in, 25
  coronary artery disease in, 28-29, 29f
  demographics of, 23, 24f
  health care disparities for, 25-26
  heart failure in, 29-31, 30f, 31t, 32f, 613,
    634-635, 635f
    acute, 586
    genetic heterogeneity and, 709
  hypertension in, 26-27, 26f, 27f, 1028,
    1029f
  hypertension therapy in, 27-28, 28f, 28t,
    1065
Afterdepolarization
  amplitude of, determinants of, 748t
  delayed, in arrhythmogenesis, 748-750,
    748f-751f
  early, in arrhythmogenesis, 748, 748f,
    750, 752f

Afterload, 530
  in acute mitral regurgitation, 1669
  contractility and, 529
  definition of, 570t
  in heart failure, 573
  in left ventricular systolic function,
    569-570, 570f
  in myocardial infarction, 1268
  preload and, relationship between, 530
  wall stress and, 531, 531f
Agatson score, for coronary calcium,
  424
Age. See also Adolescent(s); Children;
    Elderly persons; Infant(s); Neonate(s).
  cardiovascular disease and, 5, 8, 9f
  heart transplantation and, 676
  maximum heart rate and, 195
  sudden cardiac death and, 936, 937f
AGEs (advanced glycation end products),
    in diabetes mellitus, 1097-1098,
    1098f
Aggrastat. See Tirofiban (Aggrastat).
A-H interval, in atrioventricular nodal
  reentrant tachycardia, 879
Air embolism, 468, 1868
Air travel, pulmonary embolism and,
    1864, 1876
Airlines, AED deployment by, 960
Airway clearance, in cardiac arrest
  management, 959
Airway resistance, in chronic obstructive
  pulmonary disease, 1906
Ajmaline, in arrhythmias, 780t, 781t,
    782t, 786t, 788
Akt, in left ventricular response to
  mechanical stress, 536, 537f, 538
Alagille syndrome, 95, 1571, 1615
Albumin
  ischemia-modified, diagnostic
    performance of, 1199
  technetium-99m–labeled, 358
Albumin-to-creatinine ratio, 2156
Albuminuria. See also Microalbuminuria.
  definition of, 2156
  persistent, in diabetes mellitus. See
    Diabetes mellitus, nephropathy in.
Alcapa syndrome, 1571
Alcohol
  cardiovascular effects of, 1805-1808,
    1806t, 1807f
    on myocellular structure and
      function, 1805, 1806t
    on organ function, 1805-1806
  cocaine and, 1810
  hypertension and, 1028
  intake of
    arrhythmias and, 1807
    blood pressure and, 1114
    cardiovascular disease and, 1110
    coronary artery disease and, 1806-
      1807, 1807f
    in diabetes mellitus, 1807, 1807f
    holiday heart syndrome and, 948
    in hypertension, 1806
    lipid metabolism and, 1806
    sudden cardiac death and, 1807,
      1807f, 1808
  moderate consumption of
    in cardiovascular disease prevention,
      1139, 1806-1807, 1807f
    in hypertension therapy, 1052t, 1053
Alcohol septal ablation, in hypertrophic
  cardiomyopathy, 1772-1773
Alcoholic cardiomyopathy, 1744-1745
Aldactone. See Spironolactone
  (Aldactone).
Aldomet. See Methyldopa (Aldomet).

Aldosterone. *See also* Renin-angiotensin-
aldosterone system.
actions of, 2036, 2036f
in heart failure, 543-544
in hypertension, 1033-1034, 1033f
Aldosterone antagonists
in diabetes mellitus, 1556-1557
in heart failure, 38, 618t, 621t, 622-623,
623f, 624t, 630t, 633
in idiopathic pulmonary arterial
hypertension, 1896-1897
mechanisms of action of, 622-623
in myocardial infarction, 1262, 1263f
side effects of, 633
Aldosteronism
cardiovascular manifestations of,
2036-2037
glucocorticoid-suppressible, 1042
hypertension in, 1041-1042, 1041f,
1041t, 1042f
Alemtuzumab, cardiotoxicity of, 2115
Algorithms, diagnostic, 42
Aliasing, in Doppler echocardiography,
237
Alkalosis, metabolic, from diuretics, 626
Allele, 75
Allen test
before radial artery access, 469
in thromboangiitis obliterans, 1506
Allergy, radiocontrast, prophylaxis for,
442, 471-472, 472t
Aloe, 1159t
Alpha- and beta-adrenergic agonists, in
hypertension, 1061
Alpha-adrenergic agonists, central
in chronic kidney disease patients,
2165t
in hypertension, 1059
Alpha-adrenergic blocking agents
contraindications to, 1055t
in hypertension, 1059-1060
indications for, 1055t
in Prinzmetal variant angina, 1339
in pulmonary blood flow regulation,
1884
Alpha-adrenergic effects, on force-
velocity relationship, 533
Alpha-adrenergic receptors
polymorphisms in, 708t, 709-710, 710f
in pulmonary blood flow regulation,
1884
subtypes of, 520f, 521-522
Alpha$_1$-adrenergic receptors, G protein
coupling of, 522
Alpha-adrenergic signaling, 520f, 521-524,
523f, 524f
Alpha$_1$-adrenergic stimulation
cardiovascular effects of, 525t
positive inotropic effect of, 522
Alpha$_2$-agonists, preoperative use of,
2025
Alpha$_2$-antiplasmin, 2054
Alpha-galactosidase A
mutation of, in Fabry disease, 114
recombinant, in Fabry disease, 1754,
1754f
Alpha-linolenic acid, cardiovascular
disease and, 1110
Alprazolam, cardiovascular aspects of,
2132t
Alteplase. *See* Tissue plasminogen
activator (t-PA).
Alternans patterns, in
electrocardiography, 186-187, 186t,
187f, 770, 771f
Alternative medicine. *See* Complementary
and alternative medicine.

Alternative use principle, in economic
analysis, 35
Altitude, pulmonary hypertension and,
1886
Alveolar capillaries, anatomy of, 1883
Alveolar hypoventilation disorders,
pulmonary hypertension in,
1909-1910
Alveolar hypoxia, in chronic obstructive
pulmonary disease, 1906
Alveolar oxygenation, during hypoxia,
1884
Ambulatory electrocardiography. *See*
Holter monitoring.
American College of Cardiology/American
Heart Association (ACC/AHA),
guidelines and performance measures
of, 49-50, 50t-52t. *See also* Practice
guidelines.
American Indians, demographics of, 23,
24f
American Medical Association (AMA),
quality improvement measures of, 50t
Amiloride (Midamor)
in heart failure, 621t, 623
in hypertension, 1058
Aminophylline, for reversal of vasodilator
pharmacological stress, 365
4-Aminopyridine–resistant calcium-
activated chloride channel, in action
potential phase 1, 743
4-Aminopyridine–sensitive potassium
channel, in action potential phase 1,
742-743, 743f
Aminorex, pulmonary hypertension from,
1902
Amiodarone, 794-795
adverse effects of, 795
in atrial fibrillation, 873
in atrial flutter, 875
in cardiac arrest, 962, 963
in cardiac arrest prevention, 964, 969
dosage and administration of, 784t,
794
electrophysiological characteristics of,
780t, 781t, 782t, 786t, 794
empirical therapy with, 966
in heart failure, 635-636
hemodynamic effects of, 794
in hypertrophic cardiomyopathy, 1771
indications for, 794-795
in periodic paralyses, 2148
pharmacokinetics of, 784t, 794
in pregnancy, 1976t, 1977
thyroid disorders from, 2044
in ventricular fibrillation, 1279
in ventricular tachycardia, 902
Amitriptyline, cardiovascular aspects of,
2129t
Amlodipine
pharmacokinetics of, 1375t
in stable angina, 1376
in UA/NSTEMI, 1327
Ammonia, nitrogen-labeled
coronary blood flow reserve analysis
and, 362-363
in positron emission tomography, 360,
360t
Amniotic fluid embolism, 1868
Amphetamines
cardiovascular effects of, 1811
in HIV-infected patients, complications
of, 1803t
Amplatz catheter, for arteriography, 470,
470f
Amplifiers, for electrocardiography,
154-155

Amputation, risk of, in diabetes mellitus,
1095
Amrinone, postoperative, 2001
Amyl nitrate, during cardiac
catheterization, 460
Amyloidosis
cardiac, 1751-1753
clinical manifestations of, 1751-1752
diagnosis of, 1752
echocardiography in, 295-296, 295f,
297f
magnetic resonance imaging in, 403
management of, 1752-1753, 1753f
noninvasive testing in, 1752
nuclear imaging in, 385
pathology of, 1751, 1751f
physical examination in, 1752
sudden cardiac death in, 944
etiology of, 1751, 1751f
familial, 1751
systemic, senile, 1751
types of, 1751
Anacrotic arterial pulse, 133, 133f
Anaerobic threshold, in exercise stress
testing, 196-197, 196f
Analgesics
in arteriography, 470
in myocardial infarction, 1237-1238
postoperative, 1999, 2022
Anatomical reentry, 752, 755f
Anatomical variants, chest radiography
of, 331, 335
Anchoring heuristic, 46
Andersen-Tawil syndrome, 101, 2147-2148,
2147f
Anemia
after cardiac surgery, 1999
in chronic kidney disease, 2156-2158
definition of, 2156
in heart failure, 564, 594, 614, 615f
hyperviscosity syndrome from, 1568
in infective endocarditis, 1722
Anesthesia
hypertension therapy and, 1064-1065
intraoperative hemodynamics and, 2021
monitoring of, 2021
for noncardiac surgery, 2020-2021
Aneuploidy, 86
Aneurysmectomy
left ventricular, 1285, 1285f, 1399, 1399f
in ventricular tachycardia, 820f
Aneurysms
aortic, 1458-1469. *See also* Aortic
aneurysms.
aortic sinus, 1609
in atherosclerosis, 1000
atrial septal, patent foramen ovale and,
1581
coronary artery
in Kawasaki disease, 2092, 2092f
in stable angina, 1360
false. *See* Pseudoaneurysm.
genetic studies in, 95
intracranial
mycotic, 1521
in polycystic kidney disease, 94-95
left ventricular. *See* Ventricle(s), left,
aneurysm of.
mycotic, 1521, 1730
sinus of Valsalva, 299, 299f, 1609
Anger
in cardiovascular disease, 2119, 2122
in hypertension, 2123-2124
Angina pectoris. *See also* Chest pain.
in aortic stenosis, 1629
chest pain in, 1195-1196
circadian rhythm in, 1367

in congenital heart disease, 1571
demand, 1355, 1356f
differential diagnosis of, 1354-1355
in elderly persons, 1934
equivalents of, 1353
exercise effects in, 1150-1151, 1150f, 1151f
during exercise stress testing, 204, 205-206
first-effort, 1354
fixed-threshold, 1356
grading of, 1354
in left ventricular aneurysm, 1398
mechanisms of, 1354
microvascular, 1395
mixed, 1356
with normal coronary arteries, 1395-1396
orthostatic, 2175
postprandial, 1356
precipitation of, 1355
Prinzmetal variant. See Prinzmetal variant angina.
in pulmonary hypertension, 1886
recurrent, after coronary artery bypass graft surgery, 1386-1388
stable, 1353-1395
    angiography in, 1359-1360, 1361-1362, 1361f, 1362f, 1409, 1411t, 1413t
    arteriography in, 465, 466t, 501, 502t, 1359-1360
    biochemical tests in, 1356-1357
    cardiac examination in, 1355
    characteristics of, 1353-1354
    chest radiography in, 1358
    clinical presentations in, 1353
    collateral vessels in, 1360
    computed tomography in, 1358-1359
    coronary artery ectasia and aneurysms in, 1360
    coronary blood flow in, 1360
    definition of, 1319
    diagnosis of, practice guidelines for, 1405, 1405t, 1406, 1408-1409, 1409t-1410t
    diseases associated with
        antianginal therapy and, 1377-1378, 1377t
        treatment of, 1362
    electrocardiography in
        exercise, 1357-1358, 1358t, 1361
        resting, 1357
    follow-up in, practice guidelines for, 1416t, 1417
    gender differences in, 1358
    left ventricular function in, 1360
    magnetic resonance imaging in, 1359
    management of
        angiotensin-converting enzyme inhibitors in, 1365-1366, 1366f
        anti-inflammatory agents in, 1365
        antioxidants in, 1366
        approach to, 1378
        aspirin in, 1365
        beta blockers in, 1365, 1369-1371, 1370f, 1370t, 1372t-1374t, 1377-1378
        calcium channel blockers in, 1371-1376, 1374t-1375t, 1377-1378
        chelation in, 1379
        clopidogrel in, 1365
        combination therapy in, 1378
        coronary artery bypass graft surgery in, 1380-1391. See also Coronary artery bypass graft surgery.

Angina pectoris (Continued)
        counseling in, 1366-1367
        enhanced external counterpulsation in, 1378-1379
        exercise in, 1364-1365
        glycemic control in, 1363-1364
        hormone replacement therapy in, 1364
        hypertension therapy in, 1362-1363
        laser-assisted myocardial revascularization in, 1394-1395
        lifestyle changes in, 1367
        lipid-lowering therapy in, 1363
        medical, 1362-1379
        metabolic agents in, 1377
        nitrates in, 1367-1369, 1367t, 1368f, 1368t
        in patients with associated diseases, 1377-1378, 1377t
        percutaneous coronary intervention in, 1379-1380, 1380f, 1391-1392
        pharmacological, 1363-1366, 1367-1378
        practice guidelines for, 1411, 1413-1417, 1413t-1416t
        smoking cessation in, 1363
        spinal cord stimulation in, 1378
        surgical, 1380-1395
    myocardial bridging in, 1360
    myocardial metabolism in, 1360
    myocardial oxygen demand in, 1355, 1356f
    myocardial oxygen supply in, 1355-1356, 1356f
    myocardial perfusion imaging in, 371-380, 372f-379f
    noninvasive testing in, 1356-1359, 1357t-1359t, 1361
    pathophysiology of, 1355-1356, 1356f
    percutaneous coronary intervention in, 1420, 1450, 1450t-1451t
    physical examination in, 1355
    practice guidelines for, 1405-1417, 1406f-1408f, 1407t, 1409t-1416t
    revascularization in
        comparison and choice between PCI and CABG for, 1392-1394, 1392f-1394f, 1393t
        complete, need for, 1394
        in diabetic patients, 1394
        indications for, 1385-1386, 1386f, 1386t, 1387f, 1391-1392
        laser-assisted, 1394-1395
        practice guidelines for, 1415t, 1416-1417
    risk stratification in, 1358, 1359t, 1360-1362, 1360f-1362f, 1385-1386, 1386f, 1386t, 1387f, 1409-1411, 1412t, 1413t
    silent myocardial ischemia in, 1396-1397
    stress echocardiography in, 1358, 1358t, 1361
    stress myocardial perfusion imaging for, 1358, 1358t, 1361
    supply, 1355-1356, 1356f
    unstable. See UA/NSTEMI.
    variable-threshold, 1356
    during vasodilator pharmacological stress, 365
    warm-up, 1354
Anginal equivalents, 126
Angiocardiography. See Angiography.
Angiogenesis
    versus arteriogenesis, 1183
    in atherosclerotic plaque, 994-995
    in diabetes mellitus, 1555

Angiogenesis (Continued)
    gene transfer and, 81-82
    genetic disorders primarily affecting, 97-98
    interventions to improve, 1183-1184
Angiogenic growth factors, in peripheral arterial disease, 1503-1504
Angiographic stroke volume, 455
Angiography. See also Arteriography; Cardiac catheterization.
    in aortic dissection, 1478
    in aortic regurgitation, 1640
    in aortic stenosis, 1631
    in cardiac arrest survivors, 954
    cardiac output measurements with, 455
    complications of, 461-462, 461t
    computed tomography. See Computed tomography angiography.
    in constrictive pericarditis, 1844, 1844f
    diagnostic exercise testing versus, 206-207
    in dilated cardiomyopathy, 1748
    as gold standard for stress myocardial perfusion imaging, 374-375
    in heart failure, 568-569, 569t
    intravascular ultrasonography versus, 496, 496f
    magnetic resonance. See Magnetic resonance angiography.
    in mitral regurgitation, 1664
    in mitral stenosis, 1651
    in mitral valve prolapse, 1672
    in peripheral arterial disease, 1499, 1501f
    pulmonary
        in pulmonary embolism, 1870
        in pulmonary hypertension, 1888
    in pulmonic regurgitation, 1680
    quantitative, 492-494, 494t
    racial/ethnic differences in, 25
    radionuclide. See Radionuclide angiography or ventriculography.
    routine, economic analysis of, 39-40
    in stable angina, 1359-1360, 1361-1362, 1361f, 1362f, 1409, 1411t, 1413t
    in tricuspid stenosis, 1675
    in vasculitis, 2087
Angiojet thrombectomy catheter, 1308, 1425
Angioma, cerebral cavernous, 96
Angioplasty. See also Percutaneous coronary intervention.
    atherectomy-assisted. See Atherectomy.
    carotid, in elderly persons, 1941-1942
    economic analysis of, 37
    percutaneous coronary. See Percutaneous transluminal coronary angioplasty.
    percutaneous noncoronary. See Percutaneous intervention.
    in renovascular hypertension, 1040
    versus thrombolysis, 1301-1307, 1302f
Angiosarcoma, 405, 406f, 1818t, 1824-1825, 1824f
Angioscopy, in UA/NSTEMI, 1323
Angiotensin I, 542, 544f, 545f
Angiotensin II. See also Renin-angiotensin-aldosterone system.
    in heart failure, 542-543, 544f, 545f
    in hypertension, 1034, 1034f
    in pulmonary circulation, 1885-1886
    receptors for, 543
    release of, in left ventricular response to mechanical stress, 536, 536f, 537f

Angiotensin II receptor blockers
  in chronic kidney disease patients,
    2165, 2165t, 2167
  clinical use of, 1063-1064
  complications of, 629-630
  contraindications to, 1055t
  in diabetes mellitus, 1551-1552, 1556
  in elderly persons, 1931
  in heart failure
    with normal ejection fraction, 654,
      655f
    systolic, 618t, 624t, 629-630, 630t,
      631f
  in hypertension, 1063-1064
  hypertension from, 1038
  indications for, 1055t
  mechanism of action of, 1063
  in myocardial infarction, 1260, 1262,
    1262f
  in renovascular hypertension, 1040
  side effects of, 1064
  in UA/NSTEMI, 1335
Angiotensin-converting enzyme (ACE),
    542, 544f, 545f
  gene for, polymorphisms in, 62, 62t,
    708t, 709
Angiotensin-converting enzyme (ACE)
    inhibitors
  in aortic dissection, 1479
  in aortic regurgitation, 1642
  in aortic stenosis, 1633
  in cardiovascular disease prevention,
    1133-1134
  in chronic kidney disease patients,
    2165, 2165t, 2167
  clinical use of, 1062t, 1063
  complications of, 628-629
  contraindications to, 1055t
  in diabetes mellitus, 1102-1103, 1102t,
    1551, 1552, 1556
  in elderly persons, 1931, 1939
  in heart failure, 38, 559, 559t
    with normal ejection fraction, 654,
      655f
    systolic, 618t, 624t, 628-629, 629f,
      630t
  in hypertension, 1062-1063, 1062t
  hypertension from, 1038
  indications for, 1055t
  mechanism of action of, 1062-1063
  in myocardial infarction, 1260, 1261f,
    1262, 1262f
  in myocardial infarction prevention,
    1290
  in myocarditis, 1788-1789
  in peripheral arterial disease, 1501-
    1502, 1503, 1503tf
  polymorphisms associated with, 62,
    62t, 708t, 709
  in pregnancy, 1976t, 1977
  psychiatric side effects of, 2132
  in renovascular hypertension, 1040
  side effects of, 1063
  in stable angina, 1365-1366, 1366f
  in stroke prevention, 1518, 1519
  in syndrome X, 1396
  in transposition of the great arteries,
    1601
  in UA/NSTEMI, 1335
Angiotensin-converting enzyme (ACE)
    receptor system, tissue, nuclear
    imaging of, 386
Animal models
  of cardiovascular disease, 78-79, 80f
  of dilated cardiomyopathy in HIV-
    infected patients, 1797
  in gene therapy, 81-82

Anisotropic conduction, 151, 737, 737f
Anisotropic reentry, 758, 760f
Anistreplase, in myocardial infarction,
    1246
Ankle/brachial index, 131
  definition of, 1491
  in peripheral arterial disease, 1496-
    1497, 1497f
Ankylosing spondylitis, 2096
Annuloaortic ectasia, thoracic aortic
    aneurysms and, 1464, 1464f
Annuloplasty
  in aortic regurgitation, 1644-1645, 1645f
  in mitral regurgitation, 1665-1666, 1666f
  mitral valve, in dilated cardiomyopathy,
    669-671, 671f
  in tricuspid regurgitation, 1678
  tricuspid valve, in dilated
    cardiomyopathy, 671-672
Annulus, mitral, calcification of, 1650,
    1657-1658
  chest radiography in, 338, 339f
  in elderly persons, 1948
Annulus paradoxus, in constrictive
    pericarditis, 293
Anorectic drugs
  pulmonary arterial hypertension from,
    1902
  valvular heart disease from, 1704
Anoxic encephalopathy, after cardiac
    arrest, 964
ANREP effect, in contraction-relaxation
    cycle, 530
Antagonism, accentuated, 863
Anterior internodal pathway, 728
Anthracycline, cardiotoxicity of, 1813,
    2108-2110, 2110f
Antianginal agents
  exercise stress testing and, 213-214,
    1357-1358
  review of, 1368-1379
Antiapoptotic response, to myocardial
    hibernation, 1190
Antiarrhythmic agent(s), 779-801
  actions of, 779, 780t, 781t
  adenosine as, 799-800
  in atrial fibrillation, 872-873
  in atrial flutter, 875-876, 876f
  in atrial tachycardia, 877
  in atrioventricular nodal reentrant
    tachycardia, 881, 881t
  in cardiac arrest, 962, 963
  cardiac arrest from, 964
  in cardiac arrest prevention, 964,
    965-966
  in chronic kidney disease patients,
    2165t
  class IA, 779, 785-788
  class IB, 779, 788-790
  class IC, 779, 790-792
  class II, 779, 792-793
  class III, 779, 794-797
  class IV, 779, 798-799
  classification of, 779-780
  clinical usage information for, 782,
    783-784t
  digoxin as, 800-801
  electrophysiological characteristics of,
    782t, 786t
  general considerations regarding,
    779-785
  mechanisms of, 780-781, 781t
  metabolites of, 781
  in mitral stenosis, 1653
  after myocardial infarction, 1289, 1289f
  pharmacogenetics of, 781-782
  in pregnancy, 1976, 1976t

Antiarrhythmic agent(s) (Continued)
  proarrhythmic effects of, 785
  psychiatric side effects of, 2132
  reverse use-dependence of, 780
  side effects of, 782, 785
  in torsades de pointes, 905
  use-dependence of, 780
  in ventricular premature complexes,
    895
  in ventricular tachycardia, 899, 902
  in Wolff-Parkinson-White syndrome,
    891-892, 893
Antibiotics
  in HIV-infected patients, complications
    of, 1802t
  in infective endocarditis, 1723-1727,
    1723t-1726t
    monitoring of, 1727
    outpatient, 1727
    postoperative, 1729
    prophylactic, 1731-1732, 1731t, 1732f,
      1732t, 1734, 1734t
    timing of, 1727
  resistance to, 1725
  in rheumatic fever, 2085, 2085t
Anticardiolipin antibodies, in
    thromboangiitis obliterans, 1505
Anticoagulant mechanisms, in
    hemostasis, 2052-2054, 2053f, 2054f
Anticoagulant therapy. See also Direct
    thrombin inhibitors; Fondaparinux;
    Heparin; Warfarin.
  in acute aortic occlusion, 1486
  in acute ischemic stroke, 1521
  agents used in, 2062-2067
  in antiphospholipid antibody
    syndrome, 2061-2062, 2099
  in arteriography, 470
  in atheroembolism, 1511
  in atrial fibrillation, 870-872
  in atrial flutter, 875
  in cardiovascular disease prevention,
    1134
  drug/herbal interactions in, 1158, 1159t-
    1161t, 1163
  economic analysis of, 37
  in elderly persons, 1941, 1941t
  in Fontan patients, 1596
  in heparin-induced thrombocytopenia,
    2064-2065
  in hyperthyroidism with atrial
    fibrillation, 2041
  in hypertrophic cardiomyopathy, 1771
  in idiopathic pulmonary arterial
    hypertension, 1897
  infective endocarditis and, 1730
  in mitral stenosis, 1652
  in myocardial infarction prevention,
    1286, 1291, 1291f, 1292t
  in patent foramen ovale, 1581
  in pregnancy, 1973, 1979, 1981, 1981t
  in prosthetic valve replacement, 1683
  in pulmonary embolism, 1871-1876
    complications of, 1874-1875
    novel agents for, 1875
    optimal duration of, 1875-1876, 1875t
    prophylactic, 1879, 1879t
  in stroke prevention, 1516-1517, 1516f
  in UA/NSTEMI, 1331-1333
Anticoagulation clinics, 1874
Anticonvulsants, cardiovascular aspects
    of, 2131-2132, 2131t
Antidepressants
  cardiovascular aspects of, 2128-2130,
    2129t
  after myocardial infarction, in elderly
    persons, 1939

Antidepressants (Continued)
  pharmacokinetics of, 60
  tricyclic. See Tricyclic antidepressants.
Anti–double-stranded DNA, in systemic
    lupus erythematosus, 2097
Antidromic tachycardia, in Wolff-
    Parkinson-White syndrome, 888-889,
    889f, 890f
Antifungal agents, in HIV-infected
    patients, complications of, 1802t
Antihypertensive drug therapy, 1054-
    1064. See also Hypertension therapy;
    specific agents, e.g., Captopril
    (Capoten).
  algorithm for, 1056, 1056f
  in aortic dissection, 1479, 1482
  benefits of, 1049, 1050f
  in children, 1065
  in chronic kidney disease, 1039,
    2167m8
  combinations in, 1056
  in diabetes mellitus, 1065, 1102-1103,
    1102t, 1556
  in elderly persons, 1050-1051, 1065,
    1065t, 1931-1933, 1932t, 1933t
  in erectile dysfunction, 1065
  goal of, 1051-1052, 1051f
  guidelines in, 1131t, 1132
    general, 1054-1057, 1054t
    practice, 1069-1070, 1069t
  in heart failure, 1065
  initial drug in, 1055-1056, 1055t,
    1056f
  in ischemic heart disease, 1065
  once daily dosing in, 1056-1057
  parenteral, 1066, 1066t
  perioperative use of, 2014
  in peripheral arterial disease,
    1501-1502, 1503tf
  polymorphisms associated with,
    62, 62t
  in pregnancy, 1045, 1975, 1976t
  psychiatric side effects of, 2132
  in renovascular hypertension, 1040
  resistance to, 1064, 1064t
  starting dosages for, 1054-1055, 1055f
  in stroke prevention, 1518-1519, 1519f,
    1520f
  threshold for, 1049-1050, 1051f
  withdrawal of, 1064
Anti-inflammatory approaches to
    immunomodulation, in heart failure,
    712-714, 712f, 713f
Anti-inflammatory drugs. See also
    Nonsteroidal anti-inflammatory drugs
    (NSAIDs).
  in rheumatic fever, 2086
  in stable angina, 1365
Antimony, cardiovascular effects of,
    1813-1814
Antimyosin antibody imaging, in
    myocarditis, 1786
Antineutrophil cytoplasmic antibodies, in
    Churg-Strauss syndrome, 2093
Antinuclear antibodies, in systemic lupus
    erythematosus, 2097
Antioxidant systems, in heart, 544
Antioxidants, 1115-1116, 1115f
  in cardiovascular disease prevention,
    1140
  in myocardial infarction prevention,
    1292
  in stable angina, 1366
Antiparasitic agents
  in Chagas disease, 1780
  in HIV-infected patients, complications
    of, 1802t

Antiphospholipid antibody syndrome,
    2098-2099, 2099f
  cardiac surgery in patients with,
    1996
  catastrophic, 2061
  thrombosis in, 2061-2062
  venous thromboembolism in, 1864
Antiplatelet therapy. See also specific
    agent, e.g., Aspirin (acetylsalicylic
    acid).
  in acute ischemic stroke, 1521
  agents used in, 2068-2075
  in atheroembolism, 1511
  in cardiovascular disease prevention,
    1133
  in chronic kidney disease patients,
    2164, 2164t
  after coronary artery bypass graft
    surgery, 1385
  in diabetes mellitus, 1549, 1549t
  economic analysis of, 37
  in elderly persons, 1941
  mechanisms of action of, 1328f
  in myocardial infarction, 1253-1256,
    1254f-1256f
  in myocardial infarction prevention,
    1290
  in patent foramen ovale, 1581
  during percutaneous coronary
    intervention, 1436-1437
  in peripheral arterial disease, 1502,
    1503f, 1504f
  resistance to, 2071-2073, 2071f, 2072t
  sequence of events in, 2068, 2069f
  in stroke prevention, 1515-1516
Antiplatelet therapy in UA/NSTEMI,
    1327-1329, 1321f
Antipsychotic drugs
  cardiovascular aspects of, 2130-2131,
    2130t
  in hospitalized cardiac patient, 2126
Antiretroviral therapy
  cardiovascular considerations in, 1798f
  cardiovascular effects of, 1812
  complications of, 1801, 1802t
Antirheumatic therapy, 2085-2086
Antitheft devices, electromagnetic
    interference from, 850
Antithrombin III, 2052-2053, 2053f
  deficiency of, in deep vein thrombosis,
    2058-2059, 2059t
Antithrombotic mechanisms, in
    hemostasis, 2052-2054, 2053f,
    2054f
Antithrombotic therapy. See also specific
    agent, e.g., Heparin.
  agents used in, 2062-2075
  in chronic kidney disease patients,
    2164, 2164t
  in elderly persons, 1938
  in myocardial infarction, 1251-1253,
    1251f, 1252f
  in percutaneous coronary intervention,
    1437
  perioperative use of, 2005
  in UA/NSTEMI, 1327-1330
Antiviral agents, in HIV-infected patients,
    complications of, 1802t
Anxiety
  cardiovascular disease and, 2120-2121
  in convalescence and recovery phase,
    2127
  in hospitalized cardiac patient, 2126
  in hypertension, 2124
  in sudden cardiac death, 2123
Anxiolytics, in hospitalized cardiac
    patient, 2126

Aorta, 1457-1487
  abdominal, 1457
    aneurysm of. See Aortic aneurysms,
      abdominal.
    thrombosis of, 1486
  aging of, 1457-1458
  anatomy of, 1457
  aneurysms of. See Aortic aneurysms.
  anomalies of, magnetic resonance
    imaging of, 407, 407f
  arch of. See Aortic arch(es).
  atherosclerosis in, echocardiography in,
    299-300, 300f
  bacterial infection of, 1486-1487
  chest radiography of, 329, 332f, 338-339,
    339f, 340f
  coarctation of. See Coarctation of the
    aorta.
  descending, retroesophageal, 1609-1610
  dissection of. See Aortic dissection.
  embryogenesis of, 1564
  examination of, 1458
  functions of, 1457
  imaging of, 1458
    in abdominal aortic aneurysms, 1460-
      1461, 1461f
    in aortic dissection, 1474-1478,
      1475f-1478f
    in thoracic aortic aneurysms, 1465-
      1466, 1466f
  intramural hematoma of, 1483-1484,
    1484f
  normal, 1457-1458
  occlusion of, acute, 1486
  rupture of, echocardiography in, 301
  saddle embolus of, 1486
  thoracic
    aneurysm of. See Aortic aneurysms,
      thoracic.
    ascending, 1457
    computed tomography of, 432, 432f
    descending, 1457
  transesophageal echocardiography of,
    228, 236, 237f
  trauma to, aortic dissection and, 1471
  tumors of, 1487, 1487f
  ulcer of
    echocardiography in, 301
    penetrating atherosclerotic, 1484-
      1486, 1485f
Aortic aneurysms, 1458-1469
  abdominal, 1458-1464
    atherosclerosis in, 1000
    clinical manifestations of, 1459
    diagnosis and sizing of, 1460-1461,
      1461f
    etiology and pathogenesis of,
      1458-1459
    genetic studies in, 95
    hypertension in, 1037
    infrarenal, 1458
    medical management of, 1463-1464
    natural history of, 1461
    physical examination in, 1459-1460
    rupture of, 1459, 1460f, 1461
    screening for, 1460-1461
    suprarenal, 1458
    surgical treatment of, 1461-1463, 1462f
      open repair in, 1462
        risk assessment prior to, 1463
      stent-grafting in, 1462-1463, 1462f
      survival after, 1463
    echocardiography in, 299, 299f
    false, 1458
    fusiform, 1458
    infected, 1486-1487
    saccular, 1458

Aortic aneurysms (Continued)
  in Takayasu arteritis, 2088, 2088f
  thoracic, 1464-1469
    annuloaortic ectasia and, 1464, 1464f
    atherosclerosis in, 1465
    clinical manifestations of, 1465, 1465f
    cystic medial degeneration in, 1464-1465, 1464f
    diagnosis and sizing of, 1465-1466, 1466f
    etiology and pathogenesis of, 1464-1465, 1464f
    familial, 1464
    infectious aortitis and, 1465
    medical management of, 1469
    natural history of, 1466-1467
    rupture of, 1465
    surgical treatment of, 1467-1469
      complications of, 1468, 1469
      composite graft in, 1467, 1468f
      elephant trunk technique in, 1468
      multilimbed graft in, 1467, 1469f
      pulmonary autograft in, 1467
      stent-grafting in, 1468-1469
      valve-sparing procedure in, 1467
    syphilis and, 1465
  thoracoabdominal, 1464
Aortic arch(es)
  aneurysms of, repair of, 1467-1468, 1469f
  double, 1609, 1610, 1610f
  embryogenesis of, 1564
  hypoplasia of, 1608
  interruption of, 1608-1609
  normal anatomy of, 1564-1565
  right, 1609, 1610
    tetralogy of Fallot with, 1588
Aortic disease
  echocardiography in, 299-302, 299f-302f, 320, 320t
  exercise and sports in patients with, 1989
Aortic dissection, 1469-1486
  angiography in, 1478
  aortic regurgitation in, 1472, 1473f
  atypical, 1483-1486, 1484f, 1485f
  cardiac tamponade in, 1480
  chest pain in, 1196, 1355
  chest radiography in, 329f, 340
  classification of, 1470, 1470f, 1470t
  clinical manifestations of, 1471-1474
  cocaine and, 1811
  computed tomography in, 432, 432f
  cystic medial degeneration in, 1470-1471, 1470f
  duration of, 1470
  echocardiography in, 300-301, 300f, 301f
  etiology and pathogenesis of, 1470-1471, 1470f
  extension of, 1473
  genetic studies in, 95
  hypertension in, 1471, 1472, 1479, 1482
  hypotension in, 1472, 1479-1480
  imaging of, 1474-1478, 1475f-1478f
  intramural hematoma in, echocardiography in, 301, 301f
  laboratory findings in, 1473-1474, 1474f
  magnetic resonance imaging in, 409, 409f
  management of, 1479-1483
    blood pressure reduction in, 1479, 1482
    definitive therapy in, 1480-1482, 1480t, 1481f
    follow-up for, 1483
    long-term, 1482-1483

Aortic dissection (Continued)
  medical
    definitive, 1482
    immediate, 1479-1480
    percutaneous interventions in, 1481-1482
    surgical, 1480-1481, 1480t, 1481f
      complications of, 1481
      composite graft in, 1481, 1481f
      newer techniques in, 1481
  in Marfan syndrome, 92
  pain in, 1222, 1471
  physical examination in, 1471-1473, 1472f, 1473f
  pregnancy and, 1471
  pseudohypertension in, 1480
  symptoms of, 1471
  without intimal rupture, 1483-1484, 1484f
Aortic impedance, 531
Aortic isthmus, 1457
Aortic pressure, 451, 452t, 454t
Aortic pulse, evaluation of, 132
Aortic regurgitation, 1635-1646
  acute, 1645-1646
  angiography in, 1640
  in aortic dissection, 1472, 1473f
  aortic root disease in, 1636, 1644-1645, 1645f
  auscultation in, 1639
  chest radiography in, 340, 1640
  chronic, 1636-1638, 1638f-1640f
  clinical presentation in, 1638-1641
  echocardiography in, 270-272, 271f-272f, 1639-1640, 1640f, 1646
  in elderly persons, 1948
  electrocardiography in, 1640, 1646
  etiology and pathology of, 1635-1636, 1637f
  left ventricular function in, 1638, 1639f
  magnetic resonance imaging in, 1641
  with mitral regurgitation, 1681
  with mitral stenosis, 1680-1681
  murmur in, 137, 145-146
  myocardial ischemia in, 1638
  natural history of, 1641, 1641f, 1642t
  pathophysiology of, 1636-1638, 1638f-1640f
  physical examination in, 145-146, 1638-1639, 1645-1646
  practice guidelines for, 1696-1699, 1697t-1699t
  in pregnancy, 1972
  radionuclide imaging in, 1640-1641, 1646
  severity of, classification of, 1629t
  symptoms of, 145, 1638
  in thoracic aortic aneurysm, 1465
  treatment of, 1641-1645, 1643f
    acute, 1646
    medical, 1641-1643
    surgical, 672, 1643-1645, 1644f, 1645f
  valvular causes of, 1635-1636, 1637f
Aortic root, 1457
  disease of
    in aortic regurgitation, 1635, 1644-1645, 1645f
    in spondyloarthropathies, 2096
  repair of, in Marfan syndrome, 91-92
Aortic sclerosis, 145, 400
Aortic sinus
  aneurysm of, 299, 299f, 1609
  dilatation of
    genetic studies in, 95
    in Marfan syndrome, 91, 91f
  fistula of, 1609

Aortic stenosis, 1625-1635. See also Subaortic stenosis.
  angiography in, 1631
  asymptomatic, natural history of, 269
  auscultation in, 1630-1631, 1630f
  calcific, 1625-1626, 1626f, 1627f, 1633-1634
    percutaneous valvuloplasty in, 1442, 1444, 1444f
  cardiac catheterization in, 1631
  cardiac structure in, 1628
  chest radiography in, 338, 339f, 340, 340f, 1631
  clinical presentation in, 1628-1632
  computed tomography in, 1631
  congenital, 1610-1611, 1625, 1626f
  diastolic properties in, 1628
  echocardiography in, 267-269, 267f-269f, 1631
  in elderly persons, 1947-1948
  electrocardiography in, 1631
  etiology and pathology of, 1625-1626, 1626f, 1627f
  exercise and sports in patients with, 1989
  exercise stress testing in, 215
  exertional syncope in, 2178, 2179f
  with left ventricular dysfunction, 1634
  left ventricular outflow obstruction in, 1627, 1628f, 1629t
  with low aortic pressure gradient, 269, 269f
  with low gradient and low cardiac output, 1634, 1635f
  magnetic resonance imaging in, 1631
  with mitral regurgitation, 1681
  with mitral stenosis, 1681
  murmur in, 136
  myocardial function in, 1628
  myocardial ischemia in, 1628
  natural history of, 1631-1632, 1632t, 1633f
  noncardiac surgery in patients with, 2015
  pathophysiology of, 1626-1628, 1628f
  physical examination in, 145, 1630-1631, 1630f
  practice guidelines for, 1694-1696, 1695t-1696t
  in pregnancy, 1970
  pressure gradient determination in, 455-456, 456f
  pulmonary hypertension in, 1904
  rheumatic, 1626, 1626f
  severe, 268-269, 269f
  severity of, classification of, 1629t
  sudden cardiac death in, 944
  supravalvular, 1612-1614
    autosomal dominant, genetic studies in, 90
    clinical features of, 1613
    familial autosomal dominant, 1613
    interventional options and outcomes in, 1614
    laboratory studies in, 1614
    morphology of, 1612-1613
    Williams syndrome as, 1613-1614, 1613f
  symptoms of, 145, 1628-1630
  treatment of, 1633-1635, 1634f
    medical, 1633
    percutaneous, 1444-1446, 1445f
    surgical, 672, 672f, 1633-1635, 1634f
Aortic valve
  abnormalities of, in elderly persons, 1947-1949, 1947t

I-8 Aortic valve *(Continued)*
area of, calculation of, 268, 268f, 457
bicuspid, 1625, 1626f
aortic aneurysms and, 1464-1465
aortic regurgitation in, 1635
computed tomography of, 423, 424f
with dilated ascending aorta, 1699
echocardiography in, 299, 299f
genetic studies in, 119-120, 119t
calcification of, chest radiography in,
340, 340f
computed tomography of, 423, 423f
normal anatomy of, 1564
prosthetic
computed tomography of, 423, 424f
patient mismatch in, 279-280
repair of, in aortic regurgitation, 1644
replacement of
in aortic regurgitation, 1645
in aortic stenosis, 1633-1635, 1634f
percutaneous, 1444-1446, 1445f
volume of, as marker of quality of
cardiovascular care, 53f, 53t
resistance of, calculation of, 457
surgery on
in aortic disease with ventricular
dysfunction or heart failure, 672,
672f
tricuspid, aortic aneurysms and, 1465
Aortic valvotomy, in aortic stenosis, 1633
Aortic valvuloplasty, percutaneous, 1442,
1444, 1444f
Aortitis
echocardiography in, 301-302, 302f
idiopathic, 2090-2091
infectious, thoracic aortic aneurysms
and, 1465
Aortoarteritis syndromes, 1486-1487
Aortobifemoral bypass, in peripheral
arterial disease, 1505
Aortography
in abdominal aortic aneurysms, 1460
in acute aortic occlusion, 1486
in aortic dissection, 1474-1475, 1475f
in aortic penetrating atherosclerotic
ulcer, 1485
in thoracic aortic aneurysm, 1466
Aortoiliac disease
chronic, muscle atrophy in, 1495
percutaneous intervention in, 1524-
1525, 1525f, 1526f, 1526t
surgical reconstructive procedures for,
1505
Aortopulmonary window, magnetic
resonance imaging in, 407
Aortotomy, in acute aortic occlusion,
1486
Apelin, in heart failure, 549
Apex beat, 135
Apical ballooning syndrome, 258, 259f
Apical thinning, normal, on single
photon emission computed
tomography, 353, 353f
Apnea, sleep. *See* Sleep apnea.
Apnea-hypopnea index (AHI), 1915, 1916
Apolipoprotein(s)
biochemistry of, 1071-1072, 1072f
cardiovascular disease risk and, 1008,
1008f
roles of, 1072, 1074t
Apolipoprotein A1 gene, defects of, 1081
Apolipoprotein B
familial defective, 1079
in stable angina, 1356
Apolipoprotein E gene polymorphism,
cardiovascular disease risk and,
1020-1021

Apoptosis
in dilated cardiomyopathy, 1747
in heart failure, 554-555, 554f
modulators of, cardiotoxicity of, 2115
in myocardial hibernation, 1190, 1192f
nuclear imaging of, 385
Apoptosis-based theory of pulmonary
arterial hypertension, 1895f
Appetite suppressants, cardiovascular
effects of, 277, 1812
Apresoline. *See* Hydralazine (Apresoline).
Aprotinin, for postoperative bleeding,
2005
Argatroban, in chronic kidney disease
patients, 2164t
Arginine, 1159t
Arginine vasopressin, in heart failure,
545, 546f
Arm ergometry, for exercise stress testing,
197
Arrestins, 523-524, 524f
Arrhythmias, 726-930. *See also specific
types, e.g.,* Ventricular tachycardia.
in acromegaly, 2034
in acute cerebrovascular disease, 2150,
2151f-2152f
in alcoholic cardiomyopathy, 1745
alcohol-induced, 1807
artifacts simulating, 188, 188f
autonomic dysfunction and, 733
in Becker muscular dystrophy, 2137
in cancer patients, 2108
in cardiac arrest, 952
in cardiac tumors, 1816
catecholamine-dependent, sudden
cardiac death and, 945
characteristics of, 864t-865t
in chronic kidney disease, 2166
cocaine-induced, 1811, 1811t
in congenital heart disease, 1570-1571
in coronary artery disease, 1400
diagnosis of, 763-777
baroreceptor reflex sensitivity testing
in, 770
body surface mapping in, 771
electrocardiographic imaging in, 771
electrocardiography in
algorithm for, 765f
esophageal, 772
with event recorder, 768, 769f
with Holter monitor, 766-768, 769f
with implantable loop recording,
768-769, 769f
Ladder diagram in, 764, 767f
long-term, 766-770, 769f, 770f
signal-averaged, 769-770, 770f
substrate clues detected during,
764, 768f
electrophysiology in, 772-777,
773f-777f
exercise stress testing in, 765-766
heart rate turbulence in, 769
heart rate variability in, 769
history in, 763
late potentials in, 770
P waves in, 764, 766f
physical examination in, 763-764
QRS duration in, 764, 766t
QT dispersion in, 769
T wave alternans in, 770, 771f
tilt-table testing in, 771-772, 772f
in Duchenne muscular dystrophy,
2136-2137
echocardiography in, 321t, 322t, 324
in elderly persons, 1946-1947, 1947t
in Emery-Dreifuss muscular dystrophy
and associated disorders, 2144

Arrhythmias *(Continued)*
exercise and sports in patients with,
1989
exercise stress testing in, 210-213,
212f-213f, 225-226, 226t
in Fontan patients, 1595, 1596
in Friedreich's ataxia, 2146
genetics of, 101-108, 102t
in Guillain-Barré syndrome, 2149
in heart failure
management of, 635-636
with normal ejection fraction, 645
lethal
drug-induced, 964
pathophysiological mechanisms of,
949-951, 949f, 950f
management of, 779-830
ablation therapy in, 803-819
direct-current electrical cardioversion
in, 801-803, 801f
electrotherapy in, 801-819
implantable cardioverter-defibrillator
in. *See* Cardioverter-defibrillator,
implantable.
pharmacological, 779-801, 780t-784t,
786t. *See also* Antiarrhythmic
agent(s).
practice guidelines for, 823-830,
824t-830t
surgical, 819-821, 820f
in Marfan syndrome, 92
in mitral stenosis, 1652, 1653
in mitral valve prolapse, 1672, 1673
in myasthenia gravis, 2149
in myocardial infarction, 1275-1282,
1277t
hemodynamic consequences of,
1276-1277
mechanism of, 1276
pacemakers for, 1281
prophylaxis for, 1289, 1289f
reperfusion-induced, 1241
in myocarditis, 1786
in myotonic muscular dystrophy, 2139,
2141f, 2142
noncardiac surgery in patients with,
2016, 2016f
in obstructive sleep apnea, 1915-1916
versus panic attacks, 2125
in periodic paralyses, 2147, 2147f
personal and public safety issues in,
860t, 861
postoperative, 2003-2004
postshock, 802
in pregnancy, 1975-1976, 1976t
psychosocial factors in, 2122-2123
in spinal muscle atrophy, 2148
in stable angina, 1357
stress and, 2122-2123
syncope in, 977t, 978
in traumatic heart disease, 1858, 1860,
1861t
Arrhythmogenesis, 746-761, 747t
automaticity abnormalities in, 745-746,
746f, 747
conduction slowing and, 737
deceleration-dependent block in,
751
decremental conduction in, 751
delayed afterdepolarizations in, 748-
750, 748f-751f
early afterdepolarizations in, 748, 748f,
750, 752f
impulse conduction disorders in, 747t,
750-753, 754f-756f
impulse formation disorders in, 746-
750, 747t, 748f-753f

Arrhythmogenesis (Continued)
  membrane potential reduction in, 746, 746f
  parasystole in, 750, 753f
  reentry in, 751-761, 754f-760f. See also Reentry.
  sympathetic innervation in, 733
  tachycardia-dependent block in, 751
  triggered activity in, 747-750, 748f-752f, 748t
Arrhythmogenic right ventricular dysplasia/cardiomyopathy, 1759-1760, 1759f
  computed tomography in, 422-423, 423f
  diagnosis of, 1760
  echocardiography in, 288, 290f
  exercise and sports in patients with, 1989
  genetic studies in, 117, 117t, 1760
  magnetic resonance imaging in, 402
  management of, 1760
  natural history of, 1759-1760
  pathology of, 1760
  sudden cardiac death in, 944
  ventricular tachycardia in, 903-904, 903f
Arsenic, cardiovascular effects of, 1814
Arterial baroreceptors, 2171
Arterial blood gases
  in heart failure, 595
  in pulmonary embolism, 1868
Arterial bruits, 134, 1495
Arterial conduits, for coronary artery bypass graft surgery, 1382
Arterial ectasia, genetic studies in, 95
Arterial embolism, in acute limb ischemia, 1508
Arterial occlusive disease, familial, 95
Arterial pressure. See Blood pressure.
Arterial pulse
  anacrotic, 133, 133f
  in aortic regurgitation, 1638
  in aortic stenosis, 1630, 1630f
  assessment of, 132-134, 133f, 134f, 134t
  bifid, 133, 133f
  dicrotic, 133, 133f
  in mitral regurgitation, 1662
  in mitral stenosis, 1649
Arterial switch operation, in transposition of the great arteries, 1598-1599, 1599f, 1600
  reintervention after, 1601
  two-stage, 1601
Arterial tortuosity, familial, 95
Arterial ulcer, 1495, 1496f
Arteriogenesis, 81, 1183
Arteriography, 465-495. See also Angiography.
  analgesics in, 470
  angiographic views for, 473, 474f, 475f
  anticoagulation during, 470
  atherosclerotic lesion morphology on, 489-492, 491f
  brachial artery approach for, 468-469
  of branch superimposition, 495
  catheters for, 469-470, 469f-470f
  cineangiographic image technology for, 472, 472f
  complications of, 467-468, 467t
  of congenital coronary stenosis or atresia, 487
  contraindications to, 467, 467t
  contrast agents for, 471-472, 471t, 472t
  coronary, 444, 444f, 445f-447f, 446-448
  of coronary anomalies, 482-488, 483f-489f, 483t

Arteriography (Continued)
  coronary artery bypass graft catheterization in, 478-481, 482f
  of coronary artery fistula, 487, 488f, 489f
  of coronary artery spasm, 488-489, 490f-491f
  of coronary collateral circulation, 492, 493f
  of coronary perfusion, 492, 492t
  coronary segment classification systems for, 472-473, 473t
  of coronary thrombus, 492
  in dilated cardiomyopathy, 1748
  drugs used during, 470-471
  of eccentric stenoses, 494-495
  femoral artery approach for, 468, 468f
  gastroepiploic artery graft catheterization for, 480-481, 482f
  inadequate vessel opacification in, 494
  indications for, 465-467, 466t, 501-508, 502t-508t
  internal mammary artery graft catheterization for, 480, 482f
  left anterior descending artery anatomy on, 474f, 475-476
  left circumflex artery anatomy on, 474f, 476
  of left circumflex artery origin from right coronary sinus, 483, 485f-486f, 487
  left coronary artery angiographic views for, 473, 474f
  left coronary artery catheterization for, 473, 475, 476f
  of left coronary artery origin from contralateral sinus, 483, 484f, 487
  of left coronary artery origin from pulmonary artery, 482, 483f
  left coronary system dominance on, 478, 481f
  left main coronary artery anatomy on, 475, 477f, 478f
  microchannel recanalization in, 495
  of myocardial bridging, 487, 489f
  myocardial ischemia during, 470-471
  nomenclature for, 472-473, 473t
  patient preparation for, 468
  pitfalls of, 494-495
  practice guidelines for, 501-508, 502t-508t
  quantitative, 492-494, 494t
  radial artery approach for, 468-469
  right coronary artery anatomy on, 477-478
  right coronary artery angiographic views for, 473, 475f
  right coronary artery catheterization for, 476-477, 478f
  right coronary artery dominance on, 478, 479f-480f
  of right coronary artery high anterior origin, 488
  of right coronary artery origin from contralateral sinus, 483, 486f-487f, 487
  saphenous vein graft catheterization in, 478-479
  in stable angina, 1359-1360
  standardized projection acquisition for, 481-482, 483f
  superimposition of branches in, 495
  technique of, 468-470, 468f-470f
  in thromboangiitis obliterans, 1506, 1507f
  of total coronary occlusion, 492

Arteriography (Continued)
  in UA/NSTEMI, 1321f, 1323
  vascular access for, 468-469, 468f
Arteriohepatic dysplasia, 95
Arterioles
  precapillary, in coronary blood flow regulation, 1167-1177
  pulmonary, anatomy of, 1883
Arteriosclerosis
  after arterial intervention, 999. See also Restenosis.
  after heart transplantation, 999-1000, 999f, 1000f
Arteriovenous fistula
  coronary, 1620-1621
  pulmonary, 1620
Arteriovenous malformations, in hereditary hemorrhagic telangiectasia, 98
Arteritis
  coronary, in systemic lupus erythematosus, 2097
  giant cell, 2089-2090, 2090t
  septic, in infective endocarditis, 1730
  Takayasu, 2087-2089, 2088f
Artery(ies). See also Arterial entries.
  adventitia of, 988-989, 989f
  for cardiac catheterization, 443, 443f, 444f
  endothelial cells of, 987, 987f
  genetic disorders primarily affecting, 89-96
  intima of, 988, 989f
  smooth muscle cells of, 987-988, 988f
  stenosis of, in atherosclerosis, 994f, 995-996
  structure of, 987-989, 987f-990f
  tunica media of, 988, 989f
Arthritis
  exertional leg pain in, 1495
  gouty, in cyanotic congenital heart disease, 1568
  inflammatory bowel disease–associated, 2096
  postinfectious reactive, 2096
  psoriatic, 2096
  in rheumatic fever, 2083, 2086
  rheumatoid, 1851, 2094-2096
Artichoke leaf extract (Cynara scolymus), 1159t
Artificial heart, total, 691-692, 691f
Aschoff bodies, in rheumatic fever, 2081
Ascites, in heart failure, 563
Ashman beats, 172, 172f
Asian Americans
  cardiovascular mortality in, 25
  demographics of, 23, 24f
  health care disparities for, 25
Aspergillosis, pericarditis in, 1849
Aspergillus species, in infective endocarditis, 1717
Aspiration devices, in percutaneous coronary intervention, 1425, 1426f
Aspirin (acetylsalicylic acid)
  in acute ischemic stroke, 1521
  in antiphospholipid antibody syndrome, 2099
  in atrial fibrillation, 871
  after cardiac surgery, 1999
  in cardiovascular disease prevention, 1133
  in chronic kidney disease patients, 2164t
  in diabetes mellitus, 1549-1550
  in disease prevention, economic analysis of, 39
  in elderly persons, 1934, 1938

I-10 Aspirin (acetylsalicylic acid) *(Continued)*
in end-stage renal disease, 2167
in giant cell arteritis, 2090
in heart failure, 635
in Kawasaki disease, 2092
in mitral valve prolapse, 1673
in myocardial infarction, 1235-1236,
1253, 1255f, 1256
in myocardial infarction prevention,
1290
in percutaneous coronary intervention,
1436
in pericardial pain, 1284
in peripheral arterial disease, 1502,
1504f
as platelet inhibitor, 2068-2069, 2070f
in post-MI pericarditis, 1850
in pregnancy, 1976-1977, 1976t
in preoperative risk analysis, 1994
in Prinzmetal variant angina, 1339
in prosthetic valve replacement, 1683
resistance to, 2071-2073, 2071f, 2072t
in rheumatic fever, 2086
in stable angina, 1365
in stroke prevention, 1515
in UA/NSTEMI, 1327-1328, 1328f,
1329t
in women, 1960-1961
Association studies, in molecular
genetics, 76
Asthma
cardiac. *See* Paroxysmal nocturnal
dyspnea.
in Churg-Strauss syndrome, 2093
sudden death in, 948
Asymmetrical dimethylarginine (ADMA),
in diabetic vascular disease, 1097
Asymptomatic Cardiac Ischemia Pilot
(ACIP) trial protocol, for exercise
stress testing, 198
Asystole
in myocardial infarction, 1281
ventricular, in carotid sinus
hypersensitivity, 912
Asystolic cardiac arrest, 951
in acute myocardial infarction, 963
management of, 956-957, 957f
post-arrest care in, 961f, 962-963, 962f
progression in, 953
Ataxia, Friedreich's, 2145-2147, 2145f,
2146f
Atelectasis, after cardiac surgery, 1998
Atenolol (Tenormin), 792-793
in chronic kidney disease patients,
2165t
in myocardial infarction, 1260, 1261f
pharmacokinetics and pharmacology of,
1372t
in UA/NSTEMI, 1327
Atherectomy, 1420f, 1425
directional, 1425
rotational, 1422, 1423f, 1424f, 1425
Atheroembolism
cardiac surgery and, 2007
in peripheral arterial disease,
1509-1511, 1510f
Atherogenesis
focality of lesion formation in, 991-992,
992f
inflammation in
mechanisms of, 993-995, 993f-995f
systemic, diffuse nature of, 998-999
leukocyte recruitment in, 989-991, 990f,
991f
lipid accumulation in
extracellular, 989, 990f
intracellular, 990f, 992-993

Atherogenesis *(Continued)*
peripheral arterial disease risk and,
1492-1493
Atherosclerosis, 985-1022. *See also*
Arteriosclerosis; Coronary artery
disease.
in abdominal aortic aneurysms,
1458-1459
accelerated
in chronic kidney disease, 2161-2162
in Cushing syndrome, 2035
in insulin resistance, 2035
aneurysmal disease in, 1000
arterial stenosis complicating, 994f,
995-996
arteriography in, 489-492, 491t
cerebral, in diabetes mellitus, 1095
complications of, 995-999
coronary calcium as marker of, 424
diabetes-related, 1093-1103. *See also*
Cardiovascular disease, in diabetes
mellitus.
evolution of atheroma in, 993-995,
993f-995f
extracellular matrix in, 994
fatty streak of, 985, 986f
foam cell formation in, 990f, 992-993
genetic factors in, overview of, 96, 97t
graft, 999-1000, 999f, 1000f
in heart failure, 634
in HIV-infected patients, 1795t, 1800,
1800f, 1801f
immune response in, 993, 993f
infection and, 1000-1001
initiation of, 989-993, 990f-992f. *See
also* Atherogenesis.
lesions of
ACC/AHA complexity scoring of, 489,
491t
angulation of, 490, 492
bifurcation of, 492
calcification of, 492
focality of, 991-992, 992f
length of, 490
morphological characteristics of, 490,
491t, 492
ostial location of, 490
scoring systems for, 489, 491t
magnetic resonance imaging of,
400-401
noncoronary obstructive disease in,
percutaneous interventions for,
1523-1542
pathophysiology of, gender differences
in, 1955
peripheral. *See* Peripheral arterial
disease.
plaque of
angiogenesis in, 994-995
calcified, 424-426, 425f-426f, 492, 496,
995, 1020
composition of, 1209-1210, 1211f
direct imaging of, 1020
evolution of, 993-995, 993f-995f
fissuring of, 1210
sudden cardiac death and, 949
hypoechoic (soft), 495-496, 495f
intravascular ultrasonography of,
495-496, 495f
magnetic resonance imaging of,
400-401
in myocardial infarction, 1209-1210,
1211f
noncalcified, computed tomography
of, 429, 429f
potentially unstable, nuclear imaging
of, 382

Atherosclerosis *(Continued)*
rupture of
C-reactive protein (hs-CRP) level
and, 1016
in myocardial infarction, 1210
thrombosis due to, 995f, 996-997,
996f, 998f
scoring systems for, 473
superficial erosion of, thrombosis due
to, 997-998, 997f
vulnerable
in diabetes mellitus, 1547
features of, 996-997
imaging of, invasive versus
noninvasive, 498f, 499t
multiple, in acute coronary
syndromes, 1323-1324, 1324f
systemic, diffuse nature of, 998-999
risk factors for, 1003-1022. *See also*
Cardiovascular disease, risk
factor(s) for.
conventional, 1004-1012
future research on, 1020-1022, 1021t,
1022f
novel, 1012-1020, 1013f-1016f, 1013t
smooth muscle cell death in, 994
smooth muscle cell migration and
proliferation in, 993-994, 994f
in thoracic aortic aneurysms, 1465
thrombosis complicating, 996-999,
996f-998f
time course of, 985-986
vascular biology of, 985-1001
venous thromboembolism and, 1863
Atherosclerotic ulcer, penetrating, of
aorta, 1484-1486, 1485f
Atherothrombosis
genetic determinants of, 1020-1021
in UA/NSTEMI, 1319, 1320, 1321f
Athletes. *See also* Sports.
cardiac arrest in, primary prevention
of, 970
cardiovascular disease in, screening
for, 1986-1988, 1986t, 1987t
competitive versus recreational, 1984
hypertrophic cardiomyopathy in, 1768
sports participation and, 1768
sudden death in, 947, 1770f, 1985, 1985t
Athlete's heart, 537-538, 537t, 1768, 1988
Atorvastatin (Lipitor), 1083
in peripheral arterial disease, 1500,
1503f
ATP (adenosine triphosphate), in heart
failure with normal ejection fraction,
650
ATP binding pocket of myosin filament,
512, 513f, 515f
ATP potassium channel
in coronary blood flow regulation,
1174-1175
mutation of, in dilated cardiomyopathy,
115t, 116
Atretic veins, 96
Atrial appendages, isomerism of,
1593-1594
Atrial arrhythmias
in acute cerebrovascular disease, 2150
in heart failure, 635-636
noncardiac surgery in patients with,
2016, 2016f
Atrial fibrillation, 869-873
alcohol-induced, 1807
anticoagulation in, 870-872
in aortic stenosis, 1633
atrial electrical remodeling in, 755-756
cardiac surgery in patients with, 1996
characteristics of, 864t-865t

Atrial fibrillation *(Continued)*
classification of, 923
clinical features of, 869-870
in congenital heart disease, 1570
after coronary artery bypass graft surgery, 1384
disopyramide effects on, 788
in Duchenne muscular dystrophy, 2136
echocardiography in, 304-306
in elderly persons, 1946-1947, 1947t
electrocardiography in, 869
embolism in, 870-872
prevention of, 926t-927t, 930
in Emery-Dreifuss muscular dystrophy and associated disorders, 2144
exercise and sports in patients with, 1989
exercise stress testing in, 212
in Fontan patients, 1595, 1596
in Friedreich's ataxia, 2146
genes involved in, 102t
in heart failure
acute, 591-592, 596
with normal ejection fraction, 645
in hyperthyroidism, 928t-929t, 2041, 2043, 2044f
in hypertrophic cardiomyopathy, 930t, 1772
ion channel abnormalities in, 755
in mitral regurgitation, 1664, 1666
in mitral stenosis, 1652, 1653
in myocardial infarction, 927t-928t, 1282
in myotonic muscular dystrophy, 2139
obstructive sleep apnea and, 1916, 1917f
postoperative, 927t, 2003, 2016, 2016f
practice guidelines for, 923-930, 924t-930t
in pregnancy, 929t, 1976, 1979, 1980t
prevention of, pacemaker for, 833-834, 834f, 858
in pulmonary disease, 930t
quality of care indicators for, 53t
reentry in, 753, 755-756
risk factors for, 870
spatiotemporal organization and focal discharge in, 753, 755
stroke associated with, anticoagulant therapy in, 1521
treatment of
acute, 872-873
electrical cardioversion in, 801, 802
long-term, 873
radiofrequency catheter ablation in, 812-816, 812f-814f, 815t, 816f
rate control in, 923, 924t
rhythm control in, 923, 924t-925t
sinus rhythm maintenance in, 926t, 930
special considerations in, 927t-930t, 930
surgical, 819f, 820
in Wolff-Parkinson-White syndrome, 889, 892f, 928t
Atrial flutter, 873-876
atypical, 809, 810f, 874-875
characteristics of, 864t-865t
clinical features of, 875
in congenital heart disease, 1570, 1572
disopyramide effects on, 788
in Duchenne muscular dystrophy, 2136
electroanatomical map of, 777f
electrocardiography in, 873-875, 874f-876f
in Emery-Dreifuss muscular dystrophy and associated disorders, 2144
in Fontan patients, 1595, 1596

Atrial flutter *(Continued)*
in Friedreich's ataxia, 2146
in myocardial infarction, 1282
in myotonic muscular dystrophy, 2139
postoperative, 2003
prevention of, 876
reentry in, 753
treatment of, 875-876, 876f
electrical cardioversion in, 801, 802
radiofrequency catheter ablation in, 809-810, 810f-811f
typical, 873-874
Atrial myxoma, 429-430, 430f
Atrial natriuretic peptide, in heart failure, 546-547, 547f, 564, 594
Atrial pacing, postoperative, 2003, 2004
Atrial premature complexes, 867-869
clinical features of, 869
electrocardiography in, 867-868, 868f-869f
management of, 869
Atrial pressure
with cardiac catheterization, 451, 452t, 453t
right, in pulmonary hypertension, 1889-1890
Atrial pressure-volume loop, 535
Atrial reentry, 756
Atrial refractory period, postventricular, 838, 840f
Atrial septal aneurysm, patent foramen ovale and, 1581
Atrial septal defect, 1577-1580
chest radiography in, 336f
clinical features of, 1579
computed tomography in, 431f
coronary sinus, 1577, 1578f-1579f
echocardiography in, 307-308, 308f-309f, 1578f, 1579
familial, 118-119
follow-up in, 1580
interventional options and outcomes in, 1578f, 1579-1580
laboratory studies in, 1579
magnetic resonance imaging in, 408
morphology of, 1577, 1578f-1579f
natural history of, 1577, 1579
ostium primum, 1577, 1578f-1579f
ostium secundum
morphology of, 1577, 1578f-1579f
repair of, 1578f, 1579-1580
pathophysiology of, 1577
in pregnancy, 1970
pulmonary arterial hypertension in, 1900-1901
reproductive issues in, 1580
right ventricular remodeling in, 577
sinus venosus, 1577, 1578f-1579f
spontaneous closure of, 1579
Atrial septal pacing, 833
Atrial septostomy
in idiopathic pulmonary arterial hypertension, 1900
in total anomalous pulmonary venous connection, 1597
Atrial septum, lipomatous hypertrophy of, 1818t, 1820, 1821f, 1822
Atrial switch operation, in transposition of the great arteries, 1598, 1599, 1599f, 1600, 1609f, 1610f
reintervention after, 1600-1601
Atrial tachyarrhythmias, radiofrequency catheter ablation of, 810-812
Atrial tachycardia, 873-877
with block, 864t-865t
chaotic (multifocal), 877, 877f
electroanatomical map of, 777f

Atrial tachycardia *(Continued)*
focal, 876-877, 877f
macroreentrant, 873-876, 874f-876f. *See also* Atrial flutter.
radiofrequency catheter ablation of, 808-809, 809f
reentrant
in congenital heart disease, 1570, 1572
in pregnancy, 1976
radiofrequency catheter ablation of, 808-809, 809f
Atrial tumors
left, 1816, 1819, 1820f
right, 1816
Atriofascicular accessory pathways, 805
in Wolff-Parkinson-White syndrome, 884, 887, 887t, 888f
Atriohisian tracts, in Wolff-Parkinson-White syndrome, 884, 887, 887t, 888f
Atrioventricular block, 913-919
acquired
electrophysiology in, 826t, 827
pacemaker in, 831-832, 832t, 854, 855t
in carotid sinus hypersensitivity, 912
congenital, in systemic lupus erythematosus, 2098
in congenital heart disease, 1571
in Duchenne muscular dystrophy, 2136
in elderly persons, 1946
electrophysiology in, 772-773
exercise stress testing in, 212
first-degree, 864t-865t, 914, 915, 1279
in myocardial infarction, 1279-1280, 1280t
paroxysmal, 918
postoperative, 2004
in rheumatic fever, 2084
second-degree, 864t-865t, 914-917, 916f-917f
Mobitz type I (Wenckebach), 914-917, 916f
Mobitz type II, 914-917, 917f
in myocardial infarction, 1279
sudden cardiac death and, 944-945
in syncope, 981
third-degree (complete), 864t-865t, 917-919, 918f
clinical features of, 919
management of, 919
in myocardial infarction, 1279-1280
during vasodilator pharmacological stress, 365
Atrioventricular canal defect. *See* Atrioventricular septal defect.
Atrioventricular conduction for atrial tachyarrhythmias, radiofrequency catheter ablation in, 810-812
Atrioventricular connection(s)
abnormal, magnetic resonance imaging in, 407-408
normal, 1564
right, absent, 1590-1591, 1591f
Atrioventricular dissociation, 919-921
classification of, 919-920, 919f, 920f
clinical features of, 920-921
electrocardiography in, 920
management of, 921
mechanisms of, 920
Atrioventricular interval, 838, 840f, 842
Atrioventricular junctional area, 728-731, 730f-733f
tachycardias involving, nomenclature for, 878
Atrioventricular junctional reciprocating tachycardia, permanent form of, 889, 891f

Atrioventricular junctional rhythm
    characteristics of, 864t-865t
    persistence of, 911, 911f, 912f
Atrioventricular junctional tachycardia,
    nonparoxysmal, 864t-865t
Atrioventricular nodal reentrant
    tachycardia, 878-882
    characteristics of, 864t-865t
    clinical features of, 881
    dual-pathway concept in, 879-880, 880f
    electrocardiography in, 878-879, 879f
    electrophysiology in, 878f, 879-880,
        880f
    prevention of, 881-882
    radiofrequency catheter ablation of,
        806-808, 806f-808f
    retrograde atrial activation in, 880
    slow and fast pathways in, 878f, 879
    treatment of, 881-882, 881t
    variants of, 806, 807f
Atrioventricular nodal reentry, 756-757,
        757f, 758f
    in Wolff-Parkinson-White syndrome,
        889-890, 889f
Atrioventricular node
    branching portion of, 730, 733f
    cells of, 730-731
    compact portion of, 729, 730f, 731f
    conduction pattern in, 732f
    function of, 729, 732f
    innervation of, 732-733, 734f
    penetrating portion of, 729-730, 731f
    PR segment and, 157
    radiofrequency catheter ablation of,
        806-808, 806f-808f
    transmembrane potentials in, 738t
Atrioventricular pressure gradient,
    diastolic function and, 574
Atrioventricular reciprocating
    tachycardia, 757-758, 759f, 878
    orthodromic, in Wolff-Parkinson-White
        syndrome, 888-889, 889f
Atrioventricular reentrant tachycardia,
    radiofrequency catheter ablation of,
        804-806, 804f-805f
Atrioventricular septal defect, 1581-1583
    clinical issues in, 1582
    complete, 1581, 1582-1583
    follow-up in, 1583
    indications for interventions in, 1582
    interventional options and outcomes in,
        1582-1583
    laboratory studies in, 1582
    morphology of, 1581, 1581f, 1582f
    natural history of, 1581-1582
    partitioned versus complete, 1581
    pathophysiology of, 1581
    primum, 1581, 1582
    reproductive issues in, 1583
    terminology in, 1581
    unbalanced, 1581
Atrioventricular valves, normal anatomy
    of, 1564
Atrium (atria)
    activation of
        abnormal sites of, 160-161
        and P wave, 156-157
    biatrial abnormalities of,
        electrocardiography in, 162, 162f
    conduction delays in, 161
    dysfunction of, in heart failure with
        normal ejection fraction, 653
    electrical remodeling of, in atrial
        fibrillation, 755-756
    embryogenesis of, 1563
    function of, in contraction-relaxation
        cycle, 535

Atrium (atria) (Continued)
    infarction of, 179, 1214-1215
    left
        abnormalities of, electrocardiography
            in, 161-162, 161f, 162t
        appendage of, 304-305, 305f, 578
        chest radiography of, 331, 331f, 332f,
            337-338, 338f, 339f
        compliance of, in mitral
            regurgitation, 1661-1662
        enlargement of
            in heart failure with normal
                ejection fraction, 646
            in mitral regurgitation, 1664
            in mitral stenosis, 1651
            on plain chest radiography, 337-338,
                338f, 339f
        function of, 578-579, 579t
        in mitral stenosis, 1649
        myxoma of, versus mitral stenosis,
            1647, 1650
        pressure in, in mitral stenosis, 1648,
            1648f
        size and volume of, 245, 245t, 247f,
            578
    lipomatous hypertrophy of
        cardiovascular magnetic resonance
            in, 405
        echocardiography in, 304, 304f
        morphology of, magnetic resonance
            imaging of, 407
    myocytes of, 509, 510t, 738t
    normal anatomy of, 1564
    remodeling of, 535
    repolarization of, 157
    right
        abnormalities of, electrocardiography
            in, 161f, 162, 162t
        chest radiography of, 336-337
        diastolic collapse of, in cardiac
            tamponade, 1838, 1839f
        enlargement of, on plain chest
            radiography, 336-337
        thrombus of, echocardiography of,
            304, 305f
Atromid. See Clofibrate (Atromid).
Atropine
    actions of, 780t
    in atrioventricular block, 919
    in cardiac arrest, 962-963
    in carotid sinus hypersensitivity, 912
    in myocardial infarction, 1238, 1266
    in sinus bradycardia, 1279
Auscultation, 135-139
    in aortic regurgitation, 1639
    in aortic stenosis, 1630-1631, 1630f
    in congenital heart disease, 1572
    heart murmurs on, 136-139. See also
        Murmur(s).
    heart sounds on, 135-136. See also
        Heart sound(s).
    in mitral regurgitation, 1662
    in mitral stenosis, 1649-1650
    in mitral valve prolapse, 1670-1671,
        1670f
    in myocardial infarction, 1223
    in pregnancy, 1968
    of prosthetic valves, 1683f
    in pulmonic regurgitation, 1679-1680
    in rheumatic fever, 2082-2083
    in tricuspid regurgitation, 1676
Auscultatory gap, 131
Austin Flint murmur, 1639
Australia, cardiovascular disease in, 10
Authority, person or test, in decision-
    making, 46
Autoimmune autonomic failure, 2176

Autoimmune disease, in dilated
    cardiomyopathy, 1746
Automaticity
    abnormalities of
        in arrhythmogenesis, 745-746, 746f,
            747
        in ventricular tachycardia, 761
    antiarrhythmic drug effects on, 780,
        781t
    normal, 744-745, 745f
Autonomic dysfunction, 2174-2183. See
    also Orthostatic intolerance; Syncope.
    arrhythmias and, 733
    in diabetes mellitus, 2176
    in dopamine beta-hydroxylase
        deficiency, 2176
    in Guillain-Barré syndrome, 2149,
        2176
    in heart failure, 542, 543f
    in HIV-infected patients, 1795t, 1800,
        1801f
    in multiple system atrophy, 2175
    in orthostatic hypotension, 976, 976t
    parasympathetic, 2175, 2182-2183
        in heart failure, 542, 543f
        in sinus arrhythmia, 2182-2183
    in Parkinson's disease, 2175
    sympathetic, 2174-2175, 2180-2182
        bed rest and, 2182
        in heart failure, 2181, 2181f
        in hypertension, 2180
        in obstructive sleep apnea, 2182
        in panic disorder, 2180-2181
        in pheochromocytoma, 2182
        during REM sleep, 2182, 2182f
Autonomic failure
    autoimmune, 2176
    congenital, 2176
    diagnosis of, 2175-2176
    primary chronic, 2175-2176
    pure, 2175
    secondary, 2176
    treatment of, 2176
Autonomic nervous system
    cardiovascular control by, 2171-2172,
        2172f
    in elderly persons, 1925
    testing of, 2172-2174
Autonomic neuropathy, cardiovascular, in
    diabetic patients, 1558
Autophagy, in heart failure, 555
Autoreactive pericarditis, 1851
Autoregulation
    of cerebral blood flow, in hypertension,
        1046, 1046f, 1054, 1054f
    of coronary blood flow, 1168, 1169f
Autosomal dominant inheritance, 87,
    88f
Autosomal recessive inheritance, 87, 87f
Autosomes, 85
Availability heuristic, 46
Axial flow pumps, 692, 692f, 693f
AZD6140, as platelet inhibitor, 2071
Azidothymidine. See Zidovudine
    (azidothymidine).
Azimilide, in arrhythmias, 780t, 781t,
    782t, 784t, 786t, 796
Azotemia, from diuretics, 626

B

Bachmann bundle, 728, 833
Back pain
    in abdominal aortic aneurysm,
        1459
    in thoracic aortic aneurysm, 1465
Bacteremia, in infective endocarditis,
    1719, 1722

Bacterial infection
  of aorta, 1486-1487
  in myocarditis, 1778
  in pericarditis, 1847
Bad news, communication of, 718, 719t
Bainbridge reflex, 535
Balloon fenestration, in aortic dissection, 1482
Balloon flotation catheter, for cardiac catheterization, 443-444, 443f, 445f
Balloon venoplasty, in venous thrombosis, 1542
Baroreceptor reflex sensitivity testing, in arrhythmia diagnosis, 770
Baroreceptor set point, 2171
Baroreceptors
  arterial, 2171
  cardiopulmonary, 2172
  hypertension and, 1030-1031
Baroreflex
  autonomic components of, 2171-2172, 2172f
  failure of, 2178
  sensitivity of, as measure of autonomic function, 2173
Barrier contraception, 1977
Barth syndrome, dilated cardiomyopathy in, 117
Bartonella species, in infective endocarditis, 1717, 1727
Bat-plasminogen activator, 2068
Bayesian theory, 42, 44
  in exercise stress testing, 207
  in interpretation of cardiac markers, 1199, 1200f
  in single photon emission computed tomography, 350-352, 351f
Bazett formula, for correction of QT interval, 160
Bcr-Abl inhibitors, cardiotoxicity of, 2113-2114, 2114f
Becker muscular dystrophy, 2135-2137, 2136f
  arrhythmias in, 2137
  cardiovascular manifestations of, 2135-2137, 2137f
  clinical presentation in, 2135
  genetics of, 2135
  prognosis for, 2137
  treatment of, 2137
Beck's triad
  in cardiac tamponade, 1836-1837
  in traumatic heart disease, 1857
Bed rest, prolonged, autonomic tone after, 2182
Behavior, from type A to type D, 2119
Benazepril, in chronic kidney disease patients, 2165t
Benefit. See Risk-benefit analysis.
Bentall procedure, in thoracic aortic aneurysm, 1467, 1468f
Benzathine penicillin G, in rheumatic fever, 2085
Benznidazole, in Chagas disease, 1780
Benzodiazepines
  in baroreflex failure, 2178
  cardiovascular aspects of, 2132, 2132t
  in hospitalized cardiac patient, 2126
Beraprost, in idiopathic pulmonary arterial hypertension, 1899
Berlin Questionnaire, 1919
Bernoulli equation, 262, 263f
Beta blockers
  in abdominal aortic aneurysms, 1463
  in acute cerebrovascular disease, 2150
  adverse effects of, 1371

Beta blockers (Continued)
  alpha-adrenergic receptor–blocking activity of, 1371
  antiarrhythmic actions of, 1370
  in aortic dissection, 1479
  in arrhythmias, 792-793
  in atrial fibrillation, 873
  in atrioventricular nodal reentrant tachycardia, 881
  candidates for use of, 1374t
  in cardiac arrest, 962
  in cardiac arrest prevention, 965, 966
  cardioselectivity of, 1060
  in cardiovascular disease prevention, 1133
  in catecholaminergic polymorphic ventricular tachycardia, 107-108
  in Chagas disease, 1780
  in chronic fatigue syndrome, 2178
  in chronic kidney disease patients, 2165t, 2167
  classification of, 1060, 1060f
  clinical effects of, 1060
  in combination therapy, 1378
  contraindications to, 1055t, 1371
  in diabetes mellitus, 1551, 1556
  dosage of, 1371
  dyslipidemia and, 1082
  in elderly persons, 1931, 1939
  exercise stress testing and, 213-214
  in heart failure, 559, 559t
    cost-effectiveness analysis of, 38
    initiation of, 596
    systolic, 618t, 624t, 630-633, 630t, 632f
  in hypertension, 1060-1061, 1060f
  in hyperthyroidism with atrial fibrillation, 2041-2042
  in hypertrophic cardiomyopathy, 1771
  indications for, 1055t
  intrinsic sympathomimetic activity of, 1060, 1370
  lipid profile changes with, 1371
  lipid solubility of, 1060, 1370-1371
  in long QT syndrome, 103, 104f, 906
  in Marfan syndrome, 92
  mechanism of action of, 1060
  in mitral stenosis, 1653
  in mitral valve prolapse, 1673
  after myocardial infarction, 792, 792f
  in myocardial infarction, 1238, 1258-1260, 1259f, 1260t, 1261f
    contraindications to, 1260t
    prophylactic, 1290-1291
    recommendations for, 1259-1260
    selection of, 1260, 1261f
  in myocarditis, 1788-1789
  in neurally mediated syncope, 983
  in periodic paralyses, 2148
  in peripheral arterial disease, 1501
  pharmacokinetics and pharmacology of, 60, 1372t-1373t
  physiological actions of, 1369-1370, 1370f, 1370t
  polymorphisms of, 61, 62t, 708t, 709, 709f, 1371
  potency of, 1370
  in pregnancy, 1976t, 1977
  preoperative use of, 2024-2025, 2024f, 2025t, 2031t, 2032
  in Prinzmetal variant angina, 1339
  psychiatric side effects of, 2132
  relative advantages of, 1377-1378, 1377t
  selectivity of, 1370
  side effects of, 633, 1060-1061
  in silent myocardial ischemia, 1397

Beta blockers (Continued)
  in stable angina, 1365, 1369-1371, 1370f, 1370t, 1372t-1374t, 1377-1378
  in stroke prevention, 1518
  in syndrome X, 1396
  in UA/NSTEMI, 1327
  in ventricular tachycardia, 899
Beta-adrenergic agonists, in myocardial infarction, 1268-1269
Beta$_1$-adrenergic effects, 521f, 523, 523f
Beta$_2$-adrenergic effects, 524
Beta$_3$-adrenergic effects, 524
Beta-adrenergic receptor(s)
  desensitization of, 523-524, 524f
    in left ventricular remodeling in heart failure, 552-553
  polymorphisms in, 708t, 709, 709f
  in sinus node, 728
  subtypes of, 521
Beta$_1$-adrenergic receptor, 521
Beta$_2$-adrenergic receptor, 521
Beta-adrenergic signal systems, in contraction-relaxation cycle, 520-524, 520f-524f
Beta-adrenergic stimulation. See Catecholamines.
Beta-agonist receptor kinase (βARK), 523-524, 524f
  as gene therapy target, 706t, 707
  in heart failure, 553
Beta-arrestin, 523-524, 524f
  in heart failure, 553
Beta-glucosidase deficiency, in Gaucher disease, 1754
Betaxolol, 792-793, 1373t
Bevacizumab, cardiotoxicity of, 2114
Bezafibrate (Bezalip), 1083
Bezold-Jarisch reflex, during reperfusion of myocardial infarction, 1241
Bias
  in diagnostic test evaluation, 43
  referral, in myocardial perfusion imaging, 374, 375f
Biatrial technique, in heart transplantation, 677, 677f
Bicaval technique, in heart transplantation, 677-678, 677f
Bicycle ergometry, for exercise stress testing, 197, 198f
Bifascicular block
  chronic, pacemaker in, 832, 854, 855t
  electrocardiography in, 170, 171f
  in myocardial infarction, 1281
Bifid arterial pulse, 133, 133f
Bigeminy, 893
Bile acid–binding resins, in dyslipidemia, 1082-1083
Bileaflet prosthetic valves, 1682, 1682f
Biliary colic, chest pain in, 1354
Bioavailability, 59
Biochemical tests, in stable angina, 1356-1357
Biofeedback
  in hypertension, 2124
  for stress management, 1157
Bioimpedance, measurement of, in heart failure management, 600
Biological death
  definition of, 933, 934t
  progression from cardiac arrest to, 953
Biological model of sudden cardiac death, 949, 949f
Biomarkers. See Cardiac markers.
Biomechanical model of heart failure, 559
Biomedicus Biopump, 689
Bioprostheses. See Tissue prosthetic valves.

of cardiac tumors, 1817
endomyocardial. *See* Endomyocardial biopsy.
of lung
in atrioventricular septal defect, 1582
in Eisenmenger syndrome, 1569
percutaneous, in pericardial effusion, 1841-1842
pericardial, in tuberculous pericarditis, 1848
of temporal (cranial) artery, in giant cell arteritis, 2090
in vasculitis, 2087
Bipolar limb leads, 152
Birth
pulmonary vascular resistance at, 1886
transitional circulation at, 1565-1566
Birth weight, low, salt-sensitive hypertension and, 1032
Bisoprolol, 792-793
in heart failure, 624t, 630, 630t, 631
pharmacokinetics and pharmacology of, 1373t
preoperative use of, 2024
Bivalirudin, 2067
in chronic kidney disease patients, 2164t
in diabetes mellitus, 1550-1551
in myocardial infarction, 1251, 1253
in percutaneous coronary intervention, 1437
in UA/NSTEMI, 1332
Black population. *See* African Americans.
Blalock-Taussig shunt, in cyanotic congenital heart disease, 1568, 1568t
Bleeding. *See also* Hemorrhage.
after coronary artery bypass graft surgery, 1383
heparin-induced, 2063
postoperative, 2004-2005
warfarin-induced, 2066
Bleeding diathesis, in cyanotic congenital heart disease, 1568
Blood chemistry, in cardiac arrest survivors, 954
Blood cultures, in infective endocarditis, 1722
Blood flow. *See* Circulation.
Blood phobia, syncope in, 2179-2180
Blood pressure
acute heart failure treatment and, 598-599, 598t
in acute ischemic stroke, 1521-1522
in aortic dissection, 1479, 1482
cardiovascular disease risk and, 1131-1133, 1131t
J curve in, 1051, 1051f
cardiovascular mortality and, 1027, 1028f, 1029f
classification of, 1006, 1131, 1131t
coronary atheroma progression and, 1037, 1037f
dietary influences on, 1113-1115, 1114f
in elderly persons, 1050
during exercise stress testing, 204
glomerular filtration rate and, 1038, 1038f
in heart failure, 592-593
high. *See* Hypertension.
low. *See* Hypotension.
lower extremity, 131, 132f
measurement of, 130-132, 131t, 132f, 1035-1036, 1035t
home and ambulatory, 1035-1036, 1035f, 1036f

Blood pressure *(Continued)*
office, 1035, 1035t
segmental, in peripheral arterial disease, 1496, 1497f
self-, 1006
in myocardial infarction, 1222
in peripheral arterial disease, 1501-1502, 1503tf
in pregnancy, 1968, 1969f
smoking and, 1052
in stable angina, 1355
stress and, 2123
sympathetic regulation of, 1031
variability in
behavioral determinants of, 1028-1029
genetic determinants of, 1029
Blood tests
in heart failure, 564
in syncope, 979
Blood transfusion
postoperative, 2005
threshold for, in noncardiac surgery, 2026-2027
Blood urea nitrogen (BUN), in heart failure, 593
Blood viscosity, in myocardial infarction, 1220
Blood volume, in pregnancy, 1968, 1969f
Blotting techniques, in molecular biology, 73-74, 73f
Blue toe, in peripheral arterial disease, 1510, 1510f
Blunt chest injury, 1855-1856, 1857-1858, 1859, 1860. *See also* Traumatic heart disease.
BMIPP, in single photon emission computed tomography, 367, 382, 383f
BMP-2 (bone morphogenetic protein receptor type 2) gene, in familial primary pulmonary hypertension, 1894-1895, 1894f
BNP. *See* B-type natriuretic peptide.
Body mass index
apnea-hypopnea index and, 1916
racial/ethnic differences in, 24
Body surface mapping, in arrhythmia diagnosis, 771
Body temperature
in myocardial infarction, 1222
noncardiac surgery and, 2026
Bone marrow—derived stem cells, 698. *See also* Stem cells, clinical applications of.
Bonhoeffer valve, in tetralogy of Fallot, 1590
Borg scale, 217
Bortezomib, cardiotoxicity of, 2111
Bosentan
in Eisenmenger syndrome, 1570
in idiopathic pulmonary arterial hypertension, 1899
Bowditch effect, 531, 532f
Brachial artery pulse, 132
Brachial artery technique
in arteriography, 468-469
in cardiac catheterization, 447
in percutaneous coronary intervention, 1423
Sones, 447
Brachiocephalic artery, obstruction of, percutaneous interventions in, 1536-1538, 1537f
Brachytherapy, radiation, for in-stent restenosis, 1429, 1431t
Bradbury-Eggleston syndrome, autonomic failure in, 976

Bradyarrhythmia, 909-913
in acute cerebrovascular disease, 2150
after coronary artery bypass graft surgery, 1384
in myocardial infarction, 1279-1281, 1280t
syncope from, 978
Bradyarrhythmic cardiac arrest, 951
in acute myocardial infarction, 963
management of, 956-957, 957f
post-arrest care in, 961f, 962-963, 962f
progression in, 953
Bradycardia
in hypertrophic cardiomyopathy, 2179
in inferior wall myocardial infarction, 2179
in right coronary artery thrombolysis, 2179
sinus. *See* Sinus bradycardia.
Bradycardia-dependent block, 751
Bradycardia-tachycardia syndrome, 913, 915f
Bradykinin, in heart failure, 548
Braunwald clinical classification of UA/NSTEMI, 1320t
Breast cancer, radiation therapy in, cardiovascular effects of, 2115-2116
Breast tissue, on single photon emission computed tomography, 353, 353f
Bretylium tosylate, in arrhythmias, 780t, 781t, 782t, 784t, 786t, 795-796
Brevibloc. *See* Esmolol (Brevibloc).
Brockenbrough maneuver, with cardiac catheterization, 460
Broken heart syndrome (stress cardiomyopathy), 181-182, 1216, 1743, 1744f, 1811-1812
Bronchial artery(ies), anatomy of, 1883
Bronchitis, chronic, 1905. *See also* Chronic obstructive pulmonary disease.
Bronchodilators, in chronic obstructive pulmonary disease, 1908
Bronchospasm, during vasodilator pharmacological stress, 365
Bruce protocol, for exercise stress testing, 197-198, 198f, 200f
Brugada syndrome, 904, 904f
cardiac arrest in, primary prevention of, 970
clinical features of, 104-105
diagnosis of, 105, 106f
electrocardiography in, 105, 106f
genetic basis of, 102t, 105
management of, 105-106
prognosis in, 105-106
reentry mechanism in, 758
risk stratification in, 106, 106f
sudden cardiac death in, 945, 946f
Bruits, arterial, 134, 1495
B-type natriuretic peptide
conditions that influence, 595t
in dyspnea assessment, 594f
in heart failure, 253, 546-547, 547f, 564-565, 564f, 594, 594f, 595t, 600
in heart failure with normal ejection fraction, 646
in HIV-infected patients, 1793
in hypertrophic cardiomyopathy, 1771
in pulmonary hypertension, 1887
recombinant (nesiritide)
actions of, 603
in chronic kidney disease patients, 2165
in heart failure, 547, 601t, 602f, 603
in renal artery stenosis, 1533

B-type natriuretic peptide (Continued)
in stable angina, 1357
in UA/NSTEMI, 1325
Bucindolol, in heart failure, 632
Bull's eye display, in single photon emission computed tomography, 348, 350, 350f
Bumetanide, in heart failure, 620, 621t, 622, 625
Bundle branch(es), anatomy of, 730, 733f
Bundle branch block. See also Left bundle branch block (LBBB); Right bundle branch block (RBBB).
myocardial infarction and, 178-179, 179f, 180f
Bundle branch reentrant ventricular tachycardia, 908
Bundle of His
anatomy of, 729-730, 731f
innervation of, 732-733, 734f
Bupropion, cardiovascular aspects of, 2129-2130, 2129t
Burns, cardiac injuries associated with, 1856-1857
Bypass surgery. See Cardiopulmonary bypass; Coronary artery bypass graft surgery.

C

C wave
in atrial pressure, 451
normal, 128f, 130
CABG. See Coronary artery bypass graft surgery.
Cachexia, cardiac, in heart failure, 563
CACNA1C gene, 736
CACNA1G gene, 736
CAD. See Coronary artery disease.
CADASIL, 95
Cafe coronary, 948
Caffeine, hypertension and, 1028
Caged-ball prosthetic valves, 1682f, 1683
Calcific aortic regurgitation, 1635, 1637f, 1640
Calcific aortic stenosis, 1625-1626, 1626f, 1627f, 1633-1634
percutaneous valvuloplasty in, 1442, 1444, 1444f
Calcification(s)
of aortic valve, chest radiography in, 340, 340f
in atherosclerosis, 424-426, 425f-426f, 492, 496, 995, 1020
of coronary artery
in chronic kidney disease, 2161-2162
clinical significance of, 425-426
computed tomography in, 424-425, 425f-426f, 1020
pathology of, 424
metastatic, in hyperparathyroidism, 2038
of mitral annulus, 1650, 1657-1658
chest radiography in, 338, 339f
in elderly persons, 1948
myocardial, chest radiography in, 341
percutaneous coronary intervention in, 1422, 1423f, 1424f
pericardial
chest radiography in, 334f, 340-341
computed tomography in, 422, 422f
in constrictive pericarditis, 1843, 1843f
pleural, chest radiography in, 341

Calcium
abnormalities of, electrocardiography in, 184, 185f
in contraction-relaxation cycle, 510, 511f, 515-520, 517f-520f, 534
in cross-bridge cycling, 511, 512, 513, 515f
in delayed afterdepolarizations, 748-750, 750f, 751f
in diabetes mellitus, 1554
diastolic relaxation and, 649
in early afterdepolarizations, 750, 752f
equilibrium potential of, 738
in hypoxic pulmonary vasoconstriction, 1884
in initiation of electrical instability, 761
intake of, blood pressure and, 1114
myocardial concentration of, 735t
parathyroid hormone and, 2037
postoperative, 1999
release of
calcium-induced, 515, 517f
heart rate-induced, 515, 518
turn-off of, 518
in resting membrane potential, 739
sarcolemmal control of, 519-520
in sinus node automaticity, 745, 745f
storage of, in sarcoplasmic reticulum, 519
supplementation of, in hypertension therapy, 1053
thyroid hormones and, 2039
uptake of, by SERCA, 518-519, 518f
Calcium channel(s)
in action potential phase 0, 740, 742
in idiopathic pulmonary arterial hypertension, 1893
L-type, 519
in heart failure, 551
ryanodine receptor, 509, 515-517, 517f
in heart failure, 551
sarcolemmal L, 519
synopsis of, 741t
T-type, 519
voltage-gated, molecular structure of, 734f, 736
Calcium channel blockers
antiatherogenic action of, 1372-1373
in aortic dissection, 1479
in arrhythmias, 798-799
in atrial fibrillation, 873
in atrioventricular nodal reentrant tachycardia, 881
clinical use of, 1061-1062, 1062t
in combination therapy, 1378
contraindications to, 1055t
in diabetes mellitus, 1102
in elderly persons, 1931
exercise stress testing and, 213-214
first-generation, 1373-1376
in hypertension, 1061-1062, 1062t
in idiopathic pulmonary arterial hypertension, 1898
indications for, 1055t
mechanism of action of, 1061, 1372
in myocardial infarction, 1263
in myocardial infarction prevention, 1291
pharmacokinetics of, 1374t-1375t
in pregnancy, 1976t, 1977
in Prinzmetal variant angina, 1338-1339
psychiatric side effects of, 2132
relative advantages of, 1377-1378, 1377t
second-generation, 1376
side effects of, 1062
in stable angina, 1371-1376, 1374t-1375t, 1377-1378

Calcium channel blockers (Continued)
in stroke prevention, 1518
in UA/NSTEMI, 1327
Calcium chloride
in cardiac arrest, 963
postoperative, 2001
Calcium gluconate, in cardiac arrest, 962
Calcium score, in stable angina, 1359
Calcium sensitizers, in acute heart failure, 601t, 604-605
Calcium sign, in aortic dissection, 1473
Calcium signaling, as gene therapy target, 707
Calcium sparks, from sarcoplasmic reticulum, 518
Calcium transients, 530
Calcium-activated, 4-aminopyridine–resistant chloride channel, 743
Calcium-activated potassium channel, 744
Calcium-pumping ATPase, of sarcoplasmic reticulum, 518-519, 518f
Calrectulin, 519
Calsequestrin, 519
Canada, cardiovascular disease in, 6, 6f, 10
Cancer, 2105-2116. See also Tumor(s).
arrhythmias with, 2108
cardiac surgery in patients with, 1996
cardiovascular complications of
direct, 2105-2108
indirect, 2108
coronary artery disease with, 2108
after heart transplantation, 681
hyperviscosity syndrome with, 2108
pericardial involvement in, 1850-1851, 2105-2106
prior or current, heart transplantation in, 676-677
superior vena cava syndrome with, 2106-2108, 2106f, 2107f, 2107t
systolic heart failure with, 635
thrombosis and, 2060-2061
valvular heart disease with, 2108
venous thromboembolism and, 1863-1864, 1875
CANCION ventricular assist device, 690
Candesartan, in heart failure, 624t, 629, 631f, 654, 655f
Candida infection, in infective endocarditis, 1717, 1727
Candidiasis, pericarditis in, 1849
Cangrelor, as platelet inhibitor, 2071
Capecitabine, cardiotoxicity of, 2111
Capillary leak syndrome, in HIV infection, 1847
Captopril (Capoten)
in Chagas disease, 1780
in chronic kidney disease patients, 2165t
in heart failure, 624t
Capture beats, in ventricular tachycardia, 897, 897f
Carbamazepine
cardiovascular aspects of, 2131, 2131t
drug interactions of, 2133, 2133t
Carbohydrate, diet low in, 1111-1112, 1111t
CarboMedics prosthesis, 1682, 1682f
Carbon dioxide, production of, during exercise, 196, 196f
Carbon monoxide
cardiovascular effects of, 1814
diffusing capacity for, in pulmonary hypertension, 1888
vasodilator properties of, 2050

Carbonic anhydrase inhibitors, in heart failure, 623
Carbonyl stress, in diabetes mellitus, 1099
Carcinoid heart disease
  echocardiography in, 296-297
  pulmonic stenosis in, 1678, 1678f
  restrictive cardiomyopathy in, 1758-1759
  tricuspid regurgitation in, 1676, 1677f
Cardene. See Nicardipine (Cardene).
Cardiac. See also Cardiovascular entries; Coronary entries; Heart.
Cardiac action potential. See Action potential.
Cardiac anatomy, normal, 329-335, 331f-335f, 1564-1565
Cardiac arrest. See also Sudden cardiac death.
  in acute myocardial infarction, 963-964
  asystolic/bradyarrhythmic, 951
    in acute myocardial infarction, 963
    management of, 956-957, 957f
    post-arrest care in, 961f, 962-963, 962f
    progression in, 953
  in Brugada syndrome, 105-106
  in catecholaminergic polymorphic ventricular tachycardia, 107
  clinical features of, 951-971
  coronary artery pathology in, 948, 949-951, 949f, 950f
  cough-version in, 958
  definition of, 933, 934t
  in-hospital
    clinical features of, 953-954
    course of, 953-954
    with noncardiac abnormalities, 964
  in long QT syndrome, 101
  management of, 955-965
    advanced life support in, 961-963, 961f, 962f
    airway clearance in, 959
    basic life support in, 958-960, 959f, 960f
    cardiopulmonary resuscitation in
      bystander, 957
      mortality in, 952-953, 953t
      procedure for, 958-960, 959f, 960f
    circulation in, 959
    community-based, 955-957, 956f-958f
    defibrillation-cardioversion in
      definitive, 961-962, 962f
      early, 956-957, 957f, 958f, 960, 960f
    electrical mechanisms in, importance of, 955-957, 956f-958f
    external chest compression in, 959-960, 959f
    initial assessment in, 958
    long-term, 964-965, 968-969
    pharmacotherapy in, 961f, 962
    stabilization in, 963
    thumpversion in, 899, 958
    ventilatory support in, 959
  metabolic acidosis of, 962
  onset of terminal event in, 952
  out-of-hospital
    with advanced heart disease, primary prevention of, 969
    in elderly persons, 953
    emergency medical services for, 955-957, 956f-958f
    survivors of
      clinical profile of, 954, 954f
      initial management of, 964
      long-term management of, 964-965
      prognosis in, 954, 955f
      secondary prevention in, 968-969

Cardiac arrest (Continued)
  prevention of, 965-971, 966t
    ambulatory electrocardiographic monitoring in, 966
    antiarrhythmic agents in, 964, 965-966
    catheter ablation therapy in, 967
    implantable defibrillators in, 967-968, 967f, 968t, 969
    primary, 969-970
    programmed electrical stimulation in, 966-967
    secondary, 968-969
    surgical interventions in, 967
  prodromal symptoms in, 952
  progression in, 953
  public safety and, 970-971
  pulseless electrical activity after, 951, 961f, 962-963, 962f
  recurrent, 953, 954, 955f
  survivors of
    electrophysiology in, 828, 828t
    hospital course of, 953-954
    secondary prevention for, 968-969
Cardiac Arrhythmia Suppression Trial (CAST), 57
Cardiac arrhythmias. See Arrhythmias.
Cardiac asthma. See Paroxysmal nocturnal dyspnea.
Cardiac atrophy, in Addison disease, 2037, 2037f
Cardiac biomarkers. See Cardiac markers.
Cardiac cachexia, in heart failure, 563
Cardiac catheterization, 439-462. See also Angiography; Arteriography.
  in aortic sinus aneurysm and fistula, 1609
  in aortic stenosis, 1611, 1631
  arteries for, 443, 443f, 444f
  in atrioventricular septal defect, 1582
  brachial artery technique of
    percutaneous, 447
    Sones, 447
  cardiac output measurements with, 452, 454-455
    angiographic, 455
    Fick method for, 452, 454-455, 454f
    thermodilution techniques for, 452, 452f
  cardiac trauma with, 1856
  catheters for, 442-443, 443f
  complementary and alternative medicine in, 1163-1164
  complications of, 461-462, 461t
  in congenital heart disease, 1575, 1577
  in constrictive pericarditis, 1844, 1844f
  contraindications to, 440, 440t
  in coronary arteriovenous fistula, 1621
  coronary blood flow measurements with, 460
  digital imaging in, 440-441
  in dilated cardiomyopathy, 1748
  in Ebstein anomaly, 1605
  in Eisenmenger syndrome, 1569
  endomyocardial biopsy in, 448
  equipment for, 440-441, 441f
  exercise with
    dynamic, 459
    isometric, 459
  in Fontan patients, 1595
  future perspectives on, 462
  hemodynamic component of, 449-459
  heparin for, 446
  hospitalization considerations in, 440
  indications for, 439-440
  intraaortic balloon pump insertion in, percutaneous, 448-449, 450f

Cardiac catheterization (Continued)
  intracardiac echocardiography with, 460, 461f
  Judkins technique for, 444, 444f, 445f-446f, 446-447
  laboratory caseload for, 440
  laboratory facilities for, 440
  left ventricular electromechanical mapping with, 460
  left ventricular puncture in, direct transthoracic, 448
  left-heart, 444, 444f, 445f-447f, 446-448
  in mitral stenosis, 1651
  mortality in, 461-462
  pacing tachycardia with, 459-460
  patient preparation for, 441-442
  personnel for, 440
  pharmacological maneuvers with, 460
  physiological maneuvers with, 459-460
  physiological monitors for, 441
  physiological stress with, 460
  pressure gradients with
    intraventricular, 457
    in valvular stenosis, 455-457, 456f
  pressure measurements with, 449, 451-452
    abnormal, 452, 453t-454t
    equipment for, 449, 451
    normal, 451, 451f, 452t
  protocol for, 442, 442t
  in pulmonary artery stenosis, 1616
  in pulmonary hypertension, 1888-1889
  radiation safety in, 441
  radiographic equipment for, 440-441, 441f
  in restrictive cardiomyopathy, 1750
  right-heart
    indications for, 442
    techniques for, 443-444, 443f-445f
  risk of, 467t
  in shunt evaluation, 458-459
  in stable angina, 1359-1360
  in subpulmonary right ventricular outflow tract obstruction, 1618
  in syncope, 980
  technical aspects of, 440-449
  techniques for, 443-449
  in tetralogy of Fallot, 1589
  therapeutic, in congenital heart disease, 1577
  in thromboembolic pulmonary hypertension, 1910
  in transposition of the great arteries
    complete, 1600
    congenitally corrected, 1602
  transseptal, 447-448, 447f
  in tricuspid atresia, 1590-1591
  in valvular regurgitation, 457-459
  in valvular stenosis, 455-457, 456f
  vascular closure devices in, 446
  vascular resistance measurements with, 452t, 455
  veins for, 443, 443f, 444f
  in ventricular septal defect, 1584
Cardiac chambers, chest radiography of, 329, 331, 331f-334f, 335f, 336-338, 337f-339f
Cardiac checklist, for UA/NSTEMI, 1337, 1337t
Cardiac compression
  cough-induced, after cardiac arrest, 958
  external, in cardiac arrest management, 959-960, 959f
Cardiac conduction system. See Conduction system.
Cardiac contusion, 1860, 1861f

Cardiac cycle. *See* Contraction-relaxation cycle.
Cardiac dipole, 150, 150f
Cardiac drugs
    interactions of
        with HIV therapy, 1802t-1803t
        with psychotropic agents, 2132-2133, 2133t
    in pregnancy, 1976-1977, 1976t
    psychiatric side effects of, 2132
Cardiac enzymes
    in acute pericarditis, 1833
    in heart failure, 565
    in myocardial infarction, 1224-1225, 1225f, 1226t
    in traumatic heart disease, 1859
Cardiac examination. *See also* Physical examination.
    in arrhythmias, 763-764
    auscultation in, 135-139
    in heart failure, 563, 593
    heart sounds in, 135-136, 136f. *See also* Heart sound(s).
    inspection in, 134-135
    murmurs in, 136-139, 137t, 138f, 139t. *See also* Murmur(s).
    in myocardial infarction, 1223-1224
    palpation in, 134-135
    in pregnancy, 1968-1969
    in stable angina, 1355
Cardiac function assessment, 569-580
    diastolic, 573-578
    during exercise, 579-580
    left atrial, 578-579
    systolic, 561-573
Cardiac glycosides, in heart failure, 618t, 624t, 630t, 633-634
Cardiac herniation, in traumatic heart disease, 1856, 1858
Cardiac impulse, in aortic stenosis, 1630
Cardiac index, 264
    in elderly persons, 1925f
    in heart failure, 142
Cardiac injury. *See* Traumatic heart disease.
Cardiac mapping, in arrhythmia diagnosis, 776-777, 776f, 777f
Cardiac markers, 1197-1199, 1198t, 1199t, 1200f, 1201t
    of atherosclerotic risk, novel, 1012-1020, 1013f-1016f, 1013t
    in cardiovascular disease, 1141
    diagnostic performance of, 1198-1199, 1198t, 1199t
    in dilated cardiomyopathy, 1748
    in heart failure, 564-565, 564f, 594-595, 600
    of heart failure prognosis, 613-614, 614f, 615f
    in infarct size estimation, 1230
    interpretation of tests for, 1199, 1200f
    in myocardial infarction, 1224-1227, 1225f, 1226f, 1226t
        recommendations for measurement of, 1210t, 1226t, 1227
    in myocarditis, 1785-1786
    prognostic implications of, 1198t, 1199, 1199t
    in pulmonary embolism, 1871
    single, test performance of, 1199
    in stable angina, 1357
    testing strategy for, 1199-1200, 1201t
    in UA/NSTEMI, 1322-1323, 1325
Cardiac mass, echocardiography of, 302-304, 302f-305f, 320, 320t
Cardiac memory T wave, 183
Cardiac morphogenesis, principles of, 118

Cardiac myosin activators, in acute heart failure, 605
Cardiac necrosis. *See* Myocardial necrosis.
Cardiac nerves, sudden cardiac death and, 949
Cardiac output
    in aortic stenosis, 1634, 1635f
    definition of, 570t
    Doppler echocardiography of, 264
    during exercise, 195, 196f
    in heart failure, 584, 584t
    measurement of, 452, 454-455, 571
        angiographic, 455
        Fick method for, 452, 454-455, 454f
        thermodilution techniques for, 452, 452f
    patient position and, 195-196
    in pregnancy, 1968, 1969f
    in pulmonary hypertension, 1889t
    in thyroid disorders, 2040
    in traumatic heart disease, 1857
Cardiac rehabilitation, 1149-1155
    in angina pectoris, 1150-1151, 1150f, 1151f
    in coronary artery disease, 1151-1152
    education in, 1154
    in elderly persons, 1940
    exercise in
        benefits of, 1150-1152, 1150f, 1151f
        future of, 1155
        physiology of, 1149-1150, 1150t
        prescription for, 1153, 1154t
        terminology related to, 1149-1150, 1150t
        underutilization of, 1154-1155
        unsupervised, 1154
    exercise stress testing in, 1153
    in heart failure, 1152
    history of, 1149
    insurance coverage of, 1154
    lipid-lowering therapy in, 1154
    after myocardial infarction, 1286
    after percutaneous transluminal coronary angioplasty, 1152
    phases of, 1152-1153, 1153t
    psychosocial interventions in, 2128
    smoking cessation in, 1154
    staff coverage in, 1153
Cardiac resynchronization therapy, 834-835, 835f, 836f
    in heart failure, 243, 244f, 618t, 636, 636f
    with implantable cardioverter-defibrillator, 848, 848f
Cardiac rupture, in traumatic heart disease, 1855-1856, 1858
Cardiac situs, 1564
Cardiac support devices, in heart failure, 559, 559t, 674-675, 675f
Cardiac surgery, 1993-2009
    aortic dissection after, 1471
    in cardiac arrest prevention, 967
    chest radiography after, 336f, 341, 341f, 342f
    complementary and alternative medicine prior to, 1164
    delirium after, 2126
    electromagnetic interference during, 850
    herbals to avoid preoperatively, 1164
    hypertension after, 1043, 1043t
    incisions for, infection of, 2008-2009
    "normal" convalescence after, 1998-2000
        cardiovascular, 1998
        chest pain in, 1999

Cardiac surgery *(Continued)*
        chest radiograph in, 1999
        drug therapy in, 1999-2000
        electrocardiographic changes in, 1999
        hospital course in, 2000
        laboratory values in, 1999
        neurological, 1998-1999
        pulmonary, 1998
    organization of surgical program in, 1993
    postoperative morbidity after
        acute respiratory distress syndrome in, 2004
        arrhythmias in, 2003-2004
        atrial fibrillation/flutter in, 2003
        atrioventricular block in, 2004
        bleeding in, 2004-2005
        cardiovascular, 2000-2004
        cardioversion in, 2003
        cognitive impairment in, 2006
        constrictive pericarditis in, 2003
        depression in, 2007-2008
        encephalopathy in, 2007
        endocrine abnormalities in, 2009
        gastrointestinal, 2008
        hypertension in, 2001-2002
        hypotension and low output syndrome in, 2000-2001, 2000t
        infection in, 2008-2009
        mechanical circulatory support in, 2001
        myocardial infarction in, 2002
        neurological, 2006-2008
        neuropathy in, 2007
        pneumonia in, 2004
        postpericardiotomy syndrome in, 2002, 2002t
        pulmonary, 2004
        renal failure in, 2005-2006
        right ventricular failure in, 2001
        stroke in, 2006, 2007
        supraventricular tachyarrhythmias in, 2003
        ventricular arrhythmias in, 2003-2004
    in pregnancy, 1969, 1995
    preoperative evaluation for
        advanced age in, 1993
        baseline laboratory values in, 1994
        cardiovascular risk factors in, 1995
        case volume in, 1994
        drug therapy in, 1994-1995
        ethnicity/race in, 1994
        gender in, 1993-1994
        general medical condition in, 1995-1996
        reoperation in, 1994
        risk assessment models in, 1996-1998, 1997t
        surgical technique in, 1994
    quality of care in, 1993
        improvement of, 55
        volume as marker of, 52-53, 53f, 53t
    thrombosis and, 2060
    thyroid hormones after, 2045
    venous thromboembolism prophylaxis after, 1878-1879, 1879t
Cardiac syncope, 978. *See also* Syncope.
Cardiac tamponade
    in aortic dissection, 1480
    after catheter-based arrhythmia procedures, 1851
    chest radiography in, 1837-1838, 1837f
    clinical presentation in, 1836-1837
    versus constrictive pericarditis, 1835t
    echocardiography in, 289-290, 292f, 1838, 1838f-1840f

Cardiac tamponade (Continued)
electrocardiography, 1837, 1837f
etiology of, 1834
hemodynamics of, 1834-1836, 1835f, 1835t, 1836f
in hypothyroidism, 2042
laboratory examination in, 1837-1838, 1837f-1840f
low pressure, 1835
malignant, 2105-2106
pathophysiology of, 1834-1836, 1835f, 1835t, 1836f
after percutaneous coronary intervention, 1851
pulsus paradoxus in, 1835, 1835f, 1837
regional, 1835-1836
total electrical alternans in, 186-187, 186t, 187f
in traumatic heart disease, 1857, 1858, 1860
treatment of, 1840-1841
x and y descents in, 1835, 1836f, 1837
Cardiac time intervals, evaluation of cardiac function by, 251-252
Cardiac toxin(s), 1805-1814
amphetamines as, 1811
antimony as, 1813-1814
appetite suppressants as, 1812
arsenic as, 1814
carbon monoxide as, 1814
catecholamines as, 1811-1812
chemotherapeutic agents as, 1812-1813, 1813t, 2108-2115, 2109t
cobalt as, 1813
cocaine as, 1808-1811, 1808t, 1809f, 1810t, 1011t
ergotamine as, 1812
ethanol as, 1805-1808, 1806t, 1807f
inhalants as, 1812
lead as, 1813
mercury as, 1813
pergolide as, 1812
protease inhibitors as, 1812
radiation therapy as, 2115-2116
sumatriptan as, 1812
thallium as, 1814
Cardiac trauma. See Traumatic heart disease.
Cardiac tumor. See Tumor(s), cardiac.
Cardiac ultrasonography. See Echocardiography.
Cardioactive agents, ECG effects of, 184
Cardioembolic disease, echocardiography in, 321t, 324
Cardiogenic pulmonary edema, 589
Cardiogenic shock
intraaortic balloon counterpulsation in, 685
in myocardial infarction, 1218, 1218f, 1222, 1269-1270
diagnosis of, 1269
intraaortic balloon counterpulsation in, 1269-1270
medical management of, 1269
pathology of, 1269
revascularization for, 1270, 1270f
percutaneous coronary intervention in, 1306, 1306f
ventricular assist device in, 686
after myocardial infarction, 688
postcardiotomy, 687-688
Cardioinhibitory carotid sinus hypersensitivity, 912
Cardiomegaly
in acromegaly, 2034
chest radiography of, 335, 336f

Cardiomyopathy, 1739-1773
alcoholic, 1744-1745
arrhythmogenic right ventricular. See Arrhythmogenic right ventricular dysplasia/cardiomyopathy.
in Becker muscular dystrophy, 2135
Chagastic, 1779-1780, 1779f
classification of, 282, 282t, 1739, 1740f, 1740t-1742t
cobalt, 1744-1745
contractile proteins and, 514-515
in desmin-related myopathies, 2148-2149
in diabetes mellitus, 1555-1556, 1555t
dilated, 1739-1749, 1742f, 1743f
angiography in, 1748
autoimmune causes of, 1746
in Barth syndrome, 117
clinical evaluation of, 1747-1749
computed tomography in, 1748
with conduction system disease, 116
contractile proteins and, 515
in Duchenne muscular dystrophy, 117
echocardiography in, 282-284, 283f-284f, 1748
electrocardiography in, 1748
in Emery-Dreifuss muscular dystrophy and associated disorders, 2144
endomyocardial biopsy in, 1748-1749
etiology of, 1743-1747
with extracardiac manifestations, 116-117
familial, 1745-1746, 1746t
in Friedreich's ataxia, 2146, 2146f
genetic studies in, 114-117, 115t, 116f, 1745-1746, 1746t
histopathology of, 1742, 1743f
history in, 1747
in HIV-infected patients, 1793-1797, 1794t, 1796f-1798f
animal models of, 1797
in children, 1795, 1796, 1798f
pathogenesis of, 1794-1795
prognosis in, 1795-1796, 1796f
treatment of, 1796, 1797f, 1798f
idiopathic, 114, 611-612, 1740
etiology of, 1745-1747, 1746t
prognosis in, 1741
in limb-girdle muscular dystrophy, 2144, 2145
magnetic resonance imaging in, 401, 401f, 1748
in mitochondrial syndromes, 117
myocarditis leading to, 1775-1776
in myotonic muscular dystrophy, 2138, 2140f
natural history of, 1740-1741
pathology of, 1741-1742, 1743f
physical examination in, 1747
in pregnancy, 1974
prognosis in, 1741, 1743t, 1744f
radionuclide imaging in, 1748
in spinal muscle atrophy, 2148
stress myocardial perfusion imaging in, 376, 376f
sudden cardiac death in, 941t, 943
treatment of, 283-284, 284f, 1749
valve surgery in, 669-672, 671f-672f
ventricular tachycardia in, 902
viral myocarditis in, 1746
without conduction system disease, 115-116, 116f
X-linked, 117
in Duchenne muscular dystrophy, 2135, 2136, 2138f

Cardiomyopathy (Continued)
echocardiography in, 282-288, 283f-291f, 318-319, 319t
exercise and sports in patients with, 1989
future perspectives on, 1760
genetic studies in, 111-117, 112t, 115t, 116f, 117t
glycogen storage, 114, 755
in hyperthyroidism, 2041
hypertrophic, 1763-1773
apical, 286, 286f, 287f
athlete's heart versus, 287, 1768
atrial fibrillation in, 930t, 1772
bacterial endocarditis in, 1773
bifid pulse in, 133, 133f
clinical course of, 1768-1770
clinical manifestations of, 1767-1768
conditions mimicking, 287
contractile proteins and, 515
definition of, 1763
diagnosis of, 1764, 1766f
diastolic dysfunction in, 1767
echocardiography in, 284-287, 285f-287f
electrocardiography in, 1768
equilibrium radionuclide angiography or ventriculography in, 371
exercise and sports in patients with, 1989, 1990
exercise stress testing in, 215-216
family screening strategies in, 1767
in Friedreich's ataxia, 2145, 2145f
future directions in, 1773
gender differences in, 1768
genetic studies in, 111-114, 112t, 1763-1764
heart failure in, 1769, 1771-1772
histopathology of, 1765-1766, 1765f
hypertensive, 286
left ventricular hypertrophy in, 1764-1765, 1764f-1766f
left ventricular outflow obstruction in, 1766-1767, 1767f
magnetic resonance imaging in, 401-402, 402f
management of, 1770-1773
alcohol septal ablation in, 1772-1773
dual-chamber pacing in, 1772
echocardiography in, 286-287
ICD implantation in, 1770
pharmacologic, 1770-1771, 1771f
surgical, 1772, 1772f
mitral valve abnormalities in, 1765
morphology of, 1764-1766, 1764f-1766f
mortality in, 1768, 1769f
myocardial ischemia in, 1767
myocardial perfusion imaging in, 375-376, 375f
natural history of, 1768-1769, 1769f
nomenclature in, 1763
obstructive, noncardiac surgery in patients with, 2015
pacemaker in, 835
pathophysiology of, 1766-1767, 1767f
physical examination in, 1767
in pregnancy, 1773, 1974-1975, 1979
preparticipation screening for, 1768
prevalence of, 1763
pseudoinfarct patterns in, 181, 181f
racial/ethnic differences in, 1768
risk stratification in, 1769-1770, 1770f
sudden cardiac death in, 941t, 942-943, 1769-1770, 1770f

Cardiomyopathy *(Continued)*
symptoms of, 1767-1768
syncope in, 2179
ventricular tachycardia in, 902-903
iron overload, 402, 403f
ischemic
chest radiography in, 336f
coronary artery bypass graft surgery in, 665-669, 666f, 667f, 668t-670t, 670f
in coronary artery disease, 1398
definition of, 1741
mitral valve surgery in, 671
myocardial hibernation in, 1187, 1190f
ventricular tachycardia in, 902
magnetic resonance imaging in, 401-403, 401f-403f
metabolic, 114
noncompaction, 288, 291f
pacemaker in, 857t, 858
peripartum, 1743, 1974
in pregnancy, 1974-1975
primary, 1739, 1740f
after radiation therapy, 2115
restrictive, 1749-1758
in amyloidosis, 1752
in carcinoid heart disease, 1758-1759
classification of, 1749, 1749t
clinical manifestations of, 1750
versus constrictive pericarditis, 1749, 1750, 1751, 1845-1846, 1845t
echocardiography in, 288, 288f, 289f
in endomyocardial disease, 1756-1758, 1757f
in Fabry disease, 1754, 1754f
in Gaucher disease, 1754
in giant cell myocarditis, 1755-1756, 1755f
in glycogen storage disease, 1755
in hemochromatosis, 1754-1755
idiopathic, 646, 1749, 1750f
infiltrative disorders in, 1753-1759
laboratory studies of, 1750-1751
in Löffler endocarditis, 1756-1757
prognosis in, 1750, 1750f
in sarcoidosis, 1755-1756, 1755f
stress (takotsubo), 181-182, 1216, 1743, 1744f, 1811-1812
tachycardia-induced, 1744
Cardiomyoplasty, dynamic, early experiences with, 674
Cardioplegia, in coronary artery bypass graft surgery, 1382
Cardioprotection, in cardiovascular disease prevention, 1133-1134
Cardiopulmonary baroreceptors, 2172
Cardiopulmonary bypass
hemodilution during, stroke risk and, 2007
mortality risk during, factors influencing, 1552, 1552f
in pregnancy, 1969
in pulmonary embolism, 1877
systemic inflammatory response syndrome after, 1998
thyroid hormones after, 2045
Cardiopulmonary exercise testing, 196-197, 196f. *See also* Exercise stress testing.
guidelines for, 224, 225t
in heart failure, 210, 211f
in heart failure with normal ejection fraction, 646-647
heart transplantation and, 216
in pulmonary hypertension, 1888

Cardiopulmonary resuscitation (CPR)
bystander, 957
defibrillation-cardioversion in
definitive, 961-962, 962f
early, 956-957, 957f, 958f, 960, 960f
mortality in, 952-953, 953t
pharmacotherapy in, 961f, 962
physicians' orders for, 722
procedure for, 958-960, 959f, 960f
for ventricular fibrillation, 899
Cardiorenal intersection, 2155, 2156f, 2157f
Cardiorenal syndrome, in heart failure, 589, 599, 627-628
Cardiorrhaphy, 1860, 1861f
Cardiotomy. *See also* Pericardiotomy.
cardiogenic shock after, ventricular assist device in, 687-688
Cardiotrophin, in contraction-relaxation cycle, 526
Cardiovascular collapse, definition of, 934t
Cardiovascular disease. *See also* Coronary artery disease; Stroke.
age and, 5, 8, 9f
in athletes, screening for, 1986-1988, 1986f, 1987t
biomarkers in, 1141. *See also* Cardiac markers.
cancer and, 2105-2116
cardiac examination in, 134-139
chest pain in, 1195-1204
chest radiography in, 327-341, 328f-342f
complementary and alternative medicine for, 1157-1164
in diabetes mellitus, 1093-1103, 1547-1558
comprehensive risk factor modification for, 1103, 1103f
epidemiology of, 1093-1095, 1095f
life style modification for, 1099
medical therapy for, 1099-1103, 1101t, 1102t
pathophysiology of, 1096-1099, 1096f-1098f
risk assessment for, 1122-1123
scope of problem in, 1547-1548, 1548f
treatment of, 1099-1103
dietary influences on, 1107-1116
economics and, 35-40
in elderly persons, 1923-1949
versus age-associated changes, 1927t
epidemiology of, 1923-1924, 1924f
future perspectives on, 1949
pathophysiology of, 1924-1926, 1925f, 1926f, 1927t
endocrine disorders and, 2033-2046
end-stage. *See* End-stage heart disease.
epidemiological transitions in
concept of, 1-26
parallel transformations accompanying, 5-6, 5f
rate of change of, 4-5, 5f, 6
stages of, 2, 3t, 4
in United States, 6-9, 6t, 7f, 8t, 9f
worldwide variations in, 2, 3f, 9-13, 10t
exercise and sports in patients with, 1988-1990
functional classification of, 126, 126t
genetic factors in, 74-76, 75f, 76f, 85-98, 111-122
global burden of, 1-21
future challenges in, 18-21, 19t
in high-income countries, 9-10, 10t, 11t

Cardiovascular disease *(Continued)*
in low- and middle-income countries, 10t, 11-13, 12f
trends in, 14-15, 14t
global risk detection in, novel approach to, 1021-1022, 1021t, 1022f
history in, 125-126
in HIV-infected patients, 1793-1804, 1794t-1795t
in hyperthyroidism, 2040-2042, 2041t
mortality in, 1119, 1120f
blood pressure and, 1027, 1028f, 1029f
in Canada, 6, 6f
changing pattern of, 1-2, 2f
global trends in, 14-15, 14t
strategies to reduce, 18-21, 19t
in United States, 7, 7f, 8, 8t
in varied populations, 25
as multifactorial disease, 1120-1121, 1121f
murine models of, 78-79, 80f
neurological disorders and, 2135-2152
noncardiac surgery in patients with, 2013-2032
nutrition and, 1107-1116
pericardium in, passive role of, 1830
physical examination in, 127-139
pregnancy and, 1967-1981
prevention of, 1119-1145
alcohol consumption in, 1139
angiotensin-converting enzyme inhibitors in, 1133-1134
anticoagulants in, 1134
antiplatelet therapy in, 1133
aspirin in, 1133
beta blockers in, 1133
blood pressure control in, 1131-1133, 1131t
cardiac protective agents in, 1133-1134
class 1 interventions in, 1126, 1126t, 1127-1134, 1127t
class 2 interventions in, 1126t, 1127, 1127t, 1134-1139
class 3 interventions in, 1126t, 1127, 1127t, 1139-1141
complementary approaches to, 1125-1126
diet in, 1138, 1140
economic analysis of, 39, 39t
exercise in, 1137-1138, 1137t
future challenges in, 1145
glycemic control in, 1134-1135
lipid-lowering therapy in, 1128-1131, 1129f, 1130f, 1130t
multiple-risk factor intervention programs in, 1141, 1142t-1143t, 1143f
psychosocial interventions in, 1140-1141
recommendations for, 1141, 1143-1145, 1144t-1145t
smoking cessation in, 1127-1128
types of studies used in, 1119-1120, 1120t
vitamin supplementation in, 1140
weight loss in, 1136-1137, 1137t
in women, 1143, 1145
psychiatric and behavioral aspects of, 2119-2133
quality of care in, 49-56
rehabilitation in. *See* Cardiac rehabilitation.
renal disease and, 2155-2168
risk assessment in, 1121-1125, 1122f-1125f
absolute, 1122, 1122f

Cardiovascular disease (Continued)
global, 1021-1022, 1021t, 1022f
global and individual risk scores for, 1122-1124, 1123f-1124f
individual, 1122, 1122f
office-based, 1124-1125, 1125f
population-attributable, 1121-1122
risk factor(s) for, 1003-1022, 1119-1127
categories of, 1121, 1121f, 1126-1127, 1126t, 1127t
conventional, 1004-1012
C-reactive protein (hs-CRP) as, 1013-1017, 1013f-1016f, 1020
depression as, 1012, 2120
diabetes as, 1009-1010, 1134-1135
diet as, 1138
epidemiological studies on, 1119-1120, 1120t
fibrinogen and fibrin D-dimer as, 1018, 1018f
fibrinolytic function markers as, 1018-1019
future research on, 1020-1022, 1021t, 1022f
genetic, 1020-1021
high-density lipoprotein level as, 1128, 1129, 1131
homocysteine as, 1017-1018
hypercholesterolemia as, 1128-1131, 1129f, 1130f, 1130t
hyperlipidemia as, 1007-1008, 1008f
hypertension as, 1005-1007, 1005f, 1006f, 1131-1133, 1131t
hypertriglyceridemia as, 1128-1129
inflammatory markers as, 1012-1020, 1013f-1016f, 1013t
lipoprotein(a) as, 1019-1020, 1019f
in menopausal patients, 1139-1140
mental stress as, 1012
metabolic syndrome as, 1009-1010, 1010f, 1135
modifiable, interventions for. See Cardiovascular disease, prevention of.
novel, 1012-1020, 1013f-1016f, 1013t, 1141
obesity/overweight as, 1011-1012, 1136-1137, 1136f, 1137t
physical inactivity as, 1010-1012, 1011f, 1137-1138
predictive value of, 1121-1125, 1122f-1125f
psychosocial, 1140-1141
regional trends in, 15-18, 15f-17f
smoking as, 1004-1005, 1004f, 1127-1128
triglyceride-rich lipoproteins and, 1009
in varied populations, 23-24
risk of
blood pressure and, 1051, 1051f
chronic kidney disease and, 2155-2156
sleep disorders and, 1915-1920
thyroid hormone changes in, 2044-2045
in varied populations, 23-32. See also Racial/ethnic differences.
in women, 1955-1964
background on, 1955
future perspectives on, 1964
mortality in, 1955
scope of problem for, 1955, 1956t
Cardiovascular magnetic resonance. See Magnetic resonance imaging.
Cardiovascular system. See also Cardiac; Heart; specific component and function, e.g., Blood pressure.

Cardiovascular system (Continued)
autonomic control of, 2171-2172, 2172f
development of, 1563-1564
embryogenesis of, 1563-1564
nonpathological variation in, 89
in pregnancy, 1967-1968, 1968f
rheumatic disease and, 2087-2101
Cardioversion
for atrial fibrillation, 872-873, 923, 924t-925t
embolism after, 871
in mitral stenosis, 1653
for atrial flutter, 875
for atrioventricular nodal reentrant tachycardia, 881
chest thump, 803, 899, 958
echocardiography in, 305-306, 322t, 324
electrical, 801-803
complications of, 802-803
indications for, 802
mechanisms of, 801
results of, 802
technique for, 801-802, 801f
postoperative, 2003
for ventricular tachycardia, 899
Cardioverter-defibrillator, implantable, 847-852
antitachycardia pacing by, 848, 849t
automated, in end-stage heart disease, 722
in Brugada syndrome, 106
in cardiac arrest prevention, 967-968, 967f, 968t, 969
cardiac resynchronization therapy with, 848, 848f
chest radiography of, 341, 341f, 342f
clinical trial results of, 847-848
complications of, 849, 850t
computed tomography of, 430, 431f
cost-effectiveness analysis of, 38, 38t
defibrillation threshold testing for, 849
design of, 848, 849t
drug effects on, 851
electromagnetic interference with, 849-851, 850f
in Emery-Dreifuss muscular dystrophy and associated disorders, 2144
exercise stress testing and, 213
failure to deliver appropriate therapy by, 849
follow-up for, 851-852, 851f, 852f
in heart failure, 618t, 636, 637f
in hypertrophic cardiomyopathy, 1770
implantation methods for, 841, 849
inappropriate discharges by, 849, 850t
indications for, 847, 847t
in long QT syndrome, 103, 906
longevity of, 848
magnetic resonance imaging and, 394
metabolic abnormality interference with, 851
in myocardial infarction, 1289, 1289f
in myotonic muscular dystrophy, 2142
practice guidelines for, 858-861, 858t-860t
in Prinzmetal variant angina, 1339
remote monitoring of, 851-852
selection of, 848f, 849
in short QT syndrome, 108
surgery and, 850
in ventricular tachycardia, 901-902
in women, 1964
CardioWest (Jarvik) total artificial heart, 691-692, 691f

Carditis. See also Infective endocarditis; Myocarditis; Pericarditis.
in rheumatic fever, 2082, 2083, 2085-2086
Cardura. See Doxazosin (Cardura).
Caribbean, cardiovascular disease in, 10t, 13
Carney complex, 121, 1817, 2035-2036
Carney syndrome, myxoma in, 302
Carnitine, as dietary supplement, 1159t
Carotid artery disease
coronary artery disease with, 1391
in elderly persons, 1940-1942, 1941t, 1942t
Carotid artery stenosis, 1538-1541
background on, 1538
imaging of, 1538, 1538f, 1539f
treatment of
catheter-based, 1539-1541, 1540f, 1541f, 1541t
emboli protection systems in, 1539
endarterectomy in, 1538-1539, 1539t, 1941
Carotid pulse
in aortic stenosis, 1630, 1630f
evaluation of, 132, 133, 133f
jugular venous pulse versus, 128, 129t
in myocardial infarction, 1223
Carotid shudder, in aortic regurgitation, 1639
Carotid sinus hypersensitivity
cardioinhibitory, 912
clinical features of, 912
electrocardiography in, 911-912, 914f
management of, 912
pacemaker in, 833, 857t, 858
syncope from, 977-978
vasodepressor, 912
Carotid sinus massage
in arrhythmias, 764
in atrial flutter, 875
in atrioventricular nodal reentrant tachycardia, 878-879
in syncope evaluation, 977-978
Carpentier-Edwards porcine valve, 1684, 1684f
Cartelol, pharmacokinetics and pharmacology of, 1373t
Carvajal syndrome, 117, 117t
Carvallo sign, in tricuspid regurgitation, 1676
Carvedilol, 792-793
in diabetes mellitus, 1551
in heart failure, 624t, 630, 630t, 631-632, 632f
in hypertension, 1061
pharmacokinetics and pharmacology of, 1373t
Case volume
as marker of quality, 52-53, 53f, 53t
in preoperative risk analysis, 1994
Casinos, AED deployment in, 960
CASQ2 mutations, in catecholaminergic polymorphic ventricular tachycardia, 107, 748-749
Catapres. See Clonidine (Catapres).
Catecholaminergic polymorphic ventricular tachycardia, 904
autosomal dominant, 107
autosomal recessive, 107
clinical features of, 106-107, 107f
electrocardiography in, 106, 107f
genetic basis of, 102t, 107
genotype-phenotype correlation studies in, 107
management of, 107-108

Catecholamines
  arrhythmias dependent on, sudden
    cardiac death and, 945
  in cardiac arrest, 963
  cardiovascular effects of, 525t,
    1811-1812
  and force-velocity relationship, 533
  lusitropic (relaxant) effects of, 523, 523f
  in myocardial infarction, 1220
  in pheochromocytoma, 2045
  positive inotropic effects of, 521f, 523,
    523f
  in pulmonary blood flow regulation,
    1884
  thyroid hormones and, 2039-2040
Catheter(s)
  Amplatz, 470, 470f
  for arteriography, 469-470, 469f-470f
  balloon flotation, 443-444, 443f, 445f
  for cardiac catheterization, 442-443,
    443f
  fluid-filled, 449
  Judkins, 469-470, 469f
  micromanometer, 449, 451
  multipurpose, 470, 470f
  nonflotation, 444
  pigtail, 446, 446f
  transseptal, 447-448, 447f
Catheter ablation. See Radiofrequency
  catheter ablation.
Catheter-assisted embolectomy, in
  pulmonary embolism, 1877, 1877f
Catheterization, cardiac. See Cardiac
  catheterization.
Catheterization laboratory, flat-panel, 472
Cationic liposomes, in gene transfer, 81
Causal reasoning, in decision-making, 41
Cavernous angioma, cerebral, 96
CD40 ligand, as inflammatory marker,
  1017
CD11/CD18 leukocyte adhesion receptor,
  antibodies against, in myocardial
  infarction, 1264
Cell(s)
  death of
    apoptotic versus necrotic, 554
    autophagic, 555
  mammalian, anatomy of, 67-68, 68f
  survival of, in myocardial hibernation,
    1190
Cell biology, principles of, 67-70, 68f, 69f
Cell cycle, 68-70, 68f, 69f
Cell membrane
  action potential of. See Action
    potential.
  electrophysiology of, 733-736, 734f,
    735f. See also Membrane potential.
  passive electrical properties of, 745
Cell therapy. See Myocardial repair and
  regeneration; Stem cells.
Cellular telephones, electromagnetic
  interference from, 850
Centerline method of regional wall
  motion measurement, 572, 573f
Centers for Medicare and Medicaid
  Services (CMS), quality improvement
  activities of, 50t
Central Asia, cardiovascular disease in,
  10t, 11-12, 19-20
Central cyanosis, 1567, 1567t
Central nervous system
  in cyanotic congenital heart disease,
    1568
  in sudden cardiac death, 945-946,
    947f
Central sleep apnea, in heart failure, 140,
  636-638, 637f

Central venous lines, cardiac trauma
  with, 1856
Central venous obstruction, percutaneous
  interventions in, 1543, 1544f
Centrifugal pumps, as ventricular assist
  device
  extracorporeal, 689
  miniaturized, 692-693
Cerebral blood flow, autoregulation of, in
  hypertension, 1046, 1046f, 1054,
  1054f
Cerebral cavernous angioma, 96
Cerebral embolism
  in aortic stenosis, 1630
  cardiac surgery and, 2007
Cerebral hemorrhage, 1522, 2149-2150,
  2150f, 2151f-2152f. See also
  Intracranial hemorrhage.
Cerebral protection methods, for aortic
  arch surgery, 1468
Cerebral symptoms, in heart failure, 562
Cerebral venous thrombosis, prothrombin
  gene mutation and, 2058
Cerebritis, in infective endocarditis, 1721
Cerebrovascular accident. See Stroke.
Cerebrovascular disease
  acute, 2149-2150, 2150f, 2151f-2152f
  in diabetes mellitus, 1095
  in hypertension, 1037
  with peripheral vascular disease, 1500
Cerubidine. See Daunorubicin
  (Cerubidine).
Cervical radiculitis, chest pain in, 1197,
  1354
Cesarean section, hemodynamic effects
  of, 1968
CETP deficiency, 1081
Cetuximab, cardiotoxicity of, 2115
Chagas disease, 611, 1779-1780, 1779f
CHARGE association, 1571
Chelation, in stable angina, 1379
Chemical ablation, in arrhythmias, 819
Chemokines, in atherogenesis, 991
Chemoreflexes
  breathing and, 2172
  as measure of autonomic function, 2174
Chemotherapy
  cardiotoxicity of, 1812-1813, 1813t,
    2108-2115, 2109t
    with targeted therapies, 2111-2115,
      2112t, 2114f
    with traditional agents, 2108-2111,
      2110f
  heart failure from, 2116
  in HIV-infected patients, complications
    of, 1803t
Chest
  compression of, external, in cardiac
    arrest management, 959-960, 959f
  discomfort in, during exercise stress
    testing, 204, 205-206, 217
  physical examination of, 128
Chest pain. See also Angina pectoris.
  acute, 1195-1204
    algorithms for, 1201, 1202, 1202f,
      1203f
    cardiac marker assay in, 1197-1199,
      1198t, 1199t, 1200f, 1201t
    causes of, 1195-1197, 1196t
    clinical evaluation of, 1197
    clinical history in, 1200
    critical pathways for, 1202, 1203f
    early noninvasive testing in,
      1202-1204
    electrocardiography in, 1197, 1201
    exercise stress testing in, 1202, 1203t
    imaging tests in, 1202-1204

Chest pain (Continued)
    immediate management of, 1202-1204,
      1203f
    initial assessment of, 1197
    initial risk stratification in,
      1200-1201, 1202f
    physical examination in, 1197,
      1200-1201
  in angina pectoris, 1195-1196
  in aortic dissection, 1196, 1355, 1471
  in aortic regurgitation, 1638
  approach to patient with, 1195-1204,
    1406f-1408f
  arteriography in, 467, 501, 504t
  atypical descriptions of, 1195-1196
  after cardiac surgery, 1999
  causes of, 1195-1197, 1196t
  cocaine-induced, 1810
  in congenital heart disease, 1571
  differential diagnosis of, 126, 1354-
    1355, 1832
  echocardiography in, 317-318, 317t-318t,
    1202, 1203
  in elderly persons, 1938
  in gastrointestinal disorders, 1197
  in hypertrophic cardiomyopathy,
    1767-1768
  ischemic, 1195
  in mitral stenosis, 1649
  in mitral valve prolapse, 1670
  in musculoskeletal disorders, 1197
  in myocardial infarction, 1195-1196
    differential diagnosis of, 1221-1222
    nature of, 1221
  in myocardial ischemia, 1195-1196
  after noncardiac surgery, 2022
  with normal coronary arteries,
    1395-1396
  in pericardial disease, 1196
  in pericarditis, 1196
  pleuritic, 1195
  psychosocial factors in, 2125
  in pulmonary disorders, 1197
  in pulmonary embolism, 1196-1197,
    1355
  in pulmonary hypertension, 1355
  in systemic lupus erythematosus,
    2097
  in thoracic aortic aneurysm, 1465
  in UA/NSTEMI, 1319, 1326-1327
  in vascular disease, 1196-1197
  during vasodilator pharmacological
    stress, 365
  in women, 1957, 1958
Chest pain units, 1202
Chest radiography
  in acute pericarditis, 1833
  anteroposterior view for, 328
  of aorta, 329, 332f, 338-339, 339f, 340f,
    1458
  in aortic arch interruption, 1609
  in aortic dissection, 329f, 340, 1473,
    1474f
  in aortic penetrating atherosclerotic
    ulcer, 1485
  in aortic regurgitation, 340, 1640
  in aortic sinus aneurysm and fistula,
    1609
  in aortic stenosis, 338, 339f, 340, 340f,
    1631
  in aortic valve calcification, 340, 340f
  in atrial septal defect, 1579
  in atrioventricular septal defect,
    1582
  of cardiac chambers, 329, 331,
    331f-334f, 335f, 336-338, 337f-339f
  after cardiac surgery, 1999

Chest radiography *(Continued)*
  in cardiac tamponade, 1837-1838, 1837f
  of cardiomegaly, 335, 336f
  in cardiovascular disease, 327-341,
      328f-342f
  in coarctation of the aorta, 1606, 1607
  in congenital aortic stenosis, 1611
  in congenital heart disease, 1572-1573
  in constrictive pericarditis, 1843, 1843f
  in cor triatriatum, 1619
  in coronary arteriovenous fistula, 1620
  in dilated cardiomyopathy, 1748
  in double-inlet ventricle, 1593
  in Ebstein anomaly, 1605
  in Eisenmenger syndrome, 1569
  in Fontan patients, 1595
  in heart failure, 565, 595
  in hypoplastic left heart syndrome,
      1591
  image recording in, 329
  of implantable devices, 336f, 341, 341f,
      342f
  lateral
      retrosternal filling on, causes of,
          1573
      view for, 327, 328, 328f, 329, 332f
  of left atrium, 331, 331f, 332f, 337-338,
      338f, 339f
  of left ventricle, 335f, 338, 339f
  of lungs, 331, 335, 336f, 337f
  in mitral annulus calcification, 338,
      339f
  in mitral regurgitation, 337-338, 339f,
      1615, 1664
  in mitral stenosis, 337, 337f, 338f, 1614,
      1651
  in myocardial calcification, 341
  after myocardial infarction, 335f, 338
  in myocardial infarction, 1229
  normal, 329-335, 331f-335f
  in partial anomalous pulmonary
      venous drainage, 1620
  in pericardial calcification, 334f,
      340-341
  in pericardial effusion, 340, 1837-1838,
      1837f
  of pericardium, 334f, 340-341
  physics of, 328, 328f
  of pleura, 341
  in pleural calcification, 341
  portable, 328, 329f
  posteroanterior view for, 327, 328f, 329,
      331f, 333f
  in pregnancy, 1969
  of pulmonary arteries, 331, 331f, 332f,
      335, 336f, 337f, 338
  in pulmonary artery stenosis, 1616
  in pulmonary embolism, 1868
  in pulmonary hypertension, 1887
  in pulmonary vein stenosis, 1619
  in pulmonic regurgitation, 1680
  in pulmonic stenosis, 337f, 338, 1617,
      1618
  in restrictive cardiomyopathy, 1750
  of right atrium, 336-337
  of right ventricle, 337, 337f, 338f
  scatter in, 327-328
  source-imaging distance in, 327, 328f
  in stable angina, 1358
  in subpulmonary right ventricular
      outflow tract obstruction, 1618
  in supravalvular aortic stenosis, 1614
  technical considerations in, 327-329,
      328f
  in tetralogy of Fallot, 1589
  in thoracic aortic aneurysm, 1465-1466,
      1466f

Chest radiography *(Continued)*
  in total anomalous pulmonary venous
      drainage, 1597
  in transposition of the great arteries
      complete, 1600
      congenitally corrected, 1602
  in traumatic heart disease, 1858
  in tricuspid atresia, 1590
  in tricuspid regurgitation, 1677
  in tricuspid stenosis, 1675
  in UA/NSTEMI, 1323
  in vascular rings, 1610
  in ventricular septal defect, 1584
Chest thump, for ventricular tachycardia,
      803, 899, 958
Chest wall disorders, pulmonary
      hypertension in, 1909
Cheyne-Stokes respiration
  in end-stage heart disease, 723
  in heart failure, 140, 562, 1917-1918,
      1919, 1920, 1920f
Children. *See also* Adolescent(s); Infant(s);
      Neonate(s).
  complete atrioventricular block in,
      919
  congenital heart disease in. *See*
      Congenital heart disease.
  dose adjustments in, 64
  HIV infection in, 14, 1794, 1795, 1796,
      1798f, 1802
  hypertension therapy in, 1065
  infective endocarditis in, 1713
  obesity in, 1136
  prosthetic valves in, 1688
  sudden cardiac death in, 942t, 946-947
  ventricular assist device in, 695-696
China, cardiovascular disease in, 10t, 12
Chlamydia, in infective endocarditis,
      1717
Chlamydia pneumoniae infection,
      atherosclerosis and, 1000
Chlordiazepoxide, cardiovascular aspects
      of, 2132t
Chloride
  equilibrium potential of, 738
  myocardial concentration of, 735t
Chloride channel(s)
  calcium-activated, 4-aminopyridine–
      resistant, in action potential phase
      1, 743
  synopsis of, 741t
Chloroquine, cardiotoxicity of, 297
Chlorothiazide, in heart failure, 600,
      621t
Chocolate, dark, intake of, blood pressure
      and, 1115
Cholesterol
  biochemistry of, 1071, 1072f
  cardiovascular disease risk and,
      1007-1008, 1008f
  dietary management of, 1112-1113,
      1112f
  elevated. *See* Dyslipidemia;
      Hypercholesterolemia.
  HDL. *See* High-density lipoprotein
      (HDL).
  LDL. *See* Low-density lipoprotein
      (LDL).
  levels of, regional trends in, 16-17
  regulation of, 1074f, 1076, 1077f-1078f
  reverse transport of, 1074f, 1076-1077,
      1077f-1078f
  transport defects of, 1081
Cholesterol absorption inhibitors, in
      dyslipidemia, 1083
Cholesterol embolism, 1509-1511, 1510f

Cholesterol embolization
  in arteriography, 468
  in percutaneous coronary intervention,
      1423, 2158-2159
Cholesterol ester(s), 1071, 1072f
**Cholesterol ester transfer protein
      inhibitors (CETP),** 1084, 1129
Cholestyramine (Questran), in
      dyslipidemia, 1083
Cholinergic receptors, muscarinic, in
      sinus node, 728
Cholinergic signaling, in contraction-
      relaxation cycle, 524-525, 525f, 525t
Cholinergic system, in coronary blood
      flow regulation, 1175
Chordae tendinae, abnormalities of, in
      mitral regurgitation, 1658f, 1659
Chorea, in rheumatic fever, 2083, 2086
Chromatography, affinity, 78
Chromosome(s), 68, 70f, 71
  aberrations of, 86, 86t
  deletions of, 86
  duplications of, 86
  gain or loss of, 86
  karyotyping of, 85-86
  microscopic alterations in, 85-86, 86t
  rearrangements of, 86
  sex, 85
Chronic kidney disease
  accelerated atherosclerosis in,
      2161-2162
  acute coronary syndromes in
      diagnosis of, 2162-2163
      outcomes of, 2163
      prognosis and, 2163, 2163f
      treatment of, 2163-2164, 2164t
  anemia in, 2156-2158
  arrhythmias in, 2166
  cardiovascular disease risk and, 2155-
      2156, 2157f, 2158f
  classification of, 2155, 2158f
  contrast-induced nephropathy in
      pathophysiology of, 2158-2159, 2159f
      prevention of, 2159-2161, 2160f, 2161f
  definition of, 2155-2156, 2157f
  diabetic nephropathy in, 2155
  heart failure in, 2164-2166, 2165t, 2166f
      anemia and, 2156-2157
  hypertension in, 2162
  myocardial infarction in, 2162-2164,
      2163f, 2164t
  pathobiology of, 2158f
  valvular heart disease in, 2166
Chronic obstructive pulmonary disease,
      1904-1909, 1905f, 1906t, 1907f, 1908f
  definitions of, 1905
  diagnosis of, 1906-1907, 1906t
  echocardiography in, 293-294, 294f,
      1907
  electrocardiography in, 166, 166f
  management of, 1907-1909, 1908f
      lung transplantation in, 1908-1909
      lung volume reduction surgery in,
          1908
      noninvasive positive-pressure
          ventilation in, 1908
      oxygen in, 1908
      pharmacological, 1907-1908
      pulmonary rehabilitation in, 1907
      smoking cessation in, 1907
  pathogenesis of, 1905
  prognosis and predictors of survival in,
      1907, 1907f
  pulmonary hypertension in,
      pathophysiology of, 1905-1906
  risk factors for, 1905
  systemic effects of, 1905

Chronotropic incompetence, during exercise stress testing, 205
Chronotropic index, 205
Churg-Strauss syndrome, 2093
Chylomicrons and chylomicron remnants, 1072, 1073f, 1073t
  genetic disorders of, 1080
  in intestinal fat absorption, 1073, 1074f, 1075
Cigarette smoking. See Smoking.
Cilostazol
  in peripheral arterial disease, 1503, 1504f
  as platelet inhibitor, 2073
Cimetidine, for contrast reaction prophylaxis, 472
Cineangiographic image technology, for arteriography, 472, 472f
Ciprofibrate (Lypanthyl, Lipanor), 1083
Circadian rhythm
  in angina pectoris, 1367
  in myocardial infarction, 1221
Circulation
  bronchial, 1883
  in cardiac arrest management, 959
  cerebral, autoregulation of, in hypertension, 1046, 1046f, 1054, 1054f
  coronary. See Coronary blood flow.
  fetal, 1565, 1565f
    persistent pulmonary hypertension in, 1902
  pulmonary. See Pulmonary circulation.
  renal, 2155, 2156f
  systemic, pulmonary versus, 1883, 1884t
  transitional, at birth, 1565-1566
Circulatory support, mechanical. See Mechanical circulatory support.
Circumferential profile technique, in single photon emission computed tomography, 348, 350f
Circumflex artery, left
  anatomy of, 474f, 475-476
  anomalous right coronary sinus origin of, arteriography of, 483, 485f-486f, 487
Cirrhosis
  cardiac surgery in patients with, 1996
  pulmonary arterial hypertension in, 1901
Cisplatin, cardiotoxicity of, 2111
Citalopram, cardiovascular aspects of, 2129t
CK. See Creatine kinase.
Claims data, for quality measurement, 50
Claudication
  in acute limb ischemia, 1507
  in diabetes mellitus, 1095
  in fibromuscular dysplasia, 1507
  intermittent
    in elderly persons, 1942-1943, 1943t
    percutaneous interventions in, 1523-1542
    in peripheral arterial disease, 1494-1495
      differential diagnosis of, 1494-1495, 1494t
      pathophysiology of, 1493
      prevalence of, 1491, 1492f
      risk factors for, 1492, 1493f
      treatment of, 1502-1504, 1504f
    in popliteal artery entrapment syndrome, 1507
    versus pseudoclaudication, 1523, 1524t
    treatment algorithm for, 1524f

Claudication (Continued)
  in thromboangiitis obliterans, 1506
  venous, 1495
  in women, 1964
Clavicle, as reference point for jugular venous pulse, 129, 129f
Clearance, drug, 59, 60, 61t
Click(s)
  nonejection, 135, 136f
  systolic
    in mitral valve prolapse, 1670
    in pulmonic stenosis, 1617
Clinical decision-making. See Decision-making.
Clofibrate (Atromid), in dyslipidemia, 1083
Clonazepam, cardiovascular aspects of, 2132t
Clonidine (Catapres)
  in baroreflex failure, 2178
  in chronic kidney disease patients, 2165t
  in hypertension, 1059
  preoperative use of, 2025
Cloning, molecular, 73
Clopidogrel (Plavix)
  after cardiac surgery, 1999-2000
  in cardiovascular disease prevention, 1133
  in chronic kidney disease patients, 2164t
  in diabetes mellitus, 1550
  in disease prevention, economic analysis of, 39
  in elderly persons, 1938
  in myocardial infarction, 1254, 1255f, 1256, 1256f
  in myocardial infarction prevention, 1290
  in percutaneous coronary intervention, 1436
  in peripheral arterial disease, 1502, 1504f
  as platelet inhibitor, 2070
  in preoperative risk analysis, 1994-1995
  resistance to, 2071-2073, 2071f, 2072t
  in stable angina, 1365
  in stroke prevention, 1515-1516
  in UA/NSTEMI, 1328-1329, 1328f, 1329f, 1330f
Clostridial infection, myocarditis in, 1778
Clot retrieval, mechanical, in acute ischemic stroke, 1520-1521
Clozapine
  cardiovascular aspects of, 2130t, 2131
  myocarditis from, 1781
Coagulation, 2050-2052
  cascade of, 2051, 2051f
  common pathway of, 2052
  extrinsic (tissue factor) pathway of, 2051, 2051f
  inhibitors of. See Anticoagulant therapy.
  intrinsic (contact activation) pathway of, 2051-2052
  phospholipid-associated enzyme complexes in, 2052, 2052f
  thrombin in, 2056, 2057f, 2058f
Coagulation necrosis, in myocardial infarction, 1212
Coagulopathy, stroke prophylaxis in, 1516-1517
Coarctation of the aorta, 1605-1608
  in adults, 1607-1608
  in aortic arch hypoplasia, 1608
  clinical features of, 1606
  complex, 1607, 1608

Coarctation of the aorta (Continued)
  computed tomography in, 431f
  echocardiography in, 310-311, 310f
  follow-up in, 1608
  hypertension in, 1043
  in infants and children, 1607
  localized, 1606-1608
  long-term complications of, 1607
  magnetic resonance imaging in, 407, 407f
  morphology of, 1606
  in neonate, 1606-1607, 1606f
  in pregnancy, 1975, 1975f
  recoarctation in, 1607
  significant, 1607-1608
  simple, 1607
Cobalt
  cardiomyopathy from, 1744-1745
  cardiovascular effects of, 1813
Cocaethylene, 1810
Cocaine
  alcohol and, 1810
  aortic dissection and, 1811
  arrhythmias from, 1811, 1811t
  cardiovascular effects of, 1808-1811, 1808t, 1809f, 1810t, 1811t
  coronary artery disease and, 1400
  endocarditis and, 1811
  mechanisms of action of, 1808, 1809f
  myocardial dysfunction from, 1810-1811
  myocardial ischemia and infarction related to, 1808, 1809f, 1810, 1810t
  pharmacology of, 1808, 1808t
Coccidioidomycosis, pericarditis in, 1848, 1849
Cockcroft-Gault equation, for creatine clearance, 2155
Codeine, pharmacokinetics of, 60
Coenzyme Q10 (ubiquinone), 1159t
  for heart failure, 1162
  for hypertension, 1158
Cognitive errors, in therapeutic decision-making, 46
Cognitive impairment
  in hospitalized cardiac patients, 2126
  postoperative, 2006
Colchicine, in pericarditis, 1833, 1834
Colestipol (Colestid), in dyslipidemia, 1083
Collagen
  in heart failure, 555-556, 555f-557f, 557
  type III, deficiency of, aortic aneurysms and, 95
Collagenases, 557, 557t
Collateral resistance, regulation of, 1184
Collateral vessels, 1183-1184
  arteriography of, 492, 493f
  growth of
    by angiogenesis and arteriogenesis, 1183
    interventions to improve, 1183-1184
  in myocardial infarction, 1215
  in stable angina, 1360
Collimator, for single photon emission computed tomography, 345, 346f
Commotio cordis, 1985
Communication, in end-stage heart disease, 718, 719t
Community, cardiac arrest management in, 955-957, 956f-958f
Community Quality Index (CQI) study, 53-54, 53t
Compartment syndrome, exertional, 1495

Complementary and alternative medicine, 1157-1164
  aging and, 1164
  in cardiac catheterization, 1163-1164
  drug/herbal interactions in, 1158, 1159t-1161t, 1163
  for dyslipidemia, 1158, 1162
  general considerations in, 1157
  for heart failure, 1162
  herbal. See Dietary supplements.
  for hypertension, 1158
  in intensive care units, 1164
  in patients undergoing cardiac surgery, 1164
  for peripheral vascular disease and venous insufficiency, 1162
  for stress management, 1157-1158
Complement-fixation test, in Chagas disease, 1780
Complex trait analysis, in molecular genetics, 75-76, 76f
Compliance, 570t
Compression stockings, 1878, 1879
Computational flow dynamics, 497, 499
Computed radiography, 329
Computed tomography, 415-434
  in abdominal aortic aneurysms, 1460, 1461f
  in aortic dissection, 1475-1476, 1475f, 1476f
  in aortic intramural hematoma, 1483, 1484f
  in aortic penetrating atherosclerotic ulcer, 1485, 1485f
  in aortic stenosis, 1631
  of atherosclerotic plaque, 1020
  of cardiac morphology, 421
  in cardiac tumors, 429-430, 430f, 1817
  in congenital heart disease, 430, 431f
  in constrictive pericarditis, 1844-1845, 1845f
  in coronary artery calcification, 424-426, 425f-426f
  in coronary artery disease, 424-426, 425f-426f
  of coronary lumen, 426-429, 426f-429f, 427t
  in dilated cardiomyopathy, 1748
  display of, 415, 416f
  dual-source, 418, 418f
  electrocardiographic gating in, 417-418
  electron beam (cine, ultrafast), 415-416, 416f, 567
  future directions in, 418, 418f, 433-434
  of great vessels, 432-433, 432f-433f
  of heart
    artifacts in, 421, 421f
    contrast-enhanced, 419-421, 419f, 420f
    nonenhanced, 419, 419f
    radiation exposure estimates for, 419t
    special considerations in, 415
  in heart failure, 566-567, 566f, 567f
  image acquisition protocols for, 418t
  in infective endocarditis, 1722
  mechanical, 416
  in mitral valve prolapse, 1672
  multidetector, 417, 418, 418t, 426-429, 426f-429f, 427t
  multislice, 566
  in myocardial disease, 422-423, 423f
  in myocardial infarction, 1229
  of myocardial perfusion, 430
  of myocardial viability, 431, 432f
  of noncalcified coronary artery plaque, 429, 429f
  partial scan reconstruction in, 416-417, 417f

Computed tomography (Continued)
  in pericardial disease, 421-422, 422f
  in pericardial effusion and tamponade, 1838
  practice guidelines for, 436, 437t-438t
  principles of, 415-418, 416f-418f, 416t
  in pulmonary artery stenosis, 1616
  in pulmonary embolism, 432-433, 433f, 1868-1870, 1869f, 1869t
  in pulmonary hypertension, 1888
  of pulmonary veins, 432, 433f
  in renovascular hypertension, 1040
  sequential scan mode for, 416, 417f
  single photon emission. See Single photon emission computed tomography.
  spiral, 416, 417f, 566, 566f
  in stable angina, 1358-1359
  in superior vena cava syndrome, 2107, 2107f, 2107t
  of thoracic aorta, 432, 432f
  in thoracic aortic aneurysm, 1466, 1466f
  in thromboembolic pulmonary hypertension, 1910, 1911f
  in valvular disease, 423, 423f, 424f
  in vascular rings, 1610
  of ventricular function, 430, 431f
Computed tomography angiography
  in carotid artery stenosis, 1538, 1538f
  combined with positron emission tomography, 354-355, 355f
  combined with single photon emission computed tomography, 354-355, 379f, 380
  of coronary arteries, 418t, 426-429, 426f-429f, 427t
  in peripheral arterial disease, 1499, 1500f
Computed tomography coronary calcium imaging, myocardial perfusion imaging after, 379-380, 379f
Computed tomography venography, in venous thrombosis, 1869
Computer analysis, in exercise stress testing, 203
Conditional knockout mouse, 79
Conduction
  anisotropic, 151, 737, 737f
  decremental, in arrhythmogenesis, 751
  internodal, 728
  intraatrial, 728
  Mahaim, in Wolff-Parkinson-White syndrome, 884
  slowing of, arrhythmogenesis and, 737
Conduction block. See Heart block.
Conduction disorders, 747t, 750-753, 754f-756f
  in amyloidosis, 1752
  after cardiac surgery, 2004
  after coronary artery bypass graft surgery, 1384
  in dilated cardiomyopathy, 116
  genes involved in, 102t
  intraventricular. See Intraventricular conduction block.
  quinidine-induced, 786
  sudden cardiac death and, 948-949
Conduction system
  anatomy of, 727-733, 728f-734f
  intraventricular, 728-731, 730f-733f
Congenital heart disease, 1561-1621. See also specific defects, e.g., Atrial septal defect.
  in adults
    exercise stress testing in, 216, 217f
    heart failure in, 1567
    management approach to, 1566

Congenital heart disease (Continued)
    pregnancy and, 1970-1971, 1971f, 1971t
    types of, 1562, 1562t
  arrhythmias in, 1570-1571
  arteriography in, 505, 507t, 508
  auscultation in, 1572
  cardiac catheterization in, 440, 1575, 1577
  chest pain in, 1571
  chest radiography in, 1572-1573
  computed tomography in, 430, 431f
  cyanotic, 1567-1568, 1567t, 1568t
    in pregnancy, 1568, 1970-1971, 1971t
  echocardiography in, 306-311, 306f-310f, 323t-324t, 324
    intracardiac, 1575
    three-dimensional, 1575, 1577f
    transesophageal, 1575
    transthoracic, 1573-1575, 1574f, 1576f
  Eisenmenger syndrome in, 1569-1570
  electrocardiography in, 1572
  environmental factors in, 1563
  etiology of, 1563
  evaluation of, 1572-1577
  exercise and sports in patients with, 1989-1990
  fetal circulation in, 1565
  gender and, 1561-1562
  genetic factors in, 118-121, 119t, 1563
  genetic testing in, 1563
  heart failure in, 1566-1567, 1572
  in HIV-infected children, 1802
  incidence of, 1561-1562
  infective endocarditis in, 1571, 1714
  isolated, 118-120
  magnetic resonance imaging in, 407-409, 407f-408f, 1573
  management approach to, 1566
  mendelian inheritance in, 118-121, 119t
  noncardiac surgery in patients with, 2015-2016
  pathological consequences of, 1566-1571
  physical examination in, 1572
  prevention of, 1563
  pulmonary hypertension in, 1568-1569, 1900-1901
  in spinal muscle atrophy, 2148
  sudden cardiac death in, 944
  syndromes associated with, 1571
Congestive heart failure. See Heart failure.
Conivaptan, in heart failure, 605-606, 621t, 624
Conn syndrome, 2036
Connective tissue disorders
  in atherosclerosis, 994
  cardiac surgery in patients with, 1996
  in coronary artery disease, 1400
  in elderly persons, 1924-1925
  genetic, 89-94, 90t
  in heart failure, 555-556, 555f, 556f
  left ventricular diastolic stiffness and, 653
  in pregnancy, 1974
  pulmonary arterial hypertension in, 1901
Connexins
  in atrioventricular junctional area, 729, 731
  in gap junctions, 737, 737f
  in sinus node, 727, 729f
Consciousness, loss of
  nonsyncopal causes of, 975, 976t
  syncopal. See Syncope.
Constipation, after cardiac surgery, 1998

Contiguous gene syndromes. *See* Genomic disorders.
Continuity equation
  in aortic stenosis, 268, 268f
  in Doppler echocardiography, 264-265, 265f
Continuous goal assessment, in end-stage heart disease, 719
Continuous quality improvement (CQI), 55
Contraceptive methods, 1977-1978. *See also* Oral contraceptives.
Contractile cells, ultrastructure of, 509-510, 510t, 511f, 512f
Contractile proteins
  and cardiomyopathy, 514-515
  in heart failure, 552, 553f
  microanatomy of, 510-515, 511f-515f
Contractility. *See* Myocardial contractility.
Contraction band necrosis, in myocardial infarction, 1212, 1213f, 1214f
Contraction-relaxation cycle, 509-538, 569f
  adenosine in, 526
  ANREP effect in, 530
  atrial function in, 535
  beta-adrenergic signal systems in, 520-524, 520f-524f
  calcium in, 534
    cytosolic, graded effects of, 513
    ion fluxes of, 515-520, 517f-520f
  cardiotrophin in, 526
  cholinergic signaling in, 524-525, 525f, 525t
  contractility in
    versus loading conditions, 529
    measurements of, 533-534, 533f
  versus cross-bridge cycling, 514, 515f
  cyclic guanosine monophosphate in, 522, 524, 525, 525f
  cytokines in, 526
  diastole of, 529, 529t
  force transmission in, 514, 514f
  force-frequency relationship in, 531-532, 532f
  force-length relationships in, 530, 530f
  force-velocity relationship in, 533
  Frank-Starling relationship in, 513, 516f, 529-530, 530f
  future perspectives on, 538
  G protein–coupled receptors in, 522, 526, 527f
  G proteins in, 521, 521f
  interleukins in, 526
  ion exchangers and pumps in, 519-520, 520f
  isovolumic relaxation phase in, 534-535, 535f
  left ventricular contraction in, 527, 528f
  left ventricular filling phases in, 527, 528f, 529
  left ventricular relaxation in, 527, 528f
  length-dependent activation in, 513-514, 516f
  mechanical events in, 526-529, 527t, 528f
  mechanical load effects on, 535-537, 536f, 537f, 537t
  molecular basis of, 512-513, 513f, 515f
  myofilament response to hemodynamic demands in, 514
  nitric oxide in, 525-526, 525f, 526f
  opioid receptors in, 526
  oxygen uptake and, 532-533, 532f, 533f
  pressure-volume loop measurements of, 533-534, 534f

Contraction-relaxation cycle *(Continued)*
  protein kinase A in, 522-523, 522f
  protein kinase G in, 524, 525f
  sodium pump in, 520
  sodium-calcium exchanger in, 519-520, 520f
  systole of, 529, 529t
  tumor necrosis factor in, 526
  vasoconstrictive signaling in, 526, 527f
  wall stress in, 530-531, 531f
Contrast agents
  allergic reactions to, prophylaxis for, 442, 471-472, 472t
  for arteriography, 471-472, 471t, 472t
  characteristics of, 471, 471t
  for computed tomography, 419-421, 419f, 420f
  for magnetic resonance imaging, 394
  nephrotoxicity of, 2160, 2160f
  side effects of, 471
Contrast-induced nephropathy, 471
  glomerular filtration rate and, 2158, 2159f
  pathophysiology of, 2158-2159, 2159f
  in percutaneous coronary intervention, 1423
  postprocedural monitoring for, 2161
  prevention of, 2159-2161, 2160f, 2161f
  risk stratification in, 2159, 2160f, 2161
Cor bovinum, in aortic regurgitation, 1637
Cor pulmonale
  electrocardiography in, 166, 167f
  pathogenesis of, 1904t
  in pulmonary embolism, 1866, 1867f
Cor triatriatum, 1618-1619
CorAide ventricular assist device, 692
CorCap cardiac support device, 674, 675f
CoreValve revalving procedure, 1445f, 1446
Corgard. *See* Nadolol (Corgard).
Corlopam. *See* Fenoldopam (Corlopam).
Corneal arcus, in stable angina, 1355
Cornell regression equation, for left ventricular hypertrophy, 164, 164t
Cornell voltage criteria, for left ventricular hypertrophy, 164, 164t
Coronary angiography. *See* Angiography.
Coronary arteriovenous fistula, 1620-1621
Coronary arteritis, in systemic lupus erythematosus, 2097
Coronary artery(ies)
  abnormalities of
    intramural, in hypertrophic cardiomyopathy, 1765, 1765f
    sudden cardiac death in, 940, 941t, 942
  aneurysm of
    in Kawasaki disease, 2092, 2092f
    in stable angina, 1360
  anomalies of
    arteriography of, 482-488, 483f-489f
    computed tomography of, 428, 429f
    exercise and sports in patients with, 1990
    incidence of, 483t
    magnetic resonance imaging of, 409
    myocardial ischemia in, 483t
    tetralogy of Fallot with, 1588
  anterior descending, left, anatomy of, 474f, 475-476
  atresia of, congenital, arteriography of, 487
  branches of, superimposition of, arteriography of, 495
  calcification of
    in chronic kidney disease, 2161-2162
    clinical significance of, 425-426

Coronary artery(ies) *(Continued)*
  computed tomography in, 424-425, 425f-426f, 1020
  pathology of, 424
  computed tomography angiography of, 418t, 426-429, 426f-429f, 427t
  dilation of, in cyanotic congenital heart disease, 1568
  dissection of
    during percutaneous coronary intervention, 1438, 1440f
    in pregnancy, 1975
    spontaneous, in coronary artery disease, 1400
  ectasia of, in stable angina, 1360
  embolism to, sudden cardiac death and, 942
  fistula of, arteriography of, 487, 488f, 489f
  left
    angiographic views of, 473, 474f
    anomalous origin of
      from contralateral sinus, 483, 484f, 487
      from pulmonary artery, 482, 483f
      sudden cardiac death in, 942
    catheterization of, 473, 475, 476f
    dominance of, 478, 481f
    magnetic resonance angiography of, 399, 400f
    main, left, anatomy of, 475, 477f, 478f
    obstruction of
      localization of, electrocardiography in, 177-178, 178f
      sudden cardiac death and, 942
    total, arteriography of, 492
  perforation of, during percutaneous coronary intervention, 1438
  perfusion of, arteriography of, 492, 492t
  recanalization of, arteriography of, 495
  right
    anatomy of, 477-478
    angiographic views of, 473, 475f
    anomalous origin of, from contralateral sinus, 483, 486f-487f, 487
    catheterization of, 476-477, 478f
    coronary blood flow in, 1177
    dominance of, 478, 479f-480f
    high anterior origin of, arteriography of, 488
    thrombolysis of, 2179
  spasm of
    arteriography of, 488-489, 490f-491f
    coronary blood flow in, 1175-1176
    methylergonovine maleate test for, 460
    in Prinzmetal variant angina, 1338, 1339f
    sudden cardiac death and, 942, 950, 950f
  stenosis of
    in atherosclerosis, 994f, 995-996
    computed tomography of, 426, 426f, 427f, 427t, 428
    congenital, arteriography of, 487
    coronary blood flow effects of, 363, 363f
    eccentric, 494-495
    left main, coronary artery bypass graft surgery for, survival after, 1388
    maximal perfusion concept in, 1178-1182, 1179f-1181f
    physiological assessment of, 1177-1183, 1177f-1184f

I-26 Coronary artery(ies) *(Continued)*
pressure-flow relationships in, 1177-1178, 1177f, 1178f
distal coronary pressure and, 1178, 1179f
thrombosis of
in atherosclerosis, 996-999, 996f-998f
in sudden cardiac death, 949
in UA/NSTEMI, 1320, 1321f
traumatic injury to, 1860
vasculopathy of, after heart transplantation, 679, 681, 682f
vasoconstriction of
causes of, 1321-1322
cocaine-induced, 1808, 1809f
in UA/NSTEMI, 1321-1322
wall of, magnetic resonance imaging of, 399-401, 400f
Coronary artery bypass graft surgery. *See also* Cardiac surgery.
angina relief after, 1386-1388
antiplatelet therapy after, 1385
arterial conduits for, 1382
cardioplegia in, 1382
catheterization of graft after, 478-481, 482f
in chronic kidney disease patients, 2164, 2164f, 2168, 2168f
complications of, 1383-1384
computed tomography in, 428, 428f
depression after, 2120
in diabetic patients, 1391, 1394, 1552, 1553, 1558
disease progression after, 1385
distal vasculature in, 1382-1383
dyslipidemia after, 1363
economic analysis of, 37
in elderly persons, 1390, 1936-1938, 1937f, 1937t
endocrine abnormalities after, 2009
exercise stress testing after, 216
graft patency after, 1384-1385
high-dose narcotic technique in, 2020
internal mammary artery for, 1382
intraaortic balloon counterpulsation in, 685
in ischemic heart failure, 665-669
benefits of, 667-669, 668t-670t, 670f
functional improvement after, 668
left ventricular function improvement after, 667-668, 668t
versus medical therapy, 665-666, 666f, 667f
patient selection for, 666-667
risks of, 667
survival after, 668-669, 669t, 670f, 670t
in left main coronary artery stenosis, 1388
in left ventricular dysfunction, 1388-1390, 1389f, 1389t, 1390f
lipid-lowering therapy after, 1385
versus medical therapy, 1385-1386, 1386f, 1386t, 1387f
minimally invasive, 1381-1382, 1381f
minimally invasive direct, 1381
with mitral valve surgery, 1400
morbidity and mortality in, risk factors for, 1993-1995
myocardial infarction after, 1388
myocardial perfusion imaging after, 378
off-pump, 1381-1382, 1381f
operative mortality for, 1383
partial aortic clamping during, avoidance of, 2007
patient selection for, 1385-1386, 1386f, 1386t, 1387f, 1391-1392

Coronary artery bypass graft surgery *(Continued)*
versus percutaneous coronary intervention, 1392-1394, 1392f-1394f, 1393t
peripheral vascular disease and, 1391
port access, 1381
practice guidelines for, 1415t, 1416-1417
preoperative, 2022-2023
previous, percutaneous coronary intervention in patients with, 1307, 1380
in Prinzmetal variant angina, 1339
quality of care in, volume as marker of, 53f, 53t
racial/ethnic differences in, 25
radial artery for, 1382
in renal failure, 1390
reoperation after, 1391
results of, 1386-1390, 1386f-1388f, 1386t
return to employment after, 1384
right gastroepiploic artery for, 1382
smoking cessation after, 1385
in stable angina, 1380-1391
surgical outcomes of, 1383-1385
survival after, 1386f-1388f, 1386t, 1387-1388
technical considerations in, 1380-1381
in UA/NSTEMI, 1347, 1349-1350, 1350t
venous conduits for, 1382
in ventricular tachycardia, 821
in women, 1390, 1962
in younger patients, 1390
Coronary artery disease, 1353-1400
alcohol intake and, 1806-1807, 1807f
angina pectoris and, 1353-1395
arrhythmias in, 1400
in cancer patients, 2108
in cardiac arrest survivors, 965
cardiac catheterization in, 439
with carotid artery disease, 1391
classification of, 473
clinical presentations in, 1353
cocaine and, 1400
collateral pathways in, 492, 493f, 1360
computed tomography in, 424-426, 425f-426f
connective tissue disorders in, 1400
coronary artery ectasia and aneurysms in, 1360
coronary blood flow in, 1360
coronary vasculitis in, 1400
cost of, 1353
in diabetes mellitus, 1093-1095, 1095f
diagnosis of
angiography in, 1359-1360, 1361-1362, 1361f, 1362f, 1409, 1411t, 1413t
arteriography in, 1359-1360
in asymptomatic persons, 1358
biochemical tests in, 1356-1357
cardiac examination in, 1355
chest radiography in, 1358
computed tomography in, 1358-1359
in diabetes mellitus, 379
exercise stress testing in, 206-207, 206t, 207t, 221, 221t, 1357-1358, 1358t, 1361
gender differences in, 1358
high-risk findings in, 1358, 1359t
magnetic resonance imaging in, 399, 399f, 1359
noninvasive testing in, 1356-1359, 1357t-1359t, 1361
physical examination in, 1355
practice guidelines for, 1405, 1405t, 1406, 1408-1409, 1409t-1410t

Coronary artery disease *(Continued)*
stress echocardiography in, 1358, 1358t, 1361
stress myocardial perfusion imaging for, 374-379, 375f-376f, 1358, 1358t, 1361
in valvular heart disease, 378
in women, 378
diseases associated with
antianginal therapy and, 1377-1378, 1377t
treatment of, 1362
echocardiography in, 253, 255-262, 256f-261f, 317-318, 317t-318t
in elderly persons, 1934-1940
approach to, 1940t
clinical presentation in, 1934
diagnosis of, 1934
management of, 1934-1938, 1935t, 1937f, 1937t
prevalence and incidence of, 1934
exercise and sports in patients with, 1988-1989
exercise effects in, 1151-1152. *See also* Exercise, in cardiac rehabilitation.
exercise prescriptions for, 1153, 1154t
exercise stress testing in
diagnostic use of, 206-207, 206t, 207t, 221, 221t, 1357-1358, 1358t, 1361
prognostic use of, 207-210, 208f, 221-222, 222t, 223t
in familial combined hyperlipidemia, 1080
in familial hypercholesterolemia, 1079
follow-up in, practice guidelines for, 1416t, 1417
genetic factors in, overview of, 96, 97t
graft, in heart transplantation, 679, 681, 682f
heart failure in, 382-383, 383f, 611, 645, 1397-1400
hypertension and, 1027, 1028f, 1029f, 1037, 1037f
in hypothyroidism, 2042-2043
ischemic cardiomyopathy in, 1398
left ventricular aneurysm in, 1398-1399, 1398f, 1399f
left ventricular function in, 1360
magnetic resonance imaging in, 394-401, 395f-400f
magnitude of problem in, 1353
management of
angiotensin-converting enzyme inhibitors in, 1365-1366, 1366f
anti-inflammatory agents in, 1365
antioxidants in, 1366
approach to, 1378
aspirin in, 1365
beta blockers in, 1365, 1369-1371, 1370f, 1370t, 1372t-1374t, 1377-1378
calcium channel blockers in, 1371-1376, 1374t-1375t, 1377-1378
chelation in, 1379
clopidogrel in, 1365
combination therapy in, 1378
coronary artery bypass graft surgery in, 1380-1391
counseling in, 1366-1367
enhanced external counterpulsation in, 1378-1379
exercise in, 1364-1365
glycemic control in, 1363-1364
hormone replacement therapy in, 1364
hypertension therapy in, 1065, 1362-1363

Coronary artery disease (Continued)
  laser-assisted myocardial
    revascularization in, 1394-1395
  lifestyle changes in, 1367
  lipid-lowering therapy in, 1363
  medical, 1362-1379
  metabolic agents in, 1377
  nitrates in, 1367-1369, 1367t, 1368f,
    1368t
  in patients with associated diseases,
    1377-1378, 1377t
  percutaneous coronary intervention
    in, 1379-1380, 1380f, 1391-1392
  pharmacological, 1363-1366,
    1367-1378
  practice guidelines for, 1411, 1413-
    1417, 1413t-1416t
  smoking cessation in, 1363
  spinal cord stimulation in, 1378
  surgical, 1380-1395
  mitral regurgitation in, 1399-1400, 1659,
    1667, 1667f
  myocardial bridging in, 1360, 1400
  myocardial metabolism in, 1360
  myocardial oxygen demand in, 1355,
    1356f
  myocardial oxygen supply in, 1355-
    1356, 1356f
  myocardial perfusion imaging in, 371-
    380, 372f-379f
  nonatheromatous, 1400
  noncardiac surgery in patients with
    anesthesia for, 2020-2021
    preoperative risk assessment for,
      2013-2014, 2018, 2020
    risk reduction intervention in, 2022-
      2027, 2031t, 2032
  with peripheral vascular disease, 1355,
    1391, 1499-1500
  practice guidelines for, 1405-1417, 1406f-
    1408f, 1407t, 1409t-1416t
  in pregnancy, 1975
  prognosis in, exercise stress testing
    and, 207-210, 208f, 221-222, 222t,
    223t
  psychiatric and behavioral aspects of,
    2119-2122
  quality of care indicators for, 53t
  racial/ethnic differences in, 25, 28-29,
    29f
  after radiation therapy, 1400, 2115-2116
  rehabilitation in, psychological factors
    in, 2128
  revascularization in
    comparison and choice between PCI
      and CABG for, 1392-1394, 1392f-
      1394f, 1393t
    complete, need for, 1394
    in diabetic patients, 1394
    indications for, 1385-1386, 1386f,
      1386t, 1387f, 1391-1392
    laser-assisted, 1394-1395
    practice guidelines for, 1415t,
      1416-1417
  in rheumatoid arthritis, 2095
  risk factors for, 1003-1022, 1119-1127.
    See also Cardiovascular disease,
    prevention of; Cardiovascular
    disease, risk factor(s) for.
  risk stratification in, 1358, 1359t,
    1360-1362, 1360f-1362f, 1385-1386,
    1386f, 1386t, 1387f, 1409-1411,
    1412t, 1413t
  silent myocardial ischemia in,
    1396-1397
  spontaneous coronary dissection in,
    1400

Coronary artery disease (Continued)
  sudden cardiac death in
    pathology of, 948, 949-951, 949f,
      950f
    progression to, 937-938, 938f
    ventricular arrhythmias and, 939-940,
      940f
  syndrome X in, 1395-1396
  in systemic lupus erythematosus,
    2097
  Takayasu arteritis in, 1400
  valvular heart disease in, 1709, 1711t,
    1712
  ventricular tachycardia in, surgical
    management of, 820-821, 820f
  in women, 1955-1963. See also Women,
    coronary artery disease in.
Coronary blood flow
  collateral, 1183-1184. See also Collateral
    vessels.
  future perspectives on, 1191
  magnetic resonance angiography of,
    399, 400f
  measurement of, in cardiac
    catheterization laboratory, 460
  after myocardial infarction, 1184-1185,
    1185f
  in myocardial infarction, mortality and,
    1243, 1243f
  myocardial oxygen consumption and,
    during exercise, 203-204
  regulation of, 1167-1177
    acetylcholine in, 1168, 1170, 1170t
    acidosis in, 1175
    adenosine in, 1174, 1176-1177
    adenosine triphosphate (ATP)
      potassium channel in, 1174-1175
    autoregulation in, 1168, 1169f
    cholinergic, 1175
    coronary resistance vessels in,
      1171-1174, 1172f-1174f
    dipyridamole in, 1177
    endothelin in, 1170-1171
    endothelium-dependent, 1168,
      1170-1171, 1170t
    endothelium-dependent
      hyperpolarizing factor in, 1170
    extravascular compressive resistance
      in, 1171, 1172f
    hypoxia in, 1175
    metabolic, 1174-1175
    in myocardial infarction, 1218,
      1218f
    nitric oxide in, 1170
    nitroglycerin in, 1176
    papaverine in, 1177
    paracrine mediators in, 1170t, 1175
    pharmacological, 1170t, 1176-1177
    prostacyclin in, 1170
    sympathetic, 1175, 1176f
  in right coronary artery, 1177
  in stable angina, 1360
  systolic and diastolic variations in,
    1167, 1168f
Coronary blood flow reserve. See
    Coronary reserve.
Coronary care unit (CCU), for myocardial
    infarction, 1256-1258, 1258t
Coronary hyperemia
  exercise stress-induced, 363-364
  pharmacological stress-induced,
    364-367, 365f
    dobutamine for, 366-367
    heterogeneity of, 365
    vasodilators for, 364-366, 365f, 366t
Coronary lumen, computed tomography
    of, 426-429, 426f-429f, 427t

Coronary reserve
  absolute, 1178-1179, 1180f
  in coronary stenosis, 363, 363f
  definition of, 362, 1168
  fractional, 1179f, 1180f, 1181
  measurement of, 1178-1182, 1179f-1181f
  microcirculatory, pathophysiological
    states affecting, 1182-1183,
    1182f-1184f
  perfusion tracers and, 362-363, 362f
  positron emission tomography of, 363
  relative, 1179-1181, 1180f
  single photon emission computed
    tomography of, 363, 364f
  stenosis pressure-flow relationships
    and, 1178, 1179f, 1181, 1181f
Coronary resistance vessels
  in coronary blood flow regulation,
    1171-1174, 1172f-1174f
  flow-mediated regulation of, 1174, 1174f
  myogenic regulation of, 1173-1174,
    1174f
  neural control of, 1175, 1176f
  structure and function of, 1172-1173,
    1172f, 1173f
Coronary segments, classification system
    for, 472-473, 473t
Coronary sinus atrial septal defect, 1577,
    1578f-1579f
Coronary steal, 365
Coronary stents. See Stent(s), coronary.
Coronary thrombolysis. See
    Thrombolysis; Thrombolytic therapy.
Coronary tone, endothelium-dependent
    modulation of, 1168, 1170-1171, 1170t
Coronary vascular resistance,
    determinants of, 1171-1177,
    1171f-1174f
Coronary vasculitis, in coronary artery
    disease, 1400
Coronary vasodilator reserve, in
    hypertrophied hypertensive heart,
    1034
Corrigan (water-hammer) pulse, 133,
    1638
Corticosteroids
  in amiodarone-induced
    hyperthyroidism, 2044
  cardiotoxicity of, 297
  in chronic obstructive pulmonary
    disease, 1908
  in Churg-Strauss syndrome, 2093
  in constrictive pericarditis, 1846
  for contrast reaction prophylaxis, 472
  dyslipidemia and, 1082
  in giant cell arteritis, 2090
  in HIV-infected patients, complications
    of, 1803t
  in idiopathic aortitis, 2091
  in rheumatic fever, 2085-2086
  in sarcoidosis, 2101
  in systemic lupus erythematosus, 2098
  in Takayasu arteritis, 2089
  in tuberculous pericarditis, 1848
Cortisol
  actions of, 2035
  in Addison disease, 2037
  in Cushing syndrome, 2035-2036
Corynebacterium, in infective
    endocarditis, 1717, 1727
CoStar stent, 1436
Cost-effectiveness analysis. See Economic
    analysis.
Cost-effectiveness ratio, definition of, 35
Costochondritis, chest pain in, 1197
Costosternal syndrome, chest pain in,
    1354

I-28 Cough, nocturnal, in heart failure, 561
Cough-version, 958
Coumadin. *See* Warfarin.
Counseling
  after myocardial infarction, 1286
  in stable angina, 1366-1367
Coxiella burnetii, in infective
    endocarditis, 1717, 1727
Coxsackie adenoviral receptor, in
    myocarditis, 1777, 1782, 1783f
Coxsackie virus infection, myocarditis in,
    1776-1777, 1777f, 1781-1782, 1783f
Cozaar. *See* Losartan (Cozaar).
CPR. *See* Cardiopulmonary resuscitation
    (CPR).
Crackles, in heart failure, 593
Cranial artery, biopsy of, in giant cell
    arteritis, 2090
Cre transgene, 79
C-reactive protein (hs-CRP)
  in cardiovascular disease risk
      assessment, 1124, 1141
  dietary influences on, 1114f, 1115
  fibrinogen level and, 1018, 1018f
  in heart failure, 595
  in hypertension, 1032-1033
  as inflammatory marker of
      atherosclerosis, 1013-1017, 1013f-
      1016f, 1020
  in metabolic syndrome, 1009, 1010f,
      1015
  in preoperative risk analysis, 1994
  in rheumatic fever, 2084
  in stable angina, 1356-1357
  statin therapy and, 1015, 1016f
  in UA/NSTEMI, 1325
Creatine clearance
  in elderly persons, 1927-1928, 1927t
  for renal function assessment, 2155
Creatine kinase
  in heart failure, 593
  in hypothyroidism, 2042
  in myocardial infarction, 1224, 1225f,
      1226t
  in myocarditis, 1785-1786
Creatine kinase isoenzymes, in
    myocardial infarction, 1224-1225,
    1225f, 1226t
Creatine kinase isoforms, in myocardial
    infarction, 1225, 1225f, 1226t
Creatine kinase MB isoenzyme (CK-MB)
  diagnostic performance of, 1198-1199,
      1198t, 1199t
  interpretation of tests for, 1199, 1200f
  in myocardial infarction, 1224-1225,
      1225f, 1226t
  prognostic implications of, 1198t, 1199,
      1199t
  single, test performance of, 1199
  testing strategy for, 1199-1200, 1201t
  troponin versus, 1227
  in UA/NSTEMI, 1325
Creep, definition of, 570t
CREST syndrome, 1901, 2099-2100
Crestor. *See* Rosuvastatin (Crestor).
Cribier-Edwards valve, 1445-1446, 1445f
Critically ill and injured patients,
    echocardiography in, 322t-323t, 324
Cross-bridge cycling, 511, 511f
  binding states in, 511-512, 515f
  versus contraction-relaxation cycle, 514,
      515f
  cytosolic calcium in, graded effects of,
      513
  titin in, length sensing and, 511, 514f
Cross-bridge detachment, diastolic
    relaxation and, 649

Cryoablation
  in arrhythmias, 804
  in ventricular tachycardia, 820f, 821
C-statistic, 1021-1022
CT. *See* Computed tomography.
CTG repeat expansion, in myotonic
    muscular dystrophy, 2137, 2139f
Cushing disease and syndrome
  cardiovascular manifestations of,
      2035-2036
  hypertension in, 1042-1043
Cutis laxa, cardiovascular manifestations
    of, 90t
Cyanide metabolite, of nitroprusside, 602
Cyanosis
  in cardiovascular disease, pregnancy
      and, 1970-1971, 1971t
  central, 127, 1567, 1567t
  in congenital heart disease, 1567-1568,
      1567t, 1568t, 1587-1605
    clinical features of, 1567
    follow-up in, 1568
    interventional options and outcomes
        in, 1567-1568, 1568t
    management of, 1567-1568, 1568t
    pathophysiology of, 1567
    reproductive issues in, 1568
  differential, 127
    in Eisenmenger syndrome, 1569
    in Fontan patients, 1595, 1596
    in persistent truncus arteriosus, 1587
    in pulmonary hypertension, 1887
    shunt vascularity in, 1573
Cyclic adenosine monophosphate (cAMP)
  compartmentalization of, 523
  production of, 522
  protein kinase dependence on, 522-523,
      522f
Cyclic guanosine monophosphate (cGMP)
  compartmentalization of, 524-525
  in contraction-relaxation cycle, 522,
      524, 525, 525f
Cyclin(s), 68, 69f
Cyclin-dependent kinase(s) (CDKs), 68, 69f
Cyclin-dependent kinase (CDK)
    inhibitors, 69, 69f
Cyclooxygenase inhibitors, 2068-2069,
    2070f, 2071f
Cyclophosphamide
  cardiotoxicity of, 297, 2110-2111
  in Churg-Strauss syndrome, 2093
  in scleroderma, 2100
  in Takayasu arteritis, 2089
  in thromboangiitis obliterans, 1506
Cyclosporine, in heart transplantation,
    678
CYP enzyme systems
  in drug metabolism and elimination,
      60, 61t, 65t
  in elderly persons, 1928, 1929
CYPHER sirolimus-eluting stent, 1430-
    1431, 1435f
Cyst(s)
  computed tomography of, 429
  hydatid, myocarditis in, 1780
  pericardial, 1852
    computed tomography in, 422, 422f
    echocardiography in, 289, 291f
    magnetic resonance imaging in, 405
Cystatin C test, for renal function
    assessment, 2155-2156
Cystic fibrosis, pulmonary hypertension
    in, 1909
Cystic medial degeneration
  in aortic dissection, 1470-1471, 1470f
  in thoracic aortic aneurysms, 1464-
      1465, 1464f

Cytokines
  in contraction-relaxation cycle,
      526
  in dilated cardiomyopathy, 1746-1747
  in heart failure, 558-559
  in HIV-infected patients, 1795
  in metabolic traumatic heart disease,
      1857
Cytoplasm, 510
Cytoskeletal proteins, in heart failure,
    552
Cytosol, 510

D
Daily living activities, in preoperative
    risk assessment for noncardiac
    surgery, 2017, 2017t
Dallas criteria
  for cardiomyopathy, 1746
  for myocarditis, 1775, 1776f, 1787
Dalteparin, in pulmonary embolism, 1873,
    1873t
Danon disease, genetic studies in, 114
Danshen *(Salvia miltiorhiza),* 1159t
Darbopoetin-alpha, in chronic kidney
    disease, 2157-2158
Dasatinib, cardiotoxicity of, 2114
DASH diet, blood pressure and, 1113-1114,
    1114f
Daunorubicin (Cerubidine),
    cardiovascular effects of, 297,
    2108-2110
D-dimers, 2054
  in aortic dissection, 1474
  in heart failure, 595
  in pulmonary embolism, 1868
De Musset sign, in aortic regurgitation,
    1638
Death
  during arteriography, 467
  biological
    definition of, 933, 934t
    progression from cardiac arrest to,
        953
  care during last hours prior to, 723,
      723f. *See also* End-stage heart
      disease.
  preventable causes of, 1028f
  site of, 717-718
  sudden. *See also* Sudden cardiac
      death.
    noncardiac causes of, 948
    temporal definition of, 933, 934
  voodoo, 946
"Death rattle," in end-stage heart disease,
    723
Deceleration-dependent block, 172, 173f,
    751
Decision analysis, 44
Decision-making, 41-47
  diagnostic, 41-43
  diagnostic test, 42-43
  information technology/systems in, 47
  shared, 45-46
  therapeutic, 43-47
    adoption of innovation in, 47
    cognitive errors in, 46
    evidence in
      accuracy of, 46-47
      interpretation of, 44-46
Decompression sickness, patent foramen
    ovale and, 1580
Deductive inference, 41
Deep vein thrombosis. *See* Venous
    thrombosis.
Defecation syncope, 977
Defibrillation threshold testing, 849

Defibrillation-cardioversion, in cardiac arrest
  definitive, 961-962, 962f
  early, 956-957, 957f, 958f, 960, 960f
Defibrillator(s)
  external, automatic
    deployment strategies for, 956f, 960, 960f
    for ventricular fibrillation, 909
  implantable. See Cardioverter-defibrillator, implantable.
Degenerative and man-made disease age
  cardiovascular disease in, 3t, 4
  in United States, 7
Delayed degenerative disease age
  cardiovascular disease in, 3t, 4
  in United States, 8-9, 8t
Deletion, nucleotide, 75, 75f
Delirium, in hospitalized cardiac patient, 2126-2127
Demand angina, 1355, 1356f
Dementia, hypertension and, 1037
Demographic transition, cardiovascular disease and, 5
Dental procedures, endocarditis prophylaxis for, 1731, 1731t
Deoxyribonucleic acid. See DNA.
Depolarization
  diastolic, 744
    in deceleration-dependent block, 751
  early rapid, 742-743, 743f
  final rapid, 744
  rapid, 739-740, 739f, 740f, 742
Depression
  from cardiac drugs, 2132
  cardiovascular disease and, 1012, 1140-1141, 2119-2120
  in convalescence and recovery phase, 2127
  heart failure and, 591, 2124
  postinfarction, 1290, 2120, 2127
  postoperative, 2007-2008
  stable angina and, 1366-1367
  sudden cardiac death and, 2123
Dermatan sulfate, 2065
Dermatomyositis, 2100-2101
Desethylamiodarone, 794
Desflurane, for noncardiac surgery, 2020
Desipramine, cardiovascular aspects of, 2129t
Desirudin. See Hirudin (Desirudin).
Desmin-related myopathies, 2148-2149
Desmopressin acetate (DDAVP), perioperative use of, 2005
Desmosome protein, mutations of, in arrhythmogenic right ventricular cardiomyopathy, 117, 117t
Deterministic reasoning, in decision-making, 41
Device therapy, in heart failure, 618t, 628, 636, 636f, 637f
Dexrazoxane (Zinecard), in anthracycline cardiotoxicity, 2110
Dextran, in infective endocarditis, 1719
Dextroamphetamine, cardiovascular aspects of, 2130
Diabetes insipidus, after coronary artery bypass graft surgery, 2009
Diabetes mellitus, 1547-1558
  adenosine diphosphate receptor antagonists in, 1550
  adipocyte biology in, 1096, 1096f
  alcohol intake and, 1807, 1807f
  aldosterone antagonists in, 1556-1557
  angiotensin II receptor blockers in, 1551-1552, 1556

Diabetes mellitus (Continued)
  angiotensin-converting enzyme inhibitors in, 1551, 1552, 1556
  antihypertensive drug therapy in, 1102-1103, 1102t
  antiplatelet drugs in, 1549, 1549t
  aspirin in, 1549-1550
  autonomic dysfunction in, 2176
  beta blockers in, 1060, 1551, 1556
  calcium channel blockers in, 1061
  cardiac surgery and, 1995
  cardiomyopathy in, 1555-1556, 1555t
  cardiovascular disease in, 1093-1103, 1547-1558
    comprehensive risk factor modification for, 1103, 1103f
    epidemiology of, 1093-1095, 1095f
    life style modification for, 1099
    medical therapy for, 1099-1103, 1101t, 1102t
    pathophysiology of, 1096-1099, 1096f-1098f
    risk assessment for, 1122-1123
    risk factor intervention for, 1134-1135
    risk factors for, 1009-1010
    scope of problem in, 1547-1548, 1548f
    treatment of, 1099-1103
  cerebrovascular disease in, epidemiology of, 1095
  coronary artery bypass graft surgery in patients with, 1391, 1394, 1552, 1553, 1558
  coronary artery disease in
    costs of, 1093
    epidemiology of, 1093-1095, 1095f
    myocardial perfusion imaging of, 378
    in women, 1957
  diagnostic criteria for, 1093, 1094t
  direct thrombin inhibitors in, 1550-1551
  dyslipidemia in, 1082, 1100-1102, 1101f, 1101t
  endothelial dysfunction in, 1097, 1097f
  exercise stress testing in, 215
  free fatty acids in, 1096-1097, 1097f
  glycoprotein IIb/IIIa inhibition in, 1550
  heart failure in, 1553-1557
    blood pressure control in, 1556
    factors related to, 1554-1556
    glycemic control in, 1556
    medical therapy in, 1556-1557
    with normal ejection fraction, 645-646
    overview of, 1553-1554
  heart transplantation and, 676
  hyperglycemia in, 1096, 1097, 1097f, 1099-1100, 1100t
  hypertension in
    pathology of, 1555-1556
    treatment of, 1102-1103, 1102t, 1556
  hypertriglyceridemia in, 1101, 1113
  inflammation in, 1096, 1096f
  insulin resistance in, 1097, 1097f, 1100-1101, 1101f. See also Metabolic syndrome.
  management of
    glycemic control in, 1552-1553, 1553f, 1554f, 1556
    hypertension therapy in, 1065
    in patients with cardiovascular disease, 1557-1558
    in peripheral arterial disease, 1501
  metabolic abnormalities in, 1096-1097, 1100, 1100t
  myocardial infarction in, 1548-1553
    epidemiology of, 1094-1095, 1095f
    intensive glycemic control in, 1552-1553, 1553f, 1554f

Diabetes mellitus (Continued)
  medical therapy in, 1549-1552
  prognosis after, 1548, 1549f
  remodeling after, 1555
  nephropathy in, 1039, 2155
  neuropathy in, 1558
  percutaneous coronary intervention in patients with, 1380, 1394
  peripheral arterial disease in, 1095, 1492, 1501
  prevalence of, 1093, 1094f, 1134
  prevention of, 1099
  quality of care indicators for, 53t
  racial/ethnic differences in, 23
  regional trends in, 18
  revascularization in, 1557-1558
    in stable angina, 1363-1364
  statin therapy in, 1086, 1090
  stroke in, 1095
  "thrifty gene" hypothesis in, 1093
  thrombolytic therapy in, mortality and, 1244
1,2-Diacylglycerol
  in contraction-relaxation cycle, 522
  in diabetes mellitus, 1097
Diagnostic decision-making, 41-43
Diagnostic tests
  authority of, unwavering acceptance of, 47
  economic analysis of, 39-40
  evaluation of, 42-43
  ordering of, assessment prior to, 43
Dialysis. See also End-stage renal disease.
  in heart failure, 628
  in hypertensive patient, 1039
  hypotension during, 2178-2179, 2180f
  pericarditis after, 1849
  prosthetic valves in, 1688
Diaphragmatic paralysis, pulmonary hypertension in, 1909-1910
Diastasis, 648
Diastole
  coronary blood flow during, 1167, 1168f
  definition of, 529
  force transmission during, 514
  phases of, 647-648, 648f
  physiologic versus cardiologic, 529, 529t
  ventricular suction during, 535
Diastolic blood pressure, in heart failure, 592
Diastolic depolarization, 744
  in deceleration-dependent block, 751
Diastolic dysfunction. See also Ventricle(s), diastolic function of.
  in aortic stenosis, 1628
  drug-induced, 1805-1806, 1810-1811
  grade 1 (mild), 250
  grade 2 (moderate), 250-251
  grade 3-4 (severe), 251, 252f
  grading of, 249, 250f
  in heart failure. See Heart failure, with normal ejection fraction.
  in HIV-infected patients, 1797
  in hypertrophic cardiomyopathy, 1767
  indices of, 535
  left ventricular hypertrophy and, 536-537
  in myocardial infarction, 1218
  thyroid disorders and, 2039, 2040f
  ventricular relaxation and, 534, 648-650, 649f, 651f
  ventricular stiffness and, 650-653, 652f

I-30 Diastolic filling pattern
echocardiography of, 248-249, 249f, 250f
grading of, 249, 250f
normal, 249-250, 250f, 251t
tissue Doppler echocardiography and, 286
Diastolic heart failure. See Heart failure, with normal ejection fraction.
Diastolic heart sounds, 136
Diastolic murmurs, 137-138, 1650
Diastolic stress test, 262
Diazepam (Valium), cardiovascular aspects of, 2132t
Dicrotic arterial pulse, 133, 133f
Diet(s)
cardiovascular disease and, 1107-1116
clinical trials of, 1109t, 1110-1111, 1110f
observational evidence on, 1107-1108, 1108f, 1110
for prevention, 1138, 1140
risk factors related to, 16, 16f, 1111-1116, 1111t, 1112f, 1114f, 1115t, 1138
DASH, blood pressure and, 1113-1114, 1114f
in dyslipidemia, 1089
in heart failure, 620
in hypertension therapy, 1052t, 1053, 1053f
lipid-lowering, 1089, 1112-1113, 1112f, 1131
low-carbohydrate, 1111-1112, 1111t
low-fat, 1110-1111, 1111t, 1112
low-sodium
in hypertension therapy, 1052t, 1053, 1053f
in mitral stenosis, 1652
in tricuspid stenosis, 1675
Mediterranean-style, 1110, 1110f
racial/ethnic differences in, 24
Dietary supplements
cardiac surgery and, 1164
drug/herbal interactions with, 1158, 1159t-1161t, 1163
for dyslipidemia, 1158, 1162
for heart failure, 1162
herbal versus synthetic drug comparison for, 1158, 1158t
for hypertension, 1158
for peripheral vascular disease and venous insufficiency, 1162
reference sources on, 1165t-1166t
Diethylenetriaminepentaacetic acid, technetium-99m–labeled, 358
DiGeorge syndrome, 1571, 1587
Digit infarct, in infective endocarditis, 1720, 1720f
Digital imaging, in cardiac catheterization, 440-441
Digital radiography, 329
Digital subtraction angiography, in carotid artery stenosis, 1538, 1539f
Digoxin (digitalis)
in aortic regurgitation, 1642
in arrhythmias, 800-801
in atrial fibrillation, 873
in atrial flutter, 875
in atrioventricular nodal reentrant tachycardia, 881
in cardiac arrest prevention, 965
in chronic kidney disease patients, 2165t
complications of, 634
dosage and administration of, 784t, 800
drug interactions of, 2132

Digoxin (digitalis) (Continued)
electrophysiological characteristics of, 183-184, 184f, 780t, 781t, 782t, 786t, 800
in heart failure
with normal ejection fraction, 654, 655f
systolic, 618t, 624t, 630t, 633-634
in hyperthyroidism with atrial fibrillation, 2041
in idiopathic pulmonary arterial hypertension, 1896
indications for, 800
in mitral stenosis, 1652, 1653
in myocardial infarction, 1268
pharmacokinetics of, 60, 784t, 800
in pregnancy, 1976t, 1977
psychiatric side effects of, 2132
toxicity of, 800-801
in Wolff-Parkinson-White syndrome, 891-892
Dihydroxyphenylserine, in autonomic failure, 2176
Dilantin. See Phenytoin (Dilantin).
Dilated cardiomyopathy. See Cardiomyopathy, dilated.
Diltiazem
adverse effects of, 799
in aortic dissection, 1479
in arrhythmias, 798-799
in atrial flutter, 875
dosage and administration of, 784t, 798
drug interactions of, 1376
electrophysiological characteristics of, 780t, 781t, 782t, 786t, 798
in fascicular ventricular tachycardia, 907
hemodynamic effects of, 798
indications for, 798-799
in myocardial infarction, 1263
pharmacokinetics of, 784t, 798, 1374t
in stable angina, 1375-1376
in UA/NSTEMI, 1327
in Wolff-Parkinson-White syndrome, 892
Dilute Russell viper venom test, in antiphospholipid antibody syndrome, 2061
Diphenhydramine, for contrast reaction prophylaxis, 472
Diphtheria, myocarditis in, 1778
Diploid set, 68
Dipole model, in electrocardiography, 150, 150f, 151
Dipyridamole
in coronary blood flow regulation, 1177
as platelet inhibitor, 2073
for stress myocardial perfusion imaging, 364-366, 365f, 366t
in stroke prevention, 1515
Direct thrombin inhibitors, 2066-2067
advantages of, 2067
in atrial fibrillation, 872
in diabetes mellitus, 1550-1551
mechanism of action of, 2066f, 2067
in percutaneous coronary intervention, 1437
in UA/NSTEMI, 1332-1333
Direct-current electrical cardioversion. See Cardioversion.
Disability, cardiovascular, assessment of, 126, 126t
Disease management programs for heart failure, cost-effectiveness analysis of, 38-39
Disease prevention, economic analysis of, 39, 39t

Disease-modifying antirheumatic drugs (DMARDs), 2095
Disopyramide
adverse effects of, 788
in arrhythmias, 787-788
in chronic kidney disease patients, 2165t
dosage and administration of, 783t, 788
electrophysiological characteristics of, 780t, 781t, 782t, 786t, 788
hemodynamic effects of, 788
in hypertrophic cardiomyopathy, 1771
indications for, 788
pharmacokinetics of, 783t, 788
Distal embolic protection devices, in percutaneous coronary intervention, 1308, 1426, 1427f, 1428f, 1429f
Distal embolization, after myocardial infarction, 1308
Distichiasis, lymphedema associated with, 97
Distribution, drug, 59-60
volume of, 58, 59f
Diuretics
in aortic stenosis, 1633
braking phenomenon with, 625f, 626
in cardiac arrest prevention, 965
classes of, 620, 621t
clinical effects of, 1057
complications of, 625-626
contraindications to, 1055t
distal collecting tubule, in heart failure, 600, 627
dosage and choice of agent for, 1057
exercise stress testing and, 213
in heart failure, 618t, 620-628, 621f, 621t, 623f-625f
acute, 596, 600, 601t
systolic, 618t, 620-628, 621f, 621t, 623f-625f
in hypertension, 1057-1058, 1057t, 1058f
in hypertensive crises, 1066, 1066t
in hypertrophic cardiomyopathy, 1771
in idiopathic pulmonary arterial hypertension, 1896-1897
indications for, 1055t
loop, 1057t, 1058
dose-response curves for, 626, 627f
in heart failure, 600, 601t, 620, 621t, 622, 625
mechanisms of action of, 622
low-dose, benefits of, 1006
mechanisms of action of, 1057
in mitral stenosis, 1652
in myocardial infarction, 1267-1268
in myocarditis, 1788
overview of, 1058
polymorphisms associated with, 61-62, 62t
potassium-sparing, 1057t, 1058
in heart failure, 621t, 623
in pregnancy, 1977
psychiatric side effects of, 2132
renal site of action of, 621f
resistance to, 625f, 626-628, 627f
side effects of, 1057-1058, 1058f
in stroke prevention, 1518-1519
thiazide, 1057, 1057t
dyslipidemia and, 1082
in elderly persons, 1931, 1932
in heart failure, 621t, 622
mechanisms of action of, 622
thiazide-like, 622
in tricuspid stenosis, 1675
Diving reflex, 2172, 2173f

DNA
  amplification of, with polymerase chain reaction, 74, 74f
  recombinant, 72-74, 73f, 74f
  sequencing of, human genome project and, 86-87
  structure of, 70-71, 70f, 72f
DNA microarrays, in molecular genetics, 76-77, 77f
DNA polymorphisms. See Polymorphisms.
Do Not Resuscitate (DNR) order, 722
Dobutamine
  in acute heart failure, 601t, 603-604
  in acute mitral regurgitation, 1669
  in cardiac arrest, 963
  during cardiac catheterization, 460
  in magnetic resonance imaging, 397, 398f
  in myocardial infarction, 1266, 1268-1269
  in myocardial viability assessment, 261-262
  postoperative, 2000
  in stress echocardiography, 259, 260, 260f, 261
  in stress myocardial perfusion imaging, 366-367, 377
Docetaxel (Taxotere), cardiotoxicity of, 2110
Docosahexaenoic acid (DHA), 1108, 1110
Dofetilide
  in arrhythmias, 780t, 781t, 782t, 784t, 786t, 796
  in atrial fibrillation, 873
  in chronic kidney disease patients, 2165t
Dong quai (Angelica sinensis), 1159t
Dopamine
  in acromegaly, 2035
  in acute heart failure, 601t, 604
  in cardiac arrest, 963
  in myocardial infarction, 1268-1269
  postoperative use of, 2000
Dopamine beta-hydroxylase deficiency, autonomic dysfunction in, 2176
Doppler echocardiography. See Echocardiography, Doppler.
Doppler effect, 236, 237f
Doppler equation, 236
Doppler shift, 236-237, 237f
Doppler ultrasound, in peripheral arterial disease, 1498
Dor procedure, 673, 673f
Dose of physical activity, definition of, 1983
Dose-reponse curves, 1054-1055, 1055f
Double-switch procedure, in transposition of the great arteries, 1603
Down syndrome, 132, 1571, 1582
Doxazosin (Cardura), in hypertension, 1059-1060
Doxorubicin (Adriamycin)
  cardiotoxicity of, 297, 2108-2110, 2110f
    with paclitaxel, 2110
Doxycycline, in abdominal aortic aneurysms, 1459
Dressler syndrome, 1284, 1849-1850
Driving risk, in patients with syncope, 982
Dronedarone, 794
Drotrecogin alfa, 2067
Drug(s). See also specific drug or drug group.
  abuse of, infective endocarditis in, 1678, 1714-1715, 1714t

Drug(s) (Continued)
  bioavailability of, 59
  clearance of, 59, 60, 61t
  distribution of, 59-60
    volume of, 58, 59f
  dose-reponse curves for, 1054-1055, 1055f
  electrocardiographic abnormalities caused by, 183-184, 184f
  elimination half-life of, 58, 59, 59f
  excretion of, 60, 61t
  exercise stress testing effects of, 213-214, 213f
  hypertension from, 1038
  hypotensive effects of, 976, 976t
  lethal arrhythmias from, 964
  metabolism of, 60, 61t
  molecular targets of, 57-58, 58f
  myocarditis from, 1780-1781
  pericarditis from, 1851
  route of administration of, 58-59, 59f
  steady-state effects of, 59, 59f
  synthetic, herbal versus, 1158, 1158t
  teratogenicity of, 1563
  valvular heart disease from, 277, 277f
Drug therapy, 57-66
  dosage optimization principles in, 62-64, 63f
  dose adjustments in, 59, 64
  drug-drug interactions in, 64, 65t
  drug/herbal interactions, 1158, 1159t-1161t, 1163
  for elderly persons, 1926-1931, 1927t, 1928t, 1929f, 1930t
    adherence to, 1930-1931
    adverse events in, 1928, 1929t
    dose adjustments in, 1926-1928, 1928t
    guidelines for, 1928t
    inappropriate prescribing in, 1930, 1930t
    Medicare D and, 1931
    pharmacodynamic interactions in, 1929-1930
    pharmacokinetic interactions in, 1929
  future prospects in, 64, 66
  pharmacodynamic variability in, 58, 58f, 60-62, 62t
  pharmacogenetic variability in, 58, 58f, 60-62, 61t, 62t
  pharmacokinetic variability in, 58-60, 59f, 61t
  plasma concentration monitoring in, 63
  polypharmacy in, 64, 1928, 1929f
  risk versus benefit in, 57
  therapeutic ratio in, 63, 63f
  variability in drug action in, 57-58, 58f
Drug-eluting stent. See Stent(s), drug-eluting.
Dual-chamber pacing, in hypertrophic cardiomyopathy, 1772
Dual-site atrial pacemaker, 833, 834f
Duchenne muscular dystrophy, 2135-2137
  arrhythmias in, 2136-2137
  cardiomyopathy in, 2136, 2138f
  cardiovascular manifestations of, 2135-2137, 2137f, 2138f
  clinical presentation in, 2135, 2136f
  dilated cardiomyopathy in, 117
  electrocardiography in, 2136, 2138f
  genetics of, 2135
  prognosis for, 2137
  treatment of, 2137
Ductus arteriosus, patent. See Patent ductus arteriosus.

Duke Activity Scale Index, in preoperative risk assessment for noncardiac surgery, 2017, 2017t
Duke criteria for infective endocarditis, 1718t, 1721
Duke treadmill score, prognostic value of, 208-209
Duloxetine, cardiovascular aspects of, 2129t, 2130
Dunnigan lipodystrophy, 1082
DuraHeart ventricular assist device, 692
Duroziez sign, in aortic regurgitation, 1638
Dynamic exercise, 197-198, 198f
  with cardiac catheterization, 459
Dyrenium. See Triamterene (Dyrenium).
Dysautonomias. See Autonomic dysfunction.
Dysgeusia, after cardiac surgery, 1998
Dyslipidemia, 1077-1082. See also Hypercholesterolemia; Hyperlipidemia; Hyperlipoproteinemia.
  approach to, 1088-1091
  atherogenic, 1113
  definitions of, 1077-1078
  in diabetes mellitus, 1100-1102, 1101f, 1101t
  diagnosis of, 1089, 1089t
  dietary influences on, 1112-1113, 1112f
  dietary supplements for, 1158, 1162
  drug-induced, 1082
  genetic factors in, 1078-1081, 1079t
  hormonal causes of, 1081-1082
  laboratory tests in, 1089, 1089t
  lifestyle and, 1082, 1089
  in liver disease, 1082
  metabolic causes of, 1082
  after myocardial revascularization, 1363
  peripheral arterial disease risk and, 1492
  physical examination in, 1089
  from protease inhibitors, 1801, 1802t
  racial/ethnic differences in, 24
  in renal disorders, 1082
  secondary causes of, 1081-1082, 1081t
  in stable angina, 1363
  target levels in, 1089
  treatment of, 1082-1091. See also Lipid-lowering therapy.
Dysmetabolic syndrome. See Metabolic syndrome.
Dysplasia, arrhythmogenic right ventricular. See Arrhythmogenic right ventricular dysplasia/cardiomyopathy.
Dyspnea
  assessment of, B-type natriuretic peptide in, 594f
  in cardiac tamponade, 1836
  differential diagnosis of, 126
  exertional
    in aortic stenosis, 1628-1629
    in heart failure, 561
    in mitral stenosis, 1649
  in heart failure, 140, 561, 563t, 590
  in pulmonary embolism, 1866
  in pulmonary hypertension, 1886
  in recumbent position. See Orthopnea.
Dystrophin
  in Duchenne and Becker muscular dystrophies, 2135
  in limb-girdle muscular dystrophy, 2144
  mutation of, in X-linked dilated cardiomyopathy, 117

East Asia, cardiovascular disease in, 10t, 12
Eastern Europe, cardiovascular disease in, 10t, 11-12, 19-20
Ebstein anomaly, 307f, 1604-1605, 1604f, 1605f, 1971
Echinococcus, myocarditis in, 1780
Echocardiography, 227-325
  in acute chest pain, 1203
  in acute pericarditis, 1833
  A-mode, 227, 228f
  in amyloidosis, 1752
  in aortic aneurysms, 299, 299f
  in aortic arch interruption, 1609
  in aortic atherosclerotic disease, 299-300, 300f
  in aortic disease, 299-302, 299f-302f, 320, 320t
  in aortic dissection, 300-301, 300f, 301f, 1476-1477, 1476f-1478f
  in aortic regurgitation, 270-272, 271f-272f, 1639-1640, 1640f, 1646
  in aortic rupture and pseudoaneurysm, 301
  in aortic sinus aneurysm and fistula, 1609
  in aortic stenosis, 267-269, 267f-269f, 1611, 1631
  in aortic ulcer, 301
  in aortitis, 301-302, 302f
  in apical ballooning syndrome, 258, 259f
  in arrhythmias, 321t, 322t, 324
  in arrhythmogenic right ventricular dysplasia, 288, 290f
  in atrial fibrillation, 304-306
  in atrial septal defect, 307-308, 308f-309f
  in atrioventricular septal defect, 1582
  in bicuspid aortic valve, 299, 299f
  in carcinoid heart disease, 296-297
  in cardiac amyloidosis, 295-296, 295f, 297f
  of cardiac manifestations of systemic illness, 295-298, 296t
  of cardiac structures, 229f-234f
  in cardiac tamponade, 289-290, 292f, 1838, 1838f-1840f
  in cardiac tumors and masses, 302-304, 302f-305f, 320, 320t, 1817, 1820f, 1821f
  in cardioembolic disease, 321t, 324
  in cardiomyopathy, 282-288, 283f-291f, 318-319, 319t
  in cardioversion, 305-306, 322t, 324
  for chamber quantitation, 243-247, 243t-245t
  in chest pain, 255, 317-318, 317t-318t
  in chronic obstructive pulmonary disease, 1907
  clinical competence in, 325
  in coarctation of the aorta, 310-311, 310f, 1606, 1606f, 1607
  in congenital absence of pericardium, 288
  in congenital heart disease, 306-311, 306f-310f, 323t-324t, 324
    in adult, 1575
    in fetus, 1573-1574, 1574f
    intracardiac, 1575
    in neonate and infant, 1574-1575
    in older child and adolescent, 1575, 1576f
    segmental approach to, 1574, 1574f

Echocardiography (Continued)
  in constrictive pericarditis, 290, 292-295, 293f-294f, 1843-1844, 1845, 1845t
  contrast
    using agitated saline, 242
    using microbubbles, 242-243, 242f, 243f, 245f
  in cor triatriatum, 1619
  in coronary arteriovenous fistula, 1620-1621
  in coronary artery disease, 253, 255-262, 256f-261f, 317-318, 317t-318t
  in critically ill and injured patients, 322t-323t, 324
  of diastolic function, 239, 242, 248-253, 249f, 250f, 251t
  in dilated cardiomyopathy, 282-284, 283f-284f, 1748
  dobutamine, in stable angina, 1358, 1358t, 1361
  Doppler
    in aortic regurgitation, 271-272, 271f-272f, 1640, 1640f
    in aortic stenosis, 1631
    of cardiac output, 264
    in cardiac tamponade, 290, 292f, 1838, 1840f
    in carotid artery stenosis, 1538
    in chronic obstructive pulmonary disease, 293-294, 294f, 1907
    color flow, 237-238, 238f
    in constrictive pericarditis, 290, 292-295, 293f-294f, 1843-1844
    continuity equation in, 264-265, 265f
    continuous wave, 236f, 237, 238f
    of diastolic function in heart failure with normal ejection fraction, 646, 647f
    of diastolic relaxation, 649
    in dilated cardiomyopathy, 283-284, 283f-284f
    in heart failure management, 600
    for hemodynamic assessment, 262-267, 263f
    in hypertrophic cardiomyopathy, 285-286, 286f
    of intracardiac pressures, 262-263, 263f
    of left ventricular diastolic stiffness, 653
    of left ventricular end-diastolic pressure, 263
    in mitral regurgitation, 272-274, 272f-275f, 1663
    in mitral stenosis, 1650-1651
    in myocardial infarction, 1229
    of pressure gradients, 262, 263f
    pressure half-time in, 265, 265f
    principles of, 236-237, 237f, 238f
    of prosthetic valves, 277-278, 278f, 279t
    of pulmonary artery pressures, 262-263, 263f
    in pulmonary hypertension, 1887
    in pulmonic regurgitation, 1679f, 1680
    pulsed wave, 236f, 237, 238f
    rate of left ventricular pressure change in, 266-267, 267f
    of regurgitant volume, fraction, and orifice area, 265-266, 266f
    of right ventricular function, 577, 578t
    of stroke volume, 263-264, 264f
  tissue, 238-242, 239f-241f, 239t-240t

Echocardiography (Continued)
    in hypertrophic cardiomyopathy, 286
    speckle tracking in, 239, 241f
    strain and strain rate in, 239-240, 240f, 240t
    in tricuspid regurgitation, 1677, 1677f
    of vascular resistance, 267
  in double-inlet ventricle, 1593, 1593f
  in double-outlet right ventricle, 1604
  in drug-induced cardiac disease, 297
  in Ebstein anomaly, 1605, 1605f
  in Eisenmenger syndrome, 1569
  fetal, 307, 1573-1574, 1574f, 1969
  in Fontan patients, 1595
  in heart failure, 253, 254f, 566, 566t, 595
  in hemochromatosis, 297-298
  in HIV-infected patients, 1793, 1796, 1797f
  in hypereosinophilic syndrome, 298, 298f
  in hypertension, 320, 321t, 324
  in hypertrophic cardiomyopathy, 284-287, 285f-287f, 1764, 1766f
  in hypoplastic left heart syndrome, 1591-1592, 1592f
  in infective endocarditis, 280-282, 280t, 282f, 1721-1722, 1734, 1735t, 1737t
  intraoperative, 324-325, 325t
  intravascular. See Ultrasonography, intravascular.
  of left atrial size and volume, 245, 245t, 247f
  of left ventricular dimensions, 243, 243t, 245, 246f
  of left ventricular mass, 244t, 245-246
  of left ventricular volume, 242, 242f, 246-247, 247f, 248f
  in Marfan syndrome, 299, 299f
  in mitral regurgitation, 272-275, 272f-275f, 1615, 1658f, 1663-1664
  in mitral stenosis, 269-270, 270f, 271t, 1614, 1647f, 1650-1651
  in mitral valve prolapse, 273, 274f, 1671-1672, 1671f
  M-mode, 227-228, 234f-235f
    anatomical, 228, 234f-235f
  in murmurs, 314-317, 315t-316t
  in myocardial infarction, 255-257, 257f-258f, 317-318, 317t-318t, 1229
  of myocardial viability, 243, 261-262
  in myocarditis, 1786
  in myotonic muscular dystrophy, 2139
  in myxoma, 1819, 1820f, 1821f
  in neurological disease, 321t, 324
  in nonbacterial thrombotic endocarditis, 281-282, 282f
  in noncompaction cardiomyopathy, 288, 291f
  in palpitations, 321t, 324
  in partial anomalous pulmonary venous drainage, 1620
  in patent ductus arteriosus, 309-310, 310f
  in pericardial cyst, 289, 291f
  in pericardial disease, 288-295, 291f-294f, 319, 319t
  in pericardial effusion, 289-290, 292f, 1838, 1838f-1840f
  in pericardiocentesis, 290
  practice guidelines for, 314-325, 315t-325t
  of prosthetic valves, 277-280, 278f, 279t, 280f
  in pulmonary arteriovenous fistula, 1620

Echocardiography (Continued)
in pulmonary artery stenosis, 1616
in pulmonary disease, 320, 321t
in pulmonary embolism, 1870, 1870t
in pulmonary hypertension, 1887
in pulmonary vein stenosis, 1619
in pulmonic regurgitation, 276-277, 277f, 1679f, 1680
in pulmonic stenosis, 270, 1617, 1618
in radiation-induced cardiac disease, 298
in renal failure, 298
in restrictive cardiomyopathy, 288, 288f, 289f, 1750-1751
in rheumatic fever, 2083
of right ventricular dimensions, 244t, 245, 247f
in right ventricular infarction, 258, 1271
in sarcoidosis, 298
for screening, 322t, 324
in sepsis, 298
in sinus of Valsalva aneurysm, 299, 299f
stress, 259-262
in acute chest pain, 1202, 1203
diagnostic accuracy of, 260-261
diagnostic criteria for, 259-260, 260f
exercise protocol for, 259, 260f
in mitral regurgitation, 1664
pharmacological, 259, 260f, 261
preoperative, for noncardiac surgery, 2018
as prognostic indicator, 261
in stable angina, 1358, 1358t
in women, 1958, 1960f
in subpulmonary right ventricular outflow tract obstruction, 1618
in supravalvular aortic stenosis, 1614
in syncope, 322t, 324, 979
in systemic lupus erythematosus, 298
of systolic function, 247-248
in tetralogy of Fallot, 1589, 1589f
three-dimensional, 227, 231f-233f, 235f
in congenital heart disease, 1575, 1577f
harmonic real-time, of left ventricular volume and mass, 246, 247
in total anomalous pulmonary venous drainage, 1597, 1598f
transducer locations in, 227, 228f-230f
transesophageal, 228, 236, 236f, 237f
in aortic dissection, 300-301, 301f, 1476-1477, 1476f-1478f
in aortic tumors, 1487, 1487f
in atrial fibrillation, 304-306
in congenital heart disease, 307, 1575
in infective endocarditis, 280-281
in mitral regurgitation, 274-275, 275f, 1663-1664
in noncardiac surgery, 2026
in pericardial disease, 295
in pregnancy, 1969
in transposition of the great arteries
complete, 1599f, 1600, 1600f
congenitally corrected, 1602, 1602f
transthoracic
in aortic dissection, 1476
in aortic regurgitation, 1639-1640
in congenital heart disease, 1573-1575, 1574f, 1576f
in pregnancy, 1969
transthoracic two-dimensional, 227, 230f
and color flow imaging, 235f
indications for, 139, 140f

Echocardiography (Continued)
of left ventricular volume, 246-247, 247f, 248f
in myocardial infarction, 1229
in thoracic aortic aneurysm, 1466
in traumatic heart disease, 1858, 1859
in tricuspid atresia, 1590
in tricuspid regurgitation, 275-276, 276f, 1676-1677, 1677f
in tricuspid stenosis, 270, 1675
in valvular heart disease, 267-280, 314-317, 315t-316t
guidelines for, 1693, 1694t
in vascular rings, 1610
in ventricular septal defect, 308-309, 309f-310f, 1584
of wall motion abnormalities, 255, 256f
Eclampsia, 1045, 1975, 1975t
Economic analysis, 35-40
of acute coronary syndrome treatments, 36-37
alternative use principle in, 35
of anticoagulation and antiplatelet therapy, 37
of cardiovascular disease prevention, 39, 39t, 1120
of coronary artery bypass graft, 37
of coronary stenting, 37-38
developments in, 40
of diagnostic testing, 39-40
of disease prevention, 39, 39t
of heart failure therapies, 38-39
of hypertension therapy, 1132
of implantable cardioverter-defibrillator, 38, 38t
law of diminishing returns in, 35, 36f
of lipid-lowering therapy, 39, 39t
medical cost measurement in, 35-36
of percutaneous coronary intervention, 37
of smoking cessation, 1128
societal perspective in, 35
of statin therapy, 1129
of thrombolytic agents, 36-37
Economic burden, in end-stage heart disease, 721
Economic development. See High-income countries; Low- and middle-income countries.
Economic transition, cardiovascular disease and, 1551
Ectopic atrial rhythms, 161
Ectopic junctional tachycardia, radiofrequency catheter ablation of, 808
Ectopic (latent or subsidiary) pacemaker, 746-747
Edema
in heart failure, 140, 142, 593
of lower extremity, in pulmonary hypertension, 1886
pulmonary. See Pulmonary edema.
in restrictive cardiomyopathy, 1750
Edifoligide, after coronary artery bypass graft surgery, 1385
Education, in cardiac rehabilitation, 1154
Edwards stentless valve, 1684f, 1686
Effective blood flow, in shunt quantification, 458-459
Efficacy/effectiveness, in risk-benefit analysis, 45
Efficiency of work, in myocardial oxygen uptake, 533
Ehlers-Danlos syndrome
cardiovascular manifestations of, 90t
genetic studies in, 90, 93, 93f

Eicosapentaenoic acid (EPA), dietary supplementation of, 1108, 1110
Einthoven's law, 152
Eisenmenger syndrome, 1569-1570
clinical manifestations of, 1569
definition of, 1569
follow-up in, 1570
interventions in, 1569-1570
laboratory studies in, 1569
natural history of, 1569
noncardiac surgery in patients with, 2015-2016
in persistent truncus arteriosus, 1587
pulmonary arterial hypertension in, 1900-1901
sudden cardiac death in, 944
Ejection fraction, left ventricular. See Left ventricular ejection fraction.
Ejection sounds, 135
Elastance, 570t. See also Stiffness.
Elastase, in idiopathic pulmonary arterial hypertension, 1893
Elastic arteries, 989f, 1883
Elasticity, definition of, 570t
Elderly persons
anticoagulant therapy in, 1941, 1941t
antithrombotic agents in, 1938
aortic elasticity in, 1457
aortic regurgitation in, 1948
aortic stenosis in, 1947-1948
aortic valve abnormalities in, 1947-1949, 1947t
arrhythmias in, 1946-1947, 1947t
atrial fibrillation in, 1946-1947, 1947t
atrioventricular block in, 1946
blood pressure in, 1050
cardiovascular disease in, 1923-1949
versus age-associated changes, 1927t
epidemiology of, 1923-1924, 1924f
future perspectives on, 1949
pathophysiology of, 1924-1926, 1925f, 1926f, 1927t
carotid artery disease in, 1940-1942, 1941t, 1942t
carotid sinus hypersensitivity in, 978
complementary and alternative medicine in, 1164
coronary artery bypass graft surgery in, 1390, 1936-1938, 1937f, 1937t
coronary artery disease in, 1934-1940
approach to, 1940t
clinical presentation in, 1934
diagnosis of, 1934
management of, 1934-1938, 1935t, 1937f, 1937t
prevalence and incidence of, 1934
diastolic function in, 250, 251t
dose adjustments in, 64
drug therapy for, 1926-1931, 1927t, 1928t, 1929f, 1930t
adherence to, 1930-1931
adverse events in, 1928, 1929t
dose adjustments in, 1926-1928, 1928t
guidelines for, 1928t
inappropriate prescribing in, 1930, 1930t
Medicare D and, 1931
pharmacodynamic interactions in, 1929-1930
pharmacokinetic interactions in, 1929
electrocardiography in, 1938, 1946
exercise stress testing in, 214-215
giant cell arteritis in, 2089-2090, 2090t
heart failure in, 1943-1945, 1944f, 1946t
with normal ejection fraction, 645
systolic, 635
hypertension in, 1931-1933

Elderly persons (*Continued*)
approach to, 1933t
prevalence and incidence of, 1931
treatment of, 1050-1051, 1065, 1065t, 1931-1933, 1932t, 1933t
lipid-lowering therapy in, 1090-1091, 1935-1936, 1935t
mitral annular calcification in, 1948
mitral regurgitation in, 1948
mitral stenosis in, 1948
myocardial infarction in, 1306-1307, 1938-1940
mortality and, 1208, 1208f
out-of-hospital cardiac arrest in, 953
percutaneous coronary intervention in, 1306-1307, 1936-1938, 1937f, 1937t, 1939
peripheral arterial disease in, 1942-1943, 1943t
preoperative risk analysis for, 1993
pulmonary circulation in, 1886
revascularization in, 1936-1938, 1937f, 1937t, 1938-1939
sinus node dysfunction in, 1946
stroke in, 1940-1942, 1941t, 1942t
sudden cardiac death in, 936, 937f
thrombolytic therapy in, 1938, 1940
mortality and, 1244, 1245f, 1246f
valvular heart disease in, 1947-1949, 1947t, 1948t
vascular disease in, 1931-1943
ventricular arrhythmias in, 1947
ventricular function in, 1943
Electrical alternans, in cardiac tamponade, 289-290, 292f
Electrical axis of heart, 154, 155f
Electrical cardioversion. *See* Cardioversion.
Electrical injuries, 1857
Electrical stimulation, programmed
in Brugada syndrome, 106
in cardiac arrest prevention, 966-967
in tachycardias, 774
Electrocardiogram
genesis of
during activation, 149-150, 150f
during recovery, 151
interpretation of, 155
normal, 155-160, 156f-161f
P wave on, 155, 156-157, 156f, 156t
PR segment on, 155, 156f, 156t, 157
QRS axis on, 158
QRS complex on, 155, 156f, 156t, 158-159, 158f
QRST angle on, 160
QT interval on, 159-161
ST segment on, 155, 156f, 156t
ST-T wave on, 156f, 159
T wave on, 155, 156f, 156t
U wave on, 159
ventricular gradient on, 160
Electrocardiographic imaging, 771
Electrocardiography, 149-193
in acceleration-dependent block, 172, 172f, 173f
in acromegaly, 2034
in acute cerebrovascular disease, 2149, 2150f, 2151f-2152f
in acute chest pain, 1197, 1201
in acute pericarditis, 181, 182f, 182t, 1832-1833, 1832f
in Addison disease, 2037
in alcoholic cardiomyopathy, 1745
alternans patterns in, 186-187, 186t, 187f, 770, 771f

Electrocardiography (*Continued*)
ambulatory
in arrhythmia diagnosis, 766-768, 769f
in cardiac arrest prevention, 966
clinical competence in, 825
practice guidelines for, 823-825, 824t-827t
in silent myocardial ischemia, 1396-1397
in syncope, 980
amplifiers for, 154-155
in amyloidosis, 1752
in aortic arch interruption, 1609
in aortic dissection, 1473-1474
in aortic regurgitation, 1640, 1646
in aortic sinus aneurysm and fistula, 1609
in aortic stenosis, 1611, 1631
in arrhythmia diagnosis, 764-771, 771
in atrial abnormalities, 160-162, 161f, 162f, 162t
in atrial infarction, 179
in atrial septal defect, 1579
in atrioventricular septal defect, 1582
in biventricular enlargement, 166-167, 167f
in cardiac arrest survivors, 954
after cardiac surgery, 1999
in cardiac tamponade, 1837, 1837f
in chronic obstructive pulmonary disease, 166, 166f
clinical competence in, 192
in coarctation of the aorta, 1606, 1607
in congenital heart disease, 1572
in constrictive pericarditis, 1843
in cor triatriatum, 1619
in coronary arteriovenous fistula, 1620
in Cushing syndrome, 2035
in deceleration-dependent block, 172, 173f
in dilated cardiomyopathy, 1748
dipole model in, 150, 150f, 151
display systems for, 155
in double-inlet ventricle, 1593
drug-induced changes in, 183-184, 184f
in Duchenne muscular dystrophy, 2136, 2138f
in Ebstein anomaly, 1605
in Eisenmenger syndrome, 1569
in elderly persons, 1938, 1946
electrodes for, 151, 151f
in Emery-Dreifuss muscular dystrophy and associated disorders, 2144
esophageal, in arrhythmia diagnosis, 772
event recording in, 768, 769f, 980-981
exercise. *See* Exercise stress testing.
in fascicular block, 167-168, 168f, 168t
in Fontan patients, 1595
frequency domain analysis in, 770
in Friedreich's ataxia, 2146, 2146f
in heart failure, 565, 565f, 595
heart rate turbulence in, 769
heart rate variability in, 769
heart vectors in, 152-154, 154f
hexaxial reference system in, 154, 155f
in HIV-infected patients, 1793
in hypercalcemia, 184, 185f
in hyperkalemia, 184, 185f
in hypermagnesemia, 185
in hyperparathyroidism, 2038
in hypertrophic cardiomyopathy, 181, 181f, 1768
in hypocalcemia, 184, 185f
in hypokalemia, 184, 185f
in hypomagnesemia, 185

Electrocardiography (*Continued*)
in hypoplastic left heart syndrome, 1591
in hypothermia, 185, 186f
in hypothyroidism, 2042
implantable event recording in, 980-981
implantable loop recording in, 768-769, 769f
indications for, 187-188
in infarct size estimation, 1230
interpretation of, clinical issues in, 187-189
in intraventricular conduction delays, 167-172, 168f, 168t, 169f, 169t, 171f-173f
knowledge of clinical context and prior ECG findings in, 188
Ladder diagram in, 764, 767f
leads for, 151-154, 151f, 152t
augmented limb, 152, 152t, 153f
bipolar versus unipolar, 152
precordial, 152, 152t, 153f
standard limb, 152, 152t, 153f
in vectorcardiogram, 152, 154f
vectors in, 152-154, 154f
in left anterior fascicular block, 167-168, 168f, 168t
in left atrial abnormalities, 161-162, 161f, 162t
in left bundle branch block, 168-170, 169f, 169t
in left posterior fascicular block, 168, 168f, 168t
in left septal fascicular block, 168
in left ventricular hypertrophy and enlargement, 162-165, 163f, 164f, 164t
in limb-girdle muscular dystrophy, 2144
long-term monitoring in, 766-770, 769f, 770f
in mitral regurgitation, 1615, 1664
in mitral stenosis, 167f, 1614, 1651
in mitral valve prolapse, 1672
in multifascicular blocks, 170-172, 171f
in myocardial infarction, 1227-1229, 1228f, 1230
in emergency department screening, 1234, 1235, 1235t, 1237t
for evaluating coronary blood flow, 1243
in right ventricular infarction, 1271, 1271f
for risk stratification, 1287-1288
in myocardial ischemia and infarction, 172-183
in myocarditis, 1786
in myotonic muscular dystrophy, 2138-2139, 2140f
in noninfarction Q waves, 180-181, 180t, 181f
normal variants in, 160, 160f, 161f
pacemaker abnormalities on, 844-845, 845f-847f
in partial anomalous pulmonary venous drainage, 1620
in pericardial effusion, 1837, 1837f
in pheochromocytoma, 2045
practice guidelines for, 190-193, 191t-193t
principles of, 149, 150f
in Prinzmetal angina, 176, 177f
in pulmonary artery stenosis, 1616
in pulmonary embolism, 166, 167f, 1867f, 1868, 1868t
in pulmonary hypertension, 1887
in pulmonic regurgitation, 1680

Electrocardiography (Continued)
in pulmonic stenosis, 1617, 1618, 1619
reading errors in, 188-189
resting, in stable angina, 1357
in restrictive cardiomyopathy, 1750
in rheumatic fever, 2084
in right atrial abnormalities, 161f, 162, 162t
in right bundle branch block, 169f, 169t, 170
in right ventricular hypertrophy, 165-166, 165f-167f, 165t
sampling rate in, 155
for self-assessment, 189
signal-averaged, 769-770, 770f, 980
solid angle theorem in, 150-151
in subarachnoid hemorrhage, 2149, 2150f, 2151f-2152f
in subpulmonary right ventricular outflow tract obstruction, 1618
in supravalvular aortic stenosis, 1614
in syncope, 774, 980-981
T wave alternans in, 770, 771f
technical errors and artifacts in, 188, 188f
in tetralogy of Fallot, 1589
time domain analysis in, 770
in total anomalous pulmonary venous drainage, 1597
transmission factors in, 151
in transposition of the great arteries
complete, 1600
congenitally corrected, 1602
in traumatic heart disease, 1859
in tricuspid atresia, 1590
in tricuspid regurgitation, 1677
in tricuspid stenosis, 1675
in UA/NSTEMI, 1322, 1322f, 1325
in vascular rings, 1610
in ventricular hypertrophy and enlargement, 162-167, 163f-167f, 164t, 165t
in ventricular septal defect, 1584
wave fronts in, 150
waveforms and intervals in, 155-160, 156f-161f, 156t. See also specific waveform, e.g., P wave.
Electrocautery, electromagnetic interference from, 850
Electrodes, for electrocardiography, 151, 151f
Electrolyte disturbances
after cardiac surgery, 1999
electrocardiography in, 184-185, 184f-186f
in heart failure, 564, 593
pacemaker abnormalities caused by, 851
Electromagnetic interference, 849-851, 850f
Electron microscopy, in myocardial infarction, 1212, 1213f
Electronic implant, in cardiovascular magnetic resonance, 394
Electronic surveillance equipment, electromagnetic interference from, 850
Electrophysiology
in amyloidosis, 1752
of antiarrhythmic agents, 782t, 786t
in arrhythmias, 772-777, 773f-777f
in atrioventricular block, 772-773
of cardiac action potential. See Action potential.
cardiac mapping in, 776-777, 776f, 777f
clinical competence in, 828, 830
complications of, 776

Electrophysiology (Continued)
diagnostic, practice guidelines for, 825-828, 826t-828t
in intraventricular conduction disturbance, 773, 773f
in myotonic muscular dystrophy, 2139
in palpitations, 775-776
practice guidelines for, 825-830, 826t-830t
principles of, 733-746
in sinus node dysfunction, 773-774, 774f
in sudden cardiac death, 941t-942t, 944-946, 966-967
in syncope, 774-775, 981
in tachycardia, 774, 775f
therapeutic, practice guidelines for, 828-830, 829t-830t
in ventricular tachycardia, 821
Electrotherapy, for arrhythmias, 801-819
Elephant trunk technique, in thoracic aortic aneurysms, 1468
Elfin facies, in supravalvular aortic stenosis, 1613, 1613f
Elimination half-life, 58, 59, 59f
in elderly persons, 1928
Ellence. See Epirubicin (Ellence).
Ellis-van Creveld syndrome, 1571
Embolectomy, in pulmonary embolism
catheter, 1877, 1877f
surgical, 1877, 1878f
Embolic protection devices
in carotid artery interventions, 1539
in percutaneous coronary intervention, 1308, 1425-1426, 1427f-1429f
Embolic stroke, in infective endocarditis, 1721
Embolism
air, 468, 1868
amniotic fluid, 1868
atherogenic, in peripheral arterial disease, 1509-1511, 1510f
in atrial fibrillation, 870-872
prevention of, 926t-927t, 930
after cardioversion, 802-803
coronary artery, sudden cardiac death and, 942
fat, 1868
in infective endocarditis, 1720, 1721, 1729
in mitral stenosis, 1649, 1652
after myocardial infarction, 1285-1286
paradoxical, 1867-1868
pulmonary. See Pulmonary embolism.
saddle, 1486, 1864, 1865f
after ventricular assist device implantation, 693
Embolization
of cardiac myxoma, 1816
of cardiac tumors, 1816
cholesterol, in percutaneous coronary intervention, 2158-2159
Embryogenesis of cardiovascular system, 1563-1564
Embryonic stem cell–derived myocardial cells, 697
Embryonic stem cells, 697
Emergency department
cardiac trauma assessment in, 1858
exercise stress testing in, 209-210, 1202, 1203t
myocardial infarction management in, 1234-1239, 1235t, 1237t, 1239f
thoracotomy indications in, 1858

Emergency medical services
in myocardial infarction management, 1233-1234, 1235t, 1236f
for out-of-hospital cardiac arrest, 955-957, 956f-958f
Emerin, deficiency of, in Emery-Dreifuss muscular dystrophy and associated disorders, 2143
Emery-Dreifuss muscular dystrophy and associated disorders, 2142-2144, 2143f
cardiovascular manifestations of, 2143f, 2144
clinical presentation in, 2143-2144, 2143f
genetics of, 2142-2143
prognosis for, 2144
treatment of, 2144
Emetine, cardiotoxicity of, 297
Emotional state
in myocardial infarction, 1221
in sudden cardiac death, 939
Emotional stress
left ventricular dysfunction from, 617
sudden cardiac death and, 946
Emotional support, in pulmonary embolism, 1877
Emotions, negative, sudden, cardiovascular effects of, 2122
Emphysema, 166, 166f, 1905. See also Chronic obstructive pulmonary disease.
Enalapril (Vasotec)
in chronic kidney disease patients, 2165t
in heart failure, 4, 624t, 628
Enalaprilat, in aortic dissection, 1479
Encephalopathy
anoxic, after cardiac arrest, 964
in HIV-infected patients, 1793
hypertensive, 1045-1046
postoperative, 2007
Encircling endocardial ventriculotomy, in ventricular tachycardia, 820-821, 820f
Endarterectomy
carotid, 1538-1539, 1539t, 1941
in chronic pulmonary hypertension, 1878
in thromboembolic pulmonary hypertension, 1910
End-diastolic pressure-volume relationship (EDPVR), 651-652, 652f
End-diastolic volume, 455, 572
Endocardial cushion defect. See Atrioventricular septal defect.
Endocarditis
cocaine and, 1811
infective. See Infective endocarditis.
Libman-Sacks, in systemic lupus erythematosus, 2098, 2098f
Löffler, 1756-1757
nonbacterial thrombotic
in cancer patients, 2108
in HIV-infected patients, 1794t, 1799
sudden cardiac death in, 944
Endocrine system
disorders of
cardiovascular disease and, 2033-2046
hypertension in, 1043
postoperative, 2009
in myocardial infarction, 1219-1220
Endoleaks, after abdominal aortic aneurysm repair, 1462-1463
Endomyocardial biopsy
in anthracycline cardiotoxicity, 2110
complications of, 448
in dilated cardiomyopathy, 1748-1749

Endomyocardial biopsy (Continued)
  in Friedreich's ataxia, 2146
  for graft rejection surveillance, 679
  indications for, 448, 1787
  in myocarditis, 1787
  in restrictive cardiomyopathy, 1750
  risks of, 1787
  techniques for, 448
Endomyocardial disease, 1756-1758
Endomyocardial fibroelastosis, 1758
Endomyocardial fibrosis
  biventricular, 1758
  left ventricular, 1757f, 1758
  versus Löffler endocarditis, 1757
  restrictive cardiomyopathy in, 1757-1758, 1757f
  right ventricular, 1757-1758, 1757f
Endoplasmic reticulum, 67-68, 68f
Endothelial cells
  arterial, 987, 987f
  in atherosclerotic plaque, neovascularization of, 994-995
  developmental biology of, 987
  progenitors of, 698, 987, 2049
Endothelial dysfunction
  in diabetes mellitus, 1097, 1097f, 1554-1555
  exercise effects on, 1151, 1151f
  in hypertension, 1032-1033, 1032f, 1033f
  in idiopathic pulmonary arterial hypertension, 1892-1893
  magnetic resonance imaging of, 400
  myocardial perfusion imaging in, 376
  in syndrome X, 1395
Endothelin(s)
  in coronary blood flow regulation, 1170-1171
  in heart failure, 547
  in pulmonary circulation, 1885
Endothelin receptor(s), 547
Endothelin receptor antagonists
  in Eisenmenger syndrome, 1570
  in heart failure, 547, 606
  in idiopathic pulmonary arterial hypertension, 1899
Endothelium
  in hemostasis, 2049-2050, 2050f
  vasoregulation by, 2050, 2050f
Endothelium-dependent hyperpolarizing factor (EDHF), 1170
Endothelium-dependent vasodilation
  in coronary blood flow regulation, 1168, 1170-1171, 1170t
  impaired, microcirculatory coronary reserve in, 1182-1183, 1183f, 1184f
  in thromboangiitis obliterans, 1505
Endothelium-derived hyperpolarizing factor, vasodilator properties of, 2050
Endothelium-derived relaxing factor. See Nitric oxide.
Endovascular interventions, extracardiac, 1523-1544. See also Percutaneous intervention; Stent(s); Stent-grafting.
End-stage heart disease, 717-724
  advance care planning in, 719-721, 720t
  automated implantable cardioverter-defibrillator in, 722
  care during last hours in, 723, 723f
  communication in, 718, 719t
  continuous goal assessment in, 719
  domains of illness experience in, 718
  epidemiology of, 717-718
  euthanasia and physician-assisted suicide in, 722-723
  existential or spiritual needs in, 721-722
  futile care concerns in, 722

End-stage heart disease (Continued)
  interventions in, 721-722
  life-sustaining treatment in
    patient's right to refuse or terminate, 720-721
    withdrawing and withholding, 722
  mechanical ventilation in, withdrawal of, 722
  outcome measures in, 724
  palliative care in, 718, 724
  physical and psychological symptoms in, 718, 721
  prognosis in, 718-719
  resuscitation preferences in, 722
  social needs in, 718, 721
  sudden death in, 723
  whole-person assessment in, 718
End-stage renal disease
  accelerated atherosclerosis in, 2162
  acute coronary syndromes in
    diagnosis of, 2162-2163
    outcomes of, 2163
    prognosis and, 2163, 2163f
    treatment of, 2163-2164, 2164t
  arrhythmias in, 2166
  consultative approach in, 2166-2168, 2167t, 2168f
  diabetic nephropathy in, 2155
  heart failure in, 2164-2166, 2165t, 2166f
  myocardial infarction in, 2162-2164, 2163f, 2164t
  valvular heart disease in, 2166
End-systolic elastance, 571f, 572, 572f
End-systolic pressure-volume relationship (ESPVR), 571, 571f, 572f
End-systolic stiffness, 572
End-systolic volume, 455, 571
  in mitral regurgitation, 1661
Endurance training, 1983
  in cardiovascular disease, 1153, 1154t
  definition of, 1150t, 1983
  exercise prescription for, 1986t
Energetics, in myocardial hibernation, 1190
Enhanced external counterpulsation, in stable angina, 1378-1379
Enoxaparin
  in myocardial infarction, 1252-1253, 1252f
  in percutaneous coronary intervention, 1437
  in preoperative risk analysis, 1995
  in pulmonary embolism, 1873, 1873t
  in UA/NSTEMI, 1331, 1332f
  versus unfractionated heparin, 2063
Enoximone, in acute heart failure, 601t, 604
Enterococci, in infective endocarditis, 1716-1717, 1724-1725, 1724t, 1725t
Enterovirus infection, myocarditis in, 1776-1777, 1777f
Entrainment, in reentry tachycardia, 751-752, 754f
Environmental factors, in congenital heart disease, 1563
Enzymes
  cardiac. See Cardiac enzymes.
  drug-metabolizing, 60, 61t
Eosinophils
  in endomyocardial disease, 1756
  in Löffler endocarditis, 1756
Ephedra, cardiac surgery and, 1164
Epicardial catheter mapping, in radiofrequency catheter ablation, 819

Epidemiological transitions
  concept of, 1-26
  parallel transformations accompanying, 5-6, 5f
  rate of change of, 4-5, 5f, 6
  stages of, 2, 3t, 4
  in United States, 6-9, 6t, 7f, 8t, 9f
  worldwide variations in, 2, 3f, 9-13, 10t
Epidermal growth factor receptor antagonists, cardiotoxicity of, 2114
Epidural anesthesia, for noncardiac surgery, 2021
Epilepsy, 2149
Epinephrine
  in acute heart failure, 601t, 604
  in cardiac arrest, 962-963
  in pheochromocytoma, 2045
  postoperative, 2001
Epirubicin (Ellence), cardiovascular effects of, 2108-2110
Eplerenone
  in heart failure, 38, 621t, 622-623, 623f, 624t, 633
  in hypertension, 1058
  in myocardial infarction, 1262, 1263f
Epoprostenol
  in congenital heart disease, 1901
  in idiopathic pulmonary arterial hypertension, 1898-1899, 1899f
  in pulmonary hypertension, 1889
Epsilon aminocaproic acid, for postoperative bleeding, 2005
Eptifibatide (Integrilin)
  in chronic kidney disease patients, 2164t
  in diabetes mellitus, 1550
  economic analysis of, 37
  in percutaneous coronary intervention, 1436
  as platelet inhibitor, 2073
  in UA/NSTEMI, 1329
Epworth Sleepiness Scale, 1919
Equilibrium potentials, 738, 738t
Erectile dysfunction
  from diuretics, 1058
  hypertension therapy in patients with, 1065
Ergometry, for exercise stress testing, 197, 198f
Ergonovine, coronary artery spasm from, 488
Ergonovine test, in Prinzmetal variant angina, 1338
Ergotamine, cardiovascular effects of, 277, 1812
ERK (extracellular signal–regulated kinase) pathway, in left ventricular response to mechanical stress, 536, 537f
Error reduction, and quality of cardiovascular care, 51-52
Erythema marginatum, in rheumatic fever, 2084
Erythrocyte sedimentation rate
  in infective endocarditis, 1722
  in myocardial infarction, 1227
  in rheumatic fever, 2084
Erythrocyte-stimulating proteins, in chronic kidney disease, 2156-2158
Erythropoietin, in chronic kidney disease, 2156-2158
Escitalopram, cardiovascular aspects of, 2129t
E-selectin, 990

Esmolol (Brevibloc), 792-793
  in aortic dissection, 1479
  in atrial flutter, 875
  in hypertensive crises, 1066, 1066t
  pharmacokinetics and pharmacology of, 1373t
  postoperative, 2016
Esophagus
  disorders of, pain in, 1197, 1354
  electrocardiography of, in arrhythmias, 772
Estrogen
  coronary artery disease and, 1961
  dyslipidemia and, 1081-1082
  hypertension and, 1044
  Prinzmetal variant angina and, 1339
  pulmonary embolism and, 1864
  thrombosis and, 2061
Estrogen-replacement therapy (ERT). See Hormone replacement therapy.
Etanercept, in rheumatoid arthritis, 2095
Ethanol. See Alcohol.
Ether-a-go-go–related gene (HERG), in torsades de pointes, 744
Ethmozine. See Moricizine (Ethmozine).
Ethnicity. See Racial/ethnic differences.
Etomoxir, in heart failure, 710
Europe, cardiovascular disease in, 9-10, 10t, 11t
EuroSCORE, 1997-1998, 1997t
Euthanasia, in end-stage heart disease, 722-723
Euthyroid sick syndrome, after coronary artery bypass graft surgery, 2009
Eutrophic remodeling of small arteries, in hypertension, 1033, 1033f
Event recording, electrocardiographic
  in arrhythmias, 768, 769f
  in syncope, 980-981
Everolimus, in heart transplantation, 678
Everolimus-eluting stents, 1436
Evidence, in therapeutic decision-making
  accuracy of, 46-47
  interpretation of, 44-46
Evidence-based medicine. See also Quality of cardiovascular care.
  failure to comply with, errors associated with, 52
Excitation-contraction coupling
  calcium in, 511, 515f
  calcium movements and, 515, 517f
  in cross-bridge cycling, 1185-1186
  in heart failure, 550-551
Exercise, 1983-1990. See also Physical activity.
  aerobic (endurance), 1983
    in cardiovascular disease, 1153, 1154t
    definition of, 1150t, 1983
    exercise prescription for, 1986t
  benefits of, 1984-1985
  cardiac function during, 579-580
    abnormalities of, definition of, 579
    diastolic, 580
    systolic, 579-580, 579f
  in cardiac rehabilitation
    benefits of, 1150-1152, 1150f, 1151f
    future of, 1155
    physiology of, 1149-1150, 1150t
    prescription for, 1153, 1154t
    terminology related to, 1149-1150, 1150t
    underutilization of, 1154-1155
    unsupervised, 1154
    in women, 1963
  in cardiovascular disease, 1988-1990
  in cardiovascular disease prevention, 1137-1138, 1137t

Exercise (Continued)
  definition of, 1150t, 1983
  dynamic, 197-198, 198f
    with cardiac catheterization, 459
  in Eisenmenger syndrome, 1569
  future perspectives on, 1990
  in hypertension therapy, 1052-1053, 1052t
  in idiopathic pulmonary arterial hypertension, 1896
  left ventricular dysfunction from, 617
  in mitral stenosis, 1648
  myocardial infarction precipitated by, 1221
  physiology of, 195-197, 196f
  pulmonary circulation with, 1886
  pulmonary hypertension associated with, 1890
  resistance (strengthening), 1983-1984
    in cardiovascular disease, 1153, 1154t
    definition of, 1150t
  in restrictive cardiomyopathy, 1750
  risks of, 1985, 1985t
  in stable angina, 1364-1365
  static, 197
    with cardiac catheterization, 459
  submaximal, during exercise stress testing, 204
  tolerance of, in preoperative risk assessment for noncardiac surgery, 2017, 2017t
  types of, 1983-1984
  vigorous, sudden cardiac death with, 938-939, 947. See also Athletes, sudden death in.
Exercise index, 459
Exercise prescription
  in cardiac rehabilitation, 1153, 1154t
  for health and fitness, 1986, 1986t
Exercise stress testing, 195-226
  in acute chest pain, 1202, 1203t
  in acute coronary syndromes, 209
  in adult congenital heart disease, 216, 217f
  anaerobic threshold in, 196-197, 196f
  arm ergometry for, 197
  in arrhythmias, 210-213, 212f-213f, 225-226, 226t, 765-766
  in asymptomatic population, 207-208, 208f, 225, 225t
  in atrial fibrillation, 212
  in atrioventricular block, 212
  Bayesian theory in, 207
  bicycle ergometry for, 197, 198f
  blood pressure during, 204
  in cardiac arrest survivors, 954
  in cardiac rehabilitation, 1153
  chest discomfort during, 204, 205-206, 217
  chronotropic incompetence during, 205
  contraindications to, 217, 217t, 220, 221t
  after coronary artery bypass graft, 216
  coronary revascularization and, 225, 226t
  in diabetes mellitus, 215
  diagnostic use of, 206-207, 206t, 207t, 221, 221t, 1357-1358, 1358t, 1361
  drug effects on, 213-214, 213f
  in elderly persons, 214-215, 1934
  electrocardiography in, 199-206
    computer-assisted analysis of, 203
    lead systems in, 199
    ST segment displacement on
      measurement of, 200, 201f-203f, 202-203
      mechanism of, 203-204
      types of, 199-200, 199f-201f

Exercise stress testing (Continued)
  in emergency department, 209-210
  evaluation of, terms used in, 206, 206t
  in heart failure, 210, 211f, 565-566, 647
  heart rate during, 204-205
  heart rate recovery after, 205, 205f
  heart rate–systolic blood pressure product during, 205
  heart transplantation and, 216
  in hypertension, 214, 215f
  in hypertrophic cardiomyopathy, 215-216
  implantable cardioverter-defibrillators and, 213
  indications for, 206, 220-224, 222t-223t, 224f, 225t-226t
  ischemic response to, severity of, 207, 207t
  in left bundle branch block, 212, 212f
  maximal work capacity during, 204, 205f
  metabolic equivalent in, 197
  in mitral stenosis, 1650-1651
  multivariate analysis in, 207
  after myocardial infarction, 222, 223t, 224, 224f
  in myocardial infarction, 209, 1288
  nonelectrocardiographic observations in, 204-206
  pacemakers and, 213
  after percutaneous coronary intervention, 216
  performance standards for, 220, 221t
  in peripheral arterial disease, 1497
  practice guidelines for, 220-225, 221t-223t, 224f, 225t-226t
  in preexcitation syndrome, 212-213, 213f
  preoperative, in noncardiac surgery, 210, 2018, 2020
  prognostic use of, 207-210, 208f, 221-222, 222t, 223t
  protocols for, 197-199, 198f
  in pulmonary hypertension, 1888
  report of, 208t, 218
  in right bundle branch block, 212, 212f
  risks of, 216-217, 217t
  safety of, 216-217, 217t
  in sick sinus syndrome, 212
  in silent myocardial ischemia, 209
  in stable angina, 1357-1358, 1357t-1359t, 1358t, 1361
  standards for testing and training in, 220, 221t
  submaximal exercise during, 204
  in supraventricular arrhythmias, 212
  in symptomatic patients, 208-209
  in syncope, 979-980
  technique of, 198-199
  termination of, 217-218, 220, 221t
  treadmill
    in peripheral arterial disease, 1497
    protocol for, 197-198, 198f
    in pulmonary hypertension, 1888
    in women, 214, 214f
  in UA/NSTEMI, 1323
  in valvular heart disease, 215, 225, 225t
  with ventilatory gas analysis, 196, 196f, 197, 224, 225t. See also Cardiopulmonary exercise testing.
  in ventricular arrhythmias, 211-212
  walk test for, 198
  in women, 214, 214f, 225, 1958, 1959f
Exercise training
  AHA risk classification for, 1986, 1987t
  definition of, 1150t, 1983
  effects of, 1150

Exercise training (Continued)
in heart failure, 619
in peripheral arterial disease, 1504, 1504f
preparticipation screening for, 1986-1988, 1986t, 1987t
Exertional dyspnea
in aortic stenosis, 1628-1629
in heart failure, 561
in mitral stenosis, 1649
Exertional leg pain, 1494-1495, 1494t. See also Claudication, intermittent.
Exertional syncope, in aortic stenosis, 2178, 2179f
Existential needs, in end-stage heart disease, 721-722
Exons, 71
External impedance cardiography, in heart failure, 595
Extracellular matrix, disorders of. See Connective tissue disorders.
Extracellular signal–regulated kinase (ERK) pathway, in left ventricular response to mechanical stress, 536, 537f
Extracorporeal LDL lipoprotein filtration, 1090
Extracorporeal ultrafiltration, in heart failure, 628
Extravascular compressive resistance, in coronary blood flow regulation, 1171, 1172f
Extremities
blood supply to, factors influencing, 1493-1494, 1494f
cool, in heart failure, 593
examination of, in myocardial infarction, 1224
lower
blood pressure measurement in, 131, 132f
claudication of, percutaneous intervention in, 1523-1542
edema of, in pulmonary hypertension, 1886
ischemia of, in aortic dissection, 1473
pain in, in acute aortic occlusion, 1486
venous interventions in, 1542-1543, 1543f
physical examination of, 127-128
upper, venous thrombosis in, 1864
vascular disease of. See Peripheral arterial disease; Peripheral vascular disease.
Extubation, early, after cardiac surgery, 1998
Ezetimibe, in dyslipidemia, 1083

F

f wave, in atrial fibrillation, 869
Fabry disease
genetic studies in, 114
restrictive cardiomyopathy in, 1754, 1754f
Facies
elfin, in supravalvular aortic stenosis, 1613, 1613f
mitral, in mitral stenosis, 1649
Facioscapulohumeral muscular dystrophy, 2145
Factor V Leiden gene mutation
APC resistance and, 2057-2058
deep vein thrombosis in, 2056-2057, 2058f
venous thromboembolism in, 1864

Factor VIII, elevated, in venous thrombosis, 2060
Factor Xa, inhibitors of, 2067. See also Fondaparinux.
Failure to thrive, in congenital heart disease, 1572
Fainting. See Neurally mediated syncope.
Falls
postprandial, in elderly persons, 1932
versus syncope, 979
Family caregivers, in end-stage heart disease, 721
Family screening strategies, in hypertrophic cardiomyopathy, 1767
Famine, age of
cardiovascular disease in, 2, 3t, 4
in United States, 7
Fascicular block
electrocardiography in, 167-168, 168f, 168t
left anterior, 167-168, 168f, 168t
left posterior, 168, 168f, 168t
left septal, 168
in myocardial infarction, 1281
Fascicular ventricular tachycardia, 907, 908f
Fasciculoventricular connections, in Wolff-Parkinson-White syndrome, 887, 887t, 888f
Fasudil, in stable angina, 1377
Fat, dietary
intestinal absorption of, 1073, 1074f, 1075
low, 1110-1111, 1111t, 1112
regional trends in, 16, 16f
Fat embolism, 1868
Fatigue
chronic, orthostatic intolerance in, 2177-2178
in heart failure, 561, 563t, 591
Fatty acid(s)
free, in diabetes mellitus, 1096-1097, 1097f
intake of, cholesterol and, 1112-1113, 1112f
metabolism of, nuclear imaging of, 367, 382, 383f
omega-3, 1160t
intake of, cardiovascular disease and, 1108, 1108f, 1109t, 1110
Fatty acid oxidation, partial inhibitors of, in heart failure, 710-711, 711f
Fatty streak of atherosclerosis, 985, 986f
Felodipine
pharmacokinetics of, 1375t
in stable angina, 1376
in UA/NSTEMI, 1327
Femoral access site, preparation of, in percutaneous coronary intervention, 1311
Femoral artery
catheterization of, 444, 444f, 445f-446f, 446-447
intraaortic balloon pump insertion through, 448-449, 450f
left ventricular biopsy from, 448
superficial disease of, percutaneous intervention for, 1525-1530, 1527f, 1528f, 1529t
Femoral artery approach
in arteriography, 468, 468f
in percutaneous coronary intervention, 1423
Femoral artery pulse, 132-133
Femoral vein
catheterization of, 443-444, 445f
right ventricular biopsy from, 448

Femoropopliteal disease, percutaneous intervention in, 1525-1530, 1527f, 1528f, 1529t
Fenfluramine
cardiovascular effects of, 1812
pulmonary hypertension from, 1902
Feng shui, in intensive care units, 1164
Fenofibrate (Tricor, Lipidil Micro)
in diabetic patients, 1101-1102
in dyslipidemia, 1083
Fenoldopam (Corlopam), in hypertensive crises, 1066, 1066t
Fenugreek (Trigonella foenum-graecum), 1159t
Fetal alcohol syndrome, 1563
Fetal gene induction, in heart failure, 550
Fetus
cardiac circulation in, 1565, 1565f
cardiac lesions in
direct intervention for, 1574
effects of, 1565
echocardiography in, 307, 1573-1574, 1574f, 1969
heart disease of. See Congenital heart disease.
heart failure in, 1566
heart of, 1565
maternal cyanotic heart disease effects on, 1970-1971, 1971t
pulmonary circulation in, 1565, 1565f, 1886
Fever
in infective endocarditis, 1720
in myocardial infarction, 1222
rheumatic. See Rheumatic fever.
Fiber consumption, cardiovascular disease and, 1107-1108
Fibric acid derivatives/fibrates
in diabetic patients, 1101-1102
in dyslipidemia, 1083, 1086-1087
Fibrillin-1 gene mutation, in Marfan syndrome, 92-93
Fibrin D-dimer, as atherosclerotic risk factor, 1018
Fibrinogen
as atherosclerotic risk factor, 1018, 1018f
elevated, in atherothrombosis, 2060
Fibrinogen bridge, 2055-2056, 2056f
Fibrinolytic agents. See Thrombolytic therapy.
Fibrinolytic function markers, atherothrombotic risk and, 1018-1019
Fibrinolytic inhibitors, 2054
Fibrinolytic system, 2053-2054, 2054f
Fibroblasts, in heart failure, 556-557, 557f
Fibroelastoma, papillary, 1816
Fibroelastosis, endomyocardial, 1758
Fibroma, 303, 303f, 1818t, 1823
Fibromuscular dysplasia, 95, 1507
Fibronectin, in infective endocarditis, 1719
Fick method, for cardiac output measurement, 452, 454-455, 454f
Fight or flight reaction, versus heart rate-induced calcium release, 515, 518
Figure-of-8 reentry, 756f, 758
FilterWire, 1426, 1429f
Financial burden, in end-stage heart disease, 721
FINAPRES device, 2173
Finland, cardiovascular disease in, 10, 11t
Fish, intake of, cardiovascular disease and, 1108, 1108f, 1109t, 1110

Fish oils, 1160t
in cardiovascular disease prevention, 1140
in dyslipidemia, 1084
Fistula
aortic sinus, 1609
arteriovenous
coronary, 1620-1621
pulmonary, 1620
coronary artery, arteriography of, 487, 488f, 489f
intracardiac, in traumatic heart disease, 1860
Five Wishes document, 1164
FK-506. *See* Tacrolimus (FK-506).
Flamm formula, for mixed venous oxygen content, 459
Flecainide
in arrhythmias, 780t, 781t, 782t, 783t, 786t, 790-791
in atrial fibrillation, 873
in chronic kidney disease patients, 2165t
pacemaker abnormalities caused by, 851
in pregnancy, 1976t
Fludrocortisone, in autonomic failure, 2176
Fluid retention. *See* Edema; Pulmonary edema.
Fluid status management, in heart failure
device-based therapies for, 628
diuretics for, 620-628, 621f, 621t, 623f-625f
Fluid-filled catheter(s), 449
Fluoro-2-deoxyglucose, radiolabeled, in positron emission tomography, 367-368, 370f
Fluoroscopy, in pericardial effusion and tamponade, 1838
5-Fluorouracil, cardiotoxicity of, 1813, 2111
Fluoxetine, cardiovascular aspects of, 2129t
Fluvastatin (Lescol), 1083
Foam cells, formation of, in atherogenesis, 990f, 992-993, 1800f
Focused Assessment for the Sonographic Examination of the Trauma Victim (FAST), 1858
Folate/folic acid
dietary supplementation of, 1115, 1140
postoperative, 1999
Foley balloon catheter, in traumatic heart disease, 1860, 1861f
Fondaparinux
description of, 2065
in heparin-induced thrombocytopenia, 2065
in myocardial infarction, 1253
in percutaneous coronary intervention, 1437
in pulmonary embolism, 1873, 1873t
in UA/NSTEMI, 1331-1332, 1332f
Fontan obstruction, 1595, 1596
Fontan procedure
background on, 1594
clinical features after, 1595
complications and sequelae of, 1595
in Ebstein anomaly, 1605
follow-up in, 1596
laboratory studies after, 1595-1596
lesions requiring, 1590-1594
management options and outcomes in, 1596
modifications of, 1590, 1594, 1594f
pathophysiology after, 1590-1595

Force transmission, in contraction-relaxation cycle, 514, 514f
Force-frequency relationship, in contraction-relaxation cycle, 531-532, 532f
Force-length relationships, in contraction-relaxation cycle, 530, 530f
Force-velocity relationship, in contraction-relaxation cycle, 533
Foreign bodies, in traumatic heart disease, 1856
Forward stroke volume, 458
Fosinopril, in heart failure, 624t
Fractalkine, in atherogenesis, 991
Fractional coronary reserve, 1179f, 1180f, 1181
Fractional renal reserve, in renal artery stenosis, 1533
Fractional shortening, 248
Frameshift mutation, 75, 75f
Framing effects, in decision-making, 46
Framingham Heart Study, risk factor scores in, 1123
France, cardiovascular disease in, 10, 11t
Frank-Starling relationship, in contraction-relaxation cycle, 513, 516f, 529-530, 530f
Frataxin gene, in Friedreich's ataxia, 2145
Free wall rupture, 256-257, 258f, 1272-1273, 1272f, 1274f, 1275f, 1303
French paradox, 1806
Frequency domain analysis, in electrocardiography, 770
Friction rub. *See* Pericardial rub.
Friedreich's ataxia
cardiovascular manifestations of, 2145-2146, 2145f, 2146f
clinical presentation in, 2145
genetics of, 2145
prognosis in, 2147
treatment of, 2146-2147
Fruit consumption, cardiovascular disease and, 1107
Functional capacity, sudden cardiac death and, 938
Fundus (fundi), in myocardial infarction, 1223
Fungal infection
in infective endocarditis, 1717-1718
in pericarditis, 1848-1849
Furosemide (Lasix)
in heart failure, 600, 601t, 620, 621t, 622, 625
in hypertension, 1058
in hypertensive crises, 1066, 1066t
in myocardial infarction, 1267-1268
in pregnancy, 1976t
Fusion beats, in ventricular tachycardia, 897, 897f
Futile care concerns, in end-stage heart disease, 722

G
G protein(s)
in contraction-relaxation cycle, 521, 521f
inhibitory, 521, 521f
stimulatory, 521, 521f
third, 521
G protein–coupled receptors, in contraction-relaxation cycle, 522, 526, 527f
Gadolinium, in cardiovascular magnetic resonance, 394
Gallawardin phenomenon, in aortic stenosis, 1630

Gamma camera, for single photon emission computed tomography, 345, 346f
Gap junctions, 727, 736-737, 737f
Garlic *(Allium sativum)*, 1159t
for hypertension, 1158
Gastroepiploic artery graft, catheterization of, 480-481, 482f
Gastroesophageal reflux, chest pain in, 1197
Gastrointestinal bleeding
in aortic stenosis, 1630
postoperative, 2008
Gastrointestinal disorders
chest pain in, 1197
in heart failure, 562
postoperative, 2008
Gastrointestinal procedures, endocarditis prophylaxis for, 1731-1732
GATA4, mutation of, in atrial septal defect, 118-119
Gaucher disease, restrictive cardiomyopathy in, 1754
Gelatinases, 557, 557t
Gemfibrozil (Lopid), 1083
in cardiovascular disease prevention, 1128-1129
in chronic kidney disease patients, 2165t
in diabetic patients, 1101
in stable angina, 1363
Gender differences. *See also* Women.
in cardiovascular mortality, 25
in congenital heart disease, 1561-1562
in hypertrophic cardiomyopathy, 1768
in preoperative risk analysis, 1993-1994
in sudden cardiac death, 936-937, 937f
Gene(s)
chromosomes and, 70f, 71
conversion of, to proteins, 71-72, 72f
housekeeping, 72
lineage-specific, 72
mutations of
in cardiovascular disease, 75
definition of, 75
incomplete penetrance of, 88
nonpenetrant, 88
types of, 75, 75f
Gene expression. *See also* Phenotype.
serial analysis of. *See* Genomics.
variability in, 88, 89t
Gene therapy
animal models in, 81-82
clinical trials in, 82
in dyslipidemia, 1091
in heart failure, 706-708, 706t, 707f
mechanical approaches in, 706, 707f
vectors for, 706
Gene transfer, 79-81
adeno-associated viral, 81
adenoviral, 80-81
cationic liposomes in, 81
polymers in, 81
retroviral, 80
vectors for, 79-81
General anesthesia, for noncardiac surgery, 2020-2021
General appearance
in heart failure, 562
in myocardial infarction, 1222
on physical examination, 127
Genetic anticipation, in myotonic muscular dystrophy, 2137
Genetic code, 70-72, 70f, 71, 72f
Genetic compound, 87

I-40

Genetic disorders, 85-98
  due to changes in single nuclear genes, 86-87
  due to microscopic alterations in chromosomes, 85-86, 86t
  of vascular system, 89-98
Genetic heterogeneity, 88-89
Genetic studies
  in adult polycystic kidney disease, 94-95
  in arrhythmias, 101-108, 102t
  in arrhythmogenic right ventricular dysplasia, 117, 117t
  in arterial aneurysm, ectasia, or dissection, 95
  in arterial occlusive disease, 95
  in arteriohepatic dysplasia, 95
  in atherosclerosis, 96, 97t
  in atrial septal defect, 118-119
  in bicuspid aortic valve, 119-120, 119t
  in cardiac tumors, 121
  in cardiomyopathies, 111-117, 112t, 115t, 116f, 117t
  in cardiovascular disease, 74-76, 75f, 76f, 85-98, 111-122, 1956
  in congenital heart disease, 118-121, 119t, 1563
  in connective tissue disorders, 89-94, 90t
  in dilated cardiomyopathy, 114-117, 115t, 116f
  in Ehlers-Danlos syndrome, 90
  in hemiplegic migraine, 95-96
  in Holt-Oram syndrome, 120
  in hypertrophic cardiomyopathy, 111-114, 112t, 1763-1764
  in idiopathic pulmonary arterial hypertension, 1893-1895, 1895f
  in Marfan syndrome, 92-93
  in mitral valve prolapse, 93, 120
  in Noonan syndrome, 120-121
  in polycystic kidney disease, 95
  in pseudoxanthoma elasticum, 94, 94f
  in pulmonary hypertension, 96
  in sudden cardiac death, 936, 937f
  in supravalvular aortic stenosis, 90
  in transforming growth factor-ß receptor disorders, 93
  in trisomy 21 (Down syndrome), 132
  in Turner syndrome, 132
  in ventricular septal defect, 119
  in von Hippel–Lindau syndrome, 98
Genetic testing, in congenital heart disease, 1563
Genetics
  medical, principles of, 87-89, 87f, 88f, 89t
  molecular. See Molecular genetics.
Genitourinary procedures, endocarditis prophylaxis for, 1731-1732
Genome, 71
  human, 85, 86-87
  proteome and, 77, 77f
Genome-wide scans, in molecular genetics, 76
Genomic disorders, 86, 86t
Genomics, 74, 76-77, 77f
  in cardiovascular disease risk assessment, 1020-1021
  pharmacological, 58, 58f, 60-62, 61t, 62t
Genotype, 74, 75, 85
Gestational hypertension, 1044-1045, 1044t
Giant cell arteritis, 2089-2090, 2090t
Giant cell myocarditis, 1755-1756, 1755f, 1784

Ginkgo biloba, 1160t
  for peripheral vascular disease and venous insufficiency, 1162
Ginseng root, Asian, 1160t
Glenn operation, bidirectional
  in double-inlet ventricle, 1593
  in hypoplastic left heart syndrome, 1592
  in tricuspid atresia, 1591
Glenn shunt, in cyanotic congenital heart disease, 1568, 1568t
Global burden of cardiovascular disease, 1-21
  future challenges in, 18-21, 19t
  in high-income countries, 9-10, 10t, 11t
  in low- and middle-income countries, 10t, 11-13, 12f
  trends in, 14-15, 14t
Glomerular filtration rate
  blood pressure and, 1038, 1038f
  contrast-induced nephropathy and, 2158, 2159f
  in elderly persons, 1927-1928, 1927t
  in heart failure, 593-594, 599
  for renal function assessment, 2155, 2157f
Glomerular vasculature, 2155, 2156f
Glucocorticoid-suppressible aldosteronism, 1042
Glucose
  metabolism of, nuclear imaging of, 367-368, 370f
  plasma, fasting, in diagnosis of diabetes mellitus, 1093, 1094t
  postoperative, 1999
  in UA/NSTEMI, 1325
Glucose-insulin-potassium (GIK) solution, in myocardial infarction, 1264, 1309, 1552-1553, 1554f
Glycemic control
  in cardiovascular disease prevention, 1134-1135
  in diabetes mellitus
    heart failure and, 1556
    myocardial infarction and, 1552-1553, 1553f, 1554f
  in end-stage renal disease, 2167
  in stable angina, 1363-1364
Glycemic index, 1108
Glycogen storage cardiomyopathy, 114, 755
Glycolysis, anaerobic, in myocardium, 367
P-Glycoprotein, in drug metabolism and elimination, 60, 61t, 65t
Glycoprotein Ib, in platelet adhesion, 2055
Glycoprotein IIb/IIIa complex, 2055-2056, 2056f
Glycoprotein IIb/IIIa inhibition. See also specific agent, e.g., Abciximab.
  agents used in, 2073
  complications of, 2075
  in diabetes mellitus, 1550
  in elderly persons, 1938
  in myocardial infarction, with thrombolytic therapy, 1254, 1256
  in percutaneous coronary intervention, 1301, 1302, 1302f, 1307-1308, 1307f, 1436-1437, 2075
  pharmacodynamics and optimal dosing with, 2073, 2075
  thrombocytopenia and, 2074f, 2075
  and thrombolytic therapy, facilitated PCI with, 2075
  in UA/NSTEMI, 1329-1330
  in women, 1962

Glycoprotein VI, in platelet adhesion, 2055
Glycosaminoglycan-derived drugs, 2065
Glycosides, cardiac. See Digoxin (digitalis).
Golgi apparatus, 68, 68f
Gorlin formula, for orifice area calculation, 456-457
Gorlin syndrome, fibroma in, 1823
Gouty arthritis, in cyanotic congenital heart disease, 1568
Gradient-echo sequence, in cardiovascular magnetic resonance, 394
Graft coronary artery disease, in heart transplantation, 679, 681, 682f
Graft rejection, in heart transplantation, 678-679, 680f
Graham Steell murmur, 1680
Gram-negative bacteria, in infective endocarditis, 1717
Granulocyte colony-stimulating factor (G-CSF), mobilization of progenitor cells with
  in acute myocardial infarction, 703-704, 705t
  in chronic heart failure, 705
Granuloma, noncaseating, in sarcoidosis, 1755, 1755f
Granulomatosis, Wegener, 2094
Great arteries
  embryogenesis of, 1564
  transposition of. See Transposition of the great arteries.
Great vessels
  computed tomography of, 432-433, 432f-433f
  magnetic resonance angiography of, 409, 409f
  pressure of, with cardiac catheterization, 451, 452t, 454t
Green tea, 1160t
Group A streptococcal (GAS) infection, in rheumatic fever, 2080-2081, 2084-2085
Growth, impaired, in congenital heart disease, 1572
Growth factor(s)
  angiogenic
    in gene transfer research, 81-82
    in peripheral arterial disease, 1503-1504
  insulin-like
    in acromegaly, 2034-2035
    actions of, 2033-2034
  vascular endothelial
    angiogenic properties of, in gene transfer research, 81
    in hypoxic pulmonary vasoconstriction, 1884
    in peripheral arterial disease, 1503
Growth factor receptor antagonists, cardiotoxicity of, 2114-2115
Growth factor signaling pathways, in pulmonary circulation, 1884-1886, 1885f
Growth hormone
  in acromegaly, 2034-2035
  actions of, 2033-2034
Guanabenz (Wytensin), in hypertension, 1059
Guanethidine (Ismelin), in hypertension, 1059
Guanfacine (Tenex), in hypertension, 1059
Guanosine monophosphate, cyclic (cGMP)
  compartmentalization of, 524-525
  in contraction-relaxation cycle, 522, 524, 525, 525f

Guardwire distal protection balloon, 1426, 1427f
Guggulipid (Commiphora guggul), for dyslipidemia, 1158, 1162
Guided imagery
in cardiac catheterization, 1163-1164
for stress management, 1157
Guidelines. See Practice guidelines.
Guidewires, for cardiac catheterization, 442-443, 446
Guillain-Barré syndrome, 2149, 2176
Gunshot wounds, 1855, 1857, 1860

H
HAART (highly active antiretroviral therapy), complications of, 1801, 1802t
HACEK organisms, in infective endocarditis, 1717, 1726, 1726t
Half-life, drug, 58, 59, 59f
Haloperidol
cardiovascular aspects of, 2130t, 2131
in hospitalized cardiac patient, 2126
in myocardial infarction, 1257
Hamartoma, 1823
Hampton hump, in pulmonary embolism, 1868
Hancock porcine valve, 1684, 1684f
Handgrip exercise, stress myocardial perfusion imaging with, 366
Haplotype, 76
Haplotype Map (HapMap), 76, 87
Harmonic imaging, in echocardiography, 242, 246, 247
Hawthorn, 1160t
for heart failure, 1162
HCN4 gene, 736
HDL. See High-density lipoprotein (HDL).
Head
injury to, closed, 2149-2150
physical examination of, 127
Head bobbing, in aortic regurgitation, 1638
Headache, in giant cell arteritis, 2090
Head-up tilt sleeping, in neurally mediated syncope, 983
Healing touch, in cardiac catheterization, 1163-1164
Health, exercise prescription for, 1986, 1986t
Health and fitness facilities, preparticipation screening in, 1988
Health care
costs of, in United States, 42
disparities in, in varied populations, 25-26, 25f
Health care industry, growth of, 7
Health care proxy form, in end-stage heart disease, 720-721
Health care–associated infective endocarditis, 1716
Heart. See also Cardiac; Cardiovascular; Coronary; Myocardial.
apex of, fat pad surrounding, 331, 333f, 334f
artificial, total, 691-692, 691f
athlete's, 537-538, 537t, 1768, 1988
computed tomography of
artifacts in, 421, 421f
contrast-enhanced, 419-421, 419f, 420f
nonenhanced, 419, 419f
radiation exposure estimates for, 419t
special considerations in, 415
electrical axis of, 154, 155f
of fetus, 1565
iron deposition in, 1754-1755

Heart (Continued)
and kidney, communication between, 2155, 2157f
morphology of, computed tomography of, 421
normal anatomy of, 329-335, 331f-335f, 1564-1565
physical examination of. See Cardiac examination.
strangulated, 1856
Heart block
advanced, 913
atrioventricular, 913-919. See also Atrioventricular block.
classification of, 913
congenital, pacemaker in, 832
deceleration-dependent, 751
in infants of mothers with systemic lupus erythematosus, 2098
versus interference, 913
tachycardia-dependent, 751
ventricular. See Fascicular block; Left bundle branch block (LBBB); Right bundle branch block (RBBB).
Heart failure, 509-724
abdominal examination in, 563
acute, 583-607
cardiac dysfunction in, 587-588
classification of, 583-584, 584t
clinical manifestations of, 589-593
definition of, 583
diagnostic evaluation of, 593-595
epidemiology of, 584-587, 585f, 585t
future perspectives on, 607
inflammatory abnormalities in, 589
laboratory findings in, 593-595
myocardial injury in, 589
neurohormonal alterations in, 589
pathophysiology of, 587-589, 587f, 590t, 591t
physical examination in, 592-593
precipitants of, 589, 590t, 591t
renal dysfunction in, 588-589
sudden cardiac death in, 941t, 943-944
symptoms of, 590-592, 591t, 592f
treatment of, 595-606
adrenergic agonists in, 601t, 603-604
calcium sensitizers in, 601t, 604-605
clinical outcomes and prognosis for, 606-607, 606t
diuretics in, 596, 600, 601t
future perspectives on, 605-606
pharmacological, 600-605, 601t, 602f
phosphodiesterase inhibitors in, 601t, 604
stage 1 (urgent/emergent care), 596-597, 596f
stage 2 (hospitalization), 597
stage 3 (pre-discharge), 597
strategies for, 597-600, 598f, 598t
vasodilators in, 596, 600-603, 601t, 602f
vascular dysfunction in, 588
adrenomedullin in, 548-549
in African Americans, 29-31, 30f, 31t, 32f
anemia in, 614, 615f
anthracycline-induced, 2109-2110
in aortic dissection, 1471
apelin in, 549
approach to patient with, 561-569
arginine vasopressin in, 545, 546f

Heart failure (Continued)
arrhythmias in, 635-636
arteriography in, 501, 506t
asymptomatic, 561
atherosclerosis in, 634
backward versus forward, 588-589
beta-adrenergic desensitization in, 552-553
biomarkers in, 564-565, 564f, 594-595, 600
blood pressure in, 592-593
bradykinin in, 548
B-type natriuretic peptide in, 253
cardiac arrest in, 952
primary prevention of, 969
cardiac cachexia in, 563
cardiac examination in, 563, 593
cardiac rehabilitation in, 1152
cardiorenal syndrome in, 627-628
central sleep apnea in, 636-638, 637f, 1917-1918, 1919, 1920, 1920f
chemotherapy-induced, 2116
chest radiography in, 565, 595
Cheyne-Stokes respiration in, 562
chronic
acute decompensation in, 561, 619, 620t, 646
myocardial repair and regeneration in, 704-705
in chronic kidney disease, 2164-2166, 2165t, 2166f
clinical assessment of, 561-580
clinical scoring systems for, 615, 617
cold versus warm, 584, 597-598, 598f
comorbidities of, 585t, 586-587
computed tomography in, 566-567, 566f, 567f
in congenital heart disease, 1566-1567, 1572
contractile and myofilament regulatory proteins in, 552, 553f
coronary angiography in, 568-569, 569t
in coronary artery disease, 382-383, 383f, 611, 645, 1397-1400
cytoskeletal proteins in, 552
de novo, 583
decompensated, 561, 583, 584t, 591t
acute, 561, 619, 620t, 646
treatment of, 597-598, 598f
ventricular assist device in, 688
with depressed ejection fraction. See Heart failure, systolic.
in diabetes mellitus, 1553-1557
blood pressure control in, 1556
factors related to, 1554-1556
glycemic control in, 1556
medical therapy in, 1556-1557
overview of, 1553-1554
diagnostic criteria for, 617t
diagnostic laboratory tests in, 563-569, 563t
diastolic, 587-588. See also Heart failure, with normal ejection fraction.
dietary supplements for, 1162
disease management approach to, 638
dose adjustments in, 64
dry versus wet, 597-598, 598f
dyspnea in, 561, 563t, 590
echocardiography in, 253, 254f, 566, 566f, 595
edema in, 140, 142
in Eisenmenger syndrome, 1569
in elderly persons, 1943-1945, 1944f, 1946t
electrocardiography in, 565, 565f, 595
electrolytes in, 593

I-42 Heart failure *(Continued)*
endothelin in, 547
end-stage. *See* End-stage heart disease.
epidemiology of, 611, 612f, 612t, 613f
equilibrium radionuclide angiography
or ventriculography in, 371, 371f
etiology of, 382-383, 611-612, 612t
evaluation of, practice guidelines for,
657-658, 659t
excitation-contraction coupling in,
550-551
exercise and sports in patients with,
1989
exercise stress testing in, 210, 211f,
565-566
extracellular matrix in, 555-556, 555f,
556f
fatigue in, 561, 563t, 591
fibroblasts and mast cells in, 556-557,
557f
forward versus backward, 588-589
functional capacity in, sudden cardiac
death and, 943, 943f
future directions in, 559-560
general appearance in, 562, 592
heart sounds in, 141-142, 141f, 142t, 143f
hematological studies in, 594
high-output, 584, 584t
history in, 140-141, 561-562, 562t, 563t
in hypertension, 583, 584t, 588, 611,
645, 1034-1035
hypertension therapy in, 1065
in hyperthyroidism, 2041
in hypertrophic cardiomyopathy, 1769,
1771-1772
in infective endocarditis, 1721,
1727-1728
inflammatory mediators in, 558-559,
559t
jugular venous pressure in, 141, 562,
593
left ventricular dysfunction in, 573
left ventricular remodeling in, 549-559,
550f-558f, 550t
liver function tests in, 594
low-output, 584, 584t
L-type calcium channel in, 551
magnetic resonance imaging in, 567-
568, 567t, 568f
matrix metalloproteinases in, 557
myocardial alterations in, 553-556,
554f-556f
myocardial energetics in, 558
in myocardial infarction
left ventricular, 1267-1269, 1267f
mechanical causes of, 1272-1275,
1272f, 1273t, 1274f-1277f
myocardial recovery in, 559, 559t
in myocarditis, 1784
myocyte biological alterations in, 549,
550t
myocyte hypertrophy in, 549-550,
550f-552f
myocyte loss in, 553-555, 554f
natriuretic peptides in, 546-547, 547f,
594, 594f, 595t
neurohormonal alterations in, 541-549
neuropeptide Y in, 547
nitric oxide in, 548, 548f, 549f
noncardiac surgery in patients with,
2014-2015
with normal ejection fraction, 641-664
atrial dysfunction in, 653
B-type natriuretic peptide in, 646
classification of, 641, 642f
clinical features of, 644-647, 645t
comorbidity of, 644-646

Heart failure *(Continued)*
demographic features of, 644-645
diastolic dysfunction in, 647-653,
648f, 649f, 650t, 651f, 652f
left ventricular diastolic stiffness
(elastance) and, 650-653, 652f
left ventricular relaxation and,
648-650, 649f, 651f
volume overload without, 653
Doppler echocardiographic findings
in, 253, 646, 647f
echocardiography in, 248, 566t
in elderly persons, 1945
epidemiology of, 641, 642f, 643f
exercise testing in, 646-647
future perspectives on, 654, 656
historical perspective on, 641
left ventricular systolic function in,
653-654
management of, 654, 655f, 655t
morbidity in, 641, 644
mortality in, 641, 643f, 644f
natural history of, 641, 643f, 644,
644f
neurohumoral activation in, 653
nomenclature for, 641
pathophysiology of, 647-654
systolic ventricular vascular
stiffening in, 653
nuclear imaging in, 382-386, 383f-386f
of left ventricular function, 385
of myocardial viability, 383-385,
383f-385f
research directions for, 385-386,
386f
NYHA classification of, 619, 619t
obesity paradox in, 611, 613f
orthopnea in, 561-562, 563t
oxidative stress in, 30, 31f, 544, 545f
paroxysmal nocturnal dyspnea in, 140,
562, 563t
pathogenesis of, 541, 542f
pathophysiology of, 541-560
peripheral edema in, 563
peripheral vasculature in,
neurohormonal alterations in,
547-548
in persistent truncus arteriosus, 1587
physical examination in, 141-142, 562-
563, 563t
polymorphisms in, 29, 31t
population screening for, 615, 617
positron emission tomography in, 569
practice guidelines for, 657-664, 658f,
659t-664t
prevalence of, 611, 612f
prognosis for, 612-615, 614f, 614t, 615f
biomarkers and, 613-614, 614f, 615f
renal insufficiency and, 614-615,
615f
as progressive model, 541-559
psychosocial factors in, 2124-2125
pulmonary artery catheter in, 595,
599-600
pulmonary edema in, 562, 583-584,
584t, 589, 590
pulmonary examination in, 562-563
quality of care for
in hospitals, 54, 54t
measures of, 51t, 53t
radionuclide angiography in, 566
rales in, 142, 562-563, 563t, 590
refractory end-stage, 638
renal function in, 544-547, 546f, 547f,
593-594
renin-angiotensin-aldosterone system
activation in, 542-544, 544f, 545f

Heart failure *(Continued)*
right-sided, 584, 584t, 588
in constrictive pericarditis, 1843
after ventricular assist device
implantation, 694
risk factors for, 611, 612t, 613f
sarcoplasmic reticulum in, 550-551,
551t
signs of, 141
sodium-calcium exchanger in, 551
stage A (high risk with no symptoms),
615
stages of, 615, 616f
structural changes in, 557-558, 558f
surgical management of, 665-683
coronary artery bypass grafting in,
665-669, 666f, 667f, 668t-670t,
670f
future perspectives on, 683
heart transplantation in, 675-683,
676t, 677f, 680f-682f
left ventricular reconstruction in,
672-674, 673f, 674f
passive cardiac support devices in,
674-675, 675f
valve surgery in, 669-672, 671f-672f
sympathetic dysfunction in, 542, 543f,
2181, 2181f
symptoms of, 140-141, 561-562, 562t,
563t
systolic, 587, 611-639
in amyloidosis, 1752
approach to patient with, 615-617,
616f
diagnosis of, 140-141
echocardiography in, 253, 566t
in elderly persons, 1945
epidemiology of, 611, 612t, 613f
etiology of, 611-612, 612t
future perspectives on, 639
management of, 617-638
in African Americans, 634-635,
635f
aldosterone antagonists in, 618t,
624t, 630t, 633
angiotensin receptor blockers in,
618t, 624t, 629-630, 630t, 631f
angiotensin-converting enzyme
(ACE) inhibitors in, 618t, 624t,
628-629, 629f, 630t
anticoagulation in, 635
antiplatelet therapy in, 635
beta blockers in, 618t, 624t, 630-
633, 630t, 632f
in cancer patient, 635
carbonic anhydrase inhibitors in,
623
device therapy in, 618t, 628, 636,
636f, 637f
digoxin in, 618t, 624t, 630t, 633-634
diuretics in, 618t, 620-628, 621f,
621t, 623f-625f
in elderly person, 635
general measures in, 619-620, 620t
left ventricular dysfunction and,
617, 619f
in patients who remain
symptomatic, 633-634, 633f
preventing disease progression in,
628-633
stage of heart failure and, 616f, 618t
strategy in, 617-619, 618t
vasopressin antagonists in, 621t,
623-624, 624f
prognosis for, 612-615, 614f, 614t, 615f
terminology in, 561
thyroid hormones in, 2045

Heart failure (Continued)
  treatment of
    in African Americans, 30, 32t
    assisted circulation in, 685-696
    cost-effectiveness analysis of, 38-39
    emerging therapies and strategies in, 697-714
    gaps in, 638
    gene therapy in, 706-708, 706t, 707f
    immunomodulation in, 712-714, 712f, 713f
    metabolic modulation in, 710-711, 711f
    myocardial repair and regeneration in, 697-706. See also Myocardial repair and regeneration.
    pharmacogenetics in, 708-710, 708t, 709f, 710f
    urotensin II in, 547-548
  Valsalva maneuver in, 142, 144f
  vasoconstrictor activity in, 545, 546f, 547-548
  vasodilatory activity in, 545-547, 548-549, 548f, 549f
  ventricular function curves in, exercise and, 579-580, 579f
  vital signs in, 562
  warm versus cold, 584, 597-598, 598f
  wet versus dry, 584
  in women, 1963-1964, 1963f
Heart failure clinics, 638
Heart rate
  autonomic modulation of, 2172
  calcium release triggered by, versus fight or flight reaction, 515, 518
  diastolic function and, 573, 573f
  in elderly persons, 1925f
  during exercise, 195, 196, 196f, 204-205
  force-frequency relationship and, 531-532, 532f
  in hyperthyroidism, 2040
  maximum, 195
  in myocardial infarction, 1222
  myocardial oxygen consumption and, 1167-1168, 1168f
  neural control of, 2123
  perioperative myocardial ischemia and, 2021
  in pulmonary hypertension, 1889t, 1890
  sodium-calcium exchanger and, 520
  turbulence of, in arrhythmia diagnosis, 769
  vagal lowering of, 524, 525, 525f
  variability in
    analysis of, 157
    in arrhythmia diagnosis, 769
    as measure of autonomic function, 2173-2174
Heart rate recovery
  abnormal, after exercise stress testing, 205, 205f
  as measure of autonomic function, 2174
Heart rate reserve, calculation of, 205
Heart rate–systolic blood pressure product, during exercise stress testing, 205
Heart rhythm
  disorders of. See Arrhythmias.
  neural control of, 2123
Heart sound(s), 135-136. See also Murmur(s).
  in aortic regurgitation, 1639
  in aortic stenosis, 1630-1631
  in cardiac tamponade, 1836
  in congenital heart disease, 1572
  diastolic, 136

Heart sound(s) (Continued)
  ejection, 135
  first, 135
  fourth, 136
    in heart failure, 141, 141f, 142, 142t
  in heart failure, 141-142, 141f, 142t, 143f, 563, 563t, 593
  in mitral regurgitation, 1662
  in mitral stenosis, 1649
  in myocardial infarction, 1223
  in pregnancy, 1968
  prosthetic valves and, 147
  in pulmonary hypertension, 1886
  in pulmonic regurgitation, 1679-1680
  in rheumatic fever, 2082
  second, 135
    in heart failure, 142
  systolic, 135, 136f
  third, 136
    in heart failure, 141, 141f, 142, 142t, 143f
  in tricuspid regurgitation, 1676
Heart tissue, engineered, 700
Heart transplantation, 675-683
  arteriography after, 467
  arteriosclerosis after, 999-1000, 999f, 1000f
  clinical outcomes of, 679, 681f, 682f
  contraindications to, 676
  donor allocation system in, 675
  donor selection in, 675-676, 676t
  exercise stress testing and, 216
  future perspectives on, 683
  graft coronary artery disease in, 679, 681, 682f
  graft rejection in, 678-679, 680f
  in heart failure, 675-683
  heterotopic, 677f, 678
  hypertension after, 681, 683
  immunosuppression in, 678
  infection after, 681
  long-term complications of, 679, 681-683, 682f
  magnetic resonance imaging in, 403-404
  malignancy after, 681
  operative technique of, 677-678, 677f
  osteoporosis after, 683
  pacemaker after, 857t, 858
  physiology of transplanted heart in, 678
  psychosocial issues in, 677
  recipient selection in, 676-677, 676t
  renal failure after, 683
  in transposition of the great arteries, 1601, 1603
  tricuspid regurgitation after, 678
  in women, 1964
Heart valve(s). See Valve(s).
Heart vectors, in electrocardiography, 152-154, 154f
Heart work, 532-533, 533f
Heart-lung transplantation
  in Eisenmenger syndrome, 1570
  in idiopathic pulmonary arterial hypertension, 1900
HeartMate II axial flow pump, 692
HeartMate left ventricular assist device, 690-691, 690f, 694-695, 695f
HeartScore, 1123
Heart/Stroke Recognition Program, 55, 55t
Heat stroke, myocarditis in, 1781
HEDIS (Healthplan Employers Data and Information Set), cardiovascular measures in, 49, 50t
Hemangioma, 1816, 1818t, 1823
Hemangiomatosis, pulmonary capillary, 1902-1903

Hematologic disorders
  in cyanotic congenital heart disease, 1568
  in myocardial infarction, 1227
Hematological studies, in heart failure, 594
Hematoma
  intramural, of aorta, 1483-1484, 1484f
  retroperitoneal, in cardiac catheterization, 462
Hematopoietic stem cells, 698. See also Stem cells, clinical applications of.
Hemiblock, after cardiac surgery, 1999
Hemi-Fontan, in hypoplastic left heart syndrome, 1592
Hemiplegic migraine, familial, 95-96
Hemochromatosis
  echocardiography in, 297-298
  restrictive cardiomyopathy in, 1754-1755
Hemodialysis. See also End-stage renal disease.
  in hypertensive patient, 1039
  hypotension during, 2178-2179, 2180f
  prosthetic valves in, 1688
Hemodynamic monitoring
  implantable devices for, 595
  in myocardial infarction, 1264-1265, 1265t
Hemodynamic support, in myocarditis, 1790-1791
Hemodynamics
  in cardiac tamponade, 1834-1836, 1835f, 1835t, 1836f
  in constrictive pericarditis, 1845-1846, 1845t
  Doppler echocardiographic assessment of, 262-267, 263f
  in hypertension, 1029-1030, 1030f
  in idiopathic pulmonary arterial hypertension, 1893, 1896
  in mitral regurgitation, 1661, 1661f
  in myocardial infarction, 1265-1267, 1265t, 1266f
  in pericardial effusion, 1834-1836, 1835f, 1835t, 1836f
  in pregnancy, 1967-1968, 1968f
  of prosthetic valves, 1686-1687
  in thyroid disorders, 2040, 2040f, 2040t
  in tricuspid regurgitation, 1677
Hemoglobin
  in chronic kidney disease and heart failure, 2156-2157
  in heart failure, 614, 615f
  in myocardial infarction, 1219, 1227
Hemogram, in acute pericarditis, 1833
Hemopericardium, 1851
Hemoptysis, in mitral stenosis, 1649, 1652
Hemorrhage
  cerebral, 1522, 2149-2150, 2150f, 2151f-2152f
  heparin-induced, 1874
  intracranial
    in antithrombotic therapy, 1251
    familial, 95
    in infective endocarditis, 1721
    after percutaneous coronary intervention versus thrombolytic therapy, 1303
    in thrombolytic therapy, 1247, 1248f
  splinter or subungual, in infective endocarditis, 1720
  subarachnoid, 2149-2150, 2150f, 2151f-2152f
  in traumatic heart disease, 1857
  after ventricular assist device implantation, 693
  warfarin-induced, 1875

I-44 Hemorrhagic telangiectasia, hereditary, 97-98

Hemostasis
anticoagulant (antithrombotic) mechanisms in, 2052-2054, 2053f, 2054f
coagulation in, 2050-2052, 2051f, 2052f
markers of, in myocardial infarction, 1220
mechanisms of, 2049-2056
platelets in, 2054-2056, 2055f, 2056f
thrombin in, 2056, 2057f, 2058f
in UA/NSTEMI, 1320-1321, 1321f
vascular endothelium in, 2049-2050, 2050f

Henoch-Schönlein purpura, 2094
Heparan sulfate, 2065
Heparin, 2062-2065
in acute aortic occlusion, 1486
in acute limb ischemia, 1508
during arteriography, 470
in atrial fibrillation, 871
in cardiac catheterization, 446
in chronic kidney disease patients, 2164t
complications of, 1874-1875, 2063-2065, 2064f
low-molecular-weight
advantages of, 2063
in chronic kidney disease patients, 2164t
complications of, 2063-2065, 2064f
mechanism of action of, 2063, 2063f
in myocardial infarction, 1251-1253, 1252f
in percutaneous coronary intervention, 1437
in pregnancy, 1973
in pulmonary embolism, 1872-1873, 1873t
in UA/NSTEMI, 1331, 1332f
in venous thrombosis without pulmonary embolism, 1873
mechanism of action of, 2062, 2062f
in mitral stenosis, 1653
monitoring of, 2062-2063
in myocardial infarction, 1251, 1253
in percutaneous coronary intervention, 1437
in pregnancy, 1973
in pulmonary embolism, 1871-1872, 1872t
thrombocytopenia from, 1874-1875, 2063-2065, 2064f
diagnosis of, 2064
pathophysiology of, 2063-2064, 2064f
treatment of, 2064-2065
in UA/NSTEMI, 1331, 1331t
in venous thromboembolism prophylaxis, 1878-1879
warfarin overlap with, 1874
Heparin cofactor II deficiency, 2060
Heparin sulfate proteoglycan molecules, on endothelial cells, 987
Hepatic clearance, in elderly persons, 1928
Hepatic vein, Doppler echocardiography of, 293, 294f
Hepatitis C infection
heart transplantation and, 675-676
with HIV infection, complications of, 1801
myocarditis in, 1778
Hepatojugular reflux, 130
in heart failure, 141, 593
Hepatomegaly, in heart failure, 563, 593

Her2 receptor inhibitors, cardiotoxicity of, 2111-2112
Herbal medicines. See Dietary supplements.
Herceptin. See Trastuzamab (Herceptin).
Hereditary hemorrhagic telangiectasia, genetic studies in, 97-98
HERG gene, in torsades de pointes, 744
Heterogeneity, genetic, 88-89
Heuristic reasoning, in decision-making, 46
Hexaxial reference system, in electrocardiography, 154, 155f
Hibernating myocardium. See Myocardial hibernation.
High-density lipoprotein (HDL), 1072, 1073f, 1073t
cardiovascular disease risk and, 1008, 1008f, 1128, 1129, 1131
in diabetes mellitus, 1101
dietary management of, 1112f, 1113
genetic disorders of, 1081
metabolism of, 1074f, 1076-1077, 1077f-1078f
receptors for, 1073
in stable angina, 1363
High-income countries, cardiovascular disease in
global burden of, 9-10, 10t, 11t
global trends in, 14, 14t
strategies to reduce, 19
Highly active antiretroviral therapy (HAART), complications of, 1801, 1802t
High-output heart failure, 584, 584t
Hill sign, in aortic regurgitation, 145-146, 1638
Hirudin (desirudin), 2067
in myocardial infarction, 1251
His bundle
anatomy of, 729-730, 731f
innervation of, 732-733, 734f
Hispanic Americans
cardiovascular disease risk factors in, 23-24
cardiovascular mortality in, 25
demographics of, 23, 24f
health care disparities for, 25
hypertension in, 26, 26f
His-Purkinje block, procainamide-induced, 787
Histoplasma, in infective endocarditis, 1717
Histoplasmosis, pericarditis in, 1848-1849
History-taking, technique of, 125-126
HIV infection. See Human immunodeficiency virus (HIV) infection.
HLA-B-27 gene, in spondyloarthropathies, 2096
HMG CoA reductase inhibitors. See Statin therapy.
Hodgkin disease, radiation therapy in, cardiovascular effects of, 2115
Holiday heart syndrome, 948, 1745
Holter monitoring
in arrhythmia diagnosis, 766-768, 769f
in cardiac arrest prevention, 966
clinical competence in, 825
practice guidelines for, 823-825, 824t-827t
in silent myocardial ischemia, 1396-1397
in syncope, 980
Holt-Oram syndrome, 1571
gene expression in, 88
genetic studies in, 120

Homocysteine
in cardiovascular disease prevention, 1141
coronary artery disease risk and, 1017-1018
metabolism of, 2059, 2059f
plasma, dietary influences on, 1115
postoperative, 1999
in stable angina, 1356
Homocysteinemia, 2059-2060
Homocysteinuria, 2059
Homograft (allograft) prosthetic valves, 1684f, 1686
Homologue, 68
Hormone receptor, actions of, 2036, 2036f
Hormone(s)
disturbances of, hypertension in, 1043
thrombosis and, 2057, 2058, 2061
Hormone replacement therapy
cardiovascular disease risk and, 1139-1140, 1961
in elderly persons, 1939
in myocardial infarction prevention, 1291-1292
in stable angina, 1364
in syndrome X, 1396
thrombosis and, 2057
Horse chestnut, 1160t
for peripheral vascular disease and venous insufficiency, 1162
Hospice care, in end-stage heart disease, 724
Hospital(s)
admission to, for syncope, 982
discharge from
after cardiac surgery, 2000
after myocardial infarction
assessment at, 1288-1289
timing of, 1286
after UA/NSTEMI, 1349
myocardial infarction management in, 1256-1258, 1258t
quality of cardiovascular care in
for heart failure, 54, 54t
mortality and, 54, 55f
for myocardial infarction, 54, 55t
surgical volume as marker of, 52-53, 53f, 53t
UA/NSTEMI management in, 1344-1347, 1346f, 1347t, 1348t
Hostility
in cardiovascular disease, 2119, 2122
in hypertension, 2123-2124
Hounsfield scale, in computed tomography, 415, 416t
Housekeeping gene, 72
Human genome, 85
Human Genome Project, 86-87
Human immunodeficiency virus (HIV) infection
atherosclerosis in, accelerated, 1795t, 1800, 1800f, 1801f
autonomic dysfunction in, 1795t, 1800, 1801f
cardiac surgery in patients with, 1996
cardiovascular disease in, 1793-1804
algorithm for, 1797f
background on, 1793
summary of, 1794t-1795t
cardiovascular malignancy in, 1794t, 1799
in children, 1794, 1795, 1796, 1798f, 1802
cytokine alterations in, 1795
dilated cardiomyopathy in, 1793-1797, 1794t, 1796f-1798f
future perspectives on, 1803-1804

Human immunodeficiency virus (HIV)
   infection (Continued)
   infective endocarditis in, 1714, 1794t,
      1798-1799
   left ventricular diastolic dysfunction
      in, 1797
   long QT syndrome in, 1800-1801
   monitoring recommendations in, 1803
   myocarditis in, 1777, 1778, 1795
   nonbacterial thrombotic endocarditis
      in, 1794t, 1799
   nutritional deficiencies in, 1795
   pericardial disease in, 1847-1848
   pericardial effusion in, 1794t, 1797-1798
   perinatal and vertical transmission of,
      1802-1803
   pulmonary arterial hypertension in,
      1902
   pulmonary hypertension in, 1795t,
      1799-1800
   right ventricular disease in, isolated,
      1799
   in sub-Saharan Africa, 13
   treatment of
      complications of, 1801-1802,
         1802t-1803t
      immunoglobulins in, 1796, 1798f
   vasculitis in, 1795t, 1800
H-V interval
   description of, 772
   in Emery-Dreifuss muscular dystrophy
      and associated disorders, 2144
   in intraventricular conduction
      disturbance, 773, 773f
   in myotonic muscular dystrophy, 2139
   in syncope, 981
   in tachycardia, 774, 775f
   in trifascicular blocks, 171
   in Wolff-Parkinson-White syndrome,
      887
Hydatid cyst, myocarditis in, 1780
Hydralazine (Apresoline)
   in chronic kidney disease patients,
      2165t
   in hypertension, 1061
   in hypertensive crises, 1066, 1066t
   in pregnancy, 1976t
Hydration, for prevention of contrast-
   induced nephropathy, 2160
Hydrochlorothiazide, in heart failure,
   621t
Hydrocortisone, in Addison disease,
   2037
Hydrothorax, in heart failure, 593
11-Hydroxylase deficiency, 1043
17-Hydroxylase deficiency, 1043
Hydroxymethylglutaryl–coenzyme A
   reductase inhibitors. See Statin
   therapy.
11-beta-Hydroxysteroid dehydrogenase
   type 2 deficiency, 1042
Hypercalcemia
   cardiac effects of, 2038
   from diuretics, 1058
   electrocardiography in, 184, 185f
Hypercholesterolemia. See also
   Dyslipidemia.
   cardiovascular disease risk and,
      1007-1008, 1008f, 1128-1131, 1129f,
      1130f, 1130t
   familial, 1078-1079
   future challenges in, 1131
   prevalence of, 1128
   treatment of, economic analysis of, 39,
      39t
   in women, 1957
Hyperchylomicronemia, familial, 1080

Hypercoagulable states, in pulmonary
   embolism, 1864, 1864t
Hyperdynamic state, in myocardial
   infarction, 1267
Hyperemia, coronary
   exercise stress-induced, 363-364
   pharmacological stress-induced,
      364-367, 365f
      dobutamine for, 366-367
      heterogeneity of, 365
      vasodilators for, 364-366, 365f, 366t
Hypereosinophilic syndrome, 298, 298f,
   1756-1757
Hyperglycemia
   after cardiac surgery, 1999
   cardiopulmonary bypass mortality risk
      and, 1552, 1552f
   in diabetes mellitus, 1096, 1097, 1097f,
      1099-1100, 1100t
   from diuretics, 626, 1058
   myocardial infarction in patients with,
      prognosis after, 1548, 1549f
Hyperhomocysteinemia, 2059-2060
Hyperkalemia
   from aldosterone antagonists, 633
   electrocardiography in, 184, 185f
   in heart failure, 593
   pacemaker abnormalities caused by,
      851
Hyperkalemic periodic paralyses,
   2147-2148
Hyperlipidemia. See also Dyslipidemia.
   as atherosclerotic risk factor, 1007-1008,
      1008f
   from diuretics, 626
   familial combined, 1080
   posttransplantation, 681
   quality of care indicators for, 53t
   type II, 1078-1080
   in women, 1957
Hyperlipoproteinemia
   type I, 1080
   type III, 1080
   type IV, 1079-1080
Hypermagnesemia, 185
Hyperparathyroidism, 2038
Hyperpnea, central, 1917
Hypersensitive carotid sinus syndrome.
   See Carotid sinus hypersensitivity.
Hypersensitivity myocarditis, 1780-1781
Hypersensitivity vasculitis, 2094
Hypertension, 1027-1070
   accelerated-malignant, 1045-1046, 1045t,
      1046f, 1046t
   in acromegaly, 2034
   alcohol intake and, 1806
   in aortic dissection, 1471, 1472, 1479,
      1482
   baroreceptors and, 1030-1031
   in blacks, 1028, 1029f
   cardiovascular disease risk and, 1005-
      1007, 1005f, 1006f, 1131-1133, 1131t
   cardiovascular risk stratification in,
      1036-1038, 1036t, 1037f
   cerebral blood flow autoregulation in,
      1046, 1046f, 1054, 1054f
   cerebrovascular disease in, 1037
   chemoreflexes and, 2172
   chronic, pregnancy in, 1045
   in chronic kidney disease, 2162
   classification of, 1069t
   in coarctation of the aorta, 1607
   after coronary artery bypass graft
      surgery, 1383
   coronary artery disease and, 1027,
      1028f, 1029f, 1037, 1037f
   definition of, 1027, 1028f

Hypertension (Continued)
   in diabetes mellitus, 1102-1103, 1102t
      pathology of, 1555-1556
      treatment of, 1556
   diastolic, in middle age, 1029-1030
   dietary influences on, 1113-1115, 1114f
   dietary supplements for, 1158
   drug-induced, 1038
   echocardiography in, 320, 321t, 324
   in elderly persons, 1931-1933
      approach to, 1933t
      prevalence and incidence of, 1931
      treatment of, 1931-1933, 1932t, 1933t
   emergency treatment of, 1045-1046,
      1045t, 1046f, 1046t
   endothelial cell dysfunction in, 1032-
      1033, 1032f, 1033f
   exercise and sports in patients with,
      1989
   exercise stress testing in, 214, 215f
   future perspectives on, 1046
   genetic studies in, 1029
   gestational, 1044-1045, 1044t, 1975,
      1975t
   heart failure in, 583, 584t, 588, 611, 645,
      1034-1035
   after heart transplantation, 681, 683
   high-risk, definition of, 1037, 1037f
   initial evaluation of, 1035-1040
   large vessel disease in, 1037
   left ventricular hypertrophy in, 1034
   lipid-lowering therapy in patients with,
      1085t, 1086
   low-renin, 1041
   masked, 131, 1036
   measurement of, 1035-1036, 1035f,
      1035t, 1036f
   mendelian forms of, 1042, 1042f
   mineralocorticoid, 1041-1042, 1041f,
      1041t, 1042f
   in myocardial infarction, 1222
   nephrosclerosis in, 1037-1038
   neurogenic, from sleep apnea, 1031
   nocturnal, 1036, 1036f
   noncardiac surgery in patients with,
      preoperative risk assessment for,
      2014
   obesity and, 1029, 1031
   obstructive sleep apnea and, 1916
   perioperative, 1043, 1043t
   in pheochromocytoma, 2045
   poor control of, factors influencing,
      1049
   portal, pulmonary arterial hypertension
      in, 1901
   postoperative, 2001-2002
   in pregnancy, 1975, 1975t, 1976t
   pressure-natriuresis curve in, 1031-1032
   prevalence of, 1005, 1006f, 1007f, 1027-
      1028, 1028f, 1029f, 1131
   primary
      behavioral contributions to,
         1028-1029
      hemodynamic patterns in, 1029-1030,
         1030f
      hormonal mechanisms of, 1033-1034,
         1033f, 1034f
      mechanisms of, 1029-1034
      neural mechanisms of, 1030-1031
      renal mechanisms of, 1031-1032
      sympathetic nervous hyperactivity
         in, 1031
      vascular mechanisms of, 1032-1033,
         1032f, 1033f
   psychosocial factors in, 2123-2124
   pulmonary. See Pulmonary
      hypertension.

I-46 Hypertension *(Continued)*
    quality of care indicators for, 53t
    racial/ethnic differences in, 23, 26-28,
        26f-28f, 28t
    regional trends in, 17-18
    renal disease in
        acute, 1038
        chronic, 1037-1038, 1038f, 1039
    renin-angiotensin-aldosterone system
        in, 1033 1034, 1033f, 1034f
    renovascular, 1039-1040
        classification of, 1039
        diagnosis of, 1039f, 1040, 1040f
        management of, 1040
        mechanisms of, 1039-1040
    resistant, causes of, 1064, 1064t
    salt-sensitive, 1032
    secondary
        adrenal causes of, 1040-1043, 1041f,
            1041t, 1042f
        in aldosteronism, 1041-1042, 1041f,
            1041t, 1042f
        after cardiac surgery, 1043, 1043t
        in coarctation of the aorta, 1043
        in Cushing syndrome, 1042-1043
        estrogen and, 1044
        in hormonal disturbances, 1043
        oral contraceptive–induced, 1044
        in pheochromocytoma, 1043, 1043t
        in pregnancy, 1044-1045, 1044t
        in renal parenchymal disease,
            1038-1039, 1038f
        work-up for, 1038t
    sociocultural factors in, 2124
    stress and, 1157, 2123
    stroke and, 1027, 1028f, 1029f, 1037,
        1065-1066
    sudden cardiac death and, 937
    sympathetic dysfunction in, 2180
    systolic, isolated
        in elderly persons, 1050-1051
        noncardiac surgery and, 2014
        in older adults, 1030, 1030f
        in young adults, 1030
    in Takayasu arteritis, 2088, 2089
    target organ disease in, evaluation,
        1037-1038
    in thyroid disorders, 2040
    treatment of. *See* Hypertension therapy.
    vascular remodeling in, 1033, 1033f
    white coat, 131, 1035-1036
    in women, 1044-1045, 1044t, 1956-1957
Hypertension therapy, 1006-1007,
    1049-1070. *See also* Antihypertensive
    drug therapy.
    ACE inhibitors in, 1062-1063, 1062t
    adrenergic inhibitors in, 1058-1061,
        1059f, 1059t
    alcohol moderation in, 1052t, 1053
    algorithms for, 1049-1050, 1051f, 1056,
        1056f
    alpha- and beta-adrenergic agonists in,
        1061
    alpha-adrenergic blocking agents in,
        1059-1060
    anesthesia and, 1064-1065
    angiotensin II receptor blockers in,
        1063-1064
    benefits of, 1049, 1050f, 1132
    beta blockers in, 1060-1061, 1060f
    in blacks, 1065
    calcium channel blockers in, 1061-1062,
        1062t
    calcium supplementation in, 1053
    central alpha-adrenergic agonists in,
        1059
    in children, 1065

Hypertension therapy *(Continued)*
    in chronic kidney disease, 2162, 2167
    in diabetic patients, 1065
    dietary changes in, 1052t, 1053, 1053f
    diuretics in, 1057-1058, 1058f, 1058t
    economic analysis of, 1132
    in elderly persons, 1050-1051, 1065,
        1065t, 1931-1933, 1932t, 1933t
    in erectile dysfunction, 1065
    follow-up in, 1068, 1069t, 1070
    future challenges in, 1066, 1132-1133
    general considerations in, 1049-1054
    goal of, 1051-1052, 1051f
    guidelines/recommendations on, 1131t,
        1132
    in heart failure, 1065
    initial strategy in, 1068-1069, 1069t
    in ischemic heart disease, 1065
    J curve in, 1051, 1051f
    lifestyle modifications in, 1052-1054,
        1052t
    magnesium supplementation in, 1053
    peripheral arterial disease risk and,
        1492
    peripheral neuronal inhibitors in,
        1058-1059
    physical activity in, 1052-1053, 1052t
    potassium supplementation in, 1053
    practice guidelines for, 1068-1070, 1069t
    in pregnancy, 1063, 1975, 1976t
    racial/ethnic differences in, 27-28, 28f,
        28t
    relaxation techniques in, 1053
    risk stratification in, 1036-1038, 1036t,
        1131-1132, 1131t
    sodium restriction in, 1052t, 1053, 1053f
    in stable angina, 1362-1363
    threshold for, 1049-1050, 1051f
    tobacco avoidance in, 1052
    vasodilators in, 1061-1064
    weight reduction in, 1052
Hypertensive crises, 1045-1046, 1045t,
    1046f, 1046t
    postoperative, 2014
    therapy for, 1066, 1066t
Hypertensive emergencies, 1045
Hypertensive encephalopathy, 1045-1046
Hypertensive pulmonary arteriopathy, in
    idiopathic pulmonary arterial
    hypertension, 1891, 1891f, 1892t
Hypertensive urgencies, 1045
Hyperthyroidism
    amiodarone-induced, 2044
    atrial fibrillation in, 928t-929t
    cardiovascular manifestations of,
        2040-2042, 2040t, 2041t
    catecholamine sensitivity in,
        2039-2040
    subclinical, 2043-2044, 2044f
Hypertriglyceridemia
    cardiovascular disease risk and, 1009,
        1128-1129
    in diabetes mellitus, 1101
    dietary management of, 1113
    familial, 1079
Hypertrophic cardiomyopathy. *See*
    Cardiomyopathy, hypertrophic.
Hypertrophic remodeling of large arteries,
    in hypertension, 1033, 1033f
Hyperuricemia, from diuretics, 1058
Hyperventilation
    coronary artery spasm from, 489
    syncope from, 978
Hyperviscosity syndrome
    in cancer patients, 2108
    in cyanotic congenital heart disease,
        1568

Hypobetalipoproteinemia, 1079
Hypocalcemia
    cardiac effects of, 2038
    electrocardiography in, 184, 185f
Hypoglycemia, syncope in, 978
Hypokalemia
    from diuretics, 625-626, 1057
    electrocardiography in, 184, 185f
    in heart failure, 564, 593
    ventricular fibrillation and, 1278
Hypokalemic periodic paralyses,
    2147-2148
Hypomagnesemia
    from diuretics, 626, 1057
    electrocardiography in, 185
Hyponatremia
    from diuretics, 626, 1058
    in heart failure, 564, 593
Hypoparathyroidism, 2038
Hypoplastic left heart syndrome,
    1591-1592, 1592f
Hypopnea, obstructive, 1915
Hypotension
    in aortic dissection, 1472, 1479-1480
    in cardiac tamponade, 1836
    causes of, 1051
    during dialysis, 2167, 2178-2179,
        2180f
    from diuretics, 626
    during dobutamine pharmacological
        stress, 366-367
    in hypertrophic cardiomyopathy,
        2179
    in inferior wall myocardial infarction,
        2179
    in myocardial infarction
        hypovolemic, 1266-1267
        in prehospital phase, 1266
        prevention of, 1237-1238
    neurally mediated, 977, 977t
    orthostatic. *See* Orthostatic
        hypotension.
    positional, in traumatic heart disease,
        1858
    postexertional, 204
    postoperative, 2000-2001, 2000t
    in right coronary artery thrombolysis,
        2179
    in right ventricular infarction, 1272
Hypothermia
    electrocardiography in, 185, 186f
    induced
        for anoxic encephalopathy after
            cardiac arrest, 964
        during percutaneous coronary
            intervention, 1309
    myocarditis in, 1781
Hypothesis testing, 44
Hypothyroidism
    cardiovascular manifestations of, 2040t,
        2042-2043
    diagnosis of, 2043
    dyslipidemia and, 1081
    muscle disease syndromes in, 2043,
        2043t
    pericardial effusion in, 1852
    subclinical, 2043
    treatment of, 2042f, 2043
Hypotrichosis-lymphedema-telangiectasia
    syndrome, 97
Hypovolemic hypotension, in myocardial
    infarction, 1266-1267
Hypoxemia
    arterial, in pulmonary hypertension,
        1888
    in myocardial infarction, 1238
        avoidance of, 1267

Hypoxia
  alveolar, in chronic obstructive pulmonary disease, 1906
  in coronary blood flow regulation, 1175
  in pulmonary vasoconstriction, 1884
Hypoxia-inducible factor-1, 1884
Hytrin. *See* Terazosin (Hytrin).

I

Iatrogenic cardiac injuries, 1856
Ibawi procedure, in transposition of the great arteries, 1603
Ibuprofen, in pericarditis, 1833
Ibutilide
  in arrhythmias, 780t, 781t, 782t, 784t, 786t, 796-797
  in atrial flutter, 875
Idarubicin (Idamycin PFS), cardiovascular effects of, 2108-2110
Idebenone, in Friedreich's ataxia, 2146-2147
Iliac artery disease, percutaneous interventions in, 1524-1525, 1525f, 1526f, 1526t
Iloprost
  in idiopathic pulmonary arterial hypertension, 1899
  in thromboangiitis obliterans, 1506
Imatinib, cardiotoxicity of, 2113-2114, 2114f
Imipramine, cardiovascular aspects of, 2129t
Immobilization, thrombosis and, 2060
Immune adsorption therapy, in myocarditis, 1790
Immune globulin, intravenous
  in HIV-infected patients, 1796, 1798f
  in Kawasaki disease, 2092
  in myocarditis, 1790
Immune system
  in atherogenesis, 993, 993f
  in dilated cardiomyopathy, 1746
  in myocarditis, 1782-1783, 1783f, 1790
Immunization, in heart failure, 619
Immunological perturbations, with ventricular assist device, 694
Immunomodulation, in heart failure, 712-714, 712f, 713f
Immunosuppression
  dyslipidemia and, 1082
  in heart transplantation, 678
  in myocarditis, 1788f, 1789
Impella ventricular assist device, 690
Implantable cardioverter-defibrillator. *See* Cardioverter-defibrillator, implantable.
Implantable devices, chest radiography of, 336f, 341, 341f, 342f
Implantable event recording, electrocardiographic, in syncope, 980-981
Implantable hemodynamic monitors, 595
Implantable loop recording, in arrhythmias, 768-769, 769f
Impulse conduction disorders, 747t, 750-753, 754f-756f
Impulse formation disorders, 746-750, 747t, 748f-753f
Incidence, 1122
Incisions, for cardiac surgery, infection of, 2008-2009
Income, worldwide. *See* High-income countries; Low- and middle-income countries.
Incontinence, in end-stage heart disease, 723
Inderal. *See* Propranolol (Inderal).

Indicator-dilution techniques, for shunt detection, 459
Indinavir, 1801
Inductive inference, 41
Infant(s). *See also* Children; Neonate(s).
  aortic stenosis in, 1611
  coarctation of the aorta in, 1607
  congenital heart disease in
    echocardiography in, 1574-1575
    management approach to, 1566
  heart failure in, 1566-1567
  patent ductus arteriosus in, 1585, 1586
  premature, heart failure in, 1566
  pulmonic stenosis in, 1616, 1617
  sudden cardiac death in, 936, 942t, 946-947
Infection
  in abdominal aortic aneurysms, 1459
  active systemic, heart transplantation and, 677
  atherosclerosis and, 1000-1001
  bacterial
    of aorta, 1486-1487
    in myocarditis, 1778
    in pericarditis, 1847
  fungal
    in infective endocarditis, 1717-1718
    in pericarditis, 1848-1849
  after heart transplantation, 681
  mortality in, in United States, 7, 7f
  with pacemaker, 844
  postoperative, 2008-2009
  after ventricular assist device implantation, 693-694
  viral
    in dilated cardiomyopathy, 1746
    geographical distribution of, 1777f
    in myocarditis, 1778
      agents causing, 1776-1778, 1777f
      pathogenesis of, 1781-1782, 1783f
    in pericarditis, 1846-1847
Infectious agents
  in infective endocarditis, 1716-1718
  in myocarditis, 1776-1780, 1777t
Infectious aortitis, thoracic aortic aneurysms and, 1465
Infective endocarditis, 1713-1737
  acute, 1713
  in adults, 1713-1714
  anticoagulant therapy and, 1730
  in aortic regurgitation, 1635
  in aortic stenosis, 1630
  bacteremia in, 1719, 1722
  blood cultures in, 1722
  in children, 1713
  clinical features of, 1720-1721, 1720f, 1720t
  complications of, 280-281, 280t, 282f
  in congenital heart disease, 1571, 1714
  culture-negative, 1727, 1728-1729
  diagnosis of, 1718t, 1721-1722
  echocardiography in, 280-282, 280t, 282f, 1721-1722, 1734, 1735t, 1737t
  emboli in, 1720, 1721, 1729
  in end-stage renal disease, 2166
  enterococci in, 1716-1717, 1724-1725, 1724t, 1725t
  epidemiology of, 1713
  etiological microorganisms in, 1716-1718
  extracardiac complications of, 1729-1730
  fungal, 1717-1718
  future perspectives on, 1732
  gram-negative bacteria in, 1717
  HACEK organisms in, 1717, 1726, 1726t
  health care–associated, 1716

Infective endocarditis *(Continued)*
  heart failure in, 1727-1728
  in HIV-infected patients, 1714, 1794t, 1798-1799
  in hypertrophic cardiomyopathy, 1773
  in intravenous drug abusers, 1714-1715, 1714t
  laboratory testing in, 1722
  microbiology of, 1714, 1714t, 1715, 1715t, 1716-1718, 1722
  in mitral stenosis, 1652
  in mitral valve prolapse, 1713-1714
  mycotic aneurysms in, 1730
  nonbacterial thrombotic endocarditis in, 1718-1719
  pathogenesis of, 1718-1719
  pathophysiology of, 1719-1720, 1720f
  perivalvular extension of, 1728
  practice guidelines for, 1734-1737, 1734t-1736t
  predisposing conditions in, 1713, 1714t
  prophylaxis against, 1731-1732, 1731t, 1732f, 1732t, 1734, 1734t
  prosthetic valve, 1715-1716
    microbiology of, 1715, 1715t
    pathology of, 1715-1716, 1715f
    staphylococcal, 1725-1726, 1726t, 1728
    surgical treatment of, 1728
  relapse and recurrence of, 1730
  in rheumatic heart disease, 1714
  septic arteritis in, 1730
  splenic abscess in, 1729
  staphylococci in, 1717, 1719, 1720f, 1725-1726, 1726t, 1732
  streptococci in, 1716, 1719, 1723-1724, 1723t, 1724t
  stroke associated with, anticoagulant therapy in, 1521
  subacute, 1713
  treatment of, 1722-1730
    antimicrobial, 1723-1727, 1723t-1726t
      monitoring of, 1727
      outpatient, 1727
      postoperative, 1729
      timing of, 1727
    response to, 1730
    surgical, 1727-1729
      antimicrobial therapy after, 1729
      indications for, 1727-1729, 1728t
      practice guidelines for, 1736t, 1737
      techniques for, 1729
      timing of, 1729
  tricuspid, in intravenous drug abusers, 1678
  viridans streptococci in, 1716, 1723-1724, 1723t
Inferior vena cava, radiography of, 331
Inferior vena caval filters, in pulmonary embolism, 1876
Inferior wall attenuation, on single photon emission computed tomography, 353-354, 354f
Infiltrative disorders, in restrictive cardiomyopathy, 1753-1759
Inflammation
  in abdominal aortic aneurysms, 1459
  in acute heart failure, 589
  in atherogenesis
    mechanisms of, 993-995, 993f-995f
    systemic, diffuse nature of, 998-999
  in diabetes mellitus, 1096, 1096f
  myocardial. *See* Myocarditis.
  pericardial. *See* Pericarditis.
  peripheral arterial disease risk and, 1492-1493
Inflammatory bowel disease, arthritis in, 2096

Inflammatory markers
in atherosclerosis, 1012-1020, 1013f-1016f, 1013t
in chest pain, diagnostic performance of, 1198-1199
Inflammatory mediators, in heart failure, 558-559, 559t
Infliximab, in rheumatoid arthritis, 2095
Influenza, myocarditis in, 1777, 1778
Information technology/systems, in decision-making, 47
Infrainguinal disease, surgical reconstructive procedures for, 1505
Inhalants, cardiovascular effects of, 1812
Inhalation agents, for noncardiac surgery, 2020
Injuries, during exercise and sports activities, 1985
Injury phobia, syncope in, 2179-2180
Innate immunity
in atherogenesis, 993, 993f
in myocarditis, 1782-1783, 1783f
Innovation, adoption of, 47
Inositol triphosphate (IP$_3$), in contraction-relaxation cycle, 522
Inositol triphosphate (IP$_3$) receptor, in arrhythmogenesis, 749
Inotropic state. See Myocardial contractility.
Insertion, nucleotide, 75, 75f
Inspection, in cardiac examination, 134-135
Instructional directives, in end-stage heart disease, 720-721
Insulin resistance
accelerated atherosclerosis in, 2035
as atherosclerotic risk factor, 1009
in diabetes mellitus, 1097, 1097f, 1100-1101, 1101f
from diuretics, 1058
dyslipidemia of, 1100-1101, 1101f
racial/ethnic differences in, 23
Insulin therapy
in diabetic patients with myocardial infarction, 1264, 1552-1553, 1553f, 1554f
perioperative, 2009
Insulin-like growth factors
in acromegaly, 2034-2035
actions of, 2033-2034
Insulin-resistance metabolic syndrome. See Metabolic syndrome.
Insurance coverage, of cardiac rehabilitation, 1154
Integrated backscatter analysis ("virtual histology"), 497, 498f
Integrative medicine. See Complementary and alternative medicine.
Integrilin. See Eptifibatide (Integrilin).
Intensity of physical activity, definition of, 1983
Intensive care unit
complementary and alternative medicine in, 1164
after noncardiac surgery, 2021-2022
Intercalated discs, 736-737, 737f
Intercellular adhesion molecule-1 (ICAM-1), in atherogenesis, 990
Interference, heart block versus, 913
Interferon beta, in myocarditis, 1789-1790
Interleukin-6, in myxoma, 1816
Interleukin-8, in atherogenesis, 991
Interleukin(s), in contraction-relaxation cycle, 526
Intermediate coronary care unit, for myocardial infarction, 1257-1258

Intermediate-density lipoprotein(s), 1072, 1073f, 1073t
formation of, 1074f, 1075-1076
Intermittent claudication. See Claudication, intermittent.
Intermittent pneumatic compression devices, in venous thromboembolism prophylaxis, 1879
Internal cardiac crux, 306-307, 306f
Internal mammary artery graft, 1382
catheterization of, 480, 482f
patency rate for, 1385
Internal thoracic impedance, in heart failure, 595
Internal work, in myocardial oxygen uptake, 533, 533f
International normalized ratio (INR), 2066
Internodal atrial myocardium, 728
Internodal conduction, 728
Interphase, 68
Interstitial lung disease, pulmonary hypertension in, 1909
Interventional magnetic resonance imaging, 410
Intestine
clearance in, in elderly persons, 1928
lipoprotein synthesis in, 1073, 1074f, 1075
Intima
of arteries, 988, 989f
diffuse thickening of, 988, 990f
proliferation of, in idiopathic pulmonary arterial hypertension, 1893
Intraaortic balloon counterpulsation, 685-686
balloon insertion for, 685-686, 686f
balloon removal for, 686
in cardiogenic shock, 1269-1270
chest radiography in, 336f, 341
complications of, 686
indications for, 685, 686t
in myocardial infarction, 1264
postoperative, 2001
in UA/NSTEMI, 1336
Intraaortic balloon pump
complications of, 449
indications for, 449
optimal timing and arterial waveforms with, 450f
percutaneous insertion of, 448-449, 450f
Intraatrial baffles, magnetic resonance imaging of, 408
Intraatrial conduction, 728
Intraatrial shunt, contrast echocardiography of, 242
Intracardiac pressures, Doppler echocardiography of, 262-263, 263f
Intracranial aneurysms
mycotic, management of, 1521
in polycystic kidney disease, 94-95
Intracranial hemorrhage
in antithrombotic therapy, 1251
familial, 95
in infective endocarditis, 1721
after percutaneous coronary intervention versus thrombolytic therapy, 1303
in thrombolytic therapy, 1247, 1248f
Intramural hematoma
of aorta, 1483-1484, 1484f
echocardiography in, 301, 301f
Intrathoracic pressure, in obstructive sleep apnea, 1916
Intrauterine devices, 1977
Intravascular imaging, novel invasive modalities for, 497-499, 498f, 499t

Intravascular magnetic resonance imaging, 410
Intravascular ultrasonography, 495-497. See also Ultrasonography, intravascular.
Intravenous drug abusers, infective endocarditis in, 1678, 1714-1715, 1714t
Intravenous immune globulin
in HIV-infected patients, 1796, 1798f
in Kawasaki disease, 2092
in myocarditis, 1790
Intravenous rt-PA, in acute ischemic stroke, 1519-1520, 1521t
Intraventricular conduction block
concealed, 172, 172f, 173f
electrocardiography in, 167-172, 168f, 168t, 169f, 169t, 171f-173f
electrophysiology in, 773, 773f
multifascicular, 170-172, 171f
in myocardial infarction, 1280-1281
rate-dependent, 172, 172f, 173f
sudden cardiac death and, 937, 944-945
Intraventricular conduction system, 728-731, 730f-733f
Intraventricular delay, chronic, electrophysiology in, 826t, 827
Intrinsicoid deflection
in left bundle branch block, 169
in QRS complex, 159
Introns, 71
Inward currents, 742
Inwardly rectifying potassium channel, 734f, 736, 743-744
Iodixanol, in patients with chronic kidney disease, 2160-2161, 2160f
Ion channels. See also specific channel, e.g., Calcium channel(s).
in generation of resting and action potentials, 738f
molecular structure of, 734f, 736
physiology of, 733-736, 734f, 735f
voltage-gated
ion flux through, 735, 735f
molecular structure of, 734f, 736
Ion exchangers and pumps, in contraction-relaxation cycle, 519-520, 520f
Ion-exchanging proteins, electroneutral, 742t
Ionic currents
in generation of resting and action potentials, 738f
inward, 742
modulation of, principles of, 735-736
synopsis of, 741t-742t
transmembrane, during activation, 149-150, 150f
Ionic permeability ratio, 734
IP$_3$. See Inositol triphosphate (IP$_3$).
Iron
deficiency of. See Anemia.
deposition of, in heart, 1754-1755
overload of. See also Hemochromatosis.
cardiomyopathy in, 402, 403f
replacement of, in cyanotic congenital heart disease, 1568
Ischemia
limb. See Limb ischemia.
mesenteric, chronic, 1535-1536
diagnosis of, 1536, 1536f, 1537f
percutaneous interventions in, 1536, 1537f
myocardial. See Myocardial ischemia.
Ischemia-modified albumin, diagnostic performance of, 1199

Ischemic attacks, transient, in elderly persons, 1940-1942
Ischemic cardiomyopathy. See Cardiomyopathy, ischemic.
Ischemic heart disease. See Coronary artery disease.
Ischemic memory, nuclear imaging of, 382, 383f
Ischemic preconditioning, 1238
  in diabetes mellitus, 1555
Ischemic rest leg pain, 1495
Ischemic stroke, acute. See Stroke, acute ischemic.
Ismelin. See Guanethidine (Ismelin).
Isoflurane, for noncardiac surgery, 2020
Isomerism
  definition of, 1593
  of left atrial appendages, 1594
  morphology of, 1593
  of right atrial appendages, 1593-1594
Isometric contraction, and force-velocity relationship, 533
Isoproterenol
  in atrioventricular block, 919
  in cardiac arrest, 963
  during cardiac catheterization, 460
  in myocardial infarction, 1268
  postoperative, 2001
  pulmonary vascular effects of, 1884
  in torsades de pointes, 905
  in upright tilt-table testing, 771-772, 772f, 979
Isosorbide dinitrate
  in acute heart failure, 601t
  in stable angina, 1368t, 1369
Isosorbide 5-mononitrate, in stable angina, 1368t, 1369
Isotonic contraction, and force-velocity relationship, 533
Isovolumic contraction, 527, 528f, 529-530
Isovolumic index, 252
Isovolumic relaxation, 527, 528f, 534-535, 535f
Isradipine
  pharmacokinetics of, 1375t
  in stable angina, 1376
Istaroxime, in acute heart failure, 605
Italy, cardiovascular disease in, 10
Ivabradine
  in sinus tachycardia, 867
  in stable angina, 1377

J

J curve, in hypertension therapy, 1051, 1051f
J point
  in exercise stress testing, 199, 199f, 200f
  in hypothermia, 185, 186f
JAK2 inhibitors, cardiotoxicity of, 2115
Janeway lesions, in infective endocarditis, 1720
Japan, cardiovascular disease in, 9, 10-11
Jarvik 2000 axial flow pump, 692, 693f
Jaundice, in heart failure, 563
Jervell and Lange-Nielsen syndrome, 101, 104, 105f. See also Long QT syndrome.
Job strain, cardiovascular disease and, 2121
Joint Commission on Accreditation of Healthcare Organizations, 49, 50t
Jones criteria, 2080f, 2081
Judkins catheter, for arteriography, 469-470, 469f
Judkins technique, for cardiac catheterization, 444, 444f, 445f-446f, 446-447

Jugular vein, examination of, 128-130, 128f-130f, 129t
Jugular venous pressure, in congenital heart disease, 1572
Jugular venous pulse
  abnormalities of, 129-130, 130f
  in cardiac tamponade, 1836, 1837
  in constrictive pericarditis, 1843
  examination of, 128-130, 128f-130f, 129t
  in heart failure, 141, 562, 593
  in mitral stenosis, 1649
  in myocardial infarction, 1222-1223
  in pulmonary hypertension, 1886
  in restrictive cardiomyopathy, 1750
  in tricuspid regurgitation, 130, 130f, 1676
  in tricuspid stenosis, 1674-1675
Junction or J point
  in exercise stress testing, 199, 199f, 200f
  in hypothermia, 185, 186f

K

Kaposi sarcoma, in HIV-infected patients, 1799
Karyotyping, 85-86
Kasabach-Merritt syndrome, 1823
Kawasaki disease, 2091-2092, 2092f
  definition of, 2092t
  sudden cardiac death and, 942
KCNH1 gene, 736
KCNH2 gene, 736
KCNQ1 gene, 736
Kearns-Sayre syndrome, 2148
Kerberos embolic protection system, 1426
Ketoconazole, in Cushing syndrome, 2036
Kidney(s). See also Renal entries.
  disease of. See Renal disease.
  failure of. See Renal failure.
  heart and, communication between, 2155, 2157f
  structure of, 2155, 2156f
Kinetic work, in myocardial oxygen uptake, 533
Knock, pericardial, in constrictive pericarditis, 1843
Knockout mouse, 78-79, 80f
Korotkoff sounds
  in aortic regurgitation, 1638
  evaluation of, 131
KRAS, mutations of, in Noonan syndrome, 119t, 121
Krupple-like factor-2 (KLF-2), in atherogenesis, 992, 992f
Kugelberg-Welander disease, 2148
Kussmaul sign, 130, 2105
  with cardiac catheterization, 460
  in constrictive pericarditis, 1843

L

Labetalol (Normodyne, Trandate)
  in aortic dissection, 1479
  in hypertension, 1061
  in hypertensive crises, 1066, 1066t
  pharmacokinetics and pharmacology of, 1373t
Labor and delivery, 1968. See also Pregnancy.
Lactic acid accumulation, during exercise, 196
Lactic acidosis, after arteriography, 468
Ladder diagram, in electrocardiography, 764, 767f
Lambda, 745

Lamin A and C gene
  in limb-girdle muscular dystrophy, 2145
  mutation of
    in dilated cardiomyopathy, 115t, 116
    in Emery-Dreifuss muscular dystrophy and associated disorders, 2143, 2144
Lanoteplase, 2068
Lapatinib, cardiotoxicity of, 2113
Laplace law, 530, 531f, 569-570, 570f
Laser-assisted myocardial revascularization, in stable angina, 1394-1395
Lasix. See Furosemide (Lasix).
Late potentials, in arrhythmia diagnosis, 763
Latin America, cardiovascular disease in, 10t, 13
Law of diminishing returns, in economic analysis, 35, 36f
LCAT deficiency, 1081
Lead(s)
  electrocardiographic, 151-154, 151f, 152t
    augmented limb, 152, 152t, 153f
    bipolar versus unipolar, 152
    in exercise stress testing, 199
    precordial, 152, 152t, 153f
    standard limb, 152, 152t, 153f
    in vectorcardiogram, 152, 154f
    vectors in, 152-154, 154f
  pacemaker, complications related to, 843-844, 843f-844f
Lead, cardiovascular effects of, 1813
Leading circle reentry, 758, 760f
Leapfrog, 49, 50t, 1993
Leber hereditary optic neuropathy, 2148
Lecithin cholesterol acyltransferase, 1071, 1072f
  deficiency of, 1081
Left anterior fascicular block
  electrocardiography in, 167-168, 168f, 168t
  inferior wall myocardial infarction in, 179
Left axis deviation
  in congenital heart disease, 1572
  in left anterior fascicular block, 167-168
Left bundle branch block (LBBB). See also Fascicular block.
  characteristics of, 864t-865t
  clinical significance of, 169-170
  electrocardiography in, 168-170, 169f, 169t
  exercise stress testing in, 212, 212f
  incomplete form of, 169
  left ventricular hypertrophy and, 164
  in myocardial infarction, 178-179, 179f, 180f
  myocardial perfusion imaging in, 375
  pseudoinfarct patterns in, 180
Left cardiac sympathetic denervation (LCSD), in long QT syndrome, 103
Left posterior fascicular block, electrocardiography in, 168, 168f, 168t
Left ventricular assist device
  in heart failure, 559, 559t
  percutaneous, 1422
Left ventricular contractility index, in elderly persons, 1925f
Left ventricular diastolic pressure, in mitral stenosis, 1648
Left ventricular ejection fraction
  after coronary artery bypass graft surgery, 667-668, 668t
  definition of, 571

I-50 Left ventricular ejection fraction
(*Continued*)
echocardiographic measurement of,
247-248
in heart failure, 573
normal values for, 571
reduced, heart failure with, 611-639.
See also Heart failure, systolic.
sudden cardiac death and, 938, 939
Left ventricular end-diastolic pressure
(LVEDP), 263
in aortic stenosis, 1627
Doppler echocardiography of, 263
as indicator of cardiac function, 570
measurement of, 570
Left ventricular end-diastolic volume
(LVEDV)
in aortic regurgitation, 1637, 1639f
in mitral regurgitation, 1659-1660,
1660f
Left ventricular filling pressure
assessment of, 141
in heart failure, 141
Left ventricular noncompaction,
computed tomography in, 431f
Left ventricular outflow tract ventricular
tachycardia, 907
Left ventricular pressure change (dp/dt),
in Doppler echocardiography, 266-
267, 267f
Left ventricular–femoral artery pressure
gradient, 455
Left-to-right shunt(s), 1577-1587. *See also*
specific defects, e.g, Atrial septal
defect.
detection of, cardiac catheterization for,
458-459
Leg(s)
pain in
exertional, 1494-1495, 1494t. *See also*
Claudication, intermittent.
ischemic rest, 1495
segmental pressure measurement in,
1496, 1497f
ulcers in, in peripheral arterial disease,
1495, 1496f
Legumes, intake of, cardiovascular
disease and, 1108
Leiomyosarcoma, 1818t, 1825
in HIV-infected patients, 1799
Leopard syndrome, 1571
Lepirudin
in chronic kidney disease patients,
2164t
in heparin-induced thrombocytopenia,
2064
Lescol. *See* Fluvastatin (Lescol).
Leukocyte(s)
in atherogenesis, 989-991, 990f, 991f
count of
in preoperative risk analysis, 1994
in UA/NSTEMI, 1325
in myocardial infarction, 1220, 1227
Leukocyte adhesion molecules (LAMs),
in atherogenesis, 990-991
Leukocytosis, in infective endocarditis,
1722
Lever-arm model of cross-bridge cycling,
512, 515f
Levine sign, in myocardial infarction,
1222
Levitronix ventricular assist device, 692
Levosimendan, in acute heart failure,
601t, 604-605
Levothyroxine sodium, in
hypothyroidism, 2042f, 2043
Lewis cycle, 528f

Libman-Sacks endocarditis, in systemic
lupus erythematosus, 2098, 2098f
Lidocaine, 788-789
adverse effects of, 789
in cardiac arrest, 962, 963
dosage and administration of, 783t,
789
electrophysiological characteristics of,
780t, 781t, 782t, 786t, 788
in heart failure, 64
hemodynamic effects of, 788
indications for, 789
in myocardial infarction, 1278
pharmacokinetics of, 59-60, 783t,
788-789
in pregnancy, 1976t
prophylactic, for ventricular fibrillation,
1278
psychiatric side effects of, 2132
in torsades de pointes, 905
in ventricular premature complexes,
895
Life expectancy, 9, 1930, 1930t
Life support, in cardiac arrest
management
advanced, 961-963, 961f, 962f
basic, 958-960, 959f, 960f
Lifestyle
coronary artery disease in women and,
1957
dyslipidemia and, 1082, 1089
modification of
in diabetes mellitus, 1099
in hypertension therapy, 1052-1054,
1052t
in idiopathic pulmonary arterial
hypertension, 1896
in myocardial infarction prevention,
1289-1290
in stable angina, 1367
sudden cardiac death and, 938-939
Life-sustaining treatment, in end-stage
heart disease
patient's right to refuse or terminate,
720-721
withdrawing and withholding, 722
Light microscopy, of myocardial
infarction, 1212, 1213f, 1214f
Lightheadedness, in hypertrophic
cardiomyopathy, 1768
Likelihood ratios, in assessing test
performance, 42-43
Limb ischemia
acute, 1507-1509
classification of, 1507-1508, 1508t
diagnostic testing in, 1507
pathogenesis of, 1508
prognosis in, 1507-1508, 1508t
treatment of, 1508-1509, 1509f, 1509t
critical
in diabetes mellitus, 1095
in fibromuscular dysplasia, 1507
in peripheral arterial disease
classification of, 1495, 1496t
incidence of, 1491
pathophysiology of, 1493, 1494,
1494f
progression to, 1500
risk factors for, 1492
Limb-girdle muscular dystrophy,
2144-2145
Linkage analysis, in molecular genetics,
76
Linkage disequilibrium, 76
Linoleic acid, cholesterol and, 1112
Lipanor. *See* Ciprofibrate (Lypanthyl,
Lipanor).

Lipid(s)
accumulation of, in atherogenesis
extracellular, 989, 990f
intracellular, 990f, 992-993
biochemistry of, 1071-1072, 1072f
levels of
dietary influences on, 1112-1113,
1112f
in myocardial infarction, 1227
regional trends in, 16-17
in UA/NSTEMI, 1323
in women, 1957
metabolism of, alcohol intake and, 1806
Lipid screening, in stable angina, 1356
Lipidil Micro. *See* Fenofibrate (Tricor,
Lipidil Micro).
Lipid-lowering therapy
ACCORD trial in, 1086-1087
in acute coronary syndromes, 1088
ALL-HAT trial in, 1085t, 1086
approach to, 1088-1091
ASCOT trial in, 1085t, 1086
ASTEROID trial in, 1088
A-to-Z trial in, 1088
AVERT trial in, 1088
benefits of, 1128-1129, 1129f
bile acid–binding resins in, 1082-1083
BIP trial in, 1086
in cardiac rehabilitation, 1154
in cardiovascular disease prevention,
1128-1131, 1129f, 1130f, 1130t
CARDS trial in, 1086
cholesterol absorption inhibitors in,
1083
cholesterol ester transfer protein
inhibitors (CETP) in, 1084
clinical trials of, 1084-1088, 1085t,
1087f, 1087t
in combined lipoprotein disorders,
1089-1090
after coronary artery bypass graft
surgery, 1385
COURAGE trial in, 1088
in diabetic patients, 1086, 1090,
1101-1102, 1101t
diet in, 1089, 1112-1113, 1112f, 1131
drugs used for
clinical trials of, 1084-1088, 1085t,
1087t
description of, 1082-1084, 1082t
economic analysis of, 39, 39t, 1129
in elderly persons, 1090-1091,
1935-1936, 1935t
extracorporeal LDL lipoprotein
filtration in, 1090
fibric acid derivatives/fibrates in, 1083
FIELD trial in, 1086
fish oils in, 1084
future developments in, 1090
gene therapy in, 1091
guidelines on, 1129-1131, 1130f, 1130t
herbal, 1158, 1162
HPS trial in, 1085, 1085t
in hypertensive patients, 1085t, 1086
IDEAL trial in, 1087-1088, 1087t
MIRACL trial in, 1088
monitoring in, 1084
in myocardial infarction prevention,
1290
nicotinic acid (niacin) in, 1083-1084
novel approaches to, 1090
in peripheral arterial disease, 1500,
1502f, 1503f
phytosterols in, 1084
preoperative use of, 2026
for primary prevention, 1084-1088,
1085t

Lipid-lowering therapy *(Continued)*
PROSPER trial in, 1085-1086, 1085t
PROVE-IT trial in, 1088
regression studies of, 1088
versus revascularization, 1088
REVERSAL trial in, 1088
for secondary prevention, 1087-1088, 1087f, 1087t
in silent myocardial ischemia, 1397
in stable angina, 1363
statins in. *See* Statin therapy.
TNT trial in, 1087, 1087t
in UA/NSTEMI, 1335, 1335f
VA-HIT trial in, 1086
in women, 1961
Lipitor. *See* Atorvastatin (Lipitor).
Lipodystrophy, 1082
Lipoma, 1818t, 1819-1820
cardiovascular magnetic resonance in, 405, 406f
computed tomography of, 429
Lipomatous atrial hypertrophy, 1818t, 1820, 1821f, 1822
cardiovascular magnetic resonance in, 405
echocardiography in, 304, 304f
Lipoprotein(a), 1072, 1073t
as atherosclerotic risk factor, 1019-1020, 1019f
in cardiovascular disease prevention, 1141
genetic disorders of, 1079
plasma, dietary influences on, 1116
in stable angina, 1356
Lipoprotein(s)
apolipoprotein content of, 1072, 1074t
disorders of, 1077-1082. *See also*
Dyslipidemia;
Hypercholesterolemia;
Hyperlipidemia.
enzymes processing, 1075t
high-density, 1072, 1073f, 1073t
cardiovascular disease risk and, 1008, 1008f, 1128, 1129, 1131
in diabetes mellitus, 1101
dietary management of, 1112f, 1113
genetic disorders of, 1081
metabolism of, 1074f, 1076-1077, 1077f-1078f
receptors for, 1073
in stable angina, 1363
intermediate-density, 1072, 1073f, 1073t
formation of, 1074f, 1075-1076
low-density, 1072, 1073f, 1073t
cardiovascular disease risk and, 1007-1008, 1008f, 1128-1131, 1129f, 1130f, 1130t
C-reactive protein (hs-CRP) level and, 1014, 1014f
dietary management of, 1112-1113, 1112f
extracorporeal filtration of, 1090
formation of, 1074f, 1076, 1077f-1078f
genetic disorders of, 1078-1080
receptors for, 1072
small, dense particles of
in diabetes mellitus, 1101
in stable angina, 1356
subclasses of, 1008
particle size and concentration of, 1008
plasma, composition of, 1073t
receptors for, 1072-1073, 1075t
size of, 1072, 1073f
structure of, 1072, 1072f
subclasses of, 1008
target levels of, 1089

Lipoprotein(s) *(Continued)*
transport of, 1073-1077, 1074f
hepatic pathway in, 1074f, 1075-1076
intestinal pathway in, 1073, 1074f, 1075
triglyceride-rich, 1072, 1073f, 1073t
cardiovascular disease risk and, 1009
genetic disorders of, 1079
very-low-density, 1072, 1073f, 1073t
hepatic synthesis of, 1074f, 1075-1076
Lipoprotein lipase, 1075
Lipoprotein-associated phospholipase A_2, in stable angina, 1356
Lipoprotein-x, 1082
Liquid chromatography, 78
Lisinopril
in chronic kidney disease patients, 2165t
in heart failure, 624t
Lithium
cardiovascular aspects of, 2131, 2131t
in congenital heart disease, 1563
drug interactions of, 2132, 2133, 2133t
Liver
cirrhosis of
cardiac surgery in patients with, 1996
pulmonary arterial hypertension in, 1901
clearance in, in elderly persons, 1928
in constrictive pericarditis, 1843
in heart failure, 564
in lipoprotein transport, 1074f, 1075-1076
Liver disease
dose adjustments in, 64
dyslipidemia in, 1082
in Fontan patients, 1595
Liver function tests, in heart failure, 594
Living will, in end-stage heart disease, 720-721
Lixivaptan, in heart failure, 621t, 624
Löffler endocarditis, restrictive cardiomyopathy in, 1756-1757
Long QT syndrome
acquired, 906
Brugada syndrome and, 105
cardiac arrest in, primary prevention of, 970
clinical manifestations of, 101, 103, 103t, 104f, 906
early afterdepolarizations in, 748f, 750, 752f
electrocardiography in, 101, 103f, 905f, 906
genetic basis of, 101, 102t
genotype-phenotype correlation studies in, 103-104, 104f
in HIV-infected patients, 1800-1801
idiopathic (congenital), 906
management of, 906
natural history of, 104
risk stratification in, 104, 105f
sudden cardiac death in, 945
torsades de pointes in, 906
Long QT(U) syndrome, 184
Loop diuretics, 1057t, 1058
dose-response curves for, 626, 627f
in heart failure, 600, 601t, 620, 621t, 622, 625
mechanisms of action of, 622
Lopid. *See* Gemfibrozil (Lopid).
Lopressor. *See* Metoprolol (Lopressor, Toprol).
Lorazepam, cardiovascular aspects of, 2132t

Losartan (Cozaar)
in diabetes mellitus, 1102-1103, 1102t
in heart failure, 624t, 629
in Marfan syndrome, 92
Lovastatin (Mevacor), in dyslipidemia, 1083
Low- and middle-income countries, cardiovascular disease in
global burden of, 10t, 11-13, 12f
global trends in, 14-15, 14t
strategies to reduce, 19-21
Low output syndrome, postoperative, 2000-2001, 2000t
Low-density lipoprotein (LDL), 1072, 1073f, 1073t
cardiovascular disease risk and, 1007-1008, 1008f, 1128-1131, 1129f, 1130f, 1130t
C-reactive protein (hs-CRP) level and, 1014, 1014f
dietary management of, 1112-1113, 1112f
extracorporeal filtration of, 1090
formation of, 1074f, 1076, 1077f-1078f
genetic disorders of, 1078-1080
receptors for, 1072
small, dense particles of, in diabetes mellitus, 1101
subclasses of, 1008
Low-molecular-weight heparin. *See* Heparin, low-molecular-weight.
Lown-Ganong-Levine syndrome, 757-758, 884
Low-output heart failure, 584, 584t
Lumbosacral radiculopathy, exertional leg pain in, 1495
Lung(s). *See also* Pulmonary *entries*.
amiodarone toxicity to, 795
anatomy of, 1883
biopsy of
in atrioventricular septal defect, 1582
in Eisenmenger syndrome, 1569
cancer of, superior vena cava syndrome in, 2106-2107, 2107t
chest radiography of, 331, 335, 336f, 337f
physiology of, 1883-1886, 1885f
transplantation of
in chronic obstructive pulmonary disease, 1908-1909
in Eisenmenger syndrome, 1570
in idiopathic pulmonary arterial hypertension, 1900
volume reduction surgery of, in chronic obstructive pulmonary disease, 1908
Lung scan
in pulmonary artery stenosis, 1616
in pulmonary embolism, 1868, 1870
in pulmonary hypertension, 1888, 1888f
in thromboembolic pulmonary hypertension, 1910
Lung uptake, in single photon emission computed tomography, 352, 352f
Lupus anticoagulants, 2061
Lupus erythematosus. *See* Systemic lupus erythematosus.
Lutembacher syncope, 1647
Lyme disease, myocarditis in, 1778-1779
Lymphangiogenesis, 81
Lymphangioma, 1816, 1818t, 1823
Lymphatic disorders, genetic studies in, 97
Lymphedema, hereditary, 97
Lymphocyte-selective chemokines, in atherogenesis, 991

I-52

Lymphoma, 1826
  cardiac, primary, 1818t
  computed tomography of, 430, 430f
  non-Hodgkin, in HIV-infected patients, 1799
  superior vena cava syndrome in, 2107, 2107f
Lypanthyl. *See* Ciprofibrate (Lypanthyl, Lipanor).
Lysosomal protein mutations, 114
Lysosome, 68, 68f, 510t
Lysosome-associated membrane protein (LAMP2), mutation of, in Danon disease, 114

M

M cells
  in long QT syndrome, 906
  in torsades de pointes, 905
Machado-Guerreiro test, in Chagas disease, 1780
Macrophage colony-stimulating factor (M-CSF), in foam cell replication, 992-993
Magnesium
  abnormalities of, electrocardiography in, 185
  as dietary supplement, 1160t
  in eclampsia, 1045
  intake of, blood pressure and, 1114
  in myocardial infarction, 1264, 1278
  in quinidine-induced syncope, 786
  supplementation of, in hypertension therapy, 1053
  in torsades de pointes, 905
Magnesium sulfate, in cardiac arrest, 962
Magnetic resonance angiography, 394
  in abdominal aortic aneurysms, 1460
  of coronary arteries, 399, 400f
  of great vessels, 409, 409f
  in peripheral arterial disease, 1498, 1499f
  of renal arteries, 409, 410f
  in renovascular hypertension, 1040
  in thoracic aortic aneurysm, 1465f, 1466
Magnetic resonance imaging, 393-414
  in acute coronary syndromes, 397
  in amyloidosis, 1752
  in aortic dissection, 1476
  in aortic regurgitation, 1641
  in aortic stenosis, 1631
  appropriateness guidelines for, 412-414, 413t-414t
  in arrhythmogenic right ventricular cardiomyopathy, 402
  of atrial and ventricular morphology, 407
  in atrioventricular connection abnormalities, 407-408
  in cardiac amyloidosis, 403
  in cardiac tumors, 405, 406f, 1817, 1824f
  in cardiomyopathy, 401-403, 401f-403f
  in coarctation of the aorta, 1607
  in congenital heart disease, 407-409, 407f-408f, 1573
  in constrictive pericarditis, 1844-1845
  contrast agents for, 394
  in coronary artery anomalies, 409
  in coronary artery disease, 394-401, 395f-400f
  of diastolic function, 575, 576f, 577f
  in dilated cardiomyopathy, 401, 401f, 1748
  dobutamine, 397, 398f
  in Ebstein anomaly, 1605
  electromagnetic interference during, 850-851

Magnetic resonance imaging (Continued)
  in Fontan patients, 1595
  future perspectives on, 410
  gating in, 394, 567
  in great vessel abnormalities, 407, 407f
  in heart failure, 567-568, 567t, 568f
  in heart transplantation, 403-404
  in hypertrophic cardiomyopathy, 401-402, 402f, 1764, 1766f
  in infective endocarditis, 1722
  interventional, 410
  intravascular, 410
  in iron overload cardiomyopathy, 402, 403f
  late enhancement, 395, 395f, 396f, 397, 567, 568f
  in mitral regurgitation, 1664
  in mitral valve prolapse, 1672
  of myocardial hibernation, 397, 397f
  in myocardial infarction, 395, 395f-397f, 397, 1229, 1230f
  of myocardial perfusion, 397-399, 398f, 399f
  in myocardial sarcoidosis, 402-403
  of myocardial viability, 395, 397, 397f
  in myocarditis, 403, 1786-1787, 1786f
  in partial anomalous pulmonary venous drainage, 1620
  in pericardial disease, 405, 405f
  in pericardial effusion and tamponade, 1838
  principles of, 393-394
  of prosthetic valves, 405
  in pulmonary artery stenosis, 1616
  in pulmonary embolism, 1870
  in pulmonary vein stenosis, 1619, 1619f
  in pulmonic regurgitation, 1679f, 1680
  of right ventricular function, 577, 578t
  safety of, 394
  scanner for, 393-394
  in septal defects, 408-409, 408f
  sequences in, 394
  in single ventricle, 409
  in stable angina, 1359
  stress, 397, 398f
  in tetralogy of Fallot, 409, 1589
  in total anomalous pulmonary venous drainage, 1597
  in transposition of the great arteries
    complete, 1600
    congenitally corrected, 1602
  in valvular heart disease, 404-405, 404f, 409
  in vascular rings, 1610
  of ventricular volumes, mass, and function, 394-395
  in ventriculoarterial connection abnormalities, 408, 408f
Mahaim conduction, in Wolff-Parkinson-White syndrome, 884
Ma-huang, in autonomic failure, 2176
Marathon racing, risks of, 1985
Marfan syndrome, 90-93
  aortic dissection in, 92, 1470
  aortic root involvement in, 91-92, 91f
  arrhythmias in, 92
  cardiovascular manifestations of, 90t
  diagnostic criteria for, 90, 90t, 91f
  echocardiography in, 299, 299f
  exercise and sports in patients with, 1990
  forme fruste of, 1464
  genetic studies in, 92-93
  left ventricular dysfunction in, 92
  management of, 92
  mitral valve involvement in, 90-91
  multivalvular heart disease in, 1680

Marfan syndrome (Continued)
  in pregnancy, 1974
  thoracic abnormalities in, 92
  thoracic aortic aneurysm in, 1464, 1466
Mason-Likar modification, in electrocardiography, 199
Mass, cardiac, echocardiography of, 302-304, 302f-305f, 320, 320t
MASS phenotype
  cardiovascular manifestations of, 90t
  in mitral valve prolapse, 93
Mass spectrometry, 77-78, 78f
Mast cells, in heart failure, 556-557, 557f
Matrix metalloproteinases
  in abdominal aortic aneurysms, 1459
  in atherosclerosis, 994
  classes of, 557, 557t
  in heart failure, 557
  in myocarditis, 1784
Maximal velocity of contraction (V_{max}), 533
Maximal work capacity, during exercise stress testing, 204, 205f
Maximum heart rate, 195
Maximum oxygen uptake (VO_{2max}), 1149
  in heart failure, 565-566
Maze procedure, in atrial fibrillation, 812, 815t, 873
McArdle syndrome, exertional leg pain in, 1495
Meals, orthostatic hypotension after, 976
Mechanical circulatory support, 685-696.
  See also specific device, e.g.,
    Intraaortic balloon counterpulsation.
  devices for, 685-696
  future directions in, 696
  history of, 685
  postoperative, 2001
Mechanical index, in echocardiography, 242
Mechanical load, effects of, on contraction-relaxation cycle, 535-537, 536f, 537f, 537t
Mechanical myocardial protection, during percutaneous coronary intervention, 1309
Mechanical prosthetic valves
  durability of, 1683
  indications for, 1687-1688, 1687f
  thrombogenicity of, 1683
  types of, 1682-1683, 1682f
Mechanical stress, left ventricular response to, 536, 536f, 537f
Mechanical ventilation
  in cardiac arrest, 959
  in end-stage heart disease, withdrawal of, 722
Median neuropathy, after cardiac surgery, 1998
Median sternotomy, technique for, 1860, 1860f
Mediastinitis, postoperative, 2008
Medical costs, measurement of, 35-36. *See also* Economic analysis.
Medical decision-making. *See* Decision-making.
Medical genetics, principles of, 87-89, 87f, 88f, 89t
Medicare, reimbursement of cardiac rehabilitation by, 1154
Medicare D drug therapy, 1931
Meditation
  in hypertension, 2124
  for stress management, 1157
Mediterranean-style diet(s), 1110, 1110f
Medtronic Freestyle valve, 1684f, 1686
Medtronic Intact valve, 1684, 1684f

Medtronic-Hall valve, 1682, 1682f
Megestrol acetate, in HIV-infected patients, complications of, 1803t
Meige lymphedema, 97
MELAS syndrome, 2148
Membrane. See Cell membrane.
Membrane potential. See also Action potential.
  ionic fluxes regulating, 738, 738f
  loss of, in arrhythmogenesis, 745-746, 746f
  recording of, 738-739, 738f
  resting, 738, 738f, 738t, 739
    reduced, effects of, 746, 746f
Membrane-type matrix metalloproteinases, 557, 557t
Mendelian inheritance
  in congenital heart disease, 118-121, 119t
  in hypertension, 1042, 1042f
  in vascular disorders, 89-94, 90t
Mendelian phenotype, 87-88, 87f, 88f
Meningitis, in infective endocarditis, 1721
Menopause
  cardiovascular disease risk during, 1139-1140
  hormone replacement therapy after. See Hormone replacement therapy.
Mental status, altered, in heart failure, 591
Mental stress, cardiovascular disease and, 1012, 2121-2122
MERCI clot retriever, in acute ischemic stroke, 1520-1521
Mercury, cardiovascular effects of, 1813
MERRF syndrome, 2148
Mesenteric arterial disease, in women, 1964
Mesenteric ischemia
  in aortic dissection, 1473, 1482
  chronic, 1535-1536
    diagnosis of, 1536, 1536f, 1537f
    percutaneous interventions in, 1536, 1537f
Mesoangioblasts, 698
Meta-analyses, of cardiovascular disease prevention, 1120
Metabolic abnormalities
  in diabetes mellitus, 1096-1097, 1100, 1100t
  from marathon racing, 1985
  pacemaker interference by, 851
Metabolic acidosis
  in cardiac arrest, 962
  after cardiac surgery, 1999
Metabolic agents, in stable angina, 1377
Metabolic alkalosis, from diuretics, 626
Metabolic cardiac injury, 1856-1857
Metabolic cardiomyopathy, genetic studies in, 114
Metabolic equivalent
  definition of, 1983
  in exercise stress testing, 197
Metabolic modulation, in heart failure, 710-711, 711f
Metabolic syndrome
  as atherosclerotic risk factor, 1009-1010, 1010f
  components of, 1100
  C-reactive protein (hs-CRP) in, 1009, 1010f, 1015
  definition of, 1009
  dyslipidemia in, 1082
  hypertriglyceridemia and, 1113
  inflammation in, 1096, 1096f

Metabolic syndrome (Continued)
  myocardial infarction in patients with, prognosis after, 1549
  obstructive sleep apnea and, 1916
  racial/ethnic differences in, 23
  treatment of, 1099, 1100, 1135
Metabolism-perfusion match, imaging of, 367, 370f
Metallic implant, in cardiovascular magnetic resonance, 394
Metastatic calcifications, in hyperparathyroidism, 2038
Metazoal myocarditis, 1780
Metformin, in diabetic patients with cardiovascular disease, 1557
Methadone, in HIV-infected patients, complications of, 1803t
Methemoglobinemia, nitroglycerin-induced, 1263
Methotrexate, in Takayasu arteritis, 2089
Methyldopa (Aldomet)
  in baroreflex failure, 2178
  in chronic kidney disease patients, 2165t
  drug interactions of, 2133
  in hypertension, 1059
  in pregnancy, 1976t
  psychiatric side effects of, 2132
Methylene tetrahydrofolate reductase (MTHFR) gene, in homocysteinuria, 1017
Methylergonovine maleate, during cardiac catheterization, 460
Methylphenidate, cardiovascular aspects of, 2129t, 2130
Metolazone (Mykrox, Zaroxolyn)
  in heart failure, 600, 621t, 627
  in hypertension, 1058
Metoprolol (Lopressor, Toprol), 792-793
  in cardiac arrest, 962
  in heart failure, 624t, 630, 630t, 631, 632f
  in myocardial infarction, 1238, 1259, 1260, 1261f
  pharmacokinetics and pharmacology of, 1372t
  preoperative use of, 2024-2025
  in UA/NSTEMI, 1327
Mevacor. See Lovastatin (Mevacor).
Mexican Americans, cardiovascular mortality in, 25
Mexiletine
  in arrhythmias, 780t, 781t, 782t, 783t, 786t, 789
  in chronic kidney disease patients, 2165t
  in long QT syndrome, 103
  in periodic paralyses, 2148
  in torsades de pointes, 905
Microalbuminuria
  definition of, 2156
  in hypertension, 1037-1038
Microbial surface components recognizing adhesive matrix molecules, in infective endocarditis, 1719
Microcirculatory coronary reserve, pathophysiological states affecting, 1182-1183, 1182f-1184f
"Microcosting," 36
Microgravity exposure, prolonged, autonomic tone after, 2182
Micromanometer catheter(s), 449, 451
MicroMed DeBakey axial flow pump, 692, 692f
Microscopic polyangiitis, 2093
Microvascular angina pectoris, 1395

Microvascular obstruction, in critical limb ischemia, 1494, 1494f
Micturition syncope, 977
Midamor. See Amiloride (Midamor).
Middle East, cardiovascular disease in, 10t, 13
Middle internodal tract, 728
Midodrine
  in autonomic failure, 2176
  in chronic fatigue syndrome, 2178
  in neurally mediated syncope, 983
Migraine
  hemiplegic, familial, 95-96
  patent foramen ovale and, 1580
Milrinone
  in acute heart failure, 601t, 604
  in chronic kidney disease patients, 2165, 2165t
  in myocardial infarction, 1269
  postoperative, 2001
Mind-body therapy, in patients undergoing cardiac surgery, 1164
Mindfulness-based stress reduction, 1157
Mineralization, in atherosclerotic plaque, 995
Mineralocorticoid hypertension, 1041-1042, 1041f, 1041t, 1042f
Mineralocorticoid receptor, actions of, 2036, 2036f
Mineralocorticoid receptor antagonists, in heart failure, 621t, 622-623, 623f
Minipress. See Prazosin (Minipress).
Minoxidil, in hypertension, 1061
Minute ventilation, during exercise, 197
Mirtazapine, cardiovascular aspects of, 2129t, 2130
Missense mutation, 75, 75f
Missiles, intracardiac, 1856
Misuse, as error in health care, 52
Mitochondria, 68, 68f, 509, 510t
Mitochondrial disorders, 2148
Mitochondrial function, nuclear imaging of, 367
Mitochondrial inheritance, 88, 88f
Mitochondrial syndromes, dilated cardiomyopathy in, 117
Mitogen-activating protein (MAP) kinase signaling pathway, in left ventricular response to mechanical stress, 536, 536f, 537f
Mitosis, 68, 69f
Mitral annulus
  calcification of, 1650, 1657-1658
    chest radiography in, 338, 339f
    in elderly persons, 1948
  dilatation of, 1657, 1658f
  echocardiography of, 248
Mitral balloon valvuloplasty, echocardiography in, 269, 271t
Mitral facies, in mitral stenosis, 127, 1649
Mitral flow filling pattern, pseudonormalized, 250-251
Mitral regurgitation, 1657-1669
  acute, 1668-1669
  angiography in, 1664
  in antiphospholipid antibody syndrome, 2099, 2099f
  with aortic regurgitation, 1681
  with aortic stenosis, 1681
  auscultation in, 1662
  chest radiography in, 337-338, 339f, 1664
  chordae tendinae abnormalities in, 1658f, 1659
  clinical presentation in, 1662-1664
  congenital, 1614-1615
  in coronary artery disease, 1399-1400

Mitral regurgitation (Continued)
differential diagnosis of, 1662-1663
in Duchenne and Becker muscular
    dystrophies, 2136
echocardiography in, 272-275, 272f-275f,
    1658f, 1663-1664
in elderly persons, 1948
electrocardiography in, 1664
end-systolic volume in, 1661
etiology and pathology of, 1657-1659,
    1657f, 1657t
exercise and sports in patients with,
    1989
functional, 273-274, 275f
hemodynamics in, 1661, 1661f
in hypertrophic cardiomyopathy, 1766
ischemic, 256, 258
left atrial compliance in, 1661-1662
left ventricular compensation in, 1659-
    1660, 1660f
left ventricular dysfunction in, 1659
magnetic resonance imaging in, 1664
in Marfan syndrome, 91, 92
with mitral valve prolapse, 1673-1674
murmur in, 136-137, 138f
myocardial contractility in, 1660-1661
natural history of, 1664, 1665f
in papillary muscle dysfunction, 1659
in papillary muscle rupture, 1275,
    1277f
pathophysiology of, 1659-1662, 1660f,
    1661f
physical examination in, 144-145,
    1662-1663, 1663t
practice guidelines for, 1702-1704,
    1703t-1704t
in pregnancy, 1972
radionuclide angiography in, 1664
in rheumatic fever, 2082
severity of, classification of, 1629t
symptoms of, 144-145, 1662
treatment of, 1665-1669, 1668f
    acute, 1669
    medical, 1665
    percutaneous valve repair in, 1442,
        1443f
    surgical, 669-671, 671f, 1665-1668,
        1666f, 1667f
Mitral stenosis, 1646-1657
acute rheumatic fever and, interval
    between, 1651, 1651f
angiography in, 1651
with aortic regurgitation, 1680-1681
with aortic stenosis, 1681
atrial fibrillation in, 1652, 1653
auscultation in, 1649-1650
cardiac catheterization in, 1651
chest radiography in, 337, 337f, 338f,
    1651
clinical presentation in, 1649-1651
complications of, 1652
congenital, 1614, 1647
differential diagnosis of, 1650
echocardiography in, 269-270, 270f,
    271t, 1647f, 1650-1651
in elderly persons, 1948
electrocardiography in, 167f, 1651
embolism in, 1652
etiology of, 1646-1647, 1647f
exercise and sports in patients with,
    1648, 1989
exercise stress testing in, 215
infective endocarditis in, 1652
left atrial changes in, 1649
left atrial pressure in, 1648, 1648f
left ventricular diastolic pressure in,
    1648

Mitral stenosis (Continued)
murmur in, 137, 1650
natural history of, 1651-1652, 1651f,
    1652f
noncardiac surgery in patients with,
    2015
opening snap in, 136
pathophysiology of, 1647-1649, 1648f
physical examination in, 144,
    1649-1650
practice guidelines for, 1699,
    1700t-1701t
in pregnancy, 1972
pressure gradient determination in, 456,
    456f
pulmonary arterial pressure in, 1648,
    1648f
pulmonary hypertension in, 1648, 1904
rheumatic, 1441-1442, 1442f, 1646-1647,
    1647f
severity of, classification of, 1629t
symptoms of, 144, 1649
treatment of, 1652-1657, 1653f
    for arrhythmias, 1653
    medical, 1652-1653
    mitral valve replacement in,
        1656-1657
    valvotomy in
        closed, 1655-1656
        open, 1656
        percutaneous, 1653-1655, 1654f,
            1655f
        restenosis after, 1656
    with tricuspid stenosis, 1674-1675
Mitral valve
abnormalities of, in hypertrophic
    cardiomyopathy, 1765
anatomy of, 1657, 1657f
area of, calculation of, 265, 265f, 269-
    270, 457
computed tomography of, 423, 423f
leaflets of
    abnormalities of, 1657, 1658f
    myxomatous proliferation of,
        1669-1670
normal anatomy of, 1564
opening snap of, 1649-1650
reconstruction of
    in mitral regurgitation, 1665-1668,
        1666f, 1667f
    in mitral valve prolapse, 1673-1674
repair of, percutaneous, 1442, 1443f
replacement of
    in mitral regurgitation, 1666-1668,
        1666f, 1667f
    in mitral stenosis, 1656-1657
    volume of, as marker of quality of
        cardiovascular care, 53f, 53t
scallops of, identification of, 274-275,
    275f
surgery of, coronary artery bypass graft
    surgery with, 1400
systolic anterior motion of, in
    hypertrophic cardiomyopathy,
    1766
Mitral valve annuloplasty, in dilated
    cardiomyopathy, 669-671, 671f
Mitral valve prolapse, 1669-1674
angiography in, 1672
arrhythmias in, 1672, 1673
auscultation in, 1670-1671, 1670f
classification of, 1669t
clinical presentation in, 1670-1672
computed tomography in, 1672
definition of, 1669
echocardiography in, 273, 274f,
    1671-1672, 1671f

Mitral valve prolapse (Continued)
electrocardiography in, 1672
etiology of, 1669
exercise stress testing in, 215
familial, 1669
genetic studies in, 93, 120
infective endocarditis in, 1713-1714
magnetic resonance imaging in, 1672
management of, 1673-1674
in Marfan syndrome, 90-91, 92
MASS phenotype in, 93
natural history of, 1672-1673, 1672t,
    1673f
pathology of, 1669-1670
physical examination in, 1670-1671,
    1670f
practice guidelines for, 1699, 1702,
    1702t
stress myocardial perfusion imaging in,
    1672
sudden cardiac death in, 944, 1673
Mitral valvuloplasty, percutaneous, 1441-
    1442, 1442f
Mixed venous oxygen content, in shunt
    quantification, 459
MMF. See Mycophenolate mofetil (MMF).
M-mode echocardiography. See
    Echocardiography, M-mode.
Mobilization strategies, in myocardial
    repair and regeneration, 703-705,
    705t
Mobitz type I (Wenckebach)
    atrioventricular block, 914-917,
    916f
Mobitz type II atrioventricular block,
    914-917, 917f
Modification of Diet in Renal Disease
    equation, for creatine clearance,
    2155
Molecular biology, 67-82
    blotting techniques in, 73-74, 73f
    cloning and recombinant DNA in, 73
    murine models of cardiovascular
        disease in, 78-79, 80f
    polymerase chain reaction in, 74, 74f
    principles and techniques of, 72-74, 73f,
        74f
Molecular fingerprinting techniques, for
    graft rejection surveillance, 679
Molecular genetics
    association studies in, 76
    cDNA microarrays in, 76-77, 77f
    complex trait analysis in, 75-76, 76f
    future directions in, 82
    genome-wide scans in, 76
    genomics in, 76-77, 77f. See also
        Genomics.
    genotype in, 74
    identification of disease-causing genes
        in, 74-76, 75f, 76f
    linkage analysis in, 76
    of monogenic disorders, 75, 75f
    oligonucleotide microarrays in, 77
    principles of, 74-78, 75f-78f
    proteomics in, 77-78, 78f
    SAGE technique in, 77
Monocyte chemoattractant protein-1
    (MCP-1), in atherogenesis, 991
Monogenic disorders, molecular genetics
    of, 75, 75f
Monosomy, 86
Monoxidine, in heart failure, 632
Monteplase, 2068
Mood stabilizers, cardiovascular aspects
    of, 2131-2132, 2131t, 2132t
Moricizine (Ethmozine), in arrhythmias,
    780t, 781t, 782t, 783t, 786t, 791-792

Morphine
in acute heart failure, 596
in myocardial infarction, 1237
in UA/NSTEMI, 1326-1327
Morrow procedure, in hypertrophic
cardiomyopathy, 1772, 1772f
Mouse
conditional knockout, 79
genetically modified, in cardiovascular
disease modeling, 78-79, 80f
knockout, 78-79, 80f
physiology of, 79
transgenic, 78
Mouth-to-mouth respiration, after cardiac
arrest, 959
Mucocutaneous lymph node syndrome.
See Kawasaki disease.
Müller maneuver, with cardiac
catheterization, 460
Muller sign, in aortic regurgitation, 1638
Mullins transseptal catheter, 447-448,
447f
Multidetector computerized tomography,
in acute chest pain, 1203-1204
Multielectrode mapping systems, in
radiofrequency catheter ablation, 819
Multifascicular blocks,
electrocardiography in, 170-172, 171f
Multiple endocrine neoplasia (MEN)
syndrome type II, 2045
Multiple system atrophy, autonomic
dysfunction in, 2175
Multisystem organ failure, after
ventricular assist device
implantation, 694
Multivariate analysis, in exercise stress
testing, 207
Murine models, of cardiovascular disease,
78-79, 80f
Murmur(s), 136-139. See also Heart
sound(s).
in aortic regurgitation, 137, 145-146,
1472, 1639
in aortic stenosis, 136, 1630, 1630f
Austin Flint, 138, 145, 1639
in carcinoid heart disease, 1758-1759
causes of, 137t
in congenital heart disease, 1572
continuous, 138-139
in coronary artery disease, 1355
diastolic, 137-138, 1650
dynamic auscultation of, 139, 139t
echocardiography in, 139, 140f, 314-317,
315t-316t
evaluation of, strategy for, 140f
Graham Steell, 137, 146, 1680
in heart failure, 563
holosystolic, 136
in hypertrophic cardiomyopathy, 1767
in infective endocarditis, 1720
in mitral regurgitation, 136-137, 138f,
1662, 1663t
in mitral stenosis, 137, 1650
in mitral valve prolapse, 1670
in myocardial infarction, 1223
in patent ductus arteriosus, 1585
in pregnancy, 1968
prosthetic valves and, 147
in pulmonary artery stenosis, 1615-1616
in pulmonic regurgitation, 137, 146,
1679, 1680
in pulmonic stenosis, 1617
in rheumatic fever, 2082
systolic, 136-137, 138f
dynamic auscultation of, 1663t
in myocardial infarction, differential
diagnosis of, 255-256, 257f

Murmur(s) (Continued)
in tricuspid regurgitation, 136, 1676
in tricuspid stenosis, 137-138
in ventricular septal defect, 1583, 1584
Muscarinic receptor, 524
Muscle disease syndromes, in
hypothyroidism, 2043, 2043t
Muscle stiffness, 561
Muscular arteries, 989f, 1883
Muscular dystrophy, 2135-2145
Becker, 2135-2137, 2136f
Duchenne, 2135-2137, 2136f, 2137f, 2138f
Emery-Dreifuss, 2142-2144, 2143f
facioscapulohumeral, 2145
limb-girdle, 2144-2145
myotonic, 2137-2142, 2139f-2142f
X-linked, 2135-2137, 2136f, 2137f
Musculoskeletal disorders
chest pain in, 1197
in infective endocarditis, 1721
Mutations. See Gene(s), mutations of.
Myasthenia gravis, 2149
Mycophenolate mofetil (MMF), in heart
transplantation, 678
Mycotic aneurysms
in infective endocarditis, 1730
intracranial, 1521
Myeloperoxidase
as inflammatory marker, 1017
in UA/NSTEMI, 1325
Mykrox. See Metolazone (Mykrox,
Zaroxolyn).
Myocardial amyloidosis. See Amyloidosis,
cardiac.
Myocardial blood flow, imaging of. See
Myocardial perfusion imaging.
Myocardial bridging
arteriography of, 487, 489f
in coronary artery disease, 1400
in stable angina, 1360
Myocardial calcification, chest
radiography in, 341
Myocardial contractility
defects in concept of, 534
definition of, 570t
as essential concept, 534
in heart failure, 550-551
in left ventricular systolic function, 570
versus loading conditions, 529
measurements of, 533-534, 533f
in mitral regurgitation, 1660-1661
myocardial oxygen consumption and,
1167-1168, 1168f
Myocardial energetics, in heart failure,
558
Myocardial fibrosis, in heart failure, 556-
557, 557f
Myocardial hibernation
adaptation versus degeneration in, 1191
apoptosis-induced myocyte loss in,
1190, 1192f
cell survival and antiapoptotic response
to, 1190
chronic, 1187, 1189t, 1190, 1190f, 1191f
coronary artery bypass graft surgery
and, 1389-1390, 1389f, 1389t, 1390f
detection of, 1389, 1389f, 1389t
inhomogeneity in sympathetic nerve
function in, 1190-1191
in ischemic cardiomyopathy, 1398
magnetic resonance imaging of, 397,
397f
metabolism and energetics in, 1190
after myocardial infarction, 1241
myocyte cellular changes in, 1190,
1192f
pathophysiology of, 367, 368f

Myocardial hibernation (Continued)
prognostic implications of, 1389-1390,
1390f
progression from chronic myocardial
stunning to, 1190, 1191f
short-term, 1185
Myocardial infarction, 1207-1317. See also
Acute coronary syndromes.
abdominal examination in, 1223-1224
accelerated idioventricular rhythm in,
1278
in aortic regurgitation, 1472-1473
in apical ballooning syndrome, 258,
259f
arrhythmias in, 1275-1282, 1277t
hemodynamic consequences of,
1276-1277
mechanism of, 1276
pacemakers for, 1281
prophylaxis for, 1289, 1289f
reperfusion-induced, 1241
arteriography in, 466t, 467, 501, 503t
asystole in, 1281
atrial, 1214-1215
atrial fibrillation in, 927t-928t, 1282
atrial flutter in, 1282
atrioventricular block in, 915, 1279-
1280, 1280t
atypical presentations of, 1222
auscultation in, 1223
bifascicular block in, 1281
blood pressure in, 1222
body temperature in, 1222
bradyarrhythmias in, 1279-1281, 1280t
cardiac arrest in, 963-964
in cardiac catheterization, 462
cardiac examination in, 1223-1224
cardiac markers in, 1224-1227, 1225f,
1226f, 1226t, 1230
cardiac rehabilitation after, 1286
cardiac-specific troponins in, 1225-
1226, 1225f, 1226t, 1227
cardiogenic shock in, 1269-1270
diagnosis of, 1269
intraaortic balloon counterpulsation
in, 1269-1270
medical management of, 1269
pathology of, 1269
percutaneous coronary intervention
for, 1306, 1306f
revascularization for, 1270, 1270f
ventricular assist device in, 688
carotid pulse in, 1223
chest pain in, 1195-1196, 1354-1355
differential diagnosis of, 1221-1222
nature of, 1221
chest radiography in, 335f, 338, 1229
in chronic kidney disease, 2162-2164,
2163f, 2164f
circadian periodicity in, 1221
clinical features of, 1220-1230
cocaine-induced, 1808, 1809f, 1810,
1810t
collateral circulation in, 1215
complications of, echocardiography in,
255-257, 257f, 258f
computed tomography in, 1229
after coronary artery bypass graft
surgery, 1383, 1388
coronary blood flow after, 1184-1185,
1185f
creatine kinase in, 1224, 1225f, 1226t
creatine kinase isoenzymes in, 1224-
1225, 1225f, 1226t
creatine kinase isoforms in, 1225, 1225f,
1226t
definition of, revised, 1207, 1208t

I-56 Myocardial infarction (Continued)

depression after, 1290, 2120, 2127
in diabetes mellitus, 1548-1553
  epidemiology of, 1094-1095, 1095f
  intensive glycemic control in, 1552-
    1553, 1553f, 1554f
  medical therapy in, 1549-1552
  prognosis after, 1548, 1549f
  remodeling after, 1555
diagnosis of
  in chronic kidney disease, 2162-2163
  after noncardiac surgery, 2022
  requirements for, 1207, 1208t
differential diagnosis of,
  electrocardiography in, 179-180
Dressler syndrome after, 1284
dynamic nature of, 1238-1239
echocardiography in, 255-257, 257f-258f,
  259, 317-318, 317t-318t, 1229
in elderly persons, 1938-1940
  mortality and, 1208, 1208f
electrocardiography in, 172-183, 1227-
  1229, 1228f, 1230
  in emergency department screening,
    1234, 1235, 1235t, 1237t
  evolution of changes in, 174-175, 175f
  in right ventricular infarction, 1271,
    1271f
  for risk stratification, 1287-1288
exercise stress testing after, 209, 222,
  223t, 224, 224f
expansion of, 1218-1219
extremities examination in, 1224
fascicular block in, 1281
fever in, 1222
free wall rupture in, 256-257, 258f,
  1272-1273, 1272f, 1274f, 1275f, 1303
funduscopic examination in, 1223
general appearance in, 1222
genetic polymorphisms associated with,
  1956
healed
  cardiac arrest prevention in, 969
  sudden cardiac death and, 939-940,
    940f, 948
heart failure in
  left ventricular, 1267-1269, 1267f
  mechanical causes of, 1272-1275,
    1272f, 1273t, 1274f-1277f
heart rate in, 1222
hematological findings in, 1227
hemodynamic abnormalities in, 1265-
  1267, 1265t, 1266t
hemodynamic monitoring in, 1264-
  1265, 1265t
history in, 1221
hospital discharge after
  assessment at, 1288-1289
  timing of, 1286
hyperdynamic state in, 1267
hypotension in
  hypovolemic, 1266-1267
  in prehospital phase, 1266
  prevention of, 1237-1238
hypoxemia in, 1238
  avoidance of, 1267
imaging techniques in, 1229-1230
inducible myocardial ischemia after,
  381, 382f
inferior wall, 179, 2179
intraventricular block in, 1280-1281
ischemia at a distance in, 1217,
  1228-1229
jugular venous pulse in, 1222-1223
laboratory examination in, 1224-1230
in left bundle branch block, 178-179,
  179f, 180f

Myocardial infarction (Continued)

left ventricular aneurysm after, 257,
  1285, 1285f
left ventricular failure in, 1267-1269,
  1267f
left ventricular function in, 382, 1216-
  1218, 1218f, 1288
left ventricular outflow obstruction
  after, 256
left ventricular remodeling after,
  257-258
left ventricular thrombus and arterial
  embolism after, 1285-1286
lipid levels in, 1227
localization of, electrocardiography in,
  176-178, 178f
location of, 1214-1215, 1217f
magnetic resonance imaging in, 395,
  395f-397f, 397, 1229, 1230f
management of, 1233-1293
  adenosine in, 1264
  afterload reduction in, 1268
  aldosterone receptor blocker in, 1262,
    1263f
  analgesics in, 1237-1238
  angiotensin II receptor blockers in,
    1260, 1262, 1262f
  angiotensin-converting enzyme
    inhibitors in, 1260, 1261f, 1262,
    1262f
  antiplatelet therapy in, 1253-1256,
    1254f-1256f
  antithrombotic therapy in, 1251-1253,
    1251f, 1252f
  aspirin in, 1235-1236, 1253, 1255f,
    1256
  beta blockers in, 792, 792f, 1238,
    1258-1260, 1259f, 1260t, 1261f
  beta-adrenergic agonists in, 1268-1269
  calcium channel blockers in, 1263
  changing patterns in, 1207
  in chronic kidney disease, 2163-2164,
    2164t
  clopidogrel in, 1254, 1255f, 1256,
    1256f
  counseling in, 1286
  digitalis in, 1268
  diuretics in, 1267-1268
  drug-eluting stents in, 1435t
  in emergency department, 1234-1239,
    1235t, 1237t, 1239f
  emergency medical services (EMS)
    systems in, 1233-1234, 1235t,
    1236f
  exercise stress testing in, 1288
  glucose-insulin-potassium infusions
    in, 1264
  for hemodynamic abnormalities,
    1265-1267, 1265t, 1266t
  hospital, 1256-1258, 1258t
  implantable cardioverter-defibrillator
    in, 1289, 1289f
  infarct size limitation in, 1238-1239,
    1239f
  insulin infusion in, 1264
  intraaortic balloon counterpulsation
    in, 1264
  limitations of current therapy for,
    1208-1209, 1208f
  magnesium in, 1264
  myocardial regeneration
    interventions in, 1309
  myocardial repair and regeneration
    in, 701-704, 702t, 703t, 704f, 705t,
    1309
  nitrates in, 1238, 1262-1263, 1268
  oxygen in, 1238, 1239

Myocardial infarction (Continued)

pacemakers in, 1281
pain control in, 1237-1238
percutaneous coronary intervention
  in, 1249, 1301-1317
  advantages of, 1302-1303, 1302t,
    1303f
  economic analysis of, 37
  in elderly persons, 1306-1307
  future directions in, 1311
  in late presentation patients, 1307
  during later hospitalization, 1314,
    1316t
  logistic challenge of, 1304-1305
  operator and institutional volume
    considerations for, 1316
  in patients with cardiogenic shock,
    1306, 1306f
  in patients with prior coronary
    bypass surgery, 1307
  practice guidelines for, 1314-1317,
    1315t-1316t
  versus thrombolysis, 1301-1307,
    1302f, 1314, 1315t
  in thrombolytic-ineligible patients,
    1305-1306
  time delay in, mortality and, 1304,
    1304f
  time to, 1235, 1240, 1240f, 1303-
    1304, 1304f
pharmacoinvasive approach to, 1283,
  1284f, 1310
pharmacological therapy in,
  1258-1264
postconditioning in, 1240-1241, 1241f
prehospital, 1233-1234, 1234f, 1235t,
  1236f
  hypotension in, 1266
regionalized centers for, 1235
renin-angiotensin-aldosterone system
  inhibitors in, 1260-1262,
  1261f-1263f
reperfusion in
  arrhythmias from, 1241
  catheter-based, 1249
  combination pharmacological,
    1254, 1256
  complications of, 1303
  developments in, 1308-1310
  early, benefits of, 1239, 1239f
  general concepts for, 1239-1240,
    1240f
  injury in, 1240-1241, 1241f
  late, benefits of, 1215f, 1219, 1219f
  logistic challenge of, 1304-1305
  mechanical myocardial protection
    during, 1309
  options for
    assessment of, 1234-1235, 1235t,
      1237t
    comparison of, 1237t, 1249-1251,
      1250f
  pathology after, 1212-1213, 1215f,
    1216f
  pathophysiology of, 1240
  pharmacological interventions
    during, 1309
  summary of effects of, 1241, 1242f
  surgical, 1249
  temporal dynamics of, 1303-1305,
    1304f
  thrombolytic, 1241-1249
  time delay between, 1233, 1234f
  time to, 1235, 1236f, 1240, 1240f
in scleroderma, 2100
thrombolytic therapy in, 1241-1249
  agents for

Myocardial infarction (Continued)
  comparison of, 1245-1246, 1247f,
    1247t
  selection of, 1248
  complications of, 1247, 1248f
  economic analysis of, 36-37
  glycoprotein IIb/IIIa inhibition
    with, 1254, 1256
  intracoronary, 1241
  intravenous, 1242-1244, 1243f,
    1244f
  late, 1248-1249
  left ventricular function and,
    1246-1247
  mortality and, 1244-1245, 1245f,
    1246f
  myocardial perfusion evaluation of,
    1242-1244, 1243f, 1244f
  net clinical benefit of, 1248
  versus percutaneous coronary
    intervention, 1301-1307, 1302f
  prehospital, 1234
  recommendations for, 1248-1249
  TIMI flow grade and, 1242, 1242f
  TIMI frame count and, 1242, 1243f
  TIMI myocardial perfusion grade
    and, 1244, 1244f
  TIMI risk score for, 1244, 1246f
  vasodilators in, 1268
mechanical complications of, 255
mitral regurgitation after, 258
mortality in
  angiotensin-converting enzyme
    inhibitors and, 1260, 1261f
  antithrombotic therapy and, 1251
  beta blockers and, 1259, 1259f
  chronic kidney disease and, 2163,
    2163f
  coronary blood flow and, 1243, 1243f
  improvements in, 1207-1209, 1208f
  left ventricular dysfunction and,
    1267, 1267f
  thrombolytic therapy and, 1244-1245,
    1245f, 1246f
  TIMI flow grade and, 1242, 1242f
  TIMI myocardial perfusion grade
    and, 1244, 1244f
  TIMI risk score and, 1244, 1246f
myocardial hibernation after, 1241
myocardial perfusion imaging in, 361-
    362, 362f, 363, 364f, 380-382, 381-
    382, 381f, 382f, 1243
myocyte regeneration after. See
  Myocardial repair and regeneration.
myoglobin in, 1225, 1225f, 1226t
nausea and vomiting in, 1221
neuropsychiatric findings in, 1224
"no reflow" phenomenon in, 1302
nonatherosclerotic etiology of, 1209,
    1209t, 1215
noncardiac surgery after, preoperative
  risk assessment for, 2014
non–Q wave, 1209, 1228, 1228f
non–ST segment elevation (NSTEMI).
  See UA/NSTEMI.
nuclear imaging in, 1229-1230
obstructive sleep apnea and, 1916, 1917f
pacemaker in, 854, 856t
palpation in, 1223
papillary muscle rupture in, 256, 257f,
    1272f, 1273t, 1274-1275, 1276f
pathology of, 1209-1216
  acute coronary syndromes in, 1210-
    1211, 1210f, 1211f
  acute plaque change in, 1209-1210,
    1211f
  anatomy and, 1214-1215, 1217f

Myocardial infarction (Continued)
  with angiographically normal
    coronary vessels, 1209t,
    1215-1216
  apoptosis in, 1212, 1214f
  atrial involvement in, 1214-1215
  coagulation necrosis in, 1212
  collateral circulation and, 1215
  contraction band necrosis in, 1212,
    1213f, 1214f
  electron microscopy of, 1212, 1213f
  gross, 1211-1212, 1212f, 1213f
  light microscopy of, 1212, 1213f, 1214f
  myocardial necrosis patterns in, 1212,
    1213f, 1214f
  myocytolysis in, 1212
  nonatherosclerotic factors in, 1209,
    1209t, 1215
  after reperfusion, 1212-1213, 1215f,
    1216f
  right ventricular involvement in,
    1214, 1217f
  pathophysiology of, 1216-1220
    circulatory regulation in, 1218, 1218f
    diastolic function in, 1218
    endocrine function in, 1219-1220
    hematological function in, 1220
    infarct expansion in, 1218-1219
    pulmonary function in, 1219
    renal function in, 1220
    systolic function in, 1215f, 1216-1218
    ventricular dilation in, 1219, 1219f
    ventricular remodeling in, 1215f,
      1218-1219, 1219f
  after percutaneous coronary
    intervention, 1437-1438
  pericardial effusion after, 1283
  pericarditis after, 1284, 1833, 1849-1850
  physical activity in, 1257
  physical examination in, 1222-1224
  plaques in, 1209-1210, 1211f
  postoperative, 2002
    after noncardiac surgery, 2014, 2021
  predisposing factors in, 1220-1221
  in pregnancy, 1975
  premature ventricular contractions
    after, 766, 767
  prevention of, secondary, 1289-1292
    angiotensin-converting enzyme
      inhibitors in, 1290
    anticoagulants in, 1291, 1291f, 1292t
    antioxidants in, 1292
    antiplatelet agents in, 1290
    beta blockers in, 1290-1291
    calcium channel blockers in,
      1291-1292
    lifestyle modification in, 1289-1290
    lipid profile modification in, 1290
    nitrates in, 1291
    nonsteroidal anti-inflammatory drugs
      in, 1292
  prodromal symptoms in, 1221
  prognosis in, with angiographically
    normal coronary vessels, 1216
  pseudoaneurysm after, 257, 258f, 1273,
    1274f
  pulmonary artery pressure monitoring
    in, 1265
  pulmonary embolism after, 1284-1285
  Q wave, 1209, 1210, 1210f, 1228, 1228f
  Q wave in
    ECG classification of, 174
    ECG sequence with, 174-175, 175f
    left bundle branch block and, 178-
      179, 179f, 180f
  QRS changes in, 174, 176f
  QT interval in, 176

Myocardial infarction (Continued)
  quality measures for, 52t
  quality of hospital care for, 54, 54f, 54t
  rales in, 1223
  recurrent ischemia or infarction after,
    1282-1283, 1283f
    assessment of, 1288
    diagnosis of, 1282
    management of, 1282-1283, 1283f
    prognosis in, 1282
  respiration in, 1222
  in right bundle branch block, 178, 179f,
    1281
  right ventricular, 258, 1223, 1229,
    1271-1272
    diagnosis of, 1271, 1271f
    pathology of, 1214, 1217f
    treatment of, 1271-1272, 1271f
  risk stratification in, 259, 382, 1286-
    1289, 1287f, 1303
  silent, 1222
  sinus bradycardia in, 910, 1279
    reperfusion-induced, 1241
  sinus tachycardia in, 1281-1282
  size of
    estimation of, 1230
    limitation of, 1238-1239, 1239f
  ST segment elevation in, in ACS
    spectrum concept, 1210-1211, 1210f
  subacute, 1240
  subendocardial (nontransmural), 1211
  sudden cardiac death after, risk
    stratification for, 1288-1289
  supraventricular tachyarrhythmias in,
    1281-1282
  symptoms of, delay and denial of,
    2125-2126
  in systemic lupus erythematosus,
    2097
  systolic murmur in, differential
    diagnosis of, 255-256, 257f
  thyroid hormones after, 2044-2045
  transmural, 1211
  transportation options in, 1236f
  treatment of inciting pathobiology in,
    1303
  venous thrombosis after, 1284-1285
  ventricular arrhythmias in, 1277-1279
  ventricular fibrillation in, 1278-1279
  ventricular premature complexes in,
    895, 1277-1278
  ventricular remodeling in, in diabetic
    patients, 1555
  ventricular septal defect rupture in,
    1272f, 1273t, 1274, 1276f, 1277f
  ventricular tachycardia in, 902, 1278
    surgical management of, 820-821,
      820f
  in women
    age of onset and, 1955, 1956t
    cardiac rehabilitation after, 1963
    genetic polymorphisms associated
      with, 1956
    risk factors for, 1957, 1958f
    symptoms of, 1957-1958
    treatment of, 1961-1963, 1962f, 1962t
Myocardial injury
  in acute heart failure, 589
  alcohol-induced, 1805, 1806t
  markers of. See Cardiac markers.
  pseudoinfarct patterns in, 181
Myocardial instability, lethal arrhythmias
  and, 949f, 951
Myocardial ischemia
  acute
    electrophysiological effects of,
      950-951

Myocardial ischemia *(Continued)*
lethal arrhythmias in, 950, 950f
perfusion-contraction matching during, 1185, 1187f
in aortic regurgitation, 1638
in aortic stenosis, 1628
during arteriography, 470-471
arteriography in, 466t, 467
chest pain in, 1195-1196
cocaine-induced, 1808, 1809f, 1810
consequences of, metabolic and functional, 1184-1191, 1185f-1192f
in coronary artery anomalies, 483t
differential diagnosis of, electrocardiography in, 176, 178f, 179-180
at a distance, 1217, 1228-1229
electrocardiography in, 172-183
during exercise stress testing
mechanism of ST segment displacement in, 203-204
severity of, 207, 207f
future perspectives on, 1191
in heart failure with normal ejection fraction, 645
in hypertrophic cardiomyopathy, 1767
inducible, after myocardial infarction, 381, 382f
intraoperative hemodynamics and, 2021
irreversible injury in, 1184-1185, 1185f
localization of, electrocardiography in, 176-178, 178f
mental stress–induced, 2122
myocardial viability and, 367
pain associated with, 1221
potential outcomes of, 1216f
programmed cell survival in, 367
pseudoinfarct patterns in, 180-181, 180t, 181f
QT interval in, 176
reversible injury in, 1185, 1186f
functional consequences of, 1186-1191, 1188f-1192f
silent, 209, 1396-1397
ST segment abnormalities in, 172-174, 173f-175f
ST-T changes simulating, 181-182, 182f, 182t
sudden negative emotions and, 2122
in syndrome X, 1395
T wave in, 176, 177f
TQ segment in, 173
U wave in, 176
in UA/NSTEMI, 1319-1320
during vasodilator pharmacological stress, 366
Myocardial metabolism
in diabetes mellitus, 1554
imaging alterations in, 367-368, 368f, 370f
in stable angina, 1360
Myocardial necrosis
in heart failure, 553-554, 554f
markers of
in stable angina, 1357
in UA/NSTEMI, 1322-1323, 1325
patterns of, in myocardial infarction, 1212, 1213f, 1214f
wavefront of, 1185, 1185f
Myocardial oxygen consumption. *See also* Oxygen consumption.
in contraction-relaxation cycle, 532-533, 532f, 533f
determinants of, 1167-1168, 1168f
during exercise, 203-204, 1149
in silent myocardial ischemia, 1396

Myocardial oxygen requirements, increase in, angina pectoris caused by, 1355, 1356f
Myocardial oxygen supply, reduction in, angina pectoris caused by, 1355-1356, 1356f
Myocardial performance index (IMP or Tei index), 252
Myocardial perfusion, maximal, coronary reserve and, 1178-1182, 1179f-1181f
Myocardial perfusion imaging
in acute coronary syndromes, 380-382, 380f-383f
clinical questions answered by, 380
in emergency department, 380, 380f
research directions for, 382, 383f
computed tomography in, 430. *See also* Single photon emission computed tomography.
in coronary artery disease, 371-380, 372f-379f
clinical questions answered by, 371
after coronary artery bypass graft, 378
after CT coronary calcium imaging or CTA, 379-380, 379f
for dynamic assessment of prognosis, 373-374, 374f
for identification of treatment benefit, 372, 374f
patient outcomes as gold standard for, 371
after percutaneous coronary intervention, 378
for risk stratification, 371-373, 372f-374f
echocardiographic, 242-243, 242f, 243f, 245f
in heart failure, 569
irreversible defect on, 363, 364f
magnetic resonance imaging in, 397-399, 398f, 399f
in myocardial infarction, 361-362, 362f, 363, 364f, 380-382, 381f, 382f, 1243
perfusion tracers in, 376
planar, 357-358, 358f
positron emission tomography in. *See* Positron emission tomography.
at rest, 361-362, 362f
reversible defect on, 363, 364f
single photon emission computed tomography in. *See* Single photon emission computed tomography.
stress, 362-367
adenosine for, 364-366, 365f, 366t
angiography as gold standard for, 374-375
for cardiac risk assessment prior to noncardiac surgery, 386
for detection of coronary artery disease, 374-379
in asymptomatic patients, 378-379
and defining extent of disease, 377-378
in diabetic patients, 379
factors influencing, 374-376, 375f-376f
in patients with left ventricular dysfunction, 382-383, 383f
pharmacological, 376-377
submaximal exercise performance and, 377
in valvular heart disease, 378
in women, 378
for detection of myocardial infarction versus ischemia, 363, 364f

Myocardial perfusion imaging *(Continued)*
in dilated cardiomyopathy, 376, 376f, 1748
dipyridamole for, 364-366, 365f, 366t
dobutamine for, 366-367, 377
in endothelial dysfunction, 376
exercise, 363-364, 366
in hypertrophic cardiomyopathy, 375-376, 375f
incremental value of, 372, 373f
in left bundle branch block, 375
in left ventricular hypertrophy, 376
in mitral valve prolapse, 1672
normal, prognostic significance of, 372-373, 373f
perfusion tracers in, 362-363, 362f
pharmacological vasodilation for, 364-366, 365f, 366t
prognosis and, 372-373, 372f
quantification of, and detection of coronary artery disease, 376, 377f
referral bias in, 374, 375f
sensitivity and specificity of, 374-376, 375f-376f
in stable angina, 1358, 1358t, 1361
in unstable angina, 380-381, 381f
Myocardial postconditioning, 1186, 1240-1241, 1241f
Myocardial preconditioning, 1186
Myocardial recovery, in heart failure, 559, 559t
Myocardial relaxation, 249, 250
Myocardial remodeling. *See* Ventricular remodeling.
Myocardial repair and regeneration, 700-701, 702t, 703t. *See also* Stem cells.
in chronic heart failure, 704-705
future perspectives on, 705-706
mobilization strategies in combination with, 703-705, 705t
in myocardial infarction, 701-704, 702t, 703t, 704f, 705t, 1309
nuclear imaging of, 385-386, 386f
Myocardial sarcoidosis. *See* Sarcoidosis.
Myocardial stiffness, 574-575, 574f
Myocardial stunning, 1186-1187, 1189f
chronic, progression to myocardial hibernation from, 1190, 1191f
pathophysiology of, 367, 368f
Myocardial tagging, magnetic resonance, 575, 576f, 577f
Myocardial viability
computed tomography of, 431, 432f
echocardiography of, 243
magnetic resonance imaging of, 395, 397, 397f
markers of, 1389, 1389f, 1389t
myocardial ischemia and, 367
nuclear imaging of, 383-385, 383f-385f
patient selection for, 384-385
principles in, 383-384, 384f
protocols for, 384, 385f
in patients with CAD and left ventricular dysfunction, prognostic implications of, 1389-1390, 1390f
Myocarditis, 1775-1791
active, 1784
bacterial, 1778
borderline, 1775
cardiac remodeling phase in, 1784
chronic active, 1784-1785
clinical presentation in, 1784-1785
Dallas criteria for, 1775, 1776f, 1787
definition of, 1775
diagnostic approaches in, 1785-1787, 1785t, 1786f

Myocarditis (Continued)
  dilated cardiomyopathy due to, 1775-1776
  drug- or toxin-induced, 1780-1781
  endomyocardial biopsy in, 1787
  epidemiology of, 1776, 1777f
  etiological agents causing, 1776-1781, 1777t
  exercise and sports in patients with, 1989
  fulminant, 1784
  future perspectives on, 1791
  geographical distribution of, 1776, 1777f
  giant cell, 1755-1756, 1755f, 1784
  histological evaluation of, 1787
  in HIV-infected patients, 1795
  hypersensitivity, 1780-1781
  immune response in, 1782-1783, 1783f
  incidence of, 1775
  infectious causes of, 1746
  laboratory testing in, 1785-1786
  magnetic resonance imaging in, 403, 1786-1787, 1786f
  metazoal, 1780
  molecular evaluation of, 1787
  in myasthenia gravis, 2149
  nuclear imaging in, 385
  pathophysiology of, 1781-1784, 1782f, 1783f
  physical agents causing, 1781
  prevention of, 1791
  prognosis in, 1787-1788, 1788f
  protozoal, 1779-1780, 1779f
  spirochetal, 1778-1779
  sudden cardiac death in, 944
  in systemic lupus erythematosus, 2097
  treatment of, 1788-1791, 1789f
    hemodynamic support in, 1790-1791
    immune adsorption therapy in, 1790
    immune modulation in, 1790
    immunosuppression in, 1788f, 1789
    interferon beta in, 1789-1790
    intravenous immunoglobulin in, 1790
    supportive therapy in, 1788-1789
  vaccination in, 1791
  ventricular assist device in, 688
  viral
    agents causing, 1776-1778, 1777f, 1778
    pathogenesis of, 1781-1782, 1783f
    viral persistence in, 1782
    viral phase in, 1781-1782, 1783f
Myocardium
  depression of, in traumatic heart disease, 1857
  ion concentrations in, 735t
Myocyte(s)
  antiapoptotic response of, 1190
  apoptosis of
    in myocardial hibernation, 1190, 1192f
    in myocardial infarction, 1212, 1214f
  biological alterations of, in heart failure, 549, 550t
  cellular changes in, in myocardial hibernation, 1190, 1192f
  contractile proteins in, 510-515, 511f-515f
  disorganization of, in hypertrophic cardiomyopathy, 1765, 1765f
  embryonic stem cell–derived, 697
  hypertrophy of, in heart failure, 549-550, 550f-552f
  loss of, in heart failure, 553-555, 554f
  necrosis of. See Myocardial necrosis.
  regeneration of. See Myocardial repair and regeneration.

Myocyte(s) (Continued)
  ultrastructure of, 509-510, 510t, 511f, 512f
Myocytolysis, in myocardial infarction, 1212
Myofiber, 509, 511f
  inactivation of, diastolic relaxation and, 649
Myofibril, 510t
Myofilament regulatory proteins, in heart failure, 552, 553f
Myoglobin
  in myocardial infarction, 1225, 1225f, 1226t
  serum, diagnostic performance of, 1198
Myopathy
  skeletal
    dilated cardiomyopathy with, 116-117
    in peripheral arterial disease, 1494
    zidovudine-induced, 1801
  statin-induced, in elderly persons, 1935-1936
Myosin binding protein C, mutation of, in hypertrophic cardiomyopathy, 112t, 113
Myosin filament, 510, 511f
  ATP binding pocket of, 512, 513f, 515f
Myosin head, 512-513, 513f
Myosin heavy chain
  alpha-, mutations of
    in hypertrophic cardiomyopathy, 112, 112t
    in septation defects, 119, 119t
  beta-, mutations of
    in dilated cardiomyopathy, 115-116, 115t, 116f
    in hypertrophic cardiomyopathy, 112-113, 112t
Myosin heavy chain isoforms, 512, 513f
  in heart failure, 552, 553f
Myosin light chain, 512-513, 513f
  mutations of, in hypertrophic cardiomyopathy, 112t, 113
Myosin light chain isoforms, in heart failure, 552
Myosin neck, 512, 513f
Myosin-binding protein C, 513, 513f
Myositis
  exertional leg pain in, 1495
  inflammatory, 2100-2101
Myotonic muscular dystrophy, 2137-2142, 2139f-2142f
  arrhythmias in, 2139, 2141f, 2142
  cardiovascular manifestations of, 2138-2142, 2140f-2142f
  clinical presentation in, 2137-2138, 2139f
  echocardiography in, 2139
  electrocardiography in, 2138-2139, 2140f
  genetics of, 2137, 2139f
  types of, 2137
Myxoma, 121
  atrial, computed tomography of, 429-430, 430f
  in Carney complex, 1817, 2036
  characteristic clinicopathologic features of, 1818t
  clinical manifestations of, 1817, 1819
  diagnosis of, 1819
  echocardiography in, 302-303, 302f, 1819, 1820f, 1821f
  embolization of, 1816
  interleukin-6 in, 1816
  pathogenesis of, 1817
  systemic manifestations of, 1815-1816
  treatment of, 1819

Nadolol (Corgard), 792-793, 1372t
Nadroparin, in pulmonary embolism, 1873t
Naftidrofuryl, in peripheral arterial disease, 1503
NAPA, 787
Narcotic(s), high-dose, in coronary artery bypass graft, 2020
National Academy of Clinical Biochemistry (NACB) Practice Guidelines, 1199-1200, 1201t
National Committee for Quality Assurance (NCQA)
  Heart/Stroke Recognition Program of, 55, 55t
  HEDIS measures developed by, 49, 50t, 54, 55t
National Heart Attack Alert Program, 1197
National Quality Forum, 50t
Native Americans
  cardiovascular mortality in, 25
  demographics of, 23, 24f
  health care disparities for, 25
Natriuresis, braking phenomenon in, 625f, 626
Natriuretic peptides
  B-type. See B-type natriuretic peptide.
  in heart failure, 546-547, 594, 594f, 595t
  in myocardial infarction, 1220
  potential, in acute heart failure management, 605
  signaling pathway of, 546, 547f
Natural frequencies, 43
Natural products. See Dietary supplements.
Naughton protocol, for exercise stress testing, 198
Nausea, in myocardial infarction, 1221
Navigator echo sequence, in cardiovascular magnetic resonance, 394
Naxos syndrome, 117, 117t
Nebivolol, in heart failure, 632-633, 654, 655f
Neck, physical examination of, 127
Necrosis
  versus apoptosis, 554
  myocardial. See Myocardial necrosis.
  skin, warfarin-induced, 2066
Needles, for cardiac catheterization, 444, 446, 446f
Neisseria organisms, in infective endocarditis, 1717
Nelfinavir, 1801
Neonate(s). See also Children; Infant(s).
  aortic stenosis in, 1611
  coarctation of the aorta in, 1606-1607, 1606f
  congenital heart disease in
    echocardiography in, 1574-1575
    management approach to, 1566
  dose adjustments in, 64
  heart failure in, 1566
  pulmonary circulation in, 1886
  pulmonary hypertension in, persistent, 1902
  pulmonic stenosis in, 1616, 1617
Neoplasms. See Tumor(s).
Neovascularization, by stem cells, 700
Nephropathy
  calcium channel blockers in, 1062
  contrast-induced. See Contrast-induced nephropathy.

I-60 Nephropathy (Continued)
diabetic, 1039, 1558, 2155
hypertension and, 1039
unilateral renal artery stenosis and, 1535
Nephrosclerosis, in hypertension, 1037-1038
Nernst potential, 734
Nerve pain, after arteriography, 468
Nerves
of atrioventricular node, 732-733, 734f
cardiac, sudden cardiac death and, 949
of sinus node, 727-728
Nervous system. See Autonomic nervous system; Central nervous system.
Nesiritide
actions of, 603
in chronic kidney disease patients, 2165
in heart failure, 547, 601t, 602f, 603
Neurally mediated syncope, 977, 977t, 2177
exercise and sports in patients with, 1989
tilt-table testing in, 979
treatment of, 983
variants of, 2178-2180, 2179f, 2180f
Neurocardiogenic syncope. See Neurally mediated syncope.
Neurogenic hypertension, from sleep apnea, 1031
Neurogenic pseudoclaudication, 1495
Neurogenic pulmonary edema, in acute cerebrovascular disease, 2150
Neurohormonal activation
in heart failure with normal ejection fraction, 653
after left ventricular reconstruction, 674, 674f
Neurohormonal alterations
from diuretics, 626
in heart failure, 541-549, 589
Neurohumoral factors, in sudden cardiac death, 945
Neurohypophysis, cell types of, 2033
Neurological disorders
in aortic regurgitation, 1472
after cardiac surgery, 1998-1999
cardiac surgery in patients with, 1996
after coronary artery bypass graft surgery, 1383-1384
echocardiography in, 321t, 324
in infective endocarditis, 1721
postoperative, 2006-2008
Neurological tests, in syncope evaluation, 981
Neuromuscular disease, pulmonary hypertension in, 1909
Neuromuscular disorders, with cardiovascular manifestations, 2135-2152
Neuropathy
in diabetes mellitus, 1558
optic, Leber hereditary, 2148
panautonomic, 976
postoperative, 1998, 2007
Neuropeptide Y
in heart failure, 547
in sinus node, 728
Neuropsychiatric findings, in myocardial infarction, 1224
Neutral endopeptidase inhibitors, in heart failure, 546
New York Heart Association
cardiovascular disability assessment system of, 126, 126t
heart failure classification of, 619, 619t

New Zealand, cardiovascular disease in, 10
New Zealand task force risk assessment tool, 1123-1124, 1123f-1124f
Nexus, 736-737, 737f
Niacin. See Nicotinic acid (niacin).
Niaspan, 1083
Nicardipine (Cardene)
in hypertensive crises, 1066, 1066t
pharmacokinetics of, 1374t
in stable angina, 1376
Nicorandil
in myocardial infarction, 1309
in stable angina, 1377
Nicotine. See Smoking.
Nicotinic acid (niacin)
in cardiovascular disease prevention, 1129
in chronic kidney disease patients, 2165t
in dyslipidemia, 1083-1084
Niemann-Pick disease, 1081
Nifedipine (Procardia)
adverse effects of, 1374-1375
in aortic dissection, 1479
in aortic regurgitation, 1642
in myocardial infarction, 1263
pharmacokinetics of, 1374t
in stable angina, 1373-1375
in UA/NSTEMI, 1327
Nilotinib, cardiotoxicity of, 2114
Nipride. See Nitroprusside (Nipride, Nitropress).
Nisoldipine, pharmacokinetics of, 1375t
Nitinol self-expanding stent, in femoral artery disease, 1527
Nitrates
in acute heart failure, 600-601, 601t, 602f
adverse effects of, 1263, 1368
antithrombotic effects of, 1368
in combination therapy, 1378
coronary circulation effects of, 1367-1368, 1367t
dosage and administration of, 1368-1369, 1368t
drug interactions of, 1369
exercise stress testing and, 213-214
mechanism of action of, 1367, 1368, 1368f
in myocardial infarction, 1238, 1262-1263, 1268
in myocardial infarction prevention, 1291
myocardial oxygen consumption and, 1367t
preparations of, 1368-1369, 1368t
in Prinzmetal variant angina, 1339
in stable angina, 1367-1369, 1367t, 1368f, 1368t
tolerance to, 1369
in UA/NSTEMI, 1327
withdrawal from, 1369
Nitric oxide, 1170
abnormalities of, coronary flow reserve and, 1182-1183, 1183f, 1184f
antithrombotic properties of, 2050
in atherogenesis, 992
during cardiac catheterization, 460
in contraction-relaxation cycle, 525-526, 525f, 526f
in coronary blood flow regulation, 1170
deficiency of
in diabetes mellitus, 1096
heart failure and, 30, 31f
in heart failure, 548, 548f, 549f
in HIV-infected patients, 1795

Nitric oxide (Continued)
in pulmonary circulation, 1885
in pulmonary hypertension, 1889
vasodilator properties of, 2050
Nitric oxide synthase, 2050
endothelial, in idiopathic pulmonary arterial hypertension, 1892
Nitroblue tetrazolium (NBT) stain, in myocardial infarction, 1211
Nitrogen-82, in positron emission tomography, 360, 360t
Nitroglycerin
in acute heart failure, 600-601, 601t, 602f
adverse effects of, 1263
during cardiac catheterization, 460
in coronary blood flow regulation, 1176
in hypertensive crises, 1066, 1066t
in myocardial infarction, 1238, 1262-1263, 1268
postoperative, 2002
preoperative, 2025-2026
preparations of, 1368t, 1369
in stable angina, 1368-1369, 1368t
in syndrome X, 1396
in upright tilt-table testing, 979
Nitroprusside (Nipride, Nitropress)
in acute heart failure, 601-603, 601t, 602f
in acute mitral regurgitation, 1669
in baroreflex failure, 2178
cyanide metabolite of, 602
in hypertensive crises, 1066, 1066t
postoperative, 2002
NKX2-5, mutation of
in electrophysiological defects, 119, 119t
in septation defects, 119, 119t
"No reflow" phenomenon
in diabetes mellitus, 1547-1548
in myocardial infarction, 1302
in percutaneous coronary intervention, 1438
Nocturia
in heart failure, 562
in hypertension, 1031-1032
Nocturnal dyspnea, paroxysmal, in heart failure, 140, 562, 563t
Nocturnal hypertension, 1036, 1036f
Nodofascicular accessory pathways, in Wolff-Parkinson-White syndrome, 884, 887, 887f, 888f
Nodules, subcutaneous, in rheumatic fever, 2083-2084
Noetic therapies, in cardiac catheterization, 1163-1164
Nonbacterial thrombotic endocarditis, 1718-1719
echocardiography in, 281-282, 282f
in HIV-infected patients, 1794t, 1799
Noncardiac surgery, 2013-2032
anesthesia for, 2020-2021
coronary arteriography before and after, 467, 505, 507t
in Eisenmenger syndrome, 1570
exercise stress testing before, 210
hemodynamics during, myocardial ischemia and, 2021
myocardial infarction precipitated by, 1221
normothermia in, 2026
pain management after, 2022
perioperative monitoring in, 2026
postoperative management of, 2021-2022
practice guidelines for, 2028-2032, 2029f, 2030t-2031t

Noncardiac surgery (*Continued*)
preoperative risk assessment for,
2013-2020, 2028-2032, 2029f,
2030t-2031t
in arrhythmias, 2016, 2016f
in congenital heart disease, 2015-2016
in coronary artery disease, 2013-2014
diagnostic testing in, 2016-2020,
2017t, 2018t, 2019f
in heart failure, 2014-2015
in hypertension, 2014
in valvular heart disease, 2015
prosthetic valves and, 1688
risk reduction intervention(s) in, 2022-
2027, 2031t, 2032
nonpharmacological, 2026-2027
pharmacological, 2024-2026, 2024f,
2025t
revascularization as, 2022-2023
stress myocardial perfusion imaging
before, 386
surveillance of cardiac complications
after, 2022
transfusion threshold in, 2026-2027
type of, risk stratification based on,
2017, 2018t
volume of, risk stratification based on,
2017
Nonflotation catheter(s), 444
Nonne-Milroy lymphedema, 97
Nonnucleoside reverse transcriptase
inhibitors, in HIV-infected patients,
complications of, 1802t
Nonsense mutation, 75, 75f
Non–ST segment elevation myocardial
infarction (NSTEMI). *See* UA/
NSTEMI.
Nonsteroidal anti-inflammatory drugs
(NSAIDs)
in elderly persons, 1931-1932
in heart failure, 619
hypertension from, 1038
in myocardial infarction prevention,
1292
in pericarditis, 1833, 1834
as platelet inhibitors, 2069, 2071f
in rheumatic fever, 2086
Noonan syndrome, 120-121, 1571
Norepinephrine
cardiac effects of, 733
in cardiogenic shock, 1269
in heart failure, 542, 543f, 601t, 604,
613, 614f
in pheochromocytoma, 2045
postoperative, 2001
release of, 520-521, 520f, 1058, 1059f
Norepinephrine transporter deficiency,
2178
Normal test result, definition of, 43
Normodyne. *See* Labetalol (Normodyne,
Trandate).
North Africa, cardiovascular disease in,
10t, 13
Northern blotting, 73
Nortriptyline, cardiovascular aspects of,
2129t
Norwood procedure
in double-inlet ventricle, 1593
in hypoplastic left heart syndrome,
1592
NOTCH1, mutations of, in bicuspid aortic
valve, 119t, 120
Novacor left ventricular assist device, 691
NREM sleep, 1915
NSAIDs. *See* Nonsteroidal anti-
inflammatory drugs (NSAIDs).
NSTEMI. *See* UA/NSTEMI.

N-terminal (NT) pro-BNP
in heart failure, 564, 594, 646
in stable angina, 1357
Nuclear imaging, 345-391. *See also*
Myocardial perfusion imaging;
Positron emission tomography;
Radionuclide angiography or
ventriculography; Single photon
emission computed tomography.
in acute coronary syndromes, 380-382,
380f-383f
in cardiac amyloidosis, 385
in coronary artery disease, 371-380,
372f-379f
of diastolic function, 370-371, 370f, 371f
of fatty acid metabolism, 367, 382, 383f
future perspectives on, 386
of glucose metabolism, 367-368, 370f
in heart failure, 382-386, 383f-386f
of left ventricular function, 385
of myocardial viability, 383-385,
383f-385f
research directions for, 385-386, 386f
of ischemic memory, 382, 383f
of left ventricular function, 370-371,
370f
of myocardial blood flow, 361-367,
362f-365f
in myocardial infarction, 1229-1230
of myocardial metabolism and
physiology, 367-368, 368f, 370f
of myocardial viability, 383-385,
383f-385f
in myocarditis, 385
before noncardiac surgery, 386
of oxidative metabolism and
mitochondrial function, 367
of potentially unstable atherosclerotic
plaques, 382
practice guidelines for, 389-391, 390t
in right ventricular infarction, 1271
in sarcoid heart disease, 385
stress
in abdominal aortic aneurysms, 1463
preoperative, for noncardiac surgery,
2018, 2020
technical aspects of, 345-361
of ventricular function, 369-370
Nucleus, 68, 68f, 510t
Nucleus tractus solitarii, in baroreflex,
2171, 2172f
Number needed to screen (NNS), 43
Number needed to treat (NNT), 45
Nursing homes, hospice care in, 724
Nutrition. *See also* Diet(s).
cardiovascular disease and, 1107-1116
deficiencies in, in HIV-infected
patients, 1795
Nuts, intake of, cardiovascular disease
and, 1108
Nyquist frequency, in Doppler
echocardiography, 237

O
OAT trial, 1307
Obedience, blind, in decision-making, 46
Obesity/overweight
age of
cardiovascular disease in, 3t, 4
in United States, 9
cardiac surgery and, 1995
cardiovascular disease and, 1011-1012,
1136-1137, 1136f, 1137t
dietary influences on, 1111-1112, 1111t
dyslipidemia and, 1082
in heart failure with normal ejection
fraction, 645

Obesity/overweight (*Continued*)
hypertension and, 1029, 1031
obstructive sleep apnea and, 1916, 1919
paradox of, in heart failure, 611, 613f
prevalence of, 1093, 1094f, 1136, 1136f
pulmonary embolism and, 1863
racial/ethnic differences in, 23-24
regional trends in, 17, 17f
sudden cardiac death and, 938
Obstructive sleep apnea. *See* Sleep apnea,
obstructive.
Occam's razor, 46
Octreotide, in acromegaly, 2035
Odds ratios, in assessing test
performance, 44
Olanzapine, cardiovascular aspects of,
2130t, 2131
Oligonucleotide microarrays, in
molecular genetics, 77
Omega-3 fatty acids, 1160t
intake of, cardiovascular disease and,
1108, 1108f, 1109t, 1110
Omniscience valve, 1682, 1682f
Open-lung biopsy
in atrioventricular septal defect, 1582
in Eisenmenger syndrome, 1569
Opioid receptors, in contraction-
relaxation cycle, 526
Opportunity cost, 35
Optic neuropathy
after cardiac surgery, 2007
Leber hereditary, 2148
Optical coherence tomography, 497, 498f,
499t
Oral contraceptives
hypertension from, 1044
thrombosis and, 2057, 2058, 2061
Organ transplantation. *See specific organ,*
e.g., Heart transplantation.
Orqis CANCION ventricular assist device,
690
Orthodromic atrioventricular
reciprocating tachycardia, in Wolff-
Parkinson-White syndrome, 888-889,
889f
Orthopnea
in heart failure, 561-562, 563t
in pulmonary hypertension, 1886
Orthostatic angina, 2175
Orthostatic hypotension, 131. *See also*
Syncope.
in amyloidosis, 1752
from antipsychotic agents, 2128
after cardiac surgery, 1998
causes of, 976-977, 976t
definition of, 975
examination for, 2173
in heart failure, 593
symptoms of, 975-976
treatment of, 983
from tricyclic antidepressants, 2129
Orthostatic intolerance, 2176-2178
in Addison disease, 2178
in baroreflex failure, 2178
in chronic fatigue syndrome, 2177-2178
in neurally mediated syncope, 2177
in norepinephrine transporter
deficiency, 2178
in postural tachycardia syndrome,
2176-2177
Orthostatic tachycardia syndrome,
postural, 772, 867, 976-977, 2176-2177
Orthostatics, as measure of autonomic
function, 2173
Ortner syndrome
in mitral stenosis, 1649
in pulmonary hypertension, 1887

Osler maneuver, 131
Osler nodes, in infective endocarditis, 1720
Osteogenesis imperfecta
   cardiovascular manifestations of, 90t
   genetic studies in, 90
Osteoporosis, after heart transplantation, 683
Ostium primum atrial septal defect, 1577, 1578f-1579f
Ostium secundum atrial septal defect
   morphology of, 1577, 1578f-1579f
   repair of, 1578f, 1579-1580
Ototoxicity, of diuretics, 626
Outcome, in risk-benefit analysis, 45
Outcome measures
   in end-stage heart disease, 724
   for quality of cardiovascular care, 52
Outflow tract ventricular tachycardia, 906-907, 907f
Overdrive suppression, 744-745
Overuse, as error in health care, 52
Overweight. *See* Obesity/overweight.
Oxazepam, in myocardial infarction, 1257
Oxfenicine, in heart failure, 710
Oxidative phosphorylation, in
   myocardium, nuclear imaging of, 367
Oxidative stress
   in diabetes mellitus, 1096, 1099
   dietary influences on, 1115-1116, 1115f
   in heart failure, 30, 31f, 544, 545f
Oximetry
   pulse, in congenital heart disease, 1901
   for shunt detection, 458-459
Oxygen consumption
   in elderly person, 214-215
   estimation of, 198
   during exercise, 196, 196f, 197
   in Fick method, 454-455
   in heart failure, 210, 211f
   minimization of, in myocardial
      infarction, 1239
   myocardial. *See* Myocardial oxygen
      consumption.
   myocardial contractility and, 532-533, 532f, 533f
   ventilatory, 1149
Oxygen saturation
   pulmonary, in pulmonary hypertension, 1889t
   systemic arterial, in pulmonary
      hypertension, 1889t, 1890
Oxygen therapy
   in acute heart failure, 596
   in central sleep apnea, 1920
   in chronic obstructive pulmonary
      disease, 1908
   in Eisenmenger syndrome, 1570
   hyperbaric, during percutaneous
      coronary intervention, 1309
   in idiopathic pulmonary arterial
      hypertension, 1897
   in myocardial infarction, 1238, 1239
Oxygen uptake, maximum, 1149
   in heart failure, 565-566

P

P21(Cip1), 70, 787
P27(Kip1), 69-70
P. aeruginosa, in infective endocarditis, 1717, 1727
p53 gene, mutations of, 70
p value, 44
P wave, 155, 156-157, 156f, 156t
   in arrhythmia diagnosis, 764, 766f
   in atrial abnormalities, 161, 161f, 162, 162f, 162t

P wave *(Continued)*
   in atrial premature complexes, 867, 868f, 869f
   in atrial tachycardia, 876
   in atrioventricular dissociation, 920
   in atrioventricular nodal reentrant
      tachycardia, 878, 879, 879f
   in concealed accessory pathway, 882
   in first-degree atrioventricular block, 914
   normal, 863
   in potassium abnormalities, 184
   in sinoatrial exit block, 911
   in sinus tachycardia, 866, 867f
Pacemaker(s), 831-846. *See also* Cardiac
   resynchronization therapy.
   activity sensors for, 840
   for atrial fibrillation prevention, 833-834, 834f, 858
   atrial synchronous (VDD), 838, 839f
   atrial-inhibited (AAI), 838, 839f
   in atrioventricular block, 831-832, 832t, 854, 855t, 919
   atrioventricular interval in, 838, 840f, 842
   in atrioventricular nodal reentrant
      tachycardia, 881
   atrioventricular sequential, non-P-
      synchronous (DDI), 838, 839f
   biventricular, 834, 835f
   in cardiomyopathy, 857t, 858
   in carotid sinus hypersensitivity, 833, 857t, 858, 912
   chest radiography of, 341, 341f
   in chronic bifascicular and trifascicular
      block, 832, 854, 855t
   complications of, 842-844, 843f-844f
   in congenital complete heart block, 832
   drug effects on, 851
   dual-chamber, 838-839, 839f-840f
      and sensing with inhibition and
         tracking (DDD), 838-839, 840f
   dual-chamber rate-adaptive (DDDR), 839-840
   dual-sensor combinations for, 840-841
   dual-site atrial, 833, 834f
   ectopic (latent or subsidiary), 746-747
   electrocardiographic abnormalities
      with, 844-845, 845f-847f
   electromagnetic interference with, 849-851, 850f
   in Emery-Dreifuss muscular dystrophy
      and associated disorders, 2144
   exercise stress testing and, 213
   failure to capture by, 844, 845f
   failure to output by, 844-845, 845f-846f
   follow-up for, 851-852, 858
   fusion and pseudofusion beat with, 845, 847f
   in hypertrophic cardiomyopathy, 835
   implantation methods for, 841
   implant-related complications of, 842-843, 843f
   indications for, 831-835, 832t-833t
   infection with, 844
   lead-related complications of, 843-844, 843f-844f
   in long QT syndrome, 103, 906
   magnetic resonance imaging and, 394
   metabolic abnormality interference
      with, 851
   minute ventilation sensors for, 840
   in mitochondrial disorders, 2148
   mode switching in, 842, 842f
   in myocardial infarction, 854, 856t, 1281

Pacemaker(s) *(Continued)*
   in myotonic muscular dystrophy, 2139, 2142
   in neurally mediated syncope, 833, 857t, 858, 983
   nomenclature for, 831, 832t
   oversensing of, 845, 845f
   pacing mode of
      algorithms for selection of, 840, 841f
      morbidity and mortality and, 835, 837, 837t
      selection of, 835, 837, 837t, 838f, 858, 858t
      timing cycle and, 837-839, 838f-840f
   postventricular atrial refractory period
      in, 838, 840f
   practice guidelines for, 854-858, 855t-858t
   programming of, 841-842, 842f
   pulse width of, 842
   rate-adaptive
      indications for, 839-840, 841f
      programming of, 842
      sensor selection for, 840-841
      single-chamber, 839-840
   sensing abnormalities by, 845, 845f-847f
   sensors for, 840-841
   single-chamber (AAT or VVT), 837
   single-chamber rate-adaptive (AAIR or
      VVIR), 839-840
   in sinus node disease, 832-833, 833t, 854, 856t, 913
   stimulus-T or QT sensing, 840
   surgery and, 850
   for tachyarrhythmia prevention and
      termination, 833, 854, 856t-857t, 858
   undersensing of, 845, 846f
   in vasovagal syncope, 833
   ventricular avoidance, 837, 838f
   ventricular-inhibited (VVI), 837-838, 838f
   wandering, 911, 911f
Pacemaker channel, molecular structure
   of, 736
Pacemaker current, 742, 744-745, 745f
Pacemaker reentrant tachycardia, 839, 840f
Pacemaker syndrome, 837-838
Pacific Islanders
   cardiovascular disease in, 10t, 12
   cardiovascular mortality in, 25
   demographics of, 23, 24f
Pacing
   for atrioventricular nodal reentrant
      tachycardia, 881
   after cardiac arrest, 963
   in myocardial infarction, 1281
   in myocardial infarction with
      atrioventricular block, 1279-1280
   rapid atrial, for atrial flutter, 875
   in sinus bradycardia, 910
   ventricular, for ventricular tachycardia, 899
Pacing tachycardia, with cardiac
   catheterization, 459-460
Paclitaxel (Taxol), cardiotoxicity of, 1813, 2110
Paclitaxel-eluting stent, 1431
Pain. *See also* Angina pectoris; Chest
   pain.
   in abdominal aortic aneurysms, 1459
   abnormal perception of, in syndrome X, 1395
   in acute aortic occlusion, 1486
   in acute limb ischemia, 1507
   in aortic dissection, 1222, 1471

Pain (Continued)
  control of
    in myocardial infarction, 1237-1238
      after noncardiac surgery, 2022
  in esophageal disorders, 1354
  leg
    exertional, 1494-1495, 1494t
    ischemic rest, 1495
  nerve, after arteriography, 468
  pericardial, 1284, 1355
  in pericardial effusion, 1836
  in pericarditis, 1221, 1355, 1831-1832, 1834
  pleural, 1221
  in pulmonary embolism, 1221-1222
  in thoracic aortic aneurysm, 1465
Palindrome, 73
Palliative care, in end-stage heart disease, 718, 724
Palmitate, carbon-labeled, in positron emission tomography, 367
Palpation
  of aorta, 1458
  in cardiac examination, 134-135
  in myocardial infarction, 1223
Palpitations
  echocardiography in, 321t, 324
  electrophysiology in, 775-776, 828, 828t
  in heart failure, 591
  in hypertrophic cardiomyopathy, 1768
  in mitral stenosis, 1649
  psychosocial factors in, 2125
Palpography, 497, 498f
Pamiteplase, 2068
Pancreas, in myocardial infarction, 1219
Pancreatitis, chest pain in, 1197
Pandemics age, receding
  cardiovascular disease in, 3t, 4
  in United States, 7, 7f
Panic attacks, arrhythmias versus, 2125
Panic disorder
  chest pain in, 1197, 2125
  palpitations in, 2125
  sympathetic dysfunction in, 2180-2181
Papaverine, in coronary blood flow regulation, 1177
Papillary fibroelastoma, 303, 303f, 1816, 1818t, 1822
Papillary muscle
  dysfunction of, in mitral regurgitation, 1659
  rupture of
    in myocardial infarction, 256, 257f, 1272f, 1273t, 1274-1275, 1276f
    surgical treatment of, 1669
Paracor cardiac support device, 674-675
Paracrine mediators, in coronary blood flow regulation, 1170t, 1175
Paradoxical embolism, 1867-1868
Paraplegia
  after aortic dissection surgery, 1481
  after thoracic aortic aneurysm repair, 1468
Parasternal lift, 135
Parasympathetic dysfunction, 2175, 2182-2183
  in heart failure, 542, 543f
  in sinus arrhythmia, 2182-2183
Parasympathetic-sympathetic interactions, 524-525, 525f, 732
Parasystole, in arrhythmogenesis, 750, 753f
Parathyroid disease, 2037-2038
Parathyroid hormone–related peptide, 2037-2038
Parietal pericardium, 1829

Parkinson's disease, autonomic dysfunction in, 976, 2175
Paroxetine, cardiovascular aspects of, 2129t
Paroxysmal atrioventricular block, 918
Paroxysmal nocturnal dyspnea, in heart failure, 140, 562, 563t
Paroxysmal supraventricular tachycardia, 878
  in mitral valve prolapse, 1672
Paroxysmal ventricular tachycardia, 906-907, 907f
Parvovirus B19 infection, myocarditis in, 1777-1778
Passive cardiac support devices, in heart failure, 674-675, 675f
Patency rate, 1242
Patent ductus arteriosus, 1585-1586
  clinical features of, 1585
  echocardiography in, 309-310, 310f
  follow-up in, 1586
  indications for interventions in, 1585-1586
  interventional options and outcomes in, 1586
  laboratory studies in, 1585
  magnetic resonance imaging in, 407
  morphology of, 1585
  natural history of, 1585
  pathophysiology of, 1585
  in pregnancy, 1970
  reproductive issues in, 1586
Patent foramen ovale, 1580-1581
  stroke prophylaxis in, 1516
Patient outcome data, for quality measurement, 51
PCI. See Percutaneous coronary intervention.
Pectus excavatum, in Marfan syndrome, 92
Pediatric autoimmune neuropsychiatric disorder associated with streptococcal infection (PANDAs), 2083
Pegvisomant, in acromegaly, 2035
Penbutolol, pharmacokinetics and pharmacology of, 1373t
Penetrance, 88
Penetrating traumatic heart disease, 1855, 1857, 1859-1860, 1859f-1861f
Penicillin
  prophylactic, in mitral stenosis, 1652
  in rheumatic fever, 2085, 2085t
Pentamidine, in HIV-infected patients, 1801
Pentoxifylline
  in HIV-infected patients, complications of, 1803t
  in peripheral arterial disease, 1503, 1504f
Percutaneous coronary intervention, 1419-1441
  adjunctive medical therapies during, 1314
  guidelines on, 1452, 1454t
  adjunctive technologies in, guidelines on, 1451-1452, 1453t
  angiographic complications during, 1438, 1440f
  angiography after, quantitative, 492-494, 494t
  antiplatelet therapy during, 1436-1437
  antithrombotic therapy during, 1437
  aspiration devices in, 1425, 1426f
  atherectomy in, 1420f, 1425
    directional, 1425
    rotational, 1422, 1423f, 1424f, 1425

Percutaneous coronary intervention (Continued)
  balloon angioplasty in, 1425. See also Percutaneous transluminal coronary angioplasty.
  baseline lesion morphology for, 1421-1422, 1421t, 1422f-1424f
  in bifurcation lesions, 1422, 1422f
  in calcified lesions, 1422, 1423f, 1424f
  cardiac trauma in, 1856
  cholesterol embolization in, 2158-2159
  in chronic kidney disease patients, 2164, 2164f, 2168, 2168f
  in chronic total occlusions, 1421-1422
  complications of, 1437-1441
  conduct of, 1310-1311
  contrast-induced nephropathy after. See Contrast-induced nephropathy.
  versus coronary artery bypass graft surgery, 1392-1394, 1392f-1394f, 1393t
  coronary devices for, 1424-1436
  definition of, 1419
  in diabetic patients, 1380, 1394, 1557-1558
  drug-eluting stents in, 1429-1436, 1432t-1435t, 1435f. See also Stent(s), drug-eluting.
  early mortality after, 1437, 1439t
  economic analysis of, 37
  in elderly persons, 1936-1938, 1937f, 1937t, 1939
  embolic protection devices in, 1308, 1425-1426, 1427f-1429f
  exercise stress testing after, 216
  facilitated, 1309, 2075
  future directions in, 1446
  glycoprotein IIb/IIIa inhibition during, 1301, 1302, 1302f, 1307-1308, 1307f, 2075
  heparin dosage and administration in, 2062-2063
  indications for, 1419-1421, 1450, 1450t-1451t
  intravascular ultrasonography in, 496
  in left ventricular dysfunction, 1422
  management issues in, 1452, 1454t
  mechanical myocardial protection during, 1309
  versus medical therapy, 1379-1380, 1380f
  in myocardial infarction, 1249, 1301-1317
    advantages of, 1302-1303, 1302t, 1303f
    economic analysis of, 37
    in elderly persons, 1306-1307
    future directions in, 1311
    in late presentation patients, 1307
    during later hospitalization, 1314, 1316t
    logistic challenge of, 1304-1305
    operator and institutional volume considerations for, 1316
    in patients with cardiogenic shock, 1306, 1306f
    in patients with prior coronary bypass surgery, 1307
    practice guidelines for, 1314-1317, 1315t-1316t
    versus thrombolysis, 1301-1307, 1302f, 1314, 1315t
    in thrombolytic-ineligible patients, 1305-1306
    time delay in, mortality and, 1304, 1304f
    time to, 1235, 1240, 1240f, 1303-1304, 1304f

I-64 Percutaneous coronary intervention
(Continued)
  myocardial infarction after, 1437-1438
  myocardial perfusion imaging after, 378
  outcome of, 1437-1441, 1438f,
      1439t-1441t
    early clinical, 1437-1438, 1439t
    late clinical, 1441
  patient selection for, 1379, 1421-1423,
      1421t, 1422f-1424f
  in patients with left ventricular
      dysfunction, 1380
  in patients with medical comorbidities,
      1423
  in patients with previous coronary
      artery bypass graft, 1380
  in patients without options for
      revascularization, 1421
  pericardial disease and, 1851
  pharmacological interventions during,
      1309
  practice guidelines for, 1415t, 1416-1417,
      1449-1453, 1450t-1455t
  preoperative, 2023
  in Prinzmetal variant angina, 1339
  proficiency in, 1453, 1455t
  proximal occlusion devices in, 1426
  quality assessment and outcomes
      benchmarking in, 1441
  quality of care in, volume as marker of,
      53, 53f, 53t
  in renal insufficiency, 1422-1423
  rescue, 1309, 1314, 1315t
  restenosis after, 999
    guidelines on, 1452-1453, 1455t
  rheolytic thrombectomy in, 1425
  risk assessment for, 1421-1423, 1421t,
      1422f-1424f
  in saphenous vein graft, 1422, 1426,
      1427f, 1429f
  in stable angina, 1379-1380, 1380f, 1391-
      1392, 1420, 1450, 1450t-1451t
  stent thrombosis after, 1429, 1438, 1440-
      1441, 1440t, 1441t
  stents in, 1301, 1302f, 1308, 1308f, 1428-
      1429, 1430t, 1431t. See also Stent(s),
      coronary.
  stroke after, 1522
  after successful thrombolytic therapy,
      1309, 1314, 1316t
  thrombectomy during, 1308
  with thrombolytic therapy, 1309-1310,
      1314, 1315t, 2075
  in thrombus-containing lesion, 1422
  TIMI flow grade/TIMI myocardial
      perfusion grade after, 1302, 1302t,
      1303f
  in UA/NSTEMI, 1329, 1334-1335, 1347,
      1349-1350, 1350t, 1420-1421
    practice guidelines for, 1450-1451,
        1452f, 1452t
  urgent revascularization after, 1438
  vascular access in, 1423-1424
  vascular closure devices in, 1424
  without on-site cardiac surgery,
      1316-1317
  in women, 1961-1962
Percutaneous intervention
  in acute limb ischemia, 1508-1509,
      1509t
  in aortic dissection, 1481-1482
  in aortoiliac disease, 1524-1525, 1525f,
      1526f, 1526t
  in brachiocephalic artery stenosis,
      1536-1538, 1537f
  in carotid artery stenosis, 1539-1541,
      1540f, 1541f, 1541t

Percutaneous intervention (Continued)
  in chronic mesenteric ischemia, 1536,
      1537f
  coronary. See Percutaneous coronary
      intervention.
  in deep venous thrombosis, 1542-1543,
      1543f
  in femoropopliteal disease, 1525-1530,
      1527f, 1528f, 1529t
  noncoronary, 1523-1544
  in pulmonary embolism, 1877, 1877f
  in renal artery stenosis, 1533-1535,
      1533f-1536f, 1534t
  in subclavian artery stenosis, 1536-
      1538, 1537f
  in superior vena cava syndrome, 1543,
      1544f
  in tibioperoneal obstructive disease,
      1530-1532, 1530f, 1531t, 1532f
  in vertebral artery stenosis, 1542, 1542f
Percutaneous left ventricular assist
    device, 1422
Percutaneous transluminal angioplasty,
    in peripheral arterial disease,
    1504-1505
Percutaneous transluminal coronary
    angioplasty
  cardiac rehabilitation after, 1152
  coronary stents versus, 1430t
  in diabetic patients, 1557-1558
  preoperative, 2023
Percutaneous valve repair, mitral, 1442,
    1443f
Percutaneous valve replacement, aortic,
    1444-1446, 1445f
Percutaneous valvotomy, in mitral
    stenosis, 1653-1655, 1654f, 1655f
Percutaneous valvular intervention,
    1441-1446
Percutaneous valvuloplasty
  aortic, 1442, 1444, 1444f
  mitral, 1441-1442, 1442f
Performance measures, for quality of
    cardiovascular care
  guidelines and, relationship between,
      49-50, 50t
  principles for selection of, 50, 50t
Perfusion imaging. See Myocardial
    perfusion imaging.
Perfusion tracers
  coronary blood flow reserve and,
      362-363, 362f
  in myocardial perfusion imaging,
      362-363, 362f, 376
Perfusion-contraction matching, during
    acute myocardial ischemia, 1185,
    1187f
Pergolide (Permax), cardiovascular effects
    of, 277, 1812
Perhexiline
  in heart failure, 710-711
  in stable angina, 1377
Pericardial biopsy, in tuberculous
    pericarditis, 1848
Pericardial disease, 1829-1852
  chest pain in, 1196
  classification of, 1831t
  computed tomography in, 421-422, 422f
  echocardiography in, 288-295,
      291f-294f, 319, 319t
  in HIV infection, 1847-1848
  magnetic resonance imaging in, 405,
      405f
  metastatic, 1850-1851
  percutaneous coronary intervention
      and, 1851
  pericardial fluid analysis in, 1841

Pericardial disease (Continued)
  in rheumatic fever, 2082-2083
  in rheumatoid arthritis, 2095
  in scleroderma, 2100
Pericardial effusion, 1834-1842
  after catheter-based arrhythmia
      procedures, 1851
  chest radiography in, 340, 1837-1838,
      1837f
  clinical presentation in, 1836-1837
  computed tomography in, 422, 422f
  constrictive pericarditis in, 294-295
  echocardiography in, 289-290, 292f,
      1838, 1838f-1840f
  electrocardiography in, 1837, 1837f
  etiology of, 1834
  hemodynamics of, 1834-1836, 1835f,
      1835t, 1836f
  in HIV infection, 1794t, 1797-1798,
      1847-1848
  in hypothyroidism, 1852, 2042
  laboratory examination in, 1837-1838,
      1837f-1840f
  magnetic resonance imaging in, 405
  malignant, 1850, 2105
  management of, 1838, 1840-1842, 1840t
    with actual or threatened tamponade,
        1840-1841
    pericardial fluid analysis in, 1841
    pericardioscopy and percutaneous
        biopsy in, 1841-1842
    without actual or threatened
        tamponade, 1840
  after myocardial infarction, 1283
  pathophysiology of, 1834-1836, 1835f,
      1835t, 1836f
  in pregnancy, 1852
  total electrical alternans in, 186-187,
      186t, 187f
Pericardial fat pad sign, in pericardial
    effusion, 1837-1838
Pericardial fluid analysis, 1841
Pericardial friction rub. See Pericardial
    rub.
Pericardial knock, 136, 1843
Pericardial prosthetic valves
  autograft, 1684f, 1686
  xenograft, 1684f, 1686, 1686f
Pericardial reserve volume, 1830
Pericardial rub
  in acute pericarditis, 1832
  after cardiac surgery, 1998
  in myocardial infarction, 1223,
      1284
  in post-MI pericarditis, 1849
Pericardial space or sac, 1829, 1830f
Pericardial window, subxiphoid, in
    traumatic heart disease, 1858-1859
Pericardiectomy, in constrictive
    pericarditis, 1846
Pericardiocentesis
  in aortic dissection, 1480
  in bacterial pericarditis, 1847
  in cardiac tamponade, 2106
  closed, 1841
  echocardiographically guided, 290
  open, 1841
  in pericardial effusion, 1840, 1841
  in traumatic heart disease, 1859
  in tuberculous pericarditis, 1848
Pericardioscopy, in pericardial effusion,
    1841-1842
Pericardiotomy, 1850, 2002, 2002t
Pericarditis
  acute, 1830-1834
    cardiac enzymes and troponin
        measurements in, 1833

Pericarditis (Continued)
  chest radiography in, 1833
  complications of, 1833, 1833t
  differential diagnosis of, 1832
  echocardiography in, 1833
  electrocardiography in, 1832-1833, 1832f
  epidemiology of, 1830-1831
  etiology of, 1830-1831, 1831t
  hemogram in, 1833
  history in, 1831-1832
  laboratory examination in, 1832-1833, 1832f
  management of, 1833, 1833t
  natural history of, 1833
  pain in, 1221, 1355, 1831-1832, 1834
  pathophysiology of, 1831
  physical examination in, 1832
  ST segment elevation in, 181, 182f, 182t
  autoreactive, 1851
  bacterial, 1847
  after cardiac injury, 1850
  chest pain in, 1196
  constrictive, 1842-1846
    angiography in, 1844, 1844f
    cardiac catheterization in, 1844, 1844f
    cardiac tamponade versus, 1835t
    chest radiography in, 1843, 1843f
    clinical presentation in, 1843
    computed tomography in, 1844-1845, 1845f
    Doppler diagnostic criteria for, 292, 293f
    echocardiography in, 290, 292-295, 293f-294f, 1843-1844, 1845, 1845t
    electrocardiography in, 1843
    etiology of, 1842, 1842t
    hemodynamics of, 1845-1846, 1845t
    jugular venous pressure in, 130, 130f
    laboratory examination in, 1843-1845, 1843f-1845f
    magnetic resonance imaging in, 405, 405f, 1844-1845
    management of, 1846
    pathophysiology of, 1842, 1842f
    in pericardial effusion, 294-295
    physical examination in, 1843
    postoperative, 2003
    after radiation therapy, 2106
    versus restrictive cardiomyopathy, 1749, 1750, 1751, 1845-1846, 1845t
    transient, 295
  dialysis-associated, 1849
  in Dressler syndrome, 1849-1850
  drug-induced, 1851
  effusive-constrictive, 1846
  fungal, 1848-1849
  after myocardial infarction, 1284, 1833, 1849-1850
  after pericardiotomy, 1850
  in progressive systemic sclerosis, 1851
  radiation-induced, 1850
  relapsing and recurrent, 1834
  in rheumatoid arthritis, 1851, 2095
  in systemic lupus erythematosus, 1851, 2097
  tuberculous, 1841, 1848
  uremic, 1849
  viral, 1846-1847
Pericardium
  anatomy of, 1829, 1830f
  calcification of
    chest radiography in, 334f, 340-341
    computed tomography in, 422, 422f

Pericardium (Continued)
  in constrictive pericarditis, 1843, 1843f
  chest radiography of, 334f, 340-341
  congenital absence of, 1852
    echocardiography in, 288
    magnetic resonance imaging in, 405
  congenital anomalies of, 1852
  cyst of, 1852
    computed tomography in, 422, 422f
    echocardiography in, 289, 291f
    magnetic resonance imaging in, 405
  functions of, 1829-1830, 1831f
  in heart disease, passive role of, 1830
  neoplasms of, 422, 1851
  parietal, 1829
  physiology of, 1829-1830, 1831f
  pressure-volume relationships of, 1829-1830, 1831f
  properties of, in diastolic function, 575
  trauma to, 1858
  traumatic rupture of, 1856
  visceral, 1829
Perindopril, in heart failure, 624t, 654, 655f
Periodic paralyses, 2147-2148, 2147f
Peripartum cardiomyopathy, 1743
Peripheral arterial disease, 1491-1511, 1496-1499, 1500-1505. See also Peripheral vascular disease.
  algorithm for, 1505, 1506f
  ankle/brachial index in, 1496-1497, 1497f
  antiplatelet therapy in, 1502, 1503f, 1504f
  atheroembolism in, 1509-1511, 1510f
  blood pressure control in, 1501-1502, 1503tf
  classification of, 1495, 1496t
  clinical manifestations of, 1494-1495
  computed tomography angiography in, 1499, 1500f
  contrast angiography in, 1499, 1501f
  critical limb ischemia in
    classification of, 1495, 1496t
    incidence of, 1491
    pathophysiology of, 1493, 1494, 1494f
    progression to, 1500
    risk factors for, 1492
  definition of, 1491
  in diabetes mellitus, 1095, 1492, 1501
  in elderly persons, 1942-1943, 1943t
  epidemiology of, 1491, 1492f, 1492t
  exercise stress testing in, 1497
  exercise training rehabilitation in, 1504, 1504f
  intermittent claudication in, 1494-1495
    differential diagnosis of, 1494-1495, 1494t
    pathophysiology of, 1493
    percutaneous intervention for, 1523-1542
    prevalence of, 1491, 1492f
    risk factors for, 1492, 1493f
    treatment of, 1502-1504, 1504f
  lipid-lowering therapy in, 1500, 1502f, 1503f
  magnetic resonance angiography in, 1498, 1499f
  mortality in, 1500, 1502f
  pathophysiology of, 1493-1494, 1493t, 1494f
  percutaneous intervention in, 1523-1542
  percutaneous transluminal angioplasty and stents in, 1504-1505
  peripheral arterial surgery in, 1505

Peripheral arterial disease (Continued)
  pharmacotherapy in, 1502-1504, 1504f
  physical findings in, 1495
  prevalence and incidence of, 1491, 1492f, 1492t, 1493f
  prognosis for, 1499-1500, 1502f
  pulse volume recording in, 1497-1498
  risk factors for, 1491-1493, 1492t
  segmental pressure measurement in, 1496, 1497f
  signs and symptoms of, 134, 134t
  skeletal muscle in, 1494
  smoking cessation in, 1500
  ultrasonography in, 1498, 1498f, 1499f
  in women, 1964
Peripheral arterial pulse, evaluation of, 132
Peripheral blood supply, factors influencing, 1493-1494, 1494f
Peripheral edema, in heart failure, 563
Peripheral neuronal inhibitors, in hypertension therapy, 1058-1059
Peripheral vascular disease. See also Peripheral arterial disease; Venous thrombosis.
  cardiac surgery and, 1995
  coronary artery disease with, 1355, 1391
  definition of, 1491
  dietary supplements for, 1162
Peripheral vasculature, in heart failure, neurohormonal alterations in, 547-548
Peritoneal dialysis, in heart failure, 628
Permax. See Pergolide (Permax).
Permeability ratio, 734
Peroneal obstructive disease, percutaneous intervention in, 1530-1532, 1530f, 1531t, 1532f
Persistent truncus arteriosus, 1586-1587
Personal safety issues, in arrhythmias, 860t, 861
Personality, in cardiovascular disease, 2119
Pertechnetate, technetium-99m–labeled, 358
Pestilence and famine age
  cardiovascular disease in, 2, 3t, 4
  in United States, 7
PET. See Positron emission tomography.
Pet ownership, for stress management, 1157
Petechiae, in infective endocarditis, 1720
Pexelizumab, in myocardial infarction, 1264, 1309
Phage vector, 73
Pharmacodynamic variability
  in drug therapy, 58, 58f, 60-62, 62t
  in elderly persons, 1929-1930
Pharmacogenetics
  of antiarrhythmic agents, 781-782
  in heart failure, 708-710, 708t, 709f, 710f
  and variability in drug action, 58, 58f, 60-62, 61t, 62t
Pharmacogenomics, and variability in drug action, 58, 58f, 60-62, 61t, 62t
Pharmacoinvasive approach, to myocardial infarction management, 1283, 1284f, 1310
Pharmacokinetic variability
  in drug therapy, 58-60, 59f, 61t
  in elderly persons, 1929
  high-risk concept of, 60
Pharmacological maneuvers, with cardiac catheterization, 460

I-66

Pharyngeal muscles, in obstructive sleep apnea, 1915
Pharyngitis, streptococcal, in rheumatic fever, 2080-2081, 2084-2085
Phenothiazine
   cardiotoxicity of, 297
   myocarditis from, 1781
Phenotype, 75
   dominant, 87, 88f
   heterogeneity of, 88-89
   mendelian, 87-88, 87f, 88f, 89-94, 90t
   mitochondrial, 88, 88f
   pleiotropy of, 88
   recessive, 87, 87f
   variability in, 88, 89t
   X-linked, 87-88, 88f
Phentermine, cardiovascular effects of, 1812
Phentolamine (Regitine)
   in hypertensive crises, 1066, 1066t
   pulmonary vascular effects of, 1884
Phenylephrine
   during cardiac catheterization, 460
   in myocardial infarction, 1266
   postoperative, 2001
Phenytoin (Dilantin)
   in arrhythmias, 780t, 781t, 782t, 783t, 786t, 790
   pharmacokinetics of, 60
   in torsades de pointes, 905
Pheochromocytoma, 2045
   echocardiography in, 303, 303f
   hypertension in, 1043, 1043t
   sympathetic dysfunction in, 2182
Phlebography, contrast, in pulmonary embolism, 1870
Phlebotomy, in cyanotic congenital heart disease, 1568
Phobia, blood or injury, syncope in, 2179-2180
Phonocardiography, in heart failure, 595
Phosphate, postoperative, 1999
Phosphodiesterase inhibitors
   in acute heart failure, 601t, 604
   as platelet inhibitors, 2073
   postoperative, 2001
Phosphodiesterase-5 inhibitors, 524-525
   in idiopathic pulmonary arterial hypertension, 1900
Phospholamban
   diastolic relaxation and, 649
   in dilated cardiomyopathy, 115t, 116, 1745-1746
   as gene therapy target, 706t, 707
   in heart failure, 551
   in regulation of calcium uptake pump, 518-519, 518f
   thyroid hormones and, 2039
Phospholemman, 520, 520f
Phospholipid-associated enzyme complexes, in coagulation, 2052, 2052f
Phospholipids, biochemistry of, 1071-1072, 1072f
Phrenic nerve injury, in coronary artery bypass graft surgery, 2007
Physical activity. See also Exercise; Physical inactivity.
   benefits of, 1984-1985
   in cardiovascular disease prevention, 1137-1138, 1137t
   cardiovascular disease risk and, 1010-1012, 1011f
   definition of, 1150t, 1983
   dose of, 1983
   future perspectives on, 1990
   in heart failure, 619

Physical activity (Continued)
   in hypertension, 1028-1029
   in hypertension therapy, 1052-1053, 1052t
   intensity of, 1983
   in myocardial infarction, 1257
   sudden cardiac death and, 938-939, 947
Physical agents, myocarditis from, 1781
Physical examination, 127-139. See also Cardiac examination.
   of abdomen, 128
   in arrhythmias, 763-764
   of arterial pressure, 130-132, 131t, 132f
   of arterial pulse, 132-134, 133f, 134f, 134t
   of chest, 128
   in dyslipidemia, 1089
   of extremities, 127-128
   general appearance on, 127
   of head, 127
   of jugular venous pressure, 128-130, 128f-130f, 129t
   of neck, 127
   of skin, 127
   in syncope, 979
Physical fitness
   definition of, 1983
   exercise prescription for, 1986, 1986t
Physical inactivity
   age of
      cardiovascular disease in, 3t, 4
      in United States, 9
   regional trends in, 16
Physical maneuvers
   in arrhythmias, 764
   with cardiac catheterization, 459-460
   murmur response to, 139, 139t
   in neurally mediated syncope, 983
Physician-assisted suicide, in end-stage heart disease, 722-723
Physicians, quality of cardiovascular care by, 53, 54-55, 55t
Physiological monitors, for cardiac catheterization, 441
Physiological stress, with cardiac catheterization, 460
Phytosterols, in dyslipidemia, 1084
Pigtail catheter(s), 446, 446f
Pindolol, 792-793, 1372t
Pioglitazone, in diabetic vascular disease prevention, 1100
PISA (proximal isovelocity surface area) method, in Doppler echocardiography, 265-266, 266f
Pituitary gland
   adenoma of, acromegaly from, 2035
   anatomy of, 2033
   disorders of, 2033-2037
Placental circulation, 1565, 1565f
Plakoglobin, mutations of, in Naxos and Carvajal syndromes, 117, 117t
Planar myocardial perfusion imaging, 357-358, 358f
Plaque. See Atherosclerosis, plaque of.
Plasma concentration, monitoring of, 63
Plasma membrane, 67
Plasmid vector, 73
Plasmin, 2053, 2054f
Plasminogen, 2053, 2054f
Plasminogen activator(s), 2053-2054, 2054f
   tissue-type, 2054, 2068. See also Tissue plasminogen activator (t-PA).
   urokinase-type, 1246, 2054, 2068
   variants of, 2068
Plasminogen activator inhibitor-1 (PAI-1), 1018-1019, 2054

Platelet(s)
   activation of, 2055, 2055f, 2056f
   adhesion of, 2055, 2055f
   aggregation of, 2055-2056, 2055f, 2056f
   in diabetes mellitus, 1099
   in hemostasis, 2054-2056, 2055f, 2056f
   inhibitors of, 2054-2055, 2055f. See also Antiplatelet therapy.
   in myocardial infarction, 1220, 1253, 1254f
   thrombin and, 2056, 2057f, 2058f
   in UA/NSTEMI, 1320-1321, 1321f
Platypnea-orthodeoxia syndrome, patent foramen ovale and, 1580
Plavix. See Clopidogrel (Plavix).
Pleiotropy, 88
Pleura, chest radiography of, 341
Pleural effusion
   in aortic dissection, 1473
   after cardiac surgery, 1998
   in heart failure, 563, 593
   pericardial effusion versus, 290
Pleural pain, 1195, 1221
Pneumonia
   chest pain in, 1197
   postoperative, 2004
Pneumothorax, chest pain in, 1197
Point of maximal impulse, 135
Polar maps, in single photon emission computed tomography, 348, 350, 350f
Police, AED deployment by, 960, 960f
Policosanol, 1161t
   for dyslipidemia, 1162
Polyarteritis nodosa, 2093-2094, 2094f
Polycystic kidney disease, 94-95
Polymerase chain reaction, 74, 74f
Polymers, in gene transfer, 81
Polymorphic ventricular tachycardia, 905. See also Torsades de pointes.
   catecholaminergic, 102t, 106-108, 107f, 904
Polymorphisms
   single nucleotide, 75-76, 76f, 87
   and variability in drug action, 58f, 60-62, 61t, 62t
Polymyositis, 2100-2101
Polypharmacy, 64, 1928, 1929f
Polysomnography, in sleep apnea, 1919
Popliteal artery, obstructive disease of, percutaneous intervention for, 1525-1530, 1527f, 1528f, 1529t
Popliteal artery entrapment syndrome, 1507
Population-attributable risk, of cardiovascular disease, 1121-1122
Porcine prosthetic valves
   stented, 1684-1686, 1684f, 1685f, 1686f
   stentless, 1684f, 1685-1686
Portal hypertension, pulmonary arterial hypertension in, 1901
Portugal, cardiovascular disease in, 9-10, 11t
Positive airway pressure
   in acute heart failure, 596
   in central sleep apnea, 1920, 1920f
   in chronic obstructive pulmonary disease, 1908
   in obstructive sleep apnea, 1919, 1920t
Positive inotropic agents, in chronic kidney disease patients, 2165t
Positron emission tomography, 359-361
   attenuation correction in, 354
   CT, 455
   clinical applications of, 360-361, 361f
   combined with computed tomography angiography, 354-355, 355f
   of coronary blood flow reserve, 363

Positron emission tomography (Continued)
of fatty acid metabolism, 367
of glucose metabolism, 367-368, 370f
in heart failure, 569
image acquisition in, 360, 361f
image analysis in, 360
of myocardial viability, 384
perfusion tracers for, 360, 360t
in Takayasu arteritis, 2089
Postconditioning, myocardial, 1186, 1240-1241, 1241f
Posterior internodal tract, 728
Postinfectious reactive arthritis, 2096
Postpericardiotomy syndrome, 2002, 2002t
Postprandial angina, 1356
Postrepolarization refractoriness, 740
Postthrombotic syndrome, 1878
Postural orthostatic tachycardia syndrome, 772, 867, 976-977, 2176-2177
Postventricular atrial refractory period, 838, 840f
Potassium
abnormalities of. See also Hyperkalemia; Hypokalemia.
electrocardiography in, 184, 185f
depletion of, diuretic-induced, 625-626
equilibrium potential of, 738
intake of
blood pressure and, 1114
racial/ethnic differences in, 24
myocardial concentration of, 735t
postoperative, 1999
supplementation of
in heart failure, 626
in hypertension therapy, 1053
Potassium channel(s)
4-aminopyridine–sensitive, in action potential phase 1, 742-743, 743f
ATP
in coronary blood flow regulation, 1174-1175
mutation of, in dilated cardiomyopathy, 115t, 116
calcium-activated, 744
delayed rectifier, 744
in idiopathic pulmonary arterial hypertension, 1893
inwardly rectifying (Kir channels), 734f, 736, 743-744
synopsis of, 741t
voltage-gated, molecular structure of, 734f, 736
Potassium-sensitive periodic paralyses, 2147
Power production, and contractile function, 534
P-P interval
in sinoatrial exit block, 911
in sinus arrest, 910
PQ junction, in exercise stress testing, 200, 201f
PR interval
in atrial premature complexes, 867, 868f, 869f
in first-degree atrioventricular block, 914
in potassium abnormalities, 184
in supraventricular tachycardias, 893, 893t
in Wolff-Parkinson-White syndrome, 884
PR segment, 155, 156f, 156t, 157
in acute pericarditis, 181, 1832, 1832f

Practice guidelines
for ambulatory electrocardiography, 823-825, 824t-827t
for aortic regurgitation, 1696-1699, 1697t-1699t
for aortic stenosis, 1694-1696, 1695t-1696t
for arrhythmias, 823-830, 824t-830t
for arteriography, 501-508, 502t-508t
for atrial fibrillation, 923-930, 924t-930t
for cardiac catheterization, 439
for computed tomography, 436, 437t-438t
for congenital heart disease, 1561
for coronary artery bypass graft surgery, 1415t, 1416-1417
for coronary artery disease, 1405-1417, 1406f-1408f, 1407t, 1409t-1416t
for echocardiography, 314-325, 315t-325t
for electrocardiography, 190-193, 191t-193t
for electrophysiological studies, 825-830, 826t-830t
for exercise stress testing, 220-225, 221t-223t, 224f, 225t-226t
for heart failure, 618f, 619t-622t, 657-664, 658f, 659t-664t
for hypertension therapy, 1068-1070, 1069t
for implantable cardioverter-defibrillator, 858-861, 858t-860t
for infective endocarditis, 1734-1737, 1734t-1736t
for magnetic resonance imaging, 412-414, 413t-414t
for mitral regurgitation, 1702-1704, 1703t-1704t
for mitral stenosis, 1699, 1700t-1701t
for mitral valve prolapse, 1699, 1702, 1702t
for noncardiac surgery, 2028-2032, 2029f, 2030t-2031t
for nuclear imaging, 389-391, 390t
for pacemaker, 854-858, 855t-858t
for percutaneous coronary intervention, 1415t, 1416-1417, 1449-1453, 1450t-1455t
in myocardial infarction, 1314-1317, 1315t-1316t
for pregnancy and heart disease, 1979-1981, 1980t-1981t
for prosthetic valves, 1709, 1709t-1710t
for stable angina pectoris, 1405-1417, 1406f-1408f, 1407t, 1409t-1416t
for tricuspid regurgitation, 1704, 1705t
for UA/NSTEMI, 1344-1351, 1345t-1350t, 1346f
for valvular heart disease, 1693-1712, 1694t-1711t
Prasugrel, as platelet inhibitor, 2070-2071
Pravastatin (Pravachol), 1083
Prayer, distant intercessory, in cardiac catheterization, 1163-1164
Prazosin (Minipress), in Prinzmetal variant angina, 1339
Preconditioning
ischemic, 1238, 1555
myocardial, 1186
Precordial leads, 152, 152t, 153f
Precordial thump. See Thumpversion.
Prediabetes, 1135
Predictive value, test, 42
Prednisone
in amiodarone-induced hyperthyroidism, 2044
for contrast reaction prophylaxis, 472
in Dressler syndrome, 1850

Prednisone (Continued)
in pericarditis, 1833, 1834
in postpericardiotomy syndrome, 2002
Preeclampsia, 1044-1045, 1044t
Preeclampsia-eclampsia, 1975, 1975t
Preexcitation syndrome. See Wolff-Parkinson-White syndrome.
Pregnancy, 1967-1981
anticoagulant therapy in, 1979, 1981, 1981t
aortic dissection and, 1471
aortic regurgitation in, 1972
aortic stenosis in, 1970
arrhythmias in, 1975-1976, 1976t
atrial fibrillation in, 929t
atrial septal defect in, 1580, 1970
atrioventricular septal defect in, 1583
cardiac drugs in, 1976-1977, 1976t
cardiac evaluation in, 1968-1969
cardiac risk during, predictors of, 1967
cardiac surgery in, 1969, 1995
cardiomyopathies in, 1974-1975
cesarean section in, hemodynamic effects of, 1968
chronic hypertension in, 1045
coarctation of the aorta in, 1975, 1975f
complete transposition of the great arteries in, 1601
congenital heart disease in, 1970-1971, 1971f, 1971t
connective tissue disorders in, 1974
coronary artery disease in, 1975
cyanotic heart disease in, 1568, 1970-1971, 1971t
Ebstein anomaly in, 1605, 1971
hemodynamic adaptations to, 1967-1968, 1968f
high-risk, 1969-1970, 1970t
hypertension in, 1044-1045, 1044t, 1975, 1975t, 1976t
hypertension therapy in, 1063, 1975, 1976t
hypertrophic cardiomyopathy in, 1773
idiopathic pulmonary arterial hypertension and, 1896
labor and delivery in, hemodynamic changes during, 1968
Marfan syndrome and, 92, 1974
mitral regurgitation in, 1972
mitral stenosis in, 1972
myocardial infarction in, 1975
patent ductus arteriosus in, 1586, 1970
pericardial effusion in, 1852
persistent truncus arteriosus in, 1587
physical examination in, 1968-1969
practice guidelines for, 1979-1981, 1980t-1981t
prevention of, 1977-1978
prosthetic valves in, 1688, 1972-1973, 1979, 1981, 1981t
pulmonary hypertension in, 1971-1972
pulmonic stenosis in, 1970
tetralogy of Fallot in, 1971, 1971f
transposition of the great arteries in, congenitally corrected, 1971
valvular heart disease in, 1972-1973, 1979
venous thrombosis and, 2061
ventricular septal defect in, 1584, 1970
Prehypertension, 1131
Preload
afterload and, relationship between, 530
contractility and, 529
definition of, 570t
in heart failure, 573
in left ventricular systolic function, 569
wall stress and, 531

Premature closure heuristic, 46
Premature complexes. *See* Atrial premature complexes; Ventricular premature complexes.
Premature infant, patent ductus arteriosus in, 1585-1586
Preoperative evaluation. *See* Cardiac surgery, preoperative evaluation for; Noncardiac surgery, preoperative risk assessment for.
Preparticipation screening
  of competitive athletes, 1988
  for exercise and sports activities, 1986-1988, 1986t, 1987t
  in health and fitness facilities, 1988
  for hypertrophic cardiomyopathy, 1768
  in medical office setting, 1986, 1986t, 1987t, 1988
Pressor agents, in autonomic failure, 2176
Pressure gradients
  with cardiac catheterization
    intraventricular, 457
    in valvular stenosis, 455-457, 456f
  Doppler echocardiography of, 262, 263f
Pressure half-time, in Doppler echocardiography, 265, 265f
Pressure measurements, with cardiac catheterization, 449, 451-452. *See also* Cardiac catheterization.
  abnormal, 452, 453t-454t
  equipment for, 449, 451
  normal, 451, 451f, 452t
Pressure overload
  left ventricular, 1034
  right ventricular, 577-578
Pressure overload (concentric) hypertrophy, 549, 550f, 551f, 1034
Pressure-flow relationships, in coronary artery stenosis, 1177-1178, 1177f, 1178f
  distal coronary pressure and, 1178, 1179f
Pressure-natriuresis curve, in hypertension, 1031-1032
Pressure-volume area, and myocardial oxygen consumption, 532-533
Pressure-volume loops, for contractility measurement, 533-534, 534f
Pressure-volume relationships
  in constrictive pericarditis, 1842, 1842f
  end-diastolic, 651-652, 652f
  end-systolic, 571, 571f, 572f
  of pericardium, 1829-1830, 1831f
Pressure-work index, in myocardial oxygen uptake, 532-533
Prevalence, 1122
Prinzmetal variant angina, 176, 177f, 1337-1340
  arteriography in, 488-489, 490f-491f, 1338, 1339f
  clinical findings in, 1338
  electrocardiography in, 176, 177f, 1338, 1339f
  laboratory findings in, 1338, 1339f
  management of, 1338-1339
  mechanisms of, 1176, 1338
  prognosis in, 1339-1340
  provocative tests in, 1338
Priscoline. *See* Tolazoline (Priscoline).
PRKAR1α, mutation of, in Carney complex, 121
Proarrhythmic effects
  of antiarrhythmic agents, 785
  of sotalol, 796
Probabilistic reasoning, in decision-making, 41
Probabilities, natural frequencies versus, 43

Procainamide
  adverse effects of, 787
  in atrial fibrillation, 872-873
  in atrial flutter, 875
  in cardiac arrest, 962, 963
  in chronic kidney disease patients, 2165t
  dosage and administration of, 783t, 787
  electrophysiological characteristics of, 780t, 781t, 782t, 786t, 787
  hemodynamic effects of, 787
  indications for, 787
  pharmacokinetics of, 783t, 787
  in pregnancy, 1976t
  psychiatric side effects of, 2132
  in ventricular premature complexes, 895
PROCAM risk assessment algorithm, 1123
Procardia. *See* Nifedipine (Procardia).
Progesterone, depot, 1977
Programmed electrical stimulation
  in Brugada syndrome, 106
  in cardiac arrest prevention, 966-967
  in tachycardias, 774
Progressive systemic sclerosis, 1851, 2099-2100
Propafenone
  in arrhythmias, 780t, 781t, 782t, 783t, 786t, 791
  in atrial fibrillation, 873
  pacemaker abnormalities caused by, 851
  pharmacokinetics of, 60
  in pregnancy, 1976t
Propionyl L-carnitine, in peripheral arterial disease, 1503
Propofol, for noncardiac surgery, 2020-2021
Propranolol (Inderal)
  in abdominal aortic aneurysms, 1463
  adverse effects of, 793
  in aortic dissection, 1479
  in cardiac arrest, 962
  dosage and administration of, 793
  electrophysiological characteristics of, 780t, 781t, 782t, 786t, 792-793
  hemodynamic effects of, 793
  indications for, 793
  in Marfan syndrome, 92
  pharmacokinetics and pharmacology of, 59, 784t, 793, 1372t
  in ventricular premature complexes, 895
  in Wolff-Parkinson-White syndrome, 891
Prorenin, in hypertension, 1034
Prospective data collection, for quality measurement, 51
Prostacyclin
  antithrombotic properties of, 2050
  in coronary blood flow regulation, 1170
  in Eisenmenger syndrome, 1570
  in idiopathic pulmonary arterial hypertension, 1898-1899, 1899f
  pulmonary vascular effects of, 1885
  vasodilator properties of, 2050
Prostacyclin synthase, in idiopathic pulmonary arterial hypertension, 1892
Prostaglandin(s)
  in congenital aortic stenosis, 1611
  in congenital heart disease, 1566
  in pulmonary circulation, 1884-1885
Prostaglandin E$_1$
  in coarctation of the aorta, 1607
  in pulmonic stenosis, 1617
  in transposition of the great arteries, 1598

Prostaglandin E$_2$, in heart failure, 545-546
Prosthetic valves, 1682-1688
  auscultatory characteristics of, 1683f
  bileaflet, 1682, 1682f
  caged-ball, 1682f, 1683
  in children, 1688
  echocardiography of, 277-280, 278f, 279t, 280f
  in hemodialysis patients, 1688
  hemodynamics of, 1686-1687
  homograft (allograft), 1684f, 1686
  infective endocarditis of, 1715-1716
    microbiology of, 1715, 1715t
    pathology of, 1715-1716, 1715f
    staphylococcal, 1725-1726, 1726t, 1728
    surgical treatment of, 1728
  magnetic resonance imaging of, 405
  mechanical
    durability of, 1683
    indications for, 1687-1688, 1687f
    in pregnancy, 1973, 1979, 1981, 1981t
    thrombogenicity of, 1683
    types of, 1682-1683, 1682f
  noncardiac surgery and, 1688, 2015
  pericardial (autograft), 1684f, 1686
  pericardial (xenograft), 1684f, 1686, 1686f
  physical examination in patients with, 146-147
  porcine
    stented, 1684-1686, 1684f, 1685f, 1686f
    stentless, 1684f, 1685-1686
  practice guidelines for, 1709, 1709t-1710t
  in pregnancy, 1688, 1972-1973
  pulmonary autograft, 1686
  selection of, 1687-1688, 1687f
  thrombosis with, 1683
  tilting-disc, 1682-1683, 1682f
  tissue (bioprostheses)
    durability of, 1685, 1685f, 1686f
    indications for, 1687-1688, 1687f
    in pregnancy, 1972-1973
    types of, 1684-1686, 1684f, 1685f
  in tricuspid position, 1688
Protamine sulfate, for heparin reversal, 470, 2063
Protease inhibitors, 2067
  cardiovascular effects of, 1812
  complications of, 1801, 1802t
Proteasome inhibitors, cardiotoxicity of, 2111
Protein(s)
  conversion of genes to, 71-72, 72f
  C-reactive. *See* C-reactive protein (hs-CRP).
  G. *See* G protein(s).
Protein C
  activated
    recombinant, 2067
    resistance to
      factor V Leiden gene mutation and, 2057-2058
      venous thromboembolism in, 1864
    antithrombotic properties of, 2053
    deficiency of, in deep vein thrombosis, 2059, 2059t
Protein kinase, cAMP-dependent, 522-523, 522f
Protein kinase A
  in beta-adrenergic response, 522-523, 522f
  compartmentalization of, 523
Protein kinase C, in diabetes mellitus, 1097
Protein kinase G, in contraction-relaxation cycle, 524, 525f

Protein S
  antithrombotic properties of, 2053
  deficiency of, in deep vein thrombosis,
    2059, 2059t
Protein sorting (trafficking), 68
Protein Z, antithrombotic properties of,
    2053, 2053f
Protein-losing enteropathy, in Fontan
    patients, 1595, 1596
Proteoglycans, 2065
Proteomics, 74, 77-78, 77f, 78f
Prothrombin gene mutation, 2058, 2059f
  venous thromboembolism in, 1864
Protodiastole, 529
Protozoal myocarditis, 1779-1780, 1779f
Proximal isovelocity surface area method,
    in Doppler echocardiography, 265-
    266, 266f
Proximal occlusion devices, in
    percutaneous coronary intervention,
    1426
Proxis catheter, 1426
P-selectin, in atherogenesis, 990-991
Pseudoaneurysm
  versus aneurysm, 1274f
  aortic, 301, 1458
  after free wall rupture, 257, 258f
  after myocardial infarction, 1273,
    1274f
Pseudocholinesterase, in drug metabolism
    and elimination, 61t
Pseudoclaudication, 1523, 1524t
  neurogenic, 1495
Pseudohypertension, 131-132
  in aortic dissection, 1480
Pseudonormalized mitral flow filling
    pattern, 250-251
Pseudoxanthoma elasticum
  cardiovascular manifestations of, 90t
  genetic studies in, 94, 94f
Psoriatic arthritis, 2096
P-SPIKES approach, to communication of
    bad news, 718, 719t
Psychiatric care of cardiac patient,
    2126-2128
  in convalescence and recovery phase,
    2127-2128
  drug therapy in, 2128-2133. See also
    Psychotropic agents.
  in hospitalized patient, 2126-2127
  in rehabilitation, 2128
Psychiatric disorders
  chest pain and, 2125
  palpitations and, 2125
  sudden cardiac death and, 2123
  syncope in, 978
Psychological symptoms, in end-stage
    heart disease, 718, 721
Psychopharmacology, in cardiac patients,
    2128-2133
Psychosocial factors
  in arrhythmias, 2122-2123
  in cardiovascular disease, 2121
  cardiovascular disease risk and, 1140
  in chest pain, 2125
  in heart failure, 2124-2125
  in heart transplantation, 677
  in hypertension, 2123-2124
  in palpitations, 2125
  in sudden cardiac death, 939, 2123
Psychosocial interventions
  in cardiovascular disease prevention,
    1140-1141
  in postinfarction depression, 2127
  in rehabilitation, 2128
Psychostimulants, cardiovascular aspects
    of, 2129t, 2130

Psychotropic agents
  cardiovascular aspects of, 2128-2132,
    2129t-2132t
  drug interactions of, 2132-2133, 2133t
  ECG effects of, 184
PTCA. See Percutaneous transluminal
    coronary angioplasty.
PTPN11, mutations of, in Noonan
    syndrome, 119t, 121
Public health interventions, in United
    States, cardiovascular disease and,
    8
Public safety
  arrhythmias and, 860t, 861
  cardiac arrest and, 970-971
Public sites, AED deployment at, 960
Pulmonary. See also Cardiopulmonary
    entries; Lung(s).
Pulmonary angiography
  in pulmonary embolism, 1870
  in pulmonary hypertension, 1888
Pulmonary arterial hypertension. See
    also Pulmonary hypertension.
  from anorexigens, 1902
  apoptosis-based theory of, 1895f
  in congenital heart disease, 1900-1901
  in connective tissue disorders, 1901
  in heart failure, 142
  in HIV infection, 1902
  idiopathic, 1891-1900
    calcium channels in, 1893
    versus chronic thromboembolic
      pulmonary hypertension, 1912
    clinical course in, 1896
    clinical features of, 1895-1896
    elastase in, 1893
    endothelial dysfunction in,
      1892-1893
    etiology of, 1892-1893, 1892f-1894f
    familial, 1894-1895, 1894f
    genetic factors in, 1893-1895, 1895f
    hemodynamic findings in, 1893,
      1896
    left ventricular dysfunction in,
      1896
    natural history of, 1895-1896
    pathological findings in, 1891-1892,
      1891f, 1892t
    potassium channels in, 1893
    pregnancy and, 1896
    pulmonary arteriopathy in
      hypertensive, 1891, 1891f, 1892t
      thrombotic, 1891-1892
    serotonin in, 1893, 1894f
    treatment of, 1896-1900
      anticoagulants in, 1897
      atrial septostomy in, 1900
      calcium channel blockers in, 1898
      digoxin in, 1896
      diuretics in, 1896-1897
      endothelin receptor blockers in,
        1899
      heart-lung and lung transplantation
        in, 1900
      lifestyle changes in, 1896
      oxygen in, 1897
      phosphodiesterase-5 inhibitors in,
        1900
      principles of, 1897-1898
      prostacyclins in, 1898-1899, 1899f
      vasodilators in, 1898-1900, 1899f
  in portal hypertension, 1901
  in pulmonary capillary
    hemangiomatosis, 1902-1903
  in pulmonary venoocclusive disease,
    1902
  in sickle cell disease, 1902

Pulmonary arterioles, anatomy of, 1883
Pulmonary arteriopathy
  hypertensive, in idiopathic pulmonary
    arterial hypertension, 1891, 1891f,
    1892t
  thrombotic, in idiopathic pulmonary
    arterial hypertension, 1891-1892
Pulmonary arteriovenous fistula, 1620
Pulmonary arteriovenous malformations,
    in hereditary hemorrhagic
    telangiectasia, 98
Pulmonary artery(ies)
  anatomy of, 1883
  anomalies of, magnetic resonance
    imaging of, 407
  banding of, in double-inlet ventricle,
    1593
  catheterization of, 444
  chest radiography of, 331, 331f, 332f,
    335, 336f, 337f, 338
  elastic, 1883
  large central, causes of, 1573
  left coronary artery origin from, 482,
    483f
  magnetic resonance imaging of, 407
  muscular, 1883
  normal anatomy of, 1564-1565
  stenosis of
    isolated branch, 1615
    peripheral, 1615-1616
  transesophageal echocardiography of,
    236
Pulmonary artery catheter
  in heart failure, 595, 599-600
  hemodynamic monitoring with, in
    pericardial effusion, 1841
  in noncardiac surgery, 2026
Pulmonary artery end-diastolic pressure
    (PAEDP), 262
Pulmonary artery pressure, 451, 452t,
    453t-454t
  Doppler echocardiography of, 262-263,
    263f
  in mitral stenosis, 1648, 1648f
  monitoring of, in myocardial infarction,
    1265
  in pulmonary hypertension, 1889t
Pulmonary artery sling, 1610
Pulmonary atresia, tetralogy of Fallot
    with, 1588, 1589
Pulmonary autograft, in thoracic aortic
    aneurysms, 1467
Pulmonary autograft prosthetic valves,
    1686
Pulmonary blood flow/systemic blood
    flow (PBF/SBF or QP/QS ratio), in
    shunt assessment, 458-459
Pulmonary capillary hemangiomatosis,
    1902-1903
Pulmonary capillary wedge pressure
  with cardiac catheterization, 451, 452t,
    453t
  chest radiography and, 335-336
  in heart failure, 593
  in mitral stenosis, 456
  in pulmonary hypertension, 1889, 1889t
Pulmonary circulation
  aging and, 1886
  exercise effects on, 1886
  fetal, 1565, 1886
  neonatal, 1886
  normal, 1883-1886, 1885f
  versus systemic circulation, 1883, 1884t
Pulmonary disease
  atrial fibrillation in, 930t
  cardiac surgery in patients with, 1996
  chest pain in, 1197

I-70 **Pulmonary disease** (Continued)
chronic obstructive. *See* Chronic obstructive pulmonary disease.
echocardiography in, 320, 321t
postoperative, 2004
pulmonary hypertension in, 1904-1909, 1904t
Pulmonary edema
cardiogenic, 589
in heart failure, 562, 583-584, 584t, 589, 590
neurogenic, in acute cerebrovascular disease, 2150
Pulmonary embolism, 1863-1879. *See also* Venous thrombosis.
chest pain in, 1196-1197, 1355
chronic pulmonary hypertension after, 1878
clinical presentation in, 1866, 1866t, 1867f, 1867t
clinical syndromes of, 1866-1868
computed tomography in, 432-433, 433f
deep vein thrombosis and, 1864-1865, 1865f
diagnosis of, 1865-1870
arterial blood gases in, 1868
chest radiography in, 1868
computed tomography in, 1868-1870, 1869f, 1869t
contrast phlebography in, 1870
echocardiography in, 1870, 1870t
electrocardiography in, 1867f, 1868, 1868t
integrated approach to, 1870, 1871t, 1872f
lung scanning in, 1868, 1870
magnetic resonance imaging in, 1870
plasma D-dimer ELISA in, 1868
pulmonary angiography in, 1870
risk stratification in, 1870-1871, 1871t
scoring system for, 1866, 1867t
venous ultrasonography in, 1870
differential diagnosis of, 1866, 1867t
electrocardiography in, 166, 167f
epidemiology of, 1863-1864
future perspectives on, 1879
hypercoagulable states in, 1864, 1864t
management of, 1870-1878, 1872f
anticoagulation in, 1871-1876
complications of, 1874-1875
novel agents for, 1875
optimal duration of, 1875-1876, 1875t
embolectomy in
catheter, 1877, 1877f
surgical, 1877, 1878f
emotional support in, 1877
fondaparinux in, 1873, 1873t
inferior vena cava filters in, 1876
low-molecular-weight heparin in, 1872-1873, 1873t
thrombolytic therapy in, 1876-1877, 1876t
unfractionated heparin in, 1871-1872, 1872t
warfarin in, 1873-1874
massive, 1866, 1877-1878, 1878f, 1878t
moderate to large (submassive), 1866-1867
mortality in, predictors of, 1871, 1871t
after myocardial infarction, 1284-1285
nonthrombotic, 1868
pain in, 1221-1222
paradoxical, 1867-1868
pathophysiology of, 1864-1865, 1864t, 1865f, 1866f

Pulmonary embolism (Continued)
prevention of, 1878-1879, 1879t
pulmonary infarction syndrome in, 1867, 1868t
right ventricular dysfunction and, 1865, 1866f, 1871
risk factors for, 1863-1864, 1864t
small to moderate, 1867
sudden death in, 948
thromboembolic pulmonary hypertension and, 1910
venous insufficiency in, chronic, 1878
ventricular interdependency and, 1865, 1866f
Pulmonary examination, in heart failure, 562-563
Pulmonary extravascular water, in myocardial infarction, 1219
Pulmonary function, in myocardial infarction, 1219
Pulmonary function tests, in pulmonary hypertension, 1888
Pulmonary hypertension, 1883-1913
altitude and, 1886
in alveolar hypoventilation disorders, 1909-1910
in aortic stenosis, 1904
arterial. *See* Pulmonary arterial hypertension.
cardiac catheterization in, 1888-1889
chest pain in, 1355
chest radiography in, 1887
in chest wall disorders, 1909
in chronic obstructive pulmonary disease, 1904-1909, 1905f, 1906t, 1907f, 1908f
classification of, 1890, 1890t, 1891t
clinical assessment of, 1886-1890
computed tomography in, 1888
concomitant illness in, 1887
in congenital heart disease, 1568-1569
exercise and sports in patients with, 1990
in cystic fibrosis, 1909
diagnostic studies in, 1887-1890, 1887t, 1888f, 1889t
in diaphragmatic paralysis, 1909-1910
echocardiography in, 1887
in Eisenmenger syndrome, 1569
electrocardiography in, 1887
exercise stress testing in, 1888
exercise-induced, 1890
familial, 96
future perspectives on, 1913
in heart failure with normal ejection fraction, 646
histopathological classification of, 1892t
history in, 1886
in HIV-infected patients, 1795t, 1799-1800
in hyperthyroidism, 2041
irreversible, heart transplantation and, 677
laboratory tests in, 1887-1888, 1887t
lung scintigraphy in, 1888, 1888f
in mitral stenosis, 1648, 1904
in neuromuscular disease, 1909
noncardiac surgery in patients with, 2015-2016
persistent, of newborn, 1902
physical examination in, 1886-1887
in pregnancy, 1971-1972
pulmonary angiography in, 1888
pulmonary function tests in, 1888
radionuclide ventriculography in, 1887-1888

Pulmonary hypertension (Continued)
in respiratory disorders, 1904-1909, 1904t
in restrictive cardiomyopathy, 1750
right ventricular remodeling in, 577-578
in sarcoidosis, 1912
in schistosomiasis, 1912
in scleroderma, 2100
in sleep-disordered breathing, 1909
in systemic lupus erythematosus, 2098
thromboembolic, 1878, 1910-1912, 1911f
tricuspid regurgitation in, 1677-1678
types of, 1891-1912
vasodilator testing in, 1889-1890, 1889t
Pulmonary infarction syndrome, in pulmonary embolism, 1867, 1868t
Pulmonary insufficiency, after coronary artery bypass graft surgery, 1383
Pulmonary radionuclide perfusion scintigraphy. *See* Lung scan.
Pulmonary rehabilitation, in chronic obstructive pulmonary disease, 1907
Pulmonary thromboembolism, in Fontan patients, 1595
Pulmonary thromboendarterectomy
in chronic pulmonary hypertension, 1878
in thromboembolic pulmonary hypertension, 1910
Pulmonary vascular resistance, 452t, 455
at birth, 1886
Doppler echocardiography of, 267
in pulmonary hypertension, 1889t
quantification of, 1883-1884
regulation of, 1884-1886, 1885f
in thromboembolic pulmonary hypertension, 1911
Pulmonary vein(s)
ablation of, in atrial fibrillation, 812f-814f, 813, 815t, 816f
computed tomography of, 432, 433f
embryogenesis of, 1564
right, compression/obstruction of, in Fontan patients, 1595, 1596
stenosis of, 1619, 1619f
transesophageal echocardiography of, 236
Pulmonary venoocclusive disease, 1902
Pulmonary venous drainage
anomalous
magnetic resonance imaging in, 407, 408-409, 408f
partial, 1619-1620
pulmonary arterial hypertension in, 1900-1901
total, 1596-1597, 1596f, 1598f
in normal heart, 1564
Pulmonary venous hypertension, 1903-1904
Pulmonic regurgitation
angiography in, 1680
auscultation in, 1679-1680
chest radiography in, 1680
clinical presentation in, 1678-1680
echocardiography in, 276-277, 277f, 1679f, 1680
electrocardiography in, 1680
etiology and pathology of, 1678, 1679f
history and physical examination in, 146
magnetic resonance imaging in, 1679f, 1680
management of, 1680
murmur in, 137, 146
physical examination in, 1679-1680

Pulmonic stenosis
chest radiography in, 337f, 338
dysplastic, 1617-1618
echocardiography in, 270
etiology and pathology of, 1678, 1678f
history and physical examination in, 146
with intact ventricular septum, 1616-1617, 1616f, 1617f
in pregnancy, 1970
pressure gradient determination in, 456
Pulmonic valve
absent, tetralogy of Fallot with, 1588
normal anatomy of, 1564
Pulse
in acute limb ischemia, 1507
in aortic regurgitation, 1472
arterial. *See* Arterial pulse.
bounding, 133
in congenital heart disease, 1572
Corrigan (water-hammer), 133, 1638
in peripheral arterial disease, 1495
venous. *See* Jugular venous pulse.
Pulse oximetry, in congenital heart disease, 1901
Pulse pressure
cardiovascular disease risk and, 1006
in elderly persons, 1925f
in heart failure, 592-593
Pulse volume recording, in peripheral arterial disease, 1497-1498
Pulseless electrical activity, after cardiac arrest, 951, 961f, 962-963, 962f
Pulsus alternans, 133, 134f
Pulsus paradoxus, 133
in cardiac tamponade, 1835, 1835f, 1837
in constrictive pericarditis, 1843
in heart failure, 593
Pulsus parvus et tardus, 133
Purkinje cells, 510t, 730, 733f
Purkinje fibers
free-running, 730-731
terminal, 730
transmembrane potentials in, 738t
Purpura, Henoch-Schönlein, 2094
Purpuric rash, in vasculitis, 2087, 2088f

Q

Q wave, 158
in congenital heart disease, 1572
in myocardial infarction, 1209, 1210, 1210f, 1228, 1228f
ECG classification of, 174
ECG sequence with, 174-175, 175f
left bundle branch block and, 178-179, 179f, 180f
noninfarction, 180-181, 180t, 181f
in stable angina, 1357
q wave, septal, in left bundle branch block, 169
QRS axis, 158
in right bundle branch block, 170
in right ventricular hypertrophy, 165
QRS complex, 155, 156f, 156t, 158-159, 158f
in atrial premature complexes, 868
in atrioventricular dissociation, 920
in atrioventricular nodal reentrant tachycardia, 878, 879, 879f
duration of, 159
in arrhythmia diagnosis, 764, 766t
early patterns in, 158
fragmented, 181
intrinsicoid deflection in, 159
in left bundle branch block, 168, 169
in left ventricular hypertrophy, 162, 163, 163f

QRS complex *(Continued)*
low-voltage, causes of, 185-186, 186t
mid and late patterns in, 158-159
in myocardial infarction, 174-175, 175f, 176f
in potassium abnormalities, 184
in right bundle branch block, 170
terminology for, 158
in third-degree atrioventricular block, 918
in torsades de pointes, 905
in ventricular premature complexes, 893
in Wolff-Parkinson-White syndrome, 884
QRS contours, in ventricular tachycardia, 897, 897f
QRS tachycardia
narrow and wide complex, electrophysiology in, 826t, 827
wide
algorithm for diagnosis of, 898f
in Wolff-Parkinson-White syndrome, 890
QRST angle, 160
QT interval, 159-160, 159-161
in calcium abnormalities, 184
corrected, 159-160
disopyramide effects on, 788
dispersion of, 160
in arrhythmia diagnosis, 764, 766f
dofetilide effects on, 796
ibutilide effects on, 797
in left ventricular hypertrophy, 163
in myocardial infarction, 174, 176
in potassium abnormalities, 184
procainamide effects on, 787
prolongation of. *See also* Long QT syndrome.
cardiac arrest with, 964
drug-induced, 64
electrophysiology in, 826t, 827
in periodic paralyses, 2147
quinidine effects on, 786
shortening of, 102t, 108, 108f
in torsades de pointes, 905
QT(U) interval, 159
Quadrigemy, 893
Quality of cardiovascular care, 49-56
in cardiac surgery, 1993
current data on, 53-54, 53t
for hospitals, 54, 54f, 54t, 55f
for physicians, 54-55, 55t
definition of, 51-53
error reduction and, 51-52
future perspectives on, 56
improvement of, strategies for, 55-56
measurement of, 49-51
for heart failure, 51t
methodological issues in, 50-51
for myocardial infarction, 52t
organizations involved in, 49, 50t
performance measures for
guidelines and, relationship between, 49-50
principles for selection of, 50, 50t
volume as marker of, 52-53, 53f, 53t
Quality-adjusted life years, as measure of cost-effectiveness, 35
Questran. *See* Cholestyramine (Questran).
Quincke sign, in aortic regurgitation, 1638
Quinidine, 785-787
adverse effects of, 786-787
dosage and administration of, 783t, 785

Quinidine *(Continued)*
drug interactions of, 786-787
electrophysiological actions of, 780t, 781t, 782t, 785, 786t
hemodynamic effects of, 785
indications for, 785-786
pharmacokinetics of, 783t, 785
in pregnancy, 1976t
psychiatric side effects of, 2132

R

R wave, 158
in exercise stress testing, 202
in left bundle branch block, 168-169
in left ventricular hypertrophy, 162, 163f
in myocardial infarction, 174
poor progression of, factors associated with, 180-181
in right bundle branch block, 170
in right ventricular hypertrophy, 165
tall, differential diagnosis of, 176t
R′ wave, 158
r wave
in left bundle branch block, 169
in right ventricular hypertrophy, 165
Racial/ethnic differences, 23, 24f
in cardiovascular care and outcomes, 25-26, 25f
in cardiovascular disease risk factors, 23-24
in cardiovascular mortality, 25
clinical messages related to, 31-32
construct of, 31
in coronary artery disease, 25, 28-29, 29f
in diabetes mellitus, 23
in diet, 24
in dyslipidemia, 24
in heart failure, 29-31, 30f, 31t, 32f
in hypertension, 26-28, 26f-28f, 28t
in hypertension therapy, 27-28, 28f, 28t
in hypertrophic cardiomyopathy, 1768
in insulin resistance, 23
in left ventricular hypertrophy, 24, 27
in metabolic syndrome, 23
in obesity, 23-24
in preoperative risk analysis, 1994
in sudden cardiac death, 936, 937f
Radial artery approach
in arteriography, 468-469
in percutaneous coronary intervention, 1423-1424
Radial artery graft, for coronary artery bypass graft surgery, 1382, 1385
Radial artery infection, postoperative, 2008
Radial artery pulse, 132
Radiation brachytherapy, for in-stent restenosis, 1429, 1431t
Radiation injury, from arteriography, 468
Radiation safety, in cardiac catheterization, 441
Radiation therapy
cardiac disease after, echocardiography in, 298
cardiovascular effects of, 2115-2116
constrictive pericarditis after, 2106
mediastinal, coronary artery disease after, 1400
myocarditis from, 1781
pericarditis after, 1850
Radiculitis, cervical, chest pain in, 1354
Radiculopathy, lumbosacral, exertional leg pain in, 1495

Radiofrequency catheter ablation, 803-819
in accessory pathways, 804-806, 804f-805f
in atrial fibrillation, 812-816, 812f-814f, 815t, 816f, 873
in atrial flutter, 809-810, 810f-811f, 876
in atrial tachycardia, 808-809, 809f
in atrioventricular conduction for atrial tachyarrhythmias, 810-812
in atrioventricular nodal reentrant tachycardia, 806-808, 806f-808f, 881-882
in cardiac arrest prevention, 967
cooled-tip, 804
in ectopic junctional tachycardia, 808
epicardial catheter mapping in, 819
in inappropriate sinus tachycardia, 808
multielectrode mapping systems in, 819
pericardial effusion after, 1851
in premature ventricular complexes, 819
in sinus node reentrant tachycardia, 808
strategies for, 803-804, 803f, 804f
in ventricular tachycardia, 816-819, 817f-818f, 902
in Wolff-Parkinson-White syndrome, 892-893
Radiographic equipment, for cardiac catheterization, 440-441, 441f
Radiography
chest. See Chest radiography.
computed, 329
digital, 329
Radionuclide angiography or ventriculography, 358-359
in acute chest pain, 1202-1203
in amyloidosis, 1752
in aortic regurgitation, 1640-1641, 1646
in coronary artery disease, 378
for detection of coronary artery disease, 378
for diastolic function evaluation, 370-371, 370f, 371f
in heart failure, 371, 371f
in hypertrophic cardiomyopathy, 371
in dilated cardiomyopathy, 1748
equilibrium
advantages of, 359
image acquisition in, 358
image display and analysis in, 356f, 358, 359f
first-pass
advantages of, 359
image acquisition in, 358, 360
image analysis in, 358-359
in heart failure, 566
for left ventricular function quantification, 369, 370
for left ventricular volume assessment, 369-370
in mitral regurgitation, 1664
in pulmonary hypertension, 1887-1888
serial, 370
Radionuclide lung scan. See Lung scan.
RAGE (receptor for advanced glycation end products), in diabetes mellitus, 1098, 1098f, 1547
Rales
in heart failure, 142, 562-563, 563t, 590, 593
in myocardial infarction, 1223

Ramipril
in chronic kidney disease patients, 2165t
in heart failure, 624t
in peripheral arterial disease, 1501-1502, 1503tf
Ramp protocol, for exercise stress testing, 198
Randomized Evaluation of Mechanical Assistance for the Treatment of Congestive Heart Failure (REMATCH) trial, 694-695, 695f
Ranolazine
in heart failure, 711
in stable angina, 1376-1377
Raschke nomogram, 1872, 1872t
Rash, purpuric, in vasculitis, 2087, 2088f
Rastelli procedure, in transposition of the great arteries, 1599, 1600
reintervention after, 1601
Rayment model of cross-bridge cycling, revised, 512, 515f
Raynaud phenomenon, in scleroderma, 2100
Reactive arthritis, postinfectious, 2096
Reactive oxygen species
in heart failure, 544, 545f
in hypertension, 1033
as signaling molecules, 526
Reasoning, diagnostic, 41-42
Recanalization, 1242
Receding pandemics age
cardiovascular disease in, 3t, 4
in United States, 7, 7f
Receiver operating characteristic curves, in diagnostic test evaluation, 43
Receptor for advanced glycation end products (RAGE), 1098, 1098f
in diabetes mellitus, 1547
Receptors, 67
Reciprocating tachycardia, 878
atrioventricular. See Atrioventricular reciprocating tachycardia.
using accessory pathway, 864t-865t
Recombinant DNA technologies, 72-74, 73f, 74f
Red blood cell, technetium-99m–labeled, 358
Red clover, 1161t
Reentry, 751-761, 754f-760f
anatomical, 752, 755f
anisotropic, 758, 760f
antiarrhythmic drug effects on, 781, 781t
atrial, 756
atrioventricular nodal, 756-757, 757f, 758f
figure-of-8, 756f, 758
functional, 753, 756f
leading circle, 758, 760f
over concealed accessory pathway, 881-884, 882f-883f
single-circle, 758, 760f
sinus, 756
tachycardias caused by, 751-761, 754f-760f
treatment of, electrical cardioversion in, 801
Referral bias, in myocardial perfusion imaging, 374, 375f
Reflex-mediated syncope, 977-978, 977t
Regional anesthesia, for noncardiac surgery, 2021
Regitine. See Phentolamine (Regitine).
Regurgitant fraction, determination of, 265, 458

Regurgitant orifice area, Doppler echocardiography of, 265-266, 266f
Regurgitant stroke volume, 458
Regurgitant volume, Doppler echocardiography of, 265, 266f
Regurgitation. See also specific types, e.g., Mitral regurgitation.
prosthetic valve, 279
Rehabilitation
cardiac, 1149-1155. See also Cardiac rehabilitation.
in peripheral arterial disease, 1504, 1504f
pulmonary, in chronic obstructive pulmonary disease, 1907
Relative coronary reserve, 1179-1181, 1180f
Relative risk, 44
Relaxation therapy
in hypertension, 1053, 2124
in rehabilitation, 2128
REM sleep, 1915, 2182, 2182f
Remote monitoring, of implantable cardioverter-defibrillator, 851-852
Renal. See also Kidney(s).
Renal artery(ies)
magnetic resonance angiography of, 409, 410f
stenosis of
diagnosis of, 1533, 1533f, 1533t, 1534f
hypertension in, 1039-1040, 1039t, 1040f
percutaneous interventions in, 1533-1535, 1533f-1536f, 1534t
prevalence of, 1532
severity of, mortality risk and, 1532-1533, 1533t
unilateral, nephropathy and, 1535
in women, 1964
Renal artery resistive index, 1534, 1535f
Renal cell carcinoma, from diuretics, 1058
Renal clearance, in elderly persons, 1926-1928, 1927t
Renal disease
cardiovascular disease and, 2155-2168
chronic. See Chronic kidney disease.
in cyanotic congenital heart disease, 1568
dose adjustments in, 64
dyslipidemia in, 1082
end-stage. See End-stage renal disease.
in heart failure
acute, 588-589
with normal ejection fraction, 646
in hypertension
acute, 1038
chronic, 1037-1038, 1038f, 1039
in infective endocarditis, 1721
parenchymal, hypertension in, 1038-1039, 1038f
as prognostic factor in acute coronary syndromes, 2163, 2163f
Renal failure
in aortic dissection, 1473
cardiac surgery in patients with, 1995-1996
chronic. See End-stage renal disease.
after coronary artery bypass graft surgery, 1384
coronary artery bypass graft surgery in, 1390
echocardiography in, 298
heart failure prognosis and, 614-615, 615f
after heart transplantation, 683

Renal failure (Continued)
   hemodialysis for, hypotension during,
     2178-2179, 2180f
   percutaneous coronary intervention in,
     1422-1423
   postoperative, 2005-2006
Renal function
   in heart failure, 564, 593-594, 598t, 599
     neurohormonal alterations of,
      544-547, 546f, 547f
   in myocardial infarction, 1220
Renal transplantation, in hypertension,
   1039
Renin
   in hypertension, 1034, 1041
   tumors secreting, hypertension in,
     1040
Renin-angiotensin-aldosterone system
   activation of, in heart failure, 542-544,
     544f, 545f
   in cardiorenal intersection, 2155
   in hypertension, 1033-1034, 1033f, 1034f
   inhibitors of. See also Aldosterone
     antagonists; Angiotensin II receptor
     blockers; Angiotensin-converting
     enzyme (ACE) inhibitors.
     in myocardial infarction, 1260-1262,
      1261f-1263f
   in myocardial infarction, 1220
Renovascular hypertension, 1039-1040,
   1039f, 1040f
Reoperation, in preoperative risk analysis,
   1994
Reperfusion/revascularization
   in acute limb ischemia, 1508-1509,
     1509f
   after cardiac arrest, 965
   in cardiogenic shock, 1270, 1270f
   catheter-based. See Percutaneous
     coronary intervention;
     Percutaneous intervention;
     Percutaneous transluminal
     coronary angioplasty.
   in diabetes mellitus, 1557-1558
   in elderly persons, 1936-1938, 1937f,
     1937t, 1938-1939
   in end-stage renal disease, 2167-2168,
     2168f
   evaluation for, nuclear imaging in, 373,
     374f
   exercise stress testing and, 216, 225,
     226t
   injury in, after pulmonary
     thromboendarterectomy, 1910
   in ischemic cardiomyopathy, 1398
   lipid-lowering therapy versus, 1088
   in myocardial infarction
     arrhythmias from, 1241
     catheter-based, 1249
     combination pharmacological, 1254,
      1256
     complications of, 1303
     developments in, 1308-1310
     early, benefits of, 1239, 1239f
     general concepts for, 1239-1240, 1240f
     injury in, 1240-1241, 1241f
     late, benefits of, 1215f, 1219, 1219f
     logistic challenge of, 1304-1305
     mechanical myocardial protection
      during, 1309
     options for
      assessment of, 1234-1235, 1235t,
       1237t
      comparison of, 1237t, 1249-1251,
       1250f
     pathology after, 1212-1213, 1215f,
      1216f

Reperfusion/revascularization
   (Continued)
     pathophysiology of, 1240
     pharmacological interventions
      during, 1309
     summary of effects of, 1241, 1242f
     surgical, 1249
     temporal dynamics of, 1303-1305,
      1304f
     thrombolytic, 1241-1249
     time delay between, 1233, 1234f
     time to, 1235, 1236f, 1240, 1240f
   preoperative, 2022-2023
   in silent myocardial ischemia, 1397
   in stable angina
     comparison and choice between PCI
      and CABG for, 1392-1394, 1392f-
      1394f, 1393t
     complete, need for, 1394
     in diabetic patients, 1394
     indications for, 1385-1386, 1386f,
      1386t, 1387f, 1391-1392
     laser-assisted, 1394-1395
     practice guidelines for, 1415t,
      1416-1417
   surgical
     in acute limb ischemia, 1509, 1509t
     in coronary artery disease. See
      Coronary artery bypass graft
      surgery.
     in peripheral arterial disease, 1505
     in renovascular hypertension, 1040
   thrombolytic. See Thrombolytic
     therapy.
   in UA/NSTEMI, 1347, 1349-1350, 1350t
   in women, 1961-1962, 1962t
Reproductive issues. See Pregnancy.
Reserpine, in hypertension, 1058-1059
Resistance (strengthening) exercise, 1983-
   1984, 1984
   in cardiovascular disease, 1153, 1154t
   definition of, 1150t
   prescription for, 1986t
Respiration
   Cheyne-Stokes
     in end-stage heart disease, 723
     in heart failure, 1917-1918, 1919, 1920,
      1920f
     mouth-to-mouth, after cardiac arrest,
      959
     in myocardial infarction, 1222
Respiratory distress syndrome,
   postoperative, 2004
Respiratory muscle weakness, pulmonary
   hypertension in, 1909
Restenosis
   after coronary stents, 999, 1429, 1430t,
     1431t
     brachytherapy for, 1429, 1431t
     drug-eluting stents for, 1434t
   after mitral valvotomy, 1656
   after percutaneous coronary
     intervention, 999
     guidelines on, 1452-1453, 1455t
Resting membrane potential, 738, 738f,
   738t, 739
   reduced, effects of, 746, 746f
Restriction endonucleases, 72, 73
Restrictions, in patients with
   arrhythmias, 860t, 861
Restrictive cardiomyopathy. See
   Cardiomyopathy, restrictive.
Restrictive filling, 251, 252f
Resuscitation, cardiopulmonary. See
   Cardiopulmonary resuscitation (CPR).
Resuscitation preferences, in end-stage
   heart disease, 722

Reteplase (r-PA), 2068
   in myocardial infarction, 1245-1246,
     1247t, 1248, 1254, 1256
   structure of, 1247f
Retinoic acid, dyslipidemia and, 1082
Retroperitoneal hematoma, in cardiac
   catheterization, 462
Retrospective chart review, for quality
   measurement, 50-51
Retroviral gene transfer, 80
Return to employment, after coronary
   artery bypass graft surgery, 1384
Revascularization.
   See Reperfusion/revascularization.
Reversal potential, 734
Reviparin
   in myocardial infarction, 1252
   in pulmonary embolism, 1873t
Revised Cardiac Risk Index (RCRI), 2013,
   2018, 2018t
Reynolds Risk Score, 1022
Rhabdomyoma, 303, 1818t, 1822
Rhabdomyosarcoma, 1818t, 1825
Rheolytic thrombectomy, in percutaneous
   coronary intervention, 1425
Rheumatic fever, 2079-2086
   acute, mitral stenosis and, interval
     between, 1651, 1651f
   arthritis in, 2083, 2086
   carditis in, 2082, 2083, 2085-2086
   chorea in, 2083, 2086
   cutaneous manifestations of, 2083-2084
   diagnosis of, 2080f, 2081-2082
   differential diagnosis of, 2082t
   echocardiography in, 2083
   epidemiology of, 2079-2080, 2080f
   future directions in, 2086
   Jones criteria for, 2080f, 2081
   laboratory findings in, 2084-2085
   pathobiology of, 2080-2081
   pathology of, 2081
   physical examination in, 2082-2083
   prevention of, 2085
   treatment of, 2085-2086, 2085t
Rheumatic heart disease, 2087-2101
   aortic regurgitation in, 1635, 1637f
   aortic stenosis in, 1626, 1626f
   general principles in, 2087
   heart failure in, 611
   infective endocarditis in, 1714
   mitral regurgitation in, 1662-1663
   mitral stenosis in, 1441-1442, 1442f,
     1646-1647, 1647f
   tricuspid regurgitation in, 1675-1676
   tricuspid stenosis in, 1674
   vasculitis in, 2101
Rheumatoid arthritis, 1851, 2094-2096
Rheumatoid factor, in rheumatoid
   arthritis, 2094
Rhonchi, in heart failure, 593
Ribosome, 71
Right axis deviation, in congenital heart
   disease, 1572
Right bundle branch block (RBBB). See
   also Fascicular block.
   characteristics of, 864t-865t
   clinical significance of, 170
   electrocardiography in, 169f, 169t, 170
   exercise stress testing in, 212, 212f
   incomplete form of, 170
   with left anterior fascicular block, 170,
     171f
   with left posterior fascicular block, 170,
     171f
   left ventricular hypertrophy and, 164
   in myocardial infarction, 178, 179f,
     1281

I-74 Right gastroepiploic artery, for coronary
artery bypass graft surgery, 1382
Right ventricular end-diastolic pressure
(RVEDP), 262-263
Right ventricular outflow tract ventricular
tachycardia, 906-907, 907f
Right ventricular systolic pressure, 262
Right-sided valve disease, severity of,
classification of, 1629t
Right-to-left shunt, detection of, cardiac
catheterization for, 458-459
Rigler sign, 331
Risk assessment models, in cardiac
surgery, 1996-1998, 1997t
Risk factors for cardiovascular disease.
See Cardiovascular disease, risk
factor(s) for.
Risk stratification, 45
in acute chest pain, 1200-1201, 1202f
in Brugada syndrome, 106, 106f
in contrast-induced nephropathy, 2159,
2160f, 2161
exercise stress testing for
in emergency department, 209-210
before noncardiac surgery, 210
in hypertension therapy, 1036-1038,
1036t, 1131-1132, 1131t
in hypertrophic cardiomyopathy, 1769-
1770, 1770f
in long QT syndrome, 104, 105f
in myocardial infarction, 382, 1286-
1289, 1287f, 1303
myocardial perfusion imaging in, 371-
373, 372f-374f
in noncardiac surgery, 2016-2020, 2017t,
2018t, 2019f
in pulmonary embolism, 1870-1871,
1871t
in stable angina, 1358, 1359t, 1360-1362,
1360f-1362f, 1385-1386, 1386f,
1386t, 1387f, 1409-1411, 1412t,
1413t
in UA/NSTEMI, 1323-1326, 1324f
by cardiac markers, 1325
by clinical variables, 1324t, 1325
early, 1344, 1345t
by electrocardiography, 1325
later, 1347, 1348t, 1349, 1349t
methods of, 1324-1326, 1324t, 1326f
multimarker, 1326, 1326f
to target glycoprotein IIb/IIIa
inhibitors, 1330
TIMI risk score for, 1325-1326, 1326f
Risk-benefit analysis
expressions used in, 44-45
shared decision-making and, 46
Risk-treatment paradox, 45
Risperidone, cardiovascular aspects of,
2130t, 2131
Ritonavir, dyslipidemia from, 1801
Rituximab, cardiotoxicity of, 2115
RNA
messenger, 71, 72f
structure of, 71
transfer, 71
RNA polymerase, transfer, 71
Romano-Ward syndrome, 101. *See also*
Long QT syndrome.
Romhilt-Estes point score system, for left
ventricular hypertrophy, 164, 164t
Rosiglitazone, in diabetic vascular
disease prevention, 1099, 1100
Ross procedure
in congenital aortic stenosis, 1611
in thoracic aortic aneurysms, 1467
Rosuvastatin (Crestor), in dyslipidemia,
1083

RP interval
in atrial premature complexes, 867,
868f, 869f
in supraventricular tachycardias, 893,
893t
R-R interval
in atrioventricular nodal reentrant
tachycardia, 878
in ventricular premature complexes,
893
Rubella syndrome, 1563, 1571, 1615
Rubidium-82
coronary blood flow reserve analysis
and, 362-363
in positron emission tomography, 360,
360t
uptake and retention of, mechanisms
of, 369f
Rules
diagnostic, 42
of thumb, in therapeutic decision-
making, 46
Russia, cardiovascular disease in, 10t, 11
Ryanodine receptor monomer subunit
RyR2, 748, 750f
Ryanodine receptors, 509, 515-517, 517f
in heart failure, 551
RyR2 gene mutations, in
catecholaminergic polymorphic
ventricular tachycardia, 107, 748-749

S
S wave, 158
in left anterior fascicular block, 168
in left bundle branch block, 169
in left ventricular hypertrophy, 162,
163f
in right bundle branch block, 170
in right ventricular hypertrophy, 165
Saddle embolus, 1486, 1864, 1865f
SAGE technique, in molecular genetics,
77
St. John's wort (*Hypericum perforatum*),
64, 65t, 1161t
St. Jude bileaflet valve, 1682, 1682f
St. Jude Medical valve, 1684f, 1686
Salicylates, in rheumatic fever, 2086
Salt-sensitive hypertension, 1032
Saphenous vein graft
degeneration of, arteriography of, 492
lesions of, drug-eluting stents for, 1434t
percutaneous coronary intervention in,
1422, 1426, 1427f, 1429f
Saquinavir, 1801
Sarcoendoplasmic reticulum Ca++
ATPase pump. *See* SERCA
(sarcoendoplasmic reticulum Ca++
ATPase) pump.
Sarcoglycan, delta-, mutation of, in
dilated cardiomyopathy, 115t, 116-117
Sarcoglycanopathies, in limb-girdle
muscular dystrophy, 2144
Sarcoidosis, 1755-1756, 1755f, 2101
clinical manifestations of, 1755-1756
echocardiography in, 298
magnetic resonance imaging in,
402-403
management of, 1756
nuclear imaging in, 385
pathology of, 1755, 1755f
pulmonary hypertension in, 1912
sudden cardiac death in, 944
vasculitis in, 2101, 2102f
Sarcolemma, 509, 510t
Sarcoma, cardiac, 1818t, 1824-1826
Sarcomere, 510, 512f
length changes in, 530, 530f

Sarcomere proteins, mutations of
in dilated cardiomyopathy, 115-116,
115t, 116f
in hypertrophic cardiomyopathy, 111-
114, 112t
Sarcoplasmic reticulum, 510t
anatomy of, 509-510, 511f
calcium release channels of, 515-518,
517f
ryanodine receptor, 509, 515-517, 517f
calcium sparks from, 518
calcium storage in, 519
calcium-induced calcium release in,
515, 517f
calcium-pumping ATPase of, 518-519,
518f
in heart failure, 550-551, 551t
junctional, 510
longitudinal or network, 510
turn-off of calcium release by, 518
Saruplase, 2068
Satavaptan, in heart failure, 621t, 624
Scaffolding proteins, 510
SCAP (SREBP cholesterol activated
protein), 1076
Scavenger lipoprotein receptors, 1072,
1073
Scavenger receptor-A molecules, in foam
cell formation, 992
Schistosomiasis, pulmonary hypertension
in, 1912
Scimitar syndrome, 1571, 1619
Scintigraphy
in infective endocarditis, 1722
lung. *See* Lung scan.
Scleroderma, 1901, 2099-2100
Sclerosis
aortic, 145, 400
progressive systemic, 1851, 2099-2100
SCN5A gene, 736
Scoliosis, cardiovascular diseases
associated with, 1573
Screening tests, number needed to screen
and, 43
Seattle Heart Failure Model, 613
Sedation, conscious, during arteriography,
470
Seizures, versus syncope, 977t, 978-979
Seldinger's technique, modified, in
cardiac catheterization, 444, 445f, 446
Selectins, in atherogenesis, 990-991
Senile systemic amyloidosis, 1751
Sensitivity
of exercise electrocardiography, 206,
206t
of noninvasive stress testing, 1358t
of stress myocardial perfusion imaging,
374-376, 375f-376f
test, 42
Sensitization, to ventricular assist device,
694
Sepsis, echocardiography in, 298
Septal accessory pathways, 804, 804f, 882
Septal myectomy, in hypertrophic
cardiomyopathy, 1772, 1772f
Septic arteritis, in infective endocarditis,
1730
Septostomy, atrial
in idiopathic pulmonary arterial
hypertension, 1900
in total anomalous pulmonary venous
connection, 1597
Septum
ablation of, in hypertrophic
cardiomyopathy, 1772-1773
atrial, lipomatous hypertrophy of,
1818t, 1820, 1821f, 1822

Septum (Continued)
  basal, normal dropout of, on single
    photon emission computed
    tomography, 353, 353f
  defects of. See Atrial septal defect;
    Atrioventricular septal defect;
    Ventricular septal defect.
  interventricular, rupture of, traumatic,
    1855-1856, 1858
SERCA (sarcoendoplasmic reticulum
    Ca++ ATPase) pump, 510, 518-519,
    518f
  diastolic relaxation and, 649
  as gene therapy target, 706t, 707
  in heart failure, 550-551
  thyroid hormones and, 2039
Serotonin
  in coronary blood flow regulation, 1175
  in idiopathic pulmonary arterial
    hypertension, 1893, 1894f
  in pulmonary circulation, 1885
Serotonin reuptake inhibitors, selective
  cardiovascular aspects of, 2128, 2129t
  drug interactions of, 2132, 2133t
  in postinfarction depression, 2127
Serotonin transporter gene, in idiopathic
    pulmonary arterial hypertension,
    1895
Sertraline
  cardiovascular aspects of, 2129t
  in postinfarction depression, 2127
Serum cardiac markers. See Cardiac
    markers.
Sestamibi, technetium-99m–labeled, 346,
    349t
  coronary blood flow reserve and, 362,
    362f
  for myocardial viability assessment,
    384
Sevelamer, in end-stage renal disease,
    2162
Sevoflurane, for noncardiac surgery,
    2020
Sex chromosomes, 85
Sexual activity, in stable angina, 1367
Sheaths, introducer, for cardiac
    catheterization, 443
Shock, cardiogenic. See Cardiogenic
    shock.
Shone complex, 1571
Short QT syndrome, 102t, 108, 108f
Shumway-Lower biatrial technique, in
    heart transplantation, 677, 677f
Shunt(s)
  evaluation of, cardiac catheterization
    in, 458-459
  intraatrial, contrast echocardiography
    of, 242
  left-to-right, 1577-1587
  right-to-left, 458-459
  systemic-to-pulmonary
    in cyanotic congenital heart disease,
      1568, 1568t
    in tricuspid atresia, 1591
  vascularity of, in cyanosis, 1573
Shy-Drager syndrome, autonomic failure
    in, 976
Sick sinus syndrome. See Sinus node
    disease.
Sickle cell disease, pulmonary arterial
    hypertension in, 1902
SIDS (sudden infant death syndrome),
    101, 936, 942t, 946-947
Signal transduction, 67
Signal-averaged electrocardiography
  in arrhythmia diagnosis, 769-770, 770f
  in syncope, 980

Sildenafil, 525
  in Eisenmenger syndrome, 1570
  in idiopathic pulmonary arterial
    hypertension, 1900
  nitrates and, 1369
Silent myocardial ischemia, 209,
    1396-1397
Simpson method, biplane, left ventricular
    volume measurement by, 246, 247f
Simvastatin (Zocor), 39, 1083
Single nucleotide polymorphisms, 75-76,
    76f, 87
Single photon emission computed
    tomography, 345-357. See also
    Myocardial perfusion imaging.
  appropriateness criteria for, 391
  artifacts on, 350, 353-354, 353f-354f
  attenuation correction in, 354, 355f
    CT, 455
  Bayesian principles in, 350-352, 351f
  cardiovascular magnetic resonance
    versus, 395, 396f
  circumferential profile technique in,
    348, 350f
  combined with computed tomography
    angiography, 354-355, 379f, 380
  combined with computed tomography
    coronary calcium imaging, 379-380,
    379f
  in coronary artery disease
    after coronary artery bypass graft,
      378
    after percutaneous coronary
      intervention, 378
  of coronary blood flow reserve, 362,
    362f, 363, 364f
  for detection of coronary artery disease,
    377-378, 378
  equipment for, 345, 346f
  of fatty acid metabolism, 367
  gated
    of left ventricular function, 355-357,
      356f, 357f
    for left ventricular volume
      assessment, 370
  image acquisition in, 345
  image display in, 345, 347f
  image interpretation in, 348, 349f-352f,
    350-353
  lung uptake in, 352, 352f
  in myocardial infarction, 361-362, 362f,
    381, 382f
  of myocardial perfusion abnormalities,
    348, 349f-351f, 350-352
  of myocardial viability, 384, 385f
  normal variations in, 353, 353f
  perfusion tracers in, 346, 348f
    extracardiac uptake of, 352, 352f, 354
    properties of, 349t
  planar myocardial perfusion imaging
    versus, 357-358, 358f
  polar maps (bull's eye display) in, 348,
    350, 350f
  quality control in, 345-346
  quantitative analysis of, 348, 350, 350f
    for detection of coronary artery
      disease, 376, 377f
  semiquantitative visual analysis of, 348,
    349f, 350
  stress
    in coronary artery disease, 1358,
      1358t, 1361
    in women, 1958, 1960f
  transient ischemic dilation of left
    ventricle on, 352-353, 352f
Single-circle reentry, 758, 760f
Sinoatrial conduction time, 774

Sinoatrial coupling, 727, 729f
Sinoatrial exit block, 911, 911f, 912f
Sinus arrest, 910, 911f, 912-913, 914f
Sinus arrhythmia, 910, 910f
  exercise and sports in patients with,
    1989
  parasympathetic dysfunction in,
    2182-2183
  ventriculophasic, 910, 910f
Sinus bradycardia
  characteristics of, 864t-865t
  clinical features of, 909-910
  electrocardiography in, 909, 910f
  management of, 910
  in myocardial infarction, 1279
    reperfusion-induced, 1241
  pacemaker in, 832-833, 833t
Sinus exit block, 912-913, 914f
Sinus node
  anatomy of, 727-728, 728f, 729f
  automaticity in, 744-745, 745f
  cellular structure of, 727
  function of, 727
  innervation of, 727-728
  transmembrane potentials in, 738t
Sinus node disease
  in elderly persons, 1946
  electrocardiography in, 912-913,
    914f-915f
  electrophysiology in, 773-774, 774f, 825,
    826t
  exercise stress testing in, 212
  genes involved in, 102t
  management of, 913
  pacemaker in, 832-833, 833t, 854, 856t,
    913
  in syncope, 981
Sinus node recovery time, 773, 774, 774f
  in syncope, 981
Sinus node reentrant tachycardia, 808,
    867, 867f
Sinus of Valsalva. See Aortic sinus.
Sinus pause, 910, 911f
Sinus reentry, 756
Sinus rhythm, normal, 863, 864t-865t
Sinus tachycardia
  after cardiac surgery, 1998
  characteristics of, 864t-865t
  clinical features of, 865f, 866-867
  in Duchenne muscular dystrophy,
    2136
  electrocardiography in, 866, 867f
  inappropriate
    chronic, 866-867
    radiofrequency catheter ablation of,
      808
  management of, 867
  in myocardial infarction, 1281-1282
  in systemic lupus erythematosus,
    2097
Sinus venosus atrial septal defect, 1577,
    1578f-1579f
Sirolimus, in heart transplantation,
    678
Sirolimus-eluting stent, 4, 1308,
    1430-1431, 1435f
Sister chromatid, 68
Sitosterolemia, 1079, 1083
Situs ambiguus, 1564
Situs inversus, 1564
  with dextrocardia, 1573
  with levocardia, 1573
Situs solitus, 1564
  with dextrocardia, 1573
Six-minute walk test
  in heart failure, 566
  in pulmonary hypertension, 1888

I-76 Skeletal myopathy
dilated cardiomyopathy with, 116-117
in peripheral arterial disease, 1494
zidovudine-induced, 1801
Skin
lesions of, in pseudoxanthoma elasticum, 94, 94f
physical examination of, 127
warfarin-induced necrosis of, 2066
Skin stapler, in traumatic heart disease, 1860, 1861f
Sleep, physiology of, 1915
Sleep apnea, 1915-1920
central
definition of, 1917
diagnosis of, 1919
in heart failure, 1918
physiology of, 1917-1918
treatment of, 1920, 1920f
chemoreflexes and, 2172
neurogenic hypertension from, 1031
obstructive
in cardiovascular disease, 1915-1917, 1916t, 1917f, 1918f
definition of, 1915
diagnosis of, 1918-1919
physiology of, 1915
pulmonary hypertension in, 1909
screening tools for, 1919
sympathetic dysfunction in, 2182
treatment of, 1919-1920, 1920t
polysomnography in, 1919
Sleep disturbances, in heart failure, 591
Sleep-disordered breathing, pulmonary hypertension in, 1909
Sleepiness, daytime, in obstructive sleep apnea, 1918
Sleeping, head-up tilt, in neurally mediated syncope, 983
Smallpox vaccination, myocarditis from, 1780
Smoking
abdominal aortic aneurysms and, 1458
blood pressure and, 1052
cardiac surgery and, 1995
cardiovascular disease risk and, 1004-1005, 1004f, 1127-1128
in chronic obstructive pulmonary disease, 1905
hypertension and, 1028
peripheral arterial disease risk and, 1492, 1493f
prevalence of, 7, 8, 1127
regional trends in, 15-16, 15f
sudden cardiac death and, 938
in thromboangiitis obliterans, 1505
Smoking cessation
in abdominal aortic aneurysms, 1463
benefits of, 1127-1128
in cardiac rehabilitation, 1154
in cardiovascular disease prevention, 1004-1005, 1004f, 1127-1128
in chronic obstructive pulmonary disease, 1907
after coronary artery bypass graft surgery, 1385
economic analysis of, 1128
in end-stage renal disease, 2167
future challenges in, 1128
guidelines/recommendations on, 1128
in hypertension therapy, 1052
in peripheral arterial disease, 1500
in stable angina, 1363
in thromboangiitis obliterans, 1506

Smooth muscle cells
in aneurysmal disease, 1000
arterial, 987-988, 988f
in atherosclerosis
death of, 994
migration and proliferation of, 993-994, 994f
developmental biology of, 987-988, 988f
Snoring, in obstructive sleep apnea, 1918
Social disruption, cardiovascular disease and, 2121
Social factors. See Psychosocial factors.
Social isolation, cardiovascular disease and, 2121
Social support
cardiovascular disease and, 2121
in end-stage heart disease, 718, 721
in heart failure, 2124-2125
Social transition, cardiovascular disease and, 5, 5f
Societal perspective, in economic analysis, 35
Society of Thoracic Surgeons (STS) risk model for cardiac surgery, 1997
Sociocultural factors
in hypertension, 2124
in sudden cardiac death, 2123
Sociodemographic factors
in cardiovascular disease, 2121
in sudden cardiac death, 2123
Socioeconomic status
cardiovascular disease and, 40, 40f, 2121
sudden cardiac death and, 2123
Sodium
deficiency of
from diuretics, 626, 1058
in heart failure, 564, 593
equilibrium potential of, 738
intake of
in autonomic failure, 2176
blood pressure and, 1113-1114, 1114f
hypertension and, 1029
racial/ethnic differences in, 24
myocardial concentration of, 735t
renal retention of, in heart failure, 544-545, 546f
restriction of
in heart failure, 620
in hypertension therapy, 1052t, 1053, 1053f
in mitral stenosis, 1652
in tricuspid stenosis, 1675
sarcolemmal control of, 519-520
sensitivity to, in African Americans, 27
Sodium bicarbonate, in cardiac arrest, 962, 963
Sodium channel(s)
in action potential phase 0, 740, 740f
epithelial, in hypertension, 1033-1034, 1033f
mutation of, in Brugada syndrome, 105
synopsis of, 741t
voltage-gated, molecular structure of, 734f, 736
Sodium nitroprusside
in aortic dissection, 1479
during cardiac catheterization, 460
Sodium pump (NA⁺/K⁺-ATPase), 520, 739
Sodium-calcium exchanger
in action potential phase 1, 743, 743f
in contraction-relaxation cycle, 519-520, 520f
in heart failure, 551
heart rate and, 520
in resting membrane potential, 739

Sokolow-Lyon index, for left ventricular hypertrophy, 164, 164t
Solid angle theorem, 150-151
Somatic cell, 68
Somatostatin receptor agonists, in acromegaly, 2035
Sones technique, for cardiac catheterization, 447
Sorafenib, cardiotoxicity of, 2114-2115
Sotalol
in arrhythmias, 780t, 781t, 782t, 784t, 786t, 796
in atrial fibrillation, 873
in chronic kidney disease patients, 2165t
pharmacokinetics and pharmacology of, 1373t
in ventricular tachycardia, 901, 902
South Asia/India, cardiovascular disease in, 10t, 12-13
South Asian Americans, hypertension in, 26, 26f
Southern blotting, 73, 73f
Soy products, intake of
blood pressure and, 1115
cardiovascular disease and, 1140
Spain, cardiovascular disease in, 10, 11t
Spasm, coronary artery
arteriography of, 488-489, 490f-491f
coronary blood flow in, 1175-1176
methylergonovine maleate test for, 460
in Prinzmetal variant angina, 1338, 1339f
sudden cardiac death and, 942, 950, 950f
Specificity
of exercise electrocardiography, 206, 206t
of stress myocardial perfusion imaging, 374-376, 375f-376f
test, 42
Speckle tracking, in tissue Doppler echocardiography, 239, 241f
SPECT. See Single photon emission computed tomography.
Sphingomyelin, biochemistry of, 1071-1072, 1072f
Sphygmomanometer, arterial pressure measurement with, 131
Spin echo sequence, in cardiovascular magnetic resonance, 394
Spinal anesthesia, for noncardiac surgery, 2021
Spinal cord injury
after aortic dissection surgery, 1481
after thoracic aortic aneurysm repair, 1468
Spinal cord stimulation, in stable angina, 1378
Spinal muscle atrophy, 2148
Spindle, 68
Spiritual needs, in end-stage heart disease, 721-722
Spirochetal myocarditis, 1778-1779
Spirometry, in chronic obstructive pulmonary disease, 1906-1907
Spironolactone (Aldactone)
in heart failure, 621t, 622, 623f, 624t, 633
in hypertension, 1058
in idiopathic pulmonary arterial hypertension, 1896-1897
Spleen
abscess of, in infective endocarditis, 1729

Spleen *(Continued)*
enlargement of
in heart failure, 593
in infective endocarditis, 1720
Splinter hemorrhage, in infective
endocarditis, 1720
Spondylitis, ankylosing, 2096
Spondyloarthropathies, HLA-B-27–
associated, 2096
Sports. *See also* Athletes.
classification of, by dynamic/static
components, 1984t
competitive versus recreational, 1984
in patients with cardiovascular disease,
1988-1990
preparticipation screening for,
1986-1988, 1986t, 1987t
Sports cardiology, 1983-1990. *See also*
Exercise; Physical activity.
Square root sign, in restrictive
cardiomyopathy, 1750
SSRIs. *See* Serotonin reuptake inhibitors,
selective.
ST segment, 155, 156f, 156t
in acute pericarditis, 1832, 1832f
during angina episode, 1357
depression of, during vasodilator
pharmacological stress, 365
digitalis effect on, 183-184, 184f
displacement of, in exercise stress
testing
diagnostic value of, 206-207, 206t,
207t
measurement of, 200, 201f-203f,
202-203
mechanism of, 203-204
noncoronary causes of, 206t
prognostic value of, 207-210, 208f
types of, 199-200, 199f-201f
elevation of
differential diagnosis of, 181-182,
182f, 182t
in exercise stress testing, 201f, 202,
202f
in left bundle branch block, 169
in left ventricular hypertrophy, 162,
163f
monitoring of, in noncardiac surgery,
2026
in myocardial ischemia, 172-174,
173f-175f
normal variants of, 160, 161f
in potassium abnormalities, 184
in Prinzmetal variant angina, 176, 177f,
1338, 1339f
in silent myocardial ischemia,
1396-1397
in UA/NSTEMI, 1322, 1322f
upsloping, in exercise stress testing,
200f, 201f, 202
ST segment elevation myocardial
infarction (STEMI). *See also*
Myocardial infarction.
in ACS spectrum concept, 1210-1211,
1210f
Stab wounds, 1855, 1857, 1860
Stabilization, in cardiac arrest
management, 963
Staphylococci, in infective endocarditis,
1717, 1719, 1720f, 1725-1726, 1726t,
1732
Staphylokinase, in myocardial infarction,
1246
Starling's law of the heart, 529-530, 530f
Starr-Edwards prosthetic valve, 1682f,
1683
Static (isometric) exercise, 197, 459

Statin therapy
in abdominal aortic aneurysms, 1459,
1463
in acute coronary syndromes, 1088
benefits of, 1128-1129, 1129f
in calcific aortic stenosis, 1626
in cardiovascular disease prevention,
1128-1131, 1129f, 1130f, 1130t
clinical trials of
for primary prevention, 1085-1086,
1085t
for secondary prevention, 1087-1088,
1087f, 1087t
in combined lipoprotein disorders,
1090
in coronary artery disease, myocardial
perfusion imaging after, 374, 374f
C-reactive protein (hs-CRP) and, 1015,
1016f
in diabetic patients, 1086, 1090, 1101,
1101t
in dyslipidemia, 1083
economic analysis of, 39, 39t, 1129
in elderly persons, 1935-1936, 1935t
in end-stage renal disease, 2162, 2167
in hyperlipidemia, 1007
in hypertensive patients, 1085t, 1086
immunomodulation with, in heart
failure, 712-713, 712f, 713f
muscle disease syndromes from, versus
hypothyroidism-induced myopathy,
2043, 2043t
in myocardial infarction prevention,
1290
in peripheral arterial disease, 1500,
1502f, 1503, 1503f
pharmacokinetics of, 60
in posttransplantation hyperlipidemia,
681
in preoperative risk analysis, 1995
preoperative use of, 2026
regression studies of, 1088
versus revascularization, 1088
in stable angina, 1363, 1365
in stroke prevention, 1517-1518, 1517f,
1518f
in UA/NSTEMI, 1335, 1335f
in women, 1961
Statutory documents, 721
Stem cells
adult, 698-699
bone marrow–derived, 698
clinical applications of, 700-701, 702t,
703t
in acute myocardial infarction,
701-704, 702t, 703t, 704f, 705f
in chronic heart failure, 704-705
future perspectives on, 705-706
mobilization strategies in
combination with, 703-705, 705t
differentiation of, 699-700, 699t
embryonic, 697
mechanisms of action of, 699-700, 699f,
700f
neovascularization by, 700
tissue engineering with, 700
tissue-resident, 698-699
types of, 697-699, 698f
STEMI (ST segment elevation myocardial
infarction). *See also* Myocardial
infarction.
in ACS spectrum concept, 1210-1211,
1210f
Stenosis, valvular. *See also* Aortic
stenosis; Mitral stenosis; Pulmonic
stenosis; Tricuspid stenosis.
calculating area of, 266, 266f

Stenosis pressure-flow relationships,
coronary reserve and, 1178, 1179f,
1181, 1181f
Stent(s)
in aortoiliac disease, 1525, 1525f, 1526f,
1526t
carotid
in carotid artery stenosis, 1539-1541,
1540f, 1541f, 1541t
in elderly persons, 1941-1942
in chronic mesenteric ischemia, 1536,
1537f
coronary, 1301, 1302f, 1308, 1308f, 1428-
1429, 1430t, 1431t
computed tomography of, 428, 428f
economic analysis of, 37-38
kissing, for bifurcation lesions, 1422,
1422f
preoperative, 2023
versus PTCA, 1430t
restenosis after, 999, 1429, 1430t,
1431t
brachytherapy for, 1429, 1431t
thrombosis after, 1429, 1438, 1440-
1441, 1440t, 1441t
in deep venous thrombosis, 1542-1543,
1543f
drug-eluting, 1429-1436, 1432t-1435t,
1435f
for chronic total occlusions, 1433t
CoStar program in, 1436
design characteristics, 1432t
economic analysis of, 38
efficacy of, 1429-1430, 1432t-1435t
for in-stent restenosis, 1434t
intravascular ultrasonography after,
496-497, 497f
during percutaneous coronary
intervention, 1308
preoperative, 2023
for saphenous vein graft disease,
1434t
in STEMI, 1435t
in femoropopliteal disease, 1526-1530,
1527f, 1528f, 1529t
in peripheral arterial disease,
1504-1505
in pulmonary embolism, 1877
in renal artery stenosis, 1533-1535,
1533f-1536f, 1534t
in superior vena cava syndrome, 1543,
1544f, 2108
in vertebral artery stenosis, 1542,
1542f
Stent-grafting
in abdominal aortic aneurysm, 1462-
1463, 1462f
in aortic dissection, 1482
in thoracic aortic aneurysms, 1468-1469
Sternal angle, 129, 129f
Sternal wound infection, postoperative,
2008-2009
Steroid-responsive element binding
protein (SREBP), 1076
ST/heart rate index, in exercise stress
testing, 203
STICH (Surgical Treatment for Ischemic
Heart Failure) trial, 665-666, 667f
Stiffness
definition of, 570t
left ventricular diastolic, 650-653, 652f
muscle, 561
myocardial, 574-575, 574f
vascular, measurement of, 131-132
ventricular, 574, 574f, 575
Stokes-Adams attacks, syncope in, T wave
inversion after, 183

I-78 Stop codon, 71
Strain, definition of, 570t
Strain imaging, 239-240, 240f, 240t
Strength training. *See* Resistance
(strengthening) exercise.
Streptococcal infection
in infective endocarditis, 1716, 1719,
1723-1724, 1723t, 1724t
in myocarditis, 1778
in rheumatic fever, 2080-2081,
2084-2085
Streptokinase, 2068
in acute coronary syndromes, economic
analysis of, 36-37
in myocardial infarction, 1247t, 1248
Stress
arrhythmias and, 2122-2123
blood pressure and, 2123
cardiovascular disease and, 2121
emotional
left ventricular dysfunction from, 617
sudden cardiac death and, 946
in hypertension, 2123
hypertension and, 1157, 2123
management of
complementary and alternative
medicine in, 1157-1158
in hypertension, 1053, 2124
in rehabilitation, 2128
mechanical, left ventricular response
to, 536, 536f, 537f
mental, cardiovascular disease and,
1012, 2121-2122
myocardial, definition of, 570t
oxidative
in diabetes mellitus, 1096, 1099
dietary influences on, 1115-1116,
1115f
in heart failure, 30, 31f, 544, 545f
physiological, with cardiac
catheterization, 460
sudden cardiac death and, 939
wall, 530-531, 531f
and compensated left ventricular
hypertrophy, 535-536, 537f
components of, 570f
in contraction-relaxation cycle, 530-
531, 531f
definition of, 570t
myocardial oxygen uptake and, 532
Stress cardiomyopathy, 181-182, 1216,
1743, 1744f, 1811-1812
Stress echocardiography. *See*
Echocardiography, stress.
Stress magnetic resonance imaging, 397,
398f
Stress myocardial perfusion imaging. *See*
Myocardial perfusion imaging, stress;
Nuclear imaging, stress.
Stress relaxation
in cardiac catheterization, 1163-1164
definition of, 570t
Stress single photon emission computed
tomography
in coronary artery disease, 1358, 1358t,
1361
in women, 1958, 1960f
Stress testing
in abdominal aortic aneurysms, 1463
exercise. *See* Exercise stress testing.
noninvasive
sensitivity and specificity of, 1358t
in stable angina, 1357-1358, 1357t-
1359t, 1361
in UA/NSTEMI, 1323
Stress ventriculography, magnetic
resonance, 397, 398f

Stroke
acute ischemic
anticoagulant therapy in, 1521
antiplatelet therapy in, 1521
blood pressure management in,
1521-1522
endovascular therapy in, 1520-1521
intravenous rt-PA in, 1519-1520,
1521t
management of, 1519-1522
during arteriography, 467-468
atrial fibrillation and, 870-871
cryptogenic, patent foramen ovale and,
1580, 1581
in diabetes mellitus, 1095
in elderly persons, 1940-1942, 1941t,
1942t
embolic, in infective endocarditis,
1721
in Fontan patients, 1595
in HIV-infected patients, 1800
hypertension and, 1027, 1028f, 1029f,
1037, 1065-1066
obstructive sleep apnea and, 1916,
1917f
pathophysiology of, racial/ethnic
differences in, 27
after percutaneous coronary
intervention, 1522
postoperative, 2006, 2007
in pregnancy, 1979, 1980t
prevention of
anticoagulant therapy in, 1516-1517,
1516f
antihypertensive drug therapy in,
1518-1519, 1519f, 1520f
antiplatelet therapy in, 1515-1516
medical therapy in, 1515-1520
statin therapy in, 1517-1518, 1517f,
1518f
T wave in, 183, 183f
Stroke force, definition of, 570t
Stroke syndromes, 2149-2150
Stroke volume
angiographic, 455
calculation of, 571
Doppler echocardiography of, 263-264,
264f
echocardiographic measurement of,
248
forward, 458
patient position and, 195-196
regurgitant, 458
Stroke work
definition of, 570t
preload recruitable, 572
Stromelysins, 557, 557t
ST-T alternans, 187
ST-T wave, 156f, 159
abnormalities in
nonspecific, 185-186
simulating myocardial ischemia, 181-
182, 182f, 182t
in myocardial ischemia, 172-174,
173f-175f
in stable angina, 1357
in Wolff-Parkinson-White syndrome,
884
Stunned myocardium. *See* Myocardial
stunning.
Subaortic stenosis, 1611-1612
complex, 1612
discrete (fibrous and muscular),
1611-1612
focal, 1612
Subarachnoid hemorrhage, 2149-2150,
2150f, 2151f-2152f

Subclavian artery
obstruction of, percutaneous
interventions in, 1536-1538, 1537f
right, anomalous origin of, 1609, 1610
stenosis of, percutaneous interventions
in, 1536-1538, 1537f
Subclavian steal syndrome, 1536-1537
Subendocardial (nontransmural)
myocardial infarction, 1211
Subendocardial resection, in ventricular
tachycardia, 820f, 821
Subgroup analysis, of risk/benefit, 44-45
Submaximal exercise, during exercise
stress testing, 204
Sub-Saharan Africa, cardiovascular
disease in, 10t, 13
Substituted-judgment criterion, 722
Subungual hemorrhage, in infective
endocarditis, 1720
Subxiphoid pericardial window, in
traumatic heart disease, 1858-1859
Sudden cardiac death, 933-951. *See also*
Cardiac arrest.
in acute heart failure, 941t, 943-944
age and, 936, 937f
alcohol intake and, 1807, 1807f, 1808
in alcoholic cardiomyopathy, 1745
in amyloidosis, 944
in aortic stenosis, 944
in arrhythmogenic right ventricular
dysplasia, 944
in athletes, 947
biological model of, 949, 949f
in Brugada syndrome, 945, 946f
cardiac nerves and, 949
in catecholaminergic polymorphic
ventricular tachycardia, 107
causes of, 940-948, 941t-942t
central nervous system influences in,
945-946, 947f
in children, 942t, 946-947
in congenital heart disease, 944, 1571
in coronary artery abnormalities, 940,
941t, 942
in coronary artery disease
pathology of, 948, 949-951, 949f, 950f
progression to, 937-938, 938f
ventricular arrhythmias and, 939-940,
940f
definition of, 933
in dilated cardiomyopathy, 941t, 943
in Duchenne muscular dystrophy, 2137
in Eisenmenger syndrome, 944
electrophysiology in, 941t-942t, 944-
946, 966-967
in endocarditis, 944
in end-stage heart disease, 723
epidemiology of, 934-940
functional capacity and, 938
gender and, 936-937, 937f
hereditary factors in, 936, 937f
in hypertrophic cardiomyopathy, 941t,
942-943, 1769-1770, 1770f
incidence of, 934, 936
in infants, 936, 942t, 946-947
left ventricular dysfunction and, 939
lifestyle and, 938-939
in limb-girdle muscular dystrophy,
2144
in long QT syndrome, 101, 906, 945
during marathon racing, 1985
mimics of, 948
in mitral valve prolapse, 944, 1673
multivariate risk of, 939f
after myocardial infarction, 939-940,
940f, 948
risk stratification for, 1288-1289

Sudden cardiac death (Continued)
in myocarditis, 944
in myotonic muscular dystrophy, 2139, 2142
neurohumoral factors in, 945
obstructive sleep apnea and, 1916-1917, 1918f
pathology of, 948-949
pathophysiological mechanisms of, 949-951, 949f, 950f
physical activity and, 938-939, 947
population subgroups and, 934-936, 935f
prevention of, 965-971, 966t
ambulatory electrocardiographic monitoring in, 966
antiarrhythmic agents in, 964, 965-966
catheter ablation therapy in, 967
implantable defibrillators in, 847-848, 967-968, 967f, 968t, 969
primary, 969-970
programmed electrical stimulation in, 966-967
secondary, 968-969
surgical interventions in, 967
psychosocial factors in, 939, 2123
public safety and, 970-971
race and, 936, 937f
risk factors for, 937-940, 937f-940f
in sarcoidosis, 944
in scleroderma, 2100
specialized conducting system in, 948-949
terminology related to, 933, 934t
time references in, 933, 934f
time-dependent risk of, 935f, 936
in valvular heart disease, 944
ventricular arrhythmias and, 939-940, 940f
ventricular hypertrophy and, 941t, 942-943, 948
in ventricular tachycardia, 899
prevention of, 902-903
Sudden death
noncardiac causes of, 948
temporal definition of, 933, 934
Sudden infant death syndrome (SIDS), 101, 936, 942t, 946-947
Suicide, physician-assisted, in end-stage heart disease, 722-723
Sulfa sensitivity, with diuretics, 1058
Sulfonylureas, in diabetic patients with cardiovascular disease, 1557
Sumatriptan, cardiovascular effects of, 1812
Sunitinib, cardiotoxicity of, 2114-2115
Superior vena cava syndrome
anatomy of, 2106, 2106f
diagnosis of, 2107, 2107f, 2107t
differential diagnosis of, 2107
etiology of, 2106-2107, 2107f, 2107t
management of, 2107-2108
percutaneous interventions in, 1543, 1544f
symptoms of, 2106
in thoracic aortic aneurysm, 1465
Superoxide anion, in hypertension, 1033
Supply angina, 1355-1356, 1356f
Supravalvular aortic stenosis, 1612-1614, 1613f
Supraventricular arrhythmias, exercise stress testing in, 212
Supraventricular tachyarrhythmias
in myocardial infarction, 1281-1282
postoperative, 2003

Supraventricular tachycardia
definition of, 863
differential diagnosis of, 766f
electrocardiographic diagnosis of, 893, 893t
electrophysiology in, 774, 775f
exercise and sports in patients with, 1989
paroxysmal, 878
in mitral valve prolapse, 1672
in pregnancy, 1979, 1980t
syncope and, 978, 981
treatment of
electrical cardioversion in, 801, 802
surgical, 819f, 820
ventricular tachycardia versus, 863, 866, 866f, 866t, 897, 897f
Surgery. See Cardiac surgery; Noncardiac surgery; specific type, e.g., Coronary artery bypass graft surgery.
Surgical technique, in preoperative risk analysis, 1994
Sutton's law, 46
Swallowing syncope, 977
Swan-Ganz catheter, for cardiac catheterization, 443-444, 443f, 445f
Sydenham's chorea, in rheumatic fever, 2083, 2086
Sympathetic activation, cardiac effects of, 733
Sympathetic dysfunction, 2174-2175, 2180-2182
bed rest and, 2182
in central sleep apnea, 1918
in heart failure, 542, 543f, 2181, 2181f
in hypertension, 1031, 2180
in obstructive sleep apnea, 1915, 2182
in panic disorder, 2180-2181
in pheochromocytoma, 2182
during REM sleep, 2182, 2182f
Sympathetic innervation
in arrhythmogenesis, 733
intraventricular, 732, 734f
nuclear imaging of, 385
Sympathetic nervous system
in blood pressure regulation, 1031
in coronary blood flow regulation, 1175, 1176f
in myocardial hibernation, 1190-1191
Sympathetic-parasympathetic interactions, 524-525, 525f, 732
Syncope, 975-983
in aortic dissection, 1471
in aortic stenosis, 1629-1630
in arrhythmias, 977t, 978
in blood or injury phobia, 2179-2180
in Brugada syndrome, 105-106
cardiac, 978
from carotid sinus hypersensitivity, 977-978
in catecholaminergic polymorphic ventricular tachycardia, 106-107
causes of
classification of, 975-978, 976t
clinical features suggestive of, 983t
prognosis and, 978
in concealed accessory pathway, 884
defecation, 977
definition of, 975
diagnosis of, 978-982
approach to, 981-982, 982f, 983t
blood tests in, 979
cardiac catheterization in, 980
echocardiography in, 979
electrocardiography in, 980-981
electrophysiology in, 981
exercise stress testing in, 979-980

Syncope (Continued)
history in, 977t, 978-979
physical examination in, 979
tilt-table testing in, 771-772, 772f, 979
driving risk in patients with, 982
echocardiography in, 322t, 324
electrocardiography in, 774
electrophysiology in, 774-775, 828, 828t, 981
exertional, in aortic stenosis, 2178, 2179f
hospital admission for, 982
in hypertrophic cardiomyopathy, 1768, 2179
hyperventilation-induced, 978
in hypoglycemia, 978
in long QT syndrome, 101, 906
management of, 982-983
metabolic causes of, 978
micturition, 977
neurally mediated, 977, 977t, 2177
pacemaker in, 833, 857t, 858
tilt-table testing in, 979
treatment of, 983
variants of, 2178-2180, 2179f, 2180f
neurological causes of, 978, 981
orthostatic, 975-977, 976t, 983
in psychiatric disorders, 978
in pulmonary hypertension, 1886
quinidine-induced, 786
reflex-mediated, 977-978, 977t
swallowing, 977
vascular, 975-978, 976t, 977t
vasovagal, pacemaker in, 833
Syndrome X, 1395-1396
metabolic. See Metabolic syndrome.
Syphilis, thoracic aortic aneurysms and, 1465
Systemic blood flow, in shunt quantification, 458-459
Systemic inflammatory response syndrome (SIRS), after cardiopulmonary bypass, 1998
Systemic lupus erythematosus, 2096-2098, 2098f
echocardiography in, 298
pericarditis in, 1851, 2097
valvulitis in, 2098, 2098f
Systemic lupus erythematosus–like syndrome, procainamide-induced, 787
Systemic vascular resistance, 267, 452t, 455
Systemic venous connections, in normal heart, 1564
Systole
coronary blood flow during, 1167, 1168f
definition of, 529
force transmission during, 514
physiological versus cardiologic, 529, 529t
transmural perfusion during, 1171, 1172f
Systolic blood pressure, in heart failure, 592
Systolic click, in mitral valve prolapse, 1670
Systolic function. See Ventricle(s), left, systolic function of.
Systolic heart failure. See Heart failure, systolic.
Systolic hypertension, isolated, in elderly persons, 1050-1051
Systolic load, diastolic relaxation and, 649
Systolic murmur. See Murmur(s), systolic.

Systolic pressure, myocardial oxygen consumption and, 1167-1168, 1168f
Systolic sounds, 135, 136f
Systolic ventricular vascular stiffening, in heart failure with normal ejection fraction, 653

T

T cells
    in myocarditis, 1783, 1783f
    in plaque evolution, 993, 993f
T tubule, 509, 510t, 511f, 512f
T wave, 155, 156f, 156t
    abnormalities of, simulating myocardial ischemia, 182
    in acute pericarditis, 1832
    in calcium abnormalities, 184
    cardiac memory changes in, 183
    in cerebrovascular accident, 183, 183f
    in exercise stress testing, 199, 200f, 202, 203f
    inversion of, 182-183, 183f, 183t
        idiopathic global, 183
    in left bundle branch block, 169
    in left ventricular hypertrophy, 162, 163, 163f
    in myocardial infarction, 174
    in myocardial ischemia, 173, 174, 174f, 175f, 176, 177f
    normal variants of, 160, 160f, 182-183
    in potassium abnormalities, 184
    in Prinzmetal angina, 176, 177f
    pseudonormalization of, 176, 177f, 202, 203f
    in right bundle branch block, 170
    in right ventricular infarction, 1271
    in UA/NSTEMI, 1322, 1322f
    in ventricular premature complexes, 893
T wave alternans, in arrhythmia diagnosis, 770, 771f
Tachyarrhythmia(s), 863, 866-893
    atrial, radiofrequency catheter ablation of, 810-812
    lethal, pathophysiological mechanisms of, 949-951, 949f, 950f
    prevention and termination of, pacemaker for, 833, 854, 856t-857t, 858
    supraventricular
        in myocardial infarction, 1281-1282
        postoperative, 2003
    surgical management of, 819-821, 819f-820f
    in systemic lupus erythematosus, 2097
    triggered, 751f
Tachycardia
    antidromic, in Wolff-Parkinson-White syndrome, 888-889, 889f, 890f
    atrial. See Atrial tachycardia.
    atrioventricular junctional, nonparoxysmal, 864t-865t
    atrioventricular junctional reciprocating, permanent form of, 889, 891f
    atrioventricular nodal reentrant. See Atrioventricular nodal reentrant tachycardia.
    atrioventricular reciprocating, 757-758, 759f, 878
        orthodromic, in Wolff-Parkinson-White syndrome, 888-889, 889f
    atrioventricular reentrant, radiofrequency catheter ablation of, 804-806, 804f-805f
    in cardiac tamponade, 1837

Tachycardia (Continued)
    diagrammatic representations of, 878f
    ectopic junctional, radiofrequency catheter ablation of, 808
    electrical cardioversion of, 801-803
    electrophysiology in, 774, 775f
    endless-loop (pacemaker reentrant), 839, 840f
    involving atrioventricular junctional area, nomenclature for, 878
    narrow complex, 863, 866, 866f
    orthostatic, postural, 772, 867, 976-977, 2176-2177
    pacemaker reentrant, 839, 840f
    pacing, with cardiac catheterization, 459-460
    QRS
        narrow and wide complex, electrophysiology in, 826t, 827
        wide
            algorithm for diagnosis of, 898f
            in Wolff-Parkinson-White syndrome, 890
    reciprocating, 878
        using accessory pathway, 864t-865t
    reentry, 751-761, 754f-760f
    sinus. See Sinus tachycardia.
    sinus node reentrant, 808, 867, 867f
    supraventricular. See Supraventricular tachycardia.
    ventricular. See Ventricular tachycardia.
    wide complex, 863, 866, 866t
Tachycardia-dependent block, 751
Tachycardia-induced cardiomyopathy, 1744
Tachypnea, in pulmonary embolism, 1866
Tacrolimus (FK-506), in heart transplantation, 678
Tafazzin, mutation of, in Barth syndrome, 117
Tagging, in cardiovascular magnetic resonance, 394, 395
Takayasu arteritis, 1037, 2087-2089, 2088f
Takotsubo cardiomyopathy, 181-182, 1216, 1743, 1744f, 1811-1812
Tamoxifen, cardiotoxicity of, 2111
Tamponade, cardiac. See Cardiac tamponade.
TandemHeart ventricular assist device, 690
Tangier disease, 1081
Tapazole, in amiodarone-induced hyperthyroidism, 2044
Tau (time constant of relaxation), 535, 648-649, 649f, 745
Taxanes, cardiotoxicity of, 2110
Taxol. See Paclitaxel (Taxol).
Taxotere. See Docetaxel (Taxotere).
TAXUS stent, 1431, 1436
TBX5, mutations of, in Holt-Oram syndrome, 120
Teboroxime, technetium-99m–labeled, 346, 349t
Technetium-99m–labeled tracers
    coronary blood flow reserve and, 362, 362f
    lung uptake of, 352, 352f
    for myocardial viability assessment, 384
    for radionuclide angiography or ventriculography, 358
    for single photon emission computed tomography, 346, 349t
    uptake and retention of, mechanisms of, 369f

Tei index, 252
Telangiectases, hereditary, 127
Telangiectasia, hemorrhagic, hereditary, 97-98
Telemonitoring, in heart failure, 638
Temperature, body
    in myocardial infarction, 1222
    noncardiac surgery and, 2026
Temporal artery, biopsy of, in giant cell arteritis, 2090
Tenecteplase, 2068
    in myocardial infarction, 1246, 1247t, 1248, 1254, 1256, 1310
    structure of, 1247f
Tenex. See Guanfacine (Tenex).
Tenormin. See Atenolol (Tenormin).
Teratogens, in congenital heart disease, 1563
Terazosin (Hytrin), in hypertension, 1059-1060
Terfenadine, pharmacokinetics of, 60
Tests, diagnostic. See Diagnostic tests.
Tetralogy of Fallot, 1587-1590
    associated anomalies in, 1588
    clinical features of, 1588-1589
    indications for interventions in, 1589-1590
    interventional options and outcomes in, 1590
    laboratory studies in, 1589, 1589f
    magnetic resonance imaging in, 409
    morphology of, 1587-1588, 1588f
    natural history of, 1588
    pathophysiology of, 1588
    in pregnancy, 1971, 1971f
    with pulmonary atresia, 1588, 1589
    ventricular tachycardia in, 904
Tetrofosmin, technetium-99m–labeled, 346, 349t
    coronary blood flow reserve and, 362, 362f
    for myocardial viability assessment, 384
Tezosentan, in acute heart failure, 606
Thalidomide
    in congenital heart disease, 1563
    immunomodulation with, in heart failure, 713
Thallium, cardiotoxicity of, 1814
Thallium-201–labeled tracers, 346, 348f, 349t
    coronary blood flow reserve and, 362, 362f
    for myocardial viability assessment, 384, 385f
    for single photon emission computed tomography, lung uptake of, 352, 352f
    uptake and retention of, mechanisms of, 369f
Theophylline, in central sleep apnea, 1920
Therapeutic decision-making, 43-47
    adoption of innovation in, 47
    cognitive errors in, 46
    evidence in
        accuracy of, 46-47
        interpretation of, 44-46
Thermodilution techniques, for cardiac output measurement, 452, 452f
Thermography, intracoronary, 497, 499t
Thiazide diuretics, 1057, 1057t
    dyslipidemia and, 1082
    in elderly persons, 1931, 1932
    in heart failure, 621t, 622
    mechanisms of action of, 622
Thiazide-like diuretics, 622

Thiazolidinediones
in diabetic patients with cardiovascular disease, 1557
in diabetic vascular disease prevention, 1099, 1100
Thick-filament proteins, mutations of
in dilated cardiomyopathy, 115-116, 115t
in hypertrophic cardiomyopathy, 111-113, 112t
Thienopyridine derivatives
in percutaneous coronary intervention, 1436
as platelet inhibitors, 2070-2071
Thin-filament protein, mutations of
in dilated cardiomyopathy, 115t, 116
in hypertrophic cardiomyopathy, 112t, 113-114
Thiopurine methyltransferase, in drug metabolism and elimination, 61t
Thioridazine, cardiovascular aspects of, 2130
Thoracic aorta. See Aorta, thoracic.
Thoracotomy
emergency, indications for, 1858
technique for, 1859, 1859f
Thoracovertebral deformities, pulmonary hypertension in, 1909
Thoratec ventricular assist devices, 691
Thorax. See Chest.
Three-dimensional echocardiography. See Echocardiography, three-dimensional.
"Thrifty gene" hypothesis, in diabetes mellitus, 1093
Thrombectomy
in deep venous thrombosis, 1542
in percutaneous coronary intervention, 1308
rheolytic, in percutaneous coronary intervention, 1425
Thrombin
in common pathway of coagulation, 2052
in coronary blood flow regulation, 1175
formation of, 2050-2052, 2051f, 2052f
in hemostasis, 2056, 2057f, 2058f
inactivation of, 2052-2054, 2053f, 2054f
Thrombin inhibitors
in atrial fibrillation, 872
direct, 2066-2067
advantages of, 2067
in diabetes mellitus, 1550-1551
mechanism of action of, 2066f, 2067
in percutaneous coronary intervention, 1437
in UA/NSTEMI, 1332-1333
Thrombin paradox, 2056, 2058f
Thrombin-activatable fibrinolysis inhibitor, 2054
Thromboangiitis obliterans, 1505-1506, 1507f
Thrombocytopenia
after cardiac surgery, 1999
glycoprotein IIb/IIIa inhibition and, 2074f, 2075
heparin-induced, 1874-1875, 2063-2065, 2064f
diagnosis of, 2064
pathophysiology of, 2063-2064, 2064f
treatment of, 2064-2065
Thromboembolic pulmonary hypertension, 1878, 1910-1912, 1911f

Thromboembolism
venous. See Pulmonary embolism; Venous thrombosis.
after ventricular assist device implantation, 693
Thromboendarterectomy, pulmonary
in chronic pulmonary hypertension, 1878
in thromboembolic pulmonary hypertension, 1910
Thrombolectomy, in acute limb ischemia, 1509, 1509t
Thrombolysis, in deep venous thrombosis, 1542
Thrombolytic therapy. See also specific agent, e.g., Streptokinase.
in acute coronary syndromes, economic analysis of, 36-37
in acute limb ischemia, 1508-1509, 1509t
agents used in, 2067-2068
contraindications to, percutaneous coronary intervention in patients with, 1305-1306
in elderly persons, 1938, 1940
glycoprotein IIb/IIIa inhibition and, facilitated PCI with, 2075
intraarterial, 1520-1521
intracerebral hemorrhage after, 1522
intravenous, 1519-1520, 1521t
in myocardial infarction, 1241-1249
abciximab with, 1254, 1256
agents for
comparison of, 1245-1246, 1247f, 1247t
selection of, 1248
complications of, 1247, 1248f
glycoprotein IIb/IIIa inhibition with, 1254, 1256
intracoronary, 1241
intravenous, 1242-1244, 1243f, 1244f
late, 1248-1249
left ventricular function and, 1246-1247
mortality and, 1244-1245, 1245f, 1246f
myocardial perfusion evaluation of, 1242-1244, 1243f, 1244f
net clinical benefit of, 1248
versus percutaneous coronary intervention, 1301-1307, 1302f, 1314, 1315t
prehospital, 1234
recommendations for, 1248-1249
TIMI flow grade and, 1242, 1242f
TIMI frame count and, 1242, 1243f
TIMI myocardial perfusion grade and, 1244, 1244f
TIMI risk score for, 1244, 1246f
percutaneous coronary intervention with, 1309-1310, 1314, 1315t, 2075
in prosthetic valve thrombosis, 1683
in pulmonary embolism, 1876-1877, 1876t
racial/ethnic differences in, 25
successful, percutaneous coronary intervention after, 1309, 1314, 1316t
in UA/NSTEMI, 1333
in venous thrombosis, 1877
in women, 1962
Thrombomodulin
antithrombotic properties of, 2053, 2054
in endothelial cells, 987
Thrombophilia, 2056-2062
acquired, 2060-2062, 2060t
inherited, 2056-2060, 2058f, 2059t
venous thromboembolism and, 1864, 1864t, 1875-1876

Thrombosis. See also Hemostasis.
of abdominal aorta, 1486
in antiphospholipid antibody syndrome, 2061-2062
antithrombin III deficiency in, 2058-2059, 2059t
cancer and, 2060-2061
of coronary arteries
in atherosclerosis, 996-999, 996f-998f
in sudden cardiac death, 949
after coronary stents, 1429, 1438, 1440-1441, 1440t, 1441t
factor V Leiden gene mutation in, 2056-2058, 2058f
in Fontan patients, 1595
heparin-induced thrombocytopenia with, 2064, 2064f
hormone-induced, 2057, 2058, 2061
hyperhomocysteinemia in, 2059-2060
mechanisms of, 2049-2056
with prosthetic valves, 1683
protein C and S deficiencies in, 2059, 2059t
prothrombin gene mutation in, 2058, 2059f
of pulmonary arteries, in pulmonary hypertension, 1892, 1893f
risk factors for, 2060-2061, 2060t
in UA/NSTEMI, 1319, 1320, 1321f
venous. See Venous thrombosis.
Thrombosis in situ, in acute limb ischemia, 1508
Thrombotic endocarditis, nonbacterial, 1718-1719
in cancer patients, 2108
in HIV-infected patients, 1794t, 1799
Thrombotic pulmonary arteriopathy, in idiopathic pulmonary arterial hypertension, 1891-1892
Thrombotic thrombocytopenic purpura, from thienopyridine derivatives, 2070
Thromboxane
inhibitors of, 2068-2069, 2070f
pulmonary vascular effects of, 1885
Thromboxane A_2
in coronary blood flow regulation, 1175
synthesis of, 2055, 2055f
Thrombus (thrombi), coronary
arteriography of, 492
computed tomography of, 429, 430f
echocardiography of, 304, 305f
magnetic resonance imaging of, 405
in myocardial infarction, 1210, 1211f, 1285-1286
percutaneous coronary intervention in, 1422
prosthetic valve obstruction from, 278-279, 280f
Thumpversion, 803, 899, 958
Thyroid disorders. See also Hyperthyroidism; Hypothyroidism.
amiodarone-induced, 795, 2044
diastolic dysfunction and, 2039, 2040f
hemodynamic alterations in, 2040, 2040f, 2040t
in myocardial infarction, 1220
subclinical, 2043-2044, 2044f
Thyroid function testing, 1887, 2039
Thyroid gland, 2038-2045
Thyroid hormones
actions of, 2038
cardiac effects of, 2038-2039, 2038f, 2039f, 2039t
catecholamines and, 2039-2040
changes in, in cardiovascular disease, 2044-2045

Tibioperoneal obstructive disease, percutaneous intervention in, 1530-1532, 1530f, 1531t, 1532f
Ticlopidine (Ticlid)
  in chronic kidney disease patients, 2164t
  in diabetes mellitus, 1550
  as platelet inhibitor, 2070
Tietze syndrome, chest pain in, 1354
Tilt training, in neurally mediated syncope, 983
Tilting-disc prosthetic valves, 1682-1683, 1682f
Tilt-table testing
  as measure of autonomic function, 2174
  in syncope, 771-772, 772f, 979
Time domain analysis, in electrocardiography, 770
Time velocity integral, in Doppler echocardiography, 264
TIMI flow grade, 1242, 1242f
  classification of, 1302t
  after percutaneous coronary intervention, 1302, 1302t, 1303f
TIMI frame count, 492, 492t, 1242, 1243f
TIMI myocardial perfusion grade, 1244, 1244f
  classification of, 1302t
  after percutaneous coronary intervention, 1302, 1302t, 1303f
TIMI risk score, 1244, 1246f
  in UA/NSTEMI, 1325-1326, 1326f
Timolol, 792-793, 1372t
Tinzaparin, in pulmonary embolism, 1873t
Tirofiban (Aggrastat)
  in chronic kidney disease patients, 2164t
  in percutaneous coronary intervention, 1436
  as platelet inhibitor, 2073
  in UA/NSTEMI, 1329
Tissue engineering, 700
Tissue factor pathway, 2051, 2051f
Tissue factor pathway inhibitors, 2053, 2067
Tissue inhibitors of metalloproteinases, 557
Tissue plasminogen activator (t-PA), 2054, 2068. See also Thrombolytic therapy.
  in acute coronary syndromes, economic analysis of, 36-37
  in myocardial infarction, 1245, 1247t, 1248
  plasma, atherothrombotic risk and, 1018-1019
  in pulmonary embolism, 1876-1877, 1876t
  structure of, 1247f
  variants of, 1245-1246
  in venous thrombosis, 1877
Tissue prosthetic valves
  durability of, 1685, 1685f, 1686f
  indications for, 1687-1688, 1687f
  types of, 1684-1686, 1684f, 1685f
Tissue-resident stem cells, 698-699
Titin
  left ventricular diastolic stiffness and, 653
  mutation of
    in dilated cardiomyopathy, 115t, 116
    in hypertrophic cardiomyopathy, 112t, 113
  structure and functions of, 510, 511, 514f
Tobacco. See Smoking.

Toe(s), blue, in peripheral arterial disease, 1510, 1510f
Tolazoline (Priscoline), pulmonary vascular effects of, 1884
Toll-like receptors, in myocarditis, 1782, 1783f
Tolvaptan, in heart failure, 605-606, 621t, 624
Topiramate, cardiovascular aspects of, 2132
Toprol. See Metoprolol (Lopressor, Toprol).
Torcetrapib, in stable angina, 1363
Toronto SPV stentless valve, 1684f, 1686
Torsades de pointes
  in acute cerebrovascular disease, 2150, 2151f-2152f
  from azimilide, 796
  cardiac arrest with, 964
  clinical features of, 905
  from disopyramide, 788
  from dofetilide, 796
  electrocardiography in, 904-905, 905f
  electrophysiology in, 905
  from ibutilide, 797
  management of, 905-906
  in periodic paralyses, 2147
  short-coupled variant of, sudden cardiac death in, 946, 947f
  ventricular tachycardia in, 904-905, 905f
Torsemide, in heart failure, 620, 621t, 622, 625
Torsion, left ventricular, 239, 241f
Total artificial heart, 691-692, 691f
Total electrical alternans, 186-187, 186t, 187f
Touch, healing, in cardiac catheterization, 1163-1164
Toxins, cardiac. See Cardiac toxin(s).
TQ segment, in myocardial ischemia, 173
Trachea, deviation of, in thoracic aortic aneurysm, 1465
Tracheobronchitis, chest pain in, 1197
Trandate. See Labetalol (Normodyne, Trandate).
Trandolapril, in heart failure, 624t
Tranexamic acid, for postoperative bleeding, 2005
Transcendental meditation, for stress management, 1157
Transcription, 71, 72f
Transesophageal echocardiography. See Echocardiography, transesophageal.
Transfection efficiency, 79
Transforming growth factor-β receptor disorders, 93
Transforming growth factor-β signaling pathway, 1894f
Transfusion
  postoperative, 2005
  threshold for, in noncardiac surgery, 2026-2027
Transgenic mouse, 78
Transient ischemic attacks, in elderly persons, 1940-1942
Transitional cells, of atrioventricular node, 729, 730
Transitional circulation, at birth, 1565-1566
Translation, 71, 72f
Transmembrane potentials. See Action potential; Resting membrane potential.
Transmural myocardial infarction, 1211

Transplantation. See also specific organ, e.g., Heart transplantation.
  cell. See Myocardial repair and regeneration; Stem cells.
  in cyanotic congenital heart disease, 1568
  in Eisenmenger syndrome, 1570
Transportation options, in myocardial infarction, 1236f
Transposition of the great arteries
  complete, 1597-1601
    clinical features of, 1597-1598
    definition of, 1597
    follow-up in, 1601
    management of, 1598-1600, 1599f, 1600f
    morphology of, 1597
    pathophysiology of, 1597
    reinterventions in, 1600-1601
    reproductive issues in, 1601
  congenitally corrected, 1601-1603
    clinical features of, 1602
    definition of, 1601
    echocardiography in, 307f
    follow-up in, 1603
    indications for intervention and reinterventions in, 1602
    interventional options and outcomes in, 1602-1603
    laboratory studies in, 1602, 1602f
    morphology of, 1601-1602, 1601f
    pathophysiology of, 1602
    in pregnancy, 1971
  magnetic resonance imaging in, 408, 408f
Transpositional complexes, 1597-1601
Transseptal catheterization, 447-448, 447f
Transthoracic echocardiography. See Echocardiography, transthoracic two-dimensional.
Trastuzamab (Herceptin)
  cardiotoxicity of, 1813, 2111-2112
  polymorphisms associated with, 61
Traube sign, in aortic regurgitation, 1638
Traumatic heart disease, 1855-1862
  arrhythmias in, 1858, 1860, 1861t
  blunt/nonpenetrating, 1855-1856, 1857-1858, 1859, 1860
  burn-related, 1856-1857
  cardiac enzymes in, 1859
  clinical presentation and pathophysiology of, 1857-1858
  complications of, 1860, 1861t
  echocardiography in, 1858, 1859
  electrical, 1857
  electrocardiography in, 1859
  etiology and patterns of, 1855-1856, 1856t
  evaluation of, 1858-1859
  follow-up in, 1860, 1862
  foreign bodies/missiles in, 1856
  iatrogenic, 1856
  incidence of, 1855
  metabolic, 1856-1857
  penetrating, 1855, 1857, 1859-1860, 1859f-1861f
  pericardial, 1858
  pericardiocentesis in, 1859
  pericarditis after, 1850
  results of, 1860
  subxiphoid pericardial window in, 1858-1859
  treatment of, 1859-1860, 1859f-1861f
  ultrasonography in, 1858
Trazodone, cardiovascular aspects of, 2130

Treadmill ECG stress testing
  in peripheral arterial disease, 1497
  protocol for, 197-198, 198f
  in pulmonary hypertension, 1888
  in women, 214, 214f
Treadmill exercise, stress myocardial
    perfusion imaging with, 366
Trendelenburg position, reverse, in
    myocardial infarction, 1266
Trepopnea, in heart failure, 140
Treppe effect, 531, 532f
Treprostinil, in idiopathic pulmonary
    arterial hypertension, 1899
Triactive Device, 1426
Triamterene (Dyrenium)
  in heart failure, 621t, 623
  in hypertension, 1058
Triangle of Koch, 729, 731f
Trichinosis, myocarditis in, 1780
Tricor. See Fenofibrate (Tricor, Lipidil
    Micro).
Tricuspid atresia, 1590-1591, 1591f
Tricuspid position, prosthetic valves in,
    1688
Tricuspid regurgitation, 1675-1678
  auscultation in, 1676
  in carcinoid heart disease, 297, 1676,
    1677f
  chest radiography in, 1677
  clinical presentation in, 1676-1677
  congenital, 1675
  echocardiography in, 275-276, 276f,
    1676-1677, 1677f
  electrocardiography in, 1677
  etiology and pathology of, 1675-1676,
    1676t, 1677f
  after heart transplantation, 678
  hemodynamics of, 1677
  history and physical examination in,
    146
  jugular venous pressure in, 130, 130f
  management of, 671-672, 1677-1678
  murmur in, 136
  physical examination in, 1676
  practice guidelines for, 1704, 1705t
  in pulmonary hypertension,
    1886-1887
  rheumatic, 1675-1676
  right ventricular remodeling in, 577
  symptoms of, 1676
Tricuspid stenosis, 1674-1675
  angiography in, 1675
  chest radiography in, 1675
  clinical presentation in, 1674-1675,
    1674t
  echocardiography in, 270, 1675
  electrocardiography in, 1675
  etiology and pathology of, 1674
  history and physical examination in,
    146
  laboratory examination in, 1674t, 1675
  murmur in, 137-138
  pathophysiology of, 1674
  rheumatic, 1674
  treatment of, 1675
Tricuspid valve
  Ebstein anomaly of, 307f, 1604-1605,
    1604f, 1605f, 1971
  infective endocarditis of, in intravenous
    drug abusers, 1678
  normal anatomy of, 1564
  prolapse of, 1676, 1677f
  replacement of
    in transposition of the great arteries,
      1603
    in tricuspid regurgitation, 1678
    in tricuspid stenosis, 1675

Tricuspid valve annuloplasty, in dilated
    cardiomyopathy, 671-672
Tricyclic antidepressants
  cardiotoxicity of, 297
  cardiovascular aspects of, 2128-2129,
    2129t
  contraindications to, 2128
  drug interactions of, 2132, 2133t
  myocarditis from, 1781
Trifascicular block
  chronic, pacemaker in, 832, 854, 855t
  electrocardiography in, 170-171, 171f
Trigemy, 893
Triggered activity
  antiarrhythmic drug effects on, 780,
    781t
  in arrhythmogenesis, 747-750, 748f-752f,
    748t. See also Afterdepolarization.
  in ventricular tachycardia, 761
Triglyceride(s)
  biochemistry of, 1071, 1072f
  dietary management of, 1113
  elevated. See Hypertriglyceridemia.
Triglyceride-rich lipoprotein,
    cardiovascular disease risk and, 1009
Triiodothyronine
  cardiac effects of, 2038-2039, 2038f,
    2039f, 2039t
  in preoperative risk analysis, 1994
  vasodilatory effects of, 2040
Trimetazidine
  in heart failure, 711
  in stable angina, 1377
Triphenyltetrazolium chloride (TTC)
    stain, in myocardial infarction, 1211,
    1212f, 1213f
Triploidy, 86
Trisomy, 86
Trisomy 21 (Down syndrome), 132, 1571,
    1582
Tropheryma whippelii infection, in
    infective endocarditis, 1717
Tropomyosin, 512, 513f
  alpha-, mutation of, in hypertrophic
    cardiomyopathy, 112t, 114
Troponin(s)
  in acute cerebrovascular disease, 2150
  in acute pericarditis, 1833
  cardiac-specific
    versus CK-MB, 1227
    cutoff values for, 1225f, 1226
    diagnostic performance of, 1198-1199,
      1198t, 1199t
    interpretation of tests for, 1199, 1200f
    in myocardial infarction, 1225-1226,
      1225f, 1226t
    prognostic implications of, 1198t,
      1199, 1199t
    single, test performance of, 1199
    testing strategy for, 1199-1200, 1201t
  in postoperative myocardial infarction,
    2022
  in preoperative risk analysis, 1994
  in UA/NSTEMI, 1322-1323, 1325
Troponin C
  in cross-bridge cycling, 511, 512, 513,
    513f, 515f
  in heart failure with normal ejection
    fraction, 650
Troponin complex, of actin filament, 512,
    515f
Troponin I
  in chronic kidney disease, 2162
  phosphorylation of
    diastolic relaxation and, 649
    in heart failure with normal ejection
      fraction, 650

Troponin T
  mutation of, in hypertrophic
    cardiomyopathy, 112t, 113
  in myocarditis, 1785-1786
Troponin T isoforms, in heart failure,
    552
Truncus arteriosus, persistent, 1586-1587,
    1587f
Trypanosomiasis, 611, 1779-1780, 1779f
TU wave alternans, 187, 187f
Tubal sterilization, 1977-1978
Tuberculosis
  myocarditis in, 1778
  pericarditis in, 1841, 1848
  tests for, 1841
Tumor(s). See also Cancer.
  of aorta, 1487, 1487f
  cardiac, 1815-1827
    benign, 1817-1823
      incidence of, 1817
      myxomatous, 1817, 1819, 1820f,
        1821f
      nonmyxomatous, 1819-1823, 1821f
      treatment of, 1826
    cardiac manifestations of, 1816-1817
    characteristic clinicopathologic
      features of, 1818t
    clinical presentation of, 1815-1817
    computed tomography in, 429-430,
      430f, 1817
    diagnosis of, 1817, 1818t
    echocardiography in, 302-304,
      302f-305f, 320, 320t, 1817, 1820f,
      1821f
    embolization of, 1816
    future perspectives on, 1827
    genetic studies in, 121
    magnetic resonance imaging in, 405,
      406f, 1817, 1824f
    malignant, 1818t, 1824-1826
      in HIV-infected patients, 1794t,
        1799
      imaging of, 1817
      incidence of, 1824
      treatment of, 1826-1827
      types of, 1824-1826, 1824f
    metastatic, 1817, 1824, 2105
    primary, 2105
    systemic manifestations of,
      1815-1816
    treatment of, 1826-1827
  malignant
    cardiac surgery in patients with,
      1996
    echocardiography in, 303-304, 304f
  of pericardium, 422, 1851
  renin-secreting, hypertension in, 1040
Tumor necrosis factor inhibitors
  in rheumatoid arthritis, 2095
  in Takayasu arteritis, 2089
Tumor necrosis factor-alpha
  in contraction-relaxation cycle, 526
  in diabetic vascular disease, 1096,
    1096f
  in HIV-infected patients, 1795
  in left ventricular volume loading, 537
Tumor plop, 136, 1816
Tunica media, 988, 989f
Turbulence, in color Doppler, 238
Turner syndrome, 132, 1571
Two-dimensional echocardiography. See
    Echocardiography, transthoracic
    two-dimensional.
Type A behavior, 2119
Type D behavior, 2119
Tyrosine kinase inhibitors, in cancer
    therapy, 2111-2115, 2112t

U wave, 159
  in exercise stress testing, 202
  in long QT syndrome, 906
  in myocardial ischemia, 176
  in potassium abnormalities, 184
UA/NSTEMI, 1319-1340
  angioscopy in, 1323
  arteriography in, 465, 466t, 467, 501,
      503t-504t, 1321f, 1323
  cardiac checklist for, 1337, 1337t
  cardiac necrosis markers in, 1322-1323,
      1325
  classification of, 1319, 1320t, 1321f
  clinical presentation in, 1321f, 1322-
      1323, 1322f
  coronary vasoconstriction in, 1321-1322
  definition of, 1319
  electrocardiography in, 1322, 1322f,
      1325
  etiologic approach to, 1319, 1321f
  hospital discharge after, 1349
  intravascular ultrasound in, 1323
  laboratory testing in, 1323
  long-term risk following,
      pathophysiology of, 1323-1324,
      1324f
  long-term secondary prevention
      following, 1336, 1337f
  management of, 1325-1337
    acute, summary of, 1336, 1336f
    angiotensin receptor blockers in, 1335
    angiotensin-converting enzyme
        inhibitors in, 1335
    anticoagulant therapy in, 1331-1333
    antithrombotic therapy in, 1327-1330
    aspirin in, 1327-1328, 1328f, 1329t
    beta blockers in, 1327
    calcium channel blockers in, 1327
    clopidogrel in, 1328-1329, 1328f,
        1329f, 1330f
    coronary artery bypass graft in, 1329,
        1334-1335, 1347, 1349-1350,
        1350t
    critical pathways and continuous
        quality improvement in, 1337,
        1337t
    direct thrombin inhibitors in,
        1332-1333
    early invasive versus conservative
        strategy in, 1333-1334, 1334f,
        1347, 1349t
    economic analysis of, 36-37
    in emergency department, 1235
    fondaparinux in, 1331-1332, 1332f
    general measures in, 1326-1327
    glycoprotein IIb/IIIa inhibition in,
        1329-1330
    heparin in, 1331, 1331t
    hospital, 1344-1347, 1346f, 1347t,
        1348t
    intraaortic balloon counterpulsation
        in, 1336
    lipid-lowering therapy in, 1335, 1335f
    long-term, 1336, 1337f
    low-molecular-weight heparin in,
        1331, 1332f
    medical, 1325-1333
    nitrates in, 1327
    percutaneous coronary intervention
        in, 1329, 1334-1335, 1347, 1349-
        1350, 1350t, 1420-1421
      practice guidelines for, 1450-1451,
          1452f, 1452t
    registry experience with, 1336-1337
    reperfusion in, 1347, 1349-1350, 1350t
    thrombolytic therapy in, 1333

UA/NSTEMI (Continued)
    timing of invasive strategy in, 1334
    warfarin in, 1333
  mechanical obstruction in, 1322
  myocardial infarction precipitated by,
      1221
  myocardial perfusion imaging in,
      380-381, 381f
  natural history of, 1324
  pathophysiology of, 1319-1321, 1321f
  platelet activation and aggregation in,
      1320-1321, 1321f
  practice guidelines for, 1344-1351,
      1345t-1350t, 1346f
  risk stratification in, 1323-1326, 1324f
    by cardiac markers, 1325
    by clinical variables, 1324t, 1324-1325
    early, 1344, 1345t
    by electrocardiography, 1325
    later, 1347, 1348t, 1349, 1349t
    methods of, 1324-1326, 1324t, 1326f
    multimarker, 1326, 1326f
    to target glycoprotein IIb/IIIa
        inhibitors, 1330
    TIMI risk score for, 1325-1326,
        1326f
  secondary, 1322
  secondary hemostasis in, 1321
  thrombosis in, 1319, 1320, 1321f
Ubiquinone, 1159t
  for heart failure, 1162
  for hypertension, 1158
UDP-glucuronosyltransferase, in drug
    metabolism and elimination, 61t
Ulcer(s)
  of aorta
    echocardiography in, 301
    penetrating atherosclerotic,
        1484-1486, 1485f
  chest pain associated with, 1197
  neurotrophic, 1495
  in peripheral arterial disease, 1495,
      1496f
Ulnar neuropathy, after cardiac surgery,
    1998
Ultrafiltration, veno-venous, in chronic
    kidney disease patients, 2166
Ultrasonography
  in abdominal aortic aneurysms, 1460
  cardiac. See Echocardiography.
  duplex, in peripheral arterial disease,
      1498, 1498f, 1499f
  intravascular, 495-497
    arteriography with, 460, 461f
    versus conventional angiography, 496,
        496f
    after drug-eluting stents, 496-497,
        497f
    limitations of, 497
    longitudinal, 496f
    after percutaneous coronary
        intervention, 496
    during percutaneous coronary
        intervention, 496
    quantitative, 496f
    in stable angina, 1359
    technical issues in, 495
    in UA/NSTEMI, 1323
    of vessel wall composition, 495-496,
        495f
  venous, in pulmonary embolism,
      1870
Underuse, as error in health care,
    51-52
Unipolar limb leads, 152
United Network for Organ Sharing
    (UNOS), 675

United States
  cardiovascular disease in, 6-9, 6t, 7f, 8t,
      9f
  population demographics in, 23, 24f
Urbanization
  cardiovascular disease and, 5, 5f
  in United States, 7, 7f
Uremic pericarditis, 1849
Uric acid, in pulmonary hypertension,
    1887
Urinalysis
  in heart failure, 564
  in infective endocarditis, 1722
Urinary retention, after cardiac surgery,
    1998
Urokinase, 1246, 2054, 2068. See also
    Thrombolytic therapy.
Urotensin II, in heart failure, 547-548

V
V wave
  abnormal, 130, 130f
  in atrial pressure, 451
  normal, 128f, 130
VA (ventriculoatrial) interval
  in atrioventricular nodal reentrant
      tachycardia, 879-880
  in concealed accessory pathway, 882,
      883-884
Vaccination
  in myocarditis, 1791
  smallpox, myocarditis from, 1780
Vagal innervation
  intraventricular, 732, 734f
  of sinus and AV nodes, 727-728
Vagal reactivation, after exercise, 195
Vagal stimulation
  cardiac effects of, 732-733
  negative inotropic effect of, 524, 525,
      525f
Validity, 44
Valium. See Diazepam (Valium).
Valproate, cardiovascular aspects of,
    2131-2132, 2131t
Valsalva maneuver
  in arrhythmias, 764
  with cardiac catheterization, 460
  in heart failure, 142, 144f, 593
  as measure of autonomic function, 2173
  murmur response to, 139, 139t
  normal response to, 142, 143f
Valsartan
  in heart failure, 624t, 629
  in myocardial infarction, 1260, 1262,
      1262f
Valve(s). See also Aortic valve; Mitral
    valve; Pulmonic valve; Tricuspid
    valve.
  area of, calculation of, 264-266, 265f,
      266f, 456-457
  morphology of, magnetic resonance
      imaging of, 404
  papillary fibroelastoma of, 1822
  prosthetic, 1682-1688. See also
      Prosthetic valves.
Valve surgery, in dilated cardiomyopathy,
    669-672, 671f-672f
Valvotomy
  in aortic stenosis, 1633
  in mitral stenosis
    closed, 1655-1656
    open, 1656
    percutaneous, 1653-1655, 1654f, 1655f
    restenosis after, 1656
  in tricuspid stenosis, 1675
Valvular apparatus dysfunction,
    traumatic, 1860

Valvular heart disease, 1625-1712. *See also specific types, e.g.,* Aortic stenosis.
from anorectic drugs, 1704
in antiphospholipid antibody syndrome, 2099, 2099f
from appetite suppressants, 1812
arteriography in, 501, 505, 506t-507t
in cancer patients, 2108
cardiac catheterization in, 439-440
in chronic kidney disease, 2166
computed tomography in, 423, 423f, 424f
with coronary artery disease, 1709, 1711t, 1712
myocardial perfusion imaging of, 378
drug-induced, 277, 277f
echocardiography in, 314-317, 315t-316t
guidelines for, 1693, 1694t
in elderly persons, 1947-1949, 1947t, 1948t
exercise and sports in patients with, 1989
exercise stress testing in, 215, 225, 225t
history and physical examination in, 142, 144-147, 146f
magnetic resonance imaging in, 404-405, 404f, 409
multivalvular involvement in, 1680-1682
noncardiac surgery in patients with, 2015
practice guidelines for, 1693-1712, 1694t-1711t
in pregnancy, 1972-1973, 1979
after radiation therapy, 2115
severity of, classification of, 1629t
sudden cardiac death in, 944
surgical considerations in, guidelines for, 1704, 1708-1709
in systemic lupus erythematosus, 2098, 2098f
in young adults, 1704, 1705t-1708t
Valvular regurgitation
cardiac catheterization in, 457-459
in Fontan patients, 1595, 1596
magnetic resonance imaging in, 404-405, 404f
visual assessment of, 458
Valvular stenosis
cardiac catheterization in, 455-457, 456f
magnetic resonance imaging in, 404f, 405
orifice area in, 456-457
Valvulitis
in rheumatic fever, 2082
in systemic lupus erythematosus, 2098, 2098f
Vampire bat, saliva from, tissue plasminogen activator of, 2068
Variant angina. *See* Prinzmetal variant angina.
Varicose veins, 96
Vascular access
in arteriography, 468-469, 468f
needles for, 444, 446, 446f
in percutaneous coronary intervention, 1423-1424
Vascular biology, of atherosclerosis, 985-1001
Vascular cell adhesion molecule-1 (VCAM-1), in atherogenesis, 990-991
Vascular closure devices
in cardiac catheterization, 446
in percutaneous coronary intervention, 1424

Vascular complications, in cardiac catheterization, in cardiac catheterization, 462
Vascular disease
chest pain in, 1196-1197
coronary. *See* Cardiovascular disease.
in elderly persons, 1931-1943
noncoronary. *See* Peripheral arterial disease; Peripheral vascular disease.
Vascular disrupting agents, cardiotoxicity of, 2115
Vascular endothelial growth factor
angiogenic properties of, in gene transfer research, 81
in hypoxic pulmonary vasoconstriction, 1884
in peripheral arterial disease, 1503
Vascular endothelial growth factor receptor antagonists, cardiotoxicity of, 2114-2115
Vascular interventions, extracardiac, 1523-1544
Vascular mediators, in pulmonary circulation, 1884-1886, 1885f
Vascular remodeling
cellular regulation of, 69-70
in hypertension, 1033, 1033f
Vascular resistance
coronary. *See also* Coronary resistance vessels.
determinants of, 1171-1177, 1171f-1174f
Doppler echocardiography of, 267
measurement of, 452t, 455
pulmonary. *See* Pulmonary vascular resistance.
systemic, 452t, 455
Vascular rings, 407, 1609-1610, 1610f
Vascular sling, 407
Vascular stiffness, measurement of, 131-132
Vascular syncope, 975-978, 976t, 977t
Vascular system. *See also* Cardiovascular system.
in elderly persons, 1924, 1925f, 1926f
genetic disorders of, 89-98
nonpathological variation in, 89
Vasculitis, 2087-2101
diagnosis of, 2087, 2088f, 2088t
in HIV-infected patients, 1795t, 1800
hypersensitivity, 2094
of large-sized vessels, 2087-2092
primary versus secondary, 2087, 2088t
sarcoid, 2101, 2102f
of small or medium-sized vessels, 2093-2101
Vasculopathy, coronary artery, after heart transplantation, 679, 681, 682f
Vasoactive drugs, postoperative, 2000-2001, 2000t
Vasoactive intestinal peptide (VIP)
in idiopathic pulmonary arterial hypertension, 1893
in sinus node, 728
Vasoconstriction
coronary
causes of, 1321-1322
cocaine-induced, 1808, 1809f
in UA/NSTEMI, 1321-1322
in heart failure, 545, 546f, 547-548, 588
pulmonary, hypoxia in, 1884
Vasoconstrictive signaling, in contraction-relaxation cycle, 526, 527f
Vasodepressor carotid sinus hypersensitivity, 912

Vasodepressor response, in upright tilt-table testing, 771, 772f
Vasodilation
endothelium-dependent
in coronary blood flow regulation, 1168, 1170-1171, 1170t
in hypertension, 1032, 1032f
impaired, microcirculatory coronary reserve in, 1182-1183, 1183f, 1184f
pharmacological, 1170t, 1176-1177
for detection of coronary artery disease, 376-377
versus exercise stress, 366
hemodynamic effects of, 365
heterogeneity of coronary hyperemia with, 365
in myocardial perfusion imaging, 364-366, 365f, 366t
protocols for, 366, 366t
reversal of, 365-366
side effects of, 365
Vasodilator testing, in pulmonary hypertension, 1889-1890, 1889t
Vasodilator therapy
in acute heart failure, 596, 600-603, 601t, 602f
in aortic regurgitation, 1642, 1643
direct, in hypertension, 1061
in hypertension, 1061-1064
in hypertensive crises, 1066, 1066t
in idiopathic pulmonary arterial hypertension, 1898-1900, 1899f
in mitral regurgitation, 1665
in myocardial infarction, 1268
in myocarditis, 1788
in peripheral arterial disease, 1502-1503
postoperative, 2002
in Prinzmetal variant angina, 1339
in right ventricular infarction, 1272
Vasodilatory activity, in heart failure, 545-547, 548-549, 548f, 549f
Vasopressin antagonists, in heart failure, 605-606, 621t, 623-624, 624f
Vasoregulation, by endothelium, 2050, 2050f
Vasotec. *See* Enalapril (Vasotec).
Vasovagal syncope. *See* Neurally mediated syncope.
Vatalinib, cardiotoxicity of, 2114-2115
Vaughan Williams classification of antiarrhythmic agents, 779
Vectorcardiogram, 152, 154f
Vegetable consumption, cardiovascular disease and, 1107
Veins
atretic, 96
for cardiac catheterization, 443, 443f, 444f
genetic disorders primarily affecting, 96
Velocity mapping, in cardiovascular magnetic resonance, 394
Velocity of circumferential fiber shortening, 571-572
Velocity time integral, in Doppler echocardiography, 264
Venlafaxine, cardiovascular aspects of, 2129t, 2130
Venous claudication, 1495
Venous conduits, for coronary artery bypass graft surgery, 1382
Venous filling pressure, and heart volume, 529
Venous grafts, patency rate for, 1384-1385
Venous insufficiency
chronic, in pulmonary embolism, 1878
dietary supplements for, 1162

I-86

Venous obstructive disease, percutaneous interventions for, 1542-1543, 1543f, 1544f
Venous thrombosis. *See also* Pulmonary embolism.
  antiphospholipid antibody syndrome in, 2061-2062
  antithrombin III deficiency in, 2058-2059, 2059t
  cancer and, 1875
  computed tomography venography in, 1869
  contrast phlebography in, 1870
  epidemiology of, 1863
  fondaparinux in, 1873, 1873t
  future perspectives on, 1879
  heparin in, 1871-1872, 1872t
  hormone-induced, 2057, 2061
  hypercoagulable states in, 1864, 1864t
  hyperhomocysteinemia in, 2059-2060
  inferior vena caval filters and, 1876
  after myocardial infarction, 1284-1285
  paradoxical embolism in, 1867-1868
  pathophysiology of, 1864-1865, 1865f, 1866f
  percutaneous interventions in, 1542-1543, 1543f
  postoperative, 1864
  pregnancy and, 2061
  prevention of, 1878-1879, 1879t
  protein C and S deficiencies in, 2059, 2059t
  prothrombin gene mutation in, 2058, 2059f
  proximal, asymptomatic, 1863
  pulmonary embolism and, 1864-1865, 1865f
  risk factors for, 2060-2061, 2060t
  thrombolytic therapy in, 1877
  ultrasonography in, 1870
  upper extremity, 1864
  warfarin in, 1873-1874
Venous ulcer, 1495
Venous ultrasonography, in pulmonary embolism, 1870
Ventilation
  abnormalities of, in central sleep apnea, 1917
  mechanical
    in cardiac arrest, 959
    in end-stage heart disease, withdrawal of, 722
  minute, during exercise, 197
  noninvasive, in chronic obstructive pulmonary disease, 1908
  positive pressure
    in acute heart failure, 596
    in central sleep apnea, 1920, 1920f
    in chronic obstructive pulmonary disease, 1908
    in obstructive sleep apnea, 1919, 1920t
Ventilatory gas analysis, exercise stress testing with, 196, 196f, 197, 224, 225t
Ventilatory oxygen consumption (VO_2), 1149
Ventilatory threshold (VT), 1149-1150
VentrAssist ventricular assist device, 692-693
Ventricle(s). *See also* Atrioventricular *entries*; Ventricular *entries*.
  activation of, 157-158, 158f
    QRS complex and, 158-159, 158f
  autonomic innervation of, 732, 734f
  diastolic function of, 573-575
    abnormalities of. *See* Diastolic dysfunction.

Ventricle(s) (*Continued*)
    aging and, 250, 251t
    assessment of, 573-578, 576f, 577f
    cardiac time intervals and, 251-252
    chamber properties in, 574, 574f
    definitions related to, 570t
    determinants of, 573-574, 573f
    echocardiographic assessment of, 239, 242, 248-253, 249f, 250f, 251t
    during exercise, 580
    magnetic resonance imaging of, 575, 576f, 577f
    myocardial properties in, 574-575, 574f
    nuclear imaging of, 370-371, 370f, 371f
    passive elastic properties in, 574, 574f
    pericardial properties in, 575
    radionuclide angiography or ventriculography of, 370-371, 370f, 371f
    relaxation in, 574
  double-inlet, 307f, 1574, 1592-1593, 1593f
  double-outlet, 1574
  embryogenesis of, 1563-1564
  end-diastolic volume of, 455, 572
  end-systolic volume of, 455, 571
  function of
    in acute heart failure, 587-588
    in aortic stenosis, 1628
    computed tomography of, 430, 431f
    in elderly persons, 1943
    in Fontan patients, 1595, 1596
    magnetic resonance imaging of, 395
    nuclear imaging of, 369-370, 370f, 371f
  hypertrophy of
    in acromegaly, 2034
    in athletes, 537-538, 537t
    electrocardiography in, 162-167, 163f-167f, 164t, 165t
    physiological, 537-538, 537t
    sudden cardiac death and, 941t, 942-943, 948
  innervation of, 732-733, 734f
  left
    aneurysm of
      in coronary artery disease, 1398-1399, 1398f, 1399f
      detection of, 1399
      after myocardial infarction, 1285, 1285f
      true, 257
    biopsy of, 448
    chest radiography of, 335f, 338, 339f
    compensation of, in mitral regurgitation, 1659-1660, 1660f
    contraction of, 527, 528f
    diastolic filling pattern of
      echocardiography of, 248-249, 249f, 250f
      grading of, 249, 250f
      normal, 249-250, 250f, 251t
    diastolic function of
      during exercise, 580
      in myocardial infarction, 1218
      in pulmonary venous hypertension, 1904
    diastolic stiffness of, 650-653, 652f
    dimensions of, echocardiography of, 243, 243t, 245, 246f
    double-inlet, 1592, 1593, 1593f
    dysfunction of
      in aortic regurgitation, 1638, 1639f
      in aortic stenosis, 1634

Ventricle(s) (*Continued*)
    in cardiac arrest survivors, 954, 954f, 965
    coronary artery bypass graft surgery in patients with, 1388-1390, 1389f, 1389t, 1390f
    in heart failure, 573
    in HIV-infected patients, 1793-1797, 1794t, 1796f-1798f
    in idiopathic pulmonary arterial hypertension, 1896
    in Marfan syndrome, 92
    in mitral regurgitation, 1659
    in myocardial infarction, 382, 1216-1218, 1218f, 1288
    percutaneous coronary intervention in patients with, 1380, 1422
    reversible, pathophysiology of, 367, 368f
    in stable angina, 1360
    sudden cardiac death and, 939
    systolic heart failure and, 617, 619f
   ejection fraction of. *See* Left ventricular ejection fraction.
   elastic recoil of, diastolic function and, 573-574
   electromechanical mapping of, with cardiac catheterization, 460
   endomyocardial fibrosis of, 1757f, 1758
   failure of, in myocardial infarction, 1267-1269, 1267f
   filling phases of, in contraction-relaxation cycle, 527, 528f, 529
   free wall rupture of, 256-257, 258f, 1272-1273, 1272f, 1274f, 1275f, 1303
   function of
    computed tomography of, 430, 431f
    myocardial ischemia effects on, 1188
    nuclear imaging of, 369-370, 370f, 371f
    single photon emission computed tomography of, 355-357, 356f, 357f
    thrombolytic therapy and, 1246-1247
   hypertrophy of
    in aortic regurgitation, 1637, 1640f
    in aortic stenosis, 1631
    clinical significance of, 165
    compensated, wall stress and, 535-536, 537f
    diagnostic criteria for, 163-165, 164f, 164t
    diastolic dysfunction and, 536-537
    dose adjustments in, 64
    electrocardiography in, 162-165, 163f, 164f, 164t
    in heart failure, 549-550, 550f-552f, 646
    in hypertension, 1034
    in hypertrophic cardiomyopathy, 1764-1765, 1764f-1766f
    microcirculatory coronary reserve in, 1182, 1182f
    in mitral regurgitation, 1659-1660
    myocardial perfusion imaging in, 376
    physiological, 1768
    on plain chest radiography, 338, 339f
    racial/ethnic differences in, 24, 27
    in stable angina, 1357
    sudden cardiac death and, 941t, 942-943

Ventricle(s) (Continued)
  mass of, echocardiography of, 244t,
    245-246
  morphological, 1564
  opacification of, in echocardiography,
    242-243, 242f, 243f, 245f
  outflow tract hypoplasia of, 1612
  outflow tract obstruction of,
    1605-1614, 1606f
    in aortic stenosis, 1627, 1628f,
      1629t
    differential diagnosis of, 286
    in hypertrophic cardiomyopathy,
      284-285, 285f, 1766-1767, 1767f
    after myocardial infarction, 256
  pressure overload of, 1034
  pseudoaneurysm of, after free wall
    rupture, 257, 258f
  puncture of, for cardiac
    catheterization, 448
  reconstruction of, in heart failure,
    672-674, 673f, 674f
  relaxation of
    assessment of, 648-649, 649f
    in contraction-relaxation cycle, 527,
      528f
    and cytosolic calcium, 534
    and diastolic dysfunction, 534
    factors regulating, 534-535, 535f,
      649-650
    impaired, in heart failure with
      normal ejection fraction, 650,
      651f
  remodeling of
    in heart failure, 549-559, 550t
      beta-adrenergic desensitization
        in, 552-553
      contractile and myofilament
        regulatory proteins in, 552,
        553f
      cytoskeletal proteins in, 552
      excitation-contraction coupling
        in, 550-551
      fibroblasts and mast cells in,
        556-557, 557f
      inflammatory mediators in,
        558-559, 559t
      myocardial alterations in,
        553-556, 554f-556f
      myocardial energetics in, 558
      myocyte biological alterations in,
        549, 550t
      myocyte hypertrophy in, 549-550,
        550f-552f
      passive cardiac support devices
        for, 674-675, 675f
      reversibility of, 559, 559t
      structural changes in, 557-558,
        558f
    in myocardial infarction, 257-258,
      1215f, 1218-1219, 1219f
    reversal of, passive cardiac support
      devices for, 674-675, 675f
  response of, to mechanical stress,
    536, 536f, 537f
  rotational motion of, Doppler
    echocardiography of, 239, 241f
  suction effect of, in contraction-
    relaxation cycle, 535
  systolic function of, 569-572, 569f
    afterload in, 569-570, 570f
    assessment of, 571-572, 571f, 572f
    cardiac time intervals and, 251-252
    contractility in, 570
    definitions related to, 570t
    drug-induced abnormalities in,
      1805-1806, 1810-1811

Ventricle(s) (Continued)
  echocardiography of, 239, 242,
    247-248
  during exercise, 579-580, 579f
  filling pressures in, 570
  in heart failure, 573
  in heart failure with normal
    ejection fraction, 653-654
  in HIV-infected patients, 1793-1797,
    1794t, 1796f-1798f
  in myocardial infarction, 1215f,
    1216-1218
  preload in, 569
  in pulmonary venous hypertension,
    1904
  regional indices of, 572, 573f
  specific indices of, 571-572, 571f,
    572f
  thrombus of, 257
    echocardiography of, 304, 305f
    after myocardial infarction,
      1285-1286
  transient ischemic dilation of,
    on single photon emission
    computed tomography, 352-353,
    352f
  volume loading of, signals involved
    in, 537
  volume of
    echocardiography of, 242, 242f,
      246-247, 247f, 248f
    magnetic resonance imaging of,
      394-395
  wall stress of, 530-531, 531f
  mass of, magnetic resonance imaging
    of, 395
  morphology of, magnetic resonance
    imaging of, 407
  myocytes of, 509, 510t, 738t
  overload of, pseudoinfarct patterns in,
    181, 181f
  pressure of
    with cardiac catheterization, 451,
      452t, 454t
    maximum rate of rise of (dP/dt$_{max}$),
      and end-diastolic volume, 572
  recovery of
    sequence of, 159
    ST-T wave and, 156f, 159
  regional wall motion of, 572, 573f
  remodeling of. See Ventricle(s), left,
    remodeling of; Ventricular
    remodeling.
  right
    arrhythmogenic dysplasia/
      cardiomyopathy of. See
      Arrhythmogenic right ventricular
      dysplasia/cardiomyopathy.
    biopsy of, 448
    chest radiography of, 337, 337f,
      338f
    diastolic collapse of, in cardiac
      tamponade, 1838, 1839f
    dimensions of, echocardiography of,
      244t, 245, 247f
    double-chambered, 1618
    double-inlet, 1592, 1593
    double-outlet, 408, 1603-1604, 1603f
    dysfunction of
      acute ischemic, 578
      chronic, 578
      pulmonary embolism and, 1865,
        1866f, 1871
      in pulmonic regurgitation,
        1679
    endomyocardial fibrosis of, 1757-1758,
      1757f

Ventricle(s) (Continued)
  failure of
    in idiopathic pulmonary arterial
      hypertension, 1896
    postoperative, 2001
  function of, 575, 577, 577f
    assessment of, 577, 578t
    pathophysiology of, 575, 577, 577f
  hypertrophy of
    chest radiography in, 337, 337f
    in chronic obstructive pulmonary
      disease, 166, 166f
    in congenital heart disease, 1572
    diagnostic criteria for, 165, 165t
    electrocardiography in, 165-166,
      165f-167f, 165t
    in mitral stenosis, 1651
    in pulmonary embolism, 166, 167f
    in pulmonary hypertension, 1887
  infarction of. See Myocardial
    infarction, right ventricular.
  isolated disease of, in HIV-infected
    patients, 1799
  morphological, 1564
  outflow tract lesions of, 1615-1618
    subpulmonary, 1618
    supravalvular, 1616
  overload of
    pressure, 577-578
    volume, 577
  remodeling of, 577-578
  thrombus of, echocardiography of,
    304, 305f
  single, magnetic resonance imaging in,
    409
  stiffness of, 574, 574f, 575
  tumors of, 1816-1817, 1819
  volume of
    magnetic resonance imaging of,
      394-395
    venous filling pressure and, 529
Ventricular arrhythmias
  in Duchenne muscular dystrophy,
    2136-2137
  in elderly persons, 1947
  in Emery-Dreifuss muscular dystrophy
    and associated disorders, 2144
  exercise stress testing in, 211-212
  exercise-induced, 210-211
  in heart failure, 636
  in myocardial infarction, 1277-1279
  noncardiac surgery in patients with,
    2016
  postoperative, 2003-2004
  sudden cardiac death and, 939-940,
    940f
  ventricular assist device in, 688
Ventricular assist device, 686-696
  axial flow pumps as, 692, 692f, 693f
  bridge-to-bridge cohort for, 687
  bridge-to-recovery cohort for, 686-687
  bridge-to-transplantation cohort for, 687
  in cardiogenic shock, 686
    after myocardial infarction, 688
    postcardiotomy, 687-688
  centrifugal pumps as
    extracorporeal, 689
    miniaturized, 692-693
  in children, 695-696
  complications of, 693-694
  contraindications to, 689
  in decompensated chronic heart failure,
    688
  destination therapy with, 687, 694-695,
    695f
  failure rate for, 694
  future developments in, 696

Ventricular assist device (*Continued*)
history in, 685
immunological perturbations with, 694
indications for, 687-688, 687t
long-term, 690-693, 690f-693f
in myocarditis, 688
postoperative management in, 693
preoperative risk assessment for, 688, 689t
pulsatile, 690-692, 690f, 691f
rationale and treatment goals for, 686-687
selection of, 689-693
sensitization to, 694
short-term, 689-690
triage cohort for, 687
in ventricular arrhythmias, 688
Ventricular asystole, in carotid sinus hypersensitivity, 912
Ventricular ectopy, postoperative, 2003-2004
Ventricular fibrillation
cardiac arrest with
advanced life support for, 961-962, 961f
management of, 955-956, 956f
post-arrest care in, 963
characteristics of, 864t-865t
clinical features of, 909
dynamic wave break hypothesis in, 760
electrocardiography in, 908, 908f
idiopathic, 101-108, 102t, 904, 904f, 907
management of, 909
mechanisms of, 909
mother rotor hypothesis in, 759-760
in myocardial infarction, 1278-1279
reentry in, 758-761, 760f
in Wolff-Parkinson-White syndrome, 889, 892f
Ventricular flutter
characteristics of, 864t-865t
clinical features of, 909
electrocardiography in, 908, 908f
management of, 909
mechanisms of, 909
Ventricular function curves, 571, 571f, 572f
in heart failure, 579-580, 579f
Ventricular gradient, on electrocardiogram, 160
Ventricular interdependency, pulmonary embolism and, 1865, 1866f
Ventricular mapping, intraoperative, 821
Ventricular premature complexes, 893-895
with cardiac catheterization, 460
clinical features of, 895
electrocardiography in, 893-895, 894f, 895f
during exercise stress testing, 210-211
in exercise stress testing, 765-766
management of, 895
multiform, 893, 895, 895f
in myocardial infarction, 766, 767, 1277-1278
new mapping and ablation technologies for, 819
physical examination in, 895
in pregnancy, 1976
sudden cardiac death and, 939-940, 940f
Ventricular remodeling
left. *See* Ventricle(s), left, remodeling of.
in myocarditis, 1784
right, 577-578
Ventricular rhythm, disturbances of, 893-909

Ventricular septal defect, 1583-1585
clinical features of, 1583-1584
cyanosis in, with normal or decreased pulmonary vascularity, 1573
doubly committed subarterial, 1583
echocardiography in, 308-309, 309f-310f
follow-up in, 1584-1585
genetic studies in, 119
indications for interventions in, 1584
infarct-related, 255-256, 257f
interventional options and outcomes in, 1584
laboratory studies in, 1584
magnetic resonance imaging in, 408
membranous, 1583
moderately restrictive, 1583
morphology of, 1583, 1583f
muscular, 1583
natural history of, 1583, 1583f
noncommitted, double-outlet right ventricle with, 1603, 1603f, 1604
nonrestrictive, 1583
in pregnancy, 1970
reproductive issues in, 1584
restrictive, 1583
rupture of, in myocardial infarction, 1272f, 1273t, 1274, 1276f, 1277f
subaortic, double-outlet right ventricle with, 1603, 1603f, 1604
subaortic stenosis with, 1612
subpulmonary, double-outlet right ventricle with, 1603, 1603f, 1604
Ventricular tachycardia, 896-908. *See also specific types, e.g.,* Ventricular fibrillation.
in acute cerebrovascular disease, 2150, 2151f-2152f
in arrhythmogenic right ventricular dysplasia, 903-904, 903f
atrioventricular dissociation in, 897
bidirectional, 908
bundle branch reentrant, 908
capture beats in, 897, 897f
cardiac arrest with
advanced life support for, 961-962, 961f
management of, 955-956, 956f
post-arrest care in, 963
progression in, 953
characteristics of, 864t-865t
clinical features of, 898-899
in congenital heart disease, 1570
definition of, 863, 893
in dilated cardiomyopathy, 902
electrocardiography in, 896-897, 896f, 897f
electrophysiology in, 774, 775f, 896f, 897-898
exercise and sports in patients with, 1989
fascicular (left septal), 907, 908f
in Friedreich's ataxia, 2146
fusion beats in, 897, 897f
in hypertrophic cardiomyopathy, 902-903
idiopathic, 906-907, 907f, 908f
in inherited arrhythmia syndromes, 904, 904f
in ischemic cardiomyopathy, 902
in long QT syndrome, 905f, 906
monomorphic, repetitive, 906-907, 907f
in myocardial infarction, 1278
in myotonic muscular dystrophy, 2139, 2141f
nonreentrant mechanisms in, 761
nonsustained, electrophysiology in, 827t, 828

Ventricular tachycardia (*Continued*)
outflow tract, 906-907, 907f
paroxysmal, 906-907, 907f
in periodic paralyses, 2147, 2147f
polymorphic, 905. *See also* Torsades de pointes.
catecholaminergic, 102t, 106-108, 107f, 904
postinfarct, radiofrequency catheter ablation of, 818f
postoperative, 2004
in pregnancy, 1976
prevention of, long-term therapy for, 899, 901-902
prognosis for, 899
reentry in, 758, 760f
versus supraventricular tachycardia, 863, 866, 866f, 866t, 897, 897f
sustained, acute management of, 899
syncope and, 978, 981
in tetralogy of Fallot, 904
in torsades de pointes, 904-905, 905f
treatment of, 899-902, 900t-901t
chest thump cardioversion in, 803, 899, 958
electrical cardioversion in, 801
radiofrequency catheter ablation in, 816-819, 817f-818f
surgical, 820-821, 820f
Ventriculoarterial connections, normal, 1564
Ventriculoarterial discordance, in transpositional complexes, 1597
Ventriculography
left, in dilated cardiomyopathy, 1748
radionuclide. *See* Radionuclide angiography or ventriculography.
Ventriculophasic sinus arrhythmia, 910, 910f
Ventriculotomy, encircling endocardial, in ventricular tachycardia, 820-821, 820f
Venturi effect, 284-285, 285f
Verapamil
adverse effects of, 799, 1375
in aortic dissection, 1479
in arrhythmias, 798-799
in atrial flutter, 875
in chronic kidney disease patients, 2165t
dosage and administration of, 784t, 798
drug interactions of, 1375
electrophysiological characteristics of, 780t, 781t, 782t, 786t, 798
in fascicular ventricular tachycardia, 907
hemodynamic effects of, 798
in hypertrophic cardiomyopathy, 1771
indications for, 798-799
in myocardial infarction, 1263
pharmacokinetics of, 784t, 798, 1375t
in stable angina, 1375
in UA/NSTEMI, 1327
in Wolff-Parkinson-White syndrome, 891, 892
Vertebral artery stenosis, 1541-1542, 1542f
Very-low-density lipoprotein (VLDL), 1072, 1073f, 1073t
hepatic synthesis of, 1074f, 1075-1076
Viral infection
in dilated cardiomyopathy, 1746
geographical distribution of, 1777f
in myocarditis, 1778
agents causing, 1776-1778, 1777f
pathogenesis of, 1781-1782, 1783f
in pericarditis, 1846-1847

Viral persistence, in myocarditis, 1782
Viridans streptococci, in infective
    endocarditis, 1716, 1723-1724, 1723t
Visceral pericardium, 1829
Viscoelasticity, definition of, 570t
Visual symptoms, after cardiac surgery,
    1999
Vital capacity
    in myocardial infarction, 1219
    sudden cardiac death and, 937
Vital signs
    in heart failure, 562
    orthostatic, 979
Vitamin(s)
    antioxidant, 1115-1116, 1115f
    supplementation of, in cardiovascular
        disease prevention, 1140
Vitamin E, 1140, 1161t
Vitamin K, 1161t
    for warfarin-induced hemorrhage, 1875
Vitamin K cycle, warfarin inhibition of,
    2065, 2065f
VLDL. See Very-low-density lipoprotein
    (VLDL).
Vocal cord palsy, after cardiac surgery,
    2007
Voltage-gated ion channels
    ion flux through, 735, 735f
    molecular structure of, 734f, 736
Volume, as marker of quality of
    cardiovascular care, 52-53, 53f, 53t
Volume expansion
    in aortic dissection, 1479-1480
    in autonomic failure, 2176
    for hypotension in right ventricular
        infarction, 1272
Volume overload
    acute heart failure treatment and, 598-
        599, 598t
    right ventricular, 577
Volume overload (eccentric) hypertrophy,
    549-550, 550f, 551f
Volumetric method of regurgitant volume
    estimation, 265, 266f
Vomiting, in myocardial infarction, 1221
Von Hippel–Lindau syndrome, genetic
    studies in, 98
Von Willebrand factor, 2055, 2055f
Voodoo death, 946
V-slope method, of anaerobic threshold
    determination, 196, 196f

W

Walk test, for exercise stress testing, 198
Walking capacity, measurement of, 1497
Wall
    chest, disorders of, pulmonary
        hypertension in, 1909
    coronary arterial, magnetic resonance
        imaging of, 399-401, 400f
    vessel, composition of, intravascular
        ultrasonography of, 495-496, 495f
Wall motion
    abnormalities of
        echocardiography of, 255, 256f
        in heart failure with normal ejection
            fraction, 646
    regional indices of, 572, 573f
Wall motion score index (WMSI), 255
Wall stress, 530-531, 531f
    and compensated left ventricular
        hypertrophy, 535-536, 537f
    components of, 570f
    in contraction-relaxation cycle, 530-531,
        531f
    definition of, 570t
    myocardial oxygen uptake and, 532

Wandering pacemaker, 911, 911f
Warfarin, 2065-2066
    in atheroembolism, 1511
    in atrial fibrillation, 871
    complications of, 1875, 2066
    drug interactions of, 2065-2066
        with dietary supplements, 1163
        with serotonin reuptake inhibitors,
            2132
    in elderly persons, 1941
    in heart failure, 635
    heparin overlap with, 1874
    in idiopathic pulmonary arterial
        hypertension, 1897
    mechanism of action of, 2065, 2065f
    in mitral stenosis, 1653
    monitoring of, 1874, 2066
    in myocardial infarction prevention,
        1286, 1291, 1291f, 1292t
    pharmacogenetics of, 62
    pharmacogenomics of, 1874
    in pregnancy, 1973, 1976t, 1977
    in prosthetic valve replacement, 1683,
        1685
    in pulmonary embolism, 1873-1874
    reversal of, 1875
    in stroke prevention, 1516-1517, 1516f
    in UA/NSTEMI, 1333
Water
    ingestion of, in neurally mediated
        syncope, 983
    renal retention of, in heart failure, 545,
        546f
Water-hammer pulse, 133, 1638
Weber protocol, for exercise stress testing,
    198
Wegener granulomatosis, 2094
Weight gain, in heart failure, 619
Weight reduction
    blood pressure and, 1113
    in cardiovascular disease prevention,
        1011, 1136-1137, 1137t
    in chronic obstructive pulmonary
        disease, 1905
    C-reactive protein level and, 1114f, 1115
    in diabetic vascular disease prevention,
        1099
    dietary influences on, 1111-1112, 1111t
    in hypertension therapy, 1052
Welding, electromagnetic interference
    from, 850
Wenckebach atrioventricular block, 914-
    917, 916f
Werdnig-Hoffman disease, 2148
Westermark sign, in pulmonary
    embolism, 1868
Western blotting, 73
Western Europe, 10, 11t
Wheezing, in heart failure, 593
Whipple disease, myocarditis in, 1778
White blood cells. See Leukocyte(s).
White coat hypertension, 131, 1035-1036
Whole grain consumption, cardiovascular
    disease and, 1107-1108
Whole-person assessment, in end-stage
    heart disease, 718
Wide QRS tachycardias
    algorithm for diagnosis of, 898f
    in Wolff-Parkinson-White syndrome,
        890
Wiggers cycle, 528f
Williams syndrome, 1571, 1615
Wilson central terminal, in
    electrocardiography, 152
Windkessel effect, 527
Wine intake, cardiovascular disease and,
    1110

"Wire pleating," 490f-491f
Wolff-Parkinson-White syndrome,
    884-893
    accessory pathway conduction in, 888-
        889, 889f, 890f
    accessory pathway recognition in, 889
    accessory pathway variants in, 884, 887,
        887f, 887t, 888f
    atrial fibrillation in, 889, 892f, 928t
    atriofascicular accessory pathways in,
        884, 887, 887t, 888f
    atriohisian tracts in, 884, 887, 887t, 888f
    atrioventricular nodal reentry in, 889-
        890, 889f
    atrioventricular reciprocating
        tachycardia in, 757-758, 759f
    clinical features of, 890
    electrocardiography in, 884, 885f-888f
    electrophysiology in, 826t, 827, 887,
        887f-892f
    exercise stress testing in, 212-213, 213f
    fasciculoventricular connections in,
        887, 887t, 888f
    versus Lown-Ganong-Levine syndrome,
        884
    nodofascicular accessory pathways in,
        884, 887, 887t, 888f
    prevention of, 892-893
    pseudoinfarct patterns in, 180
    treatment of, 890-893
    ventricular fibrillation in, 889, 892f
    wide QRS tachycardias in, 890
Women. See also Gender differences.
    acute coronary syndromes in
        cardiac rehabilitation after, 1963
        symptoms of, 1957-1958
        treatment of, 1961-1963, 1962f, 1962t
    cardiovascular disease in, 1955-1964
        background on, 1955
        future perspectives on, 1964
        mortality in, 1955
        prevention of, 1143, 1145
        scope of problem for, 1955, 1956t
    chest pain in, 1957, 1958
    coronary artery bypass graft surgery in,
        1390
    coronary artery disease in
        age and, 1956
        age at onset of, 1955, 1956t
        diabetes and, 1957
        discordance between predicted
            probability and observed rates of,
            1958, 1959f
        family history and, 1956
        hypertension and, 1956-1957
        imaging of, 1958, 1959f, 1960f
        life style and, 1957
        lipid levels and, 1957
        myocardial perfusion imaging of, 378
        prevention of
            primary, 1960-1961
            secondary, 1961-1963
        risk factors for, 1956-1957, 1958f
        treatment of
            ACC/AHA and UA/NSTEMI ACS
                guidelines for, 1961
            evidence-based research on, 1958-
                1959, 1961f
            glycoprotein IIb/IIIa inhibition in,
                1962
            practice guidelines for, 1959-1961,
                1960f
            revascularization in, 1961-1962,
                1962t
            sex differences in, 1962-1963, 1962f
            thrombolytic therapy in, bleeding
                with, 1962

I-90 Women *(Continued)*
    exercise stress testing in, 214, 214f, 225,
        1958, 1959f
    heart failure in, 613, 1963-1964, 1963f
        acute, 586
        with normal ejection fraction, 643f,
            645
    hypertension in, 1044-1045, 1044t
    peripheral arterial disease in, 1964
    smoking prevalence in, 1004, 1004f
Women's Health Study, 1960-1961
Work, in myocardial oxygen uptake, 532-
    533, 533f
Work output, during exercise, 196, 196f
World Health Organization, pulmonary
    hypertension classification of, 1890,
    1891t
Wound healing, myocardial. *See*
    Myocardial repair and regeneration.
Wound infection, after coronary artery
    bypass graft surgery, 1383
Wytensin. *See* Guanabenz (Wytensin).

X
X descent
    in atrial pressure, 451
    in cardiac tamponade, 1835, 1836f
    normal, 128f, 130
X' descent, normal, 128f, 130
45,X karyotype, in Turner syndrome,
    121
Xanthelasma, in stable angina, 1355
Xanthoma, 127
X-linked dilated cardiomyopathy, 117
X-linked inheritance, 87-88, 88f
X-linked muscular dystrophy, 2135-2137,
    2136f, 2137f

Y
Y descent
    abnormal, 130, 130f
    in atrial pressure, 451
    in cardiac tamponade, 1835, 1836f, 1837
    in constrictive pericarditis, 1843
    normal, 128f, 130

Yohimbine, 1161t
    in autonomic failure, 2176
Younger patients, coronary artery bypass
    graft surgery in, 1390

Z
Z line, 510, 512f
Zaroxolyn. *See* Metolazone (Mykrox,
    Zaroxolyn).
Z-disc proteins, mutation of, in dilated
    cardiomyopathy, 115t, 116
Zero flow pressure, 1172
Zidovudine (azidothymidine),
    complications of, 1801
Zinc sulfate, for postoperative dysgeusia,
    1998
Zinecard. *See* Dexrazoxane (Zinecard).
Ziprasidone, cardiovascular aspects of,
    2131
Zocor. *See* Simvastatin (Zocor).
Zotarolimus-eluting stents, 1431,
    1436